DATE DUE

		PRINTED IN U.S.A.

ASHCRAFT'S
PEDIATRIC SURGERY

Content Strategist: Michael Houston
Content Development Specialist: Alexandra Mortimer
Content Coordinators: Sam Crowe/Humayra Rahman Khan
Project Managers: Srividhya Vidhya Shankar/Sukanthi Sukumar
Designer: Miles Hitchen
Illustration Manager: Jennifer Rose
Illustrator: Antbits
Marketing Manager: Abigail Swartz

ASHCRAFT'S PEDIATRIC SURGERY

SIXTH EDITION

George W. Holcomb III, MD MBA

Katharine B. Richardson Professor of Surgery
Surgeon-in-Chief
Department of Surgery
Children's Mercy Hospital
Kansas City, MO, USA

J. Patrick Murphy, MD

Professor of Surgery
Chief, Section of Urology
Department of Surgery
Children's Mercy Hospital
Kansas City, MO, USA

Daniel J. Ostlie, MD

Surgeon-in-Chief, American Family Children's Hospital
WARF Professor of Pediatric Surgery
Chief, Pediatric Surgery
Department of Surgery
University of Wisconsin
Madison, WI, USA

Associate Editor

Shawn D. St. Peter, MD

Professor of Surgery
Director, Center for Prospective Trials
Department of Surgery
Children's Mercy Hospital
Kansas City, MO, USA

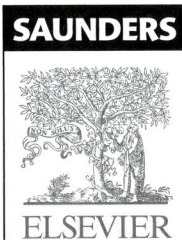

London New York Oxford Philadelphia St Louis Sydney Toronto 2014

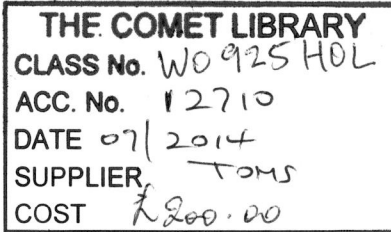

ELSEVIER
SAUNDERS

First edition 1980
Second edition 1993
Third edition 2000
Fourth edition 2005
Fifth edition 2010

Video clip 34.1 Trans Anal Pullthrough ©Cincinnati Children's Hospital Medical Center
Video clip 35.1 Rectourethral Fistula Repair ©Cincinnati Children's Hospital Medical Center

---

Notices

Knowledge and best practice in this field are constantly changing. As new research and experience broaden our understanding, changes in research methods, professional practices, or medical treatment may become necessary.

Practitioners and researchers must always rely on their own experience and knowledge in evaluating and using any information, methods, compounds, or experiments described herein. In using such information or methods they should be mindful of their own safety and the safety of others, including parties for whom they have a professional responsibility.

With respect to any drug or pharmaceutical products identified, readers are advised to check the most current information provided (i) on procedures featured or (ii) by the manufacturer of each product to be administered, to verify the recommended dose or formula, the method and duration of administration, and contraindications. It is the responsibility of practitioners, relying on their own experience and knowledge of their patients, to make diagnoses, to determine dosages and the best treatment for each individual patient, and to take all appropriate safety precautions.

To the fullest extent of the law, neither the Publisher nor the authors, contributors, or editors, assume any liability for any injury and/or damage to persons or property as a matter of products liability, negligence or otherwise, or from any use or operation of any methods, products, instructions, or ideas contained in the material herein.

ISBN: 978-1-4557-4333-9

Ebook ISBN: 978-0-323-18736-7

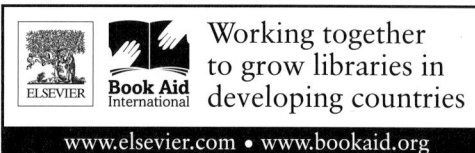

Working together
to grow libraries in
developing countries

www.elsevier.com • www.bookaid.org

Printed in China

Last digit is the print number: 9 8 7 6 5 4 3 2 1

Dedication

This book is dedicated to Dr. Ronald J. Sharp
Master Surgeon, Colleague, Friend

CONTENTS

Video Contents

PREFACE

This textbook represents the sixth edition of a textbook which was first published in 1980 under the direction of Drs. Tom Holder and Keith Ashcraft. One of the underlying tenets of this book has always been to make it as readable as possible. In the Preface of the second edition, Drs. Holder and Ashcraft wrote 'Our intent is to provide a book that has a clear explanation of a subject done in a readable style.' For this edition and previous ones, authors have been selected because of their expertise about their chapter's subject matter and their writing ability. Also, because many pediatric general surgeons outside the United States have a significant part of their practice in urology, we have continued to emphasize this subject in the sixth edition. As minimally invasive surgery (MIS) continues to weave its way more and more into mainstream pediatric surgery and urology, the MIS approach is emphasized in most of the chapters as well.

There are many new figures and tables in this edition. In addition, most of the figures and artwork are in color. There are only a few figures in which the color version is not available. We feel the color photographs and drawings add significantly to the readability of the book. In addition, there are 30 videos that accompany this edition and most depict the minimally invasive approach to a particular surgical condition. These videos are accessible via our Expert Consult website (expertconsult.com). There is a code in the front of this book that allows access to the online version of the book and the videos.

The editors would like to acknowledge the tireless efforts of our administrative assistants Linda Jankowski, Barbara Juarez, and Jeanette Whitney without whose efforts this book would not have been possible. They have done a remarkable job in helping us in so many ways with the task of editing this book. We also thank Dr. Rand O'Donnell, President/CEO of Children's Mercy Hospital, who has given us the support and resources needed to produce this book.

The editors have dedicated this edition to our former senior partner, Dr. Ron Sharp, who recently retired from practice at Children's Mercy Hospital. Ron was instrumental in the founding of our burn and trauma programs, and directed these two programs for almost thirty years. During his career, he was board certified in general surgery, pediatric surgery, and surgical critical care. He was known as the 'go to' person for advice and help with a complicated surgical problem. In addition to trauma, burns and critical care, he had a long-standing interest and expertise in the repair of pectus excavatum, and was the one who conceptualized making a small subxyphoid incision so that the surgeon can use his/her finger to direct the substernal bar across the mediastinum and help protect the heart when performing the Nuss operation. Although his talents will be missed, we have all benefitted from his association and expertise.

George W. Holcomb III, MD MBA
J. Patrick Murphy, MD
Daniel J. Ostlie, MD
Shawn D. St. Peter, MD

List of Contributors

Pablo Aguayo, MD
Assistant Professor, Department of Surgery, Children's
Mercy Hospital, Kansas City, MO, USA
Ch 30 Duodenal and Intestinal Atresia and Stenosis

D. Adam Algren, MD
Medical Toxicologist, Divisions of Clinical
Pharmacology, Medical Toxicology, Departments of
Emergency Medicine and Pediatrics, Truman
Medical Center, Children's Mercy Hospital,
University of Missouri-Kansas City School of
Medicine, Kansas City, MO, USA
Ch 12 Bites

Uri S. Alon, MD
Professor of Pediatrics, University of Missouri-Kansas
City School of Medicine; Pediatric Nephrologist;
Director, Bone and Mineral Disorders Clinic,
Children's Mercy Hospitals and Clinics, Kansas City,
MO, USA
Ch 4 Renal Impairment

Maria H. Alonso, MD
Associate Professor of Surgery; Surgical Assistant
Director, Liver Transplantation, Division of Pediatric
& Thoracic Surgery, Cincinnati Children's Hospital
Medical Center, Cincinnati, OH, USA
Ch 45 Solid Organ Transplantation in Children

Richard J. Andrassy, MD
Professor and Chairman, Department of Surgery,
University of Texas Medical School at Houston,
Surgeon-in-Chief, Memorial Hermann Hospital,
Houston, TX, USA
Ch 70 Rhabdomyosarcoma

Walter S. Andrews, MD
Professor of Pediatric Surgery, University of Missouri
School of Medicine at Kansas City; Chief, Transplant
Services, Children's Mercy Hospital, Kansas City,
MO, USA
Ch 67 Lesions of the Liver

Kelly M. Austin, MD
Program Director, Surgical Critical Care; Residency
Program; Surgical Director, Neonatal Intensive Care
Unit; Co-Surgical Director of the Intestinal Care and
Rehabilitation (ICARE) Center; Assistant Professor,
University of Pittsburgh School of Medicine,
Division of Pediatric General & Thoracic Surgery,
Pittsburgh, PA, USA
Ch 16 Abdominal and Renal Trauma

Sean J. Barnett, MD MS
Assistant Professor of Surgery and Pediatrics, Division
of Pediatric General & Thoracic Surgery, Cincinnati
Children's Hospital Medical Center, University of
Cincinnati College of Medicine, Cincinnati, OH,
USA
Ch 77 Bariatric Surgery in Adolescents

Elizabeth A. Berdan, MD MS
Senior Resident in Surgery, Department of Surgery,
University of Minnesota Medical School,
Minneapolis, MN, USA
Ch 1 Physiology of the Newborn

Martin A. Birchall, MD
Chair of Laryngology, University College London Ear
Institute, Royal National Throat, Nose and Ear
Hospital, London, UK
Ch 79 Tissue Engineering

John W. Brock III, MD
Monroe Carell Jr. Professor and Surgeon-in-Chief;
Professor of Urologic Surgery and Pediatrics;
Director of Pediatric Urology, Monroe Carell Jr.
Children's Hospital at Vanderbilt University,
Nashville, TN, USA
Ch 61 Prune-Belly Syndrome

R. Cartland Burns, MD
Co-Director, Intestinal Care and Rehabilitation Center,
Division of Pediatric General and Thoracic Surgery
View Biography, Children's Hospital of Pittsburgh of
UPMC, Pittsburgh, PA, USA
Ch 41 Inflammatory Bowel Disease

Casey M. Calkins, MD
Associate Professor; Pediatric Surgery, The Medical
College of Wisconsin, The Children's Hospital of
Wisconsin, Milwaukee, WI, USA
Ch 37 Acquired Anorectal Disorders

Patrick C. Cartwright, MD
Professor and Chief, Division of Urology, University of
Utah School of Medicine; Surgeon-in-Chief, Primary
Children's Hospital, Salt Lake City, UT, USA
Ch 56 Bladder and Urethra

Michael G. Caty, MD MMM
Robert Pritzker Professor of Surgery and Chief,
Section of Pediatric Surgery, Yale University School
of Medicine; Surgeon-in-Chief, Yale-New Haven
Children's Hospital, New Haven, CT, USA
Ch 32 Meconium Disease

Joel Cazares, MD
Research Associate, Department of Pediatric General and Urogenital Surgery, Juntendo University School of Medicine, Tokyo, Japan
Ch 43 Biliary Atresia

Nicole M. Chandler, MD
Assistant Professor of Surgery, Division of Pediatric Surgery, All Children's Hospital / Johns Hopkins University School of Medicine, St. Petersburg, FL, USA
Ch 26 The Esophagus

Paul M. Colombani, MD MBA
Robert Garrett Professor of Pediatric Surgery, The Johns Hopkins Univ School of Medicine, Baltimore, Maryland; Pediatric Surgeon-in-charge, Bloomberg Children's Center, The Johns Hopkins Hospital, Baltimore, Maryland; Chairman of Surgery, All Children's Hospital, St. Petersburg, FA, USA
Ch 26 The Esophagus

Arthur Cooper, MD MS
Professor of Surgery, Columbia University College of Physicians and Surgeons; Director of Trauma and Pediatric Surgical Services, Harlem Hospital Center, New York, NY, USA
Ch 14 Early Assessment and Management of Trauma

Douglas E. Coplen, MD
Associate Professor and Director, Department of Surgery, Division of Pediatric Urology, St Louis Children's Hospital and Washington University School of Medicine, St. Louis, MO, USA
Ch 54 Ureteral Obstruction and Malformations

M. Sidney Dassinger III, MD
Associate Professor of Surgery, Division of Pediatric Surgery, Arkansas Children's Hospital, University of Arkansas for Medical Sciences, Little Rock, AR, USA
Ch 31 Malrotation

Andrew M. Davidoff, MD
Chairman and Member, Department of Surgery, St. Jude Children's Research Hospital, Memphis, TN, USA
Ch 66 Neuroblastoma

W. Robert DeFoor, Jr. MD MPH
Associate Professor and Director of Clinical Research, Division of Pediatric Urology, Cincinnati Children's Hospital Medical Center, Cincinnati, OH, USA
Ch 55 Urinary Tract Infections and Vesicoureteral Reflux

Romano T. DeMarco, MD
Chief and Associate Professor, Division of Pediatric Urology, Department of Urology, Gainesville, FL, USA
Ch 61 Prune-Belly Syndrome

Laura K. Diaz, MD
Pediatric Anesthesiologist, Department of Anesthesiology and Critical Care Medicine, The Children's Hospital of Philadelphia; Assistant Professor of Anesthesiology and Critical Care, Perelman School of Medicine at the University of Pennsylvania, Philadelphia, PA, USA
Ch 3 Anesthetic Considerations for Pediatric Surgical Conditions

Diana L. Diesen, MD
Assistant Professor of Surgery, Division of Pediatric Surgery, UT Southwestern Medical Center, Dallas, TX, USA
Ch 76 Endocrine Disorders and Tumors

Kathleen M. Dominguez, MD
Surgical Critical Care Fellow, Nationwide Children's Hospital, Columbus, OH, USA
Ch 33 Necrotizing Enterocolitis

Peter F. Ehrlich, MD MSc
Associate Professor of Surgery, Section of Pediatric Surgery; Vice Chair Renal Tumor, Children Oncology Group, University of Michigan, Ann Arbor MI, USA
Ch 65 Renal Tumors

Jack S. Elder, MD
Chief of Urology, Henry Ford Health System; Associate Director, Vattikuti Urology Institute, Department of Urology, Children's Hospital of Michigan, Detroit, MI, USA
Ch 57 Posterior Urethral Valves

Mauricio A. (Tony) Escobar, Jr. MD
Pediatric Trauma Medical Director, Pediatric Surgery, MultiCare Health Systems, Mary Bridge Children's Hospital; Health Center Clinical Instructor, Department of Surgery, University of Washington Medicine, Tacoma, WA, USA
Ch 32 Meconium Disease

Mary E. Fallat, MD
Hirikati S. Nagaraj Professor of Surgery, Division of Pediatric Surgery, University of Louisville, Louisville, KY, USA
Ch 38 Intussusception

Steven J. Fishman, MD
Stuart and Jane Weitzman Family Chair, Department of Surgery; Co-Director, Vascular Anomalies Center, Boston Children's Hospital; Professor of Surgery, Harvard Medical School, Boston, MA, USA
Ch 72 Vascular and Lymphatic Anomalies

Alan W. Flake, MD
Ruth and Tristram C. Colket, Jr. Chair in Pediatric
    Surgery; Director, Children's Center for Fetal
    Research, Children's Hospital of Philadelphia;
    Professor of Surgery and Obstetrics, University of
    Pennsylvania, School of Medicine, Philadelphia, PA,
    USA
Ch 22 Congenital Bronchopulmonary Malformations

Jason D. Fraser, MD
Pediatric Surgery Fellow, Department of Surgery,
    Children's Mercy Hospital, Kansas City, MO, USA
Ch 50 Inguinal Hernias and Hydroceles

Samir K. Gadepalli, MD MBA
Assistant Professor, Pediatric Surgery and Surgical
    Critical Care, University of Michigan, Ann Arbor,
    MI, USA
Ch 7 Mechanical Ventilation in Pediatric Surgical Disease

Barbara A. Gaines, MD
Clinical Director, Division of General and Thoracic
    Surgery; Director of Trauma and Injury Prevention;
    Program Director, Pediatric Surgery, Children's
    Hospital of Pittsburgh of UPMC; Associate
    Professor of Surgery, University of Pittsburgh School
    of Medicine, Pittsburgh, PA, USA
Ch 16 Abdominal and Renal Trauma

Alan S. Gamis, MD MPH
Professor of Pediatrics, Division of Pediatric
    Hematology, Oncology, Children's Mercy Hospital,
    Kansas City, MO, USA
Ch 69 Lymphomas

Alejandro V. Garcia, MD
Senior Clinical Research Fellow, Division of Pediatric
    Surgery, Morgan Stanley Children's Hospital,
    Columbia University Medical Center, New York,
    NY, USA
Ch 6 Extracorporeal Membrane Oxygenation

John M. Gatti, MD
Associate Professor of Surgery, Department of Surgery,
    Children's Mercy Hospital, University of Missouri,
    Kansas City, Kansas City, MO, USA
*Ch 52 The Acute Scrotum, Ch 62 Disorders of Sexual
Differentiation*

George K. Gittes, MD
Surgeon-in-Chief, Benjamin R. Fisher Chair of
    Pediatric Surgery, Division of General and Thoracic
    Surgery, Children's Hospital of Pittsburgh of UPMC,
    Department of Surgery, University of Pittsburgh
    School of Medicine, Pittsburgh, PA, USA
Ch 46 Lesions of the Pancreas

Jeffrey Goldstein, MD
Chief, Section of Plastic and Craniofacial Surgery;
    Professor of Surgery, University of Missouri-Kansas
    City School of Medicine, Children's Mercy Hospital,
    Kansas City, MO, USA
Ch 17 Head Injury and Facial Trauma

Richard Grady, MD
Professor of Urology, Attending, Pediatric Urology;
    Fellowship Program Director, The University of
    Washington School of Medicine, Seattle Children's
    Hospital, Seattle, WA, USA
Ch 58 Bladder and Cloacal Exstrophy

Clarence S. Greene, Jr. MD
Associate Professor of Neurosurgery, University of
    Missouri–Kansas City School of Medicine; Attending
    Neurosurgeon, Children's Mercy Hospital, Kansas
    City, Missouri
Ch 19 Neurosurgical Conditions

Tracy C. Grikscheit, MD
Assistant Professor of Surgery, Division of Pediatric
    Surgery, Keck School of Medicine, The Saban
    Research Institute, Children's Hospital Los Angeles,
    Los Angeles, CA USA
Ch 79 Tissue Engineering

André Hebra, MD
H. Biemann Othersen Professor of Surgery,
    Department of Surgery, Medical University of South
    Carolina; Surgeon-in-Chief, MUSC Children's
    Hospital, Charleston, SC, USA
*Ch 21 Management of Laryngotracheal Obstruction in
Children*

Richard J. Hendrickson, MD
Associate Professor of Pediatric Surgery, University of
    Missouri School of Medicine at Kansas City;
    Director, Small Bowel Transplantation, Children's
    Mercy Hospital, Kansas City, MO, USA
Ch 67 Lesions of the Liver

Robert A. Hetz, MD
Surgical Resident and Post-doctoral Research Fellow,
    Department of Surgery, University of Texas Medical
    School at Houston, Houston, TX, USA
Ch 70 Rhabdomyosarcoma

Shinjiro Hirose, MD
Associate Professor of Surgery, Department of Surgery,
    Division of Pediatric Surgery, University of
    California, San Francisco, CA, USA
Ch 10 Fetal Therapy

Ronald B. Hirschl, MD MS
Professor and Head, Section of Pediatric Surgery,
    Department of Surgery, University of Michigan, Ann
    Arbor, MI, USA
Ch 7 Mechanical Ventilation in Pediatric Surgical Disease

George W. Holcomb III, MD MBA
Katharine B. Richardson Professor of Surgery,
  Surgeon-in-Chief, Department of Surgery, Children's
  Mercy Hospital, Kansas City, MO, USA
*Ch 28 Gastroesophageal Reflux, Ch 39 Alimentary Tract
Duplications, Ch 44 Choledochal Cyst and Gallbladder
Disease, Video 23.2 Thoracoscopic Debridement and
Decortication for Empyema, Video 23.3 Thoracoscopic
Right Middle Lobectomy, Video 25.1 Thoracoscopic Biopsy
of an Anterior Mediastinal Mass, Video 26.1 Laparoscopic
Esophagomyotomy, Video 28.1 Laparoscopic
Fundoplication: Minimal Esophageal Dissection &
Placement of Esophago-Crural Sutures, Video 28.2
Laparoscopic Thal Fundoplication, Video 28.3 The Use of
Surgisis for Hiatal Reinforcement at Re-Do Laparoscopic
Fundoplication and Antroplasty, Video 28.4 Laparoscopic
Gastrostomy, Video 29.1 Laparoscopic Repair of Pyloric
Atresia, Video 30.1 Laparoscopic Duodenal Atresia Repair
with U-clips, Video 44.1 Laparoscopic Cholecystectomy,
Video 47.2 Laparoscopic Resection of a Splenic Cyst,
Video 51.1 Two-Staged Laparoscopic Orchiopexy for a
Left Non-Palpable Testis, Video 76.1 Laparoscopic Right
Adrenalectomy*

Gregory W. Hornig, MD
Clinical Assistant Professor, University of Missouri-
  Kansas City; Chief, Section of Neurosurgery,
  Children's Mercy Hospital and Clinics, Kansas City,
  MO, USA
Ch 19 Neurosurgical Conditions

Thomas H. Inge, MD PhD
Professor of Surgery and Pediatrics, Division of
  Pediatric General & Thoracic Surgery, Cincinnati
  Children's Hospital Medical Center, Cincinnati, OH,
  USA
*Ch 77 Bariatric Surgery in Adolescents, Video 77.1
Laparoscopic Roux-En-Y Gastric Bypass*

Corey W. Iqbal, MD
Chief, Section of Fetal Surgery, Children's Mercy
  Hospital, Kansas City, MO USA
Ch 10 Fetal Therapy, Ch 28 Gastroesophageal Reflux

Saleem Islam, MD MPH
Associate Professor of Surgery, University of Florida
  College of Medicine, Gainesville, FL, USA
Ch 48 Congenital Abdominal Wall Defects

Tom Jaksic, MD PhD
W. Hardy Hendren Professor of Surgery Harvard
  Medical School, Boston Children's Hospital, Boston,
  MA, USA
Ch 2 Nutritional Support for the Pediatric Patient

David Juang, MD
Assistant Professor of Surgery; Director, Trauma, Burns
  & Surgical Critical Care Director, Surgical Critical
  Care Fellowship, Department of Surgery, Children's
  Mercy Hospital, University of Missouri—Kansas
  City, Kansas City, MO, USA
*Ch 13 Burns, Video 29.1 Laparoscopic Repair of Pyloric
Atresia*

Aviva L. Katz, MD MA
Assistant Professor of Surgery, Pediatric General and
  Thoracic Surgery; Director, Ethics Consultation
  Service, Children's Hospital of Pittsburgh of UPMC,
  Department of Surgery, University of Pittsburgh
  School of Medicine, Pittsburgh, PA, USA
Ch 80 Ethics in Pediatric Surgery

Scott J. Keckler, MD
Pediatric Surgeon, Springfield, MO, USA
Ch 39 Alimentary Tract Duplications

Robert E. Kelly, Jr. MD
Chief, Division of Pediatric Surgery, Department of
  Surgery, Children's Hospital of The King's
  Daughters; Professor of Clinical Surgery and
  Pediatrics, Eastern Virginia Medical School, Norfolk,
  VA, USA
*Ch 20 Congenital Chest Wall Deformities, Video 20.1
The Nuss Procedure*

E. Marty Knott, DO
Pediatric Surgery Fellow, Department of Surgery,
  Children's Mercy Hospital, University of Missouri—
  Kansas City, MO, USA
Ch 13 Burns

Curt S. Koontz, MD
Assistant Professor of Surgery, Department of Surgery,
  University of Tennessee College of Medicine—
  Chattanooga, Chattanooga, TN, USA
Ch 29 Lesions of the Stomach

Thomas M. Krummel, MD
Emile Holman Professor and Chair, Department of
  Surgery, Stanford University School of Medicine;
  Susan B. Ford Surgeon-in-Chief, Lucile Packard
  Children's Hospital, Palo Alto, CA, USA
Ch 9 Surgical Infectious Disease

Arlet G. Kurkchubasche, MD
Associate Professor of Surgery and Pediatrics, Division
  of Pediatric Surgery, Alpert Medical School of Brown
  University, Providence, RI, USA
Ch 71 Nevus and Melanoma

Jean-Martin Laberge, MD
Professor and Associate Chair, Department of Pediatric
  Surgery, McGill University, Division of Pediatric
  General Surgery, The Montreal Children's Hospital
  of the McGill University Health Center, Montreal,
  Quebec, Canada
*Ch 68 Teratomas, Dermoids and Other Soft Tissue
Tumors*

Kevin P. Lally, MD MS
A.G. McNeese, Chair in Pediatric Surgery; Richard J. Andrassy Distinguished Professor; Chairman and Professor, Department of Pediatric Surgery, University of Texas Medical School at Houston, Houston, TX, USA
Ch 24 Congenital Diaphragmatic Hernia and Eventration

Jacob C. Langer, MD
Professor of Surgery, Division of Pediatric General and Thoracic Surgery, University of Toronto, Toronto, Ontario, Canada
Ch 34 Hirschsprung Disease

Oliver B. Lao, MD MPH
Pediatric Surgical Fellow, Children's Hospital and Medical Center, Omaha, NE, USA
Ch 60 Circumcision

Hanmin Lee, MD
Professor of Surgery, Pediatrics, Ob-Gyn and Reproductive Health Services; Chief, Division of Pediatric Surgery; Director, Fetal Treatment Center; Surgeon-in-Chief, UCSF Benioff Children's Hospital, UCSF School of Medicine, San Francsisco, CA, USA
Ch 10 Fetal Therapy

Steven L. Lee, MD
Associate Professor of Surgery and Pediatrics, David Geffen School of Medicine at UCLA; Chief of Pediatric Surgery at Harbor-UCLA, Los Angeles, CA, USA
Ch 42 Appendicitis

J. Joy Lee, MD
Chief Resident in Urology, Department of Urology, Stanford University Medical Center, Stanford, CA, USA
Ch 51 Undescended Testes and Testicular Tumors

Philip A. Letourneau, MD
Senior Resident, Department of Surgery, University of Texas Medical School at Houston, Houston, TX, USA
Ch 70 Rhabdomyosarcoma

Daniel E. Levin, MD
Pediatric Surgery Research Fellow, Division of Pediatric Surgery, The Saban Research Institute, Children's Hospital Los Angeles, Los Angeles, CA USA
Ch 79 Tissue Engineering

Marc A. Levitt, MD
Director, Colorectal Center for Children, Cincinnati Children's Hospital Medical Center; Professor of Surgery, Division of Pediatric Surgery, Department of Surgery, University of Cincinnati, Cincinnati, OH, USA
Ch 35 Imperforate Anus and Cloacal Malformations, Ch 36 Fecal Incontinence and Constipation, Video 34.1 Trans Anal Pullthrough, Video 35.1 Rectourethral Fistula Repair, Video 36.1 Appendicostomy for Antegrade Enemas for Patients with Fecal Incontinence

Shauna M. Levy, MD
Surgical Resident and Clinical Research Fellow, Department of Surgery, University of Texas Medical School at Houston, Houston, TX, USA
Ch 70 Rhabdomyosarcoma

Karen B. Lewing, MD
Associate Professor of Pediatrics, Division of Pediatric Hematology/Oncology, Children's Mercy Hospital, Kansas City, MO, USA
Ch 69 Lymphomas

Charles M. Leys, MD MSCI
Associate Professor of Surgery, Department of Surgery, University of Wisconsin, Madison, WI, USA
Ch 40 Meckel Diverticulum

Nguyen Thanh Liem, MD PhD
Professor of Pediatric Surgery; Chair of Surgery; Director of Research Institute of Child Health, Department of Surgery, National hospital of Pediatrics, Hanoi, Vietnam
Ch 44 Choledochal Cyst and Gallbladder Disease, Video 44.2 Laparoscopic Excision Choledochal Cyst with Choledocho-Jejunostomy

Danny C. Little, MD
Surgeon in Chief, McLane Children's Hospital, Department of Surgery, Texas A&M College of Medicine, Temple, TX USA
Ch 11 Ingestion of Foreign Bodies, Video 25.1 Thoracoscopic Biopsy of an Anterior Mediastinal Mass

Jennifer A. Lowry, MD
Chief, Section of Clinical Toxicology; Associate Professor of Pediatrics, Children's Mercy Hospital University of Missouri, Kansas City School of Medicine, Kansas City, MO, USA
Ch 12 Bites

Alexandra C. Maki, MD
General Surgery Resident, Department of Surgery, University of Louisville, Louisville, KY, USA
Ch 38 Intussusception

Jeffrey E. Martus, MD
Assistant Professor of Orthopaedic Surgery and
 Pediatrics, Vanderbilt University Medical Center,
 Monroe Carell Jr. Children's Hospital at Vanderbilt,
 Nashville, TN, USA
Ch 18 Pediatric Orthopedic Trauma

Lynne G. Maxwell, MD
Senior Anesthesiologist, Department of Anesthesiology
 and Critical Care Medicine, The Children's Hospital
 of Philadelphia; Associate Professor, Anesthesiology
 and Critical Care, Perelman School of Medicine at
 the University of Pennsylvania, Philadelphia, PA,
 USA
*Ch 3 Anesthetic Considerations for Pediatric Surgical
Conditions*

Jarod McAteer, MD
Clinical Research Fellow, Department of Surgery,
 Seattle Children's Hospital, University of
 Washington School of Medicine, Seattle, WA, USA
Ch 73 Head and Neck Sinuses and Masses

Nilesh M. Mehta, MD
Associate Medical Director, Critical Care Medicine,
 Department of Anesthesiology, Pain and
 Perioperative Medicine, Boston Children's Hospital;
 Associate Professor of Anesthesia, Harvard Medical
 School, Boston, MA, USA
Ch 2 Nutritional Support for the Pediatric Patient

Gregory A. Mencio, MD
Professor and Vice Chairman, Department of
 Orthopaedics, Vanderbilt University Medical Center;
 Chief, Pediatric Orthopaedics, Monroe Carell Jr
 Children's Hospital at Vanderbilt, Nashville, TN,
 USA
Ch 18 Pediatric Orthopedic Trauma

Eugene Minevich, MD
Professor, Division Pediatric Urology, Cincinnati
 Children's Hospital Medical Center, Cincinnati, OH,
 USA
Ch 55 Urinary Tract Infections and Vesicoureteral Reflux

Michael E. Mitchell, MD
Associate Professor of Surgery; Pediatric
 Cardiothoracic Surgeon, Department of Surgery
 Medical College of Wisconsin, Division of Pediatric
 Cardiothoracic Surgery, Children's Hospital of
 Wisconsin, Milwaukee, WI, USA
Ch 58 Bladder and Cloacal Exstrophy

Takeshi Miyano, MD PhD
Professor Emeritus, Pediatric General and Urogenital
 Surgery, Juntendo University School of Medicine,
 Tokyo, Japan
Ch 43 Biliary Atresia

R. Lawrence Moss, MD
Surgeon-in-Chief, Nationwide Children's Hospital,
 The Ohio State University, College of Medicine,
 Columbus, OH, USA
Ch 33 Necrotizing Enterocolitis

J. Patrick Murphy, MD
Professor of Surgery; Chief, Section of Urology,
 Department of Surgery, Children's Mercy Hospital,
 Kansas City, MO, USA
Ch 59 Hypospadias

Don K. Nakayama, MD MBA
Milford B. Hatcher Professor and Chair, Department
 of Surgery, Mercer University School of Medicine,
 Macon, GA, USA
Ch 75 Breast Disease

Jaimie D. Nathan, MD MS
Assistant Professor of Surgery and Pediatrics,
 University of Cincinnati College of Medicine,
 Cincinnati Children's Hospital Medical Center,
 Cincinnati, OH, USA
Ch 45 Solid Organ Transplantation in Children

Donald Nuss, MBChB
Professor of Surgery; Emeritus, Department of Surgery,
 Eastern Virginia Medical School, Norfolk, VA, USA
*Ch 20 Congenital Chest Wall Deformities, Video 20.1
The Nuss Procedure*

Keith T. Oldham, MD
Professor and Chief, Division of Pediatric Surgery,
 Medical College of Wisconsin; Marie Z. Uihlein
 Chair and Surgeon-in-Chief; Clinical Vice President
 of Surgery, Children's Hospital of Wisconsin,
 Milwaukee, WI, USA
Ch 37 Acquired Anorectal Disorders

James A. O'Neill, Jr. MD
JC Foshee Distinguished Professor and Chairman;
 Emeritus, Section of Surgical Sciences, Vanderbilt
 University Medical Center, Nashville, TN, USA
Ch 63 Renovascular Hypertension

Daniel J. Ostlie, MD
Surgeon-in-Chief, American Family Children's
 Hospital, WARF Professor of Pediatric Surgery;
 Chief, Pediatric Surgery, Department of Surgery,
 University of Wisconsin, Madison, WI, USA
*Ch 13 Burns, Ch 30 Duodenal and Intestinal Atresia and
Stenosis, Video 28.2 Laparoscopic Thal Fundoplication,
Video 46.1 Laparoscopic Cyst-Gastrostomy*

H. Biemann Othersen, Jr. MD
Professor of Surgery and Pediatrics; Emeritus Head,
 Division of Pediatric Surgery, Department of
 Surgery, Medical University of South Carolina,
 Charleston, SC, USA
*Ch 21 Management of Laryngotracheal Obstruction in
Children*

Erik G. Pearson, MD
Research Fellow, Children's Center for Fetal Research,
Department of Surgery, Children's Hospital of
Philadelphia, Philadelphia, PA, USA
Ch 22 Congenital Bronchopulmonary Malformations

Alberto Peña, MD
Clinical Professor of Surgery; Founding Director,
Colorectal Center, Cincinnati Children's Hospital
Medical, University of Cincinnati School of
Medicine, Cincinnati, OH, USA
*Ch 35 Imperforate Anus and Cloacal Malformations,
Ch 36 Fecal Incontinence and Constipation, Video 35.1
Rectourethral Fistula Repair, Video 36.1 Appendicostomy
for Antegrade Enemas for Patients with Fecal
Incontinence*

Janine Pettiford, MD
Surgical Scholar Research Fellow, Department of
Pediatric Surgery, Children's Mercy Hospital and
Clinics, Kansas City, MO, USA
Ch 52 The Acute Scrotum

Pramod S. Puligandla, MD MSc
Associate Professor of Surgery and Pediatrics, McGill
University; Pediatric Surgery Program Director,
Divisions of Pediatric Surgery and Pediatric Critical
Care Medicine, The Montreal Children's Hospital of
the McGill University Health Centre, Montreal,
Quebec, Canada
*Ch 68 Teratomas, Dermoids and Other Soft Tissue
Tumors*

Stephen C. Raynor, MD
Professor of Surgery, University of Nebraska Medical
Center; Clinical Service Chief, Children's Hospital
and Medical Center, Omaha, NE, USA
Ch 60 Circumcision

Frederick J. Rescorla, MD
Professor of Surgery, Indiana University School of
Medicine; Surgeon-in-Chief, Riley Hospital for
Children, Indianapolis, IN, USA
*Ch 47 Splenic Conditions, Video 47.1 Laparoscopic
Splenectomy*

Kirsty L. Rialon, MD
Research Fellow, Boston Children's Hospital,
Department of Surgery, Boston, MA, USA
Ch 72 Vascular and Lymphatic Anomalies

Steven S. Rothenberg, MD
Clinical Professor of Surgery, Columbia University
College of Physicians and Surgeons; Chief of
Pediatric Surgery, The Rocky Mountain Hospital
For Children, Denver, CO, USA
*Ch 27 Esophageal Atresia and Tracheoesophageal Fistula
Malformations, Video 22.1 Thoracoscopic Right Lower
Lobectomy for a CCAM, Video 23.1 Thoracoscopic Lung
Biopsy Using the Endoscopic Stapler and Using a Loop
Ligature, Video 27.1 Thoracoscopic Repair of Esophageal
Atresia with Tracheoesophageal Fistula*

Alejandro R. Ruiz-Elizalde, MD
Pediatric Surgery Fellow, Division of Pediatric Surgery,
Department of Surgery, Children's Hospital at OU
Medical Center, University of Oklahoma, Oklahoma
City, OK, USA
Ch 15 Thoracic Trauma

Frederick C. Ryckman, MD
Professor of Surgery, Department of Pediatric Surgery;
Sr. Vice President—Medical Operations, Cincinnati
Children's Hospital, University of Cincinnati,
Cincinnati, OH, USA
Ch 45 Solid Organ Transplantation in Children

Daniel A. Saltzman, MD PhD
AS Leonard Endowed Chair in Pediatric Surgery;
Associate Professor of Surgery and Pediatrics; Chief,
Division of Pediatric Surgery, University of
Minnesota Medical School; Surgeon-in-Chief,
University of Minnesota Amplatz Children's
Hospital, Minneapolis, MN, USA
Ch 1 Physiology of the Newborn

Bradley J. Segura, MD PhD
Assistant Professor of Surgery and Pediatrics,
University of Minnesota Amplatz Children's
Hospital, Minneapolis, MN, USA
Ch 1 Physiology of the Newborn

Sohail R. Shah, MD MHA
Assistant Professor of Surgery, Children's Mercy
Hospital, Kansas City, MO, USA
Ch 11 Ingestion of Foreign Bodies

Robert C. Shamberger, MD
Chief of Surgery, Boston Children's Hospital; Robert
E. Gross Professor of Surgery, Harvard Medical
School, Boston, MA, USA
Ch 65 Renal Tumors

Ellen Shapiro, MD
Professor of Urology; Director, Pediatric Urology,
Department of Urology, New York University School
of Medicine, New York, NY, USA
Ch 57 Posterior Urethral Valves

Mukta Sharma, MD MPH
Assistant Professor of Pediatrics, Division of
Hematology/Oncology, Children's Mercy Hospitals
and Clinics, University of Missouri at Kansas City
School of Medicine, Kansas City, MO, USA
Ch 5 Coagulopathies and Sickle Cell Disease

Kenneth Shaw, MD
Assistant Professor, Department of Pediatric Surgery,
McGill University, Division of Pediatric General
Surgery, The Montreal Children's Hospital of the
McGill University Health Center, Montreal, Quebec,
Canada
*Ch 68 Teratomas, Dermoids and Other Soft Tissue
Tumors*

Curtis A. Sheldon, MD
Founding Director, Division of Urology, Center for
Genitourinary Reconstruction, Cincinnati Children's
Hospital Medical Center, Cincinnati, Ohio. USA
MD
Ch 55 Urinary Tract Infections and Vesicoureteral Reflux

Linda M. Dairiki Shortliffe, MD
Stanley McCormick Memorial Professor and Chair
Emerita, Department of Urology, Stanford
University School of Medicine, Stanford, CA, USA
Ch 51 Undescended Testes and Testicular Tumors

Michael A. Skinner, MD
The Edwin Ide Smith, M.D. Professorship in Pediatric
Surgery, Division of Pediatric Surgery, UT
Southwestern Medical Center, Dallas, TX, USA
Ch 76 Endocrine Disorders and Tumors

Bethany J. Slater, MD
Pediatric Surgery Fellow, Division of Pediatric Surgery,
Michael E. DeBakey Department of Surgery, Baylor
College of Medicine, Houston, TX, USA
Ch 9 Surgical Infectious Disease

Samuel D. Smith, MD
Professor of Pediatric Surgery, University of Arkansas
for Medical Sciences, Little Rock, AR, USA
Ch 31 Malrotation

Brent W. Snow, MD
Professor of Surgery and Pediatrics, Pediatric Urology
Chairman, University of Utah School of Medicine,
Salt Lake City, UT, USA
Ch 56 Bladder and Urethra

Charles L. Snyder, MD
Section Chief, Division of General and Thoracic
Surgery; Director of Clinical Research; Professor of
Surgery, Children's Mercy Hospital, Kansas City,
MO, USA
Ch 50 Inguinal Hernias and Hydroceles

Howard M. Snyder III, MD
Professor of Urology, Department of Surgery,
University of Pennsylvania School of Medicine;
Director of Surgical Teaching, Division of Pediatric
Urology, Children's Hospital of Philadelphia,
Philadelphia, PA, USA
*Ch 53 Developmental and Positional Anomalies of the
Kidneys*

Shawn D. St. Peter, MD
Professor of Surgery; Director, Center for Prospective
Trials, Department of Surgery, Children's Mercy
Hospital, Kansas City, MO, USA
*Ch 23 Acquired Lesions of the Lung and Pleura, Ch 78
Evidence-Based Medicine, Video 28.1 Laparoscopic
Fundoplication: Minimal Esophageal Dissection &
Placement of Esophago-Crural Sutures, Video 30.1
Laparoscopic Duodenal Atresia Repair with U-clips*

Heidi A. Stephany, MD
Assistant Professor of Urology, University of Pittsburgh
School of Medicine, Children's Hospital of
Pittsburgh, Pittsburgh, PA
Ch 61 Prune-Belly Syndrome

Charles J.H. Stolar, MD
Rudolph N. Schullinger Professor Emeritus of Surgery
and Pediatrics, Columbia University, College of
Physicians and Surgeons and Children's Specialty
Network, Inc., Santa Barbara, CA, USA
Ch 6 Extracorporeal Membrane Oxygenation

Julie L. Strickland, MD MPH
Professor Obstetrics and Gynaecology, University of
Missouri, Kansas City School of Medicine; Chief,
Gynecologic Surgery, Children's Mercy Hospital,
Kansas City, Missouri, USA
*Ch 74 Pediatric and Adolescent Gynecology, Video 74.1
Non-communicating Uterine Horn: A Laparoscopic
Approach, Video 74.2 Prepubertal EUA and Vaginoscopy*

Veronica F. Sullins, MD
Chief Resident, Department of Surgery, Harbor-UCLA
Medical Center; Pediatric Surgery Research Fellow,
Division of Pediatric Surgery, University of
California Los Angeles, Los Angeles, CA, USA
Ch 42 Appendicitis

Arul S. Thirumoorthi, MD
Senior Clinical Research Fellow, Division of Pediatric
Surgery, Morgan Stanley Children's Hospital,
Columbia University Medical Center, New York,
NY, USA
Ch 6 Extracorporeal Membrane Oxygenation

Gregory M. Tiao, MD
Richard G. and Geralyn Azizkhan Chair in Pediatric
Surgery; Professor of Surgery and Pediatrics, The
University of Cincinnati Department of Surgery,
Surgical Directory, Liver Transplantation, Cincinnati
Children's Hospital Medical Center, Cincinnati, OH,
USA
Ch 45 Solid Organ Transplantation in Children

Kelly S. Tieves, DO MS
Associate Professor of Pediatrics, Department of
Pediatrics, Critical Care Medicine, University of
Missouri-Kansas City School of Medicine, Pediatric
Intensivist, Children's Mercy Hospital, Kansas City,
MO, USA
Ch 17 Head Injury and Facial Trauma

Juan A. Tovar, MD PhD
Chair and Surgeon-in-Chief, Department of Pediatric
Surgery, Hospital Universitario La Paz, Universidad
Autónoma de Madrid, Madrid, Spain
Ch 25 Mediastinal Tumors

Thomas F. Tracy, Jr. MS MD
Professor of Surgery and Pediatrics; Vice Chairman,
Department of Surgery, Alpert Medical School,
Brown University; Pediatric Surgeon in Chief,
Hasbro Children's Hospital, Providence, RI, USA
Ch 71 Nevus and Melanoma

Erica J. Traxel, MD
Assistant Professor, Department of Surgery, Division of
Pediatric Urology, St Louis Children's Hospital,
Washington University School of Medicine, St.
Louis, MO, USA
Ch 54 Ureteral Obstruction and Malformations

KuoJen Tsao, MD
Associate Professor, Department of Pediatric Surgery,
University of Texas Medical School at Houston,
Houston, TX, USA
*Ch 24 Congenital Diaphragmatic Hernia and
Eventration, Video 28.3 The Use of Surgisis for Hiatal
Reinforcement at Re-Do Laparoscopic Fundoplication and
Antroplasty, Video 28.4 Laparoscopic Gastrostomy, Video
47.2 Laparoscopic Resection of a Splenic Cyst*

David W. Tuggle, MD FACS
Associate Trauma Medical Director; Clinical Professor,
Division of Pediatric Surgery, Dell Children's
Medical Center of Central Texas, Department of
Surgery, University of Texas Southwestern Medical
School, Austin, Texas
Ch 15 Thoracic Trauma

Ravindra K. Vegunta, MBBS
Chief of Pediatric Surgery, Banner of Children's
Specialists, Cardon Children's Medical Center, Mesa,
AZ; Visiting Clinical Professor of Surgery, University
of Illinois College of Medicine at Peoria, Peoria, IL,
USA
Ch 8 Vascular Access

Daniel von Allmen, MD
Director, Division of Pediatric General and Thoracic
Surgery, Cincinnati Children's Hospital Medical
Center, Cincinnati, OH, USA
*Ch 64 Principles of Adjuvant Therapy in Childhood
Cancer*

John H.T. Waldhausen, MD
Professor of Surgery, Division Chief Pediatric General
and Thoracic Surgery, Department of Surgery,
Seattle Children's Hospital, University of
Washington School of Medicine, Seattle, WA, USA
Ch 73 Head and Neck Sinuses and Masses

M. Chad Wallis, MD
Associate Professor of Surgery, Division of Urology,
University of Utah, Primary Children's Medical
Center, Salt Lake City, Utah, USA
Ch 56 Bladder and Urethra

Bradley A. Warady, MD
Professor of Pediatrics, University of Missouri-Kansas
City School of Medicine; Senior Associate Chairman,
Department of Pediatrics; Director, Pediatric
Nephrology; Director, Dialysis and Transplantation,
Children's Mercy Hospitals and Clinics, Kansas City,
MO, USA
Ch 4 Renal Impairment

Gary S. Wasserman, DO
Section of Clinical Toxicology and Professor Emeritus
of Pediatrics Children's Mercy Hospital University of
Missouri—Kansas City School of Medicine, Kansas
City, MO, USA
Ch 12 Bites

Thomas R. Weber, MD
Professor of Pediatric Surgery, Rush University School
of Medicine, Chicago, IL, USA
Ch 49 Umbilical and Other Abdominal Wall Hernias

David R. White, MD
Associate Professor; Director, Division of Pediatric
Otolaryngology Department of Otolaryngology-
Head and Neck Surgery Medical University of South
Carolina, Charleston, SC, USA
*Ch 21 Management of Laryngotracheal Obstruction in
Children*

Brian M. Wicklund, MDCM MPH
Associate Professor of Pediatrics, University of
Missouri-Kansas City, School of Medicine; Director,
Coagulation Medicine Program, Division of
Hematology/Oncology, Children's Mercy Hospitals
and Clinics, Kansas City, MO, USA
Ch 5 Coagulopathies and Sickle Cell Disease

John Wiersch, MD
Research Fellow, Division of General and Thoracic
Surgery, Children's Hospital of Pittsburgh of UPMC,
Department of Surgery, University of Pittsburgh
School of Medicine, Pittsburgh, PA, USA
Ch 46 Lesions of the Pancreas

Gerald M. Woods, MD
Division Director, Division of Hematology/Oncology/
BMT; Director, Sickle Cell Program; Professor of
Pediatrics, University of Missouri-Kansas City
School of Medicine, Children's Mercy Hospitals and
Clinics, Kansas City, MO, USA
Ch 5 Coagulopathies and Sickle Cell Disease

Hsi-Yang Wu, MD
Associate Professor of Urology, Department of
Urology, Stanford University School of Medicine;
Pediatric Urology Fellowship Program Director,
Lucile Packard Children's Hospital, Stanford, CA,
USA
*Ch 53 Developmental and Positional Anomalies of the
Kidneys*

Mark L. Wulkan, MD
Surgeon-in-Chief, Children's Healthcare of Atlanta;
Professor and Chief, Pediatric Surgery, Emory
University School of Medicine, Atlanta, GA, USA
*Ch 29 Lesions of the Stomach, Video 29.2 Laparoscopic
Pyloromyotomy*

Atsuyuki Yamataka, MD PhD
Professor & Head, Pediatric General & Urogenital
Surgery, Juntendo University School of Medicine;
Visting Co-Professor, The Third Department of
Surgery, Tokyo Medical University; Director,
Perinatal Medical Support Centre, Juntendo,
University School of Medicine, Tokyo, Japan
Ch 43 Biliary Atresia, Video 43.1 Laparoscopic Kasai

SECTION I

GENERAL

CHAPTER 1

PHYSIOLOGY OF THE NEWBORN

Elizabeth A. Berdan • Bradley J. Segura • Daniel A. Saltzman

Of all pediatric patients, the neonate possesses the most distinctive and rapidly changing physiologic characteristics. These changes are necessary because the newborn must adapt from placental support to the extrauterine environment. There is also early organ adaptation, and the physiologic demands of rapid growth and development. This chapter will emphasize the dynamic physiologic alterations of the neonate.

Newborns are classified based on gestational age vs weight, and gestational age vs head circumference and length. Preterm infants are those born before 37 weeks of gestation. Term infants are those born between 37 and 42 weeks of gestation, while post-term infants have a gestation that exceeds 42 weeks. Babies whose weight is below the 10th percentile for age are considered small-for-gestational-age (SGA). Those at or above the 90th percentile are large-for-gestational-age (LGA). The babies whose weight falls between these extremes are appropriate-for-gestational-age (AGA). Further subclassified, premature infants are characterized as moderately low birth weight if they weigh between 1501–2500 g, very low birth weight between 1001–1500 g and extremely low birth weight if less than 1000 g.

SGA newborns are thought to suffer intrauterine growth retardation (IUGR) as a result of placental, maternal, or fetal abnormalities. Conditions associated with IUGR are shown in Figure 1-1. SGA infants have a body weight below what is appropriate for their age, yet their body length and head circumference are age appropriate. To classify an infant as SGA, the gestational age must be estimated by the physical findings summarized in Table 1-1.

Although SGA infants may weigh the same as premature infants, they have different physiologic characteristics. Due to intrauterine malnutrition, body fat levels are frequently below 1% of the total body weight. This lack of body fat increases the risk of hypothermia with SGA infants. Hypoglycemia is the most common metabolic problem for neonates and develops earlier in SGA infants due to higher metabolic activity and reduced glycogen stores. The red blood cell (RBC) volume and the total blood volume are much higher in the SGA infant compared with the preterm AGA or the non-SGA full-term infant. This rise in RBC volume frequently leads to polycythemia, with an associated rise in blood viscosity. Due to an adequate length of gestation, the SGA infant has pulmonary function approaching that of an AGA or a full-term infant.

Infants born before 37 weeks of gestation, regardless of birth weight, are considered premature. The physical exam of the premature infant reveals many abnormalities.

Special problems with the preterm infant include the following:
1. Weak suck reflex
2. Inadequate gastrointestinal absorption
3. Hyaline membrane disease (HMD)
4. Intraventricular hemorrhage
5. Hypothermia
6. Patent ductus arteriosus
7. Apnea
8. Hyperbilirubinemia
9. Necrotizing enterocolitis (NEC)

SPECIFIC PHYSIOLOGIC PROBLEMS OF THE NEWBORN

Glucose Metabolism

The fetus maintains a blood glucose value 70–80% of maternal value by facilitated diffusion across the placenta. There is a build-up of glycogen stores in the liver, skeleton, and cardiac muscles during the later stages of fetal development, but little gluconeogenesis. The newborn must depend on glycolysis until exogenous glucose is supplied. Following delivery, the baby depletes its hepatic glycogen stores within two to three hours. The newborn is severely limited in his or her ability to use fat and protein as substrates to synthesize glucose. When total parenteral nutrition (TPN) is needed, the glucose infusion rate should be initiated at 4–6 mg/kg/min and advanced 1–2 mg/kg/min to a goal of 12 mg/kg/min.

Hypoglycemia

Clinical signs of hypoglycemia are nonspecific and subtle. Seizure and coma are the most common manifestations of severe hypoglycemia. Neonatal hypoglycemia is generally defined as a glucose level lower than 50 mg/dL.[1] Infants who are at high risk for developing hypoglycemia are those who are premature, SGA, and born to mothers with gestational diabetes, severe preeclampsia, and HELLP (hemolysis, elevated liver enzymes, low platelet count). Newborns that require surgical procedures are at particular risk of developing hypoglycemia; therefore, a 10% glucose infusion is typically started on admission to the hospital. Hypoglycemia is treated with an infusion of 1–2 mL/kg (4–8 mg/kg/min) of 10% glucose. If an emergency operation is required, concentrations of up to 25% glucose may be used. Traditionally, central venous access has been a prerequisite for glucose infusions exceeding 12.5%. During the first 36 to 48 hours after a major surgical procedure, it is common to see wide variations in serum glucose levels.

Hyperglycemia

Hyperglycemia is a common problem with the use of parenteral nutrition in very immature infants who are less than 30 weeks' gestation and less than 1.1 kg birth weight. These infants are usually fewer than 3 days of age and are frequently septic.[2] This hyperglycemia appears to be associated with both insulin resistance and relative insulin deficiency, reflecting the prolonged catabolism seen in very low birth weight infants.[3] Historically, neonatal hyperglycemia has been linked to intraventricular hemorrhage, dehydration, and electrolyte losses; however, a causal relationship has not been established. Congenital hyperinsulinism refers to an inherited disorder that is the most common cause of recurrent hypoglycemia in the infant. This group of disorders was previously referred to as nesidioblastosis, which is a misnomer. Nesidioblastosis is a term used to describe hyperinsulinemic hypoglycemia attributed to dysfunctional pancreatic beta cells with a characteristically abnormal histological appearance.

Calcium

Calcium is actively transported across the placenta. Of the total amount of calcium transferred across the placenta, 75% occurs after 28 weeks' gestation.[4] This observation partially accounts for the high incidence of hypocalcemia in preterm infants. Neonates are predisposed to hypocalcemia due to limited calcium stores, renal immaturity, and relative hypoparathyroidism secondary to suppression by high fetal calcium levels. Some infants are at further risk for neonatal calcium disturbances due to the presence of genetic defects, pathological intrauterine conditions, or birth trauma.[5] Hypocalcemia is defined as an ionized calcium level of less than 1.22 mmol/L (4.9 mg/dL).[6] At greatest risk for hypocalcemia are preterm infants, newborn surgical patients, and infants of complicated pregnancies, such as those of diabetic mothers or those receiving bicarbonate infusions. Calcitonin, which inhibits calcium mobilization from the bone, is increased in premature and asphyxiated infants.

Signs of hypocalcemia are similar to those of hypoglycemia and may include jitteriness, seizures, cyanosis, vomiting, and myocardial arrhythmias. Hypocalcemic infants have increased muscle tone, which helps differentiate infants with hypocalcemia from those with hypoglycemia. Symptomatic hypocalcemia is treated with 10% calcium gluconate administered IV at a dosage of 1–2 mL/kg (100–200 mg/kg) over 30 minutes while monitoring the electrocardiogram for bradycardia.[1] Asymptomatic hypocalcemia is best treated with calcium gluconate in a dose of 50 mg of elemental calcium/kg/day added to the maintenance fluid: 1 mL of 10% calcium gluconate contains 9 mg of elemental calcium. If possible, parenteral calcium should be given through a central venous line given necrosis that may occur should the peripheral IV infiltrate.

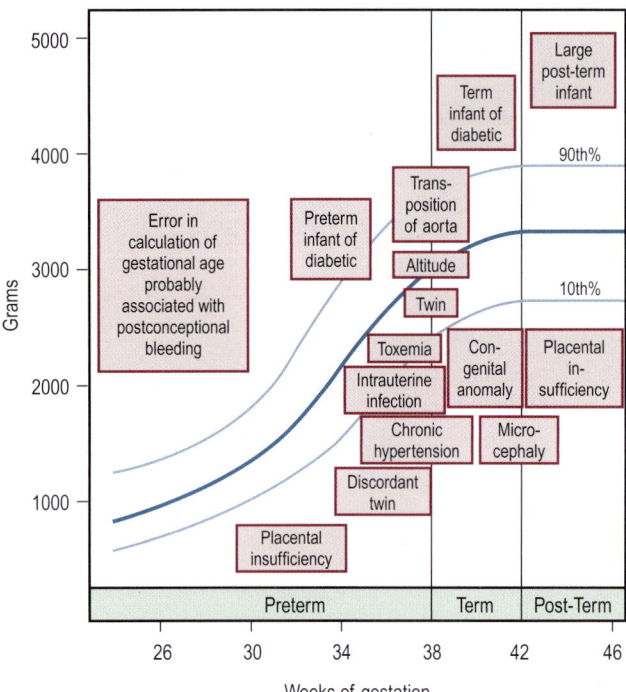

FIGURE 1-1 ■ Graph of conditions associated with deviations in intrauterine growth. The boxes indicate the approximate birth weight and gestational age at which the condition is likely to occur. (Adapted from Avery ME, Villee D, Baker S, et al. Neonatology. In: Avery ME, First LR, editors. Pediatric Medicine. Baltimore: Williams & Wilkins; 1989. p. 148.)

TABLE 1-1 **Clinical Criteria for Classification of Low Birth Weight Infants**

Criteria	36 Weeks (Premature)	37–38 Weeks (Borderline Premature)	39 Weeks (Term)
Plantar creases	Rare, shallow	Heel remains smooth	Creases throughout sole
Size of breast nodule	Not palpable to <3 mm	4 mm	Visible (7 mm)
Head hair	Cotton wool quality		Silky; each strand can be distinguished
Earlobe	Shapeless, pliable with little cartilage		Rigid with cartilage
Testicular descent and scrotal changes	Small scrotum with rugal patch; testes not completely descended	Gradual descent	Enlarged scrotum creased with rugae; fully descended testes

Adapted from Avery ME, Villee D, Baker S, et al. Neonatology. In: Avery ME, First LR, editors. Pediatric Medicine. Baltimore: William & Wilkins; 1989. p. 148.

Magnesium

Magnesium is actively transported across the placenta. Half of total body magnesium is in the plasma and soft tissues. Hypomagnesemia is observed with growth retardation, maternal diabetes, after exchange transfusions, and with hypoparathyroidism. While the mechanisms by which magnesium and calcium interact are not clearly defined, they appear to be interrelated. The same infants at risk for hypocalcemia are also at risk for hypomagnesemia. Magnesium deficiency should be suspected and confirmed in an infant who has seizures that do not respond to calcium therapy. Emergent treatment consists of magnesium sulfate 25–50 mg/kg IV every six hours until normal levels are obtained.

Blood volume

Total RBC volume is at its highest point at delivery. Estimation of blood volume for premature infants, term neonates, and infants are summarized in Table 1-2. By about 3 months of age, total blood volume per kilogram is nearly equal to adult levels as they recover from their postpartum physiologic nadir. The newborn blood volume is affected by shifts of blood between the placenta and the baby prior to clamping the cord. Infants with delayed cord clamping have higher hemoglobin levels.[7] A hematocrit greater than 50% suggests placental transfusion has occurred.

Hemoglobin

At birth, nearly 80% of circulating hemoglobin is fetal $(a_2^A\gamma_2^F)$. When infant erythropoiesis resumes at about 2 to 3 months of age, most new hemoglobin is adult. When the oxygen level is 27 mmHg, 50% of the bound oxygen is released from adult hemoglobin (P_{50} = 27 mmHg). Reduction of hemoglobin's affinity for oxygen allows more oxygen to be released into the tissues at a given oxygen level as shown in Figure 1-2.

Fetal hemoglobin has a P_{50} value 6–8 mmHg lower than that of adult hemoglobin. This lower P_{50} value allows more efficient oxygen delivery from the placenta to the fetal tissues. The fetal hemoglobin equilibrium curve is shifted to the left of the normal adult hemoglobin equilibrium curve. Fetal hemoglobin binds less avidly to 2,3-diphosphoglycerate (2,3-DPG) compared to adult hemoglobin causing a decrease in P_{50}.[8] This is somewhat of a disadvantage to the newborn because lower peripheral oxygen levels are needed before oxygen is released from fetal hemoglobin. By 4 to 6 months of age in a term infant, the hemoglobin equilibrium curve gradually shifts to the right and the P_{50} value approximates that of a normal adult.

Polycythemia

A central venous hemoglobin level greater than 22 g/dL or a hematocrit value greater than 65% during the first week of life is defined as polycythemia. After the central venous hematocrit value reaches 65%, further increases result in rapid exponential increases in blood viscosity. Neonatal polycythemia occurs in infants of diabetic mothers, infants of mothers with toxemia of pregnancy, or SGA infants. Polycythemia is treated using a partial exchange of the infant's blood with fresh whole blood or 5% albumin. This is frequently done for hematocrits greater than 65%.

Anemia

Anemia present at birth is due to hemolysis, blood loss, or decreased erythrocyte production.

Hemolytic Anemia

Hemolytic anemia is most often a result of placental transfer of maternal antibodies that are destroying the

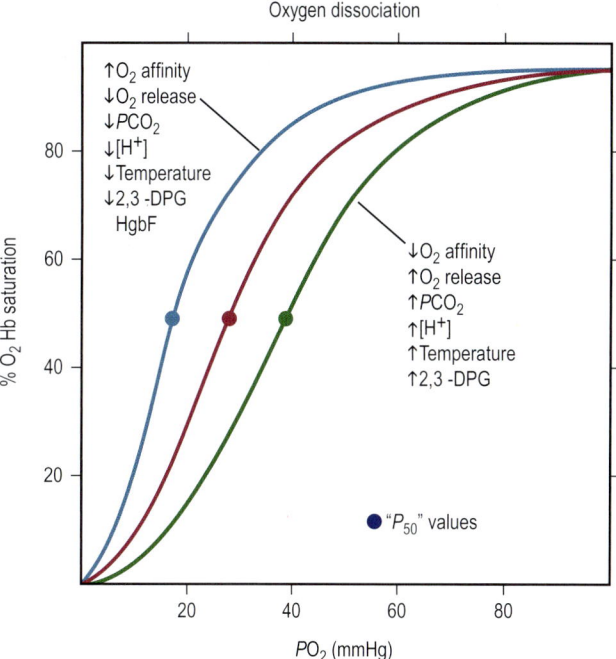

FIGURE 1-2 ■ The oxygen dissociation curve of normal adult blood is shown in red. The P_{50}, the oxygen tension at 50% oxygen saturation, is approximately 27 mmHg. As the curve shifts to the right, the affinity of hemoglobin for oxygen decreases and more oxygen is released. Increases in PCO_2, temperature, 2,3-DPG, and hydrogen ion concentration facilitates the unloading of O_2 from arterial blood to the tissue. With a shift to the left, unloading of O_2 from arterial blood into the tissues is more difficult. Causes of a shift to the left are mirror images of those that cause a shift to the right: decreases in temperature, 2,3-DPG, and hydrogen ion concentration. (Modified from Glancette V, Zipursky A. Neonatal hematology. In: Avery GB, editor, Neonatology. Philadelphia: JB Lippincott; 1986. p. 663.)

TABLE 1-2 Estimation of Blood Volume

Group	Blood Volume (mL/kg)
Premature infants	85–100
Term newborns	85
>1 month	75
3 months to adult	70

Adapted from Rowe PC, editor. The Harriet Lane Handbook. 11th eds. Chicago: Year Book Medical; 1987. p. 25.

infant's erythrocytes. This can be determined by the direct Coombs test. The most common severe anemia is Rh incompatibility. Hemolytic disease in the newborn produces jaundice, pallor, and hepatosplenomegaly. The most severely affected infants manifest hydrops. This massive edema is not strictly related to the hemoglobin level of this infant. ABO incompatibility frequently results in hyperbilirubinemia but rarely causes anemia.

Congenital infections, hemoglobinopathies (sickle cell disease), and thalassemias produce hemolytic anemia. In a severely affected infant with a positive-reacting direct Coombs test result, a cord hemoglobin level less than 10.5 g/dL, or a cord bilirubin level greater than 4.5 mg/dL, immediate exchange transfusion is indicated. For less severely affected infants, exchange transfusion is indicated when the total indirect bilirubin level is greater than 20 mg/dL.

Hemorrhagic Anemia

Significant anemia can develop from hemorrhage that occurs during placental abruption. Internal bleeding (intraventricular, subgaleal, mediastinal, intra-abdominal) in infants can also often lead to severe anemia. Usually, hemorrhage occurs acutely during delivery with the baby occasionally requiring a transfusion. Twin–twin transfusion reactions can produce polycythemia in one baby and profound anemia in the other. Severe cases can lead to death in the donor and hydrops in the recipient.

Anemia of Prematurity

Decreased RBC production frequently contributes to anemia of prematurity. Erythropoietin is not released until a gestational age of 30 to 34 weeks has been reached. These preterm infants have large numbers of erythropoietin-sensitive RBC progenitors. Research has focused on the role of recombinant erythropoietin (epoetin alpha) in treating anemia in preterm infants.[9–11] Successful increases in hematocrit levels using epoetin may obviate the need for blood transfusions and reduce the risk of blood borne infections and reactions. Studies suggest that routine use of epoetin is probably helpful for the very low birth weight infant (<750 g), but its regular use for other preterm infants is not likely to significantly reduce the transfusion rate.[9–11]

Jaundice

In the hepatocyte, bilirubin created by hemolysis is conjugated to glucuronic acid and rendered water soluble. Conjugated (also known as direct) bilirubin is excreted in bile. Unconjugated bilirubin interferes with cellular respiration and is toxic to neural cells. Subsequent neural damage is termed *kernicterus* and produces athetoid cerebral palsy, seizures, sensorineural hearing loss, and, rarely, death.

The newborn's liver has a metabolic excretory capacity for bilirubin that is not equal to its task. Even healthy full-term infants usually have an elevated unconjugated bilirubin level. This peaks about the third day of life at approximately 6.5–7.0 mg/dL and does not return to

TABLE 1-3	Causes of Prolonged Indirect Hyperbilirubinemia
Breast milk jaundice	Pyloric stenosis
Hemolytic disease	Crigler–Najjar syndrome
Hypothyroidism	Extravascular blood

Data from Maisels MJ. Neonatal jaundice. In: Avery GB, editor. Neonatology. Pathophysiology and Management of the Newborn. Philadelphia: JB Lippincott; 1987. p. 566.

normal until the tenth day of life. A total bilirubin level greater than 7 mg/dL in the first 24 hours or greater than 13 mg/dL at any time in full-term newborns often prompts an investigation for the cause. Breast-fed infants usually have serum bilirubin levels 1–2 mg/dL greater than formula-fed babies. The common causes of prolonged indirect hyperbilirubinemia are listed in Table 1-3.

Pathologic jaundice within the first 36 hours of life is usually due to excessive production of bilirubin. Hyperbilirubinemia is managed based on the infant's weight. While specific cutoffs defining the need for therapy have not been universally accepted, the following recommendations are consistent with most practice patterns.[12] Phototherapy is initiated for newborns: (1) less than 1500 g, when the serum bilirubin level reaches 5 mg/dL; (2) 1500–2000 g, when the serum bilirubin level reaches 8 mg/dL; or (3) 2000–2500 g, when the serum bilirubin level reaches 10 mg/dL. Formula-fed term infants without hemolytic disease are treated by phototherapy when levels reach 13 mg/dL. For hemolytic-related hyperbilirubinemia, phototherapy is recommended when the serum bilirubin level exceeds 10 mg/dL by 12 hours of life, 12 mg/dL by 18 hours, 14 mg/dL by 24 hours, or 15 mg/dL by 36 hours.[13] An absolute bilirubin level that triggers exchange transfusion is still not established, but most exchange transfusion decisions are based on the serum bilirubin level and its rate of rise.

Retinopathy of Prematurity

Retinopathy of prematurity (ROP) develops during the active phases of retinal vascular development from the 16th week of gestation. In full-term infants the retina is fully developed and ROP cannot occur. The exact causes are unknown, but oxygen exposure (greater than 93–95%) and extreme prematurity are two risk factors that have been demonstrated.[14] The risk and extent of ROP is probably related to the degree of vascular immaturity and abnormal retinal angiogenesis in response to hypoxia. ROP is found in 1.9% of premature infants in large neonatal units.[15] Retrolental fibroplasia (RLF) is the pathologic change observed in the retina and overlying vitreous after the acute phases of ROP subsides. Treatment of ROP with laser photocoagulation has been shown to have the added benefit of superior visual acuity and less myopia when compared to cryotherapy in long-term follow-up studies.[16–19] The American Academy of Pediatrics' guidelines recommends a screening examination for all infants who received oxygen therapy who weigh less than 1500 g and are fewer than 32 weeks' gestation, and selected infants with a birth weight between 1500 and 2000 g or gestational age of more than 32 weeks with an unstable clinical course, including those requiring cardiorespiratory support.[20]

Thermoregulation

Newborns have difficulty maintaining body temperature due to their relatively large surface area, poor thermal regulation, and small mass to act as a heat sink. Heat loss may occur owing to: (1) evaporation (wet newborn); (2) conduction (skin contact with cool surface); (3) convection (air currents blowing over newborn); and (4) radiation (non-contact loss of heat to cooler surface, which is the most difficult factor to control). Thermoneutrality is the range of ambient temperatures that the newborn can maintain a normal body temperature with a minimal metabolic rate by vasomotor control. The *critical temperature* is the temperature that requires adaptive metabolic responses to the cold in an effort to replace lost heat. Infants produce heat by increasing metabolic activity by shivering like an adult, nonshivering thermogenesis, and futile cycling of ions in skeletal muscle.[21] Brown adipose tissue (BAT) may be involved in thermoregulatory feeding and sleep cycles in the infant with an increase in body temperature signaling an increase in metabolic demand.[22] The uncoupling of mitochondrial respiration that occurs in BAT where energy is not conserved in ATP but rather is released as heat may be rendered inactive by vasopressors, anesthetic agents, and nutritional depletion.[23–25] Failure to maintain thermoneutrality leads to serious metabolic and physiologic consequences. Double-walled incubators offer the best thermoneutral environment, whereas radiant warmers cannot prevent convection heat loss and lead to higher insensible water loss. In the operating room, special care must be exercised to maintain the neonate's body temperature in the normal range.

FLUIDS AND ELECTROLYTES

At 12 weeks of gestation, the fetus has a total body water content that is 94% of body weight. This amount decreases to 80% by 32 weeks' gestation and 78% by term (Fig. 1-3). A further 3–5% reduction in total body water content occurs in the first 3 to 5 days of life. Body water continues to decline and reaches adult levels (approximately 60% of body weight) by 1½ years of age. Extracellular water also declines by 1 to 3 years of age. Premature delivery requires the newborn to complete both fetal and term water unloading tasks. Surprisingly, the premature infant can complete fetal water unloading by one week following birth. Postnatal reduction in extracellular fluid volume has such a high physiologic priority that it occurs even in the presence of relatively large variations of fluid intake.[26]

Glomerular Filtration Rate and Early Renal Function

The glomerular filtration rate (GFR) of newborns is slower than that of adults.[27] From 21 mL/min/1.73 m² at

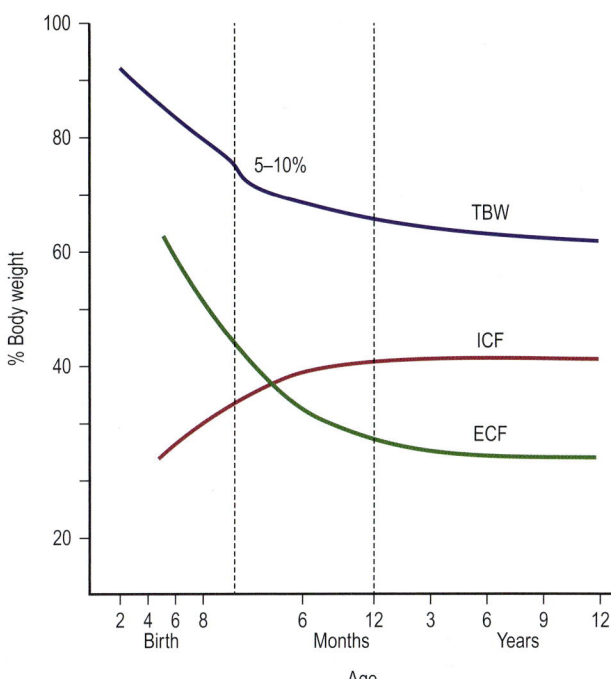

FIGURE 1-3 ■ Friss–Hansen's classic chart relating total body weight (TBW) and extracellular (ECF) and intracellular (ICF) fluid to percentage of body weight, from early gestation to adolescence. (Adapted from Welch KJ, Randolph JG, Ravitch MM, et al, editors. Pediatric Surgery. 4th ed. Chicago: Year Book Medical; 1986. p. 24.)

birth in the term infant, GFR quickly increases to 60 mL/min/1.73 m² by 2 weeks of age. GFR reaches adult levels by 18 months to 2 years of age. A preterm infant has a GFR that is only slightly slower than that of a full-term infant. In addition to this difference in GFR, the concentrating capacity of the preterm and the full-term infant is well below that of the adult. An infant responding to water deprivation increases urine osmolarity to a maximum of 600 mOsm/kg. This is in contrast to the adult, whose urine concentration can reach 1200 mOsm/kg. It appears that the difference in concentrating capacity is due to the insensitivity of the collecting tubules of the newborn to antidiuretic hormone. Although the newborn cannot concentrate urine as efficiently as the adult, the newborn can excrete very dilute urine at 30–50 mOsm/kg. Newborns are unable to excrete excess sodium, an inability thought to be due to a tubular defect. Term babies are able to conserve sodium, but premature infants are considered 'salt wasters' because they have an inappropriate urinary sodium excretion, even with restricted sodium intake.

Neonatal Fluid Requirements

To estimate fluid requirements in the newborn requires an understanding of: (1) any preexisting fluid deficits or excesses; (2) metabolic demands; and (3) losses. Because these factors change quickly in the critically ill newborn, frequent adjustments in fluid management are necessary (Table 1-4). Hourly monitoring of intake and output allows early recognition of fluid balance that

TABLE 1-4	Newborn Fluid Volume Requirements (mL/kg/24 hr) for Various Surgical Conditions		
Group	**Day 1**	**Day 2**	**Day 3**
Moderate surgical conditions (e.g., colostomies, laparotomies for intestinal atresia, Hirschsprung disease)	80 ± 25	80 ± 30	80 ± 30
Severe surgical conditions (e.g., gastroschisis, midgut volvulus, meconium peritonitis)	140 ± 45	90 ± 20	80 ± 15
Necrotizing enterocolitis with perforation	145 ± 70	135 ± 50	130 ± 40

will affect treatment decisions. This dynamic approach requires two components: (1) an initial hourly fluid intake that is safe and (2) a monitoring system to detect the patient's response to the treatment program selected. No 'normal' urine output exists for a given neonate, yet one may generally target 1–2 mL/kg/h.

After administering the initial hourly volume for four to eight hours, depending on the patient's condition, the newborn is reassessed by observing urine output and concentration. With these two factors, it is possible to determine the state of hydration of most neonates and their responses to the initial volume. In more difficult cases, changes in serial serum osmolarity, sodium (Na), creatinine, and blood urea nitrogen (BUN), along with urine osmolarity, Na, and creatinine make it possible to assess the infant's response to the initial volume and to use fluid status to guide the next 4-8 hours' fluid intake.

Illustrative Examples

Insufficient Fluid. A 1 kg premature infant, during the first eight hours postoperatively, has 0.3 mL/kg/h of urine output. Specific gravity is 1.025. Previous initial volume was 5 mL/kg/h. Serum BUN has increased from 4 mg/dL to 8 mg/dL; hematocrit value has increased from 35% to 37%, without transfusion. This child is dry. The treatment is to increase the hourly volume to 7 mL/kg/h for the next 4 hours and to monitor the subsequent urine output and concentration to reassess fluid status. Depending on the degree of dehydration and the child's underlying cardiopulmonary status, it may be prudent to bolus the child with 10–20 mL/kg 0.9% normal saline—all the while carefully monitoring physiologic responsiveness.

Inappropriate Antidiuretic Hormone Response. A 3 kg newborn with congenital diaphragmatic hernia during the first eight hours postoperatively has 0.2 mL/kg/h of urine output and a urine osmolarity of 360 mOsm/L. The previous fluid volume was 120 mL/kg/day (15 mL/h). The serum osmolarity has decreased from 300 mOsm/L preoperatively to 278 mOsm/L; BUN has decreased from 12 mg/dL to

8 mg/dL. The inappropriate antidiuretic hormone response requires reduction in fluid volume from 120 mL/kg/day to 90 mL/kg/day for the next 4-8 hours. Repeat urine and serum measurements will allow for further adjustment of fluid administration.

Over-Hydration. A 3 kg baby, 24 hours following operative closure of gastroschisis, had an average urine output of 3 mL/kg/h for the past 4 hours. During that time period, the infant received fluids at a rate of 180 ml/kg/day. The specific gravity of the urine has decreased to 1.006; serum BUN is 4 mg/dL; hematocrit value is 30%, down from 35% preoperatively. The total serum protein concentration is 4.0 mg/dL, down from 4.5 mg/dL. This child is overhydrated. The treatment is to decrease the fluids to 3 mL/kg/h for the next 4 hours and then to reassess urine output and concentration.

Renal Failure. A 5 kg infant with severe sepsis secondary to Hirschsprung enterocolitis has had a urine output of 0.1 mL/kg/h for the past 8 hours. The specific gravity is 1.012; serum sodium, 150; BUN, 25 mg/dL; creatinine, 1.5 mg/dL; urine sodium, 130; and urine creatinine, 20 mg/dL.

Fractional Na excretion (FE Na):

$$FE\ Na = \frac{Ur\ Na \times Pl\ Cr}{Pl\ Na \times Ur\ Cr} = \frac{130 \times 1.5}{150 \times 20}$$
$$= 193/3000 \times 100$$
$$= 6.5\% \ (normal = 2-3\% \ in\ newborns)$$

FE Na less than 1% usually indicates a prerenal cause of oliguria, whereas greater than 3% usually implies a renal cause (e.g., acute tubular necrosis). This patient is in acute renal failure. The plan is to restrict fluids to insensible losses plus measured losses for the next 4 hours and to then reassess the plan using both urine and serum studies. Of note, while the FE urea may be a better predictor of prerenal failure in this population, both FE urea and the FE Na have limited utility in neonates, reflecting the relative immaturity of neonatal renal function.[28]

PULMONARY SYSTEM OF THE NEWBORN

Maturation of the lungs is generally divided into five periods:
- Embryonic phase (begins approximately week 3)
- Pseudoglandular phase (5–17 weeks)
- Canalicular phase (16–25 weeks)
- Terminal saccular phase (24 weeks to full-term birth)
- Alveolar phase (late fetal phase to childhood).

Pulmonary development begins in the third week (embryonic phase) when a ventral diverticulum develops off the foregut (laryngotracheal groove), initiating tracheal development. During the pseudoglandular phase, all of the major elements of the lung form except those involved in gas exchange. The dichotomous branching of the bronchial tree that develops during the fourth week from the primitive trachea is usually completed by 17 weeks' gestation. Fetuses born during this phase are unable to survive because respiration is not possible. In the canalicular phase, respiration is made possible because thin-walled terminal sacs (primordial alveoli) have developed at the ends of the respiratory bronchioles and the lung tissue is well vascularized. No actual alveoli are seen until 24 to 26 weeks' gestation, during the terminal saccular phase. The air–blood surface area for gas diffusion is limited should the fetus be delivered at this age. The terminal saccular phase is defined by the establishment of the blood–air barrier that allows gas exchange for the survival of the fetus should it be born prematurely. Between 24 and 28 weeks, the cuboidal and columnar cells flatten and differentiate into type I (lining cells) and/or type II (granular) pneumocytes. Between 26 and 32 weeks of gestation, terminal air sacs begin to give way to air spaces. At the same time, the phospholipids that constitute pulmonary surfactant begin to line the terminal lung air spaces. Surfactant is produced by type II pneumocytes and is extremely important in maintaining alveolar stability. During the alveolar phase, further budding of these air spaces occurs and alveoli become numerous, a process that continues postnatally until the age of 3 to 8 years.[29]

The change in the ratio of the amniotic phospholipids (lecithin: sphingomyelin) is used to assess fetal lung maturity. A ratio greater than 2 is considered compatible with mature lung function. Absence of adequate surfactant leads to HMD or respiratory distress syndrome (RDS). HMD is present in 10% of premature infants. Other conditions associated with pulmonary distress in the newborn include delayed fetal lung absorption, meconium aspiration syndrome, intrapartum pneumonia, and developmental structural anomalies (e.g., congenital diaphragmatic hernia (CDH) and congenital lobar emphysema). In all of these conditions, endotracheal intubation and mechanical ventilation may be required for hypoxia, CO_2 retention, or apnea. Ventilator options and management depend on the clinical context and are further discussed in Chapter 7.

Surfactant

The development of exogenous surfactant in the 1990s has significantly advanced the field of neonatology resulting in reductions in the rates of neonatal mortality. Surfactant deficiency is the major cause of HMD. Surfactant replacement therapy reduces the surface tension on the inner surface of the alveoli preventing the alveoli from collapsing during expiration, thereby improving air exchange. Three exogenous surfactants are available: (1) surfactant derived from bovine or porcine lung; (2) synthetic surfactant without protein components; and (3) synthetic surfactant containing protein components. A human derived surfactant was tested but is not currently in use.

The most efficacious administration method is currently under investigation. The standard approach is to instill aliquots into an endotracheal tube. The indications for the use of surfactant include: (1) intubated infants with RDS; (2) intubated infants with meconium aspiration syndrome (MAS) requiring more than 50% oxygen; (3) intubated infants with pneumonia and an oxygen index great than 15; and (4) intubated infants with pulmonary hemorrhage that have clinically deteriorated. Its efficacy is uncertain in neonates with pulmonary hemorrhage and pneumonia. Worse outcomes are associated with surfactant use in CDH.[30,31]

The acute pulmonary effects of surfactant therapy are improved lung function and alveolar expansion leading to improved oxygenation, which results in a reduction in the need for mechanical ventilation and extracorporeal oxygenation.[32–34]

Two meta-analyses support the use of surfactant therapy in infants with RDS to reduce air leak syndromes, pneumothorax, bronchopulmonary dysplasia (BPD), pulmonary interstitial emphysema, and mortality.[35,36] The INSURE (INtubate, SURfactant, Extubate) technique consists of administration of surfactant followed by extubation within one hour to nasal continuous positive airway pressure (nCPAP). Another randomized trial demonstrated the reduced mortality and air leaks for infants assigned to early surfactant treatment versus nCPAP alone.[37] In large trials that reflect the current practice of treating infants at risk for the development of RDS (administration of maternal steroids and the routine stabilization on CPAP), the selective use of surfactant in infants with established RDS demonstrates a decreased risk of chronic lung disease or death when compared to infants who are more aggressively treated with prophylactic administration of surfactant.[38]

Several adverse outcomes have been associated with the use of surfactant (Table 1-5). Intraventricular hemorrhage is one of the most worrisome potential side effects. However, meta-analyses of multiple trials have not shown a statistically significant increase in this risk.[35,36]

TABLE 1-5 Adverse Effects of Surfactant Therapy

Acute Adverse Effects of Surfactant Therapy	Transient Adverse Effects of Surfactant Therapy	Minimal to Small Risk	No Differences Between Placebo and Surfactant Treated Infants
• Transient hypoxia and bradycardia from airway obstruction • Reflux of surfactant into the pharynx • Mucous plugging of the endotracheal tube	• Decrease in blood pressure • Decrease in cerebral blood flow velocity • Decrease in cerebral activity on EEG	• Pulmonary hemorrhage	• Neurodevelopment outcomes • Respiratory outcomes • Physical growth • Intraventricular hemorrhage

Monitoring

Continuous monitoring of physiologic indices provides data to assess the response to therapy. In retrospect, many episodes of 'sudden deterioration' in critically ill patients are viewed as changes in clinical condition that had been occurring for some time.

Arterial Blood Gases and Derived Indices

Arterial oxygen tension (PaO_2) is measured most commonly by obtaining an arterial blood sample and by measuring the partial pressure of oxygen with a polarographic electrode. In the term newborn, the general definition for hypoxia is a PaO_2 less than 55 mmHg, whereas hyperoxia is greater than 80 mmHg.

Capillary blood samples are 'arterialized' by topical vasodilators or heat to increase blood flow to a peripheral site. Blood flowing sluggishly and exposed to atmospheric oxygen falsely raises the PaO_2 from a capillary sample, especially in the 40–60 mmHg range.[39] Capillary blood pH and carbon dioxide tension (PCO_2) correlate well with arterial samples, unless perfusion is poor. PaO_2 is least reliable when determined by capillary blood gas. In patients receiving oxygen therapy in which arterial PaO_2 exceeds 60 mmHg, the capillary PaO_2 correlates poorly with the arterial measurement.[40,41]

In newborns, umbilical artery catheterization provides arterial access. The catheter tip should rest at the level of the diaphragm or below L3. The second most frequently used arterial site is the radial artery. Complications of arterial blood sampling include repeated blood loss and anemia. Distal extremity or organ ischemia from thrombosis or arterial injury is rare, but can be seen. Changes in oxygenation are such that intermittent blood gas sampling may miss critical episodes of hypoxia or hyperoxia. Due to the drawbacks of ex vivo monitoring, several in vivo monitoring systems have been used.

Pulse Oximetry

The noninvasive determination of oxygen saturation (SaO_2) gives moment-to-moment information regarding the availability of O_2 to the tissues. If the PaO_2 is plotted against the oxygen saturation of hemoglobin, the S-shaped hemoglobin dissociation curve is obtained (see Fig. 1-2). From this curve, it is evident that hemoglobin is 50% saturated at 27 mmHg PaO_2 and 90% saturated at 50 mmHg. Pulse oximetry has a rapid (5-7 seconds) response time, requires no calibration, and may be left in place continuously.

Pulse oximetry is not possible if the patient is in shock, has peripheral vasospasm, or has vascular constriction due to hypothermia. Inaccurate readings may occur in the presence of jaundice, direct high-intensity light, dark skin pigmentation, and greater than 80% fetal hemoglobin. Oximetry is not a sensitive guide to gas exchange in patients with high PaO_2 due to the shape of the oxygen dissociation curve. On the upper horizontal portion of the curve, large changes in PaO_2 may occur with little change in SaO_2. For instance, an oximeter reading of 95% could represent a PaO_2 between 60–160 mmHg.

A study comparing pulse oximetry with PaO_2 from indwelling arterial catheters has shown that SaO_2 greater than or equal to 85% corresponds to a PaO_2 greater than 55 mmHg, and saturations less than or equal to 90% correspond with a PaO_2 less than 80 mmHg.[42] Guidelines for monitoring infants using pulse oximetry have been suggested for the following three conditions:

1. In the infant with acute respiratory distress without direct arterial access, saturation limits of 85% (lower) and 92% (upper) should be set
2. In the older infant with chronic respiratory distress who is at low risk for ROP, the upper saturation limit may be set at 95%; the lower limit should be set at 87% to avoid pulmonary vasoconstriction and pulmonary hypertension
3. As the concentration of fetal hemoglobin in newborns affects the accuracy of pulse oximetry, infants with arterial access should have both PaO_2 and SaO_2 monitored closely. A graph should be kept at the bedside documenting the SaO_2 each time the PaO_2 is measured. Limits for the SaO_2 alarm can be changed because the characteristics of this relationship change.

Carbon Dioxide Tension

Arterial carbon dioxide tension ($PaCO_2$) is a direct reflection of gas exchange in the lungs and metabolic rate. In most clinical situations, changes in $PaCO_2$ are due to changes in ventilation. For this reason, serial measurement of $PaCO_2$ is a practical method to assess the adequacy of ventilation. It is also possible to monitor $PaCO_2$ and pH satisfactorily with venous or capillary blood samples. Therefore, many infants with respiratory insufficiency no longer require arterial catheters for monitoring.

End-Tidal Carbon Dioxide

Measuring expired CO_2 by capnography provides a noninvasive means of continuously monitoring alveolar PCO_2. Capnometry measures CO_2 by an infrared sensor either placed in-line between the ventilator circuit and the endotracheal tube or off to the side of the air flow, both of which are applicable only to the intubated patient. A comparative study of end-tidal carbon dioxide in critically ill neonates demonstrated that both sidestream and mainstream end-tidal carbon dioxide measurements approximated $PaCO_2$.[43] When the mainstream sensor was inserted into the breathing circuit, the $PaCO_2$ increased an average of 2 mmHg.

Central Venous Catheter

Indications for central venous catheter placement include: (1) hemodynamic monitoring; (2) inability to establish other venous access; (3) TPN; and (4) infusion of inotropic drugs or other medications that cannot be given peripherally. Measuring central venous pressure (CVP) to monitor volume status is frequently used in the resuscitation of a critically ill patient. A catheter placed in the superior vena cava or right atrium measures the filling pressure of the right side of the heart, which usually reflects left atrial and filling pressure of the left ventricle. Often, a wide discrepancy exists between left and right atrial pressure if pulmonary disease, overwhelming sepsis, or cardiac anomalies are present. Positive-pressure ventilation, pneumothorax, abdominal distention, or pericardial tamponade all elevate CVP.

Pulmonary Artery

The pulmonary artery pressure catheter has altered the care of the child with severe cardiopulmonary derangement by allowing direct measurement of cardiovascular variables at the bedside. With this catheter, it is possible to monitor CVP, pulmonary artery pressure, pulmonary wedge pressure, and cardiac output. The catheter is usually placed by percutaneous methods (as in the adult), except in the smallest pediatric patient in whom a cutdown is sometimes required.

When the tip of the catheter is in a distal pulmonary artery and the balloon is inflated, the resulting pressure is generally an accurate reflection of left atrial pressure because the pulmonary veins do not have valves. This pulmonary 'wedge' pressure represents left ventricular filling pressure, which is used as a reflection of preload. The monitors display phasic pressures, but treatment decisions are made based on the electronically derived mean CVP. A low pulmonary wedge pressure suggests that blood volume must be expanded. A high or normal pulmonary wedge pressure in the presence of continued signs of shock suggests left ventricular dysfunction.

Cardiac output is usually measured in liters per minute. Cardiac index represents the cardiac output divided by the body surface area. The normalized cardiac index allows the evaluation of cardiac performance without regard to body size. The normal value for cardiac index is between 3.5–4.5 L/min/m². The determination of cardiac output by the thermodilution technique is possible with a Swan–Ganz pulmonary artery catheter. Accurate cardiac output determination depends on rapid injection, accurate measurement of the injectant temperatures and volume, and absence of shunting. Because ventilation affects the flow into and out of the right ventricle, three injections should be made at a consistent point in the ventilatory cycle, typically at end-expiration.

Another study concluded that using right heart catheters in treating critically ill adult patients resulted in an increased mortality.[44] However, a consensus committee report documents the continued safety and efficacy of right heart catheters in the care of critically ill children.[45] A newer technique of deriving some of these data employs femoral arterial access and is gaining popularity in the pediatric intensive care unit: transcardiopulmonary thermodilution monitoring device (pulse contour cardiac output [PCCO]).

A proprietary PiCCO® device has been developed, and employs a standard central venous catheter and a proprietary thermistor-tipped arterial catheter to assess hemodynamic parameters via transpulmonary thermodilution. Manual calibration is required and must be performed frequently (every hour) for reasonably accurate data.[46] It is recommended to recalibrate the curve after interventions are performed.[47] This device may give incorrect thermodilution measurements if blood is either extracted from or infused back into the cardiopulmonary circulation as seen with an intracardiac shunt, aortic stenosis, lung embolism, and extracorporeal membrane oxygenation (ECMO).[48]

Venous Oximetry

Mixed venous oxygen saturation (SvO_2) is an indicator of the adequacy of oxygen supply and demand in perfused tissues. Oxygen consumption is defined as the amount of oxygen consumed by the tissue as calculated by the Fick equation:

$$O_2 \text{ consumption} = \text{Cardiac output} \times \text{Arterial} - \text{venous oxygen content difference}$$

Reflectance spectrophotometry is currently used for continuous venous oximetry. Multiple wavelengths of light are transmitted at a known intensity by means of fiber optic bundles in a special pulmonary artery or right atrial catheter. The light is reflected by RBCs flowing past the tip of the catheter. The wavelengths of light are chosen so that both oxyhemoglobin and deoxyhemoglobin are measured to determine the fraction of hemoglobin saturated with oxygen. The system requires either in vitro calibration by reflecting light from a standardized target that represents a known oxygen saturation or in vivo calibration by withdrawing blood from the pulmonary artery catheter and measuring the saturation by laboratory co-oximetry.

Mixed venous oxygen saturation values within the normal range (68–77%) indicate a normal balance between oxygen supply and demand, provided that vasoregulation is intact and distribution of peripheral blood flow is normal. Values greater than 77% are most commonly associated with syndromes of vasoderegulation, such as sepsis. Uncompensated changes in O_2 saturation, hemoglobin level, or cardiac output lead to a decrease in SvO_2. A sustained decrease in SvO_2 greater than 10% should lead to measuring SaO_2, hemoglobin level, and cardiac output to determine the cause of the decline.[49] The most common sources of error in measuring SvO_2 are calibration and catheter malposition. The most important concept in SvO_2 monitoring is the advantage of continuous monitoring, which allows early warning of a developing problem.[50]

Although most clinical experience has been with pulmonary artery catheters, right atrial catheters are more easily inserted and may thus provide better information to detect hemodynamic deterioration earlier and permit more rapid treatment of physiologic derangements.[51] A study has shown that, when oxygen consumption was monitored and maintained at a consistent level, the right atrial venous saturation was found to be an excellent monitor.[52]

SHOCK

Shock is a state in which the cardiac output is insufficient to deliver adequate oxygen to meet metabolic demands of the tissues. Cardiovascular function is determined by preload, cardiac contractility, heart rate, and afterload. Shock may be classified broadly as hypovolemic, cardiogenic, or distributive (systemic inflammatory response syndrome [SIRS]—septic or neurogenic).

Hypovolemic Shock

In infants and children, most shock situations are the result of reduced preload secondary to fluid loss, such as from diarrhea, vomiting, or blood loss from trauma. Preload is a function of blood volume. In most clinical situations, right atrial pressure or CVP is the index of cardiac preload. In situations in which left ventricular or right ventricular compliance is abnormal or in certain forms of congenital heart disease, right atrial pressure may not correlate well with left atrial pressure.

Hypovolemia results in decreased venous return to the heart. Preload is reduced, cardiac output falls, and the overall result is a decrease in tissue perfusion. The first step in treating all forms of shock is to correct existing fluid deficits. Inotropic drugs should not be initiated until adequate intravascular fluid volume has been established. The speed and volume of the infusate are determined by the patient's responses, particularly changes in blood pressure, pulse rate, urine output, and CVP. Shock resulting from acute hemorrhage is treated with the administration of 20 mL/kg of Ringer's lactate solution or normal saline as fluid boluses. If the patient does not respond, a second bolus of crystalloid is given. Type-specific or cross-matched blood is given to achieve an SvO_2 of 70%. In newborns with a coagulopathy, we provide fresh frozen plasma or specific factors as the resuscitation fluid.

The rate and volume of resuscitation fluid given is adjusted based on feedback data obtained from monitoring the effects of the initial resuscitation. After the initial volume is given, the adequacy of replacement is assessed by monitoring urine output, urine concentration, plasma acidosis, oxygenation, arterial pressure, CVP, and pulmonary wedge pressure, if indicated. When cardiac failure is present, continued vigorous delivery of large volumes of fluid may cause further increases in preload to the failing myocardium and accelerates the downhill course. In this setting, inotropic agents are given while monitoring cardiac and pulmonary function, as outlined previously.

Cardiogenic Shock

Myocardial contractility is usually expressed as the ejection fraction that indicates the proportion of left ventricular volume that is pumped. Myocardial contractility is reduced with hypoxemia and acidosis. Inotropic drugs increase cardiac contractility. Inotropes are most effective when hypoxemia and acidosis are corrected. In cases of fluid-refractory shock and cardiogenic shock, inotropic drugs are necessary. Traditionally, administration of inotropes requires the adjunct of central venous access. However, initial administration of pressors through peripheral IVs may be prudent.

Adrenergic receptors are important in regulating calcium flux, which, in turn, is important in controlling myocardial contractility. The α and β receptors are proteins present in the sarcolemma of myocardial and vascular smooth muscle cells. The $β_1$ receptors are predominantly in the heart and, when stimulated, result in increased contractility of myocardium. The $β_2$ receptors are predominately in respiratory and vascular smooth muscle. When stimulated, these receptors result in bronchodilation and vasodilation. The $α_1$-adrenergic receptors are located on vascular smooth muscle and result in vascular constriction when stimulated. The $α_2$ receptors are found mainly on prejunctional sympathetic nerve terminals. The concept of dopaminergic receptors has also been used to account for the cardiovascular effects of dopamine not mediated through α or β receptors. Activation of dopaminergic receptors results in decreased renal and mesenteric vascular resistance and, usually, increased blood flow. The most commonly used inotropic and vasoactive drugs are listed in Table 1-6.

Epinephrine

Epinephrine is an endogenous catecholamine with α- and β-adrenergic effects. At low doses, the β-adrenergic effect predominates. These effects include an increase in heart rate, cardiac contractility, cardiac output, and bronchiolar dilation. Blood pressure rises, in part, not only due to increased cardiac output but also due to increased peripheral vascular resistance, which occurs with higher doses as the α-adrenergic effects become predominant. Renal blood flow may increase slightly, remain unchanged, or decrease depending on the balance between greater cardiac output and changes in peripheral vascular resistance, which lead to regional redistribution of blood flow. Cardiac arrhythmias can be seen with epinephrine, especially with higher doses. Dosages for treating compromised cardiovascular function range from 0.05–1.0 μg/kg/min. Excessive doses of epinephrine can cause worsening cardiac ischemia and dysfunction from increased myocardial oxygen demand.

Isoproterenol

Isoproterenol is a β-adrenergic agonist. It increases cardiac contractility and heart rate, with little change in systemic vascular resistance (SVR). The peripheral vascular β-adrenergic effect and lack of a peripheral vascular α-adrenergic effect may allow reduction of left ventricular afterload. The intense chronotropic effect of isoproterenol produces tachycardia, which can limit its usefulness. Isoproterenol is administered IV at a dosage of 0.5–10.0 μg/kg/min.

Dopamine

Dopamine is an endogenous catecholamine with β-adrenergic, α-adrenergic, and dopaminergic effects. It is both a direct and an indirect β-adrenergic agonist. Dopamine elicits positive inotropic and chronotropic responses by direct interaction with the β receptor (direct effect) and by stimulating the release of norepinephrine from the sympathetic nerve endings, which interacts with the β receptor (indirect effect). At low dosages

TABLE 1-6 Vasoactive Medications Commonly Used in the Newborn

Vasoactive Agent	Principal Modes of Action	Major Hemodynamic Effects	Administration and Dosage	Indications
Epinephrine	α and β agonist	Increases heart rate and myocardial contractility by activating β_1 receptors	0.1 mL/kg of 1:10,000 solution given IV intracardial, or endotracheal 0.05–1.0 μg/kg/min IV	Cardiac resuscitation; short-term use when severe heart failure resistant to other drugs
Norepinephrine	α and β agonist	Increases BP by vasoconstriction with its greater action on β receptors	20–100 ng/kg/min initially, up to 1.0 μg/kg/min as base.	Shock state with high cardiac output and low systemic vascular resistance
Vasopressin	ADH agonist in arterioles	May replace basal vasopressin levels in cases of severe hypotension	0.018–0.12 units/kg/h used as a rescue treatment	Restoration of vascular tone in vasodilatory shock
Dopamine, low dose	Stimulates dopamine receptors	Decrease in vascular resistance in splanchnic, renal, and cerebral vessels	<5 μg/kg/min IV	Useful in managing cardiogenic or hypovolemic shock or after cardiac surgery
Dopamine, intermediate dose	Stimulates β_1 receptors; myocardial	Inotropic response	5–10 μg/kg/min IV	Blood pressure unresponsive to low dose
Dopamine, high dose	Stimulates α receptors	Increased peripheral and renal vascular resistance	10–20 μg/kg/min IV	Septic shock with low systemic vascular resistance
Dobutamine	Synthetic β_1 agonist in low doses; α and β_2 effects in higher doses	Increased cardiac output, increased arterial pressure; less increase in heart rate than with dopamine	1–10 μg/kg/min IV	Useful alternative to dopamine if increase in heart rate undesirable
Isoproterenol	β_1 and β_2 agonist	Increased cardiac output by positive inotropic and chronotropic action and increase in venous return; systemic vascular resistance generally reduced; pulmonary vascular resistance generally reduced	0.5–10.0 μg/kg/min IV	Useful in low-output situations, especially when heart rate is slow
Sodium nitroprusside	Direct-acting vasodilator that relaxes arteriolar and venous smooth muscle	Afterload reduction; reduced arterial pressure	1–10 μg/kg/min IV (for up to ten minutes); 0.5–2.0 μg/kg/min IV	Hypertensive crisis; vasodilator therapy
Milrinone	Phosphodiesterase inhibitor relaxes arteriolar and venous smooth muscle via calcium/cyclic adenosine monophosphate	Increased cardiac output, slight decreased BP, increased oxygen delivery	75 μg/kg bolus IV, then 0.75–1.0 μg/kg/min IV	Useful as an alternative or in addition to dopamine (may act synergistically) if increased heart rate undesirable

ADH, antidiuretic hormone; BP, blood pressure; IV, intravenous.
Adapted from Lees MH, King DH. Cardiogenic shock in the neonate. Pediatr Rev 1988;9:263; Yager P, Noviski N. Shock. Pediatrics in Review 2010;21:311–18; and Piastra M, Luca E, Mensi S, et al. Inotropic and Vasoactive Drugs in Pediatric ICU. Current Drug Targets 2012;13:900–5.

(<5 μg/kg/min), the dopaminergic effect of the drug predominates, resulting in reduced renal and mesenteric vascular resistance and further blood flow to these organs. The β-adrenergic effects become more prominent at intermediate dosages (5–10 μg/kg/min), producing a higher cardiac output. At relatively high dosages (10–20 μg/kg/min), the α-adrenergic effects become prominent with peripheral vasoconstriction.

Experience with the use of dopamine in pediatric patients suggests that it is effective in increasing blood pressure in neonates, infants, and children. The precise dosages at which the desired hemodynamic effects are maximized are not known. The effects of low dosages of dopamine on blood pressure, heart rate, and renal function were studied in 18 hypotensive, preterm infants.[53] The blood pressure and diuretic effects were observed at 2, 4, and 8 μg/kg/min. Elevations in heart rate were seen only at 8 μg/kg/min. Further work is needed to better characterize the pharmacokinetics and pharmacodynamics of dopamine in children, especially in newborns.

Dobutamine

Dobutamine, a synthetic catecholamine, has predominantly β-adrenergic effects with minimal α-adrenergic effects. The hemodynamic effect of dobutamine in infants and children with shock has been studied.[54] Dobutamine infusion significantly increased cardiac index, stroke index, and pulmonary capillary wedge pressure, and it decreased SVR. The drug appears more efficacious in treating cardiogenic shock than septic shock. The advantage of dobutamine over isoproterenol is its lesser chronotropic effect and its tendency to maintain systemic pressure. The advantage over dopamine is dobutamine's lesser peripheral vasoconstrictor effect. The usual range of dosages for dobutamine is 1–10 µg/kg/min. The combination of dopamine and dobutamine has been increasingly used; however, little information regarding their combined advantages or effectiveness in the neonate and infant has been published.

Milrinone

Milrinone, a phosphodiesterase inhibitor, is a potent positive inotrope and vasodilator (hence, also known as an ino-dilator) that has been shown to improve cardiac function in infants and children.[55–57] The proposed action is due, in part, to an increase in intracellular cyclic adenosine monophosphate and calcium transport secondary to inhibition of cardiac phosphodiesterase. This effect is independent of β-agonist stimulation and, in fact, may act synergistically with the β agonist to improve cardiac performance. Milrinone increases cardiac index and oxygen delivery without affecting heart rate, blood pressure, or pulmonary wedge pressure. Milrinone is administered as a 75 µg/kg bolus followed by infusion of 0.75–1.0 g/kg/min.

Distributive Shock

Distributive shock is caused by derangements in vascular tone from endothelial damage that lead to end-organ hypotension and is seen in the following clinical situations: (1) septic shock; (2) SIRS; (3) anaphylaxis; and (4) spinal cord trauma. Septic shock in the pediatric patient is discussed in further detail.

Septic Shock

Afterload represents the force against which the left ventricle must contract to eject blood. It is related to SVR and myocardial wall stress. SVR is defined as the systemic mean arterial blood pressure minus right arterial pressure divided by cardiac output. Cardiac contractility is affected by SVR and afterload. In general, increases in afterload reduce cardiac contractility, and decreases in afterload increase cardiac contractility.

Septic shock is a distributive form of shock that differs from other forms of shock. Cardiogenic and hypovolemic shock lead to increased SVR and decreased cardiac output. Septic shock results from a severe decrease in SVR and a generalized maldistribution of blood and leads to a hyperdynamic state.[58] The pathophysiology of septic shock begins with a nidus of infection. Organisms may invade the blood stream, or they may proliferate at the infected site and release various mediators into the blood stream. Substances produced by microorganisms, such as lipopolysaccharide, endotoxin, exotoxin, lipid moieties, and other products can induce septic shock by stimulating host cells to release numerous cytokines, chemokines, leukotrienes, and endorphins.

Endotoxin is a lipopolysaccharide found in the outer membrane of Gram-negative bacteria. Functionally, the molecule is divided into three parts: (1) the highly variable O-specific polysaccharide side chain (conveys serotypic specificity to bacteria and can activate the alternate pathway of complement); (2) the R-core region (less variable among different gram-negative bacteria; antibodies to this region could be cross protective); and (3) lipid-A (responsible for most of the toxicity of endotoxin). Endotoxin stimulates tumor necrosis factor (TNF) and can directly activate the classic complement pathway in the absence of antibody. Endotoxin has been implicated as an important factor in the pathogenesis of human septic shock and Gram-negative sepsis.[59] Therapy has focused on developing antibodies to endotoxin to treat septic shock. Antibodies to endotoxin have been used in clinical trials of sepsis with variable results.[60–62]

Cytokines, especially TNF, play a dominant role in the host's response. Endotoxin and exotoxin both induce TNF release in vivo and produce many other toxic effects via this endogenous mediator.[63–65] TNF is released primarily from monocytes and macrophages. It is also released from natural killer cells, mast cells, and some activated T-lymphocytes. Antibodies against TNF protect animals from exotoxin and bacterial challenge.[66,67] Other stimuli for its release include viruses, fungi, parasites, and interleukin-1 (IL-1). In sepsis, the effects of TNF release may include cardiac dysfunction, disseminated intravascular coagulation, and cardiovascular collapse. TNF release also causes the release of granulocyte–macrophage colony-stimulating factor (GM-CSF), interferon-α, and IL-1.

IL-1 is produced primarily by macrophages and monocytes. IL-1, previously known as the endogenous pyrogen, plays a central role in stimulating a variety of host responses, including fever production, lymphocyte activation, and endothelial cell stimulation, to produce procoagulant activity and to increase adhesiveness. IL-1 also causes the induction of the inhibitor of tissue plasminogen activator and the production of GM-CSF. These effects are balanced by the release of platelet-activating factor and arachidonic metabolites.

IL-2, also known as *T-cell growth factor*, is produced by activated T-lymphocytes and strengthens the immune response by stimulating cell proliferation. Its clinically apparent side effects include capillary leak syndrome, tachycardia, hypotension, increased cardiac index, decreased SVR, and decreased left ventricular ejection fraction.[68,69]

Studies in dogs have suggested that in immature animals, septic shock is more lethal and has different mechanisms of tissue injury.[70] These include more dramatic aberrations in blood pressure (more constant decline), heart rate (progressive, persistent tachycardia), blood sugar level (severe, progressive hypoglycemia), acid–base status (severe acidosis), and oxygenation (severe hypoxemia). These changes are significantly different from those seen in the adult animals that also experience an improved survival of almost 600% (18.5 vs 3.1 hours) compared with the immature animal.

The neonate's host defense can usually respond successfully to ordinary microbial challenge. However, defense against major challenges appears limited, which provides an explanation for the high mortality rate with major neonatal sepsis. As in adults, the immune system consists of four major components: cell-mediated immunity (T-cells), complement system, antibody-mediated immunity (B-cells), and macrophage–neutrophil phagocytic system. The two most important deficits in newborn host defenses that seem to increase the risk of bacterial sepsis are the quantitative and qualitative changes in the phagocytic system and the defects in antibody-mediated immunity.

The proliferative rate of the granulocyte–macrophage precursor has been reported to be at near-maximal capacity in the neonate. However, the neutrophil storage pool is markedly reduced in the newborn compared with the adult. After bacterial challenge, newborns fail to increase stem cell proliferation and deplete their already reduced neutrophil storage pool. Numerous in vitro abnormalities have been demonstrated in neonatal polymorphonuclear neutrophils, especially in times of stress or infection.[71] These abnormalities include decreased deformability, chemotaxis, phagocytosis, C3b receptor expression, adherence, bacterial killing, and depressed oxidative metabolism. Chemotaxis is impaired in neonatal neutrophils in response to various bacterial organisms and antigen–antibody complexes.[72] Granulocytes are activated by their interaction with endothelial cells followed by entry into secondary lymphoid issues via the endothelial venules. Initial adhesion of granulocytes is dependent on their expression of L-selectin, a cell adhesion molecule expressed on the granulocyte cell surface. Evaluation of cord blood has demonstrated a significantly lower expression of L-selectin on granulocyte surfaces when compared to older newborn (5 days old) and adult samples, indicating a depressed level of interaction with vascular endothelial cells at the initial stage of adhesion.[73] Although phagocytosis has additionally been demonstrated to be abnormal in neonatal phagocytes, it appears that this phenomenon is most likely secondary to decreased opsonic activity rather than an intrinsic defect of the neonatal polymorphonuclear neutrophils.[74,75] Currently, there is inconclusive evidence to support or refute the routine use of granulocyte transfusions in the prevention or treatment of sepsis in the neonate.[76]

Preterm and term newborns have poor responses to various antigenic stimuli, reduced gamma globulin levels at birth, and reduced maternal immunoglobulin supply from placental transport. Almost 33% of infants with a birth weight less than 1500 g develop substantial hypogammaglobulinemia.[77] IgA and IgM levels are also low due to the inability of these two immunoglobulins to cross the placenta. Thus, neonates are usually more susceptible to pyogenic bacterial infections because most of the antibodies that opsonize pyogenic bacterial capsular antigens are IgG and IgM. In addition, neonates do not produce type-specific antibodies because of defects in the differentiation of B-lymphocytes into immunoglobulin-secreting plasma cells and in T-lymphocyte-mediated facilitation of antibody synthesis. In the term infant, total hemolytic complement activity, which measures the classic complement pathway, constitutes approximately 50% of adult activity.[78] The activity of the alternative complement pathway, secondary to lowered levels of factor B, is also decreased in the neonate.[79] Fibronectin, a plasma protein that promotes reticuloendothelial clearance of invading microorganisms, is deficient in neonatal cord plasma.[80]

The use of intravenous immunoglobulins (IVIGs) for the prophylaxis and treatment of sepsis in the newborn, especially the preterm, low birth weight infant, has been studied in numerous trials with varied outcomes. In one study, a group of infants weighing 1500 g was treated with 500 mg/kg of IVIG each week for four weeks and compared with infants who were not treated with immunoglobulin.[81] The death rate was 16% in the IVIG-treated group compared with 32% in the untreated control group. Another recent analysis examined the role of IVIG to prevent and treat neonatal sepsis.[82] A significant (but only marginal) benefit was noted from prophylactic use of IVIG to prevent sepsis in low birth weight premature infants. However, using IVIG to treat neonatal sepsis produced a greater than 6% decrease in the mortality rate. A review of nineteen randomized control trials found a 3% decrease in the incidence of neonatal sepsis in preterm infants without a significant difference in all-cause and infection-related mortality when prophylactic IVIG was administered.[83] Based on the marginal reduction of neonatal sepsis without a reduction in mortality, routine use of prophylactic IVIG cannot be recommended.

Colony-stimulating factors (CSFs) are a family of glycoproteins that stimulate proliferation and differentiation of hematopoietic cells of various lineages. GM-CSF and granulocyte CSF (G-CSF) have similar physiologic actions. Both stimulate the proliferation of bone marrow myeloid progenitor cells, induce the release of bone marrow neutrophil storage pools, and enhance mature neutrophil effect or function.[82-84] Preliminary studies of GM-CSF in neonatal animals demonstrate enhancement of neutrophil oxidative metabolism as well as priming of neonatal neutrophils for enhanced chemotaxis and bacterial killing. Both GM-CSF and G-CSF induce peripheral neutrophilia within two to six hours of intraperitoneal administration. This enhanced affinity for neutrophils returns to normal baseline level by 24 hours.[85] Studies have confirm the efficacy and safety of G-CSF therapy for neonatal sepsis and neutropenia.[86] Other investigations have demonstrated no long-term adverse hematologic, immunologic, or developmental effects from G-CSF therapy in the septic neonate. Prolonged prophylactic treatment in the very low birth weight neonate with recombinant GM-CSF has been shown to be well tolerated and have a significant decrease in the rate of nosocomial infections.[87,88]

Unique to the newborn in septic shock is the persistence of fetal circulation and resultant pulmonary hypertension.[89] In fact, the rapid administration of fluid can further exacerbate this problem by causing left to right shunting through a patent ductus arteriosus (PDA) and subsequent congestive heart failure from ventricular overload. Infants in septic shock with a new heart murmur should undergo a cardiac echocardiogram. If present, a PDA may warrant treatment with indomethacin (prostaglandin inhibitor) or surgical ligation to achieve closure, depending on the clinical picture.

The critical care of a neonate/infant in septic shock can be extremely challenging. Septic shock has a distinctive clinical presentation and is characterized by an early compensated stage where one can see a decreased SVR, an increase in cardiac output, tachycardia, warm extremities, and an adequate urine output. Later in the clinical presentation, septic shock is characterized by an uncompensated phase where one will see a decrease in intravascular volume, myocardial depression, high vascular resistance, and a decreasing cardiac output.[90] Management of these patients is based on the principles of source control, antibiotics (broad-spectrum, institutionally based when possible and including antifungal agents as warranted), and supportive care.

Patients with severe septic shock often do not respond to conventional forms of volume loading and cardiovascular supportive medications. The administration of arginine vasopressin has been shown to decrease mortality in adult patients with recalcitrant septic shock.[91,92] Vasopressin (see Table 1-6), also known as antidiuretic hormone (ADH), is made in the posterior pituitary and plays a primary role in water regulation by the kidneys. In septic shock, vasopressin has profound effects on increasing blood pressure in intravascular depleted states. Sparked initially by a randomized, double-blinded, placebo-controlled study in adults that demonstrated a beneficial effect of vasopressin in recalcitrant septic shock, its utilization in the pediatric population has become common.[93,94] While a detailed discussion is beyond the scope of this chapter, current trends suggest that ECMO may serve as rescue therapy in select patients with profound sepsis and cardiopulmonary failure refractory to other measures (reported ELSO database newborn survival 80%, older children 50%).[94,95]

Given the difficult nature of caring for septic patients, extensive investigation has been launched in attempt to identify patients at risk.[96–98] Early serum markers such as C-reactive protein, IL-6, and procalcitonin carry promise but warrant further validation.

REFERENCES

1. Sarafoglou K, Hoffmann G, Roth K. Pediatric Endocrinology and Inborn Errors of Metabolism. China: The McGraw-Hill Companies, Inc; 2009.
2. Dweck HS, Cassady G. Glucose intolerance in infants of very low birth weight, I: Incidence of hyperglycemia in infants of birth weights 1,110 grams or less. Pediatr 1974;53:189–95.
3. Beardsall K, Dunger D. The physiology and clinical management of glucose metabolism in the newborn. Endocr Dev 2007; 12:124–37.
4. Ziegler EE, O'Donnell AM, Nelson SE, et al. Body composition of reference fetus. Growth 1976;40:329.
5. Hsu SC, Levine MA. Perinatal calcium metabolism: Physiology and pathophysiology. Semin Neonatol 2004;9:23–6.
6. Thomas TC, Smith JM, White PC, Adhikari S. Transient neonatal hypocalcemia: Presentation and outcomes. Pediatrics 2012; 129:e1461–1467.
7. Colozzi AE. Clamping of the umbilical cord. Its effect on the placental transfusion. N Engl J Med 1954;250:629.
8. Bauer C, Ludwig I, Ludwig M. Different effects of 2,3-diphosphoglycerate and adenosine triphosphate on the oxygen affinity of adult and fetal human hemoglobin. Life Sci 1968;7: 1339.
9. Asch J, Wedgwood JF. Optimizing the approach to anemia in the preterm infant: Is there a role for erythropoietin therapy? J Perinatol 1997;17:276–82.
10. Doyle JJ. The role of erythropoietin in the anemia of prematurity. Semin Perinatol 1997;21:20–7.
11. King PJ, Sullivan TM, Leftwich ME, et al. Score for neonatal acute physiology and phlebotomy blood loss predict erythrocyte transfusions in premature infants. Arch Pediatr Adolesc Med 1997;151 27–31.
12. Maisels MJ. What's in a name? Physiologic and pathologic jaundice: The conundrum of defining normal bilirubin levels in the newborn. Pediatrics 2006;118:805–7.
13. Osborn LM, Lenarsky C, Oakes RC, et al. Phototherapy in full-term infants with hemolytic disease secondary to ABO incompatibility. Pediatrics 1984;73:520–6.
14. Saugstad O. Optimal oxygenation at birth and in the neonatal period. Neonatology 2007;91:319–22.
15. Biglan AW, Cheng KP, Brown DR. Update on retinopathy of prematurity. Intern Ophthalmol Clin 1989;29:2–4.
16. National Institutes of Health. Cryotherapy for retinopathy of prematurity cooperative group. Multicenter trial of cryotherapy for retinopathy of prematurity. Arch Ophthalmol 1988;106:471–9.
17. Ng E, Connolly B, McNamara J, et al. A comparison of laser photocoagulation with cryotherapy for threshold retinopathy of prematurity at 10 years: Part 1. Visual function and structural outcome. Ophthalmol 2002;202:928–35.
18. Shalev B, Farr A, Repka M. Randomized comparison of diode laser photocoagulation versus cryotherapy for threshold retinopathy of prematurity: Seven-year outcome. Am J Ophthalmol 2002;132: 76–80.
19. Connolly B, McNamara J, Sharma S, et al. A comparison of laser phototherapy with trans-scleral cryotherapy for the treatment of threshold retinopathy. Ophthalmol 1998;105:1628–31.
20. American Academy of Pediatrics, Section on Ophthalmology, AAo Ophth, AAo Ophth/Strabismus. Screening examination of premature infants for retinopathy of prematurity. Pediatrics 2006;117: 572–6.
21. Lowell BB, Spiegelman BM. Towards a molecular understanding of adaptive thermogenesis. Nature 2000;404:652–60.
22. Chardon K, Cardot V, Leke A, et al. Thermoregulatory control of feeding and sleep in premature infants. Obesity 2006;14: 1535–42.
23. Karlberg P, Moore RE, Oliver TK. The thermogenic response of the newborn infant to noradrenaline. Acta Paediatr Scand 1962;51:284.
24. Stein J, Cheu H, Lee M, et al. Effects of muscle relaxants, sedatives, narcotics and anesthetics on neonatal thermogenesis. In: Pannell M, editor. Surgical Forum, vol. 38. Chicago: American College of Surgeons; 1987. p. 76.
25. Landsberg L, Young JB. Fasting, feeding and regulation of the sympathetic nervous system. N Engl J Med 1978;198:1295.
26. Lorenz JM, Kleinman LI, Kotagal UR, et al. Water balance in very low birth weight infants: Relationship to water and sodium intake and effect on outcome. J Pediatr 1982;101:423–32.
27. Aperia A, Broberger O, Herin P, et al. Postnatal control of water and electrolyte homeostatis in pre-term and full-term infants. Acta Paediatr Scand 1983;305:61–5.
28. Fahimi D, Mohajeri S, Hajizadeh N, et al. Comparison between fraction excretions of urea and sodium in children with acute kidney injury. Pediatr Nephrol 2009;24:2409–12.
29. Thurlbeck WM. Lung growth and development. In: Thurlbeck WM, Churg AM, editor. Pathology of the Lung. 2nd ed. New York: Thieme Medical Publishers; 1995.
30. Meurs KV, The Congenital Diaphragmatic Hernia Study Group. Is surfactant therapy beneficial in the treatment of the term newborn infant with congenital diaphragmatic hernia? J Pediatr 2004;145:312–16.
31. Lally KP, Lally PA, Langham MR, et al. Surfactant does not improve survival rate in preterm infants with congenital diaphragmatic hernia. J Pediatr Surg 2004;39:829–33.

32. Tooley WH, Clements JA, Muramatsu K, et al. Lung function in prematurely delivered rabbits treated with a synthetic surfactant. Am Rev Respir Dis 1987;136:651–6.

33. Robertson B, Enhorning G. The alveolar lining of the premature newborn rabbit after pharyngeal deposition of surfactant. Lab Invest 1974;31:54–9.

34. Shahed AI, Dargaville PA, Ohlsson A, et al. Surfactant for meconium aspiration syndrome in full term/near term infants. Cochrane Database Syst Reviews 2009:Art. No. CD002054.

35. Seger N, Soll R. Animal derived surfactant extract for treatment of respiratory distress syndrome. Cochrane Database Syst Reviews 2009;(3):Art. No. CD007636.

36. Soll R. Synthetic surfactant for respiratory distress syndrome in preterm infants. Cochrane Database Syst Reviews 2009;(3):Art. No. CD00149.

37. Rojas MA, Lozano JM, Rojas MX, et al. Very early surfactant without mandatory ventilation in premature infants treated with early continuous positive airway pressure: A randomized, controlled trial. Pediatrics 2009;123:137–42.

38. Rojas-Reyes MX, Morley CJ, Soll R. Prophylactic versus selective use of surfactant in preventing morbidity and mortality in preterm infants. Cochrane Database Syst Reviews 2012;(3):Art. No. CD000510.

39. Garg AK. 'Arterialized' capillary blood [letter]. CMAJ 1972;107:16.

40. Glasgow JF, Flynn DM, Swyer PR. A comparison of descending aortic and 'arterialized' capillary blood in the sick newborn. CMAJ 1972;106:660.

41. Siggaard-Andersen O. Acid-base and blood gas parameters—arterial or capillary blood? Scand J Clin Lab Invest 1968;21:289.

42. Reynolds GJ, Yu VYH. Guidelines for the use of pulse oximetry in the non-invasive estimation of oxygen saturation in oxygen-dependent newborn infants. Aust Paediatr J 1988;24:346–50.

43. McEvedy BAB, McLeod ME, Kirpalani H, et al. End-tidal carbon dioxide measurements in critically ill neonates: A comparison of sidestream capnometers. Can J Anaesth 1990;37:322–6.

44. Connors A. The effectiveness of right heart catheterization in the initial care of critically ill patients. JAMA 1996;276:889–97.

45. Thompson AE. Pulmonary artery catheterization in children. New Horiz 1997;5:244–50.

46. Hamzaoui O, Monnet X, Richard C. Effects of changes in vascular tone on the agreement between pulse contour and transpulmonary thermodilution cardiac output measurements within an up to 6-hour calibration-free period. Crit Care Med 2008;36:434–40.

47. Bein B, Meybohm P, Cavus E. The reliability of pulse contour-derived cardiac output during hemorrhage and after vasopressors administration. Anesth Analg 2007;105:107–13.

48. Gazit A, Cooper DS. Emerging technologies. Pediatr Crit Care Med 2011;12:S55–S61.

49. Nelson LD. Application of venous saturation monitoring. In: Civetta JM, Taylor RW, Kirby RR, editors. Critical Care. Philadelphia: JB Lippincott; 1988. p. 327–34.

50. Norfleet EA, Watson CB. Continuous mixed venous oxygen saturation measurement: A significant advance in hemodynamic monitoring? J Clin Monit Comput 1985;1:245–58.

51. Ko WJ, Chang CI, Chiu IS. Continuous monitoring of venous oxygen saturation in critically-ill infants. J Formos Med Assoc 1996;95:258–62.

52. Hirschl RB, Palmer P, Heiss KF, et al. Evaluation of the right atrial venous oxygen saturation as a physiologic monitor in a neonatal model. J Pediatr Surg 1993;28:901–5.

53. DiSessa TG, Leitner M, Ti CC, et al. The cardiovascular effects of dopamine in the severely asphyxiated neonate. J Pediatr 1981;99:772–6.

54. Perkin RM, Levin DL, Webb R, et al. Dobutamine: A hemodynamic evaluation in children with shock. J Pediatr 1982;100:977–83.

55. Osborn D, Evans N, Klucklow M. Randomized trial of dobutamine versus dopamine in preterm infants with low systemic blood flow. J Pediatr 2002;140:183–91.

56. Barton P, Garcia JK, Kitchen A, et al. Hemodynamic effects of I.V. milrinone lactate in pediatric patients with septic shock. A prospective double-blinded, randomized, placebo-controlled interventional study. Chest 1996;109:1302–12.

57. Chang AC, Am A, Wernovsky G, et al. Milrinone: Systemic and pulmonary hemodynamic effects in neonates after cardiac surgery. Crit Care Med 1995;23:1907–14.

58. Parrillo JE. Septic shock in humans. Advances in the understanding of pathogenesis, cardiovascular dysfunction, and therapy. Ann Intern Med 1990;113:227–42.

59. Danner R, Elin RJ, Hosline KM, et al. Endotoxin determinations in 100 patients with septic shock. Clin Res 1988;36:453A.

60. McCloskey RV, Straube KC, Sanders C, et al. Treatment of septic shock with human monoclonal antibody HA-1A. A randomized, double-blind, placebo-controlled trial. CHESS Trial Study Group. Ann Intern Med 1994;121:1–5.

61. Rogy MA, Moldawer LL, Oldenburg HS, et al. Anti-endotoxin therapy in primate bacteremia with HA-1A and BPI. Ann Surg 1994;220:77–85.

62. Ziegler EJ, Fisher CJ Jr, Sprung CL, et al. Treatment of gram-negative bacteremia and septic shock with HA-1A human monoclonal antibody against endotoxin. A randomized, double-blind, placebo-controlled trial. The HA-1A Sepsis Study Group. N Engl J Med 1991;324:429–36.

63. Tracey KJ, Lowry SF, Cerami A. Chachectin: A hormone that triggers acute shock and chronic cachexia. J Infect Dis 1988;157:413–20.

64. Nedwin GE, Svedersky LP, Bringman TS. Effect of interleukin-2, interferon-gamma and mitogens on the production of tumor necrosis factors alpha and beta. J Immunol 1985;135:2492–7.

65. Jupin C, Anderson S, Damais C, et al. Toxic shock syndrome toxin 1 as an inducer of human tumor necrosis factors and gamma interferon. J Exp Med 1988;167:752–61.

66. Tracey KJ, Fong Y, Hesse DG, et al. Anti-cachectin/TNF monoclonal antibodies prevent septic shock during lethal bacteraemia. Nature 1987;330:662–4.

67. Beutler B, Milsaark IW, Cerami AC. Passive immunization against cachectin/tumor necrosis factor protects mice from the lethal effects of endotoxin. Science 1981;229:869–71.

68. Rosenstein M, Ettinghausen SE, Rosenberg SA. Extravasation of intravascular fluid mediated by the systemic administration of recombinant interleukin-2. Immunology 1986;137:1735.

69. Ognibene FP, Rosenberg SA, Lotze M, et al. Interleukin-2 administration causes reversible hemodynamic changes and left ventricular dysfunction similar to those seen in septic shock. Chest 1988;94:750.

70. Pryor RW, Hinshaw LB. Sepsis/septic shock in adults and children. Pathol Immunopathol Res 1989;8:222–30.

71. Hill HR. Biochemical, structural and functional abnormalities of polymorphonuclear leukocytes in the neonate. Pediatr Res 1987;22:375–82.

72. Miller M. Chemotactic function in the human neonate: Humoral and cellular aspects. Pediatr Res 1971;5:487–92.

73. Moriguchi N, Yamamoto S, Isokawa S, et al. Granulocyte function and changes in ability with age in newborns; Report no,1: Flow cytometric analysis of granulocyte functions in whole blood. Pediatr Int 2006;48:17–21.

74. Miller ME. Phagocytosis in the newborn: Humoral and cellular factors. J Pediatr 1969;75:255–9.

75. Forman ML, Stiehm ER. Impaired opsonic activity but normal phagocytosis in low-birth-weight infants. N Engl J Med 1969;281:926–31.

76. Mohan P, Brocklehurst. Granulocyte transfusions for neonates with confirmed or suspected sepsis. Cochrane Database Syst Reviews 2003;(4):Art. No.: CD003956.

77. Cates KL, Rowe JC, Ballow M. The premature infant as a compromised host. Curr Probl Pediatr 1983;13:1–63.

78. Anderson DC, Hughes J, Edwards MS, et al. Impaired chemotaxigenesis by type III group B streptococci in neonatal sera: Relationship to diminished concentration of specific anticapsular antibody and abnormalities of serum complement. Pediatr Res 1983;17:496–502.

79. Stossel TP, Alper CH, Rosen F. Opsonic activity in the newborn: Role of properidin. Pediatr 1973;52:134–7.

80. Gerdes JS, Yoder MC, Douglas SD, et al. Decreased plasma fibronectin in neonatal sepsis. Pediatrics 1983;72:877–81.

81. Chirico G, Rondini G, Plebani A, et al. Intravenous gamma globulin therapy for prophylaxis of infection in high-risk neonates. J Pediatr 1987;110:437–42.

82. Clark SC, Kamen R. The human hematopoietic colony-stimulating factors. Science 1987;236:1229–37.

83. Ohlsson A, Lacy J. Intravenous immunoglobulin for preventing infection in preterm and or low birth weight infants. Cochrane Database Syst Reviews 2004(1):Art. No.: CD000361.

84. Sieff CA. Hematopoietic growth factors. J Clin Invest 1987;79:1549.

85. Barak Y, Leibovitz E, Mogilner B, et al. The in vivo effect of recombinant human granulocyte-colony stimulating factor in neutropenic neonates with sepsis. Eur J Pediatr 1997;156:643–6.

86. Wolach B. Neonatal sepsis: Pathogenesis and supportive therapy [Review]. Semin Perinatol 1997;21:28–38.

87. Cairo M, Seth T, Fanaroff A, et al. A double-blinded randomized placebo controlled pilot study of RhGM-CSF in low birth weight neonates (LBWN): Preliminary results demonstrate a significant reduction in nosocomial infections with Rhu-GM-CS. Pediatr Res 1996;39:294a.

88. Brancho F, Goldman S, Cairo M. Potential use of granulocyte colony-stimulating factor and granulocyte-macrophage colony-stimulating factor in neonates. Curr Opin Hematology 1998;5:315–20.

89. Carcillo JA, Fields AI, Task Force Committee Members. Clinical practice parameters for hemodynamic support of pediatric and neonatal patients septic shock. Crit Care Med 2002;30:1365–77.

90. Tobin JR, Wetzel RC. Shock and multi-organ system failure. In Handbook of Pediatric Intensive Care, Rogers and Helfaer, eds. 1999. p. 324–51.

91. Ruokonen E, Parviainen I, Usuaro A. Treatment of impaired perfusion in septic shock. Ann Med 2002;34:590–7.

92. Dellinger RP. Cardiovascular management of septic shock. Crit Care Med 2003;31:946–55.

93. Malay MB, Ashton RC, Landry DW, et al. Low-dose vasopressin in the treatment of vasodilatory septic shock. J Trauma 1999; 47:699–703.

94. Brierley J, Carcillo JA, Choong K, et al. Clinical practice parameters for hemodynamic support of pediatric and neonatal septic shock: 2007 update from the American College of Critical Care Medicine. Crit Care Med 37:666–88, 2009.

95. Yager P, Noviski N. Shock. Pediatr Rev 2010;21:311–18.

96. Srinivasan L, Harris MC. New technologies for the rapid diagnosis of neonatal sepsis. Curr Opin Pediatr 2012;24:165–71.

97. Hofer N, Zacharias E, Muller W, et al. An update on the use of C-reactive protein in early-onset neonatal sepsis: current insights and new tasks. Neonatol 2012;102:25–36.

98. Dilli D, Dilmer U. The role of interleukin-6 and C-reactive protein in non-thyroidal illness in premature infants followed in neonatal intensive care unit. J Clin Res Pediatr Endocrinol 2012;4:66–71.

CHAPTER 2

Nutritional Support for the Pediatric Patient

Nilesh M. Mehta • Tom Jaksic

Despite advances in the field of nutritional support, the prevalence of malnutrition among hospitalized patients, especially those with a protracted clinical course, has remained largely unchanged over the last two decades.[1,2] The provision of optimal nutritional therapy requires a careful assessment of energy needs and the provision of macronutrients and micronutrients via the most suitable feeding route. The profound and stereotypic metabolic response to injury places unique demands on the hospitalized child. Standard equations available for estimating energy needs have proven to be unreliable in this population.[3,4] In addition, children with critical illness have a marked net protein catabolism and often lack adequate nutritional support.[5] Ultimately, an individualized nutritional regimen should be tailored for each child and reviewed regularly during the course of illness. An understanding of the metabolic events that accompany illness and surgery in a child is the first step in implementing appropriate nutritional support.

THE METABOLIC RESPONSE TO STRESS

The metabolic response to illness due to stressors such as trauma, surgery, or inflammation has been well described. Cuthbertson was the first investigator to realize the primary role that whole-body protein catabolism plays in the systemic response to injury.[6] Based on his work, the metabolic stress response has been conceptually divided into two phases. The initial, brief 'ebb phase' is characterized by decreased enzymatic activity, reduced oxygen consumption, low cardiac output, and a core temperature that may be subnormal. This is followed by the hypermetabolic 'flow phase' characterized by increased cardiac output, oxygen consumption, and glucose production. During this phase, fat and protein mobilization is manifested by increased urinary nitrogen excretion and weight loss. This catabolic phase is mediated by a surge in cytokines and the characteristic endocrine response to trauma or operation that results in an increased availability of substrates essential for healing and glucose production.

Neonates and children share similar qualitative metabolic responses to illness as adults, albeit with significant quantitative differences. The metabolic stress response is beneficial in the short term, but the consequences of sustained catabolism are significant as the child has limited tissue stores and substantial nutrient requirements for growth. Thus the prompt institution of nutritional support is a priority in sick neonates and children. The goal of nutrition in this setting is to augment the short-term benefits of the metabolic response to injury while minimizing long-term consequences. In general, the metabolic stress response is characterized by an increase in net muscle protein degradation and the enhanced movement of free amino acids through the circulation (Fig. 2-1). These amino acids serve as the building blocks for the rapid synthesis of proteins that act as mediators for the inflammatory response and structural components for tissue repair. The remaining amino acids not used in this way are channeled through the liver where their carbon skeletons are utilized to create glucose through gluconeogenesis. The provision of additional dietary protein may slow the rate of net protein loss, but does not eliminate the overall negative protein balance associated with injury.[7]

Carbohydrate and lipid turnover are also increased several fold during the metabolic response. Although these metabolic alterations would be expected to increase overall energy requirements, data show that such an increase is quantitatively variable, modest, and evanescent. Overall, the energy needs of the critically ill or injured child are governed by the severity and persistence of the underlying illness or injury. Accurate assessment of energy requirements in individual patients allows optimal caloric supplementation and avoids the deleterious effects of both under- and overfeeding. Children with critical illness demonstrate a unique hormonal and cytokine profile characterized by an elevation in serum levels of insulin, the catabolic hormones (glucagons, cortisol, catecholamines), and specific cytokines known to interact with the inflammatory process.[8] Novel ways to manipulate these hormonal and cytokine alterations with an aim to minimize the deleterious consequences induced by the stress response are a focus of research.

BODY COMPOSITION AND NUTRIENT RESERVES

The body composition of the young child contrasts with that of the adult in several ways that significantly affect nutritional requirements. Table 2-1 lists the macronutrient stores of the neonate, child, and adult as a percentage of total body weight.[9,10] Carbohydrate stores are limited in all age groups and provide only a short-term supply of glucose. Despite this fact, neonates have a high demand

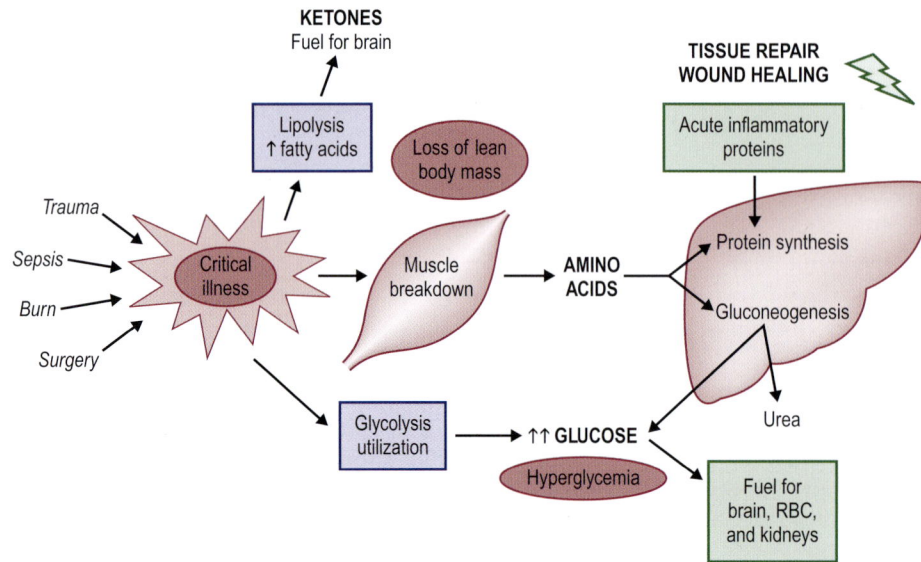

FIGURE 2-1 ■ The metabolic changes associated with the pediatric stress response to critical illness and injury. In general, net protein catabolism predominates and amino acids are transported from muscle stores to the liver, where they are converted to inflammatory proteins and glucose through the process of gluconeogenesis.

TABLE 2-1   **The Body Composition of Neonates, Children, and Adults as a Percentage of Total Body Weight**

Age	Protein (%)	Fat (%)	Carbohydrate (%)
Neonates	11	14	0.4
Children (age 10 years)	15	17	0.4
Adults	18	19	0.4

TABLE 2-2   **Estimated Requirements for Energy and Protein in Healthy Humans of Different Age Groups**

Age	Protein (g/kg/day)	Energy (kcal/kg/day)
Neonates	2.2	120
Children (age 10 years)	1.0	70
Adults	0.8	35

for glucose and have shown elevated rates of glucose turnover when compared with those of the adult.[11] This is thought to be related to the neonate's increased brain-to-body mass ratio because glucose is the primary energy source for the central nervous system. Neonatal glycogen stores are even more limited in the early postpartum period, especially in the preterm infant.[12] Short periods of fasting can predispose the newborn to hypoglycemia. Thus when infants are burdened with illness or injury, they must rapidly turn to the breakdown of protein stores to generate glucose through the process of gluconeogenesis.

Lipid reserves are low in the neonate, gradually increasing with age. Premature infants have the lowest proportion of lipid stores as the majority of polyunsaturated fatty acids accumulate in the third trimester.[13] This renders lipid less useful as a potential fuel source in the young child.[14] The most dramatic difference between adult and pediatric patients is in the relative quantity of stored protein. The protein reserve of the adult is nearly twofold that of the neonate. Thus infants cannot afford to lose significant amounts of protein during the course of a protracted illness or injury. An important feature of the metabolic stress response, unlike in starvation, is that the provision of dietary glucose does not halt gluconeogenesis. Consequently, the catabolism of muscle protein

to produce glucose continues unabated.[15] Neonates and children also share much higher baseline energy requirements. Studies have demonstrated that the resting energy expenditure for neonates is two to three times that of adults when standardized for body weight.[14,16] Clearly, the child's need for rapid growth and development is a large component of this increase in energy requirement. Moreover, the relatively large body surface area of the young child may increase heat loss and further contributes to elevations in energy expenditure.

The basic requirements for protein and energy in the healthy neonate, child, and adult, based on recent recommendations by the National Academy of Sciences, are listed in Table 2-2.[17] As illustrated, the recommended protein provision for the neonate is almost three times that of the adult. In premature infants, a minimum protein allotment of 2.8 g/kg/day is required to maintain in utero growth rates.[18] The increased metabolic demand and limited nutrient reserves of the infant mandates early nutritional support in times of injury and critical illness to avoid negative nutritional consequences.

Accurate assessment of body composition is necessary for planning nutritional intake, monitoring dynamic changes in the body compartments (such as the loss of lean body mass), and assessing the adequacy of nutritional supportive regimens during critical illness. Ongoing loss of lean body mass is an indicator of inadequate dietary supplementation and may have clinical implications in the hospitalized child. However, current methods of body composition analysis (such as anthropometry, weight and biochemical parameters) are either impractical for clinical use or inaccurate in a subgroup of hospitalized children with critical illness. One of the principal problems in critically ill children is the presence of capillary leak, manifesting as edema and large fluid shifts. These make anthropometric measurements invalid and other bedside techniques have not been validated.

ENERGY EXPENDITURE DURING ILLNESS

For children with illness or undergoing operative intervention, knowledge of energy requirements is important for the design of appropriate nutritional strategies. Dietary regimens that both under- and overestimate energy needs are associated with injurious consequences. Owing to the high degree of individual variability in energy expenditure, particularly in the most critically ill patients, the actual measurement of resting energy expenditure (REE) is recommended.

The components of total energy expenditure (TEE) for a child in order of magnitude are: resting REE, energy expended during physical activity (PA), and diet-induced thermogenesis (DIT). The sum of these components determines the energy requirement for an individual. In general, REE rates decline with age from infancy to young adulthood, at which time the rate becomes stable. In children with critical illness, the remaining factors in the determination of total energy requirement are of reduced significance as PA is low and DIT (the heat generated by the consumption of food products) may not be significant.

REE can be measured using direct or indirect methods. The direct calorimetric method measures the heat released by a subject at rest and is based on the principle that all energy is eventually converted to heat. In practice, the patient is placed in a thermally isolated chamber, and the heat dissipated is measured for a given period of time.[19] This method is the true gold standard for measured energy expenditure. Direct calorimetry is not practical for most hospitalized children and REE is often estimated using standard equations. Unfortunately, REE estimates using standardized World Health Organization (WHO) predictive equations are unreliable, particularly in underweight subjects.[19–21]

REE estimation is difficult in critically ill or postoperative children. Their energy requirements show individual variation and are dependent upon severity of injury. For instance, an infant with respiratory distress on pressure support is likely to have high energy requirement due to increased work of breathing. The same patient, when started on mechanical ventilation with muscle relaxants, is unlikely to have sustained high energy requirements. Infants with congenital diaphragmatic hernia on extracorporeal membrane oxygenation (ECMO) support have been shown to have energy expenditures of approximately 90 kcal/kg/day. Following extubation, the same patients may have energy requirements

as high as 140 kcal/kg/day. Although stress factors ranging from 1.0 to 2.7 have been applied to correct for these variations, calculated standardized energy expenditure equations have not been satisfactorily validated in critically ill children.[22–25]

Indirect calorimetry measures VO_2 (the volume of oxygen consumed) and VCO_2 (the volume of CO_2 produced), and uses a correlation factor based on urinary nitrogen excretion to calculate the overall rate of energy production.[26] The measurement of energy needs is 'indirect' because it does not use direct temperature changes to determine energy needs. Indirect calorimetry provides a measurement of the overall respiratory quotient (RQ), defined as the ratio of CO_2 produced to O_2 consumed (VCO_2 / VO_2), for a given patient. Oxidation of carbohydrate yields an RQ of 1.0, whereas fatty acid oxidation gives an RQ of 0.7. However, the role of the RQ as a marker of substrate use and as an indicator of underfeeding or overfeeding is limited. The body's ability to metabolize substrate may be impaired during illness, making assumptions invalid about RQ values and substrate oxidation.

Although RQ is not a sensitive marker for adequacy of feeding in individual cases, RQ values greater than 1.0 are generally associated with lipogenesis secondary to overfeeding.[27,28] A recent study has suggested the utility of extremes of RQ in monitoring feeding adequacy, where an RQ higher than 0.85 reliably indicates the absence of underfeeding and an RQ higher than 1.0 reliably indicates the presence of overfeeding.[29] However, numerous factors, related and unrelated to feeding, can alter the value of a measured RQ in critically ill patients, e.g., hyperventilation, acidosis, effects of cardiotonic agents and neuromuscular blocking, and an individual response to a given substrate load, injury, or disease. Furthermore, in the setting of wide diurnal and day-to-day variability of REE in critically ill individuals, the extrapolation of short-term calorimetric REE measurements to 24-hour REE may introduce errors. The use of steady-state measurements may decrease these errors. Steady state is defined by change in VO_2 and VCO_2 of <10% over a period of five consecutive minutes. The values for the mean REE from this steady-state period may be used as an accurate representation of the 24-hour TEE in patients with low levels of physical activity.[30] In a patient who fails to achieve steady state and is metabolically unstable, prolonged testing is required (minimum of 60 minutes), and 24-hour indirect calorimetry should be considered. With the advent of newer technology, the application of indirect calorimetry at the bedside for continuous monitoring shows promise.

Indirect calorimetry is not accurate in the setting of air leaks around the endotracheal tube, ventilator circuit or through a chest tube, or in subjects on ECMO. High inspired oxygen fraction (FiO_2 >0.6) will also affect indirect calorimetry. Indirect calorimetry is difficult to use in babies on ECMO because a large proportion of the patient's oxygenation and ventilation is performed through the membrane oxygenator. The use of indirect calorimetry for assessment and monitoring of nutrition intake requires attention to its limitations and expertise in the interpretation. Nonetheless, its application in children at high risk for underfeeding and overfeeding may be helpful.[31,32]

Nonradioactive stable isotope techniques have been used to measure REE in the pediatric patient. Stable isotope technology has been available for many years and was first applied for energy expenditure measurement in humans in 1982.[33,34] Both ^{13}C-labeled bicarbonate and doubly labeled water ($^2H_2^{18}O$) have been used to measure TEE in pediatric surgical patients, and have been shown to correlate well with indirect calorimetry.[31,34,35] The ^{13}C-labeled bicarbonate method allows the calculation of REE on the basis of infusion rate and the ratio of labeled to unlabeled CO_2 in expired breath samples.[35] Orally administered stable isotopes of water (^2H_2O and $H_2^{18}O$) mix with the body water and the ^{18}O is lost from the body as both water and CO_2, while the ^2H is lost from the body only as water. The difference in the rates of loss of the isotopes ^{18}O and ^2H from the body reflects the rate of CO_2 production, which can be used to calculate the TEE.[36-38] However, the doubly labeled water method has its limitations in children with active capillary leak, decreased urine output, fluid overload, and diuretic use.[36]

In general, any increase in energy expenditure during illness or after an operation is variable, and studies suggest that the increase is far less than originally hypothesized. In children with severe burns, the initial REE during the flow phase of injury is increased by 50% but then returns to normal during convalescence.[39] In neonates with bronchopulmonary dysplasia, in which the illness increases the patient's work of breathing, a 25% elevation in energy requirement is evident.[40] Newborns undergoing major surgery have only a transient 20% increase in energy expenditure that returns to baseline values within 12 hours postoperatively, provided no major complications develop.[41,42] Stable extubated neonates, five days after operation, have been shown to have REE comparable to normal infants.[43] Effective anesthetic and analgesic management may play a significant role in muting the stress response of the neonate. Studies have demonstrated no discernible increase in REE in neonates undergoing patent ductus arteriosus ligation who received intraoperative fentanyl anesthesia and postoperative intravenous analgesic regimens.[42] A retrospective stratification of surgical infants into low- and high-stress cohorts based on the severity of underlying illness found that high-stress infants undergo moderate short-term elevations in energy expenditure after operation, whereas low-stress infants do not manifest any increase in energy expenditures during the course of illness.[44] Finally, by using stable isotopic methods, it has been found that the mean energy expenditures of critically ill neonates on ECMO are nearly identical to age- and diet-matched nonstressed controls.[45]

All these studies suggest that critically ill neonates have only a small and usually short-term increase in energy expenditure. Although children have increased energy requirements from increased metabolic turnover during illness, their caloric needs may be lower than previously considered due to possible halted or slow growth,[46] and the use of sedation and muscle paralysis.[47] This could result in overfeeding when energy intake is based on presumed or estimated energy expenditure with

stress factors. On the other hand, unrecognized hypermetabolism in select individuals result in underfeeding with negative nutritional consequences.[31] The variability in energy requirements may result in cumulative energy imbalances in the intensive care unit (ICU) over a period of time.[32] A direct relationship has been reported between cumulative caloric imbalance and the mortality rate in critically ill surgical patients.[48]

For practical purposes, the recommended dietary caloric intake for healthy children may represent a reasonable starting point for the upper limit of caloric allotment in the hospitalized child.[17] However, as discussed earlier, energy requirement estimates in select groups of patients remain variable and possibly overestimated, mandating an accurate estimation using measured energy expenditure where available. Regular anthropometric measurements plotted on a growth chart to assess the adequacy of caloric provision will allow relatively prompt detection of underfeeding or overfeeding in most cases. However, some critically ill children may be too sick for regular weights or have changes in body water that make anthropometric measurements unreliable.

MACRONUTRIENT INTAKE

Protein Metabolism and Requirement During Illness

Amino acids are the key building blocks required for growth and tissue repair. The vast majority (98%) are found in existing proteins, and the remainder reside in the free amino acid pool. Proteins are continually degraded into their constituent amino acids and resynthesized through the process of protein turnover. The reutilization of amino acids released by protein breakdown is extensive. Synthesis of proteins from the recycling of amino acids is more than two times greater than from dietary protein intake. An advantage of high protein turnover is that a continuous flow of amino acids is available for the synthesis of new proteins. This allows the body tremendous flexibility in meeting ever-changing physiologic needs. However, the process of protein turnover requires the input of energy to power both protein degradation and synthesis. At baseline, infants are known to have higher rates of protein turnover than adults. Healthy newborns have a protein-turnover rate of 6–12 g/kg/day compared with 3.5 g/kg/day in adults.[49] Even greater rates of protein turnover have been measured in premature and low birth weight infants.[50] For example, it has been demonstrated that extremely low birth weight infants receiving no dietary protein can lose in excess of 1.2 g/kg/day of endogenous protein.[51] At the same time, infants must maintain a positive protein balance to attain normal growth and development, whereas the healthy adult can subsist with a neutral protein balance.

In the metabolically stressed patient, such as the child with severe burn injury or cardiorespiratory failure requiring ECMO, protein turnover is doubled when compared with normal subjects.[34,49] A study of critically ill infants and children found an 80% increase in protein turnover, which correlated with the duration of the critical illness.[52] This process redistributes amino acids from skeletal muscle to the liver, wound, and tissues taking part in the inflammatory response. The factors required for the inflammatory response (acutely needed enzymes, serum proteins, and glucose) are thereby synthesized from degraded body protein stores. The well-established increase in hepatically derived acute phase proteins (including C-reactive protein, fibrinogen, transferrin, and α-1-acid glycoprotein), along with the concomitant decrease in transport proteins (albumin and retinol-binding protein), is evidence of this protein redistribution. As substrate turnover is increased during the stress response, rates of both whole-body protein degradation and whole-body protein synthesis are accelerated. However, protein breakdown predominates, thereby leading to a hypercatabolic state with an ensuing net negative protein and nitrogen balance.[27]

Protein loss is evident in elevated levels of excreted urinary nitrogen during critical illness. For example, infants with sepsis demonstrate a severalfold increase in the loss of urinary nitrogen that directly correlates with the degree of illness.[53] Clinically, severe protein loss can be manifested by skeletal muscle wasting, weight loss, delayed wound healing, and immune dysfunction.[54] In addition to the reprioritization of protein for tissue repair, healing and inflammation, the body appears to have an increased need for glucose production during times of metabolic stress.[55] The accelerated rate of gluconeogenesis during illness and injury is seen in both children and adults, and this process appears to be accentuated in infants with low body weight.[13,54] The increased production of glucose in times of illness is necessary as glucose represents a versatile energy source for tissues taking part in the inflammatory response. For example, it has been shown that glucose utilization by leukocytes is significantly increased during the inflammatory response.[56] Unfortunately, the provision of additional dietary glucose does not suppress the body's need for increased glucose production. Therefore, net protein breakdown continues to predominate.[14,57,58]

Specific amino acids are transported from muscle to the liver to facilitate hepatic glucose production. The initial step of amino acid catabolism involves removal of the toxic amino group (NH_3). Through transamination, the amino group is transferred to α-ketoglutarate, thereby producing glutamate. The addition of another amino group converts glutamate to glutamine, which is subsequently transported to the liver. Here, the amino groups are removed from glutamine and detoxified to urea through the urea cycle. The amino acid carbon skeleton can then enter the gluconeogenesis pathway. Alternatively, in skeletal muscle, the amino group can be transferred to pyruvate, thereby forming alanine. When alanine is transported to the liver and detoxified, pyruvate is reformed and can be converted to glucose through gluconeogenesis. The transport of alanine and pyruvate between peripheral muscle tissue and the liver is termed the glucose-alanine cycle.[59] Hence the transport amino acid systems involving glutamine and alanine provide carbon backbones for gluconeogenesis, while facilitating the hepatic detoxification of ammonia by the urea cycle.

Increased muscle protein catabolism is a successful short-term adaptation during critical illness, but it is limited and ultimately harmful to the child with reduced protein stores and elevated protein demands. Unless the inciting stress is eliminated, the progressive breakdown of diaphragmatic, cardiac, and skeletal muscle can lead to respiratory compromise, fatal arrhythmia, and loss of lean body mass. Moreover, a prolonged negative protein balance may have a significant impact on the child's growth and development. Healthy, nonstressed neonates require a positive protein balance of nearly 2 g/kg/day.[48,60] In contrast, critically ill, premature neonates requiring mechanical ventilation have a negative protein balance of −1 g/kg/day.[61,62] Critically ill neonates who require ECMO have exceedingly high rates of protein loss, with a net negative protein balance of −2.3 g/kg/day.[63] It has been well established that the extent of protein catabolism correlates with morbidity and mortality in surgical patients.

Fortunately, amino acid supplementation tends to promote increased nitrogen retention and positive protein balance in critically ill patients.[59,64] The mechanism appears to be an increase in protein synthesis while rates of protein degradation remain constant.[60,61] Therefore the provision of dietary protein sufficient to optimize protein synthesis, facilitate wound healing and the inflammatory process, and preserve skeletal muscle mass is the single most important nutritional intervention in critically ill children. The quantity of protein needed to enhance protein accrual is greater in hospitalized sick children than in healthy children. Table 2-3 lists recommended quantities of dietary protein for hospitalized children. Extreme cases of physiologic stress, including the child with extensive burns or the neonate on ECMO, may necessitate additional protein supplementation to meet metabolic demands.

The influence of macronutrient intake on protein balance has been explored in a limited number of studies. A systematic review of all such studies in mechanically ventilated children showed that a minimum of 1.5 g/kg/day protein and 57 kcal/kg/day energy intake was needed to achieve a positive protein balance in this group.[62] However, it should be noted that toxicity from excessive protein administration can occur, particularly in children with impaired renal and hepatic function. The provision of protein at levels greater than 3 g/kg/day is rarely indicated and is often associated with azotemia. In

TABLE 2-3 Recommended Protein Requirements for Hospitalized Infants and Children

Age (years)	Estimated Protein Requirement (g/kg/day)
Extremely low birth weight infants	up to 3.5
Very low birth weight	up to 3.0
0–2	2.0–3.0
2–13	1.5–2.0
13–18	1.0–1.5

premature neonates, the possible beneficial effects of protein allotments of 3–3.5 g/kg/day are being actively investigated in an effort to replicate intrauterine growth rates. Studies using protein provisions of 6 g/kg/day in children have demonstrated significant morbidity, including azotemia, pyrexia, strabismus, and lower IQ scores.[64,65]

Protein Quality

In addition to the sufficient quantity of dietary protein, an increased focus has been placed on the protein quality of nutritional provisions. The specific amino acid formulation to best increase whole-body protein balance has yet to be fully determined, although numerous clinical and basic science research projects are actively focusing on this topic. It is known that infants have an increased requirement per kilogram for the essential amino acids compared to the adult.[66] In particular, neonates have immature biosynthetic pathways that may temporarily alter their ability to synthesize specific amino acids. One example is the amino acid histidine, which has been shown to be a conditionally essential amino acid in infants up to age 6 months. Data suggest that cysteine, taurine, and proline also may be limited in the premature neonate.[67–70] Interest has also been expressed in the use of arginine as an 'immunonutrient' to enhance the function of the immune system in critically ill patients. Although preliminary studies show that arginine supplementation may reduce the risk of infectious complications, its safety and efficacy in infants and children has yet to be established.[71]

The restricted availability of the amino acid cysteine may have clinical relevance in the critically ill child. Cysteine is a required substrate for the production of glutathione, the body's major antioxidant. In critically ill children, cysteine turnover is increased significantly, whereas rates of glutathione synthesis are decreased by 60%. In this way, cysteine may become a conditionally essential amino acid in the sick child. Recent experiments have demonstrated that the enteral feeding of cysteine in small quantities to rats dependent on total parenteral nutrition (TPN) significantly increases the hepatic concentration of glutathione.[72] The enteral supplementation of cysteine in a pediatric nutritional regimen warrants further basic science and clinical investigation.

Glutamine is another amino acid that has been studied extensively in both children and adults in the ICU. Glutamine is an important amino acid source for gluconeogenesis, intestinal energy production, and ammonia detoxification. In healthy subjects, glutamine is a nonessential amino acid, although it has been hypothesized that glutamine may become conditionally essential in critically ill patients. Because it is difficult to keep glutamine soluble in solution, standard TPN formulas do not include glutamine in the amino acid mixture. Although preliminary data on glutamine supplementation in the clinical setting are encouraging, numerous problems with study methodology have been noted.[73] Additional prospective, randomized trials are needed to define its utility fully in both the adult and pediatric population.

In summary, during illness and recovery from trauma or surgery, there is increased protein catabolism. The short-term adaptive benefit of this response is outweighed by the loss of protein in critical organs and the consequent morbidity seen after the exhaustion of limited protein reserves. This sustained protein breakdown cannot be stopped by increasing caloric intake alone (as is the case in starvation), but protein balance may be restored by optimal (probably individual and disease specific) quantities of protein intake during this state. Future studies may also elucidate if specific amino acid mixtures may be of benefit to select subpopulations.

Modulating Protein Metabolism

The dramatic increase in protein breakdown during critical illness, coupled with the known association between protein loss and patient mortality and morbidity, has stimulated a wide array of research efforts. The measurement of whole-body nitrogen balance through urine and stool was once the only way to investigate changes in protein metabolism, but new and validated stable isotope tracer techniques now allow precise measurement of protein turnover, breakdown, and synthesis.[74] However, the modulation of protein metabolism in critically ill patients has been difficult. Dietary supplementation of amino acids increases protein synthesis, but appears to have no effect on rates of protein breakdown. Thus investigators have recently focused on the use of alternative anabolic agents to decrease protein catabolism. Studies have used various pharmacologic tools to achieve this goal, including growth hormone, insulin-derived growth factor I (IGF-I), and testosterone, with varying degrees of success.[75–77] One of the more promising agents, however, may be the anabolic hormone insulin. Multiple studies have used insulin to reduce protein breakdown in healthy volunteers and adult burn patients.[50,78] In children with extensive burns, intravenous insulin has been shown to increase lean body mass and mitigate peripheral muscle catabolism.[79] A recent prospective, randomized trial of more than 1500 adult postoperative patients in the ICU demonstrated significant reductions in mortality and morbidity with the use of intravenous insulin.[80] Preliminary stable isotopic studies demonstrate that an intravenous insulin infusion may reduce protein breakdown by over 30% in critically ill neonates on ECMO.[81] The use of intensive insulin therapy for critically ill children and adults continues to be another active and interesting area of clinical investigation. Some recent studies examining the role of insulin for tight glycemic control in critically ill patients have been less encouraging and are discussed in the next section.

Carbohydrate Metabolism and Requirement During Illness

Glucose production and availability are a priority in the pediatric metabolic stress response. Glucose is the primary energy source for the brain, erythrocyte, and renal medulla, and is used extensively in the inflammatory response. Injured and septic adults demonstrate a threefold increase in glucose turnover, glucose oxidation, and gluconeogenesis.[16] This increase is of particular concern in neonates who have an elevated glucose turnover at baseline.[10] Moreover, glycogen stores provide only a limited endogenous supply of glucose in adults and an even smaller reserve in the neonate. Thus the critically ill neonate has a greater glucose demand and reduced glucose stores. During illness, the administration of exogenous glucose does not halt the elevated rates of gluconeogenesis, and thus net protein catabolism continues unabated.[14] It is clear, however, that a combination of dietary glucose and amino acids can effectively improve protein balance during critical illness, primarily through augmentation of protein synthesis.

In the past, nutritional support regimens for critically ill patients used large amounts of glucose in an attempt to reduce endogenous glucose production. Unfortunately, excess glucose increases CO_2 production, engenders fatty liver, and does not result in a reduction in endogenous glucose turnover.[82] Thus a surplus of carbohydrate may increase the ventilatory burden on the critically ill patient. In one study, adults in the ICU fed with high-glucose TPN demonstrate a 30% increase in oxygen consumption, a 57% increase in CO_2 production, and a 71% elevation in minute ventilation.[83] In critically ill infants, the conversion of excess glucose to fat has also been correlated with increased CO_2 production and higher respiratory rates.[84] In addition, excessive carbohydrate may play a role in the genesis of TPN-associated cholestatic liver injury. Finally, some data in critically ill neonates have shown that excess caloric allotments of carbohydrate are paradoxically associated with an increased rate of net protein breakdown.[85]

When designing a nutritional regimen for the critically ill child, excessive carbohydrate calories should be avoided. A mixed fuel system, with both glucose and lipid substrates, should be used to meet the child's caloric requirements. When the postoperative neonate is fed a high-glucose diet, the corresponding RQ is approximately 1.0, and may be higher than 1.0 in selected patients, signifying increased lipogenesis.[86] A mixed dietary regimen of glucose and lipid (at 2–4 g/kg/day) lowers the effective RQ in neonates to 0.83.[87] This approach provides the infant with full nutritional supplementation while alleviating an increased ventilatory burden and difficulties with hyperglycemia.

Administration of high caloric (glucose load) diets in the early phase of critical illness may exacerbate hyperglycemia, increase carbon dioxide generation with an increased load on the respiratory system, promote hyperlipidemia resulting from increased lipogenesis, and result in a hyperosmolar state. Several reports have linked hyperglycemia with increased mortality and established the role of insulin-assisted tight glycemic control in improving outcomes in critically ill adults.[80,88,89] A remarkable 43% reduction in mortality was reported in postcardiac surgery patients in an adult ICU by implementing strict glycemic control (arterial blood glucose levels below 110 mg/dL) and using insulin infusion in the treatment group compared with the control group (average blood glucose level of 150–160 mg/dL).[80] The precise mechanism(s) responsible for this beneficial effect of tight glycemic control with an insulin protocol remains unanswered. A recent meta-analysis of studies examining the role of tight glycemic control in adult ICUs has shown a high incidence of hypoglycemia in the treatment group and less impressive benefit.[90] Although the incidence of hyperglycemia in children is high and may be associated with increased mortality and length of stay,[91] there are no data for similar benefits of tight glycemic control in this patient population. Studies examining the role of a tight glycemic control strategy in infants and children are currently underway.

Lipid Metabolism and Requirements During Illness

Similar to protein and carbohydrate metabolism, the turnover of lipid is generally increased by critical illness, major surgery, and trauma in the pediatric patient.[92] During the early ebb phase, triglyceride levels may initially increase as the rate of lipid metabolism decreases. However, this process reverses itself in the predominant flow phase, and during this time, critically ill adults have demonstrated two- to fourfold increases in lipid turnover.[93] Also, it has been shown that critically ill children on mechanical ventilation have increased rates of fatty acid oxidation.[94] The increased lipid metabolism is thought to be proportional to the overall degree of illness. The process of lipid turnover involves the conversion of free fatty acids and their glycerol backbone into triglycerides. Approximately 30–40% of free fatty acids are oxidized for energy. RQ values may decline during illness, reflecting an increased utilization of fat as an energy source.[95] This suggests that fatty acids are a prime source of energy in metabolically stressed pediatric patients. In addition to the rich energy supply from lipid substrate, the glycerol moiety released from triglycerides may be converted to pyruvate and used to manufacture glucose. As seen with the other catabolic changes associated with illness and trauma, the provision of dietary glucose does not decrease fatty acid turnover in times of illness. The increased demand for lipid utilization in critical illness coupled with the limited lipid stores in the neonate puts the metabolically stressed infant/child at high risk for the development of essential fatty acid deficiency.[96,97] Preterm infants have been shown to develop biochemical evidence of essential fatty acid deficiency two days after the initiation of a fat-free nutritional regimen.[98]

In the human, the polyunsaturated fatty acids linoleic and linolenic acid are considered essential fatty acids because the body cannot manufacture them by desaturating other fatty acids. Linoleic acid is used by the body to synthesize arachidonic acid, an important intermediary in prostaglandin synthesis. The prostaglandin family includes the leukotrienes and thromboxanes, all of which serve as mediators in wide-ranging processes such as vascular permeability, smooth muscle reactivity, and platelet aggregation. If an individual lacks dietary linoleic acid, the formation of arachidonic acid (a tetraene) cannot occur, and eicosatrienoic acid (a triene) accumulates. Clinically, a fatty acid profile can be performed on human serum, and an elevated triene-to-tetraene ratio greater than 0.4 is characteristic of biochemical essential fatty acid deficiency, though this value is somewhat variable and dependent upon the specific laboratory assay utilized. Signs of fatty acid deficiencies include dermatitis, alopecia, thrombocytopenia, increased susceptibility to infection, and overall failure to thrive. To avoid essential fatty acid deficiency in neonates, the allotment of linoleic and linolenic acid is recommended at concentrations of 4.5% and 0.5% of total calories, respectively. In addition, some evidence exists that the long-chain fatty acid docosahexaenoic acid (DHA), a derivative of linolenic acid, also may be deficient in preterm and formula-fed infants. At present, clinical trials are actively seeking to determine whether supplementation with long-chain polyunsaturated fatty acids will be of clinical benefit in this population.

Parenterally delivered lipid solutions also limit the need for excessive glucose intake. These lipid emulsions provide a higher quantity of energy per gram than does glucose (9 kcal/g vs 4 kcal/g). This reduces the overall rate of CO_2 production, the RQ value, and the incidence of hepatic steatosis.[99] There are risks when starting a patient on intravenous lipid administration. These include hypertriglyceridemia, a possible increased risk of infection, and decreased alveolar oxygen-diffusion capacity.[100-102] Most institutions, therefore, initiate lipid provisions in children at 0.5–1.0 g/kg/day and advance over a period of days to 2–4 g/kg/day. During this time, triglyceride levels are monitored closely. Lipid administration is generally restricted to 30–40% of total caloric intake in ill children in an effort to obviate immune dysfunction, although this practice has not been validated in a formal clinical trial.

In settings of prolonged fasting or uncontrolled diabetes mellitus, the accelerated production of glucose depletes the hepatocyte of needed intermediaries in the citric acid cycle. When this occurs, the acetyl-coenzyme A (CoA) generated from the breakdown of fatty acids cannot enter the citric acid cycle and instead forms ketone bodies, acetoacetate, and b-hydroxybutyrate. These ketone bodies are released by the liver to extrahepatic tissues, particularly, skeletal muscle and the brain, where they can be used for energy production instead of glucose. During surgical illness, however, ketone body formation is relatively inhibited secondary to elevated serum insulin levels.[103] Thus in surgical patients, ketone bodies do not significantly supplant the need for glucose and do not play a major role in the metabolic management of the pediatric stress response.

In addition to their nutritional role, fatty acids profoundly influence inflammatory and immune events by changing lipid mediators and inflammatory protein and coagulation protein expression. After ingestion, n-6 and n-3 fats are metabolized by an alternating series of desaturase and elongase enzymes, transforming them into the membrane associated lipids: arachidonic acid, eicosapentaenoic acid (EPA), DHA, respectively (Figs 2-2 and 2-3).[104] Substitution of the intralipid component of parenteral nutrition (PN) (rich in proinflammatory omega-6 fatty acids) with fish oil (a source of omega-3 fatty acids) may alleviate some of the toxic hepatic effects of long-term PN.[105] The beneficial effects of omega-3 fatty acids have been shown in animal and human models and this is an area of great interest. Omega-3 fatty acids have an anti-inflammatory effect, with decreased cytokine production in some models.[104]

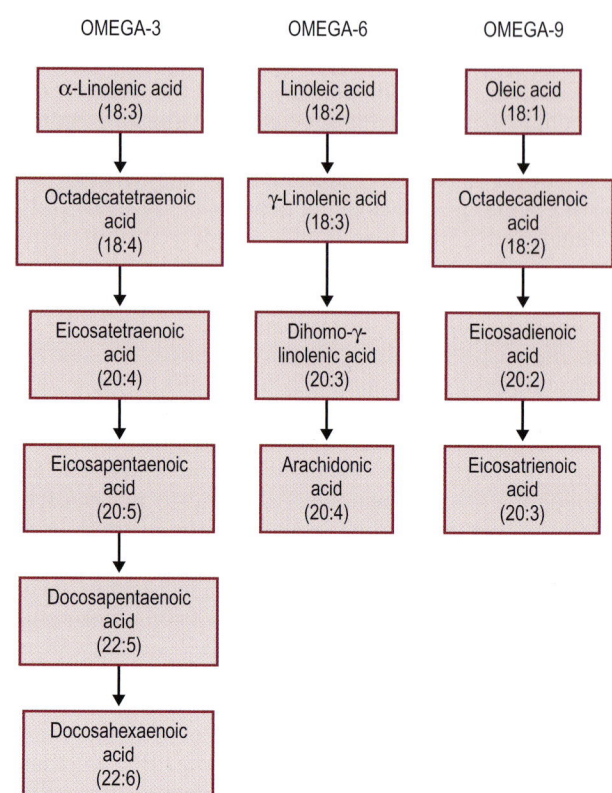

FIGURE 2-2 ■ Fatty acid synthesis from omega-3, omega-6, and omega-9 fats. (From Lee S, Gura KM, Kim S, et al. Current clinical applications of omega-6 and omega-3 fatty acids. Nutr Clin Pract 2006;21:323–41.)

More recently, a commercially available omega-3 fatty acid for parenteral administration has been administered in children with exciting results. In a cohort of PN dependent children with PN associated hyperbilirubinemia, Omegaven®, at a low lipid allocation of 1 g/kg/day, was associated with a normalization of bilirubin levels.[106] A clinical trial, in surgical neonates, to test the relative benefits of Omegaven® vs reduced omega-6 lipid allotments alone is currently underway.

ROUTES OF NUTRITIONAL PROVISION

Enteral Nutrition

Following the estimation of energy expenditure and macronutrient requirement in the hospitalized child, the next challenge is to facilitate the provision of this nutritional support. In most pediatric patients with a functioning gastrointestinal tract, the enteral route of nutrient administration is preferable to PN. Enteral nutrition (EN) is physiologic and has been shown to be more cost effective without the added risk of nosocomial infection inherent in PN. Early EN has been shown to decrease infectious episodes and decrease length of hospitalization in critically ill patients.[107] Based on level 1 and level 2 evidence in the adult critical care literature, The Canadian Clinical Practice Guidelines for Nutrition Support have strongly recommended the use of early enteral feeds

PRECURSOR OF EICOSANOIDS

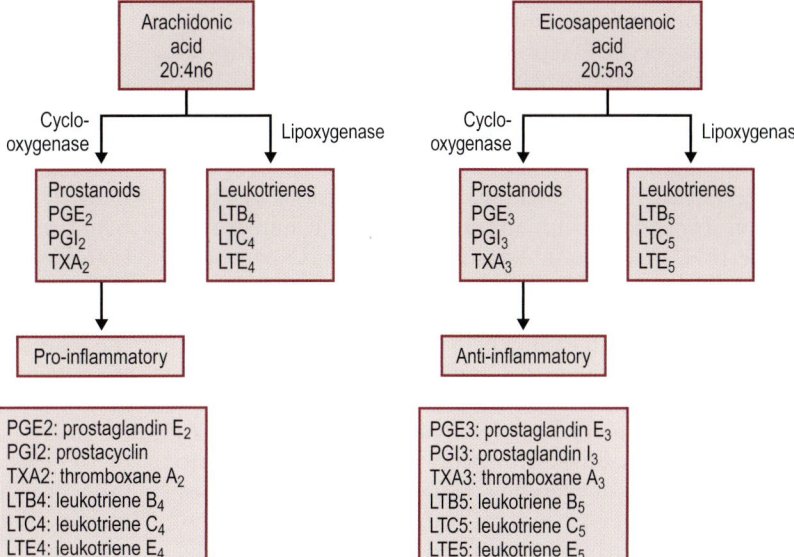

FIGURE 2-3 ■ The pro- and anti-inflammatory products that are generated from the metabolism of arachidonic acid and eicosapentaenoic acid. (From Lee S, Gura KM, Kim S, et al. Current clinical applications of omega-6 and omega-3 fatty acids. Nutr Clin Pract 2006;21:323–41.)

(within 24–48 hourrs after ICU admission).[108] The optimal route of nutrient delivery has not been systematically studied in children. In the absence of a randomized-controlled trial comparing the effects of EN vs PN, many centers have adopted institutional guidelines. Current practice includes the initiation of gastric or post-pyloric enteral feeding within 48 hrs to 72 hrs after admission. PN is being used to supplement or replace EN in those patients where EN alone is unable to meet the nutritional goal.

In children on EN, there are insufficient data to make recommendations regarding the site of enteral feeding (gastric vs postpyloric). Both enteral routes have been successfully used for nutritional support of the critically ill child.[109–111] In a study examining the role of small bowel feeding in 74 critically ill children randomized to receive either gastric or postpyloric feeds, no significant difference was observed in microaspiration, tube displacement and feeding intolerance between the two groups.[112] The study was not powered to detect differences in mortality and enteral feeds were interrupted in a large number of subjects in this study. Also, caloric goals were met in only a small percentage of the population studied. A higher percentage of subjects in the small bowel group achieved their daily caloric goal when compared to the gastric fed group. Critically ill children receiving early (less than 24 hours after ICU admission) postpyloric feeds have been shown to have better feeding tolerance (decreased incidence of abdominal distension) compared to those where post-pyloric feeding was initiated late.[113]

It may be prudent to consider postpyloric feeds in patients who do not tolerate gastric feeding or those who are at a high risk of aspiration. Transpyloric feeding may be limited by the ability to obtain small bowel access and the expertise and resources in individual ICUs are likely to be variable. Operative placement of gastrostomy or jejunostomy tubes allows long-term enteral feeding and drug administration in the ICU and after discharge. Stoma site infection, obstruction, and tube dislodgement are common complications and must be identified and managed early. Malposition of the tube is frequently encountered with any of these devices either at placement or during the course of its use. Bedside screening methods to identify tip position range from auscultation during air insufflation to ultrasound-guided localization. However, feedings should be held when malposition of tip is suspected. When in doubt, a contrast study may be needed to confirm tip position before recommencing feeds.

EN in critically ill children is often interrupted for a variety of reasons, some of which may be avoidable.[114] Children with frequent interruptions have a higher reliance on PN. Intolerance to enteral feeds may be a limiting factor and supplementation with PN in this group of patients allows for improved nutritional intake. Enteral feeds are held for a period of time before procedures such as elective endotracheal intubation, general anesthesia, procedural sedation, extubation, and other such interventions to lower the corresponding risk of aspiration. Most centers do not to use enteral feeds with patients who are on multiple vasopressor drugs for hypotension or who have evidence of bowel ischemia so as to limit the risk of small bowel necrosis associated with rapid enteral feeding.[115] In a subgroup of critically ill patients, TPN may be required for a period before initiation of enteral feeds.

Prospective cohort studies and retrospective chart reviews have reported the inability to achieve the daily caloric goal in many critically ill children.[4,116] In a recent study of mechanically ventilated children from 30 centers, energy and protein intake were found to be grossly inadequate.[117] By the end of the first week in the ICU just over 50% of the prescribed energy and protein were delivered. Patients with energy intake less than 66% of the prescribed goal had higher mortality rates. The most common reasons for suboptimal enteral nutrient delivery in these studies were fluid restriction, procedures interrupting feeds, and feeding intolerance. In a study examining the endocrine and metabolic response of children with meningococcal sepsis, goal nutrition was achieved in only 25%.[7] Similar observations have been made in a group of 95 children in a pediatric ICU (PICU) where patients received a median of 58.8% (range 0–277%) of their estimated energy requirements.[116] In this review, enteral feeding was interrupted on 264 occasions to allow clinical procedures. In another review of nutritional intake in 42 patients in a tertiary-level PICU over 458 days, actual energy intake was compared with estimated energy requirement.[4] Only 50% of patients were reported to have received full estimated energy requirements after a median of seven days. Prolonged fluid resuscitation was a major factor hindering the achievement of estimated energy requirements despite maximizing the energy content of the feedings. Protocols for use of transpyloric feeding tubes and changing from bolus to continuous feeds during brief periods of intolerance are strategies that may help achieve estimated energy goals in this population. Consistently underachieved EN goals are thought to be one of the reasons for the absence of a beneficial effect in multiple studies and meta-analyses of the efficacy of immunonutrition in preventing infection.[118] Addressing preventable interruptions in enteral feeding in critically ill children is essential to attaining goal feeds. At this time, there is not enough evidence to recommend the use of prokinetic medications, motility agents (for feeding intolerance or to facilitate enteral tube placement), prebiotics, probiotics, or synbiotics in critically ill children. Randomized studies comparing enteral feeds administered by bolus or continuously are also lacking.

In summary, EN must be initiated early in hospitalized children with bowel activity. Postpyloric EN may be utilized in children with a high risk of aspiration or when gastric feeding is either contraindicated or has failed. Enterally administered feeds meet nutritional requirements in critically ill children with a functional gastrointestinal system and have the advantages of low cost, manageability, safety, and preservation of hepatic and other gastrointestinal function. Early introduction of enteral feeds in critically ill patients helps to achieve positive protein and energy balance and restores nitrogen balance during the acute state of illness. It maintains gut integrity and elicits release of growth factors and hormones that maintain gut integrity and function.[119] Despite its perceived benefits, current practice in ICUs shows that a significant proportion of eligible patients do not receive EN.[120] Fig. 2-4 offers an algorithm for initiating and advancing EN in children admitted to the multidisciplinary ICU at Children's Hospital, Boston.

Parenteral Nutrition

PN provides intravenous administration of macronutrients and micronutrients to meet the nutritional requirements when EN is not possible. Although widespread in its application, PN is associated with mechanical, infectious, and metabolic complications and should only be used in carefully selected patients. In the setting of an

intact intestinal function, PN is not indicated if enteral feeds alone can maintain nutritional balance.

The decision to initiate PN is based on the anticipated length of fasting, the underlying nutritional status of the individual, and a careful examination of the risks associated with PN use in relation to the consequences of poor nutritional intake. If the expected period during which minimal or no EN will be provided to the child is longer than five days, the use of PN is prudent and probably beneficial. In children with underlying malnutrition, prematurity, or conditions associated with hypermetabolism, PN can be initiated earlier. The main limiting factor for provision of full nutritional support in the form of PN is the availability of central access. Administration of full PN requires a central venous catheter with its tip placed at the junction of superior vena cava and right atrium (RA). If a lower extremity central line is utilized, the tip of the catheter should be placed at the junction of the inferior vena cava and RA. The large vessel diameter and maximal blood flow rate at these sites allows for the safe administration of the hypertonic PN. To avoid the complications associated with malpositioned tips of central venous catheters, the practice at our institute is to document the location of the central venous catheter tip prior to its use. Peripheral administration of PN in the absence of an ideally located central venous catheter requires dilution (maximum 900 mosm/L) to avoid the risks of phlebitis and sclerosis. Osmolarity of the PN solution can be calculated using available online calculators or simple equations such as:

$$\{(\text{dextrose grams/L} \times 5) + (\text{protein grams/L} \times 10) + (\text{lipid grams/L} \times 1.5) + [(\text{mEq/L of Na} + \text{K} + \text{Ca} + \text{Mg}) \times 5]\}.$$

Fluid and electrolytes status will guide the initial PN prescription. The patient's hydration, size, age, and underlying disease will dictate the amount of the fluid to be administered. Fluid requirements in the pediatric age group are routinely estimated based on the Holliday–Segar method (Table 2-4). PN should not routinely be used to replace ongoing losses. Fluid shifts, increased insensible losses, drainage of bodily secretions, and renal failure can complicate electrolyte management in these patients. PN should be prescribed daily after reviewing the electrolytes (Na^+, K^+, Cl^-, HCO_3^-, Ca^{2+}) and glucose to allow adjustments in the macro- and micronutrient composition. In sick patients with significant gastrointestinal fluid loss (gastric, pancreatic, small intestinal, or bile), the measurement of electrolytes from the drained

TABLE 2-4	Daily Fluid Requirement for Infants and Children
Body Weight (kg)	**Maintenance Daily Fluid Requirement**
0–10	100 mL/kg
10–20	1000 mL + 50 mL/kg >10 kg
>20	1500 mL + 20 mL/kg >20 kg

MSICU ENTERAL FEEDING ALGORITHM

Unless contraindicated,* begin enteral nutrition support within 24 h of admission to the MSICU.

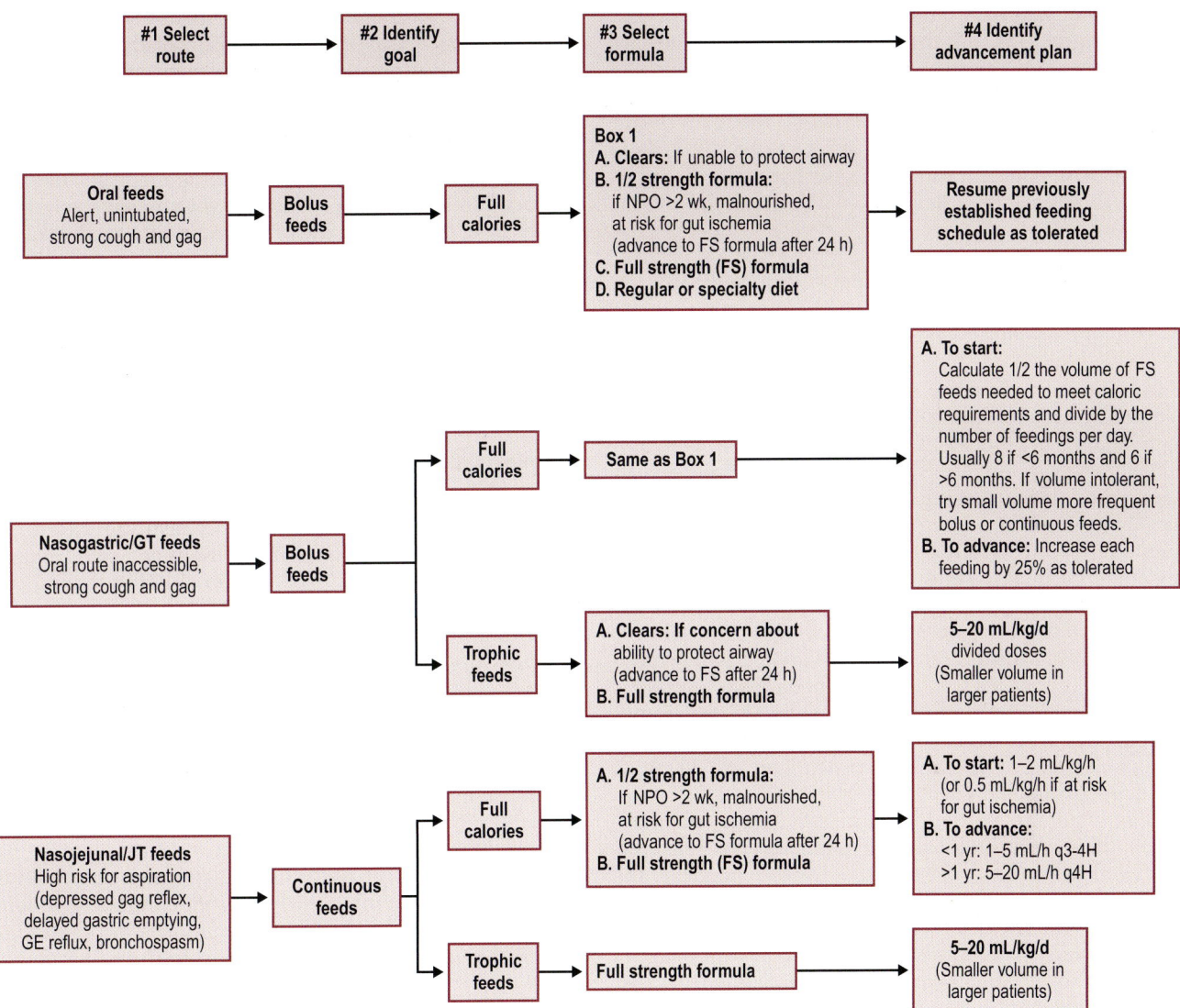

*Contraindications include potential for endotracheal intubation/extubation within 4 hours; hemodynamically unstable requiring escalation of therapy; postoperative ileus, upper gastrointestinal bleeding, at risk for NEC/intestinal ischemia, intestinal obstruction, post-allogenic BMT who have GVHD or post-BMT patients prior to gut recontamination and in patients in whom care is being redirected.

FIGURE 2-4 ■ Example of an algorithm for a feeding regimen and route for patients admitted to a multidisciplinary intensive care unit. (Courtesy of Children's Hospital, Boston.)

fluid is recommended. However, urgent changes in serum electrolytes should not be managed by changes in PN infusion rate or composition because these represent imprecise methods to treat a potentially serious electrolyte abnormality. In addition, careful attention to phosphate and magnesium levels is important. Hypophosphatemia may lead to hemolytic anemia, respiratory muscle dysfunction, and cardiac failure. A significant decrease in serum phosphate also may be seen with the re-feeding syndrome. In contrast, renal failure can result in the retention of phosphate and potassium, and nutritional allotments must be reduced accordingly. Magnesium deficiency can cause fatal cardiac arrhythmia in children and adults alike. Abnormalities of acid-base physiology also can influence the nutritional regimen of the hospitalized child. If a metabolic alkalosis from active diuresis or gastric suction occurs, chloride administration is used to correct the alkalosis. Severe, untreated alkalemia may inhibit the patient's respiratory drive, shift potassium intracellularly, decrease ionized calcium concentrations by increasing the affinity of albumin for calcium, and promote refractory cardiac arrhythmias. Metabolic acidosis is often seen in critically ill children and may be associated with hypotension, ischemia, or renal failure. In such patients, the use of acetate instead of chloride in the PN regimen may be helpful.[121]

The three main macronutrients in PN are carbohydrate, lipid, and protein. Protein is administered in the form of crystalline amino acids starting at 0.5 g/kg/day in preterm neonates and 1 g/kg/day in others. The protein intake is advanced daily in increments of 1 g/kg/day until the goal intake is achieved. Table 2-3 lists recommended quantities of dietary protein needs for hospitalized children. Dextrose provides the main source of energy in PN and is initiated at a rate of 5 mg/kg/min using 5–10% concentration. The glucose infusion rate in mg/kg/min can be calculated with the help of the equation:

$$[(\% \text{ dextrose}) \times (1\,\text{dL}/100\,\text{mL}) \times (1000\,\text{mg}/\text{L g}) \\ \times (\text{hourly rate in mL/h}) \times (1\,\text{h}/60\,\text{min}) \\ \times (1/\text{weight in kg})].$$

Infusion rates higher than 12 mg/kg/min are infrequently required and overfeeding with carbohydrate is associated with lipogenesis (RQ >1.0), hepatic steatosis, hyperglycemia, and osmotic diuresis. Three to 5% of the energy needs must be met using intravenous lipids, which are usually initiated at a rate of 1 g/kg/day, and advanced in increments to reach a maximum of 3 g/kg/day or 50% of total energy intake. Intravenous lipids prevent essential fatty acid deficiency and are a concentrated and isotonic source of energy. Triglyceride levels should be monitored and intralipid infusion rate is lowered when hypertriglyceridemia is noted. As noted previously, available evidence suggests that limiting lipids to 1g/kg/day may be indicated in patients with intestinal failure-associated PN cholestasis or in those patients who are likely to require a protracted course of PN.[122]

The vitamin and micronutrient (trace element) needs of healthy children and neonates are relatively well defined in the literature.[17] In the neonate and child, required vitamins include the fat-soluble vitamins (A, D, E, and K) as well as the water-soluble vitamins: ascorbic acid, thiamine, riboflavin, pyridoxine, niacin, pantothenate, biotin, folate, and vitamin B12. Because vitamins are not consumed stoichiometrically in biochemical reactions but instead act as catalysts, the administration of large vitamin supplements in metabolically stressed states is not logical from a nutritional standpoint. The trace elements required for normal growth and development include zinc, iron, copper, selenium, manganese, iodide, molybdenum, and chromium. Trace elements are usually used in the synthesis of the active sites of a ubiquitous and extraordinarily important class of enzymes called metalloenzymes. More than 200 zinc metalloenzymes alone exist, and both DNA and RNA polymerase are included in this group. As with vitamins, these metalloenzymes act as catalytic agents. Unless specific mineral losses occur, such as enhanced zinc loss with severe diarrhea, large nutritional requirements would not be anticipated during critical illness. Selenium and carnitine may be added after 30 days of exclusive PN administration. The addition of copper and manganese in the PN of children with cholestasis is controversial and usually the dose is halved in view of their biliary excretion. The pharmacologic use of vitamins and trace minerals in pediatric illness has not been adequately studied. Reviews of both vitamin and trace mineral toxicity clearly demonstrate that excessive intake is a health risk.[123,124]

Careful biochemical monitoring is mandatory to prevent acute and long-term complications from PN therapy. A PN profile is recommended at the initiation of therapy and then weekly. It includes serum levels of sodium, potassium, chloride, glucose, carbon dioxide, blood urine nitrogen, creatinine, albumin, magnesium, phosphate, total and direct bilirubin, and transaminases. For children requiring PN longer than 30 days, selenium, iron, zinc, copper and carnitine levels may be checked. It is essential to monitor daily vital statistics and routine anthropometry to ensure adequate growth and development. Critical care units benefit from the expertise of a dedicated nutritionist who should be consulted on a regular basis to guide the optimal nutritional intake of patients.

IMMUNE-ENHANCING DIETS

Immunomodulation is thought to play a significant role in the response to an infectious insult and impacts outcome in children with sepsis. In 1996, Bone and colleagues outlined the role of the compensatory anti-inflammatory response that follows the initial proinflammatory response engendered by trauma or infection.[125] Therapies aimed at modulating or stimulating the immune response have been a focus of many recent nutritional studies.

Unfortunately investigations examining the role of immune-enhancing diets in critically ill patients are marred by heterogeneous clinical populations, methodological flaws, and the use of nutritional formulations that often contain multiple potentially active components. Thus, studies and meta-analyses offer conflicting conclusions.[69,114,121–123] Furthermore, there are no published studies specifically evaluating the role of immunonutrition in critically ill children. Potentially promising, but unproven, additives include arginine, glutamine, cysteine, nucleic acids, and omega-3 fatty acids.

CONCLUSION

The nutritional status of children influences outcome in surgical patients. Malnutrition is associated with physiological instability and a longer ICU stay accompanied by increased utilization of resources.[126] The first step in implementing appropriate nutritional support is an understanding of the metabolic events that accompany critical illness and surgery. Individualized, quantitative assessments of protein, carbohydrate, lipid, electrolyte, vitamin and micronutrient requirements are made, and the appropriate route of nutrient delivery is determined. This nutrition regimen needs to be reviewed and amended regularly during the course of illness. The goal of nutrition therapy in sick pediatric surgical patients is to augment the short-term benefits of the metabolic stress response while minimizing any long-term consequences.

REFERENCES

1. Pollack MM, Wiley JS, Kanter R, et al. Malnutrition in critically ill infants and children. J Parenter Enteral Nutr 1982;6:20–4.
2. Hults J, Joosten K, Zimmermann L, et al. Malnutriion in critically il children: From admision to 6 months after discharge. Clin Nutr 2004;23:223–32.
3. Alexander E, Susla GM, Burstein AH, et al. Retrospective evaluation of commonly used equations to predict energy expenditure in mechanically ventilated, critically ill patients. Pharmacotherapy 2004;24:1659–67.
4. Chwals WJ, Bistrian BR. Predicted energy expenditure in critically ill children: Problems associated with increased variability. Crit Care Med 2000;28:2655–6.
5. Rogers EJ, Gilbertson HR, Heine RG, et al. Barriers to adequate nutrition in critically ill children. Nutrition 2003;19:865–8.
6. Cuthbertson D. Intensive-care-metabolic response to injury. Br J Surg 1970;57:718–21.
7. Munro HN. Nutrition and muscle protein metabolism: Introduction. Fed Proc 1978;37:2281–2.
8. de Groof F, Joosten KF, Janssen JA, et al. Acute stress response in children with meningococcal sepsis: Important differences in the growth hormone/insulin-like growth factor I axis between nonsurvivors and survivors. J Clin Endocrinol Metab 2002;87:3118–24.
9. Fomon SJ, Haschke F, Ziegler EE, et al. Body composition of reference children from birth to age 10 years. Am J Clin Nutr 1982;35:1169–75.
10. Forbes GB, Bruining GJ. Urinary creatinine excretion and lean body mass. Am J Clin Nutr 1976;29:1359–66.
11. Long CL, Spencer JL, Kinney JM, et al. Carbohydrate metabolism in man: Effect of elective operations and major injury. J Appl Physiol 1971;31:110–16.
12. Ogata ES. Carbohydrate metabolism in the fetus and neonate and altered neonatal glucoregulation. Pediatr Clin N Am 1986;33:25–45.
13. Herrera E, Amusquivar E. Lipid metabolism in the fetus and the newborn. Diabetes Metab Res Rev 2000;16:202–10.
14. Schulze KF, Stefanski M, Masterson J, et al. Energy expenditure, energy balance, and composition of weight gain in low birth weight infants fed diets of different protein and energy content. J Pediatr 1987;110:753–9.
15. Long CL, Kinney JM, Geiger JW. Nonsuppressability of gluconeogenesis by glucose in septic patients. Metabolism 1976;25:193–201.
16. Whyte RK, Haslam R, Vlainic C, et al. Energy balance and nitrogen balance in growing low birthweight infants fed human milk or formula. Pediatr Res 1983;17:891–8.
17. National Academy of Sciences. Recommended Dietary Allowances. 10th ed. Washington, DC: National Academy Press; 1989.
18. Kashyap S, Schulze KF, Forsyth M, et al. Growth, nutrient retention, and metabolic response in low birth weight infants fed varying intakes of protein and energy. J Pediatr 1988;113:713–21.
19. Seale JL, Rumpler WV. Comparison of energy expenditure measurements by diet records, energy intake balance, doubly labeled water and room calorimetry. Eur J Clin Nutr 1997;51:856–63.
20. Daly JM, Heymsfield SB, Head CA, et al. Human energy requirements: Overestimation by widely used prediction equation. Am J Clin Nutr 1985;42:1170–4.
21. Schofield WN. Predicting basal metabolic rate, new standards and review of previous work. Hum Nutr Clin Nutr 1985;39(Suppl 1):5–41.
22. Hunter DC, Jaksic T, Lewis D, et al. Resting energy expenditure in the critically ill: Estimations versus measurement. Br J Surg 1988;75:875–78.
23. Muller MJ, Bosy-Westphal A, Klaus S, et al. World Health Organization equations have shortcomings for predicting resting energy expenditure in persons from a modern, affluent population: Generation of a new reference standard from a retrospective analysis of a German database of resting energy expenditure. Am J Clin Nutr 2004;80:1379–90.
24. Elwyn DH, Kinney JM, Askanazi J. Energy expenditure in surgical patients. Surg Clin North Am 1981;61:545–56.
25. Tilden SJ, Watkins S, Tong TK, et al. Measured energy expenditure in pediatric intensive care patients. Am J Dis Child 1989;143:490–2.
26. Ferrannini E. The theoretical bases of indirect calorimetry: A review. Metabolism 1988;37:287–301.
27. Joosten KF, Verhoeven JJ, Hazelzet JA. Energy expenditure and substrate utilization in mechanically ventilated children. Nutrition 1999;15:444–8.
28. Chwals WJ. Overfeeding the critically ill child: Fact or fantasy? New Horiz 1994;2:147–55.
29. Hulst JM, van Goudoever JB, Zimmermann LJ, et al. Adequate feeding and the usefulness of the respiratory quotient in critically ill children. Nutrition 2004;21:192–8.
30. McClave SA, Spain DA, Skolnick JL, et al. Achievement of steady state optimizes results when performing indirect calorimetry. J Parenter Enteral Nutr 2003;27:16–20.
31. Mehta NM, Bechard LJ, Leavitt K, et al. Severe weight loss and hypermetabolic paroxysmal dysautonomia following hypoxic ischemic brain injury: The role of indirect calorimetry in the intensive care unit. J Parenter Enteral Nutr 2008;32:281–4.
32. Mehta NM, Bechard LJ, Leavitt K, et al. Cumulative energy imbalance in the pediatric intensive care unit: Role of targeted indirect calorimetry. J Parenter Enteral Nutr. 2009;33:336–44.
33. Schoenheimer R, Rittenberg D. Deuterium as an indicator in the study of intermediary metabolism. Science 1935;82:156–7.
34. Schoeller DA, van Santen E. Measurement of energy expenditure in humans by doubly labeled water method. J Appl Physiol 1982;53:955–9.
35. Shew SB, Beckett PR, Keshen TH, et al. Validation of a [13C] bicarbonate tracer technique to measure neonatal energy expenditure. Pediatr Res 2000;47:787–91.
36. Schoeller DA, Hnilicka JM. Reliability of the doubly labeled water method for the measurement of total daily energy expenditure in free-living subjects. J Nutr 1996;126:348S–54S.
37. Schoeller DA, Kushner RF, Jones PJ. Validation of doubly labeled water for measuring energy expenditure during parenteral nutrition. Am J Clin Nutr 1986;44:291–8.
38. Jones PJ, Winthrop AL, Schoeller DA, et al. Validation of doubly labeled water for assessing energy expenditure in infants. Pediatr Res 1987;21:242–6.
39. Jahoor F, Desai M, Herndon DN, et al. Dynamics of the protein metabolic response to burn injury. Metabolism 1988;37:330–7.
40. Weinstein MR, Oh W. Oxygen consumption in infants with bronchopulmonary dysplasia. J Pediatr 1981;99:958–61.
41. Jones MO, Pierro A, Hammond P, et al. The metabolic response to operative stress in infants. J Pediatr Surg 1993;28:1258–62.
42. Shew SB, Keshen TH, Glass NL, et al. Ligation of a patent ductus arteriosus under fentanyl anesthesia improves protein metabolism in premature neonates. J Pediatr Surg 2000;35:1277–81.
43. Pierro A, Carnielli V, Filler RM, et al. Partition of energy metabolism in the surgical newborn. J Pediatr Surg 1991;26:581–6.
44. Chwals WJ, Letton RW, Jamie A, et al. Stratification of injury severity using energy expenditure response in surgical infants. J Pediatr Surg 1995;30:1161–4.
45. Jaksic T, Shew SB, Keshen TH, et al. Do critically ill surgical neonates have increased energy expenditure? J Pediatr Surg 2001;36:63–7.
46. Briassoulis G, Venkataraman S, Thompson AE. Energy expenditure in critically ill children. Crit Care Med 2000;28:1166–72.
47. Goran MI, Kaskoun M, Johnson R. Determinants of resting energy expenditure in young children. J Pediatr 1994;125:362–7.
48. Bartlett RH, Dechert RE, Mault JR, et al. Measurement of metabolism in multiple organ failure. Surgery 1982;92:771–9.
49. Beaufrere B. Protein turnover in low-birth-weight (LBW) infants. Acta Paediatr Suppl 1994;405:86–92.
50. Denne SC, Karn CA, Ahlrichs JA, et al. Proteolysis and phenylalanine hydroxylation in response to parenteral nutrition in extremely premature and normal newborns. J Clin Invest 1996;97:746–54.
51. Hay WW Jr, Lucas A, Heird WC, et al. Workshop summary: Nutrition of the extremely low birth weight infant. Pediatrics 1999;104:1360–8.

52. Cogo PE, Carnielli VP, Rosso F, et al. Protein turnover, lipolysis, and endogenous hormonal secretion in critically ill children. Crit Care Med 2002;30:65–70.

53. Mrozek JD, Georgieff MK, Blazar BR, et al. Effect of sepsis syndrome on neonatal protein and energy metabolism. J Perinatol 2000;20:96–100.

54. Williamson DH, Farrell R, Kerr A, et al. Muscle-protein catabolism after injury in man, as measured by urinary excretion of 3-methylhistidine. Clin Sci Mol Med 1977;52:527–33.

55. Pierro A. Metabolism and nutritional support in the surgical neonate. J Pediatr Surg 2002;37:811–22.

56. Meszaros K, Bojta J, Bautista AP, et al. Glucose utilization by Kupffer cells, endothelial cells, and granulocytes in endotoxemic rat liver. Am J Physiol 1991;260:G7–12.

57. Denne SC, Karn CA, Wang J, et al. Effect of intravenous glucose and lipid on proteolysis and glucose production in normal newborns. Am J Physiol 1995;269:E361–7.

58. Mitton SG, Garlick PJ. Changes in protein turnover after the introduction of parenteral nutrition in premature infants: Comparison of breast milk and egg protein-based amino acid solutions. Pediatr Res 1992;32:447–54.

59. Felig P. The glucose-alanine cycle. Metabolism 1973;22:179–207.

60. Duffy B, Pencharz P. The effects of surgery on the nitrogen metabolism of parenterally fed human neonates. Pediatr Res 1986;20:32–5.

61. Poindexter BB, Karn CA, Leitch CA, et al. Amino acids do not suppress proteolysis in premature neonates. Am J Physiol 2001;281:E472–8.

62. Bechard LJ, Parrott JS, Mehta NM. Systematic review of the influence of energy and protein intake on protein balance in critically ill children. J Pediatr 2012;161:333–9.

63. Keshen TH, Miller RG, Jahoor F, et al. Stable isotopic quantitation of protein metabolism and energy expenditure in neonates on- and post-extracorporeal life support. J Pediatr Surg 1997;32:958–62.

64. Goldman HI, Freudenthal R, Holland B, et al. Clinical effects of two different levels of protein intake on low-birth-weight infants. J Pediatr 1969;74:881–9.

65. Goldman HI, Liebman OB, Freudenthal R, et al. Effects of early dietary protein intake on low-birth-weight infants: Evaluation at 3 years of age. J Pediatr 1971;78:126–9.

66. Imura K, Okada A. Amino acid metabolism in pediatric patients. Nutrition (Burbank, Los Angeles County, Calif 1998;14:143–8.

67. Miller RG, Jahoor F, Jaksic T. Decreased cysteine and proline synthesis in parenterally fed, premature infants. J Pediatr Surg 1995;30:953–7.

68. Miller RG, Keshen TH, Jahoor F, et al. Compartmentation of endogenously synthesized amino acids in neonates. J Surg Res 1996;63:199–203.

69. Reeds PJ, Berthold HK, Boza JJ, et al. Integration of amino acid and carbon intermediary metabolism: Studies with uniformly labeled tracers and mass isotopomer analysis. Eur J Pediatr 1997;156(Suppl 1):S50–8.

70. Zlotkin SH, Anderson GH. The development of cystathionase activity during the first year of life. Pediatr Res 1982;16:65–8.

71. Heyland DK, Novak F, Drover JW, et al. Should immunonutrition become routine in critically ill patients? A systematic review of the evidence. JAMA 2001;286:944–53.

72. Dzakovic A, Kaviani A, Eshach-Adiv O, et al. Trophic enteral nutrition increases hepatic glutathione and protects against peroxidative damage after exposure to endotoxin. J Pediatr Surg 2003;38:844–7.

73. Duggan C, Gannon J, Walker WA. Protective nutrients and functional foods for the gastrointestinal tract. Am J Clin Nutr 2002;75:789–808.

74. Liu Z, Barrett EJ. Human protein metabolism: Its measurement and regulation. Am J Physiol 2002;283:E1105–12.

75. Demling RH, Orgill DP. The anticatabolic and wound healing effects of the testosterone analog oxandrolone after severe burn injury. J Crit Care 2000;15:12–17.

76. Takala J, Ruokonen E, Webster NR, et al. Increased mortality associated with growth hormone treatment in critically ill adults. N Engl J Med 1999;341:785–92.

77. Yarwood GD, Ross RJ, Medbak S, et al. Administration of human recombinant insulin-like growth factor-I in critically ill patients. Crit Care Med 1997;25:1352–61.

78. Sakurai Y, Aarsland A, Herndon DN, et al. Stimulation of muscle protein synthesis by long-term insulin infusion in severely burned patients. Ann Surg 1995;222:283–94; 94–7.

79. Thomas SJ, Morimoto K, Herndon DN, et al. The effect of prolonged euglycemic hyperinsulinemia on lean body mass after severe burn. Surgery 2002;132:341–7.

80. van den Berghe G, Wouters P, Weekers F, et al. Intensive insulin therapy in the critically ill patients. N Engl J Med 2001;345:1359–67.

81. Agus MS, Javid PJ, Ryan DP, et al. Intravenous insulin decreases protein breakdown in infants on extracorporeal membrane oxygenation. J Pediatr Surg 2004;39:839–44.

82. Tappy L, Schwarz JM, Schneiter P, et al. Effects of isoenergetic glucose-based or lipid-based parenteral nutrition on glucose metabolism, de novo lipogenesis, and respiratory gas exchanges in critically ill patients. Crit Care Med 1998;26:860–7.

83. Askanazi J, Rosenbaum SH, Hyman AI, et al. Respiratory changes induced by the large glucose loads of total parenteral nutrition. JAMA 1980;243:1444–7.

84. Jones MO, Pierro A, Hammond P, et al. Glucose utilization in the surgical newborn infant receiving total parenteral nutrition. J Pediatr Surg 1993;28:1121–5.

85. Shew SB, Keshen TH, Jahoor F, et al. The determinants of protein catabolism in neonates on extracorporeal membrane oxygenation. J Pediatr Surg 1999;34:1086–90.

86. Forsyth JS, Murdock N, Crighton A. Low birthweight infants and total parenteral nutrition immediately after birth. III. Randomised study of energy substrate utilisation, nitrogen balance, and carbon dioxide production. Arch Dis Child 1995;73:F13–16.

87. Jones MO, Pierro A, Garlick PJ, et al. Protein metabolism kinetics in neonates: Effect of intravenous carbohydrate and fat. J Pediatr Surg 1995;30:458–62.

88. Krinsley JS. Association between hyperglycemia and increased hospital mortality in a heterogeneous population of critically ill patients. Mayo Clin Proc 2003;78:1471–8.

89. Laird AM, Miller PR, Kilgo PD, et al. Relationship of early hyperglycemia to mortality in trauma patients. J Trauma 2004;56:1058–62.

90. Wiener RS, Wiener DC, Larson RJ. Benefits and risks of tight glucose control in critically ill adults: A meta-analysis. JAMA 2008;300:933–44.

91. Srinivasan V, Spinella PC, Drott HR, et al. Association of timing, duration, and intensity of hyperglycemia with intensive care unit mortality in critically ill children. Pediatr Crit Care Med 2004;5:329–36.

92. Jeevanandam M, Young DH, Schiller WR. Nutritional impact on the energy cost of fat fuel mobilization in polytrauma victims. J Trauma 1990;30:147–54.

93. Nordenstrom J, Carpentier YA, Askanazi J, et al. Metabolic utilization of intravenous fat emulsion during total parenteral nutrition. Ann Surg 1982;196:221–31.

94. Coss-Bu JA, Klish WJ, Walding D, et al. Energy metabolism, nitrogen balance, and substrate utilization in critically ill children. Am J Clin Nutr 2001;74:664–9.

95. Powis MR, Smith K, Rennie M, et al. Effect of major abdominal operations on energy and protein metabolism in infants and children. J Pediatr Surg 1998;33:49–53.

96. Friedman Z, Danon A, Stahlman MT, et al. Rapid onset of essential fatty acid deficiency in the newborn. Pediatrics 1976;58:640–9.

97. Paulsrud JR, Pensler L, Whitten CF, et al. Essential fatty acid deficiency in infants induced by fat-free intravenous feeding. Am J Clin Nutr 1972;25:897–904.

98. Giovannini M, Riva E, Agostoni C. Fatty acids in pediatric nutrition. Pediatr Clin North Am 1995;42:861–77.

99. Van Aerde JE, Sauer PJ, Pencharz PB, et al. Metabolic consequences of increasing energy intake by adding lipid to parenteral nutrition in full-term infants. Am J Clin Nutr 1994;59:659–62.

100. Cleary TG, Pickering LK. Mechanisms of intralipid effect on polymorphonuclear leukocytes. J Clin Lab Immunol 1983;11:21–6.

101. Freeman J, Goldmann DA, Smith NE, et al. Association of intravenous lipid emulsion and coagulase-negative staphylococcal bacteremia in neonatal intensive care units. N Engl J Med 1990;323:301–8.

102. Periera GR, Fox WW, Stanley CA, et al. Decreased oxygenation and hyperlipemia during intravenous fat infusions in premature infants. Pediatrics 1980;66:26–30.

103. Birkhahn RH, Long CL, Fitkin DL, et al. A comparison of the effects of skeletal trauma and surgery on the ketosis of starvation in man. J Trauma 1981;21:513–19.

104. Lee S, Gura KM, Kim S, et al. Current clinical applications of omega-6 and omega-3 fatty acids. Nutr Clin Pract 2006;21:323–41.

105. Lee S, Gura KM, Puder M. Omega-3 fatty acids and liver disease. Hepatology 2007;45:841–5.

106. Gura KM, Duggan CP, Collier SB, et al. Reversal of parenteral nutrition-associated liver disease in two infants with short bowel syndrome using parenteral fish oil: Implications for future management. Pediatrics 2006;118:e197–201.

107. Zaloga GP. Early enteral nutritional support improves outcome: Hypothesis or fact? Crit Care Med 1999;27:259–61.

108. Heyland DK, Dhaliwal R, Drover JW, et al. Canadian clinical practice guidelines for nutrition support in mechanically ventilated, critically ill adult patients. JPEN 2003;27:355–73.

109. Briassoulis G, Zavras N, Hatzis T. Malnutrition, nutritional indices, and early enteral feeding in critically ill children. Nutrition 2001;17:548–57.

110. Briassoulis GC, Zavras NJ, Hatzis MT. Effectiveness and safety of a protocol for promotion of early intragastric feeding in critically ill children. Pediatr Crit Care Med 2001;12:113–21.

111. Chellis MJ, Sanders SV, Webster H, et al. Early enteral feeding in the pediatric intensive care unit. J Parenter Enteral Nutr 1996;20:71–3.

112. Meert KL, Daphtary KM, Metheny NA. Gastric vs. small bowel feeding in critically ill children receiving mechanical ventilation: A randomized controlled trial. Chest 2004;126:872–8.

113. Sanchez C, Lopez-Herce J, Carrillo A, et al. Early transpyloric enteral nutrition in critically ill children. Nutrition 2007;23:16–22.

114. Mehta NM, McAleer D, Hamilton S, et al. Challenges to optimal enteral nutrition in a multidisciplinary pediatric intensive care unit. J Parenter Enteral Nutr 2010;34:38–45.

115. Munshi IA, Steingrub JS, Wolpert L. Small bowel necrosis associated with early postoperative jejunal tube feeding in a trauma patient. J Trauma 2000;49:163–5.

116. Taylor RM, Preedy VR, Baker AJ, et al. Nutritional support in critically ill children. Clin Nutr 2003;22:365–9.

117. Mehta NM, Bechard LJ, Cahill N, et al. Nutritional practices and their relationship to clinical outcomes in critically ill children–an international multicenter cohort study. Crit Care Med 2012;40:2204–11.

118. Atkinson S, Sieffert E, Bihari D. A prospective, randomized, double-blind, controlled clinical trial of enteral immunonutrition in the critically ill. Guy's Hospital Intensive Care Group. Crit Care Med 1998;26:1164–72.

119. Briassoulis G, Tsorva A, Zavras N, et al. Influence of an aggressive early enteral nutrition protocol on nitrogen balance in critically ill children. J Nutr Biochem 2002;13:560.

120. Heyland DK, Cook DJ, Guyatt GH. Enteral nutrition in the critically ill patient: A critical review of the evidence. Intensive Care Med 1993;19:435–42.

121. Peters O, Ryan S, Matthew L, et al. Randomised controlled trial of acetate in preterm neonates receiving parenteral nutrition. Arch Dis Child 1997;77:F12–15.

122. Garza JJ, Shew SB, Keshen TH, et al. Energy expenditure in ill premature neonates. J Pediatr Surg 2002;37:289–93.

123. Flodin NW. Micronutrient supplements: Toxicity and drug interactions. Prog Food Nutr Sci 1990;14:277–331.

124. Marks J. The safety of the vitamins: An overview. Int J Vitam Nutr Res Suppl 1989;30:12–20.

125. Bone RC, Grodzin CJ, Balk RA. Sepsis: A new hypothesis for pathogenesis of the disease process. Chest 1997;112:235–43.

126. Pollack MM, Ruttimann UE, Wiley JS. Nutritional depletions in critically ill children: Associations with physiologic instability and increased quantity of care. J Parenter Enteral Nutr 1985;9:309–13.

CHAPTER 3

Anesthetic Considerations for Pediatric Surgical Conditions

Laura K. Diaz • Lynne G. Maxwell

Anesthetizing children is an increasingly safe undertaking. When discussing the risks and benefits of a child's operation with his or her family, surgeons should feel confident that their anesthesiology colleagues can provide an anesthetic that facilitates the procedure while ensuring the child's safety. Providing optimal perioperative care for children requires close collaboration between the surgeon and anesthesiologist on issues both large and small. This chapter is designed to inform surgeons about the considerations important to anesthesiologists.

RISKS OF ANESTHESIA

In an effort to reduce patient complications, anesthesiologists have carefully analyzed anesthetic morbidity and mortality over the past generation. Whereas anesthesia was historically considered a dangerous enterprise, serious anesthesia-related complications are now relatively rare, especially in healthy patients. The reasons for this improvement include advances in pharmacology, improved monitoring technology, increased rigor of subspecialty training, and the ability to target problems using an analysis strategy.

Quantifying the risk of pediatric anesthesia is difficult due to the difficulty in determining whether complications are attributable to the anesthetic, and if so, to what degree. The risk of cardiac arrest for children undergoing anesthesia was estimated in the 1990s to be 1:10,000.[1,2] However, these studies did not take patient co-morbidity or the surgical condition into consideration. The risk of a healthy child suffering cardiac arrest during myringotomy tube placement is significantly less than the likelihood of a child with complex cardiac disease arresting during a complex cardiac repair.[3]

A recent review of cardiac arrests in anesthetized children compared 193 events from 1998–2004 to 150 events from 1994–1997.[4] A reduction in medication-caused arrests from 37% to 18% was identified, and was attributed to the decline in halothane use (that causes myocardial depression) and the advent of using sevoflurane (that is not associated with myocardial depression). There was also a reduction in unrecognized esophageal intubation as a cause of arrest, due in large part to the advent of end-tidal carbon dioxide ($ETCO_2$) monitoring, pulse oximetry, and an increased awareness of the problem.

Recent large single center reports yield a current estimate of anesthesia-related mortality of 1:250,000 in healthy children. To put this into perspective for parents, the risk of a motor vehicle collision on the way to the hospital or surgery center is greater than the risk of death under anesthesia. However, risks of mortality and morbidity are increased in neonates and infants less than one year of age, those who are ASA (American Society of Anesthesiologists) status 3 or greater, and those who require emergency surgery.[5]

PREOPERATIVE ANESTHESIA EVALUATION

All patients presenting for operations under anesthesia benefit greatly from a thorough preanesthetic/preoperative assessment and targeted preparation to optimize any coexisting medical conditions. The ASA physical status (PS) score is a means of communicating the condition of the patient. The PS is not intended to represent operative risk and serves primarily as a common means of communication among care providers (Table 3-1). Any child with an ASA classification of 3 or greater should be seen by an anesthesiologist prior to the day of surgery. This may be modified in cases of hardship due to the distance from the surgical venue or when the patient is well known to the anesthesia service, and the child's health is unchanged. Finally, outstanding and unresolved medical issues may be significant enough to warrant cancellation of the procedure for optimization of anesthesia and/or further diagnostic workup.

Criteria for Ambulatory Surgery

Ambulatory surgery comprises 70% or more of the caseload in most pediatric centers. Multiple factors should be considered when evaluating whether a child is suitable for outpatient surgery. Some states regulate the minimum age allowed in an ambulatory surgical center. For example, the minimum age in Pennsylvania is six months. In most cases, the child should be free of severe systemic disease (ASA PS 1 or 2). Other factors that may determine the suitability of a child for outpatient surgery are family and social dynamics. Some institutions utilize a telephone screening evaluation process to determine whether a patient can have their full anesthesia history and physical on the day of surgery rather than being evaluated in a preoperative evaluation clinic prior to surgery.[6]

Well-controlled systemic illnesses do not necessarily preclude outpatient surgery, but any concerns must be

TABLE 3-1	ASA Physical Status Classification
ASA Classification	**Patient Status**
1	A normal healthy patient
2	A patient with mild systemic disease
3	A patient with severe systemic disease
4	A patient with severe systemic disease that is a constant threat to life
5	A moribund patient who is not expected to survive without the operation
6	A declared brain-dead patient whose organs are being removed for donor purposes
E	An emergency modifier for any ASA classification when failure to immediately correct a medical condition poses risk to life or organ viability

addressed in advance in a cooperative fashion between the surgical and anesthesia services. If a child has a moderate degree of impairment, but the disease is stable and the surgical procedure is of minimal insult, outpatient surgery may be acceptable.

General Principles

In addition to the physical examination, the essential elements of the preoperative assessment in all patients are listed in Box 3-1. Patients and parents may be anxious about recurrence of adverse perianesthetic events such as those listed, and they should be reassured that efforts will be made to prevent these events.

BOX 3-1	**Essential Elements of the Preoperative Assessment (In Addition to Physical Examination)**

Vital signs
  Height/weight
  Heart rate
  Respiratory rate
  Blood pressure
  Pulse oximetry (both in room air and with supplemental O_2 if applicable)
Allergies
Medications
Cardiac murmur history
Previous subspecialty encounters
Past anesthetic history including any adverse perianesthetic events
  Emergence delirium
  Postoperative nausea and vomiting
  Difficult intubation
  Difficult IV access
Past surgical history
Family history of pseudocholinesterase deficiency or malignant hyperthermia

Patient History

Documentation of allergy status is an essential part of the preoperative evaluation, particularly as prophylactic antibiotics may be administered prior to incision. Allergies to certain antibiotics (especially penicillin, ampicillin and cephalosporins) are the most common medication allergies in children presenting for surgery. Anaphylactic allergic reactions are rare, but can be life threatening if not diagnosed and treated promptly. Latex allergy is the most common etiology for an anaphylactic reaction, and children with spina bifida (myelomeningocele), bladder exstrophy, or those who have undergone multiple operations (such as repeated ventriculoperitoneal shunts) are at greatest risk for such reactions.

In general, parents should be instructed to continue routine administration of anticonvulsant medications, cardiac medications, and pulmonary medications even while the child is fasting.

The family history should be reviewed for pseudocholinesterase deficiency (prolonged paralysis after succinylcholine) or any first-degree relative who experienced malignant hyperthermia (MH). A complete review of systems is important and should focus on those areas in which abnormalities may increase the risk of adverse events in the perioperative period.

Miscellaneous Conditions

Malignant Hyperthermia Susceptibility

MH is an inherited disorder of skeletal muscle calcium channels, triggered in affected individuals by exposure to inhalational anesthetic agents (e.g., isoflurane, desflurane, sevoflurane), succinylcholine, or both in combination, resulting in an elevation of intracellular calcium. The incidence of an MH crisis is 1:15,000 general anesthetics in children. Fifty per cent of patients who have an MH episode have undergone a prior general anesthetic without complication. The resulting MH crisis is characterized by hypermetabolism (fever, hypercarbia, acidosis), electrolyte derangement (hyperkalemia), arrhythmias, and skeletal muscle damage (elevated creatine phosphokinase [CPK]). This constellation of events may lead to death if unrecognized and/or untreated. Dantrolene, which reduces the release of calcium from muscle sarcoplasmic reticulum, when given early in the course of an MH crisis, has significantly improved patient outcomes. With early and appropriate treatment, the mortality is now less than 10%. Current suggested therapy can be remembered using the mnemonic 'Some Hot Dude Better GIve Iced Fluids Fast" and is summarized in Box 3-2.[7] It should be noted that dantrolene must be prepared at the time of use by dissolving in sterile water. It is notoriously difficult to get into solution and the surgeon may be asked to help with this process.

Patients traditionally thought to be MH susceptible are those with a spectrum of muscle diseases listed in Box 3-3. However, many patients who develop MH have a normal history and physical examination. In the past, patients with mitochondrial disorders were thought to be at risk. Anesthetic gases appear safe in this population,

BOX 3-2	Treatment of Malignant Hyperthermia Crisis:

'SOME HOT DUDE BETTER GIVE ICED FLUIDS FAST'[12]

*S*top all triggering agents, administer 100% oxygen
*H*yperventilate: treat *H*ypercarbia
*D*antrolene (2.5 mg/kg) immediately
*B*icarbonate (1 mEq/kg): treat acidosis
*G*lucose and *I*nsulin: treat hyperkalemia with 0.5 g/kg glucose, 0.15 units/kg insulin
*I*ced *I*ntravenous fluids and cooling blanket
*F*luid output: ensure adequate urine output: *F*urosemide and/or mannitol as needed
*F*ast heart rate: be prepared to treat ventricular tachycardia

but succinylcholine should still be avoided as some patients may have rhabdomyolysis (elevated CPK, hyperkalemia, myoglobinuria) with hyperkalemia without having MH.

Trisomy 21

Perioperative complications occur in 10% of patients with trisomy 21 who undergo noncardiac surgery and include severe bradycardia, airway obstruction, difficult intubation, post-intubation croup, and bronchospasm. Patients may have airway obstruction due to a large tongue and mid-face hypoplasia. The incidence of obstructive sleep apnea (OSA) may exceed 50% in these patients, and may worsen after anesthesia and operation. Airway obstruction may persist even after adenotonsillectomy. Many patients with trisomy 21 have a smaller caliber trachea than children of similar age and size; therefore, a smaller endotracheal tube (ETT) may be required.

Congenital heart disease (CHD) is encountered in 40–50% of patients with trisomy 21. The most common defects are atrial and ventricular septal defects, tetralogy of Fallot, and atrioventricular (AV) canal defects. Children with a cardiac history should have records from their most recent cardiology consultation and echocardiogram available for preoperative evaluation. Recent clinical changes in their condition may warrant an assessment by their cardiologist prior to operation.

Cervical spine instability can lead to spinal cord injury in the perianesthetic period. Patients with trisomy 21 have laxity of the ligament holding the odontoid process of C2 against the posterior arch of C1. This can lead to atlanto-axial instability that occurs in about 15% of these patients. The need for preoperative screening for this condition is controversial. However, even if the radiographic examination is normal, care should be taken perioperatively to keep the neck in as neutral a position as possible, avoiding extreme flexion, extension or rotation, especially during tracheal intubation. Any patient with trisomy 21 who has neurologic symptoms such as sensory or motor changes, or loss of bladder or bowel control, should have preoperative neurosurgical consultation to exclude cervical cord compression.

Preoperative Fasting Guidelines

Violation of fasting guidelines is one of the most common causes for cancellation or delay of surgeries. Preoperative fasting is required to minimize the risk of vomiting and aspiration of particulate matter and gastric acid during anesthesia induction. While the risk of aspiration is generally small, it is a real risk that may be associated with severe morbidity or death.

Research performed at our institution has demonstrated that intake of clear liquids (i.e., liquids that print can be read through, such as clear apple juice or Pedialyte) up until two hours prior to the induction of anesthesia does not increase the volume or acidity of gastric contents.[8] Our policy is to recommend clear liquids until two hours prior to the patient's scheduled arrival time. Breast milk is allowed up to three hours before arrival for infants up to 12 months of age. Infant formula is allowed until four hours before arrival in infants less than 6 months old, and until six hours before arrival in babies 6–12 months old. All other liquids (including milk), solid food, candy, and gum are not allowed less than eight hours before induction of anesthesia. Although these are the guidelines for our institution, the surgeon should be aware that NPO (nil per os) guidelines are variable and institutionally dependent.

Mitigating circumstances for NPO rules are limited to emergency operations, in which steps are taken to protect the airway from aspiration through the use of rapid sequence intubation. Nonemergent patients at particular risk for dehydration should be scheduled as the first case of the day when possible, and administration of clear liquids by mouth until two hours prior to arrival at the surgical facility should be encouraged. Insulin-dependent diabetics, infants, and patients with cyanotic or single ventricle cardiac disease are among those requiring careful planning so that fasting times are not prolonged.

Laboratory Testing

At the time of consultation, selected laboratory studies may be ordered, but routine laboratory work is usually not indicated. Policies vary among institutions regarding the need for preoperative hemoglobin testing. In general, any patient undergoing a procedure with the potential for significant blood loss and need for transfusion should have a complete blood count (CBC) performed in the preoperative period. Certain medications, particularly anticonvulsants (tegretol, depakote), may be associated with abnormalities in blood components (white blood cells, red blood cells, platelets), making a preoperative CBC desirable.

BOX 3-3	Muscle Diseases Associated with Malignant Hyperthermia

Central core myopathy
Becker muscular dystrophy
Duchenne muscular dystrophy
Myotonic dystrophy
King–Denborough syndrome

Although serum electrolytes are not routinely screened, electrolytes may be helpful in patients on diuretics. Preoperative glucose should be monitored in insulin-dependent diabetic patients, and also in any patient who has been receiving parenteral nutrition or intravenous (IV) fluids with a dextrose concentration greater than 5% prior to surgery.

Routine screening for pregnancy in all females who have passed menarche is strongly recommended. An age-based guideline (at our institution, any female 11 years of age or older) may be preferable. Although it is easiest to perform a urine test for human chorionic gonadotropin (hCG), if a patient cannot provide a urine sample, blood can be drawn for serum hCG testing. Institutional policy may allow the attending anesthesiologist to waive pregnancy testing at their discretion.

Certain medications, particularly anticonvulsants, should be individually assessed regarding the need for preoperative blood levels. The nature of the planned operation may also require additional studies.

CLINICAL SCENARIOS AND HIGH RISK POPULATIONS

Upper Respiratory Tract Infection

One of the most common questions confronting an anesthesiologist is whether to cancel a procedure because of an upper respiratory infection (URI). It is not uncommon for some patients to spend much of their childhood catching, suffering from, or recovering from a URI, with the highest frequency occurring in children under age 6 who attend day care or preschool.[9] Patients with a current or recent URI undergoing general anesthesia are theoretically at increased risk for perioperative respiratory complications, including laryngospasm, bronchospasm, and hypoxia, with the youngest patients (<2 years of age) being at greatest risk.[10,11] However, anesthetic management may also be tailored to reduce stimulation of a potentially hyper-reactive airway. In addition, cancellation of a procedure imposes an emotional and/or economic burden on patients and families, physicians, and operating rooms. Unless the patient is acutely ill, it is often acceptable to proceed with the anesthetic. Patients with high fever, wheezing, or productive cough may actually have a lower respiratory tract infection and the planned procedure is more likely to be cancelled. Our approach is to discuss the urgency of the scheduled operation with the surgeon, and then to review the risks and benefits of proceeding versus rescheduling with the parents, taking into consideration the possibility that the child may have another URI at the time of the rescheduled procedure. Allowing the parents to participate in the decision-making process (when appropriate) usually leads to mutual satisfaction among all involved parties.

The decision to cancel or postpone a procedure (usually a delay of four to six weeks because of concern for prolonged hyperreactivity of the bronchi) should not be made lightly. Families have often sacrificed time away from work, taken children out of school, arranged child care for other children, or have planned a vacation around the scheduled surgery. These economic and social considerations deserve respectful attention. Symptoms that would tip the scales toward cancellation include the severity of illness, as measured by an intractable or productive cough, bronchospasm, malaise, fever, or hypoxia on pulse oximetry. In contrast, clear rhinorrhea with a simple cough is usually not sufficient grounds for cancellation, provided the family understands the very small chance of needing postoperative supplemental oxygen and bronchodilator therapy.

The Former Preterm Infant

Infants born prematurely (<37 weeks gestation) may exhibit sequelae such as bronchopulmonary dysplasia (BPD), gastroesophageal reflux, intraventricular hemorrhage/hypoxic–ischemic encephalopathy (IVH/HIE), or laryngo/tracheomalacia or stenosis. Preterm infants are also at increased risk for postoperative apnea after exposure to anesthetic and analgesic agents.

Respiratory and Airway Considerations

Although the incidence of BPD has fallen over the past two decades as the use of surfactant and new ventilation strategies have been introduced, it remains the most common form of chronic lung disease in infants, and significantly complicates the perioperative management of ex-premature infants. BPD is associated with airway hyper-reactivity, bronchoconstriction, airway inflammation, pulmonary edema, and chronic lung injury.

Several effects of anesthesia, together or separately, may have life-threatening consequences. After anesthetic induction, pulmonary vasoconstriction can aggravate ventilation-perfusion mismatch and lead to profound hypoxemia. Anesthetic effects on myocardial contractility can result in impaired right ventricular function, reduced cardiac output, decreased pulmonary blood flow, and profound cardiovascular compromise with hypoxemia. Increased airway reactivity during anesthetic induction or emergence from anesthesia can result in severe exacerbation of bronchoconstriction, impairing ventilation and pulmonary blood flow. Increased oral and bronchial secretions induced by the anesthetic can compromise airflow and lead to airway or endotracheal tube plugging. Because of diminished respiratory reserves in these patients, such plugging can quickly cause profound hypoxia and acute right-sided heart strain, arrhythmias, and possibly death.

Preoperative measurement of electrolytes is warranted in children taking diuretics such as furosemide and spironolactone on a chronic basis, In addition, 48–72 hours of steroid administration may provide anti-inflammatory coverage which may reduce the risk of perioperative bronchospasm. If the child has received large doses of or continuous treatment with steroids, perioperative stress doses may be necessary.

Postanesthetic Apnea

The risk of apnea is increased in ex-premature infants because of immaturity of the central and peripheral chemoreceptors with blunted responses to hypoxia and hypercapnia, even without the additional burden of anesthetic/opioid-induced respiratory depression. In addition, anesthetic agents decrease muscle tone in the upper airway, chest wall, and diaphragm, thereby further depressing the ventilatory response to hypoxia and hypercapnia. In the immediate neonatal period, immaturity of the diaphragmatic musculature causes early fatigability, which may also contribute to apnea.[12] Although postanesthetic apnea may be brief and resolve either spontaneously or with minor stimulation, in ex-premature infants even brief apnea may result in significant hypoxia. Although most apneic episodes occur within the first two hours after anesthesia, apnea can be seen up to 18 hours postoperatively.

This increased risk of apnea affects the postanesthetic care of infants born prematurely, mandating that those at risk be admitted for cardiorespiratory monitoring. Despite numerous studies on this issue, the postnatal age at which this increased risk of apnea disappears is still being debated. The results of a meta-analysis of pertinent studies indicated that a significant reduction occurred in the incidence of apnea at 52 to 54 weeks' postconceptual age.[13] A hematocrit less than 30% was identified as an independent risk factor, and it was recommended that ex-premature infants with this degree of anemia be hospitalized postoperatively for observation regardless of the postconceptual age. However, conclusions drawn from this meta-analysis have been challenged. Moreover, the sample size of this study may not have been large enough to draw valid conclusions.[14]

Until more patients are systematically studied, the choice of when a former preterm infant can undergo an outpatient operation is up to the discretion and personal bias of the anesthesiologist and surgeon. Institutional policies most commonly mention ages of 44 weeks for infants born at term (>37 weeks), and from 52 weeks to 60 weeks postconceptual age for infants born at <37weeks. Legal issues direct these practices in many institutions, but regardless of the postconceptual age at the time of surgery, an infant should be hospitalized if any safety concerns arise during the operative or recovery period.

Although the risk of apnea can be decreased with regional anesthesia and/or caffeine, our practice is to admit all at-risk patients (those with a postconceptual age of younger than 60 weeks), regardless of the anesthetic technique used, to monitored, high-surveillance inpatient units for 23 hours after anesthesia and operation. Similarly, infants born at term must be at least 1 month of age to be candidates for outpatient surgery because postanesthetic apnea has been reported in full-term infants up to 44 weeks postconceptual age.[13] Figure 3-1 shows an algorithm useful for decision making regarding eligibility for day surgery in young infants.

Anterior Mediastinal Mass

It has long been recognized that the anesthetic management of the child with an anterior mediastinal mass is very challenging and fraught with the risk of sudden airway and cardiovascular collapse. Signs and symptoms of positional airway compression and cardiovascular dysfunction may, or may not, be present. However, the absence of signs and symptoms does not preclude the possibility of life-threatening collapse of the airway or cardiovascular obstruction upon induction of anesthesia. Patients presenting with anterior mediastinal masses (e.g., lymphoma) are at particularly high risk of airway compromise and cardiovascular collapse with the induction of general anesthesia due to compression of the trachea or great vessels when intrinsic muscle tone is lost and spontaneous respiration ceases.[15-17] When this occurs, there may not be airway compromise, but rather obstruction of vascular inflow to the right atrium and/or outflow tract obstruction from the right or left ventricle.

Preoperative evaluation should begin with a careful history to elicit any respiratory symptoms. Common symptoms of tracheal compression and tracheomalacia include cough, dyspnea, wheezing, chest pain, dysphagia, orthopnea, and recurrent pulmonary infections. Cardiovascular symptoms may result from infiltration of the pericardium and myocardium or compression of the pulmonary artery or superior vena cava. The diagnostic evaluation includes chest radiographs and/or computed tomography (CT) scans. Echocardiography may be useful to assess the pericardial status, myocardial contractility, and compression of the cardiac chambers and major vessels. Flow-volume loops and fluoroscopy can provide a dynamic assessment of airway compression that other tests cannot assess. Chest CT is helpful in planning the anesthetic technique and in evaluating the potential for airway compromise during anesthesia. Tumor-associated superior vena cava syndrome develops rapidly and is poorly tolerated.

Premedication is inadvisable in most patients with an anterior mediastinal mass as any loss of airway muscle tone may upset the balance between negative intrathoracic pressure and gravity, resulting in airway collapse. Once the decision is made to sedate or anesthetize the child, maintenance of spontaneous respiration, regardless of induction technique, is paramount. It is essential to avoid the use of muscle relaxants because the subsequent airway collapse can be fatal.

Positioning the child is an important part of the anesthetic plan for these patients. The sitting position favors gravitational pull of the tumor toward the abdomen rather than allowing the tumor to fall posteriorly onto the airway and major vessels as occurs in the supine position. However, the sitting position makes intubation challenging. Thus, positioning the symptomatic child in the lateral decubitus position is recommended. Turning the child lateral or prone, or lifting the sternum, have been shown to alleviate acute deterioration in ventilation or cardiovascular collapse secondary to tumor compression.[18,19] In any patient with an increased potential for such obstruction, provision should be made for the availability of a rigid bronchoscope, the ability to move the operating room table to effect position changes, and the ability to institute cardiopulmonary bypass or extracorporeal membrane oxygenation (ECMO). Compression of greater than 50% of the cross-sectional area of the trachea on CT imaging has been suggested to identify a population at risk of airway collapse during induction of general anesthesia.[20]

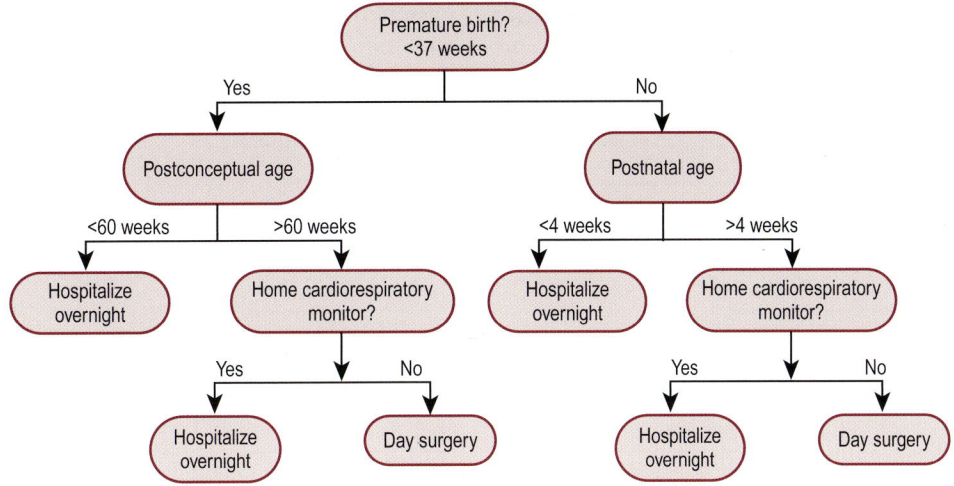

FIGURE 3-1 ■ This algorithm is useful for decision making regarding eligibility for outpatient surgery.

When possible, percutaneous biopsy of the mass using local anesthesia with or without judicious doses of sedative medication is often ideal and poses the least risk to the patient. In patients who have additional tissue sites from which a biopsy can be obtained (e.g., cervical, axillary, or inguinal lymph nodes), it may be safer to proceed with the patient in a semi-sitting position using local anesthesia and carefully titrating sedation so that spontaneous ventilation is preserved. Recently, ketamine and dexmedetomidine have been shown to provide good sedation with preservation of airway patency and spontaneous respiration in this setting.[21] If progression to general anesthesia is required and airway and/or vascular compression exists, standby ECMO capability is strongly recommended.

The inherent conflict between the need to obtain an accurate and timely tissue diagnosis and the very real concern regarding the safe conduct of the anesthetic requires an open dialogue between the anesthesiologist, surgeon, and oncologist to reach an agreement on strategies to achieve these goals. Many experts recommend the development and utilization of an algorithm for anesthetic management of the child with an anterior mediastinal mass (Fig. 3-2). The algorithm addresses assessment of signs and symptoms, evaluation of cardiopulmonary compromise, and treatment options.[18,22,23]

Patients with Congenital Heart Disease

Each year in the U.S., nearly 32,000 children are born with CHD. Extracardiac anomalies are seen in up to 30% of infants with CHD,[24,25] and may necessitate operative intervention in the neonatal period prior to repair or palliation of the cardiac lesion. Although physiologically well-compensated patients may undergo noncardiac surgery with minimal risk, certain patient groups have been identified as high risk: children less than 1 year of age, especially premature infants; patients with severe cyanosis, poorly compensated congestive failure or pulmonary hypertension; patients requiring emergency surgery and patients with multiple coexisting diseases.[26]

Preoperative Preparation and Evaluation

The spectrum of congenital and acquired cardiac lesions is so varied that formulating one set of rules for evaluation and perioperative care is nearly impossible. Children with unrepaired or palliated heart disease, children requiring operation as a result of their cardiac disease, and children undergoing emergency surgery tend to be more critically ill and require more intensive preoperative preparation and assessment.

Patients with CHD may be receiving antithrombotic therapy for a variety of reasons, including the presence of systemic-to-pulmonary shunts, mechanical or biological prosthetic heart valves, a history of thrombosis involving a conduit or a shunt, recent transcatheter interventions or device placement, treatment of Kawasaki disease, and the presence of risk factors for thromboembolic events including Fontan physiology. No specific pediatric guidelines exist for the discontinuation of antithrombotic medications prior to an elective operation, and management strategies ideally should be coordinated between the child's cardiologist, surgeon, and anesthesiologist.

An emergency operation presents additional management issues and often adds risk in several areas. There may be little time preoperatively to optimize the patient's cardiac condition, along with difficulty in quickly obtaining complete cardiology and surgical records. In these cases, the anesthetic preoperative evaluation is distilled into the most important factors, including the nature and duration of the present illness, the child's underlying cardiac disease, baseline status, and medications. Patients with cyanosis, or those who depend on shunts for pulmonary blood flow (PBF), or those with single ventricle physiology who have undergone total cavopulmonary anastomosis (Fontan procedure) require intravenous hydration prior to induction of anesthesia if they are hypovolemic. Based on the child's condition and the nature of the emergency, a decision can be made as to whether to proceed with the case with no further workup or a review of available old records, or whether new consultations and studies should be obtained prior to surgery.

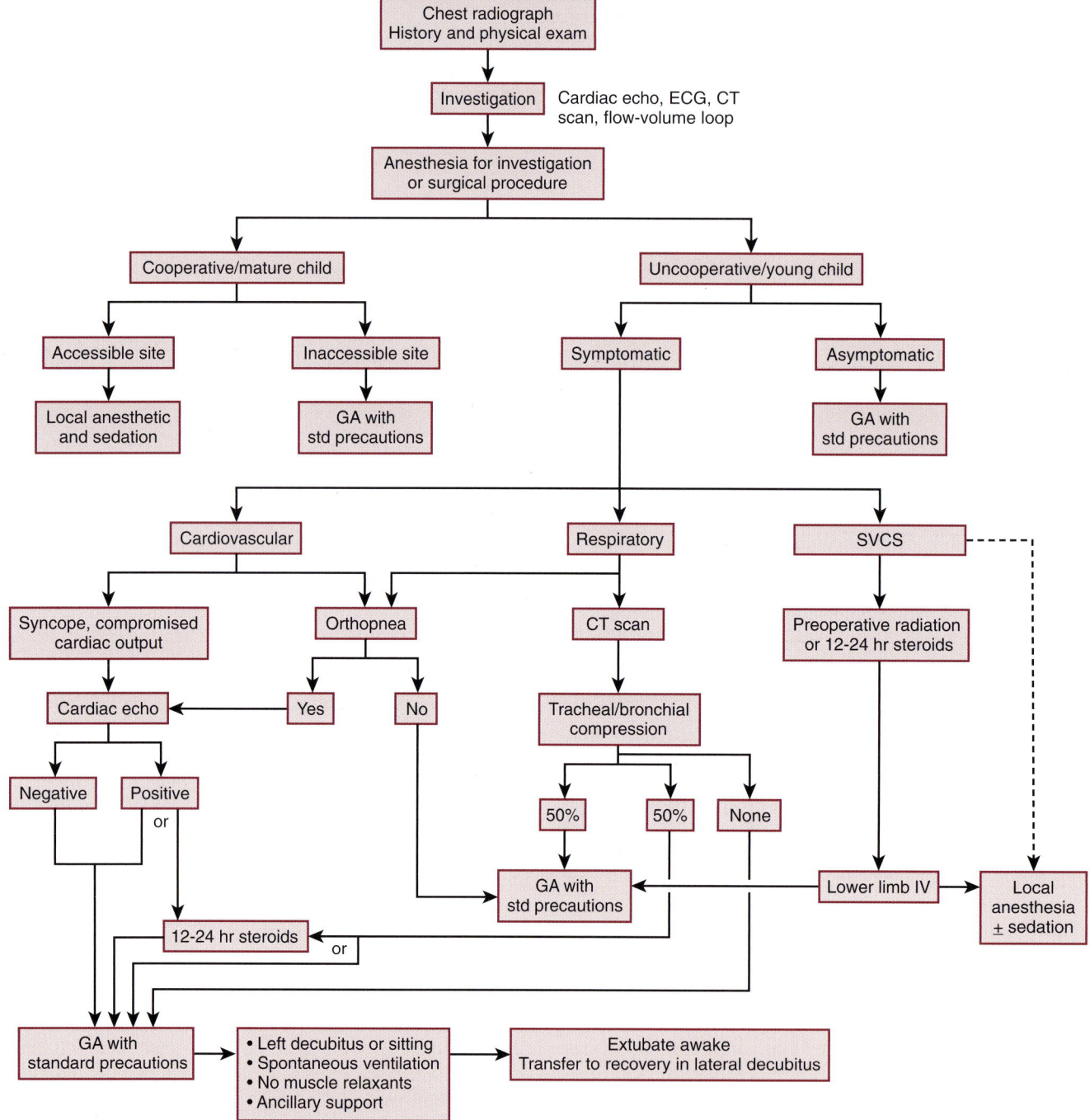

FIGURE 3-2 ■ This algorithm describes management of the patient with a large anterior mediastinal mass. GA, general anesthesia. SVCS, superior vena cava syndrome. (Adapted from Cheung S, Lerman J. Mediastinal masses and anesthesia in children. In: Riazi J, editor. The Difficult Pediatric Airway. Anesthesiol Clin North Am 1998;16:893–910.)

Endocarditis Prophylaxis

The most recent American Heart Association (AHA) guidelines for perioperative antibiotic prophylaxis emphasize evidence-based practice. Current opinion reflects the view that endocarditis is more likely to result from frequent exposure to bacteremias occurring as a consequence of activities of daily living than those due to dental, gastrointestinal, or genitourinary tract procedures.[27–30] Except for the conditions listed in Box 3-4, the AHA no longer recommends routine antibiotic

prophylaxis for any other form of CHD. For a more comprehensive discussion, the reader is referred to the original publications.[31,32]

Special Issues in Patients with CHD

Pulmonary Hypertension

Prolonged exposure of the pulmonary vascular bed to high flows secondary to left-to-right shunting, pulmonary venous obstruction, or high left atrial pressures can

BOX 3-4

Cardiac Conditions for Which Antibiotic Prophylaxis with Dental, Respiratory Tract, Gastrointestinal, and Genitourinary Procedures

Congenital heart disease (CHD)[a]
  Unrepaired cyanotic CHD, including palliative shunts and conduits
  Completely repaired congenital heart defect with prosthetic material or device, whether placed by surgery or by catheter intervention, during the first 6 months after the procedure[b]
  Repaired CHD with residual defects at the site or adjacent to the site of a prosthetic patch or prosthetic device (which inhibit endothelialization)
Cardiac transplantation recipients who develop cardiac valvopathy
Prosthetic cardiac valves
Previous infective endocarditis

[a]Except for the conditions listed above, antibiotic prophylaxis is no longer recommended for any other form of CHD.
[b]Prophylaxis is recommended because endothelialization of prosthetic material occurs within 6 months of the procedure.
Adapted from Wilson W, Taubert KA, Gewitz M, et al. Prevention of infective endocarditis. Guidelines from the American Heart Association Rheumatic Fever, Endocarditis, and Kawasaki Disease Committee, Council on Cardiovascular disease in the Young, and the Council on Clinial Cardiology, Council on Cardiovascular Surgery and Anesthesia, and Quality of Care and Outcomes Research Interdisciplinary Working Group. Circulation 2007;116:1736–54.

lead to elevated pulmonary artery (PA) pressures and the development of pulmonary veno-occlusive disease.

The pathophysiology and anesthetic implications of pulmonary hypertension have been well reviewed,[33–35] and there is no ideal sedative/anesthetic agent for these patients. A frank discussion of the high risk of anesthesia in these patients should be held with the patient's family when the anesthetic consent is obtained.

Anesthetic management strategies are guided by three considerations: (1) appropriate manipulation of factors affecting pulmonary vascular resistance (PVR); (2) the effect of anesthetic agents on PVR; and (3) maintenance of cardiac output (CO) and coronary perfusion pressures. Increases in PVR can potentially culminate in right ventricular (RV) failure if excessive.[36–38] Ventilatory strategies can profoundly alter cardiovascular pathophysiology via complex interactions influencing cardiac function and output due to alterations in RV preload and afterload. Given the propensity for desaturation and increases in PCO_2 with spontaneous ventilation, controlled ventilation is recommended intraoperatively with maintenance of lung volumes at or around functional residual capacity (FRC) with minimal positive end expiratory pressure (PEEP) and avoidance of high inspiratory pressures, hypercarbia, or hypoxemia. Normal preload should be maintained and hypotension avoided in these patients in order to optimize CO, coronary artery flow, and oxygen supply to the RV. Dopamine, epinephrine, and milrinone should be available to further improve cardiac function if necessary.

Cyanosis and Polycythemia

Cyanosis in patients with CHD can be the result of either right-to-left shunting with inadequate PBF or admixture of oxygenated and deoxygenated blood in the systemic circulation. Severe, longstanding cyanosis causes a variety of systemic derangements including hematologic, neurologic, vascular, respiratory, and coagulation abnormalities. During preoperative evaluation, the child's baseline range of hemoglobin–oxygen saturation, heart rate, and blood pressure should be noted along with any history of stroke, seizure, or pre-existing neurologic defects. Care should be taken intraoperatively to maintain normal fluid balance and cardiac function. The use of air filters in IV lines and meticulous attention to air in volume lines without filters is essential to avoid the occurrence of paradoxical emboli in children with right-to-left shunts. Controlled ventilation is recommended for all but the shortest procedures due to the ventilatory abnormalities in these patients.

One of the initial responses to cyanosis is an increase in erythropoietin levels with a subsequent increase in hemoglobin and hematocrit. At hematocrit levels greater than 65%, increased blood viscosity can result in a decrease in the delivery of oxygen to tissues. Preoperative phlebotomy is recommended only in patients who have hematocrit greater than 65%, are experiencing symptoms of hyperviscosity, and are not dehydrated. Acute onset of symptomatic hyperviscosity syndrome can be seen in cyanotic patients whose hematocrit abruptly increases due to dehydration. In these patients, rehydration is recommended rather than phlebotomy.

Increased bleeding tendencies, and a variety of associated laboratory abnormalities, have long been noted in cyanotic patients. When compared to acyanotic children a disproportionate number of cyanotic children are thrombocytopenic, with the degree of thrombocytopenia directly related to the severity of polycythemia. Abnormalities in prothrombin time, partial thromboplastin time, and individual factor deficiencies have also been described and defy simple classification.[39] Although these deficiencies may cause no symptoms other than bruising, severely cyanotic patients should have clotting studies prior to operation.

Pacemakers/Implantable Cardioverter-Defibrillators

Increasing numbers of infants and children have pacemakers or implantable cardioverter-defibrillators (ICDs). In recent years increasing numbers of children have had ICDs placed for prevention of sudden cardiac death due to congenital or acquired long QT syndrome.[40] Necessary preoperative information for these patients includes the indication for device placement, the date of last device check, and the current underlying cardiac rate and rhythm without device support. Indications for permanent pacemakers in patients with CHD include congenital or postsurgical complete heart block, and sinus node or AV node dysfunction.

The American College of Cardiology/American Heart Association (ACC/AHA) guidelines advocate pre- and postoperative interrogation of permanent pacemakers.[41] All patients with an ICD should undergo preoperative device interrogation with disabling of defibrillation capability intraoperatively and resumption in the postoperative period. Bipolar electrocautery should be utilized whenever possible in the patient with a pacemaker or ICD. If monopolar electrocautery is used, the electrocautery return pad should be placed as far away from the pacing generator as possible, and the pacemaker generator/leads axis should not be located between the operative site and the grounding pad. If the pacemaker cannot be placed in an asynchronous mode and electrocautery adversely affects it, cautery current should be applied for not more than 1 second at a time, with 10 seconds between burses of current, to allow for maintenance of CO.[42,43]

Single Ventricle Physiology

A brief review of the anatomy and physiology of patients with single ventricle (SV) abnormalities is essential to understanding the consequences of anesthesia in this population. The anatomy of patients classified as having SV physiology may include any lesion or group of lesions in which a two-ventricle cardiac repair is not feasible. Generally, either both AV valves enter a single ventricular chamber, or there is atresia of an AV or semilunar valve. Intracardiac mixing of systemic and pulmonary venous blood flow occurs, and the SV output is shared between the pulmonary and systemic circulations. Patients with relative hypoplasia of one ventricle, such as an unbalanced AV canal defect or severe Ebstein anomaly, may also undergo SV palliation operations.

A series of three separate staged palliative cardiac surgeries are generally performed for most children with SV physiology. After initial stage I palliation, patients are dependent on either a modified systemic-to-pulmonary shunt or an RV to PA conduit to provide PBF. The ratio of pulmonary to systemic blood flow is then dependent on the balance between systemic vascular resistance (SVR) and PVR, with patients vulnerable to perturbations in PO_2, PCO_2, acid–base status, temperature, and volume status. Oxygen saturations greater than 85% indicate pulmonary overcirculation and patients may exhibit symptoms of congestive heart failure (CHF). Once the patient is anesthetized and mechanically ventilated, their oxygen saturation often increases, requiring the adjustment of the FiO_2 and PCO_2 to target oxygen saturations between 75–85%. An acute drop in oxygen saturation along with the absence of a murmur indicates loss of shunt flow and is catastrophic. Immediate echocardiographic confirmation of shunt flow is crucial, with rapid institution of ECMO if necessary.

Patients usually undergo a second stage procedure, or bidirectional cavopulmonary anastomosis, at 3 to 6 months of age, with the anastomosis of the superior vena cava to the pulmonary circulation replacing the systemic-to-pulmonary shunt created during the first stage surgery. Oxygen saturations will continue to range from 75–85% as patients are still mixing oxygenated and deoxygenated blood for ejection from the SV. Ventricular function is generally improved as the volume load has been removed

from the heart. However, systemic hypertension is frequently seen in these children. At 18 months to 3 years of age, a total cavopulmonary anastomosis, or Fontan procedure, is performed. Surgeons usually choose to place a fenestration in the atrial baffle allowing right-to-left shunting to occur, and these patients often have hemoglobin-oxygen saturation of 80–90%. The presence of aorto-pulmonary collaterals or baffle leaks may also result in decreased systemic oxygen saturation.

It is clear that the patient's volume status must be assessed preoperatively. Patients with dehydration should have an IV placed and adequate hydration assured prior to induction of anesthesia. Care should be taken to avoid hypovolemia as PBF is dependent on preload. Normal sinus rhythm should be maintained if possible. Controlled ventilation is appropriate for most procedures as long as excessive airway pressures are avoided, and physiologic levels of PEEP may be used to avoid atelectasis without impairing PBF.

Although many children with SV physiology may appear well, they are uniquely susceptible to physiologic perturbations, especially hypovolemia. Laparoscopic procedures, while presenting many advantages, should be carefully undertaken in these patients

The Difficult Pediatric Airway

The patient with a 'difficult airway' may require advanced airway management techniques in order to secure his/her airway including the lighted stylet, the fiberoptic intubating stylet, the flexible fiberoptic bronchoscope, direct laryngoscopy with intubating stylet, fiberoptic rigid laryngoscopy, an anterior commissure scope, the laryngeal mask airway, cricothyrotomy, and tracheostomy. Anesthesiologists and facilities do not need availability of all of the listed techniques. When a difficult airway is anticipated, it is important to have all necessary airway equipment present in the operating room (OR) before induction of anesthesia, as well as communication of the difficult airway potential to all members of the OR team. Indirect intubation methods should be utilized rather than repeated attempts at direct laryngoscopy because airway edema and bleeding increase with each attempt, decreasing the likelihood of success with subsequent indirect methods.[44]

Patients that require additional approaches to obtain an airway require additional OR time and, in certain cases, continuation of intubation postoperatively may be necessary, mandating ICU admission. Most difficult airways in the pediatric age group can be anticipated. Unlike in adults, it is rare to encounter an unanticipated difficult airway in a normal-appearing child. Some congenital syndromes associated with difficult airway management are listed in Table 3-2.

The ASA has developed practice guidelines and an algorithm for management of the difficult airway. This guideline and algorithm are continually updated and well known to anesthesiologists.[44] Although the guidelines and algorithm are intended for use in adult patients, their emphasis on the importance of having a clear primary plan with multiple back-up contingency plans is equally applicable to infants and children.

TABLE 3-2 Syndromes and Craniofacial Abnormalities Associated with Difficult Intubation

Syndrome	Associated Features
Arthrogryposis	Limited mouth opening and cervical mobility
Beckwith–Wiedemann	Macroglossia
Freeman–Sheldon (whistling face)	Microstomia
Goldenhar syndrome (hemifacial microsomia)	Hemifacial microsomia, mandibular hypoplasia (uni- or bilateral)
Klippel–Feil	Limited cervical mobility
Mucopolysaccharidoses (e.g., Hurler)	Macroglossia, limited cervical mobility, Infiltration of tongue, supraglottis
Pierre–Robin	Micrognathia, glossoptosis, cleft palate
Treacher–Collins	Maxillary/mandibular hypoplasia
Trisomy 21 (Down)	Macroglossia, subglottic stenosis, atlanto-axial instability

INTRAOPERATIVE MANAGEMENT

Monitoring and Vascular Access

Standard monitoring in pediatric anesthesia follows the ASA 'Standards for Basic Anesthetic Monitoring'[45] and includes pulse oximetry, noninvasive automated blood pressure measurement, electrocardiography, capnography, and temperature monitoring. Temperature monitoring is indicated in most pediatric anesthetics because of the increased prevalence of both MH and, more commonly, hypothermia in infants and children exposed to ambient OR temperatures.

Oxygenation is measured indirectly by pulse oximetry with an audible and variable pitch tone and low threshold alarm. Measurement of inspired oxygen concentration is standard with the use of an anesthesia machine. Depending on the duration and magnitude of the planned operation, as well as the child's preoperative condition, more invasive monitoring with placement of an arterial or central venous line may be necessary. The surgeon should communicate his or her expectations regarding the expected duration of surgery, the potential for blood loss, and the need for invasive monitoring intraoperatively and/or postoperatively. In cases where large fluid shifts or blood loss are expected, the placement of a urinary catheter aids in assessing ongoing urine output and fluid balance.

Anesthetic Considerations for Specific Surgical Approaches

The successful application of minimally invasive techniques is now commonplace in infants and children. Anesthetic concerns center around the effects of abdominal insufflation on ventilation and hemodynamics.

Two features of laparoscopic intervention create concern in the anesthetic management of infants and children: (1) the creation of a pneumoperitoneum with the concomitant increase in intra-abdominal pressure and resultant changes in ventilatory parameters; and (2) the extremes of patient positioning that may be required for optimal exposure of intra-abdominal structures.[46] An appreciation of the physiologic, hemodynamic, and ventilatory consequences during and after a laparoscopic operation is an important part of careful patient selection.

Carbon dioxide is the gas of choice for insufflation for several reasons. Carbon dioxide is noncombustible and is cleared more rapidly from the circulation than the other options. The cardiovascular consequences of intravascular gas embolism present less risk with CO_2 than with an insoluble gas such as helium or air. However, cardiovascular collapse has been reported in several infants following insufflation, with end-tidal gas monitoring implying that these events were due to gas embolism.[47,48] Neonates and very young infants may be uniquely at risk for such events because of possible patency and large caliber of the ductus venosus. Carbon dioxide uptake may be significantly greater in children, owing to the greater absorptive area of the peritoneum in relation to body weight, and the smaller distance between capillaries and peritoneum. Regardless, hypercarbia has been demonstrated in pediatric studies during CO_2 insufflation.[49] Increases in minute ventilation by as much as 60% may be required to maintain baseline $ETCO_2$, but the goal for an appropriate CO_2 level need not be the baseline value. Instead, $ETCO_2$ can safely rise into the 50s.

Hydrocephalic patients warrant special mention in regard to CO_2 insufflation. Although patients with VP shunts have been shown to have intracranial pressure increases associated with a modest decrease in cerebral perfusion pressure at an intra-abdominal pressure of 10 mmHg or less,[50] a recent review of laparoscopic compared to open abdominal surgery in children with shunts showed no pneumocephalus or increase in the incidence of shunt infection in the laparoscopic group.[51] This is due to the fact that most VP shunts now have a one-way valve that will not allow gas entry. Interestingly, one group recently reported a case of pneumocephalus that occurred in a patient with such a shunt and valve that was inserted 20 years earlier.[52]

The increase in intra-abdominal pressure seen with laparoscopy is associated with well-documented cardiorespiratory changes. Changes in ventilatory dynamics occur due to cephalad displacement of the diaphragm. This results in a reduction in lung volume, ventilation-perfusion mismatch, and altered gas exchange. Bozkurt and coworkers demonstrated statistically significant decreases in pH and PaO_2 and increased $PaCO_2$ after 30 minutes of pneumoperitoneum.[53] These changes are additive to the 20% reduction in FRC that occurs with induction of general anesthesia. The magnitude of the pulmonary effects correlates directly with intraperitoneal pressures, and may be further exacerbated by steep Trendelenburg positioning.[54]

Significant cardiovascular changes have been demonstrated in response to increased intra-abdominal pressure and patient position. In the supine or Trendelenburg position, the venous return is less impaired when the intra-abdominal pressure is kept below 15 mmHg. The position preferred for upper abdominal procedures is reverse-Trendelenburg or supine. The head-up position reduces venous return and CO.[55] Several pediatric studies have utilized echocardiography (supine),[56] impedance cardiography (15° head-down),[57] and continuous esophageal aortic blood flow echo-Doppler (supine)[58] to assess hemodynamic changes during laparoscopic surgery. These studies demonstrated significant reductions in stroke volume and cardiac index (CI), along with a significant increase in SVR. Pneumoperitoneum was found to be associated with significant increases in left ventricular end-diastolic volume, left ventricular end-systolic volume, and left ventricular end-systolic wall stress.[56] All three studies demonstrated a decrease in cardiac performance and an increase in vascular resistance in healthy patients undergoing laparoscopy for lower abdominal procedures. The cardiovascular changes seen with pneumoperitoneum (Box 3-5) occur immediately with creation of the pneumoperitoneum and resolve on desufflation.

Thoracoscopy

Thoracoscopy has advantages over open thoracotomy, including reduced postoperative pain, decreased duration of hospitalization, improved cosmetic results, and decreased incidence of chest wall deformity.[59,60] An optimal anesthetic plan considers potential respiratory derangements including ventilation-perfusion mismatch which may result from positioning, CO_2 insufflation into the pleural cavity, and single-lung ventilation. In addition, much like insufflation during laparoscopy, hemodynamic changes during chest insufflation can compromise preload, stroke volume, CI, and blood pressure.[60]

In a study of 50 pediatric patients undergoing thoracoscopy for a variety of operations, systolic and diastolic blood pressures were significantly lower, and $ETCO_2$ was significantly higher during thoracoscopy.[60] After intrapleural CO_2 insufflation, there was a statistically significant increase in $ETCO_2$ during one-lung ventilation (OLV) compared with two-lung ventilation. On the other hand, two-lung ventilation with CO_2 insufflation was associated with a lower systolic and diastolic pressure than OLV. The increase in $ETCO_2$ correlated with the

duration of the insufflation. These factors should be considered along with any pre-existing preoperative respiratory or cardiovascular compromise in planning the operation and anesthetic management. The magnitude of the physiologic changes induced by either one-lung or two-lung ventilation with insufflation is impacted by the patient's age, underlying co-morbid conditions, and anesthetic agents utilized.

Many thoracic procedures require lung deflation and minimal lung excursion on the operative side while ventilating the contralateral lung. OLV is useful if the surgeon requires additional exposure. In the pediatric patient, there are several options for attaining unilateral lung isolation (Fig. 3-3).[61]

Complications related to anesthetic management are usually related to mechanical factors such as airway injury and malposition of the ETT. Additional problems related to physiologic alterations include hypoxemia and hypercapnia. An unusual complication was reported during attempted thoracoscopic resection of a congenital cystic adenomatoid malformation in a 3.5 kg infant.[62] During CO_2 insufflation, there was a sharp rise in $ETCO_2$ accompanied by severe hypoxemia and bradycardia. This was due to occlusion of the ETT by blood. After immediate conversion, it was discovered that there had been direct insufflation into the cyst and that the cyst communicated directly with the tracheobronchial tree.

Blood obstructing the ETT is a common occurrence during thoracic procedures, whether open or thoracoscopic, especially in infants in whom the ETT inner diameter is so small and therefore at high risk for obstruction. Ventilatory parameters, such as increasing airway pressure during volume ventilation or decreasing tidal volume during pressure ventilation, may precede desaturation and an increase in $ETCO_2$ due to compromised ventilation associated with ETT obstruction. ETT suctioning, and if necessary, ETT lavage may be required during the procedure to remove blood and/or secretions.

It is important to try to maintain a reasonable range of elevated CO_2 in neonates undergoing thoracoscopic procedures. Mukhtar and colleagues reported that permissive hypercapnia with $ETCO_2$ 50–70 mmHg was associated with improved cardiac output and arterial oxygen tension in neonates undergoing thoracoscopic ligation of patent ductus arteriosus.[63] A case series in which high-frequency oscillating ventilation (HFOV) was used in neonates undergoing thoracoscopic procedures has been reported.[64] HFOV enables better CO_2 elimination while optimizing the visualization for the surgeons.

POSTANESTHESIA CARE

The recovery period for infants and children may be more crucial than for adult patients with 3–4% of infants and children developing major complications in the recovery period, compared to only 0.5% of adults. Most of these complications occur in the youngest children (<2 years of age) and are most commonly respiratory in nature.[65]

BOX 3-5	**Physiologic Effects of Creation of a Pneumoperitoneum**

↑ Systemic vascular resistance
↑ Pulmonary vascular resistance
↓ Stroke volume
↓ Cardiac index
↑ PCO_2
↓ Functional residual capacity
↓ pH
↓ PO_2
↓ Venous return (head up)

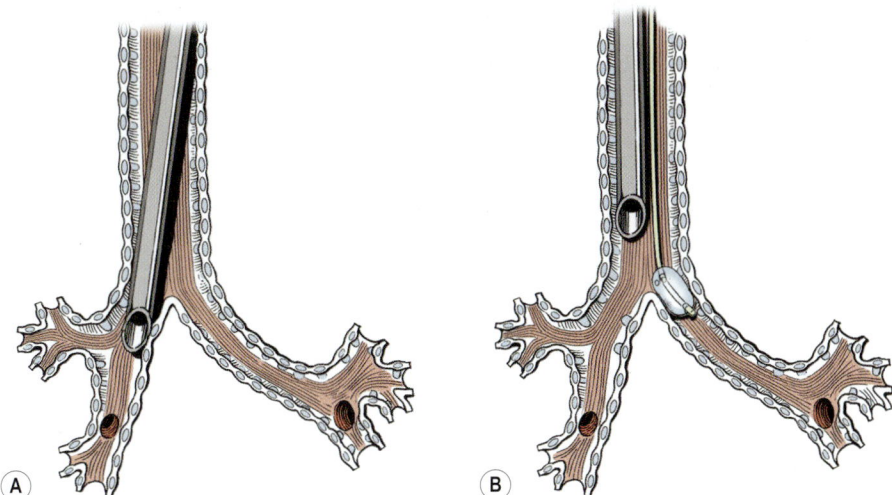

FIGURE 3-3 ■ There are several methods available for single-lung ventilation in infants and children. **(A)** The most common method is to use a conventional single-lumen endotracheal tube to intubate a main-stem bronchus. **(B)** Another technique is to position the endotracheal tube in the trachea followed by insertion of a balloon-tipped bronchial blocker that is passed along the endotracheal tube and occludes the ipsilateral main-stem bronchus. The position of the bronchial blocker is usually confirmed using fiberoptic bronchoscopy.

Common Postanesthesia Problems

Postoperative events can include pain, emergence delirium, nausea and/or vomiting, stridor which may be due to laryngospasm or subglottic edema, and hypoxia. Persistence of these conditions can delay discharge. The most common minor adverse effects of anesthesia include throat pain or discomfort from airway tubes, and postoperative nausea and vomiting (PONV). These issues should be discussed with families preoperatively, along with assurances of prophylaxis and/or treatment if necessary.

Postoperative Nausea and Vomiting

PONV is the most common cause of delayed discharge from the postanesthesia care unit (PACU) and the most common reason for unanticipated hospitalization following outpatient surgery.[66,67] Certain procedures, such as strabismus surgery, middle ear surgery, orchiopexy, and umbilical hernia repair are associated with a greater than 50% incidence of postoperative vomiting. Similarly, the perioperative use of any opioid is associated with a very high incidence of PONV, even when general anesthetic drugs associated with a lower incidence of nausea, such as propofol, are used.[68] Common approaches to treat or prevent PONV include alteration of the anesthetic technique, perioperative administration of antiemetics (either prophylactically or as treatment), and limitation of postoperative oral intake.[69,70]

Respiratory Complications

Respiratory complications are the most serious of the common problems seen postoperatively in infants and children. All respiratory complications are more common in children with a recent history of respiratory tract infection.

Postintubation croup, or postextubation subglottic edema, has been a well-recognized entity since airways were first secured with endotracheal tubes. Children are more prone to develop croup following intubation than adults because of the differences in their airway anatomy. Children have narrower laryngeal and tracheal lumens that are more easily compromised by mucosal edema. Children with trisomy 21 may be at increased risk for this complication due to the increased incidence of occult subglottic narrowing. Other contributing factors to the development of croup include traumatic or repeated intubation attempts, coughing ('bucking') on the ETT, changes in patient position after intubation, and general anesthesia in children with a current or recent upper respiratory tract infection.[71-73]

The incidence of post-intubation croup has decreased from 6% to 1% of all endotracheally intubated children.[74] This reduction has occurred because of the development and use of sterile, implant-tested ETTs, the routine intraoperative use of humidified gases, and by using an appropriately sized (air leak pressure of less than 25 cm water) ETT in children younger than 5 years of age.

Laryngospasm, while possibly life threatening, is almost always transient and treatable by early application of continuous positive airway pressure (CPAP) by mask combined, if necessary, with a small dose of propofol (1–2 mg/kg). Rescue with succinylcholine is indicated if oxygen desaturation persists despite CPAP and propofol. Laryngospasm may also occur in the OR during anesthetic induction or emergence from anesthesia. Effective maneuvers for management of laryngospasm have recently been outlined in a helpful algorithm accompanying a case scenario publication.[75] Bronchospasm is more common in children with poorly controlled asthma and those exposed to second hand smoke. It is most often managed with administration of nebulized β-agonists such as albuterol.[73]

Intraoperative Awareness

Intraoperative awareness is a rare but disturbing condition in which patients undergoing an operation and anesthesia can recall surroundings, sounds, events, and sometimes even pain. The definition of intraoperative awareness is becoming conscious during a procedure performed under general anesthesia, with subsequent explicit memory of specific events that took place during that time. A Sentinel Event Alert was issued by the Joint Commission (JC) regarding the prevention and management of intraoperative awareness in October 2004. The ASA published a *Practice Advisory for Intraoperative Awareness and Brain Functioning Monitoring* in April 2006.[76]

The incidence of intraoperative awareness in adults has been reported to be 0.1–0.9% in older studies, and 0.0068% or 1 per 14,560 patients in a 2007 report of 87,361 patients.[77] Most experts estimate the true incidence in adults to be 0.1–0.2%. There is a dearth of literature about intraoperative awareness in infants and children, but there is a 2005 study of 864 children in which the incidence was reported as 0.8%.[78] Some of these data may be confounded by the memory of entering the OR after administration of preoperative sedation or a memory of events and sensations during emergence. Certainly, the likelihood of a clear memory of a painful event during surgery is a much rarer event than the other events more commonly reported. However, there are multiple adverse consequences of intraoperative awareness, including post-traumatic stress disorder and medical-legal implications.

Pain Management

The goal of postoperative pain management should be to achieve good pain relief with minimal adverse effects. Effective pain management is associated with early mobilization, more rapid recovery, and faster return to work, school, and play.

The incidence of postoperative pain in the pediatric population, although difficult to evaluate objectively, is probably similar to that in the adult population. It is reasonable, therefore, to assume that about 75% of children will report significant pain on the first postoperative day.[79] Many studies looking at pain in hospitalized children report under-treatment in both medical and surgical patients.[80] This under-treatment may be related to: (1) inadequate analgesia provided intraoperatively; (2) underestimation of an infant's ability to experience pain (primarily in neonates who are erroneously believed to be incapable of experiencing or remembering painful experiences); (3) fear of analgesic (primarily opioid) side effects; (4) fear of addiction by both caregivers and parents; (5) inadequate knowledge or utilization of pain assessment scales in children who are either pre-verbal or unable to use numerical rating scales; (6) failure to appreciate the benefit of nonopioid analgesics in provision of effect pain relief while reducing total opioid dose and attendant adverse effects; and (7) failure to utilize basic regional analgesic techniques that are easily applied even in the ambulatory setting.

TABLE 3-3	Equianalgesic Opioid Doses	
Name	**Equipotent IV Dose (mg/kg)**	**Equipotent PO Dose (mg/kg)**
Morphine	0.1	0.3
Fentanyl	0.001	N/A
Hydromorphone	0.015	0.04
Methadone	0.1	0.1
Nalbuphine	0.1	N/A
Hydrocodone	N/A	0.1
Oxycodone	N/A	0.1

The management of pain in infants and children is hampered by the difficulty that exists in assessing pain. Many children may respond to pain by emotionally withdrawing from their surroundings, and this may be misinterpreted by the medical and nursing staff as evidence that they have no pain. In addition, when questioned as to their degree of pain, children may not volunteer useful information for fear of painful interventions (e.g., 'shots'). To circumvent these difficulties, pain assessment scales have been developed for use in infants and children that are more objective and depend on caregiver assessment of body positions, facial expression, and physiologic variables. Although there are many scales available, an institution should adopt one scale for each stage of development, and ensure that caregivers are trained so that they are used reproducibly in settings where pain is treated. Examples of these pain scales include CRIES for neonates (until 1 month of age), FLACC from 1 month to age 4 years, FACES for age 5 to 9 years and in children who are developmentally appropriate, and a numerical scale for those older than 10 years of age.[81,82]

Opioids

The mainstay in pain control remains the use of opioids, although increasingly regional analgesic techniques (epidural or peripheral nerve block) are being used in infants and children. There are many opioids available for both IV and oral administration, but they all have common adverse effects. These include dose-dependent respiratory depression as mentioned above, which may be more prominent in neonates and young infants and in patients with OSA.[12,83,84] Other side effects that vary in prevalence among drugs and patients are dysphoria, somnolence, nausea and vomiting, pruritus, constipation, and urinary retention.

Morphine remains the standard by which the potency of other opioids is measured. Equipotent analgesic doses of commonly used IV opioids are listed in Table 3-3. As the plasma concentration of morphine correlates poorly with its desired analgesic effect—a fourfold variation has been measured in the plasma concentration of morphine at which patients express the need for additional pain medication—many clinicians believe that morphine is best administered in a patient-controlled device (patient-controlled analgesia [PCA]) to allow self-titration of medication according to the level of pain experienced.

A discussion of patient selection and dosing for PCA is beyond the scope of this chapter, but can be found in many textbooks of pediatric anesthesiology and pain management.[81] Patients receiving PCA should be continuously monitored for cardiorespiratory depression by monitoring the echocardiogram, respiratory rate, and pulse oximetry.[85]

When PCA devices are not used, the intermittent bolus administration of morphine to opioid-naive children should be started at 0.05–0.1 mg/kg every two to four hours. If the treatment of pain is initiated in the PACU or intensive care setting, similar doses may be administered every five to ten minutes until the child is comfortable.

Fentanyl is a synthetic opioid that usually has a relatively short duration of action as a result of its rapid distribution into fat and muscle due to its high lipid solubility. With repeated dosing, the duration of action appears to increase.[86] When compared with morphine, fentanyl is about 100 times more potent. (Fentanyl dosages are calculated in micrograms rather than milligrams.) In controlled comparisons with equipotent dosages, morphine is generally found to provide better, more long-lasting analgesia than fentanyl, but with more side effects such as pruritus, nausea, and vomiting.[87–89] Opioids with short half-lives like fentanyl may also demonstrate the development of much more rapid tolerance to its analgesic effects than morphine or hydromorphone.

Hydromorphone is a well-tolerated alternative to morphine and fentanyl, and is felt to cause less pruritus and sedation than morphine, with the few adult studies that exist suggesting equivalence rather than superiority.[90] It is five to seven times more potent than morphine, and its duration of action is similar to morphine, and longer than fentanyl.

Nonsteroidal Anti-Inflammatory Drugs (NSAIDs)

As more and more pediatric operations are being performed on an outpatient basis, and with the goal of minimizing opioid dosing to reduce adverse effects, significant interest has developed in the role of nonopioid analgesics for management of postoperative pain. Acetaminophen is an effective analgesic for mild to moderate pain, and can be administered rectally in the perioperative period, especially to infants. Rectal absorption is variable and bioavailability is lower, mandating a higher initial dose (30–40 mg/kg) than that administered orally (10–15 mg/kg).[91,92] A rectal dose of 30 mg/kg of acetaminophen has proved to have analgesic properties similar to 1 mg/kg of ketorolac.[93] In 2011, intravenous acetaminophen was approved for use in adults and children older than 2 years of age in the U.S.

Ketorolac is an oral and parenteral NSAID shown to have excellent pain control characteristics unassociated with PONV, or respiratory depression.[94–96] Dosage recommendations are 0.5 mg/kg intravenously (maximum dose 30 mg) every 6 to 8 hours for 48 hours. Due to its effects on renal blood flow and tubular function, ketorolac is contraindicated in patients with pre-existing impairment of renal function. Likewise, it should not be administered to patients at risk for coagulopathy or a history of gastric ulcers. As NSAIDs such as ketorolac and ibuprofen affect platelet aggregation and adhesiveness, their use is limited in many patients that are at risk for postoperative bleeding, particularly children who have undergone tonsillectomy.[93,97] In addition, many orthopedic surgeons forbid the use of NSAIDS during and after operations in which new bone formation is important (fractures, spine fusions) because NSAIDS have been shown to impair osteoblastic activity.[98] The extent to which this effect is clinically important is unclear.[99,100]

Regional and Local Anesthetic Techniques

As general anesthesia is nearly universal in children, pure regional anesthesia is less common than in adults. However, pediatric patients, including outpatients, are excellent candidates for a host of regional blocks.[101–103] Some blocks require specialized equipment like a nerve stimulator or ultrasound, but others such as an ilioinguinal block can be performed by landmarks alone. Local infiltration by the surgeon is encouraged when a neuraxial or peripheral block is not performed.

Regional anesthetic techniques used concomitantly with general anesthesia have had resurgence in both adult and pediatric patients. These techniques include peripheral nerve blocks, and caudal, epidural, or spinal blocks. These blocks include the rectus sheath block for umbilical procedures, ilioinguinal block for inguinal procedures, and the transversus abdominis plane block for lower abdominal procedures.[104–106]

Clonidine has gained favor as an adjunct in regional anesthesia. A centrally acting alpha-2 agonist with antiemetic and mild sedative effects, clonidine confers an analgesic benefit as well. It has been shown to increase the analgesic duration of caudal blocks to as long as 18 hours.[107] Clonidine has also been used effectively in epidural infusions. Moreover, rather than causing nausea or pruritus, clonidine actually decreases the incidence of postoperative nausea. In higher doses (≥ 2 µg/kg) given epidurally, clonidine may cause sedation, with some authors recommending that children receiving this dose be admitted for observation. Clonidine is not recommended for use in infants under 6 months of age.

In selected cases, peripheral nerve blocks appear to be a superior pain control modality. They offer the benefit of no systemic side effects (nausea, pruritus, sedation, urinary retention) and often allow for faster recovery. It is increasingly common for these blocks to be performed under ultrasound guidance, which confers increased accuracy of placement, which in turn allows the use of reduced local anesthetic volume, greater efficacy, and improved efficiency. For orthopedic extremity surgery, some children are being discharged home with peripheral nerve catheters which are removed at home by the parents two days postoperatively.[108]

Prescribing Discharge Analgesics

The surgeon or surgeon's designee must take seriously the responsibility of prescribing pain medications to be administered by the parents at home after discharge. This

TABLE 3-4 Components of the Modified Aldrate Score

	0	1	2
Motor activity	None	Two extremities	Four extremities
Respiration	Apnea	Dyspnea	Normal
Circulation (BP)	± 50% baseline	± 20–49% baseline	± 20% baseline
Consciousness	Unresponsive	Arousable	Awake
Oxygen saturation	$SpO_2 < 90\%$ despite O_2	$SpO_2 > 90\%$ with O_2	$SpO_2 > 92\%$ in room air

is important for all patients, but especially for ambulatory surgery patients because of the rapid transition from PACU to home. It is imperative to clearly communicate with the parent/guardian regarding the nature of the medications prescribed, assessment of pain, and realistic expectations for the course of pain in the days after surgery. It is important to emphasize the same issues that are of concern when giving analgesics in the hospital: right drug, right dose, right time.

Numerous studies looking at parental home analgesic administration after surgery have shown that parents commonly do not understand that some children may become withdrawn and immobile in response to pain instead of crying.[109] In addition, many parents fail to administer prescribed pain medication even when they recognize their child is having pain, in part because of lack of specific instructions or because of fear of adverse effects, including misperceptions about the potential for 'addiction'.[110,111] Care must be taken to avoid advising time-contingent (especially around the clock) dosing of opioids because of the increased risk of nausea, vomiting, constipation, but most importantly somnolence and respiratory depression.[112]

With regard to choice of opioid, prescribers should be knowledgeable about recommended dosage and formulations available for various oral opioids. The most commonly prescribed opioid in children has been codeine (more specifically acetaminophen with codeine). A recent publication has noted concerns about a number adverse effects of codeine administration.[113] These include lack of analgesic efficacy in approximately 5–10% of the population in whom low CYP2D6 activity leads to low or no conversion of codeine to morphine in the body, which is required for analgesia.[114] More worrisome is the fact that up to a third of individuals (depending on their ethnic origin) are ultrarapid metabolizers because of increased CYP2D6 activity. Codeine administration in these individuals results in high plasma levels of morphine which can cause respiratory depression, which is especially worrisome in children and especially in children with OSA. The risk of codeine administration to children who may be unidentified ultrarapid metabolizers led the U.S. Food and Drug Administration to issue a safety alert in August, 2012 regarding the risk of adverse events or death in children given codeine after tonsillectomy and/or adenoidectomy.[115,116]

Whether undergoing an operation on an inpatient or an outpatient basis, infants and children should be afforded the most effective pain relief possible along with a minimum of adverse effects.

BOX 3-6   Criteria for Discharge Home from the Postanesthesia Care Unit

Return to preoperative level of consciousness
Normothermia (≥35.5°C)
No oxygen requirement (or return to baseline oxygen requirement)
Return to preoperative level of motor function (excepting expected effects of nerve block)
Acceptable pain control
No ongoing vomiting, minimal nausea
Absence of surgical bleeding
At least 30 minutes after last administration of opioid
Discharge acceptable to surgeon
Oral intake (if required by surgeon)

DISCHARGE CRITERIA

In general, children should be comfortable, awake, and stable, on room air or back to baseline oxygen supplementation, have age-appropriate vital signs, and be well hydrated before discharge from outpatient surgery. These variables have been quantified with the modified Aldrete score (Table 3-4), which lists the important factors taken into consideration for discharge. Most institutions require a modified Aldrete score of 9 or greater for discharge to floor, but criteria for discharge home should be stricter, comprising the elements listed in Box 3-6.

CONCLUSION

Many children who present for surgery are frightened and uncomfortable. It is the pediatric surgeon's and anesthesiologist's privilege to help calm and comfort these children and their families in addition to providing the best possible anesthetic experience. Guiding the child through an operation safely, with provision for analgesia and amnesia, are goals shared by both the anesthesiologist and surgeon alike. Open communication between surgical and anesthesia services from the time of scheduling through the peri- and postoperative periods facilitates the achievement of these goals, and helps to ensure the best possible outcome for patients and their families.

REFERENCES

1. Chopra V, Bovill JG, Spierdijk J. Accidents, near accidents and complications during anesthesia: A retrospective analysis of a 10-year period in a teaching hospital. Anaesthesia 1990;45:3–6.

2. Aubas S, Biboulet P, Daures JP, et al. Incidence and etiology of cardiac arrest occurring during the peroperative period and in the recovery room: Apropos of 102,468 anesthesia cases. Ann Fr Anesth Reanim 1991;10:436–42.

3. Odegard KC, DiNardo JA, Kussman BD, et al. The frequency of anesthesia-related cardiac arrests in patients with congenital heart disease undergoing cardiac surgery. Anesth Analg 2007;105:335–43.

4. Bhananker SM, Ramamoorthy C, Geiduschek JM, et al. Anesthesia-related cardiac arrest in children: Update from the Pediatric Perioperative Cardiac Arrest Registry. Anesth Analg 2007;105:344–50.

5. Flick RP, Sprung J, Harrison TE, et al. Perioperative cardiac arrests in children between 1988 and 2005 at a tertiary referral center. Anesthesiology 2007;106:226–37.

6. Patel RI, Hannallah RS. Preoperative screening for pediatric ambulatory surgery: Evaluation of a telephone questionnaire method. Anesth Analg 1992;75:258–61.

7. Zuckerberg AL. A hot mnemonic for the treatment of malignant hyperthermia. Anesth Analg 1993;77:1077.

8. Cook-Sather SD, Harris KA, Chiavacci R, et al. A liberalizaed fasting guideline for formula-fed infants does not increase average gastric fluid volume before elective surgery. Anesth Analg 2003;96:965–9.

9. Tait AR, Reynolds PI, Gutstein HB. Factors that influence an anesthesiologist's decision to cancel elective surgery for the child with an upper respiratory tract infection. J Clin Anesth 1995;7:491–9.

10. Parnis SJ, Barker DS, Van Der Walt JH. Clinical predictors of anaesthetic complications in children with respiratory tract infections. Paediatr Anaesth 2001;11:29–40.

11. Tait AR, Malviya S, Voepel-Lewis T, et al. Risk factors for perioperative adverse respiratory events in children with upper respiratory tract infections. Anesthesiology 2001;95:299–306.

12. Rigatto H, Brady JP. Periodic breathing and apnea in preterm infants: Evidence for hypoventilation possibly due to central respiratory depression. Pediatrics 1972;50:202–18.

13. Coté CJ, Zaslavsky A, Downes JJ, et al. Postoperative apnea in former preterm infants after inguinal herniorrhaphy: A combined analysis. Anesthesiology 1995;82:809–22.

14. Fisher D. When is the ex-premature infant no longer at risk for apnea? Anesthesiology 1995;82:807–8.

15. Hammer GB. Anaesthetic management for the child with a mediastinal mass. Paediatr Anaesth 2004;14:95–7.

16. Yamashita M, Chin I, Horigome H. Sudden fatal cardiac arrest in a child with an unrecognized anterior mediastinal mass. Resuscitation 1990;19:175–7.

17. Viswanathan S, Campbell CE, Crok RC. Asymptomatic undetected mediastinal mass: A death during ambulatory anesthesia. J Clin Anesth 1995;7:151–5.

18. Lerman J.. Anterior mediastinal masses in children. Semin Anesth 2007;26:133–40.

19. Cho Y, Suzuki S, Yokoi M, et al. Lateral position prevents respiratory occlusion during surgical procedure under general anesthesia in the patient of huge anterior mediastinal lymphoblastic lymphoma. J Thorac Cardiovasc Surg 2004;52:476–9.

20. Shamberger RC, Holzman RS, Griscom NT, et al. CT quantitation of tracheal cross-sectional area as a guide to the surgical and anesthetic management of children with anterior mediastinal masses. J Pediatr Surg 1991;26:138–42.

21. Mahmoud M, Tyler T, Sadhasivam S. Dexmedetomidine and ketamine for large anterior mediastinal mass biopsy. Paediatr Anaesth 2008;18:1011–13.

22. Cheung S, Lerman J. Mediastinal masses and anesthesia in children. Anesthesiol Clin North Am 1998;16:893–910.

23. Ricketts RR. Clinical management of anterior mediastinal tumors in children. Semin Pediatr Surg 2001;10:161–8.

24. Greenwood RD, Rosenthal A, Parisi L, et al. Extracardiac abnormalities in infants with congenital heart disease. Pediatrics 1975;55:485–92.

25. Hoffman JI, Christianson R. Congenital heart disease in a cohort of 19,502 births with long-term follow-up. Am J Cardiol 1978;42:641–7.

26. Hennein HA, Mendeloff EN, Cilley RE, et al. Predictors of postoperative outcome after general surgical procedures in patients with congenital heart disease. J Pediatr Surg 1994;29:866–70.

27. Strom BL, Abrutyn E, Berlin JA, et al. Dental and cardiac risk factors for infective endocarditis. A population based, case-control study. Ann Intern Med 1998;129:761–9.

28. Roberts GJ. Dentists are innocent! Everyday bacteremia is the real culprit: A review and assessment of the evidence that dental surgical procedures are the principal cause of endocarditis in children. Paediatr Cardiol 1999;20:317–25.

29. Seymour RA, Lowry R, Whitworth JM, et al. Infective endocarditis, dentistry and antibiotic prophylaxis; Time for a rethink? Br Dent J 2000;189:610–15.

30. Durack D. Antibiotics for prevention of endocarditis during dentistry: Time to scale back? Ann Intern Med 1998;129:829–31.

31. Horskotte D, Follath F, Gutschik E, et al. Guidelines on the prevention, diagnosis and treatment of infective endocarditis: Executive summary. The task force on infective endocarditis of the European Society of Cardiology. European Heart Journal 2004;25:267–76.

32. Danchin N, Duval X, Leport C. Prophylaxis of infective endocarditis: French recommendations 2002. Heart 2005;91:715–18.

33. Blaise G, Langleben D, Hubert B. Pulmonary arterial hypertension. Anesthesiology 2003;99:1415–32.

34. Fischer LG, Van Aken H, Burkle H. Management of pulmonary hypertension: Physiological and pharmacological considerations for anesthesiologists. Anesth Analg 2003;96:1603–16.

35. Friesen RH, Williams GD. Anesthetic management of children with pulmonary arterial hypertension. Pediatric Anesthesia 2008;18:208–16.

36. Hakim TS, Michel RP, Chang HK. Effect of lung inflation on pulmonary vascular resistance by arterial and venous occlusion. J Appl Physiol 1982;53:1110–15.

37. Luce JM. The cardiovascular effects of mechanical ventilation and positive end expiratory pressure. JAMA 1984;252:807–11.

38. Jardin F, Vieillard-Baron A. Right ventricular function and positive pressure ventilation in clinical practice: From hemodynamic subsets to respiratory settings. Intensive Care Med 2003;29:1426–34.

39. Henriksson P, Varendh G, Lundstron MR. Haemostatic defects in cyanotic congenital heart disease. Br Heart J 1979;41:23–7.

40. Silka MJ, Bar-Cohen Y. Pacemakers and implantable cardioverter-defibrillators in pediatric patients. Heart Rhythm 2006;3:1360–6.

41. Epstein AE, DiMarco JP, Ellenbogen KA, et al. ACC/AHA/HRS 2008 Guidelines for Device-Based Therapy of Cardiac Rhythm Abnormalities: A Report of the American College of Cardiology/American Heart Association Task Force on Practice Guidelines (Writing Committee to Revise the ACC/AHA/NASPE 2002 Guideline Update for Implantation of Cardiac Pacemakers and Antiarrhythmia Devices): Developed in Collaboration with the American Association for Thoracic Surgery and Society of Thoracic Surgeons. Circulation 2008;117:e350–408.

42. Madigan JD, Choudhri AF, Chen J. et al. Surgical management of the patient with an implanted cardiac device: Implications of electromagnetic interference. Ann Surg 1999;230:639–47.

43. Practice Advisory for Perioperative Management of Patients with Cardiac Rhythm Management Devices. Pacemakers and Implantable Cardioverter-Defibrillators. Anesthesiology 2005;103:186–98.

44. Litman RS. The difficult pediatric airway. In: Litman RS, editor. Pediatric Anesthesia—The Requisites in Anesthesiology. Philadelphia: Elsevier Mosby; 2004. p. 135–46.

45. Standards for basic anesthetic monitoring (Approved by the ASA House of Delegates on October 21, 1986 and last amended on October 20, 2010.

46. Pennant JH. Anesthesia for laparoscopy in the pediatric patient. Anesth Clin North Am 2001;19:69–74.

47. Kudsi OY, Jones SA, Brenn BR. Carbon dioxide embolism in a 3-week-old neonate during laparoscopic pyloromyotomy: A case report. J Pediatr Surg 2009;44:842–5.

48. Taylor SP, Hoffman GM. Gas embolus and cardiac arrest during laparoscopic pyloromyotomy in an infant. Can J Anaesth 2010;57:774–8.

49. McHoney MC, Corizia L, Eaton S, et al. Carbon dioxide elimination during laparoscopy in children is age dependent. J Pediatr Surg 2003;38:105–10.

50. Uzzo RG, Bilsky M, Mininberg DT, et al. Laparoscopic surgery in children with ventriculoperitoneal shunts: Effect of

pneumoperitoneum on intracranial pressure— preliminary experience. Pediatr Urol 1997;49:753–7.

51. Fraser JD, Aguayo P, Sharp SW, et al. The safety of laparoscopy in pediatric patients with ventriculoperitoneal shunts. J Laparoendosc Adv Surg Tech 2009;19:675–8.

52. Raskin J, Guillaume DJ, Ragel BT. Laparoscopic-induced pneumocephalus in a patient with a ventriculoperitoneal shunt. Pediatr Neurosurg 2010;46:390–1.

53. Bozkurt P, Kaya G, Altintas F, et al. Systemic stress response during operations for acute abdominal pain performed via laparoscopy or laparotomy in children. Anaesthesia 2000;55:5–9.

54. Bannister CF, Brosius KK, Wulkan M. The effect of insufflation pressure on pulmonary mechanics in infants during laparoscopic surgical procedures. Paediatr Anaesth 2003;13:785–9.

55. Joris JL, Noirot DP, Legrand MJ, et al. Hemodynamic changes during laparoscopic cholecystectomy. Anesth Analg 1993; 76:1067–71.

56. Gentili A, Iannettone CM, Pigna A, et al. Cardiocirculatory changes during videolaparoscopy in children: An echocardiographic study. Paediatr Anaesth 2000;10:399–406.

57. Kardos A, Vereczkey G, Pirot L, et al. Use of impedance cardiography to monitor haemodynamic changes during laparoscopy in children. Paediatr Anaesth 2001;11:175–9.

58. Gueugniaud P, Abisseror M, Moussa M, et al. The hemodynamic effects of pneumoperitoneum during laparoscopic surgery in healthy infants: Assessment by continuous esophageal aortic blood flow echo-Doppler. Anesth Analg 1998;86:290–3.

59. Haynes SR, Bonner S. Anaesthesia for thoracic surgery in children. Paediatr Anaesth 2000;10:237–51.

60. Gentili A, Lima M, De Rose R, et al. Thoracoscopy in children: Anaesthesiological implications and case reports. Minerva Anestesiol 2007;73:161–71.

61. Hammer GB. Single-lung ventilation in infants and children. Paediatr Anaesth 2004;14:98–102.

62. Mukhtar AM, Dessouky NM. Unusual complication during pediatric thoracoscopy. Pediatr Anesth 2006;16:986–8.

63. Mukhtar AM, Obayah GM, Elmasry A, et al. The therapeutic potential of intraoperative hypercapnia during video-assisted thoracoscopy in pediatric patients. Anesth Analg 2008;106:84–8.

64. Mortellaro VE, Fike FB, Adibe OO, et al. The use of high-frequency oscillating ventilation to facilitate stability during neonatal thoracoscopic operations. J Laparoendosc Adv Surg Tech 2011;21:877–9.

65. Murat I, Constant I, Maud'huy H. Perioperative anaesthetic morbidity in children: A database of 24,165 anaesthetics over a 30-month period. Paediatr Anaesth 2004;14:158–66.

66. Patel RI, Hannallah RS. Anesthetic complications following pediatric ambulatory surgery: A 3-year study. Anesthesiology 1988; 69:1009–12.

67. Watcha MF, White PF. Postoperative nausea and vomiting: Its etiology, treatment, and prevention. Anesthesiology 1992;77: 162–84.

68. Weir PM, Munro HM, Reynolds PI, et al. Propofol infusion and the incidence of emesis in pediatric outpatient strabismus surgery. Anesth Analg 1993;76:760–4.

69. Schreiner MS. Preoperative and postoperative fasting in children. Pediatr Clin North Am 1994;41:111–20.

70. Schreiner MS, Nicolson SC, Martin T, et al. Should children drink before discharge from day surgery? Anesthesiology 1992;76:528–33.

71. Koka BV, Jeon IS, Andre JM, et al. Postintubation croup in children. Anesth Analg 1977;56:501–5.

72. Schreiner MS, O'Hara I, Markakis DA, et al. Do children who experience laryngospasm have an increased risk of upper respiratory tract infection? Anesthesiology 1996;85:475–80.

73. von Ungern-Sternberg BS, Boda K, Chambers NA, et al. Risk assessment for respiratory complications in paediatric anaesthesia: A prospective cohort study. Lancet 2010;376:773–83.

74. Khine HH, Corddry DH, Kettrick RG, et al. Comparison of cuffed and uncuffed endotracheal tubes in young children during general anesthesia. Anesthesiology 1997;86:627–31.

75. Orliaquet GA, Gall O, Savoldelli GL, et al. Case scenario: Perianesthetic management of laryngospasm in children. Anesthesiology 2012;116:458–71.

76. Practice advisory for intraoperative awareness and brain function monitoring: A report by the American Society of Anesthesiologists Task Force on Intraoperative Awareness. Anesthesiology 2006;104:847–64.

77. Pollard RJ, Coyle JP, Gilbert RL, et al. Intraoperative awareness in a regional medical system: A review of 3 years' data. Anesthesiology 2007;106:269–74.

78. Davidson AJ, Huang GH, Czarnecki C, et al. Awareness during anesthesia in children: A prospective cohort study. Anesth Analg 2005;100:653–61.

79. Mather L, Mackie J. The incidence of postoperative pain in children. Pain 1983;15:271–82.

80. Groenewald CB, Rabbitts JA, Schroeder DR, et al. Prevalence of moderate-severe pain in hospitalized children. Paediatr Anaesth 2012;22:661–8.

81. Malviya S, Polaner DM, Berde C. Acute Pain. In: Cote CJ, Lerman J, Todres ID, editors. A Practice of Anesthesia for Infants and Children. 4th ed. Philadelphia: Saunders Elsevier; 2009. p. 939–78.

82. Merkel SI, Voepel-Lewis T, Shayevitz JR, et al. The FLACC: A behavioral scale for scoring postoperative pain in young children. Pediatr Nurs 1997;23:293–7.

83. Pasternak GW, Zhang A, Tecott L. Developmental differences between high and low affinity opiate binding sites: Their relationship to analgesia and respiratory depression. Life Sci 1980; 27:1185–90.

84. Brown KA, Laferriere A, Lakheeram I, et al. Recurrent hypoxemia in children is associated with increased analgesic sensitivity to opiates. Anesthesiology 2006;105:665–9.

85. Nelson KL, Yaster M, Kost-Byerly S, et al. A national survey of American Pediatric Anesthesiologists: Patient-controlled analgesia and other intravenous opioid therapies in pediatric acute pain management. Anesth Analg 2010;110:754–60.

86. Kay B, Rolly G. Duration of action of analgesia supplement of anesthesia: A double-blind comparison between morphine, fentanyl, and sufentanil. Acta Anaesthesiol Belg 1977;28:25–32.

87. Claxton AR, McGuire G, Chung F, et al. Evaluation of morphine versus fentanyl for postoperative analgesia after ambulatory surgical procedures. Anesth Analg 1997;84:509–14.

88. Sanford Jr. TJ, Smith NT, Dec-Silver H, et al. A comparison of morphine, fentanyl, and sufentanil anesthesia for cardiac surgery: Induction, emergence, and extubation. Anesth Analg 1986;65: 259–66.

89. Lejus C, Roussiere G, Testa S, et al. Postoperative extradural analgesia in children: Comparison of morphine with fentanyl. Br J Anesth 1994;72:156–9.

90. Rapp SE, Egan KJ, Ross BK, et al. A multidimensional comparison of morphine and hydromorphone patient-controlled analgesia. Anesth Analg 1996;82:1043–8.

91. Birmingham PK, Tobin MJ, Henthom TK, et al. Twenty-four hour pharmacokinetics of rectal acetaminophen in children. Anesthesiology 1997;87:244–52.

92. Montgomery CJ, McCormack JP, Reichert CC, et al. Plasma concentrations after high-dose (45 mg•kg-1) rectal acetaminophen in children. Can J Anaesth 1995;42:982–6.

93. Rusy LM, Houck CS, Sullivan LJ, et al. A double-blind evaluation of ketorolac tromethamine versus acetaminophen in pediatric tonsillectomy: Analgesia and bleeding. Anesth Analg 1995;80: 226–9.

94. Forrest JB, Heitlinger EL, Revell S. Ketorolac for postoperative pain management in children. Drug Saf 1997;16:309–29.

95. Gillis JC, Brogden RN. Ketorolac: A reappraisal of its pharmacodynamic and pharmacokinetic properties and therapeutic use in pain management. Drugs 1997;53:139–88.

96. Yaster M. Non-steroidal anti-inflammatory drugs. In: Yaster M, Krane EJ, Kaplan RF, Cote CJ, Lappe DG, editors: Pediatric pain management and sedation handbook. St Louis: Mosby Year Book; 1997. p. 19–27.

97. Gunter JB, Varughese AM, Harrington JF, et al. Recovery and complications after tonsillectomy in children: A comparison of ketorolac and morphine. Anesth Analg 1995;81:1136–41.

98. Chang JK, Wang GJ, Tsai ST, et al. Nonsteroidal anti-inflammatory drug effects on osteoblastic cell cycle, cytotoxicity, and cell death. Connect Tissue Res 2005;46:200–10.

99. Sucato DJ, Lovejoy JF, Agrawal S, et al. Postoperative ketorolac does not predispose to pseudoarthrosis following posterior spinal fusion and instrumentation for adolescent idiopathic scoliosis. Spine 2008;33:1119–24.

100. Li Q, Zhang Z, Cai Z. High-dose ketorolac affects adult spinal fusion: A meta-analysis of the effect of perioperative nonsteroidal anti-inflammatory drugs on spinal fusion. Spine 2011;36: E461–8.

101. Marhofer P, Ivani G, Suresh S, et al. Everyday regional anesthesia in children. Paediatr Anaesth 2012;22:995–1001.

102. Lonnqvist PA. Blocks for pain management in children undergoing ambulatory surgery. Curr Opin Anaesthesiol 2011;24: 627–32.

103. Willschke H, Marhofer P, Machata AM, et al. Current trends in paediatric regional anaesthesia. Anaesthesia 2010;65(Suppl 1):97–104.

104. Willschke H, Kettner S. Pediatric regional anesthesia: Abdominal wall blocks. Paediatr Anaesth 2012;22:88–92.

105. Gurnaney HG, Maxwell LG, Kraemer FW, et al. Prospective randomized observer-blinded study comparing the analgesic efficacy of ultrasound-guided rectus sheath block and local anaesthetic infiltration for umbilical hernia repair. Br J Anaesth 2011; 107:790–5.

106. Mai CL, Young MJ, Quraishi SA. Clinical implications of the transversus abdominis plane block in pediatric anesthesia. Paediatr Anaesth 2012;22:831–40.

107. Tripi PA, Palmer JS, Thomas S, et al. Clonidine increases duration of bupivacaine caudal analgesia for ureteroneocystostomy: A double-blind prospective trial. J Urol 2005;174:1081–3.

108. Gurnaney H, Kraemer FW, Maxwell L, et al. Ambulatory continuous peripheral nerve blocks in children and adolescents-A longitudinal eight year single center study. Anesth Analg 2013; in press.

109. Zisk RY, Grey M, Medoff-Cooper B, et al. The squeaky wheel gets the grease: Parental pain management of children treated for bone fractures. Pediatr Emerg Care 2008;24:89–96.

110. Kankkunen P, Vehvilainen-Julkunen K, Pietila AM, et al. Is the sufficiency of discharge instructions related to children's postoperative pain at home after day surgery? Scand J Caring Sci 2003;17:365–72.

111. Fortier MA, MacLaren JE, Martin SR, et al. Pediatric pain after ambulatory surgery: Where's the medication? Pediatrics 2009; 124:e588–95.

112. Sutters KA, Holdridge-Zeuner D, Waite S, et al. A descriptive feasibility study to evaluate scheduled oral analgesic dosing at home for the management of postoperative pain in preschool children following tonsillectomy. Pain Med 2012;13:472–83.

113. Baugh RF, Archer SM, Mitchell RB, et al. Clinical practice guideline: Tonsillectomy in children. Otolaryngol Head Neck Surg 2011;144:S1–30.

114. Williams DG, Patel A, Howard RF. Pharmacogenetics of codeine metabolism in an urban population of children and its implications for analgesic reliability. Br J Anaesth 2002;89:839–45.

115. Ciszkowski C, Madadi P, Phillips MS, et al. Codeine, ultrarapid-metabolism genotype, and postoperative death. NEJM 2009; 361:827–8.

116. Kelly LE, Rieder M, van den Anker J, et al. More codeine fatalities after tonsillectomy in North American children. Pediatrics 2012; 129:e1343–7.

CHAPTER 4

RENAL IMPAIRMENT

Uri S. Alon • Bradley A. Warady

BODY FLUID AND ELECTROLYTE REGULATION

Effective kidney function maintains the normal volume and composition of body fluids. Although there is a wide variation in dietary intake and nonrenal expenditures of water and solute, water and electrolyte balance is maintained by the excretion of urine, with the volume and composition defined by physiologic needs. Fluid balance is accomplished by glomerular ultrafiltration of plasma coupled with modification of the ultrafiltrate by tubular reabsorption and secretion.[1,2] The excreted urine, the modified glomerular filtrate, is the small residuum of the large volume of nonselective ultrafiltrate modified by transport processes operating along the nephron. The glomerular capillaries permit free passage of water and solutes of low molecular weight while restraining formed elements and macromolecules. The glomerular capillary wall functions as a barrier to the filtration of macromolecules based on their size, shape, and charge characteristics. The glomerular filtrate is modified during passage through the tubules by the active and passive transport of certain solutes into and out of the lumenal fluid and the permeability characteristics of specific nephron segments. The transport systems in renal epithelial cells serve to maintain global water, salt, and acid–base homeostasis.

An adequate volume of glomerular filtrate is essential for the kidney to regulate water and solute balance effectively. Renal blood flow accounts for 20–30% of cardiac output. Of the total renal plasma flow, 92% passes through the functioning excretory tissue and is known as the effective renal plasma flow. The glomerular filtration rate (GFR) is usually about one-fifth of the effective renal plasma flow, giving a filtration fraction of about 0.2.

The rate of ultrafiltration across the glomerular capillaries is determined by the same forces that allow the transmural movement of fluid in other capillary networks.[3] These forces are the transcapillary hydraulic and osmotic pressure gradients and the characteristics of capillary wall permeability. A renal autoregulatory mechanism enables the kidney to maintain relative constancy of blood flow in the presence of changing systemic arterial and renal perfusion pressures.[1] This intrinsic renal autoregulatory mechanism appears to be mediated in individual nephrons by tubuloglomerular feedback involving the macula densa (a region in the early distal tubule that juxtaposes the glomerulus) and the magnitude of resistance in the afferent and efferent arterioles,

Under normal conditions, the reabsorption of water and the reabsorption and secretion of solute during passage of the glomerular filtrate through the nephron are subservient to the maintenance of body fluid, electrolytes, and acid–base homeostasis. In the healthy, nongrowing individual, the intake and the expenditure of water and solute are equal and the hydrogen ion balance is zero. Renal function may be impaired by systemic or renal disease, and by medications such as vasoactive drugs, nonsteroidal anti-inflammatory drugs, diuretics, and antibiotics. Hypoxia and renal hypoperfusion appear to be the events most commonly associated with postoperative renal dysfunction.

RENAL FUNCTION EVALUATION

The evaluation of kidney function begins with the history, physical examination, and laboratory studies. Persistent oliguria or significant impairment in renal concentrating capacity should be evident from the history. Examination of the urinary sediment may provide evidence of renal disease if proteinuria and/or cellular casts are present. Normal serum concentrations of sodium, potassium, chloride, total CO_2, calcium, and phosphorus indicate appropriate renal regulation of the concentration of electrolytes in body fluids. The serum creatinine concentration is the usual parameter for GFR. Important limitations and caveats must be observed when using creatinine to estimate GFR. Urinary creatinine excretion reflects both filtered and secreted creatinine because creatinine is not only filtered by the glomerular capillaries, but is also secreted by renal tubular cells. As a consequence, creatinine clearance, which is calculated by using serum creatinine concentration and the urinary excretion of creatinine, overestimates true GFR measured by using inulin clearance by 10–40%.[4] Serum creatinine concentration and the rate of urinary creatinine excretion are affected by diet. The ingestion of meat, fish, or fowl, which are substances containing preformed creatinine and creatinine precursors, causes an increase in serum creatinine concentration and in urinary creatinine excretion.[5] The overestimation of GFR by creatinine clearance increases as kidney function deteriorates owing to the relative increase in the tubular component of urine creatinine. Another caveat should be applied in the case of the patient with an abnormal muscle mass. The smaller the muscle mass, the lower is the release of creatinine into the circulation resulting in lower blood levels and urine excretion rates. The opposite picture will be seen in a patient with a very large muscle mass.

During the past 15 years, the serum concentration of cystatin C, a nonglycosylated 13.3 kDa basic protein, has been shown to correlate with GFR as well as or better than serum creatinine.[6-9] From about age 12 months and up until age 50 years, normal serum cystatin C concentrations are similar in children and adults (0.70–1.38 mg/L). Currently, the measurement of cystatin C has not been incorporated into routine clinical practice. However, in the near future it may become a new tool in the assessment of GFR. In contrast, a 'bedside' equation is used to estimate GFR:

$$eGFR = 0.413 \times Height\ (cm)/serum\ creatinine\ (mg/dL)$$

has recently been developed in children with chronic kidney disease based on data generated from the measurement of GFR using the plasma disappearance of iohexol.[10] The bedside formula is most applicable to those children whose GFR is in the range of 15–75 mL/min/1.73m^2.

Urine Volume

The appropriate urine volume depends on the status of body fluids, fluid intake, extrarenal losses, obligatory renal solute load, and renal concentrating and diluting capacity. Patients with impaired renal concentrating capacity require a larger urinary volume for excretion of the obligatory renal solute load. On the other hand, patients with elevated levels of antidiuretic hormone (ADH) retain water out of proportion to solute and are prone to hyponatremia. Increased levels of ADH may occur because of physiologic factors such as hypertonic body fluids or a decrease in the effective circulatory volume (as encountered with low levels of serum albumin or with generalized vasodilatation as with sepsis). Some researchers have expressed concern that 'usual maintenance fluids' (Table 4-1) providing 2–3 mEq/L of sodium, potassium, and chloride per 100 calories metabolized may contribute to the development of hyponatremia in children hospitalized with conditions likely to be associated with ADH excess.[11] The children at risk are those with nonosmotic stimuli for ADH release, such as central nervous system disorders, the postoperative patient, pain, stress, nausea, and emesis. It has been proposed that in patients prone to develop the syndrome of inappropriate secretion of ADH, isotonic 0.9% normal saline might be a better choice for maintenance fluid therapy.[12]

Approximately 30 mOsm of obligatory renal solute/100 mL of usual maintenance water is taken as the obligatory renal solute load in children aged 2 months and older.[13] Urinary concentrating capacity increases rapidly during the first year of life and reaches the adult level of 1200–1400 mOsm/L at around year two.[14] The maximum

urinary concentrating capacity of the term infant from 1 week to 2 months of age is about 800 mOsm/L; from 2 months to 3 years, about 1000 mOsm/L; and beyond that age, about 1200 mOsm/L.

Noteworthy is the recent re-characterization of acute renal failure as acute kidney injury (AKI) to better describe renal dysfunction.[15,16] Nonoliguric AKI occurs about as frequently as oliguric AKI. It is diagnosed when the patient with normal urine output has elevated serum creatinine and urea nitrogen concentrations.

Glomerular Filtration Rate

GFR is the most useful index of renal function because it reflects the volume of plasma ultrafiltrate presented to the renal tubules. Decline in GFR is the principal functional abnormality in both acute and chronic renal failure. Assessment of GFR is important not only for evaluating the patient with respect to kidney function, but also for guiding the administration of antibiotics and other drugs. Inulin clearance, which is the accepted standard for measurement of GFR, is too time consuming and inconvenient for use in the clinical evaluation of most patients. Serum urea nitrogen concentration shows so much variation with dietary intake of nitrogen-containing foods that it is not a satisfactory index of GFR. Serum creatinine concentration and creatinine clearance have become the usual clinical measures for determining the GFR. However, precautions should be taken when creatinine alone is used for estimation of GFR because of the effect of diet as well as common medications on serum creatinine concentration and excretion rate. Ingestion of a meal containing a large quantity of animal protein increases serum creatinine levels about 0.25 mg/dL in two hours and increases the creatinine excretion rate about 75% over the next three- to four-hour period.[5] Serum creatinine concentrations are also increased by ingestion of commonly used medications such as salicylate and trimethoprim.[17,18] These agents compete with creatinine for tubular secretion through a base-secreting pathway. They do not alter GFR but do elevate the serum creatinine concentration.

Because of the difficulties in timed urine collection, several equations have been developed to estimate GFR. Historically the most commonly used equation has been the one developed by Schwartz[19-21] and is based on the serum creatinine value (as determined by the Jaffe kinetic method) and the child's height:

$$GFR\ (mL/min/1.73\,m^2) = \\ k \times Height\ (cm)/serum\ creatinine\ (mg/dL)$$

where k for low birth weight infants is 0.33, full-term infants, 0.45; males 2–12 and females 2–21 years old, 0.55: and males 13–25 years old, 0.70.

Creatinine is formed by the nonenzymatic dehydration of muscle creatinine at a rate of 50 mg creatinine/kg muscle.[4] The serum creatinine concentration in the neonate reflects the maternal level for the first three to four days of life and somewhat longer in the premature infant due to delayed maturation of kidney function. After this time, the serum creatinine concentration should

TABLE 4-1	Usual Maintenance Water Requirements
Weight Range (kg)	**Maintenance Water**
2.5–10	100 mL/kg
10–20	1000 mL + 50 mL/kg >10 kg
>20	1500 mL + 20 mL/kg >20 kg

TABLE 4-2 **Plasma Creatinine Levels at Different Ages**

Age	Height (cm)	True Plasma Creatinine[a] (mg/dL) MEAN	RANGE (±2 SD)
Fetal cord blood		0.75	0.15–0.99
0–2 weeks	50	0.50	0.34–0.66
2–26 weeks	60	0.39	0.23–0.55
26 weeks to 1 year	70	0.32	0.18–0.46
2 years	87	0.32	0.20–0.44
4 years	101	0.37	0.25–0.49
6 years	114	0.43	0.27–0.59
8 years	126	0.48	0.31–0.65
10 years	137	0.52	0.34–0.70
12 years	147	0.59	0.41–0.78
Adult male	174	0.97	0.72–1.22
Adult female	163	0.77	0.53–1.01

[a]Conversion factor: mmol/L = mg/dL × 88.4

Adapted from Changler C, Barratt TM. Laboratory evaluation. In: Holiday MA, editor. Pediatric Nephrology. 2nd ed. Baltimore: Williams & Wilkins; 1987. p. 282–99.

decrease. From age 2 weeks to 2 years, the value averages about 0.4 ± 0.04 mg/dL (35 ± 3.5 μM).[22] The serum creatinine concentration is relatively constant during this period of growth because the increase in endogenous creatinine production, which is directly correlated with muscle mass, is matched by the increase in GFR. During the first two years of life, GFR increases from 35–45 mL/min/1.73 m² to the normal adult range of 90–170 mL/min/1.73 m². The normal range for serum creatinine concentration increases from 2 years through puberty, although the GFR remains essentially constant when expressed per unit of surface area. This occurs because growth during childhood is associated with increased muscle mass and, therefore, increased creatinine production, which is greater than the increased GFR per unit of body weight.[22] Table 4-2 shows the mean values and ranges for plasma or serum creatinine levels at different ages.[23] Normative data of serum creatinine may differ from one laboratory to another, depending on the methodology used, although efforts are being made for standardization.[20,24]

Fractional Excretion of Substances

Fractional excretions (FE) are indexes of renal function that are helpful in evaluating specific clinical conditions. Conceptually, a fractional excretion is the fraction of the filtered substance that is excreted in the urine. In clinical practice, FE is calculated by obtaining simultaneous blood and urine samples for creatinine and the substance studied. The formula used to express FE as a percentage is:

$$FE = Us/Ps \times Pcr/Ucr \times 100$$

where Us is urine solute concentration, Ps is plasma solute concentration, Pcr is plasma creatinine concentration, and Ucr is urine creatinine concentration.

Fractional Excretion of Sodium

The fractional excretion of sodium (FE Na) is 2–3% in normal newborns and may be higher in premature infants. In older children it is usually less than 1%, but may be elevated with high salt intake, adaptation to chronic renal failure, and diuretic administration.[25] When a decrease in renal perfusion occurs, which is common in intravascular volume depletion or congestive heart failure, the normal renal response results in a marked increase in the tubular reabsorption of sodium leading to a decrease in sodium excretion and consequently a FE Na of less than 1%. The FE Na, is usually greater than 2% in ischemic AKI (also known as acute tubular necrosis), reflecting the impaired ability of the tubules to reabsorb sodium.

When using FE Na to aid in differentiating prerenal azotemia from AKI, it is important that diuretics have not been recently given as the FE Na will be artificially high. Also, FE Na will be elevated in a patient with a decrease in renal perfusion superimposed on chronic renal failure, as the tubules will not be able to preserve sodium despite the dehydration. However, with fluid and electrolyte replenishment, kidney function will improve to some extent. The FE Na, as well as the other diagnostic indices used to help differentiate prerenal azotemia from ischemic AKI, is not pathognomonic for either disorder. Furthermore, the FE Na is often less than 1% in cases of AKI due to glomerular disease, as tubular function remains intact.

Renal Tubular Acidosis

Renal tubular acidosis (RTA) describes a group of disorders in which metabolic acidosis occurs as a result of an impairment in the reclamation of filtered HCO_3 in the proximal tubule or from a defect in the renal hydrogen ion excretion in the distal tubule, assuming an absence of a significant reduction in GFR.[26] RTA is considered in the differential diagnosis of the patient with metabolic acidosis; a normal serum anion gap (hyperchloremic metabolic acidosis), and, other than a few exceptions, a urinary pH above 6.0. It is important to remember that an identical biochemical profile is seen in the child with diarrhea, which needs to be excluded before considering the diagnosis of RTA.

In addition to several genetic disorders such as cystinosis, proximal tubular damage is often seen in children receiving chemotherapy. The diagnosis of a defect in proximal tubular reabsorption of HCO_3 is made by showing that the fraction excretion of bicarbonate (FE HCO_3) is greater than 15% when the plasma HCO_3 concentration is normalized with alkalization. Classic distal RTA is caused by a defect in the secretion of H^+ by the cells of the distal nephron. It is characterized by hyperchloremic metabolic acidosis, urine pH greater than 6.0 at normal as well as at low serum HCO_3 concentrations, and a FE HCO_3 less than 5% when the serum HCO_3 is normal.[26,27]

Type IV RTA, a form of distal RTA associated with low urinary pH (<6.0) and hyperkalemia, is a result of decreased H^+ and K^+ secretion in the distal tubule and is related to a failure to reabsorb sodium.[26,27] Type IV RTA is probably the most commonly recognized type of RTA in both adults and children. The hyperkalemia inhibits ammonia synthesis, resulting in decreased available ammonia to serve as a urinary buffer. Therefore, a low urinary pH occurs despite decreased H^+ secretion ($NH_3 + H^+ = NH_4^+$). Type IV RTA is physiologically equivalent to aldosterone deficiency, which is one cause of the disorder. In children, it may reflect true hypoaldosteronism but it is much more common as a consequence of renal parenchymal damage, especially that due to obstructive uropathy. In children, the physiologic impairment of type IV RTA resolves in a few weeks to months after relief of an obstructive disorder.[28]

ACUTE KIDNEY INJURY

Pathophysiology

AKI is characterized by an abrupt decrease in kidney function. Because AKI is caused by a decrease in the GFR, the initial clinical manifestations are elevations in serum urea nitrogen and creatinine concentrations, and frequently a reduction in urine output. Among pediatric surgical patients, an impairment in kidney function is most common to those who are undergoing cardiopulmonary procedures.[29,30] In recent years, research has focused on the identification of biomarkers that indicate imminent kidney failure, even before a rise in serum creatinine is noted.[31] The idea is to identify urine and possibly blood proteins and enzymes released from the tubules very early in the development of AKI. A substantial amount of data has been collected in children undergoing elective heart surgery, using the biomarker neutrophil gelatinase-associated lipocalin (NGAL).[31] However, at this point, such markers have not been incorporated into routine clinical practice.[32]

The most important factor in the pathogenesis of postoperative kidney failure is decreased renal perfusion. In the early phase, the reduction in renal blood flow results in a decline in GFR. Intact tubular function results in enhanced reabsorption of sodium and water. This clinical condition is recognized as prerenal azotemia. Analysis of the patient's urine reveals a high urinary osmolality of greater than 350 mOsm/kg H_2O and a urine sodium concentration less than 10 mEq/L (20 mEq/L in the neonate).[33] The most useful index for the tubular response to renal hypoperfusion with intact tubular function is FE Na. The FE Na test is invalid if the patient received diuretics before giving the urine sample. With renal hypoperfusion and intact renal function, FE Na is less than 1% in term infants and children, and below 2.5% in premature infants.[34] In most patients with prerenal azotemia, intravascular volume depletion is clinically evident. However, in patients with diminished cardiac output (pump failure), clinical appreciation of reduced renal perfusion can be obscured because body weight and central venous pressure may suggest fluid overload. Similarly, assessment of volume status is difficult in patients with burns, edema, ascites, anasarca, or hypoalbuminemia. The reduced effective intraarterial volume might be evident from the reduced

systemic blood pressure, tachycardia, and prolonged capillary refill time.

Prerenal azotemia can be alleviated by improving renal perfusion either by repleting the intravascular fluid volume or by improving the cardiac output. The improved kidney function is recognized by increased urine output and normalization of serum urea nitrogen and creatinine concentrations. However, if renal hypoperfusion persists for a significant period or if other nephrotoxic factors are present, parenchymal kidney failure can result. Factors that may predispose the patient to AKI include preexisting congenital urinary anomalies or impaired kidney function, septicemia, hypoxemia, hemolysis, rhabdomyolysis, hyperuricemia, drug toxicity, and the use of radiocontrast agents. Also, abdominal compartmental syndrome resulting from tense ascites may impair renal perfusion. In this setting, kidney failure may be alleviated by abdominal decompression.[35]

Medical Management

The child with postoperative oliguria and an elevated serum creatinine concentration should be assessed for possible prerenal azotemia. If the child is found to be hypovolemic, an intravenous fluid challenge of 20 mL/kg of isotonic saline or plasma is commonly given. In acidotic patients, it may be physiologically advantageous to provide a solution in which bicarbonate accounts for 25–40 mEq/L of the anions in the fluid bolus (0.5 isotonic NaCl in 5% glucose, to which is added 25–40 mEq/L of 1 M $NaHCO_3$ and additional NaCl or $NaHCO_3$ to bring the solution to isotonicity). If no response is observed and the child is still dehydrated, the dose can be repeated. When the urine output is satisfactory after fluid replenishment, the child should receive appropriate maintenance and replacement fluids. Body weight, urinary volume and serum concentrations of urea nitrogen, creatinine, and electrolytes also should be monitored. As discussed below, if a solution containing alkali is used, the serum ionized calcium level should be closely monitored.

If urinary output is inadequate after the fluid challenge, an intravenous infusion of furosemide, 1 mg/kg, may be given. Patients with renal failure may require higher doses, up to 5 mg/kg. If no response occurs after the initial infusion of furosemide, a second, higher dose can be repeated after one hour. Some patients may require furosemide every four to eight hours to maintain satisfactory urinary volume. A protocol with constant furosemide infusion has been successfully used in oliguric children after cardiac surgery.[36] Furosemide is infused at 0.1 mg/kg/h, with the dose increased by 0.1 mg after two hours if the urinary volume remains less than 1 mL/kg/h. The maximum dose is 0.4 mg/kg/h. At times, urine output can be increased by the use of vasoactive agents such as dopamine. However, their efficacy in otherwise altering the course of AKI is not well established.[37,38] It is very important to maintain adequate blood pressure and effective renal plasma flow.

Careful monitoring of the patient's fluid and electrolyte status is essential. Those children who fail to respond to furosemide are at risk for fluid overload. Overzealous fluid administration during anesthesia and surgery and for the management of persistent hypoperfusion, along with decreased urinary output, can result in hypervolemia, hypertension, heart failure, and pulmonary edema. In extreme cases, fluid administration must be decreased to the minimum necessary to deliver essential medications. In less severe instances, and in euvolemic patients with impaired kidney function, total fluid intake should equal insensible water loss, urine volume, and any significant extrarenal fluid losses. Urine output must be monitored hourly and fluid management should be re-evaluated every four to 12 hours, as clinically indicated. Valuable information about the patient's overall fluid status can be obtained by carefully monitoring blood pressure, pulse, and body weight. The preoperative values of these parameters help serve as a baseline for postoperative evaluation. Ideally, the patient's hemodynamic status should be assessed continuously by using central venous pressure monitoring. In patients with complicated cardiac problems, a Swan–Ganz catheter that monitors pulmonary wedge pressure should be used.

Fluid overload can lead to hyponatremia. In most cases, because total body sodium remains normal or high, the best way to normalize serum sodium concentration is by restriction of fluid intake and enhancement of urinary volume.[39] In patients with acute symptomatic hyponatremia, careful infusion of NaCl 3% solution (512 mEq Na/L or 0.5 mEq/mL) may be given to correct hyponatremia. Rapid correction at a rate of 1–2 mEq/h over a two to three-hour period, with an increase of serum sodium level by 4–6 mEq/L, is usually well tolerated and adequate. Infusion of 6 mL/kg of 3% NaCl increases serum sodium concentration by about 5 mEq/L. Hyponatremia present for more than 24 to 48 hours should not be corrected at a rate more rapid than 0.5 mEq/L/h.

In children with AKI, hyperkalemia often develops. The early sign of potassium cardiotoxicity is peaked T waves on the electrocardiogram. Higher levels of serum potassium can cause ventricular fibrillation and cardiac asystole. The treatment of hyperkalemia is shown in Box 4-1. Emergency treatment of hyperkalemia is indicated when the serum potassium concentration reaches 7.0 mEq/L or when electrocardiographic changes are noted.

In children with AKI, metabolic acidosis rapidly develops. Owing to decreased kidney function, fewer hydrogen ions are excreted. Organic acids accumulate in the body, causing a reduction in the serum HCO_3 concentration. Although a child with uncompromised ventilatory capacity is able to hyperventilate and achieve partial compensation, a child with compromised pulmonary function or a hypercatabolic state is at risk for profound acidosis. Metabolic acidosis is usually treated by administering $NaHCO_3$. However, attention should be directed toward the excess sodium load associated with this mode of therapy. Because hypocalcemia develops in many patients with AKI, treatment with alkali should be done cautiously to protect them from hypocalcemic tetany due to a shift of ionized calcium from free to albumin-bound. It is not necessary to correct the metabolic acidosis completely to prevent the untoward effects of acidemia. Increasing

---

BOX 4-1	Treatment of Hyperkalemia

CARDIAC PROTECTION

Calcium gluconate, 10%, 0.5–1.0 mL/kg body weight injected intravenously and slowly over 5–10 min, with continuous monitoring of heart rate

SHIFT OF POTASSIUM INTO THE INTRACELLULAR COMPARTMENT

Sodium bicarbonate, 1–2 mEq/kg body weight intravenously over ten to 20 minutes, provided that salt and water overload is not a problem

Glucose, 1 g/kg body weight, and insulin, one unit per every 4 g of glucose, intravenously over 20–30 minutes

Stimulants of β_2-adrenergic receptors, such as salbutamol, intravenously or by inhalation

ELIMINATION OF EXCESS POTASSIUM

Furosemide 1 mg/kg, or higher in the face of decreased GFR

Cation exchange resin, sodium polystyrene sulfonate, 1 g/kg body weight, administered orally or rectally in 20–30% sorbitol or 10% glucose, 1 g resin/4 mL. Additional 70% sorbitol syrup may be given if constipation occurs

Dialysis

---

the serum HCO_3 concentration to 15 mEq/L is usually satisfactory.[40]

Dialysis

The inability to control the fluid and electrolyte or acid-base disorders caused by renal failure necessitates the initiation of dialysis. The indications for urgent dialysis are persistent oligoanuria, hyperkalemia, metabolic acidosis, fluid overload, severe electrolyte and mineral disturbances, and uremic syndrome.

The most common indication for postoperative dialysis in a child is hypervolemia caused by repeated attempts at fluid resuscitation, administration of medications, and total parenteral nutrition.[41] Repeated intravenous catheter flushes and endotracheal tube lavages can add a significant amount of water and solute to the total intake. Fluid overload in the postoperative patient can cause pulmonary edema and hypertension and may have a significant impact on patient recovery.[42]

Dialysis Methods. The three modes of dialysis therapy include hemodialysis (HD), peritoneal dialysis (PD), and continuous renal replacement therapy (CRRT). Although PD has historically been used most often in children, more recent data have revealed an increased use of CRRT in those centers where the expertise and resources are available.[38,41,43,44] Recognition of the needs of the patient, the resources of the treating facility, and the advantages and disadvantages of each dialytic technique dictate which modality is best (Table 4-3).[41]

The intrinsic factors that affect the efficacy of PD include peritoneal blood flow, peritoneal vascular permeability, and peritoneal surface area. Although removal of up to 50% of the peritoneal surface area does not seem to interfere with dialysis efficacy, hypoperfusion of the

TABLE 4-3　**Characteristics of Dialysis Modalities**

Variable	CRRT	PD	HD
Continuous therapy	Yes	Yes	No
Hemodynamic stability	Yes	Yes	No
Fluid balance achieved	Yes, pump controlled	Yes/no, variable	Yes, intermittent
Easy to perform	No	Yes	No
Metabolic control	Yes	Yes	Yes, intermittent
Optimal nutrition	Yes	No	No
Continuous toxin removal	Yes	No/yes, depends on the nature of the toxin (larger molecules are not well cleared)	No
Anticoagulation	Yes, requires continuous anticoagulation	No, anticoagulation not required	Yes/no, intermittent anticoagulation
Rapid poison removal	Yes/no, depending on patient size and dose	No	Yes
Stable intracranial pressure	Yes	Yes/no, less predictable than CRRT	Yes/no, less predictable than CRRT
ICU nursing support	Yes, high level of support	Yes/no, moderate level of support (if frequent, manual cycling can be labor intensive)	No, low level of support
Dialysis nursing support	Yes/no, institution dependent	Yes/no, institution dependent	Yes
Patient mobility	No	Yes, if intermittent PD used	No
Cost	High	Low/moderate. Increases with increased dialysis fluid used	High/moderate
Vascular access required	Yes	No	Yes
Recent abdominal surgery[a]	Yes	No	Yes
Ventriculoperitoneal shunt	Yes	Yes/no, relative contraindication	Yes
Prune-belly syndrome	Yes	Yes/no, relative contraindication	Yes
Ultrafiltration control	Yes	Yes/no, variable	Yes, intermittent
PD catheter leakage	No	Yes	No
Infection potential	Yes	Yes	Yes
Use in acute kidney injury: associated inborn errors of metabolism	Yes	No	Yes
Use in acute kidney injury: associated ingestions	Yes	No	Yes

CRRT, continuous renal replacement therapy; HD, hemodialysis; PD, peritoneal dialysis.
[a]Omphalocele, gastroschisis, frequent or extensive abdominal surgery. Varies, depending on the location of the hemodialysis catheter.
Adapted from Changler C, Barratt TM. Laboratory evaluation. In Holiday MA (ed): Pediatric Nephrology, 2nd ed. Baltimore, Williams & Wilkins, 1987, pp. 282–99.

peritoneal membrane vasculature renders PD ineffective.[45] PD is feasible in the postoperative patient even in the presence of peritonitis or immediately after major abdominal operations.[43,46–48] Increased intra-abdominal pressure caused by the dialysis fluid can cause respiratory embarrassment and can contribute to leakage from the incisions and the exit site of the PD catheter. If leakage persists, the smallest effective dialysis fluid volume (10–20 mL/kg) can be tried. Common complications associated with PD are peritonitis, exit site infection, dialysate leakage, catheter obstruction from omentum or fibrin, and abdominal wall hernia. Sclerosing peritonitis can also occur and is seen more commonly in females. It results in peritoneal scarring and can lead to bowel obstruction and perforation. Resection and stoma may be needed due to concerns about healing with a primary repair.

The provision of antibiotics at the time of catheter placement is recommended and may decrease the risk of peritonitis.[49,50] Also, the use of fibrin glue at the site of catheter entry into the peritoneum has been associated with a decreased incidence of dialysate leakage during the immediate postoperative period and may be particularly beneficial when PD is initiated soon after catheter placement.[51] A study in 2000 showed placement of a Tenckhoff catheter (Fig. 4-1) to be superior to the Cook catheter (Cook Medical, Bloomington, IN, USA) in terms of complication-free survival.[52] More recently, there is evidence for equal outcomes with the Cook Multipurpose Drainage catheter, a flexible catheter that is placed at the bedside, in contrast to the Tenckhoff catheter, which typically requires operative insertion.[53]

PD is performed with dialysis solutions that contain a 1.5%, 2.5%, or 4.25% glucose concentration. Dialysate with a 1.5% glucose concentration has an osmolality of 350 mOsm/kg H_2O, which is moderately hypertonic to normal plasma (280–295 mOsm/kg H_2O). Other factors being equal, the higher the tonicity of the dialysate and the greater the osmotic gradient between blood and dialysate, the greater the ultrafiltrate (fluid removed from the body). Owing to the rapid movement of water and glucose across the peritoneal membrane, the effect of PD on fluid removal is maximal when short dialysis cycles of 20 to 30 minutes are used. When solutions containing glucose concentrations higher than 1.5% are used, close monitoring of the patient's serum glucose concentration is necessary. If hyperglycemia develops with a blood glucose concentration greater than 200 mg/dL, it can be

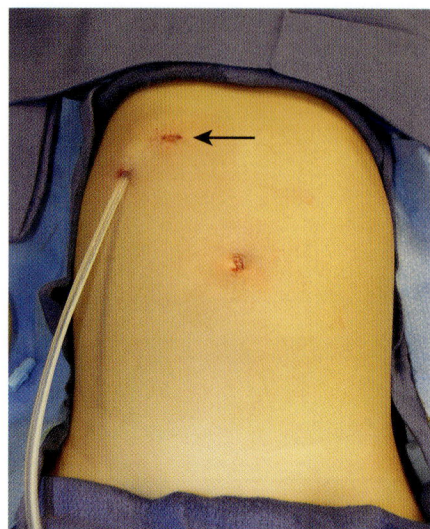

FIGURE 4-1 ■ This 4-year-old child developed hemolytic uremic syndrome related to *Escherichia coli* colitis. A peritoneal dialysis catheter was inserted laparoscopically. Note the catheter is oriented caudally at the exit site which is felt to be the optimal way the peritoneal dialysis catheter should be oriented. A 5 mm incision in the right upper abdomen (arrow) is the site where the peritoneal dialysis catheter was introduced into the abdominal cavity. A 5 mm cannula and telescope were inserted in the umbilicus for visualization.

controlled by the addition of insulin to the dialysate solution or by intravenous insulin drip. The volume of fluid removed by dialysis in a 24-hour period should generally be limited to 500 mL in the neonate, 500–1000 mL in infants and 1000–1500 mL in young children. The effect of dialysis on the removal of solutes depends mainly on the length of the dwell time of the dialysate within the peritoneal cavity and the molecular weight of the solute. The following are the relative rates of removal of common substances: urea> potassium> sodium> creatinine> phosphate> uric acid> calcium> magnesium. Standard dialysate solutions do not contain potassium. Therefore, hyperkalemia may be controlled with a few hours of effective PD.

Hemodialysis has the advantage of more rapid ultrafiltration and solute removal than either PD or CRRT. Adequate vascular access is the most important requirement, and a variety of temporary pediatric catheters are available.[54] Ideally, insertion of the dialysis catheter in the right internal jugular vein is preferred, followed by the femoral vein and the left internal jugular vein. Placement in the subclavian vein should be discouraged because of the potential development of subclavian stenosis and the subsequent inability to create a dialysis fistula in the ipsilateral arm of those patients who go on to develop endstage renal disease.[38] Fluid removal can be problematic in the patient who is hypotensive and receiving HD because of poor patient tolerance, and is better accomplished by either PD or CRRT in this clinical setting.

The types of CRRT consist of continuous venovenous hemodialysis (CVVHD), continuous venovenous hemofiltration (CVVH), and continuous venovenous hemodiafiltration (CVVHDF). CRRT is now widely practiced in many tertiary pediatric centers because of the safety and efficacy of the technique in even the sickest patients. The

choice of one method of CRRT over another depends on whether one chooses to make use of the diffusive (CVVHD) or convective (CVVH) method or a combination of the two (CVVHDF) properties of the technique. As in HD, a well-functioning vascular access catheter is crucial for CRRT. Data suggest that the optimal access is the one with the largest diameter preferably located within the internal jugular vein.[55] Likewise, large extracorporeal blood volumes are necessary for the CRRT (and HD) circuit, and require blood products in the small patient in whom the circuit volume exceeds 10% of the patient's blood volume. Particular attention must be paid to the possible development of hemofilter-related reactions that might occur with the initiation of therapy.[56,57] The predictability and efficiency of ultrafiltration and solute removal make CRRT an ideal dialytic technique for hemodynamically unstable patients. In children at risk for hemorrhage, a protocol using citrate instead of heparin as the anticoagulant has been developed.[58–60] Finally, new information has provided direction regarding the preferred timing of dialysis initiation. Fluid overload itself appears to be a significant risk factor for mortality, and its early and aggressive management with dialysis may prove particularly beneficial.[61] A recent analysis has revealed 29.6% mortality with <10% fluid overload, 43.1% with 10–20% fluid overland, and 65.6% with >20% fluid overload.[42]

ACUTE KIDNEY INJURY IN THE NEONATE

AKI occurs in as many as 24% of all patients admitted to the neonatal intensive care unit (NICU).[62,63] The definition of AKI in a term neonate has historically been considered to be a serum creatinine level above 1.5 mg/dL for more than 24 hours in the setting of normal maternal renal function.[64] On occasion, it may be diagnosed in the term infant with a serum creatinine value less than 1.5 mg/dL when it fails to decrease in a normal manner over the initial days/weeks of life.[65,66] More recently, it has been defined by an age independent increase in serum creatinine to ≥1.5 times baseline, which is known to have occurred within the past 7 days or a urine volume <0.5 mL/kg/h for 6 hours.[38] A recent proposed neonatal specific classification has characterized stage 1 AKI as an increase in serum creatinine of 0.3 mg/dL or an increase in serum creatinine of 1.5–2 times the previous value.[63] A pediatric modification (pRIFLE) of an adult AKI classification system has also been developed.[67] The limited availability of cystatin C data from the neonatal population currently precludes its routine use to define AKI.[68,69]

AKI is of the oliguric variety when the elevated serum creatinine concentration is accompanied by a urine output below 1 mL/kg/hr after the initial 24 hours of life and when urine output fails to improve in response to a fluid challenge.[70] In contrast, solute retention develops in some neonates, as evidenced by an elevated serum creatinine level, with a normal (>1.0 mL/kg/h) urine flow rate. These neonates are diagnosed as having nonoliguric AKI.[71] The nonoliguric form is particularly common in neonates with AKI secondary to perinatal asphyxia and appears to be associated with a better prognosis than does the oliguric form.[66,71] The diagnosis of nonoliguric AKI can be missed if patients at risk for developing renal insufficiency are monitored solely by the evaluation of urine output without repeated assessments of the serum creatinine concentration.

The causes of AKI in newborns traditionally have been divided into three categories: prerenal, intrinsic, and postrenal (Box 4-2). This division, based on the site of the problem, has important implications because the evaluation, treatment, and prognosis of the three groups can be quite different.

Prerenal Acute Kidney Injury

Impairment of renal perfusion is the cause of 70% of AKI during the neonatal period.[62,63,65,66] Prerenal AKI may occur in any patient with hypoperfusion of an otherwise normal kidney. Although prompt correction of the low perfusion state usually reverses this impairment, delay in fluid resuscitation may result in renal parenchymal damage.

BOX 4-2	Major Causes of Acute Renal Failure in the Neonate

PRERENAL FAILURE

- Systemic hypovolemia: fetal hemorrhage, neonatal hemorrhage, septic shock, necrotizing enterocolitis, dehydration
- Renal hypoperfusion: perinatal asphyxia, congestive heart failure, cardiac surgery, cardiopulmonary bypass/extracorporeal membrane oxygenation, respiratory distress syndrome, pharmacologic (tolazoline, captopril, enalapril, indomethacin)

INTRINSIC RENAL FAILURE

- Acute tubular necrosis
- Congenital malformations: bilateral agenesis, renal dysplasia, polycystic kidney disease
- Infection: congenital (syphilis, toxoplasmosis), pyelonephritis
- Renal vascular: renal artery thrombosis, renal venous thrombosis, disseminated intravascular coagulation
- Nephrotoxins: aminoglycosides, indomethacin, amphotericin B, contrast media, captopril, enalapril, vancomycin
- Intrarenal obstruction: uric acid nephropathy, myoglobinuria, hemoglobinuria

POSTRENAL (OBSTRUCTIVE) RENAL FAILURE

- Congenital malformations: imperforate prepuce, urethral stricture, posterior urethral valves, urethral diverticulum, primary vesicoureteral reflux, ureterocele, megacystis megaureter, Eagle–Barrett syndrome, ureteropelvic junction obstruction, ureterovesical obstruction
- Extrinsic compression: sacrococcygeal teratoma, hematocolpos
- Intrinsic obstruction: renal calculi, fungus balls
- Neurogenic bladder

Adapted from Karlowicz MG, Adelman RD. Acute renal failure in the neonate. Clin Perinatol 1992;19:139–58.

Intrinsic Acute Kidney Injury

Intrinsic AKI occurs in 6–8% of admissions to the NICU and implies the presence of renal cellular damage associated with impaired kidney function.[65] Intrinsic AKI usually falls into one of the following categories: ischemic (acute tubular necrosis), nephrotoxic (aminoglycoside antibiotics, indomethacin), congenital renal anomalies (autosomal recessive polycystic kidney disease), and vascular lesions (renal artery or vein thrombosis), especially with a solitary kidney.[72]

Postrenal Acute Kidney Injury

Postrenal AKI results from obstruction of urine flow from both kidneys or from a solitary kidney. The most common causes of postrenal AKI in neonates are posterior urethral valves (PUV), bilateral ureteropelvic junction obstruction, and bilateral ureterovesical junction obstruction.[73,74] Although these types of obstructions are characteristically reversible, neonates with long-standing intrauterine obstruction have varying degrees of permanent impairment of kidney function.[75,76] This impairment may be due not only to the presence of renal dysplasia but also to cellular damage secondary to AKI.

Clinical Presentation

The clinical presentation of the neonate with AKI often reflects the condition that has precipitated development of the renal insufficiency. Accordingly, sepsis, shock, dehydration, severe respiratory distress syndrome, and other related conditions may be present. Nonspecific symptoms related to anemia, such as poor feeding, lethargy, emesis, seizures, hypertension, and anemia, are also often found.

Diagnostic Evaluation

Evaluation of the neonate with AKI should include a thorough patient and family history and a physical examination. Suspected prerenal causes of acute oliguria are usually addressed diagnostically and therapeutically by volume expansion, with or without furosemide. If this approach does not result in increased urine output, a more extensive evaluation of renal function is indicated.

Laboratory studies are an important component of this evaluation and include the following measures: complete blood cell count and determination of serum concentrations of urea nitrogen, creatinine, electrolytes, uric acid, calcium, glucose, and phosphorus. The serum creatinine value during the first several days of life is a reflection of the maternal value. In term infants, a value of 0.4–0.5 mg/dL is expected after the first week of life. In contrast, the expected value in preterm infants is related to their gestational age, with an initial increase followed by a gradual decrease.[77,78] In all cases, a urinalysis should be obtained to check for the presence of red blood cells, protein, and casts suggestive of intrinsic renal disease.

Urine indices can help distinguish intrinsic renal failure from prerenal azotemia in the oliguric newborn.[37,79] As mentioned previously, the index usually found to be most useful is the FE Na. This factor is based on the assumption that the renal tubules of the poorly perfused kidney reabsorb sodium avidly, whereas the kidney with intrinsic renal disease and tubular damage is unable to do so. Accordingly, in most cases of neonatal oliguric renal failure secondary to intrinsic disease, the FE Na is >2.5–3.0%, a value that is different from that of the older child.[62,70] The FE Na should be measured before administering furosemide. In addition, the results should be interpreted with caution in the very premature infant who normally has an even higher (i.e., >5%) FE Na.[64,80]

Ultrasonography commonly is the initial imaging study.[81] The urinary tract should be evaluated for the presence of one or two kidneys and for their size, shape, and location. A voiding cystourethrogram (VCUG) may also be necessary, specifically when the diagnosis of PUV or vesicoureteral reflux is entertained. In most cases, a VCUG is deemed preferable to radionuclide cystography in this setting because of its superior ability to provide reliable anatomic information about the grading of vesicoureteral reflux or the appearance of the urethra.[82] Antegrade pyelography or diuretic renography with either ^{99m}Tc-dimercaptosuccinic acid (DMSA) or ^{99m}Tc-dimercaptoacetyltriglycine (MAG₃) may be needed to evaluate for ureteral obstruction. Finally, assessment of the differential kidney function may be performed with radioisotope scanning as well.

Management

The treatment of neonatal AKI should proceed simultaneously with the diagnostic workup. Bladder catheter placement is a good immediate therapy for PUV, whereas high surgical drainage may be needed for other obstructive lesions in the neonate. The fluid challenge for the neonate should consist of 20 mL/kg of an isotonic solution containing 25 mEq/L of $NaHCO_3$ infused over a one- to two-hour period. In the absence of a prompt diuresis of 2 mL or more of urine per kilogram over one to two hours, intravenous furosemide at 1–3 mg/kg may be helpful, As noted previously, the potential role of low-dose (0.5–3.0 μg/kg/min) dopamine continues to be debated, but recent guidelines recommend against its use to prevent or treat AKI.[37,38] The failure to achieve increased urinary output after volume expansion in the neonate with an adequate cardiac output and an unobstructed urinary tract indicates the presence of intrinsic kidney disease and the need to manage oliguric or anuric kidney failure appropriately.

Maintenance of normal fluid balance is of primary concern in the management of the patient with AKI. Daily fluid intake should equal insensible water loss, urine output, and fluid losses from nonrenal sources. In term infants, insensible water losses amount to 30–40 mL/kg/day, whereas premature infants may require as much as 50–100 mL/kg/day.[80,83] A frequent assessment of the neonate's body weight is essential for fluid management. The electrolyte content of the fluids administered should be guided by frequent laboratory studies. Insensible water losses are electrolyte free and should be replaced by using 5% dextrose in water.

Important systemic disturbances that may arise secondary to AKI include hyperkalemia, hyponatremia, hypertension, hypocalcemia, hyperphosphatemia, and metabolic acidosis. All exogenous sources of potassium should be discontinued in patients with AKI. Despite this restriction, elevated serum potassium levels develop in many neonates and must be treated aggressively due to the potential for cardiac toxicity.[34] Treatment should be initiated by correction of metabolic acidosis with $NaHCO_3$. A dose of 1–2 mEq/kg should be given intravenously over a ten to 20-minute period, provided that salt and water balance is not problematic. The quantity of $NaHCO_3$ to be prescribed also can be calculated in the following manner:

$$(0.3 \times \text{body weight [kg]} \times \text{base deficit [mM]}).$$

Associated hypocalcemia should be treated with the intravenous administration of 10% calcium gluconate at a dose of 0.5–1.0 mL/kg injected slowly over a five- to 15-minute period with continuous monitoring of the heart rate. If a progressive increase in the serum potassium concentration is noted, additional treatment measures may include the use of a sodium–potassium exchange resin (sodium polystyrene sulfonate in 20–30% sorbitol, 1 g/kg by enema), with recognition of its frequent ineffectiveness and/or associated complications when used in low birth weight infants.[84] The use of glucose (0.5–1.0 g/kg) followed by insulin (0.1–0.2 unit regular insulin per gram glucose over a 1-hour period) may be the preferred approach. Either intravenous salbutamol or inhaled albuterol is an additional therapeutic option.[85–87] Dialysis should be considered if these measures prove unsuccessful.[48,87,88]

Hyponatremia and systemic hypertension arc most often related to over-hydration in the infant with oliguria. These problems should be treated initially with fluid restriction or water removal with dialysis, if necessary. The addition of high-dose intravenous furosemide (5 mg/kg) may be helpful. Serum sodium levels below 125 mEq/L can be associated with seizures, and levels below 120 mEq/L should be corrected rapidly to at least 125 mEq/L by calculating the amount of sodium required in the following manner:

$$Na^+ (mEq) = ([Na^+]\,\text{Desired} - [Na^+]\,\text{Actual}) \times \text{Weight (kg)} \times 0.8$$

When serum sodium levels are less than 120 mEq/L and are associated with symptoms (e.g., seizures), prompt treatment with hypertonic (3%) saline is indicated. The provision of 10–12 mL/kg of 3% saline is generally therapeutic.

The treatment of persistent hypertension may include parenterally administered hydralazine (0.15 to 0.6 mg/kg/dose), labetalol (0.20 to 1.0 mg/kg/dose or 0.25 to 3.0 mg/kg/hr infusion), or enalapril at (5.0 to 10 μg/kg/dose). Orally administered amlodipine (0.05 to 0.3 mg/kg/dose) can be prescribed for the patient who is without symptoms. Treatment of the patient with marked or refractory hypertension can include intravenous sodium nitroprusside (0.5 to 10 μg/kg/min infusion), nicardipine (1 to 4 µg/kg/min infusion), or labetalol.[89] Caution should be exercised when initiating therapy with captopril (initial oral dose, 0.01 to 0.05 mg/kg/dose), owing to the profound hypotension that can occur in neonates in association with higher doses.[90,91]

In the infant in whom AKI does not fully resolve and becomes chronic renal failure (CKD), the development of hyperphosphatemia (serum phosphorus level > 7 mg/dL) necessitates a low phosphorus infant formula and possibly calcium carbonate (50–100 mg/kg/day) as a phosphate binder.[89] The use of aluminum hydroxide as a binder is contraindicated, owing to its association with aluminum toxicity in infants and children with renal insufficiency.[90] No experience has been published about the use of newer, noncalcium-containing phosphate-binding agents, such as sevelamer, in the neonatal population.[91,92] Hypocalcemia, as reflected by a low total serum calcium level, often occurs in AKI in association with hypoalbuminemia. Less commonly, the ionized calcium level is low and the patient is symptomatic. In these cases, intravenous 10% calcium gluconate, 0.5–1.0 mL/kg, over a five-minute period with cardiac monitoring should be given until the ionized calcium level is restored to the normal range.

Metabolic acidosis may arise as a result of retention of hydrogen ions and may require $NaHCO_3$ for correction. The dose of $NaHCO_3$ to be given can be calculated as follows:

$$NaHCO_3 (mEq) = (\text{Desired bicarbonate} - \text{Observed bicarbonate}) \times \text{Weight (kg)} \times 0.5$$

This dose may be given orally or added to parenteral fluids and infused during several hours.

Adequate nutrition should be provided, with the goal of 100–120 calories and 1–2 g of protein/kg/day, provided intravenously or orally. Additional protein may be needed to account for dialysis related losses in those patients receiving PD and CRRT.[93,94] For neonates who can tolerate oral fluids, a formula containing low levels of phosphorus and aluminum, such as Similac PM 60/40 (Abbott Labs, Abbott Park, IL), is recommended. An aggressive approach to nutrition may well contribute to kidney recovery by providing necessary energy at the cellular level.[34]

Although most neonates with AKI can be managed conservatively, occasional patients require PD or CRRT for the treatment of the metabolic complications and fluid overload.[95–97] The mortality rate in this group of patients can be exceedingly high in the setting of AKI post-cardiac surgery.[47,98–100] Apart from the need for pressor support, the procedure was well tolerated in one report on the use of CRRT in 85 children weighing less than 10 kg, with survival rates of 25% and 41% for those weighing less than 3 kg and from 3–10 kg, respectively.[97] A recent retrospective study of PD treatment of AKI post-cardiac surgery in 146 neonates and infants revealed that the mortality rate was decreased by more than 40% in those patients who received 'early PD' (day of surgery or postoperative day 1) versus 'delayed PD' (postoperative day 2 or later).[101] Finally, when AKI occurred in neonates receiving extracorporeal membrane oxygenation, the mortality rate was 3.2 times higher than in those without AKI.[102] Moreover, patients who required renal replacement therapy had 1.9 higher odds of death than those who did not receive this therapy.

OBSTRUCTIVE UROPATHY

Obstructive uropathy in the neonate is the most common renal abnormality diagnosed prenatally and is most often the result of ureteropelvic junction obstruction, PUV, or ureterovesical junction obstruction.[73] Obstruction also represents a significant cause of end-stage renal disease in children, accounting for 13% of all cases.[103] Accordingly, early recognition and treatment of these lesions are desirable because of the adverse effects that obstruction can have on kidney function.[39,40,75,76,104] Regardless, after surgical intervention and relief of obstruction, alterations of GFR, renal blood flow, and renal tubular function can still occur.[76,104,105] Specifically, injury to the renal tubule can result in an impaired capacity to reabsorb sodium, to concentrate urine, and to secrete potassium and hydrogen, all of which can have profound clinical implications. The resorption of other solutes, such as magnesium, calcium and phosphorus, may also be affected.[76,105]

The ability of the renal tubule to reabsorb salt and water after relief of the obstruction typically depends on whether the obstruction is unilateral or bilateral. In unilateral obstruction, the proximal tubules of the juxtamedullary nephrons are unable to reabsorb salt and water maximally, whereas the fractional reabsorption of salt and water is increased in the superficial nephrons.[105] However, the amount of sodium excreted by the previously obstructed kidney is not different from that of the contralateral kidney, because tubuloglomerular balance is maintained. In contrast, relief of bilateral obstruction or, on occasion, unilateral obstruction in neonates, results in a postobstructive diuresis characterized by a marked elevation in the absolute amount of sodium and water lost.[106] In part, these changes are a result of an osmotic diuresis secondary to retained solutes, such as urea.[106,107] Some contribution may also occur from atrial natriuretic factor, the plasma level of which is elevated during obstruction, as well as from enhanced synthesis of prostaglandins.[105] Decreased renal medullary tonicity and decreased hydraulic water permeability of the collecting duct in response to ADH, the latter a result of reduced aquaporin channels, contribute to the impaired concentrating ability of the kidney.[36,104]

The clinical conditions associated with prolonged salt wasting are severe volume contraction and circulatory impairment. Conditions associated with the concentrating abnormalities are secondary nephrogenic diabetes insipidus and hyponatremic dehydration. Accordingly, management must ensure the provision of adequate amounts of fluid and salt. Sodium intake should be monitored by serum and urine electrolyte determinations. Fluid intake should equal insensible losses, urine output, and nonrenal losses, and should be guided by frequent assessments of body weight.

Ureteral obstruction also can result in the impairment of hydrogen and potassium secretion and the syndrome of hyperkalemia, hyperchloremic metabolic acidosis, or type IV RTA.[108–110] This clinical situation appears to be the result of the impaired turnover of the sodium-potassium pump or a decreased responsiveness of the distal renal tubule to the actions of aldosterone. In a portion of the patients with this presentation, the FE Na is normal and the FE κ is inappropriately low, relative to the elevated serum level. Treatment is directed toward correcting the underlying obstructive abnormality as well as providing NaHCO$_3$ to alleviate the metabolic acidosis and hyperkalemia.

Finally, the outcome of obstructive uropathy in the neonate in terms of preservation of GFR is, in part, related to how promptly relief of obstruction occurs. In these patients, the serum creatinine obtained at age 12 months has been shown to be predictive of long-term kidney function.[39,40,76,104] Attempts to preserve renal function with fetal surgery in the patient with obstructive uropathy have not proven to be successful.[111]

REFERENCES

1. Brenner B, Dworkin L, Kchikawa L. Glomerular ultrafiltration. In: Brenner B, Rector F, editors. The Kidney, Vol.1. Philadelphia: WB Saunders; 1986. p. 124–44.
2. Hogg R, Stapleton F. Renal tubular function. In: Holliday M, Barratt T, Vernier R, editors. Pediatric Nephrology. Baltimore: Williams & Wilkins; 1987. p. 59–77.
3. Yared A, Ichikawa I. Renal blood flow and glomerular filtration rate. In: Holliday M, Barratt T, Vernier R, editors. Pediatric Nephrology. Baltimore: Williams & Wilkins; 1987. p. 45–58.
4. Perrone R, Madias N, Levey A. Serum creatinine as an index of renal function: New insights into old concepts. Clin Chem 1992;38:1933–53.
5. Hellerstein S, Hunter J. Warady B. Creatinine excretion rates for evaluation of kidney function in children. Pediatr Nephrol 1988;2:419–24.
6. Newman D, Thakkar H, Edwards R, et al. Serum cystatin C measured by automated immunoassay: A more sensitive marker of changes in GFR than serum creatinine. Kidney Int 1995;47:312–18.
7. Bokenkamp A, Domanetzki M, Zinck R, et al. Cystatin C serum concentrations underestimate glomerular filtration rate in renal transplant recipients. Clin Chem 1999;45:1866–8.
8. Finney H, Newman D, Price C. Adult reference ranges for serum cystatin C, creatinine and predicted creatinine clearance. Ann Clin Biochem 2000;31:49–59.
9. Fisehbach M, Graff V, Terzie J, et al. Impact of age on reference values for serum concentration of cystatin C in children. Pediatric Nephrol 2002;17:104–6.
10. Schwartz GJ, Munoz A. Schneider M, et al. New equations to estimate GFR in children with CKD. J Am Soc Nephrol 2009;20:629–37.
11. Moritz M, Ayus J. Prevention of hospital-acquired hyponatremia: A case for using isotonic saline. Pediatrics 2003;111:227–30.
12. Moritz M, Ayus J. Hospital-acquired hyponatremia—why are hypotonic parenteral fluids still being used? Nat Clin Pract Nephrol 2007;3:374–82.
13. Holliday M, Segar W. The maintenance need for water in parenteral fluid therapy. Pediatrics 1957;19:823–32.
14. Polacek B, Vocel J, Neugebauerova L, et al. The osmotic concentrating ability in healthy infants and children. Arch Dis Child 1965;40:291–5.
15. Zappitelli M, Parikh C, Akcan-Arikan A, et al. Ascertainment and epidemiology of acute kidney injury varies with definition interpretation. Clin J Am Soc Nephrol 2008;3:948–54.
16. Hui-Stickle S, Brewer E, Goldstein S. Pediatric ARF epidemiology at a tertiary care center from 1999 to 2001. Am J Kidney Dis 2005;45:96–101.
17. Burry H, Dieppe P. Apparent reduction of endogenous creatinine clearance by salicylate treatment. Br Med 1976;2:16–17.
18. Berglund F, Killander J, Pompeius R. Effect of trimethoprim-sulfamethoxazole on the renal excretion of creatinine in man. J Urol 1975;114:802–8.
19. Work D, Schwartz G. Estimating and measuring glomerular filtration rate in children. Curr Opin Nephrol Hypertens 2008;17:320–5.
20. Fadrowski J, Neu A, Schwartz GJ, et al. Pediatric GFR estimating equations applied to adolescents in the general population. Clin J Am Soc Nephrol 2011;6:1427–35.
21. Schwartz GJ, Schneider M, Maier P, et al. Improved equations estimating GFR in children with chronic kidney disease using an immunonephelometric determination of cystatin C. Kidney Inf 2012;82(4):445–53.
22. Hellerstein S, Holliday M, Grupe W, et al. Nutritional management of children with chronic renal failure. Summary of the task force on nutritional management of children with chronic renal failure. Pediatr Nephrol, 1987;l:195–211.
23. Chantler C, Barratt T. Laboratory evaluation. In: Holliday M, Barratt T, Vernier R, editors. Pediatric Nephrology. Baltimore: Williams & Wilkins; 1987. p. 282–99.
24. Srivastava T, Garg U, Alon U. Impact of standardization of creatinine methodology on the assessment of glomerular filtration rate. Pediatr Res 2008;65:113–16.
25. Steiner R. Interpreting the fractional excretion of sodium. Am J Med 1984;77:699–702.
26. Halperin M, Goldstein M, Stinebaugh B, et al. Renal tubular acidosis. In: Maxwell M, Kleeman C, Narins R, editors. Clinical Disorders of Fluid and Electrolyte Metabolism. New York: McGraw-Hill; 1987. p. 675–89.
27. Rodriguez-Soriano J, Vallo A. Renal tubular acidosis. Pediatr Nephrol 1990;4:268–75.
28. Alon U, Chan J. Inherited form of renal tubular acidosis. In: Fernandes J, Saudubray J, Tada K, editors. Inherited Metabolic Diagnosis and Treatment. New York: Springer-Verlag; 1990. p. 585–95.
29. Wedekin M, Ehrich J, Offner G, et al. Aetiology and outcome of acute and chronic renal failure in infants. Nephrol Dial Transplant 2008;23:1575–80.
30. Goldstein S. Pediatric acute renal failure: Demographics and treatment. In: Ronco C, Bellomo R, Brendolan A, editors. Sepsis, Kidney and Multiple Organ Dysfunction. Basel: Karger; 2004. p. 284–90.
31. Fadel F, Abdel Rahman A, Mohamed M, et al. Plasma neutrophil gelatinase-associated lipocalin as an early biomarker for prediction of acute kidney injury after cardiopulmonary bypass in pediatric cardiac surgery. Arch Med Sci 2012;8:250–5.
32. Devarajan P. Biomarkers for the early detection of acute kidney injury. Curr Opin Pediatr 2011;23:194–200.
33. Cohen M, Ritkind D. The pediatric abacus. Boca Raton: The Parthenon Publishing Group; 2002.
34. Gaudio K, Siegel N, Pathogenesis and treatment of acute renal failure. Pediatr Clin North Am 1987;34:771–87.
35. Bailey J, Shapiro M. Abdominal compartment syndrome. Crit Care Med 2000;4:23–9.
36. Singh N, Kissoon N, Al-Mofada S, et al. Furosemide infusion versus furosemide bolus in the postoperative pediatric cardiac patient. Pediatr Res 1990;27:35A.
37. Kellum J, Decker JM. Use of dopamine in acute renal failure: A meta-analysis. Crit Care Med 2001;29:1526–31
38. Kidney Disease: Improving Global Outcomes (KDIGO) Acute Kidney Injury Work Group, KDIGO Clinical Practice Guideline for Acute Kidney Injury. Kidney Int Suppl 2012;2:1–138.
39. Trachtman H. Sodium and water homeostasis. Pediatr Clin N Am 1995;2:1343–63.
40. Feld L, Cachero S, Springate J. Fluid needs in acute renal failure. Pediatr Clin N Am 1990;37:337–50.
41. Walters S, Porter C, Brophy P. Dialysis and pediatric acute kidney injury: Choice of renal support modality. Pediatr Nephrol 2008;24:37–48.
42. Sutherland S, Zappitelli M, Alexander S, et al. Fluid overload and mortality in children receiving continuous renal replacement therapy: The prospective pediatric continuous renal replacement therapy registry. Am J Kidney Dis 2010;55:316–25.
43. Sebestyen JF, Warady BA. Advances in pediatric renal replacement therapy. Adv Chronic Kidney Dis 2011;18:376–83.

44. Warady B, Bunchman T. Dialysis therapy for children with acute renal failure: Survey results. Pediatr Nephrol 2000;15: 11–13.

45. Alon U, Bar-Maor JA, Bar-Joseph G. Effective peritoneal dialysis in an infant with extensive resection of the small intestine. Am J Nephrol 1988;8:65–7.

46. Bonifati C, Pansini F, Torres D, et al. Antimicrobial agents and catheter-related interventions to prevent peritonitis in peritoneal dialysis using evidence in the context of clinical practice. Int J Artif Organs 2006;29:41–9.

47. Pedersen K, Hjortdal V, Christensen C, et al. Clinical outcome in children with acute renal failure treated with peritoneal dialysis after surgery for congenital heart disease. Kidney Int 2008;108: S81–6.

48. Zaritsky J, Warady B. Peritoneal Dialysis in the Newborn. In: Kiessling S, Chisthti A, Alam S, editors. Kidney and Urinary Tract Diseases in the Newborn. Springer Medical Publishing; 2012.

49. Warady BA, Bakkaloglu S, Newland J, et al. Consensus guidelines for the prevention and treatment of catheter-related infections and peritonitis in pediatric patients receiving peritoneal dialysis: 2012 update. Perit Dial Int 2012;32:S29–86.

50. Bonifati C, Pansini F, Torres D, et al. Antimicrobial agents and catheter-related interventions to prevent peritonitis in peritoneal dialysis: Using evidence in the context of clinical practice. Int J Artif Organs 2006;29:41–9.

51. Sojo E, Grosman M, Monteverde M, et al. Fibrin glue is useful in preventing early dialysate leakage in children on chronic peritoneal dialysis. Perit Dial Int 2004;24:186–90.

52. Chadha V, Warady B, Blowey D, et al. Tenckhoff catheters prove superior to Cook catheters in pediatric acute peritoneal dialysis. Am J Kidney Dis 2000;35:1111–16.

53. Auron A, Warady B, Simon S, et al. Use of the multipurpose drainage catheter for the provision of acute peritoneal dialysis in infants and children. Am J Kidney Dis 2007;49:650–5.

54. Bunchman T, Donckerwolcke R. Continuous arterial-venous diahemofiltration and continuous veno-venous diahemofiltration in infants and children. Pediatr Nephrol 1994;8:96–102.

55. Hackbarth R, Bunchman T, Chua A, et al. The effect of vascular access location and size on circuit survival in pediatric continuous renal replacement therapy: A report from the PPCRRT registry. Int J Artif Organs 2007;30:1116–21.

56. Strazdins V, Watson A, Harvey B, European Pediatric Peritoneal Dialysis Working Group. Renal replacement therapy for acute renal failure in children: European guidelines. Pediatr Nephrol 2004;19:199–207.

57. Brophy P, Mottes T, Kudelka T, et al. AN-69 membrane reactions are pH-dependent and preventable. Am J Kidney Dis 2001; 38:173–8.

58. Brophy P, Somers M, Baum M, et al. Multi-centre evaluation of anticoagulation in patients receiving continuous renal replacement therapy (CRRT). Nephrol Dial Transplant 2005;20: 1416–21.

59. Chadha V, Garg U, Warady B, et al. Citrate clearance in children receiving continuous venovenous renal replacement therapy. Pediatr Nephrol 2002;17:819–24.

60. Symons J, Chua A, Somers M, et al. Demographic characteristics of pediatric continuous renal replacement therapy: A report of the Prospective Pediatric Continuous Renal Replacement Therapy Registry. Clin J Am Soc Nephrol 2007;2:732–8.

61. Goldstein S, Somers M, Baum M, et al. Pediatric patients with multi-organ system dysfunction syndrome receiving continuous renal replacement therapy. Kidney Int 2005;67:653–8.

62. Chan J, Williams D, Roth K. Kidney failure in infants and children. Pediatr Rev 2002;23:47–60.

63. Jetton J, Askenazi D. Update on acute kidney injury in the neonate. Curr Opin Pediatr 2012;24:191–6.

64. Whyte D, Fine R. Acute renal failure in children. Pediatr Rev 2008;29:299–306.

65. Stapleton F, Jones D, Green R. Acute renal failure in neonates: Incidence, etiology and outcome. Pediatr Nephrol 1987; 1:314–20.

66. Drukker A, Guignard J. Renal aspects of the term and preterm infant: A selective update. Curr Opin Pediatr 2002;14: 175–82.

67. Akcan-Arikan A, Zappitelli M, Loftis L, et al. Modified RIFLE criteria in critically ill children with acute kidney injury. Kidney Int 2007;71:1028–35.

68. Finney H, Newman D, Thakkar H, et al. Reference ranges for plasma cystatin C and creatinine measurements in premature infants, neonates, and older children. Arch Dis Child. 2000;82:71–5.

69. Harmoinen A, Ylinen E, Ala-Houhala M, et al. Reference intervals for cystatin C in pre- and full-term infants and children. Pediatr Nephrol 2000;15:105–8.

70. Andreoli S. Acute renal failure in the newborn. Semin Perinatol 2004;28:112–23.

71. Karlowicz M, Adelman R. Nonoliguric and oliguric acute renal failure in asphyxiated term neonates. Pediatr Nephrol 1995;9: 718–22.

72. Blowey D, Ben D, Koren G. Interactions of drugs with the developing kidney. Pediatr Clin N Am 1995;42:1415–31.

73. Elder J, Duckett J. Management of the fetus and neonate with hydronephrosis detected by prenatal ultrasonography. Pediatr Ann 1988;17:19–28.

74. Saphier C, Gaddipati S, Applewhite L, et al. Prenatal diagnosis and management of abnormalities in the urologic system. Clin Perinatol 2000;27:921–45.

75. Chevalier R. Obstructive uropathy: State of the art. Pediatr Med Chir 2002;24:95–7.

76. Kemper M, Muller-Wiefel D. Renal function in congenital anomalies of the kidney and urinary tract. Curr Opin Urol 2001;11:571–5.

77. Gallini F, Maggio L, Romagnoli C, et al. Progression of renal function in preterm neonates with gestational age < 32 weeks. Pediatr Nephrol 2000;15:119–24.

78. Feldman W, Guignard J. Plasma creatinine in the first month of life. Arch Dis Child 1982;57:123–6.

79. Bellomo R, Chapman M, Finfer S, et al. Low-dose dopamine in patients with early renal dysfunction: A placebo-controlled randomised trial. Australian and New Zealand Intensive Care Society (ANZICS) Clinical Trials Group. Lancet 2000;356:2139–43.

80. Anand S. Acute renal failure. In: Taeusch H, Ballard R, Avery M, editors. Diseases of the Newborn. Philadelphia: W B Saunders; 1991. p. 894–5.

81. Mercado-Deane M, Beeson J, John S. Ultrasound of renal insufficiency in neonates. Radiographics 2002;22:1429–38.

82. Kraus S. Genitourinary imaging in children. Pediatr Clin N Am 2001;48:1381–424.

83. Roy R. Hydration of the low birth-weight infant. Clin Perinatol 1975;2:393–417.

84. Ohlsson A, Hosking M. Complications following oral administration of exchange resins in extremely low-birth-weight infants. Eur J Pediatr 1987;146:571–4.

85. Singh B, Sadiq H, Noguchi A, et al. Efficacy of albuterol inhalation in treatment of hyperkalemia in premature neonates. J Pediatr 2002;141:16–20.

86. Mildenberger E, Versmold H. Pathogenesis and therapy of nonoliguric hyperkalemia of the premature infant. Eur J Pediatr 2002;161:415–22.

87. Vemgal P, Ohlsson A. Interventions for non-oliguric hyperkalaemia in preterm neonates. Cochrane Database Syst Rev 2007;24(1):CD005257.

88. Goldstein S. Advances in pediatric renal replacement therapy for acute kidney injury. Semin Dial 2011;24:187–91.

89. Alon U, Davidai G, Bentur L, et al. Oral calcium carbonate as phosphate binder in infants and children with chronic renal failure. Miner Electrolyte Metab 1986;12:320–5.

90. American Academy of Pediatrics. Aluminum toxicity in infants and children. Pediatrics 1996;97:412–16.

91. Slatopolsky E, Burke S, Dillon M, et al. RenaGel, a nonabsorbed calcium- and aluminum-free phosphate binder, lowers serum phosphorus and parathyroid hormone. Kidney Int 1999;55:299–307.

92. Salusky I. A new era in phosphate binder therapy: What are the options? Kidney Int 2006;105:S10–15.

93. Zappitelli M, Goldstein S, Symons J, et al. Protein and calorie prescription for children and young adults receiving continuous renal replacement therapy: A report from the Prospective Pediatric Continuous Renal Replacement Therapy Registry Group. Crit Care Med 2008;36:3239–45.

94. National Kidney Foundation. KDOQI Clinical Practice Guideline for Nutrition in Children with CKD. Am J Kidney Dis 2009;53:S1–124.
95. Flynn J. Choice of dialysis modality for management of pediatric acute renal failure. Pediatr Nephrol 2002;17:61–9.
96. Golej J, Kitzmueller E, Hermon M, et al. Low-volume peritoneal dialysis in 116 neonatal and pediatric critical care patients. Eur J Pediatr 2002;161:385–9.
97. Symons J, Brophy P, Gregory M, et al. Continuous renal replacement therapy in children up to 10 kg. Am J Kidney Dis 2003;41:984–9.
98. Pedersen K, Povlsen J, Christensen S, et al. Risk factors for acute renal failure requiring dialysis after surgery for congenital heart disease in children. Acta Anaesthesiol Scand 2007;51:1344–9.
99. Blinder JJ, Goldstein SL, Lee W, et al. Congenital heart surgery in infants: Effects of acute kidney injury on outcomes. J Thorac Cardiovasc Surg 2012;143:368–74.
100. Baskin E, Saygili A, Harmanci K, et al. Acute renal failure and mortality after open-heart surgery in infants. Ren Fail 2005;27:557–60.
101. Bojan M, Gioanni S, Vouhe P, et al. Early initiation of peritoneal dialysis in neonates and infants with acute kidney injury following cardiac surgery is associated with a significant decrease in mortality. Kidney Int 2012.
102. Askenazi D, Ambalavanan N, Hamilton K, et al. Acute kidney injury and renal replacement therapy independently predict mortality in neonatal and pediatric noncardiac patients on extracorporeal membrane oxygenation. Pediatr Crit Care Med 2011;12:1–6.
103. North American Pediatric Renal Trials and Collaborative Studies (NAPRTCS). 2011 Annual Dialysis Report 2011.
104. Chevalier R, Kim A, Thornhill B, et al. Recovery following relief of unilateral ureteral obstruction in the neonatal rat. Kidney Int 1999;55:793–807.
105. Klahr S, Harris K, Purkerson M. Effects of obstruction on renal functions. Pediatr Nephrol 1992;147:430–2.
106. Boone T, Allen T. Unilateral postobstructive diuresis in the neonate. J Urol 1992;147:43–432.
107. Harris R, Yarger W. The pathogenesis of post-obstructive diuresis: The role of circulating natriuretic and diuretic factors, including urea. J Clin Invest 1975;56:880–7.
108. Rodriguez-Soriano J, Vallo A, Oliveros R, et al. Transient pseudo-hypoaldosteronism secondary to obstructive uropathy in infancy. J Pediatr 1983:103:375–80.
109. Yarger W, Buerkert J. Effect of urinary tract obstruction on renal tubular function. Semin Nephrol 1982;2:17–30.
110. Alon U, Kordoff M, Broecker B, et al. Renal tubular acidosis type IV in neonatal unilateral kidney diseases. J Pediatr 1984;104:855–60.
111. Hodges S, Patel B, McLorie G, et al. Posterior urethral valves. Scientific World Journal 2009;14:1119–26.

CHAPTER 5

Coagulopathies and Sickle Cell Disease

Mukta Sharma • Brian M. Wicklund • Gerald M. Woods

BIOCHEMISTRY AND PHYSIOLOGY OF HEMOSTASIS

The hemostatic system functions to arrest bleeding from injured blood vessels and to prevent the loss of blood from intact vessels. It also maintains a delicate balance that prevents unwanted clots from forming and dissolves blood clots that previously formed. This system, which is comprised of both thrombotic and thrombolytic proteins, platelets, and cells lining blood vessels, maintains hemostasis. Pathologic defects in this regulatory system result in either bleeding or thrombosis when too little or too much clot is formed or when dissolution of a clot is not properly regulated. Three distinct structures are involved in the process of hemostasis: blood vessels, platelets, and circulating hemostatic proteins. Together, these components form the coagulation system, the naturally occurring anticoagulation system, and the fibrinolytic system. Coagulation must act rapidly to stop the loss of blood from an injured vessel, but the clot that is formed must remain localized so that it does not interfere with the passage of blood through the intact circulation. The anticoagulation system prevents the extension of the clot beyond the site of injury. The fibrinolytic system removes excess hemostatic material that has been released into the circulation and slowly lyses the clot once it is no longer needed.

The stimulus that initially causes clot formation occurs as a consequence of disruption of endothelial cells. This leads to exposure of collagen and subendothelial tissues. The hemostatic response to tissue injury consists of four stages. First, vasoconstriction by the contraction of smooth muscle in the injured vessel wall reduces blood flow. Second, platelets adhere to the exposed endothelium, aggregate, and release their granular contents. This activity stimulates further vasoconstriction and recruits more platelets. This action results in 'primary hemostasis' that occludes the gap in the blood vessel and stops blood loss through the vessel. Third, the extrinsic and intrinsic coagulation systems are activated to form fibrin, which stabilizes the platelets and prevents disaggregation. Fourth, fibrinolysis results from the release of plasminogen activators from the injured vessel wall. These activators limit the coagulation process. Once healing has taken place, they begin dissolution of formed clot so that vascular patency can be restored.[1]

Endothelial Cells

Endothelial cells maintain the integrity of the blood vessel and prevent extravasation of blood into the surrounding tissue.[1] Passive thromboresistance is provided by endothelial proteoglycans, primarily endogenous heparin sulfate. Active thromboresistance is achieved through several mechanisms, including the synthesis and release of prostacyclin, a potent vasodilator and an inhibitor of platelet adhesion and aggregation.[1,2]

When the endothelium is injured, tissue factor (thromboplastin) is produced and rapidly promotes local thrombin formation.[3] Tissue factor binds factor VII and converts it to factor VIIa (Fig. 5-1), which is the first step in activation of the extrinsic coagulation pathway. It also activates factor IX, which is the major activator of the common pathway, resulting in fibrin formation.[4] Capillaries seal with little dependence on the hemostatic system, but arterioles and venules require the presence of platelets to form an occluding plug. In arteries and veins, hemostasis depends on both vascular contraction and clot formation around an occluding primary hemostatic plug.[5]

Platelets

In the resting state, platelets circulate as disk-shaped, anuclear cells that have been released from megakaryocytes in the bone marrow. They are 2–3 μm in size and remain in circulation for approximately five to nine days unless they participate in coagulation reactions or are removed by the spleen. Normal blood contains 150,000–400,000 platelets/μL.[5] In the resting state platelets do not bind to intact endothelium.

Platelet Adhesion

Once platelets bind to injured tissue and are activated, their discoid shape changes. They spread on the subendothelial connective tissue and degranulate releasing serotonin, adenosine diphosphate, adenosine triphosphate, and calcium, and alpha granules release factor V, fibrinogen, von Willebrand factor (FVIII:vWF), fibronectin, platelet factor 4, β-thromboglobulin, and platelet-derived growth factor.[6,7] This recruits and aggregates more platelets from the circulation onto the already adherent platelets.[7]

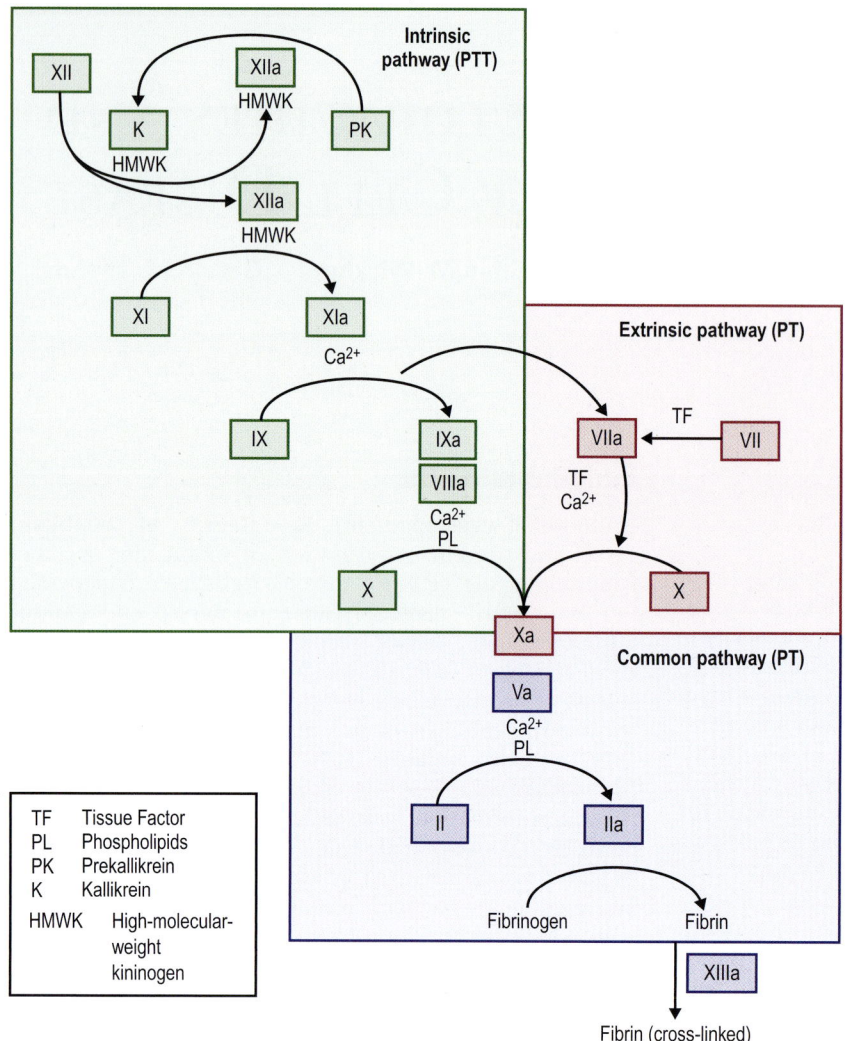

FIGURE 5-1 ▪ The coagulation cascade.

When a vessel is disrupted, platelet adhesion occurs through the binding of collagen and vWF (found in the subendothelium) to the platelet membrane (Fig. 5-2). For platelet adhesion to occur, platelets must express specific glycoprotein Ib receptors on their surface to bind the vWF complex. If this specific glycoprotein is missing, platelets are unable to adhere to areas of injury.[8] Platelets in Bernard–Soulier syndrome lack glycoprotein Ib and are unable to adhere and form the initial hemostatic plug.[9] If the vWF is defective or deficient, platelets do not adhere to sites of vascular injury. The result is von Willebrand disease, of which several specific types and subtypes have been defined.[10–12] Very high concentrations of prostacyclin also can inhibit platelet adhesion to exposed subendothelium.[5]

Platelet Aggregation

Aggregation is a complex reaction that involves platelet granule release, cleavage of membrane phospholipids by phospholipases A_2 and C, alterations in intracellular cyclic adenosine monophosphate levels, mobilization of intracellular calcium, and the expression of fibrinogen receptors on the platelet surface. If fibrinogen receptors

(glycoproteins IIb and IIIa) or fibrinogen are missing, platelets do not aggregate.[13,14] This results in Glanzmann thrombasthenia causing patients to have a serious, life-long bleeding disorder.[6]

After aggregation, platelets function to enhance thrombin formation. The platelet membrane provides specific binding sites for factors Xa and V causing effective assembly of the prothrombinase complex making thrombin.[7] Thrombin formation makes a stable hemostatic plug of adherent platelets surrounded by a network of fibrin strands.

Generation of Thrombin

Thrombin is the enzyme responsible for transforming liquid blood into a fibrin gel. The initial activation of factor VII by tissue factor results in the production of thrombin by the extrinsic system. Tissue factor is released only after injury to the endothelial cells.

The majority of thrombin production results from the activation of the intrinsic coagulation system, not the extrinsic system. Exposed subendothelium converts factor XII to factor XIIa and thereby activates the intrinsic pathway, although deficits in factor XII do not cause

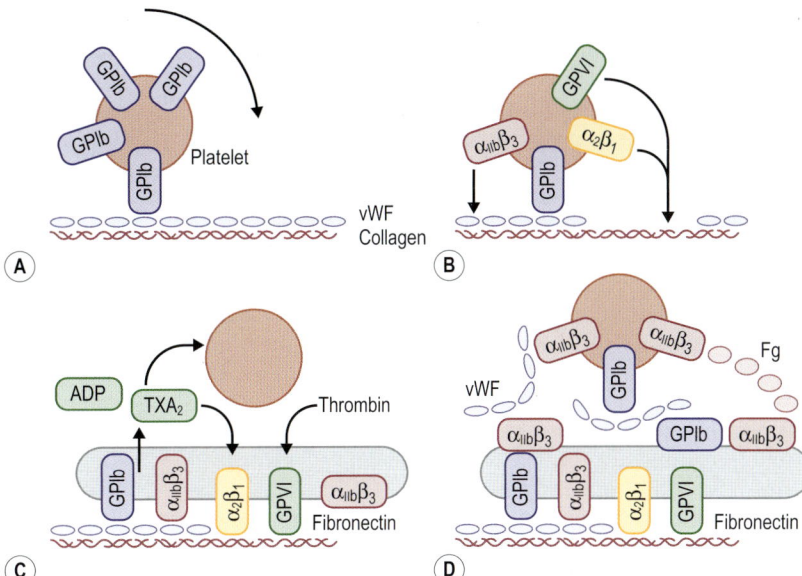

FIGURE 5-2 ■ Schematic representation of platelet adhesion and aggregation under flow conditions. **(A)** Rolling of platelets over collagen-bound vWF mediated by GPIb. **(B)** Firm attachment mediated by $\alpha_2\beta_1$ and glycoprotein VI (GP VI) binding to collagen, and by $\alpha_{IIb}\beta_3$) binding tocollagen-bound vWF. **(C)** Platelet activation, secretion, and spreading. **(D)** Aggregate formation.

a bleeding disorder. Activation of factors XI and IX follows, and activated factor IX in combination with factor VIII, calcium, and platelet phospholipid activates factor X. Activated factor VII, complexed with tissue factor, activates factor IX. Factor Xa with factor V then cleaves prothrombin into the active molecule thrombin, which can convert fibrinogen into fibrin.[4,15]

Formation of Fibrin

When thrombin acts on fibrinogen, fibrin monomers result after the proteolytic release of fibrinopeptides A and B. The monomeric fibrin then polymerizes into a gel.[4,15] With additional stabilization of the fibrin gel provided by factor XIII, fibrin surrounds and stabilizes the platelet plug. This process makes the multimeric fibrin more resistant to plasmin digestion and completes the formation and stabilization of the blood clot.[16]

Several regulatory proteins serve to localize thrombin formation to the surface of the blood vessel. Endothelial cells have receptors for protein C. Protein S is a co-factor for the activation of protein C. Thrombomodulin is an endothelial surface protein that acts in combination with thrombin to activate the bound protein C. Activated protein C then degrades factors Va and VIIIa, which inhibit thrombin formation.[17]

Heparin-like anticoagulant molecules, present on endothelial cells, act in combination with antithrombin III to inhibit factors XIIa, XIa, IXa, and Xa and thrombin. Inhibition of these factors prevents the spread of clot to uninjured adjacent vessels and the blockage of large vessels by excessive clot formation.[15,17] Endothelial cells, as mentioned previously, produce PGI_2 (prostacyclin), a potent vasodilator and inhibitor of platelet aggregation and adhesion.

Fibrinolysis

The regulatory process that dissolves fibrin and preserves vessel patency is called fibrinolysis. Circulating plasminogen is converted into plasmin by tissue plasminogen activators. These activators are released from the vessel walls at the site of blood clotting. They bind to the fibrin clot and convert plasminogen to plasmin. Plasmin enzymatically degrades fibrin, fibrinogen, and other plasma proteins, and this process results in the dissolution of formed clot.[15,17]

CLINICAL EVALUATION

There is currently no completely reliable screening test available to evaluate hemostasis in the preoperative patients. A careful history, including a full family history, remains the best means of uncovering mild bleeding problems, including von Willebrand disease or qualitative platelet abnormalities.[18] These disorders may easily escape standard laboratory screening procedures, such as prothrombin time (PT), activated partial thromboplastin time (aPTT), platelet count, and bleeding time. aPTT screening yields many false-positive results caused by both analytical problems and detection of clinically insignificant disorders. In addition, a normal aPTT may lead to a false sense of safety because it does not exclude all serious bleeding disorders. Because no method can reliably predict all bleeding complications, postoperative monitoring remains important for all patients.[19] Likewise, patients with mild disorders who have not previously undergone an operation may have no history of bleeding problems and might be identified preoperatively only if screening tests are performed.[18] It is important to consider the history as the most important component of a diagnostic strategy and to investigate thoroughly any story of unusual bleeding, even if the screening tests are normal.[20] Conversely, studies examining the utility of a screening preoperative PT and aPTT in patients undergoing tonsillectomy and adenoidectomy concluded that routine screening with a PT and aPTT for all patients regardless of history cannot be recommended.[19,21] In obtaining a history from the patient and parents, positive answers to the questions posed in Box 5-1 indicate the need for further evaluation.[18,22–24]

If there is a history of abnormal bleeding, the following points must be established. The type of bleeding (i.e., petechiae, purpura, ecchymosis, and single or generalized bleeding sites) can give an indication of the underlying defect. Petechiae and purpura are most frequently associated with platelet abnormalities, either of function or numbers. Von Willebrand disease is most frequently associated with mucosal bleeding, including epistaxis, whereas hemophilia is most often associated with bleeding into joints or soft tissue ecchymosis, or both. Bleeding when the umbilical cord separates is most often associated with a deficiency in factor XIII, as is unexplained bleeding of the central nervous system.[16,25] A single bleeding site, such as repetitive epistaxis from the same nostril, is frequently indicative of a localized, anatomic problem and not a system-wide coagulation defect.

The course or pattern of the bleeding (i.e., spontaneous or after trauma) and its frequency and duration is important, and the pattern of inheritance (i.e., X-linked or autosomal; recessive or dominant) can help narrow the differential diagnosis (e.g., hemophilia A and B are X-linked recessive diseases, whereas von Willebrand disease is autosomal dominant).

Any previous or current drug therapy must be fully documented, and a search is made for over-the-counter medications that the patient might be taking but does not consider 'medicine' and has therefore not mentioned. Aspirin, ibuprofen, cough medications containing guaifenesin, and antihistamines can lead to platelet dysfunction or uncover a previously undiagnosed bleeding disorder such as von Willebrand disease.[26,27] The presence of other medical problems including renal failure with uremia, hepatic failure, malignancies, gastrointestinal malabsorption, vascular malformations, cardiac anomalies with or without repair, and autoimmune disorders is essential to elicit because these may have associated coagulopathies.

The physical examination is used to help narrow the differential diagnosis and guide the laboratory investigation of hemostatic disorders. Petechiae and purpuric bleeding occur with platelet and vascular abnormalities. Mucocutaneous bleeding suggests a platelet disorder and includes petechiae, ecchymoses, epistaxis, and genitourinary and gastrointestinal bleeding. Bleeding into potential spaces such as joints, fascial planes, and the retroperitoneum is instead suggestive of a coagulation factor deficiency. Bleeding from multiple sites in an ill patient can be seen with disseminated intravascular coagulation (DIC) or thrombotic thrombocytopenic purpura. Hemophilia patients often have palpable purpura and deep muscle bleeding that is painful but may be difficult to detect. Findings compatible with a collagen disorder include the body habitus of Marfan syndrome; blue sclerae; skeletal deformities; hyperextensible joints and skin; and nodular, spider-like, or pinpoint telangiectasia. Organomegaly may suggest an underlying malignancy, whereas jaundice and hepatomegaly may be indicative of hepatic dysfunction.

LABORATORY EVALUATION

When the bleeding history and/or family history suggest the possibility of a bleeding disorder, or if it is impossible to obtain a history due to family or social circumstances, it is customary to proceed with a series of laboratory investigations to look for a possible bleeding diagnosis. Generally, screening tests are performed first and should include a blood cell count, PT, and aPTT (Fig. 5-3).[20] Additional tests can measure fibrinogen levels, assess the thrombin time, screen for inhibitors of specific coagulation factors, measure specific factor levels, and test for platelet function and von Willebrand disease.[20,28] Patients also can be evaluated for evidence of DIC by using multiple assays to test for the presence of various fibrinopeptides and products from the breakdown of fibrin or fibrinogen.

Platelet Count

The platelet count measures the adequacy of platelet numbers to provide initial hemostasis. Thrombocytopenia (a platelet count of $<150,000/\mu L$) is one of the most common problems that occur in hospitalized patients. As stated previously, typical manifestations include mucocutaneous bleeding. The risk of bleeding is inversely proportional to the platelet count. When the platelet count is $<50,000/\mu L$, minor bleeding occurs easily and the risk

BOX 5-1	Questions to Ask about Potential Bleeding Problems

1. Is there any history of easy bruising, bleeding problems, or an established bleeding disorder in the patient or any family members?
2. Has excessive bleeding occurred after any previous surgical procedure or dental work? Have the parents or any siblings had excessive bleeding after any surgical or dental procedures, specifically tonsillectomy or adenoidectomy?
3. Have frequent nosebleeds occurred, and has nasal packing or cautery been needed? Has bleeding without trauma occurred into any joint or muscle?
4. Does excessive bleeding or bruising occur after aspirin ingestion?
5. Does significant gingival bleeding occur after tooth brushing?
6. Has there been any significant postpartum hemorrhage?
7. Has the patient been taking any medication that might affect platelets or the coagulation system?
8. If the patient is male and was circumcised, were any problems noted with prolonged oozing after the circumcision?
9. If the patient is a child, do the parents remember any bleeding problems when the umbilical cord separated?
10. If the patient is menstruating, does she have profuse menstruation?
11. Has the patient ever received any transfusions of blood or blood products? If so, what was the reason for the transfusion?

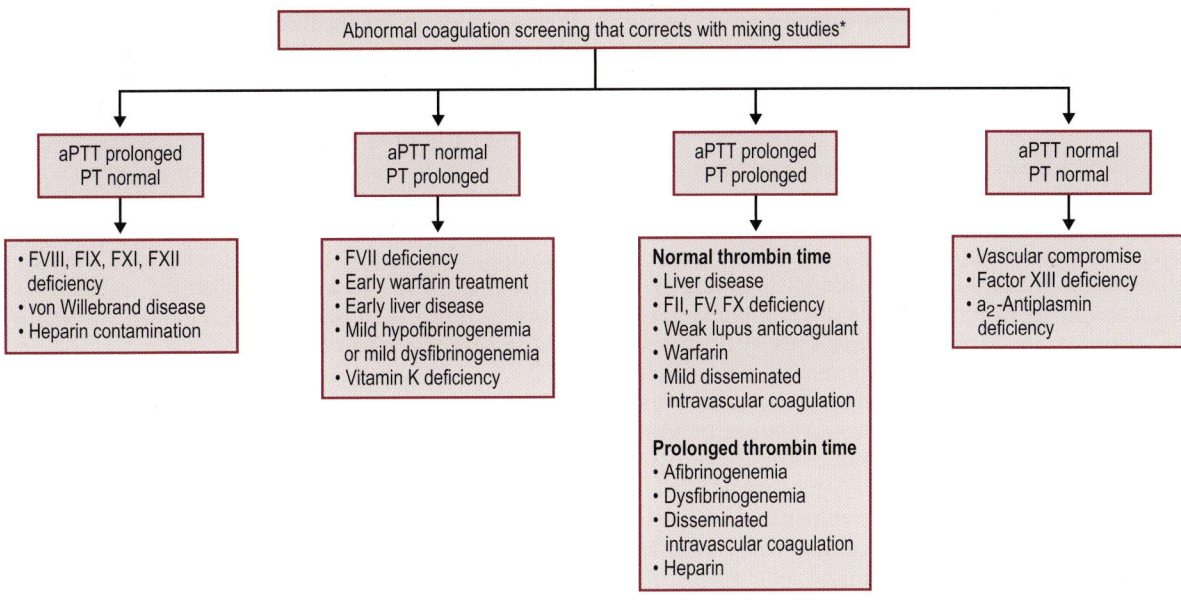

*Repeating an abnormal coagulation screening with a mixture of 1 part patient plasma and 1 part normal plasma ("mixing studies") will normalize the test if a factor deficiency is present, but the screening test will remain abnormal if an anticoagulant is present. These anticoagulants rarely are a cause of thromboembolic disease and even more rarely cause bleeding.

FIGURE 5-3 ■ Screening tests for abnormal coagulation.

of major bleeding increases. Counts between 20,000–50,000/μL predispose to bleeding with even minor trauma; with counts <20,000/μL, spontaneous bleeding may occur; with counts <5000/μL, severe spontaneous bleeding is more likely. However, patients with counts <10,000/μL may be asymptomatic for years.[29] Surgical bleeding does not usually occur until the platelet count is <50,000 platelets/μL.[30] A platelet count of <50,000/μL is considered a cut-off criterion for transfusions, and the prophylactic use of platelet transfusion is indicated for any invasive procedure. Patients with significant clinical bleeding should also be transfused with platelets.[30]

Bleeding Time and the PFA-100 Analyzer

The bleeding time is defined as the length of time required for a standardized incision to stop oozing blood that can be absorbed onto filter paper. A variety of procedures have been used, but all have variable sensitivity and have been difficult to reproduce accurately, leading many centers to drop the bleeding time from the list of approved laboratory tests.[31] The PFA-100 Analyzer (Siemans Healthcare Diagnostics, Deerfield, IL) is now widely used as a replacement for the bleeding time. It creates an in vitro high shear stress condition that results in the activation of platelet-dependent and vWF-dependent attachment and aggregation of platelets to a collagen–ADP or collagen–epinephrine surface. In most cases, the PFA-100 closure time is superior to the bleeding time in the detection of von Willebrand disease, aspirin effect, or platelet dysfunction.[31] However, test results can be influenced by the sample's hematocrit. Although the PFA-100 does not detect all platelet dysfunctions or cases of von Willebrand disease, when used in conjunction with a standardized questionnaire, it will likely detect impaired hemostasis in most cases.[31,32]

Prothrombin Time

The PT is a measure of the function of the extrinsic and common coagulation pathways. It represents the time (in seconds) for the patient's plasma to clot after the addition of calcium and thromboplastin (an activator of the extrinsic pathway).[33,34] Isolated prolongation of the PT is seen most commonly in patients who are deficient in vitamin K due to previous antibiotic treatment. It also occurs with factor VII deficiency, mild hypofibrinogenemia, dysfibrinogenemia, and warfarin therapy. The PT may also be prolonged with significant liver dysfunction.[33,34]

Partial Thromboplastin Time

The aPTT measures the function of the intrinsic and common coagulation pathways. The aPTT represents the time (in seconds) for the patient's plasma to clot after the addition of phospholipid, calcium and an intrinsic pathway activator. The aPTT detects deficiencies in factors XII, XI, IX, and VIII and in the common pathway, but mild factor deficiencies may be missed. The aPTT also is used to monitor anticoagulation with heparin.[33,34]

Several inherited disorders of coagulation are not detected by the preceding tests. Results from standard hemostatic screening tests, such as the aPTT and international normalized ratio (INR) assessments, are normal in factor XIII (FXIII) deficiency. Therefore, assessment of clot stability is the most common screening test used for FXIII deficiency with a quantitative assay required to confirm the diagnosis of FXIII deficiency.[35] Von Willebrand disease patients may have normal or prolonged aPTTs, and patients with a deficiency in α²-antiplasmin have a normal aPTT. Both the PT and aPTT are prolonged in patients with deficiencies of factors X and V, prothrombin, and fibrinogen and in patients with DIC or severe liver disease.[34,36]

Fibrinogen

The standard method for fibrinogen determination measures clottable fibrinogen by using a kinetic assay. Normal levels of fibrinogen are 150–350 mg/dL. As fibrinogen is the substrate for the final reaction in the formation of a clot and all plasma-based screening tests depend on the formation of a clot as the end point of the reaction, fibrinogen levels below 80 mg/dL prolong the PT, aPTT, and thrombin time and therefore make the results uninterpretable. Large amounts of fibrin degradation products interfere with the formation of fibrin and cause an artificially low level of measured fibrinogen. An immunologic-based assay for fibrinogen is used to measure both clottable and nonclottable fibrinogen. This test is most often used in identifying patients with a dysfibrinogenemia in whom the functional level of fibrinogen is low and the immunologic level is normal.[34,36]

Inhibitor Screening Tests

Repeating the PT or aPTT by using a 1:1 mix of patient plasma with normal plasma is a useful procedure for investigating a prolonged PT or aPTT. Normal plasma has, by definition, 100% levels of all factors. When mixed with an equal volume of patient plasma, if there is a minimum of 50% of any given factor present, the PT or aPTT should normalize. Correction of the clotting time suggests the presence of a factor deficiency whereas lack of normalization suggests the presence of an inhibitor that interferes with either thrombin or fibrin formation.[33,34]

Two types of acquired inhibitors prolong the aPTT. One blocks or inactivates one of the intrinsic factors, whereas the other is a lupus-like inhibitor that interferes with phospholipid-based clotting reactions. The first type of inhibitor occurs in 10–15% of hemophilia A patients and can occur spontaneously, but it is extremely rare in nonhemophiliac children.[37] The lupus-like inhibitor is associated not with bleeding problems but rather with an increased risk of thrombotic problems in adults. Lupus-like inhibitors are mentioned because they commonly cause prolongations of the aPTT.[38] Specific investigation of either of these situations should be referred to a coagulation reference laboratory.

Platelet Function Studies

Platelet function studies measure in vitro platelet aggregation. In this procedure, platelet-rich plasma is incubated with an agonist and then changes are noted in the amount of light transmitted through the platelet suspension. Agonists used to induce platelet aggregation include collagen, epinephrine, ADP, thrombin, and ristocetin. Three distinct phases are seen in the reaction. The first is an initial change in the shape of the platelets, leading to a temporary decrease in light transmission. Next is the first wave of aggregation, which is a reversible platelet-platelet interaction. With additional stimulation, the final phase—the second wave of aggregation—occurs and produces irreversible platelet aggregation. The second wave of aggregation is due to release of the platelet granules and thromboxane A_2 synthesis. The release reaction is blocked by aspirin and is absent in patients with an inherited storage pool defect, congenital deficiency in thromboxane A_2 synthesis, or cyclooxygenase deficiency.[7] The PFA-100 has become the test of choice to replace the bleeding time and is used to screen for a variety of disorders, but full characterization of platelet function requires traditional platelet aggregation studies in a specialized laboratory.

Specific Factor Assays

Specific factor assays are available for all known coagulation, fibrinolysis, and anticoagulation factors to quantify their levels in plasma. These tests are not indicated unless a screening test result is abnormal. The only exception involves the patient with a history that is suggestive of von Willebrand disease, factor XIII deficiency, or dysfibrinogenemia. In these cases, the aPTT may not be sensitive enough to detect the disorder. Further testing may be justified on clinical suspicion based on the patient's history.[33,34] For von Willebrand disease, the workup consists of measuring factor VIII levels, vWF antigen levels, ristocetin co-factor activity, and ristocetin-induced platelet aggregation. Analysis of the distribution of vWF multimers can be useful to the hematologist in identifying the specific type of von Willebrand disease.[10–12]

Tests for Disseminated Intravascular Coagulation

The tests that are available in most hospital laboratories for identification of DIC are semiquantitative fibrin or fibrinogen degradation product assays, which involve a slide agglutination procedure or a D-dimer assay. An increased amount of these degradation products suggests that either plasmin has circulated to lyse fibrin and fibrinogen or the patient's hepatic function is insufficient to clear the small amounts of regularly produced degradation products. The D-dimer test is a slide agglutination procedure that tests for the presence of two D subunits of fibrin that are cross-linked by factor XIII. This test provides specific evidence that plasmin has digested the fibrin clot and not fibrinogen. It is positive in patients with DIC, in patients with resolving large intravascular clots, and in patients with hepatic insufficiency. Specific assays to demonstrate the presence of soluble fibrin monomer complexes or fibrinopeptides produced by the conversion of prothrombin to thrombin are also useful in some situations and available in specialized laboratories.[34,39]

Thromboelastograph

Thromboelastograph is used as a functional measure of whole blood coagulation in pediatric cardiac surgical and liver transplant patients, and is a useful monitor in patients with major trauma and patients with coagulation deficits.[40]

HEMOPHILIA A AND B

Hemophilia A and B are X-linked recessive bleeding disorders caused by decreased levels of functional procoagulant factor VIII (FVIII) and factor IX (FIX), respectively. Approximately 80% of all hemophilia patients have FVIII deficiency, which is classic hemophilia. The remaining 20% have FIX deficiency, which is called Christmas disease. These are rare disorders, with a prevalence of only 13.4/100,000 males.[41] Until 1964, the treatment of hemophilia was limited by volume restrictions imposed by the use of whole blood or fresh frozen plasma. At that time, the FVIII-rich fraction of fresh frozen plasma (known as cryoprecipitate) was discovered.[42] Specific lyophilized FVIII concentrates have since been developed, as have prothrombin concentrates containing factors II, VII, IX, and X. Concentrates containing only FIX for the treatment of hemophilia B patients and factor VIII/vWF concentrates for the treatment of von Willebrand disease have also been developed.[43,44] The lyophilized factor concentrates have allowed storage of the clotting factor using standard refrigeration and have permitted the outpatient treatment of bleeding episodes plus the development of home self-infusion programs.[45] This treatment, combined with the development of comprehensive hemophilia treatment centers, has produced a remarkable change in the outlook for these patients who previously developed significant joint deformities in their teens to 20s and were frequently wheelchair bound in adult life. Home therapy has decreased the damage caused by hemarthroses, with hemophiliac children born since the mid-1970s having far fewer joint deformities than do older hemophilia patients. These factor concentrates have allowed operations to be performed with much less risk, even to the point that orthopedic procedures can be readily accomplished.[46] Moreover, the comprehensive hemophilia treatment system has shown a 40% reduction in mortality for hemophilia patients.[47]

Viral infections transmitted by cryoprecipitate and factor concentrates were the major problem faced by hemophilia patients in the late 1970s to mid-1980s. Approximately 60% of all hemophilia patients became human immunodeficiency virus (HIV) positive in the 1980s.[48] Hepatitis C is the other major viral infection that was transmitted by plasma-derived factor concentrates used to treat hemophilia. Estimates from the mid-1980s are that more than 90% of multiply transfused hemophiliacs were positive for non-A, non-B hepatitis and that more than 95% had been infected with hepatitis B.[49] A different study showed that 75% of HIV-negative hemophilia patients, treated with earlier plasma-derived factor concentrates, have evidence of hepatitis C infection.[50] No documented cases of HIV or hepatitis C transmission by clotting factor concentrates after 1987 are known.[48] Since 1993, recombinant-produced FVIII concentrates have been available. At present, only recombinant FVIII and FIX concentrates are used for the treatment of patients with newly diagnosed hemophilia A and B.[51]

In the future, long-acting FVIII as replacement therapy for hemophilia would significantly improve treatment options for patients. To develop factors with an extended circulating half-life, but without a reduction in activity, engineered FVIII variants with surface-exposed cysteine residues to which a polyethylene glycol polymer is conjugated are being studied in animals.[52]

Hemophilia patients are classified into three categories based on their level of circulating factor. Severe hemophiliacs (factor levels below 1%) have a high risk of bleeding and are managed with factor prophylaxis to prevent joint damage.[41,53] Bleeding occurs in areas subject to minor trauma. Hemarthroses, hematomas, and ecchymoses are common. Recurrent hemarthroses can cause pseudotumors of the bone, whereas hematomas can cause ischemic compartment syndromes. In moderate hemophiliacs (factor levels of 1–5%), spontaneous hemorrhage occurs infrequently but relatively minor trauma can cause bleeding into joints or soft tissues.

Mild hemophiliacs, with levels >5%, rarely have bleeding problems and typically have problems only with major trauma or surgical procedures.[37,41] Some mild hemophiliacs may not be diagnosed until late childhood or adulthood. Therefore, the history may not be helpful in alerting the pediatric surgeon about the risk of bleeding. Moreover, because one-third of all cases of hemophilia are caused by new mutations, there also may not be a family history to arouse suspicion of a bleeding problem.[37] Preoperative laboratory testing may be the only means by which mild hemophilia is diagnosed.

The need for surgical intervention in hemophilia patients most frequently center on areas of damage secondary to bleeding episodes. In 1985, the results of a review of 350 consecutive operations performed at the Orthopedic Hospital in Los Angeles were published.[54] As the study represented patients from before the start of home therapy and comprehensive care, it was expected that this group would have significant orthopedic problems secondary to multiple hemarthroses. Of the 350 procedures reviewed, 312 were characterized as serious and 38 of lesser intensity; 318 operations were on hemophiliacs with moderate and severe hemophilia; and 30 were on patients with mild hemophilia. As expected, musculoskeletal procedures made up two-thirds of all operations on moderate and severe hemophiliacs and half of all operations on mild hemophiliacs. Bleeding problems during operation were not observed, but 23% of all serious operations were complicated by postoperative hemorrhages. Only operations on the knee had significantly more postoperative hemorrhages (40%). Operations on other joints and soft tissue areas had similar rates of complications (15%). Most of the postoperative hemorrhages occurred with plasma factor levels greater than 30%, which is the minimum level that is considered hemostatic. The authors also noted that the incidence of postoperative hemorrhage decreased after postoperative day 11. Interestingly, other studies have found that vigorous physical therapy may cause postoperative hemorrhage and have therefore recommended the continuation of factor replacement throughout the period of physical therapy.[54,55]

The management of the hemophilic patient requires close cooperation among surgeons, hematologists, and personnel in the hemophilia center, the coagulation laboratory, and the pharmacy or blood bank. Careful preoperative planning is essential to the success of the intervention, and an adequate supply of clotting factor concentrate must be available to cover the child's needs before admission. The patient also must be screened for the presence of an inhibitor to either FVIII or FIX during the two to four weeks before the operation. A low-titer inhibitor may be overcome with increased doses of factor, but high-titer inhibitors may require the use of activated prothrombin complex concentrate (FEIBA) or recombinant activated factor VII (rFVII) to 'bypass' the effect of the antibody against either FVIII or FIX. These patients have been desensitized with daily doses of human factor concentrate over a period of months to years, restoring their response to regular infusions of factor VIII or IX.[46,56,57]

At our institution, on the day of surgery the hemophilia patient receives a bolus dose of factor (usually 50 units/kg of FVIII in hemophilia A patients), and a continuous infusion of 4–8 units/kg/h of FVIII (for the hemophilia A patient) is started to maintain a factor level greater than 80% for the next one to two days.[58] The factor level is checked immediately before the operation and is the final screen for the presence of an inhibitor. The infusion is maintained throughout the procedure and is then reduced on the second or third postoperative day to allow the plasma levels to decrease to 50%. Replacement is continued for a full ten to 14 days. Daily factor levels are necessary to ensure appropriate levels. For neurosurgical or orthopedic procedures, much longer periods of factor coverage—even four to six weeks—are utilized, especially if significant physical therapy is planned.[41,46]

Many hemophilia patients perform their own factor infusions at home supported by home care pharmacies. With the advent of home nursing services, patients are being discharged home with prolonged periods of factor coverage. Hemophilia center personnel must be closely involved in the planning of these discharges to ensure that sufficient clotting factor is available at home and that close follow-up is maintained during periods of scheduled home therapy. Hemophilia patients should not receive any compounds that contain aspirin or ibuprofen. Any minor procedures that would require factor correction should be combined with the major procedure, if possible, to save on the use of factor concentrate.

Previously, the hemophilia B patient undergoing an operation had specific problems because of the thrombogenic risk inherent in the use of older FIX concentrates. Since the advent of newer, more purified plasma-derived and recombinant-produced FIX concentrates, operative interventions in hemophilia B patients have been performed without excess thrombotic problems.[59,60]

CLOTTING FACTOR DOSING

Factor VIII is dosed differently from FIX, based on their half-lives. FVIII has an eight- to 12-hour half-life, and the infusion of 1 unit/kg of body weight increases the plasma level by 2%. If a severe hemophilia A patient weighs 50 kg, an infusion of 25 units/kg, or 1250 units, of FVIII will raise his factor level to 50%. FIX has a half-life of 24 hours and must be infused in larger amounts

than FVIII to raise the plasma level. Infusion of 1 unit/kg of FIX will raise the plasma level only by 1%. Continuous infusion of highly purified FIX, as well as FVIII, has been shown to prevent excessive peaks and troughs of factor levels, is simpler to manage, and decreases the cost by decreasing the overall amount of factor used. It has not shown to cause any problems with excess thrombosis.[61] Recombinant FIX has a marked variability in dose response to infusions, and individual recovery studies may be needed before it is used for surgical hemostasis. Often, a 20% increase in dose is needed to achieve the same factor levels as obtained by use of plasma-derived FIX.[62]

NEONATAL HEMOSTASIS

The newborn's coagulation system is not fully mature until 6 months after birth. The lower levels of procoagulant, fibrinolytic, and anticoagulant proteins in neonatal patients complicate both operations and the care of sick and preterm infants. Platelet counts are within the usual adult normal ranges. These platelets have a lower function than those of adults, but enough to produce a normal bleeding time.[62] Circulating coagulation factors do not cross the placenta, and infants with inherited deficiencies of clotting factors, fibrinolytic proteins, or natural anticoagulants may initially be seen in the neonatal period. Levels of fibrinogen, factor V, factor VIII, and vWF are within the adult normal range at birth.[63] All other procoagulants are at reduced levels, depending on gestational age. Vitamin K-dependent factors may become further depressed in infants who are breast fed and not given vitamin K at birth.[62]

Of more concern are the low levels of anticoagulant and fibrinolytic proteins. Very low levels of protein C have been associated with purpura fulminans in newborns. In sick infants, levels of antithrombin III and plasminogen may be inadequate to deal with increased levels of clot-promoting activity in the blood. Sick infants with indwelling catheters are at significant risk of thrombotic complications.[64]

DISSEMINATED INTRAVASCULAR COAGULATION

DIC is the inappropriate activation of both thrombin and fibrin. It may follow sepsis, hypotension, hypoxemia, trauma, malignancy, burns, and extracorporeal circulation. Hemorrhage due to the depletion of clotting factors as well as thrombosis due to the excess formation of clot are seen, and the end-organ damage caused by ischemia and impairment of blood flow causes irreversible disease and death.[65]

Acute DIC is associated with the consumption of factors II, V, VIII, X, and XIII, as well as fibrinogen, antithrombin III, plasminogen, and platelets. Review of the peripheral smear usually shows a microangiopathic hemolytic anemia. The PT and aPTT may both be prolonged, and the fibrinogen level ultimately decreases as the DIC worsens. The presence of D-dimers may indicate the presence of DIC, but they may also be elevated due to thrombus or hepatic dysfunction. Antithrombin III levels may be low, and the use of antithrombin III concentrates in septic shock may play a role in the future treatment of DIC. However, adult studies have not shown any improvement in mortality for patients with septicemia treated with antithrombin III.[66] At present, the major therapy for DIC is correction of the underlying disorder with fresh frozen plasma and platelet transfusions as indicated to support hemostasis. Low-dose heparin infusions have not been shown to appreciably improve the outcome.[65,67]

MANAGEMENT OF QUANTITATIVE AND QUALITATIVE PLATELET DISORDERS

Thrombocytopenias are caused by either inadequate production of platelets by the bone marrow, or by increased destruction or sequestration of the platelets in the circulation. The history and physical examination may be suggestive of a diagnosis that can be confirmed by laboratory testing. Medication use, a family history of blood disorders, a history of recent viral infection, short stature, absent thumbs or radii, or a congenital malformation may indicate a defect in platelet production. The destruction may be immunologic, as in immune thrombocytopenic purpura (ITP); mechanical, as in septicemia; or drug induced, as in patients with sensitivity to heparin or cimetidine. Establishing the cause of the thrombocytopenia determines the therapy needed to restore the platelet count in preparing the patient for operation. The clinical response to therapeutic modalities, such as a platelet transfusion, can be important tests and can help direct further investigations. In patients with immune-based platelet consumptions, such as ITP, usually no response is found to platelet transfusion. Moreover, only a very short response may be seen in patients with other causes of increased consumption. Management of the patient is then aimed at reducing the consumption and should involve consultation with a hematologist about the use of corticosteroids, the use of intravenous immunoglobulin or anti-D immunoglobulin, the discontinuation of medications, and other treatment modalities.[68]

If the thrombocytopenia is caused by a lack of production of platelets, due to either aplastic anemia, malignancy, or chemotherapy, transfusion with platelet concentrates to increase the platelet count above a minimum of 50,000/μL will allow minor procedures to be performed safely. Most surgeons and anesthesiologists prefer for the platelet count to be greater than 100,000/μL before major surgery. Continued monitoring of platelet counts is vital because further transfusions may be needed to keep the platelet count above 50,000/μL for three to five days after operation.[69]

Qualitative platelet defects can be caused by rare congenital defects such as Bernard–Soulier syndrome, Glanzmann thrombasthenia, or platelet storage pool disease. Alternatively, they can be caused by drug ingestions such as an aspirin-induced cyclooxygenase deficiency. In these situations, transfusion of normal donor platelets provides adequate hemostasis for the operation. Discontinuation

of all aspirin-containing products one week before operation permits correction of the cyclooxygenase deficiency as new platelets are produced.[6,70]

DISORDERS OF THROMBIN GENERATION AND FIBRIN FORMATION

Patients with rare deficiencies of other clotting factors, such as factors XI, X, VII, V, prothrombin, and fibrinogen, can have clinical bleeding depending on the level of deficiency. Most of these disorders are inherited in an autosomal recessive manner and can therefore affect both male and female patients. Replacement therapy with fresh frozen plasma or, in certain situations, with prothrombin complex concentrates corrects the deficiency and should be conducted under the direction of a hematologist.[46,71]

Vitamin K deficiency, both in the neonatal period and from malabsorption, can cause deficiencies of factors II, VII, IX, and X. Treatment with 1–2 mg of intravenous vitamin K may begin to correct the deficiencies within four to six hours. However, if a procedure is contemplated, fresh frozen plasma (15 mL/kg) should be given with the vitamin K, and repeated. Also, the PT should be monitored for correction of the coagulopathy before the operation. Laboratory monitoring should be maintained during the postoperative period to ensure continuation of the appropriate factor levels.[5]

Patients with factor XIII deficiency often present with delayed bleeding from the umbilical cord, rebleeding from wounds, intracranial hemorrhage, and poor wound healing. These problems may be treated with relatively small amounts of fresh frozen plasma (5–10 mL/kg). Because factor XIII has a half-life of six days, this treatment is usually needed only once to stop bleeding or at the time of operation.[16,46] Patients with dysfibrinogenemia or afibrinogenemia may be given fresh frozen plasma or cryoprecipitate.[46] There are ongoing trials looking at a fibrinogen concentrate preparation infusion for these conditions.

FIBRINOLYTIC AND THROMBOTIC DISORDERS

Failure to control excess fibrinolysis can result in a bleeding problem, and deficiencies of the naturally occurring anticoagulants may result in excess clot formation. A severe hemorrhagic disorder due to a deficiency of α^2-antiplasmin has responded to treatment with aminocaproic acid or tranexamic acid, both antifibrinolytic agents.[37] Congenital antithrombin III, protein S, and protein C deficiencies are associated with recurrent thrombosis and are usually controlled with oral anticoagulants.[37] Factor V Leiden, prothrombin G20210A, and other activated protein C resistance gene mutations will cause or add additional risk for thrombosis in proportion to their homozygous or heterozygous states.[72–74] Discontinuation of the anticoagulation is needed before an operation. The patients will require replacement therapy during the procedure and in the postoperative period until the anticoagulation can be restarted. Depending on the deficiency, antithrombin III concentrates or fresh frozen plasma can be used for replacement therapy.

RECOMBINANT ACTIVATED FACTOR VII

Recombinant activated factor VII (rFVIIa) was developed for the treatment of bleeding in patients with hemophilia A or B who had inhibitors, and was approved by the ultrasound Food and Drug Administration for this indication in 1999.[75-77] Good hemostasis with few side effects has been found in patients with intracranial hemorrhage, postlaparotomy and postpartum hemorrhage, hemorrhage into the gluteal muscles (as a complication after cholecystectomy), and for surgical prophylaxis for major and minor procedures.[78-80] Home treatment programs for those hemophilia patients who have inhibitors now use rFVIIa as front-line therapy for bleeding.[81] Children have a more rapid rate of clearance (elimination mean half-life, 1.32 hours in children vs 2.74 hours in adults).[82] They also seem to have fewer side effects with this treatment.[77,83] Although various dosages and schedules have been studied, initial recommended therapy in hemophilia A or B with inhibitors is 90 mg/kg intravenously every two hours until the bleeding is controlled.[84]

The off-label use of rFVIIa has been reported in therapy-resistant severe bleeding from other conditions such as congenital factor VII deficiency, chronic liver disease, and inherited platelet disorders.[85-87] Successes in patients without a known bleeding disorder who have trauma or postoperative hemorrhage also are described.[83,85,88,89] These reports should be interpreted with caution because rFVIIa is currently not the standard of care in any of these off-label uses and exceptional circumstances impelled its use. It is highly recommended that rFVIIa be administered under the supervision of a physician experienced in its use who can anticipate the risks and respond to the complications, particularly risks of thrombosis, which are reported in 1–3% of patients.[75,90,91] rFVIIa shows great promise in the emergency treatment of uncontrolled hemorrhage for many situations, and is becoming the standard of care for the treatment of intracranial hemorrage.[92]

SICKLE CELL DISEASE

Sickle cell disease (SCD) is the most common disorder identified by neonatal blood screening with approximately 2000 affected infants born in the ultrasound each year. Overall, the incidence of SCD exceeds that of most other serious genetic disorders, including cystic fibrosis and hemophilia.[93,94] SCD is caused by a genetic mutation that results in an amino acid change in the β-globin and the production of sickle hemoglobin (Hb S) instead of normal hemoglobin. The sickle cell gene, in combination with any other abnormal β-globin gene, results in SCD. There are many types of SCD. The most common include sickle cell anemia (Hb SS), the sickle β-thalassemias (Hb Sβ0 and Hb Sβ+), hemoglobin SC disease (Hb SC) and sickle cell/hereditary persistence of fetal hemoglobin

(S/HPFH). Sickle cell anemia is the most common and, in general, the most severe form of SCD. Sickle β0-thalassemia patients have clinical manifestations similar to patients with Hb SS disease. Sickle-C disease is the second most common form of SCD and generally has a more benign clinical course than does Hb SS or sickle β0-thalassemia. Sickle β+-thalassemia and S/HPFH patients also usually have a more benign clinical course. Patients with Hb SS disease and sickle β0-thalassemia generally have lower hemoglobin levels and present a greater risk under general anesthesia than do patients with Hb SC disease and sickle β+-thalassemia. Patients with S/HPFH may actually have hemoglobin levels that approach or are normal.

The red cell membrane is abnormal in patients with SCD, and the red cell life span is shortened by hemolysis. Intermittent episodes of vascular occlusion cause tissue ischemia, which results in acute and chronic organ dysfunction.[95] Consequently, patients with SCD require special considerations to prevent perioperative complications.

Because of the nature of the complications of SCD, people with this disorder are more likely than the general population to need an operation during their lifetime.[96] According to one study, the most common procedures were cholecystectomy; ear, nose, and throat procedures; orthopedic procedures; splenectomy; or herniorrhaphy.[97] Cholecystectomy, splenectomy, and orthopedic procedures are often required to treat complications of SCD.

Children with SCD can require surgical evaluation and treatment either because of complications of their SCD or unrelated processes. Moreover, symptoms associated with vaso-occlusive episodes, such as abdominal pain and bone pain with fever, may be difficult to distinguish from other pathologic processes, such as cholecystitis and osteomyelitis.

The differential diagnosis for acute abdominal pain in a patient with SCD includes an uncomplicated sickle cell acute pain episode ('crisis'), cholelithiasis, appendicitis, pancreatitis, ulcer, constipation, pneumonia, pericarditis, and splenic sequestration. Whereas 50% of painful crises include abdominal pain, they are usually associated with pain in the chest, back, and joints. However, although previous episodes of pain that are similar in character suggest an acute painful episode, the incidence of gallstones, peptic ulcer disease, and pyelonephritis is increased in these patients. Complications such as splenic or hepatic sequestration are unique problems in patients with this disease. Abdominal pain as a solitary symptom, especially when accompanied by fever, leukocytosis, and localized abdominal tenderness, is suggestive of pathology other than that which occurs with a sickle cell acute painful episode. A study that reviewed the presentation and management of acute abdominal conditions in adults with SCD suggested that a surgical condition is more likely if the pain does not resemble previous painful episodes and if no precipitating event is found.[98] Acute painful episodes were relieved within 48 hours with hydration and oxygen in 97% of patients, whereas no patient with a surgical disease achieved pain relief over the same period with these modalities. The leukocyte count and serum bilirubin were not helpful in establishing the correct diagnosis.

Vaso-occlusive episodes can also produce bone pain and fever, symptoms that are difficult to differentiate from those of osteomyelitis. The majority of bone pain in SCD is due to vaso-occlusion, but osteomyelitis secondary to *Salmonella* species or *Staphylococcus aureus* is not infrequent.[99,100] The presence of an immature leukocyte count or elevation of the sedimentation rate, C-reactive protein, or leukocyte alkaline phosphatase is suggestive of a bone infection and may be an indication for aspiration of the bone lesion. Radiographic studies including plain films, bone scan, or magnetic resonance imaging are generally less helpful but may be useful in arriving at the proper diagnosis when positive and combined with the appropriate clinical findings.[100]

Preoperative Assessment and Management

An optimal outcome requires careful preoperative, intraoperative, and postoperative management by a team consisting of a surgeon, anesthesiologist, and hematologist. Potential sickle cell-related complications include acute chest syndrome, pain episodes, hyperhemolytic crisis, aplastic crisis, alloimmunization with delayed transfusion reactions, and infections. The outcome of children with SCD requiring a procedure is improved by careful attention to the cardiorespiratory, hemodynamic, hydration, infectious, neurologic, and nutritional status of the child.[96,101–103] If possible, procedures should be performed when the child is in his or her usual state of health with regard to the SCD. Attention should be directed toward chronic manifestations of disease because predictors of a poor postoperative outcome include increased age, recent exacerbations of the disease, and preexisting infection and pregnancy.[104] Particular attention should be directed toward any recent history of acute chest syndrome, pneumonia, wheezing, and alloimmunization. Special efforts must be made to avoid perioperative hypoxia, hypothermia, acidosis, and dehydration because any of these events can result in serious morbidity.

Many centers perform preoperative transfusions with the aim of reducing the complications of surgery and anesthesia.[105] The largest study that examined the role of transfusion in the preoperative management of sickle cell anemia was a randomized study that compared exchange transfusion (with a goal of achieving an Hb value of >10 g/dL and Hb S value of <30%) versus simple transfusion (to achieve an Hb value of >10 g/dL).[97] This study concluded that not only was simple transfusion as effective as exchange transfusion in preventing perioperative complications, but it also provided a significantly lower rate of transfusion-related complications. The question about which procedures are safe to perform in children with SCD without preoperative transfusion remains controversial because there is a lack of randomized controlled trials to answer this question. However, transfusion only to increase the Hb level to 10 g/dL for major procedures and blood replacement for both profound anemia of less than 5 g/dL and intraoperative hemorrhage appear appropriate.[106] Several studies suggest that minor procedures can be safely undertaken without transfusion.[96,105,107]

Alloimmunization is minimized by using antigen-matched blood (matched for K, C, E, S, Fy, and Jk antigens).[103] Regardless of transfusion status, strong multidisciplinary collaboration is vital throughout the perioperative period.

Intraoperative Management

Anesthetic considerations are based more on the type of operation than on the presence of SCD because no single anesthetic technique has been shown to be the gold standard. However, regional anesthetic techniques may allow for opioid sparing postoperatively.[104] The goals of anesthetic management are to avoid factors that predispose the patient to sickling (e.g., hypoxemia, hypothermia, dehydration, and acidosis). Careful monitoring for hypoxia, hypothermia, acidosis, and dehydration is essential. Monitoring should include arterial blood gases, digital oxygen saturation, end-tidal carbon dioxide, temperature, electrocardiogram, blood pressure, and urine output.[104,108]

Postoperative Management

As with the preoperative and intraoperative periods, it is important to prevent hypothermia, hypoxia, and hypotension throughout the postoperative period. Before extubation, the patient should be awake and well-oxygenated. Once extubated, the patient should be carefully monitored with a digital oxygen saturation monitor and the pulmonary status critically assessed on a continuing basis. Continuous pulse oximetry should be provided in the early postoperative period. Assessment of fluid status should continue until the patient has resumed adequate oral intake and is able to maintain hydration without intravenous supplementation. All patients should receive incentive spirometry as well as adequate hydration and oxygenation.

Appropriate levels of analgesia (preferably by a continuous intravenous line and patient-controlled analgesia, if appropriate) should be provided so the patient is comfortable for ambulation and for vigorous pulmonary toilet. The patient must be monitored closely for the occurrence of pulmonary edema or atelectasis that can progress to acute chest syndrome.[109]

Specific Surgical Conditions

Adenotonsillectomy

Adenotonsillectomy is a fairly common procedure in children with SCD. Adenotonsillar hypertrophy, which may be associated with early functional hyposplenism and obstructive sleep apnea (OSA) secondary to enlarged adenoids, occurs somewhat frequently.[96,110,111] As with other types of surgery, preoperative transfusions should be performed before operation.[112] Clinicians should be aware that postoperative complications may be greater in patients who are younger or have OSA.[96,113]

Cholelithiasis and Cholecystectomy

Abdominal operations such as cholecystectomy and splenectomy are the most frequent abdominal procedures in patients with SCD.[96,106] Currently, there is no clear consensus regarding the appropriate management for SCD children who have cholelithiasis. The reported prevalence of cholelithiasis varies from 4–55%.[114,115] This wide variation is dependent on the ages of the study population and the diagnostic modalities used.[116] We routinely screen symptomatic children with ultrasonography and serum studies (e.g., total and direct bilirubin, serum glutamic-oxaloacetic transaminase, serum glutamate-pyruvate transaminase, alkaline phosphatase, and γ-glutamyl-transpeptidase). It is our practice to screen all SCD children for gallstones no later than age 12.

A child with SCD and symptomatic cholelithiasis should undergo cholecystectomy after appropriate preoperative preparation to avoid the increased morbidity of an emergency operation on an unprepared patient.[116–121] If indicated, intraoperative cholangiography can be performed to assess for common duct stones.[122]

The utility of laparoscopic cholecystectomy in SCD was first reported in 1990.[123] Since that time, laparoscopic cholecystectomy has been performed with increasing frequency in children with SCD.[116,124–127] The advantages of laparoscopic cholecystectomy over open cholecystectomy are decreased pain, earlier feeding, earlier discharge, earlier return to school, and improved cosmesis. The presence of common duct stones at times complicates the laparoscopic approach and may require conversion to an open operation for removal. At present, the role of extracorporeal shock wave lithotripsy as a palliative therapeutic modality is uncertain.

Splenic Sequestration and Splenectomy

Before the advent of routine newborn screening for hemoglobinopathies, acute splenic sequestration was the second most common cause of mortality in children younger than age 5 years with sickle cell anemia.[128] Splenic sequestration classically was first seen with the acute onset of pallor and listlessness, a precipitate decrease in hemoglobin, thrombocytopenia, and massive splenomegaly.[129] It now appears that parental education along with earlier recognition and immediate treatment with volume support (including red blood cell transfusions) has resulted in significantly decreased mortality for this condition. It is rare for an otherwise uncomplicated patient with Hb SS disease who is older than 6 years of age to develop acute splenic sequestration syndrome. However, patients with Hb SC and sickle β+-thalassemia disease can experience splenic sequestration at an older age.[130]

The management of the SCD child with splenic sequestration can be difficult. The rate of recurrent splenic sequestration is high and greatly influences subsequent management, which may be divided into observation only, chronic transfusion, and splenectomy. Indications for these approaches are not clearly defined.[103] The benefit of splenectomy must be balanced with the increased risk of overwhelming bacterial sepsis in the younger asplenic SCD patient.[103,131] Partial splenectomy[132,133] and, especially, laparoscopic splenectomy[134] are being performed more commonly as the number of experienced practitioners grows.

REFERENCES

1. Thompson AR, Harker LA. Manual of Hemostasis and Thrombosis, 3rd ed. Philadelphia: FA Davis; 1983.
2. Moncada S, Gryglewski R, Bunting S, et al. An enzyme isolated from arteries transforms prostaglandin endoperoxides to an unstable substance that inhibits platelet aggregation. Nature 1976;263:663–5.
3. Stern D, Nawroth P, Handley D, et al. An endothelial cell-dependent pathway of coagulation. Proc Natl Acad Sci U S A 1985;82:2523–7.
4. Esmon C. Blood coagulation. In: Nathan D, Orkin S, editors. Nathan and Oski's Hematology of Infancy and Childhood. Philadelphia: WB Saunders; 1998. p. 1532.
5. Saito H. Normal hemostatic mechanisms. In: Ratnoff O, Forbes C, editors. Disorders of Hemostasis. 2nd ed. Philadelphia: WB Saunders; 1996. p. 23–52.
6. George JN, Nurden AT, Phillips DR. Molecular defects in interactions of platelets with the vessel wall. N Engl J Med 1984;311:1084–98.
7. Marcus A. Platelets and their disorders. In: Ratnoff OD, Forbes CD, editors. Disorders of Hemostasis. 3rd ed. Philadelphia: WB Saunders; 1996.
8. Turrito V, Baumgartner H. Platelet-surface interactions. In: Coleman R, Hirsh J, Marder V, editors. Hemostasis and Thrombosis: Basic Principles and Clinical Practice. 2nd ed. Philadelphia, JB: Lippincott; 1987. p. 555.
9. Nurden AT, Didry D, Rosa JP. Molecular defects of platelets in Bernard-Soulier syndrome. Blood Cells 1983;9:333–58.
10. Castaman G, Federici AB, Rodeghiero F, et al. Von Willebrand's disease in the year 2003: Towards the complete identification of gene defects for correct diagnosis and treatment. Haematologica 2003;88:94–108.
11. Sadler J. A revised classification of von Willebrand disease. Thromb Haemost 1994;71:520–5.
12. Tuddenham EG. Von Willebrand factor and its disorders: An overview of recent molecular studies. Blood Rev 1989;3:251–62.
13. Lisman T, Weeterings C, de Groot P. Platelet aggregation: Involvement of thrombin and fibrin(ogen). Front Biosci 2005;10:2504–17.
14. Coleman R, Walsh P. Mechanisms of platelet aggregation. In: Coleman R, Hirsh J, Marder V, editors. Hemostasis and Thrombosis: Basic Principles and Clinical Practice. 2nd ed. Philadelphia, JB: Lippincott; 1987. p. 594.
15. Mackie IJ, Bull HA. Normal haemostasis and its regulation. Blood Rev 1989;3:237–50.
16. Lorand L, Losowsky MS, Miloszewski KJ. Human factor XIII: Fibrin-stabilizing factor. Prog Hemost Thromb 1980;5:245–90.
17. Rosenberg RD, Rosenberg JS. Natural anticoagulant mechanisms. J Clin Invest 1984;74:1–6.
18. Rodeghiero F, Tosetto A, Castaman G. How to estimate bleeding risk in mild bleeding disorders. J Thromb Haemost 2007;5(Suppl 1):157–66.
19. Bidlingmaier C, Sax F, Treutwein J, et al. The PTT is not enough—Preoperative coagulation screening in children. J Thromb Haemost 2007;5(Suppl 2):P-S-221.
20. Greaves M, Watson HG. Approach to the diagnosis and management of mild bleeding disorders. J Thromb Haemost 2007;5(Suppl 1):167–74.
21. Shaw PH, Reynolds S, Gunawardena S, et al. The prevalence of bleeding disorders among healthy pediatric patients with abnormal preprocedural coagulation studies. J Pediatr Hematol Oncol 2008;30:135–41.
22. Rapaport SI. Preoperative hemostatic evaluation: Which tests, if any? Blood 1983;61:229–31.
23. Sramek A, Eikenboom JC, Briet E, et al. Usefulness of patient interview in bleeding disorders. Arch Intern Med 1995;155:1409–15.
24. Rodeghiero F, Castaman G, Tosetto A, et al. The discriminate power of bleeding history for the diagnosis of type 1 von Willebrand disease: An international, multicenter study. J Thromb Haemost 2005;3:2619–26.
25. Anwar R, Minford A, Gallivan L, et al. Delayed umbilical bleeding—a presenting feature for factor XIII deficiency: Clinical features, genetics, and management. Pediatrics 2002;109:e32.

26. Shen YM, Frenkel EP. Acquired platelet dysfunction. Hematol Oncol Clin North Am 2007;21:647–61.vi

27. George JNM, Shattil SJM. The clinical importance of acquired abnormalities of platelet function. N Engl J Med 1991; 324:27–39.

28. Acosta M, Edwards R, Jaffee IM, et al. A practical approach to pediatric patients referred with an abnormal coagulation profile. Arch Pathol Lab Med 2005;129:1011–16.

29. Merck Manual Online Series: Thrombocytopenia and Platelet Dysfunction. In: Porter R, editor. Hematology and Oncology. Whitehouse Station, NJ: Merck & Co; 2008.

30. Kam PC. Anaesthetic management of a patient with thrombocytopenia. Curr Opin Anaesthesiol 2008;21:369–74.

31. Harrison P. The role of PFA-100 testing in the investigation and management of haemostatic defects in children and adults. Br J Haematol 2005;130:3–10.

32. Koscielny J, von Tempelhoff GF, Ziemer S, et al. A practical concept for preoperative management of patients with impaired primary hemostasis. Clin Appl Thromb Hemost 2004;10: 155–66.

33. Kamal AH, Tefferi A, Pruthi RK. How to interpret and pursue an abnormal prothrombin time, activated partial thromboplastin time, and bleeding time in adults. Mayo Clin Proc 2007;82:864–73.

34. Wicklund B. The bleeding child: Congenital and acquired disorders. In: Hillyer C, Strauss R, Luban N, editors. Handbook of Pediatric Transfusion Medicine. Boston: Elsevier; 2004.

35. Israels S. Factor XIII deficiency. emedicine, Omaha: WebMD; 2007.

36. Goodnight S, Hathaway W, editors. Disorders of Hemostasis and Thrombosis. New York: McGraw-Hill; 2001.

37. Lusher J. Approach to the bleeding patient. In: Nathan D, Orkin S, editors. Nathan and Oski's Hematology of Infancy and Childhood. 5th ed. Philadelphia, WB: Saunders; 1998.

38. Shapiro SS, Thiagarajan P. Lupus anticoagulants. Prog Hemost Thromb 1982;6:263–85.

39. Levi M, Ten Cate H. Disseminated intravascular coagulation. N Engl J Med 1999;341:586–92.

40. Pivalizza E, Pivalizza P, Gottschalk L, et al. Celite-Activated Thrombelastography in Children. J Clin Anesth 2001;1:20–3.

41. Soucie J, Evatt B, Jackson D. Occurrence of hemophilia in the United States. The Hemophilia Surveillance System Project Investigators. Am J Hematol 1998;59:288–94.

42. Pool JG, Gershgold EJ, Pappenhagen AR. High-potency antihaemophilic factor concentrate prepared from cryoglobulin precipitate. Nature 1964;203:312.

43. Kasper CK, Lusher JM. Recent evolution of clotting factor concentrates for hemophilia A and B. Transfusion Practices Committee. Transfusion 1993;33:422–34.

44. Mannucci PM, Chediak J. Treatment of von Willebrand disease with a high-purity factor VIII/von Willebrand factor concentrate: A prospective, multicenter study. Blood 2002;99:450–6.

45. Levine PH. Delivery of health care in hemophilia. Ann N Y Acad Sci 1975;240:201–7.

46. Hilgartner MW. Factor Replacement Therapy. In: Hilgartner MW, Pochedly C, editors. Hemophilia in the Child and Adult. New York: Raven Press; 1989. p. 1–26.

47. Soucie JM, Nuss R, Evatt B, et al. Mortality among males with hemophilia: Relations with source of medical care. The Hemophilia Surveillance System Project Investigators. Blood 2000; 96:437–42.

48. Report on the Universal Data Collection Program. Atlanta: Centers for Disease Control and Prevention; 2005.

49. Kernoff PB, Lee CA, Karayiannis P, et al. High risk of non-A non-B hepatitis after a first exposure to volunteer or commercial clotting factor concentrates: Effects of prophylactic immune serum globulin. Br J Haematol 1985;60:469–79.

50. Troisi CL, Hollinger FB, Hoots WK, et al. A multicenter study of viral hepatitis in a United States hemophilic population. Blood 1993;81:412–18.

51. MASAC Recommendations Concerning the Treatment of Hemophilia and Other Bleeding Disorders. National Hemophilia Foundation; revised.

52. Mei B, Pan C, et al. Rational design of a fully active, long-acting PEGylated factor VIII for hemophilia A treatment. Blood 2010;116(2):270–9.

53. Lusher JM, Warrier I. Hemophilia. Pediatr Rev 1991;12: 275–81.

54. Kasper CK, Boylen AL, Ewing NP, et al. Hematologic management of hemophilia A for surgery. JAMA 1985;253: 1279–83.

55. Manco-Johnson MJ, Abshire TC, Shapiro AD, et al. Prophylaxis versus episodic treatment to prevent joint disease in boys with severe hemophilia. N Engl J Med 2007;357:535.

56. Scharf R, Kucharski W, Nowak T. Surgery in hemophilia A patients with factor VIII inhibitor: 10-year experience. World J Surg 1996;20:1171–81.

57. Jimenez-Yuste V, Rodriguez-Merchan EC, Alvarez MT, et al. Controversies and challenges in elective orthopedic surgery in patients with hemophilia and inhibitors. Semin Hematol 2008;45:S64–7.

58. Montgomery RE. Hemophilia and von Willebrand disease. In: Nathan D, Orkin S, editors. Nathan and Oski's Hematology of Infancy and Childhood. 6th ed. Philadelphia: WB Saunders; 2003. p. 1547.

59. Scharrer I. The need for highly purified products to treat hemophilia B. Acta Haematol 1995;94(Suppl 1):2–7.

60. Shapiro AD, Di Paola J, Cohen A, et al. The safety and efficacy of recombinant human blood coagulation factor IX in previously untreated patients with severe or moderately severe hemophilia B. Blood 2005;105:518–25.

61. Kobrinsky N. Management of hemophilia during surgery. In: Forbes C, Aledort L, Madhok R, editors. Hemophilia. Oxford: Chapman & Hall; 1997. p. 242.

62. Shapiro AD. Coagulation factor concentrates. In: Goodnight S, Hathaway W, editors. Disorders of Hemostasis and Thrombosis: A Clinical Guide. New York: McGraw-Hill; 2001. p. 505.

63. Andrew M, Paes B, Milner R, et al. Development of the human coagulation system in the full-term infant. Blood 1987;70: 165–72.

64. Gibson B. Normal and disordered coagulation. In: Hann I, Gibson B, Letsky E, editors. Fetal and Neonatal Haematology. London: Bailliere Tindall; 1991. p. 123.

65. Bick RL. Disseminated intravascular coagulation and related syndromes: A clinical review. Semin Thromb Hemost 1988;14: 299–338.

66. van Beek EJ, von der Mohlen MA, ten Cate JW, et al. Antithrombin III concentrate in the treatment of DIC: A retrospective follow-up study. Neth J Med 1994;45:206–10.

67. Albisetti M, Andrew M. Hemostatic abnormalities. In: de Alarcon P, Werner E, editors. Neonatal Hematology. Cambridge: Cambridge University Press; 2005. p. 310–48.

68. George JN. Diagnosis, clinical course, and management of idiopathic thrombocytopenic purpura. Curr Opin Hematol 1996;3:335–40.

69. Jackson D. Management of thrombocytopenia. In: Coleman R, Hirsh J, Marder V, editors. Hemostasis and Thrombosis: Basic Principles and Clinical Practice. 2nd ed. Philadelphia: JB Lippincott; 1987. p. 530.

70. Salzman E. Hemostatic problems in surgical patients. In: Coleman R, Hirsh J, Marder V, editors. Hemostasis and Thrombosis: Basic Principles and Clinical Practice. 2nd ed. Philadelphia, JB: Lippincott; 1987.

71. Greenberg C. Hemostasis: Pathophysiology and management of clinical disorders. In: Sabiston DJ, editor. Sabiston's Essentials of Surgery. Philadelphia: WB Saunders; 1987. p. 79.

72. Bick RL. Prothrombin G20210A mutation, antithrombin, heparin co-factor II, protein C, and protein S defects. Hematol Oncol Clin North Am 2003;17:9–36.

73. Nicolaes GA, Dahlback B. Activated protein C resistance (FV[Leiden]) and thrombosis: Factor V mutations causing hypercoagulable states. Hematol Oncol Clin North Am 2003;17: 37–61, vi.

74. Whiteman T, Hassouna HI. Hypercoagulable states. Hematol Oncol Clin North Am 2000;14:355–77.viii.

75. Hay CR, Negrier C, Ludlam CA. The treatment of bleeding in acquired haemophilia with recombinant factor VIIa: A multicentre study. Thromb Haemost 1997;78:1463–7.

76. Hedner U. Recombinant coagulation factor VIIa: From the concept to clinical application in hemophilia treatment in 2000. Semin Thromb Hemost 2000;26:363–6.

77. Hedner U, Bjoern S, Bernvil SS, et al. Clinical experience with human plasma-derived factor VIIa in patients with hemophilia A and high-titer inhibitors. Haemostasis 1989;19:335–43.

78. Arkin S, Cooper HA, Hutter JJ, et al. Activated recombinant human coagulation factor VII therapy for intracranial hemorrhage in patients with hemophilia A or B with inhibitors: Results of the NovoSeven emergency-use program. Haemostasis 1998;28: 93–8.

79. Liebman HA, Chediak J, Fink KI, et al. Activated recombinant human coagulation factor VII (rFVIIa) therapy for abdominal bleeding in patients with inhibitory antibodies to factor VIII. Am J Hematol 2000;63:109–13.

80. Shapiro AD, Gilchrist GS, Hoots WK, et al. Prospective, randomised trial of two doses of rFVIIa (NovoSeven) in haemophilia patients with inhibitors undergoing surgery. Thromb Haemost 1998;80:773–8.

81. Santagostino E, Gringeri A, Mannucci PM. Home treatment with recombinant activated factor VII in patients with factor VIII inhibitors: The advantages of early intervention. Br J Haematol 1999;104:22–6.

82. Erhardtsen E. Pharmacokinetics of recombinant activated factor VII (rFVIIa). Semin Thromb Hemost 2000;26:385–91.

83. Lusher J, Ingerslev J, Roberts H, et al. Clinical experience with recombinant factor VIIa. Blood Coagul Fibrinolysis 1998; 9:119–28.

84. NovoSeven [package insert]. Princeton, NJ, Novo Nordisk, Inc., 2006.

85. Hedner U, Erhardtsen E. Potential role for rFVIIa in transfusion medicine. Transfusion 2002;42:114–24.

86. Mariani G, Testa MG, Di Paolantonio T, et al. Use of recombinant, activated factor VII in the treatment of congenital factor VII deficiencies. Vox Sang 1999;77:131–6.

87. Poon MC, d'Oiron R. Recombinant activated factor VII (Novo-Seven) treatment of platelet-related bleeding disorders. International Registry on Recombinant Factor VIIa and Congenital Platelet Disorders Group. Blood Coagul Fibrinolysis 2000; 11(Suppl 1):S55–68.

88. Martinowitz U, Kenet G, Segal E, et al. Recombinant activated factor VII for adjunctive hemorrhage control in trauma. J Trauma 2001;51:431–9.

89. McMullin NR, Kauvar DS, Currier HM, et al. The clinical and laboratory response to recombinant factor VIIA in trauma and surgical patients with acquired coagulopathy. Curr Surg 2006;63:246–51.

90. Mahmoud A, Al-Ruzzeh S, McKeague H, et al. Systemic venous thrombosis after recombinant factor VIIa in the control of bleeding after cardiac surgery. Tex Heart Inst J 2007;34:485–8.

91. O'Connell KA, Wood JJ, Wise RP, et al. Thromboembolic adverse events after use of recombinant human coagulation factor VIIa. JAMA 2006;295:293–8.

92. Broderick J, Connolly S, Feldmann E, et al. Guidelines for the Management of Spontaneous Intracerebral Hemorrhage in Adults. 2007 Update: A Guideline from the American Heart Association/American Stroke Association Stroke Council, High Blood Pressure Research Council, and the Quality of Care and Outcomes in Research Interdisciplinary Working Group; the American Academy of Neurology affirms the value of this guideline as an educational tool for neurologists. Stroke 2007;38:2001–23.

93. American Academy of Pediatrics: Health supervision for children with sickle cell disease. Pediatrics 2002;109:526–35.

94. (CORN) TCoRNfGS. National Newborn Screening Report—1992. New York, 1995.

95. Lane PA. Sickle cell disease. Pediatr Clin North Am 1996;43:639–64.

96. Buck J, Davies SC. Surgery in sickle cell disease. Hematol Oncol Clin North Am 2005;19:897–902.vii

97. Vichinsky EP, Haberkern CM, Neumayr L, et al. A comparison of conservative and aggressive transfusion regimens in the perioperative management of sickle cell disease. The Preoperative Transfusion in Sickle Cell Disease Study Group. N Engl J Med 1995;333:206–13.

98. Baumgartner F, Klein S. The presentation and management of the acute abdomen in the patient with sickle-cell anemia. Am Surg 1989;55:660–4.

99. Epps CH Jr, Bryant DD 3rd, Coles MJ, et al. Osteomyelitis in patients who have sickle-cell disease: Diagnosis and management. J Bone Joint Surg Am 1991;73:1281–94.

100. Chambers JB, Forsythe DA, Bertrand SL, et al. Retrospective review of osteoarticular infections in a pediatric sickle cell age group. J Pediatr Orthop 2000;20:682–5.

101. Sutton J, et al. Surgical management of patients with sickle cell syndromes. In: Mankad V, Moore R, editors. Sickle Cell Disease: Pathophysiology, Diagnosis, and Management. Westport, CT: Praeger; 1992. p. 364–86.

102. Ware RE, Filston HC. Surgical management of children with hemoglobinopathies. Surg Clin North Am 1992;72:1223–36.

103. Management of Sickle Cell Disease. 4th ed. NIH Publication No. 02–2117, 2002.

104. Haxby E, Flynn F, Bateman C. Anaesthesia for patients with sickle cell disease or other haemoglobinopathies. Anaesth Intensive Care Med 2007;8:217–19.

105. Amrolia PJ, Almeida A, Halsey C, et al. Therapeutic challenges in childhood sickle cell disease: I. Current and future treatment options. Br J Haematol 2003;120:725–36.

106. Koshy M, Weiner SJ, Miller ST, et al. Surgery and anesthesia in sickle cell disease. Cooperative Study of Sickle Cell Diseases. Blood 1995;86:3676–84.

107. Hirst C, Williamson L. Preoperative blood transfusions for sickle cell disease. Cochrane Database Syst Rev 2001. CD003149.

108. Mankad A. Anesthetic management of patients with sickle cell disease. In: Mankad V, Moore R, editors. Sickle Cell Disease: Pathophysiology, Diagnosis, and Management. Westport, CT: Praeger; 1992. p. 351–63.

109. Castro O, Brambilla DJ, Thorington B, et al. The acute chest syndrome in sickle cell disease: Incidence and risk factors. The Cooperative Study of Sickle Cell Disease. Blood 1994;84:643–9.

110. Kemp JS. Obstructive sleep apnea and sickle cell disease. J Pediatr Hematol Oncol 1996;18:104–5.

111. Wali YA, al Okbi H, al Abri R. A comparison of two transfusion regimens in the perioperative management of children with sickle cell disease undergoing adenotonsillectomy. Pediatr Hematol Oncol 2003;20:7–13.

112. Duke RL, Scott JP, Panepinto JA, et al. Perioperative management of sickle cell disease children undergoing adenotonsillectomy. Otolaryngol Head Neck Surg 2006;134:370–3.

113. Halvorson DJ, McKie V, McKie K, et al. Sickle cell disease and tonsillectomy. Preoperative management and postoperative complications. Arch Otolaryngol Head Neck Surg 1997;123: 689–92.

114. Lachman BS, Lazerson J, Starshak RJ, et al. The prevalence of cholelithiasis in sickle cell disease as diagnosed by ultrasound and cholecystography. Pediatrics 1979;64:601–3.

115. Sarnaik S, Slovis TL, Corbett DP, et al. Incidence of cholelithiasis in sickle cell anemia using the ultrasonic gray-scale technique. J Pediatr 1980;96:1005–8.

116. Suell MN, Horton TM, Dishop MK, et al. Outcomes for children with gallbladder abnormalities and sickle cell disease. J Pediatr 2004;145:617–21.

117. Haberkern CM, Neumayr LD, Orringer EP, et al. Cholecystectomy in sickle cell anemia patients: Perioperative outcome of 364 cases from the National Preoperative Transfusion Study. Preoperative Transfusion in Sickle Cell Disease Study Group. Blood 1997;89:1533–42.

118. Pappis CH, Galanakis S, Moussatos G, et al. Experience of splenectomy and cholecystectomy in children with chronic haemolytic anaemia. J Pediatr Surg 1989;24:543–6.

119. Stephens CG, Scott RB. Cholelithiasis in sickle cell anemia: Surgical or medical management. Arch Intern Med 1980;140: 648–51.

120. Ware R, Filston HC, Schultz WH, et al. Elective cholecystectomy in children with sickle hemoglobinopathies: Successful outcome using a preoperative transfusion regimen. Ann Surg 1988; 208:17–22.

121. Miltenburg DM, Schaffer R 3rd, Breslin T, et al. Changing indications for pediatric cholecystectomy. Pediatrics 2000;105: 1250–3.

122. Ware RE, Schultz WH, Filston HC, et al. Diagnosis and management of common bile duct stones in patients with sickle hemoglobinopathies. J Pediatr Surg 1992;27:572–5.

123. Dubois F, Icard P, Berthelot G, et al. Coelioscopic cholecystectomy: Preliminary report of 36 cases. Ann Surg 1990;211:60–2.

124. Gadacz TR, Talamini MA, Lillemoe KD, et al. Laparoscopic cholecystectomy. Surg Clin North Am 1990;70:1249–62.

125. Tagge EP, Othersen HB Jr, Jackson SM, et al. Impact of laparoscopic cholecystectomy on the management of cholelithiasis in children with sickle cell disease. J Pediatr Surg 1994;29:209–13.

126. Ware RE, Kinney TR, Casey JR, et al. Laparoscopic cholecystectomy in young patients with sickle hemoglobinopathies. J Pediatr 1992;120:58–61.

127. Curro G, Meo A, Ippolito D, et al. Asymptomatic cholelithiasis in children with sickle cell disease: Early or delayed cholecystectomy? Ann Surg 2007;245:126–9.

128. Gill FM, Sleeper LA, Weiner SJ, et al. Clinical events in the first decade in a cohort of infants with sickle cell disease. Cooperative Study of Sickle Cell Disease. Blood 1995;86:776–83.

129. Emond AM, Collis R, Darvill D, et al. Acute splenic sequestration in homozygous sickle cell disease: Natural history and management. J Pediatr 1985;107:201–6.

130. Aquino VM, Norvell JM, Buchanan GR. Acute splenic complications in children with sickle cell-hemoglobin C disease. J Pediatr 1997;130:961–5.

131. Pegelow CH, Wilson B, Overturf GD, et al. Infection in splenectomized sickle cell disease patients. Clin Pediatr 1980;19:102–5.

132. Nouri A, de Montalembert M, Revillon Y, et al. Partial splenectomy in sickle cell syndromes. Arch Dis Child 1991;66:1070–2.

133. Svarch E, Vilorio P, Nordet I, et al. Partial splenectomy in children with sickle cell disease and repeated episodes of splenic sequestration. Hemoglobin 1996;20:393–400.

134. Hicks BA, Thompson WR, Rogers ZR, et al. Laparoscopic splenectomy in childhood hematologic disorders. J Laparoendosc Surg 1996;6(Suppl 1):S31–4.

CHAPTER 6

Extracorporeal Membrane Oxygenation

Alejandro V. Garcia • Arul S. Thirumoorthi • Charles J.H. Stolar

Extracorporeal membrane oxygenation (ECMO) is a life-saving technology that employs partial heart/lung bypass for extended periods. It provides gas exchange and perfusion for patients with acute, reversible cardiac or respiratory failure. This affords the patient's cardiopulmonary system a time to 'rest,' during which the patient is spared the deleterious effects of high airway pressure, high FiO_2, traumatic mechanical ventilation, and impaired perfusion. As of 2011, the Extracorporeal Life Support Organization (ELSO) has registered approximately 40,000 neonates and children treated with ECMO for a variety of cardiopulmonary disorders. The number of centers providing extracorporeal support and reporting to ELSO continues to increase along with the total number of cases.[1]

HISTORY

The initial effort to develop extracorporeal bypass came from cardiac surgeons. Their goal was to correct intracardiac lesions and, therefore, they needed to arrest the heart, divert and oxygenate the blood, and perfuse the patient so that repair could be performed. The first cardiopulmonary bypass circuits involved cross circulation between the patient and another subject (usually the patient's mother or father) acting as both the pump and the oxygenator.[2]

The first attempts at establishing cardiopulmonary bypass and oxygenation by complete artificial circuitry were constructed with disk-and-bubble oxygenators, and were limited because of hemolysis encountered by direct mixing of oxygen and blood. The discovery of heparin and the development of semipermeable membranes (silicone rubber) capable of supporting gas exchange by diffusion were major advancements toward the development of ECMO.[3] During the 1960s and early 1970s, this silicone membrane was configured into a number of oxygenator models.[4–7]

In 1972, the first successful use of prolonged cardiopulmonary bypass was reported.[8] The patient had sustained a ruptured aorta following a motorcycle accident. Venoarterial extracorporeal bypass support was maintained for three days. A multicenter prospective randomized trial sponsored by the National Heart, Lung, and Blood Institute (a branch of the National Institutes of Health) studied the efficacy of ECMO for adult respiratory distress syndrome. In 1979, they concluded that the use of ECMO had no advantage over conventional mechanical ventilation, and the trial was stopped before completion.[9] However, Bartlett and colleagues noted that all of the patients in the study had irreversible pulmonary fibrosis before the initiation of ECMO. In 1976, they reported the first series of infants with ECMO.[10] Six (43%) of 14 babies with respiratory distress syndrome survived. Many of these infants were premature and weighed less than 2 kg. In addition, 22 patients with meconium aspiration syndrome had a 70% survival rate, although these neonates tended to be larger.

Since then, despite study design issues, three randomized controlled trials and a number of retrospective published reports have confirmed the efficacy of ECMO over conventional mechanical ventilation.[11–18] By 1996, 113 centers had ECMO programs registered with ELSO.[1] Over the next two decades, improvements in technology, a better understanding of the pathophysiology of pulmonary failure, and a greater experience using ECMO have contributed to improved outcomes for infants with respiratory failure. In 2003, the University of Michigan reported an association between ECMO volume and an observed reduction in neonatal mortality seen in that state between 1980 and 1999.[19]

ELSO, formed in 1989, is a collaboration of health care professionals and scientists with an interest in ECMO. The organization provides the medical community with guidelines, training manuals and courses, and a forum in which interested individuals can meet and discuss the future of extracorporeal life support. The group also provides a registry to investigators for the collection of data from most centers with an ECMO program throughout the world. This database provides valuable information for analysis of this life-saving biotechnology.[20,21]

CLINICAL APPLICATIONS

Neonates are the patients who benefit most from ECMO. Cardiopulmonary failure in this population secondary to meconium aspiration syndrome (MAS), congenital diaphragmatic hernia (CDH), persistent pulmonary hypertension of the newborn (PPHN), and congenital cardiac disease are the most common pathophysiologic processes requiring ECMO. In children, the most common disorders treated with ECMO are viral and bacterial pneumonia, acute respiratory distress syndrome (ARDS), acute respiratory failure (non-ARDS), sepsis, and cardiac disease. Treatment of patients who cannot be weaned from bypass after cardiac surgery and patients with end-stage ventricular failure needing a bridge to heart transplantation are areas where ECMO use is increasing.[1,22,23] Some less frequently used indications for ECMO include respiratory failure secondary to smoke inhalation,[24] severe asthma,[25] rewarming of hypercoagulopathic/hypothermic trauma patients,[26] and maintenance of an organ donor pending liver allograft harvest and transplantation.[27]

PATHOPHYSIOLOGY OF NEWBORN PULMONARY HYPERTENSION

Pulmonary vascular resistance (PVR) is the hallmark and driving force of the fetal circulation. Normal fetal circulation is characterized by PVR that exceeds systemic pressures, resulting in higher right-sided heart pressures and, therefore, preferential right-to-left blood flow. The fetal umbilical vein carries oxygenated blood from the placenta to the inferior vena cava via the ductus venosus. Because of the high PVR, the majority of the blood that reaches the right atrium from the inferior vena cava is directed to the left atrium through the foramen ovale. The superior vena cava delivers deoxygenated blood to the right atrium that is preferentially directed to the right ventricle and pulmonary artery. This blood then takes the path of least resistance and shunts from the main pulmonary artery directly to the descending aorta via the ductus arteriosus, bypassing the pulmonary vascular bed and the left side of the heart. Therefore, as a consequence of these anatomic right-to-left shunts, the lungs are almost completely bypassed during fetal circulation.

At birth, with the infant's initial breath, the alveoli distend and begin to fill with air. This is paralleled by relaxation of the muscular arterioles of the pulmonary circulation and the expansion of the pulmonary vascular bed. This leads to a rapid drop in PVR to below systemic levels that causes the left atrial pressure to become higher than the right atrial pressure. The result is closure of the foramen ovale, and all venous blood flows from the right atrium to the right ventricle and into the pulmonary artery. The ductus arteriosus also closes at this time. Therefore, all fetal right-to-left circulation ceases, completing separation of the pulmonary and systemic circulations. Anatomic closure of these structures takes several days to weeks. Thus, maintaining systemic pressure greater than the pulmonary circulation is vital to sustaining normal circulation.

Failure of the transition from fetal circulation to newborn circulation is described as PPHN or persistent fetal circulation (PFC).[28] Clinically, PPHN is characterized by hypoxemia out of proportion to pulmonary parenchymal or anatomic disease. In hypoxic fetuses and infants, the proliferation of smooth muscle in the arterioles may extend far beyond the terminal bronchioles, resulting in thickened and more reactive vessels. In response to hypoxia, these vessels undergo significant self-perpetuating vasoconstriction. Although sometimes idiopathic, PPHN can occur secondary to a number of disease processes such as MAS, CDH, polycythemia, and sepsis.

Treatment for PPHN is directed at decreasing right-to-left shunting and increasing pulmonary blood flow. Previously, most newborns were treated with hyperventilation, induction of alkalosis, neuromuscular blockade, and sedation. Unfortunately, these therapies have not reduced morbidity, mortality, or the need for ECMO. ECMO allows for the interruption of the hypoxia-induced negative cycle of increased smooth muscle tone and vasoconstriction. ECMO provides richly oxygenated blood and allows the pulmonary blood pressure to return to normal subsystemic values without the iatrogenic complications encumbered by overly aggressive 'conventional' therapy.

Data recommending permissive hypercapnia and spontaneous respirations as principles of treatment for these children have been reported.[29] Hyperventilation and neuromuscular blockade are not part of the treatment strategy. This strategy has decreased morbidity, mortality, and the need for ECMO in several centers.

PATIENT SELECTION CRITERIA

The selection of patients as potential ECMO candidates continues to remain controversial. The selection criteria are based on data from multiple institutions, patient safety, and mechanical limitations related to the equipment. The risk of performing an invasive procedure that requires heparinization of a critically ill infant or child must be weighed against the predicted mortality of the patient with conventional therapy alone. A predictive mortality of greater than 80% after exhausting all conventional therapies is the criterion most institutions follow to select patients for ECMO. These criteria are subjective and will vary between facilities based on local clinical experience and available technologies. All ECMO centers must develop their own criteria and continually evaluate their patient selection based on ongoing outcomes data.

Recommended pre-ECMO studies are listed in Box 6-1. The definition of 'conventional therapy' is not consistent for each indication. Nevertheless, ECMO is indicated when (1) there is a reversible disease process; (2) the ventilator treatment is causing more harm than good; and (3) tissue oxygenation requirements are not being met. A discussion of generally accepted selection criteria for using neonatal ECMO follows.

BOX 6-1	Recommended Pre-ECMO Studies

Head ultrasonography
Cardiac echocardiography
Chest radiography
Complete blood cell count, with platelets
Type and cross-match of blood
Electrolytes, calcium
Coagulation studies (prothrombin time, partial thromboplastin time, fibrinogen, fibrin degradation products)
Serial arterial blood gas analysis

Reversible Cardiopulmonary Disorders

The underlying principle of ECMO relies on the premise that the patient has a reversible disease process that can be corrected with either therapy (including the possibility of organ transplantation) or 'rest', and that this reversal will occur in a relatively short period of time. Prolonged exposure to high-pressure mechanical ventilation with high concentrations of oxygen can have a traumatic effect on the newborn's lungs and frequently leads to the development of bronchopulmonary dysplasia (BPD).[30] It has been suggested that BPD can result from high levels of ventilatory support for as little as four days or less.[31] The pulmonary dysfunction that follows barotrauma and oxygen toxicity associated with mechanical ventilation typically requires weeks to months to resolve. Therefore, patients who have been ventilated for a long time and in whom lung injury has developed are not amenable to a short course of therapy with ECMO. Most ECMO centers will not accept patients who have had more than ten to 14 days of mechanical ventilation, owing to the high probability of established, irreversible pulmonary dysfunction.

Echocardiography should be performed on every patient being considered for ECMO to determine cardiac anatomy and function. Treatable conditions such as total anomalous pulmonary venous return and transposition of the great vessels, which may masquerade initially as pulmonary failure, can be surgically corrected but may require ECMO resuscitation initially. Infants with correctable cardiac disease should be considered on an individual basis. Also, ECMO is an excellent bridge to cardiac and lung transplantation.

Coexisting Anomalies

Every effort should be made to establish a clear diagnosis before the initiation of ECMO. Infants with anomalies incompatible with life do not benefit from ECMO (i.e., trisomy 13 or 18). ECMO is not a resource that is intended to delay an inevitable death. Many lethal pulmonary conditions, such as overwhelming pulmonary hypoplasia, congenital alveolar proteinosis, and alveolar capillary dysplasia, may present as reversible conditions but are considered lethal.[32]

Gestational Age

The gestational age of an ECMO patient should be at least 34 to 35 weeks. In the early experience with ECMO, significant morbidity and mortality related to intracranial hemorrhage (ICH) was associated with premature infants (<34 weeks' gestation).[33] Despite modifications in the ECMO technique over the past two decades, premature infants continue to be at risk for ICH. In preterm infants, ependymal cells within the brain are not fully developed, thus making these infants susceptible to hemorrhage. Systemic heparinization necessary to maintain a thrombus-free circuit adds to this risk.

Birth Weight

Technical considerations and limitation of cannula size restrict ECMO candidates to infants weighing at least 2000 g. The smallest single-lumen ECMO cannula is 8 French, and flow through a tube is proportional to the fourth power of the radius. Small veins permit only small cannulas, resulting in flow that will be reduced by a power of four. Neonates who weigh less than 2 kg provide technical challenges in cannulation and in maintaining adequate blood flow through the small catheters.

Bleeding Complications

Infants with ongoing, uncontrollable bleeding or an uncorrectable bleeding diathesis pose a relative contraindication to ECMO.[20] Any coagulopathy should be corrected before initiating ECMO because the need for continuous systemic heparinization adds an unacceptable risk of bleeding.

Intracranial Hemorrhage

As a general rule, candidates for ECMO should not have had an ICH. A preexisting ICH may be exacerbated by the use of heparin and the unavoidable alterations in cerebral blood flow while receiving ECMO. Patients with small intraventricular hemorrhages (grade I) or small intraparenchymal hemorrhage can be successfully treated on ECMO by maintaining a lower than optimal activated clotting time in the range of 180–200 seconds. These patients should be closely observed for extension of the intracranial bleeding. Patients posing a particularly high risk for ICH are those with a previous ICH, a cerebral infarct, prematurity, coagulopathy, ischemic central nervous system injury, or sepsis. Consideration of these patients for ECMO should be individualized.[32]

Failure of Medical Management

ECMO candidates are expected to have a reversible cardiopulmonary disease process, with a predictive mortality of >80–90% with all available modalities short of ECMO. As different institutions have varying technical capabilities, opinions and expertise, 'optimal' medical management is a subjective term that varies widely. Vasoconstrictive agents, inotropic agents, pulmonary vascular smooth muscle relaxants, sedatives, and analgesics are all pharmacologic agents that are part of the medical management. Ventilatory management usually begins with conventional support but may also include the administration of surfactant, nitric oxide, inverse inspiration/expiration (I:E) ratios, or high-frequency ventilation. Ventilator and respiratory care strategies that incur significant barotrauma and other morbidity should be avoided.

With recent innovations in medical management, ECMO use has been obviated in patients who otherwise meet ECMO criteria. These innovations include the use of permissive hypercapnia with spontaneous ventilation, avoidance of muscle paralysis, and the avoidance of chest tubes. In 1978, the Children's Hospital of New York initiated a nontraditional approach to the management of patients with PPHN, which has been successfully extended to infants with CDH.[34] Hyperventilation, hyperoxia, and muscle relaxants were not used, and permissive hypercapnia in conjunction with spontaneous ventilation was emphasized. Low-pressure ventilator settings were used and a persistent $PaCO_2$ of 50–60 mmHg and a PaO_2 of 50-70 mmHg were allowed. With careful attention to maintaining a preductal oxygen saturation greater than 90% or PaO_2 of 60 mmHg or greater, 15 infants who met ECMO criteria with PPHN and in severe respiratory failure were initially treated with this approach and survived without ECMO.

Risk Assessment

Because of the invasive nature of ECMO, and the potentially life-threatening complications, investigators have worked to develop an objective set of criteria to predict which infants will have an 80% mortality without ECMO. The two most commonly used measurements for neonatal respiratory failure are the alveolar-arterial oxygen gradient ($[A – a]DO_2$) and the oxygenation index (OI), which are calculated as follows:

$$(A-a)DO_2 = (P_{atm} - 47)(FiO_2) - [(PaCO_2)/0.8] - PaO_2$$

where P_{atm} is the atmospheric pressure and FiO_2 is the inspired concentration of oxygen.

$$OI = MAP \times FiO_2 \times 100/PaO_2$$

where MAP is the mean airway pressure.

Although criteria for ECMO varies from institution and by diagnosis, it is generally accepted that, in the setting of optimal management, an $(A-a)DO_2$ greater than 625 mmHg for more than four hours, or an $(A-a)DO_2$ greater than 600 mmHg for more than 12 hours, or an OI of greater than 40 establishes both a relatively sensitive and specific predictor of mortality. Other criteria used by many institutions include a preductal PaO_2 less than 35–50 mmHg for two to 12 hours or a pH of less than 7.25 for at least two hours along with intractable hypotension. These are sustained values measured over a period of time and are not accurate predictors of mortality.[14,20,35–37] Patients with CDH are in their own category, and criteria for this disease are discussed later in this chapter.

Older infants and children do not have as well-defined criteria for high mortality risk. The ventilation index is determined by the following:

$$Respiratory\ rate \times PaCO_2 \times Peak\ inspiratory\ pressure\ /\ 1000$$

The combination of a ventilation index greater than 40 and an OI more than 40 correlates with a 77% mortality.[38] A mortality of 81% is associated with an $(A-a)DO_2$ greater than 580 mmHg and a peak inspiratory pressure of 40 cmH_2O.[38] Indications for support in patients with cardiac pathology are based on clinical signs such as hypotension despite the administration of inotropes or volume resuscitation, oliguria (urine output < 0.5 mL/kg/h), and decreased peripheral perfusion.

Congenital Diaphragmatic Hernia

Of most interest to pediatric surgeons are neonates with abdominal viscera in the thoracic cavity due to a CDH.

These patients are plagued with pulmonary hypertension and have pulmonary hypoplasia, both on the ipsilateral and contralateral sides. Often, pulmonary insufficiency ensues and a vicious cycle of hypoxia, hypercarbia, and acidosis is very detrimental. This process must be interrupted by medical management, which has vastly improved over the past two decades with the use of permissive hypercapnia/spontaneous respiration, pharmacologic therapy, and delayed elective repair.

Various other strategies have been tried to manage critically ill newborns with CDH.[39] High-frequency oscillation may have its major role in forestalling respiratory failure when used as a 'front end' strategy rather than as a 'rescue therapy'.[40] Surfactant plays no more than an anecdotal role. Nitric oxide may be helpful as a vasodilator in the treatment of pulmonary hypertension in these patients. Other pulmonary vasculature vasodilators such as epoprostenol, sildenafil, and iloprost are starting to demonstrate significant efficacy in babies with CDH. The primary indicator for ECMO in the CDH patient occurs when tissue oxygen requirements are not being met, as evidenced by progressive metabolic acidosis, mixed venous oxygen desaturation, and multiple organ failure. The other major indicator is mounting iatrogenic pulmonary injury.

The goal is to maintain preductal oxygen saturations between 90–95%. Spontaneous breathing is preserved by rigorously avoiding muscle relaxants.[41,42] Sedation is used only as needed. Meticulous attention to maintaining a clear airway and the well-being of the infant is obvious, but critical. Permissive hypercapnia with spontaneous respiration is initiated with intermittent mandatory ventilation (IMV), 30–40 breaths per minute, equal I/E time, inspiratory gas flow of 5–7 L/min, peak inspiratory pressure (PIP) of 20–22 cmH_2O, and positive end-expiratory pressure (PEEP) of 5 cmH_2O. The FiO_2 is selected to maintain preductal SaO_2 greater than 90%. If this method of ventilation is not effective, as demonstrated by severe paradoxical chest movement, severe retractions, tachypnea, inadequate or labile oxygenation (preductal O_2 saturations <80%), or $PaCO_2$ greater than 60 mmHg, then a new mode of ventilation is needed.

High-frequency ventilation would be the next option. It is delivered by setting the ventilator to IMV mode with a rate of 100, inspiratory time of 0.3 seconds, an inspiratory gas flow of 10–12 L, a PIP of 20, and a PEEP of 0 (due to auto-PEEP). The PIP is adjusted as needed based on chest excursion, trying to maintain the PIP at less than 25 mmHg. High-frequency oscillation can be instituted if the high-frequency ventilation is unable to improve the hypoxia and hypercarbia using the same parameters just mentioned, but improvement may be temporary.

Before ECMO is initiated for an infant with CDH, the baby should first demonstrate some evidence of adequate lung parenchyma. Some programs use radiographic parameters to determine adequate lung volumes. The lung-to-head ratio (LHR) is measured by prenatal ultrasonography (US).[43,44] It is defined as the product of the orthogonal diameters of the non-affected lung divided by the head circumference. Severe pulmonary hypoplasia is considered when the LHR is less than 1.0 and intermediate hypoplasia lies between 1.0–1.4.[45]

Recent data have shown that an LHR threshold of 0.85 predicted mortality with 95% sensitivity and 64% specificity.[45] The LHR is operator dependent and can only be obtained in a narrow gestational window and therefore leads to poor reproducibility across different centers.

Many centers believe the best method to evaluate pulmonary hypoplasia and predict outcome is to evaluate the patient clinically. This is assessed by having a recorded best $PaCO_2$ less than 50 mmHg and a preductal oxygen saturation greater than 90% for a sustained period of at least one hour at any time in the clinical course. With these criteria, successful ECMO should yield an overall survival rate of 75% or better. If patients with lethal anomalies, overwhelming pulmonary hypoplasia, or neurologic complications are not included, survival approaches 85%.[41,42,46]

Extracorporeal Cardiopulmonary Resuscitation

Studies demonstrate that 1–4% of pediatric intensive care unit (PICU) admissions suffer a cardiac arrest. Survival to discharge for a patient who has an arrest in the PICU ranges from 14–42%. The ELSO data demonstrate that approximately 73% of extracorporeal cardiopulmonary resuscitation (ECPR) has been used for patients with primary cardiac disease. Overall survival to discharge in this population reached 38%.[47] The American Heart Association recommends ECPR for in-hospital cardiac arrest refractory to initial resuscitation, secondary to a process that is reversible or amenable to heart transplantation. Conventional cardiopulmonary resuscitation (CPR) must have failed, no more than several minutes should have elapsed, and ECMO must be readily available. Future research needs to analyze long-term neurologic status amongst survivors and which patients will benefit the most with as little morbidity as possible.

Second Course of ECMO

Approximately 3% of patients that are treated with ECMO will require a second course. The survival rates for patients in this cohort are comparable to the first course. Negative prognostic indicators for second course ECMO patients include patients with renal impairment, higher number of first-course complications, age older than 3 years old, or a prolonged second course.[48]

METHODS OF EXTRACORPOREAL SUPPORT

The goal of ECMO support is to provide an alternate means for oxygen delivery. Three different extracorporeal configurations are used clinically: venoarterial (VA), venovenous (VV), and double-lumen single cannula venovenous (DLVV) bypass. The inception of ECMO and its early days were characterized by VA ECMO because it offered the ability to replace both cardiac and pulmonary function. Venous blood is drained from the right atrium through the right internal jugular vein, and oxygenated blood is returned via the right common carotid artery to the aorta.

VV and DLVV bypass provide pulmonary support but do not provide cardiac support. VV bypass is established by drainage from the right atrium via the right internal jugular vein with reinfusion into a femoral vein. DLVV is accomplished by means of a double-lumen catheter inserted into the right atrium via the right internal jugular vein. A major limitation of VV or DLVV ECMO is that a fraction of the infused oxygenated blood re-enters the pump and, at high flows, may limit oxygen delivery due to recirculation. A limitation specific to DLVV is catheter size, which confines use of this method of support to larger neonates, infants, and smaller children. VV and DLVV bypass have become the preferred method of extracorporeal support for all appropriate patients who do not require cardiac support.[20]

Cannulation

Cannulation can be performed with proper monitoring in the neonatal or PICU under adequate sedation and intravenous anesthesia. The infant is positioned supine with the patient's head at the foot of the bed. The head and neck are hyperextended over a shoulder roll and turned to the left. Local anesthesia is administered in the incision site. A transverse cervical incision is made along the anterior border of the sternomastoid muscle, one finger-breadth above the right clavicle. The platysma muscle is divided, and dissection is carried down with the sternomastoid muscle retracted to expose the carotid sheath. The sheath is opened, and the internal jugular vein, common carotid artery, and vagus nerve are identified (Fig. 6-1A). The vein is exposed first and encircled with proximal and distal ligatures. Occasionally it is necessary to ligate the inferior thyroid vein. The common carotid artery lies medial and posterior, contains no branches, and is mobilized in a similar fashion. The vagus nerve should be identified and protected.

The arterial cannula (usually 10 French for newborns) is measured so that the tip will lie in the ascending aorta. This is approximately one-third the distance between the sternal notch and the xiphoid. The venous cannula (usually 12–14 French for neonates) is measured so that its tip lies in the distal right atrium which is approximately half the distance between the suprasternal notch and the xiphoid process. If time permits, an activated clotting time (ACT) should be checked before heparinization. The patient is then systemically heparinized with 100 U/kg of heparin, which is allowed to circulate for two to three minutes, which should produce an ACT of more than 300 seconds. The arterial cannula is usually inserted first with VA bypass. The carotid artery is ligated cephalad. Proximal control is obtained, and a transverse arteriotomy is made near the cephalad ligature (Fig. 6-1B). To help prevent intimal dissection, fine Prolene sutures can be placed around the arteriotomy and used for retraction when introducing the arterial cannula. The saline-filled cannula is inserted to its premeasured position and secured with two silk ligatures (2-0 or 3-0). A small piece of vessel loop (bumper) may be placed under the ligatures on the anterior aspect of the carotid to protect the vessel from injury during decannulation (Fig. 6-1C).

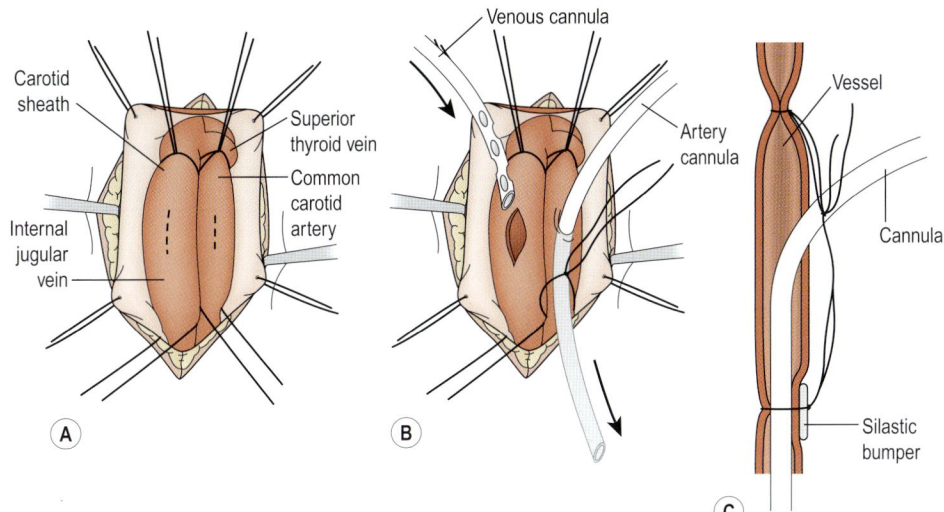

FIGURE 6-1 ■ The cannulation procedure. **(A)** The carotid sheath is exposed, the sternocleidomastoid muscle is retracted laterally, and the common carotid artery and the internal jugular vein are dissected free. **(B)** The patient is anticoagulated after the vessels are dissected and ligated cephalad. The arterial cannula is passed into the junction of the innominate artery and the aorta. The venous catheter is passed into the right atrium. **(C)** A polymeric silicone (Silastic) bumper is used to facilitate ligation of the cannulas. The two ligatures on each vessel are then tied together.

In preparation for the venous cannulation, the patient is given succinylcholine to prevent spontaneous respiration. The proximal internal jugular vein is then ligated cephalad to the site selected for the venotomy. Gentle cephalad traction on this ligature helps during insertion the venous catheter. A venotomy is made close to the ligature. The saline-filled venous catheter is inserted into the right atrium and secured in a manner similar to that used for the arterial catheter. Any air bubbles are removed from the cannulas as they are connected to the ECMO circuit. Bypass is initiated. The cannulas are then secured to the skin above the incision. The incision is closed in layers, ensuring that hemostasis is meticulous.

For VV and DLVV bypass, the procedure is exactly as just described, including dissection of the artery, which is surrounded with a vessel loop to facilitate conversion to VA ECMO should that become necessary. The venous catheter tip should be in the mid-right atrium (5 cm in the neonate) with the arterial portion of the DLVV catheter oriented medially (pointed toward the ear) to direct the oxygenated blood flow toward the tricuspid valve.

The cannula positions for VA ECMO are confirmed by chest radiograph and/or transthoracic echocardiogram. The venous catheter should be located in the inferior aspect of the right atrium, and the arterial catheter in the ascending aorta about 1–2 cm above the aortic valve. With a double-lumen venous catheter, the tip should be in the mid-right atrium with oxygenated blood flow directed toward the tricuspid valve.[49]

A challenging situation arises when one attempts to cannulate a newborn with a right-sided CDH. Anatomic distortion of the mediastinum can lead to cannulation of the azygos vein, which will then fail to provide adequate ECMO support. This is usually detected by poor pump function and echocardiography, which will not demonstrate the cannula in the superior vena cava or right atrium. In these patients, attempted manipulation of the cannula is often wrought with failure, and one should

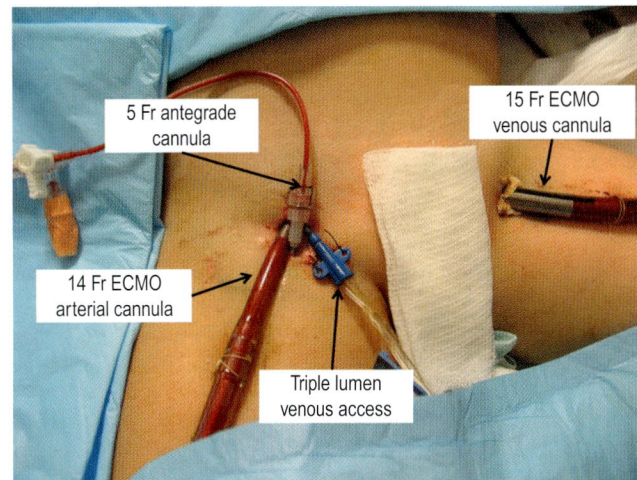

FIGURE 6-2 ■ This infant has been cannulated for ECMO using the femoral artery and vein. To prevent possible distal limb ischemia, antegrade flow has been provided via a percutaneously placed distal perfusion catheter.

consider other avenues for venous drainage, including central cannulation.[50]

The small pediatric population (ages 2–12 years of age) presents a difficult and controversial scenario with regard to cannulation. Some centers continue to perform arterial cannulation via the carotid artery. The long-term neurologic outcome is unknown in this population. Due to this concern, some centers will cannulate these patients via femoral access. However, the arterial cannula is large and can either partially or completely obstruct antegrade arterial flow. This can result in distal limb ischemia which can lead to sensory or motor deficits, tissue loss, or even limb loss. One potential way to avoid this problem is to provide antegrade flow via a percutaneously placed distal perfusion catheter (Fig. 6-2).[51]

ECMO Circuit

Venous blood is drained into a small reservoir or bladder through the cannula that is in the right atrium via the right internal jugular vein (Fig. 6-3). The bladder is a 30–50 mL reservoir that acts as a safety valve. If the venous drainage does not keep up with arterial outflow from the pump, the bladder volume will be depleted, sounding an alarm, and automatically shutting off the pump. Sensors can be placed into the circuit to measure arterial oxygen saturation, mixed venous saturation, hematocrit, and pump flow. Hypovolemia is one of the most common causes of decreased venous inflow into the circuit, but kinking and occlusion of the venous line should be suspected first. An algorithm for managing pump failure due to inadequate venous return is shown in Figure 6-4.

Two types of ECMO pumps, centrifugal and roller head, are used to pump blood through the membrane oxygenator. Centrifugal pumps are dependent on adequate preload and afterload, and have continuous flow. The revolutions per minute (RPM) are adjusted to maintain the desired flow rate. A low preload or high afterload will lead to lower flow despite a fixed RPM. Alternatively, roller pumps operate by displacing a fixed volume of blood per revolution and are afterload independent. The roller pumps are designed with microprocessors that allow for calculation of the blood flow based on the roller-head speed and tubing diameter of the circuit. The pumps are connected to continuous pressure monitoring throughout the circuit and are servoregulated if pressures within the circuit exceed preset parameters. Another safety device, the bubble detector (not depicted in Figure 6-3), is interposed between the pump and the membrane oxygenator that halts perfusion to the patient if air is detected in the circuit.

The oxygenator consists of a hollow-fiber membrane made of polymethylpentene. This provides an interface for blood and gas exchange. These oxygenators have built-in heat exchangers to maintain patient normothermia. Oxygen diffuses through the membrane into the circuit, and carbon dioxide and water vapor diffuse from the blood into the sweep gas. The size (surface area) of

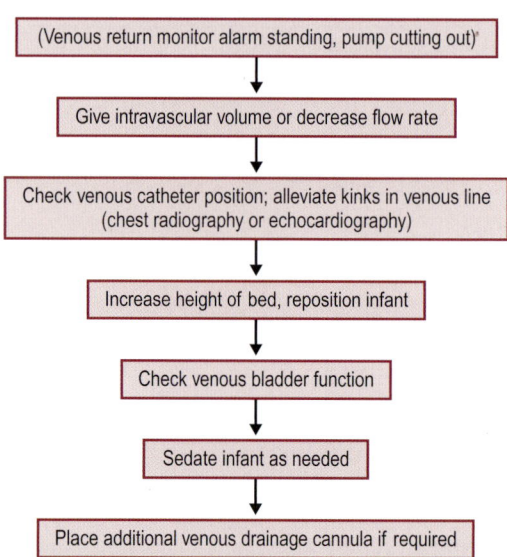

INADEQUATE VENOUS RETURN

(Venous return monitor alarm standing, pump cutting out)*

↓

Give intravascular volume or decrease flow rate

↓

Check venous catheter position; alleviate kinks in venous line (chest radiography or echocardiography)

↓

Increase height of bed, reposition infant

↓

Check venous bladder function

↓

Sedate infant as needed

↓

Place additional venous drainage cannula if required

FIGURE 6-4 ■ Suggested algorithm for the management of inadequate venous return during extracorporeal membrane oxygenation. (Adapted from DeBerry BB, Lynch J, Chung DH, Zwischenberger JB. Emergencies during ECLS and their management. In: Van Meurs K, Lally KP, Peek G, Zwischenberger JB, editors. ECMO: Extracorporeal Cardiopulmonary Support in Critical Care. 3rd ed. Ann Arbor, MI: Extracorporeal Life Support Organization; 2005. p. 133–56.)

the oxygenator is based on the patient's size with smaller infants utilizing a pediatric oxygenator and larger patients using an adult sized oxygenator.

PATIENT MANAGEMENT ON ECMO

Once the cannulas are connected to the circuit, bypass is initiated, and the flow is slowly increased to 100–150 mL/kg/min. Continuous in-line monitoring of the (prepump) SvO_2 and arterial (post-pump) PaO_2 as well as pulse oximetry is vital. The goal of VA ECMO is to maintain an SvO_2 of 37–40 mmHg and saturation of 65–70%. VV ECMO is more difficult to monitor because of recirculation, which may produce a falsely elevated SvO_2. Inadequate oxygenation and perfusion are indicated by metabolic acidosis, oliguria, hypotension, elevated liver function studies, and seizures. Arterial blood gases should be monitored closely with PaO_2 and $PaCO_2$ maintained as close to normal levels as possible. The oxygen level of the blood returning to the patient should be fully saturated. To increase a patient's oxygen delivery on ECMO, one can either increase the ECMO flow rate (~ cardiac output) or the hemoglobin can be increased to maintain hemoglobin at 15 g/dL (~ oxygen content). CO_2 elimination is extremely efficient, and it is important to adjust the sweep (gas mixing) to maintain a $PaCO_2$ in the range of 40–45 mmHg. This is important, especially during weaning, because a low $PaCO_2$ inhibits the infant's spontaneous respiratory drive. Serial monitoring allows timely adjustments. The arterial blood gas is measured hourly. As soon as these parameters are met, all vasoactive drugs are weaned and ventilator levels are adjusted to

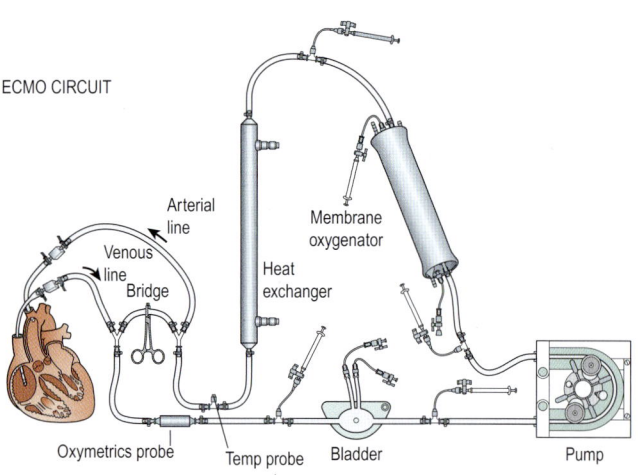

ECMO CIRCUIT

Venous line

Arterial line

Bridge

Membrane oxygenator

Heat exchanger

Oxymetrics probe

Temp probe connector

Bladder

Pump

FIGURE 6-3 ■ Venoarterial extracorporeal membrane oxygenation circuit.

'rest' settings. Gastrointestinal prophylaxis (H$_2$ antagonists or proton pump inhibitors) is initiated, and mild sedation and analgesia are provided, usually with fentanyl and midazolam. Paralyzing agents are avoided. Cefazolin is used for antimicrobial prophylaxis. Routine blood cultures should be obtained.[20,49] A daily chest radiograph is performed. Opacification or 'white out' is often noted during the early ECMO course. The reasons for this are multifactorial and include decreased ventilatory pressures (both PIP and PEEP), reperfusion of the injured lung, and exposure of the blood to a foreign surface, causing an inflammatory response with the release of cytokines. A list of typical diagnostic tests is shown in Table 6-1.

Heparin is administered (30–60 mg/kg/h) throughout the ECMO course to preserve a thrombus-free circuit. ACTs should be monitored hourly and maintained at 180–220 seconds. A complete blood cell count should be obtained every six hours and coagulation profiles obtained daily. To prevent thrombocytopenia, platelets are transfused to maintain a platelet count greater than 100,000/mm^3. The use of fibrinogen and other clotting factors is controversial. Fresh frozen plasma should be considered in infants with international normalized ratio (INR) levels >1.5 in order to replete coagulation cascade factors and allow for adequate anticoagulation. In cases of heparin resistance, anti-thrombin 3 levels should be checked and repleted as necessary. The hematocrit should remain above 40% by using red blood cell transfusions so that oxygen delivery is maximized.[20]

The volume management in patients on ECMO is very important and difficult. It is imperative that all inputs and outputs be diligently recorded and electrolytes monitored every six hours. Fluid losses should be repleted and electrolyte abnormalities corrected. Patients should receive maintenance fluids as well as adequate nutrition by using parenteral hyperalimentation. The first 48 to 72 hours on ECMO typically involve fluid extravasation into the soft tissues. The patient becomes edematous and often requires volume replacement (crystalloid, colloid, or blood products) to maintain adequate intravascular and bypass flows, appropriate hemodynamics, and urine output greater than 1 mL/kg/h. By the third day of bypass, diuresis of the excess extracellular fluid begins and can be facilitated with the use of diuretics and, if necessary, an in-line hemofilter.[20,49]

Selective hypothermia for cerebral ischemia/hypoxia may improve neurologic outcome. It is not yet clear if whole body or cap cooling provides significant improvement in ECMO outcomes. It is possible to maintain temperature of 34°C for 45 hours on ECMO without increasing morbidity.[52] The largest study to date is underway in the UK. The Neonatal ECMO Study of Temperature (NEST) is a multicenter prospective randomized control trial of mild hypothermia versus normothermia in neonates on ECMO.[53]

Operative Procedure on ECMO

Operations, such as CDH repair, can be performed while the child remains on bypass, but one must account for the continued postoperative anticoagulation. Hemorrhagic complications are a frequent morbidity associated with an operation on ECMO, and these complications increase mortality. To try to avoid these problems, the platelet count should be greater than 150,000/mm^3, the ACT can be reduced to 180–200 seconds, and ECMO flow is increased to full support. Moreover, it is imperative that meticulous hemostasis is obtained throughout the operation. The fibrinolysis inhibitor aminocaproic acid (100 mg/kg) is administered just prior to incision, and is infused continuously (30 mg/kg/h) until there is no evidence of bleeding.[20,49]

Weaning and Decannulation

As the patient improves, less blood flow is required to pass through the ECMO circuit and the flow can be weaned at a rate of 10–20 mL/h as long as the patient maintains good oxygenation and perfusion. The most important guide to VA ECMO weaning is the SvO_2. For VV ECMO, it is the SaO_2. Regardless of the cannulation format, successful weaning is marked by stable acid–base balance and good urine output. Flows should be decreased to 30–50 mL/kg/min, and the ACT should be at a higher level (200–240 seconds) to prevent thrombosis. Newer oxygenators have higher limits of allowable flow, which may limit full weaning. Adjustable shunts placed across the oxygenator allow higher overall flow to the oxygenator with a lower flow being delivered to the patient. Also, flow probes placed on the arterial cannula can be used to accurately guide weaning. Moderate conventional ventilator settings are used, but higher settings can be used if the patient needs to be weaned from ECMO urgently. If the child tolerates the low flow, all medications and fluids should be switched to vascular access on the patient. The cannulas are flushed and clamped, with the circuit bypassing the patient via the bridge. If it is possible that the child may need to be returned to bypass, then the cannulas should be flushed with heparin (2 U/mL). The

TABLE 6-1	General Studies Obtained During ECMO	
Laboratory Study	**General Frequency and Comments**
Chest radiography	Daily
Cranial ultrasonography	Only for neonates, the first three days and then as needed
Activated clotting time	Every hour, more often if outside of parameters
Preoxygenator blood gas	Every four hours
Postoxygenator blood gas	Every four hours
Patient blood gas	Every six hours
Glucose monitoring test	Every four hours
Complete blood cell count with platelets	Every six hours; include a differential daily
Chem-7	Every six hours, including magnesium, calcium, and phosphorus daily
Fibrinogen	Daily and after infusion of cryoprecipitate and fresh frozen plasma; may also include prothrombin time and D-dimer

patient is then observed for two to four hours. If this is tolerated, decannulation can be accomplished.

Decannulation is performed under sterile conditions with the patient in the Trendelenburg position. With the use of a short acting muscle relaxant to prevent air aspiration into the vein, ventilator settings should be increased. The venous catheter is typically removed first, and the jugular vein is ligated. Repair of the carotid artery is controversial. Short-term results demonstrate acceptable patency rates and equivalent short-term neurodevelopmental outcomes when compared with children undergoing carotid artery ligation.[54,55] Another study of neonates who underwent arterial repair found a 72% incidence of an occluded or highly stenotic right common carotid artery at two years of age.[56] Similar to other studies, there was no significant difference in neurologic development when compared to controls. The incision should be irrigated and closed over a small drain, which is removed 24 hours later.[20,49]

COMPLICATIONS

Mechanical Complications

Membrane Failure

Failure of the membrane oxygenator is seen with a decrease in oxygenation or retention of CO_2. The cause of such complications include a fibrin clot or water condensation, both of which diminish the oxygenator's ability to transfer oxygen and CO_2. Oxygenator failure has been reported in 21.6% of respiratory ECMO runs in the neonatal and pediatric population.[1] The oxygenator should not be subject to high pressures, which should be continuously monitored. Pressure limits are specific for different manufacturers and for the size of the membrane. Clots in the oxygenator can be seen but the extent of the clot cannot be determined. The progressive consumption of coagulation factors, such as platelets and fibrinogen, also indicates that the membrane may be progressively building clot, and the need to change the oxygenator should be considered. Another sign of impending membrane failure is rising CO_2 levels in the post-oxygenator blood.

Accidental Decannulation

Securing the cannulas properly and taping the tubing to the bed will help prevent accidental decannulation. Unexpected decannulation is an emergency, and immediate pressure should be applied to the cannula site along with discontinuation of bypass. Conventional ventilator settings should be increased simultaneously. The cervical incision must be immediately re-explored to prevent further hemorrhage and the cannulas replaced if continued bypass is needed.

Patient Complications

Air Embolism

The ECMO circuit has several potential sources for entry of air. The initial cannulation procedure can be a source of air embolism. Thus, all visible air bubbles should be removed by filling the cannulas with heparinized saline. Other entry points in the circuit include all of the connectors and stopcocks as well as the membrane oxygenator. Therefore, the circuit must be continually inspected. Air on the arterial side requires removing the patient from bypass immediately. Next, the air should be aspirated from a port until all air has been removed. Air on the venous side is not as urgent a problem, and the air can often be 'walked' into the bladder where it can be aspirated without coming off bypass.

In the event that an air embolism reaches the patient, the patient should be immediately taken off ECMO and conventional ventilator settings adjusted to best meet the patient's needs. The patient should be placed in the Trendelenburg position to prevent air from entering the cerebral circulation. Next, an attempt should be made to aspirate any accessible air out of the arterial cannula. If air enters the coronary circulation, inotropic support may be necessary. Before reinstituting ECMO, identifying and correcting the cause of the air embolus is essential.

Neurologic Complications

Neurologic complications develop in 25% of infants and children on ECMO.[1] ICH, infarct, and seizure carry significant mortality when encountered in ECMO patients. Frequent neurologic examinations should be performed and the use of paralytic agents avoided. The examination should include evaluation of alertness and interaction, spontaneous movements, eye exams, the presence of seizures, fullness of the fontanelles, tone, and reflexes. Electroencephalography (EEG) may also be helpful in the neurologic evaluation. Cranial ultrasound should be performed on all neonates before initiating ECMO to identify those patients in whom significant ICH already exists. A retrospective analysis revealed that birth weight and gestational age were the most significant correlating factors with ICH in neonates on ECMO.[33] Once the patient is placed on ECMO, ultrasound is repeated during the first three days when indicated by the clinical condition. If the examination reveals a new moderate (grade II) hemorrhage or an expanding ICH, ECMO is usually discontinued.

In the event that an ICH is suspected, or detected on cranial ultrasound, and deemed to be small in size, it is reasonable to maintain a low ACT (180–200 seconds) with a platelet count greater than 125,000–150,000/mm³. Serial head ultrasound should be performed to monitor the progression of the hemorrhage.[20]

Cannula Site or Bleeding at Other Sites

The ECMO registry reports an 8.4% incidence of cannulation site bleeding and a 13% incidence of other surgical site bleeding.[1] Contact of blood with the foreign surface of the circuit activates the coagulation cascade. The number of platelets and their function are also affected. With anticoagulation, the risk of bleeding while undergoing an operation on ECMO is considerable. To reduce this risk, meticulous hemostasis needs to be maintained during the procedure and before closure. If necessary, the surgeon should employ topical hemostatic agents. Lowering the ACT parameters to 180–200 seconds and maintaining a platelet count of at least 125,000/mm^3 can assist with hemostasis. If bleeding from the cervical incision is greater than 10 mL/h for two hours despite conservative treatment strategies, exploration may be needed.[20]

Bleeding into previous operative sites occurs frequently and must be handled aggressively. A decreasing hematocrit, an increasing heart rate, a decline in the blood pressure, or inadequate venous return are signs of ongoing hemorrhage. Treatment includes replenishing blood products, including coagulation factors, if necessary. ACT parameters should be decreased to 180 to 200 seconds and the platelet count maintained greater than 125,000/mm^3. Agents that inhibit fibrinolysis, such as aminocaproic acid, also can help prevent bleeding. The use of recombinant activated factor VII (NovoSeven, Novo Nordisk, Inc., Princeton, NJ) has been described in the management of bleeding unresponsive to conventional methods.[57] This is an off-label use, and thrombosis is a significant concern. Often, one must evacuate the hematoma and explore for the cause as is often the case in the postcardiac surgery patient with an open chest and central cannulation. If bleeding is not quickly controlled, decannulation and stopping the anticoagulation may need to be strongly considered.

Coagulation Abnormalities

ECMO patients have a coagulopathy secondary to consumption by the circuit. Removal of the source and a circuit change is a logical approach. Disseminated intravascular coagulation (DIC) occurs in approximately 2% of ECMO cases.[1] DIC is characterized by the consumption of plasma clotting factors and platelets, resulting in deposition of fibrin thrombi in the microvasculature. Once the factor levels and platelet count decrease below certain levels, bleeding will occur. Sepsis, acidosis, hypoxia, and hypotension are the most common causes which is why ECMO patients are at risk for developing DIC. The most common cause of a coagulopathy is consumption of clotting factors by the circuit and rarely is it due to sepsis or DIC.

Patent Ductus Arteriosus

The dramatic decrease in pulmonary hypertension, usually seen in the first 48 hours of an ECMO run, causes dramatic changes in the neonate's circulation. A left-to-right shunt through the patent ductus arteriosus (PDA) develops and causes less-efficient oxygenation, pulmonary edema, and poor peripheral perfusion. Usually, the PDA closes spontaneously with fluid restriction and diuresis. The use of indomethacin should be avoided because of its adverse effects on platelet function. Rarely is PDA ligation required or indicated while on ECMO.

Renal Failure

Oliguria is common in ECMO patients and is often seen during the first 24 to 48 hours. The capillary leak that occurs after placing a child on ECMO may cause decreased renal perfusion. Alternatively, it may result from the nonpulsatile blood flow that occurs with VA ECMO. Once the patient is adequately volume resuscitated, and fluid shifts have stabilized, the use of furosemide (1–2 mg/kg) can improve urine output. If the creatinine continues to rise, then renal ultrasound is recommended. The use of continuous hemofiltration, which can be added in-line to the ECMO circuit, is another mechanism to assist in managing the fluid shifts, hyperkalemia, and azotemia. Hemofiltration removes plasma water and dissolved solutes while retaining proteins and the cellular components of the intravascular space.[20]

Hypertension

The incidence of hypertension on ECMO varies from 28% to as high as 92%.[58] According to the ELSO registry, 13% of ECMO patients require pharmacologic intervention.[1] One group reported that detectable ICH occurred in 44% of their hypertensive patients and clinically significant ICH developed in 27%.[59] The patient should be assessed initially for reversible causes of hypertension, such as pain, hypercarbia, and hypoxia. Embolic renal infarction is another cause of hypertension. Medical management includes the use of hydralazine, nitroglycerin, and captopril.

Infection

The incidence of nosocomial infections during ECMO has been reported as high as 30%.[1] Associated risk factors include the duration of the ECMO course, the length of hospitalization, and procedures performed before the initiation of ECMO or during the run.[60] The ELSO registry data from July 2011 describes an 8% culture-proven infection rate in ECMO neonates and pediatric patients.[1] This is remarkably low, considering the large surface area of the circuit, the duration of bypass, and the frequency of access to the circuit. Fungal infections carry a significantly higher hospital mortality rate, and sepsis carries a higher morbidity and mortality rate in neonates.[61,62] Access to the circuit should be minimized and meticulous sterile techniques are important.

RESULTS

ECMO is a prime example of the evolution from an experimental technique to a commonly used therapeutic approach. The ELSO registry has accumulated data since the early 1980s from all registered centers throughout the world. The number of registered centers continues to rise, as does the number of ECMO cases. In 1992, over 1500 ECMO cannulations for neonatal respiratory disease were performed. In 2010, only 747 cases were reported. The decline in case volume is likely due to improvements in ventilation management and the addition of new agents including inhaled nitric oxide, smooth muscle relaxants, exogenous surfactant, and high-frequency oscillation.[1,20]

Overall survival to discharge for neonates and children is 63% for all diagnoses.[1] Higher survival rates are seen in neonates with respiratory diseases (75%) versus children with respiratory failure (56%), but older patients (48%) fair better than neonates (39%) with cardiac failure as the reason for ECMO (Table 6-2).[1] According to the 2011 ELSO Registry data, newborns with MAS who require ECMO have the best survival rate at 94%, whereas ECMO survival for infants with CDH is only 51% (Table 6-3).[1]

The pediatric population of ECMO patients represents a diverse group with regard to patient age as well as diagnoses. Almost an equal number of respiratory cases ($n = 3854$) and cardiac cases ($n = 4181$) have been reported.[1] This is in contrast to the neonatal population in which there is an almost 3:1 ratio of a primary respiratory to a primary cardiac diagnosis.[1] A higher complication rate is found in children, reflecting the longer duration of bypass required for reversal of the respiratory failure.

Feeding and Growth Sequelae

Approximately one-third of ECMO-treated infants have feeding problems.[63-65] The possible causes for the poor feeding are numerous and include tachypnea, generalized central nervous system depression, poor hunger drive, soreness in the neck from the operation, manipulation or compression of the vagus nerve during the cannulation, sore throat from prolonged intubation, and poor oral motor coordination.[66,67] Newborns with CDH have a higher incidence of feeding difficulties when compared to those with MAS. CDH children often have foregut dysmotility, which leads to significant gastroesophageal reflux, delayed gastric emptying, and feeding difficulties. Respiratory compromise and chronic lung disease add to the problem.[66-70]

Although normal growth is commonly reported in ECMO-treated patients, these children are more likely to experience problems with growth when compared to normal controls. Head circumference below the fifth percentile occurs in 10% of ECMO-treated children.[70] Growth problems are most commonly associated with ECMO patients who had CDH or have residual lung disease.[67]

TABLE 6-2 ELSO Registry Data Comparing Neonatal and Children Requiring ECMO

Indication	Number of Cases	Survival to Discharge (%)
Neonatal respiratory failure	24,344	75
Neonatal cardiac failure	4232	39
Neonatal ECPR	640	38
Pediatric respiratory failure	4771	56
Pediatric cardiac failure	5221	48
Pediatric ECPR	1220	39

ECMO CASES by Patient Group (ELSO Registry, 1980–2011). ECPR, Extracorporeal cardiopulmonary resuscitation; ELSO, Extracorporeal Life Support Organization.

TABLE 6-3 ELSO Registry Data Comparing Outcomes in Neonates Requiring ECMO

Indication	Number of Cases	Survival to Discharge (%)
Meconium aspiration syndrome	7743	94
Respiratory distress syndrome	1496	84
PPHN/PFC	4043	78
Sepsis	2635	75
Congenital diaphragmatic hernia	6147	51

Neonatal Respiratory ECMO cases (ELSO Registry, 1980–2010). ELSO, Extracorporeal Life Support Organization; PFC, persistent fetal circulation; PPHN, persistent pulmonary hypertension of the newborn.

Respiratory Sequelae

Respiratory morbidity is more likely to be iatrogenic than a consequence of congenital lung disease. Nevertheless, approximately 15% of infants require supplemental oxygen at 4 weeks of age in some series. At age 5 years, ECMO children are twice as likely to have reported cases of pneumonia as compared with controls (25% vs 13%).[70,71] These children with pneumonia are more likely to require hospitalization, and the pneumonia occurs at a younger age (half of the pneumonias were diagnosed before 1 year of life). CDH infants often have severe lung disease after ECMO and often require supplemental oxygen at the time of discharge.[67,72-75]

Neurodevelopmental Sequelae

Probably the most serious post-ECMO morbidity is neuromotor injury. The total rate of neurologic injury from 540 patients at 12 institutions was 6%, with a range from 2–18%.[70,76-89] ECMO survivors have significant developmental delay, ranging from none to 21%.[71,73] This is comparable to other critically ill, non-ECMO-treated neonates.[90-92] A single-center study using multivariate analysis identified ventilator time as the only independent predictor of motor problems at age 1 in CDH patients.[90] Auditory defects are reported in more than one-quarter of ECMO neonates at discharge.[93] These deficits are detected by brain stem auditory evoked response (BAER) testing, are considered mild to moderate, and generally resolve over time. The auditory defects may be iatrogenic, or caused by induced alkalosis, diuretics, or gentamicin ototoxicity. As a result, all patients should have a hearing screening at the time of discharge. Visual deficits are uncommon in ECMO neonates who weigh more than 2 kg.[94]

Seizures are widely reported among ECMO neonates, ranging from 20% to 70%.[95-99] However, by age 5 years, only 2% had a diagnosis of epilepsy. Seizures in the neonatal population are associated with neurologic disease and worse outcomes, including cerebral palsy and epilepsy.[99] Severe nonambulatory cerebral palsy has an incidence of less than 5% and is usually accompanied by significant developmental delay.[70,76,82] Milder cases of cerebral palsy are seen in up to 20% of ECMO survivors.

Overall, ECMO-treated neonates function within the normal range and the rate of handicap appears to be stable across studies with an average of 11%, ranging from 2% to 18%.[70,76,79–89] This morbidity reflects how desperately ill these children are and is not a direct effect of ECMO.

REFERENCES

1. Extracorporeal Life Support Organization. International Registry Report of the Extracorporeal Life Support Organization. Ann Arbor; University of Michigan Medical Center; July 2011.
2. Lillehei CW, Cohen M, Warden HE, et al. The direct-vision intracardiac correction of congenital anomalies by controlled cross circulation. Surgery 1955;38:11–29.
3. Clowes GHA Jr, Hopkins AL, Neville WE. An artificial lung dependent upon diffusion of oxygen and carbon dioxide through plastic membranes. J Thorac Surg 1956;32:630–7.
4. Kolobow T, Zapol W, Pierce JE, et al. Partial extracorporeal gas exchange in alert new born lambs with a membrane artificial lung perfused via an AV shunt for periods up to 96 hours. Trans Am Soc Artif Intern Organs 1968;14:328–34.
5. Osborn JJ, Bramson ML, Main FB, et al. Clinical experience with a disposable membrane oxygenator. Bull Soc Int Chir 1966;25:346–53.
6. Peirce EC 2d, Thebaut AL, Kent BB, et al. Techniques of extended perfusion using a membrane lung. Ann Thorac Surg 1971;12:451–70.
7. Lande AJ, Edwards L, Block JH, et al. Prolonged cardiopulmonary support with a practical membrane oxygenator. Trans Am Soc Artif Intern Organs 1970;16:352–6.
8. Hill D, O'Brien TG, Murray JJ, et al. Extracorporeal oxygenation for acute post-traumatic respiratory failure (shock-lung syndrome): Use of the Bramson Membrane Lung. N Engl J Med 1972;286:629–34.
9. Zapol WM, Snider MT, Hill JD, et al. Extracorporeal membrane oxygenation in severe respiratory failure. JAMA 1979;242:2193–6.
10. Bartlett RH, Gazzaniga AB, Jefferies MR, et al. Extracorporeal membrane oxygenation (ECMO) cardiopulmonary support in infants. Trans Am Soc Artif Intern Organs 1976;22:80–93.
11. Bartlett RH, Roloff DW, Cornell RG, et al. Extracorporeal circulation in neonatal respiratory failure: A prospective randomized study. Pediatrics 1985;76:479–87.
12. O'Rourke PP, Crone RK, Vacanti JP, et al. Extracorporeal membrane oxygenation and conventional medical therapy in neonates with persistent pulmonary hypertension of the newborn: A prospective randomized study. Pediatrics 1989;84:957–63.
13. Firmin R. United Kingdom Neonatal ECMO Study. Presented at the 7th International ELSO Conference, Dearborn, Michigan, 1995.
14. Krummel TM, Greenfield LJ, Kirkpatrick BU, et al. Extracorporeal membrane oxygenation in neonatal pulmonary failure. Pediatr Ann 1982;11:905–8.
15. Toomasion JM, Snedecor SM, Cornell RG, et al. National experience with extracorporeal membrane oxygenation for newborn respiratory failure: Data from 715 cases. Trans Am Soc Artif Intern Organs 1988;34:140–7.
16. Stolar CJH, Snedecor SM, Bartlett RH. Extracorporeal membrane oxygenation and neonatal respiratory failure: Experience from the extracorporeal life support organization. J Pediatr Surg 1991;26:563–71.
17. O'Rourke PP, Stolar CJ, Zwischenberger JB, et al. Extracorporeal membrane oxygenation: Support for overwhelming pulmonary failure in the pediatric population: Collective experience from the extracorporeal life support organization. J Pediatr Surg 1993;28:523–8.
18. Galantowicz ME, Stolar CJ. Extracorporeal membrane oxygenation for perioperative support in pediatric heart transplantation. J Thorac Cardiovasc Surg 1991;102:148–51.
19. Campbell BT, Braun TM, Schumacher RE, et al. Impact of ECMO on neonatal mortality in Michigan (1980–1999). J Pediatr Surg 2003;38:290–5.
20. In: Van Meurs K, Lally KP, Peek G, et al, editors. ECMO: Extracorporeal Cardiopulmonary Support in Critical Care. 3rd ed. Ann Arbor, MI: Extracorporeal Life Support Organization; 2005.
21. In: Van Meurs K, editor. ECMO Specialist Training Manual. 3nd ed. Ann Arbor, MI: Extracorporeal Life Support Organization; 2010.
22. Gajarski RJ, Mosca RS, Ohye RG, et al. Use of extracorporeal life support as a bridge to pediatric cardiac transplantation. J Heart Lung Transplant 2003;22:28–34.
23. Bae J, Frischer J, Waich M, et al. Extracorporeal membrane oxygenation in pediatric cardiac transplantation. J Pediatr Surg 2005;40:1051–7.
24. Lessin JS, el-Eid SE, Klein MD, et al. Extracorporeal membrane oxygenation in pediatric respiratory failure secondary to smoke inhalation injury. J Pediatr Surg 1996;31:1285–7.
25. Tobias JD, Garrett JS. Therapeutic options for severe, refractory status asthmaticus: Inhalational anesthetic agents, extracorporeal membrane oxygenation and helium/oxygen ventilation. Paediatr Anesth 1997;7:47–57.
26. Travis JA, Pranikoff T, Chang MC, et al. Extracorporeal rewarming in trauma patients. Presented at the 13th Annual ELSO Conference, Scottsdale, Arizona, 2002.
27. Johnson LB, Plotkin JS, Howell CD, et al. Successful emergency transplantation of a liver allograft from a donor maintained on extracorporeal membrane oxygenation. Transplantation 1997;63:910–11.
28. Gersony WM, Duc GV, Sinclair JC. 'PFC' syndrome (persistence of the fetal circulation). Circulation 1969;40(Suppl. 111):87.
29. Gupta A, Shantanu R, Rakesh S, et al. Inhaled nitric oxide and gentle ventilation in the treatment of pulmonary hypertension of the newborn—a single-center 5-year experience. J Perinatol 2002;22:435–41.
30. Northway WH, Rosan RC, Porter DY. Pulmonary disease following respiratory therapy of hyaline membrane disease. N Engl J Med 1967;276:357–68.
31. Kornhauser MS, Cullen JA, Baumgart S, et al. Risk factors for bronchopulmonary dysplasia after extracorporeal membrane oxygenation. Arch Pediatr Adolesc Med 1994;148:820–5.
32. Kim ES, Stolar CJ. ECMO in the newborn. Am J Perinatol 2000;17:345–56.
33. Cilley RE, Zwischenberger JB, Andrews AF, et al. Intracranial hemorrhage during extracorporeal membrane oxygenation in neonates. Pediatrics 1986;78:699–704.
34. Wung JT, James LS, Kilchevsky E, et al. Management of infants with severe respiratory failure and persistence of the fetal circulation, without hyperventilation. Pediatrics 1985;76:488–94.
35. Beck R, Anderson KD, Pearson GD, et al. Criteria for extracorporeal membrane oxygenation in a population of infants with persistent pulmonary hypertension of the newborn. J Pediatr Surg 1986;21:297–302.
36. Marsh TD, Wilkerson SA, Cook LN. Extracorporeal membrane oxygenation selection criteria: Partial pressure of arterial oxygen versus alveolar-arterial oxygen gradient. Pediatrics 1988;82:162–6.
37. Ortiz RM, Cilley RE, Bartlett RH. Extracorporeal membrane oxygenation in pediatric respiratory failure. Pediatr Clin North Am 1987;34:39–46.
38. Rivera RA, Butt W, Shann F. Predictors of mortality in children with respiratory failure possible indications for ECMO. Anaesth Intensive Care 1990;18:385–9.
39. Garcia AV, Stolar CJH. Congenital diaphragmatic hernia and protective ventilation strategies in pediatric surgery. Surg Clin N Am 2012;92:659–68.
40. Azarow K, Messineo A, Pearl R, et al. Congenital diaphragmatic hernia—a tale of two cities: The Toronto experience. J Pediatr Surg 1997;32:395–400.
41. Wung JT, Sahni R, Moffitt ST, et al. Congenital diaphragmatic hernia: Survival treated with very delayed surgery, spontaneous respiration, and no chest tube. J Pediatr Surg 1995;30:406–9.
42. Boloker J, Bateman DA, Wung JT, et al. Congenital diaphragmatic hernia in 120 infants treated consecutively with permissive hypercapnia/spontaneous respiration/elective repair. J Pediatr Surg 2002;37:357–66.
43. Metkus AP, Filly RA, Stringer MD, et al. Sonographic predictors of survival in fetal diaphragmatic hernia. J Pediatr Surg 1996;31:148–51.

44. Aspelund G, Fisher JC, Simpson LL, et al. Prenatal lung-head ratio: Threshold to predict outcome for congenital diaphragmatic hernia. J Matern Fetal Neona 2012;25:1011–16.

45. Graham G, Devine PC. Antenatal diagnosis of congenital diaphragmatic hernia. Semin Perinatol 2005;29:69–76.

46. Stolar CJH, Dillon PW, Reyes C, et al. Selective use of extracorporeal membrane oxygenation in the management of congenital diaphragmatic hernia. J Pediatr Surg 1988;23:207–11.

47. Fiser RT, Morris MC. Extracorporeal cardiopulmonary resuscitation in refractory pediatric cardiac arrest. Pediatr Clin North Am 2008;55:929–41.

48. Fisher JC, Stolar CJH, Cowles RA. Extracorporeal membrane oxygenation of cardiopulmonary failure in pediatric patients: Is a second course justified? J Surg Res 2008;148:100–8.

49. Frischer JS, Stolar CJH. Extracorporeal membrane oxygenation. In: Puri P, Hollwarth M, editors. Operative Pediatric Surgery. Heidelberg: Springer; 2006.

50. Fisher JC, Jefferson RA, Kuenzler KA, et al. Challenges to cannulation for extracorporeal support in neonates with right-sided congenital diaphragmatic hernia. J Pediatr Surg 2007;42:2123–8.

51. Haley MJ, Fisher JC, Ruiz-Elizalde AR, et al. Percutaneous distal perfusion of the lower extremity following femoral cannulation for venoarterial ECMO in a small child. J Pediatr Surg 2009;44:437–40.

52. Horan M, Ichiba S, Firmin RK, et al. A pilot investigation of mild hypothermia in neonates receiving extracorporeal membrane oxygenation (ECMO). J Pediatr 2004;144:301–8.

53. Field DJ, Firmin R, Azzopardi DV, et al. Neonatal ECMO Study of Temperature (NEST)- a randomized controlled trial. BMC Pediatr 2010;10:24.

54. Levy MS, Share JC, Fauza DO, et al. Fate of the reconstructed carotid artery after extracorporeal membrane oxygenation. J Pediatr Surg 1995;30:1046–9.

55. Cheung PY, Vickar DB, Hallgren RA, et al. Carotid artery reconstruction in neonates receiving extracorporeal membrane oxygenation: A 4-year follow-up study. J Pediatr Surg 1997;32:560–4.

56. Buesing KA, Kilian AK, Schaible T, et al. Extracorporeal membrane oxygenation in infants with congenital diaphragmatic hernia: Follow-up MRI evaluating carotid artery reocclusion and neurologic outcome. Am J Roentgenol 2007;188:1636–42.

57. Preston TJ, Olshove VF, Ayad O, et al. NovoSeven use in a noncardiac pediatric ECMO patient with uncontrolled bleeding. J Extra Corpor Technol 2008;40:123–6.

58. Boedy RF, Goldberg AK, Howell CG, et al. Incidence of hypertension in infants on extracorporeal membrane oxygenation. J Pediatr Surg 1990;25:258–61.

59. Sell LL, Cullen ML, Lerner GR, et al. Hypertension during extracorporeal membrane oxygenation: Cause, effect, and management. Surgery 1987;102:724–30.

60. Coffin SE, Bell LM, Manning M, et al. Nosocomial infections in neonates receiving extracorporeal membrane oxygenation. Infect Control Hosp Epidemiol 1997;18:93–6.

61. Douglass BH, Keenan AL, Purohit DM. Bacterial and fungal infection in neonates undergoing venoarterial extracorporeal membrane oxygenation: An analysis of the registry data of the Extracorporeal Life Support Organization. Artif Organs 1996;20:202–8.

62. Meyer DM, Jessen ME, Eberhart RC. Neonatal extracorporeal membrane oxygenation complicated by sepsis. Extracorporeal Life Support Organization. Ann Thorac Surg 1995;59:975–80.

63. Grimm P. Feeding difficulties in infants treated with ECMO. CNMC ECMO Symposium 1993;25.

64. Nield T, Hallaway M, Fodera C, et al. Outcome in problem feeders post-ECMO. CNMC ECMO Symposium 1990;79.

65. Glass P. Patient neurodevelopmental outcomes after neonatal ECMO. In: Arensman R, Cornish J, editors. Extracorporeal Life Support. Boston: Blackwell Scientific Publications; 1993. p. 241–51.

66. Tarby T, Waggoner J. Are the common neurologic problems following ECMO related to jugular bulb thrombosis? CNMC ECMO Symposium 1994;110.

67. Van Meurs K, Robbins S, Reed V, et al. Congenital diaphragmatic hernia: Long-term outcome of neonates treated with ECMO. CNMC ECMO Symposium 1991;25.

68. Pace MRD, Caruso AM, Farina F, et al. Evaluation of esophageal motility and reflux in children treated for congenital diaphragmatic hernia with the use of combined multichannel intraluminal impedance and pH monitoring. J Pediatr Surg 2011;46:1881–6.

69. Rajasingham S, Reed V, Glass P, et al. Congenital diaphragmatic hernia: Outcome post-ECMO at 5 years. CNMC ECMO Symposium 1994;35.

70. Glass P, Wagner A, Papero P, et al. Neurodevelopmental status at age five years of neonates treated with extracorporeal membrane oxygenation. J Pediatr 1995;127:447–57.

71. Gershan L, Gershan W, Day S. Airway anomalies after ECMO: Bronchoscopic findings. CNMC ECMO Symposium 1992;65.

72. Wagner A, Glass P, Papero P, et al. Neuropsychological outcome of neonatal ECMO survivors at age 5. CNMC ECMO Symposium 1994;31.

73. D'Agostino J, Bernbaum J, Gerdes M, et al. Outcome for infants with congenital diaphragmatic hernia requiring extracorporeal membrane oxygenation: The first year. J Pediatr Surg 1995;30:10–15.

74. Van Meurs K, Robbins S, Reed V, et al. Congenital diaphragmatic hernia: Long-term outcome in neonates treated with extracorporeal membrane oxygenation. J Pediatr 1993;122:893–9.

75. Atkinson J, Poon M. ECMO and the management of congenital diaphragmatic hernia with large diaphragmatic defects requiring a prosthetic patch. J Pediatr 1992;27:754–6.

76. Adolph V, Ekelund C, Smith C, et al. Developmental outcome of neonates treated with ECMO. J Pediatr Surg 1990;25:43–6.

77. Andrews A, Nixon C, Cilley R, et al. One-to-three year outcome for 14 neonatal survivors of extracorporeal membrane oxygenation. Pediatrics 1986;78:692–8.

78. Flusser H, Dodge N, Engle W, et al. Neurodevelopmental outcome and respiratory morbidity for ECMO survivors at 1 year of age. J Perinatol 1993;13:266–71.

79. Glass P, Miller M, Short BL. Morbidity for survivors of extracorporeal membrane oxygenation: Neurodevelopmental outcome at 12 years of age. Pediatrics 1989;83:72–8.

80. Griffin M, Minifee P, Landry S, et al. Neurodevelopmental outcome in neonates after ECMO: Cranial magnetic resonance imaging and ultrasonography correlation. J Pediatr Surg 1992;27:33–5.

81. Hofkosh D, Thompson A, Nozza R, et al. Ten years of ECMO: Neurodevelopmental outcome. Pediatrics 1991;87:549–55.

82. Krummel T, Greenfield L, Kirkpatrick B, et al. The early evaluation of survivors after ECMO for neonatal pulmonary failure. J Pediatr Surg 1984;19:585–90.

83. Schumacher R, Palmer T, Roloff D, et al. Follow-up of infants treated with ECMO for newborn respiratory failure. Pediatrics 1991;87:451–7.

84. Towne B, Lott I, Hicks D, et al. Long-term follow-up of infants and children treated with ECMO: A preliminary report. J Pediatr Surg 1985;20:410–14.

85. Wildin S, Landry S, Zwischenberger J. Prospective, controlled study of developmental outcome in survivors of ECMO: The first 24 months. Pediatrics 1994;93:404–8.

86. Stolar CJ, Crisafi MA, Driscoll YT. Neurocognitive outcome for neonates treated with extracorporeal membrane oxygenation: Are infants with congenital diaphragmatic hernia different? J Pediatr Surg 1995;30:366–72.

87. Davis D, Wilkerson S, Stewart D. Neurodevelopmental follow-up of ECMO survivors at 7 years. CNMC ECMO Symposium 1995;34.

88. Stanley C, Brodsky K, McKee L, et al. Developmental profile of ECMO survivors at early school age and relationship to neonatal EEG status. CNMC ECMO Symposium 1995;33.

89. Hack M, Taylor H, Klein N, et al. School-age outcomes in children with birthweights under 750 g. N Engl J Med 1994;331:753–9.

90. Friedman S, Chen C, Chapman JS, et al. Neurodevelopmental outcomes of congenital diaphragmatic hernia survivors followed in a multidisciplinary clinic at ages 1 and 3. J Pediatr Surg 2008;43:1035–43.

91. Leavitt AM, Watchko JF, Bennett FC, et al. Neurodevelopmental outcome following persistent pulmonary hypertension of the neonate. J Perinatol 1987;7:288–91.

92. Marron MJ, Crisafi MA, Driscoll JM Jr, et al. Hearing and neurodevelopmental outcome in survivors of persistent pulmonary hypertension of the newborn. Pediatrics 1992;90:392–6.

93. Desai S, Stanley C, Graziani L, et al. Brainstem auditory evoked potential screening (BAEP) unreliable for detecting sensorineural

hearing loss in ECMO survivors: A comparison of neonatal BAEP and follow-up behavioral audiometry. CNMC ECMO Symposium 1994;62.

94. Haney B, Thibeault D, Sward-Comunelli S, et al. Ocular findings in infants treated with ECMO. CNMC ECMO Symposium 1994;63.

95. Hahn J, Vaucher Y, Bejar R, et al. Electroencephalographic and neuroimaging findings in neonates undergoing extracorporeal membrane oxygenation. Neuropediatrics 1993;24:19–24.

96. Graziani L, Streletz L, Baumgart S, et al. Predictive value of neonatal electroencephalograms before and during extracorporeal membrane oxygenation. J Pediatr 1994;125:969–75.

97. Campbell L, Bunyapen C, Gangarosa M, et al. The significance of seizures associated with ECMO. CNMC ECMO Symposium 1991;26.

98. Kumar P, Bedard M, Delaney-Black V, et al. Post-ECMO electroencephalogram (EEG) as a predictor of neurological outcome. CNMC ECMO Symposium 1994;65.

99. Scher M, Kosaburo A, Beggerly M, et al. Electrographic seizures in preterm and full-term neonates: Clinical correlates, associated brain lesions, and risk for neurologic sequelae. Pediatrics 1993;91:128–34.

CHAPTER 7

MECHANICAL VENTILATION IN PEDIATRIC SURGICAL DISEASE

Samir K. Gadepalli • Ronald B. Hirschl

Amazingly, ventilation via tracheal cannulation was performed as early as 1543 when Vesalius demonstrated the ability to maintain the beating heart in animals with open chests.[1] This technique was first applied to humans in 1780, but there was little progress in positive-pressure ventilation until the development of the Fell–O'Dwyer apparatus. This device provided translaryngeal ventilation using bellows and was first used in 1887 (Fig. 7-1).[2,3] The Drinker–Shaw iron lung, which allowed piston-pump cyclic ventilation of a metal cylinder and concomitant negative-pressure ventilation, became available in 1928 and was followed by a simplified version built by Emerson in 1931.[4] Such machines were the mainstays in the ventilation of victims of poliomyelitis in the 1930s through the 1950s.

In the 1920s, the technique of tracheal intubation was refined by Magill and Rowbotham.[5,6] In World War II, the Bennett valve, which allowed cyclic application of high pressure, was devised to allow pilots to tolerate high-altitude bombing missions.[7] Concomitantly, the use of translaryngeal intubation and mechanical ventilation became common in the operating room as well as in the treatment of respiratory insufficiency. However, application of mechanical ventilation to newborns, both in the operating room and in the intensive care unit (ICU), lagged behind that for children and adults.

The use of positive-pressure mechanical ventilation in the management of respiratory distress syndrome (RDS) was described in 1962.[8] It was the unfortunate death of Patrick Bouvier Kennedy at 32 weeks gestation in 1963 that resulted in additional National Institutes of Health (NIH) funding for research in the management of newborns with respiratory failure.[9] The discovery of surfactant deficiency as the etiology of RDS in 1959, the ability to provide positive-pressure ventilation in newborns with respiratory insufficiency in 1965, and demonstration of the effectiveness of continuous positive airway pressure in enhancing lung volume and ventilation in patients with RDS in 1971 set the stage for the development of continuous-flow ventilators specifically designed for neonates.[10–12] The development of neonatal ICUs (NICUs), hyperalimentation, and neonatal invasive and noninvasive monitoring enhanced the care of newborns with respiratory failure and increased survival in preterm newborns from 50% in the early 1970s to more than 90% today.[13]

PHYSIOLOGY OF GAS EXCHANGE DURING MECHANICAL VENTILATION

The approach to mechanical ventilation is best understood if the two variables of oxygenation and carbon dioxide elimination are considered separately.[14]

Carbon Dioxide Elimination

The primary purpose of ventilation is to eliminate carbon dioxide, which is accomplished by delivering tidal volume (V_t) breaths at a designated rate. The product ($V_t \times$ rate) determines the minute volume ventilation ($\dot{V}_E$). Although CO_2 elimination is proportional to $\dot{V}_E$, it is, in fact, directly related to the volume of gas ventilating the alveoli because part of the $\dot{V}_E$ resides in the conducting airways or in nonperfused alveoli. As such, the portion of the ventilation that does not participate in CO_2 exchange is termed the dead space (V_d).[15] In a patient with healthy lungs, this dead space is fixed or 'anatomic', and consists of about one-third of the tidal volume (i.e., $V_d/V_t = 0.33$). In a setting of respiratory insufficiency, the proportion of dead space (V_d/V_t) may be augmented by the presence of nonperfused alveoli and a reduction in V_t. Furthermore, dead space can unwittingly be increased through the presence of extensions of the trachea such as the endotracheal tube, a pneumotachometer to measure tidal volume, an end-tidal CO_2 monitor, or an extension of the ventilator tubing beyond the 'Y.'

Tidal volume is a function of the applied ventilator pressure and the volume/pressure relationship (compliance), which describes the ability of the lung and chest wall to distend. At the functional residual capacity (FRC), the static point of end expiration, the tendency for the lung to collapse (elastic recoil) is in balance with the forces that promote chest wall expansion.[15] As each breath develops, the elastic recoil of both the lung and chest wall work in concert to oppose lung inflation. Therefore, pulmonary compliance is a function of both the lung elastic recoil (lung compliance) and that of the rib cage and diaphragm (chest wall compliance).

The compliance can be determined in a dynamic or static mode. Figure 7-2 demonstrates the dynamic volume/pressure relationship for a normal patient. Note that application of 25 cmH_2O of inflating pressure (ΔP)

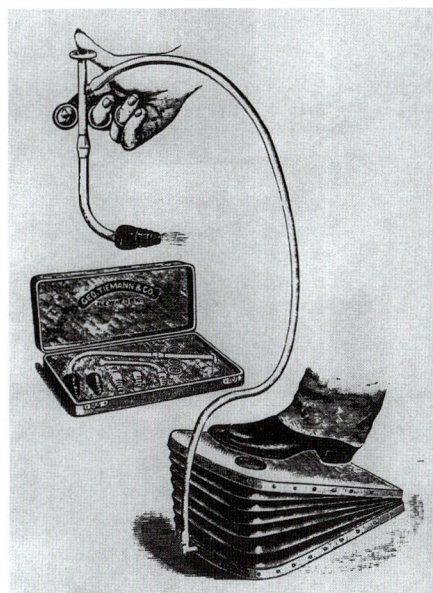

FIGURE 7-1 ■ The Fell–O'Dwyer apparatus that was first used to perform positive-pressure ventilation in newborns. (Reprinted from Matas R. Intralaryngeal insufflation. JAMA 1900;34: 1468–73.)

TABLE 7-1	Definitions and Normal Values for Respiratory Physiologic Parameters	
Variable	**Definition**	**Normal Value**
TLC	Total lung capacity	80 mL/kg
FRC	Functional residual capacity	40 mL/kg
IC	Inspiratory capacity	40 mL/kg
ERV	Expiratory reserve volume	30 mL/kg
RV	Residual volume	10 mL/kg
V_t	Tidal volume	5 mL/kg
$\dot{V}_E$	Minute volume ventilation	100 mL/kg/min
$\dot{V}_F$	Alveolar ventilation	60 mL/kg/h
V_d	Dead space	mL = wt in lb
V_d/V_t	% Dead space	0.33
C_{St}	Static compliance	2 mL/cm H_2O/kg
C_{eff}	Effective compliance	1 mL/cm H_2O/kg

above static FRC at positive end-expiratory pressure (PEEP) of 5 cmH$_2$O generates a V_t of 40 mL/kg. The lung, at an inflating pressure of 30 cmH$_2$O when compared with ambient (transpulmonary) pressure, is considered to be at total lung capacity (TLC) (Table 7-1). Note that the loop observed during both inspiration and expiration is curvilinear. This is due to the resistance that is present in the airways and describes the work required to overcome air flow resistance. As a result, at any given point of active flow, the measured pressure in the airways

is higher during inspiration and lower during expiration than at the same volume under zero-flow conditions. Pulmonary compliance measurements, as well as alveolar pressure measurements, can be effectively performed only when no flow is present in the airways (zero flow), which occurs at FRC and TLC. The change observed is a volume of 40 mL/kg and pressure of 25 cmH$_2$O or 1.6 mL/kg/cmH$_2$O. This is termed effective compliance because it is calculated only between the two arbitrary points of end inspiration and end expiration.

As can be seen from Figure 7-3, the volume/pressure relationship is not linear over the range of most inflating pressures when a static compliance curve is developed. Such static compliance assessments are most commonly performed via a large syringe in which aliquots of 1–2 mL/kg of oxygen, up to a total of 15–20 mL/kg, are instilled sequentially with 3 to 5-second pauses. At the end of each pause, zero-flow pressures are measured. By plotting the data, a static compliance curve can be generated. This curve demonstrates how the calculated compliance can change depending on the arbitrary points used for assessment of the effective compliance (C_{eff}).[16]

Alternatively, the pulmonary pressure/volume relationship can be assessed by administration of a slow constant flow of gas into the lungs with simultaneous determination of airway pressure.[17,18] A curve may be fitted to the data points to determine the optimal compliance and FRC.[19] The compliance will change as the FRC or end-expiratory lung volume (EELV) increases or decreases. For instance, as can be seen in Figure 7-3, at low FRC (point A), atelectasis is present. A given ΔP will not optimally inflate alveoli. Likewise, at a high FRC (point C), because of air trapping or application of high PEEP, the lung is already distended. Application of the same ΔP will result only in over distention and potential lung injury with little benefit in terms of added V_t. Thus, optimal compliance is provided when the pressure/volume range is on the linear portion of the static compliance curve (point B). Clinically, the compliance at a variety of FRC or PEEP values can be monitored to establish optimal FRC.[20]

Finally, it is important to recognize that a portion of the V_t generated by the ventilator is actually compression of gas within both the ventilator tubing and the airways.

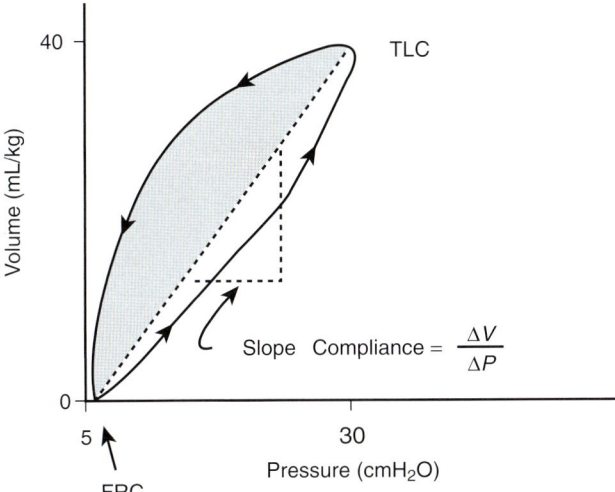

FIGURE 7-2 ■ Dynamic pressure/volume relation and effective pulmonary compliance (C_{eff}) in the normal lung. The volume at 30 cmH$_2$O is considered total lung capacity (TLC). C_{eff} is calculated by $\Delta V/\Delta P$. (Adapted from Bhutani VK, Sivieri EM. Physiological principles for bedside assessment of pulmonary graphics. In: Donn SM, editor. Neonatal and Pediatric Pulmonary Graphics: Principles and Applications. Armonk, NY: Futura Publishing; 1998.)

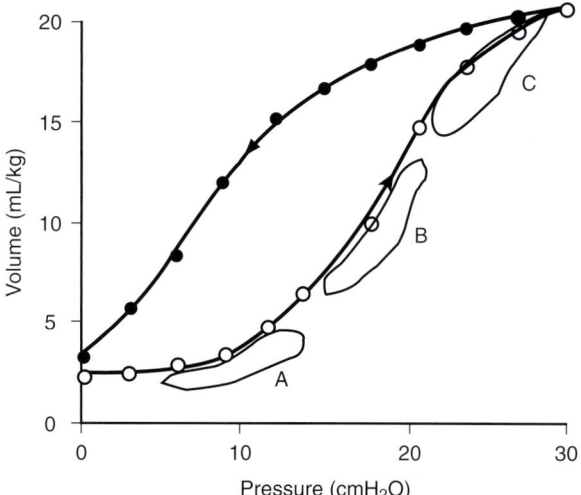

FIGURE 7-3 ■ Static lung compliance curve in a normal lung. Effective compliance would be altered depending on whether FRC were to be at a level resulting in lung atelectasis (point A) or over distention (point C). Optimal lung mechanics are observed when FRC is set on the steepest portion of the curve (point B). (Adapted from West JB. Respiratory Physiology. Baltimore: Williams & Wilkins; 1985.)

The ratio of gas compressed in the ventilator tubing to that entering the lungs is a function of the compliance of the ventilator tubing and the lung. The compliance of the ventilator tubing is 0.3–4.5 mL/cmH$_2$O.[21] A change in pressure of 15 cmH$_2$O in a 3 kg newborn with respiratory insufficiency and a pulmonary compliance of 0.4 mL/cmH$_2$O/kg would result in a lung V_t of 18 mL and an impressive ventilator tubing/gas compression volume of 15 mL if the tubing compliance were 1.0 mL/cmH$_2$O. The relative ventilator tubing/gas compression volume would not be as striking in an adult. The ventilator tubing compliance is characterized for all current ventilators and should be factored when considering V_t data. The software in many ventilators corrects for ventilator tubing compliance when displaying V_t values.

Typical ventilator rate requirements in patients with healthy lungs range from 10 breaths/min in an adult to 30 breaths/min in a newborn. The V_t is maintained at 5–10 mL/kg, resulting in a $\dot{V}_E$ of about 100 mL/kg/min in adults and 150 mL/kg/min in newborns. In healthy lungs, these settings should provide sufficient ventilation to maintain normal $PaCO_2$ levels of approximately 40 mmHg, and should generate peak inspiratory pressures between 15–20 cmH$_2$O above an applied PEEP of 5 cmH$_2$O. Clinical assessment by observing chest wall movement, auscultation, and evaluation of gas exchange determines the appropriate V_t in a given patient.

Oxygenation

In contrast to CO$_2$ determination, oxygenation is determined by the fraction of inspired oxygen (FiO_2) and the degree of lung distention or alveolar recruitment, determined by the level of PEEP and the mean airway pressure (P_{aw}) during each ventilator cycle. If CO$_2$ was not a competing gas at the alveolar level, oxygen within the

pulmonary capillary blood would simply be replaced by that provided at the airway, as long as alveolar distention was maintained. Such apneic oxygenation has been used in conjunction with extracorporeal carbon dioxide removal (ECCO$_2$R) or arteriovenous CO$_2$ removal (AVCO$_2$R), in which oxygen is delivered at the carina, whereas lung distention is maintained through application of PEEP.[22,23] Under normal circumstances, however, alveolar ventilation serves to remove CO$_2$ from the alveolus and to replenish the PO_2, thereby maintaining the alveolar/pulmonary capillary blood oxygen gradient.

Rather than depending on the degree of alveolar ventilation, oxygenation predominantly is a function of the appropriate matching of pulmonary blood flow to inflated alveoli (ventilation/perfusion [$\dot{V}/\dot{Q}$] matching).[15] In normal lungs, the PEEP should be maintained at 5 cmH$_2$O, a pressure that allows maintenance of alveolar inflation at end expiration, balancing the lung/chest wall recoil. An FiO_2 of 0.50 should be administered initially. However, one should be able to wean the FiO_2 rapidly in a patient with healthy lungs and normal $\dot{V}/\dot{Q}$ matching. Areas of ventilation but no perfusion (high $\dot{V}/\dot{Q}$), such as in the setting of pulmonary embolus, do not contribute to oxygenation. Therefore, hypoxemia supervenes in this situation once the average residence time of blood in the remaining perfused pulmonary capillaries exceeds that necessary for complete oxygenation. Normal residence time is threefold that required for full oxygenation of pulmonary capillary blood.

However, the common pathophysiology observed in the setting of respiratory insufficiency is that of minimal or no ventilation, with persistent perfusion (low $\dot{V}/\dot{Q}$), resulting in right-to-left shunting and hypoxemia. Patients with the acute respiratory distress syndrome (ARDS) have collapse of the posterior, or dependent, regions of the lungs when supine.[24,25] As the majority of blood flow is distributed to these dependent regions, one can easily imagine the limited oxygen transfer and large shunt secondary to $\dot{V}/\dot{Q}$ mismatch and the resulting hypoxemia that occurs in patients with ARDS. Attempts to inflate the alveoli in these regions, such as with the application of increased PEEP, can reduce $\dot{V}/\dot{Q}$ mismatch and enhance oxygenation.

Just as partial pressure of CO$_2$ in the pulmonary artery ($PaCO_2$) is used to evaluate ventilation, partial pressure of oxygen in pulmonary arterial blood (PaO_2) and arterial oxygen saturation (SaO_2) levels are the measures most frequently used to evaluate oxygenation. Lung oxygenation capabilities are also frequently assessed as a function of the difference between the ideal alveolar and the measured systemic arterial oxygen levels (A–a gradient), the ratio of the PaO_2 to the FiO_2 (P/F ratio), the physiologic shunt ($\dot{Q}_{ps}/\dot{Q}_t$), and the oxygen index (OI).

$$A\text{–a gradient} = (FiO_2 \times [P_B - PH_2O] - PaCO_2/RQ) - PaO_2$$

where FiO_2 is the fraction of inspired oxygen, P_B is the barometric pressure, PH_2O is the partial pressure of water, and RQ is the respiratory quotient or the ratio of CO$_2$ production ($\dot{V}CO_2$) to oxygen consumption ($\dot{V}O_2$).

$$\dot{Q}_{ps}/\dot{Q}_{t} = (C_iO_2 - C_aO_2)/(C_iO_2 - C_vO_2)$$

where C_vO_2, C_aO_2, and C_iO_2 are the oxygen contents of venous, arterial, and expected pulmonary capillary blood, respectively.

$$OI = (P_{aw} \times FiO_2 \times 100)/PaO_2$$

where P_{aw} represents the mean airway pressure.[15]

The overall therapeutic goal of optimizing oxygenation parameters is to maintain oxygen delivery (DO_2) to the tissues. Three variables determine $DO2$: cardiac output (Q), hemoglobin concentration (Hgb), and arterial blood oxygen saturation (SaO_2). The product of these three variables determines DO_2 by the relation:

$$DO_2 = Q \times CaO_2 \text{ where}$$
$$CaO_2 = (1.36 \times Hgb \times [SaO_2/100]) + (0.0031 \times PaO_2)$$

Note that the contribution of the PaO_2 to DO_2 is minimal and may be disregarded in most circumstances. If the hemoglobin concentration of the blood is normal (15 g/dL) and the hemoglobin is fully saturated with oxygen, the amount of oxygen bound to hemoglobin is 20.4 mL/dL (Fig. 7-4). In addition, approximately 0.3 mL of oxygen is physically dissolved in each deciliter of plasma, which makes the oxygen content of normal arterial blood equal to approximately 20.7 mL O_2/dL. Similar calculations reveal that the normal venous blood oxygen content is approximately 15 mL O_2/dL.

Typically, DO_2 is four to five times greater than the associated oxygen consumption (VO_2). As DO_2 increases or VO_2 decreases, more oxygen remains in the venous blood. The result is an increase in the oxygen hemoglobin saturation in the mixed venous pulmonary artery blood ($S\bar{V}O_2$). In contrast, if the DO_2 decreases or VO_2 increases, relatively more oxygen is extracted from the blood, and therefore less oxygen remains in the venous blood. A decrease in $S\bar{V}O_2$ is the result. In general, the $S\bar{V}O_2$ serves as an excellent monitor of oxygen kinetics because it specifically assesses the adequacy of DO_2 in

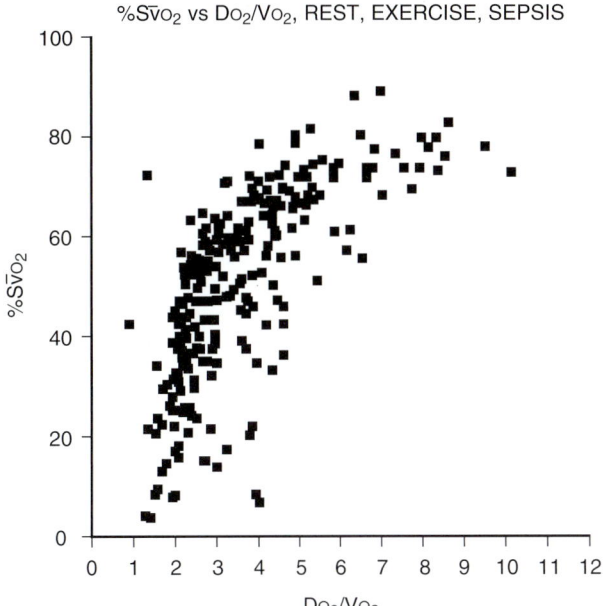

FIGURE 7-5 ■ The relation of the mixed venous oxygen saturation (SO_2) and the ratio of oxygen delivery to oxygen consumption (DO_2/VO_2) in normal eumetabolic, hypermetabolic septic, and hypermetabolic exercising canines. (Reprinted from Hirschl RB. Cardiopulmonary Critical Care and Shock: Surgery of Infants and Children: Scientific Principles and Practice. Philadelphia: Lippincott-Raven; 1997.)

relation to DO_2 (DO_2/VO_2 ratio) (Fig. 7-5).[26] Many pulmonary arterial catheters contain fiber optic bundles that provide continuous mixed venous oximetry data. Such data provides a means for assessing the adequacy of DO_2, rapid assessment of the response to interventions such as mechanical ventilation, and cost savings due to a diminished need for sequential blood gas monitoring.[26,27] If a pulmonary artery catheter is unavailable, the central venous oxygen saturation ($Sc\bar{V}O_2$) may serve as a surrogate of the $S\bar{V}O_2$.[28]

Four factors are manipulated in an attempt to improve the DO_2/VO_2 ratio: cardiac output, hemoglobin concentration, SaO_2, and VO_2. The result of various interventions designed to increase cardiac output, such as volume administration, infusion of inotropic agents, administration of afterload-reducing drugs, and correction of acid–base abnormalities, can be assessed by the effect on the $S\bar{V}O_2$. One of the most efficient ways to enhance DO_2 is to increase the oxygen-carrying capacity of the blood. For instance, an increase in hemoglobin from 7.5 g/dL to 15 g/dL will be associated with a twofold increase in DO_2 at constant cardiac output. However, blood viscosity is also increased with blood transfusion, which may result in a reduction in cardiac output.[29] The SaO_2 can often be enhanced through application of supplemental oxygen and mechanical ventilation.

Assessment of the 'best PEEP' identifies the level at which DO_2 and $S\bar{V}O_2$ are optimal without compromising compliance.[30,31] Evaluation of the best PEEP should be performed in any patient requiring an FiO_2 greater than 0.60 and may be determined by continuous monitoring of the $S\bar{V}O_2$ as the PEEP is sequentially increased from 5 cmH$_2$O to 15 cmH$_2$O over a short period. The

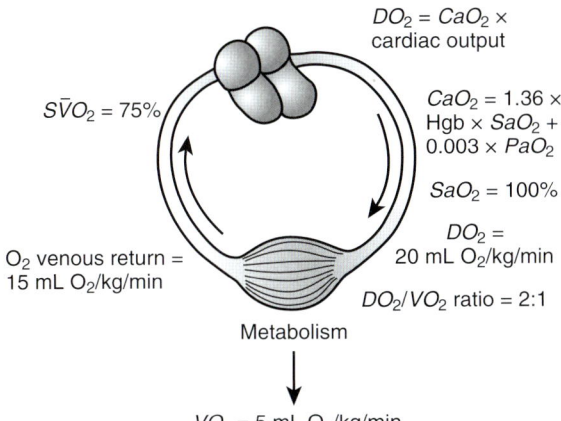

FIGURE 7-4 ■ Oxygen consumption (VO_2) and delivery (DO_2) relations. (Adapted with permission from Hirschl RB. Oxygen delivery in the pediatric surgical patients. Opin Pediatr 1994;6:341–7.)

point at which the $S\bar{V}O_2$ is maximal indicates optimal DO_2. The use of PEEP with mechanical ventilation is limited, however, by the adverse effects observed on cardiac output, the effect of barotrauma, and the risk for ventilator-induced lung injury with application of peak inspiratory pressures greater than 30–40 cmH$_2$O.[32,33] Furthermore, oxygen consumption can be elevated secondary to sepsis, burns, agitation, seizures, hyperthermia, hyperthyroidism, and increased catecholamine production or infusion. A number of interventions may be applied to reduce VO_2, such as sedation and mechanical ventilation. Paralysis may enhance the effectiveness of mechanical ventilation while simultaneously reducing VO_2.[34,35] In the appropriate setting, hypothermia may be induced with an associated reduction of 7% in VO_2 with each 1°C decrease in core temperature.[36]

MECHANICAL VENTILATION

As discussed earlier, failure of gas exchange (CO$_2$ elimination or oxygenation) may be an indication for mechanical ventilation. The ventilator can also be used to reduce the work of breathing and decrease VO_2. Finally, mechanical ventilation is used in patients who are unable to breathe independently for neurologic reasons (primary hypoventilation, traumatic brain injury, inability to protect airway).

The Mechanical Ventilator and Its Components

The ventilator must overcome the pressure generated by the elastic recoil of the lung at end inspiration plus the resistance to flow at the airway. To do so, most ventilators in the ICU are pneumatically powered by gas pressurized at 50 pounds per square inch (psi). Microprocessor controls allow accurate management of proportional solenoid-driven valves, which carefully control infusion of a blend of air or oxygen into the ventilator circuit while simultaneously opening and closing an expiratory valve.[37] Additional components of a ventilator include a bacterial filter, a pneumotachometer, a humidifier, a heater/thermostat, an oxygen analyzer, and a pressure manometer. A chamber for nebulizing drugs is usually incorporated into the inspiratory circuit. The V_t is not usually measured directly. Rather, flow is assessed as a function of time, thereby allowing calculation of V_t. The modes of ventilation are characterized by three variables that affect patient and ventilator synchrony or interaction: the parameter used to initiate or 'trigger' a breath, the parameter used to 'limit' the size of the breath, and the parameter used to terminate inspiration or 'cycle' the breath (Fig. 7-6).[38]

Gas flow in most ventilators is triggered either by time (controlled breath) or by patient effort (assisted breath). Controlled ventilation modes are time triggered: the inspiratory phase is concluded once a desired volume, pressure, or flow is attained, but the expiratory time will be the difference between the inspiratory time and the preset respiratory cycle time. In the assist mode, the ventilator is pressure or flow triggered. With the former,

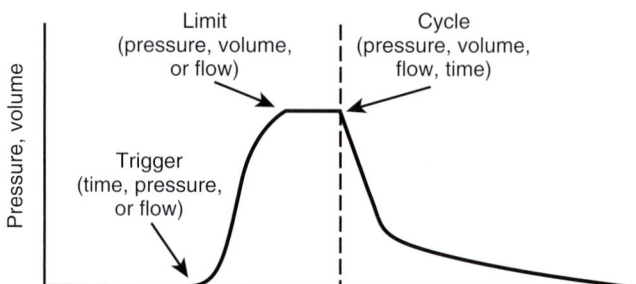

FIGURE 7-6 ■ Variables that characterize the mode of mechanical ventilation.

a pressure generated by the patient of approximately −1 cmH$_2$O will trigger the initiation of a breath. The sensitivity of the triggering device can be adjusted so that patient work is minimized. Other ventilators detect the reduction in constant ventilator tubing gas flow that is associated with patient initiation of a breath. Detection of this decrease in flow results in initiation of a positive-pressure breath.

The magnitude of the breath is controlled or limited by one of three variables: pressure, volume, or flow. When a breath is volume, pressure, or flow 'controlled,' it indicates that inspiration concludes once the limiting variable is reached. Pressure-controlled or pressure-limited modes are the most popular for all age groups, although volume-control ventilation may be of advantage in preterm newborns.[39,40] In the pressure modes, the respiratory rate, the inspiratory gas flow, the PEEP level, the inspiratory/expiratory (I/E) ratio, and the P_{aw} are determined. The ventilator infuses gas until the desired peak inspiratory pressure (PIP) is provided. Zero-flow conditions are realized at end inspiration during pressure-limited ventilation. Therefore, in this mode, PIP is frequently equivalent to end-inspiratory pressure (EIP) or plateau pressure.

In many ventilators, the gas flow rate is fixed, although some ventilators allow manipulation of the flow rate and therefore the rate of positive-pressure development. Those with rapid flow rates will provide rapid ascent of pressure to the preset maximum, where it will remain for the duration of the inspiratory phase. This 'square wave' pressure pattern results in decelerating flow during inspiration (Fig. 7-7). Airway pressure is 'front loaded,' which increases P_{aw}, alveolar volume, and oxygenation without increasing PIP.[41] However, one of the biggest advantages of pressure-controlled or pressure-limited ventilation is the ability to avoid lung over-distention and barotrauma/volutrauma (discussed later). The disadvantage of pressure-controlled or pressure-limited ventilation is that delivered volume varies with airway resistance and pulmonary compliance, and may be reduced when short inspiratory times are applied (Fig. 7-8).[42] For this reason, both V_t and $\dot{V}_E$ must be monitored carefully.

Volume-controlled or volume-limited ventilation requires delineation of the V_t, respiratory rate, and inspiratory gas flow. Gas will be inspired until the preset V_t is attained. The volume will remain constant despite changes in pulmonary mechanics, although the resulting EIP and PIP may be altered. Flow-controlled or flow-limited ventilation is similar in many respects to volume-controlled or volume-limited ventilation. A flow pattern

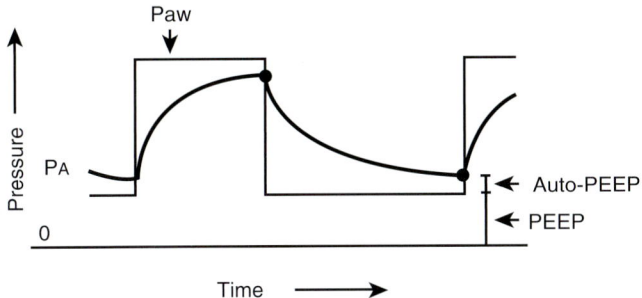

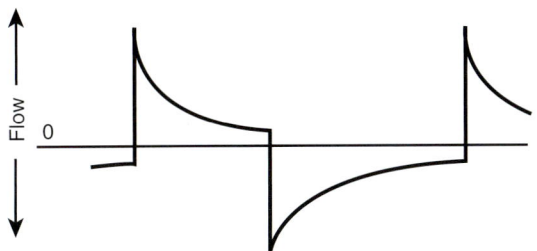

FIGURE 7-7 ■ Pressure and flow waveforms during pressure-limited, time-cycled ventilation. Decelerating flow is applied, which 'front loads' the pressure during inspiration. Auto-positive end-expiratory pressure is present when the expiratory time is inadequate for complete expiration. (Reprinted from Marini JJ. New options for the ventilatory management of acute lung injury. New Horiz 1993;1:489–503.)

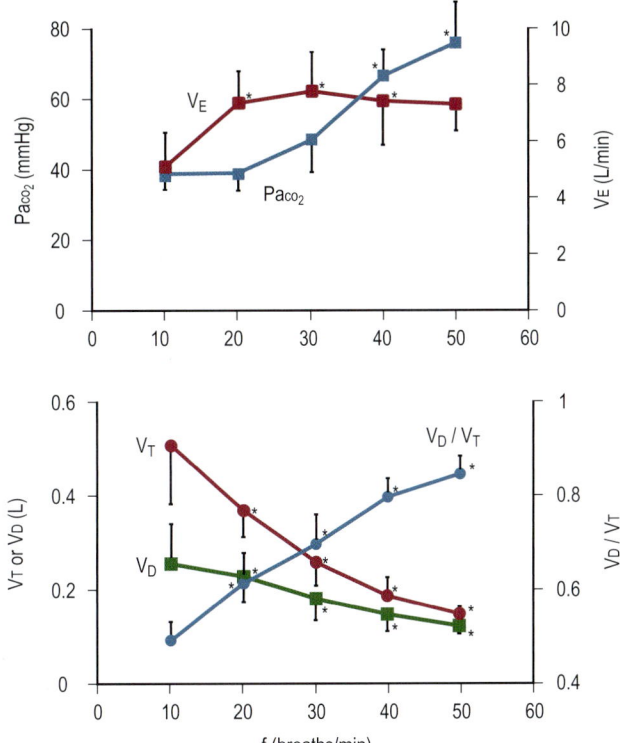

FIGURE 7-8 ■ Effect of rate on tidal volume (V_d/V_t) and minute ventilation (V_E) during pressure-limited ventilation. Note that V_E remains unchanged above 20 breaths/min. Simultaneously, V_d/V_t and $PaCO_2$ increase, despite an increase in respiratory rate. (Reprinted from Nahum A, Burke WC, Ravenscraft SA. Lung mechanics and gas exchange during pressure-control ventilation in dogs: Augmentation of CO_2 elimination by an intratracheal catheter. Am Rev Respir Dis 1992;146:965–73.)

is predetermined, which effectively results in a fixed volume as the limiting component of inspiration.

The ventilator breath is concluded based on one of four variables: volume, time, pressure, or flow. With volume-cycled ventilation, inspiration is terminated when a prescribed volume is obtained. Likewise, with time-, pressure-, or flow-cycled ventilation, expiration begins after a certain period has passed, the airway pressure reaches a certain value, or when the flow has decreased to a predetermined level, respectively.

A factor that limits inspiration suggests that the chosen value limits the level of the variable during inspiration, but the inspiratory phase does not necessarily conclude once this value is attained. For instance, during 'pressure-limited' ventilation, gas flow continues until a given pressure limit is attained. However, the inspiratory phase may continue beyond that point. The limitation only controls the magnitude of the breath but does not always determine the length of the inspiratory phase. In contrast, during pressure-controlled ventilation, both gas flow and the inspiratory phase terminate once the preset pressure is reached because pressure is used to limit the magnitude of the breath and the gas flow.

Modes of Ventilation (Table 7-2)

Controlled Mechanical Ventilation

Controlled mechanical ventilation (CMV) is time triggered, flow limited, and volume or pressure cycled. Spontaneous breaths may be taken between the mandatory breaths. However, no additional gas is provided during spontaneous breaths. Therefore, the work of breathing

is markedly increased in the spontaneously breathing patient. This mode of ventilation is no longer used.

Intermittent Mandatory Ventilation

Intermittent mandatory ventilation (IMV) is time triggered, volume or pressure limited, and either time, volume, or pressure cycled. A rate is set, as is a volume or pressure parameter. Additional inspired gas is provided by the ventilator to support spontaneous breathing when additional breaths are desired. The difference between CMV and IMV is that, in the IMV mode, inspired gases are provided to the patient during spontaneous breaths.[43] IMV is useful in patients who do not have respiratory drive such as those who are neurologically impaired or pharmacologically paralyzed. Work of breathing is still elevated with this mode in the awake and spontaneously breathing patient.

Synchronized Intermittent Mandatory Ventilation

In the SIMV mode, the ventilator synchronizes IMV breaths with the patient's spontaneous breaths (Fig. 7-9). Small, patient-initiated negative deflections in airway pressure (pressure triggered) or decreases in the constant ventilator gas flow (bias flow) passing through the exhalation valve (flow triggered) provide a signal to the

TABLE 7-2 Modes of Ventilation

Mode	Trigger	Limit	Cycle	Comment
CMV	Time	Flow	Pressure/volume	No longer used
IMV	Time	Volume/pressure	Time Volume/pressure	For no respiratory drive (neurologically impaired or paralyzed) Work of breathing elevated in spontaneously breathing patient
SIMV[a]	Pressure/flow	Volume/pressure	Time Volume/pressure	Supports limited number of breaths
ACV[a]	Pressure/flow	Volume/pressure	Time Volume/pressure	Supports all patient breaths Similar to IMV but patient controls breaths Sedation for hyperventilation and backup rate for apnea
PSV[a]	Pressure/flow	Pressure	Flow Time	Supports all patient breaths Usually partially supported to allow for weaning Time cycled when termination sensitivity for flow is off
VSV[a]	Pressure/flow	Volume	Flow Time	Similar to PSV but volume used for partial support
VAPSV	Pressureflow	Pressure	Flow Time	Maintains a desired tidal volume using both VSV and PSV Dynamically maintains tidal volume
PAV[a]	Patient	Pressure	Patient	Size of the breath is determined by patient effort

ACV, assist-control ventilation; CMV, controlled mechanical ventilation; IMV, intermittent mandatory ventilation; PAV, proportional assist ventilation; PSV, pressure support ventilation; SIMV, synchronized intermittent mandatory ventilation; VAPSV, volume-assured pressure support ventilation; VSV, volume support ventilation.
[a]Patient-controlled rate.

ventilator that a patient breath has been initiated. Ventilated breaths are timed with the patient's spontaneous respiration, but the number of supported breaths each minute is predetermined and remains constant. Additional constant inspired gas flow is provided for use during any other spontaneous breaths. Advances in neonatal ventilators have provided the means for detecting small alterations in bias flow. As such, flow-triggered SIMV can be applied to newborns, which appears to enhance ventilatory patterns and allows ventilation with reduced airway pressures and FiO_2.[44,45] SIMV may be associated with a reduction in the duration of ventilation and the incidence of air leak in newborns in general, as well as in those premature infants with bronchopulmonary dysplasia (BPD) and intraventricular hemorrhage.[46,47]

Assist-Control Ventilation

In the spontaneously breathing patient, brain stem reflexes dependent on cerebrospinal fluid levels of CO_2 and pH can be harnessed to determine the appropriate breathing rate.[15] As in SIMV, with assist-control ventilation (ACV) the assisted breaths can be either pressure triggered or flow triggered. The triggering-mechanism sensitivity can be set in most ventilators. In contrast to SIMV, the ventilator supports all patient-initiated breaths. This mode is similar to IMV but allows the patient inherently to control the ventilation and minimizes patient work of breathing in adults and neonates.[48,49] Occasionally, patients may hyperventilate, such as when they are agitated or have neurologic injury. Heavy sedation may be required if agitation is present. A minimal ventilator rate below the patient's assist rate should be established in case of apnea.

Pressure Support Ventilation

Pressure support ventilation (PSV) is a pressure- or flow-triggered, pressure-limited, and flow-cycled mode of ventilation. It is similar in concept to ACV, in that mechanical support is provided for each spontaneous breath and the patient determines the ventilator rate. During each breath, inspiratory flow is applied until a predetermined pressure is attained.[50] As the end of inspiration approaches, flow decreases to a level below a specified value (2–6 L/min) or a percentage of peak inspiratory flow (at 25%). At this point, inspiration terminates. Although it may apply full support, PSV is frequently used to support the patient partially by assigning a pressure limit for each breath that is less than that required for full support.[51] For example, in the spontaneously breathing patient, PSV can be sequentially decreased from full support to a PSV 5–10 cmH$_2$O above PEEP, allowing weaning while providing partial support with each breath.[52,53] Thus, V_t during PSV may be dependent on patient effort. PSV provides two advantages during ventilation of spontaneously breathing patients: (1) it provides excellent support and decreases the work of breathing associated with ventilation; and (2) it lowers PIP and P_{aw} while higher V_t and cardiac output levels may be observed.[50,54,55]

Pressure-triggered SIMV and PSV can be applied to newborns. Inspiration is terminated when the peak airway flow decreases to a set percentage between 5–25%. This flow cutoff for inspiration, known as the termination sensitivity, can be adjusted. The higher the termination sensitivity value, the shorter is the inspiratory time. The termination sensitivity function also may be disabled, at which point ventilation is time cycled instead of flow cycled. There is a reduction in work of breathing and sedation requirements when SIMV with pressure support is applied to newborns.

Volume Support Ventilation

Volume support ventilation (VSV) is similar to PSV except that a volume, rather than a pressure, is assigned to provide partial support. Automation with VSV is

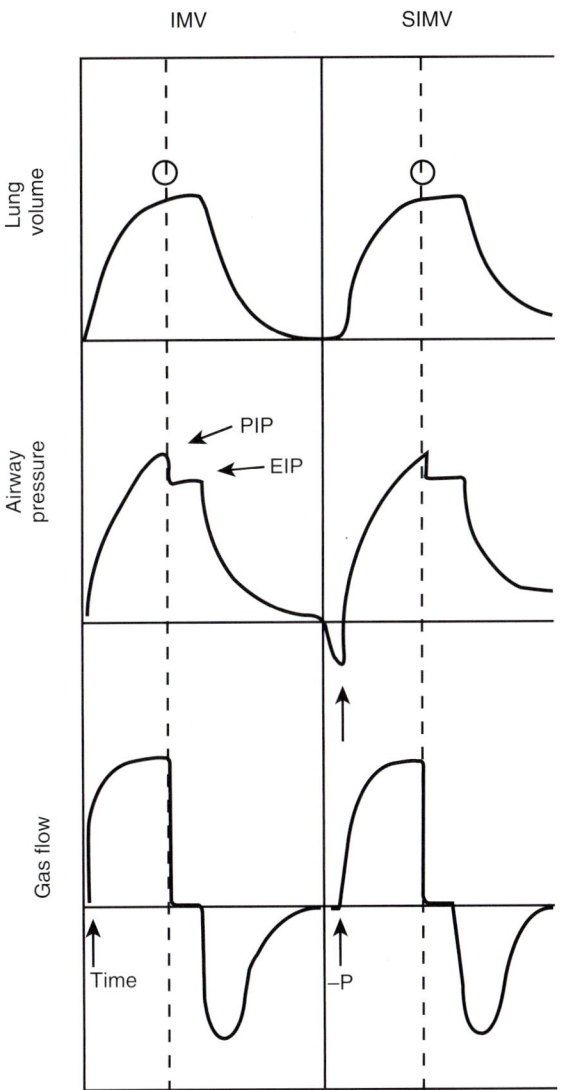

FIGURE 7-9 ■ Pressure, volume, and flow waveforms observed during intermittent mandatory ventilation (IMV) and synchronized IMV (SIMV). In this case, an end-inspiratory pause has been added. Note the difference between peak (PIP) and end-inspiratory (EIP) or plateau pressure. Arrows, triggering variables; open circles, cycling variables. (Adapted from Bartlett RH. Use of the Mechanical Ventilator: Surgery. New York: Scientific American; 1988.)

enhanced because there is less need for manual changes to maintain stable tidal and minute volume during weaning.[56] Both VSV and PSV are equally effective at weaning infants and children from the ventilator.[57]

Volume-Assured Pressure Support Ventilation

Volume-assured pressure support ventilation (VAPSV) attempts to combine volume- and pressure-controlled ventilation to ensure a desired V_t within the constraints of the pressure limit. It has the advantage of maintaining inflation to a point below an injurious PIP level while maintaining V_t constant in the face of changing pulmonary mechanics. Work of breathing may be markedly decreased while C_{eff} is increased during VAPSV.[58]

Proportional Assist Ventilation

Proportional assist ventilation (PAV) is an intriguing approach in the spontaneously breathing patient. It relies on the concept that the combined pressure generated by the ventilator (P_{aw}) and respiratory muscles (P_{mus}) is equivalent to that required to overcome the resistance to flow of the endotracheal tube/airways (P_{res}) and the tendency for the inflated lungs to collapse.[59]

With PAV, airway pressure generation by the ventilator is proportional at any instant to the respiratory effort (P_{mus}) generated by the patient. Small efforts, therefore, result in small breaths, whereas greater patient effort results in development of a greater V_t. Inspiration is patient triggered and terminates with discontinuation of patient effort. Rate, V_t, and inspiratory time are entirely patient controlled. The predominant variable controlled by the ventilator is the proportional response between P_{mus} and the applied ventilator pressure. This proportional assist (P_{aw}/P_{mus}) can be increased until nearly all patient effort is provided by the ventilator.[60] Patient work of breathing, dyspnea, and PIP are reduced.[61,62] Elastance and resistance are set, as is applied PEEP. V_t is variable, and the risk of atelectasis is present. PAV produces similar gas exchange with lower airway pressures when compared with conventional ventilation in infants.[63] Compared with preterm newborns being ventilated with the assist-control mode and with IMV, preterm newborns managed with PAV maintained gas exchange with lower airway pressures and a decrease in the oxygenation index by 28%.[64] Chest wall dynamics also are enhanced.[65] PAV represents an exciting first step in servoregulating ventilators to patient requirements. Additional studies using neutrally adjusted ventilation are also underway and certain populations (obstructive lung disease and small children) may benefit from the increased patient-ventilator synchrony.[66,67]

Continuous Positive Airway Pressure

During continuous positive airway pressure (CPAP), pressures greater than those of ambient pressure are continuously applied to the airways to enhance alveolar distention and oxygenation.[68] Both airway resistance and work of breathing may be substantially reduced. Since ventilation is unsupported, this mode requires that the patient provides all of the work of breathing and CPAP should be avoided in patients with hypovolemia, untreated pneumothorax, lung hyperinflation, or elevated intracranial pressure, and in infants with nasal obstruction, cleft palate, tracheoesophageal fistula, or untreated congenital diaphragmatic hernia. CPAP is frequently applied via nasal prongs, although it can be delivered in adult patients with a nasal mask.

Bilevel Control of Positive Airway Pressure (BiPAP)

Although sometimes used in the setting of acute lung injury, BiPAP is frequently used for home respiratory support by varying airway pressure between one of two settings: the inspiratory positive airway pressure (IPAP) and the expiratory positive airway pressure (EPAP).[69,70] With patient effort, a change in flow is detected, and the IPAP pressure level is developed. With reduced flow at end expiration, EPAP is re-established. Therefore, this device provides both ventilatory support and airway distention during the expiratory phase; however, BiPAP ventilators should be used only to support the patient who is spontaneously breathing. In fact, in a randomized trial of noninvasive ventilation (NIV) in a subset of pediatric patients with lung injury, NIV improved hypoxemia and decreased the rate of endotracheal intubation.[71] In neonates, a multicenter randomized trial demonstrated decreased days of mechanical ventilation, chronic lung disease, and mortality when early CPAP was used instead of intubation and surfactant in preterm infants.[72]

Inverse Ratio Ventilation

In the setting of respiratory failure, it would be helpful to enhance alveolar distention to reduce hypoxemia and shunt. One means to accomplish this is to maintain the inspiratory plateau pressure for a longer proportion of the breath.[73] The inspiratory time may be prolonged to the point at which the I/E ratio may be as high as $4:1$.[74] In most circumstances, however, the I/E ratio is maintained at approximately $2:1$. Inverse ratio ventilation (IRV) is usually performed during pressure-controlled ventilation (PC-IRV), although prolonged inspiratory times can be applied during volume-controlled ventilation by adding a decelerating flow pattern or an end-inspiratory pause to the volume-controlled ventilator breath.[75] One advantage of IRV is the ability to recruit alveoli that are associated with high-resistance airways that inflate only with prolonged application of positive pressure.[76] Unfortunately, IRV is associated with a profound sense of dyspnea in patients who are awake and spontaneously breathing. Therefore, heavy sedation and pharmacologic paralysis is required during this ventilator mode.

As E_t is reduced, the risk for incomplete expiration, identified by the failure to achieve zero-flow conditions at end expiration, is increased. This results in 'auto-PEEP' or a total PEEP greater than that of the preset or applied PEEP. Care should be taken to recognize the presence of auto-PEEP and to incorporate it into the ventilation strategy to avoid barotrauma.[77] IRV also may negatively affect cardiac output and, therefore, decrease DO_2.[78] Some studies using IRV revealed an increase in Paw and oxygenation while protecting the lungs by reducing PIP.[79-82] Other reports suggest that early implementation of IRV in severe ARDS enhances oxygenation and allows reduction in FiO_2, PEEP, and PIP.[83] On the contrary, a number of studies have failed to demonstrate enhanced gas exchange with this mode of ventilation. Some series have suggested that IRV is less effective at enhancing gas exchange than is application of PEEP to maintain the same mean airway pressure.[84] Overall, it appears that oxygenation is determined primarily by the mean airway pressure rather than specifically by the application of IRV. As such, the usefulness of IRV remains in question.[85]

Airway Pressure Release Ventilation

Airway pressure release ventilation (APRV) is a unique approach to ventilation in which CPAP at high levels is used to enhance mean alveolar volume while intermittent reductions in pressure to a 'release' level provide a period of expiration (Fig. 7-10). Re-establishment of CPAP results in inspiration and return of lung volume back to the baseline level. The advantage of APRV is a reduction in PIP of approximately 50% in adult patients with ARDS when compared with other more conventional modes of mechanical ventilation.[86,87] Spontaneous ventilation also is allowed throughout the cycle, which may enhance cardiac function and renal blood flow.[88,89] Some data suggest that $\dot{V}/\dot{Q}$ matching may be improved and dead space reduced.[90,91] In performing APRV, tidal volume is altered by adjusting the release pressure. Conceptually, ventilator management during APRV is the inverse of other modes of positive-pressure ventilation in that the PIP, or CPAP, determines oxygenation, while the expiratory pressure (release pressure) is used to adjust V_t and CO_2 elimination.

APRV is very similar to modes of ventilation, such as IRV, that use prolonged I/E ratios; however, APRV appears to be better tolerated when compared with IRV in patients with acute lung injury/ARDS, as demonstrated by a reduced need for paralysis and sedation, increased cardiac performance, decreased pressor use, and decreased PIP requirements.[92] APRV improved the lung perfusion, as measured by pulmonary blood flow and oxygen delivery, in infants who underwent repair of tetralogy of Fallot or cavopulmonary shunt.[93] However, the overall clinical experience with APRV is limited in the pediatric population.[94,95]

Management of the Mechanical Ventilator

IMV and SIMV may suffice for patients with normal lungs, such as when needed after an operation.[96] If the patient is spontaneously breathing and is to be ventilated for more than a brief period, a flow- or pressure-triggered assist mode, pressure support, or PAV will result in maximal support and minimal work of breathing.[48,49] Ventilator modes that allow adjustment of specific details of pressure, flow, and volume are required in the patient

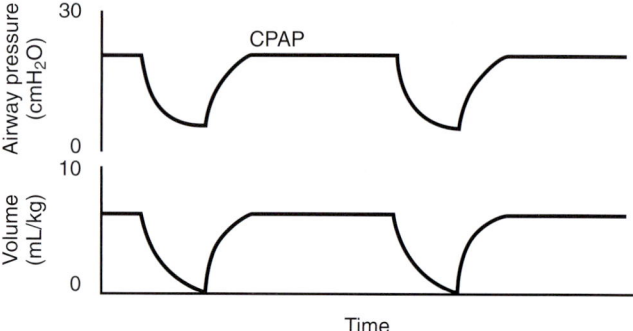

FIGURE 7-10 ■ Typical pressure and volume waveforms observed during airway pressure release ventilation (APRV).

with severe respiratory failure. With all these modes, the ventilator rate, V_t or PIP, PEEP, and either inspiratory time alone or I/E ratio (if ventilation is pressure limited) must be assigned. Other secondary controls such as the flow rate, the flow pattern, the trigger sensitivity for assisted breaths, the inspiratory hold, the termination sensitivity, and the safety pressure limit also are set on individual ventilators. The normal $\dot{V}_E$ is 100–150 mL/kg/min. The FiO_2 is usually initiated at 0.50 and decreased based on pulse oximetry. All efforts should be made to maintain the FiO_2 less than 0.60 to avoid alveolar nitrogen depletion and the development of atelectasis.[97,98] Oxygen toxicity likely is a result of this phenomenon, although free oxygen radical formation may play a role when an FiO_2 greater than 0.40 is applied for prolonged periods.[99] A short inspiratory phase with a low I/E ratio favors the expiratory phase and CO_2 elimination, whereas longer I/E ratios enhance oxygenation. In the normal lung, I/E ratios of 1:3 and inspiratory time of 0.5 to 1 second are typical.

Strategies in Respiratory Failure

Preventing Ventilator-Induced Lung Injury

A decrease in pulmonary compliance and FRC is seen in the patient with acute lung injury (PaO_2/FiO_2 ratio, 200–300) or ARDS (PaO_2/FiO_2 ratio, <200). This is secondary to alveolar collapse and a decrease in the volume of lung available for ventilation and, in turn, to decreased pulmonary compliance. As a result, higher ventilator pressures are necessary to maintain V_t and $\dot{V}_E$. However, any attempt to ventilate the patient with respiratory insufficiency due to parenchymal disease with higher pressures can result in compromise of cardiopulmonary function and the development of ventilator-induced lung injury.[100]

The concept of ventilator-induced lung injury was first identified in 1974 by demonstrating the detrimental effects of ventilation at PIP of 45 cmH$_2$O in rats.[101] Electron microscopy has been used to document an increased incidence of alveolar stress fractures in ex-vivo, perfused rabbit lungs exposed to transalveolar pressures more than 30 cmH$_2$O.[102] Other studies have demonstrated increases in albumin leak, elevation of the capillary leak coefficient, enhanced wet-to-dry lung weight, deterioration in gas exchange, and augmented diffuse alveolar damage on histology with application of increased airway pressure (45–50 cmH$_2$O) in otherwise normal rats and sheep over a 1- to 24-hour period.[31,103,104] Pulmonary exposure to high pressures may potentially worsen nascent respiratory insufficiency and, ultimately, lead to the development of pulmonary fibrosis.

Such injury may be prevented during application of high PIPs by strapping the chest, thereby preventing lung over-distention, suggesting that alveolar distention or 'volutrauma' is the injurious element, rather than application of high pressures or 'barotrauma'.[105] A low-V_t (6 mL/kg) approach to mechanical ventilation in rabbits with *Pseudomonas aeruginosa*-induced acute lung injury appears to be associated with enhancement in oxygenation, increase in pH, increase in arterial blood pressure, and decrease in extravascular lung water when compared

with a high-V_t group (15 mL/kg).[106] A relation may also exist between ventilator gas flow rate and the development of lung injury.[107] Positive blood cultures were found in five of six animals exposed to high EIP, but rarely in those with low EIP.[108]

Together, the above data suggest that the method of ventilation has an effect on lung function and gas exchange as well as a systemic effect, which may include translocation of bacteria from the lungs. As such, avoidance of high PIPs and lung over-distention should be a primary goal of mechanical ventilation. Although the animal data suggests that high PIPs and volumes may be deleterious, two multicenter studies have attempted to randomize patients with ARDS to high and low peak pressure or volume strategies. The first failed to demonstrate a difference in mortality or duration of mechanical ventilation in patients randomized to either the low-volume (7.2 ± 0.8 mL/kg) or the high-volume (10.8 ± 1.0 mL) strategy, although the applied PIP was not elevated to what would commonly be considered injurious levels in either group (low, 23.6 ± 5.8 cmH$_2$O; high, 34.0 ± 11.0 cmH$_2$O).[109] Another study found similar results, but had similar design limitations.[110] A survival increase from 38% to 71% at 28 days, a higher rate of weaning from mechanical ventilation, and a lower rate of barotrauma has been demonstrated in patients in whom a lung-protective ventilator strategy was used. This strategy consisted of lung distention to a level that prevented alveolar collapse during expiration (see later) and avoidance of high distending pressures.[111] One study identified a significant reduction over time in bronchoalveolar lavage concentrations of polymorphonuclear cells ($P < 0.001$), interleukin (IL)-1β ($P < 0.05$), tumor necrosis factor (TNF)-α ($P < 0.001$), interleukin (IL)-8 ($P < 0.001$), and IL-6 ($P < 0.005$) and in the plasma concentration of IL-6 ($P < 0.002$) among 44 patients randomized to receive a lung-protective strategy rather than a conventional approach.[112] The mean number of ventilator-free days at 28 days in the lung-protective strategy group was higher than in the control group (12 ± 11 vs. 4 ± 8 days, respectively; $P < 0.01$). However, mortality rates at 28 days from admission were not different.

The NIH's Acute Respiratory Distress Network convincingly demonstrated that mortality was reduced with the use of a low-volume (6 mL/kg, mortality of 31%) when compared with a high-volume (12 mL/kg, mortality of 39%; $P = 0.005$) ventilator approach (Fig. 7-11).[113] Interestingly, no difference was found in gas exchange or pulmonary mechanics between groups to account for the difference in mortality. The majority of clinicians are now convinced that avoidance of high PIP and support of lung recruitment, through the application of appropriate levels of PEEP (see later), should be a primary goal of any mechanical ventilatory program.

Permissive Hypercapnia

To avoid ventilator-induced lung injury, practitioners have applied the concept of permissive hypercapnia. With this approach, $PaCO_2$ is allowed to increase to levels as high as 120 mmHg as long as the blood pH is maintained

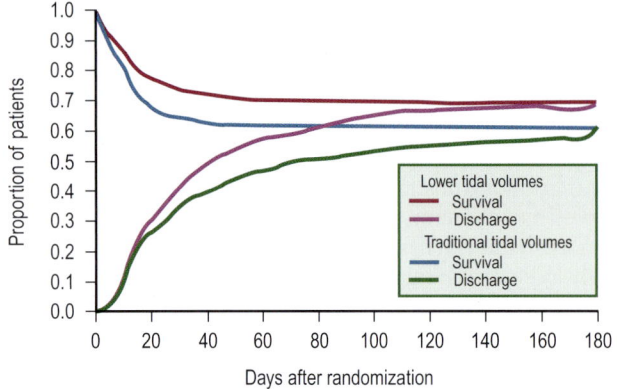

FIGURE 7-11 ■ Probability of survival and of being discharged home and breathing without assistance during the first 180 days after randomization in patients with acute lung injury and the acute respiratory distress syndrome. The status at 180 days or at the end of the study was known for all but nine patients. (From The Acute Respiratory Distress Network. Ventilation with lower tidal volumes as compared with traditional tidal volumes for acute lung injury and the acute respiratory distress syndrome. N Engl J Med 2000;342:1301–8.)

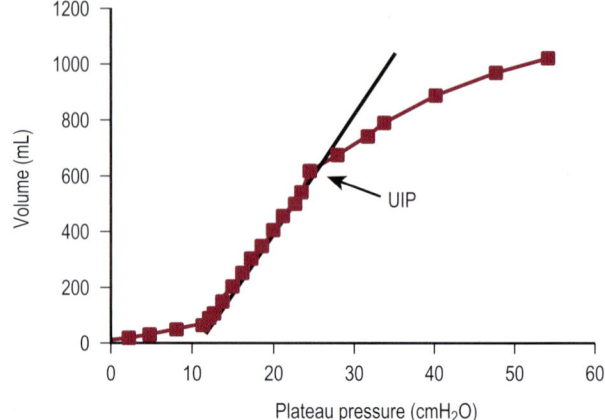

FIGURE 7-12 ■ Static pressure/volume curve demonstrating the P_{flex} point in a patient with acute respiratory distress syndrome. Positive end-expiratory pressure should be maintained approximately 2 cmH$_2$O above that point. The upper inflection point (UIP) indicates the point at which lung over distention is beginning to occur. Ventilation to points above the UIP should be avoided in most circumstances. (Reprinted from Roupie E, Dambrosio M, Servillo G. Titration of tidal volume and induced hypercapnia in acute respiratory distress syndrome. Am J Respir Crit Care Med 1995;152:121–8.)

in the 7.1–7.2 range by administration of buffers.[114] Mortality was reduced to 26% when compared with that expected (53%; $P < 0.004$) based on Acute Physiology and Chronic Health Evaluation II (APACHE II) scores when low-volume, pressure-limited ventilation with permissive hypercapnia was applied in the setting of ARDS in adults.[115] For burned children, the mortality rate was only 3.7% despite a high degree of inhalation injury when a ventilator strategy used a PIP of 40 cmH$_2$O and accepted an elevated $PaCO_2$ as long as the arterial pH was greater than 7.20.[116] Other studies suggested that a strategy of high-frequency (40–120 breaths/min) ventilation with a low V_t, low PIP, high PEEP (7–30 cmH$_2$O), and mild hypercapnia ($PaCO_2$ from 45 to 60 mmHg) enhances the survival rate in children with severe ARDS.[117]

Using Protective Effects of PEEP

Although application of high, over distending airway pressures appears to be associated with the development of lung injury, a number of studies have demonstrated that application of PEEP or high-frequency oscillatory ventilation (HFOV) may prevent lung injury by the following mechanisms: (1) recruitment of collapsed alveoli, which reduces the risk for over-distention of healthy units; (2) resolution of alveolar collapse, which in and of itself is injurious; and (3) avoidance of the shear forces associated with the opening and closing of alveoli.[118,119] In the older child with injured lungs, a pressure of 8–12 cmH$_2$O is required to open alveoli and to begin V_t generation.[111,120,121] Alveoli will subsequently close unless the end-expiratory pressure is maintained at such pressures, and cyclic opening and closing is thought to be particularly injurious because of application of large shear forces.[120] One way to avoid this process is through the application of PEEP to a point above the inflection pressure (P_{flex}), such that alveolar distention is maintained throughout the ventilatory cycle (Fig. 7-12).[122,123] In addition, as mentioned previously, it

has been demonstrated that the distribution of infiltrates and atelectasis in the supine patient with ARDS is predominantly in the dependent regions of the lung.[124] This is likely the result of compression due to the increased weight of the overlying edematous lung. It has been shown that when the superimposed gravitational pressure from the weight of the overlying lung exceeded the PEEP applied to a given region of the lung, end-expiratory lung collapse increased, resulting in de-recruitment.[125] Thus, application of PEEP may result in recruitment of these atelectatic lung regions, simultaneously enhancing pulmonary compliance and oxygenation. PEEP and prone positioning (see later) are more effective if the need for ventilation is of extrapulmonary etiology rather than pulmonary etiology.[126]

As a result of these new data and concepts, the approach to mechanical ventilation in the patient with respiratory failure has changed drastically over the past few years (Box 7-1). Time-cycled, pressure-controlled ventilation has become favored because of the ability to limit EIP to noninjurious levels at a maximum of 35 cmH$_2$O.[121] In infants and newborns, this EIP limit is set lower at 30 cmH$_2$O. The V_t should be maintained in the range of 6 mL/kg.[113] A lung-protective approach also incorporates lung distention and prevention of alveolar closure. Pressure/volume curves should be developed on each patient at least daily so that the P_{flex} can be identified and the PEEP maintained above P_{flex}. If a pressure/volume curve cannot be determined, then P_{flex} can be assumed to be in the 7–12 cmH$_2$O range, and PEEP, at that level or up to 2 cmH$_2$O higher, can be applied.[121,127,128] Recruitment maneuvers that use intermittent sustained inflations of approximately 40 cmH$_2$O for up to 40 seconds often can be beneficial by initially inflating collapsed lung regions.[129] The inflation obtained with the recruitment maneuver is then sustained by maintaining PEEP greater than P_{flex}.

BOX 7-1	Current Favored Approaches to the Treatment of ARDS

Pressure-limited ventilation
$V_t \approx 6$ mL/kg
IRV
EIP < 35 cmH$_2$O
PEEP > P_{flex} or > 12 cmH$_2$O
Permissive hypercapnia
$FiO_2 \le 0.06$
$SO_2 \ge 65\%$
$SaO_2 \ge 80-85\%$
Transfusion to hemoglobin > 13 g/dL
Diuresis to dry weight
Prone positioning
Extracorporeal support

ARDS, acute respiratory distress syndrome; V_t, tidal volume; IRV, inverse ratio ventilation; EIP, end-inspiratory pressure.

As both PIP and PEEP are increased, enhancements in compliance and reductions in V_d/V_t and shunt are to be expected. If they are not observed, then one should suspect the presence of over-distention of currently inflated alveoli instead of the desired recruitment of collapsed lung units. Application of increased levels of PEEP also may result in a decrease in venous return and cardiac output. In addition, West's zone I physiology, which predicts diminished or absent pulmonary capillary flow in the nondependent regions of the lungs at end inspiration, may be exacerbated with application of higher airway pressures. This may be especially detrimental, because it is the nondependent regions that are best inflated and to which one would wish to direct as much pulmonary blood flow as possible.[15] As a result, parameters of DO_2 should be carefully monitored during application of increased PEEP.[130] One approach for monitoring delivery is by applying close attention to the SVO_2 whenever the PEEP is increased to more than 5 cmH$_2$O.

If oxygenation remains inadequate with application of higher levels of PEEP, FiO_2 should be increased to maintain SaO_2 greater than 90%, although levels as low as 80% may be acceptable in patients with adequate DO_2. As mentioned previously, one of the most effective ways to enhance DO_2 is with transfusion. All attempts should be made to avoid the atelectasis and oxygen toxicity associated with FiO_2 levels greater than 0.60.[97] Extending FiO_2 to levels more than 0.60 often has little effect on oxygenation, because severe respiratory failure is frequently associated with a large transpulmonary shunt. If inadequate DO_2 persists, a trial increase in PEEP level should be performed or institution of extracorporeal support considered.[131] Inflation of the lungs also can be enhanced by prolonging the inspiratory time by PC-IRV. Pharmacologic paralysis and sedation are required during performance of PC-IRV, and paralysis may have the additional benefit of decreasing oxygen consumption and enhancing ventilator efficiency.[35] PaO_2 may improve with application of PC-IRV.[132,133] Monitoring the effect on DO_2 and $S\bar{V}O_2$ is critical to ensure the benefit of this intervention. The advantages of the alveolar inflation associated with a decelerating flow waveform during pressure-limited modes of ventilation also should be used.[41]

Prone Positioning

Altering the patient from the supine to the prone position appears to enhance gas exchange.[134,135] Enhanced blood flow to the better-inflated anterior lung regions with the prone position would logically appear to account for this increase in oxygenation. However, data in oleic acid lung-injured sheep suggest that the enhancement in gas exchange may be due predominantly to more homogeneous distribution of ventilation, rather than to redistribution of pulmonary blood flow, because lung distention is more uniform in the prone position.[136–138] This effect may be reversed after a number of hours. Enhanced posterior region lung inflation frequently accounts for persistent increases in oxygenation when the patient is returned to the supine position. Therefore, benefit may be seen when the prone and supine positions are alternated, usually every four to six hours.[124] A randomized, controlled, multicenter trial evaluating the effectiveness of the prone position in the treatment of patients with ARDS was recently completed.[139] One group was placed in the prone position for 6 or more hours daily for ten days while the control group remained in the supine position. Although the PaO_2/FiO_2 ratio was greater in the prone when compared with the supine group (prone, 63.0 + 66.8, vs supine, 44.6 + 68.2; $P = 0.02$), no difference in mortality was noted between groups. It is clear that some patients will not respond to altered positioning, in which case this adjunct should be discontinued. Meticulous attention to careful patient padding and avoidance of dislodgement of tubes and catheters is of the utmost importance in successful implementation of this approach.

Adjunctive Maneuvers

Another means for enhancing oxygenation is through administration of diuretics and the associated reduction of left atrial and pulmonary capillary hydrostatic pressure.[140] Diuresis results in a decrease in lung interstitial edema. In addition, reduction of lung edema decreases compression of the underlying dependent lung.[141] Collapsed dependent lung regions are thereby recruited. Although this treatment approach has not been proved in randomized clinical trials, reduction in total body fluid in adult patients with ARDS appears to be associated with an increase in survival.[142] One must be cognizant of the risks of hypoperfusion and organ system failure, especially renal insufficiency, if overly aggressive diuresis is performed. Overall, however, a strategy of fluid restriction and diuresis should be pursued in the setting of ARDS, while monitoring organ perfusion and renal function.[143] In a randomized trial, a conservative fluid management strategy improved the oxygenation index, the lung injury score, the ventilator-free days, and the number of days spent out of the ICU while the prevalence of shock and use of dialysis did not increase.[144] Although the study was limited to 60 days, the results further support keeping a patient with acute lung injury in a state of fluid balance.

Applying noninjurious PIPs and enhancing PEEP levels limits the ΔP (the amplitude between the PIP and the PEEP) and V_t, and compromises CO_2 elimination.

Therefore, the concept of permissive hypercapnia, which was discussed previously, is integral to the successful application of lung-protective strategies. $PaCO_2$ levels greater than 100 mmHg have been allowed with this approach, although most practitioners prefer to maintain the $PaCO_2$ at less than 60–70 mmHg.[115] Bicarbonate or tris-hydroxymethyl-aminomethane (THAM) can be used to induce a metabolic alkalosis to maintain the pH at greater than 7.20. Few significant physiologic effects are observed with elevated $PaCO_2$ levels as long as the pH is maintained at reasonable levels.[145] If adequate CO_2 elimination cannot be achieved while limiting EIP to noninjurious levels, then initiation of extracorporeal life support (ECLS) should be considered.

The one situation in which it may be acceptable to increase EIP to levels greater than 35 cmH$_2$O (30 cmH$_2$O in the infant and newborn) is in the patient with reduced chest wall compliance and relatively normal pulmonary compliance. As pulmonary compliance is a combination of lung compliance and chest wall compliance, a decrease in chest wall compliance, such as due to abdominal distention, obesity, or chest wall edema, can markedly reduce pulmonary compliance despite reasonable lung compliance. This situation is analogous to studies discussed previously in which the lungs remain uninjured despite application of high airway pressures because the chest is strapped to prevent lung over distention.[105] This is a frequent problem in secondary respiratory failure due to trauma, sepsis, and other disease processes observed among surgical patients, including tightly placed dressings. A cautious increase in EIP in such patients may be warranted. Finally, a simple intervention, such as raising the head of the bed, may have marked effects on FRC and gas exchange in such patients.

Weaning From Mechanical Ventilation

Once a patient is spontaneously breathing and able to protect the airway, consideration is given to weaning from ventilator support. Weaning in the majority of children should take 2 days or less.[57] The FiO_2 should be decreased to less than 0.40 before extubation. Simultaneously, PEEP should be lowered to 5 cmH$_2$O. The pressure support mode of ventilation is an efficient means for weaning because the preset inspiratory pressure can be gradually decreased while partial support is provided for each breath.[146] Adequate gas exchange with a pressure support of 7–10 cmH$_2$O above PEEP in adults and newborns is predictive of successful extubation.[147] Another study in adults demonstrated that simple transition from full ventilator support to a 'T-piece,' in which oxygen flow-by is provided, is as effective at weaning as is gradual reduction in rate during IMV or pressure during PSV.[148] In all circumstances, brief trials of spontaneous breathing before extubation should be performed with flow-by oxygen and CPAP. Prophylactic dexamethasone administration does not appear to increase the odds of a successful extubation in infants, except in 'high risk' patients who receive multiple doses starting at least four hours before extubation.[149,150] Parameters during a T-piece trial that indicate readiness for extubation include the following: (1) maintenance of the pretrial respiratory and heart

rates; (2) inspiratory force greater than 20 cmH$_2$O; (3) $\dot{V}_E$ less than 100 mL/kg/min; and (4) SaO_2 greater than 95%. If the patient's status is unclear, transcutaneous CO_2 monitoring, along with arterial blood gas analysis ($PaCO_2 < 40$ mmHg; $PaO_2 > 60$ mmHg), may help in determining whether extubation is appropriate. The weaning trial should be brief, and under no circumstances should it last longer than one hour. In most cases, the patient who tolerates spontaneous breathing through an endotracheal tube for only a few minutes will demonstrate enhanced capabilities once the tube is removed.

Frequent causes of failed extubation include persistent pulmonary parenchymal disease, interstitial fibrosis, and reduced breathing endurance. PSV is ideal for use in the difficult-to-wean patient because it allows gradual application of spontaneous support to enhance respiratory strength and conditioning (Box 7-2).[146] Enteral and parenteral nutrition should be adjusted to maintain the total caloric intake to no more than 10% above the estimated caloric needs of the patient. Excess calories will be converted to fat, with a high respiratory quotient and increased CO_2 production. Nutritional support high in glucose will have a similar effect.[150] Manipulation of feedings along with treatment of sepsis may reduce VCO_2 and enhance weaning. Pulmonary edema should be treated with diuretics. Some patients will benefit from a tracheostomy to avoid ongoing upper airway contamination, to decrease dead space and airway resistance, and to provide airway access for evacuation of secretions during the weaning process. In addition, the issue of 'extubating' the patient is removed by tracheostomy. Spontaneous breathing trials, therefore, are easy to perform, and the transition from the mechanical ventilator is a much smoother and efficient process.[151] In older patients, the tracheostomy can be performed percutaneously in the ICU.[152] Long-term complications are fairly minimal in older patients. However, in newborns and infants, the rate of development of stenoses and granulation tissue may be significant.[153,154]

NONCONVENTIONAL MODES AND ADJUNCTS TO MECHANICAL VENTILATION

High-Frequency Ventilation

The concept of high-frequency jet ventilation (HFJV) was developed in the early 1970s to provide gas exchange during procedures performed on the trachea. HFJV uses small bursts of gas through a small 'jet port' in the endotracheal tube typically at a rate of 420 breaths/min, with the range being 240–660 breaths/min.[155] The expiratory phase is passive.[156] The V_t is adjusted by controlling the PIP, which is usually initiated at 90% of conventional PIP. CO_2 removal is most affected by the ΔP. Therefore, an increase in the PIP or a decrease in the PEEP will result in enhanced CO_2 elimination. Adjusting the P_{aw}, PEEP, and FiO_2 alters oxygenation. HFJV is typically superimposed on background conventional V_t mechanical ventilation.

The utilization of HFJV has decreased in favor of HFOV, which uses a piston pump-driven diaphragm and delivers small volumes at frequencies between 3–15 Hz.[155] Both inspiration and expiration are active. Oxygenation is manipulated by adjusting P_{aw}, which controls lung inflation similar to the role of PEEP in conventional mechanical ventilation. CO_2 elimination is controlled by adjusting the tidal volume, also known as the amplitude or power. In short, only four variables are adjusted during HFOV:

1. Mean airway pressure (P_{aw}) is typically initiated at a level 1–2 cmH_2O higher in premature newborns and 2–4 cmH_2O higher in term newborns and children than that used during conventional mechanical ventilation.[156] For most disease processes, P_{aw} is adjusted thereafter to maintain the right hemidiaphragm at the rib 8 to 9 level on the anteroposterior chest radiograph.
2. Frequency (Hz) is usually set at 12 Hz in premature newborns and 10 Hz in term patients. Lowering the frequency tends to result in an increase in V_t and a decrease in $PaCO_2$.
3. Inspiratory time, which may be increased to enhance tidal volume, is usually set at 33%.
4. Amplitude or power (ΔP) is set to achieve good chest wall movement and adequate CO_2 elimination.

Gas exchange during HFOV is thought to occur by convection involving those alveoli located close to airways. For the remaining alveoli, gas exchange occurs by streaming, a phenomenon in which inspiratory gas, which has a parabolic profile, tends to flow down the center of the airways whereas the expiratory flow, which has a square profile, takes place at the periphery (Fig. 7-13).[157] Other effects may also play a role: (1) pendelluft, in which gas exchange takes place between lung units with different time constants, as some are filling while others are emptying; (2) the movement of the heart itself may enhance mixing of gases in distal airways; (3) Taylor dispersion, in which convective flow and diffusion together function to enhance distribution of gas; and (4) local diffusion.[158]

HFOV should be applied to the newborn and child for whom conventional ventilation is failing, because of either parameters of oxygenation or CO_2 elimination. The advantage of HFOV lies in the alveolar distention and recruitment that is provided while limiting exposure to potentially injurious high ventilator pressures.[159] Thus, the approach during HFOV should be to apply a mean airway pressure that will effectively recruit alveoli and

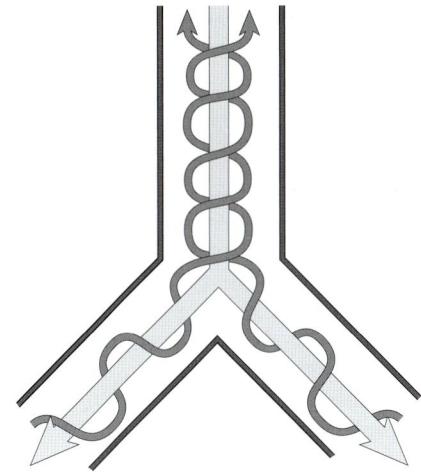

FIGURE 7-13 ■ Streaming as a mechanism of gas exchange during high-frequency ventilation. Note that the parabolic wavefront of the inspiratory gas induces central flow in the airways, whereas expiratory gas flows at the periphery.

maintain oxygenation while limiting the ΔP to that which will provide chest wall movement and adequate CO_2 elimination. CO_2 elimination at lower PIPs may be a specific advantage in patients with air leak, especially those with bronchopleural fistulas.[160] Once again, the effect on DO_2, rather than simply PaO_2, should be considered.

Although some studies with HFOV in preterm newborns have suggested that the incidence of BPD is similar to that found with conventional ventilation, other trials have found an increase in the rescue rate and a reduction in BPD with HFOV.[161–165] One multicenter, randomized trial found that 56% of preterm newborns managed with HFOV were alive without the need for supplemental oxygen at 36 weeks postmenstrual age as compared with 47% of those receiving conventional ventilation ($P = 0.046$).[166] In an additional pilot study, those preterm infants managed with HFOV were extubated earlier and had decreased supplemental oxygen requirements.[167] In addition, improved neurodevelopmental outcomes were also seen after early intervention with HFOV, especially when used in conjunction with surfactant.[168] Thus, although mixed, the data would suggest a reduction in pulmonary morbidity with the use of HFOV when compared with conventional ventilation.

In term newborns and children with respiratory insufficiency, studies suggest that the rescue rate and survival in those treated with HFOV is significantly increased when compared with conventional mechanical ventilation.[169–171] In a randomized controlled trial of HFOV and inspired (inhaled) nitrous oxide (iNO) in pediatric ARDS, HFOV with or without iNO resulted in greater improvement in the PaO_2/FiO_2 ratio than did conventional mechanical ventilation.[172] However, in contrast, one randomized controlled trial in term newborns failed to identify a significant difference in outcome between these treatment modalities.[173] In fact, a Cochrane Database review of randomized clinical trials comparing the use of HFOV versus conventional ventilation failed to show any clear advantage in the elective use of HFOV as a primary modality in the treatment of premature infants with acute pulmonary dysfunction.[174]

Inhaled Nitric Oxide Administration

Nitric oxide is an endogenous mediator that serves to stimulate guanylate cyclase in the endothelial cell to produce cyclic guanosine monophosphate (cGMP), which results in relaxation of vascular smooth muscle (Fig. 7-14).[175] NO is rapidly scavenged by heme moieties. Therefore, iNO serves as a selective vasodilator of the pulmonary circulation, but is inactivated before reaching the systemic circulation. Diluted in nitrogen and then mixed with blended oxygen and air, iNO is administered in doses of 1–80 parts per million (ppm).

Pediatric patients with respiratory failure demonstrate increases in PaO_2 with iNO at 20 ppm.[176] Unfortunately, a prospective, randomized, controlled trial investigating the effects of iNO therapy in children with respiratory failure revealed that although pulmonary vascular resistance and systemic oxygenation were acutely improved at one hour by administration of 10 ppm iNO, a sustained improvement at 24 hours could not be identified.[177]

Other studies have shown more promising results with iNO. In one study, only 40% of the iNO-treated term infants with pulmonary hypertension required ECLS when compared with 71% of controls.[178] These results were corroborated in another study by demonstrating a reduction in the need for ECLS in control newborns (ECLS, 64%) when compared with

iNO-treated newborns (ECLS, 38%; $P = 0.001$).[179] The incidence of chronic lung disease was also decreased in newborns managed with iNO (7% vs 20%). Similar results were noted for infants with persistent pulmonary hypertension of the newborn (PPHN) who were on HFOV. In another study, the need for ECLS was decreased from 55% in the control HFOV group to 14% in the combined iNO and HFOV group ($P = 0.007$).[180] In a clinical trial conducted by the Neonatal Inhaled Nitric Oxide Study (NINOS) Group, neonates born at 34 weeks or older gestational age with hypoxic respiratory failure were randomized to receive 20 ppm iNO or 100% oxygen as a control.[181] If a complete response, defined as an increase in PaO_2 of more than 20 mmHg within 30 minutes after gas initiation, was not observed, then iNO at 80 ppm was administered. Sixty-four per cent of the control group and 46% of the iNO group died within 120 days or were treated with ECLS ($P = 0.006$). No difference in death was found between the two groups (iNO, 14% vs control, 17%), but significantly fewer neonates in the iNO group required ECLS (39% vs 54%). Follow-up at age 18 to 24 months failed to demonstrate a difference in the incidence of cerebral palsy, rate of sensorineural hearing loss, and mental developmental index scores between the control and iNO patients.[182] Other studies have similarly failed to identify a difference in pulmonary, neurologic, cognitive, or behavioral outcomes between survivors managed with iNO and those in the conventional group.[183]

An associated, but separate, trial demonstrated no difference in mortality and a significant increase in the need for ECLS when neonates with congenital disphragmatic hernia (CDH) were treated with 20 or 80 ppm of iNO versus 100% oxygen as control.[184] It should be noted, however, that some investigators have suggested that the efficacy of iNO in patients with CDH may be more substantial after surfactant administration or at the point at which recurrent pulmonary hypertension occurs.[185] iNO administration also may be helpful in the moribund CDH patient until ECLS can be initiated.

Some concern has been expressed for the development of intracranial hemorrhage in premature newborns treated with iNO. More than a 25% increase in the arterial/alveolar oxygen ratio (PaO_2/PAO_2) was observed in ten of 11 premature newborns, with a mean gestational age of 29.8 weeks and severe RDS, in response to administration of 1–20 ppm iNO.[186] However, in seven of these 11 newborns, intracranial hemorrhage developed during their hospitalization. Also, a meta-analysis of the three completed studies evaluating the efficacy of iNO in premature newborns suggested no significant difference in survival, incidence of chronic lung disease, or rate of development of intracranial hemorrhage between iNO and controls.[187]

NO is associated with the production of potentially toxic metabolites. When combined with O_2, iNO produces peroxynitrates, which can be damaging to epithelial cells and also can inhibit surfactant function.[188,189] Nitrogen dioxide, which is toxic, can be produced, and hemoglobin can be oxidized to methemoglobin. Additional concerns exist about the immunosuppressive effects and the potential for platelet dysfunction.

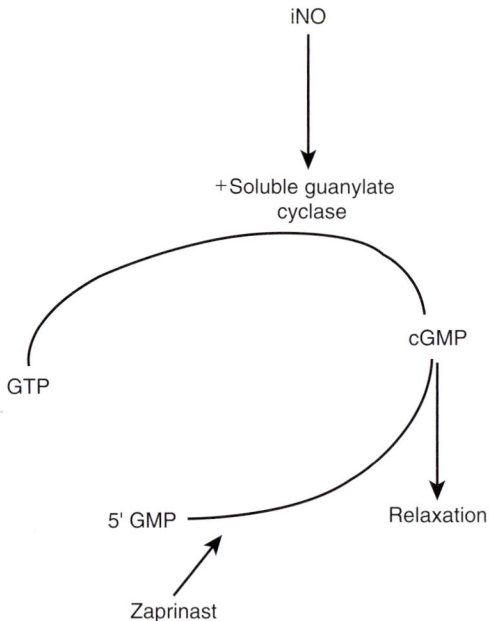

FIGURE 7-14 ■ Mechanism of action of inhaled nitrous oxide (iNO) in inducing vascular smooth muscle relaxation. Zaprinast is a phosphodiesterase inhibitor that may increase the potency and duration of the effect of iNO. GTP, guanosine triphosphate; cGMP, cyclic guanosine monophosphate. (Reprinted from Hirschl RB. Innovative therapies in the management of newborns with congenital diaphragmatic hernia. Semin Pediatr Surg 1996;5: 255–65.)

Surfactant Replacement Therapy

The use of exogenous surfactant has been responsible for a 30–40% reduction in the odds of death among very low birth weight newborns with RDS.[190,191] In addition, in those premature neonates with birth weight more than 1250 g, mortality in a controlled, randomized, blinded study decreased from 7% to 4%.[192]

A randomized, prospective, controlled trial in term newborns with respiratory insufficiency demonstrated that the need for extracorporeal membrane oxygenation (ECMO) was significantly reduced in those managed with surfactant when compared with placebo.[193] The benefit of surfactant was greatest in those with a lower oxygenation index (<23). Another randomized controlled study demonstrated the utility of surfactant in term newborns with the meconium aspiration syndrome.[194] The OI minimally decreased following the initial dose, but markedly decreased with the second and third surfactant doses from a baseline of 23.7 to 5.9 (Fig. 7-15). After three doses of surfactant, PPHN had resolved in all but one of the infants in the study group versus none in the control group. The incidence of air leaks and need for ECLS were markedly reduced in the surfactant group compared with the control infants. The neurodevelopmental outcome, however, was not affected by timing of surfactant administration. Therefore, gas exchange after intubation can be initially evaluated before surfactant is given, if needed.[195] The incidence of air leaks, chronic lung disease, and time on the ventilator seem to improve though when early surfactant administration with extubation to nasal CPAP was used.[196]

Studies have concluded that surfactant phospholipid concentration, synthesis, and kinetics are not significantly deranged in infants with CDH compared with controls, although surfactant protein A concentrations may be reduced in CDH newborns on ECMO.[197–199] Animal and human studies have suggested that surfactant administration before the first breath is associated with enhancement in *Pa*O$_2$ and pulmonary mechanics.[200,201] However, among CDH patients on ECLS, no difference was noted

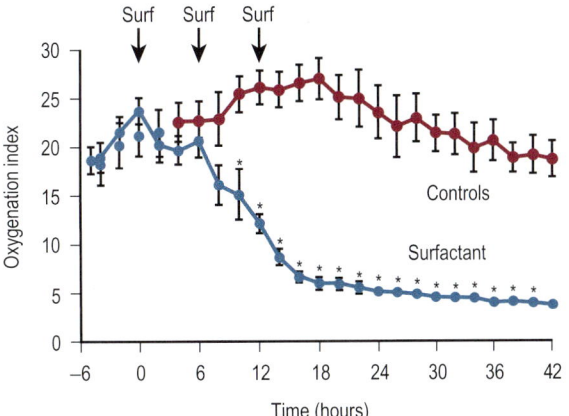

FIGURE 7-15 ■ The effect of exogenous surfactant administration on oxygen index in term newborns with meconium-aspiration syndrome. (Reprinted from Findlay RD, Taeusch HW, Walther FJ. Surfactant replacement therapy for meconium aspiration syndrome. Pediatrics 1996;97:48–52.)

BOX 7-3	NNIS/CDC Criteria for Diagnosis of Ventilator-Associated Pneumonia in Infants 1 Year or Younger

Worsening gas exchange (oxygen desaturations, increased oxygen requirements, or increased ventilator demand) and three of the following:

  Temperature instability with no other recognized cause

  New onset of purulent sputum, change in character of sputum, increased respiratory secretions, or increased suctioning requirements

  Apnea, tachypnea, nasal flaring with retraction of chest wall, or grunting

  Wheezing, rales, or rhonchi

  Cough

  Bradycardia (<100 beats/min) or tachycardia (>170 beats/min)

From NNIS/CDC—National Nosocomial Infections Surveillance System/Centers for Disease Control.

---

in terms of lung compliance, time to extubation, period of oxygen requirement, and the total number of hospital days.[197]

In summary, multiple approaches to preserve lung function should be used in patients with severe lung injury or RDS, including limiting lung volumes, recruitment maneuvers, prone positioning, APRV, high-frequency oscillation, nitric oxide, surfactant, and early ECMO use in nonresponders.[202,203]

VENTILATOR-ASSOCIATED PNEUMONIA

Ventilator-associated pneumonia (VAP), diagnosed at 48 hours or later on mechanical ventilation, is the second most common hospital-acquired infection in the neonatal and pediatric ICUs. Occurring in 3–10% of all ventilated PICU patients and up to 32% of NICU patients, VAP results in higher mean lengths of ICU stay, increased mortality rates, and increased hospital costs.[204–206] Controversies surround the definition, treatment, and prevention of VAP. Finally, many studies do not incorporate the pediatric population and the data therefore cannot be applied blindly to all patients.

Definitions for VAP differ for infants 1 year or younger (Box 7-3), children between 1 and 12 years old (Box 7-4), and those older than 12 years of age (Box 7-5). In all patients, mechanical ventilation must have been used for more than 48 hours.[204,206] Microbial confirmation is not necessary for the NNIS/CDC criteria defined in Boxes 7-3, 7-4 or 7-5, and the use of quantitative cultures for diagnosis in children and neonates is variable. The technique of fiberoptic bronchoalveolar lavage (BAL) has been described in children, but is not routinely used. Blind BAL findings of a bacterial index (defined as the log10 of the colony-forming units of microorganisms per milliliter of BAL fluid) greater than 5 are the most reliable method for diagnosing VAP in mechanically ventilated children.[207]

Investigations on the treatment of VAP focus on empirical use of antibiotics and duration of therapy.

BOX 7-4	**NNIS/CDC Criteria for Diagnosis of Ventilator-Associated Pneumonia in Children Between Ages 1 and 12 Years**

Three of the following:
Fever (>38.4°C) or hypothermia (<37°C) with no other recognized cause
Leukopenia (<4,000 white blood cells/mm³) or leukocytosis (≥15,000 white blood cells/mm³)
New onset of purulent sputum, change in character of sputum, increased respiratory secretions, or increased suctioning requirements
Rales or bronchial breath sounds
Worsening gas exchange (O_2 desaturations [pulse oximetry <94%], increased oxygen requirements, or increased ventilation demand)

From NNIS/CDC—National Nosocomial Infections Surveillance System/ Centers for Disease Control.

BOX 7-5	**NNIS/CDC Criteria for Diagnosis of Ventilator-Associated Pneumonia in Children Older Than 12 Years**

One of the following:
Fever (>38°C) with no other recognized cause
Leukopenia (<4000 white blood cells/mm³) or leukocytosis (≥12,000 white blood cells/mm³)
Two of the following:
New onset of purulent sputum, change in character of sputum, increased respiratory secretions, or increased suctioning requirements
New onset of worsening cough, dyspnea, or tachypnea
Rales or bronchial breath sounds
Worsening gas exchange ($PaO_2/FiO_2 \leq 240$, increased oxygen requirements, or increased ventilation demand)
Two or more abnormal chest radiographs (can be one if no pulmonary or cardiac disease) with one of the following:
New or progressive and persistent infiltrate
Consolidation
Cavitation
Pneumatoceles (in infants ≤1 year)

From NNIS/CDC—National Nosocomial Infections Surveillance System/ Centers for Disease Control.

Broad-spectrum, early empirical antibiotics, when appropriately chosen, have been shown to decrease mortality in adults, but overuse can increase antibiotic resistance.[208,209] Risk factors for multidrug-resistant pathogens in pediatric patients include younger age, increasing risk of mortality score, previous PICU admissions, exposure to household contacts hospitalized over the past year, intravenous antibiotic use in the past 12 months, and exposure to chronic care facilities.[210,211] Once final cultures are available, it is important to target therapy to prevent overuse of antibiotics and the breeding of multidrug-resistant organisms. The optimal duration of therapy in adults was addressed in a multicenter, randomized, controlled trial comparing eight days of antibiotics versus 15 days.[212] There was no difference in the mortality rates. Patients infected with nonfermenting

gram-negative bacilli, however, benefited from the longer duration of therapy with a reduced relapse rate. Finally, patients treated for 8 days also had a reduced incidence of multidrug-resistant pathogens on relapse when compared with those treated for 15 days.

Guidelines for the prevention of VAP have been established based on current evidence by the VAP Guidelines Committee and the Canadian Critical Care Trials Group.[205] Recommended therapeutic interventions include the orotracheal route for intubation, a ventilator circuit specific for each patient, circuit changes if soiled or damaged but no scheduled changes, change of heat and moisture exchangers every 5 to 7 days or as indicated, use of a closed endotracheal suctioning system changed for each patient and as clinically indicated, subglottic secretion drainage in patients expected to be mechanically ventilated for more than 72 hours, and the head of bed elevated at 45 degrees when possible. Consideration should be given to the use of rotating beds and oral antiseptic rinses.[213] Finally, in adult patients, a team approach and implementation of a VAP bundle encompassing all the evidence-based guidelines has been shown to improve outcomes.[214]

REFERENCES

1. Baker AB. Artificial respiration, the history of an idea. Med Hist 1971;15:336–51.
2. Matas R. Intralaryngeal insufflation for the relief of acute surgical pneumothorax: Its history and methods with a description of the latest devices for this purpose. J Am Med Assoc 1900;23: 1468–73.
3. Daily WJ, Smith PC. Mechanical ventilation of the newborn infant. I Curr Prob Pediatr 1971;1:1–37.
4. Emerson JH. The Evolution of 'Iron Lungs': 1928-78. J.H. Emerson Company; 1978.
5. Magill IW. Endotracheal Anaesthesia. Proc R Soc Med 1928;22: 83–8.
6. Rowbotham S. Intratracheal anaesthesia by the nasal route for operations on the mouth and lips. BMJ 1920;2:590–1.
7. Eckman M, Barach B. An appraisal of intermittent pressure breathing as a method of increasing altitude tolerance. J Aviat Med 1947;18:565–76.
8. Stahlman MT, Young WC, Payne G. Studies of ventilatory aids in hyaline membrane disease. Am J Dis Child 1962;104: 526.
9. Cassani VL 3rd. We've come a long way baby! Mechanical ventilation of the newborn. Neonatal Netw 1994;13:63–8.
10. Avery ME, Mead J. Surface properties in relation to atelectasis and hyaline membrane disease. Am J Dis Child 1959;97: 517–23.
11. Thomas DV, Fletcher G, Sunshine P, et al. Prolonged respirator use in pulmonary insufficiency of newborn. JAMA 1965;193: 183–90.
12. Gregory GA, Kitterman JA, Phibbs RH, et al. Treatment of the idiopathic respiratory-distress syndrome with continuous positive airway pressure. N Engl J Med 1971;284:1333–40.
13. Kössel H, Versmold H. 25 years of respiratory support of newborn infants. Perinat Med 1997;25:421–32.
14. Bartlett RH. Use of Mechanical Ventilation. In: Holcroft J, editor. Care of the Surgical Patient. New York: Scientific American Medicine; 1989.
15. West JB. Pulmonary Pathophysiology—The Essentials. Baltimore: Williams & Wilkins; 1990.
16. Gattinoni L, Mascheroni D, Basilico E, et al. Volume/pressure curve of total respiratory system in paralysed patients: Artefacts and correction factors. Intensive Care Med 1987;13:19–25.
17. Gama AM, Meyer EC, Gaudêncio AM, et al. Different low constant flows can equally determine the lower inflection point in acute respiratory distress syndrome patients. Artif Organs 2001;25:882–9.

18. Kondili E, Prinianakis G, Hoeing S, et al. Low flow inflation pressure-time curve in patients with acute respiratory distress syndrome. Intensive Care Med 2000;26:1756–63.

19. Harris RS, Hess DR, Venegas JG. An objective analysis of the pressure-volume curve in the acute respiratory distress syndrome. Am J Respir Crit Care Med 2000;161:432–9.

20. Putensen C, Baum M, Hörmann C. Selecting ventilator settings according to variables derived from the quasi-static pressure/volume relationship in patients with acute lung injury. Anesth Analg 1993;77:436–47.

21. Bartel LP, Bazik JR, Powner DJ. Compression volume during mechanical ventilation: Comparison of ventilators and tubing circuits. Crit Care Med 1985;13:851–4.

22. Gattinoni L, Pesenti A, Mascheroni D, et al. Low-frequency positive-pressure ventilation with extracorporeal CO2 removal in severe acute respiratory failure. JAMA 1986;256:881–6.

23. Zwischenberger JB, Wang D, Lick SD. The paracorporeal artificial lung improves 5-day outcomes from lethal smoke/burn-induced acute respiratory distress syndrome in sheep. Ann Thorac Surg 2002;74:1011–18.

24. Gattinoni L, D'Andrea L, Pelosi P, et al. Regional effects and mechanism of positive end-expiratory pressure in early adult respiratory distress syndrome. JAMA 1993;269:2122–7.

25. Maunder RJ, Shuman WP, McHugh JW, et al. Preservation of normal lung regions in the adult respiratory distress syndrome. Analysis by computed tomography. JAMA 1986;255:2463–5.

26. White KM. Completing the hemodynamic picture: SvO2. Heart Lung 1985;14:272–80.

27. Nelson LD. Continuous venous oximetry in surgical patients. Ann Surg 1986;203:329–33.

28. Rivers EP, Ander DS, Powell D. Central venous oxygen saturation monitoring in the critically ill patient. Curr Opin Crit Care 2001;7:204–11.

29. Jan K, Usami S, Smith JA. Effects of transfusion on rheological properties of blood in sickle cell anemia. Transfusion 1982;22:17–20.

30. Ranieri VM, Mascia L, Fiore T, et al. Cardiorespiratory effects of positive end-expiratory pressure during progressive tidal volume reduction (permissive hypercapnia) in patients with acute respiratory distress syndrome. Anesthesiology 1995;83:710–20.

31. Michaels AJ, Wanek SM, Dreifuss BA, et al. A protocolized approach to pulmonary failure and the role of intermittent prone positioning. J Trauma 2002;52:1037–47.

32. Marini JJ. Pressure-targeted, lung-protective ventilatory support in acute lung injury. Chest 1994;105:S109–15.

33. Parker JC, Townsley MI, Rippe B, et al. Increased microvascular permeability in dog lungs due to high peak airway pressures. J Appl Physiol 1984;57:1809–16.

34. Palmisano BW, Fisher DM, Willis M, et al. The effect of paralysis on oxygen consumption in normoxic children after cardiac surgery. Anesthesiology 1984;61:518–22.

35. Coggeshall JW, Marini JJ, Newman JH. Improved oxygenation after muscle relaxation in adult respiratory distress syndrome. Arch Intern Med 1985;145:1718–20.

36. Ganong WF. Ganong's Review of Medical Physiology. New York: Appleton & Lange; 1979.

37. Kacmarek RM, Hess D. Basic principles of ventilator machinery. In: Tobin MJ, editor. Principles and Practice of Mechanical Ventilation. New York: McGraw-Hill Professional Publishing; 1994. p. 65–110.

38. Pilbeam SP. Physical aspects of mechanical ventilators. In: Russell J, editor. Mechanical Ventilation: Physiological and Clinical Applications. St. Louis: Mosby; 1998. p. 62–91.

39. Piotrowski A, Sobala W, Kawczyński P. Patient-initiated, pressure-regulated, volume-controlled ventilation compared with intermittent mandatory ventilation in neonates: A prospective, randomised study. Intensive Care Med 1997;23:975–81.

40. Sinha SK, Donn SM. Volume-controlled ventilation. Variations on a theme. Clin Perinatol 2001;28:547–60.

41. Abraham E, Yoshihara G. Cardiorespiratory effects of pressure controlled ventilation in severe respiratory failure. Chest 1990;98:1445–9.

42. Nahum A, Burke WC, Ravenscraft SA, et al. Lung mechanics and gas exchange during pressure-control ventilation in dogs.

Augmentation of CO_2 elimination by an intratracheal catheter. Am Rev Respir Dis 1992;146:965–73.

43. Kirby RR. Intermittent mandatory ventilation in the neonate. Crit Care Med 1977;5:18–22.

44. Bernstein G, Mannino FL, Heldt GP, et al. Randomized multicenter trial comparing synchronized and conventional intermittent mandatory ventilation in neonates. J Pediatr 1996;128:453–63.

45. Cleary JP, Bernstein G, Mannino FL, et al. Improved oxygenation during synchronized intermittent mandatory ventilation in neonates with respiratory distress syndrome: a randomized, crossover study. J Pediatr 1995;126:407–11.

46. Chen JY, Ling UP, Chen JH. Comparison of synchronized and conventional intermittent mandatory ventilation in neonates. Acta Paediatr Jpn 1997;39:578–83.

47. Greenough A, Milner AD, Dimitriou G. Synchronized mechanical ventilation for respiratory support in newborn infants. Cochrane Database Syst Rev 2001:CD000456.

48. Leung P, Jubran A, Tobin MJ. Comparison of assisted ventilator modes on triggering, patient effort, and dyspnea. Am J Respir Crit Care Med 1997;155:1940–8.

49. Jarreau PH, Moriette G, Mussat P, et al. Patient-triggered ventilation decreases the work of breathing in neonates. Am J Respir Crit Care Med 1996;153:1176–81.

50. Dekel B, Segal E, Perel A. Pressure support ventilation. Arch Intern Med 1996;156:369–73.

51. Banner MJ, Kirby RR, Blanch PB, et al. Decreasing imposed work of the breathing apparatus to zero using pressure-support ventilation. Crit Care Med 1993;21:1333–8.

52. Kacmarek RM. The role of pressure support ventilation in reducing the work of breathing. Respir Care 1988;33:99–120.

53. Brochard L, Pluskwa F, Lemaire F. Improved efficacy of spontaneous breathing with inspiratory pressure support. Am Rev Respir Dis 1987;136:411–15.

54. Gullberg N, Winberg P, Selldén H. Pressure support ventilation increases cardiac output in neonates and infants. Paediatr Anaesth 1996;6:311–15.

55. Tokioka H, Kinjo M, Hirakawa M. The effectiveness of pressure support ventilation for mechanical ventilatory support in children. Anesthesiology 1993;78:880–4.

56. Marraro GA. Innovative practices of ventilatory support with pediatric patients. Pediatr Crit Care Med 2003;4:8–20.

57. Randolph AG, Wypij D, Venkataraman ST, et al. Effect of mechanical ventilator weaning protocols on respiratory outcomes in infants and children: A randomized controlled trial. JAMA 2002;288:2561–8.

58. Amato MB, Barbas CS, Bonassa J, et al. Volume-assured pressure support ventilation (VAPSV). A new approach for reducing muscle workload during acute respiratory failure. Chest 1992;102:1225–34.

59. Younes M. Proportional assist ventilation, a new approach to ventilatory support. Theory. Am Rev Respir Dis 1992;145:114–20.

60. Younes M. Proportional assist ventilation and pressure support ventilation: Similarities and differences. In: Ventilatory Failure (Update in Intensive Care and Emergency Medicine) 1st edition by Marini, JJ, ed. Springer; 1991. p. 361–80.

61. Younes M, Puddy A, Roberts D, et al. Proportional assist ventilation. Results of an initial clinical trial. Am Rev Respir Dis 1992;145:121–9.

62. Bigatello LM, Nishimura M, Imanaka H, et al. Unloading of the work of breathing by proportional assist ventilation in a lung model. Crit Care Med 1997;25:267–72.

63. Schulze A, Bancalari E. Proportional assist ventilation in infants. Clin Perinatol 2001;28:561–78.

64. Schulze A, Gerhardt T, Musante G, et al. Proportional assist ventilation in low birth weight infants with acute respiratory disease: A comparison to assist/control and conventional mechanical ventilation. J Pediatr 1999;135:339–44.

65. Musante G, Schulze A, Gerhardt T, et al. Proportional assist ventilation decreases thoracoabdominal asynchrony and chest wall distortion in preterm infants. Pediatr Res 2001;49:175–80.

66. Verbrugghe W, Jorens PG. Neurally adjusted ventilatory assist: A ventilation tool or a ventilation toy? Respir Care 2011;56:327–35.

67. Breatnach C, Conlon NP, Stack M, et al. A prospective crossover comparison of neurally adjusted ventilatory assist and pressure-support ventilation in a pediatric and neonatal intensive care unit population. Pediatr Crit Care Med 2010;11:7–11.

68. Gittermann MK, Fusch C, Gittermann AR, et al. Early nasal continuous positive airway pressure treatment reduces the need for intubation in very low birth weight infants. Eur J Pediatr 1997;156:384–8.

69. Padman R, Lawless ST, Kettrick RG. Noninvasive ventilation via bilevel positive airway pressure support in pediatric practice. Crit Care Med 1998;26:169–73.

70. Lofaso F, Brochard L, Hang T, et al. Home versus intensive care pressure support devices. Experimental and clinical comparison. Am J Respir Crit Care Med 1996;153:1591–9.

71. Yañez LJ, Yunge M, Emilfork M, et al. A prospective, randomized, controlled trial of noninvasive ventilation in pediatric acute respiratory failure. Pediatr Crit Care Med 2008;9:484–9.

72. Finer NN, Carlo WA, Walsh MC, et al. Early CPAP versus surfactant in extremely preterm infants. N Engl J Med 2010;362:1970–9.

73. Lain DC, DiBenedetto R, Morris SL, et al. Pressure control inverse ratio ventilation as a method to reduce peak inspiratory pressure and provide adequate ventilation and oxygenation. Chest 1989;95:1081–8.

74. Tharratt RS, Allen RP, Albertson TE. Pressure controlled inverse ratio ventilation in severe adult respiratory failure. Chest 1988;94:755–62.

75. Marcy TW, Marini JJ. Inverse ratio ventilation in ARDS. Rationale and implementation. Chest 1991;100:494–504.

76. Porembka DT. Inverse ratio ventilation. Probl Respir Care 1989;2:69–76.

77. McCarthy MC, Cline AL, Lemmon GW, et al. Pressure control inverse ratio ventilation in the treatment of adult respiratory distress syndrome in patients with blunt chest trauma. Am Surg 1999;65:1027–30.

78. Mercat A, Titiriga M, Anguel N, et al. Inverse ratio ventilation (I/E = 2/1) in acute respiratory distress syndrome: A six-hour controlled study. AM J Resp Crit Care Med 1997;155:1637–42.

79. Armstrong BW Jr, MacIntyre NR. Pressure-controlled, inverse ratio ventilation that avoids air trapping in the adult respiratory distress syndrome. Crit Care Med 1995;23:279–85.

80. Mancebo J, Vallverdú I, Bak E, et al. Volume-controlled ventilation and pressure-controlled inverse ratio ventilation: A comparison of their effects in ARDS patients. Monaldi Arch Chest Dis 1994;49:201–7.

81. Lessard MR, Guérot E, Lorino H, et al. Effects of pressure-controlled with different I:E ratios versus volume-controlled ventilation on respiratory mechanics, gas exchange, and hemodynamics in patients with adult respiratory distress syndrome. Anesthesiology 1994;80:983–91.

82. Goldstein B, Papadakos PJ. Pressure-controlled inverse-ratio ventilation in children with acute respiratory failure. AM J Crit Care 1994;3:11–15.

83. Wang SH, Wei TS. The outcome of early pressure-controlled inverse ratio ventilation on patients with severe acute respiratory distress syndrome in surgical intensive care unit. Am J Surg 2002;183:151–5.

84. Huang CC, Shih MJ, Tsai YH, et al. Effects of inverse ratio ventilation versus positive end-expiratory pressure on gas exchange and gastric intramucosal PCO(2) and pH under constant mean airway pressure in acute respiratory distress syndrome. Anesthesiology 2001;95:1182–8.

85. McIntyre RC Jr, Pulido EJ, Bensard DD, et al. Thirty years of clinical trials in acute respiratory distress syndrome. Crit Care Med 2000;28:3314–31.

86. Chiang AA, Steinfeld A, Gropper C, et al. Demand-flow airway pressure release ventilation as a partial ventilatory support mode: Comparison with synchronized intermittent mandatory ventilation and pressure support ventilation. Crit Care Med 1994;22:1431–7.

87. Rasanen J, Cane RD, Downs JV, et al. Airway pressure release ventilation during acute lung injury: A prospective multicenter trial. Crit Care Med 1991;19:1234–41.

88. Neumann P, Golisch W, Strohmeyer A, et al. Influence of different release times on spontaneous breathing pattern during airway pressure release ventilation. Intensive Care Med 2002;28:1742–9.

89. Hering R, Peters D, Zinserling J, et al. Effects of spontaneous breathing during airway pressure release ventilation on renal perfusion and function in patients with acute lung injury. Intensive Care Med 2002;28:1426–33.

90. Cane RD, Peruzzi WT, Shapiro BA. Airway pressure release ventilation in severe acute respiratory failure. Chest 1991;100:460–3.

91. Valentine DD, Hammond MD, Downs JB, et al. Distribution of ventilation perfusion with different modes of mechanical ventilation. Am Rev Respir Dis 1991;143:1262–6.

92. Kaplan LJ, Bailey H, Formosa V. Airway pressure release ventilation increases cardiac performance in patients with acute lung injury/adult respiratory distress syndrome. Crit Care (Lond) 2001;5:221–6.

93. Walsh MA, Merat M, La Rotta G, et al. Airway pressure release ventilation improves pulmonary blood flow in infants after cardiac surgery. Crit Care Med 2011;39:2599–604.

94. Martin LD, Wetzel RC, Bilenki AL. Airway pressure release ventilation in a neonatal lamb model of acute lung injury. Crit Care Med 1991;19:373–8.

95. Foland JA, Martin J, Novotny T, et al. Airway pressure release ventilation with a short release time in a child with acute respiratory distress syndrome. Respir Care 2001;46:1019–23.

96. Hollinger IB. Postoperative management: Ventilation. Int Anesth Clin 1980;18:205–16.

97. Jenkinson SG. Oxygen toxicity. New Horiz 1993;1:504–11.

98. Wolfe WG, DeVries WC. Oxygen toxicity. Annu Rev Med 1975;26:203–17.

99. Gladstone IM Jr, Levine RL. Oxidation of proteins in neonatal lungs. Pediatrics 1994;93:764–8.

100. Wung JT, James LS, Kilchevsky E, et al. Management of infants with severe respiratory failure and persistence of the fetal circulation without hyperventilation. Pediatrics 1985;76:488.

101. Webb HH, Tierney DF. Experimental pulmonary edema due to intermittent positive pressure ventilation with high inflation pressures: Protection by positive end-expiratory pressure. Am Rev Respir Dis 1974;110:556–65.

102. Fu Z, Costello ML, Tsukimoto K, et al. High lung volume increases stress failure in pulmonary capillaries. J Appl Physiol 1992;73:123–33.

103. Kolobow T, Moretti MP, Fumagalli R, et al. Severe impairment in lung function induced by high peak airway pressure during mechanical ventilation. Am Rev Respir Dis 1987;135:312–15.

104. Dreyfuss D, Basset G, Soler P, et al. Intermittent positive-pressure hyperventilation with high inflation pressures produces pulmonary microvascular injury in rats. Am Rev Respir Dis 1985;132:880–4.

105. Hernandez LA, Peevy K, Moise AA, et al. Chest wall restriction limits high airway pressure-induced lung injury in young rabbits. J Appl Physiol 1989;66:2364–8.

106. Savel R, Yao E, Gropper M. Protective effects of low tidal volume ventilation in a rabbit model of Pseudomonas aeruginosa-induced acute lung injury. Crit Care Med 2001;29:392–8.

107. Rich PB, Reickert CA, Sawada S, et al. Effect of rate and inspiratory flow on ventilator induced lung injury. J Trauma 2000;49:903–11.

108. Nahum A, Hoyt J, Schmitz L, et al. Effect of mechanical ventilation strategy on dissemination of intratracheally instilled Escherichia coli in dogs. Crit Care Med 1997;25:1733–43.

109. Stewart TE, Meade M, Cook DJ, et al. Evaluation of a ventilation strategy to prevent barotrauma in patients at high risk for acute respiratory distress syndrome. N Engl J Med 1998;338:355–61.

110. Brochard L. Low versus high tidal volumes. In: Vincent JL, editor. Acute Lung Injury. Brussels: Springer-Verlag; 1998. p. 276–81.

111. Amato MB, Barbas CS, Mederios DM, et al. Effect of a protective-ventilation strategy on mortality in the acute respiratory distress syndrome. N Engl J Med 1998;338:347–54.

112. Ranieri VM, Suter PM, Tortoralla T, et al. Effect of mechanical ventilation on inflammatory mediators in patients with acute respiratory distress syndrome. JAMA 1999;282:54–61.

113. The Acute Respiratory Distress Syndrome Network. Ventilation with lower tidal volumes as compared with traditional tidal

volumes for acute lung injury and the acute respiratory distress syndrome. N Engl J Med 2000;342:1301–8.

114. Hickling KG. Low volume ventilation with permissive hypercapnea in the adult respiratory distress syndrome. Clin Intensive Care 1992;3:67–78.

115. Hickling KG, Walsh J, Henderson S, et al. Low mortality rate in adult respiratory distress syndrome using low-volume, pressure-limited ventilation with permissive hypercapnia: A prospective study. Crit Care Med 1994;22:1568–78.

116. Sheridan R, Kacmarek R, McEttrick M, et al. Permissive hypercapnia as a ventilatory strategy in burned children: Effect on barotrauma, pneumonia, and mortality. J Trauma 1995;39:854–9.

117. Paulson TE, Spear RM, Silva PD, et al. High-frequency pressure-control ventilation with high positive end-expiratory pressure in children with acute respiratory distress syndrome. J Pediatr 1996;129:566–73.

118. McCulloch PR, Forkert PG, Forese AB. Lung volume maintenance prevents lung injury during high frequency oscillatory ventilation in surfactant-deficient rabbits. Am Rev Respir Dis 1988;137:1185–92.

119. Dreyfuss D, Sjoer P, Basset G, et al. High inflation pressure pulmonary edema: Respective effects of high airway pressure, high tidal volume, and positive end-expiratory pressure. Am Rev Respir Dis 1988;137:1159–64.

120. Lachmann B. Open up the lung and keep the lung open. Intensive Care Med 1992;18:319–21.

121. Mancebo J. PEEP, ARDS, and alveolar recruitment. Intensive Care Med 1992;18:383–5.

122. Gattinoni L, Pesenti A, Avalli L, et al. Pressure-volume curve of total respiratory system in acute respiratory failure. Am Rev Respir Dis 1987;136:730–6.

123. Roupie E, Dambrosio M, Servillo G, et al. Titration of tidal volume and induced hypercapnia in acute respiratory distress syndrome. AJRCCM 1995;152:121–8.

124. Gattinoni L, Caironi P, Pelosi P, et al. What has computed tomography taught us about the acute respiratory distress syndrome? Am J Respir Crit Care Med 2001;164:1701–11.

125. Crotti S, Mascheroni D, Caironi P, et al. Recruitment and derecruitment during acute respiratory failure: A clinical study. Am J Respir Crit Care Med 2001;164:131–40.

126. Desai SR, Wells AU, Suntharalingam G, et al. Acute respiratory distress syndrome caused by pulmonary and extrapulmonary injury: A comparative CT study. Radiology 2001;218:689–93.

127. DiRusso SM, Nelson LD, Safcsak K, et al. Survival in patients with severe adult respiratory distress syndrome treated with high-level positive end-expiratory pressure. Crit Care Med 1995;23:1485–96.

128. Nagano O, Tokioka H, Ohta Y, et al. Inspiratory pressure-volume curves at different positive end-expiratory pressure levels in patients with ALI/ARDS. Acta Anaesth Scand 2001;45:1255–61.

129. Valente Barbas CS. Lung recruitment maneuvers in acute respiratory distress syndrome and facilitating resolution. Crit Care Med 2003;31:265–71.

130. Witte MK, Galli SA, Ghatburn RL, et al. Optimal positive end-expiratory pressure therapy in infants and children with acute respiratory failure. Pediatr Res 1988;24:217–21.

131. Bartlett R, Roloff DW, Custer J, et al. Extracorporeal life support: The University of Michigan experience. JAMA 2000;283:904–8.

132. Sjostrand UH, Lichtwarch-Aschoff M, Nielsen JB, et al. Different ventilatory approaches to keep the lung open. Intensive Care Med 1995;21:310–18.

133. Papadakos PJ, Halloran W, Hessney JI, et al. The use of pressure-controlled inverse ratio ventilation in the surgical intensive care unit. J Trauma 1991;31:1211–14.

134. Pappert D, Rossaint R, Slama K, et al. Influence of positioning on ventilation-perfusion relationships in severe adult respiratory distress syndrome. Chest 1994;106:1511–16.

135. Fridrich P, Krafft P, Hochleuthner H, et al. The effects of long-term prone positioning in patients with trauma-induced adult respiratory distress syndrome. Anesth Analg 1996;83:1206–11.

136. Langer M, Mascheroni D, Marcolin R, et al. The prone position in ARDS patients: A clinical study. Chest 1988;94:103–7.

137. Albert RK, Leasa D, Sanderson M, et al. The prone position improves arterial oxygenation and reduces shunt in oleic-acid-induced acute lung injury. Am Rev Respir Dis 1987;135:628–33.

138. Wiener CM, Kirk W, Albert RK. Prone position reverses gravitational distribution of perfusion in dog lungs with oleic acid-induced injury. J Appl Physiol 1990;68:1386–92.

139. Gattinoni L, Tognoni G, Pesenti A, et al. Effect of prone positioning on the survival of patients with acute respiratory failure. N Engl J Med 2001;345:568–73.

140. Baltopoulos G, Zakynthinos S, Dimpoulos A, et al. Effects of furosemide on pulmonary shunts. Chest 1989;96:494–8.

141. Gattinoni L. Decreasing edema results in improved pulmonary function and survival in patients with ARDS. Intensive Care Med 1986;12:137.

142. Simmons RS, Berdine GG, Seidenfeld JJ, et al. Fluid balance in the respiratory distress syndrome. Am Rev Respir Dis 1987;135:924–9.

143. Schuster DP. The case for and against fluid restriction and occlusion pressure reduction in adult respiratory distress syndrome. New Horiz 1993;1:478–88.

144. Wiedemann HP, Wheeler AP, Bernard GR, et al. Comparison of two fluid-management strategies in acute lung injury. N Engl J Med 2006;354:2564–75.

145. McIntyre RC Jr, Haenel JB, Moore FA, et al. Cardiopulmonary effects of permissive hypercapnia in the management of adult respiratory distress syndrome. J Trauma 1994;37:433–8.

146. Brochard L, Rauss A, Benito SM, et al. Comparison of three methods of gradual withdrawal from ventilation support during weaning from mechanical ventilation. AJRCCM 1995;150:896–903.

147. Leitch EA, Moran JL, Grealy B. Weaning and extubation in the intensive care unit. Clinical or index-driven approach? Intensive Care Med 1996;22:752–9.

148. Esteban A, Frutos F, Tobin MJ, et al. A comparison of four methods of weaning patients from mechanical ventilation. N Engl J Med 1995;332:345–50.

149. Ferrara TB, Georgieff MK, Ebert J, et al. Routine use of dexamethasone for the prevention of postextubation respiratory distress. J Perinatol 1989;9:287–90.

150. Couser RJ, Ferrera B, Falde B, et al. Effectiveness of dexamethasone in preventing extubation failure in preterm infants at increased risk for airway edema. J Pediatr 1992;121:591–6.

151. Dries DJ. Weaning from mechanical ventilation. J Trauma 1997;43:372–84.

152. Holdgaard HO, Pedersen J, Jensen RH, et al. Percutaneous dilatational tracheostomy versus conventional surgical tracheostomy: A clinical randomised study. Acta Anaesth Scand 1988;42:545–50.

153. Rosenbower TJ, Morris JA Jr, Eddy VA, et al. The long-term complications of percutaneous dilatational tracheostomy. Am Surg 1998;64:82–7.

154. Citta-Pietrolungo TJ, Alexander MA, Cook SP, et al. Complications of tracheostomy and decannulation in pediatric and young patients with traumatic brain injury. Arch Phys Med Rehab 1993;74:905–9.

155. Biarent D. New tools in ventilatory support: High frequency ventilation, nitric oxide, tracheal gas insufflation, non-invasive ventilation. Pediatr Pulmonol Suppl 1999;18:178–81.

156. Clark RH. High-frequency ventilation. J Pediatr 1994;124:661–70.

157. Froese AB, Bryan AC. High frequency ventilation. Am Rev Respir Dis 1987;135:1363–74.

158. Krishnan JA, Brower RG. High-frequency ventilation for acute lung injury and ARDS. Chest 2000;118:795–807.

159. Rouby JJ, Simonneau G, Benhamou D, et al. Factors influencing pulmonary volumes and CO2 elimination during high-frequency jet ventilation. Anesthesiology 1985;63:473–82.

160. Baumann MH, Sahn SA. Medical management and therapy of bronchopleural fistulas in the mechanically ventilated patient. Chest 1991;97:721–8.

161. High-frequency oscillatory ventilation compared with conventional mechanical ventilation in the treatment of respiratory failure in preterm infants. The HIFI Study Group. N Engl J Med 1989;320:88–93.

162. Clark RH, Gerstmann DR, Null DMJ, et al. Prospective randomized comparison of high-frequency oscillatory and

conventional ventilation in respiratory distress syndrome. Pediatrics 1992;89:5–12.

163. Keszler M, Donn SM, Bucciarelli RL, et al. Multicenter control trial comparing high frequency jet ventilation and conventional ventilation in newborn patients with pulmonary interstitial emphysema. J Pediatr 1991;119:85–93.

164. Gerstmann DR, Minton SD, Stoddard RA, et al. The Provo multicenter early high-frequency oscillatory ventilation trial: Improved pulmonary and clinical outcome in respiratory distress syndrome. Pediatrics 1996;98:1044–57.

165. Moriette G, Paris-Llado J, Walti H, et al. Prospective randomized multicenter comparison of high-frequency oscillatory ventilation and conventional ventilation in preterm infants of less than 30 weeks with respiratory distress syndrome. Pediatrics 2001;107: 363–72.

166. Courtney SE, Durand DJ, Asselin JM, et al. High-frequency oscillatory ventilation versus conventional mechanical ventilation for very-low-birth-weight infants. N Engl J Med 2002;347:643–52.

167. Durand DJ, Asselin LM, Hudak HL, et al. Early high-frequency oscillatory ventilation versus synchronized intermittent mandatory ventilation in very low birth weight infants: A pilot study of two ventilation protocols. J Perinatol 2001;21:221–9.

168. Gerstmann DR, Wood K, Miller A, et al. Childhood outcome after early high-frequency oscillatory ventilation for neonatal respiratory distress syndrome. Pediatrics 2001;108:617–23.

169. Clark RH, Yoder BA, Sell MS. Prospective, randomized comparison of high-frequency oscillation and conventional ventilation in candidates for extracorporeal membrane oxygenation. J Pediatr 1994;124:447–54.

170. Arnold JH, Hanson JH, Toro-Figuero LO, et al. Prospective, randomized comparison of high-frequency oscillatory ventilation and conventional mechanical ventilation in pediatric respiratory failure. Crit Care Med 1994;22:1530–9.

171. Rosenberg RB, Broner CW, Peters KJ, et al. High-frequency ventilation for acute pediatric respiratory failure. Chest 1994;104:1216–21.

172. Dobyns EL, Anas NG, Fortenberry JD, et al. Interactive effects of high-frequency oscillatory ventilation and inhaled nitric oxide in acute hypoxemic respiratory failure in pediatrics. Crit Care Med 2002;30:2425–9.

173. Bhuta T, Clark RH, Henderson-Smart DJ. Rescue high frequency oscillatory ventilation vs conventional ventilation for infants with severe pulmonary dysfunction born at or near term. Cochrane Database Syst Rev 2001;CD002974-CD002974.

174. Cools F, Henderson-Smart DJ, Offringa M, et al. Elective high frequency oscillatory ventilation versus conventional ventilation for acute pulmonary dysfunction in preterm infants. Cochrane Database Syst Rev 2009;(8):CD000104-CD000104.

175. Murad F. Cyclic guanosine monophosphate as a mediator of vasodilation. J Clin Invest 1986;78:1–5.

176. Abman SH, Griebel JL, Parker DK, et al. Acute effects of inhaled nitric oxide in children with severe hypoxemic respiratory failure. J Pediatr 1994;124:881–8.

177. Day RW, Allen EM, Witte MK. A randomized, controlled study of the 1-hour and 24-hour effects of inhaled nitric oxide therapy in children with acute hypoxemic respiratory failure. Chest 1997;112:1324–31.

178. Roberts JJ, Fineman J, Morin F. Inhaled nitric oxide and persistent pulmonary hypertension of the newborn: The Inhaled Nitric Oxide Study Group. N Engl J Med 1997;336:605–10.

179. Clark R, Kueser T, Walker M, et al. Low-dose nitric oxide therapy for persistent pulmonary hypertension of the newborn. N Engl J Med 2000;342:469–74.

180. Christou H, Van Marter L, Wessel D, et al. Inhaled nitric oxide reduces the need for extracorporeal membrane oxygenation in infants with persistent pulmonary hypertension of the newborn. Crit Care Med 2000;28:3722–7.

181. The Neonatal Inhaled Nitric Oxide Study Group. Inhaled nitric oxide in full-term and nearly full-term infants with hypoxic respiratory failure. N Engl J Med 1997;336:597–604.

182. Inhaled nitric oxide in term and near-term infants: Neurodevelopmental follow-up of the neonatal inhaled nitric oxide study group (NINOS). J Pediatr 2000;136:611–17.

183. Ellington MJ, O'Reilly D, Allred E, et al. Child health status, neurodevelopmental outcome, and parental satisfaction in a randomized, controlled trial nitric oxide for persistent pulmonary hypertension of the newborn. Pediatrics 2001;107:1351–6.

184. Inhaled nitric oxide and hypoxic respiratory failure in infants with congenital diaphragmatic hernia. The Neonatal Inhaled Nitric Oxide Study Group (NINOS). Pediatrics 1997;99: 838–45.

185. Karamanoukian HL, Glick PL, Wilcox DT, et al. Pathophysiology of congenital diaphragmatic hernia. VIII: Inhaled nitric oxide requires exogenous surfactant therapy in the lamb model of congenital diaphragmatic hernia. J Pediatr Surg 1995;30: 1–4.

186. Van Meurs KP, Rhine WD, Asselin JM, et al. Response of premature infants with severe respiratory failure to inhaled nitric oxide. Preemie NO Collaborative Group. Pediatr Pulmonol 1997;24:319–23.

187. Hoehn T, Krause M, Buhrer C. Inhaled nitric oxide in premature infants: A meta-analysis. J Perinat Med 2000;28:7–13.

188. Haddad IY, Ischiropoulos H, Holm BA, et al. Mechanisms of peroxynitrite-induced injury to pulmonary surfactants. Am J Physiol 1993;265:L555–64.

189. Beckman JS, Beckman T, Chen J, et al. Apparent hydroxyl radical production by peroxynitrite: Implications for endothelial injury from nitric oxide and superoxide. Proc Natl Acad Sci U S A 1990;87:1620–4.

190. Jobe AH. Pulmonary surfactant therapy. N Engl J Med 1993;328:861–8.

191. Hallman M, Merritt TA, Jarvenpaa AL, et al. Exogenous human surfactant for treatment of severe respiratory distress syndrome: A randomized prospective clinical trial. J Pediatr 1985;106: 963–9.

192. Long W, Corbet A, Cotton R, et al. A controlled trial of synthetic surfactant in infants weighing 1250 g or more with respiratory distress syndrome: The American Exosurf Neonatal Study Group I, and the Canadian Exosurf Neonatal Study Group. N Engl J Med 1991;325:1696–703.

193. Lotze A, Mitchell BR, Bulas DI, et al. Multicenter study of surfactant (beractant) use in the treatment of term infants with severe respiratory failure. Survanta in Term Infants Study Group. J Pediatr 1998;132:40–7.

194. Findlay RD, Taeusch HW, Walther FJ. Surfactant replacement therapy for meconium aspiration syndrome. Pediatrics 1996;97:48–52.

195. Hentschel R, Dittrich F, Hilgendorff A, et al. Neurodevelopmental outcome and pulmonary morbidity two years after early versus late surfactant treatment: Does it really differ? Acta Paediatr 2009;98:654–9.

196. Stevens TP, Harrington EW, Blennow M, et al. Early surfactant administration with brief ventilation vs. selective surfactant and continued mechanical ventilation for preterm infants with or at risk for respiratory distress syndrome. Cochrane Database Syst Rev (Online) 2007;CD003063-CD003063.

197. Lotze A, Knight GR, Anderson KD, et al. Surfactant (beractant) therapy for infants with congenital diaphragmatic hernia on ECMO: Evidence of persistent surfactant deficiency. J Pediatr Surg 1994;29:407–12.

198. Cogo PE, Zimmermann LJ, Rosso F, et al. Surfactant synthesis and kinetics in infants with congenital diaphragmatic hernia. Am J Respir Crit Care Med 2002;166:154–8.

199. IJsselstijn H, Zimmermann LJ, Bunt JE, et al. Prospective evaluation of surfactant composition in bronchoalveolar lavage fluid of infants with congenital diaphragmatic hernia and of age-matched controls. Crit Care Med 1998;26:573–80.

200. Wilcox DT, Glick PL, Karamanoukian H, et al. Pathophysiology of congenital diaphragmatic hernia, V: Effect of exogenous surfactant therapy on gas exchange and lung mechanics in the lamb congenital diaphragmatic hernia model. J Pediatr 1994;124:289–93.

201. Glick PL, Leach CL, Besner GE, et al. Pathophysiology of congenital diaphragmatic hernia, III: Exogenous surfactant therapy for the high-risk neonate with CDH. J Pediatr Surg 1992; 27:866–9.

202. Ullrich R, Lorber C, Röder G, et al. Controlled airway pressure therapy, nitric oxide inhalation, prone position, and extracorporeal membrane oxygenation (ECMO) as components of an integrated approach to ARDS. Anesthesiology 1999;91:1577–86.

203. Priestley MA, Helfaer MA. Approaches in the management of acute respiratory failure in children. Curr Opin Pediatr 2004 16:293–8.

204. Foglia E, Meier MD, Elward A. Ventilator-associated pneumonia in neonatal and pediatric intensive care unit patients. Clin Microbiol Rev 2007;20:409–25.

205. Muscedere J, Dodek P, Keenan S, et al. Comprehensive evidence-based clinical practice guidelines for ventilator-associated pneumonia: Prevention. J Crit Care 2008;23:126–37.

206. Principi N, Esposito S. Ventilator-associated pneumonia (VAP) in pediatric intensive care units. Pediatr Infect Dis J 2007; 26:841–4.

207. Gauvin F, Dassa C, Chaibou M, et al. Ventilator-associated pneumonia in intubated children: Comparison of different diagnostic methods. Pediatr Crit Care Med 2003;4:437–43.

208. Iregui M, Ward S, Sherman G, et al. Clinical importance of delays in the initiation of appropriate antibiotic treatment for ventilator-associated pneumonia. Chest 2002;122:262–8.

209. Shlaes DM, Gerding DN, John JF, et al. Society for Healthcare Epidemiology of America and Infectious Diseases Society of America Joint Committee on the Prevention of Antimicrobial Resistance: Guidelines for the prevention of antimicrobial resistance in hospitals. Clin Infect Dis 1997;25:584–99.

210. Toltzis P, Hoyen C, Spinner-Block S, et al. Factors that predict preexisting colonization with antibiotic-resistant gram-negative bacilli in patients admitted to a pediatric intensive care unit. Pediatrics 1999;103:719–23.

211. Toltzis P, Yamashita T, Vilt L, et al. Colonization with antibiotic-resistant gram-negative organisms in a pediatric intensive care unit. Crit Care Med 1997;25:538–44.

212. Chastre J, Wolff M, Fagon JY, et al. Comparison of 8 vs 15 days of antibiotic therapy for ventilator-associated pneumonia in adults: A randomized trial. JAMA 2003;290:2588–98.

213. Dodek P, Keenan S, Cook D, et al. Evidence-based clinical practice guideline for the prevention of ventilator-associated pneumonia. Ann Int Med 2004;141:305–13.

214. Curley MA, Schwalenstocker E, Deshpande JK, et al. Tailoring the Institute for Health Care Improvement 100,000 Lives Campaign to pediatric settings: The example of ventilator-associated pneumonia. Pediatr Clin North Am 2006;53:1231–51.

CHAPTER 8

Vascular Access

Ravindra K. Vegunta

A peripheral intravenous (PIV) cannula is the most commonly used device for venous access in children. Although venous access is often achieved in adults with minimal distress, placement of an intravenous catheter in children can be quite traumatic to the child, the parents, and the attendant health care providers. In some situations, it can be a fairly frustrating and time-consuming procedure.[1] Particular circumstances of each child may demand specific solutions for vascular access, namely the choice of device and the site chosen for its placement (Table 8-1). Clinicians must be aware of the limitations and potential adverse effects of the various vascular access devices (VADs) that are available.

In an emergency, other options should promptly be considered after a few failed attempts at PIV cannula placement. Historically, the only available options were a venous cutdown or an emergency central venous catheter (CVC) placement. These options take considerable time and frequently require the services of a pediatric surgeon. Intraosseous (IO) needle placement has become the most common contingency method of emergency vascular access in children. The newer mechanical devices allow easier training of emergency medical personnel and have improved the success rate of IO placement in the prehospital setting. In fact, with appropriate training, an IO needle can be placed more quickly than a PIV cannula.[2] In sick neonates, umbilical vessels are frequently cannulated, but can only be used for a finite period [maximum of 5 days for an umbilical artery catheter (UAC)] and 14 days for an umbilical venous catheter (UVC).[3] Early placement of a peripherally introduced CVC (PICC) is preferable in these infants. Persistence with using PIV cannulas leads to higher complication rates and reduces the number of future PICC placement sites.

In choosing the appropriate VAD for an oncology patient, the requirements of the oncologist, the patient's age, expected activity level, expected chance of cure, number of previous VADs placed, and patency of the central veins should all be considered. The number of lumens, size of the catheter, type of catheter, and its location can all be tailored to the specific patient.[4] Long-term maintenance of central venous access in patients suffering from intestinal malabsorption is particularly challenging. Once the six conventional sites of central venous access—bilateral internal jugular, subclavian, and femoral veins—are exhausted, one must become more creative in gaining central access.

Complications that are common to all types of VADs are extravasation of infusate, hemorrhage, phlebitis, septicemia, thrombosis, and thromboembolism. Multiple studies have shown that catheter-related blood stream infections can be prevented with appropriate education and training utilizing insertion and maintenance bundles.[3,5,6]

PERIPHERAL VENOUS ACCESS

Peripheral intravenous catheter placement is the most frequently used method of gaining vascular access. In infants and children, PIV access is usually achieved by using the veins on the dorsum of the hand, forearm, dorsum of the foot, medial aspect of the ankle, and the scalp. In infants, the median vein tributaries on the ventral aspect of the distal forearm and wrist, and the lateral tributaries of the dorsal venous arch on the dorsum of the foot, may be available, but typically allow cannulation of only the finest-diameter catheters. The location of the distal long saphenous vein (anterior to the medial malleolus) is fairly constant and is frequently palpable, making it one of the most popular veins used for PIV access, particularly in infants. It allows a larger size catheter and excellent stabilization of the catheter as well. Scalp veins can be readily visible and accessible but it can be difficult to maintain access for any length of time. Similarly, external jugular vein catheters tend to get dislodged promptly in a moving patient and may only be useful for a short time.

Several techniques have been shown to be beneficial in cannulating a peripheral vein, including warming the extremity, transillumination, and epidermal vasodilators.[7] Ultrasound (US) guidance has been used to obtain access to basilic and brachial veins in the emergency department.[8] Devices utilizing near-infrared imaging of the veins up to a depth of 10 mm are being used routinely in the hospitals, as well as by emergency medical personnel in the field, to find and access peripheral veins in all age groups.[9] Unlike ultrasound, there is no physical contact with the overlying skin and hence there is no compression or distortion of the veins. Significant complications associated with PIV catheters include phlebitis, thrombosis, and extravasation with chemical burn or necrosis of surrounding soft tissue.

UMBILICAL VEIN AND ARTERY ACCESS

Neonates are often managed with catheters placed either in the umbilical vein and/or one of the umbilical arteries. They can be used for monitoring central venous or arterial pressure, blood sampling, fluid resuscitation, medication administration, and total parenteral nutrition (TPN).

TABLE 8-1 Indications for Vascular Access in Infants and Children and the Recommended Devices

Indications	PIV	PICC	IO	CVC		
				NONTUNNELED	TUNNELED	SUBCUTANEOUS PORT
Emergency venous access	X		X	X		
Short-term venous access	X			X		
Medium-term venous access	X	X		X		
Long-term venous access		X			X	X

CVC, central venous catheter; IO, intraosseous needle; PICC, peripherally introduced central venous catheter; PIV, peripheral intravenous catheter.

To minimize infectious complications, the UVCs are usually removed after a maximum of 14 days.[3,10] These catheters are typically placed by neonatal nurse practitioners or neonatologists, and require dissection of the umbilical cord stump within a few hours of birth. It is possible for the pediatric surgeon to cannulate the umbilical vessels after the umbilical stump has undergone early desiccation. A small vertical skin incision is made above or below the umbilical stump to access the umbilical vein or artery, respectively. Once the fascia is incised, the appropriate vessel is identified, isolated, and cannulated. The tip of the UVC should be positioned at the junction of the inferior vena cava (IVC) and the right atrium (RA).[11] The xiphisternum is a good landmark for the RA/IVC junction. On the chest radiograph, the tip of the UVC should be at or above the level of the diaphragm. The tip of the UAC is best positioned between the sixth and tenth thoracic vertebrae, cranial to the celiac axis (Fig. 8-1). Various calculations have been proposed to estimate the correct length of the catheter before insertion, based on weight and other biometric measures of the infant.[12,13] The long-standing argument about the safety of a 'high' versus 'low' position for the UAC tip has been laid to rest; the 'high' position just described has been shown to be associated with a low incidence of clinically significant aortic thrombosis without any increase in other adverse sequelae.[14,15] These umbilical vessel catheters have been associated with various complications. In addition to tip migration, sepsis and thrombosis can occur. UVCs have also been associated with perforation of the IVC, extravasation of infusate into the peritoneal cavity, and portal vein thrombosis.[16] UACs are associated with aortic injuries, thromboembolism of aortic branches, aneurysms of the iliac artery and/or the aorta, paraplegia, and gluteal ischemia with possible necrosis.[11] Pooled rates of bloodstream infections associated with umbilical catheters and CVCs in level III NICUs has improved over the recent years (Table 8-2).[17–19]

PERIPHERALLY INTRODUCED CENTRAL CATHETER

PICC lines provide reliable central venous access in neonates and older children without a need for directly accessing the central veins. PICC lines are suitable for infusion of fluids, medications, TPN, and blood products. Many institutions caring for sick children on a

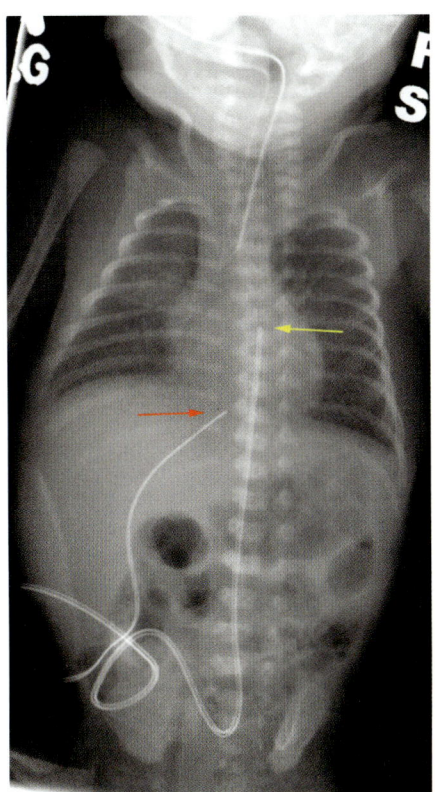

FIGURE 8-1 ■ This abdominal and chest film of a newborn shows the UAC catheter at the level of the seventh thoracic vertebral body (yellow arrow) and the umbilical venous catheter (red arrow) at the level of the diaphragm. These are the recommended positions for these catheters.

TABLE 8-2 Pooled Rates of Catheter-Associated Blood Stream Infections Shown as Occurrence Per 1000 Catheter-Days

Patient Weight	Central Venous Catheter			Umbilical Catheter	
	2007	2009	2010	2007	2009
≤750 g	6.4	4.2	2.6	6.9	4.2
751–1000 g	4.4	2.7	2.2	4.3	2.7
1001–1500 g	4.8	1.9	1.3	3.2	0.9
1501–2500 g	4.2	1.5	1.0	1.8	0.5
>2500 g	3.1	1.3	0.8	0.9	0.5

Published as part of National Healthcare Safety Network (NHSN) Report, data summary for 2007, 2009 and 2010.

routine basis have developed special teams and protocols for placement of PICC lines to reduce variations in practice and increase availability.[20] The modified Seldinger technique is used most frequently. A small peripheral intravenous catheter (about 24 gauge) is first placed, preferably with ultrasound guidance, in a suitable extremity vein such as the basilic, cephalic, or long saphenous vein. A fine guide wire is advanced through the vein, the initial catheter is removed, the track is dilated, and a peel-away PICC introducer sheath is advanced over the guide wire. The guide wire is then removed, and the PICC line is introduced through the sheath (Fig. 8-2).[21,22] The tip of the PICC should be placed at the superior vena cava (SVC)/RA junction or the IVC/RA junction. Locations peripheral to these are considered non-central and are associated with higher complications.[23] PICC lines are also eminently suitable for short- to medium-term (weeks) home intravenous therapy of antibiotics or TPN.[24] The most common complications associated with PICC lines are infections, occlusion, and dislodgement of the catheter.[25]

CENTRAL VENOUS CATHETERS

With the development of PICC teams and the increasing use of PICC lines, there has been a decline in the use of CVCs in neonates and older children.[20] Nontunneled CVCs are used for short- and medium-term indications, whereas surgically placed tunneled CVCs are used for medium- and long-term indications. In premature neonates, if PICC placement is not successful, tunneled CVCs are preferentially used because of their smaller size and durability as opposed to nontunneled CVCs. The

central veins accessed for placement of CVCs are the bilateral internal jugular veins, subclavian veins, and femoral veins. In older children and full-term neonates, the percutaneous Seldinger technique is used. In premature neonates and occasionally in older children, the relevant central vein or one of its tributaries (i.e., common facial vein or external jugular vein in the neck, cephalic vein in the deltopectoral groove, or the long saphenous vein at the groin [Fig. 8-3]), is dissected and cannulated.[26–28] In some emergency situations, percutaneous femoral vein access may be preferred as the insertion site is away from the activity centered around the head, neck, and chest. The tip of a CVC placed from the lower body should be positioned at the junction of the IVC and RA, which will ensure prompt dilution of the infusate and likely has a lower chance of thrombosis. Again, the xiphoid process is a good surface landmark to estimate the length of catheter needed. Radiographically, the tip should be positioned just above the diaphragm.

A CVC placed through an upper body vein should be positioned such that the tip is at the junction of the SVC and RA. Surface landmarks for this location are less reliable. A point about 1 cm caudal to the manubriosternal junction, at the right sternal border, gives a close estimate to the SVC/RA junction in toddlers and older children. The lower margin of the third right costosternal junction has been shown to be the best surface landmark in adults for placement of the CVC tip at the SVC/RA junction.[29] Length recommendations have been made based on a child's weight for placement of right internal jugular and right subclavian CVCs.[30] On a chest radiograph, the tip of the catheter should project about two vertebral bodies caudal to the carina. A tunneled CVC can be left in place for several months to years. The Broviac and Hickman

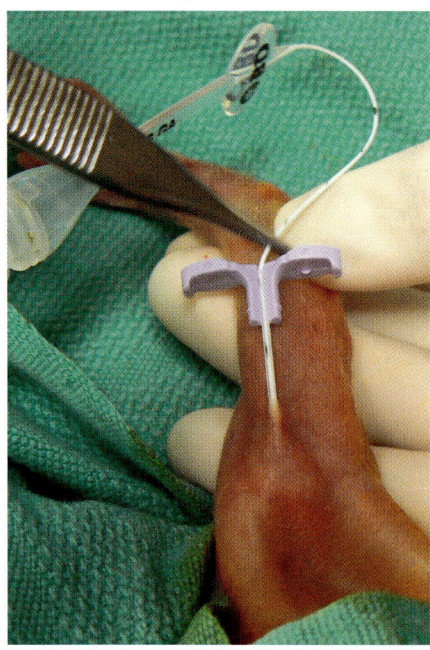

FIGURE 8-2 ■ Placement of a PICC using the modified Seldinger technique described in the text. The axillary vein is being accessed in this premature infant.

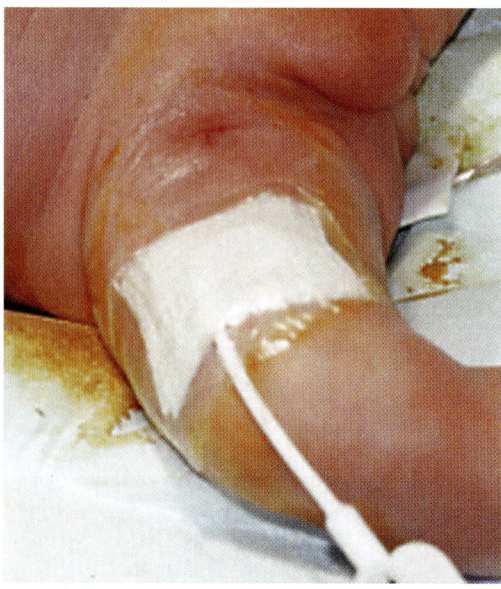

FIGURE 8-3 ■ This broviac catheter was placed through a cutdown at the groin to access the long saphenous vein close to the saphenofemoral junction. The catheter is positioned in a subcutaneous tunnel in the thigh to exit just above the knee on the anteromedial aspect.

catheters (Bard Access Systems, Salt Lake City, UT) are made of silicone and are available in various sizes, the smallest being a 2.7 French single-lumen catheter. These catheters have a Dacron cuff that promotes tissue ingrowth, resulting in anchoring of the catheter within the subcutaneous tunnel. The cuff can be placed close to the exit site of the catheter to facilitate removal by dissection through the exit site. Placement of the Dacron cuff midway between the venotomy site and the exit site has the advantage of reducing the chance of unintended removal of the catheter.

Use of ultrasound guidance for percutaneous central venous access is becoming standard of care. The benefits of ultrasound assistance include higher success rate, faster access, fewer needle passes, and fewer arterial punctures.[31-36] Real-time 2D ultrasound guidance is recommended as the preferred method when placing a CVC into the internal jugular vein (IJV) in adults and children in elective situations.[31,32,36] In a randomized controlled trial, ultrasound was shown to be beneficial in IJV catheterization in infants weighing less than 7.5 kg when compared with a ultrasound image-based skin surface marking.[33] During insertion, the ultrasound transducer is wrapped in a sterile sleeve, and sterile gel is used to obtain real-time images of the vessel being accessed. Either a short-axis view across the diameter of the vessel (Fig. 8-4) or the long axis view along the length of the vessel is used to visualize the needle approaching and entering the vessel. A guide wire is then passed into the vessel, followed by the Seldinger technique for placement of the CVC.[36] Because of the proximity of the clavicle, visualization of the subclavian vein is poor with ultrasound. Infraclavicular axillary vein cannulation has been performed with 96% success with ultrasound guidance for tunneled CVC placement into the subclavian vein.[37]

The majority of bloodstream infections in children are associated with the use of a vascular access device. Tunneled CVCs inserted in the neck veins in neonates in the NICU have been associated with a higher rate of complications than those placed in the inguinal region. Infection rates were 5.8 (neck) versus 0.7 (groin) per 1000

catheter days.[28] Urgent CVCs placed in 289 pediatric burn unit patients also resulted in higher infection rates associated with subclavian and internal jugular CVCs compared with the femoral CVCs (10 and 13.6 versus 8.2 per 1000 catheter days).[38] This is thought to be due to the higher nursing and respiratory therapy activity around the head and neck in these patients requiring intensive burn care. Ethanol lock, in addition to antibiotic therapy, has been shown to be beneficial in salvaging CVCs that become infected.[39] Ethanol lock has also been shown to be superior to heparin lock in preventing catheter infection and loss in children with intestinal failure.[40] Retained fragments of CVCs after attempted removal has been reported to occur at a rate of 2%. Leaving a ligated fragment of the catheter within the blood vessel is felt to be safer than the alternative, which involves interventional or operative removal.[41]

TOTALLY IMPLANTED CENTRAL VENOUS CATHETERS

Totally implantable intravascular devices (ports) are subcutaneous reservoirs attached to CVCs. The reservoirs are made of a metal or hard plastic shell with a central silicone septum that is penetrated for access. They provide a reliable, long-lasting solution for patients who need intermittent access to their central venous system. They are ideal for patients who desire to be involved in aquatic sports and other physical activities. They are most useful for patients with malignancies, coagulopathies, hemolytic syndromes, and renal failure, all of which require recurrent vascular access. Low profile ports with 5 or 6 French catheters are available for use in infants. Larger ports are available with dual lumens. High-flow ports are available (PowerPort-Bard Access Systems, Salt Lake City, UT) that allow high-pressure injection of intravenous contrast for radiologic imaging. Ports require special noncoring needles to keep the septum from leaking. The reservoir should be implanted in a subcutaneous pocket, over a firm base such as the chest wall. Preferred sites for port placement include the pectoral area, parasternal area, (above and medial to the areola) and the subclavicular area (medial to the anterior axillary fold). In females with a concern for cosmesis, the low presternum area and the lateral chest wall are locations that hide the scar when the port is eventually removed. In determining port placement, consideration should be given to the age of the patient, the intended activities, as well as the convenience of the caregivers. Subclavicular placement will make it easy to access the port with minimal disrobing; in obese girls and young women, it is less likely to get displaced by the highly mobile breast tissue. The presternal location will provide a very stable foundation for the port, even in the obese child. When placed over the lower sternum, it can be accessed with opening the front of a button-down top or shirt. Complications that are unique to a port include an inability to access the port, disconnection of the catheter from the reservoir with extravasation, flipping of the port, fracture and embolization of the catheter, and breakdown of the overlying skin.[42]

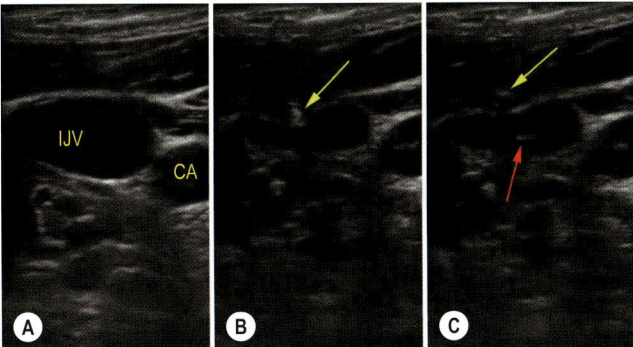

FIGURE 8-4 ■ Ultrasound short-axis image of the right internal jugular vein and carotid artery obtained with SonoSite S Series using a 13–6 MHz transducer (SonoSite Inc., Bothell, Washington) in a child. **(A)** The internal jugular vein (IJV) and the carotid artery (CA). **(B)** The yellow arrow is pointing to the needle indenting the IJV. **(C)** The red arrow points to the target sign caused by the needle in the middle of the IJV confirming correct placement.

INTRAOSSEOUS ACCESS

Several studies have been published over the past 60 years establishing the safety and effectiveness of IO access for infusion of fluids and medications in children, including neonates.[43,44] IO access has also been shown to be faster than access with a PIV[2] and safer than an emergency CVC.

Bone marrow consists of rich lattice network of vessels. Whereas the peripheral veins collapse in patients in shock, the vascular spaces in the bone marrow do not.[45] The bioavailability of resuscitative drugs administered through IO access has been well established and shown to be better than that of those administered through an endotracheal tube.[46,47] The current Pediatric Advanced Life Support (PALS) recommendation is to establish IO access promptly if PIV access cannot be attained rapidly in neonates and children of all ages who need intravenous drugs or fluids urgently.[48] In children, the long bones of the lower extremities are used preferentially for IO placement. The proximal tibia is the most common site used, followed by the distal femur. With full sterile precautions, a needle designed for bone marrow aspiration is advanced through the cortical bone to access the bone marrow. In an infant, a spinal needle may be used, but in an older child, a generic bone marrow needle or a purpose designed IO needle such as the widely used Jamshidi needle (Cardinal Health, McGraw Park, IL) is used.[47,49]

The anteromedial flat surface of the tibia, 1–3 cm distal to the tibial tuberosity, is the best site. A small skin incision is made using the tip of a pointed scalpel or a large-bore hypodermic needle. The IO needle is positioned pointing posteriorly and angled slightly caudad. It is then advanced through the cortical bone using a screwing and unscrewing motion with constant pressure. Once the needle penetrates the outer cortex, a sudden 'give' is felt. The needle is held in this position and the obturator is removed. A syringe is attached and bone marrow is aspirated to confirm correct placement. The IO needle is stabilized with a dressing. The distal femur location is accessed by placing the needle 1–3 cm cephalad to the patella, angled slightly cranial to avoid the growth plate.

Contraindications to IO placement include injury or suspected injury to the bone or soft tissue overlying the placement site. Mechanical devices such as the Bone Injection Gun (BIG, Wasimed, Caesarea, Israel), FAST1 System (Pyng Medical Corporation, Vancouver, Canada), and EZ-IO (Vidacare, San Antonio, TX) have helped to expand the use of IO access.[2,47] The first two are spring-loaded devices. The FAST1 System is designed for sternal use in adults. The EZ-IO is a power drill-assisted device that makes IO placement easier in older children and adults.

Early concerns about potential adverse effects on the growth plates of long bones used for IO access have been allayed by animal studies.[49] The overall complication rate is estimated to be about 1%.[47] Extravasation of fluid is the most common adverse event. Compartment syndrome, osteomyelitis, skin and soft tissue infection, bone fractures, and fat embolism, although rare, have also been reported.[47]

VENOUS CUTDOWN

Although the advent and eventual broader acceptance of IO infusion has almost eliminated the need for venous cutdown and reduced the role of emergency placement of CVCs, pediatric surgeons should maintain the knowledge and skills required to perform this procedure.[7] The vessel of choice is the long saphenous vein near the medial malleolus. The vein is superficial, is of satisfactory size, and there is minimal subcutaneous fat in this location. A transverse incision is made anterior and cephalad to the medial malleolus. The vein is readily identified by dissecting through the thin subcutaneous tissue and is stabilized by placing proximal and distal stay ligatures. The vein is then directly cannulated using a venous catheter of appropriate size relative to the vein, and the catheter is anchored to the adjacent skin.

ALTERNATE ROUTES FOR CENTRAL VENOUS ACCESS

Patients who have had multiple previous CVCs can have thrombosis or stenosis of the central veins that precludes successful placement of a new catheter. Doppler ultrasound or magnetic resonance angiography can be used to survey the central veins, including the brachiocephalic vein, the SVC, and the IVC.[50] When necessary, percutaneous access can be gained via a patent IVC by either by a translumbar or a transhepatic approach.[51–53] A tunneled catheter can then be inserted to reach the IVC/RA junction. Translumbar IVC catheters are quite durable while transhepatic catheters tend to get withdrawn from the vascular space owing to the constant respiratory excursions of the diaphragm. The brachiocephalic vein, if patent, can similarly be accessed through a suprasternal route. The azygos vein may be accessed through one of the intercostal veins percutaneously or surgically using a thoracotomy or thoracoscopic assistance.[54–56] Direct RA access has been used to manage patients with intestinal failure and occluded central veins for long periods, and in cardiac patients in an acute situation.[53,57]

ARTERIAL CATHETER

Intra-arterial catheters allow continuous hemodynamic monitoring and blood sampling. The radial artery at the wrist is most commonly used for intra-arterial access due to the excellent collateral circulation. The dorsalis pedis and posterior tibial arteries are other peripheral sites that may sometimes be used. Femoral arteries are frequently used by cardiologists for catheter-based cardiac interventions and occasionally for monitoring. However, in general, it is advisable not to use the main artery of an extremity for chronic arterial catheter placement to avoid thromboembolic and ischemic complications.[3] Adequacy of collateral arterial supply through the ulnar artery should be confirmed before placement of a radial arterial line by using the Allen test.[58] The right radial artery allows preductal monitoring and sampling. Percutaneous cannulation is usually successful. If unsuccessful, an arterial cutdown can be performed. Digital ischemia can result from radial artery catheters. Thromboembolism can result in limb loss if the axillary, brachial, or femoral artery is catheterized. Local infections can occur when the catheters are left for several days. A pseudoaneurysm can result from injury to the adjacent vein during placement.

HEMODIALYSIS CATHETERS

The current recommendation is to use an autologous arteriovenous fistula (AVF) as the route of choice for hemodialysis.[59] AVFs permit high-flow rates that facilitate effective dialysis. They also are reliable, durable, and, once established, have low complication rates. Because patients are often referred late, and AVFs take time to mature, there is frequently a need for CVCs for immediate dialysis. Temporary and tunneled long-term double-lumen hemodialysis catheters are placed preferentially through the right IJV, either percutaneously or by cutdown. The larger size of the vein and the straight internal path of the catheter allow a larger catheter to be placed safely through the right IJV. Additionally, use of the IJV avoids possible injury or thrombosis to the SCV which must be patent to develop a functioning AVF at the wrist. The long-term, cuffed hemodialysis catheters are precurved to allow right internal jugular placement with tunneling to the pectoral area. Flow rates achieved through hemodialysis catheters tend to be lower and they last a relatively short time. AVF is also an option for management of young children with severe hemophilia.[60]

REFERENCES

1. Stovroff M, Teague WG. Intravenous access in infants and children. Pediatr Clin North Am 1998;45:1373–93.
2. de Caen A. Venous access in the critically ill child: When the peripheral intravenous fails! Pediatr Emerg Care 2007;23:422–4.
3. O'Grady N, Alexander M, Burns LA, et al. Healthcare Infection Control Practices Advisory Committee (HICPAC) (Appendix 1). Summary of recommendations: Guidelines for the Prevention of Intravascular Catheter-related Infections. Clin Inf Dis 2011;52:1087–99.
4. Alexander N. Question 3. Do Portacaths or Hickman lines have a higher risk of catheter-related bloodstream infections in children with leukaemia? Arch Dis Child 2010;95:239–41.
5. Stevens TP, Schulman J. Evidence-based approach to preventing central line-associated bloodstream infection in the NICU. Acta Paediatrica Supplement 2012;101:11–16.
6. Holzmann-Pazgal G, Kubanda A, Davis K, et al. Utilizing a line maintenance team to reduce central-line-associated bloodstream infections in a neonatal intensive care unit. J Perinatol 2012;32: 281–6.
7. Haas NA. Clinical review: Vascular access for fluid infusion in children. Crit Care 2004;8:478–84.
8. Keyes LE, Frazee BW, Snoey ER, et al. Ultrasound-guided brachial and basilic vein cannulation in emergency department patients with difficult intravenous access. Ann Emerg Med 1999;34: 711–14.
9. Miyake RK, Zeman HD, Duarte FH, et al. Vein imaging: A new method of near infrared imaging, where a processed image is projected onto the skin for the enhancement of vein treatment. Dermatol Surg 2006;32:1031–8.
10. Butler-O'Hara M, Buzzard CJ, Reubens L, et al. A randomized trial comparing long-term and short term use of umbilical venous catheters in premature infants with birth weights of less than 1251 grams. Pediatrics 2006;118:e25–35.
11. Ramasethu J. Complications of vascular catheters in the neonatal intensive care unit. Clin Perinatol 2008;35:199–222.
12. Sritipsukho S, Sritipsukho P. Simple and accurate formula to estimate umbilical arterial catheter length of high placement. J Med Assoc Thai 2007;90:1793–7.
13. Lin MS, Lim YJ, Ho NK. A quicker simpler method of predetermination of the length of umbilical artery catheter insertion in Asian babies. J Singapore Paediatr Soc 1989;31:79–81.
14. Green C, Yohannan MD. Umbilical arterial and venous catheters: Placement, use, and complications. Neonatal Netw 1998;17:23–8.
15. Barrington KJ. Umbilical artery catheters in the newborn: Effects of position of the catheter tip. Cochrane Database Syst Rev 2000:000505.
16. Kim JH, Lee YS, Kim SH, et al. Does umbilical vein catheterization lead to portal venous thrombosis? Prospective ultrasound evaluation in 100 neonates. Radiology 2001;219:645–50.
17. Edwards JR, Peterson KD, Andrus ML, et al. National Healthcare Safety Network (NHSN) Report, data summary for 2006, issued June 2007. Am J Infect Control 2007;35:290–301.
18. Dudeck MA, Horan TC, Peterson KD, et al. National Healthcare Safety Network (NHSN) report, data summary for 2009, device-associated module. Am J Infect Control 2011;39:349–67.
19. Dudeck MA, Horan TC, Peterson KD, et al. National Healthcare Safety Network (NHSN) Report, data summary for 2010, device-associated module. Am J Infect Control 2011;39:798–816.
20. Linck DA, Donze A, Hamvas A. Neonatal peripherally inserted central catheter team. Evolution and outcomes of a bedside-nurse-designed program. Adv Neonat Care 2007;7:22–9.
21. Pettit J. Technological advances for PICC placement and management. Adv Neonat Care 2007;7:122–31.
22. Braswell LE. Peripherally inserted central catheter placement in infants and children. Tech Vasc Interv Radiol 2011;14:204–11.
23. Racadio JM, Doellman DA, Johnson ND, et al. Pediatric peripherally inserted central catheters: Complication rates related to catheter tip location. Pediatrics 2001;107:E28.
24. Earhart A, Jorgensen C, Kaminski D. Assessing pediatric patients for vascular access and sedation. J Infus Nurs 2007;30:226–31.
25. Pettit J. Assessment of infants with peripherally inserted central catheters: Part 1. Detecting the most frequently occurring complications. Adv Neonat Care 2002;2:304–15.
26. Zumbro GL Jr, Mullin MJ, Nelson TG. Catheter placement in infants needing total parenteral nutrition utilizing common facial vein. Arch Surg 1971;102:71–3.
27. Meland NB, Wilson W, Soontharotoke CY, et al. Saphenofemoral venous cutdowns in the premature infant. J Pediatr Surg 1986;21:341–3.
28. Vegunta RK, Loethen P, Wallace LJ, et al. Differences in the outcome of surgically placed long-term central venous catheters in neonates: Neck vs. groin placement. J Pediatr Surg 2005;40: 47–51.
29. Hsu JH, Wang SS, Lu DV, et al. Optimal skin surface landmark for the SVC-RA junction in cancer patients requiring the implantation of permanent central venous catheters. Anaesthesia 2007;62:818–23.
30. Andropoulos DB, Bent ST, Skjonsby B, et al. The optimal length of insertion of central venous catheters for pediatric patients. Anesth Analg 2001;93:883–6.
31. Hind D, Calvert N, McWilliams R, et al. Ultrasonic locating devices for central venous cannulation: Meta-analysis. BMJ 2003; 16:327–361.
32. Abboud PA, Kendall JL. Ultrasound guidance for vascular access. Emerg Med Clin North Am 2004;22:749–73.
33. Hosokawa K, Shime N, Kato Y, et al. A randomized trial of ultrasound image-based skin surface marking versus real-time ultrasound-guided internal jugular vein catheterization in infants. Anesthesiology 2007;107:720–4.
34. Maecken T, Grau T. Ultrasound imaging in vascular access. Crit Care Med 2007;35:S178–85.
35. Wigmore TJ, Smythe JF, Hacking MB, et al. Effect of the implementation of NICE guidelines for ultrasound guidance on the complication rates associated with central venous catheter placement in patients presenting for routine surgery in a tertiary referral centre. Br J Anaesth 2007;99:662–5.
36. Pirotte T. Ultrasound-guided vascular access in adults and children: Beyond the internal jugular vein puncture. Acta Anaesthesiol Belg 2008;59:157–66.

37. Sharma A, Bodenham AR, Mallick A. Ultrasound-guided infraclavicular axillary vein cannulation for central venous access. Br J Anaesth 2004;93:188–92.

38. Sheridan RL, Weber JM. Mechanical and infectious complications of central venous cannulation in children: Lessons learned from a 10-year experience placing more than 1000 catheters. J Burn Care Res 2006;27:713–18.

39. Valentine KM. Ethanol lock therapy for catheter-associated blood stream infections in a pediatric intensive care unit. Pediatr Crit Care Med 2011;12:e292–6.

40. Oliveira C, Nasr A, Brindle M, et al. Ethanol locks to prevent catheter-related bloodstream infections in parenteral nutrition: A meta-analysis. Pediatrics 2012;129:318–29.

41. Milbrandt K, Beaudry P, Anderson R, et al. A multiinstitutional review of central venous line complications: Retained intravascular fragments. J Pediatr Surg 2009;44:972–6.

42. Dillon PA, Foglia RP. Complications associated with an implantable vascular access device. J Pediatr Surg 2006;41:1582–7.

43. DeBoer S, Russell T, Seaver M, et al. Infant intraosseous infusion. Neonatal Netw 2008;27:25–32.

44. Engle WA. Intraosseous access for administration of medications in neonates. Clin Perinatol 2006;33:161–8.

45. Calkins MD, Fitzgerald G, Bentley TB, et al. Intraosseous infusion devices: A comparison for potential use in special operations. J Trauma 2000;48:1068–74.

46. Buck ML, Wiggins BS, Sesler JM. Intraosseous drug administration in children and adults during cardiopulmonary resuscitation. Ann Pharmacother 2007;41:1679–86.

47. Blumberg SM, Gorn M, Crain EF. Intraosseous infusion: A review of methods and novel devices. Pediatr Emerg Care 2008 quiz 57-8;24:50–6.

48. de Caen AR, Kleinman ME, Chameides L, et al. Part 10: Paediatric basic and advanced life support: 2010 International Consensus on Cardiopulmonary Resuscitation and Emergency Cardiovascular Care Science with Treatment Recommendations. Resuscitation 2010;81:e213–59.

49. Boon JM, Gorry DL, Meiring JH. Finding an ideal site for intraosseous infusion of the tibia: An anatomical study. Clin Anat 2003;16:15–18.

50. Gupta H, Araki Y, Davidoff AM, et al. Evaluation of pediatric oncology patients with previous multiple central catheters for vascular access: Is Doppler ultrasound needed? Pediatr Blood Cancer 2007;48:527–31.

51. Azizkhan RG, Taylor LA, Jaques PF, et al. Percutaneous translumbar and transhepatic inferior vena caval catheters for prolonged vascular access in children. J Pediatr Surg 1992;27:165–9.

52. Mortell A, Said H, Doodnath R, et al. Transhepatic central venous catheter for long-term access in paediatric patients. J Pediatr Surg 2008;43:344–7.

53. Rodrigues AF, van Mourik ID, Sharif K, et al. Management of end-stage central venous access in children referred for possible small bowel transplantation. J Pediatr Gastroenterol Nutr 2006;42:427–33.

54. Solomon BA, Solomon J, Shlansky-Goldberg R. Percutaneous placement of an intercostal central venous catheter for chronic hyperalimentation guided by transhepatic venography. JPEN J Parenter Enteral Nutr 2001;25:42–4.

55. Tannuri U, Tannuri AC, Maksoud JG. The second and third right posterior intercostal veins: An alternate route for central venous access with an implantable port in children. J Pediatr Surg 2005;40:e27–30.

56. Sola JE, Thompson WR. Thoracoscopic-assisted placement of azygos vein central venous catheter in a child. Am J Transplant 2008;8:715–18.

57. Oram-Smith JC, Mullen JL, Harken AH, et al. Direct right atrial catheterization for total parenteral nutrition. Surgery 1978; 83:274–6.

58. Kohonen M, Teerenhovi O, Terho T, et al. Is the Allen test reliable enough? Eur J Cardiothorac Surg 2007;32:902–5.

59. D'Cunha PT, Besarab A. Vascular access for hemodialysis: 2004 and beyond. Curr Opin Nephrol Hypertens 2004;13:623–9.

60. Mancuso ME, Berardinelli L. Arteriovenous fistula as stable venous access in children with severe haemophilia. Haemophilia 2010;16:25–8.

CHAPTER 9

SURGICAL INFECTIOUS DISEASE

Bethany J. Slater • Thomas M. Krummel

Despite improvements in antimicrobial therapy, surgical technique, and postoperative intensive care, infection continues to be a significant source of mortality and morbidity for pediatric patients. Widespread antibiotic use has brought with it the complication of resistant organisms, and the selection of the appropriate antibiotic has become increasingly complex as newer antibiotics are continually developed.[1,2] In addition, infections with uncommon organisms are becoming more frequent with diminished host resistance from immunosuppressive states such as immaturity, cancer, systemic diseases, and medications after transplant procedures. Surgical infections generally require some operative intervention, such as drainage of an abscess or removal of necrotic tissue, and seldom respond to antibiotics alone.

Two broad classes of infectious disease processes affect a surgical practice: those infectious conditions brought to the pediatric surgeon for treatment and cure, and those that arise in the postoperative period as a complication of an operation.[3]

COMPONENTS OF INFECTION

The pathogenesis of infection involves a complex interaction between the host and infectious agent. Four components are important: virulence of the organism, size of inoculum, presence of nutrient source for the organism, and a breakdown in the host's defense.

The virulence of any microorganism depends on its ability to cause damage to the host. Exotoxins, such as streptococcal hyaluronidase, are digestive enzymes released locally that allow the spread of infection by breaking down host extracellular matrix proteins. Endotoxins, such as lipopolysaccharides, are components of gram-negative cell walls that are released only after bacterial cell death. Once systemically absorbed, endotoxins trigger a severe and rapid systemic inflammatory response by releasing various endogenous mediators such as cytokines, bradykinin, and prostaglandins.[4] Surgical infections are often polymicrobial, involving various interactions among the microorganisms.

The size of the inoculum is the second component of an infection. The number of colonies of microorganisms per gram of tissue is a key determinant. Predictably, any decrease in host resistance decreases the absolute number of colonies necessary to cause clinical disease. In general, if the bacterial population in a wound exceeds 100,000 organisms per gram of tissue, invasive infection is present.[5]

For any inoculum, the presence of suitable nutrients for the organism is essential and comprises the third component of any clinical infection. Accumulation of necrotic tissue, hematoma, and foreign matter is an excellent nutrient medium for continued organism growth and spread. Of special importance to the surgeon is the concept of necrotic tissue and infection.[6] This tissue often needs to be debrided to restore the host–bacterial balance and lead to effective wound healing.[7] Neutrophils, macrophages and cytokines accumulate in necrotic tissue initiating an inflammatory secondary response.[8]

Finally, for a clinical infection to arise, the body's defenses must be overcome. Even highly virulent organisms can be eradicated before clinical infection occurs if resistance is intact. Evolution has equipped humans with numerous mechanisms of defense, both anatomic and systemic.

DEFENSE AGAINST INFECTION

Anatomic Barriers

Intact skin and mucous membranes provide an effective surface barrier to infection.[9] These tissues are not merely a mechanical obstacle. The physiologic aspects of skin and mucous membranes provide additional protection. In the skin, the constant turnover of keratinocytes, temperature of the skin, and acid secretion from sebaceous glands inhibits bacterial cell growth. The mucosal surfaces also have developed advanced defense mechanisms to prevent and combat microbial invasion. Specialized epithelial layers provide resistance to infection. In addition, mechanisms such as the mucociliary transport system in the respiratory tract and normal colonic flora in the gastrointestinal tract prevent invasion of organisms. Anything that affects the normal function of these anatomic barriers increases the host's susceptibility to infection. A skin injury or a burn provides open access to the soft tissues, and antibiotic use disrupts normal colonic flora.[10] Such breakdowns in surface barriers are dealt with by the second line of defenses, the immune system.

Immune Response

The immune system involves complex pathways and many specialized effector responses. The first line of defense is the more primitive and nonspecific innate system, which consists primarily of phagocytic cells and the complement system. The neutrophil is able to rapidly migrate to the source of the infection and engulf and destroy the infecting organisms by phagocytosis. Cytokines, low molecular weight proteins including tumor necrosis factor (TNF), and many interleukins attract and activate neutrophils, and play a significant role in mediating the inflammatory response. In addition, the complement system, when activated, initiates a sequential cascade that also enhances phagocytosis and leads to lysis of pathogens. Neonates, particularly premature infants, have an immature immune system and are helped by the protective agents in human breast milk.[11,12] The more specialized, adaptive immune system involves a highly specific response to antigens as well as the eventual production of a variety of humoral mediators.[13]

Humoral and Cell-Mediated Immunity

Specific, adaptive immunity has two major components. The humoral mechanism (B-cell system) is based on bursa cell lymphocytes and plasma cells. The cellular mechanism (T-cell system) consists of the thymic-dependent lymphocytes.[14] The adaptive immune system is an antigen-specific system that is regulated by the lymphocytes. A myriad of receptors on the T-cells that are matched to particular individual antigens create these specific responses. Furthermore, antibody production from B-cells enhances the antigen-specific interaction.

B-cell immunity is provided by antibodies. The first exposure of an antigen leads to the production of IgM antibodies, whereas subsequent exposure to the same antigen results in rapid production of IgG antibodies. Humoral antibodies may neutralize toxins, tag foreign matter to aid phagocytosis (opsonization), or lyse invading cellular pathogens. Plasma cells and non-thymic-dependent lymphocytes that reside in the bone marrow and in the germinal centers and medullary cords of lymph nodes produce the reactive components of this humoral system. These agents account for most of the human immunity against extracellular bacterial species.

The cellular or T-cell component of immunity is based on sensitized lymphocytes located in the subcortical regions of lymph nodes and in the periarterial spaces of the spleen. T-cells are specifically responsible for immunity to viruses, most fungi, and intracellular bacteria. They produce a variety of lymphokines, such as transfer factors, that further activate lymphocytes, chemotactic factors, leukotrienes, and interferons.

Immunodeficiencies

Susceptibility to infection is increased when one of the components of the host defense mechanism is absent, reduced in numbers, or curtailed in function. Some of these derangements may be congenital, although the majority are acquired as a direct result of medications, radiation, endocrine disease, surgical ablation, tumors, or bacterial toxins. Immunodeficiencies from any cause significantly increase the risk of infection both in hospitalized and postoperative patients. Mycotic infections are an increasing problem in immunocompromised pediatric patients.[15]

Systemic diseases lead to diminished host resistance. For example, in diabetes mellitus, leukocytes often fail to respond normally to chemotaxis. Therefore, more severe,

recurrent, and unusual infections often occur in diabetic patients.[16] In addition, malignancy and other conditions that impair hematopoiesis lead to alterations in phagocytosis, resulting in an increased predilection for infection. Human immunodeficiency virus (HIV) infection in children is another major source of immunodeficiency. Vertical transmission from mother to child is the dominant mode of HIV acquisition among infants and children. Finally, poor nutritional status has adverse effects on immune function owing to a wide variety of negative influences on specific defense mechanisms, including decreased production of antibodies and phagocytic function.[17]

In patients with a primary immune defect, susceptibility to a specific infection is based on whether the defect is humoral, cellular, or a combination. Primary immunodeficiencies are rare but important because prompt recognition can lead to life-saving treatment or significant improvement in the quality of life.[18] B-cell deficiencies are associated with sepsis from encapsulated bacteria, especially pneumococcus, *Haemophilus influenzae*, and meningococcus. Often a fulminating course rapidly ends in death, despite timely therapeutic measures. Although congenital agammaglobulinemia or dysgammaglobulinemia has been widely recognized, other causes of humoral defects include radiation, corticosteroid and antimetabolite therapy, sepsis, splenectomy, and starvation. Chronic granulomatous disease is caused by a deficiency in the respiratory burst action of phagocytes that leads to severe and recurrent bacterial and fungal infections in early childhood. Children with chronic granulomatous disease are prone to develop hepatic abscesses as well as suppurative adenitis of a single node or multiple nodes, both of which may require surgical drainage or excision.[19]

T-cell deficiencies are responsible for many viral, fungal, and bacterial infections. Cutaneous candidiasis is a good example of a common infection seen with a T-cell deficiency. DiGeorge syndrome is a developmental anomaly in which both the thymus and the parathyroid glands are deficient, thus increasing the risk for infection and hypocalcemic tetany during infancy.

ANTIBIOTICS

The several classes of antibiotics are based on their molecular structure and site of action. The varying classes of antibiotics may be divided into bacteriostatic, which inhibit bacterial growth, and bacteriocidal, which destroy bacteria. The early initiation and correct choice of antibiotics is essential for timely and successful treatment of infections. In addition, it is important to have knowledge of the specific susceptibility patterns in a particular hospital or intensive care unit to direct initial empirical antibiotic therapy. Finally, awareness of interactions and adverse reactions in children from commonly used medications is critical.

The pharmacokinetics and monitoring of drug dosages in infants and children is also important when treating them with antibiotics. The efficacy and safety of many drugs have not been established in the pediatric patient, especially in the newborn.[20] Dosages based on pediatric pharmacokinetic data offer the most rational approach. Dosage requirements constantly change as a function of age and body weight. Furthermore, the volume of distribution and half-life of many medicines are often increased in neonates and children compared with adults for a variety of reasons.[21,22] Knowledge of a drug's pharmacokinetic profile allows manipulation of the dose to achieve and maintain a given plasma concentration.

Newborns usually have extremely skewed drug-distribution patterns. The entire body mass can be considered as if it were a single compartment for the purposes of dose calculations. For the majority of drugs, dose adjustments can be based on plasma drug concentration. Administering a loading dose is advisable when rapid onset of drug action is required. For many drugs, loading doses (milligrams per kilogram) are generally greater in neonates and young infants than in older children or adults.[22] However, prolonged elimination of drugs in the neonate requires lower maintenance doses, given at longer intervals, to prevent toxicity. Monitoring serum drug concentrations is useful if the desired effect is not attained or if adverse reactions occur.

The neonate undergoing extracorporeal membrane oxygenation (ECMO) presents a special challenge to drug delivery and elimination. Because the ECMO circuit may bind or inactivate drugs and make them unavailable to the patient, dosing requires careful attention to drug response and serum levels. The pharmacokinetics under these conditions generally include a larger volume of distribution and prolonged elimination, with a return to baseline after decannulation.[23]

PREVENTION OF INFECTIONS

The most effective way to deal with surgical infectious complications is to prevent their occurrence. The clinician must recognize the variables that increase the risk of infection and attempt to decrease or eliminate them. A summary of the category 1 recommendations published by the Hospital Infection Control Practices Advisory Committee (HICPAC) of the Centers for Disease Control and Prevention is listed in Box 9-1.

Patient Characteristics

In adults, comorbidities often increase the risk of a surgical site infection (SSI). However, these chronic diseases are infrequently encountered in children. A prospective multicenter study of wound infections in the pediatric population found that postoperative wound infections were more likely related to factors at the operation rather than to patient characteristics.[24] In this study of more than 800 children, the only factors associated with increased SSI were contamination at the time of operation and the duration of the procedure. Other investigators have similarly found that local factors at the time of operation, such as degree of contamination, tissue perfusion, and operative technique, play a more important role in initiation of an SSI than the general condition of the patient.[25]

BOX 9-1 Guidelines for Prevention of Surgical Site Infections

- Treat remote infections before elective surgery
- Do not remove hair preoperatively unless it will interfere with operation
- Adequately control serum blood glucose levels perioperatively
- Require patients to shower or bathe with an antiseptic agent before the operative day
- Use an appropriate antiseptic agent for skin preparation
- Perform a surgical scrub for at least two to five minutes using an appropriate antiseptic
- Administer a prophylactic antimicrobial agent only when indicated
- Administer an antimicrobial agent such that bactericidal concentration of the drug is established in serum and tissues when the incision is made and maintained throughout the operation
- Sterilize all surgical instruments
- Wear a surgical mask
- Wear a cap or hood to fully cover hair on head and face[a]
- Wear sterile gloves[a]
- Use sterile gowns and drapes that are effective barriers when wet
- Handle tissue gently, maintain effective hemostasis, minimize devitalized tissue and foreign bodies, and eradicate dead space at the surgical site
- If drainage is necessary, use closed suction drain
- Protect with a sterile dressing for 24 to 48 hours postoperatively an incision that has been closed primarily

[a]Required by the ultrasound Occupational Safety and Health Administration regulations.
From Mangram AJ, Horan TC, Pearson ML, et al. Guideline for Prevention of Surgical Site Infection, 1999. Centers for Disease Control and Prevention (CDC) Hospital Infection Control Practices Advisory Committee. Am J Infect Control 1999;27:97–132.

Surgical Preparation

Preoperative preparation of the operative site and the sterility of the surgical team are very important in reducing the risk of postoperative infection. Hand scrubbing remains the most important proactive mechanism to reduce infection by reducing the number of microorganisms present on the skin during the operation. In the USA, the conventional method for scrubbing consists of a five-minute first scrub followed by subsequent two- or three-minute scrubs for subsequent cases with either 5% povidone-iodine or 4% chlorhexidine gluconate. These scrubbing protocols can achieve a 95% decrease in skin flora.[26,27] Newer alcohol-based antiseptic cleaners with shorter applications, usually 30 seconds, have been shown to be as effective as or even more effective than hand washing in decreasing bacterial contamination.[28–30] In addition, these solutions increase compliance and are less drying to the surgeon's skin.

Normothermia has also been suggested as a means to decrease the incidence of wound infections. Infants and children are at particular risk for experiencing hypothermia during surgery due to an increased area-to-body weight ratio leading to greater heat loss.[31] Intraoperative hypothermia can potentially lead to serious complications, including coagulopathy, SSIs, and cardiac complications. A prospective randomized trial of 200 adult patients undergoing colorectal surgery showed that intraoperative hypothermia caused delayed wound healing and a greater incidence of infections.[32] A number of techniques are available to warm infants and children during surgery, including warming intravenous fluids or using forced-air warming systems. In addition, supplemental oxygen given during the perioperative period in adults has been shown to decrease the rate of wound infection by as much as 40–50%.[33,34] Finally, adequate control of glucose levels perioperatively has also been demonstrated to decrease morbidity and mortality in both adult and pediatric surgical patients, particularly in those patients undergoing cardiac surgery.[35,36]

Antibiotic Prophylaxis

Operative procedures can be classified into one of four types, as outlined in Table 9-1. In adults, several well-designed prospective trials have documented a decreased incidence of infection for all types of operative procedures with established antibiotic recommendations.[37] Important points for preoperative antibiotic prophylaxis include using agents that cover the most probable intraoperative contaminants for the operation, optimal timing for the initial dose of antibiotic so that bactericidal concentrations are reached at the time of incision, and maintaining the contribution levels throughout the operation.[38] Timing of the perioperative antibiotic coverage is crucial. The first dose is generally given 30 minutes to one hour before the start of the operation. In operations that take more than the half-life of the administered drug, a second dose of prophylactic antibiotics is indicated to re-achieve adequate serum levels.[39]

Prophylaxis accounts for nearly 75% of antibiotic use on pediatric surgical services. As such, prophylaxis is the major cause of the inappropriate use of antimicrobials in children. In one study of children younger than 6 years of age undergoing surgical procedures, prophylactic antibiotics were administered inappropriately to 42% of children receiving preoperative antibiotics.[40] A more recent study demonstrated that 82% of patients received prophylactic antibiotics when indicated and that 40% of patients received antibiotics when there was no indication.[41] In pediatric surgery, it is clear that antibiotic coverage is required during clean-contaminated, contaminated, or dirty cases. Antibiotic prophylaxis in a clean case in the pediatric population is now at the discretion of the operating surgeon.

Bowel Preparation

The efficacy of bowel preparation before an elective colon operation is well documented.[42,43] Bowel preparation includes mechanical irrigation and flushing of the colon to remove stool, oral antibiotics against colonic aerobes and anaerobes, and preoperative intravenous antibiotics that cover both common skin and colonic flora.[44] The preparation can be started on an outpatient basis the day before the operation, and the parenteral drugs are added to the regimen just before the procedure. Recently, there has been debate in the adult literature regarding the necessity of mechanical bowel preparation. In infants and children, protocols for bowel preparation have largely been extrapolated from the adult colorectal literature. It appears that the majority of pediatric surgeons use bowel preparations for elective colorectal surgery.[45] Recently, others have proposed that omitting mechanical bowel preparation carries no increased risk of infectious or anastomotic complications.[46] If bowel preparation is used in the pediatric population, care must be taken to avoid dehydration.

TYPES OF INFECTION

Postoperative Surgical Site Infection

Despite meticulous technique and perioperative antibiotics, infectious complications still occur. Postoperative wound infections can be divided into superficial or deep.[47] Early diagnosis and prompt intervention help to avoid morbidity and occasional mortality. Erythema, fever, leukocytosis, tenderness, crepitus, and suppuration are diagnostic signs but are not always present. When confronted with one or more of these signs, clinical judgment is important. Treatment may include oral or intravenous antibiotics, simple incision and drainage, or extensive surgical debridement.

An abscess is a localized collection of pus in a cavity formed by an expanding infectious process (Fig. 9-1A) Pus is a combination of leukocytes, necrotic material, bacteria, and extracellular fluid. The usual cause is the staphylococcal species in combination with one or more organisms. The treatment is incision and drainage (Fig. 9-1B), followed by antibiotic therapy if associated with

TABLE 9-1	**Wound Classification**
Class	**Definition**
Clean	An uninfected operative wound in which no inflammation is encountered and the respiratory, alimentary, genital, or infected urinary tract is not entered. In addition, clean wounds are closed primarily and, if necessary, drained with closed drainage
Clean–contaminated	An operative wound in which the respiratory, alimentary, genital, or urinary tract is entered under controlled conditions and without unusual contamination
Contaminated	Open, fresh, accidental wounds. This includes operations with major breaks in sterile technique or gross spillage from the gastrointestinal tract and incisions in which acute, nonpurulent inflammation is encountered
Dirty	Old traumatic wounds with retained devitalized tissue and those that involve existing clinical infection or perforated viscera

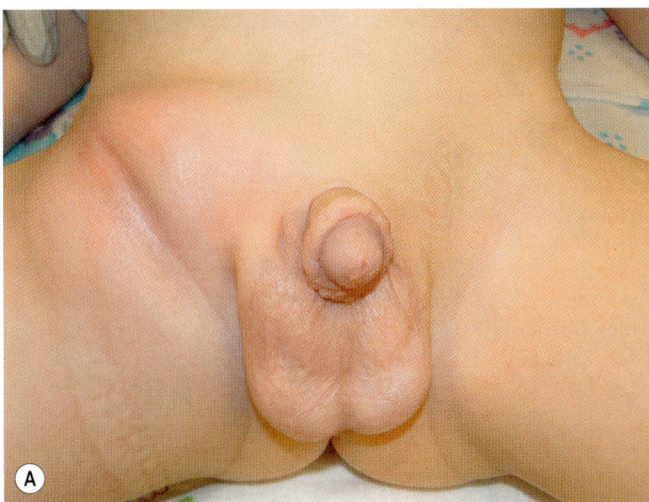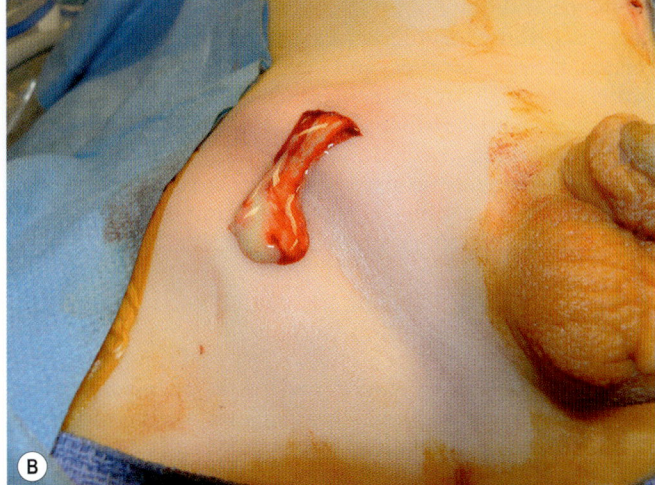

FIGURE 9-1 ■ (A) This young boy developed a large expanding right inguino-femoral abscess. (B) The abscess has been drained and the purulent fluid is seen draining from the abscess.

localized cellulitis or an immunocompromised patient. Drainage must be complete, or the abscess will reform. A phlegmon is an area of diffuse inflammation with little pus and some necrotic tissue. A phlegmon can often be treated with antibiotics, although it can progress to an abscess.

Streptococcal soft tissue infections are probably the most virulent and can arise within a few hours after surgical procedures. High fever, delirium, leukocytosis, and severe pain are hallmarks of the patient's presentation. *Bacillus* infections are the next most virulent infections. Inspection of the wound will show dark, mottled areas, as opposed to the bright pink of a streptococcal cellulitis. Less than half of the patients with *Bacillus* infections have detectable gas crepitation. Severe pain is the most telling clinical symptom of this type of infection. High doses of penicillin and operative debridement of necrotic tissue are the hallmarks of treatment for these patients.

Nosocomial Infection

Nosocomial infections are defined as those infections that are hospital acquired.[48] As such, they are a potential threat to all hospitalized patients and increase morbidity and mortality significantly. Their incidence appears to be increasing as surgical care becomes more advanced and patients survive longer. Recent focus on patient safety has made prevention of nosocomial infections increasingly important. One report describing 676 operative procedures in 608 pediatric patients showed a nosocomial infection rate of 6.2%.[48] The infectious complications included septicemia, pulmonary, urinary tract, abdominal, and diarrhea. The highest overall occurrence of infection was in the infant group. The most common isolates were *Staphylococcus epidermidis* from septic patients and gram-negative enteric bacteria from organ and wound infections. Infection was associated with impaired nutrition, multiple disease processes, and multiple operations. In addition, ECMO use has been shown to correlate with an increased incidence of nosocomial infection as does length of the preoperative stay and exposure to invasive medical devices.[49–51]

Pneumonia can be a lethal nosocomial infection, with mortality ranging from 20–70% and accounting for 10–15% of all pediatric hospital-acquired infections.[52] The mortality rate is dependent on the causative organism. The risk factors for nosocomial pneumonia in the pediatric population include serious underlying illness, immunosuppression, and length of time on a ventilator.[53] Measures to prevent ventilator-associated pneumonia in children include elevating the head of the bed, daily assessment of readiness for extubation, and age-appropriate mouth care.[54]

Clostridium difficile is a well-recognized cause of infectious diarrhea that develops after antibiotic therapy in many patients, although it likely only accounts for 20% of antibiotic-associated diarrhea. It is a very common cause of nosocomial infection, and its incidence is increasing in frequency with associated increasing mortality.[55,56] The best method of prevention is the judicious and appropriate use of antibiotics.

To decrease nosocomial infections in hospitals, the Centers for Medicare and Medicaid Services (CMS) released a proposal in 2008 to expand the list of hospital-acquired conditions that will not be reimbursed by Medicare. These have been termed 'Never Events' and include SSIs after specific elective surgeries, extreme glycemic aberrancies, ventilator-associated pneumonia, and *C. difficile*-associated diseases, among others. Under this proposal, CMS will not reimburse hospitals for treatment (medical or surgical treatment) of these nosocomial entities.

Catheter Infections

Central venous catheters (CVCs) are essential for managing critically ill patients. The use of CVCs in infants and children has increased as prolonged vascular access has become increasingly necessary to provide parenteral nutrition, chemotherapy, antimicrobial therapy, and hemodynamic monitoring. However, catheter-related infections are common, despite considerable effort to reduce their occurrence, and are associated with increased hospital costs and length of stay. Infection is manifested as erythema at the site of insertion, tachycardia, and/or leukocytosis. Rates of infection are influenced by patient-related factors, by type and severity of illness, and by catheter-related parameters (catheter type, purpose, and conditions under which it was placed).[57] Coagulase-negative staphylococci, followed by enterococci, were the most frequently isolated causes of hospital-acquired bloodstream infections in a report from the National Nosocomial Infections Surveillance System.[58] A number of factors are associated with the development of catheter-related infections, including the sterility of the insertion technique, type of solution being administered through the line, care of the catheter once inserted, proximity of the catheter to another wound, and the presence of another infection elsewhere. Updated guidelines for the prevention of intravascular catheter-related infections were published in 2011.[59] For catheters that will remain for a long time, tunneling the catheter has been shown to significantly reduce the risk of catheter-related infection.[60,61]

Absolute sterile techniques should be maintained in all instances of line insertion whenever possible. Emergency situations may necessitate less-than-sterile technique. The use of maximal sterile barriers, including sterile gown and gloves and a large sterile sheet, has been shown in adults to greatly reduce the risk of catheter-related infection.[62] Studies suggest that chlorhexidine significantly reduces the incidence of microbial colonization compared with povidone-iodine, and 0.5% chlorhexidine preparations with alcohol is now recommend for skin antisepsis.[63] The safety and efficacy of chlorhexidine is unknown in infants < 2 months.

The skin and catheter hub are the most common sources of colonization and infection. Thus, various methods have been used to combat these risks. Silver ions have broad antimicrobial activity, and the use of silver-impregnated cuffs have been tried as a preventive measure.[64,65] In addition, antimicrobial and antiseptic catheters and cuffs may decrease the incidence of catheter-related infections.[66,67] Catheters have been coated with chlorhexidine/silver sulfadiazine as well as minocycline/rifampin along with other agents. The use of these coated catheters has been approved by the ultrasound Food and Drug Administration for use in patients weighing more than 3 kg. It is likely that the efficacy for reducing infection decreases after being in place for longer than three weeks because of a decrease in the antimicrobial activity.[67] These impregnated catheters and sponge dressings can be used if the infection rate is not decreasing with other measures. Of note, no studies in adults have demonstrated a benefit for systemic antibiotic prophylaxis after insertion of a CVC. Studies in high-risk neonates and children have demonstrated conflicting results. However, concern exists for the emergence of resistance with the routine use of antimicrobial prophylaxis.[68,69]

Other Infections Requiring Surgical Care and Treatment

Although the infections discussed previously are possibly preventable and occur after operations or hospitalization, some infections are seen by the pediatric surgeon for the first time.

Necrotizing Soft Tissue Infection

Necrotizing fasciitis is a rapidly progressing infection of the fascial tissues and overlying skin. Although it can occur as a postoperative complication or as a primary infection, necrotizing fasciitis is more likely in immunocompromised patients.[70] However, in the pediatric population, necrotizing fasciitis often affects previously healthy children and infants.[71] Because the diagnosis is often not obvious, the clinician must look for clinical clues such as edema beyond the area of erythema, crepitus, skin vesicles, or cellulitis refractory to intravenous antibiotics. Skin necrosis is generally a late sign and is indicative of thrombosis of vessels in the subcutaneous tissue. Necrotizing fasciitis often occurs in the truncal region in children as opposed to adults where infection in the extremities is most common (Figs 9-2 and 9-3).[72] Although infections with a single organism often occur in adults with necrotizing fasciitis, polymicrobial infections predominate in children.[73] Prompt surgical intervention, including wide excision of all necrotic and infected tissue, along with the institution of antibiotics including penicillin, is mandatory to avoid progression and mortality. Necrotizing fasciitis can also occur as a complication of chickenpox.[74] In neonates, necrotizing fasciitis can occur as a secondary infection of omphalitis, balanitis, and fetal monitoring.[75]

Sepsis

Sepsis, by contemporary definition, defines the systemic derangements that are caused by the infectious organisms and their byproducts as opposed to those derangements that are caused by the host-systemic inflammatory response. In 1992, the Society of Critical Care Medicine published the results of a consensus conference to define accurately the terms regarding sepsis and the inflammatory response to injury and infection.[76] These definitions were updated in the 2001 Consensus Conference.[77] Although there has been a significant decrease in the mortality rate among children with sepsis, severe sepsis remains one of the leading causes of death in the pediatric population. In 2002, a group of experts gathered to focus specifically on pediatric sepsis.[78] Systemic inflammatory response syndrome (SIRS) has previously been defined in adults as the nonspecific inflammatory process after a variety of insults with sepsis specifically occurring from infection.[79] The main pediatric modifications include the inclusion of temperature or leukocyte abnormalities in addition to tachycardia and tachypnea because these last two indices are common in many pediatric disease processes. Another difference is that hypotension is not necessary for the diagnosis of septic shock, but cardiovascular dysfunction must be present. SIRS may progress to multi-organ dysfunction and death. Gram-negative organisms possess a lipopolysaccharide moiety on the cell wall that has been shown to incite most, if not all, of the toxic effects of end-organ failure.

Neonatal sepsis is defined as a generalized bacterial infection accompanied by a positive blood culture within the first month of life.[80] Neonatal sepsis occurring during the first week of life is caused primarily by maternal

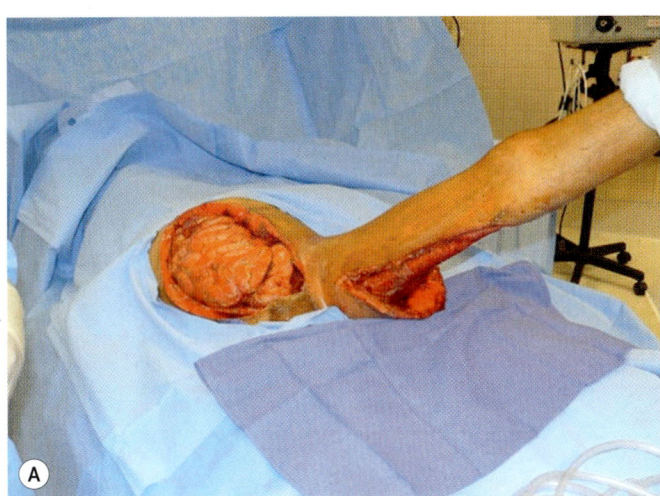 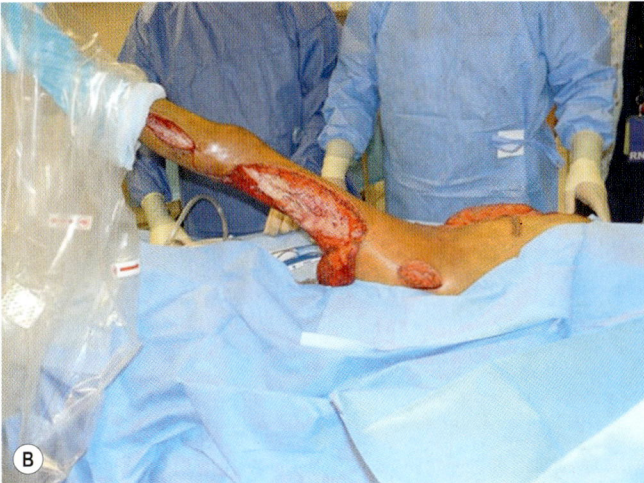

FIGURE 9-2 ■ This 15-year-old was ill for two weeks with perforated appendicitis and presented in shock. After a midline incision for exploration for a rigid abdomen, his appendix was removed. The peritoneal cavity was extensively and copiously irrigated and the abdominal incision was left open. He returned to the operating room two days later for evaluation and was found to have necrotizing fasciitis of the rectus abdominis muscles bilaterally. Eventually, despite aggressive surgical debridement, this process spread to the retroperitoneum and down the left inguinal canal through a patent processus vaginalis. One week postoperatively, he was found to have edema and erythema of the left leg that prompted exploration. The necrotizing fasciitis had progressed down all compartments of the left thigh and the lateral compartment of the left lower leg. In the upper thigh, the semimembranosus and semitendinosus muscles had to be excised due to necrotic musculature. These photographs were taken on his ninth postoperative day. **(A)** The abdomen is seen to be open and the medial aspect of the left thigh is visualized. **(B)** The incisions in the left buttock area, the left lateral thigh, and the left lateral lower leg are seen.

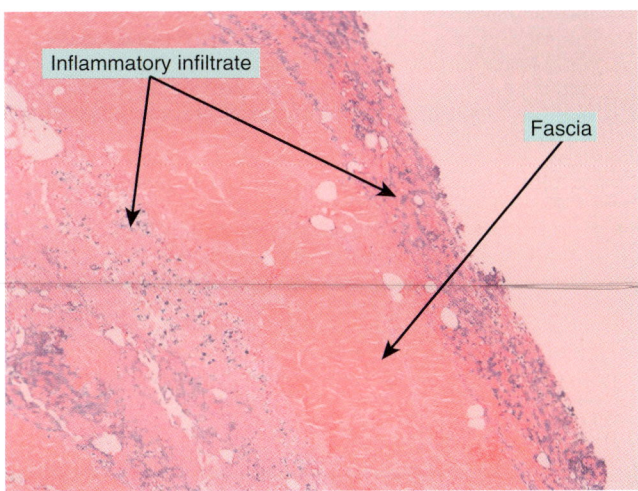

FIGURE 9-3 ■ This photomicrograph depicts the histologic findings of necrotizing fasciitis in the patient shown in Figure 9-2. Note the inflammatory infiltrate on both sides of the fascia. The fascial cultures grew *Escherichia coli.*

organisms transferred during delivery. Maternal contamination can be transmitted through the placenta to the newborn via the birth canal or by direct contamination of the amniotic fluid. The mortality of this early onset sepsis approaches 50%. Late-onset neonatal sepsis is primarily nosocomial and is most often secondary to indwelling catheters or bacterial translocation from the gut. In the surgical neonate, three factors promote bacterial translocation and sepsis: (1) intestinal bacterial colonization and overgrowth; (2) compromised host defenses; and (3) disruption of the mucosal epithelial barrier.[81] The mortality of late-onset sepsis approaches 20%. The clinician must be alert for the subtle signs and symptoms of neonatal sepsis, which include lethargy, irritability, temperature instability, and a change in respiratory or feeding pattern. Neonates may not demonstrate leukocytosis. Empirical triple antibiotic coverage may be started, pending the results of blood and other cultures.

Peritonitis

Peritonitis is defined as inflammation of the peritoneum.[82] It is divided into primary, secondary, and tertiary. Spontaneous primary peritonitis is a bacterial infection without enteric perforation. Primary peritonitis is usually caused by a single organism. An infant with primary peritonitis usually does not exhibit signs of peritonitis but may have poor feeding, lethargy, distention, vomiting, and mild to severe abdominal tenderness. Definitive treatment may require only a course of broad-spectrum antibiotics. Secondary peritonitis is associated with gastrointestinal tract disruption. This can be caused directly by intestinal perforation, bowel wall necrosis, trauma, or postoperatively as a result of iatrogenic injury or an anastomotic leak. In addition, secondary peritonitis also may result from an indwelling dialysis catheter or ventriculoperitoneal shunt.[83] These infections are generally polymicrobial. Treatment of secondary peritonitis is a combination of operative intervention, removal of any prosthetic device, and antibiotics. Tertiary peritonitis, also called recurrent peritonitis, is characterized by organ dysfunction and systemic inflammation in association with recurrent infection. The mortality rate is very high, and management is difficult.[84] Treatment consists of broad-spectrum antibiotics because the infection often includes nosocomial organisms and multidrug-resistant bacteria.

REFERENCES

1. Brueggemann AB. Antibiotic resistance mechanisms among pediatric respiratory and enteric pathogens: A current update. Pediatr Infect Dis J 2006;25:969–73.
2. Liu HH. Antibiotics and infectious diseases. Prim Care 1990;17:745–74.
3. Kosloske AM. Surgical infections in children. Curr Opin Pediatr 1994;6:353–9.
4. DeLa Cadena RA, Majluf-Cruz A, Stadnicki A, et al. Activation of the contact and fibrinolytic systems after intravenous administration of endotoxin to normal human volunteers: Correlation with the cytokine profile. Immunopharmacol 1996;33:231–7.
5. Robson MC, Stenberg BD, Heggers JP. Wound healing alterations caused by infection. Clinics in plastic surgery 1990;17:485–92.
6. Baxter CR. Immunologic reactions in chronic wounds. Am J Surg 1994;167:12S–14S.
7. Bowler PG. Wound pathophysiology, infection and therapeutic options. Ann Med 2002;34:419–27.
8. Harris BH, Gelfand JA. The immune response to trauma. Semin Pediatr Surg 1995;4:77–82.
9. Forslind B, Lindberg M, Roomans GM, et al. Aspects on the physiology of human skin: Studies using particle probe analysis. Microscopy research and technique 1997;38:373–86.
10. Godet AS, Williams RD. Postoperative clostridium difficile gastroenteritis. J Urol 1993;149:142–4.
11. Newburg DS, Walker WA. Protection of the neonate by the innate immune system of developing gut and of human milk. Pediatr Res 2007;61:2–8.
12. Newburg DS. Neonatal protection by an innate immune system of human milk consisting of oligosaccharides and glycans. J Anim Sci 2009;87:26–34.
13. Fleisher TA. Back to basics: Primary immune deficiencies: Windows into the immune system. Pediatr Rev 2006;27:363–72.
14. Fleisher TA, Bleesing JJ. Immune function. Pediatr Clin North Am 2000;47:1197–2109.
15. Hilfiker ML, Azizkhan RG. Mycotic infections in pediatric surgical patients. Semin Pediatr Surg 1995;4:239–44.
16. Menne EN, Sonabend RY, Mason EO, et al. Staphylococcus aureus infections in pediatric patients with diabetes mellitus. J Infect 2012;65:135–41.
17. Scrimshaw NS. Historical concepts of interactions, synergism and antagonism between nutrition and infection. J Nutr 2003;133:316S–21S.
18. Puck JM. Primary immunodeficiency diseases. JAMA 1997;278:1835–41.
19. Berescher E. Infectious complications of dysfunction or deficiency of polymorphonuclear and mononuclear phagocytes. 2nd ed. In: Long S, Pickering LK, Prober CG, editors. Principles and Practice of Pediatric Infectious Diseases. New York: Churchill Livingstone; 2003.
20. Musoke RN. Rational use of antibiotics in neonatal infections. East Afr Med J 1997;74:147–50.
21. Hall P, Kaye CM, McIntosh N, et al. Intravenous metronidazole in the newborn. Arch Dis Child 1983;58:529–31.
22. Routledge PA. Pharmacokinetics in children. J Antimicrob Chemother 1994;34(Suppl. A):19–24.
23. Buck ML. Pharmacokinetic changes during extracorporeal membrane oxygenation: Implications for drug therapy of neonates. Clin Pharmacokinet 2003;42:403–17.
24. Horwitz JR, Chwals WJ, Doski JJ, et al. Pediatric wound infections: A prospective multicenter study. Ann Surg 1998;227:553–8.
25. Bhattacharyya N, Kosloske AM. Postoperative wound infection in pediatric surgical patients: A study of 676 infants and children. J Pediatr Surg 1990;25:125–9.
26. Pereira LJ, Lee GM, Wade KJ. The effect of surgical handwashing routines on the microbial counts of operating room nurses. Am J Infect Control 1990;18:354–64.
27. Wheelock SM, Lookinland S. Effect of surgical hand scrub time on subsequent bacterial growth. AORN J 1997;65:1087–94.
28. Tanner J, Swarbrook S, Stuart J. Surgical hand antisepsis to reduce surgical site infection. Cochrane Database Syst Rev 2008:CD004288.
29. Parienti JJ, Thibon P, Heller R, et al. Hand-rubbing with an aqueous alcoholic solution vs traditional surgical hand-scrubbing and 30-day surgical site infection rates: A randomized equivalence study. JAMA 2002;288:722–7.
30. Girou E, Loyeau S, Legrand P, et al. Efficacy of handrubbing with alcohol based solution versus standard handwashing with antiseptic soap: Randomised clinical trial. BMJ 2002;325:360–2.
31. Serour F, Weissenberg M, Boaz M, et al. Intravenous fluids warming by mattress is simple and efficient during pediatric surgery. Acta Anaesthesiol Scand 2002;46:80–4.
32. Kurz A, Sessler DI, Lenhardt R. Perioperative normothermia to reduce the incidence of surgical-wound infection and shorten hospitalization. Study of wound infection and temperature group. N Engl J Med 1996;334:1209–15.
33. Greif R, Akça O, Horn EP, et al. Supplemental perioperative oxygen to reduce the incidence of surgical-wound infection. Outcomes Research Group. N Engl J Med 2000;342:161–7.
34. Belda FJ, Aguilera L, García de la Asunción J, et al. Supplemental perioperative oxygen and the risk of surgical wound infection: A randomized controlled trial. JAMA 2005;294:2035–42.
35. Krinsley J. Perioperative glucose control. Curr Opin Anaesthesiol 2006;19:111–16.
36. Yates AR, Dyke PC, Taeed R, et al. Hyperglycemia is a marker for poor outcome in the postoperative pediatric cardiac patient. Pediatr Crit Care Med 2006;7:351–5.
37. Nichols RL. Surgical antibiotic prophylaxis. Med Clin North Am 1995;79:509–22.
38. Mangram AJ, Horan TC, Pearson ML, et al. Guideline for Prevention of Surgical Site Infection, 1999. Centers for Disease Control and Prevention (CDC) Hospital Infection Control Practices Advisory Committee. Am J Infect Control 1999;27:97–132; quiz 3.
39. Nichols RL. Preventing surgical site infections. Clin Med Res 2004;2:115–18.
40. Kesler RW, Guhlow LJ, Saulsbury FT. Prophylactic antibiotics in pediatric surgery. Pediatrics 1982;69:1–3.
41. Rangel SJ, Fung M, Graham DA, et al. Recent trends in the use of antibiotic prophylaxis in pediatric surgery. J Pediatr Surg 2011;46:366–71.
42. Bartlett JG, Condon RE, Gorbach SL, et al. Veterans Administration cooperative study on bowel preparation for elective colorectal operations: Impact of oral antibiotic regimen on colonic flora, wound irrigation cultures and bacteriology of septic complications. Ann Surg 1978;188:249–54.
43. Debo Adeyemi S, Tai da Rocha-Afodu J. Clinical studies of 4 methods of bowel preparation in colorectal surgery. Eur Surg Res 1986;18:331–6.
44. Le TH, Timmcke AE, Gathright JB, et al. Outpatient bowel preparation for elective colon resection. South Med J 1997;90:526–30.
45. Breckler FD, Fuchs JR, Rescorla FJ. Survey of pediatric surgeons on current practices of bowel preparation for elective colorectal surgery in children. Am J Surg 2007;193:315–18.
46. Leys CM, Austin MT, Pietsch JB, et al. Elective intestinal operations in infants and children without mechanical bowel preparation: A pilot study. J Pediatr Surg 2005;40:978–82.
47. Upperman JS, Sheridan RL, Marshall J. Pediatric surgical site and soft tissue infections. Pediatr Crit Care Med 2005;6:S36–41.
48. Allen U, Ford-Jones EL. Nosocomial infections in the pediatric patient: An update. Am J Infect Control 1990;18:176–93.
49. Coffin SE, Bell LM, Manning M, et al. Nosocomial infections in neonates receiving extracorporeal membrane oxygenation. Infect Control Hosp Epidemiol 1997;18:93–6.
50. Bizzarro MJ, Conrad SA, Kaufman DA, et al. Infections acquired during extracorporeal membrane oxygenation in neonates, children, and adults. Pediatr Crit Care Med 2011;12:277–81.
51. Yogaraj JS, Elward AM, Fraser VJ. Rate, risk factors, and outcomes of nosocomial primary bloodstream infection in pediatric intensive care unit patients. Pediatrics 2002;110:481–5.
52. Stein F, Trevino R. Nosocomial infections in the pediatric intensive care unit. Pediatr Clin North Am 1994;41:1245–57.
53. Jarvis WR. The epidemiology of colonization. Infect Control Hosp Epidemiol 1996;17:47–52.
54. Sandora TJ. Prevention of healthcare-associated infections in children: New strategies and success stories. Curr Opin Infect Dis 2010;23:300–5.
55. Benson L, Song X, Campos J, et al. Changing epidemiology of Clostridium difficile-associated disease in children. Infect Control Hosp Epidemiol 2007;28:1233–5.

56. Nylund CM, Goudie A, Garza JM, et al. Clostridium difficile infection in hospitalized children in the United States. Arch Pediatr Adoles Med 2011;165:451–7.

57. O'Grady NP, Alexander M, Dellinger EP, et al. Guidelines for the prevention of intravascular catheter-related infections. The Hospital Infection Control Practices Advisory Committee, Center for Disease Control and Prevention. Pediatrics 2002;110: e51.

58. System ArftN. National Nosocomial Infections Surveillance (NNIS) System Report, data summary from January 1992 through June 2004, issued October 2004. Am J Infect Control 2004; 32:470–85.

59. O'Grady NP, Alexander M, Burns LA, et al. Summary of recommendations: Guidelines for the Prevention of Intravascular Catheter-related Infections. Clin Infect Dis 2011;52:1087–99.

60. Randolph AG, Cook DJ, Gonzales CA, et al. Tunneling short-term central venous catheters to prevent catheter-related infection: A meta-analysis of randomized, controlled trials. Crit Care Med 1998;26:1452–7.

61. Timsit JF, Sebille V, Farkas JC, et al. Effect of subcutaneous tunneling on internal jugular catheter-related sepsis in critically ill patients: A prospective randomized multicenter study. JAMA 1996;276:1416–20.

62. Raad II, Hohn DC, Gilbreath BJ, et al. Prevention of central venous catheter-related infections by using maximal sterile barrier precautions during insertion. Infect Control Hosp Epidemiol 1994;15:231–8.

63. Maki DG, Ringer M, Alvarado CJ. Prospective randomised trial of povidone-iodine, alcohol, and chlorhexidine for prevention of infection associated with central venous and arterial catheters. The Lancet 1991;338:339–43.

64. Dahlberg PJ, Agger WA, Singer JR, et al. Subclavian hemodialysis catheter infections: A prospective, randomized trial of an attachable silver-impregnated cuff for prevention of catheter-related infections. Infect Control Hosp Epidemiol 1995;16:506–11.

65. Groeger JS, Lucas AB, Coit D, et al. A prospective, randomized evaluation of the effect of silver impregnated subcutaneous cuffs for preventing tunneled chronic venous access catheter infections in cancer patients. Ann Surg 1993;218:206–10.

66. Raad I, Darouiche R, Dupuis J, et al. Central venous catheters coated with minocycline and rifampin for the prevention of catheter-related colonization and bloodstream infections. A randomized, double-blind trial. The Texas Medical Center Catheter Study Group. Ann Intern Med 1997;127:267–74.

67. Veenstra DL, Saint S, Saha S, et al. Efficacy of antiseptic-impregnated central venous catheters in preventing catheter-related bloodstream infection: A meta-analysis. JAMA 1999;281: 261–7.

68. Kacica MA, Horgan MJ, Ochoa L, et al. Prevention of gram-positive sepsis in neonates weighing less than 1500 grams. J Pediatr 1994;125:253–8.

69. Spafford PS, Sinkin RA, Cox C, et al. Prevention of central venous catheter-related coagulase-negative staphylococcal sepsis in neonates. J Pediatr 1994;125:259–63.

70. Farrell LD, Karl SR, Davis PK, et al. Postoperative necrotizing fasciitis in children. Pediatrics 1988;82:874–9.

71. Bingol-Kologlu M, Yildiz RV, Alper B, et al. Necrotizing fasciitis in children: Diagnostic and therapeutic aspects. J Pediatr Surg 2007;42:1892–7.

72. Murphy JJ, Granger R, Blair GK, et al. Necrotizing fasciitis in childhood. J Pediatr Surg 1995;30:1131–4.

73. Moss RL, Musemeche CA, Kosloske AM. Necrotizing fasciitis in children: Prompt recognition and aggressive therapy improve survival. J Pediatr Surg 1996;31:1142–6.

74. Waldhausen JH, Holterman MJ, Sawin RS. Surgical implications of necrotizing fasciitis in children with chickenpox. J Pediatr Surg 1996;31:1138–41.

75. Hsieh W-S, Yang P-H, Chao H-C, et al. Neonatal necrotizing fasciitis: A report of three cases and review of the literature. Pediatrics 1999;103:e53.

76. American College of Chest Physicians/Society of Critical Care Medicine Consensus Conference. Definitions for sepsis and organ failure and guidelines for the use of innovative therapies in sepsis. Crit Care Med 1992;20:864–74.

77. Levy MM, Fink MP, Marshall JC, et al. 2001 SCCM/ESICM/ACCP/ATS/SIS International Sepsis Definitions Conference. Intensive Care Med 2003;29:530–8.

78. Goldstein B, Giroir B, Randolph A. International pediatric sepsis consensus conference: Definitions for sepsis and organ dysfunction in pediatrics. Pediatr Crit Care Med 2005;6:2–8.

79. Bone RC, Sprung CL, Sibbald WJ. Definitions for sepsis and organ failure. Crit Care Med 1992;20:724–6.

80. Wolach B. Neonatal sepsis: Pathogenesis and supportive therapy. Semin Perinatol 1997;21:28–38.

81. Jackson RJ, Smith SD, Wadowsky RM, et al. The effect of E coli virulence on bacterial translocation and systemic sepsis in the neonatal rabbit model. J Pediatr Surg 1991;26:483–5.

82. Heemken R, Gandawidjaja L, Hau T. Peritonitis: Pathophysiology and local defense mechanisms. Hepato-gastroenterology 1997; 44:927–36.

83. Levy M, Balfe JW, Geary D, et al. Exit-site infection during continuous and cycling peritoneal dialysis in children. Perit Dial Int 1990;10:31–5.

84. Nathens AB, Rotstein OD, Marshall JC. Tertiary peritonitis: Clinical features of a complex nosocomial infection. World J Surg 1998;22:158–63.

CHAPTER 10

FETAL THERAPY

Corey W. Iqbal • Shinjiro Hirose • Hanmin Lee

A heightened awareness of fetal anomalies coupled with advances in imaging techniques have allowed clinicians to make early and accurate diagnoses of fetal anomalies. These advances in prenatal diagnosis have led to the identification of measurable parameters that now allow the clinician to prognosticate and counsel families on the likely outcomes for several prenatally diagnosed anomalies. In cases that carry a grim prognosis, the question is often asked: is in utero fetal intervention feasible and will it positively impact the outcome?

Most prenatally diagnosed anomalies are best treated expectantly, with definitive therapy performed after birth. If a condition poses a threat to the fetus (or mother) and the fetus has reached a viable gestational age, then early delivery can be performed. However, when a condition progresses to a life-threatening stage at a nonviable gestational age, then the only options become expectant management with a high likelihood of intrauterine fetal demise (IUFD) or fetal intervention, which does not carry the guarantee of a positive outcome and puts the mother at risk.

The first open fetal surgical procedure was performed at the University of California, San Francisco (UCSF) in 1982.[1] Since then, more than 515 fetal interventions have been performed at UCSF over the past 30 years without maternal mortality. Over the past 30 years, a number of advances have been developed to allow a broader application of fetal intervention. These techniques, including maternal hysterotomy, minimal-access fetoscopy, and percutaneous fetal access, were initially tested and validated in animal models. More recently, in utero therapy has shown to be beneficial for non-life-threatening conditions such as myelomeningocele (MMC). In this chapter, we will present an overview of the current state of fetal surgery and will review specific fetal problems outlining current management strategies.

GENERAL PRINCIPLES

Fetal intervention is complicated, not only by the risk to the unborn patient, but by the risk to the mother as well. Fetal intervention does not impart a health benefit to the mother, yet she is at a significant risk for morbidity and potential mortality with any fetal surgical intervention. In this light, fetal surgery should be considered only when there is a clear benefit to the fetus. To date, there have been no reported maternal deaths from fetal surgery, although significant short- and long-term maternal morbidity is possible.

The primary morbidity following fetal surgery has been, and remains, preterm labor resulting in premature delivery, usually between 25 and 35 gestational weeks. Preventing preterm labor after fetal intervention remains problematic. Complications can also arise from endotracheal intubation, general anesthesia, epidural and spinal anesthesia, blood transfusion, premature rupture of membranes, chorioamniotic separation, chorioamnionitis, and placental abruption. Long-term morbidity from the hysterotomy includes infertility, uterine rupture with the current and future pregnancies, and mandatory cesarean section with future pregnancies. Notably, in reviewing our experience, subsequent fertility following fetal intervention has been good.[2]

A crucial component contributing to the success of a fetal treatment program is a multidisciplinary approach. In addition, specific subspecialists are involved for certain cases, such as the pediatric neurosurgeon for fetal MMC repair. Multidisciplinary meetings not only cover the medical and surgical aspects of the patient's care, but also include the ethical and social considerations specific to each case. Finally, at UCSF, a special institutional fetal treatment oversight committee reviews all fetal interventions on a monthly basis. This group serves as a quality control mechanism as well as an ethical review board.

FETAL ACCESS

There are three general methods for accessing the fetus: percutaneous, fetoscopy, and open hysterotomy. In all three approaches, preoperative and intraoperative ultrasound (US) is crucial for defining the anomaly or anomalies, delineating the placental anatomy, determining the position of the fetus, detecting the location of the maternal blood vessels, and monitoring the fetal heart rate during the procedure. With percutaneous and fetoscopic procedures, ultrasound is particularly important due to the lack of visualization of the fetus, placenta, and uterus during the procedure.

The mother is positioned supine with her left side down to minimize compression of the inferior vena cava by the gravid uterus. Maternal anesthesia can be either spinal or general, depending on the nature and duration of the intervention. In addition, fetal anesthesia is needed when operating on the fetus. An intramuscular injection of an opiate and a non-depolarizing neuromuscular blocking agent are usually utilized.

Ultrasound-guided percutaneous procedures are performed through small skin incisions on the mother's abdominal wall. During these operations, real-time ultrasound is needed to visualize the fetal and maternal anatomy.[3] Catheters and shunts can be inserted into the fetus to drain cystic masses, ascites, or pleural fluid into the amniotic space. In addition, radio frequency ablation (RFA) probes can be deployed into the amniotic space to treat various twin gestational anomalies. The needles used to place these catheters, as well as the RFA device, are approximately 1.5–2 mm in diameter, minimizing morbidity to the mother and irritation of the uterus.[4,5]

Fetoscopic procedures are generally performed using a 3 mm fetoscope and instruments. Occasionally, standard 5 mm laparoscopic telescopes and instruments are used. For many fetoscopic procedures, a 3 mm fetoscope with a 1 mm working channel is sufficient. It is important to identify a 'window' in the uterus that is devoid of the placenta to reduce the risk of maternal bleeding, placental abruption, and fetal morbidity. Occasionally, the amniotic fluid is not clear enough for good visualization with the small endoscopes. In such cases, we perform amnio-exchange, using warmed crystalloid solutions to provide a clear operative view.

Open fetal procedures require general anesthesia with a combination of preoperative indomethacin and high mean alveolar concentration of inhalational agents to maintain uterine relaxation.[6–8] An epidural is also inserted for postoperative analgesia.

A low, transverse maternal incision is usually used with a vertical or transverse fascial incision, depending on the exposure needed. Preoperative and intraoperative ultrasound are crucial to map out the placenta and avoid iatrogenic injury. Uterine staplers with absorbable staples have been developed specifically for fetal surgery and allow a hemostatic hysterotomy with minimal blood loss. Absorbable staples prevent infertility as nonabsorbable materials can act as an intrauterine device and prevent future pregnancies. The uterus is stabilized within the maternal abdomen. Care is taken to minimize tension on the uterine blood vessels, which would decrease placental flow. Also, fetal exposure is limited to the specific body part in question. Most of the fetus is left inside the uterus, and great care is taken not to handle or stretch the umbilical cord as this can cause fetal ischemia from injury or vasospasm. Amniotic fluid volume is maintained using warmed, isotonic crystalloid solution. After the fetal procedure is completed, the fetus is returned to the uterus, the amniotic fluid is completely restored, and the uterus is closed in multiple layers using absorbable sutures. Postoperatively, the mother and fetus are monitored continuously for uterine contractions and heart rate, respectively. Often, the uterus is irritable and contractions require control with tocolytic agents.

Open fetal surgery requires cesarean section for future pregnancies due to the potential for uterine rupture with subsequent births. While vaginal delivery after cesarean section (VBAC) can be considered for routine, lower uterine segment hysterotomy, VBAC is not an option after hysterotomy for fetal surgery.

As previously mentioned, complications can occur after any fetal intervention. Bleeding can originate from the fetus, the placenta, the uterine wall, or the maternal abdominal wall despite identifying the uterine vessels with ultrasound and specifically avoiding them to prevent injury and minimize bleeding. Premature rupture of membranes and preterm labor remain a common problem complicating fetal surgery. These problems are often the result of inadequate membrane closure, chorioamnionitis, chorioamniotic separation, and uterine contractions.

ANOMALIES AMENABLE TO FETAL SURGERY

Congenital Diaphragmatic Hernia

Despite significant advances in neonatal respiratory support, survival for children born with congenital diaphragmatic hernia (CDH) remains only 60–70% throughout the USA. Additionally, survival for prenatally diagnosed CDH may be as low as 25% due to IUFD and stillborns that are not included in conventional postnatal survival data.[9–11] This high mortality rate has made CDH a primary area of interest for the development of effective prenatal intervention. In fact, improving outcomes specifically for CDH was a significant driving force in the genesis of fetal surgery at UCSF.

Prognostic Criteria

One of the key elements in developing fetal intervention for CDH has been identifying what factors will identify those fetuses at the greatest risk for a poor outcome. The factors most consistently associated with a poor outcome on prenatal ultrasound are (1) the presence of liver herniation into the chest; and (2) a low lung-to-head ratio (LHR). In our experience, survival has been 100% in fetuses with CDH that do not have liver herniation on prenatal ultrasound and 56% in fetuses with CDH and liver herniation into the chest.[12] The LHR is calculated as the area of the contralateral lung at the level of the cardiac atria divided by the head circumference. This LHR value has been shown to statistically correlate with survival: 100% survival with an LHR greater than 1.35, 61% survival with an LHR between 0.6 and 1.35, and 0% survival with an LHR less than 0.6.[12]

While the LHR has been a reliable predictor of outcomes at our center, other institutions have suggested the LHR does not account for discrepant growth rates between the head and lung during gestation and therefore may not be reliable at certain gestational ages.[13,14] To account for this, the observed to expected LHR (OE LHR) has been proposed. The OE LHR is represented as a percentage of what the expected LHR would be in a normal fetus of the same gestational age. For left-sided defects, an OE LHR <25% is associated with an 18% survival whereas an OE LHR >45% correlates with 89% survival.[13,15]

Magnetic resonance imaging (MRI) for volumetric measurement of the lungs is a promising modality for prognosis with CDH.[16] MRI can be used to calculate the percent-predicted lung volume (PPLV). Results for PPLV have varied. In one study, a PPLV >20% was associated with 100% survival whereas survival was only 40% when PPLV was <15%.[17] In another study, a PPLV <25% was associated with a 13% survival and a PPLV >35% correlated with 83% survival.[18] MRI can also be used to determine the percentage of liver herniation, although the prognostic value of this finding is still being investigated.[18]

Fetal Interventions

CDH and its effect on fetal lung development has been studied in animal models.[19,20] In the fetal lamb model, compression of the lungs, either with an intrathoracic balloon or by creation of a diaphragmatic hernia, results in uniformly fatal pulmonary hypoplasia. However, in utero correction of the compressing lesion leads to sufficient lung growth and development, which improves postnatal survival.[20]

This concept of early, in utero correction of CDH has been studied and applied in humans.[21,22] Fetal surgery for CDH initially involved open repair of the diaphragmatic defect. The first successful case was reported in 1990 which demonstrated the feasibility of open fetal repair using a two-step approach which involved creation of an abdominal silo to accommodate the reduced viscera and prevent compression of the umbilical vessels.[23] This initial success was followed by a prospective trial at UCSF comparing open fetal surgery to postnatal repair in severe cases of prenatally diagnosed CDH. However, in this study, there was no difference in survival or in the need for extracorporeal membranous oxygenation (ECMO) between fetal repair and postnatal repair.[22,24] Concordant with this effort, investigators at UCSF observed that fetuses with congenital high airway obstruction syndrome (CHAOS) had pulmonary hyperplasia.[25] Also, fetal tracheal occlusion had been shown to cause pulmonary hyperplasia.[26] In this condition, the lung parenchyma creates fluid that is 'exhaled' by the fetus. Occluding the trachea causes a build-up of this fluid and subsequent pulmonary hyperplasia.[27,28] The inability to improve outcomes with open fetal repair for severe cases of CDH led to an interest in this physiologic process.[29]

The first eight patients were treated with open hysterotomy and tracheal occlusion with a metallic clip.[30] This approach proved to be problematic for several reasons. First, the open hysterotomy led to significant prematurity due to premature labor. Second, the use of clips was associated with tracheal stenosis and also required a stringent delivery plan—which was later described as the ex utero intrapartum treatment (EXIT) procedure—whereby the fetus was exposed through a hysterotomy and maintained on utero–placental circulation while the clip was removed and a patent airway established prior to delivering the baby.[31] However, outcomes with this approach were poor with only a 15% survival rate.[30]

Ongoing advancements in fetal surgery led to fetoscopic balloon placement for tracheal occlusion (Fig. 10-1). This technique has the advantages of being less invasive, a lower risk of tracheal stenosis, and the balloon being much easier to remove, although still necessitating an EXIT procedure. Results in the first eight cases were favorable with a 75% survival rate compared to a 38% survival rate in historical, case-matched controls managed with postnatal repair.[32]

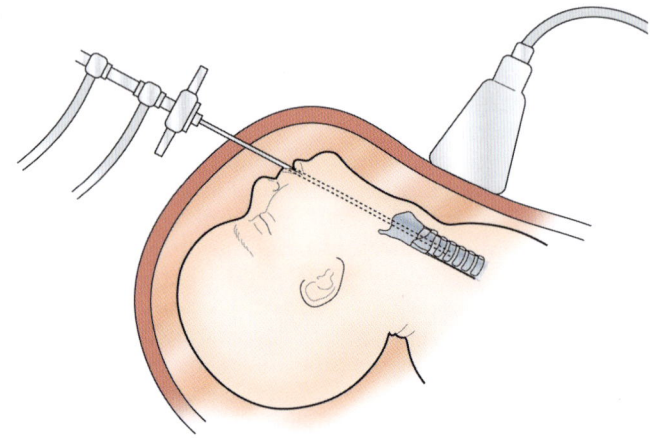

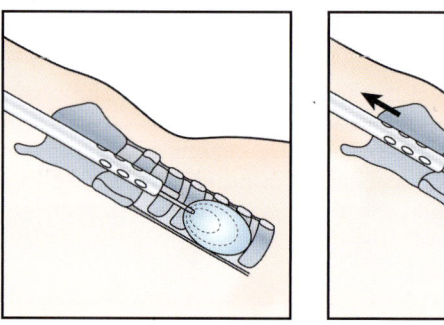

FIGURE 10-1 ■ This schematic diagram shows the method of fetoscopic tracheal occlusion. A fetoscope is placed into the fetal mouth, the airway is identified, and a balloon is inserted into the trachea by using both fetoscopic and ultrasonographic visualization.

These early results led to an National Institutes of Health (NIH) funded, prospective randomized trial comparing in utero fetoscopic tracheal occlusion to standard postnatal care for fetuses diagnosed with severe left-sided CDH (liver up and LHR <1.4) and no other detectable anomalies. However, results of the trial showed no difference in survival between the tracheal occlusion group and the standard postnatal care group (73% vs 77%, respectively).[33] Unexpectedly, the survival in the postnatal repair group was considerably greater when compared to historical controls. Although this study did not demonstrate a difference in survival between the prenatal intervention group and the postnatal group, the results of this trial demonstrate the tremendous importance of proper randomized controlled trials for novel fetal surgical procedures.

Further data regarding fetal tracheal occlusion have suggested that temporary, short-term reversible tracheal occlusion may be preferable to a longer duration of occlusion. Animal models of fetal tracheal occlusion have demonstrated that long-term tracheal occlusion can be deleterious to type II pneumocytes (the cells that secrete surfactant) and that this adverse effect is not seen with a shorter duration of tracheal occlusion.[34] To test the hypothesis that temporary fetal tracheal occlusion is better, Deprest et al. studied patients undergoing fetal tracheal balloon occlusion who also had the balloon removed prenatally to limit the duration of occlusion.[35] In this group of patients, improved lung growth was evident on fetal MRI and was also associated with improved postnatal survival. While reversal of the tracheal occlusion requires a second maternal and fetal intervention for balloon removal, it obviates the need for an EXIT procedure at birth. Early results have been favorable.[31,36]

These promising findings with temporary tracheal occlusion have led to its current application in Europe. The European FETO consortium has reported a 48% survival rate among 210 cases of severe CDH treated with temporary fetal tracheal occlusion, and the Eurofetus group is currently sponsoring a prospective fetal tracheal occlusion trial that seeks to determine the ideal time and duration for tracheal occlusion.[37] Our group at UCSF is currently offering reversible, fetal tracheal balloon occlusion for fetuses with liver herniation in the chest and an LHR of <1.0, as these babies continue to have a very high mortality.[38] This study has Food and Drug Administration oversight, and involves percutaneous placement of a fetoscopic tracheal balloon between 26 and 28 weeks gestation, with removal of the balloon via a second percutaneous fetoscopic procedure between 32 and 34 weeks.

Neoplasms

Fortunately, fetal neoplasms are rare. When they do occur, most are benign. However, if they become large enough, they can impede venous return to the heart or cause high-output heart failure via arteriovenous shunting. Such shunting can lead to non-immune fetal hydropic changes such as polyhydramnios, placentomegaly, skin and scalp edema, and pleural, pericardial, and peritoneal fluid accumulation. When only one compartment is involved, this is considered early fetal hydrops; when two or more compartments are affected, then true hydrops is present. If left untreated, hydrops is nearly always fatal.[39-40] The two most common prenatally diagnosed neoplasms that cause nonimmune fetal hydrops are congenital pulmonary airway malformations (CPAM) and sacrococcygeal teratomas (SCT).

Congenital Pulmonary Airway Malformations

CPAMs are pulmonary lesions with a broad range of clinical presentations. This new terminology includes congenital cystic adenomatoid malformations (CCAM) and bronchopulmonary sequestrations. CCAMs are much more likely than sequestrations to cause nonimmune fetal hydrops. CCAMs are characterized by an overgrowth of respiratory bronchioles with the formation of cysts of various sizes.[41-44] Most fetuses diagnosed with a CCAM develop normally, and can be followed with serial ultrasound studies. These asymptomatic patients then undergo standard, postnatal resection. A small percentage of patients with the prenatal diagnosis of CCAM will develop non-immune hydrops.[43,44]

Various measurements have been developed to predict which fetuses are at risk for developing hydrops. The most accepted measurement is the CCAM volume ratio (CVR), defined as the product of the three longest measurements of the lesion on ultrasound multiplied by the constant 0.52, and then divided by the head circumference. Crombleholme and colleagues identified a CVR of 1.6 as a cut-off for an increased likelihood of developing hydrops.[45] When the CVR is <1.6, there is only a 2% risk of developing hydrops. When the CVR is >1.6, there is an 80% chance of developing hydrops.

CCAMs that are predominantly microcystic have a more predictable course than the macrocystic ones. Microcystic or solid CCAMs undergo steady growth that tends to plateau at 26 to 28 weeks gestation. At this point, fetal growth exceeds that of the CCAM. For this reason, patients with microcystic or solid CCAMs should be followed closely up to 26 to 28 weeks gestation at which point the interval between ultrasound examinations can be lengthened if the pregnancy has been otherwise uncomplicated. In contrast, macrocystic CCAMs undergo abrupt enlargement due to rapid fluid accumulation in a dominant cyst. Therefore, macrocystic CCAMs require close follow-up with serial ultrasound throughout the duration of the pregnancy.[42,46]

If a fetus develops hydrops at a viable gestational age, early delivery should be considered. Hydropic fetuses who are not yet viable outside the uterus, and have a dominant macrocystic lesion, are appropriate candidates for a thoracoamniotic shunt.[47] Needle drainage alone has not been found to be an effective therapy as rapid re-accumulation of fluid in the cyst necessitates repeat intervention. In the largest single-center experience with thoracoamniotic shunts, shunting led to a mean 51% volume reduction in the size of the lesion and a 70% survival rate.[48] Other institutions have reported similar survival rates.[49] Despite shunting, these babies can still have significant respiratory distress at birth and should be delivered at a tertiary referral center.

Open fetal thoracotomy and CCAM resection is an option in the pre-viable fetus with a microcystic or solid lesion. This is performed through an open hysterotomy. A thoracotomy is made through the fifth intercostal space, and the lobe containing the CCAM is identified and exteriorized through the incision (Fig. 10-2). The pulmonary hilar structures are then mass ligated using an endoloop or endoscopic stapler. The thoracotomy is then closed in layers.[50-51]

In a group of 120 patients with the prenatal diagnosis of CPAM from UCSF and Children's Hospital of Philadelphia (CHOP), 79 had no evidence of hydrops.[51] Of these, 76 were followed expectantly and all survived. Three fetuses without evidence of hydrops and with large dominant cysts underwent thoracoamniotic shunting. All three fetuses survived. Twenty-five hydropic fetuses were followed with no intervention. All mothers delivered prematurely and all fetuses died perinatally. Sixteen fetuses with hydrops underwent intervention: 13 underwent open fetal surgery while three underwent thoracoamniotic shunting. Two of the three survived in the group that underwent shunt insertion and eight of 13 survived in the open fetal surgery group.

Despite positive results with open fetal resection in the hydropic fetus, there has been a shift away from this therapy in the last five years due to the efficacy of

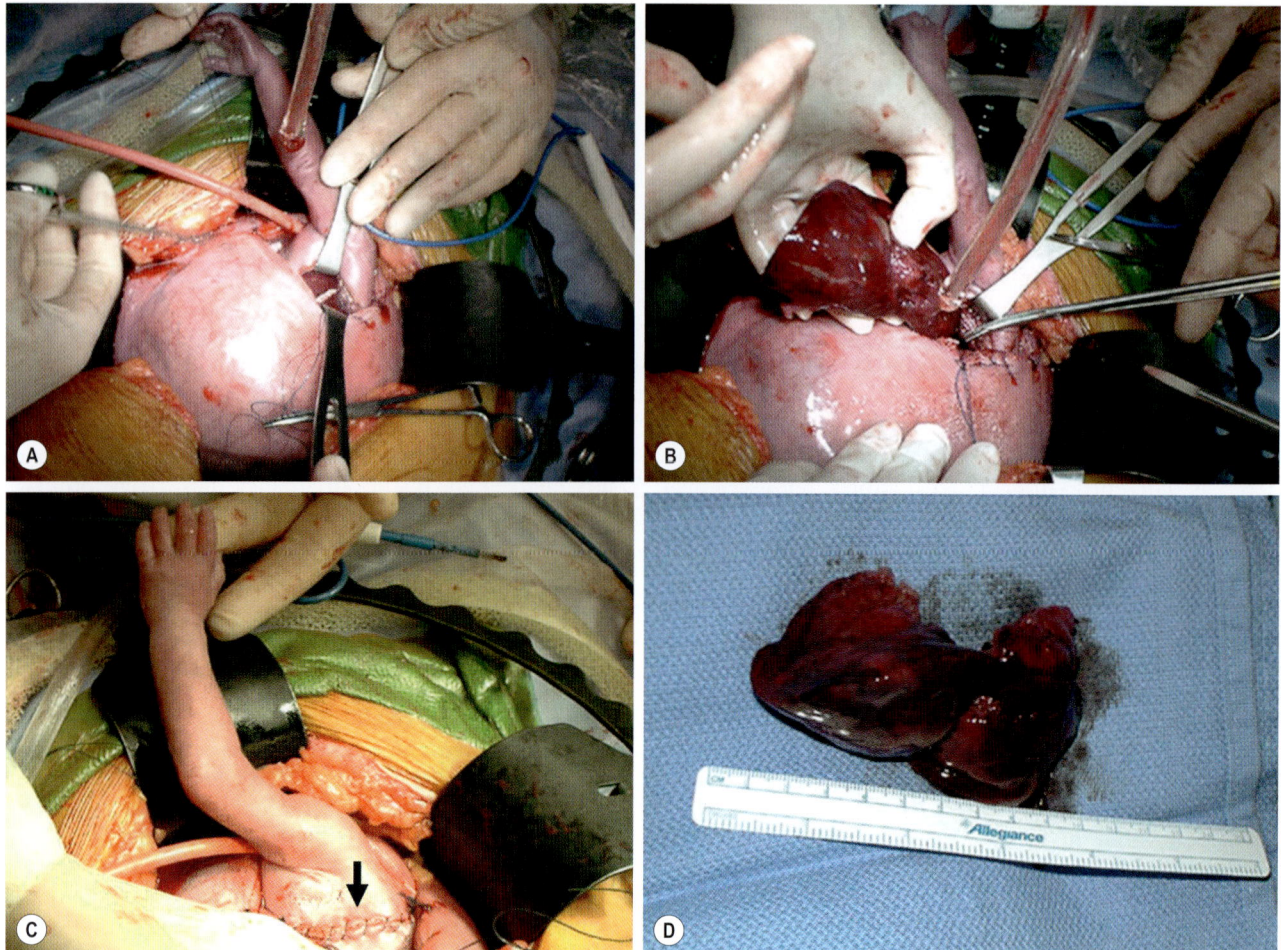

FIGURE 10-2 ■ These photographs depict an infant with a large left upper lobe CCAM undergoing in utero left lobectomy. **(A)** The infant's left arm is visualized. Note the maternal hysterotomy and the left fetal thoracotomy (with retractors inserted) through the fifth intercostal space. **(B)** The left upper lobe containing the CCAM has been identified and exteriorized through the thoracotomy incision. The pulmonary hilar structures were mass ligated using an endoloop. **(C)** The fetal thoracotomy incision (arrow) has been closed. **(D)** The left upper lobe specimen containing the CCAM is seen.

maternal steroids. This finding was discovered serendipitously at UCSF during the preparation of several hydropic fetuses for open fetal surgery.[52] In these cases, maternal steroids were administered to enhance fetal lung maturity. Preoperative ultrasound studies showed resolution of the hydrops and those fetuses survived to delivery and beyond. Thirteen patients with microcystic CCAMs, nine of which were complicated by hydrops, had an overall survival rate of 85% with resolution of hydrops in seven of nine fetuses.[53] CHOP has reported a series of 11 patients, five of which had hydrops, and all survived after receiving steroids.[54]

Currently, we recommend maternal betamethasone for fetuses with nonimmune hydrops or a CVR >1.6. Steroids can be re-dosed, but repeated administration of maternal steroids beyond three to five courses can result in untoward effects such as reduced birth weight.[55] It is widely accepted that steroids are most effective for predominantly microcystic or solid lesions as this is the component of the malformation that responds to steroids. Macrocystic lesions are less likely to respond.

Sacrococcygeal Teratoma

SCT is another rare tumor that is being diagnosed prenatally with increasing frequency, allowing for observation of the natural history of the disease and appropriate perinatal management. As with CCAM, fetuses with SCT are susceptible to IUFD. SCTs can grow to a tremendous size in relation to the fetus and can cause high-output cardiac failure and nonimmune hydrops through vascular shunting. Rarely, tumors can hemorrhage internally or externally, resulting in fetal anemia, hypovolemia, and IUFD. Other potential problems for a fetus with a large SCT are dystocia and preterm labor. Delivery can be particularly difficult when the diagnosis has not been made prenatally. A traumatic delivery can result in tumor rupture and/or hemorrhage. Most clinicians favor cesarean delivery for fetuses with large SCTs. Thus, prenatal diagnosis and careful obstetrical planning are critical in the management of these fetuses.

Recent evidence has identified the tumor volume to fetal weight ratio (TFR) as an important prognostic indicator.[56] Tumor volume is calculated using the greatest length, width, and height of the tumor as measured by ultrasound or MRI; fetal weight can be calculated by ultrasound as well. In the initial report of ten fetuses with SCT, a TFR >0.12 was associated with an 80% incidence of hydrops and a 60% mortality, whereas a TFR <0.12 was associated with 100% survival.[56] UCSF has recently presented our experience in 37 fetuses with SCT and confirmed that a TFR <0.12 was a favorable prognostic finding up to 24 weeks. Between 24–32 weeks, a TFR of <0.11 was associated with better outcomes. In addition, we also found that cystic SCTs had a more favorable prognosis than solid ones.[57]

The fetus with SCT has a high risk for mortality, especially when associated with non-immune fetal hydrops. The group at CHOP has published their experience with 30 fetuses with SCT.[58] There were 14 survivors and four pregnancies were terminated. Fifteen fetuses had solid tumors. Of those, four developed signs of hydrops and underwent fetal debulking operations. Three of the four survived. In the UCSF experience with 65 prenatally diagnosed SCTs, the overall survival was 44%.[57,59] Nineteen of these pregnancies were complicated by fetal hydrops of which eight underwent a fetal intervention and had a 38% survival. In the 11 patients with hydrops who did not undergo fetal intervention, there was only one survivor. Overall, 15 patients with SCT have undergone fetal intervention at UCSF (excluding patients who had cyst aspiration to facilitate delivery): six underwent open resection, five underwent RFA, one underwent alcohol ablation, one had therapeutic cyst aspiration to relieve urinary tract obstruction, one had RFA followed by EXIT-to-resection, and one had EXIT-to-resection alone. Overall survival was 33%. Although ten patients survived to delivery, the mean gestational age was 28.1 weeks and there was a 50% neonatal mortality rate.[57]

The most common approach for fetal SCT resection is a maternal hysterotomy with resection or debulking of the tumor (Fig. 10-3). A predominantly cystic lesion may be amenable to percutaneous drainage or placement of a shunt which may not be necessary given the favorable prognosis for cystic SCTs. However, immediate decompression of an SCT may be needed just prior to delivery to prevent dystocia or to facilitate cesarean delivery. Tumor debulking using percutaneous coagulation techniques, such as with RFA or laser coagulation, to decrease the vascular shunt are minimally invasive alternatives to open resection that may warrant further investigation.[40,60]

Abnormalities of Twin Gestations

Twin–Twin Transfusion Syndrome

Twin–twin transfusion syndrome (TTTS) is the most common complication of monochorionic twin pregnancies.[61] In such twin pregnancies, the two fetuses share a single placenta with normal vascular connections (arterial-to-venous, venous-to-arterial, and arterial–arterial) between the fetuses. TTTS occurs when these connections lead to unbalanced blood flow from one twin

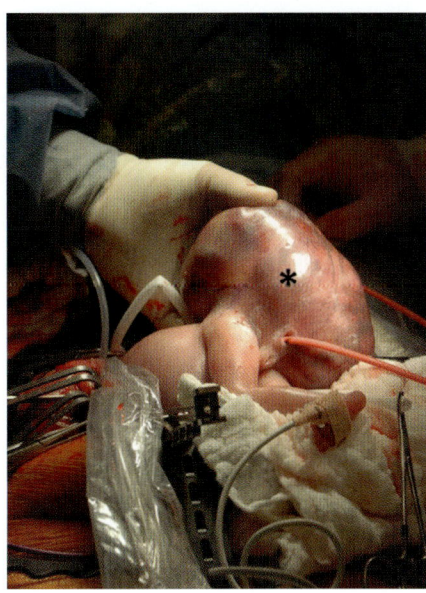

FIGURE 10-3 ■ The sacrococcygeal teratoma (asterisk) was exposed after maternal laparotomy and excised in standard fashion.

to the other. As a result of the transfusion of blood from the donor twin to the recipient twin through this unbalanced flow, hemodynamic compromise can occur in either or both twins. The donor twin suffers from a low flow state manifesting initially as oligohydramnios and possibly resulting in high-output cardiac failure or ischemia to the brain and kidneys. Conversely, the recipient twin has fluid overload (polyhydramnios), and may develop congestive heart failure and hydrops. The hallmark of TTTS is oligohydramnios in the donor twin and polyhydramnios in the recipient twin, both of which must be present to make the diagnosis. Often there is size discordance between the twins with the donor being smaller than the recipient.

Quintero described four stages of TTTS (Table 10-1).[62] Advanced stages of the disease are evidenced by progressive discordance in fluid volumes with the donor becoming 'stuck' in its amniotic sac due to a lack of amniotic fluid. This is followed by worsening cardiac changes in the recipient twin and hydrops. If left untreated, TTTS carries an 80–90% mortality rate for both twins. In addition, in monochorionic twins, if one twin dies, the other is at risk for neurologic injury due to a sump phenomenon in the placenta which leads to temporary hypotension and ischemia in the surviving twin.[63–65]

Clinicians have attempted a variety of treatments aimed at achieving improved outcome in one or both twins. Historically, high-volume amnioreduction in the polydramniotic sac has been the primary therapy. Because polyhydramnios can incite labor, the initial aim of amnioreduction is to reduce uterine volume to decrease the risk of preterm labor. In the International Amnioreduction Registry, high-volume amnioreduction resulted in a survival rate in at least one twin of almost 60%.[66]

Several groups have introduced fetoscopic guidance to laser ablate the intertwin vascular connections. This approach has largely replaced amnioreduction. This can

TABLE 10-1 **Four Stages of Twin–Twin Transfusion Syndrome**

Stage	Description
Stage I	Polyhydramnios (DVP > 8 cm) with oligohydramnios (DVP < 2 cm) with bladders present in both twins
Stage II	Bladder not visible in the donor twin
Stage III	Changes in umbilical cord or ductus venosus end-diastolic flow; tricuspid regurgitation in the recipient twin
Stage IV	Evidence of hydrops in either twin
Stage V	Fetal death

DVP, deepest vertical pocket.

be done either nonselectively by ablating all intertwin connections, or selectively by ablating only the arteriovenous connections with flow in the causative direction. Fetoscopic laser ablation is performed percutaneously using a 3 mm fetoscope with a side channel for irrigation and insertion of a laser. Two large prospective trials have compared amnioreduction to laser ablation of intertwin vessels. A European trial enrolled 70 women in the amnioreduction arm and 72 women in the laser ablation arm. The trial was stopped early after interim analysis showed a clear survival advantage for laser therapy: 76% vs 51% single survivor and 36% vs 26% for dual survivors.[67] A North American trial was also stopped early after randomizing 42 mothers (20 in the amnioreduction arm and 22 in the laser ablation cohort) because of reluctance among referring physicians to send patients to participating centers for randomization due to a strong bias for laser ablation.[68] There was no survival benefit to either intervention in this study which was under-powered due to the early termination of the trial. A Cochrane review and meta-analysis also favored laser ablation for TTTS with an overall survival of 66% for laser ablation compared to 48% for amnioreduction.[69] When laser ablation is not available or not possible for technical reasons, amnioreduction is an appropriate alternative.

Whether or not every case of TTTS requires intervention is controversial. At UCSF, favorable outcomes with expectant management for stage I TTTS have been found, and laser ablation is only offered in those cases with stage II or more advanced TTTS. In fact, we have identified that the presence of an arterial-arterial anastomosis is protective (by serving as a pop-off valve). Of 639 placentas evaluated at our center, only 5% of those with an arterial-arterial anastomosis had true TTTS.[70]

Twin Reversed Arterial Perfusion

Twin reversed arterial perfusion sequence (TRAP) is a rare disease of monochorionic twins that occurs when one normal twin acts as a 'pump' for an acardiac, acephalic twin. This occurs because of early formation of arterial-arterial anastomoses that results in flow from the umbilical arteries of the 'pump' twin into the umbilical arteries of the acardiac twin. Since the umbilical arteries connect with the iliac arteries, the acephalic, acardiac twin's upper body does not develop, but the lower extremities develop well.

The normal twin is put at risk for high-output heart failure and hydrops as it has to maintain blood flow throughout the entire placenta as well as to the acardiac twin. The vascular flow in the acardiac twin is characteristically reversed. The natural history of TRAP is greater than a 50% mortality in the pump twin due to hydrops.[71,72] The risk of hydrops increases as the mass of the acardiac twin increases relative to the normal twin. Generally, intervention is needed when there is evidence of hydrops in the pump twin, or when the estimated fetal weight of the acardiac twin is 50% or more relative to the twin functioning as the pump.

Multiple approaches have been used to separate the vascular connections in TRAP pregnancies: open hysterotomy and delivery, fetoscopic ligation, bipolar cautery, harmonic scalpel division, thermal coagulation, and laser coagulation. At UCSF, RFA is used to coagulate the umbilical cord insertion site on the acardiac twin's abdomen.[73–75] RFA was originally designed for ablation of solid tumors, but its small size and effective coagulation has been ideal for this application.[76] The most recent UCSF review identified 29 patients who underwent RFA between 18 and 24 weeks gestation.[5] Survival was 92% percent overall.

Other Complications of Monochorionic Twins

Nearly 50% of all monochorionic twin gestations will be complicated. Although TTTS is the most common complication, it only occurs in 10% of all monochorionic twin pregnancies. Thus, the clinician should be aware of other complications that can be confused with TTTS.

Unequal placental sharing occurs because there is no predetermined organization for each umbilical cord insertion to ensure that each twin has an equal share of the placenta. When one of the twins has an eccentric cord insertion, their growth can be adversely affected when their demand exceeds what their share of the placenta can provide. This results in intrauterine growth restriction (IUGR) and eventual growth discordance between the twins (defined as discordant weights >20%). In fact, the growth-restricted twin can develop oligohydramnios raising the suspicion for TTTS, but the distinction is that the normal twin will have normal amniotic fluid volume. The growth-restricted twin can become distressed leading to preterm labor and extreme prematurity which can also adversely affect the normal twin. The other scenario is IUFD. When this occurs, there is transient shunting with hypotension in the normal twin that can lead to permanent neurologic injury in 20–40% of cases. These pregnancies require close monitoring to ensure there is no evidence of TTTS and that growth is appropriate. Selective RFA of the growth-restricted twin has been offered to protect the normal twin. At UCSF, survival of the normal twin has been 87% without any reported adverse neurologic outcomes.[70]

The corollary to unequal sharing is polyhydramnios affecting a recipient-like twin (PART). In this condition, one of the twins has polyhydramnios which can raise a concern for TTTS. However, the other twin does not have oligohydramnios and therefore does not meet criteria for TTTS.[70] Similarly, pregnancies affected by PART require close surveillance. Currently, there is no fetal intervention recommended for PART, but underlying causes for the polyhydramnios should be sought and treated as needed.

Myelomeningocele

MMC, or spina bifida, is characterized by an open neural tube and exposed spinal canal elements. MMC can occur anywhere along the spine, but most commonly occurs in the lumbar or cervical vertebral levels. Complications include neurologic deficits with motor and somatosensory abnormalities which correspond to the level of the spinal defect. In addition, autonomic function is commonly affected with an inability to control bladder or bowel function. Also, nearly all patients with MMC develop the Arnold–Chiari II malformation of the hindbrain and most will require ventriculoperitoneal (VP) shunting for hydrocephalus. Unlike patients that have historically been considered for fetal intervention, fetuses with MMC are generally born alive and healthy. However, the attendant morbidity from the neurologic abnormalities is severe. Up to 30% of patients die before reaching adulthood due to respiratory, urinary, or central nervous system complications. Standard current therapy for MMC is postnatal repair of the spinal defect followed by extensive rehabilitation.[77]

The rationale for fetal intervention in MMC is the 'two-hit' hypothesis, where the first hit is the original neural tube defect that results in an open spinal canal. The second hit is postulated to be trauma to the exposed neural elements while the fetus is in utero.[78,79] It is this second hit that may be ameliorated by fetal intervention and early closure.[80] The results of animal and preliminary human studies showed improved neurologic outcomes and a decreased need for VP shunting with prenatal closure.[79,81–84] These promising findings prompted a multi-institutional prospective randomized trial known as the management of myelomeningocele study (MOMS) that compared open fetal repair with postnatal repair.[85]

Fetal repair in the MOMS trial was performed using an open hysterotomy (Fig. 10-4) with primary repair or the use of skin allografts for large defects as had been previously described.[86–89] The study's power analysis indicated 200 patients were required. However the study was terminated early, after 183 patients, because of the clear advantage to prenatal repair compared to postnatal repair for the primary outcome variable which was need for VP shunting. At 12 months, only 68% of the prenatally repaired group met study criteria for VP shunt placement compared to 98% in the postnatal group. Furthermore, neurologic function favored the prenatal repair group, with 42% walking without assistance at 30 months compared to 21% in the postnatal repair cohort.[85] Not only were these results a milestone in the evolving treatment of MMC, but this was the first nonlethal anomaly for which fetal surgery has been shown to be beneficial.

The benefit of prenatal MMC repair is associated with risks. In the MOMS trial, there was a 38% incidence of preterm labor. Also, the mean gestational age in the prenatal repair group was 34 weeks compared to 37 weeks in the postnatal group. Additionally, 46% had premature rupture of membranes contributing to earlier delivery.

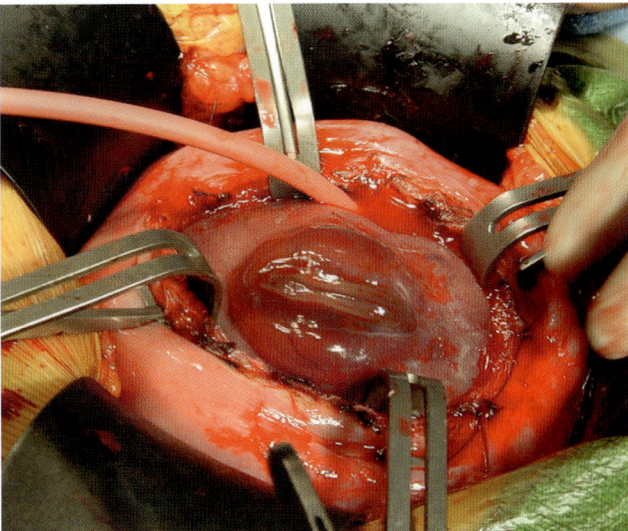

FIGURE 10-4 ■ The myelomeningocele is exposed after maternal hysterectomy. The defect is closed by pediatric neurosurgeons using an operating microscope.

There was a 10% rate of uterine dehiscence, and fetal death occurred in 3% of the prenatal repair group.[85] For these reasons, families require extensive counseling to ensure that they fully understand the risks and benefits. Currently, less invasive methods for the treatment of MMC are being pursued to minimize morbidity. One promising area may be fetoscopic coverage of the defect for temporary protection followed by definitive closure postnatally.[90]

Hydronephrosis and Low Urinary Tract Obstruction

Hydronephrosis is a common prenatal diagnosis. In most cases of minimal hydronephrosis, there will be complete resolution. However, 10% will have progression and require postnatal evaluation.[91] Therefore, in the setting of minimal hydronephrosis, an ultrasound should be obtained in the third trimester to determine if there has been resolution or progression which will help guide the need for postnatal evaluation.

More severe cases of hydronephrosis suggest a ureteropelvic junction (UPJ) obstruction, a ureterovesical junction obstruction, or an obstructing ureterocele. In these scenarios, when unilateral, there is no indication for fetal intervention. Bilateral hydronephrosis is a more significant problem which can be complicated by oligohydramnios which leads to fatal pulmonary hypoplasia. Fortunately, bilateral UPJ obstruction rarely leads to oligohydramnios and the need for fetal intervention with shunting.[92]

Lower urinary tract obstruction (LUTO) can be due to urethral atresia or, most commonly, posterior urethral valves (PUV). The fetus presents with a classic constellation of three ultrasound findings: a dilated, keyhole shaped bladder; bilateral megaureters; and bilateral hydronephrosis.[93] The fetus with LUTO is at high risk for the development of oligohydramnios and subsequent pulmonary hypoplasia that is fatal in the immediate

TABLE 10-2 Normal values for fetal urine electrolytes

Measurement	Normal Values
Osm	<210 mEq/L
Na	<100 mEq/L
Cl	<90 mEq/L
Ca	<2 mmol/L
PO$_4$	<2 mmol/L
β$_2$-microglobulin	<2 mg/L

Valid after 20 weeks gestational age

postnatal period. Additionally, the pressure that results from the obstruction leads to dysplastic changes in the kidney that predisposes the surviving neonate to at least a 20–30% risk of developing end-stage renal disease in their lifetime.[94-96] The chronic distention of the bladder also results in a 45% incidence of neurogenic bladder, although most of these babies have some degree of permanent bladder dysfunction.[96]

Oligohydramnios is an absolute indication for fetal intervention to restore the amniotic fluid volume and prevent pulmonary hypoplasia. Whether fetal intervention prevents renal dysplasia is not entirely known because it is not possible to determine if the oligohydramnios is purely due to the obstruction, or related to oliguria from poorly functioning kidneys (or both). Current fetal interventions are aimed at decompressing the urinary tract and restoring amniotic fluid volume via vesicoamniotic shunting, open fetal vesicostomy, or fetoscopic cystoscopy with ablation of the obstruction.

The timing of intervention in the absence of oligohydramnios is controversial. Imaging and fetal urine electrolyte studies are not definitive in identifying those fetuses at risk for renal dysplasia. Fetal urine electrolytes can be useful when obtained beyond 20 weeks gestation and are easily assessed by a percutaneous aspirate from the dilated fetal bladder.[97] However, the initial tap may be a misrepresentation because the urine has been in the bladder for some time. Thus, serial taps can be more helpful in determining the presence of renal dysplasia, especially if the β$_2$-microblogulin is elevated.[97] Established normal values for fetal urine electrolytes are outlined in Table 10-2.

The challenge in managing LUTO is that our current diagnostic methods detect renal dysplasia after it has already developed. There is not an effective method to identify the fetus at risk for developing dysplasia who will benefit from fetal intervention. While the presence of oligohydramnios seems to be the only definite indication for intervention, this may not be the most effective strategy for preventing renal damage. Whether intervention is undertaken or not, these pregnancies require close monitoring, especially regarding the amniotic fluid volumes. Delivery should occur in a tertiary center.

Abdominal Wall Defects

Abdominal wall defects warrant discussion in a chapter dedicated to fetal surgery because these anomalies are frequently referred to fetal treatment centers. Currently,

there are no fetal interventions for correction of abdominal wall defects that are found in utero.

Gastroschisis is often diagnosed prenatally by ultrasound and usually has an elevated maternal serum α-fetoprotein (which can also be elevated in omphalocele).[98] Attention has been given to the presence of bowel dilation or bowel wall thickening on prenatal ultrasound as an early series of ten patients indicated this represented intestinal injury.[99] However, several subsequent series since have failed to find any correlation between bowel dilation or bowel wall thickening and outcomes.[100-102] Current recommendations are not to deliver early based on the presence of bowel dilation or bowel wall thickening.

Pregnancies complicated by gastroschisis require close monitoring. Nearly three-quarters of fetuses with gastroschisis are affected by IUGR. Preterm labor may be precipitated by polyhydramnios. The risk for IUFD is as high as 10%, particularly in the third trimester.[103] Contrary to popular belief, gastroschisis is not an indication for cesarean section, and vaginal delivery should be offered in the absence of another indication for cesarean delivery.[104]

Similar to MMC, clinicians have theorized that intestinal injury and the intestinal dysmotility associated with gastroschisis may be related to injury while the bowel is exposed to the amniotic fluid. Initial investigations have centered on amnio exchange where the amniotic fluid is replaced with sterile saline.[105] While these investigators reported subjectively favorable findings of less serosal inflammation, the postnatal outcomes were not different. Currently, some investigators have applied the same principle of early coverage to gastroschisis and have proposed fetoscopic closure. This has been attempted in a lamb model, but this approach has not been well studied.[106] Given long-term follow-up data and the quality of life studies that have found that most gastroschisis patients are essentially normal by two years of age, aggressive pursuit of fetal intervention for gastroschisis will probably only benefit those patients who develop short-gut syndrome, either anatomically or functionally.[107] Unfortunately, it has not been possible to identify these patients prenatally.

STEM CELLS AND GENE THERAPY

Gene therapy for prenatally identifiable diseases is being actively pursued for specific disorders. The rationale behind in utero therapy with stem cells and/or virally directed genes includes halting the progression of disease in the fetus during gestation as well as taking advantage of the developing immune system of the fetus, thus potentially negating postnatal problems of tolerance, rejection, and graft versus host disease.[108]

Specific issues for in utero treatment of genetic diseases include the timing of diagnosis and therapy, how to deliver the stem cells or genes, the sources of the stem cells, and the longevity of treatment. With the advent of chorionic villus sampling, genetic diseases can now be identified in the first trimester. Timing of potential treatments is crucial to take advantage of the possible 'pre-immune' status of the fetus, making fetuses potentially more receptive to exogenous genes or cells. Several investigators have utilized hematopoietic stem cells (HSC) as a vector in an attempt to induce chimerism to treat the diseases.[109–111] Others have investigated the use of retroviral vectors to insert genetic material into the fetus.[112,113] This approach reduces the problem of obtaining the large numbers of stem cells needed to create even a modest amount of chimerism. Other approaches include using maternal stem cells or genetic material as studies have demonstrated early cross-trafficking of maternal cells in the fetus.

Diseases that are a candidate for this approach include hematologic, immunologic, metabolic, and neurologic abnormalities (Box 10-1). To date, there have been over 30 reports of in utero therapy utilizing HSCs with limited success. Until recently, the only durable treatment has been in patients with preexisting immunologic defects.[114,115] However a recent study from UCSF applied HSCs in the treatment of four patients with Pelizaeus–Merzbacher disease, a demyelinating leukodystrophy, with promising results in three of the patients who have demonstrated modest improvements in neurologic function as well as durable engraftment.[116]

THE FUTURE

Fetal surgery has progressed from an investigational approach to an accepted mode of therapy for select fetal diseases. Multidisciplinary teams are critical for the success of any fetal program. Some diseases that historically have had a high perinatal mortality rate have shown improved survival with fetal intervention. NIH funded, prospective trials have been performed for CDH, TTTS, and MMC which have helped clearly define the roles of fetal therapy in these cases. Current clinical trials include evaluations for the efficacy of reversible tracheal occlusion for CDH, shunting for LUTO in the absence of oligohydramnios, balloon valvuloplasty for critical aortic valve stenosis, and stem cell therapies. Historically, in order to maximize the benefit to the fetus balanced with minimizing the risk to the mother, fetal interventions have been reserved for fetuses with lethal anomalies. MMC represents the first non-lethal anomaly that has been evaluated. It is not known if the outcomes for other non-lethal anomalies can be improved through fetal intervention.

As minimal-access techniques improve, and the maternal risks are further reduced, indications for fetal intervention will continue to expand. New areas of investigation include tissue engineering, stem cell therapy, and gene therapy. Maternal safety must remain paramount, and the risk to the mother should be minimized at all times.

REFERENCES

1. Harrison MR, Golbus MS, Filly RA, et al. Fetal surgery for congenital hydronephrosis. New Engl J Med 1982;306:591–3.
2. Farrell JA, Albanese CT, Jennings RW, et al. Maternal fertility is not affected by fetal surgery. Fetal Diagn Ther 1999;14:190–2.
3. VanderWall KJ, Meuli M, Szabo Z, et al. Percutaneous access to the uterus for fetal surgery. J Laparoendosc Surg 1996;6:S65–7.
4. Sydorak RM, Feldstein V, Machin G, et al. Fetoscopic treatment for discordant twins. J Pediatr Surg 2002;37:1736–9.
5. Lee H, Wagner AJ, Sy E, et al. Efficacy of radiofrequency ablation for twin-reversed arterial perfusion sequence. Am J Obstet Gynecol 2007;196:459e1–4.
6. De Buck F, Deprest J, Van de Velde M. Anesthesia for fetal surgery. Curr Opin Anaesthesiol 2008;21:293–7.
7. Harrison MR, Anderson J, Rosen MA, et al. Fetal surgery in the primate I. Anesthetic, surgical, and tocolytic management to maximize fetal-neonatal survival. J Pediatr Surg 1982;17:115–22.
8. Rosen MA. Anesthesia for fetal procedures and surgery. Yonsei Med J 2001;42:669–80.
9. Logan JW, Rice HE, Goldberg RN, et al. Congenital diaphragmatic hernia: A systematic review and summary of best-evidence practice strategies. J Perinatol 2007;27:535–49.
10. Moya FR, Lally KP. Evidence-based management of infants with congenital diaphragmatic hernia. Semin Perinatol 2005;29:112–17.
11. Doyle NM, Lally KP. The CDH Study Group and advances in the clinical care of the patient with congenital diaphragmatic hernia. Semin Perinatol 2004;28:174–84.
12. Metkus AP, Filly RA, Stringer MD, et al. Sonographic predictors of survival in fetal diaphragmatic hernia. J Pediatr Surg 1996;31:148–52.
13. Jani J, Nicolaides KH, Keller RL, et al. Observed to expected lung area to head circumference ratio in the prediction of survival in fetuses with isolated diaphragmatic hernia. Ultrasound Obstet Gynecol 2007;30:67–71.
14. Cruz-Martinez R, Castanon M, Moreno-Alvarez O, et al. Usefulness of lung-to-head ratio and intrapulmonary Doppler in predicting neonatal morbidity in fetuses with congenital diaphragmatic hernia treated with fetoscopic tracheal occlusion. Ultrasound Obstet Gynecol 2012;41:59–65.
15. Jani JC, Benachi A, Nicolaides KH, et al. Prenatal prediction of neonatal morbidity in survivors with congenital diaphragmatic hernia: A multicenter study. Ultrasound Obstet Gynecol 2009;33:64–9.
16. Coakley FV, Lopoo JB, Lu Y, et al. Normal and hypoplastic fetal lungs: Volumetric assessment with prenatal single-shot rapid acquisition with relaxation enhancement MR imaging. Radiology 2000;216:107–11.

BOX 10-1 — Diseases for which in Utero Stem Cell or Gene Therapy may be Applicable

HEMATOLOGIC
α-Thalassemia
Fanconi anemia
Chronic granulomatous disease
Hemophilia A

IMMUNOLOGIC
Severe combined immunodeficiency (SCID) syndrome
Wiskott–Aldrich syndrome

METABOLIC
Wolman disease
Type II Gaucher disease
Pompe disease
Osteogenesis imperfecta
Cystic fibrosis

NEUROLOGIC
Lesch–Nyhan syndrome
Tay–Sachs disease
Sandhoff disease
Niemann–Pick disease
Leukodystrophies
Generalized gangliosidosis
Leigh disease

17. Barnewolt CE, Kunisaki SM, Fauza DO, et al. Percent predicted lung volumes as measured on fetal magnetic resonance imaging: A useful biometric parameter for risk stratification. J Pediatr Surg 2007;42:193–7.

18. Victoria T, Bebbington MW, Danzer E, et al. Use of magnetic resonance imaging in prenatal prognosis of the fetus with isolated left congenital diaphragmatic hernia. Prenatal Diagnosis 2012;32:715–23.

19. Adzick NS, Harrison MR, Flake AW. Experimental studies on prenatal treatment of congenital anomalies. Br J Hosp Med 1985;34:154–9.

20. Adzick NS, Outwater KM, Harrison MR, et al. Correction of congenital diaphragmatic hernia in-utero. IV. An early gestational fetal lamb model for pulmonary vascular morphometric analysis. J Pediatr Surg 1985;20:673–80.

21. Adzick NS, Harrison MR, Glick PL, et al. Diaphragmatic hernia in the fetus: Prenatal diagnosis and outcome in 94 cases. J Pediatr Surg 1985;20:357–61.

22. Harrison MR, Adzick NS, Flake AW, et al. Correction of congenital diaphragmatic hernia in-utero. VI. Hard-earned lessons. J Pediatr Surg 1993;28:1411–18.

23. Harrison MR, Adzick NS, Longaker MT, et al. Successful repair in utero of a fetal diaphragmatic hernia after removal of herniated viscera from the left thorax. New Eng J Med 1990;322:1582–4.

24. Harrison MR, Adzick NS, Bullard KM, et al. Correction of congenital diaphragmatic hernia in utero VII: A prospective trial. J Pediatr Surg 1997;32:1637–42.

25. Hedrick MH, Ferro MM, Filly RA, et al. Congenital high airway obstruction syndrome (CHAOS): A potential for perinatal intervention. J Pediatr Surg 1994;29:271–4.

26. Carmel JA, Friedman F, Adams FH, et al. Fetal tracheal ligation and lung development. Am J Dis Child 1965;109:452–7.

27. DiFiore JW, Fauza DO, Slavin R, et al. Experimental fetal tracheal ligation and congenital diaphragmatic hernia: A pulmonary vascular morphometric analysis. J Pediatr Surg 1995;30:917–24.

28. DiFiore JW, Fauza DO, Slavin R, et al. Experimental fetal tracheal ligation reverses the structural and physiological effects of pulmonary hypoplasia in congenital diaphragmatic hernia. J Pediatr Surg 1994;29:248–57.

29. Hedrick MH, Estes JM, Sullivan KM, et al. Plug the lung until it grows (PLUG): A new method to treat congenital diaphragmatic hernia in-utero. J Pediatr Surg 1994;29:612–17.

30. Harrison MR, Adzick NS, Flake AW, et al. Correction of congenital diaphragmatic hernia in utero VIII: Response of the hypoplastic lung to tracheal occlusion. J Pediatr Surg 1996;31:1339–46.

31. Hirose S, Harrison MR. The ex-utero intrapartum treatment (EXIT) procedure. Semin Neonatol 2003;8:207–14.

32. Harrison MR, Mychaliska GB, Albanese CT, et al. Correction of congenital diaphragmatic hernia in utero IX: Fetuses with poor prognosis (liver herniation and lung-to-head ratio) can be saved by fetoscopic temporary tracheal occlusion. J Pediatr Surg 1998;33:1017–23.

33. Harrison MR, Keller RL, Hawgood SB, et al. A randomized trial of fetal endoscopic tracheal occlusion for severe fetal congenital diaphragmatic hernia. New Engl J Med 2003;349:1916–24.

34. Saddiq WB, Piedboeuf B, Laberge JM, et al. The effects of tracheal occlusion and release on type II pneumocytes in fetal lambs. J Pediatr Surg 1997;32:834–8.

35. Cannie MM, Jani JC, De Keyzer F, et al. Evidence and patterns in lung response after fetal tracheal occlusion: Clinical controlled study. Radiology 2009;252:526–33.

36. Hirose S, Farmer DL, Lee H, et al. The ex-utero intrapartum treatment procedure: Looking back at the EXIT. J Pediatr Surg 2004;39:375–80.

37. Jani JC, Nicolaides KH, Gratacos E, et al. Severe diaphragmatic hernia treated by fetal endoscopic tracheal occlusion. Ultrasound Obstet Gynecol 2009;34:304–10.

38. Jelin E, Lee H. Tracheal occlusion for fetal congenital diaphragmatic hernia: The ultrasound experience. Clin Perinatol 2009;36:349–61.

39. Adzick NS, Harrison MR, Glick PL, et al. Fetal cystic adenomatoid malformation: Prenatal diagnosis and natural history. J Pediatr Surg 1985;20:483–8.

40. Adzick NS. Open fetal surgery for life-threatening fetal anomalies. Semin Fetal Neonatal Med 2010;15:1–8.

41. Schott S, Mackensen-Haen S, Wallwiener M, et al. Cystic adenomatoid malformation of the lung causing hydrops fetalis: Case report and review of the literature. Arch Gynecol Obstet 2009;280:293–6.

42. Kunisaki SM, Barnewolt CE, Estroff JA, et al. Large fetal congenital cystic adenomatoid malformations: Growth trends and patient survival. J Pediatr Surg 2007;42:404–10.

43. Ierullo AM, Ganapathy R, Crowley S, et al. Neonatal outcome of antenatally diagnosed congenital cystic adenomatoid malformations. Ultrasound Obstet Gynecol 2005;26:150–3.

44. Hsieh CC, Chao AS, Chang YL, et al. Outcome of congenital cystic adenomatoid malformation of the lung after antenatal diagnosis. Int J Gynaecol Obstet 2005;89:99–102.

45. Crombleholme TM, Coleman B, Hedrick HL, et al. Cystic adenomatoid malformation volume ratio predicts outcome in prenatally diagnosed cystic adenomatoid malformation of the lung. J Pediatr Surg 2002;37:331–8.

46. Miller JA, Corteville JE, Langer JC. Congenital cystic adenomatoid malformation in the fetus: Natural history and predictors of outcome. J Pediatr Surg 1996;31:805–8.

47. Wilson RD, Baxter JK, Johnson MP, et al. Thoracoamniotic shunts: Fetal treatment of pleural effusions and congenital cystic adenomatoid malformations. Fetal Diagn Ther 2004;19:413–20.

48. Wilson RD, Baxter JK, Johnson MP, et al. Thoracoamniotic shunts: Fetal treatment of pleural effusions and congenital cystic adenomatoid malformations. Fetal Diagn Ther 2004;19:413–20.

49. Hedrick HL, Flake AW, Crombleholme TM, et al. History of fetal diagnosis and therapy: Children's Hospital of Philadelphia experience. Fetal Diagn Ther 2003;18:65–82.

50. Adzick NS, Harrison MR. Management of the fetus with a cystic adenomatoid malformation. World J Surg 1993;17:342–9.

51. Adzick NS, Harrison MR, Flake AW, et al. Fetal surgery for cystic adenomatoid malformation of the lung. J Pediatr Surg 1993;28:806–12.

52. Tsao K, Hawgood S, Vu L, et al. Resolution of hydrops fetalis in congenital cystic adenomatoid malformation after prenatal steroid therapy. J Pediatr Surg 2003;38:508–10.

53. Curran PF, Jelin EB, Rand L, et al. Prenatal steroids for microcystic congenital cystic adenomatoid malformations. J Pediatr Surg 2010;45:145–50.

54. Peranteau WH, Wilson RD, Liechty KW, et al. Effect of maternal betamethasone administration on prenatal congenital cystic adenomatoid malformation growth and fetal survival. Fetal Diagn Ther 2007;22:365–71.

55. French NP, Hagan R, Evans SF, et al. Repeated antenatal corticosteroids: Size at birth and subsequent development. Am J Obstet Gynecol 1999;180:114–21.

56. Rodriguez MA, Cass DL, Lazar DA, et al. Tumor volume to fetal weight ratio as an early prognostic classification in fetal sacrococcygeal teratoma. J Pediatr Surg 2011;46:1182–5.

57. Shue EH, Bolouri MS, Jelin EB, et al. Tumor metrics and morphology predict poor outcome in prenatally diagnosed sacrococcygeal teratoma. J Pediatr Surg. In Press.

58. Westerburg B, Feldstein VA, Sandberg PL, et al. Sonographic prognostic factors in fetuses with sacrococcygeal teratoma. J Pediatr Surg 2000;35:322–6.

59. Hedrick HL, Flake AW, Crombleholme TM, et al. Sacrococcygeal teratoma: Prenatal assessment, fetal intervention, and outcome. J Pediatr Surg 2003;39:430–8.

60. Ruano R, Duarte S, Zugaib M. Percutaneous laser ablation of sacrococcygeal teratoma in a hydropic fetus with severe heart failure—too late for a surgical procedure? Fetal Diagn Ther 2009;25:26–30.

61. Sebire NJ, Snijders RJ, Hughes K, et al. The hidden mortality of monochorionic twin pregnancies. Br J Obstet Gynaecol 1997;104:1203–7.

62. Quintero R, Morales W, Allen M, et al. Staging of twin-twin transfusion syndrome. J Perinatol 1999;19:550–5.

63. Fusi L, Gordon H. Twin pregnancy complicated by single intrauterine death. Problems and outcome with conservative management. Br J Obstet Gynaecol 1990;97:511–16.

64. Fusi L, McParland P, Fisk N, et al. Acute twin-twin transfusion: A possible mechanism for brain-damaged survivors after intrauterine death of a monochorionic twin. Obstet Gynecol 1991; 78:517–20.

65. Berghella V, Kaufmann M. Natural history of twin-twin transfusion syndrome. J Reprod Med 2001;46:480–4.

66. Roberts D, Gates S, Kilby M, et al. Interventions for twin-twin transfusion syndrome: A Cochrane review. Ultrasound Obstet Gynecol 2008;31:701–11.

67. Senat MV, Deprest J, Boulvain M, et al. Endoscopic laser surgery versus serial amnioreduction for severe twin-to-twin transfusion syndrome. New Engl J Med 2004;351:136–44.

68. Crombleholme TM, Shera D, Lee H, et al. A prospective, randomized, multicenter trial of amnioreduction vs. selective fetoscopic laser photocoagulation for the treatment of severe twin-twin transfusion syndrome. Am J Obstet Gynecol 2007;197:396 e1–9.

69. Rossi AC, D'Addario V. Laser therapy and serial amnioreduction as therapy for twin-twin transfusion syndrome: A metaanalysis and review of literature. Am J Obstet Gynecol 2008;198:147–52.

70. Rand L, Lee H. Complicated monochorionic twin pregnancies: Updates in fetal diagnosis and treatment. Clin Perinatol 2009;36:417–30.

71. Van Allen MI, Smith DW, Shepard TH. Twin reversed arterial perfusion (TRAP) sequence: A study of 14 twin pregnancies with acardius. Semin Perinatol 1983;7:285–93.

72. Goh A, Loke HL, Tan KW. The 'TRAP' sequence–life threatening consequences to the pump twin. Singapore Med J 1994;35:329–31.

73. Quintero R, Munoz H, Hasbun J, et al. [Fetal endoscopic surgery in a case of twin pregnancy complicated by reversed arterial perfusion sequence (TRAP sequence)]. Rev Chil Obstet Ginecol 1995;60:112–17.

74. Hecher K, Hackeloer BJ, Ville Y. Umbilical cord coagulation by operative microendoscopy at 16 weeks' gestation in an acardiac twin. Ultrasound Obstet Gynecol 1997;10:130–2.

75. Tan TY, Sepulveda W. Acardiac twin: A systematic review of minimally invasive treatment modalities. Ultrasound Obstet Gynecol 2003;22:409–19.

76. Tsao K, Feldstein VA, Albanese CT, et al. Selective reduction of acardiac twin by radiofrequency ablation. Am J Obstet Gynecol 2002;187:635–40.

77. Hirose S, Farmer DL. Fetal surgery for myelomeningocele. Clin Perinatol 2009;36:431–4.

78. Heffez DS, Aryanpur J, Hutchins GM, et al. The paralysis associated with myelomeningocele: Clinical and experimental data implicating a preventable spinal cord injury. Neurosurgery 1990;26:987–92.

79. Meuli M, Meuli-Simmen C, Yingling CD, et al. Creation of myelomeningocele in-utero: A model of functional damage from spinal cord exposure in fetal sheep. J Pediatr Surg 1995;30:1028–33.

80. Walsh DS, Adzick NS, Sutton LN, et al. The rationale for in-utero repair of myelomeningocele. Fetal Diagn Ther 2001;16:312–22.

81. Meuli M, Meuli-Simmen C, Yingling CD, et al. In-utero repair of experimental myelomeningocele saves neurological function at birth. J Pediatr Surg 1996;31:397–402.

82. Bruner JP, Tulipan N, Paschall RL, et al. Fetal surgery for myelomeningocele and the incidence of shunt-dependent hydrocephalus. JAMA 1999;282:1819–25.

83. Sutton LN, Adzick NS, Bilaniuk LT, et al. Improvement in hindbrain herniation demonstrated by serial fetal magnetic resonance imaging following fetal surgery for myelomeningocele. JAMA 1999;282:1826–31.

84. Farmer DL, von Koch CS, Peacock WJ, et al. In-utero repair of myelomeningocele: Experimental pathophysiology, initial clinical experience, and outcomes. Arch Surg 2003;138:872–8.

85. Adzick NS, Thom EA, Spong CY, et al. A randomized trial of prenatal versus postnatal repair of myelomeningocele. N Engl J Med 2011;364:993–1004.

86. Hirose S, Meuli-Simmen C, Meuli M. Fetal surgery for myelomeningocele: Panacea or peril? World J Surg 2003;27:87–94.

87. Johnson MP, Sutton LN, Rintoul N, et al. Fetal myelomeningocele repair: Short-term clinical outcomes. Am J Obstet Gynecol 2003;189:482–7.

88. Bruner JP, Tulipan NE, Richards WO. Endoscopic coverage of fetal open myelomeningocele in-utero. Am J Obstet Gynecol 1997;176:256–7.

89. Bruner JP, Tulipan NB, Richards WO, et al. In-utero repair of myelomeningocele: A comparison of endoscopy and hysterotomy. Fetal Diagn Ther 2000;15:83–8.

90. Fontecha CG, Peiro SL, Sevilla JJ, et al. Fetoscopic coverage of experimental myelomeningocele in sheep using a patch with surgical sealant. Eur J Obstet Gynecol Reprod Biol 2011;156:171–6.

91. Morin L, Cendron M, Crombleholme TM, et al. Minimal hydronephrosis in the fetus: Clinical significance and implications for management. J Urol 1996;155:2047–9.

92. Flake AW, Adzick NS, Harrison MR, et al. Ureteropelvic junction obstruction. J Pediatr Surg 1986;21:1058–64.

93. Mahoney BS, Callen PW, Filly RA. Sonographic evaluation of renal dysplasia. Radiology 1984;152:143–9.

94. Heikkla J, Holmberg C, Kyllonen L, et al. Long-term risk of end-stage renal disease in patients with posterior urethral valves. J Urol 2011;186:2392–6.

95. Caione P, Nappo SG. Posterior urethral valves: Long-term outcome. Pediatr Surg Int 2011;27:1027–35.

96. Biard JM, Johnson MP, Carr MC, et al. Long-term outcomes in children treated by prenatal vesicoamniotic shunting for lower urinary tract obstruction. Obstet Gynecol 2005;106:503–8.

97. Nicolini U, Fisk NM, Rodeck CH, et al. Fetal urine biochemistry: An index of renal maturation and dysfunction. Br J Obstet Gynaecol 1992;99:46–50.

98. Carroll SG, Kuo PY, Kyle PM, et al. Fetal protein loss in gastroschisis as an explanation of associated morbidity. Am J Obstet Gynecol 2001;184:1297–301.

99. Bond SJ, Harrison MR, Filly RA, et al. Severity of fetal midgut herniation: Normal size criteria and correlation with crown-rump length. J Ultrasound Med 1993;12:251–4.

100. Lenke RR, Persutte WH, Nemes J. Ultrasonographic assessment of intestinal damage in fetuses with gastroschisis: Is it of clinical value? Am J Obstet Gynecol 1990;163:995–8.

101. Sipes SL, Weiner CP, Williamson RA, et al. Fetal gastroschisis complicated by bowel dilatation: An indication for imminent delivery? Fetal Diagn Ther 1990;5:100–3.

102. Alsulyman OM, Monteiro H, Ouzounian JG, et al. Clinical significance of prenatal ultrasonographic intestinal dilatation in fetuses with gastroschisis. Am J Obstet Gynecol 1996;175:982–4.

103. Crawford RAF, Ryan G, Wright VM, et al. The importance of serial biophysical assessment of fetal wellbeing in gastroschisis. Br J Obstet Gynaecol 1992;99:899–902.

104. Langer JC. Abdominal wall defects. World J Surg 2003;27:117–24.

105. Aktug T, Erdag G, Kargi A, et al. Amnio-allantoic fluid exchange for the prevention of intestinal damage in gastroschisis: An experimental study on chick embryos. J Pediatr Surg 1995;30:384–7.

106. Kohl T, Tchatcheva K, Stressiq R, et al. Is there a therapeutic role for fetoscopic surgery in the prenatal treatment of gastroschisis? A feasibility study in sheep. Surg Endosc 2009;23:1499–505.

107. Koivusalo A, Lindahl H, Rintala RJ. Morbidity and quality of life in adult patients with a congenital abdominal wall defect: A questionnaire survey. J Pediatr Surg 2002;37:1594–601.

108. Wagner AM, Schoeberlein A, Surbek D. Fetal gene therapy: Opportunities and risks. Adv Drug Deliv 2009;61:813–21.

109. Burt R, Testor A, Craig R, et al. Hematopoietic stem cell transplantation for autoimmune disease: What have we learned? J Autoimmun 2008;30:116–20.

110. Verda L, Kim D, Ikehara S, et al. Hematopoietic mixed chimerism derived from allogeneic embryonic stems cells prevents autoimmune diabetes mellitus in NOD mice. Stem Cells 2008;26:381–6.

111. Shizuru J, Weissman I, Kernoff R, et al. Purified hematopoietic stem cell grafts induce tolerance to alloantigens and can mediate positive and negative T cell selection. Proc Natl Acad Sci 2000;97:9555–60.

112. Moreno R, Rosal M, Cabero L, et al. Feasibility of retroviral vector-mediated in-utero gene transfer to the fetal rabbit. Fetal Diagn Ther 2005;20:485–93.

113. Ekhterae D, Crumbleholme T, Karson E, et al. Retroviral vector-mediated transfer of the bacterial neomycin resistance gene into fetal and adult sheep and human hematopoietic progenitors in vitro. Blood 1990;75:365–9.

114. Hayashi S, Flake AW. In-utero hematopoietic stem cell therapy. Yonsei Med J 2001;42:615–29.

115. Shaaban AF, Flake AW. Fetal hematopoietic stem cell transplantation. Semin Perinatol 1999;23:515–23.

116. Gupta N, Henry RG, Strober J, et al. Neural stem cell engraftment and myelination in the human brain. Sci Transl Med 2012;4:155ra137.

SECTION II

TRAUMA

CHAPTER 11

INGESTION OF FOREIGN BODIES

Sohail R. Shah • Danny C. Little

ESOPHAGEAL FOREIGN BODIES

Foreign body (FB) ingestions are a common occurrence in infants and young children. The exact incidence is unknown since many cases are not reported. In 2010, the Annual Report of the American Association of Poison Control Centers noted over 116,000 cases of FB ingestion. More than 86,000 occurred in children ≤5 years of age.[1] The vast majority of ingestions in children are accidental.[2] The most common type of FB varies by geographic region. In the USA and Europe, coins are the most common.[2,3] Other commonly ingested objects include toys, batteries, needles, straight pins, safety pins (Fig. 11-1), screws, earrings, pencils, erasers, glass, fish and chicken bones, and meat. However, in areas of the world where fish contributes a significant portion of the diet, such as in Asia, a fish bone may be the most common FB ingested in children.[2,4]

FB ingestions usually present after a witnessed event or disappearance of an object. Also, there may be heightened suspicion for an ingestion by a caregiver based on the child's description. The initial presentation can vary from the child being completely asymptomatic to a variety of symptoms including drooling, neck and throat pain, dysphagia, emesis, wheezing, respiratory distress, abdominal pain, or distention. The majority of patients will have a normal physical exam; however, the child should be evaluated for signs of complications. Physical exam findings that raise suspicion of a potential complication include oropharyngeal abrasions, crepitus, or signs of peritonitis.

The esophagus is the narrowest portion of the alimentary tract and is thus a common site for FB impaction. Within the esophagus itself, there are three areas of anatomical narrowing that are potential areas of impaction: the upper esophageal sphincter, the level of the aortic arch, and the lower esophageal sphincter. Other areas of potential impaction may be found in the esophagus of children who have underlying esophageal pathology (i.e., strictures or eosinophilic esophagitis), or prior esophageal surgery (i.e., esophageal atresia).

Symptoms of esophageal FB impaction are nonspecific and include drooling, poor feeding, neck and throat pain, vomiting, or wheezing. Radiopaque objects can be detected on the anteroposterior (AP) and lateral neck and chest radiographs (Fig. 11-2), while radiolucent objects may require further workup with a gastrografin esophagram or esophagoscopy depending on the symptoms and level of suspicion (Fig. 11-3).

The most common round, smooth object ingested that is amenable to extraction or advancement techniques is a coin. The majority of esophageal coins will appear en face in the anteroposterior view, and from the side on the lateral radiograph (see Fig. 11-2). On occasion, more than one coin will have been ingested (Fig. 11-4).

The location of the object on the radiograph is important in determining the treatment options. Approximately 60–70% of FB impactions are located in the proximal esophagus at the level of the upper esophageal sphincter or thoracic inlet.[5-7] The majority of FB impactions found in the upper or mid-esophagus will remain entrapped and require retrieval. Options for retrieval include nonemergent endoscopy (rigid or flexible) (Fig. 11-5) and Foley balloon extraction with fluoroscopy (Fig. 11-6). The Foley balloon extraction technique should be limited to round, smooth objects that have been impacted for less than one week in appropriately selected children without any evidence of complications.[8] This technique has been shown to have a success rate of 80% while significantly lowering costs. Objects that are impacted in the lower esophagus often spontaneously pass into the stomach. For this reason, certain lower esophageal impactions may be observed for a brief duration of time, or attempted to be advanced into the stomach with bougienage or a nasogastric tube in the emergency department without anesthesia.[9] Rarely, a chronic esophageal coin can cause esophageal perforation, but this will usually be contained (Fig. 11-7).

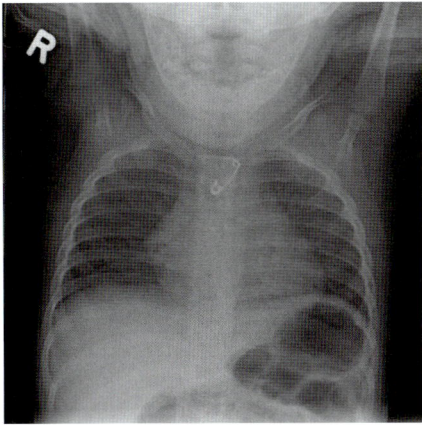

FIGURE 11-1 ■ This child accidentally ingested this open safety pin which was able to be extracted with esophagoscopy.

147

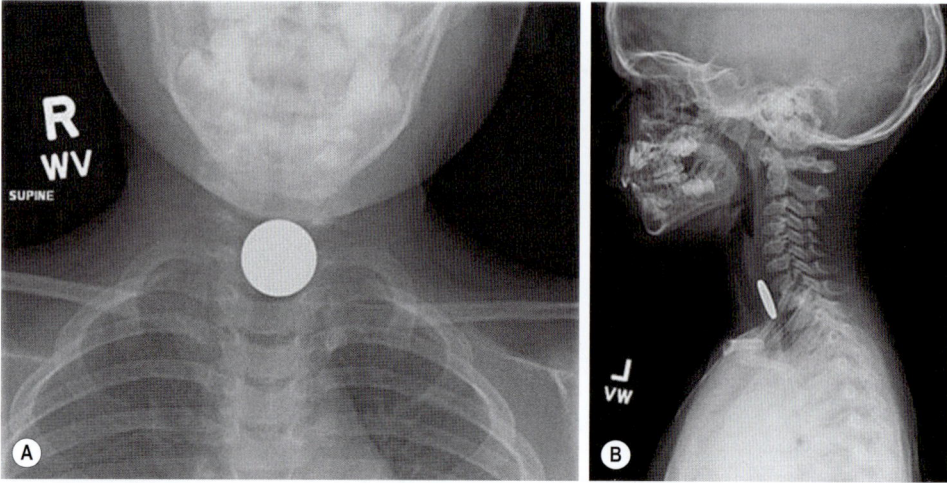

FIGURE 11-2 ■ This 3-year-old child presented with dysphagia and drooling. **(A)** The anteroposterior radiograph shows a coin that appears en face in the upper esophagus. **(B)** The lateral view shows that the coin is posterior to the trachea, confirming its esophageal location.

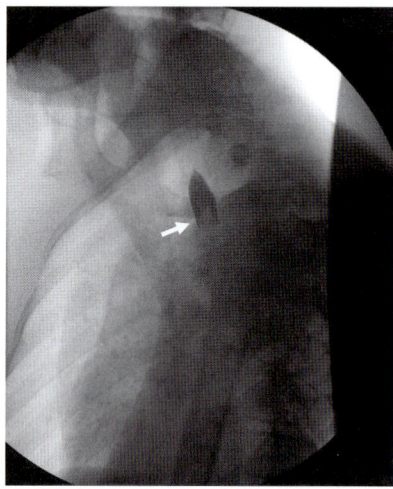

FIGURE 11-3 ■ A piece of chicken became lodged in this child's upper esophagus. The chest radiograph was normal, but the esophagram shows the foreign material (arrow) obstructing the esophagus.

GASTROINTESTINAL FOREIGN BODIES

FB ingestions that are found to be distal to the esophagus are usually asymptomatic when discovered. Signs and symptoms including significant abdominal pain, nausea, vomiting, fevers, abdominal distention, or peritonitis should alert the provider to potential complications including obstruction and/or perforation. The majority of FBs that pass into the stomach will usually pass through the remainder of the gastrointestinal tract uneventfully. These patients can be managed as an outpatient. Occasionally, a FB will remain present in the bowel after a period of observation and serial radiographs (Fig. 11-8). Prokinetic agents and cathartics have not been found to improve gut transit time and passage of the FB.[10] Often parents are instructed to strain the child's stool; however, in up to 50% of cases, the FB is not identified even with successful passage.[5,11] If the child remains asymptomatic and the FB has not been identified, a repeat abdominal

radiograph can be performed at two to three week intervals. Subsequent endoscopy is usually deferred for four to six weeks. Rarely, a chronic esophageal coin can cause esophageal perforation, but this will usually be contained (Fig. 11-8).

SPECIAL TOPIC INGESTIONS

Batteries

Battery ingestions deserve special attention due to the potential for significant morbidity associated with esophageal battery impactions. Button batteries are more commonly ingested than cylindrical batteries in young children.[12] Symptoms occur in less than 10% of cases.[12] Button batteries will appear as a round, smooth object on radiographs and are often misdiagnosed as coins. However, on close inspection, some larger button batteries will demonstrate a double contour rim (Fig. 11-9).

Esophageal batteries are associated with increased morbidity due to the tissue injury that can occur through pressure necrosis, release of a low voltage electric current, or leakage of an alkali solution, which causes a liquefaction necrosis.[11] This mucosal injury may occur in as little as one hour of contact time and may continue even after removal. Therefore, any suspected case of esophageal battery impaction warrants immediate removal. Following removal, an intraoperative esophagram may need to be considered. Early and late complications of esophageal battery impaction include esophageal perforation, tracheoesophageal fistula (Fig. 11-10), stricture and stenosis, and death.

If the battery is confirmed to be distal to the esophagus in the gastrointestinal tract, then it may be observed, similar to other gastrointestinal foreign bodies. More than 80% of batteries that are distal to the esophagus will pass uneventfully within 48 hours.[2,12]

Magnets

Magnet ingestion can be another source of significant morbidity when multiple magnets or a single magnet and

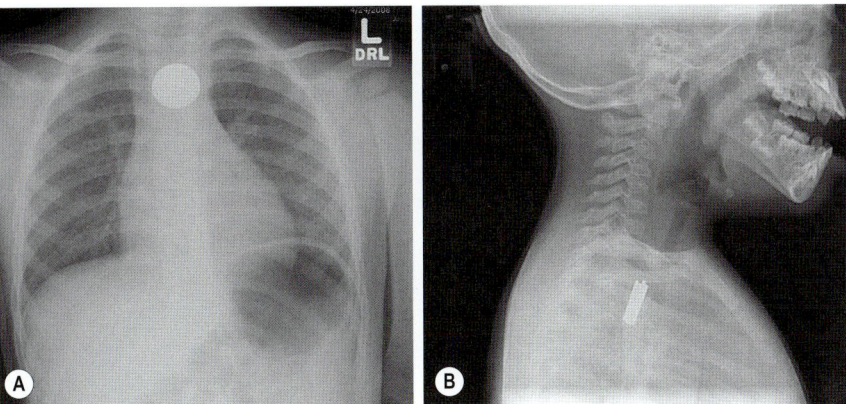

FIGURE 11-4 ■ This infant was seen in the emergency department for swallowing difficulty and drooling. **(A)** Anteroposterior radiograph shows a coin in the upper esophagus. **(B)** However, on the lateral view, there are actually four coins superimposed on one another. The lateral view is very helpful for the purpose of determining whether more than one coin has been ingested.

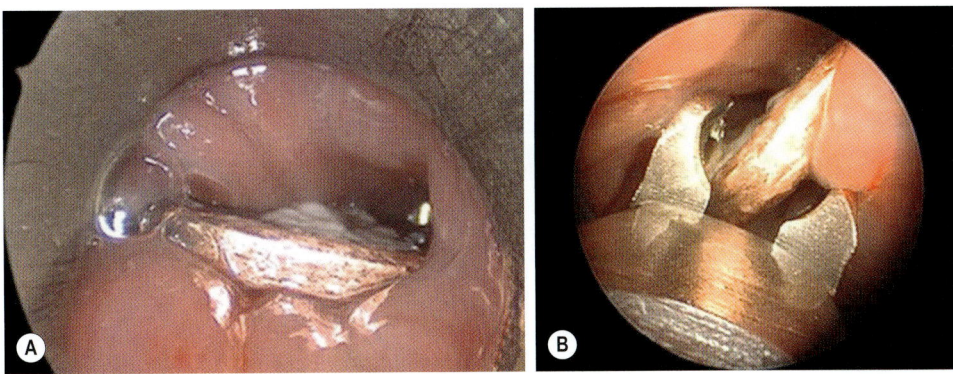

FIGURE 11-5 ■ This coin was lodged in the esophagus of a 2-year-old child. It was unclear how long the coin had been in the esophagus. Rigid esophagoscopy was performed. (A) The coin is seen through the esophagoscope. (B) The optical graspers are being used to grasp the coin and remove it. The safety and success rate for rigid esophagoscopy and coin removal approaches 100% with minimal complications. This is usually a safe and successful way to remove a coin in the esophagus of children in whom the Foley catheter technique is not appropriate.

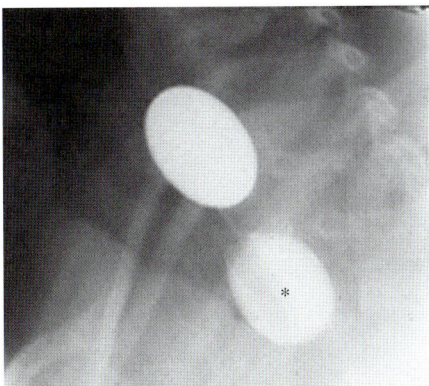

FIGURE 11-6 ■ This radiograph shows the Foley catheter technique for removing a coin lodged in the upper esophagus. Under fluoroscopy, the Foley catheter is advanced past the coin and the balloon is filled with barium (asterisk). Under fluoroscopy, the catheter is then removed, bringing the coin with it. Care must be taken to ensure the patient does not aspirate the coin during its removal. This is a very cost-efficient way to remove coins in the upper esophagus in young children.

a second metallic FB are ingested simultaneously, or within a short time of each other. These patients may also be asymptomatic when the FB is discovered, often with a plain radiograph taken for another reason. Radiographs should be interpreted with caution because multiple magnets may appear to be attached at a single point in

the gastrointestinal lumen when, in fact, they are really attached across the bowel wall from two different intestinal lumens (Fig. 11-11A). Therefore, once the ingestion is confirmed on radiographs, close observation for potential complications is important.

If the magnet is identified in the esophagus or stomach, endoscopy should be performed to prevent potential subsequent complications. Once the objects pass distal to the stomach, if separated within the gastrointestinal tract, they may attach to each other and lead to an obstruction, volvulus, perforation, or fistulization through pressure necrosis (Fig. 11-11B). Therefore, these children should be observed as an inpatient with serial abdominal exams and radiographs. At any time if the child becomes symptomatic, develops signs of obstruction on abdominal radiograph, or shows failure of the objects to progress in greater than 24 hours, then intervention is warranted.

Sharp Foreign Bodies

Ingestion of sharp foreign bodies can cause significant morbidity with an associated 15–35% risk of perforation.[5] Commonly ingested objects include nails, needles, screws, toothpicks, safety pins, and bones. Perforation is most likely to occur in narrowed portions or areas of curvature in the alimentary tract, especially the ileocecal valve. Smaller objects and straight pins are associated with lower rates of perforation and can be conservatively

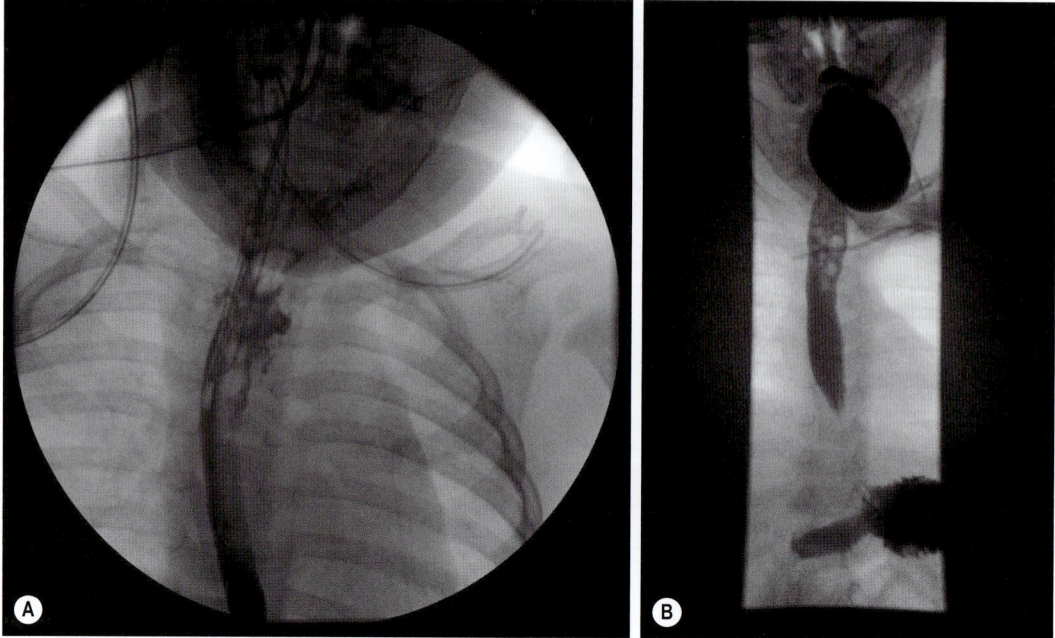

FIGURE 11-7 ■ **(A)** This child was found to have an esophageal leak after uneventful extraction of a coin. **(B)** As the leak appeared to be contained, the patient was managed conservatively, and a repeat study two weeks later showed no evidence of a leak. A central line was placed for total parenteral nutrition.

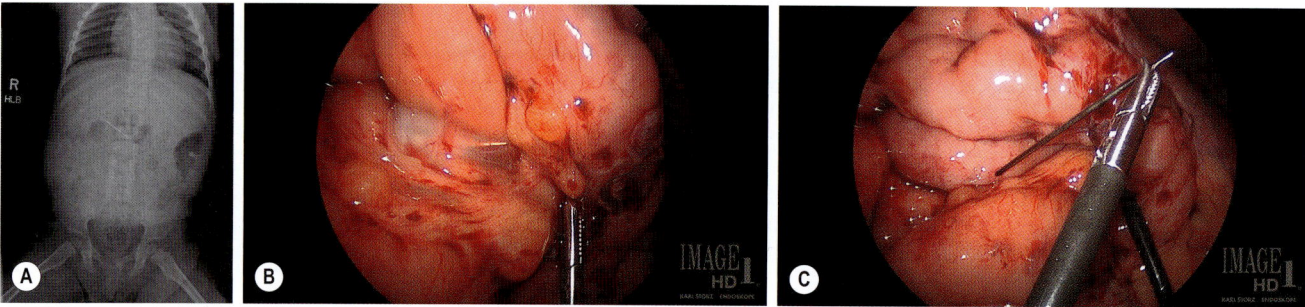

FIGURE 11-8 ■ This child began to complain of abdominal pain and the **(A)** plain film was obtained. Due to the fact that it was unclear how long ago the sewing needle was ingested and because she was exhibiting new symptoms, diagnostic laparoscopy was performed. **(B)** At laparoscopy, the sewing needle was seen to have penetrated the proximal jejunum and **(C)** was able to be extracted. A water soluble contrast study was performed a few days later. The study was unremarkable, her diet was advanced, and she recovered uneventfully.

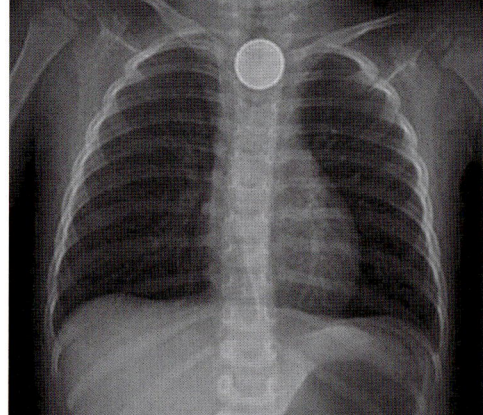

FIGURE 11-9 ■ This child presented within 12 hours of swallowing an unknown foreign body. However, the double contour rim raised suspicion of ingestion of a button battery. This was confirmed upon emergency removal of the battery via rigid esophagoscopy.

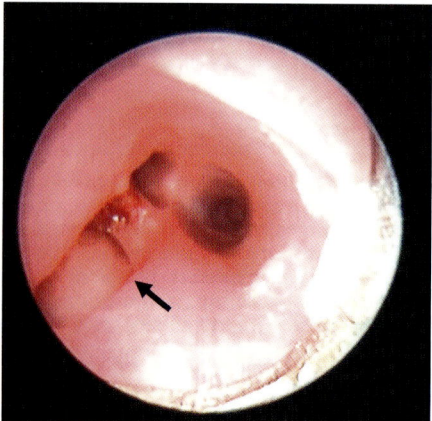

FIGURE 11-10 ■ This infant accidentally swallowed a lithium battery. The battery was removed within a few hours of its ingestion. However, 1 week later, the patient developed respiratory distress and bronchoscopy revealed this tracheoesophageal fistula (arrow).

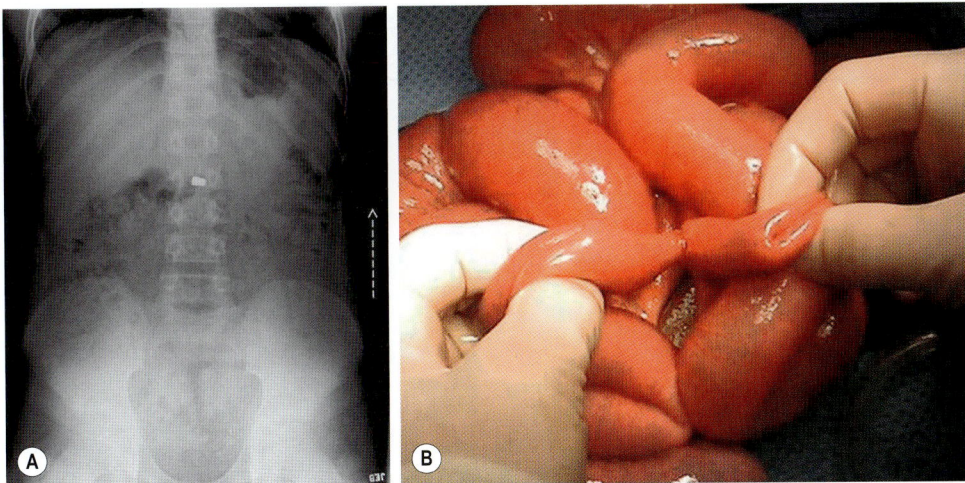

FIGURE 11-11 ■ This 11-year-old child swallowed two small magnets 24 hours prior to presentation to the emergency department. **(A)** The abdominal radiograph demonstrates an inability to detect if the two magnets are within a single intestinal lumen or attached across the bowel wall in two separate lumens. **(B)** This child underwent exploratory laparotomy for obstructive signs. The two magnets were found to be in two separate bowel lumens causing the bowel obstruction and fistulization between the two intestinal segments.

managed.[5] However, other objects should be retrieved endoscopically if possible or observed closely for potential development of complications.

Bezoars

A bezoar is a tight collection of undigested material that may often present as a gastric outlet or intestinal obstruction. These can include lactobezoars, phytobezoars, or trichobezoars. Presenting symptoms often include nausea, vomiting, weight loss, and abdominal distention. The diagnosis may be confirmed on plain radiographs, upper gastrointestinal contrast studies, or endoscopy. Often due to the size and density of the bezoar, medical management and endoscopic removal are unsuccessful, and operation is necessary (Fig. 11-12). See Chapter 29 for more information about bezoars.

AIRWAY FOREIGN BODIES

Most episodes of aspirated FBs occur while eating or playing. Proposed explanations include the fact that young children are still in the oral exploration phase of development when everything tends to go into the mouth. Additionally, children often will cry or run with objects in their mouth. Overall, these young patients tend to have immature coordination of swallowing and less developed airway protection. The average age for fatal events is 15 months, and 75% of aspiration events occur in those less than 4 years.[13] A high index of suspicion is required to make the diagnosis in these young children and especially in those who are debilitated. The annual death rates from aspiration of foreign bodies range from 350–2000 in the USA.[13]

Boys are affected twice as often as girls. Like esophageal FBs, geographical differences have been noted (Table 11-1). For example, sunflower seeds are the most common seed aspirated in the USA, yet watermelon seeds are much more common internationally.[14] A recent publication of

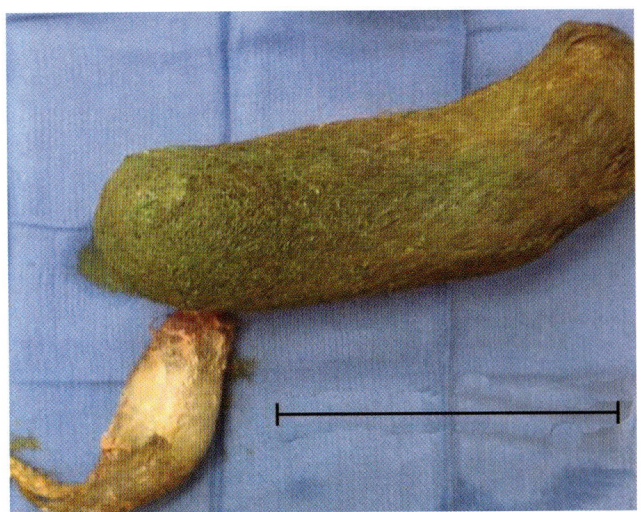

FIGURE 11-12 ■ This was a gastric bezoar with extension into the proximal duodenum found in a 12-year-old child that presented to the hospital with obstructive signs and symptoms. The size and density of the trichobezoar necessitated a laparotomy for removal. The scale bar is 15 cm.

TABLE 11-1	Commonly Aspirated Foreign Bodies in Pediatric Patients (1968–2010)	
Type of Foreign Body	**United States (%)**	**International (%)**
Nuts	41	37
Seeds	8	29
Vegetables	5	–
Beans	–	8
Popcorn	4	–
Bones	2	2
Nonfood	25	12

Adapted from Kaushal, P, Brown D, Lander L, et al. Aspirated foreign bodies in pediatric patients, 1968–2010: A comparison between the United States and other countries. Int J Pediatr Otorhinolaryngol 2011;75:1322–6.

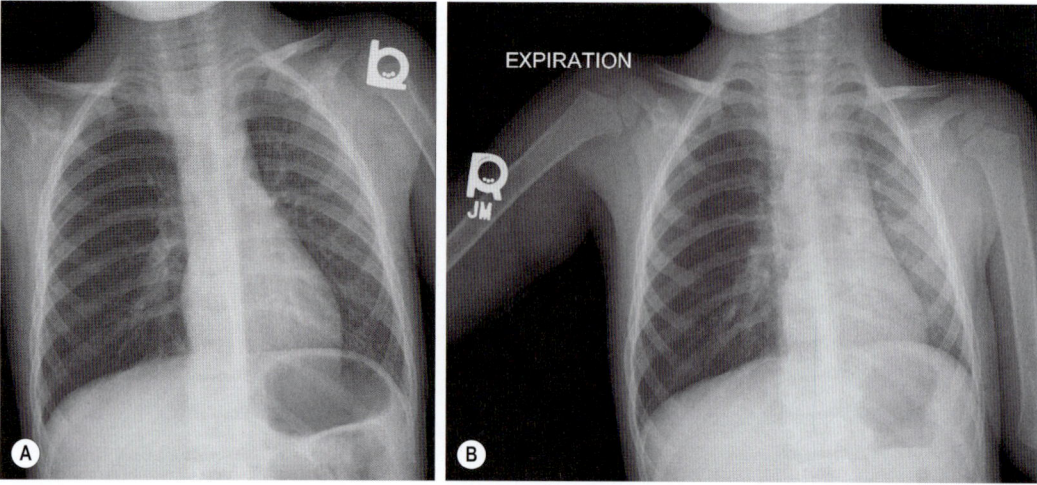

FIGURE 11-13 ■ **(A)** The anteroposterior chest radiograph shows slight hyperexpansion of the right lung in a four year old who aspirated a peanut. **(B)** On the expiratory film, note the increased lucency of the right lung compared to the left. This hyper-lucency on the right is due to air trapping from obstruction of the right main stem bronchus.

132 cases noted a high incidence of food aspirations, especially nuts, in children from non-English speaking backgrounds.[15] Therefore, there may be a role for public education in targeted communities. Victims of child abuse represent another community that is at higher risk. Caregivers should be on alert when tending to a young child with multiple FBs or multiple episodes of aspiration.[16,17]

Several anatomical differences are found in the airway of children compared to older patients. Children have a shorter airway which is smaller in caliber. The anterior position of a child's larynx can increase the difficulty with oral intubation. Additionally, the subglottic region is the narrowest part of a child's airway. The proclivity for FBs to find the right main stem bronchus is well known. Not only is the diameter of the right bronchus larger than the left and airflow generally greater to the right lung, but also the right bronchus has a smaller angle of divergence from the trachea. This important anatomical feature 'directs' the aspirated FB down into the right bronchus.

Common presenting symptoms include respiratory distress, stridor, and/or wheezing. Dysphonia may also be observed. A subtle change in voice or cry may be noted, yet many children will be asymptomatic. Many aspiration events go unwitnessed. Laryngeal pathology usually will manifest as inspiratory stridor while tracheal FBs cause expiratory stridor. Albeit rare, FBs may completely obstruct the larynx or trachea producing sudden death. Chronic FBs often masquerade as respiratory illnesses with persistent cough and atelectasis, recurrent pneumonia, or hoarseness. Other late findings include the development of granulation tissue, strictures, perforation, and bronchiectasis.

Following a detailed history, investigation usually turns to AP and lateral films of the neck and chest. If the child is cooperative, inspiratory and expiratory films are beneficial (Fig. 11-13). Review of the radiograph may reveal hyperinflation or 'air trapping' in up to 60% of children as the FB is acting as a one-way valve producing obstructive emphysema.[18] In time, mediastinal shift may develop. Decubitus views may also prove helpful since the obstructed lung will not deflate, even while in a dependent position. Interestingly, up to 56% of patients may have a normal chest film within 24 hours of aspiration.[19] Radiopaque foreign bodies are easily identified (Fig. 11-14A), but radiolucent FBs become clinically diagnosed through indirect radiographically clues such as hyperexpansion. Foreign bodies lodged in the larynx or trachea tend to have a higher radiographic detection rate (90%) than those in the bronchus (70%).[18–22] A multi-institutional review of 1269 FB events revealed that 85% were correctly diagnosed following a single physician encounter.[23] Therefore, a negative bronchoscopy rate of 10–15% is considered acceptable in order to avoid a delay in treatment with subsequent morbidity.[24] Radiographic imaging remains helpful in children with a history of choking, yet definitive diagnosis still requires bronchoscopy.

Emergent management of airway FBs can be a dramatic experience. An accurate history remains important, yet sometimes is hard to obtain from small children who are unreliable historians. The use of the flexible bronchoscope to diagnose a FB followed by a rigid bronchoscopy for removal is a common approach utilized by pediatric surgeons. General anesthesia in the operating room using spontaneous ventilation offers the best chance for safe and successful removal. Positive pressure ventilation may be required, but this technique runs the risk for further propagating the FB into the more distal passages of the airway. With severely ill children, where transportation presents a logistical risk, rigid bronchoscopy has been performed safely in the intensive care setting.[25]

Bronchoscopy

We recommend positioning the head in the 'sniffing' position with a folded towel under the shoulders. The eyes are taped and protected. Precautions to minimize secretions, laryngospasm, and hypoxia are employed. Careful laryngoscopy may reveal a FB that can be retrieved with McGill forceps. More distal evaluation

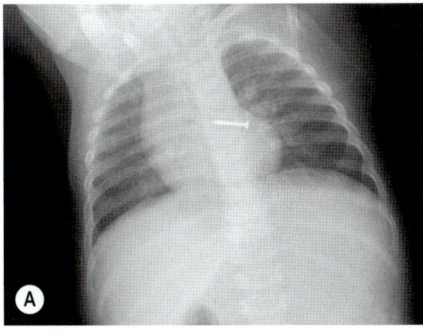
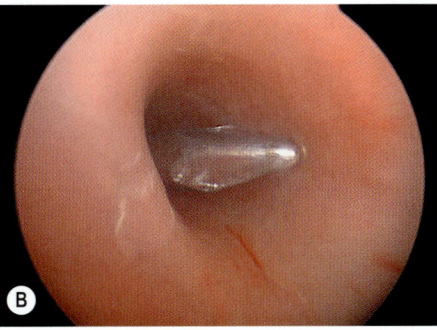
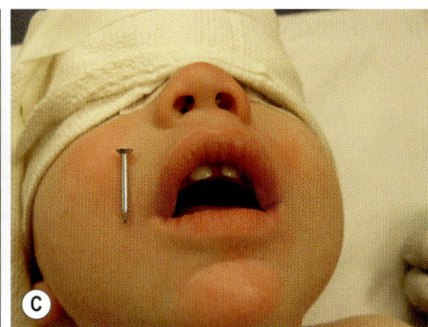

FIGURE 11-14 ■ **(A)** This young child accidentally aspirated this nail which was found to be in the left main stem bronchus on chest radiography. **(B)** At bronchoscopy, with the bronchoscope in the trachea, the nail is seen to be peering out of the left main stem bronchus. **(C)** The nail was removed, and the child recovered uneventfully. Note the size of the nail relative to the child's face and mouth.

requires direct instrumentation of the airway. Special precautions must be considered to avoid injuries to the lips, tongue, and most importantly the teeth. Once the bronchoscopy starts, the operative team must be ready for emergent intubation, or rarely, tracheostomy. Liberal use of lidocaine (4 mg/kg) applied to the glottic area may minimize laryngospasm.

There are several commercial available rigid broncho-scopes. Instruments vary in size between 2.5 cm × 20 cm and 6 × 30 cm. Length and diameter of the bronchoscope will be determined by the age and size of the child. The Doesel–Huzly bronchoscope with Hopkins rod-lens tel-escope or Holinger ventilating bronchoscope are com-monly used. Exposure is excellent with both, and the caliber of the scope allows the FB to be retracted into the scope during removal, thereby decreasing the risk of inadvertently dropping the FB during extraction (Fig. 11-14B,C). Equipment combining optics and illumina-tion while allowing the introduction of working forceps are favored in most children's hospitals.

The larynx and cords are visualized and the broncho-scope is advanced to the right of the laryngoscope and into the trachea. Inspection of the right or left main stem bronchus can be facilitated by turning the head to the opposite side. Angled scopes are generally not needed. The operative side channel allows passage of suction and retrieval instruments as well as instillation of fluids to help clear a bloody airway. The ventilation side port allows continuous ventilation during the procedure. Loose connections from any of these sites can lead to hypoventilation. Furthermore, if ventilation is impaired, the telescope can be removed, leaving the unobstructed bronchoscope for ventilation. In difficult cases, especially with FBs lodged distal to the main bronchus, a Fogarty catheter may be helpful to wedge the FB between the bronchoscope and Fogarty balloon. Partial FB removal will at times be necessary, especially with chronic foreign bodies associated with significant bleeding or airway edema. Prior to the second endoscopy,[26] the child's condi-tion can be optimized with inhaled epinephrine and intravenous corticosteroids.[27,28]

Flexible bronchoscopy remains an option, especially for diagnostic purposes. The standard pediatric flexible bronchoscope has a two way deflection tip with a range between 180–220° and a side port to allow passage of suction catheters and working instruments. Most newborns can breathe normally around this scope for brief periods of time. A face mask adapter can be used to reduce the risk of hypoxia. The ultrathin scope ('noodle scope') can be inserted through smaller caliber endotra-cheal or tracheostomy tubes while maintaining ventila-tion. However, these scopes have very limited, if any, working channels and suction capability. Overall compli-cations of rigid or flexible endoscopy include bleeding from local inflammation, laryngospasm, pneumothorax, and hypoxia with the more serious complications being found in the youngest patients.[29,30]

A lack of experience, poor visualization, and inade-quate instrumentation contribute to failure of a successful examination. Many of these cases are seen at night, and operating room personnel frequently struggle to find the required instruments. The surgeon performing the pro-cedure must ensure that all of the needed instruments are in working order before the child is brought to the oper-ating room. A preoperative 'game plan' between nursing, anesthesia, and surgical staff is also important. Bleeding that obscures visualization is common, and the introduc-tion of a small suction catheter through the working channel may be helpful. In other cases, partial FB removal is recommended with a plan to return to the operating room the next day. Rarely a thoracotomy with bron-chotomy or lobectomy is required. Following successful removal, attention to proper cleaning of the instruments is important, given that inadequate cleaning and storage may predispose to cracks in the equipment that could lead to bacterial contamination.[31]

Maintaining bronchoscopic skills remains necessary to effectively manage these difficult cases. Across under-graduate and graduate medical education, simulation continues to gain momentum. Several institutions have developed simulation courses for residents to improve psychomotor skills associated with airway FBs. Objec-tives include an understanding of the tracheobronchial anatomy, ability to adequately visualize the larynx with laryngoscopy, proficiency in rigid bronchoscopy, and familiarity with FB instrumentation. Of note, in one institution, success in assembling the needed instruments and completing assigned tasks increased after completing the course on average 81% and 43%, respectively.[32] One would expect further development of simulation exercises to be useful for initial credentialing and continued profi-ciency for both trainees and faculty.

REFERENCES

1. 2010 Annual Report of the American Association of Poison Control Centers' National Poison Data System (NPDS): 28th Annual Report.
2. Kay M, Wyllie R. Pediatric foreign bodies and their management. Curr Gastroenterol Rep 2005;7:212–18.
3. Arana A, Hauser B, Hachimi-Idrissi S, et al. Management of ingested foreign bodies in childhood and review of the literature. Eur J Pediatr 2001;160:468–72.
4. Watanabe K, Kikuchi T, Katori Y, et al. The usefulness of computed tomography in the diagnosis of impacted fish bones in the oesophagus. J Laryngol Otol 1998;112:360–4.
5. Wahbeh G, Wyllie R, Kay M. Foreign body ingestion in infants and children: Location, location, location. Clin Pediatr 2002;41:633–40.
6. Panieri E, Bass DH. The management of ingested foreign bodies in children—A review of 663 cases. Eur J Emerg Med 1995; 2:83–7.
7. Macpherson RI, Hill JG, Othersen HB, et al. Esophageal foreign bodies in children: Diagnosis, treatment, and complications. AJR Am J Roentgenol 1996;166:919–24.
8. Little DC, Shah SR, St Peter SD, et al. Esophageal foreign bodies in the pediatric population: Our first 500 cases. J Pediatr Surg 2006;41:914–18.
9. Louie MC, Bradin S. Foreign body ingestion and aspiration. Pediatr Rev 2009;30:295–301.
10. Macgregor D, Ferguson J. Foreign body ingestion in children: An audit of transit time. J Accid Emerg Med 1998;15:371–3.
11. Litovitz T, Schmitz BF. Ingestion of cylindrical and button batteries: An analysis of 2382 cases. Pediatrics 1992;89:747–57.
12. Hesham A-Kader H. Foreign body ingestion: Children like to put objects in their mouth. World J Pediatr 2010;6:301–10.
13. Cataneo AJ, Cataneo DC, Ruiz RL Jr. Management of tracheobronchial foreign body in children. Pediatr Surg Int 2008;24: 151–6.
14. Kaushal, P, Brown D, Lander L, et al. Aspirated foreign bodies in pediatric patients, 1968–2010: A comparison between the United States and other countries. Int J Pediatr Otorhinolaryngol 2011;75: 1322–6.
15. Choroomi S, Curotta J. Foreign body aspiration and language spoken at home: 10 year review. J Laryngol Otol 2011;125: 719–23.
16. Binder L, Anderson W. Pediatric gastrointestinal foreign body ingestions. Ann Emerg Med 1984;13:112–17.
17. Nolte K. Esophageal foreign bodies as child abuse: Potential fatal mechanisms. Am J Forensic Med Pathol 1993;14:323–6.
18. Zerella J, Dimler M, McGill L. Foreign body aspiration in children: Value of radiography and complications of bronchoscopy. J Pediatr Surg 1998;33:1651–4.
19. Oguz F, Citak A, Unuvar E, et al. Airway foreign body aspiration in children. Int J Pediatrc Otorhinolaryngol 2000;52:11–16.
20. Mu L, He P, Sun D. Inhalation of foreign bodies in Chinese children: A review of 400 cases. Laryngoscope 1991;101: 657–60.
21. Metrangelo S, Monetti C, Meneghini L, et al. Eight years' experience with foreign body aspiration in children: What is really important for timely diagnosis. J Pediatr Surg 1999;34:1229–31.
22. Karakoc F, Karadag B, Akbenglioflu C, et al. Foreign body aspiration: What is the outcome? Pediatr Pulmonol 2002;34: 30–6.
23. Reilly J, Thompson J, MacArthur C, et al. Pediatric aerodigestive foreign body injuries are complications related to timeliness of diagnosis. Laryngoscope 1997;107:17–20.
24. Mantor P, Tuggle D, Tunell W. An appropriate negative bronchoscopy rate in suspected foreign body aspiration. Am J Surg 1989;158:622–4.
25. Muntz H. Therapeutic rigid bronchoscopy in the neonatal intensive care unit. Ann Otol Rhinol Laryngol 1985;94:462–5.
26. Ciftci A, Bingol-Kologlu M, Senocak M, et al. Bronchoscopy for evaluation of foreign body aspiration in children. J Pediatr Surg 2003;38:1170–6.
27. Ritter F. Questionable methods of foreign body treatment. Ann Otol 1974;83:729–33.
28. Black R, Johnson D, Matlak M. Bronchoscopic removal of aspirated foreign bodies in children. J Pediatr Surg 1994;29:682–4.
29. Nussbaum E. Pediatric fiberoptic bronchoscopy. Clin Pediatr (Phila) 1995;34:430–5.
30. Wain JC. Rigid bronchoscopy: The value of a venerable procedure. Chest Surg Clin North Am 2001;11:691–9.
31. Nicolai T. Pediatric bronchoscopy. Pediatr Pulmonol 2001; 31:150–64.
32. Jabbour N, Reihsen T, Sweet R, et al. Psychomotor skills training in pediatric airway endoscopy simulation. Otolaryngol Head Neck Surg 2011;145:43–50.

CHAPTER 12

BITES

Gary S. Wasserman • Jennifer A. Lowry • D. Adam Algren

A wide variety of bites are seen in children. It is estimated that more than 1 million children are treated annually for bites (Table 12-1).[1] In this chapter we concentrate on bites of interest to the surgeon. The reader is referred elsewhere for discussions of management of venomous stings and injuries from marine life and general details of wound management.

TETANUS

The Gram-positive anaerobic organism *Clostridium tetani* is the causative agent for tetanus, a severe and often fatal disease. In 2009, there were a total of 18 cases (zero under 14 years of age) reported in the USA.[2]

There has been a low incidence rate of tetanus since a peak of 102 cases in 1975. Mortality from tetanus is associated with co-morbid conditions such as diabetes, intravenous drug use, and old age, especially when vaccination status is unknown. Infection can occur weeks after a break in the skin, even after a wound has seemed to heal. The ideal anaerobic surroundings allow spores to germinate into mature organisms producing two neurotoxins: tetanolysin and tetanospasmin.[3] The latter is able to enter peripheral nerves and travel to the brain, causing the clinical manifestations of uncontrolled muscle spasms and autonomic instability. The incubation period varies from as short as two days to several months, with most cases occurring within 14 days.[4] In general, the shorter the incubation period, the more severe the disease and the higher the fatality risk.

Initially, the diagnosis is made clinically because cultures are often negative and serology for antitoxin antibodies has a long turn-around time. So-called 'dirty' wounds (lacerations treated after 24 hours, abscesses, ulcers, gangrene, and wounds with nonviable tissue) are the most common injuries that become infected with tetanus. However, a history of trauma is not necessary for infection.

All wounds should be cleaned and debrided. Symptomatic and supportive care includes medications such as benzodiazepines to control tetanic spasms and antimicrobials for infection. Metronidazole (oral or intravenous, 30 mg/kg/day, divided into four daily doses, maximum 4 g/day) is the preferred antibiotic because it decreases the number of vegetative forms of *C. tetani*.[5] An alternate choice is parenteral treatment with penicillin G (100,000 U/kg/day every four to six hours, not to exceed 12 million units/day) for ten to 14 days. Human tetanus immune globulin (TIG) is administered to adults and adolescents as a one-time dose of 3000–6000 units

intramuscularly. Some experts recommend that children receive 500 units to decrease the discomfort from injection.[5] Infiltrating part of the dose locally is controversial. Tetanus prevention in a potentially exposed patient depends on the nature of the wound and history of immunization with tetanus toxoid (Table 12-2).

CAT, DOG, HUMAN, AND OTHER MAMMALIAN BITES

Children are frequent victims of mammalian bites. The most common complication from bites is infection: cats, 16–50%; dogs, 1–30%, and humans, 9–18%.[6] When the bite is from a cat, dog, or other mammal, the most common infectious organisms are *Streptococcus*, *Staphylococcus*, *Actinomycetes*, *Pasteurella* species, *Capnocytophaga* species, *Moraxella* species, *Corynebacterium* species, *Neisseria* species, *Eikenella corrodens*, *Haemophilus* species, anaerobes, *Fusobacterium nucleatum*, and *Prevotella melaninogenica*.[5,7,8] Human bites are a potential source not only for bacterial contamination but also for hepatitis B and, possibly, human immunodeficiency virus (HIV) infection.[9]

Recommendations for bite wound management are presented in Box 12-1. Evidence-based medicine studies concerning whether to close wounds are not conclusive. Distal extremity wounds, especially hand/fist to teeth, are at higher risk for infection. Whether minimal risk wounds require prophylactic antimicrobial therapy is also controversial. Antibiotics started within eight to 12 hours of the bite and continued for two to three days may decrease infection rate.[5] The oral drug of choice is amoxicillin-clavulanate. For penicillin-allergic patients, an extended-spectrum cephalosporin or trimethoprim-sulfamethoxazole plus clindamycin should be used.[5]

RABIES AND POSTEXPOSURE PROPHYLAXIS

Rabies is a viral disease usually transmitted through the saliva of a sick mammal (e.g., dogs, cats, ferrets, raccoons, skunks, foxes, bats, and most other carnivores). The majority of reported cases in the USA are caused by raccoons, skunks, foxes, mongooses, and bats. Small rodents such as rats, mice, squirrels, chipmunks, hamsters, guinea pigs, rabbits and gerbils are almost never infected with rabies. Over the past decade, cats have been the most common domestic animal with rabies. Rabies-related human deaths in the USA occur one to seven times per year since 1975. Modern prophylaxis has proven nearly 100% successful. Worldwide, fatalities are about

TABLE 12-1 **Bites and Envenomations to Humans: Calls to Poison Centers in 2010**

Animal	Total Calls	Age <6 Years	Age >6–19 Years	All Ages Treated at Facility	Severe Outcome/Death
Bat	663	85	120	335	0/0
Cat	814	65	136	485	2/0
Dog	2292	367	689	1704	5/1
Fox	26	0	4	21	0/0
Human	42	5	4	22	0/0
Insects	38446	6499	6499	4595	63/2
Other Mammals	929	119	189	516	1/0
Raccoon	146	10	24	112	2/0
Rodent/lagomorphs	1397	269	381	409	1/0
Skunks	12	0	2	5	0/0
Snakes	7013	398	1567	7392	189/2
Spiders	10394	1059	1488	2704	32/1

n = 2,384,825 total human poisoning calls; *n* = 61,854 (2.6% total) in the category of bites and envenomations.
Data from Bronstein AC, Spyker DA, Cantilena LR, et al, editors. 2010 Annual Report of the American Association of Poison Control Centers National Poison Data System (NPDS): 28th Report. Clin Toxicol 2011;49:910–41, Appendix.

TABLE 12-2 **Wound Tetanus Prophylaxis Guideline**

Vaccination History (Td)	Clean/minor Wounds	All Other Wounds
? or <3 doses	Td or Tdap—No TIG	Td or Tdap—TIG
≥3 doses	Td or Tdap—No TIG if ≥10 years since last dose	Td or Tdap—No TIG if ≥5 years since last dose

Td, adult type diphtheria and tetanus toxoids vaccine; TIG, tetanus immune globulin (human); Tdap, booster tetanus toxoid, reduced diphtheria toxoid, and cellular pertussis.
Data from American Academy of Pediatrics: Tetanus (lockjaw), Bite Wounds. In Pickering LK, Baker CJ, Kimberlin DW, Long SS (eds): Redbook: 2009 Report of the Committee on Infectious Diseases, 28th ed. Elk Grove Village, IL, American Academy of Pediatrics, 2009, pp 187-191, 655–60.

BOX 12-1 **Components of Bite Wound Management**

- Obtain detailed history of injury
- Evaluate injury and re-examine in 24–48 hours
  - Check for foreign bodies and possible deep structure injury in small children
- Evaluate for risk of tetanus, rabies, hepatitis B, human immunodeficiency virus
- Perform meticulous cleansing and irrigation
  - Do NOT irrigate puncture wounds
- Obtain wound culture as indicated
  - Culture is recommended if wound appears infected or is of late presentation (>8–12 hours)
- Debride necrotic tissue or contaminants not removed by irrigation
- Perform exploratory surgery as indicated
- Primary closure for selected fresh nonpuncture wounds
- Consider antimicrobial therapy

40,000–70,000. The rabies virus enters the central nervous system and causes an acute, progressive encephalomyelitis from which survival is extremely unlikely. The human host has a wide range for the incubation period from days to years (most commonly weeks to months).

Prophylactic treatment for humans potentially exposed to rabies includes immediate and thorough wound cleansing followed by passive vaccination with human rabies immune globulin and cell culture rabies vaccines, either human diploid or purified chick embryo.[10–12] Many factors help determine the risk assessment in deciding which patient benefits from post exposure prophylaxis and which regimen should be given. The risk of infection depends on the type of exposure, surveillance, epidemiology of animal rabies in the region of contact, species of animal, animal behavior causing it to bite, and availability of the animal for observation or laboratory testing for the rabies virus. The final decision for treatment with vaccines is complex. Therefore local, state, or CDC (Centers for Disease Control) experts are available for assistance. There is no single effective treatment for rabies once symptoms are evident.

SPIDER BITES

There are about 40,000 species of spiders that have been named and placed in about 3000 genera and 105 families.[13] In regard to medically relevant spiders, few are known to cause significant clinical effects. In 2010, about 11,000 calls were made to USA Poison Control Centers (PCC) regarding spider bites.[1] It is rare that a spider bite requires surgical care. Few spiders have been shown to have the ability to bite humans because their fangs cannot pierce the skin. The two most medically important spiders in the USA are Sicariidae (brown spiders) and *Lactrodectus* (widow spiders).

Brown Recluse Spiders

Loxoscelism is a form of cutaneous–visceral (necrotic–systemic) arachnidism found throughout the world with predilection for North and South America.[14] There are four species of brown spiders within the USA that are known to cause necrotic skin lesions (*Loxosceles deserta*, *L. arizonica*, *L. rufescens*, and *L. reclusa*). *L. deserta* and *L. arizonica* can be found in the southwestern USA *L. reclusa* is the most common species associated with human bites. It is usually found in the south central USA, especially Missouri, Kansas, Oklahoma, Arkansas, Tennessee, and Kentucky.[15] Spiders can be transported out of their natural habitat but rarely cause arachnidism in nonendemic areas. *L. reclusa* is tan to brown with a characteristic dark, violin-shaped marking on its dorsal cephalothorax, giving it the nickname 'fiddleback' or 'violin' spider. The spider can measure up to 1 cm in total body length with a 3 cm or longer leg span (Fig. 12-1). These spiders only have three pairs of eyes whereas most spiders have four pairs.

The incidence of *L. reclusa* bites predominantly occurs from April through October in the USA. The venom of the brown recluse spider contains at least 11 protein components. Most are enzymes with cytotoxic activity.[16] Sphingomyelinase D is believed to be the enzyme responsible for dermonecrosis and activity on red blood cell membranes.[17–19] In addition to the local effects, the venom has activity against neutrophils and the complement pathway that induces an immunologic response.[19–21] The resulting effect is a necrotic dermal lesion and the possibility that a systemic response will be life threatening.

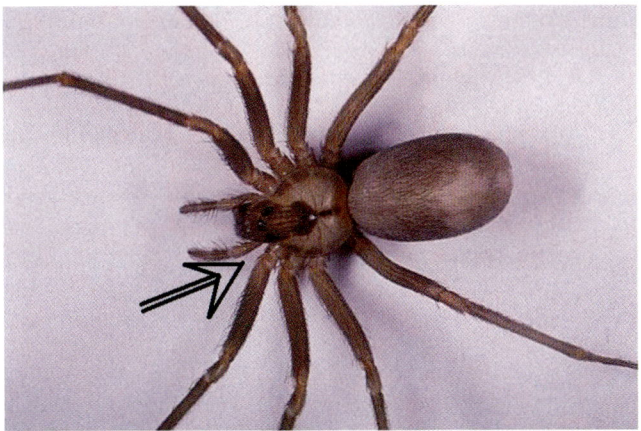

FIGURE 12-1 ■ *Loxosceles reclusa* (brown recluse, 'fiddleback') spider showing the classic violin-shaped marking on the back (dorsal side) of the cephalothorax. Note the long slender legs and oval body segment with short hairs. The arrow is pointing toward the classic violin marking. (From Ford M, Delaney K, Ling L, et al. Clinical Toxicology. Philadelphia: Elsevier; 2001.)

The prevalence of brown recluse spider envenomations is unknown. The victim may not feel the bite or may only feel a mild pinprick sensation. Many victims are bitten while they sleep and may be unaware of the envenomation until a wound develops. The majority of victims do not see the spider at the time of the bite.[22] Typically, the bite progressively begins to itch, tingle, and become ecchymotic, indurated, and edematous within several hours.[23] Often within hours, a characteristic bleb or bullae will form. The tissue under a blister is likely to become necrotic, but the extent of necrosis is not predictable. As the ischemia and inflammation progresses, the wound becomes painful and may blanch or become erythematous, forming a 'target' or 'halo' design. Inflammation, ischemia, and pain increase over the first few days after the bite as enzymes spread. Over hours to weeks, an eschar forms at the site of the bite. Eventually, this eschar sloughs, revealing an underlying ulcer that may require months to heal, usually by secondary intention (Fig. 12-2). On very rare occasions, the ulcer does not heal and may require surgical intervention.

The need for hospitalization occurs if the patient develops systemic symptoms. Two studies documented that 14% to more than 50% of patients developed systemic symptoms, with fever being the most common symptom.[10] Other common symptoms include a maculopapular rash, nausea and vomiting, headache, malaise, muscle/joint pain, hepatitis, pancreatitis, and other organ toxicity. Life-threatening systemic effects include hemolysis (intravascular and/or extravascular), coagulopathy, and multiple organ system failure. Secondary effects include sepsis, necrotizing fasciitis, and shock.[24–26] Hemolysis usually manifests within the first 96 hours. However, late presentations can occur. When hemolysis does develop, it can take four to seven days (or longer) to resolve. Complications such as cardiac dysrhythmias, coma, respiratory compromise, pulmonary edema, congestive heart failure, renal failure, and seizures can occur.

The diagnosis of a brown recluse spider envenomation is largely one of exclusion as it is rare to see or identify the spider. While the wound can look classic for an

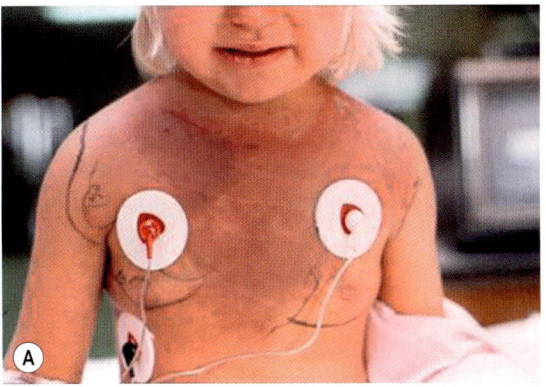 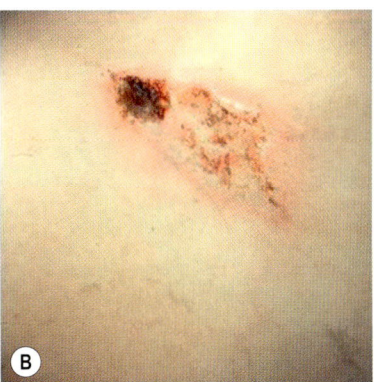 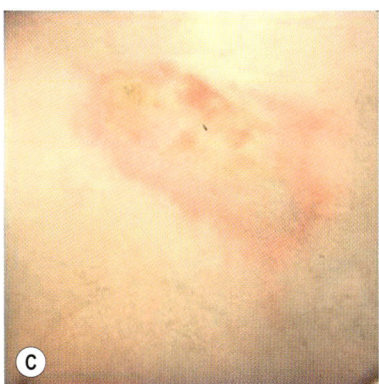

FIGURE 12-2 ■ (A) A 3-year-old girl hospitalized on the third day after a brown recluse spider bite for severe hemolytic anemia, hemoglobinuria, and ecchymosis (note the vast expansion of the ecchymosis secondary to hyaluronidase 'spreading factor' in the venom). There is no necrosis or ischemia, but a small bleb/blister is present over the right clavicle that, although not pathognomonic, is often present early in lesion progression. Also note that the cutaneous lesion is mild in comparison with this patient's systemic presentation. (B) On the 15th day after envenomation, the lesion measures 5 cm × 2 cm. Multiple small areas of necrosis have become apparent in the past week. The largest area indicates the original bite size. The lesion's edges have begun to involute with healing, and the ischemia is fading. (C) Nine months after the bite, the necrotic wound has healed with no significant scarring.

envenomation, other etiologies must be considered (Box 12-2). Certain laboratory findings can be consistent with a brown recluse spider envenomation but are not specific in making the diagnosis (Box 12-3).

Controversy surrounds the treatment of dermal and systemic symptoms of loxoscelism. Medications such as dapsone, nitroglycerin, and tetracycline have been used. Also, hyperbaric oxygen (HBO) therapy has been advocated as has excision of the necrotic wound. However, none of these has proven to be effective in treating or preventing the ulcer development. In South America, an antivenom has been developed and used in the treatment of *Loxosceles* envenomations. Unfortunately, the usual long delay in seeking medical care often leads to ineffective use of this antivenom.[27] An antivenom is not available in North America.

The use of dapsone, a leukocyte inhibitor, has been advocated in case reports and animal studies.[28-30] However, other animal studies have shown no benefit from this treatment. In an animal study,[31] piglets received venom and were randomized to receive one of four treatments: no treatment, HBO, dapsone, or dapsone with HBO.

<table>
<tr><td>**BOX 12-2**</td><td>**Differential Diagnosis of Brown Recluse Spider Envenomations**</td></tr>
</table>

Acquired hemolytic anemias
Bites from other creatures (e.g., snakes, spiders, insects) that can result in cutaneous lesions
Dermatologic conditions (e.g., pyoderma gangrenosum)
Hereditary hemolytic anemias
Infectious causes (e.g., Lyme disease, infection with *Streptococcus*, *Staphylococcus*, or *Clostridium* species)
Medical conditions causing necrotic lesions:
    Emboli
    Frostbite or thermal injuries
    Ischemic injuries
    Neoplastic wounds (e.g., ecthyma gangrenosum)
    Trauma

<table>
<tr><td>**BOX 12-3**</td><td>**Laboratory Findings Consistent with Systemic Effects of *Loxosceles* Envenomations**</td></tr>
</table>

Hemoglobinemia
Hemoglobinuria or hematuria, elevated urobilinogen
Elevated plasma free hemoglobin or decreased free haptoglobin
Leukocytosis
Anemia
Thrombocytopenia
Coagulopathy (elevated prothrombin time, decreased fibrinogen, elevated D-dimer, decreased antithrombin III)
Inflammatory markers (elevated C-reactive protein, elevated erythrocyte sedimentation rate, elevated liver and/or pancreatic enzymes), elevated lactate dehydrogenase
Immunology (positive antiglobulin tests: direct or indirect Coombs; decreased total serum complement or components; interference with blood screening or crossmatching)

Neither dapsone, HBO, nor the combination treatment reduced necrosis compared with controls. A second study compared the use of HBO, dapsone, or cyproheptadine against no treatment in decreasing the necrotic wound after envenomation with *L. deserta* venom. No statistical difference was seen with respect to lesion size, ulcer size, or histopathologic ranking.[32] In addition, the use of dapsone is not without risk, especially hypersensitivity reactions.[33] Therapeutic doses of dapsone are associated with hemolytic anemia, methemoglobinemia, and other hematologic effects in patients with and without glucose-6-phosphate dehydrogenase deficiency.

Topically applied nitroglycerin as a vasodilator had been advocated but is not effective in preventing necrosis.[34] Tetracycline has been shown to be effective. Rabbits were inoculated with *Loxosceles* venom and randomized to receive topical doxycycline, topical tetracycline, or placebo.[35] Those who received topical tetracycline had reduced progression of the dermal lesion. However, treatment was started at six hours after envenomation, which may not be realistic after a human bite. In addition, the agents used for this research study are not commercially available in the United States. Further studies need to be performed before topical tetracycline can be recommended.

HBO has been advocated for treatment to prevent progression of the necrotic wound. The initial use of HBO was based on the belief that tissue hypoxia was partially responsible for the subsequent necrosis seen after a bite. As mentioned previously, no statistical differences were noted in animal studies that compared dapsone and HBO.[31,32] Similar results have been seen in animal studies assessing the effect of HBO alone.[36,37] However, a randomized, controlled trial of HBO in a rabbit model in which standard HBO was used showed a significantly reduced wound diameter at ten days.[38] No significant change in blood flow at the wound center or 1–2 cm from the wound center was seen. HBO is expensive and not without complications. At the present time, much of the literature contradicts the benefit of HBO for brown recluse spider envenomations. As such, it is not currently recommended as a therapy for these bites, but may be helpful in patients with underlying/preexisting vascular compromise such as sickle cell anemia or diabetes.

Early surgical intervention is not helpful because the venom diffuses rapidly throughout the soft tissues surrounding the bite.[39] In addition, patients may be more at risk for delayed wound healing and excessive scarring if operation occurs within the first 72 hours of the bite.[40,41] Debridement of enlarging blebs is proposed with the theory that toxins exist within the blister fluid. However, necrosis almost always occurs beneath the blisters.[42] The question is whether surgical intervention should be advocated late after envenomations? The wound from the brown recluse spider may take two to three months to heal. Thus, skin grafting of a non-healing necrotic area should be delayed up to 12 weeks to allow for neovascularization of the demarcated area.[43]

Treatment of systemic symptoms largely involves supportive care. Patients should be monitored closely for hemolysis (and children hospitalized) if systemic symptoms such as fever and rash develop. Systemic corticosteroids seem to suppress hemolysis and may be needed for five to ten days with a subsequent tapering dose.[43] Methylprednisolone can be administered as a 1.0–2.0 mg/kg intravenous loading dose (no maximum) followed by a 0.5–1.0 mg/kg maintenance dose every six hours. Hydration to maintain good urine output is required to prevent acute renal tubular necrosis if hemolysis or hematuria occurs. Antibiotics are not generally required early in the care of these patients because the spider does not inoculate humans with bacteria. However, secondary infections can occur and lead to sepsis, toxic shock syndrome, and necrotizing fasciitis. These complications require close observation and antibiotic therapy to cover anaerobic, staphylococcal, and streptococcal infections.

Black Widow Spider

Black widow spiders (*Latrodectus mactans*) are found throughout North America.[44] They can usually be found outdoors in warm, dark places, or in a garage or basement. They are web-making spiders and usually strike when their web is disturbed. The female spider is readily recognized as she is a black spider with a red marking on her abdomen in the shape of an hourglass. Widow spiders have a neurotoxic venom that is responsible for their clinical effects. The venom, α-latrotoxin, acts on the neuromuscular junction to cause depletion of acetylcholine at motor endings and catecholamines at the postganglionic sympathetic synaptic sites, which is followed by complete blockade of the neuromediator release.[45]

In the majority of cases, a pinprick sensation may be felt at the time of a bite. A 'halo' lesion may develop, but this tends to disappear within 12 hours of envenomation. A few hours after the bite, the regional lymph nodes and affected extremity may become tender. Depending on where the bite occurs, pain usually migrates to the large muscle groups in the thigh, buttock, abdomen or chest. The most common presenting complaint is intractable abdominal, chest, back, or leg pain, depending on the site of the bite.[46] Board-like rigidity of the abdomen, shoulders, and back may develop that may lead to misdiagnosis of a surgical abdomen or other etiology. The pain generally peaks at two to three hours, but can last up to 72 hours.

Because the venom affects the autonomic nervous system, patients can present with symptoms of dysautonomia that include hypertension (sometimes severe), tachycardia, weakness, ptosis, eyelid edema, pruritus, nausea and vomiting, diaphoresis, hyperreflexia, difficulty breathing, and excessive salivation. Fatalities are rare, but have been reported. Children are more at risk for developing systemic symptoms.

Management is largely symptomatic and supportive. For the most part, treatment is focused on analgesia. For those with mild pain, oral medications are appropriate. Patients may present with severe pain requiring opioids and benzodiazepines as adjunctive therapy. Calcium gluconate was advocated in the past, but is not recommended now because of lack of consistent effects in alleviating the symptoms. Antivenom is available and generally reserved for patients who have life-threatening symptoms or for pain that is not relieved by opioids and benzodiazepines.

CROTALID SNAKE ENVENOMATIONS

In the USA, there are two major classes of poisonous snakes: crotalids and elapids. Crotalids, otherwise known as pit vipers, are indigenous to almost every state and account for the vast majority of poisonous snake bites in the USA annually. Most snake bites occur during the warm summer months when both snakes and humans are more active and thus more likely to come into contact with each other. It is thought that up to 20% of snake bites are 'dry bites' and do not result in envenomation.[47]

Crotalids can be classified into three major groups: rattlesnakes, cottonmouths (water moccasins), and copperheads. Copperheads are responsible for the majority of crotalid envenomations. In general, these bites are less severe and rarely result in systemic toxicity.[48,49] Rattlesnake envenomations more commonly produce coagulopathy and systemic toxicity.

Crotalids have several physical features that help distinguish them from nonpoisonous snakes (Fig. 12-3). Crotalids have triangular heads and elliptical pupils. Nonpoisonous snakes have round heads and pupils. Crotalids have a single row of subcaudal plates/scales distal to the anal plate, whereas nonpoisonous snakes have a double row of subcaudal plates. Most importantly, crotalids have two retractable fangs and the characteristic heat-seeking pit located between the nostril and the eye. Nonpoisonous snakes have short, pointy teeth, but no fangs.

Crotalid Venom Pharmacology/ Pathophysiology

Crotalid venom is a complex mixture of proteins, including metalloproteinases, collagenase, hyaluronidase, and phospholipase.[50] These enzymes act to destroy tissue at the site of envenomation. Damage to the vascular endothelium and basement membranes leads to edema, ecchymosis, and bullae formation. Concurrently with local tissue destruction, venom is absorbed systemically and can result in shock and coagulopathy. The potency of venom varies with the snake's age, species, diet, and time of year.[47] Even for the same snake, the composition and potency of venom can vary substantially based on these factors.

Clinical Effects

In questioning the patient, one should ascertain the circumstance and timing of the bite as well as any first aid methods that were used. Knowing what prehospital measures were instituted can be extremely helpful. Certain therapies such as incision, excision, and suction may result in significant local trauma and act to confound the assessment of local injury. The clinician should determine if the patient has previously received antivenom because sensitization can occur, thereby placing the patient at higher risk for an allergic reaction. Health care

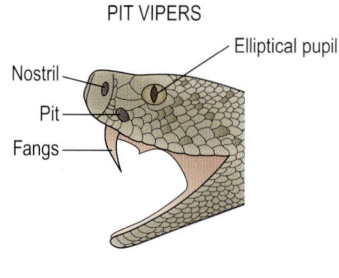

PIT VIPERS

Nostril
Pit
Fangs
Elliptical pupil

NONPOISONOUS

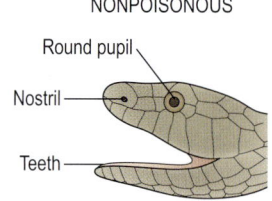

Round pupil
Nostril
Teeth

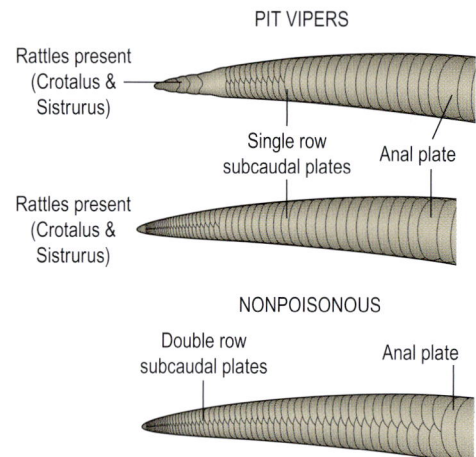

PIT VIPERS

Rattles present
(Crotalus &
Sistrurus)

Single row
subcaudal plates
Anal plate

Rattles present
(Crotalus &
Sistrurus)

NONPOISONOUS

Double row
subcaudal plates
Anal plate

FIGURE 12-3 ■ Identifying characteristics of pit vipers and non-poisonous snakes. The presence or absence of a single row of subcaudal plates may be the only identifying feature in a decapitated snake. (From Ford M, Delaney K, Ling L, et al. Clinical Toxicology. Philadelphia: Elsevier; 2001.)

TABLE 12-3	**Clinical Grading of Snake Envenomations**
Grading	**Comments**
Minimal	Mild local swelling without progression; no systemic or hematologic toxicity
Moderate	Local swelling with proximal progression and/or mildly abnormal laboratory parameters (e.g., decreased platelets, prolonged coagulation studies)
Severe	Marked swelling with progression and/or significant systemic toxicity (shock, compartment syndrome) or laboratory abnormalities (severe thrombocytopenia/coagulopathy)

Adapted from Gold BS, Dart RC, Barish RA. Bite of Venomous Snakes. N Engl J Med 2002;347:347–56.

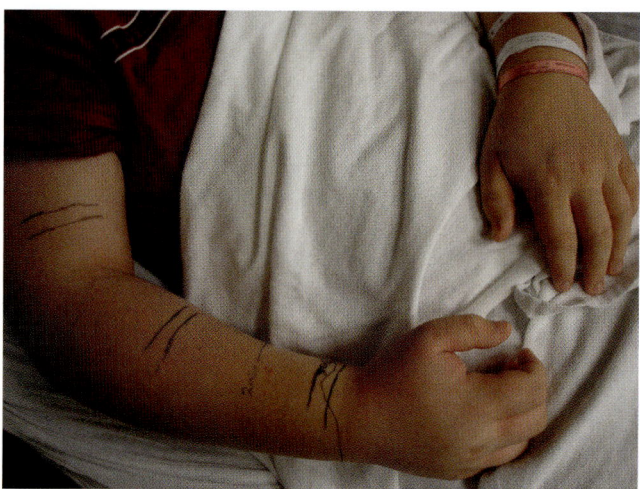

FIGURE 12-4 ■ A 15-year-old boy was bitten on his right hand by a timber rattlesnake. Note the significant swelling of the arm. Serial limb circumference measurements were documented; the lines mark the progression of the swelling. The patient did well after treatment with Fab antivenom.

providers should be cautious regarding the reliability of the victim's identification of the snake. It is often assumed that rattlesnakes will rattle their tails before biting. However, this is not always the case. Also, rattles may be absent from rattlesnakes due to shedding or trauma. Victims occasionally trap or kill the snake and bring it to the emergency department. Vigilance is necessary when examining these snakes because they are capable of biting again. Even dead snakes have been known to bite reflexively for up to an hour after they have been killed.[47]

Envenomations can result in significant local pain and swelling. The patient typically has two fang marks at the location of the bite. Often, there is mild bleeding or oozing from the wound. Swelling typically develops within one to two hours, and ecchymosis or bullae (some hemorrhagic) may appear. Several different grading systems have been developed to grade the severity of snake bites.[47,51] The minimal, moderate, severe model is a simple tool that can help assess severity and determine the need for antivenom (Table 12-3).

Serial measurements of the extremity are required to detect progression of the swelling. The local effects have traditionally been documented by drawing a line demarcating the progression of the swelling. Unfortunately, this method requires subjective interpretation and can result in measurement variability. Measurement of the limb circumference is more objective and can be easily repeated to determine any progression (Fig. 12-4). These measurements should be recorded every 15 minutes for the first two hours and then less frequently (every 30-60 minutes). In addition to measuring the limb circumference, serial neurovascular examinations can identify ischemia or evidence of compartment syndrome.

Compartment syndrome is rare (<1–2%) after snake envenomation because it is unusual for a snake's fangs to penetrate the muscle fascia.[52] The true incidence is difficult to ascertain from the literature because many of the older case series report the use of prophylactic fasciotomies without measuring the compartment pressure.[52–54] Although swelling may be severe, it is almost always localized to the subcutaneous tissue. If there is concern for compartment syndrome in the setting of severe pain and swelling, measurement of compartment pressures is needed. Even if elevated compartment pressures are found, treatment with antivenom is usually sufficient to reduce the elevated pressures and reverse the compartment syndrome.[52–56] Given the efficacy and safety of the current crotalid antivenom, prophylactic fasciotomies are not routinely indicated in the setting of an envenomation.[57] Recent evidence has shown that prophylactic fasciotomies worsen local effects and do not improve clinical outcomes.[58,59] If compartment pressures are elevated, they should be re-measured after antivenom administration and repeat antivenom should be given, if needed. If the pressures remain elevated for more than 4 hours despite antivenom, then fasciotomy is indicated (Fig. 12-5). Measurement of finger compartment pressures is not possible. If significant concern exists about the viability of the finger, a digit dermotomy is indicated.[59]

Systemic manifestations present in a variable fashion after envenomation. Nonspecific symptoms and signs include nausea, vomiting, diaphoresis, and metallic taste. Hypotension and shock can develop in severe cases. Severe rattlesnake envenomations often cause coagulopathy with a disseminated intravascular coagulation-like syndrome. Thrombocytopenia has been noted to be severe and prolonged after timber rattlesnake envenomations.[60] Canebrake rattlesnake envenomations have been associated with significant rhabdomyolysis.[61] Rarely, following envenomation, patients have been noted to have extremely rapid decompensation. In these cases, it is thought that the patient experiences either an immediate anaphylactoid-like reaction or receives a significant intravascular venom load.[62]

Management

After a crotalid bite, the victim should avoid exertion and have the involved extremity immobilized. These actions may decrease venom absorption into the systemic circulation. Rings, jewelry, and other constrictive clothing should be removed. Most importantly, the victim should be rapidly transported to the nearest emergency department.

Historically, different procedures and therapies have been advocated in the prehospital and in-hospital management of snake bites. Treatments such as cryotherapy and electric shock are associated with significant complications and are not recommended.[63] It is commonly thought that tourniquets should be applied to the affected extremity. However, their use has not been found to improve outcomes and evidence suggests they may worsen local toxicity.[64–66] Therefore, their use should be discouraged. Given the short transport times of most patients, the morbidity associated with tourniquet application (limb ischemia) outweighs any potential benefit. In those situations in which the victim is in a remote location that is hours away from an emergency department, the use of a constriction band should be considered. There are limited data to suggest that constriction bands decrease the rate of systemic venom absorption.[64] Constriction bands differ from venous tourniquets in that they serve to impede lymphatic return rather than blood flow. When placed correctly, two fingers should easily slip under a constriction band.

Pressure immobilization is another modality commonly recommended for snake bites. It involves wrapping the entire limb in an elastic compression bandage and then immobilizing the limb in extension with a splint. Although likely effective in cases of elapid envenomations,[67] their use in cases of crotalid envenomation should be discouraged despite a recent position statement supporting their use.[68] Animal models of crotalid envenomation demonstrated pressure immobilization slightly prolonged the time to death but was associated with a significant increase in extremity compartment pressures.[69,70] Additionally, it has been shown that pressure immobilization bandages are often applied incorrectly and can act as a tourniquet.[71]

Suction using a commercially available extractor device has been previously suggested. The concept is that the suction would pull the venom out of the wound if applied shortly after the bite. However, it has been demonstrated that these devices are not efficacious and remove less than 1% of injected venom.[72] Also, these devices may actually increase the amount of local tissue destruction.[73] Therefore, use of extractor devices in the prehospital or hospital setting is not recommended.

Incision therapy, often combined with suction, gained favor in the early 20th century. This procedure entailed making several parallel incisions longitudinally along the affected extremity. While early animal models demonstrated some survival improvement, subsequent human studies have failed to show any change in clinical outcomes.[74] Incising the wound also risks injury to underlying tendons, nerves, and blood vessels, and increases infection rates.[74–76]

In-hospital management should initially focus on assessing and supporting the airway, breathing, and circulation. Anaphylactic reactions have been reported after envenomation.[77] The initial evaluation should assess the

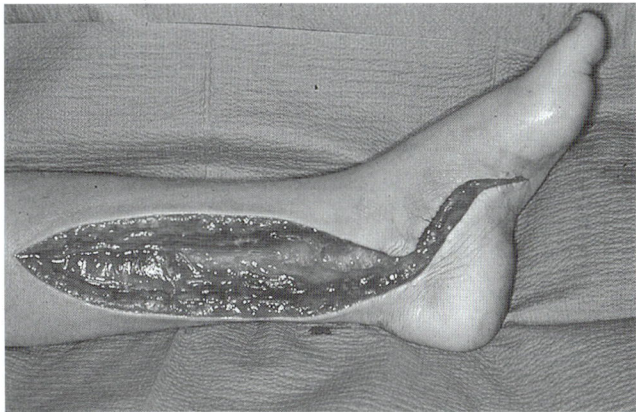

FIGURE 12-5 ■ The need for fasciotomy for compartment syndrome may be suggested by excessive swelling in the soft tissue, but compartment pressures are rarely elevated significantly. Prophylactic fasciotomy is based on the belief that it protects against compartment syndrome. Such practices are unnecessary and can be catastrophic in venom-defibrinated patients. (From Brent J, Wallace K, Burkhart K, et al. Critical Care Toxicology: Diagnosis and Management of the Critically Poisoned Patient. Philadelphia: Elsevier; 2005.)

patient for shock and hypoperfusion. Hypotension mandates aggressive resuscitation with crystalloid, antivenom (see later), and possibly vasopressors. If the patient arrives in the emergency department with a tourniquet on the extremity, it should be slowly loosened and removed over 20 to 30 minutes. Rapid removal of the tourniquet could result in a bolus of the venom into the central circulation, resulting in decompensation of the patient.[64] Intravenous access should be obtained in the noninjured extremity, with placement of a second access line in those with significant envenomation. Opioids are often required for management of pain. The patient's tetanus should be updated as needed. Prophylactic antibiotics are not warranted because the risk of infection resulting from snake bites is less than 5%.[78] Although snakes carry pathogenic bacteria in their mouths, the majority of infections are secondary to the victim's normal skin flora.

The antivenom supplies of the hospital should be assessed in all cases of snake bites, even those cases in which antivenom administration does not appear to be indicated. This is prudent because the patient's clinical condition can change rapidly in the first several hours after envenomation. It is important for the clinician to arrange for procurement of antivenom or hospital transfer while the patient is stable and not in immediate need of antivenom. A complete blood cell count, chemistries, coagulation studies, fibrinogen, and creatinine kinase are indicated in all cases of snake bites to assess systemic toxicity. Medical toxicologists and regional poison centers (1-800-222-1222) can serve as valuable resources to clinicians who are unfamiliar with the management of snake envenomations.

Antivenom is indicated for envenomations displaying more than minimal local effects (Box 12-4). The older Wyeth (Collegeville, PA) polyvalent antivenom that was introduced in the USA in 1954 is no longer manufactured. This product was a crudely purified, equine-derived IgG antibody directed against the venom of several crotalids. As it contained foreign proteins and was highly immunogenic, the incidence of immediate hypersensitivity reactions was high. Approximately 50% of recipients developed urticaria or signs of anaphylactic shock.[79] Serum sickness, a delayed immunologic reaction to the foreign proteins, was much more commonly associated with this antivenom (approximately 50% of cases treated with more than five vials of the Wyeth antivenom).[79] It typically occurs one to three weeks after antivenom administration and manifests clinically as a fever, rash, arthralgias, myalgias, and occasionally glomerulonephritis and pericarditis. It is generally self-limited and can be treated with corticosteroids and antihistamines.

Fortunately, a new polyvalent immune Fab antivenom (CroFab, Protherics, Inc., Brentwood, TN) is available that is much safer and associated with significantly fewer adverse reactions. It is a highly purified product that contains the Fab fragments of IgG antibodies. The product is sheep-derived and is effective against all North American crotalid species. The incidence of immediate hypersensitivity reactions is less than 5% to 10%.[80–84] Many of the hypersensitivity reactions are mild (urticaria) and do not prevent further antivenom administration. Anaphylaxis is uncommon. Likewise, the incidence of serum sickness is also less than 5%.[83,84] The dosing of polyvalent immune Fab is based on the clinical severity and response of the patient to the antivenom (Fig. 12-6). The dosing is not weight based. Therefore, the dosing in children is the same as in adults. Skin testing is not required. Clinical trials have demonstrated improved outcomes when regular follow-up doses of antivenom were given for recurrence (see later) of local and systemic toxicity in those who received a single dose of antivenom. This resulted in the development of the currently recommended dosing schedule. Multiple studies have demonstrated that the polyvalent immune Fab antivenom is efficacious in ameliorating the local and systemic venom toxicity. Recent analysis of pediatric data also demonstrates excellent efficacy and safety in treating children as young as 18 months of age. There were no cases of anaphylaxis in pediatric patients (>100 cases) reported in five

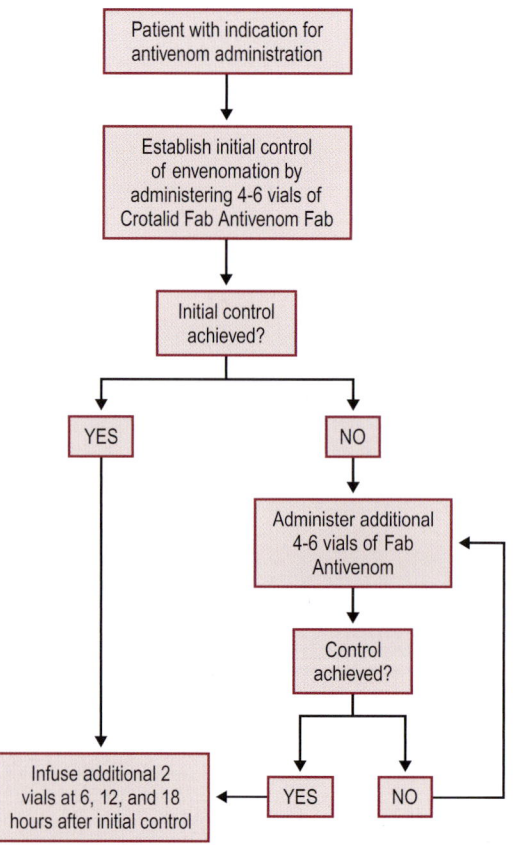

FIGURE 12-6 ■ This schematic depicts management of the patient who needs crotalid polyvalent immune Fab antivenom.

case series.[85–89] Liberal use should be considered for bites involving the hands or feet because these envenomations are associated with significant morbidity and prolonged recovery.[90]

Recurrence is defined as worsening of local and/or systemic toxicity after a period of improvement with antivenom therapy. This results from the pharmacokinetic differences between the antivenom and venom.[91] The Fab components have a low molecular weight and are small enough to be freely filtered by the kidney. This results in an elimination half-life of Fab antivenom of about 15 to 20 hours versus venom that has a half-life of approximately 40 hours.[91,92] Multiple reports have documented progression of swelling or worsening hematologic toxicity after antivenom therapy.[80,83,93] Those patients who develop hematologic toxicity during initial treatment are at highest risk for recurrence. Administration of antivenom is usually effective in treating further local progression. Although hematologic toxicity does not typically result in clinically significant bleeding, further antivenom administration is not effective in completely normalizing hematologic abnormalities.[83,94] Close monitoring is indicated, and treatment can be resumed in those with bleeding or markedly abnormal laboratory parameters.[94]

The disposition of patients who are bitten is dependent on the severity of the envenomation. Discharge after eight to 12 hours of observation can be considered in those circumstances in which it is thought that no significant envenomation occurred (dry bite).[95] There should be no appreciable local swelling, and results of initial laboratory studies and repeat laboratory studies before discharge should be normal. Patients with local swelling or evidence of systemic toxicity should be admitted for further evaluation and management. Rattlesnake bite victims from those areas in which the Mojave rattlesnake is endemic should be monitored for neurotoxicity.

CORAL SNAKE ENVENOMATION

The coral snake is the only poisonous elapid snake native to the USA. While there are several species of coral snakes in the USA, the species of greatest concern is found in Florida and southern Georgia. These snakes are brightly colored and have bands in a distinctive pattern (black, yellow, red). This order gives rise to the common phrases, 'red on yellow, kill a fellow' and 'red on black, venom lack,' that can help to differentiate a coral snake from the nonpoisonous king snake. Unlike crotalids, coral snakes have round heads and pupils. Instead of fangs, they have short teeth. Up to 25% of bites result in no significant envenomation.[96]

Unlike crotalids that produce local tissue destruction and coagulopathy, venom from elapids is associated with neurotoxicity. After a bite, local effects tend to be mild. Of greater concern is the risk of progressive weakness and resulting respiratory failure. Neurologic symptoms (cranial nerve palsies, weakness) typically develop within two hours but may be delayed up to 13 hours.[96] Given the lack of significant local effects, surgical management is not indicated.

All patients with suspected coral snake bites should be admitted for observation. Treatment is supportive with close monitoring for respiratory compromise. Traditionally it had been recommended to administer antivenom to any patient in whom there was a significant likelihood of envenomation (even if the patient was asymptomatic as the antivenom is less effective after the onset of symptoms due to its neurotoxicity). More recently, it has been recommended to administer antivenom only if symptoms develop. The initial dose is three to five vials with subsequent antivenom administration based on worsening of symptoms.

Coral snake antivenom is an equine-derived IgG. In the largest series describing USA coral snake envenomations, immediate hypersensitivity reactions occurred in 15% of patients, whereas serum sickness was reported in 10%.[96]

REFERENCES

1. Bronstein AC, Spyker DA, Cantilena LR, et al. 2010 Annual Report of the American Association of Poison Control Centers' National Poison Data System (NPDS). Clin Toxicol 2011;49:910–1011 and Appendix.
2. Centers for Disease Control and Prevention. Summary of Notifiable Diseases—United States, 2009. MMWR 2011;58:33, 36.
3. Wu DT. Tetanus. In: Wolfson AB, Hendey GW, Hendry PL, et al, editors. Harwood-Nuss' Clinical Practice of Emergency Medicine. Philadelphia: Lippincott Williams & Wilkins; 2005. p. 718–20.
4. Loscalzo LI, Ryan J, Loscalzo J, et al. Tetanus: A clinical diagnosis. Am J Emerg Med 1995;13:488–90.
5. American Academy of Pediatrics. Tetanus (lockjaw), Bite Wounds. In: Pickering LK, Baker CJ, Kimberlin DW, et al, editors. Redbook: 2009 Report of the Committee on Infectious Diseases. 28th ed. Elk Grove Village, IL: American Academy of Pediatrics; 2009. p. 187–91, 655–60.
6. Capellan O, Hollander JE. Management of lacerations in the emergency department. In: Peth HA, editor. High Risk Presentations. Emerg Med Clin North Am 2003;21:205–31.
7. Talan DA, Citron DM, Abrahamian EM, et al. Bacteriologic analysis of infected dog and cat bites. N Engl J Med 1999;340:85–92.
8. Talan DA, Abrahamian EM, Moran GJ, et al. Clinical presentation and bacteriologic analysis of infected human bites in patients presenting to emergency departments. Clin Infect Dis 2003;37:1481–9.
9. Pretty IA, Anderson GS, Sweet DJ. Human bites and risk of human immunodeficiency virus transmission. Am J Forens Med Pathol 1999;20:232–9.
10. Human rabies prevention. United States, 1999. Recommendation of the Advisory Committee on Immunization Practices (ACIP). Morb Mortal wkly Rep 1999;48(No. RR-1):1–21.
11. World Health Organization. WHO expert committee on rabies. World Health Organ Tech Rep Ser 2005;931:1–121.
12. Rabies Prevention Policy Update. New Reduced-Dose Schedule. Committee on Infectious Diseases. Pediatrics 2001;127:785–7.
13. Coddington JA, Levi HW. Systematics and evolution of spiders (Araneae). Annu Rev Ecol Syst 1991;22:565–92.
14. Sams HH, Dunnick CA, Smith ML, et al. Necrotic arachnidism. J Am Acad Dermatol 2001;44:561–73.
15. Vetter RS. Spiders of the genus Loxosceles (Araneae, Sicariidae): A review of biological, medical, and psychological aspects regarding envenomations. J Arachnol 2008;36:150–63.
16. Forrester LJ, Barrett JT, Campbell BJ. Red blood cell lysis induced by the venom of the brown recluse spider: The role of sphingomyelinase D. Arch Biochem Biophys 1978;187:355–65.
17. Rees RS, Nanney LB, Yates RA, et al. Interaction of brown recluse spider venom on cell membranes: The inciting mechanism? J Invest Dermatol 1984;83:270–5.
18. Tambourgi DV, Magnoli FC, van den Berg CW, et al. Sphingomyelinases in the venom of the spider Loxosceles intermedia are responsible for both dermonecrosis and complement-dependent hemolysis. Biochem Biophys Res Commun 1998;251:366–73.

19. Majeski JA, Stinnett JD, Alexander JW, et al. Action of venom from the brown recluse spider (Lososceles reclusa) on human neutrophils. Toxicon 1977;15:423–7.

20. Futrell JM, Morgan PN. Inhibition of human complement components by Loxosceles reclusa venom. Int Arch Allergy Appl Immunol 1978;57:275–8.

21. Kurpiewski G, Campbell JF, Forrester LJ, et al. Alternate complement pathway activation by recluse spider venom. Int J Tissue React 1981;3:39–45.

22. Wright SW, Wrenn KD, Murray L, et al. Clinical presentation and outcome of brown recluse spider bite. Ann Emerg Med 1997;30:28–32.

23. Wasserman GS. Brown recluse and other necrotizing spiders. In: Ford MD, Delaney KA, Ling LJ, et al, editors. Clinical Toxicology. Philadelphia: WB Saunders; 2001. p. 878–84.

24. Williams ST, Khare VK, Johnston GA, et al. Severe intravascular hemolysis associated with brown recluse spider envenomation. Am J Clin Pathol 1995;104:463–7.

25. Berger RS, Adelstein EH, Anderson PC. Intravascular coagulation: The cause of necrotic arachnidism. J Invest Dermatol 1973;61: 142–50.

26. de Souza AL, Malague CM, Sztajnbok J, et al. Loxosceles venom–induced cytokine activation, hemolysis and acute kidney injury. Toxicon 2008;51:151–6.

27. Pauli I, Puka J, Gubert IC, et al. The efficacy of antivenom in loxoscelism treatment. Toxicon 2006;48:123–37.

28. King LE, Rees RS. Dapsone treatment of a brown recluse bite. JAMA 1983;250:648.

29. Wesley RE, Close LW, Ballinger WH, et al. Dapsone in the treatment of presumed brown recluse spider bite of the eyelid. Ophthalmic Surg 1985;16:116–7, 120.

30. Barrett SM, Romine-Jenkins M, Fisher DE. Dapsone or electric shock therapy of brown recluse spider envenomation? Ann Emerg Med 1994;24:21–5.

31. Hobbs GD, Anderson AR, Greene TJ, et al. Comparison of hyperbaric oxygen and dapsone therapy for Loxosceles envenomation. Acad Emerg Med 1996;3:758–61.

32. Phillips S, Kohn M, Baker D, et al. Therapy of brown spider envenomation: A controlled trial of hyperbaric oxygen, dapsone and cyproheptadine. Ann Emerg Med 1995;25:363–8.

33. Wille RC, Morrow JD. Case report: Dapsone hypersensitivity syndrome associated with treatment of the bite of a brown recluse spider. Am J Med Sci 1988;296:270–1.

34. Lowry BP, Bradfield JF, Carroll RG, et al. A controlled trial of topical nitroglycerin in a New Zealand white rabbit model of brown recluse spider envenomation. Ann Emerg Med 2001;37:161–5.

35. Paixao-Cavalcante D, van den Berg CW, Goncalves-de-Andrade RM, et al. Tetracycline protects against dermanecrosis induced by. Loxosceles spider venom. J Invest Dermatol 2007;127:1410–18.

36. Strain GM, Snider TG, Tedford BL, et al. Hyperbaric oxygen effect on brown recluse spider (Loxosceles reclusa) envenomation in rabbits. Toxicon 1991;29:988–96.

37. Merchant ML, Hinton JF, Geren CR. Effect of hyperbaric oxygen on sphingomyelinase D activity of brown recluse spider (Loxosceles reclusa) venom as studied by 31P nuclear magnetic resonance spectroscopy. Am J Trop Med Hyg 1997;56:335–8.

38. Maynor ML, Moon RE, Klitzman B, et al. Brown recluse spider envenomation: A prospective trial of hyperbaric oxygen therapy. Acad Emerg Med 1997;4:184–92.

39. Gomez HF, Greenfield DM, Miller MJ, et al. Direct correlation between diffusion of Loxosceles reclusa venom and extent of dermal inflammation. Acad Emerg Med 2001;8:309–14.

40. Rees R, Shack B, Withers E, et al. Management of the brown recluse spider bite. Plast Reconstr Surg 1981;68:768–73.

41. Rees R, Altenbern DP, Lynch JB, et al. Brown recluse spider bites: A comparison of early surgical excision versus dapsone and delayed surgical excision. Ann Surg 1985;202:659–63.

42. Wasserman GS, Lowry JA. Loxosceles spiders. In: Brent J, Wallace KL, Burkhart KK, et al, editors. Critical Care Toxicology: Diagnosis and Management of the Critically Poisoned Patient. Philadelphia: Elsevier Mosby; 2005. p. 1195–203.

43. Wasserman GS, Anderson PC. Loxoscelism and necrotic arachnidism. Clin Toxicol 1983-1984;21:451–72.

44. Bond GR. Snake, spider, and scorpion envenomation in North America. Pediatr Rev 1999;20:147–51.

45. Kunkel DB. The sting of the arthropod. Emerg Med 1996; 28:136–41.

46. Clark RF, Wethern-Kestner S, Vance MV, et al. Clinical presentation and treatment of black widow spider envenomation: A review of 163 cases. Ann Emerg Med 1992;21:782–7.

47. Russell FE. Snake Venom Poisoning. Great Neck, NY: Scholium International; 1983.

48. Scharman EJ, Noffsinger NJ. Copperhead snakebites: Clinical severity of local effects. Ann Emerg Med 2001;38:55–61.

49. Thorson A, Lavonas EJ, Rouse AM, et al. Copperhead envenomations in the Carolinas. J Tox Clin Toxicol 2003;41:29–35.

50. Gold BS, Dart RC, Barish RA. Bite of venomous snakes. N Engl J Med 2002;347:347–56.

51. Dart RC, Hurlbut KM, Garcia R, et al. Validation of a severity score for the assessment of Crotalid snakebite. Ann Emerg Med 1996;27:321–6.

52. Cumpston KL. Is there a role for fasciotomy in crotaline envenomations in North America. Clin Toxicol 2011;49:351–65.

53. Shaw BA, Hosalkar HS. Rattlesnake bites in children: Antivenin treatment and surgical indications. J Bone Joint Surg Am 2002;84:1624–9.

54. Corneille MG, Larson S, Stewart RM, et al. A large single center experience with treatment of patients with Crotalid envenomations: Outcomes with and evolution of antivenin therapy. Am J Surg 2006;192:848–52.

55. Tanen DA, Danish DC, Clark RF. Crotalid polyvalent immune Fab antivenom limits the decrease in perfusion pressure of the anterior leg compartment in a porcine crotaline envenomation model. Ann Emerg Med 2003;41:384–90.

56. Gold BS, Barish RA, Dart RC, et al. Resolution of compartment syndrome after rattlesnake envenomation utilizing noninvasive measures. J Emerg Med 2003;24:285–8.

57. Tanen DA, Danish DC, Grice GA. Fasciotomy worsens the amount of myonecrosis in a porcine model of crotaline envenomation. Ann Emerg Med 2004;44:99–104.

58. Stewart RM, Page CP, Schwesinger WH, et al. Antivenin and fasciotomy/debridement in the treatment of severe rattlesnake bite. Am J Surg 1989;158:543–7.

59. Hall EL. Role of surgical intervention in the management of crotaline snake envenomation. Ann Emerg Med 2001;37:175–80.

60. Bond GR, Burkhart KK. Thrombocytopenia following timber rattlesnake envenomation. Ann Emerg Med 1997;30:40–4.

61. Carroll RR, Hall EL, Kitchens CS. Canebrake rattlesnake envenomation. Ann Emerg Med 1997;30:45–8.

62. Curry SC, O'Connor AD, Ruha AM. Rapid-onset shock and/or anaphylactoid reactions from rattlesnake bites in central Arizona [abstract]. J Med Toxicol 2010;6:241.

63. McKinney PE. Out-of-hospital and interhospital management of crotaline snakebite. Ann Emerg Med 2001;37:168–74.

64. Burgess JL, Dart RC, Egen NB, et al. Effects of constriction bands on rattlesnake venom absorption: A pharmacokinetic study. Ann Emerg Med 1992;21:1086–93.

65. Sutherland SK, Coulter AR. Early management of bites by eastern diamondback rattlesnake (Crotalus adamanteus) studies in monkeys (Macaca fascicularis). Am J Trop Med Hyg 1981;30:497–500.

66. Straight RC, Glenn JL. Effects of pressure/immobilization on the systemic and local action of venoms in a mouse tail model [abstract]. Toxicon 1985;23:40.

67. German BT, Hack JB, Brewer K, et al. Pressure-immobilization bandages delay toxicity in a porcine model of eastern coral snake (Micrurus fulvius fulvius) envenomation. Ann Emerg Med 2005;45:603–8.

68. Markenson D, Ferguson JD, Chameides L, et al. Part 17: First Aid: 2010 American Heart Association and American Red Cross Guidelines for First Aid. Circulation 2010;122(18 Suppl 3):S934–46.

69. Bush SP, Green SM, Laack TA, et al. Pressure immobilization delays mortality and increases intracompartmental pressure after artificial intramuscular rattlesnake envenomation in a porcine model. Ann Emerg Med 2004;44:599–604.

70. Meggs WJ, Courtney C, O'Rourke D, et al. Pilot studies of pressure-immobilization bandages for rattlesnake envenomations. Clin Toxicol 2010;48:61–3.

71. American College of Medical Toxicology, American Academy of Clinical Toxicology, American Association of Poison Control Centers, European Association of Poison Control Centers and Clinical Toxicologists, International Society on Toxinology, Asia

Pacific Association of Medical Toxicology. Pressure immobilization after North American Crotalinae snake envenomation. Clin Toxicol 2011;49:881–2.

72. Alberts MB, Shalit M, LoGolbo F. Suction for venomous snakebite: A study of 'mock venom' extraction in a human model. Ann Emerg Med 2004;43:181–6.

73. Bush SP, Hegewald KG, Green SM, et al. Effects of a negative pressure venom extraction device (extractor) on local tissue injury after artificial rattlesnake envenomation in a porcine model. Wilderness Environ Med 2000;11:180–8.

74. Wingert WA, Chan L. Rattlesnake bites in southern California and rationale for recommended treatment. West J Med 1988;148: 37–44.

75. Tokish JT, Benjamin J, Walter F. Crotalid envenomation: The southern Arizona experience. J Orthop Trauma 2001;15:5–9.

76. Arnold RE. Results of treatment of Crotalus envenomation. Am Surg 1975;41:643–7.

77. Brooks DE, Graeme KA, Ruha AM, et al. Respiratory compromise in patients with rattlesnake envenomation. J Emerg Med 2002;23:329–32.

78. LoVecchio F, Klemens J, Welch S, et al. Antibiotics after rattlesnake envenomation. J Emerg Med 2002;23:327–8.

79. Dart RC, McNally J. Efficacy, safety, and use of snake antivenoms in the United States. Ann Emerg Med 2001;37:181–8.

80. Dart RC, Seifert SA, Boyer LV, et al. A randomized multicenter trial of Crotalidae Polyvalent Immune Fab (ovine) antivenom for the treatment of crotaline snakebite in the United States. Arch Intern Med 2001;161:2030–6.

81. Lavonas EJ, Gerardo CJ, O'Malley G, et al. Initial experience with Crotalidae Polyvalent Immune Fab (ovine) antivenom in the treatment of copperhead snakebite. Ann Emerg Med 2004;43:200–6.

82. Dart RC, Seifert SA, Carroll L, et al. Affinity-purified, mixed monospecific crotalid antivenom ovine Fab for the treatment of crotalid venom poisoning. Ann Emerg Med 1997;30:33–9.

83. Ruha AM, Curry SC, Beuhler M, et al. Initial postmarketing experience with Crotalidae Polyvalent Immune Fab for the treatment of rattlesnake envenomation. Ann Emerg Med 2002;39:609–15.

84. Cannon R, Ruha AM, Kashani J. Acute hypersensitivity reactions associated with administration of Crotalidae Polyvalent Immune Fab antivenom. Ann Emerg Med 2008;51:407–11.

85. Pizon AF, Riley BD, LoVecchio F, et al. Safety and efficacy of Crotalidae Polyvalent Immune Fab in pediatric crotaline envenomations. Acad Emerg Med 2007;14:373–6.

86. Offerman SR, Bush SP, Moynihan JA, et al. Crotaline Fab antivenom for the treatment of children with rattlesnake envenomation. Pediatrics 2002;110:968–71.

87. Rowden AK, Holstege CP, Kirk MA. Pediatric copperhead envenomations [abstract]. Clin Toxicol 2007;45:644.

88. Rowden AK, Boylan VV, Wiley SH, et al. Crofab use for copperhead envenomation in the young [abstract]. Clin Toxicol 2006;44:696–7.

89. Feng S, Stephan M. What a bite—Review of snakebites in children [abstract]. Clin Toxicol 2005;43:712.

90. Spiller HA, Bosse GM. Prospective study of morbidity associated with snakebite envenomation. J Tox Clin Toxicol 2003;41: 125–30.

91. Seifert SA, Boyer LV. Recurrence phenomena after immunoglobulin therapy for snake envenomations: I. Pharmacokinetics and pharmacodynamics of immunoglobulin antivenoms and related antibodies. Ann Emerg Med 2001;37:189–95.

92. Seifert SA, Boyer LV, Dart RC, et al. Relationship of venom effects to venom antigen and antivenom serum concentrations in a patient with Crotalus atrox envenomation treated with a Fab antivenom. Ann Emerg Med 1997;30:49–53.

93. Bogdan GM, Dart RC, Falbo SC, et al. Recurrent coagulopathy after antivenom treatment of Crotalid snakebite. South Med J 2000;93:562–6.

94. Boyer LV, Seifert SA, Cain JS. Recurrence phenomena after immunoglobulin therapy for snake envenomations: II. Guidelines for clinical management with Crotaline Fab antivenom. Ann Emerg Med 2001;37:196–201.

95. Lavonas EJ, Ruha AM, Banner W, et al. Unified treatment algorithm for the management of crotaline snakebite in the United States: Results of an evidence-informed consensus workshop. BMC Emerg Med 2011;11:2.

96. Kitchens CS, Van Mierop LHS. Envenomation by the eastern coral snake (Micrurus fulvius fulvius). JAMA 1987;258:1615–18.

CHAPTER 13

BURNS

E. Marty Knott • Daniel J. Ostlie • David Juang

Over the past several decades, burn-related hospital admissions and deaths have decreased by 50% in large part due to advancements in burn care, introduction of topical antimicrobial agents, and a better understanding of fluid resuscitation and aggressive surgical management.[1–3] Despite these advances, nearly 100,000 children age 14 years and under were treated for burns in hospital emergency rooms in 2007. Of these, 20% occurred in children less than 4 years old.[4] Thus, burns remain a leading cause of morbidity and mortality in children. Optimal management requires a team of health care providers, therapists, and social workers.

PATHOPHYSIOLOGY

Skin is a complex, multilayer organ with a surface area ranging from 0.2–0.3 m^2 in the newborn to 1.5–2.0 m^2 in the adult. An understanding of its basic structure and regenerating ability is critical to burn management. The skin provides protection, participates in thermoregulation and vitamin D production, and is involved in sensation. The epidermis is the avascular and aneural superficial layer made up of keratinocytes (95%), melanocytes, Langerhans cells, and Merkel cells. Desquamation of cells formed at the basal layer takes 2 to 4 weeks. The entire epidermis is replaced by new cells every 48 days. The dermis has a deep reticular layer and a superficial papillary region that are connected to the epidermis via the basement membrane. Composed primarily of collagen and elastin from fibroblasts, the dermis provides support for the skin.

The mechanism of any burn plays an important role in how deep and severe the injury will extend as well as how it is treated. The extent of injury is determined by the temperature, duration of exposure, skin thickness, and specific heat of the causative agent. Grease burns result in deeper injury than water of the same temperature, since lipid has a higher specific heat. Scald burns constitute 70% of pediatric burns with the majority occurring in toddlers. Whether due to spilling hot drinks or hot tap water, they tend to be superficial dermal burns. Flame burns are more common in adolescents and can result in deep injury. Contact burns are also common in children and may be caused by touching a hot oven door, an iron, or even hot pavement.

In 1953, Jackson described the zones of burn injury that remain important to the understanding and management of burns today (Fig. 13-1).[5] The zone of coagulation occurs at the site of maximal damage and is defined by irreversible tissue loss due to protein coagulation. The zone of stasis surrounds this area and has decreased tissue perfusion, but remains salvageable with aggressive resuscitation. Outside the zone of stasis is the zone of hyperemia where tissue perfusion is increased and often survives unless faced with infection or hypotension.

The systemic response to burn injury is mediated by the release of inflammatory mediators such as thromboxane A2, bradyknin, oxidants, and cytokines which can impair flow to the zone of stasis through thrombosis, vasoconstriction, and capillary blockage.[6] The administration of antioxidants, bradykinin antagonists, and thromboxane A2 inhibitors can improve blood flow and mitigate injury.[7–9] In addition, the administration of β-glucan, through its immunomodulatory effects, antioxidant properties, and ability to reduce the inflammatory response, has been shown to improve re-epithelialization in a rat model of burn injury.[10]

The systemic effects of burn injury extend beyond these three zones and can potentially lead to multiorgan dysfunction. The cardiovascular system can experience myocardial depression and hypovolemia. Pulmonary vasoconstriction and edema lead to respiratory failure.[11] Splanchnic vasoconstriction can result in gut dysmotility and malabsorption by causing epithelial apoptosis and decreased epithelial proliferation.[12–14] This results in atrophy of small bowel mucosa, increased intestinal permeability, bacterial translocation, and sepsis.[15] Splanchnic vasoconstriction and activation of stress-induced hormones and mediators, such as angiotensin, aldosterone, and vasopressin, leads to a decrease in renal perfusion that can lead to oliguria.[16] When unrecognized, this can progress to acute tubular necrosis, renal failure, and, ultimately, death.[17,18] Finally, there is a systemic decrease in immune function due to impaired production and function of neutrophils, macrophages and T-lymphocytes, placing the patient at risk for infectious complications.[19,20]

INITIAL MANAGEMENT

The majority of pediatric burns are minor, often resulting from scald accidents and affecting less than 10% total body surface area (TBSA), or from thermal injuries isolated to the hands. Such burns are usually limited to partial-thickness injury of the skin and can be managed on an outpatient basis, which is beyond the scope of this chapter. Unfortunately, larger burns require inpatient treatment and special attention. The initial step is completion of the primary and secondary surveys.[21] Issues with airway, breathing, and circulation should be

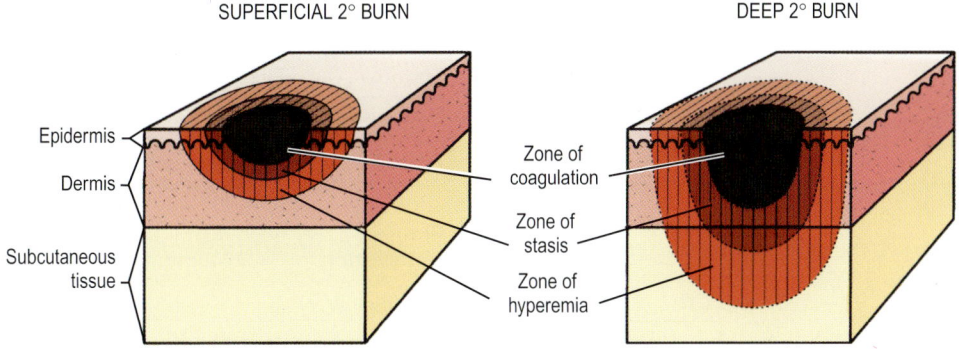

SUPERFICIAL 2° BURN DEEP 2° BURN

Epidermis
Dermis
Subcutaneous tissue

Zone of coagulation
Zone of stasis
Zone of hyperemia

FIGURE 13-1 ■ Three zones of burn injury: coagulation, stasis, and hyperemia.

addressed immediately. Signs and symptoms including increased respiratory effort, wheezing, stridor, and tachypnea should raise concern for impending loss of the airway. The decision to intubate a patient with a tenuous airway should be made early. Inhalation injury can result in edema that may worsen over the first few hours, so repeated evaluations of the airway are important. Burn injuries can have a negative effect on breathing mechanics through smoke inhalation, a blast injury causing blunt chest trauma, and the restrictive effects of a burn eschar that limits full chest expansion. Escharotomy should be performed for the latter. Patients need support with 100% supplemental oxygen. If inhalation injury is suspected, arterial blood gas analysis and carboxyhemoglobin level are needed. Two large bore IVs should be placed and aggressive fluid resuscitation is important. When extremity burns limit peripheral IV access or if there is difficulty obtaining central venous access, intraosseus access should be utilized as a temporary (<24 hours) alternate route for fluid administration. A urinary catheter should be inserted, and heart rate, blood pressure and urine output should be monitored as tachycardia and low urine output signal a low intravascular volume state.

The source of thermal injury needs to be removed from the patient as quickly as possible, even during the primary survey, if not done before. Active cooling may limit the depth of the burn but can result in hypothermia. Chemicals need to be removed from the skin and the area should be thoroughly irrigated with water. Neutralization of chemicals is not needed and may produce additional heat that could lead to a deeper burn. Care should be taken to keep the patient warm as the risk of hypothermia increases with increasing burn area.

A decision should be made after initial evaluation, resuscitation, and wound dressing as to whether or not the patient needs to be transferred to a burn center. The American Burn Association and American College of Surgeons have clear recommendation regarding which patients should be referred to these centers (Box 13-1).[22] However, a recent study raises concern that resources are often wasted by transferring less severe injuries to burn centers.[23]

There are several techniques to estimate the TBSA of the burn. The Wallace rule of nines estimates burn area fairly well for adolescents. Each upper extremity and the head represent 9% of the TBSA. The lower extremities

BOX 13-1 | **Major Burn Injury Criteria (American Burn Association)**

Second-degree burns >10% TBSA in patients younger than 10 years of age
Third-degree burns >5% TBSA
Burns involving the face, hands, feet, genitalia, perineum, and major joints
Chemical burns
Electrical burns including lightning injury
Inhalation injury
Burns with significant concomitant trauma
Burns with significant preexisting medical disorders

TBSA, total body surface area.

and the anterior and posterior trunks are 18% each. The perineum, genitalia, and neck each measures 1%. Due to differences in body proportions for infants and children, the rule of nines has been modified to more accurately determine burn area in these patients. In this modification, the head represents 18% of the TBSA and each leg is 13.5%. Other modifications have been proposed to better estimate TBSA burn in obese patients.[24] The Lund and Browder chart may provide more accurate determination of burn area in children as it compensates for variations in body shape and proportions (Fig. 13-2). For a rapid estimation of burn size, the palmar method can be used. The palmar surface is approximately 1% of the TBSA and is best used for estimating small surface area burns. First-degree burns should not be included in burn size calculations using any of these techniques. A recent study found that estimates of burn area are inaccurate in approximately 80% of children with the majority being overestimated.[25] The authors concluded that this may be due to the variety of techniques used, or inclusion of first-degree burns in the calculation. This can also lead to unnecessary transfer of patients to burn care centers as discussed previously.

A key component to the initial management of the severely burned patient includes escharotomy when indicated (Fig. 13-3). Full-thickness circumferential burns on the extremities can produce a constricting eschar which, together with the associated edema, can impede venous outflow and impair arterial flow. If pulses are absent, a bedside escharotomy should be performed with a scalpel or electrocautery along the lateral and medial aspects of

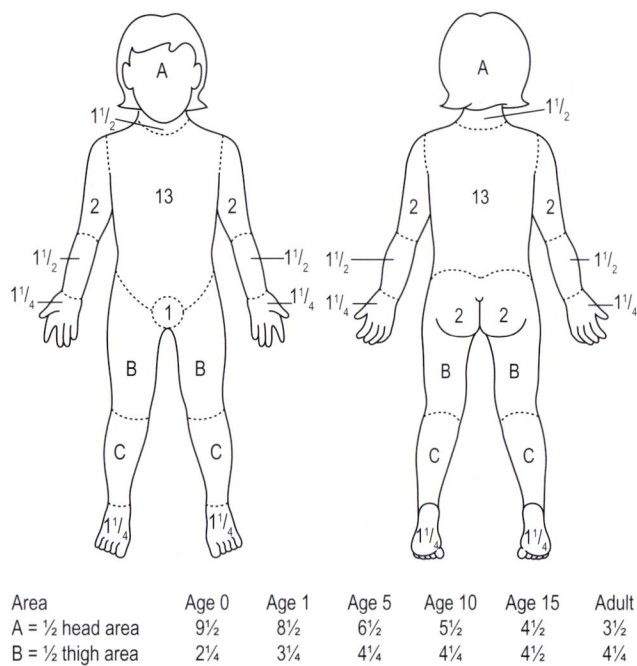

Area	Age 0	Age 1	Age 5	Age 10	Age 15	Adult
A = ½ head area	9½	8½	6½	5½	4½	3½
B = ½ thigh area	2¼	3¼	4¼	4¼	4½	4¼
C = ½ leg area	2½	2½	3	3	3¼	3½

FIGURE 13-2 ■ The Lund–Browder burn diagram is depicted for estimating the body surface area for burns in children.

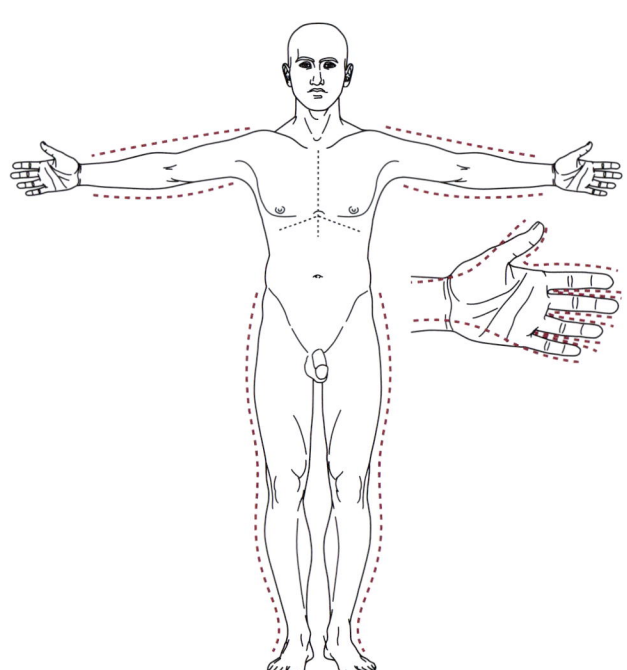

FIGURE 13-3 ■ Escharatomies. The incisions are made on the medial and lateral aspects of the extremity. Hand escharotomies are performed on the medial and lateral digits and on the dorsum of the hand. (From Eichelberger MR [ed]; Pediatric Trauma: Prevention, Acute Care, Rehabilitation. St Louis, Mosby, 1993.)

TABLE 13-1   Burn Resuscitation Formulas

Formula	First 24 Hours	Fluid Solution
Parkland	4 mL/kg per %TBSA burn	Lactated Ringer's (LR)
Brooke	1.5 mL/kg per %TBSA burn	LR + colloid 0.5 mL/kg per %TBSA burn
Shriners–Galveston	5000 mL/m² burned + 2000 mL/m² total	LR + 12.5 g albumin

TBSA, total body surface area

TABLE 13-2   Formulas for Body Surface Area (BSA)

Dubois Formula	BSA (m²) = height (cm)$^{0.725}$ × weight (kg)$^{0.425}$ × 0.007184
Jacobson Formula	BSA (m²) = [height (cm) + weight (kg) − 60]/100

compartment pressures. Although rare, fasciotomy may be necessary to relieve pressure and prevent necrosis of the underlying muscles and neurovascular bundles.

FLUID RESUSCITATION

Once adequate intravenous or intraosseous access is obtained, fluid resuscitation is initiated. There are several formulas available to guide this resuscitation (Table 13-1). The Parkland formula is the most widely used, but is not as applicable in young children because children have greater TBSA relative to their body weight than adults. As a result, weight-based formulas can under-resuscitate children with minor burns and can grossly over-resuscitate children with extensive burns.[26] TBSA-based formulas, such as the Shriners–Galveston formula, are therefore better at estimating fluid requirements in children less than 20 kg.[27] TBSA is assessed from height and weight using standard nomograms or calculated using formulas (Table 13-2). Dextrose-containing solutions, such as 5% dextrose with 0.25 to 0.5 normal saline, are used as the primary solution. Children younger than 2 years of age are susceptible to hypoglycemia due to limited glycogen stores. Therefore, lactated Ringer's solution with 5% dextrose is given during the first 24 hours in these patients.

Regardless of which formula is utilized, there must be close monitoring of the patient's physiologic response to the fluid administration. Urine output should be maintained at 1 mL/kg/h. Inadequate resuscitation can result in hypoperfusion to the zone of stasis, with subsequent deepening of the burn, as well as hypoperfusion of major organs. During the first six to 12 hours, capillary permeability is increased and fluid moves from the intravascular space to the interstitial tissues with worsening edema. Overly aggressive fluid administration can result in significant tissue edema, tissue hypoxia, and elevated compartment pressures.[28]

Several authors have shown that the addition of colloid solutions such as albumin can reduce crystalloid

the affected extremity. Incisions can be carried onto the hypothenar and thenar eminences and dorsolateral aspects of the digits if the hands or fingers are involved (Fig. 13-4). The resulting ischemia reperfusion injury and edema can cause significant increases in fascial

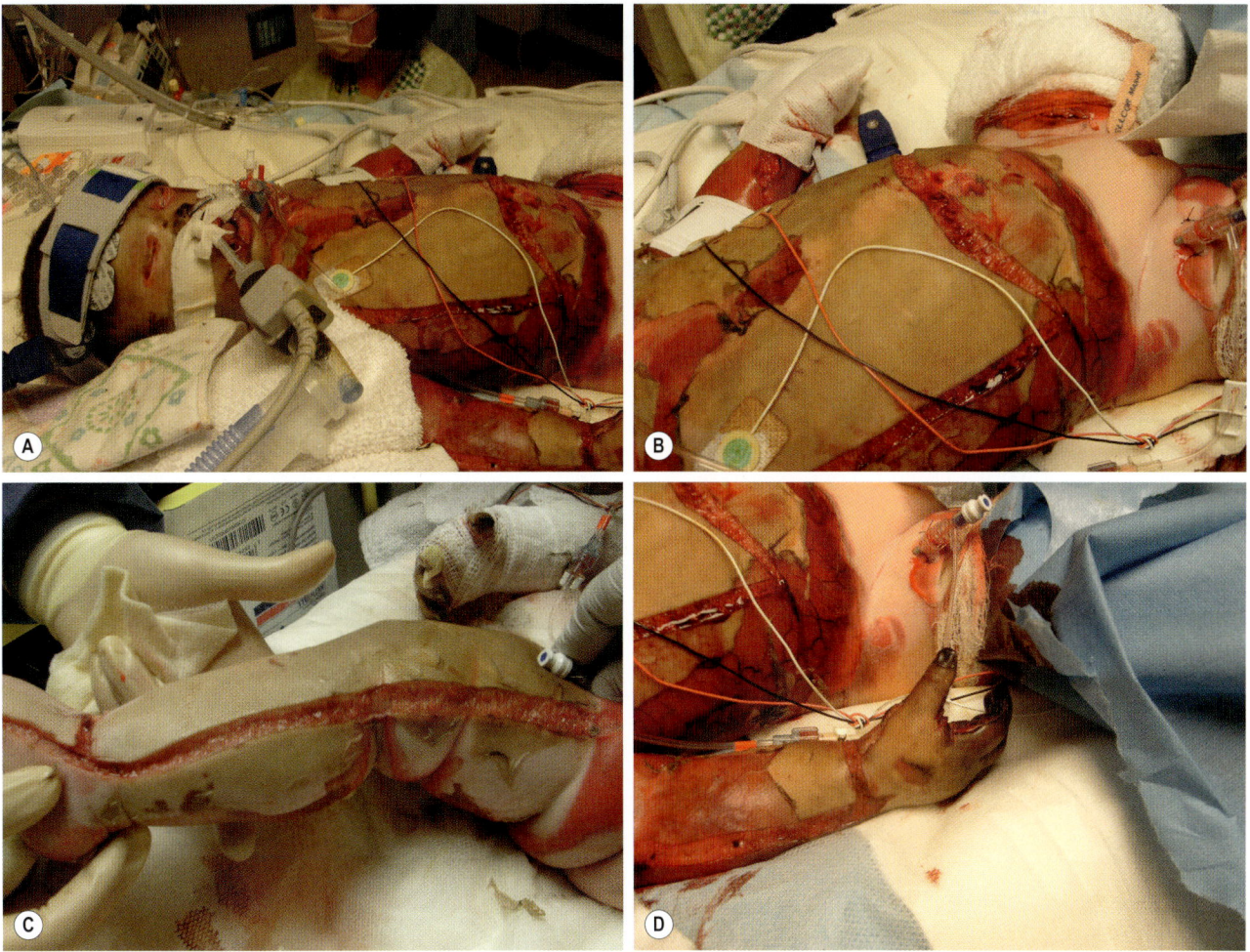

FIGURE 13-4 ■ A 3-year-old male transferred after being rescued from a house fire. He required extensive escharotomies of the **(A,B)** chest and **(C)** distal extremities during the initial resuscitation. **(D)** Incisions should be carried onto the hypothenar and thenar eminences and dorsolateral aspects of the digits if the hands or fingers are involved.

requirements and more rapidly establish a balanced fluid intake to output ratio.[29,30] However, a 2011 Cochrane database review found that albumin does not lower mortality in adults with major burns.[31] Thus, the benefit of the more expensive albumin instead of standard crystalloid solutions is questionable. Other solutions, such as hypertonic saline, have been used in an effort to provide a high osmotic pressure which is thought to keep more volume in the intravascular space. Hypertonic saline also may have anti-inflammatory effects. However, it should be used with caution as it causes hypernatremia, and has not been shown to improve outcomes for hypotensive trauma patients.[32]

Unlike adults, children do not show hemodynamic changes reflecting hypovolemia until they are significantly volume depleted. Tachycardia may be a sign of compensation for a low volume state or stress response to injury. Signs of inadequate perfusion include lethargy and decreased capillary refill with cool, clammy extremities. Laboratory tests should be performed along with serial clinical exams to follow the response to resuscitation. Resolving acidosis, for example, may serve as an objective marker of improvement. Hyponatremia is a frequent complication in pediatric burn patients after

aggressive fluid resuscitation, and correction is required to avoid severe electrolyte imbalance.

An increased incidence of pneumonia, bloodstream infection, acute respiratory distress syndrome (ARDS), multiple-organ failure, and death may be associated with over-resuscitation during the first 24 hours postburn.[33] Interestingly, 'permissive hypovolemia' helps avoid these complications and has been shown to decrease multiple-organ dysfunction.[34]

Inhalation Injury

While inhalation injury is less common in children than adults, the mortality increases to nearly 40% when it occurs.[35] The heat of inhaled gas causes upper airway injury. Inhaled toxins can result in upper airway injury in addition to causing tracheobronchial irritation and bronchoconstriction. Damaged epithelium releases vasoactive substances (thromboxanes A2, C3a, and C5a) that lead to hypoxia, increased airway resistance, decreased pulmonary compliance, increased alveolar epithelial permeability, and increased pulmonary vascular resistance.[36] Carbon monoxide (CO) is produced during combustion and can contribute to the inhalational injury by displacing oxygen from hemoglobin-binding sites. The oxyhemoglobin dissociation curve is shifted to the left as the ability of hemoglobin to unload oxygen in the tissues is decreased. Secondary injury is due to impaired ciliary clearance of airway debris. Neutrophil infiltration occurs, macrophages are destroyed, and bacteria accumulate leading to pneumonia.

An inhalation injury should be recognized early through a detailed history of the burn and the initial evaluation. On examination, patients may be found to have facial burns, singed hairs in the nose, eyebrows or head, and/or carbonaceous sputum. Patients with inhalation injury who are obtunded are likely to have a carboxyhemoglobin level greater than 10%. Additional signs of significant injury are an altered voice along with hoarseness and stridor. Airway security in these patients is imperative. Fiberoptic bronchoscopy continues to be the preferred technique for documenting inhalation injury. Inflammatory changes in the tracheal mucosa such as edema, hyperemia, mucosal ulceration, and sloughing can be visualized. A ventilation scan with xenon-133 can also identify regions of inhalation injury by assessing respiratory exchange and excretion of xenon-133 from the lungs.[37] When combined, bronchoscopy and xenon-133 scanning are over 90% accurate in the diagnosis of inhalation injury. However, the clinical applicability of xenon-133 scans remains unclear due to false positives in children with pulmonary disease.[38,39] They may also be potentially dangerous due to the need to transport a critically ill burn patient to a nuclear medicine suite. Chest radiographs are not useful as they are often normal immediately following injury.[38,40] Bedside bronchoscopy and a heightened clinical suspicion remain paramount in the diagnosis and treatment of these injuries.

After the airway is secured, an inhalation treatment protocol is utilized in the intensive care unit that focuses on the clearance of secretions and control of bronchospasm. One hundred per cent high flow, humidified oxygen should be administered to displace CO from hemoglobin. Early and aggressive pulmonary therapy

consisting of chest physiotherapy, frequent suctioning, and early mobilization of the patient should be started. Bronchodilators and racemic epinephrine are used to treat bronchospasm. Clearance of secretions can be assisted with inhalation treatments composed of heparin and acetylcysteine. Human autopsy and animal models have shown nebulized heparin (5000–10,000 units/3 mL of NS q5 hours) to reduce tracheobronchial cast formation improves minute ventilation and decreases peak inspiratory pressures after smoke inhalation.[41–43] The addition of 20% acetylcysteine (3 mL q4 hours) also improves the clearance of tracheobronchial secretions and minimizes bronchospasm. Pediatric and adult studies have shown this combination of medications to decrease reintubation rates and reduce mortality.[44–46]

ASSESSMENT OF BURN DEPTH

Burn injury may involve one or both layers of the skin and may even extend to the subcutaneous fat, muscle, and bone.[47] First-degree burns involve the epidermis. They are erythematous and very painful. Most sunburns fit this category of superficial, epidermal injury. For first-degree burns, topical ointments may be used for symptom relief and the involved areas should be kept out of the sunlight.

Superficial second-degree burns (superficial dermal burns) extend into the papillary dermis. They characteristically form blisters, but these blisters may not immediately follow the injury, making determination of depth difficult (Fig. 13-5). These wounds are painful when uncovered. The wound blanches with pressure due to increased vascularity secondary to vasodilatation. Superficial second-degree burns are managed with daily dressing changes with topical antimicrobials. They may also be treated with application of petroleum gauze or a synthetic dressing to allow for rapid spontaneous re-epithelialization. With appropriate care, these wounds will heal spontaneously within two to three weeks without the need for excision and grafting.

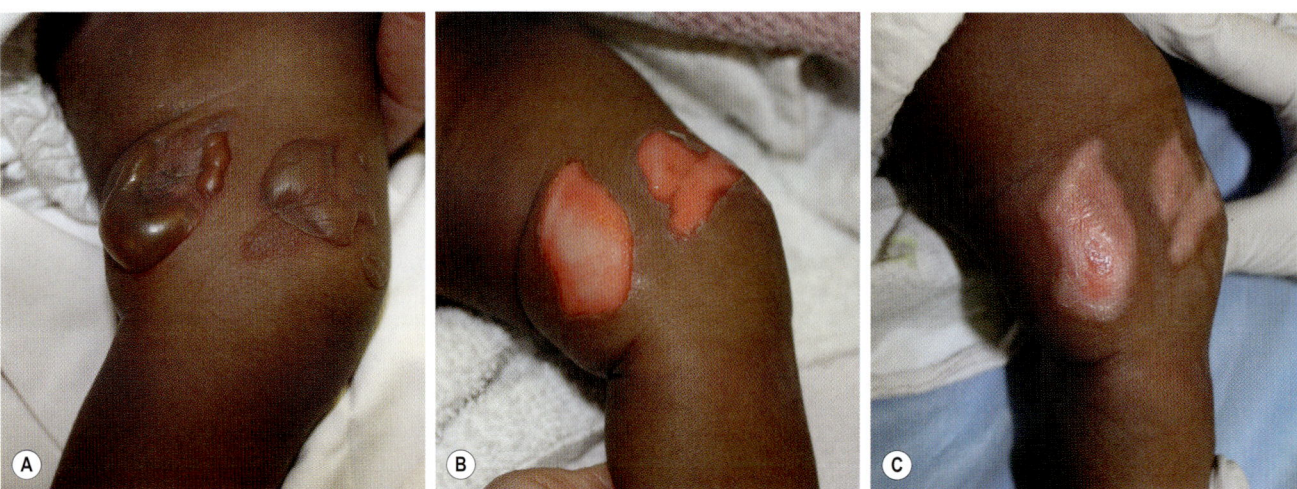

FIGURE 13-5 ■ A superficial second-degree burn of the lower extremity is shown. **(A)** The characteristic blisters seen with this degree of burn injury. **(B)** After removal of the blister, the wounds are painful and blanch when pressure is applied. **(C)** The progress of healing after several days of daily dressing changes with topical antimicrobials.

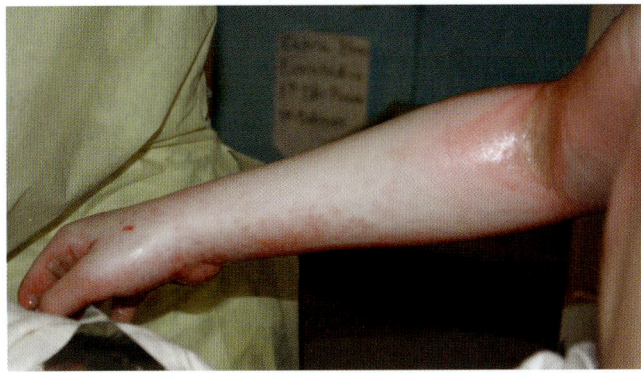

FIGURE 13-6 ■ A deep second-degree burn of the right upper extremity is seen. Note the mottled and white appearance of the extremity.

Deep second-degree burns (deep dermal burns) extend into the reticular dermis and healing takes several weeks. These burns also blister, but the surface of the wound remains mottled and white (Fig. 13-6). Blanching occurs very slowly. Patients complain of pressure and discomfort rather than pain. These burns will require operative treatment if healing does not occur by 3 weeks.

Third-degree or full-thickness burns involve the entire dermis and extend into the subcutaneous tissue. These appear charred, leathery, and firm (Fig. 13-7). Patients typically are insensate in the burned regions and may not feel pressure. Blanching does not occur when pressure is applied. Full-thickness injuries should be excised and grafted early.[48]

Determination of burn wound depth can sometimes be difficult. Initial evaluation by an experienced surgeon as to whether an indeterminate dermal burn will heal in three weeks is only about 50–70% accurate.[49–51] Scald injuries are particularly difficult to assess for depth and extent of injury. A number of techniques or tools have been described to improve accuracy. These techniques utilize the physiology of the skin and the alterations that

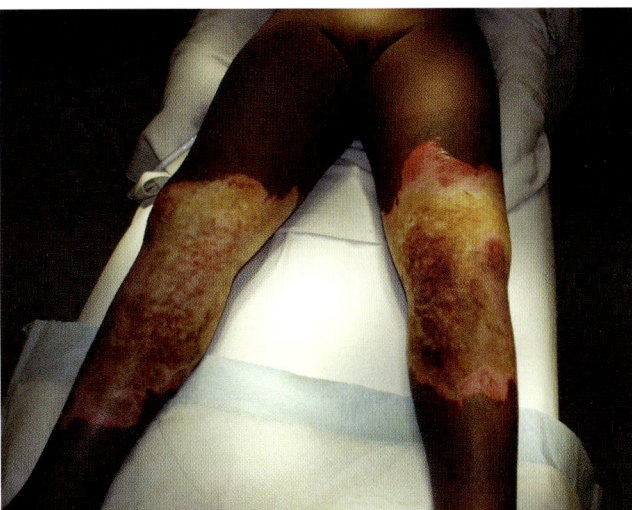

FIGURE 13-7 ■ Bilateral lower extremity burns are shown. The outside areas of the burns are second degree while the central areas are third degree with eschar. Note the 'leathery' appearance of the areas that are third degree in depth.

occur with burn injury. Detection of dead cells or denatured collagen using ultrasound, biopsy, or vital dyes has been trialed.[52–55] Other technologies such as analyzing altered blood flow using fluorescein, laser doppler imaging, and thermography have shown some promise.[56–58] Unfortunately, many of these techniques have not been adopted due to variable reproducibility. Laser Doppler imaging has been shown to increase the accuracy of burn depth assessment when compared with experienced burn surgeons.[59] Videomicroscopy has also been found to be accurate, especially when used after the first 24 hours.[60] This technique is relatively inexpensive and easy to learn.

WOUND CARE

Most partial-thickness burns can be managed nonoperatively for ten to 14 days with topical therapies and dressings. Using this strategy, the goal of burn care is to provide an optimal environment for re-epithelialization by providing a warm and moist environment, removal of exudate and potentially contaminated or necrotic material (eschar), and control of bacterial proliferation. Burns should be excised and grafted if there are no signs of healing by three weeks. Desai et al confirmed the validity of this strategy with scald injuries in a randomized trial.[61]

Antimicrobial agents

The initial treatment of partial-thickness burns is debridement and coverage with a topical agent that has antibacterial properties and allows for separation of the burn eschar.[62–64] Various topical antimicrobial agents have been used (Table 13-3). These agents decrease bacterial content, but they do not eradicate or prevent colonization. In general, quantitative wound biopsy cultures that exceed 100,000 organisms per gram are consistent with, although not diagnostic of, invasive infection.

Silver sulfadiazine (Silvadene, Monarch Pharmaceuticals Inc., Bristol, TN) is currently the most commonly used topical antimicrobial agent for burn care. It is a white, highly insoluble compound synthesized from silver nitrate and sodium sulfadiazine.[65] It has a broad spectrum of efficacy including *Staphylococcus aureus*, *Escherichia coli*, *Klebsiella*, *Pseudomonas*, and *Proteus* species. It also possesses an analgesic effect but does not penetrate eschar well. The combination of silver sulfadiazine with nystatin has significantly reduced the incidence of *Candida* infection in burned patients.[66] The most common side effect from silver sulfadiazine is leukopenia which is caused by margination of leukocytes and is usually transient.[67] It occurs somewhere between 5–15% of patients treated.[68] Changing to another topical antimicrobial agent usually resolves this side effect.

Mafenide acetate (Sulfamylon, UDC Laboratories, Inc, Rockford IL) was introduced as a topical burn agent in the mid-1960s. It is more effective in penetrating eschar and is frequently used in third-degree burns. It has broad activity against most Gram-negative and Gram-positive pathogens, but unfortunately has minimal antifungal activity.[69] The application of Sulfamylon can be

TABLE 13-3 **Burn Wound Dressings**

Dressings	Advantages	Disadvantages
Antimicrobial Salves		
Silver sulfadiazine (Silvadene)	Painless; broad spectrum; rare sensitivity	Leukopenia; some Gram-negative resistance; mild inhibition of epithelialization
Mafenide acetate (Sulfamylon)	Broad spectrum; penetrates eschar; effective against Pseudomonas	Painful; metabolic acidosis; mild inhibition of epithelialization
Bacitracin/Neomycin/Polymyxin B	Ease of application, painless, useful on face	Limited antimicrobial property
Nystatin	Effective in inhibiting fungal growth; use in combination with Silvadene, Bacitracin	Cannot use in combination with mafenide acetate
Mupirocin (Bactroban)	Effective against Staphylococcus, including MRSA	Cost; poor eschar penetration
Antimicrobial Soaks		
0.5% Silver nitrate	Painless; broad spectrum; rare sensitivity	No eschar penetration; discolors contacted areas; electrolyte imbalance; methemoglobinemia
Povidone-iodine (Betadine)	Broad-spectrum antimicrobial	Painful; potential systemic absorption; hypersensitivity
5% Mafenide acetate	Broad-spectrum antimicrobial	Painful; no fungal coverage; metabolic acidosis
0.025% Sodium hypochlorite (Dakin's solution)	Effective against most organisms	Mildly inhibits epithelialization
0.25% Acetic acid	Effective against most organisms	Mildly inhibits epithelialization
Silver Impregnated		
Aquacel, Acticoat	Broad-spectrum antimicrobial; no dressing changes	Cost
Synthetic Dressings		
Biobrane	Provides wound barrier; minimizes pain; useful for outpatient burns, hands (gloves)	Exudate accumulation risks invasive wound infection; no antimicrobial property
OpSite, Tegaderm	Provides moisture barrier; minimizes pain; useful for outpatient burns; inexpensive	Exudate accumulation risks invasive wound infection; no antimicrobial property
Transcyte	Provides wound barrier; accelerates wound healing	Exudate accumulation risks invasive wound infection; no antimicrobial property
Integra, Alloderm	Complete wound closure, including dermal substitute	No antimicrobial property; expensive; requires training, experience
Biologic Dressings		
Allograft (cadaver skin), Xenograft (pig skin)	Temporary biologic dressings	Requires access to skin bank; cost
Amniotic membrane	Minimizes dressing changes	Not widely used

MRSA, methicillin-resistant *S. aureus*.

painful which limits its practical use in the outpatient setting. Sulfamylon is a potent carbonic anhydrase inhibitor and can therefore cause metabolic acidosis.[70] This side effect can usually be avoided by limiting its use to only 20% TBSA at any given time, and rotating application sites every several hours with another topical antimicrobial agent.

Silver nitrate (0.5%) was also introduced in the mid-1960s. It is typically used to soak gauze dressings thereby avoiding frequent dressing changes with the potential loss of grafts or healing cells. Silver nitrate is painless on application and has broad coverage. Unfortunately, the compound can cause hyponatremia and hypochloremia while also creating dark gray or black stains. Another important but infrequent complication is methemoglobinemia, which occurs as a result of nitrate reduction by wound bacteria followed by the systemic absorption of the toxic nitrite. Dressings containing biologically active silver ions

(Aquacel, ConvaTec Ltd., UK; Acticoat, Smith & Nephew, London, UK) hold promise for retaining the effectiveness of silver nitrate but without its side effects. Several favorable clinical trials utilizing these products have been conducted and have found these products to be as effective as traditional dressings utilizing silver nitrate. The products were also noted to be less painful than traditional dressings when applied and removed, and also were associated with decreased burn wound cellulitis.[71–73]

Facial burns, small areas of partial-thickness burns, and healing donor sites require special mention. On superficial facial wounds, silver sulfadiazine may retard epithelialization and is not usually placed on the face.[74] An alternative is petroleum-based antimicrobial ointments. These include polymyxin B, bacitracin, and polysporin. Their application is painless and transparent which allows for easier monitoring. These agents are mostly effective against Gram-positive organisms.

Proteolytic enzymatic agents have been utilized to debride wounds, including proteases (sultilains) elaborated from *Bacillus subtilis*, collagenase, and papaine-urea. Collagen is a protein that is found normally in skin (~75% of dry weight of skin) and is the dominant protein that must be lysed to allow for eschar separation. Collagenase is an exogenous enzyme that breaks down denatured collagen but does not lyse healthy, normal collagen. Collagenase Santyl ointment (Healthpoint Biotherapeutics, Fort Worth, TX) is used in many burn units for the treatment of partial-thickness burns. A multicenter trial of 79 patients ranging in age from 5 to 60 years suggested a slight acceleration of wound closure compared to silver sulfadiazine.[75] A recent prospective randomized study in children comparing collagenase to silver sulfadiazine showed equivalent outcomes with regards to skin graft rates, hospitalization, and hospital charges.[76]

Burn Wound Dressings

The concept of an 'optimal environment' is derived from the work carried out by Winter in 1962.[77] In young pigs, he found that partial-thickness wounds that were kept moistened with polyethylene film epithelialized twice as fast as those left exposed to air. Hinman and Maiback confirmed this observation with a series of human volunteers.[78] Therefore, for 50 years, it has been felt that a burn dressing should provide an 'optimal environment' while also possessing bacterial inhibition. Typically, burn dressings consist of mesh that either contains or are placed over antimicrobial compounds. Nonadherent dressings such as Telfa (Tyco Healthcare Group LP, Mansfield, MA), Xeroform (Tyco Healthcare Group LP, Mansfield, MA), Adaptic (Johnson & Johnson, New Brunswick, NJ), or Mepitel (Molnlycke Health Care AB Gothenburg, Sweden) can be placed directly on the wound to help reduce both the pain associated with dressing changes and the friction associated damage to the wound or skin graft. The nonadherent dressing and antimicrobial compound serve to provide the 'optimal environment' for re-epithelialization.

Further advancements with burn dressings have recently led to a number of synthetic mesh products designed to adhere to wounds until epithelialization has occurred. The benefits of these dressings include less pain related to fewer dressing changes. These dressings are very effective for superficial partial-thickness wounds. Deep wounds and those with excessive drainage do not allow adherence, and therefore, negate the benefits of these synthetic dressings.

An example of a synthetic mesh product is Biobrane (UCL Laboratories, Rockford IL). It is a bilaminate thin membrane composed of thin semipermeable silicone bonded to a layer of nylon mesh, which is coated with a monomolecular layer of type I collagen of porcine origin. This dressing provides a hydrophilic coating for fibrin ingrowth which promotes wound adherence. The dressing is placed on a clean fresh superficial second-degree burn wound and can be secured using steri-strips and/or bandages. This dressing is easily removed from the wound bed as the wound epithelializes underneath it. Fluid can accumulate under the dressing and can be aspirated if needed. However, if a foul-smelling exudate is detected, the Biobrane should be removed and an antimicrobial dressing applied. Biobrane is now widely used in the management of superficial second-degree burns as it reduces pain, fluid, and electrolyte loss. These advantages make it an ideal dressing for use in the outpatient setting.[79]

Dressings that are commonly utilized for coverage of postoperative incisions may also be used as small superficial second-degree burn dressings. These alternatives include Duoderm (ER Squibb & Sons, Inc. Princeton NJ), Opsite (Smith & Nephew, London, UK), and Tegaderm (3M Pharmaceuticals, St Paul MN). Despite lacking special biological factors (collagen and growth factors), these dressings provide a cheap and transparent alternative to more expensive dressings. Also, Duoderm has been found to be less expensive than Biobrane and therefore could be a first-line treatment option for intermediate thickness burn wounds in children.[80]

The disfigurement resulting from full-thickness burns has been decreased with the advent of combined synthetic and biologic materials. Integra (Integra LifeSciences Corp, Plainsboro NJ) has an inner layer composed of a porous matrix of bovine collagen and the glycosaminoglycan chrondroitin-6-sulfate which facilitates fibrovascular ingrowth.[81] The outer layer is a polysiloxane polymer with vapor transmission characteristics similar to normal epithelium. Integra acts as a dermal replacement. It provides a matrix for the infiltration of fibroblasts, macrophages, lymphocytes, and capillaries from the wound bed, and promotes rapid neo-dermis formation. Approximately two weeks after engraftment, the outer silicone layer is removed and is replaced with an epidermal split thickness autograft (Fig. 13-8). Integra covered wounds have less scarring, but are susceptible to infection and must be monitored carefully. Its advantages were validated in a randomized study in children with large TBSA burns.[82] Children treated with Integra demonstrated significantly decreased resting energy expenditure as well as increased bone mineral content and density. Also, improved scarring was found at 24 months after burn injury.

Biological dressings include xenografts from swine and allografts from cadaver donors, such as Alloderm (LifeCell Corp., Branchburg, NJ). They are especially useful for coverage of large full-thickness burns. The dressings are eventually rejected by the patient's immune system and slough. The wound beds become excellent recipient beds for subsequent autografts. Although extremely rare, the transmission of viral diseases from the allograft is a potential concern. These dressings are useful adjuncts when autografts are not available or time is needed for donor sites to heal before being used again for grafting.

Excision and Grafting

Prompt burn excision and grafting has been shown to improve survival, decrease length of hospitalization, and reduce costs in burn patients of all ages. Children particularly have benefited from more timely and extensive operative management.[81–86] Once a burn is considered 'deep' or fails to heal with topical care, tangential excision

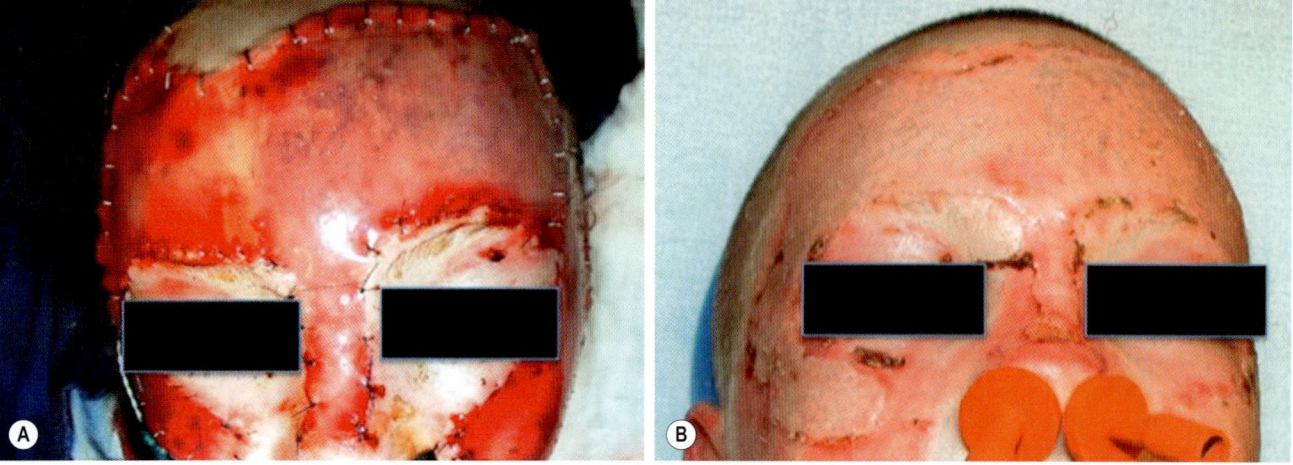

FIGURE 13-8 ■ The use of Integra for a superior cosmetic result in a child with facial burns is depicted. **(A)** The application of the Integra with the silicone layer in place. Approximately two weeks after placement, the silicone layer is removed and split thickness skin grafts are placed. **(B)** The same child after skin grafting over the Integra.

is needed. This technique was originally described by Janzekovic in 1970.[87] The eschar is sequentially shaved using a dermatome, knife blade or, more recently, a Versajet (Smith & Nephew, Inc., London, UK) water dissector until a viable tissue bed is obtained.[88] In a prospective randomized trial, the Versajet technique was shown to produce a more precise and faster excision than hand-held dermatome escharectomy.[89]

After excision, coverage is ideally completed with an autograph. Split-thickness autografts (0.008–0.010 inch thickness) are harvested and utilized as a sheet (unmeshed) or meshed graft. Sheet grafts provide better long-term aesthetic outcomes, but are complicated by the development of a seroma or hematoma and also limited coverage. Narrow meshed autografts (1:1 or 1:2) have the advantages of limiting the total surface area of donor harvest and allowing better drainage of fluid under the grafted sites. In larger burns (>20–30%), coverage may require a combination of meshed autograft and allografts. The meshed autografts (4:1 to 6:1) can be covered with meshed allograft (2:1) overlays.[90] Alternatively, grafting with sequential harvesting of split-thickness autograft from limited donor sites until the entire burn wound is covered may be needed. The use of a widely meshed graft is avoided on the face and functionally important parts of the hand. Full-thickness grafts that include both dermal and epidermal components are commonly obtained from the lower abdomen, groin, or upper arm. These grafts provide the best outcome for wound coverage with diminished contracture and a better pigment match, but their use is generally limited due to the lack of donor sites.

NONTHERMAL INJURIES

Chemical Burns

Cleaning products pose a risk for accidental exposure and chemical burns. The chemical agent responsible for the injury should be identified. Contacting poison control is often necessary. During the initial evaluation, all caustic material should be flushed from the skin with copious amounts of water. Chemicals are classified as either alkali or acid. Alkalis, such as lime, potassium hydroxide, sodium hydroxide, and bleach are the common agents involved in chemical injury and cause liquification necrosis in deep burns. Acid burns are less common and cause coagulation necrosis. Formic acid injuries are rare but can result in multiple systemic organ failure with metabolic acidosis, renal failure, intravascular hemolysis, and ARDS. Hydrofluoric acid burns are managed with copious water irrigation and neutralization of the fluoride ion using topical 2.5% calcium gluconate gel. Without this management, free fluoride ion causes liquefaction necrosis of the affected soft tissues, including bones. Because of potential hypocalcemia, patients should be closely monitored for prolonged QT intervals.

Electrical Burns

Three to 9% of all admitted burn patients are injured from electrical contact.[91] Electrical burns are categorized into low- and high-voltage injuries. Low voltage (<1000 V) injuries typically occur at home where electrical cords are bitten especially by younger children (Fig. 13-9). High-voltage (>1000 V) injuries may result from power lines or lightning strikes, and are characterized by a varying degree of local burn with destruction of deep tissues.[92] The electrical current enters the body and travels preferentially through the low resistance tissues (nerves, blood vessels, and muscles). As skin has high resistance, it is mostly spared leaving little visible evidence of injury. Primary and secondary surveys, including electrocardiography, are very important. If the initial electrocardiogram is normal, further cardiac monitoring is not needed. However, any abnormal findings require continued monitoring for 48 hours and appropriate management of dysrhythmias if detected.[93] Injuries to deep tissues and organs must be identified and treated. As tissue edema worsens, patients may develop compartment syndromes requiring fasciotomy to avoid limb loss. Myoglobinuria can lead to renal failure and should be

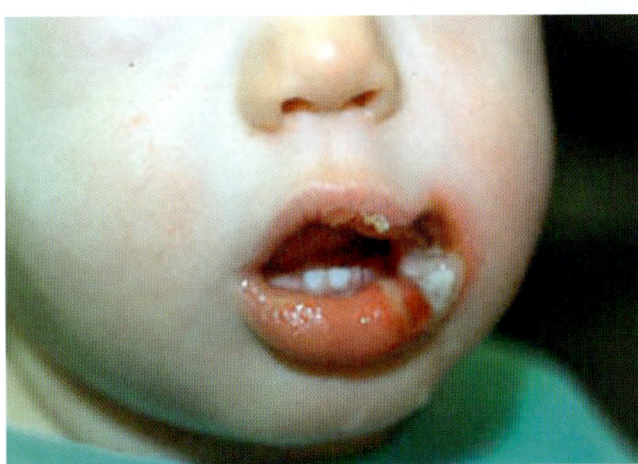

FIGURE 13-9 ■ This child suffered a full-thickness burn to the left lateral aspect of his mouth after biting into an electrical cord. These low-voltage injuries are most common in younger children.

treated with vigorous hydration with sodium bicarbonate and mannitol. Low-voltage injury is typically limited to superficial thermal burn and can be treated with topical wound care.

REFERENCES

1. Lund CC, Browder NC. The estimation of areas of burns. Surg Gynecol Obstet 1944;79:352–8.
2. Brigham PA, McLoughlin E. Burn incidence and medical care use in the United States: Estimates, trends, and data sources. J Burn Care Rehabil 1996;17:95–107.
3. Herndon DN, Gore D, Cole M, et al. Determinants of mortality in pediatric patients with greater than 70% full-thickness total body surface area thermal injury treated by early total excision and grafting. J Trauma 1987;27:208–12.
4. Hettiaratchy S, Dziewulski P. ABC of burns. Introduction. BMJ 2004;328:1366–8.
5. Jackson DM. The diagnosis of the depth of burning. Br J Surgery 1953;40:588–96.
6. Vo LT, Papworth GD, Delaney PM, et al. A study of vascular response to thermal injury on hairless mice by fiberoptic confocal imaging, laser Doppler flowmetry and conventional histology. Burns 1998;24:319–24.
7. Demling RH, LaLonde C. Early postburn lipid peroxidation: Effect of ibuprofen and allopurinol. Surgery 1990;107:85–93.
8. Nwariaku FE, Sikes PJ, Lightfoot E, et al. Effect of a bradykinin antagonist on the local inflammatory response following thermal injury. Burns 1996;22:324–7.
9. DelBeccaro EJ, Robson MC, Heggers JP, et al. The use of specific thromboxane inhibitors to preserve the dermal microcirculation after burning. Surgery 1980;87:137–41.
10. Firat C, Samdancı E, Erbatur S, et al. β-Glucan treatment prevents progressive burn ischaemia in the zone of stasis and improves burn healing: An experimental study in rats. Burns 2013;39:105–12.
11. Evers LH, Bhavsar D, Mailänder P. The biology of burn injury. Exp Dermatol 2010;19:777–83.
12. Chung DH, Evers BM, Townsend CM Jr, et al. Role of polyamine biosynthesis during gut mucosal adaptation after burn injury. Am J Surg 1993;165:144–9.
13. Chung DH, Evers BM, Townsend CM Jr, et al. Burn-induced transcriptional regulation of small intestinal ornithine decarboxylase. Am J Surg 1992;163:157–63.
14. Wolf SE, Ikeda H, Matin S, et al. Cutaneous burn increases apoptosis in the gut epithelium of mice. J Am Coll Surg 1999;188:10–16.
15. Carter EA, Gonnella A, Tompkins RG. Increased transcellular permeability of rat small intestine after thermal injury. Burns 1992;18:117–20.
16. Myers SI, Minei JP, Casteneda A, et al. Differential effects of acute thermal injury on rat splanchnic and renal blood flow and prostanoid release. Prostaglandins Leukot Essent Fatty Acids 1995;53:439–44.
17. Jeschke MG, Barrow RE, Wolf SE, et al. Mortality in burned children with acute renal failure. Arch Surg 1998;133:752–6.
18. Brusselaers N, Monstrey S, Colpaert K, et al. Outcome of acute kidney injury in severe burns: A systematic review and meta-analysis. Intensive Care Med 2010;36:915–25.
19. Gamelli RL, He LK, Liu H. Macrophage suppression of granulocyte and macrophage growth following burn wound infection. J Trauma 1994;37:888–92.
20. Hunt JP, Hunter CT, Brownstein MR, et al. The effector component of the cytotoxic T-lymphocyte response has a biphasic pattern after burn injury. J Surg Res 1998;80:243–51.
21. Hettiaratchy S, Papini R. Initial management of a major burn: I–overview. BMJ 2004;328(7455):1555–7.
22. American Burn Association/American College of Surgeons. Guidelines for the operation of burn centers. J Burn Care Res 2007;28:134–41.
23. Vercruysse GA, Ingram WL, Feliciano DV. Overutilization of regional burn centers for pediatric patients–a healthcare system problem that should be corrected. Am J Surg 2011;202:802–8.
24. Neaman KC, Andres LA, McClure AM, et al. A new method for estimation of involved BSAs for obese and normal-weight patients with burn injury. J Burn Care Res 2011;32:421–8.
25. Chan QE, Barzi F, Cheney L, et al. Burn size estimation in children: Still a problem. Emerg Med Australas 2012;24:181–6.
26. Carvajal HG. Fluid resuscitation of pediatric burn victims: A critical appraisal. Pediatr Nephrol 1994;8:357–66.
27. Ansermino JM, Vandebeek CA, Myers D. An allometric model to estimate fluid requirements in children following burn injury. Paediatr Anaesth 2010;20:305–12.
28. Du GB, Slater H, Goldfarb IW. Influences of different resuscitation regimens on acute early weight gain in extensively burned patients. Burns 1991;17:147–50.
29. Lawrence A, Faraklas I, Watkins H, et al. Colloid administration normalizes resuscitation ratio and ameliorates 'fluid creep'. J Burn Care Res 2010;31:40–7.
30. Faraklas I, Cochran A, Saffle J. Review of a fluid resuscitation protocol: 'Fluid creep' is not due to nursing error. J Burn Care Res 2012;33:74–83.
31. Roberts I, Blackhall K, Alderson P, et al. Human albumin solution for resuscitation and volume expansion in critically ill patients. Cochrane Database Syst Rev 2011;(11):CD001208.
32. Wigginton JG, Roppolo L, Pepe PE. Advances in resuscitative trauma care. Minerva Anestesiol 2011;77:993–1002.
33. Klein MB, Hayden D, Elson C, et al. The association between fluid administration and outcome following major burn: A multicenter study. Ann Surg 2007;245:622–8.
34. Arlati S, Storti E, Pradella V, et al. Decreased fluid volume to reduce organ damage: A new approach to burn shock resuscitaion? A preliminary study. Resuscitation 2007;72:371–8.
35. Herndon DN, Thompson PB, Traber DL. Pulmonary injury in burned patients. Crit Care Clin 1985;1:79–96.
36. Traber DL, Herndon DN, Stein MD, et al. The pulmonary lesions of smoke inhalation in an ovine model. Circ Shock 1986;18:311–23.
37. Moylan JA Jr, Wilmore DW, Mouton DE, et al. Early diagnosis of inhalation injury using 133 xenon lung scans. Ann Surg 1972;176:477–84.
38. Clark WR Jr. Smoke inhalation: Diagnosis and treatment. World J Surg 1992;16:24–9.
39. Chou SH, Lin SD, Chuang HY, et al. Fiberoptic bronchoscopic classification of inhalation injury: Prediction of acute lung injury. Surg Endosc 2004;18:1377–9.
40. Peitzman AB, Shires GT III, Teixidor HS, et al. Smoke inhalation injury: Evaluation of radiographic manifestations and pulmonary dysfunction. J Trauma 1989;29:1232–8.
41. Micak RP, Suman OE, Herndon DN. Respiratory management of inhalation injury. Burns 2007;33:2–13.
42. Miller AC, Rivero A, Ziad S, et al. Influence of nebulized unfractionated heparin and N-acetylcysteine in acute lung injury after smoke inhalation injury. J Burn Care Res 2009;30:249–56.
43. Cancio LC. Current concepts in the pathophysiology and treatment of inhalation injury. Trauma 2005;7:19–35.

44. Saliba MJ Jr. Heparin in the treatment of burns: A review. Burns 2001;27:349–58.
45. Desai MH, Micak R, Richardson J, et al. Reduction in mortality in pediatric patients with inhalation injury with aerosolized heparin/N-acetylcystine [correction of acetylcysteine] therapy. J Burn Care Rehabil 1998;19:210–12.
46. Brown M, Desai M, Traber LD, et al. Dimethylsulfoxide with heparin in the treatment of smoke inhalation injury. J Burn Care Rehabil 1988;9:22–5.
47. Forage AV. The history of the classification of burns (diagnosis of depth). Br J Plastic Surg 1963;16:239–42.
48. Engrav LH, Heimbach DM, Reus JL, et al. Early excision and grafting vs. nonoperative treatment of burns of indeterminate depth: A randomized prospective study. J Trauma 1983;11:1001–4.
49. Hlava P, Moserová J, Königová R. Validity of clinical assessment of the depth of a thermal injury. Acta Chir Plas 1983;25:202–8.
50. Niazi ZB, Essex TJ, Papini R, et al. New laser Doppler scanner, a valuable adjunct in burn depth assessment. Burns 1993;19:485–9.
51. Yeong EK, Mann R, Goldberg M, et al. Improved accuracy of burn wound assessment using laser Doppler. J Trauma 1996;40:956–61.
52. Ho-Asjoe M, Chronnell CM, Frame JD, et al. Immunohistochemical analysis of burn depth. J Burn Care Rehabil 1999;20:207–11.
53. Moserová J, Hlava P, Malínský J. Scope for ultrasound diagnosis of the depth of thermal damage. Preliminary report. Acta Chir Plast 1982;24:235–42.
54. Cantrell JH Jr. Can ultrasound assist an experienced surgeon in estimating burn depth? J Trauma 1984;24:S64–70.
55. Kaufman T, Hurwitz DJ, Heggers JP. The india ink injection technique to assess the depth of experimental burn wounds. Burns Incl Therm Inj 1984;10:405–8.
56. Black KS, Hewitt CW, Miller DM, et al. Burn depth evaluation with fluorometry: Is it really definitive? J Burn Care Rehabil 1986;7:313–17.
57. Pape SA, Skouras CA, Byrne PO. An audit of the use of laser Doppler imaging (LDI) in the assessment of burns of intermediate depth. Burns 2001;27:233–9.
58. Hackett ME. The use of thermography in the assessment of depth of burn and blood supply of flaps, with preliminary reports on its use in Dupuytren's contracture and treatment of varicose ulcers. Br J Plast Surg 1974;27:311–17.
59. Erba P, Espinoza D, Koch N, et al. FluxEXPLORER: A new high-speed laser Doppler imaging system for the assessment of burn injuries. Skin Res Technol 2012;18:456–61.
60. Mihara K, Shindo H, Ohtani M, et al. Early depth assessment of local burns by videomicroscopy: 24 h after injury is a critical time point. Burns 2011;37:986–93.
61. Desai MH, Rutan RL, Herndon DN. Conservative treatment of scald burns is superior to early excision. J Burn Care Rehabil 1991;12:482–4.
62. Kumar RJ, Kimble RM, Boots R, et al. Treatment of partial-thickness burns: A prospective, randomized trial using Transcyte. ANZ J Surg 2004;74:622–6.
63. Costagliola M, Agrosì M. Second-degree burns: A comparative, multicenter, randomized trial of hyaluronic acid plus silver sulfadiazine vs. silver sulfadiazine alone. Curr Med Res Opin 2005;21:1235–40.
64. Soroff HS, Sasvary DH. Collagenase ointment and polymyxin B sulfate/bacitracin spray versus silver sulfadiazine cream in partial-thickness burns: A pilot study. J Burn Care Rehabil 1994;15:13–17.
65. Fox CL Jr. Silver sulfadiazine–a new topical therapy for Pseudomonas in burns. Therapy of Pseudomonas infection in burns. Arch Surg 1968;96:184–8.
66. Desai MH, Rutan RL, Heggers JP, et al. Candida infection with and without nystatin prophylaxis. A 11-year experience with patients with burn injury. Arch Surg 1992;127:159–62.
67. Jarrett F, Ellerbe S, Demling R. Acute leukopenia during topical burn therapy with silver sulfadiazine. Am J Surg 1978;135:818–19.
68. Choban PS, Marshall WJ. Leukopenia secondary to silver sulfadiazine: frequency, characteristics and clinical consequences. Am Surg 1987;53:515–17.
69. Lindberg RB, Moncrief JA, Mason AD Jr. Control of experimental and clinical burn wounds sepsis by topical application of sulfamylon compounds. Ann N Y Acad Sci 1968;150:950–60.
70. Asch MJ, White MG, Pruitt BA Jr. Acid base changes associated with topical Sulfamylon therapy: Retrospective study of 100 burn patients. Ann Surg 1970;172:946–50.
71. Fong J, Wood F, Fowler B. A silver coated dressing reduces the incidence of early burn wound cellulitis and associated costs of inpatient treatment: Comparative patient care audits. Burns 2005;31:562–7.
72. Tredget EE, Shankowsky HA, Groeneveld A, et al. A matched-pair, randomized study evaluating the efficacy and safety of Acticoat silver-coated dressing for the treatment of burn wounds. J Burn Care Rehabil 1998;19:531–7.
73. Varas RP, O'Keeffe T, Namias N, et al. A prospective, randomized trial of Acticoat versus silver sulfadiazine in the treatment of partial-thickness burns: Which method is less painful? J Burn Care Rehabil 2005;26:344–7.
74. Muller MJ, Hollyoak MA, Moaveni Z, et al. Retardation of wound healing by silver sulfadiazine is reversed by Aloe vera and nystatin. Burns 2003;29:834–6.
75. Hansbrough JF, Achauer B, Dawson J, et al. Wound healing in partial-thickness burn wounds treated with collagenase ointment versus silver sulfadiazine cream. J Burn Care Rehabil 1995;16:241–7.
76. Ostlie DJ, Juang D, Aguayo P, et al. Topical silver sulfadiazine vs collagenase ointment for the treatment of partial thickness burns in children: A prospective randomized trial. J Pediatr Surg 2012;47:1204–7.
77. Winter GD. Formation of the scab and the rate of epithelization of superficial wounds in the skin of the young domestic pig. Nature 1962;193:293–4.
78. Hinman CD, Maibach H. Effect of air exposure and occlusion on experimental human skin wounds. Nature 1963;200:377–8.
79. Paddock HN, Fabia R, Giles S, et al. A silver-impregnated antimicrobial dressing reduces hospital length of stay for pediatric patients with burns. J Burn Care Res 2007;28:409–11.
80. Cassidy C, St Peter SD, Lacey S, et al. Biobrane versus duoderm for the treatment of intermediate thickness burns in children: A prospective, randomized trial. Burns 2005;31:890–3.
81. Tompkins RG, Burke JF. Progress in burn treatment and the use of artificial skin. World J Surg 1990;14:819–24.
82. Branski LK, Herndon DN, Pereira C, et al. Longitudinal assessment of Integra in primary burn management: A randomized pediatric clinical trial. Crit Care Med 2007;35:2615–23.
83. Herndon DN, Parks DH. Comparison of serial debridement and autografting and early massive excision with cadaver skin overlay in the treatment of large burns in children. J Trauma 1986;26:149–52.
84. Herndon DN, Gore D, Cole M, et al. Determinants of mortality in pediatric patients with greater than 70% full-thickness total body surface area thermal injury treated by early total excision and grafting. J Trauma 1987;27:208–12.
85. Muller MJ, Herndon DN. The challenge of burns. Lancet 1994;343:216–20.
86. Bull JP, Fisher AJ. A study of mortality in a burns unit: A revised estimate. Ann Surg 1954;139:269–74.
87. Janzekovic Z. A new concept in the early excision and immediate grafting of burns. J Trauma 1970;10:1103–8.
88. Klein MB, Hunter S, Heimbach DM, et al. The Versajet water dissector: A new tool for tangential excision. J Burn Care Rehabil 2005;26:483–7.
89. Gravante G, Delogu D, Esposito G, et al. Versajet hydrosurgery versus classic escharectomy for burn debridment: A prospective randomized trial. J Burn Care Res 2007;28:720–4.
90. Alexander JW, MacMillan BG, Law E, et al. Treatment of severe burns with widely meshed skin autograft and meshed skin allograft overlay. J Trauma 1981;21:433–8.
91. Celik A, Ergun O, Ozok G. Pediatric electrical injuries: A review of 38 consecutive patients. J Pediatr Surg 2004;39:1233–7.
92. Laberge LC, Ballard PA, Daniel RK. Experimental electrical burns: Low voltage. Ann Plast Surg 1984;13:185–90.
93. Robson MC, Smith DJ. Care of the thermal injured victim. In: Jurkiewicz MJ, Krizek TJ, Mathes SJ, Ariyan S, editors. Plastic Surgery: Principles and Practice. St. Louis, CV: Mosby; 1990.

CHAPTER 14

Early Assessment and Management of Trauma

Arthur Cooper

Trauma is the leading cause of morbidity and mortality in children from ages 1 to 14 years. It results in more disability and death than all other childhood diseases combined.[1] More than 10,000 pediatric patients die from trauma in the USA each year.[1] Approximately 10% of pediatric hospitalizations,[2] 15% of pediatric intensive care unit (PICU) admissions,[3] 25% of pediatric emergency department visits,[4] and 50% or more of pediatric ambulance runs are due to trauma.[5] Moreover, it also represents nearly 20% of hospitalizations for serious injury among all age groups combined.[6]

TRAUMA EPIDEMIOLOGY

Several injury severity scales exist in practice and in the literature. The large number of injury severity scales arises from the markedly different perspectives used in the application of the scales. The Abbreviated Injury Scale (AIS), primarily an anatomical measure of injury severity, was the first widely implemented scale used in practice. Criticism of the AIS included the inability to take into account multiple injuries to the same body region and the poor correlation of the AIS with severity and survival. The Injury Severity Score (ISS), New Injury Severity Score (NISS) and Pediatric Trauma Score (PTS) are just some examples of scoring systems developed to overcome the issues described. Despite the controversies in these scales, it is commonly accepted that injuries whose severity are a threat to life correspond to an ISS of 10 or higher, or a PTS of 8 or lower.[2]

The incidence of serious traumatic injury is approximately 420/100,000.[7] Although the hospital-based fatality rate is 2.4/100,000, the population-based mortality rate is 11.8/100,000, indicating that 78% of lethally injured children die before hospital admission and demonstrating the need for effective injury prevention and prehospital care.[8]

Blunt injuries outnumber penetrating injuries in children by a ratio of 12:1, a ratio that has decreased somewhat in recent years. While blunt injuries are more common, penetrating injuries are more lethal. However, despite the decline in penetrating injuries, firearm related deaths continue as one of the top three causes of death in the American youth. Most blunt trauma in childhood is sustained unintentionally, but between 5–10% of serious injuries are due to intentional physical assault (of which half are due to physical abuse).[9] Still, the leading cause of death in children is the motor vehicle, responsible for approximately 75% of all childhood deaths, which are evenly split between those due to pedestrian trauma and those resulting from occupant injuries (Table 14-1).

INJURY RISKS

The lack of adequate supervision of children during play involving possible injury hazards is recognized as a major risk factor for unintentional injury in pediatric patients. However, drug and alcohol use, obesity, poverty, and race also influence injury frequency. Toxicology screens are reportedly positive in 10–40% of injured adolescents, while obese children and adolescents appear to have more complications and require longer stays in the intensive care unit.[10–13] Socioeconomic status has also been associated with increased hospitalization and mortality following major trauma, owing to a higher frequency and more lethal mechanisms of injury, rather than injury severity.[14] Race and ethnicity affect injury risk independent of socioeconomic status, particularly among African-American children, whose rate of death from preventable injuries, head injuries, and child abuse is three to six times higher than that of white children.[15–18] Improper use of restraints may contribute to the increased fatality rates observed in African-American children, who are half as likely to be restrained as white children when involved in motor vehicle crashes (MVCs) and one-third as likely to be placed in car seats during MVCs.[19]

Analysis of the Crash Injury Research Engineering Network (CIREN) database has recently yielded valuable information about the pattern of childhood injuries after MVCs: (1) child victims in frontal crashes are more likely to suffer severe spine and musculoskeletal injuries; (2) those in lateral crashes are more likely to suffer head and chest injuries; (3) those in front seats sustain more injuries to the chest, abdomen, pelvis, and axial skeleton than those in the rear seats; (4) seat belts are especially protective against pelvic and musculoskeletal injuries; (5) children involved in high-severity, lateral-impact crashes typically sustain injuries characterized by higher ISS and lower Glasgow Coma Scale (GCS) scores.[20,21] Restraint devices have also been subjected to careful analysis in recent years: (1) they do not appear to protect young victims of MVCs as well as older victims; (2) car seats may not significantly affect injury outcome; (3) improper application may predispose to abdominal injuries, even in low-severity crashes; (4) the presence of

TABLE 14-1 **Incidence and Mortality from the Major Categories of Pediatric Trauma**

By Injury Mechanism	Incidence (%)	Mortality (%)
Blunt	92	3
Fall	32	0.3
Motor vehicle traffic	25	3
Struck by, against	11	0.5
Pedal cyclist, other	3.7	0.25
Penetrating	8	
Gunshot wound	4.5	12
Stabbing	3.5	1.3

Data from the American College of Surgeons, National Trauma Data Bank 2012.

abdominal wall bruising in restrained children, although not commonly observed, is frequently indicative of intra-abdominal injury.[22–27]

INJURY OUTCOMES

In recent years, much effort has been devoted to outcomes research in pediatric trauma with the hope that benchmarking of treatment results may lead to better care for injured children. Both historical studies and contemporary investigations indicate that children survive more frequently and recover more fully in hospitals that specialize in pediatric trauma than in other hospitals.[28–45] No less important than survival outcome is functional outcome, for which numerous studies now indicate improved outcomes in hospitals that specialize in pediatric trauma care.[32–46] However, these studies also suggest that whereas children may recover from injury more quickly than adults, physical function may not fully normalize. Even so, self-perceived long-term quality of life among seriously injured children may not be adversely affected, justifying an aggressive approach to their resuscitation.[47]

Perhaps the most important recent development for outcomes research in pediatric trauma has been the expansion of the National Trauma Data Bank™ (NTDB™) of the American College of Surgeons (ACS) to include children. Initially designed as a simple case repository, efforts continue to analyze submitted cases to provide population estimates of severe pediatric injury and develop quality benchmarks for pediatric trauma care. Preliminary data suggest that these benchmarks perform as well as existing measures.[48]

INJURY PREVENTION

Injuries are not accidents, but rather predictable events that respond to harm-reduction strategies similar to those applied for other diseases. The Haddon Factor Phase Matrix neatly depicts these in graphic form (Fig. 14-1).[49] Strategies to lessen the burden of injury are applied to the host, agent, and environment before, during, and after the traumatic event using enforcement, engineering, education, and economics as techniques to limit the adverse impact of each factor.

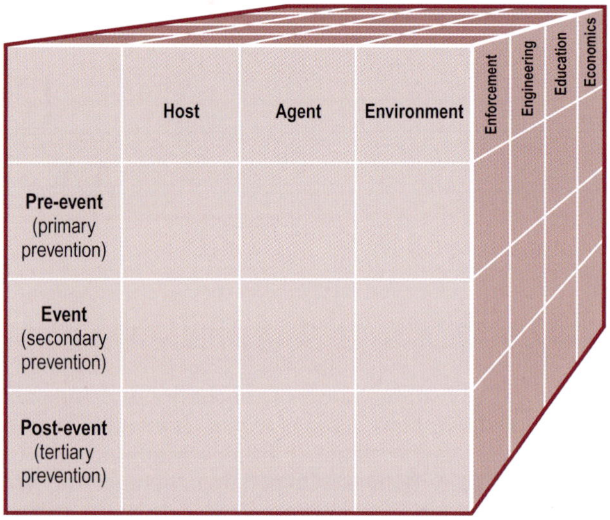

FIGURE 14-1 ■ The Haddon Factor Phase Matrix, as modified and refined to include a third strategic dimension, integrates all phases of injury control into a single system. (Adapted from Haddon W. Advances in the epidemiology of injuries as a basis for public policy. Public Health Rep 1980;95:411–21; and Runyan CW. Using the Haddon Matrix: Introducing the third dimension. Inj Prev 1998;4:302–7.)

Effective injury-prevention programs are community-based and require extensive collaboration with civic leaders, governmental agencies, community-based organizations, and neighborhood coalitions. Programs such as the National Safe Kids Campaign (http://www.safekids.org) and the Injury Free Coalition for Kids (http://www.injuryfree.org) have proven highly successful in reducing the burden of childhood injury in many communities.

INJURY PATTERNS

Injury mechanism is the main predictor of injury pattern. The body regions most frequently injured in major childhood trauma are the lower extremities, head and neck, and abdomen. In minor childhood injury, soft tissue and upper extremity injuries predominate. Motor vehicle versus pedestrian trauma results in the Waddell triad of injuries to the head, torso, and lower extremity (pelvis, femur, or tibia; Fig. 14-2). Motor vehicle accidents may cause head, face, and neck injuries in unrestrained passengers. Cervical spine injuries, bowel disruption or hematoma, and Chance fractures occur in restrained passengers (Fig. 14-3). Bicycle trauma results in head injury in the unhelmeted riders as well as upper extremity and upper abdominal injuries, the latter the result of contact with the handlebar (Fig. 14-4 and Table 14-2). Direct impact from a bicycle handlebar remains highly predictive of the need for operation.[27]

Head

Head injuries are potentially more dangerous in children than in adults for several reasons. First, developing neural

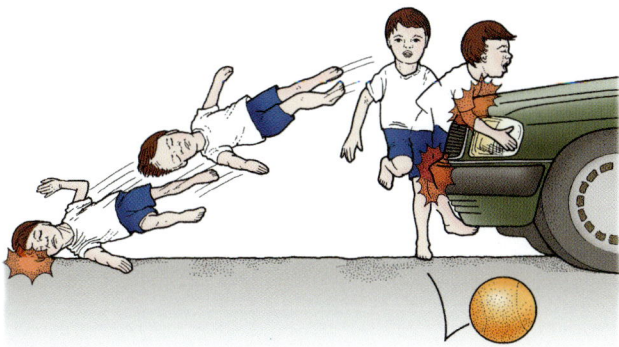

FIGURE 14-2 ■ The Waddell triad of injuries to head, torso, and lower extremity is depicted. (From Foltin G, Tunik M, Cooper A, et al, editors. Teaching Resource for Instructors of Prehospital Pediatrics. New York: Center for Pediatric Emergency Medicine; 1998. Accessed at http://www.cpem.org.)

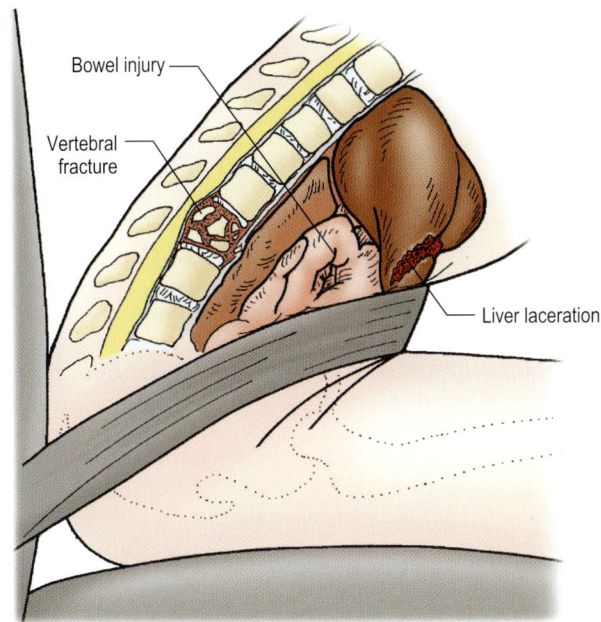

FIGURE 14-3 ■ The mechanism for the development of intestinal and vertebral injuries from lap belts is shown. (From Foltin G, Tunik M, Cooper A, et al, editors. Teaching Resource for Instructors of Prehospital Pediatrics. New York: Center for Pediatric Emergency Medicine; 1998. Accessed at http://www.cpem.org.)

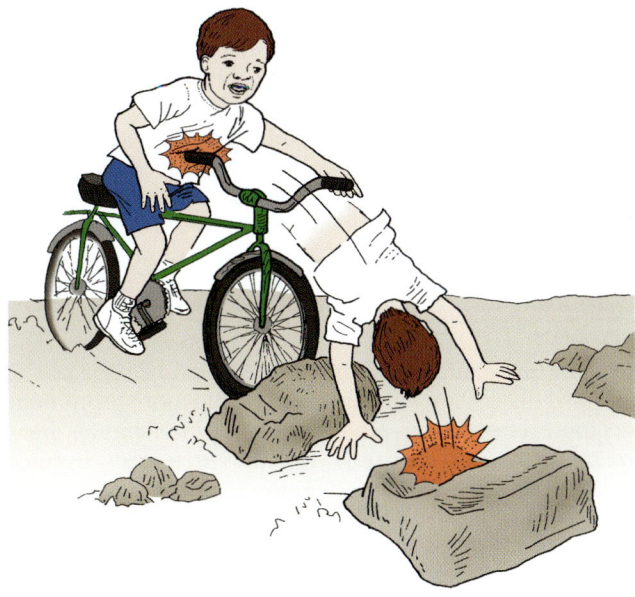

FIGURE 14-4 ■ Children riding bicycles can sustain blunt abdominal trauma after contact with handlebars or head trauma from falling off the bicycle. (From Foltin G, Tunik M, Cooper A, et al, editors. Teaching Resource for Instructors of Prehospital Pediatrics. New York: Center for Pediatric Emergency Medicine; 1998.)

TABLE 14-2 **Common Injury Mechanisms and Corresponding Injury Patterns in Childhood Trauma**

Injury Mechanism		Injury Pattern
Motor vehicle injury: occupant	Unrestrained	Head/neck injuries
		Scalp/facial lacerations
	Restrained	Internal abdomen injuries
		Lower spine fractures
Motor vehicle injury: pedestrian	Single	Lower extremity fractures
	Multiple	Head/neck injuries
		Internal chest/abdomen injuries
		Lower extremity fractures
Fall from height	Low	Upper extremity fractures
	Medium	Head/neck injuries
		Scalp/facial lacerations
		Upper extremity fractures
	High	Head/neck injuries
		Scalp/facial lacerations
		Internal chest/abdomen injuries
		Upper/lower extremity fractures
Fall from bicycle	Unhelmeted	Head/neck injuries
		Scalp/facial lacerations
		Upper extremity fractures
	Helmeted	Upper extremity fractures
	Handlebar	Internal abdomen injuries

From American College of Surgeons Committee on Trauma. Advanced Trauma Life Support® ATLS® Student Course Manual. 9th ed. Chicago: American College of Surgeons; 2012.

Neck

Cervical spine injury is a relatively uncommon event in pediatric trauma. It affects approximately 1.5% of all seriously injured children, and occurs at a rate of 1.8/100,000 population, in contrast to closed-head injury,

tissue is delicate and the softer bones of the pediatric skull allow impact forces to be transmitted directly to the underlying brain, especially at points of bony contact. Second, intracranial bleeding in infants in whom the fontanelles and sutures remain open may, on rare occasions, be severe enough to cause hypotensive shock. Third, the proportionately larger size of the head, when coupled with the injury mechanisms commonly observed in children, generally leads to head trauma with a loss of consciousness. As a consequence, the voluntary muscles of the neck lose their tone which can lead to soft tissue obstruction in the upper airway and hypoxia. Hypoxia exacerbates and potentiates the initial traumatic injury to the brain (secondary insults). See Chapter 17 for more information about head injuries.

which occurs at a rate of 185/100,000 population.[50-52] The pediatric surgeon should also be aware of normal variants of cervical spine anatomy. The greater elasticity of the interspinous ligaments and the more horizontal apposition of the cervical vertebrae also give rise to a normal anatomic variant known as pseudosubluxation, which affects up to 40% of children younger than age 7 years. The most common finding is a short (2–3 mm) anterior displacement of C2 on C3, although anterior displacement of C3 on C4 also may occur. This pseudo-subluxation is accentuated when the pediatric patient is placed in a supine position, which forces the cervical spine of the young child into mild flexion because of the forward displacement of the head by the more prominent occiput. The greater elasticity of the interspinous ligaments also is responsible for the increased distance between the dens and the anterior arch of C1 that is found in up to 20% of children.

When an injury to the cervical spine does occur, it frequently occurs at C2, C1, and the occipitoatlantal junction. The injuries are above the nerve roots that give rise to diaphragmatic innervation (C4) and predispose the afflicted child to respiratory arrest as well as paralysis. The increased angular momentum produced by movement of the proportionately larger head, the greater elasticity of the interspinous ligaments, and the more horizontal apposition of the cervical vertebrae are responsible for this spectrum of injuries. Subluxation without dislocation may cause spinal cord injury without radiographic abnormalities (SCIWORA). SCIWORA accounts for up to 20% of pediatric spinal cord injuries as well as a number of prehospital deaths that were previously attributed to head trauma.[53-55]

Chest

Serious intrathoracic injuries occur in 6% of pediatric blunt trauma victims.[56] Although thoracostomy is required in about 50%, thoracotomy is seldom needed. Lung injuries, pneumothorax and hemothorax, and rib and sternal fractures occur most frequently (Table 14-3). Injuries to the heart, diaphragm, great vessels, bronchi, and esophagus occur less frequently, but have higher mortality rates associated with them. Because blunt trauma is nearly ten times more deadly when associated with major intrathoracic injury, thoracic injury serves as a marker of injury severity, even though it is the proximate cause of death in less than 1% of all pediatric blunt trauma.[57]

The thorax of the child usually escapes major harm because the pliable nature of the cartilage and ribs allows the kinetic energy from forceful impacts to be absorbed without significant injury, either to the chest wall itself or to underlying structures. Pulmonary contusions are the typical result, but are seldom life-threatening. Pneumothorax and hemothorax, due to lacerations of the lung parenchyma and intercostal vessels, occur less frequently.

Abdomen

Serious intra-abdominal injuries occur in 8% of pediatric blunt trauma victims and are caused by crushing the solid

TABLE 14-3	**Incidence and Mortality of Injuries to Thoracic and Abdominal Organs**	
Organ	**Incidence (%)**	**Mortality (%)**
Thoracic		
Lung	52	18
Pneumothorax/hemothorax	42	17
Ribs/sternum	32	11
Heart	6	40
Diaphragm	4	16
Great vessels	2	51
Bronchi	<1	20
Esophagus	<1	43
Abdominal		
Liver	27	13
Spleen	27	11
Kidneys	25	13
Gastrointestinal tract	21	11
Great vessels	5	47
Genitourinary tract	5	3
Pancreas	4	7
Pelvis	<1	7

From Cooper A, Barlow B, DiScala C, et al. Mortality and truncal injury: The pediatric perspective. J Pediatric Surg 1994;29:33–8.

upper abdominal viscera against the vertebral column, sudden compression and bursting of the hollow upper abdominal viscera against the vertebral column, or shearing of the posterior attachments, including the vascular supply, of the upper abdominal viscera after rapid deceleration (see Table 14-3).[56,58] Injuries to the liver (27%), spleen (27%), kidneys (25%), and gastrointestinal tract (21%) occur most frequently and account for most of the deaths from intra-abdominal injury. Injuries to the great vessels (5%), genitourinary tract (5%), pancreas (4%), and pelvis (<1%) occur less frequently and account for few of the deaths that result from intra-abdominal injury. Most solid visceral injuries are successfully managed nonoperatively, especially those involving the kidneys (98%), the spleen (95%), and the liver (90%).[59-61]

The abdomen of the child is vulnerable to injury for several reasons. Flexible ribs cover only the uppermost portion of the abdomen. Thin layers of muscle, fat, and fascia provide little protection to the large solid viscera. Also, the pelvis is shallow, lifting the bladder into the abdomen. Moreover, the overall small size of the abdomen predisposes the child to multiple rather than single injuries as energy is dissipated from the impacting force. Finally, gastric dilatation due to air swallowing (which often confounds the abdominal examination by simulating peritonitis) leads to ventilatory and circulatory compromise by limiting the diaphragmatic motion, increasing the risk of pulmonary aspiration of gastric contents, and causing vagally mediated dampening of the normal tachycardic response to hypoxia caused by hypoventilation or hypovolemia.

Skeleton

Although they are the leading cause of disability, fractures are rarely an immediate cause of death from blunt trauma.

TABLE 14-4 Trauma Scores Commonly Used in Children

Pediatric Trauma Score

	+2	+1	−1
Size (kg)	>20	10–20	<10
Airway	Normal	Maintained	Unmaintained
Systolic blood pressure (mmHg)	>90	50–90	<50
Central nervous system	Awake	Obtunded	Coma
Open wound	None	Minor	Major
Skeletal trauma	None	Closed	Open-multiple

Revised Trauma Score

GLASGOW COMA SCALE	SYSTOLIC BLOOD PRESSURE (mmHg)	RESPIRATORY RATE (breaths/min)	CODE VALUE
13–15	>89	10–29	4
9–12	76–89	>29	3
6–8	50–75	6–9	2
4–5	1–49	1–5	1
3	0	0	0

They are reported to occur in 26% of serious blunt-injury cases and constitute the principal anatomic diagnosis in 22%.[9] Upper extremity fractures outnumber lower extremity fractures by 7:1, although, in serious blunt trauma, this ratio is 2:3. The most common long bone fractures sustained during pedestrian/MVCs in children are fractures of the femur and tibia. Falls are typically associated with both upper and lower extremity fractures if the fall height is significant (from the window of a high-rise dwelling or the top of a bunk bed, but not from falls from standard beds or down stairs).[62-65] Because isolated long bone and stable pelvic fractures are infrequently associated with significant hemorrhage, a diligent search must be made for another source of bleeding if signs of shock are observed.[66,67] Unstable pelvic fractures are an uncommon feature of childhood injury, but unilateral (type III) or bilateral (type IV) anterior and posterior disruptions are those most often associated with major hemorrhage and must be recognized early and treated.[68]

The pediatric skeleton is susceptible to fractures because cortical bone in childhood is highly porous whereas the periosteum is more resilient, elastic, and vascular. This results in higher percentages both of incomplete (torus and greenstick) fractures and complete, but nondisplaced fractures. Long-term growth disturbances also may complicate childhood fractures. Diaphyseal fractures of the long bones cause significant overgrowth whereas physeal (growth plate) fractures cause significant undergrowth. Both result in limb length discrepancies unless treated.

PREHOSPITAL CARE

Basic life support for the pediatric trauma patient consists of oxygen administration, airway adjuncts, bleeding control, spine stabilization, and temperature maintenance. Assisted ventilation and fracture immobilization should be provided as needed. Spinal immobilization requires both neutral positioning (which cannot be achieved without placing an approximate 2.5 cm layer of padding beneath the torso from shoulders to hips) and careful strapping (because forced vital capacity may be decreased by up to 60%).[69,70] One study suggested that cervical spine immobilization can be safely avoided in most pediatric trauma patients with minor injuries, but caution was urged in view of the known risks of SCIWORA and atlanto-axial instability.[71] Advanced life support of the pediatric trauma patient theoretically adds endotracheal intubation and volume resuscitation to this armamentarium, but neither intervention has been shown to improve outcome.[72-76]

Field triage of pediatric trauma patients to pediatric trauma centers is now well established. Regional protocols should direct ambulance transports to such centers where available. The use of scoring systems to assist in predicting the need for specialty pediatric trauma care, such as the PTS and the Revised Trauma Score (RTS), may reliably predict the need for specialty pediatric trauma care but neither is optimally sensitive nor specific (Table 14-4).[77,78] The most sensitive and specific indicators for the need for specialty pediatric trauma care are: a score of 1 in best motor response in the calculation of the GCS or a selection of 'unresponsive/unconscious' in the calculation of an AVPU Score.[79] Good results also have been achieved by using checklists to identify anatomic, physiologic, and mechanistic criteria (Box 14-1) rather than calculated scores. These checklists are currently advocated by the ACS Committee on Trauma, based upon the advice of an expert panel convened in 2011 by the United States Centers for Disease Control and Prevention (CDC).[80]

EMERGENCY CARE

Primary Survey

Early management of childhood trauma begins in the field and continues in the emergency department.[81,82] A primary survey of the *a*irway, *b*reathing, *c*irculation (see Box 14-1) and neurologic *d*isabilities (Box 14-2) should

---

BOX 14-1 | **Primary Survey, Resuscitation, and Secondary Survey**

Primary Survey

Airway: clear and maintain, protect cervical spine
Breathing: ventilate and oxygenate, fix chest wall
Circulation: control bleeding, restore volume
Disability: GCS and pupils, call the neurosurgeon
Exposure: disrobe, logroll, avoid hypothermia
Foley catheter unless contraindicated[a]
Gastric tube unless contraindicated[b]

Secondary Survey

History and physical: SAMPLE history, complete examination
Imaging studies: plain radiographs,[c] special studies[d]

[a]Meatal blood, scrotal hematoma, high-riding prostate.
[b]CSF oto-rhinorrhea, basilar skull fracture, midface instability.
[c]Chest, pelvis, lateral cervical spine; others as indicated.
[d]FAST, CT as indicated.
GCS, Glasgow Coma Scale; CSF, cerebrospinal fluid; FAST, focused assessment by sonography in trauma; CT, computed tomography.
Adapted from American College of Surgeons Committee on Trauma. Advanced Trauma Life Support® ATLS® Student Course Manual. 9th ed. Chicago: American College of Surgeons; 2012.

BOX 14-2 | **Disability/Mental Status**

Pupils: symmetry, reaction
LOC: GCS
Track and trend as a vital sign
Significant change, 2 points
Intubate for coma, GCS ≤8
Motor: strength, symmetry
Abnormality/deterioration: call neurosurgeon
Traumatic Brain Injury
Mild (GCS 13-15): observe, consider CT for history of LOC
Moderate (GCS 9-12): admit, obtain CT, repeat CT 12–24 hr
Severe (GCS 3-8): intubate, ventilate, obtain CT, repeat CT 12–24 hr

CT, computed tomography; GCS, Glasgow Coma Scale; LOC, loss of consciousness.
Adapted from American College of Surgeons Committee on Trauma. Advanced Trauma Life Support® ATLS® Student Course Manual. 9th ed. Chicago: American College of Surgeons; 2012.

---

be completed to identify and correct deficits that pose an immediate threat to life. The primary survey continues with complete exposure of the patient to ensure that no injuries are missed, taking care to avoid hypothermia. The placement of therapeutic adjuncts, such as a urinary and gastric catheter (unless contraindicated), is also completed during this initial survey. Diagnostic adjuncts, such as pulse oximetry, radiographs, and *f*ocused *a*ssessment by *s*onography in *t*rauma (FAST), facilitate the early recognition and treatment of immediate threats to vital functions (Box 14-3). The complete 'trauma series' of radiographs obtained as an adjunct to the primary survey in adults may not always be necessary in children, since the lateral cervical spine radiograph will not detect SCIWORA, and the screening pelvic radiograph seldom

---

BOX 14-3 | **Primary Survey Adjuncts**

Vital signs/pulse oximetry
Chest/pelvis/lateral cervical spine radiographs
Foley catheter/gastric tube
FAST/DPL

DPL, diagnostic peritoneal lavage; FAST, focused assessment by sonography in trauma.
Adapted from American College of Surgeons Committee on Trauma. Advanced Trauma Life Support® for Doctors Student Manual. 8th ed. Chicago: American College of Surgeons; 2008.

---

identifies a pelvic fracture. If a pelvic fracture is suspected on physical examination, a computed tomography (CT) scan should be obtained.[83,84]

Resuscitation

Any child initially seen with major trauma should receive breathing support with high-concentration oxygen by the most appropriate means. For the child with respiratory distress (increased work of breathing), a nonrebreather mask normally will suffice, provided the airway is open and breathing is spontaneous. For the child with significant respiratory distress (labored or inadequate work of breathing), assisted ventilation via face-mask or an endotracheal tube (ETT) attached to a bag-valve device should be immediately available. Endotracheal intubation with rapid-sequence induction techniques is necessary in respiratory failure.

The first step in management of the circulation is control of bleeding. Direct pressure using sterile dressings is applied to all actively bleeding external wounds. Blind clamping is avoided, owing to the potential risk of injury to neurovascular bundles. Military experience suggests that commercial arterial tourniquets, and topical hemostatic agents such as chitosan granules or powder, zeolite granules, and kaolin clay, are effective in stopping major arterial hemorrhage, and massive arteriolar, venular, and capillary oozing from large open wounds. Recent data suggests equivalent effectiveness for tourniquets in children.[85] However, because no reports of topical hemostatic agent use in children have been published to date, no recommendation can be made regarding its applicability in civilian pediatric trauma.

The child with significant trauma will require volume resuscitation if signs of hypovolemic shock are present. Intraosseous access should be used if conventional intravenous access with peripheral large bore catheters is not rapidly obtainable. Central venous catheter insertion, except in cases when venous access cannot otherwise readily be obtained, is not warranted. Simple hypovolemia usually responds to 20–40 mL/kg of warmed lactated Ringer's solution. However, frank hypotension (defined clinically by a systolic blood pressure less than 70 mmHg plus twice the age in years) typically requires 40–60 mL/kg of warmed lactated Ringer's solution followed by 10–20 mL/kg of warmed packed red blood cells. To avoid the greater mortality associated with coagulopathy and shock on hospital admission, a 1:1:1 or 2:1:1 ratio with fresh frozen plasma and platelet concentrates should be instituted when massive uncontrolled hemorrhage is present and a massive transfusion protocol is invoked.[86–88] Urinary output should be measured in all seriously injured children as an indication of tissue perfusion. The minimum urinary output that indicates adequate renal perfusion is 2 mL/kg/h in infants, 1 mL/kg/h in children, and 0.5 mL/kg/h in adolescents.

Due to the ability of a child's blood vessels to compensate vigorously for hypovolemia by intense vasoconstriction, systolic hypotension is a late sign of shock and may not develop until 30–35% of circulating blood volume is lost.[89] Thus, any child who cannot be stabilized after infusion of 40–60 mL/kg of lactated Ringer's solution and 10–20 mL/kg of packed red blood cells likely has internal bleeding and needs an operation. If a child initially is in shock, has no signs of intrathoracic, intraabdominal, or intrapelvic bleeding, but fails to improve despite seemingly adequate volume resuscitation, other forms of shock (obstructive, cardiogenic, neurogenic) should be considered. Most children in hypotensive shock are victims of unrecognized hemorrhage that can be reversed only if promptly recognized and appropriately treated by means of rapid blood transfusion and immediate intervention, particularly if major intrathoracic or intra-abdominal vessels are injured.[90–93]

Secondary Survey

Once the primary survey has been performed, and the resuscitation phase is ongoing, a secondary survey is undertaken. This consists of a 'SAMPLE' history (symptoms, allergies, medications, past illnesses, last meal, events, and environment) and a complete head-to-toe physical examination (including all body regions and organ systems). The physician's chief responsibility is to identify life-threatening injuries that may have been overlooked during the primary survey, such as a tension pneumothorax. Physical findings will also assist in determining other injuries that are not readily apparent. For example, drainage from the nose or ears, or any evidence of midface instability, suggests a basilar skull fracture (which precludes passage of a nasogastric tube) or an oromaxillofacial fracture (which may threaten the airway). All skeletal components should be palpated for evidence of instability or discontinuity, especially bony prominences such as the anterior superior iliac crests, which commonly are injured in major blunt trauma. In the absence of obvious deformities, fractures should be suspected if bony point tenderness, hematoma, spasm of overlying muscles, an unstable pelvic girdle, or perineal swelling or discoloration is found.

Selective laboratory evaluation is an integral part of the secondary survey, although routine trauma laboratory panels are of limited utility owing to their relatively low sensitivity and specificity.[94–96] Arterial blood gases are important in determining the adequacy of ventilation ($PsCO_2$), oxygenation (PsO_2), and perfusion (base deficit).[97,98] However, the critically important determinant of blood oxygen content is the blood hemoglobin concentration. Serial hemoglobin values better reflect the extent of blood loss than does the initial value. Elevations

in serum levels of transaminases or amylase and lipase suggest injury to the liver or pancreas, but the infrequency of pancreatic injury makes the latter cost ineffective versus the former.[99,100] Urine that is grossly bloody or is positive for blood by dipstick or microscopy (>50 red blood cells per high-power field) suggests kidney trauma.[101]

Selective radiologic evaluation is another important part of the secondary survey. CT of the head (without contrast) and abdomen (intravenous and oral) should be obtained as indicated. However, CT should be employed only when the short-term benefit of accurate diagnosis is felt to outweigh the long-term risk of late malignancy, particularly for body regions such as the cervical spine and the thorax for which conventional imaging is adequate. When utilized, the CT should be performed using radiation doses 'as low as reasonably achievable' (ALARA), consistent with the 'image gently®' protocols advocated by The Alliance for Radiation Safety in Pediatric Imaging.[102–108]

CT of the head should be performed whenever loss of consciousness has occurred, or if the GCS score is <15.[109] It can be safely avoided in children <2 years of age with: (1) normal mental status; (2) no scalp hematoma except frontal; (3) no loss of consciousness or loss of consciousness for less than five seconds; (4) nonsevere injury mechanism; (5) no palpable skull fracture; and (6) normal activity according to parents. Recommendations for not obtaining a head CT in children ≥2 years of age and older include: (1) normal mental status; (2) no loss of consciousness; (3) no vomiting; (4) nonsevere injury mechanism; (5) no signs of basilar skull fracture; and (6) no severe headache.[110] CT of the chest adds little to what is already known from the chest radiograph obtained during the primary survey, since the incidental pulmonary contusions identified by CT of the chest do not correlate with increased fatality.[111,112] CT of the cervical spine may facilitate earlier identification of vertebral injury, but does so at the cost of increased radiation dose.[113] CT of the abdomen should be obtained: (1) in intubated patients; (2) with signs of internal bleeding (abdominal tenderness, distention, bruising, or gross hematuria), a history of hypotensive shock (which has responded to volume resuscitation), or a hematocrit <30%; (3) if a femur fracture is evident; (4) if serum transaminase levels are elevated; (5) if significant microscopic hematuria is present, or (6) if the mechanism of injury is deemed significant.[114,115]

Sonography serves an adjunctive role in the imaging of pediatric trauma. FAST itself is most useful in detecting intra-abdominal blood, but is not sufficiently reliable to exclude blunt abdominal injury, although it does have the advantage that such injuries can be detected by repeated examination.[116–123] Therefore, like its historical predecessor diagnostic peritoneal lavage, FAST adds relatively little to the management of pediatric abdominal trauma, since unstable patients with presumed intraabdominal injuries need immediate operation, while stable patients are managed nonoperatively without regard to the presence of intra-abdominal blood.[124–128] However, diagnostic sonography has been successfully used in screening for intra-abdominal injuries when abdominal CT is unavailable or contraindicated.[129]

SPECIAL CONSIDERATIONS IN TRAUMA CARE

Definitive management of childhood trauma begins once the primary survey and resuscitation phases have concluded. This care is the responsibility not of a single individual or specialty, but from a multidisciplinary team of professionals specializing in pediatric health care led by a surgeon with experience in the care of both trauma and children. It begins with the secondary survey and re-evaluation of vital functions and progresses through the tertiary survey (a scrupulous repetition of the primary and secondary surveys conducted by the admitting team once the patient is transferred to definitive care) to ensure no injuries have been missed. It persists throughout the duration of hospitalization and concludes with rehabilitation, fully encompassing the operative, critical, acute, and convalescent phases of care. Avoidance of secondary injury (injury due to persistent or recurrent hypoxia or hypoperfusion) is a major goal of definitive management and mandates reliance on continuous monitoring of vital signs, GCS score, oxygen saturation, urinary output, and, when necessary, arterial and central venous pressure.

Definitive management of childhood trauma also depends on the type, extent, and severity of the injuries sustained. Any child requiring resuscitation should be admitted to the hospital under the care of a surgeon experienced in the management of childhood injuries. Further information and details regarding the management and treatment of traumatic injuries in children may found throughout this textbook including: vascular access (Chapter 8), burns (Chapter 13), thoracic trauma (Chapter 15), abdominal trauma (Chapter 16), traumatic brain injury (Chapter 17), and orthopedic and spinal trauma (Chapter 18).

Physical Support

The care of children with major traumatic injury also involves assessment and treatment of somatic pain. Two pain scales have now been validated.[130] In patients who are not eating, nutritional support is recommended.[131] In children who have sustained injuries resulting in hematomas, low-grade fever may develop as these are resorbed. However, high spiking fevers should prompt investigation for a source such as infected hematomas, effusions, or pelvic osteomyelitis. Children with chest tubes or long-term indwelling urinary catheters are at risk for systemic infection and should receive prophylactic or suppressive antibiotics as long as the tube or catheter is required.

Emotional Support

Efforts must be made to attend to the emotional needs of the child and family, especially for those families facing the death of a child or a sibling.[132] In addition to the loss of control over their child's destiny, parents of seriously injured children also may feel enormous guilt, whether or not these feelings are warranted. The pediatric surgeon should attempt to create as normal an environment as possible for the child and allow the parents to participate meaningfully in postinjury care, as acute stress disorder symptoms in children and parents are common after injury.[133] In so doing, treatment interventions will be facilitated as the child perceives that parents and staff are working together to ensure an optimal recovery, with the added benefit that long-term psychological effects such as posttraumatic stress disorder may be averted.[134] Even so, depression is increasingly recognized as a serious complication in adolescents after major trauma. Risk factors for depression include high injury severity, other family members injured, low socioeconomic status, and suicidal ideation or attempt prior to the current traumatic event.[135]

Nonaccidental Trauma

Nonaccidental trauma (NAT) is the underlying cause of 3–5% of significant traumatic injuries in childhood, and is a major cause of morbidity and mortality among children referred to pediatric trauma centers.[9,136] Although a detailed review of the mechanisms, patterns, presentations, and findings of NAT is beyond the scope of this chapter, NAT should be suspected when: (1) the injury remains unexplained; (2) a lengthy delay occurs in obtaining treatment; (3) the history is vague or otherwise incompatible with the observed physical findings; (4) the caretaker blames siblings or playmates or other third parties, or protects other adults rather than the child; (5) cutaneous bruises or skeletal fractures are found in multiple stages of healing or in unusual locations; (6) skeletal fractures are found in the diaphyses of long bones in infants or children too young to walk; (7) scald or contact burns are found in unusual locations or patterns; or (8) unconsciousness is said to have occurred in association with a low fall.[137,138] As with unintentional trauma, traumatic brain injury is the leading cause of death in NAT. The term 'shaken baby syndrome', characterized by the classic triad of altered mental status, bilateral subdural hematomas, and retinal hemorrhages, has largely been supplanted by the more inclusive term 'abusive head trauma'.[139,140] Although the initial assessment and medical treatment of physical injuries is no different from that for any other mechanism of injury, the sociomedicolegal management of suspected cases of NAT requires a special approach. The crucial role played by the pediatric trauma service and the pediatric trauma registry in early recognition and adequate documentation of potentially abusive injuries is paramount.[141,142] Reports of suspected NAT must be filed with local child protective services in every North American state, province, and territory, as well as in most developed nations worldwide. Still, it must be emphasized that confrontation and accusation hinder treatment and rehabilitation, and have no place in the management of the potentially abused child, regardless of the nature of the injury, or the identity of the perpetrators.

Penetrating Injuries

All penetrating wounds are contaminated and must be treated as infected. Accessible missile fragments should be removed (once swelling has subsided) to prevent the development of lead poisoning (especially those in contact with bone or joint fluid).[143] Thoracotomy is usually not required except for massive hemothorax (20 mL/kg) or ongoing hemorrhage (2–4 mL/kg/h) from the chest tube, persistent massive air leak, or food or salivary drainage from the chest tube. Laparotomy is nearly always required for gunshot wounds as well as stab wounds associated with hemorrhagic shock, peritonitis, or evisceration, although nonoperative management may be employed in carefully selected cases.[144] Thoracoabdominal injury should be suspected whenever the torso is penetrated between the nipple line and the costal margin. A diaphragmatic injury should be suspected if peritoneal irritation develops after thoracic penetration, food or chyle is recovered from the chest tube, or if injury-trajectory or imaging studies suggest the possibility of diaphragmatic penetration. Tube thoracostomy, followed by laparotomy for repair of the diaphragm and/or damaged organs, is mandated with such signs, although laparoscopy is being used with increasing frequency.[145–148]

Systems Issues

Pediatric patients, at significant risk for death from multiple and severe injuries, are best served by a fully inclusive trauma system that incorporates all appropriate health care facilities and personnel to the level of their resources and capabilities.[149,150] Unfortunately, access to specialty pediatric trauma care, including pediatric intensive care, remains highly variable.[151,152] Moreover, collaboration with local public health agencies (in programs for injury prevention and control), as well as local public health, public safety, and emergency-management agencies (in regional disaster-planning efforts) is necessary.[149,150] Although the regional trauma center is at the hub of the system, area trauma centers may be needed in localities distant from the regional trauma center. All trauma centers, whether adult or pediatric, must be capable of the initial management of the injured child or infant. This requires the immediate availability of a resuscitation team trained and credentialed for the management of pediatric trauma, for which structured review and simulation training have been shown to improve team performance, while family presence during resuscitation rarely hinders it.[153–158] All other hospitals in the region should participate as they are able, and must be fully capable of initial resuscitation, stabilization, and transfer of pediatric trauma patients. Finally, a regional trauma advisory committee should include pediatric representation that has the authority to develop and implement guidelines for triage of pediatric trauma within the system to verified pediatric-capable trauma centers.[159,160] Mature systems should expect that seriously injured pediatric patients will be primarily transported to pediatric trauma centers.[161]

Transport Issues

Pediatric victims of multisystem trauma should undergo direct primary transport from the injury scene to a pediatric-capable trauma center.[28–47,82,150] If this is not possible, additional secondary transport from the initial receiving hospital to the pediatric trauma center is needed. Transport providers must be capable of critical pediatric assessment and monitoring, and skilled in the techniques of endotracheal intubation and vascular access, as well as drug and fluid administration in children.[162,163] Specialized pediatric transport teams, staffed by physicians and nurses with advanced training in pediatric trauma and critical care treatment and transport, should be used whenever possible, as complications related to endotracheal intubation and vascular access are the leading causes of adverse events during transport, which occur twice as often as in the PICU and ten times more often without a specialized team.[164,165]

Hospital Preparedness

Regional pediatric trauma centers should be located in trauma hospitals with comprehensive pediatric services (a full-service general, university, or children's hospital) that demonstrate an institutional commitment to pediatric trauma care, including child abuse.[28–47,150] Adult trauma centers can achieve results comparable to those of pediatric trauma centers if pediatric subspecialty and nursing support (pediatric emergency, acute care, and critical care medicine) are available.[38–47,150] Finally, an organized pediatric trauma service must be available within the regional pediatric trauma center that, in addition to exemplary patient care, provides education and research in pediatric trauma, and leadership in pediatric trauma system coordination.

REFERENCES

1. National Center for Injury Prevention and Control. CDC Injury Fact Book. Atlanta: Centers for Disease Control and Prevention; 2006.
2. Buie VC, Owings MF, DeFrances CJ, et al. National Hospital Discharge Survey: 2006 Summary. National Center for Health Statistics. Vital Health Stat 2010;13(168).
3. Klem SA, Pollack MM, Glass NL, et al. Resource use, efficiency, and outcome prediction in pediatric intensive care of trauma patients. J Trauma 1990;30:32–6.
4. Krauss BS, Harakal T, Fleisher GR. The spectrum and frequency of illness presenting to a pediatric emergency department. Pediatr Emerg Care 1991;7:67–71.
5. Tsai A, Kallsen G. Epidemiology of pediatric prehospital care. Ann Emerg Med 1987;16:284–92.
6. Hale GC, Caudill SA, Hicks-Waller CM, et al. The New York State Trauma System: A Special Report on Pediatric Trauma. Albany, NY: New York State Department of Health; 2002.
7. Tepas JJ, Ramenofsky ML, Mollitt DL, et al. The pediatric trauma score as a predictor of injury severity: An objective assessment. J Trauma 1988;28:425–9.
8. Cooper A, Barlow B, Davidson L, et al. Epidemiology of pediatric trauma: Importance of population-based statistics. J Pediatr Surg 1992;27:149–54.
9. DiScala C. National Pediatric Trauma Registry Annual Report. Boston: Tufts University Rehabilitation and Childhood Trauma Research and Training Center; 2002.
10. Ehrlich PF, Brown JK, Drogonowski R. Characterization of the drug-positive adolescent trauma population: Should we, do we, and does it make a difference if we test? J Pediatr Surg 2006; 41:927–30.
11. Draus JM, Santos AP, Franklin GA, et al. Drug and alcohol use among adolescent blunt trauma patients: Dying to get high? J Pediatr Surg 2007;43:208–11.
12. Ehrlich PF, Drogonowski A, Swisher-McClure S, et al. The importance of a preclinical trial: A selected intervention program for pediatric trauma centers. J Trauma 2008;65:189–95.

13. Brown CVR, Nevill AL, Salim A, et al. The impact of obesity on severely injured children and adolescents. J Pediatr Surg 2006;41:88–91.

14. Marcin JP, Schembri MS, Jingsong H, et al. A population-based analysis of socioeconomic status and insurance status and their relationship with pediatric trauma hospitalization and mortality rates. Am J Publ Health 2003;93:461–6.

15. Falcone RA, Brown RL, Garcia VF. The epidemiology of infant injuries and alarming health disparities. J Pediatr Surg 2007;42:172–7.

16. Haider AH, Efron DT, Haut ER, et al. Black children experience worse clinical and functional outcomes after traumatic brain injury: An analysis of the National Pediatric Trauma Registry. J Trauma 2007;62:1259–63.

17. Falcone RA, Martin F, Brown RL, et al. Despite overall low pediatric head injury mortality, disparities exist between races. J Pediatr Surg 2008;43:1858–64.

18. Falcone RA, Brown RL, Garcia VF. Disparities in child abuse mortality are not explained by injury severity. J Pediatr Surg 2007;42:1031–7.

19. Rangel SJ, Martin CA, Brown RL, et al. Alarming trends in the improper use of motor vehicle restraints in children: Implications for public policy and the development of race-based strategies for improving compliance. J Pediatr Surg 2008;43:200–7.

20. Brown JK, Ying Y, Wang S, et al. Patterns of severe injury in pediatric car crash victims: Crash Injury Research Engineering Network database. J Pediatr Surg 2006;41:362–7.

21. Ehrlich PF, Brown JK, Sochor MR, et al. Factors influencing pediatric Injury Severity Score and Glasgow Coma Scale in pediatric automobile crashes: Results from the Crash Injury Research Engineering Network. J Pediatr Surg 2006;41:1854–8.

22. Zuckerbraun BS, Morrison K, Gaines B, et al. Effect of age on cervical spine injuries in children after motor vehicle collisions: Effectiveness of restraint devices. J Pediatr Surg 2004;39:483–6.

23. Hayes JR, Groner JI. Using multiple imputation and propensity scores to test the effect of car seats and seat belt usage on injury severity from trauma registry data. J Pediatr Surg 2008;43: 924–7.

24. Arbogast KB, Kent RW, Menon RA, et al. Mechanisms of abdominal organ injury in seat-belt restrained children. J Trauma 2007;62:1473–80.

25. Lutz N, Nance ML, Kallan MJ, et al. Incidence and clinical significance of abdominal wall bruising in restrained children involved in motor vehicle crashes. J Pediatr Surg 2004;39:972–5.

26. Chidester S, Rana A, Lowell W, et al. Is the 'seat belt sign' associated with serious abdominal injuries in pediatric trauma? J Trauma 2009;67:s34–36.

27. Nadler EP, Potoka DA, Shultz BL, et al. The high morbidity associated with handlebar injuries in children. J Trauma 2005; 58:1171–4.

28. Pollack MM, Alexander SR, Clarke N, et al. Improved outcomes from tertiary center pediatric intensive care: A statewide comparison of tertiary and nontertiary care facilities. Crit Care Med 1991;19:150–9.

29. Nakayama DK, Copes WS, Sacco WJ. Differences in pediatric trauma care among pediatric and nonpediatric centers. J Pediatr Surg 1992;27:427–31.

30. Cooper A, Barlow B, DiScala C, et al. Efficacy of pediatric trauma care: Results of a population-based study. J Pediatr Surg 1993;28:299–305.

31. Hall JR, Reyes HM, Meller JT, et al. Outcome for blunt trauma is best at a pediatric trauma center. J Pediatr Surg 1996;31:72–7.

32. Hulka F, Mullins RJ, Mann NC, et al. Influence of a statewide trauma system on pediatric hospitalization and outcome. J Trauma 1997;42:514–19.

33. Potoka DA, Schall LC, Gardner MJ, et al. Impact of pediatric trauma centers on mortality in a statewide system. J Trauma 2000;49:237–45.

34. Potoka DA, Schall LC, Ford HR. Improved functional outcome for severely injured children treated at pediatric trauma centers. J Trauma 2001;51:824–34.

35. Farrell LS, Hannan EL, Cooper A. Severity of injury and mortality associated with pediatric blunt injuries: Hospitals with pediatric intensive care units vs. other hospitals. Pediatr Crit Care Med 2004;5:5–9.

36. Densmore JC, Lim HJ, Oldham KT, et al. Outcomes and delivery of care in pediatric injury. J Pediatr Surg 2006;41:92–8.

37. Pracht EE, Tepas JJ, Langland-Orban B, et al. Do pediatric patients with trauma in Florida have reduced mortality rates when treated in designated trauma centers? J Pediatr Surg 2008; 43:212–21.

38. Knudson MM, Shagoury C, Lewis FR. Can adult trauma surgeons care for injured children? J Trauma 1992;32:729–39.

39. Fortune JM, Sanchez J, Graca L, et al. A pediatric trauma center without a pediatric surgeon: A four year outcome analysis. J Trauma 1992;33:130–9.

40. Rhodes M, Smith S, Boorse D. Pediatric trauma patients in an 'adult' trauma center. J Trauma 1993;35:384–93.

41. Bensard DD, McIntyre RC, Moore EE, et al. A critical analysis of acutely injured children managed in an adult level I trauma center. J Pediatr Surg 1994;29:11–18.

42. D'Amelio LF, Hammond JS, Thomasseau J, et al. 'Adult' trauma surgeons with pediatric commitment: A logical solution to the pediatric trauma manpower problem. Am Surg 1995;61:968–74.

43. Partrick DA, Moore EE, Bensard DD, et al. Operative management of injured children at an adult level I trauma center. J Trauma 2000;48:894–901.

44. Sherman HF, Landry VL, Jones LM. Should level I trauma centers be rated NC-17? J Trauma 2001;50:784–91.

45. Aaland MO, Hlaing T. Pediatric trauma deaths: A three-part analysis from a nonacademic trauma center. Am Surg 2006;72: 249–59.

46. Winthrop AL, Brasel KJ, Stahovic L, et al. Quality of life and functional outcome after pediatric trauma. J Trauma 2005;58: 468–74.

47. vanderSluis CK, Kingma J, Eisma WH, et al. Pediatric polytrauma: Short-term and long-term outcomes. J Trauma 1997;43: 501–6.

48. Burd RS, Jang TS, Nair SS. Predicting hospital mortality among injured children using a national trauma database. J Trauma 2006;60:792–801.

49. Haddon W. Advances in the epidemiology of injuries as a basis for public policy. Public Health Rep 1980;95:411–21.

50. Kokoska ER, Keller MS, Rallo MC, et al. Characteristics of pediatric cervical spine injuries. J Pediatr Surg 2001;36:100–5.

51. Patel JC, Tepas JJ, Mollitt DL, et al. Pediatric cervical spine injuries: defining the disease. J Pediatr Surg 2001;36:373–6.

52. Kewalramani LS, Kraus JF, Sterling HM, et al. Acute spinal-cord lesions in a pediatric population: Epidemiological and clinical features. Paraplegia 1980;18:206–19.

53. Pang D, Wilberger E. Spinal cord injury without radiographic abnormality in children. J Neurosurg 1982;57:114–29.

54. Bohn D, Armstrong A, Becker L, et al. Cervical spine injuries in children. J Trauma 1990;30:463–9.

55. Bosch PP, Vogt MT, Ward WT. Pediatric spinal cord injury without radiographic abnormality: The absence of occult instability and lack of indication for bracing. Spine 2002;27:2788–800.

56. Cooper A, Barlow B, DiScala C. Mortality and truncal injury: The pediatric perspective. J Pediatr Surg 1994;29:33–8.

57. Peclet MH, Newman KD, Eichelberger MR, et al. Thoracic trauma in children: An indicator of increased mortality. J Pediatr Surg 1990;25:961–6.

58. Haller JA. Injuries of the gastrointestinal tract in children: Notes on recognition and management. Clin Pediatr 1966;5:476–80.

59. Rogers CG, Knight V, MacUra KJ. High-grade renal injuries in children—is conservative management possible? Urology 2004;64:574–9.

60. Pearl RH, Wesson DE, Spence LJ, et al. Splenic injury: A 5-year update with improved results and changing criteria for conservative management. J Pediatr Surg 1989;24:121–5.

61. Galat JA, Grisoni ER, Gauderer MWL. Pediatric blunt liver injury: Establishment of criteria for appropriate management. J Pediatr Surg 1990;25:1162–5.

62. Barlow B, Niemirska M, Gandhi R. Ten years of experience with falls from a height in children. J Pediatr Surg 1983;18:509–11.

63. Selbst SM, Baker MD, Shames M. Bunk bed injuries. Am J Dis Child 1990;144:721–3.

64. Helfer RE, Slovis TL, Black M. Injuries resulting when small children fall out of bed. Pediatrics 1977;60:533–5.

65. Joffe M, Ludwig S. Stairway injuries in children. Pediatrics 1988;82:457–61.

66. Barlow B, Niemirska M, Gandhi R, et al. Response to injury in children with closed femur fractures. J Trauma 1987;27:429–30.

67. Ismail N, Bellemare JF, Mollitt D, et al. Death from pelvic fracture: Children are different. J Pediatr Surg 1996;31:82–5.

68. McIntyre RR, Bensard DD, Moore EE, et al. Pelvic fracture geometry predicts risk of life-threatening hemorrhage in children. J Trauma 1993;35:423–9.

69. Herzenberg JE, Hensinger RN, Dedrick DK, et al. Emergency transport and positioning of young children who have an injury of the cervical spine. J Bone Joint Surg Am 1989;71:15–22.

70. Schafermeyer RW, Ribbeck BM, Gaskins J, et al. Respiratory effects of spinal immobilization in children. Ann Emerg Med 1991;20:1017–19.

71. Viccellio P, Simon H, Pressman BD, et al. A prospective multicenter study of cervical spine injury in children. Pediatrics 2001;108:e20.

72. Gausche M, Lewis RJ, Stratton SJ, et al. Effect of out-of-hospital pediatric endotracheal intubation on survival and neurological outcome: A controlled clinical trial. JAMA 2000;283:783–90.

73. Cooper A, DiScala C, Foltin G, et al. Prehospital endotracheal intubation for severe head injury in children: A reappraisal. Semin Pediatr Surg 2001;10:3–6.

74. Ehrlich PF, Seidman PS, Atallah O, et al. Endotracheal intubations in rural pediatric trauma patients. J Pediatr Surg 2004;39:1376–80.

75. Cooper A, Barlow B, DiScala C, et al. Efficacy of prehospital volume resuscitation in children who present in hypotensive shock. J Trauma 1993;35:160.

76. Teach SJ, Antosia RE, Lund DP, et al. Prehospital fluid therapy in pediatric trauma patients. Pediatr Emerg Care 1995;11:5–8.

77. Tepas JJ, Mollitt DL, Talbert JL, et al. The pediatric trauma score as a predictor of injury severity in the injured child. J Pediatr Surg 1987;22:14–18.

78. Champion HR, Sacco WJ, Copes WS, et al. A revision of the trauma score. J Trauma 1989;29:623–9.

79. Hannan EL, Farrell LS, Meaker PS, et al. Predicting inpatient mortality for pediatric blunt trauma patients: A better alternative. J Pediatr Surg 2000;35:155–9.

80. Sasser SM, Hunt RC, Faul M, et al. Recommendations of the National Expert Panel on Field Triage, 2011. MMWR 2012;61(RR-1):1–21.

81. Prehospital Trauma Life Support Committee of the National Association of Emergency Medical Technicians in cooperation with the Committee on Trauma of the American College of Surgeons. PHTLS: Prehospital Trauma Life Support. 7th ed. St. Louis: Mosby Elsevier; 2010.

82. American College of Surgeons Committee on Trauma. Advanced Trauma Life Support® ATLS® Student Course Manual. 9th ed. Chicago: American College of Surgeons; 2012.

83. Rees MJ, Aickin R, Kolbe A, et al. The screening pelvic radiograph in pediatric trauma. Pediatr Radiol 2001;31:497–500.

84. Junkins EP, Stotts A, Santiago R, et al. The clinical presentation of pediatric thoracolumbar fractures: A prospective study. J Trauma 2008;65:1066–71.

85. Kragh JF, Cooper A, Aden JK, et al. Survey of trauma registry data on tourniquet use in pediatric war casualties. Pediatr Emerg Care 2012;28:1361–5.

86. Holcomb JB, Wade CE, Michalek JE, et al. Increased plasma and platelet to red cell ratios improves outcome in 466 massively transfused civilian trauma patients. Ann Surg 2008;248(3);447–58.

87. Dressler AM, Finck CM, Carroll CL, et al. Use of a massive transfusion protocol with hemostatic resuscitation for severe intraoperative bleeding in a child. J Pediatr Surg 2010;45:1530–3.

88. Patregnani JT, Borgman MA, Maegele M, et al. Coagulopathy and shock on admission is associated with mortality for children with traumatic injuries at combat support hospitals. Pediatr Crit Care Med 2012;13:273–7.

89. Schwaitzberg SD, Bergman KS, Harris BH. A pediatric model of continuous hemorrhage. J Pediatr Surg 1988;23:605–9.

90. Klinker DB, Arca MJ, Lewis BD, et al. Pediatric vascular injuries: Patterns of injury, morbidity, and mortality. J Pediatr Surg 2007;42:178–83.

91. Hammer CE, Groner JI, Caniano DA, et al. Blunt intraabdominal arterial injury in pediatric trauma patients: Injury distribution and markers of outcome. J Pediatr Surg 2008;34:916–23.

92. Anderson SA, Day M, Chen NK, et al. Traumatic aortic injuries in the pediatric population. J Pediatr Surg 2008;43:1077–81.

93. Heckman SR, Trooskin SZ, Burd RS. Risk factors for blunt thoracic injury in children. J Pediatr Surg 2005;40:98–102.

94. Isaacman DJ, Scarfone RJ, Kost SI, et al. Utility of routine laboratory testing for detecting intraabdominal injury in the pediatric trauma patient. Pediatrics 1993;92:691–4.

95. Keller MS, Coln CE, Trimble JA, et al. The utility of routine trauma laboratories in pediatric trauma resuscitations. Am J Surg 2004;188:671–8.

96. Capraro AJ, Mooney D, Waltzman ML. The use of routine laboratory studies as screening tools in pediatric abdominal trauma. Pediatr Emerg Care 2006;22:480–4.

97. Kincaid EH, Chang MC, Letton RW, et al. Admission base deficit in pediatric trauma: A study using the National Trauma Data Bank. J Trauma 2001;51:332–5.

98. Randolph LC, Takacs M, Davis KA. Resuscitation in the pediatric trauma population: Admission base deficit remains an important prognostic indicator. J Trauma 2002;53:838–42.

99. Oldham KT, Guice KS, Kaufman RA, et al. Blunt hepatic injury and elevated hepatic enzymes: A clinical correlation in children. J Pediatr Surg 1984;19:457–61.

100. Adamson WT, Hebra A, Thomas PB, et al. Serum amylase and lipase alone are not cost-effective screening methods for pediatric pancreatic trauma. J Pediatr Surg 2003;38:354–7.

101. Lieu TA, Fleisher GR, Mahboubi S, et al. Hematuria and clinical findings as indications for intravenous pyelography in pediatric blunt renal trauma. Pediatrics 1988;82:216–22.

102. Brenner DJ, Elliston CD, Berdon WE. Estimated risks of radiation-induced fatal cancer from pediatric CT. Am J Roentgenol 2001;176:289–96.

103. Fenton SJ, Hansen KW, Meyers RL, et al. CT scan and the pediatric trauma patient: are we overdoing it? J Pediatr Surg 2004;39:1877–81.

104. Kim PK, Zhu X, Houseknecht E, et al. Effective radiation dose from radiologic studies in pediatric trauma patients. World J Surg 2005;29: 1557–62.

105. Brody AS, Frush DP, Huda W, et al. Radiation risk to children from computed tomography. Pediatrics 2007;120:677–82.

106. Chwals WJ, Robinson AV, Sivit CJ, et al. Computed tomography before transfer to a level I pediatric trauma center risks duplication with associated increased radiation exposure. J Pediatr Surg 2008;43:2268–72.

107. Cook SH, Fielding JR, Phillips JD. Repeat abdominal computed tomography after pediatric blunt trauma: missed injuries, extra costs, and unnecessary radiation exposure. J Pediatr Surg 2010;45:2019–24.

108. Brunetti MA, Mahadevappa M, Nabaweesi R, et al. Diagnostic radiation exposure in pediatric trauma patients. J Trauma 2011;70:E24–8.

109. Wang MY, Griffith PR, Sterling J, et al. A prospective population-based study of pediatric trauma patients with mild alterations in consciousness (Glasgow Coma Scale score of 13–14). Neurosurg 2000;46:1093–9.

110. Kuppermann N, Holmes JF, Dayan PS, et al. Identification of children at very low risk of clinically-important brain injuries after head trauma: A prospective cohort study. Lancet 2009;374:1160–70.

111. Renton J, Kincaid S, Ehrlich PF. Should helical CT scanning of the thoracic cavity replace the conventional chest x-ray as a primary assessment tool in pediatric trauma? An efficacy and cost analysis. J Pediatr Surg 2003;38:793–7.

112. Kwon A, Sorrells DL, Kurkchubaske AG, et al. Isolated computed tomography diagnosis of pulmonary contusion does not correlate with increased morbidity. J Pediatr Surg 2006;41:78–82.

113. Keenan HT, Hollingshead MC, Chung CJ, et al. Using CT of the cervical spine for early evaluation of pediatric patients with head trauma. Am J Roentgenol 2001;177:1405–9.

114. Flood RG, Mooney DP. Rate and prediction of traumatic injuries detected by abdominal computed tomography scan in intubated children. J Trauma 2006;61:340–5.

115. Taylor GA, Eichelberger MR, O'Donnel R, et al. Indications for computed tomography in children with blunt abdominal trauma. Ann Surg 1991;213:212–18.

116. Patel JC, Tepas JJ. The efficacy of focused abdominal sonography for trauma (FAST) as a screening tool in the assessment of injured children. J Pediatr Surg 1999;34:44–7.

117. Mutabagani KH, Coley BD, Zumberge N, et al. Preliminary experience with focused abdominal sonography for trauma (FAST) in children: Is it useful? J Pediatr Surg 1999;34:48–54.

118. Pershad J, Gilmore B. Serial bedside emergency ultrasound in a case of pediatric blunt abdominal trauma with severe abdominal pain. Pediatr Emerg Care 2000;16:375–6.

119. Corbett SW, Andrews HG, Baker EM, et al. ED evaluation of the pediatric trauma patient by ultrasonography. Am J Emerg Med 2000;18:244–9.

120. Coley BD, Mutabagani KH, Martin LC, et al. Focused abdominal sonography for trauma (FAST) in children with blunt abdominal trauma. J Trauma 2000;48:902–6.

121. Soudack M, Epelman M, Maor R, et al. Experience with focused abdominal sonography for trauma (FAST) in 313 pediatric patients. J Clin Ultrasound 2004;32:53–61.

122. Suthers SE, Albrecht R, Foley D, et al. Surgeon-directed ultrasound for trauma is a predictor of intraabdominal injury in children. Am Surg 2004;70:164–8.

123. Soundappan SV, Holland AJ, Cass DT, et al. Accuracy of surgeon-performed focused abdominal sonography (FAST) in blunt paediatric trauma. Injury 2005;36:970–5.

124. Emery KH, McAneney CM, Racadio JM, et al. Absent peritoneal fluid on screening trauma ultrasonography in children: A prospective comparison with computed tomography. J Pediatr Surg 2001;36:565–9.

125. Holmes JF, London KL, Brant WE. Isolated intraperitoneal fluid on abdominal computed tomography in children with blunt trauma. Acad Emerg Med 2000;7:335–41.

126. Rathaus V, Zissin R, Werner M, et al. Minimal pelvic fluid in blunt abdominal trauma: The significance of this sonographic finding. J Pediatr Surg 2001;36:1387–9.

127. Holmes JF, Brant WE, Bond WF, et al. Emergency department ultrasonography in the evaluation of hypotensive and normotensive children with blunt abdominal trauma. J Pediatr Surg 2001;36:968–73.

128. Venkatesh KR, McQuay N. Outcomes of management in stable children with intra-abdominal free fluid without solid organ injury after blunt abdominal injury. J Trauma 2007;62:216–20.

129. Filiatrault D, Longpre D, Patriquin H, et al. Investigation of childhood blunt abdominal trauma: A practical approach using ultrasound as the initial diagnostic modality. Pediatr Radiol 1987;17:373–9.

130. Baxt C, Kassam-Adams N, Nance ML, et al. Assessment of pain after injury in the pediatric patient: Child and parent perceptions. J Pediatr Surg 2004;39:979–83.

131. Winthrop AL, Wesson DE, Pencharz PB, et al. Injury severity, whole body protein turnover, and energy expenditure in pediatric trauma. J Pediatr Surg 1987;22:534–7.

132. Oliver RC, Sturtevant JP, Scheetz JP, et al. Beneficial effects of a hospital bereavement intervention program after traumatic childhood death. J Trauma 2001;50:440–8.

133. Winston FK, Kassam-Adams N, Vivarelli-O'Neill C, et al. Acute stress disorder symptoms in children and their parents after pediatric traffic injury. Pediatrics 2002;109:e90.

134. Schreier H, Ladakokos C, Morabito D, et al. Posttrauma stress symptoms in children after mild to moderate pediatric trauma: A longitudinal examination of symptom prevalence, correlates, and parent-child symptom reporting. J Trauma 2005;58:353–63.

135. Han PP, Holbrook TL, Sise MJ, et al. Postinjury depression is a serious complication in adolescents after major trauma: Injury severity and injury-event factors predict depression and long-term quality of life deficits. J Trauma 2011;70:923–30.

136. Roaten JB, Partrick DA, Nydam TL, et al. Nonaccidental trauma is a major cause of morbidity and mortality among patients at a regional level 1 pediatric trauma center. J Pediatr Surg 2006;41:2013–15.

137. Cooper A, Floyd T, Barlow B, et al. Fifteen years' experience with major blunt abdominal trauma due to child abuse. J Trauma 1988;28:1483–7.

138. Wood J, Rubin DM, Nance ML, et al. Distinguishing inflicted versus accidental abdominal injuries in young children. J Trauma 2005;59:1203–8.

139. Duhaime A-C, Gennarelli TA, Thibault LE, et al. The shaken baby syndrome: A clinical, pathological, and biomechanical study. J Neurosurg 1987;66:409–15.

140. Christian CW, Block R, and the Committee on Child Abuse and Neglect. Abusive head trauma in infants and children. Pediatrics 2009;123:1409–11.

141. Chang DC, Knight V, Ziegfeld S, et al. The tip of the iceberg for child abuse: The critical roles of the pediatric trauma service and its registry. J Trauma 2004;57:1189–98.

142. Boyce MC, Melhorn KJ, Vargo G. Pediatric trauma documentation: Adequacy for assessment of child abuse. Arch Pediatr Adolesc Med 1996;150:730–2.

143. Selbst SM, Henretig F, Fee MA, et al. Lead poisoning in a child with a gunshot wound. Pediatrics 1986;77:413–16.

144. Cigdem MK, Onen A, Siga M, et al. Selective nonoperative management of penetrating abdominal injuries in children. J Trauma 2009;67:1284–7.

145. Chen MK, Schropp KP, Lobe TE. The use of minimal access surgery in pediatric trauma: a preliminary report. J Laparoendoscop Surg 1995;5:295–301.

146. Gandhi RR, Stringel G. Laparoscopy in pediatric abdominal trauma. J Soc Laparoendoscop Surg 1997;1:349–51.

147. Feliz A, Shultz B, McKenna C, et al. Diagnostic and therapeutic laparoscopy in pediatric abdominal trauma. J Pediatr Surg 2006;41:72–7.

148. Marwan A, Harmon CM, Georgeson KE. Use of laparoscopy in the management of pediatric abdominal trauma. J Trauma 2010;69:761–4.

149. Committee on Trauma. American College of Surgeons: Resources for Optimal Care of the Injured Patient. Chicago: American College of Surgeons; 2006.

150. Committee on Trauma. American College of Surgeons: Regional Trauma Systems: Optimal Elements, Integration, and Assessment-Systems Consultation Guide. Chicago: American College of Surgeons; 2008.

151. Nance ML, Carr BG, Branas CC. Access to pediatric trauma care in the United States. Arch Pediatr Adolesc Med 2009;163:512–18.

152. Odetola FO, Miller WC, Davis MM, et al. The relationship between the location of pediatric intensive care unit facilities and child death from trauma: A county-level ecologic study. J Pediatr 2005;147:74–7.

153. Hunt EA, Hohenhaus SM, Luo X, et al. Simulation of pediatric trauma stabilization in 35 North Carolina emergency departments: Identification of targets for performance improvement. Pediatrics 2006;117:641–8.

154. Mikrogianakis A, Osmond MH, Nuth JE, et al. Evaluation of a multidisciplinary pediatric mock trauma code educational initiative; A pilot study. J Trauma 2008;64:761–7.

155. Falcone RA, Daugherty M, Schweer L, et al. Multidisciplinary trauma team training using high-fidelity trauma simulation. J Pediatr Surg 2008;43:1065–71.

156. Popp J, Yochum L, Spinella P, et al. Simulation training for surgical residents in pediatric trauma scenarios. Connecticut Med 2012;76:159–62.

157. O'Connell KJ, Farah MM, Spandorfer P, et al. Family presence during pediatric trauma team activation: An assessment of a structured program. Pediatrics 2007;120:e565–74.

158. Dudley NC, Hansen KW, Furnival RA, et al. The effect of family presence on the efficiency of pediatric trauma resuscitation. Ann Emerg Med 2009;53:777–84.

159. Osler TM, Vane DW, Tepas JJ, et al. Do pediatric trauma centers have better survival rates than adult trauma centers? An examination of the National Pediatric Trauma Registry. J Trauma 2001;50:96–101.

160. Ehrlich PF, McClellan WT, Wesson DE. Monitoring performance: Long-term impact of trauma verification and review. J Am Coll Surg 2005;200:166–72.

161. Vavilala MS, Cummings P, Sharar SR, et al. Association of hospital trauma designation with admission patterns of injured children. J Trauma 2004;54:119–24.

162. Smith DF, Hackel A. Selection criteria for pediatric critical care transport teams. Crit Care Med 1983;11:10–12.

163. MacNab AJ. Optimal escort for interhospital transport of pediatric emergencies. J Trauma 1991;31:205–9.

164. Kanter RK, Boeing NM, Hannan WP, et al. Excess morbidity associated with interhospital transport. Pediatrics 1992;90:893–8.

165. Edge WE, Kanter RK, Weigle CGM, et al. Reduction of morbidity in interhospital transport by specialized pediatric staff. Crit Care Med 1994;22:1186–91.

CHAPTER 15

THORACIC TRAUMA

Alejandro R. Ruiz-Elizalde • David W. Tuggle

Trauma is an important cause of morbidity and mortality in children. Although it accounts for a minority of trauma injuries (4–25%), thoracic trauma is associated with a 20-fold increase in mortality when compared with injured children without thoracic trauma.[1-10] Isolated thoracic trauma in a child is associated with a mortality rate of approximately 5%, which is largely due to penetrating trauma.[1] However, children with head trauma, thoracic trauma, and abdominal trauma can have a mortality rate that approaches 40%.

Epidemiologic studies have reported a two to threefold higher incidence of thoracic trauma in boys as compared with girls.[9-15] Most injuries (80–95%) are the result of blunt trauma, typically resulting from a traffic accident in which the child is a passenger or pedestrian.[2,10] Not surprisingly, many children will have involvement of other organ systems with a high injury severity score (ISS). When penetrating trauma occurs, older children and adolescents are more likely to be the victims and there is a higher mortality rate.[5]

Contusion or laceration of the pulmonary parenchyma is the most common thoracic injury and may be associated with rib fractures and pneumothorax or hemothorax. Injuries to other organs such as the tracheobronchial tree (<1%), esophagus (<1%), aorta (<1%), diaphragm (4%), and heart (6%) are uncommon, but not insignificant.[12]

ANATOMY AND PHYSIOLOGY

Children have unique anatomic and physiologic properties that are salient to the diagnosis and management of chest injuries. As in any trauma patient, sequential management of the airway, breathing, and circulation is of primary importance. The pediatric airway may be complicated by numerous factors. The head of an infant is proportionally much larger than that of an adult, thus predisposing to neck flexion and occlusion of the airway in the supine position. The larger tongue and soft palate, as well as the more anterior glottis, can make the airway difficult to visualize. The child's trachea is shorter relative to body size, and narrower and more easily compressed compared with an adult. The subglottic region is the narrowest part of the trachea in children. Because of its small cross-sectional diameter, the pediatric airway is more susceptible to plugging with mucus or minimal airway edema.

The chest wall is more compliant in children, with less muscle mass for soft tissue protection. This allows a greater transmission of energy to underlying organs when injury occurs. The thinner chest wall also allows for easier transmission of breath sounds, which may obscure the diagnosis of a hemothorax or pneumothorax. Children are also at an increased risk for hypoxia owing to their higher oxygen consumption per unit body mass and their lower functional residual capacity to total lung volume ratio.

When assessing circulation, it is important to note that the mediastinum is more mobile in children than in older patients. This is particularly true in young children. Unilateral changes in thoracic pressure, as occurs from a pneumothorax, can lead to a tension pneumothorax. This can shift the mediastinum such that venous return is markedly reduced. The pathophysiologic effect is similar to hypovolemic shock, and this response is more pronounced than is typically seen in an adult.

Children compensate for a decrease in cardiac output by increasing their heart rate. In infants, improvement in stroke volume provides little in the way of compensation for hypotension. Infants and children also have a higher body surface area to weight ratio than adults, which predisposes them to hypothermia. This, in turn, may complicate the assessment of perfusion.

SPECIFIC INJURIES AND MANAGEMENT

Thoracic injuries in children can be categorized by location as seen in Box 15-1.

Chest Wall

Rib Fractures

Young children have a compliant thorax and do not begin to resemble adults until around 8 to 10 years of age. As a consequence, rib fractures are relatively uncommon in young children and occur more frequently in adolescents. Rib fractures are often suspected on physical examination and are identified on a chest radiograph (CXR) during the initial assessment. Independently, rib fractures are infrequently a cause of major morbidity or mortality, but are indicators of significant energy transfer.[16] If a rib fracture is found in a child younger than 3 years, nonaccidental trauma (NAT) should be considered.[17,18] Bone scans and bone surveys are useful in diagnosing remote fractures of the bony thorax in abused children, and follow-up studies improve identification of these injuries.[19] In older children, rib fractures should draw attention to the risk of an associated underlying injury. Fractures and dislocations of the bony thorax and joints may cause significant long-term pain. In addition to

CHEST WALL

Rib fracture
Flail chest
Open pneumothorax
Traumatic asphyxia

PLEURAL CAVITY/PULMONARY PARENCHYMA

Tension pneumothorax
Hemothorax
Simple pneumothorax
Pulmonary contusion/laceration
Diaphragmatic injury

MEDIASTINUM

Pericardial tamponade
Tracheobronchial injury
Great vessel injury
Cardiac contusion
Esophageal injury

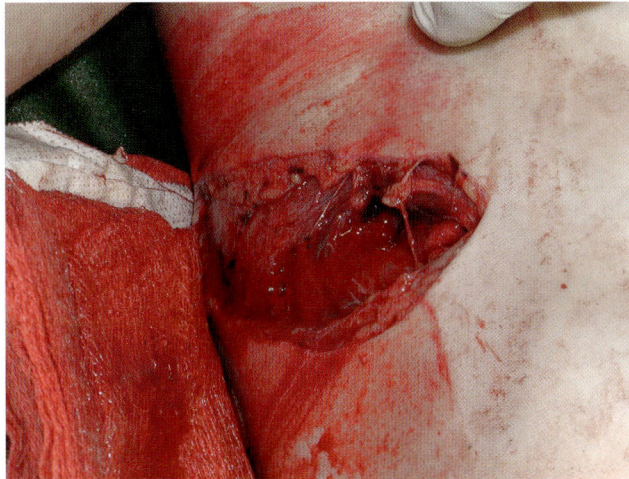

FIGURE 15-1 ■ Open pneumothorax (sucking chest wound) in a child who was impaled by a door handle along his right lateral chest wall.

pneumothorax and hemothorax, children with first rib fractures may have fractures of the clavicle, central nervous system injury, facial fractures, pelvic fractures, extremity injuries, and major vascular trauma.[20,21] When children present with multiple rib fractures, the mortality has been reported to be as high as 42%.[21] A careful survey of the child must be performed to look for significant injuries in other regions of the body.

The management of rib fractures is typically supportive. Attention to adequate pain relief will prevent atelectasis and pneumonia. Because rib fractures can be associated with a hemothorax or pneumothorax, immediate drainage of fluid, blood, or air via a chest tube or catheter is appropriate.

Flail Chest

Due to the increased pliability of the chest wall, multiple rib fractures in series (flail chest) are not commonly seen in younger children.[22] As a result of the wide age and size range, the treatment of flail chest in children, whether surgical or nonsurgical, adds a level of complexity when compared to adults. Chest wall dynamics and physiology differ significantly in infants compared to teenagers. Furthermore, flail chest has been identified in the neonatal period which increases the complexity of management of these patients.[23]

When flail chest occurs, the patient's respiratory effort can be depressed due to a paradoxical motion of the flail segment. The large force required to produce this injury invariably results in injury to the underlying lung, which contributes to the respiratory compromise. Like other thoracic injuries, treatment is tailored to avoid respiratory depression and pneumonia.[24] Adequate pain control, supplemental oxygen, chest physiotherapy, and continuous positive-pressure ventilation are non-invasive treatment modalities utilized in these patients.

In selected adults, operative correction of the flail chest has been shown to decrease morbidity, time on the ventilator, intensive care stay, and hospital costs.[25,26] Since thoracic operations can be performed in injured children with minimal morbidity and mortality, similar results should be expected.[14] Indications for operative management include failure to wean from mechanical ventilation. Other indications for thoracotomy are flail chest with no associated contusion, severe dyspnea, and severe chest deformity, among others.[27,28]

There is no standard operative approach for correction of a flail chest. Currently used techniques include wire cerclage, clamping, screw fixation, and intramedullary fixation.[29] The use of absorbable plates for rib trauma has also been described with good results.[30] The optimal surgical treatment in children is unclear given the required future growth of a child's thoracic cavity. A multidisciplinary approach between pediatric surgeons, orthopedic surgeons, and critical care physicians is important.

Open Pneumothorax

Open pneumothorax (sucking chest wound) occurs when there is a gaping defect in the chest wall, and typically is caused by a blast injury, a severe avulsion injury, or an impalement (Fig. 15-1). This is not often seen in children but can be life threatening when it occurs. The negative pressure in the pleural cavity created by spontaneous breathing sucks air into the thorax. Air trapping results in collapse of the ipsilateral lung and mediastinal shift, similar to a tension pneumothorax. Treatment requires placement of an occlusive dressing to prevent further air from entering the chest cavity as well as chest tube or catheter insertion to drain a hemo/pneumothorax that may have developed.

Traumatic Asphyxia

Traumatic asphyxia is typically caused by a large compressive force against the chest wall combined with deep inspiration against a closed glottis (Valsalva maneuver). The increased thoracic pressure compresses the right atrium, excludes blood return from the superior vena cava, and results in rupture of venules and capillaries about the face and head.[31] Patients will exhibit conjunctival hemorrhages, facial swelling, and petechial hemorrhages on the face and upper chest. Although severe cases may result in loss of vision or other permanent neurologic sequelae, the morbidity and mortality associated with traumatic asphyxia is generally related to the associated injuries. The majority of children who survive have good outcomes.[32,33]

Pleural Cavity and Pulmonary Parenchyma

Pneumothorax–Pulmonary Lacerations

Pneumothorax may occur with a penetrating injury to the chest wall or air leak into the pleural space from a pulmonary laceration or disruption of the proximal airway. It is a relatively common finding in children with blunt and penetrating thoracic trauma. The air leak may dissect under the pleura to cause pneumomediastinum and subcutaneous emphysema. A simple pneumothorax is often asymptomatic because the lack of increased intrathoracic pressure limits the recognition of symptoms. For this reason, a screening CXR is an important component in the evaluation of thoracic injury in children. Air within the pleural cavity can layer anteriorly, posteriorly, or in the subpulmonic space. A simple pneumothorax can be easily missed on chest film, but can be found on a subsequent computed tomographic (CT) scan.[34] However, a recent study analyzing the utility of CT scan as a screening modality to replace initial CXR concluded that although a CT scan is highly sensitive, it should not be used as a primary imaging tool given its cost and the acceptable sensitivity of routine CXR.[35] Ultrasonography (US) is another diagnostic modality that has been shown to be nearly as sensitive as CT in determining the presence of an occult pneumothorax and has gained wide acceptance as a screening tool.[36,37]

The need for intervention in the presence of a simple pneumothorax will depend on its severity and the child's clinical condition. Some authors have suggested that if the volume of the pneumothorax is greater than 20% of the pleural space, then drainage is needed.[38] Although insertion of a chest tube can be considered appropriate in almost every circumstance of traumatic pneumothorax, there are alternatives to conventional chest tubes, such as pigtail catheters.[39] Additionally, there may be a benefit in treating with supplemental oxygen alone. The rationale for this therapy is that atmospheric gas (78% nitrogen) comprises the majority of the entrapped air collection. If the nitrogen level in the blood is 'washed out' by increased inspired oxygen, a nitrogen gradient will be created that will cause accelerated absorption of the air. Oxygen can be delivered by way of nasal cannula, a hood, or a mask. Treatment with supplemental oxygen may be required for 24 to 48 hours.

In contrast, a tension pneumothorax is a life-threatening condition that requires expeditious decompression. A tension pneumothorax likely causes symptoms initially from hypoxemia and later from increased intrapleural pressure with subsequent decreased venous return

and cardiovascular collapse.[40] If the clinician suspects a tension pneumothorax in a patient with appropriate signs and symptoms, it is reasonable to proceed with decompression without waiting for a CXR. If rapid drainage of intrapleural air cannot be accomplished with a needle, insertion of a pigtail catheter or a chest tube should be performed. A tension pneumothorax treated initially with needle decompression will require chest tube or pigtail catheter insertion due to the continuing collection of air under pressure in the involved hemithorax. If one or both lungs have been compressed for a long time, re-expansion pulmonary edema may develop.[41]

Systemic air embolism can occur with any pulmonary parenchymal injury and increased intrabronchial pressure, creating a bronchopulmonary venous fistula.[42] This is most often seen when positive-pressure ventilation is required to support the injured patient. Sudden neurologic findings or cardiovascular decompensation may be the initial sign that air has embolized to the coronary or cerebral vessels. If this complication is recognized, steps should be taken to prevent further air embolism. If possible, the removal of the intravascular air should be considered. Treatment options include tube thoracostomy, but more often an emergency thoracotomy will provide immediate reversal of the physiology promoting the air embolism. The hilum of the lung should be occluded to prevent further escape of air into the venous system, and operative control of the bronchial–venous interface should be obtained. The mortality associated with this complication is high.

Hemothorax

Hemothorax can result from blunt or penetrating injury to any of the intrathoracic vessels, the chest wall vessels, the pleura, or the pulmonary parenchyma. Occasionally, a rib fracture can lacerate an intercostal vessel or the lung. Rarely, the aorta or vena cava may be injured by pressure or shearing. Unless the volume of blood is large, a hemothorax may be asymptomatic. Smaller volumes may be more easily detected on CT scan, which also allows for measurement of Hounsfield density to aid in the diagnosis.[43] Each hemithorax can hold approximately 40% of a child's blood volume and it is difficult to estimate the amount of blood loss on a CXR.[44] Prompt chest tube placement allows for evacuation of the blood from the pleural space and re-expansion of the lung. It also allows the surgeon to assess the volume of blood loss and whether the hemorrhage is ongoing.

There are instances in which an operation may be needed to stop ongoing intrathoracic bleeding. After tube thoracostomy, the immediate blood return of 15 mL/kg, or ongoing losses of 2–3 mL/kg/h for 3 or more hours, are indicators for thoracic exploration.[45,46] If undrained, the hemothorax can become organized with the development of a fibrothorax that can cause a restrictive lung defect. This predisposes to atelectasis, ventilation–perfusion mismatching, and subsequent pneumonia.

Residual blood is also an excellent culture medium, and empyema and sepsis can result from infection of an undrained hemothorax. Tube thoracostomy may not adequately evacuate an organizing post-traumatic hemothorax in up to 12% of patients.[47] In this situation, thoracoscopy may be useful to evacuate the residual clot. Patients who undergo early thoracoscopy may experience less morbidity.[48,49] However, there are also data to suggest that thrombolytic therapy is equally effective in treating a chronic hemothorax.[47] The use of intrapleural tissue plasminogen activator (tPA) has also been used for the treatment of traumatic residual hemothoraces and other parapneumonic processes with good results.[50,51]

Chylothorax

Chylothorax caused by injury to thoracic lymphatic channels is an uncommon complication from thoracic trauma. Chylothorax usually becomes evident three to seven days after injury. The diagnosis is made by obtaining a sample of the pleural fluid and identifying the lymphocyte and lipid content. Treatment includes drainage and either enteral feedings with medium-chain triglycerides or parenteral nutrition.

Pulmonary Contusion

One of the most common thoracic injuries in children is a pulmonary contusion, which can occur with blunt or penetrating trauma.[1] The flexible chest wall of a child allows for contusion of the lung without rib fracture, resulting in areas of lung consolidation and chest wall contusion. Microscopically, pulmonary contusions show alveolar hemorrhage, consolidation, and edema. The presence of a pulmonary contusion contributes to decreased pulmonary compliance, hypoxia, hypoventilation, and a ventilation–perfusion mismatch. A CXR taken during the initial assessment may demonstrate the pulmonary contusion. However, because this is invariably a supine film, it is sometimes difficult to differentiate fluid/blood in the pleural space from a lung contusion. To this end, a chest CT scan can show areas of pulmonary contusion not appreciated on the chest radiograph and can differentiate a parenchymal process (contusion) from free fluid.[52] However, when a contusion is seen on CXR, these children typically have a larger parenchymal volume that has been injured with a higher degree of impaired oxygenation.[53] Also, a significant percentage will require ventilatory support. When a pulmonary contusion is seen only on CT, the morbidity of the injured child does not appear to be affected when compared with children with normal CT findings.[54] The overall injury severity, associated injuries, and outcomes in these patients are similar to those seen in adults.[52] Treatment includes appropriate fluid resuscitation, supplemental oxygen, pain management, and strategies to prevent atelectasis and pneumonia.

A significant percentage of patients may develop pneumonia or acute respiratory distress syndrome (ARDS) after pulmonary contusion.[13] Occasionally, the pulmonary contusion can cause life-threatening hypoxia that cannot be supported with conventional ventilation, including high-frequency oscillation. Extracorporeal life support has been used in extreme circumstances to support patients with severe pulmonary contusions or

ARDS.[55] Children with pulmonary contusions can have prolonged changes in respiratory function and radiographic abnormalities. These changes may persist for an extended period of time after resolution of the symptoms.[56] However, these children do not appear to suffer any significant long-term sequelae.[15]

Diaphragmatic Injuries

Blunt diaphragmatic rupture is an uncommon occurrence. The left diaphragm is involved more often because of the protective effect of the right lobe of the liver. There have been occasional reports of bilateral diaphragmatic injury (Fig. 15-2).[57,58] The frequency of associated injuries, especially liver and spleen injuries, is very high.[58] Blunt injury to the diaphragm can have several manifestations, but usually include chest pain that radiates to the shoulder, shortness of breath, or abdominal pain. Breath sounds may be diminished and bowel sounds may be heard on the ipsilateral side.[59]

On imaging studies, an abnormal diaphragm contour, a high-riding diaphragm, or a questionable overlap of abdominal visceral shadows may suggest injury. Visceral herniation or the abnormal placement of a nasogastric tube into the left hemithorax should be considered diagnostic. Many diaphragmatic ruptures are not identified in the first few days after injury, and may not be detected for a considerable period of time (Fig. 15-3).[60] CXR findings may be obscured by associated contusion or atelectasis in the lung bases. In patients requiring intubation, herniation of abdominal viscera through the injury may not occur until after the patient is off positive-pressure ventilation.[61] CT has been used to establish the diagnosis, but the CT may appear normal in some patients. A heightened awareness of this injury should be present to avoid the late complications of visceral herniation or bowel complications.

When penetrating trauma is sustained below the nipple line, a diaphragmatic injury needs to be

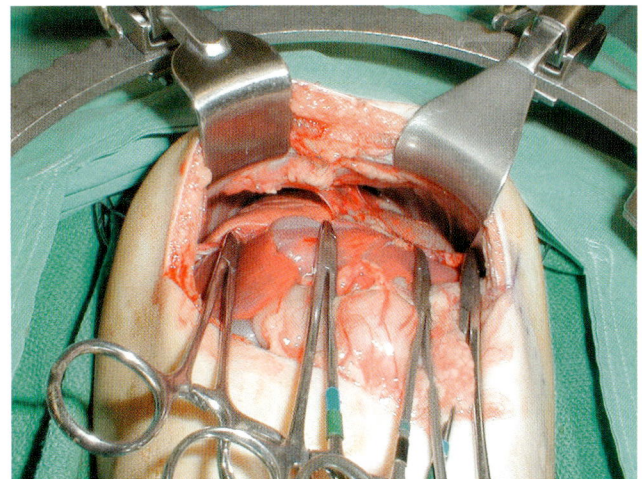

FIGURE 15-2 ■ Bilateral diaphragmatic rupture after blunt abdominal trauma. The hemostats have been placed on the lower rim of the diaphragmatic rupture.

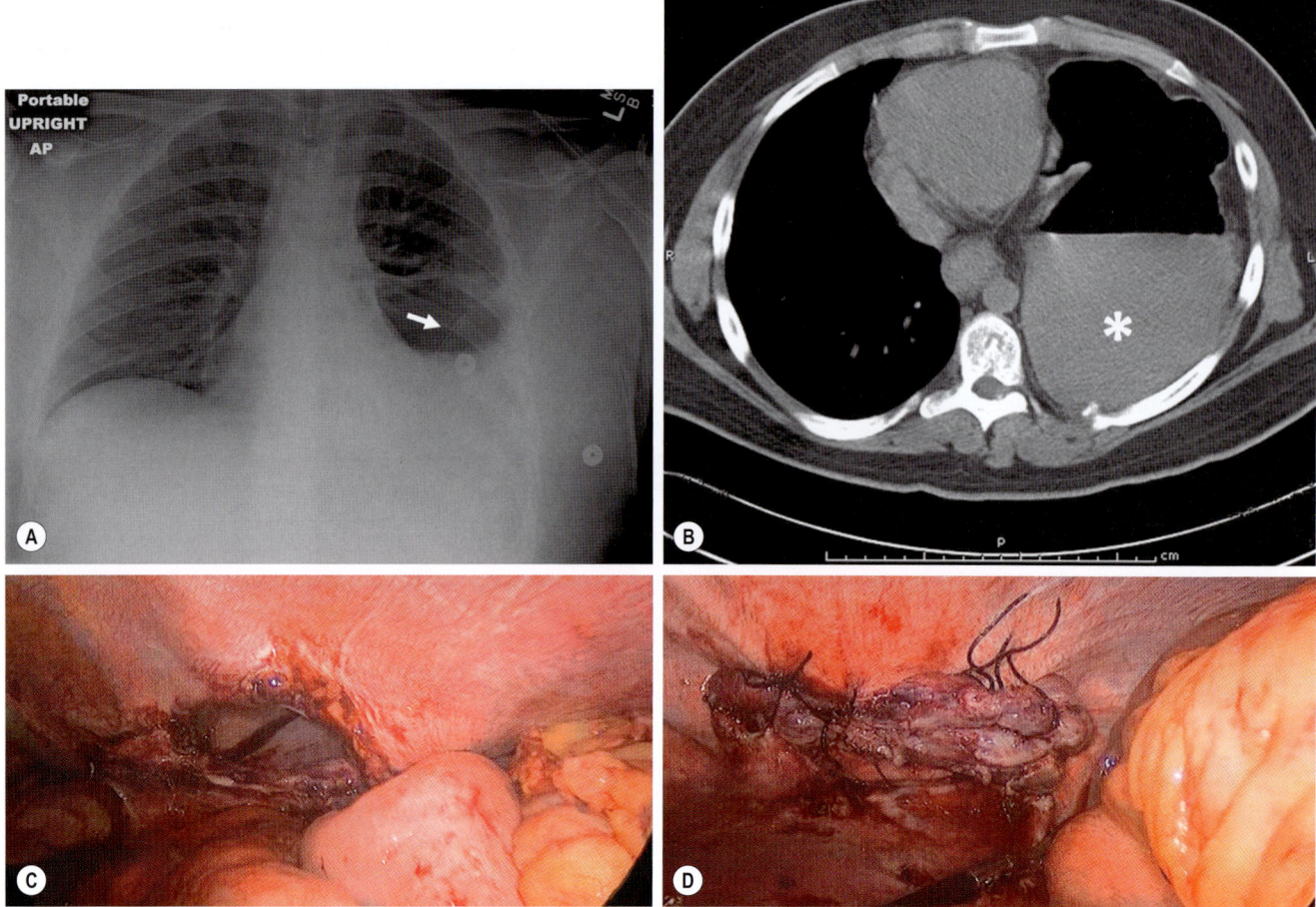

FIGURE 15-3 ■ This 16-year-old was initially admitted to another hospital following a motor vehicle accident that necessitated insertion of a left chest tube. Six weeks later, he began to develop left-sided chest discomfort and vomiting. **(A)** The patient's chest radiograph. Note the tip of the nasogastric tube in the left thoracic cavity (arrow). **(B)** A CT scan was performed at the outlying hospital which shows an air-fluid level in the stomach which is located in the left side chest cavity. The solid contents in the stomach are marked with an asterisk. **(C)** At laparoscopic exploration, the diaphragmatic defect is seen. **(D)** This defect was able to be closed laparoscopically and he was discharged two days later. He has recovered uneventfully and has not developed any postoperative problems with more than a one year follow-up.

considered. Imaging evaluation is often unreliable in this setting. Therefore after determining whether other life-threatening injuries to the heart, lung, liver, spleen, or gastrointestinal tract exist, operative exploration and repair may be needed.[59] If exploration is undertaken, laparoscopy, thoracoscopy, thoracotomy, or laparotomy have all been used with success (see Fig. 15-3C,D).

Mediastinum

Airway Injury

Injuries to the tracheobronchial tree are infrequent in children. Airway disruption may occur with penetrating injury or with blunt injury such as high-energy acceleration or deceleration. Up to three-quarters of these injuries are noted within 2 cm of the carina and almost half occur within the first 2 cm of the right main-stem bronchus.[62] Most patients with tracheal injuries have mediastinal air on CXR. More distal injuries may rupture into the pleural space and present as a tension pneumothorax. Other findings associated with a major airway injury

include a persistent large air leak from a chest tube, mediastinal air, cervical subcutaneous emphysema without pneumothorax, or florid respiratory compromise. Rarely, complete transection of a distal main-stem bronchus will appear on CXR with total lung collapse and mediastinal displacement.[63] Persistent pneumomediastinum and pneumothoraces on CXR after adequate tube thoracostomy should alert the clinician to consider an injury to the tracheobronchial tree (Fig. 15-4).

Once recognized, these injuries require prompt diagnosis and treatment. Pleural air or fluid collections should be drained until an accurate evaluation and diagnosis of the airway injury is made. Mechanical ventilation may be necessary because of respiratory failure in this setting. Fiberoptic bronchoscopy allows for evaluation of the airway and may improve the probability of successful intubation. Many airway injuries are diagnosed by rigid or flexible bronchoscopy. Chest CT with a multiple-array scanner may have a role in visualizing tracheal or bronchial injuries, especially if three-dimensional reconstructions of the airway are used (virtual bronchoscopy) (Fig. 15-5).[64,65]

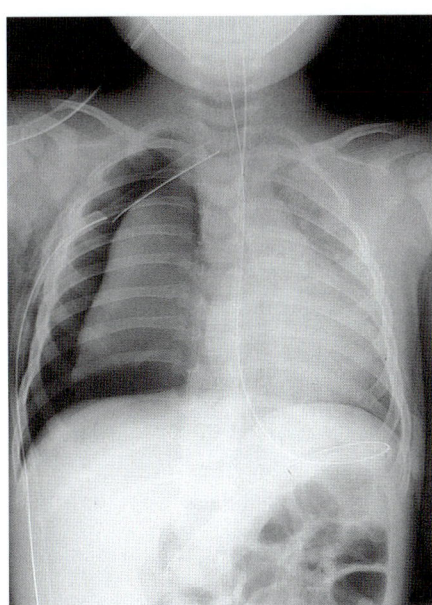

FIGURE 15-4 ■ Chest radiograph of a 2-year-old patient who was run over by an automobile. Note the persistent large right pneumothorax despite the adequate placement of a chest tube. This patient was found to have a complete disruption of the right main-stem bronchus at the orifice of the right upper lobe bronchus.

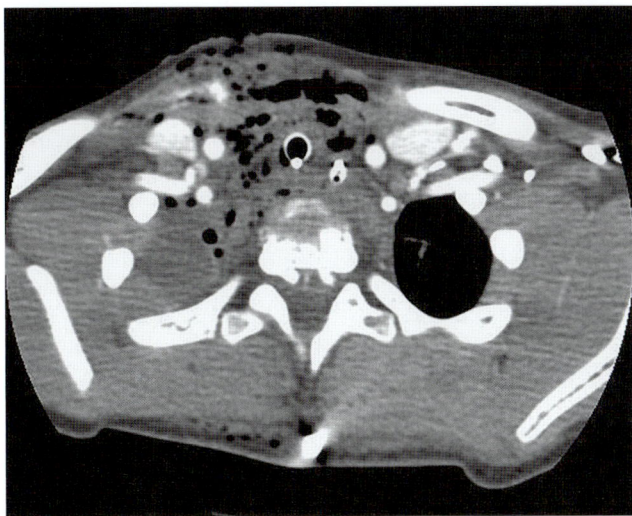

FIGURE 15-5 ■ CT scan of the chest in a child who sustained penetrating trauma. This image was taken from the upper thoracic region. Note the air in the subcutaneous tissue and mediastinum. This child was found to have a tracheal and an esophageal injury.

A delay in diagnosis is not uncommon in children. A retrospective review found that 75% of cases with a delayed diagnosis of tracheobronchial injury occurred in children younger than age 15.[66] This was thought to be related to the probability that incomplete tears in children cause minimal symptoms and the possibility that children involved in a severe accident with the loss of a family member may be reluctant to express physical complaints.

In general, when a tracheobronchial injury is identified, operative repair is usually needed. Repair may be delayed if the symptoms can be managed without significant morbidity. Repair of some bronchial injuries can be successful even a year after injury.[62] Occasionally, more distal bronchial injuries may heal with nonoperative management.[67] Distal bronchial injuries are generally well managed by pulmonary resection, whereas more proximal airway trauma is best treated by direct repair. Nonoperative management of a tracheobronchial injury may result in a high incidence of airway stenosis. When the diagnosis of a tracheobronchial injury is substantially delayed, scarring may obliterate the airway lumen and cause chronic collapse of the lung segment or lobe. The degree of injury may also play a role in determining whether a repair, as opposed to a resection, is needed. Complete transections are commonly associated with an obliterated distal bronchus, which may spare the pulmonary parenchyma from infection, thus making repair possible. Incomplete tears, on the other hand, form granulation tissue and scar that result in a patent, but narrowed lumen, predisposing the supplied lung to recurrent infection and retained secretions. This usually necessitates resection at some point. Three-dimensional reconstructions of the trachea and bronchi, taken from spiral CT images, have been found to be useful in planning

operative therapy treatment. If the esophagus and the airway are injured near one another, a traumatic tracheoesophageal fistula can occur.[68]

Great Vessel Injuries

Injuries to the heart and great vessels are rare in young children. The National Trauma Data Bank reports the incidence of blunt aortic injury to be 0.1%, but with a mortality rate of over 40%.[69] Traumatic thoracic aortic disruptions can occur in children as young as 4 years of age.[70,71] However, these injuries are more likely in the older child. Most (80%) children who sustain a thoracic aortic tear will have significant associated injuries to the lung, heart, skeletal system, abdominal organs, or central nervous system.[72] Only half of these patients will have external evidence of a thoracic injury. Most aortic injuries in children are related to falls or motor vehicle collisions, especially when children are unrestrained.

The diagnosis of an aortic injury in a child can be difficult. Findings on a chest film can include a left apical cap, pulmonary contusion, mediastinal widening, shift of the trachea to the right, downward depression of the left main-stem bronchus, and an indistinct aorta.[71] However, none of these findings is sensitive or specific enough to make the diagnosis. A normal CXR, however, is highly predictive for the absence of an aortic injury.[73] A CT scan may reveal a mediastinal hematoma or the aortic injury. Transesophageal echocardiography has also been useful for making the diagnosis.[74] Whereas thoracic CT and transesophageal echocardiography can diagnose aortic injuries, aortic angiography gives excellent anatomic detail (Fig. 15-6). The most common finding with a traumatic aortic injury is a pseudoaneurysm located at the proximal descending aorta. This is thought to occur secondary to tethering of the aorta by the ligamentum arteriosum, resulting in a tear in the aortic intima and media.[75]

There are no large collective studies of children with aortic injuries. However, of those who survive until diagnosis, more than 70% will live to discharge.[71,72] Spinal cord ischemia is a complication that can occur and may be associated with preoperative cardiovascular instability.[76] Although urgent operative repair is thought to be the best treatment option in most patients, recent experience has demonstrated the ability to delay operative intervention by using beta-adrenergic blockers while other injuries are managed.[70,76,77] This trend in management has raised the possibility of using a less invasive endovascular approach when dealing with these injuries. In adults, studies have demonstrated that it is feasible to treat aortic injuries with endovascular stents.[78] Extrapolation of this approach to children has shown that endovascular treatment in children from the ages 12 to 14 years has been successful; however, the endovascular grafts were constructed from smaller adult stent grafts.[77,79,80] In the elective setting, such as endovascular treatment of aortic coarctation, infants and teenagers alike have been managed with larger adult stents.[81–83] Currently, the youngest reported person with a traumatic aortic disruption treated with an endovascular stent is an 11-year-old child.[84] The long-term sequelae of permanent stents in children with 'growing' aortas has not been evaluated. However, newer expandable stents may allow for multiple interventions in a given patient.[85]

Cardiac Contusion

Blunt cardiac injury such as myocardial contusion, cardiac laceration, or cardiac rupture is rare, occurring in less than 5% of children with blunt thoracic trauma.[86,87] Penetrating trauma is more often a cause of cardiac and aortic injury in this age group. Cardiac contusion accounts for 95% of blunt cardiac injuries in the child, followed by valvular dysfunction and ventricular septal defect.[87] Clinical manifestations of cardiac injury after blunt thoracic trauma include arrhythmia, new-onset murmur, and heart failure. However, these findings may be absent in children, and CXR and electrocardiographic findings are generally nonspecific.[87]

The management of a cardiac contusion is supportive. Children with a cardiac contusion who are hemodynamically stable on presentation rarely have deterioration in their cardiac rhythm. Patients should be monitored with continuous electrocardiography and frequent blood pressure determinations. Echocardiography should be performed early in the evaluation of children with a significant cardiac contusion. In patients with a suspected cardiac contusion, serum cardiac troponin I levels may be useful to confirm the diagnosis.[88]

Inotropic agents are occasionally needed to provide cardiac support in the presence of a cardiac contusion. Although blunt cardiac injury with heart rupture and cardiac tamponade is very rare, only immediate diagnosis and treatment will be life-saving. This is also true for penetrating cardiac trauma. A delayed diagnosis of cardiac rupture in children has been described.[89,90] Immediate ultrasound in the emergency department may provide the clinical information necessary to identify this injury.[91] Pericardiocentesis in this setting may provide a temporary solution while operative intervention is organized. If urgent pericardiocentesis is required in a child, it should

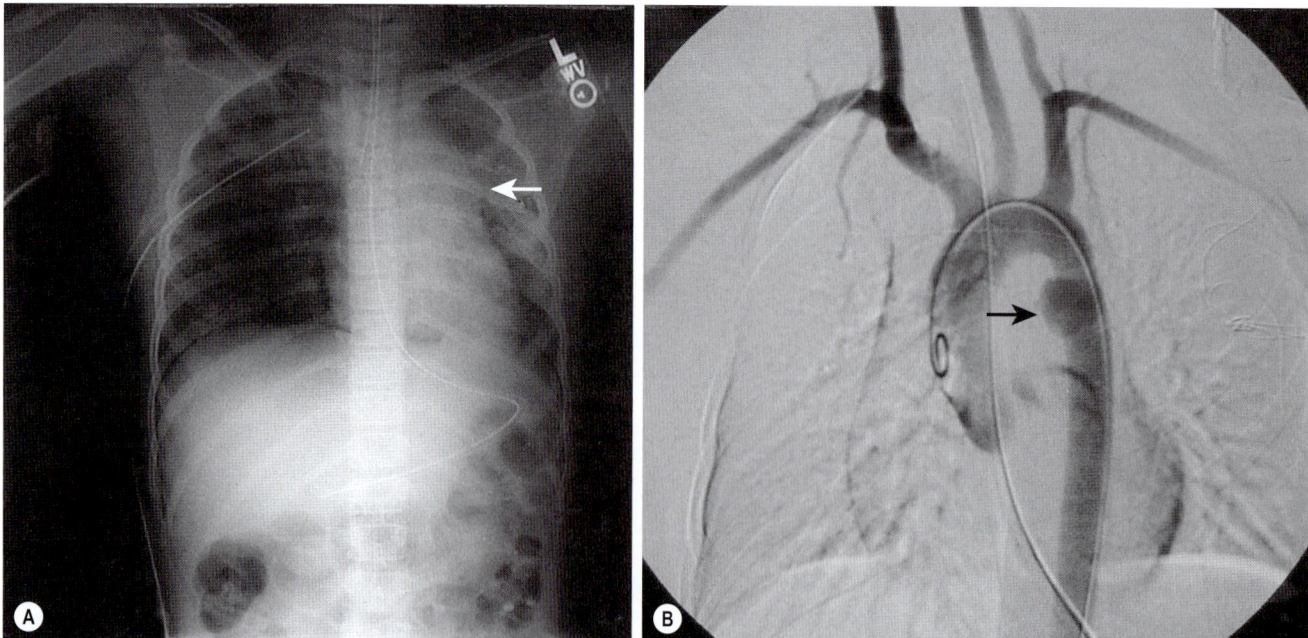

FIGURE 15-6 ■ An 8-year-old patient presented with injuries from being an unrestrained passenger in a motor vehicle accident. **(A)** On the chest radiograph, note the widened mediastinum and loss of definition of the aortic knob (*arrow*). There is also a right pneumothorax that was treated with tube thoracostomy. **(B)** An aortogram shows a pseudoaneurysm (*arrow*) at the location of the ligamentum arteriosum just distal to the left subclavian artery, representing the partial transection of the descending aorta at this point.

be remembered that the distance from the skin to the pericardium is significantly reduced in younger patients relative to adults. Undercompensating or overcompensating for chest wall thickness may lead to inadequate decompression or iatrogenic cardiac injury. Once stabilized, children with a blunt cardiac injury should be followed closely and monitored for sequelae such as valvular insufficiency or a ventricular septal defect.[87] Rarely, extracorporeal life support may be needed to manage a child with a severe blunt cardiac injury.

Commotio cordis has become a widely recognized problem in pediatric thoracic trauma.[92] Typically, a young baseball player is struck in the chest with a hit or thrown ball and collapses suddenly. Commotio cordis is characterized by the absence of cardiac contusion, coronary artery abnormalities, structural abnormalities, or conduction system pathology. It is thought that a sudden blow to the chest will result in a disorganized cardiac rhythm followed by rapid cardiovascular collapse. Although chest protective devices seem useful, they do not provide total protection against asystole.[93] Automatic electrical defibrillators may be life-saving for this rare sports-related injury.

Esophagus

Pediatric esophageal injuries are uncommon, occurring in less than 1% of children sustaining either blunt or penetrating thoracic trauma.[12,94,95] The esophagus is a relatively elastic, mediastinal structure that is largely protected by the bony thorax. This mobility is helpful when blunt force is applied as the esophagus can move, which limits the likelihood of rupture. Penetrating injuries are more likely to cause esophageal trauma. Esophageal disruption may manifest as dyspnea, dysphagia, cyanosis, mediastinal air, subcutaneous emphysema, pleural effusion, chest or epigastric pain, fever, or sepsis.[96] Initial symptoms, however, may be vague and nonspecific. Esophagography with a water-soluble contrast agent and esophagoscopy are typically the studies that will best identify an esophageal injury.

If the esophagus is ruptured or perforated, conventional management is operative repair. This is performed for the purpose of drainage and/or repair. Treatment is initiated with fluid resuscitation and parenteral antibiotics.[97] Operative repair consists of direct suture closure of the injury. If possible, pleural flap coverage and tube thoracostomy are performed. If an operation is undertaken early after injury, this treatment strategy, along with no oral intake and total parenteral nutrition (TPN), has good success. If the perforation is not identified early, treatment becomes more difficult. In perforations of more than 24 hours duration, operative closure becomes technically much more demanding owing to the degree of inflammation and the amount of contamination. Techniques used in this circumstance include attempted suture repair, esophageal isolation, multiple drain placement, gastrostomy, and TPN.

In selected cases of esophageal perforation, nonoperative management may be successful.[96] This may be the case with certain types of blunt trauma and with iatrogenic injury such as a perforation at the time of endoscopy. Nonoperative management is based on the clinical status of the patient and the injury seen on imaging studies. For example, a patient might have a small leak identified, manifested by mediastinal air or pneumothorax. If there is no fever, no effusion, and the patient looks well, nonoperative treatment with TPN and intravenous antibiotics, along with serial examinations, may be reasonable. See Chapter 26 for more information about esophageal injuries.

REFERENCES

1. Peclet MH, Newman KD, Eichelberger MR, et al. Thoracic trauma in children: An indicator of increased mortality. J Pediatr Surg 1990;25:961–6.
2. Peterson RJ, Tepas JJ, Edwards FH, et al. Pediatric and adult thoracic trauma: Age-related impact on presentation and outcome. Ann Thorac Surg 1994;58:14–18.
3. Stafford PW, Harmon CM. Thoracic trauma in children. Curr Opin Pediatr 1993;5:325–32.
4. Holmes JF, Sokolove PE, Brant WE, et al. A clinical decision rule for identifying children with thoracic injuries after blunt torso trauma. Ann Emerg Med 2002;39:492–9.
5. Black TL, Snyder CL, Miller JP, et al. Significance of chest trauma in children. South Med J 1996;89:494–6.
6. Mayer T, Matlak ME, Johnson DG, et al. The modified injury severity scale in pediatric multiple trauma patients. J Pediatr Surg 1980;15:719–26.
7. Reynolds M. Pulmonary, esophageal and diaphragmatic injuries. In: Buntain WL, editor. Management of Paediatric Trauma. Philadelphia, PA: WB Saunders; 1995. p. 238–47.
8. Woosley CR, Mayes TC. The pediatric patient and thoracic trauma. Semin Thorac Cardiovasc Surg 2008;20:58–63.
9. Smyth BT. Chest trauma in children. J Pediatr Surg 1979; 14:41–7.
10. Nakayama DK, Ramenofsky ML, Rowe MI. Chest injuries in childhood. Ann Surg 1989;210:770–5.
11. Roux P, Fisher RM. Chest injuries in children: An analysis of 100 cases of blunt chest trauma from motor vehicle accidents. J Pediatr Surg 1992;27:551–5.
12. Cooper A, Barlow B, DiScala C, et al. Mortality and truncal injury: The pediatric perspective. J Pediatr Surg 1994;29:33–8.
13. Allen GS, Cox CS Jr. Pulmonary contusion in children: Diagnosis and management. South Med J 1998;91:1099–106.
14. Balci AE, Kazez A, Eren S, et al. Blunt thoracic trauma in children: Review of 137 cases. Eur J Cardiothorac Surg 2004;26:387–92.
15. Haxhija EQ, Nöres H, Schober P, et al. Lung contusion-lacerations after blunt thoracic trauma in children. Pediatr Surg Int 2004;20:412–14.
16. Bliss D, Silen M. Pediatric thoracic trauma. Crit Care Med 2002;30:S409–15.
17. Cadzow SP, Armstrong KL. Rib fractures in infants: Red alert! The clinical features, investigations and child protection outcomes. J Paediatr Child Health 2000;36:322–6.
18. Bulloch B, Schubert CJ, Brophy PD, et al. Cause and clinical characteristics of rib fractures in infants. Pediatrics 2000;105:E48.
19. Kleinman PK, Nimkin K, Spevak MR, et al. Follow-up skeletal surveys in suspected child abuse. AJR Am J Roentgenol 1996;167:893–6.
20. Harris GJ, Soper RT. Pediatric first rib fractures. J Trauma 1990;30:343–5.
21. Garcia VF, Gotschall CS, Eichelberger MR, et al. Rib fractures in children: A marker of severe trauma. J Trauma 1990;30:695–700.
22. Lee RB, Bass SM, Morris JA Jr, et al. Three or more rib fractures as an indicator for transfer to a Level I trauma center: A population-based study. J Trauma 1990;30:689–94.
23. Gipson CL, Tobias JD. Flail chest in a neonate resulting from nonaccidental trauma. South Med J 2006;99:536–8.
24. Cannon RM, Smith JW, Franklin GA, et al. Flail chest injury: Are we making any progress? Am Surg 2012;78:398–402.
25. Tanaka H, Yukioka T, Yamaguti Y, et al. Surgical stabilization of internal pneumatic stabilization? A prospective randomized study of management of severe flail chest patients. J Trauma 2002;52: 727–32.

26. Pettiford BL, Luketich JD, Landreneau RJ. The management of flail chest. Thorac Surg Clin 2007;17:25–33.

27. Voggenreiter G, Neudeck F, Aufmkolk M, et al. Operative chest wall stabilization in flail chest–outcomes of patients with or without pulmonary contusion. J Am Coll Surg 1998;187:130–8.

28. Slater MS, Mayberry JC, Trunkey DD. Operative stabilization of a flail chest six years after injury. Ann Thorac Surg 2001;72:600–1.

29. Fitzpatrick DC, Denard PJ, Phelan D, et al. Operative stabilization of flail chest injuries: Review of literature and fixation options. Eur J Trauma Emerg Surg 2010;36:427–33.

30. Mayberry JC, Terhes JT, Ellis TJ, et al. Absorbable plates for rib fracture repair: Preliminary experience. J Trauma 2003;55:835–9.

31. Thompson A Jr, Illescas FF, Chiu RC. Why is the lower torso protected in traumatic asphyxia? A new hypothesis. Ann Thorac Surg 1989;47:247–9.

32. Gorenstein L, Blair GK, Shandling B. The prognosis of traumatic asphyxia in childhood. J Pediatr Surg 1986;21:753–6.

33. Hurtado TR, Della-Giustina DA. Traumatic asphyxia in a 6-year-old boy. Pediatr Emerg Care 2003;19:167–8.

34. Holmes JF, Brant WE, Bogren HG, et al. Prevalence and importance of pneumothoraces visualized on abdominal computed tomographic scan in children with blunt trauma. J Trauma 2001;50:516–20.

35. Renton J, Kincaid S, Ehrlich PF. Should helical CT scanning of the thoracic cavity replace the conventional chest x-ray as a primary assessment tool in pediatric trauma? An efficacy and cost analysis. J Pediatr Surg 2003;38:793–7.

36. Dente CJ, Ustin J, Feliciano DV, et al. The accuracy of thoracic ultrasound for detection of pneumothorax is not sustained over time: A preliminary study. J Trauma 2007;62:1384–9.

37. Soldati G, Testa A, Sher S, et al. Occult traumatic pneumothorax: Diagnostic accuracy of lung ultrasonography in the emergency department. Chest 2008;133:204–11.

38. Weissberg D, Refaely Y. Pneumothorax: Experience with 1,199 patients. Chest 2000;117:1279–85.

39. Dull KE, Fleisher GR. Pigtail catheters versus large-bore chest tubes for pneumothoraces in children treated in the emergency department. Pediatr Emerg Care 2002;18:265–7.

40. Barton ED, Rhee P, Hutton KC, et al. The pathophysiology of tension pneumothorax in ventilated swine. J Emerg Med 1997;15:147–53.

41. Ozlu O, Kilic A, Cengizlier R. Bilateral re-expansion pulmonary edema in a child: A reminder. Acta Anaesthesiol Scand 2000;44:884–5.

42. Rawlins R, Momin A, Platts D, et al. Traumatic cardiogenic shock due to massive air embolism. A possible role for cardiopulmonary bypass. Eur J Cardiothorac Surg 2002;22:845–6.

43. Rivas LA, Fishman JE, Múnera F, et al. Multislice CT in thoracic trauma. Radiol Clin North Am 2003;41:599–616.

44. Grisoni ER, Volsko TA. Thoracic injuries in children. Respir Care Clin N Am 2001;7:25–38.

45. Rielly JP, Brandt ML, Mattox KL, et al. Thoracic trauma in children. J Trauma 1993;34:329–31.

46. Peterson RJ, Tiwary AD, Kissoon N, et al. Pediatric penetrating thoracic trauma: A five-year experience. Pediatr Emerg Care 1994;10:129–31.

47. Kimbrell BJ, Yamzon J, Petrone P, et al. Intrapleural thrombolysis for the management of undrained traumatic hemothorax: A prospective observational study. J Trauma 2007;62:1175–9.

48. Uribe RA, Pachon CE, Frame SB, et al. A prospective evaluation of thoracoscopy for the diagnosis of penetrating thoracoabdominal trauma. J Trauma 1994;37:650–4.

49. Fabbrucci P, Nocentini L, Secci S, et al. Video-assisted thoracoscopy in the early diagnosis and management of post-traumatic pneumothorax and hemothorax. Surg Endosc 2008;22:1227–31.

50. Skeete DA, Rutherford EJ, Schlidt SA, et al. Intrapleural tissue plasminogen activator for complicated pleural effusions. J Trauma 2004;57:1178–83.

51. St. Peter SD, Tsao K, Harrison C, et al. Thoracoscopic decortication vs. tube thoracostomy with fibrinolysis for empyema in children: A prospective, randomized trial. J Pediatr Surg 2009;44:106–11.

52. Allen GS, Cox CS, Moore FA, et al. Pulmonary contusion in children: Are children different? J Am Coll Surg 1997;185:229–33.

53. Mizushima Y, Hiraide A, Shimazu T, et al. Changes in contused lung volume and oxygenation in patients with pulmonary parenchymal injury after blunt chest trauma. Am J Emerg Med 2000;18:385–9.

54. Kwon A, Sorrells DL, Kurkchubasche AG, et al. Isolated computed tomography diagnosis of pulmonary contusion does not correlate with increased morbidity. J Pediatr Surg 2006;41:78–82.

55. Weber TR, Kountzman B. Extracorporeal membrane oxygenation for nonneonatal pulmonary and multiple-organ failure. J Pediatr Surg 1998;33:1605–9.

56. Davis SL, Furman DP, Costarino AT Jr. Adult respiratory distress syndrome in children: Associated disease, clinical course, and predictors of death. J Pediatr 1993;123:35–45.

57. Karnak I, Senocak ME, Tanyel FC, et al. Diaphragmatic injuries in childhood. Surg Today 2001;31:5–11.

58. Koplewitz BZ, Ramos C, Manson DE, et al. Traumatic diaphragmatic injuries in infants and children: Imaging findings. Pediatr Radiol 2000;30:471–9.

59. Brandt ML, Luks FI, Spigland NA, et al. Diaphragmatic injury in children. J Trauma 1992;32:298–301.

60. Guth AA, Pachter HL, Kim U. Pitfalls in the diagnosis of blunt diaphragmatic injury. Am J Surg 1995;170:5–9.

61. Westra SJ, Wallace EC. Imaging evaluation of pediatric chest trauma. Radiol Clin North Am 2005;43:267–81.

62. Kiser AC, O'Brien SM, Detterbeck FC. Blunt tracheobronchial injuries: Treatment and outcomes. Ann Thorac Surg 2001;71:2059–65.

63. Nishiumi N, Maitani F, Yamada S, et al. Chest radiography assessment of tracheobronchial disruption associated with blunt chest trauma. J Trauma 2002;53:372–7.

64. Lomoschitz FM, Eisenhuber E, Linnau KF, et al. Imaging of chest trauma: Radiological patterns of injury and diagnostic algorithms. Eur J Radiol 2003;48:61–70.

65. Wan YL, Tsai KT, Yeow KM, et al. CT findings of bronchial transection. Am J Emerg Med 1997;15:176–7.

66. Ozdulger A, Cetin G, Erkmen Gulhan S, et al. A review of 24 patients with bronchial ruptures: Is delay in diagnosis more common in children? Eur J Cardiothorac Surg 2003;23:379–83.

67. Slimane MA, Becmeur F, Aubert D, et al. Tracheobronchial ruptures from blunt thoracic trauma in children. J Pediatr Surg 1999;34:1847–50.

68. Reed WJ, Doyle SE, Aprahamian C. Tracheoesophageal fistula after blunt chest trauma. Ann Thorac Surg 1995;59:1251–6.

69. Heckman SR, Trooskin SZ, Burd RS. Risk factors for blunt thoracic aortic injury in children. J Pediatr Surg 2005;40:98–102.

70. Dornhofer T, Dinkel HP, Carrel T, et al. Complex, traumatic rupture of the thoracic aorta in a child: Diagnostic findings and delayed surgery. Eur Radiol 2002;12:1459–62.

71. Lowe LH, Bulas DI, Eichelberger MD, et al. Traumatic aortic injuries in children: Radiologic evaluation. AJR Am J Roentgenol 1998;170:39–42.

72. Eddy AC, Rusch VW, Fligner CL, et al. The epidemiology of traumatic rupture of the thoracic aorta in children: A 13-year review. J Trauma 1990;30:989–91.

73. Hall A, Johnson K. The imaging of paediatric thoracic trauma. Paediatr Respir Rev 2002;3:241–7.

74. Pearson GD, Karr SS, Trachiotis GD, et al. A retrospective review of the role of transesophageal echocardiography in aortic and cardiac trauma in a level I Pediatric Trauma Center. J Am Soc Echocardiogr 1997;10:946–55.

75. Mirvis SE, Shanmuganathan K. Diagnosis of blunt traumatic aortic injury 2007: Still a nemesis. Eur J Radiol 2007;64:27–40.

76. Karmy-Jones R, Carter YM, Nathens A, et al. Impact of presenting physiology and associated injuries on outcome following traumatic rupture of the thoracic aorta. Am Surg 2001;67:61–6.

77. Karmy-Jones R, Hoffer E, Meissner M, et al. Management of traumatic rupture of the thoracic aorta in pediatric patients. Ann Thorac Surg 2003;75:1513–17.

78. Wellons ED, Milner R, Solis M, et al. Stent-graft repair of traumatic thoracic aortic disruptions. J Vasc Surg 2004;40:1095–100.

79. Hoffer EK, Karmy-Jones R, Bloch RD, et al. Treatment of acute thoracic aortic injury with commercially available abdominal aortic stent-grafts. J Vasc Interv Radiol 2002;13:1037–41.

80. Milas ZL, Milner R, Chaikoff E, et al. Endograft stenting in the adolescent population for traumatic aortic injuries. J Pediatr Surg 2006;41:e27–30.

81. Lee ML. Endovascular stent for the aortic coarctation in a 1.7-kg premie presenting intractable heart failure. Int J Cardiol 2006;113:236–8.

82. Takawira FF, Sinyangwe G, Mooloo R. Endovascular covered stent treatment for descending aorta pseudoaneurysm following coarctation of the aorta repair in an infant. Heart Lung Circ 2010;19:745–8.

83. Patnaik AN, Srinivas B, Rao DS. Endovascular stenting for native coarctation in older children and adolescents using adult self-expanding (Nitinol) iliac stents. Indian Heart J 2009;61:353–7.

84. Gunabushanam V, Mishra N, Calderin J, et al. Endovascular stenting of blunt thoracic aortic injury in an 11-year-old. J Pediatr Surg 2010;45:E15–18.

85. Chakrabarti S, Kenny D, Morgan G, et al. Balloon expandable stent implantation for native and recurrent coarctation of the aorta–prospective computed tomography assessment of stent integrity, aneurysm formation and stenosis relief. Heart 2010;96:1212–16.

86. Tiao GM, Griffith PM, Szmuszkovicz JR, et al. Cardiac and great vessel injuries in children after blunt trauma: An institutional review. J Pediatr Surg 2000;35:1656–60.

87. Dowd MD, Krug S. Pediatric blunt cardiac injury: Epidemiology, clinical features, and diagnosis. Pediatric Emergency Medicine Collaborative Research Committee: Working Group on Blunt Cardiac Injury. J Trauma 1996;40:61–7.

88. Hirsch R, Landt Y, Porter S, et al. Cardiac troponin I in pediatrics: Normal values and potential use in the assessment of cardiac injury. J Pediatr 1997;130:872–7.

89. Murillo CA, Owens-Stovall SK, Kim S, et al. Delayed cardiac tamponade after blunt chest trauma in a child. J Trauma 2002;52:573–5.

90. Rezende Neto JB, Diniz HO, Filho CS, et al. Blunt traumatic rupture of the heart in a child: Case report and review of the literature. J Trauma 2001;50:746–9.

91. Symbas NP, Bongiorno PF, Symbas PN. Blunt cardiac rupture: The utility of emergency department ultrasound. Ann Thorac Surg 1999;67:1274–6.

92. Perron AD, Brady WJ, Erling BF. Commodio cordis: An underappreciated cause of sudden cardiac death in young patients: Assessment and management in the ED. Am J Emerg Med 2001;19:406–9.

93. Maron BJ, Gohman TE, Kyle SB. Clinical profile and spectrum of commotio cordis. JAMA 2002;287:1142–6.

94. Sartorelli KH, McBride WJ, Vane DW. Perforation of the intrathoracic esophagus from blunt trauma in a child: Case report and review of the literature. J Pediatr Surg 1999;34:495–7.

95. Cotton BA, Nance ML. Penetrating trauma in children. Semin Pediatr Surg 2004;13:87–97.

96. Engum SA, Grosfeld JL, West KW, et al. Improved survival in children with esophageal perforation. Arch Surg 1996;131:604–11.

97. Asensio JA, Chahwan S, Forno W, et al. Penetrating esophageal injuries: Multicenter study of the American Association for the Surgery of Trauma. J Trauma 2001;50:289–96.

CHAPTER 16

ABDOMINAL AND RENAL TRAUMA

Barbara A. Gaines • Kelly M. Austin

While head injuries are responsible for the majority of pediatric trauma deaths, intra-abdominal and retroperitoneal injuries can still result in significant morbidity and mortality. Diagnostic uncertainty and delays in diagnosis can lead to long-term complications and adversely impact quality of life. Injuries to intra-abdominal organs occur in 10–15% of injured children.[1] The spleen is the most frequently injured organ, and low velocity mechanisms, such as falls, is the most frequent mechanism of injury. The combination of the unique anatomic and physiologic features of children and differences in mechanism result in patterns of injury unique to the pediatric population.

As just mentioned, falls are the most frequent mechanism of injury in children. However, motor vehicle crashes (MVC) are the most deadly, and are the leading cause of death for all children after the age of 1 year.[2] From the perspective of abdominal trauma, and using the spleen as a marker for intra-abdominal injury, pediatric injuries tend to be the result of lower-velocity mechanisms when compared to adults. In a study that compared splenic injuries at an adult level one trauma center and a pediatric level one trauma center, MVC accounted for 66.9% of adult injuries but only 23.7% of pediatric injuries.[3] On the other hand, 'sports mishaps' resulted in only 2.3% of the adult injuries, but 17% of injuries involving children. Even in the MVC population, pediatric injuries tend to differ from those suffered by adults. Children are less likely to be in the driver's seat (and hence less likely to suffer injuries to the thorax from the steering wheel), and are more likely to be victims of poorly fitted restraint systems. It is an important part of the initial history to ascertain whether the pediatric victims in an MVC were restrained, and the type and appropriateness of that restraint for the child's age.

Anatomically, the smaller size of children, as compared to adults, results in a closer proximity of organs. The abdominal wall, rib cage, and pelvic girdle are underdeveloped and provide less protection to the abdominal contents. In addition, children have less body fat, and hence, less 'padding' to absorb and diffuse external force.[4] From the physiologic perspective, children are generally healthy and have fewer underlying medical problems than adults. It is uncommon for children to be on medications, particularly those that potentially affect hemodynamics or hemostasis. Therefore, injured pediatric patients are better able to effectively compensate for physiologic insults such as acute blood loss. It is generally accepted that children can lose up to 45% of their circulating blood volume, and exhibit tachycardia as the only abnormal vital sign.[4] Persistent hypotension is an ominous finding, suggesting the failure of compensatory mechanisms and the potential development of irreversible shock. Complicating the evaluation of injured children is the normal variability of vital signs depending on age.

INITIAL EVALUATION AND DIAGNOSIS OF ABDOMINAL INJURIES

As the number of children with significant abdominal injuries is relatively low, but the consequences of a missed injury are high, accurate diagnosis is important. Initial assessment begins before the child arrives at the hospital. Important information from the first responders includes mechanism of injury, use of protective or restraint devices, condition of the child in the field, and, in the case of MVC, damage to vehicle. Once in the emergency department (ED), a thorough history and physical examination is essential. In most statistical models regarding the diagnosis of intra-abdominal injury, an abnormal physical examination is the highest variable.[5–8] While the examination can be challenging given the developmental level of the child, use of comfort strategies and distraction can calm an initially distraught child to a degree that he/she can reliably participate in the evaluation. Important physical findings include vital signs (particularly the presence of persistent tachycardia), abdominal contusions or abrasions, tenderness, or distention. Particular physical findings, such as the 'seat belt sign' and 'handle bar mark,' are suspicious for the presence of intra-abdominal injury (and potential spine fracture in the case of the seat belt mark) (Fig. 16-1).[9]

Laboratory Testing

Laboratory testing for the purpose of diagnosing intra-abdominal injuries has generated considerable interest and conflicting results. One study reported that the combination of an abnormal physical examination and >50 red blood cells per high power field on urinalysis was a highly sensitive screen for the presence of intra-abdominal injury.[5] The study, limited by the low number of children who actually had a documented injury (14 out of the total study population of 285), also concluded that laboratory abnormalities in this trauma population were relatively uncommon. The conclusion that routine laboratory studies add little to the evaluation has also been replicated in more recent studies.[6,7] Conversely, studies using sophisticated regression analyses have demonstrated that elevations of aspartate aminotransferase (AST) and/or alamine aminotransferase (ALT), in combination with an abnormal physical examination, correlate with the presence of an intra-abdominal injury, although the tests are

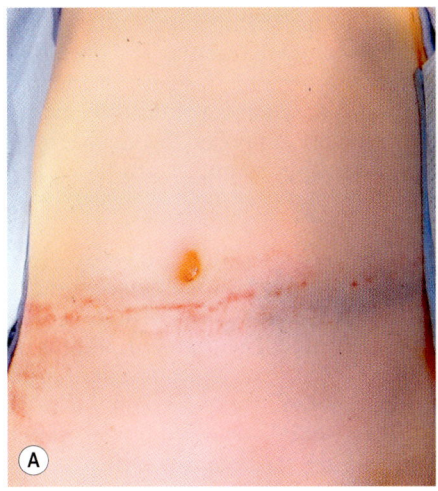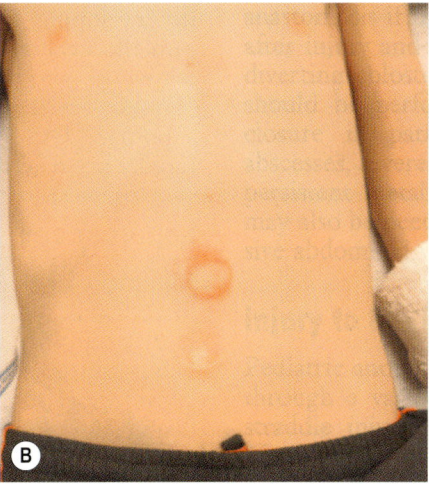

FIGURE 16-1 ■ Important physical findings that might suggest intra-abdominal injuries include the **(A)** 'seat belt sign' and the **(B)** 'handlebar mark.' With patients exhibiting the seat belt sign, there is also potential for a spine fracture. The handlebar mark may herald an underlying duodenal hematoma or pancreatic injury.

not diagnostic for a particular injured organ.[8,10–12] A clinical prediction model using a combination of physical examination findings (hypotension and abnormal examination findings) and laboratory studies (AST, amylase, hematocrit, heme-positive urinalysis) successfully predicted the presence of intra-abdominal injury in a small, single center study.[13] Interestingly, routine amylase and lipase determinations do not appear to be very reliable or cost effective screening tools.[14] In the special population of children suspected of abuse, elevations in AST or ALT, or abnormal physical examination findings (such as bruising, distention, or tenderness), may indicate the need for further abdominal imaging looking for occult injury.[15]

In summary, it appears that laboratory panels in the evaluation of children at risk for intra-abdominal injuries are best utilized in conjunction with physical examination findings and as a screen to determine those children who might require further diagnostic testing, particularly imaging.

Computed Tomography

Computed tomography (CT) with intravenous contrast (IV) is the preferred modality for the diagnosis of intra-abdominal injuries in hemodynamically stable children.[4] Newer generation scanners have excellent sensitivity and specificity, especially for the evaluation of solid organ injuries. Upwards of 95% of liver, spleen, and renal injuries can be diagnosed and staged by CT (Fig. 16-2). Injuries to the intestine and pancreas are more difficult to definitively diagnose by CT. However, with the addition of coronal reconstructions, CT provides significant information to guide the clinician regarding these injuries. Similarly, the risk of a 'missed' intra-abdominal injury in a child with a completely negative CT is very low, leading some to advocate using CT as a means to decrease the need for in-patient observation after blunt abdominal trauma.[16]

It has been suggested that in young children who lack visceral fat, the addition of oral contrast to the standard IV contrast may be helpful, especially in evaluating the duodenum and pancreatic head.[17] The use of oral contrast, however, remains controversial due to concerns regarding aspiration, and may not provide significant additional information with current, multi-detector CT imaging. Intravenous contrast, however, is essential for the evaluation of traumatic injuries. If IV contrast is contraindicated, alternative methods of abdominal evaluation should be considered.

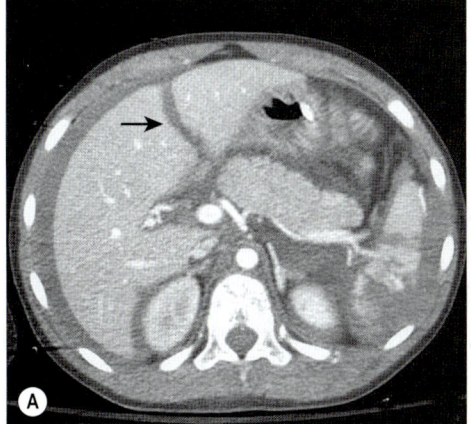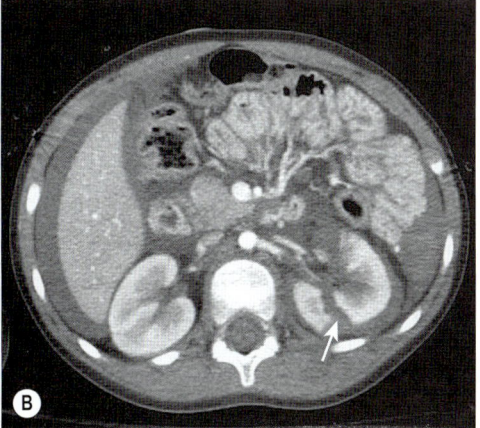

FIGURE 16-2 ■ CT scans are highly accurate in demonstrating solid organ injuries. **(A)** Hemoperitoneum with a liver laceration (arrow) and a shattered spleen is seen. **(B)** Hemoperitoneum and a left renal laceration (arrow) is shown.

The radiation exposure during CT imaging has become an area of major concern in children. The use of CT has been rapidly increasing over the past decade, with over seven million scans performed on children, mostly for the evaluation of trauma and appendicitis.[18] Using models extrapolated from radiation exposure from the atomic bomb explosions, a risk of one fatal cancer per 1000 CT scans performed in young children (above the baseline cancer risk of approximately one in four adults in the USA) has been estimated.[19] A recently published longitudinal, population-based study in Great Britain demonstrated an increased incidence of leukemia and brain cancer after repeated CT scans in children.[20] Infants and children are more sensitive than adults to the effects of radiation given their small size (larger absorbed dose per unit area) and growing organs.[21] In response, the pediatric radiology community has developed an Image Gently® campaign to address the public's concerns.[21] In addition, two recent position papers, authored by the APSA Education Committee and the American Academy of Pediatrics (AAP) Radiology Committee, have addressed the issue of CT scans in children.[22,23] Both endorse the ALARA principle (as low as reasonably achievable) and advocate for the use of scanners with pediatric dose reduction software, employing alternative imaging modalities (if available), limiting the number or phases of scans (for example with and without contrast or arterial and venous phases), and the use of limited scans. Other concepts include limiting the number of repeat scans and developing relationships with referring adult institutions to limit the number of scans performed on children prior to transfer.

Ultrasound

As concerns regarding CT have increased, there has been a renewed interest in the use of ultrasound (US) in the evaluation of pediatric abdominal trauma. The original descriptions about ultrasound in trauma centered on the rapid evaluation of the unstable adult trauma patient to determine the presence and source of life-threatening hemorrhage. The FAST (focused assessment with sonography in trauma) examination was developed to assess the presence of intra-abdominal free fluid (with examination of Morrison's pouch, the pouch of Douglas, and the left flank) or fluid within the pericardial sac (subxiphoid view), and thus indicate the need for operative exploration. In multiple studies, the traditional FAST examination has been found to have a low sensitivity and specificity for the diagnosis of injury in children.[24-27] A recently published large series directly comparing FAST examination in children to CT or laparotomy for the presence of free fluid concluded that a positive FAST suggested hemoperitoneum and associated abdominal injury, but a negative FAST adds little in decision making.[28] In addition, since the majority of pediatric solid organ injuries, even those with significant free fluid (hemoperitoneum), can be managed nonoperatively, a positive FAST examination may not be very helpful in directing clinical care. On the other hand, the use of provider-performed ultrasound has increased dramatically over the past several years in the pediatric ED, and there is significant interest

in developing algorithms that incorporate ultrasound into the evaluation of abdominal trauma.[29,30] The ultimate goal is to limit the number of CT scans. In the less common scenario of the hemodynamically unstable child, a positive FAST examination supports the decision to rapidly proceed to the operating room.

Laparoscopy

Minimally invasive approaches are now well incorporated in pediatric surgical practice so it is not surprising that laparoscopy for the evaluation of abdominal trauma is being utilized. Despite the excellent anatomic definition provided by multi-detector CT, there remain areas of diagnostic uncertainty. The child with free fluid without evidence of solid organ injury, particularly with physical examination findings of a seat belt or handlebar mark, is one example. Another scenario is the child with significant abdominal tenderness with a nondiagnostic CT scan. If the findings at laparoscopy indicate the need for a formal laparotomy, an open approach can be targeted to the specific injury. In two relatively large reviews, laparoscopy was found to be safe and beneficial by avoiding laparotomy in a significant number of patients.[31,32] Also, a number of injuries were amenable to laparoscopic repair. CT and laparoscopy now provide complementary information, with CT defining areas, such as the retroperitoneum, kidneys, and pancreas, which are difficult to assess using laparoscopy. On the other hand, laparoscopy allows for direct visualization of the bowel, mesentery, and diaphragmatic surfaces, regions that CT has traditionally not been as accurate (Fig. 16-3).

MANAGEMENT

Liver and Spleen

Close to 90–95% of injuries to the liver and spleen in children can be managed nonoperatively. It is rare for isolated low grade injuries to these organs to require blood transfusion.[33] Nonoperative management (NOM) is dependent upon the accurate diagnosis and staging of the injured organ, usually by CT imaging at present. Injuries are graded according to the American Association for the Surgery of Trauma (AAST) organ injury scale, with grade I injuries representing small lacerations or hematomas and grade V injuries indicating complete vascular disruption or massive parenchymal injury (Table 16-1).[34] In order to be a candidate for NOM, the child should have normal hemodynamics, and be monitored closely for signs of ongoing hemorrhage. Most children who fail NOM do so within four hours of injury as a result of shock, peritonitis, or persistent bleeding.[35] Late failures are often the result of peritonitis due to an evolving intestinal injury. There are published, evidence-based guidelines for NOM in a child with a liver or spleen injury.[36,37] Essentially, these guidelines recommend hospitalization for 'grade of injury plus one' days, and note that children with higher grade injuries may benefit from intensive care unit observation. Routine follow-up imaging is not indicated, and children can return to

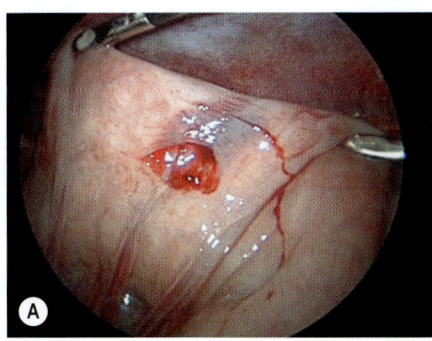
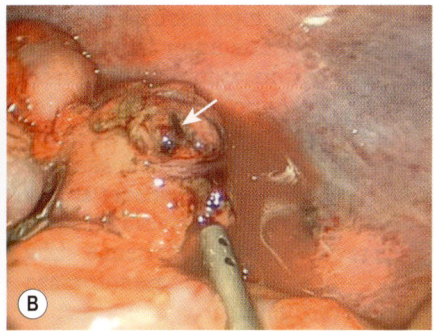

FIGURE 16-3 ■ In some patients it is not always clear whether a significant intestinal injury has occurred from either blunt or penetrating trauma. Diagnostic laparoscopy is a useful technique in these patients. **(A)** Perforation of the bowel from penetrating trauma is seen at laparoscopy. This was closed primarily. **(B)** Full-thickness injury to the colon (arrow) in a patient with blunt trauma is shown. The laparoscopic approach was converted to an open operation for treatment of this injury.

regular activity after grade of injury plus two weeks from the time of injury. More recent work challenges these recommendations, finding that more abbreviated periods of bed rest and hospitalization does not result in delayed bleeding or return to the hospital.[38] Fortunately, most splenic and hepatic injuries in children will resolve without the need for operative intervention with excellent long-term outcomes.

While bleeding from most solid organ injuries in children will stop, there are a small number in which the bleeding is significant. Tachycardia, not responsive to fluid resuscitation, is the initial sign of shock in these children. Hypotension is often a late finding and suggests significant hemorrhage. Evidence of ongoing bleeding with an abnormal abdominal examination or a positive abdominal FAST examination necessitates urgent operative exploration. Rapid transfusion protocols, while not formally validated in children, are utilized with the goal of 1:1:1 transfusion of packed red blood cells (PRBC), fresh frozen plasma (FFP), and platelets. In infants and children, this translates to 20 mL/kg of PRBC, FFP and platelets.[39] In the operating room, a rapid transfusion device and cell saver should be available in the event of rapid blood loss. The patient is prepped from neck to knees to allow for entrance into either the chest or abdomen, and to have access to the femoral vessels. Upon entrance to the abdomen, the four quadrants are packed to tamponade the bleeding and allow the anesthesiologists to 'catch-up.' The peritoneal contents are then explored in a systematic fashion. The goal of initial operative exploration is to stop bleeding and control the fecal stream (damage control).

Splenectomy easily controls bleeding in the hemodynamically unstable patient with active exsanguination from a massively damaged spleen, although at the theoretical cost of a long-term risk of postsplenectomy sepsis. Children with splenic injuries who have ongoing bleeding, but are not in shock, are potential candidates for splenic sparing operations. Partial splenectomy and mesh splenorrhaphy are techniques that can successfully save splenic parenchyma, although they may be time consuming, and are therefore not appropriate in the unstable patient.[40]

Postsplenectomy sepsis is a rare, but potentially fatal consequence of splenectomy due to overwhelming infection by encapsulated organisms. The reported incidence is around 0.23% a year, with an increased incidence in children less than 2 years of age, and those that underwent splenectomy for hematologic reasons.[41] Vaccination with the 23-valent pneumococcal vaccine, as

TABLE 16-1 Liver/Spleen Injury Grading Scale from the AAST

Grade	Injury	Description of Injury
I	Hematoma	Subcapsular, <10% surface area
	Laceration	Capsular tear, <1 cm parenchymal depth
II	Hematoma	Subcapsular, 10–50% surface area
		Intraparenchymal, <10 cm in diameter
	Laceration	Capsular tear, 1–3 cm parenchymal depth, <10 cm length
III	Hematoma	Subcapsular, >50% surface area or expanding
		Ruptured subcapsular or parenchymal hematoma
		Intraparenchymal hematoma >10 cm or expanding
	Laceration	>3 cm parenchymal depth
IV	Laceration	Parenchymal disruption involving 25–75% of hepatic lobe or 1–3 Couinaud's segments within a single lobe
V	Laceration	Parenchymal disruption involving >75% of hepatic lobe or >3
	Vascular	Juxtahepatic venous injuries: i.e., retrohepatic vena cava/central major hepatic veins
	Vascular	Couinaud's segments within single lobe
		Hepatic avulsion

From Tinkoff G, Esposito TJ, Reed J, et al. American Association for the Surgery of Trauma Organ Injury Scale I: spleen, liver, and kidney, validation based on the National Trauma Data Bank. J Am Coll Surg 2008;207:646–55.

well as vaccinations against *Haemophilus influenzae* type B and meningococcus, should be administered after splenectomy. With high grade splenic injuries managed nonoperatively, assessment of splenic function may also be indicated.

A major hepatic injury is considerably more difficult to control in the operating room. The segmental anatomy of the liver and the location of important arterial, venous, and portal structures is very important. Peitzman and Marsh recently reviewed operative techniques for the management of complex liver injury.[42] Key components of operative control of hepatic parenchymal injury include adequate exposure, an experienced co-surgeon, good anesthesia support, and supradiaphragmatic intravenous access. They recommend initial management of deep parenchymal fractures with compression, followed by suture ligation of bleeding vessels, and the avoidance of deep liver sutures. The Pringle maneuver can help differentiate between hepatic arterial bleeding (decreases when the clamp is engaged) and hepatic venous bleeding. Ideally, intermittent clamping of the porta hepatis should be performed to decrease the degree of hepatic ischemia.

Large fractures are best treated with anatomic or non-anatomic resection, assuming enough residual liver remains. Resection can be efficiently performed using mechanical staplers. While the definitive operation must control bleeding and bile leak, debride nonviable tissue, and adequately drain the resected margin, control of hemorrhage is the primary concern in an emergency operation. Temporizing maneuvers, such as packing with control of bleeding, are performed and a temporary abdominal closure is created to allow for ongoing resuscitation and to prevent abdominal compartment syndrome. Vacuum dressings have been developed specifically for this purpose, but techniques such as the 'Bogota bag' are still viable alternatives. Multiple trips to the operating room for wash-out, packing removal, and treatment of other injuries may be required before the patient is ready for formal abdominal closure.

Abdominal Compartment Syndrome

Abdominal compartment syndrome (ACS) is defined as sustained intra-abdominal hypertension (IAH) that is associated with new onset organ dysfunction or failure.[43,44] It is an uncommon, but potentially lethal condition that occurs when abdominal distension associated with IAH causes reduced perfusion to the intra-abdominal organs. The result is ischemia and refractory metabolic acidosis along with interference with cardiopulmonary function secondary to reduced preload from decreased central venous return to the heart, decreased respiratory compliance, and decreased functional residual capacity.[45] ACS is associated with a 40–60% mortality in children.[46–48]

As IAH in children is different from adults, the current proposed working definition for ACS in children is an elevated intra-abdominal pressure (IAP) of 10 mmHg or greater with the development of new or worsening multiorgan failure.[44] There are three different types of ACS: (1) primary ACS refers to ACS that occurs due to a primary intra-abdominal cause such as abdominal trauma; (2) secondary ACS or extra-abdominal compartment syndrome occurs as a result of massive bowel edema secondary to sepsis, capillary leak, and other conditions requiring massive fluid resuscitation; and (3) tertiary ACS or recurrent ACS in which ACS recurs after resolution of an earlier episode of either primary or secondary ACS.[49] IAP can be measured by using the bladder pressure. If IAH is detected, serial IAP measurements are needed. It is important to note that clinical examination is an inaccurate predictor of IAP and should not be substituted for IAP measurement.[50]

Initial management strategies in the trauma patient include improving abdominal wall compliance via adequate sedation and paralysis, evacuation of intralumenal intestinal contents, evacuation of large abdominal fluid collections, optimization of fluid administration by goal-directed therapies and correcting positive fluid balance, and optimization of abdominal perfusion pressure.[51] Over the last ten years, three major changes have led to significant reductions in the incidence and mortality from ACS in adult trauma patients. These are adoption of massive transfusion protocols and 1:1 blood to plasma transfusion strategies in trauma, the widespread use of damage control and open abdomen approaches to the polytraumatized abdominal cavity, and an increased use of plasma and colloids in the resuscitation of burn patients.[51] Similar strategies and an increased awareness of ACS in pediatric trauma patients may also result in improved outcomes.

In the unstable trauma patient who requires an emergent laparotomy and massive fluid resuscitation, maintaining an open abdomen with planned staged closure may prevent the development of ACS but often needs to be performed prophylactically (Fig. 16-4A). In patients

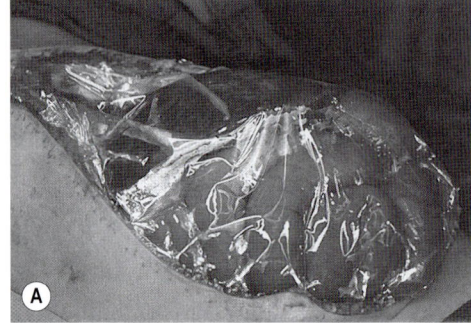 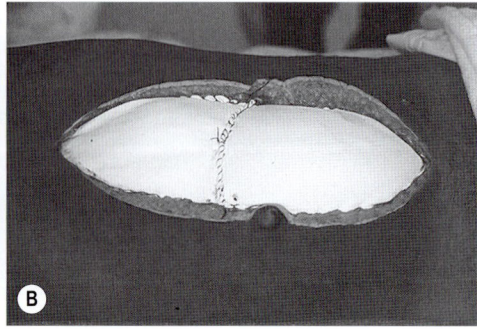

FIGURE 16-4 ◼ **(A)** Abdominal wall expansion was performed in this patient with a bowel bag. **(B)** Abdominal wall expansion in this patient was accomplished with a polytetrafluoroethylene patch.

who develop ACS, early intervention via emergent decompressive laparotomy and some form of temporary abdominal wall closure, while awaiting resolution of IAH, can be lifesaving (Fig. 16-4B).[46,48,52] The goals of operation are to decrease the elevated IAP to stop organ dysfunction, allow room for continued expansion of the viscera during ongoing resuscitation, provide temporary abdominal closure, prevent excessive fascial retraction, and allow a means for continued evacuation of fluid from the abdominal cavity.[51] Application of a negative pressure wound dressing to the open abdomen is a useful temporary dressing as well as a modality to remove edema from the abdominal cavity and intestinal wall.[53] Temporary patch abdominoplasty with a variety of materials and the placement of a silo have also been utilized in the setting of an open abdomen. However, these methods lack the capability to actively evacuate excess fluid. Subsequent staged abdominal closure with sutures or patch abdominoplasty is performed when IAH is corrected.

Role of Interventional Radiology

Angioembolization is a technique that is frequently utilized in adults with splenic or hepatic vascular injuries. The role of interventional radiology in children is less well defined. For example, embolization in adults is frequently employed for the management of a contrast blush demonstrated on CT scan. Multiple studies in children, however, demonstrate that a contrast blush is associated with the need for operative intervention in less than 20% of splenic injuries.[54–56] Long-term follow-up of large cohorts of children with splenic and hepatic injuries also reveal a very low rate of late bleeding, suggesting that the rate of bleeding from an initially unrecognized arterial pseudoaneurysm is also very low.[36,37] On the other hand, small single-center studies and case reports demonstrate that interventional radiological techniques are safe in children, and have been effective when utilized.[57–60] The population that seems most amenable to this technique are children with evidence of ongoing bleeding but are hemodynamically stable, or those that develop bleeding later in their hospital course. In our institution, we have effectively utilized angioembolization in a few cases of hepatic arterial bleeding (Fig. 16-5).

Special Considerations with Liver Injuries

The initial concern with hepatic injury is control of bleeding, but injury to the biliary system can also occur. High grade liver injuries are associated with a small (4%) risk of a significant bile leak.[61] If the patient has required operative management for the injury, it is prudent to place closed suction drains around the liver, particularly if a nonanatomic resection was performed. With nonoperative management, the development of a significant bile leak is often heralded by feeding intolerance, abdominal pain, elevations in hepatic enzymes, and fever.[62] Abdominal imaging (either ultrasound or CT) reveals the presence of a fluid collection. Initial management involves the insertion of drains, usually performed percutaneously with image guidance.

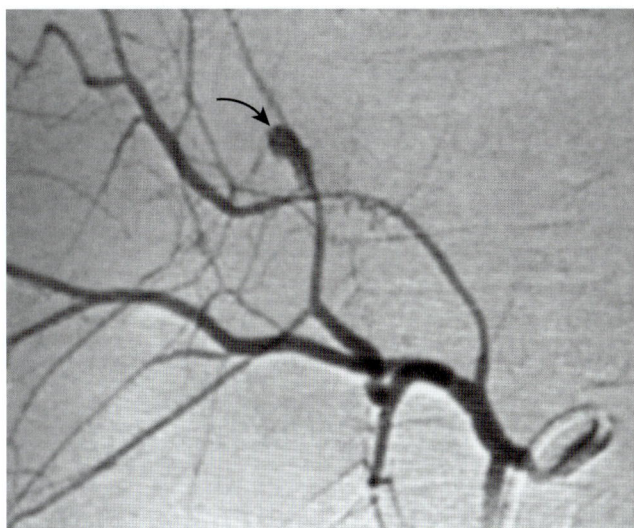

FIGURE 16-5 ■ This hepatic artery angiogram was performed in a patient with persistent hemorrhage after initial damage-control laparotomy. The site of hemorrhage is identified (arrow), and embolization was successfully performed.

Endoscopic retrograde cholangiopancreatography (ERCP) has been used to identify the location of the leak, and more importantly, with the addition of sphincterotomy, to decrease biliary pressure and promote internal drainage.[63,64] Placement of biliary stents can also be performed, both to improve drainage and to treat the ductal injury. Therapeutic ERCP requires operator expertise, and heavy sedation or general anesthesia for the procedure to be safely performed in children. In the case of stent placement, a second endoscopic procedure to remove the stent is usually necessary. Complications of ERCP include bleeding, sepsis, and stent migration or clogging.

Pancreatic Injuries

Injury to the pancreas occurs in fewer than 5% of pediatric abdominal injuries, and can be difficult to diagnose. They are most frequently the result of blunt mechanisms, such as MVC and bicycle handlebar injuries. Patients usually present with significant epigastric pain and bilious emesis, particularly in the case of injuries that have a delayed presentation. CT scan with IV contrast is the preferred imaging study, although definitive identification of these injuries can be difficult (Fig. 16-6). In unusual cases, magnetic retrograde cholangiopancreatography (MRCP) can be helpful. ERCP, if available, may be helpful in determining whether there is a major ductal injury, and may have a potential therapeutic role, but is an invasive and a technically challenging procedure.[65]

Contusions, without evidence of pancreatic ductal injury, can be managed nonoperatively with nothing by mouth. The child is followed symptomatically as an oral diet is reintroduced. Trends in serum amylase and lipase may be helpful, although the absolute value of these tests does not correlate with outcome.[66] Management of ductal transection is currently controversial. The standard approach for a distal ductal transection is a spleen

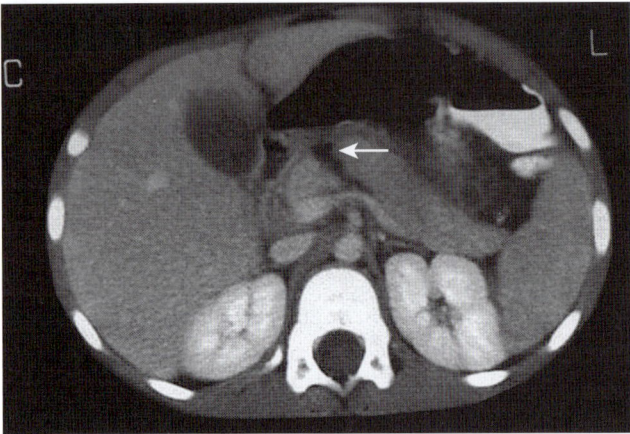

FIGURE 16-6 ■ This abdominal CT scan demonstrates blunt transection of the pancreas (arrow).

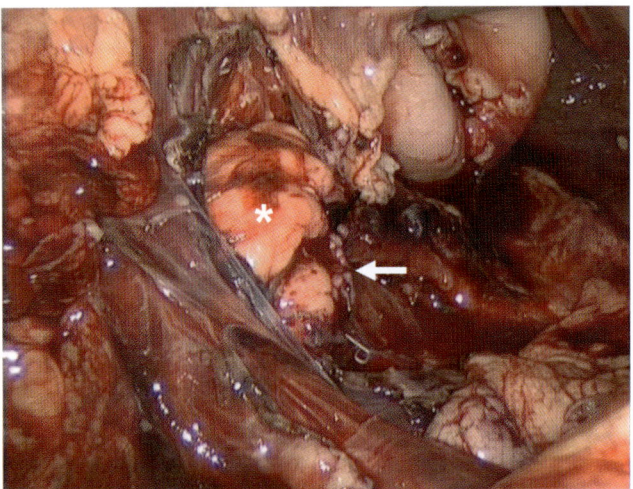

FIGURE 16-7 ■ This patient presented with a pancreatic transection just lateral to the vertebral column. He underwent laparoscopic exploration followed by a laparoscopic distal pancreatectomy with preservation of the spleen. The remaining pancreas is noted with the asterisk and the staple line is marked with the arrow.

preserving distal pancreatectomy. This procedure, which can be performed via an open laparotomy or laparoscopically (Fig. 16-7),[67,68] is generally well tolerated, and prevents pseudocyst formation. Concerns regarding late morbidity, particularly endocrine insufficiency, have led to other treatment approaches. One group has advocated for the use of Roux-en-Y distal pancreaticojejunostomy using a retrocolic jejunal limb to drain the distal pancreas.[69] Others have advocated a nonoperative approach to pancreatic ductal injuries, with percutaneous or endoscopic drainage of subsequent pseudocysts.[70,71] A recent APSA Trauma Committee retrospective review compared operative and nonoperative management, and demonstrated similar length of hospitalization, but a higher rate of pseudocyst formation and days on total parenteral nutritional (TPN) in the nonoperative group.[72] Patients undergoing NOM often require ERCP to define the ductal anatomy, perform sphincterotomy, and potentially stent the pancreatic duct, as well as percutaneous or endoscopic drainage of pseudocysts. At this time, it is unclear which patient population will benefit from a nonoperative approach for a pancreatic ductal injury. In addition, the nonoperative approach requires the availability of advanced endoscopic techniques and ERCP.

Diaphragmatic Injury

Blunt traumatic rupture of the diaphragm via massive compressive forces to the abdomen accounts for 80–90% of diaphragmatic injury in the pediatric population.[73] This injury rarely occurs in isolation, but is often associated with multiple organ injury and a high index of severity scores.[74] Abdominal contents may herniate into the thoracic cavity due to the pressure gradient between the pleura and peritoneal cavities. Right and left sided ruptures occur with equal frequency.[75] Plain radiographs may suggest the diagnosis of traumatic diaphragm rupture via an obscured or elevated hemidiaphragm, gas in herniated viscus above the diaphragm (Fig. 16-8A), tip of nasogastric tube in the thorax, the presence of an atypical pneumothorax, and plate-like atelectasis adjacent to the diaphragm.[73]

Emergent operative exploration in patients with diaphragm injury is indicated in the hemodynamically unstable patient with multiple organ injury. A thorough and systematic exploration of the entire abdomen and palpation of retroperitoneal structures is required due to the frequency of multiple organ injury. Repair of the diaphragmatic defect is typically possible after debridement of any compromised tissue. If large defects are found, a prosthetic patch may be needed to minimize the tension. Successful laparoscopic or thoracoscopic repair of diaphragmatic injuries can be performed in hemodynamically stable children and in cases with delayed diagnosis (Fig. 16-8B, C).[76-78]

Hollow Viscus Injury

Hollow viscus injury in children is typically caused by blunt trauma via crush injury from a focal or localized blow to the abdomen such as a bicycle handle bar, a punch to the abdomen, or from a seatbelt in an MVC. Distended hollow viscera are more prone to rupture with blunt trauma due to the increased intraluminal pressure.[79] Areas of mesenteric fixation such as the proximal jejunum near the ligament of Trietz, the distal ileum near the ileocecal valve, and the rectosigmoid junction are particularly vulnerable to injury via acceleration/deceleration shearing forces. Seat belt signs may also be markers of severe deceleration injury to the abdomen with an associated intra-abdominal blunt hollow viscus injury.[80] In this injury complex, the rapid deceleration from a high impact crash causes sudden flexion of the upper body around the fixed lap belt and consequent compression of the abdominal viscera between the lap belt and the spine. This injury is accentuated by using adult seat belts without booster seats in young children or using lap belts without shoulder straps. The use of age-appropriate child restraints in cars may prevent some of these injuries.[81]

Children with traumatic hollow viscus injury and perforation typically present with signs of peritoneal irritation due to the rapid contamination of the peritoneal

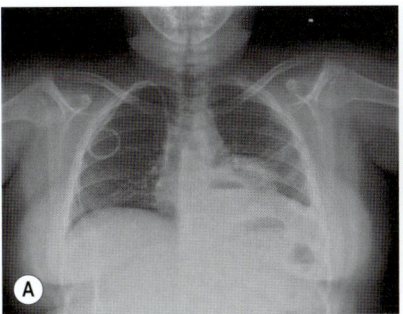 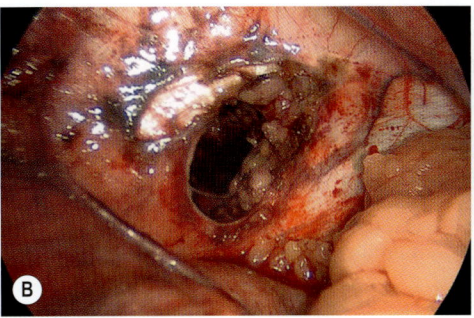 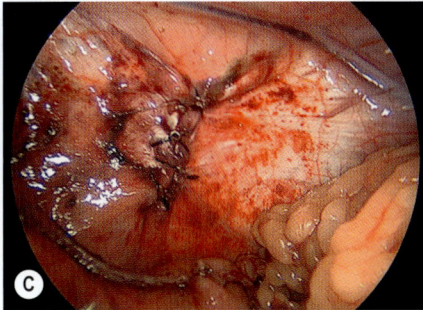

FIGURE 16-8 ■ This teenager developed respiratory symptoms several weeks after a motor vehicle accident. **(A)** The chest radiograph shows air in either the stomach or the intestine in the left chest. **(B)** At laparoscopic exploration, the traumatic diaphragmatic hernia is seen after reduction of the stomach and several loops of small intestine. **(C)** The traumatic diaphragmatic hernia was repaired laparoscopically and the patient recovered uneventfully.

cavity. In a neurologically intact patient with a perforated viscus, findings of abdominal tenderness, guarding, and rebound on initial and serial physical examinations are more specific for hollow viscus injury than abdominal ultrasound or CT findings for these injuries.[82–84] Hemodynamically unstable patients with signs and symptoms of hollow viscus injury should undergo an emergent exploratory laparotomy. In stable patients, more time can be taken for evaluation and a CT scan of the abdomen and pelvis can be performed. CT findings suggestive of hollow viscus injury include bowel wall thickening and enhancement, mesenteric stranding, and free intraperitoneal fluid in the absence of solid organ injury.[12] Despite currently available diagnostic studies, partial thickness lacerations, hematomas, or avulsions of mesenteric vessels may not initially appear significant, but can progress to full-thickness intestinal wall ischemia and perforation with leakage of intestinal content over hours to days. Some mesenteric injuries may result in an intestinal stricture or internal hernia diagnosed weeks after the accident. A recent multi-institutional retrospective review by the APSA Trauma Committee determined that delay in operative treatment up to 24 hours did not significantly affect outcome.[85]

In hemodynamically stable patients with evidence of bowel injury or in equivocal cases with concerning physical signs or symptoms, diagnostic laparoscopy is a very reasonable approach. In cases with penetrating trauma, local wound exploration to identify penetration of the anterior abdominal fascia is recommended as the initial diagnostic maneuver. If it is still unclear whether the peritoneum has been violated, then laparoscopy can be performed to determine whether there is penetration into the abdominal cavity and also to assist with the creation of a diverting stoma, if needed.[32,86,87] Whether exploration is performed laparoscopically or via an open approach, a four quadrant inspection of the abdominal cavity with meticulous examination of both the intestinal tract and mesentery should be performed. The lesser sac should be opened to evaluate the posterior gastric wall, the pancreas, and diaphragm. Regardless of the approach, principles of management of hollow viscus injury include prompt resuscitation, complete removal of devitalized tissue, reconstruction or diversion of the intestinal tract, and perioperative antibiotic coverage.

Injury to the Stomach

Penetrating injury to the stomach is more common than blunt trauma, and results in a variable presentation of local tissue destruction. Despite its rarity, blunt injury to the stomach can occur and is typically seen in the patient who has just eaten, as the full stomach is more vulnerable to burst injury.[88,89] When gastric rupture occurs, it is usually located along the greater curvature with a blow-out or stellate configuration. At exploration, the posterior wall of the stomach and the gastroesophageal junction should always be evaluated to avoid missed injuries.[89] Debridement with repair of the injury is sufficient.

Duodenal Injuries

The majority of duodenal injuries in children result from blunt mechanisms.[90,91] In younger patients, duodenal injury is often the result of nonaccidental trauma and isolated injury should raise suspicion if the history or mechanism is inconsistent with the injury.[9,92] Due to its contiguous location to many other vital structures, associated injuries are common. Also, because of its location close to the vertebral column, blow-out injuries can occur.[93] Diagnosis of a duodenal injury may be difficult due to the retroperitoneal nature of the duodenum, the poor sensitivity of plain radiographs, and the nonspecific nature of examination findings in these patients. Abdominal CT is the test of choice to evaluate for duodenal injury. Injuries to the duodenum as graded by the AAST range from hematomas involving only a portion of the duodenum (grade I) to devascularization of the duodenum or massive disruption of the duodenopancreatic complex (grade V) (Table 16-2).[94]

Duodenal hematomas may be found on CT or upper GI studies revealing transmural thickening with lumenal duodenal narrowing, or partial obstruction without evidence of extravasation of air or contrast (Fig. 16-9). They are typically managed nonoperatively with nasogastric decompression and TPN over one to three weeks.[95] Operative evacuation of the hematoma may be required if obstructive signs and symptoms do not resolve. Evacuation of the hematoma may also be performed if the duodenal hematoma is found on laparotomy or

TABLE 16-2 **Duodenal Injury Grading Scale from the AAST**

Grade	Injury	Description of Injury
I	Hematoma	Involving single portion of wall
	Laceration	Partial thickness, no perforation
II	Hematoma	Involving more than one portion
	Laceration	<50% circumference disruption
III	Laceration	Disruption 50%–75% circumference of 2nd portion
		Disruption 50%–100% circumference of 1st, 3rd, or 4th portions
IV	Laceration	Disruption of >75% circumference of 2nd portion
		Involvement of ampulla or distal common bile duct
V	Laceration	Massive disruption of duodenopancreatic complex
		Duodenal devascularization

From Moore EE, Cogbill TH, Malangoni MA, et al. Organ injury scaling, II: Pancreas, duodenum, small bowel, colon, and rectum. J Trauma 1990;30:1427–9.

laparoscopy for other injuries. CT scan findings of extravasation of air or contrast into the paraduodenal, pararenal, or retroperitoneal space is consistent with duodenal perforation.[95] Early diagnosis can simplify management and minimize morbidity, but delay in diagnosis is not uncommon due to a delay in presentation or the paucity of findings on initial imaging.[96–98] When high clinical suspicion for duodenal injury exists and initial radiographs and abdominal CT scans do not reveal significant injury, serial CT scans may be indicated to look for the delayed development of retroperitoneal air. Delay in diagnosis of greater than 24 hours is associated with established peritoneal inflammation, poor tissue integrity, and a higher leak rate following primary repair.[91]

Complications, such as fistula formation, are more common (2–14%) after repair of duodenal injuries than following operative repair for any other area of the gastrointestinal tract.[91] Several operative techniques such as serosal patch repair, transverse primary repair, duodenal diverticularization, pyloric exclusion, and gastrojejunostomy have been applied to duodenal injuries to minimize potentially significant complications.[93,95,98] Operative intervention for duodenal injuries should be made based on clinical judgment. Most full-thickness injuries with minimal tissue destruction not involving the drainage of the biliary or pancreatic ductal system can be repaired primarily.[99] In patients with a complex duodenal injury, diversion and drainage may be needed (Fig. 16-10). In these cases, a duodenostomy tube and gastrostomy may be helpful for decompression. A feeding jejunostomy is recommended for early enteral nutrition, and drains should be placed near the repair. Earlier diagnosis of duodenal injuries may make the injury more amenable to primary repair while a significant delay in diagnosis (>24 hours), or those with a grade III or greater injury, may warrant proximal drainage via a gastrojejunostomy and pyloric exclusion.[91,100]

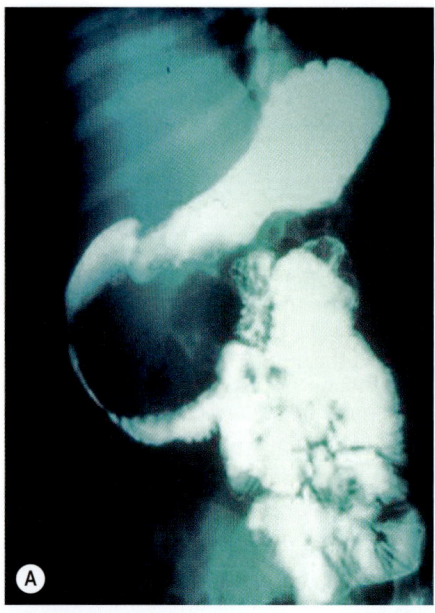

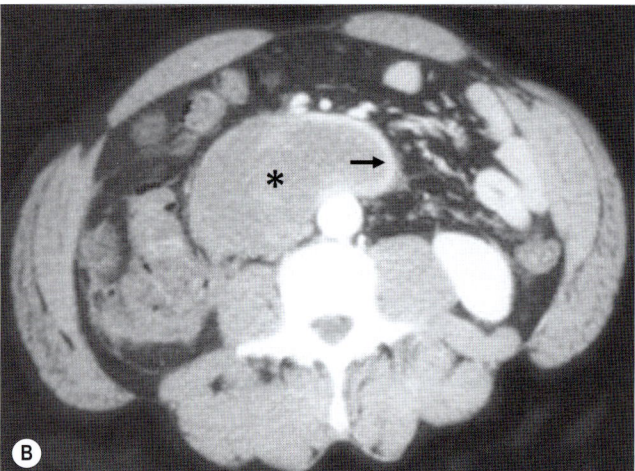

FIGURE 16-9 ■ This patient developed emesis soon after a bicycle accident. The upper gastrointestinal contrast study (**A**) shows a very narrowed duodenum due to extrinsic compression from a large mass in either the pancreas or wall of the duodenum. The CT scan (**B**) in the same patient shows a very small rim of contrast material (arrow) and a very large intramural duodenal hematoma (asterisk).

Injury to the Small Intestine and Colon

Injuries to the small intestine range from transmural hematomas, simple lacerations, complete transection, or mesenteric avulsions with segments of compromised bowel (Fig. 16-11). Even in cases of massive contamination, simple repair, debridement, or resection with primary anastomosis is usually appropriate.

Injury to the colon is infrequent but more often secondary to penetrating mechanisms than blunt injuries in pediatric patients.[101] The infrequent nature of colonic injuries in children hinders the development of guidelines, and the management principles are extracted from the adult trauma experience. Historically, concerns over peritoneal contamination with colonic injury encouraged diversion to avoid anastomotic leaks and ongoing sepsis. Currently, primary repair of early diagnosed colonic

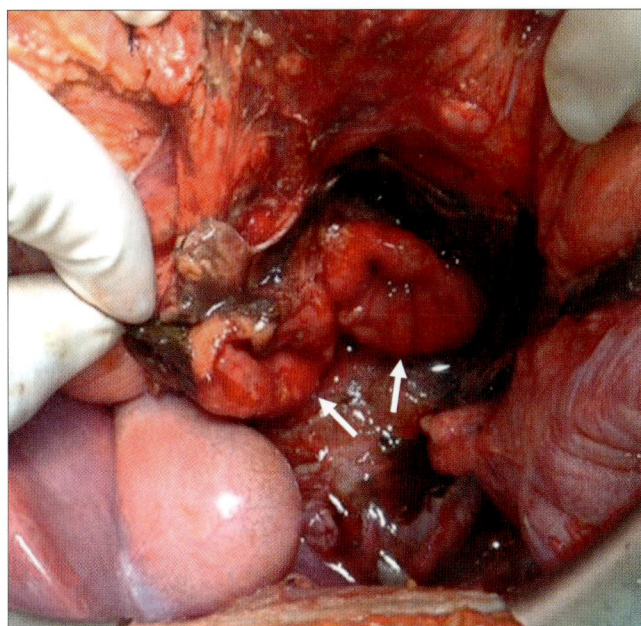

FIGURE 16-10 ■ This patient was suspected of having a duodenal injury after a CT scan showed upper abdominal fluid and retroperitoneal air adjacent to the duodenum. At operation, this patient was found to have a complete duodenal transection following a handlebar injury. As the two segments of duodenum appeared viable (arrows), a primary repair was performed. The patient recovered uneventfully.

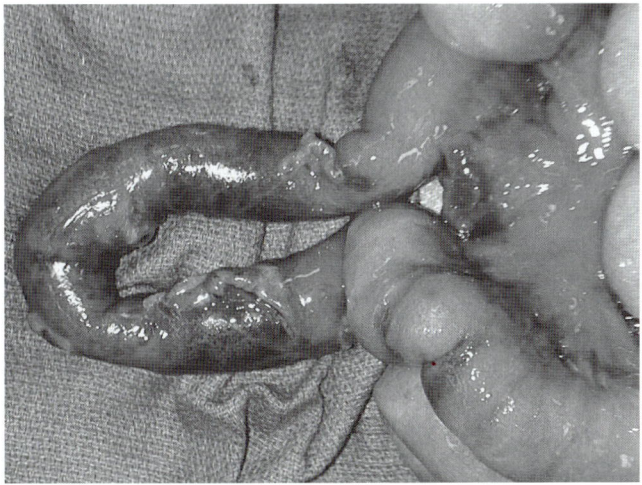

FIGURE 16-11 ■ The small bowel mesentery has been avulsed, resulting in ischemic bowel.

injuries can be performed safely and is the preferred approach, even if there is peritoneal contamination.[101,102] A Cochrane meta-analysis evaluating adult patients with colonic trauma summarizes outcomes with primary repair vs. diversion.[102] This analysis significantly favored primary repair as the optimal treatment due to the reduction in morbidity and a decrease in procedure-related costs. In the setting of significant devitalizing colonic injury in a patient in shock, initial damage-control laparotomy is recommended with delayed colonic anastomosis at the time of abdominal wall closure. In this scenario, a higher complication rate has been found with delayed

anastomosis if fascial closure occurs greater than 5 days after injury and in the case of a left colonic injury.[103] A diverting colostomy rather than a delayed anastomosis should be performed at the time of abdominal wall closure in patients with recurrent intra-abdominal abscesses, severe bowel wall edema and inflammation, or persistent metabolic acidosis.[104] A diverting colostomy may also be needed in patients with simultaneous extensive abdominal wall or perineal injury.

Injury to the Rectum

Pediatric anorectal injury is uncommon, but may occur through a variety of mechanisms, especially falls with straddle injuries, and sexual abuse.[105] Accidental falls often cause injury to the perineal body, external genitalia, urethra and anus, but rectal injury is uncommon (Fig. 16-12). Impalement on fixed objects occurs, but is typically an isolated injury. Sexual abuse often causes isolated rectal or vaginal trauma, and should be considered as a possible etiology in patients with isolated perineal injuries.[105] Blunt rectal injury secondary to MVC is often associated with multiple injuries, such as pelvic fractures and urinary tract injuries.[106] Another notable mechanism in children occurs from the use of personal watercraft (jet skis, seadoos, and wave-runners).[107–109] Passengers thrown from personal watercraft can experience significant hydrostatic force of water through the anal canal on landing, resulting in rectal injury and perforation. These hydrostatic rectal perforations, although rare, are occurring with increasing frequency, and are potentially devastating. In the USA, the National Transportation Safety Board has recommended wet suit bottoms for all children on personal watercraft as operators or passengers.[109]

In the evaluation of rectal injury, digital rectal examination is unreliable.[110] In the stable patient, abdominal and pelvic CT scans can be helpful.[111] Diagnosis of the extent of injury often requires examination under anesthesia at which time, vaginoscopy, anoscopy, proctoscopy, and possible cystoscopy are performed as necessary.[112]

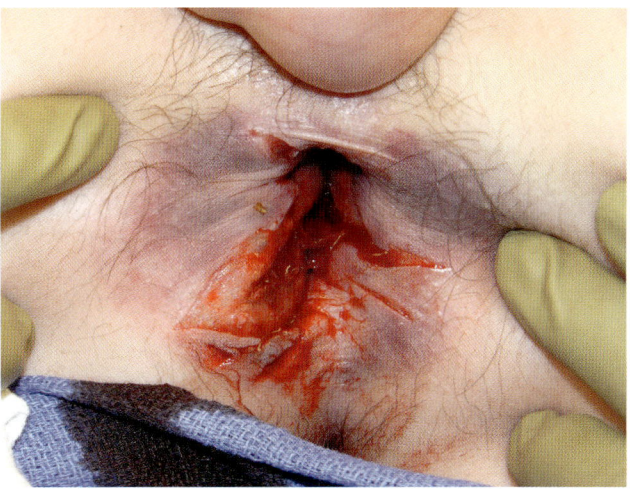

FIGURE 16-12 ■ This teenager developed this full-thickness straddle rectal injury after falling off a trampoline. It was possible to close the injury over drains placed in the perirectal tissues. He has recovered uneventfully with full continence.

Laparoscopy may be needed to evaluate for intraperitoneal extension.[106] Most vaginal, anal, and superficial perineal body injuries can be treated with primary repair. Historically, rectal trauma was managed with a diverting colostomy, drainage of the perineal wound, and rectal irrigation.[113] Currently, selective diversion has been advocated for both pediatric and adult patients with good results.[7,106]

Gallbladder Injury

The gallbladder is rarely injured in children. However, associated injuries are common.[114,115] Predisposing factors for gallbladder trauma are a thin-walled normal gallbladder, a distended gallbladder after a meal, and alcohol ingestion. If identified, a cholecystectomy is usually performed. This may be performed via laparoscopy or laparotomy.

Urinary Bladder

The bladder is the second most common genitourinary (GU) injury in children.[116,117] Bladder injuries range from grade I contusions to grade V extraperitoneal or intraperitoneal ruptures involving the bladder neck or ureteral orifices.[118] It is hypothesized that the bladder's rostral location in relation to the pelvis increases the risk of injury in children.[119] CT cystography is used to evaluate a suspected bladder injury. Prompt repair is required for intraperitoneal ruptures as incomplete drainage of intraabdominal urine can lead to infection, peritonitis, and even death.[120] Typically, a two layered closure with absorbable suture material is performed, and either transurethral or suprapubic drains are used for temporary decompression. Urethral catheter drainage is considered sufficient for uncomplicated extraperitoneal ruptures.[120]

Renal Trauma

With abdominal trauma in children, the kidney is injured in approximately 10% of patients, and is the most commonly injured GU organ.[121] The susceptibility of children for major renal trauma compared to adults appears in part secondary to the fact that the kidney occupies a relatively larger amount of the retroperitoneal space, the thoracic cage is less well ossified, the abdominal musculature is weaker, and there is less cushioning from perirenal fat.[122] Congenital renal anomalies such as hydronephrosis, tumors, or abnormal positions have been postulated to make the kidney more susceptible to trauma with relatively mild traumatic forces. However, recent studies do not support this concept.[116] Congenital abnormalities are present in approximately 1–5% of renal injuries.

Blunt trauma accounts for 80–90% of renal injuries in children. The most common mechanisms are related to MVC, falls, bicycle, and all-terrain vehicle (ATV)-related injuries.[123] In several series, the most severe grade of injury was related to dirt bikes, ATV rollovers, and bicycles.[119,123] Most children who sustain renal injury in an MVC are unrestrained.[124] ATV-related injuries suggest a unique injury mechanism such as a strike from the handlebars, collisions involving ejection, or ATV rollover. Increased awareness and use of proper safety equipment may contribute to decreased prevalence and severity, including abdominal or flank padding, to reduce blunt force and handlebar intrusion.[119]

Patients with renal trauma typically present with gross hematuria and flank pain. The diagnosis is confirmed by abdominal CT scan which is highly sensitive. Renal injuries have also been classified by the AAST (Table 16-3). This classification system has been useful in standardizing and validating treatment strategies.[125] Management goals involve maximizing functional renal parenchyma while minimizing patient morbidity.[126] Expectant NOM is widely accepted for hemodynamically stable grade I-III renal injuries which do not have urinary extravasation.[127]

Treatment for children with high grade renal injury (grade IV and grade V) remains controversial (Fig. 16-13). Urinary extravasation and urinoma continue to be relative indications for exploration in some centers.[128] Historically, patients with higher grade injury were also more likely to undergo endourologic interventions such as nephrostomies or ureteral stents.[129,130] Most current pediatric series report successful nonoperative management for grade IV and V injuries.[127] Endourologic interventions are reserved primarily for persistent extravasation or symptomatic urinomas rather than all injuries with disrupted collecting systems.[127] Selective angioembolization of renal artery branches has been successful in nearly 80% of cases with delayed hemorrhage.[131] Using individualized selective management, several studies have documented renal preservation in over 95% of children.[127,132,133] The main indications for immediate exploration in a child with a renal injury are hemodynamic

TABLE 16-3	**Renal Injury Grading Scale from the AAST**	
Grade	**Injury**	**Description of Injury**
I	Contusion	Microscopic or gross hematuria, normal urologic studies
	Hematoma	Subcapsular, nonexpanding without parenchymal laceration
II	Hematoma	Nonexpanding perirenal hematoma confined to renal retroperitoneum
	Laceration	<1.0 cm parenchymal depth of renal cortex without urinary extravasation
III	Laceration	>1.0 cm parenchymal depth of renal cortex without collecting system rupture or urinary extravasation
IV	Laceration	Parenchymal laceration extending through renal cortex, medulla and collecting system
	Vascular	Main renal artery or vein injury with contained hemorrhage
V	Laceration	Completely shattered kidney
	Vascular	Avulsion of renal hilum that devascularized kidney

From Moore EE, Shackford SR, Pachter HL, et al. Organ injury scaling: spleen, liver, and kidney. J Trauma 1989;29:1664–6.

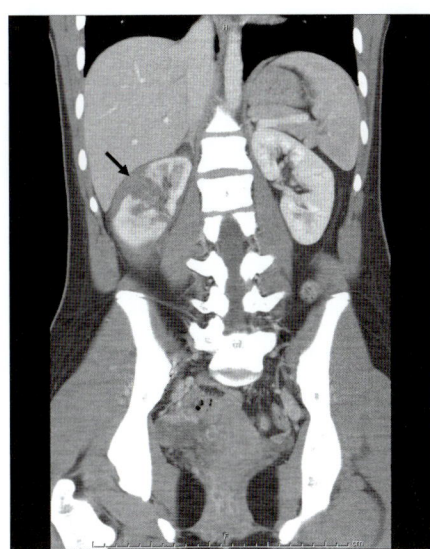

FIGURE 16-13 ■ This child developed a grade III injury to the right kidney. There is a deep laceration through the central aspect of the kidney (arrow), but no evidence of urinary extravasation or development of a urinoma. This patient was managed nonoperatively and recovered uneventfully.

instability, penetrating mechanism, and associated non-renal injuries.[132]

Stable patients with high grade injury are typically placed at bed rest with serial exams, blood counts, and close hemodynamic monitoring until the gross hematuria resolves. However, there are no evidence-based guidelines regarding length of activity restriction in these patients.[134] A multi-institutional prospective study allowing for immediate ambulation and discharge based on standard criteria, rather than resolution of gross hematuria, is currently underway to address possible guidelines.

Penetrating Renal Injury

Penetrating renal injury in children is rare, but typically requires exploration for management. Selective observation for penetrating renal trauma, however, is also being applied and can be done safely.[135,136] Hemodynamically unstable patients with penetrating injury or patients with an expanding retroperitoneal hematoma require renal exploration. During exploration, a one-shot IVP may be helpful to identify the injured area and confirm the presence of a functioning contralateral kidney.

Risk of Injury for Solitary Normal Kidney

It is not uncommon for patients with a single, normal kidney and their family to seek advice from physicians regarding the safety of participating in contact sports. As kidney injuries from sports are rare, the AAP recommends a 'qualified yes' for participation in contact or collision sports for young athletes with a single kidney.[137] Still, many physicians are reluctant to give approval.[138]

A recent prospective study, analyzing more than 4.4 million high school 'athlete exposures,' discovered that sport-related renal injuries are very rare.[139] Out of the 23,666 reported injuries in the study, only 18 involved a kidney, and none were catastrophic or required operation. This number of renal injuries is far fewer than injuries reported for other unpaired organs such as the head, neck, spine, or brain. Cycling, downhill skiing, and horseback riding (classically referred to as 'limited contact sports') are recreational activities that were found to have comparable or higher rates of renal injury in comparison with American football, yet are often not restricted by practitioners.[140]

Additionally, studies have shown that the risks of kidney injury from nonathletic pursuits are far more common than those from sport participation. MVCs alone account for two to ten times more kidney injury than sports.[141] Likewise, ATV and motorcycle use has a much greater risk of serious renal injury compared with participation in contact sports.[123]

REFERENCES

1. Gaines BA. Intra-abdominal solid organ injury in children: Diagnosis and treatment. J Trauma 2009;67:S135–139.
2. WISQARS. Centers for Disease Control and Prevention, 2008.
3. Powell M, Courcoulas A, Gardner M, et al. Management of blunt splenic trauma: Significant differences between adults and children. Surgery 1997;122:654–60.
4. Trauma AcoSCo. Advanced Trauma Life Support for Doctors, Student Course Manual. In: American College of Surgeons Committee on Trauma. Chicago; 2004. p. 251.
5. Isaacman DJ, Scarfone RJ, Kost SI, et al. Utility of routine laboratory testing for detecting intra-abdominal injury in the pediatric trauma patient. Pediatrics 1993;92:691–4.
6. Capraro AJ, Mooney D, Waltzman ML. The use of routine laboratory studies as screening tools in pediatric abdominal trauma. Pediatr Emerg Care 2006;22:480–4.
7. Haut ER, Nance ML, Keller MS, et al. Management of penetrating colon and rectal injuries in the pediatric patient. Dis Colon Rectum 2004;2004:47:1526–32.
8. Holmes JF, Sokolove PE, Brant WE, et al. Identification of children with intra-abdominal injuries after blunt trauma. Ann Emerg Med 2002;39:500–9.
9. Sokolove PE, Kuppermann N, Holmes JF. Association between the 'seat belt sign' and intra-abdominal injury in children with blunt torso trauma. Acad Emerg Med 2005;12:808–13.
10. Holmes JF, Sokolove PE, Land C, et al. Identification of intra-abdominal injuries in children hospitalized following blunt torso trauma. Acad Emerg Med 1999;6:799–806.
11. Cotton BA, Beckert BW, Smith MK, et al. The utility of clinical and laboratory data for predicting intraabdominal injury among children. J Trauma 2004;56:1068–74.
12. Flood RG, Mooney DP. Rate and prediction of traumatic injuries detected by abdominal computed tomography scan in intubated children. J Trauma 2006;61:340–5.
13. Streck CJ Jr, Jewett BM, Wahlquist AH, et al. Evaluation for intra-abdominal injury in children after blunt torso trauma: Can we reduce unnecessary abdominal computed tomography by utilizing a clinical prediction model? J Trauma Acute Care Surg 2012;73:371–6.
14. Adamson WT, Hebra A, Thomas PB, et al. Serum amylase and lipase alone are not cost-effective screening methods for pediatric pancreatic trauma. J Pediatr Surg 2003;38:354–7.
15. Lindberg D, Makoroff K, Harper N, et al. Utility of hepatic transaminases to recognize abuse in children. Pediatrics 2009;124:509–16.
16. Hom J. The risk of intra-abdominal injuries in pediatric patients with stable blunt abdominal trauma and negative abdominal computed tomography. Acad Emerg Med 2010;17:469–75.
17. Nastanski F, Cohen A, Lush SP, et al. The role of oral contrast administration immediately prior to the computed tomographic evaluation of the blunt trauma victim. Injury 2001;32:545–9.
18. Brenner DJ, Hall EJ. Computed tomography–an increasing source of radiation exposure. N Engl J Med 2007;357:2277–84.

19. Brenner D, Elliston C, Hall E, et al. Estimated risks of radiation-induced fatal cancer from pediatric CT. AJR Am J Roentgenol, 2001;176:289–96.

20. Pearce MS, Salotti JA, Little MP, et al. Radiation exposure from CT scans in childhood and subsequent risk of leukaemia and brain tumours: A retrospective cohort study. Lancet 2012;380:499–505.

21. Image Gently. www.pedrad.org/associations/5364/1g.

22. Rice HE, Frush DP, Farmer D, et al. Review of radiation risks from computed tomography: Essentials for the pediatric surgeon. J Pediatr Surg 2007;42:603–7.

23. Brody AS, Frush DP, Huda W, et al. Radiation risk to children from computed tomography. Pediatrics 2007;120:677–82.

24. Benya EC, Lim-Dunham JE, Landrum O, et al. Abdominal sonography in examination of children with blunt abdominal trauma. AJR Am J Roentgenol 2000;174:613–1616.

25. Coley BD, Mutabagani KH, Martin LC, et al. Focused abdominal sonography for trauma (FAST) in children with blunt abdominal trauma. J Trauma 2000;48:902–6.

26. Emery KH, McAneney CM, Racadio JM, et al. Absent peritoneal fluid on screening trauma ultrasonography in children: A prospective comparison with computed tomography. J Pediatr Surg 2001;36:565–9.

27. Holmes JF, Gladman A, Chang CH. Performance of abdominal ultrasonography in pediatric blunt trauma patients: A meta-analysis. J Pediatr Surg 2007;42:1588–94.

28. Fox JC, Boysen M, Gharahbaghian L, et al. Test characteristics of focused assessment of sonography for trauma for clinically significant abdominal free fluid in pediatric blunt abdominal trauma. Acad Emerg Med 2011;18:477–82.

29. Cardamore R, Nemeth J, Meyers C. Bedside emergency department ultrasonography availability and use for blunt abdominal trauma in Canadian pediatric centres. CJEM 2012;14:14–19.

30. Noble VE, Blaivas M, Blankenship R, et al. Decision rule for imaging utilization in blunt abdominal trauma–where is ultrasound? Ann Emerg Med 2010;55:487–9.

31. Feliz A, Shultz B, McKenna C, et al. Diagnostic and therapeutic laparoscopy in pediatric abdominal trauma. J Pediatr Surg 2006;41:72–7.

32. Marwan A, Harmon CM, Georgeson KE, et al. Use of laparoscopy in the management of pediatric abdominal trauma. J Trauma 2010;69:761–4.

33. Gaines BA, Ford HR. Abdominal and pelvic trauma in children. Crit Care Med 2002;30:S416–423.

34. Tinkoff G, Esposito TJ, Reed J, et al. American Association for the Surgery of Trauma Organ Injury Scale I: spleen, liver, and kidney, validation based on the National Trauma Data Bank. J Am Coll Surg 2008;207:646–55.

35. Holmes JH 4th, Wiebe DJ, Tataria M, et al. The failure of non-operative management in pediatric solid organ injury: A multi-institutional experience. J Trauma 2005;59:1309–13.

36. Stylianos S. Evidence-based guidelines for resource utilization in children with isolated spleen or liver injury. The APSA Trauma Committee. J Pediatr Surg 2000;35:164–9.

37. Stylianos S. Compliance with evidence-based guidelines in children with isolated spleen or liver injury: A prospective study. J Pediatr Surg 2002;37:453–6.

38. St Peter SD, Sharp SW, Snyder CL, et al. Prospective validation of an abbreviated bedrest protocol in the management of blunt spleen and liver injury in children. J Pediatr Surg 2011;46:173–7.

39. Dehmer JJ, Adamson WT. Massive transfusion and blood product use in the pediatric trauma patient. Semin Pediatr Surg 2010;19:286–91.

40. Jacobs LM. Splenorrhaphy. In: Jacobs LM, editor. Advanced Trauma Operative Management. Woodbury, CT; 2004. p 78–83.

41. Morgan TL, Tomich EB. Overwhelming post-splenectomy infection (OPSI): A case report and review of the literature. J Emerg Med 2012;43:758–63.

42. Peitzman AB, Marsh JW. Advanced operative techniques in the management of complex liver injury. J Trauma Acute Care Surg 2012;73:765–70.

43. Saggi BH, Sugerman HJ, Ivatury RR, et al. Abdominal compartment syndrome. J Trauma 1998;45:597–609.

44. Ejike JC, Newcombe J, Baerg J, et al. Understanding of abdominal compartment syndrome among pediatric healthcare providers. Crit Care Res Pract 2010; Article ID 876013, 6 pages.

45. Vidal MG, Ruiz Weisser J, Gonzalez F, et al. Incidence and clinical effects of intra-abdominal hypertension in critically ill patients. Crit Care Med 2008;36:1823–31.

46. Beck R, Halberthal M, Zonis Z, et al. Abdominal compartment syndrome in children. Pediatr Crit Care Med 2001;2:51–6.

47. Diaz FJ, Fernandez Sein A, Gotay F. Identification and management of abdominal compartment syndrome in the pediatric intensive care unit. P R Health Sci J 2006;25:17–22.

48. Pearson EG, Rollins MD, Vogler SA, et al. Decompressive laparotomy for abdominal compartment syndrome in children: Before it is too late. J Pediatr Surg 2010;45:1324–9.

49. Cheatham ML, Malbrain ML, Kirkpatrick A, et al. Results from the International Conference of Experts on intra-abdominal hypertension and abdominal compartment syndrome. II. Recommendations. Intensive Care Med 2007;33:951–62.

50. Sugrue M, Bauman A, Jones F, et al. Clinical examination is an inaccurate predictor of intraabdominal pressure. World J Surg 2002;26:1428–31.

51. Carr JA. Abdominal compartment syndrome: A decade of progress. J Am Coll Surg 2013;216:135–46.

52. Gutierrez IM, Gollin G. Negative pressure wound therapy for children with an open abdomen. Langenbecks Arch Surg 2012;397:1353–7.

53. Suliburk JW, Ware DN, Balogh Z, et al. Vacuum-assisted wound closure achieves early fascial closure of open abdomens after severe trauma. J Trauma 2003;55:1155–61.

54. Nwomeh BC, Nadler EP, Meza MP, et al. Contrast extravasation predicts the need for operative intervention in children with blunt splenic trauma. J Trauma 2004;56:537–41.

55. Lutz N, Mahboubi S, Nance ML, et al. The significance of contrast blush on computed tomography in children with splenic injuries. J Pediatr Surg 2004;39:491–4.

56. Davies DA, Ein SH, Pearl R, et al. What is the significance of contrast 'blush' in pediatric blunt splenic trauma? J Pediatr Surg 2010;45:916–20.

57. Puapong D, Brown CV, Katz M, et al. Angiography and the pediatric trauma patient: A 10-year review. J Pediatr Surg 2006;41:1859–63.

58. Kiankhooy A, Sartorelli KH, Vane DW, et al. Angiographic embolization is safe and effective therapy for blunt abdominal solid organ injury in children. J Trauma 2010;68:526–31.

59. Graham GP, Haan JM. Splenic artery embolization in a 7-year-old with blunt traumatic splenic rupture. Am Surg 2012;78:E297–8.

60. Yi IK, Miao FL, Wong J, et al. Prophylactic embolization of hepatic artery pseudoaneurysm after blunt abdominal trauma in a child. J Pediatr Surg 2010;45:837–9.

61. Stylianos S, Hicks BA. Abdominal and Renal Trauma. Ashcraft's Pediatric Surgery. 5th ed. Elsevier Inc.; 2010. p. 190–208.

62. Giss SR, Dobrilovic N, Brown RL, et al. Complications of non-operative management of pediatric blunt hepatic injury: Diagnosis, management, and outcomes. J Trauma 2006;61:334–9.

63. Almaramhi H, Al-Qahtani AR. Traumatic pediatric bile duct injury: Nonoperative intervention as an alternative to surgical intervention. J Pediatr Surg 2006;41:943–5.

64. Ulitsky A, Werlin S, Dua KS. Role of ERCP in the management of non-iatrogenic traumatic bile duct injuries in the pediatric population. Gastrointest Endosc 2011;73:823–7.

65. Wood JH, Partrick DA, Bruny JL, et al. Operative vs nonoperative management of blunt pancreatic trauma in children. J Pediatr Surg 2010;45:401–6.

66. Herman R, Guire KE, Burd RS, et al. Utility of amylase and lipase as predictors of grade of injury or outcomes in pediatric patients with pancreatic trauma. J Pediatr Surg 2011;46:923–6.

67. Rutkoski JD, Segura BJ, Kane TD. Experience with totally laparoscopic distal pancreatectomy with splenic preservation for pediatric trauma–2 techniques. J Pediatr Surg 2011;46:588–93.

68. Iqbal CW, Levy SM, Tsao K, et al. Laparoscopic versus open distal pancreatectomy in the management of traumatic pancreatic disruption. J Laparoendosc Adv Surg Tech A 2012;22:595–8.

69. Borkon MJ, Morrow SE, Koehler EA, et al. Operative intervention for complete pancreatic transection in children sustaining

blunt abdominal trauma: Revisiting an organ salvage technique. Am Surg 2011;77:612–20.

70. Ramesh J, Bang JY, Trevino J, et al. Endoscopic ultrasound-guided drainage of pancreatic fluid collections in children. J Pediatr Gastroenterol Nutr 2012; Epub ahead of print.

71. de Blaauw I, Winkelhorst JT, Rieu PN, et al. Pancreatic injury in children: Good outcome of nonoperative treatment. J Pediatr Surg 2008;43:1640–3.

72. Paul MD, Mooney DP. The management of pancreatic injuries in children: Operate or observe. J Pediatr Surg 2011;46:1140–3.

73. Simpson J, Lobo DN, Shah AB, et al. Traumatic diaphragmatic rupture: Associated injuries and outcome. Ann R Coll Surg Engl 2000;82:97–100.

74. Koplewitz BZ, Ramos C, Manson DE, et al. Traumatic diaphragmatic injuries in infants and children: Imaging findings. Pediatr Radiol 2000;30:471–9.

75. Ramos CT, Koplewitz BZ, Babyn PS, et al. What have we learned about traumatic diaphragmatic hernias in children? J Pediatr Surg 2000;35:601–4.

76. Meyer G, Hüttl TP, Hatz RA, et al. Laparoscopic repair of traumatic diaphragmatic hernias. Surg Endosc 2000;14:1010–14.

77. Pitcher G. Fiber-endoscopic thoracoscopy for diaphragmatic injury in children. Semin Pediatr Surg 2001;10:17–19.

78. Shehata SM, Shabaan BS. Diaphragmatic injuries in children after blunt abdominal trauma. J Pediatr Surg 2006;41:1727–31.

79. Sharma OP, Oswanski MF, Kaminski BP, et al. Clinical implications of the seat belt sign in blunt trauma. Am Surg 2009;75: 822–7.

80. Chandler CF, Lane JS, Waxman KS. Seatbelt sign following blunt trauma is associated with increased incidence of abdominal injury. Am Surg 1997;63:885–8.

81. Nance ML, Lutz N, Arbogast KB, et al. Optimal restraint reduces the risk of abdominal injury in children involved in motor vehicle crashes. Ann Surg 2004;239:127–31.

82. Ciftci AO, Tanyel FC, Salman AB, et al. Gastrointestinal tract perforation due to blunt abdominal trauma. Pediatr Surg Int 1998;13:259–64.

83. Moss RL, Musemeche CA. Clinical judgment is superior to diagnostic tests in the management of pediatric small bowel injury. J Pediatr Surg 1996;31:1178–82.

84. Jerby BL, Attorri RJ, Morton D Jr. Blunt intestinal injury in children: The role of the physical examination. J Pediatr Surg 1997;32:580–4.

85. Letton RW, Worrell V, APSA Committee on Trauma Blunt Intestinal Injury Study Group. Delay in diagnosis and treatment of blunt intestinal injury does not adversely affect prognosis in the pediatric trauma patient. J Pediatr Surg 2010;45:161–6.

86. Gaines BA, Rutkoski JD. The role of laparoscopy in pediatric trauma. Semin Pediatr Surg 2010;19:300–3.

87. Garg N, St Peter SD, Tsao K, et al. Minimally invasive management of thoracoabdominal penetrating trauma in a child. J Trauma 2006;61:211–12.

88. Tejerina Alvarez EE, Holanda MS, López-Espadas F, et al. Gastric rupture from blunt abdominal trauma. Injury 2004;35:228–31.

89. Begossi G, Danielson PD, Hirsh MP. Transection of the stomach after blunt injury in the pediatric population. J Pediatr Surg 2007;42:1604–7.

90. Asensio JA, Feliciano DV, Britt LD, et al. Management of duodenal injuries. Curr Probl Surg 1993;30:1023–93.

91. Ladd AP, West KW, Rouse TM, et al. Surgical management of duodenal injuries in children. Surgery 2002;132:748–53.

92. Gaines BA, Shultz BS, Morrison K, et al. Duodenal injuries in children: Beware of child abuse. J Pediatr Surg 2004;39:600–2.

93. Vaughan GD 3rd, Frazier OH, Graham DY, et al. The use of pyloric exclusion in the management of severe duodenal injuries. Am J Surg 1977;134:785–90.

94. Moore EE, Cogbill TH, Malangoni MA, et al. Organ injury scaling, II: Pancreas, duodenum, small bowel, colon, and rectum. J Trauma 1990;30:1427–9.

95. Shilyansky J, Pearl RH, Kreller M, et al. Diagnosis and management of duodenal injuries in children. J Pediatr Surg 1997;32: 880–6.

96. Fang JF, Chen RJ, Lin BC. Surgical treatment and outcome after delayed diagnosis of blunt duodenal injury. Eur J Surg 1999;165: 133–9.

97. Cone JB, Eidt JF. Delayed diagnosis of duodenal rupture. Am J Surg 1994;168:676–9.

98. Cogbill TH, Moore EE, Feliciano DV, et al. Conservative management of duodenal trauma: A multicenter perspective. J Trauma 1990;30:1469–75.

99. Clendenon JN, Meyers RL, Nance ML, et al. Management of duodenal injuries in children. J Pediatr Surg 2004;39:964–8.

100. Pokorny WJ, Brandt ML, Harberg FJ. Major duodenal injuries in children: Diagnosis, operative management, and outcome. J Pediatr Surg 1986;21:613–16.

101. Dokucu A, Oztürk H, Yağmur Y, et al. Colon injuries in children. J Pediatr Surg 2000;35:1799–804.

102. Nelson R, Singer M. Primary repair for penetrating colon injuries. Cochrane Database Syst Rev 2003:CD002247.

103. Weinberg JA, Griffin RL, Vandromme MJ, et al. Management of colon wounds in the setting of damage control laparotomy: A cautionary tale. J Trauma 2009;67:929–35.

104. Ordoñez CA, Pino LF, Badiel M, et al. Safety of performing a delayed anastomosis during damage control laparotomy in patients with destructive colon injuries. J Trauma 2011;71:1512–18.

105. Kadish HA, Schunk JE, Britton H. Pediatric male rectal and genital trauma: Accidental and nonaccidental injuries. Pediatr Emerg Care 1998;14:95–8.

106. Bonnard A, Zamakhshary M, Wales PW. Outcomes and management of rectal injuries in children. Pediatr Surg Int 2007;23: 1071–6.

107. Rubin LE, Stein PB, DiScala C, et al. Pediatric trauma caused by personal watercraft: A ten-year retrospective. J Pediatr Surg 2003;38:1525–9.

108. Kapur SS, Frei LW. Colorectal and vaginal injuries in personal watercraft passengers. J Trauma 2007;63:1161–4.

109. Gill RS, Mangat H, Al-Adra DP, et al. Hydrostatic rectosigmoid perforation: A rare personal watercraft injury. J Pediatr Surg 2011;46:402–4.

110. Esposito TJ, Ingraham A, Luchette FA, et al. Reasons to omit digital rectal exam in trauma patients: No fingers, no rectum, no useful additional information. J Trauma 2005;59:1314–19.

111. Leaphart CL, Danko M, Cassidy L, et al. An analysis of proctoscopy vs computed tomography scanning in the diagnosis of rectal injuries in children: Which is better? J Pediatr Surg 2006;41: 700–3.

112. Reinberg O, Yazbeck S. Major perineal trauma in children. J Pediatr Surg 1989;24:982–4.

113. Tuggle D, Huber PJ Jr. Management of rectal trauma. Am J Surg 1984;148:806–8.

114. Sharma O. Blunt gallbladder injuries: Presentation of twenty-two cases with review of the literature. J Trauma 1995;39: 576–80.

115. Jaggard MK, Johal NS, Choudhry M. Blunt abdominal trauma resulting in gallbladder injury: A review with emphasis on pediatrics. J Trauma 2011;70:1005–10.

116. McAleer IM, Kaplan GW, Scherz HC, et al. Genitourinary trauma in the pediatric patient. Urology 1993;42:563–8.

117. Deibert CM, Spencer BA. The association between operative repair of bladder injury and improved survival: Results from the National Trauma Data Bank. J Urol 2011;186:151–5.

118. Moore EE, Cogbill TH, Jurkovich GJ, et al. Organ injury scaling. III: Chest wall, abdominal vascular, ureter, bladder, and urethra. J Trauma 1992;33:337–9.

119. Kluemper C, Rogers A, Fallat M, et al. Genitourinary injuries in pediatric all-terrain vehicle trauma–a mechanistic relationship? Urology 2010;75:1162–4.

120. Gomez RG, Ceballos L, Coburn M, et al. Consensus statement on bladder injuries. BJU Int, 2004;94:27–32.

121. Peclet MH, Newman KD, Eichelberger MR, et al. Patterns of injury in children. J Pediatr Surg 1990;25:85–91.

122. Brown SL, Elder JS, Spirnak JP. Are pediatric patients more susceptible to major renal injury from blunt trauma? A comparative study. J Urol 1998;160:138–40.

123. Wu HY, Gaines BA. Dirt bikes and all-terrain vehicles: The real threat to pediatric kidneys. J Urol 2007;178:1672–4.

124. McAleer IM, Kaplan GW. Pediatric genitourinary trauma. Urol Clin North Am 1995;22:177–88.

125. Moore EE, Shackford SR, Pachter HL, et al. Organ injury scaling: spleen, liver, and kidney. J Trauma 1989;29:1664–6.

126. Santucci RA, Fisher MB. The literature increasingly supports expectant (conservative) management of renal trauma–a systematic review. J Trauma 2005;59:493–503.

127. Umbreit EC, Routh JC, Husmann DA. Nonoperative management of nonvascular grade IV blunt renal trauma in children: Meta-analysis and systematic review. Urology 2009;74:579–82.

128. Wessel LM, Scholz S, Jester I, et al. Management of kidney injuries in children with blunt abdominal trauma. J Pediatr Surg 2000;35:1326–30.

129. Russell RS, Gomelsky A, McMahon DR, et al. Management of grade IV renal injury in children. J Urol 2001;166:1049–50.

130. Philpott JM, Nance ML, Carr MC, et al. Ureteral stenting in the management of urinoma after severe blunt renal trauma in children. J Pediatr Surg 2003;38:1096–8.

131. Goffette PP, Laterre PF. Traumatic injuries: Imaging and intervention in post-traumatic complications (delayed intervention). Eur Radiol 2002;12:994–1021.

132. Nerli RB, Metgud T, Patil S, et al. Severe renal injuries in children following blunt abdominal trauma: Selective management and outcome. Pediatr Surg Int 2011;27:1213–16.

133. Broghammer JA, Fisher MB, Santucci RA. Conservative management of renal trauma: A review. Urology 2007;70:623–9.

134. Aguayo P, Fraser JD, Sharp S, et al. Nonoperative management of blunt renal injury: A need for further study. J Pediatr Surg 2010;45:1311–14.

135. Navsaria PH, Nicol AJ. Selective nonoperative management of kidney gunshot injuries. World J Surg 2009;33:553–7.

136. Wessells H, McAninch JW, Meyer A, et al. Criteria for nonoperative treatment of significant penetrating renal lacerations. J Urol 1997;157:24–7.

137. Rice SG. Medical conditions affecting sports participation. Pediatrics 2008;121:841–8.

138. Grinsell MM, Showalter S, Gordon KA, et al. Single kidney and sports participation: Perception versus reality. Pediatrics 2006;118:1019–27.

139. Grinsell MM, Butz K, Gurka MJ, et al. Sport-related kidney injury among high school athletes. Pediatrics 2012;130:e40–5.

140. Psooy K. Sports and the solitary kidney: How to counsel parents. Can J Urol 2006;13:3120–6.

141. Johnson B, Christensen C, Dirusso S, et al. A need for reevaluation of sports participation recommendations for children with a solitary kidney. J Urol 2005;174:686–9.

CHAPTER 17

HEAD INJURY AND FACIAL TRAUMA

Kelly S. Tieves • Jeffrey Goldstein

HEAD INJURY

Traumatic brain injury (TBI) is an important cause of injury-related death and disability in children.[1] In the USA, there are an estimated 1.7 million people with TBI annually, with a reported 52,000 deaths and 275,000 hospitalizations. Children ages 0 to 4 years and 15 to 19 years are most likely to suffer TBI. Nearly half a million emergency department visits annually are for children less than 14 years with TBI. Males, age 0 to 4 years, have the highest rates of TBI-related emergency department visits, hospitalizations, and deaths combined.[2]

Head trauma from child abuse remains a significant concern. In children younger than age 1 year, nonaccidental trauma (NAT) is the most common cause of fatal TBI.[3,4] Head trauma associated with NAT has a higher rate of subdural hematomas, subarachnoid hemorrhages, and retinal hemorrhages when compared with nonabusive head trauma. Public health campaigns have brought attention to the dangers of shaking a young child and have provided resources for parents and caretakers who may be at risk of harming a child.[5]

Although the reasons are not entirely clear, there has been a general trend in improved outcomes after severe TBI in children.[6] The decline in morbidity and mortality are likely due to improved prehospital care, regionalization of pediatric trauma care, adherence to evidence-based practice guidelines, more aggressive care (such as intracranial pressure [ICP] monitoring and early surgical evacuation of mass lesions), improved diagnostic imaging (computed tomography [CT], magnetic resonance imaging [MRI]), and advances in intensive care. In January 2012, the second edition of evidence-based practice guidelines was published for the acute medical management of severe TBI in infants, children, and adolescents.[7] These guidelines have allowed a decrease in variability in care across centers, but there is a striking lack of data from well-designed, randomized controlled trials.

Brain Injury Mechanisms

Nonpenetrating Cranial Trauma

Head injuries can be classified by their pathologic or morphologic descriptions. Blunt or nonpenetrating trauma occurs as the result of a direct impact on the brain and calvaria. These injuries often occur after a motor vehicle collision or fall, and account for the vast majority of TBI in the USA. This type of injury typically results in focal damage to the underlying brain (coup). In some instances, contrecoup damage occurs from the rebound movement of the viscoelastic brain within its rigid encasement. The predominant contrecoup damage occurs on the side opposite the impact. This is commonly seen with subdural hemorrhages with associated cortical contusion when the brain rebounds off the skull, causing disruption of delicate surface vessels. The inner surface of the skull at its base is irregular, ridged, and restrictive at its anterior margins. As a result, the anterior and inferior portions of the temporal and frontal lobes are often injured by abrupt brain acceleration or deceleration in the sagittal plane.

Penetrating Trauma

Penetrating injury, caused by bladed weapons and projectiles, such as handguns and rifles, cause cerebral lacerations with deleterious effects on the underlying neurons, their functional interconnections, and the cerebral vasculature at the surface of the brain. Penetrating injuries also carry a risk of increased infection, especially if foreign material is introduced into the brain.

Axonal Shearing

Axonal injury or shearing occurs as the result of changes in the angular momentum of the head. Axonal injury or shear injury is often coupled with vascular injury. Axonal shearing may occur between white matter bundles and deeper subcortical neuronal structures such as the basal ganglia and thalamus, and within the upper brain stem where the cerebrum rotates on its axis. This shearing injury, coupled with vascular injury, is classically observed as petechial hemorrhages in white matter and commonly referred to as diffuse axonal injury (DAI). The neurologic impact due to axonal shearing can present as a transient loss of consciousness or as profound and persistent neurologic deficits, even leading to death.

Concussion

The term concussion is often used to describe the constellation of symptoms that occur after mild to moderate TBI when no hematoma or other intracranial pathologic process is identified. Classic symptoms include headache, nausea, vomiting, difficulty concentrating, retrograde and/or anterograde amnesia, and personality changes. These findings are the result of neuronal dysfunction and axonal injury that can occur even after a mild TBI. Complete recovery after concussion injury is common. However, long-term consequences include impaired attention, memory, and slowed processing speed.

Pathophysiology

The intracranial contents include the brain parenchymal tissue, cerebrospinal fluid (CSF), and blood. The brain parenchyma accounts for approximately 80% of the intracranial contents, with the remainder being evenly distributed between CSF and blood. The majority of the CSF is in the subarachnoid spaces, and the remainder is in the ventricles, with the postcapillary circulation containing most of the intracranial blood.

The immature brain has some structural differences from its adult counterpart that may explain the different responses to injury often seen in children after TBI. The brain doubles in size in the first 6 months of life and reaches approximately 80% of adult size by age 2. The developing brain has a higher water content and incomplete neuronal synapse formation and arborization. In addition, incomplete myelinization and neurochemical changes result in neuronal plasticity after birth. The subarachnoid space is generally smaller and offers less protection than the mature brain, owing to less buoyancy, and thereby provides less protection to the brain parenchyma during changes in head momentum. The result is a higher incidence of diffuse cerebral edema and parenchymal injuries in children. In children with distensible skulls, some argue that the open fontanelle allows for expansion of the intracranial contents and therefore affords increased protection from elevation of ICP. However, studies have indicated that the smaller neural axis of infants and young children results in a less compliant pressure–volume relationship with an increased risk of intracranial hypertension.[8,9]

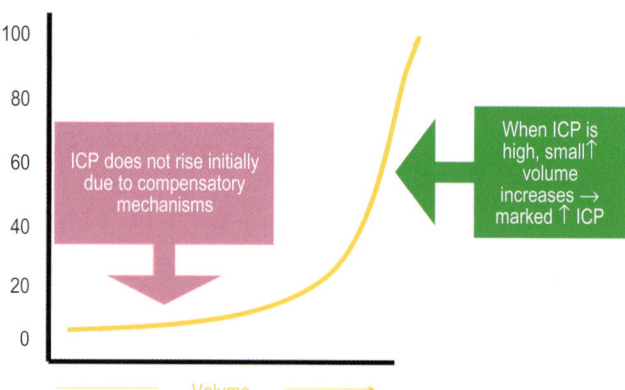

FIGURE 17-2 ■ Intracranial pressure (ICP)–volume relationship. Small increases in brain volume do not lead to immediate increase in ICP because of the ability of the cerebrospinal fluid to be displaced into the spinal canal as well as the ability the falx cerebri to stretch slightly between the hemispheres and the tentorium between the hemispheres and the cerebellum. However, once the ICP has reached around 25 mmHg, small increases in brain volume can lead to marked elevations in ICP.

The Monro–Kellie doctrine is an important concept relating to the understanding of ICP dynamics (Fig. 17-1). The Monro–Kellie doctrine uses a simple hydraulic approach to the cerebral circulation. Given that the cranium is a rigid, nonexpansile container, it states that the total volume of the intracranial contents must remain constant and any increase in the volume of one component must be at the expense of the others, assuming the intracranial volume remains constant. Thus, very early after injury, a mass such as an expanding hematoma may be enlarging while the ICP remains normal. Once the limit of displacement of CSF and intravascular blood has been reached, ICP rapidly increases (Fig. 17-2). Further work has shown that the relationship between ICP and cerebral blood flow (CBF) is much more complex and variable. Whereas simultaneous measurement of ICP and CBF would be most helpful in optimizing therapeutic strategies, the Monro–Kellie doctrine provides a reasonable basic explanation of intracranial dynamics.

CBF is defined as the velocity of blood through the cerebral circulation. In adults, the normal CBF is 50–55 mL/100g of brain tissue/minute. In children, CBF may be much higher depending on their age. At 1 year of age, it approximates adult levels, but at 5 years of age, normal CBF is approximately 90 mL/100 g/min and then gradually declines to adult levels by the mid-late teens. Brain injury severe enough to cause coma can result in a 50% reduction in CBF during the first 6 to 12 hours after injury.[10,11] It usually increases over the next 2 to 3 days, but for those patients who remain comatose, CBF remains below normal for days or weeks after injury. There is increasing evidence that such low levels of CBF are inadequate to meet the metabolic demands of the brain early after injury and that regional, if not global, cerebral ischemia results.[12–14]

Cerebral perfusion pressure (CPP) is the differential pressure of arterial flow into and venous flow out of the brain. CPP may be defined by the difference between mean arterial pressure (MAP) and ICP. CPP is

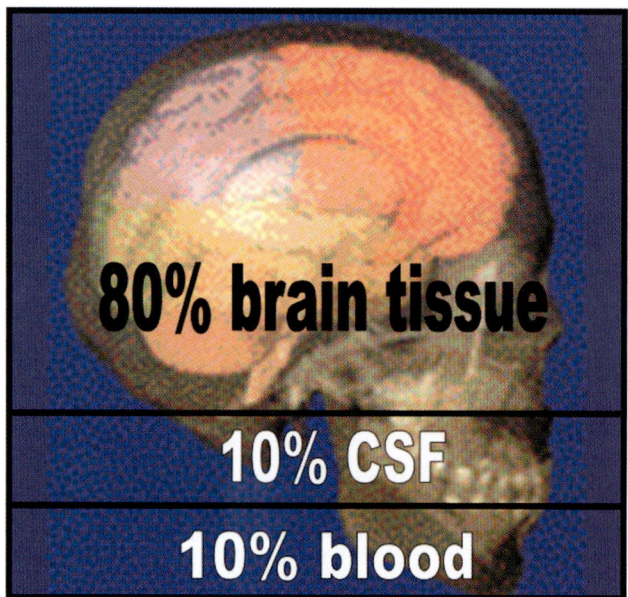

FIGURE 17-1 ■ Monro–Kellie doctrine. The Monro–Kellie doctrine states that the cranial compartment is incompressible and that the volume inside the cranium is a fixed volume. The cranium and its constituents (blood, cerebrospinal fluid [CSF], and brain tissue) create a state of volume equilibrium such that any increase in volume of one of the cranial constituents must be compensated by a decrease in volume of another.

considered the transmural pressure gradient that is ultimately the driving force required for supplying cerebral metabolic needs. As ICP increases following head injury, CPP decreases and blood flow to the brain eventually declines. At a CPP of 10 mmHg, blood vessels collapse and blood flow ceases.

Current techniques available to measure CBF, such as transcranial Doppler and Xenon-enhanced CT imaging, are still considered experimental in the management of severe TBI. Because CPP is easily determined by ICP monitoring, it has become a critical parameter for defining treatment options. Studies have shown a good correlation between CPP and CBF in patients with intact cerebral autoregulation.[13] However, cerebral autoregulation is often disrupted after severe TBI and measures of cerebral vascular resistance may be more useful in guiding therapy.[15,16]

Cerebral autoregulation refers to a homeostatic process that allows CBF to remain constant over a wide range of MAPs. Arterial vessels can dilate or constrict in response to various physiologic changes, including ICP and systemic arterial pressure, to maintain normal flow and normal brain metabolism. In healthy adult patients, CBF remains constant with a MAP between 60–160 mmHg, or a CPP between 50–150 mmHg.[17] Normally, with elevated systemic blood pressure, reflexive vasoconstriction will occur to prevent intracranial hypertension. In contrast, a moderate decrease in systemic blood pressure will paradoxically result in increased ICP because compensatory reflex vasodilatation will occur. When perfusion pressure falls below 50 mmHg, cerebral ischemia develops and compensatory cerebral arteriole vasodilatation is exhausted. When perfusion pressure exceeds 150 mmHg, cerebral arteriolar impedance is overcome, the affected vessels passively dilate, and fluid is forced through a damaged endothelium into the brain, causing diffuse vasogenic edema. Impaired cerebral autoregulation after TBI and age-related changes in CBF make the immature brain susceptible to secondary injury, both from diminished and excess CBF, and are both associated with a poor neurologic outcome.[18]

Historically, treatment protocols were principally directed toward reducing ICP. Hyperventilation and fluid restriction were important components in these older protocols. Sustained elevations in ICP above 20 mmHg are poorly tolerated by the injured brain and have been associated with poor neurologic outcome and increased mortality in pediatric patients.[19] Sustained elevation in ICP may result in cerebral ischemia if cerebral perfusion is impaired, and ultimately may result in cerebral herniation. Current treatment strategies seek to optimize CPP while reducing ICP, with little reliance on hyperventilation or fluid restriction. CPP is likely an age-related continuum, thus making it problematic to develop treatment protocols based on a single number for all age groups. To date, no study has demonstrated that active maintenance of CPP above any target threshold in infants and children following TBI improves mortality or morbidity. However, there seems to be a threshold of less than 40 mmHg that is associated with increased mortality; therefore, most treatment guidelines recommend a minimum CPP of 40 mmHg.

Primary Brain Injury

Primary brain injury occurs as a result of direct injury to the brain parenchyma due to shear forces at the time of impact. Both cortical disruption and axonal injury can occur, resulting in a cascade of events contributing to secondary brain injury, which will be discussed later. Cortical disruption, if occurring within minutes to hours, is not likely to be amenable to resuscitation.

Skull fractures occur commonly with head injury and are readily diagnosed with CT. In children, a skull fracture should prompt an evaluation of the underlying brain parenchyma given the significant impact it takes to injure the skull. Fractures of the skull vault can occur in either a linear or a stellate fashion. Fractures involving the skull base are typically associated with a greater force than simple cranial vault fractures. The classic signs of basilar skull fractures include Battle's sign (ecchymoses over the mastoid process associated with an ipsilateral skull fracture), raccoon eyes and CSF rhinorrhea (associated with a cribriform plate fracture), and otorrhea (associated with fracture of the mastoid air cells or temporal bone fracture). Meningitis associated with a basilar skull fracture occurs in up to 10% of patients.[20] Despite the risk of infection, the routine use of prophylactic antibiotics is not recommended as they have not been shown to prevent meningitis from occurring, and tend to select out for resistant organisms.[21–23] Vaccination against *Streptococcus pneumoniae* should be considered for all patients with a basilar skull fracture and CSF leak due to the increased risk of pneumococcal-associated meningitis.[24]

Post-traumatic intracranial hemorrhage includes epidural hematomas, subdural hematomas, and subarachnoid hemorrhages. Epidural hematomas usually occur in the middle fossa and are often associated with an injury to the middle meningeal artery, although they can occur in the anterior or posterior fossa. The classic CT description is a lenticular hematoma, bound by suture lines, because of the tightly bound dura (Fig. 17-3). Clot formation under the calvaria compresses the dura and can cause rapid neurologic deterioration as the brain becomes

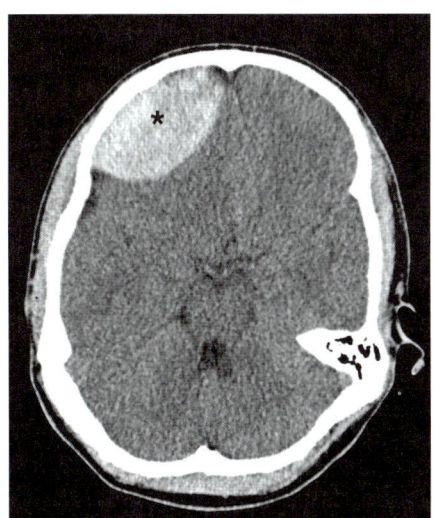

FIGURE 17-3 ■ CT scan shows an epidural hematoma (asterisk) in a 14-year-old patient. (Courtesy of Dr Lisa Lowe.)

further displaced. Skull fractures overlying the epidural hematoma are common. The classic presentation of a patient with a lucid interval followed by clinical deterioration is rare in children. Only after the hematoma enlarges is clinical evidence of elevated ICP noted. Typical symptoms include headache, lethargy, emesis, irritability, confusion, and decreased level of consciousness. Progressive deterioration results in seizures, changes in vital signs with hypertension and respiratory instability, pupillary changes, posturing, and cardiovascular compromise. Prompt neurosurgical evacuation is imperative for patient survival and good outcome. Evacuation of extremely large clots (>40 mL) in children often results in very good long-term results, provided that operative intervention is timely.

Subdural hemorrhages are classified as acute (<3 days old), subacute (3-10 days old), and chronic (>10 days old). Acute and subacute subdural hemorrhages are not infrequent in infants, and often the result of birth injury or NAT (Fig. 17-4). They usually result from lacerated bridging veins, or from associated contusions hemorrhaging into the subdural space. The superficial cortical veins in small children lack any reinforcement from arachnoidal trabeculae and are susceptible to inertial loading. Subdural hematomas tend to follow the convexities of the brain and cover the entire hemisphere. The cranial CT demonstrates hyperdense crescent-shaped blood collections at the surface of the brain, often associated with mass effect and cortical edema. Occasionally, and particularly when anemia is present, the CT findings of an acute subdural hematoma may have an isodense appearance that belies the actual hemorrhagic character later found at the time of operation.

Acute subdural hemorrhages are usually associated with a worse prognosis than patients with an epidural hematoma, primarily related to the underlying brain damage. Operation is indicated when neurologic deterioration occurs as a result of the combined effect of the subdural hemorrhage and parenchymal injury, either from the compressive effect of the subdural blood or

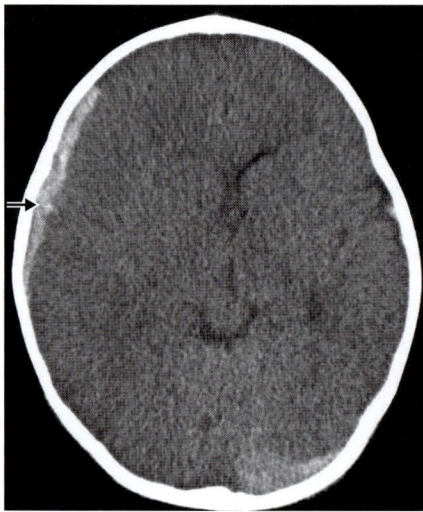

FIGURE 17-4 ■ Hyperacute subdural bleeding (arrow) is seen on this cranial CT scan of a 9-month-old patient. (Courtesy of Dr Lisa Lowe.)

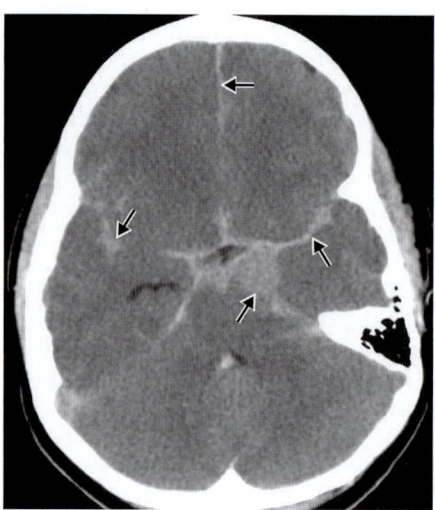

FIGURE 17-5 ■ Subarachnoid hemorrhage (arrows) is present on this cranial CT scan of a 10-year-old patient. (Courtesy of Dr Lisa Lowe.)

from the combined effect of impact forces on the entire cerebrum and diffuse bleeding. In infants, it is possible to tap the subdural space at the level of the fontanelle and produce rapid decompression. Large subdural hematomas with significant mass effect require more extensive craniotomies.

Subacute subdural hematomas in the context of trauma are much less frequent in the pediatric population. However, they will be seen in emergency settings when they are a cause of neurologic problems, and when they are considered a manifestation of previous or recurrent NAT. As with acute hematomas, subacute subdural hematomas will have a nonspecific presentation. Affected children have both the symptoms of increased ICP (coma, irritability, lethargy, emesis, seizures) and the signs of elevated ICP (frontal bossing, enlarged heads, dilated scalp veins, sun-setting eyes, papilledema, and bulging fontanelles). The CT scan often shows isodense or hypodense fluid collections at the cerebral convexities. MRI studies are helpful for making the diagnosis of these bleeding events. As with acute subdural hematomas, operative evacuation is often necessary.

Chronic subdural hematomas can cause symptomatic elevation of the ICP and may require interventions to manage cranial growth and CSF pressure. Patients present with symptoms similar to those of a subacute subdural hematoma. Management options include serial percutaneous drainage, limited craniotomies to drain and irrigate the subdural space, and subdural/peritoneal shunts.

Subarachnoid hemorrhage (SAH) in acutely traumatized children is common and is rarely the result of aneurysmal bleeding (Fig. 17-5). Subarachnoid bleeding occurs from disruption of the fragile pia-arachnoidal vasculature. This often occurs over the convexities of the brain affected by coup type injuries or the frontotemporal poles affected by contrecoup injuries. Traumatic SAH can also occur in the interhemispheric fissure and in the basilar cisterns. When SAH is an isolated finding following minor trauma, no specific therapy is indicated except symptomatic amelioration of chemical meningitis, meningismus, and photophobia. SAH can result in hydrocephalus and may require ventricular shunting to relieve the increased ICP. In patients with severe TBI, SAH is associated with a poor outcome and may also be associated with cerebral vasospasm. Transcranial Doppler imaging can be utilized to identify vasospasm. Therapy for vasospasm in adults include calcium channel blockers and neurointerventional techniques; however, these are not well studied in children and not commonly used.[25,26]

Secondary Brain Injury

The cornerstone of TBI management is the prevention of secondary injuries. Secondary brain injury includes both the evolution of damage within the brain related to a cascade of macroscopic and microscopic events, and the effects of secondary insults, including hypoxia and hypotension. Endogenous secondary brain injury involves the macroscopic cascade of edema, ischemia, necrosis, elevated ICP, and inadequate CPP.

Brain swelling traditionally has been described as either vasogenic or cytotoxic. The time course of brain edema is variable. It is thought, however, that vasogenic edema occurs early after injury and cytotoxic edema occurs in a more delayed fashion. Vasogenic swelling results from the disruption of the blood–brain barrier. The blood–brain barrier is maintained by tight junctions between endothelial cells that line the vessels of the brain. Injury to these cells allows extravasation of fluid and proteins into the interstitial space of the brain parenchyma. Disruption of these cells can occur from the primary injury or from free radical formation, cytokines, and other secondary mechanisms of brain injury. Cytotoxic edema is edema of the cells themselves, resulting from a failure of cellular ion homeostasis and membrane function.

Edema of the brain is an important marker for injury and is also a cause of secondary injury. In early (<24 hours) fatal closed-head injuries in children, CT scans often demonstrate little or no significant parenchymal bleeding. However, in children, rapid development of edema is commonly seen on serial CT scans and the diffuse brain swelling causes the obliteration of the ventricles and loss of the basilar cisterns and subarachnoid space. As swelling progresses and the compensatory mechanisms of the brain are exhausted, ICP increases markedly with small changes in intracranial volume (see Fig. 17-2). Cerebral edema typically develops early after injury, peaking at 72 to 96 hours, and then gradually resolves over the next week in survivors.[27]

Studies in adults utilizing xenon CT have shown a reduction in CBF early after severe TBI.[10,12] This hypoperfusion may be further exacerbated by hypotension and hypoxia. It is clear that this early hypoperfusion or ischemia after severe TBI is associated with a poor outcome.[28,29] Proposed mediators involved in early posttraumatic ischemia include direct vascular disruption, production of endothelin-1 (a potent vasoconstrictor), loss of endogenous vasodilators (endogenous nitric oxide synthase), and likely many other complex, interrelated, cellular and metabolic events.

The release of excitatory amino acids, such as glutamate, results in neuronal injury after TBI. Glutamate is the most abundant neurotransmitter in the brain. However, toxic levels cause neuronal cell death.[30,31] After TBI, glutamate and other excitatory amino acids are released, resulting in neuronal swelling, calcium influx, and release of cytotoxic enzymes leading to cell death. Studies have failed to demonstrate efficacy of anti-excitotoxic therapies, perhaps owing to their application in all patients with TBI rather than those with excitotoxicity, and because treatment may have been initiated too late.[32]

Oxidative stress with free radical formation is an important mechanism leading to secondary injury. Free radicals damage endothelial cells and injure the brain parenchyma. This results in disruption of the blood-brain barrier and resultant vasogenic and cytotoxic edema. Free radical scavengers, such as vitamin E, ascorbic acid, and superoxide dismutase, attempt to minimize injury by binding with the free radicals. However, these mechanisms often become overwhelmed and the process becomes self-perpetuating. Clinical studies are ongoing to identify pharmacologic free radical scavenging agents.

Apoptosis requires a cascade of intracellular events for completion of cell death and is thus termed programmed cell death. Calcium influx into the cell, oxidative stress, and energy depletion all appear to be important intracellular triggers of apoptosis. As our understanding of the complex biochemical, cellular, and molecular responses to TBI progresses, application of therapeutic strategies and agents may help halt the secondary injury processes.

Initial Evaluation and Management of Head Injury

The key principles of management after TBI rest on the foundation of the Monro–Kellie doctrine and the avoidance of secondary brain injury. Interventions that decrease CSF and hyperemia, while ensuring adequate oxygenation and blood flow, form the basis for all management strategies discussed here.

As with any trauma, the initial management and resuscitation begins with an assessment of circulation, airway and breathing (CAB). Ensuring adequate oxygenation and ventilation and promptly addressing sources of ongoing blood loss serve as the basic principles in the management of persons suspected or confirmed to have head injury. Hypotension and hypoxia in the field are proven secondary insults that are associated with poor outcomes, with hypotension being considerably more detrimental than hypoxia.[28,33] There has been no documented advantage to endotracheal intubation over effective bag-valve-mask ventilation in the field.[34,35] Providers inexperienced in pediatric airway management should defer endotracheal intubation. Efforts should be made to control bleeding, including scalp lacerations, which may be a source of shock in the child. The administration of isotonic crystalloid solution should be utilized to promptly restore the intravascular volume. Colloid solutions should be avoided. The withholding of fluid because of concerns of concomitant head injury is unjustified and may contribute to secondary brain injury with ineffective CBF. Although young children are prone to hypoglycemia, hypoglycemia occurring early after trauma is rare. Hyperglycemia may be detrimental during periods of cellular hypoxia owing to a shift to anaerobic metabolism and lactate production. Therefore, unless there is documented hypoglycemia, dextrose-containing fluids should be avoided in the early phases of resuscitation.

Current recommendations do not support ICP-directed measures in the field with the possible exception of hyperventilation and hyperosmolar therapy for signs of herniation.[7,36] Every effort should be made to transport the patient to a pediatric trauma center, or to an adult center equipped to manage pediatric trauma patients. Careful attention should be paid to cervical spine immobilization as there is an increased risk of spinal cord injury with TBI.

On arrival in the emergency department (ED), the Advanced Trauma Life Support (ATLS) protocol of the American College of Surgeons should be followed.[37] Early hospital evaluation and management is the same as that described for the prehospital setting. Endotracheal intubation should be performed in the initial hospital management, if needed. After initial stabilization and fluid resuscitation, a brief neurologic examination should be performed, preferably before the administration of sedation and neuromuscular blockade. Adjunctive diagnostic studies should be performed only after the initial resuscitation phase.

The severity of brain injury is often classified using the modified Glasgow Coma Scale (GCS) score.[38] Even with modifications, the GCS score has limitations in its use for infants and very young children (Table 17-1). In addition, the use of sedation and pharmacologic paralysis, orbital swelling impairing eye opening, endotracheal intubation making verbal responses impossible, and pre-existing conditions such as alterations in motor function further limit the use of the GCS score. Nonetheless, it is the best tool currently available to classify TBI and to share information between treating physicians.

Mild TBI: GCS 14–15

Approximately 80% of patients presenting to the ED with brain injury are categorized as having a mild brain injury. These patients may have a brief loss of consciousness and be amnestic to the events surrounding the injury. Most patients with mild TBI recover fully. However, a small percentage of patients will experience deterioration, resulting in severe neurologic dysfunction unless prompt recognition and resuscitation is performed. Adjunctive diagnostic studies should be performed as needed. Although less common in younger children, alcohol or other intoxicants can confuse the findings and make examination results unreliable. Neuroimaging is essential in the evaluation of all patients except the completely asymptomatic and neurologically normal patient. Unenhanced, or noncontrast, CT is the initial and most reliable diagnostic tool, particularly for identifying bleeding.

Patients who are asymptomatic (fully awake and alert, and neurologically normal) may be observed for several

TABLE 17-1	Modified Glasgow Coma Scale for Infants and Children	
Child	**Infant**	**Score**
Eye Opening		
Spontaneous	Spontaneous	4
To verbal stimuli	To verbal stimuli	3
To pain only	To pain only	2
No response	No response	1
Verbal Response		
Oriented, appropriate	Coos and babbles	5
Confused	Irritable cries	4
Inappropriate words	Cries to pain	3
Incomprehensible words or nonspecific sounds	Moans to pain	2
No response	No response	1
Motor Response		
Obeys commands	Moves spontaneously and purposefully	6
Localizes painful stimulus	Withdraws to touch	5
Withdraws in response to pain	Withdraws in response to pain	4
Flexion in response to pain	Decorticate posturing (abnormal flexion) in response to pain	3
Extension in response to pain	Decerebrate posturing (abnormal extension) in response to pain	2
No response	No response	1

hours and safely discharged. It is imperative that they be discharged with a reliable caretaker who understands the signs and symptoms that should prompt emergent re-evaluation. When appropriate, a follow-up visit should be scheduled with a provider who is knowledgeable with the current recommendations and treatment of post-concussive symptoms and sequelae. Admission to the hospital should be considered for patients with penetrating injuries, a history of loss of consciousness or a deteriorating level of consciousness, moderate to severe headache, intoxication, skull fracture, or lack of availability of CT. Additionally, all patients with a CSF leak or other significant associated injuries should be admitted for care.

Moderate TBI: GCS 9–13

Approximately 10% of patients presenting with TBI will fall into the moderate category. They should undergo the same initial examination as those presenting with mild TBI, but additionally will need laboratory studies and a noncontrasted CT of the head. All patients should be admitted to a facility with definitive neurosurgical care. Frequent re-evaluation of neurologic status is imperative. Approximately 90% of patients with moderate TBI will improve and will be discharged from the hospital. Ten percent experience deterioration of their condition and require management as described below for severe TBI. An emergent repeat CT should be performed in those whose condition deteriorates.

Severe TBI: GCS 3–8

The treatment of severe TBI begins with the fundamentals of resuscitation previously described including restoration of an adequate circulating blood volume, blood pressure support, appropriate ventilation, and adequate oxygenation. Patients with severe head injury often have multisystem injuries and require a multidisciplinary team to aggressively identify and treat all injuries. An evidence-based approach to resuscitation and treatment of patients with severe brain injury is presented in Figure 17-6.

Respiratory Monitoring and Management

Ensuring adequate oxygenation to avoid ongoing and worsening neuronal ischemia is essential. The airway should be secured with special attention for avoidance of hypoxia, hypercarbia, or hypocarbia. The goals of ventilation should include a target $PaCO_2$ of 35–40 mmHg. In the head-injured patient, hypercapnia ($PaCO_2$ >45 mmHg) can cause significant elevation in ICP because of CO_2-induced dilatation of the cerebral vasculature resulting in increased cerebral blood volume and

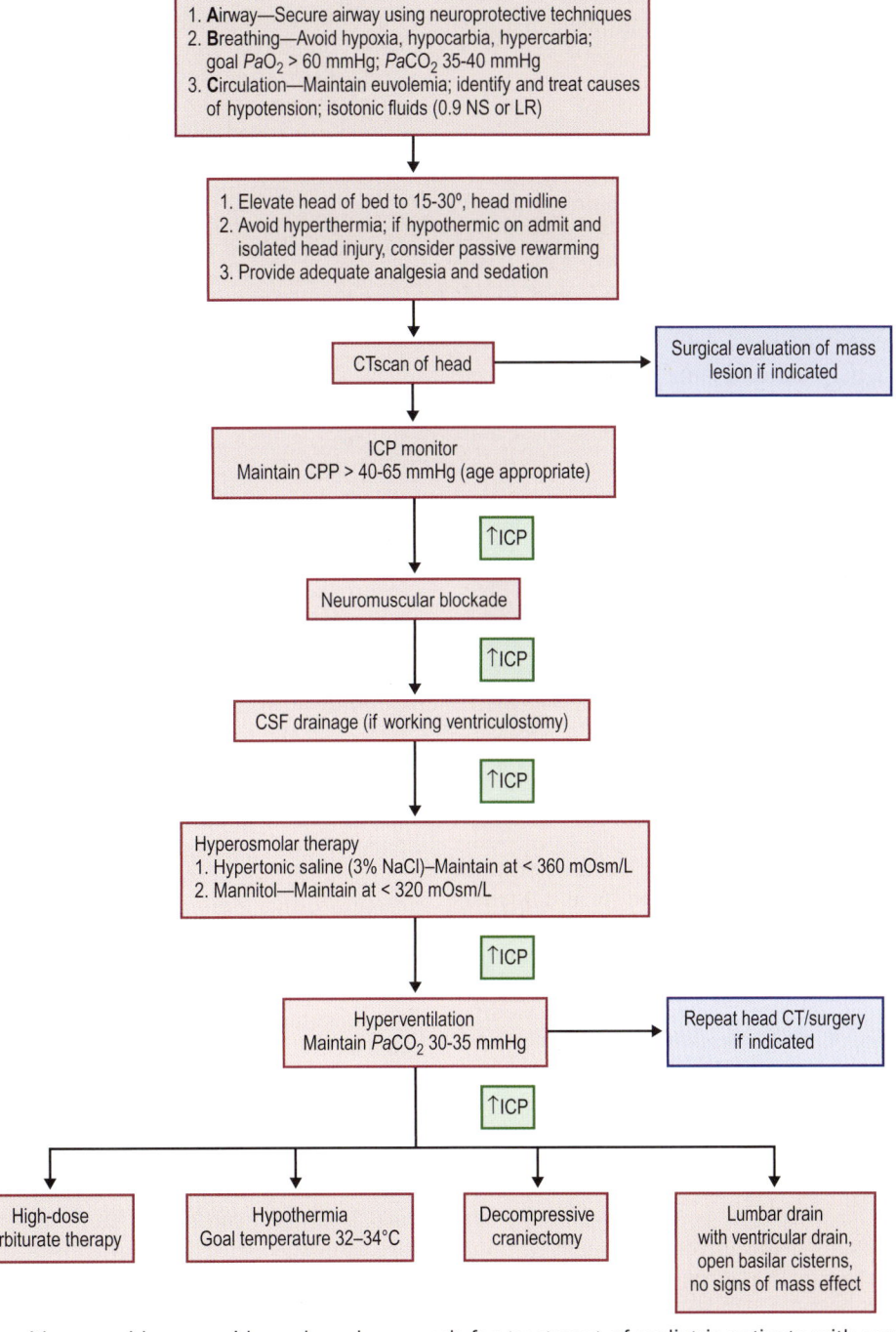

FIGURE 17-6 ■ This algorithm provides an evidence-based approach for treatment of pediatric patients with severe head trauma. NS, normal saline; LR, lactated Ringer's; ICP, intracranial pressure; CSF, cerebrospinal fluid.

flow. The immediate effect of hyperventilation is a reduction of ICP, although this response is neither universal nor sustained. Hyperventilation reduces ICP by causing cerebral vasoconstriction, with a subsequent reduction in CBF in reactive vascular beds. Hyperventilation should be reserved for those patients with obvious signs of brain stem herniation, often heralded by Cushing's triad (abnormal respiratory pattern, hypertension, and bradycardia), and nonreactive, dilated pupils.

Patient Positioning

The bed should be elevated at 15–30° and the patient's head maintained in the midline position to facilitate venous drainage from the head, thus allowing maintenance of cerebral perfusion.

Acute Surgical Management

A CT scan should be obtained in all patients with severe TBI after initial resuscitation and stabilization. Patients with intracerebral hematomas causing a mass effect need immediate neurosurgical evacuation. The traditional definition of a significant mass effect can be determined from the axial views of a noncontrasted CT scan. A line is drawn at the midline of the skull in the sagittal plane and then a perpendicular line is extended to the septum pellucidum. The basilar cisterns are also evaluated for compression. Greater than 5 mm of midline shift is considered to be significant.

Sedation and Analgesia

Sedation and analgesia are commonly used in the management of TBI. The maintenance of the airway, placement of invasive catheters or other monitoring devices, and the safe transport of the patient for diagnostic or therapeutic procedures are examples of some aspects of patient care facilitated by these medications. Sedation and analgesia may also be useful in maintaining or decreasing ICP by decreasing the metabolic rate and thereby decreasing CBF. Studies have demonstrated a two- to threefold increase in basal metabolic rate resulting from painful or stressful stimuli. Noxious stimuli, such as suctioning, can increase ICP. Painful and noxious stimuli and stress can also increase sympathetic tone, resulting in hypertension and bleeding from operative sites.[39,40] However, these medications must be used with caution, because sedative or narcotic related vasodilation may decrease CBF with resulting hypotension, or conversely may increase CBF by causing cerebral vasodilatation.

Intracranial Pressure Monitoring and Management

Despite the absence of prospective, randomized clinical trials to establish efficacy in improving outcome, the use of ICP devices has become standard in the USA for the treatment of severe head injury. There are two lines of thinking to support the use of ICP monitoring in the pediatric TBI patient. First, there is strong evidence that supports the association between intracranial hypertension and poor neurologic outcome.[41] Second, ICP monitoring and aggressive treatment of intracranial hypertension are associated with the best reported clinical outcomes.[42] The presence of open fontanelles and/or sutures in an infant does not preclude the development of intracranial hypertension or negate the utility of ICP monitoring.[7]

The treatment threshold for intracranial hypertension is typically defined as an ICP greater than 20 mmHg. Age-specific and injury mechanism–specific ICP thresholds have yet to be defined. In more recent years, the focus has switched from ICP-directed therapy to multimodal-directed therapy. Support for this change has been bolstered by a recent multicenter randomized prospective trial comparing two groups of patients ages 13 years and older. Patients were randomized into a guidelines-based management in which a protocol for monitoring intraparenchymal intracranial pressure was used (pressure-monitoring group) or a protocol in which treatment was based on imaging and clinical examination (imaging-clinical examination group).[43] The study failed to find superiority with either method in the both short and long-term outcomes of patients with severe TBI. The study authors clearly state that this study does not argue against the use of ICP monitoring, but rather indicates that more work needs to be done on interpreting and utilizing this tool in the treatment and management of TBI.

Although there is no single ICP monitoring device that is superior to the others, intraventricular devices are effective monitors that allow CSF drainage as part of the treatment for elevated ICP. However, if not inserted early after injury, placement may be difficult when damaged brain and cerebral edema have effaced the normal ventricle. Intraparenchymal monitors have fiberoptic or strain-gauge transducers that provide continuous pressure readings, and can be placed in any region of the brain. Newer monitors can measure brain tissue oxygen levels and permit manipulations to optimize regional oxygenation, including adjustments in the fraction of inspired oxygen (FiO_2) and blood transfusion. Coagulation abnormalities are a relative contraindication to the insertion of these devices. Therefore, prompt correction using plasma or activated factor VIIa should be considered before insertion.[44]

The optimal CPP for a given individual is not clear. Global and/or regional cerebral ischemia commonly complicates brain injury. Studies have consistently shown that a CPP less than 40 mmHg is associated with increased mortality.[41,45] A CPP between 40–65 mmHg likely represents an age-related continuum with inter-individual variability. Studies have suggested that avoidance of hypotension, rather than elevation of CPP, is more beneficial.[41] Efforts to increase CPP in adults to a supernormal level with the use of fluids and vasoactive infusions are associated with significant risks, including pulmonary complications, fluid overload, pressor toxicity, and renal insufficiency. Furthermore, in cases of disrupted autoregulation, exacerbation of intracranial hypertension can result.

Neuromuscular Blockade

Neuromuscular blockade is commonly used as a treatment strategy for patients with increased ICP. Neuromuscular blocking agents should be used only in those patients with a secure airway, and who are mechanically ventilated and adequately sedated. The proposed mechanisms of neuromuscular blocking agents in reducing ICP include a reduction in airway and intrathoracic pressure via facilitation of cerebral venous outflow and prevention of shivering, posturing, or breathing against the ventilator.[46] These medications have been associated with prolonged ICU stays and increased risk of nosocomial infections. Therefore, neuromuscular blockade should be reserved for the patient with increased ICP who is unresponsive to other methods such as increased sedation and/or analgesia.

Hyperosmolar Therapy

The use of hyperosmolar agents to decrease ICP was first described in the early 1900s. Hypertonic saline and mannitol were among the first agents trialed. Mannitol has become the mainstay of therapy over the past several decades. The mechanism of action of mannitol has been well studied. However, its effect on survival and functional outcome after TBI has not been well demonstrated. Mannitol requires the presence of an intact blood–brain barrier to exert its effect. Mannitol has two primary mechanisms of action. The first is an initial rheologic effect, resulting in a decrease in blood viscosity that occurs within minutes of administration. A decrease in blood vessel diameter occurs from autoregulation after reflex vasoconstriction, and leads to a decrease in cerebral blood volume and ICP.[47] Second, mannitol acts as a potent osmotic diuretic, thus pulling fluid from the interstitial space into the intravascular space. Because of its diuretic effect, intravascular volume can be depleted with the risk of decreasing cerebral perfusion, resulting in secondary brain ischemia. Careful attention must be paid to promptly replenishing intravascular volume. Finally, mannitol therapy has been associated with acute tubular necrosis. Therefore, monitoring of serum osmolarity is

recommended when using mannitol. Osmolar levels greater than 320 mOsm/L should be avoided. However, most of the reports describing the development of renal damage occurred in the era of dehydration therapy for cerebral edema. It is unclear whether the same osmolar thresholds are valid in the current era of maintaining normal intravascular volume. The beneficial effects of mannitol are best achieved with rapid bolus administration, with dosage ranging from 0.25–1.0 g/kg. Chronic administration of mannitol has been associated with a reverse osmotic shift, resulting in rebound cerebral edema and disruption of the blood–brain barrier.

More recently, hypertonic saline has re-emerged as a hyperosmolar agent and is the preferred agent in the TBI patient with hypovolemia.[48,49] Hypertonic saline includes concentrations ranging from 3 to 23.4%, with 3% hypertonic saline being the most studied in children. There is no evidence that one concentration is more effective than another for reducing intracranial hypertension. Similar to mannitol, hypertonic saline requires the presence of an intact blood-brain barrier to exert its effect. Hypertonic saline is an osmolar agent and it pulls fluid from the interstitium into the intravascular space without a strong diuretic effect, thus maintaining blood volume and cerebral perfusion. Hypertonic saline can be used as a bolus (6.5–10 mL/kg) or continuous infusion (0.1–1.0 mL/kg/h titrated to the minimum dose needed to achieve a reduction in ICP). In addition to the hyperosmolar effect, hypertonic saline has been reported to have several other potentially beneficial effects for the trauma patient, including vasoregulatory, hemodynamic, neurochemical, and immunologic properties. Serum osmolarity of 360 mOsm/L has been reported with the use of hypertonic saline and has been well tolerated in the pediatric patient with a head injury.[48] The primary theoretical concerns associated with the risk of hypertonic saline include the development of central pontine myelinolysis (rapid shrinking of the brain associated with mechanical tearing of bridging vessels leading to subarachnoid hemorrhage), renal failure, and rebound intracranial hypertension (Table 17-2).

Prophylactic administration of mannitol or other hyperosmolar therapy either in the field or in the hospital

---

TABLE 17-2   A Comparison of Mannitol and Hypertonic Saline (For Hyperosmolar Therapy)

	Mannitol	3% Hypertonic Saline
Bolus dosing guidelines	0.25–1.0 g/kg rapid bolus	3–5 mL/kg
Infusion guidelines	None	0.1–1.0 mL/kg/h
Effectiveness	May wane with repeated administration	Effective after repeated administration; effective when mannitol efficacy has waned
Augmentation of MAP	Moderate	Greater, more prolonged
Rheologic properties	Yes	Yes
Diuretic effect	Osmotic diuretic, may necessitate volume replacement to avoid hypovolemia	Diuresis through action of atrial natriuretic peptide
Maximum serum osmolarity	320 mOsm/L	360 mOsm/L
Adverse effects	Renal failure, hypotension, rebound elevation in ICP	Rebound elevation in ICP, central pontine myelinolysis, bleeding, electrolyte abnormal
Proposed beneficial effects	Antioxidant effects	Restoration of resting membrane potential and cell volume, inhibition of inflammation

ICP, intracranial pressure; MAP, mean arterial pressure.
From Knapp JM. Hyperosmolar therapy in the treatment of severe head injury in children: Mannitol and hypertonic saline. AACN Clin Issues 2005;16:199–211. Reprinted with permission.

is no longer routinely recommended. Hyperosmolar therapy should be reserved for those patients with documented intracranial hypertension or those with signs of impending herniation to avoid secondary injury and complications associated with hyperosmolar therapy.

Anticonvulsant Prophylaxis

Anticonvulsants are often administered to patients with TBI. Current clinical evidence supports their use to prevent early post-traumatic seizures which are typically defined as seizures occurring within the first 7 days after injury. Early post-traumatic seizures may further increase brain metabolic demands, increase ICP, and lead to secondary brain injury. Prophylactic anticonvulsants do not prevent late (occurring longer than seven days from injury) post-traumatic seizures.

Medically Refractory Intracranial Hypertension

It is estimated that 21–42% of children with severe TBI will develop refractory intracranial hypertension despite medical and surgical management.[7] In these patients, therapies and interventions with higher risk profiles may need to be considered. Decompressive craniectomy, high-dose barbiturate therapy, hyperventilation, lumbar drain placement, and the use of moderate hypothermia should be considered in the patient with medically refractory intracranial hypertension.

Decompressive Craniectomy

Children are more likely than adults to have diffuse brain swelling after TBI and may be more amenable to a treatment strategy utilizing early decompressive craniectomy. Decompressive craniectomy should be considered in children with severe TBI and infants with abusive head trauma and medically refractory intracranial hypertension. The main goal of decompressive craniectomy is to control ICP, thereby maintaining CPP and cerebral oxygenation. Improved outcomes have been demonstrated in several small single-center studies, and appears to be most effective when done early, before the development of extensive secondary brain injury.[50–52]

Barbiturate Therapy

High doses of barbiturates are known to reduce ICP and have been used in the management of increased ICP for decades. Their side effects limit their current use to those patients with injuries refractory to first-line therapies. Barbiturates are effective in lowering ICP by suppressing brain metabolism and altering vascular tone. In addition to the ICP-lowering benefits, barbiturates also inhibit free radical–mediated lipid peroxidation and have membrane-stabilizing effects. Small case series of children with severe TBI suggest that barbiturates may be effective in lowering ICP in the setting of refractory intracranial hypertension.[53,54] Their use is associated with myocardial depression, increased risk of hypotension, and the need for blood pressure support with intravascular fluids and inotropic infusions. It is important that barbiturates are used in the setting of systemic monitoring with the ability to rapidly detect hemodynamic instability.

Hyperventilation

Hyperventilation has been a mainstay in the management of severe TBI, but more recent concerns about its role in cerebral ischemia have lessened its use. As discussed previously, the cerebral vasculature is sensitive to changes in $PaCO_2$, with hypocarbia producing cerebral vasoconstriction and a decrease in CBF. Historically, hyperemia, or excessive CBF, was thought to be the primary mechanism resulting in cerebral edema after TBI, thus making hyperventilation a reasonable approach in the management of the patient with severe TBI. More recent studies have demonstrated that hyperemia is uncommon after severe TBI. Hyperventilation may decrease cerebral oxygenation, resulting in secondary brain ischemia.[55,56] The use of aggressive hyperventilation ($PaCO_2$ <30 mmHg) should be reserved for refractory intracranial hypertension. Monitoring of CBF, jugular venous oxygen saturation, or brain tissue oxygenation may help identify cerebral ischemia in this setting.

Lumbar Drain

Placement of a lumbar drain may be helpful in patients with refractory intracranial hypertension that is unresponsive to the first-line therapies. It is recommended that the patient has a working ventriculostomy or documentation of open basilar cisterns on CT.

Therapeutic Hypothermia

The avoidance of hyperthermia and use of therapeutic hypothermia after TBI is based on the rationale that temperature plays an important role in mechanisms contributing to secondary brain injury (excitotoxicity, free radical formation). Despite evidence in animal models demonstrating efficacy of therapeutic moderate hypothermia (32–34°C), large randomized clinical studies in both adults and children have not proven the effectiveness of hypothermia on improved outcomes after TBI.[57–61] Studies extrapolated from the adult literature indicate that hyperthermia adversely affects outcome so it may be advisable to consider passive re-warming of the mild to moderately hypothermic trauma patient with isolated head injury.[62]

FACIAL TRAUMA

The same mechanisms of injury associated with TBI (sports, motor vehicle accidents, and falls) also lead to facial trauma in infants and children. The elasticity of the facial skeleton, the enhanced facial soft tissue padding, the lack of sinuses that thin the surrounding bone, and the prominence of the skull protect the younger child's face from injury, resulting in a lower incidence of traumatic injury. As children age, develop, and become more active, the frequency of injury increases. No matter the age, the reconstructive principles remain the same: restoration of function, maximization of aesthetic results, limited visible incisions for repair, avoidance of complications, and minimal effect on later growth and development from both the trauma and the operative repair. Except for the last principle, these goals are the same as repair of facial trauma in adults. The last principle, related to later growth and development, must be understood by both the surgical team and the family as it can alter the treatment plan. Furthermore, the treatment plan can often be different for a given fracture that occurs during infancy versus childhood versus adolescence.

The aims of this portion of the chapter include an understanding of facial growth, the causes of significant facial trauma, the diagnosis and age-dependent treatment of facial injuries, and the long-term concerns and sequelae of the trauma and its repair. Because soft tissue injuries are touched on in other chapters, this discussion will focus on facial skeletal trauma and fractures.

Craniofacial Growth And Development

One cannot appropriately treat pediatric craniofacial fractures without a comprehensive understanding of facial growth and development. All infants start out 'top-heavy' with a cranial to facial proportion of 7–8 : 1. The skull and cranial vault grow rapidly, dictated by growth of the brain. The brain expands 300% in the first couple of years of life, and acts like a balloon to expand the overlying skull. The skull bones are connected by sutures and are not fused, allowing for this rapid growth to occur unimpeded. Rapid growth of the skull continues for the first four years of life. By the time children enter kindergarten, their skull is about 90 % of adult size.

Facial growth follows a different path and pattern, and varies anatomically. The upper facial bone growth is stimulated by growth of the brain and orbit. The periorbital bones are 90% of adult size by age 4 to 5 years. The frontal sinuses begin to pneumatize at age 3 to 4 years, but complete aeration is not noted until the later teenage years. Midfacial growth in the transverse, vertical, and anteroposterior planes is stimulated by dental development. The maxillary sinuses pneumatize around 12 years of age, corresponding with the eruption of permanent teeth. On the other hand, the lower facial skeleton develops more slowly. The main growth centers are the bilateral condyles. The mandible has both membranous and endochondral bone, the only major bone of the facial skeleton with that composition.

Incidence and Epidemiology

Although facial trauma is more common in children, facial fractures are less common in children, although they are likely under-diagnosed due to several factors. First, the family provides infants and younger children with a protective environment, minimizing their exposure to trauma. Second, as discussed previously, these children have a proportionally larger and protrusive skull and forehead, which protects the face by absorbing the impact at the expense of exposing the child to TBI.

Third, the infant and child's mandible is relatively retrusive compared to its adult counterpart, diminishing the incidence of impact and mandibular fracture. Fourth, pediatric facial bones are more elastic, leading to either no fracture or a greenstick fracture that does not require further treatment. Fifth, the bones still have open sutures and are more cartilaginous, decreasing the fracture rate. Lastly, the lack of sinuses strengthens the bones as compared to the adult facial structure.

As children grow, facial fracture patterns change. The face becomes relatively more prominent as craniofacial proportions change. Mixed dentition accords more teeth in the midface and less bone. The sinuses pneumatize, further weakening the bone. The facial skeleton begins to calcify, diminishing its elasticity. Thus, frontal, skull, and periorbital fractures are more common in the pre-kindergarten years while midface and mandible fractures increase in frequency as children mature. Because of its prominent anterior position, nasal fractures are the most common facial fracture, followed by mandible fractures.

The most common causes of pediatric facial fractures include MVCs, falls, and sports. As children age, assaults begin to play a causative role. The advent of air bags, mandatory use of seat belts and harnesses, mandatory use of car seats, mandatory helmeting of minors on motorcycles, and enforcement of driving under the influence laws have decreased the incidence and sequelae of MVCs. Protective helmeting and faceguards for sporting activities and bicycling have also diminished facial trauma. Safety initiatives, such as the American Academy of Pediatrics' push to deter trampoline use, should also have a positive effect on public health.

The recent popularity of extreme sports increases the susceptibility to facial trauma, especially when not appropriately protected. More significantly, the popularity of all-terrain vehicles has provided a new high-velocity mechanism for facial trauma in minors without some of the protective features seen in an MVC.

Evaluation and Diagnosis

Both evaluation and diagnosis of pediatric facial fractures can be difficult. A comprehensive understanding of the mechanism of injury is essential. The injuries may be unwitnessed, and the child may be a poor historian or too young to communicate. The child may not be able to specifically tell you what hurts, and may not be able to follow commands. Either because of age, pain, or non-compliance, the child may not be able to or does not want to participate in the examination. This is most limiting in the orbital and visual examination. The child may have an associated TBI further diminishing the ability to communicate or participate in a comprehensive evaluation. Therefore, a history of the traumatic event must often be obtained from the parents and/or the emergency medical transport team who accompany the patient.

As the mechanisms of injury leading to facial fractures mirror those of multisystem trauma, the plastic surgeon must work in tandem with the trauma team. Special attention must be given to the cervical spine, as there is an 8 to 10% incidence of spinal injury with significant craniofacial injury.

Examination should begin with an overall assessment of neurologic status and airway competency. Craniofacial fractures have a high incidence of TBI. CSF leaks may occur and neurosurgical consultation is often warranted. An unstable airway can be challenging secondary to mandibular or maxillary fractures. Teeth can be loose, free-floating, or aspirated. The cervical spine is often not cleared and the child's neck is immobilized. Intubation with a flexible endoscope may be necessary. A tracheotomy may be needed in some cases.

The craniofacial examination must be comprehensive and thorough. It should include the cervical spine, and the exam must be coordinated with that of the trauma and/or emergency room team.

The scalp/skull examination begins with observation and palpation for possible fractures. Any laceration must be cleansed and examined to insure there is no underlying skull fracture. In younger children, beware of dog bites to the scalp and associated skull punctures. Laceration examination may require sedation if not contraindicated. The forehead and supraorbital area is treated similarly. Open wounds can extend intracranially or into or through the frontal sinus if air spaces have developed. Forehead paresthesia can be related to fractures through the supraorbital nerve and ridge, or the supratrochlear area.

Periorbital trauma demands a thorough examination. Children have a higher incidence of trauma to the globe and visual damage than adults with periorbital trauma. Examination begins with visual inspection of the pupils including their size and reactivity. Symmetry of gaze and extraocular muscle motion must be assessed.

Enopthalmos or proptosis should be assessed as should upper eyelid ptosis. Subconjunctival hemorrhage is often a sign of orbital fracture. Intercanthal distance should be measured, as an increase can be a sign of bony or canthal widening and injury. Next, vision must be tested in each eye as well as a light exam of each pupil looking for afferent defects. Extraocular movement should be tested when the patient is cooperative. Forced duction tests can be performed in the unconscious patient. This test is looking for orbital muscle entrapment in fracture lines. Palpations of the orbital rims should follow, although fractures can be difficult to assess secondary to the rapid onset of swelling with periorbital trauma. Infraorbital nerve paresthesias should also be evaluated. Lastly, lacerations of the upper or lower eyelid medial to the punctum should raise suspicion for a lacrimal system injury.

Pediatric ophthalmologic consultation should be obtained in children with significant periorbital trauma. Emergent ophthalmology consultation is necessary for a patient with vision loss, superior orbital fissure syndrome, or orbital apex syndrome. Superior orbital apex syndrome consists of loss of orbital motion, upper eyelid ptosis, and supraorbital nerve paresthesia. Orbital apex syndrome includes the same constellation plus visual loss. These injuries often require emergent decompression and/or steroid administration.

Midface examination includes palpation of the orbital rims as discussed previously as well as intraoral palpation of the midfacial bones looking for step-offs. Maxillary mobility from the craniofacial skeleton is indicative of a bilateral transverse midfacial fracture, a LeFort fracture,

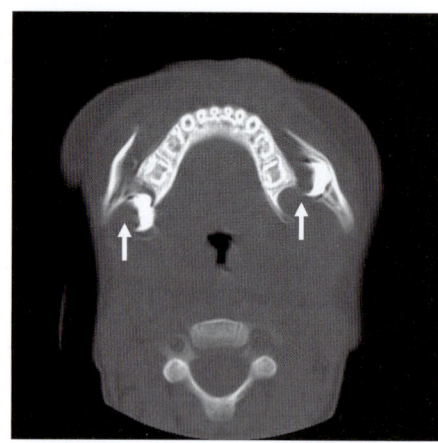

FIGURE 17-7 ■ This 18-month-old suffered a crush injury after a swing fell on his face. This CT scan shows bilateral fractures (arrows) of the body of the mandible. He required open reduction and internal fixation with intermaxillary wiring.

often accompanied by malocclusion. The zygoma and zygomatic arch must be palpated and inspected for fracture. These fractures can be associated with trismus, and decreased opening of the mouth.

Nasal examination includes an external and internal component. Externally, the bones are examined for mobility and deviation, including dorsal collapse. Internally, the septum must be examined to exclude a hematoma which might require septal drainage. Nasal drainage should raise suspicion of a CSF leak.

Mandibular examination begins by asking the patient if his or her teeth come together normally. Intraoral examination will demonstrate malocclusion. Lower lip paresthesias are indicative of fractures in the body or parasymphyseal regions of the mandible. . Gingival lacerations can also expose an underlying fracture. Dental and/or alveolar ridge injuries are also common. The clinician must palpate the mandible from temporomandibular joint to the contralateral temporomandibular joint, documenting pain if present. The older the child, the more likely they are to have two concomitant mandible fractures similar to adults (Fig. 17-7).

Diagnostic imaging is necessary for all suspicious fractures except perhaps nasal fractures. Fine-cut axial CT scans from the roof of the orbit to the bottom of the mandible accompanied by coronal and three-dimensional reconstructions will help identify facial fractures. Craniofacial fracture CT scans should include the entire skull as well. A Panorex may be useful for dental injuries and for mandibular fractures, especially condylar and proximal injuries.

Associated Injuries

When a provider encounters a pediatric patient who sustained significant facial fractures, that provider must be aware of the possibility of associated injuries. In addition, the mechanism of injury can concurrently cause injuries outside of the head and neck. A collaborative care plan with the hospital trauma team is essential for optimal care.

Cranial vault and cranial base injuries/fracture as well as intracranial trauma must be excluded. Dental trauma or intraoral bleeding can lead to aspiration. Cervical spine injuries are increased in all high-impact trauma etiology, especially with mandible fractures.

Treatment

Nasal Fractures

Nasal fractures are one of the two most common pediatric facial fractures, due to the prominence and projection of the nose from the facial skeleton. Nasal fractures increase in incidence with advancing age. The fractures not only involve the bone, but often the cartilage, most notably the septal cartilage. Septal hematomas should be drained acutely. Fracture repair can be deferred until the swelling subsists. Treatment most commonly consists of closed reduction. Even with adequate reduction, the fracture may lead to long-term growth restriction and/or distortion, which can then be addressed at skeletal maturity.

Mandible Fractures

Mandible fractures are the other of the two most common pediatric facial fractures. Treatment of mandible fractures varies by patient age, dental development, site of the fracture, and number of mandible fractures. In the young, condylar injuries are the most common. In late adolescence, fractures of the mandibular angle and body predominate. Different stages of dental development allow for different types of fixation techniques to be employed.

The goals of mandible fracture treatment are reestablishment of occlusion, bony union, and avoidance of complications including infection. Nondisplaced or minimally displaced fractures with normal occlusion can be treated with a soft diet and close observation. Often minor malocclusions can be treated the same. For patients with more than minor malocclusion, an operative approach is necessary. In younger patients with a single mandible fracture, closed reduction should be attempted. If reduction is successful, treatment should proceed with intermaxillary fixation (IMF). IMF can be difficult in the younger patients and often requires adjuvant occlusal splints and suspension wires for support. For nonreducible single fractures, an open approach with internal fixation is usually necessary. An open approach with fixation is also often needed for the treatment of multiple mandible fractures. Avoidance of open reduction with subperiosteal undermining and avoidance of internal fixation are goals of repair in the growing facial skeleton if possible.

Midfacial Fractures

Isolated midfacial fractures are rare in the young patient. The maxilla is protected by the prominence of the upper face (forehead) and the lower face (mandible/chin). The maxilla and zygoma are also fortified in the young because the midfacial sinuses have not developed. Sinus development occurs at the expense of bony weakening. Treatment of maxillary fractures again center around reestablishment of occlusion. Fractures with no or minor occlusal abnormalities can be treated with soft diet, and orthodontic intervention if necessary. As the degree of malocclusion worsens, the necessity for intermaxillary fixation and/or open reduction and internal fixation increases. Again, in the growing facial skeleton, the most successful conservative approach is advocated. In teenagers, the approach is similar to adult trauma.

Isolated displaced zygoma fractures require open reduction with fixation (Fig. 17-8). As the zygoma is a bone that constitutes part of the orbital walls and floor, the orbital floor needs to be explored and repaired at the time of zygoma fracture repair. Orbital sequelae of inadequately repaired zygoma fractures include enopthalmos, orbital dystopia, and diplopia.

Periorbital Fractures

Orbital fractures can occur in combination with zygomatic fractures or as an isolated injury. The lack of sinuses and the presence of higher maxillary tooth buds give support to the orbital bones in the young. Trapdoor fractures can occur in the floor, leading to muscle entrapment, limited orbital movement, and diplopia. The goals of repair include restoration of orbital volume, restoration of globe position and height, and elimination of any entrapment.

Unique Pediatric Concerns

Pediatric facial fractures and their repair pose long-term concerns distinct from adult trauma. The fractures themselves may inhibit long-term growth of the involved bony structures leading not only to distortion, but to asymmetry as well. Fracture repair techniques, including subperiosteal exposure of the involved bones, may further impede long-term growth. Bony fixation with permanent metallic plates also can result in growth restriction. The recent development of resorbable plates which function during the period of bony healing, and then resorb, is an attempt to eliminate this long-term concern. To date, these plates have shown great efficacy in nonweight-bearing bones, but are more limited in bones involved in

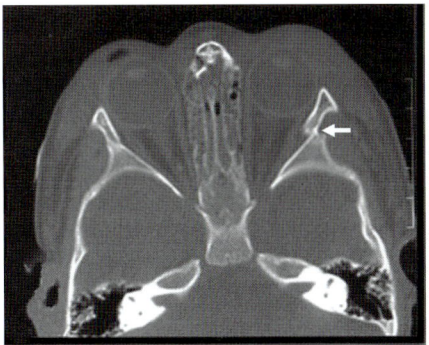

FIGURE 17-8 ■ This 7-year-old was hit by a baseball and sustained this left zygomatic fracture (arrow). He underwent open reduction and internal fixation of this displaced fracture.

mastication. Because of these concerns, because of the differences in anatomy including tooth buds and development, and because of bony elasticity and the absence of sinuses, pediatric fractures are different than adult fractures as are the philosophies for pediatric fracture repair. In addition, the fracture type and repair varies by age in this growing population.

REFERENCES

1. Adekoya N, Thurman DJ, White DD, et al. Surveillance for traumatic brain injury deaths–United States, 1989–1998. Morbidity & Mortality Weekly Report Surveillance Summaries 2002;51:1–14.
2. Langlois JA, Rutland-Brown W, Thomas KE. The incidence of traumatic brain injury among children in the United States: Differences by race. J Head Trauma Rehab 2005;20:229–38.
3. Billmire ME, Myers PA. Serious head injury in infants: Accident or abuse? Pediatr 1985;75:340–2.
4. Bruce DA, Zimmerman RA. Shaken impact syndrome. Pediatr Ann 1989;18:482–4.
5. Child Maltreatment Prevention. Center for Disease Control and Prevention; 2008 [cited 2008 May 7]; Available from: http://www.cdc.gov/ncipc/dvp/CMP/CMP-prvt-strat.htm.
6. Tilford JM, Aitken ME, Anand KJ, et al. Hospitalizations for critically ill children with traumatic brain injuries: A longitudinal analysis. Crit Care Med 2005;33:2074–81.
7. Kochanek PM, Carney N, Adelson PD, et al. Guidelines for the acute medical management of severe traumatic brain injury in infants, children, and adolescents–second edition. Pediatric Critical Care Medicine: A Journal of the Society of Critical Care Medicine and the World Federation of Pediatric Intensive and Critical Care Societies 2012;13(Suppl 1):S1–82. Epub 2012/01/11.
8. Muizelaar JP, Marmarou A, DeSalles AA, et al. Cerebral blood flow and metabolism in severely head-injured children. Part 1: Relationship with GCS score, outcome, ICP, and PVI. J Neurosurg 1989;71:63–71.
9. Shapiro K, Marmarou A. Clinical applications of the pressure-volume index in treatment of pediatric head injuries. J Neurosurg 1982;56:819–25.
10. Bouma GJ, Muizelaar JP. Evaluation of regional cerebral blood flow in acute head injury by stable xenon-enhanced computerized tomography. Acta Neur S 1993;59:34–40.
11. Bouma GJ, Muizelaar JP. Cerebral blood flow in severe clinical head injury. New Horizons 1995;3:384–94.
12. Bouma GJ, Muizelaar JP, Choi SC, et al. Cerebral circulation and metabolism after severe traumatic brain injury: the elusive role of ischemia. J Neurosurg 1991;75:685–93.
13. Cold GE. Cerebral blood flow in the acute phase after head injury. Part 2: Correlation to intraventricular pressure (IVP), cerebral perfusion pressure (CPP), $PaCO_2$, ventricular fluid lactate, lactate/pyruvate ratio and pH. Acta Anaesthesiologica Scandinavica 1981;25:332–5.
14. Jaggi J, Obrist W, Gennarelli T, et al. Relationship of early cerebral blood flow and metabolism to outcome in acute head injury. J Neurosurg 1990;72:176–82.
15. Cruz J, Jaggi JL, Hoffstad OJ. Cerebral blood flow, vascular resistance, and oxygen metabolism in acute brain trauma: Redefining the role of cerebral perfusion pressure? Crit Care Med 1995;23:1412–17.
16. Lang EW, Lagopoulos J, Griffith J, et al. Cerebral vasomotor reactivity testing in head injury: The link between pressure and flow. J Neurol Psychiatry 2003;74:1053–9.
17. Paulson OB, Strandgaard S, Edvinsson L. Cerebral autoregulation. Cerebrovas Brain Met 1990;2:161–92.
18. Vavilala MS, Muangman S, Tontisirin N, et al. Impaired cerebral autoregulation and 6-month outcome in children with severe traumatic brain injury: Preliminary findings. Dev Neurosci 2006;28:348–53.
19. Pfenninger J, Kaiser G, Lutschg J, et al. Treatment and outcome of the severely head injured child. Intens Care Med 1983;9:13–16.
20. Dagi TF, Meyer FB, Poletti CA. The incidence and prevention of meningitis after basilar skull fracture. Am J Emer Med 1983;1:295–8.
21. Rathore MH. Do prophylactic antibiotics prevent meningitis after basilar skull fracture? Pediatr Infect Dis J 1991;10:87–8.
22. Villalobos T, Arango C, Kubilis P, et al. Antibiotic prophylaxis after basilar skull fractures: A meta-analysis. Clin Infect Dis 1998;27:364–9.
23. O RB, João C, Cristina S, et al. Antibiotic prophylaxis for preventing meningitis in patients with basilar skull fractures. John Wiley & Sons, Ltd; 2011.
24. Venetz I, Schopfer K, Muhlemann K. Paediatric, invasive pneumococcal disease in Switzerland, 1985–1994. Swiss Pneumococcal Study Group. Int J Epidem 1998;27:1101–4.
25. Harders A, Kakarieka A, Braakman R. Traumatic subarachnoid hemorrhage and its treatment with nimodipine. German TSAH Study Group. J Neurosurg 1996;85:82–9.
26. Romner B, Bellner J, Kongstad P, et al. Elevated transcranial Doppler flow velocities after severe head injury: Cerebral vasospasm or hyperemia? J Neurosurg 1996;85:90–7.
27. Bareyre F, Wahl F, McIntosh TK, et al. Time course of cerebral edema aftertraumatic brain injury in rats: Effects of riluzole and mannitol. J Neurotrauma 1997;14:839–89.
28. Chestnut R, Marshall LF, Klauber MR, et al. The role of secondary brain injury in determining outcome from severe head injury. J Trauma 1993;34:216–22.
29. Gopinath SP, Robertson CS, Contant CF, et al. Jugular venous desaturation and outcome after head injury. J Neurol Psychiatry 1994;57:717–23.
30. Choi DW. Excitotoxic cell death. J Neurobiol 1992;23:1261–76.
31. Choi DW, Maulucci-Gedde M, Kriegstein AR. Glutamate neurotoxicity in cortical cell culture. J Neurosci 1987;7:357–68.
32. Koh JY, Choi DW. Selective blockade of non-NMDA receptors does not block rapidly triggered glutamate-induced neuronal death. Brain Res 1991;548:318–21.
33. Stocchetti N, Furlan A, Volta F. Hypoxemia and arterial hypotension at the accident scene in head injury. J Trauma 1996;40:764–7.
34. Cooper A, DiScala C, Foltin G, et al. Prehospital endotracheal intubation for severe head injury in children: A reaapraisal. Semin Pediatr Surg 2001;10:3–6.
35. Gausche M, Lewis R, Stratton S, et al. Effect of out-of-hospital pediatric endotracheal intubation on survival and neurological outcome: A controlled clinical trial. JAMA 2000;283:783–90.
36. Gabriel E, Ghajar J, Jagoda A, et al. Guidelines for pre-hospital management of traumatic brain injury. New York: Brain Trauma Foundation; 2000.
37. Advanced Trauma Life Support (ATLS). 7th ed. Chicago, IL: American College of Surgeons; 2004.
38. Teasdale G, Jennett B. Assessment of coma and impaired consciousness: A practical scale. Lancet 1974;2:81–4.
39. Kerr ME, Weber BB, Sereika SM, et al. Effect of endotracheal suctioning on cerebral oxygenation in traumatic brain-injured patients. Crit Care Med 1999;27:2776–81.
40. Raju TN, Vidyasagar D, Torres C, et al. Intracranial pressure during intubation and anesthesia in infants. J Pediatr 1980;96:860–2.
41. Downard C, Hulka F, Mullins RJ, et al. Relationship of cerebral perfusion pressure and survival in pediatric brain-injured patients. J Trauma 2000;49:654–8.
42. Tilford J, Aitken M, Anand K, et al. Hospitalizations for critically ill children with traumatic brain injuries: A longitudinal analysis. Crit Care Med 2005;33:2074–81.
43. Chestnut RM, Temkin N, Carney N, et al. A trial of intracranial-pressure monitoring in traumatic brain injury. N Engl J Med 2012;367:2471–81.
44. Morenski JD, Tobias JD, Jimenez DF. Recombinant activated factor VII for cerebral injury-induced coagulopathy in pediatric patients. Report of three cases and review of the literature. J Neurosurg 2003;98:611–16.
45. Elias-Jones AC, Punt JA, Turnbull AE, et al. Management and outcome of severe head injuries in the Trent region 1985–90. Arch Dis Child 1992;67:1430–5.
46. Hsiang JK, Chesnut RM, Crisp CB, et al. Early, routine paralysis for intracranial pressure control in severe head injury: is it necessary? Crit Care Med 1994;22:1471–6.
47. Muizelaar JP, Wei EP, Kontos HA, et al. Mannitol causes compensatory cerebral vasoconstriction and vasodilation in response to blood viscosity changes. J Neurosurg 1983;59:822–8.

48. Khanna S, Davis D, Peterson B, et al. Use of hypertonic saline in the treatment of severe refractory posttraumatic intracranial hypertension in pediatric traumatic brain injury. Crit Care Med 2000;28:1144–51.

49. Peterson B, Khanna S, Fisher B, et al. Prolonged hypernatremia controls elevated intracranial pressure in head-injured pediatric patients. Crit Care Med 2000;28:1136–43.

50. Guresir E, Schuss P, Seifert V, et al. Decompressive craniectomy in children: Single-center series and systematic review. Neurosurg. 2012;70:881–9.

51. Oluigbo CO, Wilkinson CC, Stence NV, et al. Comparison of outcomes following decompressive craniectomy in children with accidental and nonaccidental blunt cranial trauma. J Neuros-Pediatr 2012;9:125–32.

52. Pérez Suárez E. Decompressive craniectomy in 14 children with severe head injury: Clinical results with long-term follow-up and review of the literature. J Trauma 2011;71:133–40.

53. Kasoff SS, Lansen TA, Holder D, et al. Aggressive physiologic monitoring of pediatric head trauma patients with elevated intracranial pressure. Pediatr Neurosci 1988;14:241–9.

54. Pittman T, Bucholz R, Williams D. Efficacy of barbiturates in the treatment of resistant intracranial hypertension in severely head-injured children. Pediatr Neurosci 1989;15:13–17.

55. Skippen P, Seear M, Poskitt K, et al. Effect of hyperventilation on regional cerebral blood flow in head-injured children. Crit Care Med 1997;25:1402–9.

56. Stringer WA, Hasso AN, Thompson JR, et al. Hyperventilation-induced cerebral ischemia in patients with acute brain lesions: Demonstration by xenon-enhanced CT. Am J Neuroradiol 1993;14:475–84.

57. Adelson PD. Hypothermia following pediatric traumatic brain injury. J Neurotraum 2009;26:429–36.

58. Adelson PD, Ragheb J, Kanev P, et al. Phase II clinical trial of moderate hypothermia after severe traumatic brain injury in children. Neurosurg 2005;56:740–54.

59. Biswas AK, Bruce DA, Sklar FH, et al. Treatment of acute traumatic brain injury in children with moderate hypothermia improves intracranial hypertension. Crit Care Med 2002;30:2742–51.

60. Hutchison JS, Ward RE, Lacroix J, et al. Hypothermia Pediatric Head Injury Trial Investigators and the Canadian Critical Care Trials Group. Hypothermia therapy after traumatic brain injury in children. N Engl J Med 2008;358:2447–56.

61. Marion DW, Penrod LE, Kelsey SF, et al. Treatment of traumatic brain injury with moderate hypothermia. N Engl J Med 1997;336:540–6.

62. Jones PA, Andrews PJ, Midgley S, et al. Measuring the burden of secondary insults in head-injured patients during intensive care. J Neurosurg Anesth 1994;6:4–14.

CHAPTER 18

PEDIATRIC ORTHOPEDIC TRAUMA

Jeffrey E. Martus • Gregory A. Mencio

Musculoskeletal trauma is the most common medical emergency in children.[1] In children ages 1 to 14 years, accidents are the leading cause of death.[2] However, not all orthopedic injuries sustained by children are life threatening. The chance of a child sustaining a fracture before age 16 is 42% for boys and 27% for girls.[3] It has been estimated that between 1–2% of children present with a fracture each year.[4] As participation in sports and other recreational activities increases, the number of fractures is likely to increase. A study in 2006 looking at the impact of trauma on an urban pediatric orthopedic practice demonstrated that fracture management (both operative and nonoperative) accounted for approximately one-third of the total work-related relative value units. The most common fracture-related operations were performed on the elbow (23%), tibia (12%), femur (9.8%), forearm (5.5%), and the distal aspect of the radius (5%).[5] The same practice reported that trauma care comprised 44% of their operative volume in 2006 and 2007.[6]

Patient gender, age, climate, time of day, and social situation in the home have been shown to impact the frequency of orthopedic injuries. In children, boys sustain fractures at 2.7 times the rate of girls.[7] However, as girls become involved in more athletic events, this margin may narrow. It has been shown that fracture location varies with chronologic age, a finding that is probably due to a combination of the anatomic maturation of the child and the age-specific activities of childhood.[3] Several authors have shown that fractures are more common during the summer months when children are out of school.[4,7,8] It has also been shown that there is also a strong association between sunshine and fractures, and a negative association between rain and fractures.[9] Likewise, two studies have proven that the afternoon is the most frequent time for fractures to occur.[10,11] This correlates with the time of peak activity for children. Injuries in the home during the late afternoon and evening account for more than 83% of all injuries to children.[12] Moreover, the overall incidence of fractures occurring at home increases with the age of the child.[4,13] In a Swedish study, fracture incidence was correlated with the degree of social handicaps such as welfare or alcoholism in the family.[14] Similarly, a study from Manitoba elicited the social situation at home as a major influence of children's injuries.[15]

No discussion of pediatric orthopedic trauma is complete that does not include a discussion of nonaccidental trauma. The incidence of physical abuse to children is estimated to be 4.9 per 1,000. Of those abused, 1 of every 1,000 will ultimately die as a result.[16] Early recognition and reporting is essential because children who return home after hospitalization with unrecognized abuse have a 25% risk of serious injury and a 5% risk of death.[17] Children at highest risk for abuse are first-born children, premature infants, stepchildren, and handicapped children.[18] Most cases of child abuse involve children younger than 3 years of age. Any child presenting with fractures, particularly if they involve the long bones, should be viewed with circumspection as to cause (Table 18-1).[19,20]

PATHOPHYSIOLOGY

In the immature skeleton, longitudinal and appositional growth takes place through the physes (growth plates) that are located at the ends of the long bones, in the endplates of the vertebral bodies, or at the periphery of the round bones in the feet and hands. Thus, the physis is essential for normal skeletal growth, but is also the weakest portion of the bone in children. It is estimated that approximately 30% of fractures of the long bones include an injury to the physis.[21-23] Most fractures that involve the growth plates heal without consequence. However, some injuries can result in permanent damage with significant sequelae such as angular deformity or complete cessation of growth.

The ends of every long bone consist of an epiphysis (near the joint), physis, and metaphysis (area of newly formed bone). At the time of skeletal maturity, the physis closes, which means there is no more longitudinal growth. Fracture healing in children is rapid and the potential for remodeling is great due to the growth potential and dynamism of the immature skeleton. These characteristics allow for nonoperative treatment of some fractures in children that demand operative treatment in skeletally mature patients. Remodeling of fractures predictably occurs in the plane of primary motion of the adjacent joint (usually flexion/extension) and, to a lesser degree, in the coronal plane (varus and valgus deformities). Remodeling is virtually nonexistent in the transverse plane with rotational malalignment.[24]

Physeal fractures are classified to predict outcome and guide treatment. Currently, most orthopedic surgeons use the Salter Harris classification (Fig. 18-1).[25] Classic teaching states that type I and II injuries heal without growth abnormalities if reduced appropriately. However, some reports dispute some of this dogma.[26-28] Types III and IV injuries usually occur in older children and require anatomic realignment via open reduction to restore

TABLE 18-1 **Specificity of Musculoskeletal Radiologic Findings in Nonaccidental Trauma**

Specificity	Radiologic Finding
High	Metaphyseal corner lesions
	Posterior rib fractures
	Scapular fractures
	Spinous process fractures
	Sternal fractures
Moderate	Multiple fractures
	Fractures of different ages
	Epiphyseal separations
	Vertebral body fractures
	Digital fractures
	Complex skull fractures
Low[a]	Clavicular fractures
	Long bone shaft fractures (humerus, femur, tibia)
	Linear skull fractures

[a]Low specificity, but these findings are commonly seen in nonaccidental trauma.
Adapted from O'Connor JF, Cohen J. Dating fractures. In: Kleinman PK, editor. Diagnostic Imaging of Child Abuse. Baltimore: Williams & Wilkins, 1987. p. 6.

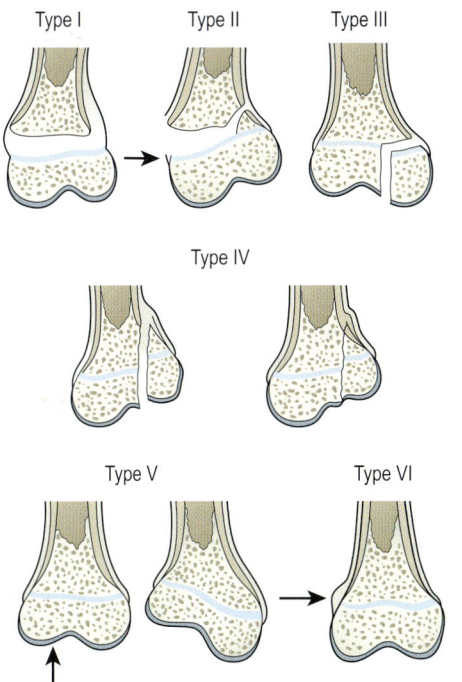

FIGURE 18-1 ■ Salter Harris classification of physeal injuries with Rang modification. (Adapted from Rang ML, editor. The Growth Plate and Its Disorders. Edinburgh: E&S Livingstone; 1969. p 139.)

congruity of the joint to minimize the risk of arthritis. Reduction also restores continuity of the physis to decrease the risk of growth disturbance. Type V are crush injuries that are not usually recognized at presentation, but have a high risk of growth arrest.[29]

TABLE 18-2 **Severity Classification for Open Fractures**

Grade	Description
I	Wound <1 cm
II	Transitional wound (1–10 cm)
III	Wound >10 cm
IIIA	Extensive soft tissue injury
IIIB	Reconstructive soft tissue injury
IIIC	Vascular injury

From Gustilo RB, Mendoza RM, Williams DN. Problems in the management of type III (severe) open fractures: A new classification of type III open fractures. J Trauma 1984;24:747–96; Gustilo RB, Anderson T. Prevention of infection in the treatment of 1025 open fractures of long bones: Retrospective and prospective analyses. J Bone Joint Surg Am 1976;50:453–58.

COMPLEX INJURIES

Children sustain injuries that are different from adults due to their size and activities. A common example is a pedestrian struck by a car. An adult will frequently sustain an injury to the tibia or knee from the car's bumper. However, the same mechanism will result in a fracture of the femur or pelvis in conjunction with a chest or head injury in a small child.[30] Motor vehicle accidents (MVAs) are the most common cause of multiple injuries to children, both as occupants and pedestrians.[30,31]

Open fractures are considered one of the true orthopedic emergencies in children.[32] These injuries usually result from high-energy mechanisms and are often seen in the setting of multiple trauma. Open fractures in children and adults are classified according to the system of Gustilo–Anderson (Table 18-2).[33–35] The four goals of treatment of open fractures are: prevention of infection, bony union, prevention of malunion, and return to function of limb and patient.[32,36] To attain these goals, open fractures must be treated by early irrigation and debridement along with broad-spectrum antibiotics.[33–35] Kindsfater and colleagues found that early treatment of tibial shaft fractures in children resulted in fewer cases of osteomyelitis when compared to those treated later.[37] As a counterpoint, data from our institution demonstrated no difference in infection or nonunion rates with delayed debridement in 390 open fractures of the lower extremities in adults.[38] Additionally, in a study of 554 pediatric open fractures, there was no difference in infection rates when debridement was within 6 hours of injury as compared to seven to 24 hours.[39] There is no consensus on the effect of delayed operative treatment of open fractures in regards to rates of infection and need for secondary surgical procedures to promote bone healing.[32,39–45] Our practice is to debride open fractures within 24 hours of presentation and more urgently if there is severe contamination.

Push and riding lawn mowers produce complex wounds and open fractures in children with an annual incidence of approximately 11 per 100,000.[46] These injuries frequently require serial debridement, internal or external fixation, and reconstruction of soft tissue defects. Unfortunately, amputation is often needed.

FRACTURES OF THE LOWER EXTREMITY

Due to the high energy required, fractures of the pelvis and proximal femur are rare but serious injuries in children. Approximately two-thirds of patients with pelvic fractures have associated injuries, and approximately one-third have residual, long-term morbidity.[47,48] Pelvic fractures rank second to head injuries in terms of complications, including life-threatening visceral injuries. The mortality rate of pelvic fractures is between 9–18%.[47] Children with multiple injuries should be checked carefully to exclude fractures of the pelvis. Some common findings of fractures of the pelvis are the presence of a hematoma beneath the inguinal ligament (Desot sign); decreased distance between the greater trochanter and anterior superior iliac spine on the affected side in lateral compression injuries (Roux sign); the presence of a bony prominence or hematoma on rectal exam (Earl sign). An anteroposterior pelvis radiograph is usually sufficient as the initial screening study, although increasingly these injuries are diagnosed by computed tomography (CT) as part of the initial trauma evaluation.[49] Most pediatric pelvic fractures, even those in which the pelvic ring is disrupted, can be treated nonoperatively with good outcomes.[48]

Fractures of the femoral neck are serious injuries that typically require operative treatment.[50–59] Osteonecrosis caused by disruption of the blood supply to the femoral epiphysis is a dreaded complication of this fracture that occurs in up to 75% of children after this injury.[50–55,59–62] The risk of developing osteonecrosis correlates with a higher anatomic location of the fracture in the femoral neck, extent of displacement, and delay in reducing the fracture. Accordingly, fractures and dislocations of the proximal femur are orthopedic emergencies. They require immediate anatomic reduction, which may be achieved by closed or open techniques, and internal fixation (Fig. 18-2).[52,56,59,63–66]

Femoral shaft fractures are common injuries in children. The incidence and mechanism of these fractures varies with patient age and gender. Child abuse accounts for up to 67% of femur fractures in children younger than age 1, but only 11% of fractures in children between ages 1 and 2 years old.[67–69] Classic teaching states that spiral fractures in preambulatory children are pathognomonic for abuse. However, studies have demonstrated that any fracture pattern can occur as the result of abuse.[68] Falls are the leading cause of femur fractures in children age 2 to 3 years, and MVAs are the most common cause in older children.[67] Although bleeding following a femur fracture can be fairly extensive, transfusion in isolated, closed injuries is rarely needed. Therefore, other causes of blood loss must be considered if there is hemodynamic instability or a falling hematocrit at 24 hours after injury in a patient with a femur fracture, especially in the setting of multiple trauma.[70]

Treatment of femur fractures also varies with age.[69] Younger children (<4 to 5 years) are usually treated nonoperatively by closed reduction and immediate spica cast immobilization.[71–74] Older children (4 to 10 years) are managed with flexible nails[75–82] or plates.[83–85] Adolescents (>10 years or >100 pounds) may be treated as adults with solid, reamed, femoral nails, which should be introduced through the tip of the greater trochanter rather than through the piriformis fossa to avoid injury to the vascular supply to the femoral head (Fig. 18-3). A recent review of rigid nails for older children and adolescents noted no cases of osteonecrosis with nail entry via the lateral aspect of the greater trochanter.[86] In contrast to adults, the timing of femur fracture stabilization in children, even in the setting of multiple trauma, does not appear to have an effect on the development of pulmonary complications.[87] The implications are that operation can be deferred until the general medical condition of the child permits, with the caveat that expeditious stabilization of femur (as well as other long bone) fracture(s) will facilitate mobilization and nursing care in the overall management of the child.

Knee injuries in children differ from those in adults. In children, the cartilage of the physes, apophyses, menisci, and articular surface are weaker than the knee ligaments and are thus more prone to injury.[88] Therefore, fractures about the knee occur more commonly than ligamentous injuries in skeletally immature individuals.[89] The distal femoral physis is the largest and fastest growing physis. It is often injured as a result of a direct blow and is a common injury in American football players. Most fractures are Salter Harris type I or II injuries. These

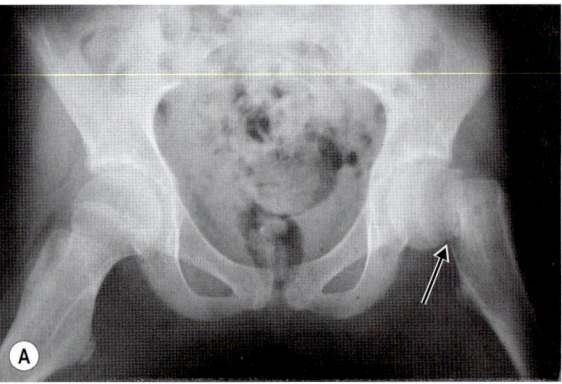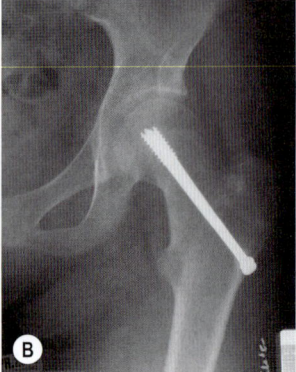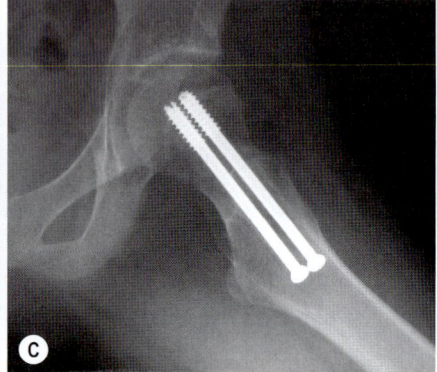

FIGURE 18-2 ■ **(A)** Anteroposterior radiograph of the pelvis of a 12-year-old female injured from a fall showing a displaced transcervical fracture of the left femoral neck (arrow). The fracture was treated emergently by closed reduction and internal fixation with two cannulated screws. **(B,C)** Radiographs one year later show healing of the fracture and no evidence of osteonecrosis.

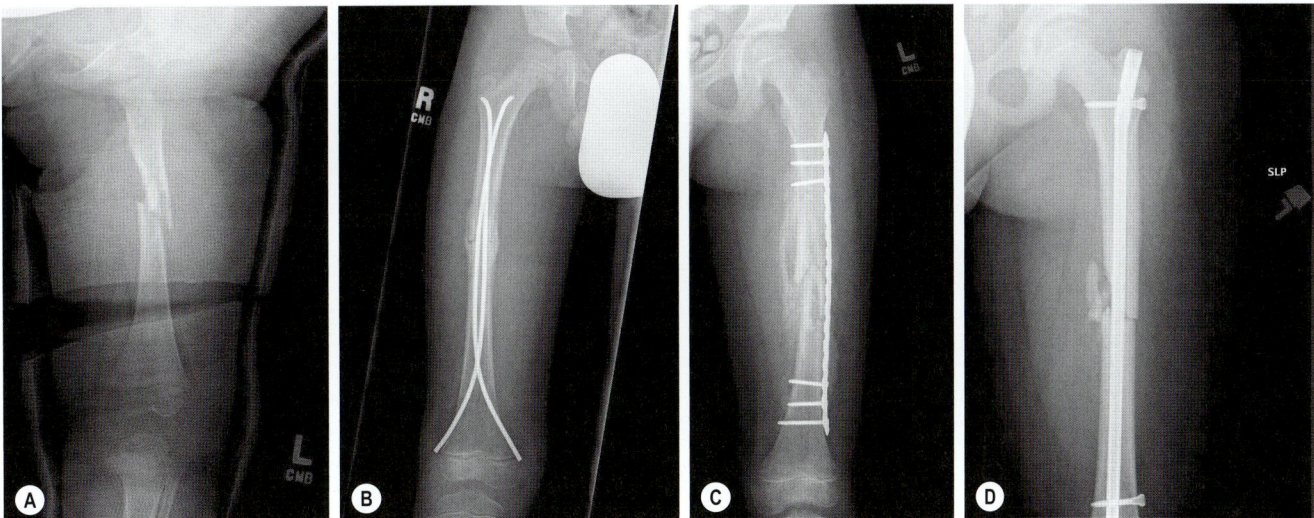

FIGURE 18-3 ■ Four methods for treatment of femoral shaft fractures in children and adolescents are shown: **(A)** spica cast in a 24-month-old; **(B)** flexible intramedullary nails in a 7-year-old; **(C)** submuscular plating in an 8-year-old with severe head injury; **(D)** rigid locked intramedullary nail in an 11-year-old.

fractures can usually be treated by closed reduction and percutaneous, cross-pin stabilization. Fractures extending into the articular surface (type III and IV injuries) require open reduction and internal fixation if displacement of the articular surface is greater than 2 mm. Because of the size of this growth plate, its complex, undulating anatomy, and the forces required for displacement, fractures of the distal femoral physis, even type I and II injuries, may result in permanent growth disturbance in up to 50% of cases.[90] All of these fractures should be followed for a minimum of 1 year to evaluate for sequelae of growth arrest.

Proximal tibial physeal injuries are uncommon due to the reinforcement provided by the knee joint capsular attachments and collateral ligaments. Vascular compromise of the lower leg due to popliteal artery injury is possible, particularly with extension-type injuries in which the proximal portion of the tibial metaphysis is displaced posteriorly. Such injuries tent the popliteal artery at the level of the physis and proximal to the trifurcation, where it is relatively tethered by the peroneal branch as it courses thru the fascia entering the anterior compartment of the leg (Fig. 18-4). Close attention to the vascular examination of the lower extremity is critical following injuries to the proximal tibia. Intra-articular knee injuries typically present with a hemarthrosis and include patellar fractures or dislocations, tibial spine/ plateau fractures, osteochondral fractures, and ligamentous/meniscal injuries. These injuries are typically not emergencies and can be splinted with delayed definitive treatment.

Nonphyseal fractures of the tibia and fibula are among the most common injuries involving the lower extremity in children.[91,92] Fortunately, most of these injuries are low energy and can be treated nonoperatively. However, one must always be cognizant of the possibility of compartment syndrome following closed or open fractures of the tibial shaft.[93] Indications for operative treatment of tibial shaft fractures include: open fractures, neurovascular

injury, impending compartment syndrome, unacceptable alignment following closed reduction, and fractures occurring in the setting of multiple trauma.

Ankle fractures are typically caused by indirect, torsional forces. Injuries to the distal tibial and fibular physes account for 25% to 38% of all children's physeal injuries.[94,95] Sports injuries account for up to 60% of physeal fractures about the ankle.[96] Nonoperative management has historically been the preferred approach, except for intra-articular fractures and those unable to be adequately reduced by closed techniques. Newer data suggests improved results with open reduction of distal tibial physeal injuries.[26] CT is very useful in defining the patho-anatomy of fractures with intra-articular involvement or unusual patterns, and is useful in making management decisions and in preoperative planning.[97] Foot fractures are uncommon and most can be treated nonoperatively with immobilization and restricted weight bearing. More complex problems that require operative intervention include fractures of the talar neck and calcaneus, fractures or dislocations of the tarsometatarsal (Lisfranc) joint, open fractures, and lawn mower injuries.[97]

SPINE INJURIES

Cervical Spine Injuries

Cervical spine injuries in children are relatively uncommon but potentially catastrophic. Accurate diagnosis requires an awareness of the injury patterns, anatomic characteristics, and radiographic variants of the immature cervical spine.[98] These injuries account for approximately 1% of all pediatric fractures and only 2% of all spine fractures.[99–101] Pediatric cervical spine injuries are fundamentally different from their adult counterparts due to the anatomic characteristics of the immature spine and, and to a lesser extent, the differences in the mechanisms of injury.[102] The cervical spine in children is

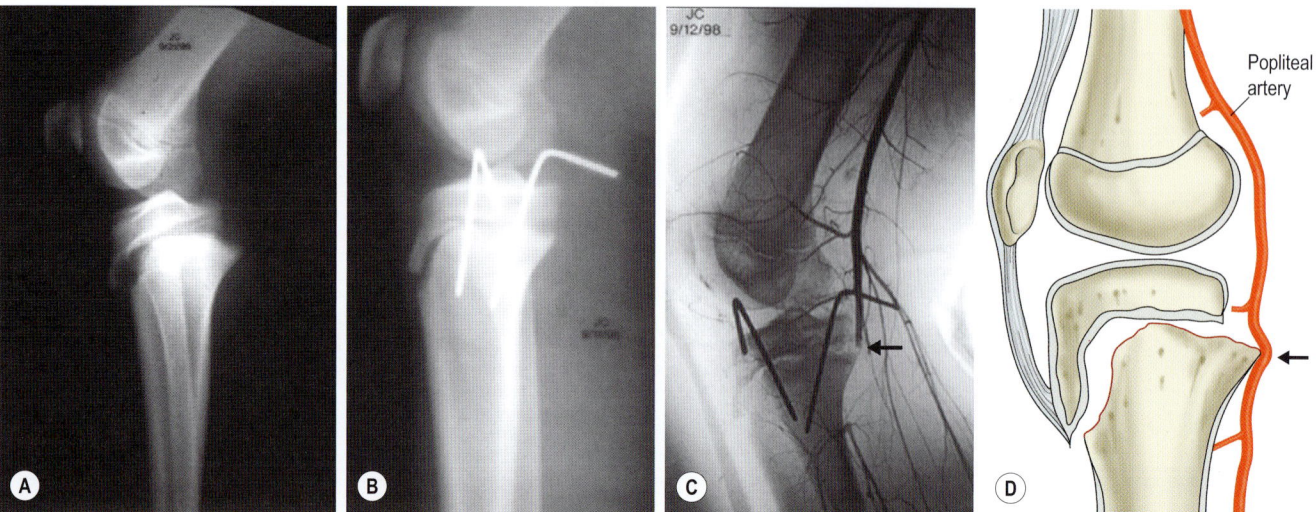

FIGURE 18-4 ■ **(A)** Anteroposterior and lateral radiographs of a 13-year-old male showing a Salter Harris type I fracture of the proximal tibial physis with posterior displacement of the distal fragment following an extension-type injury. **(B)** Distal pulses were diminished prior to and following closed reduction and stabilization of the fracture. **(C)** Arteriogram shows occlusion of the popliteal artery (arrow) at the level of the fracture. Vascular repair with an interposition graft was performed successfully. **(D)** Drawing shows the relationship of the popliteal artery to the proximal tibial physis and mechanism of vascular injury (arrow) in this fracture. (D, Adapted from Zionts LE: Fractures and Dislocations about the Knee. In Green NE, Swiontkowski MF [eds]: Skeletal Trauma in Children, 3rd Edition. Philadelphia, Saunders, 2003. 3:460)

inherently mobile because of the presence of generalized laxity of the interspinous ligaments and joint capsules, underdeveloped neck musculature, thick cartilaginous end plates, incomplete vertebral ossification (wedge-shaped vertebral bodies), and shallow-angled facet joints, particularly between the occiput and C4.[102]

In infants and young children, injuries to the upper cervical spine (above C3) predominate because the head is disproportionately large and creates a large bending moment in the upper cervical spine. In an 11-year experience with 122 pediatric neck injuries, none of the 21 patients age 8 years or less had evidence of injury below C3.[103] Also, multiple level spinal injuries are common, occurring in approximately 25% of children with cervical spine fractures.[103–106] Spinal cord injury without radiographic abnormality (SCIWORA) occurs more frequently in children than in adults.[100,102] After age 8 to 10 years, the anatomical and biomechanical characteristics of the cervical spine are more like an adult, and injuries to the cervical spine are much more likely to occur in the subaxial region (below C3). Evaluation and treatment of these injuries is essentially the same as in an adult.[98,100,102,107]

Mechanisms of injury vary somewhat with age. In neonates, birth trauma is the most common cause of cervical spine injury and occult spinal cord injury has been demonstrated at necropsy in 30% to 50% of stillborns. Excessive distraction and/or hyperextension of the cervical spine are thought to be the most common mechanisms of injury, and may be associated with abnormal intrauterine position (transverse lie) or a difficult cephalic or breech delivery.[108,109] In infants and young children, nonaccidental trauma is a significant cause of injury to the cervical spine. Avulsion fractures of the spinous processes, fractures of the pars or pedicles (most commonly C2), or compression fractures of multiple vertebral bodies are the most common patterns of injury and are thought to result from severe shaking or battering.[110,111] These

injuries may be associated with other signs of nonaccidental trauma including fractures of the skull, rib, or long bones, and superficial ecchymoses. In older children (up to about age 10), the most common causes are pedestrian-MVAs and falls. In children over 10 years of age, the most common etiologies are passenger-related MVAs, sports-related injuries, and diving accidents.

Appropriate methods of immobilizing children for transport and proper clinical and radiographic evaluation are crucial to avoid detrimental outcomes. The goal of immobilization during transport of the injured child with potential spine trauma is to avoid excessive angulation of the spinal column so as to avoid causing or exacerbating spinal cord injury. Immobilization of children less than 8 years of age on a standard spine board during emergency transportation will cause excessive flexion of the cervical spine due to the disproportionately large diameter of the head relative to the torso. It has been recommended that the child's spine board be modified by building up the area under the torso with padding to allow the head to fall back slightly or cutting out the area under the occiput to recess the skull (Fig. 18-5).[112] In addition to proper spine-board immobilization, an appropriately fitting cervical collar is necessary to achieve neutral alignment of the cervical spine after injury.[113]

Clinical evaluation of a child suspected of having an injury to the cervical spine is often hampered by an inability to obtain an accurate history and the unreliability of the physical examination.[98,100,107,114–116] Historically, overt or occult injury to the cervical spine is more likely to occur as a result of falls from a height of more than four feet, pedestrian or cyclist MVAs, and unrestrained occupant MVAs. Head or facial trauma, altered mental status and/or loss of consciousness are also risk factors. Neck pain, guarding, and torticollis are the most reliable signs of an injury to the cervical spine in children. Extremity weakness, sensory changes, bowel and bladder

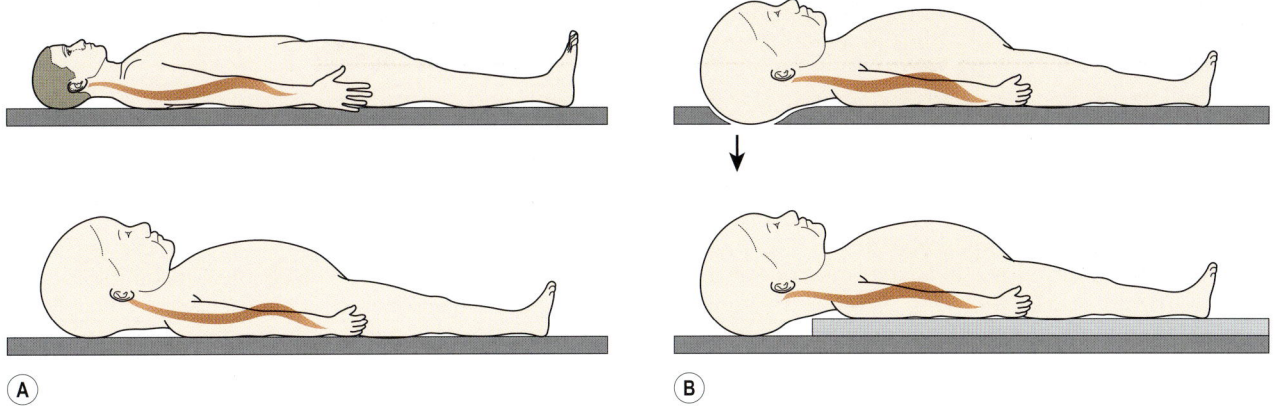

FIGURE 18-5 ■ **(A)** Drawings of an adult and a child on a normal spine board contrasting the differences in position of the head and neck during emergency transport. Because of the disproportionate head-to-body ratio in children, the child's cervical spine is flexed. **(B)** Two methods of modifying the traditional spine board for pediatric patient transport are shown. In the upper illustration, a cutout in the board allows the occiput to be recessed. In the lower illustration, the area under the thorax is built up with padding. Both methods effectively allow the head to translate posteriorly, creating more normal alignment of the cervical spine. (Adapted from Herzenberg JE, Hensiger RN, Dedrick DK. Emergency transport and positioning of young children who have an injury to the cervical spine. J Bone Joint Surg Am 1989;71:15–21.)

dysfunction, and, less frequently, headaches, seizures, syncope, and respiratory distress are signs of injury to the spinal cord.[98,99,104,117–126] When these conditions present, the cervical spine should be immobilized until imaging studies can be completed and the spine cleared.[98]

Radiographic evaluation of the cervical spine in children is hampered by the presence of normal anatomic variants that can be mistaken for trauma. Synchondroses and incompletely ossified, wedged-shaped vertebral bodies can simulate fractures.[127–130] Anterior angulation of the odontoid is a normal variant in approximately 5% of children and may be mistaken for a Salter Harris type I fracture of the dens. Physiologic subluxation of C2 on C3 or C3 on C4 of up to 3 mm is a normal variant (pseudo-subluxation) in about 40% of children younger than age 8 years and is often misinterpreted as pathologic instability.[129,131] Focal kyphosis of the mid-cervical spine is a normal variant in about 15% of children under age 16 years that can also be misinterpreted as pathologic.

Initial radiographic evaluation should include cross-table lateral and anteroposterior radiographs. On the lateral view, it is essential to see the C7–T1 disc space. Oblique radiographs provide detail of the pedicles and facet joints.[127] Open mouth odontoid radiographs are technically difficult to perform and rarely helpful.[132] CT is a much better way to image the upper cervical spine and also provides excellent definition of known fractures, confirmation of suspicious areas, and excellent visualization of the cervicothoracic level, which can be difficult to adequately image on plain radiography. CT has been shown to be more efficacious than conventional images in evaluating the cervical spine in adult and pediatric trauma and to lower institutional costs and complications in urban trauma centers.[124,133,134] Magnetic resonance imaging (MRI) is the preferred study to evaluate the spinal cord and soft tissue structures including ligaments, cartilage, and intervertebral discs.

Once a cervical collar has been placed on a child or the neck immobilized, either at the scene of an accident or in the emergency department, formal clearance of the cervical spine is necessary before immobilization is discontinued.[115] In general, the cervical spine may be cleared based on clinical examination alone if the child is awake, alert, and cooperative; if there are no signs of cervical injury; and if the mechanism of injury is not consistent with cervical trauma.[98,115] For children under age 8 to 10 years who are obtunded or otherwise unable to be examined, and all those with a profile suggestive of injury to the cervical spine, clearance may be based on a five-view cervical spine radiographic series, consisting of antero-posterior, lateral, open mouth odontoid, and two oblique views, and a CT of the axial region of the spine, from occiput to C2. In a study at our institution in which this protocol was followed, eight of 112 children were diagnosed with cervical spine injuries. Two of six children with bony injuries (33%) were diagnosed only by CT scan. No injuries were missed and cervical immobilization was discontinued in a timely fashion.[135] The rationale for CT include the predisposition for injuries to occur in the upper cervical region in children younger than 8 years old and the technical difficulty imaging this area with plain radiographs.[98] In a subsequent study from our institution, helical CT was shown to be have higher specificity, sensitivity and negative predictive value than conventional radiographs in evaluating the cervical spine in children with blunt trauma.[134]

Others have advocated for the definitive role of MRI, particularly in identifying soft tissue injury.[136–138] In a study of 79 children, MRI revealed injuries in 15 patients with normal radiographs and excluded injuries suspected on plain radiographs and CT scans in 7 and 2 patients, respectively. In 25 obtunded or uncooperative children, MRI demonstrated three with significant injuries.[136]

Halo vest immobilization is being used with increasing frequency in children with cervical spine injuries. It affords superior immobilization to a rigid cervical collar and is easier to apply and more versatile than a Minerva cast. It permits access for skin and wound care while avoiding the skin problems (maceration, ulceration) typically associated with both hard collars and casts. However, complication rates up to 70% have been reported with use of halo vests in children.[139] Pin site infections are the most common problems, but skull perforation, cerebrospinal fluid leaks, and brain abscesses have also been described.[107,139] In children younger than age 6 years, a CT scan of the skull to measure calvarial thickness can be helpful in determining optimal sites for pin placement.[140] In children older than 6 years, the standard adult halo construct utilizing four pins (two anterolaterally, two posterolaterally) inserted at standard torques of 6–8 inch-pounds generally works well (Fig. 18-6A). In younger children, more pins (up to 12) placed with lower insertional torques (2–4 inch-pounds) have been advocated (Fig. 18-6B) .[139,140] Standard pediatric halo rings fit most children, but infants and toddlers may require custom rings. Although standard pediatric halo vests are available, custom vests or body casts generally provide better immobilization.[141]

The possibility of SCIWORA should be considered in children, particularly in those younger than 8 years old. SCIWORA is defined as spinal cord injury in a patient in whom there is no visible fracture on plain radiographs or CT scan.[142–145] MRI may be diagnostic in demonstrating spinal cord edema or hemorrhage, soft tissue or ligamentous injury, or apophyseal or disc disruption, but is completely normal in approximately 25% of cases. SCIWORA is the cause of paralysis in approximately 20–30% of children with injuries of the spinal cord. Potential mechanisms of SCIWORA include hyperextension of the cervical spine, which can cause compression of the spinal cord by the ligamentum flavum, followed by flexion, which can cause longitudinal traction. Other mechanisms include transient subluxation without gross failure or unrecognized cartilaginous end plate failure (Salter Harris type I fracture).

Regardless of the specific mechanism, injury to the spinal cord occurs because of the variable elasticity of the elements of the spinal column in children.[146] Experimentally, it has been shown that the bone, cartilage and soft tissue in the spinal column can stretch about two inches without disruption but that the spinal cord ruptures after one-quarter inch.[109,145,147] Spinal cord injury occurs when deformation of the musculoskeletal structures of the spinal column exceeds the physiologic limits of the spinal cord.[146] Injury may be complete or incomplete and may occur at more than one level.[148] Partial spinal cord syndromes reported in SCIWORA include Brown–Sequard, anterior, and central cord syndromes, as well as mixed patterns of injury.[142–144,146]

Prognosis following SCIWORA is correlated to MRI findings, if any are present, and to the severity of neurological injury.[142–144,149] Effective management demands careful evaluation of the cervical spine to exclude osseous or cartilaginous injury or mechanical instability. In addition, immobilization with a rigid cervical collar for two to three months has been recommended to prevent recurrent injury.[142–145] However, the need for prolonged immobilization in the absence of radiographic or MRI evidence of instability has been challenged. In a 34-year review of SCIWORA at a single institution, recurrent injury was uncommon and of uncertain etiology. Immobilization did not prevent recurrent symptoms or improve outcomes. A full recovery occurred in all cases of recurrent SCIWORA.[149] Surgery is occasionally necessary for unstable injury patterns. The prevalence of scoliosis following infantile quadriplegia is over 90%. Therefore, long-term follow-up is necessary to monitor for vertebral column deformity. Administration of high-dose corticosteroids within the first eight hours of spinal cord injury has been shown to improve the chances of neurologic recovery in adults.[150–153] According to guidelines from the third National Acute Spinal Cord Injury Study (NASCIS), when treatment is initiated within 3 hours of injury, methylprednisolone should be administered as an intravenous bolus of 30 mg/kg over 15 minutes followed by a continuous infusion of 5.4 mg/kg/h over the next 23 hours. Also, if treatment cannot be started until more than 3 to 8 hours after injury, the corticosteroids should be given for 48 hours. After 8 hours, there is no benefit and corticosteroids should not be administered.[152,153] As the effect on younger children (<13 years old) is not known, this protocol is not universally followed at all institutions.

Thoracic, Lumbar, and Sacral Fractures

Thoracic, lumbar and sacral fractures are also relatively uncommon in children. MVAs or falls causes the majority

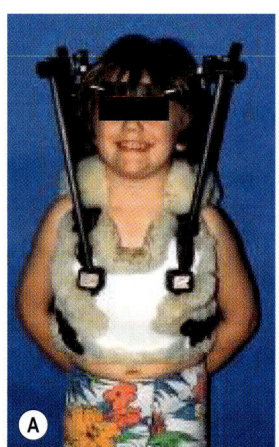
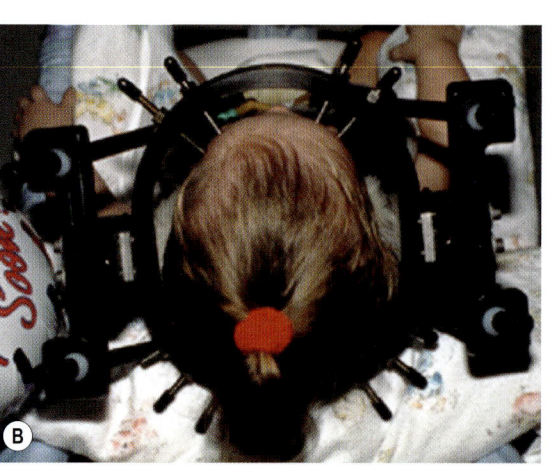

FIGURE 18-6 ■ **(A)** A 6-year-old child immobilized in standard halo construct with four pins (two anterolateral, two posterolateral) inserted at torques of 6 to 8 inch-pounds. **(B)** A 3-year-old child with halo ring with ten pins inserted at low torque, in contrast to the usual four-pin configuration used in older children and adults. (Adapted from Weiser ER, Mencio GA. Pediatric cervical spine injuries: Assessment and treatment. Semin Spine Surg 2001;13:142–51.)

of these injuries. Child abuse should be considered in younger children.[120,154–158] The most common injuries are compression fractures and flexion–distraction injuries. Compression fractures are caused by a combination of hyperflexion and axial compression. Because the disc in children is stronger than cancellous bone, the vertebral body is the first structure to fail. It is common for children to sustain multiple compression fractures. Compression rarely exceeds more than 20% of the vertebral body. In the multiply injured patient, CT has become the preferred imaging modality to diagnose and characterize these fractures.[49,159] These fractures are managed conservatively with rest, analgesics and bracing.[158]

Flexion/distraction injuries (seat-belt injuries) occur in the upper lumbar spine in children wearing a lap belt.[160–168] With sudden deceleration, the seat belt slides up on the abdomen where it provides an axis about which the spine rotates. As a result, the torso is forcibly flexed and the spinal column fails in tension, resulting primarily in disruption of the posterior column with variable patterns of extension into the middle and anterior columns (Chance fracture). These injuries may be missed on axial CT because of the transverse plane of orientation of the fracture. Widening of the interspinous distance on a lateral radiograph or CT with sagittal reconstruction are the most helpful studies in diagnosing this fracture (Fig. 18-7). Approximately two-thirds of patients have injury to a hollow viscus, a solid organ injury, or even injury to the abdominal aorta. These injuries often result in greater morbidity than the spine fracture and may be life-threatening, particularly if unrecognized initially.[165,169,170] Fortunately, neurologic injury is unusual. Lap belt injuries with mostly bony involvement and kyphosis less than 20° can be treated with hyperextension casting. Those with posterior ligamentous disruption and significant intra-abdominal injury require surgical stabilization with compression instrumentation and posterior arthrodesis.

Fracture–dislocations of the spine are unstable injuries that usually occur at the thoracolumbar junction and often are associated with neurologic deficits. These are

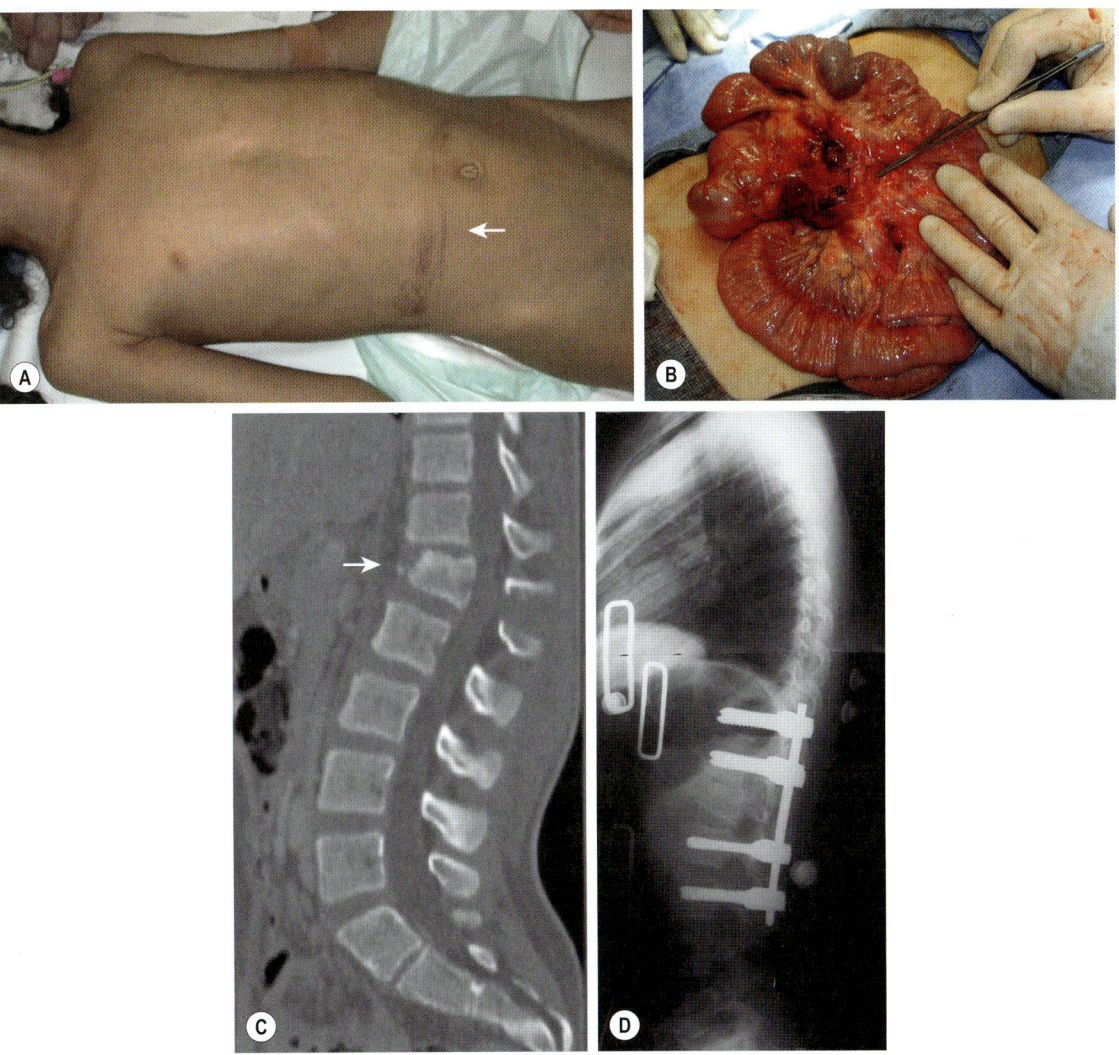

FIGURE 18-7 ■ **(A)** A 12-year-old female involved in a motor vehicle accident with ecchymosis (arrow) in the lower abdomen caused by the lap belt portion of a three-point restraint. **(B)** This child had a laceration of the mesentery discovered at laparotomy and a **(C,D)** flexion–distraction fracture of L1 (arrow) with disruption of all three columns of the spine that required operative stabilization.

rare injuries in children and require surgical stabilization and fusion. Burst fractures are also rare injuries in children that result from axial compression, and typically occur at the thoracolumbar junction or in the lumbar spine.[171] The need for operative treatment is determined by the stability of the fracture and the presence of neurologic deficits. Fractures of the sacrum are usually associated with pelvic fractures. Fractures that involve the sacral foramina or central sacral canal are associated with neurologic deficits in 28% and 50% of patients, respectively. Decompression of the sacral nerve root(s) and stabilization of the sacral fracture may be necessary to improve neurologic function. In most instances, however, fractures of the sacrum may be treated nonoperatively.

FRACTURES OF THE UPPER EXTREMITY

Fractures of the clavicle are common injuries. Clavicle shaft fractures in children are usually uncomplicated and require little, if any, treatment other than sling immobilization for comfort. Enthusiasm for internal fixation of clavicle fractures in adults has increased due to studies that have documented greater rates of nonunion, symptomatic malunion, and residual shoulder disability with nonoperative management.[172–176] In 2007, a prospective randomized trial of 132 patients with clavicle fractures aged 16 to 60 years demonstrated that internal fixation produced better outcome scores, earlier union, reduced rate of nonunions, and no malunions in comparison to nonoperative management.[177] Internal fixation of adolescent clavicle fractures remains controversial, and accepted indications include open fractures and skin compromise. Relative indications in older adolescents include multiple trauma, floating shoulder injuries, comminuted fractures, and shortened fractures. Distal clavicular fractures in the immature child may mimic acromioclavicular separation. The periosteal sleeve of the distal clavicle remains intact with the coracoclavicular ligaments attached.[23,178–180] This fracture heals rapidly and requires no treatment other than sling immobilization for comfort.

Injuries to the medial end of the clavicle are rare but potentially problematic from the standpoint of recognition and neurovascular complications. The physis of the medial clavicle is the last to close, and frequently not until after age 21.[23,180,181] The so-called 'dislocation of the sternoclavicular joint' is almost always a type I physeal fracture in children and adolescents. This injury may occur as a result of direct or indirect trauma to the shoulder. Pain and swelling is localized to the sternoclavicular joint and the shoulder is usually held forward. Although uncommon, compression of the mediastinal structures is the most devastating complication of this injury. Without treatment, the most frequent problem associated with persistent posterior displacement is dysphagia.

Diagnosis of the injury requires awareness of the injury and a CT to confirm the diagnosis. Radiographs may show the posterior dislocation, but it is most clearly seen on CT (Fig. 18-8). Closed reduction may be attempted under general anesthesia, however recurrent displacement is common.[180,182–184] When open reduction is necessary, internal fixation with large, nonabsorbable

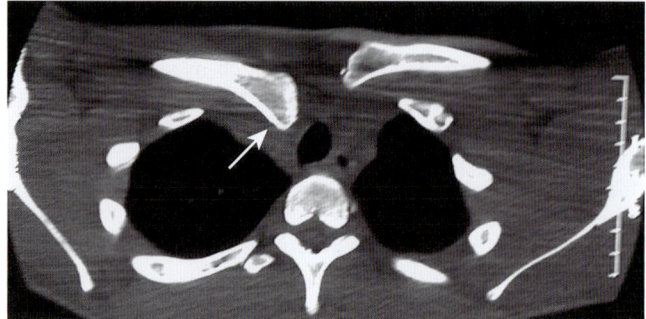

FIGURE 18-8 ■ A 16-year-old male injured his right clavicle when he was checked into the board while playing hockey. He complained of difficulty swallowing. Anteroposterior radiograph of the right clavicle appeared normal. CT scan with thin cuts through the sternoclavicular joint shows posterior displacement (arrow) of the medial end of the clavicle.

suture through the thick periosteal sleeve is usually sufficient. Smooth pins should be avoided because of the risk of migration. Open reduction should be performed in conjunction with a general, vascular or thoracic surgeon assisting or available in the event of unrecognized or iatrogenic injury of the great vessels.

Fractures about the proximal humerus can usually be treated nonoperatively. In all age groups, the tremendous arc of motion in the shoulder joint allows a fairly large margin for fracture alignment. In the younger child, the rapid growth of the proximal humeral physis, which accounts for about 80% of the length of the bone, contributes to rapid and predictable remodeling of all but the most angulated fractures. In these children, no treatment other than immobilization for comfort is necessary.[185,186] Markedly displaced fractures in the teenager, however, may not remodel because there is not sufficient remaining growth.[186–188] Most injuries in this age group are Salter Harris type II fractures, which are usually not stable in addition to being significantly angulated and displaced. These fractures need to be reduced and usually require fixation with percutaneous Steinmann pins or cannulated screws.[189,190]

Fractures about the elbow in children can be difficult to diagnose because the anatomy of the immature elbow is confusing due to the presence of numerous centers of ossification. Knowledge of the sequence of appearance and maturation of the secondary ossification centers is mandatory. A comparison radiograph of the contralateral elbow is often helpful in correctly identifying the nature of the injury.[191]

The most common fracture about the distal humerus in the child is a supracondylar fracture. These fractures are classified according to the amount of displacement. Type III fractures are the most severe, with both fragments completely displaced. The injury usually occurs from a fall on the outstretched hand. In children who are ligamentously lax, the elbow will hyperextend and shear off the distal portion of the humerus through the olecranon fossa.[192]

The major problems with this injury are swelling and nerve and/or vascular injury. In the past, it has been thought that this fracture should be treated immediately.

However, we now recognize that this fracture does not need immediate operative stabilization unless there are other extenuating circumstances, such as vascular injury, compartment syndrome, or an open wound. Currently, the general policy is to delay treatment until the next day. Initially, the elbow is splinted in less than 90° of flexion with a loose bandage over a posterior splint.[193,194] These fractures can usually be reduced by closed manipulation and stabilized by percutaneous pins (Fig. 18-9).

There has long been a controversy as to the treatment of the pulseless extremity in patients who have sustained a supracondylar fracture. Absence of the pulse with this fracture is not uncommon. It is believed that the absence of the pulse may either be the result of vascular spasm and/or direct vascular injury. However, the collateral circulation about the elbow is so rich that the circulation to the forearm and hand usually remains normal. Treatment of the vascular injury has been debated for decades in the orthopedic and vascular surgery literature. The current practice is observation as long as circulation to the hand and forearm is clinically normal.[192,193,195] It has been

shown by follow-up studies that vein grafts of vascular injuries will frequently clot because of the excellent collateral circulation about the elbow.[196] The only true indication for vascular exploration is the pulseless, ischemic extremity which is a true surgical emergency. In this instance, the fracture should be reduced and stabilized with crossed pins before vascular repair.[197,198]

Compartment syndrome is a feared complication that is uncommon in the modern era. Stabilizing the fracture with internal fixation avoids the need to immobilize the elbow in hyperflexion, which has been shown to increase the risk of vascular compression and forearm compartment swelling.[192]

The signs of compartment syndrome are well known, but the main one is pain that is out of proportion to the fracture itself. Once this fracture is stabilized, the child should be comfortable and not have significant pain. Passive extension of the fingers should be possible to a neutral position. If not, it suggests the need for investigation of a compartment syndrome by removal of the splint, palpation of the forearm compartment, and pres-

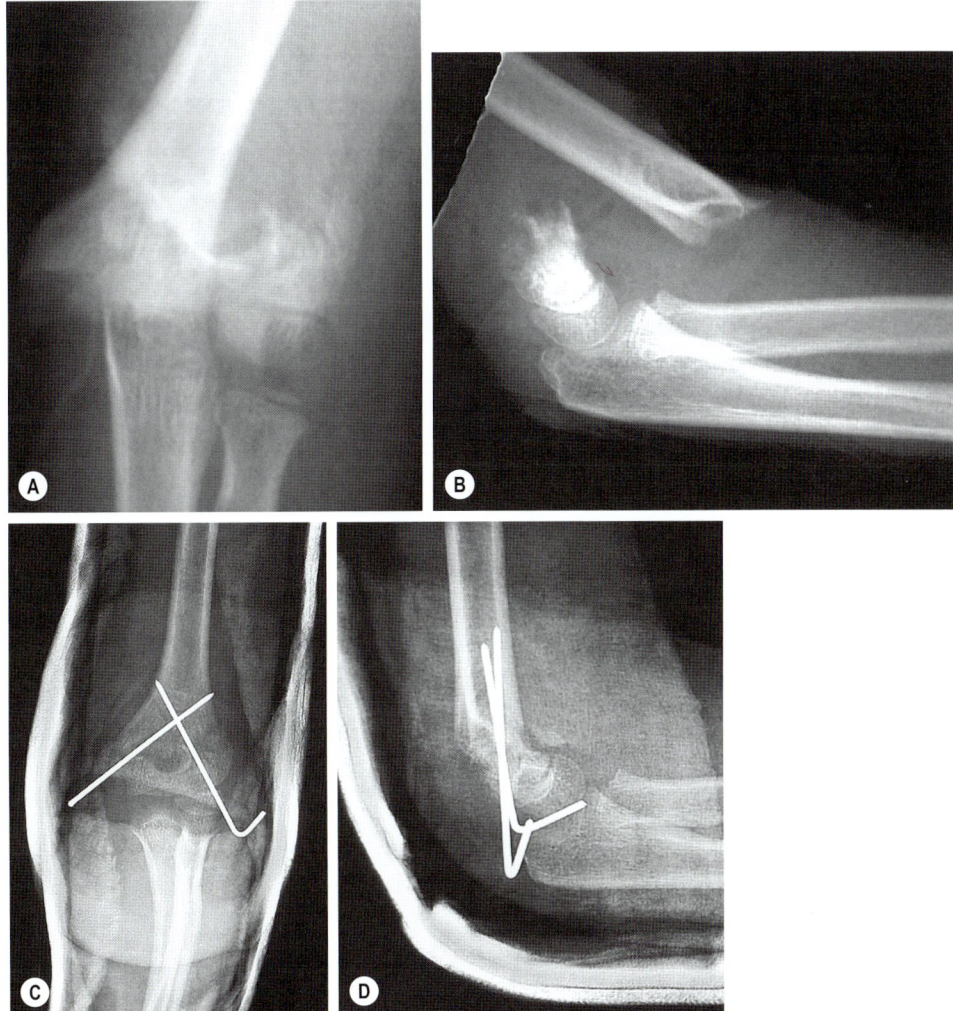

FIGURE 18-9 ■ A 6-year-old fell while horseback riding and landed on his outstretched left arm. **(A)** Anteroposterior and **(B)** lateral radiographs show a completely displaced (type III) supracondylar humerus fracture. Neurovascular status of the extremity was intact. **(C,D)** The child was treated with closed reduction and percutaneous fixation with smooth Steinmann pins.

sure measurements, if necessary. If the pressures are elevated, then fasciotomy should be urgently performed.

Salter Harris type I fractures of the distal humerus are less common than other injuries about the elbow and are frequently misdiagnosed. In very young children, this fracture often occurs as the result of nonaccidental trauma and should trigger investigation into the possibility of abuse.[199] This fracture may also occur in newborns as a result of birth trauma.[192] Unfortunately, especially in instances of nonaccidental trauma, the child is commonly seen a significant time after this injury has already begun to heal, and manipulation of the fracture is either not possible or ill advised (Fig. 18-10).

Fractures of the lateral condyle of the humerus must also be distinguished from the Salter Harris type I fractures of the distal humeral physis (Fig. 18-11). If the condylar fracture is displaced at all, it requires open reduction and pin fixation because the risk of nonunion is high when it is treated nonoperatively. Nonunion will result in a progressive valgus deformity of the elbow with an ulnar nerve palsy.[200–202]

Forearm and wrist fractures have traditionally been treated with closed manipulation and casting. Our preference is to perform closed reduction of these fractures in the emergency department with conscious sedation.[203,204] The use of a portable fluoroscopy unit is essential, both to guide reduction of the fracture and to confirm alignment following immobilization. Use of a mini-C-arm improves reduction quality, decreases need for repeat reduction, and results in less overall radiation exposure.[205] After manipulation of the fracture, the extremity is immobilized in a sugar tong splint that will allow for swelling. When swelling is no longer a concern, the sugar tong splint is incorporated into a long-arm, fiberglass cast. In general, the child should be seen weekly for the first three weeks to be certain that the alignment of the fracture is maintained. After 3 weeks, a short arm cast is applied for another 3 weeks after which progressive use and motion is started.

Fractures of the shaft of both bones of the forearm have a limited range of acceptable residual deformity to avoid loss of motion, particularly in children older than

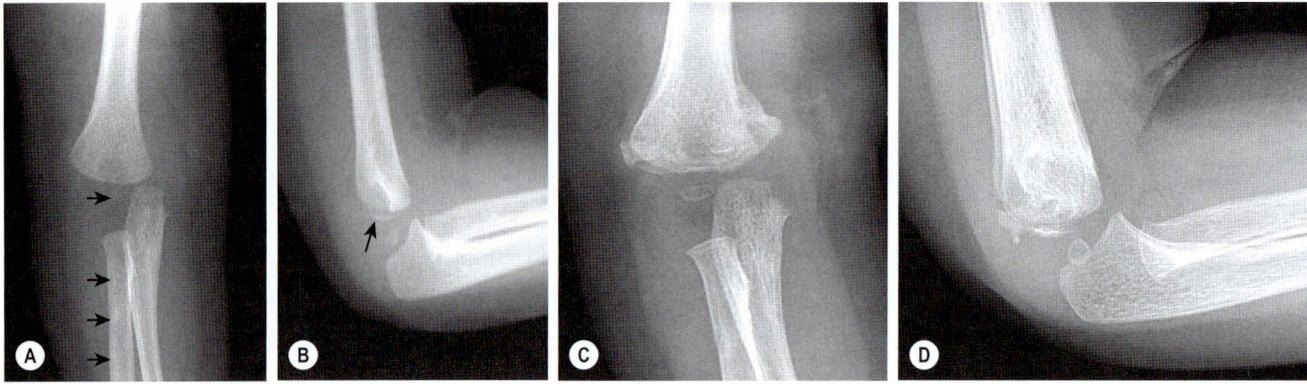

FIGURE 18-10 ■ An 11-month-old infant, ultimately determined to have been the victim of abuse, presented with a swollen arm. **(A)** On the anteroposterior radiograph of the elbow, the capitellum, the proximal radius, and the ulna are displaced from their normal positions relative to the distal humerus (*arrows*), consistent with a fracture-separation of the distal humeral epiphysis. In an elbow dislocation, the radius and ulna are displaced relative to the distal humerus but the capitellum is not displaced from its normal position in the distal humerus. **(B)** The lateral radiograph of the elbow shows a small metaphyseal fragment (*arrow*), also consistent with a fracture of the distal humeral physis and not with dislocation of the elbow. This fracture was treated with cast immobilization. **(C,D)** Note the exuberant fracture callus 3 weeks after the injury.

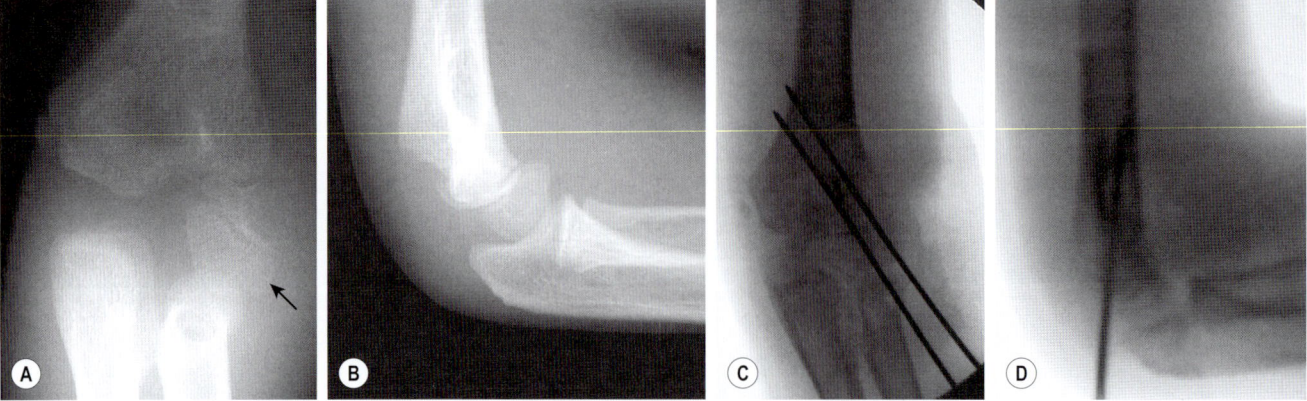

FIGURE 18-11 ■ A 7-year-old child fell from a bunk bed, resulting in a fracture of the lateral condyle of the humerus. **(A)** Anteroposterior and **(B)** lateral radiographs show displacement of the capitellum (*arrow*), whereas the radius and ulna remain aligned with the humerus. Even if they were minimally displaced, the risk of joint incongruity and nonunion is high after nonoperative treatment of this fracture. **(C)** Anteroposterior and **(D)** lateral radiographs of the elbow after open reduction and pin fixation show anatomic alignment.

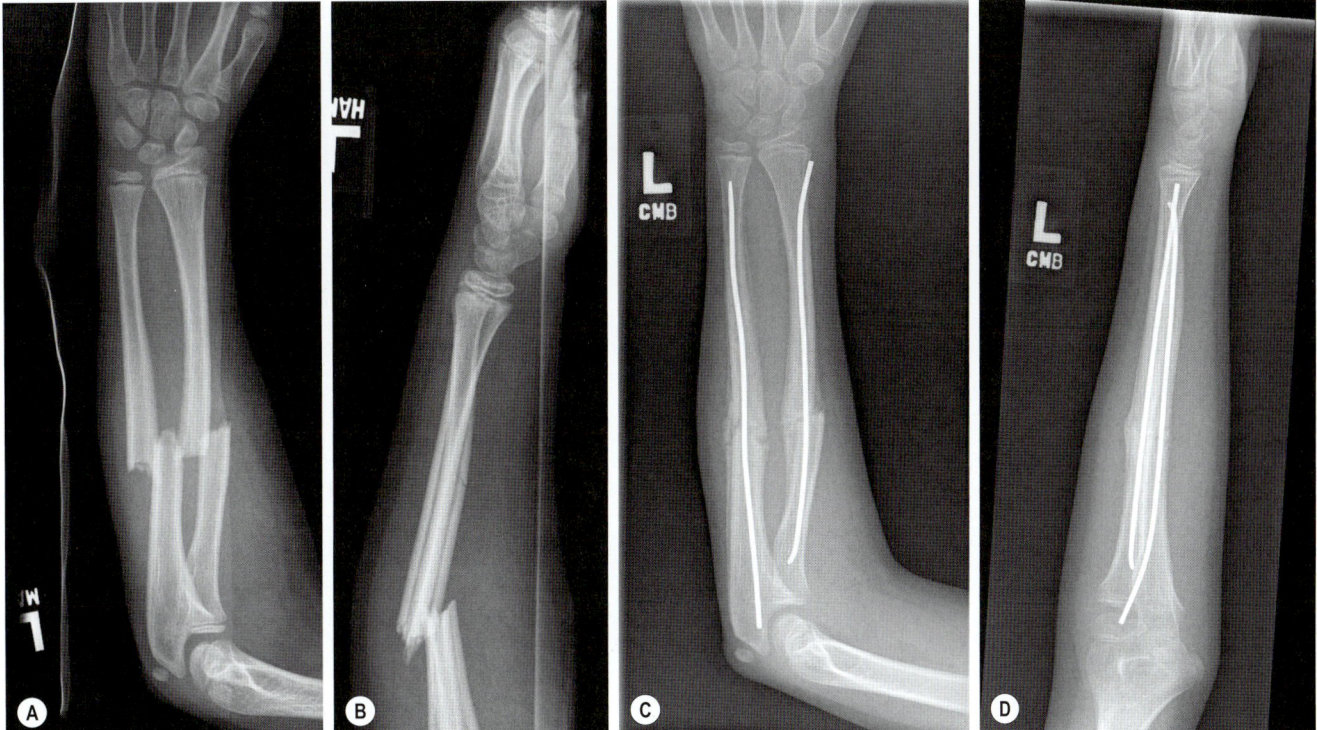

FIGURE 18-12 ■ **(A)** Anteroposterior and **(B)** lateral radiographs show grade 1 open forearm fractures in an 8-year-old. **(C,D)** Following debridement, the fracture was stabilized with flexible titanium nails inserted via 1 cm incisions, distally in the radius and proximally in the ulna, and advanced across the fracture under fluoroscopy.

the age of 8 or 9 years. It may be difficult to maintain reduction of these fractures in a cast or splint. For this reason, fractures of the shafts of the radius and ulna are being treated by internal fixation using flexible titanium nails with increasing frequency.[172,173,176,206–214] These fractures can be reduced by closed manipulation and stabilized by percutaneous insertion of titanium or stainless steel intramedullary nails, although open reduction may be required approximately in 29–44% of closed fractures (Fig. 18-12).[172,173,176]

The vast majority of wrist and hand fractures in children can be managed nonoperatively. Exceptions include open fractures or fractures that cannot be maintained in acceptable rotational or angular alignment. Phalangeal neck fractures are unstable injuries that frequently benefit from pin fixation to prevent malunion with loss of digital motion.

REFERENCES

1. Smith MD, Burrington JD, Woolf AD. Injuries in children sustained in free falls: An analysis of 66 cases. J Trauma 1975;15:987.
2. Starfield B. Childhood Morbidity: Comparisons, Clusters, and Trends. Pediatrics 1991;88:519.
3. Landin LA. Fracture patterns in children. Acta Orthop Scand 1983;54(Suppl. 202):1.
4. Worlock P, Stower M. Fracture patterns in Nottingham children. J Pediatr Orthop 1986;6:656.
5. Ward WT, Rihn JA. The impact of trauma in an urban pediatric orthopaedic practice. J Bone Joint Surg Am 2006;88:2759–64.
6. Tuason D, Hohl JB, Levicoff E, et al. Urban pediatric orthopaedic surgical practice audit: Implications for the future of this subspecialty. J Bone Joint Surg Am 2009;91:2992–8.
7. Cheng JC, Shen WY. Limb fracture pattern in different pediatric age groups: A study of 3350 children. J Orthop Trauma 1993;7:15.
8. Reed MH. Fractures and dislocations of the extremities in children. J Trauma 1977;17:351.
9. Masterson E, Borton D, Foster BK. Victims of our climate. Injury 1993;24:247.
10. Shank LP, Bagg RJ, Wagnon J, editors. Etiology of pediatric fractures: The fatigue factors in children's fractures. Indianapolis: National Conference of Pediatric Trauma; 1992.
11. Westfelt JARN. Environmental factors in childhood accidents: A prospective study in Goteborg, Sweden. Acta Paediatr Scand 1982(Suppl. 291).
12. Izant RJ, Hubay CA. The annual injury of 15,000,000 children: A limited study of childhood accidental injury and death. J Trauma 1966;6:65.
13. Ong ME, Ooi SB, Manning PG. A review of 2,517 childhood injuries seen in a Singapore emergency department in 1999–mechanisms and injury prevention suggestions. Singapore Med J 2003;44:12–19.
14. Wilkins KE. The Incidence of Fractures in Children. In: Rockwood CE Jr, Wilkins KE, Beaty JH, editors. Fractures in Children. Philadelphia: Lippincott-Raven; 1996. p. 1–17.
15. Brownell M, Friesen D, Mayer T. Childhood injury rates in Manitoba: socioeconomic influences. Can J Public Health 2002;93(Suppl 2):S50–6.
16. Johnson CF. Inflicted injury versus accidental injury. Pediatr Clin North Am 1990;37:791–814.
17. Schmitt BD, Gray JD, Britton HL. Child Abuse. In: Green M, Haggerty RJ, editors. Ambulatory. Pediatrics III: W.B. Saunders; 1984.
18. Akbarnia BA, Akbarnia NO. The role of the orthopedist in child abuse and neglect. Orthop Clin North Am 1976;7:733–42.
19. Galleno H, Oppenheim WL. The battered child syndrome revisited. Clin Orthop 1982;62:11–19.
20. O'Connor JF, Cohen J. Dating Fractures. In: Kleinman PK, editor. Diagnostic Imaging of Child Abuse. Baltimore: Williams & Wilkins; 1987. p. 6.
21. Mann DC, Rajmatra S. Distribution of physeal and non-physeal fractures of long bones in children aged 0 to 16 years. J Pediatr Orthop 1990;10:713.
22. Marcus RE, Mills MF, Thompson GH. Multiple injury in children. JBJS 1983;65:1290.

23. Ogden J. Skeletal Injury in the Child. 2nd ed. Philadelphia: Lea & Feibeger; 1990.

24. Ogden J. Complications of Fractures. Philadelphia: J.B. Lippincott; 1995.

25. Salter RB, Harris WR. Injuries involving the epiphyseal plate. JBJS Am 1963;45:587.

26. Barmada A, Gaynor T, Mubarak S. Premature physeal closure following distal tibia physeal fractures: A new radiographic predictor. J Pediatr Orthop 2003;23:733–9.

27. Kling TFJ, Bright RW, Hensinger RN. Distal tibial physeal fractures in children that may require open reduction. J Pediatr Orthop 1984;66:647–57.

28. Spiegel PG, Mast JW, Cooperman DR, et al. Epiphyseal fractures of the distal ends of the tibia and fibula. A retrospective study of two hundred and thirty-seven cases in children. JBJS Am 1978;60:1046–50.

29. Mendez AA, Bartal E, Grillot MB, et al. Compression (Salter Harris type V) physeal fracture: An experimental model in the rat. J Pediatr Orthop 1992;12:29.

30. Wilber JH, Thompson GH. The Multiply Injured Child. In: Green NE, Swiontkowski MF, editors. Skeletal Trauma in Children. 3rd ed. Philadelphia: Saunders; 2003. p. 73–101.

31. Morrison A, Stone DH, Redpath A, et al. Childhood injury mortality in Scotland, 1981-95. Health Bull (Edinb) 1999;57: 241–6.

32. Stewart DG Jr, Kay RM, Skaggs DL. Open fractures in children. Principles of evaluation and management. J Bone Joint Surg Am 2005;87:2784–98.

33. Gustillo R, Mendoza R, Williams D. Problems in the management of type III (severe) open fractures: A new classification of Type III open fractures. J Trauma 1984;24:747–96.

34. Gustilo RB, Anderson JT. Prevention of infection in treatment of 1025 open fractures of long bones: Retrospective and prospective analysis. JBJS Am 1976;58:453–8.

35. Gustilo RB, Merkow RL, Templeman D. Current Concepts Review: The Management of Open Fractures. JBJS Am 1990;72:299–304.

36. Chapman MW. The use of immediate internal fixation in open fractures. Orthop Clin North Am 1980;11:579–91.

37. Kindsfater K, Jonassen EA. Osteomyelitis in grade II and III open tibia fractures with late debridement. J Orthop Trauma 1995;9: 121–7.

38. Rohmiller MT, Kusuma S, Blanchard GM, et al, editors. Management of Open Fractures of the Lower Extremity: Does Time to Debridement and Primary Wound Closure Really Matter? OTA; 2002; Toronto, Ontario, Canada.

39. Skaggs DL, Friend L, Alman B, et al. The effect of surgical delay on acute infection following 554 open fractures in children. J Bone Joint Surg Am 2005;87:8–12.

40. Charalambous CP, Siddique I, Zenios M, et al. Early versus delayed surgical treatment of open tibial fractures: Effect on the rates of infection and need of secondary surgical procedures to promote bone union. Injury 2005;36:656–61.

41. Iobst CA, Tidwell MA, King WF. Nonoperative management of pediatric type I open fractures. J Pediatr Orthop 2005; 25:513–17.

42. Khatod M, Botte MJ, Hoyt DB, et al. Outcomes in open tibia fractures: relationship between delay in treatment and infection. J Trauma 2003;55:949–54.

43. Skaggs DL, Kautz SM, Kay RM, et al. Effect of delay of surgical treatment on rate of infection in open fractures in children. J Pediatr Orthop 2000;20:19–22.

44. Spencer J, Smith A, Woods D. The effect of time delay on infection in open long-bone fractures: a 5-year prospective audit from a district general hospital. Ann R Coll Surg Engl 2004;86: 108–12.

45. Yang EC, Eisler J. Treatment of isolated type I open fractures: is emergent operative debridement necessary? Clin Orthop Relat Res 2003(410):289–94.

46. Vollman D, Smith GA. Epidemiology of lawn-mower-related injuries to children in the United States, 1990-2004. Pediatrics 2006;118:e273–8.

47. Demetriades D, Karaiskakis M, Velmahos GC, et al. Pelvic fractures in pediatric and adult trauma patients: Are they different injuries? J Trauma 2003;54:1146–51; discussion 51.

48. Grisoni N, Connor S, Marsh E, et al. Pelvic fractures in a pediatric level I trauma center. J Orthop Trauma 2002;16:458–63.

49. Stewart BG, Rhea JT, Sheridan RL, et al. Is the screening portable pelvis film clinically useful in multiple trauma patients who will be examined by abdominopelvic CT? Experience with 397 patients. Emerg Radiol 2002;9:266–71.

50. Azouz EM, Karamitsos C. Types and complications of femoral neck fractures in children. Pediatr Radiol 1993;23:415–20.

51. Bagatur AE, Zorer G. Complications associated with surgically treated hip fractures in children. J Pediatr Orthop B 2002;11:219–28.

52. Canale ST. Fractures of the hip in children and adolescents. Orthop Clin North Am 1990;21:341–52.

53. Maeda S, Kita A, Fujii G, et al. Avascular necrosis associated with fractures of the femoral neck in children: Histological evaluation of core biopsies of the femoral head. Injury 2003;34: 283–6.

54. Moon ES, Mehlman CT. Risk factors for avascular necrosis after femoral neck fractures in children: 25 Cincinnati cases and meta-analysis of 360 cases. J Orthop Trauma 2006;20:323–9.

55. Morsy HA. Complications of fracture of the neck of the femur in children. A long-term follow-up study. Injury 2001;32:45–51.

56. Ng GP, Cole WG. Effect of early hip decompression on the frequency of avascular necrosis in children with fractures of the neck of the femur. Injury 1996;26:419–21.

57. Pape H, Krettek C, Friedrich A, et al. Long-term outcome in children with fractures of the proximal femur after high energy trauma. J Trauma 1999;46:58–64.

58. Ratliff A. Fractures of the neck of the femur in children. J Bone Joint Surg Br 1962;44:528–54.

59. Shrader MW, Jacofsky DJ, Stans AA, et al. Femoral neck fractures in pediatric patients: 30 years' experience at a level 1 trauma center. Clin Orthop Relat Res 2007;454:169–73.

60. Mirdad T. Fractures of the neck of femur in children: An experience at the Aseer Central Hospital, Abha, Saudi Arabia. Injury 2002;33:823–7.

61. Theruvil B, Kapoor V. Avascular necrosis associated with fractures of the femoral neck in children: Histological evaluation of core biopsies of the femoral head. Injury 2005;36:230–1.

62. Togrul E, Bayram H, Gulsen M, et al. Fractures of the femoral neck in children: Long-term follow-up in 62 hip fractures. Injury 2005;36:123–30.

63. Dhammi IK, Singh S. Displaced femoral neck fracture in children and adolescents: Closed versus open reduction–a preliminary study. J Orthop Sci 2005;10:173–9.

64. Flynn JM, Wong KL. Displaced fractures of the hip in children. Management by early operation and immobilization in a hip spica cast. J Bone Joint Surg Br 2002;84:108–12.

65. Forster N, Ramseier L. Undisplaced femoral neck fractures in children have a high risk of secondary displacement. J Pediatr Orthop 2006;15:131–3.

66. Song KS, Kim YS, Sohn SW, et al. Arthrotomy and open reduction of the displaced fracture of the femoral neck in children. J Pediatr Orthop B 2001;10:205–10.

67. Nork SE, Bellig GJ, Woll JP, et al. Overgrowth and outcome after femoral shaft fracture in children younger than 2 years. Clin Orthop 1998(357):186–91.

68. Scherl SA, Miller L, Lively N, et al. Accidental and nonaccidental femur fractures in children. Clin Orthop 2000(376):96–105.

69. Solga P. Pediatric femur fractures: Treatment in the year 2007. Med Health R I 2007;90:122–6.

70. Lynch JM, Gardner MJ, Gains B. Hemodynamic significance of pediatric femur fractures. J Pediatr Surg 1996;31:1358–61.

71. Cassinelli EH, Young B, Vogt M, et al. Spica cast application in the emergency room for select pediatric femur fractures. J Orthop Trauma 2005;19:709–16.

72. Czertak DJ, Hennrikus WL. The treatment of pediatric femur fractures with early 90-90 spica casting. J Pediatr Orthop 1999;19:229–32.

73. Hughes BF, Sponseller PD, Thompson JD. Pediatric femur fractures: effects of spica cast treatment on family and community. J Pediatr Orthop 1995;15:457–60.

74. Infante AF Jr, Albert MC, Jennings WB, et al. Immediate hip spica casting for femur fractures in pediatric patients. A review of 175 patients. Clin Orthop Relat Res 2000(376):106–12.

75. Flynn JM, Hresko T, Reynolds RA, et al. Titanium elastic nails for pediatric femur fractures: A multicenter study of early results with analysis of complications. J Pediatr Orthop 2001;21:4–8.

76. Flynn JM, Luedtke L, Ganley TJ, et al. Titanium elastic nails for pediatric femur fractures: Lessons from the learning curve. Am J Orthop 2002;31:71–4.

77. Heinrich SD, Drvaric D, Darr K, et al. Stabilization of pediatric diaphyseal femur fractures with flexible intramedullary nails (a technique paper). J Orthop Trauma 1992;6:452–9.

78. Ho CA, Skaggs DL, Tang CW, et al. Use of flexible intramedullary nails in pediatric femur fractures. J Pediatr Orthop 2006;26:497–504.

79. Kraus R, Schiefer U, Schafer C, et al. Elastic stable intramedullary nailing in pediatric femur and lower leg shaft fractures: Intraoperative radiation load. J Pediatr Orthop 2008;28:14–16.

80. Lee SS, Mahar AT, Newton PO. Ender nail fixation of pediatric femur fractures: A biomechanical analysis. J Pediatr Orthop 2001;21:442–5.

81. Mehlman CT, Nemeth NM, Glos DL. Antegrade versus retrograde titanium elastic nail fixation of pediatric distal-third femoral shaft fractures: A mechanical study. J Orthop Trauma 2006;20:608–12.

82. Sink EL, Gralla J, Repine M. Complications of pediatric femur fractures treated with titanium elastic nails: A comparison of fracture types. J Pediatr Orthop 2005;25:577–80.

83. Hedequist D, Bishop J, Hresko T. Locking plate fixation for pediatric femur fractures. J Pediatr Orthop 2008;28:6–9.

84. Hedequist DJ, Sink E. Technical aspects of bridge plating for pediatric femur fractures. J Orthop Trauma 2005;19:276–9.

85. Kanlic EM, Anglen JO, Smith DG, et al. Advantages of submuscular bridge plating for complex pediatric femur fractures. Clin Orthop Relat Res 2004(426):244–51.

86. MacNeil JA, Francis A, El-Hawary R. A systematic review of rigid, locked, intramedullary nail insertion sites and avascular necrosis of the femoral head in the skeletally immature. J Pediatr Orthop 2011;31:377–80.

87. Hedequist D, Starr AJ, Wilson P, et al. Early versus delayed stabilization of pediatric femur fractures: Analysis of 387 patients. J Orthop Trauma 1999;13:490–3.

88. Zobel MS, Borrello JA, Siegel MJ, et al. Pediatric knee MR imaging: pattern of injuries in the immature skeleton. Radiology 1994;190:397–401.

89. Close BJ, Strouse PJ. MR of physeal fractures of the adolescent knee. Pediatr Radiol 2000;30:756–62.

90. Riseborough EJ, Barrett IR, Shapiro F. Growth disturbances following distal femora physeal fracture-separation. JBJS Am 1983;65:885–93.

91. Karholm J, Hansson LI, Svensonn K. Incidence of tibio-fibular shaft and ankle fractures in children. J Pediatr Orthop 1982;2:386–92.

92. Shannak AO. Tibial fractures in children: Follow-up study. J Pediatr Orthop 1988;8:306–10.

93. Hope PG, Cole WG. Open fractures of the tibia in children. J Bone Joint Surg [Br] 1992;74:546–53.

94. Hynes D, O'Brien T. Growth disturbance lines after injury to the distal tibial physis. J Bone Joint Surg [Br] 1988;70:231.

95. Rogers LF. The radiography of epiphyseal injuries. Radiology 1970;96:289.

96. Goldberg VM, Aadalen R. Distal tibial epiphyseal injuries: The role of athletics in fifty-three cases. Am J Sports Med 1978;6:263.

97. Vanhoenacke FM, Bernaerts A, Gielen J, et al. Trauma of the pediatric ankle and foot. J Bone Joint Surg [Br] 2002;85:212–18.

98. Weiser ER, Mencio GA. Pediatric cervical spine injuries: Assessment and treatment. Semin Spine Surg 2001;13:142–51.

99. Eleraky M, Theodore N, Adams M, et al. Pediatric cervical spine injuries: Report of 102 cases and review of the literature. J Neurosurg 2000;92(1 Suppl):12–17.

100. Jones E, Haid R. Injuries to the pediatric subaxial cervical spine. W.B. Saunders Company; 1991.

101. McGrory B, Klassen R, Chao E, et al. Acute fractures and dislocations of the cervical spine in children and adolescents. J Bone Joint Surg [Am] 1993;75:988–95.

102. Givens T, Polley K, Smith G, et al. Pediatric cervical spine injury: A three-year experience. J Trauma 1996;41:310–14.

103. Hill S, Miller C, Kosnik E. Pediatric neck injuries: A clinical study. J Neurosurg 1984;60:700.

104. Brown RL, Brunn MA, Garcia VF. Cervical spine injuries in children: A review of 103 patients treated consecutively at a level 1 pediatric trauma center. J Pediatr Surg 2001;36:1107–14.

105. Hadden W, Gillespie W. Multiple level injuries of the cervical spine. Injury 1985;16:628–33.

106. Heilman CB, Riesenburger RI. Simultaneous noncontiguous cervical spine injuries in a pediatric patient. Neurosurg 2001;49:1017–20.

107. Jones E, Hensinger R. Injuries of the cervical spine. In: Rockwood W, Beaty, editor. Fractures in Children. Philadelphia: Lippincott-Raven; 1996. p. 1024–62.

108. Bresnam J, Adams F. Neonatal spinal cord transection secondary to intrauterine neck hyperextension in breech presentation. Fatal Neonat Med 1971;84:734.

109. Leventhal H. Birth injuries of the spinal cord. J Pediatr Orthop 1960;56:447–53.

110. Caffey J. The whiplash shaken infant syndrome. Pediatrics 1974;54:396.

111. Swischuck L. Spinal cord trauma in the battered child syndrome. Radiology 1977;92:733.

112. Herzenberg J, Hensiger R, Dedrick D, et al. Emergency transport and positioning of young children who have an injury to the cervical spine. J Bone Joint Surg [Am] 1989;71:15.

113. Curran C, Dietrich A, Bowman M, et al. Pediatric cervical spine immobilization: Achieving neutral position? J Trauma 1995;39:729–32.

114. Jaffe DM, Binns H, Radkowski MA, et al. Developing a clinical algorithm for early management of cervical spine injury in child trauma victims. Ann Emerg Med 1987;16:270–6.

115. Lee SL, Sena M, Greenholz SK, et al. A multidisciplinary approach to the development of a cervical spine clearance protocol: process, rationale, and initial results. J Pediatr Surg 2003;38:358–62; discussion -62.

116. Viccellio P, Simon H, Pressman BD, et al. A prospective multicenter study of cervical spine injury in children. Pediatrics 2001;108:E20.

117. Anderson RC, Kan P, Hansen KW, et al. Cervical spine clearance after trauma in children. Neurosurg Focus 2006;20:E3.

118. Avellino AM, Mann FA, Grady MS, et al. The misdiagnosis of acute cervical spine injuries and fractures in infants and children: The 12-year experience of a level I pediatric and adult trauma center. Childs Nerv Syst 2005;21:122–7.

119. Bayless P, Ray VG. Incidence of cervical spine injuries in association with blunt head trauma. Am J Emerg Med 1989;7:139–42.

120. d'Amato C. Pediatric spinal trauma: Injuries in very young children. Clin Orthop Relat Res 2005(432):34–40.

121. Davis J, Phreaner D, Hoyt D, et al. The etiology of missed cervical spine injuries. J Trauma 1993;34:342–6.

122. Evans D, Bethem D. Cervical spine injuries in children. J Pediatr Orthop 1989;9:563–8.

123. Finch G, Barnes M. Major cervical spine injuries in children and adolescents. J Pediatr Orthop 1998;18:811–14.

124. Grogan EL, Morris JA Jr, Dittus RS, et al. Cervical spine evaluation in urban trauma centers: Lowering institutional costs and complications through helical CT scan. J Am Coll Surg 2005;200:160–5.

125. Lewis VL, Manson PN, Morgan RF. Facial injuries associated with cervical fractures: Recognition patterns and management. J Trauma 1985;25:90–3.

126. Patel JC, Tepas JJ 3rd, Mollitt DL, et al. Pediatric cervical spine injuries: Defining the disease. J Pediatr Surg 2001;36:373–6.

127. Lally KP, Senac M, Hardin WD Jr, et al. Utility of the cervical spine radiograph in pediatric trauma. Am J Surg 1989;158:540–1; discussion 1–2.

128. Smith T, Skinner S, Shonnard N. Persistent synchondrosis of the second cervical vertebra simulating a hangman's fracture in a child. J Bone Joint Surg [Am] 1993;75:892–3.

129. Swischuck L. Anterior displacement of C2 in children. Physiologic or pathologic? Radiology 1977;122(Suppl 2):759–63.

130. Swischuck L, Swischuck P, SD J. Wedging of C3 in infants and children: Usually a normal finding not a fracture. Radiology 1993;188:523–6.

131. Cattell H, Filtzer D. Pseudosubluxation and other normal variations of the cervical spine in children. J Bone Joint Surg [Am] 1965;47:1295–309.

132. Buhs C, Cullen M, Klein M, et al. The pediatric trauma C-spine: is the 'odontoid' view necessary. J Pediatr Surg 2000;35:994–7.

133. Adelgais KM, Grossman DC, Langer SG, et al. Use of helical computed tomography for imaging the pediatric cervical spine. Acad Emerg Med 2004;11:228–36.

134. Carlan D, Bradbury T, Green N, Mencio GA, editors. The efficacy of helical CT versus conventional radiography of the cervical spine in pediatric trauma. Pediatric Orthopaedic Society of North America, Annual Meeting; 2008 May 1, 2008; Albuquerque, NM.

135. Hartley W, Mencio G, Green N. Clinical and radiographic algorithm for acute management of pediatric cervical spine trauma. Scoliosis Research Society, 32nd Annual Meeting. St. Louis, Missouri 1997. p. 138.

136. Dormans J, editor. The role of MRI in the assessment of pediatric cervical spine injuries in Evaluation and Management of Pediatric Spine Trauma. American Academy of Orthopaedic Surgeons, 67th Annual Meeting Instructional Course Lecture 321; 2000; Orlando, Florida.

137. Flynn JM, Closkey RF, Mahboubi S, et al. Role of magnetic resonance imaging in the assessment of pediatric cervical spine injuries. J Pediatr Orthop 2002;22:573–7.

138. Frank JB, Lim CK, Flynn JM, et al. The Efficacy of Magnetic Resonance Imaging in Pediatric Cervical Spine Clearance. Spine 2002;27:1176–9.

139. Dormans J, Criscitiello A, Drummond D, et al. Complications in children managed with immobilization in a halo vest. J Bone Joint Surg [Am] 1995;77:1370–3.

140. Letts M, Kaylor D, Gouw G. A biomechanical analysis of halo fixation in children. J Bone Joint Surg [Am] 1988;70B:277–9.

141. Mubarak S, Camp J, Vueltich W, et al. Halo application in the infant. J Pediatr Orthop 1989;9:612.

142. Pang D. Spinal cord injury without radiographic abnormality in children, 2 decades later. Neurosurg 2004;55:1325–42.

143. Pang D, Pollack I. Spinal cord injury without radiographic abnormality in children–the SCIWORA syndrome. J Trauma 1989;29:654–64.

144. Pang D, Wilberger J. Spinal cord injury without radiographic abnormalities in children. J Neurosurg 1982;57:114–29.

145. Sullivan A. Fractures of the Spine in Children. In: Green N, Swiontowski M, editors. Skeletal Trauma in Children. 2nd ed. Philadelphia: Saunders; 2003. p. 344–71.

146. Kriss V, Kriss T. SCIWORA (Spinal Cord Injury Without Radiographic Abnormality) in infants and children. Clin Pediatr 1996;35:119–24.

147. Copley L, Dormans J. Pediatric cervical spine problems: Developmental evaluation and congenital anomalies. J Am Acad Orthop Surg 1998;6:204–14.

148. Pollina J, Li V. Tandem spinal cord injuries without radiographic abnormalities in a young child. Pediatr Neurosurg 1999;30: 263–6.

149. Bosch PP, Vogt MT, Ward WT. Pediatric spinal cord injury without radiographic abnormality (SCIWORA): The absence of occult instability and lack of indication for bracing. Spine (Phila Pa 1976). 2002;27:2788–800.

150. Bracken M, Shepard M, Collins W, et al. A randomized, controlled trial of methylprednisolone or naloxone in the treatment of acute spinal cord injury: Results of the second national spinal cord injury study. New England J Med 1990;322:1405–11.

151. Bracken MB, Shepard MJ. Treatment of acute spinal cord injury with methylprednisolone: Results of a multicenter randomized clinical trial. J Neurtrauma 1991;8 (Suppl):47–50.

152. Bracken MB, Shepard MJ, Holford TR. Administration of methylprednisolone for 24 or 48 hours or tirilazad mesylate for 48 hours in the treatment of acute spinal cord injury: Results of the third national acute spinal cord injury randomized controlled trial- National Acute Spinal Cord Injury Study. J Am Med Assoc 1997;277:1597–604.

153. Bracken MB, Shepard MJ, Holford TR, et al. Methylprednisolone or tirilazad mesylate administration after acute spinal cord injury: 1-year follow-up: Results of the Third National Acute Spinal Cord Injury Randomized Controlled Trial. J Neurosurg 1998;1998:699–706.

154. Cirak B, Ziegfeld S, Knight V, et al. Spinal injuries in children. J Pediatr Surg 2004;39:607–12.

155. Clark CR, White AA. Fractures of the dens. J Bone Joint Surg 1985;67:1340.

156. Diamond P, Hansen CM, Christofersen MR. Child abuse presenting as a thoracolumbar spinal fracture dislocation: a case report. Pediatr Emerg Care 1994;10:83–6.

157. Reynolds R. Pediatric spinal injury. Curr Opin Pediatr 2000;12:67–71.

158. Santiago R, Guenther E, Carroll K, et al. The clinical presentation of pediatric thoracolumbar fractures. J Trauma 2006;60:187–92.

159. Hauser CJ, Visvikis G, Hinrichs C, et al. Prospective validation of computed tomographic screening of the thoracolumbar spine in trauma. J Trauma 2003;55:228–35.

160. Akbarnia BA. Pediatric spine fractures. Orthop Clin North Am 1999;30:521–36, x.

161. Banerian KG, Wang AM, Samberg LC, et al. Association of vertebral end plate fracture with pediatric lumbar intervertebral disk herniation: value of CT and MR imaging. Radiology 1990;177:763–5.

162. Greenwald TA, Mann DC. Pediatric seatbelt injuries: Diagnosis and treatment of lumbar flexion-distraction injuries. Paraplegia 1994;32:743–51.

163. Griffet J, Bastiani-Griffet F, El-Hayek T, et al. Management of seat-belt syndrome in children. Gravity of 2-point seat-belt. Eur J Pediatr Surg 2002;12:63–6.

164. Johnson DL, Falci S. The diagnosis and treatment of pediatric lumbar spine injuries caused by rear seat lap belts. Neurosurgery 1990;26:434–41.

165. Newman KD, Bowman LM, Eichelberger MR, et al. The lap belt complex: intestinal and lumbar spine injury in children. J Trauma 1990;30:1133–8; discussion 8–40.

166. Raney EM, Bennett JT. Pediatric Chance fracture. Spine 1992;17:1522–4.

167. Reid AB, Letts RM, Black GB. Pediatric Chance fractures: Association with intra-abdominal injuries and seatbelt use. J Trauma 1990;30:384–91.

168. Smith MD 2nd, Camp E 3rd, James H, Kelley HG. Pediatric seat belt injuries. Am Surg 1997;63:294–8.

169. Choit RL, Tredwell SJ, Leblanc JG, et al. Abdominal aortic injuries associated with chance fractures in pediatric patients. J Pediatr Surg 2006;41:1184–90.

170. Letts M, Davidson D, Fleuriau-Chateau P, et al.. Seat belt fracture with late development of an enterocolic fistula in a child. A case report. Spine 1999;24:1151–5.

171. Lalonde F, Letts M, Yang JP, et al. An analysis of burst fractures of the spine in adolescents. Am J Orthop 2001;30:115–20.

172. Hill JM, McGuire MH, Crosby LA. Closed treatment of displaced middle-third fractures of the clavicle gives poor results. J Bone Joint Surg Br 1997;79:537–9.

173. Lazarides S, Zafiropoulos G. Conservative treatment of fractures at the middle third of the clavicle: the relevance of shortening and clinical outcome. J Shoulder Elbow Surg 2006;15:191–4.

174. McKee MD, Pedersen EM, Jones C, et al. Deficits following nonoperative treatment of displaced midshaft clavicular fractures. J Bone Joint Surg Am 2006;88:35–40.

175. Wick M, Muller EJ, Kollig E, et al. Midshaft fractures of the clavicle with a shortening of more than 2 cm predispose to nonunion. Arch Orthop Trauma Surg 2001;121:207–11.

176. Zlowodzki M, Zelle BA, Cole PA, et al. Treatment of acute midshaft clavicle fractures: systematic review of 2144 fractures: on behalf of the Evidence-Based Orthopaedic Trauma Working Group. J Orthop Trauma 2005;19:504–7.

177. Canadian Orthopaedic Trauma Society. Nonoperative treatment compared with plate fixation of displaced midshaft clavicular fractures. A multicenter, randomized clinical trial. J Bone Joint Surg Am 2007;89:1–10.

178. Golthamer C. Duplication of the clavicle ("os claviculare"). Radiology 1957;68:576–8.

179. Twigg HL. Duplication of the clavicle. Skeletal Radiol 1981;6:281–3.

180. Webb LX, Mooney JF. Fractures and dislocations about the shoulder In: Green NE, Swiontkowski MF, editors. Skeletal Trauma in Children. Philadelphia: Saunders; 2003. p. 322–44.

181. Gray H. Anatomy of the Human Body. Philadelphia: Lea and Febiger; 1985.
182. Groh GI, Wirth MA, Rockwood CA Jr. Treatment of traumatic posterior sternoclavicular dislocations. J Shoulder Elbow Surg 2011;20:107–13.
183. Laffosse JM, Espie A, Bonnevialle N, et al. Posterior dislocation of the sternoclavicular joint and epiphyseal disruption of the medial clavicle with posterior displacement in sports participants. J Bone Joint Surg Br 2010;92:103–9.
184. Waters PM, Bae DS, Kadiyala RK. Short-term outcomes after surgical treatment of traumatic posterior sternoclavicular fracture-dislocations in children and adolescents. J Pediatr Orthop 2003;23:464–9.
185. Baxter MP, Wiley JJ. Fractures of the proximal humeral epiphysis: Their influence on humeral growth. J Bone Joint Surg [Br] 1986;68:570–3.
186. Beaty JH. Fractures of the proximal humerus and shaft in children. Instr Course Lect 1992;41:369–72.
187. Dameron TB, Reibel DB. Fractures involving the proximal humeral epiphyseal plate. J Bone Joint Surg [Am] 1969;51:289–97.
188. Smith FM. Fracture-separation of the proximal humeral epiphysis. Am J Surg 1956;91:627–35.
189. Beebe A, Bell DF. Management of severely displaced fractures of the proximal humerus in children. Tech Orthop 1989;4:1–4.
190. Loder RT. Pediatric polytrauma. Orthopaedic care and hospital course. J Orthop Trauma 1987;1:48–54.
191. Haraldsson S. On osteochondritis deformans juvenilis capituli humeri including investigation of intra-osseous vasculature in distal humerus. Acta Orthop Scand Suppl 1959;38.
192. Green NE. Fractures and dislocations about the elbow. In: Green NE, Swiontkowski MF, editors. Skeletal Trauma in Children. Philadelphia: Saunders; 2003. p. 257–322.
193. Green NE. Overnight delay in the reduction of supracondylar fractures of the humerus in children. J Bone Joint Surg [Am] 2001;93:321–2.
194. Mehlman CT, Strub WM, Roy DR. The effect of surgical timing on the perioperative complications of treatment of supracondylar humeral fractures in children. J Bone Joint Surg [Am] 2001;83:323–7.
195. Sabharwal S, Tredwell SJ, Beauchamp RD. Management of pulseless pink hand in pediatric supracondylar fractures of the humerus. J Pediatr Orthop 1997;17:303–10.
196. Sabharwal S. Role of Ilizarov external fixator in the management of proximal/distal metadiaphyseal pediatric femur fractures. J Orthop Trauma 2005;19:563–9.
197. Copley LA, Dormans JP, Davidson RS. Vascular injuries and their sequelae in pediatric supracondylar humerus fractures: Toward a goal of prevention. J Pediatr Orthop 1996;16:99–103.
198. Schoenecker PL, Delgado E, Rotman M. Pulseless arm in association with totally displaced supracondylar fracture. J Orthop Trauma 1996;10:410–15.
199. DeLee JC, Wilkins KE, Rogers LF. Fracture separation of the distal humerus epiphysis. J Bone Joint Surg [Am] 1980;62:46–51.
200. Jakob R, Fowles JV, Rang M. Observations concerning fractures of the lateral condyle in children. J Bone Joint Surg Br 1975;57:430–6.
201. Jeffrey C. Nonunion of epiphysis of the lateral condyle of the humerus. J Bone Joint Surg Am 1958;40:396–405.
202. Rutherford A. Fractures of the lateral humeral condyle in children. J Bone Joint Surg Am 1995;67:851–6, 1985:851–6.
203. McCarty EC, Mencio GA, Green NE. Ketamine sedation for the reduction of children's fractures in the emergency department. J Bone Joint Surg Am 2000;82:912–18.
204. McCarty EC, Mencio GA, Green NE. Anesthesia and analgesia for the ambulatory management of fractures in children. J Am Acad Orthop Surg 1999;2:81–91.
205. Lee MC, Stone NE 3rd, Ritting AW, et al. Mini-C-arm fluoroscopy for emergency-department reduction of pediatric forearm fractures. J Bone Joint Surg Am 2011;93:1442–7.
206. Agarwal A. Treatment of pediatric both bone forearm fractures: a comparison of operative techniques. J Pediatr Orthop 2007;27:480–1; author reply 1.
207. Flynn JM, Waters PM. Single bone fixation of both bone forearm fractures. . J Pediatr Orthop 1996;16:655–9.
208. Garg NK, Ballal MS, Malek IA, et al. Use of elastic stable intramedullary nailing for treating unstable forearm fractures in children. J Trauma 2008;65:109–15.
209. Griffet J, FeHayek T, Baby M. Intramedullary nailing of forearm fractures in children. J Pediatr Orthop Br 1999;8:88–9.
210. Kanellopoulos AD, Yiannakopoulos CK, Soucacos PN. Flexible intramedullary nailing of pediatric unstable forearm fractures. Am J Orthop 2005;34:420–4.
211. Lascombes P, Haumont T, Journeau P. Use and abuse of flexible intramedullary nailing in children and adolescents. J Pediatr Orthop 2006;26:827–34.
212. Lee S, Nicol RO, Stott NS. Intramedullary fixation for pediatric unstable forearm fractures. Clin Orthop Relat Res 2002(402):245–50.
213. Luhmann SJ, Gordon JE, Schoenecker PL. Intramedullary fixation of unstable both bone forearm fractures in children. J Pediatr Orthop 1998;18:451–6.
214. Muensterer OJ, Regauer MP. Closed reduction of forearm refractures with flexible intramedullary nails in situ. J Bone Joint Surg Am 2003;85-A:2152–5.

CHAPTER 19

Neurosurgical Conditions

Gregory W. Hornig • Clarence Greene

BRAIN TUMORS

Brain tumors are rare in the first year of life, with an incidence of 1 per 100,000 infants.[1] This incidence increases with age. By the age of 2 years, central nervous system (CNS) tumors occur in 2 to 5/100,000 children. Brain tumors represent the most common solid tumors in the pediatric population.[2]

In the group of brain tumors considered congenital, the most common are teratomas (37%), followed by primitive neuroectodermal tumors (PNETs) (12%), astrocytomas (10–15%), and choroid plexus tumors (8%).[3] In a slightly older population of children, teratomas become less frequent and other neoplasms become relatively more common, including astrocytomas (34% of brain tumors in children younger than 24 months of age), PNETs (23%), and ependymomas (11%). There is also a group of tumors that are sometimes considered non-neoplastic. These include developmental tumors, which derive from aberrant proliferative growth during embryonic brain development and include craniopharyngiomas, lipomas, dermoids, and colloid cysts.[4]

Cerebellar Astrocytomas

Low-grade astrocytomas occur throughout the CNS and constitute a fourth of all pediatric brain tumors. Cerebellar astrocytomas are common (12–17% of pediatric CNS tumors), and their treatment has the most favorable outcome of all intra-axial neoplasms in the CNS.[5] Most of these tumors are found in children younger than the age of 10 years. The symptoms of cerebellar astrocytomas include headache (80%), vomiting (80%), gait disturbance, and decreased level of consciousness. Signs include ataxia in 80%, papilledema, cranial nerve palsies (including blindness and diplopia), and dysmetria. The rapid progression of signs and symptoms is often a function of cerebrospinal fluid (CSF) obstruction because the tumor occupies the fourth ventricle or the aqueduct, and causes hydrocephalus. Treatment of the hydrocephalus is often required urgently in very sick children. Temporary diversion of CSF via external ventriculostomies or shunts often precedes removal of the tumor.

Many of the signs and symptoms of posterior fossa neoplasms have an indolent progression. It is not unusual for headache and vomiting and ataxia to continue for many months in patients who are treated for otitis, viral syndromes, gastrointestinal disorders, or failure to thrive. It is the experience of many neurosurgeons that nearly all brain tumors in young children are misdiagnosed initially, sometimes for long periods of time. The relentlessness and progression of symptomatology is the decisive factor that leads to diagnostic studies.

Operative excision of these tumors is often possible, but new neurologic deficits can occur postoperatively in 30% of patients, although at least half of these new deficits are transient.[6] Postoperative deficits occur because of the proximity of vital brain stem and delicate cranial nerve structures near the tumor, which is often large and firm. Postoperative pseudomeningoceles (the bulging of skin at the occipital incision site) and hydrocephalus are not uncommon (10–25%) and require additional treatment. Temporary continuation of postoperative CSF diversion via external ventriculostomy is favored by many surgeons to reduce the likelihood of permanent ventriculoperitoneal shunts.

The goal of operative therapy for low-grade tumors is complete removal. When total resection of these tumors is confirmed, the long-term survival without recurrence is about 90%, but much depends on the biologic aggressiveness of the tumor. Some histologic features such as mitosis, endothelial proliferation, and necrosis suggest a high-grade lesion with a much poorer prognosis. In cases of 'low-grade' astrocytomas with unanticipated rapid recurrence, additional treatment can be attempted, including further surgery and adjunctive chemotherapy and/or radiotherapy. Frequent follow-up scans are needed for at least five years after the operation.

Ependymomas

Ependymomas represent about 10% of pediatric brain tumors and are slightly less common than PNETs and astrocytomas. More than two-thirds of ependymomas in children occur in the posterior fossa (Fig. 19-1) and the symptoms they cause are similar to posterior fossa or cerebellar astrocytomas: headache, vomiting, lethargy, and ataxia. These symptoms result from a combination of compression along the dorsal brain stem and hydrocephalus. Many extend from the obex (in the inferior aspect of the fourth ventricle) and then extrude through the lateral opening of this ventricle (foramen of Luschka) into the cerebellopontine angle. Here they invade and compress cranial nerves with resulting facial weakness, diplopia, swallowing dysfunction, and hearing loss. When large, they often extend beyond the foramen magnum and can compress the cervical cord. In regard to their cell of origin, they are not limited to the ependymal layer of the ventricle but can arise from cerebellar, cerebral, or spinal cord parenchyma.

Aggressive surgical resection has been the goal of treatment of these difficult tumors, but there is high

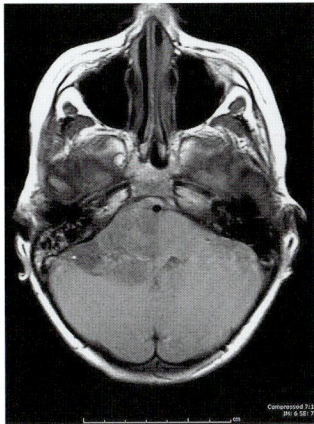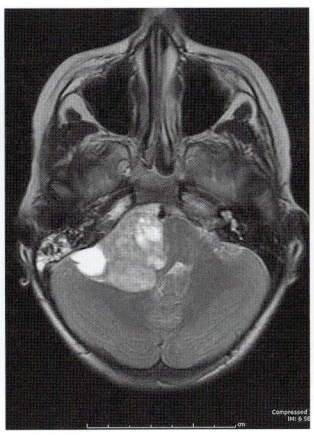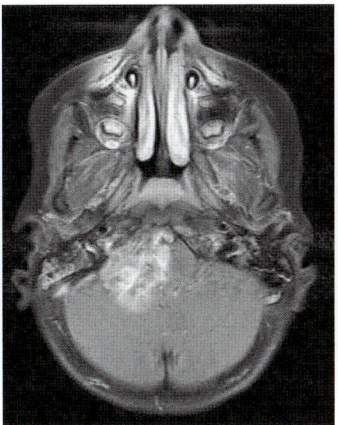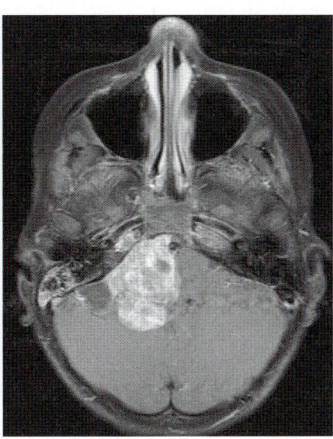

FIGURE 19-1 ■ MR image of a posterior fossa ependymoma. The tumor involves the lateral aspect of the posterior fossa and contains calcifications typical of ependymomas. The brain stem is severely distorted by the mass effect of the tumor. The tumor also compresses cranial nerves on the right side, making complete tumor removal problematic. This patient had right facial weakness, diplopia, and mild left hemiparesis postoperatively.

probability of new or worsening neurologic deficits as a result of the operative dissection. There is a correlation between postoperative residual tumor and tumor recurrence and/or progression. In the 30% of children where the tumor is totally resected, there is still a 20% to 40% possibility of recurrence, even after conventional radiotherapy.[7] In cases of near-total resection, the rate of progression-free survival falls to 30%.[8] Most of the recurrences are local and radiation therapy has become the mainstay of treatment, even with complete resection. Very small children, usually younger than age 3 years, are faced with comparatively greater morbidity from conventional radiotherapy, and radiation therapy is often deferred. Chemotherapy has been used with some success in this group of patients. The role of chemotherapy without irradiation has generally not been favorable in older age groups. Retrospective studies have failed to prove substantial benefit in survival when chemotherapy is added to surgery and radiation therapy for newly diagnosed ependymomas.

Treatment of ependymomas has remained problematic. Large, invasive tumors are clearly difficult to remove without significant risk to the patient, and residual tumors are largely refractory to chemotherapy and radiation. Some surgeons have suggested a staged operative approach with an initial subtotal debulking followed by a second aggressive operative exploration after chemotherapy. Whether this approach provides improved outcomes has not been established. Surveillance of treated patients with ependymomas must continue for many years, independent of histologic grading and extent of resection. Radiosurgery is also being used to treat focal areas of recurrent or unresectable tumor.

Medulloblastomas

Medulloblastomas are the most common malignant solid tumor in children and constitute 20% of pediatric brain tumors.[9] They are usually located in the posterior fossa and they are also referred to as PNETs because they are histologically identical to tumors (pineoblastomas, neuroblastomas, and retinoblastomas) located in other locations that are believed to have derived from progenitor subependymal neuroepithelial cells undergoing malignant transformation. Nearly half of medulloblastomas have chromosomal abnormalities, particularly the deletion of 17p chromosome that contains the tumor suppressor gene *TP53*.[10]

Hydrocephalus often occurs with medulloblastomas because of their location within the cerebellar vermis (a midline structure), often filling the fourth ventricle (Fig. 19-2). Children with this tumor often have symptoms of elevated intracranial pressure (ICP) (obtundation, headache, nausea/vomiting, irritability) and have signs suggestive of posterior fossa compression (dysmetria, ataxia, diplopia, head tilt, and papilledema). Lumbar puncture should not be done after computed tomography (CT) or magnetic resonance imaging (MRI) has established the presence of a posterior fossa tumor and obstructive hydrocephalus. CSF diversion (usually via an external drain) is usually done either before or in conjunction with craniotomy. Conversion of these temporary devices to permanent ventriculoperitoneal shunts is not uncommon in children with large tumors and marked preoperative ventriculomegaly.

Complete resection of medulloblastomas is often possible, although permanent postoperative deficits can occur.[6] The 'posterior fossa syndrome' can occur postoperatively in 10–15% of children and is characterized by mutism, drooling and swallowing difficulties, ocular palsies, and increasing ataxia.[11] These problems resolve entirely in most patients after several months. Improvement is thought to occur with resolution of swelling within the inferior vermis.

Staging is important with medulloblastomas because patients have a predictable outcome depending on age, metastases, pathology, and extent of surgical resection. Poor survival is correlated with age younger than 4 years, residual tumor measuring more than 1.5 cm,[2] and tumor dissemination, particularly 'drop' metastasis along the spinal column. After craniospinal radiation in eligible patients, survival occurs in 50–70% of patients with standard or low-risk medulloblastomas. Newer treatment protocols include chemotherapy first, which is followed

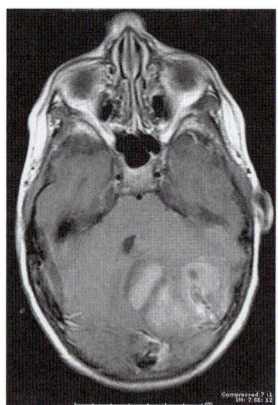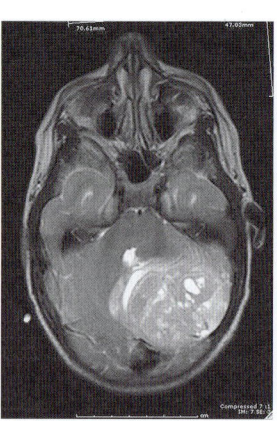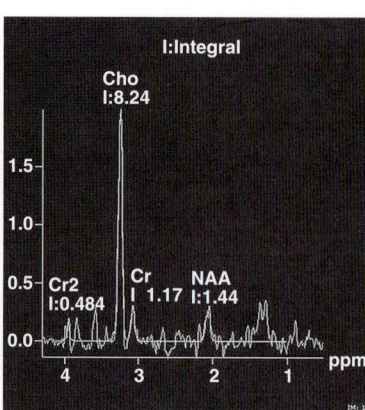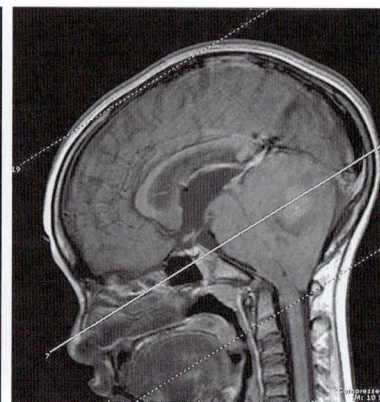

FIGURE 19-2 ■ MRI and MRS (magnetic resonance spectroscopy) of a posterior fossa medulloblastoma, with compression of fourth ventricle. The MRS profile shows a choline peak with depression of *N*-acetyl aspartate (NAA) typical of aggressive tumors.

by radiotherapy consisting of lowered cumulative cranio-spinal doses (24–36 Gy to the entire brain) with hyper-fractionated delivery, usually 1 Gy twice daily. Survival in these 'good risk' patients is nearly 90% after five years. Survival in high-risk patients is 60–65% with current multimodality therapy, with the worst outcomes in affected infants. Children younger than 3 years of age are usually treated first with chemotherapy, with irradiation deferred for 1 to 2 years. Radiation is sometimes avoided altogether in the 40% with progression-free survival.[12]

Recurrent medulloblastoma after surgery and radio-therapy is not amenable to cure, but a combination of aggressive therapies can allow remission of disease. These treatments include reoperation, radiosurgery, and high-dose chemotherapy with autologous stem cell rescue. Each of these treatments carries significant morbidity, including loss of cognitive skills, growth retardation, endocrine problems, and the risk of second tumors and vascular malformations in previously irradiated areas.

Supratentorial Nonglial and Glial Neoplasms

There are multiple nonglial tumors involving the cerebral hemisphere. Supratentorial tumors are fairly common, and the majority of these are glial in origin, usually designated in ascending order of malignancy as astrocytomas, anaplastic astrocytomas, or glioblastoma multiforme. Nonastrocytic tumors include PNETs (including cerebral neuroblastomas), choroid plexus tumors (papillomas and carcinomas), and teratomas (including dysembryoplastic neuroepithelial tumors [DNETs]), germinomas, oligodendrogliomas, meningiomas, and gangliogliomas. In this latter grouping, operative resection is the requisite initial treatment. In the last three tumors, adjunctive therapies are not recommended after gross total resection if tumor histology is benign.

Seizures are much more common with supratentorial tumors because they affect the eloquent neocortex, particularly tumors in the medial or lateral temporal cortex. Older individuals are afflicted with these tumors and can present with personality changes, cognitive difficulties, headache, and growth deficits.

Germ cell tumors are composed of germinomas and teratomas, and arise in pineal and suprasellar regions predominantly. Germ cells tumors often metastasize and cannot be surgically cured. Therefore, they are often best treated with radiation and chemotherapy. This combination of therapies is often quite successful with the majority of germ cell neoplasms.

Ependymomas that occur in the cerebral hemispheres remain problematic in terms of treatment, although hemispheric tumors generally have comparatively better outcomes. Incomplete resection (often because of diffuse involvement within critical brain regions) and leptomeningeal spread are significant adverse risk factors. Age is also a factor. Children younger than 3 years of age have significantly diminished progression-free survival (10–15%) compared with older children.[13]

As with medulloblastoma, glial and nonglial tumors often have genetic abnormalities, with chromosomal abnormalities and gene mutations. Many low-grade lesions progress to become more malignant. The pathway to this malignant progression is complex. Chromosomal translocations and mutations occur as initiating events before the amplification of deleterious genes that support tumor progression.[14–16]

With most benign tumors, there exists a strong association between extent of resection and outcome. From the neurosurgical viewpoint, maximal resection should be attempted without inordinate surgical morbidity. The advent of frameless stereotaxy for precise tumor localization, 'functional' localization with intraoperative monitoring (e.g., somatosensory evoked potential mapping to determine the location of the motor cortex), presurgical functional MRI to determine location of speech areas, and intraoperative scanning (via real-time ultrasonography [US], CT, or MRI) have each added considerably to the safety of the operation. Nonetheless, the operative approach can only achieve resection of targeted areas. Infiltrative tumors (which typically extend well beyond the target borders) cannot be ablated using current surgical technology. The roles of chemotherapy, molecular manipulation, and conformal radiation therapy remain essential to the goal of controlling high-grade brain neoplasms partially treated with operation. Unfortunately, high-grade brain lesions remain stubbornly resistant to the intensive multimodality treatments that follow surgical resection. Survival curves for highly malignant brain lesions have not changed substantially in the past several decades.

Radiotherapy for Pediatric CNS Tumors

The target for radiation therapy is cellular DNA. Ionizing radiation damages double-stranded DNA, leading to cell death. Unlike normal cells, which have a preserved ability to repair radiation damage, neoplastic cells often are replicating at abnormally high rates and radiation interferes with their mitotic or proliferative ability. With slowly growing tumors such as craniopharyngiomas, the response to radiation is subtle and such tumors may take many months to show a clinical response. The critical sublethal dose required to preserve normal tissue but damage brain tumors, the so-called therapeutic window, is quite well understood and depends on a number of factors, including vulnerability of affected tissue (which can depend on the age of the patient and locale of the target; optic nerve radiation, as an example, is poorly tolerated), tumor vulnerability, volume irradiated, total dose, fraction size, and interfraction interval. As total volume of irradiation increases, the cumulative radiation dose must necessarily decrease to reduce the morbidity of treatment. The conventional cumulative radiation dose for most pediatric CNS tumors is in the 50–60 Gy range, although some tumors (e.g., germinomas) are much more sensitive to radiation and can respond to treatment in the 30–50 Gy range.[17] Tumor type is therefore an important determinant of the effectiveness of radiation therapy, and biopsy is often a prerequisite for treatment.

Radiotherapy has enjoyed significant technologic advances with the advent of improved radiologic definition of tumors and sophisticated computer-assisted planning in three-dimensional systems. Stereotactic radiosurgery (SRS) has become routine in the USA, and single high-dose fractions can be delivered with great precision using high-energy photons produced either by linear accelerators or cobalt sources (gamma knife). Proton-beam therapy utilizes charged nuclear particles to deliver energy in discrete target points after the proton has nearly come to rest. As such, the proton can traverse normal brain without losing energy. As it comes to rest, it gives off most of its energy in less than 1 cm in the form of a Bragg 'peak,' providing a distinctively sharp rise in absorbed energy at the targeted tissue.

All these stereotactic methods are very precise and ideal for small targets, which are usually noninfiltrative lesions with well-delineated borders. The complications arising from targeting structures larger than 3.5 cm limit the radiosurgical approach. As such, the utility of treating small noninfiltrative tumors is optimal with single-fraction radiosurgery. For larger lesions in vulnerable areas of the brain (e.g., brain stem, retina, or cranial nerves), fractionation can be used with either repeat head fixation or localization systems to minimize complications of SRS therapy. In pediatric patients, SRS is mainly used as a boost to tumors that have recurred or persisted after conventional fractionated radiation therapy.

Finally, so-called conformal radiation provides the radiobiologic advantages of hyperfractionation along with the precision and control of SRS. Tumors typically treated in this manner are craniopharyngiomas, optic system tumors, and pituitary adenomas.

TREATMENT OF SPASTICITY AND MOVEMENT DISORDERS

Spasticity is defined as an abnormal response to passive muscle stretch. As the velocity of passive movement of a joint is increased, increased resistance develops. During examination of an affected extremity, there can be as little as a 'catch' to passive movement or, in more severe cases, no movement at all. Children with spastic conditions often have muscle stiffness, fatigue, and pain. If the condition is severe and chronic, muscle contractures and joint dislocation can occur, particularly in the flexor muscles and internal rotator muscles. In children with spastic quadriparesis, the typical stance is one of flexed elbows and wrists, with standing and walking on toes, the knees and hips flexed, and the legs internally rotated.

Spasticity occurs because of an imbalance of excitatory Ia afferent nerves from muscle spindles into the spinal cord and inhibitory descending impulses from the basal ganglia and cerebellum. In most children, the inhibitory impulses are diminished because of early CNS injury or injury to the spinal cord, which conducts the descending inhibitory impulses. Hence, treatment is directed toward either increasing the inhibitory neurotransmitters (usually γ-aminobutyric acid [GABA]) or reducing the afferent excitatory transmission from muscle spindles. Baclofen achieves the former, and dorsal rhizotomy (via cutting afferent nerve roots) interrupts the reflex transmission from muscle spindles.[18,19]

The children most susceptible to spasticity are those with low birth weight due to prematurity who have suffered a variety of cerebral insults, particularly hypoxic–ischemic encephalopathy with its predilection for causing periventricular white matter loss. Other affected infants have antepartum or intrapartum insults that lead to specific brain injuries that interrupt pyramidal pathways that mediate the inhibitory spinal pathways.

Treatment of spasticity should aim to improve function and facilitate care. Multidisciplinary clinics usually assess the potential candidate for surgical treatment. The best candidates for lumbosacral rhizotomy are motivated, older children (age 5 to 6 years) with spastic diplegia (affecting the legs predominantly) who lack severe contractures and have relatively good leg strength. Children with weak legs and spasticity can lose function with rhizotomy because they depend on their increased tone to maintain marginal ambulatory function. Rhizotomy can produce, to their detriment, a nonadjustable and permanent decrease in spasticity. Oral baclofen can be most useful in these very young children. Baclofen pumps are advantageous in children with severe spasticity that interferes with their care and in children with quadriplegia, often with a greater reduction of spasticity in the legs than the arms. The treatment is not permanent and non-ablative, and the dosing is amenable to adjustments. It is particularly useful in children with spinal cord insult from trauma or inflammatory processes (transverse myelitis), and in patients with familial spastic paraparesis.

Botulinum toxin produces neuromuscular blockade and thereby reduces muscle contractions and spasticity. It is typically injected into spastic muscles, and for a period of several months, will decrease spasticity and increase range of motion. These injections are often used to extend the period of time until a definitive procedure can be performed in very young children, often decreasing the risk of developing muscle contractures that become fixed deformities which are not amenable to treatment.[20]

EPILEPSY SURGERY

Epilepsy affects about 1% of the population and starts commonly in the first decade of life. Surgical management is a well-established therapy when medical treatment has not been successful. Temporal lobectomy has been a mainstay of operative care for more than 40 years, and temporal resections constitute more than half of the epilepsy operations performed in children. In a randomized, controlled trial of operation versus medical therapy, 64% of patients were free of disabling seizures after operation compared with only 8% of those in the medical group.[21] In addition, surgery may curtail the cognitive and psychosocial disabilities that can occur with medically intractable seizures, particularly in remediable syndromes that begin in infancy before the acquisition of language and social skills. The quality of life for patients with epilepsy is unambiguously related to the recurrence of seizures, and uncontrolled seizures carry a substantial risk of disability and death.

Drug-resistant epilepsy is thought to be reasonably predicted after two antiepileptic medications have proven ineffective. After the failure of a third medication, the probability of being seizure free is less than 10%. Therefore, despite the invasiveness of surgery, it is highly reasonable to consider operative intervention one or two years after the onset of disabling epileptic seizures, particularly in the 30% of epileptic children who have complex partial seizures emanating (unilaterally) from the temporal area. Surgery requires comprehensive preoperative evaluation by epilepsy specialists, along with multiple imaging and monitoring studies. Invasive monitoring is fairly common in pediatric patients, who tend to have seizures that are multilobar. Newer noninvasive modalities such as magnetoencephalography are rapidly achieving success in determining the source of the seizures.

The success of temporal lobe surgery has led to more aggressive approaches to control epilepsy originating elsewhere in the brain. The pathologic substrates of pediatric extratemporal epilepsies are quite diverse, including cortical dysplasia, developmental abnormalities of neuronal migration, gliosis, tumors, neurocutaneous disorders (e.g., Sturge–Weber syndrome, tuberous sclerosis), and inflammatory lesions. These entities are often intensely epileptogenic from an early age. In such lesions, the MRI abnormality does not strictly correlate with the source of seizures and the epileptogenic focus may, in fact, be relatively diffuse and involve eloquent cortex. Nonetheless, some series show excellent results in more than 50% of patients, particularly if there is complete resection of an epileptogenic focus, including the focal area of interictal abnormality.[22] Intelligence quotient scores tend to be stable or improved in the majority of children selected for surgery.

In some patients, seizures can be lateralized to one hemisphere by preoperative studies but not precisely localized. These patients may be considered for hemispherectomy if there is significant unilateral dysfunction. As radical as such operative resection would appear, the improvement of hemisphere disconnection procedures is in the 70% range for seizure freedom, with likely hemiparesis and hemianopia found postoperatively (although these deficits are often present before surgery). Newer techniques involve a disconnection of the hemisphere without anatomic removal of the affected hemisphere, thereby reducing some of the complications associated with volumetric removal of large portions of the brain.[23]

Corpus callosum sectioning is a palliative approach in patients who have seizures without focal onset. In patients with drop attacks, division of all or part of the corpus callosum can result in improvement in about 60% of patients by reducing the severity of their seizures and decreasing the likelihood of severe injury from falling.[24]

Vagal nerve stimulation (VNS) is useful for the treatment of partial seizures, providing about a 50% reduction in seizure frequency in patients with intractable seizures who are not candidates for resection. The morbidity of implantation of the vagal nerve stimulator is extremely small, and the efficacy of the device rivals that of new antiepileptic medications. As opposed to medications, there is no toxicity and no issues of compliance.[25]

HYDROCEPHALUS

Other than trauma, hydrocephalus is the single most common entity pediatric neurosurgeons are called on to manage. This disorder of CSF circulation and absorption accounts for 0.6% of all pediatric hospital admissions, 1.8% of all pediatric hospital days, and 3.1% of all pediatric hospital charges.[26–29] The care of hydrocephalic patients is a major health care expenditure, hovering near $1 billion in the USA per year.[30] Although hydrocephalus can afflict individuals at any age, the range of causes and manifestations are larger and often more complex in children.

CSF is a clear fluid, which is primarily secreted within the ventricles of the brain by the choroid plexus. A considerable volume may be formed by interstitial fluid from the intercellular clefts in the brain and spinal cord.[31–33] The total production of CSF has been calculated at about 500 mL/day.[34] The volume in the system turns over nearly four times per day.

The circulation of CSF is complex. CSF exits the brain through the fourth ventricle and has a pulsatile course through the subarachnoid space over the convexities of the brain, the basal cisterns, the spinal subarachnoid space, and ultimately back intracranially to the vertex of the brain. There, the CSF transits through midline arachnoid granulations into the venous system at the superior sagittal sinus. This transfer is passive from a high-pressure system into a low-pressure environment.

Escape of the CSF through alternative routes exists, although none is adequate to maintain normal nervous system function. Many mothers have observed that their children look puffy around the eyes when their shunt is malfunctioning. There is perhaps escape of CSF through the craniofacial lymphatics that might account for this observation. This transit of CSF has been confirmed in other mammals, and there is advancing evidence of this in humans.[35–37]

Congenital Hydrocephalus

Hydrocephalus may be an isolated development or be associated with many syndromes and brain maldevelopment conditions such as holoprosencephaly and schizencephaly.

The most common genetic hydrocephalus is X-linked hydrocephalus. It occurs in 1:30,000 male births and represents 2–5% of nonsyndromal cases of hydrocephalus. The aqueduct of Sylvius is narrowed, causing subsequent dilation of the third and lateral ventricles, sparing the fourth ventricle (Figs 19-3 to 19-5). In its fullest expression, other neurologic abnormalities can occur. Twenty-five percent of males with clear aqueduct stenosis will have X-linked hydrocephalus, which is very important in advising couples about future pregnancies.[38] Other causes of aqueduct stenosis can be thickening of the tectum of the midbrain from hamartoma, glioma formation, or from intrauterine infections.[39]

The Chiari II malformation includes alternation in the size and shape of the posterior fossa, descent of the midline cerebellar tonsils through the foramen magnum, and straightening of the brain stem along with a beaking appearance of the tectum or dorsal midbrain. This is the next most common etiology of hydrocephalus and is always present to some degree in children who have the spinal dysraphism of myelomeningocele or meningocele. Chiari II malformation interrupts the egress of CSF from the fourth ventricle and disrupts the pulsatile flow of CSF around the confines of the posterior fossa. Children with untreated or undertreated hydrocephalus and Chiari malformation are at risk for the development of hydromyelia or syrinx.

The Dandy–Walker malformation is next in frequency for causing hydrocephalus. In the fullest expression of this anomaly, one finds a retrocerebellar cyst, which can be quite sizable with a cleft or defect in the vermis of the cerebellum, agenesis of the corpus callosum, and extracranial anomalies such as cardiac septal defects and syndactyly. These children are at higher risk for developmental delays and epilepsy.

In Dandy–Walker malformations, the hydrocephalus is due to an alternation in CSF flow at the exit of the fourth ventricle. A Dandy–Walker malformation may be further complicated by a 'double compartment' hydrocephalus. The cyst formation may block escape of the CSF at the distal end of the aqueduct of Sylvius with resultant dilation of the third and lateral ventricles. In addition, the choroid plexus within the fourth ventricle will create CSF with no access to the subarachnoid space and subsequent enlargement of the cyst. In infants, this may lead to an unsightly distortion of the cranium and signs and symptoms of hindbrain compression. Not infrequently, additional surgical attention must be directed to the cyst, usually a CSF shunt catheter, either joined with a ventriculoperitoneal shunt or a separate shunt entirely (see Figs 19-3 and 19-4).[40,41]

Acquired Hydrocephalus

In the USA, there are more than 50,000 very low birth weight infants born each year. Almost 20% of these neonates suffer some degree of intraventricular hemorrhage, most related to bleeding within the germinal matrix adjacent to the ventricles of the brain (see

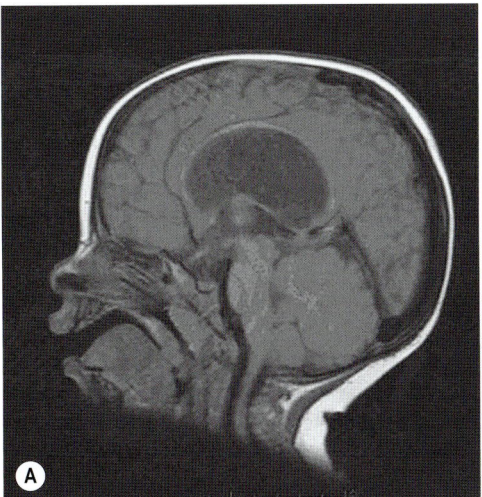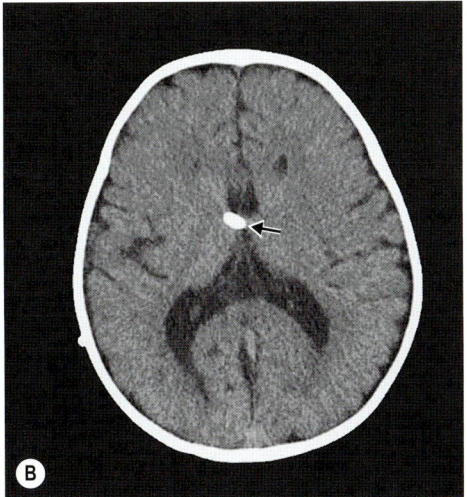

FIGURE 19-3 ■ **(A)** Sagittal MR image showing aqueduct stenosis and dilated third and lateral ventricles. **(B)** Axial CT after ventriculoperitoneal shunt (arrow).

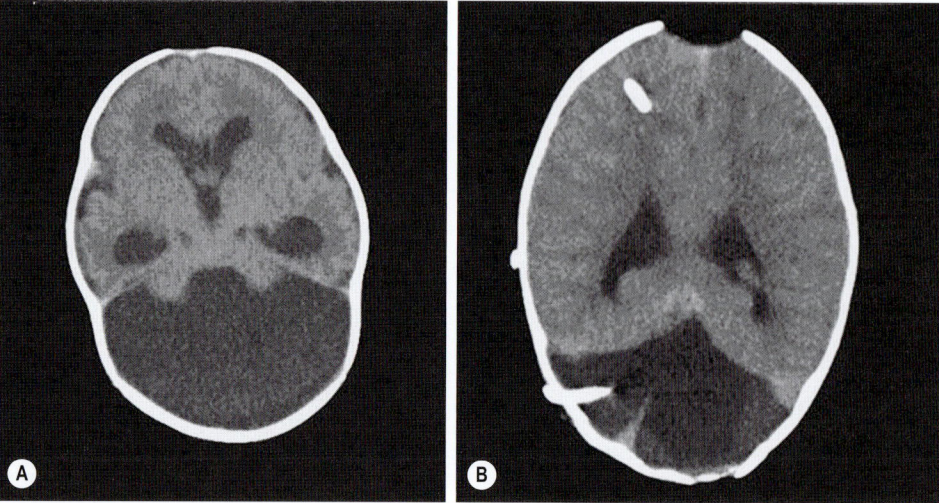

FIGURE 19-4 ■ **(A)** Axial CT scan of Dandy–Walker malformation. **(B)** The axial CT scan shows supratentorial and posterior fossa shunt catheters. The posterior fossa shunt was required after the cyst continued to expand.

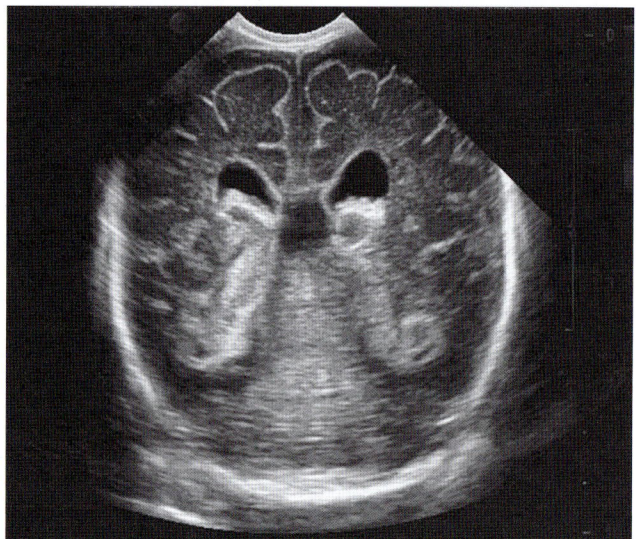

FIGURE 19-5 ■ Ultrasound image shows a grade III bilateral intraventricular hemorrhage with ventricular dilation.

	TABLE 19-1	**Grading System for Intraventricular Hemorrhage Based on Ultrasound Findings**

Grade	Cranial Ultrasound Findings
I	Hemorrhage in germinal matrix only
II	Ventricular hemorrhage without ventricular dilation
III	Ventricular hemorrhage with ventricular dilation
IV	Brain parenchymal hemorrhage

Fig. 19-5). These hemorrhages are graded on scale of I to IV (Table 19-1). At least 25% of these neonates will develop posthemorrhagic hydrocephalus.[42] Intraventricular blood is a powerful irritant to the ependymal lining of the ventricles as well as to the arachnoid membranes. The resultant inflammatory response and scarring can lead to obstruction of flow of CSF from the ventricle or, more commonly, an intense arachnoiditis with severe restriction of the CSF pathways at the base of the brain. Traumatic intracranial bleeding will manifest the same pathophysiology, leading to 'posttraumatic' hydrocephalus. In the worst cases, the resultant inflammation will be both intraventricular and in the subarachnoid space. It can lead to multiple scar septations within the ventricles and 'multiple compartments' hydrocephalus.[43]

By definition, meningitis is inflammation of the arachnoid. Fetal infection with toxoplasmosis, cytomegalovirus, and *Cryptococcus* are infrequently encountered but are devastating to the developing brain, and the concurrence of hydrocephalus is only more tragic to the infants. Finally, subdural emphysema and brain abscess may lead to altered CSF flow and subsequent hydrocephalus.

It is extremely rare to see a child with congenital hydrocephalus become shunt independent. Thus, such children need to be approached with caution in making such a diagnosis.[44,45]

Brain tumors frequently occur in the midline in children and cause CSF obstruction. In fact, it is often the signs and symptoms of hydrocephalus, not the tumor itself, which brings these children to medical attention. Fortunately, if the tumor can be excised, the hydrocephalus in the majority will resolve without additional surgical management.

There is one entity, congenital or acquired, that creates an overproduction of CSF. This condition is hyperplasia or a tumor of the choroid plexus. Choroid plexus papilloma or carcinomas (<1% of brain tumors) are not infrequently diagnosed in the neonatal period. The choroid plexus tumor is usually obvious on brain imaging studies for investigation of a large head or to delineate the type of hydrocephalus present. Hyperplasia of the plexus might not be as evident and may only become recognized when seeking why hydrocephalus treatment is not effective. Choroid plexus hyperplasia may generate excess CSF and overwhelm the absorptive capacity of a shunt terminus.

Diagnosis

Imaging for communicating hydrocephalus typically demonstrates dilation of all the ventricles of the brain and occasionally the subarachnoid space. Patients with post-meningitic hydrocephalus are a typical example. The signs and symptoms of hydrocephalus are age dependent and often relate to the rapidity of the ventricular expansion. In the neonate and young infant, there are typically few symptoms. The child often feeds well and is attentive and happy, and the only clue may be an accelerated rate of head growth.

In older children with firmer calvaria, hydrocephalus usually creates a more pronounced increase in ICP and the increased pressure will generate more symptoms. Most commonly, there is head pain or excessive irritability in the nonverbal child. Vomiting, detachment, or disinterest in play is common. Other common observations are poor school performance and easy fatigability. Visual changes such as blurriness or change in color perception can be noted by older children. Recumbence increases ICP, and therefore typically the headaches and vomiting are more pronounced in the morning. Seizures may occur, but not usually as a presenting or solitary event.

Physical findings commonly include a large head, a full but not tense anterior fontanelle, and prominent scalp veins. Peculiar to infants is the 'sunset' eye appearance. This downward and outward deviation of the eyes is a response to pressure on the superior colliculus of the midbrain by a dilated third ventricle. After treatment, this disturbance regresses. Older children may demonstrate a Parinaud sign: the failure of upward gaze, pupil unresponsiveness to light, and impairment of accommodation. Papilledema and altered visual fields often are evident.

Suspicions are to be confirmed by brain imaging studies. Ultrasonography in infants with an open fontanelle is a good screening study, but even if hydrocephalus is diagnosed with that technique, MRI or CT is required to more fully understand the etiology (Fig. 19-6).

Treatment

The first reproducibly successful treatment for hydrocephalus of any type occurred in the early 1950s. Lumboureteral shunts were successfully employed in patients with communicating hydrocephalus.[46] Success was then reported with ventricular to jugular vein shunts incorporating a miniaturized spring and ball valve.[47] As silicone replaced the earlier stiffer plastics, the ventriculoperitoneal shunt became and remains the mainstay of hydrocephalus therapy.[48]

Development of shunt hardware has matured. The quality of the silicone has improved, making the tubing more pliable and less hazardous to abdominal organs. Valves can be adjusted to various opening pressures with external magnets. Tubing that incorporates antibiotics within or coating it is available. With these mechanical advances, life expectancy of the shunt itself has improved and the complications have diminished, although only slightly. Realistically, there is little difference in the performance of one brand of shunt over another, despite the claims of the multiple vendors.[49]

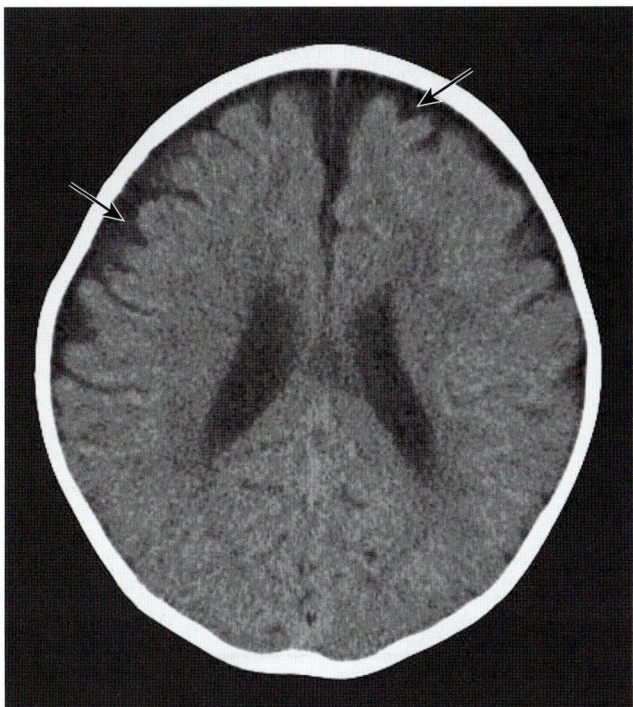

FIGURE 19-6 ■ Axial CT scan shows mildly dilated lateral ventricles and a generous subarachnoid space in the frontal and frontoparietal areas (*arrows*).

Shunt occlusions and infections are still vexing in our efforts to have these children lead a normal life. Nearly half of all shunt operations are revisions for occlusion or infection. Perioperative antibiotic usage, although not without controversy, has reduced the shunt infection rate to 8% or less in busy pediatric centers.[50] There is no consensus as to which antimicrobial agents are most efficacious.[51]

Alternatives to ventriculoperitoneal shunts are still useful, if not required in some complex cases. Lumboperitoneal shunts have regained some popularity among pediatric neurosurgeons in selected patients with communication of CSF from the intracranial compartment to the spinal subarachnoid space. The development of a Chiari I malformation from chronic CSF drainage that draws the cerebellar tonsils downward has given many neurosurgeons pause before considering this shunt in young patients.[52–54] When circumstances make the peritoneum inhospitable to CSF absorption, alternate termini for the tube include the venous system, pleural space, and even the gallbladder.[55]

An alternative to CSF shunting has re-emerged with the miniaturization of endoscopic equipment. Creating an opening in the floor of the third ventricle to look around an obstruction at the aqueduct or the outlet of the fourth ventricle is very appealing. The concept dates from 1922 but was a failure. New technology for minimally invasive surgery has given a rebirth to the idea and, today, endoscopic third ventriculostomy (ETV) is selectively done in lieu of CSF shunts (Fig. 19-7). When successful, the hydrocephalus is managed without the need for foreign body implant and without the inherent risks of infection or valve or catheter failure. This approach has been found to be successful in 60% of properly selected children.[56] The potential complications, such as uncontrollable hemorrhage, neuroendocrine dysfunction, and short-term memory loss, are severe, more so than with shunting. Nevertheless, there is great appeal in having hydrocephalus treated effectively without implanted hardware.

Shunt Malfunctions

Despite the progress in shunt design and materials, shunts will fail, and at a surprisingly high rate. Forty percent fail within the first year of implant. At 15 years, there is an 80% likelihood of failure. Again, the signs and symptoms will be age dependent. Infants may have minimal symptoms because of the expandable cranium,

whereas older children may quickly become dreadfully ill as the ICP increases. Headache, vomiting, and altered mental status predominate as symptoms. The clinical assessment typically includes a brain imaging study, a shunt survey (plain films of the shunt) to look for a fracture of the tube, a shortened end, or a migration. Although a change in the ventricular size noted on imaging is a strong clue to the diagnosis, normal ventricular size can often be a falsely reassuring sign. It is not uncommon for symptomatic children to have no dilation of their ventricles, presumably related to loss of brain compliance.[57,58] Often a percutaneous needle tap of the shunt reservoir or valve will be needed to measure pressure. Some surgeons use radioisotope or contrast flow studies (shuntograms). When in doubt, surgical exploration of the shunt is the best option.[59]

SPINAL DYSRAPHISM

There are multiple types of spinal dysraphism, or neural tube defects, in children. The most common are myelomeningocele, lipomyelomeningocele, and meningocele.

Myelomeningocele

Myelomeningocele is the most frequently encountered spinal neural tube defect. In the USA, the incidence is 0.3 per 1,000 live births, a decrease of nearly 50% since the widespread use of folic acid in women planning pregnancy or begun in the first trimester.[60] It is rarely a diagnostic problem and is now frequently discovered with fetal ultrasound or MRI.

Essentially, these are defects in the skin, fascia, posterior elements of the spine, and the conus medullaris of the cord, along with a failure in neurulation during the 26th to 28th weeks of gestation. Myelomeningocele is most frequent in the lumbar and lumbosacral area (Fig. 19-8). Often of considerable size, it might be confused with a sacral teratoma. The neonatal assessment may require MRI of the entire spinal canal to exclude concurrent anomalies. Cranial ultrasound is usually sufficient to evaluate for hydrocephalus. The surgical challenge is not so much in closing the exposed nervous system but in obtaining a tension-free cutaneous closure. At operation,

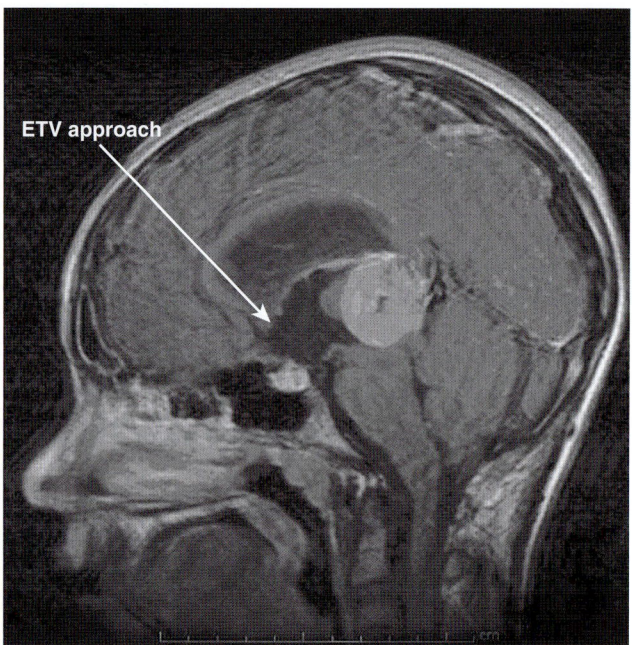

FIGURE 19-7 ■ Sagittal MRI of patient with a large tumor in the posterior third ventricle causing aqueduct occlusion. The arrow depicts the approach for an endoscopic third ventriculostomy (ETV) to bypass the obstruction and relieve the hydrocephalus. At the same operation, the tumor was sampled.

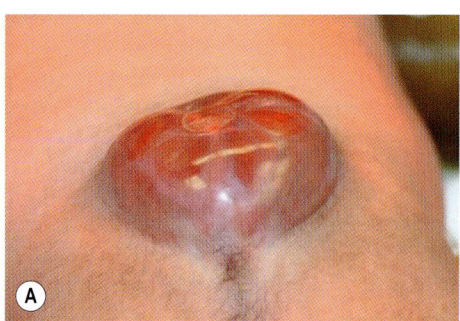
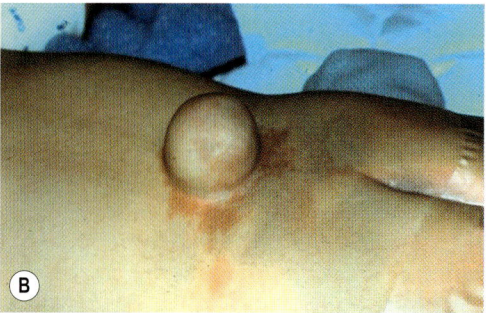

FIGURE 19-8 ■ **(A)** A typical myelomeningocele shows a small neural placode at the dome with a large CSF-filled sack and little useful skin. **(B)** A meningocele with common surrounding port-wine stains is seen.

the exposed end of the incompletely fused spinal cord is separated from the cutaneous attachments, and a pseudo-dural layer is closed over it. Not infrequently, the skin closure is the more complex segment of the operation, and plastic surgical techniques (relaxing flank incisions, skin grafts, rotational flaps) may be required to accomplish this closure.

The more rostral the defect, the more severe the neurologic deficit, and the more severe the challenges presented to the patient throughout his or her lifetime. To some degree, all of these children have a concurrent Chiari II malformation, which will lead to hydrocephalus in most patients.

Prenatal closure of the myelomeningocele defect at three designated centers has confirmed the efficacy of this intervention in highly selected patients in a recently completed trial (Management of myelomeningocele study [MOMS]).[61] The incidence of CSF shunts at one year was 40% in the prenatal surgery group vs 80% in those babies managed after birth ($p < 0.001$). Prenatal intervention also resulted in improvement in the composite score for mental development and motor function at 30 months ($p = 0.007$). Independent walking at 3 years was 42% in the prenatal group vs 21% in the postnatal surgery group ($p = 0.01$). However, prenatal operation was associated with higher rates of preterm birth, intraoperative complications, and uterine-scar defects apparent at delivery as well as a higher rate of maternal transfusion at delivery.

Lipomyelomeningocele

Lipomyelomeningocele is a complex anomaly that consists of a subcutaneous meningocele, fascia and bony defects, and a lipoma interfacing with the spinal cord, which is located dorsally, dorsolateral, or terminally. Externally, these lesions appear in the midline and can range from tiny subtle fatty lumps to large masses often accompanied by skin tags, port-wine stains, and an altered intragluteal fold (Fig. 19-9). Before the availability of CT, the connection with the spinal canal was often missed and cosmetic removal of the subcutaneous fat was performed, often with significant negative sequelae. These lesions often require tedious micro dissection with release of any tethering effect on the spinal cord to prevent neurologic (weakness, sensory loss), urologic (neurogenic bladder), or orthopedic (scoliosis, leg-length discrepancies) consequences. These children do not have Chiari malformation, sparing them the burden of hydrocephalus.

Whether to correct the asymptomatic infant with a lipomyelomeningocele is not without controversy. Unfortunately, the natural history of these anomalies is unknown. The rationale for early operation in these patients is to release any tethering on the spinal cord and prevent neurologic, urologic, or orthopedic consequences of spinal cord injury. However, a significant number of patients have suffered the same deficits postoperatively that the surgery was planned to prevent.[62,63]

Meningocele

The least common of the neural tube defects is the simplest one. A meningocele consists of a defect in the skin, fascia, posterior spine, and meninges but not the nervous system. When this anomaly occurs, it has a predilection for the lumbosacral area, although it can develop anywhere along the neural axis. Unlike the myelomeningocele, these lesions are almost always covered by nearly normal skin. Operative repair must be vigilant for cord tethering; dorsal untethering may be needed along with primary dural closure.

Tethered Spinal Cord Syndrome

With any of the spinal dysraphisms, there is a high probability the conus medullaris lies below the L2 disc space and is deemed to be 'tethered' by radiographic imaging. When constricted from free excursion, stretching of the neurons and microvascular ischemia will lead to neurologic dysfunction. This chronic injury leads to a plethora of signs and symptoms, most commonly neurogenic bladder, motor weakness or increasing tone in the lower extremities, sensory loss, and skeletal growth anomalies, including scoliosis. Operative exploration for lysis of adhesions is required. Unfortunately, the process may be recurrent throughout the child's growing years. All children with spinal dysraphism are at risk for tethered cord syndrome, and long-term follow-up is essential.

REFERENCES

1. Janisch W, Haas JF, Schreiber D, et al. Primary central nervous system tumors in stillborns and infants: Epidemiological consideration. J Neurooncol 1984;2:113–16.
2. Grabb PA, Albright AL. Brain tumors of congenital and developmental origin in infants and children: Clinical features and natural history. In: Tindall GT, Cooper PR, Barrow DL, editor. The Practice of Neurosurgery, vol. 1. Baltimore: Williams & Wilkins; 1996. p. 821–31.
3. Carmel PW. Brain tumors of disordered embryogenesis. In: Youmans JR, editor. Neurological Surgery, vol. 4. Philadelphia: WB Saunders; 1996. p. 2761–81.
4. Lieberman DM, Russo CL, Berger MS. Brain tumors during the first 2 years of life. In: Albright AL, Pollack IF, Adelson PD, editor. Principles and Practice of Pediatric Neurosurgery. New York: Thieme; 1999. p. 463–90.
5. Steinbok P, Mutat A. Cerebellar astrocytomas. In: Albright AL, Pollack IF, Adelson PD, editor. Principles and Practice of Pediatric Neurosurgery. New York: Thieme; 1999. p. 641–62.

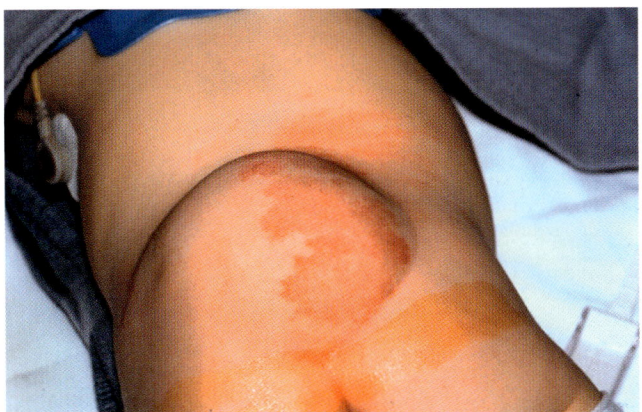

FIGURE 19-9 ■ A sizable lipomyelomeningocele is seen with cutaneous port-wine stains.

6. Cochrane DD, Gustavsson B, Poskitt KP, et al. The surgical and natural morbidity of aggressive resection for posterior fossa tumors in childhood. Pediatr Neurosurg 1994;20:19–29.

7. Pollack I. Brain tumors in children. N Engl J Med 1994;331:1500–7.

8. Sutton L, Goldwein J, Perilongo G, et al. Prognostic factors in childhood ependymomas. Pediatr Neurosurg 1990-1991;16:57–65.

9. Roberts RO, Lynch CF, Jones MP, et al. Medulloblastoma: A population-based study of 532 cases. J Neuro-pathol Exp Neurol 1991;50:134–44.

10. Raffel C, Thomas GA, Tishler DM, et al. Absence of p53 mutations in childhood central nervous system primitive neuroectodermal tumors. Neurosurgery 1993;33:301–6.

11. Pollack IF, Polinko P, Albright AL, et al. Mutism and pseudobulbar symptoms after resection of posterior fossa tumors in children: Incidence and pathophysiology. Neurosurgery 1995;37:885–93.

12. Duffner PK, Horowitz ME, Krischer JP, et al. Postoperative chemotherapy and delayed radiation in children less than 3 years of age with malignant brain tumors. N Engl J Med 1993;328:1725–31.

13. Pollack IF, Gerszten PC, Martinez AJ, et al. Intracranial ependymomas of childhood: Long-term outcome and prognostic factors. Neurosurgery 1995;37:655–67.

14. Sanai N, Alvarez-Buylla A, Berger M. Neural stem cells and the origin of gliomas. N Engl J Med 2005;353:811–22.

15. Croce CM. Oncogenes and Cancer. N Engl J Med 2008;358:502–11.

16. Esteller M. Epigenetics in cancer. N Engl J Med 2008;358:1148–59.

17. Tarbell N, Loeffler JS. Radiotherapy for pediatric brain tumors. In: Albright AL, Pollack IF, Adelson PD, editor. Principles and Practice of Pediatric Neurosurgery. New York: Thieme; 1999. p. 765–78.

18. Albright AL, Barron WB, Faick MP, et al. Continuous intrathecal baclofen infusion for spasticity of cerebral origin. JAMA 1993;270:2475–7.

19. Peacock WJ, Arens LJ, Berman B. Cerebral palsy spasticity: Selective posterior rhizotomy. Pediatr Neurosci 1987;13:61–6.

20. Jankovic J, Brin MF. Therapeutic uses of botulinum toxin. N Engl J Med 1991;324:1186–94.

21. Wiebe S, Blume WT, Girvin JP, et al. A randomized, controlled trial of surgery for temporal-lobe epilepsy. N Engl J Med 2001;345:311–18.

22. Morrison G. Extratemporal epilepsy surgery in children. In: Albright AL, Pollack IF, Adelson PD, editor. Principles and Practice of Pediatric Neurosurgery. New York: Thieme; 1999. p. 1127–46.

23. Schramm J, Kral T, Clusmann H. Transsylvian keyhole functional hemispherectomy. Neurosurgery 2001;49:891–901.

24. Black PM, Holmes G, Lombroso C. Corpus callosum section for intractable epilepsy in children. Pediatr Neurosurg 1992;18:298–304.

25. Murphy JV. Left vagal nerve stimulation in children with epilepsy. J Pediatr 1999;134:563–6.

26. Simon TD, Riva-Cambrin Srivastaua R, et al. or the hydrocephalus clinical network: Hospital care for children with hydrocephalus in the United States: Utilization, charges, comorbidities and deaths. J Neurosurg Pediatr 2008;1:131–8.

27. Cochrane DD, Kestle J. Ventricular shunting for hydrocephalus in children: Patients, procedures, surgeons, and institutions in English Canada, 1989-2001. Eur J Pediatr Surg 2002;12(1 Suppl):S6–S11.

28. Smith ER, Butler WE, Barker FG II. In-hospital mortality rates after ventricular peritoneal shunt procedures in the United States, 1998-2002: Relation to hospital and surgeon volume of care. J Neurosurg 2004;100(2 Suppl Pediatrics):90–7.

29. Berry JG, Hall MA, Sharma V, et al. A multi-institutional five year analysis of initial and multiple shunt revisions in children. Neurosurgery 2008;62:445–53.

30. Patwardham RV, Nanda A. Implanted ventricular shunts in the United States: The billion-dollar-a-year cost of hydrocephalus treatment. Neurosurgery 2005;56:139–45.

31. Milhorat TH. Cerebral Spinal Fluid and the Brain Edemas. Neuroscience Society of New York; 1987. p. 46–7.

32. Milhorat TH. Choroid plexus and CSF production. Science 1969;166:1514–16.

33. Milhorat TH, Hammock MK, Fenstermacher JD, et al. CSF production by the choroid plexus and brain. Science 1971;173:330–2.

34. Rekate HL. The treatment of hydrocephalus. In: Albright AL, Pollack EF, Adelson PD, editor. Principles and Practice of Pediatric Neurosurgery. 2nd ed. New York: Thieme; 2008. p. 103–5.

35. Boulton M, Flessner M, Armstrong D, et al. Determination of volumetric CSF absorption into extracranial lymphatics in sheep. Am J Physiol 1998;274:88–96.

36. Erlich SS, McComb JG, Hyman S, et al. Ultrastructure of the orbital pathways for CSF drainage in rabbits. J Neurosurg 1989;70:926–31.

37. Johnston M, Zakharov A, Papaiconomou C, et al. Evidence of connections between CSF and nasal lymphatic vessels in humans, non-human primates and other mammalian species. CSF Res 2004;1:2.

38. Dirks P. Genetics of hydrocephalus. In: Cinalli G, Maixner WJ, Sainte-Rose C, editor. Pediatric Hydrocephalus. New York: Springer-Verlag; 2005.

39. Barkovich AJ, Newton TH. MR of aqueductal stenosis: Evidence of a broad spectrum of tectal distortion. AJNR Am J Neuroradiol 1989;10:471–6.

40. Mohanty A, Biswas A, Satish S, et al. Treatment options for Dandy-Walker malformation. J Neurosurg 2006;105(5 Suppl Pediatrics):348–56.

41. Yüceer N, Mertol T, Arda N. Surgical treatment of 13 pediatric patients with Dandy-Walker syndrome. Pediatr Neurosurg 2007;43:358–63.

42. Boop FA. Posthemorrhagic hydrocephalus of prematurity. In: Cinalli G, Maixner WJ, Sainte-Rose C, editor. Pediatric Hydrocephalus. New York: Springer-Verlag; 2005. p. 121–6.

43. Fritsch M, Mehdorn M. Endoscopic intraventricular surgery for treatment of hydrocephalus and loculated CSF spaces in children less than one year of age. Pediatr Neurosurg 2002;36:183–8.

44. Rekate HL. The treatment of hydrocephalus. In: Albright AL, Pollack EF, Adelson PD, editor. Principles and Practice of Pediatric Neurosurgery. 2nd ed. New York: Thieme; 2008. p. 103–5.

45. Rekate HL, Nulsen FE, Mack H, et al. Establishing the diagnosis of shunt independence. Monogr Neural Sci 1982;8:223–6.

46. Matson DD. A new operation for treatment of communicating hydrocephalus. J Neurosurg 1949;6:238–47.

47. Nulsen FE, Spitz EB. Treatment of hydrocephalus by direct shunt from ventricle to jugular vein. Surg Forum (Am Coll Surg) 1952;2:399–403.

48. Ames RH. Ventricular peritoneal shunts in the management of hydrocephalus. J Neurosurg 1967;27:525–9.

49. Drake JM, Kestle JR, Milner R, et al. Randomized trial of CSF shunt valve design in pediatric hydrocephalus. Neurosurgery 1998;43:294–305.

50. Piatt JH, Carlson CV. A search of determinates of cerebrospinal fluid shunt survival: Retrospective analysis of a 14-year institutional experience. Pediatr Neurosurg 1993;19:233–42.

51. Biyani N, Grisaru-Soen G, Steinbok P, et al. Prophylactic antibiotics in pediatric shunt surgery. Childs Nerv Syst 2006;22:1465–71.

52. Welch K, Shillito J, Strand R, et al. Chiari I "malformation": An acquired disorder? J Neurosurg 1981;55:604–9.

53. Wang V, Barbaro N, Lauton M, et al. Complications of lumbar peritoneal shunts. Neurosurgery 2007;60:1045–9.

54. Dagnew E, van Loveren H, Tew J Jr. Acute foramen magnum syndrome caused by an acquired Chiari malformation after lumbar drainage of cerebral spinal fluid: Report of three cases. Neurosurgery 2002;51:823–9.

55. Aldana P, James H, Postlethwait R. Ventriculogallbladder shunts in pediatric patients. J Neurosurg Pediatr 2008;1:284–7.

56. Kadrian D, van Gelder J, Florida D, et al. Long-term reliability of endoscopic third ventriculostomy. Neurosurgery 2005;56:1271–8.

57. McNatt SA, Kim A, Hohuan D, et al. Pediatric shunt malfunction without ventricular dilation. Pediatr Neurosurg 2008;44:128–32.

58. Winston KR, Lopez JA, Freeman J. CSF shunt failure with stable normal ventricular size. Pediatr Neurosurg 2006;42:151–5.

59. Vinchon M, Fichten A, Delestret I, et al. Shunt revision for asymptomatic failures: Surgical and clinical results. Neurosurgery 2003;52:347–56.

60. Diaz M, McLone D. Myelomeningocele. In: Albright AL, Pollack IF, Adelson PD, editor. Principles and Practice of Pediatric Neurosurgery. 2nd ed. New York: Thieme; 2008. p. 338–66.

61. Adzick NS, Tom E, Spong CY, et al. A randomized trial of prenatal versus postnatal repair of myelomeningocele. N Engl J Med 2011;364:993–1004.

62. Cochrane DD, Finley C, Kestle J, et al. The patterns of late deterioration in patients with transitional lipomyelomeningocele. Eur J Pediatr Surg 2000;10(Suppl 1):13–17.

63. Cochrane DD. Occult spinal dysraphism. In: Albright AL, Pollack IF, Adelson PD, editor. Principles and Practice of Pediatric Neurosurgery. 2nd ed. New York: Thieme; 2008. p. 367–93.

SECTION III

THORACIC

CHAPTER 20

CONGENITAL CHEST WALL DEFORMITIES

Donald Nuss • Robert E. Kelly, Jr.

Congenital chest wall deformities fall into two groups: those with overgrowth of the cartilages causing either a depression or protuberance, and those with varying degrees of either aplasia or dysplasia.

Pectus excavatum, also known as an 'excavated, sunken, or funnel chest,' is the most common chest wall anomaly, constituting about 80% of deformities seen at our hospital (Table 20-1). Pectus carinatum, a chest wall protuberance, comprises approximately 12% of chest wall deformities, whereas combined excavatum/carinatum deformities are found in about 5%. Jeune syndrome, or asphyxiating chondrodystrophy, is an extreme form of mixed pectus excavatum/carinatum and is very rare.

Poland syndrome and bifid sternum represent different forms of aplasia of the anterior chest wall. Poland syndrome consists of varying degrees of dysplasia of the breast, the pectoralis muscles, and ribs. In bifid sternum, partial or complete failure of the midline fusion of the sternum is seen. This may result in ectopia cordis or varying degrees of sternal dysplasia and deficiencies of associated structures such as the heart, pericardium, diaphragm, and anterior abdominal wall (pentalogy of Cantrell).

Many of these deformities are present at birth. Some cases, such as ectopia cordis, are incompatible with life and have rarely been successfully repaired. Chest wall deformities are frequently associated with a systemic weakness of the connective tissues and with poor muscular development of the abdominal region, thorax, and spine. An association with Marfan syndrome, Ehlers–Danlos syndrome, and scoliosis, as well as with omphalocele in the case of bifid sternum, have been identified, all of which complicate the management of these patients (see Table 20-1).

PECTUS EXCAVATUM

Pectus excavatum is a depression of the anterior chest wall of variable severity and can usually be characterized as mild, moderate, or severe. The deformity may be localized and deep ('cup-shaped'; Fig. 20-1A), or diffuse and shallow ('saucer-shaped'; see Fig. 20-1B), or asymmetric (see Fig. 20-1C). The depth and extent of the depression determine the degree of cardiac and pulmonary compression, which, in turn, determines the degree of physiologic effect. Only one-third of patients referred from our own region had a deformity severe enough to require surgical correction. Even with referral of patients with a severe deformity from other centers, our ratio of operative correction has been only about 60% (Box 20-1).

This chest wall deformity may be noted at birth and usually progresses with age and growth. With rapid growth at puberty, the progression may become especially pronounced, a fact apparently unknown to many pediatricians, who mistakenly advise families of younger patients that the condition will resolve spontaneously. We have seen many families who were given this advice and missed the opportunity to have the deformity repaired before puberty while the chest was still soft and malleable and before it interfered with physical performance.

History

Pectus excavatum was recognized as early as the 16th century. Johan Schenck collected literature on the subject.[1] In 1594, Bauhinus described the clinical features of pectus excavatum in a patient who had pulmonary compression with dyspnea and paroxysmal cough, both attributed to the severe pectus excavatum.[2] The familial predisposition was first noted by Coulson in 1820, who cited a family of three brothers with pectus excavatum.[3] In 1872, Williams described a 17-year-old patient who was born with a pectus excavatum, and whose father and brother also had the condition.[4]

Numerous other case reports appeared in the 19th century, including a five-case report by Ebstein in 1882 that covered the clinical spectrum of this condition.[5] Treatment at that time was limited to 'fresh air, breathing exercises, aerobic activities, and lateral pressure'.[6,7]

Thoracic surgery remained 'forbidden territory' until the early years of the 20th century. The first attempt at correction was a tentative approach in 1911 by Meyer who removed the second and third costal cartilages on the right side without improvement.[8] Sauerbruch, one of the pioneers of thoracic surgery, used a more aggressive approach in 1913 by excising a section of the anterior chest wall, which included the left fifth to ninth costal cartilages as well as a segment of the adjacent sternum.[7] Before his operation, the patient was incapacitated by severe dyspnea and palpitations, even at rest, and was unable to work in his father's watch factory. After recovery, the heart could be seen to pulsate under the muscle flap, but the patient was able to work without dyspnea and was married three years later.

In the 1920s, Sauerbruch performed the first pectus repair that used the bilateral costal cartilage resection and sternal osteotomy technique later popularized by Ravitch.[9] He also advocated external traction to hold the sternum in its corrected position for six postoperative weeks. His technique was soon adapted by others in Europe and rapidly gained popularity in the USA. In 1939, Ochsner and DeBakey published their experience with this

TABLE 20-1	Incidence and Etiology of Congenital Chest Wall Anomalies Seen at Children's Hospital of the King's Daughters
Total children evaluated	3137
Pectus excavatum only	2512
Mixed excavatum/carinatum	163
Carinatum only	391
Poland syndrome	15
Male-female ratio	4.2 : 1
Family history of pectus excavatum	39.0%
Incidence of scoliosis	20%
Incidence of Marfan syndrome diagnosed	2.7%
Marfanoid—presumed Marfan syndrome	17.7%

Data collected from 5/18/1987 to 1/1/2012.

approach, and reviewed the entire surgical literature on the subject.[10] Also in 1939, Lincoln Brown published his experience in two patients and reviewed the literature with particular reference to the etiology of pectus excavatum.[11] He was impressed with the theory that short diaphragmatic ligaments and the pull of the diaphragm on the posterior sternum were causative factors.

Ravitch initially subscribed to the short ligament theory as well. As a result, he advocated even more radical mobilization of the sternum, with transection of all sternal attachments, including the intercostal bundles, rectus muscles, diaphragmatic attachments, and excision of the xiphisternum. In 1949, he published his experience with eight patients in which he used this radically extended modification of Sauerbruch's technique of bilateral cartilage resection and sternal osteotomy, but without external traction.[12]

The lack of external traction may have led to an increased recurrence of the condition. As a result, Wallgren and Sulamaa introduced the concept of internal support in 1956 by using a slightly curved stainless steel bar that was pushed through the caudal end of the sternum from side to side and bridged the newly created gap between the sternum and ribs.[13,14] In 1961, Adkins and Blades modified internal bracing further by passing a straight stainless steel bar behind, rather than through, the sternum.[15] This technique was rapidly adapted for patients of all ages.

As early as 1958, Welch and Gross advocated a less radical approach than that of Ravitch.[16,17] Welch showed excellent results in 75 patients without dividing all the intercostal bundles or the pectus muscle attachments. However, he still advocated performing the procedure in young patients. Conversely, Pena was very disturbed by the idea of resecting the rib cartilages from very young patients and demonstrated that asphyxiating chondrodystrophy developed in baby rabbits after cartilage resection during their growth phase.[18] Later, Haller also reported the risk of acquired asphyxiating chondrodystrophy as well.[19] As a result, many surgeons stopped performing open pectus repair in young children and waited until they had reached puberty. They also reduced the amount of cartilage resected and spoke about a 'modified Ravitch procedure,' which was really the original Sauerbruch procedure.

In 1997, we published our 10-year experience with a minimally invasive technique that did not utilize cartilage resection or sternal osteotomy, but instead relied on internal bracing made possible by the flexibility and malleability of the costal cartilages.[20] The rationale for this technique was based on the three following observations:

1. *Malleability of the chest.* Children have a soft and malleable chest. In young children, the chest is so soft that even minor respiratory obstruction can

BOX 20-1	Results from Patients Undergoing Repair of Pectus Excavatum at Children's Hospital of The King's Daughters

2512 patients evaluated for pectus excavation
1571 patients had minimally invasive pectus repair (MIPR)
1463 patients underwent primary MIPR
108 patients have had re-do MIPR:
   49 failed Ravitch procedures
   55 failed Nuss procedures
   Three failed Leonard procedures
Minimally invasive pectus repair
   Single pectus bar 68%
   Double pectus bar 38%
   Triple pectus bar 0.3%(n = 4)
   Median age 15 years
   Median Haller CT index 4.5
   Median length of stay five days

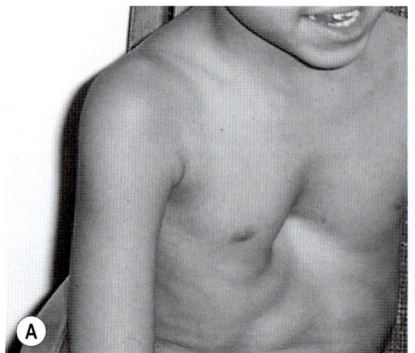 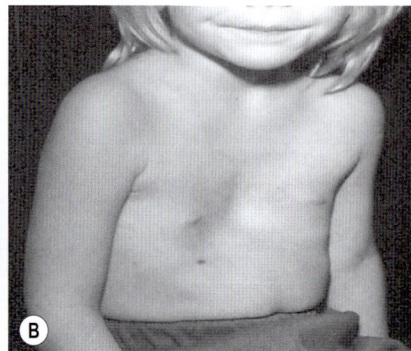 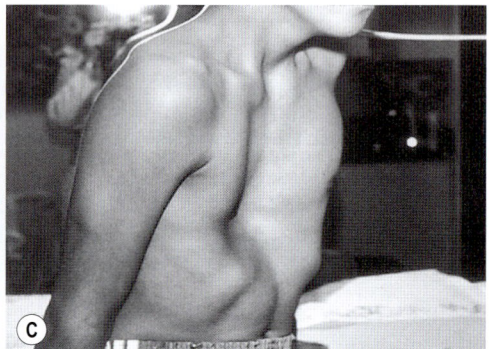

FIGURE 20-1 ■ **(A)** Localized or 'cup-shaped' pectus excavatum. **(B)** Diffuse or 'saucer-shaped' deformity. **(C)** Eccentric deformity.

cause severe sternal retraction. Trauma rarely causes rib fractures and flail chest because the chest is so soft and malleable.[21–23] Thus, the American Heart Association recommends 'using only two fingers' when performing cardiac resuscitation in young children and 'only one hand in older children' for fear of crushing the heart.

2. *Chest reconfiguration.* In middle-aged and older adults, a barrel-shaped chest configuration develops in response to chronic obstructive respiratory diseases such as emphysema. If older adults are able to reconfigure the chest wall, children and teenagers should be able to remodel as well, especially with the increased malleability of their anterior chest wall.

3. *Bracing.* The role of braces and serial casting in successfully correcting skeletal anomalies such as scoliosis, clubfoot, and maxillomandibular malocclusion by orthopedic and orthodontic surgeons is well established. The anterior chest wall, being even more malleable than the previously mentioned skeletal structures, is ideally suited for this type of correction.

INCIDENCE AND ETIOLOGY

Pectus excavatum occurs in approximately 1 in 1000 children and constitutes 80% of all chest wall deformities in our center (see Table 20-1). However, this is not the case in all countries. In Argentina, pectus carinatum is more common than pectus excavatum.[24] Pectus excavatum also is rare in African-Americans and in Africans. A genetic predisposition, already noted in the 19th century, has been found in almost 40% of our patients. We have seen families with three siblings, as well as cousins and other family members, who had a pectus deformity severe enough to require correction. We also have seen patients whose fathers and grandfathers have the deformity. The male-to-female ratio of 4:1 in our series of pectus excavatum patients is similar to that of other large series.[25] Female patients have an increased risk of associated scoliosis. Inheritance is autosomal dominant, autosomal recessive, X-linked, and multifactorial in different families.[26, 27]

The association with a connective tissue disorder is higher than in the normal population. The vast majority of our patients have an asthenic build and a definitive diagnosis of Marfan syndrome has been found in 2.7% of our patients. An additional 17% have had clinical features suggestive of Marfan syndrome. Ehlers–Danlos syndrome was present in another 0.7%. Mild scoliosis was noted in 20% of our patients. In our experience, severely asymmetric pectus excavatum tends to aggravate the postural abnormality of scoliosis. Early correction of the pectus excavatum has improved the mild scoliosis in many patients.

Clinical Features

Pectus excavatum is noted in infancy in approximately one-third of patients,[25] and usually progresses slowly as the child grows. Because young children have significant cardiac and pulmonary reserve and their chest wall is still very pliable, the majority of young children are asymptomatic. However, as they become older, the deformity becomes more severe and the chest wall becomes more rigid. Eventually, they find that they have difficulty keeping up with their peers when playing aerobic sports. A vicious cycle may develop as patients stop participating in aerobic activities because of their inability to keep up. Subsequently, their exercise capacity diminishes further. The downward spiral is further promoted by the fact that these patients, already embarrassed by their deformity, will avoid situations in which they have to remove their shirts in front of other children, inhibiting participation in school and team activities.

By withdrawing from participation in activities with their peers, they also become depressed, which may affect their schoolwork. Most pectus patients have a typical geriatric or 'pectus posture' that includes thoracic kyphosis, forward-sloping shoulders, and a protuberant abdomen (Fig. 20-2). A sedentary 'couch potato' lifestyle may aggravate this posture, and the poor posture depresses the sternum even farther. For this reason, we always recommend an aggressive pectus posture exercise and breathing program, both preoperatively and postoperatively.

Many patients have a relatively mild deformity during childhood. Because pediatricians are unaware of the potential for marked progression of the deformity as the child grows, they reassure the parents that it will resolve spontaneously or even improve. Although the deformity may not always increase in severity, it is unlikely that it will spontaneously resolve. When the patients grow rapidly during puberty, the deformity often suddenly accelerates. A mild deformity may become severe in as little as six to 12 months. These patients give a history that 'my chest suddenly caved in.' It is the rapid progression that alarms parents and stimulates them to seek consultation with a surgeon. Patients with a rapid progression of their deformity exhibit the most pronounced symptom-complex.

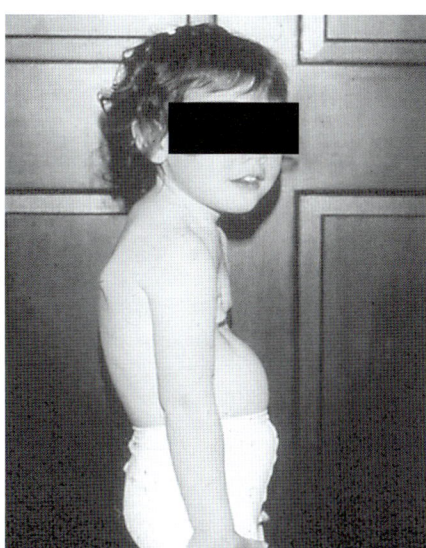

FIGURE 20-2 ■ Classic pectus posture with thoracic kyphosis, forward-sloping shoulders, and lumbar lordosis.

TABLE 20-2   **Presenting of Symptoms Patients Who Have Undergone Operative Correction of Pectus Excavatum at Children's' Hospital of the King's Daughters**

Shortness of breath, lack of endurance, exercise intolerance	81% (1197/1463)
Chest pain, with or without exercise	68% (997/1463)
Frequent respiratory infections	21% (303/1463)
Asthma/asthma-like symptoms	37% (543/1463)
Cardiology Indicators	
Cardiac compression	85% (1301/1450)
Cardiac displacement by CT	73% (1119/1419)
Murmurs	27% (314/1148)
Mitral valve prolapse	13 % (149/1148)
Pulmonary Indicators[a]	
FVC <80%	24%
FEV1% <80%	29%
FEF25–75% <80%	43%

[a]<80% defined as 2 SD below average of normal population; in a 'normal' dataset, only 2.5% of all persons.
Pulmonary Data collected from 5/18/1987 through to 10/31/2011; all data collected 5/18/1987 through to 1/1/2012.
Number of patients with echocardiograms = 1148.
Number of patients with mention of cardiac compression (or not) on CT scan = 1450.
Number of patients with mention of cardiac displacement (or not) on CT scan = 1419.

The earliest complaints are shortness of breath and lack of endurance with exercise. As the deformity progresses, chest pain and palpitations with exercise may develop, giving rise to exercise intolerance. Other symptoms include frequent and prolonged respiratory tract infections, which may lead to symptoms of asthma (Table 20-2).

A recent study showed that these patients have a poor body image, which has a major impact on their self-worth.[28] Therefore, it is important to correct the deformity before it affects their ability to function normally. Just as one would not consider leaving a child with a cleft lip untreated, one should not leave a child with a severe pectus untreated. Both have a physiologic and psychological impact on the patient.

CARDIAC AND PULMONARY EFFECTS OF PECTUS EXCAVATUM

A great deal has been written about cardiopulmonary function in patients with pectus excavatum.[29] In the last ten years, there has been increasing acknowledgement in the medical community that a severe pectus excavatum has a significant detrimental effect on cardiopulmonary function. Though studies conflict, many older studies treated the condition as either present or absent, with no quantification of the anatomic severity.[30,31] Later work demonstrated the effects more clearly, and showed that in a minority of patients there are no deleterious effects on cardiopulmonary function.[32] Several factors play a role when testing cardiopulmonary function. These include

the severity of the deformity, the inherent physical fitness of the individual patient, the patient's age, associated conditions, whether the tests are done supine or erect, and whether they are done at rest or during exercise. Recently, a study has shown statistically significant and clinically meaningful improvements in stroke volume, cardiac output, and cardiac index after minimally invasive repair of pectus excavatum.[33] Also, an improvement in exercise cardiopulmonary function has been noted as well.

Cardiac effects include decreased cardiac output, mitral valve prolapse, and arrhythmias (see Table 20-2). Compression of the heart results in incomplete filling and decreased stroke volume, which in turn, results in decreased cardiac output.[30,31,34,35] Cardiac compression may interfere with normal valve function. Mitral valve prolapse has been found in 13% of our patients and in up to 65% in other series.[36,37] Prolapse occurs in only 1% in the normal pediatric population.[38] In one study, the mitral prolapse resolved in about half of patients who underwent correction.[36] Thus, both mechanical and connective tissue derangements may be involved. Dysrhythmias, including first-degree heart block, right bundle branch block, and Wolff–Parkinson–White syndrome have been found in 16% of patients.[39]

Pulmonary effects result from poor motion of the depressed part of the chest wall. Normal chest wall motion includes 'pump handle' movement of the sternum. The lower sternum moves up and out, like the handle of a mechanical water pump. Physical examination, and now motion capture analysis, show that this motion is almost absent in the depressed area of the pectus excavatum chest. Instead, patients compensate by increased abdominal diaphragmatic breathing. Following correction, the motion is indistinguishable from normal chest wall.[40]

Pulmonary function testing shows statistically and clinically meaningful diminution in static pulmonary function tests (forced vital capacity, forced expiratory volume in one second, and others) even though most patients do not have any problem with their airways or pulmonary parenchyma (see Table 20-2).[35] These values improve after operation. Exercise pulmonary function testing also shows improvement. Stress testing has shown an increase in oxygen consumption for a given exercise when compared with that of normal patients.[41] This shows that the work of breathing is increased and explains why they lack endurance.

Evaluation and Indications for Operation

A complete history and physical examination is performed on all patients and includes documenting photographs. Younger patients with a mild to moderate deformity are treated with a posture and exercise program in an attempt to halt the progression and are followed at yearly or longer intervals (Fig. 20-3).

Patients with a severe deformity or those with documented progression also are treated with the exercise and posture program. Additionally, they undergo objective studies to evaluate whether their condition is severe enough to warrant repair. These studies include pulmonary function tests (PFTs), a thoracic computed tomography (CT), or magnetic resonance imaging (MRI) scan, and a cardiac evaluation that includes an electrocardio-gram (ECG) and an echocardiogram.

CT scans are very helpful because they clearly show the degree of cardiac compression and displacement, the degree of pulmonary compression and atelectasis,

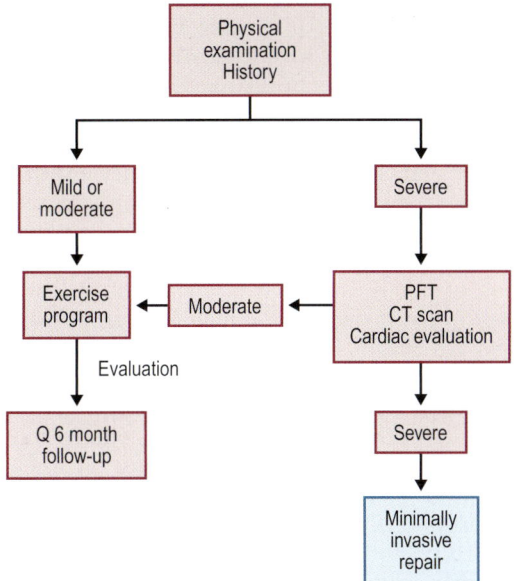

FIGURE 20-3 ■ Algorithm for evaluation and treatment of patients with pectus deformities.

asymmetry of the chest, sternal torsion, compensatory development of a barrel-chest deformity in long-standing deformities, and ossification of the cartilages in patients with previous repairs (Fig. 20-4A, B). They also are used to calculate the CT index, which gives an objective meas-urement for comparing the severity among patients. The CT index is calculated by dividing the transverse diam-eter by the anteroposterior diameter (see Fig. 20-4C).[42]

We have recently utilized MRI of the chest instead of CT scan to diminish radiation exposure. However, MRI does not give as clear a picture of the bony structures which are the central issue, and cardiac MRI, which should be able to provide the same information as echocar-diography and CT scan, remains in development.

Determination of a severe pectus excavatum and the need for repair include two or more of the following criteria: (1) a CT index greater than 3.2; (2) pulmonary function studies that indicate restrictive airway disease; (3) a cardiology evaluation in which compression is causing murmurs, mitral valve prolapse, cardiac displace-ment, or conduction abnormalities on the echocardio-gram or ECG tracings; (4) documentation of progression of the deformity with associated physical symptoms other than isolated concerns of body image; (5) a failed Ravitch procedure; or (6) a failed minimally invasive procedure. With these criteria, only about 60% of patients referred to us are found to have a deformity severe enough to warrant correction.[20,43]

The age parameters for surgical correction depend on the type of repair selected. Unlike the more invasive

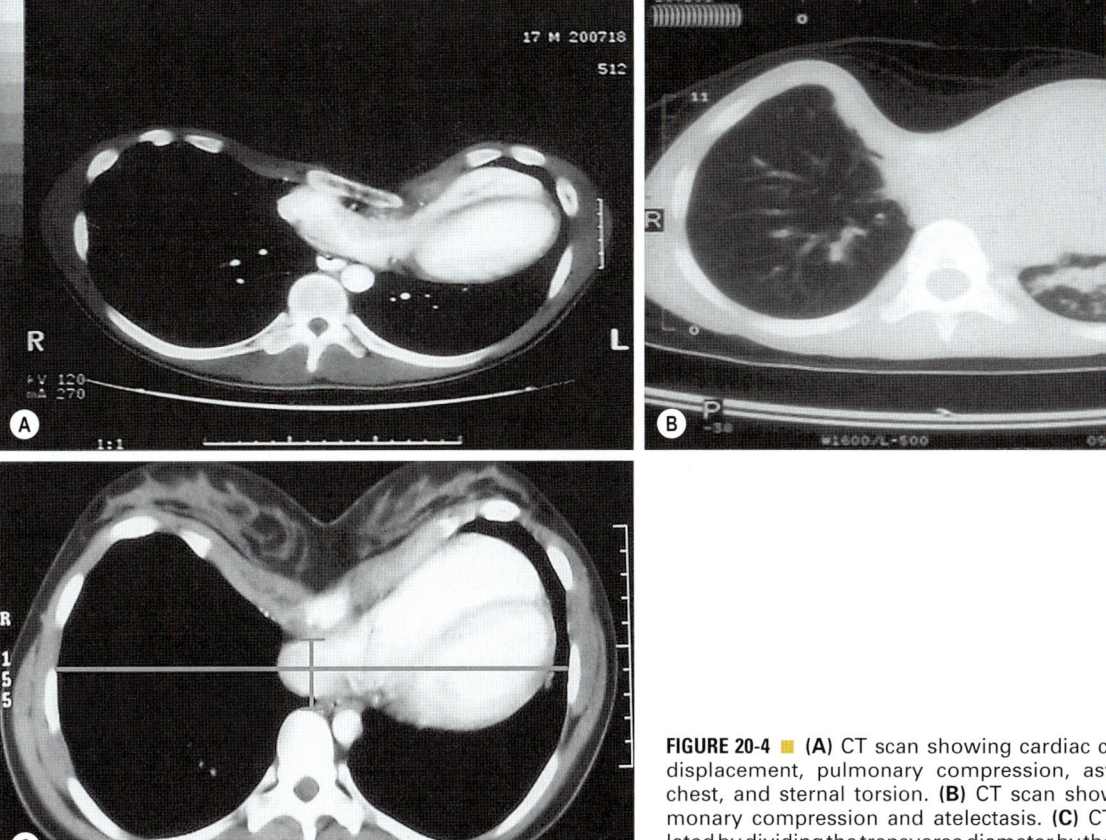

FIGURE 20-4 ■ **(A)** CT scan showing cardiac compression and displacement, pulmonary compression, asymmetry of the chest, and sternal torsion. **(B)** CT scan showing severe pul-monary compression and atelectasis. **(C)** CT index is calcu-lated by dividing the transverse diameter by the anteroposterior diameter.

procedures (e.g., Ravitch procedure, sternal turnover), there is no interference with growth plates with the minimally invasive approach. Therefore, it can be done at any age, as evidenced by the fact that we have successfully operated on patients from ages 13 months through to 31 years (Fig. 20-5). However, the concern with patients younger than 11 years is that if the procedure is performed at too young an age, many years of subsequent growth remain during which the excavatum can recur.

Our experience suggests that the optimal age for repair is 11 to 14 years. At this age, the patient is prepubertal, the chest is still soft and malleable, there is a quick recovery with a rapid return to normal activities, and results are excellent. After puberty, the flexibility of the chest wall is decreased, sometimes requiring the insertion of two bars, which makes the operation more difficult. It also takes patients longer to recover. However, patients older than 20 years have been uniformly pleased with their results. Several other centers have reported success with patients up to age 44 years.[34,44,45]

Operative Approaches

Minimally Invasive Pectus Repair

The minimally invasive pectus repair (Fig. 20-6) involves making incisions on each side of the chest and creating a subcutaneous tunnel from the lateral thoracic incision to the top of the pectus ridge on each side. At the top of the ridge, bilateral thoracostomy incisions are bluntly created, and a large introducer is inserted into the chest cavity under thoracoscopic visualization. Very carefully, the pleura and pericardium are dissected off the undersurface of the sternum and the introducer is slowly advanced across the mediastinum and exteriorized through the thoracostomy incision on the contralateral side. When the introducer is in place, the sternum is lifted out of its depressed position by the introducer. Once the sternal depression has been corrected, an umbilical tape is attached to the introducer, and the introducer is slowly

withdrawn. The pectus support bar is then attached to the umbilical tape and is slowly guided through the substernal tunnel with its convexity facing posteriorly until it emerges on the contralateral side. All the maneuvers are performed using thoracoscopy to see inside the chest.

The length of the bar is determined by measuring the distance from midaxillary line to midaxillary line and subtracting 2.5 cm (1 inch). The bar is bent to the desired configuration using a bar bender. Once the bar is positioned inside the chest with the convexity facing posteriorly, it is turned over by using specially designed bar flippers, resulting in correction of the excavatum. The bar is secured with a stabilizer on one side and sutures around the bar and underlying ribs on the other side. Alternatively, stabilizers can be used on both sides to secure the bar as well. These sutures can be placed with an EndoClose needle (Covidien, Mansfield NJ) using thoracoscopy. It is essential that the bar is well stabilized or it will become displaced. Once the bar is secure, the incisions are closed. The thoracoscope is removed, and the pneumothorax is evacuated.

The patient is discharged from the hospital, usually on the fourth or fifth day. Patients are instructed to refrain from sports or other similar activities for six weeks after operation. All patients are restarted on an exercise and posture program to facilitate chest expansion and maintain a good posture.

Pain management for both the open and closed pectus repairs is similar and designed to pre-empt the pain cascade. This is accomplished by the use of intravenous narcotics, benzodiazapenes, and nonsteroidal anti-inflammatory agents, which are started immediately before operation and continued postoperatively for three days until transition to oral medications can be accomplished. When patients are discharged, they are given prescriptions for nonsteroidal anti-inflammatory medications, muscle relaxants, and narcotic medication. Patients less than 13 years of age are generally able to stop all pain medications after 7 to 10 days while patients 13 and over may require pain medication for 10 to 14 days postoperatively.

A recent prospective randomized trial evaluated the use of a thoracic epidural catheter vs patient-controlled analgesia (PCA) with intravenous narcotics for postoperative pain management after the minimally invasive pectus repair. One hundred and ten patients were randomized with fixed protocols for each arm. The primary outcome variable was length of postoperative hospitalization with a power of 0.8 and an alpha of 0.05. No difference was found in length of hospitalization between the two treatment arms. There was a longer operative time, more calls to anesthesia, and greater hospital charges in the epidural group. Pain scores favored the epidural pathway in the first few days and the PCA pathway thereafter. Interestingly, the epidural catheter could not be placed or was removed within 24 hours in 12 patients (22%).[46]

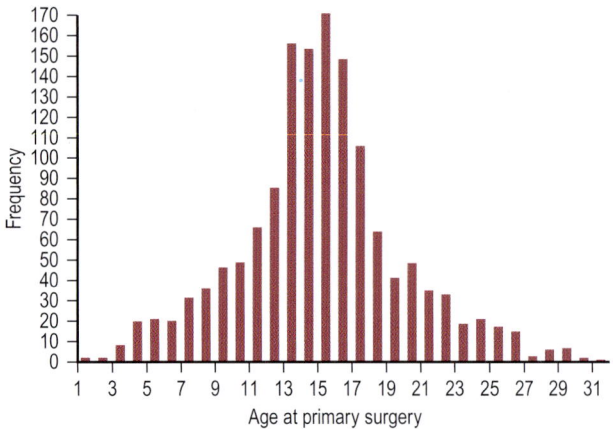

FIGURE 20-5 ■ Age distribution of the authors' primary pectus excavatum repairs (n = 1463; median age at surgery 15 years, range 1 to 31 years; data collected from 5/18/1987 through to 1/1/2012).

Open Technique

The preoperative preparation and evaluation are the same for the open approach for pectus repair as for

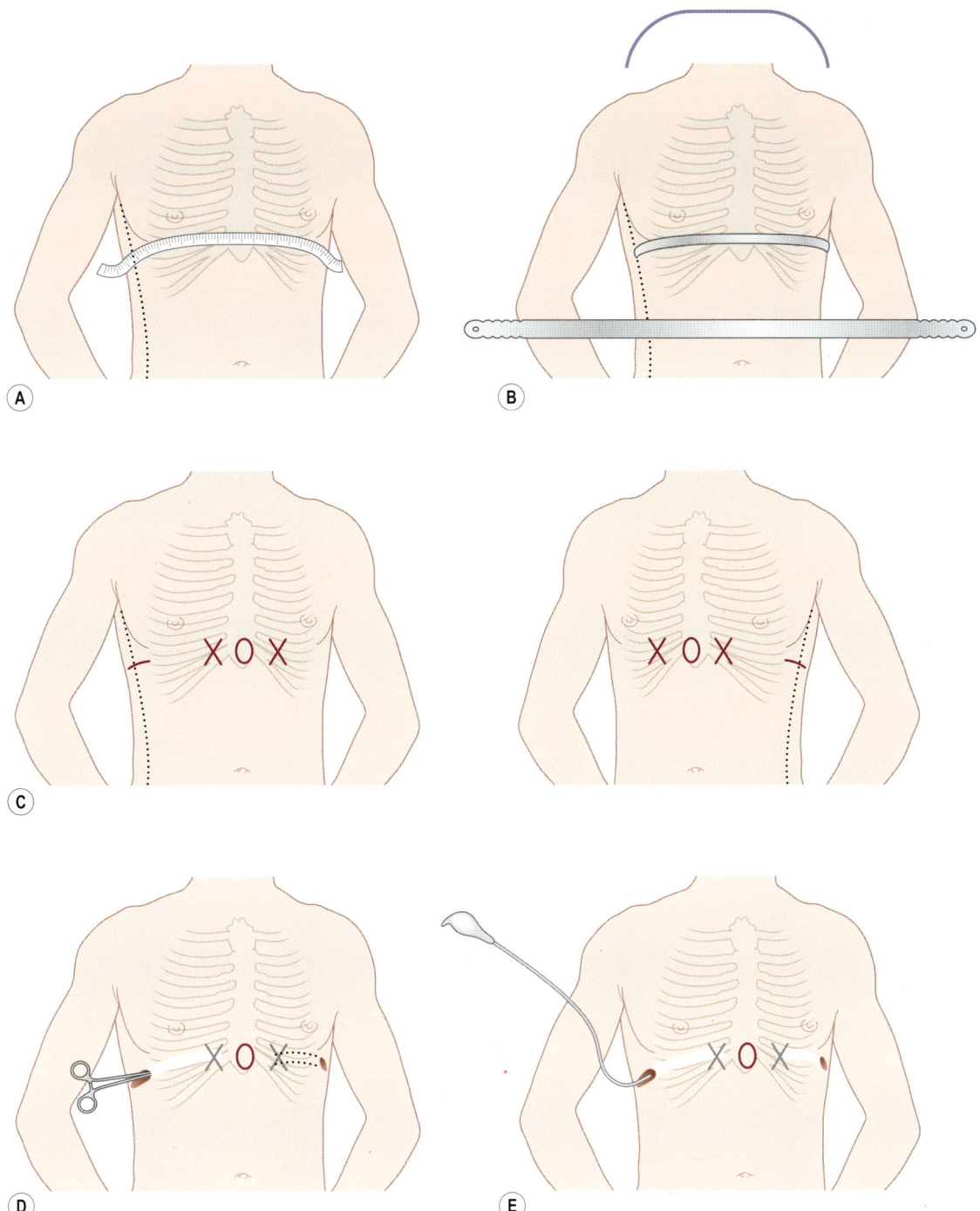

FIGURE 20-6 ■ **(A)** To calculate the length of the pectus bar, measure the distance from right to left midaxillary line and subtract 1–2 cm (1 inch). **(B)** Bend the Lorenz pectus support bar to conform to the desired chest wall curvature. **(C)** Mark the deepest point of the pectus excavatum with a circle by using a marking pen. If this point is inferior to the sternum, then move the circle superiorly to the lower end of the sternum just above the xiphoid. This point sets the horizontal plane bar for insertion. **(D)** After confirming by thoracoscopy that the internal and external anatomy match up well, make lateral thoracic skin incisions and raise skin flaps anteriorly toward the 'X' marked on the external skin at the top of the pectus ridge. **(E)** Retract skin incision anteriorly to allow visualization of the intercostal space previously marked with an 'X.' Under thoracoscopic control, insert the appropriate size Lorenz introducer through the right intercostal space at the top of the pectus ridge and at the previously marked 'X.'

Continued

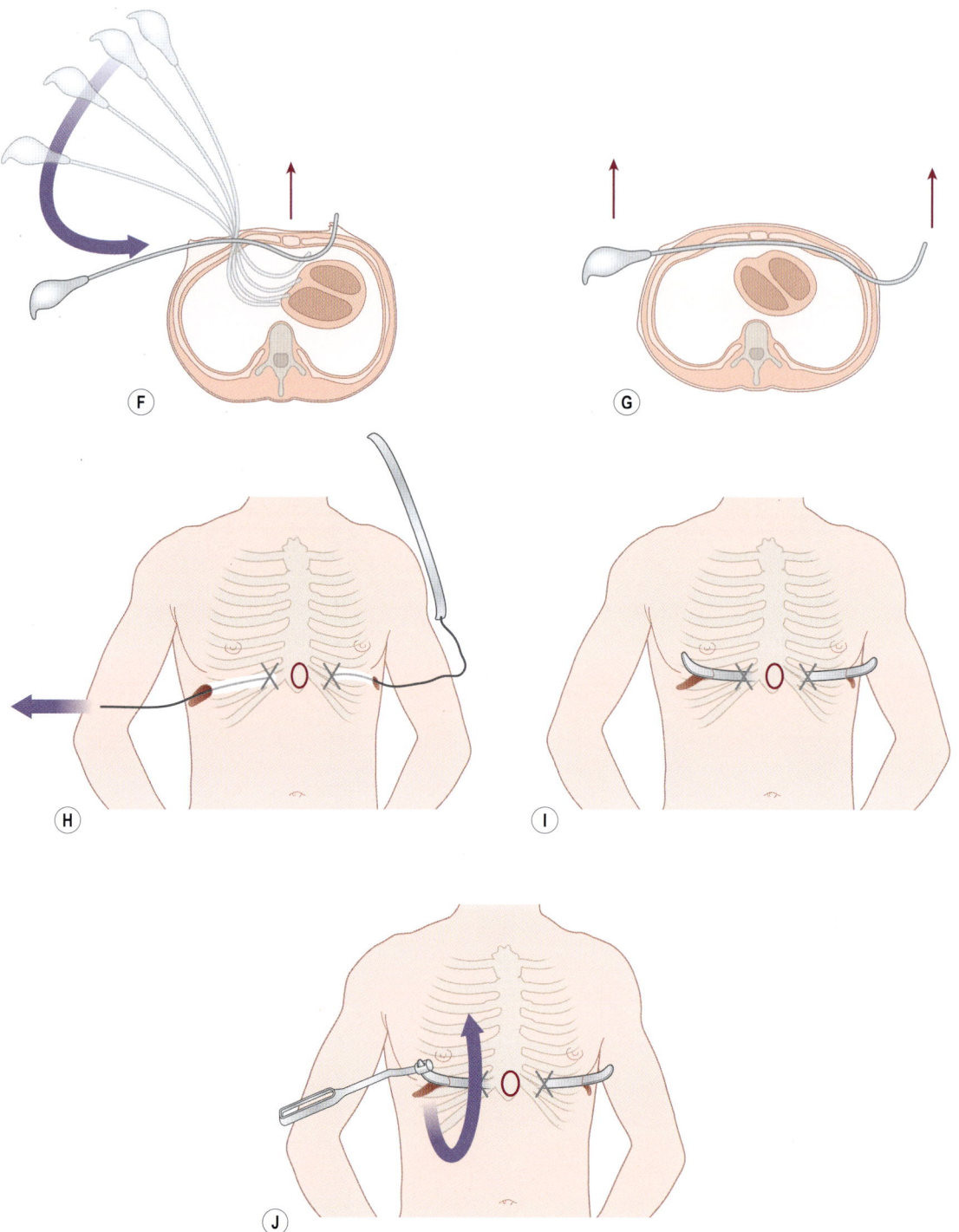

FIGURE 20-6, Cont'd ■ **(F)** When the substernal tunnel has been completed, gently push the tip of the introducer through the contralateral intercostal space at the previously marked 'X,' medial to the top of the pectus ridge on the left side. **(G)** Use the introducer to elevate the sternum. The surgeon lifts on the right side, and the assistant lifts the left side of the introducer. **(H)** Attach the previously prepared pectus bar to the umbilical tape and slowly guide the bar through the tunnel by using the umbilical tape for traction. **(I)** The bar is inserted with the convexity facing posteriorly. **(J)** When the bar is in position, use the specially designed Lorenz bar rotational instrument (bar flipper) to turn the bar over.

minimally invasive technique. However, because of the risk of interference with growth plates in young children and the development of asphyxiating chondrodystrophy, the procedure should be reserved for patients who have completed their growth.[18,19] The open procedure is best suited for the older patients, especially those who have

asymmetric or eccentric deformities, and patients with mixed pectus carinatum/excavatum deformities.

The open technique involves making an anterior thoracic incision and elevating skin and muscle flaps until all the costal cartilages from T3 to T6 are exposed. The perichondrium is then incised longitudinally, and the deformed cartilages are either partially or completely removed. Most surgeons now advocate removing only a small section (1–2 cm) of the deformed cartilages, as was originally advocated by Sauerbruch and Gross.[9,17] An anterior table, wedge-shaped, sternal osteotomy is performed at the angle of Louis. The sternum is elevated, and the osteotomy is closed with nonabsorbable sutures. Some surgeons insert a metal strut under the sternum to bridge the gap between the ribs and the sternum to prevent the sternum from sinking back into the chest. The perichondrial 'sleeves' are approximated with absorbable sutures, drains are left, the muscle flaps are sutured back into position, and the incisions are closed. Postoperative management is similar to that for the minimally invasive technique except that patients are required to refrain from contact sports for at least three months.

Results

The minimally invasive approach received rapid acceptance by the surgical community because the technique requires neither rib incision nor resection nor sternal osteotomy. The blood loss is minimal, the operating time is short, and the patient rapidly returns to regular activity.[47–53]

Although our initial report in 1998 presented a ten-year experience, the numbers were limited (42 patients) and the long-term results were affected by the early learning curve of using a support bar that was too soft.[20] Moreover, in some of these patients, the bar was removed too soon. From 1988 through December 2011, 1463 patients have had their initial operation at our institution (see Box 20-1). Since the original presentation, numerous important modifications have been made, both to the operative technique (e.g., routine use of thoracoscopy) and instruments, to minimize the risks of the procedure and facilitate insertion and stabilization of the support bar. These modifications have markedly reduced the risks and complications and have been previously reported.[43,45]

In our series of 1463 patients with pectus excavatum, only seven (0.48%) had a mixed pectus excavatum and carinatum. One (0.07%) patient had Poland syndrome, and one (0.1%) had an associated complex cardiac anomaly (atrioventricular canal). The male-to-female ratio in patients undergoing repair was more than 4:1. The median age was 15 years, with a range from 13 months to 32 years. Preoperative evaluation included CT scan with a median CT index of 4.6 (range, 2.4 to 21). Cardiac compression was noted on echocardiography or CT scan, or both, in 1,301 of 1,450 patients (89.72%). Results of PFT's are shown in Table 20-2.

In 68% of our patients, a single bar was used. Two bars were needed in 32% of the patients. The median length of stay has been five days.

Complications

Early Complications

No deaths or cardiac perforations occurred during the 1463 repairs at our institution. Pneumothorax requiring chest tube drainage developed in 56 (3.8%) repairs. Blood loss in most patients was minimal (±10 mL), with the exception of 6 (0.4%) patients in whom a hemothorax formed. Thirteen (0.9%) pleural effusions required treatment with either a chest tube or aspiration (Table 20-3).

Pericarditis requiring treatment with indomethacin occurred after 9 (0.6%) repairs. One patient required pericardiocentesis. Pneumonia developed after 13 (0.9%) procedures, and medication reactions have occurred after 36 (3.6%) operations. Wound infections developed in 22 patients (1.5%). These resulted in eventual early bar removal in 2 (0.02%) patients.

Late Complications

Eighty-four (5.7%) bars have become displaced, and 54 (3.7%) have required repositioning. In the 54 cases in which patients required repositioning of the bar, 16 occurred before stabilizers were available, a time period covering our first 105 repairs. After the introduction of stabilizers, the incidence of bar displacement decreased from 15.2% to 6.5%. When the bar and stabilizers were wired together, the incidence of bar displacement decreased to 4.3%. Since we combined placing a stabilizer on the left and polydioxanone (PDS, Ethicon, Inc., Somerville NJ) sutures around the bar and underlying rib on the right, the incidence of bar displacement has dropped to 1.5%.

In two patients, a late hemothorax developed secondary to trauma. Both underwent thoracoscopy with drainage of the hemothorax. At the time of thoracoscopy, no active bleeding was found. Therefore, an injury to an intercostal vessel was presumed. Whether hemothoraces would have developed in these patients as a result of their thoracic trauma if they had not had a bar placed in situ is unknown. We have several patients who have been involved in major automobile accidents who sustained head and musculoskeletal trauma but no chest injuries.

Thirty-nine (2.7%) of 1463 patients have had unsuspected allergies to the metal in the bar. These allergies initially presented as rashes in the area of the bar or

TABLE 20-3 Complications after Initial Pectus Excavatum Repair at Children's Hospital of the King's Daughters

Complication	Percentage (Number)
Pneumothorax w/spontaneous resolution	55.7% (815)
Pneumothorax w/chest tube	3.8% (56)
Bar displacement requiring revision	3.7% (54)
Overcorrection	3.1% (47)
Bar allergy	2.9% (39)
Suture site infection	1.2% (18)
Pneumonia	0.9% (13)
Hemothorax	0.36% (6)
Hemothorax (post-traumatic)	0.1% (2)
Pericarditis	0.6% (9)
Pleural effusion (requiring drainage)	0.9% (13)
Temporary paralysis	<0.1% (2)
Death	0%
Cardiac perforation	0%
Recurrence	0.9% (13)

Data collected from 5/18/1987 through to 1/1/2012; *n* = 1463.

stabilizer, and required revision with custom-made bars using other alloys. Mild overcorrection occurred in 47 (3.1%) patients. In four, a true carinatum deformity developed. Of the patients in whom a true carinatum deformity developed, three had Marfan syndrome and the other had Ehlers–Danlos syndrome. No patient has developed thoracic chondrodystrophy.

Overall Results and Long-Term Follow-up

Patients are evaluated six months following the operation and then yearly until the bar is removed. Long-term assessment has allowed classification of the results into excellent, good, fair, or failed categories.

An excellent repair indicates that the patient experienced complete repair of the pectus deformity and resolution of associated symptoms. A good repair is distinguished by a markedly improved but not completely normal chest wall appearance and resolution of associated symptoms. A fair result indicates a mild residual pectus excavatum without complete resolution of symptoms. A failed repair is defined as a recurrence of the pectus deformity and associated symptoms, or the need for additional surgery (or both) after final removal of the bar.

In addition, patients with ECG conduction abnormalities or mitral valve prolapse had follow-up assessments. Patients old enough to have pulmonary function studies preoperatively were reassessed with repeated studies.

It is our observation that patients who are sedentary and who do not perform the pectus breathing exercises tend to have mild recurrences over time. Therefore, we strongly emphasize these aerobic activities and deep breathing exercises.

As of December 2010, there were 972 primary repair patients who have undergone bar removal. Results were deemed excellent in 85%, good in 12%, fair in 1.1%, and failed in 1.7%. The long-term results are affected by the length of time the bar was left in place.

Bar Removal

We advise the pectus bar be left in place for two to three years. We evaluate patients on an annual basis and monitor their growth, activity level, and PFT results, and encourage them to perform their pectus exercises and participate in aerobic sports. Patients between the ages of 6 and 10 years often do not grow rapidly. Therefore, they tolerate the bar well for three or even four years. Conversely, we have had teenagers who have undergone a massive growth spurt, completely outgrowing the bar, and requiring bar removal after 2 years. We consider the exercise programs to be as important as the operation. Many children and adults lead sedentary lifestyles and never perform aerobic activities. Therefore, their lungs never expand beyond the resting tidal volume (approximately 10% of total lung capacity). Deep breathing with breath holding for ten to 15 seconds and aerobic activities, such as running (e.g., soccer, basketball) and swimming, are strongly encouraged. We have seen a mild recurrence over the long term in patients who do not follow our exercise protocol (Fig. 20-7).

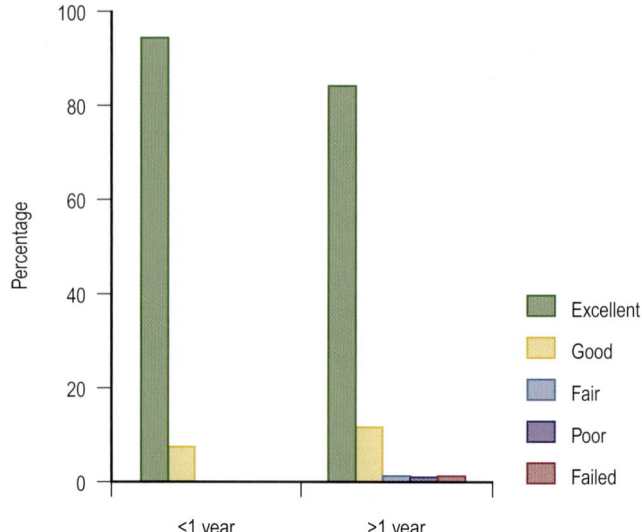

FIGURE 20-7 ■ The authors' outcomes evaluated by the length of time since bar removal.

PECTUS CARINATUM

Pectus carinatum, or protrusion deformity of the chest, occurs less frequently than does pectus excavatum in most countries. It comprises about 5% of patients with chest wall deformities.[54] The prominence may be in the upper manubrium of the sternum, which is called a chondromanubrial deformity. The most common protrusion is found in the lower segment or body of the sternum (the gladiolus) and is called chondrogladiolar (Fig. 20-8). The protrusion may be unilateral, bilateral, or mixed.[55] About 80% of patients who develop pectus carinatum are boys. Although the etiology is unknown, a genetic component of causation is suggested by the approximately 25% of patients with a family history of a chest wall defect.[53,56,57] Pectus carinatum has also been reported to occur after treatment for pectus excavatum.[58]

Pectus carinatum is usually noted in adolescence and is seen most commonly around the time of a growth spurt, rather than at birth as is often seen with pectus excavatum. Symptoms of dyspnea, reduced endurance, or tachypnea with exertion were noted in all 260 patients in one study.[59] Associated mitral valve disease has been reported as well.[60,61] Other associations include Marfan syndrome and scoliosis (in 15%[53]).

Orthotic bracing has been applied successfully in some patients with pectus carinatum. Reports have described correction or improvement in this condition by means of a brace analogous to that used for treatment of scoliosis but that exerts pressure in the anteroposterior direction.[24,62]

Following adoption of a new brace in 2009, we have seen marked improvement in success with brace treatment (Fig. 20-9). About 85% of our brace patients have been successfully treated without operation.[62] In the remainder, minimally invasive or open operation is performed.[25,55,62–66] Postoperative complications are uncommon, and recurrence rates are low in centers with a large experience.

An unusual form of pectus carinatum occurs with a short nonsegmented sternum and marked posterior angulation at the site of the normal chondromanubrial junction (Currarino–Silverman syndrome).[60] Also, congenital heart disease is often present. Although its etiology is unclear, early fusion of the sternal plates is postulated as the cause of this deformity.[67] In a large review from our hospital, we found about 1% of pectus patients had this anomaly.[68] Repair is best performed using an open technique with subparachondral resection of the second to seventh costal cartilages and a broad

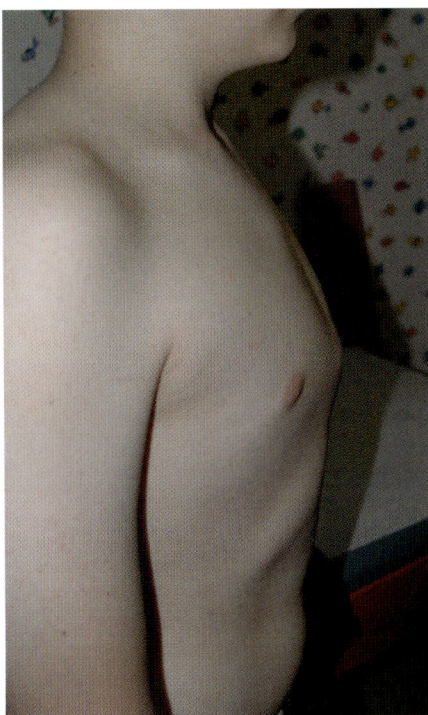

FIGURE 20-8 ■ This teenager has a chondrogladiolar pectus carinatum. This is the most common form of pectus carinatum and involves protrusion of the lower portion of the sternum (the gladiolus). In this patient, the protrusion is fairly symmetrical.

wedge-shaped osteotomy through the anterior cortex of the sternum at the point of maximal angularization. The lower sternum is then displaced anteriorly with sutures while the costal cartilages regenerate.[69] The confusing part about this anomaly is that it may appear to be a pectus excavatum deformity when, in fact, it is an uncommon variant of pectus carinatum (Fig. 20-10).

POLAND SYNDROME

Poland syndrome affects 1 in 30,000 live births and is sporadic in occurrence.[70] It is a constellation of anomalies that present in a variety of ways. Clinical manifestations can include any or all of the following: absence of the pectoralis major, pectoralis minor, serratus anterior, rectus abdominis, and latissimus dorsi muscles (Fig. 20-11). Athelia or amastia, nipple deformities, limb deformities (syndactyly, brachydactyly), absent axillary hair, and limited subcutaneous fat can also be found.

In 1841, Alfred Poland, an English medical student, published a partial description of the deformity.[71] However, the syndrome had been initially described in the French and German literature in 1826 and 1839.[72,73]

Poland syndrome does not appear to be genetic, although occasional occurrences within families have occurred. The right side is more commonly affected and is present in boys 70% of the time.[74] Approximately 15% of patients with breast hypoplasia/aplasia have Poland syndrome. The etiology is unclear, but theories include abnormal migration of the embryonic tissues forming the pectoralis muscles, hypoplasia of the subclavian artery, or in utero trauma.

No correlation has been identified between the extent of hand deformities and the chest wall anomalies. Varying degrees of either can occur with mild hypoplasia to total aplasia of muscles, ribs, and cartilage. The latter can lead to major chest wall depression and paradoxical respiratory motion.

Repair is rarely required, except in those patients with aplasia of the ribs or a major depression deformity.[74,75]

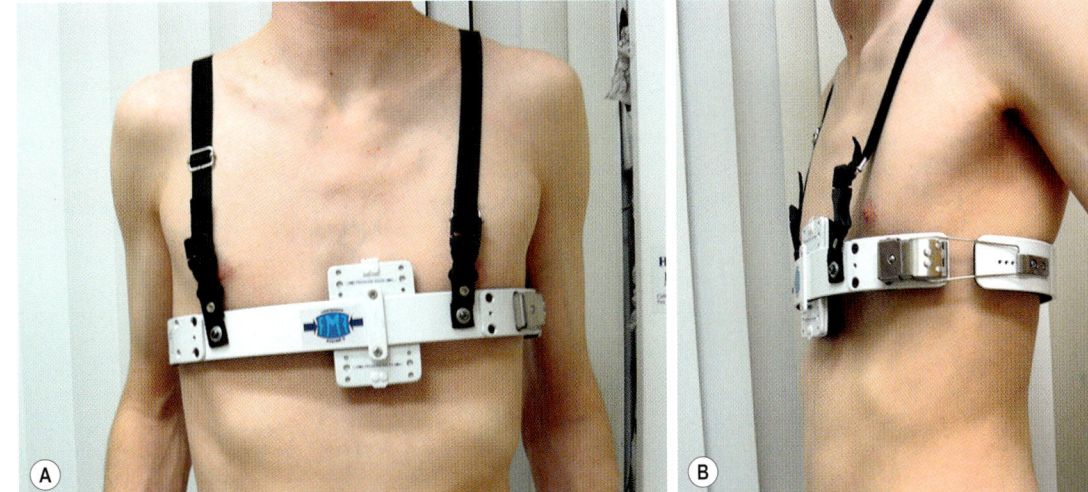

FIGURE 20-9 ■ A patient being treated with dynamic compression bracing for a prominent pectus carinatum. The advantage of this brace is that it allows a preset pressure to be used to compress the carinatum.

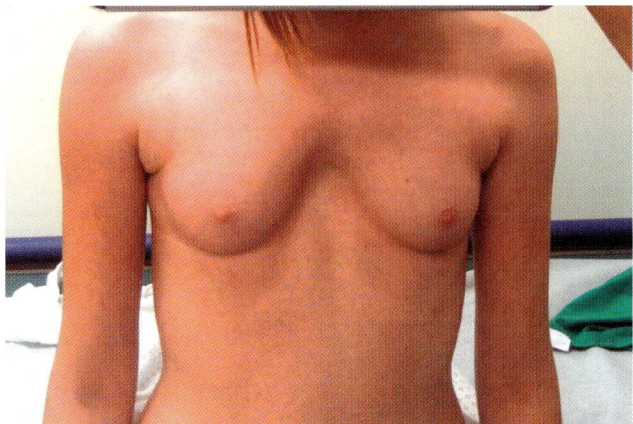

FIGURE 20-10 ■ This girl has the typical features of Currarino–Silverman syndrome. It looks like she has a pectus excavatum, but really has a variant of pectus carinatum. The sternum is short and there is marked posterior angulation at the site of the normal chondromanubrial junction. Congenital heart disease is often present.

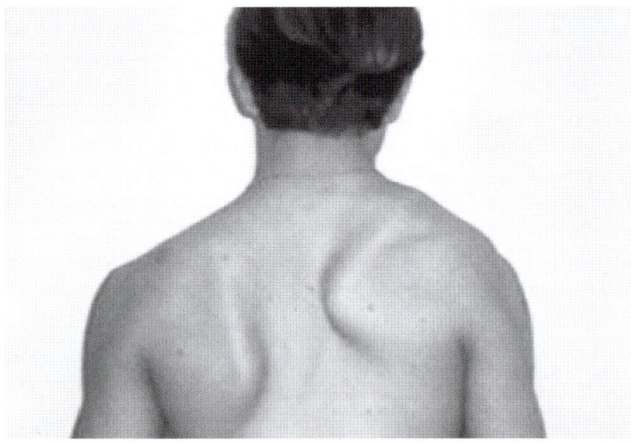

FIGURE 20-11 ■ A 12-year-old boy with Poland syndrome and absence of the serratus anterior muscles, leading to a winged scapula on the right.

When necessary, chest wall reconstruction with correction of contralateral carinatum-type protrusions can usually be performed at the same time (Fig. 20-12). Autologous rib grafts, or a variety of bioprosthetic agents, can be used with or without a latissimus dorsi flap. The use of custom-made chest wall prostheses has been associated with significant problems such as migration, erosion of local tissues, and less than optimal cosmesis. Chest wall reconstruction should be performed before breast reconstruction in a girl with hypoplasia or aplasia of the breast.

STERNAL DEFECTS

Sternal defects are found in the midline of the upper torso and range from the relatively benign sternal cleft (sternal defect without displacement of the heart) to the very rare and almost uniformly fatal thoracic ectopia cordis (the heart is out of the chest without a skin covering).

Cleft sternum (bifid sternum, partial ectopia cordis) is a rare malformation (0.15% of all chest wall malformations in some series), and is due to partial or total failure of sternal fusion at an early stage of embryonic development. Sternal clefts can be classified as either complete (the rarest form), superior, or inferior.[76]

Superior clefts are either U-shaped (proximal to the fourth cartilage) or V-shaped (reaching the xiphoid process). They are most often isolated, with only minor associated lesions. The heart is in a normal position, and cardiac anomalies are rare. Operative repair, which is usually very successful, is warranted once the diagnosis is made and can be scheduled electively. Optimally, it is performed in the neonatal period when the sternal edges can be approximated easily because of flexibility and minimal compression of mediastinal structures (Fig. 20-13). After age 1 year, primary repair is difficult and more extensive techniques may be needed, such as the use of autologous structures (costal cartilage, ribs) or prosthetic materials.[77,78]

Thoracic ectopia cordis (true ectopia cordis) is a lesion in which the heart has no overlying somatic structures. It is very rare (incidence 5.5 to 7.9 per million births) and usually occurs with some form of an abdominal wall defect, with the heart sitting on the chest and the apex pointed toward the chin (Fig. 20-14).[79] Intrinsic cardiac anomalies are frequent, especially tetralogy of Fallot, pulmonary artery stenosis, transposition of the great arteries, and ventricular septal defects (VSD). Survival in patients with thoracic ectopia cordis is rare. Most patients die because of torsion of the great vessels and compression of the heart while attempting to reduce it back in the chest. The goals of therapy are to cover the heart, prevent kinking of the great vessels, repair the associated abdominal wall defect, and stabilize the thoracic cavity so that spontaneous ventilation can be effective.[79–81]

Thoracoabdominal ectopia cordis (Cantrell pentalogy) involves lesions in which the heart is covered by an omphalocele-like membrane (Fig. 20-15).[82] Intrinsic cardiac anomalies also are common in these patients, with tetralogy of Fallot and VSDs being the most common. Cantrell's pentalogy consists of an inferior sternal cleft, ectopia cordis, midline abdominal wall defects or omphalocele, pericardial defects, and one or more cardiac defects. Repair in these patients is much more successful than in thoracic ectopia cordis. Initial management addresses the lack of skin overlying the heart and abdominal cavity. After stabilization, the goal of the first operation is to provide coverage of the midline defects, separate the abdominal and pericardial compartments, and repair the diaphragm. Various techniques for closure include flap mobilization, skin closure only, and a variety of bioprosthetic agents. The congenital heart defect is repaired at a later date.

THORACIC INSUFFICIENCY SYNDROME ASSOCIATED WITH DIFFUSE SKELETAL DISORDERS

Thoracic insufficiency syndrome may be defined as any disorder that produces the inability of the thorax to

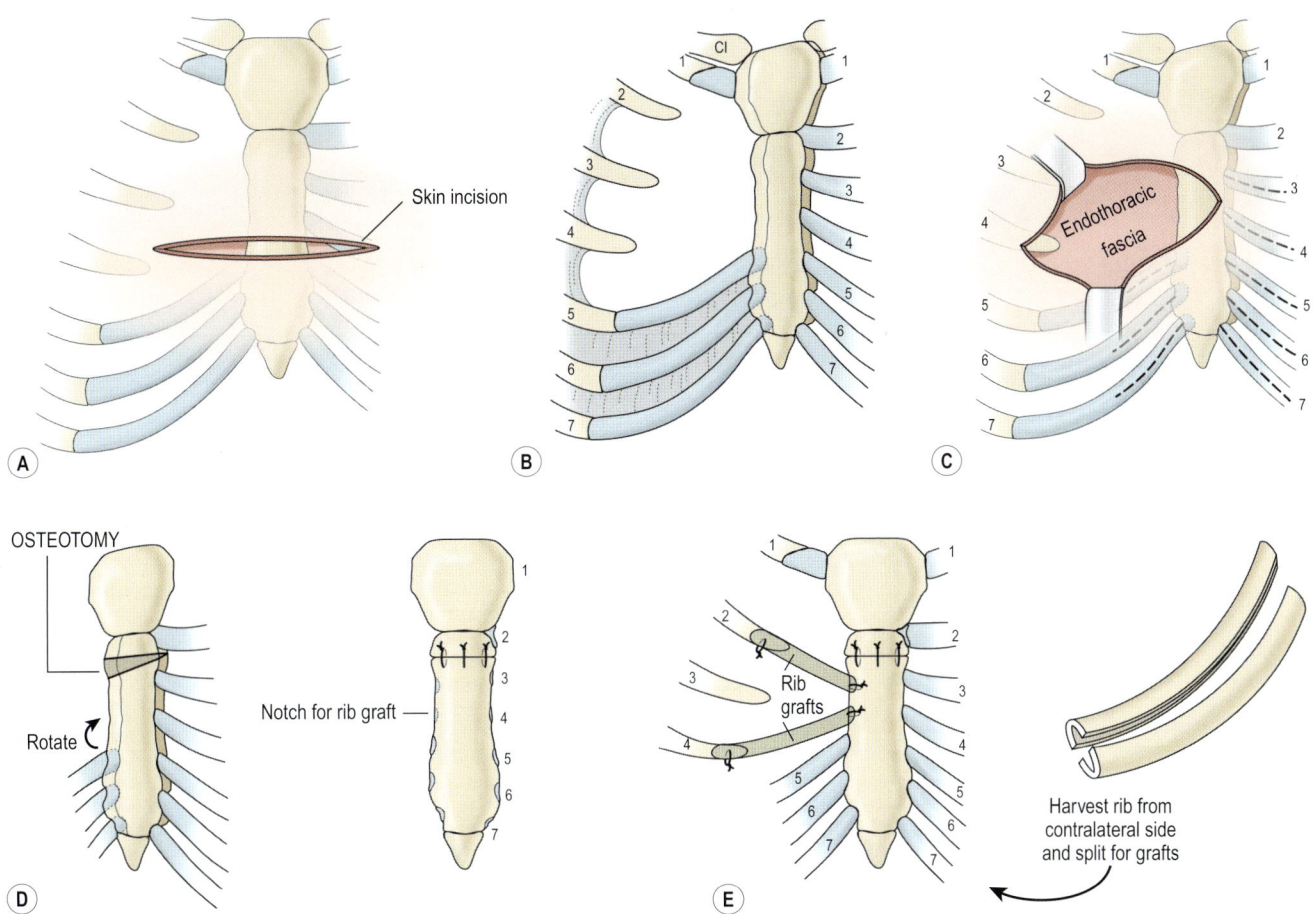

FIGURE 20-12 ■ **(A)** The transverse incision is placed below and within the nipples. In girls, it is placed in the future inframammary crease. **(B)** A schematic depiction of the deformity with rotation of the sternum, depression of the cartilages of the involved side, and carinate protrusion of the contralateral side. **(C)** In cases with aplasia of the ribs, the endothoracic fascia is encountered directly below the attenuated subcutaneous tissue and pectoral fascia. The pectoral muscle flap is elevated on the contralateral side, with the pectoral fascia, if present, on the involved side. Subperichondrial resection of the costal cartilages is carried out as shown (*dashed line*), preserving the costochondral junction. Rarely this resection must be carried to the level of the second costal cartilage. **(D)** A transverse, offset, wedge-shaped sternal osteotomy is created below the second costal cartilage. Closure of this defect with heavy silk sutures or elevation of the sternum with a strut corrects both the posterior displacement and the rotation of the sternum. **(E)** In cases with rib aplasia, rib grafts are harvested from the contralateral fifth or sixth ribs, split, and secured medially with wire sutures into notches created in the sternum and with wire to the native ribs laterally. Ribs are split as shown, along their short axes, to maintain maximal mechanical strength. (Adapted from Shamberger RC, Welch KJ, Upton J III. Surgical treatment of thoracic deformity in Poland's syndrome. J Pediatr Surg 1989;24:760–6.)

support normal respiration or lung growth.[83] It includes a spectrum of disorders including asphyxiating thoracic dystrophy (Jeune syndrome), acquired asphyxiating thoracic dystrophy (after open pectus excavatum repair), spondylothoracic dysplasia (Jarcho–Levin syndrome), congenital scoliosis with multiple vertebral anomalies and fused or absent ribs (jumbled spine), and severe kyphoscoliosis. These disorders have been viewed and treated as separate entities, with little coordinated effort between specialties. However, they are best addressed with a unified approach integrating pediatric general and orthopedic surgeons as well as pediatric pulmonologists.

Jeune syndrome is an autosomal recessive inherited osteochondrodystrophy with variable expression.[84] In mild forms, the chest may support adequate respiration. In more severe cases, the thorax is narrowed both transversely and vertically, with short, wide horizontal ribs and irregular costochondral junctions (Fig. 20-16). This chest

wall configuration produces a rigid chest with very little intercostal excursion for normal respiration, leading to ventilator dependence and eventual death from respiratory failure.[85,86] The presence or absence of intrinsic pulmonary abnormalities varies among patients. However, most have normal bronchial development with variable alveolar density.[87,88] This suggests that the extrinsic chest wall plays a significant role in the underlying hypoplasia. Other associated skeletal abnormalities in Jeune syndrome include short stubby extremities, fixed elevated clavicles, hypoplastic iliac wings, and a high incidence of C1 spinal stenosis.[89–91] These patients also have varying degrees of renal dysplasia.[92]

Spondylothoracic dysplasia (Jarcho–Levin) syndrome occurs in two forms with different inheritance patterns. Type I is an autosomal recessive deformity characterized by multiple vertebral hemivertebrae and posterior rib fusions.[93] This produces a marked shortening of the thoracic spine and a crab-like appearance of the chest on a

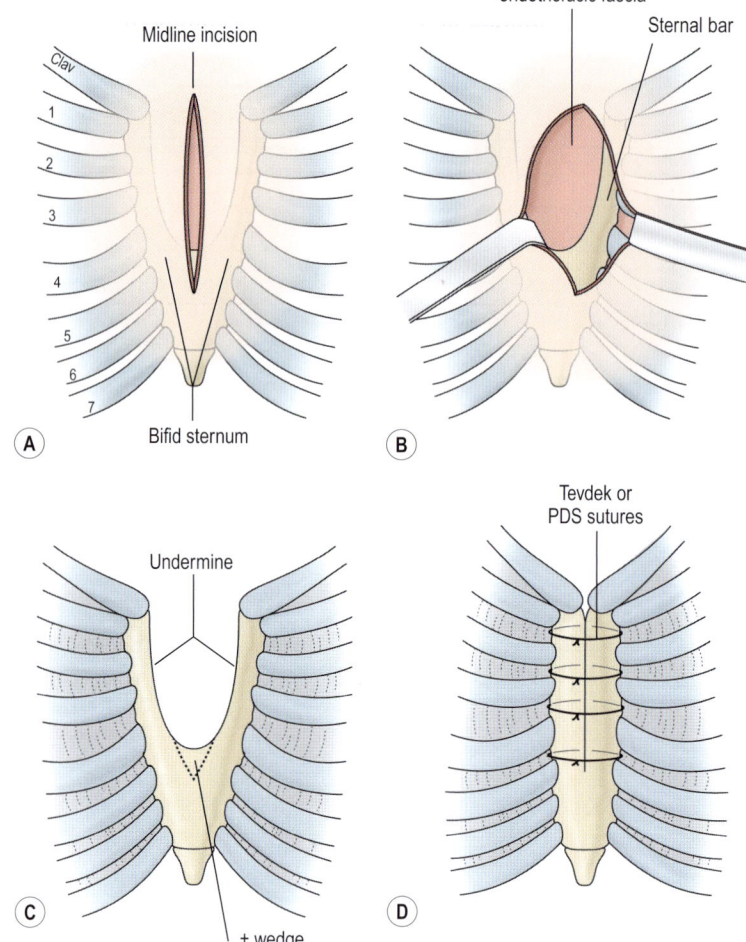

FIGURE 20-13 ■ **(A)** Repair of a bifid sternum is best performed through a longitudinal incision extending the length of the defect. These defects are characteristically cleft superiorly, as shown. **(B)** Directly beneath the subcutaneous tissues, the sternal bars are encountered, with the origin of the pectoral muscles on the lateral aspect of the bars. The endothoracic fascia and pericardium are just below these structures. **(C)** The endothoracic fascia is mobilized off the sternal bars posteriorly with blunt dissection to allow safe placement of the sutures. Approximation of the sternal bars may be facilitated by excising a wedge of cartilage inferiorly. Repair is best accomplished in the neonatal period because of the flexibility of the chest wall. **(D)** Closure of the defect is achieved with 2-0 Tevdek or polydioxanone sutures. (Adapted from Shamberger RC, Welch KJ. Sternal defects. Pediatr Surg Int 1990;5:156–64.)

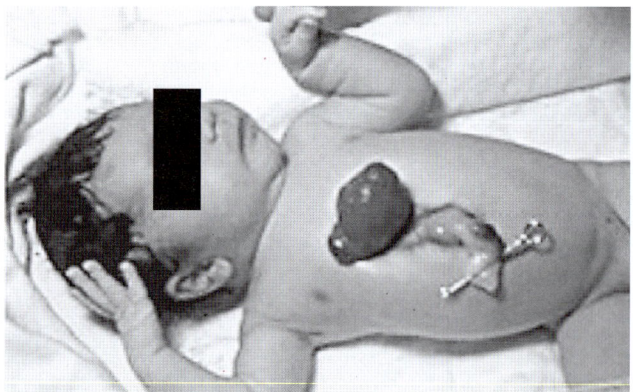

FIGURE 20-14 ■ An infant with thoracic ectopia cordis with no significant abdominal wall defect present. Note the characteristic high insertion of the umbilicus and anterior projection of the apex of the heart.

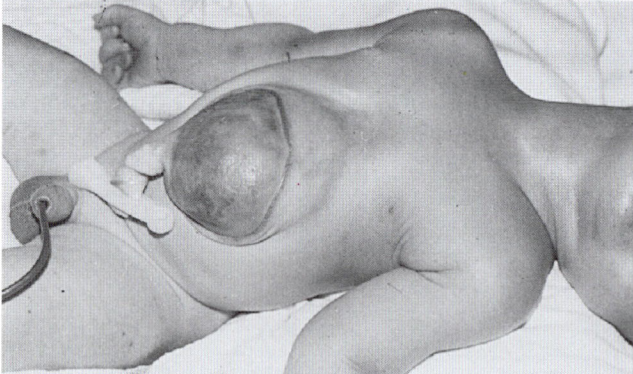

FIGURE 20-15 ■ A newborn with the external features of Cantrell pentalogy is seen. Flaring of the lower thoracic cavity is present, with a large epigastric omphalocele. The transverse septum of the diaphragm and the inferior portion of the pericardium are absent. The patient also has tetralogy of Fallot.

chest radiograph (Fig. 20-17).[94] Associated malformations are noted in 30% of patients and include cardiac and renal anomalies. This form is often fatal by age 15 months, and a high incidence is reported in Puerto Rican families.[95] Type II spondylothoracic dysplasia has an autosomal dominant inheritance pattern and is associated

with near-normal longevity. It is seen most commonly in white children.[91]

Thoracic insufficiency also may arise secondary to over-extensive Ravitch-type pectus excavation repairs or repairs performed too early in life.[19] Complex spine anomalies producing the so-called jumbled spine,

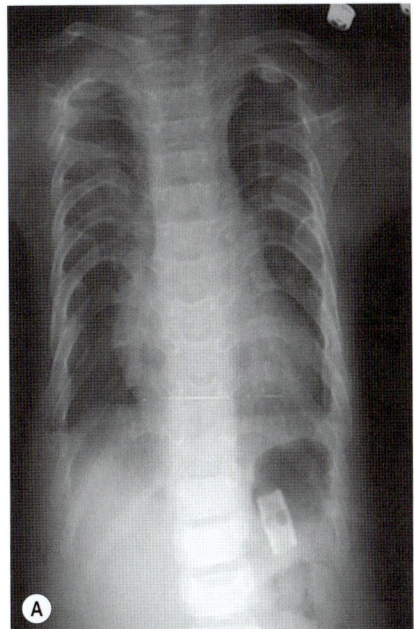

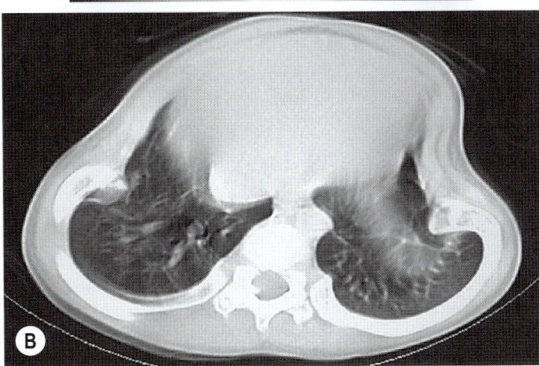

FIGURE 20-16 ■ **(A)** Chest radiograph of a patient with Jeune syndrome (asphyxiating thoracic dystrophy). The thorax is narrow, and the ribs are short and wide. **(B)** CT scan demonstrating Jeune asphyxiating thoracic dystrophy.

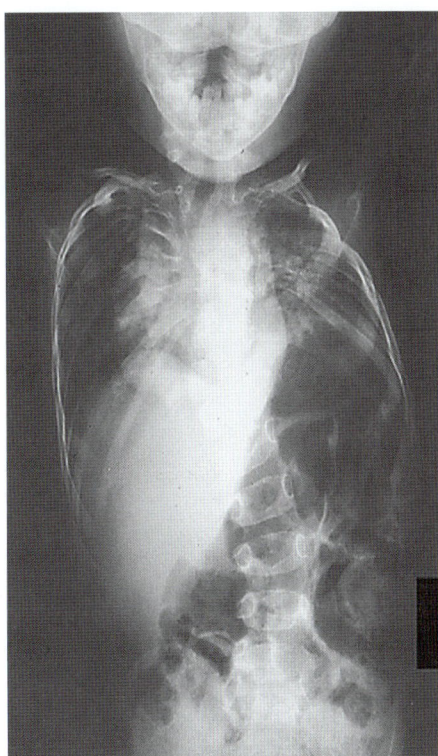

FIGURE 20-17 ■ Chest radiograph of a patient with Jarcho–Levin syndrome with a markedly shortened thoracic spine producing a crab-like appearance.

unilateral thoracic hypoplasia seen with the VACTERL (vertebral defects, anal atresia, cardiac defects, tracheo-esophageal fistula, renal anomalies, and limb abnormalities) syndrome, and kyphoscoliosis may be a cause of thoracic insufficiency as well.[96–100]

Operative techniques to correct the spectrum of these complex disorders have attempted to address the issue of thoracic volume by various approaches. In both congenital (Jeune) and acquired (post-pectus) thoracic dystrophy, one approach has been an anterior longitudinal sternal split with widening of the sternum. This has been accomplished with methylmethacrylate, bone grafts or rib, and metal plates.[101–103] A staged approach with a methylmethacrylate plate followed by secondary removal of the plate and latissimus dorsi flaps to cover the created sternal cleft also has been described.[104] In cases of acquired thoracic dystrophy, elevation of the sternum has been performed using both the open and the minimally invasive techniques used for standard pectus repair.[19,41] A lateral staged approach with staggered rib osteotomies, staggered division of the chest wall, intercostal muscles, and pleura, with transposition of alternating ribs by using metal plate

fixation, also has been described.[105] These approaches have had variable results because they are not easily revised to allow continued growth of the chest wall to allow lung expansion. The lateral thoracic expansion may also interfere with intercostal muscle function after division of multiple intercostal muscles and nerves.

A promising technique to address this problem rejoins the disciplines of pediatric general, thoracic, and orthopedic surgery. Developed by Campbell and Smith, expansion thoracoplasty and the use of a vertically expandable prosthetic titanium rib (VEPTR) addresses many of the problems found in the spectrum of these disorders. This technique allows serial expansion of the chest wall to provide continued growth of the thorax and spine until skeletal maturity is achieved. More than 300 patients with various disorders have been treated with this approach.[106] In Jeune asphyxiating thoracic dystrophy, 14 patients have undergone staged bilateral expansions.[107–109] With this technique, anterior rib osteotomies adjacent to the costochondral junction and posterior osteotomies in the 3rd to 9th ribs next to the transverse process of the spine are performed. This creates a segment of chest wall that is distracted posterolaterally and anchored to a curved VEPTR that is attached to the 2nd and 10th ribs (Fig. 20-18). The distracted segment is anchored to the VEPTR with 2 mm titanium rings, stabilizing the segment, and allowing reossification of the multiple osteotomies (Fig. 20-19). The second stage is performed three months later, and then the devices are expanded every six months.

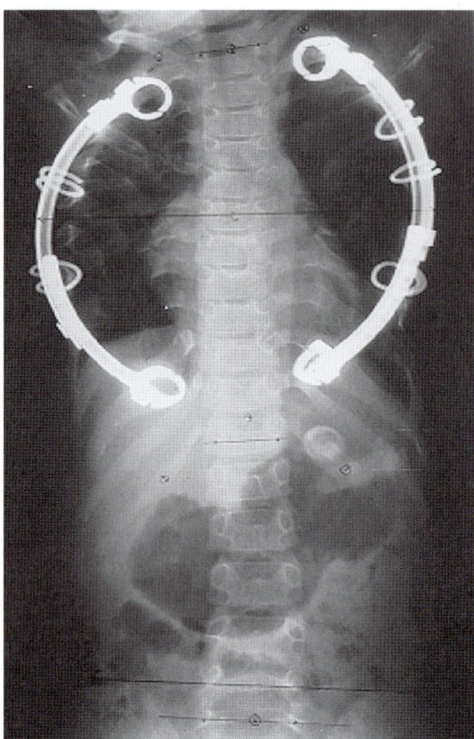

FIGURE 20-18 ■ Bilateral vertical expandable prosthetic titanium rib (VEPTR) fixed with titanium rings to ribs of the patient with Jeune's asphyxiating thoracic dystrophy seen in Figure 20-16A.

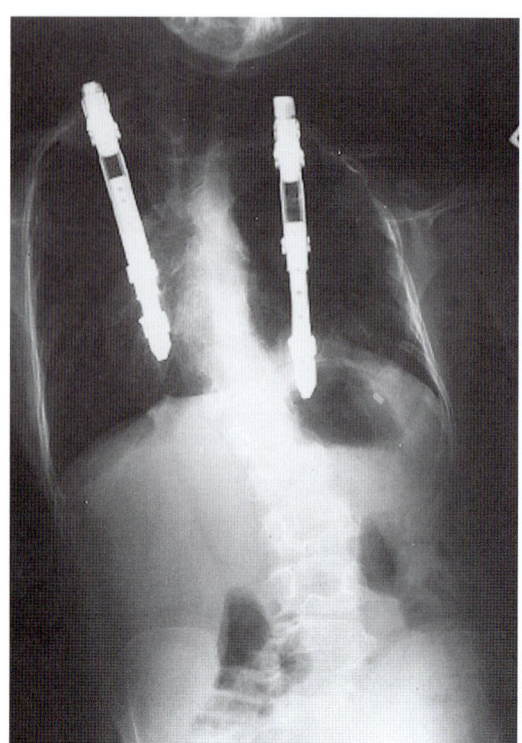

FIGURE 20-20 ■ Bilateral VEPTRs were placed in the patient in Figure 20-17 with Jarcho–Levin syndrome.

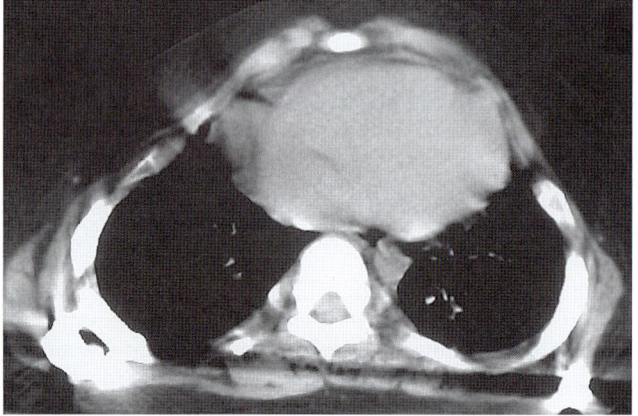

FIGURE 20-19 ■ Postoperative CT scan of the patient from Figure 20-16B after VEPTR placement, demonstrating expansion of the thorax.

In patients with fused or absent ribs and scoliosis, a wedge thoracostomy through the fused segment of ribs not only allows expansion of the chest, but also correction of the scoliosis and the rotational spinal deformity (producing a windswept thorax).[107] It also stimulates increased spinal height in both congenital scoliosis and Jarcho–Levin syndrome, in which bilateral devices are placed (Fig. 20-20).

REFERENCES

1. Ebstein E. Die Trichterbrust in ihren Beziehungen zur Konstitution. Z Konstitutionslehre 1921;8:103.
2. Bauhinus J. Observationum Medicariam. Liber II, Observ. 264, Francfurti 1600.507.
3. Coulson W. Deformities of the chest. London Med Gaz 1820;4:69–73.
4. Williams CT. Congenital malformation of the thorax: Great depression of the sternum. Trans Pathol Soc Lond 1872;24:50.
5. Ebstein W. Ueber die Trichterbrust. Dtsch Arch 1882;30:411.
6. Meade RH. A History of Thoracic Surgery. Springfield, IL: Charles C Thomas; 1961.
7. Sauerbruch F. Die Chirurgie der Brustorgane. Berlin: Springer; 1920, vol 1, p 437.
8. Meyer L. Zurchirurqishen Behandlung der augeborenen Trichterbrust. Verh Bel Med Gest 1911;42:364.
9. Sauerbruch F. Operative Beseitigung der Angeborenen Trichterbrust. Dtsch Z Chir 1931;234:760.
10. Ochsner A, DeBakey M, Chone-Chondrosternon. J Thorac Surg 1939;8:469–511.
11. Brown AL. Pectus excavatum. J Thorac Surg 1939;9:164–84.
12. Ravitch MM. The operative treatment of pectus excavatum. Ann Surg 1949;129:429–44.
13. Wallgren GR and Sulamaa M. Surgical treatment of funnel chest. Exhib. VIII, presented at the International Congress of Paediatrics 1956.32.
14. Paltia V, Parkkulainen KV, Sulamaa M, et al. Operative technique in funnel chest. Acta Chir Scand 1958/1959;116:90–8.
15. Adkins PC, Blades BA. Stainless steel strut for correction of pectus excavatum. Surg Gynecol Obstet 1961;113:111–13.
16. Welch KJ. Satisfactory surgical correction of pectus excavatum deformity in childhood. J Thorac Surg 1958;36:697–713.
17. Gross RE. The Surgery of Infancy and Childhood. Philadelphia: WB Saunders; 1953. p. 753–61.
18. Martinez D, Juame J, Stein T, et al. The effect of costal cartilage resection on chest wall development. Pediatr Surg Int 1990;5: 170–3.
19. Haller JA, Colombani PM, Humphries CT, et al. Chest wall constriction after too extensive and too early operations for pectus excavatum. Ann Thorac Surg 1996;61:1618–25.
20. Nuss D, Kelly RE Jr, Croitoru DP, et al. A 10-year review of a minimally invasive technique for the correction of pectus excavatum. J Pediatr Surg 1998;33:545–52.

21. Kelley SW. Surgical Diseases of Children: Dislocations, Congenital and Acquired. 3rd ed. St. Louis: CV Mosby; 1929. vol 1, p 537.

22. Haller JA Jr. Thoracic injuries. In: Welch KJ, Randolph JG, Ravitch MM, et al, editor. Pediatric Surgery, vol. 1. 4th ed. Chicago: Year Book Medical Publishers; 1986. p. 147.

23. Wesson DE, et al. Thoracic injuries. In: O'Neill JA Jr, Rowe MI, Grosfeld JL, editor. Pediatric Surgery, vol. 1. 5th ed. St. Louis: Mosby Grosfeld; 1998. p. 245.

24. Martinez-Ferro M, Fraire C, Bernard S. Dynamic compression system for the correction of pectus carinatum. Semin Pediatr Surg 2008;17:194–200.

25. Shamberger RC. Congenital chest wall deformities. In: Grosfeld JL, O'Neill JA Jr, Fonkalsrud EW, Coran AG, editor. Pediatric Surgery. 5th ed. Philadelphia: Elsevier; 1998. p. 787–817.

26. Creswick HA, Stacey MW, Kelly RE, et al. Family study of the inheritance of pectus excavatum. J Pediatr Surg 2006;41: 1699–703.

27. Horth L, Stacey M, Kelly RE Jr, et al. Advancing our understanding of the inheritance and transmission of pectus excavatum – Inheritance of pectus exavatum. J Pediatr Genetics. 2012: 161–73.

28. Lawson ML, Cash TF, Akers RA, et al. A pilot study of the impact of surgical repair on disease-specific quality of life among patients with pectus excavatum. J Pediatr Surg 2003;38:916–18.

29. Shamberger RC. Cardiopulmonary effects of anterior chest wall deformities. Chest Surg Clin North Am 2000;10:245–51.

30. Haller JA Jr, Peters GN, Mazur D, et al. Pectus excavatum: A 20-year surgical experience. J Thorac Cardiovasc Surg 1970;60:375–83.

31. Zhao L, Feinberg MS, Gaides M, et al. Why is exercise capacity reduced in subjects with pectus excavatum? J Pediatr 2000;136:163–7.

32. Mocchegiani R, Badano L, Lestuzzi C, et al. Relation of right ventricular morphology and function in pectus excavatum to the severity of the chest wall deformity. Am J Cardiol 1995;76: 941–6.

33. Sigalet DL, Montgomery M, Harder J, et al. Long-term cardiopulmonary effects of closed repair of pectus excavatum. Pediatr Surg Int 2007;23:493–7.

34. Coln D, Gunning T, Ramsay M, et al. Early experience with the Nuss minimally invasive correction of pectus excavatum in adults. World J Surg 2002;26:1217–21.

35. Malek MH, Berger DE, Housh TJ. Cardiovascular function following surgical repair of pectus excavatum: A meta-analysis. Chest 2006;130:506–16.

36. Shamberger RC, Welch KJ, Sanders SP. Mitral valve prolapse associated with pectus excavatum. J Pediatr 1987;111:404–7.

37. Saint-Mezard G, Duret JC, Chanudet X, et al. Mitral valve prolapse and pectus excavatum. Presse Med 1986;15:439.

38. Warth DC, King ME, Cohen JM, et al. Prevalence of mitral valve prolapse in normal children. J Am Coll Cardiol 1985;5:1173–7.

39. Park JM, Farmer AR. Wolff-Parkinson-White syndrome in children with pectus excavatum. J Pediatr Surg 1988;112:926–8.

40. Redlinger RE Jr, Wootton A, Kelly RE, et al. Optoelectronic plethysmography demonstrates abrogation of regional chest wall motion dysfunction in patients with pectus excavatum after Nuss repair. J Pediatr Surg 2012;47:160–4.

41. Haller JA Jr, Loughlin GM. Cardiorespiratory function is significantly improved following corrective surgery for severe pectus excavatum. J Cardiovasc Surg 2000;41:125–30.

42. Haller JA Jr, Kramer SS, Lietman SA. Use of CT scans in selection of patients for pectus excavatum surgery: A preliminary report. J Pediatr Surg 1987;22:904–8.

43. Croitoru DP, Kelly RE Jr, Nuss D, et al. Experience and modification update for the minimally invasive Nuss technique for pectus excavatum repair in 303 patients. J Pediatr Surg 2002;37:437–45.

44. Columbani P. Personal communication.

45. Park HJ, Lee SY, Lee CS, et al. The Nuss procedure for pectus excavatum: An evolution of techniques and results on 322 patients. Presented at the 39th annual meeting of the Society of Thoracic Surgeons, San Diego, CA, January 31 to February 2, 2003.

46. St Peter SD, Weesner KA, Weissend EE, et al. Epidural vs. patient-controlled analgesia for postoperative pain after pectus excavatum repair: A prospective, randomized trial. J Pediatr Surg 2012;47:148–53.

47. Azizkhan RG. What's new in pediatric surgery? J Am Coll Surg 1998;186:203–11.

48. Adzick NS, Nance ML. Pediatric surgery. N Engl J Med 2000;342:1651–7.

49. Hebra A, Swoveland B, Egbert M, et al. Outcome analysis of minimally invasive repair of pectus excavatum: Review of 251 cases. J Pediatr Surg 2000;35:252–8.

50. Miller KA, Woods RK, Sharp RJ, et al. Minimally invasive repair of pectus excavatum: A single institution's experience. Surgery 2001;130:652–9.

51. Molik KA, Engum SA, Rescoda FJ, et al. Pectus excavatum repair: Experience with standard and minimally invasive techniques. J Pediatr Surg 2001;36:324–8.

52. Wu PC, Knauer EM, McGowan GE, et al. Repair of pectus excavatum deformities in children: A new perspective of treatment using minimal access surgical technique. Arch Surg 2001;136: 419–24.

53. Hosie S, Sitkiewicz T, Peterson C, et al. Minimally invasive repair of pectus excavatum: The Nuss procedure: A European Multicenter Experience. Eur J Pediatr Surg 2002;12:235–8.

54. Shamberger RC, Welch KJ. Surgical correction of pectus carinatum. J Pediatr Surg 1987;22:48–53.

55. Chin EF. Surgery of funnel chest and congenital sternal prominence. Br J Surg 1957;44:360–76.

56. Robisek F, Cook JW, Daugherty HK, et al. Pectus carinatum. J Thorac Cardiovasc Surg 1979;78:52–61.

57. Pena A, Perez L, Nurka S, et al. Pectus carinatum and pectus excavatum: Are they the same disease? Am Surg 1981;47: 215–18.

58. Hebra A, Thomas PB, Tagge EP, et al. Pectus carinatum as a sequela of minimally invasive pectus excavatum repair. Pediatr Endosurg Innovat Techn 2002;6:41–4.

59. Fonkalsrud EW. Surgical correction of pectus carinatum: Lessons learned from 260 patients. J Pediatr Surg 2008;43:1235–43.

60. Currarino G, Silverman FN. Premature obliteration of the sternal sutures and pigeon breast deformity. Radiology 1958 ;70:532–40.

61. Chidambaram B, Mehta AV. Currarino-Silverman syndrome (pectus carinatum type 2 deformity) and mitral valve disease. Chest 1992;102:780–2.

62. Cohee A, Lin JR, Frantz FW, et al. Staged management of pectus carinatum. Eur J Pediatr Surg 2013;48(2):315–20.

63. Haje SA, Bowen JR. Preliminary results of orthotic treatment of pectus deformities in children and adolescents. J Pediatr Orthop 1992;12:795–800.

64. Ravitch MM. The operative correction of pectus carinatum (pigeon breast). Ann Surg 1960;151:705–14.

65. Welch KJ, Vos A. Surgical correction of pectus carinatum (pigeon breast). J Pediatr Surg 1973;8:659–67.

66. Abramson H, D'Agostino JD, Wuscovi S. A 5-year experience with a minimally invasive technique for pectus carinatum repair. J Pediatr Surg 2009;44:118–24.

67. Allwyn JS, Shetty L, Pare VS, et al. Chondro-manubrial deformity and bifid rib, rare variations seen in pectus carinatum: A radiological finding. Surg Radiol Anat 2012: Epub ahead of print.

68. Kelly RE Jr, Quinn A, Varela P, et al. Dysmorphology of chest wall deformities: Frequency distribution of subtypes of typical pectus excavatum and rare subtypes. Arch Bronconeumol 2012 Epub ahead of print.

69. Shamberger RC, Welch KJ. Surgical correction of chondromanubrial deformity (Currarino Silverman syndrome). J Pediatr Surg 1988;23:319–22.

70. Freire-Maia N, Chautard EA, Opitz JM. The Poland syndrome: Clinical and genealogical data, dermatoglyphic analysis, and incidence. Hum Hered 1973;23:97–104.

71. Poland A. Deficiency of the pectoralis muscles. Guys Hosp Rep 1841;6:191–3.

72. Froriep R. Beobachtung eines Falles Von Mangel der Brustdrüse. Notizen aus dem Gebiete der Naturund Heilkinde 1839;10: 9–14.

73. Lallemand LM. Ephermerides. Medicales de Montpellier. 1826;1:144–7.

74. Seyfer AE, Icochea R, Graber GM. Poland's anomaly: Natural history and long-term results of chest wall reconstruction in 33 patients. Ann Surg 1988;208:776–82.

75. Shamberger RC, Welch KJ, Upton J III. Surgical treatment of thoracic deformity in Poland's syndrome. J Pediatr Surg 1989;24:760–5.

76. Samarrai AR, Charmockley HA, Attr AA. Complete cleft sternum: Classification and surgical repair. Int Surg 1985;70:71–3.

77. Shamberger RC, Welch KJ. Sternal defects. Pediatr Surg Int 1990;5:156–64.

78. Knox L, Tuggle D, Knott-Craig CJ. Repair of congenital sternal clefts in adolescence and infancy. J Pediatr Surg 1994;29:1513–16.

79. Amato J, Douglas W, Desai U, et al. Ectopia cordis. Chest Surg Clin N Am 2000;10:297–316.

80. Groner JI. Ectopia cordis and sternal defects. In: Zeigler MM, Azizkhan RG, Weber TR, editor. Operative Pediatric Surgery. New York: McGraw-Hill; 2003. p. 279–93.

81. Amato U, Zelen J, Talwalker NG. Single-stage repair of thoracic ectopia cordis. Ann Thorac Surg 1995;59:518–20.

82. Engum SA. Embryology, sternal clefts, ectopia cordis, and Cantrell's pentalogy. Semin Pediatr Surg 2008;17:154–60.

83. Campbell RM, Smith MD, Mayes TC, et al. The characteristics of thoracic insufficiency syndrome associated with fused ribs and congenital scoliosis. J Bone Joint Surg Am 2003;85:399–408.

84. Jeune M, Carron R, Beraud C, et al. Polychondrodystrophie avec blocage thoracique d'evolution fatale. Pediatrie 1954;9:390–2.

85. Borland LM. Anesthesia for children with Jeune's syndrome (asphyxiating thoracic dystrophy). Anesthesiology 1987;66:86–8.

86. Tahernia AC, Stamps P. Jeune's syndrome (asphyxiating thoracic dystrophy). Chin Pediatr 1977;16:903–7.

87. Williams AJ, Vawter G, Reid LM. Lung structure in asphyxiating thoracic dystrophy. Arch Pathol Lab Med 1984;108:658–61.

88. Finegold J, Katzew H, Genieser NB, et al. Lung structure in thoracic dystrophy. Am J Dis Child 1971;122:153–9.

89. Langer LO. Thoracic pelvic phalangeal dystrophy: Asphyxiating thoracic dystrophy of the newborn, infantile thoracic dystrophy. Radiology 1968;91:447–56.

90. Oberklaid F, Danks DM, Mayne V, et al. Asphyxiating thoracic dysplasia. Arch Dis Child 1977;52:758–65.

91. Campbell RM. The incidence of proximal cervical spine stenosis in Jeune's asphyxiating dystrophy. Paper presented at the Scoliosis Research Society 2001.

92. Herdman RC, Langer LO. The thoracic asphyxiant dystrophy and renal disease. Am J Dis Child 1977;52:192–201.

93. Jarcho S, Levin PM. Hereditary malformations of the vertebral bodies. Bull Johns Hopkins Hosp 1938;62:216–26.

94. Roberts AP, Conner AN, Tolmie JL, et al. Spondylothoracic and spondylocostal dysostosis: Hereditary forms of spinal deformity. J Bone Joint Surg Br 1988;70:123–6.

95. Heilbronner DM, Renshaw TS. Spondylothoracic dysplasia. J Bone Joint Surg Am 1984;66:302–3.

96. McMaster MJ. Congenital scoliosis. In: Weinstein SL, editor. The Pediatric Spine: Principles and Practice. New York: Raven Press; 1994.

97. McMaster MJ. Congenital scoliosis caused by unilateral failure of vertebral segmentation with contralateral hemivertebrae. Spine 1998;23:998–1005.

98. McMaster MJ, David C. Hemivertebrae as a cause of scoliosis: A study of 104 patients. J Bone Joint Surg Br 1986;68:588–95.

99. Campbell RM. Congenital scoliosis due to multiple vertebrae anomalies associated with thoracic insufficiency syndrome. Spine 2000;14:209–18.

100. Campbell RM, Smith MD, Mayes T, et al. The characteristics of thoracic insufficiency syndrome associated with fused ribs and congenital scoliosis. J Bone Joint Surg 2003;85:399–408.

101. Todd DW, Tinguely ST, Norberg WJ. A thoracic expansion technique for Jeune's asphyxiating thoracic dystrophy. J Pediatr Surg 1986;21:161–3.

102. Barnes ND, Hall D, Milner AD, et al. Chest reconstruction in asphyxiating thoracic dystrophy. Arch Dis Child 1971;46:833–7.

103. Weber TR, Kurkchubasche AG. Operative management of asphyxiating thoracic dystrophy after pectus repair. J Pediatr Surg 1998;33:262–5.

104. Sharoni E, Erez E, Chorer G, et al. Chest reconstruction in asphyxiating thoracic dystrophy. J Pediatr Surg 1998;33:1578–81.

105. Davis JT, Heistein JB, Castile RG, et al. Lateral thoracic expansion for Jeune's syndrome: Mid-term results. Ann Thorac Surg 2001;72:872–8.

106. Campbell RM, Hell-Vocke AK. Growth of the thoracic spine in congenital scoliosis after expansion thoracoplasty. J Bone Joint Surg Am 2003;85:409–19.

107. Phillips JD, van Aalst JA. Jeune's syndrome (asphyxiating thoracic dystrophy): Congenital and acquired. Semin Pediatr Surg 2008;17:167–72.

108. Ramirez N, Flynn JM, Emans JB. Vertical expandable prosthetic titanium rib as treatment of thoracic insufficiency syndrome in spondylocostal dysplasia. J Pediatr Orthop 2010;30:521–6.

109. Gadepalli SK, Hirschl RB, Tsai WC, et al. Vertical expandable prosthetic titanium rib device insertion: Does it improve pulmonary function? J Pediatr Surg 2011;46:77–80.

CHAPTER 21

MANAGEMENT OF LARYNGOTRACHEAL OBSTRUCTION IN CHILDREN

David R. White • H. Biemann Othersen, Jr. • André Hebra

Pediatric surgeons are often involved in the management of acute and chronic airway obstruction. Moreover, iatrogenic injury to the pediatric airway occasionally occurs. The large number of operative techniques for the treatment of laryngotracheal stenosis shows that no single procedure or technique is universally applicable and successful. Prevention of, or prompt therapy for, injury is all important.[1,2]

PRACTICAL EMBRYOLOGY AND ANATOMY

A working knowledge of the embryonic development of the mediastinal structures aids in understanding the etiology and associated anomalies of tracheal obstruction. Malformations of the great vessels (vascular rings) should be suspected and investigated when evaluating a child with complete tracheal rings. The most common vascular malformation associated with complete tracheal rings is a pulmonary vascular sling. This anomaly occurs when the left pulmonary artery arises to the right of the trachea, around which it curves and compresses just above the carina, and then passes between the trachea and esophagus before reaching the left lung (Fig. 21-1).[3] Other vascular ring malformations may produce varying degrees of tracheal, bronchial, and esophageal compression.

SUBGLOTTIC AND TRACHEAL MALFORMATIONS

Congenital Subglottic and Tracheal Stenosis

The anatomy of the pediatric airway has been compared to an inverted cone, with the trachea fitting telescopically into the cricoid above it, the cricoid into the thyroid cartilage, and then the thyroid into the hyoid space (Fig. 21-2).[4] Congenital subglottic stenosis is the most common morphologic abnormality and presents as a narrowing of the airway at the distal end of the larynx, just at the beginning of the trachea. The subglottic region lies at the level of the cricoid cartilage, which is normally the only complete cartilaginous ring in the airway. Congenital subglottic abnormalities result in elliptical narrowing of the cricoid cartilage, the etiology of which is not known. Subglottic stenosis is exceeded only by laryngomalacia and vocal cord paralysis in the frequency of congenital airway anomalies.

When compared with an adult, the anatomy of the trachea and larynx of a child differs in several ways (Fig. 21-3). The child's epiglottis is short and small, and the valleculae are shallow. Also, the larynx points posteriorly, and the arytenoid apparatus is large in relation to the lumen of the larynx. Finally, the narrowest point of the normal pediatric airway is the subglottis. In the adult, it is the glottis.

In the normal trachea, the cartilaginous rings are horseshoe-shaped, with the posterior wall composed of connective tissue and the trachealis muscle. Thus, the lumen may change as the trachea expands or contracts with respiration. Long congenital stenotic segments in the trachea are usually the result of complete cartilaginous tracheal rings. When complete cartilaginous rings are present, the lumen is rigid and much smaller than the normal trachea. If it does not produce early respiratory distress, complete cartilaginous rings may be detected when an inflammatory process within the trachea produces mucosal edema, which further compromises the lumen and results in acute airway obstruction. Occasionally, tracheal intubation for an elective operative procedure may be difficult and the narrowed segment is discovered.

Acquired Subglottic and Tracheal Stenosis

Acquired airway malformations usually result from intrinsic injury with subsequent inflammation, ulceration, and scarring, leading to subglottic or tracheal scarring and narrowing. Occasionally, trauma is the initiating event but an iatrogenic event can exacerbate an unstable situation.[2] For example, a child with a congenitally small airway might be asymptomatic until an endotracheal tube is inserted. The tube may be appropriate in size but, because of the congenital stenosis, it will fit tightly and can lead to ulceration and stricture. Particularly difficult to treat are those injuries that occur well below the subglottic region, usually produced by an endotracheal balloon that caused compression and ulceration in the trachea. Frequently, these areas of injury are below the usual site for a tracheostomy. The cuff may even erode into overlying vessels (Fig. 21-4).

VASCULAR COMPRESSION

Compression and partial obstruction of the trachea may be caused by abnormalities of the aortic arch that impinge

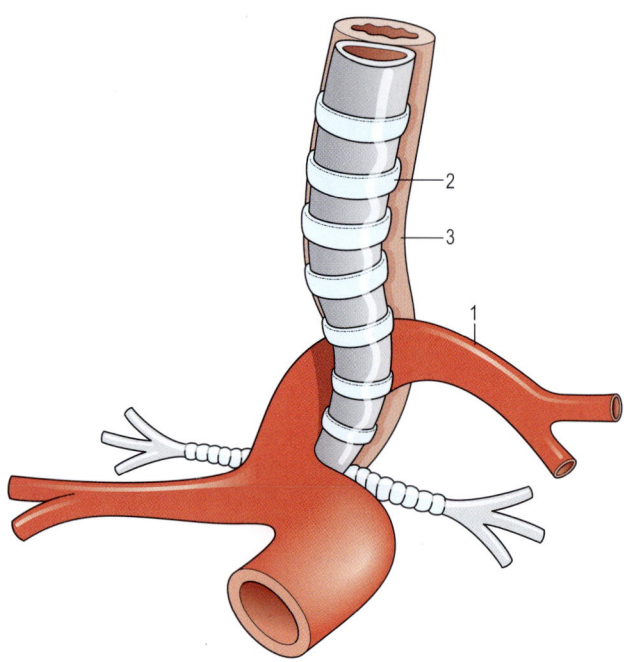

FIGURE 21-1 ■ Complete tracheal rings in distal trachea and pulmonary vascular sling. 1, Left pulmonary artery; 2, trachea; 3, esophagus.

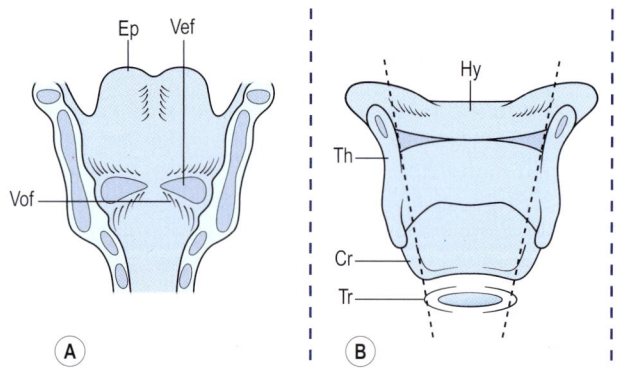

FIGURE 21-2 ■ (A) Ventral area of the larynx in the neonate viewed from behind. The ventricle, or 'third cavity,' is bounded above by the ventricular folds (Vef) and below by the vocal folds (Vof). Ep, epiglottis. (B) Laryngeal cartilages (without arytenoids). Th, thyroid; Cr, cricoid; Tr, trachea; and Hy, hyoid viewed from behind. Inner dashed lines show telescopic configuration in the neonate as opposed to the rectangular shape in the adult (outer dashed lines). (Adapted from Othersen HB Jr, editor. The Pediatric Airway. Philadelphia: WB Saunders; 1991.)

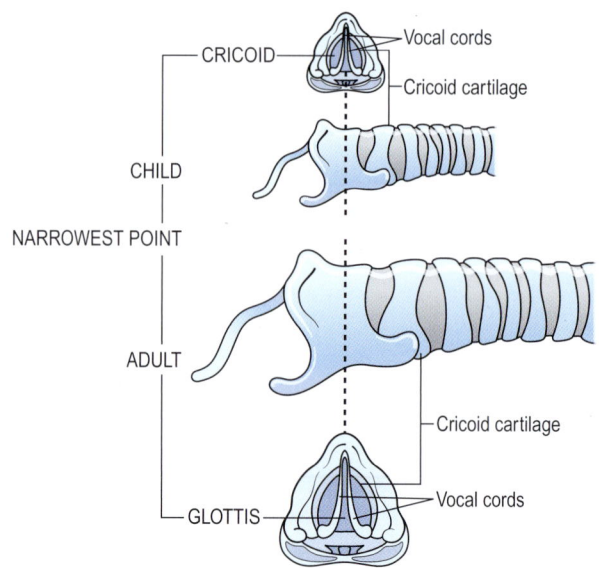

FIGURE 21-3 ■ Difference between adult and pediatric airway. (Adapted from Othersen HB Jr. Intubation injuries of the trachea in children: Management and prevention. Ann Surg 1978;189:601–6.)

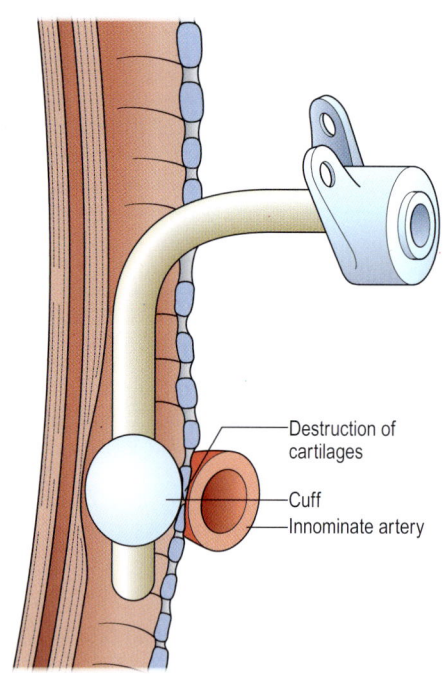

FIGURE 21-4 ■ The inflated cuff of a tracheostomy tube may erode anteriorly into the innominate artery. (Adapted from Othersen HB Jr, editor. The Pediatric Airway. Philadelphia: WB Saunders; 1991.)

on, or encircle, the trachea or esophagus, or both.[5,6] When both the trachea and esophagus are compressed, swallowing frequently produces airway compression and respiratory distress. Vascular rings are often asymptomatic in neonates and infants, yet can lead to significant airway obstruction in a child.[7]

The physiologic impingement on the trachea by a vascular ring is similar to that seen in patients after repair of esophageal atresia. The persistently distended upper esophageal pouch can displace the trachea anteriorly, producing tracheomalacia (Fig. 21-5). Particularly with swallowing, the distended esophageal pouch may compress the trachea against the innominate artery (Figs 21-6

and 21-7). Correction of this problem centers on anterior mobilization and suspension of the innominate artery (Fig. 21-8).[8–12] The treatment of a pulmonary vascular sling may require not only relocation and reimplantation of the pulmonary artery, but also repair of the stenotic distal trachea.[7,12,13]

Stridor and dyspnea are symptoms that can be produced by vascular impingement on the trachea. Patients with severe compromise from a double aortic arch are

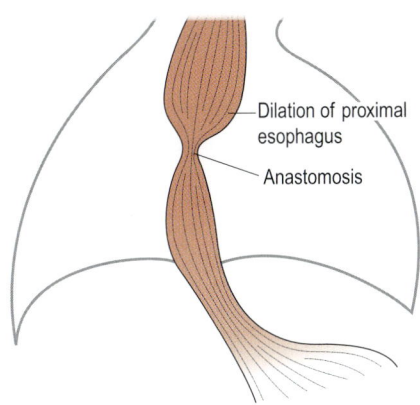

FIGURE 21-5 ■ After repair of esophageal atresia, the proximal esophagus, which is already enlarged, is further dilated by an anastomotic stricture. (Adapted from Othersen HB Jr, editor. The Pediatric Airway. Philadelphia: WB Saunders; 1991.)

usually symptomatic, but their manifestations are variable (Fig. 21-9). Some patients are seen with frequent coughing episodes and stridor accompanied by dyspnea and cyanosis, whereas small infants may have apneic episodes. The symptoms of vascular impingement on the trachea are usually more dramatic than those from compression of the esophagus.

Classically, vascular ring anomalies are diagnosed on a barium esophagogram with indentations on the esophageal column of barium and a decrease in the tracheal air column. Offset of the axis of the barium column above and below the indentation is diagnostic of a double aortic arch (Fig. 21-10A). More recently, rapid computed tomographic (CT) scans allow a graphic reconstruction of the trachea and adjacent vessels (Fig. 21-10B). Magnetic resonance imaging (MRI) enhanced with

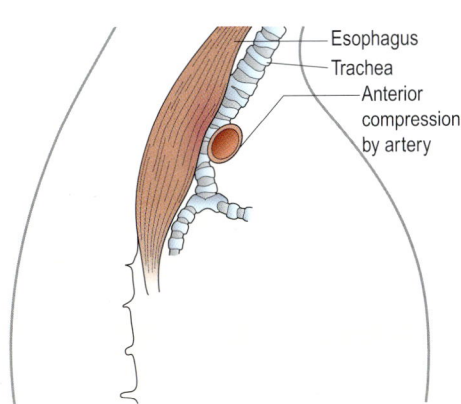

FIGURE 21-6 ■ A lateral view shows how the dilated proximal esophagus displaces the trachea and compresses it against the overlying innominate artery. (Adapted from Othersen HB Jr, editor. The Pediatric Airway. Philadelphia: WB Saunders; 1991.)

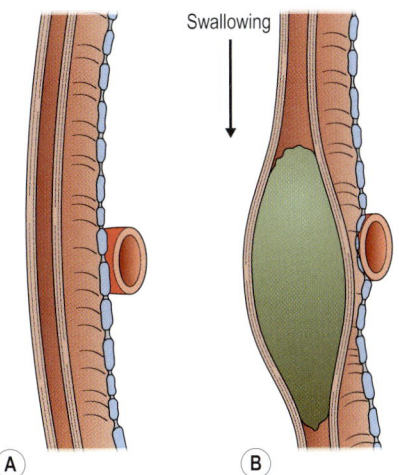

FIGURE 21-7 ■ An enlarged diagram of Figure 21-6 illustrates how the compression is increased by ingestion of food. (Adapted from Othersen HB Jr, editor. The Pediatric Airway. Philadelphia: WB Saunders; 1991.)

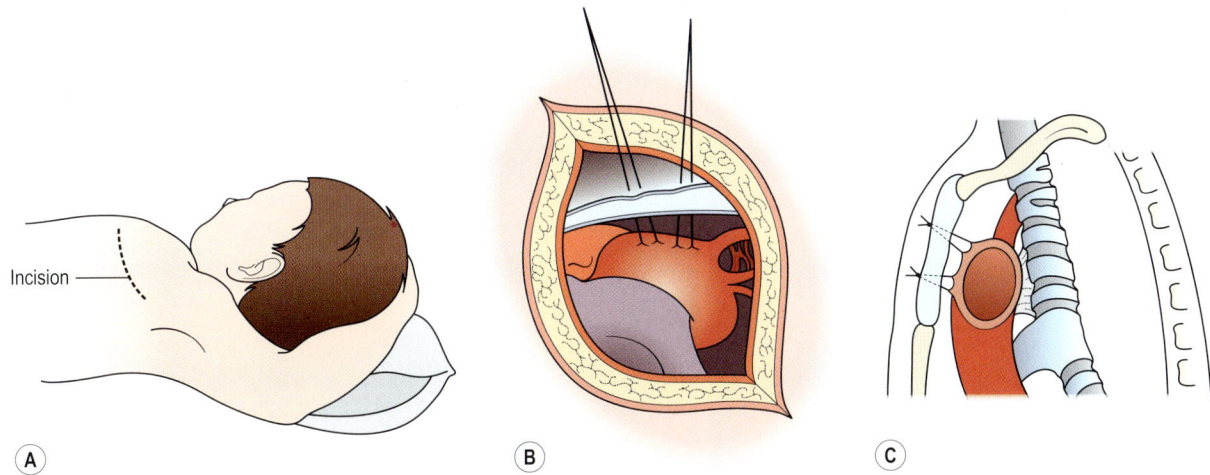

FIGURE 21-8 ■ The operative technique for aortopexy. **(A)** Anterior left thoracotomy in the third interspace. **(B)** Sutures placed into the wall of the innominate artery and the aortic arch. **(C)** Sutures passed through the sternum and tied to elevate the compressing vessels. Tracheal attachments pull the anterior wall of the trachea forward. (Adapted from Othersen HB Jr, editor. The Pediatric Airway. Philadelphia: WB Saunders; 1991.)

intravenous administration of a contrast agent allows excellent visualization of the trachea and vessels as well.

Occasionally, a child will appear with acute airway obstruction or other medical problems requiring intensive care, during which endotracheal intubation and a concomitant nasogastric tube are inserted. The presence of tubes in both airway and esophagus makes detection of a vascular ring difficult and can generate complications. In a child who is already intubated, performance of contrast radiographic procedures may not be possible. Ultrasonography (US), or CT, or contrast-enhanced MRI may delineate the vascular abnormality. When both tracheal and esophageal intubations are necessary in a patient with a double aortic arch, the encircling vessels

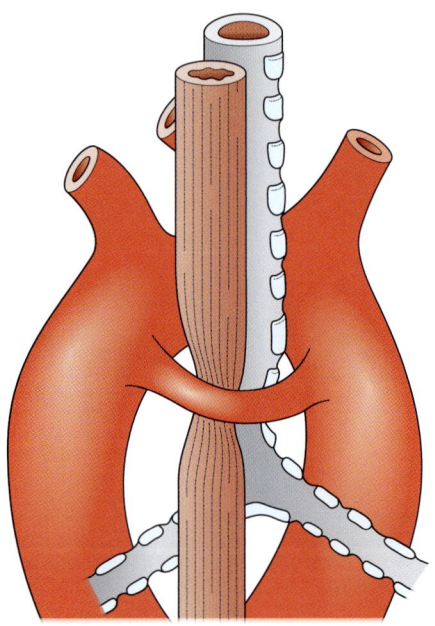

FIGURE 21-9 ■ Both trachea and esophagus are compressed by a double aortic arch. (Adapted from Othersen HB Jr, editor. The Pediatric Airway. Philadelphia: WB Saunders; 1991.)

may sustain pressure necrosis. Erosion into the aortic arch can produce an aortoesophageal fistula that may not be manifest until either the endotracheal or the esophageal tube is removed. A sentinel hemorrhage may occur before a massive, and often fatal, hemorrhage occurs into the esophagus. The passage of a Sengstaken–Blakemore tube with inflation of the esophageal balloon can be lifesaving by tamponading the fistula.[14] Because no reliable diagnostic study is available to demonstrate an aortoesophageal fistula, the observation of a sentinel hemorrhage in such a patient with ultrasound confirmation of a double aortic arch is a clear indication for urgent cardiopulmonary bypass and repair.[14]

Vascular rings cause airway constriction and not vascular problems. Thus, simple division of the vascular ring is often not enough to relieve tracheal compression. Following division of a vascular ring, if part of the ring continues to compress the airway, it should not be dissected away from the trachea but suspended anteriorly, often to the back of the sternum. The vascular-tracheal attachments will lift the anterior tracheal wall and enlarge the lumen (see Fig. 21-8). Traditionally, an open operation has been used for vascular ring repair. Significant numbers of patients are now being treated by the thoracoscopic approach.[15] Regardless of the approach, whether from the right or from the left,[16] or other technical variations,[17] the recurrent laryngeal and phrenic nerves need to be identified and protected. Flexible endoscopic observation of the trachea during these maneuvers can corroborate relief of the compression.[6]

TRACHEOMALACIA

Often, tracheomalacia is produced by constant pressure from a cardiovascular structure. Thus it is almost always necessary to suspend the offending vessel and utilize its attachments to the trachea to expand the tracheal lumen. Tracheomalacia can be primary in nature without evidence of compression. In these cases, suspension of the large mediastinal vessels may enlarge the tracheal lumen,

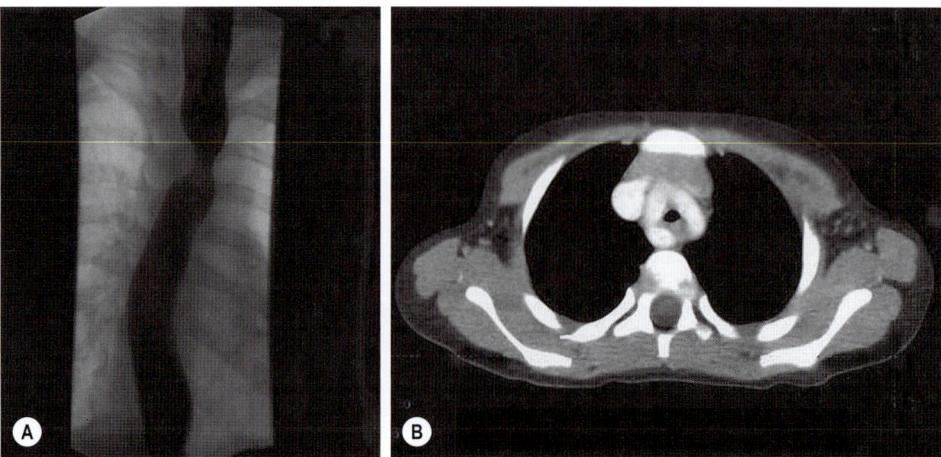

FIGURE 21-10 ■ This infant presented with stridor. There was a suggestion of tracheal indentation on the chest radiograph. Therefore, a barium esophagogram was performed **(A)** and shows the double indentations diagnostic of a double aortic arch. **(B)** A CT scan shows contrast in the double arch that is encircling the trachea and esophagus (collapsed).

or the peritracheal fascia can be suspended to the sternum to overcome collapse of the airway.[18–21] In the UK (Scotland), guidelines have been promulgated for the use of thoracoscopic aortopexy to treat severe primary tracheomalacia. Interestingly, the National Health Service believed that these guidelines were necessary because individual surgeons would operate infrequently on infants and children who are good candidates for operative correction.

INFLAMMATORY OBSTRUCTIONS

Viral laryngotracheitis (croup), bacterial or membranous tracheitis, and epiglottitis are inflammatory conditions that occasionally require operative intervention. In cases of inflammatory obstruction, endotracheal intubation is preferred instead of tracheostomy if possible. It is important to distinguish croup and bacterial tracheitis from epiglottitis because the treatments are quite different (Table 21-1).

Children with epiglottitis characteristically tolerate endotracheal intubation without airway injury because the inflammation and edema are supraglottic and not circumferential. Conversely, with viral or bacterial laryngotracheitis, the inflammatory process involves the entire circumference of the airway and prolonged intubation may lead to permanent scarring.[1,22] In the past, many hospitals had strict protocols requiring diagnostic laryngoscopy in the operating room with anesthesia standby for suspected cases of epiglottitis because an emergency tracheostomy was occasionally necessary. Fortunately, the widespread introduction of *Haemophilus influenza* type B vaccination has nearly eliminated pediatric epiglottitis in the U.S.[22]

Croup characteristically occurs during viral seasons in children age 3 months to 3 years. Children in whom the classic 'croupy' cough develops frequently have a history of an antecedent respiratory infection, usually with a high fever.[23] Bacterial tracheitis, a nonviral infectious disease, is seen with fever and rapid development of upper airway obstruction, characterized by copious mucopurulent secretions.

Fortunately, most of these inflammatory processes are now controlled with antibiotics and respiratory care without the need for operation. Treatment includes oxygen with increased humidification and inhalation of racemic epinephrine. Endotracheal intubation is well tolerated in epiglottitis. However, in cases of viral or bacterial tracheitis, even brief (24–48 hours) intubation may cause ulceration in a trachea that is already acutely inflamed and swollen. Croup is more easily treated without intubation using racemic epinephrine inhalation combined with dexamethasone.

INJURIES

Intrinsic Injuries

Most intrinsic laryngotracheal injuries are iatrogenic and produced by inappropriate introduction of an endotracheal tube from instrumentation of the airway. Another intrinsic injury is a thermal burn. The inhalation of hot gases, steam, and toxic smoke produces acute injury that can lead to inflammation and edema in addition to burn necrosis.[24,25] When an endotracheal tube is passed through an inflamed glottis and upper trachea, early tracheostomy should be considered. With more extensive involvement, prolonged stenting with a T-shaped tracheostomy or T-tube with open proximal and distal limbs may be required.[24] Also, the overaggressive use of lasers or cautery may produce direct tissue thermal injury or may lead to an airway fire. Reconstruction after an airway burn injury should be delayed until the stenosis has matured.[26]

Extrinsic Injuries

Extrinsic injury to the larynx and trachea may occur when an unrestrained child in an automobile strikes his or her neck on the dashboard or the back of the front seat (Fig. 21-11). A blow directly to the neck from a wire when falling or when riding a bicycle ('clothesline injury') may damage the larynx or trachea (Fig. 21-12). Transection of both the trachea and esophagus can occur without visible external neck injuries beyond slight erythema. Crepitus may be present. A good history is essential in determining the mechanism of injury.[27] In these instances, and particularly in conjunction with severe craniofacial injuries,

---

TABLE 21-1 **Characteristics of Laryngotracheobronchitis and Epiglottitis**

Characteristic	Laryngotracheobronchitis	Epiglottitis
Incidence	Common	Uncommon
Etiology	Viral	*Haemophilus influenzae* type b
Age	6 months to 3 years	2–6 years
Clinical picture	Gradual onset, preceding upper respiratory tract infection, barking cough	Rapid onset, fever, drooling, dysphagia
Physical examination	Respiratory distress, inspiratory stridor, low-grade temperature	Anxious, muffled voice, chin forward, drooling, high temperature
Laboratory studies	WBC usually <10,000/mm³ with lymphocytosis; radiograph shows narrowing of subglottic region	WBC often >10,000/mm³ with band cells increased; radiograph shows swollen epiglottis

WBC, white blood cell count.
Adapted from McLain LG: Croup syndrome. Am Fam Physician 1987;36:213.

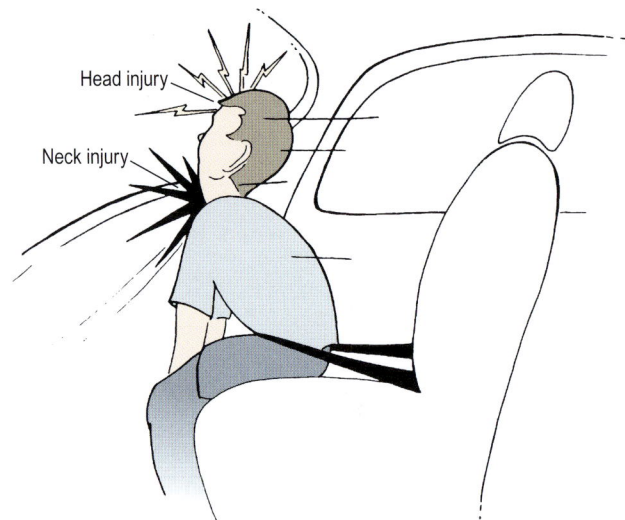

FIGURE 21-11 ■ Mechanism of head injury. With a padded dashboard, external evidence of injury is minimal. (Adapted from Othersen HB Jr. Cardiothoracic injuries. In: Touloukian RJ, editor. Pediatric Trauma. New York: John Wiley & Sons; 1978.)

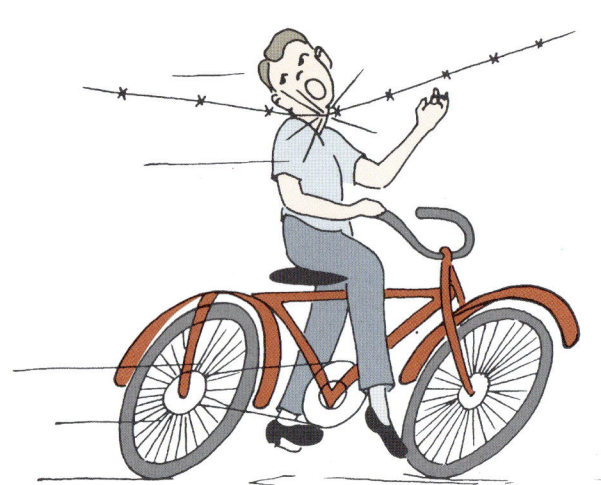

FIGURE 21-12 ■ A 'clothesline' injury may produce fracture or transection of the airway with little evidence of skin injury. (Adapted from Othersen HB Jr. Cardiothoracic injuries. In: Touloukian RJ, editor. Pediatric Trauma. New York: John Wiley & Sons; 1978.)

a tracheostomy performed under general anesthesia but without endotracheal intubation is usually advisable, because attempts at intubation may further compromise the tenuous airway. Penetrating injuries in children are infrequent, but the same general principles used for management in adults should be followed.[28]

ENDOTRACHEAL INTUBATION

Endotracheal intubation may be difficult in small children. The preferred laryngoscopic blade for infants and children is a straight blade, such as the Miller or the Wis–Hipple. Otolaryngologic laryngoscopes, such as the Parsons and Benjamin–Lindholm laryngoscopes, provide even better exposure. The child's head should be in the neutral position and not extended. With the infant's head in the neutral, or 'sniffing,' position, the laryngoscope blade is introduced and the tongue and floor of the mouth lifted to expose the epiglottis. Once the epiglottis is seen, extension or flexion of the head and neck may be needed.

For infants and children, a commonly applied formula to determine the correct endotracheal tube size is (age + 16)/4 or age/4 + 4. If a child needs to be rapidly intubated with a tube that fits snugly and allows no air leak, this fact should be noted and documented. At the earliest possible opportunity, the snugly fitting tube should be changed to a smaller size. If intubation is required for a long period (usually longer than two to three weeks), tracheostomy may be considered. An air leak is generally an indication that the tube is not too snug.

Usually a cuffed endotracheal tube is not necessary in children because compensation for air leaks can be accomplished by increasing the volume of air delivered by the ventilator. However, with massive craniofacial injuries and bleeding, or with significant gastroesophageal reflux, a cuff may be necessary to prevent aspiration of blood or gastric contents. Otherwise, it is best not to use a cuff to prevent damage to the subglottic trachea.[29,30] Indications for tracheostomy are summarized in Table 21-2.

TRACHEOSTOMY

Tracheostomy is best performed with an endotracheal tube in place so that the airway is controlled. A transverse

---

TABLE 21-2 Indications for Endotracheal Intubation and Tracheostomy

Clinical Situation	Endotracheal Intubation	Tracheostomy
Emergencies	Always, except →	Severe craniofacial or head and neck injuries
Neonates and infants <6 months	Oral intubation unless no hope of extubation →	When long-term intubation is required or when there is difficulty in maintaining intubation because of activity
Infants >6 months and children	Maintain for 7–14 days and then →	When long-term intubation or ventilatory support is required for conditions such as severe head injuries
Epiglottitis	Until infection has cleared	Usually not necessary
Croup or other severe glottic inflammatory diseases	If does not respond to inhalations of racemic epinephrine or with airway obstruction as a temporary measure before →	When glottic edema and inflammation are severe

TABLE 21-3 Tracheostomy Tube Specifications

Tube Type	French Size	ID	OD	Length (mm)
Shiley: Neonatal	00			
	0	3.4	5.0	32
	1	3.7	5.5	34
Shiley: Pediatric	00	3.1	4.5	39
	0	3.4	5.0	40
	1	3.7	5.5	41
	2	4.1	6.0	42
	3	4.8	7.0	44
	4	5.5	8.0	46
Argyle (Dover)	000	2.5	4.0	32
	00	3.0	4.7	34
	0	3.5	5.4	36
	1	4.0	6.0	36
	2	4.5	6.6	40
	3	5.0	7.3	46
	4	5.5	7.8	50
	5	6.0	8.5	54
Silastic (Dow Corning)	1	3.0	5.5	35
	3	4.0	7.0	40
	4½	5.0	8.0	43
	6	7.0	10.0	46

ID, inside diameter; OD, outside diameter.

incision made in the lower neck approximately one finger-breadth above the sternal notch is deepened to allow lateral retraction of the strap muscles after the midline is opened. In infants, the subcutaneous fibrofatty tissue superficial to the strap muscles is generally removed to improve exposure. After the strap muscles are retracted, dissection is then carried down to the trachea. The thyroid isthmus is then elevated off the trachea and divided. In small children, palpation of the ridges of the tracheal rings with a small hemostat is frequently more valuable than visualization for determining the appropriate level of tracheotomy. Our experience is that a vertical midline linear tracheal incision through the third and fourth rings, without excising any of the anterior wall of the trachea, is the preferred technique (Fig. 21-13). Cruciate incisions should not be used because the flaps may become inverted and narrow the lumen. The tracheostomy tube specifications are listed in Table 21-3. Traction sutures of polypropylene, left long and labeled 'left' and 'right,' allow easier reintubation in the event of accidental dislodgement within the first week. Skin may be sewn to the trachea in four quadrants to allow better exposure of the tracheal incision. If the tracheostomy has been in place for longer than two weeks, bronchoscopy is recommended before decannulation. A suprastomal granuloma commonly develops at the superior rim of the tracheostomy stoma and may need excision.

TRACHEAL REPAIR

Congenital Stenosis

Many congenital stenotic lesions are asymptomatic until an acute event occurs, such as an injury, acute tracheal inflammation, or endotracheal intubation. Historically, congenital tracheal stenosis was managed with pericardial patch reconstruction or with an endoscopic procedure using either the KTP (potassium titanyl phosphate) or CO_2 laser to divide each complete cartilaginous ring in the posterior midline followed by long-term stenting.[31] With a short segment of complete rings, resection and anastomosis is effective, but short-segment congenital tracheal stenosis is very uncommon.[32]

More recently, these methods have been replaced by slide tracheoplasty.[33] An improvement on standard resection techniques, slide tracheoplasty allows reconstruction without tension.[34] The narrowed segment is transected in its midportion, and the remaining stenotic segments are incised. One end of the trachea is opened in the posterior midline, and the other is incised in the anterior midline. The diameter of the resulting anastomosis is broad enough to avoid airway narrowing. Long-term evaluation has shown excellent survival rates with a lower need for airway stenting.[35]

Acquired Stenosis

When an endotracheal tube is removed, tracheal injury may be manifested by stridor or dyspnea. Diagnosis is made with microlaryngoscopy and bronchosopy. Prompt therapy may allow the trachea to heal without stenosis. The patient is initially treated with high doses of systemic corticosteroids (dexamethasone 0.8–1 mg/kg/day) in an attempt to soften the dense scar. The trachea may require dilation using balloon dilators. Balloons dilate with radial forces. Rigid dilators can produce more injury, because even though they dilate they also impart a shearing force to the tracheal mucosa. Dexamethasone is continued in the dose of 0.8–1 mg/kg/day for at least 72 hours. Longer treatment may be necessary for more severe injuries. If intubation is required, a tube small enough to allow an air leak is preferred. The endotracheal tube is removed once the patient is stable and spontaneously breathing without ventilatory assistance.

If a dense stenosis has already occurred, the previously described techniques may not be effective. Acquired tracheal obstruction can be classified as granulomatous, inflammatory, fibrous, or calcific. Congenital obstructions are usually cartilaginous. With dense fibrous and calcific strictures, open resection and reconstruction is usually necessary. However, endoscopic laser incision of the stricture with gradual and gentle balloon expansion of the lumen, combined with insertion of an endotracheal stent, may allow a functional airway to remodel over a period of time. Some authors advocate treatment of tracheal granulation tissue with mitomycin-C.[36] If stenosis recurs when the stent is removed, the stent can be reinserted and balloon dilation performed with the stent in situ.

In the past, T-tubes have been used effectively as stents in both children and adults.[24] Newer expandable metal stents are now frequently used in adults. Some of these nickel-titanium (nitinol)-coated stents have been used in children in selected cases.[37] However, these stents may not be appropriate for children because the child will grow and the metal stent does not. Removal of the stent is then necessary and can be problematic. Moreover, the ingrowth of granulation tissue through the interstices of the metal stent may produce obstruction in itself and lead to severe hemorrhage when removal is attempted. Finally, the medical conditions for which the stents are placed are often different in children from those in adults. Stent use in adults is often due to neoplastic conditions that are associated with a short life expectancy. However, in children, a stent may be required for years.

Silicone rubber stents have been successfully used in adults, but fixation to the trachea using projections from the circumference of the tube is necessary to prevent migration.[38,39] The small diameter of a child's trachea makes these stents impractical. A T-shaped tube inserted through a tracheotomy with proximal and distal tracheal extensions can be readily inserted into a child's airway and will not migrate.

Open Laryngotracheoplasty

There are variations in the operative techniques used for tracheal reconstruction in infants and children.[40,41] An

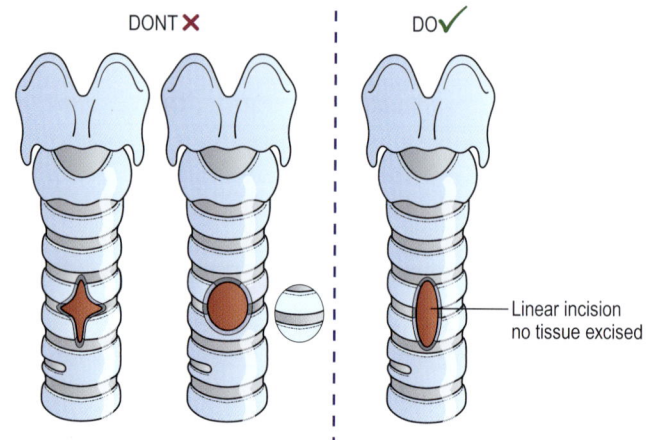

FIGURE 21-13 ■ Two techniques of tracheostomy to be avoided in children and the preferred linear incision. (Adapted from Othersen HB Jr. Intubation injuries of the trachea in children: Management and prevention. Ann Surg 1979;189:601–6.)

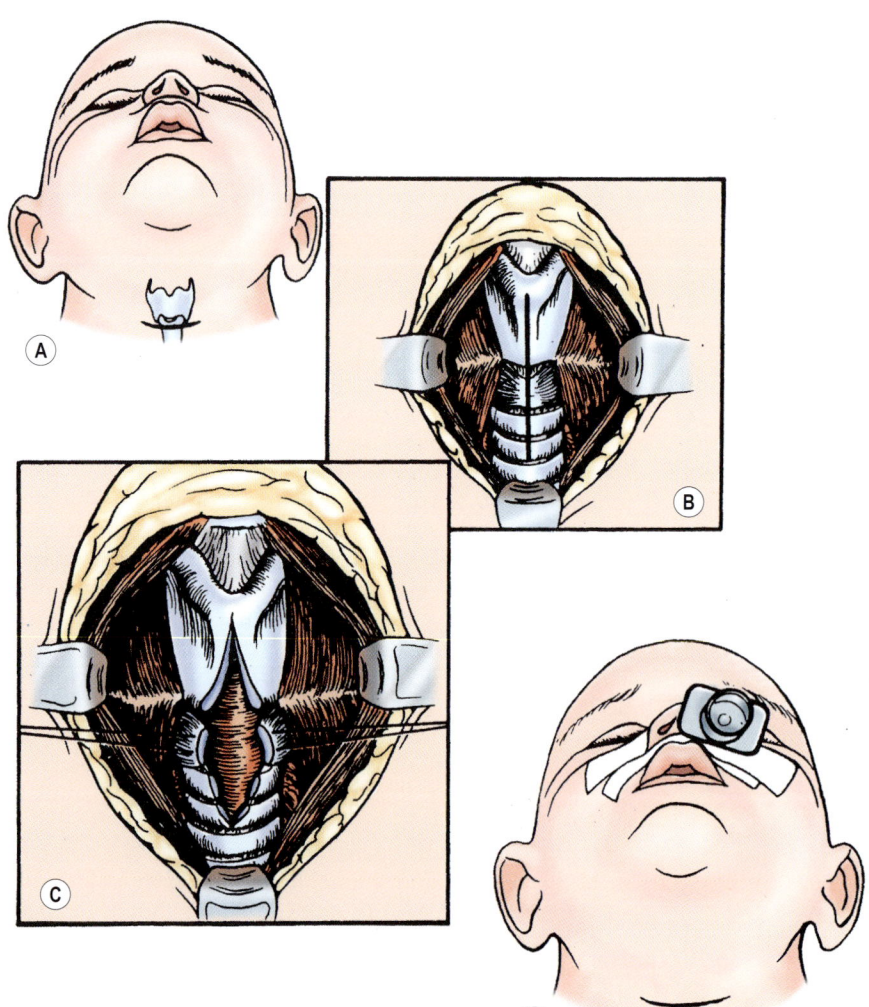

FIGURE 21-14 ■ The anterior cricoid split procedure. **(A)** Make a horizontal incision over the cricoid cartilage. **(B)** Use a combination of sharp and blunt dissection to expose the larynx and upper trachea. **(C)** Split the lower portion of the thyroid cartilage, the cricoid cartilage, and upper tracheal rings. **(D)** Close the wound loosely over a drain with the airway stented by a nasotracheal tube. (Adapted from Othersen HB Jr, editor. The Pediatric Airway. Philadelphia: WB Saunders; 1991.)

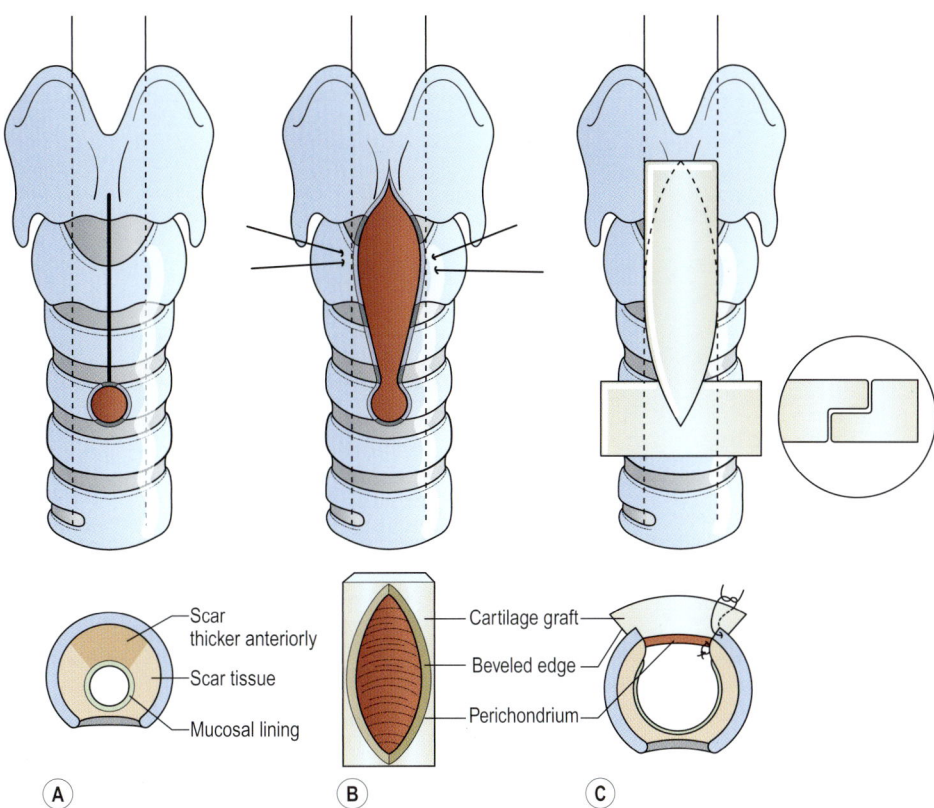

Scar thicker anteriorly
Scar tissue
Mucosal lining

Cartilage graft
Beveled edge
Perichondrium

(A)   (B)   (C)

FIGURE 21-15 ■ An autogenous costal cartilage graft reconstruction. **(A)** Expose the larynx and upper trachea. **(B)** Incise the afore-mentioned region, remaining superior to the tracheostomy stoma if the stenosis does not involve this site. **(C)** Sew the costal cartilage to the incised edges of the larynx and trachea, placing the perichondrium internally. (Adapted from Othersen HB Jr, editor. The Pediatric Airway. Philadelphia: WB Saunders; 1991.)

open procedure can be done with or without cardiopul-monary bypass.[42] Recently, there has been a tendency to avoid bypass and use only endotracheal anesthesia. Second, the repair can be performed with or without an augmentation graft. Possible graft options include tra-cheal allografts or autografts, costal cartilage, cartilage from other sites such as thyroid or alar cartilage, autolo-gous or allogeneic pericardium, or skin. Third, a stent can be used to maintain the lumen and can remain for hours, days, months, or years.

The anterior cricoid split procedure is useful in treat-ing moderate subglottic stenosis in neonates and young infants.[43,44] Infants selected for this procedure should weigh more than 1500 g and require assisted ven-tilation or inspired oxygen of more than 35%. They should also not be in cardiac failure. This technique is illustrated in Figure 21-14.[45] Proper selection of patients for the anterior cricoid split is crucial. After undergoing the anterior cricoid split, infants who can be successfully extubated have excellent long-term outcomes, while those who continue to need intubation usually require tracheostomy.

The classic laryngotracheoplasty utilizes a cartilage graft (Fig. 21-15).[46,47] An omental flap may help a long cartilaginous graft survive.[48] The cartilage is inserted anteriorly after incising the stenotic segment.[49,50] Carti-lage inserts also can be placed posteriorly and laterally as well. Ciliated mucosa has been found on the surface of a mature costal cartilage graft if the perichondrium faces

the airway lumen.[51] Another option is resection of the stenotic tracheal segment and primary end-to-end anas-tomosis.[52] A slide tracheoplasty technique can also be used.[53,54]

A fifth option for repair of tracheal stenosis utilizes an anterior tracheal incision with closure of the defect using pericardium. These pericardial patch operations are performed with cardiopulmonary bypass.[55] However, experience at some centers has not been as favorable because of complications secondary to patch collapse.[56] The original proponents of pericardial patching have now reported improved results with a free tracheal autograft in which the excised stenotic segment is flat-tened and used as a free anterior autograft to expand the tracheal lumen.[57]

Silicone T-tubes can be used as an internal stents to maintain the tracheal lumen and allow tracheal remod-eling following tracheoplasty.[58] These tubes can be placed temporarily to maintain the airway lumen while the airway heals following tracheoplasty. Alternatively, T-tubes can be effective as a permanent stent for the dif-ficult airway stenosis or in cases of failed tracheoplasty. In very complicated and difficult cases, we have utilized custom-made T-tubes. One such custom T-tube is shown in Figure 21-16. This tube was necessary for the treat-ment of tracheomalacia at the carina. As a bifurcated Y-tube is difficult to insert, in this case, a bronchial arm extended into one bronchus and a hole allowed aeration of the other lung.

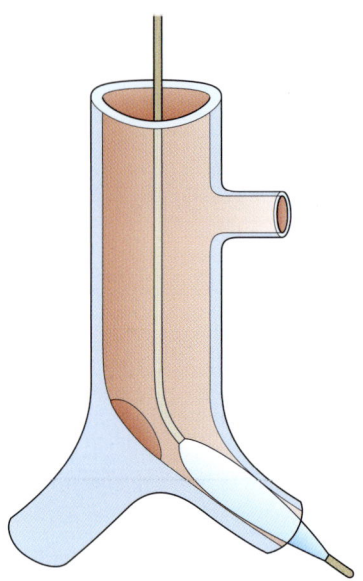

FIGURE 21-16 ■ Diagram of a custom bifurcated T-tube with extension into the left main stem bronchus and a hole to allow ventilation for the right main-stem bronchus. A guide wire is placed with visualization by a flexible scope and a balloon catheter passed over it. With the balloon inflated, introduction of the stent is facilitated.

REFERENCES

1. Othersen HB Jr. Intubation injuries of the trachea in children. Management and prevention. Ann Surg 1979;189:601–6.
2. Weber TR, Connors RH, Tracy TF Jr. Acquired tracheal stenosis in infants and children. J Thorac Cardiovasc Surg 1991;102:29–35.
3. Macpherson RI. Radiologic aspects of airway obstruction. In: Othersen HB Jr, editor. The Pediatric Airway. Philadephia: WB Saunders, 1991. p. 30–65.
4. De Vries PA, De Vries CR. Embryology and Development. In: Othersen HB Jr, editor. The Pediatric Airway. Philadelphia: WB Saunders; 1991. p. 3–16.
5. Erwin EA, Gerber ME, Cotton RT. Vascular compression of the airway: Indications for and results of surgical management. Int J Pediatr Otorhinolaryngol 1997;40:155–62.
6. Roberts CS, Othersen HB Jr, Sade RM, et al. Tracheoesophageal compression from aortic arch anomalies: Analysis of 30 operatively treated children. J Pediatr Surg 1994;29:334–7; discussion 337–8.
7. Braunstein PW, Sade RM. Vascular malformations with airway obstruction. In: Othersen HB Jr, editor. The Pediatric Airway. Philadelphia: WB Saunders; 1991. p. 81–96.
8. Adler SC, Isaacson G, Balsara RK. Innominate artery compression of the trachea: Diagnosis and treatment by anterior suspension. A 25-year experience. Ann Otol Rhinol Laryngol 1995;104:924–7.
9. Clevenger FW, Othersen HB Jr, Smith CD. Relief of tracheal compression by aortopexy. Ann Thorac Surg 1990;50:524–9.
10. Corbally MT, Spitz L, Kiely E, et al. Aortopexy for tracheomalacia in oesophageal anomalies. Eur J Pediatr Surg 1993;3:264–6.
11. Kamerkar DR, Gladstone DJ. Innominate artery compression of the trachea. A simplified technique for anterior suspension of the innominate artery. J Cardiovasc Surg (Torino) 1994;35:549–52.
12. Pasic M, von Segesser L, Carrel T, et al. Anomalous left pulmonary artery (pulmonary sling): Result of a surgical approach. Cardiovasc Surg 1993;1:608–12.
13. Ziemer G, Heinemann M, Kaulitz R, et al. Pulmonary artery sling with tracheal stenosis: Primary one-stage repair in infancy. Ann Thorac Surg 1992;54:971–3.
14. Othersen HB Jr, Khalil B, Zellner J, et al. Aortoesophageal fistula and double aortic arch: Two important points in management. J Pediatr Surg 1996;31:594–5.
15. Koontz CS, Bhatia A, Forbess J, et al. Video-assisted thoracoscopic division of vascular rings in pediatric patients. Am Surg 2005;71:289–91.
16. Kane TD, Nadler EP, Potoka DA. Thoracoscopic aortopexy for vascular compression of the trachea: Approach from the right. J Laparoendosc Adv Surg Tech A 2008;18:313–16.
17. Jensen AR, Le D, Albanese CT. Utilization of a transsternal spinal needle for retrograde sternal passage during thoracoscopic aortopexy. Pediatr Endosurg Innovative Tech 2004;8:333–8.
18. Decou JM, Parsons DS, Gauderer MWL. Thoracoscopic aortopexy for severe tracheomalacia. Pediatr Endosurg Innovative Tech 2001;4:205–8.
19. Durkin ET, Krawiec ME, Shaaban AF. Thoracoscopic aortopexy for primary tracheomalacia in a 12-year-old. J Pediatr Surg 2007;42:E15–17.
20. Schaarschmidt K, Kolberg-Schwerdt A, Pietsch L, et al. Thoracoscopic aortopericardiosternopexy for severe tracheomalacia in toddlers. J Pediatr Surg 2002;37:1476–8.
21. van der Zee DC, Bax NM. Thoracoscopic tracheoaortopexia for the treatment of life-threatening events in tracheomalacia. Surg Endosc 2007;21:2024–5.
22. Othersen HB Jr. Medical diseases of the airway: A surgeon's role. In: Othersen HB Jr, editor. The Pediatric Airway. Philadelphia: WB Saunders; 1991. p. 64–70.
23. Mauro RD, Poole SR, Lockhart CH. Differentiation of epiglottitis from laryngotracheitis in the child with stridor. Am J Dis Child 1988;142:679–82.
24. Gaissert HA, Grillo HC, Mathisen DJ, et al. Temporary and permanent restoration of airway continuity with the tracheal T-tube. J Thorac Cardiovasc Surg 1994;107:600–6.
25. Gaissert HA, Lofgren RH, Grillo HC. Upper airway compromise after inhalation injury. Complex strictures of the larynx and trachea and their management. Ann Surg 1993;218:672–8.
26. White DR, Preciado DA, Stamper B, et al. Airway reconstruction in pediatric burn patients. Otolaryngol Head Neck Surg 2005;133:362–5.
27. Slimane MA, Becmeur F, Aubert D, et al. Tracheobronchial ruptures from blunt thoracic trauma in children. J Pediatr Surg 1999;34:1847–50.
28. Huh J, Milliken JC, Chen JC. Management of tracheobronchial injuries following blunt and penetrating trauma. Am Surg 1997;63:896–9.
29. Cooper JD, Grillo HC. The evolution of tracheal injury due to ventilatory assistance through cuffed tubes: A pathologic study. Ann Surg 1969;169:334–48.
30. Othersen HB Jr. Subglottic tracheal stenosis. Semin Thorac Cardiovasc Surg 1994;6:200–5.
31. Othersen HB Jr, Hebra A, Tagge EP. A new method of treatment for complete tracheal rings in an infant: Endoscopic laser division and balloon dilation. J Pediatr Surg 2000;35:262–4.
32. Brown JW, Bando K, Sun K, et al. Surgical management of congenital tracheal stenosis. Chest Surg Clin N Am 1996;6:837–52.
33. Acosta AC, Albanese CT, Farmer DL, et al. Tracheal stenosis: The long and the short of it. J Pediatr Surg 2000;35:1612–16.
34. Grillo HC. Slide tracheoplasty for long-segment congenital tracheal stenosis. Ann Thorac Surg 1994;58:613–21.
35. Grillo HC, Wright CD, Vlahakes GJ, et al. Management of congenital tracheal stenosis by means of slide tracheoplasty or resection and reconstruction, with long-term follow-up of growth after slide tracheoplasty. J Thorac Cardiovasc Surg 2002;123:145–52.
36. Ward RF, April MM. Mitomycin-C in the treatment of tracheal cicatrix after tracheal reconstruction. Int J Pediatr Otorhinolaryngol 1998;44:221–6.
37. Prasad M, Bent JP, Ward RF, et al. Endoscopically placed nitinol stents for pediatric tracheal obstruction. Int J Pediatr Otorhinolaryngol 2002;66:155–60.
38. Puma F, Ragusa M, Avenia N, et al. The role of silicone stents in the treatment of cicatricial tracheal stenoses. J Thorac Cardiovasc Surg 2000;120:1064–9.
39. Vergnon JM, Costes F, Polio JC. Efficacy and tolerance of a new silicone stent for the treatment of benign tracheal stenosis: Preliminary results. Chest 2000;118:422–6.
40. Ein SH, Friedberg J, Williams WG, et al. Tracheoplasty: A new operation for complete congenital tracheal stenosis. J Pediatr Surg 1982;17:872–8.

41. Matute JA, Villafruela MA, Delgado MD, et al. Surgery of subglottic stenosis in neonates and children. Eur J Pediatr Surg 2000;10:286–90.

42. Loukanov T, Sebening C, Springer W, et al. Simultaneous management of congenital tracheal stenosis and cardiac anomalies in infants. J Thorac Cardiovasc Surg 2005;130:1537–41.

43. Cotton RT, Seid AB. Management of the extubation problem in the premature child. Anterior cricoid split as an alternative to tracheotomy. Ann Otol Rhinol Laryngol 1980;89:508–11.

44. Silver FM, Myer CM 3rd, Cotton RT. Anterior cricoid split. Update 1991. Am J Otolaryngol 1991;12:343–6.

45. Myer CM 3rd, Cotton RT. Cricoid split and cartilage tracheoplasty. In: Othersen HB Jr, editor. The Pediatric Airway. Philadelphia: WB Saunders; 1991. p. 117–24.

46. Kimura K, Mukohara N, Tsugawa C, et al. Tracheoplasty for congenital stenosis of the entire trachea. J Pediatr Surg 1982;17:869–71.

47. Tsugawa C, Kimura K, Muraji T, et al. Congenital stenosis involving a long segment of the trachea: Further experience in reconstructive surgery. J Pediatr Surg 1988;23:471–5.

48. Tsugawa C, Nishijima E, Muraji T, et al. The use of omental pedicle flap for tracheobronchial reconstruction in infants and children. J Pediatr Surg 1991;26:762–5.

49. Forsen JW Jr, Lusk RP, Huddleston CB. Costal cartilage tracheoplasty for congenital long-segment tracheal stenosis. Arch Otolaryngol Head Neck Surg 2002;128:1165–71.

50. Gustafson LM, Hartley BE, Liu JH, et al. Single-stage laryngotracheal reconstruction in children: A review of 200 cases. Otolaryngol Head Neck Surg 2000;123:430–4.

51. Oue T, Kamata S, Usui N, et al. Histopathologic changes after tracheobronchial reconstruction with costal cartilage graft for congenital tracheal stenosis. J Pediatr Surg 2001;36:329–33.

52. Har-El G, Shaha A, Chaudry R, et al. Resection of tracheal stenosis with end-to-end anastomosis. Ann Otol Rhinol Laryngol 1993;102:670–4.

53. Lipshutz GS, Jennings RW, Lopoo JB, et al. Slide tracheoplasty for congenital tracheal stenosis: A case report. J Pediatr Surg 2000;35:259–61.

54. Lang FJ, Hurni M, Monnier P. Long-segment congenital tracheal stenosis: Treatment by slide-tracheoplasty. J Pediatr Surg 1999;34:1216–22.

55. Backer CL, Mavroudis C, Gerber ME, et al. Tracheal surgery in children: An 18-year review of four techniques. Eur J Cardiothorac Surg 2001;19:777–84.

56. Houel R, Serraf A, Macchiarini P, et al. Tracheoplasty in congenital tracheal stenosis. Int J Pediatr Otorhinolaryngol 1998;44:31–8.

57. Backer CL, Mavroudis C, Dunham ME, et al. Repair of congenital tracheal stenosis with a free tracheal autograft. J Thorac Cardiovasc Surg 1998;115:869–74.

58. Huang CJ. Use of the silicone T-tube to treat tracheal stenosis or tracheal injury. Ann Thorac Cardiovasc Surg 2001;7:192–6.

CHAPTER 22

CONGENITAL BRONCHOPULMONARY MALFORMATIONS

Erik G. Pearson • Alan W. Flake

Congenital bronchopulmonary malformations (BPMs) represent a continuum of abnormalities of the bronchopulmonary unit for which classification and management remain in evolution. An improved understanding of the molecular mechanisms underlying the embryologic development of the lung and the pathogenesis of BPMs suggests that these lesions may have similar mechanistic origins that differ in developmental timing or location in the bronchopulmonary tree.[1] From a clinical perspective, improvements in prenatal imaging and increasing observational experience have resulted in a better understanding of the natural history of these anomalies, and a better predictive capacity for pre-, peri-, and postnatal events. Finally, postnatal treatment for the majority of lesions has improved with advances in neonatal care, and the development of thoracoscopic surgery. This chapter discusses the prenatal and postnatal management of the major congenital BPMs with an emphasis on utilizing the thoracoscopic approach for management.

EMBRYOLOGY AND DEVELOPMENT OF THE BRONCHOPULMONARY TREE

Embryological development of the human lung transitions through six separate stages to form a bronchial tree with greater than 1×10^5 conducting and 1×10^7 respiratory airways.[2] These stages include embryonic, pseudoglandular, canalicular, saccular, alveolar, and microvascular. The progression of each stage is a highly coordinated process guided by mesenchymal–epithelial interactions under the influence of a number of regulatory growth factors.

Briefly, the embryonic phase of lung development begins with the formation of the laryngotracheal bud from the anterior portion of the primitive gut. Beginning at week 5 in the pseudoglandular phase, the preacinar airways and blood vessels develop, followed by growth of the bronchial tree until all bronchial divisions are completed by 16 weeks gestation.[3] The cannalicular stage follows, and is characterized by capillary growth towards the respiratory epithelium which marks the future blood–air interface.[2] The transition to the saccular stage at 24 weeks is marked by the widening of peripheral air spaces distal to the terminal bronchioles with septa formation. The final stages of lung development include the alveolar stage, defined by the formation of secondary septa and budding alveoli, and followed by the microvascular stage with significant alveolar development and

maturation. During this complex process, the timing of congenital BPMs and their pathogenesis can be related to specific time points in each of the six developmental stages (Fig. 22-1).

PRENATAL DIAGNOSIS AND CLASSIFICATION OF CONGENITAL BRONCHOPULMONARY MALFORMATIONS

Malformations

Prenatal diagnosis and fetal therapy for congenital lung malformations have evolved significantly since Adzick et al. described the near universal mortality of congenital pulmonary airway malformation (CPAM)-induced fetal hydrops almost three decades ago.[4] Congenital BPMs represent 90% of lung lesions seen in clinical practice and include CPAMs, (formally called congenital cystic adenomatoid malformation or CCAM), bronchopulmonary sequestration (BPS), and congenital lobar emphysema (CLE).[5] Other less common malformations are varied and are included in the classification system described by Langston et al.[6] (Box 22-1), but will not be discussed in this chapter.

Prenatal ultrasonography (US) functions as a window into fetal development and is the most common mode of prenatal diagnosis of congenital thoracic abnormalities (Box 22-2). We routinely supplement ultrasound with magnetic resonance imaging (MRI) as a complementary method to further define the anatomy of the lesion and overall fetal morphology.[7,8] In combination, the two modalities allow accurate prenatal diagnosis of the different types of BPMs and exclude other anatomic anomalies.

Congenital Pulmonary Airway Malformation

CPAMs are the most commonly diagnosed BPM. The best estimate of the incidence of CPAM is 0.66 per 10,000 live births, but better studies are needed based on high quality prenatal imaging of all pregnancies in a study population.[9] This heterogeneous group of congenital cystic and noncystic lung masses is characterized by an extensive overgrowth of immature primary bronchioles localized to a segment of the bronchial tree (Fig. 22-2).[10]

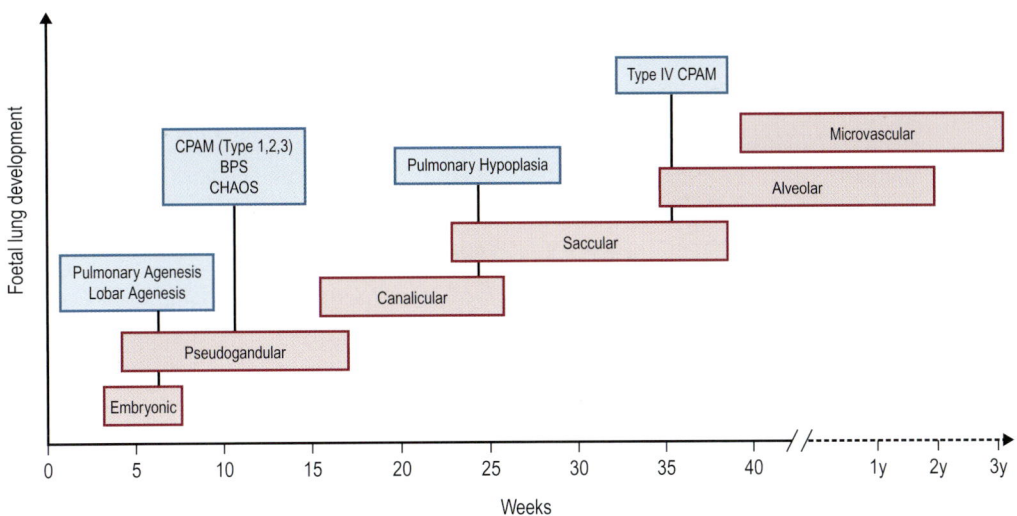

FIGURE 22-1 ■ This graphic depicts milestones in fetal lung development and the timing for development of congenital bronchopulmonary malformations. CPAM, congenital pulmonary airway malformation; BPS, bronchopulmonary sequestration; CHAOS, congenital high airway obstruction syndrome.

BOX 22-1 **Classification of Congenital Lung Lesions**

Bronchopulmonary malformation
  Bronchogenic cyst
  Bronchial atresia
  Congenital pulmonary airway malformation (Stocker type 1 and 2)
  Bronchopulmonary sequestration
Pulmonary hyperplasia and related lesions
  Laryngeal atresia
  Congenital pulmonary airway malformation (Stocker type 3)
  Polyalveolar lobe
Congenital lobar emphysema
Other cystic lesions
  Lymphatic/lymphangiomatous cysts
  Enteric cysts
  Mesothelial cysts
  Simple parenchymal cysts
  Low-grade cystic pleuropulmonary blastoma

Adapted from Langston C. New concepts in the pathology of congenital lung malformations. Semin Pediatr Surg 2003;12:17–37.

BOX 22-2 **Benefits of Prenatal Ultrasonography in the Evaluation of Bronchopulmonary Malformations**

Early diagnosis of the entire spectrum of congenital lung lesions
Serial monitoring of the size and secondary effects of the mass (polyhydramnios, mediastinal shift, and hydrops)
Planning for prenatal and perinatal treatment and delivery strategies

---

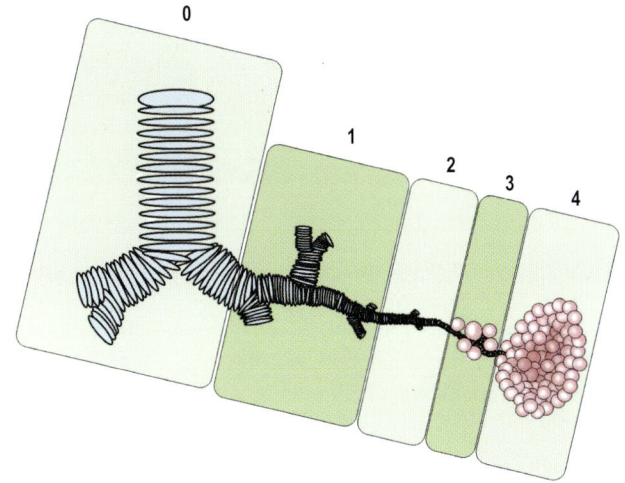

FIGURE 22-2 ■ This CPAM classification schematic is based on the location of the development of the malformation. Type 0, tracheobronchial; 1, bronchial/bronchiolar; 2, bronchiolar; 3, bronchiolar/alveolar; 4, distal acinar. Adapted from Stocker (2009).[63]

The current classification system defined by Stocker classifies CPAMs into five types that differ by location, cystic structure, size, and epithelial lining (Table 22-1). However, from a practical perspective, the prenatal classification of CPAMs is divided into two categories based on prenatal ultrasound findings: (1) macrocystic lesions containing a single or multiple cysts that are 5.0 mm in diameter or greater; and (2) microcystic lesions presenting as a solid echogenic mass on prenatal ultrasound (Fig. 22-3).[4]

In the prenatal period, ultrasound will usually demonstrate an area of hyperechogenic tissue with or without hypoechoic cysts that vary in number and size. Signs of mass effect may be seen, such as mediastinal shift, diaphragmatic eversion, and polyhydramnios. With very large lesions, heart failure (hydrops) due to mediastinal shift and cardiac compression can occur.[11] CPAMs receive their blood supply from the pulmonary artery and have pulmonary venous drainage. However, there is a subset of CPAMs, known as hybrid lesions, where the blood supply also includes an anomalous systemic artery.[12] These lesions demonstrate anatomic and histologic features of both CPAMs and BPS.

TABLE 22-1   Stocker Classification: Congenital Pulmonary Airway Malformations

Type	Incidence	Single/Multiple Cysts	Size of Cysts	Lining of Cysts
0	<2%	Multiple	Variable	Pseudostratified ciliated columnar epithelium
1	60–70%	Single or Multiple	>2 cm	Cilated pseudostratified columnar epithelium
2	15–20%	Multiple	<1 cm	Cilated cuboidal or columnar epithelium
3	5–10%	Solid or Multiple scattered thin-walled cysts	<2 cm	Low cuboidal epithelium
4	10%	Single or Multiple	Variable	Type 1 and 2 alveolar cells

From Stocker JT, Madewell JE, Drake RM. Congenital cystic adenomatoid malformation of the lung. Classification and morphologic spectrum. Hum Pathol 1977;8:155–71.

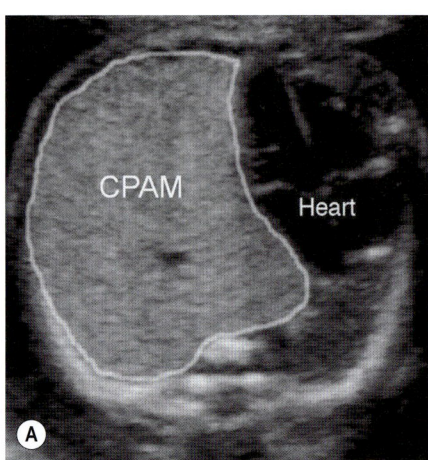 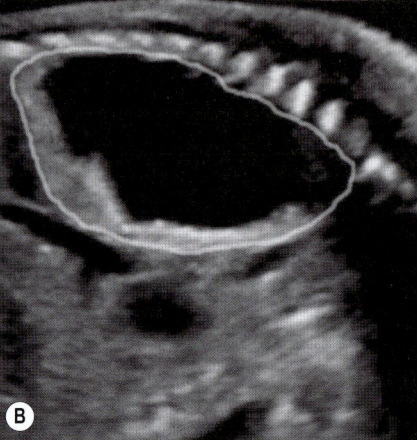

FIGURE 22-3 ■ These two prenatal ultrasounds depict a practical prenatal classification for congenital pulmonary airway malformations (CPAM). **(A)** The prenatal ultrasound study finds microcystic lesions presenting as a solid echogenic mass. **(B)** macrocystic lesions contain either a large cyst or multiple cysts that are greater than 5.0 mm diameter.

TABLE 22-2   Pitfalls in Ultrasonography in the Diagnosis of CPAM

Anomaly	Misdiagnosis
Right-sided congenital diaphragmatic hernia	Large right sided microcystic CPAM: similar echogenicity of liver to microcystic CPAM
Lung agenesis	Large microcystic CPAM: appearance of mediastinal shift with a large echogenic lung
Congenital high airway obstruction syndrome	Bilateral large microcystic CPAM: bilateral large echogenic lungs with diaphragmatic eversion
Main stem bronchial, lobar, or segmental atresia	Microcystic CCAM: hyperplasia of distal lung and increased echogenicity

The diagnosis of CPAMs by an experienced sonographer is usually straightforward. However, there are specific entities that are commonly misdiagnosed (Table 22-2). A skilled sonographer can usually easily differentiate these lesions by understanding the blood supply (congenital diaphragmatic hernia [CDH], lung agenesis, BPS), observation of bowel peristalsis (CDH), documentation of the absence of one lung (lung agenesis), or visualization of bronchial dilation (bronchial atresia, congenital high airway obstruction syndrome [CHAOS]). MRI is also a useful adjunct for differentiating these entities. In our opinion, it should be applied routinely in fetal diagnostic centers.

Bronchopulmonary Sequestration

Bronchopulmonary sequestrations comprise approximately 10% of prenatally diagnosed BPMs, and are characterized by a portion of the lung that does not connect to the tracheobronchial tree. These lesions have a systemic arterial supply that can arise from the aorta or various systemic arterial branches above or below the diaphragm, and may have systemic or pulmonary venous return. Two different types of sequestration are described: intralobar (ILS) and extralobar (ELS) which differ in their prenatal and postnatal characteristics. An ILS shares visceral pleural investment with normal lung and drains into the pulmonary venous system while an ELS has a separate pleural investment and may have either systemic or pulmonary venous drainage.[13,14]

ELS is seen as a homogeneous hyperechoic mass in a paraspinal location, most often in the left lower thorax (Fig. 22-4). The pathogenesis is related to a supernumerary lobe developing from abnormal budding early in foregut embryogenesis.[15] If the bud arises before the development of the pleura, it is invested with the adjacent lung and becomes an ILS. If the bud develops after visceral pleural formation, it grows separately and acquires its own pleural covering.[14] It is important to appreciate that ELS can be found at any level in the pleural space and are also found within or beneath the diaphragm (see Fig. 22-4B).[15] The major feature that helps discriminate an ELS from a CPAM is the blood supply derived from the systemic circulation with systemic venous drainage identified by Doppler ultrasound or MRI. However, it is important to appreciate that some anatomic ELSs can

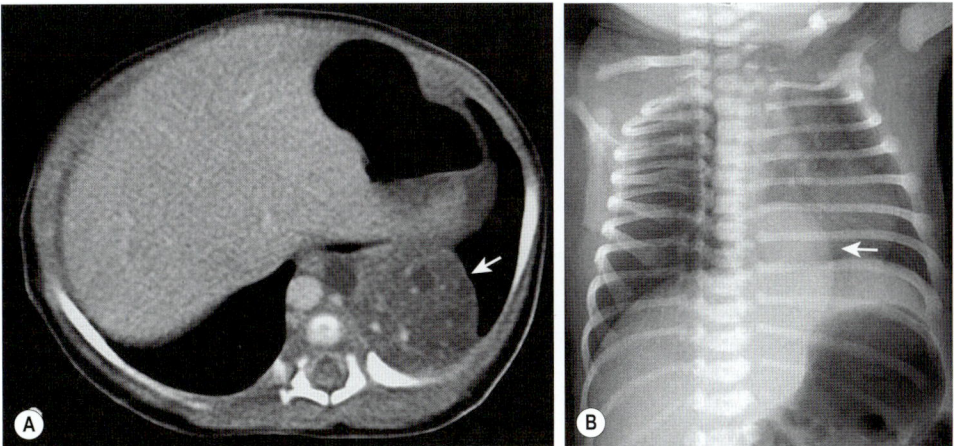

FIGURE 22-4 ■ **(A)** The CT scan demonstrates an extralobar sequestration in the typical basilar location of the left chest (arrow). **(B)** In a different patient, the chest radiograph shows a large transdiaphragmatic extralobar sequestration (arrow).

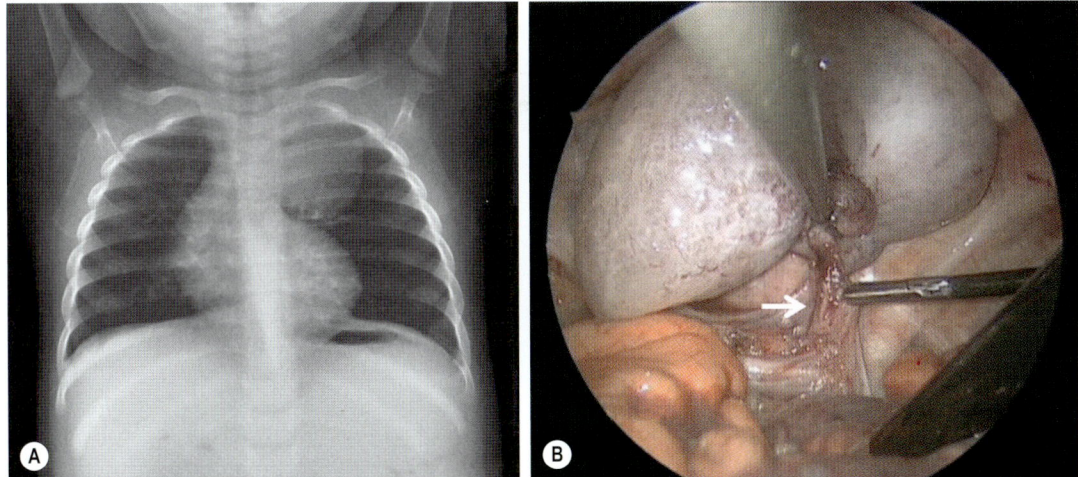

FIGURE 22-5 ■ This 9-month-old developed an upper respiratory infection and a chest radiograph was performed. **(A)** The chest radiograph shows a left apical mediastinal mass. **(B)** After her infection resolved, she was found to have this extrapulmonary mass at thoracoscopy, along with a feeding vessel (arrow). The vessel was ligated and the mass removed, and she recovered uneventfully. Histologic examination showed the mass to an extralobar sequestration associated with a microcystic congenital pulmonary airway malformation.

contain visible cysts that ultimately are shown to have CPAM histology (Fig. 22-5). In addition, an ELS can occasionally have venous drainage via a large venous channel draining directly into a pulmonary vein that is usually identified as aberrant venous drainage by imaging studies.

In contrast to ELS, ILS routinely has pulmonary venous drainage and has variable degrees of hyperechogenicity by ultrasound or MRI. They are uniformly associated with the lower lobes and are distinguishable from the microcystic hybrid lesions described previously only by the absence of pulmonary arterial inflow. Careful Doppler ultrasound identification of the arterial inflow to these lesions is required to definitively distinguish between a microcystic hybrid CPAM and an ILS prenatally. Finally, an ILS can be difficult to distinguish from a systemic to pulmonary vascular malformation where the bronchial anatomy and pulmonary parenchyma are relatively normal, but there is an aberrant systemic blood supply coursing through a vascular network within normal parenchyma with venous drainage into the

pulmonary vein. The subtleties of prenatal diagnosis of these lesions are consistent with a continuum of developmental pathogenesis. It should be emphasized that postnatal computed tomography (CT) should be obtained in all patients to confirm the anatomy and to aid in management. The final diagnosis will depend on the anatomy found at postnatal resection as well as the histologic analysis, and is frequently a combination of the classifications previously described.

Congenital Lobar Emphysema

CLE is a condition characterized by overinflation and distension of one or more pulmonary lobes with compression of the adjacent lung. In 50% of cases, the cause is unknown. In the remaining 50%, it may result from dysplastic bronchial cartilage, endobronchial obstruction, extrinsic compression from aberrant cardiopulmonary vasculature, or diffuse bronchial abnormalities related to infection.[16] In the fetus, amniotic fluid trapping is analogous to air trapping and can lead to lobar expansion. The left upper lobe is the most frequently affected, followed by right middle and upper lobes, with rare bilateral or multifocal involvement. CLE is most commonly diagnosed in the neonate or infant presenting with respiratory distress.

Prenatal discrimination between CLE and CPAM or bronchial atresia may be difficult, but the absence of a systemic vascular supply differentiates this lesion from an ELS. Although complications such as polyhydramnios and hydrops have not been reported with CLE, perinatal respiratory distress correlates with the prenatal size of the lesion as manifest by mediastinal shift or compression of adjacent lung parenchyma.[17]

Bronchogenic Cysts and Bronchial Atresia/Stenosis

Bronchogenic cysts develop from abnormal budding of the tracheal diverticulum or the ventral aspect of the primitive foregut, which is not followed by bronchial development or branching. The result is a cavity that may or may not communicate with the airway and can be found in a variety of locations depending on the location of abnormal budding during foregut development. Histologically, these lesions are thin walled and have a bronchial epithelial lining, and are filled with mucus.[18] Prenatal diagnosis of these lesions is usually made by ultrasound where they may be seen as an isolated cystic structure in the mediastinum, or causing bronchial obstruction with findings of bronchial dilation and lung hyperplasia distal to the point of obstruction. Bronchial atresia without a bronchogenic cyst also results in hyperplasia distal to the level of obstruction and is frequently associated with mucocele formation. The presence of dilated bronchi indicates a diagnosis of atresia rather than microcystic CPAM. The more proximal the atresia, the greater the potential for mass effect manifest by mediastinal shift, and ultimately, fetal hydrops. Segmental bronchial stenosis/atresia is a relatively recently recognized abnormality characterized by an echogenic segment of lung on ultrasound that is indistinguishable from and usually diagnosed as a microcystic CPAM.[19]

PRENATAL AND PERINATAL MANAGEMENT OF BRONCHOPULMONARY MALFORMATIONS

Congenital Pulmonary Airway Malformation

Experience with serial imaging of large numbers of fetuses with CPAMs has clarified the pre- and perinatal natural history of this anomaly. There is a typical pattern of growth of a CPAM with a period of growth relative to the size of the fetus until approximately 26 weeks gestation at which time growth plateaus. After 28 weeks, the CPAM typically gets smaller relative to the size of the fetus as measured by the CPAM volume ratio or CVR. The CVR is calculated by dividing the volume of the CPAM (length × height × width × 0.52) by the head circumference. In addition, the CVR has proven on retrospective and prospective assessment to be the most useful predictor for the development of hydrops.[20] A CVR of <1.6 in a CPAM without a dominant cyst predicts a risk of developing hydrops of less than 3%. If the CVR is >1.6, the risk of hydrops is around 75%. We have found the CVR very useful in counseling parents, determining the intensity of serial follow-up, and determining which patients to preemptively treat with steroids. Other parameters such a mass–thorax ratio, cystic predominance of the lesion, and eventration of the diaphragm, while associated with large lesions, do not add independent predictive value to the CVR.[21]

Based on the type of CPAM, the prenatal CVR, and gestational age, a management strategy can be formulated to optimize outcome. In recent years, the prenatal treatment of large microcystic CPAMs with a CVR of >1.6 and/or the presence of hydrops at less than 32 weeks gestation has changed. Whereas open fetal surgery and lobectomy were once the primary option at fetal treatment centers, the majority of these patients will respond to steroid treatment, with inhibition of further CPAM growth and/or regression of hydrops. The mechanism for the steroid effect is speculative, but the phenomenon has been documented by multiple fetal treatment centers with very few open resections performed since this strategy was implemented.[22–25] In a recent study at our institution, we were able to achieve 100% survival in fetuses either with hydrops (5/5) or a CVR >1.6 at the time of steroid administration.[27] This compares to a mortality rate of 100% in fetuses with hydrops and a 56% mortality rate in fetuses with a CVR >1.6 among historical controls. In contrast to microcystic CPAMs, macrocystic CPAMs do not consistently respond to steroid treatment. Also, if hydrops is evolving, the fetus is best treated by thoracoamniotic shunting (Fig. 22-6).

Our algorithm for the prenatal management of CPAM at the Children's Hospital of Philadelphia (CHOP) is shown in Figure 22-7. Three common clinical scenarios in the management of CPAM are generally apparent by 32 to 34 weeks gestation (Table 22-3) and guide recommendations for site and mode of delivery. As gestation proceeds, it is not unusual for previously hyperechoic lesions to become isoechoic with surrounding lung parenchyma (the so called 'disappearing CPAM'). This is due to increasing echogenicity of the surrounding lung tissue and rib shadowing that occurs during the third trimester. However, it is important to realize that, in essentially all such cases, a postnatal CT scan will confirm persistence of the lesion.

Future options for treatment of CPAM in the hydropic fetus may include minimally invasive ablative or vascular occlusion therapy. Thus far, however, techniques such as radiofrequency or laser thermal ablation have been associated with excessive collateral damage due to the difficulty with controlling the energy dispersion in the high fluid content fetus. Sclerotherapy has been described but the patient selection must be questioned and the advisability of injecting highly caustic agents into the fetal bloodstream is concerning and needs further research investigation.[26–28]

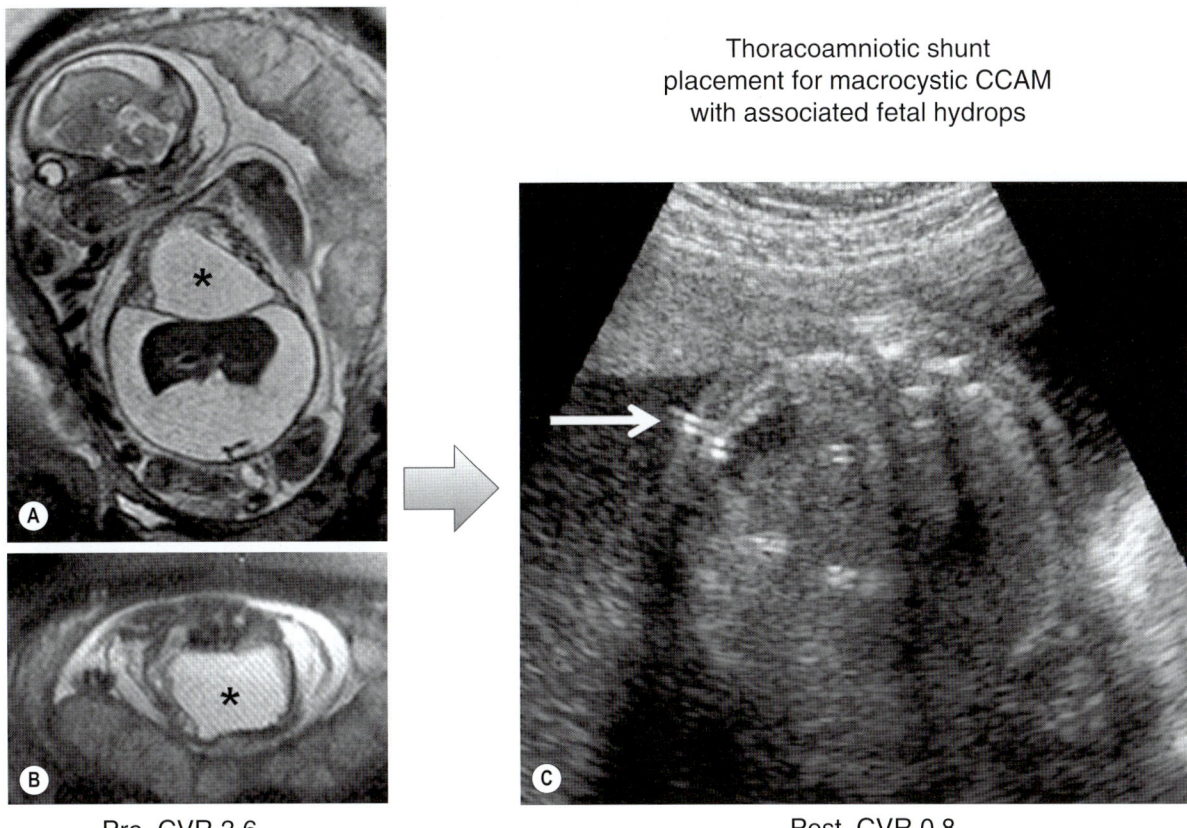

Thoracoamniotic shunt
placement for macrocystic CCAM
with associated fetal hydrops

Pre–CVR 3.6

Post–CVR 0.8

FIGURE 22-6 ■ This fetus was found to have a large cystic mass complicated by a fetal hydrops. **(A,B)** The mass is marked with an asterisk. Prior to intervention, the CPAM volume ratio (CVR) was calculated at 3.6. This carries almost 100% mortality. **(C)** A thoracoamniotic shunt (arrow) was placed. After shunting, the CVR was measured at 0.8.

TABLE 22-3	Common Clinical Scenarios in The Management of Congenital Pulmonary Airway Malformation
Scenario	**Management**
CPAM regresses or remains small without mediastinal shift	Delivery at any facility with Level II nursery, discharged home with mother, postnatal CT scan at 4–6 weeks of age and elective resection prior to 3 months of age.
CPAM with some mediastinal shift without diaphragmatic eversion or extreme compression of contralateral lung	Delivery at tertiary center with resection performed in first few days of life
CPAM that remains massive with extreme mediastinal shift or that induces hydrops after 32 weeks	Transfer to fetal center or tertiary center with EXIT to ECMO capability

CPAM, congenital pulmonary airway malformation; ECMO, extracorporeal membrane oxygenation; EXIT, ex-utero intrapartum treatment.

Bronchopulmonary Sequestration

The prenatal manifestations of BPS differ between ELS and ILS. In general, ILS have few if any prenatal manifestations and generally do not cause significant morbidity. Theoretically, the systemic arterial to pulmonary venous circuit could cause high output cardiac failure in the fetus, but the earliest this has been observed is in the neonatal period.[29] In contrast, ELS can present as a large mass with a mediastinal shift and frequently an associated pleural effusion. It has been our experience that an ELS that causes a mass effect is usually an edematous lesion with narrow vascular pedicles that presumably develops lymphatic or venous congestion and a secondary pleural effusion. Most ELS will regress in size during the third trimester. The occasional case of ELS-induced fetal hydrops is usually related to mediastinal shift from the associated pleural effusion rather than the ELS itself, and can be treated by thoracoamniotic shunting followed by postnatal resection. However, the vast majority of ELS and ILS cause no fetal compromise and are best treated after birth.

Congenital Lobar Emphysema, Bronchogenic Cysts, Bronchial Atresia

From the perspective of prenatal pathophysiology, these lesions can be grouped under the pathogenesis

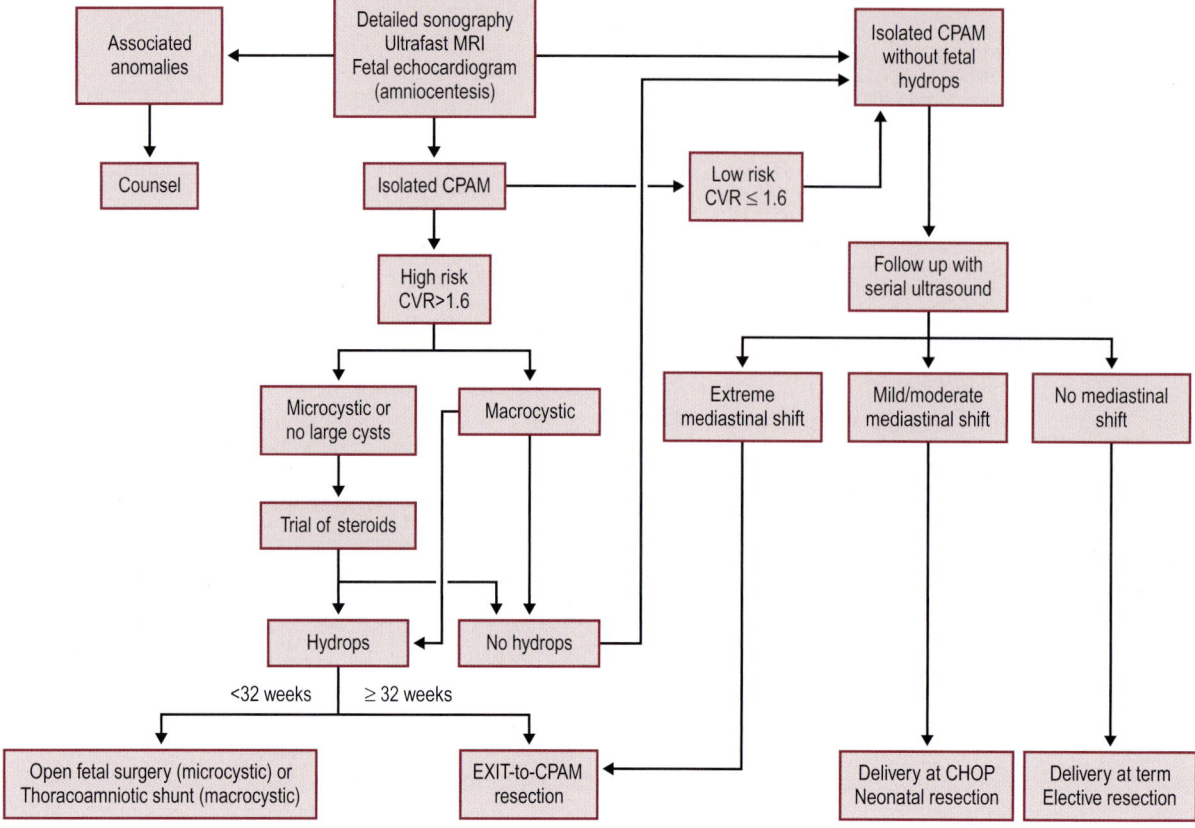

FIGURE 22-7 ■ This algorithm depicts our current management strategy at Children's Hospital of Philadelphia for a fetus with a congenital pulmonary airway malformation (CPAM). CHOP, Children's Hospital of Philadelphia; CVR, CPAM volume ratio; MRI, magnetic resonance imaging; US, ultrasound.

of bronchial stenosis or atresia. CLE and segmental bronchial stenosis are not associated with significant prenatal pathophysiology. CLE can enlarge prenatally due to fluid trapping, presumably by a similar mechanism to postnatal air trapping, though at most this has been found to cause moderate mediastinal shift. Bronchial atresia, also known as bronchial mucocele, is a condition resulting from focal obliteration or stenosis of a segmental, subsegmental, or lobar bronchus at or near its origin.[30] Bronchial atresia can result in hydrops and fetal or neonatal death when located proximally. This is due to the hyperplastic growth response induced by the bronchial obstruction that can lead to massive lung or lobar expansion. Findings of severe mediastinal shift with diaphragmatic eversion and evolution of hydrops have been uniformly fatal in cases of main stem bronchial atresia due to either fetal demise or neonatal death due to the inability to ventilate the infant. Fetuses with lobar hyperplasia resulting in fetal hydrops prior to 30 weeks gestation may be offered open fetal surgery and lobectomy. After 30 weeks gestation, delivery utilizing the ex-utero intrapartum treatment (EXIT) approach followed by resection is performed. In our experience, these lesions have not been responsive to steroid therapy. An interesting recent case of fetal bronchoscopic decompression of a right bronchus intermedius obstruction has been described which may be applicable to a subset of proximal bronchial obstructions.[31] Fortunately, cases requiring fetal intervention are rare, and most infants with lobar

bronchial atresia can be treated in the early postnatal period.

POSTNATAL MANAGEMENT OF BRONCHOPULMONARY MALFORMATIONS

Congenital Pulmonary Airway Malformation

The postnatal clinical spectrum of CPAM ranges from the neonate requiring mechanical ventilation, to the child presenting with an infected CPAM, to the asymptomatic adult. The treatment of the neonate with a symptomatic CPAM is immediate resection of the involved lobe by an open or thoracoscopic approach. Lobectomy is preferred over attempts at lung preserving surgery, such as segmental or wedge resection, due to the inability to accurately ascertain the borders of the lesion, the higher complication rate related to segmentectomy, and the compensatory lung growth that occurs in the remaining lobe or lobes that results in normal long-term pulmonary function following infant lobectomy.[32] When multiple lobes are involved (1% of CPAMs), segmentectomy should be considered if anatomically feasible. As noted previously, very large lesions with significant mediastinal shift and diaphragmatic displacement should be delivered using the EXIT procedure and resected on placental support.

With these very large masses, care must be exercised to avoid rupturing the CPAM or tearing the fragile hilar vessels during attempts at exposure when retracting the CPAM. A thoracoabdominal incision can be helpful with large CPAMs to aid in the safe delivery of the lobe and to provide additional space for the hilar dissection. In contrast to CDH, extracorporeal membrane oxygenation (ECMO) is rarely required for CPAM-related pulmonary hypoplasia, presumably because of the lesion's slow growth and the relatively late onset of pulmonary compression. Outside the neonatal period, a symptomatic CPAM should be treated by lobectomy when recognized. Babies may present with air trapping in the first few months of life, infection of the CPAM in the first several years of life, and occasionally spontaneous pneumothorax related to the lesion.[33,34] Infection in CPAMs may be difficult to clear with antibiotics and resection should be performed once the patient has improved following antibiotic therapy.

In contrast to large and symptomatic CPAMs, there is controversy regarding the treatment of the asymptomatic CPAM. In the era of prenatal diagnosis, the majority of patients are asymptomatic. The arguments for resection are that CPAMs do not completely regress and that they put the patient at risk for future infection, pneumothorax, and malignancy. There is also the risk that the mass is really a pleuropulmonary blastoma (PPB), a lesion that is rare, but indistinguishable from CPAM on pre- and post-natal imaging studies.[35] The controversy is related to the belief by some that many lesions regress and disappear, as well as the unknown frequency of infection and malignant deterioration in the asymptomatic patient. Infection in CPAMs is well documented, particularly before the era of prenatal diagnosis. CPAMs can develop infection anytime between a few weeks of age until adulthood. Infections can be severe and life threatening, difficult to clear with antibiotics, associated with complications of abscess, empyema, and other secondary complications, and in neglected or unrecognized cases, may increase the risk of lobectomy. There are no well-designed prospective studies that provide an accurate assessment of the risk of infection in a CPAM during one's lifetime, much less in the first 10 years of life. In a long-term retrospective study in which 21 patients were initially diagnosed as asymptomatic (including eight that were prenatally diagnosed) and followed, 18 developed symptoms (median age 2 years, range 1 month–13 years) and required operation. Symptoms included pneumonia with or without an infected CPAM (43%), respiratory distress (14%), and spontaneous pneumothorax (14%). Eight patients underwent multiple hospital encounters with complications related to the CPAM.[36]

There is also a clear association between CPAM and malignancy. A review of children with lung neoplasms demonstrated that 9% had a history of cystic lung malformations.[37] The mucinous cells in a type I CPAM produce gastric mucins that are important in the pathogenesis of bronchioloalveolar carcinoma.[38] The association with PPB is also clear, although resection of a CPAM does not preclude the development of PPB.[39] Type II CPAM has been demonstrated to exhibit skeletal muscle differentiation as found in PPB and rhabdomyosarcoma.

As the frequency of malignant transformation of a CPAM is unknown, it is not possible to predict which patients will develop cancer. Moreover, there is no imaging modality that can be safely used to serially image patients during a lifetime. This risk of malignancy may represent the strongest argument for resection of asymptomatic lesions.

At CHOP, we strongly advocate early resection of an asymptomatic CPAM due to the considerations outlined, the extremely low rate of complications of resection at our center, and the negligible impact on long-term pulmonary function associated with infant lobectomy. We see no surgical or anesthetic benefit to waiting and feel that resection, whether thoracoscopic or open, is easier at an early age (less adenopathy, perihilar fat, and inflammation related adhesion) than later in life. In addition, recovery, and the potential for compensatory lung growth and restoration of normal pulmonary function is likely higher in younger infants. With this policy, we have had no major complications and a combined minor complication (persistent air leak, need for transfusion, late pneumothorax, chylothorax) rate under 10% following either open or thoracoscopic resection of asymptomatic CPAMs.

While a nonoperative approach to CPAMs was evaluated in a small number of patients demonstrating a low risk of adverse events, the mean follow-up was only three years.[40] In addition, a nonoperative approach requires serial surveillance by CT scanning and exposes the patient to a significant risk of cumulative radiation with significant long-term consequences.[41] Waiting until the lesion becomes symptomatic places the patient at risk for developing complications when operating in an inflammatory or infectious field. Our data supports lobectomy between the ages of 1–3 months as the optimal management for the asymptomatic CPAM.[42,43] We prefer the thoracoscopic approach, but this recommendation is dependent on an experienced surgeon. If that is not the case, then open lobectomy using a muscle sparing thoracotomy is recommended.

Bronchopulmonary Sequestration

An increasing number of BPS are prenatally diagnosed and postnatal therapy can be planned based on the anticipated risk of postnatal complications. For ELS, the treatment depends on the size of the lesion, blood flow, associated pleural effusion, and location. Our indications for resection of ELS are defined in Box 22-3. In both an ELS and ILS that has large systemic feeding vessels, vascular flow can be anticipated to increase, not decrease, over time due to the low resistance of the vascular bed with the end result being high flow cardiac physiology and ultimately cardiac failure as the child grows. Anatomical BPS with cystic areas on imaging likely contain CPAM elements within the BPS,[44] and this may be responsible for the sporadic reports of malignancy occurring in both ILS and ELS, but more frequently in ELS. The malignancies that have been reported in association with ELS include lymphoepithelial carcinoma, PPB, squamous cell carcinoma, carcinoid, and mesothelioma.[45–48] Within ILS, benign sclerosing hemangioma can be found. Because ELS do not communicate with the tracheobronchial tree, infection is rare. However, in ILS, air enters by tracking through the pores of Kohn. Thus, with stasis of mucous and the absence of bronchial clearance, infection is a frequent complication.

The differential diagnosis of subdiaphragmatic ELS in the fetus or neonate includes neuroblastoma and adrenal hemorrhage, and these lesions can be differentiated on serial ultrasound imaging. Finally, an ELS in close proximity to the esophagus, particularly if difficult to separate, may have an esophageal bronchus that needs to be identified and closed during excision. There is debate regarding the postnatal management of a small intrathoracic or subdiaphragmatic ELS. A small ELS can remain asymptomatic throughout life, have been reported to spontaneously regress, and carry a low risk of infection or malignancy. This has led some surgeons to observe these lesions if the lesion is not visible on plain radiography, or if it is small, or does not have a significant systemic arterial blood supply.[49,50] We feel that the ELS treatment should be individualized with specific indications for resection as shown in Box 22-3.

The surgical management of ELS involves division of the systemic blood supply and removal of the mass (see Fig. 22-5). This must be done with care as systemic vessels arising from the abdominal aorta may cross the diaphragm and lead to difficult-to-control bleeding if not adequately ligated. However, ELS are generally straightforward lesions for thoracoscopic resection and patients are usually able to be discharged the next day. Percutaneous coil embolization of the feeding systemic artery to ELS has been performed in children and adults. In most cases there is little reason to favor this approach over resection.[51] In contrast to resection, embolization carries the potential for vascular injury at the catheter insertion site, embolic occlusion of other vessels, and the potential for dysplastic residual tissue that may persist with possible future malignant transformation.

In our opinion, all cases of ILS should be resected, because of the risk of infection and evolution of high output physiology. Thoracoscopic lobectomy is our preferred approach. Segmentectomy for ILS has been reported in the literature with success.[52,53] However, trying to avoid performing a lobectomy may carry a higher risk as these lesions usually do not have normal segmental anatomy, share pleural investment, can have significant internal blood flow, and can be difficult to distinguish from adjacent lung tissue which risks leaving residual disease.

Congenital Lobar Emphysema

Asymptomatic children with CLE or those with only mild symptoms can be safely managed without resection.[54] In neonates or infants presenting with respiratory distress and pulmonary lobar hyperinflation, open lobectomy is our preferred option (Fig. 22-8). These patients have unique and difficult anesthetic challenges from air trapping and cardiovascular compromise that may prevent successful single lung ventilation. Therefore, consideration for thoracoscopic resection should be highly selective and requires careful preoperative review by the anesthetic and surgical team.[55] Symptomatic patients usually present with respiratory distress within the first 6 months of life with 25% of patients presenting at birth and 50% presenting prior to one month of age. The severity of disease is dependent on the size of the affected lobe and compression of adjacent lung tissue. The mainstay of management for CLE is resection of the affected lobe. However, whether pre- or intraoperatively, care must be taken to avoid progressive air trapping with resulting lobar tension emphysema from positive pressure ventilation.[16]

BOX 22-3	Indications for Resection of Extralobar Bronchupulmonary Sequestration

Large systemic vascular supply
Large lesions with significant compression of surrounding lung parenchyma or mediastinal shift
Lesions with cystic abnormality on prenatal ultrasound or postnatal CT scan as this likely represents CPAM elements within BPS
Growth of an ELS on serial imaging
Lesions in or under the diaphragm near the esophageal hiatus causing obstructive symptoms

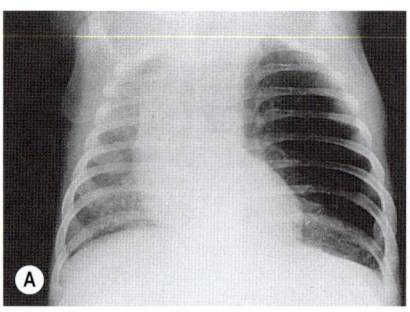 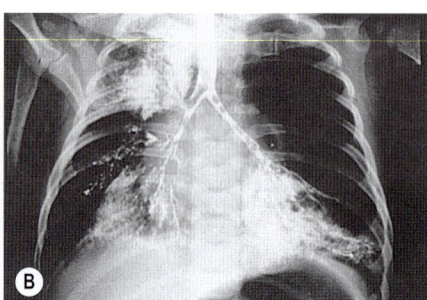 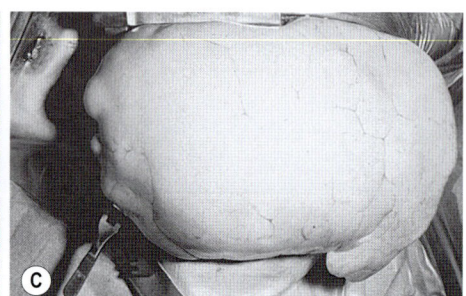

FIGURE 22-8 ■ **(A)** Chest radiograph demonstrates the characteristic changes in an infant with congenital lobar emphysema (CLE). Marked overdistention of the left upper lobe caused the mediastinal shift, flattening of the left diaphragm, and likely subsequent respiratory distress. **(B)** Bronchogram shows the absence or occlusion of the left upper lobe bronchus, producing the typical findings in CLE. **(C)** Operative photograph demonstrates the dramatic herniation of an emphysematous lobe through the thoracotomy incision.

Bronchogenic Cysts and Bronchial Atresia

Bronchogenic cysts are now frequently prenatally diagnosed by ultrasound. Postnatally, they are often diagnosed by a mass on a chest film, either incidentally or in association with respiratory symptoms. CT can confirm the presence of a bronchogenic cyst as well as its relation to adjacent mediastinal structures. Mass effect from these lesions is typically mild, but lesions identified below the carina can cause life threatening airway compromise.[56] Complications associated with bronchogenic cysts include infection, malignancy, hemoptysis, hemothorax, and pneumothorax. For these reasons, all bronchogenic cysts should be resected regardless of the clinical presentation or age at diagnosis. Symptomatic neonates or infants may require immediate resection or aspiration of the cysts as a temporizing measure for extreme duress. Asymptomatic newborns with a bronchogenic cyst identified on imaging may be followed as an outpatient and scheduled for resection after 1 month of age. Older patients should undergo resection of the bronchogenic cyst soon after it is identified, though the clinical presentation of pneumonia may complicate resection. These lesions may be safely resected using a thoracoscopic technique with equivalent outcomes to the open approach (see Fig 25-7).[57] When the cyst cannot be completely resected, the mucosal layer should be excised leaving behind only peripheral connective tissue to eliminate the risk of recurrence and malignant transformation.[58] In our opinion, all cysts associated with bronchial atresias should be excised because of the increased risk of infection. When a bronchogenic cyst is associated with bronchial obstruction, there is inevitably irreversible damage to the bronchus and lobectomy is needed.

THORACOSCOPIC LOBECTOMY

The benefits of thoracoscopy include less postoperative pain, more rapid recovery, less hospitalization, and an improved functional and cosmetic result compared to traditional thoracotomy.[59,60] However, despite these obvious advantages and the development of appropriate instrumentation for infants, the use of thoracoscopy for congenital lung lesions has been relatively limited. This is likely due to the infrequency of these anomalies, and the technical challenges inherent in learning the technique. Nevertheless, adequate experience has been accumulated in a number of centers to validate the approach and demonstrate safety and efficacy that mimics traditional thoracotomy.[59,61]

The challenges unique to infant thoracoscopic lobectomy can be separated into anesthesia, anatomic, and technical. The anesthetic challenges relate to single lung ventilation in infants and require a committed anesthesia staff. Main stem bronchial intubation can be easily achieved by the use of a 3-0 micro-cuffed tube introduced using fluoroscopy.[62] This approach is much faster than using bronchoscopy to correctly position the endotracheal tube. For left-sided lobectomies in particular, it is important to introduce the tube deep enough in the right main stem bronchus to avoid inadvertent displacement into the left main stem bronchus or trachea with dissection around the hilum during the procedure, but not so deeply to lose right upper lobe ventilation. In general, the cuff does not need to be inflated to achieve single lung ventilation in the less than 3-month-old infant, and bronchial blockers or other methods described for larger patients are not needed. With appropriate tube placement, a transient period of desaturation into the 80–92% range is expected as is resolution when positioning the patient with the ventilated lung down and redistribution of blood flow. Adjustments to the peak ventilator pressure and rate to maintain end tidal CO_2 in the 50s Torr range are usually required.

Anatomic challenges relate to the thoracoscopic perspective on pulmonary anatomy and the variations inherent with CBMs. The optimal approach is through the major fissure. Therefore, a detailed understanding of vascular and bronchial anatomy viewed through the fissure is essential (Figs 22-9 and 22-10). Working through the fissure from anterior to posterior, the sequence that structures are encountered are the arteries, bronchus, and vein in that order. The correct anatomic orientation can be significantly altered by the CPAM or lobar hyperplasia from bronchial atresia. A systematic approach in each patient is needed to identify the important structures. The anatomy can also be obscured to varying degrees by incomplete fissure formation which can be problematic for inexperienced surgeons.

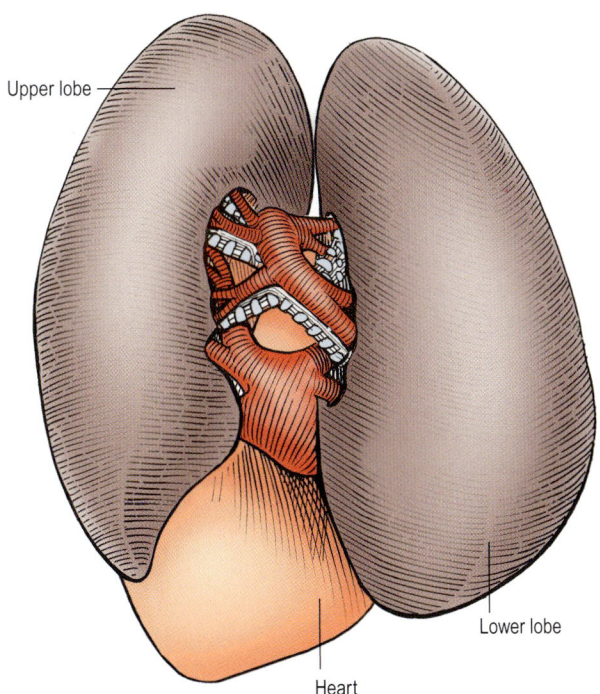

FIGURE 22-9 ■ This is the anatomy seen by the surgeon when the contents of the fissure between the left upper and lower lobes are exposed at thoracoscopy. The arteries are visualized first within the fissure and the bronchial structures are behind the arteries. The pulmonary veins exit from the inferior portion of these lobes and drain into the heart. (From Holcomb GW III, Georgeson KE, Rothenberg SS. Atlas of Pediatric Laparoscopy and Thoracoscopy. Philadelphia: Elsevier; 2008.)

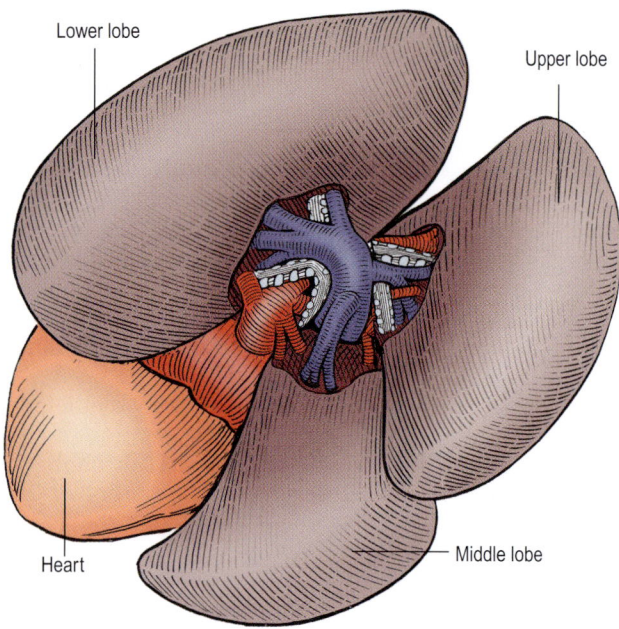

Lower lobe

Upper lobe

Heart

Middle lobe

FIGURE 22-10 ■ This is the anatomy as seen by the surgeon when performing a thoracoscopic lobectomy on the right side. Again, the arteries are the first structure seen in the fissure and the bronchial structures are behind the arteries. The pulmonary veins are inferior to the arteries and drain into the heart. (From Holcomb GW III, Georgeson KE, Rothenberg SS. Atlas of Pediatric Laparoscopy and Thoracoscopy. Philadelphia: Elsevier; 2008.)

Technical challenges are primarily related to operating in a much smaller space than is found with infant laparoscopy. When combined with the movement of the structures from ventilation and cardiac activity, thoracoscopic lobectomy can be challenging. Also, the 5 mm vascular sealing devices such as the Ligasure (Covidien, Inc., Mansfield NJ) or endoscopic clips are grossly oversized in the infant chest. It is important to be facile with endocorporeal knot tying in very small spaces. On occasion, under adverse circumstances, it may become the fall back technique at any time. With experience, thoracoscopic lobectomy, even in infants, can become a straightforward procedure that is better in many ways than open thoracotomy. However, it remains the most advanced of infant thoracoscopic procedures and should only be performed by trained individuals in centers with a reasonable volume of these procedures.

REFERENCES

1. Gonzaga S, Henriques-Coelho T, Davey M, et al. Cystic adenomatoid malformations are induced by localized FGF10 overexpression in fetal rat lung. Am J Respir Cell Mol Biol 2008;39:346–55.
2. Correia-Pinto J, Gonzaga S, Huang Y, et al. Congenital lung lesions–underlying molecular mechanisms. Semin Pediatr Surg 2010;19:171–9.
3. Biyyam DR, Chapman T, Ferguson MR, et al. Congenital lung abnormalities: Embryologic features, prenatal diagnosis, and postnatal radiologic-pathologic correlation. Radiographics 2010;30:1721–38.
4. Adzick NS, Harrison MR, Glick PL, et al. Fetal cystic adenomatoid malformation: Prenatal diagnosis and natural history. J Pediatr Surg 1985;20:483–8.
5. Epelman M, Kreiger PA, Servaes S, et al. Current imaging of prenatally diagnosed congenital lung lesions. Semin Ultrasound CT MR 2010;31:141–57.
6. Langston C. New concepts in the pathology of congenital lung malformations. Semin Pediatr Surg 2003;12:17–37.
7. Hubbard AM, Adzick NS, Crombleholme TM, et al. Congenital chest lesions: Diagnosis and characterization with prenatal MR imaging. Radiology 1999;212:43–8.
8. Quinn TM, Hubbard AM, Adzick NS. Prenatal magnetic resonance imaging enhances fetal diagnosis. J Pediatr Surg 1998;33:553–8.
9. Dolk H. EUROCAT: 25 years of European surveillance of congenital anomalies. Arch Dis Child Fetal Neonatal Ed 2005;90:F355–358.
10. Stocker JT, Madewell JE, Drake RM. Congenital cystic adenomatoid malformation of the lung. Classification and morphologic spectrum. Hum Pathol 1977;8:155–71.
11. Mahle WT, Rychik J, Tian ZY, et al. Echocardiographic evaluation of the fetus with congenital cystic adenomatoid malformation. Ultrasound Obstet Gynecol 2000;16:620–4.
12. Cass DL, Crombleholme TM, Howell LJ, et al. Cystic lung lesions with systemic arterial blood supply: A hybrid of congenital cystic adenomatoid malformation and bronchopulmonary sequestration. J Pediatr Surg 1997;32:986–90.
13. Savic B, Birtel FJ, Tholen W, et al. Lung sequestration: Report of seven cases and review of 540 published cases. Thorax 1979;34:96–101.
14. Stocker JT. Sequestrations of the lung. Semin Diagn Pathol 1986;3:106–21.
15. Rosado-de-Christenson ML, Frazier AA, Stocker JT, et al. From the archives of the AFIP. Extralobar sequestration: Radiologic-pathologic correlation. Radiographics 1993;13:425–41.
16. Olutoye OO, Coleman BG, Hubbard AM, et al. Prenatal diagnosis and management of congenital lobar emphysema. J Pediatr Surg 2000;35:792–5.
17. Usui N, Kamata S, Sawai T, et al. Outcome predictors for infants with cystic lung disease. J Pediatr Surg 2004;39:603–6.
18. Eraklis AJ, Griscom NT, McGovern JB. Bronchogenic cysts of the mediastinum in infancy. N Engl J Med 1969;281:1150–5.
19. Peranteau WH, Merchant AM, Hedrick HL, et al. Prenatal course and postnatal management of peripheral bronchial atresia: Association with congenital cystic adenomatoid malformation of the lung. Fetal Diagn Ther 2008;24:190–6.
20. Crombleholme TM, Coleman B, Hedrick H, et al. Cystic adenomatoid malformation volume ratio predicts outcome in prenatally diagnosed cystic adenomatoid malformation of the lung. J Pediatr Surg 2002;37:331–8.
21. Vu L, Tsao K, Lee H, et al. Characteristics of congenital cystic adenomatoid malformations associated with nonimmune hydrops and outcome. J Pediatr Surg 2007;42:1351–6.
22. Loh KC, Jelin E, Hirose S, et al. Microcystic congenital pulmonary airway malformation with hydrops fetalis: Steroids vs. open fetal resection. J Pediatr Surg 2012;47:36–9.
23. Morris LM, Lim FY, Livingston JC, et al. High-risk fetal congenital pulmonary airway malformations have a variable response to steroids. J Pediatr Surg 2009;44:60–5.
24. Peranteau WH, Wilson RD, Liechty KW, et al. Effect of maternal betamethasone administration on prenatal congenital cystic adenomatoid malformation growth and fetal survival. Fetal Diagn Ther 2007;22:365–71.
25. Tsao K, Hawgood S, Vu L, et al. Resolution of hydrops fetalis in congenital cystic adenomatoid malformation after prenatal steroid therapy. J Pediatr Surg 2003;38:508–10.
26. Bruner JP, Jarnagin BK, Reinisch L. Percutaneous laser ablation of fetal congenital cystic adenomatoid malformation: Too little, too late? Fetal Diagn Ther 2000;15:359–63.
27. Milner R, Kitano Y, Olutoye O, et al. Radiofrequency thermal ablation: A potential treatment for hydropic fetuses with a large chest mass. J Pediatr Surg 2000;35:386–9.
28. Oepkes D, Devlieger R, Lopriore E, et al. Successful ultrasound-guided laser treatment of fetal hydrops caused by pulmonary sequestration. Ultrasound Obstet Gynecol 2007;29:457–9.
29. Millendez MB, Ridout E, Pole G, et al. Neonatal hyperreninemia and hypertensive heart failure relieved with resection of an intralobar pulmonary sequestration. J Pediatr Surg 2007;42:1276–8.

30. Keswani SG, Crombleholme TM, Pawel BR, et al. Prenatal diagnosis and management of mainstem bronchial atresia. Fetal Diagn Ther 2005;20:74–8.
31. Martinez JM, Prat J, Gomez O, et al. Decompression through tracheobronchial endoscopy of bronchial atresia presenting as massive pulmonary tumor: A new indication for fetoscopic surgery. Fetal Diagn Ther 2012.
32. Muller CO, Berrebi D, Kheniche A, et al. Is radical lobectomy required in congenital cystic adenomatoid malformation? J Pediatr Surg 2012;47:642–5.
33. Choudhury SR, Chadha R, Mishra A, et al. Lung resections in children for congenital and acquired lesions. Pediatr Surg Int 2007;23:851–9.
34. Lujan M, Bosque M, Mirapeix RM, et al. Late-onset congenital cystic adenomatoid malformation of the lung. Embryology, clinical symptomatology, diagnostic procedures, therapeutic approach and clinical follow-up. Respiration 2002;69:148–54.
35. Oliveira C, Himidan S, Pastor AC, et al. Discriminating preoperative features of pleuropulmonary blastomas (PPB) from congenital cystic adenomatoid malformations (CCAM): A retrospective, age-matched study. Eur J Pediatr Surg 2011;21:2–7.
36. Wong A, Vieten D, Singh S, et al. Long-term outcome of asymptomatic patients with congenital cystic adenomatoid malformation. Pediatr Surg Int 2009;25:479–85.
37. Hancock BJ, Di Lorenzo M, Youssef S, et al. Childhood primary pulmonary neoplasms. J Pediatr Surg 1993;28:1133–6.
38. Lantuejoul S, Nicholson AG, Sartori G, et al. Mucinous cells in type 1 pulmonary congenital cystic adenomatoid malformation as mucinous bronchioloalveolar carcinoma precursors. Am J Surg Pathol 2007;31:961–9.
39. Papagiannopoulos KA, Sheppard M, Bush AP, et al. Pleuropulmonary blastoma: Is prophylactic resection of congenital lung cysts effective? Ann Thorac Surg 2001;72:604–5.
40. Aziz D, Langer JC, Tuuha SE, et al. Perinatally diagnosed asymptomatic congenital cystic adenomatoid malformation: To resect or not? J Pediatr Surg 2004;39:329–34.
41. Pearce MS, Salotti JA, Little MP, et al. Radiation exposure from CT scans in childhood and subsequent risk of leukaemia and brain tumours: A retrospective cohort study. Lancet 2012;380:499–505.
42. Adzick NS, Flake AW, Crombleholme TM. Management of congenital lung lesions. Semin Pediatr Surg 2003;12:10–16.
43. Tsai AY, Liechty KW, Hedrick HL, et al. Outcomes after postnatal resection of prenatally diagnosed asymptomatic cystic lung lesions. J Pediatr Surg 2008;43:513–17.
44. Conran RM, Stocker JT. Extralobar sequestration with frequently associated congenital cystic adenomatoid malformation, type 2: Report of 50 cases. Pediatr Dev Pathol 1999;2:454–63.
45. Hekelaar N, van Uffelen R, van Vliet AC, et al. Primary lymphoepithelioma-like carcinoma within an intralobular pulmonary sequestration. Eur Respir J 2000;16:1025–7.

46. Olgac G, Peirovi F, Yilmaz A, et al. Giant carcinoid tumor mimicking pulmonary sequestration. Ann Thorac Surg 2007;84:1375–6.
47. Priest JR, McDermott MB, Bhatia S, et al. Pleuropulmonary blastoma: A clinicopathologic study of 50 cases. Cancer 1997;80:147–61.
48. Westphal FL, Lima LC, Lima Netto JC, et al. Carcinoid tumor and pulmonary sequestration. J Bras Pneumol 2012;38:133–7.
49. Laberge JM, Puligandla P, Flageole H. Asymptomatic congenital lung malformations. Semin Pediatr Surg 2005;14:16–33.
50. Samuel M, Burge DM. Management of antenatally diagnosed pulmonary sequestration associated with congenital cystic adenomatoid malformation. Thorax 1999;54:701–6.
51. Chien KJ, Huang TC, Lin CC, et al. Early and late outcomes of coil embolization of pulmonary sequestration in children. Circ J 2009;73:938–42.
52. Johnson SM, Grace N, Edwards MJ, et al. Thoracoscopic segmentectomy for treatment of congenital lung malformations. J Pediatr Surg 2011;46:2265–9.
53. Peiry B, De Buys Roessingh A, Francini K, et al. Thoracoscopic segmentectomy: One vessel may hide a second one. J Pediatr Surg 2012;47:e11–13.
54. Mei-Zahav M, Konen O, Manson D, et al. Is congenital lobar emphysema a surgical disease? J Pediatr Surg 2006;41:1058–61.
55. Tempe DK, Virmani S, Javetkar S, et al. Congenital lobar emphysema: Pitfalls and management. Ann Card Anaesth 2010;13:53–8.
56. Laje P, Liechty KW. Postnatal management and outcome of prenatally diagnosed lung lesions. Prenat Diagn 2008;28:612–18.
57. Tolg C, Abelin K, Laudenbach V, et al. Open vs. thoracoscopic surgical management of bronchogenic cysts. Surg Endosc 2005;19:77–80.
58. Calzada AP, Wu W, Salvado AR, et al. Poorly differentiated adenocarcinoma arising from a cervical bronchial cyst. Laryngoscope 2011;121:1446–8.
59. Rothenberg SS. First decade's experience with thoracoscopic lobectomy in infants and children. J Pediatr Surg 2008;43:40–5.
60. Rothenberg SS, Kuenzler KA, Middlesworth W, et al. Thoracoscopic lobectomy in infants less than 10 kg with prenatally diagnosed cystic lung disease. J Laparoendosc Adv Surg Tech A 2011;21:181–4.
61. Vu LT, Farmer DL, Nobuhara KK, et al. Thoracoscopic versus open resection for congenital cystic adenomatoid malformations of the lung. J Pediatr Surg 2008;43:35–9.
62. Cohen DE, McCloskey JJ, Motas D, et al. Fluoroscopic-assisted endobronchial intubation for single-lung ventilation in infants. Paediatr Anaesth 2011;21:681–4.
63. Stocker JT. Cystic lung disease in infants and children. Fetal Pediatr Pathol 2009;28(4):155–84.

CHAPTER 23

Acquired Lesions of the Lung and Pleura

Shawn D. St. Peter

EMPYEMA

Empyema is defined as the accumulation of pus in a body cavity and is derived from the Greek word *empyein* which means to 'put pus in'. In medical terminology, it refers to pus in the pleural space. The most common etiology is a reaction to an adjacent pneumonia. However, other sources include reaction to a subphrenic abscess as well as extension of mediastinal, retropharyngeal, or paravertebral infections. Empyema can also develop secondary to infection after thoracic surgery or trauma.

Epidemiology

Although overall rates of bacterial pneumonia have been declining in children, the incidence of complications such as parapneumonic effusions and empyema has increased.[1] In the USA, pneumonia in children occurs at an estimated rate of 30–40 per 100,000.[2] Parapneumonic effusions (PPE) can complicate pediatric pneumonia in 28–53% of patients.[3,4] In children less than two years of age, the incidence of empyema doubled over a 10-year span, increasing from 3.5/100,000 in 1996–1998 to 7/100,000 in 2005–2007.[5] Similarly, in patients between 2 to 4 years age, empyema rates nearly tripled from 3.7/100,000 to 10.3/100,000 during the same time period. While empyema in children is less serious compared to adults where mortality can approach 20%, it still poses a considerable burden on hospitals and families.

Pathogenesis

The natural progression of parapneumonic pleural disease has been outlined with three to four stages of increasing complexity.[6–8] The pre-collection stage involves pleuritis and inflammation. This is followed by the exudative stage, which is a simple PPE, and is characterized by clear, free-flowing pleural fluid with a low white cell count. The fibrinopurulent stage is a complicated PPE (empyema) marked by the deposition of fibrin and purulent material in the pleural space and an increase in the leukocyte count of the fluid. Septations and fibrin strands begin to develop. These result from decreased fibrinolytic activity allowing increased fibrin deposition. The result is a procoagulant environment that leads to the development of solid material in the form of septations followed by loculations of purulent fluid (Fig. 23-1).[9] The most advanced state is termed the organized stage when a thick peel is established. This peel can entrap the lung and result in chronic restrictive lung disease. While these stages are outlined in sequential progression, there is no certainty that each stage will progress to the next. Although outlined as a simple progression, the degree of patient illness may not correspond with these stages, depending on the extent of the concomitant parenchymal disease or the inflammatory response to the infectious processes.

As the stages advance, the chemistry of the parapneumonic fluid changes: glucose decreases, pH decreases, and lactate dehydrogenase (LDH) rises. The Light criteria for complicated PPE include pH <7.2, lactate dehydrogenase >1000 units, glucose <40 mg/dL or < 25% of the blood glucose, Gram stain or culture positive, and loculations or septations documented with imaging.[10] Retrospective data suggests that a prolonged fever, a low pleural fluid pH and glucose along with a high LDH pleural/serum ratio are associated with more severe disease.[11] Another study, using multivariate logistic analysis of a retrospective dataset, found that a pleural fluid pH less than 7.27 was the only significant factor for the formation of fibrin with/without septations.[12] A third study suggested that a tumor necrosis factor level greater than 80 pg/mL in the pleural fluid suggests a complicated effusion.[13]

In a 1995 review, Light proposed a detailed classification which defines seven different stages from nonsignificant PPEs to a complex empyema. Recommendations on appropriate therapy were also described, which ranged from observation to thoracoscopic debridement/decortication (Table 23-1).[14] A consensus statement from the American College of Chest Physicians in 2000 noted that more interventional therapy was needed as the stage of effusion progressed.[15] Similarly, in another retrospective study, a pleural fluid pH less than 7.1 was found to result in a sixfold increase in the likelihood of operative intervention.[16] While all these criteria may document the physiologic progression of disease, the clinical relevance of a patient's pleural fluid analysis may not be that important because once symptoms develop and fluid with or without septations are found, intervention is needed.

Diagnosis

The diagnosis is usually a progressive clinical picture beginning with pneumonia. Patients with an empyema almost always demonstrate some degree of respiratory

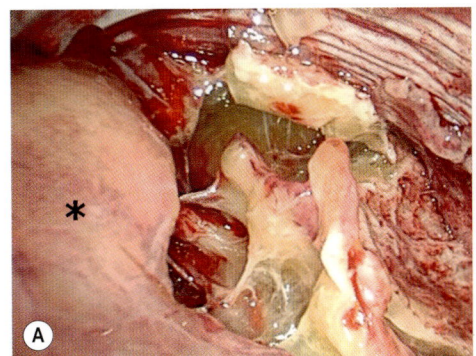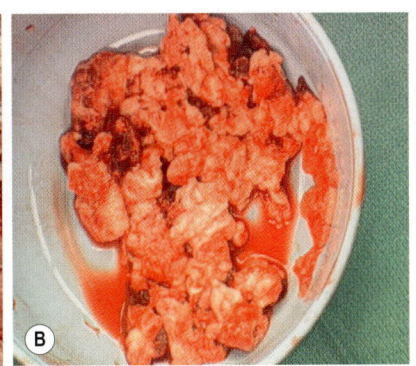

FIGURE 23-1 ■ (A) The thoracoscopic view shows the inflammatory septations that can develop with empyema. The collapsed lung is marked with an asterisk. (B) Note the thick, solid purulent material that is often found in these patients.

TABLE 23-1	**Classification Scheme for Parapneumonic Effusions and Empyema**
Categorization	**Pleural Fluid Findings**
Class 1 Nonsignificant parapneumonic effusion	Small <10 mm thick on decubitus X-ray
Class 2 Typical parapneumonic effusion	>10 mm thick Glucose >40 mg/dL, pH>7.20 Gram stain and culture negative
Class 3 Borderline complicated parapneumonic effusion	7.00<pH<7.20 and/or LDH>1,000 and glucose >40 mg/dL Gram stain and culture negative
Class 4 Simple complicated parapneumonic effusion	pH<7.00 and/or glucose <40 mg/dL and/or Gram stain or culture positive Not loculated, no frank pus
Class 5 Complex complicated parapneumonic effusion	pH<7.00 and/or glucose <40 mg/dL and/or Gram stain or culture positive Multiloculated
Class 6 Simple empyema	Frank pus present Single locule or free flowing
Class 7 Complex empyema	Frank pus present Multiple locules

Modified from Light RW. A new classification of parapneumonic effusions and empyema. Chest 1995;108:299–301.

distress, malaise, persistent fever, or pleuritic chest pain.[17–20] Diminished breath sounds with dullness to percussion on the affected side are found on examination. An ileus is common as is a lack of appetite.

Initial imaging is a chest radiograph (CXR) which shows poor penetration on the affected side. However, it is often difficult to distinguish between parenchymal consolidation and pleural fluid on a plain film.[21] In a retrospective review of over 300 adult patients, CXR missed all effusions that were significant enough to warrant drainage when compared with subsequent computed tomography (CT) scans (Fig. 23-2A).[22] Decubitus films may be helpful in distinguishing between nonloculated and loculated effusions.[21]

Ultrasonography (US) is portable, relatively inexpensive, and does not involve radiation (Fig. 23-2B). It is very sensitive in diagnosing loculated fluid and can be used to guide percutaneous drainage and catheter placement.[23,24] Some authors suggest that ultrasound is superior to CT in the identification of pleural debris or loculations.[25,26] ultrasound can reliably differentiate between parenchymal and pleural based processes.[6] A post hoc review of a prospective trial in children found that in 31 patients in whom both CT and ultrasound were performed, there was no advantage of CT over ultrasound in most cases.[1] Two independent series reviewed the implementation of an algorithm using initial ultrasound in children with complicated pneumonia.[27,28] Both demonstrated a significant reduction in hospitalization and a decrease in the use of CT without an increase in the rate of operative management or pleural drainage. A small retrospective review comparing ultrasound and CT found that CT had no advantage in most cases and suggested that CT should be used in complex cases only, such as patients undergoing operation or thought to have parenchymal abscesses or a bronchopleural fistula.[26] CT has been found to be inferior to ultrasound at demonstrating fibrin strands or septations within the pleural fluid.[25] Neither CT nor ultrasound is completely reliable in differentiating the specific stages of parapneumonic disease.[1,25,26] The main disadvantages of ultrasound appear to be lack of 24-hour ultrasound availability and being operator dependent.

With pleural space disease, CT with intravenous contrast can differentiate between parenchymal and pleural processes, identifying pleural thickening and loculations.[25] CT radiation exposure has raised the concern for a long-term cancer risk.[29] Currently, chest CT scans can

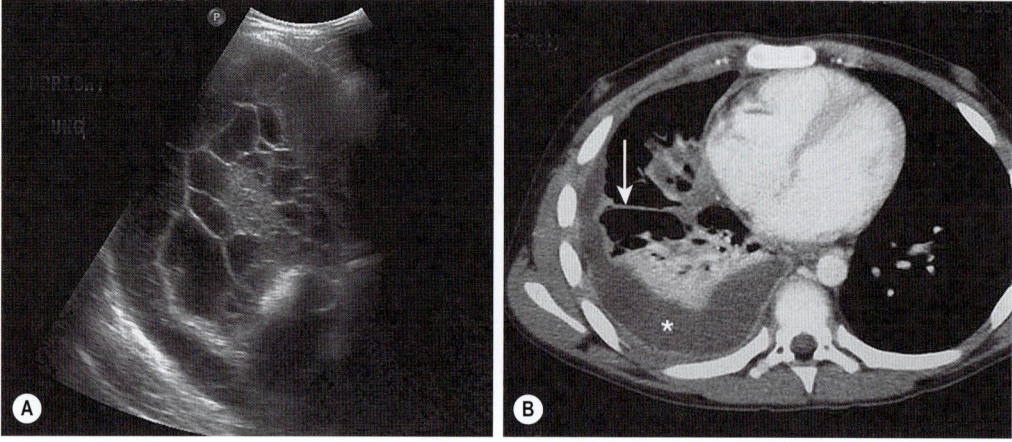

FIGURE 23-2 ■ Ultrasonography and/or CT of the chest are helpful during the initial evaluation of children with a pleural effusion and possible empyema. **(A)** In the ultrasound study, note the loculations identified in the pleural fluid. **(B)** On the CT scan, a large pleural effusion (*asterisk*) is noted. Also there is collapse of the underlying lung parenchyma as well as septations (*arrow*).

be performed effectively with the use of automatic dose modulation software that limit the radiation dose.[25] Despite this ability to limit radiation exposure with CT scan, consensus statements are clear in their recommendations for performing CT only when needed, such as preoperative planning in some cases.[6,7]

Management

Parapneumonic Effusion

After the diagnosis of PPE is made, the first branch in the management algorithm depends on the nature of the fluid. With a free-flowing effusion and no solid components or signs of frank pus, the nature of the intervention will depend on the size of the effusion and the symptoms. Classifying the size is difficult to define precisely. However, in general, small effusions are defined as having ≤1 cm rim of fluid, moderate effusions have a 1–2 cm rim, and large effusions have ≥2 cm rim on decubitus films. A recently published twelve year retrospective study in children classified small effusions as less than a quarter hemithorax opacification, moderate effusions as a quarter to a half opacification, and large effusions as more than half opacification based on upright films.[30] In this study, the authors found that small and most moderately sized effusions could be effectively managed without drainage and without an increase in the length of hospitalization or other complications. The authors suggest that interventions should be based on symptoms, not the size of the effusion alone.

Symptoms leading to intervention generally are feeding intolerance, tachypnea, and an increasing oxygen requirement. A retrospective case series in children found respiratory distress on presentation was related to prolonged stay and a higher likelihood for intervention.[31]

After deciding to drain the effusion, options include single or multiple thoracentesis versus tube thoracostomy or catheter drainage. A prospective, nonrandomized pediatric series compared treatment with repeated ultrasound-guided needle aspirations vs tube thoracostomy. There was a mean 2.4 drainages/patient in the aspiration group, but similar length of stay.[32] While this approach may be reasonable in an older child who can tolerate the procedure with local anesthesia, it would likely not be appropriate in younger children. The British Thoracic Society guidelines recommend a chest tube for cases in which the first thoracentesis fails to adequately drain the effusion in order to avoid multiple thoracentesis attempts.[6] A retrospective series compared 33 children who underwent chest tube placement on the basis of effusion size and/or thoracentesis fluid analysis vs 32 who were treated conservatively with tube thoracostomy only for progressive symptoms or mediastinal shift.[33] The authors found no difference in duration of hospitalization and suggested frugal use of chest tubes.[3] In a series of 405 adult patients, 266 had a chest tube smaller than 14 French compared to 139 with larger tubes.[34] There was no difference in the ability to drain the effusion. Furthermore, smaller caliber tubes did not hinder the use of fibrinolytics. In a retrospective series of 20 children treated with standard chest tubes compared to 12 treated with pigtail tubes, no outcome differences were found.[35] In patients with pleural effusions or empyema, we exclusively use 12 French Thal-Quick chest tubes (Cook Critical Care, Bloomington, Indiana, USA) that are inserted using the Seldinger technique (Fig. 23-3). We have not felt it necessary to use image guidance in the majority of patients.

Empyema

Empyema is diagnosed by identifying solid components in the pleural fluid on imaging studies or pus during thoracentesis or tube catheter placement. The definitive management for empyema has traditionally been operative debridement, which is currently performed via video-assisted thoracoscopy surgery (VATS).[36–40] VATS has resulted in earlier and more complete resolution of empyema than chest tube drainage alone in both retrospective and prospective studies, translating into shorter hospitalization with VATS as the initial therapy.[41–44] A retrospective series of 89 children undergoing primary thoracoscopic debridement/decortication found a 12% risk for needing another procedure to address ongoing disease or a complication.[45] However, the superiority of operative mechanical debridement as a definitive management strategy has been increasingly challenged by chemical debridement with fibrinolysis.

Examples of fibrinolytics include urokinase, streptokinase, and tissue plasminogen activator (tPA). Since fibrin is a predominant component of the extracellular matrix upon which septations and solid debris develop, fibrinolysis has been shown to be superior to tube thoracostomy alone in retrospective and prospective studies.[46–52] These studies include direct comparisons between the two treatment options as well as the use of fibrinolytic therapy after failure of tube thoracostomy.

Two prospective, randomized trials have been conducted independently comparing fibrinolysis to VATS for empyema in children.[53,54] The studies were conducted in the UK and USA in 60 and 36 patients, respectively. Both studies compared the instillation of three intrathoracic doses of fibrinolytic agents to thoracoscopy as the initial therapy for empyema. The first fibrinolytic dose in both studies was given at the time of diagnosis and/or chest tube insertion followed by two additional doses in 24-hour increments to complete the fibrinolytic course over a 48-hour period. The results were highly concordant as both studies found no difference in duration of hospitalization between the two interventions. The common parameters between the two studies are outlined in Table 23-2. The USA study found no difference in days of tube drainage, days of fever, doses of analgesics, or oxygen requirements.[54] Both studies documented thoracoscopic debridement was more expensive and both utilized an intention-to-treat analysis so the length of stay and total charges included the patients who failed fibrinolysis and subsequently required VATS. The failure rate for fibrinolysis was 16.6% in both studies. This failure rate was similar to previous studies investigating the utility of fibrinolysis.[48,55–59] An example of a first-line fibrinolytic approach is outlined Figure 23-4. A similar algorithm has been proposed based on a review of the literature.[60]

One of the groups that performed the prospective randomized trial comparing fibrinolysis to thoracoscopic debridement recently reported their data using an evidence-based algorithm with primary fibrinolytic therapy. One hundred and two consecutive patients were treated with fibrinolysis following completion of the prospective randomized trial and 16 patients (15.7%)

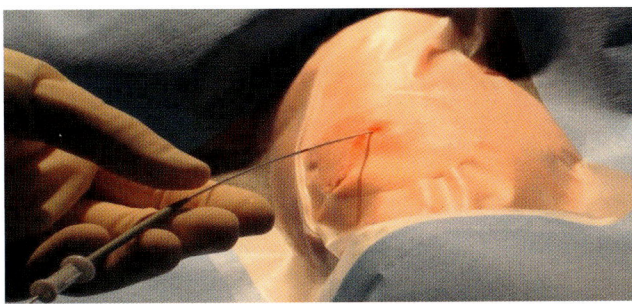
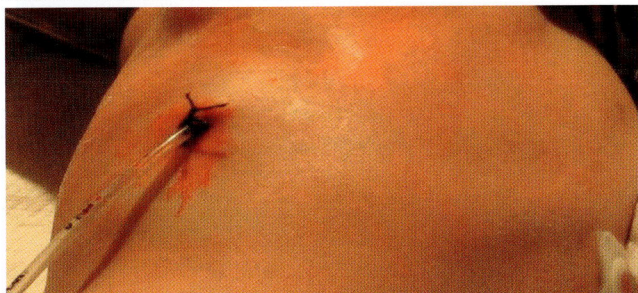

FIGURE 23-3 ■ The Seldinger technique for placement of a small chest tube for fibrinolytic therapy.

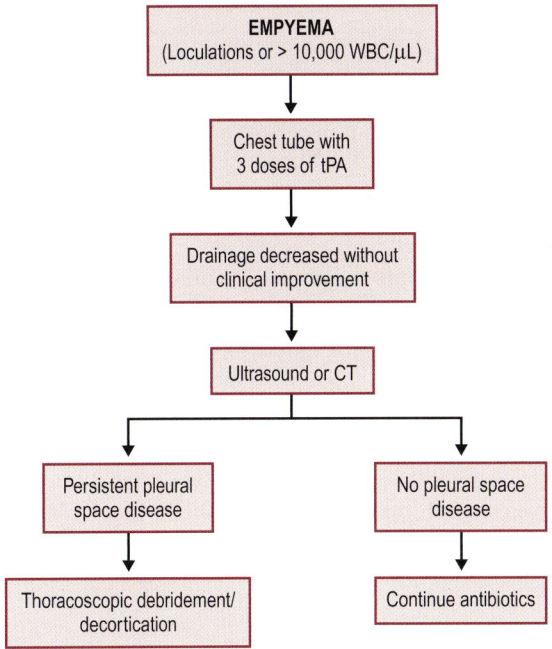

FIGURE 23-4 ■ Treatment algorithm for empyema is shown.

TABLE 23-2	Common Outcome Variables Reported between the Two Prospective Trials Comparing Fibrinolysis to VATS in Children					
Study	United Kingdom 2006[53]			United States 2009[54]		
Study variable	Urokinase	VATS	P value	tPA	VATS	P value
Mean length of stay (days)	6	6	0.33	6.8	6.9	0.96
Mean procedure charges[a]	9.1K	11.3K	<0.001	7.5K	11.6K	0.01
Failure rate for fibrinolysis	16.6%			16.6%		

[a]Charges are in thousands of British pounds and thousands of ultrasound dollars.
VATS, video-assisted thoracoscopic surgery; tPA, tissue plasminogen activator.

required subsequent thoracoscopic debridement and decortication. The length of hospitalization with fibrinolysis was 6.1 ± 2.5 days. In those patients that failed fibrinolytic therapy, the length of hospitalization after thoracoscopic debridement was 5.9 ± 3.7 days. Factors correlating with the need for thoracoscopy included age, gender, and initial drain output. However, none of these variables were independent predictors.[61]

When comparing fibrinolysis to VATS, the burden to the patient should be considered as one therapy is a nonoperative intervention requiring a single sedation and the other is an operation under general anesthesia. Available evidence suggests that thoracoscopic debridement is neither superior nor inferior to fibrinolytic therapy as a primary treatment modality. Therefore, if performed at the time of diagnosis, VATS remains an equivalent option to facilitate early recovery when fibrinolysis is not feasible, given individual hospital and physician resources. This may be particularly relevant if an anesthetic is required for tube placement to administer the fibrinolysis.

LUNG ABSCESS

Pulmonary abscess is often assumed to develop as a primary process in a previously normal lung, usually as a result of a necrotizing pneumonia. However, a pulmonary abscess in a child without an antecedent history ought to be considered as a secondary abscess which arises in an infected pulmonary anomaly such as a cystic pulmonary adenomatoid malformation, bronchogenic cyst, or foreign body. Most primary lung abscesses are located in the posterior segment of the right upper lobe and the superior segments of the right and left lower lobes (Fig. 23-5). In contrast, secondary and/or recurrent collections may be found in multiple locations with no specific anatomic predilection.

In the patient with known pneumonia, the nonresponding patient who develops a suspicious lesion on chest film should undergo CT to evaluate for an abscess. The treatment of a lung abscess in an infant or child follows the same basic principles of postural drainage and pulmonary toilet used in adults, but it is more often ineffective, secondary to the small size of the airway.[62,63]

In general, an operation should be avoided as abscesses can usually be successfully treated with antibiotics alone.[64,65] CT-guided drainage or catheter placement is usually needed if the lesion is peripheral and not connected to the airway, .[66–68] Retrospective data suggests that drainage shortens hospitalization and facilitates earlier recovery.[69] A recent series of 11 children with pulmonary abscess treated with thoracoscopic drainage fared well without complications which may be a good option when less invasive maneuvers fail.[70] Alternatively, pulmonary resection may be required for abscesses that are more centrally located and resistant to medical management.[62,71] Patients with fungal isolates and immunocompromised patients generally require early and aggressive pulmonary resection. However, as a general statement, patience should be employed in managing pulmonary abscesses.

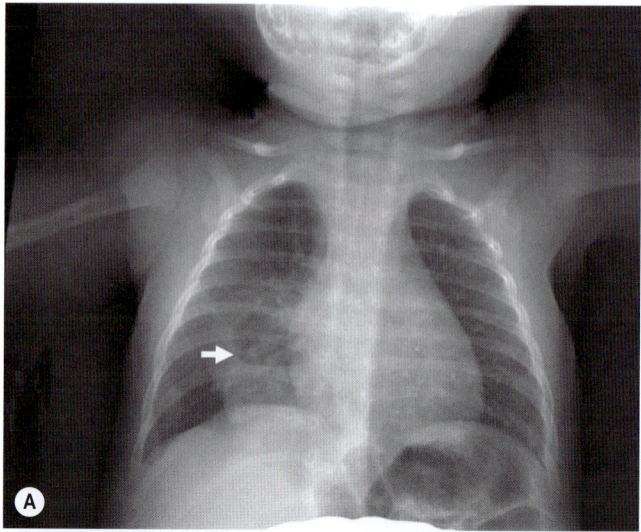

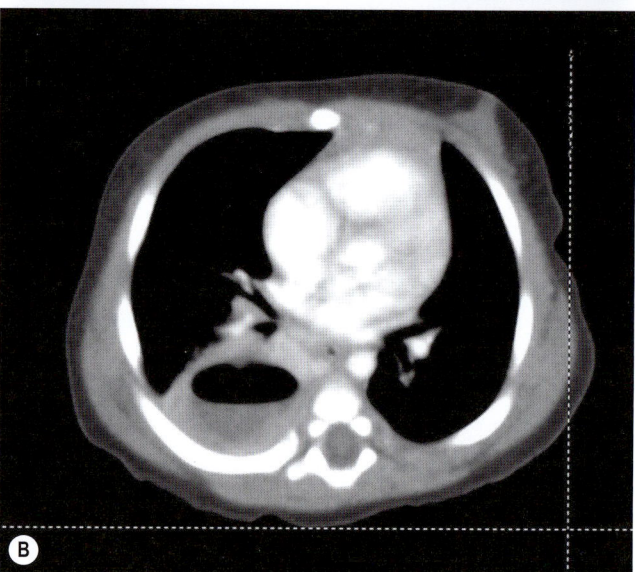

FIGURE 23-5 ■ **(A)** This young infant was found to have this lung abscess in the right lower lobe on chest radiograph. Note the air-fluid level (arrow). **(B)** The lesion is seen on the CT as well. Workup did not reveal an associated congenital pulmonary airway malformation and she recovered with antibiotic therapy.

PNEUMATOCELE

Pneumatoceles are thin-walled, air-filled, intraparenchymal pulmonary cysts. They typically occur secondary to an underlying bacterial pneumonia, a treated abscess, or as a result of trauma. Pneumatoceles are the result of a severe inflammatory reaction and the subsequent destruction of the alveolar and interstitial architecture. With an infectious etiology, the release of bacterial exotoxins has been postulated.[72] Although pneumatoceles have been associated with a variety of underlying bacterial organisms, the majority appear to be the result of staphylococcal pneumonia.[72–74] Other pathogens that have been identified as being associated with pneumatocele formation include *Streptococcus, Haemophilus influenzae, Klebsiella, Escherichia coli,* and *Pseudomonas.* In addition, pneumatoceles have been found in cases of pulmonary tuberculosis and measles.[73]

Additional complications associated with pneumatoceles include the development of secondary infections, empyema, and bronchopleural fistulas.[75]

Management

Most pneumatoceles will involve over time, and do not require any specific therapy other than supportive care and appropriate antibiotic coverage. In the case of a rapidly enlarging and/or tension pneumatocele, resulting in respiratory compromise, urgent decompression may be needed. In addition to closed-tube thoracostomy or cystostomy, percutaneous catheter drainage using fluoroscopy and ultrasound, has been reported to be an effective means of decompression.[76,77] Open drainage with decortication and oversewing of the cyst wall is rarely necessary.

The majority of pneumatoceles decrease in size and resolve over a period of several weeks to months, assuming that the underlying infectious cause is adequately treated. In uncomplicated cases, no residual pulmonary compromise or radiologic sequelae are likely.

BRONCHIECTASIS

Bronchiectasis is defined as a permanent dilatation of segmental airways, initially described almost 200 years ago.[78] A significant number of deaths from respiratory insufficiency due to bronchiectasis continue to occur. Bronchiectasis is not a pathophysiologic process, but is an architectural abnormality resulting from any pathologic process that causes persistent pulmonary inflammation and airway damage. Decreased epithelial and mucociliary integrity results in poor airway clearance leading to a predisposition for further infections. Three pathologic forms have been described: saccular, cylindrical, and fusiform or varicose.[79] Saccular bronchiectasis tends to occur in third- and fourth-order bronchioles, whereas cylindrical bronchiectasis occurs in sixth- to seventh-order bronchioles. The fusiform variety is an intermediate type.

Bronchiectasis can be categorized based on the source of the respiratory injury (Table 23-3).[80] As might be expected, congenital abnormalities are more likely to result in diffuse distribution with bilateral disease whereas acquired bronchiectasis is more likely to be focal. Focal disease is more common in the left lower lobe, lingula, or right middle lobe. Many cases remain idiopathic without an explanation for the source of the parenchymal or airway damage. Retrospective reports indicate that about 50% of patients, in whom a specific cause is determined, experience their first pulmonary insult before age 14.[81,82]

Presentation and Diagnosis

Patients typically present with nonspecific symptoms such as cough, sputum production, and lethargy. Classically, patients develop a three-layer sputum consisting of a foamy outer layer, a mucous middle layer, and a viscous purulent bottom layer. This three-layer sputum

TABLE 23-3 Etiology of Bronchiectasis

Category	Cause
Post-infection	Viral
	Bacterial
	Fungal
	Atypical mycobacteria
ABPA	
COPD	
Idiopathic traction	Post-tuberculous fibrosis
	Radiation fibrosis
	Pulmonary fibrosis
Aspiration	Foreign body aspiration
Obstruction	Benign tumors
	Enlarged lymph nodes
Amyloidosis	
Celiac disease	
Yellow nail syndrome	
Young syndrome	
Immunological defects	*Primary:*
	CVID
	Agammaglobulinemia
	Hyper-IgE syndrome
	Secondary:
	Chemotherapy
	Immunosuppressant therapy
	Tumor
Congenital defects	*Anatomical:*
	Scoliosis
	Marfan syndrome
	Tracheobronchomegaly
	Others:
	Primary ciliary dyskinesia
	Kartagener syndrome
	Alpha-1-antitrypsin deficiency
	Defect ENaC protein
Diffuse panbronchiolitis	
Rheumatoid arthritis	
Systemic lupus erythematodes	
Chronic bowel disease	

ABPA, allergic bronchopulmonary aspergillosis; CVID, common variable immunodeficiency; COPD, chronic obstructive pulmonary disease; ENaC, epithelial sodium channel.
Modified from: Rademacher J, Welte T. Bronchiectasis-Diagnosis and Treatment. Dtsch Arztebl Int 2011;108:809–15.

is considered pathognomonic, but is not often seen. Patients with more advanced disease present with hemoptysis, chest pain, weight loss, bronchospasm, dyspnea, and impaired physical performance.[83] Patients can be symptom free most of the time, but can become symptomatic during exacerbations. Physical examination usually reveals coarse inspiratory crackles and expiratory wheezes. The diagnosis is often delayed due to the lack of few specific signs and the low incidence of this disease.

A chest radiograph may show focal density and crowding of interstitial markings (Fig. 23-6). Historically, bronchography was the best diagnostic test, but high-resolution CT is now the preferred study.[81,82] There is a high correlation between bronchographic and CT findings,[84] particularly bronchi within 1 cm of the visceral pleural surface (Fig. 23-7).[85] Ventilation/perfusion scans may be

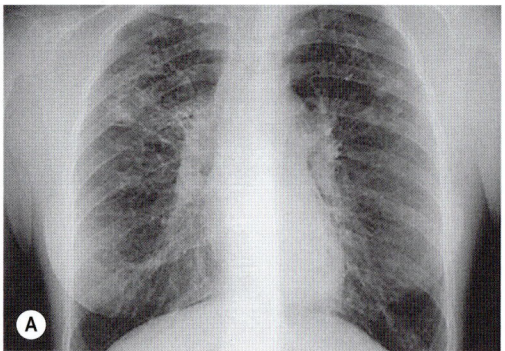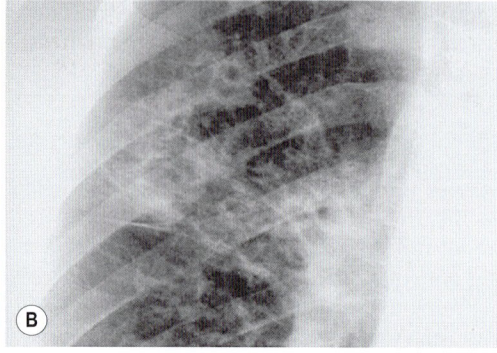

FIGURE 23-6 ■ **(A)** Chest radiograph demonstrating the classic appearance of bronchiectasis in a pediatric patient with cystic fibrosis. **(B)** Magnified view of the patient demonstrating honeycombed appearance.

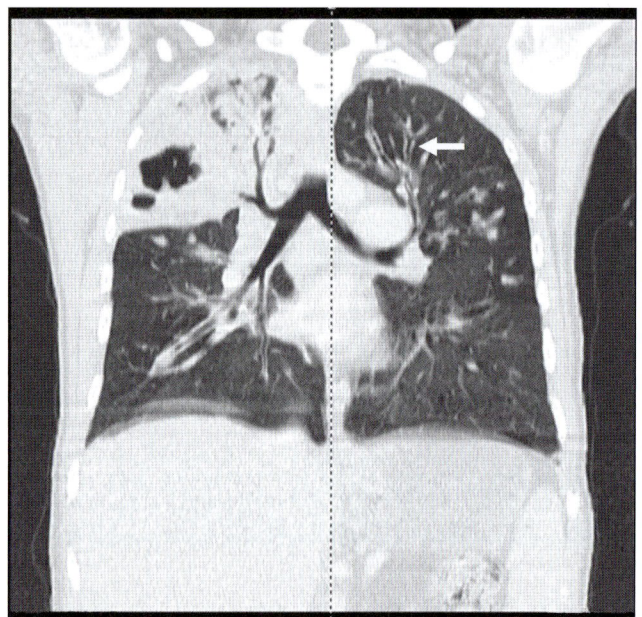

FIGURE 23-7 ■ High-resolution CT demonstrates severe bronchiectasis. On the patient's left side, dilated bronchi (arrow) are seen throughout the lung. Apically, they extend to near the pleural surface. On the patient's right, the dilated bronchi are seen extending into an upper lobe complicated by infection and consolidation which can be a recurring problem in patients with bronchiectasis.

helpful to delineate the presence of ventilation-perfusion mismatching.

Management

The surgeon is not typically involved until irreversible bronchiectasis develops. Clearly the best outcomes are obtained when the underlying process is controlled to minimize disease progression. If a foreign body is found, it may be possible to remove it at bronchoscopy. However, for a long-standing foreign body, a resection likely will be needed. Resection is also needed in children with repeated localized involvement despite nonoperative therapy. The absence of vascular perfusion indicates end-stage disease and resection will likely be needed.[85] Occasionally, massive hemoptysis will be the indication for resection, although embolization of bronchial vessels may be a viable option if hospital resources are available.

The principles of operative treatment should be to preserve as much uninvolved pulmonary parenchyma as possible using segmental resections.[86] In a retrospective series of open resection in 35 children with bronchiectasis, two-thirds had cylindrical bronchiectases.[87] Sixty-five per cent of the children became asymptomatic and 24% were clinically improved. A little over 10% did not have clinical improvement. The authors stress the importance of careful selection of patients and complete resection of the disease. Another series of 58 resections in 54 children included lobectomy (63%), pneumonectomy (18.5%), lobectomy with segmentectomy (11.1%), segmentectomy (3.7%), and bilobectomy (3.7%).[88] There were 23 patients (43%) who were clinically well, another 23 (43%) who were improved, and 5 (10%) who were the same or worse. Three patients died. In a recent series of 19 thoracoscopic lobectomies for bronchiectasis, there were no conversions and minimal complications.[89]

CHYLOTHORAX

Chylothorax is a chylous effusion or the presence of lymphatic fluid within the pleural space. Invariably there is a leak at some level within the lymphatic drainage system. Since most of the thoracic duct courses through the right chest, the majority of chyle leaks will occur on the right side. Injuries to the thoracic duct at or above the aortic arch may result in a chylothorax on the left.

The cause of a lymphatic leak into the pleural space can be broadly classified as traumatic or atraumatic. Nontraumatic causes include congenital abnormalities such as lymphatic malformations or lymphangiomatosis. Venous thromboses have been associated with chylous effusions. Infiltration of the chest and mediastinum by infection or malignancy can also result in a chyle leak. Gorham syndrome, which is a primary osteolytic process where spontaneous bone resorption occurs, is often associated with a refractory and debilitation chyle leak when ribs are involved. Congenital chylothorax occurs spontaneously in the neonatal period. It is most frequently idiopathic but has been described with some dysmorphic syndromes.[90,91] These cases are presumed to result from a structural defect in the lymphatic drainage system. By far, the most common cause is an injury to the thoracic duct or a major tributary. The incidence of chyle leak has been reported as high as 1% after cardiac operations in infants and children.[92]

Presentation and Diagnosis

As with any pleural effusion, chylothorax can present with respiratory symptoms. Congenital cases may be suspected during routine prenatal ultrasound. In postoperative patients, it will present with milky drainage from the chest drain/tube. The drainage may seem like normal pleural fluid until enteral nutrition is resumed and the drainage becomes chylous. Analysis of the fluid confirms the diagnosis. Chyle typically demonstrates a total fat content greater than 400 mg/dL, triglycerides greater than 200 mg/dL, or a specific gravity greater than 1.012. In addition, Gram stain demonstrates the presence of more than 90% lymphocytes and Sudan red staining may reveal the presence of chylomicrons.[93]

Pseudochylothorax (also termed cholesterol pleurisy or chyliform effusion) is a rare condition that is characterized by a cholesterol-rich pleural effusion and is commonly associated with chronic inflammatory disorders such as tuberculosis or rheumatoid arthritis. These are often long-standing effusions which are distinguished from chylothorax by the lack of triglycerides and chylomicrons.

Management

There are physiologic consequences from the chylothorax. Protein and fat losses can result in acute malnutrition. Lymphocyte losses result in immunosuppression. The net fluid losses can cause dehydration. Therefore, it is important to understand these losses so vigorous monitoring and replacement can occur concomitant with maneuvers to stop the leak. Initially, nonoperative maneuvers should be attempted based on the goals of reducing the amount of chyle produced while still providing adequate nutrition. This begins with limiting fat intake. As medium-chain fatty acids are carried through the portal venous system (as opposed to the intestinal lymphatic network), it is reasonable to start with a fat-restricted diet rich in medium-chain fatty acids. The next step would be to stop oral intake and begin total parenteral nutrition. As many as 80% of patients respond to this management strategy.[92]

In addition to dietary manipulations, several authors have reported success with the use of somatostatin analogs', such as octreotide, whether the chyle leak is spontaneous or post-traumatic.[94–98] Some authors recommend utilizing octreotide early in the plan of care.[97]

Nonoperative therapy is typically recommended for one to two weeks prior to considering operative options.[93] The goal of the operation begins with stopping the leak. This is straightforward if the leak is visualized and can be closed or obliterated. Thoracic duct ligation proximal to the leak is usually curative. If neither of these options can be accomplished, pleurodesis can be attempted.[99] These cases can be approached with thoracoscopy. Right thoracoscopy with occlusion of the thoracic duct as it crosses

the diaphragm has been shown to be a useful technique in patients with a traumatic leak.[100,101] Others have described direct suture of the area of chylous leak followed by the application of fibrin glue.[102] In adults, a minimally invasive technique of percutaneous injection of the cisterna chyli with platinum coil embolization of the thoracic duct has been shown to be successful in over two-thirds of patients with high-output chylothorax in whom nonoperative management has failed.[103,104] In cases that are refractory after an operation, use of a pleuroperitoneal shunt has been described (Fig. 23-8).[105] In these patients, the chyle in the pleural space is manually pumped into the peritoneal cavity where it is absorbed, presumably into the venous system. These shunts can remain open for several months until the chylous leak seals.

DIFFUSE INTERSTITIAL DISEASE

The interstitium of the lung is the tissue around and between the airway and vascular system. A persistent lung injury results in a reparative process which causes scarring and inflammation. The lung may be permanently damaged, with inflamed interstitial tissue replacing the normal capillaries, alveoli, and healthy interstitium. This condition is known as chronic interstitial lung disease (ILD). It may be the result of myriad processes, some of which are listed in Table 23-4.[106–108] The clinical consequence is restrictive lung physiology and abnormal gas exchange which produces considerable morbidity and mortality. The clinical disease patterns range from a chronic, slowly progressive picture in a relatively stable patient to one of acute pulmonary decompensation, requiring emergency life-saving maneuvers.

The role of the surgeon is to help establish the diagnosis, usually with a lung biopsy, after imaging demonstrates a diffuse pulmonary process (Fig. 23-9).

TABLE 23-4	Infectious and Noninfectious Processes Associated with the Development of Chronic Interstitial Lung Disease
Infectious	**Noninfectious**
Pneumocystis	Hypersensitivity pneumonitis
Cryptococcus	Sarcoidosis
Aspergillus	Neoplasms
Streptococcus	Systemic lupus erythematosus
Chlamydia	Graft-vs.-host disease
Mycoplasma pneumoniae	Radiation pneumonitis
Rickettsia	Adult respiratory distress syndrome
Adenovirus	
Parainfluenzavirus	Aspiration pneumonitis (gastroesophageal reflux disease)
Respiratory syncytial virus	
Cytomegalovirus	Chemotherapeutic agents
Varicella-zoster virus	Fat embolism
Herpes simplex virus	Allergic alveolitis
	Pulmonary hemosiderosis

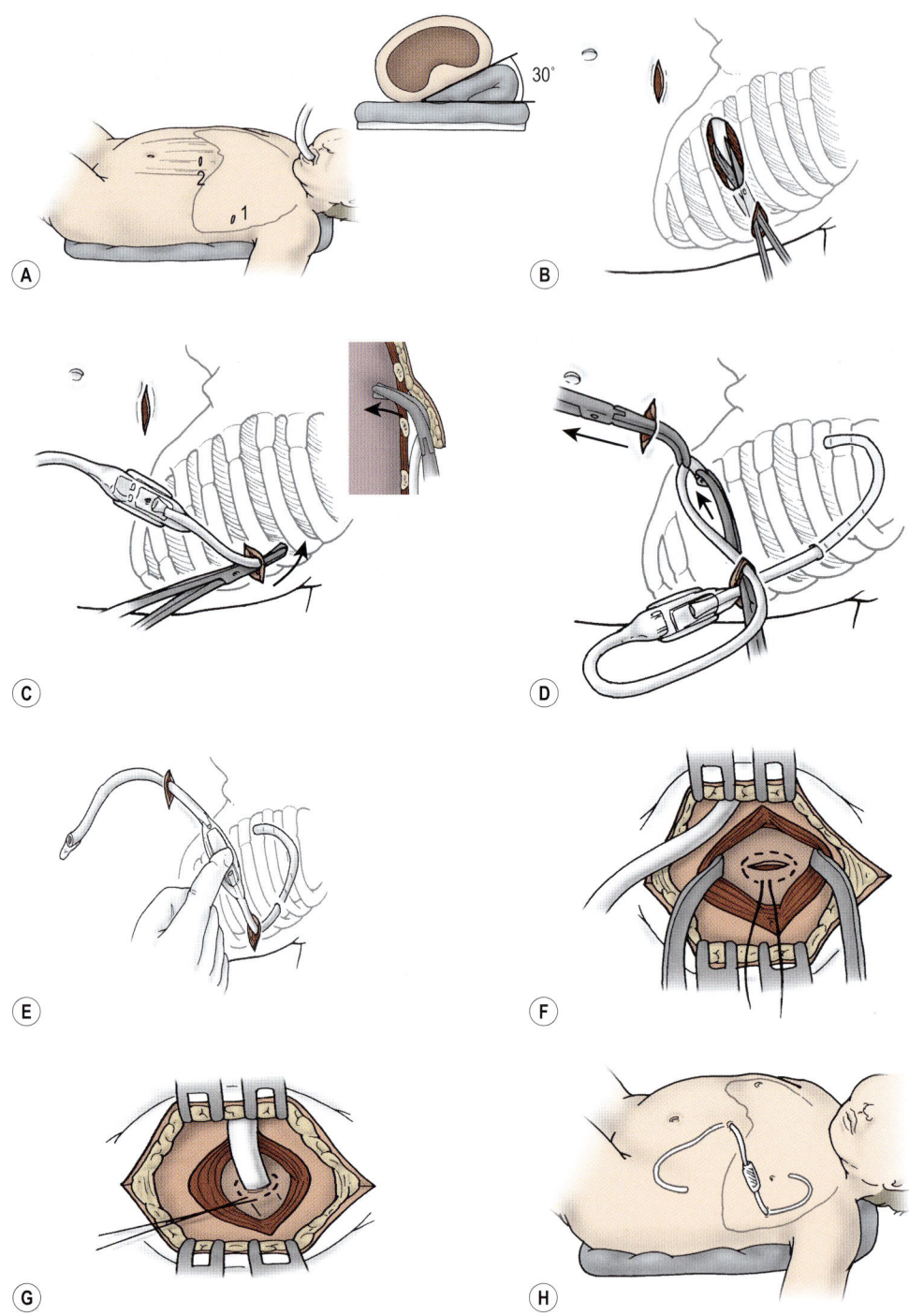

FIGURE 23-8 ◼ Insertion of pleuroperitoneal shunt. **(A)** The affected hemithorax is elevated 30°. The two incisions are planned to allow the pump chamber to rest on the costal margin. **(B)** A small incision is made over the rib in the anterior axillary line, and a deep subcutaneous pocket is created inferiorly. **(C)** Insertion of pleuroperitoneal shunt into the pleural space is done with a large curved clamp. The pleural catheter is tunneled 2–3 cm and bluntly passed through the intercostal space. The catheter must be carefully passed through the intercostal muscle at an angle to avoid kinking. **(D)** A second small incision is made overlying the rectus muscle, and the peritoneal catheter is tunneled through this incision. The distal end of the shunt device is delivered to the second incision, as shown. The pumping chamber is drawn into the subcutaneous pocket by traction on the peritoneal catheter. **(E)** The flow of chyle is confirmed before the distal catheter is inserted into the peritoneum. **(F,G)** A purse-string suture is used to secure the peritoneal catheter at the level of the posterior rectus fascia. **(H)** Both incisions should be closed with an absorbable suture, leaving a totally implanted system. (Adapted from Murphy M, Newman B, Rodgers B. Pleuroperitoneal shunts in the management of persistent chylothorax. Ann Thorac Surg 1989;48:195–200.)

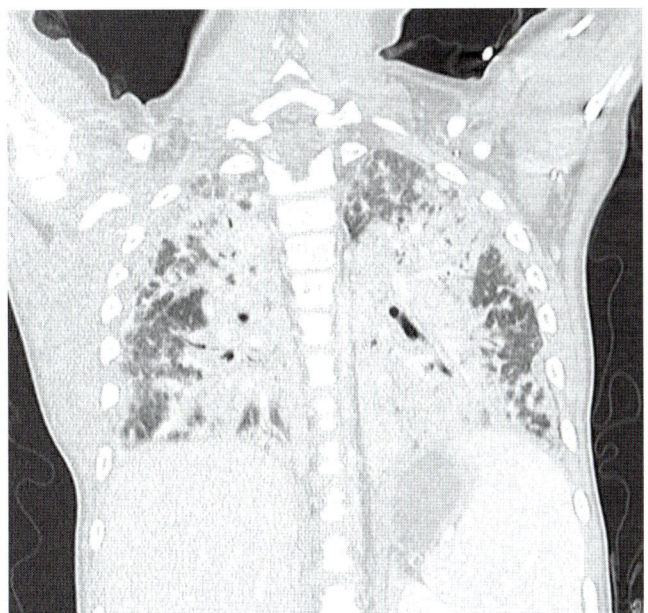

FIGURE 23-9 ■ High-resolution CT demonstrates severe diffuse bilateral parenchyma disease on a patient referred for lung biopsy.

Unfortunately, the results of bronchoalveolar lavage (BAL) are disappointing in this disease. In a prospective analysis of children with ILD undergoing BAL, a definitive primary diagnosis could be made in only 17%.[107]

Lung biopsy is currently the most definitive diagnostic maneuver, and an urgent lung biopsy may be needed to guide management. These can be performed open or with thoracoscopy. In the case of an extremely unstable patient, thoracoscopy and/or mini-thoracotomy may be needed in the intensive care unit to obtain the necessary tissue.

The Childhood Interstitial Lung Disease Pathology Co-operative Group has published guidelines about handling the biopsy tissue.[109] The principles of biopsy begin with obtaining tissue from a region of heavy involvement based on imaging. If there is diffuse lung involvement, any site is reasonable, except the tip of the right middle lobe or the tip of the lingula where the changes are often disproportionate and may lead to a faulty impression of the disease severity. If it is not obvious from the imaging studies which is the more diseased area, biopsies should be taken from more than one area. A lung biopsy in a child should yield a specimen at least 1 cm × 1 cm × 1 cm. The biopsy specimen should be a wedge with its apex extending at least 1 cm into the lung parenchyma. An elongated or elliptical shaped biopsy obtained by shaving off the margin of a lobe should be avoided. In an older child where space allows, a stapler may be the most reliable means of parenchymal division and sealing. We have had success in smaller children using the Ligasure (Covidien, Inc., Mansfield, MA). However, this often requires a deflated lung. Also, the diseased lung may not seal well and it may be necessary to oversew the lung edge. The patient on a high-frequency oscillating ventilator can be problematic. The constant distal airway pressure makes it very difficult to obtain a seal by any means. Thus,

oversewing the edge of the biopsy is usually needed. We have also used fibrin glue to help prevent an air leak. Once the biopsy is obtained, a piece should be sent for microbiologic analysis under sterile conditions prior to handing the specimen off the operative field.

RIGHT MIDDLE LOBE SYNDROME

Right middle lobe (RML) syndrome refers to a picture of persistent atelectasis in the right middle lobe. Similar to bronchiectasis, the syndrome is a clinical diagnosis resulting from a variety of underlying causes. In a large review of the literature encompassing over 900 cases, the etiologic causes of RML syndrome were inflammation in 47%, bronchiectasis in 15%, malignant tumors in 22%, benign tumors in 2%, tuberculosis in 9%, aspiration in 2%, and miscellaneous in the remaining 3%.[110] It is felt there is a predisposition for the RML to develop atelectasis because of the narrow diameter and acute take-off of the RML bronchus. Also, the relative anatomic isolation of the RML with poor collateral ventilation reduces the chance of reinflation once atelectasis develops.[111]

The clinical presentation usually consists of nonspecific respiratory symptoms. On plain chest radiograph, the diagnosis is suggested by a wedge-shaped density that extends anteriorly and inferiorly from the hilum of the lung. This finding is best visualized on the lateral view. However, plain films may be inadequate and a high-resolution CT may be needed to delineate the bronchial anatomy and the presence of bronchiectasis.[112] Bronchoscopy is a useful initial step in diagnosis as it can document stenosis or obstruction of the RML bronchus from a variety of causes such as granulation tissue, tumor, or foreign body. Clearing secretions and obtaining specimens for microbiological analysis may also guide management.

Complete bronchial obstruction, the presence of bronchiectasis, and persistent or recurrent disease despite medical management are an indication for lobectomy.[113] Given the relatively small contribution of the RML to normal ventilation along with the ineffectiveness of ventilation in the presence of this disease, the operation usually results in little morbidity to the patient and an excellent clinical outcome. In a series of 20 children, 17 were asymptomatic after RML lobectomy with an additional two being improved.[113] Therefore, it may be reasonable to consider lobectomy early in the disease course prior to chronic debilitation.

SPONTANEOUS PNEUMOTHORAX

The development of a spontaneous pneumothorax is thought to be due to ruptured apical bullae or blebs (Fig. 23-10). The incidence of spontaneous pneumothorax is thought to be 4 per 100,000 males and 1.1 per 100,000 females.[114,115] Although the etiology is unclear, this disorder appears to be more prevalent in patients with asthma, cystic fibrosis, or connective tissue disorders.

Patients can develop symptoms both at rest and with any maneuvers that increase intrathoracic pressure, such

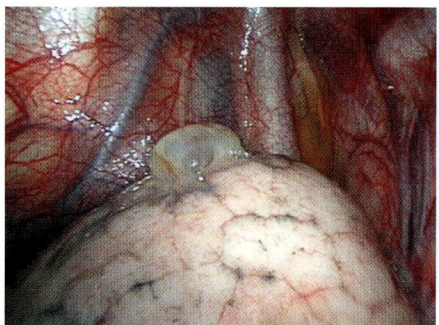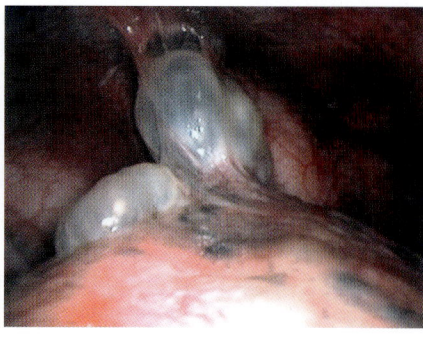

FIGURE 23-10 ■ A spontaneous pneumothorax generally develops from rupture of apical bullae. These bullae were found in two different patients at thoracoscopy for spontaneous pneumothorax.

as lifting or straining. Chest pain and shortness of breath are the most common symptoms. In a small number of patients, there can be an emergency presentation with tension pneumothorax. Tube thoracostomy is needed immediately in these patients.

Treatment is based on the patient's presentation. A small pneumothorax (10–15%) in a stable patient may be watched for a few hours followed by a repeat chest radiograph. Larger pneumothoraces require a chest tube or a small pigtail catheter for evacuation. Our protocol has been to try to manage the initial event nonoperatively using a small pigtail catheter. Assuming that the air leak resolves and the patient is asymptomatic, the patient is discharged. If the air leak does not resolve, then thoracoscopic exploration is necessary. Also, for patients presenting with a second episode, thoracoscopy is utilized for management as well. Often, these patients will be taken from the emergency room to the operating room if they are stable and bypass the need for a tube thoracoscopy as their initial intervention.

Some clinicians value a CT scan in the management of patients with a spontaneous pneumothorax. A recent study from our hospital looked at the management of 34 patients over three years.[116] The mean age was 16 years and there was an average of 1.7 pneumothoraces per patient before operation. CT scans were performed in 26 cases and blebs were found on eight studies. However, of the 18 negative scans, 14 patients (78%) were found to have blebs at thoracoscopy. In this study, the sensitivity of CT scan for identifying blebs was 36%. The authors concluded that the decisions for operation should be based on clinical judgment without the use of CT scans.

The optimal approach for management in these patients is thoracoscopy. If a bleb is identified, then it can be ligated and excised. Also, pleurodesis can be performed with a variety of measures including the use of the electrocautery scratch pad to abrade the cupola of the lung. Talc poudrage has also been found to have a high success rate in treatment of spontaneous pneumothorax and a very low morbidity.[117]

An interesting observation is that a number of children who develop a spontaneous pneumothorax on one side will present at some point with similar findings on the other side. Our feeling is that each side is managed separately. An operation is reserved for a second recurrence on each side rather than the development of a new spontaneous pneumothorax on the contralateral side.

REFERENCES

1. Jaffe A, Calder AD, Owens CM, et al. Role of routine computed tomography in paediatric pleural empyema. Thorax 2008; 63:897–902.
2. McIntosh K. Community-acquired pneumonia in children. N Engl J Med 2002;346:429–37.
3. Byington CL, Spencer LY, Johnson TA, et al. An epidemiological investigation of a sustained high rate of pediatric parapneumonic empyema: Risk factors and microbiological associations. Clin Infect Dis 2002;34: 434–40.
4. Tan TQ, Mason EO Jr, Wald ER, et al. Clinical characteristics of children with complicated pneumonia caused by Streptococcus pneumoniae. Pediatrics 2002;110:1–6.
5. Grijalva CG, Nuorti JP, Zhu Y, et al. Increasing Incidence of Empyema Complicating Childhood Community Acquired Pneumonia In The United States. CID 2010:50:805–13.
6. Balfour-Lynn IM, Abrahamson E, Cohen G, et al. BTS guidelines for the management of pleural infection in children. Thorax 2005;60(Suppl. 1):i1–21.
7. Bradley JS, Byington CL, Shah SS, et al. Executive Summary: The management of community acquired pneumonia in infants and children older than 3 months of age: Clinical practice guidelines by the Pediatric Infectious Disease Society and the Infectious Disease Society of America. Clin Infect Dis 2011;53: 617–30.
8. Hamm H, Light RW. Parapneumonic effusion and empyema. Eur Respir J 1997;10:1150–6.
9. Idell S, Girard W, Koenig KB, et al. Abnormalities of pathways of fibrin turnover in the human pleural space. Am Rev Respir Dis 1991;144:187–94.
10. Light RW. Parapneumonic effusions and empyema. Clin Chest Med 1985;6:55–62.
11. Picard E, Joseph L, Goldberg S, et al. Predictive factors of morbidity in childhood parapneumonic effusion-associated pneumonia: A retrospective study. Pediatr Infect Dis J 2010;29:840–3.
12. Padman R, King KA, Iqbal S, et al. Parapneumonic effusion and empyema in children: Retrospective review of the duPont experience. ClinPediatr (Phila) 2007;46:518–22.
13. Porcel J, Vives M, Esquerda A. Tumor necrosis factor-α in pleural fluid: A marker of complicated parapneumonic effusions. Chest 2004;125:160–4.
14. Light RW. A new classification of parapneumonic effusions and empyema. Chest 1995;108:299–301
15. Colice GL, Curtic A, Deslauriers J, et al. Medical and surgical treatment of parapneumonic effusions: An evidence based guideline. Chest 2000;118:1158–71
16. Wong KS, Lin TY, Huang YC, et al. Scoring system for empyema thoracis and help in management. Indian J Pediatr 2005;72: 1025–8.
17. Buckingham S, King M, Miller M. Incidence and etiologies of complicated parapneumonic effusions in children. Pediatr Infect Dis 2003;22:499–504.
18. McLaughlin F, Goldman D, Rosenbaum D, et al. Empyema in children: Clinical course and long-term follow-up. Pediatrics 1984;73:587–93.
19. Goeman A, Kipur N, Toppare M, et al. Conservative treatment of empyema in children. Respiration 1993;60:182–5.

20. Schultz KD, Fan L, Pinsky J, et al. The changing face of pleural empyemas in children: Epidemiology and management. Pediatrics 2004;113:1735–40.
21. King S, Thomson A. Radiological perspectives in empyema. Br Med Bull 2002;61:203–14.
22. Brixey AG, Luo Y, Skouras V, et al. The efficacy of chest radiographs in detecting parapneumonic effusions. Respirology 2011;16:1000–4.
23. Balik M, Plasil P, Waldauf P, et al. Ultrasound estimation of volume of pleural fluid in mechanically ventilated patients. Intensive Care Med 2006;32:318–21.
24. Eibenberger KL, Dock WI, Ammann ME, et al. Quantification of pleural effusions: Sonography versus radiography. Radiology 1994;191:681–4.
25. Calder A, Owens CM. Imaging of parapneumonic pleural effusions and empyema in children. Pediatr Radiol 2009;39:527–37.
26. Kurian J, Levin TL, Han BK, et al. Comparison of ultrasound and CT in the evaluation of pneumonia complicated by parapneumonic effusion in children. AJR Am J Roentgenol 2009;193:1648–54.
27. Pillai D, Song X, Pastor W, et al. Implementation and impact of a consensus diagnostic and management algorithm for complicated pneumonia in children. J Investig Med 2011;59:1221–7.
28. Shomaker KL, Weiner T, Esther CR Jr. Impact of an evidence-based algorithm on quality of care in pediatric parapneumonic effusion and empyema. Pediatr Pulmonol 2011;46:722–8.
29. Brenner DJ, Hall EJ. Computed tomography–an increasing source of radiation exposure. N Engl J Med 2007;357:2277–84.
30. Carter E, Waldhausen J, Zhang W, et al. Management of children with empyema: Pleural drainage is not always necessary. Pediatr Pulmonol 2010;45:475–80.
31. Soares P, Barreira J, Pissarra S, et al. Pediatric parapneumonic pleural effusions: Experience in a university central hospital. Rev Port Pneumol 2009;15: 241–59.
32. Shoseyov D, Bibi H, Shatzberg G, et al. Short-term course and outcome of treatments of pleural empyema in pediatric patients: Repeated ultrasound-guided needle thoracocentesis vs chest tube drainage. Chest 2002;121:836–40.
33. Epaud R, Aubertin G, Larroquet M, et al. Conservative use of chest tube insertion in children with pleural effusion. Pediatr Surg Int 2006;22:357–62.
34. Rahman NM, Maskell NA, Davies CW, et al. The relationship between chest tube size and clinical outcome in pleural infection. Chest 2010;137:536–43.
35. Lin CH, Lin WC, Chang JS. Comparison of pigtail catheter with chest tube for drainage of parapneumonic effusion in children. Pediatr Neonatol 2011;52:337–41.
36. Wurnig PN, Wittmer V, Pridun NS, et al. Video-assisted thoracic surgery for pleural empyema. Ann Thorac Surg 2006;81:309–13.
37. Hope WW, Bolton WD, Stephenson JE. The utility and timing of surgical intervention for parapneumonic empyema in the era of video-assisted thoracoscopy. Am Surg 2005;71:512–14.
38. Olgac G, Fazlioglu M, Kutlu CA. VATS decortication in patients with stage 3 empyema. Thorac Cardiovasc Surg 2005;53:18–20.
39. Cheng G, Vintch JR. A retrospective analysis of the management of parapneumonic empyemas in a county teaching facility from 1992 to 2004. Chest 2005;128:3284–90.
40. Tsao K, St Peter SD, Sharp SW, et al. Current application of thoracoscopy in children. J Laparoendosc Adv Surg Tech A 2008;18:131–5.
41. Kurt BA, Winterhalter KM, Connors RH, et al. Therapy of parapneumonic effusions in children: Video assisted thoracoscopic surgery versus conventional thoracostomy drainage. Pediatrics 2006;118:e547–553.
42. Gates RL, Hogan M, Weinstein S, et al. Drainage, fibrinolytics, or surgery: A comparison of treatment options in pediatric empyema. J Pediatr Surg 2004;39:1638–42.
43. Aziz A, Healey JM, Qureshi F, et al. Comparative analysis of chest tube thoracostomy and video-assisted thoracoscopic surgery in empyema and parapneumonic effusion associated with pneumonia in children. Surg Infect (Larchmt) 2008;9:317–23.
44. Chiu CY, Wong KS, Huang YC, et al. Echo-guided management of complicated parapneumonic effusion in children. Pediatr Pulmonol 2006;41:1226–32.
45. Freitas S, Fraga JC, Canani F. Thoracoscopy in children with complicated parapneumonic pleural effusion at the fibrinopurulent stage: A multi-institutional study. J Bras Pneumol 2009;35:660–8.
46. Yao CT, Wu JM, Liu CC, et al. Treatment of complicated parapneumonic pleural effusion with intrapleural streptokinase in children. Chest 2004;125:566–71.
47. Ekingen G, Guvenc BH, Sozubir S, et al. Fibrinolytic treatment of complicated pediatric thoracic empyemas with intrapleural streptokinase. Eur J Cardiothorac Surg 2004;26:503–7.
48. Misthos P, Sepsas E, Konstantinou M, et al. Early use of intrapleural fibrinolytics in the management of postpneumonic empyema. A prospective study. Eur J Cardiothorac Surg 2005;28:599–603.
49. Kiliç N, Celebi S, Gürpinar A, et al. Management of thoracic empyema in children. Pediatr Surg Int 2002;18:21–3.
50. Cochran JB, Tecklenburg FW, Turner RB. Intrapleural instillation of fibrinolytic agents for treatment of pleural empyema. Pediatr Crit Care Med 2003;4:39–43.
51. Ulku R, Onat S, Kiliç N. Intrapleural fibrinolytic treatment of multiloculated pediatric empyemas. Minerva Pediatr 2004;56: 419–23.
52. Bouros D, Antoniou KM, Chalkiadakis G, et al. The role of video-assisted thoracoscopic surgery in the treatment of parapneumonic empyema after the failure of fibrinolytics. Surg Endosc 2002;16: 151–4.
53. Sonnappa S, Cohen G, Owens CM, et al. Comparison of urokinase and video-assisted thoracoscopic surgery for treatment of childhood empyema. Am J Respir Crit Care Med 2006;174: 221–7.
54. St. Peter SD, Tsao K, Spilde TL, et al. Thoracoscopic decortication vs tube thoracostomy with fibrinolysis for empyema in children: A prospective, randomized trial. J Pediatr Surg 2009; 44:106–11.
55. Zuckerman DA, Reed MF, Howington JA, et al. Efficacy of intrapleural tissue-type plasminogen activator in the treatment of loculated parapneumonic effusions. J Vasc Interv Radiol 2009;20:1066–9.
56. Cohen E, Weinstein M, Fisman DN. Cost-effectiveness of competing strategies for the treatment of pediatric empyema. Pediatrics 2008;121:e1250–1257.
57. Kalfa N, Allal H, Lopez M, et al. Thoracoscopy in pediatric pleural empyema: A prospective study of prognostic factors. J Pediatr Surg 2006;41:1732–7.
58. Bouros D, Schiza S, Tzanakis N, et al. Intrapleural urokinase versus normal saline in the treatment of complicated parapneumonic effusions and empyema. A randomized, double-blind study. Am J Respir Crit Care Med 1999;159:37–42.
59. Diacon AH, Theron J, Schuurmans MM, et al. Intrapleural streptokinase for empyema and complicated parapneumonic effusions. Am J Respir Crit Care Med 2004;170:49–53.
60. Proesmans M, De Boeck K. Clinical practice: Treatment of childhood empyema. Eur J Pediatr 2009;168:639–45.
61. Gasior AC, Knott EM, Sharp SW, et al. Experience with an evidence-based protocol using fibrinolysis as first-line treatment for empyema in children. J Pediatr Surg 2013;48:1312–15.
62. Kosloske AM, Ball WS, Butler C, et al. Drainage of pediatric lung abscess by cough, catheter or complete resection. J Pediatr Surg 1986;21:596–60.
63. Tseng Y, Wu M, Lin M. Surgery for lung abscess in immunocompetent and immunocompromised children. J Pediatr Surg 2001;36:470–3.
64. Estera AS, Platt MR, Mills LJ, et al. Primary lung abscess. J Thorac Cardiovasc Surg 1980;79: 275–82.
65. Chidi CC, Mendelsohn HJ. Lung abscess. A study of the results of treatment based on 90 consecutive cases. J Thorac Cardiovasc Surg 1974;68:168–72.
66. Lorenzo RL, Bradford BF, Black J, et al. Lung abscesses in children: Diagnostic and therapeutic needle aspiration. Radiology 1985;157: 79–80.
67. Ball BS, Bisset GS, Towbin RB. Percutaneous drainage of chest abscesses in children. Radiology 1989;171: 431–4.
68. Hoffer FA, Bloom DA, Colin AA, et al. Lung abscess versus necrotizing pneumonia: Implications for interventional therapy. Pediatr Radiol 1999;29:87–91.

69. Patradoon-Ho P, Fitzgerald DA. Lung abscesses in children. Paediatr Respir Rev 2007;8:77–84.
70. Nagasawa KK, Johnson SM. Thoracoscopic treatment of pediatric lung abscesses J Pediatr Surg 2010;45:574–8.
71. Ayed AK, Al-Rowayeh A. Lung resection in children for infectious pulmonary diseases. Pediatr Surg Int 2005;21:604–8.
72. Quigley MJ, Fraser RS. Pulmonary pneumatocele: Pathology and pathogenesis. AJR Am J Roentgenol 1988;150:1275–7.
73. Oviawe O, Ogundipe O. Pneumatoceles associated with pneumonia: Incidence and clinical course in Nigerian children. Trop Geogr Med 1985;37:264–9.
74. Glustein JZ, Kaplan M. Enterobacter cloacae causing pneumatocele in a neonate. Acta Pediatr 1994;83:990–1.
75. Zuhdi MK, Bradley JS, Spear RM, et al. Fatal air embolism as a complication of staphylococcal pneumonia with pneumatoceles. Pediatr Infect Dis J 1995;14:811–12.
76. Zuhdi MK, Spear R, Worthen M, et al. Percutaneous catheter drainage of tension pneumatocele, secondarily infected pneumatocele and lung abscess in children. Crit Care Med 1996;42:330–3.
77. Kogutt M, Lutrell C, Pulau F, et al. Decompression of pneumatocele in a neonate by percutaneous catheter placement. Pediatr Radiol 1999;29:488–9.
78. Laënnec RTH. De l'Auscultation Médiaté on Traite du Diagnostic des Maladies des Poumons et du Coeur, Fondé Principalement sur ce Noveau Moyer d'Exploration. Paris: Brosson et Claude; 1819.
79. Reid LM. Reduction in bronchial subdivision in bronchiectasis. Thorax 1950;5:233–47.
80. Rademacher J, Welte T. Bronchiectasis-Diagnosis and Treatment. Dtsch Arztebl Int 2011;108: 809–15
81. McGuinnea G, Naidich DP. CT of airways disease and bronchiectasis. Radiol Clin North Am 2002;40:1–19.
82. Agasthian T, Deschamps C, Trastek VF, et al. Surgical management of bronchiectasis. Ann Thorac Surg 1996;62:976–80.
83. Goeminne P, Dupont L. Non-cystic fibrosis bronchiectasis: Diagnosis and management in 21st century. Postgrad Med J 2010;86:493–501.
84. Kumar NA, Nguyen B, Maki D. Bronchiectasis: Current clinical and imaging concepts. Semin Roentgenol 2001;36:41–50.
85. Smevik B. Complementary investigations in bronchiectasis in children. Monaldi Arch Chest Dis 2000;55:420–6.
86. Ashour M, Al-Kattan K, Rafay MA, et al. Current surgical therapy for bronchiectasis. World J Surg 1999;23:1096–1104.
87. Haciibrahimoglu G, Fazliogu M, Olcmen A, et al. Surgical management of childhood bronchiectasis due to infectious disease. Gen Thorac Surg 2004;127:1361–5.
88. Otgün I, Karnak I, Tanyel FC, et al. Surgical treatment of bronchiectasis in children. J Pediatr Surg 2004;39:1532–6.
89. Rothenberg SS, Kuenzler KA, Middlesworth W. Thoracoscopic lobectomy for severe bronchiectasis in children. J Laparoendosc Adv Surg Tech A 2009;19:555–7.
90. Dubin P, King I, Gallagher P. Congenital chylothorax. Curr Opin Pediatr 2000;12:505–9.
91. Beghatti M, La Scala G, Belli D, et al. Etiology and management of pediatric chylothorax. J Pediatr 2000;8:136–8.
92. Allen EM, Van Heeckeren DW, Spector ML, et al. Management of nutritional and infectious complications of postoperative chylothorax in children. J Pediatr Surg 1991;26:1169–74.
93. Bond SJ, Guzzetta PC, Snyder ML, et al. Management of pediatric postoperative chylothorax. Ann Thoracic Surg 1993;56:469–73.
94. Sharkey AJ, Rao JN. The successful use of octreotide in the treatment of traumatic chylothorax. Tex Heart Inst J 2012;39:428–30.
95. Luca R, Bini R, Chessa M, et al. The effectiveness of octreotide in the treatment of postoperative chylothorax. Eur J Pediatr 2002;161:149–50.
96. Rodgers B, Michalsky MP, Kattwinkel J. The use of octreotide to treat congenital chylothorax. J Pediatr Surg 2006;41:845–7.
97. Au M, Weber TR, Flemmin RE. Successful use of octreotide in a case of neonatal chylothorax. J Pediatr Surg 2003;38:1106–7.
98. Benedix F, Schulz HU, Scheidbach H, et al. Successful conservative treatment of chylothorax following oesophagectomy - a clinical algorithm. S Afr J Surg 2010;48:86–8.
99. Valentine VG, Raffin TA. The management of chylothorax. Chest 1992;102:586–91.
100. Buchan K, Amir-Reza H, Ritchie A. Thoracoscopic thoracic duct ligation for traumatic chylothorax. Ann Thorac Surg 2001;72:1366–7.
101. Graham DD, McGahren ED, Tribble CG, et al. Use of video-assisted thoracic surgery in the treatment of chylothorax. Ann Thorac Surg 1994;57:1507–11.
102. Fahimi H, Casselman F, Mariani M, et al. Current management of postoperative chylothorax. Ann Thorac Surg 2001;71:448–51.
103. Cope C. Management of chylothorax via percutaneous embolization. Curr Opin Pulmon Med 2004;10:311–14.
104. Cope C, Kaiser LR. Management of unremitting chylothorax by percutaneous embolization and blockage of retroperitoneal lymphatic vessels in 42 patients. J Vasc Interv Radiol 2002;13:1139–48.
105. Wolff AB, Silen ML, Kokoska ER, et al. Treatment of refractory chylothorax with externalized pleuroperitoneal shunts in children. Ann Thorac Surg 1999;68:1053–7.
106. Turner-Warwick M. Interstitial lung disease. Semin Respir Med 1984;6:1–102.
107. Fan L, Langston C. Chronic interstitial lung disease in children. Pediatr Pulmonol 1993;16:184–96.
108. Bokulic RE, Hilman BC. Interstitial lung disease in children. Pediatr Clin North Am 1994;41:543–67.
109. Langston C, Patterson K, Dishop MK, et al. Child Pathology Co-operative Group. A protocol for the handling of tissue obtained by operative lung biopsy: Recommendations of the child pathology co-operative group. Pediatr Dev Pathol 2006;9:173–80.
110. Wagner RB, Johnston MR. Middle lobe syndrome. Ann Thorac Surg 1983;35:679–86.
111. Saha SP, Mayo P, Long GA, et al. Middle lobe syndrome: Diagnosis and management. Ann Thorac Surg 1982;33:28–31.
112. Yung K, Aspestrand F, Kolbenstvedt A. High-resolution CT and bronchography in the assessment of bronchiectasis. Acta Radiol 1991;32:439–41.
113. Sehitoqullari A, Sayir F, Cobanaglu U, et al. Surgical treatment of right middle lobe syndrome in children. Ann Thorac Med 2012;7:8–11.
114. Healthcare Cost and Utilization Project (HCUP). Kids' Inpatient Database (KID). 1997, 2000, 2003, 2006. Available at: http://www.hcup-us.ahrq.gov/kidoverview.jsp. Accessed October 15, 2010.
115. United States Census Bureau. Your Gateway to Census 2000. Available at http://www.census.gov/main/www/cen2000.html. Accessed October 15, 2010.
116. Laituri CA, Valusek PA, Rivard DC, et al. The utility of computed tomography in the management of patients with spontaneous pneumothorax. J Pediatr Surg 2011;46:1523–5.
117. Cardillo G, Carleo F, Giunti R, et al. Videothoracoscopic talc poudrage in primary spontaneous pneumothorax: A single-institution experience in 861 cases. J Thorac Cardiovasc Surg 2006;131:322–8.

CHAPTER 24

CONGENITAL DIAPHRAGMATIC HERNIA AND EVENTRATION

KuoJen Tsao • Kevin P. Lally

The management and treatment of congenital diaphragmatic hernia (CDH) remains a challenge. Despite advances in prenatal diagnosis, operative management, and neonatal critical care, infants born with CDH still have a significant mortality and long-term disability. The relatively rare incidence of the disease and wide spectrum of disease severity results in clinical challenges for individual practitioners and institutions. The large majority of centers will treat less than 10 CDH infants per year.[1] Thus, broad clinical experience, especially in cases of the most severe disease, is difficult to achieve.

The morbidity and mortality associated with CDH is largely due to pulmonary hypoplasia and pulmonary vascular hypertension (PHTN).[2,3] Over the last 25 years, clinical efforts to avoid lung injury, including extracorporeal membrane oxygenation (ECMO), high-frequency oscillating ventilation (HFOV), and permissive hypercapnia, have improved overall survival, but significant variation remains amongst institutions.[2,4] Reported survival ranges from 50–90%.[3,5]

EPIDEMIOLOGY

The incidence of CDH has been reported as high as 1 in 2000 births.[6] In the USA, approximately 1,000 CDH infants are born with a prevalence of 2.4 per 10,000 live births.[6,7] One-third of infants with CDH die as stillbirths, often associated with other congenital anomalies.[8] However, the overall incidence of CDH may be underestimated. Proportions of fetuses are prenatally diagnosed with CDH and will die in utero or shortly after birth. Thus, many may never been seen or accounted for in a tertiary referral center. Presumed to be the most severe of all CDH infants, these patients contribute to the 'hidden mortality' of CDH.[9–12]

Infants with isolated CDH are typically male and one-third are associated with a major congenital anomaly.[7] Approximately 80% are left sided. Bilateral defects are rare and are associated with other major anomalies.[13] Although the exact etiology remains unknown, mothers that are thin or underweight may have an increased risk of bearing an infant with CDH.[14]

Genetics

CDH is no longer thought of as a sporadic isolated anomaly in all cases. A first-degree relative has an expected occurrence rate of approximately 2%.[15] All types of structural chromosomal abnormalities including deletions, translocations, and trisomies have been identified.[16–21] In addition, a gene distal to the 15q21 locus has been identified for the normal development of the diaphragm.[17,18]

CDH has been associated with over 70 syndromes.[19] In some cases, the diaphragmatic malformation is the predominant defect, as in Fryns and Donnai–Barrow syndromes.[20,21] In other syndromes, CDH only occurs in a small percentage, but still greater than the general population, as in Simpson–Golabi–Behmel and Beckwith–Wiedermann syndromes. The inheritance patterns for these syndromes include dominant and recessive as well as autosomal and X-linked variants.[22] Identifying the patterns of non-hernia-related anomalies associated with CDH and recognizing genetic syndromes help determine the prognosis, treatments, counseling, and outcomes.[16] If the antenatal diagnosis of CDH is made, amniocentesis with karyotype and chromosomal analysis is indicated.

Associated Anomalies

The posterolateral 'Bochdalek' hernia accounts for 90% of all diaphragmatic hernia cases.[23] The remainder are the anterior 'Morgagni' hernia along with defects of the central septum transversum. The majority of posterolateral CDH are left sided (85%), with right sided (13%) and bilateral (2%) accounting for the rest.[23–25]

Approximately 50% of CDH are isolated defects with the others associated with anomalies of the cardiovascular (27.5%), urogenital (17.7%), musculoskeletal (15.7%), and central nervous (9.8%) systems (CNS).[26] Many conditions, such as lung hypoplasia, intestinal malrotation, some cardiac malformations, and patent ductus arteriosus (PDA) are considered to be consequences of the diaphragmatic defect. Non-CDH-related defects are estimated to occur in 40–60% of cases and can involve the cardiovascular, CNS, gastrointestinal, and genitourinary systems, and may be a consequence of an underlying field defect of unknown etiology.[27,28]

The impact of associated anomalies on prognosis and outcome cannot be overstated. Ninety-five per cent of stillborn infants with CDH have an associated major anomaly.[29] Greater than 60% of infants who do not survive the immediate neonatal period have associated anomalies.[30] In contrast, infants that survive preoperative stabilization and come to operative repair have less than 10% additional anomalies.[30] Although the severity of pulmonary hypoplasia and hypertension are the major determinants of overall survival, there is a significant survival advantage for infants with isolated CDH (43.7% vs 7.1%).[27] Due to this dismal outcome, the emphasis on detailed and accurate prenatal diagnosis has influenced the management and treatment of CDH. Twenty per cent of prenatally diagnosed CDH infants have chromosomal anomalies, with 70% having an associated structural malformation. In contrast, only 35% of postnatally diagnosed CDH infants have an associated anomaly.[27] This difference may be the result of lethal chromosomal anomalies and/or may reflect parental decisions for termination in high-risk infants with anomalies that portend significant morbidity.

Common cardiac defects include atrial septal defects (ASDs), ventricular septal defects (VSDs), and other outflow tract anomalies (transposition of the great vessels, tetralogy of Fallot, double-outlet right ventricle, and aortic coarctation).[30–32] In a review of 4,268 infants with CDH, approximately 18% of infants had an associated cardiac defect. Major cardiac lesions (excluding patent foramen ovale, atrial septal defects, PDA) was 8% with an overall survival of 36% compared to infants with minor anomalies (67% survival) and those without cardiac defects (73% survival).[33]

Cost

Despite improvements in outcomes and advances in treatment, the cost of caring for CDH infants continues to increase. Data from the Kids' Inpatient Database has projected the annual national costs to range between $264 and $400 million based on 60% overall survival.[34] The utilization of ECMO was the highest single factor associated with cost with a 2.4-fold increase in expenditures from 1997 to 2006. The highest median cost were ECMO patients at $156,499.90/patient, constituting 28.5% of the total national costs.[34] Single-center reports

have documented expenses as high as $250,000 per CDH case with an estimated annual cost of $230 million, and estimated cost of $98,000 for non-ECMO survivors compared with $365,000 for ECMO survivors.[35]

EMBRYOLOGY

Diaphragm development and CDH pathogenesis

The development of the human diaphragm is a complex, multicellular, multi-tissue interaction that is poorly understood. Precursors to the diaphragm begin to form during the fourth week of gestation. Historically, the diaphragm was thought to develop from the fusion of four embryonic components: anteriorly by the septum transversum, dorsolaterally by the pleuroperitoneal folds (PPF), dorsally by the crura from the esophageal mesentery, and posteriorly by the body wall mesoderm (Fig. 24-1).[36,37] As the embryo begins to form, the septum transversum migrates dorsally and separates the pleuro-pericardial cavity from the peritoneal cavity. At this point, the pleural and peritoneal cavities still communicate. The septum transversum interacts with the PPF and mesodermal tissue surrounding the developing esophagus and other foregut structures, resulting in the formation of primitive diaphragmatic structures. Bound by pericardial, pleural, and peritoneal folds, the paired PPFs now separate the pleuropericardial and peritoneal cavities. Eventually, the septum transversum develops into the central tendon.[36,37] As the PPF develops during the sixth week of gestation, concurrently, the pleuroperitoneal membranes close and separate the pleural and abdominal cavities by the eighth week of gestation. Typically, the right side closes before the left. Ultimately, the phrenic axons and myogenic cells destined for neuromuscularization

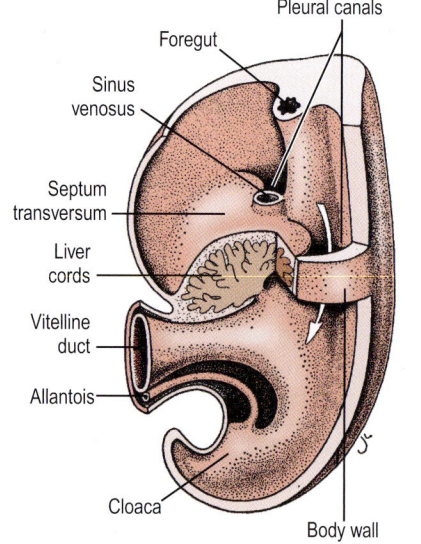
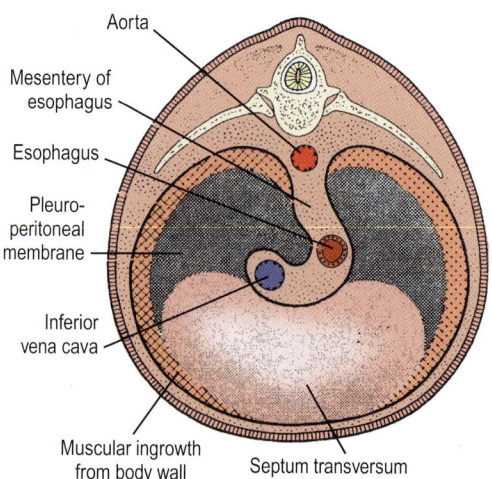

FIGURE 24-1 ■ Historically, the diaphragm has been thought to develop from fusion of its four embryologic components. According to this theory, the septum transversum fuses posteriorly with the mediastinal mesenchyme. The pleuroperitoneal canals (arrow) allow free communication between the pleural and peritoneal cavities. Closure of these canals is completed as the pleuroperitoneal membranes develop. The four embryologic components of the developing diaphragm are shown in cross section. (From Skandalakis IJ, Colborn GL, Skandalakis JE. In: Nyhus LM, Baker RJ, Fischer JE, editors. Mastery of Surgery. 3rd ed. Boston: Little, Brown; 1996.)

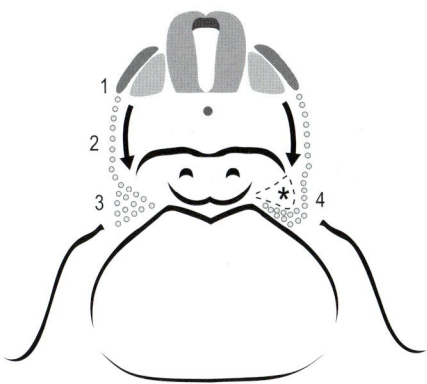

1. Muscle precursor cells delaminate from the lateral dermo-myotomal lip
2. Delaminated cells migrate through the lateral body wall
3. MPC's arrive in the PPF, from which point they spread out to populate the growing diaphragm
4. In CDH, the dorsolateral region of the PPF is missing (*) and MPC's are concentrated in the remaining tissue, ultimately leading to thickening of the diaphragm around the defect

FIGURE 24-2 ■ This schematic depicts a different embryologic pathway for diaphragmatic development and CDH formation than seen in Figure 24-1. On the left side, (1–3) is the proposed normal pathway for diaphragm development. On the right side, (4) is the pathway for CDH formation. MPC, muscle precursor cells; PPF, pleuroperitoneal fold. (From Clugston RD, Greer JJ. Diaphragm development and congenital diaphragmatic hernia. Semin Pediatr Surg 2007;16:94–100.)

migrate to the PPF and form the mature diaphragm.[38] The muscularization of the primitive diaphragm is a separate, but inter-related process. Historically, the primitive fetal diaphragm is thought to muscularize from the inner thoracic musculature as the diaphragm closes.[39] Others have implicated a progressive development of the pleuroperitoneal membrane[40] or the posthepatic mesenchymal plate (PHMP) interacting with the PPF.[41]

Another theory for CDH development is a failure of muscularization of the future diaphragm prior to complete closure of the canal (Fig. 24-2).[42] Inadequate closure of the pleuroperitoneal canal allows the abdominal viscera to enter the thoracic cavity when it returns from the extraembryonic coelom as well as the liver to herniate into the chest. Consequently, the limited intrathoracic space, due to the visceral herniation, results in pulmonary hypoplasia.

Although traditional theories suggest that the lung hypoplasia is secondary to the diaphragmatic malformation, others have postulated that the primary disturbance may be abnormal lung development that causes the diaphragmatic defect.[36] According to this theory, disturbances in lung bud formation subsequently impair the PHMP development, and results in failure of diaphragm fusion/muscularization.

The nitrofen murine model has led to improved understanding of abnormal pulmonary development in CDH.[43] Nitrofen (2,4-dichloro-phenyl-*p*-nitrophenyl ether) is an environmental teratogen that is relatively harmless to adult mice. However, if given during pregnancy, it can cause pulmonary, cardiac, skeletal, and diaphragmatic abnormalities.[44] Diaphragmatic defects

resulting from the administration of nitrofen in mice are very similar to the diaphragmatic defects seen in babies with CDH in regards to size, location, and herniation of abdominal viscera.[45,46] The side of the CDH depends on the time of nitrofen exposure during gestation. In nitrofen-exposed fetal mice, a defect is clearly seen in the posterolateral portions of the PPF.[47] In addition, nitrofen exposure appears to affect muscularization of the PPF (see Fig. 24-2).[48] Finally, the offspring will exhibit features of pulmonary hypoplasia including reduced airway branching, surfactant deficiency, pulmonary vascular abnormalities, and respiratory failure at birth.[49,50]

Other teratogens structurally similar to nitrofen have been shown to induce CDH in animal models as well. Although the exact etiology of CDH is unknown, these teratogens commonly affect the retinoic acid synthesis pathway by inhibiting retinol dehydrogenase-2 and causing similar diaphragmatic defects.[51] Several clinical observations and molecular studies have supported the importance of the retinoic acid pathways in CDH development. Vitamin A-deficient rodents will produce offspring with CDH of variable severity.[52] Retinoic acid receptor knockout mice produce fetuses with CDH.[53] Failure to convert retinoic acid to retinaldehyde following administration of nitrofen produces posterolateral diaphragmatic defects in rats.[51] Lower plasma levels of retinoic acid and retinol binding protein in infants with CDH have been found compared to controls.[54]

Lung Development and Pulmonary Hypoplasia

Lung development is recognized as a complex programmed event regulated by genetic signals, transcription factors, growth factors, and hormones. These events control the temporal and spatial interactions between epithelium and endothelium. Early transcription signals, such as thyroid transcription factor-1 and hepatocyte nuclear factor-3β, regulate pulmonary development from the primitive foregut mesenchyme. Other pathways of pulmonary development include sonic hedgehog, transforming growth factor-β, Notch-delta pathway, and Wingless-Int.[22,55] In addition, glucocorticoids, thyroid hormone, and retinoic acid have all been shown to regulate pulmonary organogenesis.[50]

Fetal lung development is divided into five overlapping stages.[56] (1) The *embryonic stage* begins during the third week of gestation as a caudal diverticulum from the laryngotracheal groove. The primary lung buds and trachea form from this diverticulum by the fourth week and lobar structures are seen by the sixth week. (2) The *pseudoglandular stage* occurs between the fifth and 17th weeks of gestation with the formation of formal lung buds as well as the main and terminal bronchi. (3) During the *canalicular stage*, the pulmonary vessels, respiratory bronchioles, and alveolar ducts develop between weeks 16 and 25 weeks with the appearance of type 1 pneumocytes and type 2 pneumocyte precursors. At this stage, functional gas exchange is possible. (4) *The saccular stage* continues from 24 weeks to term with the maturation of alveolar sacs. Airway dimensions and surfactant synthesis capabilities continue to mature as well. (5) Finally, the *alveolar stage* begins after birth with a continued increase and development of functional alveoli.

Concomitantly, fetal pulmonary vascular development occurs in concordance with the associated lung development and follows the pattern of airway and alveolar maturation. A functional unit known as the acinus consists of the alveolus, alveolar ducts, and respiratory bronchioles. The pulmonary vasculature develops as these acinar units multiply and evolve during the canalicular stage. The preacinar structures consist of the trachea, major bronchi, lobar bronchi, and terminal bronchioles. The pulmonary vascular development for the preacinus is typically completed by end of the pseudoglandular stage.[57-59] In theory, any impedance to normal pulmonary development will concurrently hinder pulmonary vascular development.

Pulmonary hypoplasia is characterized by a decrease in bronchial divisions, bronchioles, and alveoli. The alveoli and terminal saccules exhibit abnormal septations that impair the air–capillary interface limiting gas exchange.[60] At birth, the alveoli are thick-walled with intra-alveolar septations. These immature alveoli have increased glycogen content leading to thickened secretions which further limit gas exchange. Animal models of CDH have demonstrated pulmonary hypoplasia with decreased levels of total lung DNA and protein. In addition, the pulmonary vasculature appears to be less compliant with abnormally thick-walled arterioles.[61] Surfactant levels are also decreased which may result in immature functioning lungs.[62] Endogenous surfactant synthesis has been found to be decreased in CDH infants that required ECMO compared with non-CDH ventilated neonates without significant lung disease.[63] Interestingly, the contralateral lung also exhibits the structural abnormalities of pulmonary hypoplasia.

Pulmonary Vascular Development and Pulmonary Hypertension

Normal fetal cardiopulmonary circulation transitions to it postnatal state rapidly with a tenfold increase in pulmonary blood flow shortly after birth. Fetal pulmonary blood flow is characterized as a low-flow, high-resistance circuit due to medial and adventitial hypertrophy of the vasculature.[64] Normally, the pulmonary vascular resistance quickly decreases as the distal small pulmonary arteries and arterioles remodel over the first few months of life, resulting in a low-resistance, high-flow postnatal circulation.[65,66] However, this process appears to be arrested in CDH newborns, and the fetal circulation persists resulting in PHTN. In fact, the abnormal fetal pulmonary circulation in CDH fetuses appears to occur in early gestation. The pulmonary arteries exhibit a decrease in density per unit of lung parenchyma as well as an increase in muscularization that extends to the vasculature at the acinar level.[67] In fetal lamb models of surgically created CDH as well as human fetuses with CDH, there is a relative decrease in lung parenchyma.[68,69] This impaired lung growth and development has been speculated to be related to impaired vascular development.[70] As a result, PHTN appears to develop in utero, which may cause a reduction in pulmonary artery

growth, proper alveolar development, and normal lung growth.[71]

Utilizing fetal Doppler ultrasound (US), fetuses with CDH exhibit a decrease in the overall pulmonary blood flow and vascularity.[72] The modified McGoon Index, a ratio of the combined diameter of the proximal pulmonary arteries to the descending aorta, may help predict the degree of PHTN that correlates with death. A modified McGoon Index of ≤1.3 has an 85% sensitivity and 100% specificity for mortality.[73] An index <1.25 and birth weight <2755 g has been shown to result in 80% mortality, with a sensitivity of 73% and a specificity of 78%.[74] The arterial adventitia and medial wall thickness are increased in postmortem CDH infants compared to controls.[75,76] In addition, the adventitial thickness and area were greater in CDH stillborns and newborns when compared to live born non-CDH infants, suggesting that increased muscularization of the pulmonary vasculature occurs in utero and fails to appropriately remodel after birth.

In a retrospective study, CDH infants who developed normal pulmonary artery pressures during the first 3 weeks of life were found to have a 100% survival rate.[77] In this same study, an intermediate reduction in elevated pulmonary pressures after birth were seen in 34% of infants with a 75% survival. Mortality was 100% in CDH infants that failed to normalize their pulmonary pressures despite therapy. Although contemporary outcomes for infants with pulmonary hypertension have improved, these data underscore the importance of PHTN in CDH.

DIAGNOSIS

Prenatal Diagnosis

Due to the wide discrepancy of disease severity and potential fetal therapies, accurate and timely prenatal diagnosis of CDH is important. The differential diagnosis for CDH include other pulmonary anomalies, such as congenital pulmonary airway malformations (CPAM), bronchogenic cysts, bronchial atresia, or bronchopulmonary sequestrations, as well as mediastinal lesions, including enteric, neuroenteric, or thymic cysts. In these conditions, the normal intra-abdominal anatomy is not disturbed. In addition, diaphragmatic eventration can be misinterpreted for CDH. Although this differentiation from CDH can be difficult, this distinction is important as diaphragmatic eventration portends a much better prognosis and requires different management. Eventration are typically isolated lesions, but may be associated with pleural and/or pericardial effusions.[78]

The diagnosis of CDH can be made by ultrasound as early as 11 weeks' gestation, although most are not seen until after 16 weeks (Fig. 24-3).[79] Although most CDH can be detected during the second trimester, some sonographic features may not manifest until later in pregnancy.[80] Approximately 50–70% of CDH are diagnosed during pregnancy.[79,81] However, for some tertiary centers, 90% of CDH newborns may have been diagnosed in utero.[82] Fetal ultrasound features include polyhydramnios, bowel loops within the chest, an echogenic chest mass, and/or an intrathoracic stomach. Left-sided CDH

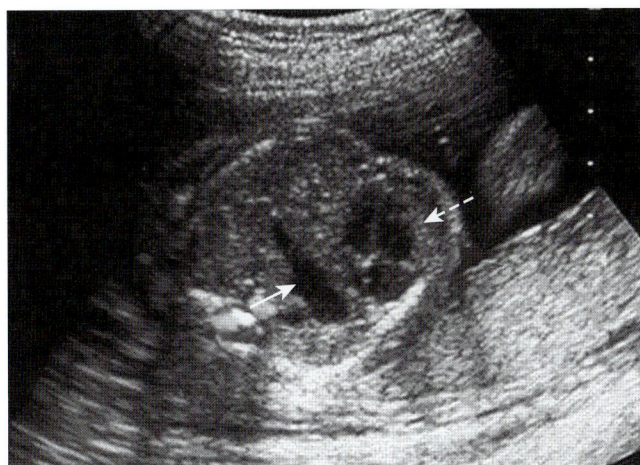

FIGURE 24-3 ■ Fetal ultrasound image at the level of the four-chamber heart (dotted arrow). Gastric bubble (solid arrow) at the level of the four-chamber heart suggests CDH. This is the level used to calculate the lung-to-head ratio.

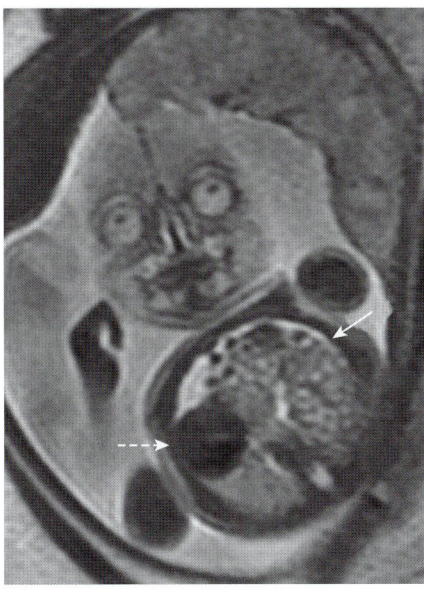

FIGURE 24-4 ■ Fetal MR image of a left-sided CDH at 28 weeks' gestation. A large CDH with herniation of the small bowel and stomach is found within the left hemithorax (solid arrow). There is dextroposition of the fetal heart (dotted arrow). There is no evidence of liver herniation.

typically feature mediastinal/cardiac shift to the right as well as herniation of stomach, intestines, and/or spleen. The liver may herniate but its echogeneity is often similar to the lung, and may be more difficult to differentiate. In right-sided CDH, the right lobe of the liver is herniated, with a left-sided mediastinal shift.

Ultrasound of the fetal chest is best performed in the axial plane. Fetal lung circumference, used to determine the lung-to-head ratio (LHR), is measured at the level of the four-chambered view of the heart (see Fig. 24-3). However, measurements of the fetal chest require an understanding of the dynamic growth of the fetal thorax which mostly occurs during the first trimester. During this time, the heart-to-thorax ratio is variable. However, after the first trimester, the heart-to-thorax ratio is generally 1:3 and remains unchanged thereafter.[83] The fetal diaphragm can be seen as early as the first trimester as a thin hypoechogenic line in the sagittal view.

Although independent sonographic features of CDH have not been shown to be accurate predictors for a poor prognosis, severe or advanced CDH may exhibit an intrathoracic 'liver up' (liver in the chest), mediastinal shift to the contralateral thoracic cavity, or features consistent with hydrops fetalis.[84] Two distinct ultrasound features have been commonly utilized to risk stratify: (1) LHR and (2) liver herniation into the chest. Predicting survival of CDH fetuses based on LHR has been statistically supported: 100% survival with LHR > 1.35, 61% with LHR between 1.35–0.6, and no survival with LHR < 0.6 in one series.[85] Survival based on liver herniation alone is 56%, compared to 100% survival without liver herniation.[86] The combination of liver herniation and low LHR (LHR < 1.0) has a 60% mortality in prenatally diagnosed CDH.[87–89] Although fetal ultrasound is the most reliable modality for prognosis, its inconsistent utilization and inter-rater variability has created variable results.[90,91]

Although the heart-to-thorax ratio is consistent after the first trimester, the effects of gestational age can influence the LHR. The fetal lung increases 16-fold, compared to a fourfold increase in head circumference, between 12 and 32 weeks gestational age. This

gestational age differential can be ameliorated by using the LHR as a function of observed or measured to the expected or mean of the same lung (O/E LHR). The definition of severe CDH as measured by O/E LHR is <25%. In one series, survival for severe CDH using this definition was approximately 10% with liver up and 25% with liver down. There were no survivors when O/E LHR was <15% with liver up.[92] The total fetal lung volume (TFLV) as determined by three-dimensional ultrasound may be more accurate than O/E LHR as it includes the contralateral lung.[93–95] Similar to the LHR, the effects of gestational age on fetal lung growth can be accounted for by using biometric measurements, total fetal body volume, or normal/expected total fetal lung volume, expressed as O/E TFLV.[96–98] Early work suggests that O/E TLFV in utero correlates well with outcome.[99,100]

Fetal magnetic resonance imaging (MRI) has become widely utilized in the prenatal diagnosis of CDH (Fig. 24-4). Due to the high water content, fetal lungs exhibit high signal intensity on T_2-weighted images which produces a stark contrast to the fetal chest and other organs. In addition, fetal MRI is an excellent modality for morphologic and volumetric measurements of the fetal lung. It is especially advantageous for oligohydramnios and maternal obesity. Utilizing an image thickness between 2–4 mm, the combination of T_2- and T_1-weighed images can help to differentiate and outline other organs, such as liver and intestine, as well as calculate MRI TFLV. The correlation between ultrasound and MRI-based measurements has been evaluated, but with limited results. The contralateral fetal lung volume (FLV) on ultrasound appears to correlate with TFLV measured by fetal MRI, irrespective of gestational age, side of defect, or liver herniation.[101] One study showed that ultrasound O/E LHR correlated well with the O/E contralateral FLV and TFLV by MRI ($R^2 = 0.44, P < 0.001; R^2 = 0.37, P < 0.001$,

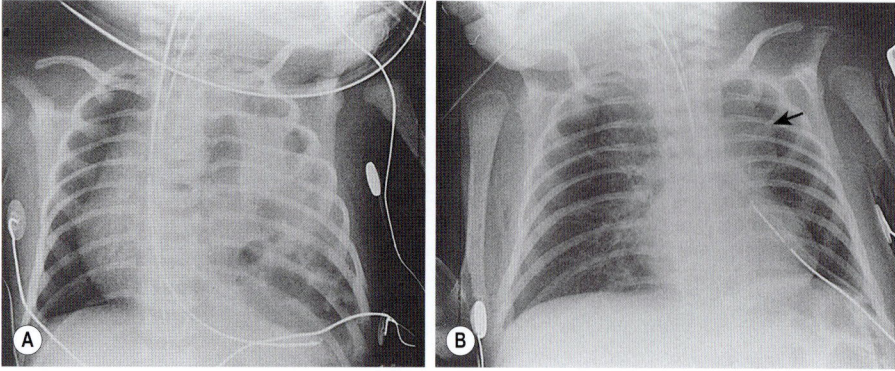

FIGURE 24-5 ■ (A) Anteroposterior chest radiograph in a neonate with a CDH demonstrating air-filled loops of bowel within the left chest. The heart and mediastinum are shifted to the right, and the hypoplastic left lung can be seen medially. (B) Postoperative radiograph demonstrating hyperexpansion of the right lung with shift of the mediastinum to the left. The edge of the severely hypoplastic left lung is again easily visualized (arrow).

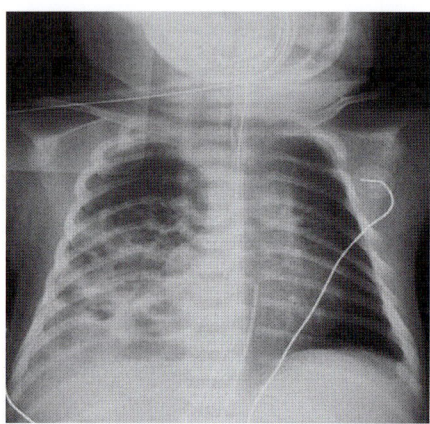

FIGURE 24-6 ■ This infant presented with respiratory distress and a right-sided CDH.

respectively).[102] When the MRI-based O/E TFLV is less than 25%, there is a significant decrease in postnatal survival.[100]

Clinical Presentation

Newborns with CDH typically present with respiratory distress. Clinical scenarios at birth range from immediate respiratory distress with associated low Apgar scores to an initial stable period and a delay in respiratory distress for 24 to 48 hours. Initial signs associated with respiratory distress include tachypnea, chest wall retractions, grunting, cyanosis, and pallor. On physical examination, infants will often have a scaphoid abdomen and an increased chest diameter. The point of maximal cardiac impulse is often displaced, suggesting mediastinal shift. Bowel sounds may be auscultated within the chest cavity with a decrease in breath sounds bilaterally. Chest excursion may be reduced, suggesting a lower tidal volume.

The diagnosis of CDH is typically confirmed by a chest radiograph demonstrating intestinal loops within the thorax (Fig. 24-5). The abdominal cavity may have minimal to no gas. Right-sided CDH is often more difficult to diagnosis (Fig. 24-6). Salient features, such as intestinal and gastric herniation, may not be seen. The herniated right lobe of the liver can be mistaken for a right diaphragmatic eventration. Occasionally, features of

lung compression may be the only radiographic sign, which can cause confusion with CPAMs, pulmonary sequestrations, bronchopulmonary cysts, neurogenic cysts, or cystic teratomas.

Although most infants with CDH will be diagnosed within the first 24 hours of life, as many as 20% may present outside the neonatal period.[103] These patients present with milder respiratory symptoms, chronic pulmonary infections, pleural effusions, pneumonias, feeding intolerance, or gastric volvulus.[104] As CDH is invariably associated with abnormal intestinal rotation and fixation, some children may present with intestinal obstruction or volvulus. Occasionally, CDH may be completely asymptomatic and is only discovered incidentally.[43,105] Older patients who present later in life have a much better prognosis due to milder or absent associated complications, such as pulmonary hypoplasia and hypertension.

TREATMENT

Prenatal Care

The prenatal diagnosis of CDH has improved with the increased use and refinement of fetal ultrasound examinations. After initial screening, an advanced ultrasound helps to determine discordant size and dates, associated anomalies (cardiovascular and neurological) as well as signs of fetal compromise (i.e., hydrops fetalis). Once diagnosed, chromosomal screening should be performed. Optimally, the mother and fetus should be referred to a tertiary perinatal center with advanced neonatal critical care capabilities, such as ECMO, inhaled nitric oxide (iNO) therapy, and oscillating ventilators.[5] A prenatal diagnosis allows the mother and family to be properly informed of treatment options and outcomes.

Prenatal Glucocorticoids

In animal models, the hypoplastic lungs of CDH infants are structurally and functionally immature. Biochemical markers for lung maturity demonstrate decreased total lung DNA, total lung protein, and desaturated phosphatidylcholine in addition to a deficiency of surfactant.[61] In one study, prenatal administration of glucocorticoids demonstrated a reduction in alveolar septal thickness, increased DNA synthesis, and increased total lung protein production.[106,107] Initial results from small patient series seemed promising in that antenatal administration of glucocorticoids suggested improved lung function.[108,109] However, a prospective randomized trial failed to demonstrate any benefit for CDH.[110] At this point, no data exist on proper dosing or timing of steroid administration in the setting of CDH. As such, prenatal steroids are not currently recommended for CDH.

Resuscitation and Stabilization

After confirming the diagnosis, initial postnatal therapy is targeted at resuscitation and stabilization of the infant in cardiopulmonary distress. A rapid overall assessment is important to determine hemodynamic stability and the severity of disease. In severe cases, prompt endotracheal intubation and mechanical ventilatory support is likely to be required. A nasogastric tube should be inserted to avoid gastric and intestinal distention. Arterial and venous catheters assist in resuscitative maneuvers. Acid–base balance and oxygenation-ventilation status should be carefully monitored.

Invasive monitoring is important in accurately assessing the infant's overall perfusion and the severity of pulmonary hypertension and hypoplasia. Umbilical venous catheters may be helpful and, if possible, should be positioned in the right atrium to measure central venous pressures. In addition, an approximation of cerebral perfusion should be available using preductal oxygen content and/or saturation via either a right radial arterial catheter or a transcutaneous saturation probe.

Targets for initial resuscitation include preductal arterial saturation (SaO_2) between 85–95% with a minimal amount of positive airway pressures. In order to maintain lower peak inspiratory pressures (PIP), a moderate level of hypercarbia ($PaCO_2$, 45–60 mmHg) is accepted without a compensatory acidosis and lactate of 3–5 mmol/L. Occasionally, higher levels of $PaCO_2$ are tolerated as long as the pH > 7.2 is maintained. Failure to provide adequate tissue oxygenation can result in metabolic acidosis which may exacerbate the PHTN. Pulmonary vascular resistance (PVR) is increased by hypoxia and acidosis, which should be avoided or corrected. If severe ductal shunting develops, iNO can be tried, although PHTN in association with CDH is less responsive to iNO than other causes of PHTN.

Depending on the degree of PHTN and associated cardiac anomalies, hemodynamic stability can be difficult to achieve. PHTN may be exhibited by a different pre- and postductal SaO_2. However, echocardiography can better characterize the degree of PHTN. Sonographic findings of PHTN include poor contractility of the right ventricle, flattening of the interventricular septum, enlarged right heart chambers, and tricuspid valve regurgitation. There may be right-to-left or bidirectional shunting across the ductus arteriosus.

Almost all infants with CDH and severe PHTN exhibit some left ventricular dysfunction. Vasopressor agents such as dopamine, dobutamine, and milrinone may be needed in hemodynamically unstable patients.

These inotropic agents can augment left ventricular output and increase systemic pressures in order to ameliorate right-to-left ductal shunting.

Mechanical Ventilation

Mechanical ventilation is a critical component in the care of infants with respiratory failure secondary to CDH. However, the physiologic limits of the hypoplastic lung make mechanical ventilation a challenge. Hypoplastic lungs in CDH infants are characterized by a decreased number of airways and smaller airspaces. Also, the pulmonary vasculature exhibits decreased vascular branching as well as increased adventitia and medial wall thickness.[111,112] This combination results in varying degrees of respiratory failure and PHTN. Fortunately, pulmonary and vascular development continues after birth and these pulmonary sequelae of CDH can improve.[113,114] Because of this ongoing maturation, mechanical ventilation strategies have trended towards less aggressive approaches with the goal of maintaining oxygenation while limiting the risks of ventilator-induced lung injury, a major contributor to mortality.[115]

The optimal type of mechanical ventilation in infants with CDH is individual clinician preference, but most cases of CDH can be managed using a pressure-cycled mode. A fractional inspired oxygen (FiO_2) of 1.0 is initially utilized to maintain adequate SaO_2. Typically, higher respiratory rates and lower peak airway pressures (18–22 cmH$_2$O) are employed while titrating the FiO_2 to a preductal PaO_2 greater than 60 mmHg, or the preductal SaO_2 > 85% and a $PaCO_2$ less than 60 mmHg. Maintaining an acceptable pH and $PaCO_2$ are important in managing PHTN.[116,117] The ventilation strategy of induced respiratory alkalosis with hyperventilation to reduce ductal shunting has been abandoned in most centers.[118–121] Initial conventional mechanical ventilation settings should include pressure-limited ventilation rates between 40–60 breaths per minute with PIP < 25 cmH$_2$O to minimize barotrauma.[118,122] The initial PIP can be weaned to minimal settings, but should be done with caution. While targeting a $PaCO_2$ < 45 mmHg, rapid reduction in mechanical support may allow transient periods of stability, but may also produce potential refractory exacerbations of PHTN. Spontaneous respirations are maintained by avoiding neuromuscular paralysis and minimal ventilation rates. This combination of spontaneous respiration and permissive hypercapnia has been a well-documented preoperative stabilization strategy in some centers with survival rates of almost 90% in patients with isolated CDH.[118–120]

If conventional ventilation fails to reverse hypercapnia and hypoxemia, HFOV strategies can be tried to avoid ventilatory-induced lung injury by preserving end-expiratory lung volume without overdistending the lung parenchyma. As the understanding of the CDH lungs continues to evolve, HFOV strategies have also changed. Initially used in a high-pressure, lung recruitment mode, this strategy demonstrated no benefit due to the nonrecruitable nature of these hypoplastic lungs.[123,124] High-frequency strategies as a rescue therapy for infants with profound hypoxia and refractory hypercapnia on conventional ventilators have also not been successful.[4,125] As the concept of preoperative stabilization became better defined, HFOV began to be used as means to avoid barotrauma early in the treatment course prior to refractory respiratory failure. In fact, some institutions have utilized HFOV as primary therapy.[5,126,127] These strategies of preoperative stabilization to prevent lung injury along with delayed operation, regardless of ventilator modalities, have resulted in improved survival.[5,115,126–128]

In order to achieve lower peak airway pressures, HFOV should be considered when PIP exceeds 25 cmH$_2$O with conventional ventilation. Initial HFOV settings include a mean airway pressure between 13–15 cmH$_2$O, 10–12 Hz, amplitude between 30–50 cmH$_2$O, and inspiration to expiration ratio of 50%. The initial $PaCO_2$ should be maintained in the range of 40–55 mmHg and can be weaned by decreasing the amplitude. Eight rib expansion of the contralateral hemithorax can be used as a guide to achieve optimal lung expansion without overdistention.[126,127] Tidal volumes are directly related to the amplitude and inversely related to frequency. As such, significant increases in tidal volume can be seen when frequencies are below 10 Hz. This can result in hyperinflation which, in turn, may adversely affect the pulmonary vasculature by impeding venous return. Constant assessment of acid-base status and end-organ perfusion is necessary as lung compliance can change before and after CDH repair.

Surfactant

Animal studies of CDH have demonstrated altered surfactant levels and composition.[129,130] Experimentally, surfactant decreases PVR, improves pulmonary blood flow, and reduces ductal shunting.[131] However, supporting data are not definite.[62] Initial reports demonstrated surfactant administration augmented iNO delivery and improved gas exchange, leading to its empiric utilization.[132] However, clinical evidence in term and preterm infants with CDH has not shown benefit.[133] Van Meurs et al. suggested that surfactant therapy in term infants with CDH was associated with an increased use of ECMO, increased incidence of chronic lung disease, and higher mortality.[134] Similar findings were found in preterm infants despite adjusting for Apgar scores and gestational age.[133] Even as a rescue therapy in CDH infants on ECMO, surfactant failed to demonstrate a survival advantage.[135,136] Despite the lack of proven efficacy, exogenous surfactant therapy continues to be used with unclear risks and benefits. Proponents of this therapy argue that the clinical evidence is based on a heterogeneous population of disease severity, and that the lack of clinical evidence to support its efficacy is due to its use in the most severe CDH infants. Given the current clinical data, surfactant therapy should only be used in the setting of clinical research.

Pulmonary Vasodilators

PHTN is a common consequence in CDH infants. Even if asymptomatic, the initial management in the CDH newborn is directed at reducing PVR. With increased PVR, patients often display super-systemic pressures leading to right-to-left shunting in both the pre- and postductal circulations. This can cause right heart failure with increases in preductal desaturation, narrowing of the pre- and postductal SaO_2, and, ultimately, systemic hypotension and decreased perfusion. In previously stable neonates, signs of poor perfusion may indicate closure of a PDA. In response, prostaglandin E$_1$ (PGE$_1$) can be instituted to re-open the ductus and improve right ventricle (RV) pressures.[122] In infants that demonstrate significant PHTN and RV dysfunction, left ventricular filling/function and overall perfusion may improve by off-loading the RV to improve the geometry of the interventricular septum.[137] Preductal SaO_2 > 85% should be maintained to ensure adequate cerebral perfusion.[118] As the RV is unloaded, systolic blood pressure may decrease, especially in the setting of left ventricular dysfunction. Adequate preload should be maintained with volume loading or vasopressor support, such as epinephrine, to ensure ventricular function and coronary artery perfusion. Increasing the systemic pressure may decrease the degree of right-to-left shunting. In a small study, CDH infants with persistent PHTN and right-to-left shunting through the ductus, despite PGE$_1$ use, had an 80% mortality.[138]

iNO is a potent pulmonary vasodilator that has been shown to have tremendous benefit in the treatment of persistent pulmonary hypertension of the neonate (PPHN).[4,139–142] Typically, iNO is utilized in the setting of echocardiographic evidence of right-to-left shunting and RV pressures greater than two-thirds systemic pressures. In clinical studies, iNO has been shown to improve oxygenation and decrease the need for ECMO in infants with respiratory failure secondary to PPHN.[142,143] However, the efficacy of iNO as a rescue therapy for PHTN secondary to CDH by either decreasing the need for ECMO or a reduction in mortality has not been supported.[144] In the Neonatal Inhaled Nitric Oxide Study Group trial, the CDH subgroup had a greater likelihood for ECMO or death.[145] The response to iNO is variable and unpredictable in infants with CDH. The initial improvement in oxygenation in CDH infants suggest that iNO could be utilized as a bridge for transport or until ECMO can be initiated.[122] Some infants may demonstrate a rebound PHTN that is more difficult to control than the initial disease.[146,147] Also, the effect appears to be transient and does not obviate the need for ECMO.[77,148] A meta-analysis of iNO utilization for persistent PHTN did not show benefit in CDH infants, and recommended its use only in hypoxic respiratory failure infants without CDH.[149]

Phosphodiesterase (PDE) inhibitors are cyclic guanosine monophosphate (cGMP) modulators that target vascular remodeling by limiting smooth muscle cell proliferation.[150] Type 5 PDEs (dipyridamole and sildenafil) are the most active on visceral and vascular smooth muscle and have been utilized with iNO for the treatment of PHTN in patients with and without CDH. In limited case reports, dipyridamole produces a transient improvement in oxygenation which may allow weaning of ventilatory support and may avoid escalation of therapy to ECMO.[151–153] Sildenafil has been shown to improve oxygenation and decrease PVR when used independently or in combination with iNO.[146,154,155] Sildenafil has been used in oral or intravenous forms for congenital heart disease and CDH-associated PHTN.[146,148,156,157] Similar to dipyridamole, utilization of sildenafil may have benefit in improving oxygenation and avoiding ECMO in the setting of refractory iNO.[146,158] However, despite its approval for use in adults, the USA Food and Drug Administration has warned against using sildenafil for pediatric pulmonary hypertension between ages 1 and 17 years due to a potential increase in mortality during long-term therapy.[159] Other vasodilators have been utilized in infants with CDH, but the experience to date is limited.[160–174]

Extracorporeal Membrane Oxygenation

CDH accounts for approximately one-quarter of all infants requiring ECMO for respiratory failure.[175–178] ECMO utilization for CDH was first introduced as a rescue therapy for infants who had severe ventilator-associated lung injury.[179] Prior to the era of preoperative stabilization, ECMO was associated with only a modest improvement in survival in high-risk CDH infants.[180–182] Since then, ECMO has evolved as a treatment modality to prevent ventilator-induced barotrauma.[183,184] In combination with other adjunctive treatments such as HFOV, ECMO is now routinely used for preoperative stabilization.[185] The strategy of stabilization with ECMO and delay in operative correction has been shown to be beneficial with a reported survival of 67% in high-risk patients.[8,186]

Although results are dependent on patient selection and disease severity, survival has been reported between 60–90% for CDH patients requiring ECMO.[5,118,139,175,187] Without ECMO, the predicted mortality in the high-risk cohort reaches 80%.[175] Despite these data, the benefits of ECMO for CDH are not universally accepted. Some authors report no survival advantage with ECMO,[188,189] while others report as high as 80% survival without using ECMO.[190,191]

Initially, strict criteria were established as indications for ECMO use in CDH. These included an oxygenation index >40 and persistent alveolar–arterial O_2 gradient >610 mmHg.[177,192] Today, those criteria have eased and the most common indication for ECMO is a 'failure to respond' to other therapy. In efforts to maintain lung-protective ventilation, clinicians have opted for ECMO rather than escalation of positive airway pressures. Relative contraindications include significant congenital anomalies, lethal chromosomal anomalies, intracranial hemorrhage, birth weight <2 kg, and gestational age <34 weeks. See Chapter 6 for more information about ECMO.

SURGERY

Timing of Operation

With an improved understanding of its pathophysiology, repair of CDH is no longer considered an emergency procedure. However, the optimal timing for repair remains unclear. Historically, early repair was thought to improve ventilation by reducing intrathoracic pressures after reduction of the herniated viscera. However, this strategy often led to urgent procedures being performed on unstable infants.[193] A paradigm shift in management to delay the operative repair until the infant is stable became widely adopted in the early 1990s.[121,122,194] Several studies have shown no difference in mortality rate or the need for ECMO in infants undergoing early vs late repairs,[195–197] including two randomized trials of early (<12 hours) versus delayed repair (after 24 hours[197] and after 96 hours[195]). Today, repair of CDH is usually delayed until cardiopulmonary stability is achieved, although the definition of physiologic stability remains highly variable and inconsistent amongst centers.[127,194,196–200]

In 1995, Wung et al. reported advantages with a delayed repair strategy for CDH.[121] Comparing three eras of treatment strategies, the study contrasted an early period of emergency surgery to the most recent era of delayed repair and 'gentle ventilation,' where infants with CDH were managed with a lung-preserving ventilation strategy. Repair was not performed until the pre- and postductal SpO_2 gradient equalized and right-to-left shunting on echocardiogram had resolved. With an average of 4.2 days after birth before operation, survival was 94% with only one patient requiring ECMO. From the same institution in 2002, 120 consecutive patients were treated with permissive hypercapnia, spontaneous respiration, and elective repair after 36 hours of life with an overall survival of 84%.[118] Of note, only 13.3% of patients needed ECMO and only 7% of infants required a prosthetic patch, suggesting a relatively small proportion of infants with large diaphragmatic defects. A different group reported similar results from a center that did not offer ECMO.[201] In this study, all high-risk patients (defined as assisted ventilation within two hours of life) were divided in three historical cohorts with the most recent group being managed by permissive hypercapnia, gentle ventilation, and delayed repair until hemodynamic stability was achieved ($PaCO_2$ < 60 mmHg, PaO_2 > 40 mmHg, SaO_2 > 85% with a FiO_2 < 50%) for at least 48 consecutive hours. Overall survival in this recent cohort was 90%. Despite the benefits of preoperative stabilization and delayed repair, the specific parameters that define hemodynamic stability and timing of operation remain unanswered.

According to data from the Congenital Diaphragmatic Hernia Registry (CDHR) and Extracorporeal Life Support Organization (ELSO) over a recent 15 year period, one-third of infants with CDH required ECMO during their initial hospitalization, during which 85% of these infants underwent early CDH repair on ECMO.[202] In this study, survival was 71% with only 9% requiring operative intervention for bleeding complications following CDH repair on ECMO compared to survival of 49% and a 14.7% bleeding complication rate from the CDH and ELSO registries. The authors attributed the better outcomes after early repair on ECMO to less body wall edema and a quicker recovery following operation which led to fewer total days on ECMO (11.7 vs 13.3 days). In another study, among infants who underwent repair of a unilateral CDH, 47.6% were repaired on ECMO, 45.8% were repaired after ECMO, and only 6.6% were repaired before ECMO.[203]

Bleeding remains the most significant complication following CDH repair on ECMO including both surgical site bleeding and intracranial hemorrhage. These risks may be minimized with early repair on ECMO prior to the development of a coagulopathy and significant edema,[177,202] as well as repair when PHTN has resolved, but prior to decannulation to allow reinstitution of ECMO if respiratory failure and/or PHTN recur.[204] Although rare, recurrent PHTN can develop after repair requiring a second ECMO run.[205] In addition, use of aminocaproic acid (Amicar®), a fibrinolysis inhibitor, has significantly decreased bleeding complications. One group reported no changes in intracranial hemorrhage rates, but a significant decrease in surgical site bleeding from 12% to 7% ($P < 0.05$) with Amicar®.[176] Amicar® should be used prior to operation and for two to three days after repair. Additional strategies include ECMO without heparinization, fresh ECMO circuits, minimal diaphragmatic muscular dissection, fibrin or thrombin sealants, and utilization of recombinant factor VII for established bleeding.

Operative Approach

Open repair of CDH can be performed using a thoracic or abdominal approach. Advantages to laparotomy include easier reduction of intrathoracic viscera, the ability to mobilize the posterior rim of diaphragm, easier management of intestinal rotational anomalies, and avoidance of thoracotomy-associated musculoskeletal sequelae. The vast majority of neonatal repairs for CDH are through a subcostal incision (91%).[206,207] Less than 10% are performed via a thoracotomy. The intra-abdominal contents should be reduced out of the thorax with careful attention to the spleen that can be caught and lacerated on the rudimentary rim of diaphragm. A true hernia sac, which is present less than 20% of the time, should be excised.[208] The thoracic and abdominal cavities should be inspected for an associated pulmonary sequestration.

Despite this 'gold standard' abdominal approach, the morbidity and respiratory sequelae of open CDH repair remain a concern. In addition to pulmonary hypoplasia and hypertension, respiratory compliance is significantly reduced after open repair. Mortality significantly increases when compliance decreases by >50% which can occur as a result of a tight abdominal wall closure.[193,209] Careful attention should be paid to the peak airway pressures as the abdominal fascia is closed. Respiratory compromise should alert the surgeon to leave the abdomen open. This approach is more often needed in CDH infants on ECMO.[210] Temporary closure can be achieved using just the skin or a prosthetic silo. Delayed closure, especially in those infants on ECMO, should be attempted after the generalized edema has resolved or the intra-abdominal domain has enlarged.[211]

The routine use of chest tubes after CDH repair to drain pleural fluid has been abandoned.[118,121,201] One concern is that the chest tube can cause ipsi- and contra-lateral lung injury secondary to mediastinal shift, especially if connected to suction. The thoracic space will eventually fill with fluid, and the lung will gradually grow. Tube thoracostomy should only be used for postoperative chylothorax or pleural fluid causing hemodynamic compromise.[212] If a chest tube is needed, it is positioned in the thoracic cavity prior to final closure of the diaphragm. Chest tubes should be placed to water seal rather than suction. Symptomatic pleural fluid can be treated with repeated thoracentesis. If used, chest tubes should be removed early to avoid infectious complications.

Minimally Invasive Techniques

The respiratory sequelae and other morbidity seen after open CDH repair has prompted surgeons to adopt minimally invasive surgical (MIS) approaches. Both thoracoscopic and laparoscopic repairs have been performed.[207,213–216] Data from the CDHR show that laparoscopic and thoracoscopic strategies are being used worldwide, and have been utilized in 20% of centers since 1995.[207] MIS techniques have been used for primary repair as well as prosthetic patch closure with suggested advantages of less postoperative pain, avoidance of thoracotomy-associated complications, and an overall reduction of surgical stress.[216,217]

The sensitivity of CDH infants to hypercapnia and acidosis has drawn concerns regarding the utilization of MIS. The overall benefits of MIS are questioned because: (1) CDH neonates may absorb the CO_2 insufflation;[218,219] and (2) insufflation with CO_2 can raise intracavity pressures that may limit venous return, end-organ perfusion, and tidal volume. The combination of CDH-related pulmonary hypoplasia, PHTN, and labile pulmonary vascular reactivity may be detrimental during MIS operations. Although increases in CO_2 absorption during MIS are generally well tolerated in infants, CDH neonates specifically demonstrate greater changes in end-tidal CO_2 ($ETCO_2$) and impaired elimination of CO_2 during thoracoscopy and laparoscopy.[220,221] Hypercapnia and the associated acidosis may result in increased pulmonary shunting.

Patient selection is paramount for successful completion of an MIS repair as well as for minimizing operative morbidity. Historically, MIS was reserved for stable infants with anticipated small defects. Utilizing anatomic markers such as stomach herniation, surgeons have attempted to predict which defects might be amenable to MIS repairs.[215] Initially, the radiographic presence of the nasogastric tube within the abdomen and minimal respiratory compromise (PIP < 24 mmHg) were thought to predict a successful thoracoscopic repair. One group reported 95% success rates with thoracoscopic repairs when patients did not have a significant congenital cardiac anomaly or the need for preoperative ECMO, and had a PIP ≤ 26 cmH$_2$O, and an oxygenation index ≤5 on the day of surgery.[222] Another group has advocated for strict preoperative selection criteria for thoracoscopic repair, including minimal ventilatory support (PIP < 24 mmHg), no clinical or sonographic evidence of PHTN, and an intra-abdominal stomach.[215] On the other hand, infants requiring preoperative ECMO have undergone successful repair with an MIS approach.[218,223] Large defects that require patch repairs[218,222,224] and right-sided defects are no longer contraindications to MIS.[225] However, patients undergoing MIS repair of CDH should have stringent intraoperative monitoring of $ETCO_2$ and $PaCO_2$.[226]

Although success with laparoscopic[216,227] and thoracoscopic[213,224] repairs have been reported, comparative evidence between MIS and open approaches has been limited to single-institution experiences or retrospective analyses.[213,228,229] A recent single-institution review of 54 neonates undergoing unilateral CDH repair between 2006–2010 was published.[228] Thirty-five neonates underwent attempted thoracoscopic repair with 26 being successfully completed. During the same time interval, 19 open CDH repairs were performed. Recurrence was higher after the thoracoscopic repair (23% vs 0%). There were no individual factors that were found to be predictive of recurrence with the thoracoscopic approach. In another report, a systematic review and meta-analysis of neonatal endosurgical CDH repairs identified only three eligible studies comparing open to endosurgical repair.[230] The cumulative risk ratio for death was 0.33 (95% CI:0.10–1.13) in favor of the MIS approach and recurrence was 3.21 (95% CI:1.11–9.29) in favor of the open repair. The overall survival rate for MIS patients was significantly higher compared with patients undergoing open repair (82.9% open and 98.7% MIS, $P < 0.01$) with a risk-adjusted odds ratio (OR) of survival for MIS repairs of 5.57 (95% CI:1.34–23.14).[222] These results suggest a significant survival advantage for the MIS approach, even after risk-adjustment. However, the data are more likely the result of selection bias based on surgeon preference regarding which patients were good candidates for MIS.

Although the ability to perform MIS repair of CDH has been shown, the short- and long-term outcomes regarding the durability and recurrence rates for an MIS approach are less clear. The reported overall recurrence rates for MIS repair range from 5–23.1%,[218,222,224,225] with early recurrences as high as 23–33%.[228,229] In another study, MIS repairs were performed in only 3.4% infants with CDH, but had a significantly higher in-hospital recurrence rate compared to open (7.9% vs 2.7%, $P < 0.05$).[207] The true risks and benefits of the MIS approach for CDH repair, including the impact of re-operations, remain unclear. At the very least, recurrence seems to be higher.

Robotic CDH repair has been demonstrated to be feasible and safe.[231-233] Proponents of robotic CDH repair tout the increased degrees of freedom of the articulating instruments for suturing.

Diaphragmatic Replacements

Repair of large diaphragmatic defects is a challenge, usually requiring diaphragmatic replacement with a prosthetic patch or autologous tissue. In one large study, 48.3% of infants undergoing CDH repair required diaphragmatic replacement.[207] Comparative studies between patch and primary repairs have consistently shown increased morbidity and mortality in the patch groups, most likely due to the large defect size and the associated severity of the pulmonary hypoplasia.[234,235] In many studies, patch repair has been utilized as a surrogate for defect size and disease severity (i.e., larger the defect = increased severity of disease).

Nonabsorbable Synthetic Patches

Synthetic patches such as polytetrafluoroethylene (PTFE or Gore-Tex®) or composite polypropylene (Marlex®) represent the majority of the mesh replacements used in neonates with a large CDH.[236] Advantages to synthetic patches include: (1) immediate availability; (2) minimal preparation time; (3) easily cut to fit the diaphragmatic defect; and (4) less tissue dissection, reducing the risk of hemorrhage, especially during repair on ECMO. However, there are several disadvantages to synthetic patches for CDH repair. PTFE, anchored to the chest wall, can potentially produce a tethering point for creating a pectus-type deformity.[237] There is an increased incidence of bowel obstruction, need for splenectomy, patch infections, and abdominal wall deformities.[236,238] The overall recurrence rate has been reported to be as high as 50% with a bimodal distribution showing early recurrence in the first months after repair and late recurrence years later.[236] Early recurrences for defects requiring a patch are most likely due to lack of tissue adhesion or scarring and an incomplete muscular rim which then requires anchoring the patch to the ribs or esophagus. PTFE tends to scar and retract over time, which may lead to late recurrences in the growing child. In an effort to prevent CDH recurrence, one group described a cone-shaped, double-fixed PTFE patch to allow expansion over time.[239] The recurrence rate decreased from 46% to 9% at one year after repair. Similar results have been seen with a mesh plug and patch technique in the setting of a recurrent CDH.[240] Another group described a double-sided composite patch consisting of PTFE and type-1 monofilament, macroporous Marlex. Utilizing a pledgeted, nonabsorbable running suture, the recurrence rate was 2.2% with a mean follow-up of 49 months.[241]

Absorbable Biosynthetic Patches

Absorbable biosynthetic materials have been utilized as an alternative replacement to synthetic patches. They have been reported to decrease complications by offering a lower risk of infection and the ability of the patch to grow with the patient. Surgisis® (SIS) is an acellular, bioengineered porcine intestinal submucosal matrix that consists of a type I collagen lattice with embedded growth factors. This non-crosslinked biological matrix promotes fibroblast migration and cellular differentiation.[242] First described for repair of incisional, inguinal, and paraesophageal hernias,[243-245] SIS® has also been utilized for CDH repair.[216,246] Permacol® is an acellular porcine dermal collagen patch consisting of collagen fibers with cross-linked lysine and hydroxylysine. By promoting an inflammatory response in a manner similar to wound healing, the neodiaphragm is more pliable and, subsequently, less prone to recurrence. One group reported no recurrences observed with a median follow-up of 20 months, while recurrences were noted in 2% of patients with primary repair and 28% with PTFE.[247] AlloDerm® is an acellular human cadaveric dermal patch that is

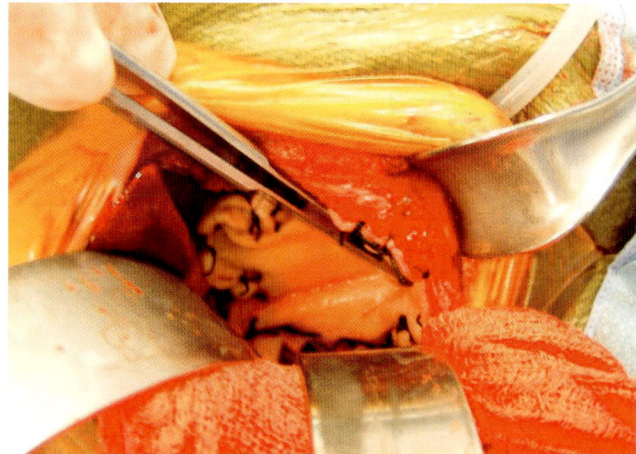

FIGURE 24-7 ■ A large left posterolateral diaphragmatic hernia was approached through a subcostal incision. After reduction of the abdominal viscera, the large defect was closed using a biosynthetic patch (Alloderm®).

cross-linked for rapid revascularization (Fig. 24-7). Animal studies have demonstrated revascularization and cell repopulation within one month.[248] Surgimend® is an acellular fetal bovine interwoven dermal collagen that promotes increased type III collagen. Because there is no cross-linking, there is increased collagen resistance leading to greater durability. Poly-lactic-co-glycolic acid (PLGA) is a collagen scaffold that promotes neovascularization and autologous tissue regeneration. Animal studies have demonstrated ingrowth of fibroblasts resulting in a thicker neodiaphragm.[249]

Despite the theoretical advantages, these absorbable biosynthetic patches remain imperfect as diaphragmatic substitutes. Thinning of the patch and incomplete muscular ingrowth, especially in large defects where native diaphragmatic muscle is absent, have been found.[250] These biosynthetic patches are also prone to recurrences, similar to nonabsorbable patches.[251] In addition, organ adherence may be required for neovascularization, and these organs often include the small bowel, spleen, or liver.[238,252] Subsequently, biologic patches can be associated with adhesive bowel obstruction.[234,238,251]

Autologous Tissue Patches

Complications with synthetic and biosynthetic patches have prompted some surgeons to advocate for primary or staged repair with autologous muscle flaps for large diaphragmatic defects.[253–258] Muscle flaps offer the advantage of using a vascularized tissue that will grow with the infant and has a minimal inflammatory response. In 1962, Meeker and Snyder first described using the anterior abdominal wall for CDH repair.[259] A few years later came the description of a split abdominal wall muscle flap used to repair a large defect in a newborn.[253] More recently, another group described using a split abdominal muscle flap consisting of the internal oblique and transversus abdominis muscles for primary repair of large defects.[254] Another approach is to use a lower abdominal incision and the transversus abdominis muscle for repair on ECMO.[255] Due to the avascular dissection plane between the muscle layers, this approach may minimize the risk of bleeding while on ECMO. In a recent report, the recurrence rate for split abdominal wall muscle flaps was only 4.3%, while the recurrence rate for patch repair was 50%.[256]

Chest wall muscles, such as the latissimus dorsi muscle, have also been used as diaphragmatic substitutes.[257] For very large defects, such as agenesis of the diaphragm, the combination of the latissimus dorsi and serratus anterior muscles has been described.[258,260] The disadvantage with using local chest wall muscle flaps is the resulting body wall deformity.[261] Consequently, chest wall muscle flaps have been primarily reserved for patients with a recurrent CDH. Although autologous muscle flaps are vascularized and tend to grow with the child, these diaphragmatic reconstructions with latissimus dorsi/serratus muscle flaps have been shown to atrophy over time due to denervation of the graft.[260] In addition, the lack of innervation prevents the natural physiologic movement of the diaphragm. As a result, the reverse latissimus dorsi flap with a microneural anastomosis of the phrenic nerve to the thoracodorsal nerve has been tried to prevent muscle atrophy and to allow physiological muscle movement.[260,262]

Tissue Engineered Patches

The ideal diaphragmatic replacement remains elusive in the operative treatment of CDH. Advances in regenerative medicine may provide the solution. Tissue engineered muscle may provide a replacement for functional skeletal muscle and does not atrophy. Although the supporting three-dimensional scaffold is a key component of tissue engineering, skeletal muscle regeneration relies on a cell source with myogenic potential.[263,264] Amniotic fluid is an abundant source of stem cells with myogenic potential.[265] Tissue engineering strategies could utilize amniotic stem cells collected at the time of amniocentesis to develop a muscular patch used during postnatal repair. Fauza and colleagues have developed a fetal tissue-based diaphragm engineered from mesenchymal amniocytes.[266] In preclinical studies, these bioengineered diaphragms demonstrated improved mechanical and functional outcomes when compared to acellular bioprosthetic patches.[267]

Fetal Therapy

The impetus for fetal therapy for CDH coincided with advances in prenatal diagnosis. Fetal ultrasound has allowed a better understanding of the true natural history of CDH. In the late 1980s, open fetal repair for left-sided CDH without liver and stomach herniation before 24 weeks gestation was conceptualized and performed.[86] In a more recent prospective study, fetuses undergoing in utero repair had a higher complication rate, including prematurity, with an average gestation of 32 weeks without an improvement in survival.[268] Surprisingly, better than expected survival was found in the standard postnatal management patients and there were higher rates of complications in the fetal surgery group. Consequently, open fetal surgery has been abandoned as a therapeutic option for CDH.

The concept of tracheal occlusion originated from the observation that infants with congenital high airway obstructions developed hyperplastic lungs. Several groups have demonstrated increases in total lung protein and DNA, alveolar space, overall lung weight, and cross-sectional area of the pulmonary vasculature as well as better lung compliance following prenatally placed tracheal balloons in sheep.[269–272] However, it has been noted that long-term tracheal occlusion decreases the number of type 2 pneumocytes and surfactant production. This finding has led to the concept of temporary in utero tracheal occlusion for CDH.[131,273]

It is known that liver herniation and LHR < 1.0 are fetal parameters that portend the worst outcomes.[274] Current in utero techniques involve endoscopic insertion of an occlusive balloon in the fetal trachea without maternal laparotomy or general anesthesia.[275] These balloons are inserted percutaneously with ultrasound guidance between 24–28 weeks' gestations and are deflated at 34 weeks. This strategy of temporary tracheal occlusion avoids the need for an ex-utero intrapartum treatment (EXIT) procedure at delivery, although emergent airway access may be needed at delivery for any patient who undergoes in utero tracheal occlusion.

In 2003, an NIH-sponsored randomized trial comparing fetal tracheal occlusion versus standard postnatal care was reported.[276] Criteria for randomization was LHR < 1.4 and liver in the chest. After 24 cases (11 with tracheal occlusion), the study was terminated early due to comparable survival outcomes (77% by postnatal care, 73% by tracheal occlusion). The hazard ratio (HR) for mortality associated with tracheal occlusion, as compared to conventional postnatal therapy, was 1.2 (95% CI:0.29–4.67). However, when stratified based on LHR, survival was significantly better for LHR greater than 0.9 with a HR for death with tracheal occlusion being 0.13 (95% CI:0.03–0.64).

In 2004, the European Fetal Endoscopic Tracheal Occlusion (FETO) task group reported on 21 fetuses undergoing tracheal occlusion.[277] This nonrandomized study of fetuses with a severe CDH (liver up and LHR < 1) showed improved survival (64%) in the last 11 patients compared to the first 10 (30%). In 2009, the FETO group reported their results in 210 patients utilizing a minimal access approach under regional and local anesthesia.[278] This FETO study also included fetuses with liver herniation and an O/E LHR < 1.0. The median time to insert the balloon was 10 minutes. Successful balloon placement was achieved in 97% at the first procedure. Ninety-seven per cent of the babies were live born and the overall survival until discharge was 48%. The mean gestational age at birth was 35.3 weeks. When these outcomes were compared to the CDH registry, fetuses with a left-sided CDH, liver up, and an O/E LHR < 1, who were treated with fetal tracheal occlusion, had a survival of 49.1% vs 24.1% in the registry. Survival increased from 0% in the registry to 35% in similar fetuses with a right CDH who underwent fetal tracheal occlusion.[278]

In 2012, Ruano et al. reported on a randomized controlled trial between FETO and conventional postnatal care for isolated, severe CDH (LHR < 1.0 and liver up) between 22 and 26 weeks.[279] With an intention-to-treat analysis, overall survival was 50% in the fetal tracheal occlusion group compared to 4.8% in controls (RR 10.5;95%CI:1.5–74.7). The mean gestational age at delivery was 35.6 ± 2.4 weeks in the treated group and 37.4 ± 1.9 weeks in controls (P < 0.01). Despite these positive results, one limitation of this study was that it did not utilize some of the currently accepted prenatal and postnatal treatment strategies. Tracheal balloons were removed at the time of delivery through an EXIT procedure, thus discarding the temporary tracheal occlusion concept. In addition, ECMO was not available in the study institution for postnatal care in both arms.

Currently, the European FETO group is conducting a multicenter randomized trial for severe, isolated CDH cases in patients with O/E LHR < 25% and liver in the chest. Short-term tracheal occlusion is performed with balloon insertion between 27 and 30 weeks gestation and removal at 34 weeks. There is a standardized postnatal management protocol as well as a standardized technique for emergent and elective balloon removal. Until definitive evidence-based practice is established, fetal tracheal occlusion for CDH remains an unproven therapy.

OUTCOMES

Clinical outcomes for the treatment and management of infants with CDH have traditionally been difficult to generalize due to the low incidence of disease and single institutions reports. Patient characteristics and clinical practices are different, and each institution's ability to offer state-of-the-art neonatal critical care is highly variable. Survival analyses for CDH remain difficult to interpret due to variations in patient, disease, management strategies, and operative techniques. Unique to individual institutions are differences in ventilation strategies, availability and entry criteria for ECMO, and operative timing. As a result, survival rates for CDH vary between institutions, even when risk adjusted, and range from 25–83%.[6] In an attempt to ameliorate these difference, the CDH Study Group (CDHSG) was the first to publish risk-stratified outcomes.[280] Multivariate analysis demonstrated birth weight and 5-minute Apgar scores to be the most significant predictors of outcome.

Volume-Based Outcomes for CDH

Outcomes for CDH appear better in centers that treat a higher volume of CDH infants. The Canadian Pediatric Surgery Network (CAPSNet) grouped centers into low (<12 cases/year) and high (≥12 cases/year) volume.[281] Low volume centers had a higher mortality (23% vs 10%). In a recent follow-up report, CAPSNet found that significant differences between centers was found at six cases per year.[282] After risk-adjustment, low-volume centers demonstrated 33% mortality compared to 15% in high-volume centers. Recent data from the Pediatric Health Information System (PHIS) administrative database showed the average yearly hospital CDH volume varies from 1.4 to 17.5 cases per year among the 42 institutions.[283] After being grouped into low (≤6 cases/year), medium (6–10 cases), and high volume (>10 cases) centers, medium and high volume centers were found to have a significant lower mortality compared to low volume hospitals.

Risk Stratification for CDH

Congenital heart defects occur in 10–35% of CDH infants.[33,284,285] Categorized into major (hemodynamically significant) and minor lesions (such asymptomatic ASD, VSD, or PDA), in one study, the overall survival was 73% without any cardiac anomalies, 67% with minor defects, and 36% with major anomalies.[33] When compared to infants without structural cardiac anomalies, the adjusted risk in-hospital mortality was 2.2 times higher in infants with major heart defects while there was no statistical difference among infants with minor lesions.

Defined as delivery <38 weeks gestation, preterm birth occurs in approximately 30% of infants with CDH.[286,287] The overall survival is approximately 53% for all preterm CDH infants.[286] However, mortality significantly increases with younger gestational age. In a recent study, infants born less than 28 weeks gestational age were found to have a survival rate of 31.6%, while survival increased to 73.1% for those born at 37 weeks.[286] After adjusting for comorbidities and disease severity, prematurity had an increased OR of 1.68 for death.

Risk stratification by defect size appears to correlate with disease severity. In two reviews, the overall mortality for patients with agenesis of the diaphragm was 43% with an OR of 14.07 compared to defects that could be repaired primarily.[288,289] The association between defect size and disease severity has prompted development of a universal grading system to define CDH defect size.[1] Based on intraoperative findings, the four classifications range from small defects which could be repaired primarily to total diaphragmatic agenesis (Fig. 24-8). Utilizing other variables of comorbidity and disease severity, the CDHSG is attempting to provide an evidence-based risk-stratification classification for CDH.

Follow-Up Guidelines

Although many survive to discharge, the sequelae and ongoing health needs of CDH infants that require medical care after discharge is significant. Despite many single institution reports, the standard follow-up care for infants with CDH has not been established.[290,291] Pulmonary, neurological, gastrointestinal, and musculoskeletal complications necessitate a multidisciplinary team of surgical, medical, and developmental specialists. In 2008, the Section on Surgery and Committee on Fetus and Newborn for the American Academy of Pediatrics established follow-up guidelines for the care of infants with CDH.[292] The recommendations begin before discharge and extend through age 16 years (Table 24-1).

Pulmonary Outcomes

Prior to the era of ECMO and lung-protective ventilation, long-term survivors were usually reported as healthy children without any respiratory disease.[59,293] However, with improved care, more severely affected CDH infants are surviving and exhibiting functional and radiographic evidence of chronic lung disease.[291,294] Pulmonary function has been reported to be normal in 50–70% of CDH survivors with the remainder exhibiting some form of restrictive or obstructive respiratory symptoms.[295,296] Approximately 25% of children beyond the age of 5 have signs of obstructive airway disease. In a review of 100 consecutive CDH survivors, disease severity (defined as the need for ECMO and patch repair) was found to be predictive of pulmonary outcome.[295] While only 16% of the infants required oxygen at discharge, 53% required at least transient usage of bronchodilators within the first year. Similarly, 41% were either dependent on or intermittently needing steroids during their first year.

Respiratory infections appear to have a higher prevalence in children with CDH.[295,297,298] Respiratory syncytial virus (RSV) is the most common pathogen seen in

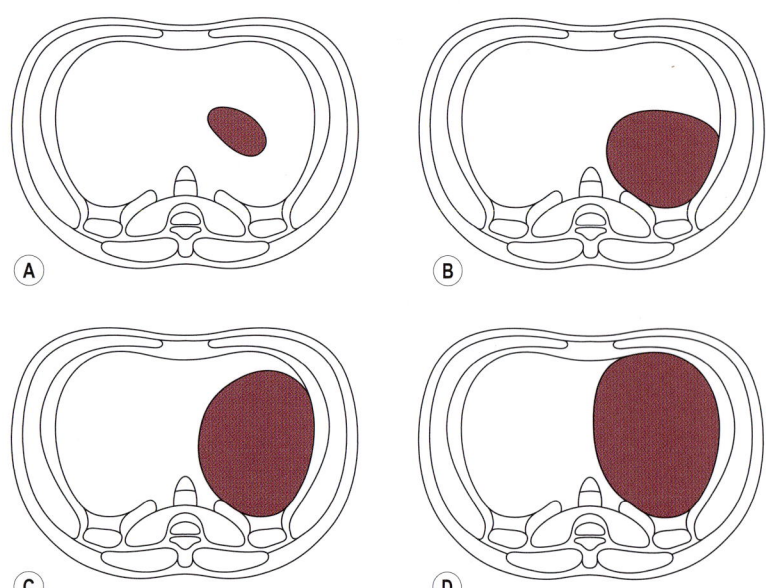

FIGURE 24-8 ■ Classification of CDH based on intraoperative defect size.[1] Diagrams are drawn with the diaphragmatic defect on the patient's left from an abdominal perspective.

TABLE 24-1   Recommended Schedule of Follow-Up for Infants with CDH

Follow-Up Guideline	Prior to Discharge	1–3 Months of Age	4–6 Months of Age	9–12 Months of Age	15–18 Months of Age	Annually through to 16 Years of Age
General Health and Prophylaxis						
Weight, length, occipital-frontal circumference	X	X	X	X	X	X
Childhood immunizations	Per childhood guidelines	X	X	X	X	X
RSV prophylaxis	At RSV season during first two years after birth, if evidence of chronic lung disease	X	X	X	X	X
Neurodevelopmental Testing						
Head computed tomography or MRI	If abnormal finding on head ultrasound, seizures, abnormal neurologic findings, or ECMO, or patch repair	If indicated	If indicated	If indicated	If indicated	If indicated
Hearing evaluation	Auditory brainstem evoked response or otoacoustic emissions screen	X	X	X	X	Every 6 months to 3 years of age, then annually to 5 years of age
Developmental screening evaluation	X	X	X	X		Annually to 5 years of age
Neurodevelopmental evaluation	X					Annually to 5 years of age
Gastrointestinal testing Oral aversion screening	X	X	If oral feeding problems persist	If oral feeding problems persist Consider for all patients	If oral feeding problems persist	If oral feeding problems persist
Upper gastrointestinal study, pH probe, and/or gastric scintiscan	Consider for all patients	If symptomatic	If symptomatic	If symptoms or if abnormal gastrointestinal evaluations	If symptomatic	If symptomatic
Esophagoscopy		If symptomatic	If symptomatic	If symptomatic	If symptomatic	If symptomatic
Cardiac Testing						
Echocardiogram and cardiology follow-up	X	If previously abnormal or if on supplemental oxygen	If previously abnormal or if on supplemental oxygen	If previously abnormal or if on supplemental oxygen	If previously abnormal or if on supplemental oxygen	If previously abnormal or if on supplemental oxygen
Pulmonary Testing						
Chest radiograph	X	If patched	If patched	If patched	If patched	If patched
Pulmonary function tests			If patched		If patched	If patched
Musculoskeletal Testing						
Scoliosis and chest wall deformity screening (physical examination, CXR, and/or CT chest)				X		X

Adapted from Lally KP, Engle W. Post-discharge follow-up of infants with CDH. Pediatrics 2008;121:627–32.

children less than 3 years of age, suggesting a need for RSV prophylaxis.[295] Recurrent pneumonias have been reported in 26–39% of CDH survivors with at least 10 years of follow-up.[114,297]

Obstructive pulmonary disease is commonly reported in surviving children with CDH. Asthma and general symptoms of bronchospasm and wheezing are well documented.[183,298,299] Although symptoms appear to improve with age, most CDH children will exhibit some combination of obstructive and restrictive pulmonary function as well as increased reactivity to pharmacological agents.[298,299] This reduced pulmonary function is most likely due to lower functional volumes rather than primary obstruction of the airways.[299]

Although lung development begins early in gestation, alveolar maturation continues after birth. In CDH, lung hypoplasia affects both lungs with a reduction in airway and pulmonary artery branching.[49,300] Based on ventilation/perfusion $(\dot{V}/\dot{Q})$ radionuclide scans, pulmonary hypoplasia will persist despite continued lung growth.[299,301] These $\dot{V}/\dot{Q}$ mismatches are due to abnormal lung perfusion. Although increases in lung volume continues during early childhood, there is not an associated increase in lung perfusion. In a review of 137 CDH infants, 61% had $\dot{V}/\dot{Q}$ mismatching with the strongest correlation in children that underwent patch repair and ECMO.[302] Even though $\dot{V}/\dot{Q}$ scans in CDH children have provided valuable information, its predictive value for chronic lung disease in CDH survivors remains to be determined.

Neurological Outcomes

Although most children with CDH may resolve their pulmonary or gastrointestinal conditions, residual neurologic morbidities may be harder to detect. Complications associated with the disease and initial treatment, such as seizure disorders, cerebral palsy, and hemorrhagic or ischemic strokes, occur with a very low prevalence.[303,304] However, neurodevelopmental conditions, such as learning disabilities, fine and gross motor skill deficits, behavior problems, and visual-motor coordination may be more common than initially prevalence.[290,305,306]

Most longitudinal data have been limited to early development (<3 years of age). Overall, only 54–58% of CDH children demonstrate normal neurodevelopment with 23–25% demonstrating suspected delays, and 17–23% showing marked delays.[305,307] Utilizing the Bayley Scales of Infant Development (BSID)-II, some neuromotor delay was seen in 77% of infants with a 19 month median follow-up.[305] The severity of neurological problems seem to be related to the severity of disease with mild to moderate developmental delay in 37% of CDH survivors, including 72% that had undergone ECMO.[291] The largest series of CDH survivors (41 patients) demonstrated mild and severely delayed cognitive and language skills in 17% and 15%, respectively.[306] With a median age at 24 months, psychomotor skills were normal, mildly delayed, and severely delayed in 46%, 23%, and 31%, respectively.

Neurodevelopment outcomes beyond 3 years of age are limited. Among preschool children born with CDH,

one study showed normal, mildly delayed, and severely delayed neuromotor testing in 58%, 29%, and 13%, respectively.[308] In a prospective cohort of ECMO survivors, only 38% of preschool children scored in the normal range.[309] Thirty-four per cent demonstrated mild motor delays only, 6% showed mild delay in motor, cognitive, and/or behavior development, while 16% were severely delayed in at least two of the three domains.

Neurological delays may continue beyond preshool age. An age-matched controlled study that compared CDH and normal children for neurocognitive, visual, and fine motor outcomes found significant differences.[310] With an average age of 13 years, the mean score for full IQ, verbal IQ, and performance IQ were similar between groups. However, 13% of CDH children were significantly delayed, with 15% scoring below average for Full-IQ and Verbal-IQ while 23% were delayed for performance-IQ. In addition, the CDH cohort had a significantly higher proportion with oral-motor programming and visual-motor deficits compared to normal controls. Furthermore, approximately 45% of CDH children had below average IQ scores at 10 years of age.[311]

ECMO use, disease severity with prolonged hypoxia, and prolonged hospitalizations have all been implicated in the poor neurologic outcomes. In a study of 82 CDH children that required ECMO, developmental delay at 1 year post-repair was significantly more prevalent compared to children needing ECMO for other indications.[303] Abnormal neuroimaging in CDH children with neurodevelopmental delays that underwent ECMO has also been found.[312] However, ECMO has not been a significant risk factor for neurological deficits in other studies.[313,314] Certainly, other comorbidities, such as low socio-economic status and prematurity, may contribute to the poor neurological outcomes as well.[315–317]

Hearing impairment is a recognized sequelae of CDH with an overall incidence exceeding those of other neonatal intensive care infants (2%) and the general population (0.1–0.2%).[183,318] The prevalence of sensorineural hearing loss (SNHL) ranges from none in some series to 100% in others.[304,318] SNHL has been detected in as many as 50% of CDH children that initially tested as normal.[318] The etiology of SNHL is unclear. One study suggested a relationship between SNHL and ECMO and hyperventilation.[291] While several studies have suggested a causal relationship between ECMO and SNHL,[183,318,319] others have suggested that SNHL occurs regardless of ECMO use.[317,320] Several ototoxic medications, including diuretics, antibiotics, and muscle relaxants, are routinely used in the acute and chronic care of infants with CDH.[319] Another study suggested that severe hypoxia and acidosis may be linked to SNHL.[317] Most likely, SNHL is due to a combination of treatments and severity of disease. Because of the increased risk of SNHL in CDH children, audiological testing is warranted as early as 6 months of age.[292]

Gastrointestinal Outcomes

Gastroesophageal reflux disease (GERD) occurs in two-thirds of all CDH survivors with approximately half requiring fundoplication.[320–322] Long-term symptoms can persist with 63% of patients requiring GERD medications after 2 years in one study.[323] The etiology of CDH-association GERD is unclear. Certainly, anatomical changes following CDH repair can contribute to GERD. Esophageal ectasia may occur due to the mediastinal shift which results in an abnormal lower esophageal sphincter.[324] An intrathoracic stomach due to herniation can cause loss of the angle of His.[325,326] The CDH may also cause a differential growth pattern and a shortening of the intra-abdominal esophagus.[327] Distortion of the esophageal hiatus and increased intra-abdominal pressure from reducing the viscera have also been implicated as post-surgical causes of GERD.[314] Due to the frequency of symptomatic GERD, fundoplication has been recommended at the time of CDH repair by some surgeons, especially in patients with large diaphragmatic defects, but without proven benefit.[304]

Musculoskeletal Outcomes

Musculoskeletal development and chest wall deformities, such as pectus deformities, chest asymmetry, and scoliosis, are common in CDH children with an estimated incidence between 21–48%.[291,296] Scoliosis can be severe and can progress until adulthood. These musculoskeletal abnormalities may be due to tension on the diaphragm after repair, or result from a thoracotomy without muscle sparing techniques, or result from a small hemithorax due to hypoplastic lungs.[11,296] Most patients are asymptomatic and do not require operative intervention.

ANTERIOR HERNIAS OF MORGAGNI

An anterior diaphragmatic Morgagni hernia accounts for less than 2% of all CDH. The foramen of Morgagni hernia results from failure of fusion of the crural and sternal portions of the diaphragm. This can occur on either side at the junction of the septum transversum and thoracic wall where the superior epigastric artery (internal mammary artery, intrathoracically) traverses the diaphragm. These are usually large anterior midline defects. Typically, a hernia sac is present containing omentum, small intestine, and/or colon. Rarely these hernias will contain liver and/or spleen. The majority of children with a Morgagni hernia are asymptomatic and are rarely diagnosed during the neonatal period. Symptoms typically include general epigastric discomfort or sometimes vomiting and coughing due to intermittent obstruction.[328,329] An acute presentation may be due to intestinal ischemia with necrosis and perforation as well as gastric volvulus. Herniation into the pericardium causing tamponade has also been described.[330]

The chest radiograph may exhibit a well-defined air-fluid level in the midline of the chest and visceral herniation in the retrosternal space (Fig. 24-9). Small hernias may require a contrast radiograph or CT scan to confirm the diagnosis. Operative repair usually entails reduction of the herniated viscera, excision of the hernia sac, and approximation of the diaphragm to the posterior rectus sheath at the costal margin. These repairs can be performed laparoscopically (Fig. 24-10).[331,332] Although most defects can be repaired primarily, large defects may require patch closure.[213,216] The long-term outcome regarding recurrence is yet to be defined.

An anterior diaphragmatic hernia may be found in association with a pentalogy of Cantrell due to a failure in the development of the septum transversum.[333] Pentalogy of Cantrell is a rare cluster of congenital anomalies which includes omphalocele, cardiac defects, ectopic cordis, and an anterior diaphragmatic defect extending into the pericardium. The cardiac defect is the most severe problem and is the main cause of mortality.

DIAPHRAGMATIC EVENTRATION

Eventration is an abnormal elevation of the diaphragm which results in a paradoxical motion during respiration and interferes with normal pulmonary mechanics and function.[334,335] Congenital eventration results from the incomplete development of the central tendon or

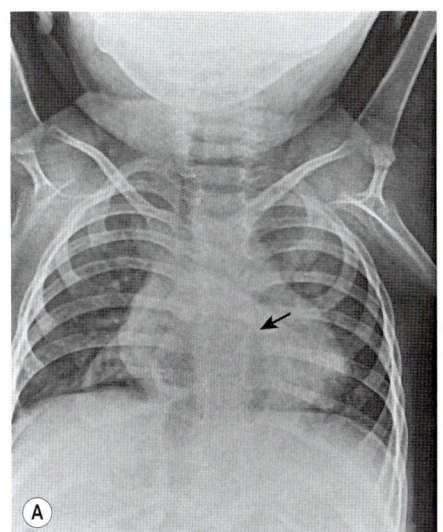
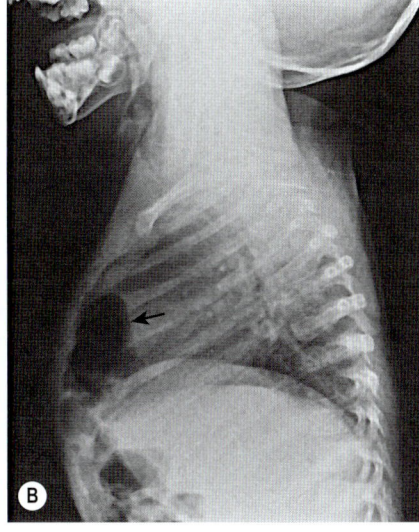

FIGURE 24-9 ■ (A) Chest radiograph in a neonate with a retrosternal hernia. Antero-posterior film demonstrates air-filled loops of bowel above the diaphragm and posterior to the sternum (arrow). **(B)** Lateral projection confirms the retrosternal position of the herniated viscera (arrow).

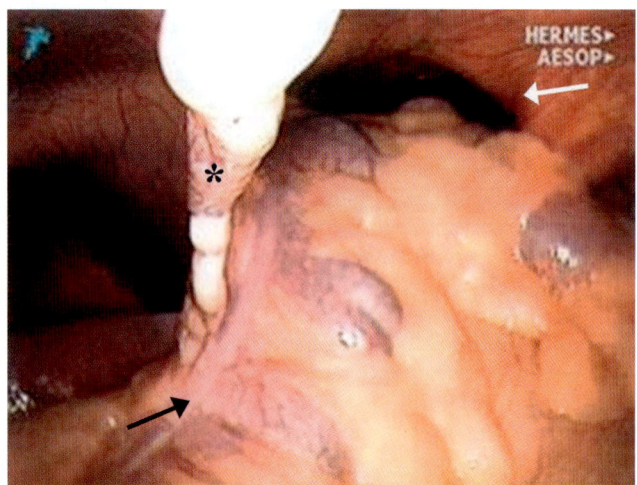

FIGURE 24-10 ■ Laparoscopic view of a Morgagni hernia. This anterior hernia (white arrow) is to the left of the falciform ligament (asterisk) with a deep sac that was excised. The large bowel (black arrow) was reduced from the hernia defect, and the defect was closed with a biosynthetic patch. (From Holcomb GW III, Ostlie DJ, Miller KA. Laparoscopic patch repair of diaphragmatic hernias with Surgisis. J Pediatr Surg 2005;40:e1–5.)

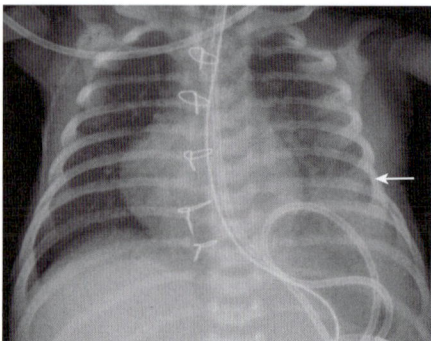

FIGURE 24-11 ■ Anteroposterior chest radiograph of a 4-week-old male neonate demonstrates a left-sided diaphragmatic eventration (arrow) after repair of total anomalous pulmonary–venous return. The abdominal viscera remain beneath an intact left hemidiaphragm.

muscular portion of the diaphragm. While commonly left-sided, bilateral congenital eventrations have been described.[336] The diaphragm muscle is typically present, but does not move in a coordinated fashion. It is usually thin, and may be indistinguishable from a hernia sac seen in CDH. Large eventrations can interfere with lung development due to the paradoxical motion and decreased thoracic space. Similar to CDH, congenital eventration can result in lung hypoplasia, although this is uncommon. Persistent fetal circulation and PHTN are usually not seen with eventration. Acquired diaphragmatic eventration can occur due to paralysis of the phrenic nerve secondary to mediastinal tumors, congenital heart surgery, or birth trauma. Its incidence after congenital cardiac surgery has been reported to be approximately 5% with the highest proportion after Fontan and Blalock–Taussig shunt procedures.[337,338]

Diaphragmatic eventration may present acutely with respiratory distress and tachypnea in the newborn, or may have a more indolent course with recurrent respiratory infections and wheezing. Neonates can have feeding intolerance due to discoordinated sucking and breathing. Older children may demonstrate exercise intolerance. Both lungs are usually affected by the paradoxical motion. With inspiration, the eventrated diaphragm rises which causes the mediastinum to shift and compress the contralateral lung.

Eventration is typically suspected on a plain chest film showing an elevated hemidiaphragm (Fig. 24-11). The diagnosis is subsequently confirmed by ultrasound or fluoroscopy. Motion studies demonstrate a paradoxical movement of the diaphragm and a mediastinal shift during respiration.[339] Occasionally, a CT scan is required to distinguish eventration from pleural effusions, mediastinal tumors, bronchogenic cysts, or pulmonary sequestrations.

Small eventrations may be observed as the child will eventually overcome and compensate for the abnormal diaphragmatic dynamics. When needed, initial treatment should include respiratory support, but mechanical ventilation is usually not necessary. However, larger defects that cause functional pulmonary impairment or promote recurring infections require repair. Neonates with large eventrations benefit from early repair rather than a course of conservative treatment.[339,340] Acquired eventrations often require repair in order to be weaned from mechanical ventilation.

Repair can be accomplished through the chest or abdomen. The eventrated diaphragm is plicated with a series of nonabsorbable sutures. Sutures should imbricate generous amounts of the diaphragmatic tissue without injuring the phrenic nerve. The edges of the diaphragm should overlap until the plicated muscle is taut. Subsequently, the diaphragm becomes immobilized which results in an increased tidal volume and prevents mediastinal shift. Minimally invasive techniques have been well described using thoracoscopy or laparoscopy.[341–343]

REFERENCES

1. Tsao K, Lally KP. The Congenital Diaphragmatic Hernia Study Group. A voluntary international registry. Semin Pediatr Surg 2008;17:90–7.
2. Moyer V, Moya F, Tibboel R, et al. Late versus early surgical correction for congenital diaphragmatic hernia in newborn infants. Cochrane Database Syst Rev (Online) 2002:CD001695.
3. Wilson JM, Lund DP, Lillehei CW, et al. Congenital diaphragmatic hernia–a tale of two cities: the Boston experience. J Pediatr Surg 1997;32:401–5.
4. Bohn DJ, Pearl R, Irish MS, et al. Postnatal management of congenital diaphragmatic hernia. Clin Perinatol 1996;23:843–72.
5. Frenckner B, Ehren H, Granholm T, et al. Improved results in patients who have congenital diaphragmatic hernia using preoperative stabilization, extracorporeal membrane oxygenation, and delayed surgery. J Pediatr Surg 1997;32:1185–9.
6. Langham MR Jr, Kays DW, Ledbetter DJ, et al. Congenital diaphragmatic hernia. Epidemiology and outcome. Clin Perinatol 1996;23:671–88.
7. Dott MM, Wong LY, Rasmussen SA. Population-based study of congenital diaphragmatic hernia: Risk factors and survival in Metropolitan Atlanta, 1968–1999. Birth Defects Res A Clin Mol Teratol 2003;67:261–7.
8. Wenstrom KD, Weiner CP, Hanson JW. A five-year statewide experience with congenital diaphragmatic hernia. Am J Obstet Gynecol 1991;165:838–42.

9. Ontario Congenital Anomalies Study Group. Apparent truth about congenital diaphragmatic hernia: A population-based database is needed to establish benchmarking for clinical outcomes for CDH. J Pediatr Surg 2004;39:661–5.

10. Harrison MR, Adzick NS, Estes JM, et al. A prospective study of the outcome for fetuses with diaphragmatic hernia. Jama 1994;271:382–4.

11. Lund DP, Mitchell J, Kharasch V, et al. Congenital diaphragmatic hernia: The hidden morbidity. J Pediatr Surg 1994;29:258–62.

12. Stege G, Fenton A, Jaffray B. Nihilism in the 1990s: The true mortality of congenital diaphragmatic hernia. Pediatrics 2003;112:532–5.

13. Neville HL, Jaksic T, Wilson JM, et al. Bilateral congenital diaphragmatic hernia. J Pediatr Surg 2003;38:522–4.

14. Waller DK, Tita AT, Werler MM, et al. Association between prepregnancy maternal body mass index and the risk of having an infant with a congenital diaphragmatic hernia. Birth Defects Res A Clin Mol Teratol 2003;67:73–6.

15. Lipson AH, Williams G. Congenital diaphragmatic hernia in half sibs. J Med Genet 1985;22:145–7.

16. Witters I, Legius E, Moerman P, et al. Associated malformations and chromosomal anomalies in 42 cases of prenatally diagnosed diaphragmatic hernia. Am J Med Genet 2001;103:278–82.

17. Schlembach D, Zenker M, Trautmann U, et al. Deletion 15q24-26 in prenatally detected diaphragmatic hernia: Increasing evidence of a candidate region for diaphragmatic development. Prenat Diagn 2001;21:289–92.

18. Aviram-Goldring A, Daniely M, Frydman M, et al. Congenital diaphragmatic hernia in a family segregating a reciprocal translocation t(5;15)(p15.3;q24). Am J Med Genet 2000;90:120–2.

19. Slavotinek AM. Single gene disorders associated with congenital diaphragmatic hernia. Am J Med Genet C Semin Med Genet 2007;145C:172–83.

20. Langer JC, Winthrop AL, Whelan D. Fryns syndrome: A rare familial cause of congenital diaphragmatic hernia. J Pediatr Surg 1994;29:1266–7.

21. Neville HL, Jaksic T, Wilson JM, et al. Fryns syndrome in children with congenital diaphragmatic hernia. J Pediatr Surg 2002;37:1685–7.

22. Scott DA. Genetics of congenital diaphragmatic hernia. Semin Pediatr Surg 2007;16:88–93.

23. Torfs CP, Curry CJ, Bateson TF, et al. A population-based study of congenital diaphragmatic hernia. Teratology 1992;46:555–65.

24. Pober BR. Genetic aspects of human congenital diaphragmatic hernia. Clin Genet 2008;74:1–15.

25. van Loenhout RB, Tibboel D, Post M, et al. Congenital diaphragmatic hernia: Comparison of animal models and relevance to the human situation. Neonatology 2009;96:137–49.

26. Stoll C, Alembik Y, Dott B, et al. Associated malformations in cases with congenital diaphragmatic hernia. Genet Couns 2008;19:331–9.

27. Bollmann R, Kalache K, Mau H, et al. Associated malformations and chromosomal defects in congenital diaphragmatic hernia. Fetal Diagn Ther 1995;10:52–9.

28. Tibboel D, Gaag AV. Etiologic and genetic factors in congenital diaphragmatic hernia. Clin Perinatol 1996;23:689–99.

29. Butler N, Claireaux AE. Congenital diaphragmatic hernia as a cause of perinatal mortality. Lancet 1962;1:659–63.

30. Sweed Y, Puri P. Congenital diaphragmatic hernia: Influence of associated malformations on survival. Arch Dis Child 1993;69:68–70.

31. Eghtesady P, Skarsgard ED, Smith BM, et al. Congenital diaphragmatic hernia associated with aortic coarctation. J Pediatr Surg 1998;33:943–5.

32. Migliazza L, Xia H, Alvarez JI, et al. Heart hypoplasia in experimental congenital diaphragmatic hernia. J Pediatr Surg 1999;34:706–10.

33. Menon SC, Tani LY, Weng HY, et al. Clinical characteristics and outcomes of patients with cardiac defects and congenital diaphragmatic hernia. J Pediatr 2013;162:114–9.

34. Raval MV, Wang X, Reynolds M, et al. Costs of congenital diaphragmatic hernia repair in the United States-extracorporeal membrane oxygenation foots the bill. J Pediatr Surg 2011;46:617–24.

35. Metkus AP, Esserman L, Sola A, et al. Cost per anomaly: What does a diaphragmatic hernia cost? J Pediatr Surg 1995;30:226–30.

36. Iritani I. Experimental study on embryogenesis of congenital diaphragmatic hernia. Anat Embryol (Berl) 1984;169:133–9.

37. Kluth D, Keijzer R, Hertl M, et al. Embryology of congenital diaphragmatic hernia. Semin Pediatr Surg 1996;5:224–33.

38. Babiuk RP, Zhang W, Clugston R, et al. Embryological origins and development of the rat diaphragm. J Comp Neurol 2003;455:477–87.

39. Skandalakis JE, Gray SE, Ricketts RR. The Diaphragm. In: Skandalakis JE, Gray SE, editors. Embryology for Surgeons. Baltimore, MD: Williams and Wilkens; 1994. p. 491–539.

40. Jenkinson EL. Absence of half of the diaphragm (thoracic stomach; diaphragmatic hernia). Am J Roentgenol 1931;26:899.

41. Bremer JL. The diaphragm and diaphragmatic hernia. Arch Pathol 1943;36:539.

42. Greer JJ, Allan DW, Babiuk RP, et al. Recent advances in understanding the pathogenesis of nitrofen-induced congenital diaphragmatic hernia. Pediatr Pulmonol 2000;29:394–9.

43. Wiseman NE, MacPherson RI. 'Acquired' congenital diaphragmatic hernia. J Pediatr Surg 1977;12:657–65.

44. Noble BR, Babiuk RP, Clugston RD, et al. Mechanisms of action of the congenital diaphragmatic hernia-inducing teratogen nitrofen. Am J Physiol Lung Cell Mol Physiol 2007;293:L1079–87.

45. Migliazza L, Otten C, Xia H, et al. Cardiovascular malformations in congenital diaphragmatic hernia: Human and experimental studies. J Pediatr Surg 1999;34:1352–8.

46. Migliazza L, Xia H, Diez-Pardo JA, et al. Skeletal malformations associated with congenital diaphragmatic hernia: Experimental and human studies. J Pediatr Surg 1999;34:1624–9.

47. Clugston RD, Klattig J, Englert C, et al. Teratogen-induced, dietary and genetic models of congenital diaphragmatic hernia share a common mechanism of pathogenesis. Am J Pathol 2006;169:1541–9.

48. Allan DW, Greer JJ. Pathogenesis of nitrofen-induced congenital diaphragmatic hernia in fetal rats. J Appl Physiol 1997;83:338–47.

49. Chinoy MR. Pulmonary hypoplasia and congenital diaphragmatic hernia: Advances in the pathogenetics and regulation of lung development. J Surg Res 2002;106:209–23.

50. Chinoy MR. Lung growth and development. Front Biosci 2003;8:d392–415.

51. Mey J, Babiuk RP, Clugston R, et al. Retinal dehydrogenase-2 is inhibited by compounds that induce congenital diaphragmatic hernias in rodents. Am J Pathol 2003;162:673–9.

52. Wilson JG, Roth CB, Warkany J. An analysis of the syndrome of malformations induced by maternal vitamin A deficiency. Effects of restoration of vitamin A at various times during gestation. Am J Anat 1953;92:189–217.

53. Mendelsohn C, Lohnes D, Decimo D, et al. Function of the retinoic acid receptors (RARs) during development (II). Multiple abnormalities at various stages of organogenesis in RAR double mutants. Development 1994;120:2749–71.

54. Major D, Cadenas M, Fournier L, et al. Retinol status of newborn infants with congenital diaphragmatic hernia. Pediatr Surg Int 1998;13:547–9.

55. Miniati D. Pulmonary vascular remodeling. Semin Pediatr Surg 2007;16:80–7.

56. Weibel ER, Gomez DM. A principle for counting tissue structures on random sections. J Appl Physiol 1962;17:343–8.

57. Hislop A, Reid L. Intra-pulmonary arterial development during fetal life-branching pattern and structure. J Anat 1972;113:35–48.

58. Hislop A, Reid L. Pulmonary arterial development during childhood: branching pattern and structure. Thorax 1973;28:129–35.

59. Reid IS, Hutcherson RJ. Long-term follow-up of patients with congenital diaphragmatic hernia. J Pediatr Surg 1976;11:939–42.

60. Dibbins AW. Congenital diaphragmatic hernia: Hypoplastic lung and pulmonary vasoconstriction. Clin Perinatol 1978;5:93–104.

61. Suen HC, Catlin EA, Ryan DP, et al. Biochemical immaturity of lungs in congenital diaphragmatic hernia. J Pediatr Surg 1993;28:471–5.

62. Moya FR, Thomas VL, Romaguera J, et al. Fetal lung maturation in congenital diaphragmatic hernia. Am J Obstet Gynecol 1995; 173:1401–5.

63. Janssen DJ, Zimmermann LJ, Cogo P, et al. Decreased surfactant phosphatidylcholine synthesis in neonates with congenital diaphragmatic hernia during extracorporeal membrane oxygenation. Intensive Care Med 2009;35:1754–60.

64. Wagenvoort CA, Neufeld HN, Edwards JE. The structure of the pulmonary arterial tree in fetal and early postnatal life. Lab Invest 1961;10:751–62.

65. Allen K, Haworth SG. Human postnatal pulmonary arterial remodeling. Ultrastructural studies of smooth muscle cell and connective tissue maturation. Lab Invest 1988;59:702–9.

66. Haworth SG. Pulmonary vascular remodeling in neonatal pulmonary hypertension. State of the art. Chest 1988;93:S133–8.

67. Roubliova X, Verbeken E, Wu J, et al. Pulmonary vascular morphology in a fetal rabbit model for congenital diaphragmatic hernia. J Pediatr Surg 2004;39:1066–72.

68. Lipsett J, Cool JC, Runciman SI, et al. Morphometric analysis of preterm fetal pulmonary development in the sheep model of congenital diaphragmatic hernia. Pediatr Dev Pathol 2000;3:17–28.

69. Sokol J, Bohn D, Lacro RV, et al. Fetal pulmonary artery diameters and their association with lung hypoplasia and postnatal outcome in congenital diaphragmatic hernia. Am J Obstet Gynecol 2002;186:1085–90.

70. Jakkula M, Le Cras TD, Gebb S, et al. Inhibition of angiogenesis decreases alveolarization in the developing rat lung. Am J Physiol Lung Cell Mol Physiol 2000;279:L600–7.

71. Grover TR, Parker TA, Balasubramaniam V, et al. Pulmonary hypertension impairs alveolarization and reduces lung growth in the ovine fetus. Am J Physiol Lung Cell Mol Physiol 2005;288: L648–54.

72. Ruano R, Aubry MC, Barthe B, et al. Quantitative analysis of fetal pulmonary vasculature by 3-dimensional power Doppler ultrasonography in isolated congenital diaphragmatic hernia. Am J Obstet Gynecol 2006;195:1720–8.

73. Suda K, Bigras JL, Bohn D, et al. Echocardiographic predictors of outcome in newborns with congenital diaphragmatic hernia. Pediatrics 2000;105:1106–9.

74. Casaccia G, Crescenzi F, Dotta A, et al. Birth weight and McGoon Index predict mortality in newborn infants with congenital diaphragmatic hernia. J Pediatr Surg 2006;41:25–8.

75. Taira Y, Yamataka T, Miyazaki E, et al. Comparison of the pulmonary vasculature in newborns and stillborns with congenital diaphragmatic hernia. Pediatr Surg Int 1998;14:30–5.

76. Taira Y, Yamataka T, Miyazaki E, et al. Adventitial changes in pulmonary vasculature in congenital diaphragmatic hernia complicated by pulmonary hypertension. J Pediatr Surg 1998;33: 382–7.

77. Dillon PW, Cilley RE, Mauger D, et al. The relationship of pulmonary artery pressure and survival in congenital diaphragmatic hernia. J Pediatr Surg 2004;39:307–12.

78. Jeanty C, Nien JK, Espinoza J, et al. Pleural and pericardial effusion: A potential ultrasonographic marker for the prenatal differential diagnosis between congenital diaphragmatic eventration and congenital diaphragmatic hernia. Ultrasound Obstet Gynecol 2007;29:378–87.

79. Garne E, Haeusler M, Barisic I, et al. Congenital diaphragmatic hernia: Evaluation of prenatal diagnosis in 20 European regions. Ultrasound Obstet Gynecol 2002;19:329–33.

80. Vettraino IM, Lee W, Comstock CH. The evolving appearance of a congenital diaphragmatic hernia. J Ultrasound Med 2002;21:85–9.

81. Dillon E, Renwick M, Wright C. Congenital diaphragmatic herniation: Antenatal detection and outcome. Br J Radiol 2000;73: 360–5.

82. Benjamin DR, Juul S, Siebert JR. Congenital posterolateral diaphragmatic hernia: Associated malformations. J Pediatr Surg 1988;23:899–903.

83. DeVore GR, Horenstein J, Platt LD. Fetal echocardiography. VI. Assessment of cardiothoracic disproportion—a new technique for the diagnosis of thoracic hypoplasia. Am J Obstet Gynecol 1986;155:1066–71.

84. Wilcox DT, Irish MS, Holm BA, et al. Prenatal diagnosis of congenital diaphragmatic hernia with predictors of mortality. Clin Perinatol 1996;23:701–9.

85. Metkus AP, Filly RA, Stringer MD, et al. Sonographic predictors of survival in fetal diaphragmatic hernia. J Pediatr Surg 1996;31:148–51.

86. Harrison MR, Adzick NS, Flake AW, et al. Correction of congenital diaphragmatic hernia in utero: VI. Hard-earned lessons. J Pediatr Surg 1993;28:1411–7.

87. Keller RL, Glidden DV, Paek BW, et al. The lung-to-head ratio and fetoscopic temporary tracheal occlusion: Prediction of survival in severe left congenital diaphragmatic hernia. Ultrasound Obstet Gynecol 2003;21:244–9.

88. Laudy JA, Van Gucht M, Van Dooren MF, et al. Congenital diaphragmatic hernia: An evaluation of the prognostic value of the lung-to-head ratio and other prenatal parameters. Prenat Diagn 2003;23:634–9.

89. Lipshutz GS, Albanese CT, Feldstein VA, et al. Prospective analysis of lung-to-head ratio predicts survival for patients with prenatally diagnosed congenital diaphragmatic hernia. J Pediatr Surg 1997;32:1634–6.

90. Ba'ath ME, Jesudason EC, Losty PD. How useful is the lung-to-head ratio in predicting outcome in the fetus with congenital diaphragmatic hernia? A systematic review and meta-analysis. Ultrasound Obstet Gynecol 2007;30:897–906.

91. Heling KS, Wauer RR, Hammer H, et al. Reliability of the lung-to-head ratio in predicting outcome and neonatal ventilation parameters in fetuses with congenital diaphragmatic hernia. Ultrasound Obstet Gynecol 2005;25:112–8.

92. Deprest JA, Flemmer AW, Gratacos E, et al. Antenatal prediction of lung volume and in-utero treatment by fetal endoscopic tracheal occlusion in severe isolated congenital diaphragmatic hernia. Semin Fetal Neonatal Med 2009;14:8–13.

93. Peralta CF, Cavoretto P, Csapo B, et al. Lung and heart volumes by three-dimensional ultrasound in normal fetuses at 12–32 weeks' gestation. Ultrasound Obstet Gynecol 2006;27: 128–33.

94. Ruano R, Benachi A, Martinovic J, et al. Can three-dimensional ultrasound be used for the assessment of the fetal lung volume in cases of congenital diaphragmatic hernia? Fetal Diagn Ther 2004;19:87–91.

95. Ruano R, Martinovic J, Dommergues M, et al. Accuracy of fetal lung volume assessed by three-dimensional sonography. Ultrasound Obstet Gynecol 2005;26:725–30.

96. Cannie MM, Jani JC, Van Kerkhove F, et al. Fetal body volume at MR imaging to quantify total fetal lung volume: Normal ranges. Radiology 2008;247:197–203.

97. Coakley FV, Lopoo JB, Lu Y, et al. Normal and hypoplastic fetal lungs: Volumetric assessment with prenatal single-shot rapid acquisition with relaxation enhancement MR imaging. Radiology 2000;216:107–11.

98. Rypens F, Metens T, Rocourt N, et al. Fetal lung volume: Estimation at MR imaging-initial results. Radiology 2001;219:236–41.

99. Cannie M, Jani J, Meersschaert J, et al. Prenatal prediction of survival in isolated diaphragmatic hernia using observed to expected total fetal lung volume determined by magnetic resonance imaging based on either gestational age or fetal body volume. Ultrasound Obstet Gynecol 2008;32:633–9.

100. Gorincour G, Bouvenot J, Mourot MG, et al. Prenatal prognosis of congenital diaphragmatic hernia using magnetic resonance imaging measurement of fetal lung volume. Ultrasound Obstet Gynecol 2005;26:738–44.

101. Jani J, Cannie M, Done E, et al. Relationship between lung area at ultrasound examination and lung volume assessment with magnetic resonance imaging in isolated congenital diaphragmatic hernia. Ultrasound Obstet Gynecol 2007;30:855–60.

102. Sandaite I, Claus F, De Keyzer F, et al. Examining the relationship between the lung-to-head ratio measured on ultrasound and lung volumetry by magnetic resonance in fetuses with isolated congenital diaphragmatic hernia. Fetal Diagn Ther 2011;29:80–7.

103. Manning PB, Murphy JP, Raynor SC, et al. Congenital diaphragmatic hernia presenting due to gastrointestinal complications. J Pediatr Surg 1992;27:1225–8.

104. Paut O, Mely L, Viard L, et al. Acute presentation of congenital diaphragmatic hernia past the neonatal period: A life threatening emergency. Can J Anaesth 1996;43:621–5.

105. Weber TR, Tracy T Jr, Bailey PV, et al. Congenital diaphragmatic hernia beyond infancy. Am J Surg 1991;162:643–6.

106. Losty PD, Suen HC, Manganaro TF, et al. Prenatal hormonal therapy improves pulmonary compliance in the nitrofen-induced CDH rat model. J Pediatr Surg 1995;30:420–6.

107. Oue T, Shima H, Guarino N, et al. Antenatal dexamethasone administration increases fetal lung DNA synthesis and RNA and protein content in nitrofen-induced congenital diaphragmatic hernia in rats. Pediatr Res 2000;48:789–93.

108. Kay HH, Bird IM, Coe CL, et al. Antenatal steroid treatment and adverse fetal effects: What is the evidence? J Soc Gynecol Investig 2000;7:269–78.

109. Smith GN, Kingdom JC, Penning DH, et al. Antenatal corticosteroids: Is more better? Lancet 2000;355:251–2.

110. Lally KP, Bagolan P, Hosie S, et al. Corticosteroids for fetuses with congenital diaphragmatic hernia: Can we show benefit? J Pediatr Surg 2006;41:668–74.

111. Levin DL. Morphologic analysis of the pulmonary vascular bed in congenital left-sided diaphragmatic hernia. J Pediatr 1978;92:805–9.

112. Shehata SM, Sharma HS, van der Staak FH, et al. Remodeling of pulmonary arteries in human congenital diaphragmatic hernia with or without extracorporeal membrane oxygenation. J Pediatr Surg 2000;35:208–15.

113. Beals DA, Schloo BL, Vacanti JP, et al. Pulmonary growth and remodeling in infants with high-risk congenital diaphragmatic hernia. J Pediatr Surg 1992;27:997–1002.

114. Okuyama H, Kubota A, Kawahara H, et al. Correlation between lung scintigraphy and long-term outcome in survivors of congenital diaphragmatic hernia. Pediatr Pulmonol 2006;41:882–6.

115. Sakurai Y, Azarow K, Cutz E, et al. Pulmonary barotrauma in congenital diaphragmatic hernia: A clinicopathological correlation. J Pediatr Surg 1999;34:1813–7.

116. Drummond WH, Gregory GA, Heymann MA, et al. The independent effects of hyperventilation, tolazoline, and dopamine on infants with persistent pulmonary hypertension. J Pediatr 1981;98:603–11.

117. Rudolph AM, Yuan S. Response of the pulmonary vasculature to hypoxia and H+ ion concentration changes. J Clin Invest 1966;45:399–411.

118. Boloker J, Bateman DA, Wung JT, et al. Congenital diaphragmatic hernia in 120 infants treated consecutively with permissive hypercapnea/spontaneous respiration/elective repair. J Pediatr Surg 2002;37:357–66.

119. Kays DW, Langham MR Jr, Ledbetter DJ, et al. Detrimental effects of standard medical therapy in congenital diaphragmatic hernia. Ann Surg 1999;230:340–8.

120. Langham MR Jr, Kays DW, Beierle EA, et al. Twenty years of progress in congenital diaphragmatic hernia at the University of Florida. Am Surg 2003;69:45–52.

121. Wung JT, Sahni R, Moffitt ST, et al. Congenital diaphragmatic hernia: Survival treated with very delayed surgery, spontaneous respiration, and no chest tube. J Pediatr Surg 1995;30:406–9.

122. Bohn D. Congenital diaphragmatic hernia. Am J Respir Crit Care Med 2002;166:911–15.

123. Azarow K, Messineo A, Pearl R, et al. Congenital diaphragmatic hernia–a tale of two cities: The Toronto experience. J Pediatr Surg 1997;32:395–400.

124. Paranka MS, Clark RH, Yoder BA, et al. Predictors of failure of high-frequency oscillatory ventilation in term infants with severe respiratory failure. Pediatrics 1995;95:400–4.

125. Hirschl RB. Innovative therapies in the management of newborns with congenital diaphragmatic hernia. Semin Pediatr Surg 1996;5:256–65.

126. Desfrere L, Jarreau PH, Dommergues M, et al. Impact of delayed repair and elective high-frequency oscillatory ventilation on survival of antenatally diagnosed congenital diaphragmatic hernia: First application of these strategies in the more 'severe' subgroup of antenatally diagnosed newborns. Intensive Care Med 2000;26:934–41.

127. Reyes C, Chang LK, Waffarn F, et al. Delayed repair of congenital diaphragmatic hernia with early high-frequency oscillatory ventilation during preoperative stabilization. J Pediatr Surg 1998;33:1010–6.

128. Cacciari A, Ruggeri G, Mordenti M, et al. High-frequency oscillatory ventilation versus conventional mechanical ventilation in congenital diaphragmatic hernia. Eur J Pediatr Surg 2001;11:3–7.

129. Cogo PE, Simonato M, Danhaive O, et al. Impaired surfactant protein b synthesis in infants with congenital diaphragmatic hernia. Eur Respir J 2012;Epub ahead of print.

130. Cogo PE, Zimmermann LJ, Rosso F, et al. Surfactant synthesis and kinetics in infants with congenital diaphragmatic hernia. Am J Respir Crit Care Med 2002;166:154–8.

131. O'Toole SJ, Karamanoukian HL, Morin FC 3rd, et al. Surfactant decreases pulmonary vascular resistance and increases pulmonary blood flow in the fetal lamb model of congenital diaphragmatic hernia. J Pediatr Surg 1996;31:507–11.

132. Karamanoukian HL, Glick PL, Wilcox DT, et al. Pathophysiology of congenital diaphragmatic hernia. VIII: Inhaled nitric oxide requires exogenous surfactant therapy in the lamb model of congenital diaphragmatic hernia. J Pediatr Surg 1995;30:1–4.

133. Lally KP, Lally PA, Langham MR, et al. Surfactant does not improve survival rate in preterm infants with congenital diaphragmatic hernia. J Pediatr Surg 2004;39:829–33.

134. Van Meurs K. Is surfactant therapy beneficial in the treatment of the term newborn infant with congenital diaphragmatic hernia? J Pediatr 2004;145:312–6.

135. Colby CE, Lally KP, Hintz SR, et al. Surfactant replacement therapy on ECMO does not improve outcome in neonates with congenital diaphragmatic hernia. J Pediatr Surg 2004;39:1632–7.

136. Lotze A, Knight GR, Anderson KD, et al. Surfactant (beractant) therapy for infants with congenital diaphragmatic hernia on ECMO: Evidence of persistent surfactant deficiency. J Pediatr Surg 1994;29:407–12.

137. Buss M, Williams G, Dilley A, et al. Prevention of heart failure in the management of congenital diaphragmatic hernia by maintaining ductal patency. A case report. J Pediatr Surg 2006;41:e9–11.

138. Tanabe M, Yoshida H, Iwai J, et al. Doppler flow patterns through the ductus arteriosus in patients with congenital diaphragmatic hernia. Eur J Pediatr Surg 2000;10:92–5.

139. Finer NN, Barrington KJ. Nitric oxide in respiratory failure in the newborn infant. Semin Perinatol 1997;21:426–40.

140. Kinsella JP, Abman SH. Inhalational nitric oxide therapy for persistent pulmonary hypertension of the newborn. Pediatrics 1993;91:997–8.

141. Kinsella JP, Ivy DD, Abman SH. Inhaled nitric oxide improves gas exchange and lowers pulmonary vascular resistance in severe experimental hyaline membrane disease. Pediatr Res 1994;36:402–8.

142. Roberts JD, Polaner DM, Lang P, et al. Inhaled nitric oxide in persistent pulmonary hypertension of the newborn. Lancet 1992;340:818–9.

143. Kinsella JP, Neish SR, Shaffer E, et al. Low-dose inhalation nitric oxide in persistent pulmonary hypertension of the newborn. Lancet 1992;340:819–20.

144. Clark RH, Kueser TJ, Walker MW, et al. Low-dose nitric oxide therapy for persistent pulmonary hypertension of the newborn. Clinical Inhaled Nitric Oxide Research Group. N Engl J Med 2000;342:469–74.

145. The Neonatal Inhaled Nitric Oxide Study Group (NINOS). Inhaled nitric oxide and hypoxic respiratory failure in infants with congenital diaphragmatic hernia. The Neonatal Inhaled Nitric Oxide Study Group (NINOS). Pediatrics 1997;99:838–45.

146. Keller RL, Hamrick SE, Kitterman JA, et al. Treatment of rebound and chronic pulmonary hypertension with oral sildenafil in an infant with congenital diaphragmatic hernia. Pediatr Crit Care Med 2004;5:184–7.

147. Ivy DD, Kinsella JP, Ziegler JW, et al. Dipyridamole attenuates rebound pulmonary hypertension after inhaled nitric oxide withdrawal in postoperative congenital heart disease. J Thorac Cardiovasc Surg 1998;115:875–82.

148. Kinsella JP, Ivy DD, Abman SH. Pulmonary vasodilator therapy in congenital diaphragmatic hernia: Acute, late, and chronic pulmonary hypertension. Semin Perinatol 2005;29:123–8.

149. Finer NN, Barrington KJ. Nitric oxide for respiratory failure in infants born at or near term. Cochrane Database Syst Rev (Online) 2006;CD000399.

150. Bender AT, Beavo JA. Cyclic nucleotide phosphodiesterases: Molecular regulation to clinical use. Pharmacol Rev 2006;58:488–520.

151. Buysse C, Fonteyne C, Dessy H, et al. The use of dipyridamole to wean from inhaled nitric oxide in congenital diaphragmatic hernia. J Pediatr Surg 2001;36:1864–5.

152. Kinsella JP, Torielli F, Ziegler JW, et al. Dipyridamole augmentation of response to nitric oxide. Lancet 1995;346:647–8.

153. Thebaud B, Saizou C, Farnoux C, et al. Dypiridamole, a cGMP phosphodiesterase inhibitor, transiently improves the response to inhaled nitric oxide in two newborns with congenital diaphragmatic hernia. Intensive Care Med 1999;25:300–3.

154. Filan PM, McDougall PN, Shekerdemian LS. Combination pharmacotherapy for severe neonatal pulmonary hypertension. J Paediatr Child Health 2006;42:219–20.

155. Noori S, Friedlich P, Wong P, et al. Cardiovascular effects of sildenafil in neonates and infants with congenital diaphragmatic hernia and pulmonary hypertension. Neonatology 2007;91:92–100.

156. De Luca D, Zecca E, Vento G, et al. Transient effect of epoprostenol and sildenafil combined with iNO for pulmonary hypertension in congenital diaphragmatic hernia. Paediatr Anaesth 2006;16:597–8.

157. Steinhorn RH, Kinsella JP, Pierce C, et al. Intravenous sildenafil in the treatment of neonates with persistent pulmonary hypertension. J Pediatr 2009;155:841–7.

158. Hunter L, Richens T, Davis C, et al. Sildenafil use in congenital diaphragmatic hernia. Arch Dis Child Fetal Neonatal Ed 2009;94:F467.

159. Abman SH, Kinsella JP, Rosenzweig EB, et al. Implications of the FDA warning against the use of Sildenafil for the treatment of pediatric pulmonary hypertension. Am J Respir Crit Care Med 2013;187:572–5.

160. Barst RJ. Recent advances in the treatment of pediatric pulmonary artery hypertension. Pediatr Clin North Am 1999;46:331–45.

161. Barst RJ, Ivy D, Dingemanse J, et al. Pharmacokinetics, safety, and efficacy of bosentan in pediatric patients with pulmonary arterial hypertension. Clin Pharmacol Ther 2003;73:372–82.

162. Rosenzweig EB, Barst RJ. Pulmonary arterial hypertension in children: A medical update. Curr Opin Pediatr 2008;20:288–93.

163. Terragno NA, Terragno A. Prostaglandin metabolism in the fetal and maternal vasculature. Fed Proc 1979;38:75–7.

164. Leffler CW, Hessler JR, Green RS. Mechanism of stimulation of pulmonary prostacyclin synthesis at birth. Prostaglandins 1984;28:877–87.

165. Leffler CW, Hessler JR, Green RS. The onset of breathing at birth stimulates pulmonary vascular prostacyclin synthesis. Pediatr Res 1984;18:938–42.

166. Yanagisawa M, Kurihara H, Kimura S, et al. A novel potent vasoconstrictor peptide produced by vascular endothelial cells. Nature 1988;332:411–5.

167. Buchan KW, Magnusson H, Rabe KF, et al. Characterisation of the endothelin receptor mediating contraction of human pulmonary artery using BQ123 and Ro 46-2005. Eur J Pharmacol 1994;260:221–6.

168. Ziegler JW, Ivy DD, Kinsella JP, et al. The role of nitric oxide, endothelin, and prostaglandins in the transition of the pulmonary circulation. Clin Perinatol 1995;22:387–403.

169. Ivy DD, Kinsella JP, Abman SH. Physiologic characterization of endothelin A and B receptor activity in the ovine fetal pulmonary circulation. J Clin Invest 1994;93:2141–8.

170. de Lagausie P, de Buys-Roessingh A, Ferkdadji L, et al. Endothelin receptor expression in human lungs of newborns with congenital diaphragmatic hernia. J Pathol 2005;205:112–8.

171. Keller RL, Tacy TA, Hendricks-Munoz K, et al. Congenital diaphragmatic hernia: Endothelin-1, pulmonary hypertension, and disease severity. Am J Respir Crit Care Med 2010;182:555–61.

172. Kobayashi H, Puri P. Plasma endothelin levels in congenital diaphragmatic hernia. J Pediatr Surg 1994;29:1258–61.

173. Ivy DD, Rosenzweig EB, Lemarie JC, et al. Long-term outcomes in children with pulmonary arterial hypertension treated with bosentan in real-world clinical settings. Am J Cardiol 2010;106:1332–8.

174. Rosenzweig EB, Ivy DD, Widlitz A, et al. Effects of long-term bosentan in children with pulmonary arterial hypertension. J Am Coll Cardiol 2005;46:697–704.

175. The Congenital Diaphragmatic Hernia Study Group. Does extracorporeal membrane oxygenation improve survival in neonates with congenital diaphragmatic hernia? J Pediatr Surg 1999;34:720–5.

176. Downard, C. Impact of Amicar on hemorrhagic complications of ECMO: A ten-year review. J Pediatr Surg 2003;38:1212–6.

177. Lally KP. Extracorporeal membrane oxygenation in patients with congenital diaphragmatic hernia. Semin Pediatr Surg 1996;5:249–55.

178. Somaschini M, Locatelli G, Salvoni L, et al. Impact of new treatments for respiratory failure on outcome of infants with congenital diaphragmatic hernia. Eur J Pediatr 1999;158:780–4.

179. German JC, Gazzaniga AB, Amlie R, et al. Management of pulmonary insufficiency in diaphragmatic hernia using extracorporeal circulation with a membrane oxygenator (ECMO). J Pediatr Surg 1977;12:905–12.

180. Heiss K, Manning P, Oldham KT, et al. Reversal of mortality for congenital diaphragmatic hernia with ECMO. Ann Surg 1989;209:225–30.

181. Sawyer SF, Falterman KW, Goldsmith JP, et al. Improving survival in the treatment of congenital diaphragmatic hernia. Ann Thorac Surg 1986;41:75–8.

182. Weber TR, Connors RH, Pennington DG, et al. Neonatal diaphragmatic hernia. An improving outlook with extracorporeal membrane oxygenation. Arch Surg 1987;122:615–8.

183. Davis PJ, Firmin RK, Manktelow B, et al. Long-term outcome following extracorporeal membrane oxygenation for congenital diaphragmatic hernia: The UK experience. J Pediatr 2004;144:309–15.

184. Langham MR Jr, Krummel TM, Greenfield LJ, et al. Extracorporeal membrane oxygenation following repair of congenital diaphragmatic hernias. Ann Thorac Surg 1987;44:247–52.

185. Lally KP, Lally PA, Van Meurs KP, et al. Treatment evolution in high-risk congenital diaphragmatic hernia: Ten years' experience with diaphragmatic agenesis. Ann Surg 2006;244:505–13.

186. Lally KP, Paranka MS, Roden J, et al. Congenital diaphragmatic hernia. Stabilization and repair on ECMO. Ann Surg 1992;216:569–73.

187. Reickert CA, Hirschl RB, Atkinson JB, et al. Congenital diaphragmatic hernia survival and use of extracorporeal life support at selected level III nurseries with multimodality support. Surgery 1998;123:305–10.

188. Keshen TH, Gursoy M, Shew SB, et al. Does extracorporeal membrane oxygenation benefit neonates with congenital diaphragmatic hernia? Application of a predictive equation. J Pediatr Surg 1997;32:818–22.

189. O'Rourke PP, Lillehei CW, Crone RK, et al. The effect of extracorporeal membrane oxygenation on the survival of neonates with high-risk congenital diaphragmatic hernia: 45 cases from a single institution. J Pediatr Surg 1991;26:147–52.

190. Al-Shanafey S, Giacomantonio M, Henteleff H. Congenital diaphragmatic hernia: Experience without extracorporeal membrane oxygenation. Pediatr Surg Int 2002;18:28–31.

191. Pusic AL, Giacomantonio M, Pippus K, et al. Survival in neonatal congenital hernia without extracorporeal membrane oxygenation support. J Pediatr Surg 1995;30:1188–90.

192. Skarsgard ED, Harrison MR. Congenital diaphragmatic hernia: The surgeon's perspective. Pediatr Rev 1999;20:e71–8.

193. Harting M. Surgical management of neonates with congenital diaphragmatic hernia. Semin Pediatr Surg 2007;16:109–14.

194. Sakai H, Tamura M, Hosokawa Y, et al. Effect of surgical repair on respiratory mechanics in congenital diaphragmatic hernia. J Pediatr 1987;111:432–8.

195. de la Hunt MN, Madden N, Scott JE, et al. Is delayed surgery really better for congenital diaphragmatic hernia?: A prospective randomized clinical trial. J Pediatr Surg 1996;31:1554–6.

196. Langer JC, Filler RM, Bohn DJ, et al. Timing of surgery for congenital diaphragmatic hernia: Is emergency operation necessary? J Pediatr Surg 1988;23:731–4.

197. Nio M, Haase G, Kennaugh J, et al. A prospective randomized trial of delayed versus immediate repair of congenital diaphragmatic hernia. J Pediatr Surg 1994;29:618–21.

198. Al-Hathal M, Crankson SJ, Al-Harbi F, et al. Congenital diaphragmatic hernia: Experience with preoperative stabilization and delayed surgery without ECMO and inhaled nitric oxide. Am J Perinatol 1998;15:487–90.

199. Breaux CW Jr, Rouse TM, Cain WS, et al. Improvement in survival of patients with congenital diaphragmatic hernia utilizing a strategy of delayed repair after medical and/or extracorporeal membrane oxygenation stabilization. J Pediatr Surg 1991;26: 333–8.

200. West KW, Bengston K, Rescorla FJ, et al. Delayed surgical repair and ECMO improves survival in congenital diaphragmatic hernia. Ann Surg 1992;216:454–62.

201. Bagolan P, Casaccia G, Crescenzi F, et al. Impact of a current treatment protocol on outcome of high-risk congenital diaphragmatic hernia. J Pediatr Surg 2004;39:313–8.

202. Dassinger MS, Copeland DR, Gossett J, et al. Early repair of congenital diaphragmatic hernia on extracorporeal membrane oxygenation. J Pediatr Surg 2010;45:693–7.

203. Levy SM, Lally PA, Lally KP, et al. The impact of chylothorax on neonates with repaired congenital diaphragmatic hernia. J Pediatr Surg 2013;48:724–9.

204. Sigalet DL, Tierney A, Adolph V, et al. Timing of repair of congenital diaphragmatic hernia requiring extracorporeal membrane oxygenation support. J Pediatr Surg 1995;30:1183–7.

205. Meehan JJ, Haney BM, Snyder CL, et al. Outcome following recannulation and a second ECMO course. J Pediatr Surg 2002;37:845–50.

206. Clark RH, Hardin WD Jr, Hirschl RB, et al. Current surgical management of congenital diaphragmatic hernia: a report from the Congenital Diaphragmatic Hernia Study Group. J Pediatr Surg 1998;33:1004–9.

207. Tsao K, Lally PA, Lally KP. Minimally invasive repair of congenital diaphragmatic hernia. J Pediatr Surg 2011;46:1158–64.

208. Puri P. Congenital diaphragmatic hernia. Curr Probl Surg 1994;31:787–846.

209. Kyzer S, Sirota L, Chaimoff C. Abdominal wall closure with a silastic patch after repair of congenital diaphragmatic hernia. Arch Surg 2004;139:296–8.

210. Schnitzer JJ, Kikiros CS, Short BL, et al. Experience with abdominal wall closure for patients with congenital diaphragmatic hernia repaired on ECMO. J Pediatr Surg 1995;30:19–22.

211. Rana AR, Khouri JS, Teitelbaum DH, et al. Salvaging the severe congenital diaphragmatic hernia patient: Is a silo the solution? J Pediatr Surg 2008;43:788–91.

212. Cheah FC, Noraida MH, Boo NY, et al. Chylothorax after repair of congenital diaphragmatic hernia–a case report. Singapore Med J 2000;41:548–9.

213. Arca MJ, Barnhart DC, Lelli JL Jr, et al. Early experience with minimally invasive repair of congenital diaphragmatic hernias: Results and lessons learned. J Pediatr Surg 2003;38:1563–8.

214. Nguyen TL, Le AD. Thoracoscopic repair for congenital diaphragmatic hernia: Lessons from 45 cases. J Pediatr Surg 2006;41:1713–5.

215. Yang EY, Allmendinger N, Johnson SM, et al. Neonatal thoracoscopic repair of congenital diaphragmatic hernia: Selection criteria for successful outcome. J Pediatr Surg 2005;40:1369–75.

216. Holcomb GW III, Ostlie DJ, Miller KA. Laparoscopic patch repair of diaphragmatic hernia with Surgisis. J Pediatr Surg 2005;40:E1–7.

217. Shah SR, Gittes GK, Barsness KA, et al. Thoracoscopic patch repair of a right-sided congenital diaphragmatic hernia in a neonate. Surg Endosc 2008;23:215.

218. McHoney M, Giacomello L, Nah SA, et al. Thoracoscopic repair of congenital diaphragmatic hernia: Intraoperative ventilation and recurrence. J Pediatr Surg 2010;45:355–9.

219. Pacilli M, Pierro A, Kingsley C, et al. Absorption of carbon dioxide during laparoscopy in children measured using a novel mass spectrometric technique. Br J Anaesth 2006;97:215–9.

220. Bliss D, Matar M, Krishnaswami S. Should intraoperative hypercapnea or hypercarbia raise concern in neonates undergoing thoracoscopic repair of diaphragmatic hernia of Bochdalek? J Laparoendosc Adv Surg Tech A 2009;19 (Suppl. 1):S55–8.

221. McHoney M, Corizia L, Eaton S, et al. Carbon dioxide elimination during laparoscopy in children is age dependent. J Pediatr Surg 2003;38:105–10.

222. Gourlay DM, Cassidy LD, Sato TT, et al. Beyond feasibility: A comparison of newborns undergoing thoracoscopic and open repair of congenital diaphragmatic hernias. J Pediatr Surg 2009;44:1702–7.

223. Kim AC, Bryner BS, Akay B, et al. Thoracoscopic repair of congenital diaphragmatic hernia in neonates: Lessons learned. J Laparoendosc Adv Surg Tech A 2009;19:575–80.

224. Cho SD, Krishnaswami S, McKee JC, et al. Analysis of 29 consecutive thoracoscopic repairs of congenital diaphragmatic hernia in neonates compared to historical controls. J Pediatr Surg 2009;44:80–6; discussion 6.

225. Shah SR, Wishnew J, Barsness K, et al. Minimally invasive congenital diaphragmatic hernia repair: A 7-year review of one institution's experience. Surg Endosc 2009;23:1265–71.

226. McHoney MC, Corizia L, Eaton S, et al. Laparoscopic surgery in children is associated with an intraoperative hypermetabolic response. Surg Endosc 2006;20:452–7.

227. Taskin M, Zengin K, Unal E, et al. Laparoscopic repair of congenital diaphragmatic hernias. Surg Endosc 2002;16:869.

228. Gander JW, Fisher JC, Gross ER, et al. Early recurrence of congenital diaphragmatic hernia is higher after thoracoscopic than open repair: A single institutional study. J Pediatr Surg 2011; 46:1303–8.

229. Keijzer R, van de Ven C, Vlot J, et al. Thoracoscopic repair in congenital diaphragmatic hernia: patching is safe and reduces the recurrence rate. J Pediatr Surg 2010;45:953–7.

230. Lansdale N, Alam S, Losty PD, et al. Neonatal endosurgical congenital diaphragmatic hernia repair: a systematic review and meta-analysis. Ann Surg 2010;252:20–6.

231. Knight CG, Gidell KM, Lanning D, et al. Laparoscopic Morgagni hernia repair in children using robotic instruments. J Laparoendosc Adv Surg Tech A 2005;15:482–6.

232. Meehan JJ, Sandler A. Robotic repair of a Bochdalek congenital diaphragmatic hernia in a small neonate: Robotic advantages and limitations. J Pediatr Surg 2007;42:1757–60.

233. Slater BJ, Meehan JJ. Robotic repair of congenital diaphragmatic anomalies. J Laparoendosc Adv Surg Tech A 2009;19 (Suppl. 1): S123–7.

234. Grethel E, Cortes R, Wagner A, et al. Prosthetic patches for congenital diaphragmatic hernia repair: Surgisis vs Gore-Tex. J Pediatr Surg 2006;41:29–33.

235. Hajer GF, vd Staak FH, de Haan AF, et al. Recurrent congenital diaphragmatic hernia; which factors are involved? Eur J Pediatr Surg 1998;8:329–33.

236. Moss RL, Chen CM, Harrison MR. Prosthetic patch durability in congenital diaphragmatic hernia: A long-term follow-up study. J Pediatr Surg 2001;36:152–4.

237. Lally KP, Cheu HW, Vazquez WD. Prosthetic diaphragm reconstruction in the growing animal. J Pediatr Surg 1993;28: 45–7.

238. St Peter SD, Valusek PA, Tsao K, et al. Abdominal complications related to type of repair for congenital diaphragmatic hernia. J Surg Res 2007;140:234–6.

239. Loff S, Wirth H, Jester I, et al. Implantation of a cone-shaped double-fixed patch increases abdominal space and prevents recurrence of large defects in congenital diaphragmatic hernia. J Pediatr Surg 2005;40:1701–5.

240. Saltzman DA, Ennis JS, Mehall JR, et al. Recurrent congenital diaphragmatic hernia: A novel repair. J Pediatr Surg 2001;36: 1768–9.

241. St Peter SD, Shah SR, Little DC, et al. Bilateral congenital diaphragmatic hernia with absent pleura and pericardium. Birth Defects Res A Clin Mol Teratol 2005;73:624–7.

242. Sandusky GE Jr, Badylak SF, Morff RJ, et al. Histologic findings after in vivo placement of small intestine submucosal vascular grafts and saphenous vein grafts in the carotid artery in dogs. Am J Pathol 1992;140:317–24.

243. Oelschlager BK, Barreca M, Chang L, et al. The use of small intestine submucosa in the repair of paraesophageal hernias: Initial observations of a new technique. Am J Surg 2003;186:4–8.

244. Franklin ME Jr, Gonzalez JJ Jr, Michaelson RP, et al. Preliminary experience with new bioactive prosthetic material for repair of hernias in infected fields. Hernia 2002;6:171–4.

245. St. Peter SD, Holcomb GW III. The use of biosynthetic mesh to enhance hiatal repair at the time of re-do Nissen fundoplication. J Pediatr Surg 2007;42:1298–301.

246. Smith MJ, Paran TS, Quinn F, et al. The SIS extracellular matrix scaffold-preliminary results of use in congenital diaphragmatic hernia (CDH) repair. Pediatr Surg Int 2004;20:859–62.

247. Mitchell IC, Garcia NM, Barber R, et al. Permacol: A potential biologic patch alternative in congenital diaphragmatic hernia repair. J Pediatr Surg 2008;43:2161–4.

248. Menon NG, Rodriguez ED, Byrnes CK, et al. Revascularization of human acellular dermis in full-thickness abdominal wall reconstruction in the rabbit model. Ann Plast Surg 2003;50:523–7.

249. Urita Y, Komuro H, Chen G, et al. Evaluation of diaphragmatic hernia repair using PLGA mesh-collagen sponge hybrid scaffold: An experimental study in a rat model. Pediatr Surg Int 2008;24:1041–5.

250. Sandoval JA, Lou D, Engum SA, et al. The whole truth: Comparative analysis of diaphragmatic hernia repair using 4-ply vs 8-ply small intestinal submucosa in a growing animal model. J Pediatr Surg 2006;41:518–23.

251. Laituri CA, Garey CL, Valusek PA, et al. Outcome of congenital diaphragmatic hernia repair depending on patch type. Eur J Pediatr Surg 2010;5.

252. Kimber CP, Dunkley MP, Haddock G, et al. Patch incorporation in diaphragmatic hernia. J Pediatr Surg 2000;35:120–3.

253. Simpson JS, Gossage JD. Use of abdominal wall muscle flap in repair of large congenital diaphragmatic hernia. J Pediatr Surg 1971;6:42–4.

254. Scaife ER, Johnson DG, Meyers RL, et al. The split abdominal wall muscle flap–a simple, mesh-free approach to repair large diaphragmatic hernia. J Pediatr Surg 2003;38:1748–51.

255. Brant-Zawadzki PB, Fenton SJ, Nichol PF, et al. The split abdominal wall muscle flap repair for large congenital diaphragmatic hernias on extracorporeal membrane oxygenation. J Pediatr Surg 2007;42:1047–50.

256. Barnhart DC, Jacques E, Scaife ER, et al. Split abdominal wall muscle flap repair vs patch repair of large congenital diaphragmatic hernias. J Pediatr Surg 2012;47:81–6.

257. Bianchi A, Doig CM, Cohen SJ. The reverse latissimus dorsi flap for congenital diaphragmatic hernia repair. J Pediatr Surg 1983;18:560–3.

258. Samarakkody U, Klaassen M, Nye B. Reconstruction of congenital agenesis of hemidiaphragm by combined reverse latissimus dorsi and serratus anterior muscle flaps. J Pediatr Surg 2001;36:1637–40.

259. Meeker IA Jr, Snyder WH Jr. Surgical management of diaphragmatic defects in the newborn infant. A report of twenty infants each less than one week old (1956–1961). Am J Surg 1962;104:196–203.

260. Sydorak, R. Reversed latissimus dorsi muscle flap for repair of recurrent congenital diaphragmatic hernia. J Pediatr Surg 2003;38:296–300.

261. Bekdash B, Singh B, Lakhoo K. Recurrent late complications following congenital diaphragmatic hernia repair with prosthetic patches: a case series. J Med Case Reports 2009;3:7237.

262. Barbosa RF, Rodrigues J, Correia-Pinto J, et al. Repair of a large congenital diaphragmatic defect with a reverse latissimus dorsi muscle flap. Microsurgery 2008;28:85–8.

263. Ferrari G, Cusella-De Angelis G, Coletta M, et al. Muscle regeneration by bone marrow-derived myogenic progenitors. Science 1998;279:1528–30.

264. Rossi CA, Pozzobon M, Ditadi A, et al. Clonal characterization of rat muscle satellite cells: Proliferation, metabolism and differentiation define an intrinsic heterogeneity. PLoS One 2010;5:e8523.

265. De Coppi P, Bartsch G Jr, Siddiqui MM, et al. Isolation of amniotic stem cell lines with potential for therapy. Nat Biotechnol 2007;25:100–6.

266. Fuchs JR, Kaviani A, Oh JT, et al. Diaphragmatic reconstruction with autologous tendon engineered from mesenchymal amniocytes. J Pediatr Surg 2004;39:834–8; discussion 8.

267. Turner CG, Klein JD, Steigman SA, et al. Preclinical regulatory validation of an engineered diaphragmatic tendon made with amniotic mesenchymal stem cells. J Pediatr Surg 2011;46:57–61.

268. Harrison MR, Adzick NS, Bullard KM, et al. Correction of congenital diaphragmatic hernia in utero VII: A prospective trial. J Pediatr Surg 1997;32:1637–42.

269. Harrison MR, Bressack MA, Churg AM, et al. Correction of congenital diaphragmatic hernia in utero. II. Simulated correction permits fetal lung growth with survival at birth. Surgery 1980;88:260–8.

270. DiFiore JW, Fauza DO, Slavin R, et al. Experimental fetal tracheal ligation reverses the structural and physiological effects of pulmonary hypoplasia in congenital diaphragmatic hernia. J Pediatr Surg 1994;29:248–56; discussion 56–57.

271. Hedrick MH, Estes JM, Sullivan KM, et al. Plug the lung until it grows (PLUG): A new method to treat congenital diaphragmatic hernia in utero. J Pediatr Surg 1994;29:612–7.

272. Lipsett J, Cool JC, Runciman SI, et al. Effect of antenatal tracheal occlusion on lung development in the sheep model of congenital diaphragmatic hernia: A morphometric analysis of pulmonary structure and maturity. Pediatr Pulmonol 1998;25:257–69.

273. Bin Saddiq W, Piedboeuf B, Laberge JM, et al. The effects of tracheal occlusion and release on type II pneumocytes in fetal lambs. J Pediatr Surg 1997;32:834–8.

274. Jani JC, Nicolaides KH, Gratacos E, et al. Fetal lung-to-head ratio in the prediction of survival in severe left-sided diaphragmatic hernia treated by fetal endoscopic tracheal occlusion (FETO). Am J Obstet Gynecol 2006;195:1646–50.

275. Deprest J, Jani J, Van Schoubroeck D, et al. Current consequences of prenatal diagnosis of congenital diaphragmatic hernia. J Pediatr Surg 2006;41:423–30.

276. Harrison MR, Keller RL, Hawgood SB, et al. A randomized trial of fetal endoscopic tracheal occlusion for severe fetal congenital diaphragmatic hernia. N Engl J Med 2003;349:1916–24.

277. Deprest J, Gratacos E, Nicolaides KH. Fetoscopic tracheal occlusion (FETO) for severe congenital diaphragmatic hernia: Evolution of a technique and preliminary results. Ultrasound Obstet Gynecol 2004;24:121–6.

278. Jani JC, Nicolaides KH, Gratacos E, et al. Severe diaphragmatic hernia treated by fetal endoscopic tracheal occlusion. Ultrasound Obstet Gynecol 2009;34:304–10.

279. Ruano R, Yoshisaki CT, da Silva MM, et al. A randomized controlled trial of fetal endoscopic tracheal occlusion versus postnatal management of severe isolated congenital diaphragmatic hernia. Ultrasound Obstet Gynecol 2012;39:20–7.

280. The Congenital Diaphragmatic Hernia Study Group. Estimating disease severity of congenital diaphragmatic hernia in the first 5 minutes of life. J Pediatr Surg 2001;36:141–5.

281. Javid PJ, Jaksic T, Skarsgard ED, et al. Survival rate in congenital diaphragmatic hernia: The experience of the Canadian Neonatal Network. J Pediatr Surg 2004;39:657–60.

282. Grushka JR, Laberge JM, Puligandla P, et al. Effect of hospital case volume on outcome in congenital diaphragmatic hernia: The experience of the Canadian Pediatric Surgery Network. J Pediatr Surg 2009;44:873–6.

283. Bucher BT, Guth RM, Saito JM, et al. Impact of hospital volume on in-hospital mortality of infants undergoing repair of congenital diaphragmatic hernia. Ann Surg 2010;252:635–42.

284. Cohen MS, Rychik J, Bush DM, et al. Influence of congenital heart disease on survival in children with congenital diaphragmatic hernia. J Pediatr 2002;141:25–30.

285. Graziano JN. Cardiac anomalies in patients with congenital diaphragmatic hernia and their prognosis: A report from the Congenital Diaphragmatic Hernia Study Group. J Pediatr Surg 2005;40:1045–9; discussion 9–50.

286. Tsao K, Allison ND, Harting MT, et al. Congenital diaphragmatic hernia in the preterm infant. Surgery 2010;148:404–10.

287. Levison J, Halliday R, Holland AJ, et al. A population-based study of congenital diaphragmatic hernia outcome in New South Wales and the Australian Capital Territory, Australia, 1992–2001. J Pediatr Surg 2006;41:1049–53.

288. Rygl M, Pycha K, Stranak Z, et al. Congenital diaphragmatic hernia: onset of respiratory distress and size of the defect: Analysis of the outcome in 104 neonates. Pediatr Surg Int 2007;23:27–31.

289. Lally KP, Lally PA, Lasky RE, et al. Defect size determines survival in infants with congenital diaphragmatic hernia. Pediatrics 2007;120:e651–7.

290. Danzer E, Hedrick HL. Neurodevelopmental and neurofunctional outcomes in children with congenital diaphragmatic hernia. Early Hum Dev 2011;87:625–32.

291. Nobuhara KK, Lund DP, Mitchell J, et al. Long-term outlook for survivors of congenital diaphragmatic hernia. Clin Perinatol 1996;23:873–87.

292. Lally KP, Engle W. Postdischarge follow-up of infants with congenital diaphragmatic hernia. Pediatrics 2008;121:627–32.
293. Wohl ME, Griscom NT, Strieder DJ, et al. The lung following repair of congenital diaphragmatic hernia. J Pediatr 1977;90:405–14.
294. Falconer AR, Brown RA, Helms P, et al. Pulmonary sequelae in survivors of congenital diaphragmatic hernia. Thorax 1990;45:126–9.
295. Muratore CS, Kharasch V, Lund DP, et al. Pulmonary morbidity in 100 survivors of congenital diaphragmatic hernia monitored in a multidisciplinary clinic. J Pediatr Surg 2001;36:133–40.
296. Vanamo K, Rintala R, Sovijarvi A, et al. Long-term pulmonary sequelae in survivors of congenital diaphragmatic defects. J Pediatr Surg 1996;31:1096–9; discussion 9–100.
297. Kamata S, Usui N, Kamiyama M, et al. Long-term follow-up of patients with high-risk congenital diaphragmatic hernia. J Pediatr Surg 2005;40:1833–8.
298. Trachsel D, Selvadurai H, Bohn D, et al. Long-term pulmonary morbidity in survivors of congenital diaphragmatic hernia. Pediatr Pulmonol 2005;39:433–9.
299. Marven SS, Smith CM, Claxton D, et al. Pulmonary function, exercise performance, and growth in survivors of congenital diaphragmatic hernia. Arch Dis Child 1998;78:137–42.
300. Bargy F, Beaudoin S, Barbet P. Fetal lung growth in congenital diaphragmatic hernia. Fetal Diagn Ther 2006;21:39–44.
301. Arena F, Baldari S, Centorrino A, et al. Mid- and long-term effects on pulmonary perfusion, anatomy and diaphragmatic motility in survivors of congenital diaphragmatic hernia. Pediatr Surg Int 2005;21:954–9.
302. Hayward MJ, Kharasch V, Sheils C, et al. Predicting inadequate long-term lung development in children with congenital diaphragmatic hernia: An analysis of longitudinal changes in ventilation and perfusion. J Pediatr Surg 2007;42:112–6.
303. Bernbaum J, Schwartz IP, Gerdes M, et al. Survivors of extracorporeal membrane oxygenation at 1 year of age: The relationship of primary diagnosis with health and neurodevelopmental sequelae. Pediatrics 1995;96:907–13.
304. Jaillard SM, Pierrat V, Dubois A, et al. Outcome at 2 years of infants with congenital diaphragmatic hernia: A population-based study. Ann Thorac Surg 2003;75:250–6.
305. Chen C, Jeruss S, Chapman JS, et al. Long-term functional impact of congenital diaphragmatic hernia repair on children. J Pediatr Surg 2007;42:657–65.
306. Danzer E, Gerdes M, Bernbaum J, et al. Neurodevelopmental outcome of infants with congenital diaphragmatic hernia prospectively enrolled in an interdisciplinary follow-up program. J Pediatr Surg 2010;45:1759–66.
307. Van Meurs KP, Robbins ST, Reed VL, et al. Congenital diaphragmatic hernia: Long-term outcome in neonates treated with extracorporeal membrane oxygenation. J Pediatr 1993;122:893–9.
308. van der Cammen-van Zijp MH, Gischler SJ, Mazer P, et al. Motor-function and exercise capacity in children with major anatomical congenital anomalies: An evaluation at 5 years of age. Early Hum Dev 2010;86:523–8.
309. Nijhuis-van der Sanden MW, van der Cammen-van Zijp MH, Janssen AJ, et al. Motor performance in five-year-old extracorporeal membrane oxygenation survivors: A population-based study. Crit Care 2009;13:R47.
310. Jakobson LS, Frisk V, Trachsel D, et al. Visual and fine-motor outcomes in adolescent survivors of high-risk congenital diaphragmatic hernia who did not receive extracorporeal membrane oxygenation. J Perinatol 2009;29:630–6.
311. Bouman NH, Koot HM, Tibboel D, et al. Children with congenital diaphragmatic hernia are at risk for lower levels of cognitive functioning and increased emotional and behavioral problems. Eur J Pediatr Surg 2000;10:3–7.
312. McGahren ED, Mallik K, Rodgers BM. Neurological outcome is diminished in survivors of congenital diaphragmatic hernia requiring extracorporeal membrane oxygenation. J Pediatr Surg 1997;32:1216–20.
313. Masumoto K, Nagata K, Uesugi T, et al. Risk factors for sensorineural hearing loss in survivors with severe congenital diaphragmatic hernia. Eur J Pediatr 2007;166:607–12.
314. Qi B, Soto C, Diez-Pardo JA, et al. An experimental study on the pathogenesis of gastroesophageal reflux after repair of diaphragmatic hernia. J Pediatr Surg 1997;32:1310–3.
315. Stolar CJ, Crisafi MA, Driscoll YT. Neurocognitive outcome for neonates treated with extracorporeal membrane oxygenation: Are infants with congenital diaphragmatic hernia different? J Pediatr Surg 1995;30:366–71; discussion 71–72.
316. Colvin J, Bower C, Dickinson JE, et al. Outcomes of congenital diaphragmatic hernia: A population-based study in Western Australia. Pediatrics 2005;116:e356–363.
317. Nield TA, Langenbacher D, Poulsen MK, et al. Neurodevelopmental outcome at 3.5 years of age in children treated with extracorporeal life support: Relationship to primary diagnosis. J Pediatr 2000;136:338–44.
318. Robertson CM, Tyebkhan JM, Hagler ME, et al. Late-onset, progressive sensorineural hearing loss after severe neonatal respiratory failure. Otol Neurotol 2002;23:353–6.
319. Fligor BJ, Neault MW, Mullen CH, et al. Factors associated with sensorineural hearing loss among survivors of extracorporeal membrane oxygenation therapy. Pediatrics 2005;115:1519–28.
320. Bagolan P, Morini F. Long-term follow up of infants with congenital diaphragmatic hernia. Semin Pediatr Surg 2007;16:134–44.
321. Muratore CS, Utter S, Jaksic T, et al. Nutritional morbidity in survivors of congenital diaphragmatic hernia. J Pediatr Surg 2001;36:1171–6.
322. Vanamo K, Rintala RJ, Lindahl H, et al. Long-term gastrointestinal morbidity in patients with congenital diaphragmatic defects. J Pediatr Surg 1996;31:551–4.
323. Cortes RA, Keller RL, Townsend T, et al. Survival of severe congenital diaphragmatic hernia has morbid consequences. J Pediatr Surg 2005;40:36–45; discussion-6.
324. Stolar CJ, Levy JP, Dillon PW, et al. Anatomic and functional abnormalities of the esophagus in infants surviving congenital diaphragmatic hernia. Am J Surg 1990;159:204–7.
325. Kieffer J, Sapin E, Berg A, et al. Gastroesophageal reflux after repair of congenital diaphragmatic hernia. J Pediatr Surg 1995;30:1330–3.
326. Koot VC, Bergmeijer JH, Bos AP, et al. Incidence and management of gastroesophageal reflux after repair of congenital diaphragmatic hernia. J Pediatr Surg 1993;28:48–52.
327. Nagaya M, Akatsuka H, Kato J. Gastroesophageal reflux occurring after repair of congenital diaphragmatic hernia. J Pediatr Surg 1994;29:1447–51.
328. Kimmelstiel FM, Holgersen LO, Hilfer C. Retrosternal (Morgagni) hernia with small bowel obstruction secondary to a Richter's incarceration. J Pediatr Surg 1987;22:998–1000.
329. Sarihan H, Imamoglu M, Abes M, et al. Pediatric Morgagni hernia. Report of two cases. J Cardiovasc Surg (Torino) 1996;37:195–7.
330. de Fonseca JM, Davies MR, Bolton KD. Congenital hydropericardium associated with the herniation of part of the liver into the pericardial sac. J Pediatr Surg 1987;22:851–3.
331. Dutta S, Albanese CT. Use of a prosthetic patch for laparoscopic repair of Morgagni diaphragmatic hernia in children. J Laparoendosc Adv Surg Tech A 2007;17:391–4.
332. Ponsky TA, Lukish JR, Nobuhara K, et al. Laparoscopy is useful in the diagnosis and management of foramen of Morgagni hernia in children. Surg Laparosc Endosc Percutan Tech 2002;12:375–7.
333. Cantrell JR, Haller JA, Ravitch MM. A syndrome of congenital defects involving the abdominal wall, sternum, diaphragm, pericardium, and heart. Surg Gynecol Obstet 1958;107:602–14.
334. Symbas PN, Hatcher CR Jr, Waldo W. Diaphragmatic eventration in infancy and childhood. Ann Thorac Surg 1977;24:113–9.
335. Wayne ER, Campbell JB, Burrington JD, et al. Eventration of the diaphragm. J Pediatr Surg 1974;9:643–51.
336. Elberg JJ, Brok KE, Pedersen SA, et al. Congenital bilateral eventration of the diaphragm in a pair of male twins. J Pediatr Surg 1989;24:1140–1.
337. Akay TH, Ozkan S, Gultekin B, et al. Diaphragmatic paralysis after cardiac surgery in children: Incidence, prognosis and surgical management. Pediatr Surg Int 2006;22:341–6.
338. Joho-Arreola AL, Bauersfeld U, Stauffer UG, et al. Incidence and treatment of diaphragmatic paralysis after cardiac surgery in children. Eur J Cardiothorac Surg 2005;27:53–7.

339. Yazici M, Karaca I, Arikan A, et al. Congenital eventration of the diaphragm in children: 25 years' experience in three pediatric surgery centers. Eur J Pediatr Surg 2003;13:298–301.

340. Smith CD, Sade RM, Crawford FA, et al. Diaphragmatic paralysis and eventration in infants. J Thorac Cardiovasc Surg 1986;91:490–7.

341. Becmeur F, Talon I, Schaarschmidt K, et al. Thoracoscopic diaphragmatic eventration repair in children: About 10 cases. J Pediatr Surg 2005;40:1712–5.

342. Guvenc BH, Korkmaz M, Avtan L, et al. Thoracoscopic diaphragm plication in children and indications for conversion to open thoracotomy. J Laparoendosc Adv Surg Tech A 2004; 14:302–5.

343. Huttl TP, Wichmann MW, Reichart B, et al. Laparoscopic diaphragmatic plication: Long-term results of a novel surgical technique for postoperative phrenic nerve palsy. Surg Endosc 2004;18:547–51.

CHAPTER 25

MEDIASTINAL TUMORS

Juan A. Tovar

The mediastinum can be divided into three compartments (Fig. 25-1). The anterior one contains the thymus, vessels, lymphoid structures, and nerves. The middle one contains the trachea, main-stem bronchi, the heart and great vessels, and the hilar lymph nodes. The posterior mediastinum accommodates the aorta, the thoracic esophagus, and the sympathetic nerve chains.

The tracheobronchial tree derives from the embryonic foregut that is innervated by neural crest cells that form the sympathetic chains. Embryonal germ cells migrate toward their final settlement in the gonads through the anterior mediastinum. The thymus primordia from the third pharyngeal pouches migrate into the anterior mediastinum and fuse to form a single organ. Finally, huge vascular structures develop in the mediastinum. All these embryonal events explain the nature of the tumors located in each compartment. Their most frequent location is summarized in Table 25-1.

CLINICAL FEATURES

Mediastinal tumors and cysts are occasionally diagnosed before birth and may even benefit from prenatal instrumentation.[1] However, most of them remain silent during infancy and are discovered serendipitously. Respiratory embarrassment, orthopnea, stridor, wheezing, severe distress, and superior vena cava syndrome are occasionally seen. Large anterior tumors may cause sternal bulging. Recurrent laryngeal or phrenic nerve palsies or Horner syndrome may also lead to diagnosis. Sudden paraplegia can occur in dumbbell tumors involving the spinal cord. Finally, secretion of catecholamines, α-fetoprotein, or gonadotropins may also uncover the tumor.

DIAGNOSTIC METHODS

Plain radiographs of the thorax or ultrasonography may show widening of the superior mediastinal shadow or masses in either hemithorax.[2,3] Computed tomography (CT) provides information about the location of the tumor, its cystic or solid nature, depicting calcifications, necrotic areas, and widening of the spinal foramina in cases with intraspinal extension. Calcifications are suggestive of neuroblastoma or teratoma, but other tumors, such as lymphangiomas or histiocytoses, can also have calcified areas.[4,5] CT is crucial for assessing the patency of the airway and the risks of anesthesia.[6] Magnetic resonance imaging (MRI) is used to better define the nature of the masses of vascular origin, and also for evaluating intraspinal invasion.[7,8]

For many tumors, histology, cell markers, and molecular biology features can be identified before undertaking operative therapy. Cells can be obtained by biopsy of cervical or suprasternal lymph nodes, by fine needle aspiration (FNA), or by pleural or pericardial fluid aspiration.[9–11] When this is not feasible, operative biopsy or excision is required. Thoracoscopy[12,13] or anterior mini-thoracotomy through the bed of the second or third rib (the Chamberlain approach)[14,15] may provide material for biopsy or for complete removal. Mediastinoscopy is rarely used in children.[16]

PRINCIPLES OF MANAGEMENT

Children with anterior mediastinal masses can undergo respiratory collapse after induction of anesthesia. Ventilation can be critically difficult, particularly in children with lymphoma. Cross-sectional surfaces of the tracheal lumen decreased by 50% or more on CT scan carry a high anesthetic risk.[14] These patients also have marked reductions in the maximum expiratory flow rates, and special modalities of anesthesia (e.g., spontaneous ventilation, laryngeal mask, rigid tubes) may be necessary.[6]

Except for lymphomas that respond to chemotherapy and/or radiotherapy and in which surgery is usually adjuvant, mediastinal tumors should be removed. Median sternotomy[17] or standard thoracotomy are the preferred approaches. Sternotomy extended to the neck allows safe approach for large cervicothoracic masses (Fig. 25-2).[18] Thoracoscopy is an alternative approach, and should respect the principles of oncologic surgery, avoiding spillage of tumor cells or fluids (particularly true for germ cell tumors).[17,19,20] Robotic surgery has also been described.[21]

LYMPHOMA

Non-Hodgkin Lymphoma (NHL)

This systemic disease is one of the more frequent mediastinal tumors characterized by massive proliferation of lymphoblasts in the lymph nodes. These cells can ontogenically differentiate into B-cells (related to humoral immunity and produced in the bone marrow) and T-cells (involved in cellular immunity and processed in the thymus). In children, B-cells cause undifferentiated Burkitt or non-Burkitt lymphomas, which together constitute about 50% of all lymphomas. T-cells cause lymphoblastic lymphomas (about 40%) that are generally found in the thymus and/or anterior mediastinal lymph nodes. The remaining 10% correspond to large cell

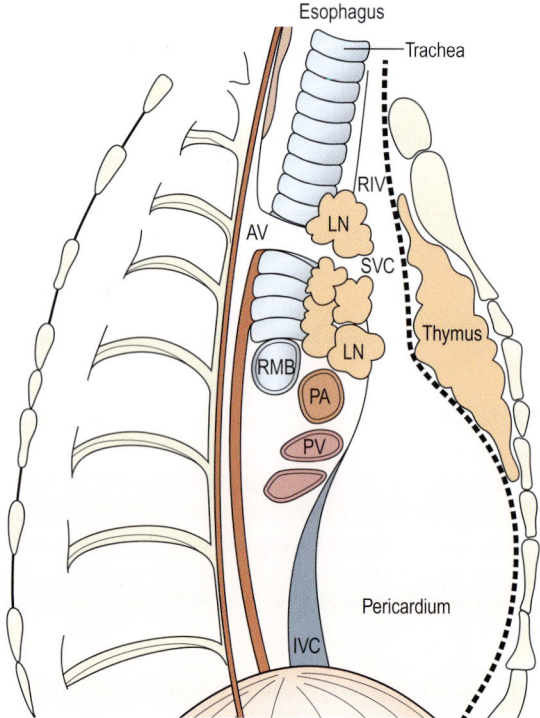

FIGURE 25-1 ■ Anatomic division of the mediastinum: anterior compartment extends from the sternum to the dotted line anterior to the pericardium. Middle mediastinum extends posteriorly to the anterior border of the vertebrae (solid line). AV, azygous vein; IVC, inferior vena cava; LN, lymph node; PA, pulmonary artery; PV, pulmonary vein; RMB, right main-stem bronchus; RIV, right internal jugular vein; SVC, superior vena cava.

lymphomas. These are similar to undifferentiated tumors, but may be of T- or B-cell origin and appear on either side of the diaphragm.

Undifferentiated lymphomas express surface IgM and CD19 and CD20 antigens, whereas lymphoblastic lymphomas contain the enzyme TdT (terminal deoxynucleotidyl transferase) and express T-cell markers such as CD5 and CD7.[22] Burkitt-type lymphomas often have 8:14, and less often 8:22 or 2:8 translocations, involving the *MYCC* proto-oncogene, whereas T-cell lymphomas occasionally have 14q11 translocations.[15,23]

At the time of diagnosis, NHLs are usually spread beyond the original site and involve the regional nodes and distant organs such as the pleural or pericardial spaces or the bone marrow. (In this case, they are indistinguishable from acute lymphoblastic leukemia.)

TABLE 25-1   Location of Mediastinal Tumors

Compartment	Benign	Malignant
Anterior	Teratoma	Non-Hodgkin lymphoma
	Thymic hyperplasia	Hodgkin lymphoma
	Thymic cysts (rare)	Thymic tumors (rare)
Middle	Lymphangioma	Non-Hodgkin lymphoma
	Foregut cysts and duplications	Hodgkin lymphoma
Posterior	Ganglioneuroma	Neuroblastoma

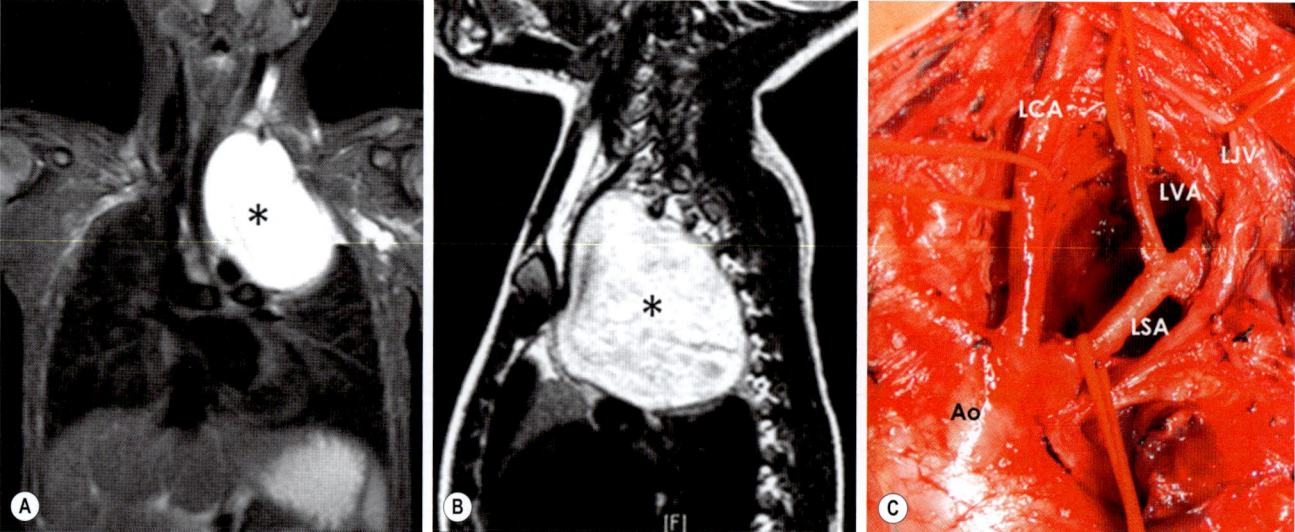

FIGURE 25-2 ■ **(A,B)** Coronal and sagittal views from an MRI of a 5-year-old girl with a high mediastinal ganglioneuroma (asterisk) extending from the hilum of the lung to the neck and involving the vessels and nerves of this area. **(C)** This was safely excised through a cervico-transternal approach seen after removal of the mass. Ao, aorta; LCA, left carotid artery; LSA, left subclavian artery; LVA, left vertebral artery; LJV, left jugular vein.

Rapid growth of mediastinal lymphomas may cause respiratory distress, wheezing, orthopnea, cervicofacial edema, and jugular ingurgitation. Systemic symptoms are possible, and bone marrow invasion causes hematologic disturbances. Enlarged lymph nodes may become palpable in the neck, axillae, and supraclavicular or suprasternal regions.

Imaging depicts an enlarged mediastinum and airway involvement. Pleural or pericardial fluid can often be obtained for cytologic analysis.[11] If neither peripheral lymph nodes nor fluids are available for biopsy or cytology, FNA or biopsy by thoracoscopy or the anterior Chamberlain approach may be necessary. In all cases, the anesthetic risks and precautions should be emphasized.[24]

Mediastinal NHL cases are stage III except when bone marrow and/or central nervous system are involved (stage IV).[25] Gallium-67 isotopic scanning may be helpful for staging.[26,27] The role of combined positron emission tomography (PET) and CT in children is still undefined.

Mediastinal NHL respond well to chemotherapy and corticosteroids, and the contribution of surgery is limited to retrieval of biopsy material for cytologic assessment. Chemotherapy leads to long-term survival in more than 80% of these children.[25,28]

Hodgkin Lymphoma

Mediastinal Hodgkin lymphoma is less frequent and occurs more often in adolescents. The main feature is the Reed–Sternberg cell, the malignant counterpart of the dendritic interdigitating cell that has a role in antigen presentation. These cells are embedded in lymph nodes in which the proportions of fibrous stroma, lymphocytes, and plasma cells are variable, allowing classification into lymphocyte predominant, lymphocyte depleted, mixed cellularity, and nodular sclerosis types. Most children with Hodgkin lymphoma have the nodular sclerosis type, but the youngest ones may have lymphocyte predominant or mixed cellularity varieties.[29] Hodgkin lymphoma originates in one group of lymph nodes and spreads to contiguous or distant nodes. Accurate staging is imperative before selection of the treatment protocol. The Ann Arbor classification of four stages with subgroups, according to the presence or absence of systemic symptoms, remains the most widely used system, but mapping of the involved organs or lymph node groups requires refined imaging tools.

Hodgkin lymphoma may be localized primarily in the mediastinum and may cause the same compressive effects as NHL (Fig. 25-3). Biopsies of extrathoracic nodes are sometimes possible. If not, the Chamberlain operation or thoracoscopy should be used. The preference for chemotherapy over radiotherapy has limited the use of staging laparotomy in children. This should be reserved for cases with thoracic stage II cases in which localized radiotherapy as the sole treatment requires excluding transdiaphragmatic involvement.[30] PET/CT seems promising as a noninvasive staging modality.[29,31]

Surgery is not usually the primary treatment of Hodgkin lymphoma, except in very localized cases. However, it may occasionally be needed in children.[32]

GERM CELL TUMORS

The primitive germ cells may produce various types of tumors. Gonadal germ cells cause seminoma or dysgerminoma whereas totipotential cells can cause yolk sac tumors and choriocarcinoma (extraembryonic) or teratomas (embryonic). In fact, these different components can be found in the same tumor.

Teratomas

These comprise only 8–16% of the tumors in this region and are uncommon in children.[33,34] They consist of solid or organoid masses containing tissues derived from all three blastodermic layers. Their histologic features are heterogeneous and may include cystic or solid areas as well as mature and immature components. Their incidence is higher in individuals with Klinefelter syndrome.[35,36]

Mediastinal teratomas originate most often from the thymus or pericardium and are therefore anterior. They

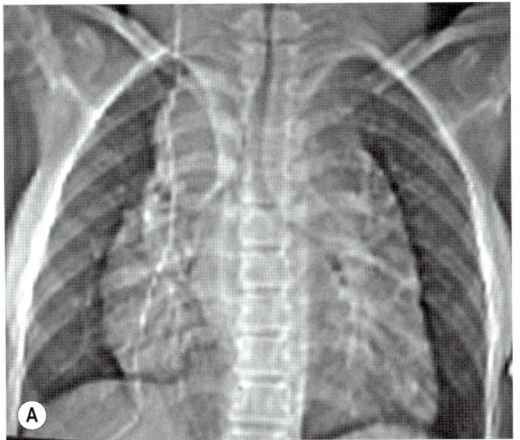
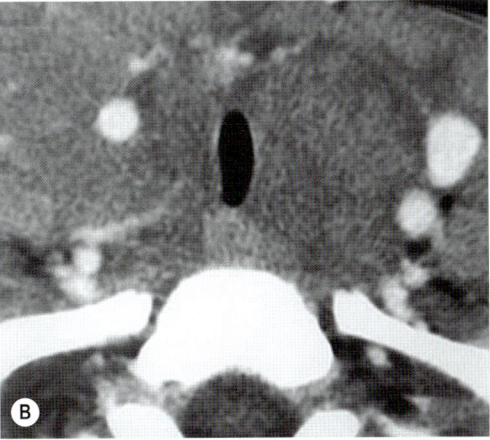

FIGURE 25-3 ■ Imaging studies in an 11-year-old boy with Hodgkin lymphoma. **(A)** Widening of the mediastinum is accompanied by compression of the upper trachea that is seen on the chest radiograph. **(B)** Transverse section on a CT scan of the upper mediastinum shows the extent of this tracheal compression by adenopathy that displaces the vessels laterally.

are as frequent in girls as in boys, in contrast to the situation in adults in whom there is a clear male predominance.[37,38] They develop relatively early in fetal life, and may cause hydrops and fetal demise.[1,39] These masses can be diagnosed prenatally (Fig. 25-4), but they are more often detected after birth because of respiratory distress or later in life because of vague symptoms (thoracic or cervical pain, dyspnea). The diagnosis is often incidental. Mediastinal teratomas should be suspected whenever a mass with or without calcifications is detected in the anterior mediastinal compartment. However, this diagnosis often is not made until the operation. Most mediastinal teratomas are benign in children, but the prognosis is definitely worse if they contain elements of yolk sac, embryonal carcinoma, seminoma, germinoma, or choriocarcinoma.[35,40,41] Some of these lesions may induce precocious puberty or detectable pancreatic secretions.[35,42]

Operative excision is the treatment of choice. Median sternotomy allows excellent exposure, but lateral thoracotomies may be preferred when the tumor extends into either hemithorax. Thoracoscopy has also been used.[43] Chemotherapy with carboplatin, bleomycin, and etoposide may allow for complete removal after tumor shrinkage in cases that cannot be initially excised.[35] Although wide adherence to adjacent tissues usually makes a complete resection difficult, it is essential to avoid recurrence. In fact, these tumors have an excellent prognosis when resection is complete. α-Fetoprotein is a good tumor marker because it is usually elevated in malignant and immature tumors and very seldom in mature ones.[44]

Nonteratomatous Germ Cell Tumors

Very rarely, pure extraembryonal germ cell tumors (seminoma/dysgerminoma, embryonal carcinoma, yolk sac tumor, or choriocarcinoma) may develop in the

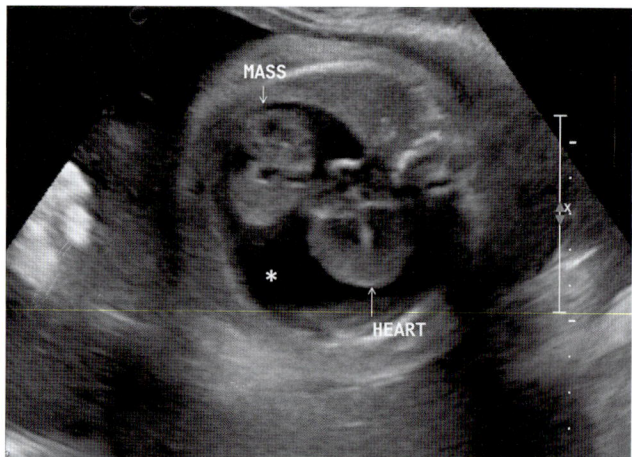

FIGURE 25-4 ■ This fetal echocardiogram is on a 30 week gestational age baby shows a 4 cm × 4 cm intrapericardial teratoma (MASS) which is closely associated with the aortic root. The bulk of the mass is in the right chest and is in direct contact with the right atrium, but does not cause any right atrial compression or systemic venous inflow or outflow obstruction. There is a large pericardial effusion (asterisk) around both the heart and the tumor. Following delivery, the baby was taken to the operating room for excision of the teratoma and has recovered uneventfully.

anterior mediastinum. These are malignant and require complete removal and chemotherapy, as explained earlier for the malignant components of teratomas.[35,44]

TUMORS AND CYSTS OF THE THYMUS

During their migration, the thymic primordia leave behind thymopharyngeal ducts that progressively obliterate. Epithelial tumors and cysts are therefore possible in this organ along with lymphocytic and mesenchymal tumors.

Thymic Hyperplasia

The thymus participates in the development of cellular immunity during infancy. Therefore, it is larger at this age and subsequently shrinks. Thymic hyperplasia may be confounded with a tumor. However, the absence of symptoms and some radiologic features (e.g., the absence of compression of the airway or the 'boat sail' shape of the inferior boundaries of the organ) rule out this suspicion. Treatment with corticosteroids achieves thymic regression, and observation may be enough.

Thymic Cysts

Cysts derived from the thymopharyngeal ducts may appear in the anterior mediastinum and/or in the neck. They are lined by pharyngeal or ciliated epithelium. They have secretory and thymic elements (Hassall's corpuscles) and may be inflamed or infected. When they reach a certain size, they become palpable (in the neck) or detected on imaging of the mediastinum.[45–47] They may also cause respiratory symptoms by compression.[48] Thymic cysts can also be found in rare instances of malignant lymphoma and in patients with human immunodeficiency virus (HIV) infection in whom they can be multilocular.[32,49]

Malignant Thymic Tumors

In contrast with adults, malignant neoplasia of the thymus is exceedingly rare in children. However, some instances of malignant thymoma with or without myasthenia gravis and thymic carcinoma have been reported.[50–52]

VASCULAR TUMORS AND ANOMALIES

Modern classifications of vascular anomalies and tumors has allowed an understanding of their unpredictable clinical course. Vascular tumors like noninvoluting (NICH) and rapidly involuting (RICH) congenital hemangioma, kaposiform hemangioendothelioma, and the capillary, venous, arteriovenous, or lymphatic vascular malformations have different clinical behaviors and require an individualized approach.[53] These conditions may occasionally locate in the mediastinum where they may pose difficult therapeutic problems.[54] (See Chapter 72 for more information about vascular tumors and anomalies.)

FIGURE 25-5 ■ This 7-year-old was found to have a cervico-thoracic lymphangioma following imaging evaluation for a left cervical soft tissue mass. **(A)** On the chest radiograph, a mass effect is noted in the left superior mediastinum with displacement of the trachea to the right. **(B)** The CT scan shows a low density soft tissue mass (asterisk) with splaying of the vasculature. Again, the tracheal deviation is noted. **(C)** Axial and **(D)** coronal T$_2$ fat saturated MRI images are seen. Both reveal a multicystic soft tissue mass which is classic for a lymphatic malformation. An asterisk is noted in a macrocyst.

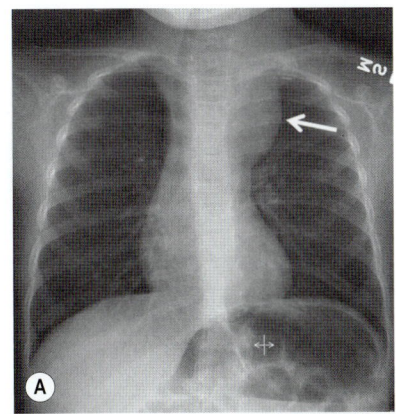

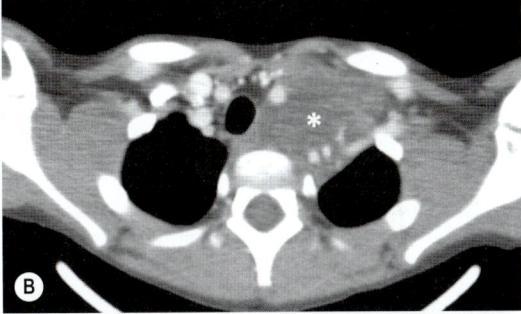

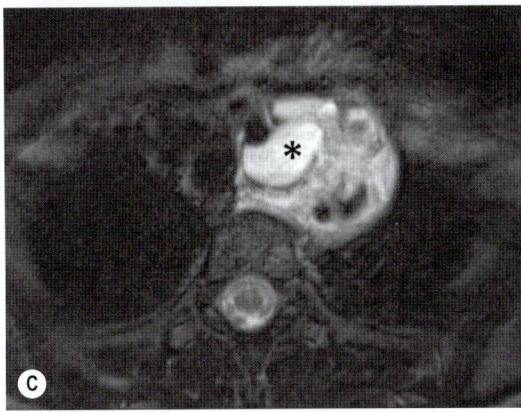

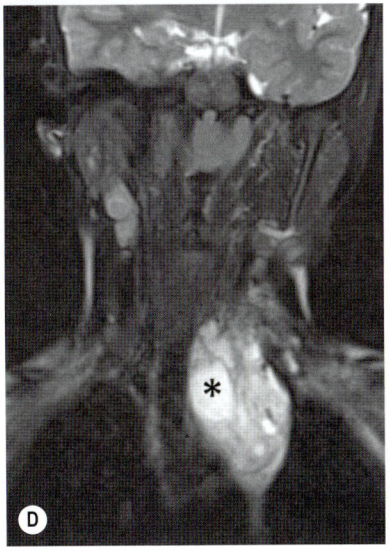

Vascular Tumors

Most hemangiomas located in the anterior mediastinum are in continuity with cervicofacial components that sometimes cause respiratory compromise when they extend into the airway. If they are asymptomatic, they should not be treated because they tend to regress over time. However, if airway compression is present, active anti-angiogenic treatment with corticosteroids and/or interferon-2α or vincristine have been used. Interferon-2α has been found to cause severe neurologic complications.[53] Propranolol, which induces rapid regression of hemangiomas, has also been used with success in mediastinal locations.[55]

Kaposiform hemangioendothelioma may be accompanied by a Kasabach–Merritt syndrome with massive platelet trapping and risks of hemorrhage. These tumors involve the thoracic wall and often the mediastinum. Full anti-angiogenic therapy together with close hematologic monitoring and eventually surgery are required. This tumor has a mortality rate close to 20%.[53]

Vascular Malformations

Venous and arteriovenous malformations, and particularly lymphangiomas, are occasionally located near the confluences of large venous and lymphatic collectors in the mediastinum.[56,57] The tumor may extend into either hemithorax and eventually into the neck and the base of the mouth. Lymphangiomas are usually multicystic and infiltrate the anatomic structures. Reaction to local infections may make the mass swell or even suppurate. Respiratory symptoms may arise in cases with airway compromise.[58] MRI in the best imaging method for diagnosis.

Mediastinal lymphangiomas do not tend to involute. Treatment strategies must take into account that they are benign, that total removal is often impossible, and that a too radical operation may endanger nerve trunks or other structures (Fig. 25-5).[59,60] Sclerosis with OK-432 or bleomycin is an alternative or a complement in cases in which incomplete removal has already reduced the volume of the tumor.[53] Only in cases of single, wide cysts is the result of sclerosing procedures generally satisfactory.[61] For masses with multiple infiltrating cysts of small size, partial debulking may be needed to reduce symptoms.[60]

FOREGUT CYSTS AND DUPLICATIONS

Abnormal branching of the tracheobronchial anlage may create closed spaces lined by either esophageal or bronchial

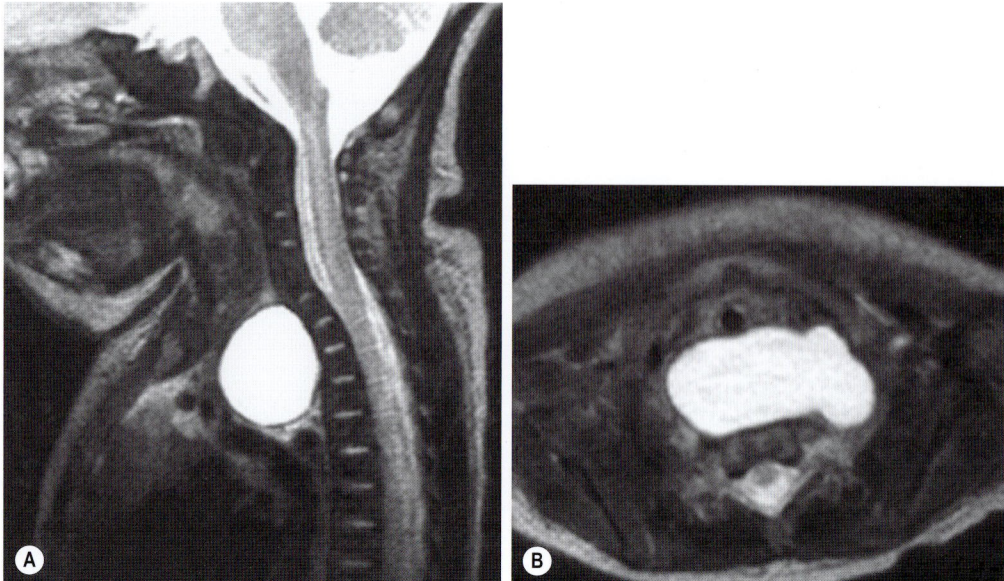

FIGURE 25-6 ■ This newborn with the prenatal diagnosis of an upper mediastinal cyst had respiratory distress at birth. These T$_2$-weighted MR images show a large prevertebral mucus cyst that **(A)** displaces the trachea forward and **(B)** extends to both sides. In A, deformation of the anterior vertebral bodies due to prolonged prenatal compression can be seen. This bronchogenic cyst was successfully removed thoracoscopically.

mucosa. These cysts are in close contact with either the trachea and main-stem bronchi or the esophagus. The secreting mucosa progressively enlarges the cysts, which can then become symptomatic. In rare instances, the foregut malformation is more extensive and involves both the respiratory and digestive tracts, and combines esophageal duplications with airway malformations.[62,63] When the foregut cyst is due to a persistence of the embryonic neuroenteric communication, it involves both the foregut and the neural tube. It splits the notochord and, as a consequence, is accompanied by split vertebral bodies. This rare variety is termed a neuroenteric cyst.[64–66]

Prenatal detection of mediastinal cysts is possible.[67] However, most cases are diagnosed at birth or later in life because of symptoms of respiratory or gastrointestinal compression (Fig. 25-6). Very seldom, mediastinal cysts may bleed due to mucosal ulceration.

The cysts located close to the trachea and main-stem bronchi are lined by ciliated epithelium and are termed 'bronchogenic cysts' (Fig. 25-7).[68,69] Those located in

contact or within the wall of the esophagus are lined by esophageal or mixed epithelium and are known as 'esophageal duplication cysts.'

Plain chest radiographs may show paramediastinal round opacities, and esophagrams depict external esophageal compression or intraluminal imprinting by the cyst. CT and/or MRI demonstrate the size and location of the cysts and the nature of their content. Endoscopy may be useful when the cyst is within the wall of the esophagus, and it can demonstrate external compression in other cases.

Foregut cysts and duplications should be excised because of their secretory nature. Prenatal diagnosis may allow intrauterine treatment.[70] Thoracoscopy has become the preferred approach.[71–74] Most esophageal duplications and bronchogenic cysts can be removed by this approach. Dissection from the esophageal wall may be delicate, but because these cysts generally do not communicate with the esophageal lumen, they can be mobilized without damage to the mucosa. As in other duplications, it is essential to completely remove the secreting mucosa to

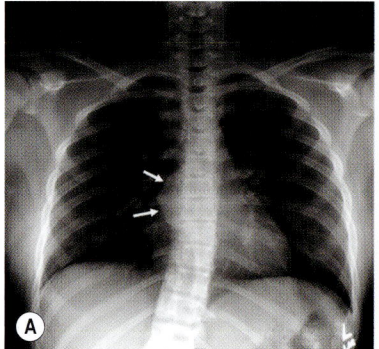
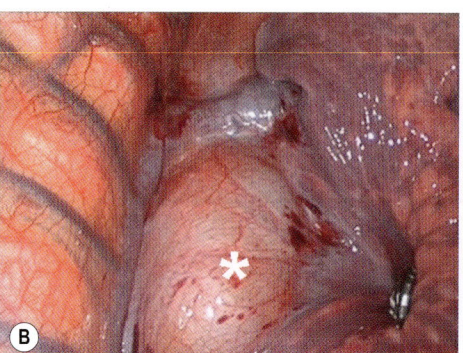
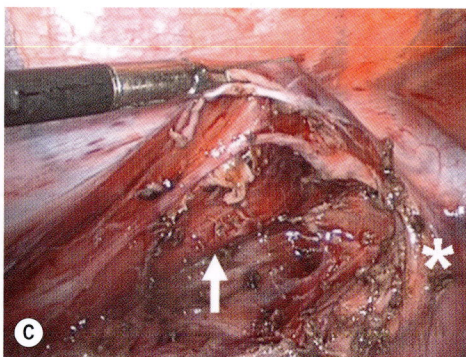

FIGURE 25-7 ■ **(A)** This 12-year-old developed some respiratory distress that prompted the chest radiograph that shows a right bronchogenic cyst (arrows). **(B)** The lesion (asterisk) is seen at thoracoscopy. **(C)** After removal of the cyst, the esophagus (arrow) is seen to lie in the posterior bed of the resection. The cyst was intimately adherent to the right main-stem bronchus (asterisk).

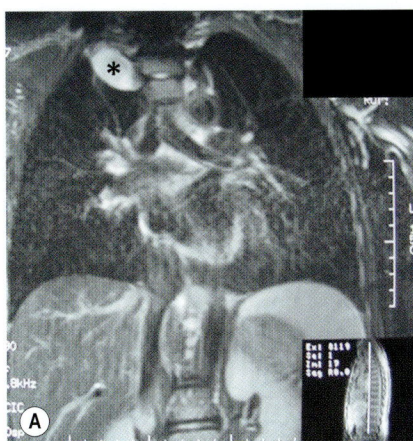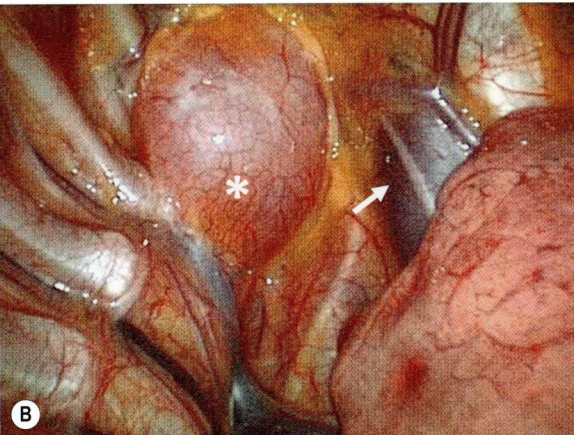

FIGURE 25-8 ■ A 16-year-old presented with Horner syndrome and was found to have a right superior mediastinal mass. **(A)** MR image of the mass showing the ganglioneuroma (asterisk). **(B)** At thoracoscopy, the mass (asterisk) can be visualized cephalad to the azygous vein and just lateral to the superior vena cava (arrow). This ganglioneuroma was able to be removed thoracoscopically.

prevent recurrence or cancer later in adulthood.[68] (See Chapter 39 for more information about duplications.)

NEURAL TUMORS

These tumors originate from the sympathetic chains located on both sides of the spine and may exhibit different degrees of differentiation, ranging from malignant neuroblastomas to mature ganglioneuromas that may appear intermixed in the same tumor (Fig. 25-8). For unknown reasons, thoracic neural tumors are less malignant than abdominal ones and tend to behave less aggressively.[75] The proportion of stages 1 and 2 and the favorable histologic patterns are definitely higher than in other locations. Moreover, these tumors often have less *MYCN* amplification.[75–78] The tumors involve the sympathetic trunks, and can extend into the spinal canal through one or several foramina (dumbbell- or hourglass-shaped tumors).[79,80] The upper or apical tumors may extend to the neck and often involve the stellate ganglion. The lower ones can extend into the abdomen through the posterior diaphragmatic insertions and/or the aortic hiatus. The aorta and the esophagus on the left side and the azygos vein on the right may be in close contact with the tumor, which sometimes passes across the midline. Intercostal arteries and veins are often intratumoral.

Horner syndrome and/or heterochromia of the iris may lead to the diagnosis.[81,82] Paraplegia due to spinal cord compression can occur suddenly.[83] However, most cases are silent and are discovered by imaging procedures for concurrent conditions or vague symptoms. Secreting tumors and paraneoplastic symptoms such as hypertension and diarrhea are rare in this location. A limited number of malignant tumors spread from the primary site and metastasize to distant regions such as the bone marrow or the bones.[78]

Imaging reveals a round or fusiform mass with sometimes hemorrhagic, necrotic, or calcified areas. The ribs and the spinal pedicles may be distorted and the foramina enlarged. In dumbbell tumors, the intraspinal component is better depicted by MRI (Fig. 25-9).[79]

All tests required for neuroblastoma workup (e.g., meta-iodine-benzyl-guanidine scan, catecholamine metabolite excretion) should be used for tumors in this location.

In cases with paraplegia, emergency laminectomy or laminotomy with removal of the intraspinal extension is generally preferred, although some groups advise chemotherapy initially.[83–85] Except in very extensive tumors and in those with bone metastases in which chemotherapy should precede surgical removal, mediastinal neural tumors are primarily excised.[86] This operation can be difficult, particularly when the tumor extends beyond the midline or into the neck, the spinal canal, or below the diaphragm. Mobilization of the aorta with division of several intercostal vessels may be required. Clearance of the tumor should be as complete as possible, although in many cases minimal macroscopic residual disease is unavoidable. In cases of thoracoabdominal tumors, splitting the diaphragm and dissecting the retroperitoneal mass from above at the same operative setting is advantageous. Thoracoscopic excision is being increasingly utilized.[19,20,87]

Irrespective of their histology, the survival of patients with thoracic neuroblastoma is encouraging and always better than that of abdominal primaries. Some sequelae are unavoidable. Paraplegia may persist when the cord has been permanently damaged (this happens in tumors that cause prenatal compression).[88,89]

Permanent paraplegia may rarely occur due to intraoperative spinal cord ischemia.[90] Division of the segmental vessels may cause localized paralysis of upper abdominal or thoracic muscles. Removal of the stellate ganglion usually leads to permanent Horner syndrome. Finally, scoliosis can develop after laminectomies.

OTHER RARE MEDIASTINAL TUMORS

Rarely, other mediastinal tumors have been reported in children. These include pseudoinflammatory tumor, Langerhans' cell histiocytosis with calcification, thymolipoma, sarcoma, and liposarcoma.[91–95]

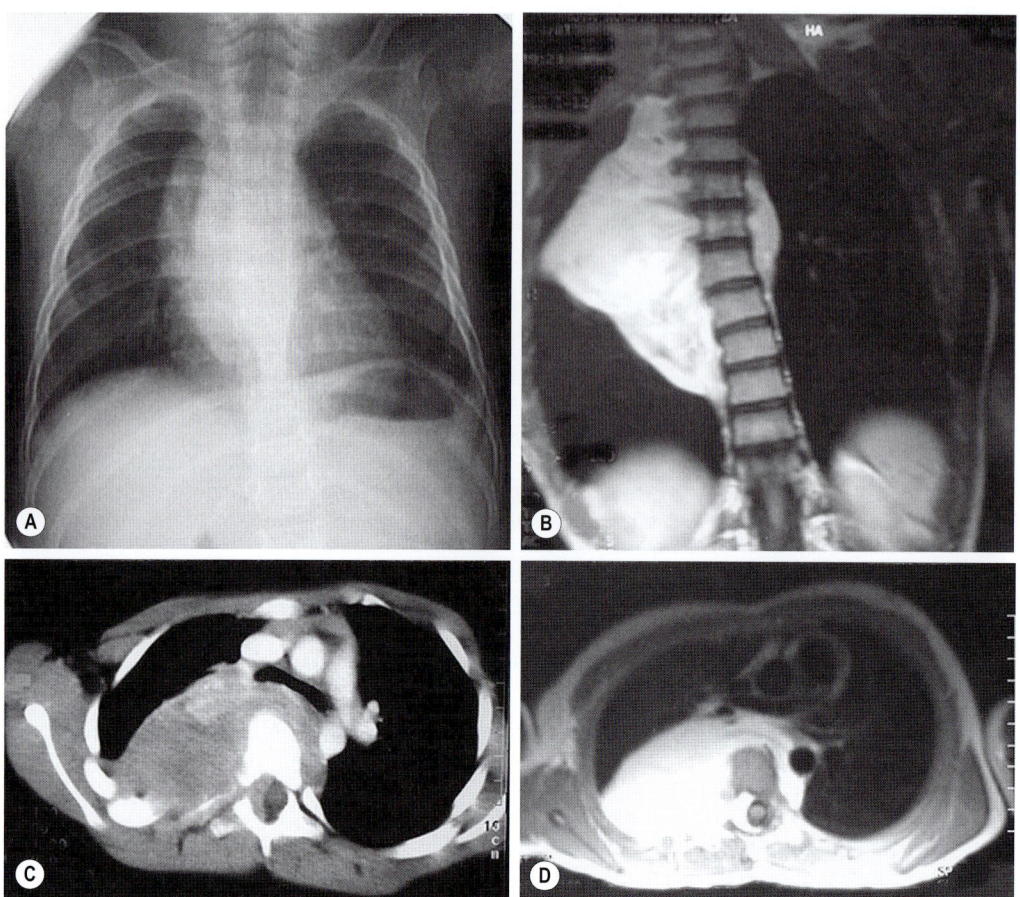

FIGURE 25-9 ■ This 7-year-old patient had a long-standing history of neuroblastoma that was treated with chemotherapy but the lesion was not resected. The tumor is seen as a fusiform mass extending to both sides of the thorax on the **(A)** plain radiograph and **(B)** and MR image. **(C)** CT scan shows rib and vertebral body deformations with widening of the foramina and displacement of the great vessels. **(D)** MR image depicts the dumbbell-shaped nature of the tumor, which invaded the spinal canal, although without paraplegia. Combined spinal and right thoracotomy approaches allowed complete resection of the mass.

REFERENCES

1. Sbragia L, Paek BW, Feldstein VA, et al. Outcome of prenatally diagnosed solid fetal tumors. J Pediatr Surg 2001;36:1244–7.
2. Lemaitre L, Leclerc F, Marconi V, et al. Ultrasonographic findings in thymic lymphoma in children. Eur J Radiol 1987;7:125–9.
3. Borecky N, Gudinchet F, Laurini R, et al. Imaging of cervicothoracic lymphangiomas in children. Pediatr Radiol 1995;25: 127–30.
4. Ichikawa T, Ohtomo K, Araki T, et al. Ganglioneuroma: Computed tomography and magnetic resonance features. Br J Radiol 1996; 69:114–21.
5. Wyttenbach R, Vock P, Tschappeler H. Cross-sectional imaging with CT and/or MRI of pediatric chest tumors. Eur Radiol 1998;8:1040–6.
6. Shamberger RC, Holzman RS, Griscom NT, et al. CT quantitation of tracheal cross-sectional area as a guide to the surgical and anesthetic management of children with anterior mediastinal masses. J Pediatr Surg 1991;26:138–42.
7. Castellote A, Vazquez E, Vera J, et al. Cervicothoracic lesions in infants and children. Radiographics 1999;19:583–600.
8. Zhang Y, Nishimura H, Kato S, et al. MRI of ganglioneuroma: Histologic correlation study. J Comput Assist Tomogr 2001;25: 617–23.
9. Motoyama T, Yamamoto O, Iwamoto H, et al. Fine needle aspiration cytology of primary mediastinal germ cell tumors. Acta Cytol 1995;39:725–32.
10. Shabb NS, Fahl M, Shabb B, et al. Fine-needle aspiration of the mediastinum: A clinical, radiologic, cytologic, and histologic study of 42 cases. Diagn Cytopathol 1998;19:428–36.
11. Chaignaud BE, Bonsack TA, Kozakewich HP, et al. Pleural effusions in lymphoblastic lymphoma: A diagnostic alternative. J Pediatr Surg 1998;33:1355–7.
12. Rothenberg SS. Thoracoscopy in infants and children. Semin Pediatr Surg 1998;7:194–201.
13. Tsao K, St Peter SD, Sharp SW, et al. Current application of thoracoscopy in children. J Laparoendosc Adv Surg Tech A 2008;18:131–5.
14. Shamberger RC. Preanesthetic evaluation of children with anterior mediastinal masses. Semin Pediatr Surg 1999;8:61–8.
15. Glick RD, Pearse IA, Trippett T, et al. Diagnosis of mediastinal masses in pediatric patients using mediastinoscopy and the Chamberlain procedure. J Pediatr Surg 1999;34:559–64.
16. Gun F, Toker A, Kaya S, et al. Cervical mediastinoscopy for paratracheal masses in pediatric patients. Pediatr Hematol Oncol 2008;25:393–7.
17. Koga H, Yamataka A, Kobayashi H, et al. Median sternotomy provides excellent exposure for excising anterior mediastinal tumors in children. Pediatr Surg Int 2005;21:864–7.
18. Grosfeld JL, Weber TR, Vane DW. One-stage resection for massive cervicomediastinal hygroma. Surgery 1982;92:693–9.
19. Partrick DA, Rothenberg SS. Thoracoscopic resection of mediastinal masses in infants and children: An evaluation of technique and results. J Pediatr Surg 2001;36:1165–7.
20. Petty JK, Bensard DD, Partrick DA, et al. Resection of neurogenic tumors in children: Is thoracoscopy superior to thoracotomy? J Am Coll Surg 2006;203:699–703.
21. Meehan JJ, Sandler AD. Robotic resection of mediastinal masses in children. J Laparoendosc Adv Surg Tech A 2008;18: 114–19.

22. Long JC, McCaffrey RP, Aisenberg AC, et al. Terminal deoxynucleotidyl transferase positive lymphoblastic lymphoma: A study of 15 cases. Cancer 1979;44:2127–39.

23. Kaneko Y, Variakojis D, Kluskens L, et al. Lymphoblastic lymphoma: Cytogenetic, pathologic, and immunologic studies. Int J Cancer 1982;30:273–9.

24. Ricketts RR. Clinical management of anterior mediastinal tumors in children. Semin Pediatr Surg 2001;10:161–8.

25. Marky I, Bjork O, Forestier E, et al. Intensive chemotherapy without radiotherapy gives more than 85% event-free survival for non-Hodgkin lymphoma without central nervous involvement: A 6-year population-based study from the Nordic Society of Pediatric Hematology and Oncology. J Pediatr Hematol Oncol 2004;26:555–60.

26. Drossman SR, Schiff RG, Kronfeld GD, et al. Lymphoma of the mediastinum and neck: Evaluation with Ga-67 imaging and CT correlation. Radiology 1990;174:171–5.

27. Hamrick-Turner JE, Saif MF, Powers CI, et al. Imaging of childhood non-Hodgkin lymphoma: Assessment by histologic subtype. Radiographics 1994;14:11–28.

28. Goubin A, Auclerc MF, Auvrignon A, et al. Survival in France after childhood acute leukaemia and non-Hodgkin's lymphoma (1990–2000). Eur J Cancer 2006;42:534–41.

29. Donaldson SS. Pediatric Hodgkin's disease–up, up, and beyond. Int J Radiat Oncol Biol Phys 2002;54:1–8.

30. Tebbi CK, Mendenhall N, London WB, et al. Treatment of stage I, IIA, IIIA1 pediatric Hodgkin disease with doxorubicin, bleomycin, vincristine and etoposide (DBVE) and radiation: A Pediatric Oncology Group (POG) study. Pediatr Blood Cancer 2006;46:198–202.

31. Metwally H, Courbon F, David I, et al. Coregistration of prechemotherapy PET-CT for planning pediatric Hodgkin's disease radiotherapy significantly diminishes interobserver variability of clinical target volume definition. Int J Radiat Oncol Biol Phys 2011;80:793–9.

32. Nogues A, Tovar JA, Sunol M, et al. Hodgkin's disease of the thymus: A rare mediastinal cystic mass. J Pediatr Surg 1987;22:996–7.

33. Weidner N. Germ-cell tumors of the mediastinum. Semin Diagn Pathol 1999;16:42–50.

34. Takeda S, Miyoshi S, Ohta M, et al. Primary germ cell tumors in the mediastinum: A 50-year experience at a single Japanese institution. Cancer 2003;97:367–76.

35. Billmire D, Vinocur C, Rescorla F, et al. Malignant mediastinal germ cell tumors: An intergroup study. J Pediatr Surg 2001;36:18–24.

36. Beresford L, Fernandez CV, Cummings E, et al. Mediastinal polyembryoma associated with Klinefelter syndrome. J Pediatr Hematol Oncol 2003;25:321–3.

37. Grosfeld JL, Billmire DF. Teratomas in infancy and childhood. Curr Probl Cancer 1985;9:1–53.

38. Moran CA, Suster S. Primary germ cell tumors of the mediastinum: I. Analysis of 322 cases with special emphasis on teratomatous lesions and a proposal for histopathologic classification and clinical staging. Cancer 1997;80:681–90.

39. Froberg MK, Brown RE, Maylock J, et al. In utero development of a mediastinal cystic teratoma: A second-trimester event. Prenat Diagn 1994;14:884–7.

40. Lakhoo K, Boyle M, Drake DP. Mediastinal teratomas: Review of 15 pediatric cases. J Pediatr Surg 1993;28:1161–4.

41. De Backer A, Madern GC, Hakvoort-Cammel FG, et al. Mediastinal germ cell tumors: Clinical aspects and outcomes in 7 children. Eur J Pediatr Surg 2006;16:318–22.

42. Kallis P, Treasure T, Holmes SJ, et al. Exocrine pancreatic function in mediastinal teratomata: An aid to preoperative diagnosis? Ann Thorac Surg 1992;54:741–3.

43. Feo CF, Chironi G, Porcu A, et al. Videothoracoscopic removal of a mediastinal teratoma. Am Surg 1997;63:459–61.

44. Dehner LP. Germ cell tumors of the mediastinum. Semin Diagn Pathol 1990;7:266–84.

45. Samuel M, Spitz L, Deleval M, et al. Mediastinal thymic cysts in children. Pediatr Surg Int 1995;10:146–7.

46. Sturm-O'Brien AK, Salazar JD, Byrd RH, et al. Cervical thymic anomalies—the Texas Children's Hospital experience. Laryngoscope 2009;119:1988–93.

47. De Caluwe D, Ahmed M, Puri P. Cervical thymic cysts. Pediatr Surg Int 2002;18:477–9.

48. Wagner CW, Vinocur CD, Weintraub WH, et al. Respiratory complications in cervical thymic cysts. J Pediatr Surg 1988;23:657–60.

49. Kontny HU, Sleasman JW, Kingma DW, et al. Multilocular thymic cysts in children with human immunodeficiency virus infection: Clinical and pathologic aspects. J Pediatr 1997;131:264–70.

50. Takeda S, Miyoshi S, Akashi A, et al. Clinical spectrum of primary mediastinal tumors: A comparison of adult and pediatric populations at a single Japanese institution. J Surg Oncol 2003;83:24–30.

51. Yaris N, Nas Y, Cobanoglu U, et al. Thymic carcinoma in children. Pediatr Blood Cancer 2006;47:224–7.

52. Stachowicz-Stencel T, Bien E, Balcerska A, et al. Thymic carcinoma in children: A report from the Polish Pediatric Rare Tumors Study. Pediatr Blood Cancer 2010;54:916–20.

53. Fishman SJ. Vascular anomalies of the mediastinum. Semin Pediatr Surg 1999;8:92–8.

54. Moran CA, Suster S. Mediastinal hemangiomas: A study of 18 cases with emphasis on the spectrum of morphological features. Hum Pathol 1995;26:416–21.

55. Fulkerson DH, Agim NG, Al-Shamy G, et al. Emergent medical and surgical management of mediastinal infantile hemangioma with symptomatic spinal cord compression: Case report and literature review. Childs Nerv Syst 2010;26:1799–805.

56. Ratan J, Bhatnagar V, Mitra DK. Mediastinal cystic hygroma in infancy and childhood. Pediatr Surg Int 1992;7:380–1.

57. Wright CC, Cohen DM, Vegunta RK, et al. Intrathoracic cystic hygroma: A report of three cases. J Pediatr Surg 1996;31:1430–2.

58. Sumner TE, Volberg FM, Kiser PE, et al. Mediastinal cystic hygroma in children. Pediatr Radiol 1981;11:160–2.

59. Glasson MJ, Taylor SF. Cervical, cervicomediastinal and intrathoracic lymphangioma. Prog Pediatr Surg 1991;27:62–83.

60. Alqahtani A, Nguyen LT, Flageole H, et al. 25 years' experience with lymphangiomas in children. J Pediatr Surg 1999;34:1164–8.

61. Okazaki T, Iwatani S, Yanai T, et al. Treatment of lymphangioma in children: Our experience of 128 cases. J Pediatr Surg 2007;42:386–9.

62. Kitano Y, Iwanaka T, Tsuchida Y, et al. Esophageal duplication cyst associated with pulmonary cystic malformations. J Pediatr Surg 1995;30:1724–7.

63. Horwitz JR, Lally KP. Bronchogenic and esophageal duplication cyst in a single mediastinal mass in a child. Pediatr Pathol Lab Med 1996;16:113–18.

64. Almog B, Leibovitch L, Achiron R. Split notochord syndrome—prenatal ultrasonographic diagnosis. Prenat Diagn 2001;21:1159–62.

65. Schurink M, van Herwaarden-Lindeboom MY, Coppes MH, et al. Neurenteric cyst—a case report of this rare disorder. J Pediatr Surg 2007;42:E5–7.

66. Kumakura A, Takahara T, Asada J, et al. Split notochord syndrome with congenital unilateral Horner's sign. Pediatr Neurol 2008;38:47–9.

67. Kawahara H, Kamata S, Nose K, et al. Congenital mediastinal cystic abnormalities detected in utero: Report of two cases. J Pediatr Gastroenterol Nutr 2001;33:202–5.

68. Suen HC, Mathisen DJ, Grillo HC, et al. Surgical management and radiological characteristics of bronchogenic cysts. Ann Thorac Surg 1993;55:476–81.

69. Ribet ME, Copin MC, Gosselin B. Bronchogenic cysts of the mediastinum. J Thorac Cardiovasc Surg 1995;109:1003–10.

70. Martinez Ferro M, Milner R, Voto L, et al. Intrathoracic alimentary tract duplication cysts treated in utero by thoracoamniotic shunting. Fetal Diagn Ther 1998;13:343–7.

71. Schier F, Waldschmidt J. Thoracoscopy in children. J Pediatr Surg 1996;31:1640–3.

72. Michel JL, Revillon Y, Montupet P, et al. Thoracoscopic treatment of mediastinal cysts in children. J Pediatr Surg 1998;33:1745–8.

73. Merry C, Spurbeck W, Lobe TE. Resection of foregut-derived duplications by minimal-access surgery. Pediatr Surg Int 1999;15:224–6.

74. Engum SA. Minimal access thoracic surgery in the pediatric population. Semin Pediatr Surg 2007;16:14–26.

75. Suita S, Tajiri T, Sera Y, et al. The characteristics of mediastinal neuroblastoma. Eur J Pediatr Surg 2000;10:353–9.

76. Morris JA, Shcochat SJ, Smith EI, et al. Biological variables in thoracic neuroblastoma: A Pediatric Oncology Group study. J Pediatr Surg 1995;30:296–302.

77. La Quaglia MP, Kushner BH, Su W, et al. The impact of gross total resection on local control and survival in high-risk neuroblastoma. J Pediatr Surg 2004;39:412–17.

78. Escobar MA, Grosfeld JL, Powell RL, et al. Long-term outcomes in patients with stage IV neuroblastoma. J Pediatr Surg 2006;41: 377–81.

79. Shadmehr MB, Gaissert HA, Wain JC, et al. The surgical approach to 'dumbbell tumors' of the mediastinum. Ann Thorac Surg 2003; 76:1650–4.

80. Takeda S, Miyoshi S, Minami M, et al. Intrathoracic neurogenic tumors—50 years' experience in a Japanese institution. Eur J Cardiothorac Surg 2004;26:807–12.

81. Jaffe N, Cassady R, Petersen R, et al. Heterochromia and Horner syndrome associated with cervical and mediastinal neuroblastoma. J Pediatr 1975;87:75–7.

82. McRae D Jr, Shaw A. Ganglioneuroma, heterochromia iridis, and Horner's syndrome. J Pediatr Surg 1979;14:612–14.

83. Mam MK, Mathew S, Prabhakar BR, et al. Mediastinal enterogenic cyst presenting as paraplegia—a case report. Indian J Med Sci 1996;50:337–9.

84. Akwari OE, Payne WS, Onofrio BM, et al. Dumbbell neurogenic tumors of the mediastinum. Diagnosis and management. Mayo Clin Proc 1978;53:353–8.

85. Plantaz D, Rubie H, Michon J, et al. The treatment of neuroblastoma with intraspinal extension with chemotherapy followed by surgical removal of residual disease. A prospective study of 42 patients—results of the NBL 90 Study of the French Society of Pediatric Oncology. Cancer 1996;78:311–19.

86. Kang CH, Kim YT, Jeon SH, et al. Surgical treatment of malignant mediastinal neurogenic tumors in children. Eur J Cardiothorac Surg 2007;31:725–30.

87. Sue K, Yamanaka K, Nakamura M. Thoracoscopic resection of a ganglioneuroma in the posterior mediastinum of 3-year-old boy. Pediatr Surg Int 1998;14:151.

88. Rothner AD. Congenital 'dumbbell' neuroblastoma with paraplegia. Clin Pediatr (Phila) 1971;10:235–6.

89. Shimada Y, Sato K, Abe E, et al. Congenital dumbbell neuroblastoma. Spine 1995;20:1295–300.

90. Boglino C, Martins AG, Ciprandi G, et al. Spinal cord vascular injuries following surgery of advanced thoracic neuroblastoma: An unusual catastrophic complication. Med Pediatr Oncol 1999;32: 349–52.

91. Gorospe L, Fernandez-Gil MA, Torres I, et al. Misleading lead: Inflammatory pseudotumor of the mediastinum with digital clubbing. Med Pediatr Oncol 2000;35:484–7.

92. Lee BH, George S, Kutok JL. Langerhans cell histiocytosis involving the thymus. A case report and review of the literature. Arch Pathol Lab Med 2003;127:e294–7.

93. Moran CA, Rosado-de-Christenson M, Suster S. Thymolipoma: Clinicopathologic review of 33 cases. Mod Pathol 1995;8:741–4.

94. Burt M, Ihde JK, Hajdu SI, et al. Primary sarcomas of the mediastinum: Results of therapy. J Thorac Cardiovasc Surg 1998; 115:671–80.

95. Plukker JT, Joosten HJ, Rensing JB, et al. Primary liposarcoma of the mediastinum in a child. J Surg Oncol 1988;37:257–63.

CHAPTER 26

THE ESOPHAGUS

Nicole M. Chandler • Paul M. Colombani

The esophagus is a hollow muscular tube connecting the pharynx to the stomach. It is positioned in the posterior mediastinum and travels through the esophageal hiatus to the cardia of the stomach. Two sphincters control passage of contents into the gastrointestinal tract: an anatomic upper esophageal sphincter (UES) and a physiologic lower esophageal sphincter (LES). The UES consists of the cricopharyngeus and inferior pharyngeal constrictors. The LES is histologically similar to the muscular component of the esophagus.

Embryologically, the trachea and esophagus are intimately related. The trachea and esophagus both develop from the foregut as a median ventral diverticulum. Familiarity with the embryologic development of the esophagus and trachea is important to understand the congenital abnormalities that arise from these structures. The classic description of these malformations proposes impairment in the process of septation of the trachea and esophagus.[1]

In humans, normal development of the foregut begins during the fourth week of gestation. At 22 days' gestation, the foregut endoderm differentiates into a ventral respiratory part and a dorsal esophageal part. The separation of the respiratory part from the esophageal part is achieved by the formation of lateral longitudinal tracheoesophageal folds. The trachea and esophagus elongate first distally and then proximally. At 6 to 7 weeks' gestation, the separation of the esophagus and trachea is complete. At birth, the esophagus is 8–10 cm in length.[2] The length of the esophagus will double in the first few years of life.

The esophageal wall is composed of mucosa, submucosa, muscularis propria, and adventia. The esophagus lacks a distinct serosa. The mucosa is lined by nonkeratinizing, stratified squamous epithelium. The muscularis mucosa is the deepest layer of the mucosa and contains longitudinal smooth muscle fibers. The submucosa contains the venous and lymphatic plexuses. The muscularis propria contains the internal circular and external longitudinal muscle layers. The upper third of the esophagus is composed primarily of striated muscle fibers under voluntary control. The middle third is mixed striated and smooth muscle fibers, and the lower third of the esophagus contains only smooth muscle fibers. These two lower segments are under anatomic control. The mucosa is the strongest layer of the esophageal wall. When the esophagus is divided, the mucosa will retract proximally and distally. Meticulous approximation of the esophageal mucosa is essential for a technically sound anastomosis.

The blood supply to the proximal esophagus is derived from the fourth brachial arch. The fourth brachial arch gives rise to the subclavian artery and its branches, including the inferior thyroid artery, which supplies the cervical esophagus. The thoracic esophagus is supplied directly from branches of the aorta. The abdominal esophagus has a generous blood supply from the phrenic branches and gastric vessels. The excellent submucosal plexus of the proximal esophagus allows for extensive mobilization without compromise to the blood supply, whereas caution should be taken distally because of the segmental lower esophageal blood supply.

Lesions of the upper esophagus are best approached through the right chest to avoid problems with the aortic arch. The azygos vein should be ligated and divided where it crosses the esophagus. As long as the superior vena cava is patent, the azygos vein can be divided without consequence. Lesions of the lower esophagus can be explored through either the right or left chest. To expose the distal esophagus via the left chest, the inferior pulmonary ligament must be divided, taking care not to injure the inferior pulmonary vein that runs in the upper aspect of the pulmonary ligament.

ENDOSCOPY

In current pediatric practice, diagnostic esophagoscopy is frequently used to evaluate dysphagia and gastroesophageal reflux (GER). Therapeutic esophagoscopy is used to dilate esophageal strictures, evaluate for trauma, aid in sclerotherapy for bleeding esophageal varices, and place gastrostomy tubes. Both rigid and flexible esophagoscopes are available for use in children of all ages.

Flexible endoscopy is the technique of choice for routine diagnostic esophagoscopy. The rigid esophagoscope is more versatile and provides a larger diameter that allows for better visualization and a larger channel for biopsies. It also does not require air insufflation of the esophagus, which is important in the setting of trauma because air will not be forced through a perforation into the mediastinum.

The main value of rigid esophagoscopy in current pediatric practice is for therapeutic procedures such as dilation of an esophageal stricture or removal of a foreign body. Rigid esophagoscopy requires general anesthesia with endotracheal intubation and muscle relaxation. The child is positioned supine with a roll under the shoulders to extend the neck. With care taken to protect the teeth, the esophagoscope, with its bevel up, is introduced into the oral cavity along the hard and soft palates to identify the cricopharyngeus muscle and enter the esophagus. Once the most distal aspect of evaluation is reached, it is easy to examine the esophagus fully when withdrawing the scope to identify any lesions or foreign bodies missed on insertion.

Flexible endoscopes are now available for upper endoscopy in premature infants all the way to adolescents in a reliable, safe, and efficient manner. Endoscopy with a flexible scope can be performed under sedation or general anesthesia. The endoscope is passed though the pharynx and cricopharynx into the upper esophagus. This is most safely done under direct vision. The scope should be advanced down the esophagus carefully, making sure to always maintain visualization of the esophageal lumen. The endoscope should never be advanced blindly. If the lumen is not apparent, the scope should be withdrawn slightly with gentle insufflation until the lumen is identified. Once the stomach is entered, it should be insufflated to allow inspection of the mucosa. In small infants, over-distention of the stomach may lead to respiratory distress.

Complications related to passage of a rigid or flexible endoscope are typically at the level of the cricopharyngeus muscle. Perforation of the cricopharyngeus occurs in about 0.093% with flexible endoscopy and 0.074% in rigid esophagoscopy.[3] Perforation during diagnostic esophagoscopy is exceedingly rare.

A more thorough description of pediatric esophagoscopy and emerging therapeutic endoscopic techniques can be found elsewhere.[4-7]

FOREIGN BODY ESOPHAGEAL INJURY

Coins are the most frequently ingested foreign body.[8,9] When foreign bodies become lodged in the esophagus, they may cause serious complications. Between 10–20% of foreign bodies may lodge in the esophagus and place the patient at risk for developing complications such as aortoesophageal fistula,[10] esophageal perforation,[11] esophageal stricture,[12] tracheoesophageal fistula,[13] and respiratory distress.[14] There are four sites of physiologic narrowing in the esophagus: (1) the cricopharyngeus of the UES; (2) the aortic notch; (3) the left main-stem bronchus; and (4) the LES. The cricopharyngeus is the narrowest point in the gastrointestinal tract. Endoscopic removal has been the preferred approach in many referral centers and has been highly successful with low complication rates.

Key principles of endoscopic management of esophageal foreign bodies are to protect the airway, maintain control of the object during extraction, and avoid causing additional damage. Children are more likely than adults to be asymptomatic and have an increased frequency of respiratory symptoms. There should be a high suspicion of foreign body ingestion in infants with excessive drooling, refusal of food, and unexplained coughing or gagging. Anteroposterior and lateral chest radiographs are the best diagnostic tests for radiopaque objects. The flat surface of a coin is best seen on the anteroposterior view when it is lodged in the esophagus, whereas the lateral view will show the flat surface when it is lodged in the trachea (Fig. 26-1).

Rigid esophagoscopy has long been considered the gold standard for removal of retained foreign bodies. This procedure has been proven to be highly successful with low complication rates. Other approaches have been described to treat esophageal coins including flexible endoscopy,[15] bougienage,[16, 17] Foley balloon extraction under fluoroscopy,[8] and brief observation trials.[17,18]

There is much more concern for serious injury with the ingestion of button batteries. There are four mechanisms of injury caused by batteries: (1) the toxic effect due to absorption of substances, particularly batteries containing mercuric oxide; (2) electrical discharge and mucosal burn; (3) pressure necrosis; and (4) caustic injury from leakage. Severe esophageal damage may occur in as little as four hours after ingestion and perforation in as little as six hours after ingestion.[19] Emetics should not be given, owing to their ineffectiveness and possible reflux of a battery back into the esophagus.

There were 20 reported cases of esophageal injury from ingested button batteries from 1979 to 2004.[19] Undoubtedly, there are many more unreported incidents. Complications from the ingestion of button batteries include death from vascular invasion and uncontrollable

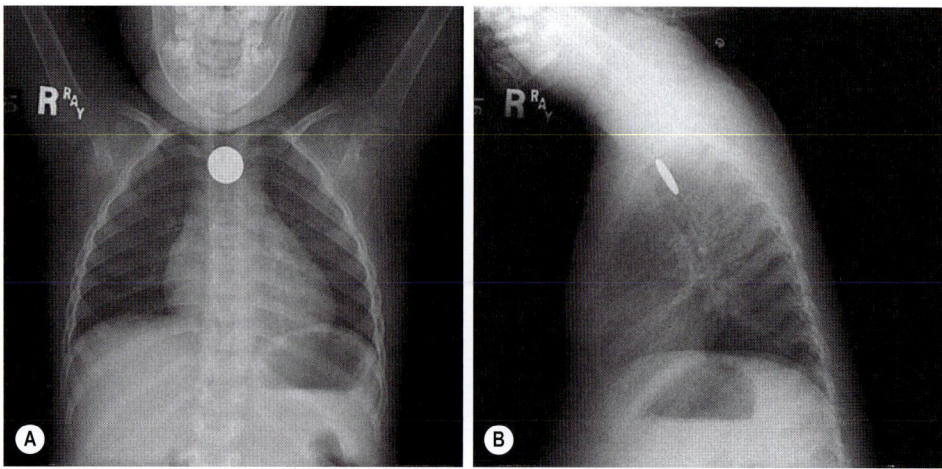

FIGURE 26-1 ■ **(A)** Anteroposterior and **(B)** lateral radiographs demonstrate a coin lodged at the cricopharyngeus muscle. Note that coins will most often orient with the flat surface facing anteroposteriorly.

hemorrhage,[20] esophageal perforation,[21] tracheoesophageal fistula (see Fig. 11-4),[22,23] and bilateral vocal cord paralysis.[24]

Further information about esophageal foreign bodies can be found in Chapter 11.

CHEMICAL ESOPHAGEAL INJURIES

In 2010, the American Association of Poison Control Centers reported that 50% of all human exposures occurred in children under the age of 6 years.[25] Household cleaning substances are the third most frequent exposure in children, accounting for 116,000 ingestions per year. In children, ingestions are primarily accidental. The mean age for ingestions is 3.7 years, and 60% of patients are male.[26]

The extent of injury is dependent on several factors including the composition of the substance, volume, concentration, and duration of contact. Acidic injury results in immediate pain and coagulative necrosis with eschar formation, which likely limits tissue penetration and injury depth. Acidic ingestions most commonly cause gastric injury. Alkali ingestions more commonly result in esophageal injury. Alkalis combine with tissue proteins to cause liquefactive necrosis and saponification, and generally penetrate deeper into tissues, potentially leading to full-thickness damage to the esophageal wall. Alkali absorption leads to vascular thrombosis, further impeding blood flow to damaged tissues. Ingestion of granular products may result in more serious injuries due to prolonged contact time with the esophageal mucosa.

Alkali ingestions have three phases of injury: liquefactive necrosis, reparative phase, and scar retraction. In liquefactive necrosis, the injury rapidly penetrates the deep layers of the esophagus until the alkali is buffered by tissue fluids. Between five days and two weeks is considered the reparative phase. Sloughing of the necrotic debris is followed by the development of granulation tissue and collagen deposition. The esophageal wall is thinnest during this subacute phase and at highest risk for perforation. Scar formation begins after two weeks. During this time, there is deposition of collagen, resulting in possible esophageal stricture formation.

Caustic injuries are classified similar to burns (Table 26-1). The classification of injury is based on endoscopic evaluation and is used clinically to help predict subsequent clinical outcomes and course. First-degree caustic injuries are superficial and will result in edema and erythema. The esophageal mucosa will slough, but no stricture will form. Second-degree injuries involve the mucosa, submucosa, and muscle layers. They result in deep ulceration and granulation tissue after which collagen deposition and contraction occur. If there is circumferential injury, a stricture may develop. Third-degree injuries are transmural with deep ulcerations that result in a black appearance to the lining of the esophagus. These injuries can result in esophageal perforation. Patients with grade 2b or 3 will develop strictures in 70–100% of cases.[27,28] Endoscopic grading of mucosal injury directly predicts risk of complications with a ninefold increase in morbidity with each incremental increase in injury grade.[29] Patients who present with peritonitis, mediastinitis, disseminated intravascular coagulation, or shock may require emergency resection of the damaged esophageal tissue.

Following a corrosive ingestion, patients may be asymptomatic or may present with nausea, vomiting, dysphagia, odynophagia, drooling, abdominal pain, chest pain, or stridor. There are no conclusive data to correlate laboratory values or symptoms with degree of injury. The absence of symptoms or oropharyngeal lesions does not exclude esophageal injury. In fact, 12% of patients who are asymptomatic and 61% of patients without oral injury will be found to have esophageal injury at endoscopy.[26,30,31] In symptomatic patients, the presence of three or more symptoms is an important predictor of severe esophageal injury.[28]

Initial management of these patients should focus on airway management and volume resuscitation. Direct laryngoscopy can be useful for identifying laryngeal edema. Inducing emesis should be discouraged because additional exposure to the substance can cause increased mucosal damage. A chest and abdominal radiograph should be obtained to look for signs of perforation. Computed tomography (CT) of the chest can also be used in selected cases.

Endoscopic evaluation should be carried out in the first 24 to 48 hours after ingestion. Contraindications to endoscopy include shock, respiratory distress, peritonitis, mediastinitis, or evidence of perforation. Endoscopy should not be performed after five days, once the reparative phase has begun, because the esophagus is at its thinnest and the risk of perforation is highest. Once the degree of injury is identified, further evaluation of the distal esophagus also increases the risk of perforation.

There is some controversy regarding whether all patients with a history of corrosive ingestion need to undergo endoscopy. Some authors advocate that all patients with suspected corrosive ingestion undergo endoscopy as part of the medical evaluation because even asymptomatic patients may have esophageal injury.[27,32] However, these injuries are typically mild, require no further acute treatment, and are at low risk for long-term complications. There is some evidence that asymptomatic patients may not benefit from routine endoscopy.[28,33] Certainly all patients who are symptomatic require endoscopic evaluation of the esophagus.

Patients found to have grade 1 or 2a injury on endoscopy can be allowed oral intake and are discharged once symptoms have resolved. Patients with grade 2b and 3

Grade	Endoscopic Findings
1	Mucosal edema and erythema
2a	Friability, hemorrhage, blisters, erosions, erythema, white exudate
2b	Findings of grade 2a plus deep or circumferential ulceration
3a	Small and scattered area of necrosis
3b	Extensive necrosis

TABLE 26-1 Classification of Caustic Esophageal Injuries

injuries should be observed for 24 to 48 hours and then may have their diets slowly advanced. Because of the frequency with which strictures occur in grades 2b and 3 injuries, these patients should have a barium swallow on day 21 after injury to evaluate for stricture (Fig. 26-2). Once a stricture is identified, gradual dilations are initiated. Strictures refractory to dilation may need operative resection.

There is no standardized acute management protocol for caustic esophageal injuries. There are several authors who advocate the use of antibiotics, steroids, and proton pump inhibitors in the treatment of severe esophageal injury.[27,31,32] Prospective studies have shown no benefit for the use of steroids in the treatment of caustic esophageal injuries in children.[34] There have been no rigorous studies evaluating the use of antibiotics or proton pump inhibitors in these patients. Because of the heterogeneous nature of ingestions and the various substances, location, and degree of injury, the optimal management remains unclear.

Treatment modalities for esophageal strictures include bougienage, esophageal stent placement, intralesional corticosteroid injection, and endoscopic dilations after stricture formation. Multiple dilations may be required for strictures to resolve. Operative intervention may be necessary if these treatments fail, if malignant transformation occurs, or if lengthy or tight strictures develop. Esophageal carcinoma is a late but serious complication of severe caustic injuries. The incidence is 1000 times the expected occurrence rate of patients of a similar age.[35] Long-term surveillance for development of esophageal malignancy in severe injuries is important.

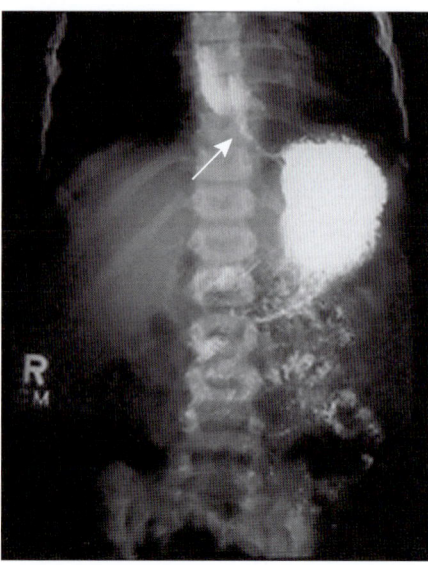

FIGURE 26-3 ■ This barium study was performed in a child with dysphagia and pain. There is marked narrowing (arrow) of the distal esophagus secondary to gastroesophageal reflux and a peptic stricture.

ESOPHAGEAL STRICTURES

In general, esophageal strictures in children do not involve malignancies. The causes of benign esophageal strictures in childhood include reflux esophagitis, corrosive ingestion, and anastomotic scarring. Anastomotic and corrosive strictures may be aggravated by GER. The incidence of stricture in patients with GER approaches 15%.[36] Management includes relief of the obstruction as well as correction of the reflux. Anastomotic strictures tend to be discrete and short, whereas corrosive strictures are more likely to be irregular and long. Peptic esophageal strictures are short and usually located in the lower third of the esophagus (Fig. 26-3).

Uncontrolled GER can result in esophageal stricture as a consequence of repeated insults to the esophageal mucosa. Vomiting and failure to thrive are present in nearly all patients with GER strictures. Many patients will also have concomitant pulmonary disease. In addition, a hiatal hernia may also be present. The majority of strictures are located in the lower third of the esophagus and less frequently in the middle third.

Treatment of strictures includes medical therapy, bouginage, fundoplication, stricture resection, and interposition grafting. Most commonly, the initial treatment of strictures is balloon catheter dilation with aggressive medical management of the GER. The theoretical advantage of balloon dilation over bouginage is that the stricture is gradually dilated by uniform radial force whereas bouginage exerts an abrupt shearing force that may cause injury to the mucosa leading to further scarring and stricture. Patients may need several dilations over several months. The perforation rate with balloon dilation is less than 2%.[37,38] Strategies to prevent perforation include choosing a balloon size that is not greater than the size of the patient's esophagus, not overinflating the balloon, and gradually increasing the size of the balloon over several sessions for tight strictures.

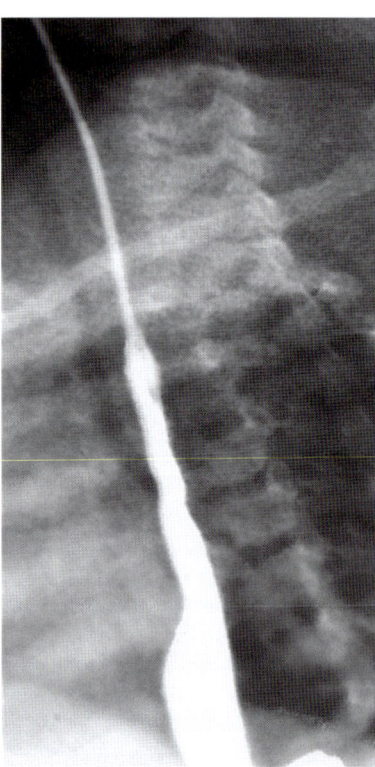

FIGURE 26-2 ■ This barium swallow was performed three weeks after lye ingestion. Note the significant narrowing in the proximal two-thirds of the esophagus.

GER-associated strictures are treated with a combination of preoperative dilations and antireflux procedures.[39] Preoperative management includes proton pump inhibitors, maximal nutritional support, and optimization of respiratory status. Fundoplication is delayed until nutritional optimization is met, esophagitis has resolved, and the stricture has been dilated. Most patients undergo three to five dilations prior to fundoplication. Postoperative dilations are then performed until the stricture is resolved. Almost 90% of patients have complete resolution of the stricture and the associated GER with this management protocol.

ESOPHAGEAL PERFORATION

Esophageal perforation is a rare but life-threatening event in children. Iatrogenic injuries, as a result of nasogastric tube placement, stricture dilations, and endotracheal intubation are the most common reasons found in infants and children. Due to the fact the esophagus lacks a serosal layer, a perforation allows bacteria and digestive enzymes to leak into the mediastinum. The surrounding loose areolar connective tissue is unable to contain the spread of infection and inflammation, and may lead to mediastinitis, empyema, abscess, and sepsis.[40]

Esophageal perforations may be iatrogenic, or result from ingestion of a foreign body, caustic substances, spontaneous, infectious, or traumatic. In the pediatric literature, nearly 80% of esophageal perforations are attributable to iatrogenic causes.[41–43] In children, the most common cause of iatrogenic esophageal perforation is from stricture dilation. The most common location of

perforation in children is the thoracic esophagus. Typically, a perforation in the upper thoracic esophagus will result in findings in the left thorax, whereas perforations in the distal thoracic esophagus will present with right-sided thoracic findings. This is in contrast to the neonate, where the pharyngoesophgeal junction is the most common site of perforation. This is likely due to the fact this region is the narrowest area of the esophagus.

Patients with thoracic esophageal perforations may present with respiratory distress, dysphagia, fever, chest pain, or subcutaneous emphysema. It is important that any child who is symptomatic following an endoscopic or esophageal dilation be evaluated for esophageal perforation. The initial study is a chest radiograph in the anteroposterior and lateral views. Findings suggestive of esophageal perforation include pneumothorax, pleural effusion, subcutaneous emphysema, pneumopericardium, or pneumomediastinum. A contrast esophagram is the preferred diagnostic study to determine the presence of an esophageal perforation. Frequently, water-soluble contrast is used initially and followed by barium if no leak is initially seen. There is a 10% false-negative rate with esophogography.[44] Chest CT can also suggest esophageal perforation, with findings such as mediastinal air, fluid, or esophageal thickening.

Treatment is guided by the type and extent of injury as well as the clinical status of the child. Most patients with esophageal perforation can be successfully managed with an aggressive conservative approach (Fig. 26-4). Patients are started on broad-spectrum antibiotics. If feasible, a nasogastric tube is inserted beyond the perforation into the stomach. This allows enteral alimentation during the healing process. Otherwise, parenteral

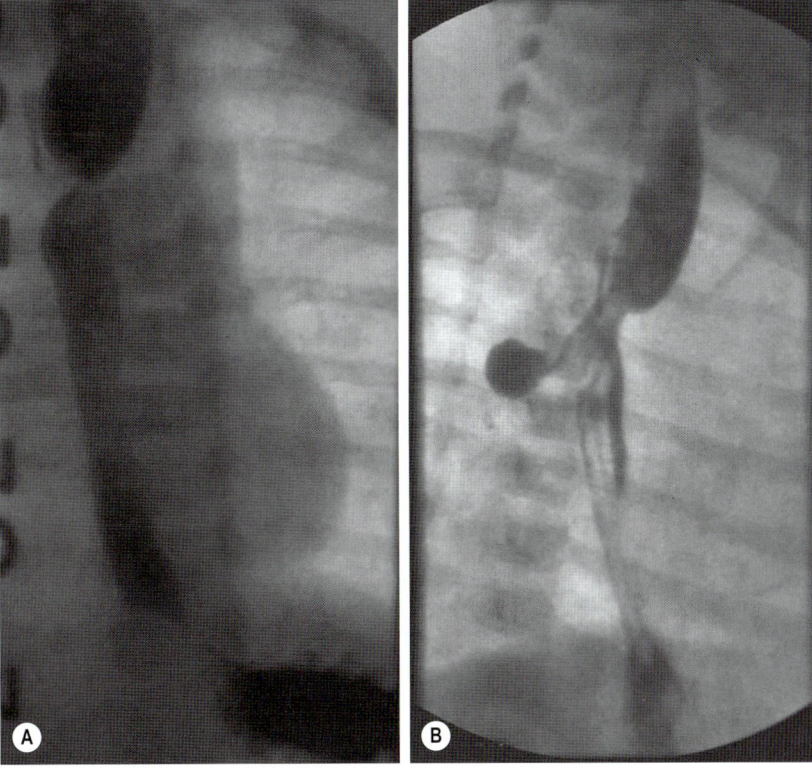

FIGURE 26-4 ■ (A) This infant developed a stricture at the anastomosis after esophageal atresia repair. Multiple balloon dilations were required. (B) Unexpectedly, at the time of one of these dilations, an esophageal perforation developed. Note the contrast leak through the esophageal perforation. This child was managed nonoperatively, and the perforation eventually sealed without the need for operative intervention.

nutrition is started. Drainage of thoracic air or fluid is performed to control the leak. It is likely the esophageal perforation will heal spontaneously, once drainage is established, sepsis is controlled, and adequate nutritional support is provided.

If the patient shows signs of clinical deterioration, has persistence of esophageal leak despite treatment, or has extensive intrapleural spillage, then operative exploration may be needed. Primary repair of the perforation may be possible if it is recognized within 24 hours. The perforation is closed in a single layer with reinforcement with pericardial fat, pleura, stomach, diaphragm, or omentum. If the perforation is large and diagnosed after 24 hours, there is typically widespread mediastinal inflammation. In this setting, the esophagus is friable and will not hold sutures. Historically, this has been managed with cervical esophagostomy and gastrostomy. However, even with extensive inflammation, conservative management with wide drainage and gastrostomy has resulted in spontaneous healing of the perforation.[43]

Morbidity and mortality of esophageal perforation is directly related to delay in the diagnosis and treatment. Complications of esophageal perforation are typically pulmonary in nature, such as pneumonia or atelectasis. There is a fivefold increase in complications following a delay in diagnosis of greater than 24 hours.[42] The mortality of esophageal perforation in the pediatric population is 4%, which is lower than reported for adults.[42]

CONGENITAL ESOPHAGEAL STENOSIS

Congenital esophageal stenosis (CES) is a rare childhood condition with an incidence of 1 in 25,000 to 50,000 live births.[45,46] It is associated with esophageal atresia in one-third of patients. The remaining are considered to be isolated cases.[47,48] Three histopathologic variants are seen: tracheobronchial remnants, membranous diaphragms or webs, and diffuse fibrosis of the muscularis and submucosa.[49] Most infants have normal physical findings at birth. As a result, CES is rarely diagnosed in the neonatal period. The onset of symptoms, most commonly vomiting, dysphagia, and failure to thrive, typically develop with the introduction of solid food at ages 4 to 10 months. Respiratory symptoms are found in about 10% of patients.[50] An esophagogram may show an abrupt or tapered stenosis, commonly at the junction of the middle and distal third of the esophagus (Fig. 26-5). Additional evaluation, including pH probe and endoscopy, is necessary to exclude the more common diagnosis of GER-associated stricture and esophagitis. When associated with esophageal atresia, the stenosis is usually found in the distal one-third of the esophagus.[50,51]

The absence of esophagitis will be confirmed on esophagoscopy. However, tracheobronchial remnants can be missed on biopsy specimens that are taken too superficially.[51] Endoscopic ultrasonography has been shown to be helpful in differentiating tracheobronchial remnants as the cause of the stenosis from stricture due to reflux.[52,53]

Dilatation of a CES does not provide long-term benefit. Case reports have described successful treatment

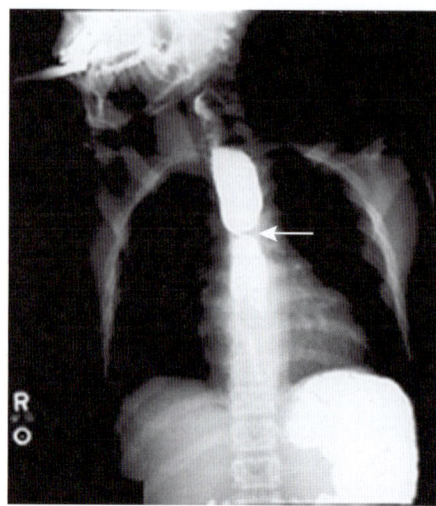

FIGURE 26-5 ■ This child presented with significant dysphagia and weight loss. An esophagogram revealed marked narrowing of the mid esophagus (arrow) due to congenital esophageal stenosis. This child underwent resection of the stenosis and primary repair of the esophagus.

with endoscopic electrocauterization and balloon dilation.[54] However, limited resection of the stenosis through the left chest (either open or thoracoscopically[48]) with primary end-to-end anastomosis is the preferred treatment for long-term relief.

ESOPHAGEAL DUPLICATION

Congenital esophageal duplication is a rare anomaly of the esophagus, with an incidence of 1 in 8000 births, accounting for 10–15% of all gastrointestinal duplications.[55] Histologic criteria for diagnosis include attachment to the esophagus, enclosure of the duplication by two muscle layers, and lining of the duplication by epithelium. Patients tend to present with respiratory symptoms, vomiting, regurgitation, and a possible neck mass. Diagnosis can be made by contrast esophagography. Because the duplication may increase in size with time and compress surrounding structures, operative resection is the treatment of choice. This can be approached via posterolateral thoracotomy or thoracoscopy. Operative guidelines include preserving the vagus and phrenic nerves, and reconstructing the muscular wall of the esophagus. Air insufflation of the esophagus intraoperatively with endoscopy or with a nasogastric tube is helpful to assess the integrity of the esophageal wall after resection. See Chapter 39 for further information about esophageal duplications.

ACHALASIA

Achalasia is a chronic motility disorder of the esophagus characterized by absent or poor esophageal peristalsis and failure of the LES to relax during swallowing. The specific etiology is unknown. In children, this has been associated with various syndromes, including trisomy 21 and triple A syndrome (achalasia, alacrima, and adrenocorti-cotropic hormone [ACTH] insensitivity).

Data obtained from the Healthcare Cost and Utiliza-tion Project (HCUP) from 1997 to 2006 found an annual hospitalization rate of 0.25/100,000 for patients with achalasia under the age of 18 years.[56] Symptoms of acha-lasia are age dependent. Infants present with frequent regurgitation, choking, pneumonia, and failure to thrive. Symptoms in older children are similar to those seen in adults and include dysphagia, vomiting, and weight loss.

The presenting symptoms are often attributed to GER; however, symptoms persist following initiation of antireflux medication. A barium esophagogram will show aperistalsis of the esophagus, a dilated esophagus, and no or minimal opening of the LES, known as the 'bird's beak' sign (Fig. 26-6). Esophageal manometry is the standard diagnostic test for achalasia and typical find-ings include an elevated LES pressure, failure of the sphincter to relax with swallowing, and low-amplitude, nonprogressive, or absent peristaltic contractions in the esophageal body.

There is no cure for the underlying pathology. The aims of therapy are to reduce the LES pressure to facili-tate esophageal emptying, and improve symptoms. Treat-ment has utilized several approaches: pharmacologic agents, mechanical dilation, and esophagomyotomy.

Pharmacologic treatment with nitrates or calcium-channel blockers can result in a decrease in the LES pressure, but the response is temporary. The need for long-term medicine limits its usefulness in children. Intersphincteric injection of *Botulinum* toxin (Botox) has been used in recent years for the treatment of achalasia.[57] Botox is a neurotoxin that binds to presynaptic choliner-gic terminals in skeletal muscle, inhibiting the release of acetylcholine at the neuromuscular junction, which creates a chemical denervation. While initially effective, there is a high recurrence rate that also limits its

applicability in children. Because of the limited success of these therapies, they not used for primary therapy but they may be considered in children unable to undergo general anesthesia.

Forceful dilation of the LES is accomplished with a balloon dilator specifically designed for the treatment of achalasia. Pneumatic dilation reduces the LES pressure by partially disrupting the sphincter muscle complex. Immediate relief of symptoms can be expected in the majority of patients following pneumatic dilation but recurrence of symptoms can be as high as 100%.[58] Sec-ondary procedures, such as repeat pneumatic dilation or surgical esophagomyotomy, may be required in 80–93% of patients.[58,59] Approximately half of these patients choose to undergo additional dilations and half proceed to surgical repair.[58,59] The perforation rate with pneu-matic dilation is about 5%[60, 61] and may be managed conservatively, or with immediate myotomy based on the patient's clinical status.

A large, multicenter, prospective, randomized trial comparing serial pneumatic dilation to primary laparo-scopic esophagomyotomy with Dor fundoplication in adults was recently conducted.[62] A minimal two-year follow-up (mean 43 months) was attained in 95 patients who underwent dilation and 106 who underwent myotomy. At two years, there was no difference in lower esophageal pressure, esophageal emptying, abnormal esophageal acid exposure, or quality of life. The authors concluded that myotomy did not offer superior therapeu-tic success and thus dilation could be considered as first-line treatment. These data may represent a paradigm shift in the treatment for achalasia, although longer follow-up is needed as are data in children.

The goal of esophagomyotomy is to disrupt the LES enough to eliminate dysphagia without causing complica-tions of excessive reflux. This can be accomplished with a thoracic or abdominal approach, open or minimally invasively, with or without a concomitant antireflux pro-cedure. Excellent results have been reported in 70–93% patients at more than five years of follow-up, either with[59,63] or without[64,65] a fundoplication. In long-term follow-up studies, manometry has shown low LES pres-sures, but no significant increase in the amplitude of the esophageal contractions.[66]

Two areas of controversy in the operative management of achalasia include the length of the myotomy and per-formance of a concomitant antireflux procedure. It is believed that an extended myotomy past the LES results in postoperative GER. Surgeons who do not routinely perform an antireflux procedure advocate for a shorter distal myotomy, extending approximately 5 mm past the gastroesophageal junction to maintain a higher pressure at the LES to prevent GER.[65] However, in patients treated with myotomy alone, the postoperative occur-rence of GER can be as high as 47%.[61,66] In addition, postoperative dysphagia occurs in 25%.[63,64] These find-ings may indicate that not only does a limited myotomy not prevent postoperative GER, but also suggest it may not always relieve the symptoms.

In adults, there is good evidence to support a longer myotomy combined with a partial fundoplication. A pro-spective randomized controlled study in adults showed a

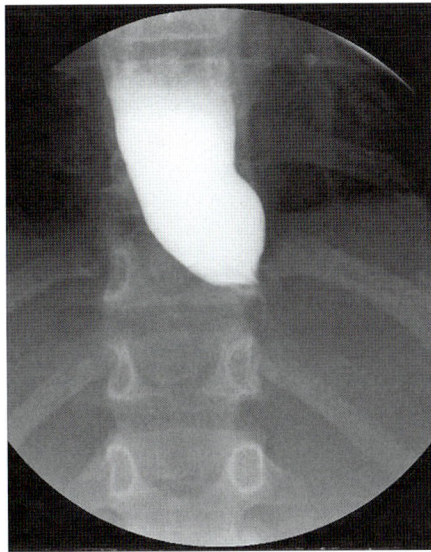

FIGURE 26-6 ■ This barium swallow was performed in a 16-year-old patient with dysphagia secondary to achalasia. The classic 'bird's beak' narrowing of the distal esophagus at the level of the spastic, contracted esophagus is seen. Also, note the dilated esophagus proximal to the lower esophageal sphincter.

fundoplication decreases the incidence of postoperative reflux from 47% to 9.1%.[66] In addition to an antireflux procedure, it has been recognized in adults that a longer myotomy, extending for 2.5–3 cm onto the gastric wall, reduces postoperative dysphagia from 17% to 5%.[67] There has also been good success reported in children undergoing an extended myotomy with partial fundoplication.[68] As a result of these findings, the most commonly utilized operation is the laparoscopic esophagomyotomy with Dor fundoplication with extension of the esophageal myotomy 4–6 cm above and 2–3 cm distal to the gastroesophageal junction.

Persistence or recurrence of dysphagia following myotomy is thought to be the result of incomplete disruption of the muscle fibers of the distal esophagus. Adjunctive techniques to improve the adequacy of the myotomy have included intraoperative endoscopy and intraoperative mamometry.[69,70] Intraoperative endoscopy correctly identifies the squamocolumnar transition at the esophagogastric junction to determine the distal extent of myotomy. Intraoperative manometery has been used to confirm reduction of LES pressures following myotomy. In one study, intraoperative manometry following myotomy showed residual high pressure in 34%, prompting extension of the myotomy.[69] The use of intraoperative manometry in children has been shown to reduce recurrence of symptoms at one year to 0%.[70]

It is important to remember that achalasia is a chronic condition. Even following operation for achalasia, children have significantly lower quality of life (QOL) scores than children with inflammatory bowel disease and have QOL scores that are comparable to children with chronic constipation.[71] Population-based studies have found a 16-fold risk of development of esophageal cancer following treatment for achalasia.[72] However, the absolute risk of esophageal cancer remains relatively low, and there is no consensus regarding the need for routine surveillance in patients with achalasia.

ESOPHAGEAL REPLACEMENT

The most common indications for esophageal replacement in infants and children are long-gap esophageal atresia, failed primary repair of esophageal atresia, and strictures related to reflux or corrosive injury.[73–75] The colon was the first conduit used as an esophageal replacement and remains the most commonly used technique in practice today. Other alternatives that have been used with success include gastric tube, gastric transposition, and jejunal interposition graft. Which conduit is best for any given patient depends on multiple factors, including the location and length of the native remaining esophagus, the original diagnosis, the patient's size and age, and previous procedures on the esophagus, stomach, or colon.

Regardless of the conduit used, there are several important principles. First, the esophagus is the optimal conduit, provided it functions relatively normally and has no malignant potential (e.g., Barrett esophagus). Second, a short straight tract is best because almost all conduits function as passive tubes rather than by means of intrinsic peristaltic activity. The posterior mediastinum is often the

shortest and straightest route. Third, the prevention of reflux into any conduit is important. An interposition procedure that incorporates the distal normal esophagus with its gastroesophageal junction may have an advantage in preventing reflux complications. Fourth, persistence is exceedingly important. Anastomotic dilatations should not be necessary except during the healing phase. Strictures should be revised (Fig. 26-7). Complex interpositions that do not function well should be revised to provide the straightest, lowest resistance conduit possible.

Gastric Tube Esophageal Replacement

Gastric tubes have become popular because they can be created rapidly with a stapling device. The gastric tube is constructed from the greater curve of the stomach with the blood supply based on the left gastroepiploic artery. These tubes can be created from the antrum up, or from the fundus down, and can be constructed so that there is enough gastric tube to reach the neck (Fig. 26-8). The advantages of a gastric tube are its reliable blood supply, its resistance to ulceration from gastric acid reflux, and its ability to bridge long gaps. The tube is also resilient and does not become tortuous or dilated over time. Theoretical disadvantages are a long suture line, continued acid production by the tube, and reduced stomach capacity.

Complications include anastomotic leak, stricture formation requiring dilation, temporary dumping syndrome, and the development of Barrett esophagus above the anastamosis.[73,74] Control studies have shown normal swallowing and manometry has shown mass contractions

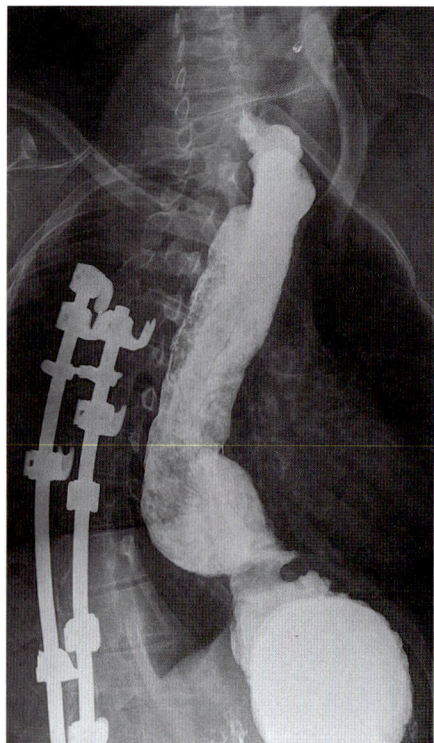

FIGURE 26-7 ■ Barium swallow of a 28-year-old patient after successful left colon interposition for isolated esophageal atresia. The patient developed bleeding and dysphagia from peptic ulceration at the distal anastomosis, requiring revision.

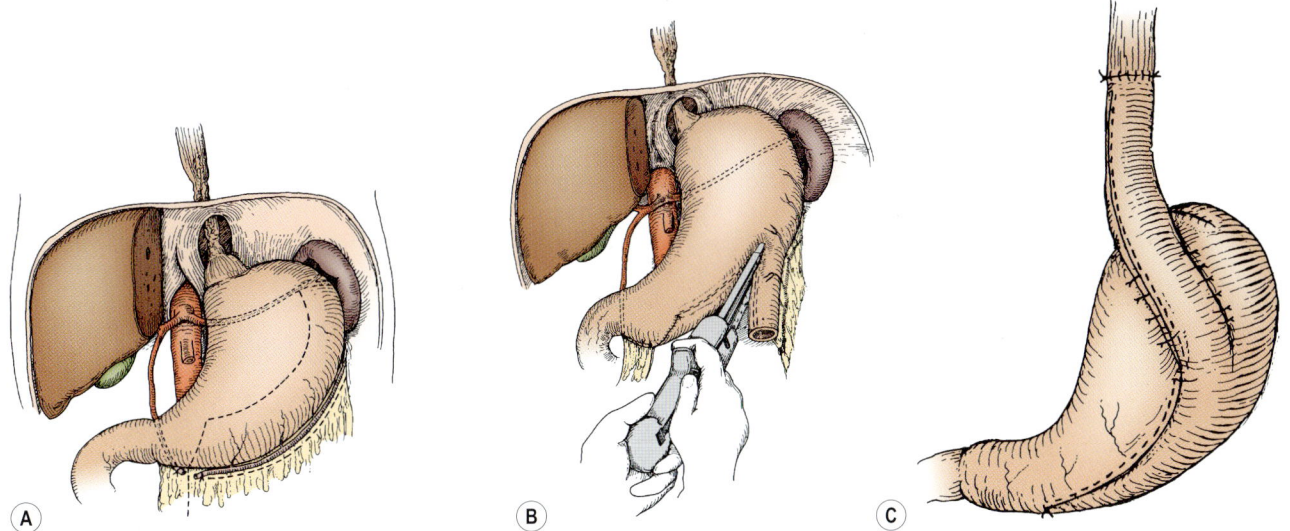

FIGURE 26-8 ■ Graphic depiction of the technique to create a reversed gastric tube for esophageal replacement. **(A)** Inspection of the blood supply to the stomach and preservation of the gastroepiploic artery for creating the tube. **(B)** The use of a stapler to create the tube along the greater curvature of the stomach. **(C)** The completed reversed tube is brought up to the chest for the esophageal anastomosis.

in about two-thirds of patients.[74] Overall, about 80% of patients report enjoying a normal diet.

Gastric Transposition

The gastric transposition (or pull-up procedure) is performed by mobilizing the entire stomach on a vascular pedicle, relocating the entire stomach into the mediastinum, and creating an anastomosis to the cervical esophagus in the neck. In addition, many surgeons will perform a pyloroplasty to prevent gastroparesis. The advantages of this approach include that it is technically straightforward, the stomach has an excellent blood supply, only one anastomosis is needed, and that the entire esophagus can be replaced with a low risk of necrosis, leak, or stricture. Complications following gastric transposition have included anastomotic leak, stricture, and significant swallowing problems. Mortality has been reported to be 4.6%.[75] Death following gastric transposition is typically due to respiratory failure. Gastric transposition may not be the ideal substitution in patients with borderline respiratory function as a bulky stomach in the chest may contribute to further respiratory compromise. Figure 26-9 depicts a postoperative barium study after a gastric pull-up procedure for an extensive stricture following lye ingestion.

The long-term outcome is considered good to excellent in 90%, although many patients prefer eating small frequent meals. There has been no documented evidence of deterioration in the function of the gastric transposition in 72 patients who were observed for longer than ten years.[75]

In older patients who have had multiple procedures, the blood supply to the stomach may be compromised and a long gastric tube is not advised. These patients also may not have adequate stomach length to reach the cervical esophagus. In such patients, a gastric pull-up, combined with a short gastric tube, may be used to

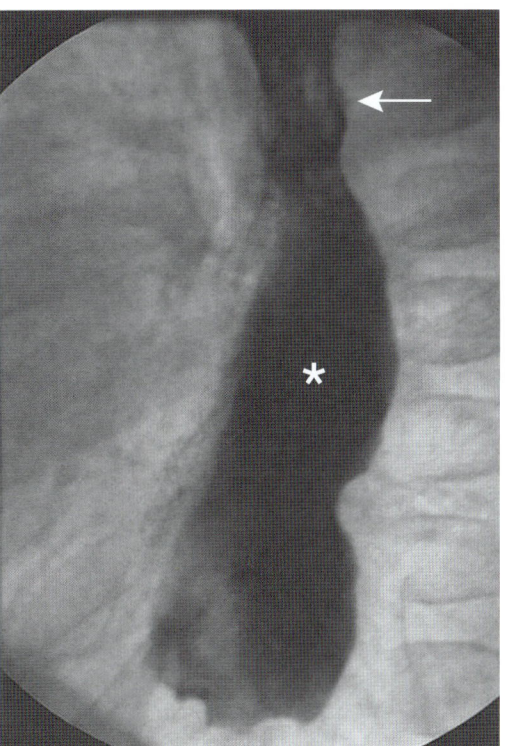

FIGURE 26-9 ■ This infant underwent a gastric pull-up after a failed colonic interposition for isolated esophageal atresia. The native esophagus is identified by the arrow, and the gastric pull-up is marked with an asterisk.

create the additional stomach length required to reach the neck.

Colon Interposition

The right, transverse, or left colon on its vascular pedicle has been used as an esophageal replacement, either in an isoperistaltic or an antiperistaltic direction. It can be placed retrosternal or in a transhiatal posterior mediastinal location. The left colon and its vascular pedicle, based on the left colic artery, is most commonly used.[76] The colon is pulled up into the neck, and an end-to-side or end-to-end esophagocolic anastomosis is performed. The gastrocolic anastomosis is then performed, followed by a fundoplication and pyloroplasty. The steps involved

with a right colon interposition for esophageal atresia are seen in Figure 26-10, and the operative steps for a left or transverse colon interposition are seen in Figure 26-11.

A colon interposition is a relatively straightforward procedure, and the colon is readily positioned into the thorax without causing respiratory compromise. Disadvantages of this approach include the need for

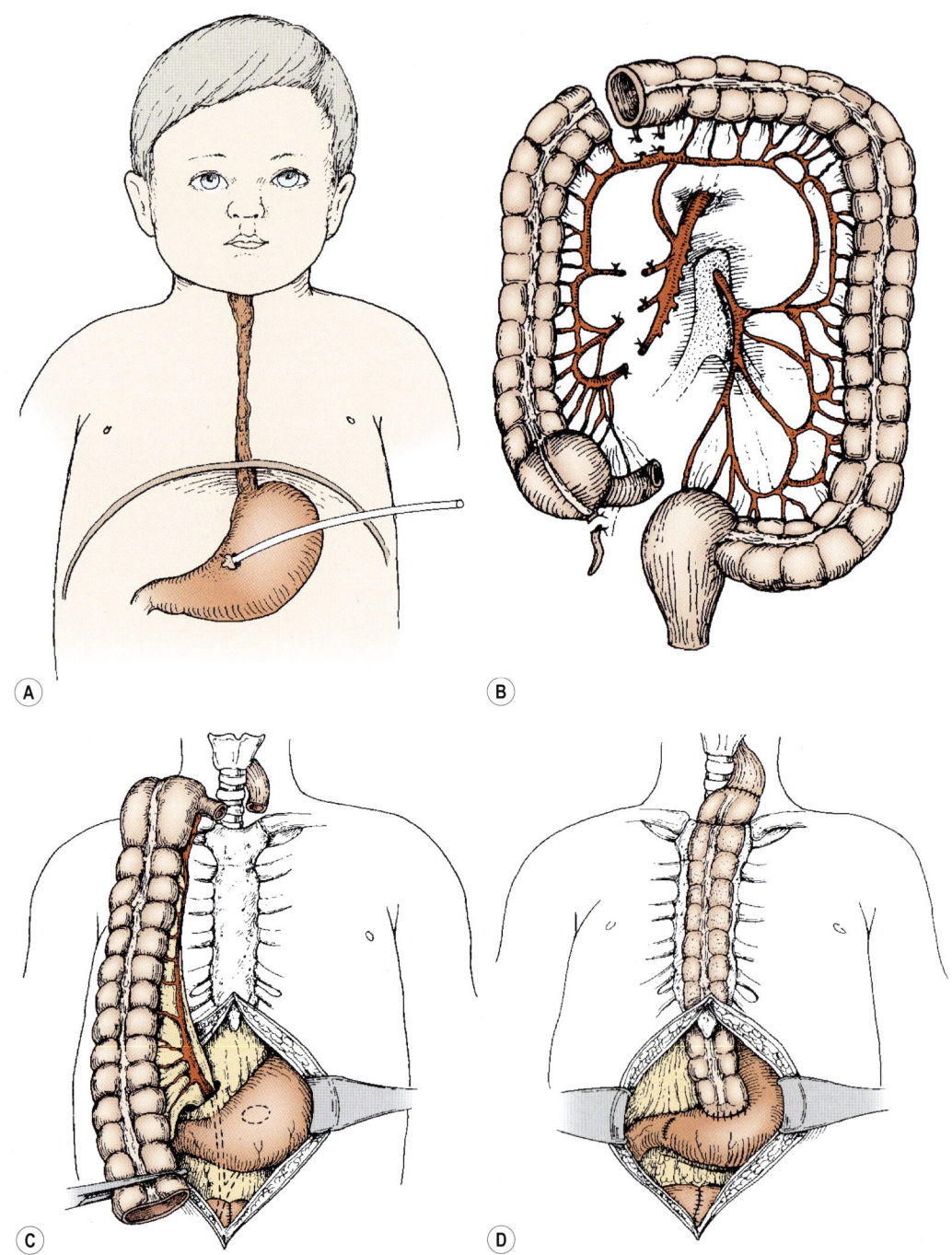

FIGURE 26-10 ■ **(A)** For any esophageal lesion in which a substitution procedure may be anticipated, the gastrostomy should be placed on the lesser curve at about the level of the incisura, so that a right or left colon or gastric tube interposition can be carried out without compromising the blood supply. **(B)** The right colon and terminal ileum are isolated, based on blood supply from the arcades and from the middle colic artery. **(C)** The colon on its pedicle is brought up through the lesser sac and positioned substernally in an isoperistaltic fashion. **(D)** Most frequently, excision of the terminal ileum and cecum is accomplished. Careful tailoring of the distal end allows a straight conduit to be anastomosed to the antrum. Pyloroplasty may or may not be added to the procedure. The incidence of significant gastrocolic reflux is reduced by a drainage procedure.

three anastomoses, an increased risk for anastomotic leak, strictures at the esophagocolic anastomosis, and tortuosity or redundancy of the graft over time.

Graft necrosis or ischemia can be prevented by meticulous attention to the blood supply. Assuring that the graft has a dual blood supply from the left colic artery and from the marginal arcade will help prevent ischemia or necrosis. Careful attention not to disrupt the vascular supply to the cervical esophagus and performing a wide anastamosis will help avoid anastomotic leak and stenosis. The addition of a partial fundoplication may decrease the incidence of GER into the graft and resultant ulceration. An accurate measurement of the graft length and excision of excess length before anastamosis should prevent redundancy.

Timing of Colon Interposition

In those patients in whom esophageal atresia has developed without a distal fistula, and in whom attempts at stretching are successful, the colon can be interposed in the newborn period. Several authors report performing colonic interposition once the patient is 3 months of age or 5 kg in weight.[77–79] Many pediatric surgeons, however, prefer a cervical esophagoscopy and gastrostomy, and wait to perform the colon interposition when the patient is walking, usually over the age of 1 year. Both approaches have theoretical and practical advantages. Most reported experience has been in patients who are 12 to 18 months of age and are walking to allow the upright position to counteract reflux into the graft and allow for passive emptying of the neoesophagus.[80] During the period from esophagostomy to colon interposition, it is important to provide sham feedings to develop oral–motor coordination. If sham oral feedings accompany gastrostomy feedings, the patient may then associate a full stomach with swallowing.

Jejunal Substitution

The jejunum has been used as an esophageal substitute much more commonly in adults than in children.

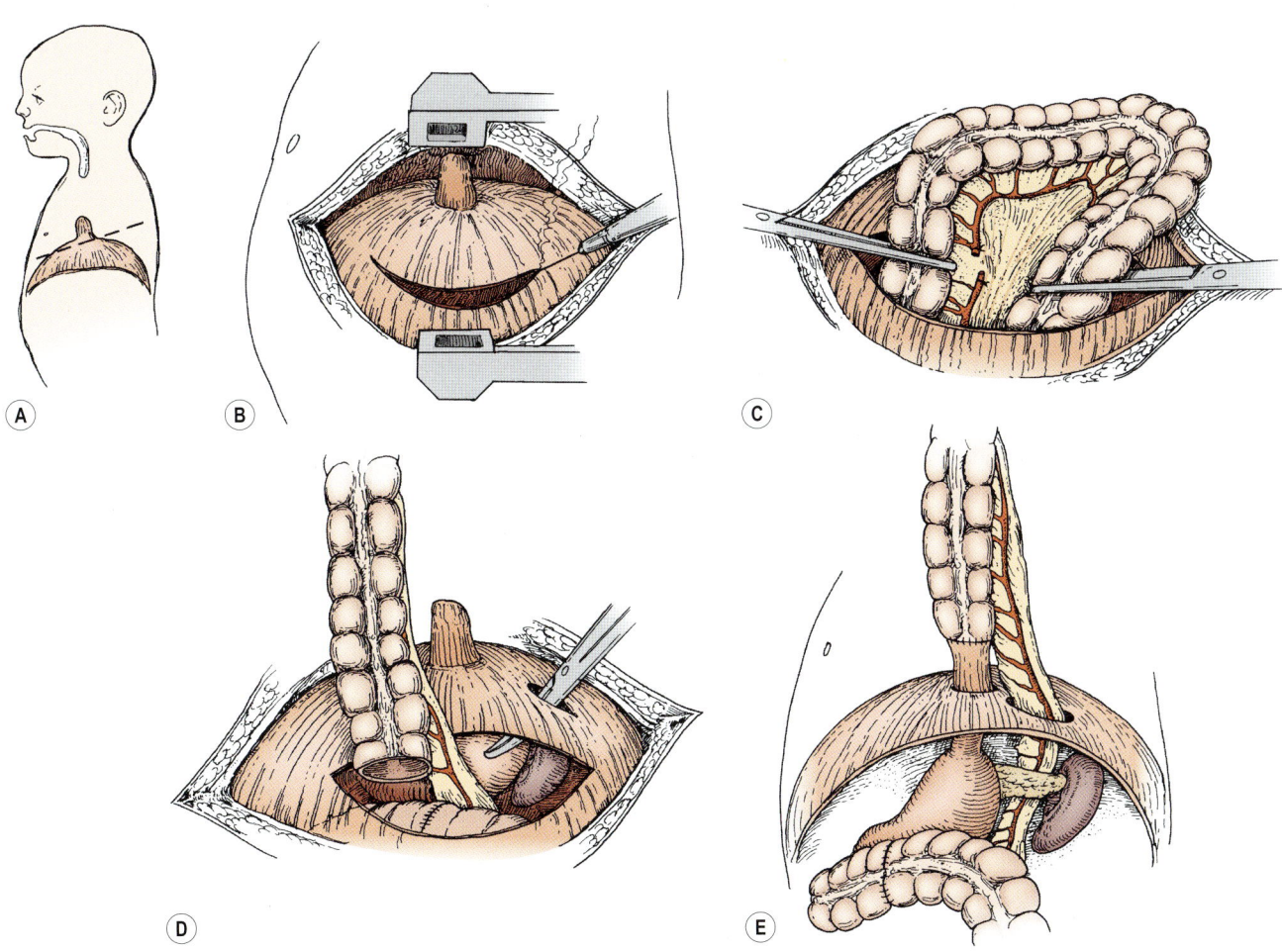

FIGURE 26-11 ■ The left colon or transverse colon substitution described by Waterston is illustrated in this patient with isolated esophageal atresia. However, it works equally well for other lesions requiring esophageal replacement. **(A)** A standard posterolateral left thoracotomy at about the sixth intercostal space. **(B)** Incision of the diaphragm peripherally. **(C)** A section of colon is isolated and its vascular pedicle is developed, usually based on the left colic artery. It may be necessary to base it on the middle colic artery, in which case, this interposed colon is placed in an antiperistaltic manner. **(D)** The colon and its vascular pedicle are delivered behind the spleen and pancreas and through a separate posterior opening in the diaphragm, so that the abdominal viscera do not stretch or otherwise obstruct the blood supply to this colon segment. **(E)** The distal anastomosis may be made to the remnant of the distal esophagus (as is depicted) or to the posterior aspect of the stomach.

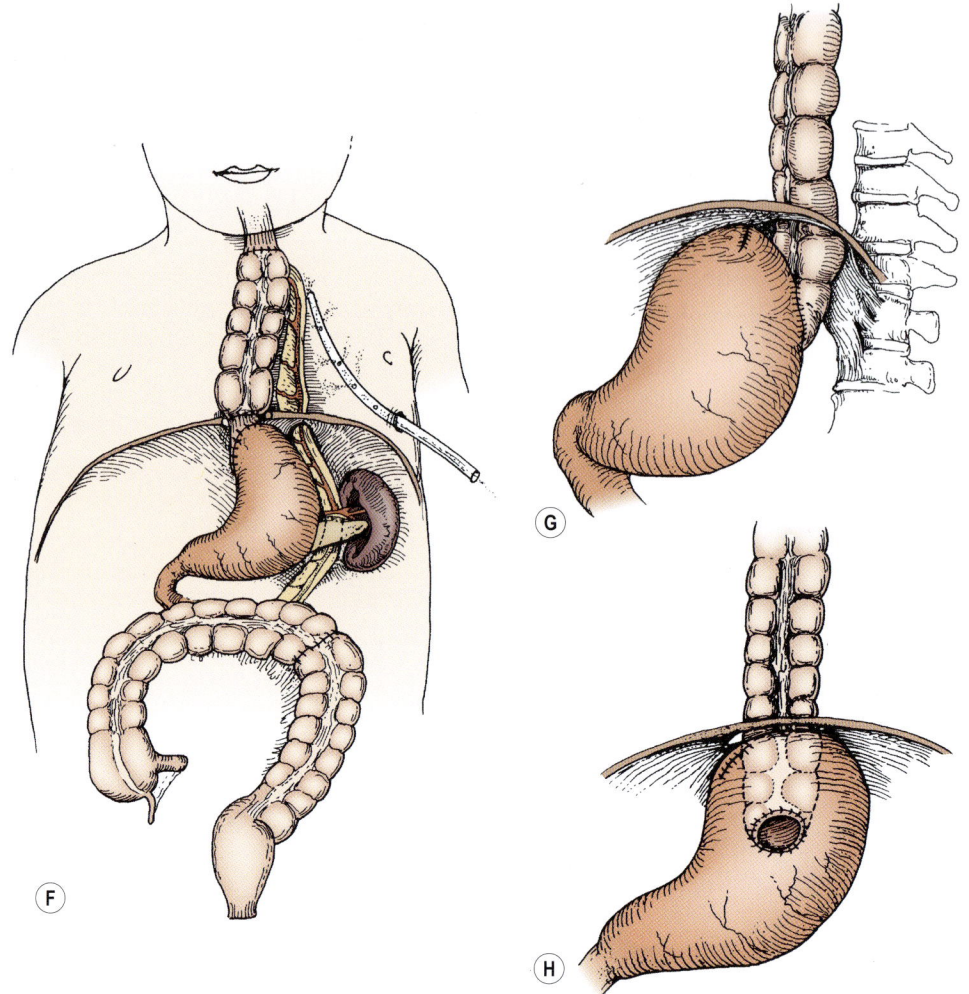

FIGURE 26-11, Cont'd ■ **(F)** The upper anastomosis is made to the esophagus either within the mediastinum or within the neck. Adequate drainage of the pleura is necessary to prevent empyema. A fundoplication after the method of Thal also may be added to this procedure, if the distal esophagus is used. This technique reduces the amount of reflux that can interfere with the healing or that can produce ulcers in the colon. **(G)** A lateral view of an alternative method of cologastrostomy with Waterston's procedure. **(H)** The segment of colon is shown within the abdominal cavity, which may possibly reduce the incidence of gastrocolic reflux.

Advantages to using jejunum include a diameter that is similar to the esophagus and does not occupy much space in the thoracic cavity. Also, the jejunum retains its peristaltic activity. Significant disadvantages include the precarious vascular supply of a pedicled jejunal graft. Also, a tension-free anastomosis may be difficult to achieve.

Esophageal substitution with free and pedicled jejunal grafts has resulted in significant perioperative morbidity, including intraoperative repeat interpositions for immediate graft loss, early postoperative graft loss, anastomotic leaks, late anastomotic strictures, and graft redundancy.[81,82] Less than 50% of patients are able to achieve a completely oral diet without reliance on gastrostomy feeds.[81] In spite of technically sound outcomes, it is known that significant complications exist, including death, graft necrosis, ischemia, and strictures.

Complications of Esophageal Substitution

Regardless of the conduit used, substitution of the esophagus carries a number of predictable complications. The most serious one is vascular insufficiency with necrosis of the interposition. This complication is most commonly seen when using the jejunum or colon and is recognized at the time of interposition as a blue, pulseless graft. Adjustment of the graft to relieve tension or twisting of the pedicle may be effective in improving the blood supply. Intraoperative hypotension may result in the graft taking on the appearance of vascular insufficiency. If the geometry of the graft and the patient's blood pressure are both satisfactory, the graft must be abandoned because its vascularity will rarely improve after completion of the operation.

Interposition of a well-vascularized graft is sometimes followed several days later by fever, increased leukocytosis, and drainage from the proximal anastomosis. An anastomotic leak from tension or mild ischemia can be managed expectantly if the conduit appears viable. A contrast study, however, may demonstrate that the mucosal pattern of the interposed segment is ischemic. The interposition must be inspected and removed if it is necrotic. In this case, a cervical esophagostomy should be established and a different form of substitution planned. Many investigators have reported using the left colon after

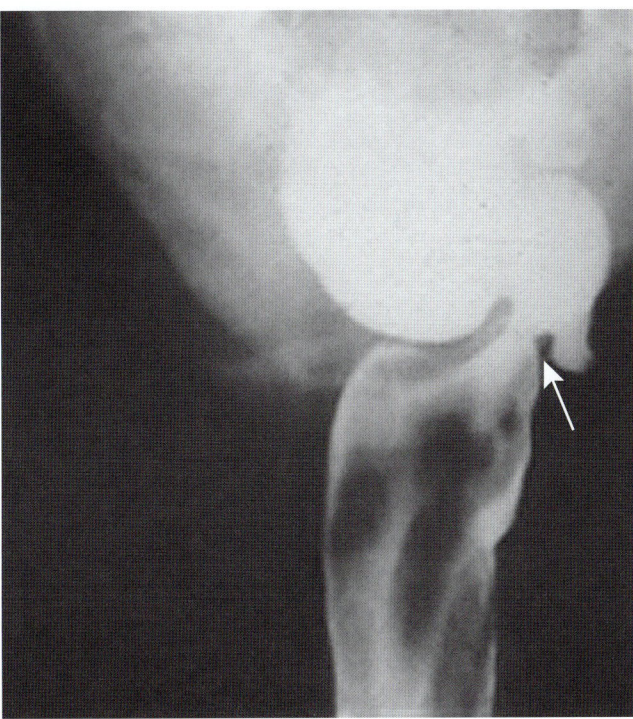

FIGURE 26-12 ■ A stricture (arrow) developed at the esophago-colonic anastomosis after colon interposition for esophageal substitution. The likely cause was vascular insufficiency.

failure of the right colon. Others may not be inclined to sacrifice additional colon and would perform a gastric tube or gastric transposition.

Proximal strictures between the esophagus and the interposition usually are the result of insufficient blood supply to the interposition (Fig. 26-12). Anastomosis to a scarred esophagus also results in stricture. After a reasonable healing period, persistent strictures should be revised rather than repeatedly dilated.

Ulceration in either a gastric tube or interposed colon is probably the result of reflux and stasis, which may be caused by kinks in the interposition or by delayed gastric emptying. The latter can be a complication of vagal injury either from the original caustic ingestion or from attempts at previous esophageal reconstruction. Whether a pyloroplasty is necessary in all interpositions is a matter of opinion. Certainly, the elimination of 'sink-trap' kinks in the interposition is important to prevent ulceration. Revision of the lower end of the interposed colon to eliminate redundancy must be performed with great care to prevent damage to the vascular pedicle and loss of the entire graft.

In the authors' experience, we prefer performing a gastric tube in younger patients and gastric transposition in older patients. We feel these options are technically straightforward, do not result in redundancy over time, and are acid resistant. If the stomach is not available for replacement, then the colon can be used.

REFERENCES

1. Kluth D, Fiegel F. The embryology of the foregut. Semin Pediatr Surg 2003;12:3–9.
2. Skandalakis JE, Ellis H. Embryologic and anatomic basis of esophageal surgery. Surg Clin North Am 2000;80:85–155.
3. Michel L, Grillo HC, Malt RA. Esophageal perforation. Ann Thorac Surg 1982;33:203–10.
4. Lloyd DA. Rigid endoscopy of the esophagus—basic technique. In: Najmaldin A, editor. Operative Endoscopy and Endoscopic Surgery in Infants and Children. London: Hodder Arnold; 2005. p. 117–20.
5. Crabbe DCG. Upper gastrointestinal endoscopy–basic techniques. In: Najmaldin A, editor. Operative Endoscopy and Endoscopic Surgery in Infants and Children. London: Hodder Arnold; 2005. p. 121–6.
6. Lee KK, Anderson MA, Baron TH, et al. Modifications in endoscopic practice for pediatric patients. Gastrointest Endosc 2008;67:1–9.
7. Isaza N, Garcia P, Dutta S. Advances in pediatric minimal access therapy: A cautious journey from therapeutic endoscopy to transluminal surgery based on the adult experience. JPGN 2008;46:359–69.
8. Little DC, Shah SR, St Peter SD, et al. Esophageal foreign bodies in the pediatric population: Our first 500 cases. J Pediatr Surg 2006;41:914–18.
9. Tokar B, Cevik AA, Ilhan H. Ingested gastrointestinal foreign bodies: Predisposing factors for complications in children having surgical or endoscopic removal. Pediatr Surg Int 2007;23:135–9.
10. McComas BC, van Miles P, Katz BE. Successful salvage of an 8-month-old child with and aortoesophageal fistula. J Pediatr Surg 1991;26:1394–5.
11. Raval MV, Campbell BT, Phillips JD. Case of the missing penny: Thoracoscopic removal of a mediastinal coin. J Pediatr Surg 2004;39:1758–60.
12. Uchida K, Inoue M, Konishi N, et al. Esophageal stricture with a pseudodiverticulum caused by the unrecognized ingestion of a small foreign body in a child: Report of a case. Surg Today 2005;35:774–7.
13. Hammond P, Jaffray B, Hamilton L. Tracheoesophageal fistula secondary to disk battery ingestion: A case report of gastric interposition and tracheal patch. J Pediatr Surg 2007;42:E39–E41.
14. Miller RS, Willging JP, Rutter MJ, et al. Chronic esophageal foreign bodies in pediatric patients: A retrospective review. Int J Pediatr Otorhinolaryngol 2004;68:265–72.
15. Popel J, El-Hakim H, El-Matary W. Esophageal foreign body extraction in children: Flexible versus rigid endoscopy. Surg Endosc 2011;25:919–22.
16. Dahshan AH, Donovan GK. Bougienage versus endoscopy for esophageal coin removal in children. J Clin Gastroenterol 2007;41:454–6.
17. Soprano JV, Mandl KD. Four strategies for the management of esophageal coins in children. Pediatrics 2000;105:e5.
18. Waltzman ML, Baskin M, Wypij D, et al. A randomized clinical trial of the management of esophageal coins in children. Pediatrics 2005;116:614–19.
19. Yardeni D, Yardeni H, Coran AG, et al. Severe esophageal damage due to button battery ingestion: Can it be prevented? Pediatr Surg Int 2004;20:496–501.
20. Stuth EAE, Stucke AG, Cohen RD, et al. Successful resuscitation of a child after exsanguination due to aortoesophageal fistula from undiagnosed foreign body. Anesthesiology 2001;95:1025–6.
21. Samad L, Ali M, Ramzi H. Button battery ingestion: Hazards of esophageal impaction. J Pediatr Surg 1999;34:1527–31.
22. Slamon NB, Hertzog JH, Penfil SH, et al. An unusual case of button battery-induced traumatic tracheoesophageal fistula. Pediatr Emerg Care 2008;24:313–16.
23. Imamoglu M, Cay A, Kosucu P, et al. Acquired tracheo-esophageal fistulas caused by button battery lodged in the esophagus. Pediatr Surg Int 2004;20:292–4.
24. Bernstein JM, Burrows SA, Saunders MW. Lodged oesophageal button battery masquerading as a coin: An unusual case of bilateral vocal cord paralysis. Emerg Med J 2007;24:e15.
25. Bronstein AC, Spyker DA, Cantilena LR, et al. 2010 Annual report of the American Association of Poison Control Centers' National Poison Data System (NPDS): 28th Annual Report. Clinical Toxicology 2011;49:910–41.
26. Dogan Y, Erkan T, Cokugras FC, et al. Caustic gastroesophageal lesions in childhood: An analysis of 473 cases. Clin Pediatr 2006;45:435–8.
27. Baskin D, Urganci N, Abbasoglu L, et al. A standardized protocol for the acute management of corrosive ingestion in children. Pediatr Surg Int 2004;20:824–8.

28. Betalli P, Falchetti D, Giuliani S, et al. Caustic ingestion in children: is endoscopy always indicated? The results of an Italian multicenter observational study. Gastrointest Endosc 2008;68:434–9.

29. Poley JW, Steyerberg EW, Kuipers EJ, et al. Ingestions of acid and alkaline agents: Outcome and prognostic value of early upper endoscopy. Gastrointest Endosc 2004;60:372–3.

30. Gaudreault P, Parent M, McGuigan MA, et al. Predictability of esophageal injury from signs and symptoms: A study of caustic ingestion in 378 children. Pediatrics 1983;71:767–70.

31. Riffat F, Cheng A. Pediatric caustic ingestion: 50 consecutive cases and a review of the literature. Dis Esophagus 2009;22:89–94.

32. Broto J, Asensio M, Soler C, et al. Conservative treatment of caustic esophageal injuries in children: 20 years of experience. Pediatr Surg Int 1999;15:323–25.

33. Gupta SK, Croffie JM, Fitzgerald JF. Is esophagogastroduodenoscopy necessary in all caustic ingestions? JPGN 2001;32:50–3.

34. Anderson KD, Rouse TM, Randolph KG. A controlled trial of corticosteroids in children with corrosive injury of the esophagus. N Engl J Med 1990;323:637–40.

35. Kay M, Wyllie R. Caustic ingestions in children. Curr Opin Pediatr 2009;21:651–4.

36. O'Neill AJ, Betts J, Ziegler MM, et al. Surgical management of reflux strictures of the esophagus in childhood. Ann Surg 1982;196:453–60.

37. Lan LC, Wong KK, Lin SC, et al. Endoscopic balloon dilation of esophageal strictures in infants and children: 17 years' experience and a literature review. J Pediatr Surg 2003;38:1712–15.

38. Said M, Mekki M, Golli M, et al. Balloon dilatation of anastomotic structures secondary to surgical repair of oesophageal atresia. Br J Radiol 2003;76:26–31.

39. Numanoglu A, Millar AJ, Brown RA, et al. Gastroesophageal reflux strictures in children, management and outcome. Pediatr Surg Int 2005;21:631–4.

40. Panieri E, Millar AJ, Rode RA, et al. Iatrogenic esophageal perforations in children: Patterns of injury, presentation, management and outcome. J Pediatr Surg 1996;31:890–5.

41. Peng L, Quan X, Zongzheng J, et al. Videothoracoscopic drainage for esophageal perforation with mediastinitis in children. J Pediatr Surg 2006;41:514–17.

42. Engum SA, Gosfeld JL, West KW, et al. Improved survival in children with esophageal perforation. Arch Surg 1996;31:604–11.

43. Martinez L, Rivas S, Hernandez F, et al. Aggressive conservative treatment of esophageal perforations in children. J Pediatr Surg 2003;38:685–9.

44. Gander JW, Berdon WE, Cowls RA. Iatrogenic esophageal perforation in children. Pediatr Surg Int 2009;25:395–401.

45. Amae S, Nio M, Kamiyama T, et al. Clinical characteristics and management of congenital esophageal stenosis: A report on 14 cases. J Pediatr Surg 2003;38:565–70.

46. Vasudevan SA, Kerendi F, Lee H, et al. Management of congenital esophageal stenosis. J Pediatr Surg 2002;37:1024–6.

47. Ibrahim AHM, Al Malki TA, Hamaza AF, et al. Congenital esophageal stenosis associated with esophageal atresia: New concepts. Pediatr Surg Int 2007;23:533–7.

48. Martinez-Ferro M, Rubio M, Piaggio L, et al. Thoracoscopic approach for congenital esophageal stenosis. J Pediatr Surg 2006;41:E5–E7.

49. Murphy SG, Yazbeck S, Russo P. Isolated congenital esophageal stenosis. J Pediatr Surg 1995;30:1238–41.

50. Takamizawa S, Tsugawa C, Mouri N, et al. Congenital esophageal stenosis: Therapeutic strategy based on etiology. J Pediatr Surg 2002;37:197–201.

51. Sneed WF, LaGarde DC, Kogutt MS, et al. Esophageal stenosis due to cartilaginous tracheobronchial remnants. J Pediatr Surg 1979;14:786–8.

52. Kouchi K, Yoshida H, Matsunaga T, et al. Endosonographic evaluation in two children with esophageal stenosis. J Pediatr Surg 2002;37:934–6.

53. Usui N, Kamata S, Kawahara H, et al. Usefulness of endoscopic ultrasonography in the diagnosis of congenital esophageal stenosis. J Pediatr Surg 2002;37:1744–6.

54. Chao H, Chen S, Kong M. Successful treatment of congenital esophageal web by endoscopic electrocauterization and balloon dilation. J Pediatr Surg 2008;43:E13–15.

55. Achildi O, Grewal H. Congenital anomalies of the esophagus. Otolaryngol Clin North Am 2007;40:219–44.

56. Sonnenberg A. Hospitalization for achalasia in the United States 1997–2006. Dig Dis Sci 2009;54:1680–5.

57. Walton JM, Tougas G. Botulinum toxin use in pediatric achalasia: A case report. J Pediatr Surg 1997;32:916–17.

58. Lee CW, Kays DW, Chen MK, et al. Outcomes of treatment of childhood achalasia. J Pediatr Surg 2010;45:1173–7.

59. Pastor AC, Mills J, Marcon MA, et al. A single center 26-year experience with treatment of esophageal achalasia: Is there an optimal method? J Pediatr Surg 2009;44:1349–54.

60. Speiss AE, Kahrilas PJ. Treating achalasia. From whalebone to laparoscope. JAMA 1998;280:638–42.

61. Csendes A, Braghetto I, Henriques A, et al. Late results of a prospective randomized study comparing forceful dilatation and oesophagomyotomy in patients with achalasia. Gut 1989;30:299–304.

62. Boeckxstaens GE, Annese V, Bruley des Varannes S, et al. Pneumatic dilation versus laparoscopic Heller's myotomy for idiopathic achalasia. N Engl J Med 2011;364:1807–16.

63. Morris-Stiff G, Foster M E, Khan R, et al. Long-term results of surgery for childhood achalasia Ann R Coll Surg Engl 1997;79:432–4.

64. Karnak I, Senocak ME, Tanyet FC, et al. Achalasia in childhood: Surgical treatment and outcome. Eur J Pediatr Surg 2001;11:223–9.

65. Vaos G, Demetriou L, Velaoras C, et al. Evaluating long-term results of modified Heller limited esophagomyotomy in children with esophageal achalasia. J Pediatr Surg 2008;43:1262–9.

66. Richards WO, Torquati A, Holzman MD, et al. Heller myotomy versus Heller myotomy with Dor fundoplication for achalasia. A prospective randomized double-blind clinical trial. Ann Surg 2004;240:405–15.

67. Wright AS, Williams CW, Pellegrini CA, et al. Long-term outcomes confirm the superior efficacy of extended Heller myotomy with Toupet fundoplication for achalasia. Surg Endosc 2007;21:713–18.

68. Patti MG, Albanese C, Holcomb GW III, et al. Laparoscopic Heller myotomy and Dor fundoplication for esophageal achalasia in children. J Pediatr Surg 2001;36:1248–51.

69. Chapman JR, Joehl RJ, Murayama KM, et al. Achalasia treatment. Improved outcome of laparoscopic myotomy with operative manometry. Arch Surg 2004;139:508–13.

70. Jafri M, Alonso M, Kaul A, et al. Intraoperative manometry during laparoscopic Heller myotomy improves outcome in pediatric achalasia. J Pediatr Surg 2008;43:66–70.

71. Marlais M, Fishman JR, Fell JM, et al. Health-related quality of life in children with achalasia. J Paediatr Child Health 2011;47:18–21.

72. Sandler RS, Nyren O, Ekbom A, et al. The risk of esophageal cancer in patients with achalasia. A population-based study. JAMA 1995;274:1359–62.

73. Borgnon J, Tounian P, Auber F, et al. Esophageal replacement in children by an isoperistaltic gastric tube: A 12-year experience. Pediatr Surg Int 2004;20:829–33.

74. Gupta L, Bhatnagar V, Gupta AK, et al. Long-term follow-up of patients with esophageal replacement by reversed gastric tube. Eur J Pediatr Surg 2011;21:88–93.

75. Spitz L. Gastric transposition in children. Semin Pediatr Surg 2009;18:30–3.

76. Burgos L, Barrena S, Andres AM, et al. Colonic interposition for esophageal replacement in children remains a good choice: 33-year median follow-up of 65 patients. J Pediatr Surg 2010;45:341–5.

77. Arul GS, Parikh D. Oesophageal replacement in children. Ann R Coll Surg Engl 2008;90:7–12.

78. Cowles RA, Coran AG Gastric transposition in infants and children. Pediatr Surg Int 2010;26:1129–34.

79. Hamza AF Colonic replacement in cases of esophageal atresia. Semin Pediatr Surg 2009;18:40–3.

80. Tannuri U, Tannuri CA Should patients with esophageal atresia be submitted to esophageal substitution before they start walking? Dis Esophagus 2011;24:25–9.

81. Cauchi JA, Buick RG, Gornall P, et al. Oesophageal substitution with free and pedicled jejunum: Short- and long-term outcomes. Pediatr Surg Int 2007;23:11–19.

82. Bax KM. Jejunum for bridging long-gap esophageal atresia. Semin Pediatr Surg 2009;18:34–9.

CHAPTER 27

ESOPHAGEAL ATRESIA AND TRACHEOESOPHAGEAL FISTULA MALFORMATIONS

Steven S. Rothenberg

Esophageal atresia (EA) and tracheoesophageal fistula (TEF) anomalies present the pediatric surgeon with a unique and complex congenital disease, which tests both the diagnostic and technical skill of the surgeon. Most pediatric surgeons consider the surgical correction of these malformations to be the height of neonatal surgical care. In 1959, Dr Willis Potts wrote, 'To anastomose the ends of an infant's esophagus, the surgeon must be as delicate and precise as a skilled watchmaker. No other operation offers a greater opportunity for pure technical artistry.'[1] While this statement still remains true, improvements in anesthetic and neonatal intensive care have made repair of these anomalies and their postoperative management much more routine so that a good outcome can be achieved in most cases. Technical advances, including the application of the minimally invasive approach, have also decreased the morbidity from these operations.

The first report of EA was by Durston in 1670,[2] who found a blind upper pouch in one of a pair of thoracopagus conjoined twins, but the initial classic description was by Thomas Gibson in 1697.[3] However, it was not until 1939 when a baby with EA/TEF survived following successful staged repairs described separately by Leven and Ladd.[4,5] In 1940, Haight described the first survival following primary anastomosis.[6] By the mid-1980s, most neonatal centers were performing primary repair and reporting successful outcomes in up to 90%.[7–10]

EMBRYOLOGY

The embryology of the foregut is still subject to controversy.[11] What is known, however, is that during the fourth week of gestation the foregut starts to differentiate into a ventral respiratory part and a dorsal esophageal part. The laryngotracheal diverticulum then invaginates ventrally into the mesenchyme. The traditional theory postulates that the ventral respiratory system separates from the esophagus by the formation of lateral tracheoesophageal folds that fuse in the midline and create the tracheoesophageal septum. At 6 to 7 weeks of gestation, the separation between trachea and esophagus is complete. Incomplete fusion of the folds results in a defective tracheoesophageal septum and abnormal connection between the trachea and esophagus.

This theory of longitudinal tracheoesophageal folds merging to form a septum has been challenged.[12,13] In chick embryo studies, these folds could not be demonstrated. Instead, cranial and caudal folds were found in the region of tracheoesophageal separation. According to this theory, EA/TEF would then be due to an imbalance in the growth of these folds. Furthermore, rat studies suggest that EA/TEF results from disturbances in either epithelial proliferation or apoptosis.[14]

More recent studies show that ectopic expression of sonic hedgehog occurs in the tissues between the notochord and the gut. Knockout mice models have helped elucidate the functions of different genes in the development of the foregut aberrations such as EA/TEF.[15] Also, the relationship between BMP4 (bone morphogenic protein) and *Nog*, the gene encoding noggin (which is a BMP antagonist), may also have an impact on the development of TEF.[16–18]

EPIDEMIOLOGY

The birth incidence of EA/TEF varies between 1 in 2500 to 3000 live births.[19–21] There is a slight male preponderance of 1.26:1. There is no evidence for a link between EA/TEF and maternal age when chromosomal cases are excluded.[22] The risk for a second child with EA/TEF among parents of one affected child is 0.5–2%, increasing to 20% when more than one child is affected. The empirical risk of an affected child born to an affected person is 3–4%.[23] The relative risk for EA/TEF in twins is 2.56 when compared with singletons.[24] The concordance rate in twins is low, but the risk among twins of the same gender is high.[25]

Environmental factors that have been implicated include the use of methimazole in early pregnancy, prolonged use of contraceptive pills, progesterone and estrogen exposure, maternal diabetes, and thalidomide exposure.[26–30] EA is occasionally seen in the fetal alcohol syndrome and in maternal phenylketonuria.[31,32]

Chromosomal anomalies are found in 6–10% of the patients.[33–35] The total number of trisomy 18 cases exceeds the total number of trisomy 21 cases. As the incidence of trisomy 18 is higher, it would seem to indicate that trisomy 18 is a greater risk for EA development. Three separate genes have been associated with EA/TEF:

MYCN haploinsufficiency in Feingold syndrome, *CHD*7 in CHARGE syndrome, and *SOX2* in the anophthalmia–esophageal–genital (AEG) syndrome.[34-37]

EA may occasionally be part of the Opitz G/BB syndrome, Fanconi anemia, oculo-auriculo-vertebral syndrome, Bartsocas–Papas syndrome, or Frijns syndrome.[38]

ASSOCIATED ANOMALIES

The factor or factors responsible for the early disturbance in organogenesis causing EA may affect other organs or systems that are developing at the same time. EA can be divided clinically into isolated EA and syndromic EA, occurring at roughly the same rate.[38]

The most frequent associated malformations encountered in syndromic EA are:

- Cardiac (13–34%)
- Vertebral (6–21%)
- Limb (5–19%)
- Anorectal (10–16%)
- Renal (5–14%).

Vertebral anomalies are confined mainly to the thoracic region. An earlier claim that the presence of 13 pairs of ribs is a good indicator of long-gap EA has not been substantiated.[39]

Nonrandom associations have been documented as well. Two of these are the VACTERL association (*v*ertebral, *a*norectal, *c*ardiac, *t*racheo-*e*sophageal, *r*enal, and *l*imb abnormalities) and the CHARGE association (*c*oloboma, *h*eart defects, *a*tresia of the choanae, developmental *r*etardation, *g*enital hypoplasia, and *e*ar deformities). In 1973, VACTERL was originally described as VATER, an acronym made up of *v*ertebral defects, *a*nal atresia, *t*racheo-*e*sophageal fistula with EA, and *r*adial dysplasia.[40] It was later extended with the C for cardiac anomalies and the L for limb anomalies. In a cohort of 463 patients with EA, 107 (23%) had at least two additional VACTERL defects.[41] Seventeen of these patients had a chromosomal defect or a syndrome without a known genetic defect. Interestingly, as many as 70% of the remaining 90 patients had additional defects other than VACTERL anomalies.

CLASSIFICATION

EA and TEF present in many forms and various classification systems have been used to describe them. It is clear that EA should be thought of as a spectrum of anomalies (Fig. 27-1).[42] The original classification system was devised by Vogt in 1929.[43] Ladd put forth his own classification in 1945[5] and Gross revised this in 1953.[44] These classifications tend to be confusing, as the same subclasses are named differently. For clarity, it seems much better to give descriptive names to the major subtypes.

Esophageal Atresia with Distal Fistula (Gross Type C)

This is the most common subtype, accounting for about 85% of EA anomalies.[45] The very dilated proximal esophagus has a thickened wall and descends into the superior mediastinum usually to the third or fourth thoracic vertebrae. The distal esophagus is slender and has a thin wall. It enters the trachea posteriorly either at the level of the carina or 1–2 cm higher. The distance between the esophageal ends varies from very small to quite wide. Very rarely, the distal fistula may be occluded, leading to the misdiagnosis of EA without distal fistula.[46]

Pure Esophageal Atresia without TEF (Gross Type A)

Pure EA has an incidence of about 7%. The proximal and distal esophagus end blindly in the posterior mediastinum. The proximal end is dilated and has a thickened wall as in the more common EA/TEF. If there is no

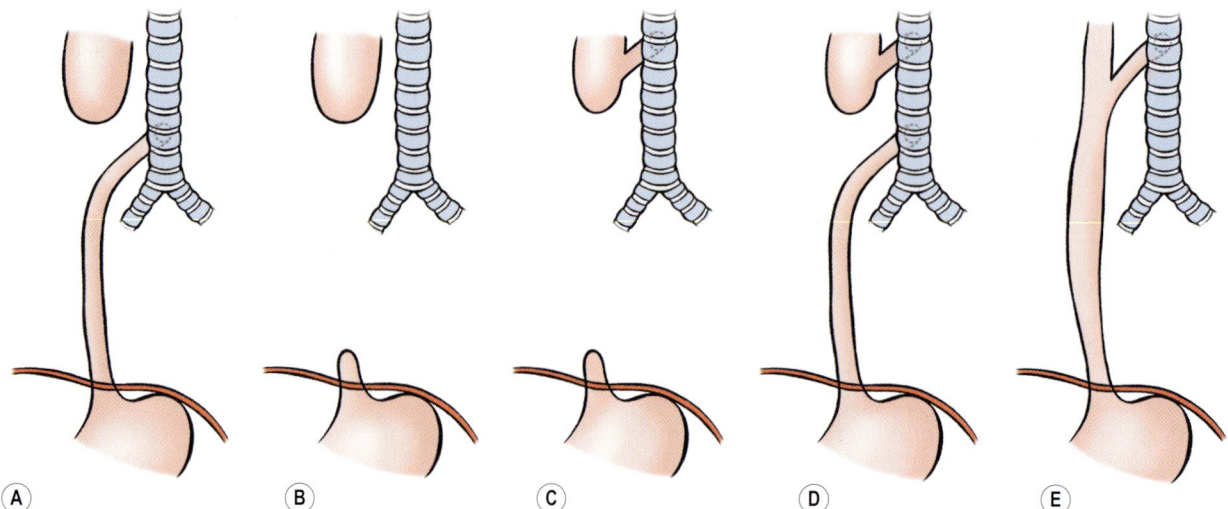

FIGURE 27-1 ■ Classification of EA and/or TEF: **(A)** esophageal atresia with distal tracheoesophageal fistula: Vogt IIIb, Ladd III, Gross C; **(B)** esophageal atresia without fistula: Vogt II, Ladd I, Gross A; **(C)** esophageal atresia with proximal fistula: Vogt IIIa, Ladd II, Gross B; **(D)** esophageal atresia with proximal and distal fistulas: Vogt IIIc, Ladd V, Gross D; **(E)** tracheoesophageal fistula (H-type) without atresia: Vogt IV, Gross E.

concomitant proximal fistula, the upper esophagus ends at the level of the azygos vein. The distal esophagus is short and often suspended by a fibrotic band. The distance between the two segments is considerable, usually precluding immediate anastomosis.

H-type Fistula without Esophageal Atresia (Gross Type E)

H-type TEF without atresia is usually discussed together with EA because it may be part of the VACTERL association. It occurs with an incidence of about 4%. The fistula starts from the membranous trachea and runs caudad to enter the esophagus. Normally it is short, although the diameter may be variable. The fistula is usually situated at the thoracic aperture or higher in the neck.[47]

Esophageal Atresia with Proximal Fistula (Gross Type B)

The association of a proximal fistula in a patient with pure EA is generally thought to be about 2%, but may be higher than is generally appreciated. In a recent series of 13 children without distal fistula, a proximal fistula was found in seven.[48] An upper esophageal fistula is usually not found at the end of the pouch. This fistula is similar to the H-type starting proximally on the trachea and ending distally in the dilated proximal esophagus. Usually, there is only one proximal fistula, but two or three have been described.[49] The fistula is usually located at the thoracic aperture or higher in the neck. Although limited in length, its diameter may vary from tiny to large. If not diagnosed preoperatively, it may be suspected during operative repair when bubbles are seen when opening the proximal esophagus.

Esophageal Atresia with Proximal and Distal Fistulas (Gross Type D)

The incidence of EA with proximal and distal fistulas is thought to be less than 1%. EA with one distal fistula and two proximal fistulas has also been described.[49] Also reported is a near-complete membranous obstruction of the esophagus in conjunction with a single TEF at the level of the membrane, communicating with both parts of the esophagus.[50]

DIAGNOSIS

Antenatal Diagnosis

The prenatal diagnosis of EA/TEF relies, in principle, on two nonspecific signs: polyhydramnios and an absent or small stomach bubble. Polyhydramnios is associated with a wide range of fetal abnormalities and is nonspecific. Similarly, the ultrasonographic (US) absence of a stomach bubble may point to a variety of fetal anomalies. The combination of a small stomach together with a dilated cervical esophagus (the pouch sign) has been confirmed to be diagnostic for pure EA in a number of patients.[51–53] Nevertheless, it is encountered in only a few patients.

Current ultrasound technology does not allow for the certain diagnosis of EA/TEF. Therefore, definitive counseling of the parents should be guarded.[54] The application of 3D power Doppler imaging seems promising, both antenatally and postnatally. Aortic arch anomalies, for example, have been diagnosed using this modality.[55,56]

Magnetic resonance imaging (MRI) has been used to identify other fetal thoracic lesions, and may be beneficial in patients deemed to be at risk on prenatal ultrasound. Sensitivity in various studies is between 60–100% and the diagnosis is made by the lack of visualization of the thoracic esophagus.[57–59]

Postnatal Diagnosis

If pregnancy was complicated by polyhydramnios, passage of a tube or catheter into the stomach should be performed to assess esophageal patency. The same holds true when the child presents with anomalies that fit the VACTERL association (e.g., radial aplasia).

As EA prevents the passage of saliva down the esophagus, saliva accumulates in the proximal esophagus and mouth, and feeding should be withheld until esophageal continuity is confirmed. This is best done with a stiff 10 French catheter inserted either through the nose or mouth. A chest film is then obtained with downward pressure on the tube. With EA, the tip of the tube is found to be slightly curled in the blind upper pouch around T2–T4 (Fig. 27-2). This technique not only

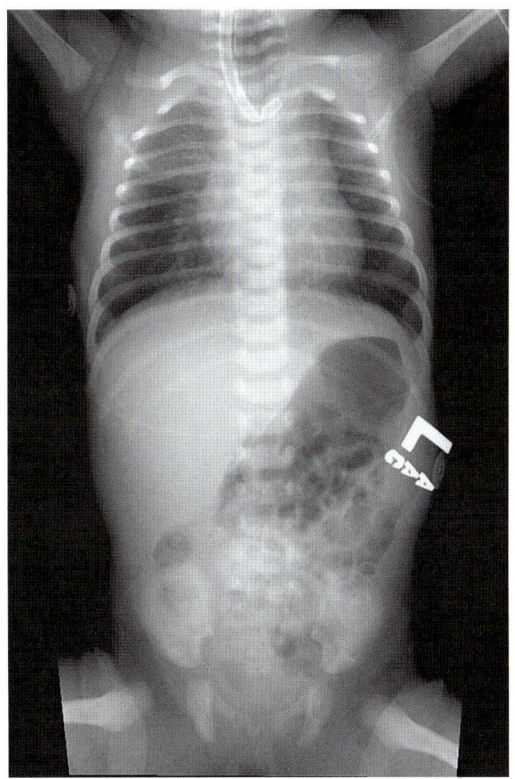

FIGURE 27-2 ■ This plain radiograph depicts the classic features seen in an infant with EA and TEF. A nasoesophageal tube is seen in the upper pouch and has kinked a little at the end of the pouch. There is air in the stomach and bowel, which signifies the presence of a distal TEF.

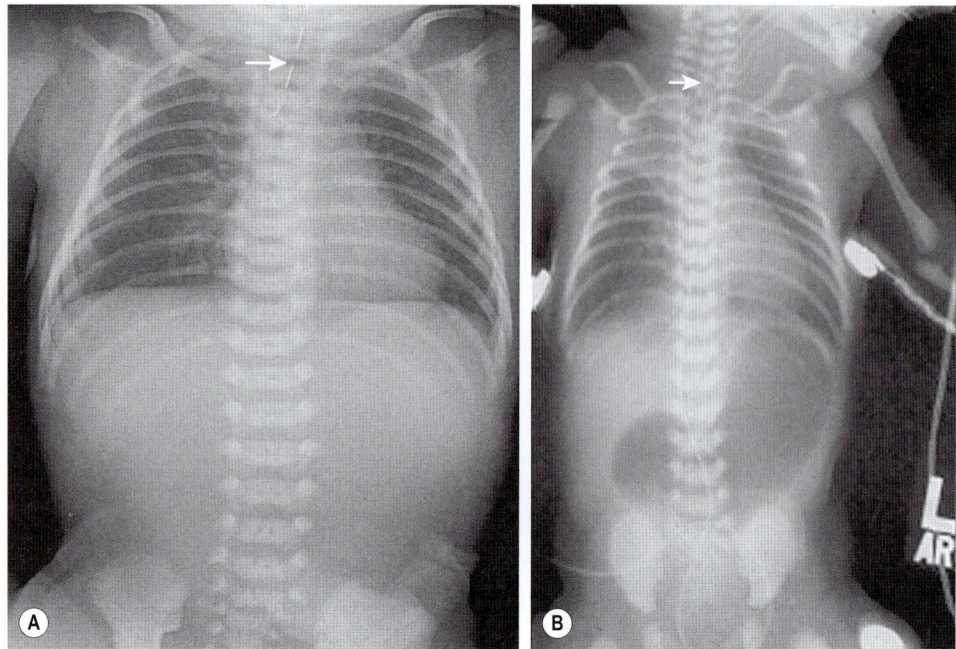

FIGURE 27-3 ■ These two radiographs depict less common presentations of EA. **(A)** Isolated EA. The nasoesophageal tube (arrow) is seen in the proximal pouch. There is no air in the gastrointestinal tract. **(B)** This patient has EA with distal TEF and duodenal atresia and has been endotracheally intubated. A nasoesophageal catheter (arrow) sits in the upper esophageal pouch. An endotracheal tube is also seen. The stomach and bulbous duodenum are distended with air but no air is seen distal to the duodenum.

identifies the atresia but gives some clue to the length of the upper pouch. Often, the dilated upper esophageal pouch is visualized by air within it. Air in the stomach signifies the presence of a distal TEF. If the tip of the catheter passes beyond the level of the carina, then the diagnosis of EA should be questioned. Esophageal stenosis, tracheal rings, and iatrogenic perforation of the esophagus can be confused with EA.[60,61] If there is any question about the diagnosis, a small amount of contrast can be dripped into the upper pouch, but this needs to be done with fluoroscopy and under direction of the surgeon to assure that the contrast is not aspirated.

Radiographs may reveal associated anomalies such as vertebral and rib anomalies, or other problems such as duodenal atresia (Fig. 27-3). The absence of air in the stomach points to EA without distal fistula (see Fig. 27-3A). Mediastinal ultrasound has been suggested as a helpful adjunct in the diagnosis of pure EA.[62]

The length of the esophageal gap is usually not known preoperatively. Absence of air in the stomach has been linked with a long gap, but has also been described in association with a distal fistula occluded with mucus.[46] Even in true long-gap EA (atresia without distal fistula), the gap length varies. In newborns with isolated EA, the first procedure is generally a gastrostomy, which allows for enteral feeding and also allows for assessment of the length and location of the lower pouch. It can be identified radiologically, either with metal bougies, a small gastroscope, or with a contrast injected through the gastrosomy.[63] This can be done at the time of the initial gastrostomy or more routinely seven to ten days later. If bougies or a telescope are introduced into the distal esophagus, the amount of pressure on these instruments

will affect the measurement of the gap between the two esophageal segments and may under- or over-estimate the gap length. In one report by an experienced surgeon, operative management was linked to the measured gap length: less than two vertebrae, then primary anastomosis; two to six vertebrae, then delayed primary anastomosis; more than six vertebrae, then esophageal replacement.[64] In the era of thoracoscopy, an initial thoracic exploration can be considered if the upper pouch appears fairly long. If the lower pouch is identified and seen to be of adequate length, a primary repair can be attempted. If not, then a gastrostomy can be placed and delayed repair planned.[65]

In EA/TEF, a longer gap between the two esophageal ends should be expected when the distal fistula is found at the carina.[66] Combined with a short upper pouch, this can mean a long gap exists between the two esophageal segments and may not be amenable to an initial primary repair. Unfortunately this may not fully be appreciated until the time of exploration. However since it is usually necessary to ligate the fistula in the early postnatal period, the gap length can be assessed at that time. A thoracoscopic approach in this scenario allows for minimal morbidity if the decision is to ligate the fistula only without reconstruction. Bronchoscopy can also be performed prior to exploration, not only to assess the site of the distal fistula, but to also look for an upper pouch fistula. Echocardiography should be performed prior to operation as it may reveal cardiac and/or aortic arch anomalies. A right descending aorta, which occurs in about 2.5% of the cases, may make a left-sided thoracic approach preferable.[67] Renal ultrasound and spine radiographs should be obtained as well. Because EA may be

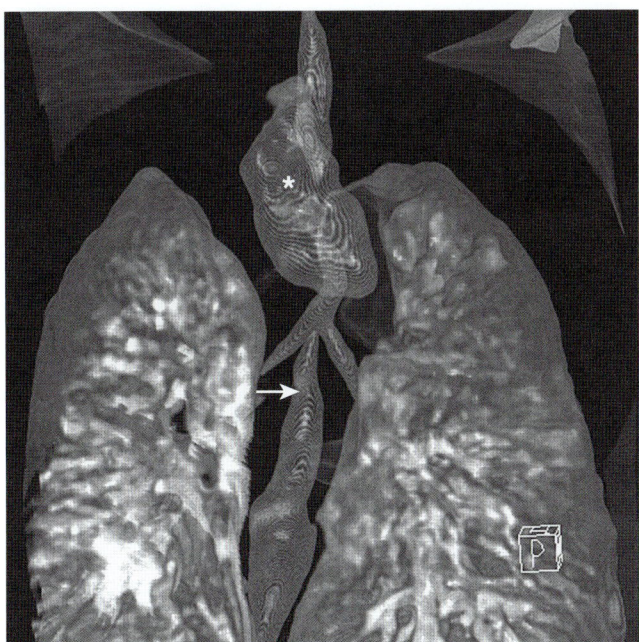

FIGURE 27-4 ■ This preoperative CT scan reconstruction shows EA with a distal TEF. The distal TEF (arrow) originates at the carina. The upper esophageal pouch is very dilated (asterisk). The distance between the upper pouch and lower esophagus is relatively short.

part of a syndrome, consultation by a geneticist is recommended at some point.

There is little doubt that better preoperative imaging of the neck and chest allows for better preoperative planning. At present, the two best imaging modalities are CT and MRI. Although MRI would certainly be preferable for its absence of radiation exposure, it requires general anesthesia. On the other hand, MRI is better for diagnosing cardiac and aortic arch anomalies.[68] CT has also been performed in children with EA/TEF (Fig. 27-4).[69–72]

MANAGEMENT

Preoperative

Once the diagnosis of EA has been established, the baby, if not delivered in a maternal/fetal/neonatal center, should be transferred to a pediatric surgical center. A 10 French Replogle tube is placed in the upper esophagus and set to continuous suction.[73] The child is positioned head-up and on his or her side. Intravenous access is important, and the vital signs are monitored.

If the child is in respiratory distress, endotracheal intubation and ventilation may be needed. Forceful ventilation will over distend the stomach, possibly causing diaphragmatic splinting and even gastric rupture.[74,75] Gentle low-pressure ventilation is therefore essential. In these cases, some feel high-frequency ventilation is advantageous. However, on occasion, emergency ligation of the fistula may be needed as a life-saving maneuver.[64,74–76] After ligation of the fistula, a delayed primary repair can be performed when the infant is more stable.

Some recommend not postponing longer than seven to 14 days because recanalization of the fistula can occur.[64,77,78] In these patients, we have performed thoracoscopic fistula ligation followed by repair two to six weeks later. We have not seen recanalization in our experience. If the infant is extremely unstable, then an emergency gastrostomy to decompress the stomach may be the best option. However this can result in a significant loss of tidal volume and may create respiratory issues as well.

Generally, the operative treatment of EA/TEF is not regarded as an emergency procedure. Thus, there is usually time to confirm the diagnosis and to assess for associated anomalies.

OPERATIVE REPAIR

Esophageal Atresia with Distal Fistula

The operation is performed with the patient under general anesthesia and with adequate venous access. An arterial line is occasionally beneficial depending on the baby's clinical status. Generally, a pulse oximeter and end tidal CO_2 monitor are adequate. The operation can be performed through a thoracotomy or using a thoracoscopic approach. The side of entrance into the chest is opposite the turn of the aortic arch: right for a left descending aorta, left for a right descending aorta. If a right-sided aortic arch is not detected until the operation has begun, change to the left side is appropriate if the thoracoscopic approach was initially chosen. If a thoracotomy has been performed, an anastomosis from the right chest should be attempted, but there is a higher morbidity in this setting.[67]

Preoperative Bronchoscopy

The value of routine preoperative rigid bronchoscopy is much debated because the incidence of a simultaneous proximal and distal fistula is less than 1%.[63] With the availability of small-diameter flexible fiberscopes, tracheobronchoscopy can now be performed after intubation through the endotracheal tube.[79,80] Forceful ventilation must be avoided, not only to avoid lung damage,[81] but also to prevent gastric distention and gastric perforation with insufflation through the distal fistula. Bronchoscopy may reveal abnormalities such as a second proximal fistula, a laryngotracheoesophageal cleft, tracheal stenosis, or a tracheal bronchus to the right upper lobe.[82–84] The entrance of the distal fistula is usually well seen (Fig. 27-5). Its distance to the carina provides a clue as to the gap between the esophageal segments: the closer the fistula is to the carina, the longer the distance. An indication of the severity of tracheomalacia is only possible when the child is breathing spontaneously. The problem with bronchoscopy is that it may prolong the procedure and the infant can decompensate prior to ligation of the fistula.[85–88] The surgeon and the anesthesiologist should discuss the advantages/disadvantages in each individual case. Following intubation, it may be helpful to position the endotracheal tube distal to the fistula, assuming the fistula is not at the carina.

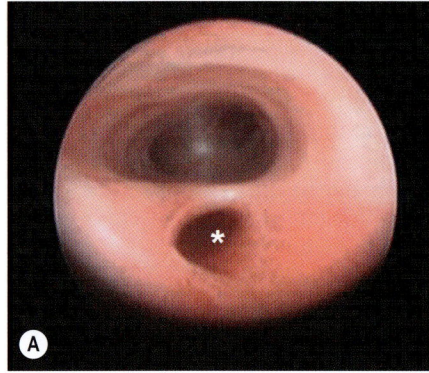
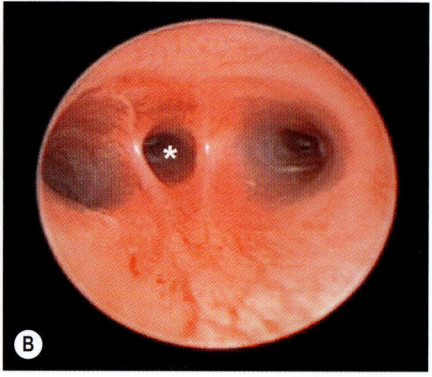

FIGURE 27-5 ■ These two photographs depict the distal TEF entering the trachea at different levels. **(A)** The fistula (asterisk) enters in the mid-trachea. **(B)** The fistula (asterisk) enters at the carina.

Repair via Thoracotomy

In a baby with a left descending aorta, the child is placed in a left lateral decubitus position. A small axillary role is placed under the chest to enlarge the right-sided intercostal spaces. The surgeon stands to the right of the patient (the infant's back) with the assistant opposite. With a right descending aorta, the baby is placed in a right lateral decubitus position close to the left edge of the table. The surgeon then stands on the left side of the table with the assistant on the right.

The patient's arm is positioned over the head (Fig. 27-6). Suction is removed from the Replogle tube, but the tube is left in place so that it can be advanced during the operation to aid in identifying the proximal pouch.

A slightly curved 4–5 cm long incision is made 1 cm below the inferior tip of the scapula. With the use of a muscle-sparing approach, the auscultatory triangle is opened and the muscles are retracted (i.e., the latissimus dorsi posteriorly and the serratus anterior anteriorly).[89,90] If the serratus muscle needs to be transected, this should be done as low as possible to preserve the long thoracic nerve. The fourth or fifth intercostal space is then entered.

An extrapleural approach has been suggested to protect the pleural space in case of an anastomotic leak, but there is no evidence that it is better than a transpleural one.[91,92] However an extrapleural approach does aid in exposure as it is easier to retract the lung when it is incased in the pleura. With the extrapleural approach, the pleura is gently pushed away from the endothoracic fascia, first in the middle of the incision so that an infant rib spreader can be inserted and opened (see Fig. 27-6B). With the rib spreader opened even farther, the pleura is carefully pushed away posteriorly until the posterior mediastinum is exposed.

The distal fistula may start from the trachea directly underneath the azygos vein, in which case the azygos vein is transected between 3-0 or 4-0 absorbable ligatures or simply cauterized and divided (Fig. 27-7). If the distal fistula originates more cephalad on the trachea, the vein can be left intact. Recently, a relationship between azygos vein transection and anastomotic leak has been suggested.[93,94]

The distal esophagus is easily found because it distends with each inspiration and the vagus nerve is intimately attached. Once identified, the distal segment should be

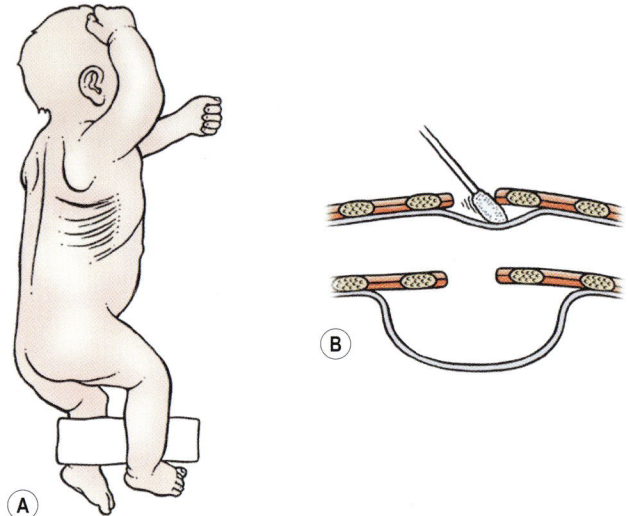

FIGURE 27-6 ■ **(A)** The infant is positioned for a right thoracotomy. The ipsilateral arm is positioned over the head of the patient. A 4–5 cm incision is made 1 cm below the tip of the scapula. **(B)** This schematic depicts a peanut or sterile cotton swab being used to gently push the pleura away from the chest wall.

followed proximally to locate where the fistula enters the trachea. The fistula should be dissected and mobilized close to the trachea, which will spare as many vagal nerve branches as possible (see Fig. 27-7B). The fistula can be encircled with a vessel loop or suture to aid in exposure. There are several ways to ligate the fistula on the tracheal side. Ligation in continuity can result in a higher recanalization rate.[95,96] We prefer to divide the fistula sharply after placing traction sutures at each end. A series of 5-0 PDS (Ethicon, Inc, Sommerville NJ) sutures are then used to close the tracheal side taking care not to compromise the tracheal lumen (Fig. 27-8). Another option is to apply a single 5mm clip across the fistula where it connects to the membranous trachea. We have found this technique to be simple and efficient, and results in a smaller pouch remnant on the posterior tracheal wall. However, there are anecdotal reports of clip migration using this technique. The tracheal closure can be checked by irrigating with warm water and applying a higher ventilation pressure to assess for an air leak.

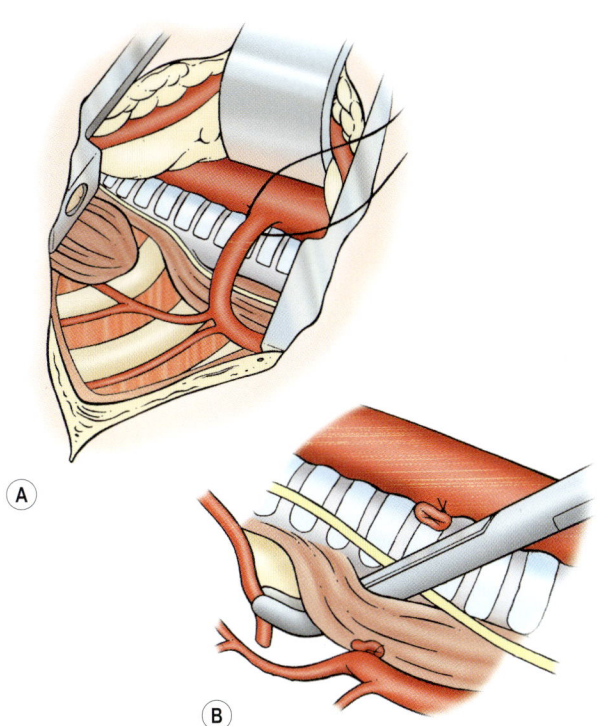

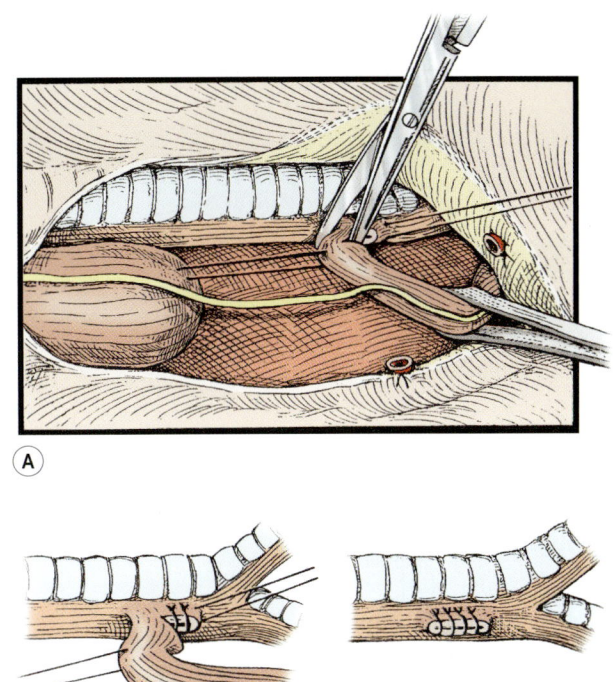

FIGURE 27-7 ■ **(A)** Ligation of the azygos vein. **(B)** The distal fistula is being mobilized from its insertion in the trachea.

FIGURE 27-8 ■ The distal esophagus is identified, looped, and carefully dissected up to its junction with the trachea, meticulously sparing the segmental vessels from the aorta. **(A)** Traction sutures may be placed for gentle handling of the segments. The fistula is divided close to the trachea without narrowing its lumen. **(B)** The tracheal end of the tracheoesophageal fistula is closed with continuous or interrupted sutures. Adjacent tissue, if available, is tacked over the closure. (From Holder TM, Manning PB. Esophageal atresia and tracheoesophageal fistula. Surg Rounds 1991;14:492–502.)

Attention is then turned to the proximal esophagus which can be identified by asking the anesthesiologist to push on the Replogle tube. A traction suture, taking a good bite of the muscular wall, is placed in the most distal part of the proximal pouch. Using the traction suture, the proximal pouch can be freed posteriorly and laterally by blunt dissection. Anteriorly, however, the pouch may be adherent to the membranous trachea. Usually, it can be dissected sharply, staying on the esophageal side to avoid entrance into the membranos trachea. Extensive dissection is not warranted, unless there is a long gap, because the dissection can damage the tracheal or esophageal walls and may interfere with innervation to the upper esophagus.[97] Extensive dissection of the proximal pouch searching for a proximal fistula should not be performed routinely because the incidence of a proximal fistula in combination with a distal one is only about 1%. If a proximal fistula is present, it is usually of the H-type. If missed at birth and diagnosed after repair of the EA, it can usually be repaired through the neck at a later date. If the trachea is entered during the dissection of the proximal pouch, one should be wary that a proximal fistula may have been opened as well. There should not be a common wall between the trachea and esophagus.

After mobilization of the proximal pouch, the tip is now amputated so that the lumen and mucosa become visible. An end-to-end anastomosis is performed with 5-0 absorbable sutures starting in the middle of the back wall of each esophageal segment (Fig. 27-9). It is important to include both the mucosa and the muscular wall with each suture. The sutures in the back wall of the anastomosis are tied intralumenally. Then, the front part of the anastomosis is performed with sutures tied on the outside.

Before finishing the anastomosis, an 8 French or 10 French tube is passed into the stomach. This protects from inadvertent closure of the lumen and for gastric decompression. Others feel the placement of an intralumenal tube or stent causes an increased risk of stricture or leak, and choose not to use it.

The use of a chest drain is also optional.[98,99] We use one until a contrast study is obtained on day 4 or 5. The chest incision is then closed in layers. The ribs should be approximated with one 3-0 absorbable suture. This suture should be tied gently so that the intercostal space is not obliterated. If a muscle-sparing approach was used, the muscles are allowed to fall back into their normal position and the skin is closed with a 5-0 absorbable subcuticular suture.

Thoracoscopic Repair

The first successful repair was reported in 2000 and the first series reported in 2002.[100,101] Since then, there have been several retrospective reports describing experience with the thoracoscopic approach.[102–105] During this early experience, attempts were made to obtain single lung ventilation by intubating the left mainstem bronchus. However, this proved time consuming and often unsuccessful so now the endotracheal tube is usually left in the trachea just above the carina and right lung collapse is

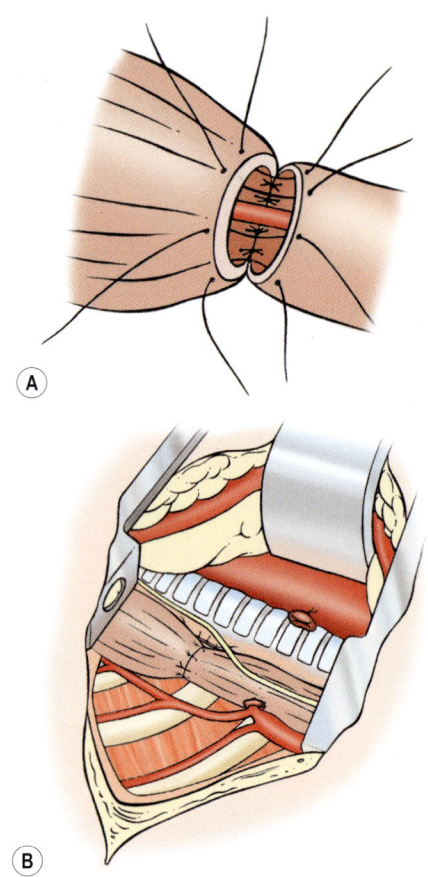

FIGURE 27-9 ■ Esophageal anastomosis. **(A)** The back wall of the anastomosis has been sutured from the inside, and a small nasogastric tube has been passed through the anastomosis. The front part of the anastomosis is being sutured with knots on the outside. **(B)** Completed anastomosis.

achieved with CO_2 insufflation alone.[106] Others have described using the oscillating ventilator to effect lung collapse and negate the adverse effects of prolonged hypercarbia.[107]

Positioning. Once the endotracheal tube is secure, the patient is placed in a modified prone position with the right side elevated approximately 30° (Fig. 27-10). The patient is placed near the edge of the table so that the handles of the instruments do not collide with the table. (If there is a right-sided arch, then a left-sided approach is used.) This positioning gives the surgeon access to the area between the anterior and posterior axillary lines for port placement while allowing gravity to retract the lung away from the posterior mediastinum. This arrangement allows excellent exposure of the fistula and esophageal segments without the need for an extra instrument or lung retractor. The assistant should not be placed on the opposite side of the table as this will place him/her at a complete paradox with the telescope. The scrub nurse can be on either side of the baby depending on the room layout. Because of the fine manipulation necessary, the surgeon and the assistant

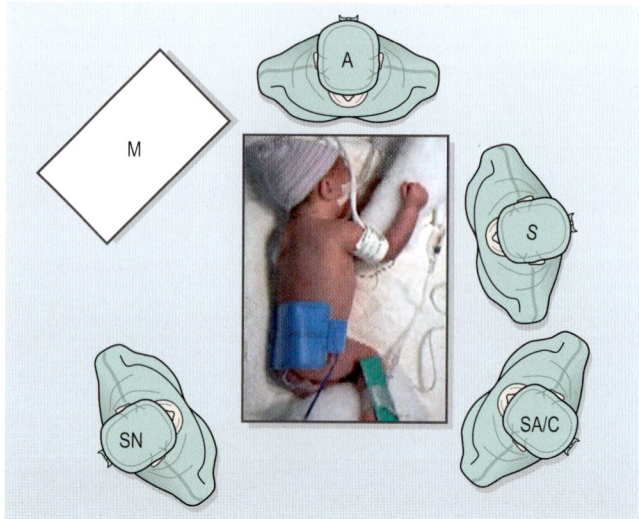

FIGURE 27-10 ■ This infant is positioned more prone than lateral for right thoracoscopic repair. The surgeon (S) stands on the left side of the operating table when the aortic arch turns to the left. The surgeon, operative field, and screen are in-line. The assistant and camera holder (SA/C) is situated to the left of the surgeon when the surgeon is right-handed. The scrub nurse (SN) stands to the right of the operating table. M, monitor; A, anesthesiologist. (From Holcomb GW, Rothenberg SS, Georgeson KE. Atlas of Pediatric Laparoscopy and Thoracoscopy. Elsevier; 2009.)

should position themselves so that they are in the most ergonomic and comfortable position.

Port placement is extremely important because of the small chest cavity and the intricate nature of the dissection and reconstruction. Usually three ports are satisfactory, but a fourth one can be used if needed (Fig. 27-11).

The initial port (3 mm or 4 mm) is placed in the fifth intercostal space behind the tip of the scapula. This is the telescope and camera port and allows excellent visualization of the posterior mediastinum. An angled telescope

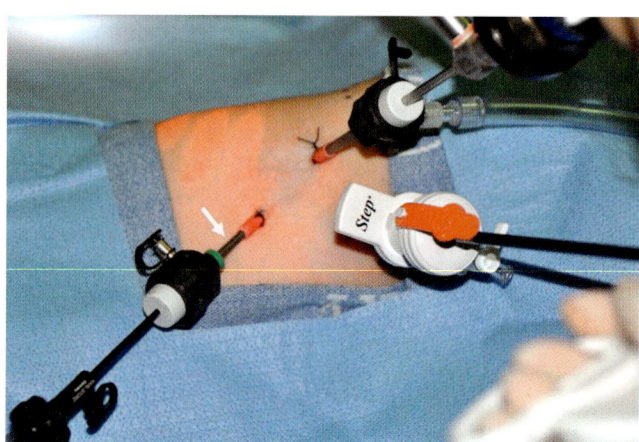

FIGURE 27-11 ■ Optimal port positions for a thoracoscopic repair are seen. The ports are inserted in triangulation to allow the working instruments to meet at 90°. The camera port is inserted just below and posterior to the tip of the scapula. It is also the site for insufflation. One working port (Step, in photograph) is inserted in the midaxillary line in the axilla. The second working port (arrow) is introduced in the posterior axillary line. (From Holcomb GW, Rothenberg SS, Georgeson KE. Atlas of Pediatric Laparoscopy and Thoracoscopy. Elsevier; 2009.)

(30° or 45°) is essential. The two instrument ports are then introduced. The first is in the midaxillary line one or two interspaces above the telescope port in the axilla. This cephalad port is 5 mm for the clip applier and needle driver/suture. The lower port is 3 mm and is located in the posterior axillary line two interspaces below the telescope port. Ideally, these ports are positioned so that the instrument tips will approximate a 90° angle at the level of the fistula which will facilitate performing the anastomosis.

Once the lung is collapsed, the surgeon should first identify the fistula. In most cases, the fistula is attached to the membranous portion of the trachea just above the carina which is usually in the area of the azygos vein.

After the azygos is identified, it is mobilized for a short segment and then cauterized and divided with a small hook cautery. As mentioned earlier, some advocate leaving the azygos intact and this is an option.

With the vein divided, the lower esophageal segment is identified and followed proximally to the fistula. Because of the magnification afforded by the thoracoscopic approach, it is easy to visualize exactly where the distal fistula enters the back wall of the trachea (Fig. 27-12). A 5 mm endoscopic clip can then be applied safely. Care should be taken to avoid the vagus nerve. A single clip is usually sufficient. The fistula is then divided with scissors. As the distal segment can retract, making it difficult to visualize, it may be preferable to wait until the upper pouch is mobilized before completely dividing the fistula. The tracheal opening can also be suture ligated, but this requires delicate suturing at a time when an air leak from the opened fistula may be causing respiratory compromise.

Attention is now turned to the thoracic inlet. Again, the anesthesiologist places pressure on the Replogle tube to help identify the upper pouch. The pleura overlying the pouch is incised sharply and the pouch is mobilized using blunt and sharp dissection. The plane between the esophagus and trachea is easily seen and the two are separated. Mobilization of the upper pouch can be carried to the thoracic inlet.

Once adequate mobilization is achieved, the distal tip of the pouch is resected, exposing the mucosa. With the two esophageal segments mobilized, the anastomosis is performed using a 4-0 or 5-0 suture on a small tapered needle. The sutures are placed one at a time in an interrupted fashion, back wall first, and then the front after the nasogastric tube is advanced, as described for the open procedure (Fig. 27-13). Once the anastomosis is complete, a chest drain is introduced through the lower port site and its tip is positioned near the anastomosis. The other ports are removed and the sites are closed with absorbable suture.

Esophageal Atresia without Distal Fistula

Initial Treatment

A gasless abdomen is the signature of EA without distal fistula. Very rarely, a blocked distal fistula is responsible for the lack of air of the abdomen.[46] One should be aware

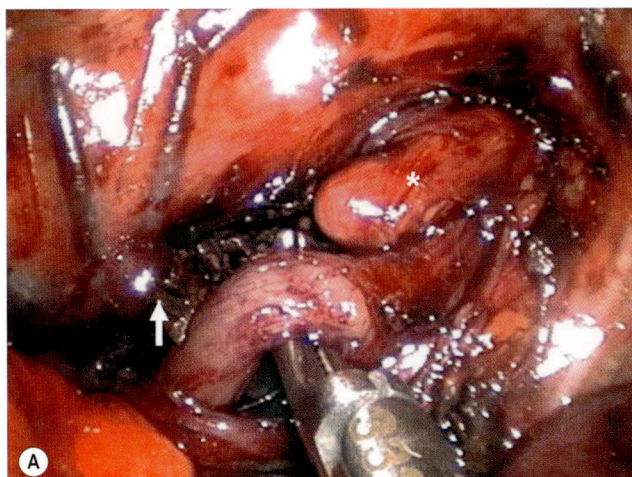
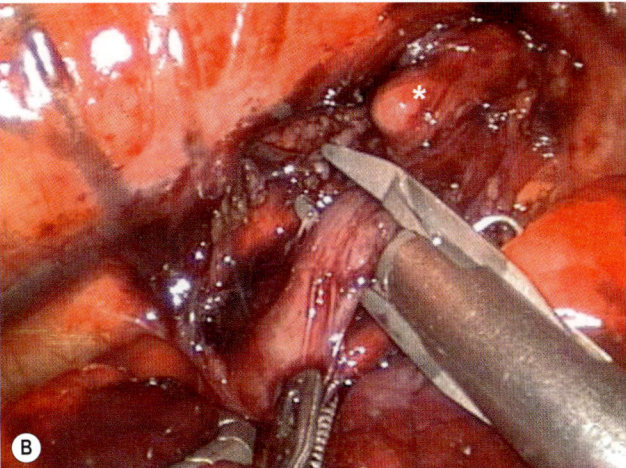

FIGURE 27-12 ■ **(A)** After ligation and division of the azygos vein (arrow), the tracheoesophageal fistula has been mobilized and is being encircled with an angled dissecting instrument. The upper esophageal pouch (asterisk) was mobilized before ligation and division of the fistula. **(B)** The tracheoesophageal fistula is being ligated with a 5 mm endoscopic clip applier. Two clips are usually applied and the fistula is divided distal to the second clip. The upper esophageal pouch is marked with an asterisk. (From Holcomb GW III, Rothenberg SS, Georgeson KE. Atlas of Pediatric Laparoscopy and Thoracoscopy. Elsevier; 2009.)

that the incidence of a proximal fistula, in the absence of a distal fistula, is relatively high.

The initial treatment is a gastrostomy with laryngotracheobronchoscopy during the same anesthesia, aimed at excluding a proximal fistula and other associated tracheobronchial anomalies. In EA without a distal fistula and in the absence of a duodenal obstruction, the stomach is usually small, which can make insertion of the gastrostomy difficult. Once placed, bolus feedings should be instituted to enlarge both the small stomach and the distal pouch.

Esophageal Reconstruction

The timing of the esophageal reconstruction is debatable and often depends on the gap length. A period of a few weeks to three months has been used.[64,108–112] During this waiting period, the proximal esophagus is emptied by continuous suction on a transnasally placed 10 French

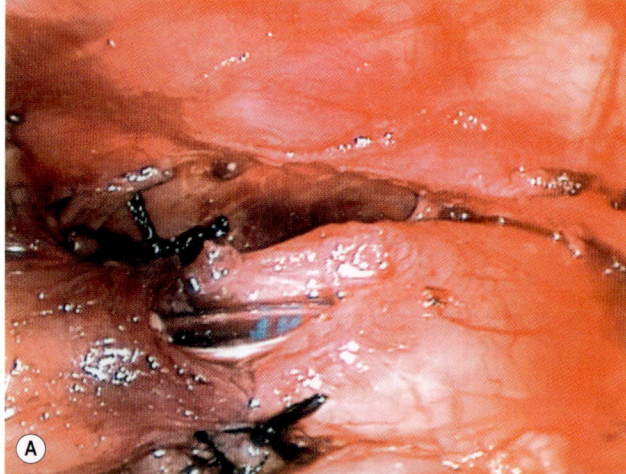

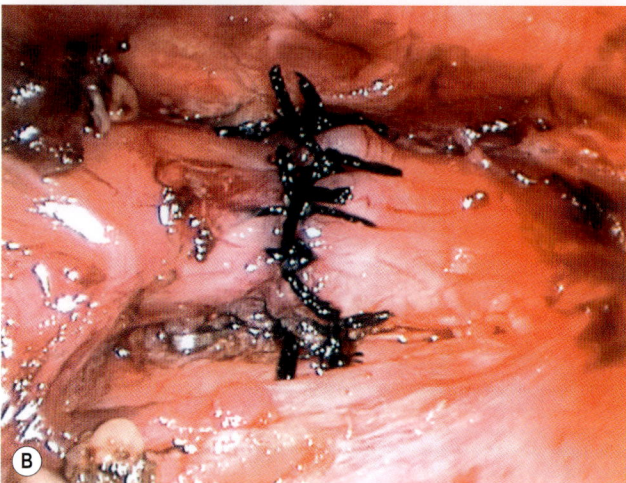

FIGURE 27-13 ■ **(A)** Esophageal anastomosis. The posterior suture line has been completed with interrupted sutures. A small silastic tube introduced through the nose is guided through the anastomosis and into the stomach. **(B)** The completed anastomosis is seen.

BOX 27-1 | **Maneuvers for lengthening the esophagus in long-gap esophageal atresia**

NONOPERATIVE MANEUVERS (IN COMBINATION WITH DELAYED PRIMARY ANASTOMOSIS)

Spontaneous growth
Bougienage
    Proximal[113,114]
    Proximal and distal[115]
    Magnetic[116]

OPERATIVE MEASURES

Using the native esophagus
    Upper pouch mobilization
    Myotomy of the upper pouch[117]
    Flap lengthening of the upper pouch[118,119]
    Multistaged extrathoracic elongation of the proximal pouch[120]
    Using thoracoscopy[121]
        Lower pouch mobilization[122,123]
        Myotomy of the lower pouch[124]
        Myotomy of the upper and lower pouch[125]
    Traction sutures[120,121]
        Thoracoscopic placement[115]
    Transluminal thread with olives[126,127]
        Thoracoscopic assistance
    Lower pouch hydrostatic distention[128]
    Elongation of the lesser curvature[129,130]
Using esophageal replacement
    Colon[131]
    Stomach
        Gastric tube[132,133]
        Gastric transposition[134]
            Laparoscopic assistance[135]
    Jejunum
        Pedicle graft[136,137]
        Free graft[138]
    Ileum[139]

Replogle tube. If the child has persistent respiratory problems, a proximal fistula should again be considered. Cervical esophagostomy should be avoided as this will likely jeopardize the ability to perform a primary esophago-esophagostomy in the future. Home care during the waiting period has been advocated, but most of the reported patients have required a long time in the hospital before they were sent home.[111,112]

The gap between the esophageal segments should be periodically measured and is usually expressed in terms of the number of vertebral bodies, thus taking the child's length into account. This can be done with a simultaneous contrast study of the upper and lower esophagus, or by insertion of a metal bougie transorally into the upper esophagus and through the gastrostomy into the lower esophagus. The metal bougie ends should overlap before attempting a primary anastomosis.

At the time of definite repair, several techniques to lengthen the native esophagus have been described, including esophageal myotomy or extensive mobilization of the proximal and distal esophagus (see Box 27-1). There is little doubt that all these maneuvers damage the esophagus and that the long-term results may be less than optimal. If a delayed primary anastomosis with or without lengthening is not feasible, an alternative procedure should be considered, such as a gastric pull-up or a jejunal, ileal, or colonic interposition. An alternative option is to attempt esophageal growth and lengthening by placing trans-thoracic traction sutures, but the results are variable.[140,141]

Thoracoscopy is ideal to evaluate the gap length to be bridged (Fig. 27-14). Moreover, the ends can be dissected and mobilized as well. An anastomosis can also be performed thoracoscopically. In one series, all long gaps were successfully closed.[142] Also, a thoracoscopic Foker procedure can be performed.

Postoperative Management

Mechanical ventilation with muscle relaxation for five days has been advocated after an anastomosis is performed under considerable tension.[143–145] Evidence for the effectiveness of this approach is lacking.[146] A chest drain is optional and feedings can be started early through the nasogastric tube if there is no evidence of a leak or concern about significant gastroesophageal reflux (GER).

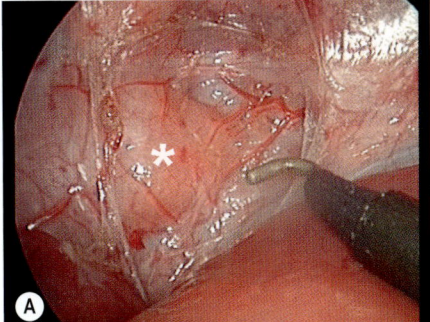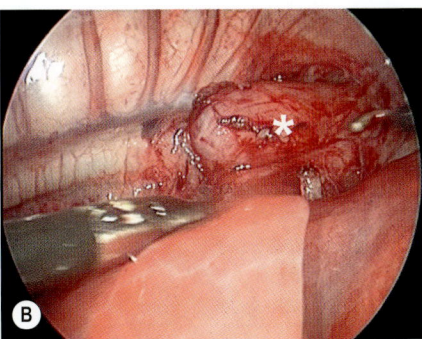

FIGURE 27-14 ■ Thoracoscopic view of esophageal atresia without fistula in a 3-month old neonate. **(A)** The short distal esophageal segment (asterisk) is seen in the inferior portion of the mediastinum. **(B)** The proximal pouch (asterisk) reaches to the azygos vein, which has been coagulated and transected.

COMPLICATIONS

Anastomotic Leaks

An overall leak rate of 3.5–17% has been reported by several authors.[9,147,148] Major leaks which require active intervention occur much less frequently—3.5% in the first study and 4.5% in the more recent one, which confirms the statement that most leaks will close spontaneously. In the largest thoracoscopic report, the leak rate was 7.6%,[103] but this was an multi-institutional study and early in each institution's experience. Published reports often include all types of EA and do not always mention whether the leak was detected at routine esophagography or how it was identified.

Anastomotic Stricture

As with anastomotic leaks, no uniform definition is used for an anastomotic stricture. It has been defined as a narrowing of more than 50% of the lumen[149] or as a narrowing detected on a contrast study, or at esophagoscopy in combination with symptoms.[150] Reported incidences range from 17–60%.[150–152] Four of 104 patients (3.8%) undergoing thoracoscopic repair developed a stricture, which was defined on the initial esophagogram.[103] Routine dilatation is not indicated because many patients never require dilatation. Anastomotic tension, anastomotic leakage, and GER have been implicated as risk factors.[153–155] Strictures usually respond well to dilation. Resection of the stricture is rarely required. Balloon dilatation seems superior, but there is no hard evidence.

Recurrent Tracheoesophageal Fistula

The reported incidence of a recurrent TEF varies between 3–15%. In one study, the 10% incidence in the period 1986 to 1995 had dropped to 5% in the period 1996 to 2005.[7] In the large multi-institution study of thoracoscopic repairs, the incidence was 1.9%.[103] The etiology of a recurrent fistula is almost certainly secondary to an anastomotic leak.

A recurrent fistula is suspected when the child starts to cough during feeding, has apneic or cyanotic episodes, or has repeat respiratory infections. The diagnosis can sometimes be made by an esophagram using a water-soluble contrast medium (Fig. 27-15) but bronchoscopy is usually needed to confirm the diagnosis.

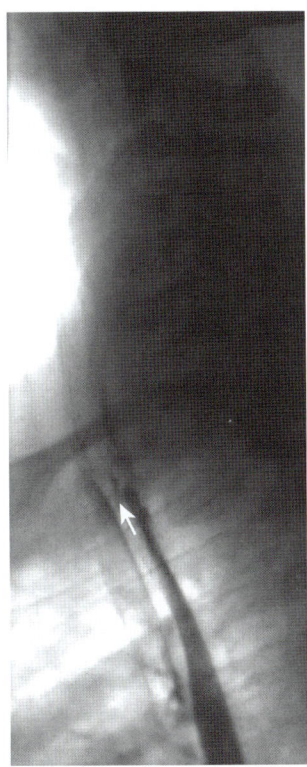

FIGURE 27-15 ■ On this water-soluble contrast study, a recurrent TEF (arrow) is seen.

Treatment of a recurrent TEF can be difficult. Thus, attempts at prevention have been described. Interposition of a biosynthetic patch between the tracheal closure and esophageal anastomosis has been described for this purpose (Fig. 27-16).[156] Native tissue such as pleura, pericardium, or intercostal muscle can also be used.

Once developed, attempts at endoscopic management with cautery, fibrin glue, and small intestine submucosa have been described (Fig. 27-17).[157–159] The results are mixed with success rates reported between 20–80%.

Tracheomalacia

Tracheomalacia is a generalized or localized weakness of the trachea that allows the anterior and posterior walls to come together during expiration or coughing.[15] The area of collapse is usually in the region of the fistula.[160] The cartilage of the rings is softened, and the length of the

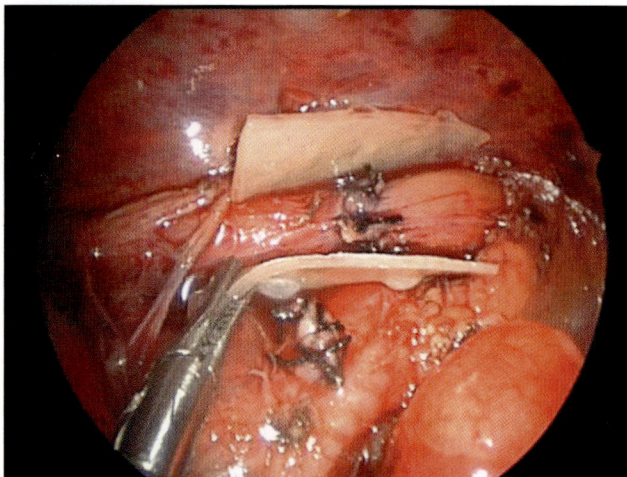

FIGURE 27-16 ■ After thoracoscopic repair of esophageal atresia and distal fistula in this infant, Surgisis was interposed between the tracheal closure and esophageal anastomosis to help prevent a recurrent TEF. (From St. Peter SD, Calkins CM, Holcomb GW III. The use of biosynthetic mesh to separate the anastomoses during the thoracoscopic repair of esophageal atresia and tracheoesophageal fistula. J Laparoendosc Adv Surg Tech 2007;17:380–2. Reprinted with permission.)

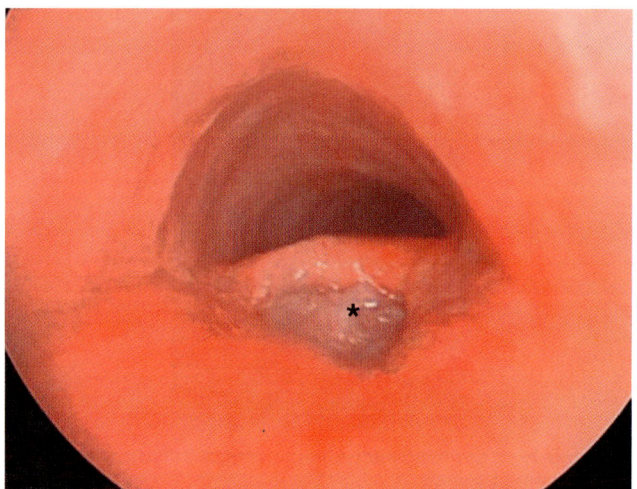

FIGURE 27-17 ■ This bronchoscopic view shows Surgisis (asterisk) placed into a recurrent TEF. In this patient, the fistula was successfully occluded using this technique.

transverse muscle is increased. As a result, the airway collapses during expiration, which produces expiratory stridor varying from a hoarse barking cough to acute life-threatening episodes of cyanosis or apnea.[161] In EA without fistula, tracheomalacia does not seem to occur very often.[162]

Treatment is required in severely symptomatic infants. The therapy of choice is aortopexy.[163–168] The principle behind this operation is that if ascending aorta and arch are suspended against the posterior surface of the sternum, the anterior wall of the trachea, which is loosely attached to the aorta, is suspended as well. This anterior aortic suspension opens the tracheal lumen. Aortopexy is classically performed through a left anterolateral thoracotomy or median sternotomy, but can also be performed

through a low cervical incision and partial sternal split,[169] or thoracoscopically either from the left[170,171] or from the right.[172] It is best to check the effect of the suspension by simultaneous tracheoscopy.

Disordered Peristalsis/ Gastroesophageal Reflux/ Esophageal Cancer

Disturbed motility of the esophagus in EA patients has been recognized for a long time.[173–176] Symptoms included dysphagia, episodes of foreign body impaction, heartburn, vomiting, and various respiratory disorders.[177–179] The oral phase of swallowing is normal, but the pharyngeal and esophageal phases are abnormal in all patients, both on video-fluoroscopy[180,181] and with manometry.[182–187]

Whether the cause of these disturbed motility problems is congenital or acquired has been a long-standing debate. Whatever the cause, it brings with it several problems, not the least of which is GER. While GER tends to improve during the first year of life in most infants, this is not the case in infants with EA. The incidence of significant reflux in patients with EA has been stated to be up to 50%, and about half of these will require antireflux surgery.[103,188–190] A considerable number of patients with EA have complaints in adult life pointing toward GER as the etiology including Barrett's esophagitis.[189] Early normal pH values in the esophagus do not exclude significant reflux on follow-up.[190] Antireflux medication, including gastric acid suppression, is successful in only about half of the cases.[191] Antireflux operations in patients with repaired EA have a higher failure rate than in non-EA patients,[192] but there seems to be no other alternative. While some surgeons have advocated partial wraps because of concerns over dysmotility,[193] there is little evidence to support this practice. The question remains whether adults with repaired EA as an infant should be screened as there may be a higher incidence of squamous cell carcinoma.[194]

Vocal Cord Dysfunction

Another complication which is becoming more recognized is injury to the recurrent laryngeal nerves during EA repair. In a retrospective review of 150 patients undergoing repair of EA and associated anomalies, five patients (3%) were found to have vocal fold paralysis on subsequent evaluation.[195] Bilateral paralysis was found in three patients and two patients had unilateral paralysis. In this study, the etiology of the paralysis was difficult to assess. However, the authors recommend preoperative laryngoscopy or bronchoscopy to identify infants with congenital vocal fold paralysis prior to operative repair. This is especially true for patients requiring revision surgery. An older review found a 12% incidence of vocal cord injury following EA repair.[196]

Respiratory Morbidity

Respiratory morbidity after EA repair is high.[197,198] In a series of 334 patients aged 1 to 37, just under half were subsequently hospitalized with a respiratory illness.[197] Two-thirds of the admissions were before 5 years of age. Also, a high proportion of the adult patients reported respiratory symptoms. These symptoms can be attributed to tracheomalacia and GER. Aortopexy is effective in preventing further life-threatening spells, but does not prevent the increased susceptibility to respiratory infections.[199]

Thoracotomy-Related Morbidity

Thoracotomy, especially in the newborn, can lead to significant morbidity, such as winged scapula, elevation or fixation of the shoulder, asymmetry of the chest wall, rib fusion, scoliosis, and breast and pectoral muscle maldevelopment.[200–207] Moreover, chronic pain after thoracic surgery is a serious problem, at least in adults, and has been reported in more than 50% of patients.[208,209] These negative consequences of a thoracotomy can be alleviated by using the thoracoscopic approach.

H-TYPE FISTULA

The incidence of H-type TEF is about 4%.[14,15] Isolated TEF is associated with the same anomalies as seen in EA, although at lower incidences.[210] The fistula runs from the trachea downward to the esophagus, typically intramurally, and is short (see Fig. 27-1). In a series of 20 children, the fistula was at C5–C6 in two, C6–C7 in three, C7–T1 in eight, T1–T2 in three, and T2–T3 in one.[47] Rarely, there is a second fistula.[211]

Respiratory symptoms, especially choking, often occur immediately after birth with feeding. Sometimes, there are unexplained cyanotic spells. Symptoms subside when the child is fed by a nasogastric tube. Often the abdomen is distended with air, and flatulence may be present. Older children can present with recurrent pneumonia. Symptoms can often be traced back to the neonatal period. On occasion, symptoms develop later in life.[212,213]

It can be difficult to diagnose an H-type fistula even if there is a high degree of suspicion. A water-soluble, low osmolar contrast study seems to be the best initial investigation and demonstrates the fistula in many cases (Fig. 27-18). Bronchoscopy (usually rigid) is another diagnostic modality, but even then, the fistula can be missed.[214] CT esophagography is another option but has the disadvantage of radiation exposure.[215]

A cervical approach can be used in most (80%) cases.[216] With the use of a small feeding tube or guide wire placed through the fistula at tracheoscopy and pulled out of the esophagus, most lower H-type fistulas can be pulled up and approached through the neck as well.[217,218] The classic approach is through a small low right cervical incision (Fig. 27-19). The sternal head of the sternocleidomastoid muscle may need transection. The esophagus is easily identified and separated from the trachea, taking care not to injure the recurrent laryngeal nerve. The left recurrent laryngeal nerve is vulnerable as well. The proximal esophagus, as well as the fistula, is encircled with separate vessel loops and so is the distal esophagus. Traction sutures are placed at the upper and lower ends of the

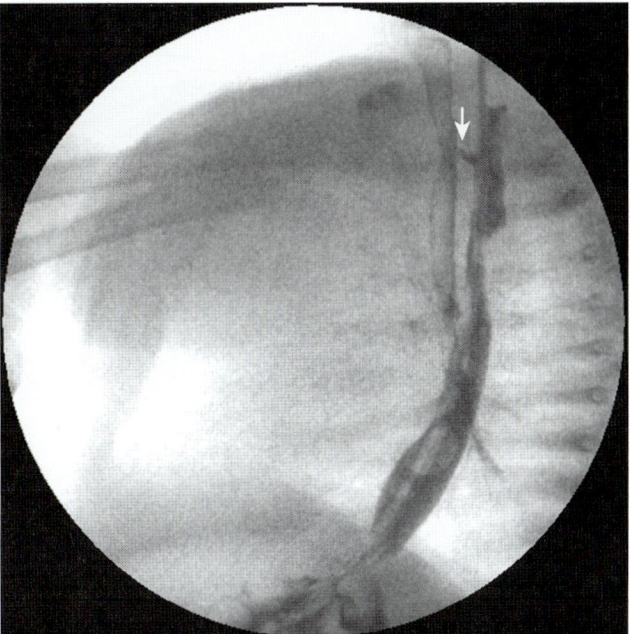

FIGURE 27-18 ■ Imaging for an H-type TEF. A contrast swallow is performed using a low osmolar, water-soluble medium. The fistula (arrow) is clearly seen on the lateral chest film. The fistula is at the level of the thoracic inlet. Contrast material entered the trachea and bronchial tree.

fistula, which is transected close to the esophagus. The trachea is closed longitudinally and the esophagus transversely with interrupted absorbable sutures. To eliminate a recurrent fistula, the sternal head of the sternocleidomastoid muscle can be interposed between the cut ends of the fistula.

It is evident that less trauma is inflicted when a thoracotomy can be avoided. The availability of thoracoscopy obviates the need for a thoracotomy, thus making a cervical approach for the extremely low H-fistulas less imperative. Several reports of thoracoscopically repaired H-fistulas have been described.[219–221] Whether a fistula should be approached from the neck or the chest depends on the location of the fistula based on preoperative imaging, and the surgeon and patient preference.

LARYNGEAL AND LARYNGOTRACHEOESOPHAGEAL CLEFT

Laryngeal and laryngotracheoesophageal clefts are rare congenital anomalies with an incidence of approximately 1 in 10,000 to 20,000 live births.[222] The cleft consists of a midline communication of the larynx, trachea, and rarely bronchus with the pharynx and upper esophagus. Its embryology is poorly understood. Originally, it was thought to be the consequence of a failure of the tracheoesophageal septum to fuse in the caudocranial direction. However, as previously mentioned, this theory of tracheoesophageal separation by fusion of a tracheoesophageal septum has been challenged.[11–18]

Many congenital malformations can coexist, including congenital heart disease, gastrointestinal and

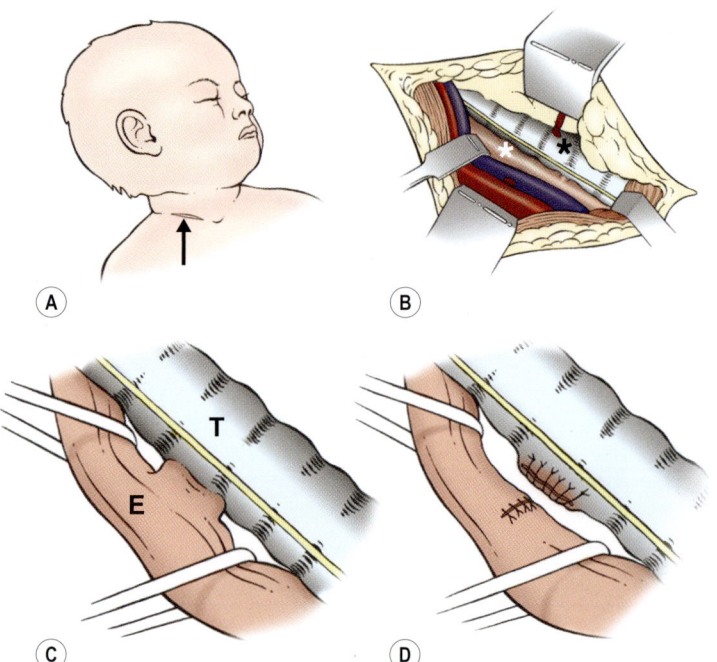

FIGURE 27-19 ■ Cervical approach used to repair an H-fistula. **(A)** Low right transverse cervical incision (arrow). **(B)** The esophagus (white asterisk) is approached medial to the carotid artery and jugular vein. Care is taken not to injure the recurrent laryngeal nerve on either side. The trachea is marked with a black asterisk. **(C)** The esophagus (E) is encircled both above and below the fistula. The fistula will be transected close to the trachea (T). **(D)** The tracheal opening is closed vertically, and the esophageal defect is closed transversely.

genitourinary tract abnormalities, and midline defects.[223] Familial occurrence has been described.[224] Clefts may be part of the Opitz–Frias syndrome and the Pallister–Hall syndrome.[225] TEFs have been found in 20–37% of these patients. Several classifications have been described (Fig. 27-20) and can be seen in Table 27-1.[226–228]

Symptoms vary according to the extension of the cleft. Patients may be symptomatic immediately from birth as a result of drowning in their saliva. Secretions are increased, and there may be choking and cyanosis. Hoarseness is common. Drinking aggravates the symptoms, and recurrent aspiration pneumonia can occur. The clinical picture may be blurred by associated anomalies, such as EA with distal fistula.

Contrast radiographs may be diagnostic, although it can be difficult to differentiate between overflow and aspiration. Tracheobronchoscopy is diagnostic (Fig. 27-21). The diagnosis can be missed, especially in less severe cases. A high degree of suspicion is often required to make the diagnosis. Often pressure applied to the scope while sitting on the arytenoids will open the cleft.

Management varies according to the type of cleft and the associated anomalies. Aspiration can be avoided by nasogastric feeding, antireflux medication, or gastrostomy in combination with antireflux surgery.

Using the Myer classification system,[228] LI may need no treatment other than antireflux therapy. If still symptomatic, these patients may need an open or endoscopic repair. LII, LIII, and LTEI are best managed through anterior laryngotomy. LTEII and LTEIII appear best treated by a combined cervical and thoracic approach.[229] A lateral cervical approach provides suboptimal access.[230] An anterior approach under cardiopulmonary bypass has also been used,[231,232] and may be the best option in some cases.

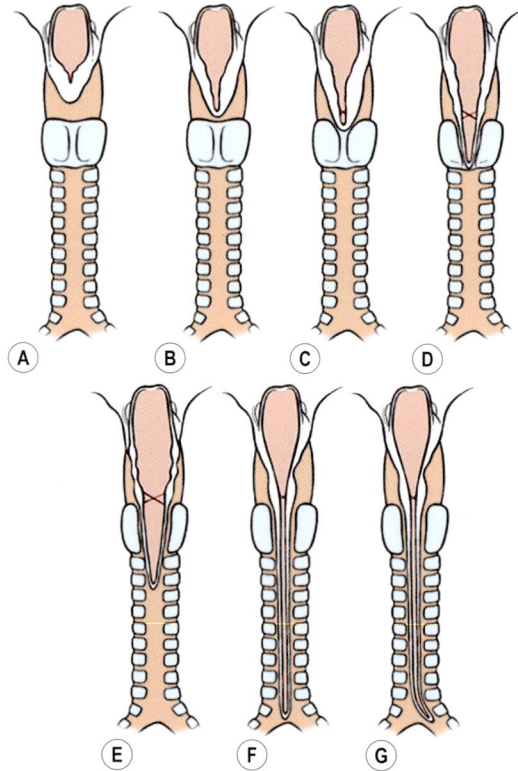

FIGURE 27-20 ■ This schematic depicts the classification of laryngotracheoesophageal clefts described by Myer and colleagues.[228] The laryngoesophageal clefts are seen in the top row, and the laryngotracheoesophageal clefts are seen on the bottom row. **(A)** Normal anatomy. **(B)** Interarytenoid cleft (LI). **(C)** Partial cricoid cleft (LII). **(D)** Complete cricoid cleft (LIII). **(E)** Cleft extends into trachea (LTEI). **(F)** Cleft extends into the carina (LTEII). **(G)** Cleft extends into the bronchus (LTEIII, proposed).

TABLE 27-1	Three Classification Systems for Laryngotracheoesophageal Clefts	
Pettersson[226]	**Ryan et al.**[227]	**Myer et al.**[228]

I: Cleft limited to the cricoid
 	
II: Cleft extending beyond the cricoid into the trachea
 	
III: Cleft involving the whole cricoid and trachea
	As described by Pettersson but with the addition of:
	IV: Cleft extending the whole way down into one of the main bronchi
		Laryngeal clefts:
		  Interarytenoid (LI)
		  Partial cricoid (LII)
		  Complete cricoid (LIII)
		Laryngotracheoesophageal:
		  Into trachea (LTEI)
		  To carina (LTEII)

Comment: The classification of Myer and colleagues seems best suited because it is more specific regarding the anatomic region involved. Extension into the bronchus, however, is not part of this classification. It could be added as LTEIII.

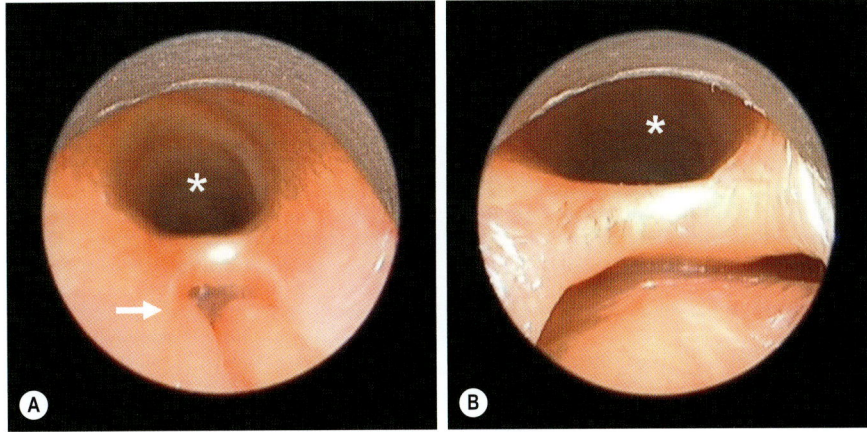

FIGURE 27-21 ■ This newborn began to have respiratory distress shortly after birth. Clinically, it was felt that the baby might have a tracheoesophageal fistula without esophageal atresia as a small nasogastric tube was able to be passed into the stomach. The bronchoscopic examination is shown. In both figures, the trachea is identified with the asterisk. **(A)** The laryngotracheoesophageal cleft is visualized. The esophagus is marked with the arrow. **(B)** The distal end of the laryngotracheoesophageal cleft is easily seen with the trachea anteriorly (asterisk) and the esophagus posteriorly. According to the classification of laryngotracheoesophageal clefts described by Meyer, this would be an LTE1 (see Fig. 27-20E).

This is a rare anomaly, and reported series are small. Tracheal instability, tracheomalacia, and GER with recurrent aspiration have been noted. The anastomotic leak rate is high, and hospitalization is often prolonged.

REFERENCES

1. Potts WJ. The Surgeon and the Child. W. B. Saunders Co; 1959.
2. Durston W. A Narrative of a Monstrous Birth in Plymouth, Oct. 22, 1670; together with the Anatomical Observations, taken thereupon by William Durston Doctor in Physick, and communicated to Dr. Tim. Clerk. Philos Trans (London) 1670;5:2096–8.
3. Gibson T. Anatomy of Humane bodies Epitomized. 5th ed. London: printed by TW for Awnsham and John Churchill, at the Black Swan in Pater-Noster-Row, and sold by Timothy Childe, at the White-Hart, the West end of St. Paul's Church Yard; 1697.
4. Levin NL. Congenital atresia of the esophagus with tracheo-esophageal fistula. J Thorac Cardiovasc Surg 1941;10:648–57.
5. Ladd WE. The surgical treatment of esophageal atresia and tracheoesophageal fistulas. N Engl J Med 1944;230:625–37.
6. Haight C, Towsley HA. Congenital atresia of the esophagus with tracheoesophageal fistula: Extrapleural ligation of fistula and end-to-end anastomosis. Surg Gynecol Obstet 1943;76:672–88.
7. Lilja HE, Wester T. Outcome in neonates with esophageal atresia treated over the last 20 years. Pediatr Surg Int 2008;24:531–6.
8. Spitz L, Kiely EM, Morecroft JA, et al. Oesophageal atresia: At-risk groups for the 1990s. J Pediatr Surg 1994;29:723–5.
9. Tonz M, Kohli S, Kaiser G. Oesophageal atresia: What has changed in the last 3 decades? Pediatr Surg Int 2004;20:768–72.
10. Orford J, Cass DT, Glasson MJ. Advances in the treatment of oesophageal atresia over three decades: The 1970s and the 1990s. Pediatr Surg Int 2004;20:402–7.
11. Felix JF, Keijzer R, van Dooren MF, et al. Genetics and developmental biology of oesophageal atresia and tracheo-oesophageal fistula: Lessons from mice relevant for paediatric surgeons. Pediatr Surg Int 2004;20:731–6.
12. Zaw-Tun HA. The tracheo-esophageal septum—fact or fantasy? Origin and development of the respiratory primordium and esophagus. Acta Anat (Basel) 1982;114:1–21.
13. Kluth D, Fiegel H. The embryology of the foregut. Semin Pediatr Surg 2003;12:3–9.
14. Qi BQ, Beasley SW. Stages of normal tracheo-bronchial development in rat embryos: Resolution of a controversy. Dev Growth Differ 2000;42:145–53.
15. Felix JF, Keijzer R, van Dooren MF, et al. Genetics and developmental biology of oesophageal atresia and tracheo-oesophageal fistula: Lessons from mice relevant for paediatric surgeons. Pediatr Surg Int 2004;20:731–6.
16. Que, J Choi M, Zeil JW, et al. Morphogenesis of the trachea and esophagus; current players and new roles for Noggin and BMPS. Differentiation 2006;74:422–37.
17. Que J, Okinbo T, Goldenring JR, et al. Multiple dose-dependent roles for Sox2 in pathway and differentiation of the anterior foregut endoderm. Development 2009;134:2521–31.
18. Jacobs J, Ku WY, Que J. Genetic and cellular mechanisms regulating anterior foregut and esophageal development. Dev Biol 2012;1:54–64.
19. Depaepe A, Dolk H, Lechat MF. The epidemiology of tracheo-oesophageal fistula and oesophageal atresia in Europe. EUROCAT Working Group. Arch Dis Child 1993;68:743–8.
20. Robert E, Mutchinick O, Mastroiacovo P, et al. An international collaborative study of the epidemiology of esophageal atresia or stenosis. Reprod Toxicol 1993;7:405–21.
21. Harris J, Kallen B, Robert E. Descriptive epidemiology of alimentary tract atresia. Teratology 1995;52:15–29.

22. Shaw-Smith C. Oesophageal atresia, tracheo-oesophageal fistula, and the VACTERL association: Review of genetics and epidemiology. J Med Genet 2006;43:545–54.

23. Pletcher BA, Friedes JS, Breg WR, et al. Familial occurrence of esophageal atresia with and without tracheoesophageal fistula: Report of two unusual kindreds. Am J Med Genet 1991;39:380–4.

24. Mastroiacovo P, Castilla EE, Arpino C, et al. Congenital malformations in twins: An international study. Am J Med Genet 1999;83:117–24.

25. Robert E, Mutchinick O, Mastroiacovo P, et al. An international collaborative study of the epidemiology of esophageal atresia or stenosis. Reprod Toxicol 1993;7:405–21.

26. Clementi M, Di Gianantonio E, Pelo E, et al. Methimazole embryopathy: Delineation of the phenotype. Am J Med Genet 1999;83:43–6.

27. Ramirez A, Espinosa de los Monteros A, Parra A, et al. Esophageal atresia and tracheoesophageal fistula in two infants born to hyperthyroid women receiving methimazole (Tapazol) during pregnancy. Am J Med Genet 1992;44:200–2.

28. Szendrey T, Danyi G, Czeizel A. Etiological study on isolated esophageal atresia. Hum Genet 1985;70:51–8.

29. Nora AH, Nora JJ. A syndrome of multiple congenital anomalies associated with teratogenic exposure. Arch Environ Health 1975;30:17–21.

30. Chen H, Goei GS, Hertzler JH, et al. Family studies in congenital esophageal atresia with and without tracheoesophageal fistula. In: Epstein CJ, Curry CJR, Packman S, editors. Risks, Communication, and Decision Making in Genetic Counseling. New York: Alan R. Liss for the National Foundation March-of-Dimes; 1979.

31. Martinez-Frias ML, Rodriguez-Pinilla E. Tracheoesophageal and anal atresia in prenatal children exposed to a high dose of alcohol. Am J Med Genet 1991;40:128.

32. Lipson A, Beuhler B, Bartley J, et al. Maternal hyperphenylalaninemia fetal effects. J Pediatr 1984;104:216–20.

33. Depaepe A, Dolk H, Lechat MF. The epidemiology of tracheo-oesophageal fistula and oesophageal atresia in Europe. EUROCAT Working Group. Arch Dis Child 1993;68:743–8.

34. Torfs CP, Curry CJ, Bateson TF. Population-based study of tracheoesophageal fistula and esophageal atresia. Teratology 1995;52:220–32.

35. van Bokhoven H, Celli J, van Reeuwijk J, et al. MYCN haploinsufficiency is associated with reduced brain size and intestinal atresias in Feingold syndrome. Nat Genet 2005;37:465–7.

36. Vissers LE, van Ravenswaaij CM, Admiraal R, et al. Mutations in a new member of the chromodomain gene family cause CHARGE syndrome. Nat Genet 2004;36:955–7.

37. FitzPatrick DR, Magee A, Friedler Z, et al. Mutations in SOX2 cause Rogers syndrome (anophthalmia, tracheoesophageal fistula, and genitourinary anomalies). Presented before the American Society of Human Genetics annual meeting, 2004(session 54), p 190.

38. Genevieve D, de Pontual L, Amiel J, et al. An overview of isolated and syndromic oesophageal atresia. Clin Genet 2007;71:392–9.

39. Kulkarni B, Rao RS, Oak S, et al. 13 pairs of ribs—a predictor of long gap atresia in tracheoesophageal fistula. J Pediatr Surg 1997;32:1453–4.

40. Quan L, Smith DW. The VATER association: Vertebral defects, Anal atresia, T-E fistula with esophageal atresia, Radial and Renal dysplasia: A spectrum of associated defects. J Pediatr 1973;82:104–7.

41. de Jong EM, Felix JF, Deurloo JA, et al. Non–VACTERL-type anomalies are frequent in patients with esophageal atresia/tracheo-esophageal fistula and full or partial VACTERL association. Birth Defects Res A Clin Mol Teratol 2008;82:92–7.

42. Kluth D. Atlas of esophageal atresia. J Pediatr Surg 1976;11:901–19.

43. Vogt EC. Congenital esophageal atresia. Am J Roentgenol 1929;22:463–5.

44. Gross RE. The Surgery of Infancy and Childhood. Philadelphia: WB Saunders; 1953.

45. Harmon C, Coran GC. Congenital anomalies of the esophagus. In: Grosfeld J, O'Neill JA, Coran AG, editors. Pediatric Surgery. 6th ed. Philadelphia: Mosby; 2006. p. 1051–81.

46. Goh DW, Brereton RJ, Spitz L. Esophageal atresia with obstructed tracheoesophageal fistula and gasless abdomen. J Pediatr Surg 1991;26:160–2.

47. Laffan EE, Daneman A, Ein SH, et al. Tracheoesophageal fistula without esophageal atresia: Are pull-back tube esophagograms needed for diagnosis? Pediatr Radiol 2006;36:1141–7.

48. Bax KN, Roskott AM, van der Zee DC. Esophageal atresia without distal tracheoesophageal fistula: High incidence of proximal fistula. J Pediatr Surg 2008;43:522–5.

49. Kane T, Atri P, Potoka DA. Triple fistula: Management of a double tracheoesophageal fistula with a third H-type proximal fistula. J Pediatr Surg 2007;42:e1–e3.

50. Touloukian RJ. Membranous esophageal obstruction simulating atresia with a double tracheoesophageal fistula in a neonate. J Thorac Cardiovasc Surg 1973;65:191–4.

51. Centini G, Rosignoli L, Kenanidis A, et al. Prenatal diagnosis of esophageal atresia with the pouch sign. Ultrasound Obstet Gynecol 2003;21:494–7.

52. Has R, Gunay S. Upper neck pouch sign in prenatal diagnosis of esophageal atresia. Arch Gynecol Obstet 2004;270:56–8.

53. Kalache KD, Chaoui R, Mau H, et al. The upper neck pouch sign: A prenatal sonographic marker for esophageal atresia. Ultrasound Obstet Gynecol 1998;11:138–40.

54. Houben CH, Curry JI. Current status of prenatal diagnosis, operative management and outcome of esophageal atresia/tracheoesophageal fistula. Prenat Diagn 2008;28:667–75.

55. Chaoui R, Schneider MB, Kalache KD. Right aortic arch with vascular ring and aberrant left subclavian artery: Prenatal diagnosis assisted by three-dimensional power Doppler ultrasound. Ultrasound Obstet Gynecol 2003;22:661–3.

56. Sivaprakasam MC, Vettukattil JJ. 3-D echocardiographic imaging of double aortic arch. Eur J Echocardiogr 2006;7:476–7.

57. Levine D, Barnewolt CE, Mehta TS, et al. Fetal thoracic abnormalities: MR imaging. Radiology 2003;228:379–88.

58. Matsuoka S, Takeuchi K, Yamanaka Y, et al. Comparison of magnetic resonance imaging and ultrasonography in the prenatal diagnosis of congenital thoracic abnormalities. Fetal Diagn Ther 2003;18:447–53.

59. Langer JC, Hussain H, Khan A, et al. Prenatal diagnosis of esophageal atresia using sonography and magnetic resonance imaging. J Pediatr Surg 2001;36:804–7.

60. Eklof O, Lohr G, Okmian L. Submucosal perforation of the esophagus in the neonate. Acta Radiol Diagn (Stockh) 1969;8:187–92.

61. Sapin E, Gumpert L, Bonnard A, et al. Iatrogenic pharyngoesophageal perforation in premature infants. Eur J Pediatr Surg 2000;10:83–7.

62. Gassner I, Geley TE. Sonographic evaluation of oesophageal atresia and tracheoesophageal fistula. Pediatr Radiol 2005;35:159–64.

63. Gross ER, Reichstein A, Gander JW, et al. The role of fiberoptic endoscopy in the evaluation and management of long gap esophageal atresia. Pediatr Surg Int 2010;45:1223–7.

64. Spitz L. Esophageal atresia: Lessons I have learned in a 40-year experience. J Pediatr Surg 2006;41:1635–40.

65. Rothenberg SS. Thoracoscopic repair of tracheoesophageal fistula. Semin Pediatr Surg 2005;14:2–7.

66. Gupta DK, Arora M, Srinivas M. Azygos vein anomaly: The best predictor of a long gap in esophageal atresia and tracheoesophageal fistula. Pediatr Surg Int 2001;17:101–3.

67. Babu R, Pierro A, Spitz L, et al. The management of oesophageal atresia in neonates with right-sided aortic arch. J Pediatr Surg 2000;35:56–8.

68. Cantinotti M, Hedge S, Bell A, et al. Diagnostic role of magnetic resonance imaging in identifying aortic arch anomalies. Congent Heart Dis 2008;3:117–23.

69. Tam PK, Chan FL, Saing H. Diagnosis and evaluation of esophageal atresia by direct sagittal CT. Pediatr Radiol 1987;17:68–70.

70. Ratan SK, Varshney A, Mullick S, et al. Evaluation of neonates with esophageal atresia using chest CT scan. Pediatr Surg Int 2004;20:757–61.

71. Ou P, Seror E, Layouss W, et al. Definitive diagnosis and surgical planning of H-type tracheoesophageal fistula in a critically ill

neonate: First experience using air distension of the esophagus during high-resolution computed tomography acquisition. J Thorac Cardiovasc Surg 2007;133:1116–17.

72. Islam S, Cavanaugh E, Honeke R, et al. Diagnosis of a proximal tracheoesophageal fistula using three-dimensional CT scan: A case report. J Pediatr Surg 2004;39:100–2.

73. Replogle RL. Esophageal atresia: Plastic sump catheter for drainage of the proximal pouch. Surgery 1963;54:296–7.

74. Holcomb GW 3rd. Survival after gastrointestinal perforation from esophageal atresia and tracheoesophageal fistula. J Pediatr Surg 1993;28:1532–5.

75. Maoate K, Myers NA, Beasley SW. Gastric perforation in infants with esophageal atresia and distal tracheo-oesophageal fistula. Pediatr Surg Int 1999;15:24–7.

76. Beasley SW, Myers NA, Auldist AW. Management of the premature infant with esophageal atresia and hyaline membrane disease. J Pediatr Surg 1992;27:23–5.

77. Holmes S, Keily EM, Spitz L. Tracheo-oesophageal atresia and the respiratory distress syndrome. Pediatr Surg Int 1987;2: 16–18.

78. Malone PS, Kiely EM, Brain AJ, et al. Tracheo-oesophageal fistula and pre-operative mechanical ventilation. Aust N Z J Surg 1990;60:525–7.

79. Atzori P, Iacobelli BD, Bottero S, et al. Preoperative tracheobronchoscopy in newborns with esophageal atresia: Does it matter? J Pediatr Surg 2006;41:1054–7.

80. Usui N, Kamata S, Ishikawa S, et al. Anomalies of the tracheobronchial tree in patients with esophageal atresia. J Pediatr Surg 1996;31:258–62.

81. Iannoli ED, Litman RS. Tension pneumothorax during flexible fiberoptic bronchoscopy in a newborn. Anesth Analg 2002;94: 512–13.

82. Holzki J. Bronchoscopic findings and treatment in congenital tracheoesophageal fistula. Paediatr Anaesth 1992;2:297–303.

83. Johnson AM, Rodgers BM, Alford B, et al. Esophageal atresia with double fistula: The missed anomaly. Ann Thorac Surg 1984;38:195–200.

84. Katsura S, Shono T, Yamanouchi T, et al. Esophageal atresia with double tracheoesophageal fistula—a case report and review of the literature. Eur J Pediatr Surg 2005;15:354–7.

85. Bikhazi G, Davis PJ. Anesthesia for neonates and premature infants. In: Motoyama E, editor. Anesthesia for Infants and Children. St. Louis: Mosby; 1990. p. 450–3.

86. Salem MR, Wong AY, Lin YH, et al. Prevention of gastric distention during anesthesia for newborns with tracheoesophageal fistulas. Anesthesiology 1973;38:82–3.

87. Schwartz N, Eisenkraft JB. Positioning the endotracheal tube in an infant with tracheoesophageal fistula. Anesthesiology 1988;69: 289–90.

88. Alabbad SI, Shaw K, Puligandla PS, et al. The pitfalls of endotracheal intubation beyond the fistula in babies with type C esophageal atresia. Semin Pediatr Surg 2009;18(2):116–18.

89. Soucy P, Bass J, Evans M. The muscle-sparing thoracotomy in infants and children. J Pediatr Surg 1990;27:1257–8.

90. Rothenberg SS, Pokorny WJ. Experience with a total muscle sparing approach for thoracotomies in neonates, infants and children. J Ped Surg 1992;27:1157–60.

91. McKinnon LJ, Kosloske AM. Prediction and prevention of anastomotic complications of esophageal atresia and tracheoesophageal fistula. J Pediatr Surg 1990;25:778–81.

92. Bishop PJ, Klein MD, Philippart AI, et al. Transpleural repair of esophageal atresia without a primary gastrostomy: 240 patients treated between 1951 and 1983. J Pediatr Surg 1985;20:823–8.

93. Sharma S, Sinha SK, Rawat JD, et al. Azygos vein preservation in primary repair of esophageal atresia with tracheoesophageal fistula. Pediatr Surg Int 2007;23:1215–18.

94. Upadhyaya VD, Gangopadhyaya AN, Gopal SC, et al. Is ligation of azygos vein necessary in primary repair of tracheoesophageal fistula with esophageal atresia? Eur J Pediatr Surg 2007; 17:236–40.

95. Touloukian RJ, Pickett LK, Spackman T, et al. Repair of esophageal atresia by end-to-side anastomosis and ligation of the tracheoesophageal fistula: A critical review of 18 cases. J Pediatr Surg 1974;9:305–10.

96. Poenaru D, Laberge JM, Neilson IR, et al. A more than 25-year experience with end-to-end versus end-to-side repair for esophageal atresia. J Pediatr Surg 1991;26:472–8.

97. Davies MR. Anatomy of the extrinsic motor nerve supply to mobilized segments of the oesophagus disrupted by dissection during repair of oesophageal atresia with distal fistula. Br J Surg 1996;83:1268–70.

98. McCallion WA, Hannon RJ, Boston VE. Prophylactic extrapleural chest drainage following repair of esophageal atresia: Is it necessary? J Pediatr Surg 1992;27:561.

99. Kay S, Shaw K. Revisiting the role of routine retropleural drainage after repair of esophageal atresia with distal tracheoesophageal fistula. J Pediatr Surg 1999;34:1082–5.

100. Rothenberg SS. Thoracoscopic repair of tracheoesophageal fistula in a newborn. Ped Endosurg Innovative Tech 2000;289–94.

101. Rothenberg SS. Thoracoscopic repair of tracheoesophageal fistula in newborns. J Pediatr Surg 2002;37:869–72.

102. Bax KM, van Der Zee DC. Feasibility of thoracoscopic repair of esophageal atresia with distal fistula. J Pediatr Surg 2002;37: 192–6.

103. Holcomb GW 3rd, Rothenberg SS, Bax KM, et al. Thoracoscopic repair of esophageal atresia and tracheoesophageal fistula: A multi-institutional analysis. Ann Surg 2005;242:422–30.

104. van der Zee DC, Bax NM. Thoracoscopic repair of esophageal atresia with distal fistula. Surg Endosc 2003;17:1065–7.

105. Bax N, van der Zee DC, et al. The thoracoscopic approach to esophageal atresia with distal fistula. In: Bax N, Georgeson KE, Rothenberg SS, editors. Endoscopic Surgery in Infants and Children. Heidelberg: Springer; 2008. p. 199–205.

106. Rothenberg SS. Thoracoscopic repair of esophageal atresia and tracheoesophageal fistula in neonates: Evolution of a technique. J Laparoendosc Adv Surg Tech A 2012;195–9.

107. Mortellaro VE, Fike FB, Adibe OO, et al. The use of high-frequency oscillating ventilation to facilitate stability during neonatal thoracoscopic operations. J Laparoendosc Adv Surg Tech 2011;A 21:877–9.

108. Puri P, Blake N, O'Donnell B, et al. Delayed primary anastomosis following spontaneous growth of esophageal segments in esophageal atresia. J Pediatr Surg 1981;16:180–3.

109. Puri P, Ninan GK, Blake NS, et al. Delayed primary anastomosis for esophageal atresia: 18 months' to 11 years' follow-up. J Pediatr Surg 1992;27:1127–30.

110. Spitz L, Kiely E, Brereton RJ, et al. Management of esophageal atresia. World J Surg 1993;17:296–300.

111. Aziz D, Schiller D, Gerstle JT, et al. Can 'long-gap' esophageal atresia be safely managed at home while awaiting anastomosis? J Pediatr Surg 2003;38:705–8.

112. Hollands CM, Lankau CA Jr, Burnweit CA. Preoperative home care for esophageal atresia—a survey. J Pediatr Surg 2000; 35:279–82.

113. Howard R, Myers NA. Esophageal atresia: A technique for elongating the upper pouch. Surgery 1965;58:725–7.

114. Mahour GH, Woolley MM, Gwinn JL. Elongation of the upper pouch and delayed anatomic reconstruction in esophageal atresia. J Pediatr Surg 1974;9:373–83.

115. Hays DM, Woolley MM, Snyder WH Jr. Changing techniques in the management of esophageal atresia. Arch Surg 1966;92: 611–16.

116. Hendren WH, Hale JR. Electromagnetic bougienage to lengthen esophageal segments in congenital esophageal atresia. N Engl J Med 1975;293:428–32.

117. Livaditis A, Radberg L, Odensjo G. Esophageal end-to-end anastomosis: Reduction of anastomotic tension by circular myotomy. Scand J Thorac Cardiovasc Surg 1972;6:206–14.

118. Kate JT. Method of suturing operations for congenital oesophageal atresia. Arch Chir Neerland 1952;4:43–7.

119. Gough MH. Esophageal atresia—use of an anterior flap in the difficult anastomosis. J Pediatr Surg 1980;15:310–11.

120. Kimura K, Soper RT. Multistaged extrathoracic esophageal elongation for long gap esophageal atresia. J Pediatr Surg 1994;29:566–8.

121. Martinez-Ferro M, et al. Thoracoscopic repair of esophageal atresia without fistula. In: Bax N, Georgeson KE, Rothenberg SS, editors. Endoscopic surgery in infants and children. Heidelberg: Springer; 2008. p. 207–19.

122. Davison P, Poenaru D, Kamal I. Esophageal atresia: Primary repair of a rare long gap variant involving distal pouch mobilization. J Pediatr Surg 1999;34:1881–3.

123. Lessin MS, Wesselhoeft CW, Luks FI, et al. Primary repair of long-gap esophageal atresia by mobilization of the distal esophagus. Eur J Pediatr Surg 1999;9:369–72.

124. Lai JY, Sheu JC, Chang PY, et al. Experience with distal circular myotomy for long-gap esophageal atresia. J Pediatr Surg 1996;31: 1503–8.

125. Giacomoni MA, Tresoldi M, Zamana C, et al. Circular myotomy of the distal esophageal stump for long gap esophageal atresia. J Pediatr Surg 2001;36:855–7.

126. Rehbein F, Schweder N. Reconstruction of the esophagus without colon transplantation in cases of atresia. J Pediatr Surg 1971;6: 746–52.

127. Okmian L, Booss D, Ekelund L. An endoscopic technique for Rehbein's silver olive method. Z Kinderchir 1975;16:212–15.

128. Vogel AM, Yang EY, Fishman SJ. Hydrostatic stretch-induced growth facilitating primary anastomosis in long-gap esophageal atresia. J Pediatr Surg 2006;41:1170–2.

129. Schaerli A. Esophageal reconstruction in very long atresia by elongation of the lesser curvature. Pediatr Surg Int 1992;7: 101–5.

130. Rao KL, Menon P, Samujh R, et al. Fundal tube esophagoplasty for esophageal reconstruction in atresia. J Pediatr Surg 2003;38: 1723–5.

131. Waterston D. Colonic replacement of the esophagus (intrathoracic). Surg Clin North Am 1994;44:.

132. Anderson KD, Randolph JG. The gastric tube for esophageal replacement in children. J Thorac Cardiovasc Surg 1973;66: 333–42.

133. Heimlich HJ, Winfield JM. The use of a gastric tube to replace or by-pass the esophagus. Surgery 1955;37:549–59.

134. Spitz L, Kiely E, Pierro A. Gastric transposition in children—a 21-year experience. J Pediatr Surg 2004;39:276–81.

135. Ure BM, Jesch NK, Sumpelmann R, et al. Laparoscopically assisted gastric pull-up for long gap esophageal atresia. J Pediatr Surg 2003;38:1661–2.

136. Bax NM, van der Zee DC. Jejunal pedicle grafts for reconstruction of the esophagus in children. J Pediatr Surg 2007;42:363–9.

137. Ring WS, Varco RL, L'Heureux PR, et al. Esophageal replacement with jejunum in children: An 18 to 33 year follow-up. J Thorac Cardiovasc Surg 1982;83:918–27.

138. Saitua F, Madrid A, Capdeville F, et al. Pharyngoesophageal reconstruction by free jejunal graft and microvascular anastomosis in a 10-year-old girl. J Pediatr Surg 2004;39:e10–12.

139. Bax NM, Van Renterghem KM. Ileal pedicle grafting for esophageal replacement in children. Pediatr Surg Int 2005;21:369–72.

140. Foker JE, Linden BC, Boyle EM Jr, Marquardt C. Development of a true primary repair for the full spectrum of esophageal atresia. Ann Surg 1997;226:533–41.

141. Foker JE, Kendall Krosch TC, Catton K, et al. A flexible approach to achieve a true primary repair for all infants with esophageal atresia. Semin Pediatr Surg 2009;18:23–9.

142. van der Zee DC, Vieirra-Travassos D, Kramer WL, et al. Thoracoscopic elongation of the esophagus in long gap esophageal atresia. J Pediatr Surg 2007;42:1785–8.

143. Spitz L, Kiely E, Brereton RJ, et al. Management of esophageal atresia. World J Surg 1993;17:296–300.

144. MacKinlay G, Burlles R. Oesophageal atresia: Paralysis and ventilation management of the wide gap. Pediatr Surg Int 1987;2: 10–12.

145. Lyall P, Bao-Quan Q, Beasley S. The effect of neck flexion on oesophageal tension in the pig and its relevance to repaired oesophageal atresia. Pediatr Surg Int 2001;17:193–5.

146. Beasley SW. Does postoperative ventilation have an effect on the integrity of the anastomosis in repaired oesophageal atresia? J Paediatr Child Health 1999;35:120–2.

147. Chittmittrapap S, Spitz L, Kiely EM, et al. Anastomotic leakage following surgery for esophageal atresia. J Pediatr Surg 1992;27: 29–32.

148. Yanchar NL, Gordon R, Cooper M, et al. Significance of the clinical course and early upper gastrointestinal studies in predicting complications associated with repair of esophageal atresia. J Pediatr Surg 2001;36:815–22.

149. Said M, Mekki M, Golli M, et al. Balloon dilatation of anastomotic strictures secondary to surgical repair of oesophageal atresia. Br J Radiol 2003;76:26–31.

150. Spitz L, et al. Oesophageal atresia and tracheoesophageal fistula. In: Freeman NV, editor. Surgery of the Newborn. New York: Churchill Livingstone; 1994. p. 353–73.

151. Chittmittrapap S, Spitz L, Kiely EM, et al. Anastomotic stricture following repair of esophageal atresia. J Pediatr Surg 1990;25: 508–11.

152. Koivusalo A, Turunen P, Rintala RJ, et al. Is routine dilatation after repair of esophageal atresia with distal fistula better than dilatation when symptoms arise? Comparison of results of two European pediatric surgical centers. J Pediatr Surg 2004;39: 1643–7.

153. Ashcraft KW, Goodwin C, Amoury RA, et al. Early recognition and aggressive treatment of gastroesophageal reflux following repair of esophageal atresia. J Pediatr Surg 1977;12:317–21.

154. Fonkalsrud EW. Gastroesophageal fundoplication for reflux following repair of esophageal atresia: Experience with nine patients. Arch Surg 1979;114:48–51.

155. Pieretti R, Shandling B, Stephens CA. Resistant esophageal stenosis associated with reflux after repair of esophageal atresia: A therapeutic approach. J Pediatr Surg 1974;9:355–7.

156. St. Peter SD, Calkins CM, Holcomb GW III. The use of biosynthetic mesh to separate the anastomoses during the thoracoscopic repair of esophageal atresia and tracheoesophageal fistula. J Laparoendosc Adv Surg Tech 2007;17:380–2.

157. Richter GT, Ryckman F, Brown RL, et al. Endoscopic management of recurrent tracheoesophageal fistula. J Pediatr Surg 2008;43:238–45.

158. Keckler SJ, St. Peter SD, Calkins CM, et al. Occlusion of a recurrent tracheoesophageal fistula. J Pediatr Surg 2008;18: 465–8.

159. Meier JD, Sulman CG, Almond PS, et al. Endoscopic management of recurrent congenital tracheoesophageal fistula: A review of techniques and result. Int J Pediatr Otorhinolaryngol 2007;71:691–7.

160. Wailoo MP, Emery JL. The trachea in children with tracheoesophageal fistula. Histopathology 1979;3:329–38.

161. Cohen B, Glasson M. Tracheomalacia in association with congenital tracheoesophageal fistula. Surgery 1978;79:504–8.

162. Rideout DT, Hayashi AH, Gillis DA, et al. The absence of clinically significant tracheomalacia in patients having esophageal atresia without tracheoesophageal fistula. J Pediatr Surg 1991; 26:1303–5.

163. Delius RE, Wheatley MJ, Coran AG. Etiology and management of respiratory complications after repair of esophageal atresia with tracheoesophageal fistula. Surgery 1992;112:527–32.

164. Gross RE, Neuhauser EBD. Compression of the trachea by an anomalous innominate artery: An operation for its relief. Am J Dis Child 1948;75:570–4.

165. Schwartz MZ, Filler RM. Tracheal compression as a cause of apnea following repair of tracheoesophageal fistula: Treatment by aortopexy. J Pediatr Surg 1980;15:842–8.

166. Applebaum H, Woolley MM. Pericardial flap aortopexy for tracheomalacia. J Pediatr Surg 1990;25:30–2.

167. Koyluoglu G, Gunay I, Ceran C, et al. Pericardial flap aortopexy: An easy and safe technique in the treatment of tracheomalacia. J Cardiovasc Surg (Torino) 2002;43:295–7.

168. Blair GK, Cohen R, Filler RM. Treatment of tracheomalacia: Eight years' experience. J Pediatr Surg 1986;21:781–5.

169. Vaishnav A, MacKinnon AE. New cervical approach for tracheopexy. Br J Surg 1986;73:441–2.

170. DeCou JM, Parsons DS, Gauderer MWL. Thoracoscopic aortopexy for severe tracheomalacia. Pediatr Endosurg Innov Tech 2001;5:205–8.

171. Bax N, van der Zee DC, et al. Aortosternopexy for tracheomalacia. In: Bax N, Georgeson KE, Rothenberg SS, editors. Endoscopic Surgery in Infants and Children. Heidelberg: Springer; 2008. p. 157–62.

172. Kane T, Nadler EP, Potoka DA. Thoracoscopic aortopexy for vascular compression of the trachea: Approach from the right. J Laparoendosc Adv Surg Tech A 2008;18:313–16.

173. Kirkpatrick JA, Cresson SL, Pilling GP 4th. The motor activity of the esophagus in association with esophageal atresia and tra-

cheoesophageal fistula. Am J Roentgenol Radium Ther Nucl Med 1961;86:884–7.

174. Lind JF, Blanchard RJ, Guyda H. Esophageal motility in tracheoesophageal fistula and esophageal atresia. Surg Gynecol Obstet 1966;123:557–64.

175. Shermeta DW, Whitington PF, Seto DS, et al. Lower esophageal sphincter dysfunction in esophageal atresia: Nocturnal regurgitation and aspiration pneumonia. J Pediatr Surg 1977;12:871–6.

176. Tovar JA, Diez Pardo JA, Murcia J, et al. Ambulatory 24-hour manometric and pH metric evidence of permanent impairment of clearance capacity in patients with esophageal atresia. J Pediatr Surg 1995;30:1224–31.

177. Deurloo JA, Ekkelkamp S, Bartelsman JF, et al. Gastroesophageal reflux: Prevalence in adults older than 28 years after correction of esophageal atresia. Ann Surg 2003;238:686–9.

178. Zigman A, Yazbeck S. Esophageal foreign body obstruction after esophageal atresia repair. J Pediatr Surg 2002;37:776–8.

179. Hormann M, Pokieser P, Scharitzer M, et al. Videofluoroscopy of deglutition in children after repair of esophageal atresia. Acta Radiol 2002;43:507–10.

180. Dutta HK, Rajani M, Bhatnagar V. Cineradiographic evaluation of postoperative patients with esophageal atresia and tracheoesophageal fistula. Pediatr Surg Int 2000;16:322–5.

181. Montgomery M, Witt H, Kuylenstierna R, et al. Swallowing disorders after esophageal atresia evaluated with videomanometry. J Pediatr Surg 1998;33:1219–23.

182. Dutta HK, Grover VP, Dwivedi SN, et al. Manometric evaluation of postoperative patients of esophageal atresia and tracheoesophageal fistula. Eur J Pediatr Surg 2001;11:371–6.

183. Kawahara H, Kubota A, Hasegawa T, et al. Lack of distal esophageal contractions is a key determinant of gastroesophageal reflux disease after repair of esophageal atresia. J Pediatr Surg 2007;42:2017–21.

184. Shono T, Suita S, Arima T, et al. Motility function of the esophagus before primary anastomosis in esophageal atresia. J Pediatr Surg 1993;28:673–6.

185. Shono T, Suita S. Motility studies of the esophagus in a case of esophageal atresia before primary anastomosis and in experimental models. Eur J Pediatr Surg 1997;7:138–42.

186. Cheng W, Poon KH, Lui VC, et al. Esophageal atresia and achalasia-like esophageal dysmotility. J Pediatr Surg 2004;39:1581–3.

187. Tibboel D, Pattenier JW, Van Krutgen RJ, et al. Prospective evaluation of postoperative morbidity in patients with esophageal atresia. Pediatr Surg Int 1988;4:252–5.

188. Koch A, Rohr S, Plaschkes J, et al. Incidence of gastroesophageal reflux following repair of esophageal atresia. Progr Pediatr Surg 1986;19:103–13.

189. Koivusalo A, Pakarinen MP, Rintala RJ. The cumulative incidence of significant gastroesophageal reflux in patients with oesophageal atresia with a distal fistula—a systematic clinical, pH-metric, and endoscopic follow-up study. J Pediatr Surg 2007;42:370–4.

190. Koivusalo A, Pakarinen M, Rintala RJ, et al. Does postoperative pH monitoring predict complicated gastroesophageal reflux in patients with esophageal atresia? Pediatr Surg Int 2004;20:670–4.

191. Van Biervliet S, Van Winckel M, Robberecht E, et al. High-dose omeprazole in esophagitis with stenosis after surgical treatment of esophageal atresia. J Pediatr Surg 2001;36:1416–18.

192. Wheatley MJ, Coran AG, Wesley JR. Efficacy of the Nissen fundoplication in the management of gastroesophageal reflux following esophageal atresia repair. J Pediatr Surg 1993;28:53–5.

193. Snyder CL, Ramachandran V, Kennedy AP, et al. Efficacy of partial wrap fundoplication for gastroesophageal reflux after repair of esophageal atresia. J Pediatr Surg 1997;32:1089–92.

194. Sistonen SJ, Koivusalo A, Lindahl H, et al. Cancer after repair of esophageal atresia: Population-based long-term follow-up. J Pediatr Surg 2008;43:602–5.

195. Mortellaro VE, Pettiford JN, St. Peter SD, et al. Incidence, diagnosis and outcomes of vocal fold immobility after esophageal atresia (EA) and/or tracheoesophageal fistula (TEF) repair. Eur J Pediatr Surg 2011;21:386–8.

196. Robertson JR, Birck HG. Laryngeal problems following infant esophageal surgery. Laryngoscope 1976;86:965–70.

197. Chetcuti P, Phelan PD. Respiratory morbidity after repair of esophageal atresia and tracheoesophageal fistula. Arch Dis Child 1993;68:167–70.

198. Malmström K, Lohi J, Lindahl H, et al. Longitudinal follow-up of bronchial inflammation, respiratory symptoms, and pulmonary function in adolescents after repair of esophageal atresia with tracheoesophageal fistula. J Pediatr Surg 2008;153:396–401.

199. Vazquez-Jimenez JF, Sachweh JS, Liakopoulos OJ, et al. Aortopexy in severe tracheal instability: Short-term and long-term outcome in 29 infants and children. Ann Thorac Surg 2001;72:1898–901.

200. Durning RP, Scoles PV, Fox OD. Scoliosis after thoracotomy in tracheoesophageal fistula patients: A follow-up study. J Bone Joint Surg Am 1980;62:1156–9.

201. Jaureguizar E, Vazquez J, Murcia J, et al. Morbid musculoskeletal sequelae of thoracotomy for tracheoesophageal fistula. J Pediatr Surg 1985;20:511–14.

202. Cherup LL, Siewers RD, Futrell JW. Breast and pectoral muscle maldevelopment after anterolateral and posterolateral thoracotomies in children. Ann Thorac Surg 1986;41:492–7.

203. Westfelt JN, Nordwall A. Thoracotomy and scoliosis. Spine 1991;16:1124–5.

204. Chetcuti P, Dickens DR, Phelan PD. Spinal deformity in patients born with oesophageal atresia and tracheo-oesophageal fistula. Arch Dis Child 1989;64:1427–30.

205. Chetcuti P, Myers NA, Phelan PD, et al. Chest wall deformity in patients with repaired esophageal atresia. J Pediatr Surg 1989;24:244–7.

206. Emmel M, Ulbach P, Herse B, et al. Neurogenic lesions after posterolateral thoracotomy in young children. Thorac Cardiovasc Surg 1996;44:86–91.

207. Schier F, Korn S, Michel E. Experiences of a parent support group with the long-term consequences of esophageal atresia. J Pediatr Surg 2001;36:605–10.

208. Perttunen K, Tasmuth T, Kalso E. Chronic pain after thoracic surgery: A follow-up study. Acta Anaesthesiol Scand 1999;43:563–7.

209. Rogers ML, Duffy JP. Surgical aspects of chronic post-thoracotomy pain. Eur J Cardiothorac Surg 2000;18:711–16.

210. Haller JO, Berdon WE, Levin TL, et al. Tracheoesophageal fistula (H-type) in neonates with imperforate anus and the VATER association. Pediatr Radiol 2004;34:83–5.

211. Fordham LA. Imaging of the esophagus in children. Radiol Clin North Am 2005;43:283–302.

212. Azoulay D, Regnard JF, Magdeleinat P, et al. Congenital respiratory-esophageal fistula in the adult: Report of nine cases and review of the literature. J Thorac Cardiovasc Surg 1992;104:381–4.

213. Garand SA, Kareti LR, Dumont TM, et al. Thoracoscopic repair of tracheoesophageal fistula in a septuagenarian. Ann Thorac Surg 2006;81:1899–901.

214. Crabbe DC. Isolated tracheo-oesophageal fistula. Paediatr Respir Rev 2003;4:74–8.

215. Nagata K, Kamio Y, Ichikawa T, et al. Congenital tracheoesophageal fistula successfully diagnosed by CT esophagography. World J Gastroenterol 2006;12:1476–8.

216. LaSalle AJ, Andrassy RJ, Ver Steeg K, et al. Congenital tracheoesophageal fistula without esophageal atresia. J Thorac Cardiovasc Surg 1979;78:583–8.

217. Garcia NM, Thompson JW, Shaul DB. Definitive localization of isolated tracheoesophageal fistula using bronchoscopy and esophagoscopy for guide wire placement. J Pediatr Surg 1998;33:1645–7.

218. Ko BA, Frederic R, DiTirro PA, et al. Simplified access for division of the low cervical/high thoracic H-type tracheoesophageal fistula. J Pediatr Surg 2000;35:1621–2.

219. Rothenberg SS. Experience with thoracoscopic tracheal surgery in infants and children. J Laparoendosc Adv Surg Tech A 2009;19:671–4.

220. Allal H, Montes-Tapia F, Andina G, et al. Thoracoscopic repair of H-type tracheoesophageal fistula in the newborn: A technical case report. J Pediatr Surg 2004;39:1568–70.

221. Aziz GA, Schier F. Thoracoscopic ligation of a tracheoesophageal H-type fistula in a newborn. J Pediatr Surg 2005;40:e35–e36.

222. Roth B, Rose KG, Benz-Bohm G, et al. Laryngo-tracheo-oesophageal cleft: Clinical features, diagnosis and therapy. Eur J Pediatr 1983;140:41–6.

223. Walner DL, Stern Y, Collins M, et al. Does the presence of a tracheoesophageal fistula predict the outcome of laryngeal cleft repair? Arch Otolaryngol Head Neck Surg 1999;125:782–4.

224. Phelan PD, Stocks JG, Williams HE, et al. Familial occurrence of congenital laryngeal clefts. Arch Dis Child 1973;48:275–8.

225. Tyler DC. Laryngeal cleft: Report of eight patients and a review of the literature. Am J Med Genet 1985;21:61–75.

226. Pettersson G. Inhibited separation of larynx and the upper part of trachea from oesophagus in a newborn: Report of a case successfully operated upon. Acta Chir Scand 1955;110:250–4.

227. Ryan DP, Muehrcke DD, Doody DP, et al. Laryngotracheoesophageal cleft (type IV): Management and repair of lesions beyond the carina. J Pediatr Surg 1991;26:962–9.

228. Myer CM 3rd, Cotton RT, Holmes DK, et al. Laryngeal and laryngotracheoesophageal clefts: Role of early surgical repair. Ann Otol Rhinol Laryngol 1990;99:98–104.

229. Donahoe PK, Gee PE. Complete laryngotracheoesophageal cleft: Management and repair. J Pediatr Surg 1984;19:143–8.

230. Mathur NN, Peek GJ, Bailey CM, et al. Strategies for managing Type IV laryngotracheoesophageal clefts at Great Ormond Street Hospital for Children. Int J Pediatr Otorhinolaryngol 2006;70:1901–10.

231. Moukheiber AK, Camboulives J, Guys JM, et al. Repair of a type IV laryngotracheoesophageal cleft with cardiopulmonary bypass. Ann Otol Rhinol Laryngol 2002;111:1076–80.

232. Geiduschek JM, Inglis AF Jr, O'Rourke PP, et al. Repair of a laryngotracheoesophageal cleft in an infant by means of extracorporeal membrane oxygenation. Ann Otol Rhinol Laryngol 1993;102:827–33.

CHAPTER 28

Gastroesophageal Reflux

Corey W. Iqbal • George W. Holcomb III

Gastroesophageal reflux (GER) is a disease that is commonly encountered in infants and children. In general, the episodes of GER that are seen in infants and children are not clinically significant and will have no identifiable etiology. In addition, 60–65% of children with GER will undergo spontaneous symptom resolution by 2 years of life, regardless of any medical treatment.[1] However, some children will have pathologic gastroesophageal reflux disease (GERD) that will result in either failure to grow appropriately, respiratory complications, or apparent life-threatening events (ALTE). This is the population that will require medical and/or surgical intervention.

HISTORY

The effects of GERD in pediatric patients have been reported for over a century.[2–6] Before the introduction of proton pump inhibitors (PPIs) in the 1990s, the medical management of GERD in children and adults was relatively ineffective and based on antacids and histamine antagonists. Due to the limited spectrum of medical management in the 1950s and 1960s, several surgeons developed operative approaches for GERD management. Lortat–Jacob, Hill, Belsey, Nissen, Rosetti, and Thal all contributed greatly to the surgical management of GERD.[7–14]

These antireflux procedures were initially developed in adults and were effective in controlling GERD. Subsequently, they were applied to infants and children with good success.[7,14,15] The overall management of GERD has progressed significantly over the past two decades with more effective PPIs and refinement in the surgical technique. One of the most important surgical advances occurred in 1991 when Dallemagne reported his experience with laparoscopic fundoplication.[16] An expected evolutionary cascade led to the use of laparoscopy in children by Georgeson[17] and Lobe.[18] It is due to these pioneers, and the many researchers that followed, that we now know that laparoscopic fundoplication is safe and effective in treating GERD with acceptable morbidity and excellent control of symptoms in infants and children. The most daunting task currently is how to identify those children who will benefit from a fundoplication. As our diagnostic tools are being further evaluated and newer methods are being introduced, there has been renewed skepticism about who should have a fundoplication. At the same time, ongoing refinement of the operative approach has yielded even better outcomes.

PATHOPHYSIOLOGY

GERD is defined as the pathologic effects of involuntary passage of gastric contents into the esophagus. Ultimately, the pathophysiologic alteration that is responsible for the development of GERD is incompetence of the antireflux barriers that exist between the lower esophagus and the stomach. The result of this incompetence is the presence of gastric refluxate in direct contact with the esophageal mucosa. While initially felt to be purely acidic, research in the utility of the pH probe as a diagnostic tool has shown this is not true.[19] In fact, adult literature has implicated alkaline bile reflux as a causative factor in the development of Barrett esophageal metaplasia.[20] The pathologic events that occur because of GERD are due to one or multiple failures of the normal physiologic barriers that exist to prevent gastric contents from entering the esophagus, or to limit injury to the esophagus as a result of gastric refluxate, or to clear the refluxate that enters the esophagus (Table 28-1).

In adults, the consequence of this refluxate in the esophagus is primarily limited to erosive esophagitis, esophageal stricture, and Barrett esophagitis. In children, its detrimental effects are much broader. Associated physiologic, anatomic, and developmental abnormalities coexist in children that make GERD and its consequences much more complex. Many children with GERD have significant neurologic impairment. These children can have increased spasticity with retching and related increased abdominal pressures. Poor swallowing mechanisms lead to gagging and choking, which add to this intermittent increased abdominal pressure. Sometimes, a hiatal hernia develops (Fig. 28-1), further predisposing to GERD. Congenital anomalies such as esophageal atresia with or without tracheoesophageal fistula (EA/TEF), duodenal and proximal small bowel atresias, congenital diaphragmatic hernia (CDH), and gastroschisis/omphalocele all predispose to the development of GERD. The consequences of GERD in children lead to the same complications seen in adults (erosive esophagitis, stricture, and Barrett esophagitis), but also include pulmonary effects (reactive airway disease and pneumonia), potential malnutrition secondary to the inability to maintain adequate caloric intake, and apneic episodes leading to ALTE spells.

Barriers against GERD

The most important factor for preventing reflux of gastric contents into the esophagus is the lower esophageal

TABLE 28-1	Mechanisms That Either Prevent Gastroesophageal Reflux, Limit the Esophageal Injury, or Clear the Refluxate	
Prevent Gastric Reflux	**Limit Esophageal Injury**	**Clear Esophageal Refluxate**
Lower esophageal sphincter	Saliva	Esophageal peristalsis
Angle of His	Amount of gastric acid	Saliva
Length of intra-abdominal esophagus	Pepsin	Gravity
Elevated intra-abdominal pressure	Trypsin	
	Bile acids	

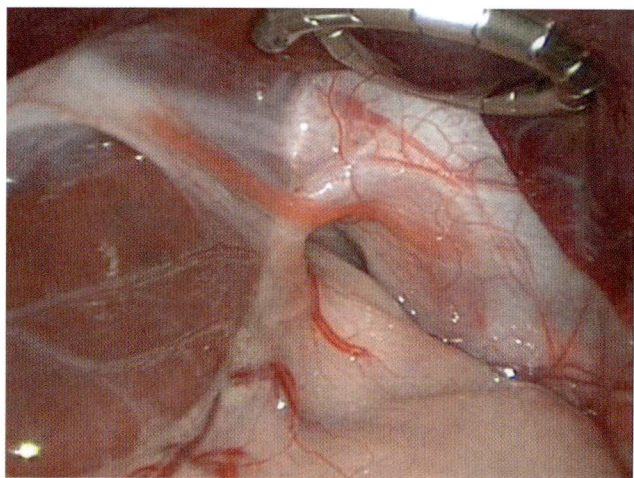

FIGURE 28-1 ■ This intraoperative photograph depicts a de novo hiatal hernia in a 13-month-old infant. Note the enlarged hiatus. A portion of the upper stomach has herniated into the chest.

sphincter (LES). Embryologically, the LES arises from the inner circular muscle layer of the esophagus, which is asymmetrically thickened in the distal esophagus. This thickened muscle layer creates a high-pressure zone that can be measured manometrically. In addition, this muscular thickening extends onto the stomach more prominently on the greater than lesser curvature.[21] The phrenoesophageal membrane, arising from the septum transversum of the diaphragm and the collar of Helvetius, holds the LES in position. The result is an LES that lies partially in the chest and partially in the abdomen. This positioning is important for the normal barrier function against GER. Esophageal manometry can identify this transition (which is known as the respiratory inversion point) from the thoracic to the abdominal esophagus.

The LES is an imperfect valve that creates a pressure gradient in the distal esophagus. The ability to prevent GER is directly proportional to the LES pressure and its length, provided that LES relaxation is normal. In an adult study, LES pressures greater than 30 mmHg prevented GER, as documented by 24-hour pH study, whereas pressures between 0–5 mmHg correlated with abnormal pH studies in more than 80% of patients.[22] Also, GER is statistically significantly more likely to develop in adults if the LES pressure falls below 6 mmHg at the respiratory inversion point or if the overall LES length is 2 cm or less.[23] As noted previously, the LES is relatively fixed across the esophageal hiatus by its surrounding attachments. Malposition of the LES, which can occur with a hiatal hernia or abnormal development, causes loss of the protective function of the LES, resulting in GER. Finally, LES relaxation occurs with esophageal peristalsis initiated by the swallowing mechanism. This relaxation is normal and must occur. Inappropriate LES relaxations, referred to as transient LES relaxations, have been shown to occur sporadically, unassociated with the swallowing mechanism. Interestingly, when children with symptoms of GER were studied with pH and manometry simultaneously, reflux episodes rarely correlated with decreased LES pressures. Rather, the majority of reflux episodes occurred during transient LES relaxations, and no reflux episodes were identified during LES relaxation after swallowing with normal peristaltic sequence.[24,25] There continues to be growing support that these transient LES relaxations are the primary mechanism for GER.

In summary, although the barrier function of the LES is imperfect, it can be highly effective. Short LES length, abnormal smooth muscle function, increased frequency of transient LES relaxations, and LES location within the chest can contribute individually (or in combination) to LES failure and GER.

Another barrier to the development of symptomatic GER is the intra-abdominal length of the esophagus.[26] Although no absolute effective intra-abdominal esophageal length has been identified that prevents GER, correlation between several lengths and GER have been identified. In one report, an intra-abdominal length of 3–4.5 cm in adults with normal abdominal pressure provided LES competency 100% of the time.[22] A length of 3 cm was sufficient in preventing reflux in 64% of individuals, whereas less than 1 cm of intra-abdominal esophagus resulted in reflux in 81% of patients. It is believed that failure to mobilize adequate esophageal length for intra-abdominal positioning during antireflux operations can lead to less than successful results or recurrent GER in adults. However, we now know these data are not applicable in infants and children and that complete mobilization of the esophagus, in the absence of a hiatal hernia, is detrimental in infants and children through the results of a multicenter, prospective, randomized trial.[27]

A third barrier to reflux is the angle of His, which is the angle at which the esophagus enters the stomach. The usual orientation is that of an acute angle, which creates a flap valve at the gastroesophageal junction. Although the actual functional component of the angle of His is not well known, it has been shown to provide resistance to GER. Experimentally, when this angle is more obtuse, GER is more prone to develop. Conversely, accentuation of the angle inhibits GER.[28]

The ability of the angle of His to prevent GER may be diminished as a result of abnormal development or may be iatrogenic, as occurs after gastrostomy placement.

When a normal angle of His is present, there is a convoluted fold of mucosa present at the gastroesophageal junction. This mucosa creates a rosette-like configuration that collapses on itself with increases in intragastric pressure or negative pressure in the thoracic esophagus, thus acting as an additional weak antireflux valve.[29,30]

Patients with increased abdominal pressure as a result of neurologically related retching, physiologic effects (obesity, ascites, peritoneal dialysis), or anatomic abnormalities (gastroschisis, omphalocele, CDH) are at increased risk for developing GERD owing to the effects of chronic pressure from the abdomen into the thorax.[31–37] Finally, certain congenital defects such as congenital short esophagus, congenital hiatal hernia, and EA/TEF predispose to GERD. In patients with EA/TEF, the esophagus has abnormal peristalsis and the LES is incompetent. It has been reported that up to 30% of these patients will require antireflux surgery after repair of their EA/TEF.[38–40] Regarding CDH, anatomic abnormalities of the esophageal hiatus and the esophagus predispose to GERD, with 15–20% of surviving patients undergoing an antireflux operation for GERD.[35–37]

Once the barrier to GER has been overcome (or failed), mechanisms for esophageal clearance become important in preventing damage associated with exposure of the esophageal mucosa to the gastric refluxate. The primary mechanism for esophageal clearance remains esophageal motility. However, gravity and saliva contribute to the ability of the esophagus to clear the refluxate.[41,42] There are three types of esophageal contractions: primary, secondary, and tertiary. Primary contraction waves are initiated with swallowing and are responsible for the clearance of refluxed contents in 80–90% of reflux episodes. Secondary waves occur when material is refluxed into the esophagus and clearance is required, especially when the reflux occurs during sleep.[43,44] Tertiary waves have nothing to do with esophageal clearance and are sporadic, non-propagating contractions. When impaired esophageal motility is present as a result of abnormal smooth muscle function, impaired vagal stimulation, or obstruction, refluxed gastric contents are not moved caudad into the stomach in a timely manner. This prolonged exposure can lead to esophageal mucosal injury and can potentiate the motility disturbance due to vagal and/or smooth muscle inflammation or injury. Saliva neutralizes refluxed material, and patients with GERD have been found to have decreased salivary function. It has also been shown that positional effects of GERD treatment may be related to gravity assisting in the clearance of esophageal refluxate.[45–48]

The final element for prevention of esophageal injury related to GERD is the ability to limit injury once refluxed contents have reached the esophagus. In addition to functioning as a neutralizing agent, saliva also aids in lubricating the esophageal contents, thus making it easier to clear any retained refluxate. Acid exposure has traditionally been postulated to cause the most significant injury, but more recent data has also implicated alkaline bile reflux as well.[20,49] Some pediatric patients with documented GERD have been shown to have increased acid secretion.[50,51] To this end, the role of PPIs in controlling GERD in this population is very important because they have the dual effect of increasing the gastric pH while simultaneously decreasing the acid volume.[52–54] However, it is now recognized that some children with GERD have normal pH probe studies and acid reflux with esophageal injury is not as big an issue for this subset of patients as is poor nutrition and pulmonary complications. Other substances that increase esophageal mucosal injury include bile salts, pepsin, and trypsin. When combined with acid, bile salts are injurious to the esophageal mucosa by increasing the permeability of the esophageal mucosa to existing acid, thus further potentiating injury.[55,56] Pepsin and trypsin are both proteolytic enzymes that can injure the esophageal mucosa. Both of these enzymes are more toxic at lower pH levels and, hence, are more injurious in the presence of acid.[57,58]

CLINICAL MANIFESTATIONS

The presentation of GERD in infants and children is variable and depends on the patient's age and overall medical condition. The surgeon must consider both this variability and the patient characteristics when evaluating a child with symptoms for possible GERD. Although the symptoms of GERD are variable for each patient, the actual frequency of symptoms seen in infants who have required surgical intervention for GERD has been reported (Table 28-2).[59]

When considering the symptoms associated with GERD, persistent regurgitation is the most common complaint reported by parents of children with GERD.[60] However, in infants, vomiting is often physiologic and can be 'normal.' This type of vomiting is termed *chalasia of infancy* and is seen early in life, usually during burping, after feeding, or when placed in the recumbent position.[61] Chalasia does not interfere with normal growth or development and rarely leads to other complications. It is a self-limited process with most infants transitioning to being asymptomatic by 2 years of age or near the time of initiating solid foods.[1] No treatment is necessary in patients who have chalasia, and no diagnostic evaluation should be pursued. However, when persistent regurgitation is the result of GER, it can lead to complications, including significant malnutrition and growth failure due to insufficient caloric intake.

In infants, another presenting symptom is irritability due to pain. Painful esophagitis can be the result of the acid refluxate. Discomfort leads to crying despite consoling measures.[62,63] Occasionally, small volumes of feeds

---

TABLE 28-2 Frequency of Symptoms in Patients with Gastroesophageal Reflux

Symptom	Frequency (%)
Regurgitation/vomiting	81
Pulmonary symptoms	41
Dysphagia/pain	30
Hemorrhage	7

Adapted from Tovar JA, Olivares P, Diaz M, et al. Functional results of laparoscopic fundoplication in children. J Pediatr Gastroenterol Nutr 1998;26:429–31.

briefly assist in alleviating pain. However, this is generally not a lasting effect.[24,25] In contrast to infants, children with GERD more often present with complaints of pain. As in adults, the pain is retrosternal in nature, and often described as heartburn. Long-standing GERD with esophagitis can lead to chronic inflammation or even ulcer formation with eventual scarring and stricture. Dysphagia develops as a result of a narrowed esophageal lumen, as well as possible esophageal dysmotility secondary to long-standing mucosal inflammation. Obstructive symptoms and pain are the two most common associated complaints when an esophageal stricture is present.[64,65]

Barrett esophagitis is a premalignant condition that is associated with prolonged GERD. It occurs when metaplasia develops in the esophageal squamous epithelium that is replaced with columnar epithelium. In adults, it is thought to be the result of chronic esophageal injury. Whether it develops from gastric acid injury or exposure to alkaline bile reflux is currently a controversial topic.[66-68] Although uncommon in infants and children, when it does develop, serious complications often result. In addition to the increased risk for adenocarcinoma, approximately 50% of these patients will develop stricture and many patients will develop ulcers.[69,70] Aggressive GERD management, along with vigilant long-term surveillance via yearly esophagogastroscopy, must be pursued to minimize these often difficult and possibly fatal complications.

Respiratory symptoms are commonly seen in infants and children. Delineating the role of GER as an etiologic agent for ongoing respiratory complaints can be difficult because of the similarity of the symptoms that are seen with other pulmonary diseases and the fact that primary aspiration from oropharyngeal dysmotility may be the inciting factor not GER. Chronic cough, wheezing, choking, apnea, or near sudden infant death syndrome (SIDS) can all be symptoms attributable to GER. Recurrent bronchitis or pneumonia can occur from aspiration of the refluxate.[71] Esophageal stimulation via acidification of the esophageal mucosa causes vagally mediated laryngospasm and bronchospasm, which clinically presents as apnea or choking or mistakenly as asthma.[72,73] Esophageal inflammation, as seen with esophagitis, likely enhances this mechanism.[74,75] The effects of GER on premature infants with respiratory problems have been studied.[76] Most of these infants were intubated for varying periods owing to respiratory distress syndrome or bronchopulmonary dysplasia. In the former group, GERD was responsible for a deteriorating pulmonary status requiring intubation. In the latter, deterioration of pulmonary status plus failure to thrive and anorexia led to the diagnosis of GERD. All improved with correction of the GERD.[77]

Although uncommon, hemorrhage can be a presenting symptom of GERD. Esophagitis, gastritis, and ulcer formation can lead to hematochezia or melena in a small percentage of infants or children.[59]

DIAGNOSTIC EVALUATION

As noted in the previous section, the clinical history is an invaluable asset when evaluating for the presence of GERD and determining the need for antireflux therapy. Once the concern for GER as the etiologic cause of the patient's complaints has been raised, diagnostic evaluation should be initiated. The aim is not only to determine the presence or absence of GERD, but to also ensure that there are no other etiologies such as oropharyngeal dysmotility, esophageal dysmotility, esophageal web, gastric outlet obstruction, or food allergies.

Upper gastrointestinal radiography is the most frequent initial study employed. Evidence for reflux is seen in up to 50% of the examinations.[78,79] However, the absence of reflux is an extremely poor indicator of GERD as a cause of the patient's symptoms. Furthermore, the presence of reflux on an upper gastrointestinal series does not necessarily indicate pathologic GER. The contrast study is most useful for delineating the anatomy of the esophagus and esophagogastric junction. It also evaluates esophageal clearance and assesses esophageal and gastric motility. The contrast study can identify the presence of esophageal strictures, webs, or distal obstructions, such as duodenal obstruction, antral web, or malrotation, as the cause of the reflux symptoms—which may be the case in 4% of patients.[80] These correctable, anatomic causes for GER are critical to rule out before pursuing further studies.

Twenty-four hour pH probe monitoring has been considered the gold standard in diagnosing GERD since the 1980s when DeMeester established scores that correlated with the presence or absence of GERD.[81-83] Boix-Ochoa later proposed a revised score that was applicable to pediatric patients aged 2 months to 3 years old that is still used today.[84] Currently, the 24-hour pH probe monitoring study is recommended in infants with respiratory symptoms, especially ALTE spells or apneic events; infants who are irritable with intractable crying and anorexia; infants and children with reactive airway disease or recurrent pneumonia; and children unresponsive to medical measures in whom GER is suspected. Special considerations should be given to those children who become symptomatic after fundoplication. Conversely, the study generally is not useful or necessary for infants with uncomplicated regurgitation, children with esophagitis already diagnosed by endoscopy and biopsy, and children with dysphagia or heartburn thought to be caused by GER.

The pH study is performed by placing an electrode 2–3 cm proximal to the gastroesophageal junction and measuring the pH in the distal esophagus. The accuracy of the pH examination is dependent on the cessation of all antireflux medication: PPIs should be withheld for seven days, and histamine receptor blockers are stopped 48 hours before the study. A reflux episode is considered to have occurred if the esophageal pH is recorded as less than 4. Ideally, the examination should occur over an uninterrupted 24-hour period. The pH is continuously monitored via the esophageal electrode while the patient's position (upright, supine, prone) and activities (awake, asleep, eating) are simultaneously recorded. The final score is calculated based on the percent of total time that the pH was less than 4, the total number of reflux episodes, the number of episodes lasting longer than 5 minutes, and the longest reflux episode.[85,86]

Data from the pH probe monitoring has increased our understanding of GER and taught us that not all GER is acidic. Three patterns of reflux have been described in symptomatic infants, as determined by extended esophageal pH monitoring: continuous, discontinuous, and mixed.[87] Those infants with the discontinuous type rarely required an antireflux operation, whereas approximately half of those with the other two types did. One should keep in mind that medical treatment at the time of this study was much less effective than it is currently. Nonetheless, this study indicates that pH monitoring can be useful in sorting out infants with GER who may or may not require an antireflux procedure.[88,89] Incidentally, all of the infants in this study, including the 'normal controls,' experienced reflux frequently in the first two hours after being given apple juice.

It has been assumed that the retrograde flow of acid/pepsin material from the stomach into the esophagus is the basic pathologic event of reflux disease. It is becoming clear that the situation is not this straightforward which suggests that pH probe monitoring may not be diagnostic in all cases of GERD. Attempts to correlate symptoms (other than spitting up and vomiting) to pH probe-detected reflux episodes have been particularly problematic. For example, in infants with spells of choking or colic, a close association between pH probe-detected acid reflux and these symptoms cannot be routinely demonstrated. Some spells coincide with reflux episodes, but many do not. Similar questions can be raised when looking at pH probe data on the relation between acid reflux episodes and apnea/bradycardia spells of premature infants or between wheezing, coughing, dental erosion, sleep disturbance, and all the other myriad symptoms attributed to reflux.

The etiology for this non-acid reflux is likely to be due to the infant diet and buffering. The infant is not capable of acidifying their gastric secretions to the extent that older children and adults are.[90,91] Probe data from infants showed that gastric pH was <4 for 15% of the time in infants compared to a pH <4 for 42% of the time in older children.[92] Furthermore, the infant's milk-based diet serves as a buffer altering the pH of the gastric contents. This effect was investigated by measuring gastric pH after feeds whereby the gastric pH was >4 for a mean time of 130 minutes post-feeding.[93]

By using one 'old' diagnostic technique and one 'new' one, some of the disparities between pH probe observations and 'events' may be better understood. This is based on the observation that some reflux of acid into the lower esophagus occurs while the intraesophageal pH is still less than 4 due to a traditional acid reflux episode. This is called 'acid re-reflux' (ARR) and will be missed by using only pH-monitoring techniques.[94] ARR is most likely to occur in patients with severe esophagitis, postprandially, and in the recumbent posture. It is now thought to be a common cause of prolonged acid contact. Detecting ARR provides a better estimation of the incompetence of the antireflux barrier than does traditional pH probe evaluations.

Two methods may be used to evaluate ARR. The first is scintigraphy, which directly measures radiolabeled liquid gastric contents flowing into the esophagus, independent of the pH of the refluxate or the esophageal lumen. The second is multichannel intraluminal impedance (MII), a method that recognizes the flow of gastric contents into the esophagus by detecting decreases in impedance from high (the esophagus) to low (the stomach) values across electrode pairs placed throughout the esophagus and in the stomach. The presence of acid, therefore, is also completely irrelevant with this diagnostic tool which can be performed at the same time as pH probe monitoring. Furthermore, MII also can distinguish liquid from gas refluxate.[95–97]

Recent studies using MII support the concept that measuring acid reflux (pH study) may not be the best method of evaluating GERD.[98–101] These studies reaffirm that the pH probe does not simultaneously detect the majority of reflux events as defined by impedance monitoring, presumably because the re-reflux boluses are not acidic. When MII and pH monitoring are used simultaneously, there are significant reflux episodes that are not identified with pH monitoring alone because the episodes are actually non-acid reflux episodes with a pH greater than 4.[99] These nonacid reflux episodes are less common in untreated GERD patients than in normal patients. MII has shown that GERD patients more commonly have liquid-type reflux events, whereas non-GERD patients generally have more gas-type reflux events.[100] Additionally, MII data suggest that treatment with PPIs does not decrease the amount of reflux but rather converts the reflux to non-acid or weakly acidic in nature.[101]

Although essential in adults, esophageal manometry is infrequently utilized in the pediatric population. When employed, the study measures the motility of the esophagus and the pressure at the LES via a multiple-port pressure transducer placed in the esophagus and traversing the LES. The clinical data accumulated in adult patients have revealed several important points that are likely applicable to infants and children with GERD. First, it has been shown that pharyngeal swallowing and primary peristaltic contractions are responsible for the majority of the esophageal clearance of refluxed gastric contents, rather than by secondary and tertiary peristalsis as previously believed.[102] Additionally, through the use of a concomitant 24-hour pH study and esophageal manometry, it has been shown that there is a direct relationship between worsening esophagitis secondary to GERD and deterioration of esophageal motility. Manometric evaluation has been particularly useful in documenting abnormal distal esophageal motility in infants after repair of EA/TEF.[103] It is hoped that, as technology continues to provide more appropriately sized instruments for sophisticated manometric studies in infants and children, the usefulness and feasibility of such studies will increase our knowledge of the physiology and abnormalities associated with GERD in this population.

Endoscopic evaluation of the esophagus and stomach is occasionally needed in the diagnosis of GERD in infants and children. Hematemesis, dysphagia, irritability in infants, or dysphagia with or without heartburn in children, should prompt esophagogastroscopy to determine if esophagitis is present. Other complications, such as ulcer formation, esophageal stricture, and Barrett esophagus, can also be diagnosed during the endoscopic examination. Mucosal biopsy should be performed to stage the severity of esophagitis or to histologically exclude dysplasia or malignancy in Barrett esophagus.[104,105]

The relationship between delayed gastric emptying (DGE) and GERD in infants and children has been extensively studied and continues to be one of the more controversial aspects of antireflux surgery. The evaluation for DGE is undertaken using radionuclide scanning via a technetium-99-labeled meal. When documented preoperatively, DGE has not been shown to significantly improve when an emptying procedure is performed at the time of an antireflux procedure.[106] In fact, one study evaluating patients with DGE undergoing fundoplication showed significantly improved gastric emptying for both solids and liquids after fundoplication alone.[107] Neurologically impaired children with GERD have been shown to have DGE more often than neurologically normal children. Conflicting data regarding the benefit and complication rates for these patients undergoing emptying procedures at the time of their fundoplication have been reported as well.[108] Based on these data, it is not recommended that an emptying procedure be performed for a patient with DGE and GERD unless a second operative intervention would place the patient at significant morbidity or mortality.

At our institution, the evaluation for GERD usually includes an upper gastrointestinal contrast study to evaluate for normal anatomy and no evidence of malrotation. We are moving away from using the pH probe in favor of clinical symptoms of GER, even utilizing nasogastric feeding trials with close clinical observation. If there is still uncertainty about the diagnosis, a pH probe/impedance study is performed. The main exception is the baby with significant underlying airway disease in the neonatal intensive care unit who needs a gastrostomy for feeding and for whom the intensivists request a fundoplication to protect the airway from aspiration. The neurologically impaired infant requiring a gastrostomy may be another exception. Esophagogastroscopy and esophageal manometry are employed only when circumstances suggest that the information they will provide will dictate changes in the operative management. An example of this situation is the patient with symptoms of GER but a normal pH study. When esophagitis or other complications of GERD are found after esophagogastroscopy or manometry, surgical intervention is usually recommended. Preoperative gastric emptying studies are not performed on a routine basis, primarily owing to the improvement that has been seen and reported in gastric emptying after fundoplication.[106,107] If symptoms of DGE persist after antireflux surgery, gastric emptying studies can be performed with a subsequent emptying procedure, if necessary. However, all patients requiring a second fundoplication undergo an emptying study to be sure their recurrent symptoms are not exacerbated by DGE.

TREATMENT

Once GERD has been diagnosed, the question becomes: should medical or surgical treatment be applied?[15] This

decision needs to be individualized based on the patient's age, anatomic information, disease severity, and social environment (which will affect compliance with a treatment regimen). In the majority of cases, nonoperative treatment is the initial therapy of choice.

Medical Management

Position and Feeding

Nonoperative therapy for GERD in infants and children has been based on postural changes and dietary modification for many years. It is important to know the caloric needs of the patient so that a reduction in feeding volume in an attempt to limit reflux does not result in caloric deprivation. Postural and dietary modifications alone will result in clinical improvement in the vast majority of infants with GERD.[109,110] In older children, dietary alterations should include a diet low in fat and the elimination of chocolate, coffee, tea, carbonated drinks, and spicy foods.

The seated semi-upright position (approximately 45°) for an infant with reflux has been recommended since the 1950s. In the 1960s, Carré showed that 60% of children with GERD treated in this way improved by approximately 2 years of age and an additional 30% improved by age 4 years.[1,111]

Failure of postural therapy may be related to social problems, chronic infections, or impaired gastric clearance. In older patients, postural treatment is impractical because of the virtual impossibility of maintaining the desired semi-sitting posture for sleep. Close attention to the details of postural therapy by the family members is most important to its success.[112]

Pharmacologic Therapy

If symptoms persist despite a well-monitored program of postural therapy and dietary modifications, pharmacologic measures should be added. Medical therapy includes the administration of one or more drugs that increase esophageal peristalsis, increase LES pressure, increase gastric emptying, or lessen gastric acid production.

Prokinetic Agents

Historically, prokinetic agents have been utilized in an attempt to increase LES pressure, enhance esophageal peristalsis, and accelerate gastric emptying. The use of cisapride and, more recently, metoclopramide has been questioned with regard to their safety.[113-115] In fact, cisapride is no longer available due to safety concerns. Both randomized controlled trials and meta-analyses have shown no clinically relevant improvement in children receiving cisapride or metoclopramide.[113,114,116,117] Therefore, the current recommendation regarding prokinetic agents in the management of GERD is that there is no beneficial effect and their use is not advantageous.

Acid Alteration

Measures to reduce gastric acidity should be undertaken for patients with complicated acid reflux, especially with esophagitis.[118] Alterations in gastric acid may be accomplished by neutralization with antacids, by competition with histamine-2 (H$_2$)-receptor antagonists, or by PPIs. Because of the superiority of PPIs in controlling acid production, H$_2$-receptor antagonists or antacids are being utilized less frequently.

PPIs inhibit the final step of gastric acid secretion by blocking proton production by bonding and deactivating H$^+$, K$^+$-ATPase (or proton pump) by traversing the parietal cell membrane and accumulating in the secretory canaliculi.[119] The PPI omeprazole has been demonstrated to reduce gastric acid production to zero.[120–122] It is a very powerful medicine that affects gastric acid production for 72 hours after cessation of administration. A prospective study determined that, within the therapeutic dose range (0.7–3.5 mg/kg/day), omeprazole was both efficacious and safe for children.[121] In this study, omeprazole was found to be highly effective in severe (grade IV) esophagitis and patients refractory to other medical therapy. A dosage of 0.7 mg/kg/day healed 45% of patients, and 1.4 mg/kg/day healed another 30%. On a body weight basis, the dosages required in children are generally higher than those in adults.[122] For children unable to swallow the whole capsule, it is suggested to open the capsule and give the granular contents in a weakly acidic vehicle such as orange juice, yogurt, or cranberry juice. The granules are stable in acid but are degraded in a neutral or alkaline pH. Multiple PPIs are now available. However, the use of PPIs is limited to acid reflux and will have no benefit for the patient with non-acid reflux.

Operative Management

Operative management usually follows failed medical management for growth failure (failure to thrive or gain weight appropriately), most respiratory symptoms, and other symptoms such as pain and esophagitis. However, in selected circumstances, it may be best to proceed with fundoplication without a trial of medical therapy. These select situations include the previously mentioned patient in an intensive care unit with underlying respiratory disease who requires gastrostomy and possibly the neurologically impaired patient with a similar need for gastrostomy and concern for aspiration. This latter scenario is commonly seen in infants and children, and the decision for or against fundoplication at the time of gastrostomy should be individualized. For example, in a 2- or 3-year-old (or older) neurologically impaired patient who begins to have difficulty with oral intake and requires tube feedings but has no reflux symptoms, gastrostomy alone without fundoplication is very reasonable. On the other hand, a neurologically impaired infant who cannot swallow and requires tube feedings in the intensive care unit due to respiratory disease probably should have a fundoplication in addition to a gastrostomy. We have found that a trial of nasogastric feeds can be helpful in determining which neurologically impaired patient, with the need for gastrostomy due to poor oral intake, would also benefit from a fundoplication. With the laparoscopic placement of gastrostomy buttons, we have not found any particular difficulties in performing a laparoscopic fundoplication later if needed.

Another scenario is the infant who presents with an ALTE spell and GER is documented but no other etiology is identified. This patient may be best served with a fundoplication as the initial therapy. In a review from our institution involving 81 infants presenting with ALTE, their symptoms resolved with fundoplication in 78.[123] The median follow-up in this study was 1,738 days. Two required a second fundoplication when their symptoms recurred, and one needed a pyloromyotomy. Interestingly, 96.3% of these patients had been treated with antireflux mediation and 87.7% were taking antireflux medications at the time of their ALTE. Therefore, medical management may not be effective in this population.

Barrett esophagitis and esophageal stricture are the two other conditions in which initial operative therapy is recommended. The changes of Barrett esophagus will usually resolve in adolescents after fundoplication, although life-long postoperative endoscopic surveillance is still needed. Regarding a stricture, dilation can be performed at the time of fundoplication. Subsequent dilations may be needed in severe cases. Finally, children with a known hiatal hernia and symptomatic GER are not likely to respond to medical management. Initial fundoplication is a reasonable choice in these patients.

Laparoscopic Nissen Fundoplication

The patient is placed at the end of the operating table so that the surgeon can stand at the foot of the bed and the assistant to his or her right. The scrub nurse stands to the surgeon's left (Fig. 28-2). For infants, the legs should be placed in a frog-leg position. For older children, the lithotomy position can be used with stirrups. Neurologically impaired children may have contractures that preclude lithotomy, and careful consideration should be given to ensure they have appropriate padding of their pressure points. Although a single monitor placed over the patient's head is usually sufficient, two monitors, placed to the right and the left of the patient's head, can be used as well. An orogastric tube is introduced by the anesthesiologist to decompress the stomach. The bladder is usually emptied using a Credé maneuver.

After prepping and draping, a 5 mm vertical incision is made in the center of the umbilicus and carried down through the umbilical fascia. A Step sheath (Covidien, Mansfield, MA) is gently introduced into the abdominal cavity, followed by introduction of a cannula with a blunt-tipped trocar through the sheath. By using this open technique, injury to the underlying viscera should be extremely rare. The sheath can be secured to the umbilical skin for stabilization should the surgeon desire. A pneumoperitoneum is created to a pressure of 12–15 mmHg, and diagnostic laparoscopy is performed with a 5 mm, 45°-angled telescope. Four stab incisions are then placed in infants, and three stab incisions and a 5 mm port for the ultrasonic scalpel are utilized in children older than 5 years of age. The arrangement of these cannulas is seen in Figure 28-3. A liver retractor is introduced through the lateral right port. The two main working sites are the instruments positioned on either side of the midline. The assistant's instrument is in the patient's left lateral abdomen.

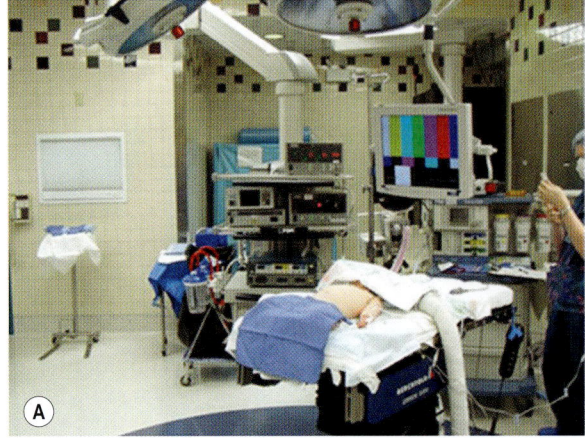

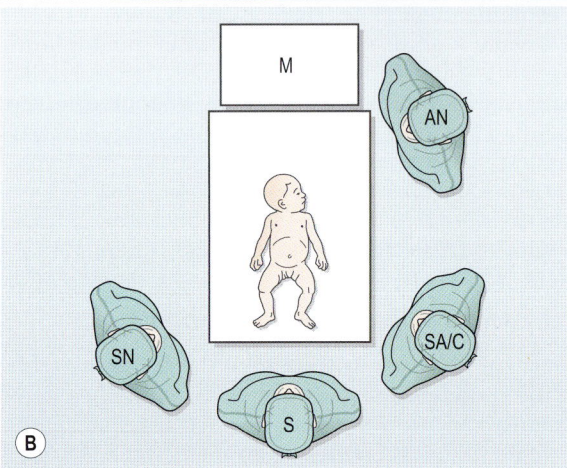

FIGURE 28-2 ■ For laparoscopic fundoplication, the patient is placed supine on the operating table. Infants and young children are positioned at the foot of the bed in a frog-leg position and the foot of the bed is dropped. The surgeon (S) and surgical assistant/camera holder (SA/C) stand next to the patient at the end of the bed. The scrub nurse (SN) is to the surgeon's left. A single monitor (M) is placed over the patient's head. AN, anesthesiologist. (Adapted from Holcomb GW III. Laparoscopic Nissen fundoplication. In: Holcomb GW, Georgeson KE, Rothenberg SS, editors. Atlas of Pediatric Laparoscopy and Thoracoscopy. Philadelphia: Elsevier; 2008. p. 15–20.)

We have standardized our technique and have utilized it for the past 12 years.[124–129] Initially, the superior short gastric vessels are ligated and divided. Electrocautery connected to a Maryland dissecting instrument is used in the younger patients. As previously mentioned, the ultrasonic scalpel is used in older children. The retroesophageal window is initially made from the patient's left side because it is easy to accomplish after mobilization and ligation of the superior short gastric vessels. We do not mobilize the esophagus very much to help reduce postoperative transmigration of the fundoplication wrap. (This will be discussed later.) Once the left side of the patient's gastroesophageal junction has been identified, the stomach is flipped to the patient's left and attention is turned toward the right aspect of the esophagus and upper stomach. The gastrohepatic ligament is incised to expose the esophagus and stomach on the right side. Great care must be taken to always know the location of the left gastric artery. It is imperative that the fundoplication wrap is positioned above the left gastric artery rather than inferior to it. The opening in the retroesophageal window is then completed from the right side so that the fundus can be brought through posteriorly for the Nissen fundoplication. Again, as little esophageal mobilization as possible is performed at the gastroesophageal junction (Fig. 28-4).

At this point, usually a single suture is placed posterior to the esophagus to close a small hiatal hernia that may have either been present initially or created during the dissection. This is usually accomplished with a 2-0 silk suture. After placement of this suture and tying it, a small bite of the esophagus at the 7 o'clock position is then taken with the same needle and tied to help obliterate the space between the posterior esophagus and the posterior crural closure. Next, esophagocrural sutures are then created with 3-0 silk at the 8, 11, 1, and 5 o'clock positions to further obliterate the space between the esophagus and the crura to prevent transmigration of the fundoplication wrap (Fig. 28-5).[127] However, the utility

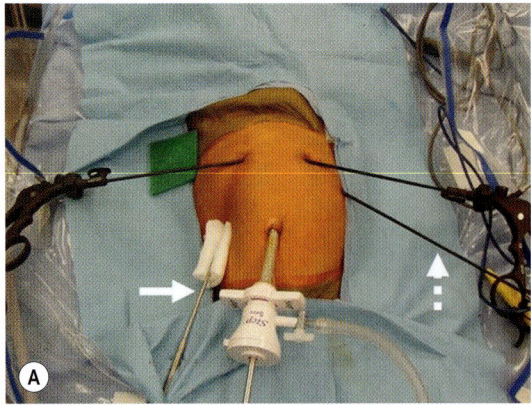
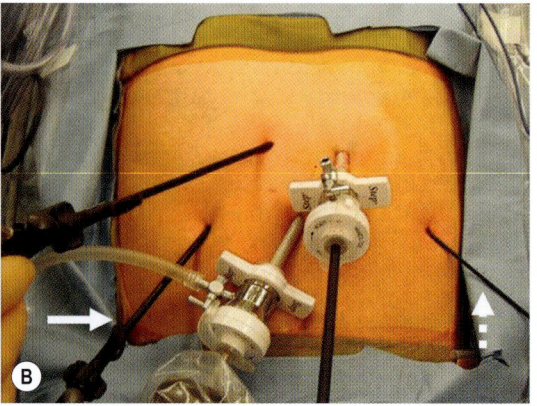

FIGURE 28-3 ■ There are a number of ways to orient the instruments when performing a laparoscopic fundoplication. With our technique, a 45°-angled, 5 mm telescope is introduced after insertion of the 5 mm umbilical cannula. The liver retractor is introduced in the patient's right subcostal region (solid arrow). The two main working ports are in the left and right epigastrium. The main working port for the surgeon is the one in the patient's left epigastric region. It is through this incision that dissecting instruments, needle holder, and suture are introduced. The instrument utilized by the surgical assistant is in the patient's left subcostal region (dotted arrow). The stab incision technique can be utilized for both **(A)** infants and **(B)** adolescents. (From Holcomb GW III. Laparoscopic Nissen fundoplication. In: Holcomb GW, Georgeson KE, Rothenberg SS, editors. Atlas of Pediatric Laparoscopy and Thoracoscopy. Philadelphia: Elsevier; 2008. p. 15–20.)

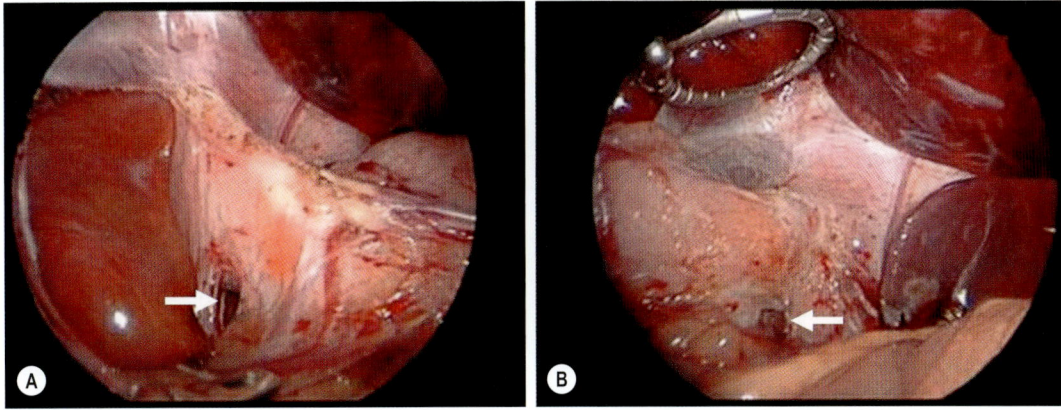

FIGURE 28-4 ■ If an adequate length of intra-abdominal esophagus is present, then as little dissection as possible is performed to help prevent migration of the fundoplication wrap through an enlarged esophageal hiatus. The phrenoesophageal ligament is kept intact on both the patient's **(A)** right side and **(B)** left side of the esophagus. Note creation of the retroesophageal window has been initiated (*arrows*). (From Holcomb GW III. Laparoscopic Nissen fundoplication. In: Holcomb GW, Georgeson KE, Rothenberg SS, editors. Atlas of Pediatric Laparoscopy and Thoracoscopy. Philadelphia: Elsevier; 2008. p. 15–20.)

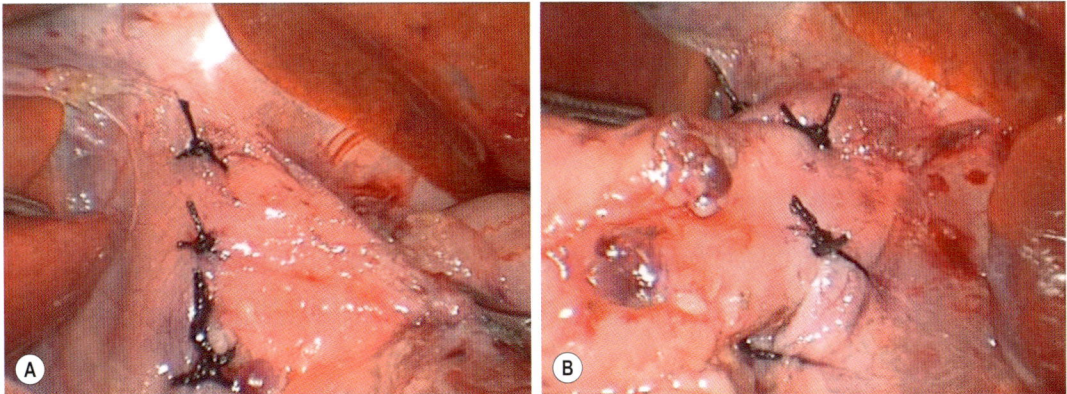

FIGURE 28-5 ■ Following closure of the esophageal hiatus with a 2-0 silk suture placed posterior to the esophagus, esophagocrural sutures are placed at the 8, 11, 1, and 5 o'clock positions around the esophagus. These photographs show the **(A)** right and **(B)** left sides of the patient's esophagus. The purpose of these sutures is to secure the esophagus in the intra-abdominal position to reduce the incidence of postoperative reflux and also to obliterate the space between the esophagus and crura in an effort to prevent transmigration of the fundoplication wrap.

of these stitches is not known if the phrenoesophageal membrane is preserved. After placement of these crural sutures, the bougie is then introduced. A table describing the appropriate bougie size for neonates weighing less than 15 kg has been developed and validated (Table 28-3).[124] The fundoplication is then performed using a standard Nissen technique. Usually, three 2-0 sutures are utilized to perform the fundoplication. The most superior suture also incorporates a small portion of the anterior esophagus to anchor the wrap around the intra-abdominal esophagus. The length of the fundoplication is measured. Usually a length of approximately 2 cm is desired.[124] For older children, 2.5–3.0 cm may be appropriate.

Bupivacaine is instilled in the incisions, and the umbilical fascia and skin are closed. Steri-strips are usually utilized for closure of the stab incisions.

Gastrostomy

If a gastrostomy is also needed, the stab incision or cannula site in the patient's left mid-epigastric area is the

TABLE 28-3 Recommended Bougie Size for Esophageal Calibration in Patients Weighing Less Than 15 kg

Weight (kg)	Bougie Size
2.5–4.0	20–24
4.0–5.5	24–28
5.5–7.0	28–32
7.0–8.5	32–34
8.5–10.0	34–36
10.0–15.0	36–40

From Ostlie DJ, Miller KA, Holcomb GW III. Effective Nissen fundoplication length and bougie diameter size in young children undergoing laparoscopic Nissen fundoplication. J Pediatr Surg 2002;37:1664–6.

one utilized for exteriorization of the gastrostomy button. If a fundoplication has not been performed, then the same site is used for locating the button. In either event, this site is marked before insufflation so as not to distort its location when the abdomen is distended with CO_2 to keep the gastrostomy off of the costal margin.

A red rubber catheter is introduced by the anesthesiologist into the stomach which is then insufflated with 30–60 mL of air to prevent incorporating the back wall of the stomach with the suture utilized to secure the stomach to the anterior abdominal wall. The anterior wall of the stomach is grasped with a locking grasper and brought toward the anterior abdominal wall. The technique for laparoscopic gastrostomy is seen in Figure 28-6. Two 2-0 PDS sutures (Ethicon, Inc., Somerville, NJ) are placed through the anterior abdominal wall cephalad to the grasper, through the stomach, and out through the anterior abdominal wall inferior to the instrument that has been used to grasp the stomach. Next, a needle followed by a guide wire is introduced through the abdominal wall and stomach in the center of the square formed by the two PDS sutures. Dilators from a Cook Vascular Dilator Set (Cook, Inc., Bloomington, IN) are used to serially dilate the anterior abdominal wall and gastrotomy. In infants, a 16 French dilator is usually the largest needed. In older children, the 20 French dilator may be required. The gastrostomy button is then placed over the guide wire and into the stomach. Under visualization, the balloon on the Mic-Key (Ballard Medical Products, Draper, UT) gastrostomy button is inflated. Attention must be paid to be sure that the button is, in fact, in the stomach and not external to the stomach (Fig. 28-7). This can also be confirmed with the angled telescope by looking around each side of the stomach with the button in place. The PDS sutures are then secured over the button to prevent its dislodgement. Our protocol is to cut these sutures in five days. Others may cut them sooner. This technique was initially described by Georgeson and Owings, and details about complications have been published.[130,131]

Postoperative Care

Postoperatively, if a gastrostomy button was placed with the fundoplication (or if a button was placed primarily), feedings are usually started several hours later and advanced over the evening and the next morning. Most (90%) patients are ready for discharge the day after the operation. The parents will have been instructed on the use of the gastrostomy during the patient's 24-hour hospitalization and can advance the feedings as needed. The patient can also be seen in the clinic should further questions or issues arise.

If the patient did not need a gastrostomy, then liquids are allowed several hours after the procedure. It is very important to mention to the family that there is initial

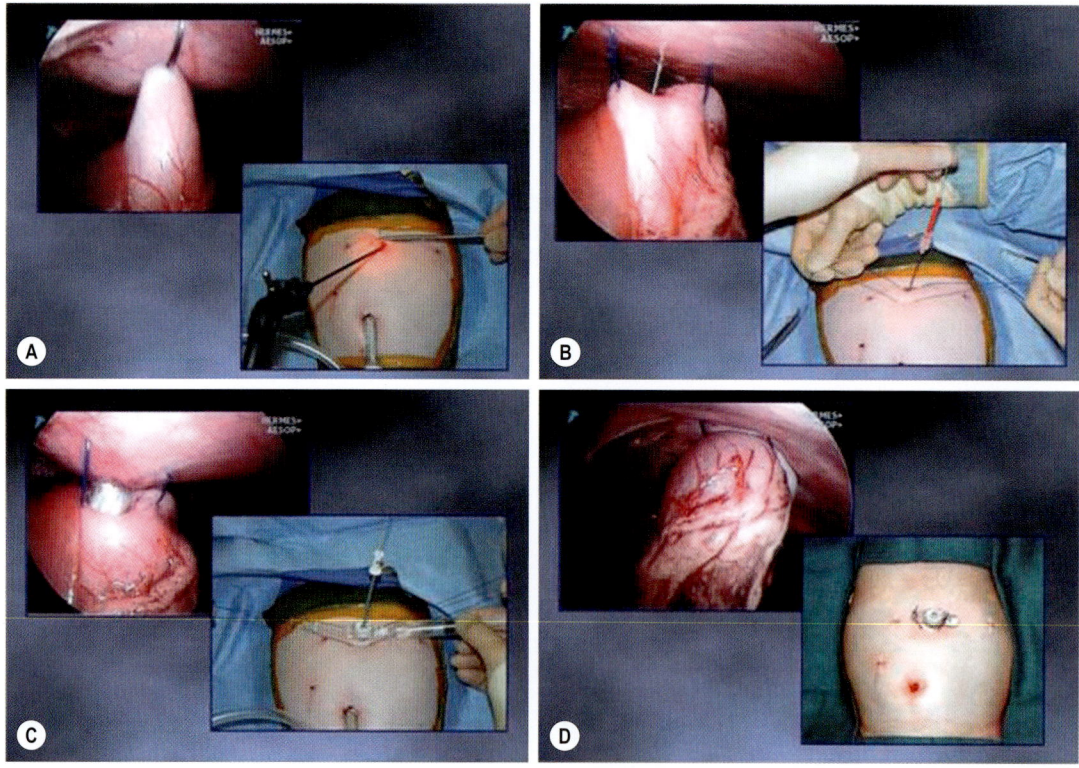

FIGURE 28-6 ■ **(A)** After approximation of the stomach to the anterior abdominal wall, two sutures of 2-0 or 0 PDS (depending on the patient's age) are placed extracorporeally through the abdominal wall, through the stomach, and out through the abdominal wall inferior to the gastrostomy. **(B)** After placing the extracorporeal sutures, an 18 gauge needle is introduced through the left epigastric incision and into the stomach under direct visualization. Following a rush of air through the needle, a guide wire is inserted through the needle and the needle is removed. With the guide wire in place, the tract is serially dilated using the Cook Vascular Dilator Set (Cook, Inc., Bloomington IN). These dilators come in 8, 12, 16, and 20 French sizes. **(C)** After dilating the tract and gastrostomy with the 20 French dilator, the 8 French dilator is placed through the Mic-Key gastrostomy button and is introduced over the guide wire and into the stomach. **(D)** After placement of the button within the stomach, the balloon on the button is inflated, the guide wire and dilator are removed, and the extracorporeal sutures are tied over the button to secure it to the anterior abdominal wall. (From Holcomb GW III. Gastroesophageal reflux in infants and children. In: Fischer JE, editor. Mastery of Surgery. 5th ed. Philadelphia: Lippincott Williams & Wilkins; 2007. p. 650–1.)

edema around the fundoplication. Therefore, for the first three weeks, especially in older children, the diet should be a mechanical soft diet that has the consistency of pudding, apple sauce, mashed potatoes, and so on. Essentially, meats and pizza should not be allowed because these food substances can become lodged above the fundoplication wrap. After three weeks, the edema usually resolves and small portions of meats and pizza can be added to the diet.

Patients are seen 2 weeks, 3 months, 6 months, and 1 year after the operation. An upper gastrointestinal contrast study is performed at 1 year to evaluate for transmigration of the wrap or any other abnormalities.

Outcomes

Our group has been interested in the efficacy of laparoscopic fundoplication for the past 12 years. A number of articles have been published from our institution detailing our thoughts about indications, complications, the operative technique, and ways to improve our results.[123-129,132-137] Also, there have been several articles published in the last few years looking at long-term outcomes.[138-142]

In early 2002, in looking at our outcomes from January 2000, through March 2002, we believed that the need for repeat fundoplication was higher than desired.[127] In 130 patients undergoing laparoscopic Nissen fundoplication

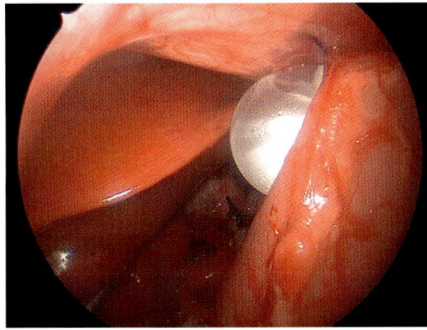

FIGURE 28-7 ■ After the button is introduced into the stomach and inflated, it is very important to insure that the button is, in fact, in the gastric lumen. Often, it is helpful to take an angled telescope (70°) to look around the portion of the stomach that is adherent to the anterior abdominal wall so that one can feel secure that the button is not outside the stomach. In this patient, the button was deflated and removed, and then reinserted correctly.

during that time, the incidence of repeat fundoplication was 12%. All patients who required a repeat operation had transmigration of the fundoplication wrap. During that time period, the esophagus was being extensively mobilized to try to create at least a 2 cm length of intra-abdominal esophagus. Moreover, there was no attempt to obliterate the space between the esophagus and the crura. These principles derived from prior training as well as literature reports in adults.[22,23] Although the operations proceeded nicely and no conversions were needed, this 12% incidence of re-do procedures seemed high. However, historical reports for the open operation have also documented a relatively high incidence of repeat fundoplications from 6–12% (Table 28-4).[60,143-146]

In an attempt to reduce the incidence of postoperative transmigration of the wrap, two modifications were made in our operative technique beginning in April, 2002. First, there was minimal mobilization of the esophagus. It was believed that the main reason for wrap transmigration was that the esophagus was being mobilized and a space was being created between the esophagus and crura to allow for the transmigration to occur. Therefore, the phrenoesophageal membrane was kept intact to obliterate this space. Second, to further reinforce this space, sutures were placed between the esophagus and crura. Initially, only two sutures were used, but eventually four sutures have come to be placed for the purpose of further obliterating this space (see Fig. 28-5). No other modifications in the operative technique were made. In looking at the results from April, 2002, through December, 2004, the incidence of transmigration was reduced to 5%.[121] This was actually reduced even further when looking at the patients in whom four esophageal crural sutures were utilized rather than two or three.

In 2005, conversations with Georgeson and colleagues at the University of Alabama–Birmingham, prompted a prospective, randomized trial looking at the operative technique.[27] It was believed that the efficacy of esophageal mobilization should be evaluated. The primary endpoint was transmigration of the wrap. A power analysis based on the difference between the 12% and 5% repeat fundoplication rate previously mentioned was made, and the study was powered at 360 patients. The patients were randomized on the day of the surgery. One group was randomized to receive minimal esophageal mobilization with placement of four esophagocrural sutures. The other group was randomized to extensive esophageal mobilization to create a 2 cm length of intra-abdominal esophagus along with the four esophagocrural sutures.

TABLE 28-4 Operative Results after Open Operations for Management of GERD

Study	Number of Patients	% Reoperation	Herniation	Wrap Dehiscence	Other
Dedinsky et al. (Indiana)[143] 1975–1985	429	6.7% (29)	29	0	0
Caniano et al. (Ohio State)[144] 1976–1988	358	6% (21)	16	2	3
Wheatley et al. (Michigan)[145] 1974–1989	242	12% (29)	3	14	3
Fonkalsrud et al. (UCLA)[146] 1976–1996	7467	7.1%	Not mentioned	Not mentioned	Not mentioned

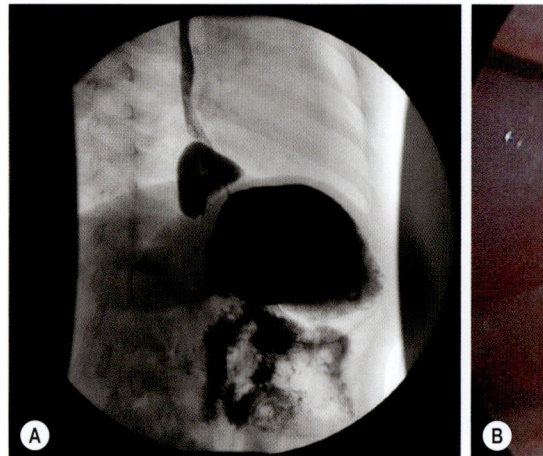
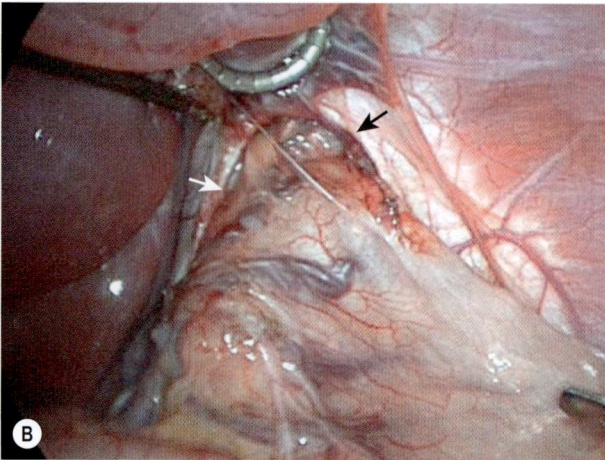

FIGURE 28-8 ■ In 5–10% of patients undergoing laparoscopic fundoplication, reoperation becomes necessary. **(A)** In our experience, almost all reoperations are due to transmigration of the fundoplication wrap, which is seen on this upper gastrointestinal study. **(B)** The intraoperative photograph shows a large esophageal hiatus (arrows) with transmigration of the fundoplication wrap and upper stomach into the lower mediastinum. Note the significant lack of adhesions after the initial laparoscopic fundoplication. (From Ostlie DJ, Holcomb GW III. Reiterative surgery for gastroesophageal reflux. Semin Pediatr Surg 2007;16:252–8.)

Also, patients were randomized according to neurological status. In addition, all patients received an upper gastrointestinal series at one-year postoperatively to evaluate for transmigration of the fundoplication wrap.[27]

The study was stopped early after 177 patients had been entered because the primary outcome overwhelmingly favored minimal esophageal mobilization with an 8% transmigration rate in the minimal dissection group compared to a 30% rate in the maximal dissection group ($p = 0.002$). Neurological status did not impact these outcomes. Furthermore, reoperation rates were higher in the maximal dissection group compared to the minimal dissection group (18% versus 3%, $p = 0.006$).[27] It is clear that minimal dissection in the pediatric patient without a hiatal hernia is important to prevent postoperative transmigration of the fundoplication wrap. The need for the four reinforcing esophagocrural stitches is currently being investigated in a prospective, randomized trial at our center.

Repeat Fundoplication

As mentioned previously, the goal of the initial fundoplication is to control GERD but also to prevent the need for a second operation.[147] In 2006, our group looked at our experience with re-do fundoplications.[148,149] Of 273 patients who underwent laparoscopic fundoplication by the senior surgeon (GWH) between January 2000 and April 2006, 21 required a re-do fundoplication (Fig. 28-8).[148] The re-do operative technique generally fell into two groups. In one group, it was performed laparoscopically without the use of mesh to reinforce the large hiatal closure that had developed after transmigration of the wrap. In the other group, acellular small intestinal submucosa (Surgisis [SIS], Cook, Inc, Bloomington IN) was used to reinforce the hiatal closure because it was believed that a great deal of tension was needed to close the large muscular defect (Fig. 28-9). Initially four-ply SIS was used, but eight-ply SIS was employed when it became

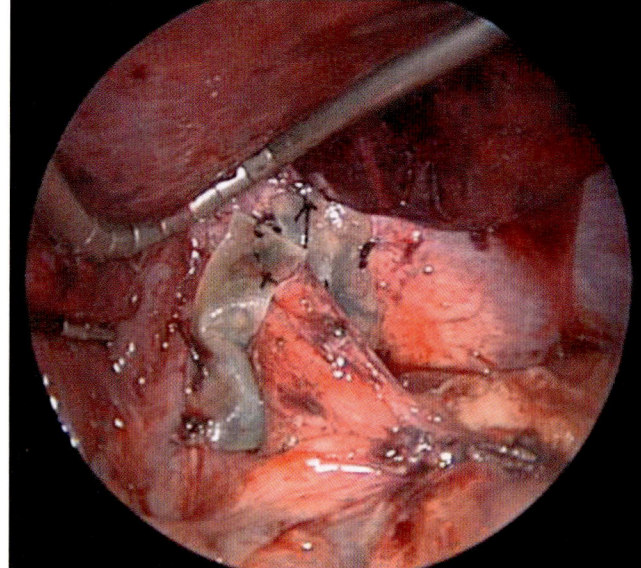

FIGURE 28-9 ■ This intraoperative photograph shows the eight-ply Surgisis that has been wrapped around the esophagus and is overlapped anterior to the esophagus. The eight-ply Surgisis is secured to the esophagus medially and the diaphragm laterally with interrupted 3-0 silk sutures. It is employed to help reinforce the closure of the crura at the time of repeat fundoplication.

available. In the patients undergoing the second operation without Surgisis, three required a second re-do or third overall fundoplication. To date, no patient has required another repeat operation in which SIS was placed at the time of the initial repeat procedure.[148]

At the same time as our concept developed about reinforcing the hiatal closure with Surgisis, a multi-institution, prospective randomized trial was being performed in adults.[149] The investigators were looking at the efficacy of placing 4-ply Surgisis at the time of initial repair of a large paraesophageal hernia defect to help prevent recurrence. This trial also closed early because of the marked disparity in results favoring the use of Surgisis to help close the large diaphragmatic defect. The primary outcome variable was recurrence of the paraesophageal hernia. The study closed at 108 total patients because, at the time of interim review, 12 patients (24%) had developed a recurrence in the arm in which Surgisis was not used, and only four patients (9%) had a recurrent paraesophageal hernia in the Surgisis arm.

Laparoscopic fundoplication has evolved into the preferred technique for surgical management of GERD. Although the Nissen operation is generally performed, similar results have been noted with the Thal operation.[150-153] It is only through critical evaluation of one's experience that advances are made in improving the results. There is no doubt that patients have less discomfort and earlier discharge from the hospital after the laparoscopic operation.[136] Moreover, there is a faster return to regular activities as well. However, the operative technique continues to need ongoing evaluation with proper data collection and critical analysis to improve these results.

REFERENCES

1. Carré IJ. The natural history of the partial thoracic stomach in children. Arch Dis Child 1959;34:344–53.
2. Fonkalsrud EW, Foglia RP, Ament ME, et al. Operative treatment for the gastroesophageal syndrome in children. J Pediatr Surg 1989;24:525–9.
3. Billard P. Maladie des Enfants Nouveau-Nés. París; 1828.
4. Allison PR, Johnston AS, Royce GB. Short esophagus with simple peptic ulceration. J Thorac Cardiovasc Surg 1943;12:432.
5. Tileston W. Peptic ulcer of the esophagus. Am J Med Sci 1906;132:240.
6. Winkelstein A. Peptic esophagitis: A new clinical entity. JAMA 1935;104:906.
7. Thal AP. A unified approach to surgical problems of the esophagogastric junction. Ann Surg 1968;168:542–9.
8. Lortat-Jacob JL. Le traitement chirurgical des maladies du reflux gastroesophagienne. Presse Med 1957;65:457.
9. Hill LD. An effective operation for hiatal hernia: An eight-year appraisal. Ann Surg 1967;166:681.
10. Hill LD. Surgery and gastroesophageal reflux. Gastroenterology 1972;63:183.
11. Belsey R. Surgery of the diaphragm. In: Brown JM, editor. Surgery of Children. Baltimore: Williams & Wilkins; 1963:762.
12. Belsey R. Gastroesophageal Reflux and Hiatal Hernia. Boston: Little, Brown; 1972.
13. Nissen R, Rossetti M. Die Behandlung von Hiatushernie und Reflux-oesophagitis mit Gastropexie und Fundoplication. Stuttgart:Georg Thieme Verlag; 1959.
14. Nissen R. Gastropexy and fundoplication in surgical treatment of hiatal hernia. Am J Dig Dis 1961;6:954–61.
15. Boix-Ochoa J. The physiologic approach to the management of gastric esophageal reflux. J Pediatr Surg 1986;21:1032–9.
16. Dallemagne B, Weerts JM, Jehaes C, et al. Laparoscopic Nissen fundoplication: Preliminary report. Surg Laparosc En dosc 1991;1:138–43.
17. Georgeson KE. Laparoscopic gastrostomy and fundoplication. Pediatr Ann 1993;92:675–7.
18. Lobe TE, Schropp KP, Lunsford K. Laparoscopic Nissen fundoplication in childhood. J Pediatr Surg 1993;28:358–61.
19. Fike FB, Mortellaro VE, Pettiford JN, et al. Diagnosis of gastroesophageal reflux disease in infants. Pediatr Surg Int 2011;27:791–7.
20. Yen CJ, Izzo JG, Lee DF, et al. Bile acid exposure up-regulates tuberous sclerosis complex 1/mammalian target of rapamycin pathway in Barrett's-associated esophageal adenocarcinoma. Cancer Res 2008;68:2632–40.
21. Liebermann-Meffert D, Allgower M, Schmid P, et al. Muscular equivalent of the lower esophageal sphincter. Gastroenterology 1979;76:31–8.
22. DeMeester TR, Wernly JA, Bryant GH, et al. Clinical and in vitro analysis of determinants of gastroesophageal competence. Am J Surg 1979;137:39–46.
23. Branton SA, Hinder RA, Floch NR, et al. Surgical treatment of gastroesophageal reflux disease. In: Castell DO, Richter JE, editors. The Esophagus. 3rd ed. Philadelphia: Lippincott Williams & Wilkins; 1999. p. 511–25.
24. Werlin SL, Dodds WJ, Hogan WJ, et al. Mechanisms of GER in children. J Pediatr 1980;97:244–9.
25. Cucchiara S, Bartolotti M, Minella R, et al. Fasting and postprandial mechanisms of GER in children with GERD. Dig Dis Sci 1993;38:86–92.
26. Winans CS, Harris LD. Quantitation of lower esophageal sphincter competence. Gastroenterology 1967;52:773–8.
27. StPeter SD, Barnhart DC, Ostlie DJ, et al. Minimal vs extensive esophageal mobilization during laparoscopic fundoplication: A prospective randomized trial. J Pediatr Surg 2011;46:163–8.
28. Thor KB, Hill LD, Mercer DD, et al. Reappraisal of the flap valve mechanism in the gastroesophageal junction. Acta Chir Scand 1987;153:25–8.
29. Altschuler SM, Boyle JT, Nixon TE, et al. Simultaneous reflex inhibition of lower esophageal sphincter and crural diaphragm in cats. Am J Physiol 1985;249:586–91.
30. Roussos C, Macklem PT. The respiratory muscles. N Engl J Med 1982;307:786–97.
31. Barak N, Ehrenpreis ED, Harrison JR, et al. Gastro-oesophageal reflux disease in obesity: Pathophysiological and therapeutic considerations. Obes Rev 2002;3:9–15.
32. Min F, Tarlo SM, Bargman J, et al. Prevalence and causes of cough in chronic dialysis patients. Adv Perit Dial 2000;16:129–33.
33. Navarro-Rodriguez T, Hashimoto CL, Carrilho FJ, et al. Reduction of abdominal pressure in patients with ascites reduces gastroesophageal reflux. Dis Esophagus 2003;16:77–82.
34. Koivusalo A, Rintala R, Lindahl H. Gastroesophageal reflux in children with a congenital abdominal wall defect. J Pediatr Surg 1999;34:1127–9.
35. Jaillard SM, Pierrat V, Dubois A, et al. Outcome at 2 years of infants with congenital diaphragmatic hernia: A population-based study. Ann Thorac Surg 2003;75:250–6.
36. Kamiyama M, Kawahara H, Okuyama H, et al. Gastroesophageal reflux after repair of congenital diaphragmatic hernia. J Pediatr Surg 2002;37:1681–4.
37. Fasching G, Huber A, Uray E, et al. Gastroesophageal reflux and diaphragmatic motility after repair of congenital diaphragmatic hernia. Eur J Pediatr Surg 2000;10:360–4.
38. Bergmeijer JH, Tibboel D, Hazebroek FW. Nissen fundoplication in the management of gastroesophageal reflux occurring after repair of esophageal atresia. J Pediatr Surg 2000;35:573–6.
39. Kubiak R, Spitz L, Kiely EM, et al. Effectiveness of fundoplication in early infancy. J Pediatr Surg 1999;34:295–9.
40. Schalamon J, Lindahl H, Saarikoski H, et al. Endoscopic follow-up in esophageal atresia—for how long is it necessary? J Pediatr Surg 2003;38:702–4.
41. Cadiot G, Bruhat A, Rigaud D, et al. Multivariate analysis of pathophysiological factors in reflux oesophagitis. Gut 1997;40:167–74.
42. Ho SC, Chang CS, Wu CY, et al. Ineffective esophageal motility is a primary motility disorder in gastroesophageal reflux disease. Dig Dis Sci 2002;47:652–6.
43. Holloway RH. Esophageal body motor response to reflux events: Secondary peristalsis. Am J Med 2000;108(Suppl):205–65.
44. Jeffery HE, Ius D, Page M. The role of swallowing during active sleep in the clearance of reflux in term and preterm infants. J Pediatr 2000;137:545–58.
45. Allen ML, Zamani S, Dimarino AJ Jr. The effect of gravity on esophageal peristalsis in humans. Neurogastroenterol Motil 1997;9:71–6.
46. Orenstein SR. Effects on behavior state of prone versus seated positioning for infants with gastroesophageal reflux disease. Pediatrics 1990;85:765–7.
47. Vandenplas Y, Hassall E. Mechanisms of gastroesophageal reflux and gastroesophageal reflux disease. J Pediatr Gastroenterol Nutr 2002;35:119–36.

48. Vandenplas Y, Sacre-Smits L. Seventeen-hour continuous esophageal pH monitoring in the newborn: Evaluation of the influence of position in asymptomatic and symptomatic babies. J Pediatr Gastroenterol Nutr 1985;4:356–61.

49. Richter JE. Importance of bile reflux in Barrett's esophagus. Dig Dis Sci 2001;18:208–16.

50. Collen MJ, Ciarleglio CA, Stanczak VJ, et al. Basal gastric acid secretion in children with atypical epigastric pain. Am J Gastroenterol 1988;83:923–6.

51. Kalach N, Badran AM, Jaffray P, et al. Correlation between gastric acid secretion and severity of acid reflux in children. Turk J Pediatr 2003;45:6–10.

52. Boyle JT. Acid secretion from birth to adulthood. J Pediatr Gastroenterol Nutr 2003;37:S12–16.

53. Gibbons TE, Gold BD. The use of proton pump inhibitors in children: A comprehensive review. Paediatr Drugs 2003;5: 25–40.

54. Gold BD, Freston JW. Gastroesophageal reflux in children: Pathogenesis, prevalence, diagnosis, and role of proton pump inhibitors in treatment. Paediatr Drugs 2002;4:673–85.

55. Penagini R. Bile reflux and oesophagitis. Eur J Gastroenterol Hepatol 2001;13:1–3.

56. Todd JAQ, de Caestecker J, Jankowski J. Gastro-esophageal reflux disease and bile acids. J Pediatr Gastroenterol Nutr 2003;36: 172–4.

57. Richter JE. Duodenogastric reflux-induced (alkaline) esophagitis. Curr Treat Options Gastroenterol 2004;7:53–58.

58. Vaezi MF, Singh S, Richter JE. Role of acid and duodenogastric reflux in esophageal mucosal injury: A review of animal and human studies. Gastroenterology 1995;108:1897–907.

59. Tovar JA, Olivares P, Diaz M, et al. Functional results of laparoscopic fundoplication in children. J Pediatr Gastroenterol Nutr 1998;26:429–31.

60. Fonkalsrud EW, Ashcraft KW, Coran AG, et al. Surgical treatment of gastroesophageal reflux in children: A combined hospital study of 7,467 patients. Pediatrics 1998;101:419–22.

61. Neuhauser EBD, Berenberg W. Cardio-esophageal relaxation as cause of vomiting in infants. Radiology 1947;48:480–3.

62. Luostarinen M. Nissen fundoplication for reflux esophagitis: Long-term clinical and endoscopic results in 109 of 127 consecutive patients. Ann Surg 1993;217:329–37.

63. Richardson JD, Kuhns JG, Richardson RL, et al. Properly conducted fundoplication reverses histologic evidence of esophagitis. Ann Surg 1983;197:763–70.

64. O'Neill JA Jr, Betts J, Ziegler MM, et al. Surgical management of reflux strictures of the esophagus in childhood. Ann Surg 1982;196:453–60.

65. Hyman PE. Gastroesophageal reflux: One reason why baby won't eat. J Pediatr 1994;125(Suppl):S103–9.

66. Kountourakis P, Ajani JA, Davila M, et al. Barrett's esophagus: A review of biology and therapeutic approaches. Gastrointest Cancer Res 2012;5:49–57.

67. Wiseman EF, Ang YS. Risk factors for neoplastic progression in Barrett's esophagus. World J Gastroenterol 2011;17: 3672–83.

68. Quante M, Bhagat G, Abrams JA, et al. Bile acid and inflammation activate gastric cardia stem cells in a mouse model of Barrett-like metaplasia. Cancer Cell 2012;21:36–51.

69. Hassall E, Weinstein WM, Ament ME. Barrett's esophagus in childhood. Gastroenterology 1985;89:1331–7.

70. Othersen HB Jr, Ocampo RJ, Parker EF, et al. Barrett's esophagus in children. Ann Surg 1993;217:676–81.

71. Lundell L, Myers JC, Jamieson GG. The effect of antireflux operations on lower oesophageal sphincter tone and postprandial symptoms. Scand J Gastroenterol 1993;28:725–31.

72. Halper LM, Jolley SG, Tunnell WP, et al. The mean duration of gastroesophageal reflux during sleep as an indicator of respiratory symptoms from gastroesophageal reflux in children. J Pediatr Surg 1991;26:686–90.

73. Foglia RP, Fonkalsrud EW, Ament ME, et al. Gastroesophageal fundoplication for the management of chronic pulmonary disease in children. Am J Surg 1980;140:72–9.

74. del Rosario JF, Orenstein SR. Evaluation and management of gastroesophageal reflux and pulmonary disease. Curr Opin Pediatr 1996;8:209–15.

75. Jolley SG, Herbst JJ, Johnson DG, et al. Esophageal pH monitoring during sleep identifies children with respiratory symptoms from gastroesophageal reflux. Gastroenterology 1981;80:1501–6.

76. Hrabovsky EE, Mullett MD. Gastroesophageal reflux and the premature infant. J Pediatr Surg 1986;21:583–7.

77. Orenstein SA. An overview of reflux-associated disorders in infants: Apnea, laryngospasm, and aspiration. Am J Med 2001; 111:60S–63S.

78. Suwandhi E, Ton MN, Schwarz TS. Gastroesophageal reflux in infancy and childhood. Pediatr Ann 2008;35:259–66.

79. Ramenofsky ML, Powell RW, Curreri PW. Gastroesophageal reflux: pH probe-directed therapy. Ann Surg 1986;203:531–5.

80. Valusek PA, St. Peter SD, Keckler SJ, et al. Does an upper gastrointestinal study change operative management for gastroesophageal reflux? J Pediatr Surg 2010;45:1169–72.

81. Spencer J. Prolonged pH recording in the study of gastroesophageal reflux. Br J Surg 1969;56:912–14.

82. Johnson LF, DeMeester TR. Twenty-four hour pH monitoring of the distal esophagus. A quantitative measure of gastroesophageal reflux. Am J Gastroenterol 1974;62:325–32.

83. DeMeester TR, Johnson LF, Joseph GJ, et al. Patterns of gastroesophageal reflux in health and disease. Ann Surg 1976; 184:459–69.

84. Boix-Ochoa J, Lafuente JM, Gil-Vernet JM. Twenty-four hour esophageal pH monitoring in gastroesophageal reflux. J Pediatr Surg 1980;15:74–8.

85. Koch A, Gass R. Continuous 20–24 hour esophageal pH monitoring in infancy. J Pediatr Surg 1981;16:109–13.

86. Stein HJ, DeMeester TR. Indications, technique, and clinical use of ambulatory 24-hour esophageal motility monitoring in a surgical practice. Ann Surg 1993;217:128–37.

87. Jolley SG, Herbst JJ, Johnson DG, et al. Patterns of postcibal gastroesophageal reflux in symptomatic infants. Am J Surg 1979;138:946–50.

88. Jamieson JR, Stein HJ, DeMeester TR, et al. Ambulatory 24-hour esophageal pH monitoring: Normal values, optimal thresholds, specificity, sensitivity, and reproducibility. Am J Gastroenterol 1992;87:1102–11.

89. Colletti RB, Christie DL, Orenstein SR. Indications for pediatric esophageal pH monitoring. J Pediatr Gastroenterol Nutr 1995; 21:253–62.

90. Harada T, Hyman PE, Everett S, et al. Meal-stimulated gastric acid secretion in infants. J Pediatr 1984;104:534–8.

91. Kelly EJ, Newell SJ, Brownlee KG, et al. Gastric acid secretion in preterm infants. Early Hum Dev 1993;35:215–20.

92. Sondheimer JM, Clark DA, Gervaise EP. Continuous gastric pH measurement in young and older healthy preterm infants receiving formula and clear liquid feedings. J Pediatr Gastroenterol Nutr 1985;4:352–5.

93. Mitchell DJ, McClure BG, Tubman TRJ. Simultaneous monitoring of gastric and oesophageal pH reveals limitations of conventional oesophageal pH monitoring in milk fed infants. Arch Dis Child 2001;84:273–6.

94. Shay SS, Johnson LF, Richter JE. Acid rereflux. Dig Dis Sci 2003;48:1–9.

95. Wenzl TC, Moroder C, Trachterna M, et al. Esophageal pH monitoring and impedance measurement: A comparison of two diagnostic tests for gastroesophageal reflux. J Pediatr Gastroenterol Nutr 2002;34:519–23.

96. Vela MF, Camacho-Lobato L, Srinivasan R, et al. Simultaneous intraesophageal impedance and pH measurement of acid and non-acid gastroesophageal reflux: Effect of omeprazole. Gastroenterology 2001;120:1599–606.

97. Sifrim D, Holloway RH, Silny J, et al. Acid, non-acid and gas reflux in patients with gastroesophageal reflux disease during 24-hr ambulatory pH-impedance recordings. Gastroenterology 2001;120:1588–98.

98. Kahrilas P. Will impedance testing rewrite the book on GERD? Gastroenterology 2001;120:1862–64.

99. Vela MF. Multichannel intraluminal impedance and pH monitoring in gastroesophageal reflux disease. Expert Rev Gastroenterol Hepatol 2008;2:665–72.

100. Lopez-Alonso M, Moya MJ, Cabo JA, et al. Twenty-four-hour esophageal impedance-pH monitoring in healthy preterm neonates: Rate and characteristics of acid, weakly acidic, and

weakly alkaline gastroesophageal reflux. Pediatrics 2006;118: e299–308.

101. Wise JL, Murray JA. Utilising multichannel intraluminal impedance for diagnosing GERD: A review. Dis Esophagus 2007; 20:83–8.

102. Bremner RM, Hoeft SF, Costantini MD, et al. Pharyngeal swallowing. Ann Surg 1993;218:364–70.

103. Shepard R, Fenn S, Seiber WK. Evaluation of esophageal function in postoperative esophageal atresia and tracheoesophageal fistula. Surgery 1966;59:608–17.

104. Biller JA, Winter HS, Grand RJ, et al. Are endoscopic changes predictive of histologic esophagitis in children? J Pediatr 1983;103:215–18.

105. Meyers WF, Roberts CC, Johnson DG, et al. Value of tests for evaluation of gastroesophageal reflux in children. J Pediatr Surg 1985;20:515–20.

106. Brown RA, Wynchank S, Rode H, et al. Is a gastric drainage procedure necessary at the time of antireflux surgery? J Pediatr Gastroenterol Nutr 1997;25:377–80.

107. Maddern GJ, Jamieson GG. Fundoplication enhances gastric emptying. Ann Surg 1985;201:296–9.

108. Maxson RT, Harp S, Jackson RL, et al. Delayed gastric emptying in neurologically impaired children with gastroesophageal reflux: The role of pyloroplasty. J Pediatr Surg 1994;29:726–9.

109. Katz PO. Treatment of gastroesophageal reflux disease: Use of algorithms to aid in management. Am J Gastroenterol 1999; 94:3–10.

110. Orenstein SR, Whitington PF, Orestein DM. The infant seat as a treatment for gastroesophageal reflux. N Engl J Med 1983;309: 760–3.

111. Carré IJ. Postural treatment of children with a partial thoracic stomach (hiatus hernia). Arch Dis Child 1960;35:569–80.

112. Ponsonby AL, Dwyer T, Gibbons LE, et al. Factors potentiating the risk of sudden infant death syndrome associated with the prone position. N Engl J Med 1993;329:377–82.

113. Augood C, MacLennan S, Gilbert R, et al. Cisapride treatment for gastro-oesophageal reflux in children. Cochrane Database Syst Rev 2003;(4):CD002300.

114. Dalby-Payne JR, Morris AM, Craig JC. Meta-analysis of randomized controlled trials on the benefits and risks of using cisapride for the treatment of gastroesophageal reflux in children. J Gastroenterol Hepatol 2003;18:196–202.

115. Enger C, Cali C, Walker AM. Serious ventricular arrhythmias among users of cisapride and other QT-prolonging agents in the United States. Pharmacoepidemiol Drug Saf 2002;11:477–86.

116. Machida HM, Forbes DA, Gall DG, et al. Metoclopramide in gastroesophageal reflux of infancy. J Pediatr 1988;112:483–7.

117. Rudolph CD, Mazur LJ, Liptak GS, et al. Guidelines for evaluation and treatment of gastroesophageal reflux in infants and children. Recommendations of the North American Society for Pediatric Gastroenterology and Nutrition. J Pediatr Gastroenterol Nutr 2001;32:S1–31.

118. Dimand RJ. Use of H2-receptor antagonists in children. Ann Pharmacother 1990;24(Suppl):42–6.

119. Wolfe MM, Sachs G. Acid suppression: Optimizing therapy for gastroduodenal ulcer healing, gastroesophageal reflux disease, and stress-related erosive syndrome. Gastroenterology 2000;118: S9–31.

120. Zimmermann AE, Walters JK, Katoma BG, et al. A review of omeprazole use in the treatment of acid-related disorders in children. Clin Ther 2001;2385:660–79.

121. Hassall E, Israel D, Shepherd R, et al. Omeprazole for treatment of chronic erosive esophagitis in children: A multicenter study of efficacy, safety, tolerability and dose requirements. International Pediatric Omeprazole Study Group. J Pediatr 2000;137: 800–7.

122. Andersson T, Hassall E, Lundborg P, et al. Pharmacokinetics of orally administered omeprazole in children. International Pediatric Omeprazole Pharmacokinetic Group. Am J Gastroenterol 2000;95:3101–6.

123. Valusek PA, St. Peter SD, Tsao K, et al. The use of fundoplication for prevention of apparent life-threatening events. J Pediatr Surg 2007;42:1022–5.

124. Ostlie DJ, Miller KA, Holcomb GW III. Effective Nissen fundoplication length and bougie diameter size in young children

undergoing laparoscopic Nissen fundoplication. J Pediatr Surg 2002;37:1664–6.

125. Ostlie DJ, Miller KA, Woods RK, et al. Single cannula technique and robotic telescopic assistance in infants and children who require laparoscopic Nissen fundoplication. J Pediatr Surg 2003;38:111–15.

126. Ostlie DJ, Holcomb GW III. Laparoscopic fundoplication in infants and children. In: Langer JC, Albanese CT, editors. Pediatric Minimal Access Surgery: A Principle and Evidence Based Approach. New York: Marcel Dekker; 2005. p. 167–90.

127. St. Peter SD, Valusek PA, Calkins CM, et al. Use of esophagocrural sutures and minimal esophageal dissection reduces the incidence of postoperative transmigration of laparoscopic Nissen fundoplication wrap. J Pediatr Surg 2007;42:25–30.

128. Holcomb GW III. Gastroesophageal reflux in infants and children. In: Fischer JE, editor. Mastery of Surgery. 6th ed. Philadelphia: Lippincott Williams & Wilkins; 2012. p. 769–80.

129. Holcomb GW III. Laparoscopic Nissen fundoplication. In: Holcomb GW III, Rothenberg SS, Georgeson KW III, editors. Atlas of Pediatric Laparoscopy and Thoracoscopy. Philadelphia: Elsevier; 2008. p. 15–20.

130. Aprahamian CJ, Morgan TL, Harmon CM, et al. U-stitch laparoscopic gastrostomy technique has a low rate of complications and allows primary button placement: Experience with 461 pediatric procedures. J Laparoendosc Adv Surg Tech A 2006;16: 643–9.

131. Georgeson K, Owings E. Surgical and laparoscopic techniques for feeding tube placement. Gastrointest Endosc Clin North Am 1998;8:581–92.

132. Ostlie DJ, Holcomb GW III, et al. Clinical principles of abdominal surgery. In: Oldham KT, Colombani PM, Foglia RP, editors. Surgery of Infants and Children. 2nd ed. Philadelphia: Lippincott Williams & Wilkins; 2005. p. 1067–86.

133. Ostlie DJ, Holcomb GW III. Laparoscopic fundoplication with gastrostomy. Semin Pediatr Surg 2002;11:196–204.

134. Holcomb GW III. Laparoscopic fundoplication in an infant. Surg Endosc 2003;17:1319.

135. St. Peter SD, Holcomb GW III. Gastroesophageal reflux disease and fundoplication in infants and children. Ann Pediatr Surg 2007;3:1–10.

136. Ostlie DJ, St. Peter SD, Snyder CL, et al. A financial analysis of pediatric laparoscopic versus open fundoplication. J Laparoendosc Adv Surg Tech 2007;17:493–6.

137. Barsness KA, St. Peter SD, Holcomb GW 3rd, et al. Laparoscopic fundoplication after previous open abdominal operations in infants and children. J Laparoendosc Adv Surg Tech A 2009;1: S47–9.

138. Davis CS, Baldea A, Johns JR, et al. The evolution and long-term results of laparoscopic antireflux surgery for the treatment of gastroesophageal reflux disease. JSLS 2010;14:332–41.

139. Rhee D, Zhang Y, Chang DC, et al. Population-based comparison of open vs laparoscopic esophagogastric fundoplication in children: Application of the Agency for Healthcare Research and Quality pediatric quality indicators. J Pediatr Surg 2011;46: 648–54.

140. Mauritz FA, van Herwaarden-Lindeboom MY, Stomp W, et al. The effects and efficacy of antireflux surgery in children with gastroesophageal reflux disease: A systematic review. J Gastrointest Surg 2011;15:1872–8.

141. Esposito C, De Luca C, Alicchio F, et al. Long-term outcome of laparoscopic Nissen Procedure in pediatric patients with gastroesophageal reflux disease measured using the modified QOSG Roma III European Society for Pediatric Gastroenterology and Hepatology and Nutrition's Questionnaire. J Laparoendosc Adv Surg Tech 2012;22:937–40.

142. Kubiak R, Andrews J, Grant HW. Long-term outcome of laparoscopic Nissen fundoplication compared with laparoscopic Thal fundoplication in children: A prospective, randomized study. Ann Surg 2011;253:44–9.

143. Dedinsky GK, Vane DW, Black T, et al. Complications and reoperation after Nissen fundoplication in childhood. Am J Surg 1987;153:177–83.

144. Caniano DA, Ginn-Pease ME, King DR. The failed antireflux procedure: Analysis of risk factors and morbidity. J Pediatr Surg 1990;25:1022–5.

145. Wheatley MJ, Coran AG, Wesley JR, et al. Redo fundoplication in infants and children with recurrent gastroesophageal reflux. J Pediatr Surg 1991;26:758–61.

146. Fonkalsrud WE, Ashcraft KW, Coran AG, et al. Surgical treatment of gastroesophageal reflux in children: A combined hospital study of 7467 patients. Pediatrics 1998;101:419–22.

147. Ostlie DJ, Holcomb GW III. Reiterative laparoscopic surgery for recurrent gastroesophageal reflux. Semin Pediatr Surg 2007; 16:252–8.

148. St. Peter SD, Ostlie DJ, Holcomb GW III. The use of biosynthetic mesh to enhance hiatal repair at the time of redo Nissen fundoplication. J Pediatr Surg 2007;42:1298–301.

149. Oelschlager BK, Pellegrini CA, Hunter J, et al. Biologic prosthesis reduces recurrence after laparoscopic paraesophageal hernia repair. Ann Surg 2006;244:481–90.

150. Esposito C, Montupet P, van der Zee D, et al. Long-term outcome of laparoscopic Nissen, Toupet, and Thal antireflux procedures for neurologically normal children with gastroesophageal reflux disease. Surg Endosc 2006;20:855–8.

151. van der Zee DC, Bax KN, Ure BM, et al. Long-term results after laparoscopic Thal procedure in children. Semin Laparosc Surg 2002;9:168–71.

152. Esposito C, Becmeur F, Centonze A, et al. Laparoscopic reoperation following unsuccessful antireflux surgery in childhood. Semin Laparosc Surg 2002;9:177–9.

153. Esposito C, van der Zee DC, Settimi A, et al. Risks and benefits of surgical management of gastroesophageal reflux in neurologically impaired children. Surg Endosc 2003;17:708–10.

CHAPTER 29

LESIONS OF THE STOMACH

Curt S. Koontz • Mark L. Wulkan

The stomach forms from the foregut and is recognizable by the fifth week of gestation. It then elongates, descends, and dilates to form its familiar structure by the seventh week of gestation. The vascular supply to the stomach is very robust, and ischemia of the stomach is rare. The stomach is supplied by the right and left gastric arteries along the lesser curvature, the right and left gastroepiploic arteries along the greater curvature, and the short gastric vessels from the spleen. There is also contribution from the posterior gastric artery, which is a branch of the splenic artery, as well as the phrenic arteries.

In this chapter, we discuss common and unusual conditions of the stomach that are treated surgically. Some topics relevant to the stomach, such as gastroesophageal reflux and obesity, are covered elsewhere.

HYPERTROPHIC PYLORIC STENOSIS

Hypertrophic pyloric stenosis (HPS) is one of the most common surgical conditions of the newborn.[1-9] It occurs at a rate of 1 to 4 per 1,000 live births in Caucasian infants, but is seen less often in non-Caucasian children.[1-4] Males are affected more often with a 4:1 male-to-female ratio. Risk factors for HPS include family history, gender, younger maternal age, being a first-born infant, and maternal feeding patterns.[4,9,10] Premature infants are diagnosed with HPS later than term or post-term infants.[4]

Etiology

The cause of HPS is unknown, but genetic and environmental factors appear to play a large role in the pathophysiology. Circumstantial evidence for a genetic predisposition includes race discrepancies, the increased frequency in males, and the birth order (first-born infants with a positive family history). Environmental factors associated with HPS include the method of feeding (breast vs formula), seasonal variability, exposure to erythromycin, and transpyloric feeding in premature infants.[5-7] Additionally, there has been interest in several gastrointestinal peptides or growth factors that may facilitate pyloric hypertrophy. Some of these include excessive substance P, decreased neurotrophins, deficient nitric oxide synthase, and gastrin hypersecretion.[8,9] Thus, the etiology of HPS is likely multifactorial with environmental influences.

Diagnosis

The classic presentation of HPS is nonbilious, projectile vomiting in a full-term neonate who is between 2 and 8 weeks old. Initially, the emesis is infrequent and may appear to be gastroesophageal reflux disease. However, over a short period of time, the emesis occurs with every feeding and becomes forceful (i.e., projectile). The contents of the emesis are usually the recent feedings, but signs of gastritis are not uncommon ('coffee-ground' emesis). On physical examination, the neonate usually appears well if the diagnosis is made early. However, depending on the duration of symptoms and degree of dehydration, the neonate may be gaunt and somnolent. Visible peristaltic waves may be present in the mid to left upper abdomen. The pylorus may be palpable in 72–89% of patients.[11,12] To palpate the hypertrophied pylorus, the baby must be relaxed. Techniques for relaxing the infant include bending the knees and flexing the hips, and using a pacifier with sugar water. These techniques should be attempted after the stomach has been decompressed with a 10 French to 12 French orogastric tube. After palpating the liver edge, the examiner's fingertips should slide underneath the liver in the midline. Slowly, the fingers are pulled back and down, trying to trap the 'olive.' Palpating the hypertrophied pylorus requires patience and an optimal examination setting. If palpated, no further studies are needed. If the pylorus cannot be palpated, ultrasound (US) should be performed.

Ultrasound has become the standard technique for diagnosing HPS and has supplanted the physical examination at most institutions. The diagnostic criteria for pyloric stenosis is a muscle thickness greater than or equal to 4 mm and a pyloric channel length greater than or equal to 16 mm (Fig. 29-1).[12] A thickness of more than 3 mm is considered positive if the neonate is younger than 30 days of age.[13] The study is dependent on the expertise of the ultrasound technician and radiologist.

There are reports of non-radiologists performing ultrasound for HPS, which would obviously reduce the need for the ultrasound technician.[14,15] If the ultrasound findings are equivocal, then an upper gastrointestinal series can be helpful in confirming the diagnosis (Fig. 29-2).

In the past, the diagnosis was often delayed and profound dehydration with metabolic derangements was common. Today, however, primary care physicians are more aware of the problem and the availability of ultrasound facilitates an earlier diagnosis and treatment. However, the complete differential diagnosis for nonbilious vomiting should be considered. This includes medical causes such as gastroesophageal reflux, gastroenteritis, increased intracranial pressure, and metabolic disorders. Anatomic causes include an antral web, foregut duplication cyst, gastric tumors, or a tumor causing extrinsic gastric compression.

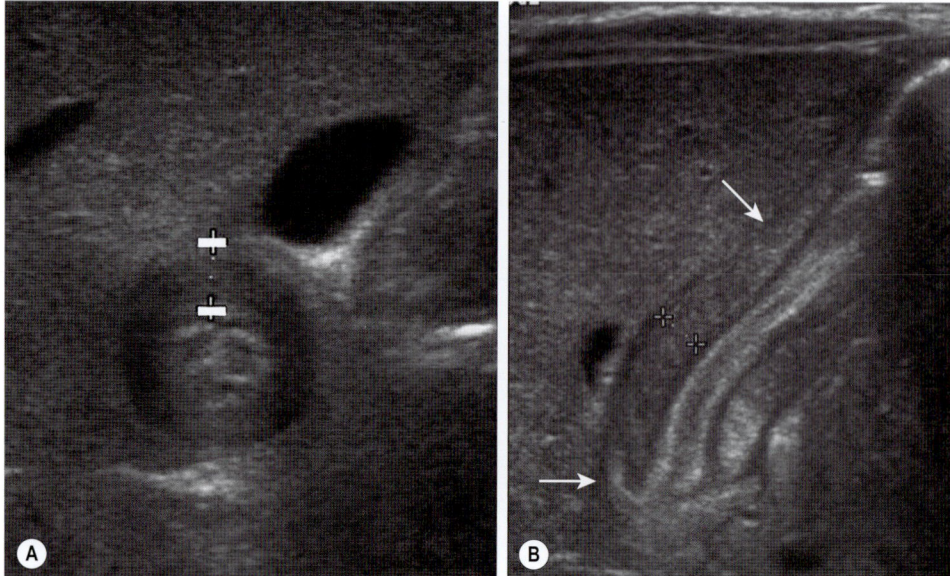

FIGURE 29-1 ■ Ultrasonography has become the standard imaging study for diagnosing pyloric stenosis and has supplanted physical examination at most institutions. The **(A)** transverse and **(B)** longitudinal views of hypertrophic pyloric stenosis are seen here. Muscle thickness greater than or equal to 4 mm on the transverse view or a length greater than or equal to 16 mm on the longitudinal view is diagnostic of pyloric stenosis. On this study, the pyloric wall thickness was 5 mm and the length (arrows) was 20 mm.

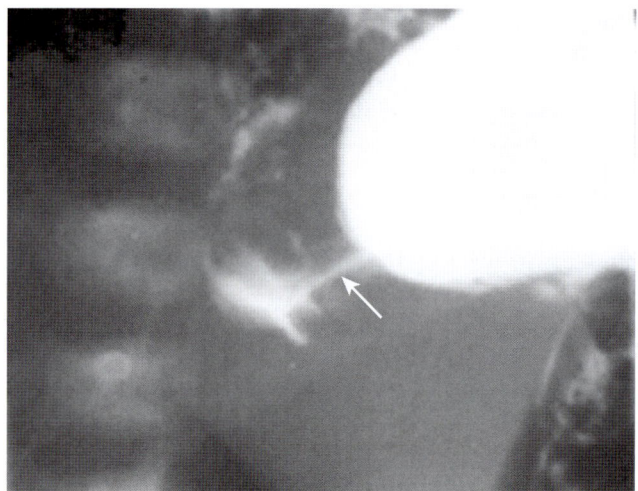

FIGURE 29-2 ■ At some hospitals outside of urban centers, ultrasound technicians and radiologists proficient in performing an ultrasound study for pyloric stenosis are not available. Also, in some instances, an ultrasound study can be equivocal. An upper gastrointestinal series can be helpful in making the diagnosis of pyloric stenosis or confirming an equivocal ultrasound study. In this upper gastrointestinal study, note the 'string sign' indicating a markedly diminished pyloric channel (arrow) and subsequent gastric outlet obstruction. It is important to evacuate the contrast material after this study to reduce the risk of aspiration and pulmonary complications.

Treatment

The mainstay of therapy is typically resuscitation followed by pyloromyotomy. There are reports of medical treatment with atropine and pyloric dilation, but these treatments require long periods of therapy and are often not effective.[16–20]

Once the diagnosis of HPS is made, feedings should be withheld. Gastric decompression is usually not necessary but occasionally may be required for extreme cases. If a barium study was performed, it is important to remove all of the contrast material from the stomach to prevent aspiration and pulmonary complications.

The hallmark metabolic derangement of hypochloremic, hypokalemic metabolic alkalosis is usually seen to some degree in most patients. Profound dehydration is rarely seen today, and correction is usually achieved in less than 24 hours after presentation. A basic metabolic panel should be ordered and the resuscitation should be directed toward correcting the abnormalities. Most surgeons use the serum carbon dioxide (<30 mmol/L), chloride (>100 mmol/L), and potassium (4.5–6.5 mmol/L) levels as markers of resuscitation. Initially, a 10–20 mL/kg bolus of normal saline should be given if the electrolytes are abnormal. Then, D5/1/2NS with 20–30 mEq/L of potassium chloride is started at a rate of 1.25 to 2 times the calculated maintenance rate. Electrolytes should be checked every six hours until they normalize and the alkalosis has resolved. Subsequent fluid boluses are given if the electrolytes remain abnormal. It is important to appreciate that HPS is not a surgical emergency and resuscitation is the initial priority. Inadequate resuscitation can lead to postoperative apnea due to a decreased respiratory drive secondary to metabolic alkalosis.

The pyloromyotomy can be performed by the standard open technique or by the minimally invasive approach. The anesthesiologist should pass and leave a suction catheter in the stomach for decompression and for instilling air after the pyloromyotomy to check for a mucosal leak.

The Open Approach

Several incisions have been described for the open approach. The typical right upper quadrant transverse incision seems to be used most commonly (Fig. 29-3). An alternate more cosmetically pleasing incision involves

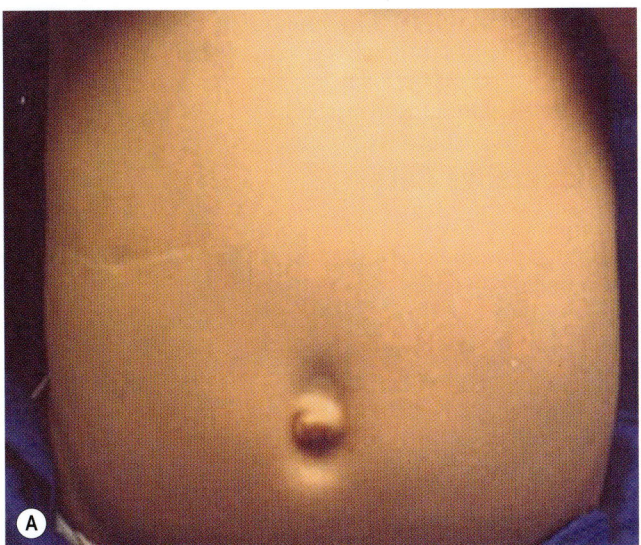

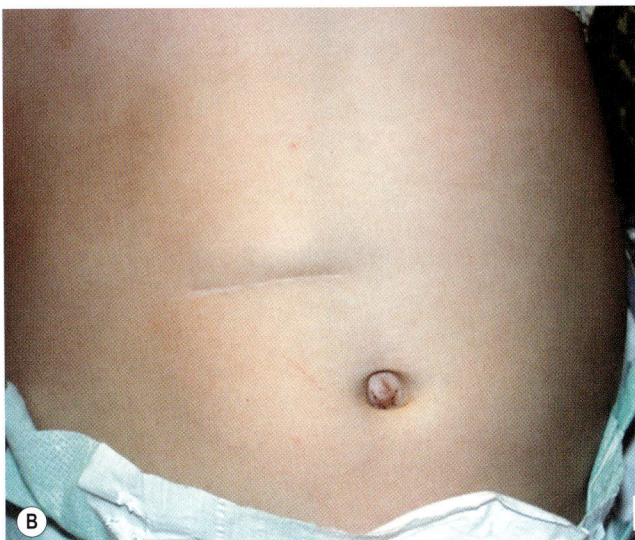

FIGURE 29-3 ■ These two children underwent open pyloromyotomy through a right upper quadrant transverse incision. Over time, the cosmetic appearance of their incision is not as attractive as that seen after the laparoscopic operation.

an omega-shaped incision around the superior portion of the umbilicus followed by incising the linea alba cephalad. With either incision, the pylorus is exteriorized through the incision. A longitudinal serosal incision is made in the pylorus approximately 2 mm proximal to the junction of the duodenum and is carried onto the anterior gastric wall for approximately 5 mm. Blunt dissection is used to initially divide the firm pyloric fibers. This can be performed using the handle of a scalpel. Once a good edge of fibers has been developed, a pyloric spreader or hemostat can be used to spread the fibers until the pyloric submucosal layer is seen. The pyloromyotomy is then completed by ensuring that all fibers are divided throughout the entire length of the pyloromyotomy. This is confirmed by visualizing the circular muscle of the stomach proximally as well as a slight protrusion of the submucosa. The most common point of mucosal entry is at the distal part of the incision at the duodenal–pyloric junction. Therefore, care must be exercised when dividing the

fibers in this region. The pyloromyotomy can be evaluated for completeness by rocking the superior and inferior edges of the myotomy back and forth to ensure independent movement. The mucosal integrity can be checked by instilling air through the previously placed suction catheter. If there are no leaks, the air should be suctioned. Minor bleeding is common and should be ignored because it will cease after the venous congestion is reduced when the pylorus is returned to the abdominal cavity. The abdominal incision is then closed in layers.

The Laparoscopic Operation

Neonatal laparoscopy has grown in popularity with the refinement in technique and smaller instruments. The first reported laparoscopic pyloromyotomy in the English language was in 1991 (the authors had reported the first case in the French literature in 1990).[21] Since then, this procedure has been accepted by most pediatric surgeons. Critics of this approach argue that laparoscopic pyloromyotomy exposes the patient to undue risks compared with the open technique. However, recent randomized prospective trials have not shown any difference in complication rates.[22,23] Operative times can vary depending on the experience of the surgeon. The minimally invasive approach for pyloromyotomy is similar to laparoscopic appendectomy in terms of acceptance and has become the standard technique for pyloromyotomy in many centers.

The technique involves entering the abdomen through an umbilical incision. A Veress needle is inserted at the base of the umbilicus between the umbilical arteries. It is paramount to ensure proper placement of the Veress needle before insufflation. This can be done by several simple methods, including the 'blind man's cane' sweep and the water drop test. Alternatively, an open approach can be used to introduce the umbilical cannula. The abdomen is then insufflated to a pressure of 10 mmHg and a 3 mm or 5 mm port is introduced for the telescope and camera. Two stab incisions are made. One incision is in the right paramedian side of the abdomen at the level of the umbilicus, and the other is in the left paramedian side of the abdomen just superior to the umbilicus.

Local anesthesia is instilled at all incisions. An atraumatic bowel grasper is inserted through the patient's right incision, and a pylorotome or spatula cautery tip is introduced through the patient's left incision (Fig. 29-4). The duodenum is grasped firmly just distal to the pylorus, and the pylorus is maneuvered into view. Occasionally, a transabdominal stay suture wrapping around the falciform ligament is helpful to elevate the liver away from the pylorus. A longitudinal pyloromyotomy is then made with the knife or cautery in a similar manner as the open technique (Fig. 29-5). Initially, a retractable arthrotomy knife was used; however, it is no longer available in the USA. Thus, most USA pediatric surgeons now use an unguarded arthrotomy knife or the cautery. Once the seromuscular layer is incised, a laparoscopic pyloric spreader or a box-type grasper is inserted to perform the myotomy. Completeness of the myotomy and mucosal integrity are checked in a similar manner as the open technique. Omentum can be placed over the myotomy to

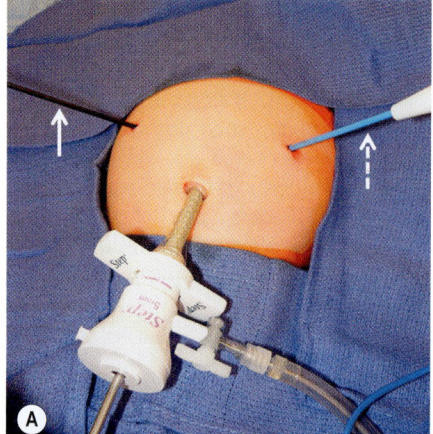

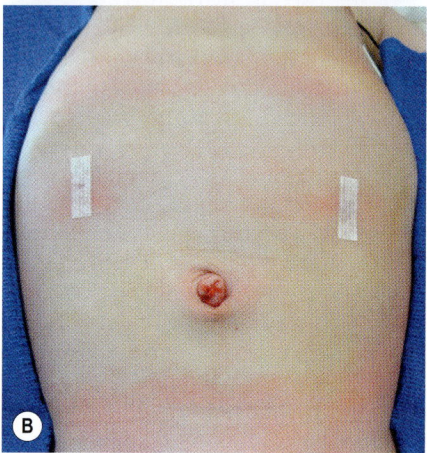

FIGURE 29-4 ■ Laparoscopic pyloromyotomy has become a common approach for pyloric stenosis in infants. In the USA, the sheathed arthrotomy knife is no longer available. Therefore, other techniques are now utilized. **(A)** The atraumatic grasper that is holding the duodenum is seen on the patient's right (solid arrow). In the patient's left upper abdomen, a spatula tipped cautery (dotted arrow) has been introduced to incise the serosa of the stomach . The 5 mm cannula has been placed in the umbilicus through which an angled telescope is introduced for visualization. **(B)** The stab incisions have been closed with steri-strips.

help with hemostasis. The pneumoperitoneum is evacuated after the instruments are removed. The umbilicus is closed with absorbable suture, and the stab incisions are closed with skin adhesive (see Fig. 29-4B).

Postoperative Care

Postoperative care is similar for both operative approaches, assuming the mucosal integrity of the stomach is intact. Complicated feeding regimens have been advocated in the past. However, more recent studies support the use of ad libitum feedings in the early postoperative period. This results in a faster time to full feeding and earlier discharge.[24,25] In many centers, if postoperative emesis is encountered, it is suggested to 'feed through it.' At our institution, we limit the feedings to a maximum of 3 oz every three hours. There are data to suggest that the degree and duration of preoperative metabolic derangement affects the postoperative feeding schedule. Babies who required more complicated resuscitation tend to take longer to reach full feeding and discharge.[26]

A survey about postoperative feeding regimens in pediatric surgery residency training centers in North America was recently performed. Thirty-two of the 47 institutions responded to the survey. The average time from operation to initiation of feedings was 4.3 hours. There was a wide variability in responses, but 26 of the 32 responding programs employ a protocol-based feeding regimen.[27]

A prospective randomized trial recently compared a protocol-based feeding regimen to ad libitum feeding after laparoscopic pyloromyotomy.[28] Feeding was begun two hours after laparoscopic pyloromyotomy in both groups. The ad libitum group was allowed formula or breast milk two hours after the operation and was considered ready for discharge after tolerating three consecutive feeds without emesis. The babies who underwent feeding via protocol were given Pedialyte two hours after the operation followed by another round of Pedialyte, which was followed by two rounds of half strength formula or breast milk, followed by two rounds of full strength formula or breast milk, followed by the home feeding regimen. The baby was discharged on the home feeding regimen if doing well. With a power of 0.9

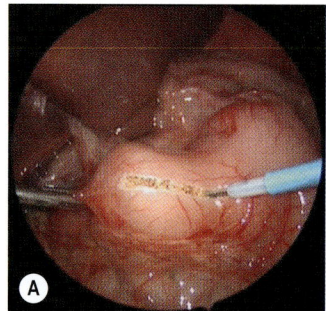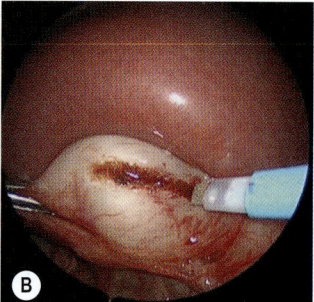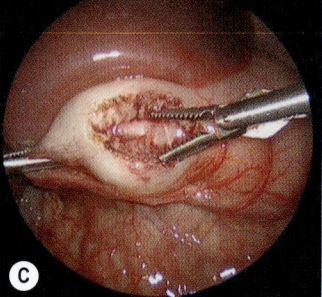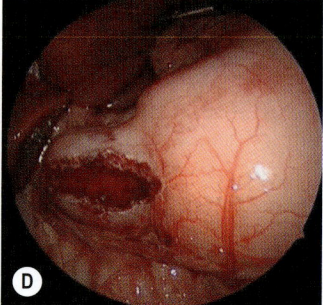

FIGURE 29-5 ■ These intraoperative photographs depict a laparoscopic pyloromyotomy. **(A)** The spatula tipped cautery is being used to incise the serosa and outer muscular layer of the hypertrophied pylorus. **(B)** The tip of the cautery is introduced into the hypertrophied muscle and twisted to break up the muscle fibers and create a space for insertion of the pyloric spreader. **(C)** The pyloric spreader is introduced into the muscle and gently opened to split the hypertrophied muscle fibers. The submucosa is visualized through the myotomy. **(D)** Air is introduced into the stomach to assess the integrity of the mucosa.

and an alpha of 0.05, a sample size of 150 patients was calculated. There were no differences in patient characteristics at presentation. The ad libitum group reached goal feeding sooner than the group who were fed via protocol (Table 29-1). However, this did not translate into a difference in length of postoperative hospitalization. There were more patients with emesis in the ad libitum group after reaching goal feedings. There was no difference in readmission rates, as two patients in each group were readmitted after discharge.[28]

Postoperatively, pain is usually controlled with acetaminophen. Most infants are ready for discharge on the first postoperative day.

Complications

The major complications of pyloromyotomy include mucosal perforation, wound infection, incisional hernia, prolonged postoperative emesis, incomplete myotomy, and duodenal injury. There are prospective randomized trials that do not show any difference in complication rates between the laparoscopic and open techniques.[22,23]

Mucosal perforation occurs in 1–2% of cases.[22,23] If the disruption occurs at the duodenopyloric junction, a simple interrupted absorbable suture can be used to close the defect and a patch of omentum can be positioned over the closure. This can be accomplished laparoscopically depending on the surgeon's experience. Otherwise, the laparoscopic procedure should be converted to open. If the perforation is large or in the middle of the myotomy, then the myotomy should be closed with absorbable suture. A new myotomy can then be made 90–180° from the original incision. Feedings should be held for 24 hours and then restarted. A water-soluble contrast study can be performed if desired.

Duodenal injuries also can occur with either the laparoscopic or open approach. In a 25-year retrospective review of 901 open pyloromyotomies performed between 1969 and 1994, there were 39 duodenal perforations that were recognized intraoperatively and repaired. There were no unrecognized duodenal perforations that developed after the operation.[29]

Wound infections also occur in 1–2% of cases.[22,23] There are no data to support the use of prophylactic perioperative antibiotics because a pyloromyotomy is considered a clean procedure. Local wound care is usually sufficient to treat these infections.

Incisional hernias and wound dehiscence occurs in approximately 1% of cases.[22] Most hernias require repair at some point. Laparoscopically, port site hernias usually involve omentum protruding through the incision. This can sometimes be managed at the bedside by cleansing the area with povidone-iodine, ligating and trimming the extracorporeal omentum, elevating the abdominal wall to get the omentum back into the peritoneal cavity, and using fine absorbable suture to close the skin.

Postoperative emesis is common, occurring in most infants to some degree. Prolonged emesis is less common and ranges in incidence from 2–26%. Most commonly, this is due to gastroesophageal reflux but can occur secondary to an incomplete myotomy. It has been suggested that the laparoscopic approach may be a risk factor for inadequate myotomy, but this is likely related to the surgeon's experience with this technique.[24]

Outcomes

In the past, the mortality from pyloric stenosis was considerable and approached 50%. Today, however, mortality is nearly zero with improvement in neonatal resuscitation and anesthesia as well as surgical techniques. Morbidity is also significantly lower than in the past, with an overall complication rate between 1–2%. Additionally, with more pyloromyotomies being performed laparoscopically, the cosmetic advantage of the minimally invasive technique cannot be overemphasized.

PYLORIC ATRESIA

Pyloric atresia is a rare disease (1:100,000 live births) and presents with symptoms of gastric outlet obstruction. The disease is difficult to characterize because it is so rare. However, several generalizations can be made from looking

---

TABLE 29-1 Preoperative and Postoperative Data from a Prospective Randomized Trial Comparing Ad Libitum Feeding to Feeding Using a Standardized Protocol after Laparoscopic Pyloromyotomy[28]

Variable	Ad lib fed (n = 75; Mean ± Standard Deviation)	Protocol fed (n = 75; Mean ± Standard Deviation)	P value
Age (days)	39.9 ± 19.08	39.75 ± 14.90	0.93
Pre-op pyloric thickness (mm)	4.44 ± 0.84	4.43 ± 0.89	0.93
Pre-op pyloric length (mm)	19.56 ± 3.44	19.97 ± 3.64	0.48
Operating time (minutes)	20.63 ± 10.64	18.19 ± 7.99	0.11
Postoperative emesis pre-goal feed (number)	1.04 ± 2.16	0.57 ± 0.99	0.09
Number of patients with pre-goal feed emesis	45 (60%)	51 (68%)	0.40
Post-goal feed emesis (number)	1.05 ± 2.26	0.47 ± 2.79	0.16
Number of patients with post-goal feed emesis	31 (41%)	11 (14.6%)	**0.0000**
Doses of analgesia (number)	1.47 ± 1.38	1.56 ± 1.40	0.68
Time to goal feeds (hours)	9.15 ± 7.02	16.58 ± 7.86	**0.0000**
Length of stay after goal (hours)	16.18 ± 14.65	9.20 ± 6.15	**0.0002**
Length of stay after operation (hours)	25.39 ± 15.41	25.78 ± 10.05	0.85
Readmission for emesis	2 (2.6%)	2 (2.6%)	1.0

at relatively large series. Other congenital anomalies are found in up to 40% of patients with pyloric atresia.[30–32] The most common associated condition is epidermolysis bullosa.[33–36] There is a suggestion of autosomal recessive transmission in patients with familial disease.[30]

Three anatomic variants have been described. With type I, there is a mucosal membrane or web. In type II, the pyloric channel is a solid cord (Fig. 29-6). In type III, there is a gap between the stomach and the duodenum.[31] These babies present with nonbilious emesis and have similar electrolyte abnormalities to infants with HPS. A 'single bubble' is usually found on an abdominal radiograph (see Figure 29-6). If necessary, the diagnosis can be confirmed with a contrast study. The differential diagnosis includes malrotation with volvulus, proximal duodenal atresia, gastric volvulus, pyloric duplication, retrograde duodenal gastric intussusception, and aberrant pancreatic tissue plugging the pylorus.[37,38]

The operative management depends on the type of atresia. Excision of the web or membrane with Heinecke–Mikulicz pyloroplasty is usually possible for a type I atresia. However, for types II or III, often a Billroth I gastroduodenostomy is needed if the solid core or gap is long (see Fig 29-6). There is also a report of successful treatment with gastroduodenal mucosal advancement for this condition.[39] Gastrojejunostomy is not recommended as there is a reported 60% failure rate and mortality rate of 50%.[40] Laparoscopic repair for a type II atresia was recently described.[41]

Generally, long-term outcomes are very good. Morbidity and mortality are usually related to the associated anomalies. Patients with pyloric atresia and epidermolysis bullosa often die due to septicemia, electrolyte imbalance, protein loss, or failure to thrive due to the exudative skin lesions. However, there are reports of long-term survival in neonates with pyloric atresia and

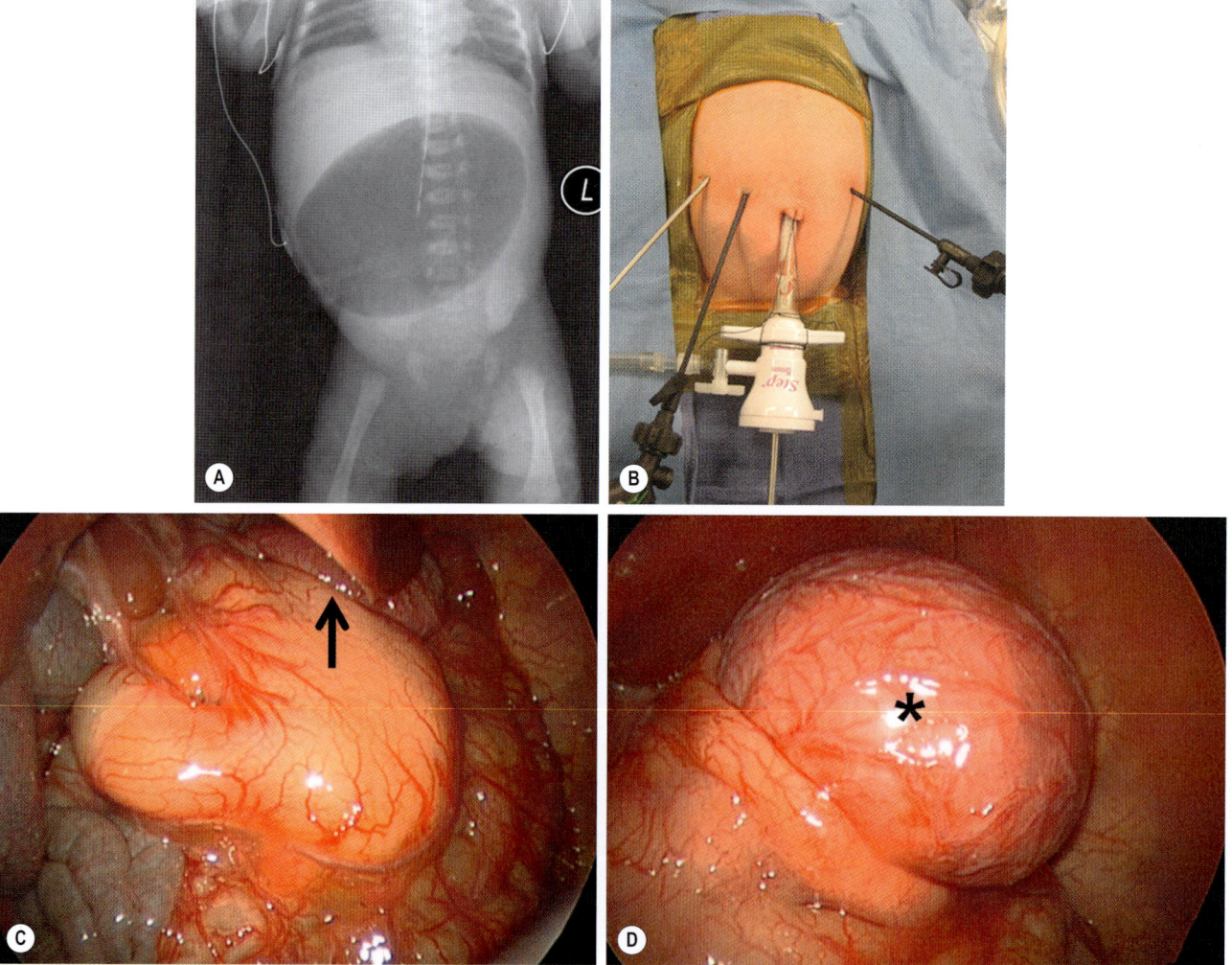

FIGURE 29-6 ■ This baby developed nonbilious emesis shortly after birth. **(A)** An abdominal film shows a single bubble. This is classic for pyloric atresia. **(B)** The baby underwent laparoscopic repair and the position of the instruments is shown. **(C)** At operation, the pylorus was a solid core (type II). On close inspection, note a gastric duplication in the superior aspect of the greater curve of the stomach (arrow). This gastric duplication is better seen in **(D)** and was resected. The baby has recovered nicely and has not developed any problems two years later.

epidermolysis bullosa so aggressive surgical intervention for these patients should not be withheld.[42]

GASTRIC PERFORATION

The causes of gastric perforation include spontaneous perforation in the newborn, iatrogenic perforation from instrumentation, peptic ulcer disease, and trauma. Gastric perforation usually presents with abdominal distention and signs of sepsis or shock. The diagnosis is suspected when a large amount of extraluminal air is seen on an abdominal radiograph.

Neonatal gastric perforations most commonly occur in premature infants. About half of neonatal perforations are spontaneous, and the other half are iatrogenic from instrumentation.[43] Prematurity is associated with an increased mortality.[44] The perforations are usually managed with laparotomy or laparoscopy. The perforation can usually be closed primarily with or without an omental patch.

Gastric perforation due to peptic ulcer disease in infants and children is very rare. Typically, perforation occurs at the site of a prepyloric ulcer. Again, this may be repaired primarily via laparotomy or laparoscopy with or without an omental patch.[45]

PEPTIC ULCER DISEASE

Peptic ulcer disease and its complications are rarely seen in children. However, there have been reports of neonatal and childhood perforated ulcers as well as gastric outlet obstruction in children due to peptic ulcer disease.[45–47] Peptic ulcer disease appears to be associated with *Helicobacter pylori* in the majority of pediatric cases. Treatment is primarily directed at acid reduction and eradication of *H. pylori*. Triple therapy with a proton pump inhibitor, amoxicillin, and clarithromycin is typically used initially. For strains that are resistant to clarithromycin, metronidazole is substituted.[48] Operative treatment is usually reserved for complications of peptic ulcer disease, such as perforation or gastric outlet obstruction (Fig. 29-7). If ulcer perforation is suspected, it is reasonable to start with exploratory laparoscopy because there are reports of successful laparoscopic treatment in children.[46] A gastric resection operation is not usually needed due to effective proton pump inhibitors.

GASTRIC DUPLICATIONS

Gastric duplications are rare anomalies that generally occur along the greater curvature (see Fig. 29-6D). If the lesion is near the pylorus, the presentation may be very similar to HPS. The diagnosis can be differentiated from pyloric stenosis by ultrasound. The lesion rarely communicates with the lumen. If it does, the patient may present with hematemesis or melena. Gastric duplications represent approximately 4% of all gastrointestinal duplications. Approximately half are discovered in the neonatal period and are seen when the neonate presents

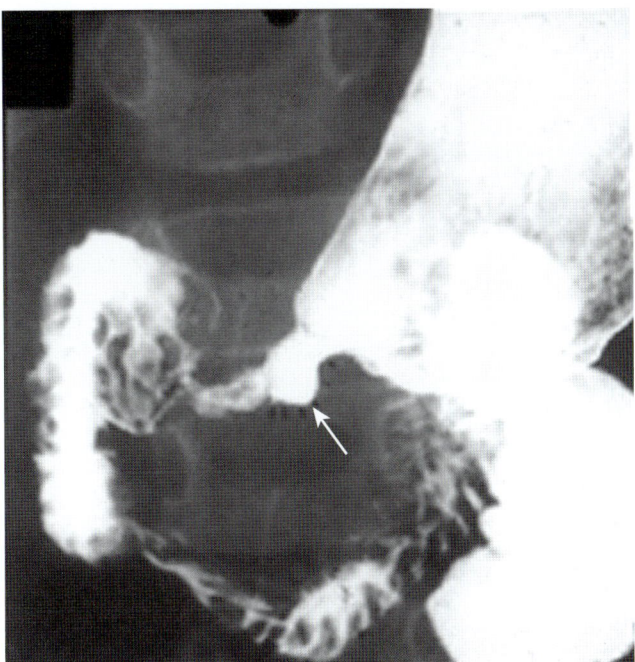

FIGURE 29-7 ■ A 10-year-old presented with abdominal pain and vomiting. She was found to have a prepyloric ulcer (arrow) on the upper gastrointestinal study. In addition, there was evidence of gastric outlet obstruction. She underwent antrectomy and Billroth I reconstruction.

with vomiting, poor feeding, and an epigastric mass.[49] Ectopic gastric mucosa is common in other duplications throughout the gastrointestinal tract. These are not considered gastric duplications.

Treatment of gastric duplications is complete resection. Gastric duplications have been found associated with pancreatic ductal abnormalities.[50] In this instance, care must be taken during the dissection not to injure normal pancreas, although it may be necessary to resect an accessory pancreas.

MICROGASTRIA

Congenital microgastria is a rare disorder that usually occurs in conjunction with other congenital anomalies or, more rarely, alone (Fig. 29-8). Associated anomalies include the VACTERL association (vertebral anomalies, anorectal atresia, cardiac anomalies, tracheoesophageal fistula and esophageal atresia, renal and limb anomalies), tracheoesophageal cleft, malrotation, and asplenia. There are currently only three reported cases of isolated microgastria.[51,52] Microgastria is usually temporized with jejunal feedings. Operative intervention consists of jejunal feeding tubes and Hunt–Lawrence gastric augmentation. There are a few patients who have been reported with successful follow-up after a Hunt–Lawrence pouch.[51,53,54]

ANTRAL WEB

The first modern description of an antral web was in 1969.[55] Early case reports in children described

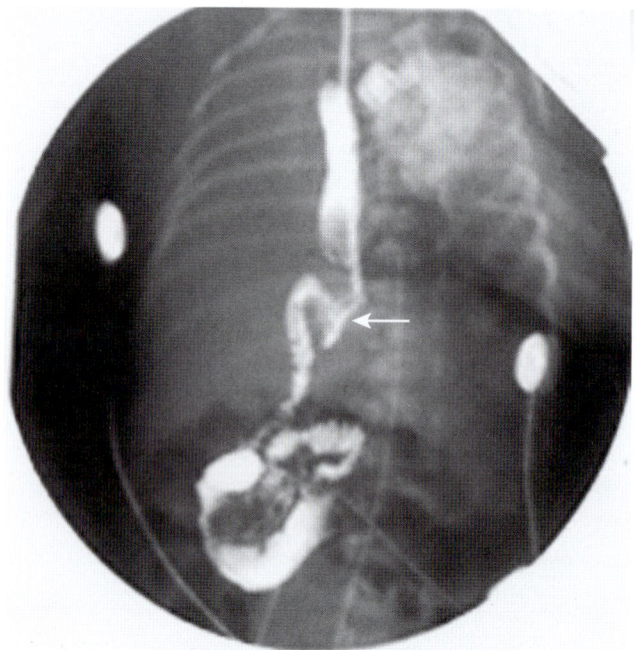

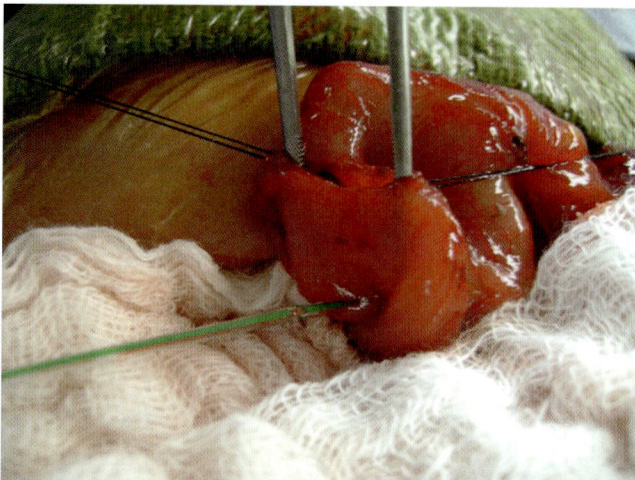

FIGURE 29-9 ■ This neonate developed nonbilious emesis shortly after birth and was thought to have an antral web. At laparotomy, the antral web is visualized. The forceps are proximal to the web and the feeding tube (arrow) has been placed through the web. After resection of the web, the patient recovered uneventfully and has not developed any further problems.

FIGURE 29-8 ■ This neonate was born with congenital microgastria. Note the dilated esophagus and the extremely small stomach (arrow). There is also malrotation. The patient underwent creation of a Hunt–Lawrence pouch and was doing well at one-year follow-up.

incomplete gastric outlet obstruction due to an antral web.[56–59] The etiology is unknown and is generally thought to be congenital or the result of an inflammatory process. In adults there is a case report that strongly suggested peptic ulcer disease led to an antral web.[60] These patients typically present with gastric outlet obstruction. In the infant, an antral web may be confused with HPS. The baby with an antral web may have a normal abdominal sonogram. The abdominal examination may be normal. However, an upper gastrointestinal series will show the lesion.

Treatment of an antral web consists of resuscitation (see earlier section on HPS) and operative correction which can be performed via laparotomy or laparoscopy (Fig. 29-9). This is a diagnosis that may be amenable to endoluminal treatment in the future.

GASTRIC VOLVULUS

Gastric volvulus can occur from primary or secondary causes. Primary gastric volvulus is thought to be due to laxity of the gastric ligaments. Secondary disease may occur due to a paraesophageal hernia or other diaphragmatic hernia. The presenting symptoms can be intermittent or complete gastric obstruction, ischemia, pain, and/or bleeding. The most common signs and symptoms of gastric volvulus in children include acute abdominal pain, intractable retching, and the inability to pass a nasogastric tube into the stomach lumen.[61,62]

The average age at presentation is 2.5 years. Equal numbers of males and females are affected.[61] Gastric volvulus is classified based on the axis of gastric rotation.

Mesenteroaxial gastric volvulus is rotation about the gastric short axis, transecting the greater and lesser curvatures. Organoaxial gastric volvulus is rotation around the long axis of the stomach (Figs 29-10 and 29-11).

The principles of treatment are patient resuscitation, nasogastric decompression, and operative correction. Diaphragmatic defects, if found, are repaired in secondary gastric volvulus. A gastropexy is then performed. This has traditionally been accomplished with a gastrostomy tube or button. However, there are recent reports of successful laparoscopic gastropexy in which the anterior stomach, along the greater curvature, is sutured to the abdominal wall.[63]

FOREIGN BODIES AND BEZOAR

Foreign bodies in the stomach can be generally ignored. If the foreign body passed through the esophagus, it will likely pass out the rectum. Even razor blades and other sharp objects usually pass safely. The exception would be button batteries, which have a high incidence of leakage and should be removed if they have not passed through the pylorus. Otherwise, watchful waiting is a reasonable strategy. Occasionally larger coins, such as quarters, can remain in the stomach and cause intermittent gastric outlet obstruction. It is also reasonable to remove the object in this circumstance. Most gastric foreign bodies are removed endoscopically with a snare, grasper, or bag. The surgeon should consider using an overtube to extract large sharp objects that may injure the esophagus upon withdrawal.

Gastric bezoars are relatively uncommon causes of gastric outlet obstruction and chronic abdominal pain in children. Phytobezoars are made up of vegetable matter. Trichobezoars are made up of hair that is swallowed. This is referred to as the Rapunzel syndrome.[64] The hair

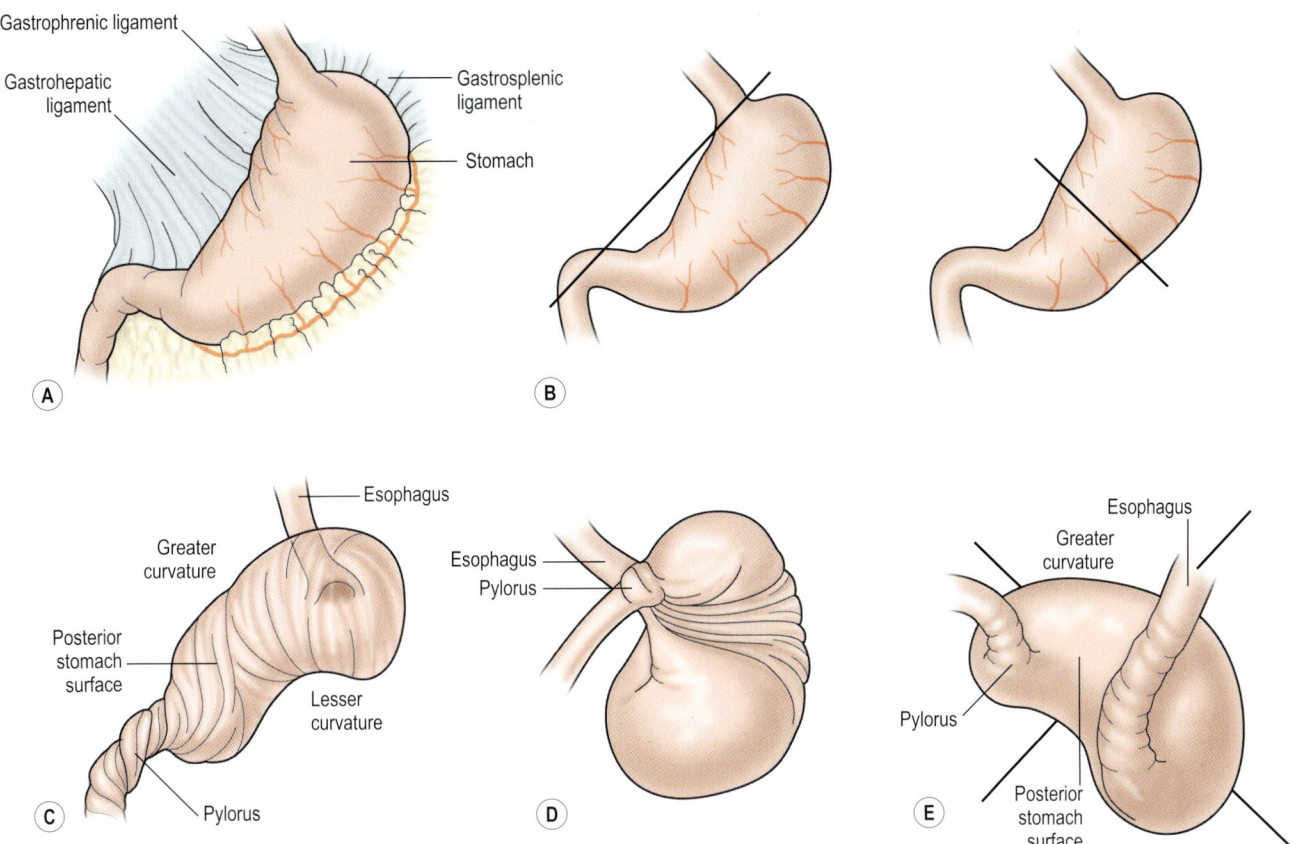

FIGURE 29-10 ■ These drawings depict the development of a gastric volvulus. **(A)** Normal anatomy. **(B)** The axis of rotation for an organoaxial volvulus is seen on the left and a mesoaxial volvulus is on the right. **(C)** Demonstration of an organoaxial volvulus. **(D)** Demonstration of a mesoaxial volvulus. **(E)** Combined mesoaxial and organoaxial volvulus. (Adapted from Cribbs RK, Gow KW, Wulkan ML. Gastric volvulus in infants and children. Pediatrics 2008;122:e752–62.)

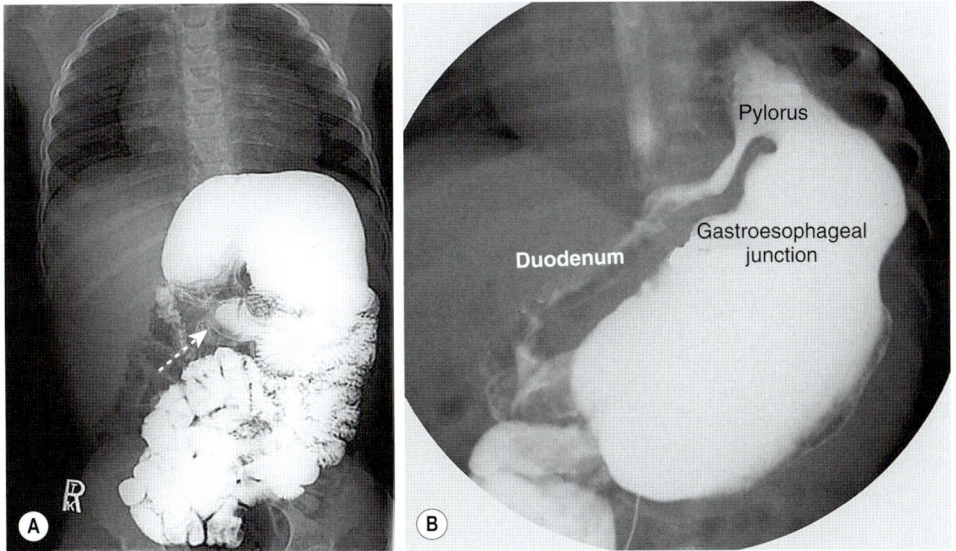

FIGURE 29-11 ■ These two contrast studies depict a gastric volvulus. **(A)** This contrast study depicts an organoaxial volvulus in which the stomach has rotated on its long axis. Note the relatively normal position of the pylorus (arrow). **(B)** This contrast study shows a mesoaxial volvulus. In this study, the pylorus is in the left upper abdomen due to rotation around the short axis of the stomach. In both studies, the gastroesophageal junction is in a relatively normal position.

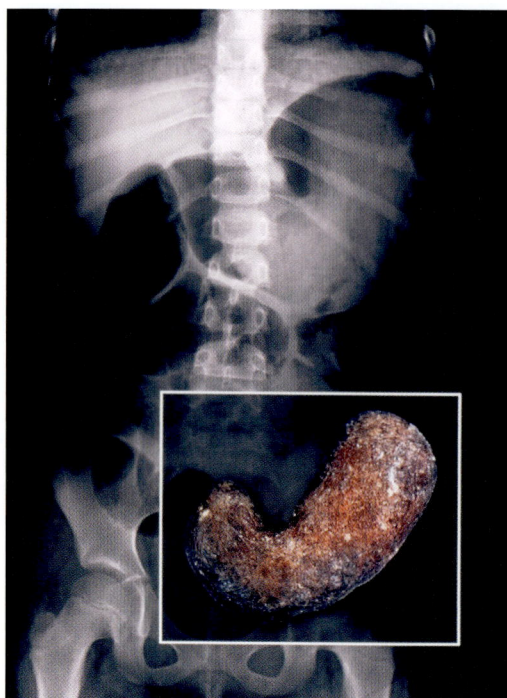

FIGURE 29-12 ■ A young girl presented with gastric outlet obstruction and was found to have a trichobezoar. The preoperative radiograph shows the outline of the bezoar in the stomach. Inset, The bezoar after removal.

usually fills the stomach and extends into the duodenum. However, it can extend to the ileum. Attempts at gastroscopic removal are usually futile, except in cases of small bezoars. The bezoar has been typically removed through a gastrotomy at laparotomy. However, there are recent reports of laparoscopic removal.[65,66] At our institution, we recently removed a large gastric trichobezoar laparoscopically with the aid of an endoscopic bag (Fig. 29-12).

REFERENCES

1. Pedersen RN, Garne E, Loane M, et al. Infantile hypertrophic pyloric stenosis: A comparative study of incidence and other epidemiological characteristics in seven European regions. J Matern Fetal Neonatal Med 2008;21:599–604.
2. Sommerfield T, Chalmers J, Youngson G, et al. The changing epidemiology of infantile hypertrophic pyloric stenosis in Scotland. Arch Dis Child 2008;93:1007–11.
3. Persson S, Ekbom A, Granath F, et al. Parallel incidences of sudden infant death syndrome and infantile hypertrophic pyloric stenosis: A common cause? Pediatrics 2001;108:E70.
4. Schechter R, Torfs CP, Bateson TF. The epidemiology of infantile hypertrophic pyloric stenosis. Paediatr Perinat Epidemiol 1997; 11:407–27.
5. Honein MA, Paulozzi LJ, Himelright IM, et al. Infantile hypertrophic pyloric stenosis after pertussis prophylaxis with erythromycin: A case review and cohort study. Lancet 1999;354:2101–5.
6. Mitchell LE, Risch N. The genetics of infantile hypertrophic pyloric stenosis: A re-analysis. Am J Dis Child 1993;147:1203–11.
7. Rasmussen L, Green A, Hansen LP. The epidemiology of infantile hypertrophic pyloric stenosis in a Danish population, 1950-84. Int J Epidemiol 1989;18:413–17.
8. Spitz L, Zail SS. Serum gastrin levels in congenital hypertrophic pyloric stenosis. J Pediatr Surg 1976;11:33–5.
9. Vanderwinden JM, Mailleux P, Schiffmann SN, et al. Nitric oxide synthase activity in infantile hypertrophic pyloric stenosis. N Engl J Med 1992;327:511–15.
10. White MC, Langer JC, Don S, et al. Sensitivity and cost minimization analysis of radiology versus olive palpation for the diagnosis of hypertrophic pyloric stenosis. J Pediatr Surg 1998;33:913–17.
11. Breaux CW Jr, Georgeson KE, Royal SA, et al. Changing patterns in the diagnosis of hypertrophic pyloric stenosis. Pediatrics 1988;81:213–17.
12. Keller H, Waldmann D, Greiner P. Comparison of preoperative sonography with intraoperative findings in congenital hypertrophic pyloric stenosis. J Pediatr Surg 1987;22:950–2.
13. Lamki N, Athey PA, Round ME, et al. Hypertrophic pyloric stenosis in the neonate—diagnostic criteria revisited. Can Assoc Radiol J 1993;44:21–4.
14. Malcom GE 3rd, Raio CC, Del Rios M, et al. Feasibility of emergency physician diagnosis of hypertrophic pyloric stenosis using point-of-care ultrasound: A multi-center case series. J Emerg Med 2009;37:283–6.
15. Boneti C, McVay MR, Kokoska ER, et al. Ultrasound as a diagnostic tool used by surgeons in pyloric stenosis. J Pediatr Surg 2008;43:87–91.
16. Meissner PE, Engelmann G, Troeger J, et al. Conservative treatment of infantile hypertrophic pyloric stenosis with intravenous atropine sulfate does not replace pyloromyotomy. Pediatr Surg Int 2006;12:1021–4.
17. Kawahara H, Takama Y, Yoshida H, et al. Medical treatment of infantile hypertrophic pyloric stenosis: Should we always slice the "olive"? J Pediatr Surg 2005;40:1848–51.
18. Kawahara H, Imura K, Nishikawa M, et al. Intravenous atropine treatment in infantile hypertrophic pyloric stenosis. Arch Dis Child 2002;87:71–4.
19. Ogawa Y, Higashimoto Y, Nishijima E, et al. Successful endoscopic balloon dilatation for hypertrophic pyloric stenosis. J Pediatr Surg 1996;31:1712–14.
20. Yusuf TE, Brugge WR. Endoscopic therapy of benign pyloric stenosis and gastric outlet obstruction. Curr Opin Gastroenterol 2006;22:570–3.
21. Alain JL, Grousseau D, Terrier G. Extramucosal pylorotomy by laparoscopy. J Pediatr Surg 1991;26:1191–2.
22. St. Peter SD, Holcomb GW, Calkins CM, et al. Open versus laparoscopic pyloromyotomy for pyloric stenosis: A prospective, randomized trial. Ann Surg 2006;244:363–70.
23. Leclair MD, Plattner V, Mirallie E, et al. Laparoscopic pyloromyotomy for hypertrophic pyloric stenosis: A prospective, randomized controlled trial. J Pediatr Surg 2007;42:692–8.
24. Adibe OO, Nichol PF, Lim FY, et al. Ad libitum feeds after laparoscopic pyloromyotomy: A retrospective comparison with a standardized feeding regimen in 227 infants. J Laparoendosc Adv Surg Tech A 2007;17:235–7.
25. Georgeson KE, Corbin TJ, Griffen JW, et al. An analysis of feeding regimens after pyloromyotomy for hypertrophic pyloric stenosis. J Pediatr Surg 1993;28:1478–80.
26. St. Peter SD, Tsao K, Sharp SW, et al. Predictors of emesis and time to goal intake after pyloromyotomy: Analysis from a prospective trial. J Pediatr Surg 2008;43:2038–41.
27. Juang D, Adibe OO, Laituri CA, et al. Distribution of feeding styles after pyloromyotomy among pediatric surgical training programs in North America. Eur J Pediatr Surg 2012;22:409–11.
28. Adibe OO, Iqbal CS, Sharp SW, et al. Protocol versus ad lib feeds after laparoscopic pyloromyotomy: A prospective randomized trial. 2012 (accepted for publication).
29. Hulka F, Harrison MW, Campbell TJ, et al. Complications of pyloromyotomy for infantile hypertrophic pyloric stenosis. Am J Surg 1997;173:450–2.
30. Ilce Z, Erdogan E, Kara C, et al. Pyloric atresia: 15-year review from a single institution. J Pediatr Surg 2003;38:1581–4.
31. Okoye BO, Parikh DH, Buick RG, et al. Pyloric atresia: Five new cases, a new association, and a review of the literature with guidelines. J Pediatr Surg 2000;35:1242–5.
32. Al-Salem AH. Congenital pyloric stenosis and associated anomalies. Pediatr Surg Int 2007;23:559–63.
33. Almaani N, Liu L, Dopping-Hepenstal PJ, et al. Autosomal dominant junctional epidermolysis bullosa. Br J Dermatol 2009;160:1094–7.
34. Birnbaum RY, Landau D, Elbedour K, et al. Deletion of the first pair of fibronectin type III repeats of the integrin beta-4 gene is associated with epidermolysis bullosa, pyloric atresia and aplasia

cutis congenita in the original Carmi syndrome patients. Am J Med Genet A 2008;146:1063–6.

35. Nakamura H, Sawamura D, Goto M, et al. Epidermolysis bullosa simplex associated with pyloric atresia is a novel clinical subtype caused by mutations in the plectin gene (PLEC1). J Mol Diagn 2005;7:28–35.

36. Samad L, Siddiqui EF, Arain MA, et al. Pyloric atresia associated with epidermolysis bullosa: Three cases presenting in three months. J Pediatr Surg 2004;39:1267–9.

37. Moore CC. Congenital gastric outlet obstruction. J Pediatr Surg 1989;24:1241–6.

38. Bronsther B, Nadeau MR, Abrams MW. Congenital pyloric atresia: A report of three cases and a review of the literature. Surgery 1971;69:130–6.

39. Dessanti A, Iannuccelli M, Dore A, et al. Pyloric atresia: An attempt at anatomic pyloric sphincter reconstruction. J Pediatr Surg 2000;35:1372–4.

40. Kourolinka CW, Steward JR. Pyloric atresia. Am J Dis Child 1978;132:903–5.

41. Juang D, Holcomb GW III. Laparoscopic repair of pyloric atresia. Video presentation, 2012 American College of Surgeons meeting.

42. Hayashi AH, Galliani CA, Gilis DA. Congenital pyloric atresia and junctional epidermolysis bullosa: A report of long-term survival and a review of the literature. J Pediatr Surg 1991;26:1341–5.

43. Abadir J, Emil S, Nguyen N. Abdominal foregut perforations in children: A 10-year experience. J Pediatr Surg 2005;40:1903–7.

44. Lin CM, Lee HC, Kao HA, et al. Neonatal gastric perforation: Report of 15 cases and review of the literature. Pediatr Neonatol 2008;49:65–70.

45. Edwards MJ, Kollenberg SJ, Brandt ML, et al. Surgery for peptic ulcer disease in children in the post-histamine2-blocker era. J Pediatr Surg 2005;40:850–4.

46. Wong BP, Chao NS, Leung MW, et al. Complications of peptic ulcer disease in children and adolescents: Minimally invasive treatments offer feasible surgical options. J Pediatr Surg 2006;41:2073–5.

47. Hua MC, Kong MS, Lai MW, et al. Perforated peptic ulcer in children: A 20-year experience. J Pediatr Gastroenterol Nutr 2007;45:71–4.

48. Kato S, Konno M, Maisawa S, et al. Results of triple eradication therapy in Japanese children: A retrospective multicenter study. J Gastroenterol 2004;39:838–43.

49. Cooper S, Abrams RS, Carbaugh RA. Pyloric duplications: Review and case study. Am Surg 1995;61:1092–4.

50. Muraoka A, Tsuruno M, Katsuno G, et al. A gastric duplication cyst with an aberrant pancreatic ductal system: Report of a case. Surg Today 2002;32:531–5.

51. Jones VS, Cohen RC. An eighteen-year follow-up after surgery for congenital microgastria—case report and review of literature. J Pediatr Surg 2007;42:1957–60.

52. Kroes EJ, Festen C. Congenital microgastria: A case report and review of literature. Pediatr Surg Int 1998;13:416–18.

53. Velasco AL, Holcomb GW, Templeton JM, et al. Management of congenital microgastria. J Pediatr Surg 1990;25:192–7.

54. Neifeld JP, Berman WF, Lawrence W, et al. Management of congenital microgastria with a jejunal reservoir pouch. J Pediatr Surg 1980;15:882–5.

55. Banks PA, Waye JD. The gastroscopic appearance of antral web. Gastrointest Endosc 1969;15:228–9.

56. Hait G, Esselstyn CB Jr, Rankin GB. Prepyloric mucosal diaphragm (antral web): Report of a case and review of the literature. Arch Surg 1972;105:486–90.

57. Campbell DP, Vanhoutte JJ, Smith EI. Partially obstructing antral web—a distinct clinical entity. J Pediatr Surg 1973;8:723–8.

58. Patnaik DN, Sun S, Groff DB. Newborn gastric outlet obstruction caused by an antral web. J Med Soc N J 1976;73:736–7.

59. Bell MJ, Ternberg JL, McAlister W, et al. Antral diaphragm—a cause of gastric outlet obstruction in infants and children. J Pediatr 1977;90:196–202.

60. Huggins MJ, Friedman AC, Lichtenstein JE, et al. Adult acquired antral web. Dig Dis Sci 1982;27:80–3.

61. Miller DL, Pasquale MD, Seneca RP, et al. Gastric volvulus in the pediatric population. Arch Surg 1991;126:1146–9.

62. Heldrich FJ, Kumarasena D, Hakim J, et al. Acute gastric volvulus in children: A rare disorder. Pediatr Emerg Care 1993;9:221–3.

63. Cribbs RK, Gow KW, Wulkan ML. Gastric volvulus in infants and children. Pediatrics 2008;122:e752–62.

64. Naik S, Gupta V, Naik S, et al. Rapunzel syndrome reviewed and redefined. Dig Surg 2007;24:157–61.

65. Shami SB, Jararaa AA, Hamade A, et al. Laparoscopic removal of a huge gastric trichobezoar in a patient with trichotillomania. Surg Laparosc Endosc Percutan Tech 2007;17:197–200.

66. Nirasawa Y, Mori T, Ito Y, et al. Laparoscopic removal of a large gastric trichobezoar. J Pediatr Surg 1998;33:663–5.

CHAPTER 30

Duodenal and Intestinal Atresia and Stenosis

Pablo Aguayo • Daniel J. Ostlie

Congenital intestinal obstruction occurs in approximately 1:2000 live births and is a common cause of admission to a neonatal surgical unit, accounting for up to one-third of all admissions.[1] Morphologically, congenital defects related to continuity of the intestine can be divided into either atresia or stenosis. Together, they constitute one of the most common etiologies of neonatal intestinal obstruction.[2–4] See Chapter 29 for information about pyloric atresia.

DUODENAL ATRESIA AND STENOSIS

Congenital duodenal atresia and stenosis is a frequent cause of intestinal obstruction and occurs in 1 per 5000 to 10,000 live births, affecting boys more commonly than girls.[5] More than 50% of affected patients have associated congenital anomalies, with trisomy 21 occurring in approximately 30% of patients.[6,7] Operative correction is accomplished via a duodenoduodenostomy, with or without tapering duodenoplasty. This can be performed either laparoscopically or open. Early postoperative survival rates of greater than 90% should be expected.[7–11]

Etiology

Congenital duodenal obstruction can occur due to an intrinsic or extrinsic lesion.[12] The most common cause of duodenal obstruction is atresia.[7] This intrinsic lesion is most commonly believed to be caused by a failure of recanalization of the fetal duodenum resulting in complete obstruction. Early in the fourth week of gestation, the duodenum begins to develop from the distal foregut and the proximal midgut. During the fifth and sixth weeks of gestation, the duodenal lumen temporarily obliterates due to proliferation of its epithelial cells. Vacuolation due to degeneration of the epithelial cells during the 11th week of gestation then leads to duodenal recanalization.[13] An embryologic insult during this period can lead to an intrinsic web, atresia, or stenosis. The extrinsic form of duodenal obstruction is due to defects in the development of neighboring structures such as the pancreas, a preduodenal portal vein, or malrotation and Ladd's bands.[14,15]

Annular pancreas as an etiology for duodenal obstruction warrants special mention as this form of obstruction is likely due to failure of duodenal development rather than a true constricting lesion. Thus, the presence of an annular pancreas is simply a visible indication of an underlying atresia or stenosis.[16] Between the fourth and eighth week of gestation, the pancreatic buds merge. In annular pancreas, the tip of the ventral pancreas becomes fixed to the duodenal wall forming a nondistensible, ring-like or annular portion of pancreatic tissue surrounding the descending part of the duodenum.[13] In annular pancreas associated with duodenal obstruction, the distal biliary tree is often abnormal and may open proximal or distal to the atresia or stenosis.[17,18] Other reported biliary abnormalities associated with duodenal obstruction include biliary atresia, gallbladder agenesis, stenosis of the common bile duct, choledochal cyst, and immune deficiency.[19–24]

Classification

Anatomically, duodenal obstructions are classified as either atresias or stenoses. An incomplete obstruction, due to a fenestrated web or diaphragm, is considered a stenosis. Most stenoses involve the third and/or fourth part of the duodenum. Atresias, or complete obstruction, are further classified into three morphologic types (Fig. 30-1). Type I atresias account for more than 90% of all duodenal obstructions and contain a lumenal diaphragm that includes mucosal and submucosal layers. A diaphragm that has ballooned distally (windsock) is a type I atresia.[25,26] It is important to understand that the anatomy of the windsock may lead to a portion of the dilated duodenum actually being distal to the actual obstruction (Fig. 30-2). Type II atresias are characterized by a dilated proximal and collapsed distal segment connected by a fibrous cord. Type III atresias have an obvious gap separating the proximal and distal duodenal segments.[27]

More than 50% of affected patients with duodenal atresia have associated congenital anomalies.[28] Approximately 30% are associated with trisomy 21, 30% with isolated cardiac defects, and 25% with other gastrointestinal (GI) anomalies.[29,30] Approximately 45% of patients are premature, and about one-third exhibit growth retardation.[6,7]

Pathology

The obstruction can be classified as either preampullary or postampullary, with approximately 85% of obstructions located distal to the ampulla.[30] With complete or almost complete obstruction, the stomach and proximal duodenum become significantly dilated. The pylorus is usually distended and hypertrophic. The bowel distal to

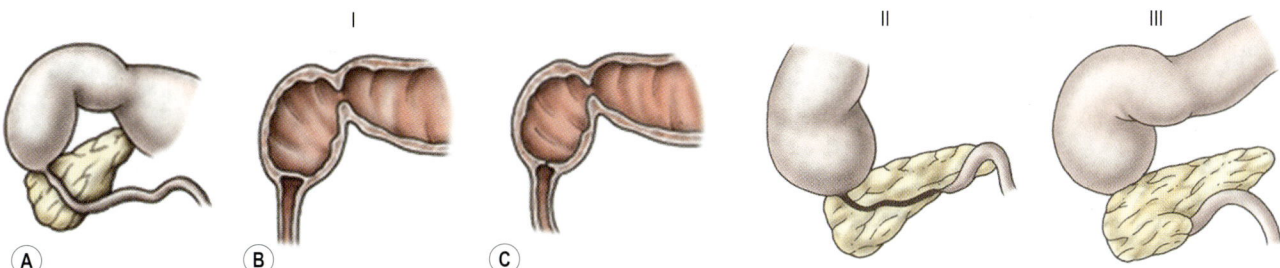

FIGURE 30-1 ■ Duodenal atresia (and stenosis) is depicted. In type I (A), either a membrane (B) or web (C) causes the intrinsic duodenal obstruction. There is no fibrous cord and the duodenum remains in continuity. Type II is characterized by complete obliteration of a segment of the duodenum with the proximal and distal portions attached via a fibrous cord. Type III is associated with complete separation of the dilated proximal duodenum from the collapsed distal duodenum.

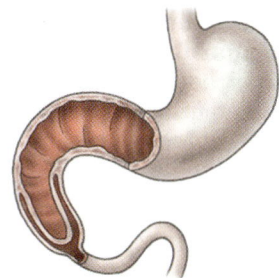

FIGURE 30-2 ■ Illustration of the 'windsock' deformity, a variant of type I duodenal atresia. Note the actual position of the origin of the web in relation to the extent of proximal duodenal dilation and the distal collapsed duodenum.

the obstruction is collapsed, except in the case of a windsock deformity in which the distal bowel is dilated to a variable length depending on the length of the windsock (see Fig. 30-2). In most cases of duodenal obstruction, the gastrointestinal tract can be decompressed proximally. With complete obstruction of the duodenum, the incidence of polyhydramnios ranges from 32–81%.[1,31–34] Growth retardation is also common, presumably from nutritional deprivation from the swallowed amniotic fluid.

Diagnosis

There are multiple benefits to the antenatal diagnosis of duodenal obstruction, including parental counseling. The diagnosis can often be suggested by prenatal ultrasound (US). Sonographic evaluation in fetuses of mothers with a history of polyhydramnios can detect two fluid-filled structures consistent with a double bubble in up to 44% of cases.[35–37] Despite duodenal obstruction usually occurring by week 12, the reason for failure of early prenatal detection is not entirely clear. Most cases of duodenal atresia are detected between 7 and 8 months gestation.[38] It is currently believed that immature gastric emptying in-utero may contribute to low gastric pressures, failing to dilate the proximal duodenum until later in gestation. While both circular and longitudinal muscle layers are present in the stomach by week 8 of gestation, pressure amplitudes at 25 weeks are only 60% of term gastric pressures.[39,40]

The presentation of the neonate with duodenal obstruction varies depending on whether the obstruction is complete or incomplete, and the location of the ampulla of Vater in relation to the obstruction. The classic presentation is that of bilious emesis within the first hours of life in an otherwise stable neonate. In about 10% of cases, however, the atresia is pre-ampullary and the emesis is nonbilious.[15] Abdominal distention may or may not be present. In neonates with duodenal atresia, the abdomen is scaphoid. Aspiration via a nasogastric (NG) tube of more than 20 mL of gastric contents in a newborn suggests intestinal obstruction, as normal aspirate is less than 5 mL.[41] For patients with stenosis, the diagnosis is often delayed until the neonate has started on enteral feeds and feeding intolerance develops with emesis and gastric distention.

In antenatally suspected cases of duodenal obstruction, as well as in neonates with a clinical presentation consistent with a proximal bowel obstruction, an upright abdominal radiograph is usually sufficient to confirm the diagnosis of duodenal atresia. The diagnostic radiographic presentation of duodenal atresia is that of a double bubble sign with no distal bowel gas (Fig. 30-3). The proximal left-sided bubble represents the air and fluid-filled stomach while the dilated proximal duodenum represents the second bubble to the right of midline.[42] In almost all cases of duodenal atresia, the distal bowel is gasless. However, the presence of distal gas does not necessarily exclude the diagnosis of atresia as there are reports of bifed common bile ducts with insertion of one of the ducts proximal and the other distal to the atretic segment which allows the air to bypass the atresia.[43] In neonates whose stomach has been decompressed by either NG aspiration or vomiting, 40–60 mL of instilled air into the stomach will reproduce the double bubble.[27] Rarely, the biliary tree is air filled, and a variety of pancreatic and biliary anomalies have been demonstrated (Fig. 30-4).[43] At our institution, neonates who present with bilious emesis and a decompressed stomach on plain abdominal films receive a limited upper GI contrast study to exclude malrotation and volvulus. With duodenal stenosis, a double bubble sign is often not present and the diagnosis is usually made with a contrast study (Fig. 30-5).

Management

After the diagnosis is made, appropriate resuscitation is required with correction of fluid balance and electrolyte abnormalities, in addition to gastric decompression. At our institution, all neonates diagnosed with duodenal obstruction receive a complete metabolic profile, complete blood count, coagulation studies, an abdominal and spinal ultrasound, and two-dimensional echocardiography prior to any operation. An emergency operation is only performed in cases where malrotation with concurrent volvulus cannot be excluded.

Prior to the mid-1970s, duodenojejunostomy was the preferred technique for correcting duodenal atresia or stenosis.[7,44,45] Since then, the various techniques utilized include side-to-side duodenoduodenostomy, diamond-shaped duodenoduodenostomy, partial web resection with Heineke–Mickulicz-type duodenoplasty, and tapering duodenoplasty.[44–46] The long side-to-side duodenoduodenostomy, although effective, is associated with a high incidence of anastomotic dysfunction and prolonged

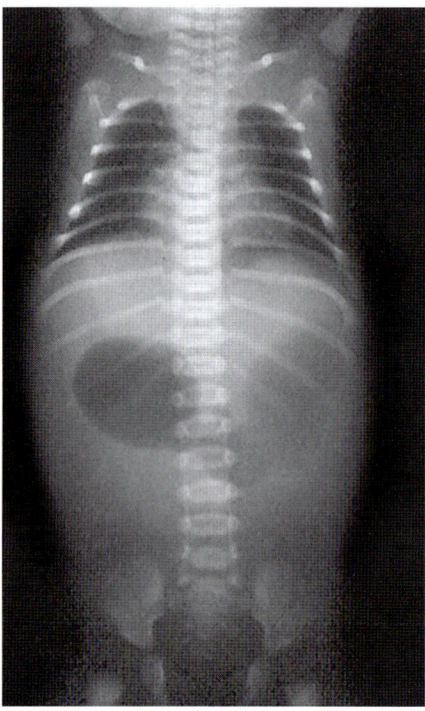

FIGURE 30-3 ■ Classic 'double bubble' sign. This abdominal radiograph in a newborn shows a markedly distended stomach and duodenal bulb without evidence of distal intestinal air.

obstruction.[30] Blind-loop syndrome appears to be more common in patients treated with duodenojejunostomy.[47] Gastrojejunostomy should not be performed as it is associated with a high incidence of marginal ulceration and bleeding.[27]

Currently, the preferred technique is either laparoscopic or open duodenoduodenostomy.[9–11,30] Originally, a side-to-side anastomosis was performed. A proximal transverse to distal longitudinal (diamond-shaped) anastomosis is now preferred.[7,44,45,48–50] For the open approach, either a right upper quadrant supraumbilical transverse incision or an umbilical crease incision is utilized.[49] After mobilizing the ascending and transverse colon to the left, the duodenal obstruction is readily exposed. Malrotation should be evaluated at this point as it can occur in association with congenital duodenal obstruction in up to 30% of patients.[1] A sufficient length of duodenum distal to the atresia is mobilized to allow for a tension-free anastomosis. A transverse duodenotomy is made in the anterior wall of the distal portion of the dilated proximal duodenum and a similar length duodenotomy is made in a vertical orientation on the antimesenteric border of the distal duodenum. The anastomosis is then fashioned by approximating the end of each incision to the appropriate mid-portion of the other incision (Fig. 30-6). Tapering duodenoplasty is generally not necessary as the proximal duodenal dilation usually resolves after relief of the obstruction. Muscular continuity of the duodenal wall suggests a windsock deformity or diaphragm. This finding should precipitate extra vigilance in the operative correction because the dilated and collapsed bowel are both distal to the windsock, and have been anastomosed in error.[26,51]

The laparoscopic approach was first described by Rothenberg in 2002.[9] The standard laparoscopic approach begins with the patient supine and the abdomen is insufflated through the umbilicus. Two other instruments are inserted, one in the baby's right lower quadrant and one in the right mid-epigastric region, respectively. A liver retractor can be placed in the right or left upper quadrant if necessary. Alternatively, the liver can be elevated by placing a transabdominal wall suture around the falciform ligament and tying it outside the abdomen (Fig. 30-7). The duodenum is mobilized and the location of obstruction is identified. Using the same principles that have been described for the open approach, a standard

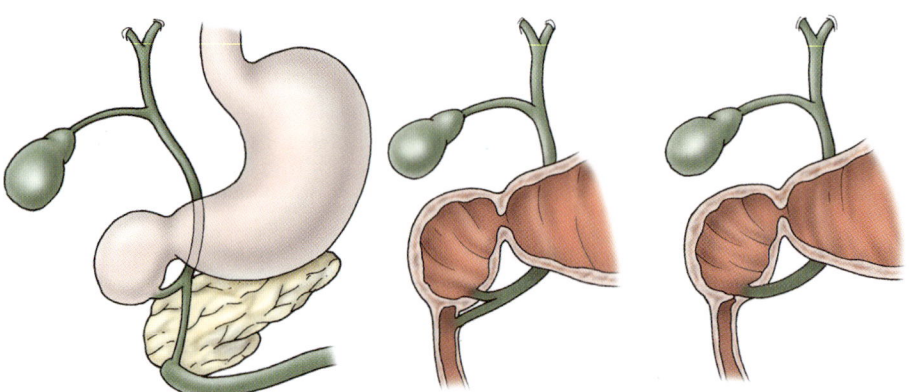

FIGURE 30-4 ■ This schematic depicts several of the variations in biliary ductal anatomy seen in babies with duodenal atresia.

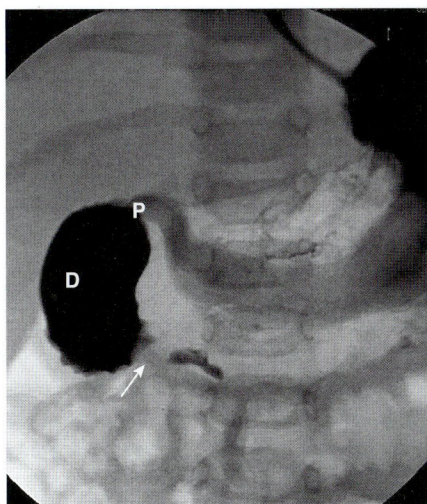

FIGURE 30-5 ■ An upper gastrointestinal contrast study is shown illustrating a duodenal web. Contrast medium outlines the markedly dilated proximal duodenum (D) with a collapsed distal segment. Note the absence of contrast agent at the location of the tiny web (arrow). P, pylorus.

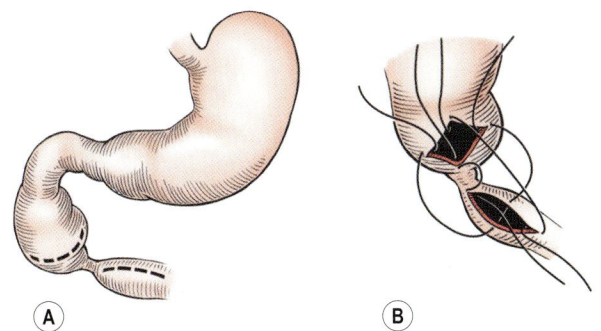

FIGURE 30-6 ■ The technique of duodenoduodenostomy. A diamond-shaped anastomosis is created via the proximal transversely oriented and distal vertically oriented duodenotomies.

diamond-shaped anastomosis is created. Although some surgeons will perform the laparoscopic anastomosis with interrupted sutures, this can be technically demanding because of the significant number of sutures required and the thin nature of the distal duodenum. We reported our results using Nitinol U-clips (Medtronic, Minneapolis, MN) to create the duodenoduodenostomy with no leaks and more rapid initiation of feeds when compared to the traditional open approach (Fig. 30-8).[10,11] Although the U-clips are no longer commercially available, this study highlighted the advantages of early feeding. The historical approach to enteral feeding following duodenal atresia repair involved a period of waiting for the gastric output to become less bilious and the volume of gastric drainage to decrease, indicating return of intestinal function. This report showed that the time spent waiting for the gastric output to decrease is likely not necessary as all of the patients undergong the laparoscopic duodenoplasty had initiation of feeds without adverse events after an upper gastrointestinal contrast study on day 5 revealed no leak. When compared to infants undergoing an open operation with the historical postoperative management mentioned previously, there was a marked reduction in hospitalization for the laparoscopically corrected infants, primarily due to the early feeding.

Historically, during repair of duodenal atresia, it has been emphasized that inspecting the entire small bowel to identify a second atresia is important. Given that duodenal atresia and jejunoileal atresia do not share common embryologic etiologies, a multi-institutional review of duodenal atresia patients was undertaken to quantify the incidence of jejunoileal atresia in this population.[52] In the largest series to date, the rate of concomitant jejunoileal atresia in patients with duodenal atresia was less than 1%. With the low incidence of a concomitant distal atresia, extensive inspection of the entire bowel does not appear necessary.

Early postoperative mortality for duodenal atresia repair has been reported to be as low as 3–5% with the

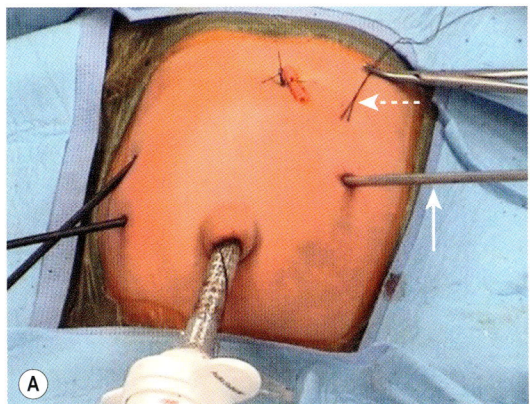
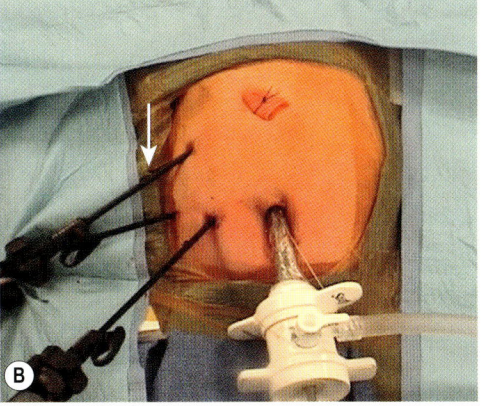

FIGURE 30-7 ■ Two approaches to placement of the instruments for a laparoscopic duodenal atresia repair. **(A)** The two right-sided instruments are the primary working sites for the surgeon. The liver retractor (arrow) has been placed in the left midepigastric region. The falciform ligament has been elevated by a suture placed under it and tied over the red rubber catheter, which is used as a bolster. The suture (dotted arrow) exteriorized in the infant's left upper abdomen was placed in the dilated proximal duodenum so that it could be easily manipulated. **(B)** This is a similar configuration except the instrument elevating the liver (arrow) is placed in the infant's right upper abdomen rather than the left upper abdomen. The suture that was placed through the proximal dilated duodenum in A was not needed in this particular case.

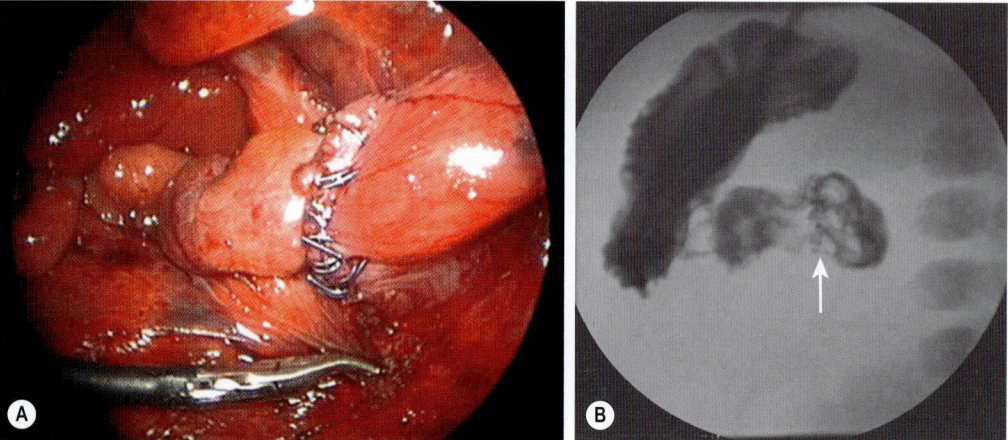

FIGURE 30-8 ■ **(A)** Laparoscopic view of a completed duodenoduodenostomy using the Nitinol U-clips. **(B)** A postoperative contrast study at five days showed no evidence of obstruction or leak at the anastomosis. The U-clips (arrow) can be seen marking the anastomosis.

majority of deaths occurring secondary to complications related to associated congenital abnormalities.[53,54] Long-term survival approaches 90%.[7,53–55] Long-term complications have been noted following repair and include delayed gastric emptying, severe gastroesophageal reflux, bleeding peptic ulcer, megaduodenum, duodenogastric reflux, gastritis, blind-loop syndrome and intestinal obstruction related to adhesions.[30]

JEJUNOILEAL ATRESIA AND STENOSIS

Etiology

Jejunoileal atresia occurs in approximately 1 in 5,000 live births. It occurs equally in males and females, and about one in three infants is premature.[56] Although the majority of cases are thought to occur sporadically, familial cases of intestinal atresias have been described.[57] It is generally accepted that jejunoileal atresia occurs as a result of an intrauterine ischemic insult to the midgut, affecting single or multiple segments of the already developed intestine.[13,58–61] Intrauterine vascular disruption can lead to ischemic necrosis of the bowel with subsequent resorption of the affected segment or segments (Fig. 30-9).

The hypothesis that most cases of jejunoileal atresia occur secondary to vascular disruption during fetal life is derived from experimental as well as clinical evidence. Isolated mesenteric vascular insults and interference with the segmental blood supply to the small intestine were created in fetal dogs, and resulted in different degrees and patterns of intraluminal obstruction, reproducing the spectrum of stenosis and atresia found in humans.[62–64] Moreover, the presence of bile, lanugo hair, and squamous epithelial cells from swallowed amniotic fluid distal to an atresia suggests that the atresia occurs subsequent to some event, but that at some time in gestation the intestinal lumen was patent, thus allowing passage of these contents. Additionally, atresias seen in association with other intrauterine vascular insults such as fetal intussusception, midgut volvulus, thromboembolic occlusions, transmesenteric internal hernias, and

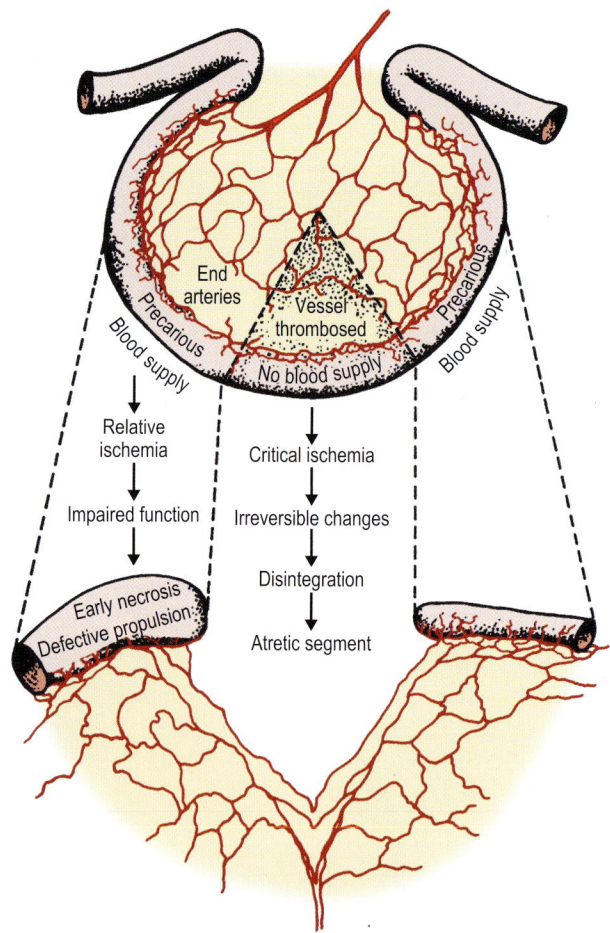

FIGURE 30-9 ■ The proposed mechanism of vascular compromise and subsequent development of jejunoileal atresias is depicted.

incarceration or snaring of bowel in an omphalocele or gastroschisis have contributed to wide acceptance of this hypothesis.[58,64–68]

The presence of associated extra-abdominal organ abnormalities in jejunoileal atresia is low (<10%) due to its occurrence later in fetal life and the localized nature of the vascular insult.[69] Rarely, jejunoileal atresia has been found in patients with Hirschsprung disease, cystic fibrosis, malrotation, Down syndrome, anorectal and vertebral anomalies, neural tube defects, congenital heart disease, and other GI atresias.[56,69,70] Methylene blue, previously used for amniocentesis in twin pregnancies, has been implicated in causing small bowel atresia.[71]

Although jejunoileal atresias are usually not hereditary, there is a well-documented autosomal recessive pattern of inheritance of multiple atresias.[72] In these cases, intestinal rotation was normal, mesenteric defects were never observed, and lanugo hairs and squamous cells were not identified distal to the most proximal atresia. All these findings suggest an early intrauterine event. Survival is poor in these infants, even with successful bowel resection.

No correlations have been found between jejunoileal atresia and parental or maternal disease. However, the use of maternal vasoconstrictive medications, as well as maternal cigarette smoking in the first trimester of pregnancy, has been shown to increase the risk of small bowel atresia.[73] Chromosomal abnormalities are seen in less than 1% of the patients with jejunoileal atresia.[74]

Pathology

The Grosfeld classification system separates these defects into four groups, with an additional consideration for type III(b) (Fig. 30-10).[4] This classification has significant prognostic and therapeutic value as it emphasizes the importance of associated loss of intestinal length, abnormal collateral intestinal blood supply, and concomitant atresia or stenosis.[75] Regarding classification, the most proximal atresia determines whether the atresia is classified as jejunal or ileal atresia. Multiple atresias are found in up to 30% of patients.[56,76]

Stenosis

Stenosis is defined as a localized narrowing of the intestinal lumen without disruption in the intestinal wall or a defect in the mesentery (see Fig. 30-10A). At the stenotic site, a short, narrow, somewhat rigid segment of intestine with a small lumen is found. Often the muscularis is irregular and the submucosa is thickened. Stenosis may also take the form of a type I atresia with a fenestrated web. Patients with jejunoileal stenosis usually have a normal length of small intestine.

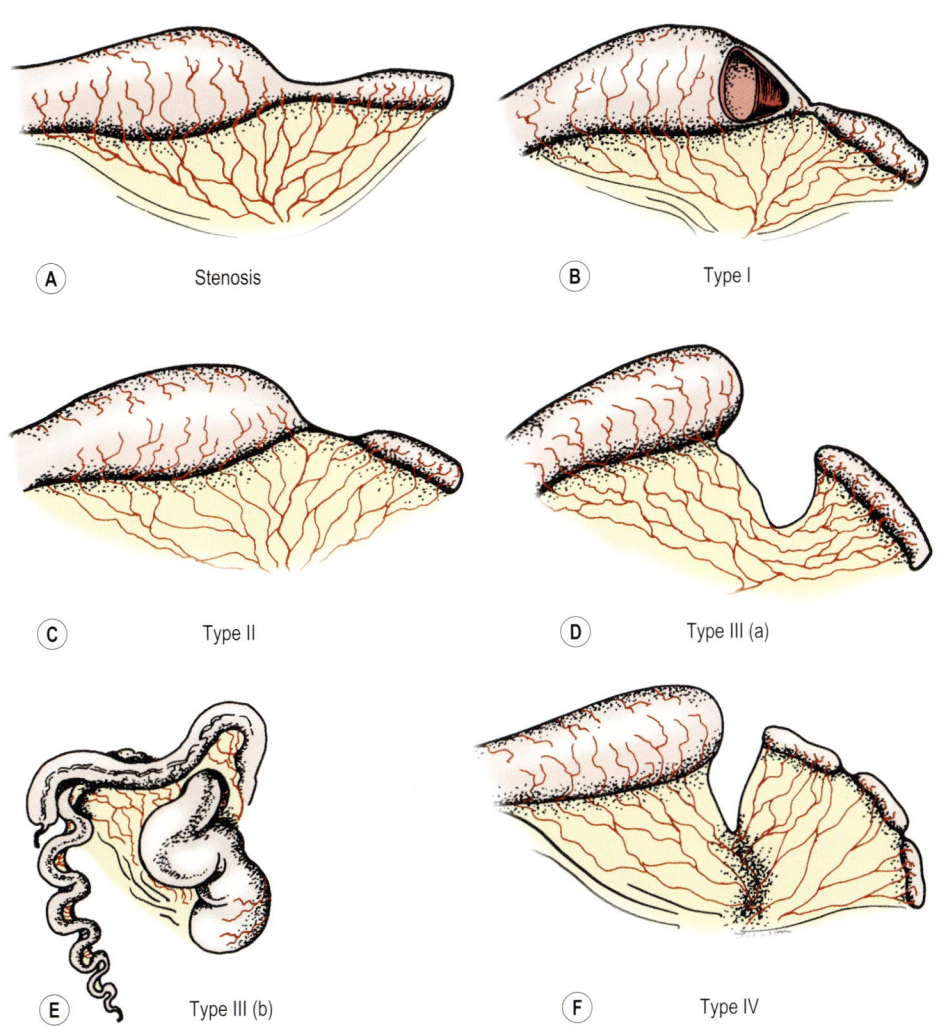

(A) Stenosis (B) Type I

(C) Type II (D) Type III (a)

(E) Type III (b) (F) Type IV

FIGURE 30-10 ■ The classification system for jejunoileal atresia and stenosis is seen.

Type I Atresia

In type I jejunoileal atresia, the intestinal obstruction occurs secondary to a membrane or web formed by both mucosa and submucosa, while the muscularis and serosa remain intact (see Figs 30-10B and 30-11). On gross inspection, the bowel and its mesentery appear to be in continuity. However, the proximal bowel is dilated while the distal bowel is collapsed. With the increased intraluminal pressure in the proximal bowel, bulging of the web into the distal intestine can create a windsock effect. As with stenosis, there is no foreshortening of the bowel in type I atresias.

Type II Atresia

The clinical findings of a type II atresia are a dilated, blind-ending proximal bowel loop connected by a fibrous cord to the collapsed distal bowel with an intact

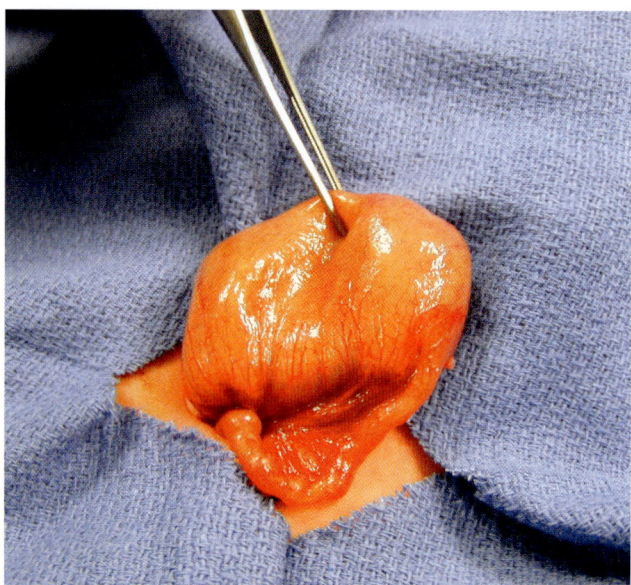

FIGURE 30-11 ■ In this infant with abdominal distention and evidence of a congenital bowel obstruction, a type I jejunal atresia was found. Note the mesentery is intact and the small, distal jejunum is connected to the very dilated, proximal jejunum.

mesentery (see Fig. 30-10C). Increased intraluminal pressure in the dilated and hypertrophied proximal bowel may lead to focal proximal small bowel ischemia. The distal collapsed bowel commences as a blind end, which sometimes assumes a bulbous appearance owing to the remains of an intussusception. Again, the total small bowel length is usually normal.

Type III(a) Atresia

In type III(a) atresia, the proximal bowel ends blindly with no fibrous connecting cord to the distal intestine. A V-shaped mesenteric defect of varying size is present between the two ends of intestine (see Figs 30-10D and 30-12). The dilated, blind-ending proximal bowel is often aperistaltic and frequently undergoes torsion or becomes overdistended, with subsequent necrosis and perforation occurring as a secondary event.[77] In this scenario, the total length of the small bowel is variable (but usually less than normal), owing to intrauterine resorption of the affected bowel.

Type III(b) Atresia

Type III(b) atresia (apple-peel, Christmas tree, or Maypole deformity) consists of a proximal jejunal atresia, absence of the superior mesenteric artery beyond the origin of the middle colic branch, agenesis of the dorsal mesentery, a significant loss of intestinal length, and a large mesenteric defect (see Fig. 30-10E). The decompressed distal small bowel lies free in the abdomen and assumes a helical configuration around a single perfusing vessel arising from the ileocolic or right colic arcades (Fig. 30-13). Occasionally, additional type I or type II atresias are found distal to the initial atresia. Also, the vascularity of the distal bowel is often impaired. This type of atresia has been found in families with a pattern suggestive of an autosomal recessive mode of inheritance. It also has been encountered in siblings with identical lesions and in twins.[77–80]

The occurrence of intestinal atresia in other siblings, the association of multiple atresias (15%), and the discordance in a set of apparently monozygotic twins may point to more complex genetic transmission with an

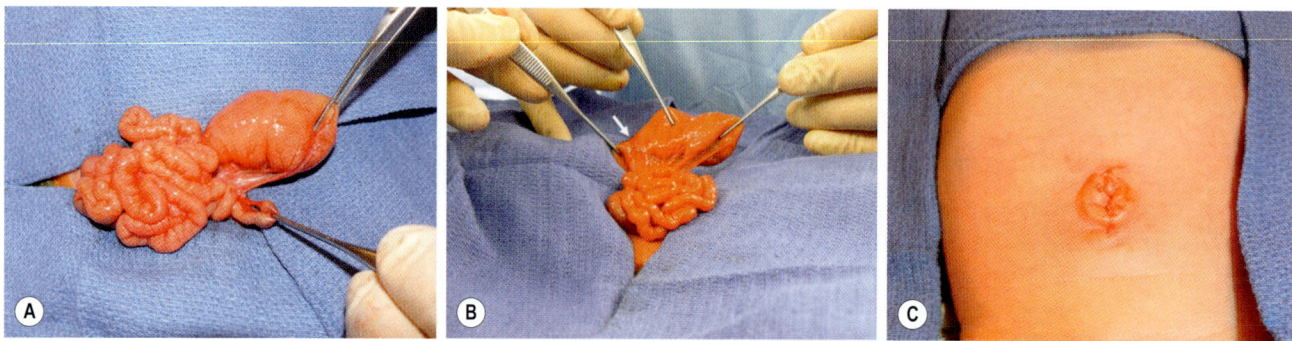

FIGURE 30-12 ■ This baby was suspected of having a proximal jejunal atresia based on symptoms of bilious emesis and the abdominal film. **(A, B)** At operation, this type III(a) jejunal atresia was found. Note the V-shaped mesenteric defect between the dilated proximal atretic bowel and the distal decompressed bowel. Due to the size discrepancy between the two ends of the intestine, the proximal dilated bowel was resected at the arrow and an end-to-side anastomosis was performed. **(C)** The operation was performed through a slightly extended umbilical incision. The baby recovered nicely and no complications developed.

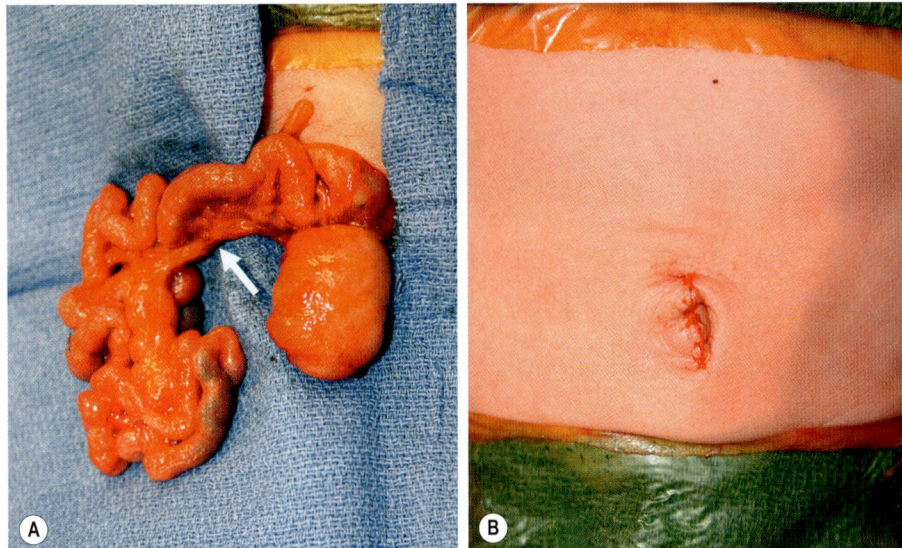

FIGURE 30-13 ■ **(A)** The operative findings in neonate with a type III(b) intestinal atresia are seen. Note the classic 'apple-core' or 'Christmas tree' deformity as well as the wide mesenteric gap between the proximal dilated bowel and distal decompressed ileum. Also, the colon and distal small bowel are perfused through a single artery (arrow) running through the mesentery of the distal bowel. **(B)** This operation was performed through a small umbilical incision. This baby recovered nicely and has not developed any complications.

overall recurrence rate of 18%.[78,81,82] Infants with this anomaly are often premature, and up to 50% may have malrotation. Short bowel syndrome is present in nearly 75% of cases. Accordingly, there is increased morbidity (63%) and mortality (54%) in this population.[78,83] Type III(b) atresias are most likely the result of a proximal superior mesenteric arterial occlusion with extensive infarction of the proximal segment of the midgut. Also, it can develop from a midgut volvulus.[58,84] Primary failure of development of the distal superior mesenteric artery has also been suggested as an etiologic factor. However, this is unlikely because meconium is usually found in the bowel distal to the atresia. This finding indicates that the atresia develops after bile secretion begins, which occurs around week 12 of intrauterine life. The superior mesenteric artery develops much earlier than 12 weeks.[85]

Type IV atresia

Multiple-segment atresias or a combination of types I to III are classified as type IV (see Fig. 30-10F). Twenty to 35% of infants affected with jejunoileal atresia present with multiple atresias.[56,76] The majority of cases of multiple-segment atresias are sporadic with no other family history of intestinal abnormalities. They are likely a result of multiple vascular insults to the mesentery, intrauterine inflammatory processes, or a malformation of the GI tract occurring during embryonic development.[76,86] Embolic material from a nonviable fetus to a living monochorionic twin through placental vascular connections could also account for single or multiple intestinal atresias.[87] Associated defects, particularly abnormalities of the central nervous system, have been noted in approximately 25% of nonfamilial multiple intestinal atresia patients.[76] Multiple atresias have also been seen in association with severe immunodeficiency.[23]

A familial form of multiple intestinal atresia (FMIA) involving the stomach, duodenum, and both the small and large bowel has been described.[72,88] It is associated with prematurity and shortened bowel length. To date, it has been uniformly fatal. It is associated with type I and II atresias, with type II predominating. An autosomal recessive mode of transmission has been suggested for this familial condition because it is unlikely that an isolated prenatal vascular accident is responsible for such extensive involvement of the GI tract. In addition, infants affected with this familial form are found to have long segments of completely occluded small or large intestine without a recognizable lumen.[88–90] Another pathognomonic feature seen in FMIA is the sieve-like appearance of the intestine on histologic examination where multiple lumina are surrounded by epithelial cells and muscularis mucosa.[88]

Pathophysiology

The vascular and subsequent ischemic insult not only causes morphologic abnormalities but also adversely influences the structure and subsequent function of the remaining proximal and distal bowel.[58,59,91] The blind-ended proximal bowel is dilated and hypertrophied with histologically normal villi, but without effective peristaltic activity. A deficiency of mucosal enzymes and muscular adenosine triphosphatase has also been found.[92] At the level of the atresia, the ganglia of the enteric nervous system are atrophic with minimal acetylcholinesterase activity. These changes are most likely secondary to local ischemia. Obstruction alone can elicit similar, but less severe, morphologic and functional abnormalities.[92]

Experimental studies showing that the intestinal atresia results from ischemic necrosis of the intestine also imply that there is a precarious blood supply to the proximally dilated bowel. This has been confirmed with postmortem injection of barium sulfate into the mesenteric vessels.[58,59,85] However, it has also been postulated that the intestine is not ischemic at birth, but rather becomes so only with swallowing air. Distention and increased intraluminal pressure or torsion can then occur. The good results obtained with tapering procedures without resection of the bulbous portion would support the contention that the blood and nerve supply to the bowel adjacent to the atresia is normal.[58] However, this ischemic insult may interfere with mucosal and neural function. Defective peristalsis is commonly noticed in the atretic area, thus supporting resection of the dilated bulbous proximal end for better function.[93] Because the proximal end of the distal atretic bowel has been subjected to a similar insult, a small portion of it should be resected at the time of operative correction as well.

Clinical Manifestations

Prompt recognition of intestinal obstruction in the neonate is paramount due to the possibility of midgut volvulus or an internal hernia with subsequent ischemia. Although prenatal ultrasound is more reliable at detecting duodenal atresia, in recent years it has become useful in diagnosing jejunoileal atresia as well. The ultrasound findings include dilated loops of bowel and polyhydramnios, which may not be present early in gestation or only with very distal obstructions. A fetus with these abnormal findings should elicit a search for familial GI abnormalities as well as referral for prenatal evaluation. The vast majority of patients with jejunoileal atresia will not be diagnosed prenatally.

In neonates with atresia or stenosis, the presenting symptoms are consistent with bowel obstruction, including bilious emesis and abdominal distention. Although

the meconium may appear normal, it is more common to see gray plugs of mucus passed via the rectum. Occasionally, if the distal bowel in type III(b) atresia is ischemic, blood may be passed through the rectum.

Intestinal stenosis is more likely to create diagnostic difficulty when compared to intestinal atresia. Intermittent partial obstruction or malabsorption may improve without treatment. Clinical investigations can initially be normal. However, these babies usually develop failure to thrive and ultimately progress to complete intestinal obstruction and require exploration.

Diagnosis

The diagnosis of jejunoileal atresia can usually be made by radiographic examination of the abdomen using swallowed air as contrast. Swallowed air reaches the proximal bowel by one hour and the distal small bowel by three hours in a normal vigorous infant in whom its passage is blocked, but this pattern may be delayed in premature or sick infants with poor sucking.[94,95] Jejunal atresia patients can have a few gas-filled and fluid-filled loops of small bowel, but the remainder of the abdomen is gasless (Fig. 30-14). When the atresia is associated with cystic fibrosis, fewer air-fluid levels are evident, and the typical ground-glass appearance of inspissated meconium is seen. A limited-contrast study may be useful if intestinal stenosis is suspected.

As haustral markings are rarely seen in neonates, distal ileal atresia may be difficult to differentiate from colonic atresia (Fig. 30-15). A contrast enema will reveal an unused appearance to the colon. Reliance on intraoperative injection of saline into the large bowel to confirm

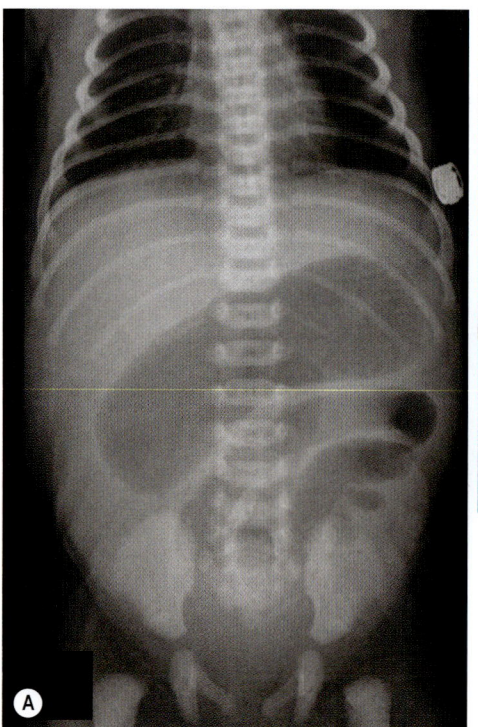
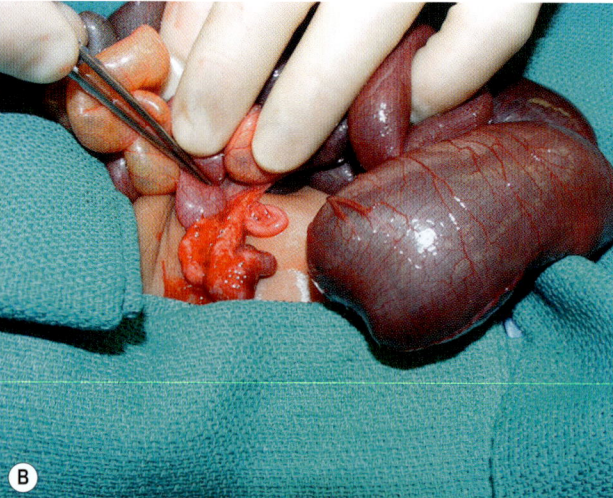

FIGURE 30-14 ■ **(A)** The abdominal radiograph in this neonate shows several proximally dilated intestinal loops consistent with jejunal atresia. **(B)** A type III(a) distal atresia was found at operation.

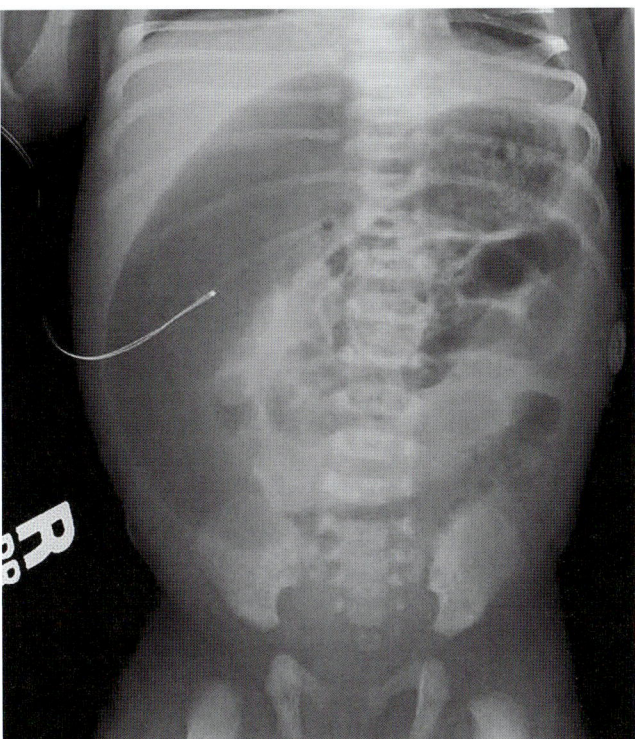

FIGURE 30-15 ■ The diagnosis of colonic atresia can be difficult on the plain abdominal radiograph. This radiograph shows multiple dilated intestinal loops and appears similar to the findings shown in Figure 30-14. At operation, the infant was found to have atresia of the transverse colon (see Fig. 30-16).

distal bowel patency may fail to identify an associated colonic or rectal atresia.[96,97] If the small bowel atresia occurred late in gestation, the bowel distal to the atresia may have a more normal caliber. Occasionally, air and meconium can accumulate proximal to an atresia, mimicking the radiologic appearance of meconium ileus. Additionally, total colonic aganglionosis may be difficult to differentiate from small bowel atresia.

Ten per cent of babies with jejunoileal atresia present with meconium peritonitis.[4] The intestinal perforation usually occurs proximal to the obstruction, near the bulbous blind end. The radiologic appearance of a meconium pseudocyst containing a large air/fluid level is related to the late intrauterine bowel perforation. Intraluminal calcification of meconium or intramural calcification in the form of diffuse punctate or rounded aggregations have been reported with intestinal stenosis or atresia.[98] Meconium calcification in patients with hereditary FMIA produces a 'string of pearls,' which is pathognomonic of this condition.[72,88]

The clinical and radiologic picture of jejunoileal stenosis is determined by the level and degree of stenosis, and the diagnosis may be delayed for years. Morphologic and functional changes in the proximal obstructed intestine vary depending on the degree of obstruction.

Differential Diagnosis

Diseases that mimic jejunoileal atresia include colonic atresia, midgut volvulus, meconium ileus, duplication cysts, internal hernias, ileus due to sepsis, birth trauma,

maternal medications, prematurity, and hypothyroidism.[4,99,100] Special investigations including an upper GI contrast study, contrast enema, rectal biopsy, and a delta F508 gene deletion assay or sweat test to exclude associated cystic fibrosis may be needed.[99,101]

Management

Delay in diagnosis may lead to impairment of intestinal viability (50%), frank necrosis and perforation (10–20%), fluid and electrolyte abnormalities, and sepsis. Preoperative management should include gastric decompression and fluid resuscitation to correct electrolyte abnormalities and hypovolemia. Antibiotics should be initiated if there is suspicion for perforation or infection.

Surgical Considerations

The operative management of intestinal atresias is based on the location of the lesion, anatomic findings, associated conditions noted at operation, and the length of the remaining instestine.[56] Resection of the dilated and hypertrophied proximal bowel (see Fig. 30-12B), with primary end-to-end anastomosis with or without tapering of the proximal bowel, is the most common technique.[4,77,100]

As recently as the 1950s, the surgical mortality for newborns with intestinal atresia was 80% to 90%.[56,99] This high mortality rate was mostly related to late presentation and dysmotility of the proximal dilated bowel which led to complications related to chronic obstruction and inanition. Fortunately, the current survival rate is greater than 90%.[56] The understanding that the proximal bowel is dysfunctional, improvements in the anastomotic technique and suture material, and the development of total parenteral nutrition (TPN) are the primary reasons for this significantly improved survival in recent years. Currently, only infants with severe associated congenital abnormalities or short bowel syndrome should not have a good prognosis.

Operative Considerations

The repair of small intestinal atresia can be undertaken via several approaches. One option is to evaluate using a laparoscopic approach, with subsequent resection and anastomosis performed in an extra-corporeal fashion. Although this approach seems attractive, it can be difficult to identify the atresia due to the markedly dilated small intestine and the small working space of the neonate's abdominal cavity. To overcome these limitations, we explore the abdomen through the umbilicus. With this technique, the umbilical skin is incised and the fascia is opened vertically in the midline to the extent allowed by the umbilical skin incision. The small intestine can be exteriorized relatively easy through the umbilical incision (see Figs 30-12C and 30-13B). In a retrospective report, a circumumbilical incision for neonatal surgery was found to as effective as the transverse abdominal incision with less morbidity and better cosmetic results.[102] The traditional transverse supra- or infraumbilical incision is also appropriate. Regardless of the approach, access to the entire intestine and peritoneal cavity is necessary. Careful inspection of the entire bowel is performed and the site and type of obstruction should be noted as well as any other abnormalities. In addition, the length of bowel should be assessed. The most distal limb of the atretic bowel can then be cannulated with a red rubber catheter and irrigated with warm saline to evaluate for distal obstruction. Continuity of the colon can be established preoperatively by a contrast enema or with a prepositioned transrectal catheter placed prior to prepping.[103] Failure to adequately evaluate for distal obstruction or stenosis can lead to postoperative complications, including an anastomotic leak. If present, malrotation should be corrected with a Ladd procedure. Because the length of functional bowel has important prognostic significance, and determines the most appropriate method of repair, the length of functional bowel should be carefully measured along the antimesenteric border and documented in the operative report.

Delayed intestinal function in the blind proximal atretic segment as well as functional obstruction after performance of a side-to-side anastomosis without resection of the dilated proximal atretic bowel have been described.[100] Therefore, if the length of functional bowel is adequate, the bulbous hypertrophied proximal bowel should be resected to approximately normal caliber bowel. Ultimately, the goal is to restore bowel continuity while maintaining both intestinal function and length. Intestinal imbrication has also been shown to be an effective method to reduce the caliber of the dilated bowel while maintaining mucosal absorptive surface.[104] Regarding the distal segment, a short length (4–5 cm) of bowel is obliquely resected, leaving the mesenteric side longer than the antimesenteric aspect. An incision along the antimesenteric border to create a 'fish mouth' may be needed to create an adequate distal enterotomy for the anastomosis.

Although there are multiple techniques for the anastomosis, we generally perform a one-layer modification of the end-to-back technique using 5-0 or 6-0 sutures. Once the anastomosis is completed, the suture line is tested for leaks, and reinforcing sutures are placed as needed. The mesenteric defect is repaired with careful attention to avoid rotation or kinking of the anastomosis, or injury to the blood supply. A temporary enterostomy should be performed if there is a question of bowel viability.[56] However, neither decompressive gastrostomy nor transanastomotic stents are usually needed.[105,106]

Similar techniques are used for stenosis and jejunoileal membranes. Procedures such as transverse enteroplasty, excision of the membrane, and bypassing techniques are not recommended primarily because they fail to remove the abnormal segments of bowel, and may produce blind-loop syndromes.

Prognostic Factors

The normal small bowel length in term neonates is approximately 250 cm. In preterm infants, it ranges from 160–240 cm. With the development of TPN, special enteral diets and pharmacologic management of short gut syndrome, previous estimates that a small bowel length of 100 cm or more is necessary to sustain oral intake and survival may no longer be applicable. Preservation of bowel length at the expense of a poorly functioning anastomosis should be avoided.

If proximal resection will lead to significant, or unacceptable bowel loss, tapering or plication of the dilated bowel is a useful technique.[104,107] Tapering enteroplasty as far proximal as the second portion of the duodenum can be accomplished by resecting an antimesenteric strip of the dilated proximal bowel.[108] During tapering duodeno-jejunoplasty, particularly with type III atresias, the duodenum is de-rotated, thus allowing a direct caudal descent from the stomach which decreases the risk for obstruction. Additionally, the mesentery should be maximally opened, while meticulously protecting the small bowel blood supply. During this process, the cecum can be mobilized to the left which results in a broader mesentery and also allows the anastomosis to lie in manner that will help avoid kinking.[109] The tapering can be safely performed up to 35 cm.[107] The tapered bowel may then be anastomosed to the distal bowel or exteriorized as a stoma.

A primary anastomosis may be contraindicated in cases of peritonitis, volvulus with vascular compromise, meconium ileus, or type III(b) atresia.[110,111] Under these circumstances, exteriorization of both ends of the atresia may be needed.

Intestinal atresia encountered in a baby with gastroschisis may be single or multiple, and may be located in either the small or large bowel. In a series from our institution, 12.6% of 199 patients with gastroschisis had an associated atresia.[112] The most common location for the atresia was jejunoileal and most were type III(a). Our current management algorithm for patients with gastroschisis and atresia is to first assess the extent of reactive change (peel) on the intestine. If there is minimal peel, primary anastomosis may be an option. This is rare and should be considered only in the most optimal situations. In nearly all instances, the atresia should be left undisturbed at the initial operation. After fascial closure is accomplished, management should include gastric decompression and TPN support with subsequent atresia repair four to six weeks later.

With type III(b) atresia, restricting bands along the free edge of the distal coiled and narrow mesentery should be divided to optimize the blood supply. The bowel should be returned to the abdomen with careful inspection of the mesentery to prevent torsing the single marginal artery and vein. In cases of questionable intestinal viability, improved long-term results have been achieved with resection and tapering of the dilated proximal bowel with limited resection of the distal bowel.[113,114]

Bowel-length conservation methods, such as multiple anastomoses for multiple atresias, may result in increased morbidity. A silicone (Silastic) catheter stent can be used with multiple primary anastomoses and serves as a conduit for radiologic evidence of anastomotic integrity, luminal patency, and enteral feeding.[115] If multiple atresias are grouped closely together and there is adequate bowel length, a single resection and anastomosis can be performed.

No attempt at any bowel lengthening procedures should be entertained at the initial operation. However, such procedures may ultimately obviate the need for prolonged TPN in patients with short gut syndrome.

Postoperative Care

Parenteral nutrition is mandatory and should begin as soon as possible, and should continue until the infant is tolerating full enteral feeds.

Enteral feedings can be initiated when the gastric aspirate is clear, output is minimal, and the infant is stooling. At our institution, enteral feeding is usually started through a feeding tube at a rate of 20 mL/kg/day of breast milk or formula in a continuous fashion. The feeds are increased by 20–30 mL/kg/day. Oral intake is started when the baby is alert, able to suck, and tolerating at least 8 mL of tube feeds per hour.

Transient GI dysfunction is frequently observed in infants with jejunal and ileal atresia, and its etiology is multifactorial.[4,116] Lactose intolerance, malabsorption (owing to stasis with bacterial overgrowth), and diarrhea may be significant in infants who have undergone repair of type III(b) atresia, or in those with short bowel syndrome after surgery for multiple atresias. Regular monitoring for clinical signs of intestinal overload or intolerance is required. Water-loss stools, increasing frequency of stooling, hematochezia, fecal-reducing substances, or a decreased stool pH warrant biochemical evaluation of the stool for disaccharide or monosaccharide intolerance.[117] Unintentional injury to the mucosa can be caused by sugars, high-osmolarity feeds, oral medications, and bacterial or viral infections. Pharmacologic control of altered GI function may hasten adaptation. Loperamide hydrochloride decreases intestinal peristaltic activity and cholestyramine is effective in binding bile salts.[117,118] Cholestyramine should not be given unless water-loss stools are evident. Vitamin B12 and folic acid should be given regularly to the patient without a terminal ileum to prevent megaloblastic anemia.

Functional outcome ultimately depends on the following factors: (1) the location of the atresia (the ileum adapts to a greater degree than the jejunum); (2) the maturity of the intestine (the small intestine in a premature infant still has time for maturation and growth); and (3) the length of the small intestine, which can be difficult to determine accurately after birth.[119] The ileocecal valve is critically important as it allows for more rapid intestinal adaptation when the residual small bowel length is short.

COLONIC ATRESIA

Colonic atresia (CA) is a rare cause of intestinal obstruction and comprises 1.8–15% of all GI atresias.[120,121] The reported incidence of CA varies greatly from 1 : 5000 to 1 : 60,000 live births.[122–125] The accepted incidence is approximately 1 in 20,000 live births. Although it is most commonly reported as an isolated anomaly, approximately one-third of babies have associated congenital lesions.[123,124,126] There are various classifications of CA, but the one most commonly used divides CA into three

types. Type I consists of mucosal atresia with an intact bowel wall and mesentery. In type II, the atretic ends are separated by a fibrous cord. In type III, the atretic ends are separated by a V-shaped mesenteric gap (Fig. 30-16). Type III lesions are the most commonly occurring lesions overall, while types I and II are seen more commonly distal to the splenic flexure.[122,127]

The rate of associated anomalies with CA is much smaller when compared to other atresias. CAs have been found in approximately 2.5% of neonates with gastroschisis.[112] There are less than 25 published cases of CA and Hirschsprung disease (HD).[126] Complex urologic abnormalities, multiple small intestinal atresias, an unfixed mesentery, and skeletal anomalies have also been reported with CA.[122,127–129] Similar to small bowel atresias, a vascular insult to the colon continues to be the accepted etiology for all types of CA.[130,131]

The characteristic clinical features of CA are abdominal distention, bilious emesis, and failure to pass meconium. On plain radiographs, air-fluid levels are usually appreciated as well as dilated intestinal loops of large bowel often associated with a 'ground-glass' appearance of meconium mixed with air. Occasionally, the dilation can be so massive that it mimics pneumoperitoneum (Fig. 30-17). The diagnosis is made with a contrast enema showing a small diameter distal colon that comes to an abrupt halt at the level of the obstruction (Fig. 30-18).

The diagnosis of CA is an indication for urgent operative management as the risk for perforation is higher than is seen in jejunoileal atresias. The operative approach depends on the clinical status of the patient, the level of

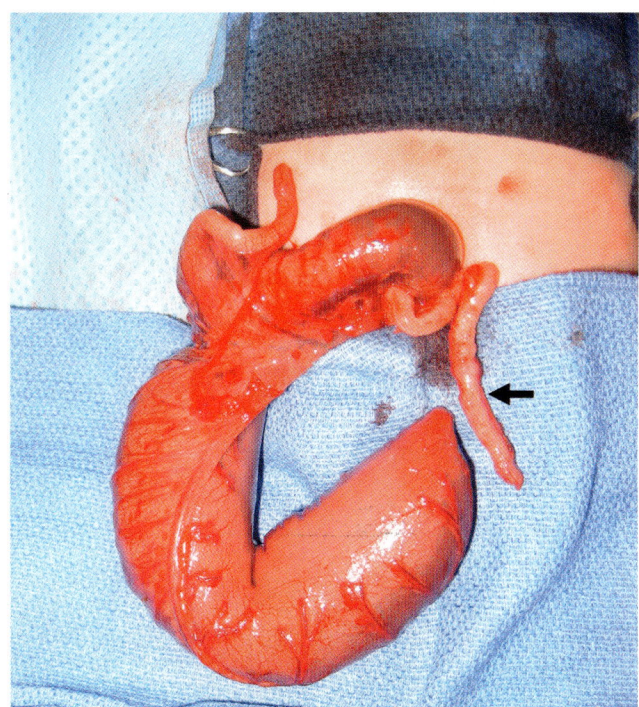

FIGURE 30-16 ■ A type III colonic atresia was found at operation in this infant with intestinal obstruction. Note the cecum and appendix and the very dilated right colon. Also, note the extremely small distal colon (arrow). A colostomy was performed as the initial procedure in this infant.

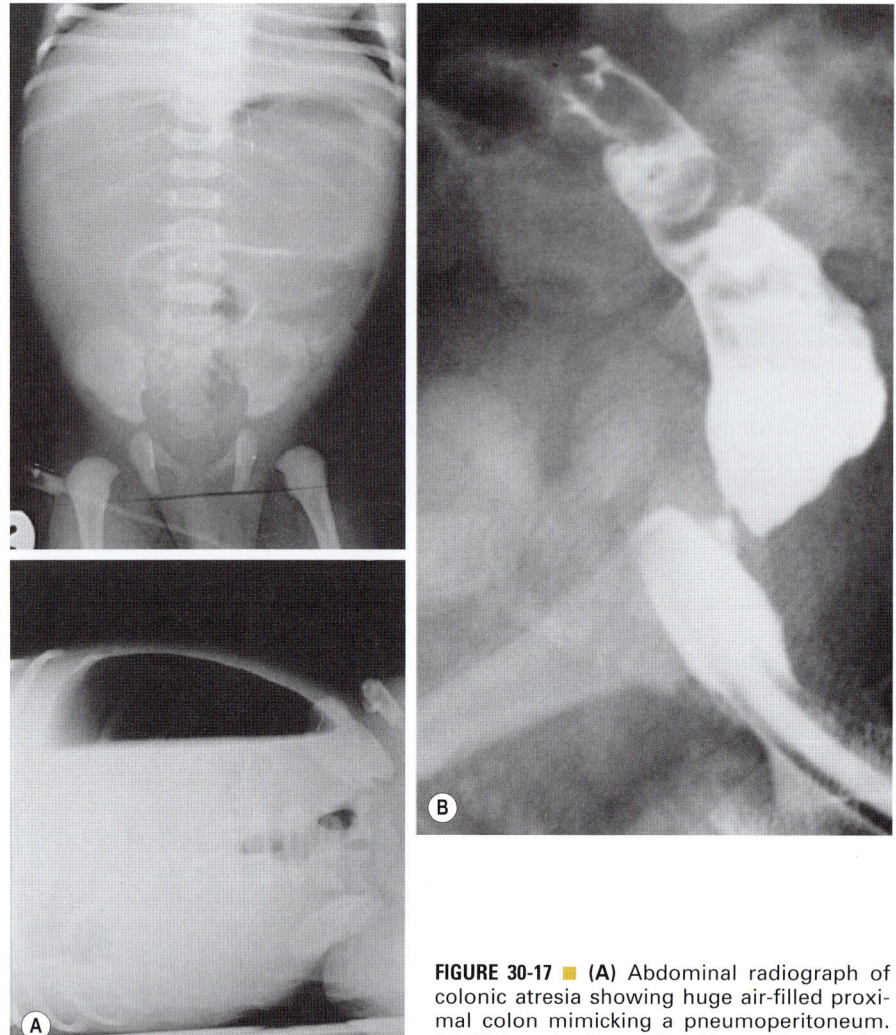

FIGURE 30-17 ■ **(A)** Abdominal radiograph of colonic atresia showing huge air-filled proximal colon mimicking a pneumoperitoneum. **(B)** Right colonic atresia with rectal stenosis.

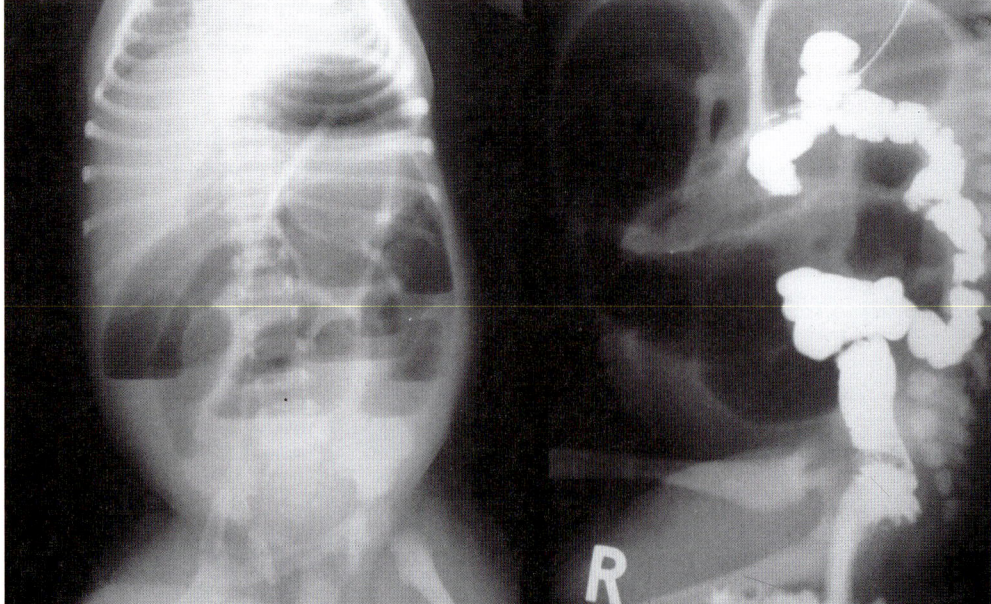

FIGURE 30-18 ■ The contrast enema on the right in a patient with a distal intestinal obstruction (left) shows a small colon and failure of the contrast to move proximally past the mid-transverse colon.

the atresia, any associated small intestinal atresias, and the patency of the bowel distal to the atresia. It is important to exclude other intestinal atresias and stenoses at the time of operation as they occur with some frequency.[132] A diagnosis of associated HD, although rare, must be made by frozen section analysis of rectal biopsies during the initial surgery as unrecognized HD can lead to an anastomotic leak or functional obstruction.

A staged approach consisting of colostomy with mucous fistula is generally preferred for CA. Because the proximal and distal ends adjacent to the atresia are abnormal in both innervation and vascularity, resection of the bulbous proximal colon as well as a portion of the distal microcolon is suggested.[133,134] Primary resection with anastomosis has a higher incidence of complications, usually due to undiagnosed distal pathology.[124,135]

A recent report of a small case series of rectal and sigmoid atresias described a transanal approach for the repair of the atresias.[136] An initial colostomy at birth was performed followed by a transanal approach three to six months later. Closure of the colostomy was then carried out one to two months later.

In the absence of other serious co-morbidities, the prognosis in CA is excellent. If diagnosed early, the overall mortality is less than 10%.[126] A delay in diagnosis beyond 72 hours, however, may result in a mortality of greater than 60%.[129] This high mortality is due, in part, to the formation of a closed loop obstruction between an intact ileocecal valve and the atresia, leading to massive colonic distention and perforation.

REFERENCES

1. Irving IM. Duodenal atresia and stenosis: Annular pancreas. In: Lister J, Irving IM, editors. Neonatal Surgery. 3rd ed. London: Butterworths; 1990. p. 424.
2. Adeyemi D. Neonatal intestinal obstruction in a developing tropical country: Patterns, problems, and prognosis. J Trop Pediatr 1989;35:66–70.
3. Cywes S, Davies MRQ, Rode H. Congenital jejuno-ileal atresia and stenosis. S Afr Med J 1980;57:630–9.
4. Grosfeld JL. Jejunoileal atresia and stenosis, section 3: The small intestine. In: Ravitch MM, Welch KJ, Benson CD, et al, editors. Pediatric Surgery. Chicago: Year Book Medical; 1986. p. 838.
5. Kimura K, Loening-Baucke V. Bilious vomiting in the newborn: Rapid diagnosis of intestinal obstruction. Am Fam Physician 2000;61:2791–8.
6. Chhabra R, Suresh BR, Weinberg G, et al. Duodenal atresia presenting as hematemesis in a premature infant with Down syndrome. Case report and review of the literature. J Perinatol 1992;12:25–7.
7. Grosfeld JL, Rescorla FJ. Duodenal atresia and stenosis: Reassessment of treatment and outcome based on antenatal diagnosis, pathologic variance, and long-term follow-up. World J Surg 1993;17:301309.
8. Adzick NS, Harrison MR, de Lorimier AA. Tapering duodenoplasty for megaduodenum associated with duodenal atresia. J Pediatr Surg 1986;21:311–12.
9. Rothenberg SS. Laparoscopic duodenoduodenostomy for duodenal obstruction in infants and children. J Pediatr Surg 2002;37:1088–9.
10. Valusek PA, Spilde TL, Tsao K, et al. Laparoscopic duodenal atresia repair using surgical U-clips: A novel technique. Surg Endosc 2007;21:1023–4.
11. Spilde TL, St Peter SD, Keckler SJ, et al. Open vs. laparoscopic repair of congenital duodenal obstructions: A concurrent series. J Pediatr Surg 2008;43:1002–5.
12. Ladd WE. Congenital obstruction of the duodenum in children. N Engl J Med 1931;206:277–83.
13. Moore KL, Persaud TVN. The digestive system. In: The Developing Human. 8th ed. Philadelphia: WB Saunders; 2007. p. 218, 233.
14. Schnaufer L. Duodenal atresia, stenosis and annular pancreas. In: Welch RJ, Randolph JG, et al, editors. Pediatric Surgery. Chicago: Year Book Medical; 1986. p. 929.
15. Shawis R, Antao B. Prenatal bowel dilatation and the subsequent postnatal management. Early Hum Dev 2006;82:297–303.
16. Elliot GB, Kliman R, Elliot KA. Pancreatic annulus: A sign or a cause of duodenal obstruction? Can J Surg 1968;11:357.
17. Gourevitch A. Duodenal atresia in the newborn. Ann R Coll Surg Engl 1971;48:141–58.
18. Jona JZ, Belin RP. Duodenal anomalies and the ampulla of Vater. Surg Gynecol Obstet 1976;143:565–9.
19. Irving IM, Rickham PP. Duodenal atresia and stenosis: Annular pancreas. In: Rickham PP, Lister J, Irving IM, editors. Neonatal Surgery. 2nd ed. Boston: Butterworths; 1978. p. 355.
20. Brereton RJ, Cudmore RE, Bouton JM. Double atresia of the duodenum. Z Kinderchir 1980;31:60–5.
21. Coughlin JP, Rector FE, Klein MD. Agenesis of the gallbladder in duodenal atresia: Two case reports. J Pediatr Surg 1992;27:1304.
22. Davenport M, Saxena R, Howard E. Acquired biliary atresia. J Pediatr Surg 1996;31:1721–3.
23. Moore SW, de Jongh G, Bouic P, et al. Immune deficiency in familial duodenal atresia. J Pediatr Surg 1996;31:1733–5.
24. Mali V, Wagener S, Sharif K, et al. Foregut atresias and bile duct anomalies: Rare, infrequent or common?! Pediatr Surg Int 2007;23:889–95.
25. Bill AH Jr, Pope WM. Congenital duodenal diaphragm. Surgery 1954;35:482–6.
26. Rowe M, Buckner D, Clatworthy HW Jr. Wind sock web of the duodenum. Am J Surg 1968;116:444–9.
27. Magnuson DK, Schwartz MZ. Stomach and duodenum. In: Oldham KT, Colombani PM, Foglia RP, et al, editors. Principles and Practice of Pediatric Surgery. Philadelphia: Lippincott Williams & Wilkins; 2004. p. 1149.
28. Kimble RM, Harding J, Kolbe A. Additional congenital anomalies in babies with gut atresia or stenosis: When to investigate, and which investigation. Pediatr Surg Int 1997;12:565–70.
29. Mustafawi AR, Hassan ME. Congenital duodenal obstruction in children: A decade's experience. Eur J Pediatr Surg 2008;18:93–7.
30. Escobar MA, Ladd AP, Grosfeld JL, et al. Duodenal atresia and stenosis: Long-term follow-up over 30 years. J Pediatr Surg 2004;39:867–71.
31. Fonkalsrud EW, DeLorimier AA, Hays DM. Congenital atresia and stenosis of the duodenum: A review compiled from the members of the Surgical Section of the American Academy of Pediatrics. Pediatrics 1969;43:79–83.
32. al-Salem AH, Khwaja S, Grant C, et al. Congenital intrinsic duodenal obstruction: Problems in the diagnosis and management. J Pediatr Surg 1989;24:1247–9.
33. Longo MF, Lynn HB. Congenital duodenal obstruction: Review of 29 cases encountered in a 30-year period. Mayo Clin Proc 1967;42:423–30.
34. Kimble RM, Harding JE, Kolbe A. Does gut atresia cause polyhydramnios? Pediatr Surg Int 1998;13:115–17.
35. Stubbs TM, Horger EO. Sonographic detection of fetal duodenal atresia [Letter]. Obstet Gynecol 1989;73:146.
36. Akhtar J, Guiney EJ. Congenital duodenal obstruction. Br J Surg 1992;79:133–5.
37. Bittnecourt DG, Barini R, Marba S, et al. Congenital duodenal obstruction: Does prenatal diagnosis improve the outcome? Pediatr Surg Int 2004;20:582–5.
38. Lawrence MJ, Ford WD, Furness ME, et al. Congenital duodenal obstruction: Early antenatal ultrasound diagnosis. Pediatr Surg Int 2000;16:342–5.
39. Dumont RC, Rudolph CD. Development of gastrointestinal motility in the infant and child. Gastroenterol Clin North Am 1994;23:655–71.
40. Berseth CL. Gestational evolution of small intestinal motility in preterm and term infants. J Pediatr 1989;115:646–51.
41. Britton JR, Britton HL. Gastric aspirate volume at birth as an indicator of congenital intestinal obstruction. Acta Paediatr 1995;84:945–6.

42. Traubici J. The double bubble sign. Radiology 2001;220:463–4.
43. Kassner EG, Sutton A, De Groot TJ. Bile duct anomalies associated with duodenal atresia: Paradoxical presence of small bowel gas. Am J Roentgenol Radium Ther Nucl Med 1972;116:577–83.
44. Kimura K, Mukohara N, Nishijima E, et al. Diamond-shaped anastomosis for duodenal atresia: An experience with 44 patients over 15 years. J Pediatr Surg 1990;25:977–9.
45. Weber TR, Lewis JE, Mooney D, et al. Duodenal atresia: A comparison of techniques of repair. J Pediatr Surg 1986;21:1133–6.
46. Singh SJ, Dickson R, Baskaranathan S, et al. Excision duodenoplasty: A new technique for congenital duodenal obstruction. Pediatr Surg Int 2002;18:75–8.
47. Rescorla FJ, Grosfeld JL. Duodenal atresia in infancy and childhood: Improved survival and long-term follow-up. Contemp Surg 1988;33:22–7.
48. Takayashi Y, Tajiri T, Masumoto K, et al. Umbilical crease incision for duodenal atresia achieves excellent cosmetic results. Pediatr Surg Int 2010;26:963–6.
49. Ein SH, Kim PC, Miller HA. The late nonfunctioning duodenal atresia repair-A second look. J Pediatr Surg 2000;35:690–1.
50. Kimura K, Tsugawa C, Ogawa K, et al. Diamond-shaped anastomosis for congenital duodenal obstruction. Arch Surg 1977;112:1262–3.
51. Richardson WR, Martin LW. Pitfalls in the surgical management of the incomplete duodenal diaphragm. J Pediatr Surg 1969;4:303–12.
52. St. Peter SD, Little DC, Barsness KS, et al. Should we be concerned about jejunoileal atresia during repair of duodenal atresia? J Laparoendoscopic Adv Surg Tech 2010;20:773–5.
53. Feggetter S. A review of the long-term results of operations for duodenal atresia. Br J Surg 1969;56:68–72.
54. Stauffer UG, Irving I. Duodenal atresia and stenosis–long-term results. Prog Pediatr Surg 1977;10:49–60.
55. Kokkonen ML, Kalima T, Jaaskelainen J, et al. Duodenal atresia: Late follow-up. J Pediatr Surg 1988;23:216–20.
56. Dalla Vecchia LK, Grosfeld JL, West KW, et al. Intestinal atresia and stenosis: A 25-year experience with 277 cases. Arch Surg 1998;133:490–6.
57. Kumaran N, Shankar KR, Lloyd DA, et al. Trends in the management and outcome of jejuno-ileal atresia. Eur J Pediatr Surg 2002;12:163–7.
58. Louw JH. Congenital intestinal atresia and stenosis in the newborn. Observations on its pathogenesis and treatment. Ann R Coll Surg Engl 1959;25:209–34.
59. Louw JH, Barnard CN. Congenital intestinal atresia: Observations on its origin. Lancet 1955;269:1065–7.
60. Abrams JS. Experimental intestinal atresia. Surgery 1968;64:185–91.
61. Puri P, Fujimoto T. New observations on the pathogenesis of multiple intestinal atresias. J Pediatr Surg 1988;23:221–5.
62. Koga Y, Hayashida Y, Ikeda K, et al. Intestinal atresia in fetal dogs produced by localized ligation of mesenteric vessels. J Pediatr Surg 1975;10:949–53.
63. Tibboel D, van der Kamp AW, Molenaar JC. An experimental study of the effect of an intestinal perforation at various developmental stages. Z Kinderchir 1982;37:62–6.
64. Khen N, Jaubert F, Sauvat F, et al. Fetal intestinal obstruction induces alteration of enteric nervous system development in human intestinal atresia. Pediatr Res 2004;56:975–80.
65. Amoury RA, Ashcraft KW, Holder TM. Gastroschisis complicated by intestinal atresia. Surgery 1977;82:373–81.
66. Grosfeld JL, Clatworthy HW Jr. The nature of ileal atresia due to intrauterine intussusception. Arch Surg 1970;100:714–17.
67. Murphy DA. Internal hernias in infancy and childhood. Surgery 1964;55:311–16.
68. Vassy LE, Boles ET Jr. Iatrogenic ileal atresia secondary to clamping of an occult omphalocele. J Pediatr Surg 1975;10:797–800.
69. Sweeney B, Surana R, Puri P. Jejunoileal atresia and associated malformations: Correlation with timing of in-utero insult. J Pediatr Surg 2001;36:774–6.
70. Moore SW, Rode H, Millar AJW, et al. Intestinal atresia and Hirschsprung's disease. Pediatr Surg Int 1990;5:182–4.
71. Nicolini U, Monni G. Intestinal obstruction in babies exposed in-utero to methylene blue. Lancet 1990;336:1258–9.
72. Guttman FM, Braun P, Garance PH, et al. Multiple atresias and a new syndrome of hereditary multiple atresias involving the gastrointestinal tract from stomach to rectum. J Pediatr Surg 1973;8:633–40.
73. Werler MM, Sheehan JE, Mitchell AA. Association of vasoconstrictive exposures with risks of gastroschisis and small intestinal atresia. Epidemiology 2003;14:349–54.
74. Cywes S, Davies MR, Rode H. Congenital jejuno-ileal atresia and stenosis. S Afr Med J 1980;57:630–9.
75. Davies MR, Louw JH, Cywes S, et al. The classification of congenital intestinal atresias [letter]. J Pediatr Surg 1982;17:224.
76. Baglaj M, Carachi R, Lawther S. Multiple atresia of the small intestine: A 20-year review. Eur J Pediatr Surg 2008;18:13–18.
77. Louw JH. Congenital intestinal atresia and severe stenosis in the newborn. S Afr J Clin Sci 1952;3:109–29.
78. Seashore JH, Collins FS, Markowitz RI, et al. Familial apple peel jejunal atresia: Surgical, genetic, and radiographic aspects. Pediatrics 1987;80:540–4.
79. Mishalany HG, Der Kaloustian VM. Familial multiple-level intestinal atresias: Report of two siblings. J Pediatr 1971;79:124–5.
80. Weitzman JJ, Vanderhoof RS. Jejunal atresia with agenesis of the dorsal mesentery with "Christmas tree" deformity of the small intestine. Am J Surg 1966;111:443–9.
81. Zerella JT, Martin LW. Jejunal atresia with absent mesentery and a helical ileum. Surgery 1976;80:550–3.
82. Smith MB, Smith L, Wells JW, et al. Concurrent jejunal atresia with "apple peel" deformity in premature twins. Pediatr Surg Int 1991;6:425–8.
83. DeLorimier AA, Fonkalsrud EW, Hays DM. Congenital atresia and stenosis of the jejunum and ileum. Surgery 1969;65:819–27.
84. Dickson JA. Apple peel small bowel: An uncommon variant of duodenal and jejunal atresia. J Pediatr Surg 1970;5:595–600.
85. Jimenez FA, Reiner L. Arteriographic findings in congenital abnormalities of the mesentery and intestines. Surg Gynecol Obstet 1961;113:346–52.
86. Tsujimoto K, Sherman FE, Ravitch MM. Experimental intestinal atresia in the rabbit fetus. Sequential pathological studies. Johns Hopkins Med J 1972;131:287–97.
87. Komuro H, Amagai T, Hori T, et al. Placental vascular compromise in jejunoileal atresia. J Pediatr Surg 2004;39:1701–5.
88. Bilodeau A, Prasil P, Cloutier R, et al. Hereditary multiple intestinal atresia: Thirty years later. J Pediatr Surg 2004;39:726–30.
89. Hasegawa T, Sumimura J, Nose K, et al. Congenital multiple intestinal atresia successfully treated with multiple anastomoses in a premature neonate: Report of a case. Surg Today 1996;26:849–51.
90. Puri P, Guiney E, Carroll R. Multiple gastrointestinal atresias in three consecutive siblings: Observations on pathogenesis. J Pediatr Surg 1985;20:22–4.
91. Baglaj SM, Czernik J, Koryszko J, et al. Natural history of experimental intestinal atresia: Morphologic and ultrastructural study. J Pediatr Surg 2001;36:1428–34.
92. Pickard LR, Santoro S, Wyllie RG, et al. Histochemical studies of experimental fetal intestinal obstruction. J Pediatr Surg 1981;16:256–60.
93. Doolin EJ, Ormsbee HS, Hill JL. Motility abnormalities in intestinal atresia. J Pediatr Surg 1987;22:320–4.
94. Cremin BJ, Cywes S, Louw JH. Small intestine. In: Cremin BJ, Cywes S, Louw JH, editors. Radiological Diagnosis of Digestive Tract Disorders in the Newborn: A Guide to Radiologists, Surgeons, and Paediatricians. London: Butterworths; 1973. p. 62.
95. Wasch MG, Marck A. The radiographic appearance of the gastrointestinal tract during the first day of life. J Pediatr 1948;32:479–89.
96. Benson CD, Lofti MW, Brogh AJ. Congenital atresia and stenosis of the colon. J Pediatr Surg 1968;3:253–7.
97. Jackman S, Brereton RJ. A lesson in intestinal atresias. J Pediatr Surg 1988;23:852–3.
98. Aharon M, Kleinhaus U, Lichtig C. Neonatal intramural intestinal calcifications associated with bowel atresia. AJR Am J Roentgenol 1986;130:999–1000.
99. Hays DM. Intestinal atresia and stenosis. In: Ravitch M, editor. Current Problems in Surgery. Chicago: Year Book Medical; 1969. p. 3.

100. Louw JH. Resection and end-to-end anastomosis in the management of atresia and stenosis of the small bowel. Surgery 1967;62:940–50.

101. Blanck C, Okmian L, Robbe H. Mucoviscidosis and intestinal atresia. A study of four cases in the same family. Acta Paediatr Scand 1965;54:557–65.

102. Suri M, Langer JC. A comparison of circumbilical and transverse abdominal incisions for neonatal abdominal surgery. J Pediatr Surg 2011;46:1076–80.

103. McKee MA. Jejunoileal Atresia. In: Oldham KT, Colombani PM, Foglia RP, et al, edsitors. Principles and Practice of Pediatric Surgery. Philadelphia: Lippincott Williams & Wilkins; 2004. p. 1149.

104. de Lorimier AA, Harrison MR. Intestinal plication in the treatment of atresia. J Pediatr Surg 1983;18:734–7.

105. Holder TM, Gross RE. Temporary gastrostomy in pediatric surgery. Experience with 187 cases. Pediatrics 1960;26:36–41.

106. Howard ER, Othersen HB. Proximal jejunoplasty in the treatment of jejunoileal atresia. J Pediatr Surg 1973;8:685–90.

107. Ramanujan TM. Functional capability of blind small bowel loops after intestinal remodeling techniques. Aust N Z J Surg 1984;54:145–50.

108. Kimura K, Perdzynski W, Soper RT. Elliptical seromuscular resection for tapering the proximal dilated bowel in duodenal or jejunal atresia. J Pediatr Surg 1996;31:1405–6.

109. Kling K, Applebaum H, Dunn J, et al. A novel technique for correction of intestinal atresia at the ligament of Treitz. J Pediatr Surg 2000;35:353–5.

110. Grosfeld JL, Ballantine TV, Shoemaker R. Operative management of intestinal atresia and stenosis based on pathologic findings. J Pediatr Surg 1979;14:368–75.

111. Touloukian RJ. Intestinal atresia. Clin Perinatol 1978;5:3–18.

112. Snyder CL, Miller KA, Sharp RJ, et al. Management of intestinal atresia in patients with gastroschisis. J Pediatr Surg 2001;36:1542–5.

113. Festen S, Brevoord JC, Goldhoorn GA, et al. Excellent long-term outcome for survivors of apple peel atresia. J Pediatr Surg 2002;37:61–5.

114. Waldhausen JH, Sawin RS. Improved long-term outcome for patients with jejunoileal apple peel atresia. J Pediatr Surg 1997;32:1307–9.

115. Chaet MS, Warner BW, Sheldon CA. Management of multiple jejunoileal atresias with an intraluminal Silastic stent. J Pediatr Surg 1994;29:1604–6.

116. Haller JA Jr, Tepas JJ, Pickard LR, et al. Intestinal atresia. Current concepts of pathogenesis, pathophysiology, and operative management. Am Surg 1983;49:385–91.

117. Dowling RH. Small bowel adaptation and its regulation. Scand J Gastroenterol Suppl 1982;17:53–74.

118. Remmington M, Malagelada JR, Zinsmeister A, et al. Abnormalities in gastrointestinal motor activity in patients with short bowels: Effect of a synthetic opiate. Gastroenterology 1983;85:629–36.

119. Rode H, Millar AJW. Jejuno-ileal atresia and stenosis. In: Puri P, editor. Newborn Surgery. 2nd ed. London: Hodder Arnold; 2003. p. 445.

120. Boles ET Jr, Vassy LE, Ralston M. Atresia of the colon. J Pediatr Surg 1976;11:69–75.

121. Benson CD, Lotfi MW, Brogh AJ. Congenital atresia and stenosis of the colon. J Pediatr Surg 1968;3:253–7.

122. Powell RW, Raffensperger JG. Congenital colonic atresia. J Pediatr Surg 1982;17:166–70.

123. Croaker GD, Harvey JG, Cass DT. Hirschsprung's disease, colonic atresia, and absent hand: A new triad. J Pediatr Surg 1997;32:1368–70.

124. Kim PC, Superina RA, Ein S. Colonic atresia combined with Hirschsprung's disease: A diagnostic and therapeutic challenge. J Pediatr Surg 1995;30:1216–17.

125. Davenport M, Bianchi A, Doig CM, et al. Colonic atresia: Current results of treatment. J R Coll Surg Edinb 1990;35:25–8.

126. Williams MD, Burrington JD. Hirschsprung's disease complicating colon atresia. J Pediatr Surg 1993;28:637–9.

127. Karnak I, Ciftci AO, Senocak ME, et al. Colonic atresia: Surgical management and outcome. Pediatr Surg Int 2001;17:631–5.

128. Sui KL, Kwok WK, Lee WY, et al. A male newborn with colonic atresia and total colonic aganglionosis. Pediatr Surg Int 1999;15:141–2.

129. Cox SG, Numanoglu A, Millar AJ, et al. Colonic atresia: Spectrum of presentation and pitfalls in management. A review of 14 cases. Pediatr Surg Int 2005;21:813–18.

130. Louw JH. Investigations into the etiology of congenital atresia of the colon. Dis Colon Rectum 1964;7:471–8.

131. Santulli TV, Blanc WA. Congenital atresia of the intestine: Pathogenesis and treatment. Ann Surg 1961;154:939–48.

132. Rescorla FJ, Grosfeld JL. Intestinal atresia and stenosis: Analysis of survival in 120 cases. Surgery 1985;98:668–76.

133. Watts AC, Sabharwal AJ, Mackinlay GA, et al. Congenital colonic atresia: Should primary anastomosis always be the goal? Pediatr Surg Int 2003;19:14–17.

134. DeFore WW, Garcia-Rinaldi R, Mattox KL, et al. Surgical management of colon atresia. Surg Gynecol Obstet 1976;143:767–9.

135. Pohlson EC, Hatch EI Jr, Glick PL, et al. Individualized management of colonic atresia. Am J Surg 1988;155:690–2.

136. Hamzaoui M, Ghribi A, Makni W, et al. Rectal and sigmoid atresia: Transanal approach. J Pediatr Surg 2012;47:E41–4.

CHAPTER 31

MALROTATION

M. Sidney Dassinger III • Samuel D. Smith

Normal rotation of the intestine requires transformation from a simple, straight alimentary tube into the mature fixed and folded configuration normally present at birth. Through precise embryologic events, the duodenojejunal junction becomes fixed in the left upper abdomen while the cecum is anchored in the right lower quadrant. The midgut, defined as the portion of the intestine supplied by the superior mesenteric artery (SMA), is thus suspended from a wide mesenteric base. In children with malrotation, the bowel is not fixed adequately and is thus held by a precariously narrow-based mesentery. Rotational anomalies create a spectrum of anatomic conditions with critical importance to the pediatric surgeon. Clinical disorders may arise when intestinal rotation either fails to occur or is incomplete. Rotational anomalies may be isolated or occur as an intrinsic component of gastroschisis, omphalocele, or congenital diaphragmatic hernia. Additionally, malrotation may present as an incidental, subtle finding discovered during the radiographic evaluation for another diagnosis or with shock from a catastrophic midgut volvulus.

The earliest descriptions of intestinal development were from Mall in 1898, and later expanded upon by Frazer and Robbins in 1915.[1,2] Eight years later, Dott translated these preliminary embryologic observations into problems encountered clinically.[3] In his 1932 landmark paper, Ladd described the evaluation and operative treatment of malrotation.[4] He described a relatively simple solution to a complicated problem.[5] Over 200 postmortem studies had been reported previous to Ladd's paper, yet he was the first to emphasize the importance of placing the duodenum along the right abdominal wall, widening the mesenteric base, and moving the cecum to the left upper abdomen. With the exception of the laparoscopic approach, Ladd's original technique has remained relatively unchanged.

EMBRYOLOGY

The development of the midgut begins with the differentiation of the primitive intestinal tract into the foregut, midgut, and hindgut at the fourth week of gestation.[6] The mature alimentary tract and all associated digestive organs are formed from this primitive tube. The most accepted model of midgut maturation involves four distinct stages: (1) herniation; (2) rotation; (3) retraction; and (4) fixation. Normal fixation of the duodenum and colon is illustrated in Figure 31-1. The intestinal loop can be divided into the cephalic (duodenojejunal) limb and the caudal (cecocolic) limb, which rotate separately but in parallel. The SMA serves as the fulcrum with the

omphalomesenteric duct at the apex. Due to the disproportional growth and elongation of the midgut during the fourth gestational week, the intestinal loop herniates into the extraembryonic coelom. Next, the bowel enters a critical period of rotation when the prearterial and postarterial limbs make three separate 90° turns, all in the counterclockwise direction around the SMA. The first 90° rotation occurs outside the abdomen. The second 90° turn commences during the return of the intestine into the abdominal cavity during the 10th gestational week. The duodenojejunal junction now passes posterior to the SMA. The last rotation occurs in the abdomen. The primitive intestine has thus completed a 270° counterclockwise rotation, allowing the duodenojejunal limb to be positioned to the left of the SMA while the cecocolic limb is on the right. Fixation of the ascending and descending colon then occurs. Disruption of any of these vital steps leads to the spectrum of malrotation encountered clinically.

The most common forms of rotational disorders include nonrotation (Fig. 31-2), incomplete rotation (Fig. 31-3), and reversed rotation. Right and left mesocolic hernias can also occur. In nonrotation, there is failure of the normal intestinal 270° counterclockwise rotation around the SMA. Thus, the duodenojejunal limb lies in the right hemi-abdomen with the cecocolic limb in the left hemi-abdomen. Midgut volvulus due to a narrow mesenteric pedicle and extrinsic duodenal obstruction secondary to abnormally positioned cecal attachments are the most common symptomatic consequences. In cases of incomplete rotation, normal rotation has been arrested at or near 180°. The cecum will usually reside in the right upper abdomen. Obstructing peritoneal bands over the duodenum are present. With reversed rotation, an errant 90° clockwise rotation occurs, which leaves a tortuous transverse colon to the right of the SMA, passing through a retroduodenal tunnel dorsal to the artery and in the small bowel mesentery.[7,8] The duodenum will assume an anterior position. Reverse rotation with volvulus may occur with obstruction of the transverse colon. Paraduodenal hernias are rare and result from failure of the right or left mesocolon to fuse to the posterior body wall. A potential space is created. Subsequently, the small intestine may become sequestered and potentially obstructed.

PRESENTATION

The incidence of malrotation has been estimated at 1 in 6000 live births. An increased incidence of 0.2% has been found in barium swallow studies,[9] whereas autopsy studies

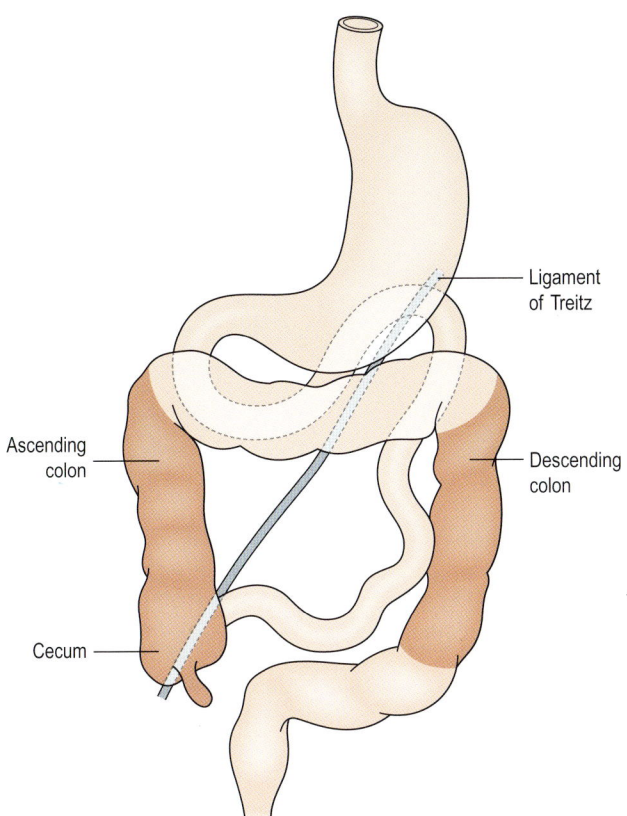

FIGURE 31-1 ■ Normal intestinal anatomy results in fixation of the duodenojejunal junction in the left upper quadrant and the cecum in the right lower quadrant. This allows a wide breadth to the mesentery of the small bowel.

Labels: Ligament of Treitz; Ascending colon; Descending colon; Cecum

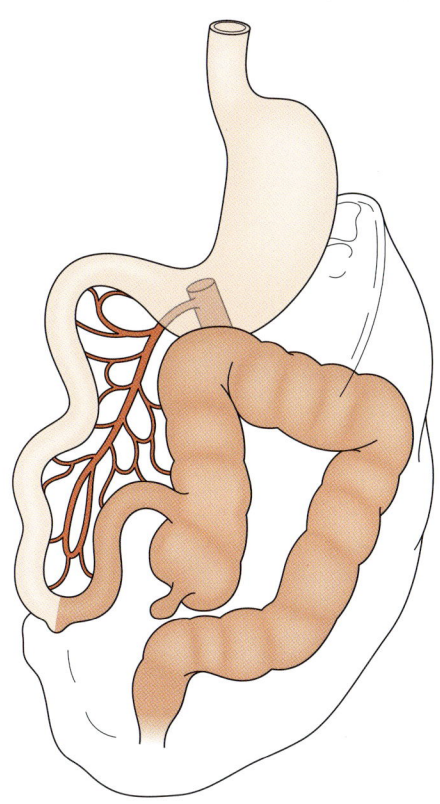

FIGURE 31-2 ■ Nonrotation. The prearterial midgut (lightly shaded) is found on the right side of the abdomen, while the postarterial midgut (darkly shaded) remains on the left. Neither segment has undergone appropriate rotation. Volvulus is a risk.

estimate that the true incidence may be as high as 1% of the total population.[10] Associated anomalies are common (Table 31-1).[11]

Classic malrotation with midgut volvulus is often discovered in a previously healthy term neonate. Up to 75% of patients present during the first month of life, while another 15% will present within the first year.[12–14] However, volvulus and mortality have been reported at all ages.[15] Sudden onset of bilious vomiting is the cardinal sign of neonatal intestinal obstruction, and malrotation with volvulus must be the presumed diagnosis until proven otherwise. Physical examination findings will vary. Initially, the patient may have a scaphoid abdomen or only mild upper abdominal distension. However, if vascular compromise to the completely obstructed bowel develops, the abdomen will become progressively more distended and peritonitis will ensue. Late signs include abdominal wall erythema and shock. Similarly, laboratory data are often nonspecific and of limited diagnostic value. Thus, the clinician must have a high index of suspicion in a previously healthy baby who presents with bilious emesis. Furthermore, if signs of bowel ischemia are present, operative intervention must occur without delay.

Patients with chronic obstruction will present less dramatically. Nonspecific presenting problems such as failure to thrive, gastroesophageal reflux, early satiety, and mild abdominal discomfort are often seen. Partial volvulus can

TABLE 31-1 Incidence of associated anomalies with malrotation

Associated Anomaly	Incidence
Intestinal atresia	5–26%
Imperforate anus	0–9%
Cardiac anomalies	7–13%
Duodenal web	1–2%
Meckel diverticulum	1–4%
Hernia	0–7%
Trisomy 21	3–10%

Rare: esophageal atresia, biliary atresia, mesenteric cyst, craniosynostosis, Hirschsprung disease, intestinal duplication.

lead to mesenteric venous and lymphatic obstruction and subsequently impaired nutrient absorption. The diagnosis becomes even more challenging with the older child or teenager because the symptoms are often vague and may sometimes seem unrelated to the abdomen.[16]

DIAGNOSIS

Radiologic studies play a critical role in establishing a diagnosis of intestinal malrotation. Initial evaluation will usually begin with a plain anteroposterior abdominal

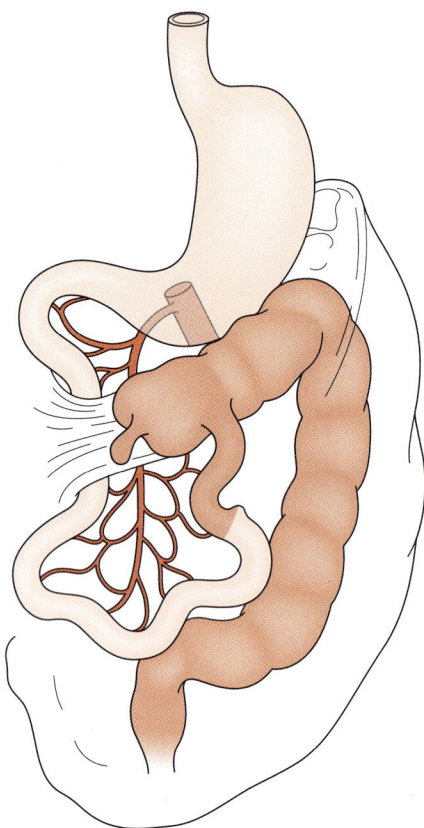

FIGURE 31-3 ■ Incomplete rotation. Both the prearterial (lightly shaded) and postarterial (darkly shaded) segments have undergone partial, yet not complete, rotation. Ladd's bands are seen attaching the cecum to the right posterior abdominal wall. The duodenum becomes compressed and possibly obstructed. Volvulus is a risk.

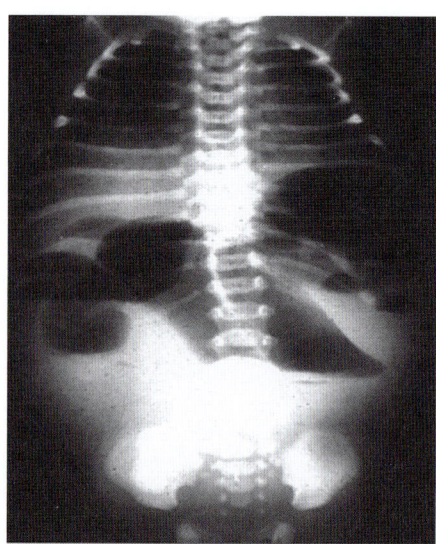

FIGURE 31-4 ■ Upright abdominal film in an infant demonstrating proximal small bowel dilatation. This infant had a midgut volvulus.

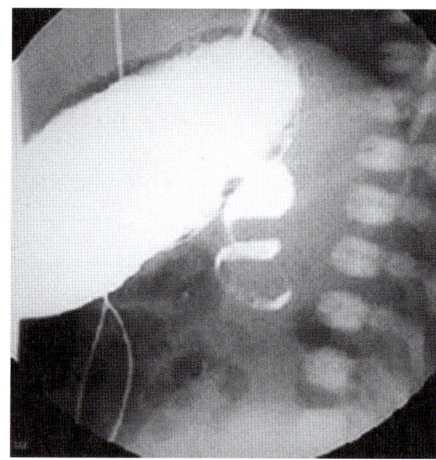

FIGURE 31-5 ■ Lateral image on upper gastrointestinal series in an infant with malrotation and midgut volvulus showing the 'corkscrew' appearance of the obstructed duodenum.

film combined with a lateral decubitus or upright view (Fig. 31-4). Nonspecific findings ranging from gastric distention to a gasless abdomen are common. Upper gastrointestinal contrast study remains the gold standard and is needed to document the position of the ligament of Treitz to the left of the spinal pedicles, and rising to the level of the gastric outlet. Additionally, the lateral film will show the duodenum in a retroperitoneal, posterior position.[17] Findings of abnormal rotation include a low-lying ligament of Treitz or failure of the ligament of Treitz to be located left of the spine. If volvulus exists, the contrast study may show the 'coil spring' or 'corkscrew' configuration with incomplete obstruction and the "beak" appearance in the duodenum with complete obstruction (Figs 31-5 and 31-6).

In some institutions, ultrasound (US) is being trialed to make the diagnosis of malrotation. Color Doppler ultrasound imaging may reveal a dilated duodenum with inversion of the SMA and vein (the whirlpool sign) in cases of acute volvulus.[18–21] Additionally, Yousefzadeh and colleagues have proposed that ultrasound be used to diagnose malrotation without volvulus based on the position of the duodenum and the SMA. Because the third portion of the duodenum assumes a retroperitoneal position anterior to the aorta and posterior to the SMA in individuals with normal intestinal rotation, verification of this position by ultrasound potentially obviates the need for further imaging. This group prospectively validated this technique in 33 neonates at their institution.[22] However, application of this technique prospectively in multiple institutions is likely needed prior to widespread acceptance.

MANAGEMENT

Preoperative

Patients with suspected or confirmed midgut volvulus may be dehydrated and demonstrate electrolyte imbalances. They should be aggressively resuscitated, given intravenous broad-spectrum antibiotics, and taken to the operating room for immediate exploration. Delaying operative intervention for further confirmatory testing or prolonged resuscitation is discouraged when suspicion is high on clinical grounds alone.

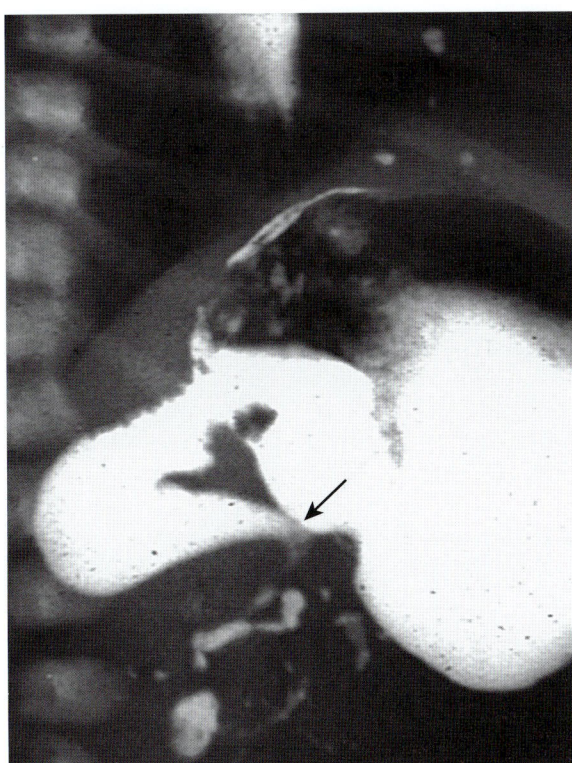

FIGURE 31-6 ■ Lateral image on upper gastrointestinal series in infant with malrotation and midgut volvulus showing the 'beak' (arrow) appearance of the obstructed duodenum. Note that a small amount of contrast agent has progressed through the volvulus.

BOX 31-1	Six key elements in operative correction of malrotation

1. Entry into abdominal cavity and evisceration (open)
2. Counterclockwise detorsion of the bowel (acute cases)
3. Division of Ladd cecal bands
4. Broadening of the small intestine mesentery
5. Incidental appendectomy
6. Placement of small bowel along the right lateral gutter and colon along the left lateral gutter

Open Approach

There has been little change from Ladd's original description of the operative technique for correction of malrotation with or without volvulus. The six steps are summarized in Box 31-1. A right upper abdominal transverse incision is typically used. Chylous ascites secondary to lymphatic obstruction and rupture of mesenteric lacteals is often initially found. The bowel and mesentery should then be completely eviscerated. In patients with volvulus, the surgeon will commonly encounter two or three complete clockwise revolutions. Prompt, gentle counterclockwise detorsion is performed (Fig. 31-7). Once detorsion has been accomplished, warm soaked lap pads are placed on the bowel, and the surgeon should patiently observe for reperfusion. If perfusion remains in question, the surgeon has several options, including

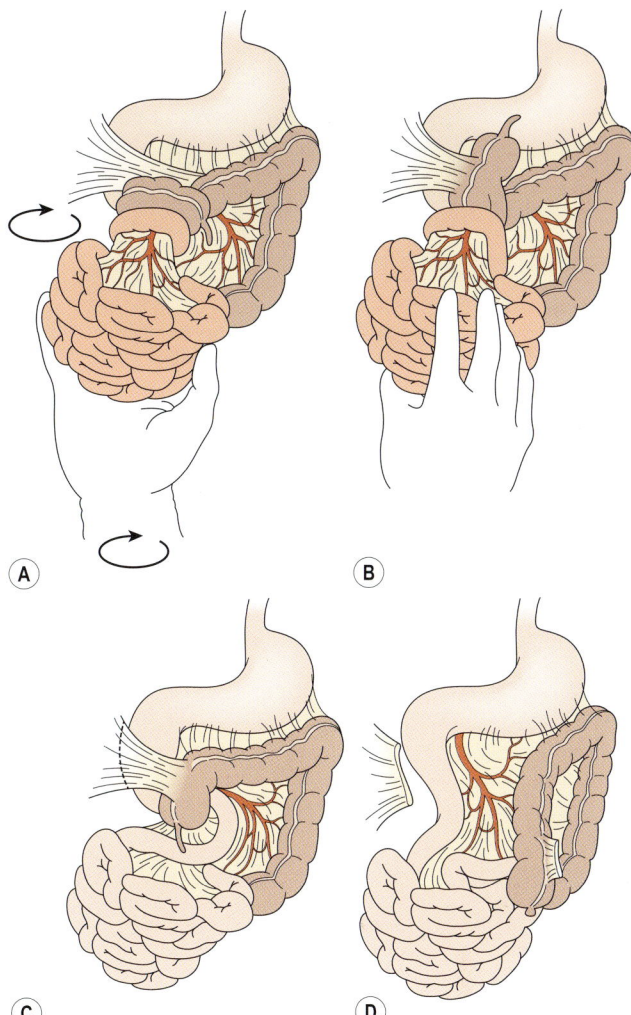

FIGURE 31-7 ■ Open correction of malrotation. (A,B) Initial appearance of the malrotated bowel during exploration. The surgeon first will perform counterclockwise detorsion of the midgut. (C) Next, Ladd bands from the cecum to the right abdominal wall are divided. (D) Last is the critical step of broadening the small bowel mesentery. An appendectomy is also performed.

assessment of the antimesenteric vascular integrity with the use of a Doppler probe and intravenous administration of fluorescein with Wood's lamp evaluation.

Bowel that is frankly necrotic should be resected. However, when longer segments are of questionable viability, a temporary closure or silo should be placed and the patient re-evaluated at a second-look operation 24 to 48 hours later. Unfortunately, an occasional patient will have complete infarction of the midgut (Fig. 31-8). Closure of the abdomen without bowel resection may be a reasonable choice after intraoperative discussion with the family. However, the development and sophistication of intestinal and multi-visceral transplantation makes the best option much less clear.

Once the bowel has been detorsed, the breadth of the mesentery must then be widened. This goal is accomplished by first dividing the Ladd bands traversing the duodenum (Fig. 31-9). Next, a generous Kocher maneuver is performed to straighten the duodenum. It is

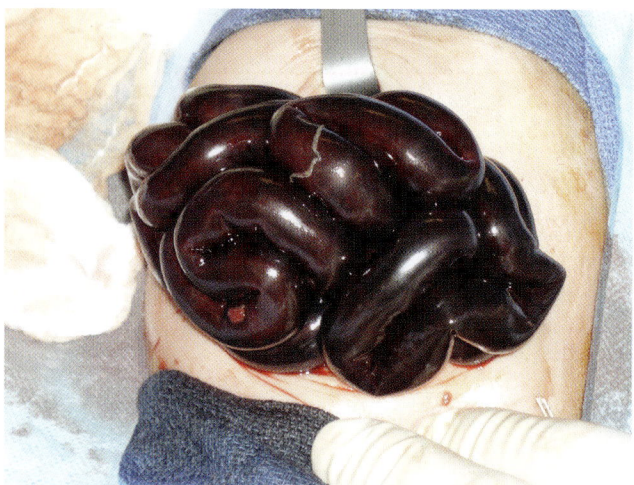

FIGURE 31-8 ■ Unfortunately, on occasion, complete infarction of the midgut due to malrotation and volvulus will be found. Management options vary depending on surgeon and the wishes of the parents.

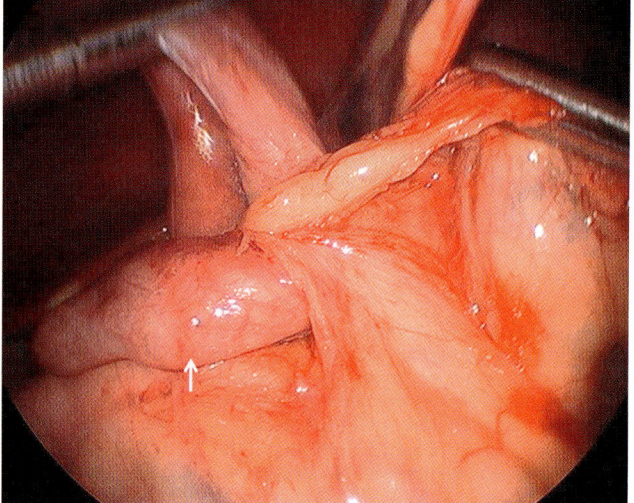

FIGURE 31-9 ■ Laparoscopic view of retroperitoneal bands extending from the cecum and partially obstructing the distal duodenum and proximal jejunum (arrow).

imperative that a nasogastric tube is passed through the now straightened duodenum so that intrinsic obstruction can be ruled out. The dissection then continues to the base of the SMA and vein by incising the anterior mesenteric leaflet. When properly opened, the mesentery is maximally broadened and the possibility of postoperative volvulus is presumably reduced, although not completely eliminated.

Most surgeons will complete the procedure with an appendectomy, owing to the subsequent malposition of the cecum to the left side of the abdomen. Standard or inversion appendectomy are equally acceptable. Finally, the duodenum and small intestine are positioned toward the right abdomen with the colon on the left. Suture fixation of the bowel to the lateral abdominal wall is not recommended.[23,24]

Laparoscopic Approach

The laparoscopic treatment for intestinal rotation anomalies in neonates, infants, and children with or without midgut volvulus was first proposed by van der Zee and colleagues in 1995.[25] Subsequent publications have been primarily single-institution case reports or small case series.[26–36] Clinical outcomes for the laparoscopic technique have generally been favorable.

The patient is placed supine in the reversed Trendelenburg position and on a shortened operating room table, if available. The surgeon will stand at the child's feet with the assistant positioned to the surgeon's left. An oro- or nasogastric tube is inserted. A port is introduced at the umbilicus and insufflation is established to a pressure of 8–12 mmHg.[26–28] The surgeon will work with two instruments while the assistant may use one to help with exposure. The surgeon's first goal is to determine if malrotation is actually present and thus confirm the preoperative imaging studies (Figs 31-10 and 31-11). Tilting the table may help identify the ligament of Treitz and the ileocecal junction. Findings of malrotation include a high and medial cecal position, an elongated, tortuous duodenum, and a malpositioned ligament of Treitz. Although there are no specific guidelines established to predict whether a future volvulus will occur, a mesenteric base

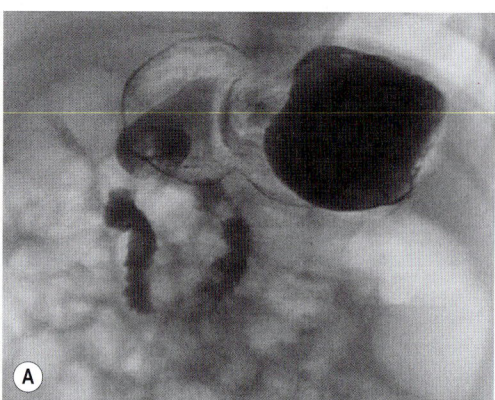
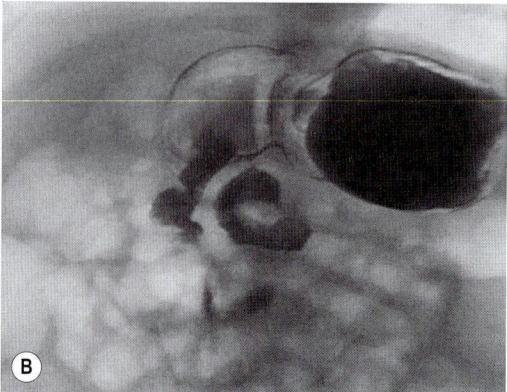

FIGURE 31-10 ■ An upper gastrointestinal study was performed in this infant who presented with vomiting. The radiologic interpretation was that the duodenum was entirely on the patient's right side and the ligament of Treitz was at the level of pylorus. Also, the ligament of Treitz did not cross the midline. There was no evidence of obstruction. This patient underwent diagnostic laparoscopy and was found to have normal anatomy with correct positioning of the ligament of Treitz and the cecum (see Fig. 31-11).

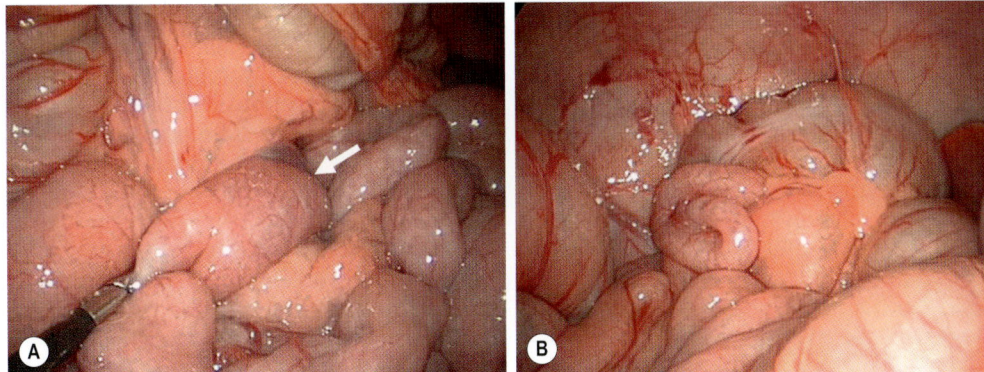

FIGURE 31-11 ■ At times, the upper gastrointestinal study can be equivocal for possible malrotation (see Fig. 31-10). In such patients, diagnostic laparoscopy is a useful technique to ascertain whether the patient actually has malrotation. **(A)** The ligament of Treitz (arrow) is seen to be to the left of the patient's midline. **(B)** In addition, the location of the cecum in the right lower quadrant also helps verify that the patient does not have malrotation.

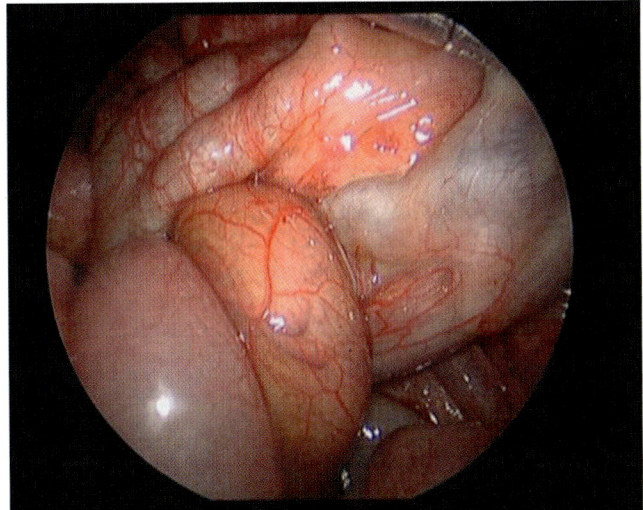

FIGURE 31-12 ■ At laparoscopy, a midgut volvulus is noted. The bowel appears healthy. The operation was converted and an open Ladd procedure was performed.

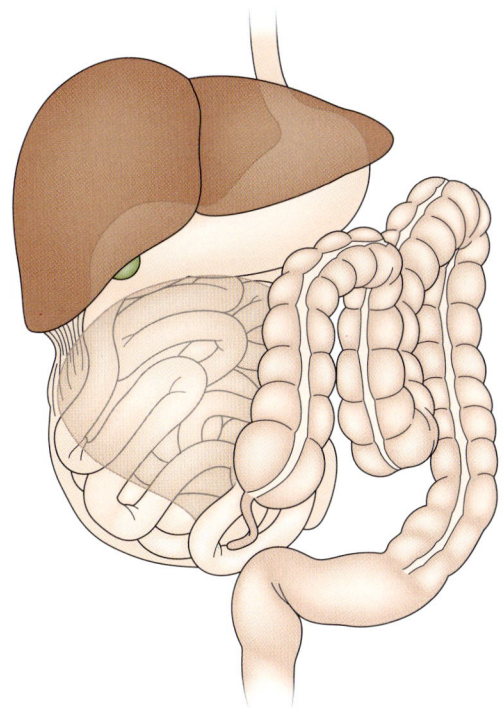

FIGURE 31-13 ■ In older children with long-standing partial obstruction or internal herniation, the Ladd bands may cause the bowel to form into a cocoon-like deformity. (From Moir CR. Laparoscopic Ladd procedure. In: Holcomb GW III, Georgeson KE, Rothenberg SS, editors. Atlas of Pediatric Laparoscopy and Thoracoscopy. Philadelphia: Elsevier; 2008. p. 55–60.)

extending more than half the diameter of the abdomen is generally sufficient to prevent volvulus.[29] If a rotational anomaly is felt to be present, the operation is then performed in the same stepwise fashion as the open Ladd procedure.

Laparoscopy for malrotation can present unique challenges. If volvulus is encountered (Fig 31-12), the surgeon may continue laparoscopically provided rapid detorsion can be achieved. However, dilated bowel may make visualization and proper orientation difficult. Further, dilated bowel can be injured by laparoscopic instruments. A second scenario occurs in older children with long-standing duodenal obstruction. In these children, the proximal bowel may be molded into a cocoon-like deformity (Fig. 31-13), which may also make laparoscopic repair challenging.[27] Lastly, appendectomy may be performed either extracorporeally via the umbilicus (Fig. 31-14) or intracorporeally using endoloops or a stapling device. Instruments are then removed under direct visualization, and the incisions are closed with absorbable suture. Postoperative management is similar to that for the open approach. Most children may begin clear liquids on the day of surgery. Discharge on day 1 or 2 is expected.[28]

Since van der Zee's initial report, other authors have described variations in technique and have published their positive results.[29–32] Successful laparoscopic management of a 15-day-old with acute midgut volvulus has been described.[33] However, the majority of patients undergoing laparoscopic repair of intestinal malrotation have been elective cases without volvulus.[30,31,34] Operative times have been reported to average 110 to 120 minutes.[31,35] In one report, the time to a regular diet was

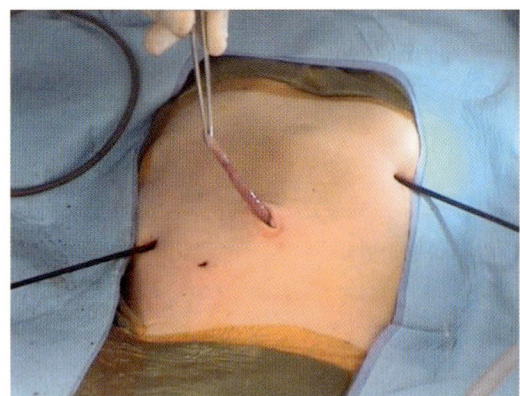

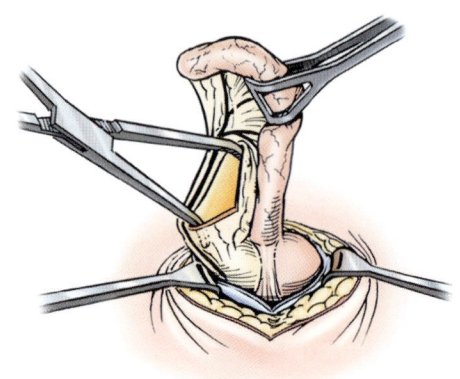

FIGURE 31-14 ■ When performing a laparoscopic Ladd procedure, an extracorporeal appendectomy eliminates the need for a large port for the endoscopic stapler. The appendix is grasped with one of the intracorporeal instruments and brought into view through the umbilical fascial defect, where it is grasped and exteriorized. (From Moir CR. Laparoscopic Ladd procedure. In: Holcomb GW III, Georgeson KE, Rothenberg SS, editors. Atlas of Pediatric Laparoscopy and Thoracoscopy. Philadelphia: Elsevier; 2008. p. 55–60.)

two days (median) and resolution of symptoms was found in five of seven patients at 15 months.[30]

In another series, 12 neonates and infants, weighing 3–7 kg, underwent a three-port laparoscopic Ladd procedure.[29] Presentation included intermittent upper intestinal obstruction, and the diagnosis was eventually confirmed by contrast study. Three 3.5 mm ports were placed in the infraumbilical ring and in the right and left abdomen. Operative time was equivalent to published open results, ranging from 35 to 120 minutes (mean, 58 minutes). Feedings were started on postoperative day 1 or 2, and the patients were discharged at a mean of two days. All symptoms resolved on postoperative evaluation.

The formation of intra-abdominal adhesions has generally been viewed as necessary to prevent postoperative volvulus. Through open exploration and direct manipulation of the bowel, adhesions are created. Concerns have been raised that adhesion formation may be limited with laparoscopy, as is seen in other laparoscopic procedures. Initial reports have not validated these concerns. In fact, in a retrospective study which compared open and laparoscopic Ladd procedures, the only patients in which postoperative volvulus occurred were in the open group.[36]

Laparoscopic correction of malrotation is an accepted procedure but still can be a technical challenge. In patients with acute volvulus, the working space may be limited owing to bowel edema and chylous ascites, and the surgeon should have a low threshold to convert to laparotomy, which can be done by slightly extending the umbilical incision.[36] Although the current literature supports consideration of laparoscopy (especially in older patients with malrotation as an incidental finding), further prospective studies with large sample sizes, possible randomization, and long-term follow-up should be conducted to confirm the proper role for the laparoscopic approach.

POSTOPERATIVE MANAGEMENT

In patients without evidence of volvulus or obstruction, a nasogastric tube is not generally used. Bowel function generally returns in 1 to 5 days. However, older patients with chronic obstruction are likely to have a prolonged ileus, and thus nasogastric drainage and parenteral support may be required. Antibiotics are not uniformly needed. Feedings can be advanced per the surgeon's discretion. Patients with extended or subtotal small bowel resection pose special problems. Total parenteral nutrition is essential to sustain these patients until adaptation and compensatory growth of the residual bowel can occur.[37] Small bowel or multiple-viscera transplantation should be considered. Postoperative intussusception has been noted in 3.1% of all patients who underwent a Ladd procedure, compared with 0.05% following other laparotomies.[38] The incidence of recurrent volvulus is low. At the author's institution, the recurrent volvulus rate has approximated 1%. Finally, up to 10% of patients may develop a postoperative adhesive small bowel obstruction requiring an operation.[23,24,39]

SPECIAL CONSIDERATIONS

The Older Patient

Malrotation is occasionally diagnosed in the teenager. The presenting symptoms are often vague, including vomiting, diarrhea, early satiety, bloating, and dyspepsia.[40–43] The patient may have undergone multiple imaging modalities, including contrast studies, computed tomography (Fig. 31-15), and magnetic resonance imaging. The imaging modalities may, however, help delineate vascular and/or hepatobiliary anatomic irregularities that are associated with rotational disorders.[44] Patients who are found to have symptoms from rotational anomalies should undergo operative intervention. Patients and their families should be cautioned, though, that when compared with younger patients, older patients (>16 years of age) endured a higher percentage of postoperative complications and required a higher percentage of reoperation.[45]

The question arises whether the incidental discovery of malrotation in the older child or young adult should be repaired at all. The principle of 'watchful waiting' has

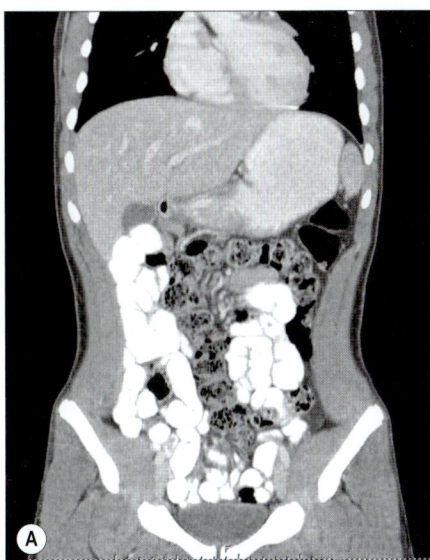

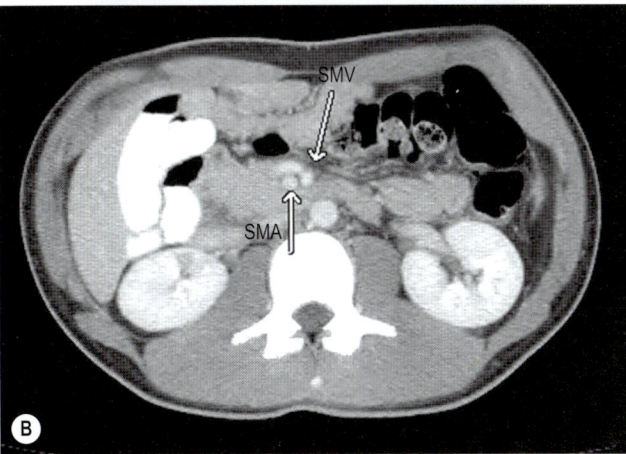

FIGURE 31-15 ■ This 15-year-old presented with chronic abdominal pain and underwent a CT scan for diagnosis. **(A)** On this coronal view, the small bowel is filled with contrast and most of it is located along the right paracolic gutter. **(B)** On transverse section, note that the superior mesenteric artery (SMA) and superior mesenteric vein (SMV) are malpositioned, and are reversed in orientation to each other. This patient underwent a laparoscopic Ladd procedure with resolution of her symptoms.

been suggested.[46] However, up to 20% of adult patients undergoing operative repair of malrotation will have an acute volvulus or bowel ischemia, both potentially life-threatening presentations.[47] Furthermore, even in patients who are believed to be asymptomatic, preoperative symptoms attributable to malrotation have retrospectively been noted to improve or resolve.[31,43,48] Thus, operative correction in the asymptomatic older patient is currently recommended.

Atypical Malrotation

The dilemma arises when an abnormality is discovered on imaging, and the child is labeled as a 'malrotation variant.' To exclude malrotation, the duodenojejunal flexure must be located to the left of the spine at the level of the duodenal bulb. Defined as the ligament of Treitz, this flexure can be in an equivocal position. Symptoms

are generally mild and can easily be attributed to other diagnoses such as gastroesophageal reflux. Volvulus or internal hernia is usually not seen with malrotation variants. This clinical scenario leaves the surgeon with the dilemma of deciding whether the symptoms are due to the radiographic abnormality. Given the higher rate of persistence of symptoms after intervention and an overall increase in postoperative complications, close observation or repeated contrast study has been suggested in these equivocal cases.[49,50] If operative intervention is decided upon, laparoscopy is an ideal approach.

Heterotaxy

Rotational disorders are known to coexist with heterotaxy syndrome (HS).[51] Thus, in many institutions, screening upper gastrointestinal contrast studies are performed. Patients that are symptomatic from these anomalies should undergo a Ladd operation. However, management of the asymptomatic patient remains controversial with literature available to support either observation or elective operation. Recently, a retrospective study documented a higher morbidity rate when heterotaxy patients, who underwent prophylactic Ladd procedure, were compared to those without heterotaxy. Despite the small sample size, they concluded that asymptomatic patients should be observed.[52] Conversely, a group from Boston noted similar outcomes when HS patients were compared to patients without HS that underwent Ladd procedures.[53] Interestingly, 27% of the HS patients that had abdominal symptoms were found to have volvulus at exploration, emphasizing the potential hazards of observational management. Multi-institutional, prospective studies are needed to make more definitive recommendations for this challenging group of patients.

REFERENCES

1. Mall FP. Development of the human intestine and its position in the adult. Johns Hopkins Hosp Bull 1898;9:197–208.
2. Frazer TE, Robbins RF. On the factors concerned in causing rotation of the intestine in man. J Anat Physiol 1915;50:74–110.
3. Dott NM. Anomalies of intestinal rotation: Their embryology and surgical aspects, with the report of five cases. Br J Surg 1923;11: 251–86.
4. Ladd W. Congenital obstruction of the duodenum in children. N Engl J Med 1932;206:277–83.
5. Ladd WE, Gross RE. Intestinal obstruction resulting from malrotation of the intestines and colon. Abdominal Surgery of Infancy and Childhood. Philadelphia: WB Saunders; 1941. p. 53–70.
6. Kluth D, Jaeschke-Melli S, Fiegel H. The embryology of gut rotation. Semin Pediatr Surg 2003;12:275–9.
7. Kanazawa T, Kasugai K, Miyata M, et al. Midgut malrotation in adulthood. Intern Med 2000;39:626–31.
8. Wang C, Welch CE. Anomalies of intestinal rotation in adolescents and adults. Surgery 1963;54:829–54.
9. Warner BR. Malrotation. In: Oldham KT, Colombani PM, Foglia RP, editors. Surgery of Infants and Children. Philadelphia: Lippincott-Raven; 1996. p. 1229–40.
10. Kapfer SA, Rappold JF. Intestinal malrotation—not just the pediatric surgeon's problem. J Am Coll Surg 2004;199:628–35.
11. Aiken JJ, Oldham KT. Malrotation. In: Ashcraft KW, Holcomb GW III, Murphy JP, editors. Pediatric Surgery. Philadelphia: Elsevier Saunders; 2005. p. 435–47.
12. Gross RE. Malrotation of the intestine and colon. In: Gross R.E., editor. The Surgery of Infancy and Childhood. Philadelphia: WB Saunders; 1953. p. 192–203.

13. Ford EG, Senac MO Jr, Srikanth MS, et al. Malrotation of the intestine in children. Ann Surg 1992;212:172–8.

14. Stewart DR, Colodny AL, Daggett WC. Malrotation of the bowel in infants and children: A 15-year review. Surgery 1976;79: 716–20.

15. Powell DM, Othersen HB, Smith CD. Malrotation of the intestine in children: The effect of age on presentation and therapy. J Pediatr Surg 1989;24:777–80.

16. Maxson RT, Franklin PA, Wagner CW. Malrotation in the older child: Surgical management, treatment, and outcome. Am Surg 1995;61:135–8.

17. Sizemore AW, Rabbani KZ, Ladd A, et al. Diagnostic performance of the upper gastrointestinal series in the evaluation of children with clinically suspected malrotation. Pediatr Radiol 2008;38: 518–28.

18. Shimanuki Y, Aihara T, Takano H. Clockwise whirlpool sign at color Doppler ultrasound: An objective and definite sign of midgut volvulus. Radiology 1996;199:261–4.

19. Pracros JP, Sann L, Genin G, et al. Ultrasound diagnosis of midgut volvulus: The "whirlpool" sign. Pediatr Radiol 1992;22:18–20.

20. Chao JC, Kong MS, Chen JY, et al. Sonographic features related to volvulus in neonatal intestinal malrotation. J Ultrasound Med 2000;19:371–6.

21. Orzech N, Navarro OM, Langer JC. Is ultrasonography a good screening test for intestinal malrotation? J Pediatr Surg 2006;41:1005–9.

22. Yousefzadeh DK, Kang L, Tessicini L. Assessment of retromesenteric position of the third portion of the duodenum: An ultrasound feasibility study in 33 newborns. Pediatr Radiol 2010;40:1476–84.

23. Stauffer UG, Herman P. Comparison of late results in patients with corrected intestinal malrotation with and without fixation of the mesentery. J Pediatr Surg 1980;15:9–12.

24. Rescorla FJ, Shedd FJ, Grosfeld JL, et al. Anomalies of intestinal rotation in childhood: Analysis of 447 cases. Surgery 1990; 108:710–15.

25. van der Zee DC, Bax NMA. Laparoscopic repair of acute volvulus in a neonate with malrotation. Surg Endosc 1995;9:1123–4.

26. Bax K, van der Zee DC. Intestinal malrotation. In: Klaas N, Bax MA, Georgeson KE, et al, editors. Endoscopic Surgery in Infants and Children. New York: Springer; 2007. p. 299–304.

27. Moir CR. Laparoscopic Ladd procedure. In: Holcomb GW III, Georgeson KE, Rothenberg SS, editors. Atlas of Pediatric Laparoscopy and Thoracoscopy. Philadelphia: WB Saunders; 2008. p. 55–60.

28. McLean SE, Minkes RK. Intestinal Rotation Abnormalities. In: Langer JC, Albanese CT, editors. Pediatric Minimal Access Surgery. Boca Raton, FL: Taylor & Francis; 2005. p. 271–83.

29. Bass KD, Rothenberg SS, Chang JH. Laparoscopic Ladd's procedure in infants with malrotation. J Pediatr Surg 1998;33:279–81.

30. Mazziotti MV, Strasberg SM, Langer JC. Intestinal rotation abnormalities without volvulus: The role of laparoscopy. J Am Coll Surg 1997;185:172–6.

31. Lessin MS, Luks FI. Laparoscopic appendectomy and duodenocolonic dissociation (Ladd) procedure for malrotation. Pediatr Surg Int 1998;13:184–5.

32. Gross E, Chen MK, Lobe TE. Laparoscopic evaluation and treatment of intestinal malrotation in infants. Surg Endosc 1996; 10:936–7.

33. Martinez-Ferro M, Bignon H, Figueroa M. Ladd laparoscopic procedure in the neonate. Cir Pediatr 2006;19:182–4.

34. Draus JM Jr, Foley DS, Bond SJ. Laparoscopic Ladd procedure: A minimally invasive approach to malrotation without midgut volvulus. Am Surg 2007;73:693–6.

35. Waldhausen JH, Sawin RS. Laparoscopic Ladd's procedure and assessment of malrotation. J Laparoendosc Surg 1996;6: S103–5.

36. Fraser JD, Aguayo P, Sharp SW, et al. The role of laparoscopy in the management of malrotation. J Surg Res 2009;156:80–2.

37. Georgeson KE, Breaux CW Jr. Outcome and intestinal adaptation in neonatal short-bowel syndrome. J Pediatr Surg 1992;27: 344–50.

38. Kidd J, Jackson R, Wagner C, et al. Intussusception following the Ladd procedure. Arch Surg 2000;135:713–15.

39. Murphy FL, Sparnon AL. Long-term complications following intestinal malrotation and the Ladd's procedure: A fifteen-year review. Pediatr Surg Int 2006;22:326–9.

40. Hsu SD, Yu JC, Chou SJ, et al. Midgut volvulus in an adult with congenital malrotation. Am J Surg 2008;195:705–7.

41. Gamblin TC, Stephens RE Jr, Johnson RK, et al. Adult malrotation: A case report and review of the literature. Curr Surg 2003;60:517–20.

42. von Flue M, Herzog U, Ackermann C, et al. Acute and chronic presentation of intestinal nonrotation in adults. Dis Colon Rectum 1994;37:192–8.

43. Fu T, Tong WD, He YJ, et al. Surgical management of intestinal malrotation in adults. World J Surg 2007;31:1797–803.

44. Pickhardt PJ, Bhalla S. Intestinal malrotation in adolescents and adults: Spectrum of clinical and imaging features. AJR Am J Roentgenol 2002;179:1429–35.

45. Durkin ET, Lund DP, Shaaban AF, et al. Age-related differences in diagnosis and morbidity of intestinal malrotation. J Am Coll Surg 2008;206:658–63.

46. Malek MM, Burd RS. The optimal management of malrotation diagnosed after infancy: A decision analysis. Am J Surg 2006;191:45–51.

47. Malek NM, Burd RS. Surgical treatment of malrotation after infancy: A population-based study. J Pediatr Surg 2005;40: 285–9.

48. Rao KM, Kiran PR. Midgut malrotation presenting in adult life. Br J Surg 1994;81:1173–4.

49. McVay MR, Kokoska ER, Jackson RJ, et al. The changing spectrum of intestinal malrotation: Diagnosis and management. Am J Surg 2007;194:712–17.

50. Smith SD. Disorders of intestinal rotation and fixation. In: Grosfeld JL, O'Neill JA Jr, Fonkalsrud EW, Coran AG, editors. Pediatric Surgery. 6th ed. Philadelphia: Mosby; 2006. p. 1342–57.

51. Chang J, Brueckner M, Touloukian RJ. Intestinal rotation and fixation abnormalities in heterotaxia: Early detection and management. J Pediatr Surg 1993;28:1281–4.

52. Pockett CR, Dicken B, Rebeyka IM, et al. Heterotaxy Syndrome: Is a prophylactic Ladd procedure necessary in asymptomatic patients? Pediatr Cardiol 2013;34:59–63.

53. Yu DC, Thiagarajan RR, Laussen PC, et al. Outcomes after the Ladd procedure in patients with heterotaxy syndrome, congenital heart disease, and intestinal malrotation. J Pediatr Surg 2009;44: 1089–95.

CHAPTER 32

MECONIUM DISEASE

Michael G. Caty • Mauricio A. Escobar, Jr.

Intestinal obstruction is one of the most common admitting diagnoses to the neonatal intensive care unit, accounting for as many as one-third of all admissions.[1] Failure to pass meconium within the first 24 to 48 hours of life, feeding intolerance, abdominal distension, and bilious emesis are hallmarks of intestinal obstruction in the newborn, and evoke a differential diagnosis of obstruction based on anatomic, metabolic, and functional considerations. The term meconium disease refers to meconium ileus and meconium plug syndrome. These conditions are considered separately from functional or anatomic causes of neonatal intestinal obstruction, such as Hirschsprung disease, intestinal atresia, and anorectal malformations.

MECONIUM ILEUS

Meconium ileus (MI) is one of the most common causes of intestinal obstruction in the newborn, accounting for 9–33% of neonatal intestinal obstructions.[2] It is characterized by extremely viscid, protein-rich, inspissated meconium causing an intraluminal obstruction in the distal ileum, usually at the ileocecal valve. It is often the earliest clinical manifestation of cystic fibrosis (CF), occurring in approximately 16% of patients with CF.[3] Although MI can occur with other uncommon conditions such as pancreatic aplasia and total colonic aganglionosis, it is often considered pathognomonic for CF.[4,5] MI may be an early indication of a more severe phenotype of cystic fibrosis, as suggested by significantly diminished pulmonary function found in children with a history of MI compared to age- and gender-matched children with CF who did not have MI.[6]

Due to abnormalities of exocrine mucus secretion and pancreatic enzyme deficiency, the meconium in MI differs from normal meconium. Meconium in MI has less water content (65% vs 75%) when compared to normal meconium, lower sucrase and lactase levels, increased albumin, and decreased pancreatic enzymes.[7–9] Additionally, concentrations of sodium, potassium, magnesium, heavy metals, and carbohydrates in MI meconium are reduced in CF. Concentrations of protein nitrogen are increased and composed of abnormal mucoproteins.[10–12] Therefore, more viscous intestinal mucus in the absence of degrading enzymes results in thick, dehydrated meconium that obstructs the intestine.[13]

CYSTIC FIBROSIS

An understanding of CF is important for all clinicians involved in the management of MI patients. CF is the most common, potentially lethal genetic defect affecting Caucasians. Each year 1,200 infants are born with CF (1:2500 live births), and 30,000 children and young adults live with CF in the USA.[4] It is an inherited autosomal recessive disease with a 4–5% carrier rate.[14] The incidence of CF is much lower in non-Caucasian populations: 1 in 10,500 Native American Aleut (Eskimo) births, 1 in 13,500 in Hispanic–Caucasian births, 1 in 15,000 African–American births (much lower in native Africans), and 1 in 31,000 in Asian–American births.

Genetics

In 1989, the CF locus was localized through linkage analysis to human chromosome 7q31, and it was discovered that mutations in the CF transmembrane (conductance) regulator (CFTR) gene result in CF.[15–18] The cell membrane protein coded by *CFTR* is a 3′–5′-cyclic adenosine monophosphate (cAMP)-induced chloride channel, which also regulates the flow of other ions across the apical surface of epithelial cells. The alteration in CFTR results in an abnormal electrolyte content in the environment external to the apical surface of epithelial membranes. This leads to desiccation and reduced clearance of secretions from tubular structures lined by affected epithelia.

The most common mutation of the *CFTR* gene, F508del (previously known as ΔF508), is a three base-pair deletion that results in the removal of a phenylalanine residue at amino acid position 508 of the CFTR. Although there are currently 1,903 mutations listed in the CFTR database, the F508del mutation is responsible for approximately 70% of abnormal CF genes.[15,16,18,19] In families with MI, there is a significantly higher occurrence rate than the expected 25% for an autosomal recessive genetic disorder.[20,21] In one series, 79% of CF patients with the F508del mutation presented with abdominal complaints (including MI) rather than pulmonary complaints.[4] However, there is no evidence of distinct allelic frequencies or haplotypic variants in CF patients with MI compared with those without[22] or in CF patients with significant liver disease.[23,24]

Gastrointestinal Pathophysiology

Cystic fibrosis is characterized by mucoviscidosis of exocrine secretions throughout the body resulting from abnormal transport of chloride ions across apical membranes of epithelial cells.[4,25–27] Abnormal bicarbonate transport also affects mucin formation in CF.[28] The clinical result is chronic obstruction and infection of the respiratory tract, insufficiency of the exocrine pancreas, and elevated sweat chloride levels.[29] Other clinical variants, such as patients with chronic sinusitis or adult males with congenital bilateral absence of the vas deferens (CBAVD), who typically have little other clinical involvement, have been described (Fig. 32-1).[30–32] In patients with CBAVD, the CFTR genotype usually includes at least one mild mutation not typical of CF patients. The mild-mutation allele is frequently associated with a severe mutation on the other allele, such as the F508del mutation.[6,33] CBAVD has been described in a patient with F508del and G551D mutations , both of which were categorized as severe.[34] The allele G551D is the third most common CF-associated mutation, and patients affected by this mutation may have pancreatic insufficiency, pulmonary symptoms, and an episode of MI equivalent, indicating CBAVD may be associated with a more severe CF phenotype.[7,35]

Development of both the pancreas and intestinal tract in fetuses with CF is abnormal. In patients with CF, abnormal pancreatic secretions obstruct the ductal system leading to autodigestion of the acinar cells, fatty replacement of pancreatic parenchyma, and fibrosis. Although this process begins in utero, it occurs variably over time. Regardless, pancreatic insufficiency is prevalent in young infants with CF and has a significant impact on growth and nutrition.[23]

Pancreatic insufficiency plays a central role in the pathogenesis of MI. Congenital stenosis of the pancreatic ducts is associated with meconium-induced bowel obstruction.[36] This is further supported by the fact that two-thirds of infants found to have CF by neonatal screening are pancreatic insufficient at birth.[37] However, approximately 10% of patients with CF are pancreatic sufficient and tend to have a milder course. Also, pancreatic lesions are variable at birth and become more severe in CF children older than age 1.[38] This finding suggests that pancreatic insufficiency is not the leading cause of abnormal meconium in MI. It appears that a prevalence of intestinal glandular abnormalities contribute more significantly to the production of abnormal meconium.[39] The lack of concordance between MI and the severity of pancreatic disease and the preponderance of intestinal glandular lesions implies that intraluminal intestinal factors contribute more to the development of MI than the absence of pancreatic secretions.[9,11,12,36–43]

Abnormal intestinal motility may also contribute to the development of MI. Some patients with CF have prolonged small intestinal transit times.[44,45] Also, the CFTR ion channel defect results in an exocrine secretion that is rich in sodium and chloride which can lead to further dehydration of the intraluminal contents, resulting in impaired clearance.[6] Non-CF diseases associated with abnormal gut motility, such as Hirschsprung disease and chronic intestinal pseudo-obstruction, have been associated with MI-like disease, signifying that decreased peristalsis may allow for increased reabsorption of water, thus favoring the development of abnormal meconium.[46–48]

Prenatal Diagnosis and Screening

The American College of Obstetrics and Gynecology recommends all women of reproductive age should be offered CF carrier screening.[14] Based on the results of CF screening, the antenatal diagnosis of MI can be made in two different groups: a high-risk group and a low-risk group. In the low-risk group, the diagnosis is suspected when the sonographic appearances of MI are found on routine prenatal ultrasound in a mother with a negative CF carrier screen. Sonographic findings consistent with MI in a fetus with parents who are known carriers of CF, and pregnancies subsequent to the birth of a CF-affected child, are considered high risk. Parents of a child with CF are considered to be obligate carriers of a CF mutation.

An algorithm has been established which may be useful in decision making and management of the fetus suspected of having MI (Fig. 32-2).[49–51] If both parents are carriers, evaluation of the fetus should be made by chorionic villus sampling or amniocentesis. In a pregnancy where CF is suspected, sonographic examinations are performed monthly until delivery. This evaluation allows the early detection of potential complications and prepares the clinicians for special or urgent medical or surgical needs upon delivery.

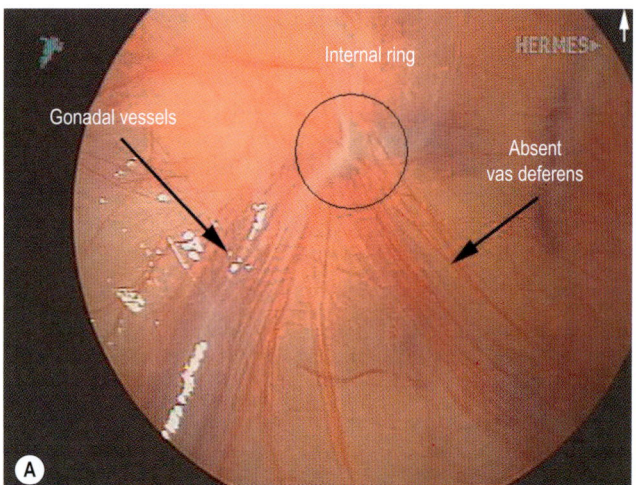

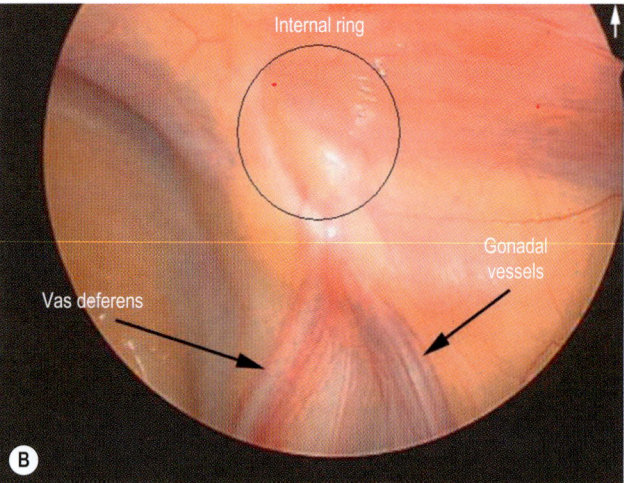

FIGURE 32-1 ■ Congenital bilateral absence of the vas deferens (CBAVD). **(A)** Laparoscopic view of a patient's left internal ring. **(B)** Compare with a laparoscopic view of a similar-aged patient's right internal ring with a normal vas deferens. (From Escobar MA, Lau ST, Glick PL. Congenital bilateral absence of the vas deferens. J Pediatr Surg 2008;43:1222–3.)

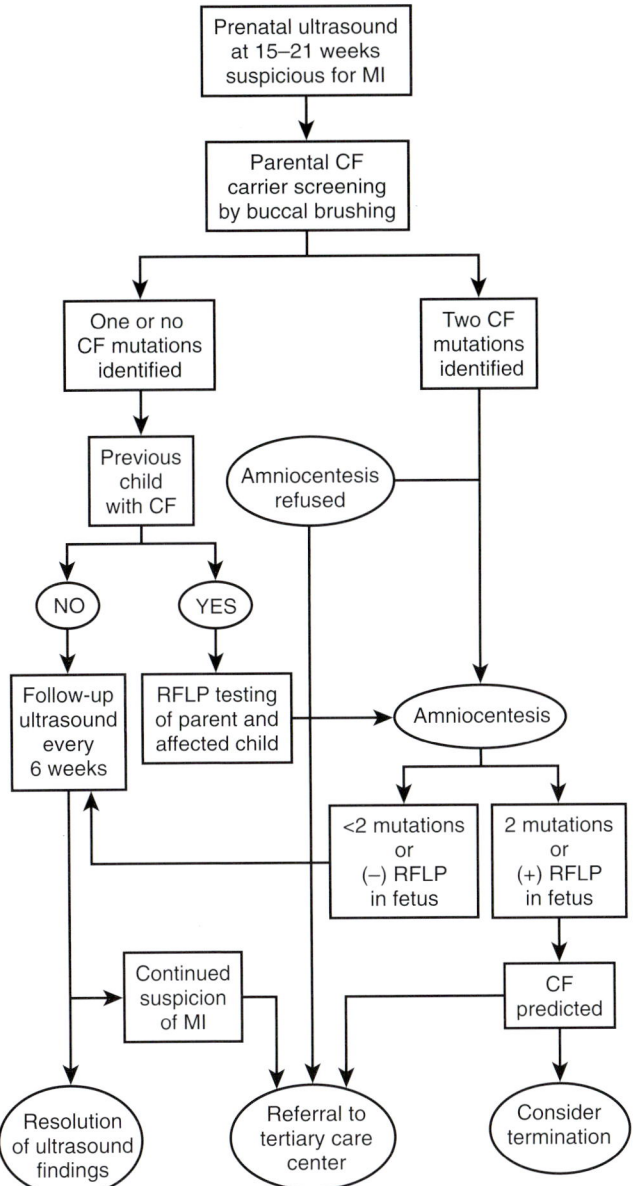

FIGURE 32-2 ■ Suggested algorithm for antenatal management of suspected meconium ileus (MI) and cystic fibrosis (CF). US, ultrasonography; RFLP, restriction fragment length polymorphism. (Adapted from Irish MS, Ragi JM, Karamanoukian H, et al. Prenatal diagnosis of the fetus with cystic fibrosis and meconium ileus. Pediatr Surg Int 1997;12:434–6.)

Sonographic Evaluation

Sonographic characteristics associated with MI include a hyperechoic, intra-abdominal mass (inspissated meconium) (Fig. 32-3), dilated bowel, and nonvisualization of the gallbladder.[52] Normal fetal meconium, when visualized in the second and third trimesters, is usually hypoechoic or isoechoic to adjacent abdominal structures.[52–57] The sensitivity of intra-abdominal echogenic masses in the detection of MI/CF is reported to be between 30–70%.[57] In addition to MI , hyperechoic bowel has been reported with Down syndrome, intrauterine growth retardation , prematurity, in utero cytomegalovirus infection, intestinal atresia, abruptio placenta, and fetal demise.[52–55,58–64] The importance of hyperechoic fetal

bowel is related to gestational age at detection, ascites, calcification, volume of amniotic fluid, and the presence of other fetal anomalies.[57] The positive predictive value of hyperechoic masses in a high-risk fetus is estimated to be 52%, but is only 6.4% in the low-risk fetus.[52] It is important to note that hyperechoic bowel has been found to be a normal variant in both the second and third trimesters.[56,57,65]

The finding of dilated bowel on prenatal ultrasound (US), in association with a family history of CF, has been reported less frequently than that of hyperechoic bowel. In MI, bowel dilation is caused by obstruction from meconium, but mimics findings in midgut volvulus, congenital bands, intestinal atresia, intestinal duplication, internal hernia, meconium plug syndrome, and Hirschsprung disease.[66] The correlation of dilated fetal bowel and MI suggests that dilated fetal bowel warrants parental testing for CF and continued sonographic surveillance of the fetus.

The inability to visualize the gallbladder on fetal ultrasound has also been associated with CF.[67] Combined with other sonographic features, nonvisualization of the gallbladder can be useful in the prenatal detection of the disease. However, caution should be exercised in the interpretation of an absent gallbladder as the differential diagnosis also includes biliary atresia, omphalocele, diaphragmatic hernia, chromosomal abnormalities, and a normal pregnancy.

Clinical Presentation

MI is categorized as either simple or complicated. The thickened meconium begins to form in utero. As it obstructs the mid-ileum, proximal bowel dilatation and thickening, along with congestion, occur. Approximately one-half of these neonates present with simple uncomplicated obstruction.[4] The remaining patients present with complications of MI, including volvulus, gangrene, atresia, and/or perforation, which may result in meconium peritonitis and giant cystic meconium peritonitis.[68–73]

Simple Meconium Ileus

In simple MI, the terminal ileum is filled with firm concretions. The bowel in this area is small in diameter and molds around the inspissated lumps of meconium. The ileum becomes dilated and is filled with thick sticky meconium with gas and fluid found within the small bowel proximal to this area.[4] Newborns with uncomplicated MI often appear healthy immediately after birth. However, within 1 to 2 days, they develop abdominal distension and bilious emesis. Normal meconium will not be passed. Eventually, dilated loops of bowel become visible on exam and have a 'doughy' character that indent on palpation. The rectum and anus are often narrow, a finding that may be misinterpreted as anal stenosis. The presentation of the baby with MI is similar to many types of neonatal small bowel obstruction. Therefore, the clinician should simultaneously consider malrotation, small intestinal atresia, colonic atresia, and meconium plug syndrome. The history, physical examination, and contrast enema help distinguish between these entities.

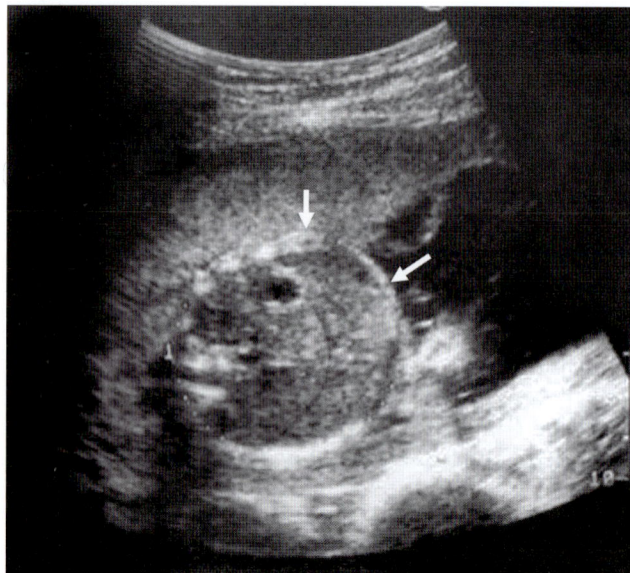

FIGURE 32-3 ■ Ultrasound image of a 22-week gestation demonstrating a 2 cm × 3 cm intraluminal (distal ileum) mass (arrows) consistent with meconium inspissation (meconium ileus). (From Irish MS, Ragi JM, Karamanoukian H, et al. Prenatal diagnosis of the fetus with cystic fibrosis and meconium ileus. Pediatr Surg Int 1997;12:434–6.)

Complicated Meconium Ileus

Infants with complicated MI present with symptoms within 24 hours of birth. Some newborns are symptomatic immediately after birth as a result of in utero perforation or bowel compromise. Signs of peritonitis, including distension, tenderness, abdominal wall edema and erythema, and clinical evidence of sepsis may be found on the initial neonatal exam. Abdominal distension can be so severe as to cause immediate respiratory distress. A palpable mass suggests pseudocyst formation, which results from in utero bowel perforation.[74,75] The neonate may present in extremis and need urgent resuscitation and operative exploration.

Historically, segmental volvulus was reported to be the most common complication of MI.[68,69] Prenatal volvulus of the meconium-distended segment of ileum may lead to interruption of the mesenteric blood flow, which can result in ischemic necrosis, intestinal atresia with an associated mesenteric defect, or perforation. When an in utero perforation occurs, most of the sterile meconium is reabsorbed with trace amounts becoming calcified. Atretic segments are common in MI and the affected bowel may appear viable, showing no evidence of perforation or gangrene. 12–17% of neonates born with jejunoileal atresia have CF.[4,76,77] Therefore, all neonates with jejunoileal atresia and an abnormal meconium presentation (MI, meconium plug syndrome, giant cystic meconium peritonitis, etc.) should undergo a sweat chloride test.[4]

The incidence of CF in neonates with meconium peritonitis is reported to be 15–40%.[78] Four types of meconium peritonitis have been recognized including: adhesive meconium peritonitis, giant cystic meconium peritonitis or pseudocyst, meconium ascites, and infected

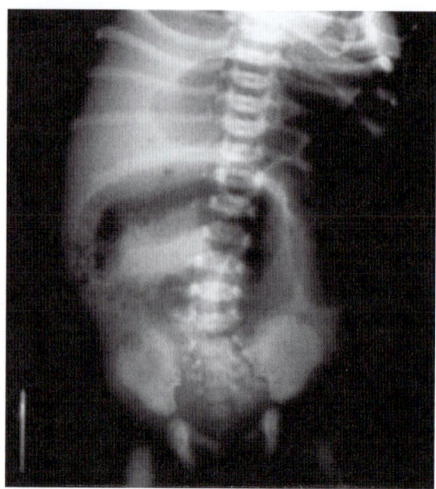

FIGURE 32-4 ■ This abdominal radiograph in a neonate with meconium ileus shows the typical ground-glass appearance in the right lower abdomen. Also note the different-sized loops of distended small bowel.

meconium peritonitis.[79] In addition to MI, other causes of in utero bowel perforation must also be considered (atresia, stenosis, colonic disorders, imperforate anus) in this clinical setting. The differences in clinical presentation are secondary to the timing of the perforation and whether or not the perforation sealed spontaneously. The site of perforation is usually closed by birth. Not surprisingly, mortality is increased in cases where the perforation remains open.[79] Initially, meconium peritonitis is a nonbacterial, chemical, and foreign body peritonitis occurring during gestation. As meconium escapes the obstructed bowel, a sterile chemical peritonitis ensues. After delivery, bacterial superinfection may occur with colonization of the gastrointestinal tract. It is important to note that meconium peritonitis can also occur without MI and is not pathognomonic for CF.[4,75,79]

Radiographic Features

Simple MI is characterized by a pattern of unevenly dilated loops of bowel on an abdominal radiograph with the variable presence of air–fluid levels.[69,80,81] The absence of air–fluid levels is due to the viscosity of the meconium not allowing an air interface with the fluid. As swallowed air mixes with the tenacious meconium, bubbles of gas may be seen. This soap bubble appearance (Fig. 32-4) depends on the viscosity of the meconium and is not a constant feature.[71,80,81] While each of these features alone is not diagnostic of MI, collectively with a family history of CF, they strongly suggest the diagnosis.

Radiographic findings in complicated MI vary with the complication. Prenatal ultrasound findings include ascites, intra-abdominal cystic masses, dilated bowel, and calcification.[82] Neonatal radiographic findings may include peritoneal calcifications, free air, and/or air–fluid levels (related to atresia).[4] Air–fluid levels may be minimally present or absent, misleading the clinician to make an incorrect diagnosis of uncomplicated MI. Speckled calcification on abdominal plain films is highly suggestive of intrauterine intestinal perforation and meconium peritonitis. Radiographic findings of obstruction and a large dense mass with a rim of calcification imply a pseudocyst (Fig. 32-5). These calcium deposits are linear and course along the parietal peritoneum and serosal surface of the visceral organs.[83] Interestingly, one-third of cases of complicated MI have no radiologic findings that suggest a complication.[84]

A contrast enema should be performed in all cases of low intestinal obstruction in the newborn. We advocate an initial water-soluble contrast enema for both diagnosis and treatment. In MI, contrast instillation is monitored fluoroscopically and demonstrates a colon of small caliber, described as the 'microcolon of disuse,' often containing small, inspissated rabbit pellets (scybala) of meconium (Fig. 32-6). The enema also identifies cecal position, indicating whether malrotation is present. In complicated cases, such as atresia, a microcolon with reflux into a decompressed terminal ileum may be noted.[4] If contrast cannot be refluxed into the dilated small bowel, operative exploration is required for diagnosis and therapy.

Diagnostic Testing

The diagnosis of CF is established with a sweat test. A sodium concentration of 60 mmol/L in 100 mg of sweat is diagnostic of CF with 40–60 mmol/L being intermediate (but more likely to be diagnostic in infants) and less than 40 mmol/L being normal.[85] The test is typically performed at several weeks of life to obtain an adequate sample size. Neonatal CF screening programs using the Guthrie blood spot test for raised concentrations of immunoreactive trypsinogen is available in many countries, but must be confirmed in a two-stage approach incorporating *CFTR* mutation analysis.[86,87] Genetic testing for *CFTR* mutations is available, however, commercial assays test for a limited number of mutations. Most regional laboratories will provide the results for the four or five most common mutations for the relevant ethnic group or geographical region in their area using the amplification refractory mutation system (ARMS) technique. Stool analyses for albumin, trypsin, and chymotrypsin are available, and abnormal values coupled with operative findings suggest CF.[37]

Neonates with MI who fail to respond to nonoperative measures may be treated by appendectomy and irrigation with water-soluble contrast into the small bowel via the small bowel or appendiceal stump.[88] The appendix (or other intestinal biopsy) may be sent for histologic analysis. Pathognomonic findings or histology for CF include goblet cell hyperplasia and accumulated secretions within crypts or lumen.[89]

Nonoperative Management of Simple Meconium Ileus

Neonates should initially be managed as any other newborn with intestinal obstruction. This management

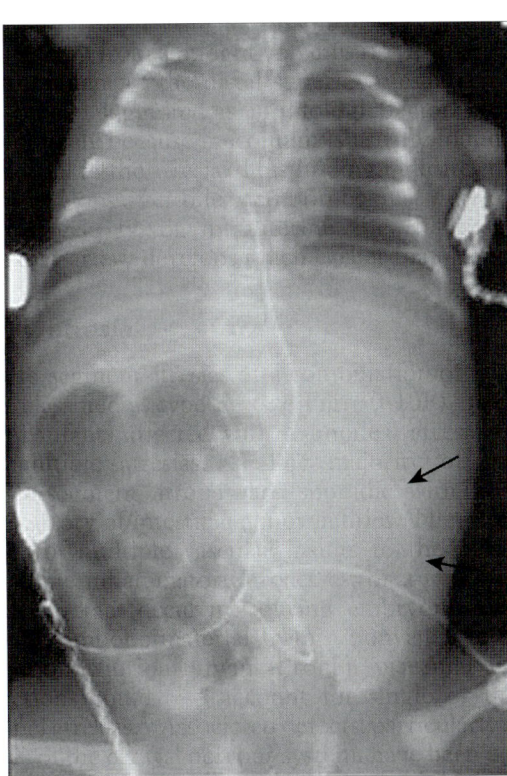

FIGURE 32-5 ■ This neonate presented with evidence of meconium peritonitis. A mass effect in the left abdomen with a rim of calcification (arrows) implies in utero perforation and a pseudocyst.

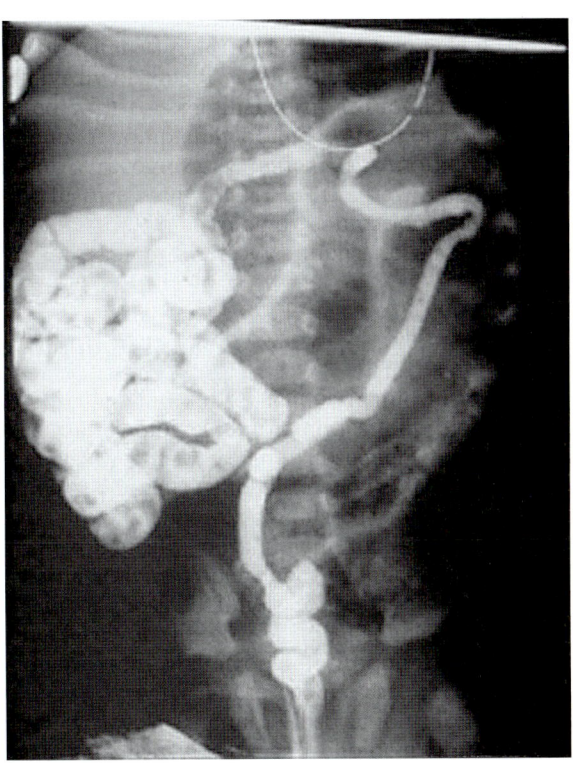

FIGURE 32-6 ■ Classic radiographic findings of meconium ileus are seen on this retrograde contrast study. First, a 'microcolon of disuse' is seen. The colon is extremely small and unused. Second, inspissated pellets (filling defects) of meconium are seen in the more proximal small bowel. Third, note there is a small bowel obstruction as the contrast material has not reached the markedly dilated loops of small bowel.

should include volume resuscitation and ventilator support as necessary. Gastric decompression to prevent progressive abdominal distension, aspiration, and pulmonary compromise is important. In addition, correction of any coagulation disorders and empiric broad-spectrum antibiotic coverage should be initiated.

The majority of newborns with MI can be managed nonoperatively. As noted above, the initial management should include an isotonic water-soluble contrast enema under fluoroscopic control. The water-soluble enema will also exclude other causes of neonatal intestinal obstruction. Prior to performing the water-soluble enema, the neonate should receive adequate intravenous fluid to correct and avoid hypovolemia, receive appropriate electrolyte repletion, and be normothermic.

Under fluoroscopic control, the water-soluble contrast material is slowly infused at low hydrostatic pressure through a catheter inserted into the rectum. Inflation of the catheter balloon should be avoided to minimize the risk of perforation. Upon completion, the catheter is withdrawn and an abdominal radiograph is obtained to evaluate for perforation. The infant is then returned to the neonatal care unit for intensive monitoring and fluid resuscitation. Usually there is rapid passage of meconium pellets followed by semi-liquid meconium, which continues in the ensuing 24–48 hours. Upon instillation of the enema, extraluminal fluid is drawn into the intestinal lumen, hydrating and softening the meconium mass. Warm saline enemas containing 1% N-acetylcysteine (Mucomyst; Apothecon, Princeton, New Jersey) may be given to help complete the evacuation.[73] Radiographs should be obtained as clinically indicated to confirm evacuation of the obstruction and to exclude late perforation. If evacuation is incomplete, or if the first attempt at contrast enema evacuation does not reflux contrast into dilated bowel, a second enema may be necessary. However, if progressive distension, signs of peritonitis, or clinical deterioration occur, operative exploration is indicated. After two failed attempts at nonoperative water-soluble enemas, operative intervention is likely warranted.

Following successful evacuation and resuscitation, 5 mL of a 10% N-acetylcysteine solution may be administered every six hours through a nasogastric tube to liquefy the upper gastrointestinal secretions. Feedings with supplemental pancreatic enzymes for those infants confirmed with CF may be initiated when signs of obstruction have subsided. In the past, the success rate of patients with uncomplicated MI, treated with Gastrografin® enemas, has ranged between 63–83%.[90,91] However, more recent reports indicate a much lower success rate likely secondary to the use of isotonic enema fluid.[4,92]

Several potential complications exist with the use of enemas in treating MI. The risk of rectal perforation can be avoided by careful placement of the catheter under fluoroscopic guidance and by not inflating the balloon-tipped catheter. A 23% perforation rate has been demonstrated in patients when inflated balloon catheters were used, and the risk of perforation increases with repeated enemas.[93,94] Late perforation, occurring between 12 and 48 hours following the enema, can occur as well.

Potential causes for late perforation include severe bowel distension by fluid osmotically drawn into the intestine or by injury to the bowel mucosa by the contrast medium.[94] Lower perforation rates have been reported more recently, possibly related to less aggressive enema attempts and isotonic enema agents.[4,52] Hypovolemic shock is a risk when delivering hypertonic enemas. Ischemia caused by overdistension is worsened by hypoperfusion caused by hypovolemia due to inadequate fluid resuscitation.[95]

Operative Management

Simple Meconium Ileus

The indications for operative management of simple MI are inadequate meconium evacuation or a complication from the contrast enema (e.g., perforation). Failure of nonoperative treatment with the contrast enema may result from the inability to advance the column of enema fluid into the ileum or from an unsuspected associated intestinal atresia. If the enema fails to promote passage of meconium within 24 to 48 hours, or two attempts at washout are unsuccessful, operative intervention is indicated.

At laparotomy, manual evacuation of the inspissated meconium can be aided by intraoperative instillation of 2% or 4% N-acetylcysteine or saline solutions. These fluids can be passed antegrade through a nasogastric tube, retrograde through the appendiceal stump, or directly into the meconium through an enterotomy. A purse-string suture is placed in the antimesenteric wall of the bowel and a red rubber catheter is inserted through a small incision within the purse-string. This is followed by gentle instillation of the solution into the proximal bowel and terminal ileum to avoid perforation. Often the thick tenacious meconium can be removed directly through the enterotomy (Fig. 32-7). The dissolved meconium and pellets can be either removed directly or milked into the colon. It is important that the surgeon avoids exposure of the meconium to the peritoneum. Once the meconium is cleared, the enterotomy or appendiceal stump is closed. If necessary, an indwelling intestinal catheter or a T-tube may be left through the enterotomy for the purpose of postoperative bowel irrigation, decompression, pancreatic enzyme instillation, and/or feeding.[96] The enterostomy tube should be positioned at the junction of the proximal dilated bowel and collapsed distal ileum. The irrigations are begun in the early postoperative period and after successful clearance of meconium, the tubes are removed and the enterocutaneous fistula is allowed to close spontaneously.[96–100]

Although uncommon, resection with primary anastomosis is occasionally required and was first described in 1962.[101] Anastomotic leakage complicated early attempts with this approach, but improved results have been recently reported.[102–104] Successful outcome following resection with primary anastomosis depends on adequate resection of compromised bowel, complete proximal and distal evacuation of meconium, and preservation of an adequate blood supply.

Other surgical approaches involve resection, anastomosis, and temporary enterostomy through which postoperative irrigations can be delivered (Fig. 32-8). Several stomas have been used: the Mikulicz double-barreled enterostomy, the Bishop-Koop distal chimney enterostomy, and the Santulli and Blanc proximal enterostomy.[98,104] Disadvantages of these and other procedures employing resection and stoma(s) include potential high-volume stoma output, bowel length loss due to resection, and the need for a second procedure to re-establish intestinal continuity.

Complicated Meconium Ileus

Operative management is almost always required in cases of complicated MI. One exception is the rare in utero spontaneously sealed perforation with intact intestinal continuity and extraluminal intraperitoneal calcified meconium.[68] Late findings include calcified meconium identified in a patent processus vaginalis during herniorrhaphy or incidentally on abdominal radiographs. Indications for operation include peritonitis, persistent intestinal obstruction, enlarging abdominal mass, and ongoing sepsis. Surgical management includes debridement of necrotic material, pseudocyst resection, diverting stoma(s), antibiotics, and meticulous postoperative care.[73] Creation of an ostomy is usually the fastest and safest operative course, alleviating concern over bowel

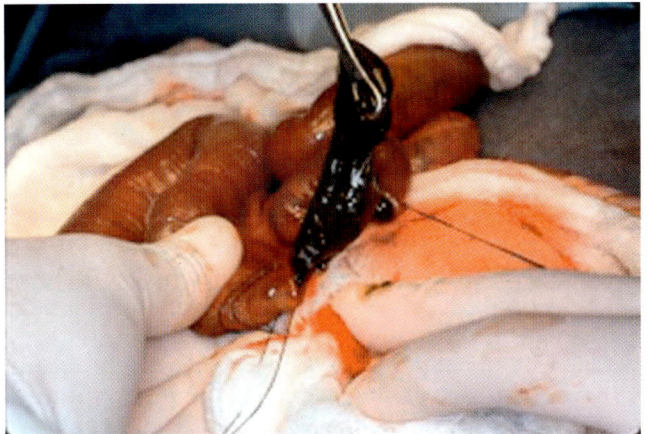

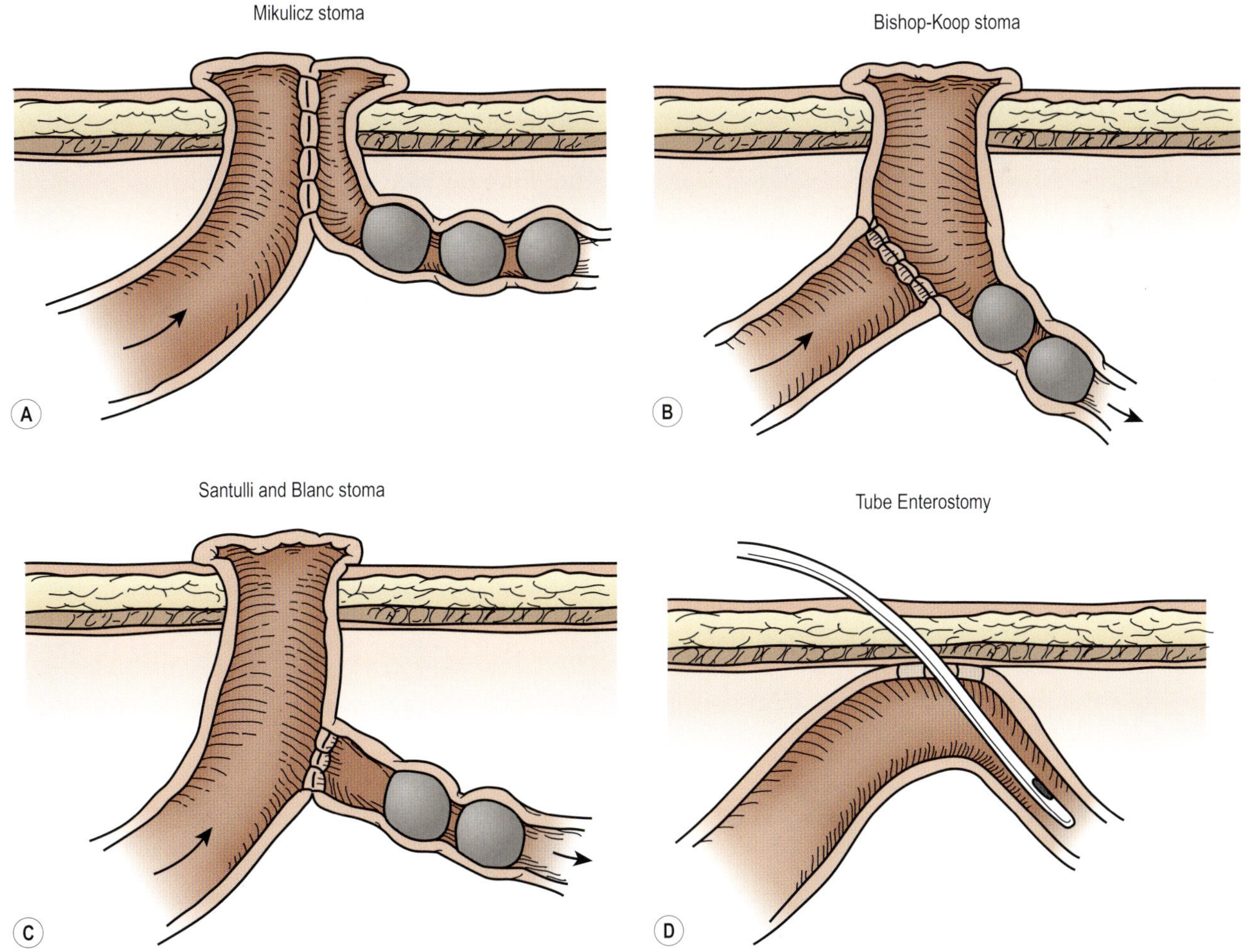

FIGURE 32-7 ■ At operation, the meconium in a neonate with cystic fibrosis is very thick and tenacious.

Mikulicz stoma

Bishop-Koop stoma

Santulli and Blanc stoma

Tube Enterostomy

(A) (B) (C) (D)

FIGURE 32-8 ■ There are a number of options for surgical management of a neonate with meconium ileus. Options for creation of an ileostomy include the **(A)** double-barrel ileostomy (Mikulicz enterostomy), **(B)** the Bishop-Koop ileostomy, and **(C)** the Santulli ileostomy. Both the Bishop-Koop and Santulli ileostomies require an intra-abdominal anastomosis. **(D)** Another option is to place a red rubber catheter into the uninvolved proximal small bowel for postoperative irrigations.

discrepancy, anastomotic leak/obstruction, and return of bowel activity. In cases with pseudocyst formation, decortication of the cyst wall is recommended if possible.[74]

Although meconium peritonitis is best managed with an enterostomy, segmental volvulus and intestinal atresia (without peritoneal contamination) in stable patients may be managed with resection, bowel irrigation, and primary anastomosis depending on the state of the intestine. Ultimately, the goal of operative management is the relief of intestinal obstruction and the preservation of maximal intestinal length.

Postoperative Management

Postoperative management requires ongoing resuscitation, including maintenance fluids and replacement of insensible and gastrointestinal fluid losses, (nasogastric suction and ileostomy). Instillation of 2% or 4% N-acetylcysteine via a nasogastric tube, enterostomy tube, or via an ileostomy or mucous fistula will help solubilize residual meconium. In the patient with fetal or neonatal bowel obstruction, diagnostic tests to evaluate for CF should be performed. Stomas should be closed when possible (four to six weeks) to avoid prolonged problems with fluid, electrolyte, nutritional losses, and cholestatic jaundice.

Nutritional Management

Enteral feeds in infants with uncomplicated MI and CF may be initiated with breast milk or infant formula, along with supplemental pancreatic enzymes and vitamins.[105,106] Caution must be used when prescribing enteric enzyme medication to patients with MI/CF. Treatment failures and complications include fibrosing colonopathy from excessive enzyme doses and MI equivalent, or distal intestinal obstruction syndrome (DIOS) from inadequate enzyme therapy or generic substitutions for proprietary medications.[48,105,107–109] Often patients with a complicated postoperative course will require either continuous enteral feeds or total parenteral nutrition (TPN). Dilation of the small bowel by the obstructing meconium may lead to mucosal damage that could contribute to poor peristalsis or malabsorption. In patients with complicated MI or in those with significant loss of intestinal length, initiating the enteral feeding with a predigested, diluted formula at low continuous volumes is best. If this is well tolerated, the concentration should be increased followed by the volume. Pancreatic enzymes should be given with enteral feeds (even with predigested formula) starting at 2,000–4,000 lipase units per 120 mL of full strength formula. Capsules containing enteric-coated microspheres can be opened and the contents mixed with formula or applesauce in older infants. The microcapsules should not be crushed as this will expose the enzymes to the acid of the stomach where they will be destroyed. Uncrushed pancreatic enzymes should be given even with MCT-oil containing formulas.[110]

Infants with MI are at increased risk for cholestasis, particularly if they have had or are receiving TPN. Alkaline phosphatase, alanine aminotransferase (ALT), aspartate aminotransferase (AST), and bilirubin should be monitored weekly. The fluid and nutritional status of infants who have had significant bowel resection (greater than one-third) may be difficult to manage. In addition, the presence of an ileostomy may lead to excessive losses of fluid and sodium. If access to the distal, defunctionalized bowel is possible, drip feeds of glutamine-enriched formula or instillation of the effluent from the proximal stoma may be given at low volumes to enhance bowel growth and help prevent bacterial translocation.

Gastric acid hypersecretion is seen in patients who have short bowel syndrome.[111] An acidic intestinal environment inactivates pancreatic enzymes and prevents dissolution of enteric-coated microcapsules. H_2-receptor antagonists or proton pump inhibitors may be used as an adjunct with pancreatic enzyme therapy in patients who have had significant bowel resections. Patients with excessive sweat and intestinal sodium losses may develop a total body sodium deficit. Urine sodium should be measured in infants with ileostomies, especially when there is growth failure, even if serum sodium levels are normal. Those with a urine sodium less than 10 mEq/L will need sodium (and possibly bicarbonate) supplementation.[107,112]

Pulmonary Management

Although clinical lung disease is usually a delayed complication, mucous plugging and atelectasis can be seen. Prophylactic pulmonary care with chest physiotherapy should be initiated early in the postoperative period. The head-down position should not be used as this increases the risk of gastroesophageal reflux (GER) and aspiration. Infants should receive nebulized albuterol twice daily followed by chest physiotherapy. Prophylactic antibiotics are contraindicated, and antibiotic therapy should be directed by respiratory cultures, if needed.

Prognosis

The prognosis for infants with MI was uniformly poor, despite operative treatment, prior to the mid-1900s. Early series reported mortality rates of 50–67%.[98,99] The improved survival in infants with MI can be attributed to many factors. Advances in prenatal diagnosis, pulmonary and neonatal intensive care, nutrition, antibiotics, anesthesia, operative management, and an improved understanding of the pathophysiology and treatment of the CF complications have resulted in dramatic prognostic improvement for infants with both complicated and simple MI.[22,113] Survival rates of 85 to 100% have been reported in uncomplicated MI, and up to 93% in complicated cases.[4,84,113]

Previously, it was thought that patients with CF presenting with MI have worse outcomes than those without MI. However, it is no longer clear if this is accurate. Several long-term follow-up studies of patients with MI report pulmonary function at age 13 years to be no different between those born with and those without MI.[114,115] However, a recent prospective study found children with MI have worse lung function and more obstructive lung disease than those with CF but without MI.[111]

Furthermore, comparison of the nutritional status of a similar population of patients with CF suggests that those who presented with MI suffer long-term nutritional complications and other problems.[116]

MECONIUM PLUG SYNDROME

The meconium plug syndrome (MPS) was first described in 1956.[117] It was hypothesized initially that either colonic motility or the character of the meconium was altered, thereby preventing its normal passage and subsequent decompression of the colon in the newborn period. Under normal conditions, the terminal two centimeters of neonatal meconium is firm in texture, forming a whitish cap. Most newborns pass this meconium cap before, during, or shortly after delivery. One in 500 newborns will have a longer, more tenacious obstructive plug. Failure to pass this plug results in MPS, and the term 'plugged-up babies' was coined.

The presentation of MPS is similar to that of MI. Signs and symptoms include failure to pass meconium, bilious vomiting, and abdominal distention with an obstructive pattern on plain abdominal films. Often, the meconium plug becomes dislodged following digital stimulation of the anus and rectum. Fortunately, colon function is generally preserved and returns to normal following passage of the plug. Ultimately, most of these infants are found to be healthy.

Pathologic causes of MPS include CF, small left colon syndrome, and Hirschsprung disease.[117–120] Less common causes include congenital hypothyroidism, maternal narcotic addiction, and neuronal intestinal dysplasia. A contrast enema may be therapeutic as well as diagnostic. Following resolution, a sweat test should be performed to exclude CF and a thryroid-stimulating hormone level should be obtained. A rectal biopsy should be performed to evaluate for Hirschsprung disease if there is a dysfunctional stooling pattern after resolution of the plug.[73,118,119]

COMPLICATIONS OF MECONIUM ILEUS AND CYSTIC FIBROSIS

Gastroesophageal Reflux Disease

GER occurs with increased prevalence in patients with CF. Aspiration in CF children may aggravate failure to thrive, adversely affect pulmonary function, and may account for the predilection of CF lung disease in the right upper lobe.[121,122] Pathological reflux with endoscopic and histological esophagitis is present in more than 50% of CF patients and the incidence of GER in patients with CF is approximately 80% in patients younger than 5 years.[123] It is clear that early diagnosis and treatment of GER is of prime importance if its complications are to be minimized and respiratory function maximized.

Antireflux medications, modification of chest physiotherapy, and eliminating the 30° head-down tilt may all decrease the incidence of GER in this population.[124] Children unresponsive to medical management should undergo evaluation for an antireflux procedure. Our preferred approach is the laparoscopic Nissen fundoplication. Recent data suggests that a fundoplication may improve respiratory function (improved FEV1 slope) in CF children with mild versus moderate disease.[125] Patients with symptomatic GER requiring an antireflux procedure may benefit from concurrent placement of a gastrostomy if inadequate caloric intake is problematic.

Barrett esophagus, a rare finding in children, has been reported in older children with CF.[4,126] Although an antireflux procedure may halt the advancement of metaplasia, if dysplasia is present, the malignant potential remains.[127] In cases with metaplasia, endoscopic monitoring is the same for patients with CF as those without.[127] In adults, if high-grade dysplasia is confirmed by two pathologists and aggressive medical therapy fails to eliminate the dysplasia, esophagectomy is recommended. With so little data available in children with CF, at a minimum, it is reasonable that patients who have dysplastic esophageal changes should be evaluated for an antireflux procedure.

Biliary Tract Disease

Multiple macroscopic cysts may replace the pancreas in CF.[27] Although it has been thought that hepatic and pancreatic dysfunction occurred together, hepatic dysfunction may occur in patients with normal pancreatic function.[128] The most common hepatic complications of CF are steatosis, fibrosis, biliary cirrhosis, atretic gallbladder, cholelithiasis, sclerosing cholangitis, and biliary dyskinesia. Obstruction of intrahepatic biliary ductules by abnormal mucoid secretions or inspissated bile, resulting from the absence of functional CFTR in bile duct epithelial cells, results in the development of cirrhosis in patients with CF.[128] When biopsied, the classic liver histology in CF is focal biliary fibrosis with progression to multilobular, biliary cirrhosis. Prolonged cholestatic liver disease in CF patients may lead to cirrhosis, portal hypertension, and ultimately liver failure and death without liver transplantation.

Though more common in older patients with CF, intrahepatic cholestasis can be seen in the neonate. In extreme forms, this process can be associated with a marked decrease in ductal diameter, varying from hypoplasia to atresia. Additionally, these neonates are at increased risk for cholestatic jaundice when they are not being fed enterally. Cholestatic jaundice is suggested by prolonged jaundice unresponsive to choleretics, nondilated bile ducts and gallbladder on ultrasound, absent biliary excretion on nuclear scan, and characteristic liver biopsy.[129–131]

End-stage liver disease (ESLD) is manifest by loss of synthetic function, growth failure, or portal hypertension presenting as variceal hemorrhage.[132] Although abnormal liver function tests have been noted in 13% of CF patients, only 4.2% manifest overt liver disease (although the prevalence is as high as 37% depending on the definition of liver disease).[133] Portosystemic shunts, transjugular intrahepatic portosystemic shunts (TIPS), partial splenectomy, and endoscopic injection sclerotherapy have been advocated in treating CF patients with portal hypertension.[134] Other surgical options for these patients are direct ligation of the varices, esophageal transection, or the Sugiura procedure (gastric devascularization).[135,136] These procedures are all palliative, with the only curative treatment for portal hypertension and end-stage liver disease being orthotopic liver transplantation (OLT).

Liver transplantation has been successfully carried out in CF patients with ESLD who did not have respiratory failure.[137,138] There are several successful reports of combined liver and intestinal transplantation, combined liver and pancreas transplant, kidney transplant after combined heart and lung transplants, and triple organ transplant (pancreas, liver and kidney) in patients with exocrine pancreatic insufficiency and insulin-dependent diabetes related to CF.[4,139,140] Long-term studies are demonstrating preservation or maintenance of respiratory function and nutritional status following OLT in patients with CF.[137,138]

Gallbladder disease is prevalent in the CF population, including cholelithiasis in up to 24%, and abnormal cholecystograms in 46%.[136,141,142] Other abnormalities include microgallbladder, atretic cystic duct , and hyperviscous mucus. Many CF patients with gallstones are asymptomatic, with the incidence of symptomatic gallbladder disease in CF reported to be approximately 4%.[143] Because the stones are radiolucent, ultrasound rather than computed tomography (CT) is recommended in patients with CF.[136,144] Bile in patients with CF is not cholesterol supersaturated; hence the stones are composed of protein and calcium bilirubinate.[141]

CF patients with symptomatic gallbladder disease (symptomatic cholelithiasis and/or acute cholecystitis) should undergo prompt cholecystectomy.[144,145] Although of historical interest only, the complication rate with open cholecystectomy was quite low with aggressive pulmonary toilet.[146,147] The laparoscopic approach is now the accepted standard.[4] Due to the low incidence of common bile duct (CBD) stones in CF patients, routine intraoperative cholangiograms or preoperative endoscopic retrograde cholangiopancreatography (ERCP) are not needed.[4,147] In fact, the biliary tract abnormalities often encountered in patients with CF make penetration of radiocontrast dye into the biliary tract during ERCP difficult.[136] Intraoperative cholangiography is recommended if jaundice, pancreatitis, cholangitis, dilated CBD, or palpable stones in the CBD are present.[4]

Distal Intestinal Obstruction Syndrome

DIOS (formerly called MI equivalent) is a recurrent, partial or complete intestinal obstruction unique to teenage and young adult patients with CF that occurs secondary to abnormally viscid mucofeculent material in the distal ileum and right colon.[148–151] The etiology of DIOS is unclear, but these patients are more likely to have a history of steatorrhea from pancreatic exocrine insufficiency despite adequate enzyme therapy. A number of aspects particular to gastrointestinal function in the CF patient may help to explain this syndrome. In addition to inherently slow intestinal motility, other contributing factors may include thickening of chyme secondary to the presence of undigested protein and fat, precipitation of undigested protein and bile acids in duodenal fluid with reduced pH, lower water content of pancreatic and duodenal secretions, hyperviscosity of mucus resulting from abnormal ion and water transport, abnormal regulation of mucin secretion, and altered biochemical properties of mucus glycoprotein.[152–154] Precipitating factors include sudden withdrawal of (or noncompliance with) enzyme supplementation, immobilization, dehydration, respiratory tract infections, and recovery from surgery. However, in the majority of cases, no identifiable cause will be found.[4]

DIOS occurs in 15–37% of patients with CF, and is seen particularly in those with associated pancreatic insufficiency with malabsorption and severe pulmonary limitation.[148,149,151] One study noted a 12% incidence in children with CF, with the majority (63%) having MI as an infant.[4] Children with normal fat absorption are rarely affected.

Patients with DIOS present with crampy abdominal pain, often localized to the right lower quadrant, and decreased frequency of defecation. They may complain of insidious, debilitating abdominal pain. Physical examination in uncomplicated DIOS usually reveals abdominal distension and a tender mass in the right lower quadrant with no evidence of peritonitis. Typically, there is no fecal impaction on rectal examination and the stool is guaiac negative. Different degrees of obstruction can occur, ranging from partial (most common) to complete with vomiting, abdominal distension, and obstipation.

A supine and erect abdominal film is the most useful initial investigation when DIOS is suspected (Fig. 32-9). This will show distended small bowel with scattered air-fluid levels and a granular, bubbly pattern of intestinal gas representing the mixing of air and inspissated meconium in the right lower quadrant, similar to infants with MI.

Inspissated material in the right colon and distal ileum can be demonstrated with a water-soluble contrast enema. With this study, an ileocolic intussusception, which can also be seen in CF patients, can be excluded, and the contrast study itself may prove therapeutic in some cases.

The diagnosis of DIOS should take into consideration other potential causes of abdominal pain and intestinal obstruction in CF patients. This constellation of signs and symptoms has historically been a diagnostic dilemma in these patients. Intussusception, mechanical small bowel obstruction due to adhesions, appendicitis, Crohn disease, and biliary tract disease may present similarly.

In the absence of mechanical small bowel obstruction due to adhesions, intussusception, or appendiceal disease, a trial of medical management aimed at relieving the inspissated distal bowel obstruction is suggested. After adequate volume resuscitation and colonic enema washout, a balanced polyethylene glycol-electrolyte solution, such as GoLytely® or Colyte®, can be given orally or by nasogastric tube.[155] The dose is 20–40 mL/kg/h with a maximum of 1200 mL/h. Alternatively, ingestion of a nonabsorbable intestinal lavage solution may produce the most striking results.[156] Younger patients will usually require nasogastric tube placement whereas older children may be able to ingest sufficient volumes of lavage solution to relieve the impacted material.

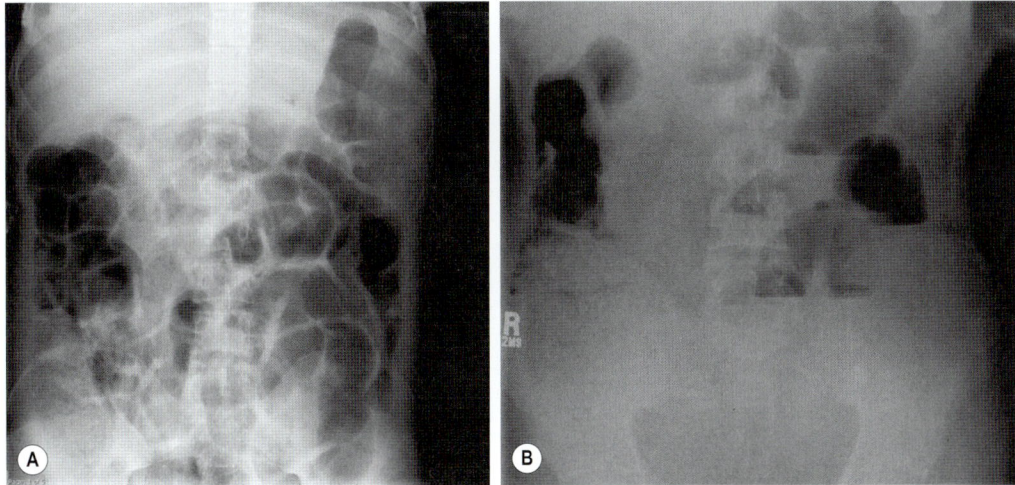

FIGURE 32-9 ■ This 18-year-old with cystic fibrosis presented with crampy abdominal pain that was localized to the right lower abdomen. In addition, he also had a decreased frequency of defecation. **(A)** The ground-glass appearance in the loops of bowel on the right side are typical findings in a patient with distal intestinal obstruction syndrome. **(B)** The upright abdominal film shows air-fluid levels. This patient responded well to a contrast enema with relief of his symptoms.

The passage of stool, resolution of symptoms, and the disappearance of a previously palpable right iliac fossa mass imply successful treatment. Sequential abdominal radiographs will help to document the resolution of DIOS, but if symptoms persist then the differential diagnosis must be re-considered. Some authors have recommended DIOS prophylaxis with use of scheduled laxatives and high dietary fiber.[148]

When there is complete obstruction or evidence of peritonitis, an operation is necessary and oral or rectal therapies are contraindicated. A nasogastric tube should be passed for decompression and adequate resuscitative measures initiated. At laparotomy, the bowel wall will feel thickened and filled with tenacious material. It can be decompressed and irrigated via a small catheter placed through the appendiceal stump, as previously described for uncomplicated MI. It is also possible to leave an irrigating tube in situ to irrigate the bowel postoperatively. Some children may require lysis of adhesions and/or bowel resections with either primary anastomosis or creation of an ostomy.[4]

Appendicitis

Abdominal pain is a common complaint of patients with CF. As they are often already being treated with antibiotics and steroids, the classical clinical signs and symptoms of appendicitis are often masked, and the diagnosis can be missed. This results in an increased incidence of perforation and substantial morbidity in this patient group. Despite the blunting of clinical signs, there may still be fever and leukocytosis. Depending on the location of the appendix, a contrast enema may show deformity of the cecum with an associated mass effect and lack of typical inspissated material features of DIOS. With appendiceal perforation, abdominal ultrasound or CT scan will show free fluid or an abscess in the region of the cecum. In cases of perforated appendicitis, initial treatment should be percutaneous drainage of the abscess

and interval appendectomy. Appendectomy is required in acute nonperforated appendicitis. If the diagnosis is still in doubt, diagnostic laparoscopy can be utilized. Many surgeons perform incidental appendectomy during other abdominal operations in CF patients.

Intussusception

Intussusception occurs in approximately 1% of children with CF with the average age of onset of 9.5 years.[151] In contrast, the average age of onset in children with idiopathic intussusception in the general pediatric population is 6–18 months.[121] Toddlers and older children presenting with intussusception and a history of recurrent pulmonary infections should be tested for CF. The most common site for intussusception is ileocolic, but it may be ileoileal, cecocolic, or colocolic.[122] The abnormally thick stool adheres to the bowel wall and acts as a lead point.[157] The appendix may also be a lead point.[158] Controversy exists over conservative management of intussusception in CF patients. Some report high rates of successful hydrostatic reduction, while others report less optimal results.[157,159] If the intussusception is unable to be reduced operatively, a bowel resection with anastomosis is required. The appendix should be removed at operation in patients with an intussusception.

Fibrosing Colonopathy

Fibrosing colonopathy is a result of colonic strictures, and presents with signs and symptoms of DIOS.[105–107,160,161] Histologic findings include colonic strictures with histopathologic changes of post-ischemic ulcer repair, erythematous cobblestone appearance to the mucosa, mucosal and submucosal fibrosis, and destruction of the muscularis mucosa. A change from conventional enteric-coated pancreatic enzymes to high-strength products 12–15 months before presentation has been described.[105] In the largest case-control study reported, the absolute dose of pancreatic enzymes, rather than the type of enzyme, was the strongest predictor of fibrosing colonopathy.[105]

The diagnosis of fibrosing colonopathy should be considered in CF patients who have been exposed to high doses of pancreatic enzymes and present with symptoms of abdominal pain, distension, chylous ascites, change in bowel habit, or failure to thrive. Continued diarrhea may also be a prominent feature, which unfortunately may prompt the family to increase supplemental enzymes further. On occasion, the diarrhea may be bloody. A barium enema may reveal mucosal irregularity, loss of haustral markings with a foreshortened colon, and varying degrees of stricture formation. In some cases, the entire colon is involved. Colonoscopy may show an erythematous mucosa with areas of narrowing, from which it is advisable to take multiple biopsies.[73]

Initial management should include reduction of the enzyme dosage to 500–2500 lipase units/kg per meal. This should be accompanied with adequate nutritional supplementation which may be enteral elemental feeding or even TPN temporarily. Those patients who show signs of unrelenting failure to thrive, obstruction, uncontrollable diarrhea, or chylous ascites will need operative intervention.

When exploration is planned electively for patients with intractable symptoms, a gentle bowel preparation may be given preoperatively. The aim of operative intervention is to resect the affected bowel and perform a primary anastomosis. Unfortunately, this is not possible with total colonic or rectal involvement, and the patient may require an ileostomy or colostomy. It is also not clear if this condition completely resolves by reducing the enzyme dosage and resecting the involved colon. Therefore, these patients also require regular follow-up for signs of recurrence.

OUTLOOK

The operative mortality in patients with CF has decreased considerably in the past three decades. The mortality rate for meconium ileus and peritonitis was 55% in the 1960s and 1970s.[159] Moreover, there was a significant decrease in survival in the first year of life for these infants compared to those patients with CF who did not have MI.[121] After the first year of life, survival among infants with MI approached that of other infants with CF. Recently, these statistics have improved dramatically. There are now reports documenting a 100% early survival and 86% late survival in patients with MI, and a 91.6% survival for uncomplicated MI and 85% for complicated cases at 1 year.[113,114] Recently, survival for patients with simple MI was found to be 93% (early 100%, late 93%) and complicated 89% (early 96%, late 93%).[4]

Discussing the long-term needs of the patient with MI means discussing the long-term needs of the patient with CF. A multidisciplinary approach to the management of the surgical patient with CF including respiratory care, nutrition support, and pancreatic enzyme therapy allows for a low operative morbidity and mortality. Children with MI need long-term follow-up as they are prone to

develop DIOS and fibrosing colonopathy. Furthermore, patients may be more prone to develop mechanical bowel obstructions later in life if operated on as an infant for MI.[4] Other late complications of MI such as gallstones, cirrhosis, and male sterility may also be viewed as late complications of CF in general. Many patients with CF are now surviving into the third and even fourth decades of life. Hence, many of the surgical complications of CF occur later in life.

REFERENCES

1. Lister J. Intestinal obstruction: General considerations. Neonatal Surgery, vol. 3. London: Butterworth; 1990. p. 421–3.
2. DeLorimier AA, Fonkalsrud EW, Hays DM. Congenital atresia and stenosis of the jejunum and ileum. Surgery 1969;65: 819–27.
3. FitzSimmons SC. The changing epidemiology of cystic fibrosis. J Pediatr 1993;122:1–9.
4. Escobar MA, Grosfeld JL, Burdick JJ, et al. Surgical considerations in Cystic Fibrosis: A 32-year evaluation of outcomes. Surgery 2005;138:560–72.
5. Stringer MD, Brereton RJ, Drake DP, et al. Meconium ileus due to extensive intestinal aganglionosis. J Pediatr Surg 1994;23: 501–3.
6. Evans AK, Fitzgerald DA, McKay KO. The impact of meconium ileus on the clinical course of children with cystic fibrosis. Eur Respir J 2001;18:784–9.
7. Antonowicz I, Lebenthal E, Schwachman H. Disaccharidase activities in small intestinal mucosa in patients with cystic fibrosis. J Pediatr 1978;92:214–19.
8. Schwachman H, Antionowicz I. Studies on meconium. In: E Lebenthal, editor. Gastroenterology and Nutrition in Infancy. New York: Raven Press; 1981. p. 83–93.
9. Emery J. Laboratory observations of the viscidity of meconium. Arch Dis Child 1954;29:34–7.
10. Di Sant'Agnese PA, Dische Z, Danilczenko A. Physiochemical differences of mucoproteins in duodenal fluid of patients with cystic fibrosis of the pancreas and controls. Pediatrics 1957;19:252–60.
11. Green M, Clarke J, Shwachman H. Studies in cystic fibrosis of the pancreas: Protein pattern in meconium ileus. Pediatrics 1958;21:635–41.
12. Stephan U, Busch EW, Kollberg H, et al. Cystic fibrosis detection by means of a test-strip. Pediatrics 1975;55:35–8.
13. Eggermont E, De Boeck K. Small-intestinal abnormalities in cystic fibrosis patients. Eur J Pediatr Surg 1991;150:824–8.
14. American College of Obstetricians and Gynecologists Committee on Genetics. ACOG Committee Opinion No. 486: Update on carrier screening for cystic fibrosis. Obstet Gynecol 2011;117: 1028–31.
15. Rommens JM, Iannuzzi MC, Kerem BS, et al. Identification of the cystic fibrosis gene: Chromosome walking and jumping. Science 1989;245:1059–65.
16. Kerem BS, Rommens JM, Buchanan JA, et al. Identification of the cystic fibrosis gene: Genetic analysis. Science 1989;245: 1073–80.
17. Welsh MJ, Anderson MP, Rich DP, et al. Cystic fibrosis transmembrane conductance regulator: A chloride channel with novel regulation. Neuron 1992;8:821–9.
18. Riordan JR, Rommens JM, Kerem B, et al. Identification of the cystic fibrosis gene: Cloning and characterization of complementary DNA [published erratum appears in Science 1989; 245:1437. Science 1989;245:1066–73.
19. Cystic fibrosis mutation database statistics [Internet]. Toronto: Cystic Fibrosis Centre at the Hospital for Sick Children in Toronto; 2012—[cited February 8, 2012]. Available from: http://www.genet.sickkids.on.ca/StatisticsPage.html.
20. Mornet E, Simon-Bouy B, Serre JL, et al. Genetic differences between cystic fibrosis with and without meconium ileus. Lancet 1988;1:376–8.
21. Fanconi G, Uehlinger E, Knauer C. Das Coeliakiesyndrom bei angeborener zystischer pancreasfibromatose und bronchiektasien. Wien Med Wochenschr 1936;27/28:753–6.

22. Kerem E, Corey M, Kerem B, et al. Clinical and genetic comparisons of patients with cystic fibrosis, with or without meconium ileus. J Pediatr 1989;114:767–73.

23. Bronstein MN, Sokol RJ, Abman SH, et al. Pancreatic insufficiency, growth, and nutrition in infants identified by newborn screening as having cystic fibrosis. J Pediatr 1992;120:533–40.

24. Duthie A, Doherty DG, Williams C, et al. Genotype analysis for delta F508, G551D and R553X mutations in children and young adults with cystic fibrosis with and without chronic liver disease. Hepatology 1992;15:660–4.

25. Wilmott RW, Tyson SL, Dinwiddie R, et al. Survival rates in cystic fibrosis. Arch Dis Child 1983;38:835–6.

26. Rescorla FJ, Grosfeld JL. Contemporary management of meconium ileus. World J Surg 1993;17:318–25.

27. Westwood ATR, Ireland JD, Bowie MD. Surgery in cystic fibrosis—a 20-year review. S Afr J Surg 1997;35:181–4.

28. Quinton PM. Cystic fibrosis: Impaired bicarbonate secretion and mucoviscidosis. Lancet 2008;372:415–17.

29. Boat T, Welsh M, Beaudet A. Cystic Fibrosis. In: Scriver C, Beaudet A, Sly W, Valle D, editors. The Metabolic Basis of Inherited Disease. New York: McGraw-Hill; 1989. p. 2649–80.

30. Dohle GR, Veeze HJ, Overbeek SE, et al. The complex relationships between cystic fibrosis and congenital bilateral absence of the vas deferens: Clinical, electrophysiological and genetic data. Hum Reprod 1999;14:371–4.

31. Jarvi K, McCallum S, Zielenski J, et al. Heterogeneity of reproductive tract abnormalities in men with absence of the vas deferens: Role of cystic fibrosis transmembrane conductance regulator gene mutations. Fertil Steril 1998;70:724–8.

32. Shin D, Gilbert F, Goldstein M, et al. Congenital absence of the vas deferens: Incomplete penetrance of cystic fibrosis gene mutations. J Urol 1997;158:1794–9.

33. Daudin M, Bieth E, Bujan L, et al. Congenital bilateral absence of the vas deferens: Clinical characteristics, biological parameters, cystic fibrosis transmembrane conductance regulator gene mutations, and implications for genetic counseling. Fertil Steril 2000;74:1164–74.

34. Escobar MA, Lau ST, Glick PL. Congenital bilateral absence of the vas deferens. J Pediatr Surg 2008;43:1222–3.

35. Bompadre SG, Sohma Y, Li M, Hwang TC. G551D and G1349D, two CF-associated mutations in the signature sequences of CFTR, exhibit distinct gating defects. J Gen Physiol 2007;129:285–98.

36. Farber S. The relation of pancreatic achylia to meconium ileus. J Pediatr 1944;24:387–92.

37. Kerem E, Corey M, Kerem BS, et al. The relation between genotype and phenotype in cystic fibrosis–analysis of the most common mutation (delta F508). N Engl J Med 1990;323:1517–22.

38. Hinen E. Meconium ileus with no pancreatic abnormality. Arch Dis Child 1950;25:99–100.

39. Thomaidis TS, Arey JB. The intestinal lesions in cystic fibrosis of the pancreas. J Pediatr 1963;63:444–53.

40. Glanzmann E. Dysporia entero-bronco-pancreatica congenita familiaris. Ann Paediat 1946;166:289.

41. Buchanan D, Rapoport S. Chemical comparison of normal meconium and meconium from patients with meconium ileus. Pediatrics 1952;9:304–10.

42. Bodian M, editor. Fibrocystic Disease of the Pancrease: Congenital disorder of mucous production-mucosis. New York: Grune and Stratton, Inc.; 1953.

43. Foulkes AG, Harris A. Localization of expression of the cystic fibrosis gene in human pancreatic development. Pancreas 1993;8:3–6.

44. Bali A, Stableforth DE, Asquith P. Prolonged small-intestinal transit time in cystic fibrosis. Br Med J (Clin Res Ed) 1983;287:1011–13.

45. Dalzell AM, Freestone NS, Billington D, et al. Small intestinal permeability and orocaecal transit time in cystic fibrosis. Arch Dis Child 1990;65:585–8.

46. Toyosaka A, Tomimoto Y, Nose K, et al. Immaturity of the myenteric plexus is the aetiology of meconium ileus without mucoviscidosis: A histopathologic study. Clin Auton Res 1994;4:175–84.

47. Emery JL. Colonic retention syndrome (megacolon) associated with immaturity of intestinal intramural plexus. Proc R Soc Med 1973;66:222–3.

48. Wilcox DT, Borowitz DS, Stovroff MC, et al. Chronic intestinal pseudo-obstruction with meconium ileus at onset. J Pediatr 1993;123:751–2.

49. Irish MS, Gollin Y, Borowitz DS, et al. Meconium Ileus: Antenatal diagnosis and perinatal care. Fetal Matern Med Rev 1996;8:79–83.

50. Irish MS, Ragi JM, Karamanoukian H, et al. Prenatal diagnosis of the fetus with cystic fibrosis and meconium ileus. Pediatr Surg Int 1997;12:434–6.

51. Irish M, Boriwitz DS, Glick PL. Meconium Ileus. In: Ziegler MM, Azizkhan RG, Gauderer MWL, Weber TR, editors. Operative Pediatric Surgery. Stamford: Appleton & Lange, Co.; 2003.

52. Dicke JM, Crane JP. Sonographically detected hyperechoic fetal bowel: Significance and implications for pregnancy management. Obstet Gynecol 1992;80:778–82.

53. Denholm TA, Crow HC, Edwards WH, et al. Prenatal sonographic appearance of meconium ileus in twins. AJR Am J Roentgenol 1984;143:371–2.

54. Caspi B, Elchalal U, Lancet M, et al. Prenatal diagnosis of cystic fibrosis: Ultrasonographic appearance of meconium ileus in the fetus. Prenat Diagn 1988;8:379–82.

55. Benacerraf BR, Chaudhury AK. Echogenic fetal bowel in the third trimester associated with meconium ileus secondary to cystic fibrosis. A case report. J Reprod Med 1989;34:299–300.

56. Fakhry J, Reiser M, Shapiro LR, et al. Increased echogenicity in the lower fetal abdomen: A common normal variant in the second trimester. J Ultrasound Med 1986;5:489–92.

57. Lince DM, Pretorius DH, Manco-Johnson ML, et al. The clinical significance of increased echogenicity in the fetal abdomen. AJR Am J Roentgenol 1985;145:683–6.

58. Goldstein RB, Filly RA, Callen PW. Sonographic diagnosis of meconium ileus in utero. J Ultrasound Med 1987;6:663–6.

59. Boue A, Muller F, Nezelof C, et al. Prenatal diagnosis in 200 pregnancies with a 1-in-4 risk of cystic fibrosis. Hum Genet 1986;74:288–97.

60. Bromley B, Doubilet P, Frigoletto FD, Jr, et al. Is fetal hyperechoic bowel on second-trimester sonogram an indication for amniocentesis? Obstet Gynecol 1994;83:647–51.

61. Nyberg DA; Resta RG, Luthy DA, et al. Prenatal sonographic findings of Down syndrome: Review of 94 cases. Obstet Gynecol 1990;76:370–7.

62. Gollin Y, Shaffer W, Gollin G, et al. Increased abdominal echogenicity in utero: A marker for intestinal obstruction. Am J Obstet Gynecol 1993;168:349.

63. Bahado-Singh R, Morotti R, Copel JA, Mahoney MJ. Hyperechoic fetal bowel: The perinatal consequences. Prenat Diagn 1994;14:981–7.

64. Forouzan I. Fetal abdominal echogenic mass: An early sign of intrauterine cytomegalovirus infection. Obstet Gynecol 1992;80:535–7.

65. Paulson EK, Hertzberg BS. Hyperechoic meconium in the third trimester fetus: An uncommon normal variant. J Ultrasound Med 1991;10:677–80.

66. De Backer AI, De Schepper AM, Deprettere A, et al. Radiographic manifestations of intestinal obstruction in the newborn. JBR-BTR 1999;82:159–66.

67. Duchatel F, Muller F, Oury JF, et al. Prenatal diagnosis of cystic fibrosis: Ultrasonography of the gallbladder at 17–19 weeks of gestation. Fetal Diagn Ther 1993;8:28–36.

68. Rescorla FJ, Grosfeld JL, West KJ, et al. Changing patterns of treatment and survival in neonates with meconium ileus. Arch Surg 1989;124:837–40.

69. Donnison AB, Shwachman H, Gross RE. A review of 164 children with meconium ileus seen at the Children's Hospital Medical Center, Boston. Pediatrics 1966;37:833–50.

70. Holsclaw DS, Eckstein JB, Nixon HH. Meconium ileus: 20 year review of 109 cases. AMA M J Dis Child 1965;109:101–13.

71. Leonidas JC, Berdon WE, Baker DH, et al. Meconium ileus and its complications. A reappraisal of plain film roentgen diagnostic criteria. Am J Roentgenol Radium Ther Nucl Med 1970;108:598–609.

72. Santulli T, Blanc W. Congenital atresia of the intestine: Pathogenesis and treatment. Ann Surg 1961;154:939–48.

73. Rescorla FJ, Grosfeld JL. Contemporary management of meconium ileus. World J Surg 1993;17:318–25.

74. Careskey JM, Grosfeld JL, Weber TR, et al. Giant cystic meconium peritonitis (GCMP): Improved management based on clinical and laboratory observations. J Pediatr Surg 1982;17:482–9.

75. Andrassy R, Nirgiotis J. Meconium disease of infancy: Meconium ileus, meconium plug syndrome,and meconium peritonitis. In: Holder T, Ashcraft K, editors. Pediatric Surgery. Philadelphia: W. B. Saunders; 1990. p. 331–40.

76. Rescorla FJ, Grosfeld JL. Intestinal atresia and stensosis: Analysis of survival in 120 cases. Surgery 1985;98:668–76.

77. Dalla Vecchia LK, Grosfeld JL, West KW, et al. Intestinal atresia and stenosis: a 25-year experience with 277 cases. Arch Surg 1998;1333:490–7.

78. Lloyd D. Meconium ileus. In: Welch K, Randolph J, Ravitch M, et al, editors. Pediatric Surgery. 4th ed. Chicago: Year Book Medical Publishers, Inc.; 1986. p. 849–58.

79. Martin LW. Meconium peritonitis. In: Ravitch MM, Welch KJ, Benson CD, et al, editors. Pediatric Surgery. Chicago: Year Book Medical Publishers; 1979. p. 952–5.

80. Speck CR, Moore TC, Stout FE. Antenatal roentgen diagnosis of meconium peritonitis. Am J Radiol 1962;88:566–70.

81. Herson R. Meconium ileus. Radiology 1957;68: 568–71.

82. Foster MA, Nyberg DA, Mahony BS, et al. Meconium peritonitis: Prenatal sonographic findings and their clinical significance. Radiology 1987;165:665–8.

83. White H. Meconium ileus: A new roentgen sign. Radiology 1956;66:567–71.

84. Ziegler MM. Meconium ileus. Curr Probl Surg 1994;31:731–77.

85. Gibson LE, Cooke RE. A test for concentration of electrolytes in sweat in cystic fibrosis of the pancreas utilizing pilocarpine by iontophoresis. Pediatrics 1959;23:545–9.

86. Wallis C. Diagnosing cystic fibrosis: Blood, sweat, and tears. Arch Dis Child 1997;76:85–8.

87. Southern KW, Munck A, Pollitt R, et al. A survey of newborn screening for cystic fibrosis in Europe. J Cyst Fibros 2007;6:57–65.

88. Fitzgerald R, Conlon K. Use of the appendix stump in the treatment of meconium ileus. J Pediatr Surg 1989;24:899–900.

89. Oppenheimer EH, Easterly JR. Pathological evidence of cystic fibrosis patients with meconium ileus. Pediatr Res 1973;7:339.

90. Noblett H. Meconium Ileus. In: Ravtch M, Welch K, Benson C, et al, editors. Pediatric Surgery. 3rd ed. Chicago: Year Book Medical Publishers; 1979. p. 943–51.

91. Rowe MI, Furst AJ, Altman DH, et al. The neonatal response to gastrografin enema. Pediatrics 1971;48:29–35.

92. Copeland DR, St Peter SD, Sharp SW, et al. Diminishing role of contrast enema in simple meconium ileus. J Pediatr Surg 2009;44:2130–2.

93. Ein S, Shandling B, Reilly B, et al. Bowel perforation with nonoperative treatment of meconium ileus. J Pediatr Surg 1987;22:146–7.

94. Rowe MI, Seagram G, Weinberger M. Gastrografin-induced hypertonicity. The pathogenesis of a neonatal hazard. Am J Surg 1973;125:185–8.

95. Lutzger LG, Factor SM. Effects of some water-soluble contrast media on the colonic mucosa. Radiology 1976;118:545–8.

96. Steiner Z, Mogilner J, Siplovich L, et al. T-tubes in the management of meconium ileus. Pediatr Surg Int 1997;12:140–1.

97. Jawaheer J, Khalil B, Plummer T, et al. Primary resection and anastomosis for complicated meconium ileus: A safe procedure? Pediatr Surg Int 2007;23:1091–3.

98. Bishop H, Koop C. Management of meconium ileus: Resection, Roux-en-Y anastomosis and ileostomy irrigation with pancreatic enzymes. Ann Surg 1957;145:410–14.

99. Gross R. The surgery of infants and childhood. Philadelphia: W. B. Saunders Co.; 1953.

100. Harberg FJ, Senekjian EK, Pokorny WJ. Treatment of uncomplicated meconium ileus via T-tube ileostomy. J Pediatr Surg 1981;16:61–3.

101. Swenson O. Pediatric Surgery. 2nd ed. New York: Appelton-Century-Crofts; 1962.

102. Mabogunje OA, Wang CI, Mahour H. Improved survival of neonates with meconium ileus. Arch Surg 1982;117:37–40.

103. Chappell JS. Management of meconium ileus by resection and end-to-end anastomosis. S Afr Med J 1977;52:1093–4.

104. Santulli T. Meconium ileus. In: Holder T, Ashcraft K, editors. Pediatric Surgery. Philadelphia: W. B. Saunders; 1980.

105. FitzSimmons SC, Burkhart GA, Borowitz D, et al. High-dose pancreatic-enzyme supplements and fibrosing colonopathy in children with cystic fibrosis. N Engl J Med 1997;336:1283–9.

106. Borowitz DS, Grand RJ, Durie PR. Use of pancreatic enzyme supplements for patients with cystic fibrosis in the context of fibrosing colonopathy. Consensus Committee. J Pediatr 1995;127:681–4.

107. Coates AJ, Crofton PM, Marshall T. Evaluation of salt supplementation in CF infants. J Cystic Fibrosis 2009;8:382–5.

108. Hendeles L. Use bioequivalency rating to select generics [letter]. Am Pharm 1989;NS29:6.

109. Hendeles L, Dorf A, Stecenko A, et al. Treatment failure after substitution of generic pancrelipase capsules. Correlation with in vitro lipase activity. JAMA 1990;263:2459–61.

110. Durie PR, Newth CJ, Forstner GG, et al. Malabsorption of medium-chain triglycerides in infants with cystic fibrosis: Correction with pancreatic enzyme supplement. J Pediatr 1980;96:862–4.

111. Li Z, Lai HJ, Kosorok MR, et al. Longitudinal pulmonary status of cystic fibrosis children with meconium ileus. Pediatr Pulmonol 2004;38:277–84.

112. Bower TR, Pringle KC, Soper RT. Sodium deficit causing decreased weight gain and metabolic acidosis in infants with ileostomy. J Pediatr Surg 1988;23:567–72.

113. McPartlin JF, Dickson JA, Swain VA. Meconium ileus. Immediate and long-term survival. Arch Dis Child 1972;47:207–10.

114. Efrati O, Nir J, Fraser D, et al. Meconium ileus in patients with cystic fibrosis is not a risk factor for clinical deterioration and survival: The Israeli Multicenter Study. JPGN 2010;50:173–8.

115. Johnson J, Bush A, Buchdahl R. Does presenting with meconium ileus affect the prognosis of children with cystic fibrosis? Pediatr Pulmonol 2010;45:951–8.

116. Lai HC, Kosorok MR, Laxova A, et al. Nutritional status of patients with cystic fibrosis with meconium ileus: A comparison with patients without meconium ileus and diagnosed early through neonatal screening. Pediatrics 2000;105:53–61.

117. Clatworthy H, Howard W, Lloyd J. The meconium plug syndrome. Surgery 1956;39:131–42.

118. Flake AW, Ryckman FC. Meconium plug syndrome. In: Fanaroff AA, Martin RJ, editors. Neonatal-Perinatal Medicine, Disease of the Fetus and Infant. 5th ed. St. Louis: Mosby-Year Book; 1992. p. 1054–5.

119. Keckler SJ, St Peter SD, Spilde TL, et al. Current significance of meconium plug syndrome. J Pediatr Surg 2008;43:896–8.

120. Stewart DR, Mixon GW, Johnson DG, et al. Neonatal small left colon syndrome. Ann Surg 1977;186:741–95.

121. Gross K, Desanto A, Grosfeld JL, et al. Intra-abdominal complications of cystic fibrosis. J Pediatr Surg 1985;20:431–5.

122. Beierle EA, Vinocur CD. Gastrointestinal surgery in cystic fibrosis. Curr Opin Pulm Med 1998;4:319–25.

123. Malfroot A, Dab I. New insights on gastro-oesophageal reflux in cystic fibrosis by longitudinal follow up. Arch Dis Child 1991;66:1339–45.

124. Button BM, Heine RG, Catto-Smith AG, et al. Postural drainage and gastro-oesophageal reflux in infants with cystic fibrosis. Arch Dis Child 1997;76:148–50.

125. Boesch RP, Acton JD. Outcomes of fundoplication in children with cystic fibrosis. J Pediatr Surg 2007;42:1341–4.

126. Hassall E, Isreal DM, Davidson AG, et al. Barrett's esophagus in children with cystic fibrosis: Not a coincidental association. Am J Gastroenterol 1993;88:1934–8.

127. McDonald ML, Trastek VF, Allen MS, et al. Barrett's esophagus: Does an antireflux procedure reduce the need for endoscopic surveillance? J Thorac Cardiovasc Surg 1996;111:1135–8.

128. Cohn JA, Strong TV, Picciotto MR, et al. Localization of the cystic fibrosis transmembrane conductance regulator in human bile duct epithelial cells. Gastroenterol 1993;105:1857–64.

129. Shapira R, Hadzic N, Francavilla R, et al. Retrospective review of cystic fibrosis presenting as infantile liver disease. Arch Dis Child 1999;81:125–8.

130. Greenholz SK, Krishnadasan B, Marr C, et al. Biliary obstruction in infants with cystic fibrosis requiring Kasai portoenterostomy. J Pediatr Surg 1997;32:175–80.

131. Oppenheimer EH, Esterly JR. Hepatic changes in young infants with cystic fibrosis: possible relation to focal biliary cirrhosis. J Pediatr 1975;86:683–9.

132. Scott-Jupp R, Lama M, Tanner MS. Prevalence of liver disease in cystic fibrosis. Arch Dis Child 1991;66:698–701.

133. Roy CC, Weber AM, Morin CL, et al. Hepatobiliary disease in cystic fibrosis: A survey of current issues and concepts. J Pediatr Gastroenterol Nutr 1982;1:469–78.

134. Debray D, Lykavieris P, Frédéric G, et al. Outcome of cystic fibrosis-associated liver cirrhosis: Management of portal hypertension. J Hepatol 1999;31:77–83.

135. Karrer FM. Portal hypertension. Semin Pediatr Surg 1992;1:134–44.

136. Williams SGJ, Westaby D, Tanner MS, et al. Liver and biliary problems in cystic fibrosis. Br Med Bull 1992;48:877–92.

137. Dowman JK, Watson D, Loganathan S, et al. Long-term impact of liver transplantation on respiratory function and nutritional status in children and adults with cystic fibrosis. Am J Transplant 2012;12:954–64.

138. Miller MR, Sokol RJ, Narkewicz MR, et al. Pulmonary function in individuals with cystic fibrosis from the USA cystic fibrosis foundation registry who had undergone liver transplant. Liver Transpl 2012;18:585–93.

139. Fridell JA, Mazariegos GV, Orenstein RS, et al. Liver and intestinal transplantation in a child with cystic fibrosis: A case report. Pediatr Transplant 2003;7:240–2.

140. Stern RC, Mayes JT, Weber FL Jr. Restoration of exocrine pancreatic function following pancreas-liver-kidney transplantation in a cystic fibrosis patient. Clin Transplant 1994;8:1–4.

141. Angelico M, Gandin C, Canuzzi P, et al. Gallstones in cystic fibrosis: A critical reappraisal. Hepatology 1991;14:768–75.

142. Rovsing H, Sloth K. Micro-gallbladder and biliary calculi in mucoviscidosis. Acta Radiol 1973;14:588–92.

143. L'heureux PR, Isenberg JN, Sharp HL, et al. Gallbladder disease in cystic fibrosis. AJR Am J Roentgenol 1977;128:953–6.

144. Stern RC, Rothstein FC, Doershunk CF. Treatment and prognosis of symptomatic gallbladder disease in patients with cystic fibrosis. J Pediatr Gastroenterol Nutr 1986;5:35–40.

145. Snyder CL, Ferrell KL, Saltzman DA, et al. Operative therapy of gallbladder disease in patients with cystic fibrosis. Am J Surg 1989;157:557–61.

146. Anagnostopoulos D, Tsagari N, Noussia-Arvanitaki S, et al. Gallbladder disease in patients with cystic fibrosis. Eur J Pediatr Surg 1993;3:348–51.

147. Saltzman DA, Johnson EM, Feltis BA, et al. Surgical experience in patients with cystic fibrosis: A 25-year perspective. Pediatr Pulmonol 2002;33:106–10.

148. Hanly JG, Ritzgerald MX. Meconium ileus equivalent in older patients with cystic fibrosis. Br Med J 1983;286:1411–13.

149. Dalzell AM, Heaf DP, Carty H. Pathology mimicking distal intestinal obstruction syndrome in cystic fibrosis. Arch Dis Child 1990;65:540–1.

150. Matseshe JW, Go VLW, Dimagno E. Meconium ileus equivalent complicating cystic fibrosis in post-neonatal children and young adults. Gastroenterology 1972;72:732–6.

151. Van der Doef HP, Kokke FT, van der Ent CK, et al. Intestinal obstruction syndromes in cystic fibrosis: Meconium ileus, distal intestinal obstruction syndrome, and constipation. Curr Gastroenterol Rep 2011;12:265–70.

152. Wilschanski M, Rivlin J, Cohen S, et al. Clinical and genetic risk factors for cystic fibrosis-related liver disease. Pediatrics 1999;103:52–7.

153. Marino CR, Gorelick FS. Scientific advances in cystic fibrosis. Gastroenterology 1992;103:681–93.

154. Kopelman H, Corey M, Gaskin K, et al. Impaired chloride secretion, as well as bicarbonate secretion, underlies the fluid secretory defect in the cystic fibrosis pancreas. Gastroenterology 1988;95:349–55.

155. O'Halloran SM, Gilbert J, McKendrick OM, et al. Gastrografin in acute meconium ileus equivalent. Arch Dis Child 1986;61:1128–30.

156. Cleghorn GJ, Forstner GG, Stringer DA, et al. Treatment of distal intestinal obstruction syndrome in cystic fibrosis with a balanced intestinal lavage solution. Lancet 1986;1:8–11.

157. Holsclaw DS, Rocmans C, Shwachman H. Intussusception in patients with cystic fibrosis. Pediatrics 1971;48:51–8.

158. Coughlin JP, Gauderer MWL, Stern RC, et al. The spectrum of appendiceal disease in cystic fibrosis. J Pediatr Surg 1990;25:835–9.

159. Olsen MM, Gauderer MWL, Girz MK, et al. Surgery in patients with cystic fibrosis. J Pediatr Surg 1987;22:613–18.

160. Lloyd-Still JD, Beno DW, Kimura RM. Cystic fibrosis colonopathy. Curr Gastroenterol Rep 1999;1:231–7.

161. Serban DE, Florescu P, Miu N. Fibrosing colonopathy revealing cystic fibrosis in a neonate before any pancreatic enzyme supplementation. J Pediatr Gastroenterol Nutr 2002;35:356–9.

CHAPTER 33

NECROTIZING ENTEROCOLITIS

Kathleen M. Dominguez • R. Lawrence Moss

Necrotizing enterocolitis (NEC) is not a new disease. Reports of a disease fitting the clinical characteristics of NEC date to the 1820s in France.[1] The earliest reports in the USA occurred in the early 1960s, when Santulli and colleagues published the first significant surgical experience with NEC.[2,3] They described a disease of low birth weight infants with a high mortality rate, which requires early, aggressive surgical management. Many investigators have devoted careers to better define this challenging disease and improve strategies for treatment and prevention. Despite these efforts, NEC remains a difficult and elusive disease. It remains unclear which premature infants are most at risk and what are the optimal prevention and treatment strategies. Long-term sequelae are easily overlooked in the acute setting, but contribute substantially to the subsequent morbidity and mortality.

EPIDEMIOLOGY

Several large population-based studies have found the incidence of NEC to be approximately 1 per 1000 live births. In select populations, such as infants under 1500 g, the incidence rises to between 2.3–11% (Table 33-1). Both the incidence and case fatality rate of NEC are inversely associated with birth weight.[4-9] Several studies have identified an increased incidence of NEC in black infants, particularly males, a difference that holds true even when adjusting for birth weight. Hispanic infants also show an increased incidence, though to a lesser degree.[4,10]

Despite improvements in other areas of neonatal care, rates of NEC have remained stable for very low birth weight infants (VLBW) infants.[11] Mortality remains high, with rates ranging from 15–30%.[4,5,9,10,12] Higher fatality rates are associated with lower birth weight and younger gestational age.[12,13] In a study summarizing trends for mortality and NEC in the USA between 1979 and 1992, the death rate was 12.4 deaths per 100,000 live births.[13] The highest mortality rate was seen in VLBW infants who were black and male.[4,10,13]

Although most cases of NEC are managed medically, 20–40% will require operative intervention.[5,7,12,14] Mortality increases up to 50% when surgery is necessary, and has not changed significantly over the past 30 years. The highest risk for mortality in this subgroup is also in the lowest birth weight and youngest gestational age infants.[15]

Long-term outcomes in patients requiring operation are worse, with increased complications such as neurodevelopmental delay, growth delay and chronic gastrointestinal problems.[16]

Though over 90% of cases are seen in preterm infants, there are occasional reports of NEC developing in full-term infants. Although the clinical and pathologic findings are similar, the initiating factors are likely different. Term infants who develop NEC are more likely to have predisposing risk factors such as congenital heart disease, sepsis, respiratory disease, or reported hypoxic events.[17-20] The common feature of these predisposing conditions is reduced mesenteric perfusion.[18] The incidence of NEC in term or near term infants is approximately 0.5 per 1000 live births.[20] The mortality rate for term infants with NEC appears to be similar to that of preterm infants with NEC.[18]

The morbidity associated with NEC translates into considerable economic burden. In one study, infants with NEC were hospitalized 60 days longer than unaffected preterm infants if operation was needed, and 20 days longer if medical treatment was successful.[21] In this study, the mean hospital costs were $186,200 greater for surgically treated patients than controls and $73,700 greater for medically treated patients. In addition to the high costs associated with the initial hospitalization, these children often have significant long-term health care needs. The mean cost of care for a child with short bowel syndrome over a five-year period exceeds $1.6M.[22]

PATHOPHYSIOLOGY

Despite decades of research into the pathogenesis of NEC, a complete understanding of its pathophysiology remains elusive. Classic histologic findings include inflammation, bacterial overgrowth, and coagulation necrosis, and are present in over 90% of surgical specimens.[23] Radiographic findings provide insight into the pathologic process that is unfolding. Pneumatosis intestinalis, or air within the intestinal wall, is thought to be due to gas produced by overgrowth of enteric bacteria.[24] Progression to portal venous or lymphatic gas suggests extension of this process along vessels draining the affected intestine. Pneumoperitoneum indicates necrosis with complete disruption of the intestinal wall.

As our understanding of the pathophysiology of NEC evolves, a working model of the multifactorial nature of this disease has emerged. The unifying concept is that NEC represents an exaggerated inflammatory response to an insult. The nature of this insult is not well defined, and may vary among affected infants. It may be a global ischemic insult from congenital heart disease, an infectious insult from abnormal bacterial colonization, an insult related to formula feeding or lack of enteral feeding,

TABLE 33-1 **Population-Based Epidemiologic Studies on Necrotizing Enterocolitis**

Author	Year	Population	Number Studied	Number NEC	%	Rate per 1000 Live Births	Fatality Rate
Llanos[4]	2002	New York State	117,892 live births	85	3.3% VLBW	0.72	19%
Guthrie[5]	2003	Pediatrix Medical Group	15,072 (23–34 weeks gestation)	390	3% preterm infants		12%
Sankaran[7]	2004	Canadian Neonatal Network	18,234 (3628 VLBW)	336	7% VLBW	1.8	
Luig & Lui[12]	2005	New South Wales NICU Study	4649 (24–31 weeks gestation)	178	4% preterm infants		30%
Guillet[9]	2006	NIHCD Neonatal Research Network	11,936 VLBW	787	7% VLBW		24%
Holman[10]	2006	Hospital discharges in USA: 2000—children inpatient database	Sample of all neonatal hospitalizations (4,058,814 live births)	4464		1.1	15%
Stoll[8]	2010	NICHD Neonatal Research Network	9575 (infants 22–28 weeks gestation and 401–1500 g)		11% VLBW		
Thompson	2011	Yale New Haven Children's Hospital	14,075 (infants 36 weeks gestational age or younger)	328 (Bell's stage II or greater)	2.3% preterm infants		

VLBW, very low birth weight.

or simply the response of translocation of normal bacterial flora in a genetically predisposed host.

Whatever the insult, it leads to a disruption of the intestinal epithelial barrier followed by translocation of bacteria. There is an exaggerated or inappropriate immune response, likely owing to the immature nature of the intestine and immune system. Stress pathways become activated, and pathways that normally suppress the immune system are inhibited. The end result is activation of the host immune system and release of cytokines, leading to a global, detrimental inflammatory response.

The Intestinal Barrier

The pathologic features of NEC suggest that failure of the intestinal barrier is either a cause or result of disease progression. The normal intestinal barrier is composed of both mechanical and non-mechanical factors. The mechanical factors include intestinal peristalsis, the mucous coat, and tight junctions between epithelial cells. Non-mechanical factors include immunologic defenses and cellular homeostasis and regeneration.

Intestinal Motility and Digestion

Intestinal motility develops during the third trimester of pregnancy but may not be fully mature until the eighth month of gestation.[25–28] In premature infants, immature motility leads to increased epithelial exposure to potentially noxious substances, and poor clearance of bacteria with subsequent overgrowth. Additionally, the immature intestine has decreased digestion and absorption, which may lead to direct epithelial injury through a lowered pH.[29–31] Newborns have reduced gastric acidity and pancreatic enzyme activity, which may further contribute to impaired digestion of macromolecules and bacterial proliferation.[32]

An increased ileal bile acid level may play a role in the pathogenesis of NEC. Bile acids are known to be cytotoxic, resulting in the development of mucosal injury.[33] In premature infants, levels of ileal bile acid-binding protein are lower, leading to increased levels of bile acids in the intestinal lumen and in enterocytes.[34] Another risk factor which may contribute is formula feeding, which elicits more toxic bile acids than breast feeding.[35]

The Mucous Coat

The mucous coat overlying the intestinal epithelium plays a key role in the barrier function. This layer is composed of water, mucin, lipids, and peptides.[36] Mucin, a glycoprotein, is secreted by goblet cells in the epithelial layer and concentrates enzymes near the intestinal surface.[37,38] Mucin aids in lubrication, mechanical protection, protection against the acidity of gastric and duodenal secretions,[39] and fixation of pathogens.[40] The effectiveness of mucin is related to maturity.[39] Mature mucins have higher viscosity, better pH buffering, and resistance to bacterial breakdown.[39–41] Mucin production and composition changes with gestational age, bacterial challenges, and colonization by commensal organisms.[42–44] Deficits in the production or composition of mucin may contribute to the ability of bacteria to invade the intestinal epithelium and thus contribute to the pathogenesis of NEC.[32,36,37,45–47]

Tight Junctions

Tight junctions create fusion points between epithelial cells, forming an intact yet semipermeable barrier. Mature tight junctions are composed of the transmembrane proteins occludin, claudin, and junctional adhesion protein; these normally present a barrier to diffusion of large molecules.[32,48] Tight junctions are not static, but may be altered by disease processes.[49] Immaturity in the composition of tight junctions likely plays a role in the increased permeability of the epithelium of the newborn intestine.[50]

Cytokines are produced in response to bacteria, and may interfere with tight junctions, promoting the translocation of bacteria.[51] Inflammatory mediators such as tumor necrosis factor, interferon (IFN)-γ, and interleukin (IL)-1β further cause epithelial dysfunction by upregulating inducible nitric oxide synthase (iNOS) leading to the overproduction of nitric oxide (NO), and the generation the reactive nitrogen intermediate peroxynitrite (ONOO$^-$). This process has been associated with increased epithelial cell apoptosis and death.[52] NO has been shown to play a role in mediating the decrease in the localization and expression of tight junction proteins.[49,53] Disruption of tight junctions may lead to increased intestinal permeability, allowing bacterial translocation and activation of the immune system.

Immunologic Defenses of the Gastrointestinal Tract

The gastrointestinal tract contains the largest amount of lymphoid tissue in the body and coordinates the immunologic mechanisms of the adaptive and innate immune systems.[54] Gut-associated lymphoid tissue consists of several cell types which work in concert to perform antigen presentation and processing[37,55]

In neonates, antigen processing and presentation is less efficient, reducing the ability of the immune system to respond to pathogenic organisms. Peyer patches are fewer, smaller, and lack germinal centers.[36] Paneth cell activation by bacteria or components of bacterial cell walls leads to secretion of a variety of antibacterial substances, including α-defensins and lysozyme.[56,57] Production of these peptides is decreased in premature infants, and may predispose to bacterial overgrowth, allowing NEC to develop. Following recovery from NEC, Paneth cell hyperplasia occurs, suggesting these cells play an important role in NEC.[56]

IgA is normally synthesized by plasma cells of the lamina propria and secreted into the mucin layer where it binds bacteria and viruses, inhibiting attachment to the epithelium. The newborn lamina propria is largely devoid of the IgA-secreting plasma cells, resulting in deficient secretion until several weeks of age.[58,59] Neonates can obtain IgA through passive transfer from breast milk,[49] but infants who do not receive breast milk lack this important immunoglobulin and its protective effects.

Regenerating the Intestinal Barrier

The pathologic findings of NEC arise not only from alterations in the integrity of the intestinal barrier but also from an impaired ability to regenerate.[60] Premature infants have a reduced capacity for intestinal repair, likely contributing to the pathogenesis of NEC.

Lipopolysaccharide

Lipopolysaccharide (LPS) is the endotoxin portion of the Gram-negative bacterial cell wall, and is one of the most abundant proinflammatory stimuli. LPS is seen in high levels in NEC.[24] LPS impairs intestinal barrier function by inhibiting repair and promoting the release of signaling molecules and proinflammatory mediators such as NO, IFN-γ, cyclooxygenase-2 (COX-2) and RhoA from enterocytes which promote intestinal injury.[49,60–62] LPS causes increased expression and function of integrins on the cell surface, resulting in increased cell adhesion to the basement membrane,[63] and compounds the effects of platelet-activating factor (PAF).[64,65]

Nitric Oxide

NO is a key mediator of numerous physiologic and pathologic systems, but has been shown to have a paradoxical role in NEC. Low levels of NO are important for maintaining vasodilation; conversely, sustained overproduction of NO can have profound cytopathic effects. The cytopathic effects of NO are believed to be due to toxic nitrogen intermediates, such as ONOO$^-$.[32]

NO is a highly reactive free radical formed by the conversion of arginine to citrulline by NO synthase (NOS) which exists in three forms: the constitutive form (nNOS), the inducible isoform (iNOS), and the constitutive endothelial isoform (eNOS).[66] The presence of the constitutive forms of NOS in the gastrointestinal tract suggests that NO has a normal physiologic role in gut function. The eNOS isoform maintains intestinal homeostasis by enhancing mucosal blood flow and maintaining microvascular tone.[67]

When produced by iNOS under inflammatory conditions, the NO level increases up to a million fold,[67] which can lead to cellular damage and failure of the intestinal barrier. Excess NO overwhelms local scavenging mechanisms and reacts with superoxide anion (O_2^-) to produce the highly toxic ONOO$^-$.[67–69] These effects may be compounded in the presence of high levels of LPS, which leads to increased iNOS expression and function within the intestine.[69–70] Studies have linked NO with the pathogenesis of NEC. The expression of iNOS has been shown to be upregulated in critically ill patients and in patients with NEC.[52] Conversely, expression is down regulated by the anti-inflammatory cytokine interleukin-10.[71] Excess NO may also inhibit intestinal restitution by blocking enterocyte migration and proliferation.[32,49,72]

Platelet-Activating Factor

PAF is potent phospholipid inflammatory mediator that is produced by most cells and tissues.[73,74] The cytotoxic effects of PAF are due to initiation of the inflammatory cascade. PAF-induced bowel injury is associated with the production of oxygen-derived free radicals as well as leukocyte migration, activation, and capillary leakage resulting in apoptosis in affected enterocytes.[75]

Various studies have shown the importance of PAF in the pathogenesis of NEC. Higher concentrations of PAF have been found in NEC patients compared with controls.[75–77] PAF-acetylhydrolase (AH) activity has been shown to be deficient in sick infants with NEC, and the administration of PAF-AH or a PAF receptor antagonist in animal models of NEC reduces the degree of intestinal injury.[74,76,78] PAF-AH is present in maternal breast milk, which may contribute to the protective effect against NEC it provides.[74]

Maintaining Intestinal Barrier Homeostasis

Epidermal Growth Factor

Epidermal growth factor (EGF) is a peptide secreted into the intestinal lumen.[79] It plays an important role in the development, maturation, and maintenance of gut homeostasis, being active in processes from intestinal repair and adaptation to cell movement and prevention of bacterial translocation.[80-86] EGF has been shown to support maintenance of the intestinal barrier, as well as being active in the down regulation of inflammatory cytokines.[79,86]

EGF is believed to play an important role in the pathogenesis of NEC. Decreased levels of EGF have been demonstrated in the saliva and serum of premature infants with NEC.[87] Furthermore, studies have shown that salivary levels of EGF in the first two weeks of preterm life may have a predictive value for the occurrence of NEC.[88] A potentially therapeutic role for EGF was reported in an infant suffering from intestinal necrosis resembling NEC who received a continuous infusion of EGF resulting in complete recovery of the damaged intestine.[89] These investigators subsequently treated a small group of neonates with stage II and III NEC in a randomized, double-blind, prospective trial with recombinant EGF and found that repair of the intestinal epithelium was seen at four, seven, and 14 days.[90]

Heparin-binding EGF (HB-EGF) is a member of this family of growth factors, and is found in amniotic fluid and breast milk.[91] In animal models of NEC, administration of HB-EGF has been shown to reduce the incidence of bowel injury by 50%, more than double survival,[92-95] and preserve the integrity of the intestinal barrier.[96] Animals with overexpression of HB-EGF have decreased susceptibility to NEC,[97] while animals with deletion of the HB-EGF gene have increased susceptibility.[86,97] These effects seem to be at least in part due to the cytoprotective effects of HB-EGF, which serves to protect intestinal stem cells from injury.[86]

EGF and HB-EGF have a role as a potential preventive strategy for NEC. These compounds may have a protective effect by altering the balance of pro- and anti-inflammatory cytokines in the pathogenesis of NEC, and may also play a role in decreasing bacterial translocation from the intestine. Active research is ongoing.

Neonatal Vasculature and the Pathogenesis of NEC

Newborn intestinal circulation is characterized by a low resting vascular resistance.[98,99] This results in increased blood flow and oxygen delivery. Control of vascular resistance involves intrinsic and extrinsic control mechanisms.[100] Extrinsic mechanisms are mediated by the autonomic nervous system. The intrinsic regulation is mediated by two vascular effector mechanisms produced

and released within the intestine—one vasoconstrictive and one vasodilatory.[101,102] Endothelin (ET)-1 is the primary vasoconstrictor stimulus in the newborn intestine and is produced by the endothelium.[103,104] Although constitutively produced, it can also be stimulated by decreased flow, hypoxia, and various inflammatory cytokines.[105-107] The production of ET-1 is age specific, being greater in younger subjects.[103]

NO is the primary vasodilator stimulus.[98,99] eNOS is also continuously produced, but like ET-1 the rate of production can be increased in response to a variety of stimuli.[101] In the neonate, the balance of these two products favors vasodilation, generating the characteristic low vascular resistance. In disease states, endothelial dysfunction leads to ET-1 mediated vasoconstriction, causing compromised blood flow, intestinal ischemia, and injury. The vasoconstrictor ET-1 has been linked to intestinal tissue injury in several studies.[103,108] Increased expression of ET-1 has been found in intestine removed from infants with NEC, and the amount of ET-1 increased proportionally to the degree of intestinal injury.[102]

In summary, the intestinal circulation of the newborn is unique, with a dynamic balance between constrictor (ET-1) and dilator (NO) stimuli maintaining basal vascular resistance. Disruption of the intestinal endothelial function can alter the delicate balance, favoring vasoconstriction over the normal state of vasodilation, leading to significant intestinal ischemia and tissue injury.

Bacterial Colonization

NEC is most commonly diagnosed during the second week of life, after intestinal colonization has been established. Bacteria likely play a role in the pathogenesis of NEC, though studies have not identified a single infectious agent. NEC likely arises from an unfavorable balance between commensal and pathogenic bacteria.

Abnormal colonization may alter the balance of pathogenic and beneficial bacteria, favoring an increase in pathogenic bacteria and resulting in a loss of the beneficial role of commensal bacteria. Furthermore, the immature immune system of premature infants may not be able to respond appropriately to normal colonization of bacteria, much less abnormal flora.[109]

CLINICAL DIAGNOSIS

The diagnosis of NEC is based on clinical and radiographic findings. The clinical course can vary from a slow, indolent process to a rapid fatal progression. Early signs are nonspecific, including apnea, bradycardia, lethargy, and temperature instability. Feeding intolerance, demonstrated by high gastric residuals, is the most common gastrointestinal symptom of NEC. The most common presenting sign is abdominal distention. Gross or occult blood in the stool may be found.

Gastrointestinal signs progress from abdominal distention to tenderness suggestive of peritoneal irritation (Fig. 33-1). Palpable loops of intestine may become evident. Localized disease may progress to generalized peritonitis or may worsen in a focal area, including

TABLE 33-2   **Modified Bell's Staging for Necrotizing Enterocolitis**

Stage	Clinical Findings	Radiographic Findings	Gastrointestinal Findings
I: Suspected	Apnea, bradycardia, temperature instability	Gas pattern of mild ileus	Increased gastric residuals, occult blood in stool, mild abdominal distention
IIa: Definite	Apnea, bradycardia, temperature instability	Ileus gas pattern with one or more dilated loops, focal pneumatosis	Grossly bloody stools, prominent abdominal distention, absent bowel sounds
IIb	Thrombocytopenia, mild metabolic acidosis	Widespread pneumatosis, ascites, portal venous gas	Abdominal wall edema with palpable loops and tenderness
IIIa: Advanced	Mixed acidosis, oliguria, hypotension, coagulopathy	Prominent bowel loops, worsening ascites, no free air	Worsening wall edema, erythema and induration
IIIb	Shock, deterioration in laboratory values and vital signs	Pneumoperitoneum	Perforated bowel

discoloration of the skin and the development of an abdominal mass. When present, the findings of a fixed abdominal mass and erythema of the abdominal wall are strongly predictive of dead bowel; however, these findings occur in only 10% of patients with NEC.[110] A sudden need for increased ventilatory support may also serve as a harbinger of NEC.[111] This is due to increased metabolic requirements combined with increased intra-abdominal pressure.

Confirmation of the diagnosis of NEC combines signs and symptoms with radiologic findings. These findings have been combined into the clinical staging system proposed by Bell that aids in describing the severity of disease (Table 33-2).[112,113]

Laboratory Studies

Laboratory studies reveal nonspecific indicators of an inflammatory or infectious process such as leukocytosis with bandemia. Thrombocytopenia and metabolic acidosis are also common. A rapid fall in platelet count is a poor prognostic factor.[114]

Several studies have tried to identify an accurate biochemical marker to identify neonates at risk for NEC, avoiding prolonged periods without enteral nutrition as well as the use of unnecessary tests and antibiotics.[115] Serum acute phase proteins and cytokines have been investigated for an association between high levels and the severity of NEC. Increased levels of IL-6, IL-10, and C-reactive protein (CRP) have been documented in premature infants with NEC, with the highest levels of IL-10 in those patients who did not survive.[116] CRP has also been associated with NEC when the levels rose quickly after the diagnosis was suspected. A failure of the levels to return to normal has been found to be associated with complications, including abscesses, strictures, and sepsis.[117] In a prospective study, CRP levels were elevated in infants with stage II and III NEC and may be useful in discriminating between stage II NEC and other gastrointestinal disorders.[118]

Multiple other potential markers have been studied—gastrointestinal tonometry, urinary D-lactate levels, exhaled breath hydrogen, endotoxin elevations in stool, plasma intestinal fatty acid-binding proteins—but none of these has yielded the sensitivity or specificity required for a diagnostic tool.[61,119–121] Currently, no biochemical markers have been adequately predictive of the patient's clinical course or outcome to be clinically useful.

Radiographic Findings

Plain Films

The cornerstone of the radiographic diagnosis of NEC relies on plain radiographs. The most specific radiographic finding is pneumatosis intestinalis, as seen in Figure 33-2. Other radiographic findings include air–fluid levels, gas-filled loops of bowel, persistently dilated loops of bowel, thickened bowel walls, portal venous gas, and pneumoperitoneum. Although most commonly seen in NEC, pneumatosis intestinalis has also been reported in cases of Hirschsprung enterocolitis, severe diarrhea, and carbohydrate intolerance. Portal venous gas (Fig. 33-3) is a less common radiographic finding but is generally considered a poor prognostic sign. This finding is associated with twice the incidence of diffuse or 'pan' necrosis and a significantly lower survival rate.[122] Nevertheless, many patients with portal venous gas recover fully with medical management.

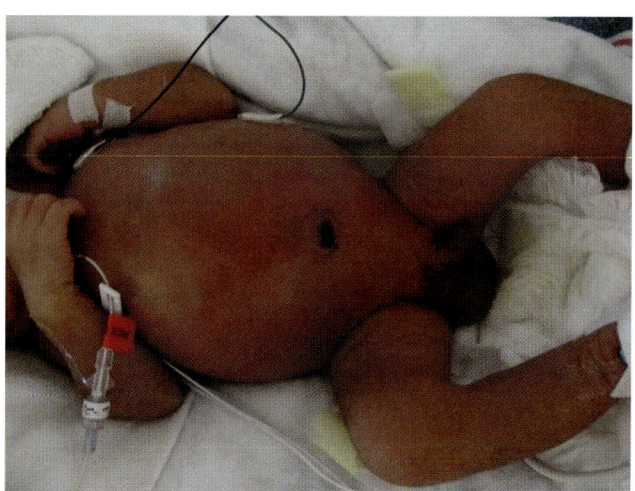

FIGURE 33-1 ■ This infant has NEC. Note the abdominal distension and abdominal wall erythema.

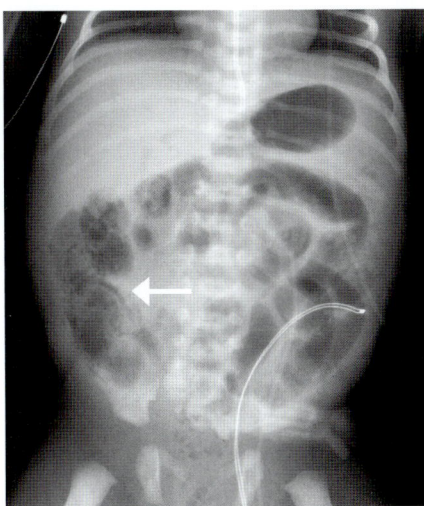

FIGURE 33-2 ■ Pneumatosis intestinalis is the classic radiographic finding in NEC. This finding may be cystic or linear (arrow), and may be seen in a focal intestinal segment or diffusely throughout the bowel.

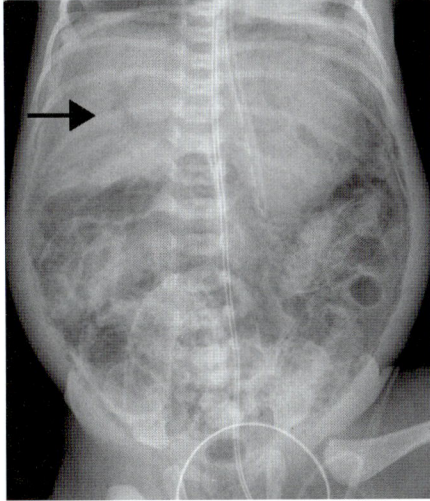

FIGURE 33-3 ■ Portal venous gas (arrow) is demonstrated on this abdominal radiograph. This finding is considered a poor prognostic sign. This baby also has widespread pneumatosis intestinalis.

Other Imaging Modalities

Studies have examined ultrasonography (US) as an adjunctive measure for the diagnosis and management of infants with NEC. Abdominal ultrasound evaluation emerged as a potential modality in the treatment of NEC after a report in 2005 that assessed bowel viability using color Doppler imaging in neonates with NEC.[123] This publication established critical data for bowel wall thickness, echogenicity, peristalsis, and perfusion in both normal neonates and those with NEC. Additional studies corroborated the usefulness of ultrasound as a means of diagnosing NEC.[124,125] ultrasound offers some potential advantages over plain films in that it can depict bowel wall thickness and echogenicity, free and focal fluid collections, peristalsis, and the presence or absence of bowel wall perfusion by using Doppler imaging.[126,127]

The presence of pneumatosis on plain abdominal radiographs helps clinch the diagnosis, but mild findings, such as the lack of intramural gas, makes the diagnosis more difficult. ultrasound may be a useful adjunct in this population because it may allow detection of small amounts of intramural gas not visible on plain films or changes in bowel wall thickness, peristalsis, or perfusion that could confirm or exclude the diagnosis of NEC.[128] The time frame for when to perform ultrasound initially or when to use it during follow-up has not been established.

In addition to assisting with the diagnosis in difficult cases, ultrasound has been suggested as an adjunct modality in two other groups of patients: those in whom the evolution of changes in the radiographs does not match the clinical course and those whose condition is deteriorating without evidence of pneumatosis on plain films.[128] Finally, ultrasound may be useful in helping to decide the appropriate time to re-initiate and advance feeding.[123] However, at this time, ultrasound does not yet have a well-defined or established role in the management of NEC.

In the acute setting, contrast examinations of the gastrointestinal tract, computed tomography, and magnetic resonance imaging have not been found to be useful modalities in clinical practice.[129–133]

DIFFERENTIAL DIAGNOSIS

The most clinically relevant differential diagnosis in a premature infant with abdominal distention is distinguishing between NEC and sepsis with ileus. In the absence of clinical signs of peritonitis or radiographic signs of NEC, the two conditions may be indistinguishable and only differentiated after observing the clinical course. The differential diagnosis also includes other conditions that may cause abdominal distention, such as Hirschsprung disease, ileal atresia, volvulus, meconium ileus, and intussusception.

A subset of premature infants presents with bowel perforation while not exhibiting other symptoms of NEC nor pneumatosis on radiographs. Some investigators have defined this as spontaneous, isolated, or focal intestinal perforation (FIP). FIP tends to occur in low birth weight infants, usually the first seven to ten days of life, and is sometimes associated with indomethacin treatment.[134–140] Whether these infants have a limited form of NEC or a distinct entity is controversial. Some reports contend that FIP is a different disease than NEC, but definitive evidence is lacking.[139–142] As expected, neonates with an isolated bowel perforation have better outcomes in the absence of extensive disease.[138,143–145]

MEDICAL MANAGEMENT

Medical management of NEC begins with bowel rest, gastric decompression, intravenous fluid resuscitation, and broad-spectrum antibiotic therapy, including anaerobic coverage. Blood, urine, and sputum cultures should be obtained before the initiation of antibiotic therapy. A critical component of medical management is ongoing close observation with serial abdominal examinations and radiographs. As long as the clinical situation is stable or improving, expectant management can continue. Clinical deterioration or worsening radiographic features may indicate the need to consider surgical intervention.

Experimental Medical Treatments: HB-EGF

Endogenous HB-EGF is increased in response to hypoxia, stress, and during wound healing.[146–151] HB-EGF mRNA is induced after intestinal ischemia/reperfusion injury in vivo[152] and is involved in epithelial cell repair, proliferation, and regeneration in the early stages after injury.[153] Based on these findings, it has been theorized that exogenous HB-EGF may also play a role protecting the intestinal mucosa from injury.

Multiple studies have demonstrated that exogenous administration of HB-EGF can protect cells and organs from injury both in vitro and in vivo. HB-EGF can protect enterocytes from proinflammatory cytokine-induced apoptosis.[154] Intestinal epithelial cells pretreated with HB-EGF before hypoxia showed less necrosis with maintenance of the cytoskeletal structure and improved recovery ability.[155] HB-EGF also downregulates the production of NO[156,157] and blocks NF-κB activation in intestinal epithelial cells after cytokine stimulation.[157] In a neonatal rat model of NEC, the administration of HB-EGF reduced the severity and incidence of NEC with preservation of gut barrier integrity.[92] Studies have also shown that treatment with HB-EGF decreases the overproduction of IL-18 and increases the production of anti-inflammatory IL-10.[158] HB-EGF is the only compound with imminent plans for investigation in humans. A host of other therapeutic agents have shown promise but not yet reached the stage of clinical testing.

SURGICAL MANAGEMENT

Although many infants can be managed medically, 20–40% will require operative intervention. In some cases, indication for operation develops during the medical management, while in others it is found at presentation. The only absolute indication for drainage or exploration is evidence of intestinal perforation either on an abdominal radiograph (Fig. 33-4) or via paracentesis that is positive for stool or bile.[159] Relative indications for operation include deterioration in the infant's clinical

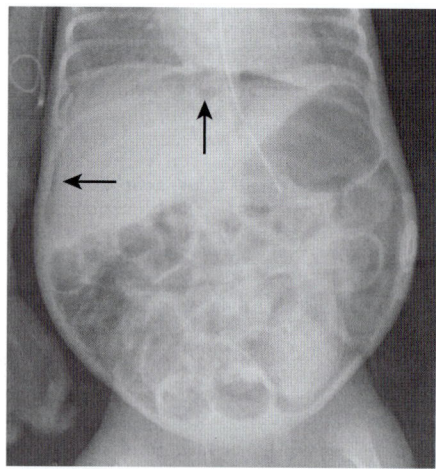

FIGURE 33-4 ■ Free air (arrows) is seen on this radiograph. This finding is an indication of perforation, and is considered an absolute indication for intervention, whether drainage or exploration.

condition despite maximal medical management. Such signs can include oliguria, hypotension, worsening metabolic acidosis, worsening thrombocytopenia, leukopenia or leukocytosis, and ventilatory failure. Relative radiographic indicators for operation include portal venous gas or persistently abnormal 'fixed' loops of bowel on serial radiographs.

Ideally, surgical intervention would occur when intestinal gangrene is imminent but before actual perforation or necrosis actually occurs. However, this ideal time for intervention is often difficult to identify. One study has tried to evaluate the sensitivity and specificity of 12 different findings to identify early indicators for operation.[110] Three findings had a specificity and positive predictive value (PPV) close to 100% with prevalence greater than 10%. These findings were deemed the 'best' indications and included portal venous gas and a positive paracentesis (Table 33-3). Three indicators had specificity and PPV close to 100% but prevalence less than 10% and were considered 'good' indicators, including a fixed loop on an abdominal radiograph, erythema of the abdominal wall, and a palpable abdominal mass. One indicator, severe pneumatosis, was deemed fair because it had a specificity and PPV above 90% and 20% prevalence. The five remaining indicators were considered poor because the specificities were less than 90% and the PPVs less than 80%. This probability analysis may be

TABLE 33-3	Probability Analysis of Various Indications for Operation in Necrotizing Enterocolitis		
Indication	Sensitivity (%)	Specificity (%)	Positive predictive Value (%)
Pneumoperitoneum	48	100	100
Portal venous gas	24	100	100
Fixed loop (on radiograph)	12.5	100	100
Fixed abdominal mass	12.5	100	100
Erythema of abdomen	8	100	100
Positive paracentesis	87	100	97
Severe pneumatosis	31	94	91
Clinical deterioration	39	89	78

useful in the complex decision-making process when an operation is being considered.

NEC can affect any segment of the gastrointestinal tract. Most commonly, both large and small bowel are involved.[23] Isolated small intestinal lesions occur with the next greatest frequency. It is as common to have a single affected area as to have multiple-segment disease.[23,160,161] A small subgroup of NEC patients develop massive necrosis of the entire intestine, known as 'NEC totalis.'[160]

Traditional operative management has consisted either of laparotomy with limited resection of the affected bowel with creation of stomas or of primary peritoneal drainage. Much of the attention of surgical investigators of NEC has focused on the relative benefits of these approaches.

Peritoneal drainage was first reported in 1977 as salvage treatment for perforation in VLBW infants who were believed to be too unstable for laparotomy (Fig. 33-5).[162] Initially intended as a temporizing procedure in the sickest and smallest patients, this treatment has evolved into a widely utilized option as primary treatment of perforated NEC. After many years of conflicting results comparing outcomes of the two approaches, a meta-analysis was attempted to synthesize these disparate data. This study found such significant bias in the assignment of patients to one treatment or another that the two options could not be adequately compared.[163] A need existed for a prospective randomized controlled trial.

Three prospective studies have compared laparotomy to peritoneal drainage. The NICHD Neonatal Research Network conducted a prospective observational cohort study at 16 centers.[164] This study included 156 infants with either NEC or FIP. Overall 50% (n = 78) of the patients died and 72% (n = 112) either died or had some

element of neurologic impairment at 18 to 22 months. The babies in this study were not randomized to their treatment groups. The treating surgeons and neonatologists chose which therapy to use for each infant. However, unlike other nonrandomized studies, extensive prospective data were collected, allowing for risk-adjusted multivariable regression analyses. This strategy enabled the investigators to account for the differences between the treatment groups. The odds ratio for death after adjusting for differences in the two treatment groups was 0.97 for laparotomy compared with peritoneal drainage (95% confidence interval [CI]: 0.43–2.20). The odds ratio for the combined outcome of death or neurodevelopmental impairment at 18 to 22 months was 0.44 for laparotomy compared with drainage (95% CI: 0.16–1.2). Although not statistically significant, there is some suggestion in this study that overall outcomes at 18 to 22 months of age may be improved by laparotomy rather than drainage.

The first randomized trial evaluating laparotomy versus peritoneal drainage was the NECSTEPS trial.[165] In this trial, 117 VLBW infants at 15 North American tertiary care centers were randomized to either treatment group. The primary outcome variable was mortality at 90 days. There was no difference in mortality at 90 days between the two treatment groups (34.5% vs 35.5%). Need for parenteral nutrition at 90 days and the length of hospitalization were also similar between the two groups. This study focused on short-term outcomes; within those limits, results suggest that the method of surgical intervention does not impact the outcome.

The second randomized trial comparing laparotomy and peritoneal drainage in infants with perforated NEC was the NET trial.[166] This trial was a multinational trial

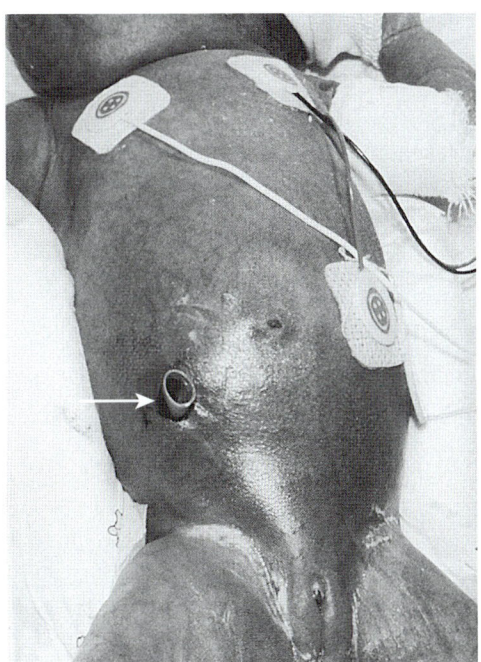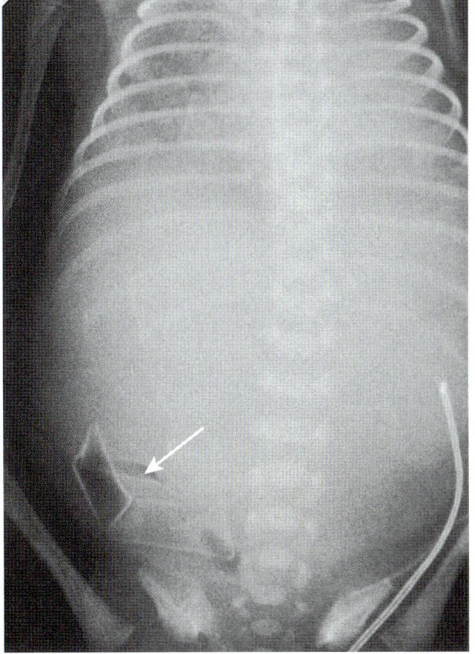

FIGURE 33-5 ■ A micropremature infant with NEC and perforation is shown with her corresponding abdominal radiograph. A percutaneous drain (arrows) has been placed in the right lower quadrant for drainage of the intestinal perforation. Note that the drain is placed at a position below the level of the umbilicus to avoid injury to the lower edge of the right lobe of the liver.

conducted at 31 centers in 13 countries. The primary outcome variable was mortality at 1 and 6 months. Sixty-nine patients weighing less than 1000 g were enrolled and randomized. There was a trend toward better survival in the laparotomy group (65% survival) compared with the drainage group (51%), with a relative risk of mortality of 0.5 (95% CI: 0.2–1.5). These findings were not statistically significant. The authors concluded that there was no evidence from the trial to support the benefit of primary peritoneal drainage in extremely low birth weight (LBW) infants with intestinal perforation.

Overall, both of these randomized trials suggest that the method of surgical management does not affect the ultimate outcome of infants with perforated NEC. The impact of choice of operation on the outcome of infants, who underwent operation for an indication other than perforation, is not known. Most commonly, these infants are treated with laparotomy.

An additional randomized trial is currently underway. The NEST trial is designed to compare long-term outcomes in extremely LBW infants (≤1000 g) with necrotizing enterocolitis or isolated intestinal perforation treated by either laparotomy or peritoneal drainage. The primary outcome is death or neurodevelopmental impairment at 18–22 months corrected gestational age. Results are expected in the fall of 2015.[167]

When laparotomy is performed, stomas are usually created. Because of concerns about the high morbidity associated with enterostomies (Box 33-1), a few centers have advocated primary anastomosis at the time of initial laparotomy. The data to support such management are nonrandomized and retrospective. In actuality, the majority of stomal complications are easily managed and early closure is well tolerated.[168] One study found that survival was 72% with intestinal diversion but only 48% in those undergoing primary anastomosis.[169]

Diffuse intestinal involvement poses the most difficult situation for the surgeon. Those infants who survive may develop short bowel syndrome and have some level of dependency on total parenteral nutrition given the extensive amount of affected bowel. Surgical strategies focus on trying to preserve as much intestine as possible while still resecting enough bowel to stabilize the patient. Second-look laparotomies have been proposed as a way to minimize the amount of bowel resected.[170] The 'clip and drop-back' technique is another option with a similar strategy.[171] All nonviable intestine is resected initially but no ostomies or anastomoses are created. Blind-ending

segments are left in the abdomen, and continuity is restored or ostomies are created on re-exploration in 48 to 72 hours. Proximal diversion alone has also been used to treat 'pan' necrosis without reported worsened survival and with recovery of much of the bowel by the time of ostomy closure.[172] None of these approaches has been prospectively evaluated; therefore, no single technique can be strongly advocated.

OUTCOMES

Recurrence

NEC recurs in approximately 5% of cases.[173,174] There is no apparent correlation between the site of disease and the site of recurrence. Usually recurrent disease can be managed nonoperatively.[159,174–179]

Length of Hospitalization

Hospital stays are longer for infants who suffer from NEC when compared with other infants of the same gestational age. Furthermore, those who require operation tend to have even longer hospitalization. Several studies have shown hospitalizations averaging two to three months for medically treated NEC and four to five months for surgically treated NEC.[180–182] There was no difference in length of hospitalization between the two treatment groups in the NECSTEPS trial.[165]

Mortality

Estimates of mortality from NEC have remained steady over the past two decades at 15–30% despite the fact that the postsurfactant era has led to a rise in the incidence of disease.[4,5,9,10,12,13,180,181,183,184] Operative mortality has improved with a decline from 70% mortality in the 1960s[185] to more recent rates of 20–50%.[5,10,13,180,183,186,187] The main predictor of mortality in NEC is gestational age. The highest mortality occurs in the youngest, smallest infants, and black male VLBW infants are at greatest risk. Additionally, infants with a greater extent of bowel affected by the disease tend to also have a higher mortality rate.[188,189]

Gastrointestinal Outcomes

Short Bowel Syndrome

NEC is the leading disease responsible for short bowel syndrome (SBS) in children, accounting for half of all pediatric cases. Furthermore, SBS develops in a fourth of all patients who suffer from NEC.[190] SBS develops when an infant is left with inadequate functional intestine to absorb the nutrients required for growth. This can result from resection at the time of operation or from poor function of the remaining intestine. Traditional teaching based on early reports suggests that a minimum of 40 cm of small intestine is required for a patient to have a chance of weaning from total parenteral nutrition.[191] Despite these observations, experience has shown that the

BOX 33-1	Enterostomal Complications

Prolapse
Stricture
Retraction
Wound separation or dehiscence
Wound infection
Parastomal hernia
Intestinal obstruction
Intestinal torsion
Fistula formation

function of the intestine is much more important to this disease than the specific length of intestine.

The portion of intestine resected is also important for subsequent gastrointestinal functioning. Patients with ileal or jejunal disease have a higher mortality rate than those with colonic disease.[187,188,192,193] Patients with extensive jejunal resection fare better than those with extensive ileal resection. This is due to the differing abilities of the intestinal regions to undergo adaptation. The ileum has the greatest capacity to adapt and increase its absorptive capacity.

Preservation of the ileocecal valve has been considered important for minimizing the risk of SBS.[194] Some studies have suggested that dependence on parenteral nutrition is lessened when the ileocecal valve was preserved,[195–198] but others have found no difference.[180,199–202] It appears that the actual length and functional capacity of the remaining ileum is far more important than the presence of the valve itself.

Stoma Complications

Creation of a properly constructed stoma can be lifesaving in the management of NEC. Stomas are used for both decompression and diversion. Enterostomies can be fraught with early and late complications. A number of strategies have been proposed for optimal stoma creation, including what type of stoma to create as well as how to exteriorize the stoma. End stomas, double-barrel (Mikulicz) stomas, and loop enterostomy have all been advocated. Small studies comparing complication rates between these various strategies have not found differences in complications, including retraction, prolapse, hernias, or wound infections.[203–205] Many surgeons exteriorize the stoma and mucous fistula through the incision, some at one end, others at opposite ends of the incision. Others advocate a separate incision, citing concerns about increased wound infection and difficulties attaching stoma appliances. Another consideration for a separate incision is whether the stoma needs to remain for a prolonged period of time. Most surgeons do not recommend maturing a stoma owing to potential interference with an already tenuous blood supply.[203]

Stomal complications can lead to significant morbidity. Studies have shown complication rates exceeding 50%.[187,206–209] The most serious complications include prolapse, stricture, and retraction, all of which may require surgical intervention. Proximal jejunostomies can cause significant electrolyte and fluid losses that can lead to problems with fluid balance and weight gain.[194,210] Fluid losses from jejunostomies can also cause peristomal skin complications. Despite these problems, with an aggressive approach to fluid and electrolyte replacement and meticulous skin care, proximal jejunostomies can be a viable option for the management of NEC.[194,211]

The timing of enterostomy closure remains controversial. Recommendations vary from as early as one month to as late as four months after operation.[212–215] Most suggest waiting one to two months after the initial operation, and until a weight of 2000 g is reached, as long as adequate feeding and growth is being maintained.[194,210,213] Earlier closure may be necessary with very proximal stomas due to fluid and electrolyte losses and the inability to gain weight. Coexisting medical problems must also be considered in determining the optimal time for closure.

Intestinal Strictures

Intestinal strictures are a common occurrence after NEC. The incidence of stricture has been reported from 12–35%, and occurs in patients who have been managed medically or surgically.[131,207,216–221] This incidence does not differ between patients treated by primary anastomosis or enterostomies.[159,186,187,199,206,207,212,215–227] In one series of patients treated for severe NEC by proximal diverting enterostomy, the incidence was 55%.[217] Most post-NEC strictures occur in the colon, specifically the left colon (Fig. 33-6).[160,212,219,226,228]

Resection of strictures is usually needed, although not all lesions are symptomatic and spontaneous resolution has been reported.[131,224,229,230] Other approaches have been proposed, including close radiographic follow-up of asymptomatic patients.[131] Balloon dilatation is an option for focal, nonobstructing lesions, but has not been widely utilized.[230]

Patients treated by laparotomy and stoma for NEC should undergo routine imaging of the distal intestine before enterostomy closure to evaluate for a possible stricture. Patients managed medically, by peritoneal drainage, or with primary anastomosis may also develop strictures. Some patients remain asymptomatic and others present acutely in distress due to perforation.[219] Thus, some surgeons advocate contrast studies in all NEC patients.[131,218,219,221] The potential for false-negative results and the invasiveness of the procedure prevent this practice from being commonly used.

Little is known about the long-term impact of stricture formation after NEC. Infants who require ostomy closure may have strictures addressed at that time. For those managed without ostomies, stricture resection requires a new operation with subsequent prolongation

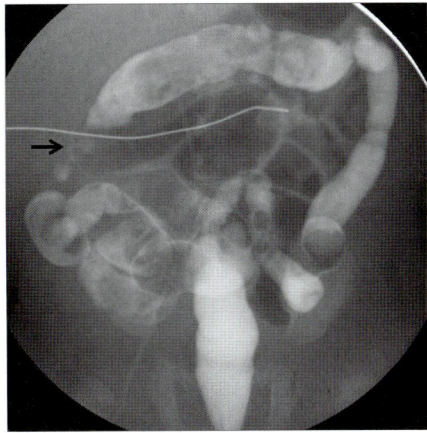

FIGURE 33-6 ■ This contrast enema demonstrates a stricture (arrow) in the ascending colon after nonoperative management for NEC. NEC strictures may occur anywhere in the intestinal tract, but are most common in the left colon. These can develop whether the baby was treated medically or surgically.

of recovery and time to full enteral feeding. Resection of additional bowel may also ultimately impact gastrointestinal outcomes.

Growth

Several small observational studies have shown that children treated for NEC fall below the 50th percentile for height and weight even into their grade-school years.[231–233] This growth retardation seems particularly to affect those who suffered from stage III NEC.[234,235] The problem is much more severe in children who develop SBS as a result of NEC. Long-term evaluations of growth are required to evaluate the impact that birth weight, NEC severity, operative strategy, and subsequent outcomes may play in ultimate growth outcomes for these children.

Neurodevelopmental Outcomes

In infants surviving NEC, adverse neurodevelopmental outcomes remain an important challenge. In 1980, a groundbreaking study reported that less than half of children surviving NEC were neurodevelopmentally normal at three-year follow-up.[236] Subsequently, multiple observational studies have cited intellectual delays,[237] moderate-to-severe developmental delay with speech and motor impairment,[183] developmental delay requiring special educational classes,[231] and delays in locomotor, hearing and speech, intellectual performance, and social skills.[234]

A large multicenter cohort study from the NICHD Neonatal Research Network evaluated neurodevelopmental outcomes in 1100 extremely LBW survivors.[238] This study confirmed that NEC is associated with increased odds of having a delayed score on psychomotor developmental assessment as well as increased odds of cerebral palsy. This study found that almost all of these abnormalities occurred in patients who required an operation for NEC.[239]

Two systematic reviews have confirmed the increased risk of neurodevelopmental impairment in VLBW infants who develop NEC (Fig. 33-7).[240,241] The risk for those treated surgically is nearly twice the risk for those treated medically. Most infants with NEC who are treated medically develop like age-matched premature infants without NEC, whereas those requiring an operation have an increased risk of poor neurodevelopmental outcomes.

PREVENTION

Prevention of NEC has become a major focus of research because management strategies have had little impact on mortality. Prevention has focused on two main aspects of care: feeding strategies and infectious characteristics of the gastrointestinal tract.

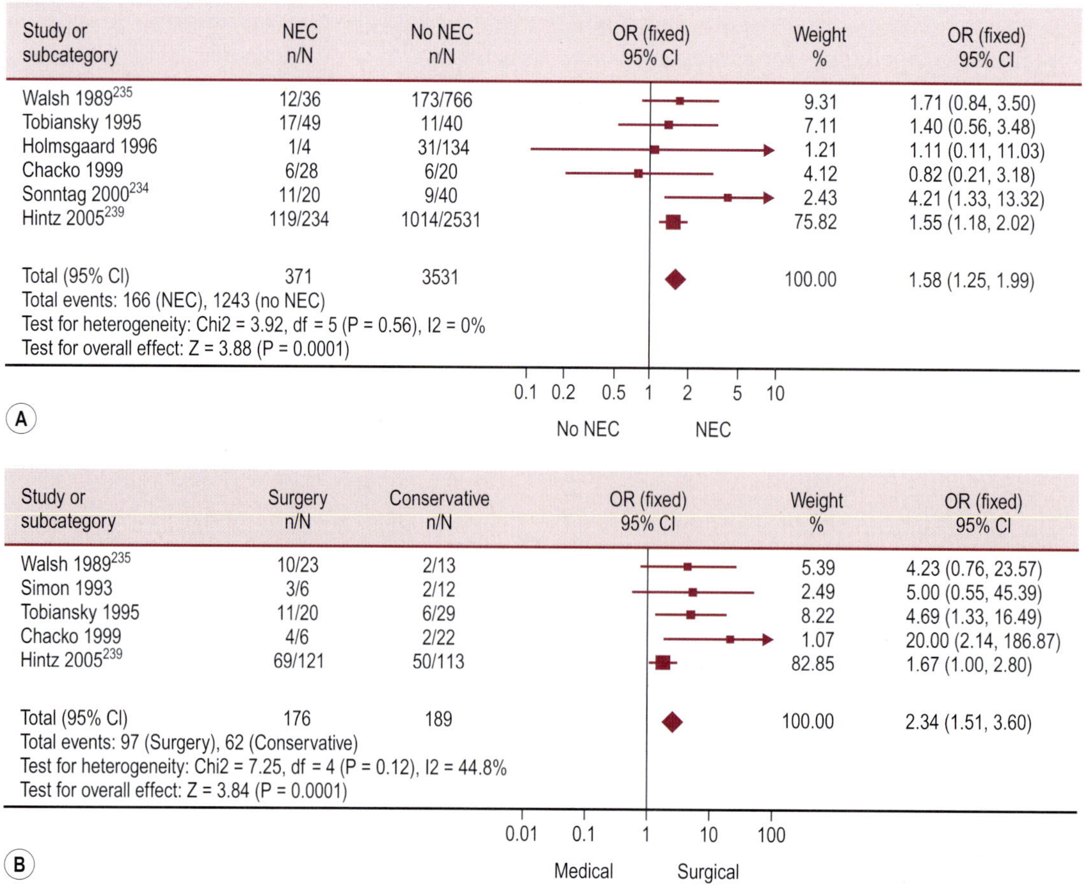

FIGURE 33-7 ■ Summary data from systematic reviews examining the relationship between NEC and neurodevelopmental outcome.

Human Milk

Human milk has a variety of antimicrobial, anti-inflammatory, and immunomodulating properties. Additionally, it furnishes the mucosa with IgA antibodies as well as macrophages, lactoferrin, and EGF. Because of these properties, it has been postulated that breast milk is protective against developing NEC. There are major challenges in evaluating the efficacy of human milk in preventing this disease. One difficulty lies in a lack of standardization of what is considered human milk: maternal preterm milk, donor preterm milk, donor term milk, and unfortified or fortified human milk. Another lies in the fact that many infants receive supplementation with formula or donor milk when there is insufficient maternal milk. Thus, determining how much human milk is fed and what constitutes human milk feeding versus formula feeding can be difficult. In addition, recent practices in the neonatal intensive care unit (NICU) often involve fortifying human milk to increase the caloric and nutritional content.

Four small (n = 36–81 patients) randomized or quasi-randomized studies in the 1980s evaluated the incidence of NEC in infants fed either human milk or formula.[242–245] None of these studies showed a statistically significant difference in NEC between the two groups, though all had a lower incidence in infants who received human milk.

Another randomized study was done as part of a larger prospective observational trial in the UK.[246] The study included 159 infants who were fed exclusively either donor breast milk or preterm formula. The incidence of NEC was slightly lower in the breast milk group, but the odds ratio did not reach significance. These investigators looked at all 926 patients who were part of the prospective observational study. They divided the patients into three groups based on what they had been fed: formula only, formula plus mother's milk, and human milk only. The formula group had a 10% incidence of NEC versus 4% in the human milk only group. When only considering confirmed cases of NEC, the formula group had 7% versus 1% in the human milk group.

Two systematic reviews and meta-analyses have subsequently been published which found that human milk reduces the risk of NEC with findings of a relative risk of 0.21 (95% CI: 0.06–0.76) in one and 0.25 (95% CI: 0.06–0.98) in the other.[247,248] However, these findings must be evaluated with some caution. The studies included in the meta-analyses had significant variation in the incidence of NEC (0–20%), the type of human milk (donor, maternal, term, or preterm), and the timing of feeding. Furthermore, one of the included studies was not truly randomized but used an alternate assignment allocation and none of the studies was blinded to allocation or outcome. Also, the criteria for NEC was not uniform among the studies.

More recently, a randomized multi-institutional study compared a human milk-based diet with a bovine milk-based diet in preterm infants. Mother's milk was used when available. Otherwise donor breast milk was used and fortified with human milk fortifier when enteral intake reached either 40 mL/kg/day or 100 mL/kg/day.

These infants were compared to infants receiving bovine milk-based formula, with fortification started once intake was 100 mL/kg/day. A total of 207 infants were enrolled. Duration of parenteral nutrition, length of hospital stay, sepsis and growth were not significantly different between groups; however, the incidence of NEC was significantly lower with a human milk-based diet (5.8% vs 15.9%, p = 0.02). The odds ratio for developing NEC on an exclusively human milk-based diet was 0.23 (95% CI 0.8–0.66; p = 0.007) or a relative risk reduction of 77%.[249] Other significant findings included a lower combined risk of death or NEC, and a lower risk of NEC requiring operation with human milk.

Fortification of human milk is commonly practiced to improve caloric and nutrient content of the human milk received. Fortification has been shown to result in increases in weight, length, and head circumference. A Cochrane review did not show an increase in NEC in the group fed fortified milk.[250] Different proprietary preparations of fortifier exist, and little research has been done to compare outcomes or to determine the optimal composition of fortifiers.

Feeding Strategies

Early initiation of enteral feedings in preterm infants helps to promote growth and decreases the need for parenteral nutrition. There have been concerns that early feeding may be associated with an increased risk of NEC. A systematic review found only two small, randomized studies with a total of 82 infants.[251] In these studies, early feeding had no effect on the incidence of NEC. Given the small sample size, important effects of either strategy may have been missed. In one large prospective study, early feeding of human milk appeared protective against NEC while early feeding of formula was linked to an increased incidence.[246] These investigators found that for each day earlier formula feeds were started, the risk of developing NEC increased 20%. Among those infants who received breast milk, there was no association between the day of life that feeding was initiated and the risk of NEC.

After starting enteral feeding, the rate at which to advance feeds is another controversy. Rapid advancement is advocated by some for infants to quickly regain their birth weight and achieve full enteral nutrition.[252] In one randomized trial, the study was terminated early due to a higher incidence of NEC in the group that had their feeds rapidly advanced.[253] Results from this study were confounded by a questionable randomization model, an unusually high incidence of NEC, early termination of the study, and exclusion of four patients who died or developed intestinal perforation. A systematic review of rapid versus slow advancement of feeds examined 372 patients in three separate trials and did not find any difference in the relative risk of developing NEC.[252] The ideal rate of feeding advancement remains unclear.

Amino Acid Supplementation

Arginine is the sole substrate for nitric oxide synthase. NO plays an important role in proper functioning of the gastrointestinal tract. Supplementation with arginine has been considered as a potential preventive measure for avoiding NEC. One randomized controlled trial of 152 preterm infants found a significant reduction in NEC in those infants receiving this supplementation.[254] This small study was unable to evaluate stage II and III NEC independently; further research on this possible preventive measure needs to be performed to confirm these results.[255]

A deficiency of serum glutamine has also been correlated with NEC.[256] Glutamine is fuel for enterocytes and promotes the growth and integrity of the intestinal epithelium. Glutamine has also been postulated as having protective effects against NEC. Two large multicenter randomized trials have failed to show a benefit for those who received glutamine.[257,258] A Cochrane systematic review of five trials also did not show any benefit to the infants receiving glutamine.[259]

Oral Antibiotics

Given the role of bacteria in the pathogenesis of NEC, enteral antibiotics have been considered as possible NEC prophylaxis. The use of antibiotics also increases the potential for the development of resistant bacteria. Five randomized trials have examined the effects of prophylactic therapy with enteral antibiotics. No individual study found a significant reduction in NEC; however, when the five were combined together in a meta-analysis, there was a significant reduction in the incidence of NEC in those who received the antibiotics.[260] Unfortunately, these studies did not report on the potential harmful effects of this use of enteral antibiotics. Without sufficient evidence regarding the safety of using enteral antibiotics as prophylaxis, an endorsement for this prophylactic measure cannot be made.

Probiotics

Probiotics are live microbial supplements that colonize the gastrointestinal tract. They have been proposed as a means of protecting against NEC. These supplements contain potentially beneficial bacteria or yeasts, most commonly *Lactobacillus*, *Bifidobacterium*, and *Streptococcus* strains.[261] They can enhance the mucosal barrier by reducing permeability, increasing mucus production, inhibiting bacterial translocation, and strengthening tight junctions.[42,262–267] Colonization with these organisms can reduce the ability of pathogenic bacteria to adhere to the intestinal mucosa.[268,269] Probiotics have also been shown to increase the production of mucosal IgA and short-chain fatty acids that help the immature immune system.[270–272] Additionally, they decrease intestinal inflammation through the reduction of proinflammatory cytokines, the increase of anti-inflammatory cytokines, and the increase of cytokine production by T-cells.[273–276]

Studies have examined the ability of probiotics to normalize intestinal flora and to prevent NEC. One randomized controlled trial showed that administration of *Bifidobacterium breve* within the first 24 hours and continued for 28 days can change the intestinal colonization rates, with increased levels of *Lactobacillus* and decreased counts of *Enterobacter*.[277] Another study showed that administering *Bifidobacterium* probiotics to preterm infants lowered the levels of pathogenic species such as *Enterobacter* and *Clostridium* in their intestines compared with controls who did not receive the probiotics.[278] These studies all suggest that the use of probiotic supplementation can influence intestinal colonization.

Once it was shown that such changes in intestinal flora could be manipulated, the next step lay in determining what clinical effect this might have on these preterm infants. One large prospective cohort study using historical controls evaluated whether newborns given *Lactobacillus acidophilus* and *Bifidobacterium infantis* would have reduced rates of NEC.[279] They studied 1237 infants over one year with a mean gestational age of 35 weeks and mean birth weight of 2040 g. These infants were treated with each probiotic daily until discharge. The results were compared with historical controls from the preceding year. During the treatment year, the incidence of NEC was 3% compared with 6.6% the year before ($p < 0.0002$). Furthermore, no side effects were noted.

Subsequently, there have been many studies analyzing the effects of probiotic supplementation in preterm infants. The first meta-analysis in 2007 reviewed seven randomized controlled trials involving a total of 690 infants who received no treatment and 703 who received probiotics (Table 33-4).[280] The relative risk for NEC in the group that received probiotics was 0.36 (95% CI: 0.20–0.65). These results must be considered with caution because this meta-analysis combined studies that had many significant differences. This heterogeneity normally would preclude the method of meta-analysis.[291] Considerable variability among the studies in the demographics of the patients, the age at commencement of treatment, and the type, dose, and duration of probiotic treatment existed. Though this meta-analysis found no increased risk of sepsis in the treatment group, side effects of probiotics were not adequately addressed due to lack of power to detect serious infections. Given the high-risk population in which these probiotics would be used, the issue of safety is crucial.

A 2012 meta-analysis included 20 studies with a total of 3816 patients. For preterm VLBW patients receiving probiotic supplements, the incidence of stage II or higher NEC was 3% compared to 7.4% in the placebo group, with a RR of 0.33 (95% CI, .024–0.46; $p < 0.00001$).[292] Due to differences in the type of probiotics used in the studies, subgroup analysis was performed; the three main probiotic agents (*Bifidobacteria*, *Lactobacillus*, and *Bifidobacteria* and *Lactobacillus*) all showed a significant risk reduction. Overall mortality was reduced in the group receiving probiotics as well: RR of 0.56 (95% CI 0.43–0.73; $p < 0.0001$). In regards to safety of probiotics, fourteen of the trials reported data for culture positive sepsis. In VLBW infants receiving probiotics, there was no difference in the risk of culture positive sepsis.

These studies suggest that probiotics are safe and effective in reducing the incidence of NEC and mortality without increasing the risk of sepsis. Despite the many studies available in the literature, there is heterogeneity in type of probiotic, timing of therapy, and dosing.

TABLE 33-4 **Clinical Trials Evaluating Probiotics and The Incidence of Necrotizing Enterocolitis[a]**

Study (First Author)	Population	Number	Probiotic	Incidence of NEC STUDY GROUP	CONTROL	p Value	Comment
Dani[281]	<33 weeks or <1500 g	585	LBG	4/295 (1.4%)	8/290 (2.8%)		
Lin[282]	<1500 g	367	LBA, BI	2/180 (1.1%)	10/187 (5.3%)	0.04	
Bin–Nun[283]	≤1500 g	145	BI, BBB, ST	3/72 (4%)	12/73 (16.4%)	0.031	
Kitajima[284]	<1500 g	91	BB	0/45	0/46	1	NEC a secondary outcome measure
Costalos[285]	28–32 weeks	87	SB	5/51 (9.8%)	6/36 (16%)	0.5	NEC a secondary outcome measure
Manzoni[286]	<1500 g	80	LBC	1/39	3/41	0.51	NEC a secondary outcome measure
Mohan[287]	<37 weeks	38	BBL	2/21	1/17		NEC a secondary outcome measure
Manzoni[288]	<1500 g	319	BLF or BLF plus LGG	3/153 (1.9%); 0/151 (0%)	10/168 (6%)	0.09; 0.002	NEC a secondary outcome measure
Braga[289]	<1500 g	231	BB, LBC	0/119	4/112		
Lin[290]	<1500 g	434	BBB, LBA	4/217	20/217	0.002	

BB, *Bifidobacterium breve*; BBB, *Bifidobacterium bifidus*; BBL, *Bifidobacterium lactis*; BI, *Bifidobacterium infantis*; BLF, bovine lactoferrin; LBA, *Lactobacillus acidophilus*; LBC, *Lactobacillus casei*; LBG, locust bean gum; LGG, *Lactobacillus rhamnosus* GG; SB, *Saccharomyces boulardii*; ST, *Streptococcus thermophilus*.
[a]See references for further information.

Long-term effects are also not well studied. While probiotics are a very promising preventative strategy, questions still need to be addressed.

Epidermal Growth Factor

As discussed earlier, EGF plays an important role in the pathogenesis of NEC. Premature infants in general, and infants with NEC specifically, have been shown to have decreased salivary concentrations of EGF.[87] Because EGF is known to support the maintenance of the intestinal barrier and downregulate proinflammatory cytokines,[122] its use has been postulated to help prevent NEC. A preliminary study of neonates diagnosed with NEC has shown that administration of EGF will promote the repair of the intestinal epithelium. In animal models, supplementation with EGF has decreased the incidence of NEC.[293] HB-EGF has been shown to have similar effects. Trials to test both EGF and HB-EGF as preventive strategies are planned.[294]

CONCLUSION

Despite many advances in the care of premature infants, NEC remains a challenging disease with a relatively constant incidence rate over the past four decades. The only clearly established risk factor is prematurity. Insight has been gained into the pathophysiology of this disease, with a unifying hypothesis emerging: an excessive and uncontrolled inflammatory response by the neonatal intestine after exposure to an inciting event. Future research efforts will focus on further elucidating the underlying causes and the molecular mechanisms that occur early in this pathogenic process. Because clinical parameters alone have not helped identify which children are at risk for developing the disease and progressing to serious

disease,[295] advanced approaches using proteomic and genomic techniques should be considered to compare those who develop NEC with those who do not, as well as those who progress to severe disease with those who have a mild course. Novel treatment strategies such as growth factors should be evaluated. Any trial of treatment should include evaluation of both short- and long-term outcomes. Finally, because no treatment for NEC will be uniformly effective once the disease is established, research efforts should focus on approaches to prevent this disease.

REFERENCES

1. Obladen M. Necrotizing enterocolitis–150 years of fruitless search for the cause. Neonatology 2009;96:203–10.
2. Santulli TV, Schullinger JN, Heird WC, et al. Acute necrotizing enterocolitis in infancy: A review of 64 cases. Pediatrics 1975;55:376–87.
3. Touloukian RJ, Berdon WE, Amoury RA, et al. Surgical experience with necrotizing enterocolitis in the infant. J Pediatr Surg 1967;2:389–401.
4. Llanos AR, Moss ME, Pinzon MC, et al. Epidemiology of neonatal necrotising enterocolitis: A population-based study. Paediatr Perinat Epidemiol 2002;16:342–9.
5. Guthrie SO, Gordon PV, Thomas V, et al. Necrotizing enterocolitis among neonates in the United States. J Perinatol 2003;23:278–85.
6. Horbar JD, Badger GJ, Carpenter JH. Trends in mortality and morbidity for very low birth weight infants, 1991-1999. Pediatrics 2002;110:143–51.
7. Sankaran K, Puckett B, Lee DS, et al. Variations in incidence of necrotizing enterocolitis in Canadian neonatal intensive care units. J Pediatr Gastroenterol Nutr 2004;39:366–72.
8. Stoll BJ, Hansen NI, Bell EF, et al. Neonatal outcomes of extremely preterm infants from the NICHD Neonatal Research Network. Pediatrics 2010;126:443–56.
9. Guillet R, Stoll BJ, Cotten CM, et al. Association of H2-blocker therapy and higher incidence of necrotizing enterocolitis in very low birth weight infants. Pediatrics 2006;117:e137–e42.
10. Holman RC, Stoll BJ, Curns AT, et al. Necrotising enterocolitis hospitalisations among neonates in the United States. Paediatr Perinat Epidemiol 2006;20:498–506.

11. Lemons JA, Bauer CR, Oh W, et al. Very low birth weight outcomes of the National Institute of Child health and human development neonatal research network, January 1995 through December 1996. NICHD Neonatal Research Network. Pediatrics 2001;107:E1.

12. Luig M, Lui K, NICUS group, et al. Epidemiology of necrotizing: enterocolitis: II. Risks and susceptibility of premature infants during the surfactant era: A regional study. J Pediatr Child Health 2005;41:174–9.

13. Holman RC, Stoll BJ, Clarke MJ, et al. The epidemiology of necrotizing enterocolitis infant mortality in the United States. Am J Public Health 1997;87:2026–31.

14. Sharma R, Hudak ML, Tepas JJ 3rd, et al. Impact of gestational age on the clinical presentation and surgical outcome of necrotizing enterocolitis. J Perinatol 2006;26:342–7.

15. Blakely ML, Lally KP, McDonald S, et al. Postoperative outcomes of extremely low birth-weight infants with necrotizing enterocolitis or isolated intestinal perforation: A prospective cohort study by the NICHHD Neonatal Research Network. Ann Surg 2005;241:984–94.

16. Blakely ML, Gupta H, Lally KP. Surgical management of necrotizing enterocolitis and isolated intestinal perforation in premature neonates. Semin Perinatol 2008;32:122–6.

17. Ng S. Necrotizing enterocolitis in the full-term neonate [see comment]. J Paediatr Child Health 2001;37:1–4.

18. Lambert DK, Christensen RD, Henry E, et al. Necrotizing enterocolitis in term neonates: Data from a multihospital health-care system [see comment]. J Perinatol 2007;27:437–43.

19. Ostlie DJ, Spilde TL, St Peter SD, et al. Necrotizing enterocolitis in full-term infants. J Pediatr Surg 2003;38:1039–42.

20. Bolisetty S, Lui K. Necrotizing enterocolitis in full-term neonates [comment]. J Pediatr Child Health 2001;37:413–14.

21. Bisquera JA, Cooper TR, Berseth CL. Impact of necrotizing enterocolitis on length of stay and hospital charges in very low birth weight infants. Pediatrics 2002;109:423–8.

22. Spencer AU, Kovacevich D, McKinney-Barnett M, et al. Pediatric short-bowel syndrome: the cost of comprehensive care. Am J Clin Nutr 2008;88:1552–9.

23. Ballance WA, Dahms BB, Shenker N, et al. Pathology of neonatal necrotizing enterocolitis: A ten-year experience. J Pediatr 1990;117:S6–13.

24. Hsueh W, Caplan MS, Qu XW, et al. Neonatal necrotizing enterocolitis: Clinical considerations and pathogenetic concepts. Pediatr Dev Pathol 2003;6:6–23.

25. Sanderson I. The physicochemical environment of the neonatal intestine. Am J Clin Nutr 1999;69:1028S–345.

26. Berseth CL. Gestational evolution of small intestine motility in preterm and term infants. J Pediatr 1989;115:646–51.

27. Berseth CL. Gastrointestinal motility in the neonate. Clin Perinatol 1996;23:179–90.

28. Milla PJ. Intestinal motility during ontogeny and intestinal pseudo-obstruction in children. Pediatr Clin North Am 1996;43:511–32.

29. Lebenthal A, Lebenthal E. The ontogeny of the small intestinal epithelium. J Parenter Enteral Nutr 1999;23(Suppl. 5):S3–6.

30. Di Lorenzo M, Bass J, Krantis A. An intraluminal model of necrotizing enterocolitis in the developing neonatal piglet. J Pediatr Surg 1995;30:1138–42.

31. Lin J. Too much short chain fatty acids cause neonatal necrotizing enterocolitis. Med Hypotheses 2004;62:291–3.

32. Ford HR. Mechanism of nitric oxide-mediated intestinal barrier failure: Insight into the pathogenesis of necrotizing enterocolitis. J Pediatr Surg 2006;41:294–9.

33. Halpern MD, Holubec H, Saunders TA. Bile acids induce ileal damage during experimental necrotizing enterocolitis. Gastroenterology 2006;130:359–72.

34. Halpern MD, Dvorak B. Does abnormal bile acid metabolism contribute to NEC? Semin Perinatol 2008;32:114–21.

35. Hammons JL, Jordan WE, Stewart RL. Age and diet effects on fecal bile acids in infants. J Pediatr Gastroenterol Nutr 1988;7:30–8.

36. Hunter CJ, Upperman JS, Ford HR, et al. Understanding the susceptibility of the premature infant to necrotizing enterocolitis. Pediatr Res 2008;63:117–23.

37. McElroy SJ, Prince LS, Weitkamp JH, et al. Tumor necrosis factor receptor 1-dependent depletion of mucus in immature small intestine: A potential role in neonatal necrotizing enterocolitis. Am J Physiol Gastrointest Liver Physiol 2011;301:G656–66.

38. Strous GJ, Dekker J. Mucin-type glycoproteins. Crit Rev Biochem Mol Biol 1992;27:57–92.

39. Allen A, Bell A, Mantle M. The structure and physiology of gastrointestinal mucus. Adv Exp Med Biol 1982;144:115–33.

40. Montagne L, Piel C, Lalles JP. Effect of diet on mucin kinetics and composition: Nutrition and health implications. Nutr Rev 2004;62:105–14.

41. Rhodes JM. Colonic mucus and mucosal glycoproteins: The key to colitis and cancer? Gut 1989;30:1660–6.

42. Deplancke B, Gaskins HR. Microbial modulation of innate defense: Goblet cells and the intestinal mucus layer. Am J Clin Nutr 2001;73:1131S–41S.

43. Hackam DJ, Upperman JS, Grishin A, et al. Disordered enterocyte signaling and intestinal barrier dysfunction in the pathogenesis of necrotizing enterocolitis. Semin Pediatr Surg 2005;14:49–57.

44. Ryley HC, Rennie D, Bradley DM. The composition of a mucus glycoprotein from meconium of cystic fibrosis, healthy pre-term and full-term neonates. Clin Chim Acta 1983;135:49–56.

45. Corfield AP, Myerscough N, Longman R, et al. Mucins and mucosal protection in the gastrointestinal tract: New prospects for mucins in the pathology of gastrointestinal disease. Gut 2000;47:589–94.

46. Kyo K, Muto T, Nagawa H, et al. Associations of distinct variants of the intestinal mucin gene MUC3A with ulcerative colitis and Crohn's disease. J Hum Genet 2001;46:5–20.

47. Vieten D, Corfield A, Carroll D, et al. Impaired mucosal regeneration in neonatal necrotizing enterocolitis. Pediatr Surg Int 2005;21:153–60.

48. Liu Z, Li N, Neu J. Tight junctions, leaky intestines, and pediatric diseases. Acta Paediatr 2005;94:386–93.

49. Anand RJ, Leaphart CL, Mollen KP, et al. The role of the intestinal barrier in the pathogenesis of necrotizing enterocolitis. Shock 2007;27:124–33.

50. Muresan Z, Paul DL, Goodenough DA. Occludin 1B, a variant of the tight junction protein occludin. Mol Biol Cell 2000;11:627–34.

51. Shen L, Turner JR. Role of epithelial cells in initiation and propagation of intestinal inflammation. Eliminating the static: Tight junction dynamics exposed. Am J Physiol Gastrointest Liver Physiol 2006;290:G577–G82.

52. Ford H, Watkins S, Reblock K, et al. The role of inflammatory cytokines and nitric oxide in the pathogenesis of necrotizing enterocolitis. J Pediatr Surg 1997;32:275–82.

53. Han X, Fink MP, Delude RL. Proinflammatory cytokines cause NO-dependent and independent changes in expression and localization of tight junction proteins in intestinal epithelial cells. Shock 2003;3:220–37.

54. Mowat AM, Viney JL. The anatomical basis of intestinal immunity. Immunol Rev 1997;156:145–66.

55. Neutra MR, Mantis NJ, Kraehenbuhl JP. Collaboration of epithelial cells with organized mucosal lymphoid tissues. Nat Immunol 2001.1004–9.

56. Puiman PJ, Burger-Van Paassen N, Schaart MW, et al. Paneth cell hyperplasia and metaplasia in necrotizing enterocolitis. Pediatr Res 2011;69:217–23.

57. Ayabe T, Satchell DP, Wilson CL, et al. Secretion of microbicidal alpha-defensins by intestinal Paneth cells in response to bacteria. Nat Immunol 2000;1:113–18.

58. Mayer L. Mucosal immunity. Pediatrics 2003;111:1595–600.

59. Ogra SS, Weintraub D, Ogra PL. Immunologic aspects of human colostrum and milk: III. Fate and absorption of cellular and soluble components in the gastrointestinal tract of the newborn. J Immunol 1977;119:245–8.

60. Cetin S, Ford HR, Sysko LR, et al. Endotoxin inhibits intestinal epithelial restitution through activation of Rho-GTPase and increased focal adhesions. J Biol Chem 2004;279:24592–600.

61. Duffy LC, Zielezny MA, Carrion V, et al. Concordance of bacterial cultures with endotoxin and interleukin-6 in necrotizing enterocolitis. Dig Dis Sci 1997;42:359–65.

62. Forsythe RM, Xu DZ, Lu Q, et al. Lipopolysaccharide-induced enterocyte-derived nitric oxide induces intestinal monolayer permeability in an autocrine fashion. Shock 2002;17:180–4.

63. Grishin A, Wang J, Hackam DJ, et al. p38 MAP kinase mediates endotoxin-induced expression of cyclooxygenase-2 in enterocytes. Surgery 2004;136:329–35.

64. Gonzalez-Crussi F, Hsueh W. Experimental model of ischemic bowel necrosis: The role of platelet-activating factor and endotoxin. Am J Pathol 1983;112:127–35.

65. Hsueh W, Gonzalez-Crussi F, Arroyave JL. Platelet-activating factor-induced ischemic bowel necrosis: The effect of PAF antagonists. Eur J Pharmacol 1986;123:79–83.

66. Levy RM, Prince JM, Billiar TR. Nitric oxide: A clinical primer. Crit Care Med 2005;33:S492–S5.

67. Chokshi N, Guner Y, Hunter CJ, et al. The role of nitric oxide in intestinal epithelial injury and restitution in neonatal necrotizing enterocolitis. Semin Perinatol 2008;32:92–9.

68. Beckman JS. Ischaemic injury mediator. Nature 1990;345:27–8.

69. Upperman JS, Potoka DA, Grishin A. Mechanisms of nitric oxide mediated intestinal barrier failure in necrotizing enterocolitis. Semin Pediatr Surg 2005;14:159–66.

70. Hoffman RA, Zhang G, Nussler NC. Constitutive expression of inducible nitric oxide synthase in the mouse ileal mucosa. Am J Physiol 1997;272(2Pt1):G383–G92.

71. Emami CN, Chokshi N, Wang J, et al. Role of interleukin-10 in the pathogenesis of necrotizing enterocolitis. Am J Surg 2012;203:428–35.

72. Chokshi N, Guner Y, Hunter CJ, et al. The role of nitric oxide in intestinal epithelial injury and restitution in neonatal necrotizing enterocolitis. Semin Perinatol 2008;32:92–9.

73. Snyder F. Platelet-activating factor and related acetylated lipids as potent biologically active cellular mediators. Am J Physiol 1990;259:C697–C708.

74. Frost BL, Jilling T, Caplan MS. The importance of proinflammatory signaling in neonatal necrotizing enterocolitis. Semin Perinatol 2008;32:100–6.

75. Caplan MS, Simon D, Jilling T. The role of PAF, TLR, and the inflammatory response in neonatal necrotizing enterocolitis. Semin Pediatr Surg 2005;14:145–51.

76. Caplan M, Hsueh W, Kelly A, et al. Serum PAF acetylhydrolase increases during neonatal maturation. Prostaglandins 1990;39:705–14.

77. Rabinowitz SS, Dzakpasu P, Piecuch S, et al. Platelet-activating factor in infants at risk for necrotizing enterocolitis. J Pediatr 2001;138:81–6.

78. Caplan MS, Lickerman M, Adler L, et al. The role of recombinant platelet-activating factor acetylhydrolase in a neonatal rat model of necrotizing enterocolitis. Pediatr Res 1997;42:779–83.

79. Coursodon CF, Dvorak B. Epidermal growth factor and necrotizing enterocolitis. Curr Opin Pediatr 2012;24:160–4.

80. Dvorak B, Philips AF, Koldovsky O. Milk-borne growth factors and gut development. In: Zeigler E, Lucas A, Moro G, editors. Nutrition of the Very Low Birthweight Infant. Philadelphia: Lippincott Williams and Wilkins; 1999. p. 245–55.

81. Pollack PF, Goda T, Colony PC. Effects of enterally fed epidermal growth factor on the small and large intestine of the suckling rat. Regul Pept 1987;17:121–32.

82. Playford R, Wright N. Why is epidermal growth factor present in the gut lumen. Gut 1996;38:303–5.

83. Barnard JA, Beauchamp D, Russel W. Epidermal growth factor-related peptides and their relevance to gastrointestinal pathophysiology. Gastroenterology 1995;108:564–80.

84. Warner B, Warner B. Role of epidermal growth factor in the pathogenesis of neonatal necrotizing enterocolitis. Semin Pediatr Surg 2005;14:175–80.

85. Hirai C, Ichiba H, Saito M. Trophic effect of multiple growth factors in amniotic fluid or human milk on cultured human fetal small intestinal cells. J Pediatr Gastroenterol Nutr 2002;34:524–8.

86. Chen CL, Yu X, James IO, et al. Heparin-binding EGF-like growth factor protects intestinal stem cells from injury in a rat model of necrotizing enterocolitis. Lab Invest 2012;92:331–44.

87. Shin CE, Falcone RA Jr, Stuart L, et al. Diminished epidermal growth factor levels in infants with necrotizing enterocolitis. J Pediatr Surg 2000;35:173–7.

88. Warner B, Ryan A, Seeger K. Ontogeny of salivary epidermal growth factor and necrotizing enterocolitis. J Pediatr 2007;150:358–63.

89. Sullivan PB, Brueton MJ, Tabara ZB. Epidermal growth factor in necrotising enteritis. Lancet 1991;338:53–4.

90. Sullivan PB, Lewindon PJ, Cheng C. Intestinal mucosal remodeling by recombinant human EGF in neonates with severe necrotizing enterocolitis. J Pediatr Surg 2007;42:462–9.

91. Christensen RD, Gordon PV, Besner GE. Can we cut the incidence of necrotizing enterocolitis in half–today? Fetal Pediatr Pathol 2010;29:185–98.

92. Feng J, El-Assal O, Besner GE. Heparin-binding EGF-like growth factor (HB-EGF) and necrotizing enterocolitis. Semin Pediatr Surg 2005;14:167–74.

93. Feng J, Besner GE. Heparin-binding epidermal growth factor-like growth factor promotes enterocyte migration and proliferation in neonatal rats with necrotizing enterocolitis. J Pediatr Surg 2007;42:214–20.

94. Feng J, El-Assal ON, Besner GE. Heparin-binding epidermal growth factor-like growth factor reduces intestinal apoptosis in neonatal rats with necrotizing enterocolitis. J Pediatr Surg 2006;41:742–7.

95. Feng J, El-Assal ON, Besner GE. Heparin-binding epidermal growth factor-like growth factor decreases the incidence of necrotizing enterocolitis in neonatal rats. J Pediatr Surg 2006;41:144–9.

96. Radulescu A, Yu X, Orvets ND, et al. Deletion of the heparin-binding epidermal growth factor-like growth factor gene increases susceptibility to necrotizing enterocolitis. J Pediatr Surg 2010;45:729–34.

97. Radulescu A, Zhang HY, Yu X, et al. Heparin-binding epidermal growth factor-like growth factor overexpression in transgenic mice increases resistance to necrotizing enterocolitis. J Pediatr Surg 2010;45:1933–9.

98. Nankervis CA, Nowicki P. Role of nitric oxide in regulation of vascular resistance in postnatal intestine. Am J Physiol 1995;268:G949–G58.

99. Reber KM, Mager GM, Miller CE. Relationship between flow rate and NO production in postnatal mesenteric arteries. Am J Physiol 2000;280:G43–G50.

100. Nowicki P. Intestinal ischemia and necrotizing enterocolitis. J Pediatr 1990;117:S14–S19.

101. Reber KM, Nankervis CA, Nowicki PT. Newborn intestinal circulation. Physiology and pathophysiology. Clin Perinatol 2002;29:23–39.

102. Nowicki P. Ischemia and necrotizing enterocolitis: Where, when and how. Semin Pediatr Surg 2005;14:152–8.

103. Nankervis CA, Dunaway DJ, Nowicki P. Role of endothelin-1 in regulation of the postnatal intestinal circulation. Am J Physiol 2000;278:G367–G75.

104. Yanagisawa M, Kurihara H, Kimura S. A novel potent vasoconstrictor peptide produced by vascular endothelial cells. Nature 1998;332:411–15.

105. Kuchan MJ, Frangos JA. Shear stress regulates endothelin-1 release via protein kinase C and cGMP in cultured endothelial cells. Am J Physiol 1993;264:H150–H6.

106. Kourembanas S, Marsden PA, McQuillan LP. Hypoxia induces endothelin gene expression and secretion in cultured human endothelium. J Clin Invest 1991;88:1054–7.

107. Woods M, Mitchel JA, Wood EG. Endothelin-1 is induced by cytokines in human vascular smooth muscle cells: Evidence for intracellular endothelin converting enzyme. Mol Pharmacol 1999;55:902–9.

108. Ito Y, Doelle S, Clark JA. Intestinal microcirculatory dysfunction during the development of experimental necrotizing enterocolitis. Pediatr Res 2007;61:180–4.

109. Lin PW, Nasr TR, Stoll BJ. Necrotizing enterocolitis: Recent scientific advances in pathophysiology and prevention. Semin Perinatol 2008;32:70–82.

110. Kosloske AM. Indications for operation in necrotizing enterocolitis revisited. J Pediatr Surg 1994;29:663–6.

111. Dolgin SE, Shlasko E, Levitt MA, et al. Alterations in respiratory status: Early signs of severe necrotizing enterocolitis. J Pediatr Surg 1998;33:856–8.

112. Bell MJ. Neonatal necrotizing enterocolitis. N Engl J Med 1978;298:281–2.
113. Kliegman RJ, Walsh MC. Neonatal necrotizing enterocolitis: Pathogenesis, classification and spectrum of disease. Curr Probl Pediatr 1987;26:327–44.
114. Kafetzis DA, Skevaki C, Costalos C. Neonatal necrotizing enterocolitis: An overview. Curr Opin Infect Dis 2003;16:349–55.
115. Noerr B. Current controversies in the understanding of necrotizing enterocolitis: I. Adv Neonatal Care 2003;3:107–20.
116. Romagnoli C, Frezza S, Cingolani A, et al. Plasma levels of interleukin-6 and interleukin-10 in preterm neonates evaluated for sepsis. Eur J Pediatr 2001;160:345–50.
117. Isaacs D, North J, Lindsell D, et al. Serum acute phase reactants in necrotizing enterocolitis. Acta Paediatr Scand 1987;76:923–7.
118. Pourcyrous M, Korones S, Yang W, et al. C-reactive protein in the diagnosis, management, and prognosis of neonatal necrotizing enterocolitis. Pediatrics 2005;116:1064–9.
119. Edelson MB, Bagwell CE, Rozycki HJ. Circulating pro- and counterinflammatory cytokine levels and severity in necrotizing enterocolitis. Pediatrics 1999;103:766–71.
120. Kosloske AM. Epidemiology of necrotizing enterocolitis. Acta Paediatr Suppl 1994;396:2–7.
121. Chandler JC, Hebra A. Necrotizing enterocolitis in infants with very low birth weight. Semin Pediatr Surg 2000;9:63–72.
122. Kennedy J, Holt CL, Ricketts RR. The significance of portal vein gas in necrotizing enterocolitis. Am Surg 1987;53:231–4.
123. Faingold R, Daneman A, Tomlinson G. Necrotizing enterocolitis: Assessment of bowel viability with color Doppler ultrasound. Radiology 2005;235:587–94.
124. Kim WY, Kim WS, Kim IO, et al. Sonographic evaluation of neonates with early-stage necrotizing enterocolitis. Pediatr Radiol 2005;35:1056–61.
125. Kim WY, Kim IO, Kim WS. Bowel sonography in necrotizing enterocolitis: Histopathologic correlation in experimental studies. Pediatr Radiol 2005;35(Suppl):S51.
126. Azarow K, Connolly B, Babyn P, et al. Multidisciplinary evaluation of the distended abdomen in critically ill infants and children: The role of bedside sonography. Pediatr Surg Int 1998;13:355–9.
127. Silva CT, Daneman A, Navarro OM, et al. Correlation of sonographic findings and outcome in necrotizing enterocolitis. Pediatr Radiol 2007;37:274–82.
128. Epelman M, Daneman A, Navarro OM, et al. Necrotizing enterocolitis: Review of state-of-the-art imaging findings with pathologic correlation. RadioGraphics 2007;27:285–305.
129. Buonomo C. The radiology of necrotizing enterocolitis. Radiol Clin North Am 1999;37:1187–98.vii.
130. Kao SC, Smith WL, Franken EA Jr, et al. Contrast enema diagnosis of necrotizing enterocolitis. Pediatr Radiol 1992;22:115–17.
131. Schwartz MZ, Hayden CK, Richardson CJ, et al. A prospective evaluation of intestinal stenosis following necrotizing enterocolitis. J Pediatr Surg 1982;17:764–70.
132. Rencken IO, Sola A, al-Ali F, et al. Necrotizing enterocolitis: Diagnosis with CT examination of urine after enteral administration of iodinated water-soluble contrast material. Radiology 1997;205:87–90.
133. Maalouf EF, Fagbemi A, Duggan PJ, et al. Magnetic resonance imaging of intestinal necrosis in preterm infants. Pediatrics 2000;105:510–14.
134. Meyer CL, Payne NR, Roback SA. Spontaneous, isolated intestinal perforations in neonates with birth weight less than 1,000 g not associated with necrotizing enterocolitis. J Pediatr Surg 1991;26:714–17.
135. Mintz AC, Applebaum H. Focal gastrointestinal perforations not associated with necrotizing enterocolitis in very low birth weight neonates. J Pediatr Surg 1993;28:857–60.
136. Aschner JL, Deluga KS, Metlay LA, et al. Spontaneous focal gastrointestinal perforation in very low birth weight infants. J Pediatr 1988;113:364–7.
137. Azarow KS, Ein SH, Shandling B, et al. Laparotomy or drain for perforated necrotizing enterocolitis: Who gets what and why? Pediatr Surg Int 1997;12:137–9.
138. Rovin JD, Rodgers BM, Burns RC, et al. The role of peritoneal drainage for intestinal perforation in infants with and without necrotizing enterocolitis. J Pediatr Surg 1999;34:143–7.
139. Okuyama H, Kubota A, Oue T, et al. A comparison of the clinical presentation and outcome of focal intestinal perforation and necrotizing enterocolitis in very-low-birth-weight neonates. Pediatr Surg Int 2002;18:704–6.
140. Tarrado X, Castanon M, Thio M, et al. Comparative study between isolated intestinal perforation and necrotizing enterocolitis. Eur J Pediatr Surg 2005;15:88–94.
141. Pumberger W, Mayr M, Kohlhauser C, et al. Spontaneous localized intestinal perforation in very-low-birth-weight infants: A distinct clinical entity different from necrotizing enterocolitis. J Am Coll Surg 2002;195:796–803.
142. Buchheit JQ, Stewart DL. Clinical comparison of localized intestinal perforation and necrotizing enterocolitis in neonates [see comment]. Pediatrics 1994;93:32–6.
143. Cass DL, Brandt ML, Patel DL, et al. Peritoneal drainage as definitive treatment for neonates with isolated intestinal perforation. J Pediatr Surg 2000;35:1531–6.
144. Lessin MS, Luks FI, Wesselhoeft CW. Peritoneal drainage as definitive treatment for intestinal perforation in infants with extremely low birth weight (<750 gms). J Pediatr Surg 1998;33:370–2.
145. Gordon PV, Swanson JR, Attridge JT, et al. Emerging trends in acquired neonatal intestinal disease: Is it time to abandon Bell's criteria. J Perinatol 2007;27:661–71.
146. Cribbs RK, Harding PA, Luquette MH. Endogenous production of heparin-binding EGF-like growth factor during murine partial thickness burn wound healing. J Burn Care Rehabil 2002;23:116–25.
147. Jin K, Mao XO, Sun Y. Heparin-binding epidermal growth factor-like growth factor: Hypoxia-inducible expression in vitro and stimulation of neurogenesis in vitro and in vivo. J Neurosci 2002;22:5365–73.
148. Frank GD, Mifune M, Inagami T. Distinct mechanisms of receptor and nonreceptor tyrosine kinase activation by reactive oxygen species in vascular smooth muscle cells: Role of metalloprotease and protein kinase C-delta. Mol Cell Biol 2003;23:1581–9.
149. Kayanoki Y, Higashiyama S, Suzuki K. The requirement of both intracellular reactive oxygen species and intracellular calcium elevation for the induction of heparin-binding EGF-like growth factor in vascular endothelial cells and smooth muscle cells. Biochem Biophys Res Commun 1999;259:50–5.
150. Marikovsky M, Breuing K, Liu PY. Appearance of heparin-binding EGF-like growth factor in wound fluid as a response to injury. Proc Natl Acad Sci U S A 1993;90:3889–93.
151. McCarthy DW, Downing MT, Brigstock DR. Production of heparin-binding epidermal growth factor-like growth factor (HBEGF) at sites of thermal injury in pediatric patients. J Invest Dermatol 1996;106:49–56.
152. Xia G, Rachfal AW, Martin AE. Upregulation of endogenous heparin-binding EGF-like growth factor (HB-EGF) expression after intestinal ischemia reperfusion injury. J Invest Surg 2003;16:57–63.
153. El-Assal O, Besner GE. Heparin-binding epidermal growth factor-like growth factor and intestinal ischemia-reperfusion injury. Semin Pediatr Surg 2004;13:2–10.
154. Michalsky MP, Kuhn A, Mehta V. Heparin-binding EGF-like growth factor decreases apoptosis in intestinal epithelial cells in vitro. J Pediatr Surg 2001;36:1130–5.
155. Pillai SB, Turman MA, Besner GE. Heparin-binding EGF-like growth factor is cytoprotective for intestinal epithelial cells exposed to hypoxia. J Pediatr Surg 1998;33:973–8.
156. Lara-Marquez ML, Mehta V, Michalsky MP. Heparin-binding EGF-like growth factor down regulates proinflammatory cytokine-induced nitric oxide and inducible nitric oxide synthase production in intestinal epithelial cells. Nitric Oxide 2002;6:142–52.
157. Mehta VB, Besner GE. Inhibition of NF-kappa B activation and its target genes by heparin-binding epidermal growth factor-like growth factor. J Immunol 2003;171:6014–22.
158. Halpern M, Dominguez JA, Dvorakova K. Ileal cytokine dysregulation in experimental necrotizing enterocolitis is reduced

by epidermal growth factor. J Pediatr Gastroenterol Nutr 2003;36:126–33.

159. Ricketts RR, Jerles ML. Neonatal necrotizing enterocolitis: Experience with 100 consecutive surgical patients. World J Surg 1990;14:600–5.

160. Albanese CT, Rowe MI. Necrotizing enterocolitis. Semin Pediatr Surg 1995;4:200–6.

161. Grosfeld JL, Cheu H, Schlatter M, et al. Changing trends in necrotizing enterocolitis: Experience with 302 cases in two decades. Ann Surg 1991;214:300–7.

162. Ein SH, Marshall DG, Girvan D. Peritoneal drainage under local anesthesia for perforations from necrotizing enterocolitis. J Pediatr Surg 1977;12:963–7.

163. Moss RL, Dimmitt RA, Henry MC, et al. A meta-analysis of peritoneal drainage versus laparotomy for perforated necrotizing enterocolitis. J Pediatr Surg 2001;36:1210–13.

164. Blakely ML, Tyson JE, Lally KP, et al. Laparotomy versus peritoneal drainage for necrotizing enterocolitis or isolated intestinal perforation in extremely low birth weight infants: Outcomes through 18 months adjusted age. Pediatrics 2006;117:e680–e7.

165. Moss RL, Dimmitt RA, Barnhart DC, et al. Laparotomy versus peritoneal drainage for necrotizing enterocolitis and perforation [see comment] [erratum appears in N Engl J Med. 2006 Aug 24;355(8):856]. N Engl J Med 2006;354:2225–34.

166. Rees C M, Eaton S, Khoo AK. Peritoneal drainage or laparotomy in neonatal bowel perforation? A randomized controlled trial. Presented at the American Pediatric Surgical Association, Orlando, FL, 38th Annual Meeting, May 2007.

167. Laparotomy vs. Drainage for Infants With Necrotizing Enterocolitis (NEST). 2012; Available at: http://www.clinicaltrial.gov/ct2/show/NCT01029353. Accessed 06/24, 2012.

168. Nadler EP, Upperman JS, Ford HR. Controversies in the management of necrotizing enterocolitis. Surg Infect 2001;2:113–20.

169. Cooper A, Ross AJ 3rd, O'Neill JA Jr, et al. Resection with primary anastomosis for necrotizing enterocolitis: A contrasting view. J Pediatr Surg 1988;23:64–8.

170. Weber TR, Lewis JE. The role of second-look laparotomy in necrotizing enterocolitis. J Pediatr Surg 1986;21:323–5.

171. Vaughan WG, Grosfeld JL, West K, et al. Avoidance of stomas and delayed anastomosis for bowel necrosis: The 'clip and drop-back' technique. J Pediatr Surg 1996;31:542–5.

172. Luzzatto C, Previtera C, Boscolo R, et al. Necrotizing enterocolitis: Late surgical results after enterostomy without resection. Eur J Pediatr Surg 1996;6:92–4.

173. Lee JS, Polin RA. Treatment and prevention of necrotizing enterocolitis. Semin Neonatol 2003;8:449–59.

174. Stringer MD, Brereton RJ, Drake DP, et al. Recurrent necrotizing enterocolitis. J Pediatr Surg 1993;28:979–81.

175. Frantz ID 3rd, L'Heureux P, Engel RR, et al. Necrotizing enterocolitis. J Pediatr 1975;86:259–63.

176. Vollman JH, Smith WL, Tsang RC. Necrotizing enterocolitis with recurrent hepatic portal venous gas. J Pediatr 1976;88:486–7.

177. Mollitt DL, Golladay ES. Postoperative neonatal necrotizing enterocolitis. J Pediatr Surg 1982;17:757–63.

178. Oldham KT, Coran AG, Drongowski RA, et al. The development of necrotizing enterocolitis following repair of gastroschisis: A surprisingly high incidence. J Pediatr Surg 1988;23:945–9.

179. Shanbhogue LK, Tam PK, Lloyd DA. Necrotizing enterocolitis following operation in the neonatal period. Br J Surg 1991;78:1045–7.

180. Ladd AP, Rescorla FJ, West KW, et al. Long-term follow-up after bowel resection for necrotizing enterocolitis: Factors affecting outcome. J Pediatr Surg 1998;33:967–72.

181. Bisquera JA, Cooper TR, Berseth CL. Impact of necrotizing enterocolitis on length of stay and hospital charges in very low birth weight infants. Pediatrics 2002;109:423–8.

182. Limpert JN, Limpert PA, Weber TR, et al. The impact of surgery on infants born at extremely low birth weight. J Pediatr Surg 2003;38:924–7.

183. Patel JC, Tepas JJ 3rd, Huffman SD, et al. Neonatal necrotizing enterocolitis: The long-term perspective. Am Surg 1998;64:575–80.

184. Kliegman RM, Fanaroff AA. Necrotizing enterocolitis. N Engl J Med 1984;310:1093–103.

185. Touloukian RJ. Neonatal necrotizing enterocolitis: An update on etiology, diagnosis, and treatment. Surg Clin North Am 1976;56:281–98.

186. Kurscheid T, Holschneider AM. Necrotizing enterocolitis (NEC)—mortality and long-term results. Eur J Pediatr Surg 1993;3:139–43.

187. Horwitz JR, Lally KP, Cheu HW, et al. Complications after surgical intervention for necrotizing enterocolitis: A multicenter review. J Pediatr Surg 1995;30:994–9.

188. de Souza JC, da Motta UI, Ketzer CR. Prognostic factors of mortality in newborns with necrotizing enterocolitis submitted to exploratory laparotomy. J Pediatr Surg 2001;36:482–6.

189. Cikrit D, Mastandrea J, West KW, et al. Necrotizing enterocolitis: Factors affecting mortality in 101 surgical cases. Surgery 1984;96:648–55.

190. Ricketts RR. Surgical treatment of necrotizing enterocolitis and the short bowel syndrome. Clin Perinatol 1994;21:365–87.

191. Wilmore DW. Factors correlating with a successful outcome following extreme intestinal resection in newborn infants. J Pediatr 1972;80:88–95.

192. Fasching G, Hollwarth ME, Schmidt B, et al. Surgical strategies in very-low-birthweight neonates with necrotizing enterocolitis. Acta Paediatr Suppl 1994;396:62–4.

193. Beasley SW, Auldist AW, Ramanjuan TM. The surgical management of neonatal necrotizing enterocolitis: 1975-1984. Pediatr Surg Int 1994;1:210–17.

194. Albanese CT, Rowe MI, et al. Necrotizing enterocolitis. In: O'Neill JA Jr, Rowe MI, Grosfeld J, editors. Pediatric Surgery. St. Louis: Mosby; 1998. p. 1297–320.

195. Thompson JS, Quigley EMM, Adrian TE. Effect of intestinal tapering and lengthening on intestinal structure and function. Am J Surg 1995;169:111–19.

196. Goulet OJ, Revillon Y, Jan D, et al. Neonatal short bowel syndrome. J Pediatr 1991;119:18–23.

197. Georgeson KE, Breaux CW Jr. Outcome and intestinal adaptation in neonatal short-bowel syndrome. J Pediatr Surg 1992;27:344–50.

198. Chaet MS, Farrell MK, Ziegler MM, et al. Intensive nutritional support and remedial surgical intervention for extreme short bowel syndrome. J Pediatr Gastroenterol Nutr 1994;19:295–8.

199. Fasoli L, Turi RA, Spitz L, et al. Necrotizing enterocolitis: Extent of disease and surgical treatment. J Pediatr Surg 1999;34:1096–9.

200. Andorsky DJ, Lund DP, Lillehei CW, et al. Nutritional and other postoperative management of neonates with short bowel syndrome correlates with clinical outcomes. J Pediatr 2001;139:27–33.

201. Cooper A, Floyd TF, Ross AJ 3rd, et al. Morbidity and mortality of short-bowel syndrome acquired in infancy: An update. J Pediatr Surg 1984;19:711–18.

202. Weber TR, Tracy T Jr, Connors RH. Short-bowel syndrome in children: Quality of life in an era of improved survival. Arch Surg 1991;126:841–6.

203. Gauderer MW, et al. Stomas of the small and large intestine. In: O'Neill JA Jr, Rowe MI, Grosfeld J, editors. Pediatric Surgery. St. Louis, CV: Mosby; 1998. p. 1349–59.

204. Musemeche CA, Kosloske AM, Ricketts RR. Enterostomy in necrotizing enterocolitis: An analysis of techniques and timing of closure. J Pediatr Surg 1987;22:479–83.

205. Alaish SM, Krummel TM, Bagwell CE, et al. Loop enterostomy in newborns with necrotizing enterocolitis. J Am Coll Surg 1996;182:457–8.

206. O'Connor A, Sawin RS. High morbidity of enterostomy and its closure in premature infants with necrotizing enterocolitis. Arch Surg 1998;133:875–80.

207. Lemelle JL, Schmitt M, de Miscault G, et al. Neonatal necrotizing enterocolitis: A retrospective and multicentric review of 331 cases. Acta Paediatr Suppl 1994;396:70–3.

208. Haberlik A, Hollwarth ME, Windhager U, et al. Problems of ileostomy in necrotizing enterocolitis. Acta Paediatr Suppl 1994;396:74–6.

209. Cogbill TH, Millikan JS. Reconstitution of intestinal continuity after resection for neonatal necrotizing enterocolitis. Surg Gynecol Obstet 1985;160:330–4.

210. Gertler JP, Seashore JH, Touloukian RJ. Early ileostomy closure in necrotizing enterocolitis. J Pediatr Surg 1987;22:140–3.

211. Sugarman ID, Kiely EM. Is there a role for high jejunostomy in the management of severe necrotizing enterocolitis? Pediatr Surg Int 2001;17:122–4.

212. Ricketts RR. Surgical therapy for necrotizing enterocolitis. Ann Surg 1984;200:653–7.

213. O'Neill JA Jr, Holcomb GW Jr. Surgical experience with neonatal necrotizing enterocolitis (NNE). Ann Surg 1979;189:612–19.

214. Rowe MI. Necrotizing enterocolitis. In: Welch KJ, Randolph JG, Ravitch MM, editors. Pediatric Surgery. Chicago: Year Book Medical; 1986. p. 944–58.

215. Gobet R, Sacher P, Schwobel MG. Surgical procedures in colonic strictures after necrotizing enterocolitis. Acta Paediatr Suppl 1994;396:77–9.

216. Schullinger JN, Mollitt DL, Vinocur CD, et al. Neonatal necrotizing enterocolitis: Survival, management, and complications: A 25-year study. Am J Dis Child 1981;135:612–14.

217. Schimpl G, Hollwarth ME, Fotter R, et al. Late intestinal strictures following successful treatment of necrotizing enterocolitis. Acta Paediatr Suppl 1994;396:80–3.

218. Radhakrishnan J, Blechman G, Shrader C, et al. Colonic strictures following successful medical management of necrotizing enterocolitis: A prospective study evaluating early gastrointestinal contrast studies. J Pediatr Surg 1991;26:1043–6.

219. Hartman GE, Drugas GT, Shochat SJ. Post-necrotizing enterocolitis strictures presenting with sepsis or perforation: Risk of clinical observation. J Pediatr Surg 1988;23:562–6.

220. Butter A, Flageole H, Laberge JM. The changing face of surgical indications for necrotizing enterocolitis. J Pediatr Surg 2002;37:496–9.

221. Kosloske AM, Burstein J, Bartow SA. Intestinal obstruction due to colonic stricture following neonatal necrotizing enterocolitis. Ann Surg 1980;192:202–7.

222. Weber TR, Tracy TF Jr, Silen ML, et al. Enterostomy and its closure in newborns. Arch Surg 1995;130:534–7.

223. Bell MJ, Ternberg JL, Askin FB, et al. Intestinal stricture in necrotizing enterocolitis. J Pediatr Surg 1976;11:319–27.

224. Schwartz MZ, Richardson CJ, Hayden CK, et al. Intestinal stenosis following successful medical management of necrotizing enterocolitis. J Pediatr Surg 1980;15:890–9.

225. Kosloske AM. Surgery of necrotizing enterocolitis. World J Surg 1985;9:277–84.

226. Janik JS, Ein SH, Mancer K. Intestinal stricture after necrotizing enterocolitis. J Pediatr Surg 1981;16:438–43.

227. Robertson JF, Azmy AF, Young DG. Surgery for necrotizing enterocolitis. Br J Surg 1987;74:387–9.

228. Born M, Holgersen LO, Shahrivar F, et al. Routine contrast enemas for diagnosing and managing strictures following nonoperative treatment of necrotizing enterocolitis. J Pediatr Surg 1985;20:461–3.

229. Tonkin IL, Bjelland JC, Hunter TB, et al. Spontaneous resolution of colonic strictures caused by necrotizing enterocolitis: Therapeutic implications. AJR Am J Roentgenol 1978;130:1077–81.

230. Ball WS Jr, Kosloske AM, Jewell PF, et al. Balloon catheter dilatation of focal intestinal strictures following necrotizing enterocolitis. J Pediatr Surg 1985;20:637–9.

231. Stanford A, Upperman JS, Boyle P, et al. Long-term follow-up of patients with necrotizing enterocolitis. J Pediatr Surg 2002;37:1048–50.

232. Orellana CB, Orellana FA, Friesen C. Long-term follow-up: Neurodevelopmental outcome and gastrointestinal function in infants < 801 grams diagnosed with necrotizing enterocolitis. Pediatr Res 2003;54:773–82.

233. Whiteman L, Wuethrich M, Egan E. Infants who survive necrotizing enterocolitis. Matern Child Nurs J 1985;14:123–33.

234. Sonntag J, Grimmer I, Scholz T, et al. Growth and neurodevelopmental outcome of very low birthweight infants with necrotizing enterocolitis. Acta Paediatr 2000;89:528–32.

235. Walsh MC, Kliegman RM, Hack M. Severity of necrotizing enterocolitis: Influence on outcome at 2 years of age. Pediatrics 1989;84:808–14.

236. Stevenson DK, Kerner JA, Malachowski N, et al. Late morbidity among survivors of necrotizing enterocolitis. Pediatrics 1980;66:925–7.

237. Cikrit D, West KW, Schreiner R, et al. Long-term follow-up after surgical management of necrotizing enterocolitis: Sixty-three cases. J Pediatr Surg 1986;21:533–5.

238. Castro L, Yolton K, Haberman B, et al. Bias in reported neurodevelopmental outcomes among extremely low birth weight survivors. Pediatrics 2004;114:404–10.

239. Hintz SR, Kendrick DE, Stoll BJ, et al. Neurodevelopmental and growth outcomes of extremely low birth weight infants after necrotizing enterocolitis. Pediatrics 2005;115:696–703.

240. Schulzke SM, Deshpande GC, Patole SK. Neurodevelopmental outcomes of very low-birth-weight infants with necrotizing enterocolitis: A systematic review of observational studies [review]. Arch Pediatr Adolesc Med 2007;161:583–90.

241. Rees CM, Pierro A, Eaton S. Neurodevelopmental outcomes of neonates with medically and surgically treated necrotizing enterocolitis [review]. Arch Dis Child Fetal Neonatal Ed 2007; 92:F193–F8.

242. Svenningsen N, Lindroth M, Lindquist B. A comparative study of varying protein intake in low birth weight infant feeding. Acta Paediatr Scand Suppl 1982;296:28–31.

243. Gross S. Growth and biochemical response of preterm infants fed human milk or modified infant formula. N Engl J Med 1983;308:237–41.

244. Tyson JE, Lasky RE, Mize CE. Growth, metabolic response, and development in very-low-birth-weight infants fed banked human milk or enriched formula. J Pediatr 1983;103:95–104.

245. Cooper PA, Rothberg AD, Pettifor J. Growth and biochemical response of premature infants fed pooled preterm milk or special formula. J Pediatr Gastroenterol Nutr 1984;3:749–54.

246. Lucas A, Cole T. Breast milk and neonatal necrotising enterocolitis. Lancet 1990;336:1519–23.

247. Boyd CA, Quigley MA, Brocklehurst P. Donor breast milk versus infant formula for preterm infants: Systematic review and meta-analysis [see comment]. Arch Dis Child Fetal Neonatal Ed 2007;92:F169–F75.

248. McGuire W, Anthony MY. Donor human milk versus formula for preventing necrotizing enterocolitis in preterm infants. Arch Dis Child Fetal Neonatal Ed 2003;88:F11–F15.

249. Sullivan S, Schanler RJ, Kim JH, et al. An exclusively human milk-based diet is associated with a lower rate of necrotizing enterocolitis than a diet of human milk and bovine milk-based products. J Pediatr 2010;156:562–7.

250. Kuschel CA, Harding JE. Multicomponent fortified human milk for promoting growth in preterm infants. Cochrane Database Syst Rev CD000343, 2002.

251. Kennedy KA, Tyson JE. Early versus delayed initiation of progressive enteral feedings for parenterally fed low birth weight or preterm infants. Cochrane Database Syst Rev CD001970, 2000

252. Kennedy KA, Tyson JE. Rapid versus slow rate of advancement of feedings for promoting growth and preventing necrotizing enterocolitis in parenterally fed low-birth-weight infants. Cochrane Database Syst Rev CD001241, 1998.

253. Berseth CL, Bisquera JA, Paje VU. Prolonging small feeding volumes early in life decreases the incidence of necrotizing enterocolitis in very low birth weight infants [see comment]. Pediatrics 2003;111:529–34.

254. Amin HJ, Zamora SA, McMillan DD, et al. Arginine supplementation prevents necrotizing enterocolitis in the premature infant [see comment]. J Pediatr 2002;140:425–31.

255. Shah P, Shah V. Arginine supplementation for prevention of necrotising enterocolitis in preterm infants. Cochrane Database Syst Rev CD004339, 2011

256. Becker RM, Wu G, Galanko JA, et al. Reduced serum amino acid concentrations in infants with necrotizing enterocolitis [see comment]. J Pediatr 2000;137:785–93.

257. Vaughn P, Thomas P, Clark R. Enteral glutamine supplementation and morbidity in low birth weight infants. J Pediatr 2003;142:662–8.

258. Poindexter BB, Ehrenkranz RA, Stoll BJ. Parenteral glutamine supplementation does not reduce the risk of mortality or late-onset sepsis in extremely low birth weight infants. Pediatrics 2004;113:1209–15.

259. Tubman TRJ, Thompson SW, McGuire W. Glutamine supplementation to prevent morbidity and mortality in preterm infants. Cochrane Database Syst Rev CD001457, 2008.

260. Bury RG, Tudehope D. Enteral antibiotics for preventing necrotising enterocolitis in low birthweight or preterm infants. Cochrane Database Syst Rev 2001.CD000405, 2001.

261. Martin CR, Walker WA. Probiotics: Role in pathophysiology and prevention in necrotizing enterocolitis. Semin Perinatol 2008;32:127–37.

262. Panigrahi P, Gupta S, Gewolb IH, et al. Occurrence of necrotizing enterocolitis may be dependent on patterns of bacterial adherence and intestinal colonization: Studies in Caco-2 tissue culture and weanling rabbit models. Pediatr Res 1994;36:115–21.

263. Mack DR, Michail S, Wei SH. Probiotics inhibit enteropathogenic E. coli adherence in vitro by inducing intestinal mucin gene expression. Am J Physiol 1999;276:G941–G50.

264. Madsen KL, Cornish A, Soper P. Probiotic bacteria enhance murine and human intestinal epithelial barrier function. Gastroenterology 2001;121:580–91.

265. Kennedy RJ, Kirk SJ, Gardiner K. Mucosal barrier function and the commensal flora. Gut 2002;50:441–2.

266. Orrhage K, Nord CE. Factors controlling the bacterial colonization of the intestine in breastfed infants. Acta Paediatr Suppl 1999;88:47–57.

267. Stratiki Z, Costalos C, Sevastiadou S. The effect of a Bifidobacter-supplemented bovine milk on intestinal permeability of preterm infants. Early Hum Dev 2007;83:575–9.

268. Bernet MF, Brassart D, Neeser JR. Lactobacillus acidophilus LA 1 binds to cultured human intestinal cell lines and inhibits cell attachment and cell invasion by enterovirulent bacteria. Gut 1994;35:483–9.

269. Collins MD, Gibson G. Probiotics, prebiotics and synbiotics: Approaches for modulating the microbial ecology of the gut. Am J Clin Nutr 1999;69:1052S–7S.

270. Sudo N, Sawamura S, Tanaka K. The requirement of intestinal bacterial flora for the development of an IgE production system fully susceptible to oral tolerance induction. J Immunol 1997;159:1739–45.

271. Fukushima Y, Kawata Y, Hara H. Effect of a probiotic formula on intestinal immunoglobulin A production in healthy children. Int J Food Microbiol 1998;42:39–44.

272. Schiffrin EJ, Rochat F, Link-Amster H. Immunomodulation of human blood cells following the ingestion of lactic acid bacteria. J Dairy Sci 1995;78:491–7.

273. Marin ML, Tejada-Simon MV, Lee JH. Stimulation of cytokine production in clonal macrophage and T-cell models by Streptococcus thermophilus: Comparison with Bifidobacterium sp. and Lactobacillus bulgaricus. J Food Prot 1998;61:859–64.

274. Murch SH. Toll of allergy reduced by probiotics. Lancet 2001;357:1057–9.

275. Klinman DM, Yi AK, Beaucage SL. CpG motifs present in bacteria DNA rapidly induce lymphocytes to secrete interleukin 6, interleukin 12 and interferon gamma. Proc Natl Acad Sci U S A 1996;93:2879–81.

276. Fujii T, Ohtsuka Y, Lee T. Bifidobacterium breve enhances transforming growth factor beta1 signaling by regulating Smad7 expression in preterm infants. J Pediatr Gastroenterol Nutr 2006;43:83–8.

277. Kitajima H, Sumida Y, Tanaka R. Early administration of Bifidobacterium breve to preterm infants: Randomized controlled trial. Arch Dis Child Fetal Neonatal Ed 1997;76:F101–F7.

278. Mohan R, Koebnick C, Schildt J. Effects of Bifidobacterium lactis B12 supplementation on intestinal microbiota of preterm infants: A double-blind, placebo-controlled, randomized study. J Clin Microbiol 2006;44:4025–31.

279. Hoyos AB. Reduced incidence of necrotizing enterocolitis associated with enteral administration of Lactobacillus acidophilus and Bifidobacterium infantis to neonates in an intensive care unit. Int J Infect Dis 1999;3:197–202.

280. Deshpande G, Rao S, Patole S. Probiotics for prevention of necrotising enterocolitis in preterm neonates with very low birthweight: A systematic review of randomised controlled trials. Lancet 2007;369:1614–20.

281. Dani C, Biadaioli R, Bertini G, et al. Probiotics feeding in prevention of urinary tract infection, bacterial sepsis and necrotizing enterocolitis in preterm infants. A prospective double-blind study. Biol Neonate 2002;82:103–8.

282. Lin HC, Su BH, Chen AC, et al. Oral probiotics reduce the incidence and severity of necrotizing enterocolitis in very low birth weight infants. Pediatrics 2005;115:1–4.

283. Bin-Num A, Bromiker R, Wilschanski M, et al. Oral probiotics prevent necrotizing enterocolitis in very low birth weight neonates. J Pediatr 2005;147:192–6.

284. Kitajima H, Sumida Y, Tanaka R, et al. Early administration of Bifidobacterium breve to preterm infants: Randomized conrolled trial. Arch Dis Child 1997;76:F101–7.

285. Costalos C, Skouteri V, Gounaris A, et al. Enteral feeding of premature infants with Saccharomyces boulardii. Early Hum Dev 2003;74:89–96.

286. Manzoni P, Mostert M, Leonessa ML, et al. Oral supplementation with Lactobacillus casei subspecies rhamnosus prevents enteric colonization by Candida species in preterm neonates: A randomized study. Clin Infect Dis 2006;42:1735–42.

287. Mohan R, Koebnick C, Schildt J, et al. Effects of Bifidobacterium lactis Bb12 supplementation on intestinal microbiota of preterm neonates: A double placebo controlled, randomized study. J Clin Microbiol 2006;44:4025–31.

288. Manzoni P, Rinaldi M, Cattani S, et al. Bovine lactoferrin supplementation for prevention of late-onset sepsis in very low-birth-weight neonates: A randomized trial. JAMA 2009 7;302: 1421–8.

289. Braga TD, da Silva GA, de Lira PI, et al. Efficacy of Bifidobacterium breve and Lactobacillus casei oral supplementation on necrotizing enterocolitis in very-low-birth-weight preterm infants: a double-blind, randomized, controlled trial. Am J Clin Nutr 2011;93:81–6.

290. Lin HC, Hsu CH, Chen HL, et al. Oral probiotics prevent necrotizing enterocolitis in very low birth weight preterm infants: a multicenter, randomized, controlled trial. Pediatrics 2008;122: 693–700.

291. Barclay AR, Stenson B, Simpson JH, et al. Probiotics for necrotizing enterocolitis: A systematic review. J Pediatr Gastroenterol Nutr 2007;45:569–76.

292. Wang Q, Dong J, Zhu Y. Probiotic supplement reduces risk of necrotizing enterocolitis and mortality in preterm very low-birth-weight infants: An updated meta-analysis of 20 randomized, controlled trials. J Pediatr Surg 2012;47:241–8.

293. Nair RR, Warner BB, Warner BW. Role of epidermal growth factor and other growth factors in the prevention of necrotizing enterocolitis. Semin Perinatol 2008;32:107–13.

294. Grave GD, Nelson SA, Walker WA, et al. New therapies and preventive approaches for necrotizing enterocolitis: Report of a research planning workshop. Pediatr Res 2007;62:510–14.

295. Moss RL, Kalish LA, Duggan C, et al. Clinical parameters do not adequately predict outcome in necrotizing enterocolitis: Results from a prospective multi-institutional study. J Perinatol 2008;28: 657–64.

CHAPTER 34

HIRSCHSPRUNG DISEASE

Jacob C. Langer

Hirschsprung disease (HD), also known as 'congenital megacolon' is characterized by the absence of ganglion cells in the myenteric and submucosal plexuses of the intestine. The first known description of this condition was by ancient Hindu surgeons in the Shushruta Samheta,[1] and the first descriptions in the modern medical literature were from the 17th century.[2] In 1887, Harald Hirschsprung, a pediatrician from Copenhagen, described two cases of the condition that ultimately bore his name.[3] At that time most children with congenital megacolon died from malnutrition and enterocolitis. As the underlying pathological basis of the disease was unknown, surgeons removed the massively dilated proximal bowel and created a colostomy. Attempts at re-anastomosis were uniformly unsuccessful.[4]

Although the absence of ganglion cells in the distal colon of a child with HD was first noted by Tittel in 1901[5] and subsequent publications repeated this observation, it took many decades for clinicians caring for these children to become aware. The first recognition of aganglionosis by a surgeon as the cause of congenital megacolon was by Ehrenpreis in 1946.[6] This was followed in 1949 by Swenson's first description of a reconstructive operation for HD.[7] Although Swenson's operation was originally performed without a colostomy, technical difficulties in small infants and the debilitated and malnourished state in which many children presented were reasons most surgeons adopted a multi-staged approach with colostomy as the initial step.[8] In recent years, improvements in operative technique and earlier diagnosis have resulted in an evolution toward one-stage and minimal access procedures. These advances have resulted in significantly improved morbidity and mortality in infants with HD.

INCIDENCE AND SPECTRUM OF DISEASE

HD occurs in approximately 1:5,000 live births. Approximately 80% of children have a 'transition zone' in the rectum or rectosigmoid colon. Another 10% have more proximal colonic involvement, and about 5–10% have total colonic aganglionosis with variable involvement of the distal small intestine. Rarely, babies are afflicted with near-total intestinal aganglionosis.

A number of syndromes are associated with HD including trisomy 21, congenital central hypoventilation syndrome, Goldberg–Shprintzen syndrome, Smith–Lemli–Opitz syndrome, neurofibromatosis, and neuroblastoma (Box 34-1).

ETIOLOGY AND GENETIC BASIS OF DISEASE

Ganglion cells are derived from the neural crest. By 13 weeks post-conception, the neural crest cells have migrated from proximal to distal through the gastrointestinal tract, after which they differentiate into mature ganglion cells.[9] There are two main theories why this process is disturbed in children with HD. The first possibility is that the neural crest cells never reach the distal intestine due to early maturation or differentiation into ganglion cells. Data supporting this theory come from animal models showing spontaneous aganglionosis[10,11] and from studies of normal neural crest cell migration performed in chick embryos and human fetuses.[12,13] The second possibility is that the neural crest cells reach their destination, but fail to survive or differentiate into ganglion cells due to an inhospitable microenvironment.[14,15] It is likely that HD is actually a heterogeneous group of diseases with multiple genetic causes and etiologies.

A genetic basis for HD has long been suspected because of the presence of a family history in many cases and the known association with trisomy 21 and other genetically based conditions. Over the past two decades, an increasing number of researchers have made significant progress in identifying and elucidating the complex array of genetic mutations and mechanisms responsible for this disease.[16–18] The first and most common gene to be identified is the *RET* proto-oncogene, which encodes a tyrosine kinase receptor. Many mutations of this gene and related genes, such as neurturin and glial cell line-derived neurotrophic factor (GDNF), have been described. It remains unclear how these mutations result in aganglionosis, but there is evidence that early neuronal cell death may be a prominent mechanism.[19,20] RET abnormalities are most commonly found in patients with familial and long-segment involvement. Mutations in the endothelin family of genes, particularly endothelin-3 and the endothelin-B receptor, are also commonly associated with HD. Many of these children have other neurocristopathies such as dysfunction of melanocytes, congenital deafness, central hypoventilation, and neuroblastoma. From animal models, there is evidence that mutations in the endothelin and SOX-10 genes may produce early maturation or differentiation of neural crest cells, which decreases the number of available progenitor cells and prevents the neural crest cells from migrating any further.[21,22] Other genes associated with HD include *S1P1* (now known as *ZFHX1B*), *Phox2B*, and the Hedgehog/Notch complex.[23]

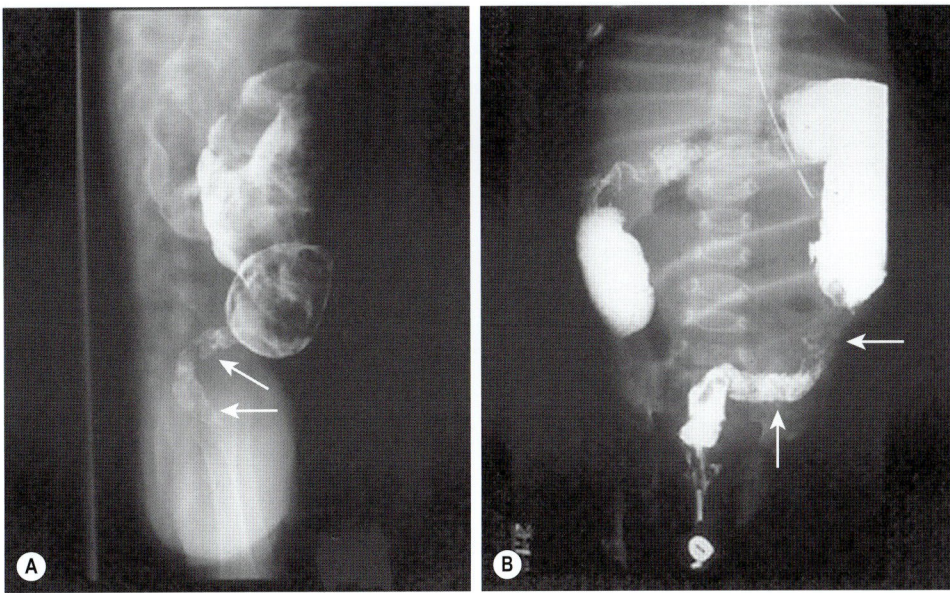

FIGURE 34-1 ■ These two barium enema examinations in different infants demonstrate Hirschsprung disease. The aganglionic rectum (arrows) in both studies is small and contracted. The proximal ganglionic colon is dilated. A transition zone between the aganglionic and ganglionic colon is nicely seen in both studies.

BOX 34-1	Congenital Anomalies and Conditions Commonly Associated with Hirschsprung Disease

Down syndrome (trisomy 21)
Neurocristopathy syndromes
   Waardenberg–Shah syndrome
   Yemenite deaf-blind-hypopigmentation
   Piebaldism
   Other hypopigmentation syndromes
Goldberg–Shprintzen syndrome
Smith–Lemli–Opitz syndrome
Multiple endocrine neoplasia 2
Congenital central hypoventilation syndrome (Ondine's curse)
Isolated congenital anomalies
   Congenital heart disease
   Malrotation
   Urinary tract anomalies
   Central nervous system anomalies
   Other

CLINICAL PRESENTATION AND DIAGNOSIS

Prenatal diagnosis of HD is rare, and is usually due to total colonic disease resulting in ultrasound (US) findings of fetal intestinal obstruction.[24] Most affected patients present during the neonatal period with abdominal distension, bilious vomiting, and feeding intolerance. Delayed passage of meconium beyond the first 24 hours is present in approximately 90%. Occasionally, cecal or appendiceal perforation may be the initial event.[25] Plain radiographs characteristically show dilated bowel loops throughout the abdomen. The next step is a water-soluble contrast enema. The pathognomonic finding of HD is a

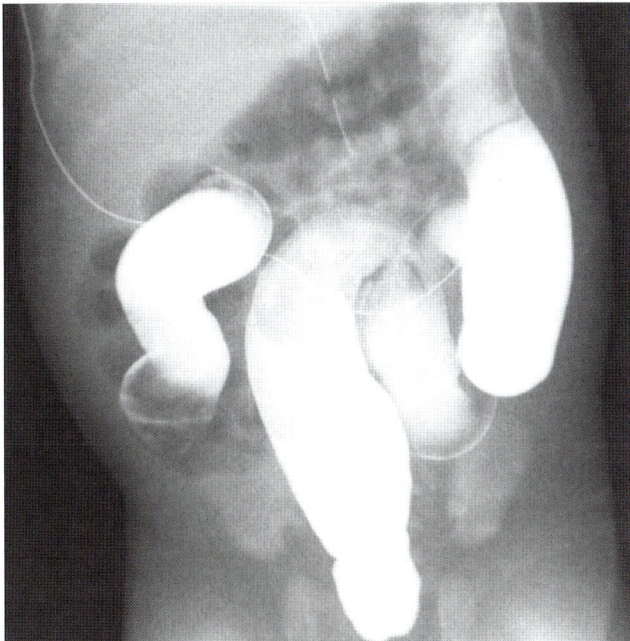

FIGURE 34-2 ■ Retention of contrast is seen on this post-evacuation film which was obtained 24 hours after the contrast enema.

transition zone between the normal and aganglionic bowel (Fig. 34-1), although approximately 10% of neonates with HD may not have a demonstrable radiological transition zone.[26] Occasionally, false positive studies occur.[27] It is also important to obtain a plain radiograph 24 hours later. Retention of the contrast is very suggestive for HD (Fig. 34-2). It is also important to use a water-soluble material as the enema potentially may be a definitive treatment for other conditions in the differential diagnosis, such as meconium ileus and meconium plug syndrome. Once the diagnosis of HD is suspected, the diagnosis must be confirmed by rectal biopsy, which in the neonate can be done at the bedside without sedation and using a suction technique.

Patients presenting later in childhood have chronic severe constipation. As constipation is common in children, it can be difficult to differentiate HD from more common causes. Clinical features pointing to the diagnosis include delayed passage of meconium at birth, failure to thrive, abdominal distention, and dependence on enemas without significant encopresis.[28] Although a contrast enema usually demonstrates a transition zone in older children, a false negative study may be due to massive rectal distension in combination with a very short aganglionic segment. Reversal of the usual rectosigmoid ratio and retention of contrast on a 24-hour postevacuation film also support the diagnosis. Anorectal manometry is another useful screening technique, in which the presence of a recto-anal inhibitory reflex (reflex relaxation of the internal anal sphincter in response to balloon distension of the rectum) essentially rules out HD (Fig. 34-3). In older children, the suction rectal biopsy may be less reliable because of a higher risk of sampling error. Full-thickness biopsies, usually under general anesthesia, may be necessary in these patients.

Approximately 10% of neonates with HD present with fever, abdominal distention, and diarrhea due to Hirschsprung-associated enterocolitis (HAEC), which can be life-threatening. Since HD characteristically causes constipation rather than diarrhea, this presentation may be confusing and the diagnosis may not be considered. A careful history, including a history of delayed passage of meconium and intermittent stooling, should lead to an investigation for HD.

The gold standard for the diagnosis is the absence of ganglion cells in the submucosal and myenteric plexuses on histological examination (Fig. 34-4A). Most patients will also have evidence of hypertrophied nerve trunks (Fig. 34-4B), although this finding is not always present, particularly in children with total colonic disease or a very short aganglionic segment. As there is normally a paucity of ganglion cells in the area 0.5–1.0 cm above the dentate line, the rectal biopsy should be taken at least 1.0–1.5 cm above it. However, a biopsy too proximal may miss a short aganglionic segment. In addition to hematoxylin and eosin, many pathologists also stain for acetylcholinesterase, which has a characteristic pattern in the submucosa and mucosa in children with HD (Fig. 34-5). Recently, it has been shown that immunochemical staining for calretinin is almost always absent in patients with HD (Fig. 34-6).[29]

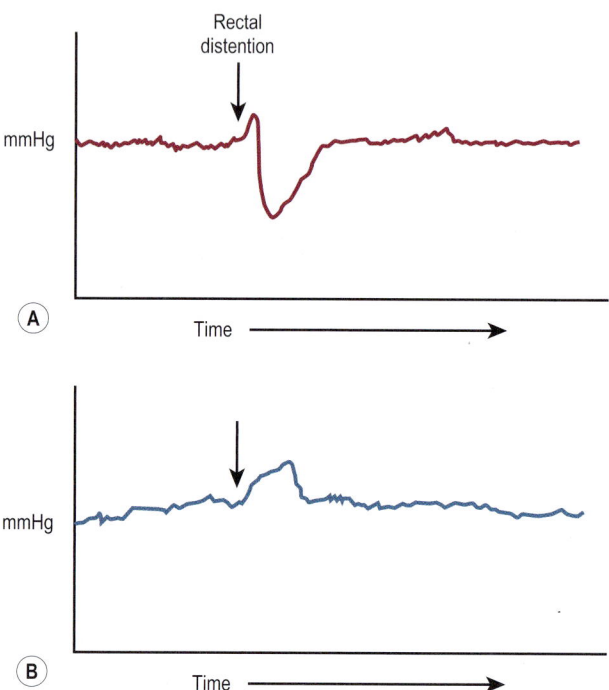

FIGURE 34-3 ■ **(A)** In the child without Hirschsprung disease undergoing anorectal manometry, the recto-anal inhibitory reflex is normal. Note the drop in the internal sphincter pressure with rectal distention. **(B)** A child with Hirschsprung disease is seen to have abnormally increased contraction of the anal canal and no relaxation of the internal sphincter with rectal distention. (The arrow points to the initiation of rectal distention in both A and B.)

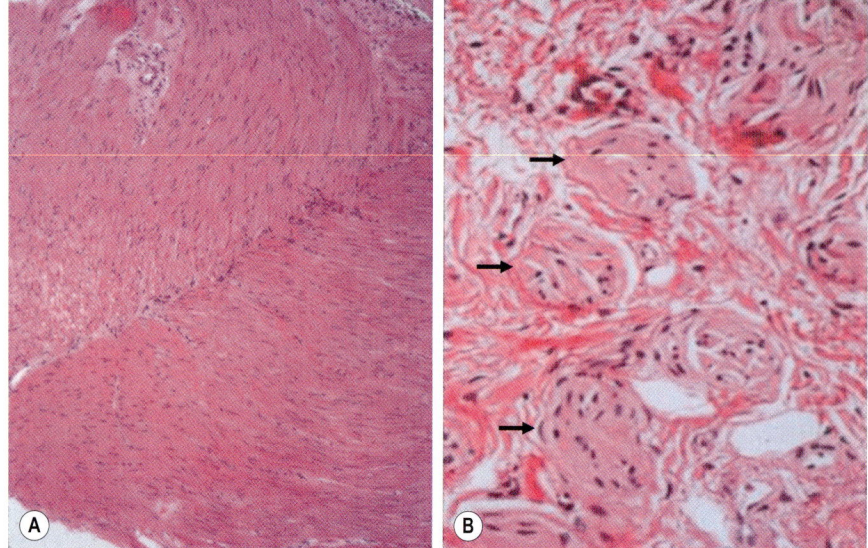

FIGURE 34-4 ■ Histological findings in children with Hirschsprung disease. **(A)** Absence of ganglion cells in the myenteric plexus. **(B)** Hypertrophied nerve trunks are marked with arrows.

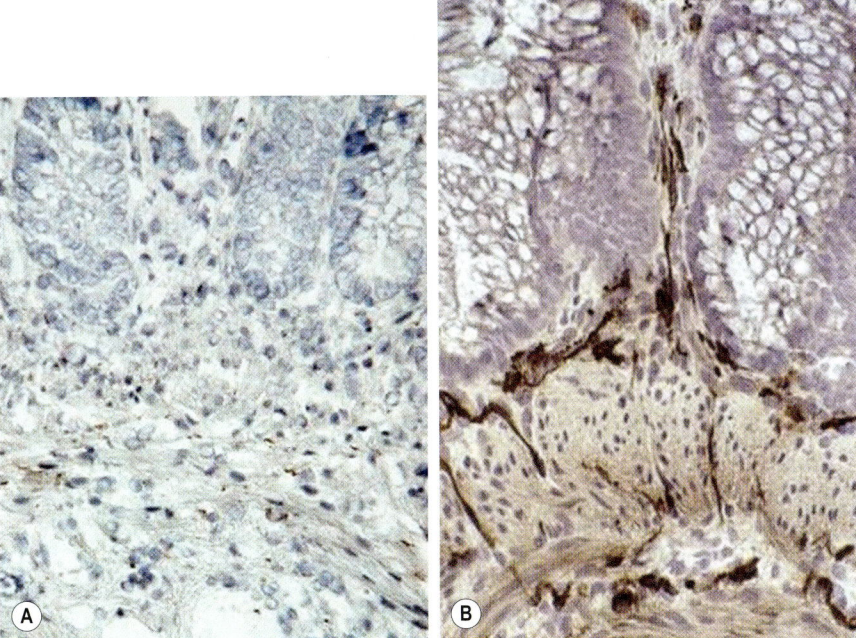

FIGURE 34-5 ■ Cholinesterase staining in **(A)** normal colon and **(B)** colon affected by Hirschsprung disease.

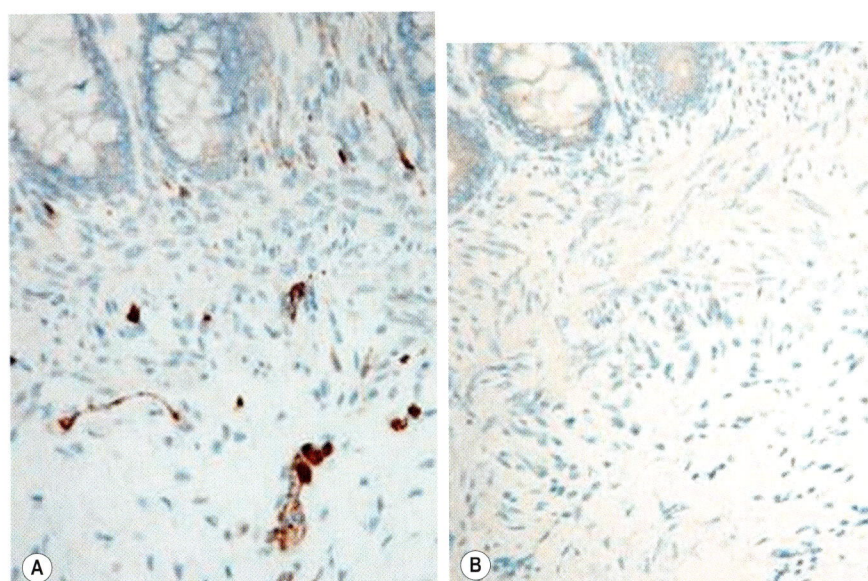

FIGURE 34-6 ■ Calretinin staining in **(A)** normal colon and **(B)** colon affected by Hirschsprung disease.

PREOPERATIVE PREPARATION

Once the diagnosis of HD is made, the child should be appropriately resuscitated with intravenous fluids and treated with broad-spectrum antibiotics, nasogastric drainage, and rectal decompression using rectal stimulation and/or irrigation. Patients with associated abnormalities such as cardiac disease or congenital central hypoventilation syndrome must be thoroughly evaluated prior to operative correction.

Once the infant or child has been resuscitated and stabilized, the operation can be done semi-electively. While waiting, many infants can be discharged home on breast milk or an elemental formula, in combination with rectal stimulations or irrigations. In the older child with an extremely dilated colon, pull-through should be delayed until the diameter of the colon has decreased sufficiently to perform a safe procedure. Weeks or months of irrigations may occasionally be needed. Some of these children may need an initial colostomy to adequately decompress the dilated colon.

Some physicians have advocated nonoperative long-term management of short segment HD using enemas and laxatives. Others have suggested that simple myectomy may be adequate.[30] However, these approaches do not provide a good quality of life for most infants and children with HD, and most pediatric surgeons recommend a pull-through procedure even for short segment disease.

SURGICAL MANAGEMENT

The goals of surgical management for HD are to remove the aganglionic bowel and reconstruct the intestinal tract by bringing the normally innervated bowel down to the anus while preserving normal sphincter function. The most commonly performed operations are the Swenson, Duhamel and Soave procedures, although a number of other operations, such as the Rebhein and State procedures, have been described and are still performed in some centers.[31] As there are very few prospective studies comparing operations, the best operation for an individual patient is the one that the surgeon has been trained to do and does frequently.

Although Swenson's operation was initially developed as a one-stage procedure, the relatively high incidence of stricture, leak, and other adverse outcomes led to the adoption of a routine preliminary colostomy, with definitive pull-through performed three to 12 months later.[32] In the 1980s, a number of surgeons reported series of single-stage pull-through operations even in small infants.[33,34] Over the following ten to 15 years, many reports suggested that a one-stage approach was safe, avoided the morbidity of stomas in infants, and was more cost effective.[35–37] However, a stoma may still be needed for infants and children with severe enterocolitis, perforation, malnutrition, or massively dilated proximal bowel, and in situations when it is not possible to reliably identify the transition zone on frozen section.

Swenson Procedure

The goal of the Swenson pull-through is to remove the entire aganglionic colon, with an end-to-end anastomosis above the anal sphincter. The operation was originally performed via a laparotomy, with the anastomosis being performed from the perineum after everting the aganglionic rectum (Fig. 34-7). It is important to keep the dissection in the correct plane along the rectal wall to avoid injury to the deep pelvic nerves, vessels and other structures such as the vagina, prostate, vas deferens, and seminal vesicles. Despite the theoretical risks inherent in the deep pelvic dissection, long-term functional outcomes after the Swenson procedure are excellent.[38]

Soave Procedure

The Soave procedure, subsequently modified by Boley, was designed to avoid the risk of injury to important pelvic structures by performing a submucosal endorectal dissection and positioning the pull-through bowel within an aganglionic muscular 'cuff' (Fig. 34-8). Despite concerns by some that the Soave procedure may result in long-term constipation due to incomplete excision of the aganglionic rectum,[39] most late follow-up studies have reported similar outcomes between the Soave and Swenson operation.[40]

Duhamel Procedure

The Duhamel procedure involves bringing the normal colon down through the bloodless plane between the rectum and sacrum, and joining the two walls with a linear stapler to create a new lumen which is aganglionic anteriorly and normally innervated posteriorly (Fig. 34-9). The Duhamel operation is felt by many surgeons to be easier and safer than the Swenson or Soave procedures. Also, it results in a very large anastomosis, which reduces the risk of stricture. Reported long term results of the Duhamel procedure have been similar to those with the other two operations, although recent studies suggest that outcomes from the Duhamel procedure are inferior to those of the transanal pull-through.[41,42]

Laparoscopic Pull-through

Georgeson first described the laparoscopic approach for HD in 1995.[43] With this technique, a biopsy is initially performed to identify the transition zone, the rectum is mobilized below the peritoneal reflection, and a short mucosal dissection is performed through a perineal

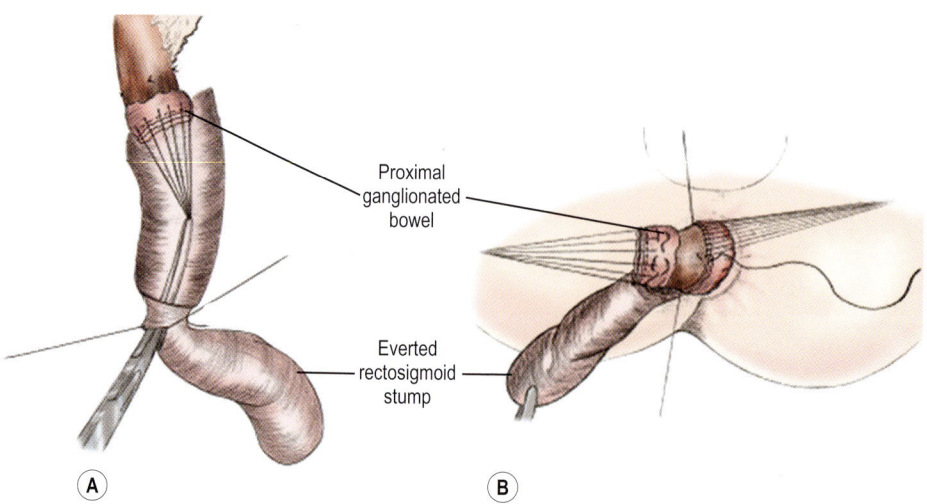

Proximal ganglionated bowel

Everted rectosigmoid stump

(A)   (B)

FIGURE 34-7 ■ The principles of the Swenson pull-through procedure are seen in these drawings. **(A)** The proximal ganglionated bowel is grasped through an incision in the prolapsed rectosigmoid stump. **(B)** The ganglionated bowel is then sewn to the anus.

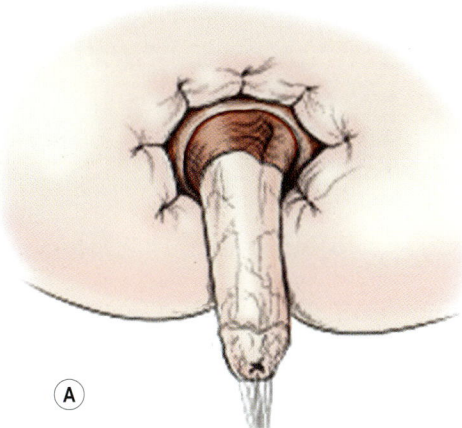

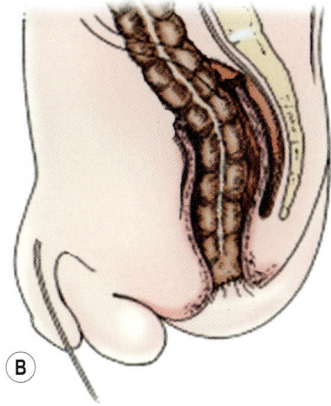

(A)

(B)

FIGURE 34-8 ■ **(A)** For the Soave operation, there is extramucosal dissection of the rectum after circumferential incision of the rectal mucosa. **(B)** The ganglionated colon is pulled through the aganglionic rectal cuff, and a coloanal anastomosis is performed.

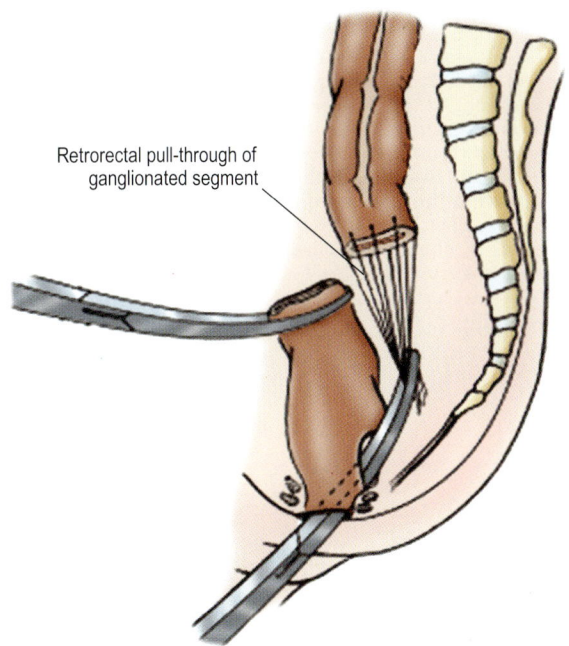

Retrorectal pull-through of ganglionated segment

FIGURE 34-9 ■ With the Duhamel technique, the ganglionated bowel is delivered through an incision in the posterior aspect of the native aganglionic rectum and sewn to the anus. The septum between the ganglionated pull-through colon and the aganglionic native rectum is then divided using a stapler.

approach (Figs 34-10 to 34-14). The rectum is then prolapsed through the anus and the anastomosis performed from below. This procedure is associated with a shorter time in the hospital, and both early and mid-term results appear to be equivalent to those reported for the other procedures.[44] Laparoscopic approaches have been also described for the Duhamel and Swenson operations, with excellent short term results.[45,46]

Transanal (Perineal) Pull-through

The transanal approach was first described by de la Torre in 1998[47] and by Langer in 1999,[48] and has been adopted and reported by an increasing number of surgeons. The

operation can be performed in the prone or lithotomy positions.[49] A mucosal incision is made 0.5–1.0 cm above the dentate line, depending on the size of the child, and the mucosa is stripped from the underlying muscle as in the Soave operation. The length of the submucosal dissection varies according to surgeon, although a shorter rectal cuff may be associated with a lower incidence of enterocolitis and the need for dilatation.[50] Some surgeons do not perform any submucosal dissection, and effectively perform a transanal Swenson procedure.[51]

The rectal muscle is incised circumferentially, and the dissection is continued on the rectal wall, dividing the vessels as they enter the rectum. The entire rectum and part of the sigmoid colon can be delivered through the anus. When the transition zone is reached, the anastomosis is performed from below (Fig. 34-15). In patients with a more proximal transition zone (usually above the proximal sigmoid colon), laparoscopy or a small umbilical incision is needed to mobilize the left colon and/or splenic flexure to achieve an adequate length of ganglionated colon for pull-through.[52] A transanal approach can also be used if the patient has already had a colostomy by using the stoma as the end of the pull-through bowel and performing the rectal excision using the transanal approach.

There is controversy around whether the histological transition zone should be defined prior to beginning the anal dissection. This controversy centers on the fact that approximately 8–10% of children who have a rectosigmoid transition zone on contrast study actually have a more proximal histological transition zone.[53,54] This concern is particularly important for surgeons who perform a different operation for long-segment disease than for rectosigmoid disease. A preliminary biopsy does not have a deleterious effect on postoperative outcomes such as time to feeding, pain, or length of hospitalization.[50,55]

The transanal approach has a low complication rate, requires minimal postoperative analgesia, and is associated with early feeding and discharge.[55,56] Although there have not been any studies comparing the transanal and laparoscopic approaches, the transanal pull-through can be accomplished by most pediatric surgeons, including

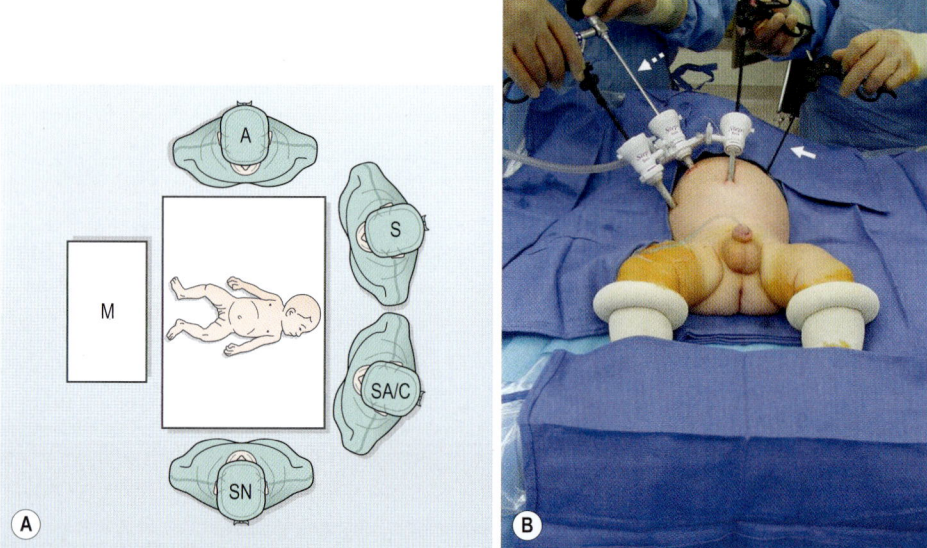

FIGURE 34-10 ■ **(A)** The surgeon (S) and surgical assistant/camera holder (SA/C) stand above the patient's head with the monitor (M) positioned beyond the infant's feet. The scrub nurse (SN) can be positioned according to the surgeon's preference, although being positioned at the foot of the operating table appears to be ideal. A, anesthesiologist. **(B)** The photograph shows port placement for this operation. Usually three or four ports are required. The umbilical port is inserted using an open technique, and the other ports are introduced under direct visualization. The telescope (dotted arrow) is placed through the 5 mm port in the right upper abdomen. The surgeon's two primary working ports are the umbilical port for the left hand and the right lower abdominal port for the right hand. A retracting instrument (solid arrow) is often helpful and can be inserted through a stab incision in the infant's left upper abdomen. A urinary catheter has been introduced to help decompress the bladder. (From Morowitz MJ, Georgeson KE. Laparoscopic assisted pull-through for Hirschsprung's disease. In: Holcomb GW, Georgeson KE, Rothenberg SS, editors. Atlas of Pediatric Laparoscopy and Thoracoscopy. Philadelphia: Elsevier; 2008. p. 101–108. Reprinted with permission.)

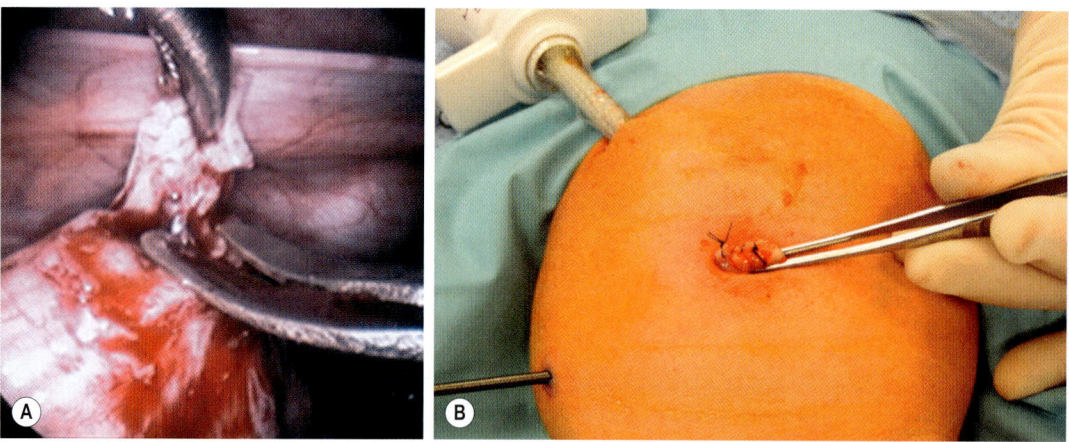

FIGURE 34-11 ■ **(A)** An intracorporeal biopsy is being performed on the sigmoid colon. A fine-tipped grasping forceps has been used to grasp the biopsy site, and Metzenbaum scissors are used to obtain the biopsy specimen. **(B)** This biopsy was performed through the umbilical incision. One port and another instrument have been introduced through the infant's abdominal wall. A site on the colon for the biopsy was visualized and delivered just under the umbilical cannula. The umbilical cannula was removed, and this portion of the colon was grasped and exteriorized. An extracorporeal biopsy was obtained and the biopsy site was closed. This is an alternative means for obtaining the biopsy. (From Morowitz MJ, Georgeson KE. Laparoscopic assisted pull-through for Hirschsprung's disease. In: Holcomb GW, Georgeson KE, Rothenberg SS, editors. Atlas of Pediatric Laparoscopy and Thoracoscopy. Philadelphia: Elsevier; 2008. p. 101–108. Reprinted with permission.)

those without laparoscopic skills, and by pediatric surgeons in parts of the world where access to laparoscopic equipment is limited.

Long-Segment Aganglionosis

Long-segment HD is usually defined as a transition zone which is proximal to the mid-transverse colon. The most common form is total colonic aganglionosis, which usually also includes some of the distal ileum (Fig. 34-16). In rare cases of near-total intestinal aganglionosis, most of the small bowel is aganglionic as well. Most neonates with long-segment disease present with a distal small bowel obstruction, although occasionally children with long-segment disease may not present until after weaning from breast milk. The contrast enema typically shows a shortened, relatively narrow 'question mark' colon (Fig. 34-17).[57] There may also be a transition zone in the small

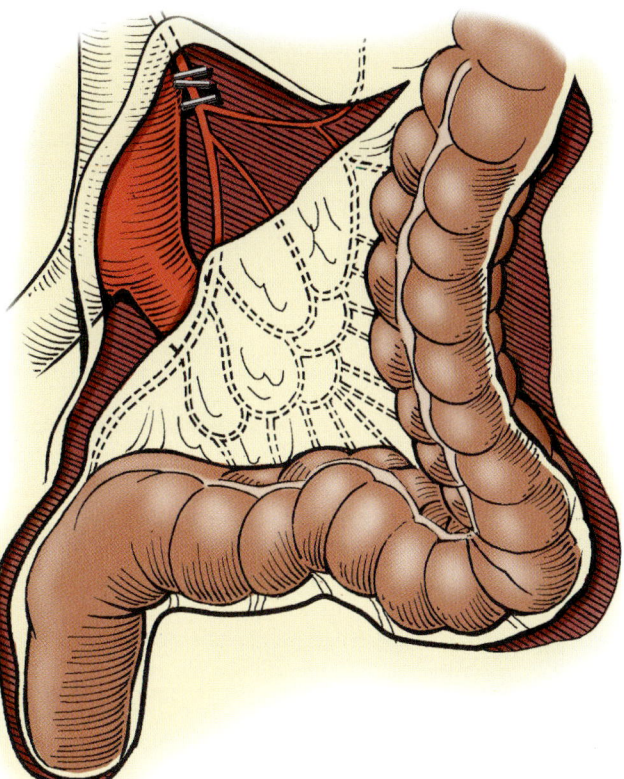

FIGURE 34-12 ■ When the transition zone is proximal to the mid-sigmoid colon, a pedicled colon flap must be developed for the endorectal pull-through. In this situation, the pull-through colon will derive its vascular supply from the marginal artery. Therefore, to mobilize the descending colon and splenic flexure, it is necessary to ligate and divide either the inferior mesenteric artery just distal to its origin from the aorta (as seen in this drawing) or the left colic artery just after it arises from the inferior mesenteric artery. By ligating these vessels at these sites, the arterial supply through the marginal artery is not compromised. (From Morowitz MJ, Georgeson KE. Laparoscopic assisted pull-through for Hirschsprung's disease. In: Holcomb GW, Georgeson KE, Rothenberg SS, editors. Atlas of Pediatric Laparoscopy and Thoracoscopy. Philadelphia: Elsevier; 2008. p. 101–108. Reprinted with permission.)

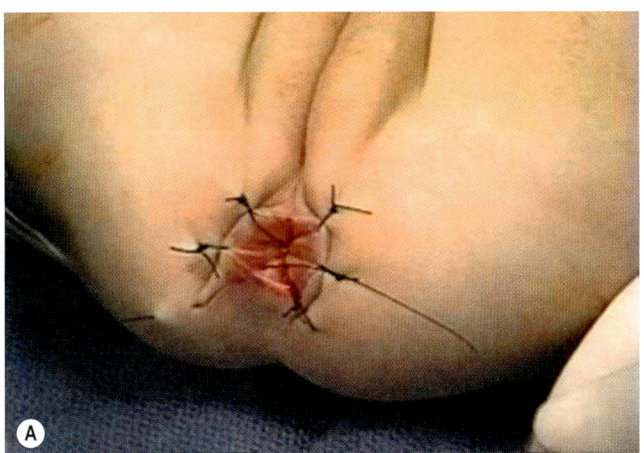

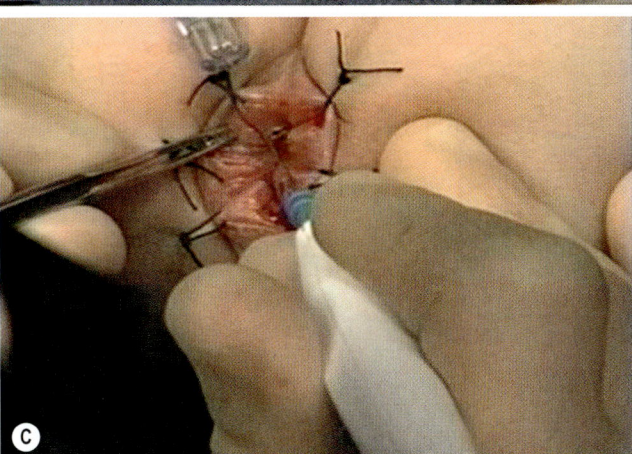

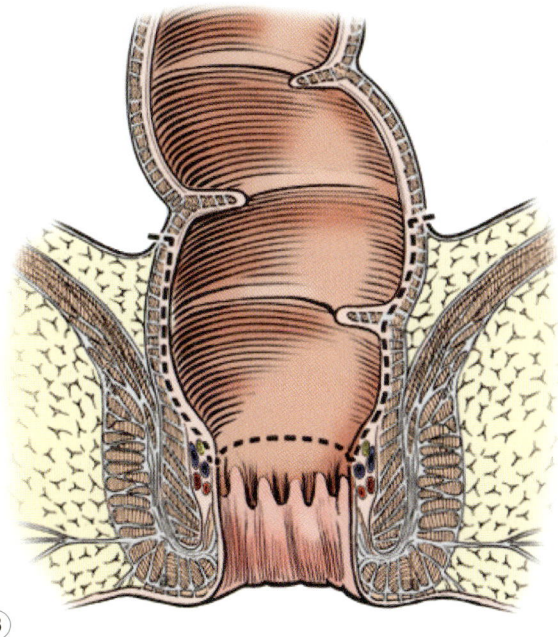

FIGURE 34-13 ■ **(A)** The perineal dissection begins with the placement of circumferential 2-0 silk traction sutures from the dentate line to the perineum 2 to 3 cm outward from the anus. **(B, C)** A needle-tipped electrocautery is used to circumferentially incise the rectal mucosa approximately 5 mm proximal to the anal columns. Fine silk traction sutures are then placed in the rectal mucosa to help retract the mucosa during circumferential dissection. (From Morowitz MJ, Georgeson KE. Laparoscopic assisted pull-through for Hirschsprung's disease. In: Holcomb GW, Georgeson KE, Rothenberg SS, editors. Atlas of Pediatric Laparoscopy and Thoracoscopy. Philadelphia: Elsevier; 2008. p. 101–108. Reprinted with permission.)

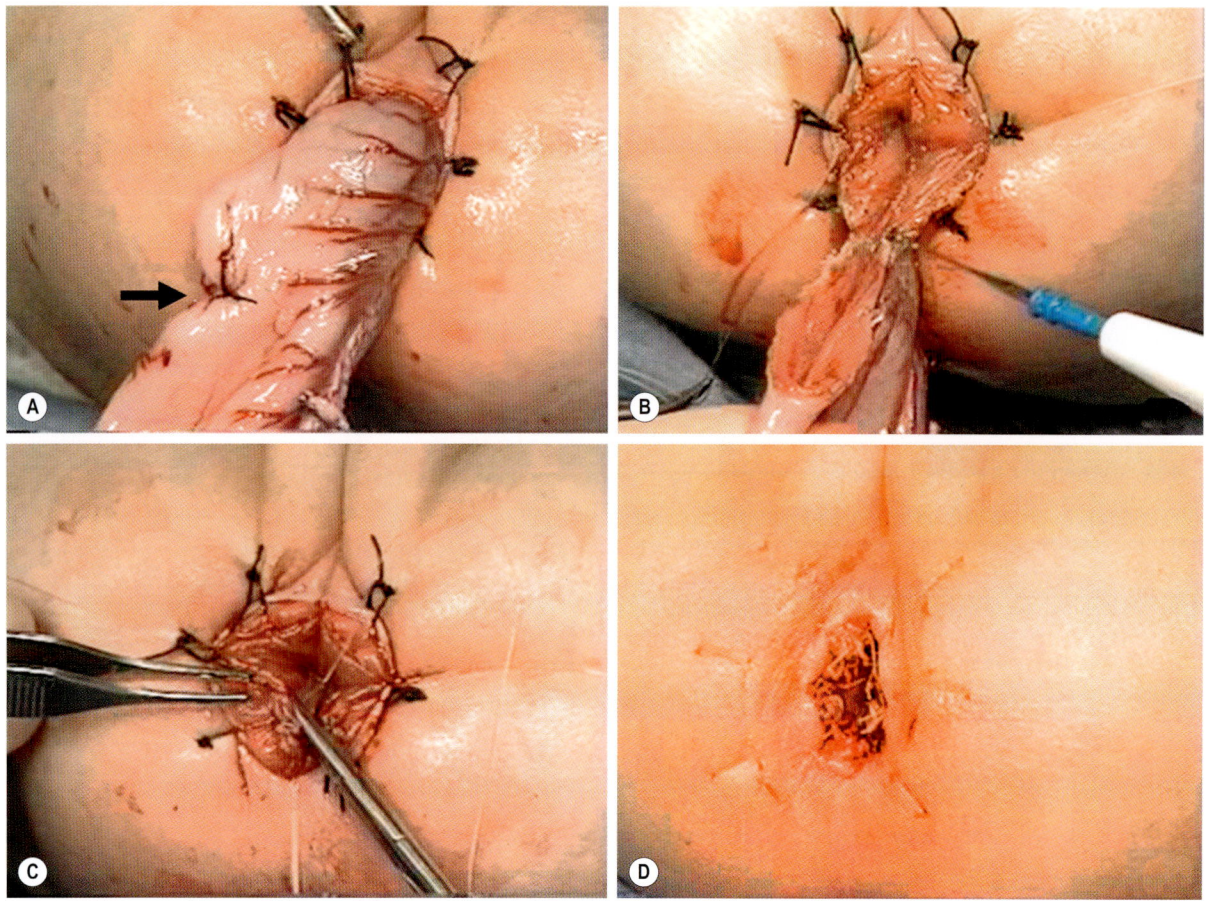

FIGURE 34-14 ■ **(A)** The muscular cuff of the rectum has been divided and the ganglionic colon has been exteriorized through the anal canal. Note that the anastomosis will be performed proximal to the biopsy site (arrow). **(B)** The pull-through colon is being completely transected above the biopsy site and made ready for the coloanal anastomosis. **(C)** The anastomosis is being performed with interrupted 4-0 absorbable sutures. **(D)** The everting stay sutures have been cut, allowing the anastomosis to retract cephalad. (From Morowitz MJ, Georgeson KE. Laparoscopic assisted pull-through for Hirschsprung's disease. In: Holcomb GW, Georgeson KE, Rothenberg SS, editors. Atlas of Pediatric Laparoscopy and Thoracoscopy. Philadelphia: Elsevier; 2008. p. 101–108. Reprinted with permission.)

bowel. The rectal biopsy shows absence of ganglion cells, but in many cases there are no hypertrophic nerves or abnormalities on acetylcholinesterase staining.

The initial operative approach involves sequential colonic biopsies looking for ganglion cells on frozen section. These biopsies can be performed via laparotomy or laparoscopy, or through an umbilical incision. Using the appendix for the initial biopsy can result in a false positive diagnosis of total colonic aganglionosis as there may be a paucity of ganglion cells in the appendix in children with shorter segment disease.[58] Thus, a biopsy of the cecum is preferable. Once the level of aganglionosis is identified, most surgeons create a stoma, wait for permanent sections, and perform the definitive reconstructive procedure later. Although primary pull-through without ileostomy for total colonic disease has been performed, this approach requires a high degree of confidence in the pathologist, since it requires performing a total colectomy on the basis of frozen section analysis alone. In addition, there are many reports of 'skip' areas in children with total colonic aganglionosis so that permanent sections are advisable before considering total colectomy.[59] Finally, some surgeons believe that the

outcomes following pull-through are better once the stool has thickened, which usually occurs after the first few months of life.

There are three types of operations available for children with long-segment disease: straight pull-through using one of the standard techniques (Swenson, Duhamel, or Soave), colon patch using either the left colon (Martin) (Fig. 34-18) or the right colon (Kimura) (Fig. 34-19), and ileal J-pouch. There are no prospective or well-controlled series reporting long-term results of operations for long-segment HD. Although the colon patch procedures theoretically result in decreased stool output due to better water absorption, the aganglionic colon tends to dilate and many of these patients develop severe enterocolitis, requiring removal of the patch or a permanent stoma. Children undergoing a straight pull-through tend to experience gradually decreasing stool frequency over time, with an acceptable quality of life.[60–62]

Rarely, almost the entire intestinal tract is aganglionic, usually leaving 10–40 cm of normally innervated jejunum. These children require total parenteral nutrition (TPN) from birth. At the time of the first exploration, the goal is to determine the extent of aganglionosis based on

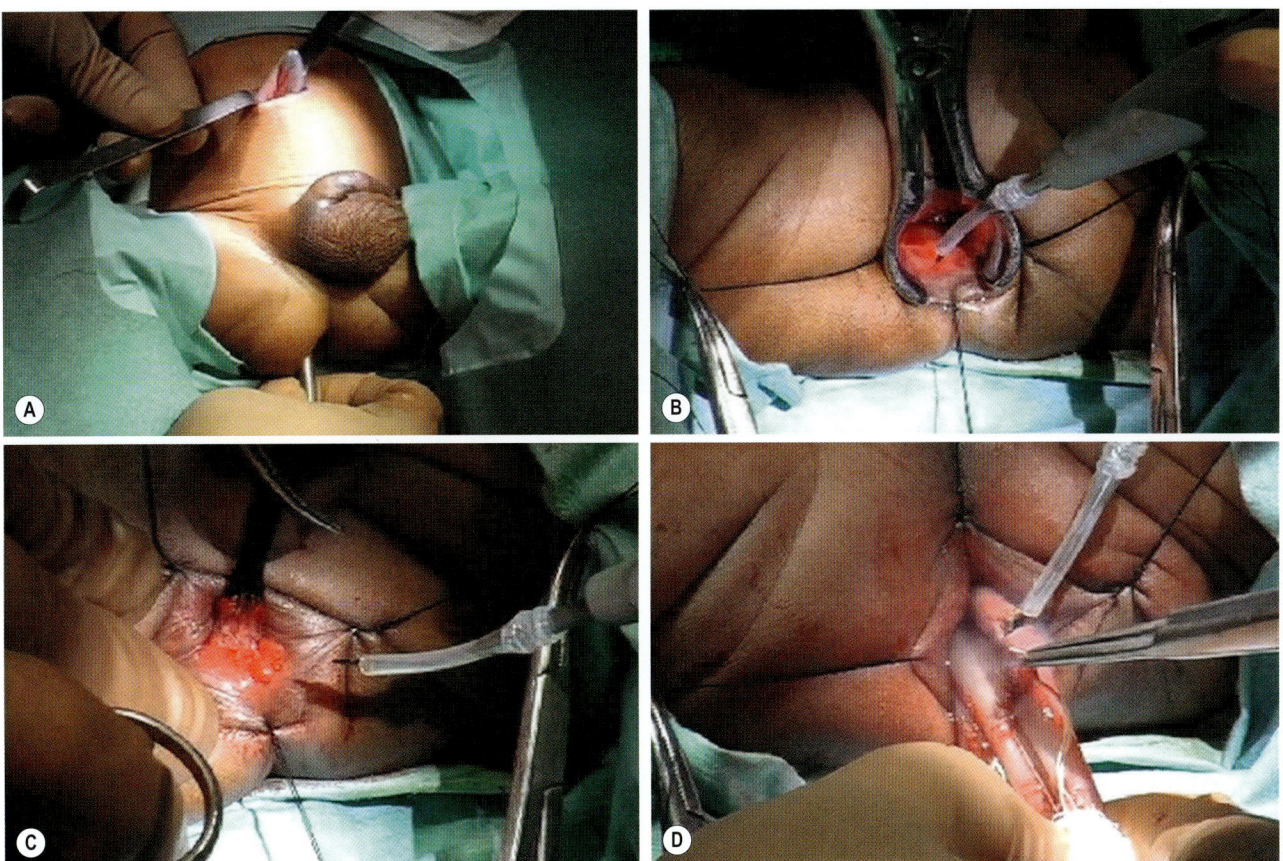

FIGURE 34-15 ■ The salient points for a transanal Soave pull-through are depicted. **(A)** An umbilical incision is used for a preliminary biopsy. A Hegar dilator is used to push the sigmoid colon into the umbilical incision. **(B)** Eversion sutures are placed in the anus, and a nasal speculum is used to provide exposure to the anal canal. A circumferential incision is made 5 mm above the dentate line. **(C)** The submucosal dissection is carried 2–3 cm. **(D)** The pull-through bowel is divided at least 2 cm above the biopsy site that has ganglion cells, and the anastomosis is performed. Care must be taken to perform the anastomosis to the rectal mucosa, not to the transitional epithelium. Otherwise, normal sensation will be lost and the risk of incontinence will be increased.

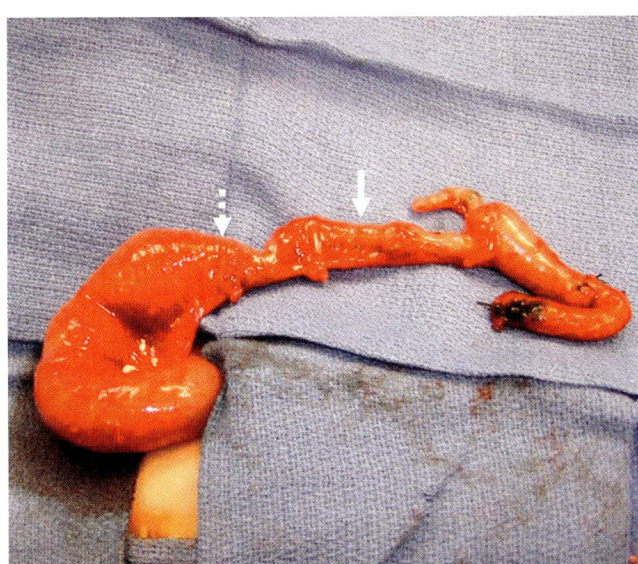

FIGURE 34-16 ■ This neonate has total colon aganglionosis. The solid arrow marks the contracted aganglionic terminal ileum and the transition zone to ganglionated ileum is marked by the dotted arrow.

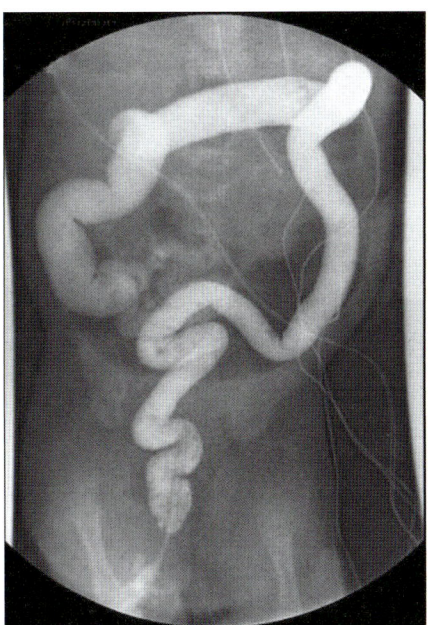

FIGURE 34-17 ■ This contrast enema was performed in a child with total colonic aganglionosis. There is no transition zone in the colon, and the colon is foreshortened with a 'question mark' configuration.

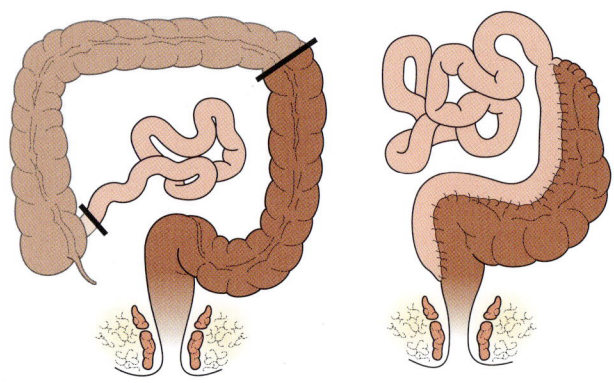

FIGURE 34-18 ■ This diagram depicts the Martin procedure for total colon aganglionosis.

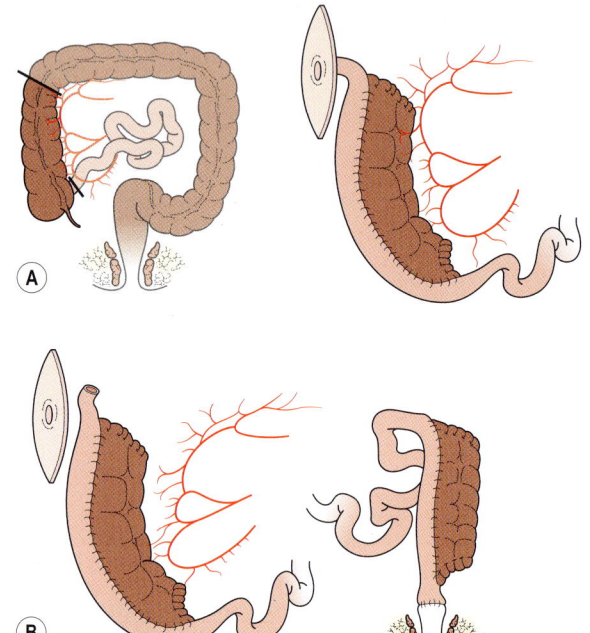

FIGURE 34-19 ■ These drawings show the salient points with the Kimura procedure.

frozen sections, and to create a stoma either at the most distal point that has normally innervated bowel or more distally with aganglionic bowel.[63] A central venous catheter should be inserted for TPN, and a gastrostomy should be considered for continuous feeding of breast milk or elemental formula.

These children are best managed by a multidisciplinary group focused on intestinal failure.[64] Strict attention to prevention of sepsis, treatment of bacterial overgrowth, use of trophic feedings, and prevention of TPN-related cholestasis using a variety of strategies including omega-3 lipids are all important.[65]

Subsequent management must be individualized, depending on the length of normally innervated bowel and the clinical status of the child.[66] For infants and children who develop significant dilatation of the normally innervated bowel, tapering, imbrication, or bowel lengthening procedures such as the Bianchi or serial transverse enteroplasty (STEP) procedure may be helpful.[67,68] The 'myectomy–myotomy' procedure popularized by Zeigler

Mechanical obstruction
Recurrent or residual aganglionosis
Motility disorder involving the ganglionated bowel
Internal anal sphincter achalasia
Functional megacolon (stool-holding behavior)

involves myectomy of a length of aganglionic small bowel distal to the transition zone.[69] For some of these patients, small bowel or combined small bowel-liver transplantation may offer the only chance for survival.[70]

POSTOPERATIVE MANAGEMENT

Most children undergoing a laparoscopic or transanal pull-through can be fed immediately and discharged within 24–48 hours. The anastomosis is calibrated with an appropriately sized dilator or finger one to two weeks after the procedure. Although most surgeons instruct the parents to perform daily dilatations, a program of weekly calibration by the surgeon is less traumatic and is associated with similar outcomes.[71] The parents should be instructed to protect the buttocks with barrier cream to prevent perineal skin breakdown. In addition, the family and the primary care physician should be educated about the signs and symptoms of postoperative enterocolitis, since this can result in rapid severe illness and even death in a few patients.[72]

LONG-TERM OUTCOMES

Long-term problems in children with HD include ongoing obstructive symptoms, soiling, and enterocolitis.[73] It is important for the surgeon to follow these children closely, at least until they are through the toilet training process, in order to identify and provide timely treatment for these problems.[40,74,75]

Obstructive Symptoms

Obstructive symptoms may take the form of abdominal distension, bloating, vomiting, or ongoing severe constipation. There are five major reasons for these symptoms following a pull-through: mechanical obstruction, recurrent or acquired aganglionosis, disordered motility in the residual colon or small bowel, internal sphincter achalasia, or functional megacolon caused by stool-holding behavior (Box 34-2). The clinician will have much greater success in managing these difficult patients if an organized approach is taken. One proposed algorithm is shown in Figure 34-20.[76]

Mechanical Obstruction

The most common cause of mechanical obstruction after a pull-through operation is a stricture. This problem is more common after a Swenson or Soave operation (Fig. 34-21A). Patients undergoing a Duhamel procedure may have a retained 'spur' consisting of the anterior aganglionic bowel, which may fill with stool and obstruct the pulled-through bowel (Fig. 34-21B). In other cases, there may be obstruction secondary to a twist in the pulled-through bowel (Fig. 34-21C), or narrowing due to a long muscular cuff in children who have had a Soave operation.

Obstruction can be discovered with digital rectal examination and a contrast enema. Initial management of

an anastomotic stricture consists of repeated dilatation using a finger, dilator, or balloon. For recalcitrant strictures, antegrade dilatation using Tucker dilators,[77] intralesional steroid,[78] or topical mitomycin C[79] can be tried. In some cases, revision of the pull-through is necessary.[80-82] Duhamel spurs can be resected from above or managed by extending the staple line from below. Twisted pull-throughs and narrow muscular cuffs usually require a repeat pull-through, although a muscular cuff can occasionally be divided laparoscopically.

Persistent or Acquired Aganglionosis

This problem may be due to an error in histological analysis,[83] a transition zone pull-through,[84,85] or loss of ganglion cells,[86] and can be diagnosed by performing a biopsy above the colo-anal anastomosis.[87] The specimen from the original operation should be reviewed and further sections should be taken circumferentially at the resection margin since the transition zone can be asymmetrical in children with HD.[88] In most cases, the best treatment for persistent or acquired aganglionosis is a repeat pull-through, which can be accomplished using either a Soave or a Duhamel approach.[81]

Motility Disorder

Children with HD often have abnormal motility throughout the intestinal tract, including gastroesophageal reflux and delayed gastric emptying.[89] These abnormalities may be focal, usually involving the left colon, or may be generalized, and may or may not be associated with other histological abnormalities such as intestinal neuronal dysplasia (IND). Techniques for diagnosing motility disorders include radiological shape study,[90] radionuclide colon transit study,[91] colonic manometry,[92] and laparoscopic biopsies looking for evidence of IND.[93] If a focal abnormality is found, resection with repeat pull-through using normal bowel is needed. Diffuse dysmotility is best treated with bowel management, which may include antegrade enemas through a cecostomy,[94] and the use of prokinetic agents.

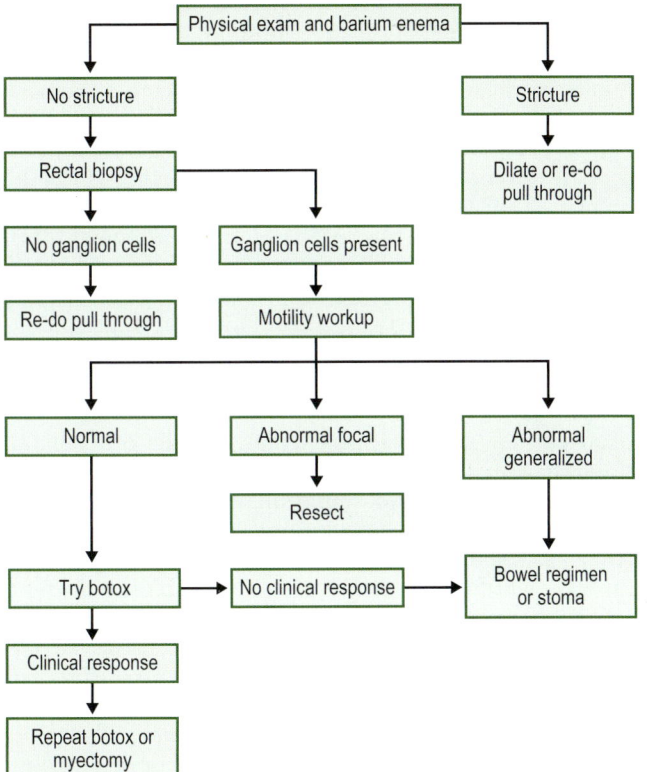

FIGURE 34-20 ■ Algorithm for the investigation and management of the child with obstructive symptoms following a pull-through.

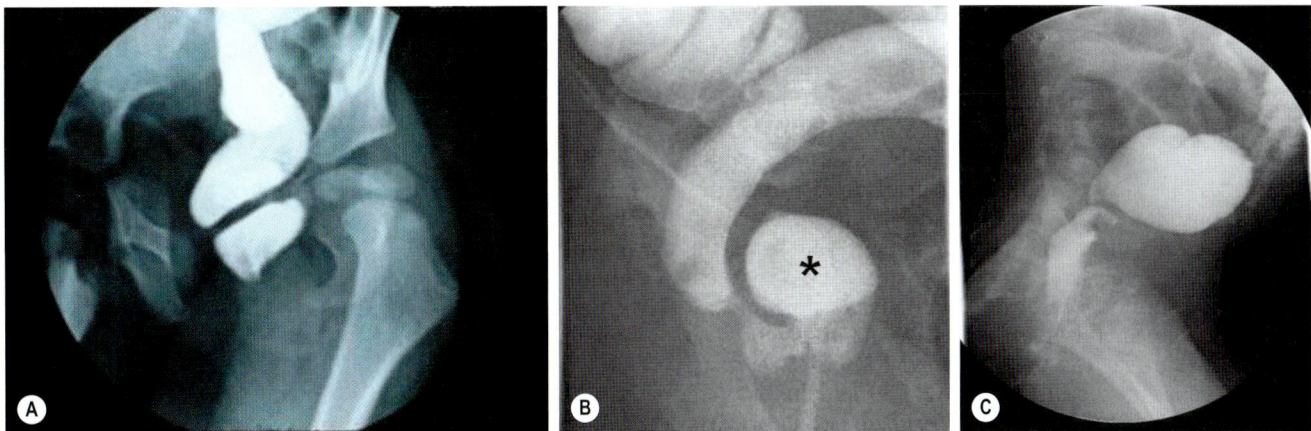

FIGURE 34-21 ■ Causes of mechanical obstruction after a pull-through are shown. **(A)** Stricture following a Soave procedure. **(B)** Anterior aganglionic 'spur' (asterisk) following a Duhamel procedure. **(C)** Twisted transanal pull-through.

Internal Sphincter Achalasia

This term refers to obstructive symptoms caused by the lack of a normal recto-anal inhibitory reflex which is found in all children with HD (see Fig. 34-3). Most children eventually 'grow out' of this problem over time, usually by the age of 5 years. The diagnosis can be confirmed by demonstrating a clinical response to intrasphinteric botulinum toxin.[95] The traditional operative approach for internal sphincter achalasia has been internal sphincterotomy or myectomy.[96,97] However, since this problem may resolve on its own, and there is concern about sphincter-cutting operations impacting continence, we prefer to use chemical sphincterotomy with intrasphincteric botulinum toxin.[98–100] In many cases, repeated injection of botulinum toxin, or applications of nitroglycerine paste or topical nifedipine, are necessary while waiting for resolution of the problem.

Functional Megacolon

Functional megacolon is the result of stool-holding behavior, which is very common in normal children.[101] This behavior may be even more common in children with HD because of their predisposition to constipation.[102] This problem is best treated with a bowel management regimen consisting of laxatives and behavior modification strategies. In severe cases, the child may require a cecostomy for antegrade enemas, or even a proximal stoma. In many cases, the cecostomy or stoma can be reversed when the child reaches adolescence.

Fecal Soiling

There are three broad causes for soiling after a pull-through: abnormal sphincter function, abnormal sensation, or 'pseudo-incontinence' (Box 34-3). Abnormal sphincter function may be due to sphincter injury during the pull-through or to a previous myectomy or sphincterotomy, and can usually be identified using anorectal manometry or endorectal ultrasound. There are two forms of abnormal sensation. The first is lack of sensation of a full rectum, which can also be identified using anorectal manometry, and the other is an inability to detect the difference between gas and stool. This problem is usually due to loss of the transitional epithelium because the anastomosis was performed below the dentate line. This distinction is usually evident on physical examination. Neither sphincter weakness nor abnormal sensation

---

BOX 34-3	Causes of Soiling following Surgery for Hirschsprung Disease

Abnormal sensation
  Inability to feel rectal distension
  Loss of transitional epithelium
Abnormal sphincter function
'Pseudo-incontinence'
  Associated with severe constipation
  Associated with hyperperistalsis of the pulled-through
  bowel

---

are amenable to a surgical solution. Most of these children are best managed using a bowel routine which may include a constipating diet, stimulant laxatives, and rectal or antegrade enemas. Biofeedback training has been advocated, especially for those children with sphincter weakness. In some cases, the child is best served by a colostomy.

If both the sphincter and sensation are intact, the most likely cause of soiling after a pull-through is pseudo-incontinence.[103] This may be caused by severe obstipation with a massively distended rectum and overflow of liquid stool. Other patients leak small amounts of stool through the day, creating 'skid marks' in the underwear on a constant basis. Other children can suffer from hyperperistalsis of the pulled-through bowel, which results in the inability of the anal sphincter to achieve control despite normal sphincter function.[92]

Successful management of soiling in a child with HD depends on a clear understanding of the reasons for the soiling. Evaluation requires a careful history and physical examination, and investigations such as abdominal films, barium enema, anorectal manometry, and in some cases, colonic manometry. Children with severe constipation will benefit from laxative therapy. However, if the sphincter and/or sensation are inadequate, passive laxatives such as lactulose or PEG 3300 will make the problem worse, and the child instead should be treated with stimulant laxatives such as senna, or enemas. On the other hand, children with stool-holding behavior who have normal sphincter function and sensation will often experience exacerbation of the behavioral problem by enemas or any other kind of anal manipulation. Children without constipation who have hyperperistalsis of the pulled-through bowel or abnormal sphincter function or sensation will benefit from a constipating diet and medications such as loperamide. On the other hand, children with slow transit constipation or stool-holding behavior will benefit from a high-fiber diet and passive laxative therapy. The treatment of soiling must be based on a clear understanding of the child's underlying problem.

Enterocolitis

The etiology of HAEC is unknown, and is probably multi-factorial. Stasis caused by functional obstruction permits bacterial overgrowth with secondary infection. Infectious agents such as *Clostridium dificile* or rotavirus have been postulated as being causative, but there are few data to support a specific pathogen.[104] There is some evidence implicating alterations in intestinal mucin production and the mucosal production of immunoglobulins, which presumably results in loss of intestinal barrier function and allows bacterial invasion.[105,106]

Enterocolitis may be present both before and after operative correction, and can range in severity from mild to life-threatening. HAEC is more common in younger children,[107] longer segment disease, and trisomy 21. Clinical presentation includes fever, abdominal distention, diarrhea, elevated leukocyte count, and evidence of intestinal edema on an abdominal film. Because there is overlap between HAEC and other conditions such as gastroenteritis, the true incidence is unknown. A HAEC

TABLE 34-1 Hirschsprung-associated enterocolitis (HAEC) score

Criteria	Score
History	
Diarrhea with explosive stool	2
Diarrhea with foul smelling stool	2
Diarrhea with bloody stool	1
Previous history of enterocolitis	1
Physical Examination	
Explosive discharge of gas and stool on rectal exam	2
Distended abdomen	2
Decreased peripheral perfusion	1
Lethargy	1
Fever	1
Radiology	
Multiple air fluid levels	1
Dilated loops of bowel	1
Sawtooth appearance with irregular mucosal lining	1
Cutoff sign in rectosigmoid with absence of distal air	1
Pneumatosis	1
Laboratory	
Leukocytosis	1
Shift to left	1
Total	**20**

A score of 10 or higher was associated with a positive diagnosis of HAEC by an international panel of experts.

score has recently been developed, which may be useful in the future in both the clinical and research settings (Table 34-1).[108]

The treatment of postoperative HAEC involves nasogastric drainage, intravenous fluids, broad-spectrum antibiotics, and decompression of the rectum and colon using rectal stimulation or irrigations. The risk of HAEC may be decreased by using preventive measures such as routine irrigations[109] or chronic administration of metronidazole or probiotic agents, particularly in those who are thought to be at higher risk for this problem based on clinical or histological grounds. Since enterocolitis is the most common cause of death in children with HD (Fig. 34-22) and can occur postoperatively even in children who did not have it preoperatively, it is very important that the surgeon educates the family about the risk of this complication and urges early return to the hospital if the child develops concerning symptoms.[72]

Despite the relatively common occurrence of postoperative problems, most resolve after the first five years of life. Studies of teenagers and adults with HD suggest that sexual function, social satisfaction, and quality of life all appear to be relatively normal in the vast majority of patients once they reach their late teens.[74,110] Exceptions include children with long-segment disease, who have a higher risk of enterocolitis, incontinence, and dehydration than children with shorter segment disease, children with trisomy 21 who have a greater risk of enterocolitis and incontinence,[111–113] and children with other co-morbidities such as those with congenital central hypoventilation syndrome, congenital heart disease, and syndromes that are associated with mental retardation or other forms of disability.[114]

VARIANT HIRSCHSPRUNG DISEASE

Variant HD is the term often used to describe children who present with a clinical picture suggestive of HD, but with ganglion cells on rectal biopsy.[115] There is a significant amount of controversy surrounding the definitions and features of many of these conditions.[116] In some cases, their existence has even been questioned.

Intestinal Neuronal Dysplasia (IND)

This condition was first described by Meier-Ruge in 1971.[117] Two types are usually described.[118] Type A is less common and is characterized by diminished or absent sympathetic innervation of the myenteric and submucosal plexuses, along with hyperplasia of the myenteric plexus. Type B consists of dysplasia of the submucous plexus with thickened nerve fibers and giant ganglia, increased acetylcholinesterase staining, and identification of ectopic ganglion cells in the lamina propria. Type B can occur independently or concomitant with HD. In addition, IND may be either diffuse or focal.

Despite multiple publications, the topic of IND continues to stimulate a lot of controversy among pediatric surgeons and pediatric pathologists.[119,120] Sophisticated histological techniques, including special stains and the use of thick sections, are often necessary for an accurate diagnosis.[116] In addition, there is some evidence that the histological finding of IND may in some cases be secondary to chronic obstruction rather than the cause of it. In many cases, there may not be good correlation between the histological finding of IND and the bowel motility.[121]

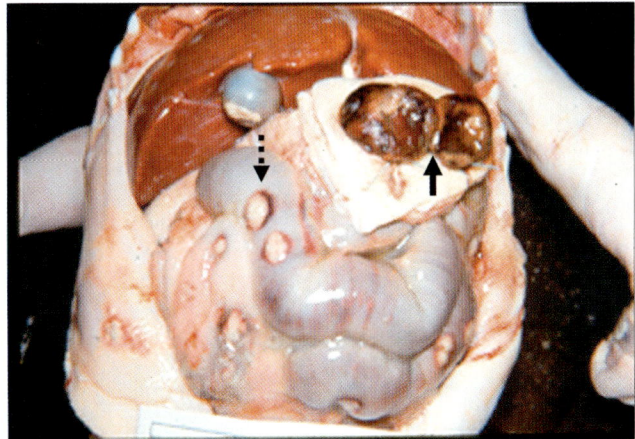

FIGURE 34-22 ■ Enterocolitis can be a major cause of morbidity and mortality, both before any operative procedure for Hirschsprung disease and in the postoperative period. Most of the deaths in the postoperative period are related to enterocolitis. In this autopsy specimen, note the several areas of perforation (dotted arrow) along the colon due to significant enterocolitis. Also note that the patient had undergone a diverting colostomy and had a mucous fistula (solid arrow).

Hypoganglionosis

Hypoganglionosis is characterized by sparse and small ganglia, usually in the distal bowel, often associated with abnormalities in acetylcholinesterase distribution. The appropriate treatment is resection of the abnormal colon with a pull-through procedure as one would do for a child with HD.[122] This condition must be differentiated from immature ganglia, which are seen in preterm children, and should not be treated surgically.[123]

Internal Sphincter Achalasia

There are some children who have normal ganglion cells on rectal biopsy, but who lack the recto-anal inhibitory reflex on anorectal manometry and develop symptoms of HD. This condition has been termed internal sphincter achalasia.[124] The initial treatment is a bowel management regimen consisting of diet, laxatives, and enemas or irrigations. If this is unsuccessful, some have advocated anal sphincter myectomy.[125,126] Because the constipation associated with this condition usually improves over the first five years of life, treatment includes temporary or reversible sphincter-relaxing measures such as botulinum toxin,[127] nitroglycerine paste,[128] or topical nifedipine, as previously discussed.

'Ultra-short Segment' Hirschsprung Disease

Some surgeons use this term to describe children with normal ganglion cells on rectal biopsy, but with absence of the recto-anal inhibitory reflex, which is synonymous with the definition of internal sphincter achalasia. We prefer to reserve it for children who have a documented aganglionic segment of less than 3–4 cm. In children with this condition, the findings of hypertrophic nerves and abnormal cholinesterase staining may be absent.[129] The treatment of ultra-short segment HD is controversial. Some authors advocate simple anal sphincter myectomy,[130,131] whereas others prefer excision of the aganglionic segment with a pull-through.

Desmosis Coli

This is a rare condition characterized by chronic constipation associated with total or a focal lack of the connective tissue net in the circular and longitudinal muscles and the connective tissue layer of the myenteric plexus, without any abnormalities in the enteric nervous system.[132] One family has been described in which HD and desmosis coli coexisted,[133] although in most cases they are separate entities.

FUTURE DIRECTIONS

There are a number of areas in which future research could potentially improve outcomes for children with HD. Perhaps the most important is our rapidly increasing understanding of the genetic basis for aganglionosis, and the tremendous variability in genetic mutations that may result in the full spectrum of clinical disease. The formation of large multidisciplinary research groups like the Hirschsprung Disease Research Collaborative [https://hdrcstudy.org/home] will lead to better correlation between genetic information and pathological and clinical outcomes. This understanding will ultimately lead to more personalized approaches to children with HD, tailoring the operative and postoperative management more precisely to the specific form of the disease.

Another exciting area of future work is the concept of repopulating the aganglionic bowel with neuronal stem cells.[134] There is some preliminary work using in vitro systems[135] and animal models.[136] This research may result in clinical application of this technology, which may be particularly helpful for children with near-total or total intestinal aganglionosis.

REFERENCES

1. Raveenthiran V. Knowledge of ancient Hindu surgeons on Hirschsprung disease: Evidence from Sushruta Samhita of circa 1200-600 BC. J Pediatr Surg 2011;46:2204–8.
2. Fiori MG. Domenico Battini and his description of congenital megacolon: A detailed case report one century before Hirschsprung. J Peripher Nerv Syst 1998;3:197–206.
3. Jay V. Legacy of Harald Hirschsprung. Pediatr Devel Pathol 2001;4:203–4.
4. Fraser J. Surgery of Childhood. New York: William Wood and Company; 1926.
5. Ehrenpreis T. Hirschsprung's Disease. Chicago: Year Book Medical Publishers; 1970.
6. Ehrenpreis T. Some newer aspects on Hirschsprung's disease and allied disorders. J Pediatr Surg 1966;1:329–37.
7. Swenson O, Rheinlander HF, Diamond I. Hirschsprung's disease: A new concept in etiology-operative results in 34 patients. N Engl J Med 1949;241:551–6.
8. Gross RE. Congenital megacolon (Hirschsprung's disease). In: Gross RE, editor. The Surgery of Infancy and Childhood. Philadelphia, PA: W.B. Saunders; 1953. p. 330–47.
9. Gariepy C. Developmental disorders of the enteric nervous system: Genetic and molecular bases. J Pediatr Gastroent Nutr 2004;39:5–11.
10. Webster W. Embryogenesis of the enteric ganglia in normal mice and in mice that develop congenital aganglionic megacolon. J Embryol Exp Morphol 1973;30:573–85.
11. Miyahara K, Kato Y, Koga H, et al. Visualization of enteric neural crest cell migration in SOX10 transgenic mouse gut using time-lapse fluorescence imaging. J Pediatr Surg 2011; 46:2305–8.
12. Le Douarin NM, Teillet M-A. The migration of neural crest cells to the wall of the digestive tract in avian embryo. J Embryol Exp Morph 1973;30:31–48.
13. Paran TS, Rolle U, Puri P. Enteric nervous system and developmental abnormalities in childhood. Pediatr Surg Int 2006;22:945–59.
14. Langer JC, Betti PA, Blennerhassett MG. Smooth muscle from aganglionic bowel in Hirschsprung's disease impairs neuronal development in vitro. Cell Tiss Res 1994;276:181–6.
15. Rauch U, Schafer K-H. The extracellular matrix and its role in cell migration and development of the enteric nervous system. Eur J Pediatr Surg 2003;13:158–62.
16. Parisi MA, Kapur RP. Genetics of Hirschsprung disease. Curr Opin Pediatr 2000;12:610–7.
17. Amiel J, Lyonnet S. Hirschsprung disease, associated syndromes, and genetics: A review. J Med Genet 2001;38:729–39.
18. Moore SW. The contribution of associated congenital anomalies in understanding Hirschsprung's disease. Pediatr Surg Int 2006;22:305–15.
19. Bordeaux MC, Forcet C, Granger L, et al. The RET proto-oncogene induces apoptosis: A novel mechanism for Hirschsprung disease. EMBO J 2000;19:4056–63.

20. Uesaka T, Nagashimada M, Yonemura S, et al. Diminished Ret expression compromises neuronal survival in the colon and causes intestinal aganglionosis in mice. J Clin Invest 2008;118: 1890–8.

21. Paratore C, Eichenberger C, Suter U, et al. Sox10 haploinsufficiency affects maintenance of progenitor cells in a mouse model of Hirschsprung disease. Hum Mol Genet 2002;11:3075–85.

22. Gershon MD. Endothelin and the development of the enteric nervous system. Clin Exp Pharmacol Physiol 1999;26:985–8.

23. Ngan ES, Garcia-Barcelo MM, Yip BH, et al. Hedgehog/Notch-induced premature gliogenesis represents a new disease mechanism for Hirschsprung disease in mice and humans. J Clin Invest 2011;121:3467–78.

24. Belin B, Corteville JE, Langer JC. How accurate is prenatal sonography for the diagnosis of imperforate anus and Hirschsprung's disease? Pediatr Surg Int 1995;10:30–2.

25. Newman B, Nussbaum A, Kirkpatrick JA Jr. Bowel perforation in Hirschsprung's disease. AJR 1987;148:1195–7.

26. Smith GHH, Cass D. Infantile Hirschsprung's disease—is barium enema useful? Pediatr Surg Int 1991;6:318–21.

27. Diamond IR, Casadiego G, Traubici J, et al. The contrast enema for Hirschsprung disease: Predictors of a false-positive result. J Pediatr Surg 2007;42:792–5.

28. Lewis NA, Levitt MA, Zallen GS, et al. Diagnosing Hirschsprung's disease: Increasing the odds of a positive rectal biopsy result. J Pediatr Surg 2003;38:412–6.

29. Kapur RP, Reed RC, Finn LS, et al. Calretinin immunohistochemistry versus acetylcholinesterase histochemistry in the evaluation of suction rectal biopsies for Hirschsprung Disease. Pediatr Dev Pathol 2009;12:6–15.

30. Kaymakcioglu N, Yagci G, Can MF, et al. Role of anorectal myectomy in the treatment of short segment Hirschsprung's disease in young adults. Int Surg 2005;90:109–12.

31. Visser R, van de Ven TJ, van Rooij IA, et al. Is the Rehbein procedure obsolete in the treatment of Hirschsprung's disease? Pediatr Surg Int 2010;26:1117–20.

32. Swenson O. Hirschsprung's disease: A review. Pediatrics 2002;109:914–8.

33. So HS, Schwartz DL, Becker JM, et al. Endorectal 'pull-through' without preliminary colostomy in neonates with Hirschsprung's disease. J Pediatr Surg 1980;15:470–1.

34. Cass DT. Neonatal one-stage repair of Hirschsprung's disease. Pediatr Surg Int 1990;5:341–6.

35. Langer JC, Fitzgerald PG, Winthrop AL, et al. One vs two stage Soave pull-through for Hirschsprung's disease in the first year of life. J Pediatr Surg 1996;31:33–7.

36. Hackam DJ, Superina RA, Pearl RH. Single-stage repair of Hirschsprung's disease: A comparison of 109 patients over 5 years. J Pediatr Surg 1997;32:1028–31.

37. Bufo AJ, Chen MK, Shah R, et al. Analysis of the costs of surgery for Hirschsprung's disease: One-stage laparoscopic pull-through versus two-stage Duhamel procedure. Clin Pediatr 1999;38: 593–6.

38. Sherman JO, Snyder ME, Weitzman JJ, et al. A 40-year multinational retrospective study of 880 Swenson procedures. J Pediatr Surg 1989;24:833–8.

39. Swenson O. Hirschsprung's disease–a complicated therapeutic problem: Some thoughts and solutions based on data and personal experience over 56 years. J Pediatr Surg 2004;39:1449–53.

40. Moore SW, Albertyn R, Cywes S. Clinical outcome and long-term quality of life after surgical correction of Hirschsprung's disease. J Pediatr Surg 1996;31:1496–502.

41. Giuliani S, Betalli P, Narciso A, et al. Outcome comparison among laparoscopic Duhamel, laparotomic Duhamel, and transanal endorectal pull-through: A single-center, 18-year experience. J Laparosc Adv Surg Tech 2011;21:859–63.

42. Gunnarsdottir A, Larsson LT, Arnbjornsson E. Transanal endorectal vs. Duhamel pull-through for Hirschsprung's disease. Eur J Pediatr Surg 2010;20:242–6.

43. Georgeson KE, Fuenfer MM, Hardin WD. Primary laparoscopic pull-through for Hirschsprung's disease in infants and children. J Pediatr Surg 1995;30:1017–21.

44. Georgeson KE, Cohen RD, Hebra A, et al. Primary laparoscopic-assisted endorectal colon pull-through for Hirschsprung's disease: A new gold standard. Ann Surg 1999;229:678–83.

45. de Lagausie P, Berrebi D, Geib G, et al. Laparoscopic Duhamel procedure. Management of 30 cases. Surg Endosc 1999;13: 972–4.

46. Hoffmann K, Schier F, Waldschmidt J. Laparoscopic Swenson's procedure in children. Eur J Pediatr Surg 1996;6:15–7.

47. De la Torre-Mondragon L, Ortega-Salgado JA. Transanal endorectal pull-through for Hirschsprung's disease. J Pediatr Surg 1998;33:1283–6.

48. Langer JC, Minkes RK, Mazziotti MV, et al. Transanal one-stage Soave procedure for infants with Hirschsprung disease. J Pediatr Surg 1999;34:148–52.

49. De La Torre L, Langer JC. Transanal endorectal pull-through for Hirschsprung disease: Technique, controversies, pearls, pitfalls, and an organized approach to the management of postoperative obstructive symptoms. Semin Pediatr Surg 2010;19:96–106.

50. Nasr A, Langer JC. Evolution of the technique in the transanal pull-through for Hirschsprung disease: Effect on outcome. J Pediatr Surg 2007;42:36–9.

51. Sookpotarom P, Vejchapipat P. Primary transanal Swenson pull-through operation for Hirschsprung's disease. Pediatr Surg Int 2009;25:767–73.

52. Sauer CJE, Langer JC, Wales PW. The versatility of the umbilical incision in the management of Hirschsprung's disease. J Pediatr Surg 2005;40:385–9.

53. Proctor ML, Traubici J, Langer JC, et al. Correlation between radiographic transition zone and level of aganglionosis in Hirschsprung's disease: Implications for surgical approach. J Pediatr Surg 2003;38:775–8.

54. Muller CO, Mignot C, Belarbi N, et al. Does the radiographic transition zone correlate with the level of aganglionosis on the specimen in Hirschsprung's disease? Pediatr Surg Int 2012;28: 597–601.

55. Langer JC, Durrant AC, de la Torre ML, et al. One-stage transanal Soave pullthrough for Hirschsprung disease: A multicenter experience with 141 children. Ann Surg 2003;238:569–76.

56. Kim AC, Langer JC, Pastor AC, et al. Endorectal pull-through for Hirschsprung's disease-a multicenter, long-term comparison of results: Transanal vs transabdominal approach. J Pediatr Surg 2010;45:1213–20.

57. Stranzinger E, DiPietro MA, Teitelbaum DH, et al. Imaging of total colonic Hirschsprung disease. Pediatr Radiol 2008;38: 1162–70.

58. Anderson KD, Chandra R. Segmental aganglionosis of the appendix. J Pediatr Surg 1986;21:852–4.

59. Burjonrappa S, Rankin L. 'Hop the skip' with extended segment intestinal biopsy in Hirschsprung's disease. Intern J Surg Case Reports 2012;3:186–9.

60. Shen C, Song Z, Zheng S, et al. A comparison of the effectiveness of the Soave and Martin procedures for the treatment of total colonic aganglionosis. J Pediatr Surg 2009;44:2355–8.

61. Barrena S, Andres AM, Burgos L, et al. Long-term results of the treatment of total colonic aganglionosis with two different techniques. Eur J Pediatr Surg 2008;18:375–9.

62. Marquez TT, Acton RD, Hess DJ, et al. Comprehensive review of procedures for total colonic aganglionosis. J Pediatr Surg 2009;44:257–65.

63. Travassos DV, van der Zee DC. Is complete resection of the aganglionic bowel in extensive total aganglionosis up to the middle ileum always necessary? J Pediatr Surg 2011;46:2054–9.

64. Diamond IR, de Silva N, Pencharz PB, et al. Neonatal short bowel syndrome outcomes after the establishment of the first Canadian multidisciplinary intestinal rehabilitation program: Preliminary experience. J Pediatr Surg 2007;42:806–11.

65. Diamond IR, Sterescu A, Pencharz PB, et al. The rationale for the use of parenteral omega-3 lipids in children with short bowel syndrome and liver disease. Pediatr Surg Int 2008;24: 773–8.

66. Ruttenstock E, Puri P. A meta-analysis of clinical outcome in patients with total intestinal aganglionosis. Pediatr Surg Int 2009;25:833–9.

67. Wales PW. Surgical therapy for short bowel syndrome. Pediatr Surg Int 2004;20:647–57.

68. Wales PW, de Silva N, Langer JC, et al. Intermediate outcomes after serial transverse enteroplasty in children with short bowel syndrome. J Pediatr Surg 2007;42:1804–10.

69. Ziegler MM, Royal RE, Brandt J, et al. Extended myectomy-myotomy. A therapeutic alternative for total intestinal aganglionosis. Ann Surg 1993;218:504–9.

70. Sauvat F, Grimaldi C, Lacaille F, et al. Intestinal transplantation for total intestinal aganglionosis: A series of 12 consecutive children. J Pediatr Surg 2008;43:1833–8.

71. Temple S, Shawyer AC, Langer JC. Is daily dilatation by parents necessary after surgery for Hirschsprung disease and anorectal malformations? J Pediatr Surg 2012;47:209–12.

72. Marty TL, Matlak ME, Hendrickson M, et al. Unexpected death from enterocolitis after surgery for Hirschsprung's disease. Pediatrics 1995;96:118–21.

73. Dasgupta R, Langer JC. Evaluation and management of persistent problems after surgery for Hirschsprung disease in a child. J Pediatr Gastroenterol Nutr 2008;46:13–9.

74. Yanchar NL, Soucy P. Long term outcomes of Hirschsprung's disease: The patients' perspective. J Pediatr Surg 1999;34:1152–60.

75. Rintala RJ, Pakarinen MP. Outcome of anorectal malformations and Hirschsprung's disease beyond childhood. Semin Pediatr Surg 2010;19:160–7.

76. Langer JC. Persistent obstructive symptoms after surgery for Hirschsprung disease: Development of a diagnostic and therapeutic algorithm. J Pediatr Surg 2004;39:1458–62.

77. Langer JC, Winthrop AL. Antegrade dilatation over a string for the management of anastomotic complications after a pull-through procedure. J Am Coll Surg 1996;183:411–2.

78. Lucha PA Jr, Fticsar JE, Francis MJ. The strictured anastomosis: Successful treatment by corticosteroid injections–report of three cases and review of the literature. Dis Colon Rectum 2005;48:862–5.

79. Mueller CM, Beaunoyer M, St-Vil D. Topical mitomycin-C for the treatment of anal stricture. J Pediatr Surg 2010;45:241–4.

80. van Leeuwen K, Teitelbaum DH, Elhalaby EA, et al. Long-term follow-up of redo pull-through procedures for Hirschsprung's disease: Efficacy of the endorectal pull-through. J Pediatr Surg 2000;35:829–33.

81. Langer JC. Repeat pullthrough surgery for complicated Hirschsprung disease: Indications, techniques, and results. J Pediatr Surg 1999;34:1136–41.

82. Pena A, Elicevik M, Levitt MA. Reoperations in Hirschsprung disease. J Pediatr Surg 2007;42:1008–13.

83. Shayan K, Smith D, Langer JC. Reliability of intraoperative frozen sections in the management of Hirschsprung disease. J Pediatr Surg 2004;39:1345–8.

84. Ghose SI, Squire BR, Stringer MD, et al. Hirschsprung's disease: Problems with transition-zone pull-through. J Pediatr Surg 2000;35:1805–9.

85. Coe A, Collins MH, Lawal T, et al. Reoperation for Hirschsprung disease: Pathology of the resected problematic distal pull-through. Pediatr Dev Pathol 2012;15:30–8.

86. West KW, Grosfeld JL, Rescorla FJ, et al. Acquired aganglionosis: A rare occurrence following pull-through procedures for Hirschsprung's disease. J Pediatr Surg 1990;25:104–8.

87. Friedmacher F, Puri P. Residual aganglionosis after pull-through operation for Hirschsprung's disease: A systematic review and meta-analysis. Pediatr Surg Int 2011;27:1053–7.

88. White FV, Langer JC. Circumferential distribution of ganglion cells in the transition zone of children with Hirschsprung disease. Pediatr Dev Pathol 2000;3:216–22.

89. Medhus AW, Bjornland K, Emblem R, et al. Liquid and solid gastric emptying in adults treated for Hirschsprung's disease during early childhood. Scand J Gastroenterol 2007;42:34–40.

90. Zaslavsky C, da Silveira TR, Maguilnik I. Total and segmental colonic transit time with radio-opaque markers in adolescents with functional constipation. J Pediatr Gastroenterol Nutr 1998;27:138–42.

91. Southwell BR, Clarke MC, Sutcliffe J, et al. Colonic transit studies: Normal values for adults and children with comparison of radiological and scintigraphic methods. Pediatr Surg Int 2009;25:559–72.

92. Di Lorenzo C, Solzi GF, Flores AF, et al. Colonic motility after surgery for Hirschsprung's disease. Am J Gastroenterol 2000;95:1759–64.

93. Mazziottti MV, Langer JC. Laparoscopic full-thickness intestinal biopsies in children. J Pediatr Gastroenterol Nutr 2001;33:54–7.

94. Yagmurlu A, Harmon CM, Georgeson KE. Laparoscopic cecostomy button placement for the management of fecal incontinence in children with Hirschsprung's disease and anorectal anomalies. Surg Endosc 2006;20:624–7.

95. Minkes RK, Langer JC. A prospective study of botulinum toxin for internal anal sphincter hypertonicity in children with Hirschsprung's disease. J Pediatr Surg 2000;35:1733–6.

96. Abbas Banani S, Forootan H. Role of anorectal myectomy after failed endorectal pull-through in Hirschsprung's disease. J Pediatr Surg 1994;29:1307–9.

97. Wildhaber BE, Pakarinen M, Rintala RJ, et al. Posterior myotomy/myectomy for persistent stooling problems in Hirschsprung's disease. J Pediatr Surg 2004;39:920–6.

98. Koivusalo AI, Pakarinen MP, Rintala RJ. Botox injection treatment for anal outlet obstruction in patients with internal anal sphincter achalasia and Hirschsprung's disease. Pediatr Surg Int 2009;25:873–6.

99. Jiang da P, Xu CQ, Wu B, et al. Effects of botulinum toxin injection on anal achalasia after pull-through operations for Hirschsprung's disease: A 1-year follow-up study. Inter J Colorectal Dis 2009;24:597–8.

100. Patrus B, Nasr A, Langer JC, et al. Intrasphincteric botulinum toxin decreases the rate of hospitalization for postoperative obstructive symptoms in children with Hirschsprung disease. J Pediatr Surg 2011;46:184–7.

101. Di Lorenzo C. Constipation. In: Hyman PE, editor. Pediatric Gastrointestinal Motility Disorders. New York, NY: Academy Professional Information Services; 1994. p. 129–44.

102. Blum NJ, Taubman B, Nemeth N. During toilet training, constipation occurs before stool toileting refusal. Pediatrics 2004;113:e520–2.

103. Levitt M, Pena A. Update on pediatric faecal incontinence. Eur J Pediatr Surg 2009;19:1–9.

104. Wilson-Storey D, Scobie WG, McGenity KG. Microbiological studies of the enterocolitis of Hirschsprung's disease. Arch Dis Child 1990;65:1338–9.

105. Mattar AF, Coran AG, Teitelbaum DH. MUC-2 mucin production in Hirschsprung's disease: Possible association with enterocolitis development. J Pediatr Surg 2003;38:417–21.

106. Imamura A, Puri P, O'Briain DS, et al. Mucosal immune defence mechanisms in enterocolitis complicating Hirschsprung's disease. Gut 1992;33:801–6.

107. Haricharan RN, Seo JM, Kelly DR, et al. Older age at diagnosis of Hirschsprung disease decreases risk of postoperative enterocolitis, but resection of additional ganglionated bowel does not. J Pediatr Surg 2008;43:1115–23.

108. Pastor AC, Osman F, Teitelbaum DH, et al. Development of a standardized definition for Hirschsprung's-associated enterocolitis: A Delphi analysis. J Pediatr Surg 2009;44:251–6.

109. Marty TL, Seo T, Sullivan JJ, et al. Rectal irrigations for the prevention of postoperative enterocolitis in Hirschsprung's disease. J Pediatr Surg 1995;30:652–4.

110. Menezes M, Corbally M, Puri P. Long-term results of bowel function after treatment for Hirschsprung's disease: A 29-year review. Pediatr Surg Int 2006;22:987–90.

111. Caniano DA, Teitelbaum DH, Qualman SJ. Management of Hirschsprung's disease in children with trisomy 21. Am J Surg 1990;159:402–4.

112. Morabito A, Lall A, Gull S, et al. The impact of Down's syndrome on the immediate and long-term outcomes of children with Hirschsprung's disease. Pediatr Surg Int 2006;22:179–81.

113. Travassos D, van Herwaarden-Lindeboom M, van der Zee DC. Hirschsprung's disease in children with Down syndrome: A comparative study. Eur J Pediatr Surg 2011;21:220–3.

114. Moore SW, Tshifularo N. Hirschsprung's disease in the neurologically challenged child. Intern J Adolesc Med Health 2011;23:223–7.

115. Puri P. Variant Hirschsprung's disease. J Pediatr Surg 1997;32:149–57.

116. Feichter S, Meier-Ruge WA, Bruder E. The histopathology of gastrointestinal motility disorders in children. Sem Pediatr Surg 2009;18:206–11.

117. Meier-Ruge W. Casuistic of colon disorder with symptoms of Hirschsprung's disease. Verh Dtsch Ges Pathol 1971;55:506–10.

118. Ryan DP. Neuronal intestinal dysplasia. Sem Pediatr Surg 1995;4:22–5.

119. Csury L, Pena A. Intestinal neuronal dysplasia: Myth or reality? Pediatr Surg Int 1995;10:441–6.

120. Koletzko S, Jesch I, Faus-Kebler T, et al. Rectal biopsy for diagnosis of intestinal neuronal dysplasia in children: A prospective multicentre study on interobserver variation and clinical outcome. Gut 1999;44:853–61.

121. Kapur RP. Neuronal dysplasia: A controversial pathological correlate of intestinal pseudo-obstruction. Am J Med Gen 2003;122A: 287–93.

122. Zhang HY, Feng JX, Huang L, et al. Diagnosis and surgical treatment of isolated hypoganglionosis. World J Pediatr 2008;4: 295–300.

123. Tatekawa Y, Kanehiro H, Kanokogi H, et al. The evaluation of meconium disease by distribution of cathepsin D in intestinal ganglion cells. Pediatr Surg Int 2000;16:53–5.

124. Davidson M, Bauer CH. Studies of distal colonic motility in children IV: Achalasia of the distal rectal segment despite presence of ganglia in the myenteric plexuses of this area. Pediatrics 1958;21:746–61.

125. De Caluwe D, Yoneda A, Akl U, et al. Internal anal sphincter achalasia: Outcome after internal sphincter myectomy. J Pediatr Surg 2001;36:736–8.

126. Heikkinen M, Lindahl HG, Rintala RJ. Long-term outcome after internal sphincter myectomy for internal sphincter achalasia. Pediatr Surg Int 2005;21:84–7.

127. Messineo A, Codrich D, Monai M, et al. The treatment of internal anal sphincter achalasia with botulinum toxin. Pediatr Surg Int 2001;17:521–3.

128. Millar AJ, Steinberg RM, Raad J, et al. Anal achalasia after pull-through operations for Hirschsprung's disease—preliminary experience with topical nitric oxide. Eur J Pediatr Surg 2002;12: 207–11.

129. Meier-Ruge W. Ultrashort segment Hirschsprung disease. An objective picture of the disease substantiated by biopsy. Z Kinderchir 1985;40:146–50.

130. Osifo OD, Okolo CJ. Outcome of trans-anal posterior anorectal myectomy for the ultrashort segment Hirschsprung's disease–Benin City experience in five years. Niger Postgrad Med J 2009;16:213–7.

131. Meier-Ruge WA, Bruder E, Holschneider AM, et al. Diagnosis and therapy of ultrashort Hirschsprung's disease. Eur J Pediatr Surg 2004;14:392–7.

132. Meier-Ruge WA. Desmosis of the colon: A working hypothesis of primary chronic constipation. Eur J Pediatr Surg 1998;8: 209–303.

133. Marshall DG, Meier-Ruge WA, Chakravarti A, Langer JC. Chronic constipation due to Hirschsprung's disease and desmosis coli in a family. Pediatr Surg Int 2002;18:110–4.

134. Hotta R, Natarajan D, Thapar N. Potential of cell therapy to treat pediatric motility disorders. Sem Pediatr Surg 2009;18:263–73.

135. Zhang D, Brinas IM, Binder BJ, et al. Neural crest regionalization for enteric nervous system formation: Implications for Hirschsprung's disease and stem cell therapy. Dev Biol 2010;339: 280–94.

136. Tsai YH, Murakami N, Gariepy CE. Postnatal intestinal engraftment of prospectively selected enteric neural crest stem cells in a rat model of Hirschsprung disease. Neurogastroenterol Motil 2011;23:362–9.

CHAPTER 35

IMPERFORATE ANUS AND CLOACAL MALFORMATIONS

Marc A. Levitt • Alberto Peña

'Imperforate anus' has been a well-known condition since antiquity.[1-3] For many centuries, physicians, as well as individuals who practiced medicine, have tried to help these children by creating an orifice in the perineum. Many patients survived, most likely because they suffered from a type of defect that is now recognized as 'low.' Those with a 'high' defect did not survive. In 1835, Amussat was the first to suture the rectal wall to the skin edges which was the first actual anoplasty.[2] Stephens made a significant contribution by performing the first anatomic studies in human specimens. In 1953, he proposed an initial sacral approach followed by an abdominoperineal operation, if needed.[4] The purpose of the sacral stage of this procedure was to preserve the puborectalis sling, considered a key factor in maintaining fecal incontinence. Over the next 25 years, different surgical techniques were described, with the common denominator being the protection and use of the puborectalis sling.[5-8]

The posterior sagittal approach for the treatment of imperforate anus was performed first in 1980, and its description was published in 1982.[9] With this approach, the unique opportunity arose to correlate the external appearance of the perineum with the operative findings and, subsequently, with the clinical results.

INCIDENCE, TYPES OF DEFECTS, AND TERMINOLOGY

An anorectal malformation occurs in one out of every 4000 to 5000 newborns and is slightly more common in males.[10-12] The estimated risk for a couple having a second child with an anorectal malformation is approximately 1%.[13-17] The most frequent defect in males is imperforate anus with a rectourethral fistula.[18] In females, it is a rectovestibular fistula.[18] Imperforate anus without a fistula is a rather unusual defect, occurring in about 5% of the entire group of malformations, and is associated with Down syndrome.[18,19] Historically, a cloaca has been considered an unusual defect, whereas a high incidence of rectovaginal fistula has been reported in the literature.[20] In retrospect, we now know that a cloaca is the third most common defect in female patients after vestibular and perineal fistulas, whereas a rectovaginal fistula is actually a rare defect, present in less than 1% of all cases.[21,22] It is likely that most females with a persistent cloaca were erroneously thought to have a rectovaginal fistula. Many of these patients underwent repair of the rectal component but were left with a persistent urogenital sinus.[21,23] Additionally, most rectovestibular fistulas were erroneously called 'rectovaginal fistula'.[21] A rectobladderneck fistula in males is the only true supralevator malformation and occurs in about 10%.[18] As it is the only malformation in males in which the rectum is unreachable through a posterior sagittal incision, it requires an abdominal approach (via laparoscopy or a laparotomy) in addition to the perineal approach.

Anorectal malformations represent a wide spectrum of defects. The terms 'low,' 'intermediate,' and 'high' are arbitrary and not useful in current therapeutic or prognostic terminology. A therapeutic and prognostically oriented classification is depicted in Box 35-1.[24]

MALE ANORECTAL DEFECTS

Rectoperineal Fistulas

Rectoperineal fistula is the lowest defect. The rectum is located within most of the sphincter mechanism. Only the lowest part of the rectum is anteriorly mislocated (Fig. 35-1). Sometimes, the fistula does not open into the perineum but rather follows a subepithelial midline tract, opening somewhere along the midline perineal raphe, scrotum, or even at the base of the penis (Fig. 35-2). This diagnosis is established by perineal inspection. No further investigations are required. Usually, the anal fistula opening is stenotic. The terms *covered anus, anal membrane, anteriorly mislocated anus*, and *bucket-handle malformations* all refer to rectoperineal fistulas.

Rectourethral Fistulas

Imperforate anus with a rectourethral fistula is the most common defect in males.[18] The fistula may be located at the lower (bulbar) (Fig. 35-3A) or the higher (prostatic) part of the urethra (Fig. 35-3B).

Immediately above the fistula, the rectum and urethra share a common wall. The lower the fistula, the longer is the common wall. This is an important anatomic fact, which guides the operation. The rectum is usually distended and surrounded laterally and posteriorly by the levator muscle. Between the rectum and the perineal skin, a portion of striated voluntary muscle called the muscle complex is present. The contraction of these muscle fibers elevates the skin of the anal dimple. At the level of the skin, a group of voluntary muscle fibers, called

BOX 35-1	Classification of Infants with Anorectal Malformations

MALES

Rectoperineal fistula
Rectourethral bulbar fistula
Rectourethral prostatic fistula
Rectobladderneck fistula
Imperforate anus without fistula
Rectal atresia/rectal stenosis

FEMALES

Rectoperineal fistula
Rectovestibular fistula
Cloaca
Complex malformations
Imperforate anus without fistula
Rectal atresia/rectal stenosis

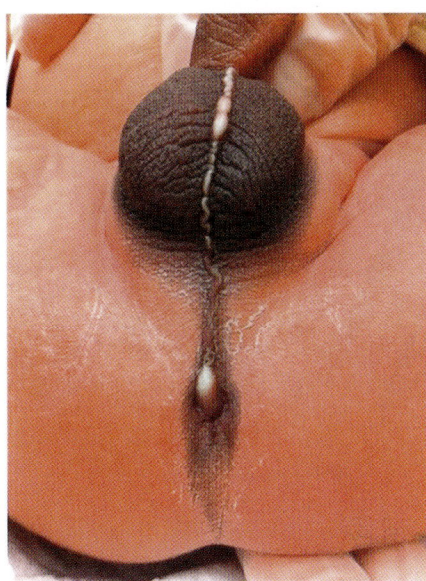

FIGURE 35-2 ■ This male infant has a rectoperineal fistula with a subepithelial tract filled with either mucus or meconium that extends into the scrotal raphe.

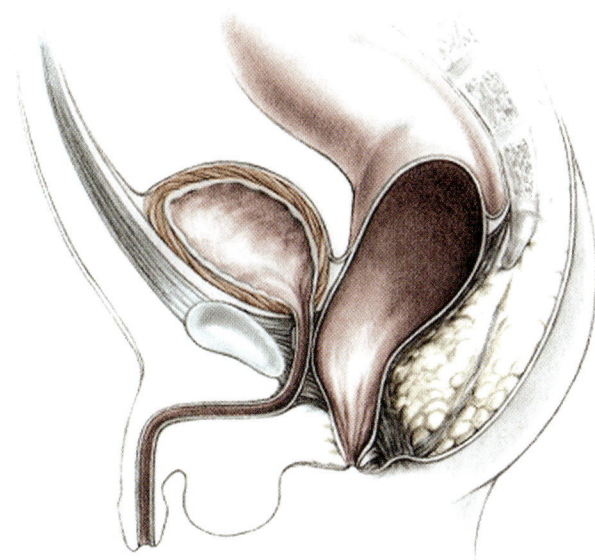

FIGURE 35-1 ■ This drawing shows the course of a perineal fistula in a male. The rectum is located within most of the muscle complex. Only the most distal aspect of the rectum is misplaced.

parasagittal fibers, are located on both sides of the midline. Lower urethral fistulas are usually associated with good-quality muscles, a well-developed sacrum, a prominent midline groove, and a prominent anal dimple. Higher urethral fistulas are more frequently associated with poor-quality muscles, an abnormally developed sacrum, a flat perineum, a poor midline groove, and a barely visible anal dimple. Of course, exceptions to these rules exist. Occasionally, the infant passes meconium through the urethra, which is an unequivocal sign of a rectourinary fistula.

Rectobladderneck Fistulas

In this defect, the rectum opens into the bladder neck (Fig. 35-4). The patient usually has poor prognosis for bowel control because the levator muscles, the striated

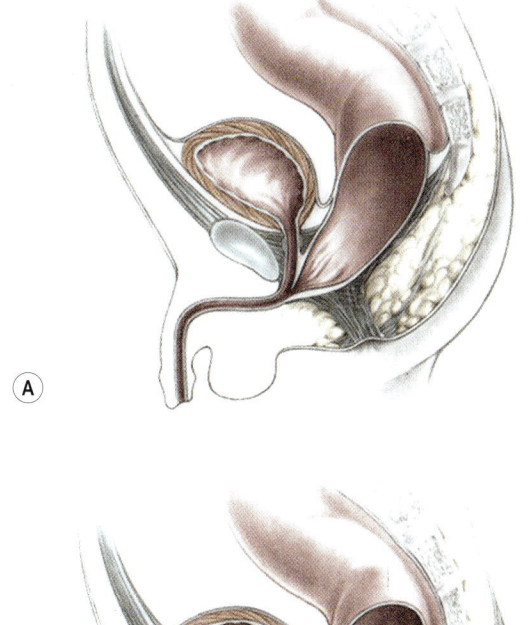

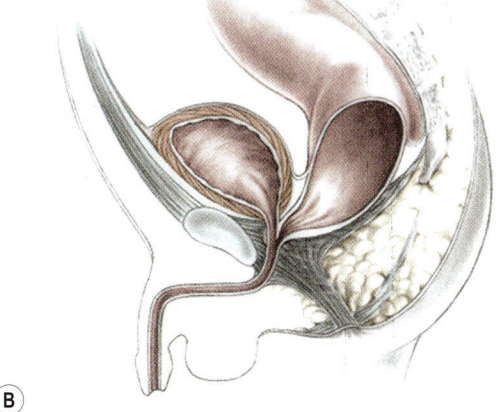

FIGURE 35-3 ■ Anorectal atresia with rectourethral fistulas. **(A)** Rectourethrobulbar fistula; **(B)** rectourethroprostatic fistula.

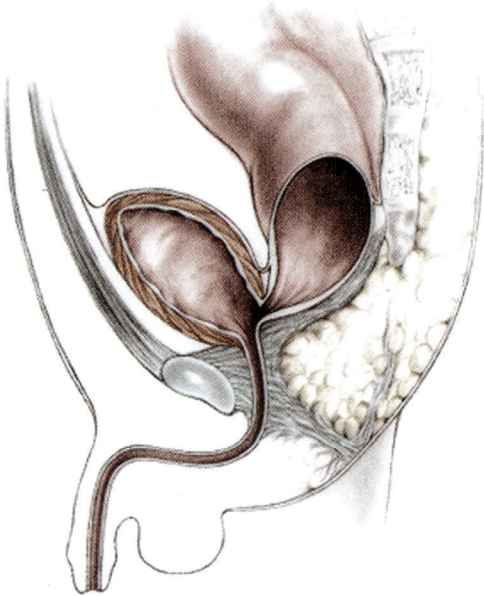

FIGURE 35-4 ■ Schematic representation of a rectobladder neck fistula. Note that the fistula enters into the bladder neck near the junction between the urethra and the bladder.

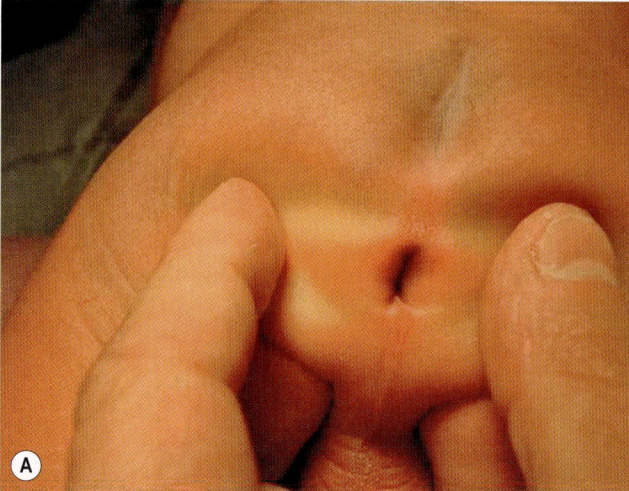

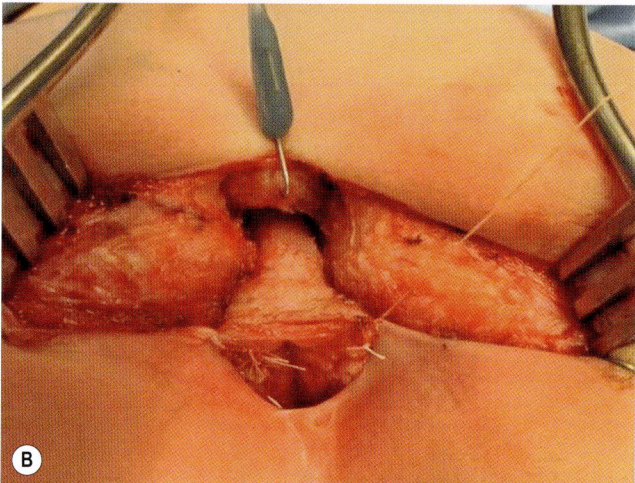

FIGURE 35-5 ■ This newborn was found to have rectal atresia. **(A)** Note the normal anal position and short depth of the anal canal. **(B)** Operative repair. The anastomosis is to the distal anal canal, preserving the dentate line which becomes the anterior 180° of the anoplasty.

muscle complex, and the external sphincter frequently are poorly developed. The sacrum is often deformed and short. In fact, the entire pelvis seems to be underdeveloped. The perineum is often flat, which is evidence of poor muscle development. About 10% of males fall into this category.[18]

Imperforate Anus without Fistula

Interestingly, most patients with this unusual defect have a well-developed sacrum and good muscles, and have a good prognosis in terms of bowel function.[18,19] The rectum usually terminates approximately 2 cm from the perineal skin. Although the rectum and urethra do not communicate, these two structures are separated only by a thin common wall. About half of the patients with no fistula also have Down syndrome, and more than 90% of patients with Down syndrome and imperforate anus have this specific defect, suggesting a chromosomal link.[17–19] The fact that these patients have Down syndrome does not seem to interfere with their good prognosis for bowel control.[19]

Rectal Atresia/Rectal Stenosis

In this unusual defect in male patients (less than 1% of the entire group of malformations), the lumen of the rectum is totally (atresia) or partially (stenosis) interrupted.[18] The upper pouch is represented by a dilated rectum, whereas the lower portion empties into a small anal canal that is in the normal location and is 1–2 cm long (Fig. 35-5A). These two rectal structures may be separated by a thin membrane or by dense fibrous tissue. The repair involves a primary anastomosis between the upper pouch and lower anal canal, and is ideally approached posterosagittally with splitting of the anal

canal longitudinally (Fig.35-5B). Patients with this defect have all the necessary elements for continence and have an excellent functional prognosis because they have a well-developed anal canal, normal sensation in the anorectum, and normal voluntary sphincters. These patients must be screened for a presacral mass.[25]

FEMALE ANORECTAL DEFECTS

Rectoperineal Fistulas

From the therapeutic and prognostic viewpoint, this common defect is equivalent to the perineal fistula described in the male patient.[18] The rectum is well positioned within the sphincter mechanism, except for its lower portion, which is anteriorly located. The rectum and vagina are well separated (Fig. 35-6). The key anatomic issues are the anal opening in relation to the sphincter mechanism, and the length of the perineal body.

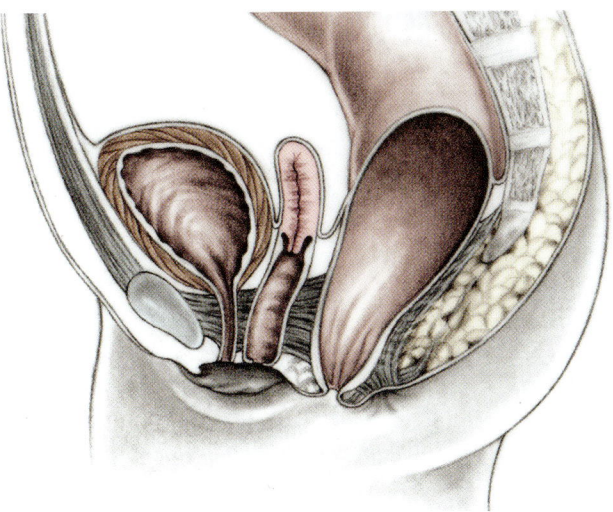

FIGURE 35-6 ■ Schematic drawing of a perineal fistula in a female. Most of the rectum is in the muscle complex. Only the most distal aspect of the rectum is anteriorly positioned.

Rectovestibular Fistulas

Rectovestibular fistula is the most common defect in females and has an excellent functional prognosis. The diagnosis is based on clinical examination. A meticulous inspection of the newborn's genitalia allows the clinician to observe a normal urethral meatus and a normal vagina, with a third hole in the vestibule, which is the rectovestibular fistula (Fig. 35-7). About 5% of these patients will have two hemivaginas with a vaginal septum.[26]

This defect can be repaired without a protective colostomy by experienced surgeons.[27–29] The advantage of this approach is that it avoids the potential morbidity of a colostomy and reduces the number of operations to one from as many as three (colostomy, main repair, and colostomy closure). Many patients do very well with a primary neonatal operation without a protective colostomy. However, a perineal infection followed by dehiscence of the anal anastomosis or perineal body, or recurrence of the fistula provokes severe fibrosis that may interfere with the sphincter function. If these complications occur, the patient may have lost the best opportunity for an optimal functional result because secondary operations do not render the same prognosis as a successful primary operation.[30] Thus, a protective colostomy is still the best way to avoid these complications for most surgeons. The decision to perform a colostomy or primary repair in these cases must be made individually by the surgeon based on experience and the clinical condition of the patient. At our institution, neonates without significant associated defects undergo repair without a colostomy.

Imperforate Anus without Fistula

This defect in female patients carries the same therapeutic and prognostic implications as described for male patients.

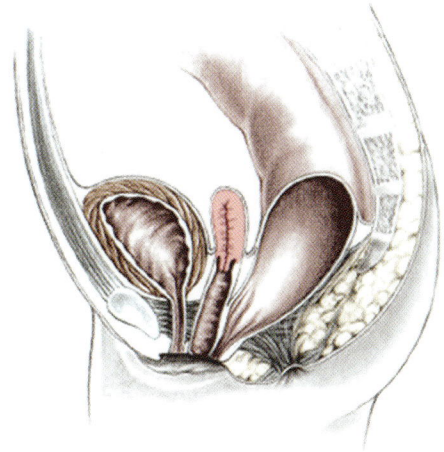

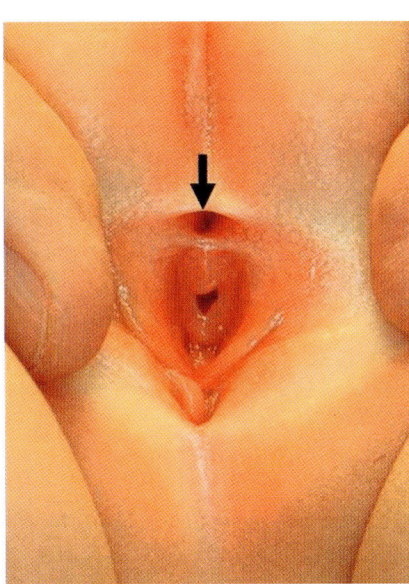

FIGURE 35-7 ■ **(A)** Schematic drawing of a rectovestibular fistula. **(B)** Female neonate with a rectovestibular fistula is in the prone position. The rectal fistula (arrow) is located in the posterior aspect of the vestibule.

Persistent Cloaca

This group of defects represents the extreme in the spectrum of complexity of female malformations. A cloaca is a defect in which the distal portions of the rectum, vagina, and urinary tract fuse and create a single common perineal channel. The diagnosis of a cloaca is a clinical one. This defect should be suspected in a female born with imperforate anus and small-looking genitalia. Careful separation of the labia discloses a single perineal orifice. The length of the common channel varies from 1–7 cm, and is very important for operative and prognostic implications (Fig. 35-8). A common channel of less than 3 cm usually means that the defect can be repaired with a posterior sagittal operation without opening the abdomen. Common channels longer than 3 cm are more complex, mobilization of the vagina is often difficult, and some form of vaginal replacement may be needed during the definitive repair. When the rectum opens high into the

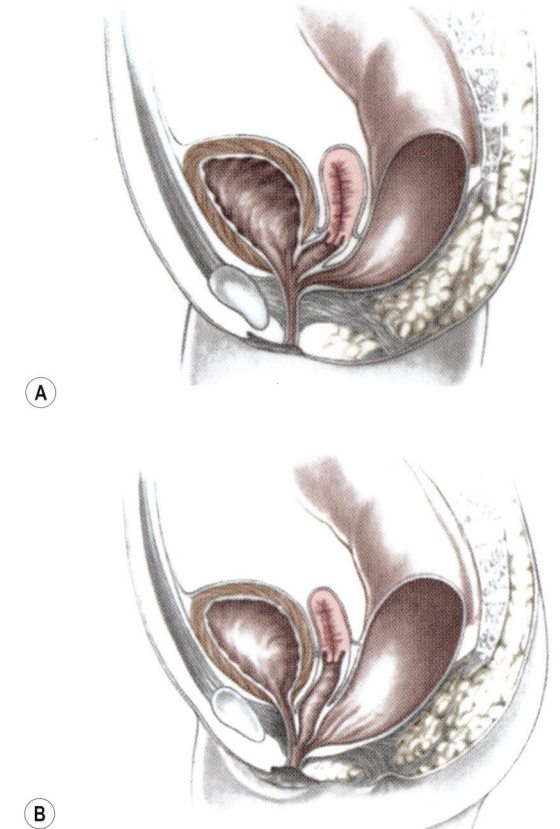

(A)

(B)

FIGURE 35-8 ■ **(A)** Schematic diagram of a long common channel in a female with a cloacal anomaly. **(B)** The more commonly encountered short common channel cloaca is depicted.

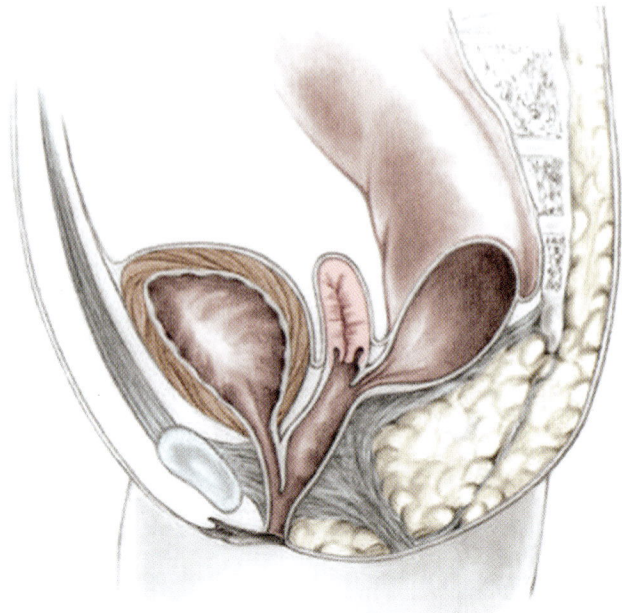

FIGURE 35-9 ■ A schematic diagram of the rectum inserting high into the posterior vagina with a short common urethral and vaginal channel is shown.

dome of the vagina (Fig. 35-9), an abdominal approach must be utilized to mobilize the bowel.

Frequently, the vagina is abnormally distended and full of secretions (hydrocolpos) (Fig. 35-10A). The distended vagina compresses the trigone and interferes with drainage of the ureters, and is frequently associated with hydronephrosis. This condition may be diagnosed prenatally.[31,32] The dilated vagina can also become infected (pyocolpos) and may lead to perforation and peritonitis. Such a large vagina may represent a technical advantage for the repair as there is more vaginal tissue to facilitate the reconstruction. A frequent finding in cloacal malformations is the presence of different degrees of vaginal and uterine septation or duplication (Fig. 35-10B). In these cases, the rectum usually enters between the two hemivaginas. Rarely, patients have cervical atresia. During puberty, a variety of anatomic anomalies may mean that they are unable to drain menstrual blood through the vagina, can accumulate menstrual blood in the peritoneal cavity, and sometimes require emergency operations.[26,33] An evaluation of the patient's Müllerian anatomy, either at the time of the definitive repair or at colostomy closure, is very important and can prevent future problems.[26] Short common channel cloacal malformations (<3 cm) are usually associated with a well-developed sacrum, a normal-appearing perineum, and adequate muscles and nerves. Therefore, a good functional prognosis can be expected.

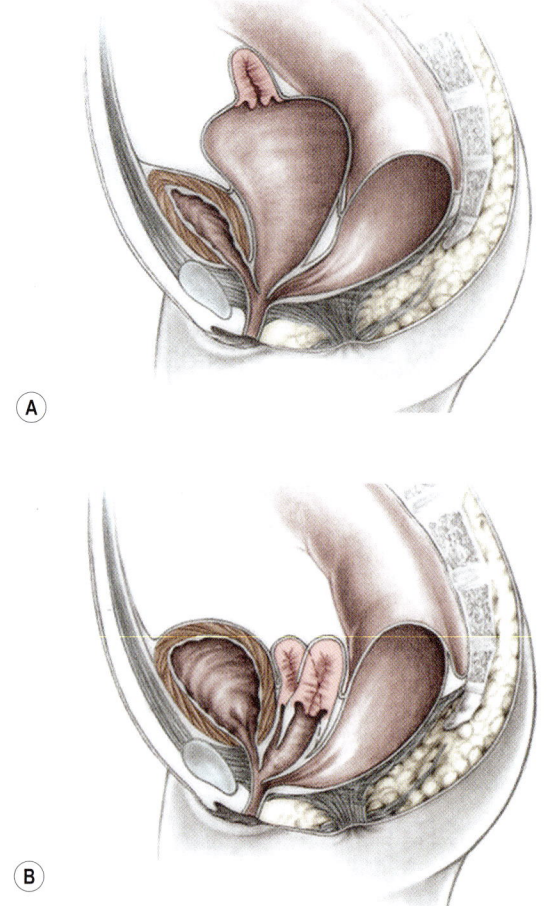

(A)

(B)

FIGURE 35-10 ■ **(A)** Schematic depiction of a cloacal anomaly with insertion of the rectum into the common channel and subsequent vaginal obstruction with hydrocolpos. **(B)** Schematic depiction of a cloacal anomaly and uterine duplication. The rectum is shown entering between the two hemivaginas.

ASSOCIATED DEFECTS

Sacrum and Spine

Sacral deformities are the most frequently associated defect.[34] One or several sacral vertebrae may be missing. A single missing vertebrae does not seem to have important prognostic implications.[18] However, more than two absent sacral vertebrae represent a poor prognostic sign in terms of bowel continence and, sometimes, urinary control, and is consistent with caudal regression. A hemisacrum is usually associated with a presacral mass and poor bowel control.[25] Other sacral abnormalities, such as spinal hemivertebra, have negative implications for bowel control.

A sacral ratio is an objective evaluation of the sacrum (Fig. 35-11). The sacral ratio can range from 0.0 to 1.0. The normal sacral ratio in children is 0.77. Children with anorectal malformations suffer varying degrees of poor sacral development. We have never seen a patient have bowel control with a sacral ratio of less than 0.3. Greater than 0.7 is usually associated with good bowel control.

A tethered cord is frequently associated with anorectal malformations, and its presence has been assumed to be associated with a poor functional prognosis.[35–44] Although it is true that most of these children have a poor prognosis, the presence of a tethered cord is usually found in patients with a very high defect, very abnormal sacrum, or spina bifida. Therefore, it is difficult to know whether the tethered cord itself is responsible for the poor prognosis. Although it is unclear whether the operation to release the tethered cord changes the functional bowel prognosis of the patient, it does seem to improve urinary function and certainly avoids motor and sensory deterioration of the lower extremeties.[41,44]

The reported frequency of associated genitourinary defects varies from 20–54%.[45–57] The accuracy and thoroughness of the urologic evaluation may account for the reported variation.

In our experience, half of patients have an associated genitourinary anomaly. These figures may not reflect the real incidence of genitourinary defects because our hospital is a referral center where we see a high proportion of complex malformations that are not necessarily representative of the entire spectrum of defects.

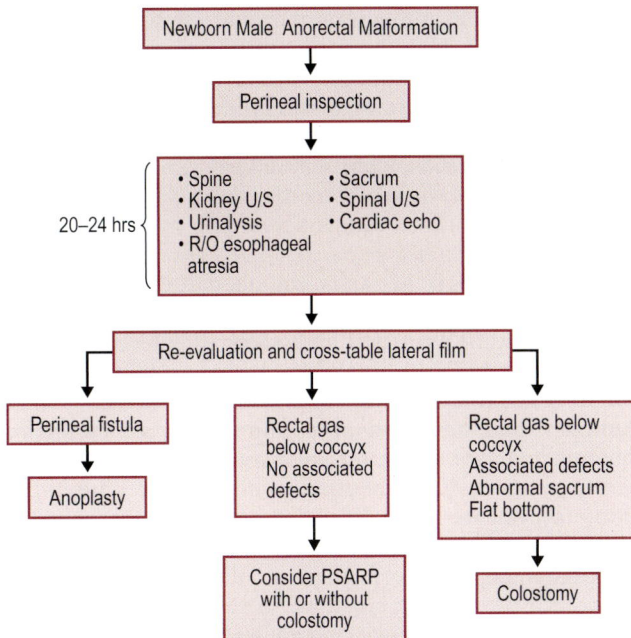

FIGURE 35-12 ■ Algorithm for the management of male newborns with anorectal malformations based on the physical examination and radiographs. PSARP, posterior sagittal anorectoplasty; U/S, ultrasonography; R/O, rule out.

It is clear that the higher the malformation, the more frequent are the associated urologic abnormalities. Patients with persistent cloacas or rectobladderneck fistulas have a 90% chance of having an associated genitourinary abnormality.[51] Conversely, children with low defects such as perineal fistulas have less than a 10% chance of having an associated urologic defect. Hydronephrosis, urosepsis, and metabolic acidosis from poor renal function represent the main sources of morbidity. Thus, a thorough urologic investigation is particularly important in patients with high defects. The evaluation in every child with imperforate anus must include an ultrasound (US) of the kidneys and abdomen to evaluate for the presence of hydronephrosis or any other urologic obstructive process. In patients with a cloaca, this study is especially important to exclude the presence of hydrocolpos. Further urologic investigations after this initial screening may also be necessary.

NEWBORN MANAGEMENT

A decision-making algorithm for the initial management in male infants is seen in Figure 35-12.

When asked to evaluate a male newborn with an anorectal malformation, a thorough perineal inspection must be performed. It is important not to make a decision about a colostomy or a primary operation before 24 hours of life. The reason is that significant intraluminal pressure is required for the meconium to be forced through a perineal fistula. If meconium is seen on the perineum, a rectoperineal fistula is present. If there is meconium in the urine, a rectourinary fistula exists.

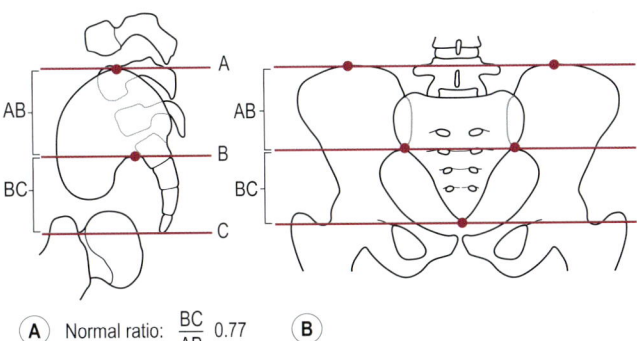

FIGURE 35-11 ■ Drawings with landmarks necessary for the calculation of the sacral ratio. **(A)** Lateral view. **(B)** Anteroposterior view. The normal ratio is 0.77.

Radiographic evaluations may not show the correct anatomy before 24 hours because the rectum is collapsed. It takes a significant amount of intraluminal pressure to overcome the muscle tone of the sphincters that surround the lower part of the rectum. Therefore, imaging studies before 24 hours most likely will show a 'very high rectum' and may lead to an incorrect diagnosis. Historically, an invertogram was used to identify whether the anomaly is 'high' or 'low'.[58]

During the first 24 hours, the neonate should receive intravenous fluids, antibiotics, and nasogastric decompression, and be evaluated for associated defects that may represent a threat to life. These include cardiac malformations, esophageal atresia, and urinary defects.[34,59] A radiograph of the lumbar spine and the sacrum should be obtained as well as a spinal ultrasound to evaluate for a tethered cord. Renal/abdominal ultrasound should be done to evaluate for hydronephrosis.

If the neonate has signs of a rectoperineal fistula, an anoplasty can be performed in the newborn period without a protective colostomy. After 24 hours, if there is no meconium on the perineum, we recommend obtaining a cross-table lateral radiograph with the patient in the prone position (Fig. 35-13A). If air in the rectum is seen distal to the coccyx (Fig. 35-13B), and the patient is in good condition with no significant associated defects, one may consider performing a posterior sagittal operation without a protective colostomy. A more conservative alternative would be to perform the posterior sagittal repair and a protective colostomy at the same stage.

Conversely, if the rectal gas does not extend beyond the coccyx, or the patient has meconium in the urine, an abnormal sacrum, or a flat bottom, we recommend a colostomy. This allows for a future distal colostogram, which will delineate the distal rectal anatomy. We will then perform a posterior sagittal anorectoplasty two to three months later, provided the neonate is gaining weight appropriately.

Performing the definitive repair early in life has important advantages including less time with an abdominal stoma, less size discrepancy between the proximal and distal bowel at the time of colostomy closure, and easier anal dilation (because the infant is smaller). In addition, at least theoretically, placing the rectum in the right location early in life potentially may represent an advantage in terms of acquired local sensation.[60]

All of these potential advantages of an early operation must be weighed against the possible disadvantages of an inexperienced surgeon who is not familiar with the anatomic structures of an infant's pelvis. Operating on patients with anorectal malformations primarily without a protective colostomy has been done successfully, but may have negative consequences if the surgeon does not have the necessary preoperative evaluation and experience.[29,61,62]

A temptation to repair these defects without a protective colostomy always exists.[27,61,62] Repair without a colostomy does not allow a distal colostogram which may be very helpful to the surgeon. The worst complications involve infants who undergo repair without a colostomy or a properly performed distal colostogram.[63] Proceeding with the posterior sagittal approach looking blindly for the rectum has resulted in a spectrum of serious complications, including damage to the urethra, complete division of the urethra, pull-through of the urethra, pull-through of the bladder neck, injury to the ureters, and division of the vas deferens or seminal vesicles.[63]

A decision-making algorithm for the initial management of newborn females is shown in Figure 35-14. Again, the perineal inspection is the most important step to guide diagnosis and decision making. The first 24 hours should also be used to evaluate for associated defects, as previously described. Perineal inspection may show the presence of a single perineal orifice, which establishes the diagnosis of a cloaca and carries a high risk of an associated urologic defect. Also, it should prompt a complete urologic evaluation, including abdominal and pelvic ultrasound, to look for hydronephrosis and hydrocolpos.

Patients with a cloaca require a colostomy. It is important to perform the divided sigmoid colostomy in such a manner as to leave enough redundant, distal rectosigmoid colon to allow for the subsequent pull-through (Fig. 35-15). When performing the colostomy for a cloaca, it is important to drain a hydrocolpos when present. This can be achieved with a curled catheter. Because a significant number of these patients have two hemivaginas, the surgeon must be certain that both hemivaginas are drained. Occasionally, a vaginovaginostomy in the vaginal septum needs to be created to drain both hemivaginas with one catheter. At times, the hydrocolpos is so large that it may produce respiratory distress. Also, the hydrocolpos can compress the trigone and cause hydronephrosis, and drainage of the hydrocolpos allows for decompression of the urologic system. Rarely, if the common channel is very narrow and does not allow the

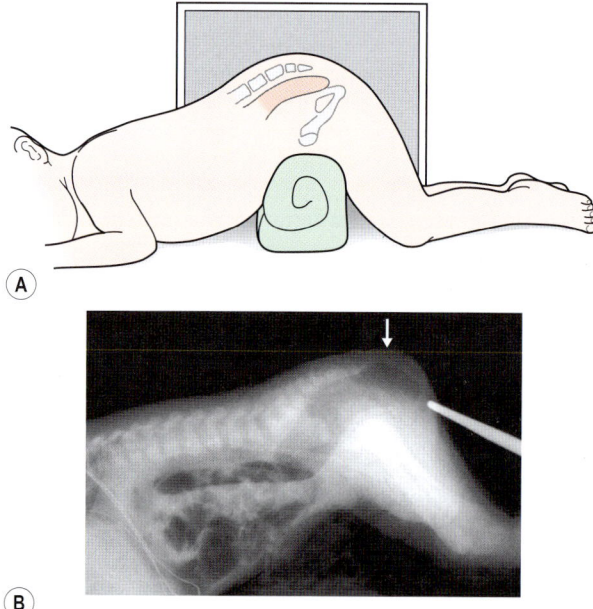

FIGURE 35-13 ■ Technique for a cross-table lateral radiograph. **(A)** A roll has been placed beneath the hips of the infant to elevate the buttocks and allow air to migrate superiorly to the end of the rectum. **(B)** Actual cross-table lateral radiograph. Air is visualized distal to the coccyx (arrow).

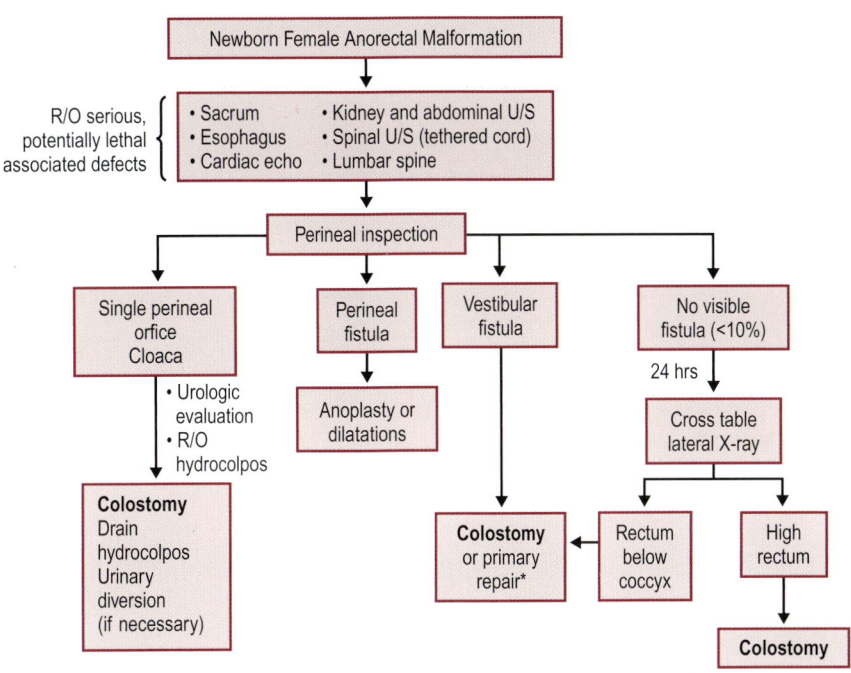

FIGURE 35-14 ■ Decision-making algorithm for female newborns with anorectal malformations. U/S, ultrasonography; R/O, rule out.

* Depending on the experience of the surgeon and general condition of the patient

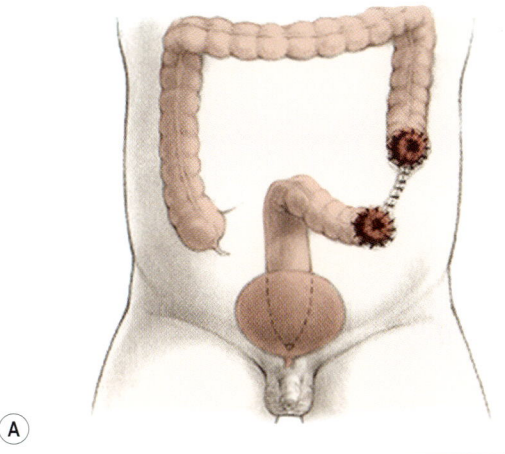

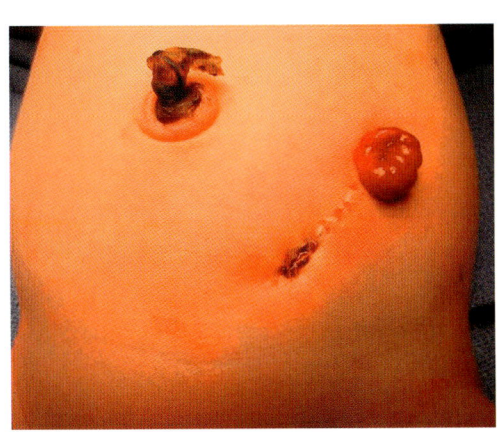

FIGURE 35-15 ■ An ideal colostomy for infants with high anorectal malformations is seen in (A) the drawing and (B) infant. Note the colostomy and mucous fistula are separated and that adequate distal colonic length remains for the subsequent rectal pull-through.

bladder to drain, the neonate may require a vesicostomy or suprapubic cystostomy to decompress the bladder. However, in most cases, drainage of the hydrocolpos is all that is required. Endoscopic examination of the cloaca is recommended to delineate the anatomy. This evaluation is best done several months later during a separate anesthetic because the neonatal perineum is swollen and endoscopy is difficult in the newborn.

The presence of a vestibular fistula represents the most common finding in female infants (see Fig. 35-7). When newborns with a vestibular fistula undergo primary repair at our institution, we hospitalize the patient for seven days with no oral intake, and use concentrated dextrose intravenous nutrition. When the patient undergoes a primary repair of a vestibular fistula or perineal fistula without colostomy later in life, we are particularly strict about preoperative bowel preparation to ensure that the intestine is completely clean.

If the perineal inspection shows a rectoperineal fistula, we recommend performing a primary anoplasty without a colostomy. In fewer than 5% of girls, there is no visible fistula and there is no evidence of meconium after 24 hours of observation. This small group of patients requires a cross-table lateral prone radiograph (see Fig. 35-13). If the radiograph shows gas in the rectum very close to the skin, it means that the baby likely has a very narrow perineal fistula or has no fistula defect. If the baby is in stable condition, one can perform a primary operation without a colostomy, depending on the surgeon's experience. Most of these patients without a fistula also have Down syndrome.[19] If associated conditions make the rectal repair not feasible in the newborn period, a colostomy should be performed, with definitive repair later.

Occasionally, if the infant with a rectoperineal or rectovestibular fistula has significant associated defects or is unstable, the surgeon may elect to dilate the fistula to

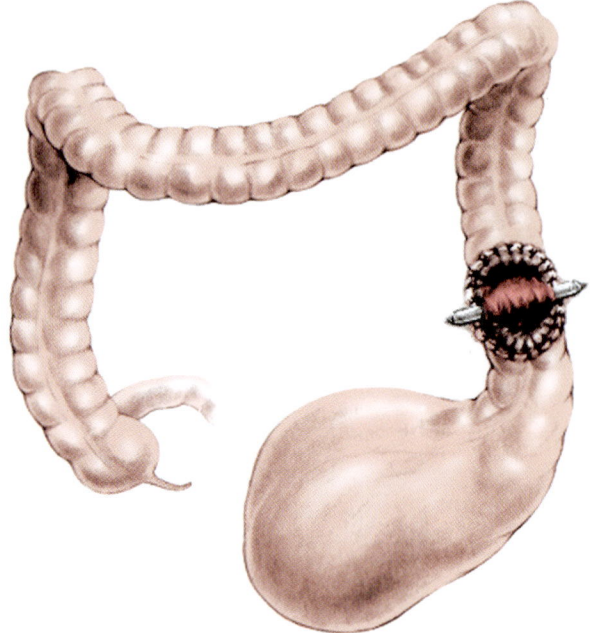

FIGURE 35-16 ■ A markedly dilated distal rectal pouch secondary to fecal impaction. (Adapted from Prem Puri. In: Newborn Surgery. 3rd ed. Hodder Arnold; 2012. p. 580.)

facilitate emptying of the colon while these other issues are addressed. Definitive repair can be performed in a few months.

A divided descending colostomy is ideal for the management of anorectal malformations when diversion is needed (see Fig. 35-15). The completely diverting colostomy provides bowel decompression as well as protection for the final reconstruction. In addition, the colostomy is used for the distal colostogram, which is the most accurate diagnostic study to determine the detailed distal anatomy.[64–66]

The descending or upper sigmoid colostomy has definitive advantages over a right or transverse colostomy.[65] It is important to have a relatively short segment of defunctionalized distal colon, but not too short as to interfere with the subsequent pull-through. The ideal location is just at the point where the proximal sigmoid comes off the left retroperitoneum. Mechanical cleansing of the distal colon at the time of colostomy is much less difficult when the colostomy is located in the descending portion of the colon. In the case of a large rectourethral fistula, the patient may pass urine into the colon. A more distal colostomy allows urine to escape through the distal stoma without significant absorption. With a more proximal colostomy, the urine remains in the colon and is absorbed, leading to metabolic acidosis. A loop colostomy permits the passage of stool from the proximal stoma into the distal bowel. This can lead to urinary tract infections, distal rectal pouch dilation, and fecal impaction (Fig. 35-16). Prolonged distention of the rectal pouch may produce a megarectosigmoid, leading to severe constipation later in life. Also, the problem of colostomy prolapse is more frequent with loop colostomies.[65] The most common error is a colostomy established too distal in the rectosigmoid that will interfere

with mobilization of the rectum during the pull-through (Fig. 35-17).

To perform the reconstruction, the patient is placed in prone position with the pelvis elevated. An electrical stimulator is used to elicit muscle contraction during the operation. The contraction serves to keep the incision in the midline, leaving an equal amount of muscle on both sides. The length of the incision varies with the type of defect and can be extended to achieve the exposure needed to result in a satisfactory repair. Thus, a perineal

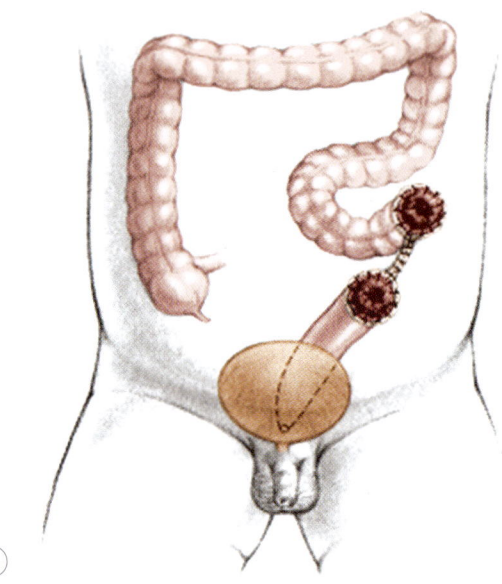

(A)

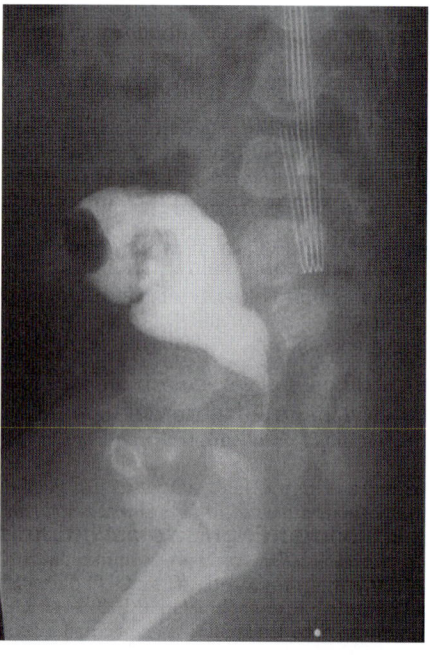

(B)

FIGURE 35-17 ■ **(A)** It is important not to create the colostomy too distal because there will not be sufficient rectal length to allow for pull-through. **(B)** This problem is seen on the lateral view of the barium enema, where there is insufficient distal rectal length for the pull-through. This is because of an inappropriately placed colostomy and mucous fistula.

fistula requires a minimal posterior sagittal incision (2 cm) whereas higher defects may require a full posterior sagittal incision that runs from the lower portion of the sacrum toward the base of the scrotum in the male or to the single perineal orifice in females with a cloaca. The incision includes the skin and subcutaneous tissue and splits the parasagittal fibers, muscle complex, and levator muscles in the midline. With perineal and vestibular fistulas, the incision divides only the parasagittal fibers and the muscle complex in the midline. It is not usually necessary to open the levator muscle. Once the sphincter mechanism is divided, the next most important step of the operation is the separation of the rectum from the urogenital structures. This is the most delicate part of the procedure. Any blind maneuver at this point exposes the patient to the possibility of serious injury.[63]

About 90% of defects in boys can be repaired via a posterior sagittal approach without entering the abdomen. Each case has individual anatomic variants that mandate technical modifications. An example is the size discrepancy frequently seen between an ectatic rectum and the space available for the pull-through. If the discrepancy is significant, the surgeon must tailor the rectum to fit. As repairs are being performed earlier in life and patients are receiving adequate colostomies, rectal dilatation is less commonly seen and tapering is less frequently required.

If a colostomy has been created, the posterior sagittal approach should never be attempted without a technically adequate high-pressure distal colostogram to determine the exact position of the rectum and the fistula (Fig. 35-18).[64] Attempting the repair without this critical information significantly increases the potential damage to the seminal vesicles, ureters, vas deferens, prostate, urethra, and innervation to the bladder.[63]

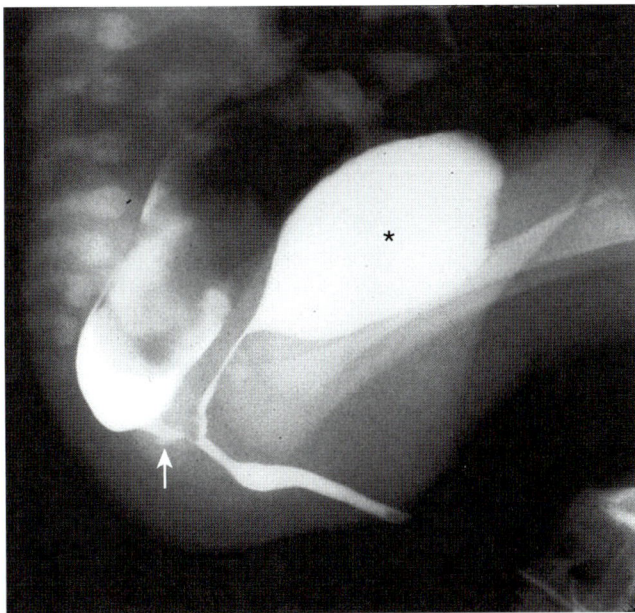

FIGURE 35-18 ■ A lateral view of a high-pressure, distal colostogram shows a rectobulbar urethral fistula (arrow). The bladder (asterisk) also filled during the study.

REPAIR OF SPECIFIC DEFECTS IN MALE INFANTS

Rectoperineal Fistula

The operation in these infants is performed in the prone position with the pelvis elevated. A urinary catheter should be inserted preoperatively. Multiple 6-0 silk stitches are placed in the fistula orifice. An incision is created dividing the sphincter mechanism located just posterior to the fistula. The incision usually measures about 2 cm in length. The sphincter is divided, and the posterior rectal wall is identified by its characteristic whitish appearance. Dissection of the rectum continues laterally following this specific plane. The last part of the dissection consists of separating the anterior rectal wall from its intimate relation to the urethra. The most common and serious complication in these relatively straightforward operations involves injury to the urethra.[63] The best way to avoid urethral injury is to understand the fact that the common wall has no plane of dissection and that the surgeon must create two walls out of one.

Rectourethral Fistulas

A urinary catheter is inserted. Sometimes the catheter goes into the rectum rather than into the bladder. Under these circumstances, the surgeon may attempt the bladder catheterization again using a Coudé catheter or catheter guide, or can relocate the catheter into the bladder under direct visualization during the operation.

A posterior sagittal incision is made (Fig. 35-19). The parasagittal fibers, muscle complex, and levator muscle fibers are completely divided in the midline. Sometimes, the coccyx can be split in the midline or dissected on each side with cautery, particularly in those cases of a rectoprostatic fistula when the surgeon requires more exposure in the upper part of the incision. The higher the malformation, the deeper the levator muscle. With the entire sphincter mechanism divided, the surgeon should identify the rectum. It is at this point that the importance of a good high-pressure distal colostogram cannot be overstated. If the colostogram showed the presence of a bulbourethral fistula (see Fig. 35-18), the rectum is going to be found just below the levators, with little risk of inadvertent injury to the urinary tract. In this situation, the rectum actually bulges through the incision when the sphincter mechanism is divided (Fig. 35-20). Minimal mobilization of the rectum is needed because only a short gap exists between the rectum and perineum. The anterior rectal wall must be adequately dissected free of the urethra so as not to leave behind the rectourethral fistula.

Conversely, if the preoperative distal colostogram shows a rectoprostatic fistula (Fig. 35-21), the surgeon must be particularly careful because the rectum joins the urinary tract much higher. The initial search for the rectum should be near the coccyx. Looking for the rectum lower than the coccyx risks injury to the urethra. If the colostogram shows a rectobladderneck fistula (Fig. 35-22), the posterior sagittal approach is not appropriate as a means of identifying the distal bowel. The rectum

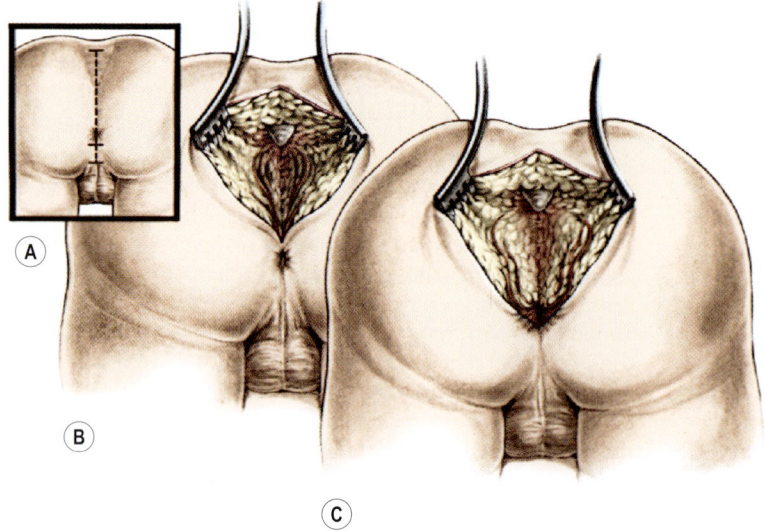

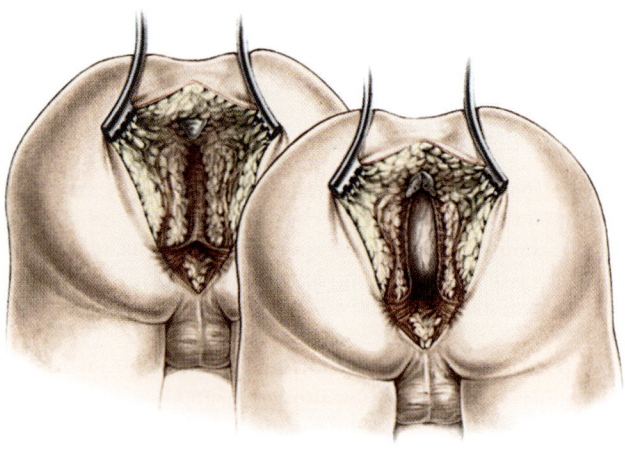

FIGURE 35-19 ■ This drawing shows a posterior sagittal incision in a male patient with a rectourethral fistula. Separation of the parasagittal fibers and exposure of the muscle complex are shown.

FIGURE 35-20 ■ Schematic drawing of the posterior sagittal approach. The muscle complex and the levator muscles have been divided, and the rectum is visualized below the levator muscle complex.

should be identified and separated from the urinary bladder through an abdominal approach (via laparoscopy or laparotomy). This is also true for a high rectoprostatic fistula.

In all cases in which the rectal fistula is approached via a posterior sagittal incision, silk traction sutures are placed in the posterior rectal wall on both sides and the rectum is opened in the midline. The incision in the rectum is extended distally, exactly in the midline, down to the fistula. Additional silk traction sutures are placed around the edges of the opened posterior rectal wall. When the fistula is visualized, silk sutures are situated around the orifice of the fistula as well.

The anterior rectal wall above the fistula is part of a common wall, with no natural plane of separation between the urinary tract and the rectum. A plane of separation must be created in the common wall. For this, multiple 6-0 silk traction stitches are positioned in the rectal mucosa immediately above the fistula orifice. The rectal mucosa is then separated from the urethra for 5–10 mm above the fistula using a submucosal dissection (Fig.

35-23). It is this dissection that is the source of the most serious complications during this repair. We recommend creating a lateral plane of dissection on either side of the rectum to help delineate the rectal wall from the urethra and prostate. The rectum is covered by a thin fascia which contains fat, vessels, and nerves that must be preserved on the back side of the bladder. This tissue should be completely stripped from the rectum to be sure that one is working as close as possible to the rectal wall, which is the only way to prevent denervation of the bladder or injury to the vas deferens. Once the rectum is fully separated from the deep structures of the urinary tract, a circumferential perirectal dissection is performed to gain enough rectal length to reach the perineum.

In babies with a rectoprostatic fistula, the perirectal dissection is considerably longer and more difficult, yet

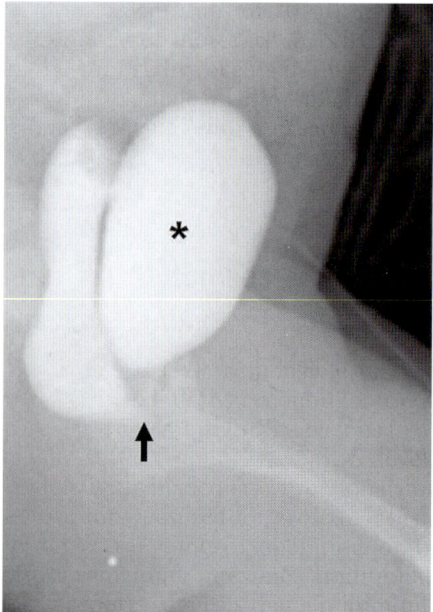

FIGURE 35-21 ■ This distal colostogram shows the rectum entering the prostatic urethra (rectoprostatic urethral fistula) (arrow). Note filling of the bladder (asterisk) as well.

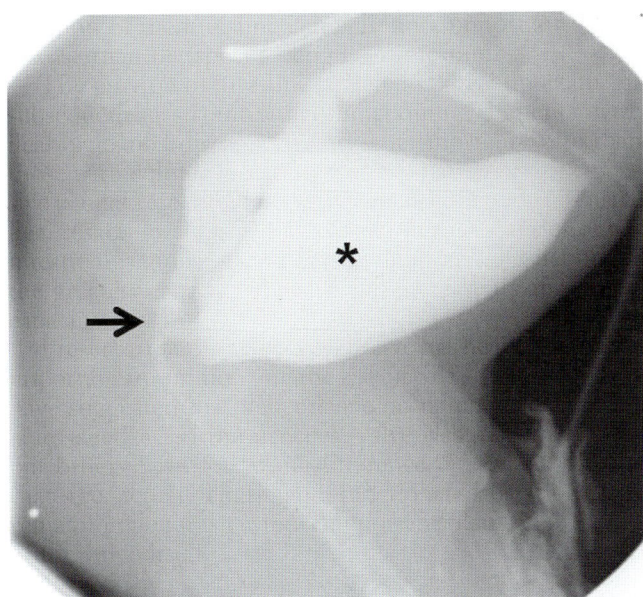

FIGURE 35-22 ■ This distal colostogram shows a rectobladder-neck fistula (arrow). The bladder is marked with an asterisk.

the separation from the posterior urethra is easier. During this dissection, uniform traction is applied on the multiple silk traction sutures that were placed on the rectal edges and also on the mucosa above the fistula. Uniform traction helps expose the rectal wall and allows identification of fibrous bands and vessels that hold the rectum in the pelvis. These bands must be carefully separated from the rectal wall using cautery because they contain vessels that tend to retract into the pelvis once divided. The dissection should be performed as close as possible to the rectal wall without injuring the wall. Laparoscopy can also be used here instead of a posterior sagittal dissection.[62,67–69]

At the completion of the dissection in prostatic fistula cases, many of the extrinsic vessels that supply the rectum have been sacrificed. The rectum should be viable, however, provided the intramural blood supply was preserved. One might think that this denervation would provoke a motility disorder, leading to severe constipation, but this has not been our experience. Patients with lower defects (who undergo less dissection) are bothered by more severe postoperative constipation than are patients with higher defects.[70] There seems to be an inherent motility disorder that is more prevalent in lower defects.

The circumferential dissection of the rectum must continue until the surgeon feels that enough length has been gained to allow for a tension-free rectoperineal anastomosis. At this point, the size of the rectum can be evaluated and compared with the available space. If necessary, the rectum can be tapered, removing part of the posterior wall (opposite the side adjacent to the urethral repair), and closing it with two layers of interrupted long-lasting absorbable stitches. The anterior rectal wall is frequently thinned to some degree as a consequence of the mucosal separation between the rectum and urethra. To reinforce this wall, both smooth muscle layers can be approximated with interrupted 5-0 absorbable stitches. The urethral fistula is closed with the same suture material.

The limits of the sphincter mechanism are electrically determined and marked with temporary silk stitches at the skin level. Sometimes, in patients with a good sphincter mechanism, these limits are easily visible, even without electrical stimulation. The limits of the sphincter are represented by the crossing of the muscle complex with the parasagittal fibers. One can use an electrical stimulator or a bipolar cautery to show the muscle contraction. These are the voluntary muscles that run from the levator all the way down to the skin parallel with the direction of the rectum. This muscle structure crosses the parasagittal fibers that run perpendicular and lateral to the muscle complex and parallel to the posterior sagittal incision. The perineal body is reconstructed, bringing together the anterior limits of the sphincter. The rectum must then be positioned in front of the levator and within the limits of the muscle complex (Fig. 35-24). Long-lasting 5-0 absorbable stitches are used to bring together the posterior edge of the levator muscle.

The posterior limit of the muscle complex is then reapproximated behind the rectum. These sutures should incorporate part of the rectal wall to anchor it and help avoid rectal prolapse.[71] An anoplasty is performed with 16 interrupted long-lasting absorbable stitches. The ischiorectal fossa and the subcutaneous tissue are then reapproximated, and the wound is closed with subcuticular 5-0 absorbable monofilament suture (Fig. 35-25).

All these infants have a urinary catheter inserted before the beginning of the operation that remains for seven days. The infant receives broad-spectrum antibiotics for 24 hours. These patients can be fed after recovery from anesthesia because they have a diverting colostomy.

Rectobladderneck Fistulas

In these patients, the rectum enters the bladder neck approximately 2 cm below the peritoneal reflection. A very important anatomic feature is that the higher the malformation, the shorter the common wall between the rectum and the urinary tract. In such cases, this means that the rectum joins with the urinary tract at nearly a

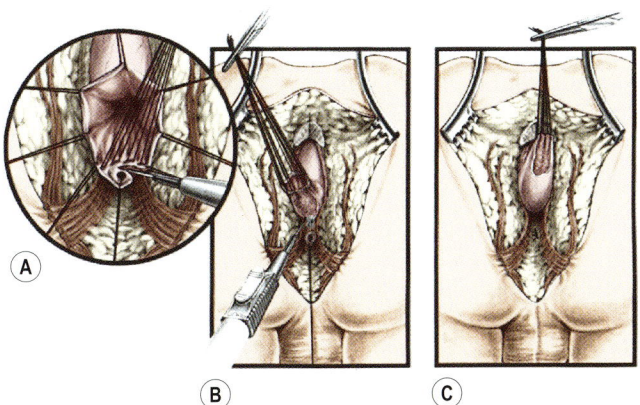

FIGURE 35-23 ■ A schematic representation of the separation of the rectal fistula from the urethra is shown. **(A)** Separation of the rectum from the urethra using silk traction stitches in the rectum. **(B)** Proximal dissection of the rectum from the urethra. **(C)** Depiction of the rectum completely separated from the underlying urethra.

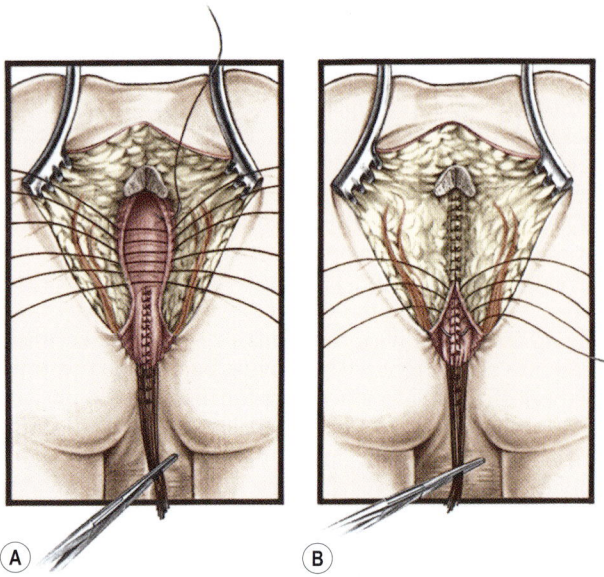

FIGURE 35-24 ■ Position of the rectum after separation from the urethra is shown. **(A)** Technique of passing the rectum in front of the levator muscle complex. **(B)** Technique of anchoring the rectal wall to the levator complex to avoid rectal prolapse.

right angle, with little common wall. Thus, separation of the rectum from the bladder is much easier. The laparoscopic approach provides an excellent view of the peritoneal reflection, the ureters, and the vas deferens, which must be visualized to prevent injury.

For this repair, a total body preparation is performed. The entire lower part of the patient's body is included in the sterile field. The operation is begun laparoscopically by dividing the peritoneum around the distal rectum to create a plane of dissection to be followed distally. The dissection should occur on the rectal wall. The rectum rapidly narrows as it reaches its communication with the bladder neck (Fig. 35-26). We use as a reference the 3 mm Maryland, which should be able to completely cross

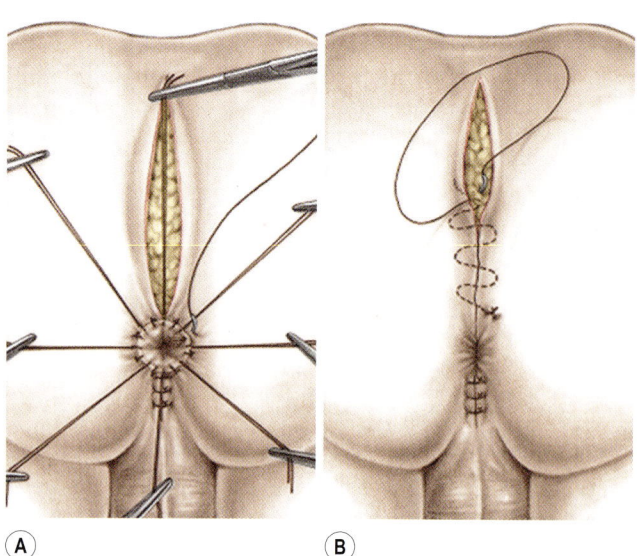

FIGURE 35-25 ■ **(A)** Technique of anoplasty. Four quadrant stay sutures are placed followed by three sutures between each quadrant. **(B)** Subcuticular skin closure.

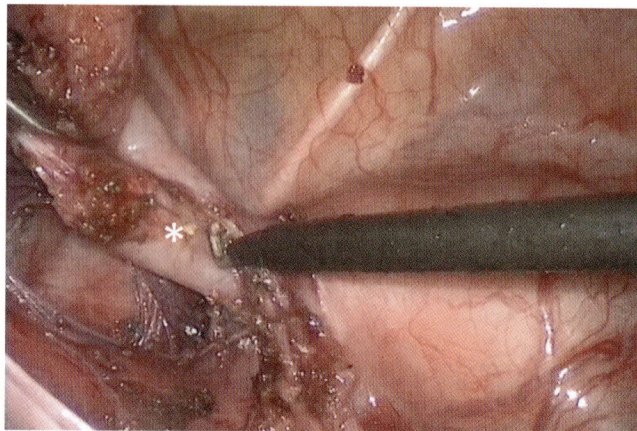

FIGURE 35-26 ■ This laparoscopic photograph shows the rectum narrow (asterisk) as it enters the bladder neck.

the distal rectal fistula. At this point, the fistula is divided and the bladder side of the fistula is sutured or ligated with an endoloop. The vessels that supply the distal rectum are divided until there is enough length to pull the rectum comfortably down to the perineum. These vessels should be divided close to the rectal wall, preserving the inferior mesenteric artery trunk because the arcade may have been disrupted by the initial colostomy. This dissection preserves perfusion to the rectum because the rectum has an excellent intramural blood supply. In these cases, the distal rectum can be ectatic and may require tapering. If the colostomy was created too distal in the sigmoid, it may interfere with this mobilization. Once the rectum is mobile, the legs are lifted up, a small midsagittal incision is made, and a clamp is gently passed through the perineum, just anterior to the coccyx. This space is much easier to see with the opened perineum afforded by the posterior sagittal incision. Great care must be taken to avoid passing the clamp too anteriorly because injury to the bladder neck or ectopic ureters can occur. The distal rectum is grasped and pulled through to be situated in the center of the sphincter mechanism. Often, in these patients, the center of the sphincter is quite anterior, near the base of the scrotum. Traction on the rectum from below can help demonstrate further lines of tension that must be divided laparoscopically to allow the rectum to reach the perineum. The posterior edges of the muscle complex are visualized and tacked to the posterior rectal wall to help avoid prolapse.[71]

Imperforate Anus without Fistula

In these cases, the blind end of the rectum is usually located at the level of the bulbar urethra and easily reachable from the posterior sagittal approach. The rectum must be carefully separated from the urethra because these structures have a common wall, even though no fistula is present. The rest of the repair is performed as described for the rectourethral fistula defect.

Rectal Atresia and Rectal Stenosis

The approach to these malformations is also posterior sagittal. The upper rectal pouch is opened and the distal anal canal is split in the posterior midline. An end-to-end anastomosis is performed (see Fig. 35-5B). If a presacral mass is identified, it is removed with presacral dissection at the same time.

REPAIR OF SPECIFIC DEFECTS IN FEMALE INFANTS

Rectoperineal Fistulas

This defect is repaired in the same way as described for male newborns. The rectum is not usually attached to the vagina and the chance of a vaginal injury is low.

Rectovestibular Fistulas

The complexity of this defect is frequently underestimated. Multiple 5-0 silk sutures are placed at the mucocutaneous junction of the fistula. The incision is shorter than the one used to repair the male rectourethral fistula, and continues down to and around the fistula into the vestibule. Once the sphincter mechanism is divided, the surgeon identifies the posterior rectal wall by its characteristic whitish appearance. The fascia that surrounds the rectum must be removed to ensure that the dissection is as close as possible to the rectal wall. The dissection is aided by working along each side of the rectum, while applying tension on the silk traction sutures. A long common wall exists between the vagina and the rectum, and two walls must be created out of one using meticulous, delicate technique. The dissection continues cephalad until the rectal and vaginal walls are fully separated and an areolar plane between the two is encountered (Fig. 35-27). If the rectum and the vagina are not completely separated, a tense anal anastomosis predisposes the patient to dehiscence, retraction, and stricture.[30,72]

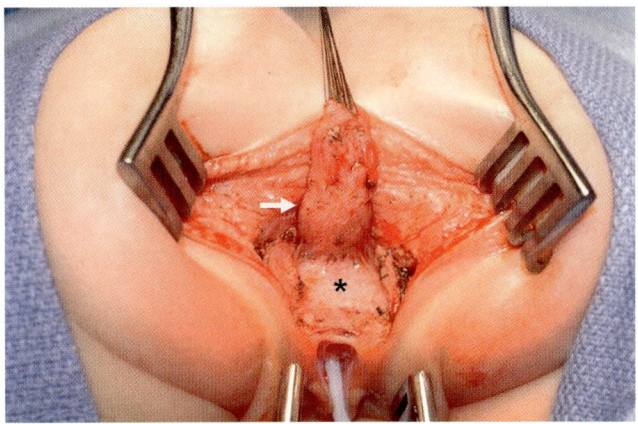

FIGURE 35-27 ■ In this operative photograph of a female patient undergoing repair of a rectovestibular fistula, note the complete separation of the rectum (arrow) from the anteriorly positioned vagina (asterisk). A catheter has been inserted into the vagina.

Once the dissection is complete, the perineal body is repaired (Fig. 35-28). The anterior edge of the muscle complex is reapproximated as previously described. The sutures include the posterior edge of the muscle complex and the posterior rectal wall to avoid rectal prolapse.[71] The anoplasty is performed as previously described for males.

Cloaca Repair

Before undertaking repair of a cloaca, the surgeon should perform an endoscopic study to determine the length of the common channel. Our review of 490 patients identified two well-characterized groups of patients with cloaca.[73] These two groups have different technical challenges and must be recognized preoperatively. The first

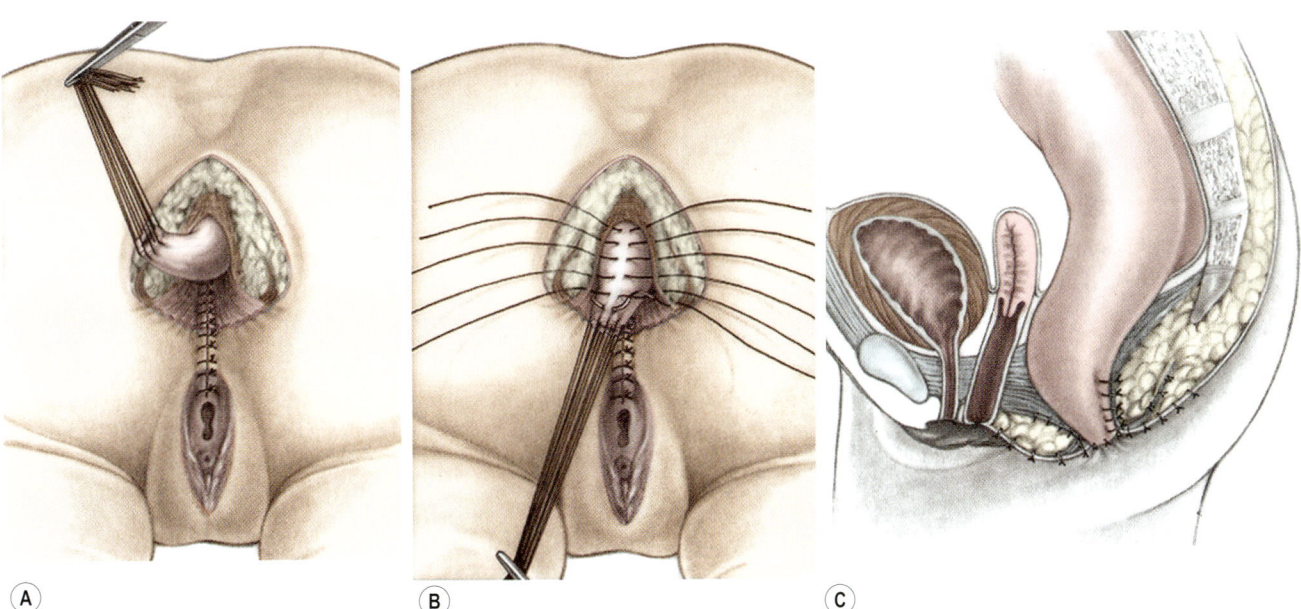

FIGURE 35-28 ■ Schematic drawings of the final stages of the repair of a rectovestibular fistula in a female. **(A)** Reconstruction of the perineal body. **(B)** Positioning the rectum in front of the levator muscle complex. **(C)** Sagittal view of the completed operation.

is represented by patients who are born with a common channel shorter than 3 cm. Fortunately, these patients comprise the majority and they can usually undergo repair with a posterior sagittal approach alone, avoiding a laparotomy. The operation to repair this particular variant is reproducible and can be accomplished by most pediatric surgeons. The second group is represented by patients with a long common channel (>3 cm). These patients usually need a laparotomy, and the intraoperative decision making requires a large experience, often a vaginal replacement, and special training in urology. Therefore, referral to a specialized center is recommended.

Cloacas with a Common Channel Shorter than 3 cm

The incision extends from the middle portion of the sacrum down to the single perineal orifice (Fig. 35-29). The sphincter mechanism is divided in the midline. The first structure that the surgeon finds after division of the sphincter mechanism is the rectum. However, because of the complexity of these malformations, bizarre anatomic arrangements of the rectum and vagina are sometimes encountered. The rectum is opened in the midline, and silk sutures are introduced along the edges of the posterior rectal wall. A mosquito clamp placed in the single perineal orifice facilitates extension of the incision through the posterior wall of the common channel. The entire common channel is exposed, which allows for measurement and visual confirmation of its length. The separation of the rectum from the vagina, which share a common wall, is performed as described for the repair of a rectovestibular fistula.

Once the rectum has been completely separated from the vagina, the total urogenital mobilization begins (Fig. 35-30), which consists of bringing both vagina and

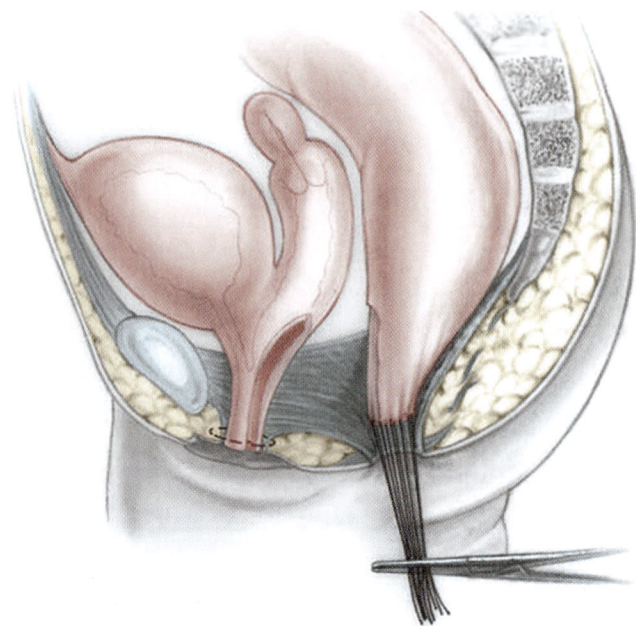

FIGURE 35-30 ■ A schematic representation of total urogenital sinus mobilization with separation of the rectum from the vagina. (Adapted from Peña A. Total urogenital mobilization: An easier way to repair cloacas. J Pediatr Surg 1997;32:263–8.)

urethra to the perineum as a single unit.[74] After the rectum has been mobilized from the urogenital complex, multiple silk traction sutures are placed at the edge of the vagina and the common channel in order to apply uniform traction on the urogenital sinus as it is mobilized. Another series of fine traction sutures is placed transversely approximately 5 mm proximal to the clitoris (Fig. 35-31). The urogenital sinus is transected between the last row of silk stitches and the clitoris. The anterior aspect is dissected full thickness from the pubic symphysis, taking advantage of the natural plane that exists between it and the pubis. This dissection is usually bloodless. At the upper edge of the pubis, there are fibrous, avascular suspensory ligaments that give support to the vagina and bladder. While applying traction to the multiple urogenital sinus sutures, the suspensory ligaments are divided, providing 2–3 cm of additional mobilization. Lateral and posterior dissection of the urogenital sinus will provide an additional 0.5–1.0 cm in length, allowing for complete urogenital mobilization (Fig. 35-32). Both the urethral meatus and the vaginal introitus can then be anastomosed to the perineum in the appropriate positions, which requires splitting of the common channel up to the urethra. Approximately 60% of all cloacas can be satisfactorily repaired with this technique, which has the additional advantage of preserving an excellent blood supply to both the urethra and vagina while placing the urethral opening and the smooth-walled urethra in a visible location to facilitate intermittent catheterization when necessary (Fig. 35-33). The common channel creates two lateral flaps that are sutured to the skin, creating the new labia. The vaginal edges are mobilized to reach the skin to create a surprisingly natural-looking introitus. The limits of the rectal sphincter are electrically determined, and the perineal body is reconstructed, bringing together

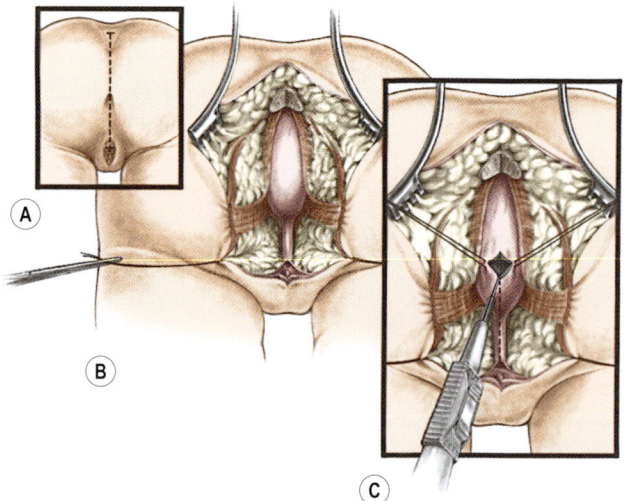

FIGURE 35-29 ■ Drawings of the initial steps of the posterior sagittal approach for cloacal repair. **(A)** The incision extends from the sacral prominence to the common orifice. **(B)** The exposure of the rectum and common channel above the levator complex. **(C)** The technique of opening the rectum and placement of traction sutures in the rectal opening.

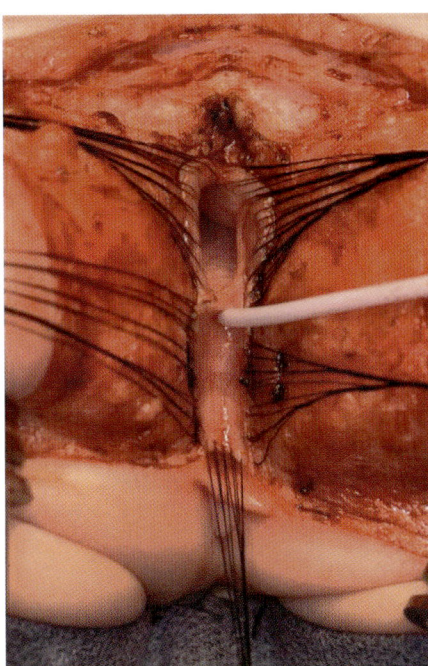

FIGURE 35-31 ■ Total urogenital mobilization. The patient is in the prone position. Silk sutures have been placed around the vagina (top) and transversely across the dissection plane near the clitoris (bottom). A catheter has been inserted in the urethra. (From Peña A, Levitt, Treatment of Cloacas. In: Anorectal Malformations in Children. Ch 22 Holschneider AM, Hutson J, editors. Heidelberg: Springer; 2006. p. 307–14.)

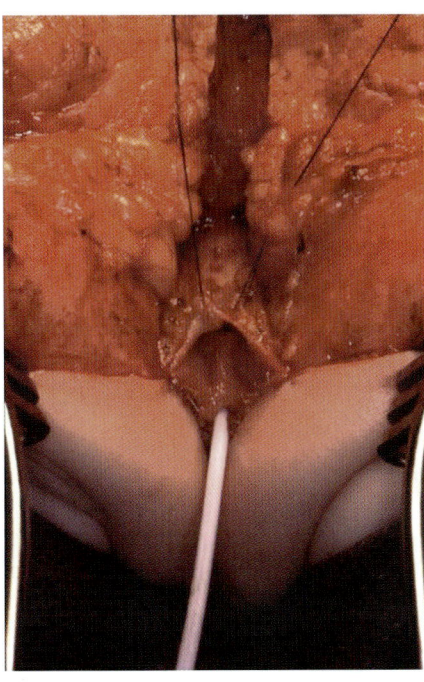

FIGURE 35-33 ■ A nearly completed cloacal repair. The urethral meatus (with catheter) and vaginal introitus have been anastomosed to the perineum in their appropriate positions. The patient is in the prone position. (From Peña A, Levitt. In Imperforate Anus and Cloacal Malformations. In: Pediaric Surgery. 4th ed. Ashcraft, Whitfield and Murphy, editors. Philadelphia: Elsevier Saunders; 2005. p. 496–517.)

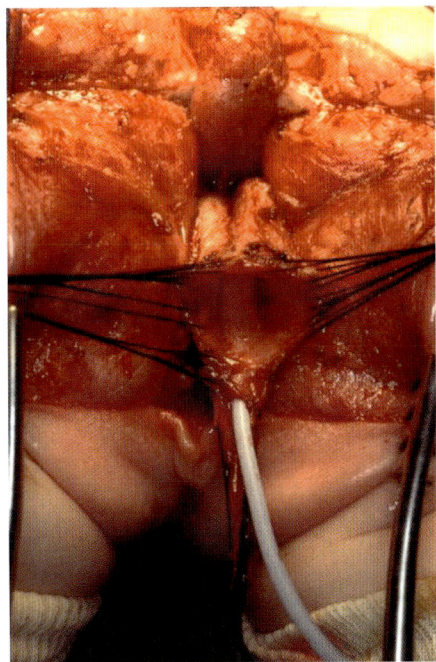

FIGURE 35-32 ■ In this female infant with a cloaca who is in the prone position, the urogenital sinus has been fully mobilized and freed from all of its lateral, anterior, and posterior attachments. The catheter is in the urethra. (From Peña A, Levitt, Treatment of Cloacas. In: Anorectal Malformations in Children. Ch 22 Holschneider AM, Hutson J, editors. Heidelberg: Springer; 2006. p. 307–14.)

the anterior limits of the sphincter. The rectum is placed within the margins of the sphincter (Fig. 35-34). As they have a colostomy, these neonates can eat the same day, and their pain is usually easily controlled. They are discharged 48 hours after surgery with their urinary catheter left for ten to 14 days.

Cloacas with a Common Channel Longer than 3 cm

When endoscopy shows that the patient has a long common channel, the surgeon must be prepared to face a significant technical challenge. In the presence of a long common channel, the patient should be prepped so that the entire lower body is accessible because it is likely that the patient will require a laparotomy after initial exploration via the posterior sagittal approach. As described previously, the rectum is separated and the length of the common channel of the urogenital sinus is determined. If the vagina is low in the pelvis, a total urogenital mobilization is performed. However, if further dissection around the urogenital complex fails to gain adequate length, the urinary tract and genital tract must be separated. To accomplish this safely, a midline laparotomy is performed. The bladder is opened in the midline, and feeding tubes are placed into the ureters to protect them. The ureters run through the common wall between the vagina and bladder, and the ureteral stents allow for their identification during the difficult dissection of the vagina from the bladder neck. Sometimes, though, delivering

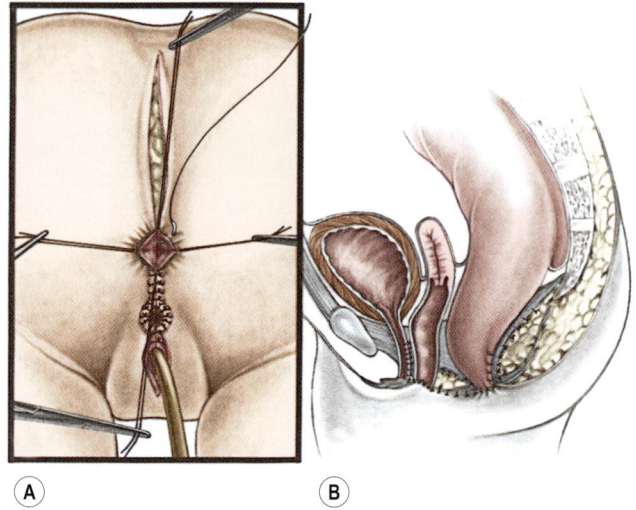

(A)   (B)

FIGURE 35-34 ■ Drawings showing the final stages of cloacal repair. **(A)** The repaired urethra and vagina and the anoplasty are being completed. **(B)** Sagittal depiction of the finished cloacal repair. (Adapted from Peña A. Atlas of Surgical Management of Anorectal Malformations. New York: Springer-Verlag; 1990. p. 69.)

the mobilized urogenital complex up into the abdomen allows for enough dissection to get it to reach. If further dissection does not allow it to reach then the vagina can be separated from the urinary tract and the urethra tubularized.

The patency of the Müllerian structures can be checked by injecting saline through a 3 French feeding tube through the fimbriae of the fallopian tubes. If one of the tubes is not patent, we recommend excising it, along with its hemiuterus if the system is bifid, and the ovary and its blood supply are preserved.[26]

When both Müllerian structures are atretic, we recommend leaving both in place, and following the patient. Once the patient develops breast buds, menstruation usually occurs one to two years thereafter and ultrasound is used to follow the size of these pelvic structures. At that point, laparoscopic inspection or intervention for nondraining structures can be done if needed.

With the abdomen open, operative decisions are based on the anatomic findings. In the presence of a single vagina of normal size, the surgeon must separate the vagina from the urinary tract, being sure to preserve its blood supply that comes from the uterine vessels. It is brought to the perineum, and the introitus is constructed. When the vagina is found to be too short, the patient requires some form of vaginal replacement that can be performed using the rectum, colon, or small bowel.

The presence of a common channel longer than 5 cm means that total urogenital mobilization from below will not be enough to repair the malformation. Therefore in this scenario, it is advisable to leave the common channel intact for use as the urethra, which will eventually be used for intermittent catheterization. The vagina is separated from the urinary tract, and the posterior wall of the previous common channel is closed with interrupted absorbable sutures. This is a very delicate maneuver best started posterosagittally and then continued via laparotomy.

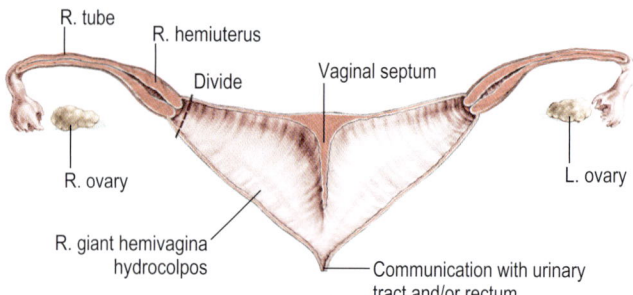

FIGURE 35-35 ■ Diagram shows the constellation of persistent cloaca with hydrocolpos in the presence of hemivaginas and hemiuterus. Bilateral hydrocolpos is present with a very high vagina. This circumstance is the ideal anatomy for a subsequent repair via a vaginal switch maneuver. (Adapted from Kiely EM, Peña A. Anorectal malformations. In: O'Neil JA, Rowe MI, Grosfeld JL, et al, editors: Pediatric Surgery. St. Louis: Mosby–Year Book; 1998. p. 1442.)

Vaginal Switch Maneuver

There is a specific group of patients who are born with hydrocolpos and two hemivaginas. The hemivaginas are very large, and the two hemiuteri are separated (Fig. 35-35). The distance between one hemiuterus and the other is longer than the vertical length of both hemivaginas. In these cases, it is ideal to perform a maneuver called a 'vaginal switch' (Fig. 35-36), whereby one of the uteri and its fallopian tube are resected, preserving the ovary and its blood supply. The blood supply of the ipsilateral hemivagina must be sacrificed, but collateral vessels from the opposite vagina should support both. The vaginal septum is resected, creating a single long vagina. The cut end of the ipsilateral vagina is turned down to the perineum. This is an excellent technique for constructing a viable and functional vagina.

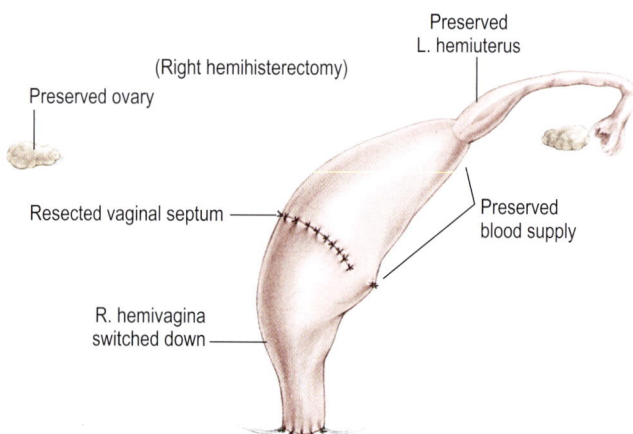

FIGURE 35-36 ■ Technique of vaginal reconstruction using a vaginal switch maneuver. (Adapted from Kiely EM, Peña A. Anorectal malformations. In: O'Neil JA, Rowe MI, Grosfeld JL, et al, editors. Pediatric Surgery. St. Louis: Mosby–Year Book; 1998. p. 1442.)

Vaginal Augmentation and/or Replacement

A short vagina can be augmented or a totally absent vagina constructed from a bowel segment. The intestinal choices are rectum, colon, or small bowel:

1. *Vaginal reconstruction with rectum.* The vagina can be constructed with the rectum when the patient has a megarectum that can be divided longitudinally, preserving the mesenteric blood supply (Fig. 35-37). Occasionally, when there is adequate length, the rectum can be divided transversely, maintaining vascular pedicles for both the rectum and vagina. The blood supply of the rectum will be provided transmurally from branches off the inferior mesenteric vessels.

2. *Vaginal replacement with colon.* The colon is an ideal substitute for the vagina. When available, the left colon is preferable. This most mobile portion of the colon usually has a long mesentery. When the patient has internal genitalia or a little cuff of vagina or cervix, the upper part of the bowel used for replacement must be sutured to the vaginal cuff. When the patient has no vagina and no uterus, the neovagina is closed at its upper end and is used only for sexual purposes (Fig. 35-38).

3. *Vaginal reconstruction with small bowel.* If a colon segment is not available, the most mobile portion of the small bowel is utilized for vaginal reconstruction. Generally, the ileum located approximately 15 cm proximal to the ileocecal valve (Fig. 35-39) is isolated and pulled down, preserving its blood supply.

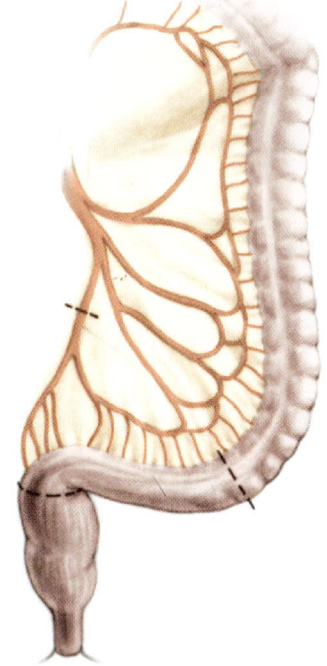
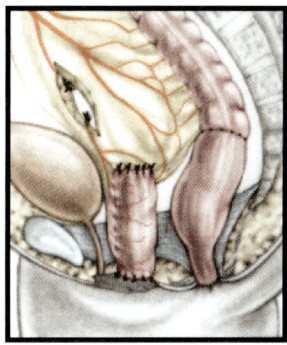

FIGURE 35-38 ■ Schematic representation of a vaginal replacement using sigmoid colon.

The most difficult type of cloacal malformation is one in which two little hemivaginas are attached to the bladder neck or even to the trigone. In these cases, the rectum also opens into the bladder neck/trigone (Fig. 35-40). Separation of these structures is performed in the abdomen, and the patient is frequently left with a nonfunctional bladder neck. The operative decision now lies between an attempt to reconstruct the bladder neck or to close it permanently. In the first situation, most of the patients will need intermittent catheterization to empty the bladder. If permanent closure of the bladder neck is elected, a vesicostomy is created, delaying a continent diversion until the patient is 3 to 4 years old. With this type of malformation, vaginal replacement should be performed using one of the substitutes described previously. Alternatively, the common channel can be left untouched, the vaginas separated from it, and the common channel then left as the catheterizable urethra.

POSTOPERATIVE MANAGEMENT AND COLOSTOMY CLOSURE

Postoperatively, these infants generally have a smooth course. Pain is rarely a complaint except for those who have undergone a laparotomy. After cloaca repair, the urinary catheter remains for ten to 14 days until the perineum is no longer swollen, and the patient can be recatheterized, if necessary. In very complex malformations, as with a bladder neck reconstruction, we prefer to leave a suprapubic tube or create a vesicostomy. Male infants with repaired rectourethral fistulas should have urinary catheter drainage for seven days. If the catheter

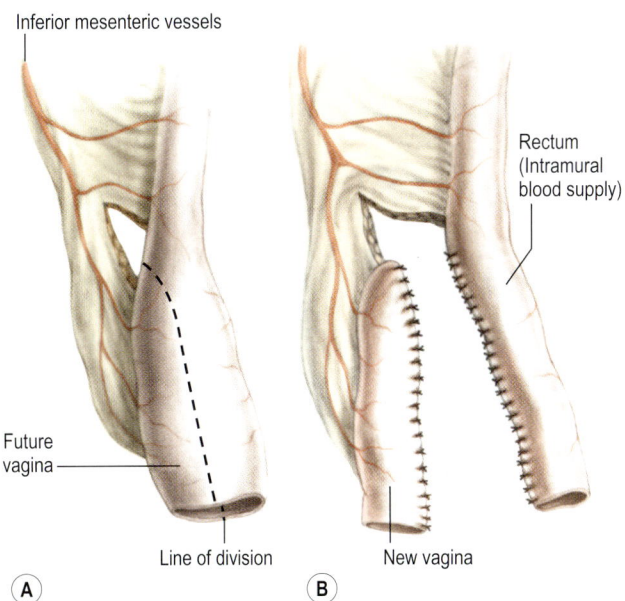

Inferior mesenteric vessels

Rectum (Intramural blood supply)

Future vagina

Line of division

New vagina

(A) **(B)**

FIGURE 35-37 ■ The technique of vaginal replacement using the rectum is depicted. The presence of a megarectum is necessary for successful vaginal reconstruction. **(A)** The portion of the existing rectum that will become the vagina. **(B)** Division of the rectum and creation of the vagina and remaining rectum.

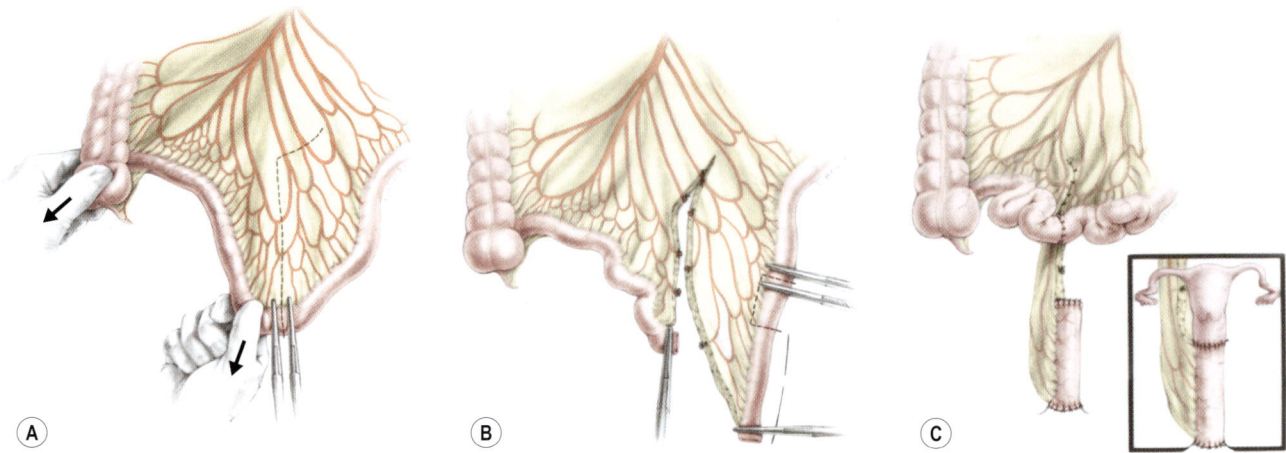

FIGURE 35-39 ■ Technique of vaginal replacement using small bowel. **(A)** A segment of small bowel is chosen that has adequate mesenteric length for transposition to the pelvis. **(B)** The mesentery has been divided, the segment of small bowel chosen for vaginal reconstruction is identified, and the blood supply is evaluated to ensure adequate perfusion. **(C)** The completed anastomosis.

becomes dislodged, the patients often can void without difficulty and do not require catheter replacement. Intravenous antibiotics are administered for 24 hours and antibiotic ointment is applied to the perineal sutures for 7 days. Most patients are discharged two days after posterior sagittal repair and 3 to 4 days if laparoscopy or laparotomy was needed.

Anal dilatations are started two weeks after repair with a dilator that fits gently into the anus. Dilation is performed twice daily by the parents at home, and the size of the dilator is increased weekly until the rectum reaches the desired size, which depends on the patient's age (Table 35-1). Once this desired size is reached, the colostomy can be closed. The frequency of dilatation can be reduced once there is no resistance using the final dilator size. After that, the parents follow a tapering dilatation

TABLE 35-1	Size of Dilator According to Age
Age	**Hegar Dilator (Number)**
1–4 months	12
4–12 months	13
8–12 months	14
1–3 years	15
3–12 years	16
>12 years	17

schedule that is once a day for one month, every third day for one month, twice a week for one month, once a week for one month, and once a month for three months. Anal strictures develop when the blood supply to the distal rectum is insufficient, or when the anoplasty was performed under tension.[30,72]

At the time of colostomy closure in patients who have undergone cloacal repair, endoscopy should be performed to evaluate the repair. After the colostomy is closed, the patient may have multiple bowel movements and may develop perineal excoriation. A constipating diet may be helpful in treating this problem. After several weeks, the number of bowel movements decreases and most patients will develop constipation and need laxatives.[70] After one to three months, the patient develops a more regular bowel movement pattern. A good prognosis can usually be predicted in a patient who has one to three bowel movements per day, remains clean between bowel movements, and shows evidence of feeling or pushing during bowel movements. This type of patient can be toilet trained. A patient with multiple bowel movements or one who passes stool constantly without showing any signs of sensation or pushing usually has a poor functional prognosis.

In our experience, about 20% of the patients with a cloacal malformation and a common channel shorter than 3 cm require intermittent catheterization to empty their bladder.[73] Patients with common channels longer than 3 cm require intermittent catheterization 70% to

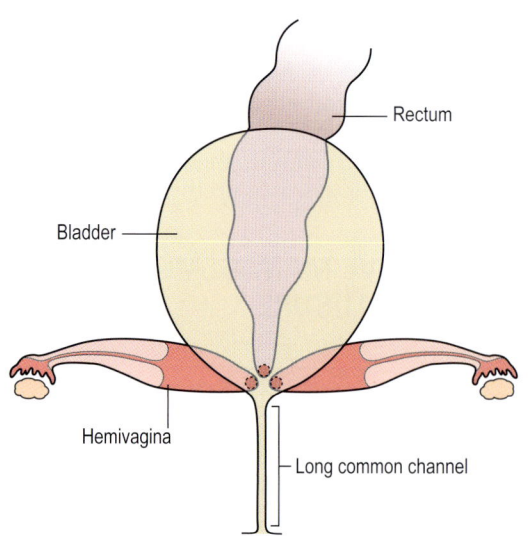

FIGURE 35-40 ■ This diagram shows the association between a cloaca with an extremely long channel with hemivaginas and the rectum entering the bladder neck. Drawing by George Rodriguez.

80% of the time. Upon removal of the urinary catheter, the patient is observed to see if the patient is capable of spontaneous bladder emptying. A kidney and bladder ultrasound can assess this emptying and should be performed two to three weeks after the catheter is removed and repeated every several months. If she cannot pass urine, or does not empty her bladder well, the parents need to learn how to perform intermittent catheterization.

Most patients with persistent cloaca have a flaccid, smooth, large bladder that does not empty completely.[75] Fortunately, most patients with cloacas have a competent bladder neck. The combination of a competent bladder neck with a flaccid bladder makes these patients ideal candidates for intermittent catheterization, which keeps them completely dry. Two exceptions to this rule exist. One is the patient with a very long common channel and the hemivaginas attached to the bladder neck, leading to bladder neck damage during the reconstruction. The other is the rare baby born with separated pubic bones, a condition that can be described as a 'covered exstrophy'.[76,77] These patients have congenital absence of the bladder neck and will eventually require a continent urinary diversion.

FUNCTIONAL DISORDERS AFTER REPAIR OF ANORECTAL MALFORMATIONS

Most patients who undergo repair of an anorectal malformation suffer from some degree of a functional defecating disorder.[78,79]

Fecal continence depends on three main factors:

1. *Voluntary muscle structures.* These structures are represented by the levator muscle, the striated muscle complex, and the external sphincter. Normally, they are used only for brief periods when the rectal fecal mass, pushed by the involuntary peristaltic contraction of the rectosigmoid, reaches the anorectal area. This contraction occurs only in the minutes prior to defecation. The voluntary muscle structures that close around the anus are used only occasionally during the rest of the day and night. Patients with anorectal malformations have abnormal voluntary striated muscles with varying degrees of hypodevelopment. Voluntary muscles can be used only when the patient feels that it is necessary to use them.

2. For that sensation, the patient needs information that can only be derived from an intact *sensory mechanism*, a mechanism lacking in many patients with anorectal malformations. Exquisite sensation in normal individuals resides in the anal canal. Except for patients with rectal atresia and stenosis, most patients with anorectal malformations are born without an anal canal. Therefore, sensation does not exist or is rudimentary. Distention of the rectum, however, can be felt in many of these patients, provided the rectum has been located accurately within the muscle structures. This proprioception seems to be a consequence of stretching of the voluntary muscle. The most important clinical implication is that liquid or soft fecal material may not be felt by the patient with anorectal malformations as the rectum is not distended. Thus, to achieve some degree of sensation and bowel control, the patient must be able to (or helped to) form solid stool.

3. *Bowel motility.* Perhaps the most important factor in fecal continence is bowel motility. In a normal individual, the rectosigmoid remains quiet for variable periods of time (one to several days), depending on an individual's defecation habits. During that time, anorectal sensation and voluntary muscle structures are almost unnecessary because the stool remains in the rectosigmoid if it is solid.

The patient normally feels the rectosigmoid's peristaltic contraction. Voluntarily, the normal individual can relax the striated muscles, which allows the rectal contents to migrate down into the highly sensitive area of the anal canal. There, accurate information is provided concerning the consistency and quality of the stool. The voluntary muscles are used to push the rectal contents back up into the rectosigmoid and hold them if desired until the appropriate time for evacuation. At the time of defecation, the voluntary muscle structures relax, allowing the fecal mass to pass into and through the anorectum.

The main factor that initiates emptying of the rectosigmoid is an involuntary peristaltic contraction that is helped sometimes by a Valsalva maneuver. Most patients with an anorectal malformation have a disturbance of this sophisticated bowel motility mechanism. Patients who have undergone a posterior sagittal anorectoplasty or any other type of sacroperineal approach, in which the most distal part of the bowel was preserved, often show evidence of an overefficient bowel reservoir (megarectum) (Fig. 35-41). The main clinical manifestation of this is constipation, which seems to be more severe in patients with lower defects.[70] The enormously dilated

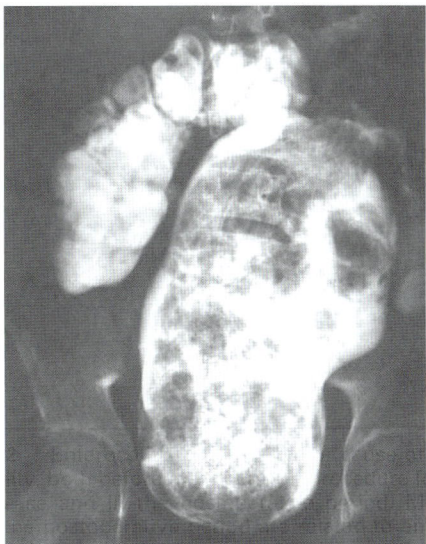

FIGURE 35-41 ■ A contrast enema is shown in a patient with a megarectum. Note the markedly dilated rectum in relation to the more proximal normal-sized colon.

TABLE 35-2   **Global Functional Results in Patients Undergoing Repair of Anorectal Malformations**

	Voluntary Bowel Movements		Soiling		Totally Continent		Constipated	
	NO. OF PATIENTS	%	NO. OF PATIENTS	%	NO. OF PATIENTS	%	NO. OF PATIENTS	%
Rectal atresia/rectal stenosis	14/14	100	4/10	40	6/10	60	9/12	75
Rectoperineal fistula	62/64	97	10/59	17	44/55	80	43/74	58
Rectovestibular fistula	144/160	90	52/140	37	87/142	61	84/152	55
Imperforate anus without fistula	35/43	81	21/40	53	18/41	44	21/42	50
Rectourethral bulbar fistula	93/117	79	52/107	49	47/108	44	69/114	61
Cloaca: short common channel (< 3cm)	68/101	67	55/92	60	33/94	35	38/97	39
Rectourethral prostatic fistula	74/112	66	84/109	77	19/110	17	47/110	43
Rectovaginal fistula	2/4	50	3/4	75	1/4	25	1/4	25
Cloaca: long common channel (> 3cm)	27/73	37	45/56	80	6/67	9	17/58	29
Rectobladderneck fistula	12/53	23	46/61	90	2/52	4	9/51	18

rectosigmoid has normal ganglion cells, but behaves like it has a hypomotility disorder. The overflow fecal incontinence based on rectosigmoid constipation in patients with potential for bowel control can be managed with the appropriate dose of stimulant laxatives. Those with a poor sacrum, poor muscles, and thus with no potential for bowel control are treated with a daily enema.[78]

Those patients treated with older techniques in which the most distal part of the bowel was resected (abdominoperineal pull-through) behave clinically as individuals without a rectal reservoir (Fig. 35-42). This is a situation equivalent to a perineal colostomy. Depending on the amount of colon resected, the patient may have loose stools. In these cases, medical management consisting of a daily enema and a constipating diet, with medications to slow down the colonic motility, is indicated.[78] See Chapter 36 for more information on bowel management.

EVALUATION OF RESULTS

Each defect described in this chapter has a different prognosis. The patients with lower defects usually have excellent results, except when technical errors have been made, or if they have associated sacral or spinal problems.

Tables 35-2 and 35-3 show our results. The patients with a sacral ratio of less than 0.3 and flat perineums have fecal incontinence regardless of the type of malformation or quality of the repair. Associated spinal anomalies negatively affect progress for bowel control.

As persistent cloacas represent another spectrum of defects, they must be subclassified on the basis of potential for bowel and bladder control. The length of the common channel seems to be the most important prognostic factor.

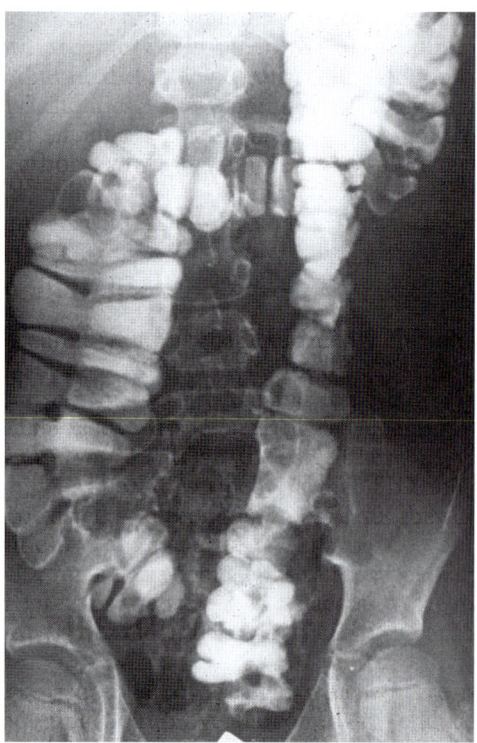

FIGURE 35-42 ■ This contrast enema was performed in a patient who has had the rectosigmoid colon resected. Note the straight position of the colon to the anus with no evidence of a rectal reservoir.

TABLE 35-3   **Urinary Continence in Patients Undergoing Repair of Anorectal Malformations**

	Urinary Continence	
	NO. OF PATIENTS	%
Rectal atresia/rectal stenosis	11/11	100
Rectoperineal fistula	56/57	98
Imperforate anus without fistula	37/39	95
Rectovestibular fistula	131/139	94
Rectourethral bulbar fistula	98/105	93
Rectourethral prostatic fistula	94/103	91
Rectobladderneck fistula	43/54	80
Recotvaginal fistula	3/4	75
Cloaca: short common channel (<3 cm)[a]	78/111	70
Coaca: long common channel (>3 cm)[a]	28/89	31

[a]Cloacas with urinary incontinence are dry via intermittent catheterization.

Complications

There are several complications related to the operative repair of anorectal malformations. Wound infection in the immediate postoperative period can occur and, fortunately, usually affects only the skin and subcutaneous tissue. These usually heal secondarily without functional sequelae. Sometimes a wound separation can be resutured in the immediate postoperative period. Anal strictures may be the consequence of failure to follow the protocol of dilatations or leaving the anoplasty under tension and/or with inadequate blood supply. When trying to prevent discomfort for the patient, some surgeons only dilate the anus once a week, frequently under anesthesia. This protocol can eventually create a severe, intractable fibrous stricture.[72] Constipation is the most common functional disorder observed in patients who undergo a posterior sagittal anorectoplasty.[70] Patients with the best prognosis for bowel control have the highest incidence of constipation. Patients with a poor prognosis, such as those with bladder neck fistula, have a low incidence of constipation and a high rate of incontinence. Colostomies that do not allow cleaning and irrigation of the distal colon can lead to megarectum. Patients require proactive aggressive treatment of constipation after colostomy closure to avoid significant problems.[70] Rectal prolapse occurs on occasion and is more prevalent in higher malformations with poor sphincters and is worsened by postoperative constipation.[71] Finally, transient femoral nerve palsy can occur as a consequence of excessive pressure on the groin during the prone position. This problem can be avoided by adequate cushioning.

Specific to cloacal repairs, urethrovaginal fistulas had been the most common and feared complication prior to the introduction of the total urogenital mobilization technique.[74] In cases in which vaginal mobilization and separation from the neourethra result in opposing suture lines, 90° rotation of the vagina can decrease the incidence of a postoperative fistula. Fibrosis of the vagina can develop secondary to an excessive dissection during the mobilization of a high vagina.[72]

In males, a review of over 500 patients showed significant urologic injuries.[63] Failure to obtain a good distal colostogram to delineate the anatomy precisely was the most important reason for these complications. Neurogenic bladder in males, as a result of the anorectal malformation or the repair itself, must be extremely unusual because it only happens in patients with an abnormal sacrum or spine.[75] Otherwise, it may reflect a poor operative technique with denervation of the bladder and bladder neck during the repair.[63]

Finally, fecal incontinence is a very common sequelae of any anorectal malformation repair and is discussed further in Chapter 36.

REFERENCES

1. Aegineta P. On the imperforate anus. In: Adams F (trans): The Seven Books (book 6). London: Sydenham Society; 1844. p. 405–6.
2. Amussat JZ. Gustiure d'une operation d'anus artifical practique avec success par un nouveau procede. Gaz Med Paris 1835;3:735–58.
3. Roux de Brignoles JN. De l'imperforation de l'anus chez les nouveaux-nex: Rapport et discussion sur l'opération à tenter dans ces cas. Gaz Med Paris 1834;2:411–12.
4. Stephens FD. Imperforate rectum: A new surgical technique. Med J Aust 1953;1:202–6.
5. Kiesewetter WB. Imperforate anus: II. The rationale and technique of sacroabdominoperineal operation. J Pediatr Surg 1967;2:106–17.
6. Louw JH, Cywes S, Cremin BJ. The management of anorectal agenesis. S Afr J Surg 1971;9:21–30.
7. Rehbein F. Imperforate anus: Experiences with abdominoperineal and abdomino sacroperineal pull-through procedures. J Pediatr Surg 1967;2:99–105.
8. Soave F. Surgery of the rectal anomalies with preservation of the relationship between the colonic muscular sleeve and puborectal muscle. J Pediatr Surg 1969;4:705–12.
9. Peña A, deVries P. Posterior sagittal anorectoplasty: Important technical considerations and new applications. J Pediatr Surg 1982;17:796–881.
10. Brenner EC. Congenital defects of the anus and rectum. Surg Gynecol Obstet 1915;20:579–88.
11. Santulli TV. Treatment of imperforate anus and associated fistulas. Surg Gynecol Obstet 1952;95:601–14.
12. Trusler GA, Wilkinson RH. Imperforate anus: A review of 147 cases. Can J Surg 1962;5:169–77.
13. Mundt E, Bates M. Genetics of Hirschsprung disease and anorectal malformations. Semin Pediatr Surg 2010;19:107–17.
14. Anderson RC, Read SC. The likelihood of recurrence of congenital malformations. Lancet 1954;74:175–6.
15. Cozzi F, Wilinson AW. Familial incidence of congenital malformations. Lancet 1954;74:175–6.
16. Murken JD, Albert A. Genetic counseling in cases of anal and rectal atresia. Progr Pediatr Surg 1976;9:115–18.
17. Falcone RA, Levitt MA, Peña A, et al. Increased heritability of certain phenotypes. J Pediatr Surg 2007;42:124–8.
18. Levitt MA, Peña A. Anorectal Malformations. In: Orphanet, [serial online] http://www.OJRD.com/content/2/1/33
19. Torres P, Levitt MA, Tovilla JM, et al. Anorectal malformations and Down syndrome. J Pediatr Surg 1998;33:1–5.
20. Stephens FD, Smith ED. Incidence, frequency of types, etiology. In: Stephens FD, Smith ED, Paul NW, editors. Anorectal Malformations in Children. Chicago: Year Book Medical; 1971. p. 160–71.
21. Rosen NG, Hong AR, Soffer SZ, et al. Recto-vaginal fistula: A common diagnostic error with significant consequences in female patients with anorectal malformations. J Pediatr Surg 2002;37:961–5.
22. Bill AH, Hall DG, Johnson RJ. Position of rectal fistula in relation to the hymen in 46 girls with imperforate anus. J Pediatr Surg 1975;10:361–5.
23. Levitt MA, Peña A. Pitfalls in the management of newborn cloacas. Pediatr Surg Int 2005;21:264–9.
24. Holschneider A, Hutson J, Peña A, et al. Preliminary report on the international conference for the development of standards for the treatment of anorectal malformations. J Pediatr Surg 2005;40:1521–6.
25. Lee SC, Chen YS, Jung SE, et al. Currarino triad: Anorectal malformation, sacral bony abnormality, and presacral mass—A review of 11 cases. J Pediatr Surg 1997;32:58–61.
26. Breech L. Gynecological concerns in patients with anorectal malformations. Semin Pediatr Surg 2010;19:139–45.
27. Moore TC. Advantages of performing the sagittal anoplasty operation for imperforate anus at birth. J Pediatr Surg 1990;25:276–7.
28. Upadhyaya VD, Gopal SC, Gangopahyaya AN, et al. Single stage repair of anovestibular fistula in neonate. Pediatr Surg Int 2007;23:737–40.
29. Menon P, Rao KL. Primary anorectoplasty in females with common anorectal malformations without colostomy. J Pediatr Surg 2007;42:1103–6.
30. Peña A, Grasshoff S, Levitt A. Reoperations for anorectal malformations. J Pediatr Surg 2007;42:318–25.
31. Bianchi DW, Crombleholme TM, D'Alton ME, et al. Cloacal exstrophy. In: Fetology: Diagnosis and Management of the Fetal Patient. 2nd ed. New York: McGraw-Hill; 2010. p. 446–53.
32. Livingston J, Eliçevik M, Crombleholme T, et al. Prenatal diagnosis of persistent cloaca: A 10-year review. Am J Obstet Gynecol 2006;195:S63.
33. Levitt MA, Stein DM, Peña A. Gynecological concerns in the treatment of teenagers with cloaca. J Pediatr Surg 1998;33:188–93.

34. Stoll C, Alembik Y, Dott B. Associated malformations in patients with anorectal anomalies. Eur J Med Genet 2007;50:281–90.

35. Karrer FM, Flannery AM, Nelson MD Jr, et al. Anorectal malformations: Evaluation of associated spinal dysraphic syndromes. J Pediatr Surg 1988;23:45–8.

36. Davidoff AM, Thompson CV, Grimm JK, et al. Occult spinal dysraphism in patients with anal agenesis. J Pediatr Surg 1991;26:1001–5.

37. Daskiewicz P, Barszsc S, Roskowski M, et al. Tethered cord syndrome in children—impact of surgical treatment on functional neurological and urological outcome. Neurol Neurochir Pol 2007;41:427–35.

38. Bui CJ, Tubbs RS, Oakes WJ. Tethered cord syndrome in children: A review. Neurosurg Focus 2007;23:1–9.

39. Tsuda T, Iwai N, Kimura O, et al. Bowel function after surgery for anorectal malformations in patients with tethered spinal cord. Pediatr Surg Int 2007;23:1171–4.

40. Kuo MF, Tsai Y, Hsu WM, et al. Tethered spinal cord and VACTERL association. J Neurosurg 2007;106:201–4.

41. Steinbok P, Garton HJ, Gupta N. Occult tethered cord syndrome: A survey of practice patterns. J Neurosurg 2006;104:309–13.

42. Drake JM. Occult tethered cord syndrome: Not an indication for surgery. J Neurosurg 2006;104:305–8.

43. Seldon NR. Occult tethered cord syndrome: The case for surgery. J Neurosurg 2006;104:302–4.

44. Levitt MA, Patel M, Rodriguez G, et al. The tethered spinal cord in patients with anorectal malformations. J Pediatr Surg 1997;32:462–8.

45. Belman BA, King LR. Urinary tract abnormalities associated with imperforate anus. J Urol 1972;108:823–4.

46. Hoekstra WJ, Scholtmeijer RJ, Molenar JC, et al. Urogenital tract abnormalities associated with congenital anorectal anomalies. J Urol 1983;130:962–3.

47. Munn R, Schillinger JF. Urologic abnormalities found with imperforate anus. Urology 1983;21:260–4.

48. Parrott TS. Urologic implications of anorectal malformations. Urol Clin North Am 1985;12:13–21.

49. Wiener ES, Kiesewetter WB. Urologic abnormalities associated with imperforate anus. J Pediatr Surg 1973;8:151–7.

50. William DI, Grant J. Urological complications of imperforate anus. Br J Urol 1969;41:660–5.

51. Rich MA, Brock WA, Peña A. Spectrum of genitourinary malformations in patients with imperforate anus. Pediatr Surg Int 1988;3:110–13.

52. Stephens FD, Smith ED. Incidence, frequency of types, etiology. In: Stephens FD, Smith ED, editors. Anorectal Malformations in Children. Chicago: Year Book Medical; 1971. p. 289–92.

53. Spence HM. Anomalies and complications of the urogenital tract associated with congenital imperforate anus. J Urol 1954; 71:453–63.

54. Smith ED. Urinary anomalies and complications in imperforate anus and rectum. J Pediatr Surg 1968;3:337–42.

55. Carcassonne M, Monfort G, Isman H. Les problemes urologiques des malformations ano-rectales. Arch Fr Pediatr 1971;28: 723–39.

56. Boemers TM. Neurogenic bladder in infants born with anorectal malformations: Comparison with spinal and urologic status. J Pediatr Surg 1999;34:1889–90.

57. Boemers TM, de Jong TP, van Gool JD, et al. Urologic problems in anorectal malformations: II. Functional urologic sequelae. J Pediatr Surg 1996;31:534–7.

58. Wangensteen OH, Rice CO. Imperforate anus: A method of determining the surgical approach. Ann Surg 1930;92:77–81.

59. Shaul DB, Harrison EA. Classification of anorectal malformations—initial approach, diagnostic tests, and colostomy. Semin Pediatr Surg 1997;6:187–95.

60. Freeman NV, Burge DM, Soar JS, et al. Anal evoked potentials. Z Kinderchir 1980;31:22–30.

61. Albanese CT, Jennings RW, Lopoo JB, et al. One-stage correction of high imperforate anus in the male neonate. J Pediatr Surg 1999;34:834–6.

62. Vick LR, Gosche JR, Boulanger SC, et al. Primary laparoscopic repair of high imperforate anus in neonatal males. J Pediatr Surg 2007;42:1877–81.

63. Hong AR, Rosen N, Acuña MF, et al. Urological injuries associated with the repair of anorectal malformations in male patients. J Pediatr Surg 2002;37:339–44.

64. Gross GW, Wolfson PJ, Peña A. Augmented-pressure colostogram in imperforate anus with fistula. Pediatr Radiol 1991;21:560–3.

65. Peña A, Migotto-Krieger M, Levitt MA. Colostomy in anorectal malformations: A procedure with serious but preventable complications. J Pediatr Surg 2006;41:748–56.

66. Wilkins S, Peña A. The role of colostomy in the management of anorectal malformations. Pediatr Surg Int 1988;3:105–9.

67. Sydorak RM, Albanese CT. Laparoscopic repair of high imperforate anus. Semin Pediatr Surg 2002;11:217–25.

68. Georgeson K. Laparoscopic-assisted anorectal pull-through. Semin Pediatr Surg 2007;16:266–9.

69. Georgeson KE, Inge TH, Albanese CT. Laparoscopically assisted anorectal pull-through for high imperforate anus: A new technique. J Pediatr Surg 2000;35:927–31.

70. Levitt MA, Kant A, Peña A. The morbidity of constipation in patients with anorectal malformations. J Pediatr Surg 2010; 45:1228–33.

71. Belizon A, Levitt MA, Shoshany G, et al. Rectal prolapse following posterior sagittal anorectoplasty for anorectal malformations. J Pediatr Surg 2005;40:192–6.

72. Levitt MA, Peña A. Reoperations in Anorectal Malformations. In: Teich S, Caniano D, editors. Reoperative Pediatric Surgery. Totowa: Humana Press; 2008. p. 311–26.

73. Levitt MA, Peña A. Cloacal malformations: Lessons learned from 490 cases. Semin Pediatr Surg 2010;19:128–38.

74. Peña A. Total urogenital mobilization—An easier way to repair cloacas. J Pediatr Surg 1997;32:263–8.

75. Peña A, Levitt MA. Neurogenic bladder and anorectal malformations. In: Esposito C, Guys JM, Gough D, et al, editors. Pediatric Neurogenic Bladder Dysfunction. Berlin: Springer; 2006. p. 85–8.

76. Peña A. New concepts in bowel reconstruction in cloacal exstrophy. Dialog Pediatr Urol 2000;23:3–4.

77. Levitt MA, Mak GA, Falcone RA, et al. Cloacal exstrophy—pull through or permanent stoma? A review of 53 patients. J Pediatr Surg 2008;43:164–70.

78. Levitt MA, Peña A. Pediatric fecal incontinence: A surgeon's perspective. Pediatr Review 2010;31: 91–101.

79. Peña A, Levitt MA. Colonic inertia disorders. Curr Prob Surg 2002;39:661–730.

CHAPTER 36

FECAL INCONTINENCE AND CONSTIPATION

Marc A. Levitt • Alberto Peña

Fecal incontinence can prevent a person from becoming socially accepted, which, in turn, provokes serious psychological sequelae. It is a problem that impacts more children than previously thought, affecting those born with anorectal malformations and Hirschsprung disease as well as children with spinal cord problems or spinal injuries.

True fecal incontinence must be distinguished from overflow pseudoincontinence. Children with true fecal incontinence can include some surgical patients with anorectal malformations (ARMs), those with Hirschsprung disease, and those with spinal problems, either congenital or acquired. In patients with pseudoincontinence, who have the potential for bowel control but who soil, their problem usually results from severe constipation (encopresis) and sometimes from hypermotility.

Most patients who require repair of an ARM suffer from some degree of a functional defecation disorder. All have some degree of an abnormality in their fecal continence mechanisms. One-quarter of them are deficient enough to the point that they are fecally incontinent and cannot have a voluntary bowel movement.[1] The majority are capable of having voluntary bowel movements but may require treatment of an underlying dysmotility disorder, which most often manifests as constipation.[2,3] A small, yet significant, number of patients with Hirschsprung disease suffer from fecal incontinence because of a lost anal canal or damaged sphincters that occurred during operative repair.[4–6] To varying degrees, patients with spinal problems[7,8] or injuries[9] can lack the capacity for voluntary bowel movements.

Patients with true fecal incontinence require artificial means to be kept clean. This regimen is termed *bowel management* and involves a daily enema.[10] On the other hand, patients with pseudoincontinence require proper medical treatment for either constipation or loose stools. This involves finding the right consistency for the stool so that they can have a bowel movement that they voluntarily control. Understanding this major differentiation is the key to deciding the correct bowel management program.

MECHANISM OF CONTINENCE

Fecal continence depends on three factors: voluntary sphincter muscles, anal canal sensation, and colonic motility.[2]

Voluntary Muscle Structures

In the normal continent patient, the voluntary muscle structures are represented by the levators, the muscle complex, and the parasagittal fibers. Normally, they are used only for brief periods of time when the fecal mass, pushed by the involuntary peristaltic contraction of the rectosigmoid colon, reaches the anorectal area. This voluntary contraction keeps the stool in the rectum by closing the anus around the time of defecation. These muscles are used only occasionally during the rest of the day and night.

Patients with ARMs have abnormal voluntary striated muscles with different degrees of hypodevelopment. Some patients are close to normal whereas some patients do not have any voluntary sphincter muscles. Also, patients with Hirschsprung disease may have suffered damage to this sphincter mechanism at the time of pull-through, and patients with spinal abnormalities may have deficient innervation of these muscles.

Anal Canal Sensation

Voluntary muscles are used only when the patient has the sensation that determines that it is necessary to use them. To appreciate that sensation, the patient needs feedback that is derived from an intact anal sensory mechanism.

Exquisite sensation in normal individuals resides in the anal canal. Except for patients with rectal atresia, most patients with ARMs are born without an anal canal. Therefore, sensation does not exist or is rudimentary. Patients with spinal conditions may lack this anal canal sensation as well.[7,8] Those with Hirschsprung disease are born with a normal anal canal, but this can be injured if not meticulously preserved at the time of their pull-through (Fig. 36-1).[5,6] Also, perineal trauma may result in an injured or destroyed anal canal.[9]

It seems that most individuals can perceive distention of the rectum. This point is important for patients undergoing pull-through procedures for imperforate anus as the distal rectum and anus must be placed precisely within the sphincter mechanism. This sensation seems to be a consequence of stretching of the voluntary muscles (proprioception). The most important clinical implication of this point is that patients might not feel liquid or soft fecal material because such stool consistency does not distend the rectum. Thus, to achieve some degree of sensation and bowel control, the patient must have the

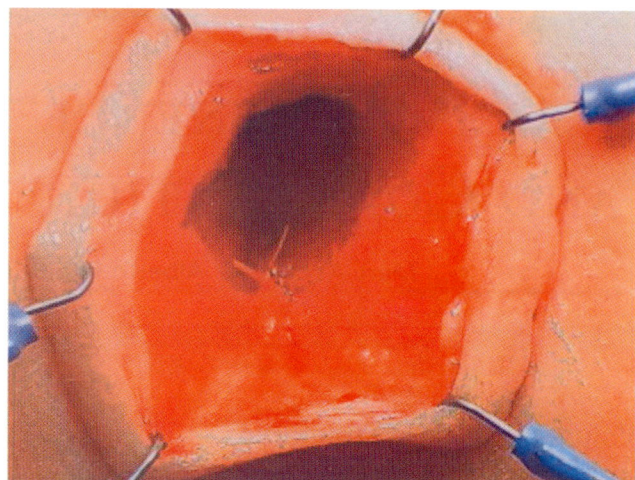

FIGURE 36-1 ■ Loss of the anal canal (with no visible dentate line) is seen after a Soave pull-through operation. In this patient, the anal dissection was begun too distally.

capacity to form solid stool. This is especially important in a patient without a good anal canal to give sensory cues. This point is relevant in children with ulcerative colitis who have undergone an ileoanal pull-through procedure. They can suffer from varying degrees of incontinence due to their incapacity to form solid stool, but their normal sphincter muscles and anal canal allow them to overcome this problem. Most need treatments that bulk up the stool.

Bowel Motility

In a normal individual, the rectosigmoid colon may remain quiet for up to several days, depending on defecation habits or dietary consumption. During that time, the previously mentioned sensation and voluntary muscle structures are not active because the stool, if it is solid, remains inside the colon. The patient can feel the peristaltic contraction of the rectosigmoid that occurs before defecation. Voluntarily, the normal individual can then relax the striated rectal muscles, which allows the rectal contents to migrate down into the highly sensitive area of the anal canal. There, the anal canal provides feedback concerning stool consistency. The voluntary muscles are used to push the rectal contents back up into the rectosigmoid and to hold them until the appropriate time for evacuation. At the time of defecation, the voluntary muscle structures relax, and the stool exits the anus helped by gravity, rectal contraction, and abdominal wall muscles.

Most patients with an ARM suffer from some disturbance of this sophisticated bowel motility mechanism. Patients who have undergone a posterior sagittal anorectoplasty (PSARP) or any perineal approach in which the most distal part of the bowel was preserved can develop an overefficient bowel reservoir (megarectosigmoid) (Fig. 36-2). The main clinical manifestation is constipation, which seems to be more severe in patients with lower defects.[3] Constipation that is not aggressively treated, combined with an ectatic distended colon, eventually leads to more severe constipation. A vicious cycle ensues,

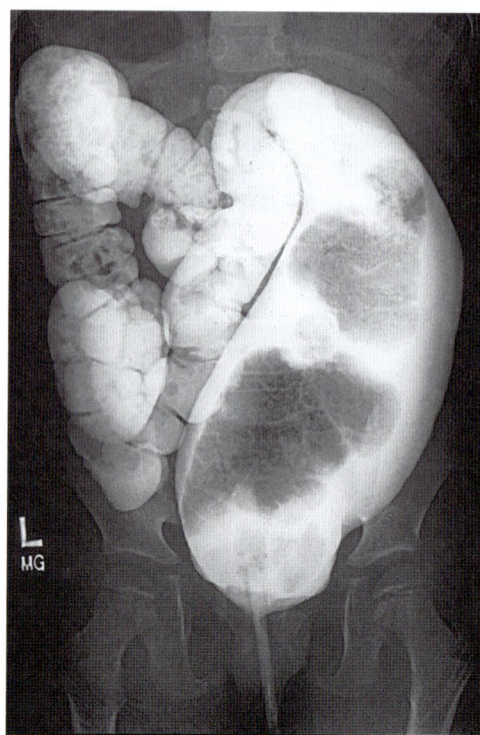

FIGURE 36-2 ■ This contrast enema shows a megarectosigmoid colon. (From Peña A, Levitt M. Colonic inertia disorders in pediatrics. Curr Prob Surg 2002;39:681.)

with worsening constipation leading to more rectosigmoid dilation, leading to more severe constipation, and then to overflow incontinence.

Patients with an ARM, who are managed with operations in which the most distal part of the bowel was resected (Fig. 36-3), behave clinically as individuals without a rectal reservoir. Depending on the amount of colon removed, the patient may have loose stools. In these cases, medical management consists of enemas, a constipating diet, and medications to slow down the colonic motility. Patients with Hirschsprung disease undergo operative resection of the distal aganglionic colon and rectum. However, their normal anal canal and sphincter mechanism (if properly preserved) allows the vast majority of them to be continent despite the lack of a rectal reservoir. Some patients with Hirschsprung disease have bowel hypermotility and need medications to slow the colon. Amazingly, some patients with an injured anal canal can be continent if their motility is normal because the regular contraction of the rectosigmoid can translate into a successful voluntary bowel movement.

TRUE FECAL INCONTINENCE

True fecal incontinence means the patient cannot have voluntary bowel movements and therefore requires an artificial mechanism to empty the colon. We have found that the ideal approach is a bowel management program consisting of teaching the patient and the parents how to clean the colon once daily with an enema so they stay completely clean for 24 hours until the next enema. This is achieved by keeping the colon quiet between enemas.

Laxatives will make such a patient soil more. The program, although simplistic, is ideally implemented by trial and error over a period of one week.[10] The patient is seen each day and an abdominal radiograph is obtained to look for the amount and location of any stool left in the colon. The presence or absence of stool in the underwear is also noted. The decision as to whether the type

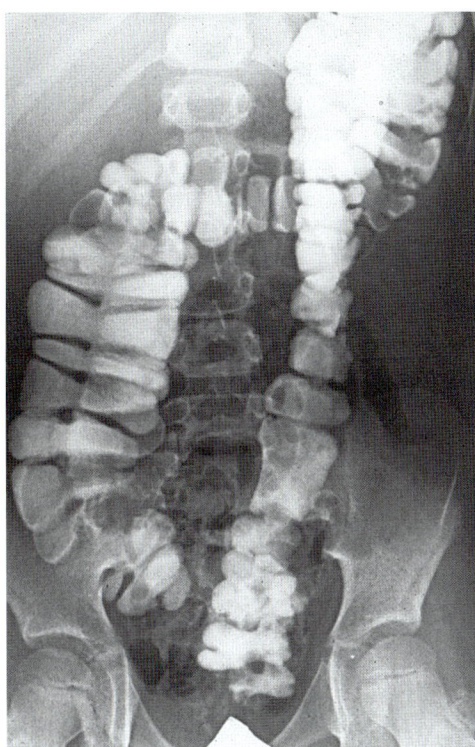

FIGURE 36-3 ■ This contrast enema was performed in a patient who had resection of the rectosigmoid colon. Often these patients act like they do not have a rectal reservoir. (From Levitt MA, Peña A. Treatment of chronic constipation and resection of the inert rectosigmoid. In: Anorectal Malformations in Children. Heidelberg: Springer; 2006. p. 417.)

and/or quality of the enemas should be modified, as well as any changes in diet and/or medication, is made each day (Fig. 36-4).[10]

Which Children Have True Fecal Incontinence?

In children with ARMs, 75% who have undergone a correct and successful operation have voluntary bowel movements after the age of 3 years.[1] About half of these patients occasionally soil their underwear. These episodes of soiling are usually related to constipation. When the constipation is treated properly, the soiling frequently disappears. Thus, approximately 40% overall have voluntary bowel movements and no soiling, and behave normally. Children with good bowel control still may suffer from temporary episodes of fecal incontinence, especially when they experience diarrhea.

Some 25% of all patients with ARMs suffer from true fecal incontinence, and are the patients who need bowel management to be kept clean. As previously noted, certain patients with Hirschsprung disease and those with spinal problems can suffer from true fecal incontinence as well. For these patients, similar principles of bowel management learned from treatment of patients with ARMs can be applied.[10]

For children with ARMs, the surgeon should be able to predict in advance which patient will likely have a good functional prognosis and which child will have a poor prognosis. Table 36-1 shows the most common indicators for a good or poor prognosis. After primary repair and colostomy closure, it is possible to establish a functional prognosis (Table 36-2). Parents should be given the information regarding their child's realistic chances for bowel control to avoid needless frustration at the age of toilet training.

Once the diagnosis of the specific anorectal defect is established, the functional prognosis can be predicted. If the child's defect is associated with a good prognosis such

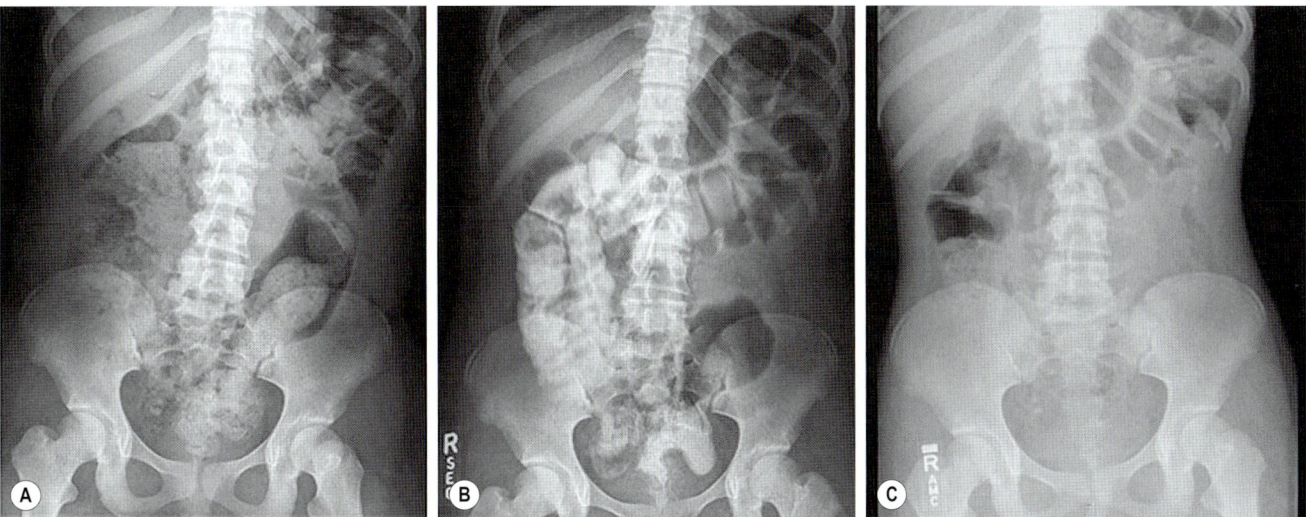

FIGURE 36-4 ■ **(A,B)** This series of abdominal radiographs was obtained during inpatient bowel management showing progression toward a completely clean colon with daily adjustment of the enema. **(C)** After five days, a postcontrast abdominal film shows minimal evidence of retained fecal material.

TABLE 36-1 Prognostic Signs in Patients with Anorectal Malformations

Good Prognosis Signs	Poor Prognosis Signs
Good bowel movement patterns: one to two bowel movements per day, no soiling in between	Constant soiling and passing of stool
Evidence of sensation with passing stool (pushing, making faces)	No sensation (no pushing)
Urinary control	Urinary incontinence, dribbling of urine

TABLE 36-2 Predictors of Prognosis in Patients with Anorectal Malformations

Good Prognostic Signs	Poor Prognostic Signs
Normal sacrum	Abnormal sacrum
Prominent midline groove (good muscles)	Flat perineum (poor muscles)
Some types of anorectal malformations:	Some types of anorectal malformations:
Rectal atresia	Rectal/bladder neck fistula
Vestibular fistula	Cloacas with a common channel >3 cm
Imperforate anus without a fistula	Complex malformations
Cloacas with a common channel <3 cm	
Less complex malformations: perineal fistula	

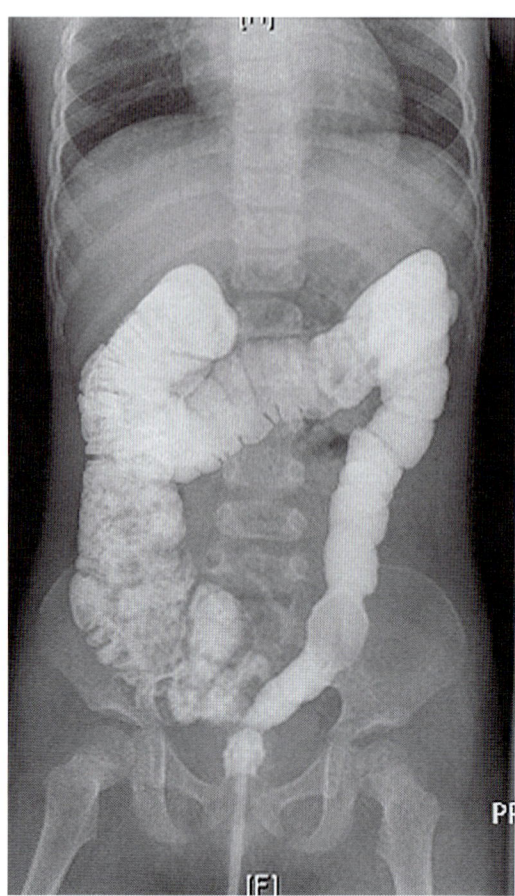

FIGURE 36-5 ■ This contrast study shows a nondilated colon.

as a vestibular fistula, perineal fistula, rectal atresia, rectourethral bulbar fistula, or imperforate anus with no fistula, one should expect that the child will have voluntary bowel movements by the age of 3 years provided the sacrum and spine are normal. These children will need careful attention to avoid fecal impaction, constipation, and soiling.[3]

If the child's defect is associated with a poor prognosis, such as a very high cloaca with a common channel longer than 3 cm, a rectobladder neck fistula, an associated myelomeningocele, or a very hypodeveloped sacrum, the child will most likely need a bowel management program with enemas to remain clean. This should be implemented at 3 to 4 years of age and before starting school. Children with a rectoprostatic fistula have a 50% chance of having voluntary bowel movements and continence. In these children, an attempt should be made to achieve toilet training by the age of 3 years. If this proves unsuccessful, bowel management should be implemented. The ability to toilet train can be reassessed each summer after school has ended.

In patients who have undergone repair of an imperforate anus and who have fecal incontinence, reoperation to relocate a misplaced rectum or repair a rectal prolapse should be considered if the child was born with a good sacrum, a good sphincter mechanism, and a malformation with good functional prognosis. A repeat PSARP can be performed and the rectum relocated within the sphincter mechanism.[11]

Children with an ARM who have reached the age for a bowel management program can be divided into two well-defined groups that require individualized treatment plans. The first and larger group has fecal incontinence and a tendency toward constipation. The second group has fecal incontinence with a tendency toward loose stools. Patients with fecal incontinence after operations for Hirschsprung disease and those with spinal disorders usually have a tendency toward constipation. A small group of Hirschsprung patients fall into the hypermotile group. These patients have multiple daily stools and a nondilated colon seen on a contrast enema (Fig. 36-5; see also Fig. 36-3). Interestingly, because of abnormal innervation of the colon, patients with spinal diseases can have severe constipation, yet have a nondilated colon.

Children with True Fecal Incontinence and Constipation (Colonic Hypomotility)

Patients with true fecal incontinence and a tendency toward constipation should not be treated with laxatives, but instead need an enema program. In these children, the motility of the colon is slow. The basis of their bowel management program is to clean the colon once a day with an enema. No special diet or medications are necessary. The fact that they suffer from constipation (hypomotility) is useful because it helps them to remain clean between enemas. The real challenge is to find the appropriate enema capable of evacuating the colon. Definitive evidence that the rectosigmoid colon is empty after an enema requires a plain abdominal radiograph (see Fig. 36-4). Soiling episodes or 'accidents' occur when there is incomplete colonic evacuation with progressive enlargement of the stool followed by leakage around the stool.

Children with True Fecal Incontinence and Loose Stools (Colonic Hypermotility)

The great majority of children with ARMs who suffer from this problem were repaired before the introduction of the PSARP technique. The older procedures frequently included a rectosigmoid resection.[12,13] Therefore, these children have an overactive colon because they lack a rectal reservoir (see Fig. 36-3). Rapid transit of stool results in frequent episodes of diarrhea. This means that even when an enema cleans their colon rather easily, stool keeps passing fairly quickly from the cecum to the descending colon and out the anus. To manage this situation, a constipating diet and/or medications (loperamide and water-soluble fiber) to slow down the colon are necessary. Also, eliminating foods that loosen bowel movements will help the colon slow down (Table 36-3). A small subset of patients with Hirschsprung disease (see Fig. 36-5) behaves like they have hypermotility and can be managed similarly.

The keys to the success of a bowel management program are dedication and sensitivity from the medical team. The basis of the program is to clean the colon and keep it quiet, thus keeping the patient clean for the 24 hours after the enema. It is an ongoing process that needs to be responsive to the individual patient and differs for each child. It is usually successful within a week, during which time the family, patient, physician, and nurse undergo a process of trial and error, tailoring the regimen to the specific patient. More than 95% of the children who follow this program are artificially kept clean for the whole day and can have a completely normal life.[10]

TABLE 36-3	Food Products and Stool Consistency
Foods that Produce Loose Stools	**Foods that Promote Constipation**
Milk or milk products	Apple sauce
Fats	Apple without skin
Fried foods	Rice
Fruits	White bread
Vegetables	Bagels
Spices	Soft drinks
Fruit juices	Banana
French fries	Pasta
Chocolate	Pretzels
	Tea
	Potato
	Jelly (not jam)
	Boiled, broiled, baked meat, chicken or fish

BOWEL MANAGEMENT: KEY STEPS

The first step is to perform a contrast enema with water-soluble material, never with barium. It is very important to obtain a postevacuation film. This contrast study shows the type of colon that is present: dilated-constipated (see Fig. 36-2) or nondilated-tendency toward loose stool (see Figs 36-3 and 36-5). The enema volume and type can also be estimated from this contrast study.

The bowel management program is then implemented according to the patient's type of colon, and the results are evaluated daily. Changes in the volume and content of the enema are made until the colon is successfully cleaned. For this, an abdominal radiograph that is obtained every day is invaluable in determining whether the colon is empty (see Fig. 36-4).

There are different types of solutions to use for enemas. Some can be bought in a drugstore. The use of phosphate enemas is convenient because they are available in prepared containers. However, saline enemas are often just as effective, and some families find them easier and less expensive. A 0.9% saline can be made at home by adding 1.5 teaspoons of salt to 1000 mL of water. Occasionally, children will complain of cramping with the phosphate enema while the saline enemas are usually well tolerated. Children should never receive more than one phosphate enema a day because of the risk of phosphate intoxication, and patients with impaired renal function should avoid them entirely. The saline enema (350–750 mL) can be mixed with glycerin (10–40 mL) and/or soap (10–40 mL) to make it more effective.

The daily enema should result in a bowel movement within 30 to 45 minutes, followed by a period of 24 hours of complete cleanliness. If the chosen enema does not radiographically clean the colon, or if the child keeps soiling, then a more voluminous or concentrated enema is needed. Administering the enema through a catheter with a balloon helps prevent leakage (Fig. 36-6). The right enema is the one that can empty the child's colon and allow him or her to stay clean for the following 24 hours. This can be only determined by trial and error.

Children with loose stools have an overactive colon, and usually do not have a rectal reservoir. This means that even when an enema cleans their colon easily, new stool passes quickly from the cecum to the descending colon and anus. To prevent this, a constipating diet, bulking agents, and/or medications to slow down the colon can be used. Eliminating foods that loosen bowel movements will help decrease the colonic motility (see Table 36-3).

Such patients should be provided with a list of constipating foods and a list of laxative foods to avoid. The constipating diet is rigid: banana, apple, baked bread, white pasta with no sauce, boiled meat, etc. Fried foods, dairy products and sugary drinks should be avoided (see Table 36-3). Most parents learn which meals provoke loose stools and which constipate their child. To determine the right combination, treatment is initiated with enemas, a very strict diet, loperamide, and a water-soluble fiber such as pectin. Most children respond to this aggressive management within one to two weeks. The child should remain on a strict diet until clean for 24 hours for

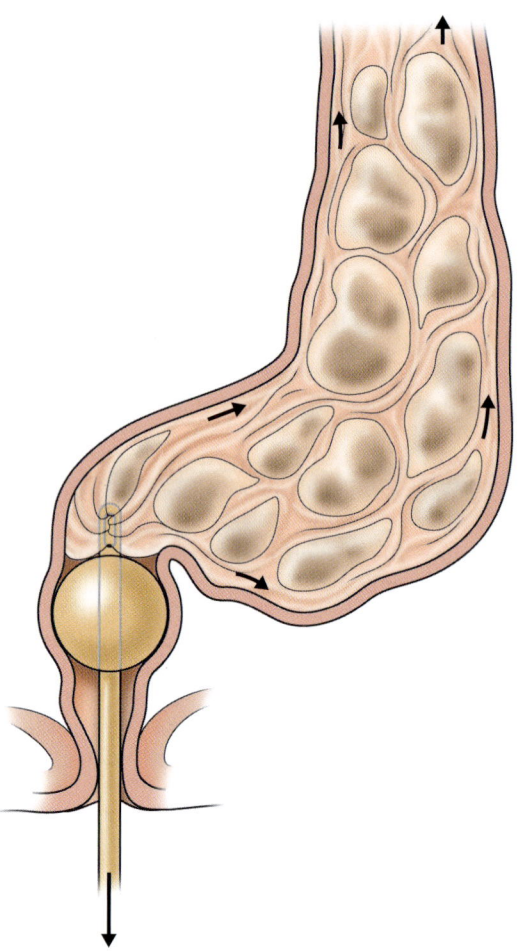

FIGURE 36-6 ■ Note that inflation of the balloon on the catheter helps prevent enema leakage.

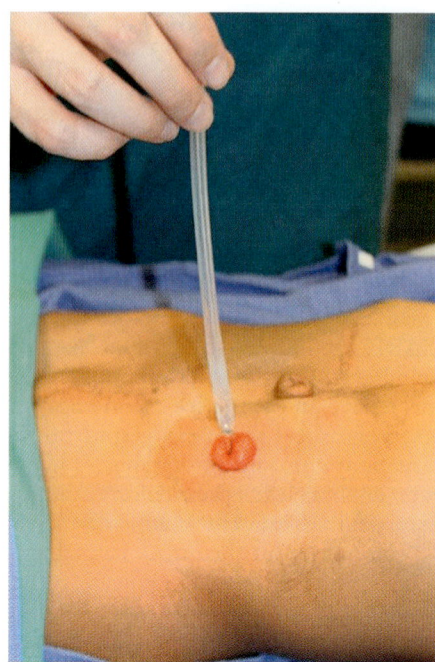

FIGURE 36-7 ■ Some patients have the capacity to have good bowel control with a daily enema administered through their colostomy.

two to three days in a row. Then they can choose one new food every two to three days and the effect of this new food on the child's colonic activity is observed. If the child soils after eating a newly introduced food, that food must be eliminated from the diet. Over several months, the most liberal diet possible should be sought. If the child remains clean with a liberal diet, the dose of loperamide can gradually be reduced to the lowest effective dose that keeps the child clean for 24 hours.

In children in whom a successful bowel management program has been implemented, the parents frequently ask if this program will be needed for life. The answer is yes for those patients born with no potential for bowel control. However, because there is a spectrum of defects, there are patients with some degree of bowel control. These patients participate in the bowel management program to avoid embarrassing accidents of uncontrolled bowel movements. As time goes by, the child becomes more cooperative and more interested in his or her problem. It is conceivable that later in life, a child may be able to stop using enemas and remain clean by following a specific regimen of a disciplined diet with regular meals (three meals per day and no snacks) to stimulate bowel movements at a predictable time. Every summer, children with some potential for bowel control can try to find out how well they can control their bowel

movements without the help of enemas. Such trials are attempted during vacations to avoid accidents at school or during a time that they can stay home and try some of the toilet training strategies. It is also facilitated by daily abdominal films to ensure they are adequately emptying (see Fig. 36-4).

A key question for patients with a colostomy, who are predicted to have minimal or no potential for bowel control, is whether to perform a pull-through operation or leave them with a permanent stoma. We believe that if the patient has the capacity to form solid stool, a pull-through procedure should be performed and a daily enema given thereafter to keep them clean. A successful bowel management program will then provide a better quality of life compared with a permanent stoma. The bowel management can be initiated with a daily enema via the stoma (Fig. 36-7). If the stoma remains quiet for 24 hours between enemas, then that stoma could be pulled through or closed, and a daily enema using the antegrade Malone technique utilized.

Most preschool and school-age children enjoy a good quality of life while undergoing the bowel management program. However, when they are older, many express dissatisfaction. They believe that their parents are intruding on their privacy by giving them enemas. It is feasible, but rather difficult, for them to administer the enema themselves. For this specific group of children, a continent appendicostomy or Malone procedure is ideal (Fig. 36-8).[14,15] Using the appendix, a valve mechanism is created and connected to the umbilicus. The appendicostomy can be catheterized to administer the enema fluid. If the child has had the appendix removed, it is possible to create a new one from a colonic flap: a continent neo-appendicostomy. The Malone procedure is just another way to administer an enema. Therefore, before

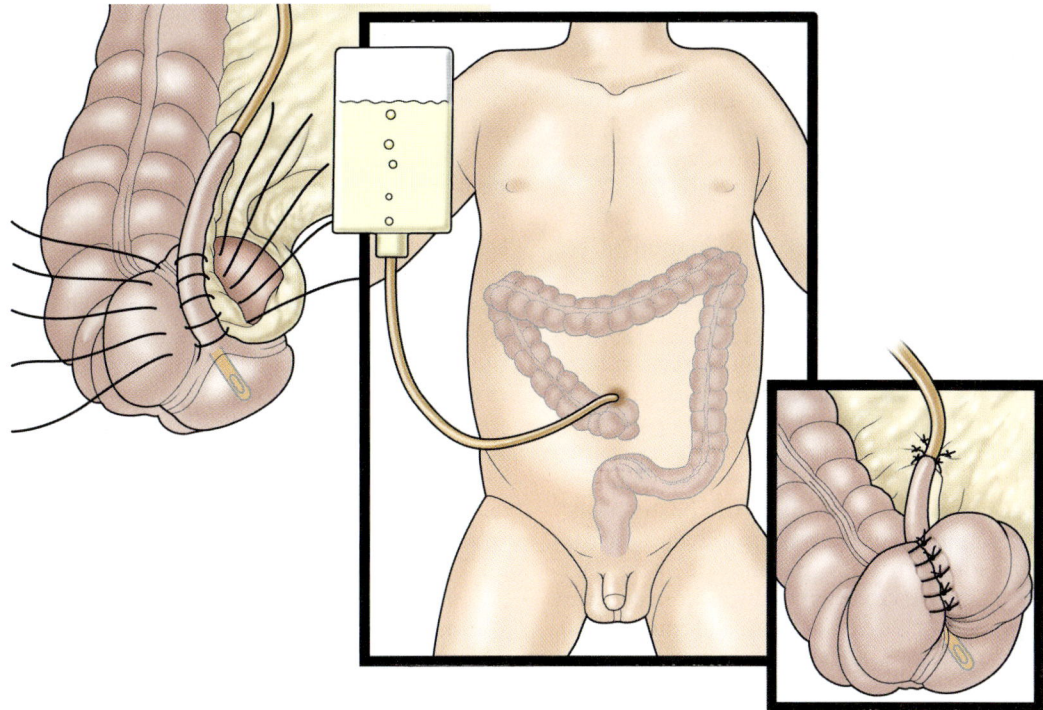

FIGURE 36-8 ■ Some patients are able to have bowel continence with a daily prograde enema administered through an appendicostomy. (Adapted from Levitt MA, Soffer SZ, Peña A. Continent appendicostomy in the bowel management of fecal incontinent children. J Pediatr Surg 1997;32:1631.)

performing it, the child should be completely clean through a bowel management regimen.

CONSIPATION

Pseudoincontinence occurs when a patient behaves like he or she is fecally incontinent but really has severe constipation and overflow soiling. Once the disimpaction is treated and the patient receives enough laxatives to avoid constipation, he or she starts having voluntary bowel movements.

The colon absorbs water from the stool and serves a reservoir function. These processes depend on colonic motility, which is an area of physiology that is not well understood and for which treatments are limited. Every 24 to 48 hours, the colon develops active peristaltic waves, indicating that it is time to empty. A normal individual feels this sensation and decides when to tighten and relax the voluntary sphincter mechanism.

If a child has potential to be fecally continent, then management involves treatment of constipation, using stimulant laxatives to provoke peristalsis and overcome the dysmotility. Stool softeners should be avoided as they can exacerbate overflow incontinence. Patients who have undergone successful surgery for Hirschsprung disease or for low ARMs with a normal spine should be fecally continent.

Constipation in children with ARMs is extremely common, particularly in the more benign types.[1,3] It is also common in patients after successful surgery for Hirschsprung disease and occurs in a large group of patients considered to have idiopathic constipation.[2] When left untreated, constipation can be extremely incapacitating.[3] Although diet affects colonic motility, its therapeutic value is negligible in the most serious forms of constipation. While it is true that many patients with severe constipation suffer from psychological disorders, a psychological origin for the constipation cannot explain the severe forms, because it is not easy to voluntarily retain stool when an autonomous rectosigmoid undergoes peristalsis. Passage of large, hard pieces of stool may provoke pain and make the patient behave like a stool retainer. This may complicate the problem of constipation, but it is not the original cause.

Constipation is a self-perpetuating disease. A patient who suffers from a certain degree of constipation and is not treated adequately will only partially empty the colon, leaving larger and larger amounts of stool inside the rectosigmoid. This results in greater degrees of distal colonic enlargement. Dilation of a hollow viscus results in poor peristalsis. This explains why constipation leads to fecal retention culminating in megacolon, which exacerbates the constipation. In addition, the passage of large, hard pieces of stool may produce anal fissures, leading to painful stooling and reluctance to have bowel movements.

The clinician must decide which type of patient is being treated. Patients with ARMs and Hirschsprung disease with good prognosis for bowel control are those more likely to have constipation. In these patients, an aggressive, proactive treatment of their constipation is the best approach. Of course, the child must be capable of being fecally continent and having the capacity for voluntary bowel movements before initiating treatment for constipation because laxatives will make an incontinent child worse.

When children with ARMs and Hirschsprung disease are managed early with aggressive treatment of constipation, children with a good prognosis should toilet train without difficulty. When constipation is not managed properly, they behave much like children with idiopathic constipation and may have overflow pseudoincontinence.[3] Because of a hypomotility disorder that interferes with complete emptying of the rectosigmoid, most of these patients suffer from different degrees of dilation of the rectum and sigmoid, a condition known as megarectosigmoid (see Fig. 36-2).[2] Often, these children were born with a good prognosis type of anorectal defect and underwent a technically correct operation, but did not receive appropriate treatment for constipation. Subsequently they developed fecal impaction and overflow pseudoincontinence. These may also be children with severe idiopathic constipation without a prior operation, who have a dilated rectosigmoid because of years of constipation.

First, the impaction needs to be removed with enemas and colonic irrigations to clean the megarectosigmoid. Fecal impaction is a stressful event resulting from retained stool for several days or weeks, crampy abdominal pain, and sometimes tenesmus. When laxatives are prescribed to such a patient, the result is exacerbation of the crampy abdominal pain and sometimes vomiting, a consequence of increased colonic peristalsis produced by the laxative acting against a fecally impacted colon. Therefore, disimpaction, proven by radiograph, must precede initiation of laxative therapy. Then, once the colon is clean, the constipation is treated with the administration of large doses of stimulant laxatives. Stool softeners should be avoided as they only soften the stool, and do not help

evacuate it. The dosage of the laxative is increased daily until the right amount is reached to completely empty the colon every day. Water soluble fiber is added which provides stool bulk and makes the laxative more efficient.

If medical treatment proves to be difficult because the child has a severe megasigmoid and requires an enormous amount of laxatives to empty, the surgeon can offer a segmental resection of the colon (Fig. 36-9). After the resection, the amount of laxatives required to treat these children can be significantly reduced or even eliminated. Before performing this operation, however, it is mandatory to confirm that the child is definitely suffering from overflow pseudoincontinence rather than true fecal incontinence with constipation. Failure to make this distinction may lead to an operation in which a fecally incontinent, constipated child is changed to one with a tendency to have loose stool, which will make the patient's condition much more difficult to manage.

The dysmotility of the colon in patients with Hirschsprung disease, even after a successful operation to remove the aganglionic bowel, is not well understood. These patients can also benefit from proactive medical treatment of their constipation.

Some clinicians treat these patients with colostomies or colonic washouts via a catheterized stoma or button device, and monitor the improvement of colonic dilation with contrast studies.[16] Once the distal colon regains a normal caliber, the physician assumes that the patient is cured and discontinues the washouts or closes the colostomy. Unfortunately, these patients' symptoms quickly recur. We have found that washouts are often

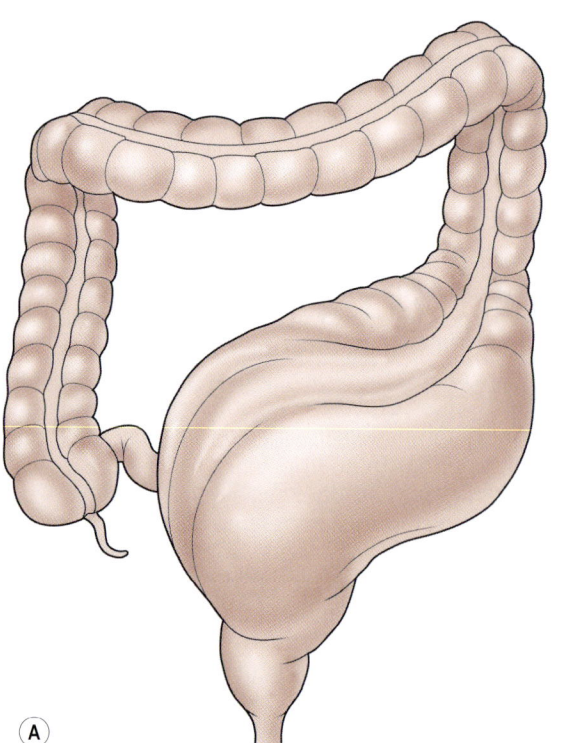
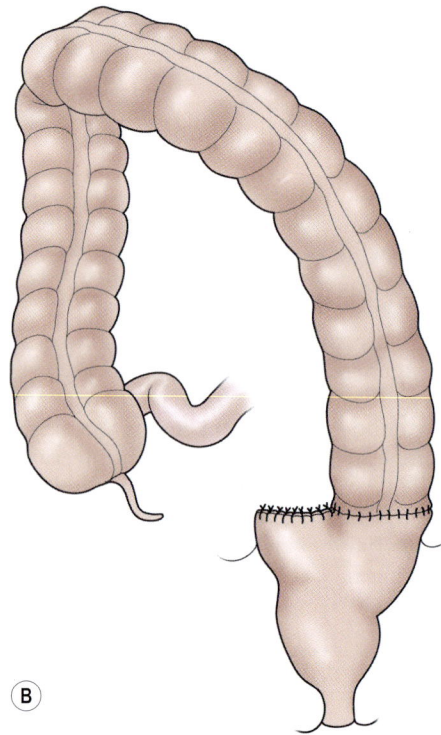

FIGURE 36-9 ■ Resection of a dilated sigmoid colon, which can be very effective in select patients with an anorectal malformation and severe constipation.

ineffective in such patients because they simply retain the fluid and believe they are really only for patients with true fecal incontinence who are incapable of having voluntary bowel movements. On the other hand, a patient with pseudoincontinence is capable of emptying their colon with the help of adequate doses of laxatives and thus does not need washouts at all.

Determining which patient the clinician is managing can be a challenge. If the patient is incontinent, washouts with a bowel management regimen are appropriate. If the patient is continent, then aggressive management of the constipation after ensuring disimpaction is the optimal treatment.

Soiling of the underwear is an ominous sign of severe constipation. A patient who is old enough to have bowel control, but soils the underwear day and night and does not have spontaneous bowel movements, may have overflow pseudoincontinence. These patients behave similarly to fecally incontinent individuals. When the constipation is treated adequately, the great majority of these pseudoincontinent children regain bowel control. Of course, this clinical presentation may also occur in a patient with true fecal incontinence. When uncertain, the clinician can start the 3- to 4-year-old who is having trouble with toilet training on a daily enema. Once clean with this regimen, and if the child has the potential for bowel control, then an attempt at a laxative program can be tried.

A contrast enema with water-soluble material is an extremely valuable study. In the constipated patient, it usually shows a megarectosigmoid with dilation of the colon all the way down to the anus (see Fig. 36-2). There is usually a dramatic size discrepancy between a normal transverse and descending colon and the dilated megarectosigmoid which is the exact opposite of Hirschsprung disease. The size of the colon guides the dosing of the laxatives. It seems that the more localized the dilatation of the rectosigmoid, the better the results of a colonic resection in reducing or eliminating the laxative requirement.

Colonic manometry is sometimes useful in the evaluation of these patients. Manometry is performed by placing balloons at different levels in the colon and recording the waves of contraction or the electrical activity.[17,18] Scintigraphy has also been used to assess colonic motility,[19] but unfortunately does not yet help guide therapeutic decisions. The key information the surgeon needs to know is if and where a colonic resection would prove beneficial to the patient who requires enormous doses of laxatives to empty the colon.

Histologic studies of the colon in these patients mainly show hypertrophic smooth muscle in the area of the dilated colon and normal ganglion cells. In the near future, it is hoped that more sophisticated histopathologic research will enhance our knowledge about colonic dysmotility.

Treatment

Patients with ARMs, severe constipation, and the potential for bowel control, as well as those with severe idiopathic constipation in whom dietary measures or gentle laxatives do not work, require a more aggressive regimen.

Drugs (containing senna) that are designed to increase the colonic motility are better when compared with stool softeners. Softening of the stool without improving the colonic motility will likely make the patient worse, because with soft stool they will no longer have control, whereas they do reasonably well with solid stool that allows them to feel rectal distention. This is a common misconception, and the switch from stool softener to laxative usually makes a significant difference.

In many cases, the laxative regimen we employ uses the same medications that have been tried previously, but were unsuccessful. Success is based on starting with a radiographically clean colon and adapting the dosage to the patient's response. The response is monitored daily with an abdominal radiograph with the laxative dose adjusted, if necessary. The colon is emptied with an enema whenever 24 hours has passed without a bowel movement. Almost always, the patient previously had received a lower dose than what was really needed.

Disimpaction

The disimpaction process is a vital and often neglected step. This includes the administration of enemas three times a day until the patient is radiographically clean. The contrast enema using water-soluble material not only shows the anatomy, but also is a helpful tool for cleaning the colon. If the patient remains impacted after three days, then he or she is given a balanced electrolyte solution via a nasogastric tube in the hospital and the enema regimen is continued. If this is unsuccessful, manual disimpaction under anesthesia may be necessary.

Determining the Laxative Requirement

Once the patient has been disimpacted, a specific amount of senna-based laxative predicted from the contrast study is begun. An empiric dose is given, and the patient is observed for the next 24 hours. If the patient does not have a bowel movement in the 24 hours after giving the laxative, it means the laxative dose was not strong enough and must be increased. An enema is also required to remove the stool produced during the previous 24 hours. In these extremely constipated patients, stool should never remain in the rectosigmoid for more than 24 hours.

The routine of increasing the amount of laxatives and giving an enema, if needed, is continued every night until the child has a voluntary bowel movement and empties the colon completely. Ideally, this routine is checked with a daily radiograph. Each day that the patient has a bowel movement, a radiograph should confirm that the bowel movement was effective, meaning that the patient completely emptied the rectosigmoid. If the patient passed stool but did not empty completely, the dose of laxative should be increased. If the patient passed stool and successfully emptied the colon, then that laxative dose should be continued each day. If the patient passed multiple stools and the abdominal film is clean, then the laxative dose can be reduced slightly.

It is important to remember that constipation covers a wide spectrum and patients may have laxative requirements that are much larger than the manufacturer's recommendation. Occasionally, in the process of increasing the amount of laxatives, patients vomit, or feel nauseated and complain of abdominal cramping before reaching any positive effect. In these patients, a different medication can be tried. Some patients vomit all kinds of laxatives and are unable to tolerate the amount of laxative that produces a bowel movement that empties the colon. Others empty but have significant symptoms from the laxatives. Such a patient is considered to have an intractable condition and is a candidate for an operation. Usually, however, the dosage that the patient needs to radiographically empty the colon can be achieved. At that dose, the patient stops soiling because he or she is successfully emptying the colon each day. Because the colon is empty, the patient remains clean until the next voluntary bowel movement.

At this point, the patient and parents have the opportunity to evaluate the quality of life that they have with this treatment, understanding that this treatment will most likely be life-long. For many of these patients, a sigmoid or rectosigmoid resection can provide symptomatic improvement leading to significant reduction or complete elimination of laxatives.[20]

Rectosigmoid Resection

The megarectosigmoid is resected and the descending colon is anastomosed to the rectum (see Fig. 36-9).[21] This can be done laparoscopically and ideally only leaves a small rectal cuff. These patients must be followed closely because the condition is not cured by the operation. The remaining rectum is most likely abnormal. Without careful follow-up and treatment of constipation, the colon can re-dilate.

In patients with ARMs, it is particularly vital to keep the rectum intact because they need it for continence. It is their reservoir in which they feel the distention of the stool. In contrast, patients with idiopathic constipation who have not undergone an operation and have a normal anal canal and sphincters, the rectum and sigmoid can be resected with preservation of fecal continence. This is only done in the rare case that the rectum is significantly dilated. Resection of the rectosigmoid down to the pectinate line can be performed in a similar manner as used for patients with Hirschsprung disease with anastomosis of the nondilated colon to the rectum above the pectinate line.[22] It seems that a laparoscopic low anterior resection is best to avoid over-stretching the sphincters, leaving behind a small cuff of rectum. Dramatic improvement in the patient's ability to empty the colon has resulted.

The most dilated part of the colon is resected because it seems to be the most seriously affected and the nondilated part of the colon is assumed to have a more normal motility. Unfortunately, we lack a more scientific way to assess the dysmotile anatomy. Perhaps emerging colonic motility technology will help with operative planning. It seems that the patients who improve the most are those who have a more localized form of megarectosigmoid. Patients with more generalized dilation of the colon do not respond as well and may require a more extensive resection that includes the left and transverse colon, sometimes accompanied by a Malone appendicostomy.

REFERENCES

1. Peña A. Anorectal malformations. Semin Pediatr Surg 1995;4: 35–47.
2. Peña A, Levitt MA. Colonic inertia disorders. Curr Prob Surg 2002;39:666–730.
3. Levitt MA, Kant A, Peña A. The morbidity of constipation in patients with anorectal malformations. J Pediatr Surg 2010;45: 1228–33.
4. Bax KMA. Duhamel Lecture: The incurability of Hirschsprung's disease. Eur J Pediatr Surg 2006;16:380–4.
5. Levitt MA, Martin C, Olesevich M, et al. Hirschsprung's disease and fecal incontinence: Diagnostic and management strategies. J Pediatr Surg 2009;44:271–7.
6. Levitt MA, Dickie B, Peña A. Evaluation and treatment of the patient with Hirschsprung disease who is not doing well after a pull-through procedure. Semin Pediatr Surg 2010;19:146–53.
7. Smith GK. The history of spina bifida, hydrocephalus, paraplegia, and incontinence. Pediatr Surg Int 2001;17:424–32.
8. Eire PF, Cives RV, Gago MC. Faecal incontinence in children with spina bifida: The best conservative treatment. Spinal Cord 1998;36: 774–6.
9. Hayden DM, Weiss EG. Fecal incontinence: Etiology, evaluation, and treatment. Clin Colon Rectal Surg 2011;24:64–70.
10. Bischoff A, Levitt MA, Peña A. Bowel management for the treatment of pediatric fecal incontinence. Pediatr Surg Int 2009;25: 1027–42.
11. Levitt MA, Peña A. Reoperations in Anorectal Malformations. In: Teich S, Caniano D, editors. Reoperative Pediatric Surgery. Totowa: Humana Press; 2008. p. 311–26.
12. Kiesewetter WB. Imperforate anus II: The rationale and technique of the sacro-abdomino-perineal operation. J Pediatr Surg 1967;2: 106–10.
13. Rehbein F. Imperforate anus: Experiences with abdomino-perineal and abdomino-sacro-perineal pull-through procedures. J Pediatr Surg 1967;2:99–105.
14. Rangel SJ, Lawal TA, Bischoff A, et al. The appendix as a conduit for antegrade continence enemas in patients with anorectal malformations: Lessons learned from 163 cases treated over 18 years. J Pediatr Surg 2011;46:1236–42.
15. Lawal TA, Rangel SJ, Bischoff A, et al. Laparoscopic assisted Malone appendicostomy in the management of fecal incontinence in children. J Laparoendosc Adv Surg Tech A, 2011;21:455–9.
16. Marshall J, Hutson JM, Anticich N, et al. Antegrade continence enemas in the treatment of slow-transit constipation. J Pediatr Surg 2001;36:1227–30.
17. DeLorenzo C, Flores AF, Reddy SN, et al. Use of colonic manometry to differentiate causes of intractable constipation in children. J Pediatr 1992;120:690–5.
18. Sarna SK, Bardakjian BL, Waterfall WE, et al. Human colonic electric control activity (ECA). Gastroenterology 1980;78: 1526–36.
19. Cook BJ, Lim E, Cook D. Radionuclear transit to assess sites of delay in large bowel transit in children with chronic idiopathic constipation. J Pediatr Surg 2005;40:478–83.
20. Peña A, El-Behery M. Megasigmoid—a source of pseudo-incontinence in children with repaired anorectal malformations. J Pediatr Surg 1993;28:1–5.
21. Levitt MA, Pena A. Surgery and constipation: When, how, yes, or no? J Pediatr Gastroenterol Nutr 2005;41(Suppl. 1):S58–60.
22. Levitt MA, Martin CA, Falcone RA, et al. Transanal rectosigmoid resection for severe intractable idiopathic constipation. J Pediatr Surg 2009;44:1285–91.

ACQUIRED ANORECTAL DISORDERS

Casey M. Calkins • Keith T. Oldham

PERIANAL AND PERIRECTAL ABSCESS

Perianal or perirectal abscesses are often encountered during infancy. The abscess typically presents as a fluctuant, tender mass in the perianal region (Fig. 37-1). A history of stool abnormalities is typically not elicited. Perianal abscesses are much more common in male infants and are infrequent in toddlers and older children.[1] Crohn disease, immunodeficiency, glucose intolerance, and perianal trauma can be causative stimuli in the older child. It is unusual to find complex ischiorectal abscesses in children unless associated with inflammatory bowel disease (IBD).

For the infant, sitz baths are prescribed if the abscess does not appear to be fluctuant. Approximately one-third of abscesses thus treated resolve without recurrence.[2] Approximately two-thirds require incision and drainage. Although drainage can be accomplished in the infant without general or topical anesthesia, we prefer a brief inhalational anesthetic to allow for adequate drainage and optimal patient comfort. Considerable debate exists with regard to making an effort to delineate a fistula at the time of abscess drainage, yet we prefer simple abscess drainage as the initial step.[3,4] The patient begins sitz baths on the first postoperative day, and oral antibiotics are not needed once the abscess has been drained.

FISTULA-IN-ANO

As many as 50% of perianal abscesses progress to a fistula-in-ano.[5] The child is usually seen after two or more 'flare ups' of a perianal abscess that either continues to drain or forms a small pustule that ruptures, only to form again (Fig. 37-2).[6] The fistula is commonly located lateral to the anus rather than in the midline. An intriguing theory has been suggested that fistula-in-ano results from infection in abnormally deep crypts that are under the influence of androgens. The fact that fistula-in-ano rarely follows a perianal abscess in female infants lends credence to this theory.[7]

Our preferred operative technique for a fistula-in-ano is fistulotomy which is described within the caption of Figure 37-3. Following the procedure, we instruct the parents to place the infant in a sitz bath after each bowel movement, at least twice daily, and to separate the skin edges of the fistulotomy during bathing to promote healing by secondary intention. We reserve cryptectomy for patients with recurrence, which is rare after an adequate fistulotomy.

ANAL FISSURE

An anal fissure commonly develops in a toddler whose diet changes from liquid to solid and whose stool consistency changes from soft to firm. A period of constipation results in a posterior midline tear in the anoderm below the mucocutaneous junction. The discomfort with defecation leads to further constipation, which aggravates the fissure and prevents healing. The diagnosis is made with a history of hematochezia, the child's crying during bowel movements, and the recognition of a split in the anoderm. Operative interventions such as lateral internal sphincterotomy or fissurectomy are rarely necessary.[8,9] We prefer sitz baths and an osmotic stool softener, such as polyethylene glycol, which usually results in healing.

For older children without evidence of IBD, topical 0.2% nitroglycerin ointment can be used. However, the collective evidence for utilizing topical glyceryl trinitrate suggests that this treatment is no better than placebo.[10] Chemical sphincterotomy using *Botulinum* toxin is employed when nonoperative interventions have failed. We prefer a total of 25–50 units of *Botulinum* toxin A prepared in sterile saline. This volume is divided into four aliquots and injected into the sphincter complex in four circumferential quadrants.

An anal fissure in an older child or a teenager may be associated with Crohn disease.[11] Immunomodulatory treatment of Crohn disease typically results in healing of the fissure.[12,13] Topical application of tacrolimus ointment is a promising relatively new therapy.[14] Internal sphincterotomy appears to be a relatively safe undertaking in this patient population, but only when local measures and immunomodulator therapy have failed.[15]

ANAL SKIN TAGS, HEMORRHOIDS, AND OTHER PERIANAL VASCULAR LESIONS

A perianal skin tag is rarely an indication of other disease, although it may result from a healed fissure (Fig. 37-4). Although it is generally of no consequence, when large enough it can be bothersome and can affect adequate perianal hygiene. In these cases, local excision is reasonable.

Hemorrhoids are uncommon in the pediatric population, and rarely is operative therapy a necessary aspect of treatment. External hemorrhoids are located in the distal one-third of the anal canal and covered by anoderm. Symptoms from external hemorrhoids are generally due to thrombosis, and examination reveals a tender, bluish

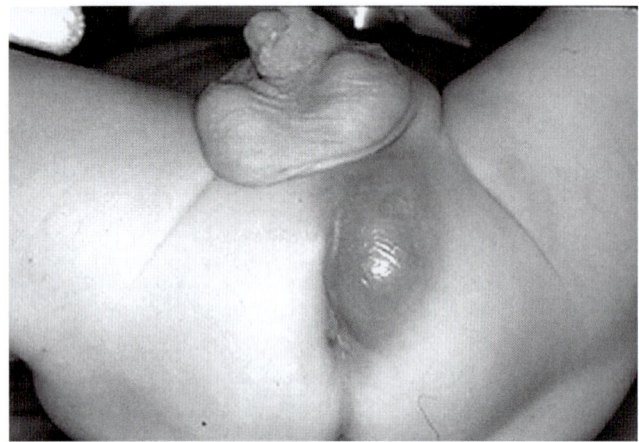

FIGURE 37-1 ■ Perianal abscesses are often seen in male infants. The abscess typically presents as a fluctuant, tender mass in the perianal region. Incision and drainage is the initial management of these abscesses.

mass at the mucocutaneous junction (Fig. 37-5). Treatment consists of incision of the hemorrhoid and extrusion of the clot with subsequent sitz baths, dietary modification (fiber supplementation), and stool softeners. Internal hemorrhoids are extremely rare in children unless associated with portal hypertension. The treatment for bleeding from internal hemorrhoids due to portal hypertension should be aimed at decreasing portal pressure, either pharmacologically or surgically. In patients without portal hypertension, initial treatment of internal hemorrhoids should be focused on conservative measures such as the provision of stool bulking agents and topical treatment (sitz baths and topical pharmaceutical preparations). Rubber band ligation or operative hemorrhoidectomy is performed when conservative measures fail.

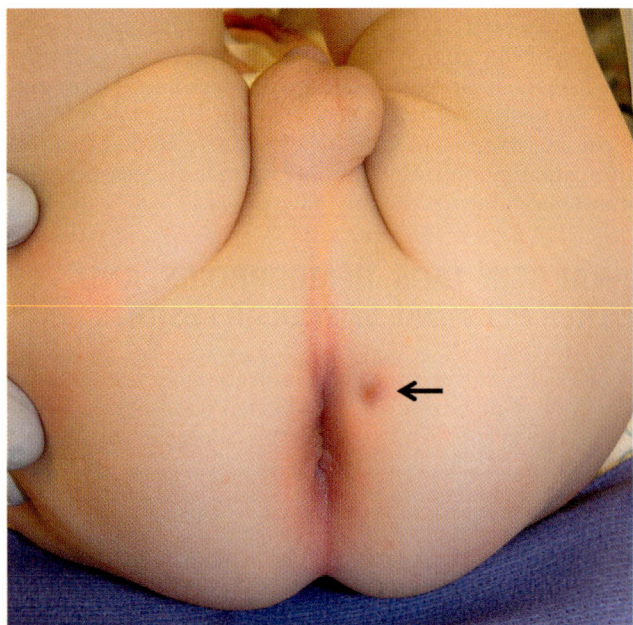

FIGURE 37-2 ■ As many as one-half of the perianal abscesses progress to a fistula-in-ano. In this photograph, the fistula is seen at 1 o'clock when the infant is in the lithotomy position.

Albeit rare, vascular malformations of the hindgut can present a diagnostic and therapeutic challenge. The vast majority of clinically significant malformations in this anatomic region are venous malformations. The typical patient presents with recurrent hematochezia, and the lesion may be initially confused with a hemorrhoid, or the latter may be present as the result of the malformation. Endoscopy is classically not helpful, as dilated vessels are rarely visible. Pelvic magnetic resonance imaging (MRI) is typically the best diagnostic method to delineate the extent of disease. Interventional vascular techniques may be utilized to control acute bleeding or embolize large feeding vessels prior to definitive therapy, which generally requires complete bowel resection. In these cases, endorectal pull-through with coloanal anastomosis has been our preferred approach.

RECTAL PROLAPSE

Rectal prolapse is a relatively common problem in young children and causes great distress to both child and parent. Prolapse can range from intermittent mucosal prolapse that reduces spontaneously to full-thickness prolapse, which often requires manual reduction. Regardless, prolapse should be reduced promptly to prevent vascular compromise. Rectal prolapse in children is likely precipitated by weakness of the pelvic levator musculature and a loose attachment of the rectal submucosa to the underlying muscularis. The latter often improves with time, whereas a weak and dilated pelvic floor may not.[16] Straining during stooling, and long periods of sitting on the toilet, allows stretching of the pelvic diaphragm and other less well-defined rectal suspensory structures which results in prolapse.[17] Up to 20% of cases of rectal prolapse diagnosed between 6 months and 3 years of age are associated with cystic fibrosis.[18]

The diagnosis is usually made by noting a rosette of mucosa when the child complains of discomfort while defecating (Fig. 37-6). Bleeding is occasionally noted, and rarely is it a source of significant disability. Unfortunately, it is uncommon for the child to be able to produce the prolapse in the examining room. We will ask the child to sit on the commode during an office visit in an attempt to demonstrate the prolapse. Often, it may be helpful to have the parents take a digital photograph during an episode so it can be viewed later at an office visit. Sometimes what appears to be rectal prolapse is an intussusception of the sigmoid colon.[19] In these cases, an intact rectal suspension system exists but a dilated levator mechanism, coupled with a redundant sigmoid colon, allows for its intussusception. It is often difficult to differentiate between prolapse and intussusception clinically. Regardless, the entity must be reduced promptly to prevent vascular compromise.

Nonoperative treatment is the primary course of action in most cases. A change in defecation habits and provision of stool softeners may allow the pelvic musculature to resume its normal tone. We advocate that patients be restricted from spending prolonged periods of time on the commode. In addition, a child-specific commode or a step stool in front of an adult commode

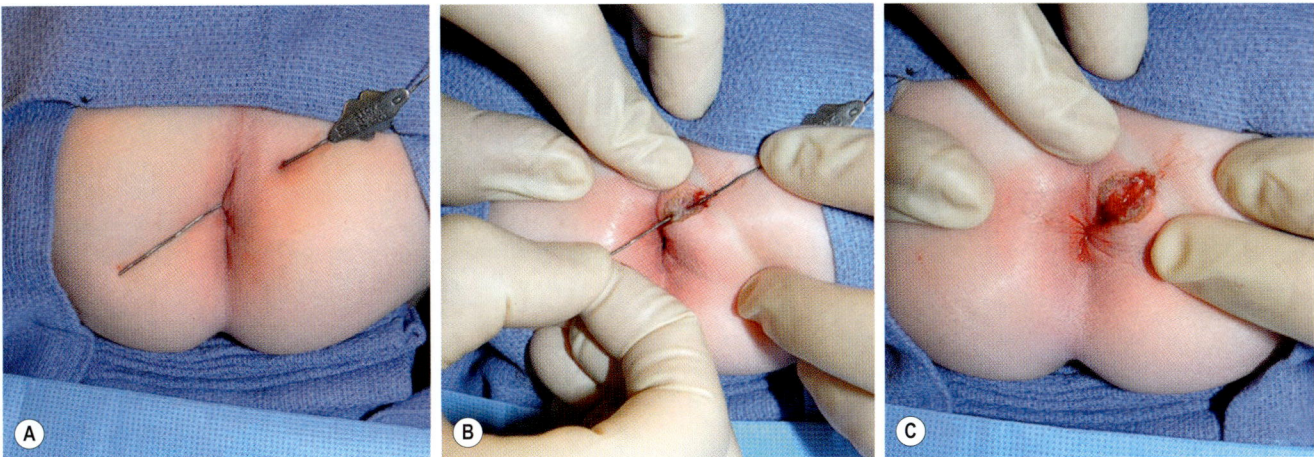

FIGURE 37-3 ■ **(A)** At the time of operation, a small, fine, malleable probe is inserted through the fistula and can usually be gently advanced until it is visualized to exit the base of the involved crypt. **(B)** An incision is then made along the probe and is deepened through the superficial portion of the external sphincter. **(C)** After complete unroofing of the tract, the incision is usually left open, which may provide some distress on the part of the parents but usually does not cause much discomfort for the child.

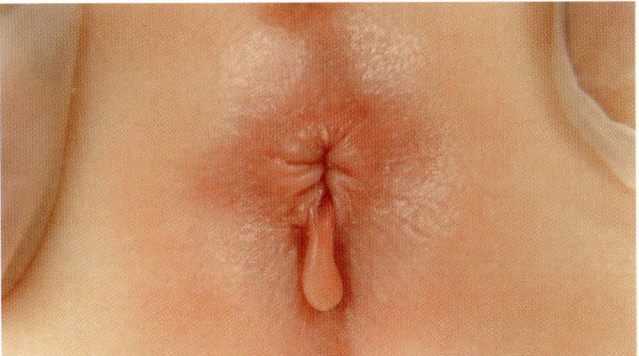

FIGURE 37-4 ■ This 1-year-old developed this anal skin tag secondary to constipation. Due to its size, it was excised.

may eliminate straining-like behaviors. In patients who are identified with cystic fibrosis, enzymatic supplementation and improving malnutrition may be all that is required to eliminate episodes of prolapse.[20]

There are a number of operative approaches. Perianal cerclage tightens the anal outlet and prevents prolapse from recurring while the musculature of the pelvic floor re-establishes its normal anatomic relationship.[21] The cerclage procedure is often effective, although one must be cautious to avoid making the cerclage too tight. This can be prevented by tying the cerclage over an appropriately sized Hegar dilator.[22] Sclerotherapy with any number of compounds (30% saline, Deflux, 25% glucose, 5% sodium morrhuate) injected into the submucosal or retrorectal space produces an inflammatory response that theoretically prevents the rectum from sliding

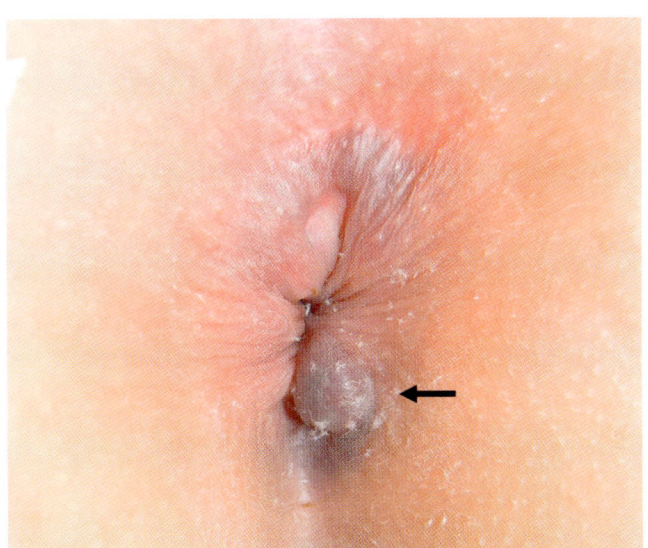

FIGURE 37-5 ■ The external hemorrhoid (arrow) is a tender, bluish mass at the mucocutaneous junction.

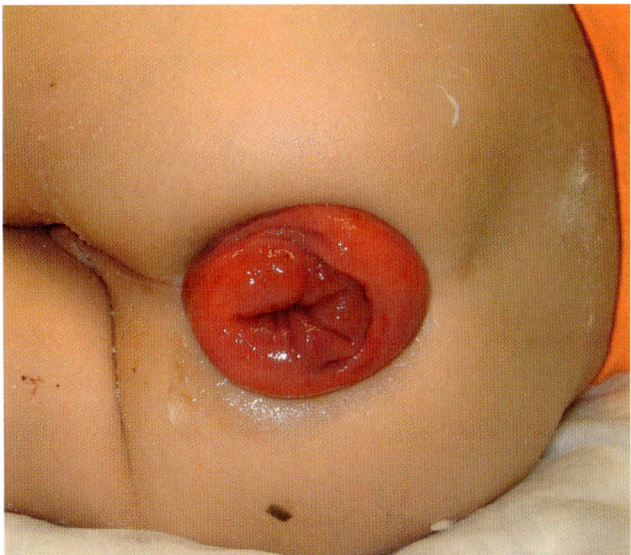

FIGURE 37-6 ■ This 2-year-old developed persistent rectal prolapse. The prolapse occurred several times daily and was not responsive to medical management. The child underwent submucosal sclerotherapy with 5% sodium morrhuate and the prolapse resolved.

downward.[23–27] We have found submucosal injection of 5% sodium morrhuate to be especially effective in children with mucosal prolapse unresponsive to nonoperative therapy. An open sclerosing procedure, in which the retrorectal space is developed and packed with gauze, is currently not routinely performed.[28,29] Endorectal cauterization or mucosal stripping may be effective; however, there is little evidence that rectal prolapse is due to mucosal 'overabundance,' and we do not recommend this as primary surgical therapy.[30,31]

In patients with full-thickness prolapse, or for those who have failed nonoperative therapy, operative fixation techniques can be used. Transanal suture fixation of the rectum (Ekehorn rectopexy) has recently been used in a group of children with good success.[32,33] Its benefit probably derives from the inflammation and adhesions that are produced by the mattress sutures. An extensive

plication or reefing of the posterior rectal wall via a coccygectomy incision has been reported to have good results, but the morbid potential for a rectocutaneous fistula makes this a technique that we do not routinely employ.[34] Laparoscopic rectopexy is an alternative to standard open rectopexy and is performed with two operating ports and a port for laparoscopic visualization.[35,36] The rectum is mobilized and sutured to the periosteum of the sacral promontory in multiple locations with nonabsorbable suture. The operation has been successfully completed in children as young as 10 months of age, and results are encouraging. Open posterior rectopexy is yet another technique for rectal prolapse.[37] Through a natal cleft incision, the coccyx is removed, the muscular hiatus is narrowed, and the rectum is suspended from the cut edge of the sacrum so that it cannot slide downward (Fig. 37-7). This maneuver immediately re-establishes the

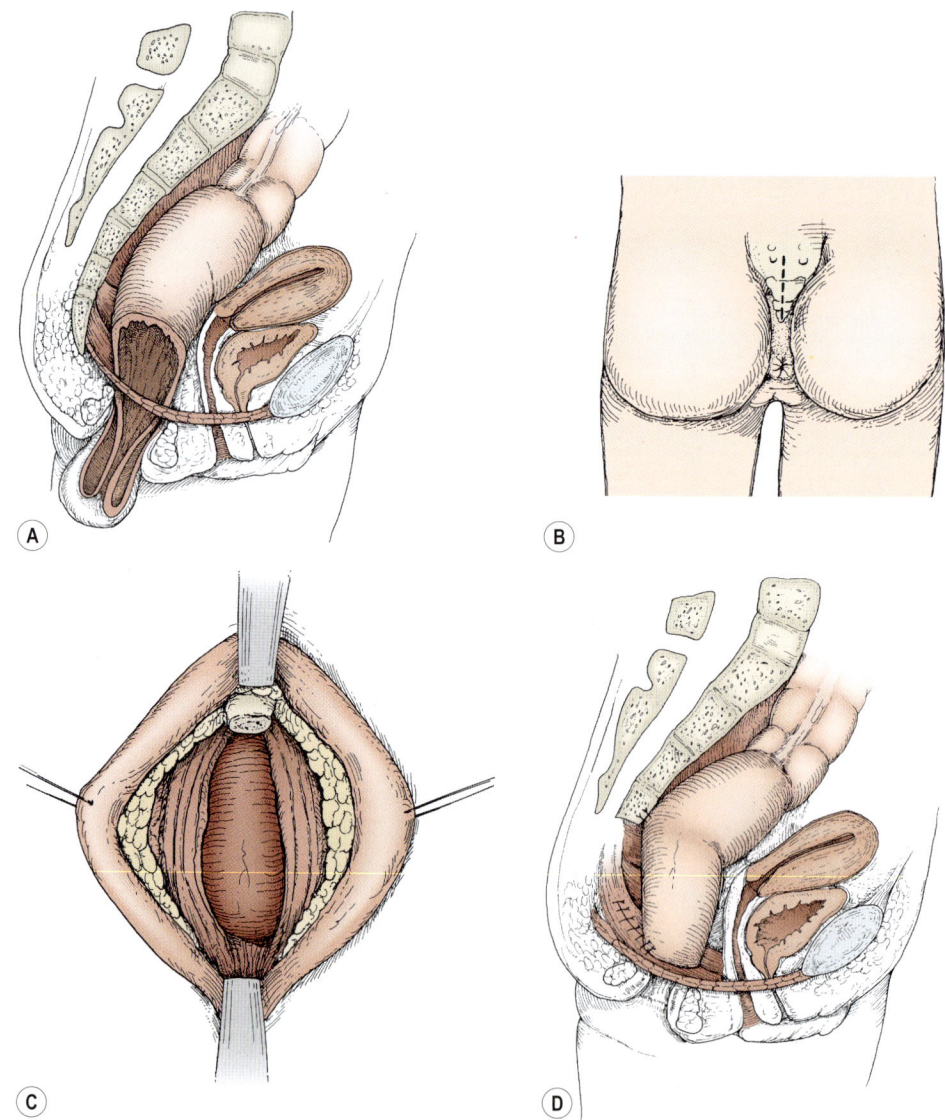

FIGURE 37-7 ■ **(A)** A cut-away sagittal view illustrates the failure of the rectal suspensory mechanism to hold the rectum within the pelvis. **(B)** The posterior sagittal incision is depicted. **(C)** The coccyx has been removed and the posterior rectal wall exposed. **(D)** The pelvic diaphragm is closed posterior to the reduced rectum. The rectum is sutured laterally to the pelvic diaphragm. The rectum is further suspended from the cut edge of the sacrum. (A and D adapted from Ashcraft KW, Amoury RA, Holder TM. Levator repair and posterior suspension for rectal prolapse. J Pediatr Surg 1977;12:241–5; B and C from Ashcraft KW. Atlas of Pediatric Surgery. Philadelphia: WB Saunders; 1994. p. 217.)

levator ani suspensory mechanism and narrows the anorectal hiatus. Successful resolution of rectal prolapse in 42/46 patients utilizing this technique over a 17-year period has been described.[38]

RECTAL TRAUMA

Rectal trauma in pediatric patients generally occurs by one of two mechanisms. The first is from penetrating trauma after an accidental impalement injury or, occasionally, a gunshot (Fig. 37-8). The second, and more common, occurs as the result of sexual abuse. The most common clinical presentation is that of a chronic stellate laceration of the anus with edema (Fig. 37-9). Perianal condylomata are common sequelae in cases of sexual abuse. Careful questioning may reveal that a male member of the immediate family has penile condylomata. However, 25% of males who carry papillomavirus in the urethra have no external evidence of disease.[39]

The patient with an accidental injury to the anus is typically seen immediately after the incident. Sexual abuse is suspected when an inconsistent history of the mechanism of injury is elucidated or there is a delay in presentation. As with other forms of sexual abuse, difficulty is often encountered in obtaining an adequate history from the victim owing to fear, threats of retaliation, or guilt. Unexplained injuries to the rectum must be considered a manifestation of sexual abuse until proven

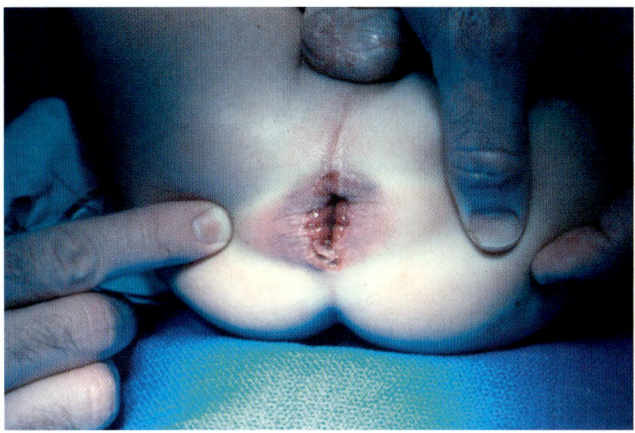

FIGURE 37-9 ■ This male child was the victim of chronic sexual abuse and shows the typical stellate lacerations of the anal mucosa and skin.

otherwise, and should be investigated through the appropriate social service authorities.[40–42]

The child who has a traumatic rectal injury is usually difficult to examine. An impalement injury often requires rectal examination and/or sigmoidoscopy under general anesthesia (Fig. 37-10). This allows a complete assessment of the injury and also allows appropriate operative treatment if necessary. Photographs should be obtained to document the injury for medicolegal purposes. A retrograde urethrogram and/or voiding cystourethrography should be obtained when there is suspicion of injury to the lower urinary tract.

Treatment of penetrating rectal injuries often requires a diverting colostomy.[43] However, primary repair without fecal diversion can be performed safely in select cases.[44,45] When in doubt, one should divert the fecal stream to avoid the consequences of perineal infection. In general, isolated intraperitoneal rectal injuries can be treated with primary repair. Inaccessible or severe distal extraperitoneal rectal injuries should be treated by fecal diversion

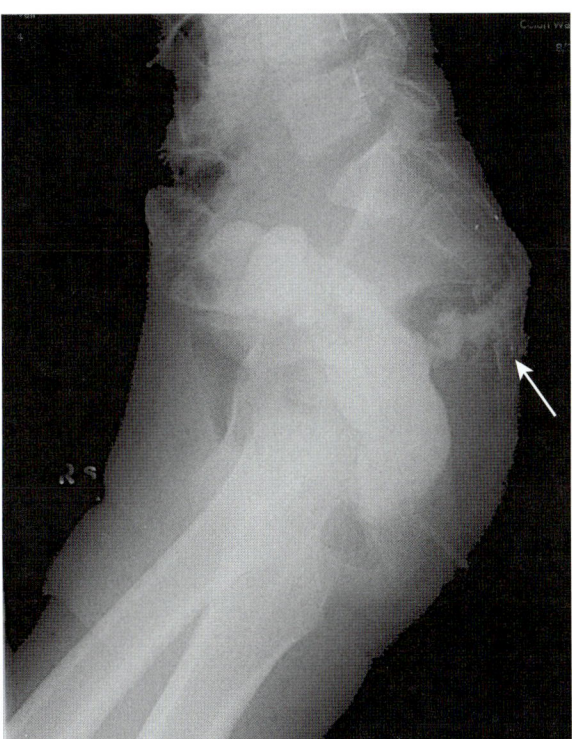

FIGURE 37-8 ■ This teenager sustained a gunshot wound to the buttocks with a suspected injury to the rectum. He underwent sigmoidoscopy followed by a diverting colostomy. Several days postoperatively, this contrast study was performed and revealed extravasation (*arrow*) from the rectal injury.

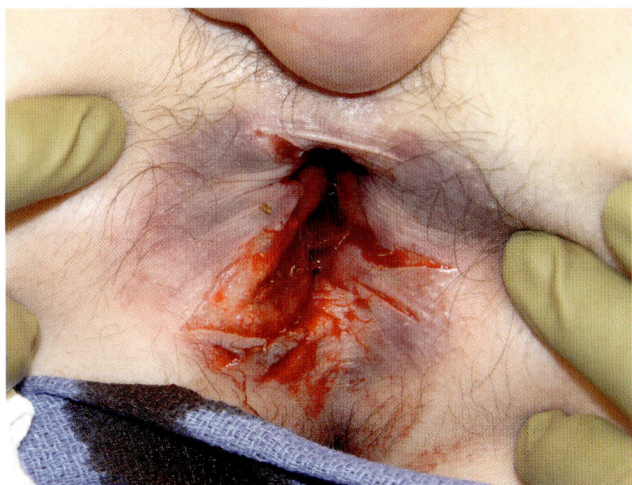

FIGURE 37-10 ■ This 14-year-old suffered a straddle injury after falling off a trampoline. He required examination under anesthesia. The perineal and rectal injuries were closed in layers without the need for colostomy.

and presacral drainage.[46] Accessible injuries to the distal rectum and anal canal can be repaired with the intent of reapproximating the underlying sphincter muscle mechanism and the overlying mucosa. In the victim who is found to have an acute laceration extending up the rectal wall, it is rarely necessary to perform a diverting colostomy, because these lacerations are not usually full thickness. However, patients with full-thickness injury should be managed by repair and diverting colostomy. When present, treatment of condylomata depends on the extent of disease. Although small lesions may be responsive to repeated applications of topical agents such as podophyllin or imiquimod, more extensive lesions require excision. Intralesional interferon may be a useful adjunct for recurrent disease.[47]

Treatment of sexual abuse involves interruption of the abuse pattern. Immediate consultation with child protective services or the local equivalent is mandatory.

REFERENCES

1. Fitzgerald RJ, Harding B, Ryan W. Fistula-in-ano in childhood: A congenital etiology. J Pediatr Surg 1985;20:80–1.
2. Rosen NG, Gibbs DL, Soffer SZ, et al. The nonoperative management of fistula-in-ano. J Pediatr Surg 2000;35:938–9.
3. Murthi GV, Okoye BO, Spicer RD, et al. Perianal abscess in childhood. Pediatr Surg Int 2002;18:689–91.
4. Stites T, Lund DP. Common anorectal problems. Semin Pediatr Surg 2007;16:71–8.
5. Poenaru D, Yazbeck S. Anal fistula in infants: Etiology, features, management. J Pediatr Surg 1993;28:1194–5.
6. Ross ST. Fistula in ano. Surg Clin North Am 1988;68:1417–26.
7. al-Salem AH, Laing W, Talwalker V. Fistula-in-ano in infancy and childhood. J Pediatr Surg 1994;29:436–8.
8. Cohen A, Dehn TC. Lateral subcutaneous sphincterotomy for treatment of anal fissure in children. Br J Surg 1995;82:1341–2.
9. Lambe GF, Driver CP, Morton S, et al. Fissurectomy as a treatment for anal fissures in children. Ann R Coll Surg Engl 2000;82:254–7.
10. Tankova L, Yoncheva K, Kovatchki D, et al. Topical anal fissure treatment: Placebo-controlled study of mononitrate and trinitrate therapies. Int J Colorectal Dis 2009;24:461–4.
11. Sweeney JL, Ritchie JK, Nicholls RJ. Anal fissure in Crohn's disease. Br J Surg 1988;75:56–7.
12. Buchmann P, Keighley MR, Allan RN, et al. Natural history of perianal Crohn's disease. Ten year follow-up: A plea for conservatism. Am J Surg 1980;140:642–4.
13. Strong SA. Perianal Crohn's disease. Semin Pediatr Surg 2007;16:185–93.
14. Hart AL, Plamondon S, Kamm MA. Topical tacrolimus in the treatment of perianal Crohn's disease: Exploratory randomized controlled trial. Inflamm Bowel Dis 2007;13:245–53.
15. Fleshner PR, Schoetz DJ Jr, Roberts PL, et al. Anal fissure in Crohn's disease: A plea for aggressive management. Dis Colon Rectum 1995;38:1137–43.
16. Severijnen R, Festen C, van der Staak F, et al. Rectal prolapse in children. Neth J Surg 1989;41:149–51.
17. Corman ML. Rectal prolapse in children. Dis Colon Rectum 1985;28:535–9.
18. Park RW, Grand RJ. Gastrointestinal manifestations of cystic fibrosis: A review. Gastroenterology 1981;81:1143–61.
19. Theuerkauf FJ Jr, Beahrs OH, Hill JR. Rectal prolapse. Causation and surgical treatment. Ann Surg 1970;171:819–35.
20. Shwachman H, Redmond A, Khaw KT. Studies in cystic fibrosis. Report of 130 patients diagnosed under 3 months of age over a 20-year period. Pediatrics 1970;46:335–43.
21. Zempsky WT, Rosenstein BJ. The cause of rectal prolapse in children. Am J Dis Child 1988;142:338–9.
22. Touloukian RJ. Anorectal Prolapse, Abscess, and Fissure. In: Ziegler MM, Azizkhan RG, Weber TR, editors. Operative Pediatric Surgery. New York: McGraw-Hill Professional; 2003. p. 735–8.
23. Abes M, Sarihan H. Injection sclerotherapy of rectal prolapse in children with 15 percent saline solution. Eur J Pediatr Surg 2004;14:100–2.
24. Chan WK, Kay SM, Laberge JM, et al. Injection sclerotherapy in the treatment of rectal prolapse in infants and children. J Pediatr Surg 1998;33:255–8.
25. Fahmy MA, Ezzelarab S. Outcome of submucosal injection of different sclerosing materials for rectal prolapse in children. Pediatr Surg Int 2004;20:353–6.
26. Shah A, Parikh D, Jawaheer G, et al. Persistent rectal prolapse in children: Sclerotherapy and surgical management. Pediatr Surg Int 2005;21:270–3.
27. Zganjer M, Cizmic A, Cigit I, et al. Treatment of rectal prolapse in children with cow milk injection sclerotherapy: 30-year experience. World J Gastroenterol 2008;14:737–40.
28. Balde I, Mbumbe-King A, Vinand P. [The Lockhart-Mummery technique in the treatment of the total rectal prolapse among children. Concerning 25 cases (author's transl)]. Chir Pediatr 1979;20:375–7.
29. Scheye T, Marouby D, Vanneuville G. [Total rectal prolapse in children. Modified Lockhart-Mummery operation]. Presse Med 1987;16:123–4.
30. El-Sibai O, Shafik AA. Cauterization-plication operation in the treatment of complete rectal prolapse. Tech Coloproctol 2002;6:51–4.
31. Hight DW, Hertzler JH, Philippart AI, et al. Linear cauterization for the treatment of rectal prolapse in infants and children. Surg Gynecol Obstet 1982;154:400–2.
32. Sander S, Vural O, Unal M. Management of rectal prolapse in children: Ekehorn's rectosacropexy. Pediatr Surg Int 1999;15:111–14.
33. Schepens MA, Verhelst AA. Reappraisal of Ekehorn's rectopexy in the management of rectal prolapse in children. J Pediatr Surg 1993;28:1494–7.
34. Tsugawa C, Matsumoto Y, Nishijima E, et al. Posterior plication of the rectum for rectal prolapse in children. J Pediatr Surg 1995;30:692–3.
35. Koivusalo A, Pakarinen M, Rintala R. Laparoscopic suture rectopexy in the treatment of persisting rectal prolapse in children: A preliminary report. Surg Endosc 2006;20:960–3.
36. Tsugawa K, Sue K, Koyanagi N, et al. Laparoscopic rectopexy for recurrent rectal prolapse: A safe and simple procedure without a mesh prosthesis. Hepatogastroenterology 2002;49:1549–51.
37. Ashcraft K. Acquired Anorectal Disorders. In: Ashcraft K, Holcomb GI, Murphy J, editors. Pediatric Surgery. 4th ed. Philadelphia: Elsevier Saunders; 2005.
38. Ashcraft KW, Amoury RA, Holder TM. Levator repair and posterior suspension for rectal prolapse. J Pediatr Surg 1977;12:241–5.
39. Rosemberg SK, Husain M, Herman GE, et al. Sexually transmitted papillomaviral infection in the male: VI. Simultaneous urethral cytology-ViraPap testing of male consorts of women with genital human papillomaviral infection. Urology 1990;36:38–41.
40. Adams JA. Medical evaluation of suspected child sexual abuse: It's time for standardized training, referral centers, and routine peer review. Arch Pediatr Adolesc Med 1999;153:1121–2.
41. Geist RF. Sexually related trauma. Emerg Med Clin North Am 1988;6:439–66.
42. Kadish HA, Schunk JE, Britton H. Pediatric male rectal and genital trauma: Accidental and nonaccidental injuries. Pediatr Emerg Care 1998;14:95–8.
43. Haut ER, Nance ML, Keller MS, et al. Management of penetrating colon and rectal injuries in the pediatric patient. Dis Colon Rectum 2004;47:1526–32.
44. Bonnard A, Zamakhshary M, Wales PW. Outcomes and management of rectal injuries in children. Pediatr Surg Int 2007;23:1071–6.
45. Levine JH, Longo WE, Pruitt C, et al. Management of selected rectal injuries by primary repair. Am J Surg 1996;172:575–9.
46. Weinberg JA, Fabian TC, Magnotti LJ, et al. Penetrating rectal trauma: Management by anatomic distinction improves outcome. J Trauma 2006;60:508–14.
47. Congilosi SM, Madoff RD. Current therapy for recurrent and extensive anal warts. Dis Colon Rectum 1995;38:1101–7.

CHAPTER 38

INTUSSUSCEPTION

Alexandra C. Maki • Mary E. Fallat

Intussusception is the most frequent cause of bowel obstruction in infants and toddlers. It is an acquired invagination of the proximal bowel (intussusceptum) into the distal bowel (intussuscipiens). It was first described in 1674 by Paul Barbette of Amsterdam, defined by Treves in 1899, and operated on successfully in 1873 by John Hutchinson.[1,2]

PATHOPHYSIOLOGY

The intussusceptum telescopes into the distal bowel by peristaltic activity. There may or may not be a lead point. As the mesentery of the proximal bowel is drawn into the distal bowel, it is compressed, resulting in venous obstruction and bowel wall edema. If reduction of the intussusception does not occur, arterial insufficiency will ultimately lead to ischemia and bowel wall necrosis. Although spontaneous reduction can occur, the natural history of an intussusception is to progress to bowel ischemia and necrosis unless the condition is recognized and treated appropriately.

Primary Intussusception

The vast majority of cases do not have a lead point and are classified as primary or idiopathic intussusceptions. The cause is generally attributed to hypertrophied Peyer patches within the bowel wall.[3] Intussusception occurs frequently in the wake of an upper respiratory tract infection or an episode of gastroenteritis, providing an etiology for the hypertrophied lymphoid tissue. Adenoviruses in children older than age two, and to a lesser extent rotaviruses, have been implicated in up to 50% of cases.[4,5] Other contributing evidence that viruses may play a role in intussusception includes the rise in cases during seasonal respiratory viral illnesses and the increased risk associated with previous rotavirus immunization.[6] The newest immunization formulas available in the USA, RotaTeq® and Rotarix®, have not been associated with intussusception in both pre- and post-marketing studies.[6–10]

Secondary Intussusception

An intussusception may have an identifiable lesion that serves as a lead point, drawing the proximal bowel into the distal bowel by peristaltic activity. The incidence of a lead point varies from 1.5% to 12% and the presence of a lead point increases in proportion with age.[11,12] The most common lead point is a Meckel diverticulum followed by polyps and duplications. Other benign lead points include the appendix, hemangiomas, carcinoid tumors, foreign bodies, ectopic pancreas or gastric mucosa, hamartomas from Peutz–Jeghers syndrome (Fig. 38-1), and lipomas. Malignant causes, although rare, increase in incidence with age and include lymphomas and small bowel tumors.[13] Systemic diseases, including Henoch–Schönlein purpura and cystic fibrosis, have been associated with intussusception. Other rare diseases related to intussusception are celiac disease and *Clostridium difficile* colitis.[14]

INCIDENCE

Idiopathic intussusception can occur at any age. Most patients are well-nourished, healthy infants, and approximately two-thirds are boys. The highest incidence occurs in infants between ages 4 and 9 months,[15] and it is also the most common cause of small bowel obstruction in this age group.[16] Intussusception is uncommon below 3 months and after 3 years of age. The condition has been described in premature infants where it has been postulated as the cause of small bowel atresia in some cases.[17]

CLINICAL PRESENTATION

The classic presentation is an infant or a young child with intermittent, crampy abdominal pain associated with 'currant jelly' stools and a palpable mass on physical examination, although this triad is seen in less than a fourth of children.[18] The abdominal pain is sudden and the child may stiffen and pull the legs up to the abdomen. The pain can also be associated with hyperextension, writhing, breath holding and vomiting. The attack often ceases as suddenly as it started. Between attacks, the child may appear comfortable but eventually will become lethargic. Small or normal bowel movements will stop as the obstruction progresses and becomes associated with bilious emesis and increasing abdominal distention. Stools may be blood tinged as impending ischemia causes mucosal sloughing and compression of mucous glands leading to evacuation of dark, red mucoid clots or 'currant jelly' stools. This is often a late sign as are laboratory derangements. A pitfall is to wait for the currant jelly stool, leukocytosis, and electrolyte abnormalities that are often hallmarks of ischemic bowel.

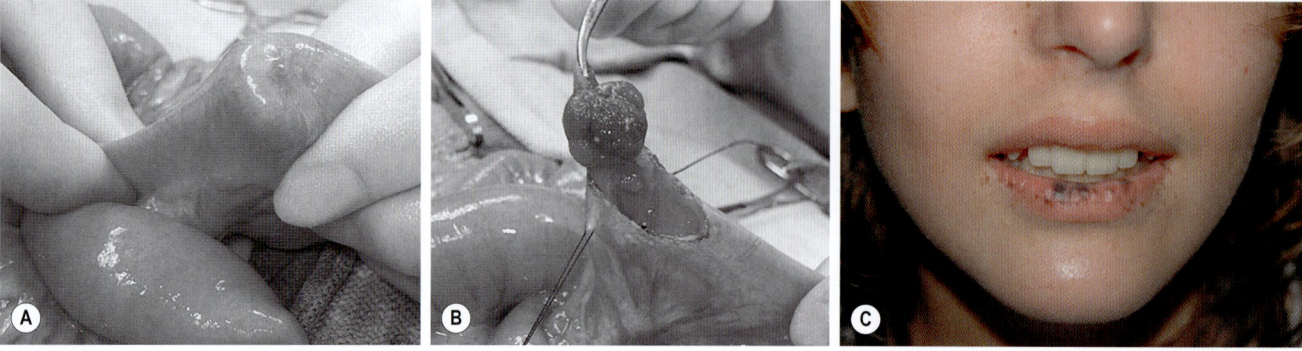

FIGURE 38-1 ■ **(A)** Operative view of the outside of the jejunum shows a palpable mass as the lead point of a reduced intussusception. **(B)** A hamartomatous polyp is characteristic of Peutz–Jeghers syndrome. **(C)** Mucocutaneous macular lesions are seen in this patient with Peutz–Jeghers syndrome. Note extension of the pigmentation beyond the vermilion border.

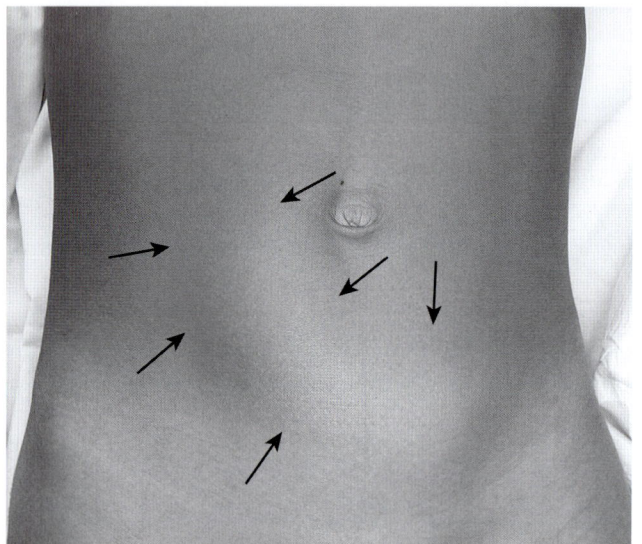

FIGURE 38-2 ■ This 10-year-old boy has a palpable sausage-shaped mass (arrows) due to an intussusception.

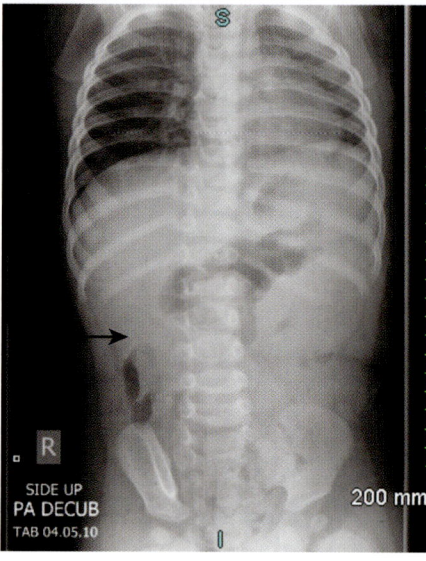

FIGURE 38-3 ■ This abdominal radiograph in a patient with intussusception shows dilated loops of small bowel in the right lower quadrant and a right upper quadrant soft tissue mass density in the vicinity of the transverse colon near the hepatic flexure (arrow).

PHYSICAL EXAMINATION

The child's vital signs are usually normal early in the disease course. During painless intervals, the child may appear comfortable and the physical examination may be unremarkable. However, the cramping episodes usually occur every 15 to 30 minutes and re-examination may prove difficult. There may be audible peristaltic rushes, and a sausage-shaped or curved mass might be palpable anywhere in the abdomen or even visualized if the child is relatively thin (Fig. 38-2). The right lower abdominal quadrant can appear flat or empty (Dance sign) as the intussuscepted mass is drawn cephalad. On rectal examination, bloodstained mucus or blood may be encountered as a later sign. If the obstructive process worsens and bowel ischemia occurs, dehydration, fever, tachycardia, and hypotension can develop in quick succession as a result of bacteremia and bowel necrosis.

Prolapse of the intussusceptum through the anus is a grave sign, particularly when the intussusceptum is ischemic. The greatest danger in a case of prolapsed intussusceptum is that the examiner will misdiagnose the condition as a rectal prolapse and attempt reduction.

Careful physical examination is mandatory and done by inserting a lubricated tongue blade along the side of the protruding mass before reduction. If the blade can be inserted more than 1–2 cm into the anus along the side of the mass, the diagnosis of intussusception should be considered.

DIAGNOSIS

Abdominal Radiography

In half of cases, the diagnosis of intussusception can be suspected on plain flat and upright abdominal radiographs (Fig. 38-3). Suggestive radiographic abnormalities include an abdominal mass, abnormal distribution of gas and fecal contents, sparse large bowel gas, and air-fluid levels in the presence of bowel obstruction. However, plain films have limited value in confirming the diagnosis and are not used as the sole diagnostic test. They are best utilized as a screening tool when one of the abnormal findings listed above is found.[19]

Ultrasonography

The use of abdominal ultrasound (US) for the evaluation of intussusception was first described in 1977.[20] Since then, most institutions have adopted it as a screening tool because of the lack of radiation exposure, ability to identify pathologic lead points, and decreased cost.[21,22] The characteristic finding on ultrasound has been referred to as a 'target' or 'doughnut' lesion (Fig. 38-4), which consists of alternating rings of low and high echogenicity representing the bowel wall and mesenteric fat within the intussusceptum in a transverse plane. The 'pseudo-kidney' sign is seen on longitudinal section (Fig. 38-5). This pattern is secondary to the edematous walls of the intussusceptum within the intussuscipiens. Ultrasonography can also guide the therapeutic reduction of an intussusception.[21] Equivocal findings using this modality should mandate a conventional contrast or air enema.[23]

Computed Tomography and Magnetic Resonance Imaging

Neither computed tomography (CT)[24] nor magnetic resonance imaging (MRI) are routinely used in the evaluation of a patient with intussusception, although either may confirm this diagnosis and/or pathologic causes for intussusception, such as a malignancy (i.e., lymphoma). The characteristic CT finding is a 'target' or 'doughnut' sign (Fig. 38-6). Transient small bowel intussusceptions that are discovered on CT or MRI are usually not clinically significant.[21] Radiographic or operative treatment

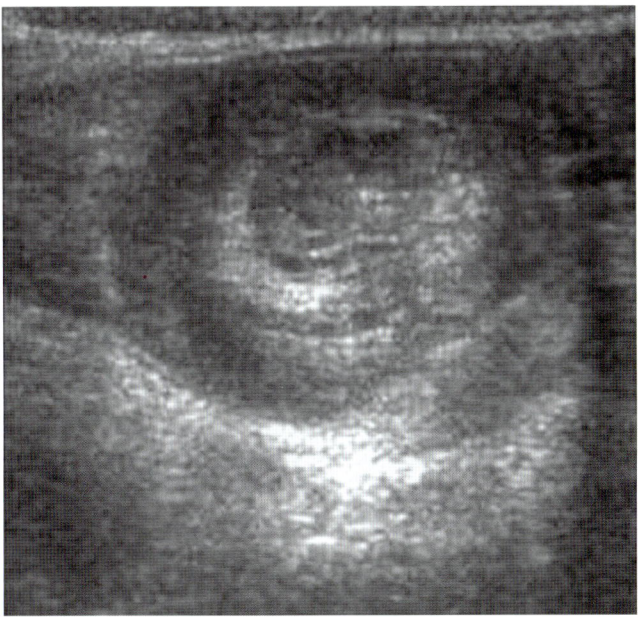

FIGURE 38-4 ■ This transverse sonographic image shows the alternating rings of low and high echogenicity due to an intussusception. This finding has been called a 'target' sign.

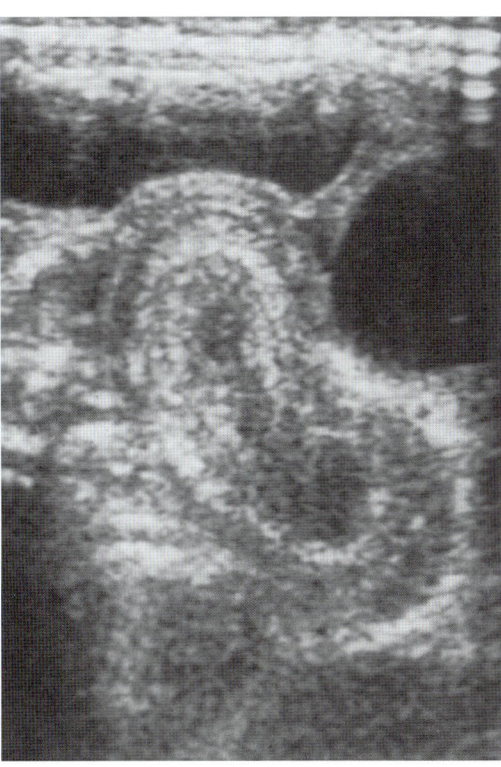

FIGURE 38-5 ■ Sonogram showing the 'pseudokidney' sign seen with intussusception on longitudinal section.[24]

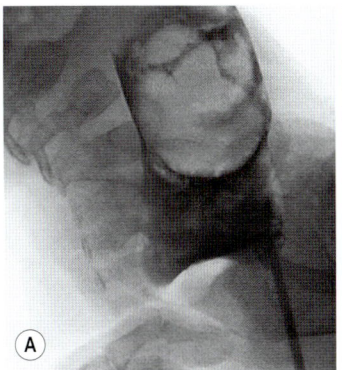
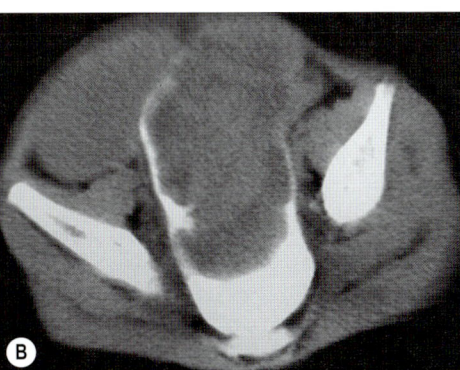
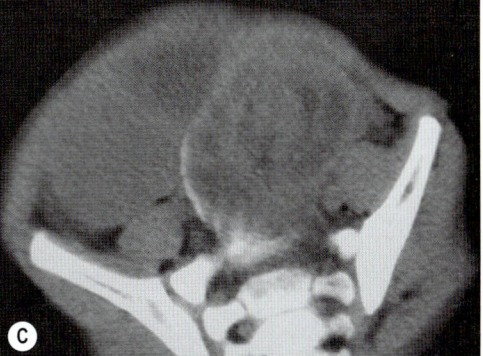

FIGURE 38-6 ■ Concurrent contrast enema and pelvic CT images of an intussusception. (A) Contrast study showing the intussusception low in pelvis. (B) CT image of the intussusception. (C) CT image of the 'layered' intussuscepted mass. This is the 'target sign' on CT.

should be based on clinical findings in symptomatic patients.[25] Laparoscopy is an excellent means to evaluate these patients if surgical intervention is needed.

NONOPERATIVE MANAGEMENT

If the diagnosis of intussusception is suspected, a nasogastric tube may be helpful to decompress the stomach. Bowel rest and intravenous fluid resuscitation should be initiated. A complete blood cell count and serum electrolytes are obtained. An air or contrast enema is first-line treatment as long as there are no contraindications to nonoperative reduction. Contraindications include intestinal perforation (free intra-abdominal air), peritonitis, or persistent hypotension. The advantages of nonoperative reduction are decreased morbidity, cost, and length of hospitalization.

Hydrostatic and Pneumatic Reduction

The methodology for hydrostatic reduction has not changed significantly since its first description in 1876.[26] Hydrostatic reduction with barium under fluoroscopic guidance has historically been used.[27] More recently, children's hospitals have transitioned to air or water-soluble isotonic contrast because of the potential hazard of barium peritonitis in patients with intestinal perforation[16,28]. Successful reduction (Fig. 38-7) in uncomplicated patients is seen in about 85% of cases and ranges from 42% to 95%.[29]

Pneumatic reduction was first described in 1897.[30] It gained popularity in the late 1980s. Since then, many institutions have adopted pneumatic decompression because it is quicker, safer, less messy, and decreases the exposure time to radiation.[31] The procedure is fluoroscopically monitored as air is insufflated into the rectum (Fig. 38-8). The maximum safe air pressure is 80 mmHg

for younger infants and 110–120 mmHg for older infants. Potential drawbacks of pneumatic reduction include the possibility of developing tension pneumoperitoneum, and poor visualization of lead points and/or the intussusception reduction process, resulting in false-positive reductions.[32–34] Rates of perforation range from 0.4–2.5% with the most recent publications citing an average rate of 0.8%.[16,35]

Tension pneumoperitoneum is best treated with immediate cessation of the procedure and immediate release of the pneumoperitoneum using a 14, 16, or 18-gauge needle or angiocatheter above or below the umbilicus. This should be followed by immediate operative exploration.[36]

For unsuccessful reduction, several studies have shown improved reduction rates using a second attempt after waiting between 30 minutes to 24 hours after the initial attempt.[28] In some instances, this is done in the operating room prior to laparoscopy or in conjunction with laparoscopic reduction.[37]

If nonoperative reduction is successful either by hydrostatic or pneumatic technique, the patient should be admitted for observation, receive a short period of bowel rest, and given intravenous fluids. Any clinical signs of abdominal pain after reduction could be a sign of ischemic bowel or recurrent intussusception and repeat ultrasound is necessary.

OPERATIVE MANAGEMENT

Open Approach

An operation is needed when nonoperative reduction is unsuccessful or incomplete, for signs of peritonitis, the presence of a lead point, or radiographic evidence of pneumoperitoneum. Preoperative preparation includes administration of broad-spectrum antibiotics, intravenous

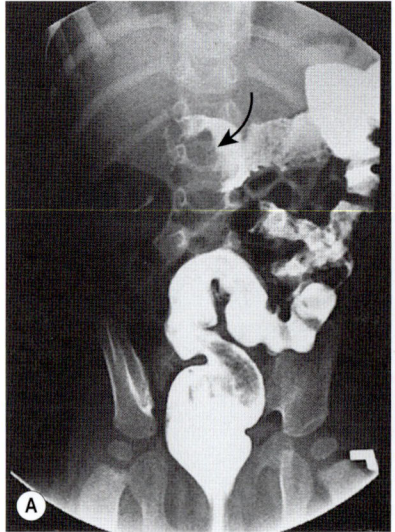 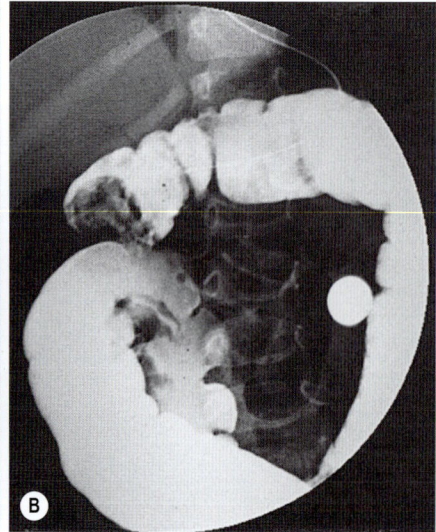 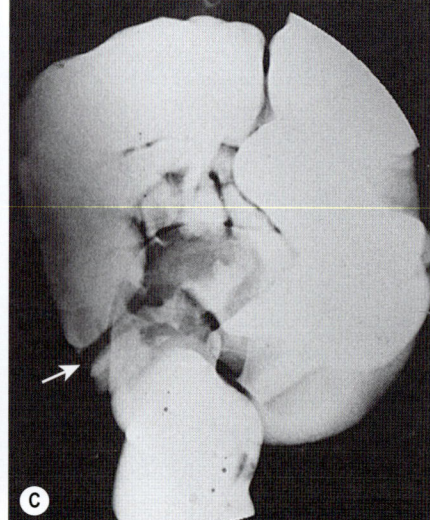

FIGURE 38-7 ■ Fluoroscopic examination using isotonic contrast for hydrostatic reduction of intussusception. **(A)** Intussusception (arrow) seen in midtransverse colon. **(B)** Reduction has occurred to the hepatic flexure. **(C)** Complete reduction with reflux of contrast medium into the terminal ileum. Note the edematous ileocecal valve (arrow).

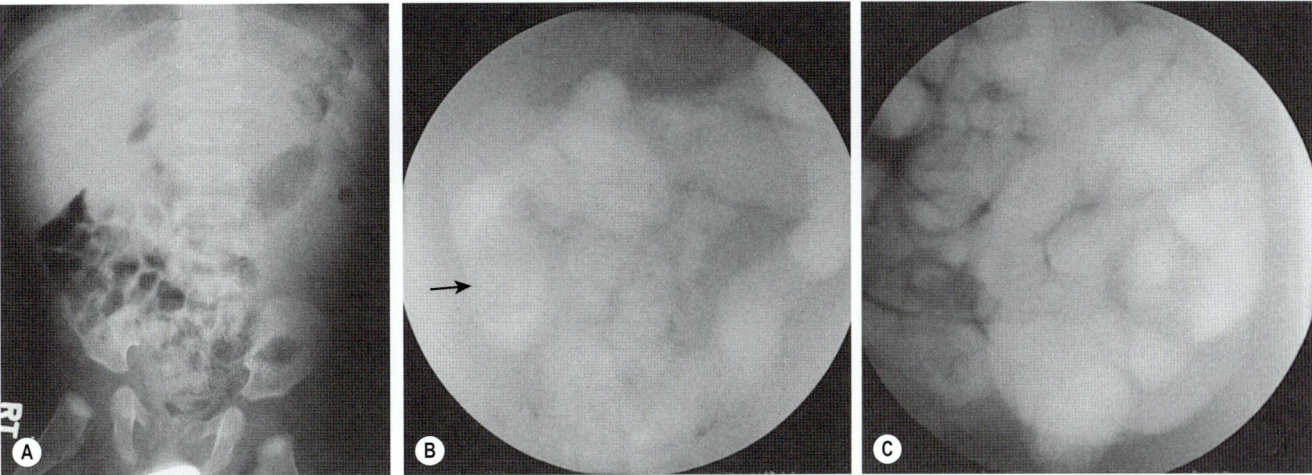

FIGURE 38-8 ■ Plain radiography and fluoroscopic examination using air for pneumatic reduction of an intussusception. **(A)** Plain radiograph showing a mass effect in the right upper quadrant. **(B)** Pneumatic reduction to the vicinity of the cecum with the intussusception still present (arrow). **(C)** Complete reduction with reflux of air into multiple loops of small intestine. (Courtesy of Charles Maxfield, MD.)

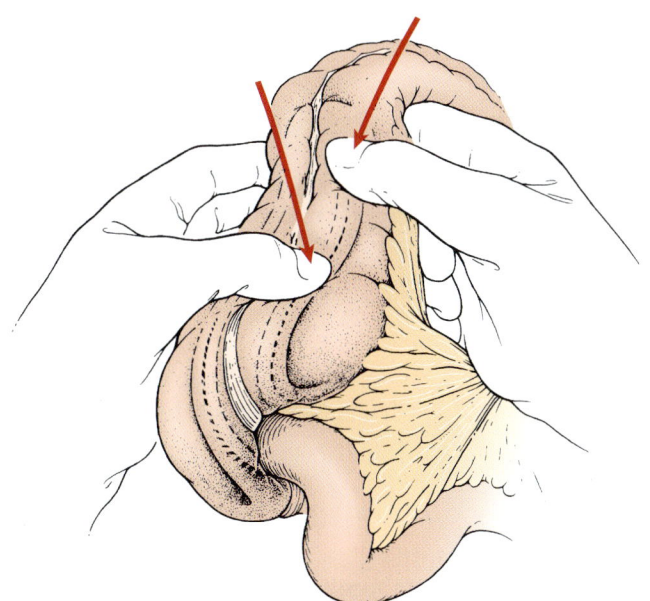

FIGURE 38-9 ■ A right lower quadrant muscle-splitting incision allows delivery of the intussusception through the incision. Gentle and continuous massage from distal to proximal usually results in reduction of the intussusception.

fluid resuscitation, insertion of a urinary catheter, and placement of a nasogastric tube for gastric decompression. Most commonly, the cecum and terminal ileum are involved, and can be delivered through the traditional right lower abdominal incision (Fig. 38-9). It is important to evaluate the extent of the intussusceptum before delivering it as it can extend into the rectosigmoid region in severe cases which usually requires extension of the incision.

Once the leading edge of the intussusceptum is identified, it is gently manipulated back toward its normal position in the terminal ileum. Excessive force or pulling is avoided to prevent injury or perforation of the bowel. Inability to manually reduce the intussusception, the finding of ischemic bowel, or identification of a lead point requires resection and bowel anastomosis or diversion, depending on the condition of the bowel and child. Ileopexy has been described in patients with recurrent intussusception after operative reduction.[38] However, in a series of 278 patients, this technique was not shown to reduce re-intussusception rates when compared to operative reduction and resection of the affected area.[39]

If surgical reduction is possible, the bowel is then evaluated for viability, perforation, or a lead point. Questionable ischemic bowel can be warmed with saline-soaked laparotomy pads and re-evaluated. After complete reduction of the intussusception, an incidental appendectomy is often performed because the location of the abdominal scar is similar to an open appendectomy incision.

Laparoscopic Approach

Initially, the use of laparoscopy in the operative management of intussusception was strictly diagnostic, or was used in cases with equivocal radiographic studies or in patients with suspected lead points, and was associated with conversion rates in up to 70% of cases.[40] More recently, there has been increased success with laparoscopic reduction with some studies showing conversion rates as low as 5.4%[41] but more in the range of 12–40%.[37,42–44]

Where laparoscopy fits into a surgeon's therapeutic algorithm is a topic frequently discussed. It would be beneficial to identify any preoperative risk factors. No study to date has specifically addressed this topic although some have noted an increased conversion rate associated with lead points. Recently, a retrospective analysis of 65 cases found that in patients unable to be reduced laparoscopically, 33% had a lead point that necessitated conversion to open (Fig. 38-10).[45] Contraindications to laparoscopy include peritonitis, hemodynamic instability, and severe bowel distension that precludes adequate visualization.[41]

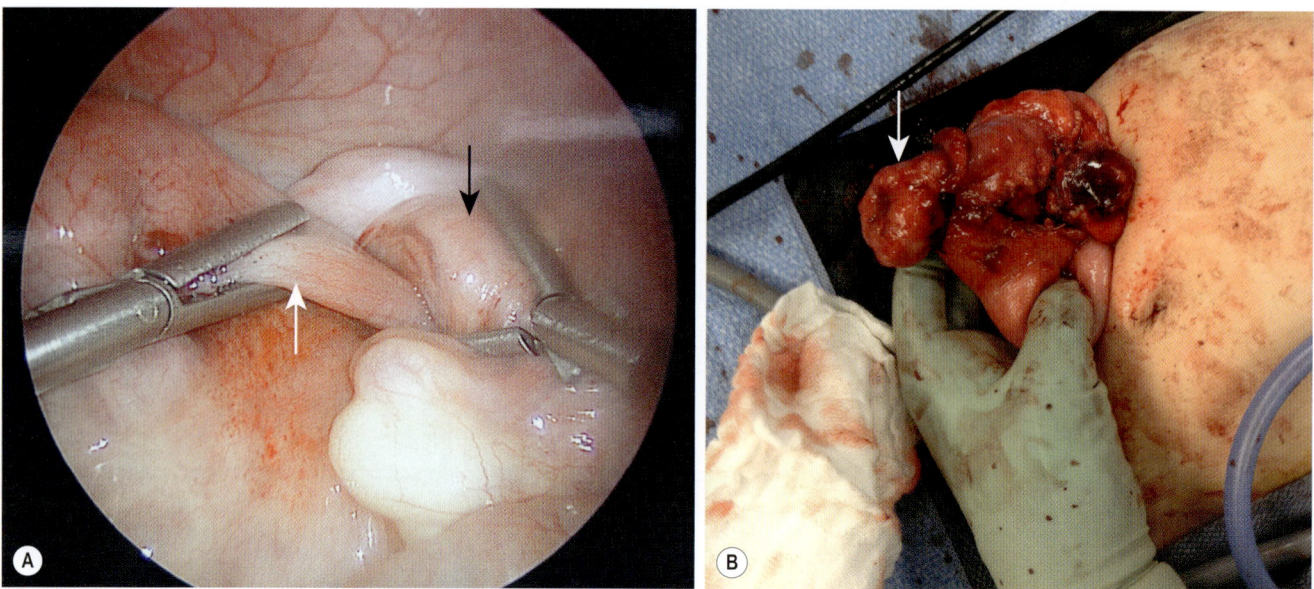

FIGURE 38-10 ■ **(A)** This laparoscopic photograph shows an incompletely reduced intussusception with the intussusceptum (white arrow) telescoping into the intussuscipiens (black arrow). **(B)** A pathologic lead point due to a Burkitt lymphoma was found requiring conversion to open.

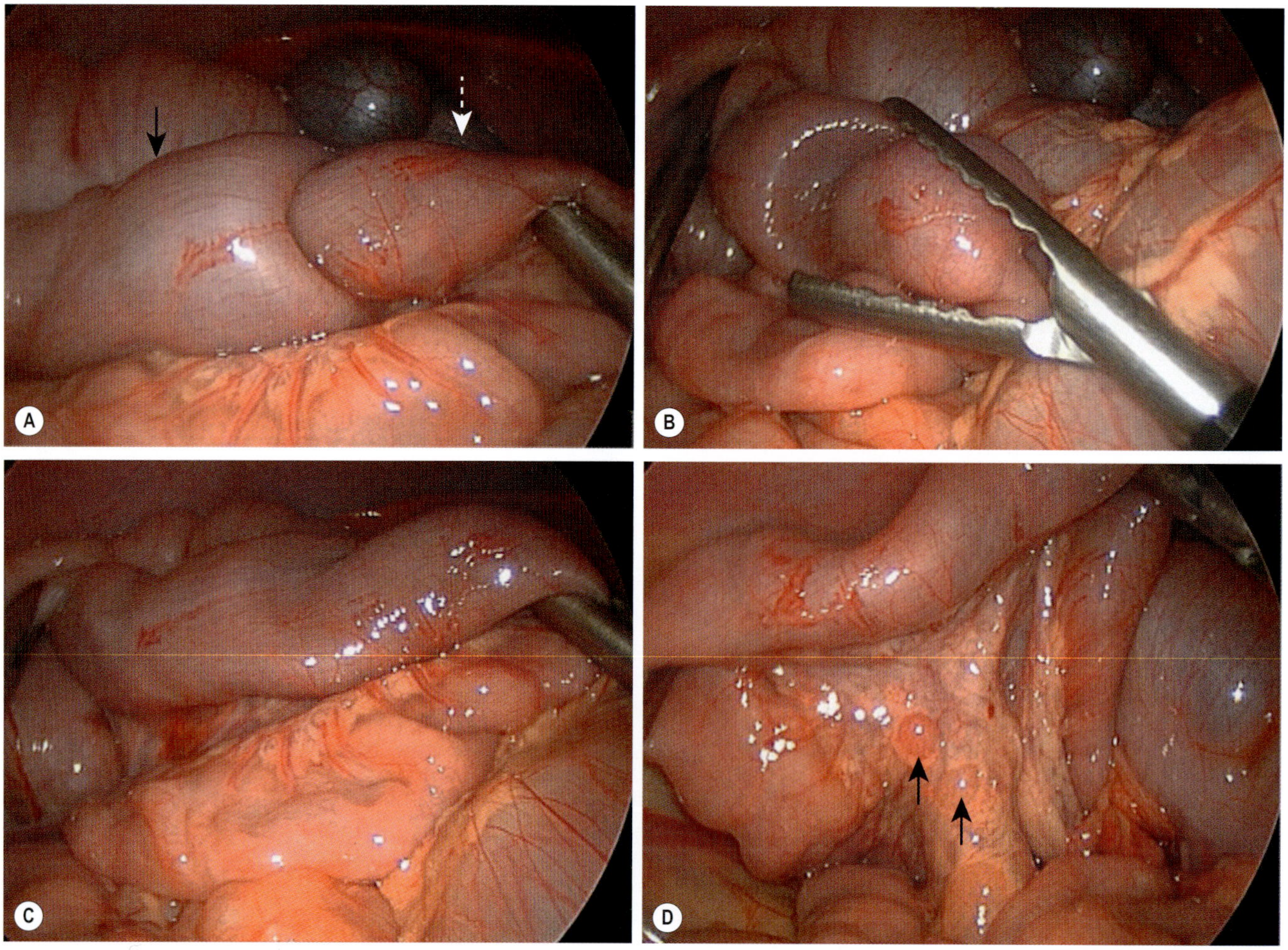

FIGURE 38-11 ■ Laparoscopic reduction of intussusception with hypertrophied lymph nodes is depicted in these four operative photographs. **(A)** Intussusceptum (white arrow) is seen telescoping into the intussuscipiens (black arrow). **(B)** The intussusception has almost been completely reduced. **(C)** This intussusception has been completely reduced and the bowel appears viable. **(D)** Hypertrophied mesenteric lymphadenopathy (arrows) is seen. This lymphadenopathy may reflect a recent viral illness.

The majority of minimally invasive approaches describe the use of three abdominal ports: one in the infraumbilical region with two other ports along the left side of the abdomen. Laparoscopic reduction is accomplished by applying gentle pressure distal to the intussusceptum using atraumatic graspers. Although counterintuitive to the conventional open method, traction is usually required proximal to the intussuscipiens to complete the reduction (Figs. 38-11). Appendectomy is not routinely performed with laparoscopic reduction and up to the surgeon's discretion. Careful inspection of the bowel is performed to evaluate for any signs of ischemia, necrosis, or perforation. A criticism of laparoscopic reduction is the loss of tactile sense that can lead to missed pathology. If resection is required, this can often be accomplished by exteriorizing the bowel by enlarging the periumbilical incision. If this is not possible, the operation should be converted to a laparotomy.

RECURRENT INTUSSUSCEPTION

Recurrent intussusception has been described in association with nonoperative intervention in 10–15% of cases, with about one-third occurring within 24 hours and the majority within 6 months of the initial episode.[46] Recurrences are less likely to occur after operative reduction or resection.[47] After laparoscopic reduction, a recurrence rate as high as 10% has been reported.[37]

Patients with recurrent intussusception tend to be seen earlier in their course because their parents are more aware of how to recognize the signs and symptoms. Success rates with enema reduction after one recurrence are comparable to those with the first episode and are better if the child did not previously require operative reduction. This finding has led to a nonoperative approach for initial management of recurrence in most patients as long as they are not toxic or show signs of peritonitis or hemodynamically instability.[29,46] A concern in recurrent intussusception is occult malignancy. Unfortunately, the clinical findings or pattern of recurrence do not predict the presence of a malignant lead point and radiographic reduction with ultrasound is recommended to look for an occult pathology.[48,49]

POSTOPERATIVE INTUSSUSCEPTION

Postoperative intussusception is a rare clinical entity that has been described after ileocolic intussusception reduction and resection, retroperitoneal dissections, long intra-abdominal procedures, a Ladd procedure, or extra-abdominal operations.[50,51] It accounts for 3% to 10% of cases of postoperative bowel obstruction and most often occurs in the initial 10 days following a procedure.[52,53] Ileus and adhesive obstruction are more frequently encountered as a cause for intestinal obstruction in the postoperative patient. Thus, an index of suspicion is needed and ultrasound is a useful diagnostic tool.[51] Most postoperative intussusceptions are ileoileal and respond to operative reduction without resection.

REFERENCES

1. Barbette P. Oeuvres Chirurgiques et Anatomiques. Geneva: Francois Miege; 1674.
2. Hutchinson J. A successful case of abdominal section for intussusception. Proc R Med Chir Soc 1873;7:195–8.
3. Stringer MD, Pablot SM, Brereton RJ. Paediatric intussusception. Br J Surg 1992;79:867–76.
4. Okimoto S, Hyodo S, Yamamoto M, et al. Association of viral isolates from stool samples with intussusception in children. Int J Infect Dis 2011;15:e641–645.
5. Bines JE, Liem NT, Justice FA, et al. Risk factors for intussusception in infants in Vietnam and Australia: Adenovirus implicated, but not rotavirus. J Pediatr 2006;149:452–60.
6. Belongia EA, Irving SA, Shui IM, et al. Real-time surveillance to assess risk of intussusception and other adverse events after pentavalent, bovine-derived rotavirus vaccine. Pediatr Infect Dis J 2010;29:1–5.
7. Shui IM, Baggs J, Patel M, et al. Risk of intussusception following administration of a pentavalent rotavirus vaccine in ultrasound infants. JAMA 2012;307:598–604.
8. Buttery JP, Danchin MH, Lee KJ, et al. Intussusception following rotavirus vaccine administration: Post-marketing surveillance in the National Immunization Program in Australia. Vaccine 2011;29:3061–6.
9. Ruiz-Palacios GM, Perez-Schael I, Velazquez FR, et al. Safety and efficacy of an attenuated vaccine against severe rotavirus gastroenteritis. N Engl J Med 2006;354:11–22.
10. Vesikari T, Matson DO, Dennehy P, et al. Safety and efficacy of a pentavalent human-bovine (WC3) reassortant rotavirus vaccine. N Engl J Med 2006;354:23–33.
11. Blakelock RT, Beasley SW. The clinical implications of non-idiopathic intussusception. Pediatr Surg Int 1998;14:163–7.
12. West KW, Grosfeld JL. Intussusception in Infants and Children. Philadelphia: WB Saunders; 1999.
13. Rampone B, Roviello F, Marrelli D, et al. Late recurrence of malignant melanoma presenting as small bowel intussusception. Dig Dis Sci 2006;51:1047–8.
14. Park JH. CMH. Intussusception associated with pseudomembranous colitis [Letter to the Editor]. J Pediatr Gastroenterol Nutr 2008;46:470–1.
15. Huppertz HI, Soriano-Gabarro M, Grimprel E, et al. Intussusception among young children in Europe. Pediatr Infect Dis J 2006;25(Suppl. 1):S22–9.
16. Applegate KE. Clinically suspected intussusception in children: Evidence-based review and self-assessment module. AJR Am J Roentgenol 2005;185(Suppl. 3):S175–83.
17. Kong FT, Liu WY, Tang YM, et al. Intussusception in infants younger than 3 months: A single center's experience. World J Pediatr 2010;6:55–9.
18. Kaiser AD, Applegate KE, Ladd AP. Current success in the treatment of intussusception in children. Surgery 2007;142:469–77.
19. Weihmiller SN, Buonomo C, Bachur R. Risk stratification of children being evaluated for intussusception. Pediatrics 2011;127:e296–303.
20. Burke LF, Clark E. Ileocolic intussusception–a case report. J Clin Ultrasound 1977;5:346–7.
21. Henrikson S, Blane CE, Koujok K, et al. The effect of screening sonography on the positive rate of enemas for intussusception. Pediatr Radiol 2003;33:190–3.
22. Navarro O, Daneman A. Intussusception. Part 3: Diagnosis and management of those with an identifiable or predisposing cause and those that reduce spontaneously. Pediatr Radiol 2004;34:305–12.
23. Gu L, Zhu H, Wang S, et al. Sonographic guidance of air enema for intussusception reduction in children. Pediatr Radiol 2000;30:339–42.
24. Fecteau A, Flageole H, Nguyen LT, et al. Recurrent intussusception: Safe use of hydrostatic enema. J Pediatr Surg 1996;31:859–61.
25. Kornecki A, Daneman A, Navarro O, et al. Spontaneous reduction of intussusception: Clinical spectrum, management and outcome. Pediatr Radiol 2000;30:58–63.
26. Hirschsprung H. Et Tilfaelde af suakat Tarminvagination. Hospitals-Tidende 1876;3:321–7.
27. Ravitch MM. Intussusception in Infants and Children. Springfield, IL; 1959.

28. Daneman A, Navarro O. Intussusception. Part 1: A review of diagnostic approaches. Pediatr Radiol 2003;33:79–85.

29. Navarro OM, Daneman A, Chae A. Intussusception: the use of delayed, repeated reduction attempts and the management of intussusceptions due to pathologic lead points in pediatric patients. AJR Am J Roentgenol 2004;182:1169–76.

30. Holt LE. The Diseases of Infancy and Childhood: For the Use of Students and Practioners of Medicine. New York: Appleton; 1897.

31. Guo JZ, Ma XY, Zhou QH. Results of air pressure enema reduction of intussusception: 6,396 cases in 13 years. J Pediatr Surg 1986;21:1201–3.

32. Kirks DR. Air intussusception reduction: 'the winds of change'. Pediatr Radiol 1995;25:89–91.

33. Peh WC, Khong PL, Chan KL, et al. Sonographically guided hydrostatic reduction of childhood intussusception using Hartmann's solution. AJR Am J Roentgenol 1996;167:1237–41.

34. Maoate K, Beasley SW. Perforation during gas reduction of intussusception. Pediatr Surg Int 1998;14:168–70.

35. Tareen F, Ryan S, Avanzini S, et al. Does the length of the history influence the outcome of pneumatic reduction of intussusception in children? Pediatr Surg Int 2011;27:587–9.

36. Sohoni A, Wang NE, Dannenberg B. Tension pneumoperitoneum after intussusception pneumoreduction. Pediatr Emerg Care 2007;23:563–4.

37. Kao C, Tseng SH, Chen Y. Laparoscopic reduction of intussusception in children by a single surgeon in comparison with open surgery. Minim Invasive Ther Allied Technol 2011;20:141–5.

38. Waldhausen JH. Intussusception. In: Mattei P, editor. Fundamentals of Pediatric Surgery. New York: Springer; 2011.

39. Koh CC, Sheu JC, Wang NL, et al. Recurrent ileocolic intussusception after different surgical procedures in children. Pediatr Surg Int 2006;22:725–8.

40. van der Laan M, Bax NM, van der Zee DC, et al. The role of laparoscopy in the management of childhood intussusception. Surg Endosc 2001;15:373–6.

41. Bailey KA, Wales PW, Gerstle JT. Laparoscopic versus open reduction of intussusception in children: A single-institution comparative experience. J Pediatr Surg 2007;42:845–8.

42. Kia KF, Mony VK, Drongowski RA, et al. Laparoscopic vs open surgical approach for intussusception requiring operative intervention. J Pediatr Surg 2005;40:281–4.

43. Burjonrappa SC. Laparoscopic reduction of intussusception: An evolving therapeutic option. JSLS 2007;11:235–7.

44. Bonnard A, Demarche M, Dimitriu C, et al. Indications for laparoscopy in the management of intussusception: A multicenter retrospective study conducted by the French Study Group for Pediatric Laparoscopy (GECI). J Pediatr Surg 2008;43:1249–53.

45. Hill SJ, Langness SM, Wulkan ML. Laparoscopic versus Open Reduction of Intussusception in Children: Experience Over a Decade. Poster presented at Southeastern Surgical Congress Feb 2012 Birmingham, AL, 2012.

46. Niramis R, Watanatittan S, Kruatrachue A, et al. Management of recurrent intussusception: Nonoperative or operative reduction? J Pediatr Surg 2010;45:2175–80.

47. Mirza B. Recurrent intussusception: Management options. APSP J Case Rep 2011;2:9.

48. Champoux AN, Del Beccaro MA, Nazar-Stewart V. Recurrent intussusception. Risks and features. Arch Pediatr Adolesc Med 1994;148:474–8.

49. Navarro O, Dugougeat F, Kornecki A, et al. The impact of imaging in the management of intussusception owing to pathologic lead points in children. A review of 43 cases. Pediatr Radiol 2000;30:594–603.

50. Holcomb GW III, Ross AJ III, O'Neill JA Jr. Post-operative intussusception: Increasing frequency or increasing awareness? South Med J 1991;84:1334–9.

51. Bai YZ, Chen H, Wang WL. A special type of postoperative intussusception: Ileoileal intussusception after surgical reduction of ileocolic intussusception in infants and children. J Pediatr Surg 2009;44:755–8.

52. Linke F, Eble F, Berger S. Postoperative intussusception in childhood. Pediatr Surg Int 1998;14:175–7.

53. Laje P, Stanley CA, Adzick NS. Intussusception after pancreatic surgery in children: A case series. J Pediatr Surg 2010;45:1496–9.

CHAPTER 39

ALIMENTARY TRACT DUPLICATIONS

Scott J. Keckler • George W. Holcomb III

Alimentary tract duplications are relatively rare congenital anomalies found anywhere from the mouth to the anus, and can present with obstruction or be discovered incidentally. While most duplications are benign, ectopic gastric mucosa and the potential for malignant degeneration remain concerns. Most duplications are discovered by 2 years of age. However, with the increased use of prenatal ultrasound (US), more are being diagnosed in utero.

The goal of operative management is to remove the duplication and prevent its recurrence. Since most share a common blood supply to the native alimentary tract, simple resection is usually adequate. Long tubular or thoracoabdominal duplications may present a more difficult scenario as radical resection can carry significant morbidity or even mortality. Overall prognosis is generally favorable but associated malformations or the presenting illness can factor into the final outcome.

Alimentary tract duplications have been described for hundreds of years and multiple terms have been used in the literature. The current term *duplication of the alimentary tract* and a common description of the congenital malformation was applied by William Ladd in 1937.[1] Three common findings were described: a well-developed smooth muscle coat, an epithelial lining, and attachment to the alimentary tract. The first large series to appear in the literature by Gross et al. in 1952 supported these findings as well.[2]

EMBRYOLOGY

The incidence of duplications has been reported to be 1 in 4500 births.[3] Two types are encountered: cystic and tubular, with cystic being the most common. Duplications are considered congenital malformations thought to arise from disturbances in embryologic development. Multiple theories have been postulated to account for their development. A persistent embryonic diverticulum from the alimentary tract was the first theory reported in the literature[4], while a defect in the recanalization of the lumen of the alimentary tract was proposed years later.[5] The coincidental finding of colonic and genitourinary duplications and similar findings in conjoined twins led to the partial twinning theory.[6,7] The 'split notochord' theory was proposed because of the association of enteric duplications and spinal anomalies[8], and relatively recent literature supports the notochord as being important in the development of both foregut and hindgut duplications.[9,10] Fetal hypoxia has also been implicated in the development of duplications.[11,12]

The associated findings of vertebral, spinal cord, and genitourinary malformations as well as malrotation and intestinal atresia suggest a multifactorial process in the development of alimentary tract duplications.[2,13,14] No single theory has been described to account for these heterogeneous malformations.

CLINICAL PRESENTATION AND DIAGNOSIS

Alimentary tract duplications present with a wide range of symptoms including abdominal distension and/or pain, obstruction, bleeding, respiratory compromise, or a painless mass. Generally, the symptoms are related to size, location, type of duplication, and presence of heterotopic mucosa. Most (80%) present before 2 years of age; prenatal ultrasound is detecting duplications as early as 16 weeks gestational age.[13-15] The majority of duplications are cystic and the remaining are tubular (Fig. 39-1). The jejunum/ileum is the most common location followed by the esophagus (Table 39-1). The epithelial lining is usually native to the surrounding lesion but heterotopic mucosa is found in 25–30% of duplications.[14] Gastric tissue is the most common type of ectopic mucosa encountered followed by both exocrine and endocrine pancreatic tissue. Ectopic gastric mucosa may lead to peptic ulceration with subsequent hemorrhage or perforation (Fig. 39-2).

Multiple imaging modalities are utilized to make the diagnosis. Plain radiographs may reveal a mediastinal mass, suggesting an esophageal duplication. Contrast studies may show a mass effect or communication with the alimentary tract. ultrasound is radiation free and noninvasive, making it a useful test, particularly for intra-abdominal duplications.[16] A typical sonographic appearance of duplications demonstrates an inner hyperechoic rim of muscosa–submucosa and an outer hypoechoic muscular layer (Fig. 39-3).[17] A history of anemia or bleeding with a suspected duplication suggests ectopic gastric mucosa, and technetium-99m (^{99m}Tc) scintigraphy is a useful imaging modality.[18,19] In cases where a combined thoracoabdominal duplication is suspected, computed tomography (CT) may aid in diagnosis. The presence of vertebral abnormalities and esophageal duplications is best investigated with magnetic resonance imaging (MRI).[20]

CLASSIFICATION AND TREATMENT BY LOCATION

To better understand the wide presentation and surgical treatment of duplications, they will be discussed according to anatomic location. A compilation of major case

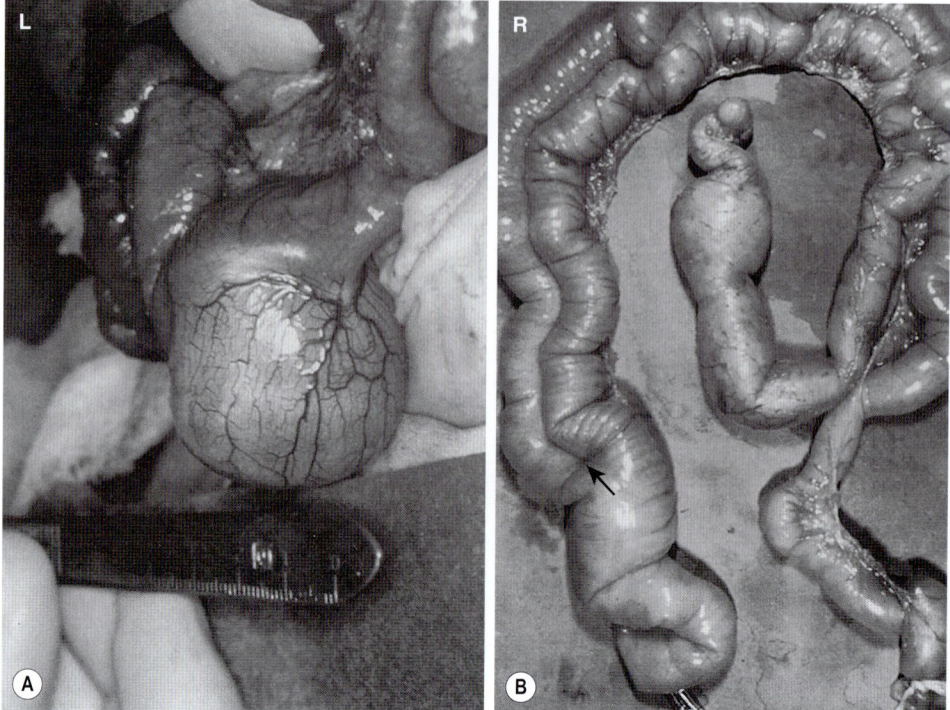

FIGURE 39-1 ■ **(A)** Most alimentary tract duplications are cystic. **(B)** A tubular duplication is seen. Note that the native bowel is bifurcated (arrow) into the tubular duplication and native intestine.

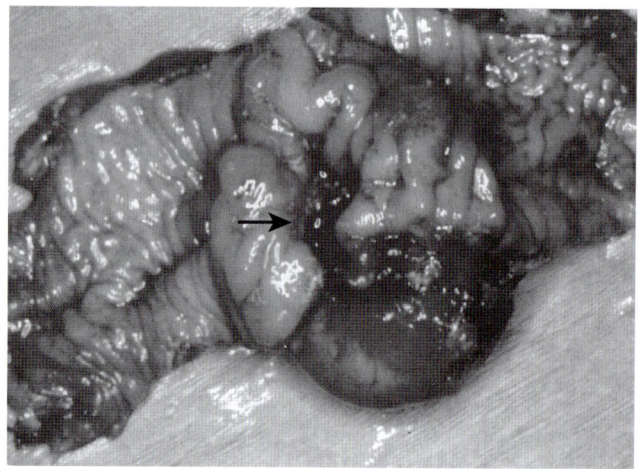

FIGURE 39-2 ■ Most intestinal bleeding from duplications is caused by tubular duplications with communication to the intestine. However, in this case, the bleeding was due to mucosal ulceration (solid arrow) secondary to an adjacent cystic duplication. (From Holcomb GW III, Gheissari A, O'Neill JA, et al. Surgical management of alimentary tract duplications. Ann Surg 1989;209:167–74.)

series reported in the last 60 years from 16 different institutions is seen in Table 39-1.[2,13–14,21–32] The report with the largest number of patients described 101 duplications in 96 patients.[14]

Esophageal Duplications

Approximately 20% of duplications arise from the esophagus. While cervical duplications do occur, the majority are located on the right side of the thoracic esophagus. Most are cystic and do not share a common muscular wall or communicate with the esophageal lumen. Clinical presentation will depend upon mass effect. Duplications impinging upon the trachea may lead to respiratory distress or pneumonia. In older patients, dysphagia may develop. Duplications should be in the differential diagnosis for any patient presenting with a mediastinal mass. Almost half of all esophageal duplications contain ectopic gastric mucosa so peptic ulceration leading to anemia or hematemesis can be seen (Table 39-2). Communication with the spinal canal is seen in 20% of patients.[14] Once a duplication is suspected on chest radiography or esophagography, further imaging with either CT or MRI should be performed (Fig. 39-4). It is important to evaluate for synchronous abdominal duplications as a 25% incidence has been described.[14] With the increased use of thoracoscopy, many esophageal duplications are being resected with a minimally invasive approach rather than the traditional thoracotomy.[33,34]

Thoracoabdominal Duplications

Extension of an esophageal duplication into the abdomen is known as a thoracoabdominal duplication. These are quite rare accounting for approximately 3% of all duplications. The length of extension can vary from the stomach to the jejunum, with jejunal connections being the most common.[13,14] These duplications are all tubular and ectopic gastric mucosa is found in a high percentage. Clinical presentation can range from asymptomatic to hemorrhage or ulceration from ectopic gastric mucosa. A

TABLE 39-1 Alimentary Tract Duplications by Location as Described in Literature Reports

First Author	Institution	No. D (No. Pts)	Oral	Esophagus	Thoracoabdominal	Stomach	Duodenum	Jejunum/ileum	Colon	Rectum	Other
Gross, 1952[2]	Children's, Boston	68 (67)	1	13	3	2	4	32	10	3	0
Basu, 1960[21]	A. H. Children's, Liverpool	33 (28)	0	7	0	1	3	16	4	2	0
Grosfeld, 1970[22]	Children's, Columbus	23 (23)	0	4	2	1	0	9	7	0	0
Favara, 1971[12]	Children's, Denver	39 (37)	1	6	0	3	4	20	4	0	1
Bower, 1978[23]	Children's, Pittsburgh	78 (64)	0	15	1	6	6	34	12	2	2
Hocking, 1981[24]	RHSC, Glasgow	60 (53)		8	2	8	1	32	4	5	0
Ildstad, 1988[25]	Children's, Cincinnati	20 (17)	0	6	0	1	0	5	8	0	0
Bissler, 1988[26]	Children's, Akron	11 (11)	0	1	0	1	2	4	2	1	0
Holcomb, 1989[14]	Children's, Philadelphia	101 (96)	0	21	3	8	2	47	15	5	0
Pinter, 1992[27]	Hungary	30 (28)		6	2	4	3	9	3	3	0
Bajpai, 1994[28]	IIMS, New Delhi, India	15 (14)	0	8	1	0	1	1	3	1	0
Stringer, 1995[13]	Hospital for Sick Children, London	77 (72)	2	15	6	10	3	21	10	6	4
Iyer, 1995[29]	Children's, Los Angeles	29 (27)	2	0	0	3	1	9	8	6	0
Yang, 1996[30]	NTUH, Taipei, China	20 (17)	0	2	0	1	0	14	3	0	0
Karnak, 2000[31]	Ankara, Turkey	42 (38)	1	7	2	1	3	17	9	2	0
Puligandla, 2003[32]	Montreal Children's	73 (73)			0	6	7	51	5	4	0
TOTALS		719 (665)	7 (1%)	119 (17%)	22 (3%)	56 (8%)	40 (6%)	321 (45%)	107 (15%)	34 (6%)	7 (1%)

No. D, number of duplications; No. Pts, number of patients.

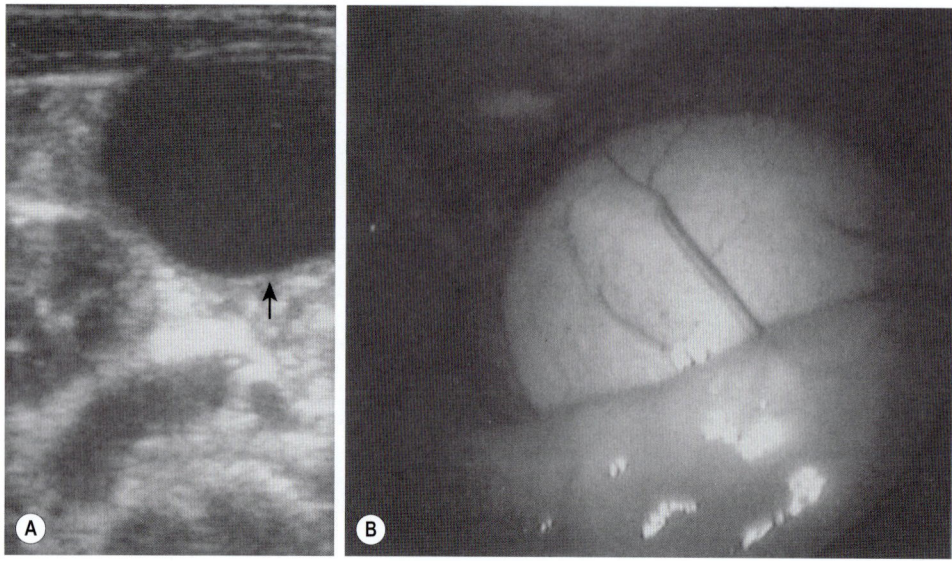

FIGURE 39-3 ■ Ultrasonography is a frequent imaging modality for diagnosing abdominal duplications. **(A)** This ultrasound image shows a cystic mass (arrow) in an infant with symptoms of intestinal obstruction. **(B)** The laparoscopic view in this same patient shows a cystic duplication of the ileum.

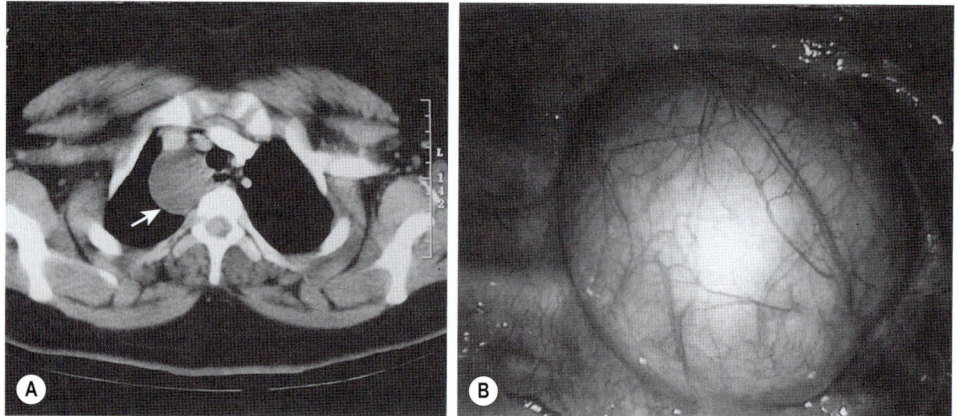

FIGURE 39-4 ■ This 16-year-old was found to have a posterior mediastinal mass on a chest radiograph. **(A)** CT scan shows the duplication (arrow) to be adjacent to the trachea and the esophagus. **(B)** View of the duplication as seen at thoracoscopy.

TABLE 39-2	Ectopic Gastric Mucosa by Location		
First Author	**Esophageal**	**Small Bowel**	**Colorectal**
Gross, 1952[2]	7/16	8/36	0/10
Favara, 1971[12]	3/6	6/24	0/4
Bower, 1978[23]	7/16	5/40	0/14
Hocking, 1981[24]	5/10	21/33	2/9
Ildstad, 1988[25]	2/6	5/13	0/8
Holcomb, 1989[14]	8/24	12/49	1/20
Bajpai, 1994[28]	9/9	2/2	1/4
Stringer, 1995[13]	9/21	7/24	0/16
Puligandla, 2003[32]		30/58	3/9
TOTALS	50/108 (46%)	96/279 (34%)	7/94 (7%)

higher incidence of vertebral anomalies (88%) in these patients warrants either CT or MRI to exclude neuroenteric communication (Fig. 39-5).[13,14] The current treatment is a one-stage combined thoracoabdominal approach for resection.

Gastric Duplications

Gastric duplications account for 8% of alimentary tract duplications and usually become symptomatic early in life, frequently presenting with pain, emesis, or melena. Unlike other duplications, a female predilection is seen.[6] Most are cystic and arise from the greater curvature and no intraluminal connection is seen (Figs 39-6 and 39-7). Peptic ulceration with hemorrhage or perforation may occur if an intraluminal connection is present. Abdominal ultrasound can usually diagnose the duplication, but pancreatic pseudocysts or choledochal cysts may have the

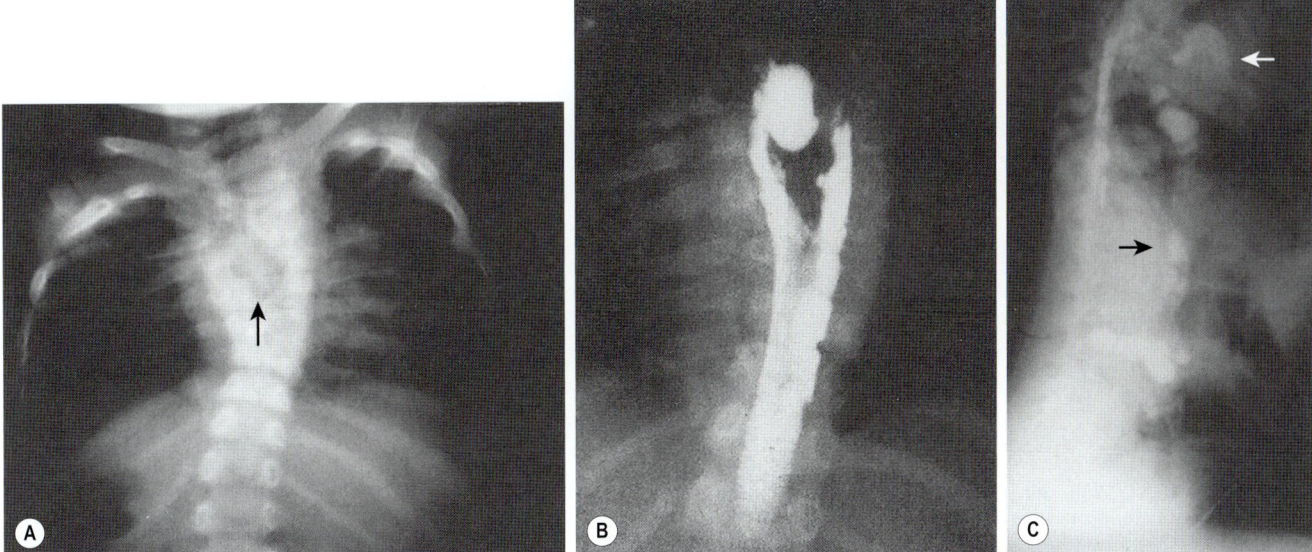

FIGURE 39-5 ■ A 3-year-old was found to have a right paravertebral mass. **(A)** A large anterior defect in the vertebral bodies of the upper thoracic spine (arrow) is seen. **(B)** This myelogram shows the filling defect caused by a neuroenteric cyst. **(C)** The contrast agent from the myelogram is seen in the neuroenteric cyst (upper arrow) with extension subdiaphragmatically (lower arrow) into the distal small intestine. (From Holcomb GW III, Gheissari A, O'Neill JA, et al. Surgical management of alimentary tract duplications. Ann Surg 1989;209:167–74.)

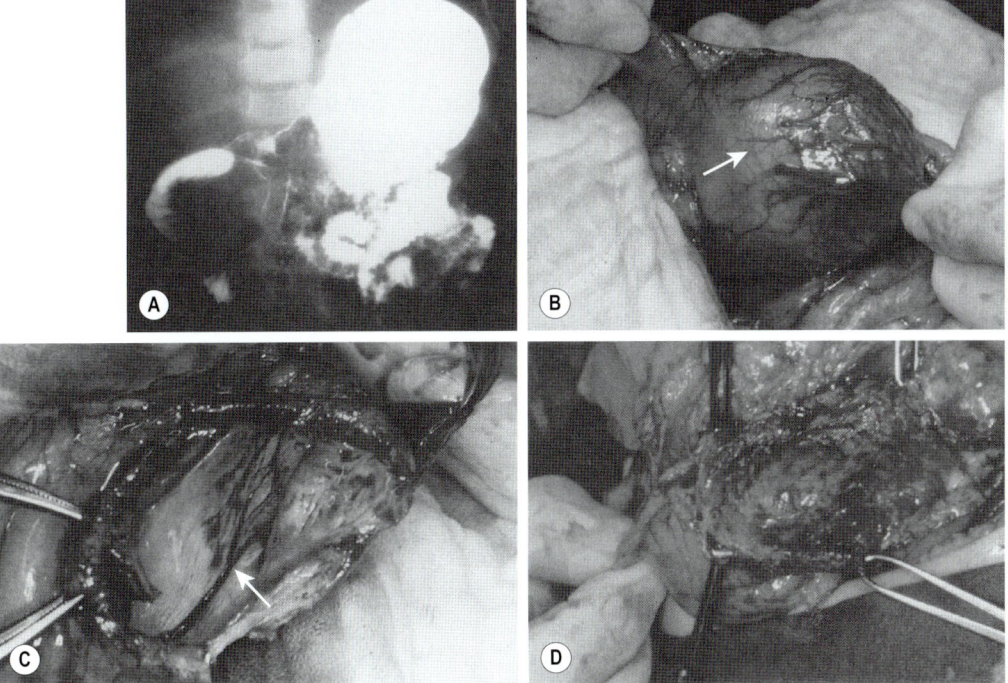

FIGURE 39-6 ■ **(A)** This patient had nonbilious emesis and was found to have a mass effect on the antrum with extrinsic compression of the second portion of the duodenum on this contrast study. **(B)** A gastric duplication (arrow) was found emanating from the inferior aspect of the greater curvature of the gastric antrum at operation. It was thought best to marsupialize the duplication, because a significant partial gastrectomy would be required to remove this lesion completely. **(C)** The duplication has been marsupialized, and the mucosa (arrow) of the duplication lying on the common wall with the stomach is seen. **(D)** The mucosa has been stripped, leaving intact the common wall between the duplication and the gastric antrum. (From Holcomb GW III, Gheissari A, O'Neill JA, et al. Surgical management of alimentary tract duplications. Ann Surg 1989;209:167–74.)

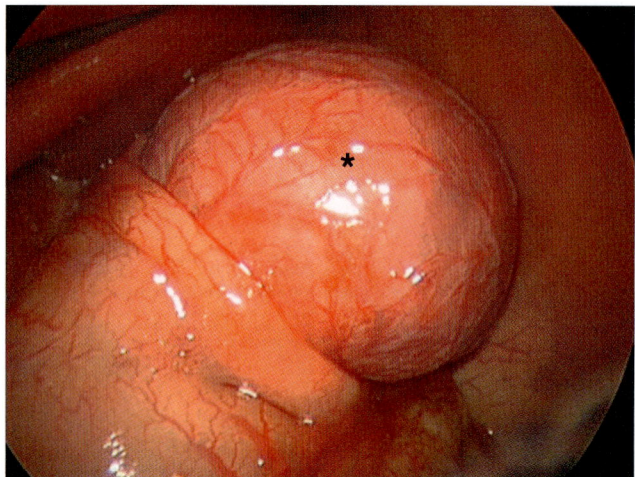

FIGURE 39-7 ■ A neonate was found to have pyloric atresia and underwent laparoscopic correction. At laparoscopy, a large gastric duplication (asterisk) was seen emanating from the greater curvature of the stomach. The duplication was excised and the greater curvature closed. The patient recovered uneventfully and did not develop any postoperative problems.

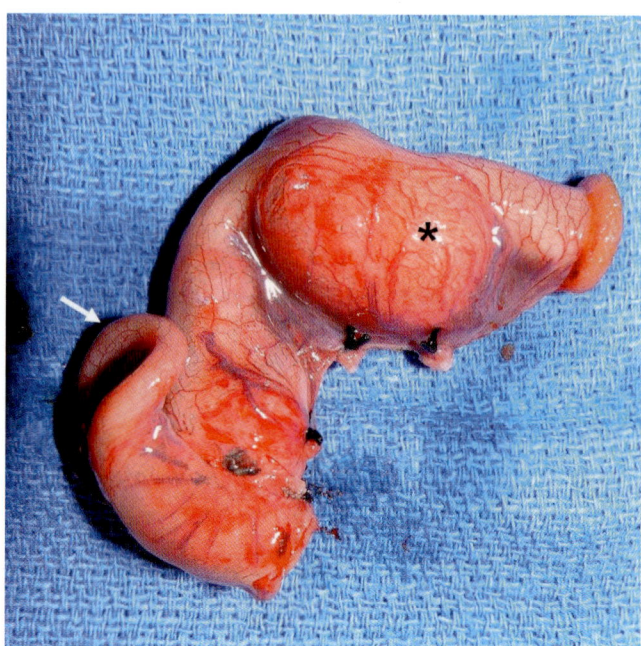

FIGURE 39-8 ■ This small bowel duplication (asterisk) was located in the terminal ileum and required removal of the terminal ileum as well as the cecum. Note the appendix (arrow) attached to the cecum. A primary anastomosis was performed.

same appearance. A contrast upper gastrointestinal series or CT can help clarify the anatomy.

Regardless of symptoms, all gastric duplications should be excised to prevent potential hemorrhagic complications. Complete excision without violating the lumen is the preferred approach. However, large duplications may require partial gastrectomy or mucosal stripping.

Duodenal and Pancreatic Duplications

Duodenal duplications account for 6% of all duplications and may be asymptomatic, or may present with intestinal obstruction secondary to cyst secretions or hemorrhage related to ectopic gastric mucosa which is found in 13% of specimens.[35] Most are cystic and noncommunicating with the lumen, but occasionally tubular variants are seen.[36] The anatomic locations of these duplications may obstruct the biliopancreatic ducts and cause jaundice or pancreatitis. Abdominal ultrasound or CT scan are commonly used for diagnosis.

The anatomic location and tenuous blood supply of these duplications dictate the operative approach. Simple excision is preferred, but the intimate relationship to the biliary or pancreatic ducts may warrant Roux-en-Y cystjejunosotomy.[37] Recently, the use of endoscopy for the treatment of duodenal duplications has been described in the literature.[38]

Pancreatic duplications are the rarest type of alimentary tract duplication. Commonly presenting with abdominal pain, nausea/vomiting, or a palpable mass, they can easily be mistaken for a pancreatic pseudocyst. The pancreatic head is involved in half of cases (51%). Intraoperative frozen section evaluation will differentiate a duplication from a pseudocyst. Simple cyst resection is

preferred but the location may dictate a more complex resection.[39]

Small Bowel Duplications

Small bowel duplications account for almost half (45%) of all reported duplications. They may be cystic or tubular (Fig. 39-8). Tubular duplications vary in size from a few centimeters to the entire length of bowel. Small bowel duplications may share a common wall or be entirely separate from the native intestine. They arise from the mesenteric side and share a common blood supply. The most common location is the ileum (34%).[13,14,23]

Small bowel duplications are frequently seen in childhood secondary to a palpable mass, obstruction, or hemorrhage. The duplication may lead to volvulus, which is sometimes seen in neonates. In older children intussusception is more common with the duplication acting as the lead point.[14] Abdominal ultrasound is usually the initial imaging study to evaluate these duplications. Additional studies such as CT or small bowel contrast study are usually less helpful and lead to unnecessary radiation exposure. The presence of ectopic gastric mucosa is found in 80% of tubular and 20% of cystic duplications.[32] Also these duplications can be mistaken for a Meckel diverticulum on technetium scanning. Laparoscopy is increasingly being used for both diagnosis and treatment of duplications, thereby eliminating open exploration and decreasing hospital stay.[32,40]

Operative treatment of small bowel duplications will vary based on the type and size. Small cystic duplications can be enucleated provided the native blood supply can be left intact. Small bowel resection with primary anastomosis is the usual approach. Long tubular duplications may pose a challenge because of the intimate blood supply to the native bowel. Resections of large lengths of bowel increase complications and may lead to short bowel syndrome. In this situation, mucosal stripping through multiple enterotomies will preserve bowel length and decrease the risk of ulceration or hemorrhage from ectopic gastric mucosa.[41]

Colonic Duplications

Colonic duplications account for approximately 15% of all duplications. Typically found on the mesenteric side of the bowel, most occur in the cecum and are cystic. However tubular duplications are seen, and vary in length and complexity (Fig. 39-9). Large bowel obstruction secondary to compression, intussusceptions, and volvulus are the usual presenting symptoms. Since colonic duplications rarely contain ectopic gastric mucosa, gastrointestinal bleeding is infrequent. However a higher number of associated anomalies are present with long tubular duplications. With total colonic tubular duplications, other duplicate structures such as bladder, vagina, and external genitalia are described, supporting the partial twinning theory of embryogenesis.[42,43] To better categorize tubular duplications, a classification system has been described.[44] Type I colonic duplications are limited to the colon, whereas type II have associated genital or urinary tract duplications.

Diagnosing colonic duplications can require more advanced imaging as plain radiographs may be nonspecific. Abdominal ultrasound, CT, or contrast enema are helpful based on symptoms. A contrast enema may demonstrate a communication with the native lumen if one is present.

The treatment of colonic duplications will vary depending on the type and size. As with small cystic duplications, enucleation is possible but resection and anastomosis is usually needed. Long tubular duplications present a difficult challenge. If resection is deemed too aggressive, a distal communication with native bowel can be created to relieve the obstruction (Fig. 39-10). Since colonic duplications rarely contain ectopic gastric mucosa, mucosal stripping is rarely needed. Long tubular duplications with distal communication are often treated conservatively with stool softeners. If a fistulous tract to the bladder or uterus is present, it should be excised.

Rectal Duplications

Rectal duplications account for approximately 6% of duplications, and are commonly found in the presacral space posterior to the rectum (Fig. 39-11). Chronic constipation is commonly found secondary to the posterior mass effect. Digital rectal examination may reveal a mass, leading to contrast enema for diagnosis. A perineal fistula should raise the suspicion for a perirectal abscess. Treatment of rectal duplications can vary from a transanal approach for marsupialization, or division of the septum between the duplication and the native rectum. A posterior sagittal approach is an alternative for more extensive duplications. Some patients may require an initial colostomy for large or complicated duplications.

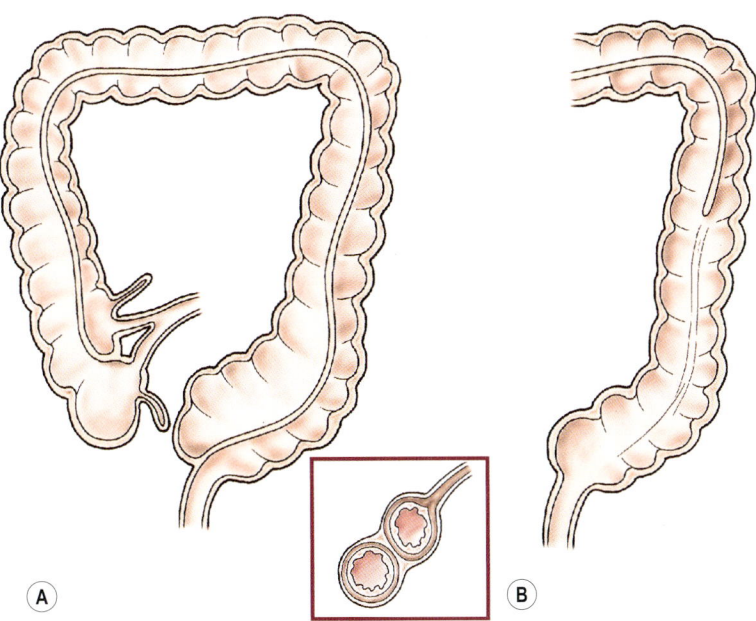

(A)   (B)

FIGURE 39-9 ■ Ileal and colonic tubular duplications vary in length and complexity. **(A)** The terminal ileum is seen to bifurcate into native colon and duplicated colon, which is medial to the native colon. In this scenario the duplicated colon ends blindly in the upper rectum. **(B)** In this drawing, the duplicated colon communicates with the native colon and forms a common descending colon.

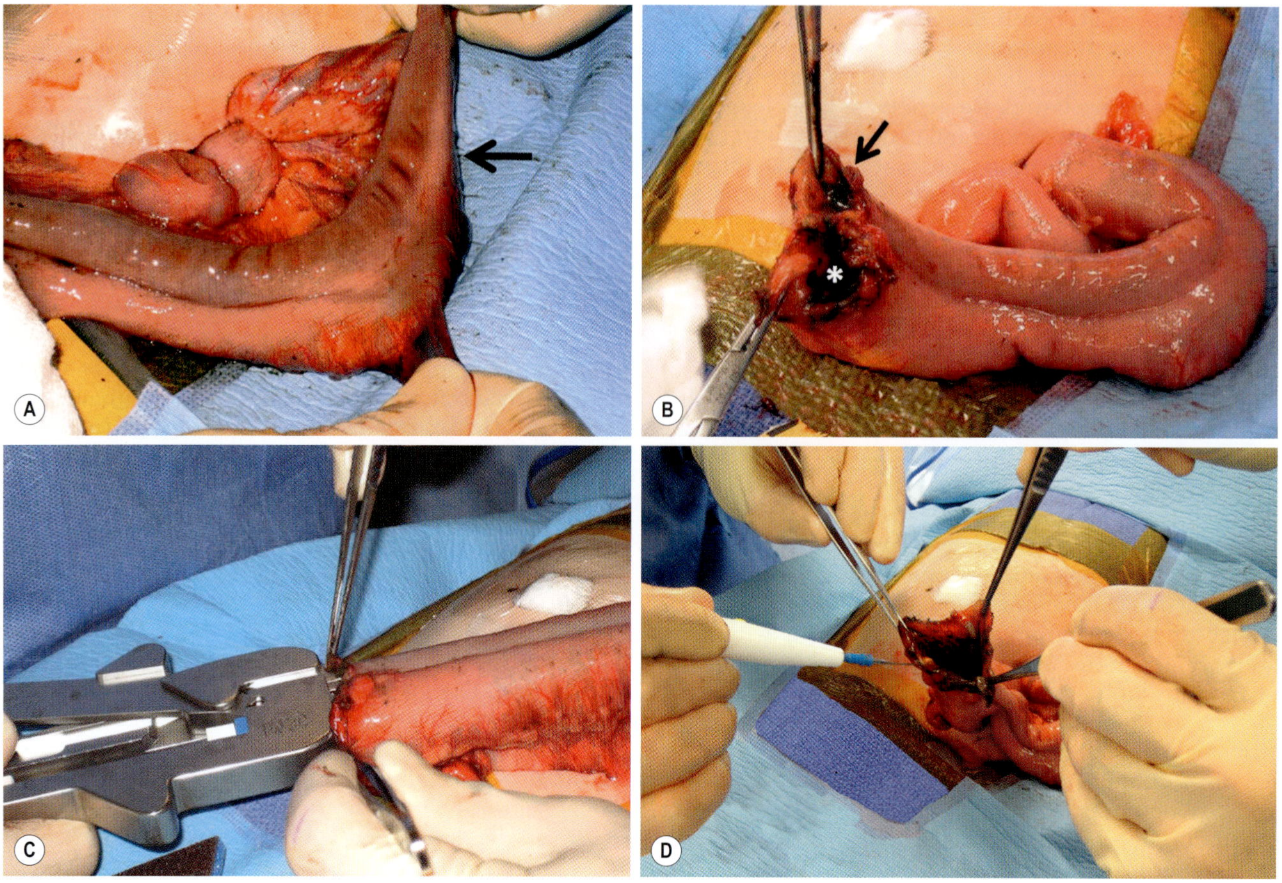

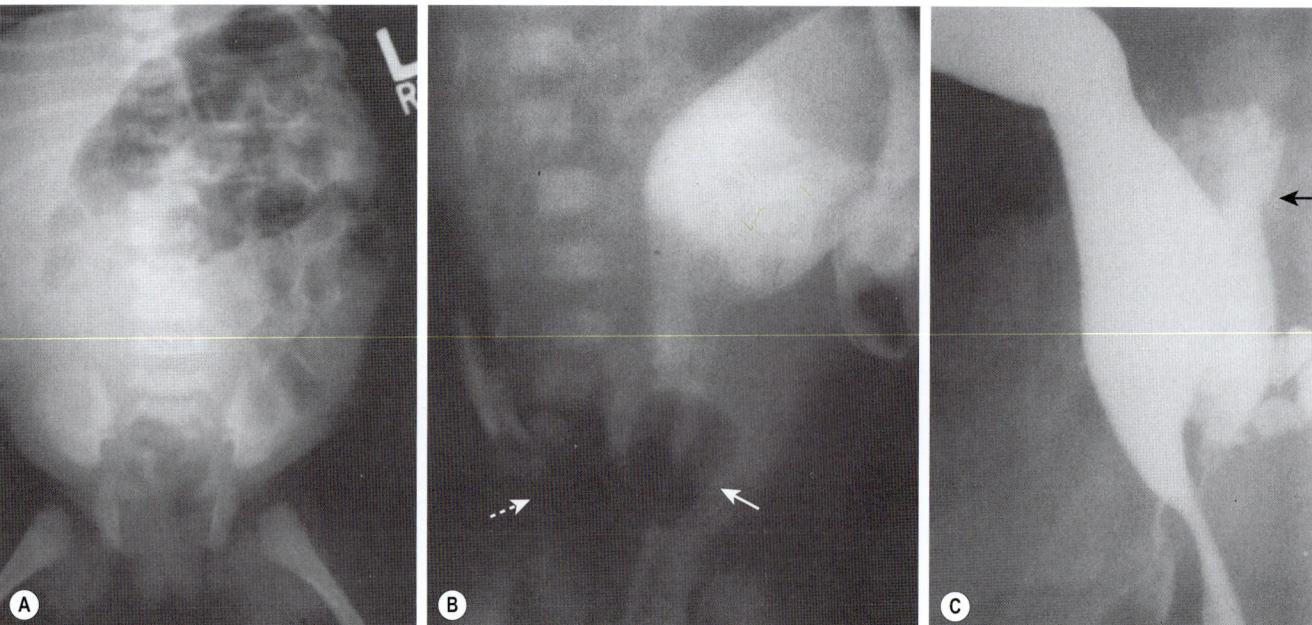

FIGURE 39-10 ■ This female infant was born with high imperforate anus and a duplicate vagina, and underwent initial colostomy. At the time of the colostomy, it was noted that she had a tubular colonic duplication. **(A)** Note where the tubular colonic duplication starts in the transverse colon (arrow). **(B)** After takedown of the colostomy, the two lumens of the colonic duplication are seen (asterisk and arrow). **(C)** A stapler is utilized to create a common channel between the two lumens. Note the dressing on the umbilicus as laparoscopy was used to completely mobilize the colon. **(D)** This end-on view shows a single lumen created after using the stapler to create the common lumen. This lumen was then anastamosed to the rectum.

FIGURE 39-11 ■ **(A)** Radiograph of a neonate with abdominal distention and evidence of a pelvic mass. On rectal examination, a mass was palpable posterior to the rectum. **(B)** A contrast study in which an 8-Fr Foley catheter was introduced into the rectum, and the balloon was inflated with air (*solid arrow*). Posterior to the rectum and compressing it is a rectal duplication with air (*dotted arrow*), indicating communication to the gastrointestinal tract. A colostomy was initially performed because of the rectal obstruction. **(C)** A barium enema was performed at age 6 months in this patient. On this lateral radiograph, filling of the posterior rectal mass is seen (*arrow*). (From Holcomb GW III, Gheissari A, O'Neill JA, et al. Surgical management of alimentary tract duplications. Ann Surg 1989;209:167–74.)

REFERENCES

1. Ladd WE. Duplications of the alimentary tract. South Med J 1937;30:363–71.
2. Gross RE, Holcomb GW, Farber S. Duplications of the alimentary tract. Pediatrics 1952;9:449–67.
3. Schalamon J, Schleef J, Hollworth ME. Experience with gastrointestinal duplications in childhood. Langenbeck's Arch Surg 2000;385:402–5.
4. Lewis FT, Thyng FW. Regular occurrence of intestinal diverticula in embryos of pig, rabbit, and man. Am J Anat 1908;7:505–19.
5. Bremer JL. Diverticula and duplications of the intestinal tract. Arch Pathol 1944;38:132–40.
6. Smith ED. Duplication of the anus and genitourinary tract. Surgery 1969;66:909–21.
7. Lewis PL, Holder T, Feldman M. Duplication of the stomach: Report of a case and review of the English literature. Arch Surg 1961;82:634–40.
8. Bentley JFR, Smith JR. Developmental posterior enteric remnants and spinal malformations: The split notochord syndrome. Arch Dis Child 1960;35:76–86.
9. Qi BQ, Beasley SW, Williams AK. Evidence of a common pathogenesis for foregut duplications and esophageal atresia with tracheo-esophageal fistula. Anat Rec 2001;264:93–100.
10. Qi BQ, Beasley SW, Frizelle FA. Evidence that the notochord may be pivotal in the development of sacral and anorectal malformations. J Pediatr Surg 2003;38:1310–16.
11. Mellish RWP, Koop CE. Clinical manifestations of duplication of the bowel. Pediatrics 1961;27:397–407.
12. Favara BE, Franciosi RA, Akers DR. Enteric duplications: Thirty-seven cases: A vascular theory of pathogenesis. Am J Dis Child 1971;35:501–6.
13. Stringer MD, Spitz L., Abel R, et al. Management of alimentary tract duplication in children. Br J Surg 1995;82:74–8.
14. Holcomb GW III, Gheissari A, O'Neill JA, et al. Surgical management of alimentary tract duplications. Ann Surg 1989;209:167–74.
15. Laje P, Flake AW, Adzick NS. Prenatal diagnosis and postnatal resection of intraabdominal enteric duplications. J Pediatr Surg 2010;45:1554–8.
16. Hur J, Yoon CS, Kim MJ, et al. Imaging features of gastrointestinal tract duplications in infants and children: From oesophagus to rectum. Pediatr Radiol 2007;37:691–9.
17. Barr LL, Hayden CK Jr, Stansberry SD, et al. Enteric duplication cysts in children: Are their ultrasonographic wall characteristics diagnostic? Pediatr Radiol 1990;20:326–8.
18. Lecouffe P, Spyckerelle C, Venel H, et al. Use of pertechnetate 99mTc abdominal scanning in localizing an ileal duplication cyst: Case report and review of the literature. Eur J Nucl Med 1992;19:65–7.
19. Kumar R, Tripathi M, Chandrashekar N, et al. Diagnosis of ectopic gastric mucosa using 99mTc pertechnetate: A spectrum of scintigraphic findings. Br J Radiol 2005;78:714–20.
20. Haddon MJ, Bowen A. Bronchopulmonary and neuroenteric forms of foregut anomalies: Imaging for diagnosis and management. Radiol Clin North Am 1991;29:241–54.
21. Basu R, Forshall I, Rickham PP. Duplications of the alimentary tract. Br J Surg 1960;47:477–84.
22. Grosfeld JL, O'Neill JA, Clatworthy HW. Enteric duplications in infancy and childhood: An 18-year review. Ann Surg 1970;172:83–90.
23. Bower RJ, Sieber WK, Kiesewetter WB. Alimentary tract duplications in children. Ann Surg 1978;188:669–74.
24. Hocking M, Young DG. Duplications of the alimentary tract. Br J Surg 1981;68:92–6.
25. Ildstad ST, Tollerud DJ, Weiss RG, et al. Duplications of the alimentary tract. Ann Surg 1988;208:184–9.
26. Bissler JJ, Klein RL. Alimentary tract duplications in children: Case and literature review. Clin Pediatr 1988;27:152–7.
27. Pinter AB, Schubert W, Szemledy F, et al. Alimentary tract duplications in infants and children. Eur J Pediatr Surg 1992;2:8–12.
28. Bajpai M, Mathur M. Duplication of the alimentary tract: Clues to the missing links. J Pediatr Surg 1994;29:1361–5.
29. Iyer CP, Mahour GH. Duplications of the alimentary tract in infants and children. J Pediatr Surg 1995;30:1267–70.
30. Yang MC, Duh YC, Lai HC, et al. Alimentary tract duplications. J Formos Med Assoc 1996;95:406–9.
31. Karnak I, Ocal T, Senocak ME, et al. Alimentary tract duplications in children: Report of 26 years' experience. Turk J Pediatr 2000;42:118–25.
32. Puligandla PS, Nguyen LT, St-Vil D, et al. Gastrointestinal duplications. J Pediatr Surg 2003;38:740–4.
33. Bratu I, Laberge JL, Flageole H, et al. Foregut duplications: Is there an advantage to thoracoscopic resection? J Pediatr Surg 2005;40:138–41.
34. Merry C, Spurbeck W, Lobe TE. Resection of foregut-derived duplications by minimal-access surgery. Pediatr Surg Int 1999;15:224–6.
35. Vertruyen M, Cadiere GB, Jacobvitz D, et al. A propos de 2 cas de duplication duodenale. Acta Chir Belg 1991;91:140–4.
36. Merrot T, Anastasescu R, Pankevych T, et al. Duodenal duplications: Clinical characteristics, embryological hypotheses, histological findings, treatment. Eur J Pediatr Surg 2006;16:18–23.
37. Leenders EL, Odsman MZ, Sukarochana K. Treatment of duodenal duplication with international review. Am Surg 1970;36:368–71.
38. Romeo E, Torroni F, Foschia F, et al. Surgery or endoscopy to treat duodenal duplications in children. J Pediatr Surg 2011;40:874–8.
39. Hunter CJ, Connelly ME, Ghaffari N, et al. Enteric duplication cysts of the pancreas: A report of two cases and review of the literature. Pediatr Surg Int 2008;24:227–33.
40. Schalamon J, Schleef J, Höllwarth ME. Experience with gastrointestinal duplications in childhood. Langenbecks Arch Surg 2000;385:402–5.
41. Wrenn EL Jr. Tubular duplication of the small intestine. Surgery 1962;52:494–8.
42. Smith ED, Stephens FD. Duplication and vesicointestinal fissure. Birth Defects Orig Artic Ser 1988;24:551–80.
43. Ravitch MM. Hind gut duplication-doubling of colon and genital urinary tracts. Ann Surg 1953;137:588–601.
44. Kottra JJ, Dodds WJ. Duplication of the large bowel. AJR Am J Roentgenol 1971;113:310–15.

CHAPTER 40

MECKEL DIVERTICULUM

Charles M. Leys

Wilhelm Fabricius Hildanus, a German surgeon, first described the presence of a small bowel diverticulum in 1598.[1] However, the diverticulum is named for Johann Meckel, a German anatomist, who further described the anatomy and embryology in 1809.[2] Meckel diverticulum is a remnant of the embryologic vitelline (omphalomesenteric) duct that connects the fetal gut with the yolk sac and normally involutes between the fifth and seventh weeks of gestation. Failure of duct regression results in a variety of abnormalities arising from persistence of the remnant (Fig. 40-1). The most common anomaly (90%) is the classic Meckel diverticulum. It is a true diverticulum, consisting of all normal layers of the bowel wall. Clinical symptoms and complications can arise from small bowel obstruction, bleeding, inflammation, umbilical abnormalities, or neoplasia.

EPIDEMIOLOGY

The true incidence of Meckel diverticulum is unknown, since most patients are asymptomatic. While the incidence is typically estimated at approximately 2%, a recent systematic review of autopsy studies found an incidence of 1.2%.[3] The incidence may be increased in patients with major anomalies of the umbilicus, alimentary tract, nervous system, or cardiovascular system.[4] An estimated 4% of patients with Meckel diverticulum will become symptomatic, and the risk of developing symptoms decreases with age.[5] A recent report based on data from the Pediatric Health Information System database found that 53% of Meckel diverticulectomies are performed before 4 years of age, with a male:female ratio of 2.3:1 overall and 3:1 in symptomatic patients.[6] The commonly cited 'rule of 2s' regarding the diverticulum is: occurs in 2% of the population, has a 2:1 male:female ratio, usually discovered by 2 years of age, located 2 feet (60 cm) from the ileocecal valve, commonly 2 cm in diameter and 2 inches (5 cm) long, and can contain two types of heterotopic mucosa.[7] Gastric is the most common type of heterotopic mucosa, followed by pancreatic (Fig. 40-2).[8] More rarely, it may contain duodenal, colonic, or endometrial tissue.

CLINICAL PRESENTATION

A variety of symptoms can develop depending on the configuration of the remnant structure and the presence of ectopic mucosa. The three most common presentations in children are intestinal bleeding (30–56%), intestinal obstruction (14–42%), and diverticular inflammation (6–14%).[8–10] Other less common signs include a cystic abdominal mass[11] and a newborn with an umbilical fistula resulting from a patent vitelline duct (Fig. 40-3). A Littré hernia refers to a Meckel diverticulum found incarcerated in a hernia which may be located at the inguinal, femoral, umbilical or Spigelian sites.[12] In adults, especially the elderly, neoplasia can develop within the Meckel diverticulum. Carcinoid is the most common tumor, but other malignancies include adenocarcinoma, leiomyosarcoma, gastrointestinal stromal tumors, and lymphoma.[13] Neonatal presentation of a Meckel diverticulum is uncommon and typically is due to perforation or obstruction.[14]

Bleeding

Episodic painless rectal bleeding in a young child is the classic presentation of a bleeding Meckel diverticulum. A Meckel accounts for nearly 50% of all lower gastrointestinal bleeding in children. The stool may be bright red, dark or maroon red, or less commonly tarry. The bleeding is often associated with anemia, and many children will require transfusion, though life-threatening hemorrhage is rare. Physical exam is typically unremarkable. The bleeding may also be slow and not clinically evident, presenting solely as unexplained anemia. Thus, any child presenting with hemoglobin-positive stools and chronic anemia should be evaluated for a Meckel diverticulum.

Bleeding is generally attributed to the presence of heterotopic mucosa. Gastric mucosa is present in up to 80% of Meckel diverticula that bleed.[15] Gastric acid produces mucosal ulceration, typically at the junction of the ectopic mucosa and the normal ileal mucosa. The ulcer may also be located within the ectopic mucosa or even on the mesenteric side of the normal ileum, opposite the diverticulum. While *Helicobacter pylori* is associated with many ulcers in the duodenum and stomach, studies have shown that *H. pylori* is rarely present in a bleeding Meckel diverticulum.[16,17]

Obstruction

A Meckel diverticulum can cause intestinal obstruction through several mechanisms, but most commonly intussusception or volvulus. The diverticulum can act as a lead point for an obstructing ileo-ileal and subsequent ileocolic intussusception. A volvulus can occur if bowel twists or kinks around a vitelline remnant with a fibrous cord between the diverticula and umbilicus (see Fig. 40-1). An internal hernia can result due to a mesodiverticular artery, coursing from the base of the mesentery to the

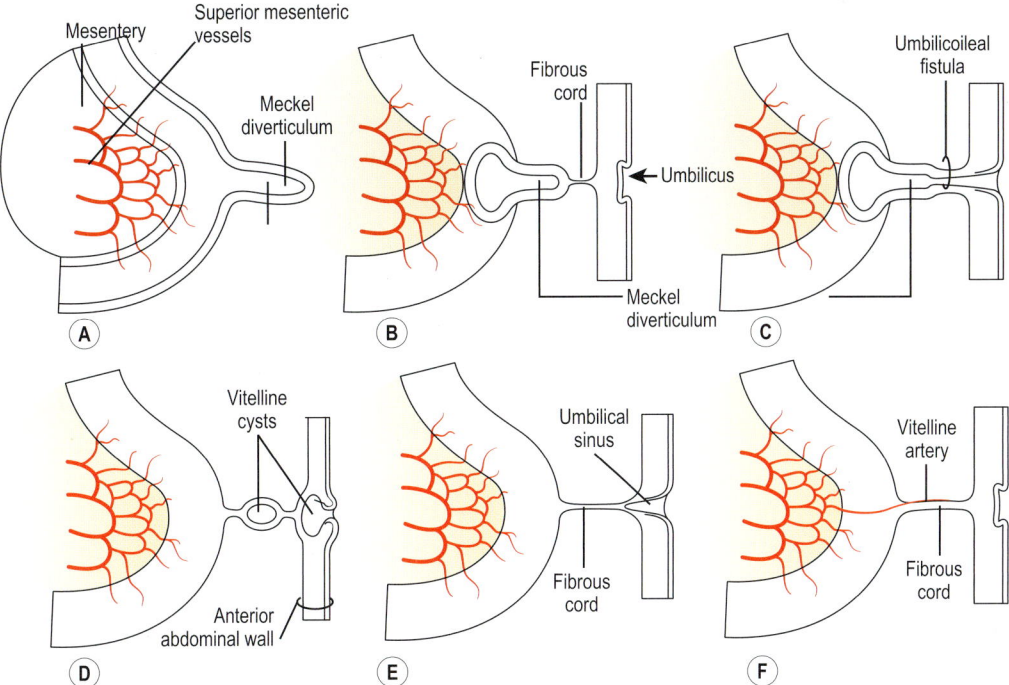

FIGURE 40-1 ■ Drawings illustrating Meckel diverticulum and other remnants of the yolk sac. (From Moore KL. *The Developing Human.* Philadelphia: WB Saunders; 1988.)

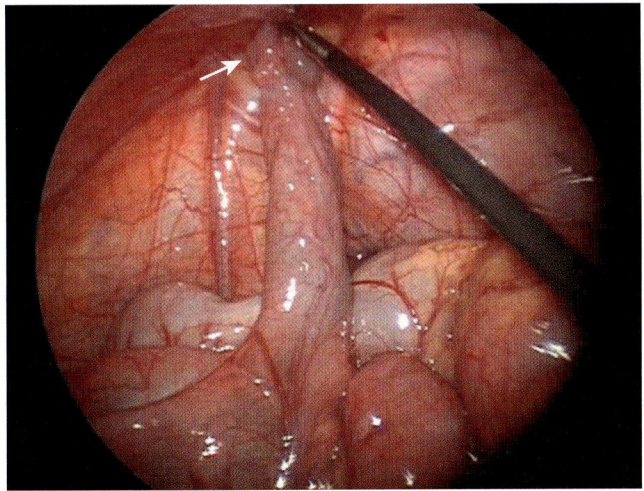

FIGURE 40-2 ■ This laparoscopic view shows a long Meckel diverticulum emanating from the antimesenteric border of the ileum. This is a true diverticulum and contains ectopic mucosa at the tip of the diverticulum (arrow).

diverticulum, under which the small bowel becomes entrapped and incarcerated. Other rare obstructing mechanisms include an incarcerated Littré hernia, and a long diverticulum that may knot on itself or twist around its base.

Patients presenting with obstruction will usually demonstrate typical signs of crampy abdominal pain, bilious vomiting, and obstipation. In the setting of intussusception, the child may pass currant-jelly stools and physical exam may demonstrate a palpable abdominal mass. If a volvulus progresses to ischemia, the patient will develop signs of peritonitis and may present in-extremis.

Inflammation

Inflammation of the diverticulum is often attributed to the presence of heterotopic gastric or pancreatic tissue. Obstruction of the diverticular lumen can also produce inflammation, similar to the mechanism for appendicitis. Lumenal obstruction can occur due to stasis of enteric contents within the diverticulum, the presence of an enterolith or foreign body, or even parasitic infections.[18–20] Meckel diverticulitis is often misdiagnosed as appendicitis due to similar presenting symptoms, including periumbilical pain that may be associated with nausea, vomiting, and fever. The point of maximal tenderness on physical exam may migrate within the abdomen. Given the possibility of misdiagnosis, the intraoperative finding of a normal appendix in a child suspected of having appendicitis should lead to a careful search for a Meckel diverticulum. Due to variability in the location of the diverticulum, at least 5 feet of distal small bowel should be examined, starting at the terminal ileum and working proximally. Meckel diverticulitis can also result in perforation, intra-abdominal abscess, and obstructive signs and symptoms.

DIAGNOSIS

In patients presenting with obstruction or inflammation, the diagnosis of a Meckel diverticulum is not typically determined preoperatively. On the other hand, in a child older than 5 years of age who has not undergone an abdominal operation and presents with signs and symptoms of small bowel obstruction, a Meckel diverticulum should be strongly considered as the etiology. The diagnosis of intussusception is often confirmed by ultrasound

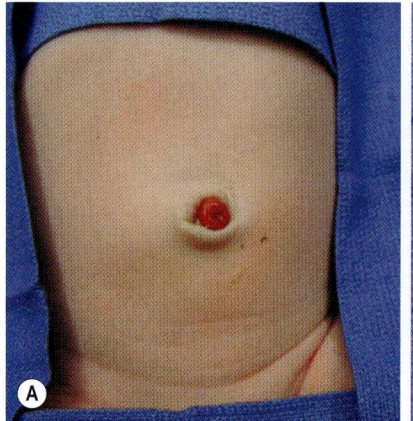 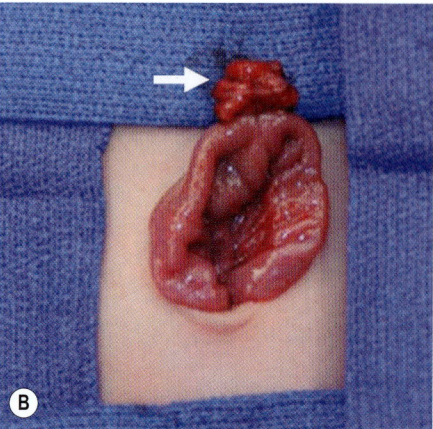 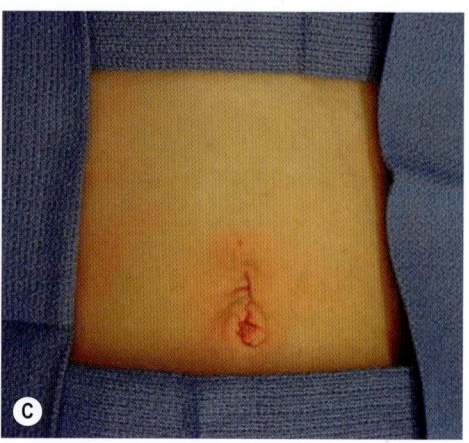

FIGURE 40-3 ■ This neonate was born with an obvious patent omphalomesenteric duct. **(A)** Meconium was seen to emanate from the stoma. **(B)** A circumumbilical incision was made, and the duct (arrow) was dissected to its connection with the ileum. **(C)** The duct was amputated from the ileum and the umbilical incision closed. The patient recovered uneventfully and has not developed any further problems.

(US) or air enema, but rarely identifies a pathologic lead point, such as a Meckel diverticulum. Air enema may reduce the ileocolic portion of the intussusception, but often the ileo-ileal component is not successfully reduced. If it is reduced, symptoms will often recur. When present, the diverticulum will be discovered either intraoperatively or when the resected segment of intestine is examined. An inflamed Meckel diverticulum is often misdiagnosed as appendicitis and found intraoperatively after a normal appendix is removed. In some cases, a preoperative computed tomography scan or ultrasound may find an inflamed midline mass with a normal appendix, suggesting the correct diagnosis.

Preoperative studies can often determine the etiology in patients presenting with lower gastrointestinal bleeding. In addition to a Meckel diverticulum, the differential diagnosis includes anal fissure, intestinal polyps, inflammatory bowel disease, intestinal duplications, hemangiomas, and arteriovenous malformations. A complete history and physical can help exclude some potential bleeding sources. Placement of a nasogastric tube can exclude an upper gastrointestinal source as well. The preferred radiologic test is the technetium-99m pertechnetate radionuclide study ('Meckel scan'). This imaging study relies on the fact that most bleeding Meckel diverticula contain ectopic gastric mucosa. The intravenously injected technetium-99m pertechnetate is taken up and secreted by the tubular gland cells of gastric mucosa. Scintigraphy can then visualize focal accumulation of the tracer in the diverticulum (Fig. 40-4).

Active bleeding is not required to achieve a positive result with scintigraphy, unlike angiography or tagged red blood cell scan. However, false negatives can occur if the diverticulum does not contain gastric mucosa or if it is lying low in the pelvis and obscured by the bladder. Other types of ectopic mucosa will not take up the radiotracer. False positives can also occur as a result of intestinal duplications, bowel obstruction or inflammation, intussusception, arteriovenous malformations, ulcers, and some neoplasms.[21] Pharmacologic uptake enhancement with the use of pentagastrin or histamine-2 blockers may improve the accuracy of the study. However, the

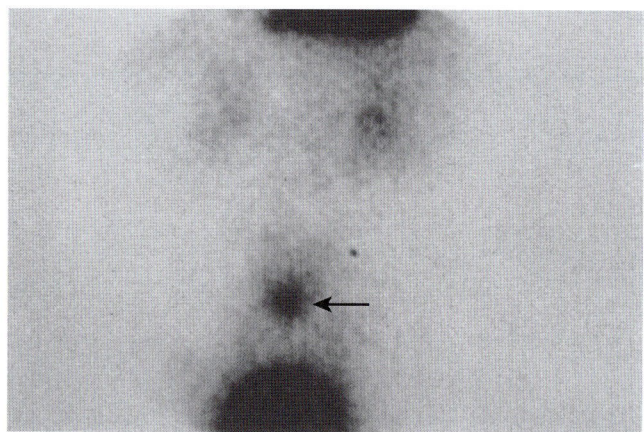

FIGURE 40-4 ■ Technetium-99m pertechnetate scan of a patient with a Meckel diverticulum. Note the blush (arrow) above the bladder. (Courtesy of Kyo Lee, MD.)

high rate of false negatives raises some concerns. Also, while the positive predictive value of scintigraphy is near 100% and specificity is over 95%, the sensitivity may be as low as 60%, with a negative predictive value of 75%.[15] Therefore, a negative scan does not exclude the possibility of a Meckel diverticulum, and several authors have recommended diagnostic laparoscopy for definitive evaluation, especially in cases with anemia and high clinical suspicion for a bleeding diverticulum.[15,22]

Other tests useful in the evaluation of intestinal bleeding include mesenteric angiography and a technetium-99m tagged red blood cell scan. Angiography is limited to cases with significant acute hemorrhage as it is invasive and requires active bleeding of at least 0.5 ml/min. A tagged red cell scan requires bleeding of at least 0.1 mL/min and may be more sensitive but less specific for localizing the bleeding source. Upper and lower endoscopy will not allow visualization of a Meckel diverticulum, but these tests are helpful to evaluate for other disorders that may produce rectal bleeding. Wireless capsule endoscopy and double-balloon enteroscopy techniques have also been utilized to identify a Meckel diverticulum.[23,24] While these modalities are not used regularly, they may be helpful when all other tests have failed to identify the site of bleeding.

TREATMENT

The treatment for a symptomatic Meckel diverticulum consists of resection using either an open or laparoscopic approach. Preoperative preparation should include rehydration with intravenous fluids, correction of electrolyte abnormalities, antibiotics, gastric decompression if the patient has a bowel obstruction, and transfusion in cases of bleeding with significant anemia.

Resection may be accomplished by either simple diverticulectomy or segmental ileal resection with anastomosis. In patients with obstruction, simple diverticulectomy is often sufficient, but all ectopic tissue should be removed. If a Meckel diverticulum is discovered after reduction of an intussusception, diverticulectomy may be possible, though segmental ileal resection may be safer depending on the appearance of the bowel (Fig. 40-5). In cases of bleeding, an ulcer may be present at the base of the diverticulum or on the mesenteric side of the ileum. Therefore, segmental resection is typically regarded as the safest approach to ensure removal of the bleeding source and avoid the risk of recurrent bleeding. The specimen should be opened after resection to confirm that it contains the ulcer.

Laparoscopy is now commonly utilized for resection of a Meckel diverticulum as it can be both diagnostic and therapeutic.[22,25] The diverticulum may be resected with either an intracorporeal technique, or grasped and exteriorized through the umbilicus for an extracorporeal diverticulectomy or segmental resection (Fig. 40-6). Port placement for the intracorporeal approach is similar to the set-up for laparoscopic appendectomy, with a 12 mm umbilical cannula and two 5 mm cannulas in the left lower quadrant. Laparoscopic-assisted extracorporeal resection is generally preferred in infants and small children, due to limited intra-abdominal working space,

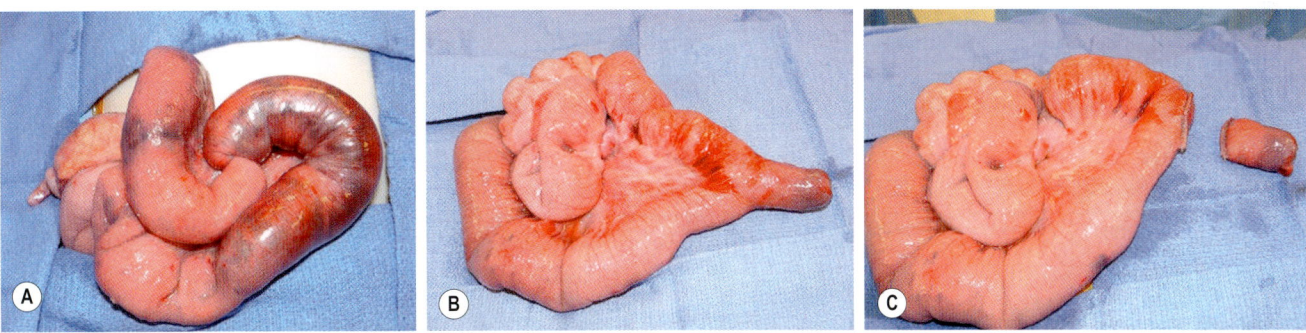

FIGURE 40-5 ■ A 4-year-old child presented with an irreducible intussusception and required an operative reduction. **(A)** Note the small bowel intussuscepted into the large bowel. **(B)** After reduction of the ileum, a Meckel diverticulum was found to be the lead point for the intussusception. **(C)** The diverticulum was excised with an endoscopic stapler.

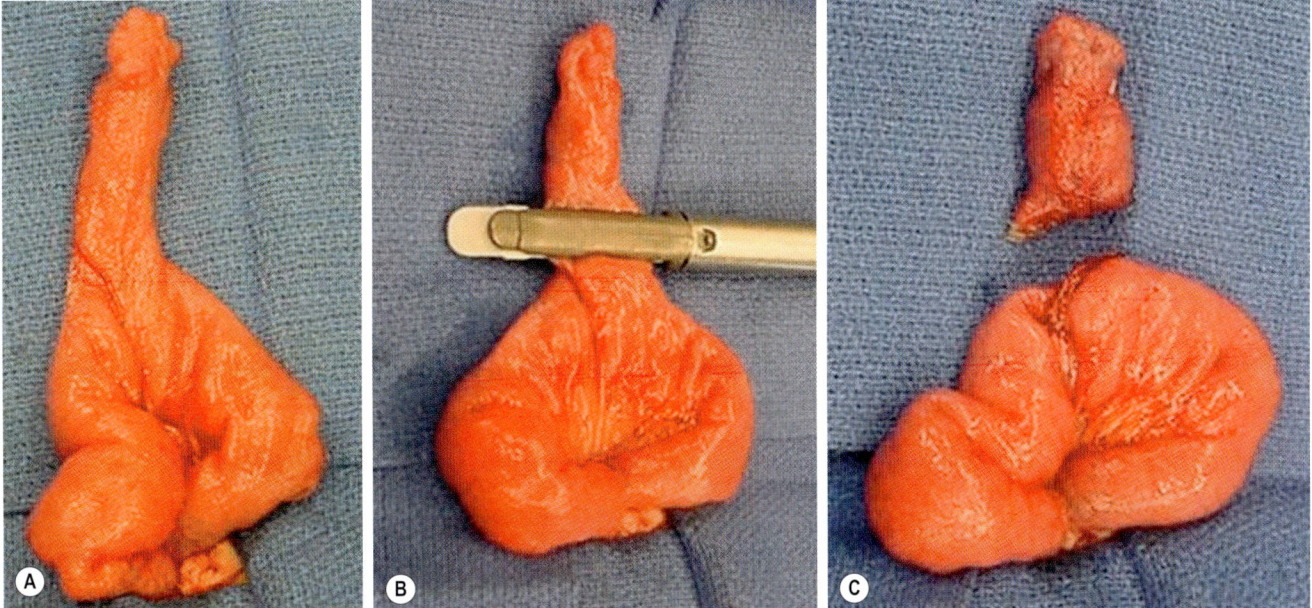

FIGURE 40-6 ■ This is the patient identified in Figure 40-2. **(A)** When diagnosed, Meckel diverticulum can be managed either totally intracorporeally or exteriorized through the umbilical incision. **(B, C)** The diverticulum and a small segment of the ileum just proximal and distal to the diverticulum were exteriorized through the umbilicus and the diverticulum was excised using the endoscopic stapler. The excision was done in an oblique direction to avoid narrowing the ileum at the site of the diverticulectomy.

which makes the use of staplers cumbersome. Segmental resection is also more easily accomplished extracorporeally. More recently, reports have described a single-incision laparoscopic approach.[26,27]

Management of an asymptomatic incidentally found diverticulum remains controversial. Operative intervention is not indicated for an asymptomatic diverticulum discovered incidentally on imaging studies. When a Meckel diverticulum is found intraoperatively, several reports recommend resection due to the risk of malignancy or other future complications.[9,13,28] However, other studies conclude that the risk of complications is less than the risk of complications following resection.[2,4] Still others recommend a selective approach, depending on characteristics of the diverticulum, such as length >2 cm, presence of ectopic mucosa, male gender, and age younger than 50 years.[8] Given the lack of clear consensus, the decision to resect an incidentally discovered Meckel diverticulum should be based on the surgeon's clinical judgment.

REFERENCES

1. Daniels IR. Historical perspectives on health: Johann Friendrich Meckel the younger and his diverticulum. J R Soc Promot Health 2000;120:125–6.
2. Meckel J. Uber die divertikel am darmkanal. Arch Physiol 1809;9:421.
3. Zani A, Eaton S, Rees CM, et al. Incidentally detected Meckel diverticulum: To resect or not to resect? Ann Surg 2008;247:276–81.
4. Simms MH, Corkery JJ. Meckel diverticulum: Its association with congenital malformation and the significance of atypical morphology. Br J Surg 1980;67:216–19.
5. Soltero MJ, Bill AH. The natural history of Meckel diverticulum and its relation to incidental removal: A study of 202 cases of diseased Meckel diverticulum found in King County, Washington, over a fifteen-year period. Am J Surg 1976;132:168–73.
6. Ruscher KA, Fisher JN, Hughes CD, et al. National trends in the surgical management of Meckel diverticulum. J Pediatr Surg 2011;46:893–6.
7. Pepper VK, Stanfill AB, Pearl RH. Diagnosis and management of pediatric appendicitis, intussusception, and Meckel diverticulum. Surg Clin N Am 2012;92:505–26.
8. Park JJ, Wolff BG, Tollefson MK, et al. Meckel Diverticulum: The Mayo Clinic experience with 1476 patients (1950–2002). Ann Surg 2005;241:529–33.
9. St-Vil D, Brandt ML, Panic S, et al. Meckel diverticulum in children: A 20-year review. J Pediatr Surg 1991;26:1289–92.
10. Menezes M, Tareen F, Saeed A, et al. Symptomatic Meckel diverticulum in children: A 16-year review. Pediatr Surg Int 2008;24:575–7.
11. Oguzkurt P, Strlic M, Kayaselcuk F, et al. Cystic Meckel diverticulum: A rare cause of cystic pelvic mass presenting with urinary symptoms. J Pediatr Surg 2001;36:1855–8.
12. Skandalakis PN, Zoras O, Skandalakis JE, et al. Littre hernia: Surgical anatomy, embryology, and technique of repair. Am Surg 2006;72:238–43.
13. Thirunavukarasu P, Sathaiah M, Sukumar S, et al. Meckel Diverticulum—A high-risk region for malignancy in the ileum. Ann Surg 2011;253:223–30.
14. Aguayo P, Fraser JD, St. Peter SD, et al. Perforated Meckel diverticulum in a micropremature infant and review of the literature. Pediatr Surg Int 2009;25:539–41.
15. Swaniker F, Soldes O, Hirschl RB. The utility of technetium 99m pertechnetate scintigraphy in the evaluation of Meckel diverticulum. J Pediatr Surg 1999;34:760–5.
16. Ergun O, Celik A, Akarca US, et al. Does colonization of Helicobacter pylori in the heterotopic gastric mucosa play a role in bleeding of Meckel diverticulum? J Pediatr Surg 2002;37:1540–2.
17. Tuzun A, Polat Z, Kilciler G, et al. Evaluation for Helicobacter pylori in Meckel diverticulum by using real-time PCR. Dig Dis Sci 2010;55:1969–74.
18. Pantongrag-Brown L, Levine MS, Buetow PC, et al. Meckel enteroliths: Clinical, radiologic, and pathologic findings. AJR 1996;167:1447–50.
19. Weissberg D. Foreign bodies within a Meckel diverticulum. Arch Surg 1992;127:864.
20. Chirdan LB, Yusufu LM, Ameh EA, et al. Meckel diverticulum due to Taenia saginata: Case report. East Afr Med J 2001;78:107–8.
21. Sfakianakis GN, Conway JJ. Detection of ectopic gastric mucosa in Meckel diverticulum and in other aberrations by scintigraphy: ii. Indications and methods—a 10-year experience. J Nucl Med 1981;22:732–8.
22. Shalaby RY, Soliman SM, Fawy M, et al. Laparoscopic management of Meckel diverticulum in children. J Pediatr Surg 2005;40:562–7.
23. Fritscher-Ravens A, Scherbakov P, Bufler P, et al. The feasibility of wireless capsule endoscopy in detecting small intestinal pathology in children under the age of 8 years: A multicentre European study. Gut 2009;58:1467–72.
24. Uchiyama S, Sannomiya I, Hidaka H, et al. Meckel diverticulum diagnosed by double-balloon enteroscopy and treated laparoscopically: Case report and review of the literature. Surg Laparosc Endosc Percutan Tech 2010;20:278–80.
25. Chan KW, Lee KH, Mou JWC, et al. Laparoscopic management of complicated Meckel diverticulum in children: A 10-year review. Surg Endosc 2008;22:1509–12.
26. Clark J, Koontz C, Smith L, et al. Video-assisted transumbilical Meckel diverticulectomy in children. Am Surg 2008;74:327–9.
27. Garey CL, Laituri CA, Ostlie DJ, et al. Single-incision laparoscopic surgery in children: Initial single-center experience. J Pediatr Surg 2011;46:904–7.
28. Onen A, Cigdem MK, Ozturk H, et al. When to resect and when not to resect an asymptomatic Meckel diverticulum: An ongoing challenge. Pediatr Surg Int 2003;19:57–61.

CHAPTER 41

INFLAMMATORY BOWEL DISEASE

R. Cartland Burns

Inflammatory bowel disease (IBD) is the broad term that encompasses Crohn disease (CD), chronic ulcerative colitis (UC), and indeterminate colitis. Regardless of which specific disease entity is present, the pediatric surgeon and physicians caring for the patient are faced with difficult medical and surgical challenges. Clinical, radiographic, and pathologic features typically distinguish CD from UC. However, in up to 25% of patients with IBD, the diagnosis cannot be specified, leading to a diagnosis of indeterminant colitis.[1] While medical therapies for all variants of IBD share similar strategies, the surgical care is driven by very different philosophical foundations. The surgical approach to UC is one of curative extirpation, rendering the patient free of disease through the removal of the affected intestine, generally with a proctocolectomy. The philosophy directing the operative approach to CD is much more humble, and is centered on treating the complications, but without cure. The fact that intervention is not curative must be communicated very clearly to families and patients prior to operation for CD, as the child will likely remain on medical therapy after the procedure and may require further surgical treatment at some point in the future.

ULCERATIVE COLITIS

UC is a mucosal-based inflammatory disease limited to the colon, and has a risk of malignancy.[2] The understanding that UC could be cured by removal of all colonic mucosa led to the development of operative treatment using total colectomy and proctectomy. The surgical approach has progressed from proctocolectomy with permanent ileostomy to restorative proctocolectomy, and is now routinely performed with minimally invasive techniques with or without a protective temporary ileostomy.[3]

Epidemiology

UC was described first in 1875 by Wilks and Moxon in the classic 'Lectures on Pathologic Anatomy'.[4] UC is predominantly diagnosed after the second decade of life. However, UC is being seen in increasing frequency in younger patients, with as many as 20% of patients becoming symptomatic before the age of 18 years.[5] The incidence of UC has reportedly increased over the past three decades, and is currently reported to occur in 3.1 children per 100,000.[6] Males and females are diagnosed with equal frequency. Western and Jewish societies are diagnosed with UC four times more frequently than Eastern cultures and developing countries, although this finding seems to be changing recently.[7,8]

Etiology

While there is much research surrounding UC and strides have been made in its underlying mechanisms, the exact etiology remains unclear.[9,10] Myriad theories have been proposed including infectious etiologies, genetic relationships, immunologic disturbances, and psychologic factors. To date, none of these, either independently or in combination, has adequately explained the disease. However, each of these factors may account for certain characteristics of the disease. The genetic relationship helps to explain the racial and ethnic distribution of the disease. For instance, the relative risk for siblings with disease is 16%,[11] and patients with extraintestinal manifestations have a high incidence of expression of the major antigen HLA-W27.[12] Also, antineutrophil cytoplasmic antibodies have been associated with UC. Unfortunately, evidence that these are present in unaffected family members of UC patients raises doubt about the relationship.[13,14] Finally, there are genetic predictors of disease severity. Recently, NOD-2insC polymorphism has been linked to worse outcome in patients following ileoanal pull-through.[15] Additionally, a single nucleotide polymorphism in chromosome 4q27,[16] and mucin abnormalities have been implicated in poor outcomes in UC patients.[17]

An infectious etiology for the basis of UC has become a rich area for investigation as evidence increases that the balance of microbial flora plays a key role in the regulation of the normal healthy intestine.[18,19] While the balance of bacterial flora may have a critical role in UC, there does not appear to be a specific infectious agent that is responsible for causing the disease.

Since UC is primarily a disease of autoimmune dysregulation, it is logical that investigation would center on the immune function of those affected. The mucosal T-cell and its regulation is the primary target of immunologic research. In addition, cytokine expression is another area of active interest. Interleukin (IL)-1, IL-6 and IL-1 receptor agonists all show imbalances in the UC population.[20]

Pathology

UC is a mucosal-based chronic inflammatory process that involves the rectum and extends proximally to include varying amounts of colon, often in a contiguous fashion.[21] The rectum is essentially always involved, and in cases of pancolitis, the rectum is usually the most severely affected. The characteristic microscopic findings include acute inflammation with crypt abscesses, mucosal bridging, and pseudopolyp formation. As the disease becomes more chronic in nature, the thin, distended colon becomes thickened, stiff, and foreshortened.

Clinical Presentation

As noted previously, UC is most commonly diagnosed in young adults, but 4% have onset of symptoms before age 10 years and 17% present between ages 10 and 20 years.[22] The initial presentation is one of persistent diarrhea, progressing to hematochezia with mucus and purulence in the stool. Tenesmus, anorexia, weight loss, and growth retardation are also common (Box 41-1). As the disease becomes more chronic, children may exhibit signs of depression and withdrawal from social and physical activities. Emotional stress has been identified as a precipitating factor in patients with relapsing disease.[23] Most patients experience chronic colitis with periods of quiescence and episodic recurring exacerbations. Only a small fraction (10%) of patients have a single exacerbation followed by longstanding remission. Unfortunately, as many as 80% of children become refractory to medical therapy, and ultimately require colectomy. Fifty per cent of children diagnosed with UC in childhood will require a colectomy before age 18 years.[24]

In about 15% of children, the presentation is fulminant with profuse bloody diarrhea, severe cramping, and abdominal pain, fever and sepsis. Aggressive medical management will control these symptoms initially in most cases; however, 5% of patients will require urgent colectomy in the face of toxic megacolon.[25]

BOX 41-1	**Clinical Findings in Ulcerative Colitis**

SIGNS/SYMPTOMS

Abdominal pain
Diarrhea
Hematochezia
Mucus in stool
Purulent exudates in stool
Tenesmus
Anorexia
Weight loss

EXTRAINTESTINAL MANIFESTATIONS

Chronic fatigue
Growth retardation
Delayed sexual maturation
Depression/emotional distress
Arthralgia
Pyoderma gangrenosum
Erythema nodosum
Oral ulceration
Anemia
Liver disease (primary sclerosing cholangitis)
Nephrolithiasis
Osteoporosis
Uveitis

Colorectal carcinoma has been reported to occur in 3% of patients in the first ten years after the initial diagnosis, and the incidence increases to 20% per decade after the first decade. Quiescent disease does not protect from the development of cancer. In fact, young age at initial UC diagnosis may be a risk factor for colorectal carcinoma.[26–28]

The extraintestinal manifestations of UC are outlined in Box 41-1 and occur in 60% of children.[29] Growth retardation and delayed bone growth is associated with the chronicity of inflammation in UC, while delayed sexual maturation has been shown to be related to low gonadotropin levels.[30,31] Since chronic inflammation has direct effects on growth and development, adequate control of disease can relieve the growth complications that would otherwise develop.[32] Arthralgias occur in about a quarter of UC patients and the knees, ankles and wrists are the most commonly affected joints. The joint symptoms often complicate the diagnostic evaluation, and may cause the child to be erroneously diagnosed with rheumatoid arthritis before the gastrointestinal symptoms become obvious.

Erythema nodosum occurs primarily on the trunk and manifests as tender, red, subcutaneous nodules. Pyoderma gangrenosum is usually seen on the lower legs and presents as chronic deep ulcerations of the skin. Although much more common in adults, both may occur in children and usually resolve with treatment of the primary disease.[33]

Liver function testing is associated with abnormalities in up to 10% of children with UC. When abnormal liver function is identified, the patient requires close observation for the possible manifestations of primary sclerosing cholangitis.[34] Anemia is common and is usually due to blood loss in the stool, but may also be related to anemia of chronic disease. Osteoporosis and malacia may be related to decreased calcium absorption associated with poor absorption of fat-soluble vitamins and/or to increased urinary loss from chronic glucocorticoid therapy. Nephrolithiasis can develop and is likely due to chronic oliguria related to inadequate intake and increased water loss in the stool.

The emotional and psychological ramifications of UC should not be dismissed. Those caring for these children will spend a great deal of time counseling, supporting, and encouraging them, and the care team should include a mental health care worker.[35]

Diagnosis

As diarrhea is usually the initial symptom, evaluation begins with investigation for infectious causes of diarrhea including *Salmonella*, *Shigella*, *Campylobacter*, *Clostridium dificile*, and *Entamoeba histolytica*. Anemia from blood loss, elevated C-reactive protein, increased sedimentation rate, and hypoalbuminemia are commonly found at the initial presentation. Additionally, the prothrombin time may be prolonged.

Although work continues on many potential candidates, serum markers for IBD have not proven to be reliable as yet. Perinuclear antineutrophil cytoplasmic antibody (pANCA) has been shown to be specific for UC and absent in controls. However, it is not predictive of disease severity or course.[36] Pancreatic autoantibodies, such as NOD2/CARD15 and PAB, have also been shown to correlate with disease.[37]

The improved visualization and characterization of disease found on computed tomography (CT) and magnetic resonance imaging (MRI) have enhanced their accuracy, and these two imaging modalities have replaced the contrast enema as a diagnostic standard.[38–41] Characteristic findings have been described as a 'lead pipe' appearance to the colon, loss of haustral markings, and a narrow lumen (Fig. 41-1). Pseudopolyps can develop in chronic UC and may be seen on both imaging studies. Upper gastrointestinal series are only helpful to assist in differentiating UC from CD with small bowel disease.

Endoscopy is useful to confirm the diagnosis, and for surveillance to monitor response to therapy. Typical endoscopic findings include a friable, inflamed mucosa with fibrinous exudate covering the surface. Ulcers may be seen as well. Biopsies may offer histologic proof of diagnosis. However, with severe inflammation, biopsies are often nonspecific and experienced endoscopists often rely on the endoscopic appearance alone.

Medical Management

Pediatric UC is characterized as mild, moderate, or severe based on the number of stools per day, and the presence of fever, anemia, nutritional depletion, and abdominal pain. These classifications are useful to characterize the disease and to monitor the success of therapies. Prior to institution of any medical therapy, a thorough medication history must be obtained, including homeopathic remedies, as many of the patients and families will have sought herbal, dietary, or alternative forms of treatment prior to diagnosis.

Maintenance therapy for UC is based on immunosuppressive and anti-inflammatory strategies. Treatment algorithms are based on severity of disease. Mild disease can often be controlled with 5-ASA (aminosalicylic acid) preparations such as sulfasalazine or mesalamine. Although it has not been proven to be beneficial, metronidazole is frequently added to this regimen.[42] Moderate disease requires a more aggressive medical regimen to attain remission. In general, 5-ASA medications are used in conjunction with glucocorticoids, with or without 6-mercaptopurine or azathioprine. The prolonged use of steroids has severe implications, especially for children. Therefore, alternate forms of therapy are appropriate to avoid steroid dependence.[43]

Severe exacerbations are treated with bowel rest, intravenous fluid resuscitation or nutrition, and antibiotics. Although less frequently seen than mild or moderate disease, a small number of patients will present with acute, fulminant colitis that in some cases is associated with pancolitis and sepsis. Toxic megacolon refers to this acute, fulminant, septic colitis with massive distention of the entire colon. It is usually manifested by a distended air-filled transverse colon on plain films. High dose parenteral steroids are generally started, and cyclosporine and antitumor necrosis factor (TNF) antibodies should be considered. The approach to these patients is one of 'rescue therapy,' with the ultimate rescue therapy being achieved by colectomy.[44,45] Perforation is an absolute indication for emergent operation, but failure to improve must be reviewed critically and objectively by the entire team to avoid allowing these children to become too sick prior to surgical intervention.

A multidisciplinary approach to the care of these children, including medical and surgical specialists, a psychologist, social worker, and nutrition specialist, is valuable in monitoring the course of therapy. Nonoperative therapy can have morbidity as well as malnutrition, growth failure, delayed sexual maturation, poor control of inflammation with persistence of symptoms, and psychological complications related to frequent stooling, fatigue, and the side effects of medications. Additionally, the immunomodulating medications that are currently most effective for controlling IBD carry their own risk of malignancy, primarily lymphoma.[27] A multidisciplinary team is less likely to become invested in a specific form of therapy, and more willing to consider alternatives than a single provider working in isolation.

Surgical Management

The understanding that UC is limited to the colon, and is cured by removing the colon, has led those caring for children with this disease to consider earlier operation. In the past, the morbidity associated with proctocolectomy and permanent ileostomy was responsible for delay in seeking surgical options until after the child was severely ill and undernourished, and carried significant operative risk. As operations have become less morbid and more refined, and are associated with a better lifestyle afterwards, the threshold for colectomy has become more relaxed. Currently, operative alternatives are considered safe and effective when compared to medical therapies. With this in mind, they should be seriously considered in all children with UC, but especially those that are not responding adequately to the medical

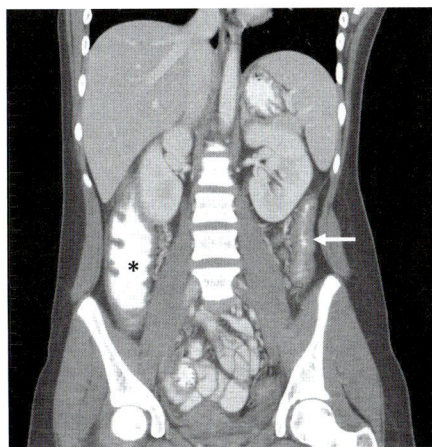

FIGURE 41-1 ■ This 13-year-old child has chronic ulcerative colitis and will undergo proctocolectomy and ileal pouch–anal anastomosis. This coronal CT image shows a 'lead pipe' appearance to the descending colon with diffuse thickening of the colon wall and a very narrowed lumen (arrow). There is also significant thickening of the wall of the cecum and ascending colon (asterisk).

TABLE 41-1 **Current Issues Surrounding Operative Intervention in Ulcerative Colitis**

Issue	Advantages	Disadvantages
Laparoscopy (compared with open)	Reduced time of recovery, less adhesions, improved scarring, less pain	Advanced laparoscopic skills needed
Mucosectomy (compared with stapled ileorectal anastomosis)	Complete resection of mucosa, no future surveillance	Higher incidence of incontinence and soiling rate, need for hand-sewn anastomosis
Pouch (compared with straight pull-through)	Improved reservoir, decreased stooling frequency and soiling, especially after operation	Pouchitis, requires surveillance
Temporary stoma (compared with single stage operation)	Fewer early postoperative complications	Second operation for closure

therapies. Although already mentioned, it is important to emphasize that the chronic inflammatory state of the intestinal mucosa is a risk factor for development of cancer, and youth does not protect against this risk.[26–28]

Preoperative Considerations

Once a decision is made for operative intervention, the preoperative preparation is important. Nutritional deficiencies must be addressed and may require a delay in the operative procedure, assuming an emergency operation is not needed. A reduction in immunosuppressive medications may be possible, although recent evidence suggests that immunosuppression is not necessarily associated with worse surgical outcomes.[46] The use of a preoperative mechanical bowel preparation was once considered standard, but has recently been questioned.[47–49] Currently, the need for mechanical bowel prep for colorectal surgery is not supported by the literature, although some authors continue to use it as part of their preoperative preparation. If a mechanical bowel prep is used, careful attention must be paid to the fluid and electrolyte status during the prep, as children are prone to dehydration.

Perioperative intravenous antibiotics are important and should provide broad-spectrum coverage. The surgeon and anesthesiologist should be mindful of the preoperative use of corticosteroids and prescribe stress dose regimens as appropriate. The placement of a urinary catheter is helpful for all operations, and consideration should be given to the use of regional anesthetics for perioperative pain management. Prophylaxis for deep vein thrombosis should be instituted in the IBD patient as the chronic inflammatory state is a known risk for a thromboembolic event.

Operative management of UC has undergone tremendous progress over the past 100 years. The earliest treatment was diversion with sigmoid colostomy. Later, ileostomy alone was advocated. These diversions accomplished little for the inflamed colon, and it was not until the 1940s that total colectomy was attempted. Unfortunately, there were countless ileostomy stomal complications until Brooke described the everted stoma that today bears his name.[50] This technical modification allowed patients to enjoy a functional stoma, although the fluid and electrolyte derangements associated with an ileostomy continued to pose problems.

In 1947, Ravitch and Sabiston reported a restorative procedure that utilized the mucosectomy technique.[51]

Although this report documented the possibility of a restorative procedure, their results were sufficiently complicated to cause others to search for alternative approaches. Hence, various catheterizable pouches and stomas became the standard form of treatment after total colectomy, with or without proctectomy, and remained so until Martin described an adaptation of Soave's endorectal pull-through used for Hirschsprung disease.[52] The results following Martin's adaptation for UC were significantly improved, but were still associated with significant issues related to stooling frequency and incontinence.[53] Subsequent investigators have described differing pouch structures in attempt to create a reservoir to reduce stool frequency and continence.[54–58] The current operative techniques for restorative proctocolectomy have resulted in significantly improved outcomes, and the current debate is centered on the issues outlined in Table 41-1.

The surgical options offered to patients with UC are based on the clinical condition of the patient at the time of consultation. The limitations relate to the emergent or elective nature of the operation, the comfort and experience of the individual surgeon, and the clinical setting in which the procedure is being performed. A final consideration is the preference of the patient and family, which is very important if the clinical situation will allow flexibility.

Emergency Operation

When faced with emergent indications for operation such as hemorrhage, perforation, or toxic megacolon, the surgical options are simplified. The standard operative procedure in this situation is total abdominal colectomy with end ileostomy. This approach is relatively fast, avoids the potential complications of creating a pouch, and allows for delayed proctectomy. It is generally performed via a laparoscopic approach, and the rectum is controlled by stapling the proximal rectum above the peritoneal reflection to simplify the subsequent proctectomy.

Elective Operation

The goal of all operative interventions for UC is to render the patient free of disease with the best possible functional outcome. The quality of the outcome is determined by the patient and family, as well as the clinical

TABLE 41-2 **Advantages and Disadvantages of a Single Operation Vs a Staged Operative Approach in Patients with Ulcerative Colitis**

Approach	Operation	Indication	Advantages	Disadvantages
Three Stage	(1) Colectomy with stoma (2) Completion proctectomy with IAPT (3) Stoma closure	Urgent/emergent Malnourished patient Infection concerns	Low risk of complications Quick initial operation Time to improve clinical status prior to pelvic dissection	Three operations and multiple admissions
Two Stage	(1) Proctocolectomy with IAPT and stoma (2) Stoma closure	Elective operation, desire to protect pouch–anal anastomosiswith proximal ostomy	Standard approach, safe, allows time for pouch and pouch–anal anastomosis to heal	Two operations, readmission for stoma closure
One Stage	(1) Proctocolectomy with IAPT	Elective operation, good nutritional status, excellent anatomy	Avoids multiple operations	Reports of poor long-term pouch function Pelvic sepsis with leak from pouch and pouch–anal anastomosis

IAPT, ileoanal pull-through.

situation. However, the goal in most instances is restoration of nearly normal anatomy and function.

While the philosophical goals for the surgical management of UC have not changed in the past 50 years, the operative approaches have continued to be refined. Table 41-2 outlines the advantages and disadvantages of a single operation versus a staged approach. The experience and familiarity of the treating surgeon with these various approaches directs much of the decision-making process. The first procedure described to have good functional results was the straight ileal pull-through.[59] However, the straight pull-through procedure is known to be associated with persistent high–pressure peristaltic contractions associated with urgency and soiling.[60] Due to this problem, most surgeons have avoided the ileal pull-through and have opted for creation of an ileal reservoir, of which the J-pouch is the most common.

Open Proctocolectomy with Ileoanal Pull-through Procedure

The most common restorative procedure for children with UC is currently a proctocolectomy with ileoanal pull-through. Historically, this operation was performed via a laparotomy. The patient is positioned in the lithotomy position, with special attention taken to avoid pressure on the lateral portion of the upper calf where the peroneal nerve courses around the tibia. Pressure induced injury to this nerve results in foot drop. Thromboembolism prevention is instituted with sequential compression devices (SCD) applied to the legs. The abdomen and perineum are prepped into a single field, and a urinary catheter is inserted on the sterile field.

The abdomen is entered through a vertical midline approach. The ileum is divided at its junction with the cecum and the entire colon is mobilized. The posterior rectal dissection is then performed outside the mesorectum as this plane allows easier dissection. When distal to the peritoneal reflection, the anterior dissection should be carried out on the rectal wall to avoid injury to the vas deferens, seminal vesicles, or vaginal wall. The dissection proceeds distally along the rectum to approximately 5 cm

from the pelvic floor. Attention is then turned to the anal portion of the procedure. The transanal mucosectomy is usually performed with a self-retaining, peri-anal retractor exposing the dentate line. The submucosa can be injected with an epinephrine solution (1 : 100,000 units) to help separate the mucosal and submucosal layers, and to assist with hemostasis. A circumferential mucosal incision approximately 1–2 cm above the anal pillars (dentate line) is created using the fine-point cautery. Multiple fine silk traction sutures are placed circumferentially around the mucosal flap, decreasing undue trauma, and making the specimen easier to handle during the dissection. The mucosa is separated from the submucosal layer in a circumferential manner from distal to proximal for approximately 5 cm. At this point, the dissection transitions to the full-thickness plane, moving outside the rectal wall, taking care to stay immediately adjacent to the rectum. The dissection is continued proximally until the transanal dissection meets the dissected tissues from the pelvis, and the rectum and colon are then removed from the abdomen.

Attention is now turned to creation of the ileal J-pouch. The distal 15 cm of ileum is identified and turned back on itself. The adjacent limbs are secured to one another and the distal tip (the J limb) is opened. A linear stapling device is used to divide and secure the common wall between the two loops, thus creating the J-pouch. The pouch is oriented carefully to avoid a twist in its mesentery. In most children, the mesentery will reach easily to the pelvis if the ileal mesentery is mobilized up to the origin of the superior mesenteric artery. If necessary, the peritoneal leaflets lining the mesentery can be opened, with care taken to avoid injury to the underlying mesenteric vasculature, to allow more length on the mesentery to facilitate the pouch reaching the pelvis. Stay sutures are placed on the ileal enterotomy through which the stapler was fired. These stay sutures are delivered through the pelvis to the anus. The pouch is positioned within the rectal muscular cuff, and an end-to-end handsewn, single layer, interrupted pouch–anal anastomosis is completed using absorbable sutures (Fig. 41-2). A convenient loop of ileum is chosen to avoid tension on the

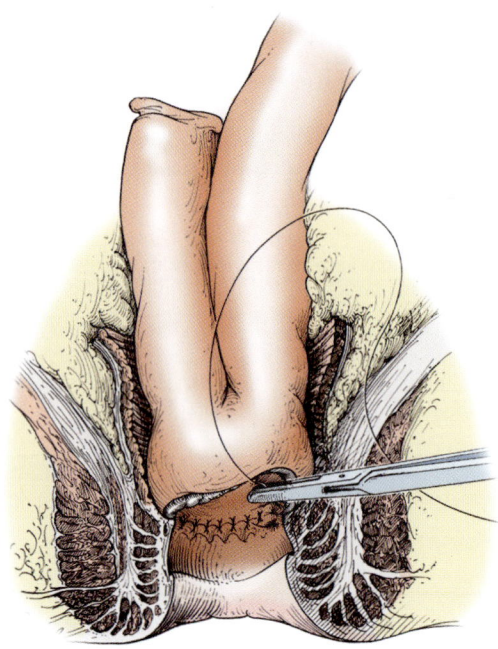

FIGURE 41-2 ■ In small patients, the double-stapled ileoanal anastomosis using the endoscopic circular stapler may not be possible. Also, some surgeons prefer the hand-sewn ileoanal anastomosis. The rectal mucosectomy begins approximately 5 mm above the dentate line and continues proximally to the completed pelvic dissection. The J-pouch is then pulled through the muscle cuff and anastomosed to the anal mucosa, just above the dentate line with interrupted sutures. (Copyrighted and used with permission of Mayo Foundation for Medical Education and Research, all rights reserved.)

distal anastomosis to create the loop ileostomy. Some authors prefer a completely divided end ileostomy, although reports indicate that a loop ileostomy is associated with lower complication rates at the time of later stomal closure.[61] Although recent studies have shown that the procedure can be performed in a single stage without a stoma, it is our preference that this should be reserved for only the most select cases. Thus, we prefer to protect the pouch, and the pouch–anal anastomosis, with a stoma for six to eight weeks.[62,63]

Standard postoperative care includes bowel rest without gastric decompression, SCDs, early mobilization, and stomal teaching. Patients undergo a retrograde contrast study at six to eight weeks postprocedure to evaluate for a leak, adequacy of the reservoir, and the ability to clear injected contrast. If there are no concerns, the child is scheduled for stoma closure. We perform rigid sigmoidoscopy to evaluate the pouch at the time of stoma closure. This 'pouchoscopy' is useful to evaluate the anastomosis for stricture and the pouch for signs of inflammation.

Proctocolectomy with Ileoanal Pull-through with Stapled Anastomosis

Recently, surgeons have modified the mucosectomy and hand-sewn pouch–anal anastomosis technique to take advantage of newer stapling technologies, including the circular end-to-end devices.[64,65] This technique is applicable for both the open and laparoscopic approaches.[66] The open operation is conducted in a similar fashion as just described. The abdominal colectomy is completed to the level of the peritoneal reflection, and the rectum is transected with a stapler. The extraperitoneal dissection is then continued to the pelvic floor, leaving a short rectal cuff of approximately 3–5 cm. The remaining rectum is then everted through the anus and out to the perineum, where it is again transected with a stapling device as close to the anus as possible, with great care taken not to injure the sphincter complex. This technique avoids the need to place the stapler into the pelvis, which universally results in a longer rectal cuff. This technique also typically leaves less than 3 cm of rectum above the dentate line. The J-pouch is created as previously described and the end-to-end circular stapler is prepared. The anvil is secured into the distal tip of the J-pouch and the pouch is positioned into the pelvis, taking care to preserve proper orientation. The hand piece of the stapler is inserted into the anus and joined to the anvil from the J-pouch (Fig. 41-3). The stapler is deployed, and the anastomosis and mucosal rings are inspected to ensure a complete anastomosis. The pelvis is filled with water, and the pouch is inflated with air to evaluate for an anastomotic leak. As there is a small amount of rectal mucosa remaining, lifelong surveillance is needed.

Laparoscopic Technique

Although performed laparoscopically, the steps of the laparoscopic proctocolectomy are conducted in a similar fashion to the above description from the open operation.[66] The ports can be placed in a variety of locations, and is largely determined by surgeon preference (Fig. 41-4). Although not utilized by many surgeons, recent reports have described a single site approach for this procedure.[67] A typical laparoscopic approach is performed with a 10–12 mm cannula inserted in the umbilicus for a 10 mm camera. A 12 mm port is placed in the right lower quadrant at the future site of the diverting ileostomy. Usually two additional 5 mm ports, in the suprapubic and left lower quadrant, are also inserted. In very small patients in whom a stapler will not fit into the pelvis, the rectal mobilization is completed laparoscopically, and the proximal rectum is divided above the pelvis. At this point, the rectum can be everted through the anus and divided with the stapler on the outside, with great care taken to avoid injury to the sphincter complex.

A few technical pearls are important. The colorectal dissection should be started distally, and the proximal rectum should be divided early to allow stool to be mobilized proximally (Fig. 41-5). This helps preserve a pristine pelvic dissection. The mesocolon can usually be transected using an energy source, either the ultrasonic scalpel or Ligasure. When a stapler can be introduced into the pelvis, the distal rectum is similarly transected with a stapling device, leaving just enough rectum to place the head of an end-to-end circular stapler.

After mobilizing the colon, the specimen can then be exteriorized through the 12 mm right lower quadrant port site (Fig. 41-6). The J-pouch can be created through the intended stoma site or the umbilicus (Fig. 41-7), and

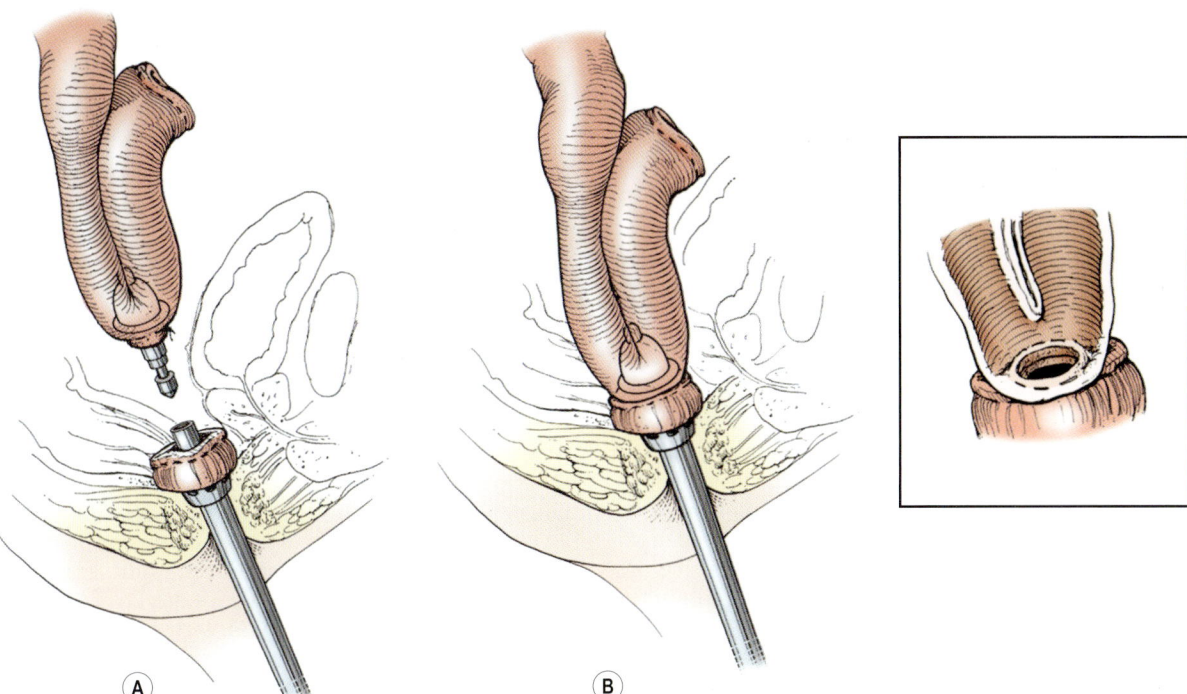

Ⓐ Ⓑ

FIGURE 41-3 ■ The double-stapled technique for the pouch/anal anastomosis has shown similar results as the hand-sewn technique. **(A)** The anvil has been placed into the pouch and is being brought close to the circular stapler, which has been introduced through the anus. **(B)** The anus and pouch have been approximated and the circled, stapled anastomosis performed (inset). There is usually about a 5 mm to 1 cm cuff of native rectal mucosa remaining that requires lifetime surveillance. (Copyrighted and used with permission of Mayo Foundation for Medical Education and Research, all rights reserved.)

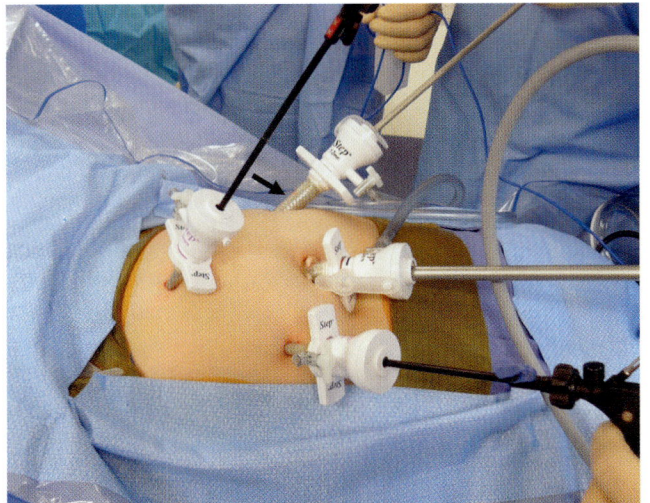

FIGURE 41-4 ■ This 8-year-old child is undergoing a laparoscopic proctocolectomy with ileal pouch–anal anastomosis and temporary ileostomy. This view from the patient's left side depicts placement of the ports for the operation. Note a 12 mm port is in the umbilicus through which a 10 mm, 45° angled telescope is inserted. In the right lower quadrant is another 12 mm cannula (arrow) which will become the site of the temporary ileostomy. Two 5 mm ports are in the left suprapubic area and the left mid-abdomen, and are working ports for the surgeon and the assistant.

is then positioned into the pelvis for an end-to-end circular stapled anastomosis (see Fig. 41-3). If an anorectal mucosectomy and hand-sewn pouch–anal anastomosis are planned with the laparoscopic approach, the laparoscopic dissection can be efficiently and safely carried to the pelvic floor, which makes for a quick and simple mucosectomy from below. This is always the back-up plan if the stapler tears the pouch or the stapled anastomosis is not secure. If desired, an ileostomy can be created according to the surgeon's preference.

Recently, this procedure has been described using robotic technology with excellent results, and may become more popular as experience grows.[68,69] This approach may be especially applicable for the completion proctectomy following emergency subtotal colectomy.

Outcomes

Children undergoing operation for UC can be expected to have excellent outcomes.[70–72] The preoperative medical therapies are tapered or discontinued appropriately. These children will predictably have five to eight stools per day until their pouch becomes functional. This stool frequency is managed with scheduled loperamide and diphenoxylate/atropine. Patients are advised to avoid caffeine, high sugar foods, and spicy foods to reduce the diarrhea. Metamucil®, or an equivalent soluble fiber, is helpful to thicken the stool to make it more controllable, and to decrease perineal irritation. Additionally, patients

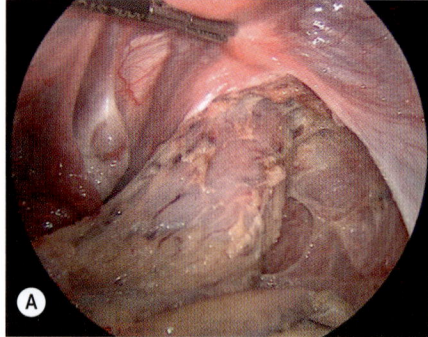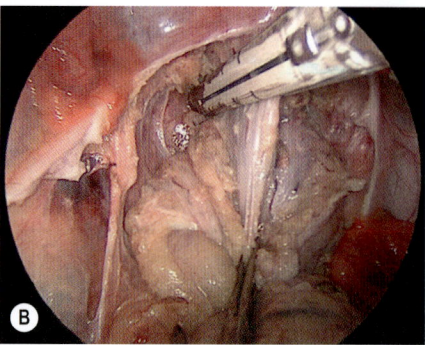

FIGURE 41-5 ■ The dissection usually starts distally on the rectum and proceeds proximally. (**A**) The mesorectum has been divided and the rectal wall has been skeletonized for several centimeters below the peritoneal reflection. (**B**) An articulating endoscopic stapler is placed across the rectum to ligate and divide it. Following ligation and division of the distal rectum, the rectum is mobilized proximally and is then exteriorized out the site of the ileostomy.

may be started on probiotics after continuity is reestablished to decrease the risk of pouchitis. These children should be advised to use the toilet frequently to avoid soiling. The stooling frequency is expected to improve rapidly over the first six months, but will continue to decrease over the first year. Patients are encouraged to work on holding the stool at first sensation to improve the interval between stools, and to strengthen their sphincter control, which can help decrease nocturnal leakage. Most children will eventually experience approximately four bowel movements per day, but some will continue to have nighttime bowel activity. Night-time soiling is predictable until stool frequency decreases, but unfortunately persists in a small number of patients. Long-term continence rates are over 95%, and the ability to delay a bowel movement reaches 90 minutes in many cases.

The restorative proctocolectomy is not without complications. Perioperative complications ranging from wound infection to bowel obstruction occur in as many 40% of patients. Most of these will not require operative intervention, but in one study, 7% required operation for intestinal obstruction, 14% required dilation for an ileoanal stricture, and 16% developed pouchitis requiring treatment.[72]

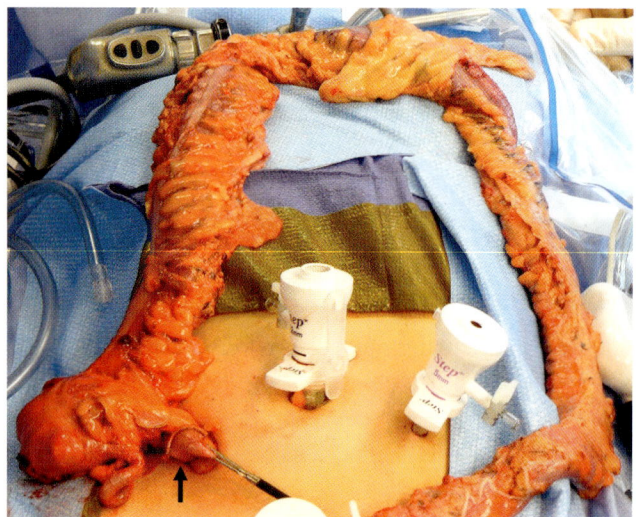

FIGURE 41-6 ■ After ligation and division of the distal rectum, the colon has been mobilized using the ultrasonic scalpel and has been exteriorized through the right lower quadrant 12 mm port site (arrow). After the colon is separated from the ileum, the J-pouch will be reconstructed extracorporeally (see Fig. 41-7).

These patients require close observation and should be followed annually with pouchoscopy, unless symptomatic in the interim. Surveillance of the remnant rectal mucosa for dysplasia, and the pouch for evidence of pouchitis, should occur yearly, and biopsies should be taken at each occasion. Pouchitis is a common problem after ileoanal pull-through procedures, and is reported to some degree in nearly half of patients.[70,73] Pouchitis manifests as lower abdominal pain with increased frequency of watery, foul-smelling stools and fever. It is typically a clinical diagnosis, but in some cases, pouchoscopy will be diagnostic. Contrast studies are usually not helpful. Treatment consists of metronidazole or ciprofloxacin, and in some cases, topical steroid applications. Early recurrence after stopping antibiotics is an indication for suppressive therapy with daily metronidazole or ciprofloxacin. Various scoring strategies are available to help with evaluation and management of patients with pouchitis. The most prominent system is the Heidelberg Pouchitis Activity Score.[74] When pouchitis is severe or recurrent, anatomic causes should be considered, including technical problems, that can be evaluated by endoscopy, CT, MRI, or contrast study. Biopsies may also reveal evidence of CD that has only become evident after the ileoanal reconstruction. Indeed, of pouches that have to be abandoned due to poor function, at least half are diagnosed as CD.[72] Although 15% of patients with a diagnosis of UC who undergo total proctocolectomy and reconstruction may end up with the subsequent diagnosis of CD, most of these patients can be managed without permanent ileostomy.[75]

CROHN DISEASE

In 1932, Crohn and colleagues described the regional ileitis that now bears his name.[76] It was originally believed to be isolated to the terminal ileum, but has now been described as occurring 'anywhere from mouth to anus'.[77] CD generally presents before 35 years of age, and is most common in western countries. There has been a steady increase in its incidence since the 1950s, most prominently in developing countries and in children.[78,79] The disease occurs equally in males and females, is five times more common in Caucasians than African Americans, and has a significantly higher incidence in the Jewish population.[80] This relationship between ethnic and racial groups is strong evidence for a genetic predisposition for

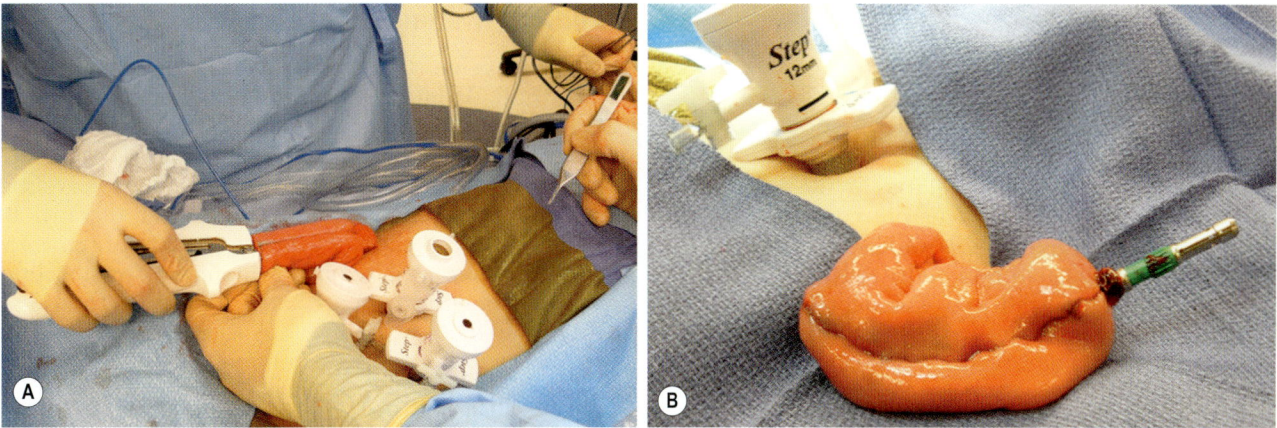

FIGURE 41-7 ■ The creation of a J-pouch. **(A)** The J-pouch is created extracorporeally using the conventional stapler. **(B)** The J-pouch has been created and the anvil has been secured into the distal tip of the J-pouch in preparation for a stapled pouch–anal anastomosis.

CD. However, other studies show a more random distribution of disease with little ethnic, racial, or socioeconomic relationships, raising the possibility for an environmental factor.[81] CD is more common in children than UC. Moreover, the surgeon must be cognizant of the fact that this disease is lifelong, not cured by resection, and will, in most cases, require subsequent operations.

Etiology

While UC and CD have been a source of tremendous investigation, the cause of CD also remains elusive and is most likely multifactorial. The chronic, relapsing nature of the disease suggests there may be an inciting or predisposing event, as well as a factor that causes persistence of the inflammatory stimulus. The presence of an environmental factor in the susceptible host is a popular concept.[82] Consideration of the intestinal microbiome as playing a causative role has gained popularity recently, and may prove to explain the increasing disease incidence in light of the increasing use of antibiotics and antimicrobial agents.[83] The relationship between genetic mutations, in particular NOD2/CARD15, seems to be related to particular manifestations such as early disease onset.[84] The multiplicity of theories and investigative threads lends strong support to the concept that CD is a multifaceted disease.

Pathologic Findings

CD differs from UC in several very important aspects. As opposed to a mucosal-based disease, CD is a transmural inflammatory disorder that is characterized by granuloma formation and intestinal wall thickening. Typical findings are submucosal edema, fibrosis, and lymphatic dilation. Fissures and ulcerations are common and there may be interspersed areas of normal mucosa. The ulcers frequently penetrate deep into the muscularis, and may progress to perforation with formation of sinus tracts, fistulas, or chronic abscesses. Granulomas are characteristic, and help to differentiate CD from UC. The granulomas most commonly occur in the submucosa, but may

TABLE 41-3 Symptom Comparison in Patients with Crohn Disease and Ulcerative Colitis

Symptom	Crohn Disease (%)	Ulcerative Colitis (%)
Weight loss	90	50
Abdominal pain	75	75
Diarrhea	67	75
Growth impairment	30	6
Perirectal disease	25	0
Extraintestinal findings	20	10

extend into the muscularis and can also be found in adjacent lymph nodes.

Clinical Presentation

CD is typically diagnosed in young adulthood. However, its incidence in children is increasing, with approximately 20% of new cases diagnosed in children less than 15 years of age.[79] In contrast to UC where diarrhea is the most common presenting symptom, the predominant presenting symptom in CD is weight loss (90%). Although acute pain may not be the symptom that prompts investigation due to its indolent onset, its presence can be elicited in up to 75% patients. The pain is typically nonspecific and is persistent. A palpable mass in the right lower quadrant may be associated with ileocolic disease, and is due to phlegmon or fibrosis. Diarrhea is present in 70% of patients, and may or may not be bloody. Hematochezia associated with CD is generally indicative of colonic disease. Growth impairment is found in a third of patients and may be multifactorial. Perirectal disease is present in 25% of patients and may be manifest as deep, nonhealing fissures, abscesses, fistulas, or large skin tags. Fistulas are often encountered and are most commonly enterocutaneous fistulas, but they can involve any site including the bladder, vagina, psoas muscle, or an adjacent loop of small or large intestine.[85–87] The typical findings associated with CD and UC are outlined in Table 41-3. The extraintestinal manifestations encountered in UC may also be seen in CD, including weight loss, growth retardation, delayed puberty, skin lesions, liver disease, uveitis, arthritis, anemia and stomatitis.

Diagnosis

The diagnosis of CD may be delayed by the nonspecific nature of the presentation. Regardless, patients with a suspicious constellation of gastrointestinal (GI) symptoms should be evaluated by a pediatrician familiar with the diagnosis, or referred to a gastroenterologist. The physical findings are typically related to growth failure and abdominal pain and tenderness, many times with a mass in the right lower quadrant. Perianal disease is not uncommon and may be quite dramatic. A thorough search for extraintestinal manifestations should be conducted and can help to direct further evaluation. Laboratory studies reveal a typical microcytic, hypochromic anemia. Hypoalbuminemia is common, as is an elevated sedimentation rate and C-reactive protein. Similar to UC, CD patients will also exhibit abnormalities in pANCA and antibodies to *Saccharomyces cerevisiae* and to *Escherichia coli* outer-membrane porin.

As with all patients with IBD, endoscopy is important, and a normal rectum is more suspicious of CD than UC. Children with CD and rectal involvement will have linear ulcerations that are less friable than those in UC, and biopsy may demonstrate granuloma formation. Both upper and lower endoscopy with biopsies is needed in children suspected of CD. These endoscopic findings are often very helpful in differentiating CD from UC.

Radiographic evaluation can be very helpful in directing therapy. For example, contrast upper gastrointestinal series with small bowel follow-through can identify strictures, some with proximal dilation (Fig. 41-8). CT with water density contrast (CT enterography) has proven to be effective at evaluating CD. Recently, MR enterography has become more popular as it avoids radiation and can detect aperstilatic segments of the midgut inaccessible by endoscopy.[88,89]

Medical Management

The management of CD is neither entirely medical or surgical. While the mainstay of therapy for CD is medical, many children will eventually require an operation and the families should be counseled at an early stage of disease for this possibility. Surgical intervention does not represent a failure of medical therapy, but rather another method of achieving a state of remission. These children will require a lifetime of medications, and psychological support should begin at the outset. The goal of medical therapy is to achieve a quiescent state of disease and the Pediatric Crohn Disease Activity Index is a reliable method for following the response to therapy.[90]

The modern approach to medical treatment of CD is changing rapidly. The initial therapy still includes glucocorticoids in an effort to forestall the inflammatory mechanism of the disease. This initial treatment is not used for maintenance therapy, and every attempt should be made to wean steroids by 30 days. Of those unable to wean in the first 30 days, many require operation to achieve disease quiescence.[91]

Aminosalicylates are used in both UC and CD, and are most effective in colonic disease to decrease mucosal inflammation. Unfortunately, due to the fact these medications are most helpful in colonic disease, they are less useful in CD than in UC. Azathioprine, 6-mercaptopurine, and methotrexate are commonly used as initial therapy when steroids do not induce remission. These drugs are known to induce remission and reduce dependence on steroids.[92–94]

Metronidazole is commonly used in patients with CD, especially patients with rectal or fistulous disease. Also, it is conceptualized that metronidazole is helpful for maintaining remission after resection of involved intestine. Interestingly, in one study, 75% of adults experienced relapse after discontinuing this antibiotic.[95] Thus, many clinicians prefer to continue metronidazole after resection.

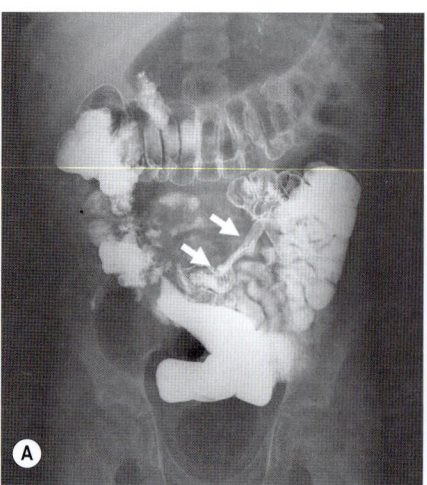 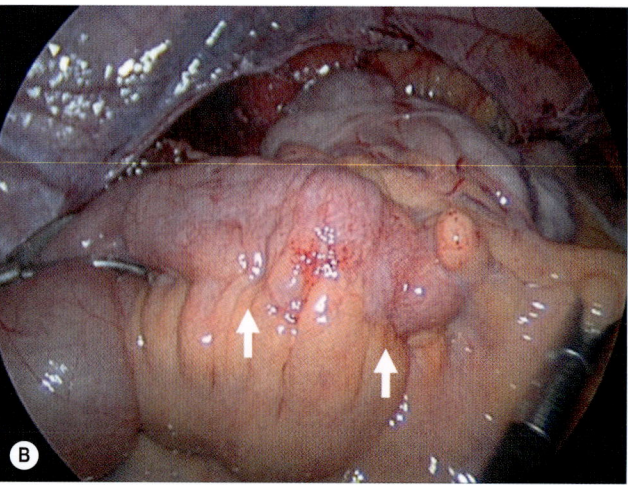

FIGURE 41-8 ■ **(A)** This upper gastrointestinal and small bowel follow-through contrast study shows a significant stricture (arrows) in the terminal ileum in a patient with persistent and symptomatic Crohn disease despite medical therapy. **(B)** The laparoscopic view shows active inflammation with creeping fat (arrows) along the terminal ileum in this patient.

Monoclonal antibodies are the newest form of therapy against CD. The most popular monoclonals are directed at TNF-α. Infliximab (a mouse-human chimeric antibody), adalimumab (a human monoclonal antibody), and certolizumab are available, and are known to control steroid resistant disease. These medications can also be helpful in treating some patients with fistulous disease. More recently, agents that are more specific against CD have been developed and natalizumab (recognizing alpha-4 integrin) has shown improved efficacy.[96] A top-down approach, beginning with infliximab and progressing through adalimumab, certolizumab, and natalizumab, has been suggested and is gaining favor with many gastroenterologists.[97]

Surgical Management

Operative approaches to CD are restricted to the treatment of complications from the disease. These complications are primarily perforation, fistula formation, obstruction, stricture, bleeding, and failure of medical therapy to achieve quiescence. It is important that the surgeon is sensitive that persistent disease may be manifest by protean findings such as growth failure, delayed puberty, complications of medications, compliance, and psychosocial complications. Surgical consultation should occur early in the course of the disease and, in many cases, can reduce the anxiety that the patient and family have about the specter of operative intervention.

The operative approach to CD may be either open or laparoscopic, although laparoscopy has become the most popular approach since the outcomes are similar with improved cosmesis and perhaps less anxiety for the patient and family.[98–100] At operation, the stepwise goal is to confirm the areas of active disease that were identified by preoperative imaging studies (see Fig. 41-8). If the disease is localized, the operative plan can be tailored to the site of disease. Options include resection of the diseased bowel with a primary anastomosis, resection with diversion, or strictureplasty. It is important to note that the primary focus of operation in CD is complete resection while preserving intestinal length, since CD is a common cause of short bowel syndrome in the adult population. The surgeon should approach any operation in a patient with CD with the goal of removing only grossly involved bowel as there is no benefit from attaining a histologic negative margin.

The most common operation performed for CD is ileocecectomy due to the distribution of the disease. This is typically performed as a laparoscopic-assisted approach using a 12 mm port in the umbilicus and two 5 mm ports in the left lower quadrant (Fig. 41-9A). The ileocecal junction is identified and the bowel is inspected proximally to the ligament of Treitz to confirm the affected areas. The cecum is freed from the lateral abdominal wall and, if necessary, the hepatic flexure is also mobilized. The umbilical incision can then be enlarged to a sufficient extent to exteriorize the ileocecum (Fig. 41-9B). The resection and anastomosis is then performed extracorporally and the mesenteric defect is closed. The bowel is returned to the abdomen and the incisions are closed (Fig. 41-9C). Many authors prefer a stapled anastomosis, while others feel that end-to-end anastomosis is best.[101] Additionally, ileocolectomy has been performed via the single incision approach with excellent results.[102]

Short segment small bowel disease may not require resection, but can be managed with a bowel-preserving strictureplasty (Fig. 41-10). The operation is conducted in a similar fashion to the ileocecectomy previously described, but the area of the small bowel stricture is identified and exteriorized through the umbilicus. The strictureplasty is performed with a longitudinal incision

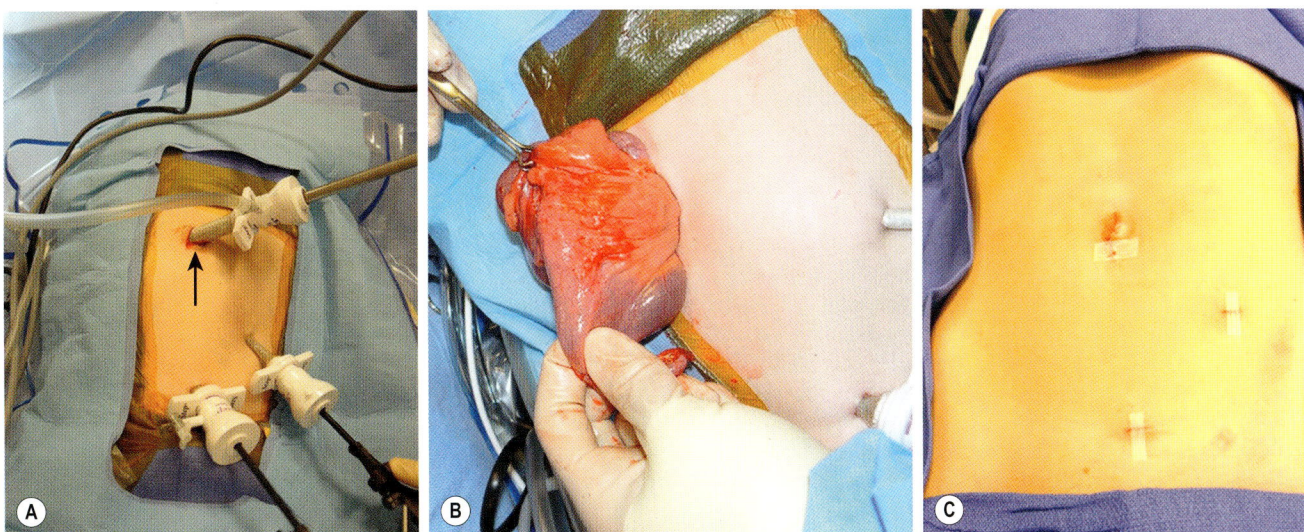

FIGURE 41-9 ■ **(A)** The port placement for a patient undergoing a laparoscopic ileocecectomy is seen. A 12 mm port is placed in the umbilicus (arrow), and two 5 mm ports are introduced in the left lower abdomen and suprapubic area. **(B)** The diseased small bowel has been exteriorized through the umbilicus for an extracorporeal resection and anastomosis. Note the inflamed bowel and creeping fat in the exteriorized portion of the small bowel. **(C)** The appearance of the incisions after the laparoscopic ileocecectomy. The intestinal resection and anastomosis was performed extracorporeally through the umbilical incision.

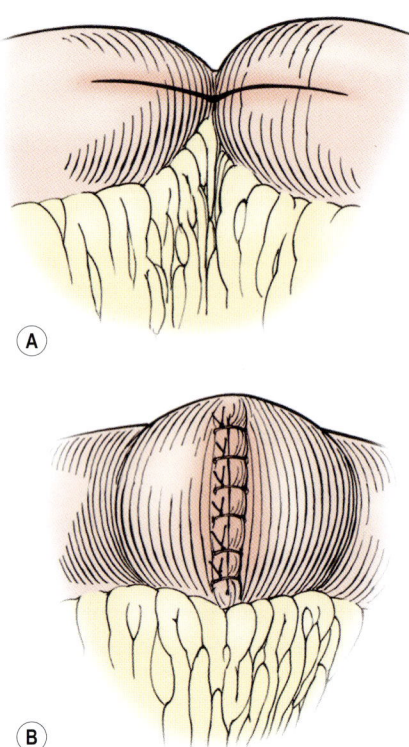

FIGURE 41-10 ■ This schematic depicts a Heineke–Mikulicz strictureplasty for a very short segment of active disease or for fibrotic strictures in a patient with multicentric Crohn disease. The incision that transverses the stricture (A) is then closed in a vertical direction (B) to enlarge the intestinal lumen.

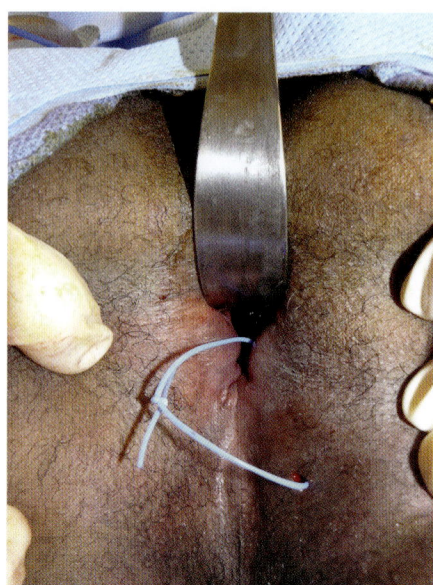

FIGURE 41-11 ■ This teenager with refractory Crohn disease developed a perianal abscess that was quite painful. Examination under anesthesia confirmed the fistula and underlying abscess that was drained. A soft, noncutting silicon vessel loop (seton) was then placed. This technique allows excellent control of the perianal disease and leads to healing in most circumstances.

through the stricture and then closing the enterotomy transversely, creating a wide repair of the stricture. The bowel is then replaced into the abdomen.

Extensive colonic disease has traditionally been treated with colectomy and permanent ileostomy. Recently, surgeons have reported segmental colectomy and anastomosis followed by more aggressive medical therapy.[103,104] Pancolitis, or rectal disease, presents fewer options, since pelvic reconstruction in this setting has been associated with a high risk of complications.[103] In those patients with extensive colitis or with rectal involvement, subtotal colectomy with Brooke ileostomy may be the least morbid approach, and may result in the fastest recovery and return to a healthy state. In patients with extensive colitis and rectal sparing, colectomy and an ileorectal anastomosis may be reasonable.[105,106] Also, if the rectum and colon need to be removed, consideration for anal reconstruction using an ileal J-pouch is not unreasonable.

Fistulous disease can be managed directly or by diversion in the most severe cases. These lesions may be quite extensive, and CT or MRI are helpful in delineating the extent of disease. Perirectal abscesses should be drained, and fistulas are controlled with fistulotomy for the most simple cases, or a noncutting seton for the more complex (Fig. 41-11). The seton will usually control the recurring abscesses and provide symptom relief, and may be left for quite some time if it is not causing any discomfort. In patients with severe perianal manifestations, proctectomy, rectosigmoid resection, or proctocolectomy with

ileostomy may be required. Simple diversion is not usually effective for healing of the affected bowel.

Outcomes

The postoperative recovery is usually good although recurrence rates increase with time and can reach 33% in long-term follow–up.[107] Perioperative complications are not uncommon, and include wound infection and bowel obstruction in as many as 25%.[108] Despite the inability to cure CD, the surgeon should approach the problem with optimism and embrace the opportunity to provide the patient with a period free from the symptoms.

INDETERMINATE COLITIS

Indeterminate colitis (IC) is a distinct clinical and pathologic entity which is diagnosed in approximately 10% of IBD patients. Over time, these patients will generally be found to have either UC or CD, with differentiation to CD more likely than to UC.[7,109] Not surprisingly, there is greater morbidity after colectomy and pouch–anal anastomosis in patients with the diagnosis of IC, which is due to the increased likelihood that they will eventually differentiate to CD. Additionally, adults with indeterminate colitis undergoing colectomy and pouch-anal anastomosis have a two to three times increased risk of serious postoperative complications compared to patients with UC, but still less than patients with CD.[110,111] The long-term success of colectomy and pouch–anal reconstruction for indeterminate colitis is 73–85% compared with 89% for UC.[112] Although these results support the consideration of performing colectomy and pouch–anal anastomosis in the setting of uncontrolled indeterminate colitis, the IC patient with features favoring CD may benefit from delayed pouch–anal reconstruction, six to 12 months after colectomy. Ultimately, operative decisions are based on the age of the patient, severity of disease, and the urgency of the operation. Children younger than age 8 years with IC should undergo colectomy and the surgeon should proceed cautiously before reconstruction is performed.

REFERENCES

1. Malaty HM, Fan X, Opekun AR, et al. Rising incidence of inflammatory bowel disease among children: A 12-year study. J Pediatr Gastroenterol Nutr 2010;50:27–31.
2. Pohl C, Hombach A, Kruis W. Chronic inflammatory bowel disease and cancer. Hepatogastroenterology 2000;47:57–70.
3. Mattioli G, Buffa P, Martinelli M, et al. Laparoscopic approach for children with inflammatory bowel diseases. Pediatr Surg Int 2011;27:839–46.
4. Wilks S, Moxon W. Lectures on Pathologic Anatomy. Longdon: Longmans, Green and Co; 1875.
5. Mamula P, Telega GW, Markowitz JE, et al. Inflammatory bowel disease in children 5 years of age and younger. Am J Gastroenterol 2002;97:2005–10.
6. Jakobsen C, Paerregaard A, Munkholm P, et al. Pediatric inflammatory bowel disease: increasing incidence, decreasing surgery rate, and compromised nutritional status: A prospective population-based cohort study 2007–2009. Inflamm Bowel Dis 2011;17:2541–50.
7. Abraham BP, Mehta S, El-Serag HB. Natural history of pediatric-onset inflammatory bowel disease: A systematic review. J Clin Gastroenterol 2012;46:581–9.
8. Prideaux L, Kamm MA, De Cruz PP, et al. Inflammatory bowel disease in Asia: A systematic review. J Gastroenterol Hepatol 2012;27:1266–80.
9. Ament ME, Berquist W, Vargas J. Advances in ulcerative colitis. Pediatrician 1988;15:45–57.
10. Haller C, Markowitz J. A perspective on inflammatory bowel disease in the child and adolescent at the turn of the millennium. Curr Gastroenterol Rep 2001;3:263–71.
11. Selby WS, Griffin S, Abraham N, et al. Appendectomy protects against the development of ulcerative colitis but does not affect its course. Am J Gastroenterol 2002;97:2834–8.
12. Bouma G, Crusius JB, García-González MA, et al. Genetic markers in clinically well defined patients with ulcerative colitis (UC). Clin Exp Immunol 1999;115:294–300.
13. Shanahan F, Duerr RH, Rotter I, et al. Neutrophil autoantibodies in ulcerative colitis: Familial aggregation and genetic heterogeneity. Gastroenterology 1992;103:456–61.
14. Locht H, Skogh T, Wiik A. Characterisation of autoantibodies to neutrophil granule constituents among patients with reactive arthritis, rheumatoid arthritis, and ulcerative colitis. Ann Rheum Dis 2000;59:898–903.
15. Tyler AD, Milgrom R, Stempak JM, et al. The NOD2insC polymorphism is associated with worse outcome following ileal pouch-anal anastomosis for ulcerative colitis. Gut 2012.
16. Glas J, Stallhofer J, Ripke S, et al. Novel genetic risk markers for ulcerative colitis in the IL2/IL21 region are in epistasis with IL23R and suggest a common genetic background for ulcerative colitis and celiac disease. Am J Gastroenterol 2009;104:1737–44.
17. Tysk C, Riedesel H, Lindberg E, et al. Colonic glycoproteins in monozygotic twins with inflammatory bowel disease. Gastroenterology 1991;100:419–23.
18. Zella GC, Hait EJ, Glavan T, et al. Distinct microbiome in pouchitis compared to healthy pouches in ulcerative colitis and familial adenomatous polyposis. Inflamm Bowel Dis 2011;17:1092–100.
19. Michail S, Durbin M, Turner D, et al. Alterations in the gut microbiome of children with severe ulcerative colitis. Inflamm Bowel Dis 2012;18:1799–808.
20. Casini-Raggi V, Kam L, Chong YJ, et al. Mucosal imbalance of IL-1 and IL-1 receptor antagonist in inflammatory bowel disease.

21. Finkelstein SD, Sasatomi E, Regueiro M. Pathologic features of early inflammatory bowel disease. Gastroenterol Clin North Am 2002;31:133–45.
22. Coulson WF. Pathological features of inflammatory bowel disease in childhood. Semin Pediatr Surg 1994;3:8–14.
23. Mackner LM, Greenley RN, Szigethy E, et al. Psychosocial Issues in Pediatric Inflammatory Bowel Disease: A Clinical Report of the North American Society for Pediatric Gastroenterology, Hepatology and Nutrition. J Pediatr Gastroenterol Nutr 2013.
24. Falcone RA Jr, Lewis LG, Warner BW. Predicting the need for colectomy in pediatric patients with ulcerative colitis. J Gastrointest Surg 2000;4:201–6.
25. Benchimol EI, Turner D, Mann EH, et al. Toxic megacolon in children with inflammatory bowel disease: Clinical and radiographic characteristics. Am J Gastroenterol 2008;103:1524–31.
26. Jess T, Rungoe C, Peyrin-Biroulet L. Risk of colorectal cancer in patients with ulcerative colitis: A meta-analysis of population-based cohort studies. Clin Gastroenterol Hepatol 2012;10:639–45.
27. Cucchiara S, Escher JC, Hildebrand H, et al. Pediatric inflammatory bowel diseases and the risk of lymphoma: Should we revise our treatment strategies? J Pediatr Gastroenterol Nutr 2009;48:257–67.
28. Markowitz JM, McKinley E, Kahn L, et al. Endoscopic screening for dysplasia and mucosal aneuploidy in adolescents and young adults with childhood onset colitis. Am J Gastroenterol 1997;92:2001–6.
29. Lagercrantz R, Winberg J, Zetterstrom R. Extra-colonic manifestations in chronic ulcerative colitis. Acta Paediatr 1958;47:675–87.
30. Brain CE, Savage MO. Growth and puberty in chronic inflammatory bowel disease. Baillieres Clin Gastroenterol 1994;8:83–100.
31. Ballinger AB, Savage MO, Sanderson IR. Delayed puberty associated with inflammatory bowel disease. Pediatr Res 2003;53:205–10.
32. Ezri J, Marques-Vidal P, Nydegger A. Impact of disease and treatments on growth and puberty of pediatric patients with inflammatory bowel disease. Digestion 2012;85:308–19.
33. Tavarela Veloso F. Review article: Skin complications associated with inflammatory bowel disease. Aliment Pharmacol Ther 2004;20(Suppl 4):50–3.
34. Knight C, Murray KF. Hepatobiliary associations with inflammatory bowel disease. Expert Rev Gastroenterol Hepatol 2009;3:681–91.
35. Szigethy E, McLafferty L, Goyal A. Inflammatory bowel disease. Child Adolesc Psychiatr Clin N Am 2010;19:301–18.
36. Ruemmele FM, Lachaux A, Cezard JP, et al. Diagnostic accuracy of serological assays in pediatric inflammatory bowel disease. Gastroenterology 1998;115:822–9.
37. Kovacs M, Lakatos PL, Papp M, et al. Pancreatic autoantibodies and autoantibodies against goblet cells in pediatric patients with inflammatory bowel disease. J Pediatr Gastroenterol Nutr 2012;55:429–35.
38. Gore RM, Balthazar EJ, Ghahremani GG, et al. CT features of ulcerative colitis and Crohn's disease. AJR Am J Roentgenol 1996;167:3–15.
39. da Luz Moreira A, Vogel JD, Baker M, et al. Does CT influence the decision to perform colectomy in patients with severe ulcerative colitis? J Gastrointest Surg 2009;13:504–7.
40. Das CJ, Makharia GK, Kumar R, et al. PET/CT colonography: A novel non-invasive technique for assessment of extent and activity of ulcerative colitis. Eur J Nucl Med Mol Imaging 2010;37:714–21.
41. Kilickesmez O, Soylu A, Yasar N, et al. Is quantitative diffusion-weighted MRI a reliable method in the assessment of the inflammatory activity in ulcerative colitis? Diagn Interv Radiol 2010;16:293–8.
42. Parlak E, Dagli U, Ulker A, et al. Comparison of 5-amino salicylic acid plus glucocorticosteroid with metronidazole and ciprofloxacin in patients with active ulcerative colitis. J Clin Gastroenterol 2001;33:85–6.
43. Timmer A, McDonald JW, Tsoulis DJ, et al. Azathioprine and 6-mercaptopurine for maintenance of remission in ulcerative colitis. Cochrane Database Syst Rev 2012;(9):CD000478.

44. Chang JC, Cohen RD. Medical management of severe ulcerative colitis. Gastroenterol Clin North Am 2004;33:235–50.

45. Hart AL, Ng SC. Review article: The optimal medical management of acute severe ulcerative colitis. Aliment Pharmacol Ther 2010;32:615–27.

46. Schaufler C, Lerer T, Campbell B, et al. Preoperative immunosuppression is not associated with increased postoperative complications following colectomy in children with colitis. J Pediatr Gastroenterol Nutr 2012;55:421–4.

47. Eskicioglu C, Forbes SS, Fenech DS, et al. Preoperative bowel preparation for patients undergoing elective colorectal surgery: A clinical practice guideline endorsed by the Canadian Society of Colon and Rectal Surgeons. Can J Surg 2010;53:385–95.

48. Zmora O, Mahajna A, Bar-Zakai B, et al. Colon and rectal surgery without mechanical bowel preparation: A randomized prospective trial. Ann Surg 2003;237:363–7.

49. Ram E, Sherman Y, Weil R, et al. Is mechanical bowel preparation mandatory for elective colon surgery? A prospective randomized study. Arch Surg 2005;140:285–8.

50. Brooke BN. The management of an ileostomy, including its complications. Lancet 1952;2:102–4.

51. Ravitch MM, Sabiston DC Jr. Anal ileostomy with preservation of the sphincter: A proposed operation in patients requiring total colectomy for benign lesions. Surg Gynecol Obstet 1947;84:1095–9.

52. Martin LW, LeCoultre C, Schubert WK. Total colectomy and mucosal proctectomy with preservation of continence in ulcerative colitis. Ann Surg 1977;186:477–80.

53. Martin LW, LeCoultre C. Technical considerations in performing total colectomy and Soave endorectal anastomosis for ulcerative colitis. J Pediatr Surg 1978;13:762–4.

54. Parks AG, Nicholls RJ, Belliveau P. Proctocolectomy with ileal reservoir and anal anastomosis. Br J Surg 1980;67:533–8.

55. Utsunomiya J, Yamamura T, Kusunoki M, et al. J-pouch: Change of a method over years. Z Gastroenterol Verh 1989;24:249–51.

56. Wong WD, Rothenberger DA, Goldberg SM. Ileoanal pouch procedures. Curr Probl Surg 1985;22:1–78.

57. Gemlo BT, Wong WD, Rothenberger DA, et al. Ileal pouch-anal anastomosis. Patterns of failure. Arch Surg 1992;127:784–7.

58. Nicholls RJ, Pezim ME. Restorative proctocolectomy with ileal reservoir for ulcerative colitis and familial adenomatous polyposis: A comparison of three reservoir designs. Br J Surg 1985;72:470–4.

59. Morgan RA, Manning PB, Coran AG. Experience with the straight endorectal pullthrough for the management of ulcerative colitis and familial polyposis in children and adults. Ann Surg 1987;206:595–9.

60. Fonkalsrud EW, Loar N. Long-term results after colectomy and endorectal ileal pullthrough procedure in children. Ann Surg 1992;215:57–62.

61. Lane JS, Kwan D, Chandler CF, et al. Diverting loop versus end ileostomy during ileoanal pullthrough procedure for ulcerative colitis. Am Surg 1998;64:979–82.

62. Mennigen R, Senninger N, Bruwer M, et al. Impact of defunctioning loop ileostomy on outcome after restorative proctocolectomy for ulcerative colitis. Int J Colorectal Dis 2011;26:627–33.

63. Ryan DP, Doody DP. Restorative proctocolectomy with and without protective ileostomy in a pediatric population. J Pediatr Surg 2011;46:200–3.

64. Mattioli G, Buffa P, Martinelli M, et al. All mechanical low rectal anastomosis in children. J Pediatr Surg 1998;33:503–6.

65. Griffen FD, Knight CD Sr, Knight CD Jr. Results of the double stapling procedure in pelvic surgery. World J Surg 1992;16:866–71.

66. Duff SE, Sagar PM, Rao M, et al. Laparoscopic restorative proctocolectomy: Safety and critical level of the ileal pouch anal anastomosis. Colorectal Dis 2012;14:883–6.

67. Fichera A, Zoccali M, Gullo R. Single incision ('scarless') laparoscopic total abdominal colectomy with end ileostomy for ulcerative colitis. J Gastrointest Surg 2011;15:1247–51.

68. Pedraza R, Patel CB, Ramos-Valadeza DI, et al. Robotic-assisted laparoscopic surgery for restorative proctocolectomy with ileal J pouch-anal anastomosis. Minim Invasive Ther Allied Technol 2011;20:234–9.

69. McLemore EC, Cullen J, Horgan S, et al. Robotic-assisted laparoscopic stage II restorative proctectomy for toxic ulcerative colitis. Int J Med Robot 2012;8:178–83.

70. Seetharamaiah R, West BT, Ignash SJ, et al. Outcomes in pediatric patients undergoing straight vs J pouch ileoanal anastomosis: A multicenter analysis. J Pediatr Surg 2009;44:1410–17.

71. Durno C, Sherman P, Harris K, et al. Outcome after ileoanal anastomosis in pediatric patients with ulcerative colitis. J Pediatr Gastroenterol Nutr 1998;27:501–7.

72. Fonkalsrud EW, Thakur A, Beanes S. Ileoanal pouch procedures in children. J Pediatr Surg 2001;36:1689–92.

73. Fonkalsrud EW. Long-term results after colectomy and ileoanal pull-through procedure in children. Arch Surg 1996;131:881–6.

74. Heuschen UA, Allemeyer EH, Hinz U, et al. Diagnosing pouchitis: Comparative validation of two scoring systems in routine follow-up. Dis Colon Rectum 2002;45:776–88.

75. Mortellaro VE, Green J, Islam S, et al. Occurrence of Crohn's disease in children after total colectomy for ulcerative colitis. J Surg Res 2011;170:38–40.

76. Crohn BB, Ginzburg L, Oppenheimer GD. Landmark article Oct 15, 1932. Regional ileitis. A pathological and clinical entity. By Burril B. Crohn, Leon Ginzburg, and Gordon D. Oppenheimer. JAMA 1984;251:73–9.

77. Brooke BN. Granulomatous diseases of the intestine. Lancet 1959;2:745–9.

78. Perminow G, Brackmann S, Lyckander LG, et al. A characterization in childhood inflammatory bowel disease, a new population-based inception cohort from South-Eastern Norway, 2005–07, showing increased incidence in Crohn's disease. Scand J Gastroenterol 2009;44:446–56.

79. Benchimol EI, Turner D, Mann EH, et al. Epidemiology of pediatric inflammatory bowel disease: A systematic review of international trends. Inflamm Bowel Dis 2011;17:423–39.

80. Rogers BH, Clark LM, Kirsner JB. The epidemiologic and demographic characteristics of inflammatory bowel disease: An analysis of a computerized file of 1400 patients. J Chronic Dis 1971;24:743–73.

81. Kugathasan S, Judd RH, Hoffmann RG, et al. Epidemiologic and clinical characteristics of children with newly diagnosed inflammatory bowel disease in Wisconsin: A statewide population-based study. J Pediatr 2003;143:525–31.

82. Fiocchi C. Inflammatory bowel disease: Etiology and pathogenesis. Gastroenterology 1998;115:182–205.

83. Bernstein CN. Why and where to look in the environment with regard to the etiology of inflammatory bowel disease. Dig Dis 2012;30(Suppl 3):28–32.

84. Rosenstiel P, Sina C, Franke A, et al. Towards a molecular risk map–recent advances on the etiology of inflammatory bowel disease. Semin Immunol 2009;21:334–45.

85. Heikenen JB, Werlin SL, Brown CW, et al. Presenting symptoms and diagnostic lag in children with inflammatory bowel disease. Inflamm Bowel Dis 1999;5:158–60.

86. El Mouzan MI, Al Mofarreh MA, Assiri AM, et al. Presenting features of childhood-onset inflammatory bowel disease in the central region of Saudi Arabia. Saudi Med J 2012;33:423–8.

87. North American Society for Pediatric Gastroenterology, Hepatology, and Nutrition; Colitis Foundation of America, Bousvaros A, Antonioli DA, Colletti RB, et al. Differentiating ulcerative colitis from Crohn disease in children and young adults: Report of a working group of the North American Society for Pediatric Gastroenterology, Hepatology, and Nutrition and the Crohn's and Colitis Foundation of America. J Pediatr Gastroenterol Nutr 2007;44:653–74.

88. Stuart S, Conner T, Ahmed A, et al. The smaller bowel: Imaging the small bowel in paediatric Crohn's disease. Postgrad Med J 2011;87:288–97.

89. Bruining DH, Siddiki HA, Fletcher JG, et al. Benefit of computed tomography enterography in Crohn's disease: Effects on patient management and physician level of confidence. Inflamm Bowel Dis 2012;18:219–25.

90. Otley A, Loonen H, Parekh N, et al. Assessing activity of pediatric Crohn's disease: Which index to use? Gastroenterology 1999;116:527–31.

91. Faubion WA Jr, Bousvaros A. Medical therapy for refractory pediatric Crohn's disease. Clin Gastroenterol Hepatol 2006;4: 1199–213.

92. Mahadevan U, Sandborn WJ. Evolving medical therapies for Crohn's disease. Curr Gastroenterol Rep 2001;3:471–6.

93. Mack DR, Young R, Kaufman SS, et al. Methotrexate in patients with Crohn's disease after 6-mercaptopurine. J Pediatr 1998;132: 830–5.

94. Ruemmele FM, Lachaux A, Cezard JP, et al. Efficacy of infliximab in pediatric Crohn's disease: A randomized multicenter open-label trial comparing scheduled to on demand maintenance therapy. Inflamm Bowel Dis 2009;15:388–94.

95. Rutgeerts P, Hiele M, Geboes K, et al. Controlled trial of metronidazole treatment for prevention of Crohn's recurrence after ileal resection. Gastroenterology 1995;108:1617–21.

96. Bousvaros A. Use of immunomodulators and biologic therapies in children with inflammatory bowel disease. Expert Rev Clin Immunol 2010;6:659–66.

97. Yang LS, Alex G, Catto-Smith AG. The use of biologic agents in pediatric inflammatory bowel disease. Curr Opin Pediatr 2012;24:609–14.

98. Diamond IR, Gerstle JT, Kim PC, et al. Outcomes after laparoscopic surgery in children with inflammatory bowel disease. Surg Endosc 2010;24:2796–802.

99. von Allmen D, Markowitz JE, York A, et al. Laparoscopic-assisted bowel resection offers advantages over open surgery for treatment of segmental Crohn's disease in children. J Pediatr Surg 2003; 38:963–5.

100. Gardenbroek TJ, Tanis PJ, Buskens CJ, et al. Surgery for Crohn's disease: New developments. Dig Surg 2012;29:275–80.

101. Resegotti A, Astegiano M, Farina EC, et al. Side-to-side stapled anastomosis strongly reduces anastomotic leak rates in Crohn's disease surgery. Dis Colon Rectum 2005;48:464–8.

102. Laituri CA, Fraser JD, Garey CL, et al. Laparoscopic ileocecectomy in pediatric patients with Crohn's disease. J Laparoendosc Adv Surg Tech A 2011;21:193–5.

103. Makowiec F, Paczulla D, Schmidtke C, et al. Long-term follow-up after resectional surgery in patients with Crohn's disease involving the colon. Z Gastroenterol 1998;36:619–24.

104. Tekkis PP, Purkayastha S, Lanitis S, et al. A comparison of segmental vs subtotal/total colectomy for colonic Crohn's disease: A meta-analysis. Colorectal Dis 2006;8:82–90.

105. Cattan P, Bonhomme N, Panis Y, et al. Fate of the rectum in patients undergoing total colectomy for Crohn's disease. Br J Surg 2002;89:454–9.

106. Davies G, Evans CM, Shand WS, et al. Surgery for Crohn's disease in childhood: Influence of site of disease and operative procedure on outcome. Br J Surg 1990;77:891–4.

107. Papi C, Spurio FF, Margagnoni G, et al. Randomized controlled trials in prevention of postsurgical recurrence in Crohn's disease. Rev Recent Clin Trials 2012;7:307–13.

108. Patel HI, Leichtner AM, Colodny AH, et al. Surgery for Crohn's disease in infants and children. J Pediatr Surg 1997;32:1063–8.

109. Guindi M, Riddell RH. Indeterminate colitis. J Clin Pathol 2004;57:1233–44.

110. Prudhomme M, Dehni N, Dozois RR. Causes and outcomes of pouch excision after restorative proctocolectomy. Brit J Surg 2006;93:82–6.

111. Yu CS, Pemberton JH, Larson D. Ileal pouch anal anastomosis in patients with indeterminate colitis: Long-term results. Dis Colon Rectum 2000;43:1487–96.

112. Wolff BG. Is ileoanal the proper operation for indeterminate colitis: The case for. Inflam Bowel Dis 2002;8:362–9.

CHAPTER 42

APPENDICITIS

Veronica F. Sullins • Steven L. Lee

Appendicitis is one of the most common surgical emergencies in children. Over 70,000 cases are seen in the USA each year.[1,2] The lifetime risk of appendicitis is 9% in boys and 7% in girls. Unfortunately, there is a lack of general consensus regarding its diagnosis and management.[3]

PATHOPHYSIOLOGY

The spectrum of appendicitis ranges from simple inflammation to gross perforation. This concept was initially described by van Zwalenberg in 1905 and confirmed in an experimental model by Wangensteen in 1939.[4,5] Obstruction of the lumen can occur from multiple causes including fecal material (fecalith), lymphoid hyperplasia, foreign body, or parasites. Fecaliths are present in roughly 20% of children with acute appendicitis and 30–40% of children with perforated appendicitis.[6,7] Fecaliths and appendicitis are more common in developed countries with low-fiber diets compared to developing countries with high-fiber diets.[8] Hyperplasia of the lymphoid tissue near the base of the appendix is also a common cause of appendiceal obstruction in children. Interestingly, the incidence of appendicitis closely resembles the amount of appendiceal lymphoid follicles present.[9] Organisms such as *Yersenia*, *Salmonella*, and *Shigella* can cause a local or generalized reaction of the lymphoid tissue leading to obstruction. In similar fashion, parasitic infestations from *Entamoeba*, *Strongyloides*, *Enterobius*, *Schistosoma*, or *Ascaris* species and viral infections such as mumps virus, coxsackie virus B, cytomegalovirus, and adenovirus can lead to luminal obstruction secondary to lymphoid hyperplasia.[10–18] In children with cystic fibrosis, obstruction may be due to abnormal production of mucus leading to painful distention with or without inflammation.[19] Appendicitis in neonates is rare and warrants evaluation for cystic fibrosis and Hirschsprung disease.[20] It is difficult to distinguish neonatal appendicitis from necrotizing enterocolitis confined to the appendix.[21]

Following obstruction, the appendix becomes distended from the accumulation of mucus and proliferation of bacteria. As intraluminal pressure increases, lymphatic and venous drainage are impaired resulting in local edema. A further increase in pressure will limit arterial inflow, thus jeopardizing tissue integrity and ultimately leading to tissue necrosis and perforation. Although the natural history of untreated appendicitis is usually perforation and abscess, not all patients will progress in this fashion. Resolution of untreated appendicitis has been described and may be the mechanism behind the clinical phenomenon of relapsing or chronic appendicitis.[22,23]

Historically, appendicitis has been considered a somewhat time-sensitive condition such that a significant delay in treatment may lead to an increased risk of perforation. It is for this reason that young children have a higher appendiceal perforation rate compared to older children.[24] Younger children have less ability to understand or articulate their developing symptoms. As a result, perforation rates have been reported to be as high as 82% in children younger than 5 years and nearly 100% in 1-year olds.[25]

Age is not the only factor accounting for delays in treatment and therefore higher perforation rates. One of the biggest concerns contributing to this delay is the lack of access to health care. It follows that patients with poor access to health care will have higher perforation rates. Indeed, children with no insurance or public insurance have higher rates of appendiceal perforation compared to children with private insurance.[26–29] Minorities also have higher perforation rates compared to whites.[26–29] Encouragingly, settings in which patients have equal access to health care or a well-established primary care network eliminate these racial, ethnic, and socioeconomic differences.[30,31]

CLINICAL PRESENTATION

The clinical presentation of appendicitis closely correlates with the pathophysiology of the disease process. The most common initial symptom is vague abdominal pain. This pain is due to activation of the visceral pain fibers from distention of the appendix following obstruction. Pain is vague, nonspecific, and commonly located in the periumbilical region as with distention of all midgut derivatives. As the appendiceal distention progresses, symptoms of nausea, vomiting, diarrhea, and anorexia often follow. The appearance of these symptoms prior to the onset of pain makes the diagnosis of appendicitis less likely. Intermittent, crampy pain is also less commonly associated with appendicitis.

Fever, tachycardia, and leukocytosis develop as a consequence of systemic inflammatory mediators released by ischemic tissues, white blood cells, and bacteria. The inflamed appendix then irritates the overlying peritoneum, typically by direct contact. This leads to focal peritonitis and localized right lower quadrant pain. This process explains the typical migrating pain from the umbilicus to the right lower quadrant. Any movement of the peritoneum will lead to an exacerbation of the pain. Thus, children will often demonstrate voluntary guarding of the right lower quadrant during the exam. Furthermore, children will usually resist walking and jumping due to the increased pain associated with such movement.

The most common finding on physical examination is focal tenderness in the right lower quadrant. Typically in children, only gentle pressure is required to elicit wincing, moving, or guarding. Applying pressure to a stethoscope while listening to the abdomen is a subtle way to palpate the abdomen in frightened children in whom it is difficult to obtain an accurate exam. Narcotic analgesics improve the comfort level of the patient, but do not alter the inflammatory process. Thus, tenderness will persist in patients receiving narcotics. Attempts to illicit rebound tenderness in children are uncomfortable, inaccurate, and should be avoided. An easier and more accurate method for determining the degree of peritoneal irritation is to ask the patient to walk or jump. Palpating a mass is difficult and often impossible due to the level of discomfort and guarding. Masses are more easily detected after induction of anesthesia. It is important to remember that localized tenderness is dependent on peritoneal irritation. Therefore, obesity, a retrocecal appendix, or an appendix that is walled off by omentum, mesentery, or small bowel may not be associated with localized tenderness, making the diagnosis more challenging.

Laboratory studies often show a mild leukocytosis. A markedly elevated leukocyte count suggests perforation or another diagnosis. Patients with appendicitis will have higher leukocyte counts compared to patients without appendicitis.[32] However a broad range of sensitivity (52–96%) exists, which limits the usefulness of this laboratory value alone. A left-shifted differential count may be a better diagnostic indicator, but a wide range in sensitivity (39–96%) also can lead to misinterpretation.[33–35] Other inflammatory markers including C-reactive protein (CRP), procalcitonin, and D-lactate have also been investigated. Of these markers, only CRP has been shown to be useful. A value greater than 3 mg/dL has been associated with the definitive diagnosis of appendicitis when compared to children with abdominal pain from a different etiology.[32] The combination of elevated leukocyte count and CRP level has the highest correlation of definitively diagnosing appendicitis.[32,36] Although normal values of both leukocyte count and CRP make the diagnosis of appendicitis less likely, the clinical signs and symptoms should be carefully considered as appendicitis cannot be excluded based on normal laboratory values. A urine analysis is typically obtained and is usually free of bacteria, but a few or moderate number of red or white blood cells may be found as the inflammatory process of the appendix may locally affect the bladder or ureter.

The typical presentation of appendicitis as described previously is found in roughly 50% of patients.[37] Children with appendicitis often present with wide deviations from this classic picture making for a challenging diagnosis. In patients with an atypical presentation of appendicitis, clinical scoring systems have been used to aid in making the diagnosis.[38,39] Accuracy of these scoring systems has been inconsistent which limits their usefulness over clinical judgment.[40–42] They have, however, been shown to decrease the use of computed tomography (CT) scans.[43] Recent studies have stratified patients into risk categories based on history, physical examination, and laboratory studies to determine which patients should have surgical consultation (high risk), additional imaging studies (medium risk), or be discharged (low risk).[38–42] This is the most applicable use of a scoring system or clinical pathway at the present time.

IMAGING STUDIES

Misdiagnosing appendicitis can lead to significant delays in treatment. Children are often diagnosed with gastroenteritis and parents are reassured that their child will improve, which may delay them from seeking further care. Epidemiologic data have shown the risk of a missed diagnosis in children to be higher in hospitals with a volume of less than one pediatric appendectomy per week.[44] Historically, negative appendectomy rates of 10% to 20% were not only considered appropriate but advisable to minimize the number of patients with a missed diagnosis and to decrease perforation rates. Some authors have questioned this philosophy, citing the risk and expense of an avoidable operation.[45] Appropriate use of diagnostic imaging can minimize both the negative appendectomy and perforation rates. Currently, the negative appendectomy rate from high-volume children's hospitals is 3–4%.[46–48] Despite the increased use of imaging studies, correctly diagnosing children less than 5 years of age continues to be challenging with negative appendectomy rates ranging from 13–17%.[48]

Plain radiography can show fecaliths in 10–20% of patients and can contribute to the diagnosis if the history and physical exam findings are consistent. Other helpful findings on plain films include lumbar scoliosis and obliteration of the psoas shadow. In general, plain films may be more useful to evaluate for other disease processes when the suspicion for appendicitis is low.

Ultrasonography (US) offers the advantages of being an efficient bedside technique that is noninvasive, requires no contrast, and emits no radiation. Thus, ultrasound should be the first imaging study utilized in patients with atypical presentations of appendicitis. Common ultrasound findings include a fluid-filled, noncompressible appendix, a diameter greater than 6 mm (Fig. 42-1), appendicolith, periappendiceal or pericecal fluid, and increased periappendiceal echogenicity caused by inflammation.[49,50] Most studies demonstrate a sensitivity greater than 85% and specificity greater than 90%.[51,52] However, ultrasound is operator dependent and results of published studies may not be similar to results obtained in many clinical settings. Patient factors such as bowel gas pattern, obesity, and guarding or movement can affect the accuracy. False-positive results may be due to a large appendix or another tubular structure being mistaken for the appendix. When a normal appendix is identified, it is a reliable study to rule out appendicitis. Unfortunately, only 10–50% of children with normal appendices can be identified.[52–54] When a normal appendix is not seen, there is still a risk of appendicitis despite an otherwise normal ultrasound study.[55] Graded compression ultrasound places pressure on the transducer to displace bowel loops and identify the appendix. The pressure is felt adequate if the psoas muscle and the iliac vessels are identified, which assure the range of view is posterior to the appendix. Furthermore, data from a large series employing upward graded compression, posterior manual compression, left oblique lateral decubitus position, and a low frequency convex transducer demonstrated that nearly all appendices could be identified with over 98% accuracy for correctly diagnosing appendicitis.[56] Contrast-enhanced power Doppler ultrasound imaging demonstrated similar accuracy in a small study.[57]

When ultrasound is unable to exclude or confirm appendicitis, additional imaging or observation with serial examinations is warranted. In order to avoid hospitalization for observation, many physicians obtain a CT scan. The findings of an enlarged appendix (>6 mm), appendiceal wall thickening (>1 mm), periappendiceal fat stranding, and appendiceal wall enhancement are useful diagnostic criteria (Fig. 42-2).[58,59] For the most part, the sensitivity and specificity of CT are around 95%.[60–66]

These values are significantly lower in diagnosing perforated appendicitis.[67] The perceived improved diagnostic accuracy of CT has led to a dramatic increase in the number of CT scans performed in children even though there is not good evidence that supports its routine use for the diagnosis of appendicitis.[68–71]

There are, however, several concerns with CT. Some protocols require a delay in the emergency department for contrast administration, and younger children may require sedation. Recently, the ease of rapid helical CT has led to an estimated 200% increase in pediatric CT scans, significantly increasing radiation exposure in young patients.[72] This has become a growing concern because although no direct connection between CT scan and malignancy has been made, lifetime radiation exposure has been linked to an increased risk of malignancy.[73] It has been estimated that a complete abdominal CT scan is equivalent to 25.7 months of natural background radiation exposure.[74] Developing tissues are more sensitive to the effects of radiation as evidenced by an increased risk of radiation-induced malignancy in patients exposed at a younger age.[73,75] The risk of a fatal radiation-induced malignancy is estimated at 0.18% for a 1-year-old child. In other words, one death due to malignancy would result from an abdominal CT scan done on 555 1-year-old patients, whereas about twice as many 15-year-olds would need to be scanned to equal that risk. Although this estimate seems significant, it represents only a 0.35% increase in overall risk compared to the risk of cancer mortality with natural background radiation.[76] Use of a staged imaging protocol, performing CT scan only if ultrasound findings are equivocal, has shown a reduction in the number of CT scans performed and therefore overall radiation exposure without sacrificing diagnostic sensitivity and specificity.[77] In addition, international guidelines on radiation protection have implemented the ALARA principle (as low as reasonably achievable), thus decreasing radiation exposure in children by 30-50%.[72,75,77] Although the overall increase in risk may be miniscule, it is important to attempt to limit radiation exposure when evaluating children with acute appendicitis.

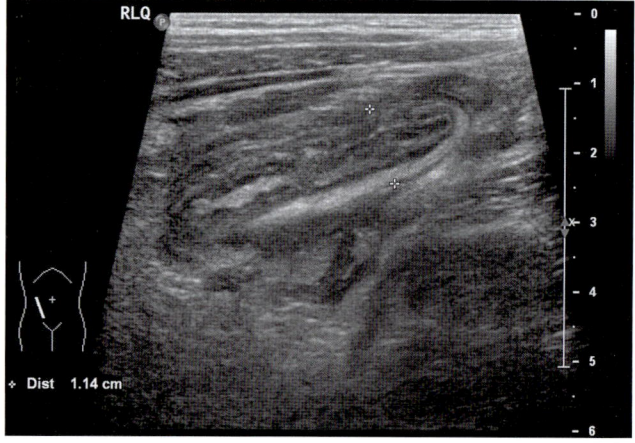

FIGURE 42-1 ■ This longitudinal view of an ultrasound in a patient with acute appendicitis shows an enlarged appendix measuring 11 mm. in diameter.

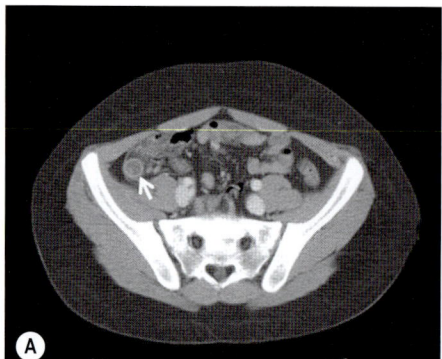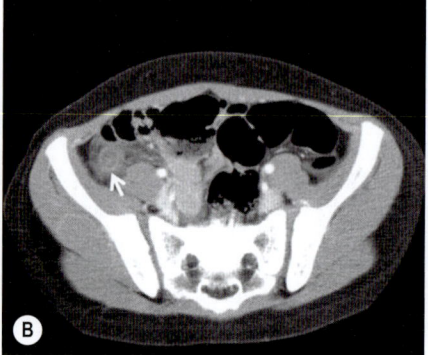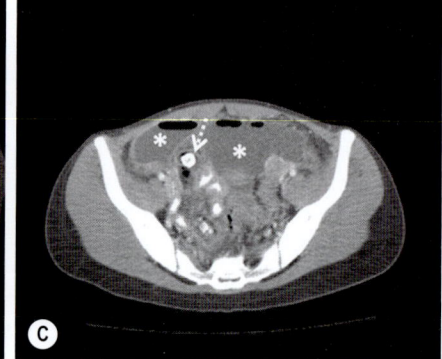

FIGURE 42-2 ■ These three CT scans show differing presentations for appendicitis. **(A)** The appendix (arrow) is enlarged and has a thickened wall. There are no inflammatory changes such as periappendiceal fat stranding seen on this study. **(B)** The appendix (arrow) is enlarged and there is free fluid and inflammatory changes medially indicating likely perforation. **(C)** The patient presented with a one week history of pain and the appendix has perforated with the development of two abscesses (asterisks). In addition, a fecalith is seen medially (dotted arrow). This patient was initially managed nonoperatively with drainage of the abscesses and intravenous antibiotics. She underwent laparoscopic interval appendectomy 10 weeks following the initial admission.

Magnetic resonance imaging (MRI) is an intriguing nonradiation alternative to CT and is extremely accurate in diagnosing appendicitis.[78] The current version of this technology makes it impractical for widespread application, but future generations of scanners could allow it to be the preferred diagnostic imaging modality.

DIFFERENTIAL DIAGNOSIS

Acute appendicitis can mimic virtually any intra-abdominal process and should be high on the differential diagnosis in children with abdominal pain.[79] Causes of acute right lower quadrant pain that are often indistinguishable from appendicitis include tubo-ovarian pathologic processes, Crohn disease, mesenteric adenitis, cecal diverticulitis, Meckel diverticulitis, constipation, viral gastroenteritis, and regional bacterial enteritis (*Yersinia* and *Campylobacter* in particular). Lower abdominal pain or vague nonfocal pain can result from a urinary tract infection, kidney stone, ureteropelvic junction obstruction, uterine pathologic process, right lower lobe pneumonia, sigmoid diverticulitis, cholecystitis, pancreatitis, gastroenteritis, vasculitis, bowel obstruction, and malignancy (lymphoma). The most common diagnosis made in the presence of missed appendicitis is reported to be gastroenteritis.[80] Although many of these conditions may seem easily distinguishable, they each possess a spectrum of presentation that overlaps with appendicitis.

TREATMENT

The treatment of appendicitis begins with intravenous fluids and broad-spectrum antibiotics to provide coverage of enteric organisms. Management after initiating antimicrobial therapy depends on the severity of inflammation and the discussion must therefore be separated into uncomplicated (nonperforated) and complicated (perforated appendicitis). This distinction, however, is not always clear. Diagnostic imaging may help but cannot accurately diagnose perforation and many patients will not undergo preoperative imaging.[61] Even intraoperative assessment showed high rates of discordance when compared to histologic evaluation of gangrenous and/or ruptured appendicitis.[81] Surgeons polled with photographs showed extreme incongruence on which patients had perforation,[82] and a survey of American Pediatric Surgical Association members revealed that most surgeons base their practice patterns on individual preferences.[3] For this reason, the literature focusing on perforated appendicitis must be viewed with caution.

In reality, appendicitis presents as a spectrum of disease and it is important to distinguish which patients are at higher risk of complications. The data comparing outcomes of nonperforated versus perforated appendicitis is extensive, but most studies fail to use a strict definition of perforation. One prospective study showed that defining perforation as a visible hole in the appendix or a fecalith in the abdomen effectively identified those with greater risk of developing intra-abdominal abscesses (Fig. 42-3).[83] In addition, outcomes in gangrenous appendicitis are similar to acute appendicitis and many patients may actually be over-treated.[84] Thus, in the following discussion, the management of uncomplicated appendicitis will include acute, suppurative, and gangrenous appendicitis whereas complicated appendicitis will be synonymous with perforated appendicitis.

Uncomplicated Appendicitis

After intravenous fluids and administration of broad-spectrum antibiotics, the current standard of care for uncomplicated appendicitis is appendectomy. Prophylactic antimicrobial agents should be given for 24 hours or less. In fact, a single preoperative dose of antibiotics has shown to decrease the risk of wound infection and abscess.[85,86] Following appendectomy, patients are typically discharged within 24 hours. Additional postoperative antibiotics for acute appendicitis are not necessary or recommended.[85,87] However, it may be reasonable to administer additional antibiotics for patients with suppurative or gangrenous appendicitis during the first 24 hours after appendectomy or longer based on the patient's clinical status.

Recent data in adults suggests that administration of antibiotics without appendectomy may be sufficient to treat uncomplicated appendicitis. Multiple prospective randomized trials in adults have demonstrated similar outcomes from acute appendicitis treated with antibiotics alone with success rates ranging from 44% to 85%.[88–92] Adults managed nonoperatively demonstrated fewer complications and less pain, although recurrence rates were high, ranging from 14% to 37%.[93] There have been no prospective, randomized trials in children comparing antibiotics alone to appendectomy. Regardless of

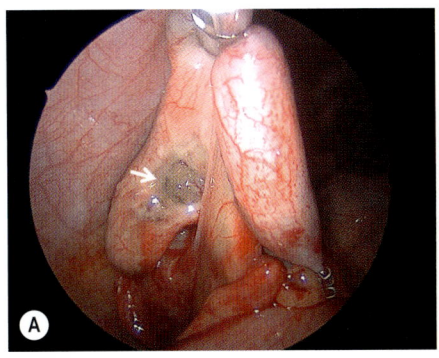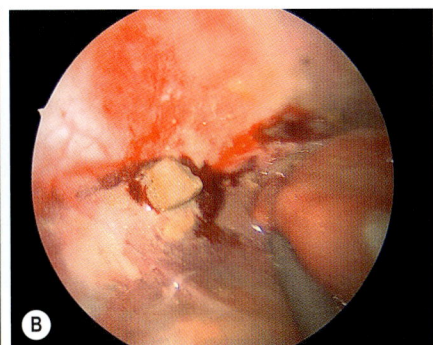

FIGURE 42-3 ■ These two images depict the definition of perforation used in a prospective randomized trial.[103] This definition of either **(A)** a hole in the appendix (arrow) or **(B)** stool in the abdomen was subsequently validated.[83] An objective definition of perforation allows surgeons to compare outcomes data more accurately about perforated appendicitis.

treatment modality, once antibiotics have been initiated, appendectomy is no longer considered to be an emergency and may even be considered somewhat elective.[88,89,93–98] Until there is enough prospective randomized data in pediatric patients proving the efficacy of primary antibiotic treatment, appendectomy remains the standard of care for uncomplicated appendicitis. However, the need for operation may not be as urgent as previously thought.

Complicated Appendicitis

Patients with perforated appendicitis should receive postoperative antibiotics until clinical resolution has occurred. The antibiotic regimen employed for perforated appendicitis has traditionally been triple antibiotic therapy (ampicillin, gentamicin, and clindamycin or metronidazole). However recently there has been a shift towards more simple antibiotic regimens. Single agent therapy with piperacillin/tazobactam or cefotaxime, or double agent therapy with ceftriaxone and metronidazole, has been shown to be as efficacious as triple antibiotic therapy but is more cost effective.[99–103] Several authors have highlighted a decrease in antibiotic expense with once daily dosing of ceftriaxone compared with multi-dose monotherapeutic agents. In addition, a prospective randomized study confirmed that single daily dosing of ceftriaxone and metronidazole is equal to and more cost effective than traditional triple antibiotic therapy in the treatment of perforated appendicitis.[103] Therefore, current best evidence suggests once-a-day dosing with ceftriaxone at 50 mg/kg/day and metronidazole at 30 mg/kg/day provides the simplest and least expensive regimen.

Although the length of antibiotic course for perforated appendicitis is not yet standardized, current findings from multiple systematic reviews recommend continuation of antibiotics until resolution of clinical symptoms.[85,102] This includes normalization of leukocyte count and differential, full return of gastrointestinal function, resolution of fever, and normalization of physical exam. In addition, if the duration of intravenous antibiotic therapy is less than 5 days, patients can be discharged safely on oral antibiotics to complete a 7-day course.[104] A patient who is clinically well by postoperative day three is unlikely to develop an abscess.[105] However, if a patient's clinical symptoms have not resolved, it should raise the suspicion of an intra-abdominal abscess and intravenous antibiotics should be continued.

After initial intravenous fluid administration and antibiotics, the management of complicated appendicitis can be separated into nonoperative and operative treatment. Choice of treatment depends on identification of patients at high risk for treatment failure. It is also important to consider that many patients will not be diagnosed with perforated appendicitis preoperatively. Risk factors for failure of nonoperative management include greater than 15% band forms on the white blood cell differential count, disease that extends beyond the right lower quadrant, absence of a well-defined abscess, or presence of an appendicolith on imaging.[106–108] Conversely, a large meta-analysis comparing appendectomy versus conservative treatment for complicated appendicitis as defined by

abscess or phlegmon on presentation demonstrated higher rates of overall complications, wound infections, and intra-abdominal abscesses in those who had immediate appendectomy.[109]

The concept of managing complicated appendicitis with antibiotics alone is to decrease the significant local and regional inflammation that may make an immediate operation very difficult and potentially more dangerous. Once treated, most surgeons will perform interval appendectomy after six to ten weeks. However, some advocate that the interval appendectomy is not necessary as recurrence rates are low, ranging from 8–14%.[110,111] One problem with these studies is the relatively short length of follow-up. A recent systematic review found a 20.5% overall risk of recurrent appendicitis with a range of 0–42%. However, nearly all studies were retrospective and thus only included patients specifically selected for nonoperative management.[112] Some studies showed high rates of pathologic findings in interval appendectomy specimens.[113,114] Although there is a lack of long-term data to accurately predict the rates of recurrence in both adults and children, some studies suggest that most recurrences will occur within three years and the majority within one to six months.[110–112] For these reasons, most pediatric surgeons perform interval appendectomy in patients with complicated appendicitis who were initially managed nonoperatively.[3]

The majority of patients who present with a well-formed abscess on initial imaging are managed nonoperatively (see Fig. 42-2C). Historically, immediate appendectomy in this patient population was difficult, required a larger incision, and had a high morbidity. Primary treatment of the abscess with antibiotics alone, or antibiotics and percutaneous drainage with or without drain placement for larger fluid collections, is a widely accepted treatment strategy. Interval appendectomy is then performed after the inflammation has subsided.[3,115–119] Although treatment with percutaneous drainage and interval appendectomy has inherent risk of complications, success rates have been reported to be as high as 88%.[107] A recent pilot randomized trial comparing initial laparoscopic appendectomy versus antibiotics, percutaneous drainage and subsequent interval laparoscopic appendectomy in patients presenting with perforated appendicitis and abscess demonstrated no difference in the rate of recurrent abscess, length of hospital stay, or hospital charges.[120] Patients undergoing immediate appendectomy had longer operations and a longer time to return of bowel function. Alternately, patients who had interval appendectomies had more CT scans. Quality of life surveys at presentation, 2 weeks, and 12 weeks in both groups from this study showed that families experience significant parenting distress related to disruption in the child's quality of life until the appendectomy is performed.[121]

The majority of patients with complicated appendicitis can be safely managed with appendectomy. Specifically, patients with a phlegmonous mass, appendicolith, or absence of a well-formed abscess on imaging have a higher risk of failure of nonoperative management.[107,122] These patients can safely and reliably undergo immediate laparoscopic appendectomy.[123,124] In patients with perforated appendicitis without abscess, a recent prospective randomized trial demonstrated lower rates of adverse events, shorter length of hospitalization, and earlier return to normal activity with early appendectomy.[122] In addition, mean total hospital charges and resource use were significantly higher in patients undergoing interval appendectomy, likely due to the increased number of adverse events.[125]

The choice of nonoperative versus operative treatment depends on the preoperative diagnosis of perforation. As mentioned previously, it is difficult to interpret data on perforated appendicitis because a strict definition of perforation has not uniformly been used. Currently, patients are initially managed operatively or nonoperatively based on disease severity and surgeon preference. Although evidence suggests that the majority of patients can safely undergo early appendectomy, the optimal management of complicated appendicitis still remains unclear.

Operative Technique

First described in 1893 by McBurney, the traditional method of appendectomy was a muscle-splitting, right lower quadrant incision.[126] The cecum is delivered through the incision, the mesoappendix is divided, and the appendix is ligated at its base. In the laparoscopic approach, both surgeon and first assistant stand on the patient's left facing a video monitor positioned on the right (Fig. 42-4A).[127] The patient is positioned supine on the operating table, and the abdomen is prepped widely. After insertion of a 10–12 mm umbilical cannula, pneumoperitoneum is established. Two 5 mm ports are then placed, one in the left lower quadrant and one in the left suprapubic area (Fig 42-4B). A 5 mm 30° or 45° telescope is introduced through the left lower quadrant port, and the other two ports are the working ports. This allows effective triangulation of instruments to maximize utility in a small space, a core principle of endoscopic surgery. Diagnostic laparoscopy is initially performed. If present, abscesses are opened and purulent fluid is aspirated from the pelvis, perihepatic space and paracolic gutters. The appendix is located by following the taenia of the cecum inferiorly. After grasping the appendix and retracting it inferiorly, a window is created in the mesoappendix close to the cecum. The endoscopic stapler is inserted through the 12 mm umbilical cannula and used to divide the appendix and mesoappendix (Fig. 42-5). The appendix is usually divided first, followed by division of the mesoappendix. On occasion, however, it may be more expedient to ligate the mesoappendix first. If the appendix can be delivered through the cannula, an endoscopic bag is not used. However, if the appendix is too large for the cannula, an endoscopic bag is employed to avoid dragging the appendix through the umbilical incision. Drains are not routinely utilized for advanced disease.

Since the introduction of laparoscopic appendectomy 25 years ago, there has been an abundance of data comparing open and endoscopic techniques. Initial advantages of the open approach seemed to be a shorter length of operation and fewer postoperative intra-abdominal abscesses.[128–130] However, as expected, there were higher rates of wound infections, presumably due to contamination of the incision when delivering an infected appendix through the wound (Fig. 42-6). Advantages of the laparoscopic approach are multiple. It allows better visualization of the entire abdomen, which is especially beneficial in obese patients who would otherwise require a larger incision, and fertile females who may have other intra-abdominal pathology.[131–133] Laparoscopy also allows lysis of interloop abscesses and aspiration of purulent fluid, and it facilitates dissection in obese patients in whom open appendectomy would be challenging. Use of laparoscopy has been associated with a higher negative appendectomy rate.[134] However, this discrepancy may be explained by the increased use of diagnostic laparoscopy in patients whose diagnosis is not clear, specifically teenage females who may have gynecologic findings. Open appendectomy may be easier in younger patients due to lack of space in the peritoneal cavity relative to the size of the laparoscopic instruments.

The use of laparoscopy has increased from about 20% in 1998 to 70% in 2007.[135–137] In the past decade, there have been multiple prospective randomized trials, large retrospective studies, and meta-analyses comparing outcomes in open versus the laparoscopic approach. While early studies found increased operating times for laparoscopy, more recent studies have shown no difference in length of operation.[138–142] A few studies actually demonstrated shorter operating times with laparoscopy.[139–140]

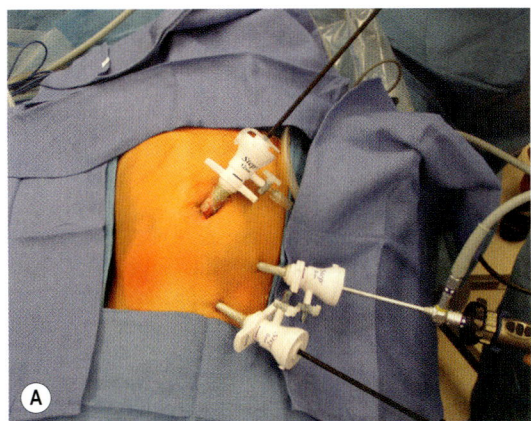
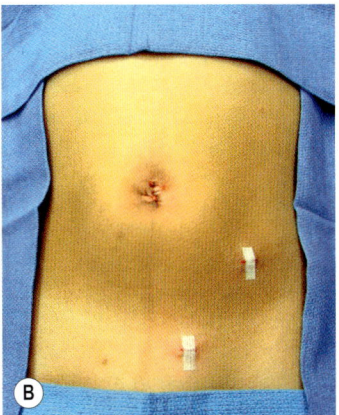

FIGURE 42-4 ■ **(A)** Port positions for a laparoscopic appendectomy. Typically three cannulas are used, with the endoscopic stapler introduced through the 12 mm umbilical port. The appendix is removed through this site as well. **(B)** Postoperative appearance.

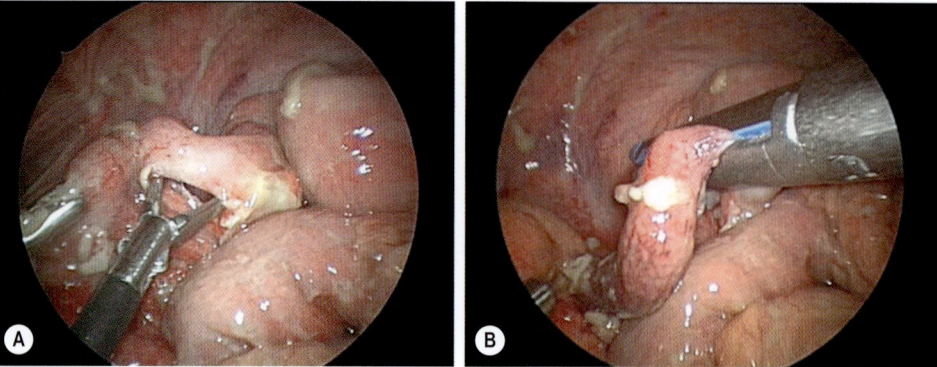

FIGURE 42-5 ■ **(A)** Initially, a window is made in the mesoappendix. **(B)** Usually, the appendix is ligated and divided with the stapler first, followed by ligation/division of the mesoappendix.

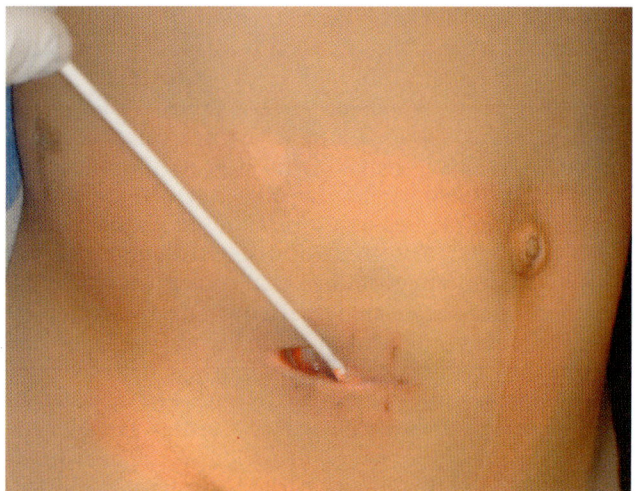

FIGURE 42-6 ■ This child underwent open appendectomy through a right lower abdominal incision and developed a wound infection which is being treated. The significant reduction in the incidence of wound infections is one of the benefits of the laparoscopic approach, especially for perforated appendicitis.

Laparoscopic appendectomy is also associated with shorter hospitalization, fewer postoperative outpatient visits, decreased time off work, and earlier return to routine activity.[134–136,138,142–144] One study suggested increased inpatient costs but lower outpatient costs for the laparoscopic approach, while a large national database review found increased costs in uncomplicated appendicitis but similar costs for complicated appendicitis.[137,142] A prospective randomized double-blind study demonstrated that patients who underwent laparoscopic appendectomy had an improved quality of life at two weeks.[145]

Overall complication rates are less than 3% for uncomplicated appendicitis and 16% to 18% for complicated appendicitis with many studies showing the same if not lower rates after laparoscopy.[131,135,137,138,144] One of the more common complications following appendectomy is an intra-abdominal abscess. Rates of postoperative abscess are estimated to be less than 1% in uncomplicated appendicitis and 1–15% in complicated appendicitis. However, in many of these studies, there is not uniform definition of perforation. When a uniform definition is used, rates

as high as 20% have been reported.[83,105,120,137] One group found an increase in abscess rate from 19% to 46% when comparing non-obese to obese patients.[146] A decade ago, a few groups reported a higher incidence of postoperative abscesses in patients who had a laparoscopic appendectomy.[128–130] However, there is now an abundance of level 1, 2, and 3 evidence showing no difference in rates of intra-abdominal abscesses.[136–138,144,147–155] In fact, the most recent national database review evaluated 212,958 pediatric patients and found a higher rate of postoperative abscess in patients who underwent open appendectomy for both uncomplicated and complicated appendicitis.[137] This discrepancy may be due to increasing surgeon experience with laparoscopy, more advanced endoscopic equipment, or possibly using an endobag for removal of the perforated appendix.[156]

Regardless of whether laparoscopic or open appendectomy is performed, culture of the fluid has not been shown to be helpful at the time of the initial operation.[157,158] One study demonstrated that children whose antibiotic treatment was based on the cultures did somewhat worse than those whose fluid was not cultured.[158] Peritoneal lavage with either saline or antibiotic solution has also not been shown to decrease the incidence of abdominal abscesses.[159] Similarly, the use of drains has not proved useful except in cases of walled-off abscess cavities.[160,161]

With respect to wound infections, this complication occurs in less than 1% of patients with uncomplicated appendicitis. In contrast, patients with complicated appendicitis may have up to 16% incidence of wound infection.[144] Most recent studies have found that laparoscopy has a lower rate of surgical site infections.[24,135–138,143,144] The use of laparoscopy has also demonstrated a nearly fourfold decrease in postoperative bowel obstructions.[162,163] Other less common postoperative complications include urinary tract infection and pneumonia.

The concept that higher complication rates accompany the laparoscopic approach is outdated. It is now widely accepted that laparoscopic appendectomy should be the procedure of choice in both uncomplicated and complicated appendicitis, except in centers without laparoscopic experience.

Recently, the use of single-site laparoscopic surgical techniques have been reported.[164–171] In single-incision

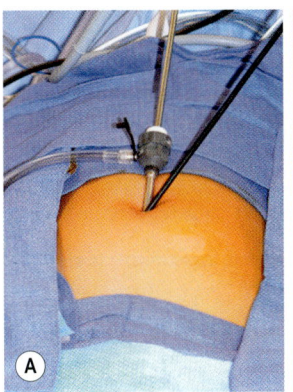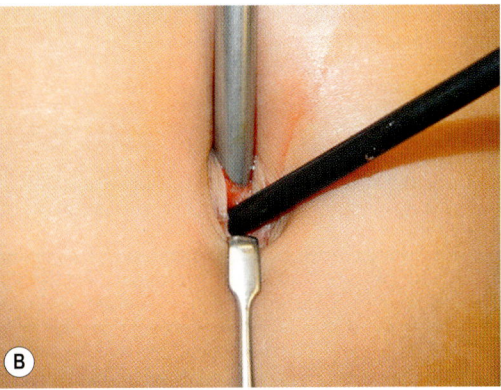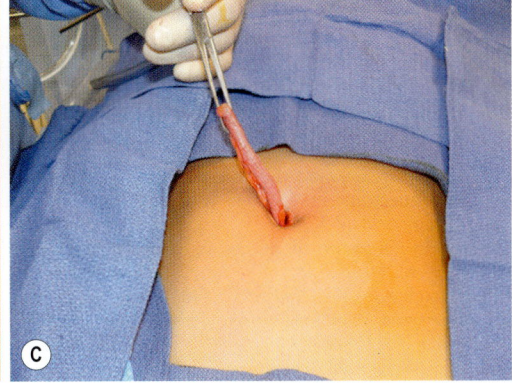

FIGURE 42-7 ■ This 10-year-old underwent a transumbilical laparoscopic-assisted appendectomy. **(A)** A 5 mm reusable cannula was introduced in the cephalad aspect of the umbilical fascia followed by insertion of a 5 mm grasping forceps inferior to the cannula for mobilization of the cecum and appendix..**(B)** Close-up view of the separate fascial incisions for introduction of the cannula and instrument. Note the fascial bridge between the instrument and the cannula. This bridge prevents escape of CO_2 around the instruments. **(C)** Following mobilization of the cecum and appendix, an extracorporeal appendectomy was then performed.

laparoscopic appendectomy (SILA), a single transumbilical incision is made and a 5 mm or 12 mm port is placed. One or two additional ports are placed through the same incision using multi-port devices or separate fascial incisions. Subsequent dissection and appendectomy are identical to the traditional three-port procedure. Advantages of this technique are thought to be shorter length of hospitalization, better cosmesis, and lower hospital costs. Technically the procedure can be more challenging as close approximation of instruments limits range of motion and narrows the visual field.[172] Theoretically a larger fascial incision may result in increased postoperative pain and higher rates of incisional hernias although preliminary evidence is limited. Hybrid procedures such as laparoscopic-assisted single-port appendectomy (SPA) and transumbilical laparoscopic-assisted appendectomy (TULAA) are other described techniques that combine a laparoscopic single-incision approach for dissection followed by extracorporeal removal of the appendix through the umbilicus as in the traditional open procedure (Fig. 42-7). Early retrospective reviews have shown no difference in postoperative complication rates and similar or even decreased hospital costs when compared to open and other laparoscopic techniques.[167,168,170] A recent prospective randomized trial comparing single site to traditional three-port appendectomy in patients with nonperforated appendicitis demonstrated no difference in postoperative wound infection or abscess rates, length of hospital stay, or hospital charges.[164] This particular study found a longer operative time (in minutes) for the single-incision approach, but this was not clinically relevant.

REFERENCES

1. Sivit CJ, Siegel MJ, Applegate KE, et al. When appendicitis is suspected in children. RadioGraphics 2001;21:247–62.
2. Wagner JM, McKinney WP, Carpenter JL. Does this patient have appendicitis? JAMA 1996;276:1589–94.
3. Chen C, Botelho C, Cooper A, et al. Current practice patterns in the treatment of perforated appendicitis in children. J Am Coll Surg 2003;196:212–21.
4. van Zwalenburg C. The relation of mechanical distention to the etiology of appendicitis. Ann Surg 1905;41:437–50.
5. Wangensteen OH, Dennis C. Experimental proof of obstructive origin of appendicitis. Ann Surg 1939;110:629–47.
6. Curran TJ, Meunchow SK. The treatment of complicated appendicitis in children using peritoneal drainage: Results from a public hospital. J Pediatr Surg 1993;28:204–8.
7. Stringel G. Appendicitis in children: A systematic approach for a low incidence of complications. Am J Surg 1987;154:631–5.
8. Jones BA, Demetriades D, Segal I. The prevalence of appendiceal fecoliths in patients with and without appendicitis: A comparative study from Canada and South Africa. Ann Surg 1985;202:80–2.
9. Burkitt DP. The aetiology of appendicitis. Br J Surg 1971;58:695–9.
10. Attwood SE, Mealy K, Cafferkey MT, et al. Yersinia infection and acute abdominal pain. Lancet 1987;1:529–33.
11. Rabau MY, Avigad I, Wolfstein I. Rubella and acute appendicitis. Pediatrics 1980;66:813.
12. Rodgers B, Karn G. Yersinia enterocolitis. J Pediatr Surg 1975;10:497–9.
13. Sanders DY, Cort CR, Stubbs AJ. Shigellosis associated with appendicitis. J Pediatr Surg 1972;7:315–17.
14. Adebamowo CA, Akang EE, Ladipo JK, et al. Schistosomiasis of the appendix. Br J Surg 1991;78:1219–21.
15. Nadler S, Cappell MS, Bhatt B, et al. Appendiceal infection by Entamoeba histolytica and Strongyloides stercoralis presenting like acute appendicitis. Dig Dis Sci 1990;35:603–8.
16. Schnell VL, Yandell R, Van Zandt S, et al. Enterobius vermicularis salpingitis: A distant episode from precipitating appendicitis. Obstet Gynecol 1992;80:553–5.
17. Kwong MS, Dinner M. Neonatal appendicitis masquerading as necrotizing enterocolitis. J Pediatr 1980;96:917–18.
18. Valerdiz-Casasola S, Pardo-Mindan FJ. Cytomegalovirus infection of the appendix in patient with the acquired immunodeficiency syndrome. Gastroenterology 1991;101:247.
19. Coughlin JP, Gauderer MW, Stern RC, et al. The spectrum of appendiceal disease in cystic fibrosis. J Pediatr Surg 1990;25:835–9.
20. Martin LW, Perrin EV. Neonatal perforation of the appendix in association with Hirschsprung's disease. Ann Surg 1967;166:799–802.
21. Stiefel D, Stallmach T, Sacher P. Acute appendicitis in neonates: Complication or morbus sui generis? Pediatr Surg Int 1998;14:122–3.
22. Heller MB, Skolnick LM. Ultrasound documentation of spontaneously resolving appendicitis. Am J Emerg Med 1993;11:51–3.
23. Mattei P, Sola JE, Yeo CJ. Chronic and recurrent appendicitis are uncommon entities often misdiagnosed. J Am Coll Surg 1994;178:385–9.
24. Lee SL, Stark R, Yaghoubian A, et al. Does age affect the outcomes and management of pediatric appendicitis? J Pediatr Surg 2011;46:2342–5.

25. Nance ML, Adamson WT, Hedrick HL. Appendicitis in the young child: A continuing diagnostic challenge. Pediatr Emerg Care 2000;16:160–2.

26. Jablonski KA, Guagliardo MF. Pediatric appendicitis rupture rate: A national indicator of disparities in healthcare access. Popul Health Metr 2005;3:4–9.

27. Ponsky TA, Huang ZJ, Kittle K, et al. Hospital- and patient-level characteristics and the risk of appendiceal rupture and negative appendectomy in children. JAMA 2004;292:1977–82.

28. Gadmonski A, Jenkins P. Ruptured appendicitis among children as an indicator of access to care. Health Serv Res 2001;36:129–42.

29. Guagliardo MF, Teach SJ, Huang ZJ, et al. Racial and ethnic disparities in pediatric appendicitis rupture rate. Acad Emerg Med 2003;10:1218–27.

30. Lee SL, Shekherdimian S, Chiu VY, et al. Perforated appendicitis in children: Equal access to care eliminates racial and socioeconomic disparities. J Pediatr Surg 2010;45:1203–7.

31. Nwomeh BC, Chisolm DJ, Caniano DA, et al. Racial and socioeconomic disparity in perforated appendicitis among children: Where is the problem? Pediatrics 2006;117:870–5.

32. Kwan KY, Nager AL. Diagnosing pediatric appendicitis: Usefulness of laboratory markers. Am J Emerg Med 2010;28:1009–15.

33. Bolton JP, Craven ER, Croft RJ, et al. An assessment of the value of the white-cell count in the management of suspected acute appendicitis. Br J Surg 1975;62:906–8.

34. Doraiswany NV. Leucocyte counts in the diagnosis and prognosis of acute appendicitis in children. Br J Surg 1979;66:782–4.

35. Hoffman J, Rasmussen OO. Aids in the diagnosis of acute appendicitis. Br J Surg 1989;76:774–9.

36. Stefanutti G, Ghirado V, Gamba P. Inflammatory markers for acute appendicitis in children: Are they helpful? J Pediatr Surg 2007;42:773–6.

37. Rothrock SG, Skeoch G, Rush JJ, et al. Clinical features of misdiagnosed appendicitis in children. Ann Emerg Med 1991;20:45–50.

38. Alvarado A. A practical score for the early diagnosis of acute appendicitis. Ann Emerg Med 1986;15:557–64.

39. Samuel M. Pediatric appendicitis score. J Pediatr Surg 2002;37:877–81.

40. Macklin CP, Radcliffe GS, Merei JM, et al. A prospective evaluation of the modified Alvarado score for acute appendicitis in children. Ann R Coll Surg Engl 1997;79:203–5.

41. McKay R, Shepherd J. The use of the clinical scoring system by Alvarado in the decision to perform computed tomography for acute appendicitis in the ED. Am J Emerg Med 2007;25:489–93.

42. Escriba A, Gamell AM, Fernandez Y, et al. Prospective validation of two systems of classification for the diagnosis of acute appendicitis. Pediatr Emer Care 2011;27:165–9.

43. Rezak A, Hussain MA, Abbas A, et al. Decreased use of computed tomography with a modified clinical scoring system in diagnosis of pediatric acute appendicitis. Arch Surg 2011;146:64–7.

44. Smink DS, Finkelstein JA, Kleinman K, et al. The effect of hospital volume of pediatric appendectomies on the misdiagnosis of appendicitis in children. Pediatrics 2004;113:18–23.

45. Flum DR, Koepsell T. The clinical and economic correlates of misdiagnosed appendicitis: Nationwide analysis. Arch Surg 2002;137:799–804.

46. Newman K, Ponsky T, Kittle K, et al. Appendicitis 2000: Variability in practice, outcomes, and resource utilization at thirty pediatric hospitals. J Pediatr Surg 2003;38:372–9.

47. Smink DS, Finkelstein JA, Garcia Peña BM, et al. Diagnosis of acute appendicitis in children using a clinical practice guideline. J Pediatr Surg 2004;39:458–63.

48. Bachur RG, Hennelly K, Callahan MJ, et al. Diagnostic imaging and negative appendectomy rates in children: Effects of age and gender. Pediatrics 2012;129:877–84.

49. Hayden CK Jr, Kuchelmeister J, Lipscomb TS. Sonography of acute appendicitis in childhood: Perforation versus nonperforation. J Ultrasound Med 1992;11:209–16.

50. Hahn HB, Hoepner FU, Kalle T, et al. Sonography of acute appendicitis in children: 7 years' experience. Pediatr Radiol 1998;28:147–51.

51. Yacoe ME, Jeffrey RB. Sonography of appendicitis and diverticulitis. Radiol Clin North Am 1994;32:899–912.

52. Trout AT, Sanchez R, Ladino-Torres MF, et al. A critical evaluation of ultrasound for the diagnosis of pediatric acute appendicitis in a real-life setting: How can we improve the diagnostic value of sonography? Pediatr Radiol 2012; March 9 Online Springer-Verlag.

53. Weyant MJ, Eachempati SR, Maluccio MA, et al. Is imaging necessary for the diagnosis of acute appendicitis. Adv Surg 2003;37:327–45.

54. Sivit CJ, Applegate KE. Imaging of acute appendicitis in children. Semin Ultrasound CT MR 2003;24:74–82.

55. Jaremko JL, Crockett A, Rucker D, et al. Incidence and significance of inconclusive results in ultrasound for appendicitis in children and teenagers. Can Assoc Radiol, 2011;62:197–202.

56. Chen SC, Chen KM, Wang SM, et al. Abdominal sonography screening of clinically diagnosed or suspected appendicitis before surgery. World J Surg 1998;22:449–52.

57. Horton MD, Counter SF, Florence MG, et al. A prospective trial of computed tomography and ultrasonography for diagnosing appendicitis in the atypical patient. Am J Surg 2000;179:379–81.

58. Gwynn LK. Appendiceal enlargement as a criterion for clinical diagnosis of acute appendicitis: Is it reliable and valid? J Emerg Med 2002;23:9–14.

59. Choi D, Park H, Lee YR, et al. The most useful findings for diagnosing acute appendicitis on contrast-enhanced helical CT. Acta Radiol 2003;44:574–82.

60. Lowe LH, Penney MW, Stein SM, et al. Unenhanced limited CT of the abdomen in the diagnosis of appendicitis in children: Comparison with sonography. AJR Am J Roentgenol 2001;176:31–5.

61. Peña BM, Taylor GA, Fishman SJ, et al. Costs and effectiveness of ultrasonography and limited computed tomography for diagnosing appendicitis in children. Pediatrics 2000;106:672–6.

62. Garcia Peña BM, Mandl KD, Kraus SJ, et al. Ultrasonography and limited computed tomography in the diagnosis and management of appendicitis in children. JAMA 1999;282:1041–6.

63. Pickuth D, Spielmann RP. Unenhanced spiral CT for evaluating acute appendicitis in daily routine: A prospective study. Hepatogastroenterology 2001;48:140–2.

64. Funaki B, Grosskreutz SR, Funaki CN. Using unenhanced helical CT with enteric contrast material for suspected appendicitis in patients treated at a community hospital. AJR Am J Roentgenol 1998;171:997–1001.

65. Weltman DI, Yu J, Krumenacker J Jr, et al. Diagnosis of acute appendicitis: Comparison of 5- and 10-mm CT sections in the same patient. Radiology 2000;216:172–7.

66. Jacobs JE, Birnbaum BA, Macari M, et al. Acute appendicitis: Comparison of helical CT diagnosis focused technique with oral contrast material versus nonfocused technique with oral and intravenous contrast material. Radiology 2001;220:683–90.

67. Fraser JD, Aguayo P, Sharp SW, et al. Accuracy of computed tomography in predicting appendiceal perforation. J Pediatr Surg 2010;45:231–5.

68. Brenner DJ. Estimating cancer risks from pediatric CT: Going from the qualitative to the quantitative. Pediatr Radiol 2002;32:228–33.

69. Garcia Pena BM, Cook EF, Mandl KD. Selective imaging strategies for the diagnosis of appendicitis in children. Pediatrics 2004;113:24–8.

70. Pena BM, Taylor GA, Fishman SJ, et al. Effect of an imaging protocol on clinical outcomes among pediatric patients with appendicitis. Pediatrics 2002;110:1088–93.

71. Martin AE, Vollman D, Adler B, et al. CT scans may not reduce the negative appendectomy rate in children. J Pediatr Surg 2004;39:886–90.

72. Linton OW, Mettler FA Jr. National Council on Radiation Protection and Measurements. National conference on dose reduction in CT, with an emphasis on pediatric patients. AJR Am J Roentgenol 2003;181:321–9.

73. Brody AS, Frush DP, Huda W, et al. Radiation risk to children from computed tomography. Pediatrics 2007;120:677–82.

74. Brennan GD. Pediatric appendicitis: Pathophysiology and appropriate use of diagnostic imaging. CJEM 2006;8:425–32.

75. Ware DE, Huda W, Mergo PJ, et al. Radiation effective doses to patients undergoing abdominal CT examinations. Radiology 1999;210:645–50.

76. Brenner DJ, Elliston CD, Hall EJ, et al. Estimated risks of radiation-induced fatal cancer from pediatric CT. Br J Radiol 2008;81:362–78.

77. Krishnamoorthi R, Ramarajan N, Wang N, et al. Effectiveness of a staged ultrasound and CT protocol for the diagnosis of pediatric appendicitis: Reducing radiation exposure in the age of ALARA. Radiology 2011;259:231–9.

78. Horman M, Paya K, Eibenberger K, et al. MR imaging in children with nonperforated acute appendicitis: Value of unenhanced MR imaging in sonographically selected cases. AJR Am J Roentgenol 1998;171:467–70.

79. Cope Z. Appendicitis and the differential diagnosis of acute appendicitis. In: Silen W, editor. Cope's Early Diagnosis of the Acute Abdomen. New York: Oxford University Press; 1991.

80. Cappendijk VC, Hazebroek FW. The impact of diagnostic delay on the course of acute appendicitis. Arch Dis Child 2000;83: 64–6.

81. Bliss D, McKee J, Cho D, et al. Discordance of the pediatric surgeon's intraoperative assessment of pediatric appendicitis with the pathologists report. J Pediatr Surg 2010;45:1398–403.

82. Ponsky T, Hafi M, Heiss K, et al. Interobserver variation in the assessment of appendiceal perforation. J Laparoendosc Adv Surg Tech A 2009;19(Suppl. 1):S15–18.

83. St Peter SD, Sharp SW, Holcomb GW, et al. An evidence-based definition for perforated appendicitis derived from a prospective randomized trial. J Pediatr Surg 2008;43:2242–5.

84. Emil S, Gaied F, Lo A, et al. Gangrenous appendicitis in children: A prospective evaluation of definition, bacteriology, histopathology, and outcomes. J Surg Res 2012; Accepted.

85. Nadler EP, Gaines BA. Therapeutic Agents Committee of the Surgical Infection Society: The Surgical Infection Society guidelines on antimicrobial therapy for children with appendicitis. Surg Infect (Larchmt) 2008;9:75–83.

86. Andersen BR, Kallehave FL, Andersen HK. Antibiotics versus placebo for prevention of postoperative complications after appendicectomy. Cochrane Database of Systematic Reviews 2005, Issue 3. Art. No.: CD001439. DOI: 10.1002/14651858.CD001439. pub2.

87. Mui LM, Ng CS, Wong SK, et al. Optimum duration of prophylactic antibiotics in acute non-perforated appendicitis. Aust NZ J Surg 2005;75:425–8.

88. Eriksson S, Granström L. Randomized controlled trial of appendicectomy versus antibiotic therapy for acute appendicitis. Br J Surg 1995;82:166–9.

89. Struyd J, Eriksson S, Nilsson I, et al. Appendectomy versus antibiotic treatment in acute appendicitis. A prospective multicenter randomized controlled trial. World J Surg 2006;30: 1033–7.

90. Hansson J, Körner U, Khorram-Manesh A, et al. Randomized clinical trial of antibiotic therapy versus appendicectomy as primary treatment of acute appendicitis in unselected patients. Br J Surg 2009;96:473–81.

91. Vons C, Barry C, Maitre S, et al. Amoxicillin plus clavulanic acid versus appendicectomy for treatment of acute uncomplicated appendicitis: An open-label, non-inferiority, randomised controlled trial. Lancet 2011;377(9777):1573–9.

92. Wilms IM, de Hoog DE, de Visser DC, et al. Appendectomy versus antibiotic treatment for acute appendicitis. Cochrane Database Syst Rev 2011;(11):CD008359.

93. Varadhan KK, Neal KR, Lobo DN. Safety and efficacy of antibiotics compared with appendicectomy for treatment of uncomplicated acute appendicitis: Meta-analysis of randomized controlled trials. BMJ 2012;344:e2156 doi: 10.1136/bmj.e2156.

94. Liu K, Ahanchi S, Pisaneschi M, et al. Can acute appendicitis be treated by antibiotics alone? Am Surg 2007;73:1161–5.

95. Friedell ML, Perez-Izquierdo M. Is there a role for interval appendectomy in the management of acute appendicitis? Am Surg 2000;66:1158–62.

96. Surana R, Quinn F, Puri P. Is it necessary to perform appendectomy in the middle of the night in children? BMJ 1993;306: 1168.

97. Yardeni D, Hirschl RB, Drongowski RA, et al. Delayed versus immediate surgery in acute appendicitis: Do we need to operate during the night? J Pediatr Surg 2004;39:464–9.

98. Stahlfeld K, Hower J, Homitsky S, et al. Is acute appendicitis a surgical emergency? Am Surg 2007;73:626–9.

99. Results of the North American trial of piperacillin/tazobactam compared with clindamycin and gentamicin in the treatment of severe intra-abdominal infections. Investigators of the Piperacillin/Tazobactam Intra-abdominal Infection Study Group. Eur J Surg Suppl 1994;573:61–6.

100. Nadler EP, Reblock KK, Ford HR, et al. Monotherapy versus multi-drug therapy for the treatment of perforated appendicitis in children. Surg Infect (Larchmt) 2003;4:327–33.

101. Maltezou HC, Nikolaidis P, Lebesii E, et al. Piperacillin/tazobactam versus cefotaxime plus metronidazole for treatment of children with intra-abdominal infections requiring surgery. Eur J Clin Microbiol Infect Dis 2001;20:643–6.

102. Lee SL, Islam S, Cassidy LD, et al. Antibiotics and appendicitis in the pediatric population: An American Pediatric Surgical Association outcomes and clinical trials committee systematic review. J Pediatr Surg 2010;45:2181–5.

103. St Peter SD, Tsao K, Spilde TL, et al. Single daily dosing of ceftriaxone and metronidazole vs. standard triple antibiotic regimen for perforated appendicitis in children: A prospective randomized trial. J Pediatr Surg 2008;43:981–5.

104. Fraser JD, Aguayo P, Leys CM, et al. A complete course of intravenous antibiotics vs a combination of intravenous and oral antibiotics for perforated appendicitis in children: A prospective, randomized trial. J Pediatr Surg 2010;45:1198–202.

105. Henry MC, Walker A, Silverman BL, et al. Risk factors for the development of abdominal abscess following operation for perforated appendicitis in children: A multicenter case-control study. Arch Surg 2007;142:236–41.

106. Kogut KA, Blakely ML, Schropp KP, et al. The association of elevated percent bands on admission with failure and complications of interval appendectomy. J Pediatr Surg 2001;36:165–8.

107. Aprahamian CJ, Barnhart DC, Bledsoe SE, et al. Failure in the nonoperative management of pediatric ruptured appendicitis: predictors and consequences. J Pediatr Surg 2007;42:934–8.

108. Levin T, Whyte C, Borzykowski R, et al. Nonoperative management of perforated appendicitis in children: Can CT predict outcome? Pediatr Radiol 2007;37:251–5.

109. Simillis C, Symeonides P, Shorthouse AJ, et al. A meta-analysis comparing conservative treatment versus acute appendectomy for complicated appendicitis (abscess or phlegmon). Surgery 2010; 147:818–29.

110. Ein SH, Shandling B. Is interval appendectomy necessary after rupture of an appendiceal mass? J Pediatr Surg 1996;31: 849–50.

111. Puapong D, Lee SL, Haigh PI, et al. Routine interval appendectomy in children is not indicated. J Pediatr Surg 2007;42: 1500–3.

112. Hall NJ, Jones CE, Eaton S, et al. Is interval appendectomy justified after successful nonoperative treatment of an appendix mass in children? A systematic review. J Pediatr Surg 2011;46:767– 71.

113. Gahukamble DB, Gahukamble LD. Surgical and pathological basis for interval appendectomy after resolution of appendicular mass in children. J Pediatr Surg 2000;35:424–7.

114. Mazziotti MV, Marley EF, Winthrop AL, et al. Histopathologic analysis of interval appendectomy specimens: Support for the role of interval appendectomy. J Pediatr Surg 1997;32:806–9.

115. Janik JS, Ein SH, Shandling B, et al. Nonsurgical management of appendiceal mass in late presenting children. J Pediatr Surg 1980;15:574–6.

116. Muehlstedt SG, Pham TQ, Schmeling DJ. The management of pediatric appendicitis: A survey of North American Pediatric Surgeons. J Pediatr Surg 2004;39:875–9.

117. Morrow SE, Newman KD. Current management of appendicitis. Semin Pediatr Surg 2007;16:34–40.

118. Owen A, Moore O, Marven S, et al. Interval laparoscopic appendectomy in children. J Laparoendosc Adv Surg Tech 2006; 16:308–11.

119. Weiner DZ, Katz A, Hirschl RB, et al. Interval appendectomy in perforated appendicitis. Pediatr Surg Int 1995;10:82–5.

120. St Peter SD, Aguayo P, Fraser JD, et al. Initial laparoscopic appendectomy versus initial nonoperative management and interval appendectomy for perforated appendicitis with abscess: A prospective, randomized trial. J Pediatr Surg 2010;45:236–40.

121. Schurman JV, Cushing CC, Garey CL, et al. Quality of life assessment between laparoscopic appendectomy at presentation and interval appendectomy for perforated appendicitis with abscess: Analysis of a prospective, randomized trial. J Pediatr Surg 2011;46:1121–5.

122. Blakely ML, Williams R, Dassinger MS, et al. Early vs. interval appendectomy for children with perforated appendicitis. Arch Surg 2011;146:660–5.

123. Goh BK, Chui CH, Yap TL, et al. Is early laparoscopic appendectomy feasible in children with acute appendicitis presenting with an appendiceal mass? A prospective study. J Pediatr Surg 2005;40:1134–7.

124. Senapathi PS, Bhattacharya D, Ammori BJ. Early laparoscopic appendectomy for appendicular mass. Surg Endosc 2002;16:1783–5.

125. Myers AL, Williams RF, Giles K, et al. Hospital cost analysis of a prospective randomized trial of early vs interval appendectomy for perforated appendicitis in children. J Am Coll Surg 2012;214:427–34.

126. McBurney C. The incision made in the abdominal wall in cases of appendicitis, with a description of a new method of operating. Ann Surg 1894;20:38–43.

127. Semm K. Endoscopic appendectomy. Endoscopy 1983;15:54–64.

128. Lintula H, Kokki H, Vanamo K, et al. Laparoscopy in children with complicated appendicitis. J Pediatr Surg 2002;37:1317–20.

129. Horwitz JR, Custer MD, May BH, et al. Should laparoscopic appendectomy be avoided for complicated appendicitis in children? J Pediatr Surg 1997;32:1601–3.

130. Eypasch E, Sauerland S, Lefering R, et al. Laparoscopic versus open appendectomy: Between evidence and common sense. Dig Surg 2002;19:518–22.

131. Nataraja RM, Teague WJ, Galea J, et al. Comparison of intraabdominal abscess formation after laparoscopic and open appendectomies in children. J Pediatr Surg 2012;47:317–21.

132. Varela JE, Hinojosa MW, Nguyen NT. Laparoscopy should be the approach of choice for acute appendicitis in the morbidly obese. Am J Surg 2008;196:218–22.

133. Corneille MG, Steigelman MB, Myers JG, et al. Laparoscopic appendectomy is superior to open appendectomy in obese patients. Am J Surg 2007;194:877–80.

134. Esposito C, Borzi P, Valla JS, et al. Laparoscopic versus open appendectomy in children: A retrospective comparative study of 2,332 cases. World J Surg 2007;31:750–5.

135. Jen HC, Shew SB. Laparoscopic versus open appendectomy in children: Outcomes comparison based on a statewide analysis. J Surg Res 2010;161:13–17.

136. Lee SL, Yaghoubian A, Kaji A. Laparoscopic versus open appendectomy in children: Outcomes comparison based on age, sex, and perforation status. Arch Surg 2011;146:1118–21.

137. Masoomi H, Mills S, Dolich MO, et al. Comparison of outcomes of laparoscopic versus open appendectomy in children: Data from the nationwide inpatient sample (NIS), 2006–2008. World J Surg 2012;36:573–8.

138. Aziz O, Athanasiou T, Tekkis PP, et al. Laparoscopic versus open appendectomy in children: A meta-analysis. Ann Surg 2006;243:17–27.

139. Yau KK, Siu WT, Tang CN, et al. Laparoscopic versus open appendectomy for complicated appendicitis. J Am Coll Surg 2007;205:60–5.

140. Olmi S, Magnone S, Bertolini A, et al. Laparoscopic versus open appendectomy in acute appendicitis: A randomized prospective study. Surg Endosc 2005;19:1193–5.

141. Moberg AC, Berndsen F, Palmquist I, et al. Randomized clinical trial of laparoscopic versus open appendicectomy for confirmed appendicitis. Br J Surg 2005;92:298–304.

142. Carbonell AM, Burns JM, Lincourt AE, et al. Outcomes of laparoscopic versus open appendectomy. Am Surg 2004;70:759–65.

143. Sauerland S, Jaschinski T, Neugebauer EA. Laparoscopic versus open surgery for suspected appendicitis. Cochrane Databse Syst Rev 2010:CD001546.

144. Taqi E, Hadher SA, Ryckman J, et al. Outcome of laparoscopic appendectomy for perforated appendicitis in children. J Pediatr Surg 2008;43;893–5.

145. Katkhouda N, Mason RJ, Towfigh S, et al. Laparoscopic versus open appendectomy: A prospective randomized double-blind study. Ann Surg 2005;242:439–48.

146. Garey CL, Laituri CA, Little DC, et al. Outcomes of perforated appendicitis in obese and non-obese children. J Pediatr Surg 2011;46:2346–8.

147. Menezes M, Das L, Alagtal M, et al. Laparoscopic appendectomy is recommended for the treatment of complicated appendicitis in children. Pediatr Surg Int 2008;24:303–5.

148. Paterson HM, Qadan M, de Luca SM, et al. Changing trends in surgery for acute appendicitis. Br J Surg 2008;95:363–8.

149. Khan MN, Fayyad T, Cecil TD, et al. Laparoscopic versus open appendectomy: The risk of postoperative infectious complications. JSLS 2007;11:363–7.

150. Lin HF, Wu JM, Tseng LM, et al. Laparoscopic versus open appendectomy for perforated appendicitis. J Gastrointest Surg 2006;10:906–10.

151. Ikeda H, Ishimaru Y, Takayasu H, et al. Laparoscopic versus open appendectomy in children with uncomplicated and complicated appendicitis. J Pediatr Surg 2004;39:1680–5.

152. Guller U, Hervey S, Purves H, et al. Laparoscopic versus open appendectomy: Outcomes comparison based on a large administrative database. Ann Surg 2004;239:43–52.

153. Marzouk M, Khater M, Elsadek M, et al. Laparoscopic versus open appendectomy: A prospective comparative study of 227 patients. Surg Endosc 2003;17:721–4.

154. Nadler EP, Reblock KK, Qureshi FG, et al. Laparoscopic appendectomy in children with perforated appendicitis. J Laparoendosc Adv Surg Tech 2006;16:159–63.

155. Fraser JD, Aguayo P, Sharp SW, et al. Physiologic predictors of postoperative abscess in children with perforated appendicitis: Subset analysis from a prospective randomized trial. Surgery 2010;147:729–32.

156. Yagmurlu A, Vernon A, Barnhart DC, et al. Laparoscopic appendectomy for perforated appendicitis: A comparison with open appendectomy. Surg Endosc 2006;20:1051–4.

157. Bilik R, Burnweit C, Shandling B. Is abdominal cavity culture of any value in appendicitis? Am J Surg 1998;175:267–70.

158. Kokoska ER, Silen ML, Tracy TF, et al. The impact of intraoperative culture on treatment and outcome in children with perforated appendicitis. J Pediatr Surg 1999;34:749–53.

159. Sherman JO, Luck SR, Borger JA. Irrigation of the peritoneal cavity for appendicitis in children: A double-blind study. J Pediatr Surg 1976;11:371–4.

160. Kokoska ER, Silen ML, Tracy TF, et al. Perforated appendicitis in children: Risk factors for the development of complications. Surgery 1998;124:619–25.

161. David IB, Buck JR, Filler RM. Rational use of antibiotics for perforated appendicitis in childhood. J Pediatr Surg 1982;17:494–500.

162. Kaselas C, Molinaro F, Lacreuse I, et al. Postoperative bowel obstruction after laparoscopic appendectomy in children: A 15-year experience. J Pediatr Surg 2009;44:1581–5.

163. Tsao KJ, St Peter SD, Valusek PA, et al. Adhesive small bowel obstruction after appendectomy in children: Comparison between the laparoscopic and open approach. J Pediatr Surg 2007;42:939–42.

164. St Peter SD, Adibe OO, Juang D, et al. Single incision versus standard 3-port laparoscopic appendectomy: A prospective randomized trial. Ann Surg 2011;254:586–90.

165. Langness SM, Hill SJ, Wulkan ML. Single-site laparoscopic appendectomy: A comparison to traditional laparoscopic technique in children. Am Surg 2011;77:961–4.

166. Muensterer OJ, Puga Nouges C, Adibe OO, et al. Appendectomy using single-incision pediatric endosurgery for acute and perforated appendicitis. Surg Endosc 2010;24:3201–4.

167. Sesia SB, Haecker FM, Kubiak R, et al. Laparoscopy-assisted single-port appendectomy in children: Is the postoperative complication rate different? J Laparoendosc Adv Surg Tech 2010;20:867–71.

168. Shekherdimian S, DeUgarte D. Transumbilical laparoscopic-assisted appendectomy: An extracorporeal single-incision

alternative to conventional laparoscopic techniques. Am Surg 2011;77:557–60.

169. Guana R, Gesmundo R, Maiullari E, et al. Treatment of acute appendicitis with one-port transumbilical laparoscopic appendectomy: A six-year, single-centre experience. Afr J Paediatr Surg 2010;7:169–73.

170. Stanfill AB, Matinsky DK, Kalvakuri K, et al. Transumbilical laparoscopically assisted appendectomy: An alternative minimally invasive technique in pediatric patients. J Laparoendosc Adv Surg Tech 2010;20:873–6.

171. Ohno Y, Morimura T, Hayashi S. Transumbilical laparoscopically assisted appendectomy in children: The results of a single-port, single-channel procedure. Surg Endosc 2012;26:523–7.

172. Garey CL, Laituri CA, Ostlie DJ, et al. A review of single site minimally invasive surgery in infants and children. Pediatr Surg Int 2010;26:451–6.

CHAPTER 43

BILIARY ATRESIA

Atsuyuki Yamataka • Joel Cazares • Takeshi Miyano

Biliary atresia is a relatively rare obstructive condition of the bile ducts causing neonatal jaundice. There is a variable incidence around the world (eg, Europe, 1 in 18,000 live births; France, 1 in 19,500 live births; the UK and Ireland, 1 in 16,700 live births; Sweden, 1 in 14,000 live births; and Japan, 1 in 9640 live births),[1–6] with the highest recorded incidence in French Polynesia (1 in 3124 live births).[7] There is a slight female predominance.

Biliary atresia first appeared as a distinct entity in the Edinburgh Medical Journal in 1891.[8] The concept of 'correctable' and 'noncorrectable' forms was introduced in 1916.[9] Despite the first successful surgical treatment for the correctable type being reported in 1928, there were only a few long-term survivors over the next three decades, all with the correctable type.[10–12]

In the 1950s and 60s, a variety of procedures for 'noncorrectable' disease were developed, but none provided consistent biliary decompression.[13–17] Also, the timing of operative intervention was controversial, with reports of 'spontaneous' cures, and second-look explorations for the rather mystical belief that a totally fibrotic extrahepatic ductal system might subsequently become patent.[18–22]

In 1959, the now common Kasai hepatic portoenterostomy procedure was first described and ended a long, hopeless era for patients with the noncorrectable-type disease.[23] Kasai's original report was in Japanese and received little attention until it was published in English in 1968.[24] Although effective bile drainage could be achieved after portoenterostomy in about 50% of patients, early repair was crucial and needed to be performed before the age of 2 months. Conversely, effective bile drainage was observed in only 7% of patients if correction was performed after the age of 4 months.[25] Kasai's portoenterostomy procedure gradually gained popularity in the USA, and by the 1990s, more than 90% of infants with biliary atresia had undergone this procedure.[26]

Since liver transplantation has become a viable treatment option for liver failure in the pediatric population, biliary atresia has become the most common indication for liver transplantation in children. Infants whose jaundice does not resolve after portoenterostomy, or those with complications associated with end-stage chronic liver disease related to biliary atresia, will usually require liver transplantation within the first few years of life.

The combination of hepatic portoenterostomy and liver transplantation has transformed a disease that was nearly universally fatal in the 1960s into one with an overall five-year survival of about 90%. Despite the debate over whether hepatic portoenterostomy or primary liver transplantation should be performed as the initial procedure for biliary atresia, the consensus among pediatric surgeons around the world is that hepatic portoenterostomy is the most reasonable first choice.

Recently, the authors had an opportunity to review an original video of Professor Kasai performing his own portoenterostomy.[27] Interestingly, his original portal dissection was actually quite shallow and limited, resulting in a narrow portoenterostomy anastomosis, with sutures placed shallowly at 2 and 10 o'clock where the native right and left bile ducts would have been, probably to minimize microscopic bile duct injury. Although not supported by research, the original technique as performed by Kasai may result in superior outcomes as it focuses specifically on the physiologic and anatomic characteristics of the liver in biliary atresia. The authors currently perform a modified version of Kasai's original portoenterostomy (KOPE) using the minimally invasive approach.

PATHOGENESIS

Various etiologic mechanisms for biliary atresia have been postulated, including intrauterine or perinatal viral infection, genetic mutations, abnormal ductal plate remodeling, vascular or metabolic insult to the developing biliary tree, pancreaticobiliary ductal malunion, and immunologically mediated inflammation. However, despite intensive interest and investigation, the cause of biliary atresia remains unknown and there is no ideal animal model.

There are syndromic and nonsyndromic forms of biliary atresia.[28] Syndromic biliary atresia (also known as the embryonic type) is associated with other congenital anomalies, including interrupted inferior vena cava, preduodenal portal vein, intestinal malrotation, situs inversus, cardiac defects, and polysplenia.[29] Syndromic biliary atresia accounts for 10–20% of all cases, and is likely to be due to a developmental insult occurring during differentiation of the hepatic diverticulum from the foregut of the embryo. A possible relation between syndromic biliary atresia and maternal diabetes has been reported.[28] Nonsyndromic biliary atresia (also known as the perinatal type) may have its origins later in gestation, and may have a different clinical course, with biliary obstruction being progressive.

Reovirus type 3 infection, rotavirus, cytomegalovirus (CMV), papillomavirus, and Epstein–Barr virus have all been proposed as possible etiologic agents, but conclusive evidence is lacking. In one report, CMV infection was found in four of ten patients with biliary atresia,[30] and reovirus infection has been found in the livers of up to 55% of biliary atresia patients versus 10–20% in a control group.[31] The identification of viruses in children with biliary atresia is inconsistent in the literature, and several viruses have been used to create animal models that may be valuable for assessing the pathogenesis and treatment of biliary atresia.

Generally, biliary atresia is not considered an inherited disorder. However, genetic mutations that result in defective morphogenesis may be important in syndromic biliary atresia. Transgenic mice with a recessive deletion of the inversin gene have situs inversus and an interrupted extrahepatic biliary tree.[32] Mutations of the *CFC1* gene, which is involved in left–right axis determination in humans, have been identified in a few patients with syndromic biliary atresia.[33] The importance of the macrophage migration inhibitory factor gene, which is a pleiotropic lymphocyte and macrophage cytokine in biliary atresia pathogenesis, has also been reported.[34] Other studies have identified abnormalities in laterality genes in a small number of patients with biliary atresia, including the transcription factor ZIC3.[35] A high incidence of polymorphic variants in the jagged-1, keratin-8, and keratin-18 genes have also been described in a series of 18 children with biliary atresia.[36,37] Taken together, the increased incidence of nonhepatic anomalies in children with biliary atresia and genetic mutations reported in subsets of patients with laterality defects suggest that multiple genes are involved, each affecting a small number of patients.

Intrahepatic bile ducts are derived from primitive hepatocytes that form a sleeve (the ductal plate) around the intrahepatic portal vein branches and associated mesenchyme early in gestation. Remodeling of the ductal plate in fetal life results in the formation of the intrahepatic biliary system. This is supported by similarities in cytokeratin immunostaining between biliary ductules in biliary atresia and normal first-trimester fetal bile ducts.[38] These findings suggest that nonsyndromic biliary atresia might be caused by a failure of bile duct remodeling at the hepatic hilum, with persistence of fetal bile ducts poorly supported by mesenchyme.

Several studies have investigated whether bile duct epithelial cells are susceptible to an immune/inflammatory attack because of abnormal expression of human leukocyte antigen (HLA) antigens or intracellular adhesion molecules on their surfaces.[39,40] A greater than threefold increase in HLA-B12 antigen has been found in babies with biliary atresia compared with controls, particularly in those with no associated malformations.[41] Aberrant expression of class II HLA-DR antigens on biliary epithelial cells and damaged hepatocytes in patients with biliary atresia may render these tissues more susceptible to immune-mediated damage by cytotoxic T-cells or locally released cytokines.[42] Increased expression of intercellular adhesion molecule-1 (ICAM-1) has been noted on bile duct epithelium in patients with biliary atresia, a finding that may play a role in immune-mediated damage.[40] Strong expression of ICAM-1 also has been found on proliferating bile ductules, endothelial cells, and hepatocytes in biliary atresia. A direct relationship exists between the degree of ductal expression of ICAM-1 and disease severity, suggesting that ICAM-1 might be important in the development of cirrhosis.[43]

Interest has also focused on co-stimulatory molecules. Two processes are involved in the activation of T lymphocytes by antigen-presenting cells (APC). One relates to the expression of major histocompatibility complex class II molecules, which interact directly with T-cell receptors. The other depends on the expression of B7 antigens on APC, and provides the second (co-stimulatory) signal to T-lymphocytes through CD28.[44] In postoperative biliary atresia patients with good liver function, co-stimulatory antigens (B7-1, B7-2, and CD40) are expressed only on bile duct epithelial cells, whereas in patients with failing livers these markers are found on the surfaces of Kupffer cells, dendritic cells, and sinusoidal endothelial cells and in the cytoplasm of hepatocytes.[45] This suggests that the biliary epithelium and hepatocytes in biliary atresia are susceptible to immune recognition and destruction. Agents that block or prevent co-stimulatory pathways might offer a new therapeutic approach for reducing liver damage.

Two studies have involved comprehensive molecular and cellular surveys of liver biopsies and found a proinflammatory gene expression signature, with increased activation of interferon-γ, osteopontin, tumor necrosis factor-α, and other inflammatory mediators.[46,47] These studies may prove to be helpful in delineating the molecular networks responsible for the proinflammatory response and autoimmunity thought to be involved in the pathogenesis of biliary atresia. However, none of these mechanisms appears to be mutually exclusive. Moreover, it is not clear which signs and symptoms are primary and which are secondary.

In summary, the etiology of nonsyndromic biliary atresia is hypothesized to involve a viral or other toxic insult to the bile duct epithelium that induces the expression of new antigens on the surfaces of biliary epithelial cells.[48] Coupled with a genetically predetermined susceptibility that is mediated via histocompatibility antigens, these neoantigens are recognized by circulating T-lymphocytes, resulting in an immune cell mediated, fibrosclerosing response.

CLASSIFICATION

Biliary atresia can be classified by using macroscopic appearance and cholangiography findings into three main categories: atresia of the common bile duct (CBD) (type I), atresia of the common hepatic duct (type IIa) or atresia of the CBD and the common hepatic duct (type IIb), and atresia of all extrahepatic bile ducts up to the porta hepatis (type III) (Fig. 43-1). Most patients have type III. In patients with a patent CBD and cystic duct (correctable type) (5% of cases), the gallbladder can be anastomosed to the porta hepatis, (gallbladder Kasai). In more than 90% of cases, however, no patent extrahepatic ductal structures are found at the porta hepatis (i.e., 'noncorrectable' type).[49]

HISTOPATHOLOGY

Early in the course of biliary atresia, the liver becomes enlarged, firm, and green. The gallbladder may be small

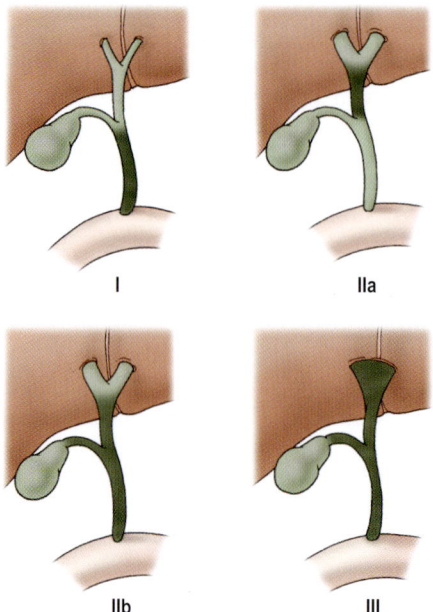

FIGURE 43-1 ■ Morphologic classification of biliary atresia based on macroscopic and cholangiographic findings. Type I, occlusion of common bile duct; type IIa, obliteration of common hepatic duct; type IIb, obliteration of common bile duct, hepatic and cystic ducts, with cystic dilatation of ducts at the porta hepatis, and no gallbladder involvement; type III, obliteration of common, hepatic, and cystic ducts without anastomosable ducts at porta hepatis. (From Lefkowitch JH. Biliary atresia. Mayo Clin Proc 1998;73:90–5.)

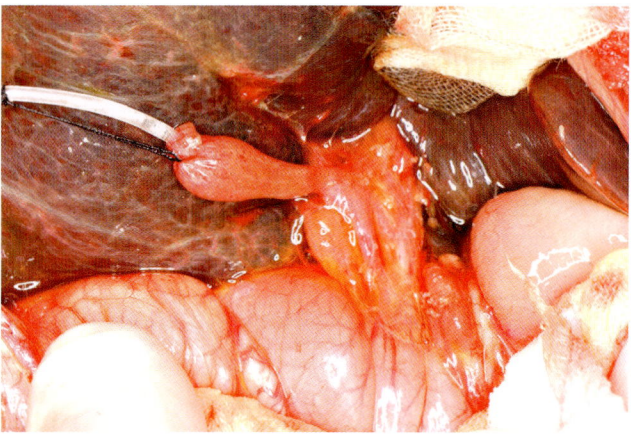

FIGURE 43-2 ■ Type III biliary atresia with an enlarged, firm, green liver and hypoplastic small gallbladder was found in this infant.

and filled with white mucus, or it may be completely atretic (Fig. 43-2). Microscopically, the biliary tracts contain inflammatory and fibrous cells surrounding miniscule ducts, which are probably remnants of the original embryonic duct system. The liver parenchyma is fibrotic and shows signs of cholestasis. Proliferation of biliary neoductules is seen (Fig. 43-3). This process develops into end-stage cirrhosis if adequate biliary drainage cannot be achieved. These early changes are often nonspecific and may be confused with neonatal hepatitis and metabolic diseases.

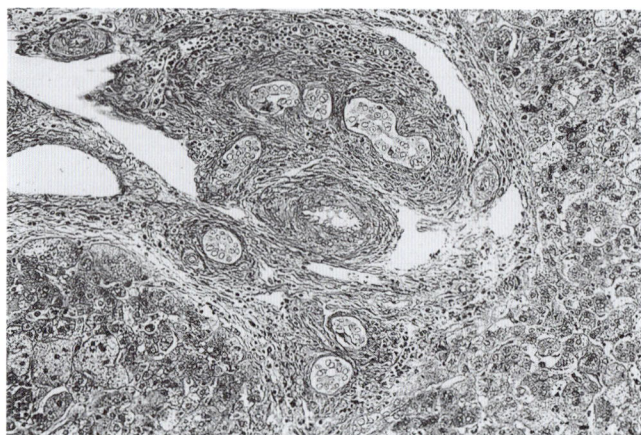

FIGURE 43-3 ■ Photomicrograph of the portal tract of the liver in a 60-day-old infant with biliary atresia. Ductal plate malformation can be seen in the center of the portal space with portal fibrosis. Note ductal metaplasia of hepatocytes (Azan stain, ×100).

It is generally accepted that the pathologic changes seen in biliary atresia are panductal, affecting the intrahepatic biliary tree as well as the extrahepatic bile duct system. Moreover, the intrahepatic bile ducts can be narrowed, distorted in configuration, or irregular in shape.[50–52] However, some authors believe that secondary damage occurs only to the extrahepatic biliary system as a result of obliteration of extrahepatic bile ducts during liver formation.[53] This theory is strongly supported by the fact that outcome is better if the portoenterostomy is performed early.

The intrahepatic biliary tree is important not only pathologically, but also clinically. The degree of damage that has already occurred in the intrahepatic biliary system is actually responsible for much of the morbidity after hepatic portoenterostomy. Intrahepatic bile duct proliferation likely results from disturbances in formation of the ductal plate as well as ductular metaplasia of hepatocytes.[54,55]

Certain substances can act as prognostic factors in biliary atresia. Serum levels of interleukin (IL)-6, IL-1ra, insulin-like growth factor-1 (IGF-1), vascular cell adhesion molecule-1 (VCAM-1), and ICAM-1 correlate with liver dysfunction in postoperative biliary atresia patients.[43,56,57] Immunohistochemically, a reduction in the expression of CD68 and ICAM-1 at the time of portoenterostomy is associated with a better prognosis.[58] The presence of ductal plate malformation in the liver predicts poor bile flow after hepatoportoenterostomy in infants with biliary atresia.[59] Growth failure and poor mean weight z-scores three months after hepatoportoenterostomy are also associated with a poor clinical outcome.[60]

DIAGNOSIS

The cardinal signs and symptoms of biliary atresia are jaundice, clay-colored stools, and hepatomegaly. However, meconium staining is normal in most patients. In the neonatal period, feces are yellow in more than half of patients.[61] The newborn's urine becomes dark brown. Although the neonates are active, and their growth is usually normal for the first few months, anemia, malnutrition, and growth retardation develop gradually because of malabsorption of fat-soluble vitamins. Jaundice that persists beyond two weeks should no longer be considered physiologic, particularly if the elevation in bilirubin is mainly in the direct fraction. Neonatal hepatitis and interlobular biliary hypoplasia are most likely to be confused with biliary atresia. Conventional liver function tests alone are useless for establishing a definitive diagnosis of biliary atresia.

Although a number of diagnostic protocols have been published, the emphasis must always be on early diagnosis (Box 43-1).[62,63] The definitive diagnosis of biliary atresia requires further investigations, including special biochemical studies, tests to confirm the patency of the extrahepatic bile ducts, and needle biopsy of the liver. Several authors consider liver biopsy to be the most reliable test for establishing the diagnosis.[64,65] Serum lipoprotein-X is positive in all patients with biliary atresia, although it also is positive in 20–40% of patients with neonatal hepatitis. Serum bile acid levels increase in infants with cholestatic disease, but both the total bile acid level and the ratio of chenodeoxycholic acid to cholic acid have no value for differentiating biliary atresia from other cholestatic diseases.[66] Hyaluronic acid, which has been considered a serum marker for liver function, has also been reported to be a biochemical marker for evaluating infants with biliary atresia.[67] Duodenal aspiration is an easy, noninvasive, and rapid test because biliary atresia can be excluded if bilirubin-stained fluid is aspirated.[68]

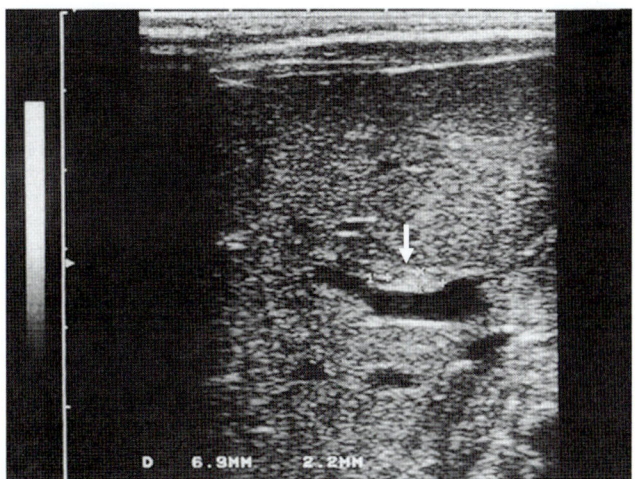

FIGURE 43-4 ■ Ultrasonography shows a well-defined triangular area of high echogenicity (arrow) at the porta hepatis, corresponding to fibrotic ductal remnants (the 'triangular cord' sign).

Hepatobiliary scintigraphy with technetium-labeled agents is widely used for differentiating biliary atresia from other cholestatic diseases. In biliary atresia, nucleotide uptake by hepatocytes is rapid, but excretion into the bowel is absent, even on delayed images. In hepatocellular jaundice, isotope uptake is delayed owing to parenchymal disease. Excretion into the intestine may or may not be seen.

Ultrasonography (US) should be performed on all jaundiced infants. Hepatobiliary ultrasound will exclude other surgical causes of jaundice such as choledochal cyst and inspissated bile syndrome. In biliary atresia, the intrahepatic ducts are not dilated on ultrasound because they are affected by the inflammatory process. Various sonographic features have been targeted in an attempt to distinguish biliary atresia from other causes of conjugated hyperbilirubinemia in infants.[69–73] In biliary atresia, the gallbladder is small, shrunken, and noncontractile, and there is increased echogenicity of the liver. The presence of other associated anomalies of the polysplenia syndrome is pathognomonic of biliary atresia.[74] Differentiation from choledochal cyst and type I biliary atresia also is rapid and simple with ultrasound.[75] Irrespective of interobserver variation, failure to visualize the CBD is not diagnostic of biliary atresia because a patent distal CBD can be found in up to 20% of biliary atresia cases. However, an absent gallbladder or one with an irregular outline is suggestive of biliary atresia.[73] In some cases, a well-defined triangular area of high reflectivity is seen at the porta hepatis, corresponding to fibrotic ductal remnants (the 'triangular cord' sign) (Fig. 43-4).[70,71]

Nonvisualization of the fetal gallbladder may indicate abnormalities ranging from gallbladder agenesis to biliary atresia.[76] Amniotic fluid digestive enzymes, which are synthesized by the biliary epithelium, gradually decrease until 24 weeks of gestation. As it is no longer possible to differentiate between abnormally low and physiologically low levels of the enzymes after 24 weeks of gestation, the prenatal diagnosis of biliary atresia is difficult.[77]

Most patients with biliary atresia can be correctly diagnosed by using an appropriate combination of the

---

BOX 43-1	**Clinical Findings and Examination for Diagnosis of Biliary Atresia**

Routine Examinations

Color of stool
Consistency of the liver
Conventional liver function tests, including test for γ-glutamyl transpeptidase
Coagulation times (PT, aPTT)

Special Examinations

Special biochemical studies
  Hepatitis A, B, C serologic studies
  TORCH titers
  α1-Antitrypsin level
  Serum lipoprotein-X
  Serum bile acid
Confirmation of patency of extrahepatic bile ducts
  Duodenal fluid aspiration
  Ultrasonography
  Hepatobiliary scintigraphy
  Endoscopic retrograde cholangiopancreatography
  Near-infrared reflectance spectroscopy
Needle biopsy of the liver for histopathologic studies
Laparoscopy
Surgical cholangiography

aPTT, activated partial thromboplastin time; PT, prothrombin time; TORCH, toxoplasmosis, other viruses, rubella, cytomegalovirus, and herpes simplex virus.

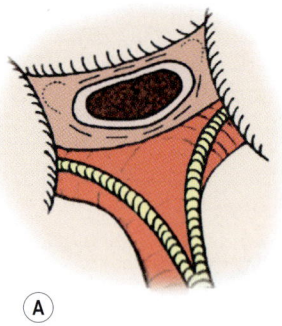 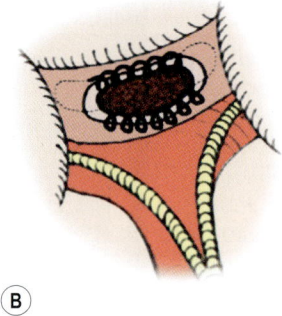 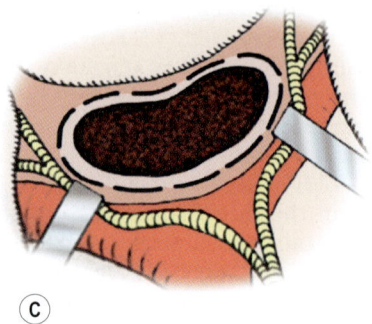

Ⓐ   Ⓑ   Ⓒ

FIGURE 43-5 ■ Salient features of three portoenterostomy procedures are depicted. **(A)** Modified Kasai portoenterostomy: Interrupted shallow sutures (thin broken lines) are placed in the liver parenchyma around the transected biliary remnant, except at the 2 and 10 o'clock positions, where the right and left bile ducts should be. If sutures are necessary at the 2 and 10 o'clock positions to prevent an anastomotic leak, shallow interrupted sutures (thin dotted lines) are placed only in the connective tissue near the right and left hepatic arteries or the hepatoduodenal ligament at the porta hepatis. **(B)** Kasai's original portoenterostomy:[23,25] A continuous suture (looped line) is placed in the side of the transected biliary remnant, except at the 2 and 10 o'clock positions, where sutures (dotted lines) are placed in the connective tissue. **(C)** Extended portoenterostomy: Deep interrupted sutures (bold broken lines) are placed in the liver parenchyma, even at the 2 and 10 o'clock positions. (From Nakamura H, Koga H, Wada M, et al. Reappraising the portoenterostomy procedure according to sound physiological/anatomic principles enhances postoperative jaundice clearance in biliary atresia. Pediatr Surg 2012;28:205; and From Yamataka A, Lane GJ, Cazares J. Laparoscopic surgery for biliary atresia and choledochal cyst. Sem Pediatr Surg 2012;21:201.)

investigations just outlined. However, to accurately differentiate biliary atresia, biliary hypoplasia, and severe neonatal hepatitis, cholangiography is usually required.

Recently, laparoscopy-assisted cholangiography has been used to display the anatomic structure of the biliary tree.[78] Also, percutaneous cholecystocholangiography may be a useful option to prevent unnecessary laparotomy in infants whose cholestasis is caused by diseases other than biliary atresia.[79]

OPERATIVE MANAGEMENT

Open Surgical Technique

Prior to operative exploration, daily doses of vitamin K should be given for several days, and broad-spectrum antibiotics are administered preoperatively.

The portoenterostomy procedure for biliary atresia has been repeatedly modified to achieve better rates of jaundice clearance and survival, and hardly resembles Kasai's original portoenterostomy (Fig. 43-5B). The current favored technique involves an extended lateral dissection around the porta hepatis with a very wide anastomosis (extended portoenterostomy, or EPE) (Fig. 43-5C).[80,81]

EPE is the most widely used open approach for treating biliary atresia. The patient is placed supine on an operating table with the capability for intraoperative cholangiography. An extended right subcostal incision, dividing the muscle layers, is used to expose the inferior margin of the liver. After division of the falciform and triangular ligaments, the liver is delivered from the abdominal cavity. This maneuver provides an excellent operative field for dissection of the porta hepatis. Cholangiography is recommended to identify the anatomy (Fig. 43-6). The fundus of the gallbladder is mobilized from the liver bed, and a 4–6 French feeding tube is passed

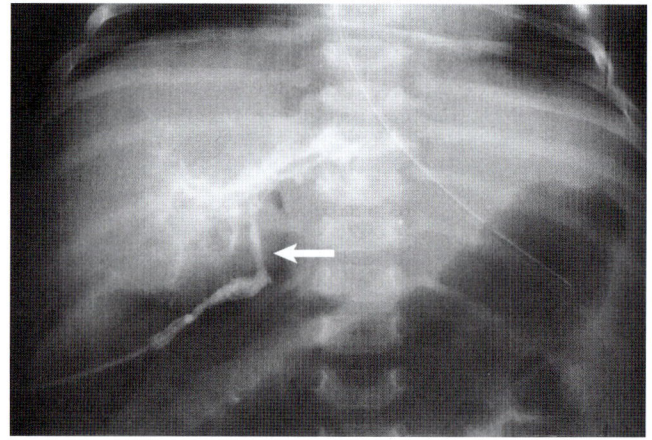

FIGURE 43-6 ■ Intraoperative cholangiogram, type III biliary atresia. Note the almost atretic common bile duct (arrow).

into the gallbladder through a small cholecystotomy incision. If bile is detected on aspiration from the gallbladder, a small amount of contrast material is injected. However, in most patients with biliary atresia, the lumen of the atrophic gall bladder is already obstructed, and it is impossible to insert even a 4 French catheter. Thus, cholangiography cannot be performed. Unless normal anatomy of the intrahepatic biliary system can be confirmed, hepatic portoenterostomy is performed.[24,82]

The cystic artery is ligated and divided and the gallbladder is dissected from the liver bed. The mobilized gallbladder is used as a guide for locating the fibrous remnant of the CBD. After the caudal end of the CBD is ligated and divided at the upper border of the duodenum, the cephalad portion of the CBD with the gallbladder attached is dissected above the bifurcation of the portal vein. The portal vein and the hepatic arteries are exposed along their entire course. For better portal dissection, the right and left hepatic arteries and the right and left portal branches are individually encircled with vessel loops (Fig. 43-7A). The hepatic ducts usually form a cone-shaped fibrous mass anterior to the bifurcation of the portal vein. Several small vessels connecting the portal vein to the fibrous cone are divided after being ligated. The posterior aspect of the fibrous cone is freed completely. The anterior aspect of the fibrous cone and the quadrate lobe of the liver are then exposed. The fibrous biliary plate should be dissected as far as the entrance of the anterior branch of the right hepatic artery on the right side and as far left as the entrance of the obliterated umbilical vein into the left portal vein. The fibrous cone is sharply transected at the level of the posterior surface of the portal vein with scissors or a scalpel, and is removed. The fibrous cone should have an extensive transected surface that allows a wide anastomosis. In other words, in EPE, dissection of the porta hepatis is not confined just to the area around the base of the fibrous ductal plate.[83,84] As much of the transected hilar surface as possible, including all potentially usable remnants of the intrahepatic ducts in the area between and beneath the branches of the right and left portal veins, is incorporated in the anastomosis. Also, the right and left portal veins and hepatic arteries must be retracted to

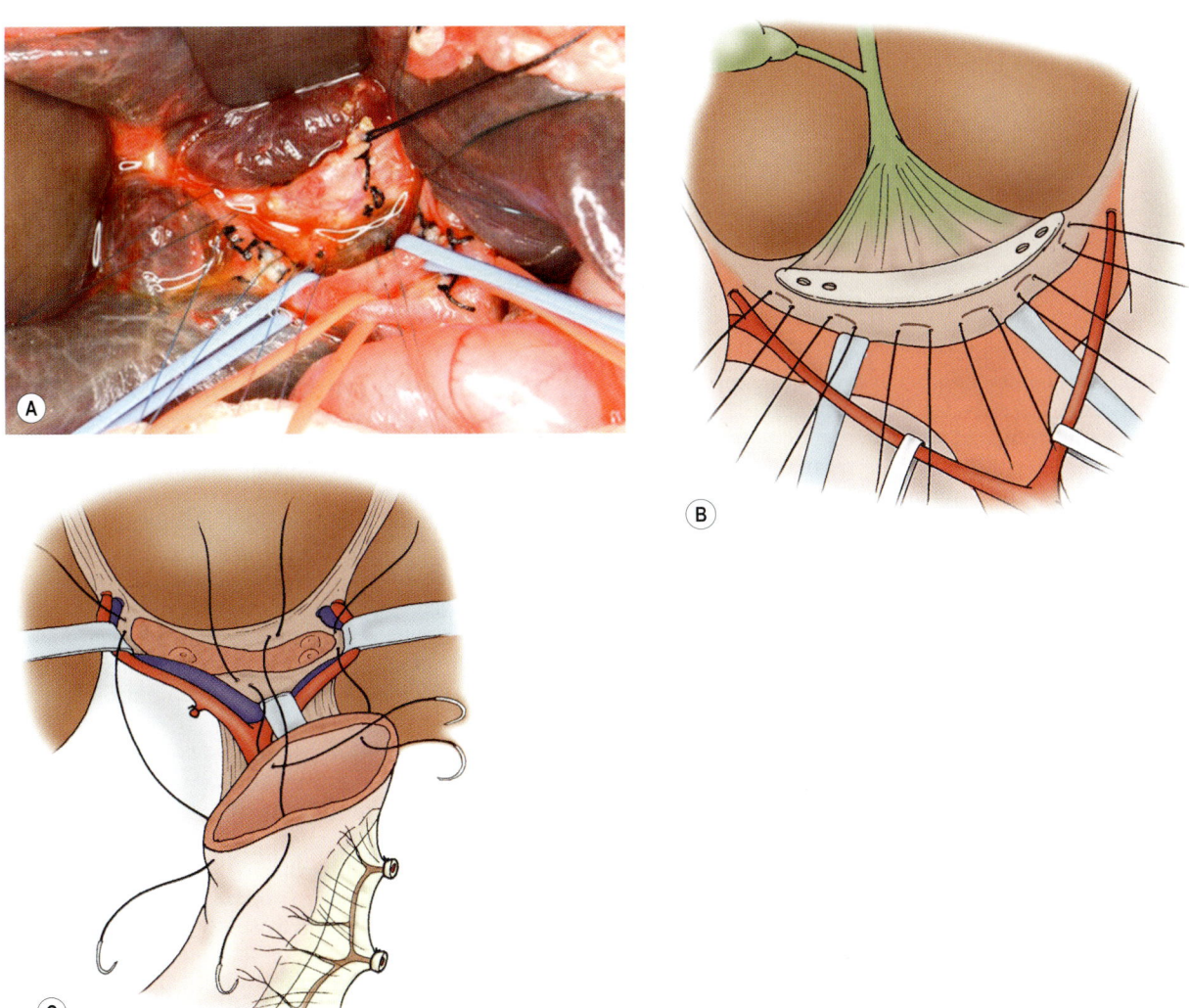

FIGURE 43-7 ■ The current favored technique for a portoenterostomy involves an extended lateral dissection around the porta hepatis with a very wide anastomosis. **(A)** Photograph of the initial mobilization of the gallbladder and atretic bile ducts and dissection/ exposure of the porta hepatis. After the common bile duct remnants are severed from the duodenal side, the dissection proceeds cephalad and the portal bile duct remnants are freed from the underlying structures. The portal vein and hepatic artery have been encircled with vessel loops. Several small vessel branches between the portal vein to the fibrous remnant can be identified and divided between ligatures. **(B)** The portal bile duct remnants must be dissected 5 or 6 mm proximal to the anterior branch of the right hepatic artery on the right side and as far left as the entrance of the obliterated umbilical vein into the left portal vein. The fibrous cone is sharply transected at the level of the posterior surface with scissors or a scalpel, and is removed. The fibrous cone should have an extensive transected surface, which allows a wide anastomosis. **(C)** The end of the Roux-en-Y limb is anastamosed around the transected end of the fibrous remnant. Sutures should not be placed into the transected surface of the bile duct remnant, because minute bile ducts may be present. As much of the transected hilar surface as possible, including all potentially usable remnants of the intrahepatic ducts in the area between and beneath the branches of the right and left portal veins, is incorporated in the anastomosis. It is important to retract the right and left portal veins and hepatic arteries to allow extensive reception of the biliary remnant and a wide portoenterostomy.

allow extensive resection of the biliary remnant and a wide portoenterostomy.

During the dissection, 5-0 or 6-0 absorbable monofilament sutures are usually placed in the liver surface posterior and caudal to the fibrous plate before transecting it (Fig. 43-7B). It is important to have adequate distance between these sutures and the remnant fibrous plate because it will be difficult to transect the fibrous plate if the sutures are too close to it. Bleeding points are controlled by packing with gauze. Diathermy should not be used as it can cause damage to any microscopic patent bile ducts. A liver biopsy should be performed on the right lobe to obtain histopathologic data for prognostic purposes. Also, if intraoperative histology of the transected portal fibrous plate does not identify microscopic (110–150 μm) patent bile duct structures at the transected surface, further cephalad dissection and transection of the portal fibrous plate is needed.[85-87]

A Roux loop of 30–40 cm is prepared by dividing the jejunum approximately 15 cm downstream from the ligament of Treitz. The distal end may be oversewn or left open, and is passed in a retrocolic position to the hepatic hilum. Small bowel continuity is re-established with an end-to-side enteroenterostomy. The hepatic portoenterostomy is performed in an end-to-side or end-to-end fashion using interrupted 5-0 or 6-0 sutures. Using the 5-0 or 6-0 sutures that were previously placed posterior to the fibrous plate, the posterior aspect of the portoenterostomy is performed first (Fig. 44-7C). Next, the anterior edge of the jejunum is anastomosed to the liver parenchyma anterior to the transected fibrous hilar remnant with interrupted 5-0 or 6-0 monofilament absorbable sutures, including the 2 and 10 o'clock positions. There should be adequate space between the anterior margin and the remnant fibrous plate as well. A small drain is positioned in the foramen of Winslow through a separate stab incision in the right abdominal wall and the incision is closed.

Modified Kasai Original Portoenterostomy

In contrast to the EPE technique just described, in both Kasai's original portoenterostomy (KOPE) and our preferred modified KOPE (M-KOPE), dissection of the porta hepatis is confined to the area around the base of the fibrous biliary plate which is not transected very deep.[27,88,89] As a result, the portoenterostomy anastomosis is not as wide as in the EPE technique. We place interrupted sutures in the liver parenchyma around the outer edge of the transected biliary remnant except at the 2 and 10 o'clock positions. At the 2 and 10 o'clock positions, where the right and left hepatic ducts should be, sutures are placed very shallow in the connective tissue near the right and left hepatic arteries or the hepatoduodenal ligament at the porta hepatis, and not to the side of the transected biliary remnant.[27,89] These sutures are placed shallow, especially at the 2 and 10 o'clock positions, to minimize microscopic bile duct injury, but deep enough to prevent leakage at the portoenterostomy. See Figure 43-5 for a comparison of M-KOPE (Fig. 43-5A), KOPE (Fig. 43-5B), and EPE (Fig. 43-5C).

Hepaticojejunostomy

Kimura reported that in correctable biliary atresia, although a wide and deep portal dissection is not required, excision of the patent CBD cephalad to the liver hilum is important.[90] Any cyst-like structure should be excised and should not be used for anastomosis to the intestine. Failure to remove all abnormal CBD or hepatic duct tissue may result in anastomotic stricture or cholangitis.

Nio reported on 323 biliary atresia patients undergoing operation between 1953 and 2004.[91] Fifty patients were classified as type I. In these 50 patients, 28 underwent portoenterostomy and 22 underwent hepaticoenterostomy. The overall survival rate for type I patients who did not require liver transplantation was significantly better than type II/III patients (52% vs 33%). However, the authors also found a higher incidence of cholangitis in type I patients, but this difference was not statistically significant.

Recently, in a review of 200 patients from 1963–2008 at one institution, the authors reported excellent long-term outcomes in 12 patients who had a hilar cyst and underwent hepaticojejunostomy (type I cyst: 9 cases and a subtype of type II: 3 cases).[92] The overall survival with the patient's native liver was 83.3%.

Minimally Invasive Kasai Operation

The first laparoscopic Kasai (lap-Kasai) procedure was described in 2002.[93] Since that report, there have been few others performed, probably because the procedure itself is technically complicated. Moreover, it may be associated with an increased incidence of postoperative complications and a worse early clinical outcome.[94] It has been suggested that the pneumoperitoneum compromises liver perfusion with subsequent liver cell damage.[95] In a rat model, it was shown that elevated intra-abdominal pressure can decrease hepatocyte proliferation and induce liver cell apoptosis.[96] One report found there was no measurable benefit of laparoscopy compared with open portoenterostomy regarding the amount of scarring and adhesions at the time of liver transplantation.[97] On the other hand, one recent study found relatively good outcomes at a median follow-up of 72 months (range: 33–89 months) after lap-Kasai, with 50% (eight cases) of the patients being jaundice-free with normal bilirubin levels.[98] Also, recently, a prospective study compared lap-Kasai to conventional Kasai and found that lap-Kasai was technically feasible.[99] However, the study also found worse survival after 24 months in the 12 infants who had lap-Kasai compared with infants who had conventional surgery.

The authors began performing the M-KOPE via laparoscopy in 2009.[100] During lap-Kasai, the Ligasure is used to divide portal vein branches draining into the caudate lobe at the porta hepatis. The Ligasure generates much less heat laterally when compared to monopolar hook diathermy that can cause thermal injury to the microscopic bile ductules in the fibrous plate during dissection.[101,102] The Roux limb is created by exteriorizing the jejunum through the umbilical port. The length of

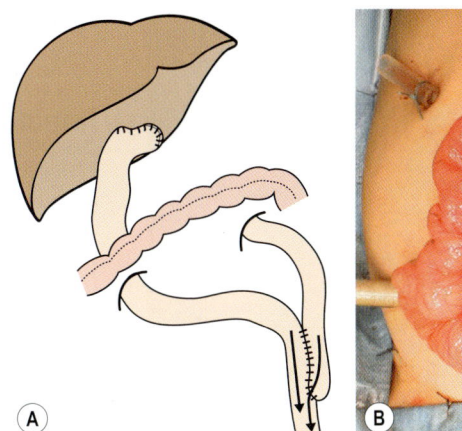
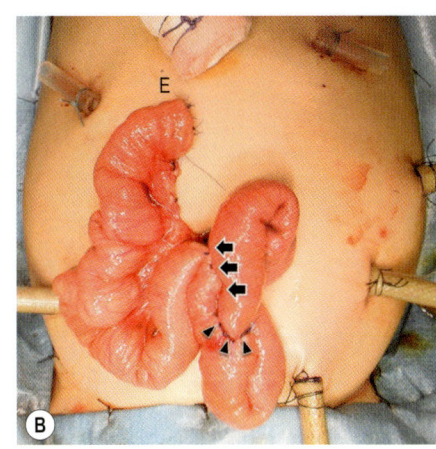

FIGURE 43-8 ■ The length of the Roux-en-Y (RY) limb is determined by exteriorizing the jejunal loop through the umbilicus and measuring the distal end (E) of the limb to be 3 cm above the xiphoid process. The jejunojejunostomy (arrowheads) will then fit naturally into the splenic flexure after anastomosis. Arrows show where the RY limb has been approximated to the native jejunum for 8 cm cranially to streamline flow into the distal jejunum and eliminate reflux into and stasis in the RY limb. (From Yamataka A, Lane GJ, Cazares J. Laparoscopic surgery for biliary atresia and choledochal cyst. Sem Pediatr Surg 2012;21:201.)

the Roux limb is customized by measuring it to reach just above the xiphoid process (Fig. 43-8). The Roux limb tends to be shorter than with the open approach. The jejuno-jejunostomy is performed extracorporeally. The portoenterostomy is then performed as described using the M-KOPE technique.

Repeated Hepatic Portoenterostomy

Bile drainage after reoperation is significant only in patients with good bile excretion after the initial surgery.[103,104] As liver transplantation is a good option, repeated hepatic portoenterostomy should only be considered for selected patients in whom good bile flow suddenly ceases, or in those patients who might benefit from a delay in transplantation.[105]

POSTOPERATIVE MANAGEMENT

Most centers have standardized protocols for postoperative corticosteroid, antibiotic, and choleretic usage. Corticosteroids are used routinely both for their choleretic effect and to decrease scarring at the anastomosis site.[106,107] Ursodeoxycholic acid may be useful in augmenting bile flow, but only in the presence of patent bile ductules. Fat-soluble vitamins (A, D, E, and K) and formula feeding enriched with medium-chain triglycerides are also used.

The authors' postoperative management protocol includes decreasing the dose of intravenous prednisolone once the C-reactive protein level falls below 1.0 mg/dL.[88] Each dose is given for three days, commencing with an initial dose of 4 mg/kg/day, then 3, 2, 1 mg/kg/day, and finishing with 0.5 mg/kg/day. This 15 day cycle can be repeated up to four to five times if jaundice persists (total bilirubin >1.2 mg/dL) and if there is evidence of clinical benefit (ie, lower serum bilirubin or improvement in stool color). However, if jaundice persists without clinical improvement, then only three cycles are administered and the patient is considered for liver transplantation. Also, if stools begin to turn pale, the cycle is either restarted from the beginning, or the previous dose is re-administered. Double agent antibiotic therapy, usually a cephalosporin and an aminoglycoside, is routine and stopped once the C-reactive protein is less than 0.3 mg/dL. An intravenous

cholagog (usually dehydrocholic acid) is begun on day 2 after portoenterostomy and continued until jaundice clears. Oral choleretics such as ursodeoxycholic acid or aminoethylsulfonic acid are administered once oral feeding is started and continued thereafter.

COMPLICATIONS

Cholangitis

Cholangitis, defined as an elevated serum bilirubin (7.5 mg/dL), leukocytosis, and normal to acholic stools in a febrile patient (>38.5°C), is the most frequent complication occurring after portoenterostomy, and most commonly occurs during the first 2 years. Cholestasis is the main risk factor because all patients with biliary atresia have very small ducts and all conduits become colonized within a month of operation.

Approximately 40% of infants develop cholangitis. Patients present initially with fever, decreased quantity and quality of bile excretion, elevation in serum bilirubin, and signs of infection. Prompt treatment is necessary because recurring attacks cause progressive liver damage. After initial blood cultures, broad-spectrum antibiotics with good Gram-negative coverage are started, and a favorable response usually results. If stools become acholic, a pulse of corticosteroids is given. To decrease the risk for cholangitis, Roux-en-Y biliary reconstruction has been modified by various maneuvers, including lengthening the Roux-en-Y limb from 50 cm to 70 cm, total diversion of the biliary conduit, creation of an intestinal valve, and the use of a physiologic intestinal valve.[108-112] The antireflux intussusception valve may be the best modification, and may result in a reduced rate of cholangitis. A gallbladder conduit is not recommended when the lumen of the patent duct is narrow or when pancreaticobiliary anomalies are demonstrated on cholangiography. Stomas complicate liver transplantation, which may be required later.

Cessation of Bile Flow

Loss of bile pigment in the stool in a patient with an apparent well-functioning portoenterostomy is an

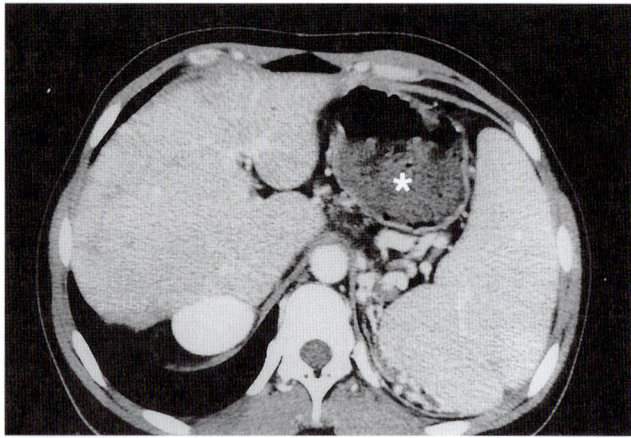

FIGURE 43-9 ■ CT scan of a 20-year-old woman in whom severe portal hypertension developed. Note marked atrophy of the left lobe of the liver, severe splenomegaly, and varices (asterisk) around the stomach.

ominous sign, and parents should be encouraged to report changes in stool color or signs of cholangitis immediately. Prompt re-establishment of bile flow is imperative to avoid liver damage. If bile flow ceases, a corticosteroid pulse is given as corticosteroids both augment bile flow and reduce inflammation.[106,107] If bile flow is re-established, then the corticosteroid dose is reduced. If bile flow is not re-established, the corticosteroids are stopped. If bile flow was initially good, it is reasonable to consider reoperation in selected cases. However, multiple attempts at reoperation generally increase the technical difficulty of subsequent transplantation.

Portal Hypertension

Portal hypertension is common after portoenterostomy, even in infants with good bile flow. The basic inflammatory process affecting the extrahepatic ducts also damages the intrahepatic branches. Persistent hepatic fibrosis has been found in some children despite successful portoenterostomy.[113] Clinical manifestations of portal hypertension include esophageal varices, hypersplenism, and ascites (Fig. 43-9). Over time, the susceptibility to complications from portal hypertension seems to decrease, resulting in reduced frequency and severity of variceal bleeding. This observation is difficult to explain and may be related to improvement in hepatic histology or the development of spontaneous portosystemic shunts. This observation justifies a nonsurgical approach to the portal hypertension as long as hepatic function is preserved (i.e., the patient remains anicteric with no coagulopathy and normal serum albumin level). However, in the presence of poor hepatic function, complications from portal hypertension are an indication for liver transplantation.

Intrahepatic Cysts

Biliary cysts, or 'lakes,' can develop within the livers of long-term survivors, and cause recurring attacks of cholangitis (Fig. 43-10).[114] Prolonged antibiotics and ursodeoxycholic acid may be helpful in preventing

cholangitis, but unremitting infection is an indication for liver transplantation.

Hepatopulmonary Syndrome

Diffuse intrapulmonary shunting can occur as a complication of chronic liver disease in children with biliary atresia. This shunting is likely a result of vasoactive compounds from the mesenteric circulation that are not deactivated in the liver. This syndrome is characterized by cyanosis, dyspnea on exertion, hypoxia, and finger clubbing. It appears to be more prevalent in children with syndromic biliary atresia. The diagnosis is confirmed by using a combination of arterial blood gas analysis with and without inspired oxygen, radionuclide lung scans with macroaggregated albumin to quantify the degree of shunting, and contrast bubble echocardiography. This complication is progressive and can usually be reversed by liver transplantation. Pulmonary hypertension is an uncommon complication, but can also develop in long-term survivors after portoenterostomy.

Hepatic Malignancy

Rarely, malignant changes (hepatocellular carcinoma or cholangiocarcinoma) complicate long-standing biliary cirrhosis after portoenterostomy. A case of hepatocellular carcinoma has been reported in a 19-year-old post-Kasai male biliary atresia patient, indicating the need for a high index of suspicion for the development of carcinoma, even in young patients.[115]

Other Complications

Due to the presence of residual hepatic disease, metabolic problems associated with malabsorption of fat, protein, vitamins, and trace minerals can occur postoperatively because of impairment of bile flow to the gut.[116,117] Weight gain after portoenterostomy may be retarded if hepatic dysfunction persists. Essential fatty acid deficiencies and rickets are common problems related to metabolic derangements.[118] Long-term monitoring of clinical

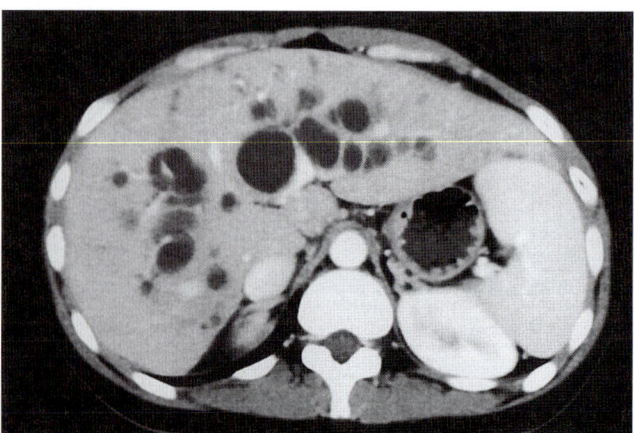

FIGURE 43-10 ■ CT scan of a 17-year-old with biliary atresia. Multiple biliary cysts or 'lakes' have developed within the liver of this long-term survivor and caused recurrent attacks of cholangitis.

symptoms and adequate nutritional supplementation are needed. Ectopic intestinal variceal bleeding and pulmonary arteriovenous fistulas are sometimes seen in long-term survivors with incomplete relief of impaired liver function.[119,120]

As more postoperative biliary atresia patients are now reaching adulthood, the issue of pregnancy in females is becoming more common. In nontransplanted corrected biliary atresia patients, preterm cesarean delivery at around the 34th week appears to be reasonable because this is a high risk pregnancy in a patient with poor hepatic reserve. Conversely, delivery at full term may be possible for selected mothers with good liver function.[121]

RESULTS AND PROGNOSIS

Without question, the Kasai hepatic portoenterostomy has greatly improved outcomes of infants with biliary atresia, and the results of surgical treatment have improved steadily over the past 30 years. Classically, the major determinants of satisfactory outcome after portoenterostomy are (1) age at initial operation; (2) successful achievement of postoperative bile flow; (3) presence of microscopic ductal structures at the hilum; (4) the degree of parenchymal disease at diagnosis; and (5) technical factors at the anastomosis. Age at portoenterostomy is the single most widely quoted prognostic variable. A favorable outcome is expected if the procedure is performed before 60 days of age, because cirrhosis will develop by 3 to 4 months of age. However, a wide discrepancy exists in reported long-term results. One study from Japan found postoperative outcome to be excellent, with a ten-year survival rate of more than 70%, if the portoenterostomy was performed before 60 days of age.[122] However, a nationwide survey of the Surgical Section of the American Academy of Pediatrics found that long-term survival was only 25%.[26] Other reported 10-year survival rates include 40–50% from the UK and 68% from France.[1,123] Outcomes are considerably worse if the infant is older than 100 days at the time of portoenterostomy because obliterative cholangiopathy and hepatic fibrosis have already developed.[123,124]

The impact of age at portoenterostomy on long-term outcome, especially in patients with type III biliary atresia, was recently evaluated.[125] Age at portoenterostomy was found to have a significant impact on jaundice clearance, but not on long-term survival in type III biliary atresia, suggesting that age at portoenterostomy might be less significant as a prognostic factor over time. In another study from Hong Kong, portoenterostomies performed beyond the age of 60 days was not associated with worse outcome, and a high percentage of patients could still achieve good bile flow and a normal bilirubin postoperatively.[126] Of particular interest is a report by Kuroda et al, who reviewed postoperative biliary atresia patients in relation to pregnancy and found that age at portoenterostomy may not necessarily influence long-term outcome.[127] However, liver function at puberty may be a useful indicator and may be predictive for the safety of pregnancy. Also, management strategies may need to be revised accordingly after puberty.

The presence of microscopic ducts at the hilum is somewhat controversial.[128,129] Some authors have suggested that duct size is important, but there is not universal agreement. Types I and II biliary atresia generally have a good prognosis if treated early. In the more typical type III disease, the presence of larger bile ductules at the porta hepatis (>150 µm in diameter) is associated with a better prognosis. The subgroup of infants with syndromic biliary atresia have worse outcomes in terms of both clearance of jaundice and survival.[1,28] The latter is related to associated malformations (particularly congenital heart disease), a predisposition to developing hepatopulmonary syndrome, and possible immune compromise from functional hyposplenism. Personal experience suggests that infants with concomitant CMV infection fare less well after a portoenterostomy.

The importance of surgeon experience was shown in a British survey in which patients who underwent portoenterostomy at centers treating one case per year had significantly worse outcomes than patients who were treated at centers performing more than five cases per year.[130] Since 1999, the management of biliary atresia has been centralized to three centers in England and Wales that are able to offer both portoenterostomy and transplantation. In 2011, the results of this policy change were reported, and it was found that outcomes were better than previously reported.[131] These improved outcomes may be due to centralization of surgical and medical resources.

Recently, outcomes in infants enrolled in the prospective Childhood Liver Disease Research and Education Network who underwent portoenterostomy were reported. Liver anatomy, splenic malformation, presence of ascites, liver nodularity at portoenterostomy, and early postoperative clearance of jaundice were found to be significant predictors of transplant-free survival.[132]

Irrespective of age and other factors related to the timing of portoenterostomy, a significant decrease in serum bilirubin and signs of good bile excretion in the stool may be predictive of good long-term outcome.[133] Due to the possibility of sudden hepatic deterioration and the constant concern for cholangitis and portal hypertension, recent reports about long-term outcomes in biliary atresia patients consistently emphasize lifelong follow-up.[134,135]

LIVER TRANSPLANTATION

The indications for liver transplantation following portoenterostomy are: (1) lack of bile drainage; (2) signs of developmental retardation or their sequelae; and (3) complications/side effects being socially unacceptable.

A high hepatic artery resistance index measured on Doppler ultrasound is an indication for relatively urgent transplantation.[136] Deterioration in hepatic status may be precipitated by adolescence or pregnancy. However, as many as 20% of patients undergoing portoenterostomy will remain healthy and reach adulthood with good liver function.

The dramatic improvement in survival with the use of cyclosporine and tacrolimus immunosuppression after liver transplantation raises the question of transplantation becoming a more conventional form of treatment for biliary atresia. The donor supply is always a problem, alleviated to some extent by reduced-size liver transplantation. Five-year survival after liver transplantation for biliary atresia is currently 80–90%, and techniques such as split-liver grafting and living-related liver transplantation have decreased waiting times.[137] Furthermore, long-term studies of post-transplant biliary atresia patients have shown that survivors have an acceptable to good quality of life.[138,139]

A recent study summarized the largest series ($n = 464$) of postportoenterostomy patients who had undergone living-related liver transplantation.[140] The outcome of living-related liver transplantation in adults with biliary atresia was significantly worse than in infants and children. The overall five- and ten-year survival rates were 70% and 56% in adults versus 87% and 81% in pediatric patients, respectively. On the other hand, there is a report concluding that living-related liver transplantation after portoenterostomy can be performed safely in adults with a long-term survival rate equivalent to that for pediatric patients.[141] Longer immunosuppression might ultimately lead to increased morbidity, including higher rates of cancer, infection, and metabolic diseases later in life. In addition, in living-related liver transplantation, the risk to the donor is always a concern.[142] The optimal timing of transplantation in postportoenterostomy patients has yet to be established.

REFERENCES

1. Chardot C, Carton M, Spire-Bendelac N, et al. Prognosis of biliary atresia in the era of liver transplantation: French national study from 1986 to 1996. Hepatology 1999;30:606–11.
2. McKiernan PJ, Baker AJ, Kelly DA. The frequency and outcome of biliary atresia in the UK and Ireland. Lancet 2000;355:25–9.
3. Yoon PW, Bresee JS, Olney RS, et al. Epidemiology of biliary atresia: A population-based study. Pediatrics 1997;99:376–82.
4. Fischler B, Haglund B, Hjern A. A population-based study on the incidence and possible pre- and perinatal etiologic risk factors of biliary atresia. J Pediatr 2002;141:217–22.
5. Petersen C, Harder D, Abola Z, et al. European biliary atresia registries: Summary of a symposium. Eur J Pediatr Surg 2008;18:111–16.
6. Nio M, Ohi R, Miyano T, et al. Five- and 10-year survival rates after surgery for biliary atresia: A report from Japanese biliary atresia registry. J Pediatr Surg 2003;38:997–1000.
7. Vic P, Gestas P, Mallet EC, et al. Biliary atresia in French Polynesia: Retrospective study of 10 years. Arch Pediatr 1994;1:646–51.
8. Thomson J. On congenital obliteration of the bile ducts. Edinburgh Med J 1891;37:523–31, 604–16, 724–35.
9. Holmes JB. Congenital obliteration of the bile ducts: Diagnosis and suggestions for treatment. Am J Dis Child 1916;11:405–31.
10. Ladd WE. Congenital atresia and stenosis of the bile ducts. JAMA 1928;91:1082–5.
11. Bill AH. Biliary atresia. World J Surg 1987;2:557–9.
12. Gross RE. The Surgery of Infancy and Children. Philadelphia: WB Saunders; 1953. p. 508–23.
13. Sterling JA. Experiences with Congenital Biliary Atresia. Springfield, IL: Charles C Thomas; 1960. p. 3–68.
14. Potts WJ. The Surgeons and the Child. Philadelphia: WB Saunders; 1959. p. 137–43.
15. Longmire WP, Sanford MC. Intrahepatic cholangiojejunostomy with partial hepatectomy for biliary obstruction. Surgery 1948;24:264–76.
16. Fonkalsrud EW, Kitagawa S, Longmire WP. Hepatic drainage to the jejunum for congenital biliary atresia. Am J Surg 1966;112:188–94.
17. Williams LF, Dooling JA. Thoracic duct-esophagus anastomosis for relief of congenital biliary atresia. Surg Forum 1963;14:189–91.
18. Swenson O, Fisher JH. Utilization of cholangiogram during exploration for biliary atresia. N Engl J Med 1952;249:247–8.
19. Thaler MM, Gellis SS. Studies in neonatal hepatitis and biliary atresia: II. The effect of diagnostic laparotomy on long-term prognosis of neonatal hepatitis. Am J Dis Child 1968;116:262–70.
20. Kanof A, Donovan EJ, Berner H. Congenital atresia of the biliary system: Delayed development of correctability. Am J Dis Child 1953;86:780–7.
21. Kravetz LJ. Congenital biliary atresia. Surgery 1960;47:453–67.
22. Carlson E. Salvage of the 'non-correctable' case of congenital extrahepatic biliary atresia. Arch Surg 1960;81:893–8.
23. Kasai M, Suzuki S. A new operation for non-correctable biliary atresia: Hepatic portoenterostomy. Shujutu 1959;13:733–9.
24. Kasai M, Kimura S, Asakura Y, et al. Surgical treatment of biliary atresia. J Pediatr Surg 1968;3:665–75.
25. Kasai M. Treatment of biliary atresia with special reference to hepatic portoenterostomy and its modification. Progr Pediatr Surg 1974;6:5–52.
26. Karrer FM, Lilly JR, Stewart BA, et al. Biliary atresia registry, 1976–1989. J Pediatr Surg 1990;25:1076–81.
27. Kasai M. Surgery for biliary atresia, Japan Surgical Society Video library: No.78-07.
28. Perlmutter DH, Shepherd RW. Extrahepatic biliary atresia: A disease or a phenotype? Hepatology 2002;35:1297–304.
29. Davenport M, Savage M, Mowat AP, et al. The biliary atresia splenic malformation syndrome. Surgery 1993;113:662–8.
30. Morecki R, Glaser JH, Cho S, et al. Biliary atresia and reovirus type 3 infection. N Engl J Med 1984;310:1610.
31. Tyler KL, Sokol RJ, Oberhaus SM, et al. Detection of reovirus RNA in hepatobiliary tissues from patients with extrahepatic biliary atresia and choledochal cysts. Hepatology 1998;27:1475–82.
32. Mazziotti MV, Willis LK, Heuckeroth RO, et al. Anomalous development of the hepatobiliary system in the Inv mouse. Hepatology 1999;30:372–8.
33. Jacquemin E, Cresteil D, Raynaud N, et al. CFC1 gene mutation and biliary atresia with polysplenia syndrome. J Pediatr Gastroenterol Nutr 2002;34:326–7.
34. Arikan C, Berdeli A, Ozgenc F, et al. Positive association of macrophage migration inhibitory factor gene-173G/C polymorphism with biliary atresia. J Pediatr Gastroenterol Nutr 2006;42:77–82.
35. Ware SM, Peng J, Zhu L, et al. Identification and functional analysis of ZIC3 mutations in heterotaxy and related congenital heart defects. Am J Hum Genet 2004;74:93–105.
36. Kohsaka T, Yuan ZR, Guo SX, et al. The significance of human jagged 1 mutations detected in severe cases of extrahepatic biliary atresia. Hepatology 2002;36:904–12.
37. Ku NO, Darling JM, Krams SM, et al. Keratin 8 and 18 mutations are risk factors for developing liver disease of multiple etiologies. Proc Natl Acad Sci U S A 2003;13:6063–8.
38. Tan CEL, Driver M, Howard ER, et al. Extrahepatic biliary atresia: A first-trimester event? Clues from light microscopy and immunohistochemistry. J Pediatr Surg 1994;29:808–14.
39. Seidman SL, Duquesnoy RJ, Zeevi A, et al. Recognition of major histocompatibility complex antigens on cultured human biliary epithelial cells by alloreactive lymphocytes. Hepatology 1991;13:239–46.
40. Dillon P, Belchis D, Tracy T, et al. Increased expression of intercellular adhesion molecules in biliary atresia. Am J Pathol 1994;145:263–7.
41. Silveira TR, Salzano FM, Donaldson PT, et al. Association between HLA and extrahepatic biliary atresia. J Pediatr Gastroenterol Nutr 1993;16:114–17.
42. Kobayashi H, Puri P, O'Brian DS, et al. Hepatic overexpression of MHC class II antigens and macrophage-associated antigen (CD68) in patients with biliary atresia of poor prognosis. J Pediatr Surg 1997;32:590–3.

43. Kobayashi H, Horikoshi K, Li L, et al. Serum concentration of adhesion molecules in postoperative biliary atresia patients: Relationship to disease activity and cirrhosis. J Pediatr Surg 2001;36:1297–301.

44. Allison JP. CD28-B7 interactions in T-cell activation. Curr Opin Immunol 1994;6:414–19.

45. Kobayashi H, Li Z, Yamataka A, et al. Role of immunologic co-stimulatory factors in the pathogenesis of biliary atresia. J Pediatr Surg 2003;38:892–6.

46. Bezerra JA, Tiao G, Ryckman FC, et al. Genetic induction of proinflammatory immunity in children with biliary atresia. Lancet 2002;23:1653–9.

47. Mack CL, Tucker RM, Sokol RJ, et al. Biliary atresia is associated with CD4+ Th1 cell-mediated portal tract inflammation. Pediatr Res 2004;56:79–87.

48. Sokol RJ, Mack C. Etiopathogenesis of biliary atresia. Semin Liver Dis 2001;21:517–24.

49. O'Neill JA, Rowe MI, Grosfeld JL, et al. Pediatric Surgery. 5th ed. St. Louis: Mosby–Year Book; 1998.

50. Ito T, Horisawa M, Ando H. Intrahepatic bile ducts in biliary atresia: A possible factor determining the prognosis. J Pediatr Surg 1983;18:124–30.

51. Raweily EA, Gibson AAM, Burt AD. Abnormalities of intrahepatic bile ducts in extrahepatic biliary atresia. Histopathology 1990;17:521–7.

52. Lilly JR, Altman RP. Hepatic portoenterostomy (the Kasai operation) for biliary atresia. Surgery 1975;78:76–86.

53. Ohi R, Chiba T, Endo N. Morphologic studies of the liver and bile ducts in biliary atresia. Acta Paediatr Jpn 1987;29:584–9.

54. Desmet VJ. Intrahepatic bile ducts under the lens. J Hepatol 1987;1:545–59.

55. Sherlock S. The syndrome of disappearing intrahepatic bile ducts. Lancet 1987;2:493–6.

56. Phavichitr N, Theamboonlers A, Poovorawan Y. Insulin-like growth factor-1 (IGF-1) in children with postoperative biliary atresia: A cross-sectional study. Asian Pac J Allergy Immunol 2008;26:57–61.

57. Kobayashi H, Yamataka A, Lane GJ, et al. Levels of circulating anti-inflammatory cytokine interleukin-1 receptor antagonist and proinflammatory cytokines at different stages of biliary atresia. J Pediatr Surg 2002;37:1038–41.

58. Davenport M, Gonde C, Redkar R, et al. Immunohistochemistry of the liver and biliary tree in extrahepatic biliary atresia. J Pediatr Surg 2001;36:1017–25.

59. Shimadera S, Iwai N, Deguchi E, et al. Significance of ductal plate malformation in the postoperative clinical course of biliary atresia. J Pediatr Surg 2008;43:304–7.

60. DeRusso PA, Ye W, Shepherd R, et al. Growth failure and outcomes in infants with biliary atresia: A report from the Biliary Atresia Research Consortium. Hepatology 2007;46:1632–8.

61. Chiba T, Ohi R, Kamiyama T, Nio M, Ibrahim M. Japanese biliary atresia registry: Biliary atresia. Tokyo: Icom Assoc; 1991.

62. Altman RP, Levy J. Biliary atresia. Pediatr Ann 1985;14:481–5.

63. Okazaki T, Kobayashi H, Yamataka A, et al. Long-term post surgical outcome of biliary atresia. J Pediatr Surg 1998;34:312–15.

64. Balistreri WF. Neonatal cholestasis. J Pediatr 1985;106:171–84.

65. Brough H, Houssin D. Conjugated hyperbilirubinemia in early infancy: A reassessment of liver biopsy. Hum Pathol 1974;5:507–16.

66. Javitt NB, Keating JP, Grand RJ, et al. Serum bile acid patterns in neonatal hepatitis and extrahepatic biliary atresia. J Pediatr 1977;90:736–9.

67. Ukarapol N, Wongsawasdi L, Ong-Chai S, et al. Hyaluronic acid: Additional biochemical marker in the diagnosis of biliary atresia. Pediatr Int 2007;49:608–11.

68. Faweya AG, Akinyinka OO, Sodeinde O. Duodenal intubation and aspiration test: Utility in the differential diagnosis of infantile cholestasis. J Pediatr Gastroenterol Nutr 1991;13:290–2.

69. Azuma T, Nakamura T, Moriuchi T, et al. Preoperative ultrasonographic diagnosis of biliary atresia with reference to the presence or absence of the extrahepatic bile duct. Paper presented at the 38th Annual Congress of the Japanese Society of Pediatric Surgeons. Tokyo, Japan, June 2001.

70. Park WH, Choi SO, Lee HJ. The ultrasonographic 'triangular cord' coupled with gallbladder images in the diagnostic prediction of biliary atresia from infantile intrahepatic cholestasis. J Pediatr Surg 1999;34:1706–10.

71. Kotb MA, Kotb A, Sheba MF, et al. Evaluation of the triangular cord sign in the diagnosis of biliary atresia. Pediatrics 2001;108:416–20.

72. Tan Kendrick AP, Ooi BC, Tan CE. Biliary atresia: Making the diagnosis by the gallbladder ghost triad. Pediatr Radiol 2003;33:311–15.

73. Farrant P, Meire HB, Mieli-Vergani G. Ultrasound features of the gallbladder in infants presenting with conjugated hyperbilirubinaemia. Br J Radiol 2000;73:1154–8.

74. Abramson SJ, Berdon WE, Altman RP, et al. Biliary atresia and noncardiac polysplenia syndrome: Ultrasound and surgical consideration. Radiology 1987;163:377–9.

75. Han BK, Babcock DS, Gelfand MM. Choledochal cyst with bile duct dilatation: Sonographic and 99mTc-IDA cholescintigraphy. AJR Am J Roentgenol 1981;136:1075–9.

76. Ochshorn Y, Rosner G, Barel D, et al. Clinical evaluation of isolated nonvisualized fetal gallbladder. Prenat Diagn 2007;27:699–703.

77. Boughanim M, Benachi A, Dreux S, et al. Nonvisualization of the fetal gallbladder by second-trimester ultrasound scan: Strategy of clinical management based on four examples. Prenat Diagn 2008;28:46–8.

78. Okazaki T, Miyano G, Yamataka A, et al. Diagnostic laparoscopy-assisted cholangiography in infants with prolonged jaundice. Pediatr Surg Int 2006;22:140–3.

79. Nwomeh BC, Caniano DA, Hogan M. Definitive exclusion of biliary atresia in infants with cholestatic jaundice: The role of percutaneous cholecysto-cholangiography. Pediatr Surg Int 2007;23:845–9.

80. Nio M, Ohi R. Biliary atresia. Semin Pediatr Surg 2000;9:177–86.

81. Davenport M. Surgery for biliary atresia. In: Spitz L, Coran AG, editors. Operative pediatric surgery. New York: Hodder Arnold; 2006. p. 661–72.

82. Miyano T, Fujimoto T, Ohya T, et al. Current concept of the treatment of biliary atresia. World J Surg 1993;17:332–6.

83. Kobayashi H, Yamataka A, Urao M, et al. Innovative modification of the hepatic portoenterostomy. Our experience of treating biliary atresia. J Pediatr Surg 2006;41:19–22.

84. Miyano T, Ohya T, Kimura K, et al. Current state of the treatment of congenital biliary atresia (in Japanese). J Jpn Surg Soc 1989;90:1343–7.

85. Kobayashi H, Horikoshi K, Yamataka A, et al. Alpha-glutathione-S-transferase as a new sensitive marker of hepatocellular damage in biliary atresia. Pediatr Surg Int 2000;16:302–5.

86. Kobayashi H, Horikoshi K, Yamataka A, et al. Hyaluronic acid: A specific prognostic indicator of hepatic damage in biliary atresia. J Pediatr Surg 1999;34:1791–4.

87. Miyano T, Suruga K, Tsuchiya H, et al. A histopathological study of the remnant of extrahepatic bile duct in so-called uncorrectable biliary atresia. J Pediatr Surg 1977;12:19–25.

88. Nakamura H, Koga H, Wada M, et al. Reappraising the portoenterostomy procedure according to sound physiological/anatomic principles enhances postoperative jaundice clearance in biliary atresia. Pediatr Surg Int 2012;28:205–9.

89. Kasai M. Treatment of biliary atresia with special reference to hepatic porto-enterostomy and its modifications. Prog Pediatr Surg 1974;6:5–52.

90. Kimura K, Tsugawa C, Matsumoto T, et al. The surgical management of the unusual forms of biliary atresia. J Pediatr Surg 1979;14:653–60.

91. Nio M, Sano N, Ishii T, et al. Long-term outcome in type I biliary atresia. J Pediatr Surg 2006;41:1973–5.

92. Takahashi Y, Matsuura T, Saeki I, et al. Excellent long-term outcome of hepaticojejunostomy for biliary atresia with a hilar cyst. J Pediatr Surg 2009;44:231–2315.

93. Esteves E, Clemente Neto E, Ottaiano Neto M, et al. Laparoscopic Kasai portoenterostomy for biliary atresia. Pediatr Surg Int 2002;18:737–40.

94. Wong KK, Chung PH, Chan KL, et al. Should open Kasai portoenterostomy be performed for biliary atresia in the era of laparoscopy? Pediatr Surg Int 2008;24:931–3.

95. Kuebler JF, Kos M, Jesch NK, et al. Carbon dioxide suppresses macrophage superoxide anion production independent of extracellular pH and mitochondrial activity. J Pediatr Surg 2007; 42:244–8.

96. Mogilner JG, Bitterman H, Hayari L, et al. Effect of elevated intraabdominal pressure and hyperoxia on portal vein blood flow, hepatocyte proliferation and apoptosis in a rat model. Eur J Pediatr Surg 2008;18:380–6.

97. Von Sochaczewski OC, Petersen C, Ure BM, et al. Laparoscopic versus conventional Kasai portoenterostomy does not facilitate subsequent liver transplantation in infants with biliary atresia. J Laparoendosc Adv Surg Tech 2012;22:408–11.

98. Chan KWE, Lee KH, Mou JWC, et al. The outcome of laparoscopic portoenterostomy for biliary atresia in children. Pediatr Surg Int 2011;27:671–4.

99. Ure BM, Kueblaer JF, Schukfeh N, et al. Survival with the native liver after laparoscopic versus conventional Kasai portoenterostomy in infants with biliary atresia. A prospective trial. Ann Surg 2011;253:826–30.

100. Koga H, Miyano G, Takahashi T, et al. Laparoscopic portoenterostomy for uncorrectable biliary atresia using Kasai's original technique. J Laparoendosc Adv Surg Tech A 2011;21:291–4.

101. Yamataka A, Lane GJ, Cazares J. Laparoscopic surgery for biliary atresia and choledochal cyst. Semi Pediatr Surg 2012;21:201–10.

102. Davenport M, Yamataka A. Surgery for biliary atresia. In: Spitz L, Goran AG, editors. Operative Pediatric Surgery. 7th ed. Florida: CRC Press; 2013. p. 655–66.

103. Freitas L, Gauthier F, Valayer J. Second operation for repair of biliary atresia. J Pediatr Surg 1987;22:857–60.

104. Ibrahim M, Ohi R, Chiba T, et al. Indication and Results of Reoperation for Biliary Atresia. Tokyo: Icom Association; 1991.

105. Bondoc AJ, Taylor JA, Alonso MH, et al. The beneficial impact of revision of Kasai portoenterostomy for biliary atresia. Ann Surg 2012;255:570–6.

106. Muraji T, Higashimoto Y. The improved outlook for biliary atresia with corticosteroid therapy. J Pediatr Surg 1997;32: 1103–7.

107. Karrer FM, Lilly JR. Corticosteroid therapy in biliary atresia. J Pediatr Surg 1985;20:693–5.

108. Suruga K, Miyano T, Kimura K, et al. Reoperation in the treatment of biliary atresia. J Pediatr Surg 1982;17:1–6.

109. Sawaguchi, S., Y. Akiyama, M. Saeki, Y. Ohta. The treatment of congenital biliary atresia with special reference to hepatic portoenteroanastomosis. Paper presented at the fifth annual meeting of the Pacific Association of Pediatric Surgeons, Tokyo, 1972.

110. Nakajo T, Hashizume K, Saeki M, et al. Intussusception-type antireflux valve in Roux-en-Y loop to prevent ascending cholangitis after hepatic portojejunostomy. J Pediatr Surg 1990;25: 311–14.

111. Tanaka K, Shirahase I, Utsunomiya H, et al. A valved hepatic portoduodenal intestinal conduit for biliary atresia. Ann Surg 1990;213:230–5.

112. Endo M, Katsumata K, Yokoyama J, et al. Extended dissection of the porta hepatis and creation of an intussuscepted ileocolic conduit for biliary atresia. J Pediatr Surg 1983;12:784–93.

113. Altman RP, Chandra R, Lilly JR. Ongoing cirrhosis after successful portoenterostomy with biliary atresia. J Pediatr Surg 1975;10:685–91.

114. Bu LN, Chen HL, Ni YH, et al. Multiple intrahepatic biliary cysts in children with biliary atresia. J Pediatr Surg 2002;37:1183–7.

115. Hol L, van den Bos IC, Hussain SM, et al. Hepatocellular carcinoma complicating biliary atresia after Kasai portoenterostomy. Eur J Gastroenterol Hepatol 2008;20:227–31.

116. Andrews WS, Pau CM, Chase HP, et al. Fat soluble vitamin deficiency in biliary atresia. J Pediatr Surg 1981;16:284–90.

117. Greene HL, Helinek GL, Moran R, et al. A diagnostic approach to prolonged obstructive jaundice by 24-hour collection of duodenal fluid. J Pediatr Surg 1979;95:412–14.

118. Barkin RM, Lilly JR. Biliary atresia and the Kasai operation: Continuing care. J Pediatr Surg 1980;96:1015–19.

119. Raffensperger JG. A long-term follow-up of three patients with biliary atresia. J Pediatr Surg 1991;26:176–7.

120. Agarwal GS, Saxena A, Bhatnagar V. The development of intrapulmonary arteriovenous shunts as a poor prognostic factor following surgery for biliary atresia. Trop Gastroenterol 2009;30: 110–12.

121. Kuroda T, Saeki M, Morikawa N, et al. Biliary atresia and pregnancy: Puberty may be an important point for predicting the outcome. J Pediatr Surg 2005;40:1852–5.

122. Kasai M, Mochizuki I, Ohkohchi N, et al. Surgical limitation for biliary atresia: Indication for liver transplantation. J Pediatr Surg 1989;24:851–4.

123. Davenport M, Kerkar N, Mieli-Vergani G, et al. Biliary atresia: The King's College Hospital experience (1974–1995). J Pediatr Surg 1997;32:479–85.

124. Chardot C, Carton M, Spire-Bendelac N, et al. Is the Kasai operation still indicated in children older than 3 months diagnosed with biliary atresia? J Pediatr Surg 2001;138:224–8.

125. Nio M, Sasaki H, Wada M, et al. Impact of age at Kasai operation on short- and long-term outcomes of type III biliary atresia at a single institution. J Pediatr Surg 2010;45:2361–3.

126. Wong KKY, Chung PHY, Chan IHY, et al. Performing Kasai portoenterostomy beyond 60 days of life is not necessarily associated with a worse outcome. J Pediatr Gastroenterol Nutr 2010;51:631–4.

127. Kuroda T, Saeki M, Morikawa N, et al. Management of adult biliary atresia patients: Should hard work and pregnancy be discouraged? J Pediatr Surg 2007;42:2106–9.

128. Chandra RS, Altman RP. Ductal remnants in extrahepatic biliary atresia: A histopathologic study with clinical correlation. J Pediatr Surg 1978;93:196–200.

129. Tan EL, Davenport M, Driver M, et al. Does the morphology of the extrahepatic biliary remnants in biliary atresia influence survival? A review of 205 cases. J Pediatr Surg 1994;29:1459–64.

130. McClement JW, Howard ER, Mowat AP. Results of surgical treatment for extrahepatic biliary atresia in the United Kingdom, 1980–1982. BMJ 1985;290:345–7.

131. Davenport M, Ong E, Sharif K, et al. Biliary atresia in England and Wales: Results of centralization and new benchmark. J Pediatr Surg 2011;46:1689–94.

132. Superina RS, Magee JC, Brandt ML, et al. The anatomic pattern of biliary atresia identified at time of Kasai hepatoportoenterostomy and early postoperative clearance of jaundice are significant predictors of transplant-free survival. Ann Surg 2011;254: 577–85.

133. Ohhama Y, Shinkai M, Fujita S, et al. Early prediction of long-term survival and the timing of liver transplantation after the Kasai operation. J Pediatr Surg 2000;35:1031–4.

134. Kumagi T, Drenth JPH, Guttman O, et al. Biliary atresia and survival into adulthood without transplantation: A collaborative multicenter clinic review. Liver Int DOI:10.1111/j.1478-3231 2011.02668.x.

135. Shinkai M, Ohhama Y, Take H, et al. Long-term outcome of children with biliary atresia who were not transplanted after the Kasai operation: > 20-year experience at a children's hospital. J Pediatr Gastroenterol Nut 2009;48:443–50.

136. Broide E, Farrant P, Reid F, et al. Hepatic artery resistance index can predict early death in children with biliary atresia. Liver Transplant Surg 1997;3:604–10.

137. Tanaka K, Uemoto S, Tokunaga Y, et al. Surgical techniques and innovations in living related liver transplantation. Ann Surg 1993;217:82–91.

138. Howard ER, MacClean G, Nio M, et al. Biliary atresia: Survival patterns after portoenterostomy and comparison of a Japanese with a UK cohort of long-term survivors. J Pediatr Surg 2001;36: 892–7.

139. Bucuvalas JC, Britto M, Krug S, et al. Health-related quality of life in pediatric liver transplant recipients: A single-center study. Liver Transplant 2003;9:62–71.

140. Uchida Y, Kasahara M, Egawa H, et al. Long-term outcome of adult-to-adult living donor liver transplantation for post-Kasai biliary atresia. Am J Transplant 2006;6:2443–8.

141. Kyoden Y, Tamura S, Sugawara Y, et al. Outcome of living donor liver transplantation for post-Kasai biliary atresia in adults. Liver Transpl 2008;14:186–92.

142. Trotter JF, Adam R, Lo CM, et al. Documented deaths of hepatic lobe donors for living donor liver transplantation. Liver Transpl 2006;12:1485–8.

CHAPTER 44

CHOLEDOCHAL CYST AND GALLBLADDER DISEASE

Nguyen Thanh Liem • George W. Holcomb III

CHOLEDOCHAL CYST

Choledochal cyst is a congenital dilatation of the biliary tract. The dilatation can be found along any portion of the biliary tract. However, the most common site is the choledochus. The diameter of the bile duct varies according to the child's age.[1-3] Normal diameter of the common bile duct (CBD) is seen in Table 44-1.[2] Any diameter of the bile duct greater than the upper limit should be considered abnormal.

Classification

Different classifications have been proposed for choledochal cyst.[4-8] However Todani's classification has been the most widely accepted (Fig. 44-1).[5] According to this classification, choledochal cyst (CC) are classified into five types:

- Type I
  - Ia: cystic dilatation of the CBD
  - Ib: fusiform dilatation of the CBD
- Type II: diverticulum of the CBD
- Type III: choledochocele (dilatation of the terminal CBD within the duodenal wall)
- Type IV
  - IVa: multiple cysts of the extrahepatic and intrahepatic ducts
  - IVb: multiple extrahepatic duct cysts
- Type V—intrahepatic duct cyst (single or multiple, as in Caroli disease).

Forme fruste is a special variant of choledochal cyst characterized by pancreaticobiliary malunion, but little or no dilatation of the extrahepatic bile duct.[8-12] Children present with symptoms similar to those in patients with a CC. Excision of the extrahepatic bile duct is recommended in children because of the likely eventual development of cancer due to chronic pancreaticobiliary reflux.

Type I CCs predominate. Together with type IVa cysts, they account for more than 90% of cases. Caroli disease is characterized by segmental saccular dilatation of the intrahepatic bile ducts. It may affect the liver diffusely or be localized to one lobe.[13-15]

Etiology

There are many theories to explain the development of a CC. However, none of these can explain the formation of the five different types of CC. Choledochal cysts seem to be either congenital or acquired. Congenital cysts develop during fetal life.[16] These appear to develop as a result of a prenatal structural defect in the bile duct. Shimotake found that the total number of ganglion cells within the wall of these CCs is significantly lower than in control specimens.[17] Also, smooth muscle fibers are more abundant in the cystic type than in the fusiform type.[18]

Choledochal cysts which develop later in life are considered 'acquired'.[16] The theory of the long common biliopancreatic channel proposed by Babit has been widely accepted to explain the formation of this type.[19] Normally, the terminal CBD and pancreatic duct unite to form a short common channel, which is well surrounded by Oddi's sphincter. This normal anatomic arrangement prevents the reflux of pancreatic fluid into the bile duct. If this common channel is long and part of it is not surrounded by the normal sphincter, pancreatic secretions can reflux into the biliary tree (Fig. 44-2). Proteolytic enzymes from the pancreatic fluid are activated and can cause epithelial and mural damage that leads to mural weakness and dilatation of the choledochus. This theory is supported by the fact that high concentrations of activated pancreatic amylase and/or lipase have been found in patients with CC and long pancreaticobiliary channels.[16,20-22] In an experimental study, CC was produced by creating a choledochopancreatic end-to-side ductal anastomosis.[23] Also, a high incidence of a common channel has been detected in CC patients.[24]

Obstruction at the level of the pancreaticobiliary junction may be an associated causal factor in choledochal dilatation. An experimental model for the study of cystic dilatation of the extrahepatic biliary system has been produced by ligation of the distal end of the CBD in the newborn lamb.[25] High biliary pressure in patients with CC have also been recorded during operative correction.[26]

In adults, an anomalous union of the pancreaticobiliary duct is defined when the common pancreaticobiliary channel is longer than 15 mm,[3,27] or when its extraduodenal portion is more than 6 mm.[28] In a study of 264 infants and children undergoing endoscopic retrograde cholangiopancreatography (ERCP), the maximal length of the common channel was found to be 2–7 mm among children ≤ 3 years old, 4 mm among children 4 to 9 years old, and 5 mm between 10 and 15 years old.[29]

An inflammatory reaction within the CC is noted in most cases. It is minimal in infants and gradually becomes more marked as the patient gets older. The degree of mucosal ulcerations and pericystic inflammation

TABLE 44-1	The Mean Common Bile Duct Diameter and the Range According to a Patient's Age	
Age (Years)	**Range (mm)**	**Mean (mm)**
≤4	2–4	2.6
4–6	2–4	3.2
6–8	2–6	3.8
8–10	2–6	3.9
10–12	3–6	4.0
12–14	3–7	4.9

Adapted from Witcombe JB, Cremin BJ. The width of the common bile duct in childhood. Pediatr Radiol 1978;7:147–9.

becomes more severe after repeated bouts of cholangitis. Stones or debris may be found in the CC, along with a dilated intrahepatic bile duct and a common biliopancreatic channel. Liver histology varies from normal to cirrhosis, depending on the patient's age and degree of cholangitis.

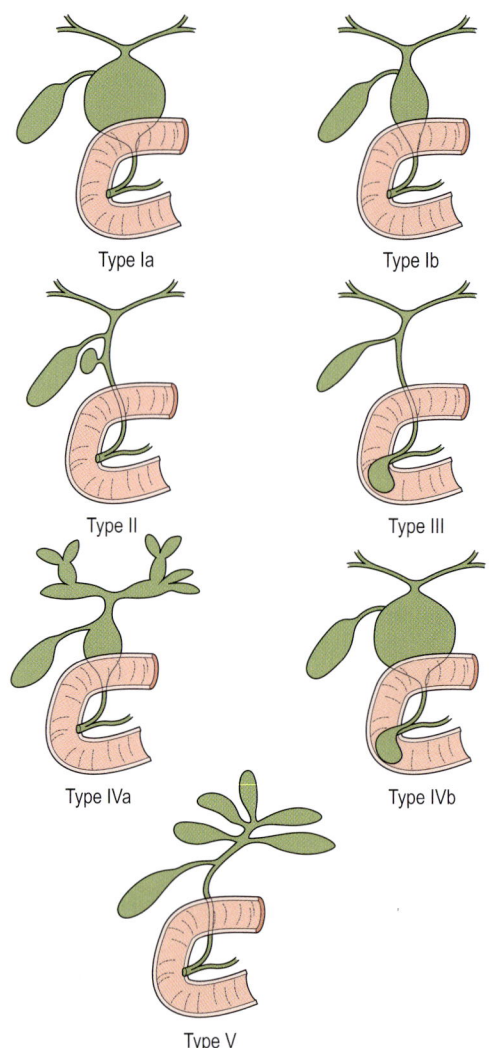

FIGURE 44-1 ■ These diagrams depict the five classifications for choledochal cyst according to Todani. (From Todani T, Watanabe Y, Narusue M, et al. Congenital bile duct cyst: Classification, operative procedure, and review of 37 cases including cancer arising from choledochal cyst. Am J Surg 1977;134:263–9.)

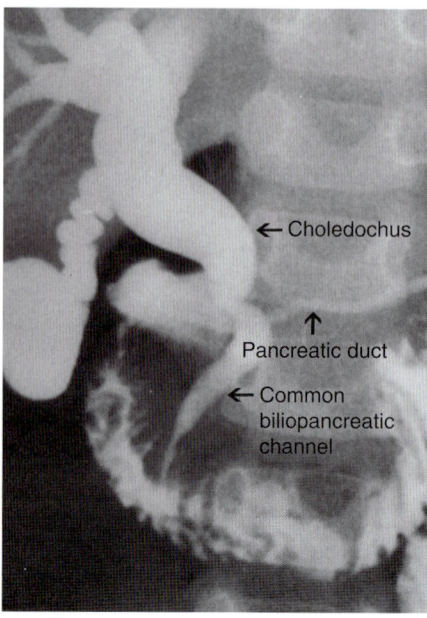

FIGURE 44-2 ■ This contrast study depicts a long common biliopancreatic channel which allows reflux of pancreatic secretions into the biliary tree. A long common biliopancreatic channel is thought to be the etiology of an acquired choledochal cyst.

Clinical Features

Females are affected more often than males. In our series of 400 cases, the female to male ratio was 3.2 to 1.[30] Clinical presentations differ according to the age of onset and the type of cyst. An abdominal mass or jaundice is a common finding in an infant with CC, whereas abdominal pain is more often seen in older children.[16,31–33] The cystic form usually presents with an abdominal mass whereas the fusiform type is usually found in patients presenting with abdominal pain. Choledochal cysts diagnosed antenatally are more likely cystic in nature.[16]

Clinical manifestations among our 400 cases included: abdominal pain (88%), vomiting (46%), fever (28%), icterus (25%), discolored stool (12%), abdominal tumor (7%), and the classic triad (2%).[30]

Complications such as perforation and hemobilia are rare;[34,35] however pancreatitis is common.[16,31] Malignant change is a late complication, mostly seen in adults.[36–39]

Imaging

Ultrasonography (US) is the initial imaging method of choice (Fig. 44-3A). Contour and position of the cyst, the status of the proximal ducts, vascular anatomy, and hepatic echotexture can all be evaluated on ultrasound.

ERCP allows excellent definition of the cyst as well as the entire anatomy, including the pancreatobiliary junction. However, this investigation is invasive and has complications such as pancreatitis, perforation of the duodenal or biliary tracts, hemorrhage, and sepsis.[40,41]

Magnetic resonance cholangiopancreatography (MRCP) is highly accurate in the detection and classification of the cysts. (Fig. 44-3B) The overall detection rate of MRCP for a CC is very high (96–100%) and

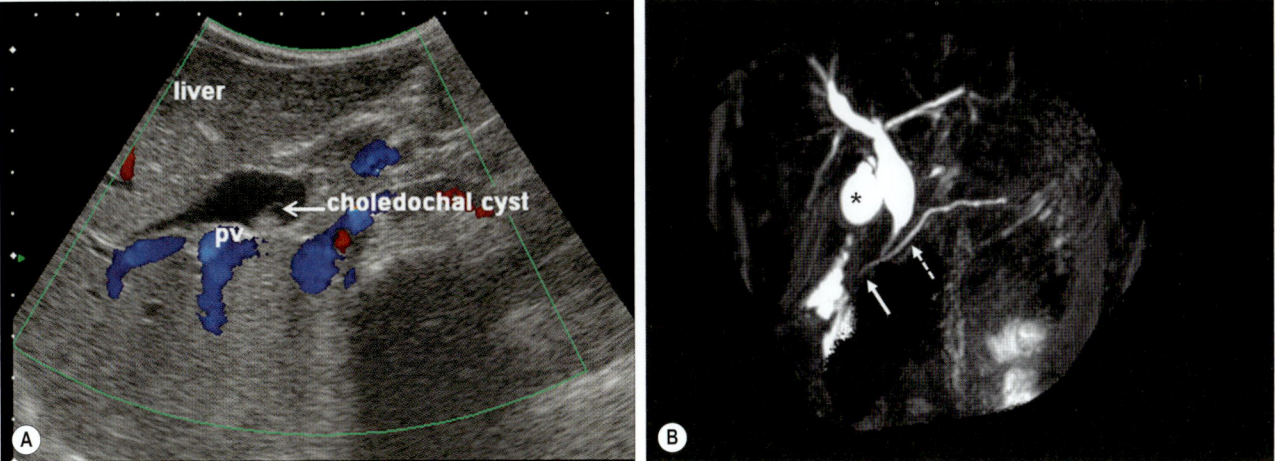

FIGURE 44-3 ■ **(A)** Ultrasound is the initial imaging method of choice for identifying a choledochal cyst. The cyst is identified as well as the portal vein (PV) lying posterior to it. **(B)** MRCP is highly accurate in the detection and classification of the cyst. On this MRCP image, note the fusiform choledochal cyst as well as the pancreatic duct (dotted arrow) and long common channel (solid arrow). The gallbladder is marked with an asterisk.

should be considered a first-choice imaging technique for evaluation.[42–44]

Intraoperative cholangiography is indicated when the anatomic detail of the biliary tract cannot be demonstrated by MRCP or ERCP (Fig. 44-4). Contrast-enhanced CT may be indicated in some patients with pancreatitis or if an associated tumor is suspected.

Surgical Techniques

General Principles

Cystoduodenostomy and cystojejunostomy have been abandoned due to cholangitis, stone formation, and

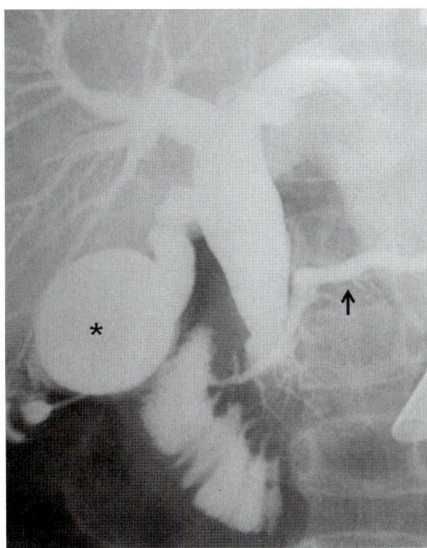

FIGURE 44-4 ■ In this patient, neither an MRCP nor ERCP were helpful preoperatively. Thus, an intraoperative cholangiogram was performed to identify the anatomic detail within the biliary tract. The distended gallbladder is marked with an asterisk. The enlarged choledochal cyst is seen and the pancreatic duct is identified with a solid arrow.

malignant degeneration.[6,45–47] External drainage is indicated for a perforated cyst in patients whose condition is too unstable to perform cystectomy and a bilio-enteric anastomosis.[34,35]

Cyst excision and a bilio-enteric anastomosis is the preferred approach for most patients. The cyst should be excised at the level of the common biliopancreatic channel orifice at its distal end and approximately 5 mm from the confluence of the right and left hepatic ducts at the proximal end. Postoperative malignancy in a residual cyst on either hepatic duct side or from the distal part has been reported.[48,49] A review from the English language and Japanese literature of 23 patients with carcinomas of the bile duct developing after CC excision found that malignancy developed in the intrapancreatic remnant of the bile duct or CC in six patients, in the remnant of the CC at the hepatic side in three patients, in the hepatic duct at or near the anastomosis in eight patients, and in the intrahepatic duct in six patients.[48] Abdominal pain and pancreatitis due to leaving a remnant of the cyst in the pancreatic head has also been described.[50]

Operative correction can be performed safely in all age groups.[30,51–53]

Preoperative Preparation

Biliary infection should be treated before operation. A prolonged prothrombin time secondary to cholestasis should be corrected with intravenous vitamin K. Drugs for elimination of ascaris are given in areas where ascaris is prevalent.

Bilio-Enteric Anastomosis after Cystectomy

Many surgeons use hepaticojejunostomy[54–59] while others prefer hepaticoduodenostomy.[60–64] Fat malabsoption and duodenal ulcer are the main concerns with a hepaticojejunostomy. In addition, the operative time is longer in comparison with hepaticoduodenostomy. Complications after Roux-en-Y hepaticojejunostomy such as a twist of the Roux limb, intestinal obstruction, and duodenal ulcers have been reported.[65–68] On the other hand, cholangitis and gastritis due to bilious reflux are the main concerns with hepaticoduodenostomy.[69,70] However, the operative time is shorter in comparison with hepaticojejunostomy. A hepaticoduodenostomy is considered more physiologic because the bile drains directly into the duodenum. This anastomosis is performed above the transverse colon mesentery which may help prevent intestinal obstruction from adhesions.

Laparoscopic Approach

Endotracheal intubation general anesthesia is standard. Epidural analgesia can provide excellent postoperative pain relief. Broad spectrum intravenous antibiotics are best given at induction of anesthesia and continued for five days postoperatively. A nasogastric tube, rectal tube, and urinary catheter are used to decompress the stomach, colon, and bladder. The patient is placed in a 30° lithotomy position (Fig. 44-5). The surgeon stands at the lower end of the operating table between the patient's legs.

The first laparoscopic operation for CC was reported in 1995.[71] This approach quickly became popular and has become a routine procedure in many centers.[30,72–84] The laparoscopic approach is preferred for most types of CC: I, II, and IV. Relative contraindications are in patients with perforation, previous biliohepatic surgery, or especially newborns with damaged hepatic functions.

A 10 mm cannula is inserted through the umbilicus for the telescope. Three additional 5 or 3 mm ports are introduced for the working instruments: one in the right flank, another in the left flank, and one in the left hypochondrium (Fig. 44-6). Carbon dioxide pneumoperitoneum is maintained at a pressure of 8–12 mmHg. The liver is secured to the abdominal wall with a suture placed around the round ligament (Fig. 44-7A). The cystic artery and the cystic duct are identified, clipped, and divided. A second traction suture is placed at the junction

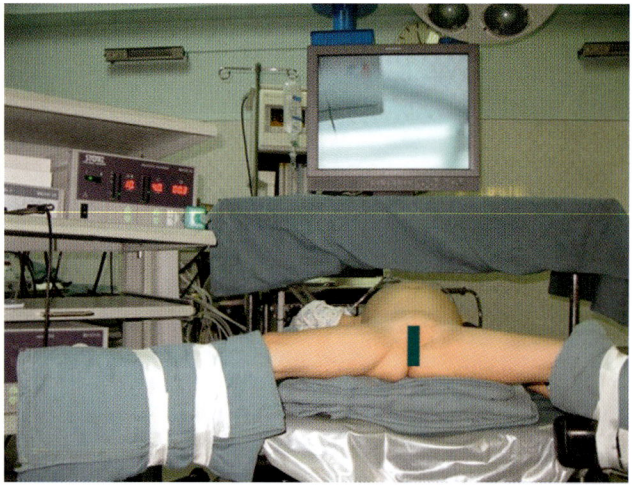

FIGURE 44-5 ■ Older patients are placed in the lithotomy position and smaller patients are moved to the end of the bed. It is helpful for the surgeon to stand either between the patient's legs (in older patients) or at the end of the operating table (in younger patients) for laparoscopic choledochal cyst repair.

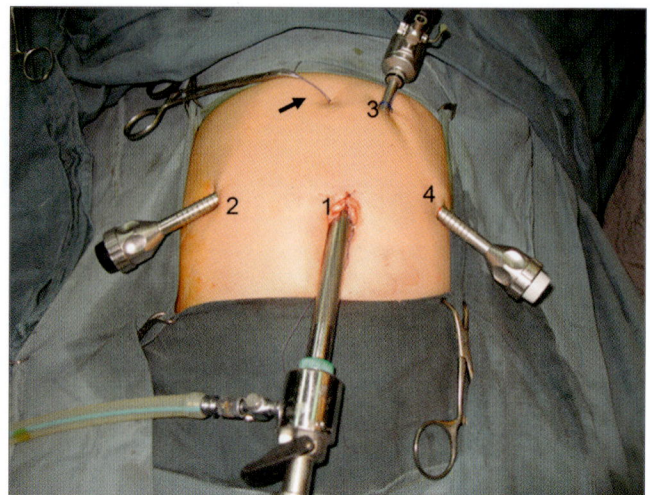

FIGURE 44-6 ■ This operative photograph depicts placement of the ports for laparoscopic repair of a choledochal cyst. A 10 mm cannula (1) is introduced through the umbilicus for the telescope. Three additional 5 mm or 3 mm ports are then used for the working instruments (2,3,4). Note the liver has been elevated anteriorly with a suture placed around the round ligament and exteriorized in the epigastric region (arrow).

of distal cystic duct and gallbladder fundus to elevate the liver and expose the hepatic hilum (Fig. 44-7B).

The appearance of the cyst, liver and spleen are noted. Intraoperative cholangiography via the gallbladder should be performed if the anatomy has not been clearly defined preoperatively. With a large cyst, bile is aspirated through a catheter, which reduces the cyst size to facilitate the pericystic dissection.

The duodenum is retracted downward using a dissector inserted through the left lower port. The mid-portion of the cyst is dissected circumferentially. Separation of the cyst from the hepatic artery and portal vein is meticulously performed until a dissector can be passed through the space between the posterior cyst wall and the portal vein going from left to right. The cyst is then divided at this site.

The inferior part of the cyst is separated from the pancreatic tissue down to the common biliopancreatic duct using a 3 mm dissector for cautery and dissection. Protein plugs or calculi within the cyst and common channel are washed out and removed. The inferior part of the cyst is opened longitudinally and inspected to identify the orifice of the common biliopancreatic channel. A small catheter is then inserted into the common channel. Irrigation with normal saline via this catheter is performed to eliminate protein plugs until clear fluid returns and the catheter can be passed down into the duodenum (Fig. 44-8A). A cystoscope can be used to remove protein plugs in the common channel if its diameter permits.[85,86] The distal CC is then clipped and divided at the level of the orifice of the common channel (Fig. 44-8B).

The cephalad portion of the cyst is further dissected to the common hepatic duct. The cyst is initially divided at the level of the cystic duct. After identifying the orifice of the right and left hepatic ducts, the rest of the cyst is removed, leaving a stump approximately 5 mm from the bifurcation of the hepatic ducts. Irrigation with normal

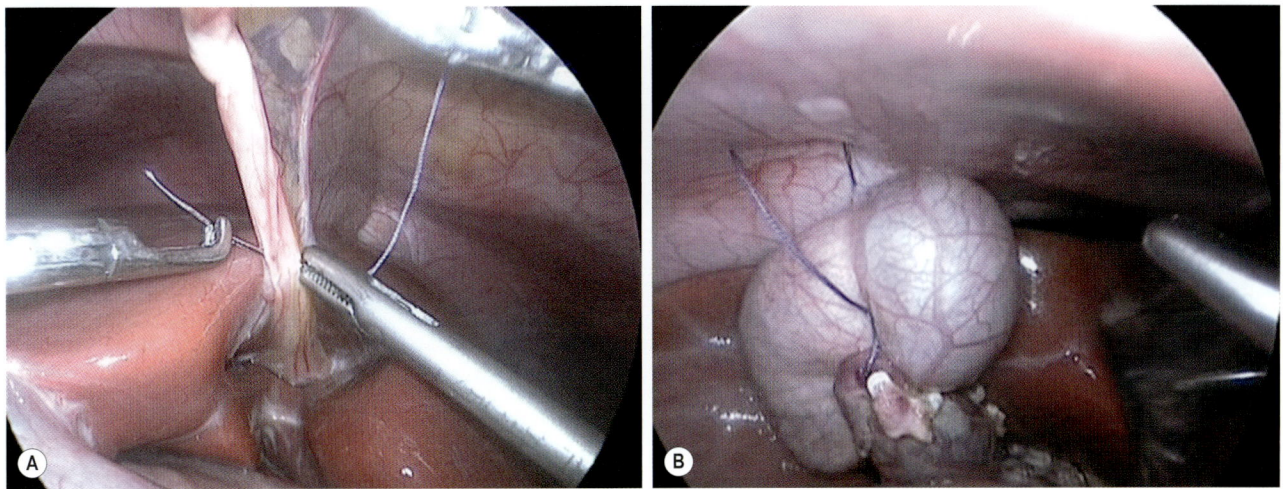

FIGURE 44-7 ■ **(A)** Suture has been placed through the round ligament and will be exteriorized in the epigastrium in order to help elevate the liver for exposure of the choledochal cyst. **(B)** A second traction suture has been positioned at the junction of the distal cystic duct and gallbladder fundus to further elevate the liver anteriorly and expose the hepatic hilum.

saline through a small catheter inserted into the right and then into the left hepatic duct is performed to wash out protein plugs or calculi until the effluent is clear.

If the cyst is intensely inflamed with extensive pericystic adhesions, the cyst is opened by a transverse incision on the anterior wall. The dissection of the cyst wall from the portal vein is then carefully performed while viewing the cyst from inside and outside. After dividing the mid-portion of the cyst, the upper and lower parts of the cyst are removed as previously described.

Hepaticojejunostomy

The ligament of Treitz is identified. A 5-0 silk suture is placed 10 cm distal to the ligament of Treitz in the newborn, 20 cm in infants, and 30 cm in children. A second suture (5-0 PDS, Ethicon, Inc., Somerville, NJ) is placed 2 cm below the first suture to mark the jejunal limb which will be anastomosed to the hepatic duct. The

jejunal segment containing the two sutures is grasped with a locking instrument. The previously-made transumbilical vertical incision is extended 1.0 cm cephalad. The jejunum is then exteriorized, and the jejunojejunostomy is performed extracorporeally. The jejunum is then returned into the abdominal cavity. The extended umbilical incision is closed and the laparoscopic instruments are reinserted.

The Roux limb is passed through a window in the transverse mesocolon to the porta hepatis. The jejunum is opened longitudinally on its antimesenteric border a few millimeters from the end of the Roux limb to avoid the creation of a significant blind pouch as the child grows. The hepaticojejunostomy is fashioned using two running sutures of 5-0 PDS (interrupted sutures are used when the diameter of the common hepatic duct is less than 1 cm). The anastomosis is performed from left to right using 3 mm instruments. If the diameter of the common hepatic duct is too small, ductoplasty is

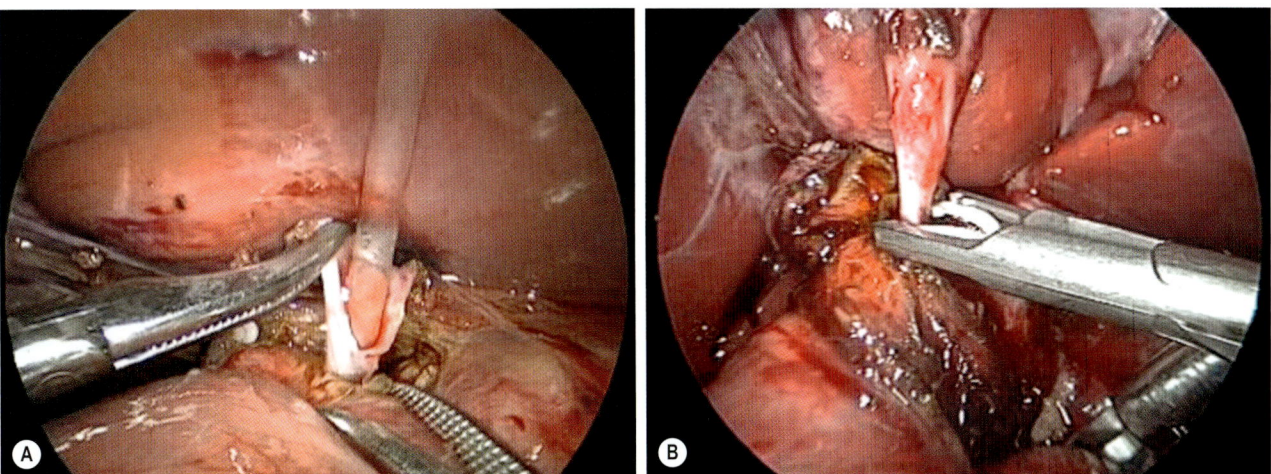

FIGURE 44-8 ■ **(A)** After opening the inferior part of the cyst to identify the orifice of the common biliopancreatic channel, a small catheter is inserted into the common channel for irrigation and elimination of protein plugs. **(B)** After irrigating the common channel, the distal choledochal cyst is being ligated with an endoscopic clip and will subsequently be divided at the level of the orifice of the common channel.

performed by opening the common hepatic duct and incising the left hepatic duct longitudinally for a variable distance.

Mesenteric defects in the transverse mesocolon and the small bowel mesentery are closed. The gallbladder is detached from its bed and the cyst and gallbladder are removed through the umbilicus. The operative field is washed with warm saline and a subhepatic closed suction drain is left.

Hepaticoduodenostomy

Following cyst resection, the duodenum is mobilized as much as possible, and a hepaticoduodenostomy is constructed 2–3 cm from the pylorus using two running sutures of 5-0 PDS. As noted previously, interrupted sutures are used when the diameter of the common hepatic duct is less than 1.0 cm. The rest of the operation is performed as previously described.

Open Operation

The open technique is used in patients with a perforated cyst, previous hepatobiliary operation, or if the surgeon does not feel comfortable with the laparoscopic approach.

A high transverse upper quadrant incision is used. The operative technique then follows that described for the laparoscopic approach. The cyst is mobilized as previously described, divided and removed, and either a hepaticojejunostomy or hepaticoduodenostomy are performed.

Alternative Operative Techniques

An alternative biliary reconstruction technique is an end-to-end hepaticojejunostomy (in contrast to end-to side). This should only be performed if there is no significant size discrepancy between the hepatic duct and Roux limb. A hepaticoduodensotomy with jejunal interposition can be performed if desired. The robotic approach has also been described.[87,88] This technique appears safe and effective, but the operative time is quite long.

Intraoperative Complications

Injury to the Portal Vein. This complication can be prevented by keeping the dissection as close to the cyst wall as possible. When severe pericystic inflammation and adhesions are present, opening the cyst on its anterior wall and carefully separating the left and posterior walls of the cyst from the portal vein, while viewing internally and externally, can help prevent injury to the portal vein.

Transection of Both Hepatic Ducts. This situation can happen when the hepatic bifurcation is low and away from the liver hilum. This complication can be avoided by identifying the orifice of the right and left hepatic ducts by internal inspection before excising the cyst from the hepatic duct.

Injury to the Pancreatic Duct. Understanding the anatomy of the common biliopancreatic channel via MRCP, ERCP or perioperative cholangiography is important. Internal inspection of the distal choledochus to identify the orifice of the common biliopancreatic duct helps the surgeon decide where the distal part of the cyst should be divided.

Postoperative Care

Oral feeding is initiated after the fluid from the gastric tube becomes clear, usually by postoperative day 2 or 3. The abdominal drain is removed on day 5 if there is no evidence of leak from the biliary-enteric anastomosis.

Complications from the laparoscopic approach are similar or lower when compared to the open operation.[89,90] Early postoperative complications include bleeding, anastomotic leak, pancreatic fistula, and intestinal obstruction. The anastomotic leak and pancreatic fistula often resolve with drainage, intravenous antibiotics, nasogastric decompression, and parenteral nutrition (TPN).

Significant late complications included cholangitis, anastomotic stricture, intrahepatic calculi, and bowel obstruction.[91] Cholangitis without anastomotic stricture or intrahepatic calculi is treated with antibiotics, whereas endoscopic maneuvers or reoperation are used for anastomotic stricture or intrahepatic calculi.

Caroli Disease and Choledochocele

Partial hepatectomy is indicated for the localized type of Caroli disease and liver transplantation is usually needed for diffuse disease.[14,15] Endoscopic unroofing of a choledochocele with sphincterotomy of the CBD, or sphincterotomy alone, are considered the preferred treatment for choledochocele.[92,93]

Outcomes

From January 2007 to June 2011, we performed laparoscopic correction in 400 patients with CC at the National Hospital of Pediatrics, Hanoi, Vietnam.[30] A total of 238 patients underwent laparoscopic cystectomy plus hepaticoduodenostomy, and 162 had cystectomy plus hepaticojejunostomy. The mean operative time for hepaticoduodenostomy was 164.8 ± 51 minutes and 212 ± 61 minutes for hepaticojejunostomy. Conversion to an open operation was required in two patients. Intraoperative complications included bleeding from the right portal vein in one patient and injury to the right hepatic duct in another. Repair was successful in both patients via laparoscopy. Early postoperative complications included biliary fistula in eight patients (2%), with one patient requiring reoperation. Pancreatic fistula developed in four patients (1.1%), but none of these required reoperation.

The mean postoperative hospital stay was 6.4 ± 3 days for hepaticoduodenostomy and 6.7 ± 0.5 days for hepaticojejunostomy. Follow-up from five to 57 months was obtained in 342 patients (85.5%). Five patients had cholangitis (1.5%) in the hepaticoduodenostomy group and one in hepaticojejunostomy group. Gastritis due to bilious reflux was 3.8% in the hepaticoduodenostomy group. Duodenal bleeding from an ulcer occurred in one patient who underwent a hepaticojejunostomy. Two patients required reoperation, one due to an anastomotic stricture and another due to stenosis at the bifurcation of hepatic ducts.

GALLBLADDER DISEASE

Over the past 15 years, gallbladder disease has become a very common problem for older children and young adolescents, especially in the U.S. Historically, gallbladder disease has been confined to children with hemolytic cholelithiasis. However, biliary dyskinesia is now the most common reason for laparoscopic cholecystectomy in many centers.[94,95]

Biliary Dyskinesia

Biliary dyskinesia is now a commonly seen condition in children.[94–100] In this disease, there is poor gallbladder contractility and cholesterol crystals are often seen in the bile. This disorder may have a similar pathophysiology to other diseases with increased numbers of mast cells in the gastrointestinal tract, such as eosinophilic gastroenteritis. A significant increase in mucosal mast cells have been noted in the gallbladder mucosa in patients with biliary dyskinesia when compared with patients with stone disease.[101,102]

These patients often present with a spectrum of symptoms that are found with gallbladder disease (nausea, vomiting, right upper abdominal pain), but they can also have atypical symptoms. In patients with this disorder, an ultrasound is usually normal. Therefore, a radionuclide study with cholecystokinin (CCK) injection or Lipomul is often needed to make this diagnosis.[96,103] Patients often complain of pain at the time the CCK is injected. Most surgeons use a gallbladder ejection fraction of less than 35% as an indicator for cholecystectomy in a patient with symptoms.[95,98,104,105] However, not all patients with an ejection fraction of less than 35% will have resolution of symptoms. Symptom resolution seems more likely the lower the gallbladder ejection fraction. In one report, unless children had an ejection fraction of less than 15%, there was not predictable relief of symptoms.[106] Thus, a careful discussion with the family is needed in these patients to inform them that their symptoms may not completely resolve following cholecystectomy.

Cholelithiasis

Historically, cholelithiasis has been the primary reason for cholecystectomy in children. Also, in the past, most adolescents with cholelithiasis had hemolytic disease, especially sickle cell disease (SCD) or hereditary spherocytosis (HS). Other reasons for the development of cholelithiasis include long-term TPN, dehydration, cystic fibrosis, short bowel syndrome, ileal resection, use of oral contraceptives, and obesity.[107–114] Nonhemolytic stones in adults are primarily cholesterol-based. In younger children, many stones have predominantly calcium carbonate.[115–117]

Classic symptoms for cholelithiasis include right upper abdominal pain following a fatty meal with associated nausea and vomiting. However, many children do not exhibit these classic symptoms and can have atypical symptoms. In younger children especially, the abdominal pain may be vague and poorly localized. Complications of cholelithiasis are increasingly being reported.[118–120] For this reason, cholecystectomy is recommended once cholelithiasis is identified. In patients with SCD, sludge has been felt to be an indication for cholecystectomy as well, even if stones are not present.[121] In a study of 35 patients with SCD and sludge, 23 (65.7%) proceeded to develop gallstones at some point.[122]

In evaluating children with gallbladder symptoms from cholelithiasis, rarely is a plain abdominal film helpful. Ultrasound is the usual initial study and has an accuracy approaching 95%.[123] In addition, the ultrasound can document involvement of the common and hepatic ducts, gallbladder inflammation, and other abnormalities in the liver and pancreas. Acute cholecystitis is usually diagnosed using a nuclear medicine study. In patients with acute cholecystitis, the radioactive analogs are excreted in the liver, but do not pass into the gallbladder due to obstruction of the cystic duct.

Special Considerations

There are four special considerations when evaluating the child with gallbladder disease. The first is the sickle cell child. Historically, it has been felt that these patients needed preoperative transfusion.[124–128] Many centers still require a hemoglobin greater than 10 mg/dl. However, some centers now stress the importance of adequate hydration in these patients rather than transfusion.

The second circumstance arises in the patient with HS who is undergoing splenectomy. In such patients, an ultrasound should be performed as it is relatively straightforward to remove the gallbladder at the same time if gallstones are noted. In a study of 17 patients with spherocytosis, but not cholelithiasis, none of these patients developed cholelithiasis with a mean follow-up of 15 years.[129] Thus, it is probably not necessary to prophylactically remove the gallbladder in HS patients undergoing splenectomy.

Another area of uncertainty is whether or not one should routinely perform a cholangiogram in all patients undergoing a laparoscopic cholecystectomy. Early in the development of minimally invasive surgery, it was felt best to perform a cholangiogram for surgeon training purposes. Now, however, it does not appear necessary to perform a cholangiogram unless there is a concern about the anatomy or it is unclear whether or not common duct stones are present.

A fourth situation involves the child or adolescent who presents with known or suspected choledocholithiasis. In adults, this situation is usually handled by ERCP with sphincterotomy and stone extraction either before or after the laparoscopic cholecystectomy. ERCP with sphincterotomy has become a routine aspect of adult care and is almost always successful in removing the stone(s). However, in children, many pediatric gastroenterologists are not trained in this technique and many children's

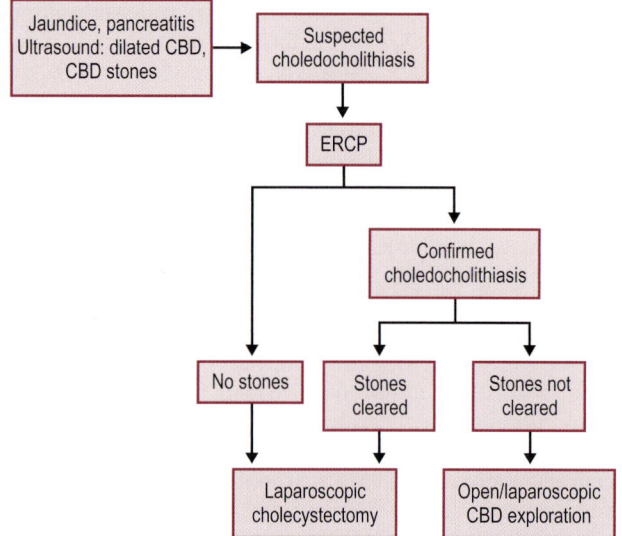

FIGURE 44-9 ■ This algorithm shows one approach for managing children with suspected choledocholithiasis. With this approach, an ERCP is performed prior to the laparoscopic cholecystectomy in a child with suspected choledocholithiasis. If stones are identified and the ERCP and sphincterotomy are successful, then the surgeon can proceed with the laparoscopic cholecystectomy soon thereafter. However, if the ERCP and sphincterotomy are not successful, the surgeon will know at the time of the laparoscopic cholecystectomy whether or not choledochal exploration is needed.

hospitals require the help of an adult endoscopist. Thus, the best approach in children depends on the institutional resources.

One approach in children with suspected CBD stones is to perform the ERCP and sphincterotomy before performing the laparoscopic cholecystectomy (Fig. 44-9).[130–133] If successful, then the surgeon can proceed with the laparoscopic cholecystectomy soon thereafter. However, if the ERCP and sphincterotomy are not successful, the surgeon will know at the time of the laparoscopic cholecystectomy whether or not choledochal exploration is needed. This can be performed laparoscopically for experienced surgeons and with an open approach for those who are not as experienced.

Surgical Techniques

Laparoscopic Cholecystectomy

The revolution in minimally invasive surgery began with the laparoscopic approach for cholecystectomy.[134–137] Recently, the four-port technique has been modified to a single incision approach through the umbilicus. Currently, there is no objective evidence that the single incision approach has advantages over the four-port technique. The most obvious presumed advantage is cosmesis. However, the small incisions utilized for the four-port technique heal very nicely and the cosmetic benefit appears marginal if there is a benefit at all. Only through prospective randomized trials with patient satisfaction surveys will this cosmetic benefit be determined.

Regardless of whether the patient is undergoing the four-port technique or a single incision approach, the patient is placed supine on the operating table and two video monitors are positioned at the head of the table. An orogastric tube is inserted for decompression of the stomach and the bladder is emptied using a Credé maneuver. For the single incision approach, some surgeons prefer to stand between the patient's legs, whereas the surgeon stands on the patient's left side for the four-port technique. Regardless of the operative approach, the patient is prepped and draped widely.

Four-Port Technique

Four small incisions are generally used for the traditional laparoscopic cholecystectomy. A 10 mm port is introduced in the umbilicus and a 10 mm telescope is introduced. (Although the optics are satisfactory with a 5 mm telescope, it is helpful to have a 10 mm port in the umbilicus to extract the gallbladder, especially if it is inflamed, so there is no real benefit to using a 5 mm umbilical port and telescope.) A 5 mm cannula is inserted in the epigastrium to the patient's right of the midline which becomes the main operating site for the surgeon. Two instruments are then placed on the patient's right side, one in the right mid-abdomen and one in the right lower abdomen (Fig. 44-10). A stab incision technique is often possible for these two right lateral instruments as they are not exchanged during the operation. Also, 3 mm instruments can be utilized in younger patients at these two sites as well.

The patient is then rotated into reverse Trendelenburg and to the left. The gallbladder is grasped using the right lower abdominal instrument and rotated cephalad over the liver to expose the triangle of Calot. The surgeon then utilizes the right upper abdominal instrument and the epigastric instrument to perform the procedure.

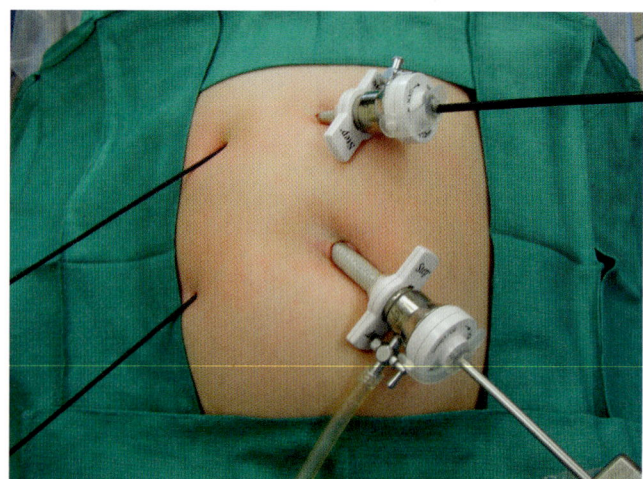

FIGURE 44-10 ■ The traditional laparoscopic cholecystectomy technique utilizes four ports. The umbilical cannula is 10 mm (as seen here) or 5 mm depending on the size of the telescope. A 5 mm cannula is inserted in the epigastrium which becomes the main operating site for the surgeon. Two instruments can often be placed through stab incisions on the patient's right side, one in the mid-abdomen and one in the lower abdomen. These two lateral instruments are not exchanged during the operation so the stab incision technique often works well. Also, in small patients, as depicted in this photograph, 3 mm instruments can be used on the patient's right side.

Initial attention is directed towards lysing adhesions to the infundibulum. Dissection follows to identify the cystic duct and cystic artery. At this point, lateral retraction of the infundibulum is essential to orient the cystic duct at 90° to the CBD to help prevent misidentification of these two structures. It is important to visualize the critical view of safety to correctly identify the anatomy. This initial view is bounded by the CBD medially, the cystic duct inferiorly, the gallbladder laterally, and the liver superiorly (Fig. 44-11A).[138] After the cystic duct and common duct have been correctly identified, two options exist. A cholangiogram can be performed if the anatomy is unclear or if there is suspicion of common duct stones. If the anatomy is clear and there is no suspicion of choledocholithiasis, then it is appropriate to ligate the cystic duct with endoscopic clips and then divide it (Fig. 44-11B). Similarly, the cystic artery is ligated and divided (Fig. 44-11C). Once these two structures have been ligated and divided, the gallbladder is then detached from the liver using retrograde dissection with cautery (Fig. 44-11D). Either the hook cautery, spatula cautery, or Maryland dissecting instrument connected to cautery can be used for this purpose. Prior to complete detachment of the gallbladder from the liver, the area of dissection should be inspected to ensure hemostasis, and then the gallbladder is completely detached. If there is little to no inflammation, the gallbladder can usually be exteriorized through the umbilical incision without using an endoscopic bag. However, for inflamed gallbladders, it is best to remove the specimen using a bag.

Single-Site Laparoscopic Cholecystectomy

For single site umbilical laparoscopic cholecystectomy (SSULS), it is necessary to use an umbilical incision of approximately 2 cm in length. In the U.S., a pre-manufactured port is often utilized. The two main devices used are the SILS Port (Covidien, Norwalk CT) or the TriPort (Olympus America, Center Valley PA). The SILS Port is a foam port with three working channels. The fourth instrument can usually be placed along the left side of the port (Fig. 44-12A). Although the TriPort is designed for three instruments, a fourth 3 mm instrument can often be inserted through one of the insufflation channels (Fig. 44-12B). It is helpful to have a long telescope so that the telescope holder is standing out of the way of the operating surgeon.

Outside the U.S., many surgeons place a single port in the umbilicus with instruments inserted through the fascia surrounding the umbilicus. Sometimes, low profile, 5 mm individual ports are utilized. Regardless of the technique and orientation of the instruments through the umbilicus, the principles of the procedure are the same as for the traditional four-port laparoscopic cholecystectomy. Lateral retraction of the infundibulum is important for visualization of the triangle of Calot and critical view

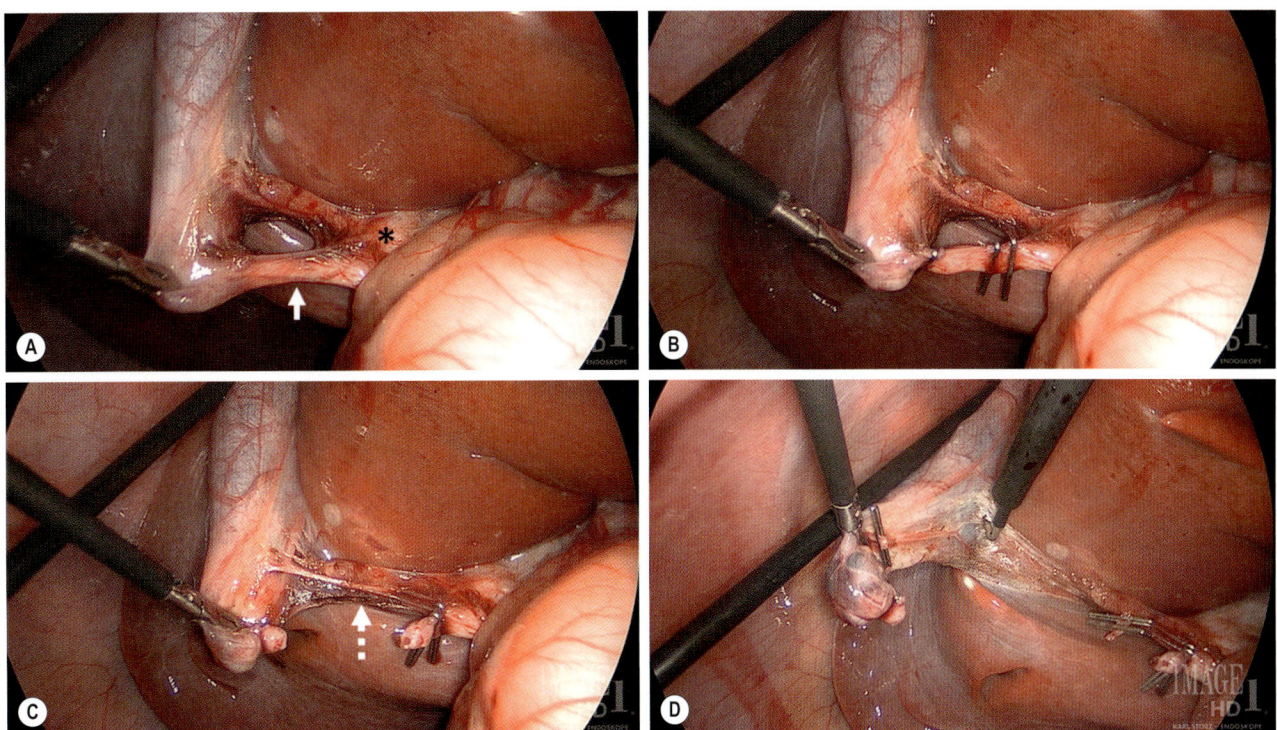

FIGURE 44-11 ■ These four figures depict the salient points for a laparoscopic cholecystectomy. **(A)** The gallbladder infundibulum is retracted laterally to orient the cystic duct (solid arrow) in relationship to the common duct (asterisk). Note the critical view of safety is identified. In this view, the liver is seen through the opened space bounded by the cystic duct inferiorly, gallbladder laterally and the liver superiorly. **(B)** The cystic duct has been ligated with endoscopic clips. Two clips are placed on the medial aspect of the duct which will remain following duct division. **(C)** The cystic duct has been divided and the cystic artery (dotted arrow) is visualized. **(D)** Following ligation and division of the cystic artery, the gallbladder is being dissected away from its liver bed using the hook cautery.

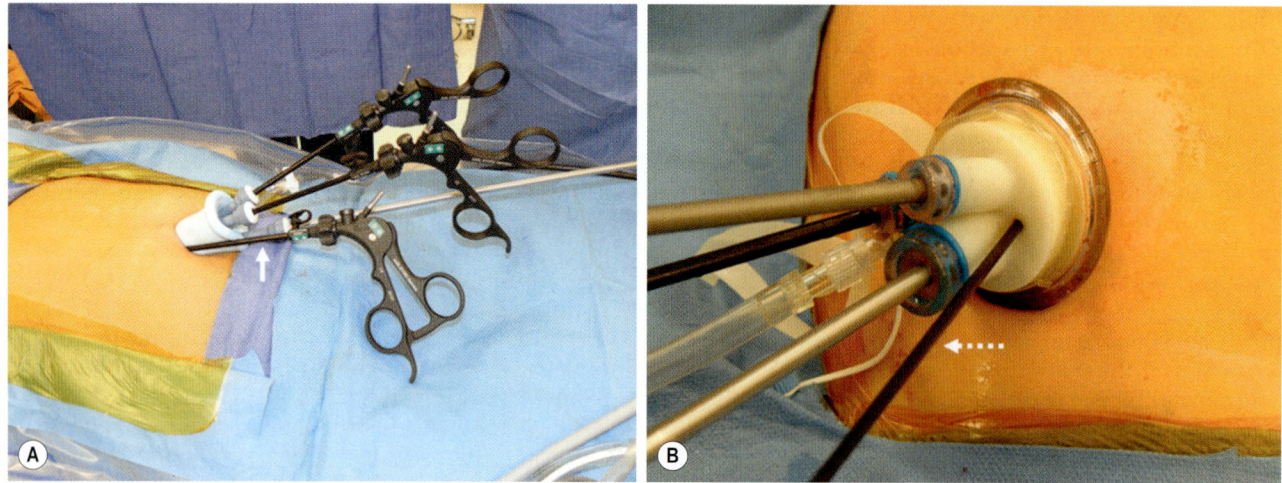

FIGURE 44-12 ■ In the United States, a pre-manufactured port is often utilized for a single site umbilical laparoscopic cholecystectomy. The two main devices used are the SILS Port (Covidien, Norwalk CT) seen on the left and the TriPort (Olympus America, Center Valley PA) on the right. In **(A)** there are three working channels in this SILS Port. A fourth instrument (solid arrow) can be inserted along the left side of the port. **(B)** The TriPort is designed for three instruments. However, a fourth 3 mm instrument (dotted arrow) can be inserted through one of the two insufflation channels.

TABLE 44-2 **Patients Undergoing Laparoscopic Cholecystectomy at Children's Mercy Hospital (September 2000–June 2006)**

Symptomatic gallstones (hemolytic disease)	166 (29)	Mean age (years)	12.9 (0–21)
Biliary dyskinesia	35	Mean Weight (kg)	58.3 (3–121)
Gallstone pancreatitis	7	Mean operating time (minutes)	77 (30–285)
Concomitant splenectomy	6		
Calculous cholecystitis	5		
Miscellaneous	5		
TOTAL	224		

From St. Peter SD, Keckler SJ, Nair A, et al. Laparoscopic cholecystectomy in the pediatric population. J Laparoendosc Adv Surg Tech A 2008;18:127–30.

of safety. The cystic duct and cystic artery are similarly ligated and divided as with the 4-port technique. One difference between the two approaches is that it is best to irrigate and suction all the fluid prior to exteriorizing the gallbladder as gallbladder removal entails removing the pre-manufactured port (if utilized). It can often be difficult to reinsert these ports so it is important to irrigate and suction prior to extracting the gallbladder. After removing the gallbladder and umbilical port, the umbilical fascia is closed with either interrupted or continuous 0-absorbable suture. The skin is approximated with interrupted 5-0 plain sutures.

Children's Mercy Hospital Experience

There are surprising few reports in the literature describing laparoscopic cholecystectomy in more than 100 children.[94,105,118,120,134] Our group at Children's Mercy Hospital (CMH) reported a six year experience between September 2000 and June 2006 with 224 patients undergoing laparoscopic cholecystectomy (Table 44-2).[98] In this study, the mean age was 12.9 years and the mean weight was 58.3 kg. Symptomatic gallstones were found in 166 children and biliary dyskinesia was diagnosed in 35 children. Seven patients presented with gallstone pancreatitis

and five had calculous cholecystitis. Six patients required splenectomy and were found to have gallstones. Only 29 patients had hemolytic disease with 18 patients having SCD and 11 having HS. The mean operating time was 77 minutes which excluded patients undergoing a concomitant splenectomy.

ERCP was performed preoperatively in 17 patients and stones were removed endoscopically in eight of these patients. An intraoperative cholangiogram was performed in 38 patients and choledocholithiasis was found in nine patients. CBD stones were cleared intraoperatively in five patients and the other four required postoperative endoscopy and sphincterotomy for stone retrieval. In this series, there were no conversions, ductal injuries, bile leaks or mortality, but one sickle cell patient required an emergency laparotomy for postoperative hemorrhage.

Recently, our group at CMH completed a prospective randomized trial comparing SSULS cholecystectomy and four-port laparoscopic cholecystectomy.[139] The primary outcome variable was operative time which was based on our own operative times for SSULS cholecystectomy and four-port cholecystectomy. Using an alpha of 0.05 and power of 0.80, 60 patients were enrolled in the study. Patients with signs of inflammation,

TABLE 44-3 Outcome Data Between Patients Randomized to Single Incision or Four-Port Laparoscopic Cholecystecomy

Outcome Variable	Single Incision (*n* = 30)	Four-Port (*n* = 30)	*P*-Value
Operative time (minutes)	68.6 ± 22.1	56.1 ± 22.1	**0.03**
Difficulty rating (1–5)	2.7 ± 1.0	1.9 ± 0.8	**0.005**
Total analgesic doses	16.4 ± 17.8	10.1 ± 4.3	0.06
Postoperative length of stay (hours)	22.7 ± 6.2	22.2 ± 6.8	0.44
Hospital charges ($)	29.7K ± 27.3K	20.6K ± 6.9K	0.08

From Ostlie DJ, Adibe OO, Juang D, et al. Single incision versus 4-port laparoscopic cholecystectomy: A propsective randomized trial. J Pediatr Surg 2013;48(1):209–14.

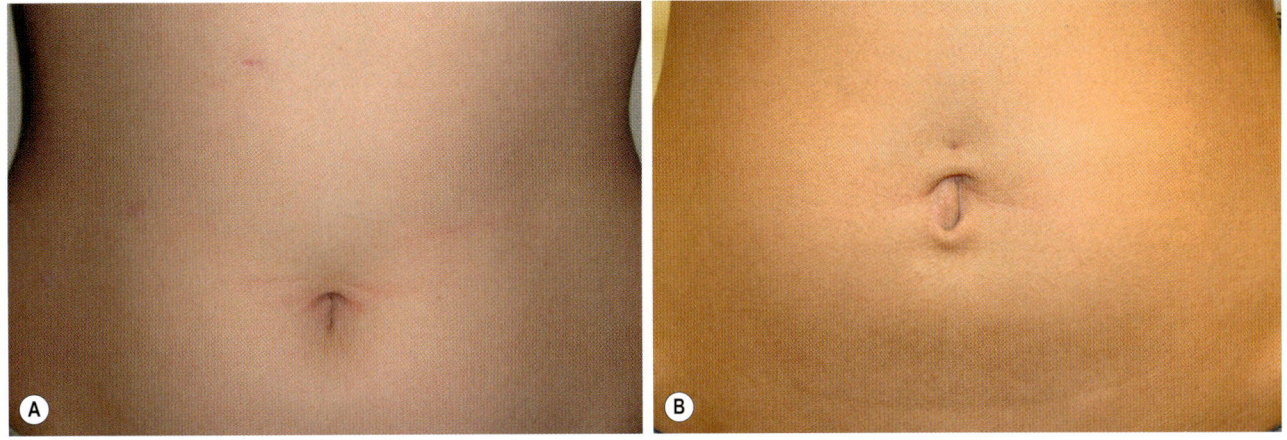

FIGURE 44-13 ■ These two patients both underwent a laparoscopic cholecystectomy. **(A)** The patient underwent a laparoscopic cholecystectomy using four ports. **(B)** The patient underwent a single site umbilical laparoscopic cholecystecotmy. To date, the main advantage of the SSULS approach appears to be cosmesis, but this advantage is marginal in most patients.

complicated disease, or weight over 100 kg were excluded. Also, surgeons participating in this study were asked to rate the degree of technical difficult from 1 (easy) to 5 (difficult). There were no differences in patient characteristics preoperatively.

Regarding the outcome data (Table 44-3), the operative time and degree of difficulty as determined by the surgeon were statistically significantly greater for the single incision approach. There were more doses of analgesics and greater hospital charges in the SSULS group which trended toward significance. The postoperative length of hospitalization was not clinically or statistically different between the two approaches. At present, cosmesis appears to be the sole advantage for the SSULS approach compared with the four-port technique (Fig. 44-13). However, the cosmetic advantage appears marginal, at best.

REFERENCES

1. Hernanz-Schulman M, Ambrosino MM, Freeman PC, et al. Common bile duct in children: Sonographic dimensions. Radiology 1995;195:193–5.
2. Witcombe JB, Cremin BJ. The width of the common bile duct in childhood. Pediatr Radiol 1978;7:147–9.
3. Kim HJ, Kim MH, Lee SK, et al. Normal structure, variations, and anomalies of the pancreaticobiliary ducts of Koreans: A nationwide cooperative prospective study. Gastrointest Endosc 2002;55:889–96.
4. Alonso-Lej F, Rever WB, Pessagno DJ. Congenital choledochal cyst, with a report of two cases, and analysis of 94 cases. Surg Gynecol Obstel 1959;108:1–30.
5. Todani T, Watanabe Y, Narusue M, et al. Congenital bile duct cyst: Classification, operative procedure, and review of 37 cases including cancer arising from choledochal cyst. Am J Surg 1977;134:263–9.
6. Thu NX, Cung HB, Liem NT, et al. Surgical treatment of congenital cystic dilatation of the biliary tract. Acta Chir Scand 1986;152:669–74.
7. Liem TL, Valayer J. Dilatation congenitale de la voie biliaire principale chez l'enfant. Etude d'une series de 52 cas. La Presse Med 1994;23:1565–8.
8. Miyano T, Ando K, Yamataka A, et al. Congenital biliary dilatation. Semin Pediatr Surg 2000;9:187–95.
9. Lilly JR, Stellin GP, Karrer FM. Forme fruste choledochal cyst. Pediatr Surg 1985;20:449–51.
10. Myanio T, Ando K, Yamataka A, et al. Pancreaticobiliary maljunction associated with nondilatation or minimal dilatation of the common bile duct in children: Diagnosis and treatment. Eur J Pediatr Surg 1996;6:334–7.
11. Shimotakahara A, Yamataka A, Kobayashi H, et al. Forme fruste choledochal cyst: Long-term follow-up with special reference to surgical technique. J Pediatr Surg 2003;38:1833–6.
12. Thomas S, Sen S, Zachariah N, et al. Choledochal cyst sans cyst-experience with six 'forme fruste' cases. Pediatr Surg Int 2002;18:247–51.
13. Caroli J, Soupault R, Kossakowski J, et al. La dilatation polykystique congénitale des voies biliaires intrahépatiques: Essai de classification. Sem Hop Paris 1958;34:128–35.
14. Madjov R, Chervenkov P, Madjova V, et al. Caroli's disease. Report of 5 cases and review of literature. Hepatogastroenterology 2005;52:606–9.
15. Kassahun WT, Kahn T, Wittekind C, et al. Caroli's disease: Liver resection and liver transplantation. Experience in 33 patients. Surgery 2005;138:888–9.
16. Davenport M, Stringer MD, Howard ER. Biliary amylase and congenital choledochal dilatation. J Pediatr Surg 1995;30:474–7.

17. Shimotake T, Iwai N, Yanagihara J, et al. Innervation patterns in congenital biliary dilatation. Eur J Pediatr Surg 1995;5:265–70.

18. Imazu M, Ono S, Kimura O, et al. Histological investigations into the difference between cystic and fusiform types of congenital biliary dilatation. Eur J Pediatr Surg 2003;13:16–20.

19. Babbitt DP. Congenital choledochal cysts: New etiological concept based on anomalous relationships of the common bile duct and pancreatic bulb. Ann Radiol 1969;12:231–40.

20. Jeong IH, Jung YS, Kim H, et al. Amylase level in extrahepatic bile duct in adult patients with choledochal cyst plus anomalous pancreatico-biliary ductal union. World J Gastroenterol 2005; 11:1965–70.

21. Ochiai K, Kaneko K, Kitagawa M, et al. Activated pancreatic enzyme and pancreatic stone protein (PSP/reg) in bile of patients with pancreaticobiliary maljunction/choledochal cyst. Dig Dis Sci 2004;49:1953–6.

22. Jung SM, Seo JM, Lee SK. The relationship between biliary amylase and the clinical features of choledochal cysts in pediatric patients. World J Surg 2012;36:2098–101.

23. Yamashiro Y, Miyano T, Suruga K, et al. Experimental study of the pathogenesis of choledochal cyst and pancreatitis, with special reference to the role of bile acids and pancreatic enzymes in the anomalous choledocho-pancreatico ductal junction. J Pediatr Gastroenterol Nutr 1984;3:721–7.

24. Komi N, Tamura T, Miyoshi Y, et al. Nationwide survey of cases of choledochal cyst. Analysis of coexistent anomalies, complications and surgical treatment in 645 cases. Surg Gastroenterol 1984;3:69–73.

25. Spitz L. Experimental production of cystic dilatation of the common bile duct in neonatal lambs. J Pediatr Surg 1977;12:39–42.

26. Davenport M, Basu R. Under pressure: Choledochal malformation manometry. J Pediatr Surg 2005;40:331–5.

27. Kimura K, Ohoto M, Ono T, et al. Congenital cystic dilatation of the common bile duct : Relationship to anomalous pancreatico-biliary ductal union. Am J Reoengenol 1977;128:571–7.

28. Ono J, Sakoda K, Akita H. Surgical aspect of cystic dilatation of the bile duct. An anomalous junction of the pancreaticobiliary tract in adults. Ann Surg 1982;195:203–8.

29. Guelrud M, Morera C, Rodriguez M, et al. Normal and anomalous pancreaticobiliary union in children and adolescents. Gastrointest Endosc 1999;50:189–93.

30. Liem NT, Hien PD, Son TN, et al. Early and intermediate outcomes of laparoscopic surgery for choledochal cyst with 400 patients. J Laparoendosc Adv Surg Tech A 2012;22:599–603.

31. Lai HS, Duh YC, Chen WJ, et al. Manifestations and surgical treatment of choledochal cyst in different age group patients. J Formos Med Assoc 1997;96:242–6.

32. Shukri N, Hasegawa T, Wasa M, et al. Characteristics of infantile cases of congenital dilatation of the bile duct. J Pediatr Surg 1998;33:1794–7.

33. Okada A, Nakmura R, Higaki J, et al. Congenital dilatation of the bile duct in 100 instances and its relationship with anomalous junction. Surg Gynecol Obstet 1991;172:291–8.

34. Ando K, Miyano T, Kohno S, et al. Spontaneous perforation of choledochal cyst: A study of 13 cases. Eur J Pediatr Surg 1998;8:23–5.

35. Ahmed I, Sharma A, Gupta A, et al. Management of rupture of choledochal cyst. Indian J Gastroenterol 2011;30:94–6.

36. Voyles CR, Smadja C, Shands WC, et al. Carcinoma in choledochal cysts. Age-related incidence. Arch Surg 1983;118:986–8.

37. Imazu M, Iwai N, Tokiwa K, et al. Factors of biliary carcinogenesis in choledochal cysts. Eur J Pediatr Surg 2001;11:24–7.

38. Kimura K, Ohto M, Saisho H, et al. Association of gallbladder carcinoma and anomalous pancreaticobiliary ductal union. Gastroenterology 1985;89:1258–65.

39. Todani T, Watanabe Y, Toki A, et al. Carcinoma related to choledochal cysts with internal drainage operation. Surg Gynecol Obstet 1987;164:61–4.

40. Jang JY, Yoon CH, Kim KM. Endoscopic retrograde cholangiopancreatography in pancreatic and biliary tract disease in Korean children. World J Gastroenterol 2010;16:490–5.

41. Otto AK, Neal MD, Slivka AN, et al. An appraisal of endoscopic retrograde cholangiopancreatography (ERCP) for pancreaticobiliary disease in children: Our institutional experience in 231 cases. Surg Endosc 2011;25:2536–40.

42. Park DH, Kim MH, Lee SK, et al. Can MRCP replace the diagnostic role of ERCP for patients with choledochal cysts? Gastrointest Endosc 2005;62:360–6.

43. Huang CT, Lee HC, Chen WT, et al. Usefulness of magnetic resonance cholangiopancreatography in pancreatobiliary abnormalities in pediatric patients. Pediatr Neonatol 2011;52:332–6.

44. Irie H, Honda H, Jimi M, et al. Value of MR cholangiopancreatography in evaluating choledochal cysts. AJR Am J Roentgenol 1998;171:1381–5.

45. Saing H, Tam PKH, Lee JMH, et al. Surgical management of choledochal cysts: A review of 60 cases. J Pediatr Surg 1985;20:443–8.

46. Shi LB, Peng SY, Meng XK, et al. Diagnosis and treatment of congenital choledochal cyst: 20 years' experience in China. World J Gastroenterol 2011;7:732–47.

47. Fu M, Wang YX, Zhang JZ. Evolution in the treatment of choledochal cyst. J Pediatr Surg 2000;335:1344–7.

48. Watanabe Y, Toki A, Todani T. Bile duct cancer developed after cyst excision for choledochal cyst. J Hepatobiliary Pancreat Surg 1999;6:207–12.

49. Kobayashi S, Asano T, Yamasaki M, et al. Risk of bile duct carcinogenesis after excision of extrahepatic bile ducts in pancreaticobiliary maljunction. Surgery 1999;126:939–44.

50. Koshinaga T, Hoshino M, Inoue M, et al. Pancreatitis complicated with dilated choledochal remnant after congenital cyst excision. Pediatr Surg Int 2005;21:936–8.

51. Lee SC, Kim HY, Jung SE, et al. Is excision of a choledochal cyst in the neonatal period necessary? J Pediatr Surg 2006; 41:1984–6.

52. Burnweit CA, Birken GA, Heiss K. The management of choledochal cysts in the newborn. Pediatr Surg Int 1996;11:130–3.

53. Howell CG, Templeton JM, Weiner S, et al. Antenatal diagnosis and early surgery for choledochal cysts. J Pediatr Surg 1983; 18:387–93.

54. Ohi R, Yaota S, Kamiyama T, et al. Surgical treatment of congenital dilatation of the bile duct with special reference to late complications after total cyst excision operation. J Pediatr Surg 1990; 25:613–17.

55. Miyano T, Yamataka A, Kato Y, et al. Hepaticoenterostomy after excision of choledochal cyst in children: A 30-year experience with 180 cases. J Pediatr Surg 1996;31:1417–21.

56. Edil BH, Cameron JL, Reddy S, et al. Choledochal cyst disease in children and adults: A 30-year single-institution experience. J Am Coll Surg 2008;206:1000–5.

57. She W, Chung HY, Lan LCL, et al. Management of choledochal cyst: 30 years of experience and results in a single center. J Pediatr Surg 2009;44:2307–11.

58. Stringer MD. Wide hilar hepaticojejunostomy: The optimum method of reconstruction after choledochal cyst excision. Pediatr Surg Int 2007;23:529–32.

59. Ono S, Fumino S, Shimadera S, et al. Long-term outcomes after hepaticojejunostomy for choledochal cyst: A 10–27 year follow-up. J Pediatr Surg 2010;45:376–8.

60. Todani T, Watanabe Y, Mizuguchi T, et al. Hepaticoduodenostomy at the hepatic hilum after excision of choledochal cyst. Am J Surg 1981;142:584–7.

61. Oweida SW, Ricketts RR. Hepatico-jejuno-duodenostomy reconstruction following excision of choledochal cysts in children. Am Surg 1989;55:2–6.

62. Cosentino CM, Luck SR, Raffensperger JG, et al. Choledochal duct cyst resection with physiologic reconstruction. Surgery 1992;112:740–7.

63. Santore MT, Behar BJ, Blinman TA, et al. Hepaticoduodenostomy vs. hepaticojejunostomy for reconstruction after resection of choledochal cyst. J Pediatr Surg 2011;46:209–13.

64. Mukhopadhyay B, Shukla RM, Mukhopadhyay M, et al. Choledochal cyst: A review of 79 cases and the role of hepaticodochoduodenostomy. J Indian Assoc Pediatr Surg 2011;16:54–7.

65. Bismuth H, Franco D, Corlette MB, et al. Long term results of Roux-en-Y hepaticojejunostomy. Surg Gynecol Obstet 1978; 146:161–7.

66. Martino A, Noviello C, Cobellis G, et al. Delayed upper gastrointestinal bleeding after laparoscopic treatment of form fruste

choledochal cyst. J Laparoendosc Adv Surg Tech A 2009;19:457–9.

67. Malhotra RS, Jain A, Prabhu RY, et al. Ischemic stricture of Roux-en-Y intestinal loop and recurrent cholangitis. Indian J Gastroenterol 2005;24:76–7.

68. Houben CH, Chan M, Cheung G, et al. A hepaticojejunostomy: Technical errors with 'twists and turns'. Pediatr Surg Int 2006;22:841–4.

69. Shimotakahara A, Yamataka A, Yanai T, et al. Roux-en Y hepaticojejunostomy or hepaticoduodenostomy for biliary reconstruction during the surgical treatment of choledochal cyst: Which is better? Pediatr Surg Int 2005;21:5–7.

70. Takada K, Hamada Y, Watanabe K, et al. Duodenalgastric reflux following biliary reconstruction after excision of choledochal cyst. Pediatr Surg Int 2005;21:1–4.

71. Farello GA, Cerofolini A, Rebonato M, et al. Congenital choledochal cyst: Video-guided laparoscopic treatment. Surg Laparosc Endosc 1995;5:354–8.

72. Tanaka M, Shimizu S, Mizumoto K, et al. Laparoscopically assisted resection of choledochal cyst and Roux-en-Y reconstruction. Surg Endosc 2001;15:545–52.

73. Tan HL, Shankar KR, Ford WD. Laparoscopic resection of type I choledochal cyst. Surg Endosc 2003;17:1495.

74. Li L, Feng W, Jing-Bo F, et al. Laparoscopic-assisted total cyst excision of choledochal cyst and Roux-en Y hepatoenterostomy. J Pediatr Surg 2004;39:1663–6.

75. Lee H, Hirose S, Bratton B, et al. Initial experience with complex laparoscopic biliary surgery in children: Biliary atresia and choledochal cyst. J Pediatr Surg 2004;39:804–7.

76. Jang JY, Kim SW, Han HS, et al. Totally laparoscopic management of choledochal cyst using a four-hole method. Surg Endosc 2006;20:1762–5.

77. Laje P, Questa H, Bailez M. Laparoscopic leak-free technique for the treatment of choledochal cyst. J Laparoendosc Adv Surg Tech A 2007;17:519–21.

78. Aspelund G, Ling SC, Ng V, et al. A role for laparoscopic approach in the treatment of biliary atresia and choledochal cysts. J Pediatr Surg 2007;42:869–73.

79. Hong L, Wu Y, Yan Z, et al. Laparoscopic surgery for choledochal cyst in children: A case review of 31 patients. Eur J Pediatr Surg 2008;18:67–71.

80. Liem NT, Dung LA, Son TN. Laparoscopic complete cyst excision and hepaticoduodenostomy for choledochal cyst: Early results in 74 cases. J Laparoendos Adv Surg Tech 2009;19:s87–90.

81. Liem NT, Hien PD, Dung LA, et al. Laparoscopic repair for choledochal cyst: Lessons learned from 190 cases. J Pediatr Surg 2010;45:540–4.

82. Chokshi NK, Guner YS, Aranda A, et al. Laparoscopic choledochal cyst excision: Lessons learned in our experience. J Laparoendosc Adv Surg Tech A 2009;19:87–91.

83. Lee KH, Tam YH, Yeung CK, et al. Laparoscopic excision of choledochal cyst in children: An intermediate-term report. Pediatr Surg Int 2009;25:355–60.

84. Kirschner HJ, Szavay PO, Schaefer JF, et al. Laparoscopic Roux-en-Y hepaticojejunostomy in children with long common pancreaticobiliary channel: Surgical technique and functional outcome. J Laparoendosc Adv Surg Tech A 2010;20:L485–8.

85. Diao M, Li L, Zhang JS, et al. Laparoscopic-assisted clearance of protein plugs in the common channel in children with choledochal cysts. J Pediatr Surg 2010;45:2099–102.

86. Miyano G, Koga H, Shimotakahara A, et al. Intralaparoscopic endoscopy: Its value during laparoscopic repair of choledochal cyst. Pediatr Surg Int 2011;27:463–6.

87. Woo R, Le D, Albanese CT, Kim SS. Robot-assisted laparoscopic resection of a type I choledochal cyst in a child. J Laparoendosc Adv Surg Tech A 2006;16:179–83.

88. Meehan JJ, Elliots S, Sandler A. The robotic approach to complex hepatobiliary anomalies in children: Preliminary report. J Pediatr Surg 2007;42:2110–14.

89. Liem NT, Pham HD, Vu HM. Is the laparoscopic operation as safe as open operation for choledochal cyst in children? J Laparoendosc Adv Surg Tech A 2011;21:367–70.

90. Diao M, Li L, Cheng W. Laparoscopic versus open Roux-en-Y hepaticojejunostomy for children with choledochal cysts:

Intermediate-term follow-up results. Surg Endosc 2011;25:1567–73.

91. Yamataka A, Ohshiro K, Okada Y, et al. Complications after cyst excision with hepaticoenterostomy for choledochal cysts and their surgical management in children versus adults. J Pediatr Surg 1997;32:1097–102.

92. Martin RF, Biber BP, Bosco JJ, et al. Symptomatic choledochoceles in adults. Endoscopic retrograde cholangiopancreatography recognition and management. Arch Surg 1992;127:536–8.

93. Dohmoto M, Kamiya T, Hünerbein M, et al. Endoscopic treatment of a choledochocele in a 2-year-old child. Surg Endosc 1996;10:1016–18.

94. Hofeldt M, Richmond B, Huffman K, et al. Laparoscopic cholecystectomy for treatment of biliary dyskinesia is safe and effective in the pediatric population. Am Surg 2008;74:1069–72.

95. Siddiqui S, Newbrough S, Alterman D, et al. Efficacy of laparoscopic cholecystectomy in the pediatric population. J Pediatr Surg 2008;43:109–13.

96. Vegunta RK, Raso M, Pollock J, et al. Biliary dyskinesia: The most common indication for cholecystectomy in children. Surgery 2005;138:726–33.

97. Cay A, Imamoglu M, Kosucu P, et al. Gallbladder dyskinesia: A cause of chronic abdominal pain in children. Eur J Pediatr Surg 2003;13:302–6.

98. St. Peter SD, Keckler SJ, Nair A, et al. Laparoscopic cholecystectomy in the pediatric population. J Laparoendosc Adv Surg Tech A 2008;18:127–30.

99. Halata MS, Berezin SH. Biliary dyskinesia in the pediatric patient. Curr Gastroenterol Rep 2008;10:332–8.

100. Campbell BT, Narasimhan NP, Golladay ES, et al. Biliary dyskinesia: A potentially unrecognized cause of abdominal pain in children. Pediatr Surg Int 2004;20:579–81.

101. Rau B, Friesen CA, Daniel JF, et al. Gallbladder wall inflammatory cells in pediatric patients with biliary dyskinesia and cholelithiasis: A pilot study. J Pediatr Surg 2006;41:1545–8.

102. Friesen CA, Neilan N, Daniel JF, et al. Mast cell activation and clinical outcomes in pediatric cholelithiasis and biliary dyskinesia. BMC Research Notes 2011;4:322:1–8.

103. Hadigan C, Fishman SJ, Connolly LP, et al. Stimulation with fatty meal (Lipomul) to assess gallbladder emptying in children with chronic acalculous cholecystitis. J Pediatr Gastroenterol Nutr 2003;37:178–82.

104. Brugge WR, Brand DL, Atkins HL, et al. Gallbladder dyskinesia in chronic acalculous cholecystitis. Dig Dis Sci 1986;31:461–7.

105. Kaye AJ, Jatia M, Mattei P, et al. Use of laparoscopic cholecystectomy for biliary dyskinesia in the child. J Pediatr Surg 2008;43:1057–9.

106. Carney DE, Kokoska ER, Grosfeld JL, et al. Predictors of successful outcome after cholecystectomy for biliary dyskinesia. J Pediatr Surg 2004;39:813–16.

107. Roy CC, Belli DC. Hepatobiliary complications associated with TPN: An enigma. J Am Coll Nutr 1985;4:651–60.

108. El-Shafie M, Mah CL. Transient gallbladder distention in sick premature infants: The value of ultrasonography and radionuclide scintigraphy. Pediatr Radiol 1986;16:468–71.

109. Manji N, Bistrian BR, Mascioli EA, et al. Gallstone disease in patients with severe short bowel syndrome dependent on parenteral nutrition. J Parent Enter Nutr 1989;13:461–4.

110. Quigley EM, Marsh MN, Shaffer JL, et al. Hepatobiliary complications of total parenteral nutrition. Gastroenterology 1993;104:286–301.

111. Lindberg MC. Hepatobiliary complications of oral contraceptives. J Gen Intern Med 1992;7:199–209.

112. Shocket E. Abdominal abscess from gallstones spilled at laparoscopic cholecystectomy. Surg Endosc 1995;9:344–7.

113. Stern RC, Rothstein FC, Doershuk CF. Treatment and prognosis of symptomatic gallbladder disease in patients with cystic fibrosis. J Pediatr Gastroenterol Nutr 1986;5:35–40.

114. Kaechele V, Wabitsch M, Thiere D, et al. Prevalence of gallbladder stone disease in obese children and adolescents: Influence of the degree of obesity, sex, and pubertal development. J Pediatr Gastroenterol Nutr 2006;42:66–70.

115. Stringer MD, Taylor DR, Soloway RD. Gallstone composition: Are children different? J Pediatr 2003;142:435–40.

116. Stringer MD, Soloway RD, Taylor DR, et al. Calcium carbonate gallstones in children. J Pediatr Surg 2007;42:1677–82.

117. Sayers C, Wyatt J, Soloway RD, et al. Gallbladder mucin production and calcium carbonate gallstones in children. Pediatr Surg Int 2007;23:219–23.

118. Holcomb GW III, Morgan WM III, Neblett WW III, et al. Laparoscopic cholecystectomy in children: Lessons learned from the first 100 patients. J Pediatr Surg 1999;34:1236–40.

119. Kumar R, Nguyen K, Shun A. Gallstones and common bile duct calculi in infancy and childhood. Aust N Z J Surg 2000;70:188–91.

120. Waldhausen JHT, Graham DD, Tapper D. Routine intraoperative cholangiography during laparoscopic cholecystectomy minimizes unnecessary endoscopic retrograde cholangiopancreatography in children. J Pediatr Surg 2001;36:881–4.

121. Winter SS, Kinney TR, Ware RE. Gallbladder sludge in children with sickle cell disease. J Pediatr 1994;125:747–9.

122. Al-Salem AH, Qaisruddin S. The significance of biliary sludge in children with sickle cell disease. Pediatr Surg Int 1998;13:14–16.

123. Cooperberg PL, Burhenne HJ. Real-time ultrasonography: Diagnostic treatment of choice in calculous gallbladder disease. N Engl J Med 1980;302:1277–9.

124. Haberkern CM, Neumayr LD, Orringer EP, et al. Cholecystectomy in sickle cell anemia patients: Perioperative outcome of 364 cases from the National Preoperative Transfusion Study. Preoperative Transfusion in Sickle Cell Disease Study Group. Blood 1997;89:1533–42.

125. Wales PW, Carver E, Crawford MW, et al. Acute chest syndrome after abdominal surgery in children with sickle cell disease: Is a laparoscopic approach better? J Pediatr Surg 2001;36:718–21.

126. Bhattacharyya N, Wayne AS, Kevy SV, Shamberger RC. Perioperative management for cholecystectomy in sickle cell disease. J Pediatr Surg 1993;28:72–5.

127. Sandoval C, Stringel G, Ozkaynak MF, et al. Perioperative management of children with sickle cell disease undergoing laparoscopic surgery. JSLS 2002;6:29–33.

128. Ware R, Filston HC, Schultz WH, et al. Elective cholecystectomy in children with sickle hemoglobinopathies. Ann Surg 1988;208:17–22.

129. Sandler A, Winkel G, Kimura K, et al. The role of prophylactic cholecystectomy during splenectomy in children with hereditary spherocytosis. J Pediatr Surg 1999;34:1077–8.

130. Mah D, Wales P, Njere I, et al. Management of suspected common bile duct stones in children: Role of selective intraoperative cholangiogram and endoscopic retrograde cholangiopancreatography. J Pediatr Surg 2004;39:808–12.

131. Newman KD, Powell DM, Holcomb GW III. The management of choledocholithiasis in children in the era of laparoscopic cholecystectomy. J Pediatr Surg 1997;32:1116–19.

132. Shah RS, Blakely ML, Lobe TE. The role of laparoscopy in the management of common bile duct obstruction in children. Surg Endosc 2001;15:1353–5.

133. Zargar SA, Javod G, Khan BA, et al. Endoscopic sphincterotomy in the management of bile duct stones in children. Am J Gastroenterol 2003;98:586–9.

134. Muhe E. Die erste cholecystectomy durch das laparoscope. Langenbecks Arch Chir 1986;369:804–6.

135. Dubois F, Berthelot G, Levard H. Cholecystectomy by coelioscopy (in French). Presse Med 1989;18:980–2.

136. Reddick EJ, Olsen DO. Laparoscopic laser cholecystectomy. A comparison with mini-lap cholecystectomy. Surg Endosc 1989;3:131–3.

137. McKernan JB. Laparoscopic cholecystectomy. Am Surg 1991;57:309–12.

138. Strasberg SM, Hertl M, Soper NJ. An analysis of the problem of biliary injury during laparoscopic cholecystectomy. J Am Coll Surg 1995;180:101–25.

139. Ostlie DJ, Adibe OO, Juang D, et al. Single incision versus 4-port laparoscopic cholecystectomy: A propsective randomized trial. J Pediatr Surg 2013;48(1):209–14.

CHAPTER 45

SOLID ORGAN TRANSPLANTATION IN CHILDREN

Frederick C. Ryckman • Maria H. Alonso • Jaimie D. Nathan • Gregory M. Tiao

The ability to successfully perform solid organ transplantation in children has led to a remarkable improvement in survival and quality of life. In this chapter each of the solid organ transplant procedures will be discussed, including the indications, operative procedure, and postoperative complications relevant to the practicing pediatric surgeon.

LIVER TRANSPLANTATION

Few subspecialties have undergone the dramatic improvements in survival that have occurred in pediatric liver transplantation (LT). In the early 1980s, survival rates of 30% limited the enthusiasm for this costly and work-intensive endeavor. The introduction of more effective immunosuppression along with refinements in the operative and postoperative management of infants and children has led to survival rates greater than 90%. Challenges remain, including the need for donor organs suitable for pediatric recipients of all ages and sizes, the optimization of the pretransplant patient physiology to increase peritransplant survival, and the improvement in long-term quality of life.

Indications for Transplantation

The most common clinical presentations prompting transplant evaluation in children can be classified as follows: (1) primary liver disease with the expected outcome of hepatic failure; (2) stable liver disease with significant morbidity or known mortality; (3) hepatic-based metabolic disease; (4) fulminant hepatic failure; and (5) hepatic malignancy, particularly hepatoblastoma, where the lesion is not resectable by conventional means. In addition, children with diffuse and extensive arteriovenous anomalies or benign vascular tumors leading to irreversible heart failure should also be considered for transplantation.

Table 45-1 reviews the leading diagnoses that lead to LT. These disease entities define the bimodal age distribution of pediatric transplant recipients. Infants and children with biliary atresia and, occasionally, rapidly progressive hepatic failure secondary to metabolic abnormalities, such as neonatal tyrosinemia, hemochromatosis, or neonatal hepatic vascular tumors, are the patients who require transplantation early in life. Patients with hepatic tumors, metabolic disturbances, fulminant hepatic failure,

and cirrhosis present as older children and adolescents requiring LT.

Biliary Atresia

Children with extrahepatic biliary atresia constitute at least 50% of the pediatric LT population. Successful biliary drainage achieving an anicteric state following the Kasai portoenterostomy is the most important factor affecting preservation of liver function and long-term survival.[1] Primary transplantation without portoenterostomy is not recommended in patients with biliary atresia unless the initial presentation is greater than 120 days of age and the liver biopsy shows advanced cirrhosis.[2,3] We believe that the Kasai portoenterostomy should be the primary surgical intervention for all other infants with extrahepatic biliary atresia. Patients with progressive disease following a Kasai procedure should be offered early orthotopic liver transplantation (OLT). The sequential use of these two procedures optimizes overall survival and organ use.[3]

Patients with extrahepatic biliary atresia who are seen for transplantation form several cohorts. Infants with a failed Kasai have recurrent cholangitis, ascites, rapidly progressive portal hypertension, malnutrition, and progressive hepatic synthetic failure, and often require OLT within the first two years of life. Children with the successful establishment of biliary drainage have an improved prognosis, but this alone does not preclude the development of cirrhosis and portal hypertension leading to hypersplenism, variceal hemorrhage, ascites, and occasionally hepatopulmonary syndrome. These patients may require LT later in childhood. Patients with mild hepatocellular enzyme and bilirubin elevation, and mild portal hypertension can be observed with ongoing medical therapy. Approximately 20% of all patients with biliary atresia will not require OLT at some point in their life.[4,5]

Alagille Syndrome

Alagille syndrome (angiohepatic dysplasia) is an autosomal dominant genetic disorder that manifests as bile duct paucity which leads to progressive cholestasis and pruritus, xanthomas, malnutrition, and growth failure. Liver failure occurs late, if at all. Specific criteria for LT are difficult to quantify. Preoperative evaluation must include assessment for congenital cardiac disease and renal insufficiency, both of which are associated with this syndrome. Hepatocellular carcinoma (HCC) has also been seen in occasional patients.[6,7]

Experience using external biliary diversion or internal ileal bypass accompanied by ursodeoxycholic acid therapy has demonstrated a significant decrease in both pruritus and complications of hypercholesterolemia.[8] Both of these procedures may ameliorate or decrease the rate of ongoing parenchymal destruction and cirrhosis, obviating the need for LT. Quality of life issues such as intractable pruritus, hypercholesterolemia, severe growth retardation, and intractable bone disease are criteria for consideration for LT.[9–11]

Metabolic Disease

An important indication for hepatic transplantation in older children is hepatic-based metabolic disease. In these patients, LT is not only lifesaving but also accomplishes phenotypic and functional cure. A review of these diseases and their mode of presentation are given in Box 45-1 and Table 45-2.

Hepatic replacement to correct the metabolic defect should be considered before other organ systems are affected, and before complications develop that would preclude transplantation, such as in patients with tyrosinemia, in whom there is a high risk of HCC.[12] Although results of transplantation are excellent in the metabolic disease subgroup, replacement of the entire liver in order to correct single enzyme deficiencies is an inefficient, but presently necessary procedure. Current research centers around hepatocyte transplantation and gene therapy.[13–17] These efforts may better serve this patient population in the future. Patients with primarily extrahepatic manifestations of their disease, such as cystic fibrosis, are occasionally helped by LT, although their prognosis is most often determined by their primary illness.[18]

Fulminant Hepatic Failure

Patients with fulminant hepatic failure without recognized antecedent liver disease present diagnostic and prognostic difficulties. Rapid clinical deterioration frequently makes establishment of a definitive diagnosis impossible before there is an urgent need for transplantation. Acute viral hepatitis of undefined etiology makes up the largest group, followed by drug toxicity and toxin exposure. Previously unrecognized metabolic disease must also be considered. Recently, an immune-based defect has been recognized as a cause of fulminant liver failure.[19] This population needs to be identified as these children may require a combination of bone marrow and LT to achieve long-term survival. When acceptable clinical and metabolic stability make liver biopsy safe, diagnostic information allowing directed treatment of the primary liver disease is helpful. The presence of ongoing coagulopathy often dictates the need for an open approach to biopsy.

The prognosis of patients with fulminant liver failure is difficult to predict, and neurologic outcome is potentially suboptimal.[16,20,21] Use of intracranial pressure (ICP) monitoring in patients with progressive encephalopathy has allowed early recognition and treatment for increased ICP. Monitoring should be instituted for patients with advancing grade III encephalopathy, and in all patients with grade IV encephalopathy. Intracranial monitoring is continued intraoperatively and for 24 to 48 hours after

TABLE 45-1 Indications for Liver Transplantation at Cincinnati Children's Hospital Medical Center, 1986–2007

Primary Diagnosis	Number of Patients	Percentage Total
Biliary atresia	173	42.5
Fulminant liver failure	62	15.2
α1-Antitrypsin deficiency	38	9.3
Hepatoblastoma/tumor	16	3.9
Cryptogenic cirrhosis	16	3.9
Alagille syndrome	11	2.7
Tyrosinemia	11	2.7
Autoimmune hepatitis	11	2.7
Urea cycle defects	10	2.5
Primary sclerosing cholangitis	10	2.5
Glycogen storage disease	5	1.2
Neonatal hepatitis	5	1.2
TPN cholestasis/short gut	5	1.2
Primary hyperoxaluria	4	1.0
Cystic fibrosis	3	0.7
Wilson disease	3	0.7
Gastroschisis	2	0.5
Hemangioendothelioma	2	0.5
Neonatal hemochromatosis	2	0.5
Other	18	4.4
Total primary transplants	**407**	
Retransplantation	50	
Second allograft	42	
Third allograft	5	
Primary transplant elsewhere	3 (one each of 2nd, 3rd, 4th allograft)	
Total transplants	**457**	

BOX 45-1 Indications for Transplantation for Metabolic Disease in Children

Wilson disease
α1-Antitrypsin deficiency
Crigler–Najjar syndrome (type I)
Tyrosinemia
Cystic fibrosis
Glycogen storage disease type IV
Branched-chain amino acid catabolism disorders
Hemophilia A
Protoporphyria
Homozygous hypercholesterolemia
Urea cycle enzyme deficiencies
Primary hyperoxaluria
Iron storage disease

Reprinted from Balistreri WF, Ohi R, Todani T, et al. Hepatobiliary, Pancreatic and Splenic Disease in Children: Medical and Surgical Management. Amsterdam: Elsevier Science; 1997. p. 395–9.

TABLE 45-2 **Mode of Presentation**[a]

Cirrhosis	Liver Tumor	Life-Threatening Progressive Liver Disease	Failure of Secondary Organ, Normal Liver
α1-Antitrypsin deficiency	Tyrosinemia	Urea cycle defect	Type 1 hyperoxalosis
Wilson disease	GSD type I	Protein C deficiency	Hypercholesterolemia
Hemochromatosis	Galactosemia	Crigler–Najjar syndrome type 1	
Byler disease	FHD	Niemann–Pick disease	
Cystic fibrosis	Hemochromatosis	Hemochromatosis	
Tyrosinemia	α1-Antitrypsin deficiency	Tyrosinemia	
GSD type IV		BCAA	
FHD			
EPP			

[a]Classification of inherited metabolic disorders according to clinical modes of presentation.
BCAA, branched-chain amino acid catabolism disorders; EPP, erythropoietic protoporphyria; FHD, fumaryl hydrolase deficiency; GSD, glycogen storage disease.
Reprinted from Balistreri WF, Ohi R, Todani T, et al. Hepatobiliary, Pancreatic and Splenic Disease in Children: Medical and Surgical Management. Amsterdam: Elsevier Science; 1997. p. 395–9.

OLT, because significant increases in ICP can develop postoperatively. Failure to maintain a cerebral perfusion pressure greater than 50 mmHg and an ICP less than 20 mmHg has been associated with very poor neurologic outcomes.[21] Also, survival following LT is significantly decreased in patients who reach grade IV encephalopathy. Efforts to identify and perform LT in children before this deterioration occurs are of utmost importance. When candidates are identified before they develop irreversible neurologic abnormalities, the results of transplantation are dramatically improved.

Liver Tumors

Transplantation for hepatoblastoma is recommended for individuals who, after the administration of several cycles of chemotherapy, have a neoplasm confined to the liver that is unresectable.[22,23] Children who had prior isolated metastasis that disappeared while undergoing preoperative chemotherapy can be considered in select instances.[24] A favorable response to pretransplant chemotherapy suggests a more favorable long-term outcome.[25] In the current Children's Oncology Group (COG) trial AHEP 0731, early referral for transplant evaluation is being evaluated for children who present with large lesions that appear unresectable.

Transplantation for HCC is complicated by less successful chemotherapy options and frequent extrahepatic involvement. The reported two-year survival rates are only 20–30%.[26] Most deaths are due to recurrent HCC within the allograft or to extrahepatic tumor involvement. When primary HCC is discovered incidentally within the cirrhotic native liver at the time of hepatectomy, the overall prognosis is unaffected by the tumor.[27]

Vascular tumors represent a group of patients with diffuse pathology who can benefit from transplantation. Children with progressive, intractable congestive heart failure, even when caused by non-neoplastic arteriovenous malformations or diffuse hemangiomas, offer a unique opportunity for complete removal of the vascular malformation and correction of congestive heart failure. Transplantation in these instances in our experience offers significantly better long-term survival compared to embolization or hepatic artery occlusion which can precipitate sudden and widespread hepatic necrosis. Pretransplant biopsy is essential in large or complex lesions to exclude angiosarcoma.

Contraindications

Contraindications to LT include (1) extrahepatic unresectable malignancy; (2) malignancy metastatic to the liver; (3) progressive terminal nonhepatic disease; (4) uncontrolled systemic sepsis; and (5) irreversible neurologic injury.

Relative contraindications to LT that need to be individually evaluated include (1) advanced or partially treated systemic infection; (2) advanced hepatic encephalopathy (grade IV); (3) severe psychosocial difficulties; (4) portal venous thrombosis extending throughout the mesenteric venous system; and (5) serology positive for HIV.

Donor Considerations

Donor Options

The single factor limiting the availability of LT is the supply of donor organs. The number of patients awaiting LT has increased by eleven fold since 1991.[28,29] Available donor resources have not kept pace. As a consequence, the waiting time to transplant for all pediatric age groups has increased significantly, with young children and infants most affected (Figs 45-1 and 45-2). This severely limited supply of available donor organs has driven the advancement of many innovative liver transplant surgical procedures. The development of reduced-size LT allowed significant expansion of the donor pool for infants and small children. This not only improved the availability of donor organs but also allowed access to donors with improved stability and organ function. Evolution of these operative techniques has resulted in the development of both split-LT and live donor (LD) transplantation.

In the hands of experienced transplant teams, these procedures all have similar success to whole organ

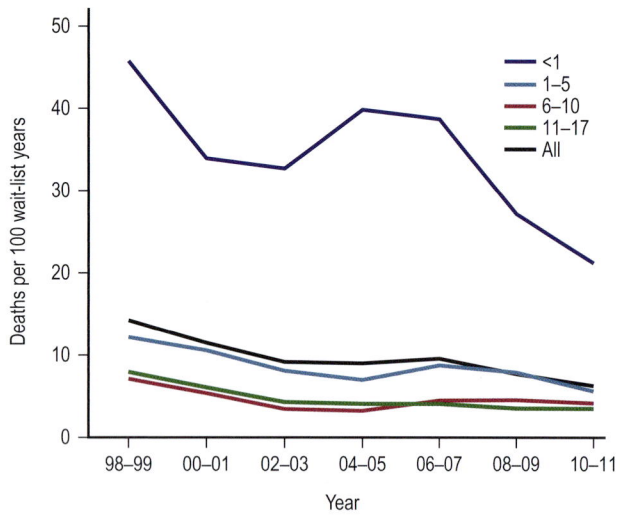

FIGURE 45-1 ■ Graph depicting the mortality rate for adults and children on the liver transplant waiting list from 1999–2010. Note the largest number of deaths occur in infants less than 1 year of age. The numbers represent the age of the patient (in years). (Source: Scientific Registry Transplant Recipients—2011 Annual Report).

transplantation. Furthermore, access to these donor options has reduced the waiting list mortality rate to less than 5%.

Organ Allocation

In 1998, the 'final rule' established by the Health Resources and Service Administration (HRSA) mandated the formation of a system for candidate stratification based on a continuous severity score reflecting 90 day waiting list mortality, i.e., outcome.[30] The system for pediatric patients, the Pediatric End-Stage Liver Disease (PELD) score, was created using an analysis of the prospective registry of children listed for transplantation by the consortium Studies of Pediatric Liver Transplantation (SPLIT).[31] The parameters selected included total bilirubin, international normalized ratio (INR), albumin,

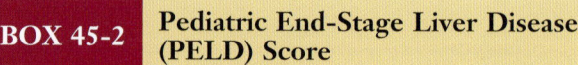

BOX 45-2	Pediatric End-Stage Liver Disease (PELD) Score

PELD score = $0.436 \times$ (age) $- 0.687 \log_e$ (albumin [g/dL]) $+ 0.480 \log_e$ (total bilirubin [mg/dL]) $+ 1.857 \log_e$ (INR) $+ 0.667$ (growth failure)

Age: Age <1, score = 1; age >1, score = 0.

Growth failure: Growth >2 standard deviations below mean, score = 1; growth <2 standard deviations below mean, score = 0.

Equation based on age, growth, and serum total bilirubin, INR, and albumin.

INR, International normalized ratio.

age <1 year, and evidence of failure to thrive (Box 45-2). The primary function of PELD is the stratification of candidates for LT by risk of 90 day waiting list mortality, allowing optimal use of donor organs. When death rates for all children listed were analyzed, PELD was an accurate predictor of mortality risk and demonstrated progressive risk until high scores were reached (>35) (Fig. 45-3).[32]

Donor Selection

Assessment of donor organ suitability is undertaken by evaluating clinical information, static biochemical tests, and dynamic tests of hepatocellular function. Static biochemical tests identify preexisting functional abnormalities or organ trauma, but do not serve as good benchmarks to differentiate among acceptable and poor donor allografts. Donor liver biopsy is helpful in questionable cases to identify preexisting liver disease or donor liver steatosis. The shortage of donor organs has led to expanded efforts to use individuals of advanced age and marginal stability, termed 'extended criteria donors' (ECD).[33] The evolving donor risk index (DRI) is used as a guide that quantifies relative risk of graft failure.[34] In the future, organ allocation may be based on maximal life years gained, an approach being utilized in kidney allocation.[35]

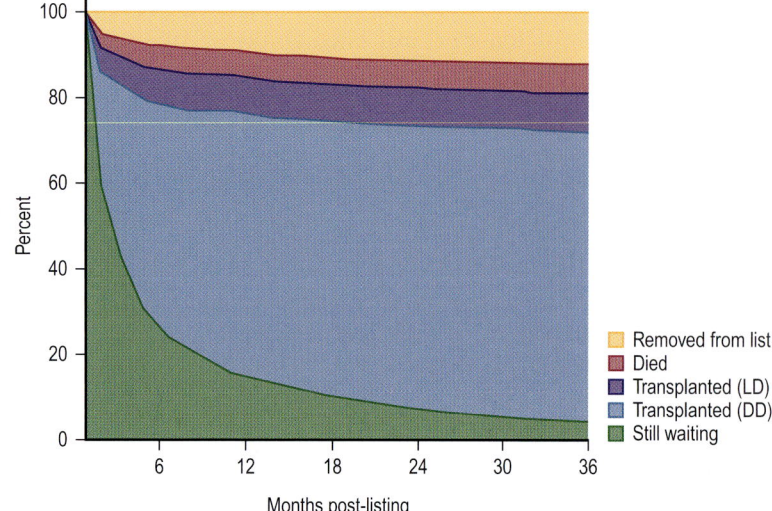

FIGURE 45-2 ■ This diagram describes what has happened to children who have been listed for liver transplantation. Fortunately, most of the patients have undergone either live donor (LD) or deceased donor (DD) transplantation, although about 5% of patients are still on the transplant list after 36 months. (Source: Scientific Registry Transplant Recipients—2011 Annual Report).

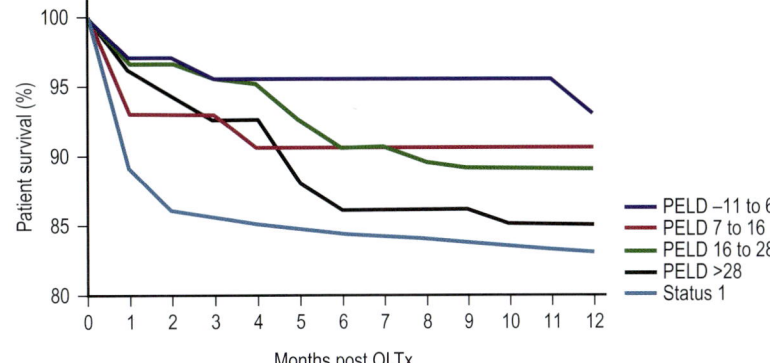

FIGURE 45-3 ■ Pediatric End-Stage Liver Disease score predictive of survival after transplantation. (Redrawn from Barshes NR, Lee TC, Udell IW, et al. The PELD model as a predictor of survival benefit and of post transplant survival in pediatric liver transplant recipients. Liver Transpl 2006;12:475–80.)

Anatomic replacement of the native liver in the orthotopic position requires selection or surgical preparation of the donor liver to fill, but not exceed available space in the recipient. When using full-sized allografts, a donor weight range from 50–125% of the recipient weight is usually appropriate, taking into consideration body habitus and factors that would increase the abdominal size in the recipient such as ascites and hepatosplenomegaly. The right lobe graft, using segments 5 to 8, and the right trisegmentectomy graft using segments 4 to 8 can be accommodated when the weight difference is no greater than 2:1 between the donor-to-recipient (D:R). The thickness of the right lobe makes this allograft of limited usefulness in small recipients. Right lobe grafts from LDs have become widely used in adults. The left lobe, using segments 1 to 4, is applicable with a D:R disparity from 2.5:1 to 5:1, and a left lateral segment (segments 2 and 3) can be used with up to a 10:1 D:R weight difference.

Although whole organ allografts are preferred, technical variant grafts are commonly employed. Preoperative preparation of variant liver allografts is based on the anatomy of the hepatic vasculature and bile ducts. In the past, reduced-size grafts were common, but because of the donor shortage, split-liver transplantation has become widespread using either ex situ or an in situ approach. The result is two transplantable grafts. The ex situ split procedure divides the right lobe allograft (segments 5 to 8) from the left lateral segment allograft (segments 2 and 3) after the whole donor organ has been procured. As this division is undertaken under hypothermic conditions without hepatic perfusion, the vascular integrity of segment 4 is difficult to assess and is frequently discarded. Conventional techniques for implanting the respective allografts are then used.

The successful experience with in situ division of the living donor left lateral segment is a basis for the in situ split procedure. Two variations of the procedure are utilized depending on the needs of the recipients, a right–left lobe split or a right trisegmentectomy–left lateral segment split. For the right trisegmentectomy–left lateral segment split, the left lateral segment is prepared similar to a living related donor graft. The viability of segment 4 can be examined at the time of the division and is usually incorporated with the right lobe graft to increase the cellular mass of the allograft. For a left-right lobe graft, the parenchymal resection follows the anatomic lobar plane through the gallbladder fossa to the vena cava.[36,37] A crush and tie technique is preferred to achieve good closure of the vascular and biliary structures. The bile duct, portal vein, and hepatic artery are divided at the right or left confluence. The vena cava is left incorporated with the allograft in both right and left lobe preparation. Vena caval reduction by posterior caval wall resection and closure is occasionally necessary. Resection of the inferior protruding portion of the caudate lobe is necessary during left lobe preparation to reduce the likelihood of arterial angulation, which can result in arterial thrombosis. This also facilitates shortening of the inferior vena cava to fit in a small recipient.[38] When using left lateral segment (LLS) allografts, the parenchymal dissection follows the right margin of the falciform ligament with preservation of the left hilar structures. Direct implantation of the left hepatic vein into the combined orifice of the right and middle/left hepatic veins in the recipient vena cava is preferred; the donor vena cava is not retained with this segmental allograft. Further reduction of the LLS graft to a monosegmental graft may be necessary in very small recipients. Resection of the distal LLS is technically easier than an anatomic segment II/III division. Because this procedure adds considerably to the donor procurement time, and the necessary skill of the donor team, it is more demanding and occasionally difficult to successfully orchestrate. This technique is, however, despite these considerations, the preferred method for split-liver donor preparation.[39,40]

The benefits of split-liver transplantation are best achieved when ideal donors are selected. Strict restrictions on age, vasopressor administration, pre-donation hepatic function, and limited donor hospitalization have been used to select optimal donor candidates. When these donors are selected, the results from both in situ and ex-situ techniques are similar, with both techniques now having patient survival for both allografts of 90–93% and graft survival rates of 86–89%.[41]

The use of LDs has increased as the safety and success of this approach has been demonstrated (Fig. 45-4).[42–44] One of the critical elements of LD transplantation is the proper selection of a donor, usually a parent or relative. This procedure is performed on the assumption that donor safety can be assured and that the donor's liver function is normal. Careful attention to proper living donor consent is important. Parental concerns to help their ill child make true informed consent are a challenge.

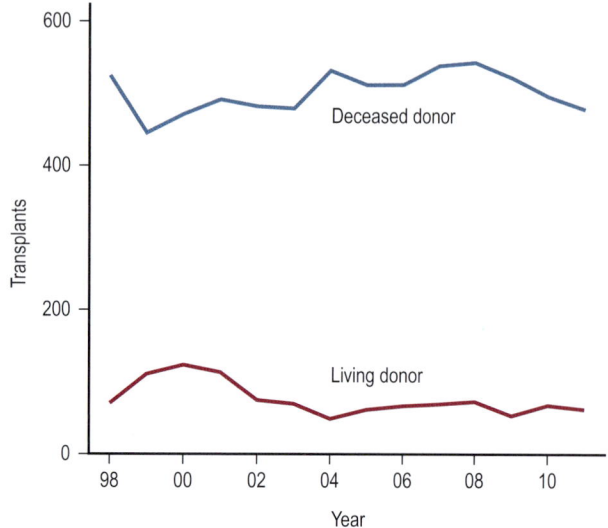

FIGURE 45-4 ■ The number of living donor and deceased donor liver transplants in infants and children performed between 1998–2011. (Source: Scientific Registry Transplant Recipients—2011 Annual Report).

A dedicated 'donor advocate' not directly associated with the transplant team should assist with this process. Independent medical assessment of the donor is essential. United Network Organ Sharing (UNOS) has recently established clear criteria for this process.[45] After a satisfactory medical and psychological examination by a physician not directly involved with the transplant program, computed tomography (CT) scanning is used to measure the volume of the potential donor segment to assure that it will meet the metabolic needs, but not exceed the space available in the recipient. If acceptable, CT angiography or arteriography is undertaken to assess the hepatic arterial anatomy, thereby excluding potential donors with multiple arteries to segments 2 and 3, and facilitating minimal hilar vascular dissection at the time of LT. Experience has shown that, when donors were deemed unacceptable, 90% of patients were excluded on the basis of history, examination, laboratory screening, and ABO type. Donor safety has been excellent in all pediatric LD series.[46–48]

In most pediatric cases, the LLS donated from an adult is used as the graft. In situ dissection of the LLS, preserving the donor vascular integrity until the parenchymal division is completed, is undertaken. At the time of harvest, the left hepatic vein is divided from the vena cava, and the left branch of the portal vein and hepatic artery are removed with the allograft.[46] Vascular continuity of the hepatic arterial branches to segment 4 is maintained, if possible. Increased experience has been gained using the right lobe as an LD allograft for larger recipients such as adolescents and adults.[42,49,50] This more extensive operation has proven to be a challenge to the donor and recipient alike, with complication and mortality rates significantly exceeding that of left lateral segmentectomy. The number of right lobe LD recipients now greatly exceeds the number of children receiving LD grafts;[51] however, several publicized donor deaths and increased interest in 'split-liver' cadaveric procurement have slowed the enthusiasm and growth of right lobe donation.

The selection of a donor segment with an appropriate parenchymal mass for adequate function is critical to success. However, the minimal mass necessary for recovery is not yet established. Any calculation must take into account loss of function following preservation damage, acute rejection, and technical problems. When the D:R weight range falls within the normal 8:1 to 10:1 ratio, risk is minimal. Estimates of donor graft to recipient body weight ratio (GRWR) may prove to be a more accurate predictor of adequate graft volume. When the GRWR is less than 0.7%, overall allograft and patient survival suffered. In extreme cases in which small-for-size grafts are used, excessive portal flow can lead to hemorrhagic necrosis of the graft. Large-for-size allografts (GRWR >5.0%) have a less deleterious effect.[52] A review of these donor anatomic options is shown in Figure 45-5.

Preoperative Preparation

Efforts to correct abnormalities noted during candidate evaluation decrease both the operative risk and postoperative complications. Complications of portal hypertension and malnutrition are treated. Assessment of prior viral exposure and meticulous attention to the delivery of all normal childhood immunizations, particularly the live-virus vaccines, are imperative, if time allows, before LT. Additionally, patients receive a one-time inoculation with pneumococcal vaccine, as well as appropriate administration of hepatitis B vaccine. Preoperative assessment of cardiopulmonary reserve and hepatic vascular anatomy is also important.

The Transplant Procedure

The transplant procedure is carried out through a bilateral subcostal incision with midline extension. Meticulous ligation of portosystemic collaterals and vascularized adhesions is necessary to avoid slow but relentless hemorrhage. Dissection of the hepatic hilum, with division of the hepatic artery and portal vein above their bifurcation, allows maximal recipient vessel length to be achieved. The bile duct, when present, is divided high in the hilum to preserve the length and vasculature of the distal duct in case it is needed for primary reconstruction in older recipients. Preservation of the Roux-en-Y limb in biliary atresia patients who have undergone Kasai portoenterostomy simplifies later biliary reconstruction. Complete mobilization of the liver, with dissection of the suprahepatic vena cava to the diaphragm and the infrahepatic vena cava to the renal veins, completes the hepatectomy.

In children with serious vascular instability who cannot tolerate caval occlusion, or when an LLS graft is being used, 'piggy-back' implantation is necessary. In this procedure, the recipient vena cava is left intact and partial caval occlusion allows end-to-side implantation of a combined donor hepatic vein patch. Access to the infrarenal aorta to implant the celiac axis of the donor liver or iliac artery vascular conduits, provided by mobilizing the right colon and duodenum, is our preference for arterial reconstruction in complex allograft recipients.

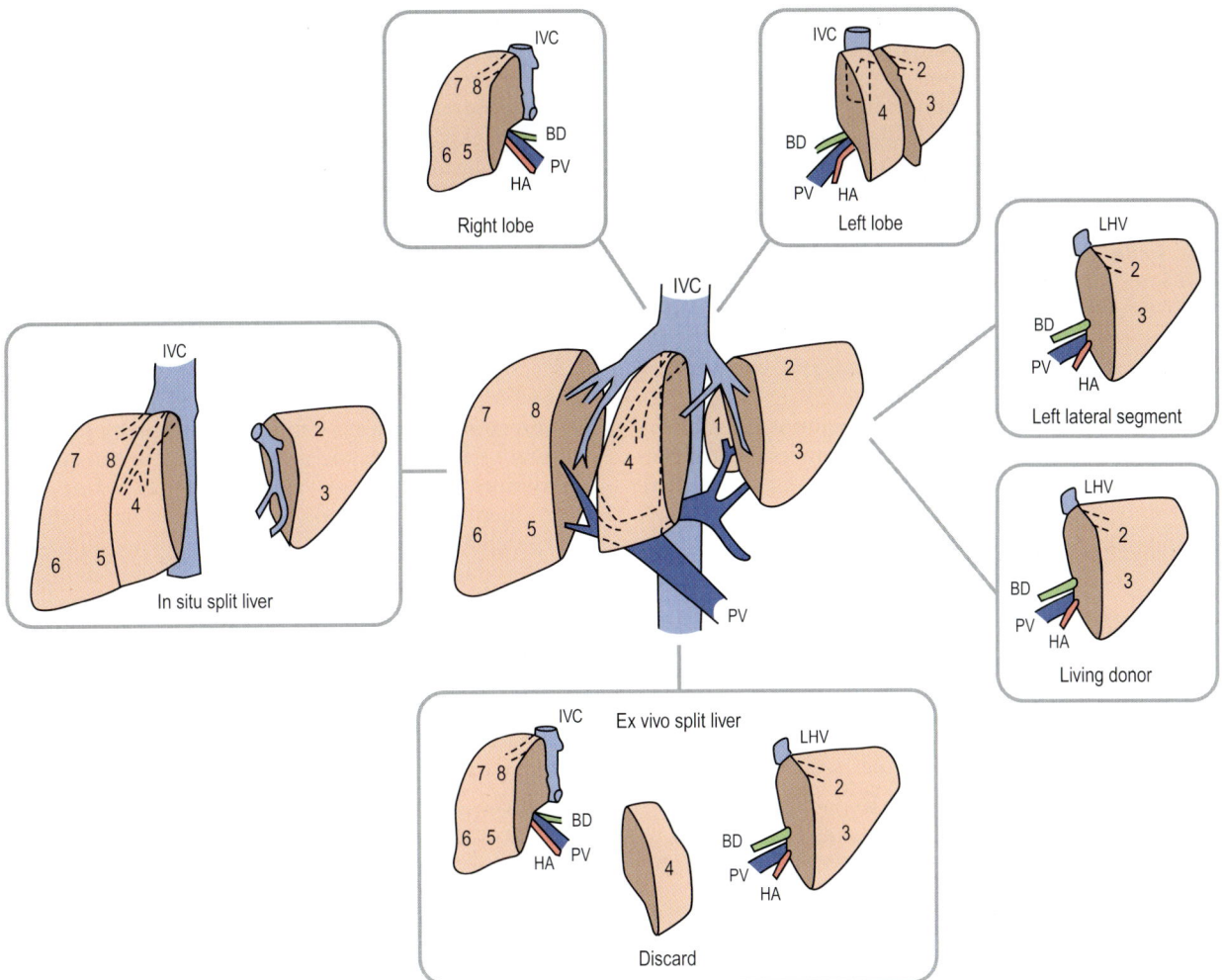

FIGURE 45-5 ■ Anatomic donor options available through surgical reduction. The numbers correlate to the segmental hepatic anatomy as defined by Couinaud. BD, bile duct; HA, hepatic artery; IVC, inferior vena cava; LHV, left hepatic vein; PV, portal vein.

Control of hemorrhage is essential during the recipient hepatectomy, requiring meticulous technique. Coagulation factor assays (V, VII, VIII, fibrinogen, platelets, prothrombin time, partial thromboplastin time) allow specific blood product supplementation to improve clotting function. Use of venovenous bypass is reserved for recipients >40 kg who demonstrate hemodynamic instability at the time of venous interruption.

Removal of the diseased liver is performed after vascular isolation is achieved. Retroperitoneal hemostasis is achieved before implanting the donor liver. In standard LT, the suprahepatic vena cava is prepared by suture ligation of any large phrenic orifices and creating one caval lumen from the confluence of the inferior vena cava and hepatic vein orifices. The donor liver is implanted using conventional vascular techniques and monofilament suture for the vascular anastomosis. In small recipients, interrupted suture techniques, monofilament dissolving suture material, and a 'growth factor' knot has been used to allow for vessel growth. When LLS grafts are used, the left hepatic vein orifice is anastomosed directly to the anterolateral surface of the infradiaphragmatic inferior vena cava using the combined right–middle hepatic vein orifices. The LLS allograft is later fixed when necessary

to the undersurface of the diaphragm to prevent torsion and venous obstruction of this anastomosis. Similar fixation is not necessary with right or left lobe allografts or with whole organ transplants.

Before completing the vena caval anastomosis, the hyperkalemic preservation solution is flushed from the graft using 500–1000 mL of hypothermic normokalemic intravenous (IV) solutions. When using full-sized grafts in older patients, we prefer to complete all venous anastomoses before constructing the hepatic artery anastomosis IV. In reduced-size allografts and in small recipients where we prefer direct aortic vascular inflow reconstruction, the hepatic arterial anastomosis is completed before the portal vein anastomosis to improve visibility of the infrarenal aorta without placing traction on the portal vein anastomosis. We prefer to complete all anastomoses using vascular isolation before organ reperfusion, although some transplant teams re-perfuse after the venous reconstruction is complete.

Before re-establishing circulation to the allograft, anesthetic adjustments must be made to address the large volume of blood needed to refill the liver as well as hypothermic solutions released upon reperfusion. Inotropic support using dopamine (5–10 μg/kg/min) is also started.

Calcium and sodium bicarbonate are administered to combat the effects of hyperkalemia from any remaining preservation solution or from systemic acidosis due to aortic and vena caval occlusion. Sufficient blood volume expansion, administered as packed red blood cells to raise the central venous pressure (CVP) to 15–20 cmH$_2$O and the hematocrit to 40%, minimizes the development of hypotension on unclamping and prevents dilutional anemia. Cooperative communication between the surgical and anesthesia teams facilitates a smooth sequential reestablishment of vena caval, portal venous, and then arterial recirculation to the allograft.

Biliary tract reconstruction in patients with biliary atresia or in those weighing less than 25 kg is achieved through an end-to-side choledochojejunostomy using interrupted dissolving monofilament sutures. A multifenestrated Silastic internal biliary stent is placed before completing the anastomosis (Fig. 45-6). In most cases,

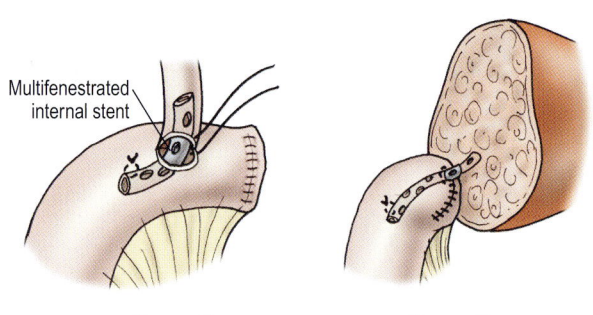

FIGURE 45-6 ■ Bile duct reconstruction is shown using the common hepatic duct in whole organ transplants (left) and segmental hepatic ducts into a Roux-en-Y intestinal limb for reduced-sized liver transplants (right). An internal multifenestrated stent is used in both situations. (From Ryckman F. Liver transplantation. In: Ziegler MM, Azizkhan RG, Weber T, editors. Operative Pediatric Surgery. New York: McGraw-Hill; 2003. p. 1275.)

the prior Roux-en-Y limb can be used, with a 30–35 cm length being preferred. Primary bile duct reconstruction without stenting is used in older patients with whole organ allografts.

When closing the abdomen, increased intra-abdominal pressure should be avoided. In many cases, the abdominal fascia is not closed and mobilized skin flaps and running monofilament skin closure are used. Formal musculofascial abdominal closure can be completed before patient discharge.

Immunosuppressive Management

Most centers use an immunosuppressive protocol based on the administration of multiple complementary medications. All use corticosteroids and cyclosporine or tacrolimus. Additional antimetabolites (azathioprine, mycophenolate) are used when more intensive treatment is needed. Prior protocols using polyclonal or monoclonal induction therapy have been abandoned in most cases due to the extent of the immunosuppressive potency. A sample protocol is given in Table 45-3.

Postoperative Complications

Most postoperative complications present with cholestasis, increasing hepatocellular enzyme levels, and on occasion fever, lethargy, and anorexia. Therapy directed at the specific causes of the allograft dysfunction is essential. Empiric therapy for presumed complications is fraught with misdiagnoses, morbidity, and mortality. A flow diagram outlining this evaluation is shown in Figure 45-7.

Primary Nonfunction

Primary nonfunction (PNF) of the hepatic allograft implies the absence of metabolic and synthetic activity

TABLE 45-3	Immunosuppression Protocol Utilized for Liver Transplantation		
Day/Week	Methylprednisolone (mg/kg/day)	Tacrolimus (mg/kg/day)	Tacrolimus Target Level
Intraoperative	15	0	
Day 1	10	0.3	
Day 2	8	0.3	
Day 3	6	0.3	
Day 4	4	0.3	12–18
Day 5	3	0.3	
Day 6	2	0.3	
Day 7	1	0.3	
Week 2	0.9	Adjust as needed	12–18
Week 3	0.8		
Week 4	0.7		
Week 5	0.6		8–14
Week 6	0.5		
Week 7	0.4		
Week 8	0.3		
Week 9	0.2		
Week 10	0.1		
Week 11	0.1		
Week 12	D/C		6–12
>1 year			3–7

D/C, discontinue.

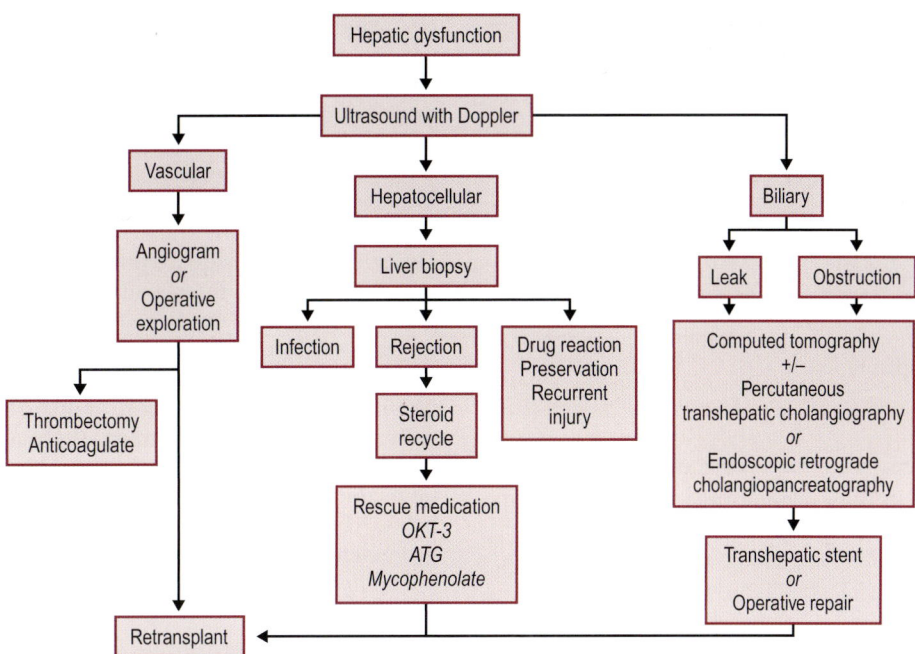

FIGURE 45-7 ■ Schematic flow diagram for management of postoperative liver allograft dysfunction. ATG, antithymocyte globulin; OKT-3, monoclonal antibody.

<table>
<tr><td colspan="2">BOX 45-3   Factors Related to Primary Nonfunction</td></tr>
</table>

BOX 45-3 | **Factors Related to Primary Nonfunction**

DONOR FACTORS

Preexisting disease or injury to donor, anemia, hypoxia, hypotension before organ harvest
Donor organ steatosis (>60% macrovesicular fat)

TRANSPLANT FACTORS

Prolonged cold ischemic storage (>8–12 hours)
Prolonged warm ischemic time at implantation
Complex vascular anastomosis requiring surgical revision
Significant size discrepancy between donor and recipient

RECIPIENT FACTORS

Post-reperfusion hypotension
Vascular thrombosis
Immunologic factors
ABO incompatible, positive cross-match

following LT. Complete nonfunction requires immediate retransplantation before irreversible coagulopathy and cerebral edema occur. Lesser degrees of allograft dysfunction occur more frequently, and are associated with several donor, recipient, and operative factors (Box 45-3). The status of the donor liver contributes significantly to the potential for PNF. Ischemic injury secondary to anemia, hypotension, hypoxia, or trauma is often difficult to ascertain in the history of multiple trauma victims. Donor liver steatosis has also been recognized as a factor contributing to severe dysfunction or nonfunction in the donor liver.[53,54] Macrovesicular steatosis on donor liver biopsy is somewhat more common in adult than pediatric

donors and, when severe, is recognized grossly by the enlarged yellow, greasy consistency of the donor liver. The risk of PNF increases as the degree of fatty infiltration increases.[54] Histologic findings are classified as mild if less than 30% of the hepatocytes have fatty infiltration, moderate if 30 to 60% are involved, and severe if more than 60% of the hepatocytes have fatty infiltration. Livers with severe fatty infiltration should be discarded, and donors with moderate involvement are used with some concern, with the degree of steatosis and the condition of the recipient determining use of the allograft.

The use of ABO-incompatible donors has been controversial. Allograft and patient survival rates in adult recipients have not been comparable to those achieved using ABO-identical or compatible donors.[55,56] However, pediatric recipients of ABO-incompatible allografts have achieved survival rates equivalent to those using ABO-compatible and ABO-identical donors with either cadaveric donors (CDs) or LDs.[57–59]

Vascular Thrombosis

Hepatic artery thrombosis (HAT) occurs in children three to four times more frequently than in adult transplant series, occurring most often within the first 30 days following transplantation.[60,61] Factors influencing the development of HAT are listed in Box 45-4. HAT presents with a variable clinical picture that may include: (1) fulminant allograft failure; (2) biliary disruption or obstruction; or (3) systemic sepsis. Doppler ultrasound (US) imaging has been accurate in identifying arterial thrombosis, and is used as the primary screening modality to assess vascular flow following transplantation or whenever complications arise. Acute HAT with allograft failure most often requires immediate retransplantation. Successful thrombectomy and allograft salvage is possible if

<table>
<tr><td colspan="2" style="background:#6b1414;color:white;">BOX 45-4</td><td style="background:#d9b44a;">Factors Affecting Vascular Thrombosis</td></tr>
</table>

BOX 45-4   Factors Affecting Vascular Thrombosis

DONOR/RECIPIENT AGE/WEIGHT ALLOGRAFT TYPE

Whole organ > reduced size
Living donor ≥ reduced size

ANASTOMOTIC ANATOMY

Primary hepatic artery > direct aortic

ALLOGRAFT EDEMA—INCREASED VASCULAR RESISTANCE

Ischemic injury secondary to prolonged preservation; prolonged implantation
Rejection
Fluid overload

RECIPIENT HYPOTENSION AND/OR HYPERCOAGULABILITY

Administration of coagulation factors, fresh-frozen plasma
Procoagulant factor deficiencies

---

reconstruction is undertaken before allograft necrosis.[62] Biliary complications are particularly common following HAT. Ischemic injury to the biliary tree or anastomosis can result in intraparenchymal biloma formation or cholestasis. The development of septicemia or multifocal abscesses in sites of ischemic necrosis secondary to gram-negative enteric bacteria, *Enterococcus*, anaerobic bacteria, or fungi can also occur. Antibiotic therapy directed toward these organisms, along with operative or percutaneous drainage, is indicated when specific abscesses are identified. Drainage and biliary stenting may control bile leakage and infection until retransplantation is undertaken.

Late HAT can be asymptomatic or present with slowly progressive bile duct stenosis. Rarely, allograft necrosis occurs. Arterial collaterals from the Roux-en-Y limb can provide a source of revascularization through hilar collaterals. These collateral channels develop during the first postoperative months, often making late thrombosis a clinically silent event. Conversely, disruption of this collateral supply during operative reconstruction of the central bile ducts in patients who later develop HAT can precipitate hepatic ischemia and parenchymal necrosis. When HAT is asymptomatic, careful observation alone is indicated.

Prevention of HAT requires meticulous arterial reconstruction at the time of transplantation. Anatomic reconstruction is preferred in whole organ allografts; direct implantation of the celiac axis into the infrarenal aorta is recommended for all reduced-size liver allografts. All complex vascular reconstructions of the donor hepatic artery should be undertaken ex vivo whenever possible using microsurgical techniques before transplantation. When vascular grafts are required, they should also be implanted onto the infrarenal aorta.[63] No systemic anticoagulation is routinely used by our group, but aspirin (20–40 mg/day) is administered to all children for 100 days.

Portal vein thrombosis (PVT) is uncommon in whole organ allografts unless prior portosystemic shunting has altered the flow within the splanchnic vascular bed or unless severe portal vein stenosis in the recipient has impaired flow to the allograft. Preexisting PVT in the recipient can be overcome by thrombectomy, portal vein replacement, or extra anatomic venous bypass. In biliary atresia recipients, portal vein hypoplasia is best corrected by anastomosis of the portal vein to the confluence of the splenic and superior mesenteric veins in the recipient. When there is inadequate portal vein length on the donor organ, iliac vein interposition grafts are used. Early thrombosis following LT requires immediate anastomotic revision and thrombectomy. Discrepancies in venous size imposed by reduced-size allografts can be modified to allow anastomotic construction.[64,65] Deficiencies of anticoagulant proteins, such as protein C and S, and antithrombin III deficiency in the recipient must also be excluded as a contributing cause for vascular thrombosis.[66] Failure to recognize PVT can lead to either allograft demise or, on a more chronic basis, to significant portal hypertension with hemorrhagic sequelae or intractable ascites.

Biliary Complications

Complications related to biliary tract reconstruction occur in approximately 10% of pediatric liver transplant recipients. Their spectrum and treatment is determined by the status of the hepatic artery and the type of allograft used. Although whole and reduced-size allografts have an equivalent risk of biliary tract complications, the spectrum of complications differs.[67,68]

Primary bile duct reconstruction is the preferred biliary tract reconstruction in adults, but it is less commonly used in children. It has the advantage of preserving the sphincter of Oddi, decreasing the incidence of enteric reflux and subsequent cholangitis, and not requiring an intestinal anastomosis. Experience using primary choledocho-choledochostomy without a T-tube has been favorable.[69] Late complications following any type of primary ductal reconstruction include anastomotic stricture, biliary sludge formation, and recurrent cholangitis. Endoscopic dilation and internal stenting of anastomotic strictures has been successful in early postoperative cases. Roux-en-Y choledochojejunostomy is the preferred treatment for recurrent stenosis or postoperative leak.

Roux-en-Y choledochojejunostomy is the reconstruction of choice in small children and is required in all patients with biliary atresia. Recurrent cholangitis, a theoretical risk, suggests anastomotic narrowing or an intrahepatic biliary stricture or small bowel obstruction within the Roux limb or distal to the Roux-en-Y anastomosis. In the absence of these complications, cholangitis is uncommon.

Reconstruction of the bile ducts in patients with reduced-size allografts is more challenging. Division of the bile duct in close proximity to the cut-surface margin of the allograft, with careful preservation of the biliary duct collateral circulation, decreases but does not eliminate a ductal stricture secondary to ischemia. In our early experience, in 14% of patients with left lobe reduced-size allografts, a short segmental stricture developed requiring anastomotic revision (Fig. 45-8). Operative revision

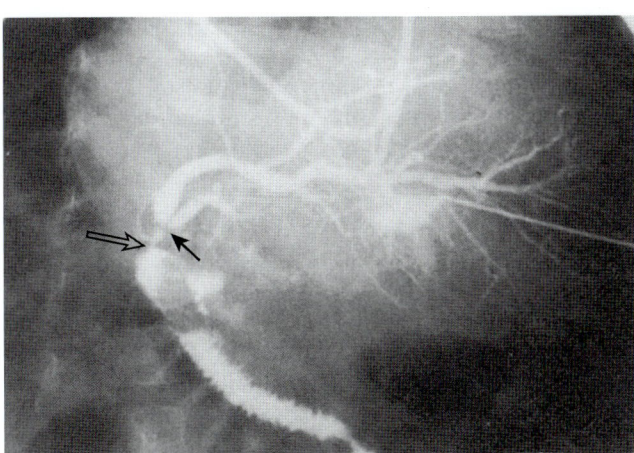

FIGURE 45-8 ■ Segmental bile duct stricture at the junction of the left lateral and left medial segmental bile ducts in a left lobe reduced-size allograft. *Solid arrow*, bile duct stricture; *open arrow*, Roux-en-Y loop and bile duct anastomosis. (From Ryckman FC. Liver transplantation in children. In: Suchy FJ, editor. Liver Disease in Children. St. Louis: CV Mosby; 1994. p. 941.)

of the biliary anastomosis and reimplantation of the bile ducts into the Roux-en-Y is necessary. Percutaneous transhepatic cholangiography is essential to define the intrahepatic ductal anatomy before operative revision, and temporary catheter decompression of the obstructed bile ducts promotes treatment of cholangitis and allows elective reconstruction. Operative reconstruction is accompanied by transhepatic passage of exteriorized multifenestrated biliary ductal stents, which remain in place until reconstructive success is documented. Late stenosis is unlikely. Dissection away from the vasobiliary sheath in the donor has significantly decreased the incidence of this complication.

Biliary complications have been seen with an increased frequency following LD in children. The LLS 2 and 3 bile ducts are frequently separate at the plane of parenchymal division. The need for individual drainage of these small biliary ducts makes the development of late anastomotic stenosis more frequent. Individual segmental strictures may not lead to jaundice in the recipient, but rather are identified by elevated gamma glutamyl transferase (GGT) or through ultrasound surveillance. Reoperation after ductal dilatation from the stricture allows for easier reconstruction due to the increased caliber of the segmental bile duct.

Acute Cellular Rejection

Allograft rejection is characterized by the histologic triad of endothelialitis, portal triad lymphocyte infiltration with bile duct injury, and hepatic parenchymal cell damage.[70] Allograft biopsy is essential to establish the diagnosis before treatment. The rapidity of the rejection process and its response to therapy dictates the intensity and duration of antirejection treatment.

Acute rejection occurs in approximately two-thirds of patients following LT.[71] The primary treatment is a short course of high-dose steroids. Bolus doses administered over several days with a rapid taper to baseline therapy is

successful in 80% of cases.[72] When refractory or recurrent rejection occurs, antilymphocyte therapy using the monoclonal antibody OKT-3® or thymoglobulin® is successful in 90% of cases.[38]

Chronic Rejection

Uniform diagnosis and management of chronic rejection is complicated by the lack of a consistent definition or clinical course. Chronic rejection occurs in 5–10% of transplanted patients. Its incidence appears to be decreasing in all transplant groups, perhaps related to better overall immunosuppressive strategies. There is some suggestion that the use of tacrolimus based immunosuppression is a key element in this apparent decrease.[73,74] Risk factors for its development are many, and no factor predicts the outcome of treatment. The chronic rejection rate is significantly lower in recipients of LD grafts compared with cadaveric grafts.[75] In that study, African-American recipients had a significantly higher rate of chronic rejection than did Caucasian recipients. In addition, the number of acute rejection episodes, transplantation for autoimmune disease, occurrence of post-transplant lymphoproliferative disease (PTLD), and cytomegalovirus (CMV) infection were also significant risk factors for chronic rejection. The primary clinical manifestation is a progressive increase in biliary ductal enzymes (alkaline phosphatase, GGT) and progressive cholestasis. Chronic rejection can be initially asymptomatic or may follow unsuccessful treatment for acute rejection. It can occur within weeks of transplantation or later in the postoperative course.

Chronic rejection usually follows one of two clinical forms.[76] In the first, the injury is primarily to the biliary epithelium and the clinical course is slowly progressive with preservation of synthetic function. Histologically, either interlobular bile duct destruction in the absence of ischemic injury or hepatocellular necrosis is seen. In full expression, this form is characterized as acute *vanishing bile duct syndrome* when severe ductopenia is seen in at least 20 portal tracts.[77,78] The eventual spontaneous resolution in up to one-half of affected patients with tacrolimus therapy has led to the development of enhanced immunosuppression protocols for this patient subgroup.[76] Retransplantation is occasionally necessary, but it is rarely needed emergently.

The second subtype is characterized by the early development of progressive ischemic injury to both bile ducts and hepatocytes, leading to ductopenia and ischemic necrosis with fibrosis. The clinical picture of cholestasis is accompanied by significant synthetic dysfunction with superimposed vascular thrombosis or biliary stricture formation. The vascular endothelial injury responsible for the progressive ischemic changes is characterized by the development of subintimal foam cells or fibrointimal hypertrophy. The clinical course is relentlessly progressive, and nearly always requires retransplantation. Unfortunately, recurrence of chronic rejection in the retransplanted allograft is common.[77]

Recent studies have focused on donor specific antibody mediated abnormalities that may be the pathophysiologic basis for chronic rejection.[79] The immunologic nature of this process is emphasized by the primary target role of the biliary and vascular endothelium, the only tissues in the liver that express class II antigen. Other interdependent cofactors such as CMV infection, human leukocyte antigen (HLA) mismatching, positive B-cell crossmatching, and differing racial demographics of the donor to recipient have all failed to show consistent correlation with the development of chronic rejection.[76,77]

Renal Insufficiency

The long-term success of LT has been related to the effective immunosuppression with calcineurin inhibitors (CNI), such as cyclosporine and tacrolimus. However, nephrotoxicity associated with their long-term use has become a major problem which can affect up to 70% of all nonrenal transplant recipients. Renal insufficiency can present in many ways following CNI administration and LT. When this occurs during the initial post-transplant weeks, it is most often related to transient excessive blood levels, and is reversible with appropriate dose correction. Impaired glomerular filtration rate (GFR) seen in pediatric recipients with stable graft function represents a more serious problem. Up to 20% may have a drop in their GFR to below 50 mL/min/1.73m^2, and 5% may progress to end-stage renal disease (ESRD). Adult studies have shown a progressive increase in chronic renal failure from 0.9% at year 1 to 8.6% at year 13 post OLTx.[80] Similarly, ESRD rose from 1.6% at year 1 to 9.5% at year 13 after LT, yielding a total incidence of renal dysfunction of 18%. The presence of an elevated serum creatinine pre-LT, at one-year post-transplant, and the presence of hepato-renal syndrome prior to transplant were all identified risk factors.[80,81] Cyclosporine and tacrolimus both appear to be similar in risk.

In a review from our program, in children who were more than three years post-LT, we found that 32% had a GFR <70 mL/minute/1.73 m^2.[82] The factors primarily related to lower GFR were the presence of an elevated creatinine at one year after LT and the length of time following transplantation. Our data supported the concept of a continued decline in renal function following LT.[83,84] Considering the expected long survival for children undergoing LT, the possibility of progressive asymptomatic renal insufficiency leading to severe kidney disease poses a significant challenge.

Efforts to reverse ongoing renal insufficiency using protocols that include instituting non-nephrotoxic agents, such as mycophenolate mofetil (MMF) while decreasing the CNI dose, have shown limited success in improving GFR while protecting against the risks of acute rejection at the time of immunosuppressive drug conversion.[85] Efforts have also been undertaken to use the new class of monoclonal anti-CD25 antibodies for induction therapy coupled with MMF and steroids in an effort to avoid administration of CNI during the first post-transplant week. These agents appear to afford sufficient protection against rejection to successfully allow the late administration of CNI. Whether these efforts will prevent the later development of renal insufficiency is yet unproven.[86] Efforts to completely eliminate CNI use have been complicated by acute or ductopenic rejection. Current efforts

suggest that earlier staged reduction of CNI prior to the development of severe GFR reduction will decrease, but not eliminate this complication. Once established, chronic renal failure does not appear to resolve with CNI dose adjustment. Although CNI toxicity is now well appreciated, the association of both hepatic and renal disease in many metabolic diseases of childhood may also contribute to the GFR abnormalities seen after LT.

Infection

Infectious complications have become the most common source of morbidity and mortality following LT. Multiple organism infection is common as are concurrent infections by different agents.

Bacterial infections occur in the immediate post-transplant period and are most often caused by Gram-negative enteric organisms, *Enterococcus*, or *Staphylococcus* species. Intra-abdominal abscesses or infected collections of serum along the cut surface of the reduced-size allograft are best addressed with extraperitoneal, abdominal, or percutaneous drainage. Intrahepatic abscesses suggest hepatic artery stenosis or thrombosis, and treatment is directed toward the vascular status of the allograft and associated bile duct abnormalities. Sepsis originating at sites of invasive monitoring lines can be minimized by replacing or removing all intraoperative lines soon after transplantation. Antibacterial prophylaxis are discontinued as soon as possible to prevent the development of resistant organisms.

Fungal sepsis represents a significant potential problem in the early post-transplant period. Aggressive protocols for pretransplant prophylaxis are based on the concept that fungal infections originate from organisms colonizing the recipient's gastrointestinal (GI) tract. In two studies, selective bowel decontamination was successful in eliminating pathogenic Gram-negative bacteria from the GI tract in 87% of adult patients.[87,88] Also, in all cases, *Candida* was eliminated. However, these protocols have not been practical in pediatric recipients because there is a long waiting time for pediatric organs and the taste of the antibiotics is not well accepted. However, these regimens are commonly used in the preoperative preparation for combined liver/small intestinal transplantation. Fungal infection most often occurs in patients requiring multiple operative procedures and those who have had multiple antibiotic courses. Development of fungemia or urosepsis requires retinal, cardiac, and renal investigation, and antifungal therapy should be promptly initiated. Severe fungal infection has a mortality rate greater than 80%, making early treatment essential. All patients undergoing LT should receive antifungal prophylaxis with fluconazole.

The majority of early and severe viral infections are caused by viruses of the Herpesviridae family, including Epstein–Barr virus (EBV), CMV, and herpes simplex virus (HSV). CMV transmission dynamics are well studied and serve as a prototype for herpesvirus transmission in the transplant population. The likelihood that CMV infection will develop is influenced by the preoperative CMV status of the donor and recipient.[89,90] Seronegative recipients receiving seropositive donor organs are at greatest risk, with seropositive donor-to-recipient combinations at the next greatest risk. Use of various immune-based prophylactic protocols including IV IgG or hyper immune anti-CMV IgG, coupled with acyclovir or ganciclovir/valganciclovir, have all achieved success in decreasing the incidence of symptomatic CMV infection, although seroconversion in seronegative recipients from seropositive donor organs inevitably occurs.

The clinical diagnosis of CMV infection is suggested by the development of fever, leukopenia, maculopapular rash, hepatocellular abnormalities, respiratory insufficiency, or GI hemorrhage. Hepatic biopsy or endoscopic biopsy of colonic or gastroduodenal sites allows early diagnosis with immunohistochemical evaluation. Rapid blood and urine assays for CMV can also expedite the diagnosis. In suspected cases, treatment should be instituted while awaiting culture or biopsy results owing to the potential rapidity and severity of this infection in a previously seronegative child. The treatment of CMV has been greatly improved by the development of ganciclovir. Early treatment with IV IgG and ganciclovir is successful in most cases.

EBV infection occurring in the perioperative period represents a significant risk to the pediatric recipient.[91] It has a varying presentation including a mononucleosis-like syndrome, hepatitis-simulating rejection, extranodal lymphoproliferative infiltration with bowel perforation, peritonsillar or lymph node enlargement, and encephalopathy. In small children, its primary portal of entry is often the tonsils, making asymptomatic tonsillar hypertrophy a common initial presentation.[92] EBV infection can occur as a primary infection or following reactivation of a past infection. When serologic evidence of active infection exists, an acute reduction in immunosuppression is indicated. It has become clear that continuous surveillance is necessary as the presentation is often nonspecific and the prognosis is related to early diagnosis. Screening using quantitative PCR testing to determine the EBV blood viral load appears to be the best current predictor of risk. However, viral loads have been identified in asymptomatic patients and patients recovering from PTLD, limiting the specificity of this approach. The balance between viral load measured by quantitative PCR and specific cellular immune response, perhaps mediated by CD8 T-cells specific to EBV, may explain this lack of specificity to viral load alone.[93–95]

Many pediatric transplant centers now use serially measured quantitative EBV DNA PCR as an indication for primary immunosuppression modulation. We recommend monthly EBV DNA PCR counts to monitor increased genomic expression. Increasing viral load levels warrant more frequent monitoring on a weekly or every two week schedule. In the EBV seronegative pretransplant patients, >40 genomes/10^5 peripheral blood leukocytes (PBL), and >200 genomes/10^5 PBL identify patients needing reduction in primary immunosuppression by 25 to 100%. Institution of antiviral therapy with ganciclovir and CMV IgG is also used in most cases, although only nonrandomized observational studies support their use. Both agents are active in vitro against linear replicating forms of the EBV, but have no activity against the circular episome in immortalized B-cells. Treatment should be

continued until symptoms of lymphadenopathy have resolved and viral EBV DNA PCR has returned to baseline.[91,96] It should however be cautioned that PTLD can develop and progress without increases in EBV-PCR viral load.[97]

PTLD, a potentially fatal abnormal proliferation of B-lymphocytes, can occur in any situation in which immunosuppression is used. The importance of PTLD in pediatric LT is a result of the intensity of the immunosuppression required, its lifetime duration, and the absence of prior exposure to EBV infection in 60–80% of pediatric recipients. PTLD is the most common tumor in children following transplantation representing 50% of all tumors compared to 15% in adults. About 80% of cases occur within the first two years following transplantation.[94] Multiple studies analyzing immunosuppressive therapy and the development of PTLD have shown a progressive increase in its incidence with (1) the increase in total immunosuppressive load; (2) EBV naïve recipients; and (3) the intensity of active viral load.[98] No single immunosuppressive agent has been directly related to PTLD, although high-dose cyclosporine, tacrolimus, polyclonal antilymphocyte sera (MALG, ALG), and monoclonal antibodies (OKT-3) have all been implicated. Prolonged treatment with anti–T-cell agents and the increased duration, intensity, and total immunosuppressive load are the origin of the immunity that creates the background for neoplasia.

The second pathogenic feature influencing PTLD appears to be EBV infection. Primary or reactivation infections usually precede the recognition of PTLD. Active EBV infection, whether primary or reactivation, involves B-cell proliferation. A simultaneous increase in cytotoxic T-cell activity is the normal host's mechanism for preventing EBV dissemination. Loss of this natural protection as a result of the administration of T-cell inhibitory immunotherapy allows polyclonal B-cell proliferation to progress following EBV viral replication and release. These EBV proliferating cells express specific viral antigens which represent possible targets for the immune system, thereby explaining the well described regression of PTLD after immunosuppressive tapering. With time, transformation of a small population of cells results in a malignant monoclonal aggressive B-cell lymphoma.[93,99–101]

Most tumors seen in children are large cell lymphomas, 80% being of B-cell origin. Extranodal involvement, uncommon in primary lymphomas, is seen in 70% of PTLD cases. Extranodal sites include central nervous system, 27%; liver, 23%; lung, 22%; kidney, 21%; intestine, 20%; and spleen, 13%. Allograft involvement is common and can mimic rejection. T-cell and B-cell immunohistochemical markers of the infiltrating lymphocyte population define the B-cell infiltrate and assist in establishing an early diagnosis.

Treatment of PTLD is stratified according to the immunologic cell typing and clinical presentation.[102] Documented PTLD requires an immediate decrease or discontinuation of immunosuppression and institution of anti-EBV therapy. We prefer to use IV ganciclovir for initial antiviral therapy owing to the high incidence of concurrent CMV infection. Acyclovir is used for long-term treatment. The development of newer antiviral alternatives such as valganciclovir may offer better long-term options in the future.[103] Patients with polyclonal B-cell proliferation frequently show regression with this treatment.[91,96] If tumor cells express B-cell marker CD 20 on histology, the anti-CD 20 monoclonal antibody Rituximab can be administered weekly. Although associated in many cases with significant reduction in tumor mass, patients have frequently experienced reversible neutropenia requiring granulocyte colony stimulating factor (GCSF) and hypogammaglobulinemia requiring supplementation.[104] Acute liver rejection has frequently been seen during Rituximab treatment. Patients with aggressive monoclonal malignancies have poor survival even with immunosuppressive reduction, acyclovir, and conventional chemotherapy or radiation therapy. These additional treatment modalities often precipitate the development of fatal systemic infection. Efforts to reconstitute the EBV specific cellular immunity using partially HLA matched EBV specific cytotoxic T-cells may offer improved treatment outcome for advanced cases. The future development of anti-EBV vaccine may decrease the present significant risks of this unique complication of pediatric transplantation.[105] When treatment is successful, careful follow-up to identify recurrent disease or delayed central nervous system involvement is essential.

Retransplantation

The vast majority of retransplantation procedures in infants and children are done as a result of acute allograft demise caused by HAT or PNF. Acute rejection, chronic rejection, and biliary complications are more uncommon causes. Many of these complications are associated with concurrent sepsis, which further complicates reoperation and compromises success. Survival following transplantation is directly related to prompt identification of appropriate patients and acquisition of a suitable organ. When retransplantation is promptly undertaken for early graft failure, patient survival rate, in our experience, is good (73%). However, when retransplantation is undertaken for chronic allograft failure, often complicated by multiple organ system insufficiency, the survival rate is lower (45%).[106]

Similar findings were reported by UNOS Region I in their combined experience. Patients undergoing retransplantation for acute organ failure experienced twice the overall survival rate as those undergoing retransplantation for chronic disease.[107] In addition, acute retransplantation survival was significantly influenced by the time to acquire a retransplant organ, with a greater than three-day wait decreasing the survival rate from 52% to 20%. The overall incidence of retransplantation is 15% in our series and ranges in others' experience from 8–29%. This incidence is similar for primary whole organ allografts and reduced-size allografts. Reduced-size allografts are frequently used when retransplantation is required in view of their greater availability and their decreased incidence of allograft-threatening complications.[38,108,109] These findings emphasize the need for early identification of children requiring retransplantation and

---

BOX 45-5 **Factors Affecting Transplant Survival**

Medical status at orthotopic liver transplantation
Primary diagnosis
Age and size
Comorbid conditions
Encephalopathy
Infection
Multiple organ dysfunction

expeditious reoperation before the development of multisystem organ failure or sepsis.

Outcome Following Transplantation

Although complications following LT are frequent and severe, the overall results are rewarding. Improvements in organ preservation, operative management, immunosuppression, and treatment of postoperative complications have all contributed to the excellent survival rate that is currently seen. Factors influencing the survival of children undergoing transplantation are detailed in Box 45-5. Most successful transplant programs have reached overall one-year survival rates of 90%, with greatly decreased risk thereafter.[110,111] Similar if not better results have resulted from LD transplantation, especially for small recipients.[112–114] Improved survival in these small recipients likely results from a decrease in life-threatening and graft-threatening complications, such as HAT and PNF, in the reduced-size donor organ.

Patients with fulminant hepatic failure have an overall survival rate that is significantly lower than other diagnostic groups, with metabolic disease having the highest survival rate. Prior operations and multiple episodes of subacute bacterial peritonitis prior to LT influence the development of complications, especially bowel perforation, but do not adversely affect overall survival in most cases. However, the most important factor determining survival is the severity of the patient's illness at the time of initial transplantation.[38,115] When stratified for illness by PELD scores, Pediatric Risk of Mortality (PRISM) score, and the UNOS score, the PRISM score was the most accurate in predicting both survival and morbidity during the perioperative period.[116] Current efforts to use technical variant grafts have experienced similar survival rates as those for whole organ recipients (Fig. 45-9).[108,117]

The significant success now achieved following LT cannot overshadow the need for improved management of post-transplant consequences of immunosuppression and pre-LT chronic disease. The most significant factors contributing to long-term failure of the allograft or patient death in our and others' program are consequences of immunosuppressive medications: late infection, PTLD, and chronic rejection.[111,118–120] Our ability to overcome these challenges will determine the life-long success of transplantation for our youngest recipients. The overriding objective of LT in children is complete rehabilitation with improved quality of life. Factors contributing to successful achievement of this goal include

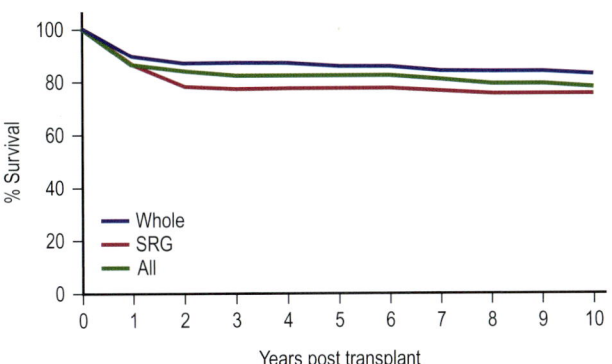

FIGURE 45-9 ■ Ten-year patient and allograft survival subdivided by whole and surgically reduced grafts (SRG). (Data from Cincinnati Children's Hospital Medical Center, Liver Care Center.)

an improved nutritional status with appropriate growth and development, as well as enhanced motor and cognitive skills that allow social reintegration.

Optimal postoperative nutrition significantly facilitates recovery and rehabilitation. This initially requires 100–130 calories/kg/day in recipients weighing less than 10 kg. Hepatic synthetic function, gut absorption, and appetite all improve following successful pediatric LT. Despite these improvements, growth disturbances do not immediately resolve.[121–123] In the first year after transplantation, very little catch-up growth occurs. During the second and third year, patients usually show significant catch-up growth, with the potential for catch-up growth being directly correlated with the degree of preoperative growth retardation. Decreased corticosteroid administration enhances this growth. Also, growth is further improved by the use of alternate-day steroids or complete steroid withdrawal in patients with stable allograft function two years following LT.[124] The 'steroid-sparing' effects of new immunosuppressive agents, such as tacrolimus, could diminish this unwanted consequence of immune modulation.

Although most pediatric LT recipients are returning to normal age-appropriate activities, recent studies indicate that they may experience subtle functional difficulties.[125–127] Neuropsychological function studies of children following transplantation demonstrate multiple deficits involving learning and memory, abstraction, concept formation, visual–spatial function, and motor function. The well-documented neurologic and cerebral abnormalities associated with chronic cirrhosis precede transplantation, but certainly influence these results.[126,128–130]

The long-term impact that transplantation has on the psychosocial and financial health of the entire family unit is also the subject of much investigation. Long-term pediatric LT survivors need in-depth, multicenter longitudinal studies to clarify these issues. Health Related Quality of Life (HRQOL) surveys of families after LT demonstrate improved health and physical perception compared to the pretransplant status.[131] However, as can be imagined, the overall impact on the family is significant. The health and quality of life in pediatric LT recipients was lower in these surveys than that reported for healthy children, but similar to that for children with other chronic illness. Age at transplantation, the time elapsed since transplantation, hospitalizations within the previous year, maternal education, and race were significant predictors of physical health. Age at transplantation and maternal education predicted psychosocial function. Both younger children and adolescents continue to have self-confidence and body image concerns, and their participation in family activities and sports is often limited. Caregivers and mothers are heavily impacted by the need for care of their chronically ill children prior to transplant and during their recovery. Many have experienced job losses, career changes, and significant family stress. The importance in providing these caregivers with critical support and psychological help is essential for the entire family to survive and flourish following the difficult times that inevitably follow LT.[131]

INTESTINAL TRANSPLANTATION

Intestinal failure can be a significant problem in the pediatric population. Total parenteral nutrition (TPN) remains the first-line therapy in children who have a loss of enteral autonomy. However, complications of long-term TPN, such as cholestatic liver disease, venous thromboses, and recurrent catheter sepsis, may preclude its continued use. When complications of long-term TPN become life threatening and the bowel length is too short for enteral alimentation, the alternative becomes intestinal transplantation. Although the exact incidence of intestinal failure in children is unclear, over two-thirds of the patients who are currently on the national intestinal transplantation waiting list are children, with the majority of active patients being 5 years of age or younger.[132]

Advances in immunosuppressive regimens, the technical aspects of the transplant operation, and the surveillance and treatment of transplant-related complications have continued to improve the outcome of patients who have required intestinal transplantation.[133,134] With the improved outcomes, the role of intestinal transplantation has evolved from a heroic last effort to salvage patients with no remaining treatment options to a standard part of the armamentarium in the management of patients with intestinal failure. Since the initial approval of federal reimbursement for intestinal transplantation by the Centers for Medicare and Medicaid Services in October 2000,[135] continued success with intestinal transplantation in children has shifted focus from short-term patient survival to optimizing long-term allograft function and patient survival.

Indications for Transplantation

The causes of intestinal failure can be divided into three broad categories: short bowel syndrome (SBS), intestinal dysmotility syndromes, and absorptive disorders. SBS, usually caused by the loss of intestinal length due to an intra-abdominal catastrophe or in the setting of a congenital gastrointestinal disorder, is the most common cause in children. Disease processes necessitating an operation that result in SBS range from necrotizing enterocolitis, intestinal atresia, and gastroschisis in the newborn to Crohn disease and traumatic injury to the main intestinal blood supply in the older population. Midgut volvulus, another frequent cause of SBS, can occur at any age, although the majority of cases occur in infants.

The intestinal dysmotility syndromes include total intestinal aganglionosis (Hirschsprung disease) and the constellation of disorders known as chronic idiopathic intestinal pseudo-obstruction. Absorptive disorders lead to intractable diarrhea due to impaired enterocyte absorption, and include congenital epithelial mucosal diseases, such as microvillus inclusion disease, tufting enteropathy, and autoimmune enteritis. Although these latter disorders are rare, affected children face life-long difficulty with gastrointestinal absorptive function and require TPN for long-term survival.

TPN is the standard treatment for patients who experience acute intestinal failure. Bowel rehabilitation should be aggressively pursued because intestinal adaptation can result in eventual enteral autonomy. Intestinal rehabilitation programs that utilize a combination of TPN, gradual re-introduction of enteral feeds, intestinal antimotility agents, and treatment of small bowel bacterial overgrowth, in association with hepatoprotective lipid minimization strategies and ethanol lock usage to reduce the incidence of catheter-related bloodstream infections, are successful in achieving enteral autonomy in many patients.[136,137] Autologous intestinal reconstruction procedures, such as the serial transverse enteroplasty (STEP) and longitudinal intestinal lengthening and tailoring (LILT), may be beneficial in selected patients. In general, survival and complete return of gastrointestinal function may be predicted when the post-resection length of the intestine exceeds 5% of normal for gestational age if the ileocecal valve is present, or is greater than 10% of normal if the ileocecal valve is absent.[138]

The current Medicare-approved indications for intestinal transplantation are shown in Box 45-6.[135] Progressive liver dysfunction and TPN-associated cholestatic liver disease result in significant mortality. Unless the

TPN can be stopped, liver failure is a strong indication for combined liver/intestinal or multivisceral transplantation. Studies have shown that the presence of hyperbilirubinemia greater than 3 mg/dL or bridging fibrosis and cirrhosis found on liver biopsy in an infant dependent on TPN is associated with a 1-year survival of less than 30%.[139] The remaining criteria of limited central venous access, multiple catheter-related bloodstream infections, and frequent episodes of severe dehydration reflect complications from chronic TPN use, and in the absence of significant concurrent liver dysfunction, are indications for isolated intestinal transplantation.

Currently, with improved outcomes after intestinal transplantation, some centers advocate early intestinal transplantation before the onset of TPN-induced complications.[140] These groups propose that patient and graft survival after intestinal transplantation will be optimized if recipients undergo transplantation prior to the onset of secondary organ damage, especially liver disease. Furthermore, the quality of life in patients who have undergone successful intestinal transplantation may be better than that of patients who require long-term TPN administration. This issue remains controversial and requires further study because TPN is a well-established and effective means of treatment for patients with intestinal failure. In addition, with recent advances in hepatoprotective approaches to TPN administration and improved care related to central venous catheters, children with intestinal failure on TPN are now able to be maintained complication-free for longer periods of time, thereby allowing further delay in the need for intestinal transplantation. Despite the lack of consensus with regard to optimal timing of intestinal transplantation, it has become clear that early and timely patient referral for pretransplant evaluation is critical to ensuring the best opportunity for long-term survival.[141]

Contraindications

The contraindications to intestinal transplantation are similar to those for any other solid organ transplantation. The presence of severe cardiopulmonary dysfunction, an active nonresectable malignancy, severe neurologic disabilities, or life-threatening extraintestinal illness or infection precludes intestinal transplantation.

Operative Considerations

The three types of intestinal allografts include multivisceral, liver-small bowel composite, and isolated small bowel. The type of intestinal transplant utilized is dictated by the needs of each patient. The biggest limitation to intestinal transplantation in the pediatric population is the need for size-matched grafts. Patients with intestinal failure generally have limited abdominal domain (due in part to a lack of intestine volume), which necessitates near-identical-size donors. Advances in the use of reduced-size liver allografts have been applied to the liver-small bowel composite allograft as a means of increasing the flexibility of donor-to-recipient size matching.[142] However, nearly 50% of patients on the intestinal transplant waiting list die before undergoing

---

BOX 45-6	**Medicare-Approved Indications for Intestinal Transplantation**

1. Impending or overt liver failure due to TPN-induced liver injury. Liver failure defined as increased serum bilirubin or liver enzyme levels (or both), splenomegaly, thrombocytopenia, gastroesophageal varices, coagulopathy, stomal bleeding, hepatic fibrosis, or cirrhosis
2. Thrombosis of two or more central veins (subclavian, jugular, or femoral)
3. The development of two or more episodes of systemic sepsis secondary to line infection that requires hospitalization, or a single episode of line-related fungemia, or septic shock and/or acute respiratory distress syndrome
4. Frequent episodes of severe dehydration despite intravenous fluid supplementation in addition to TPN

TPN, total parenteral nutrition.

transplantation owing to the lack of appropriate donors, and the highest risk subgroup are children less than 1 year old.[143] In the past, it was believed that recipients who were CMV-negative should not receive intestinal grafts from CMV-positive donors because of a high incidence of severe, potentially life-threatening CMV infection after transplantation.[144] However, with current antiviral therapy regimens, it appears this barrier has been overcome.[145] In early series, a higher risk of infectious complications was reported in patients receiving allografts that included donor colon. More recently, however, morbidity and mortality rates in recipients of colon-inclusive allografts have not been found to be higher.[146] Children with total intestinal aganglionosis and chronic idiopathic intestinal pseudo-obstruction most commonly receive colon-inclusive allografts.

An ileostomy is created in all recipients so that surveillance endoscopy and biopsy of the small bowel mucosa can be performed to monitor the allograft for rejection. If not already present, a gastrostomy is placed at the time of transplantation for gastric decompression and for access to the upper gastrointestinal tract. A particular challenge of intestinal transplantation in the pediatric recipient is closure of the abdominal incision due to pretransplant loss of domain and size discrepancy between allograft and recipient intra-abdominal space. A variety of techniques have been utilized for abdominal wall closure, including staged abdominal closure, acellular dermal matrix patches, nonvascularized rectus sheath fascia allografts, and abdominal wall transplantation.

The Transplant Procedure

Multivisceral Allograft

Multivisceral transplantation consists of transplantation of the stomach, pancreaticoduodenal complex, and intestine, either with (multivisceral allograft) or without (modified multivisceral allograft) the liver. In the pediatric population, the primary indications for multivisceral transplantation are the intestinal dysmotility syndromes. On occasion, a giant desmoid tumor of the mesentery that extensively infiltrates the mesentery may require this form of transplantation. Exenteration of the native intra-abdominal viscera is followed by transplantation of the multivisceral graft using arterial inflow through the donor celiac and superior mesenteric artery (SMA). Venous outflow for the multivisceral allograft occurs via the transplanted liver placed in the standard orthotopic position. For the modified multivisceral allograft, portal venous return is via an anastomosis with the recipient's native portal vein. Gastrointestinal continuity is completed via a gastrogastric anastomosis proximally and an ileocolic anastomosis distal to the ileostomy.

Liver–Small Bowel Composite Allograft

A liver–small bowel composite allograft is a modification of the multivisceral allograft in which the stomach is removed during procurement. This form of transplantation is indicated in patients with intestinal failure and impending or overt TPN-induced liver failure, and is the

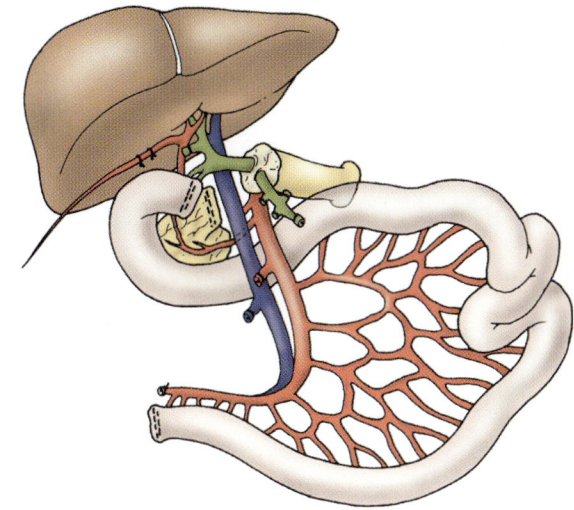

FIGURE 45-10 ■ Schematic diagram of liver/intestine composite allograft. (From Abu-Elmagd K, Reyes J, Todo S, et al. Clinical intestinal transplantation: New perspectives and immunologic considerations. J Am Coll Surg 1998;186:512–27.)

most common type of intestinal transplant currently utilized in children (Fig. 45-10). The recipient's liver and residual small intestine are removed, while the native stomach, duodenum, pancreas, and spleen are left intact. A portocaval shunt from the native portal vein to the inferior vena cava is necessary to provide venous outflow from the recipient's foregut organs (Fig. 45-11). As in the multivisceral allograft, the donor celiac artery and SMA are the source of arterial inflow to the transplanted organs. The donor portal vein and biliary tree remain intact, having not undergone dissection during procurement. As a result, no portal vein or bile duct reconstruction is needed. The pancreas is also left intact to protect the peri-biliary ductal vessels and to prevent the possibility of pancreatic leak from a divided surface. Venous outflow from the transplanted organs is once again provided by the donor liver placed in a standard orthotopic position. If the liver is too large, an ex vivo hepatic lobectomy can be performed, usually removing the right lobe of the liver (Fig. 45-12). Gastrointestinal continuity from the patient's native stomach and duodenum to the newly transplanted small bowel is achieved by anastomosis of the native duodenum to the donor jejunum. If the recipient has any colon remaining, a donor ileum to recipient colon anastomosis is created distal to the ileostomy.

Isolated Small Bowel Allograft

Transplantation of the small intestine alone entails procurement of only the jejunum and ileum. During procurement, the SMA and vein are divided just below the third portion of the duodenum at the root of the mesentery, generating an allograft of jejunum and ileum (Fig. 45-13). This type of transplant is indicated in patients with intestinal failure, but without liver dysfunction. Arterial inflow is provided by anastomosis of the SMA to the recipient's aorta. Venous drainage of the transplanted intestines is either into the inferior vena cava or to the native superior mesenteric vein. Initially it was believed

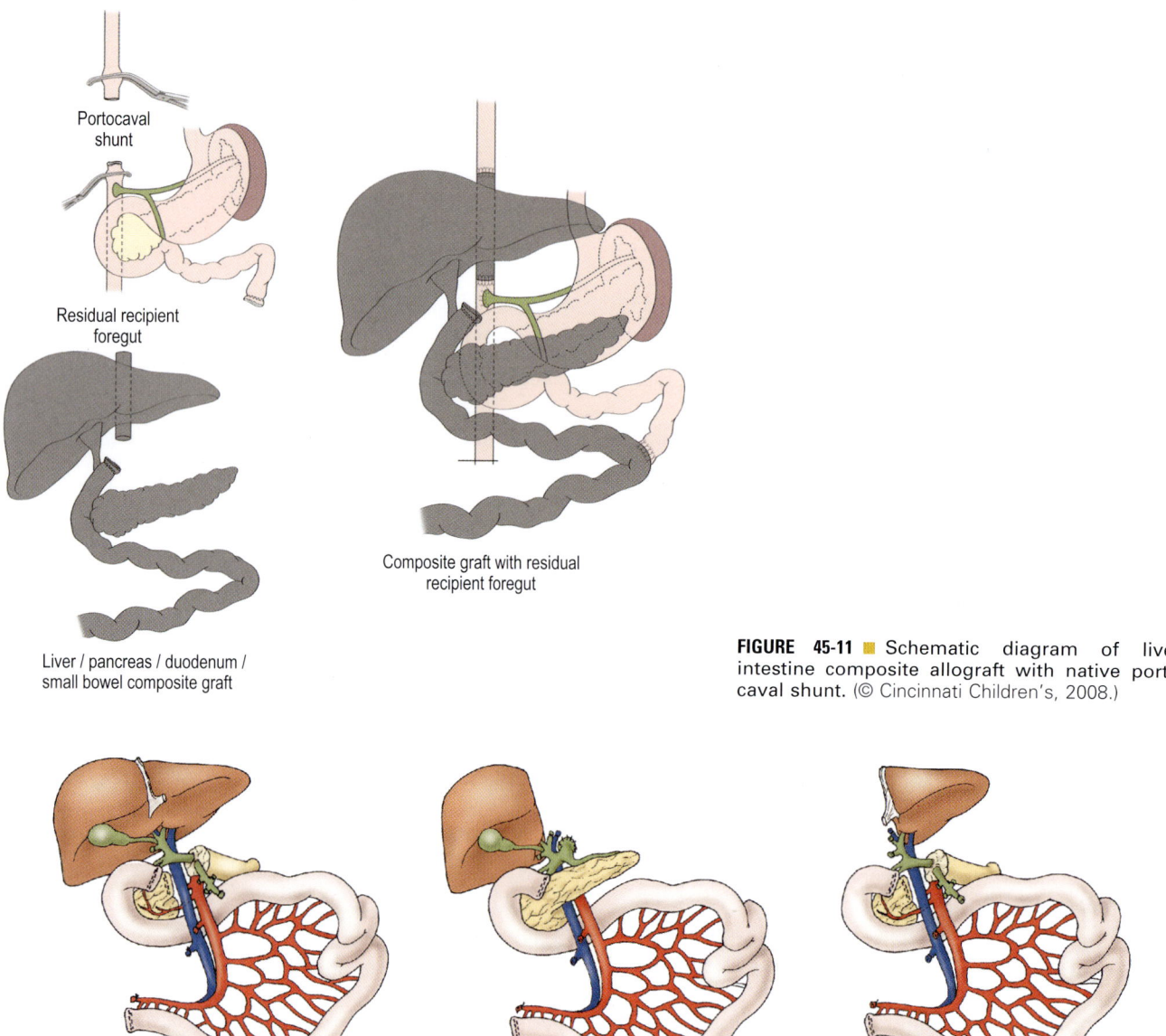

Portocaval shunt

Residual recipient foregut

Liver / pancreas / duodenum / small bowel composite graft

Composite graft with residual recipient foregut

FIGURE 45-11 ■ Schematic diagram of liver/intestine composite allograft with native portocaval shunt. (© Cincinnati Children's, 2008.)

FIGURE 45-12 ■ Schematic diagram of reduced-size liver/intestine composite allograft. (From Reyes J, Mazariegos GV, Bond GMD, et al. Pediatric intestinal transplantation: Historical notes, principles and controversies. Pediatr Transplant 2002;6:193–207.)

that venous drainage into the native portal circulation was beneficial to the liver, but recent studies suggest minimal benefit.[147] Therefore, currently, the most common approach to venous reconstruction is an end-to-side anastomosis of the donor superior mesenteric vein to the native inferior vena cava. Gastrointestinal continuity is restored by anastomosis of the recipient's native proximal bowel to the transplanted jejunum. Once again, if residual colon is present, a donor ileum to native colon anastomosis is created downstream from the ileostomy.

Postoperative Complications

Although the outcomes of intestinal transplantation continue to improve, postoperative complications are not uncommon. A breakdown of intestinal integrity

either at sites of anastomosis or in areas of mucosal injury from ischemic reperfusion injury often necessitate re-exploration. Bowel perforation can also occur following surveillance endoscopy and biopsy. Patients with a significant amount of peritoneal contamination after intestinal perforation may require serial operative explorations to clear foci of intra-abdominal infection. Postoperative bleeding is frequent, especially in patients who undergo transplantation with liver–small bowel composite allografts, because preexisting portal hypertension results in varices throughout the abdominal cavity. Chylous leaks are also frequent because lymphatic drainage may be disrupted during both the procurement and the recipient operative procedure. Most chylous leaks can be managed conservatively. A high percentage of patients who undergo intestinal transplantation will require re-exploration at some point in the postoperative period.

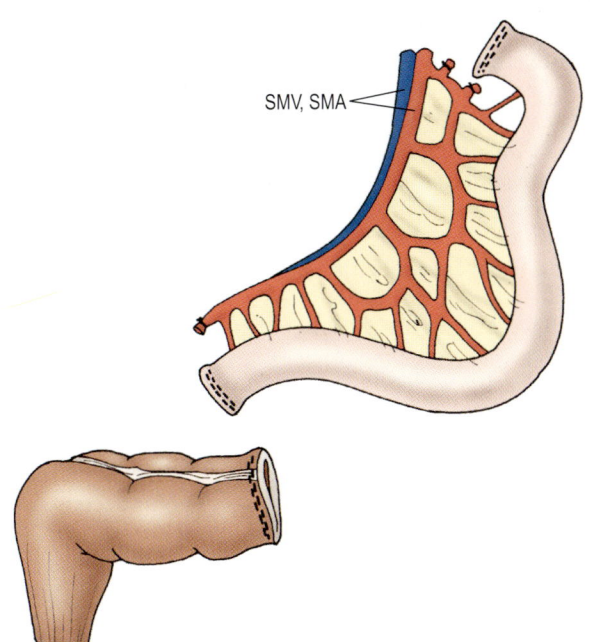

FIGURE 45-13 ■ Schematic diagram of isolated small intestinal transplant. SMV, superior mesenteric vein; SMA, superior mesenteric artery. (Adapted from Abu-Elmagd K, Fung J, Bueno J, et al. Logistics and technique for procurement of intestinal, pancreatic, and hepatic grafts from the same donor. Ann Surg 2000; 232:680–7.)

SMV, SMA

Immunosuppression and Allograft Rejection

The most significant recent advances in the management of intestinal transplant recipients have occurred in the development of immunosuppression regimens. Rejection remains the most common complication after intestinal transplantation, and acute rejection occurs in approximately 60% of pediatric recipients within the first three months after transplantation.[134] Overwhelming rejection was one of the most frequent causes of allograft loss during the early transplant experience due, in part, to the limited number of immunosuppressive agents available. Prior to the development of tacrolimus as a maintenance immunosuppression approach, high-dose immunosuppression was necessary to prevent rejection. Infections, PTLD, and adverse effects related to high-dose immunosuppression were frequent causes of a poor outcome. The goal of current immunosuppressive regimens is to use just enough immunosuppression to prevent rejection, but not so much that infections and PTLD occur. In an effort to achieve tolerance, many centers utilize a lymphocyte-depleting strategy, such as thymoglobulin or alemtuzumab, to induce early elimination of graft-specific T-lymphocytes. The management of immunosuppression in patients who undergo intestinal transplantation remains the most challenging aspect of the postoperative care.

Surveillance endoscopy and biopsy is initiated within five days of transplantation to evaluate for acute rejection, and is performed twice per week for the first month. Significant progress in the definition of the histologic characteristics of acute small bowel rejection has been achieved.[148] If acute rejection is diagnosed, a short course

of high-dose corticosteroids is administered. If rejection is severe or persists despite high-dose corticosteroid administration, antilymphocyte antibody agents (thymoglobulin or alemtuzumab) are required. Chronic rejection remains the most common cause of late allograft dysfunction and failure.

Infection

Owing in large part to the high level of immunosuppression needed after intestinal transplantation, bacterial and fungal infections are common. Patients with intestinal failure are frequently colonized with antibiotic-resistant bacteria due to recurrent infections while on TPN. As mentioned previously, because intestinal perforation is common, peritonitis is a frequent complication often requiring repeat abdominal explorations to completely clear foci of infection.

CMV, EBV, adenovirus, and calicivirus are the most frequent viral pathogens found in the postoperative period, and many can masquerade as acute rejection. PTLD remains a significant problem because most infants are EBV-negative at the time of transplantation. Surveillance for CMV and EBV using PCR, followed by aggressive treatment when detected, has diminished the impact of these dangerous pathogens on patient outcome. All patients are maintained on prophylactic antiviral agents after intestinal transplantation.

Graft-versus-Host Disease (GVHD)

GVHD occurs in approximately 5–10% of intestinal transplant recipients, most commonly in the youngest pediatric recipients. Its high incidence is related to the large burden of donor lymphocytes that are cotransplanted with the allograft. Acute GVHD characteristically affects the skin, native liver, and native gastrointestinal tract, and carries a high mortality. Monitoring of donor-derived T-cell chimerism is being utilized to identify patients at risk for GVHD. Management strategies for GVHD after intestinal transplantation include high-dose corticosteroids and lymphocyte depletion with alemtuzumab.[149]

Outcome Following Transplantation

Early outcomes of patients who underwent intestinal transplantation was poor with few long-term survivors. With advances in operative techniques, immunosuppression strategies, allograft surveillance, and monitoring and treatment of infections and other transplant-related complications, significant improvements in patient survival have occurred in the past 15 years. Currently, according to the *ultrasound Scientific Registry of Transplant Recipients*, approximately 80% of pediatric recipients survive 1 year and 65% survive 3 years after transplantation. Short-term allograft survival has likewise increased significantly. Despite improvements in short-term outcomes, the long-term outcomes have remained largely unchanged over the past decade. Current impediments to long-term allograft survival are primarily related to chronic rejection, particularly in isolated small bowel transplantation.

Chronic rejection is responsible for the greatest proportion of allograft loss 2 years after transplantation.[134] Further advances in surveillance and immunosuppressive strategies are needed to optimize long-term allograft function and survival.

RENAL TRANSPLANTATION

Acute renal failure in infants is most often the consequence of hemodynamic instability, with poor perfusion or hypoxia resulting in acute tubular necrosis (ATN). Most of these patients either recover sufficient renal function for normal long-term survival or die of multisystem failure.

Chronic renal failure is uncommon in infants. The estimate incidence of ESRD in infants is 0.2 per million total population of infants younger than 1 year of age.[150,151] Renal aplasia/dysplasia, obstructive and complex urological malformations, and focal segmental glomerulosclerosis (FSGS) are the most common causes of ESRD in children younger than 5 years of age (Table 45-4). In the

TABLE 45-4 Primary Diagnoses in Children Requiring Renal Transplantation

Primary Diagnosis	Number of Patients	Percentage
Aplasia/hypoplasia/dysplasia kidney	1,681	14.5
Obstructive uropathy	1,630	14.0
Focal segmental glomerulosclerosis	1,246	10.7
Reflux nephropathy	549	4.7
Chronic glomerulonephritis	340	2.9
Polycystic disease	323	2.8
Medullary cystic disease	287	2.5
Congenital nephrotic syndrome	277	2.4
Hemolytic uremic syndrome	273	2.4
Prune belly	268	2.3
Familial nephritis	241	2.1
Cystinosis	221	1.9
Membranoproliferative glomerulonephritis—type I	186	1.6
Pyelo/interstitial nephritis	184	1.6
Idiopathic crescentic glomerulonephritis	181	1.6
SLE nephritis	159	1.4
Renal infarct	140	1.2
Berger (IgA) nephritis	135	1.2
Henoch–Schönlein nephritis	113	1.0
Membranoproliferative glomerulonephritis—Type II	85	0.7
Wegener's granulomatosis	66	0.6
Wilms tumor	56	0.5
Drash syndrome	55	0.5
Oxalosis	55	0.5
Membranous nephropathy	47	0.4
Other systemic immunologic disease	34	0.3
Sickle cell nephropathy	16	0.2
Diabetic glomerulonephritis	11	0.1
Other	1,110	9.5
Unknown	663	5.7
Total	**11,603**	**100.0**

Data from the North American Pediatric Renal Transplant Cooperative Study 2010 Annual Report.

past antenatal renal failure caused by obstructive malformations resulted in fetal demise or pulmonary insufficiency incompatible with post natal survival. With the evolution of fetal diagnosis and in-utero therapy, the pulmonary insufficiency can be attenuated, resulting in a population of neonates with adequate pulmonary reserve, but perinatal renal insufficiency.

Glomerulonephritis and lupus nephritis, as well as recurrent pyelonephritis, are the common causes of ESRD in older children.[152] As the number of patients who have undergone renal transplantation in childhood has increased, chronic rejection following renal transplantation has recently become a cause of ESRD.

Knowledge of the etiology of the ESRD is important to allow assessment of the potential for recurrence within a transplant allograft and consideration of LD transplantation. Patients with a 'structural/congenital' etiology, without an immunologic component, also enjoy better graft survival rates than those patients with glomerulonephritis.[153]

Pretransplant Management

Pretransplant management is critical in infants and children with ESRD. Children with ESRD beginning in infancy or early childhood experience significant complications from growth retardation, renal osteodystrophy, and neuropsychiatric developmental delay. Recent advances in dialysis regimens, nutritional supplementation, and recombinant human erythropoietin and growth hormone have significantly improved the pretransplant management of these patients.

Dialysis

Dialysis is indicated when complications of ESRD occur despite optimal medical management, specifically hyperkalemia, volume overload, acidosis, intractable hypertension, and uremic symptoms such as vomiting and fatigue. In older children, lethargy and poor school performance can signal the need for more aggressive treatment. In addition, dialysis may be necessary to facilitate the administration of adequate protein as part of an extensive nutritional resuscitation plan.

When dialysis is undertaken, the use of peritoneal dialysis is preferred for the following reasons: (1) it avoids the multiple blood transfusions associated with hemodialysis; (2) it allows a gradual correction of electrolyte abnormalities, preventing cerebral disequilibrium syndrome in small infants; (3) it allows for easier control of osteodystrophy; (4) it optimizes nutrition; and (5) it is easy to perform.

Hemodialysis can be used when there is an unsuitable peritoneal cavity due to prior surgery or multiple peritoneal infections. However, the construction and maintenance of adequate long-term vascular access sites in small infants and children is difficult. Use of central venous catheters rather than arteriovenous fistulas is our preferred mode for temporary hemodialysis access in infants and small children, although infection and vascular thromboses complicate this therapy. Access via the internal jugular veins is preferred over subclavian routes to avoid obstruction of the venous outflow from the upper extremity, which compromises future arteriovenous fistula sites. Although dialysis and its complications, such as infection, have a great influence on the complexity of care, they do not affect the ultimate results of renal transplantation.[154]

Nutritional Support

The need for vigorous nutritional support of the infant with uremia is well demonstrated by the growth retardation seen in infants and children with ESRD. The etiology of this growth disturbance is multifactorial, including anorexia that leads to protein and calorie insufficiency, renal osteodystrophy, aluminum toxicity, uremic acidosis, impaired somatomedin activity, and growth hormone and insulin resistance.[155] Because the most intense period of a child's growth occurs during the first 2 years of life, careful nutritional support during that time is essential.

The mean weight at the time of renal transplantation has improved from 2.2 SD to 1.6 SD below the appropriate age-adjusted and gender-adjusted mean for normal children in a recent North American Pediatric Renal Transplant Cooperative Study (NAPRTCS). This growth deficit was greater (2.8 SD) in children younger than 5 years of age. Transplantation afforded a 0.8 SD increase in growth over the first post-transplant year. However, this growth then reached a stable plateau. After 2 to 3 years, the mean weight values were comparable to those of normal children.[152] Children 6 years of age and older showed no improvement in their height deficit 5 years after transplantation.[156,157] These limitations to 'catch-up' growth emphasize the need for early transplantation in young ESRD patients. If epiphyseal closure has occurred (bone age >12 years), additional bone growth is often not achieved.[151,158,159] Normalization of growth rarely occurs with hemodialysis or peritoneal dialysis.

The importance of efforts to normalize nutritional parameters is emphasized by the adverse impact of uremia on the infant's developing nervous system. The significance of this problem was emphasized in a study in which progressive encephalopathy, developmental delay, microcephaly, hypotonia, seizures, and dyskinesia developed in 20 of 23 children with ESRD before 1 year of age.[160] All of these patients had significant growth impairment. Monitoring of the head circumference has been suggested to identify the infant at risk, with the intent to initiate dialysis, nutritional support, or transplantation if this parameter deviates from the normal curve.[151]

Preoperative Preparation

In preparation for renal transplantation, an extensive evaluation of the urinary tract and immunologic status of the patient is important. The increased frequency of urinary tract abnormalities as the primary cause of ESRD in infants and children necessitates the investigation of the urinary tract for sites of obstruction, the presence of ureteral reflux, and the functional state and capacity of the urinary bladder.[161] This investigation is best accomplished by obtaining an ultrasound or intravenous pyelogram evaluating the upper urinary tract and a VCUG to assess the bladder and reflux. Any concerns about bladder function or structure requires urodynamics and cystoscopy.

In patients with long-standing oliguric ESRD, the bladder may be very small. In the absence of obstructive or neuromuscular pathology, enlargement of the bladder with normal urinary production is expected. Any operative correction of urethral obstruction or augmentation of bladder size should be performed well in advance of transplantation. Preoperative sterilization of the urinary tract and the development of unobstructed urinary outflow should be the ultimate goals of evaluation and reconstruction. Although complex anomalies of the urogenital tract often require many operative procedures to augment, reconstruct, or create an acceptable lower urinary tract, most children can undergo successful reconstruction with continent urinary reservoirs without the need for intestinal conduits.[162]

Immunologic assessment includes tissue typing and panel reactive antibody analysis. Patients should be monitored periodically for the development of a positive cross-match to their potential LD or a positive cytotoxic antibody to a panel of random donors. In addition, reactivity to CMV, EBV, HSV, and hepatitis should also be performed. Childhood immunizations should be current, and immunization against hepatitis B virus is important. Any immunizations with live-virus vaccines should be given well in advance of transplantation because their use is contraindicated in the early post-transplant period.

Selection of the appropriate donor source for transplantation is a decision for the transplant team and family to consider together. A related immediate family member has the advantage of a low incidence of postoperative ATN, improved histologic matching, and extended organ function. In addition, any operative procedures required for preparation of the recipient, as well as the transplant procedure, can be scheduled around the needs of the patient, simplifying preoperative care and potentially avoiding the complications of dialysis. Parents form the majority of donors. The 2010 NAPRTCS report indicates that 40% of children receive an LD kidney from a parent.[153] Thorough evaluation of the potential donor to exclude intrinsic renal anomalies, vascular anomalies, and systemic illness is important.

Deceased donor (DD) kidneys are currently used for 49% of renal transplants.[153] The unpredictability of donor organ availability and the need to establish a negative antibody cross-match for DD transplantation make surgical planning impossible. The size of a potential allograft, DD or related LD, is also important. Kidneys from small adult donors can be transplanted into infants as small as 5 kg with good success.[163] DD organs from pediatric donors 5 years of age or older also result in an excellent survival rate. However, a progressive decrease in one-year graft survival has been noted when kidneys from donors younger than 3 to 4 years of age are used.[164,165] This decrease in graft and patient survival is related to the donor organ source. Children 2 to 5 years of age have a similar survival rate as the overall pediatric population when LDs are used. Recognition of this potential risk has led to reluctance by most centers to use donors younger than 2 years of age. An effect of donor age on graft survival has been attributed to an increased rate of both graft thrombosis and acute rejection.[152]

In the past, the decision to use a DD as opposed to an LD was influenced by the possibility of disease recurrence within the transplanted kidney. The incidence of disease recurrence following transplantation and the risk of graft loss are listed in Table 45-5.[166] With new treatment strategies for recurrent disease, the risk of graft loss has been attenuated, and as a result, LD kidneys are now preferred. This decision to favor LD kidneys is influenced by the recent improvements in outcomes which show similar one-year graft survival for DD and LD for all age groups.

Pre-emptive Transplantation

The desire to perform preemptive renal transplantation before undertaking dialysis is often fueled by the patient's or parents' desire to avoid the dialysis procedures, potential infections, or cardiovascular complications, and the psychological impairment inherent with dialysis. A NAPRTCS review found 26% of primary transplantations were performed without prior dialysis.[167] Most cases used LDs rather than DDs. There was no difference in patient or graft survival in this group when compared with patients who underwent dialysis before transplantation. Pre-emptive transplantation is not possible when uncontrolled hypertension, massive proteinuria, or recurrent infection require prior native kidney removal, or when oliguric renal failure requires immediate dialysis.

Transplant Procedure

Preparation for transplantation should include placing adequate large-bore IV lines and the largest urinary catheter possible. Central venous lines are used in all infants and children to ensure vascular access, hemodynamic monitoring, and a route for postoperative immunosuppressive delivery. Perioperative prophylactic antibiotics are administered. Arterial pressure monitoring lines are only necessary in small infants and patients with hemodynamic compromise, allowing preservation of future hemodialysis access sites.

Renal transplantation in infants and small children can be undertaken through a generous retroperitoneal approach or a transabdominal approach with placement of the allograft posterior to the right or left colon. An extraperitoneal approach to the retroperitoneum allows the possibility for peritoneal dialysis and should be used if possible. The arterial anastomosis is constructed end-to-side into the distal aorta or common iliac artery, and venous outflow of the allograft is via the inferior vena cava or common iliac vein. Ureteral implantation using the Lich extravesical ureteroneocystostomy avoids the need for a cystotomy and minimizes postoperative blood clots within the bladder, which can obstruct the urinary catheter. When larger donor kidneys are used in small recipients, the vessels must be shortened to avoid redundancy when the kidney is positioned in the retroperitoneum. The internal iliac artery is not used in children so that pelvic blood flow is preserved (Fig. 45-14). Ureteral 'double-J' stents are used when small ureter size may lead to obstruction.

Anesthetic management of the infant and small child during kidney transplantation is complicated by preexisting electrolyte abnormalities and the large fluid fluxes that occur in the operating room. In the past, perfusion of the allograft with hypothermic lactated Ringer's solution before implantation to remove any remaining UW preservation solution was necessary to avoid massive potassium infusion when the allograft was perfused. This problem has been obviated by the use of HTK solution which has a lower potassium concentration. Volume loading to a CVP of 10–12 cmH$_2$O and administration of bicarbonate, calcium, and low-dose vasopressors (dopamine 5 µg/kg/min) is important prior to reperfusion of the graft.

Postoperative Management

Post-transplant management requires careful observation for technical complications, rejection, recurrence of the primary renal disease, and prevention of immunosuppression-related complications. Frequent fluid and electrolyte monitoring is necessary immediately following transplantation because larger kidneys can excrete the equivalent of the infant's blood volume within a single hour. Careful attention to serum concentrations of calcium, phosphorus, magnesium, and electrolytes is also needed. Urine output is initially replaced isovolumetrically, then tapered as the high-output state decreases. Glucose-free replacement fluids minimize hyperglycemia

---

TABLE 45-5 Recurrence Rates and Graft Loss from Recurrent Disease in Children

Disease	Recurrence Rate (%)	Clinical Severity	Percentage of Those with Recurrence Whose Graft Failed
FSGS	25–30	High	40–50
MPGN type I	70	Mild	12–30
MPGN type II	100	Low	10–20
SLE	5–40	Low	5
HSP	55–85	Low/mild	5–20
HUS (classic)	12–20	Moderate	0–10
HUS (atypical)	±25	High	40–50

FSGS, focal segmental glomerulosclerosis; HSP, Henoch–Schönlein purpura; HUS, hemolytic uremic syndrome; MPGN, membranoproliferative glomerulonephritis; SLE, systemic lupus erythematosus.
From Fine RN, Ettenger R. In: Morris PJ, editor. Kidney Transplantation: Principles and Practice. 4th ed. Philadelphia: WB Saunders; 1994. p. 418.

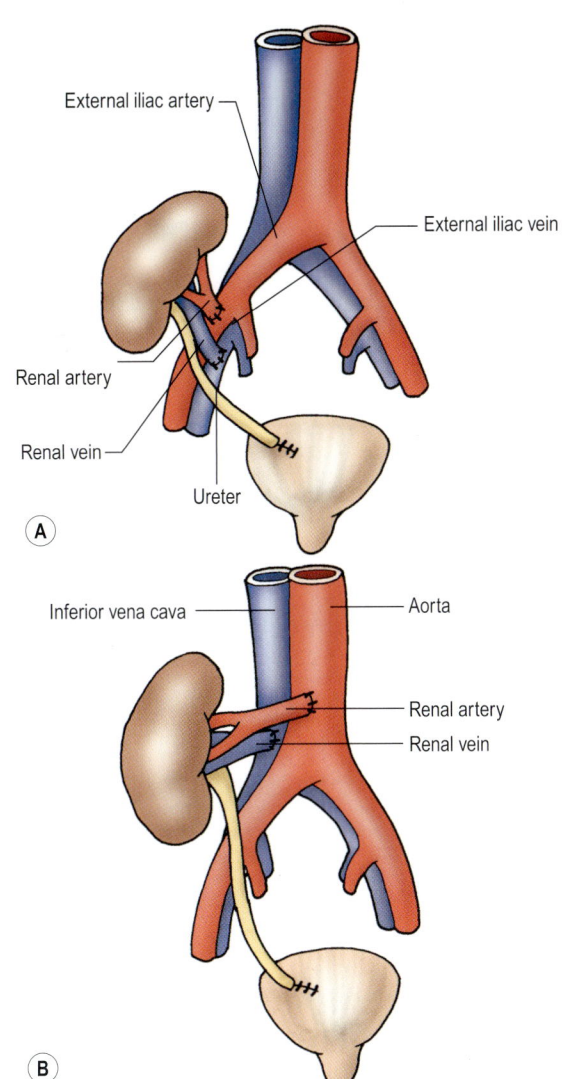

External iliac artery

External iliac vein

Renal artery

Renal vein

Ureter

(A)

Inferior vena cava

Aorta

Renal artery

Renal vein

(B)

FIGURE 45-14 ■ Schematic diagram showing the transplant arterial and venous anastomosis to the **(A)** iliac vessels or the **(B)** aorta and vena cava. Ureteral implantation using the Lich extravesical ureteroneocystostomy is preferred.

and osmotic diuresis in the recipient. Selection of appropriate electrolyte concentrations is guided by urinary electrolyte excretion. Central venous filling pressures should be maintained at 7–10 cmH$_2$O to ensure adequate intravascular volume. In patients with high-output renal failure, urine losses from both the native and transplant kidneys need to be replaced to avoid hypoperfusion and thrombosis. Maintenance of catheter patency is essential, and any episode of decreased urinary output should be rapidly investigated to exclude urinary catheter occlusion and bladder distention. An algorithm for the evaluation of early postoperative oliguria is shown in Figure 45-15.

Postoperative Complications

Vascular thrombosis still accounts for graft loss in up to 13% of initial transplants and 19% of repeat transplants in children.[166] Graft thrombosis is significantly more frequent in children younger than 2 years of age and is

directly related to the age of both the donor and the recipient. In addition, prolonged cold ischemic preservation time (>24 hours) and the related presence of ATN with delayed graft function also increase this risk. Prior transplantation and more than five pretransplant blood transfusions have also been shown to be independent risk factors.[166] Immediate post-transplant Doppler ultrasound vascular imaging is helpful in confirming suitable allograft blood flow following abdominal closure, especially when large allografts are implanted into small recipients. Adequate hydration is important to maintain perfusion. Anticoagulation has not been used in most series.

Urinary leak, most often at the neocystostomy site, presents with oliguria and persisting uremia. Ultrasound or nuclear imaging can be useful for identifying an extravesical fluid collection. Operative repair is necessary to prevent urinoma formation and its potential infectious complications. Urinary collections should be differentiated from lymphoceles at the transplant site. Lymphoceles that do not resolve are best opened into the peritoneal cavity using laparoscopy.

Hypertension

Hypertension following renal transplantation is common. One month after transplantation, 72% of all patients require treatment, although this percentage decreases to 53% at 30 months.[168] Careful attention to the pretransplant control of hypertension and dietary management improves the post-transplant management. Hypertension presents a significant risk to renal function when using small allografts. Hypertension in the early postoperative period is most often due to fluid overload or acute rejection, but it can also originate in the native kidneys.

Preexisting hypertension is augmented by the immunosuppressive drugs cyclosporine, tacrolimus, and prednisone. The development of hypertension more than three months after transplantation suggests possible renal artery stenosis and warrants ultrasound Doppler flow studies for initial evaluation. Arteriography may be needed in unclear cases. Transluminal angioplasty has been successful in alleviating the majority of these stenosis. Operative correction is reserved for angioplasty failures and vessels with complex arterial anastomoses.

Infection

Much like liver and intestinal transplantation, the highest risks for infectious complications arise within the first 6 months post-transplant. During this time, immunosuppression is intense and susceptibility to life-threatening infection is increased. In infants and children who are seronegative, use of organs from donors who have had prior exposure to CMV and EBV enhances the risk of these specific infections. Expanded use of antiviral prophylaxis using ganciclovir and acyclovir has decreased the intensity of these infections and their associated morbidity or mortality.

Immunosuppression

Many immunosuppressive regimens are available and all share similar strategy. Most regimens

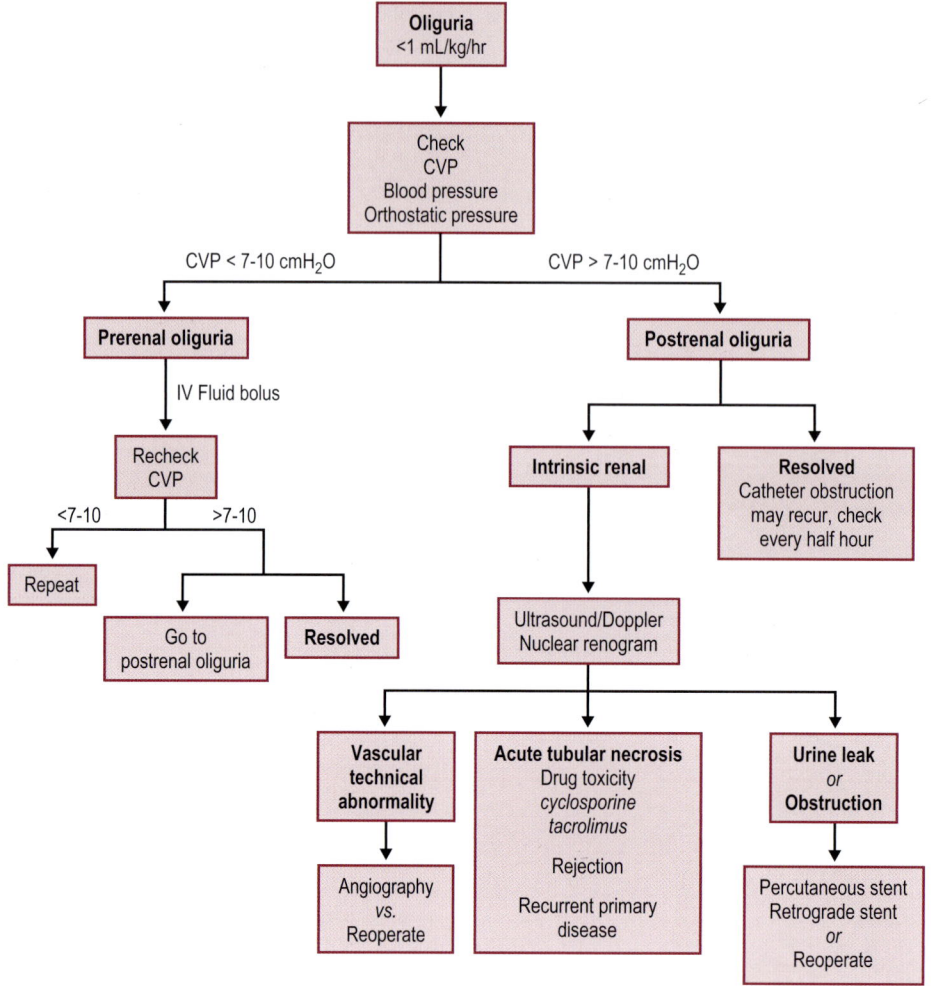

FIGURE 45-15 ■ Algorithm for the evaluation of early postoperative oliguria after pediatric renal transplant. CVP, central venous pressure.

include corticosteroids, cyclosporine or tacrolimus, and azathioprine or MMF. Polyclonal or monoclonal anti-lymphocyte antibodies are used when ATN is anticipated or for retransplantation in highly pre-sensitized patients. Significant efforts to decrease or discontinue steroids have been attempted to enhance growth and development. At four years after transplantation, 31% of LD and 23% of DD recipients were receiving alternate-day prednisone.[152]

Overall, there has been a decrease in the frequency of acute rejection with 12 month probabilities in LD of 32% and DD of 36%. The risk of rejection is similar for LD and DD recipients in the first few post-transplant weeks. Factors that increase the likelihood of rejection or long-term graft loss include receiving a graft from a DD rather than a related LD, receiving a graft from a donor younger than 5 years of age, having the graft in cold storage for more than 24 hours, being an African-American recipient, and delayed graft function from ATN.[152] The ability to treat rejection has also improved with complete reversal of acute rejection in 65% of episodes. The rate of success in treating rejection declines with each successive rejection episode, increased recipient age, and late rejection episodes.[152] Most rejection episodes can be treated with

steroid administration alone (78%); monoclonal anti–T-cell agents such as orthoclone OKT-3 are needed in 32%. In patients who remain rejection free for the 1st post-transplant year, the risk of rejection in the following year is 20%.[154]

Outcome Following Transplantation

The overall results of renal transplantation in children are steadily improving. Overall one-year transplant graft survival rates of 88–100% have been reported for LD allografts, with results for DD allografts being 50 to 72%.[151,163–166] In the a recent report, 1-, 2-, and 5-year graft survival rates were as follows: DD, 78%, 72%, and 59%; LD, 90%, 86%, and 85%, respectively (Fig. 45-16).[154]

Chronic rejection has become the most common cause of graft failure, accounting for 27% of all graft losses.[157] With improved immunosuppressive treatments, acute rejection accounts for only 15% of failures. Recurrence of the original disease caused graft failure in 6%, and vascular thrombosis accounted for 12% of graft failures. Long-term graft survival following pediatric renal transplantation continues to deteriorate after 10 years despite

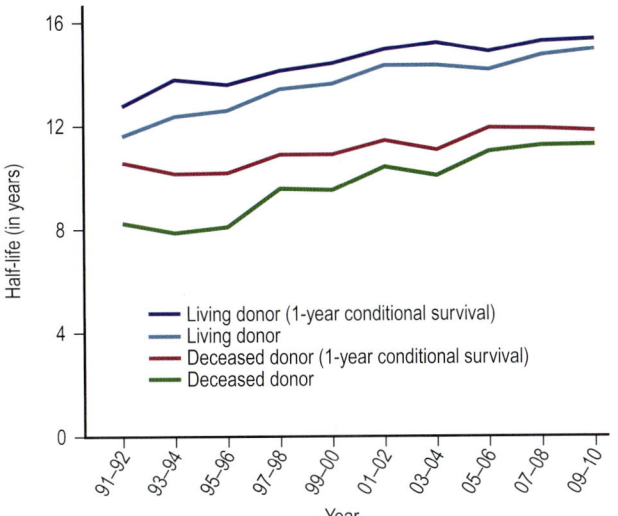

FIGURE 45-16 ■ This graph demonstrates the allograft survival characteristics over 5 years in children as measured by half lives in years versus year transplanted comparing living donor and deceased donor renal transplants. One-year conditional survival is the half-life after the recipient survives the first year. This parameter eliminates patients with early graft failure from any cause. (Source: Scientific Registry Transplant Recipients—2011 Annual Report.)

low patient mortality rates. Death of the recipient with a functioning graft is an uncommon problem. In one study, when this did occur, death resulted primarily from infection (40%) or cardiovascular causes (21%).[169] Young recipients (0 to 1 year of age) and patients with early graft failure were at the highest risk. Progressive loss of renal function may be secondary to complications of hypertension, hyperfiltration, hypercholesterolemias, chronic indolent immunologic damage leading to chronic rejection, and progressive primary renal disease, which all contribute to long-term graft loss.[153,166]

In the latest NAPRTCS report, the overall half-life of pediatric renal transplants was about 25 years for LD and 16 years for DD grafts. Most recipients will require a second transplant in their lifetime. Overall graft survival for second transplants using LDs was equivalent to primary DD allografts. The factor exerting negative influence on survival in DD grafts was donor age younger than 6 years. Better donor recipient matching improves graft survival. The rapidity of first allograft loss, immunologic protocol at retransplant, and race of recipient were not significant factors.

PANCREAS TRANSPLANATION

Children have rarely been candidates for pancreas transplantation. In the past, the results following pancreas transplantation have not justified the risks associated with immunosuppression and operation. However, recent improvements in the operative technique and follow-up have improved. Overall, 1-year patient survival rate exceeds 90%, and graft survival with complete insulin independence exceeds 70% in patients in whom combined kidney and pancreas transplantation is undertaken.

The survival rate is approximately 50% in isolated pancreas transplantation.[170,171]

The addition of pancreas transplantation with kidney replacement for diabetic nephropathy does not subject the patient to additional immunosuppressive risks, and it is better accepted. The use of isolated pancreas transplantation is reserved for patients who have extremely labile glucose control or experience hypoglycemic unawareness syndrome.[170] As the results of this operation improve in the future, its role in children will need to be reviewed.

Pancreatic islet transplantation is also possible in children. However, its role in the treatment of juvenile diabetes in childhood is still limited. This procedure has been undertaken in children following pancreatic resection when the cellular autotransplant does not require immunosuppressive treatment, with excellent results.[172] Further expansion of this approach awaits evidence that hypoglycemic correction retards the systemic complications of diabetes.

REFERENCES

1. DeRusso PA, Ye W, Shepherd R, et al. Growth failure and outcomes in infants with biliary atresia: A report from the Biliary Atresia Research Consortium. Hepatology 2007;46:1632–8.
2. Kasai M, Mochizuki I, Ohkohchi N, et al. Surgical limitation for biliary atresia: Indication for liver transplantation. J Pediatr Surg 1989;24:851–4.
3. Ryckman F, Fisher R, Pedersen S, et al. Improved survival in biliary atresia patients in the present era of liver transplantation. J Pediatr Surg 1993;28:382–5.
4. Zitelli BJ, Malatack JJ, Gartner JC Jr, et al. Evaluation of the pediatric patient for liver transplantation. Pediatrics 1986;78: 559–65.
5. Nio M, Ohi R, Hayashi Y, et al. Current status of 21 patients who have survived more than 20 years since undergoing surgery for biliary atresia. J Pediatr Surg 1996;31:381–4.
6. Ryckman FC. New issues concerning the etiology of an old problem. J Am Coll Surg 1996;183:637–9.
7. Reily D. Familial Intrahepatic Cholestasis Syndromes. In: Suchy FJ, editor. Liver Disease in Children. 1st ed. St. Louis: CV Mosby; 1994. p. 443–59.
8. Ng VL, Ryckman FC, Porta G, et al. Long-term outcome after partial external biliary diversion for intractable pruritus in patients with intrahepatic cholestasis. J Pediatr Gastroenterol Nutr 2000;30:152–6.
9. Cardona J, Houssin D, Gauthier F, et al. Liver transplantation in children with Alagille syndrome—a study of twelve cases. Transplantation 1995;60:339–42.
10. Hoffenberg EJ, Narkewicz MR, Sondheimer JM, et al. Outcome of syndromic paucity of interlobular bile ducts (Alagille syndrome) with onset of cholestasis in infancy. J Pediatr 1995;127:220–4.
11. Tzakis AG, Reyes J, Tepetes K, et al. Liver transplantation for Alagille's syndrome. Arch Surg 1993;128:337–9.
12. Ryckman FC, Alonso MH, editors. Transplantation for Hepatic Malignancy in Children. 1st ed. Philadelphia: WB Sanders; 1996.
13. Jan D, Poggi F, Laurent J, et al. Liver transplantation: New indications in metabolic disorders? Transplant Proc 1994;26:189–90.
14. Mito M, Kusano M, Kawaura Y. Hepatocyte transplantation in man. Transplant Proc 1992;24:3052–3.
15. Jan D, Laurent J, Lacaille F, et al. Liver transplantation in children with inherited metabolic disorders. Transplant Proc 1995; 27:1706–7.
16. Strom S, Fisher R. Hepatocyte transplantation: New possibilities for therapy. Gastroenterology 2003;124:568–71.
17. Strom SC, Fisher RA, Rubinstein WS, et al. Transplantation of human hepatocytes. Transplant Proc 1997;29:2103–6.
18. Fridell JA, Bond GJ, Mazariegos GV, et al. Liver transplantation in children with cystic fibrosis: A long-term longitudinal review of a single center's experience. J Pediatr Surg 2003;38:1152–6.

19. Stapp J, Wilkerson S, Stewart D, et al. Fulminant neonatal liver failure in siblings: Probable congenital hemophagocytic lymphohistiocytosis. Pediatr Dev Pathol 2006;9:239–44.

20. Strom SC, Fisher RA, Thompson MT, et al. Hepatocyte transplantation as a bridge to orthotopic liver transplantation in terminal liver failure. Transplantation 1997;63:559–69.

21. Lidofsky SD, Bass NM, Prager MC, et al. Intracranial pressure monitoring and liver transplantation for fulminant hepatic failure. Hepatology 1992;16:1–7.

22. Reyes JD, Carr B, Dvorchik I, et al. Liver transplantation and chemotherapy for hepatoblastoma and hepatocellular cancer in childhood and adolescence. J Pediatr 2000;136:795–804.

23. Tiao GM, Bobey N, Allen S, et al. The current management of hepatoblastoma: A combination of chemotherapy, conventional resection, and liver transplantation. J Pediatr 2005;146:204–11.

24. Perilongo G, Brown J, Shafford E, et al. Hepatoblastoma presenting with lung metastases: treatment results of the first cooperative, prospective study of the International Society of Paediatric Oncology on childhood liver tumors. Cancer 2000;89:1845–53.

25. Pimpalwar AP, Sharif K, Ramani P, et al. Strategy for hepatoblastoma management: Transplant versus nontransplant surgery. J Pediatr Surg 2002;37:240–5.

26. Austin MT, Leys CM, Feurer ID, et al. Liver transplantation for childhood hepatic malignancy: A review of the United Network for Organ Sharing (UNOS) database. J Pediatr Surg 2006;41: 182–6.

27. Iwatsuki S, Gordon RD, Shaw BW Jr, et al. Role of liver transplantation in cancer therapy. Ann Surg 1985;202:401–7.

28. Davies DB, Harper A. The OPTN waiting list, 1988–2003. Clin Transpl 2004;27–40.

29. Austin MT, Feurer ID, Pinson CW. Access to pediatric liver transplantation: Does regional variation play a role? J Gastrointest Surg 2006;10:387–94.

30. Organ Procurement and Transplantation Network—HRSA. Final rule with comment period. Fed Regist 1998;63:16296–338.

31. McDiarmid SV, Anand R, Lindblad AS. Development of a pediatric end-stage liver disease score to predict poor outcome in children awaiting liver transplantation. Transplantation 2002;74: 173–81.

32. Barshes NR, Lee TC, Udell IW, et al. The pediatric end-stage liver disease (PELD) model as a predictor of survival benefit and posttransplant survival in pediatric liver transplant recipients. Liver Transpl 2006;12:475–80.

33. Tector AJ, Mangus RS, Chestovich P, et al. Use of extended criteria livers decreases wait time for liver transplantation without adversely impacting posttransplant survival. Ann Surg 2006; 244:439–50.

34. Schaubel DE, Sima CS, Goodrich NP, et al. The survival benefit of deceased donor liver transplantation as a function of candidate disease severity and donor quality. Am J Transplant 2008;8: 419–25.

35. Wolfe RA, McCullough KP, Leichtman AB. Predictability of survival models for waiting list and transplant patients: Calculating LYFT. Am J Transplant 2009;9:1523–7.

36. Broelsch CE, Emond JC, Whitington PF, et al. Application of reduced-size liver transplants as split grafts, auxiliary orthotopic grafts, and living related segmental transplants. Ann Surg 1990; 212:368–75.

37. Emond JC, Whitington PF, Thistlethwaite JR, et al. Reduced-size orthotopic liver transplantation: Use in the management of children with chronic liver disease. Hepatology 1989;10:867–72.

38. Ryckman FC, Flake AW, Fisher RA, et al. Segmental orthotopic hepatic transplantation as a means to improve patient survival and diminish waiting-list mortality. J Pediatr Surg 1991;26:422–7.

39. Emond JC, Whitington PF, Thistlethwaite JR, et al. Transplantation of two patients with one liver. Analysis of a preliminary experience with 'split-liver' grafting. Ann Surg 1990;212:14–22.

40. Reyes J. Adaptation of split liver grafts in pediatric patients. Pediatr Transplant 2001;5:148–52.

41. Deshpande RR, Bowles MJ, Vilca-Melendez H, et al. Results of split liver transplantation in children. Ann Surg 2002;236: 248–53.

42. Broelsch CE, Frilling A, Testa G, et al. Living donor liver transplantation in adults. Eur J Gastroenterol Hepatol 2003;15:3–6.

43. Broelsch CE, Burdelski M, Rogiers X, et al. Living donor for liver transplantation. Hepatology 1994;20:49S–55S.

44. Rogiers X, Burdelski M, Broelsch CE. Liver transplantation from living donors. Br J Surg 1994;81:1251–3.

45. Klein AS, Messersmith EE, Ratner LE, et al. Organ donation and utilization in the United States, 1999–2008. Am J Transplant 2010;10:973–86.

46. Broelsch CE, Whitington PF, Emond JC, et al. Liver transplantation in children from living related donors. Surgical techniques and results. Ann Surg 1991;214:428–37.

47. Otte JB. Auxiliary partial orthotopic liver transplantation for acute liver failure in children. Pediatr Transplant 1999;3:252–6.

48. Otte JB. Donor complications and outcomes in live-liver transplantation. Transplantation 2003;75:1625–6.

49. Tissieres P, Prontera W, Chevret L, et al. The pediatric risk of mortality score in infants and children with fulminant liver failure. Pediatr Transplant 2003;7:64–8.

50. Fan ST, Lo CM, Liu CL. Technical refinement in adult-to-adult living donor liver transplantation using right lobe graft. Ann Surg 2000;231:126–31.

51. Humar A, Beissel J, Crotteau S, et al. Whole liver versus split liver versus living donor in the adult recipient: An analysis of outcomes by graft type. Transplantation 2008;85:1420–4.

52. Lo CM, Fan ST, Liu CL, et al. Minimum graft size for successful living donor liver transplantation. Transplantation 1999;68: 1112–16.

53. Zamboni F, Franchello A, David E, et al. Effect of macrovescicular steatosis and other donor and recipient characteristics on the outcome of liver transplantation. Clin Transplant 2001;15: 53–7.

54. Imber CJ, St Peter SD, Handa A, et al. Hepatic steatosis and its relationship to transplantation. Liver Transpl 2002;8:415–23.

55. Mor E, Skerrett D, Manzarbeitia C, et al. Successful use of an enhanced immunosuppressive protocol with plasmapheresis for ABO-incompatible mismatched grafts in liver transplant recipients. Transplantation 1995;59:986–90.

56. Farges O, Kalil AN, Samuel D, et al. The use of ABO-incompatible grafts in liver transplantation: a life-saving procedure in highly selected patients. Transplantation 1995;59:1124–33.

57. Tanaka A, Tanaka K, Kitai T, et al. Living related liver transplantation across ABO blood groups. Transplantation 1994;58:548–53.

58. Cacciarelli TV, So SK, Lim J, et al. A reassessment of ABO incompatibility in pediatric liver transplantation. Transplantation 1995;60:757–60.

59. Yandza T, Lambert T, Alvarez F, et al. Outcome of ABO-incompatible liver transplantation in children with no specific alloantibodies at the time of transplantation. Transplantation 1994;58:46–50.

60. Warnaar N, Polak WG, de Jong KP, et al. Long-term results of urgent revascularization for hepatic artery thrombosis after pediatric liver transplantation. Liver Transpl 2010;16:847–55.

61. Kim HB. Urgent revascularization for hepatic artery thrombosis: Maybe good for the few, definitely good for the many. Liver Transpl 2010;16:812–14.

62. Langnas AN, Marujo W, Stratta RJ, et al. Hepatic allograft rescue following arterial thrombosis. Role of urgent revascularization. Transplantation 1991;51:86–90.

63. Stevens LH, Emond JC, Piper JB, et al. Hepatic artery thrombosis in infants. A comparison of whole livers, reduced-size grafts, and grafts from living-related donors. Transplantation 1992;53: 396–9.

64. Kirsch JP, Howard TK, Klintmalm GB, et al. Problematic vascular reconstruction in liver transplantation. Part II. Portovenous conduits. Surgery 1990;107:544–8.

65. Stieber AC, Zetti G, Todo S, et al. The spectrum of portal vein thrombosis in liver transplantation. Ann Surg 1991;213: 199–206.

66. Harper AM, Edwards EB, Ellison MD. The OPTN waiting list, 1988-2000. Clin Transpl 2001;73–85.

67. Peclet MH, Ryckman FC, Pedersen SH, et al. The spectrum of bile duct complications in pediatric liver transplantation. J Pediatr Surg 1994;29:214–19.

68. Heffron TG, Emond JC, Whitington PF, et al. Biliary complications in pediatric liver transplantation. A comparison of reduced-size and whole grafts. Transplantation 1992;53:391–5.

69. Rouch DA, Emond JC, Thistlethwaite JR Jr, et al. Choledochocholedochostomy without a T tube or internal stent in transplantation of the liver. Surg Gynecol Obstet 1990;170:239–44.

70. Snover DC, Sibley RK, Freese DK, et al. Orthotopic liver transplantation: A pathological study of 63 serial liver biopsies from 17 patients with special reference to the diagnostic features and natural history of rejection. Hepatology 1984;4:1212–22.

71. Mor E, Solomon H, Gibbs JF, et al. Acute cellular rejection following liver transplantation: Clinical pathologic features and effect on outcome. Semin Liver Dis 1992;12:28–40.

72. Adams DH, Neuberger JM. Treatment of acute rejection. Semin Liver Dis 1992;12:80–8.

73. Jain A, Mazariegos G, Pokharna R, et al. The absence of chronic rejection in pediatric primary liver transplant patients who are maintained on tacrolimus-based immunosuppression: A long-term analysis. Transplantation 2003;75:1020–5.

74. Jain A, Mazariegos G, Kashyap R, et al. Pediatric liver transplantation. A single center experience spanning 20 years. Transplantation 2002;73:941–7.

75. Gupta P, Hart J, Cronin D, et al. Risk factors for chronic rejection after pediatric liver transplantation. Transplantation 2001;72:1098–102.

76. Freese DK, Snover DC, Sharp HL, et al. Chronic rejection after liver transplantation: A study of clinical, histopathological and immunological features. Hepatology 1991;13:882–91.

77. Ludwig J, Wiesner RH, Batts KP, et al. The acute vanishing bile duct syndrome (acute irreversible rejection) after orthotopic liver transplantation. Hepatology 1987;7:476–83.

78. Demetris A, Adams D, Bellamy C, et al. Update of the International Banff Schema for Liver Allograft Rejection: Working recommendations for the histopathologic staging and reporting of chronic rejection. An International Panel. Hepatology 2000;31:792–9.

79. O'Leary JG, Kaneku H, Susskind BM, et al. High mean fluorescence intensity donor-specific anti-HLA antibodies associated with chronic rejection Postliver transplant. Am J Transplant 2011;11:1868–76.

80. Gonwa TA, Mai ML, Melton LB, et al. End-stage renal disease (ESRD) after orthotopic liver transplantation (OLTX) using calcineurin-based immunotherapy: Risk of development and treatment. Transplantation 2001;72:1934–9.

81. Fisher NC, Nightingale PG, Gunson BK, et al. Chronic renal failure following liver transplantation: A retrospective analysis. Transplantation 1998;66:59–66.

82. Campbell K, Yazigi N, Ryckman F, et al. Renal Function in Long-Term Pediatric Liver Transplant Survivors. American Transplantation Congress 2003.

83. Campbell K, Ng V, Martin S, et al. Glomerular filtration rate following pediatric liver transplantation—the SPLIT experience. Am J Transplant 2010;10:2673–82.

84. Campbell KM, Yazigi N, Ryckman FC, et al. High prevalence of renal dysfunction in long-term survivors after pediatric liver transplantation. J Pediatr 2006;148:475–80.

85. Aw MM, Samaroo B, Baker AJ, et al. Calcineurin-inhibitor related nephrotoxicity- reversibility in paediatric liver transplant recipients. Transplantation 2001;72:746–9.

86. Heffron TG, Pillen T, Smallwood GA, et al. Pediatric liver transplantation with daclizumab induction. Transplantation 2003;75:2040–3.

87. Wiesner RH, Hermans PE, Rakela J, et al. Selective bowel decontamination to decrease gram-negative aerobic bacterial and Candida colonization and prevent infection after orthotopic liver transplantation. Transplantation 1988;45:570–4.

88. Andrews W, Siegel J, Renaro T. Prevention and treatment of selected fungal and viral infections in pediatric liver transplant recipients. Clin Transplant 1991;5:204–7.

89. Patel R, Snydman DR, Rubin RH, et al. Cytomegalovirus prophylaxis in solid organ transplant recipients. Transplantation 1996;61:1279–89.

90. Fox AS, Tolpin MD, Baker AL, et al. Seropositivity in liver transplant recipients as a predictor of cytomegalovirus disease. J Infect Dis 1988;157:383–5.

91. Holmes RD, Sokol RJ. Epstein-Barr virus and post-transplant lymphoproliferative disease. Pediatr Transplant 2002;6:456–64.

92. Broughton S, McClay JE, Murray A, et al. The effectiveness of tonsillectomy in diagnosing lymphoproliferative disease in pediatric patients after liver transplantation. Arch Otolaryngol Head Neck Surg 2000;126:1444–7.

93. Smets F, Latinne D, Bazin H, et al. Ratio between Epstein-Barr viral load and anti-Epstein-Barr virus specific T-cell response as a predictive marker of posttransplant lymphoproliferative disease. Transplantation 2002;73:1603–10.

94. Smets F, Sokal EM. Epstein-Barr virus-related lymphoproliferation in children after liver transplant: Role of immunity, diagnosis, and management. Pediatr Transplant 2002;6:280–7.

95. Sokal EM, Antunes H, Beguin C, et al. Early signs and risk factors for the increased incidence of Epstein-Barr virus-related posttransplant lymphoproliferative diseases in pediatric liver transplant recipients treated with tacrolimus. Transplantation 1997;64:1438–42.

96. Holmes RD, Orban-Eller K, Karrer FR, et al. Response of elevated Epstein-Barr virus DNA levels to therapeutic changes in pediatric liver transplant patients: 56-month follow up and outcome. Transplantation 2002;74:367–72.

97. Axelrod DA, Holmes R, Thomas SE, et al. Limitations of EBV-PCR monitoring to detect EBV associated post-transplant lymphoproliferative disorder. Pediatr Transplant 2003;7:223–7.

98. Penn I. Post-transplant malignancy: The role of immunosuppression. Drug Saf 2000;23:101–13.

99. Sokal EM, Caragiozoglou T, Lamy M, et al. Epstein-Barr virus serology and Epstein-Barr virus-associated lymphoproliferative disorders in pediatric liver transplant recipients. Transplantation 1993;56:1394–8.

100. Jabs WJ, Hennig H, Kittel M, et al. Normalized quantification by real-time PCR of Epstein-Barr virus load in patients at risk for posttransplant lymphoproliferative disorders. J Clin Microbiol 2001;39:564–9.

101. Guthery SL, Heubi JE, Bucuvalas JC, et al. Determination of risk factors for Epstein-Barr virus-associated posttransplant lymphoproliferative disorder in pediatric liver transplant recipients using objective case ascertainment. Transplantation 2003;75:987–93.

102. Hanto DW, Frizzera G, Gajl-Peczalska KJ, et al. Epstein-Barr virus, immunodeficiency, and B cell lymphoproliferation. Transplantation 1985;39:461–72.

103. Bueno J, Ramil C, Green M. Current management strategies for the prevention and treatment of cytomegalovirus infection in pediatric transplant recipients. Paediatr Drugs 2002;4:279–90.

104. Serinet MO, Jacquemin E, Habes D, et al. Anti-CD20 monoclonal antibody (Rituximab) treatment for Epstein-Barr virus-associated, B-cell lymphoproliferative disease in pediatric liver transplant recipients. J Pediatr Gastroenterol Nutr 2002;34:389–93.

105. Haque T, Wilkie GM, Taylor C, et al. Treatment of Epstein-Barr-virus-positive post-transplantation lymphoproliferative disease with partly HLA-matched allogeneic cytotoxic T cells. Lancet 2002;360:436–42.

106. Tiao GM, Alonso M, Bezerra J, et al. Liver transplantation in children younger than 1 year—the Cincinnati experience. J Pediatr Surg 2005;40:268–73.

107. Washburn WK, Bradley J, Cosimi AB, et al. A regional experience with emergency liver transplantation. Transplantation 1996;61:235–9.

108. Langnas AN, Marujo WC, Inagaki M, et al. The results of reduced-size liver transplantation, including split livers, in patients with end-stage liver disease. Transplantation 1992;53:387–91.

109. Esquivel CO, Nakazato P, Cox K, et al. The impact of liver reductions in pediatric liver transplantation. Arch Surg 1991;126:1278–85.

110. Studies of Pediatric Liver Transplantation (SPLIT). Year 2000 outcomes. Transplantation 2001;72:463–76.

111. Fridell JA, Jain A, Reyes J, et al. Causes of mortality beyond one year after primary pediatric liver transplant under tacrolimus. Transplantation 2002;74:1721–4.

112. Mack CL, Ferrario M, Abecassis M, et al. Living donor liver transplantation for children with liver failure and concurrent multiple organ system failure. Liver Transpl 2001;7:890–5.

113. Emre S. Living-donor liver transplantation in children. Pediatr Transplant 2002;6:43–6.

114. Bucuvalas JC, Ryckman FC. The long- and short-term outcome of living-donor liver transplantation. J Pediatr 1999;134:259–61.

115. Bilik R, Greig P, Langer B, et al. Survival after reduced-size liver transplantation is dependent on pretransplant status. J Pediatr Surg 1993;28:1307–11.

116. PRCarroll CL, Goodman DM, Superina RA, et al. Timed Pediatric Risk of Mortality Scores predict outcomes in pediatric liver transplant recipients. Pediatr Transplant 2003;7:289–95.

117. Otte JB, de Ville de Goyet J, Sokal E, et al. Size reduction of the donor liver is a safe way to alleviate the shortage of size-matched organs in pediatric liver transplantation. Ann Surg 1990;211: 146–57.

118. Ryckman FC, Alonso MH, Bucuvalas JC, et al. Long-term survival after liver transplantation. J Pediatr Surg 1999;34:845–9.

119. Wallot MA, Mathot M, Janssen M, et al. Long-term survival and late graft loss in pediatric liver transplant recipients—a 15-year single-center experience. Liver Transpl 2002;8:615–22.

120. Sudan DL, Shaw BW Jr, Langnas AN. Causes of late mortality in pediatric liver transplant recipients. Ann Surg 1998;227:289–95.

121. Sarna S, Sipila I, Jalanko H, et al. Factors affecting growth after pediatric liver transplantation. Transplant Proc 1994;26: 161–4.

122. Sarna S, Sipila I, Vihervuori E, et al. Growth delay after liver transplantation in childhood: Studies of underlying mechanisms. Pediatr Res 1995;38:366–72.

123. Balistreri WF, Bucuvalas JC, Ryckman FC. The effect of immunosuppression on growth and development. Liver Transpl Surg 1995;1:64–73.

124. Chin SE, Shepherd RW, Cleghorn GJ, et al. Survival, growth and quality of life in children after orthotopic liver transplantation: A 5 year experience. J Paediatr Child Health 1991;27:380–5.

125. Zitelli BJ, Miller JW, Gartner JC Jr, et al. Changes in life-style after liver transplantation. Pediatrics 1988;82:173–80.

126. Stewart SM, Hiltebeitel C, Nici J, et al. Neuropsychological outcome of pediatric liver transplantation. Pediatrics 1991;87: 367–76.

127. Stewart SM, Uauy R, Waller DA, et al. Mental and motor development, social competence, and growth one year after successful pediatric liver transplantation. J Pediatr 1989;114:574–81.

128. Tarter RE, Hays AL, Sandford SS, et al. Cerebral morphological abnormalities associated with non-alcoholic cirrhosis. Lancet 1986;2:893–5.

129. Bernthal P, Hays A, Tarter RE, et al. Cerebral CT scan abnormalities in cholestatic and hepatocellular disease and their relationship to neuropsychologic test performance. Hepatology 1987;7: 107–14.

130. Tarter RE, Sandford SL, Hays AL, et al. Hepatic injury correlates with neuropsychologic impairment. Int J Neurosci 1989;44: 75–82.

131. Bucuvalas JC, Britto M, Krug S, et al. Health-related quality of life in pediatric liver transplant recipients: A single-center study. Liver Transpl 2003;9:62–71.

132. Mazariegos GV, Steffick DE, Horslen S, et al. Intestine transplantation in the United States, 1999–2008. Am J Transplant 2010;10: 1020–34.

133. Mazariegos GV, Squires RH, Sindhi RK. Current perspectives on pediatric intestinal transplantation. Curr Gastroenterol Rep 2009;11:226–33.

134. Nayyar N, Mazariegos G, Ranganathan S, et al. Pediatric small bowel transplantation. Semin Pediatr Surg 2010;19:68–77.

135. (HCFA) HCFA. 'Combined Liver and Intestinal and Multivisceral Transplantation (#CAG-00036) Decision Memorandum'. 2000.

136. Youssef NN, Mezoff AG, Carter BA, et al. Medical update and potential advances in the treatment of pediatric intestinal failure. Curr Gastroenterol Rep 2012;14:243–52.

137. Ching YA, Gura K, Modi B, et al. Pediatric intestinal failure: nutrition, pharmacologic, and surgical approaches. Nutr Clin Pract 2007;22:653–63.

138. Touloukian RJ, Smith GJ. Normal intestinal length in preterm infants. J Pediatr Surg 1983;18:720–3.

139. Bueno J, Ohwada S, Kocoshis S, et al. Factors impacting the survival of children with intestinal failure referred for intestinal transplantation. J Pediatr Surg 1999;34:27–32.

140. Fishbein TM, Matsumoto CS. Intestinal replacement therapy: Timing and indications for referral of patients to an intestinal rehabilitation and transplant program. Gastroenterol 2006;130: S147–51.

141. Avitzur Y, Grant D. Intestine transplantation in children: Update 2010. Pediatr Cl N Am 2010;57:415–31.

142. de Ville de Goyet J, Mitchell A, Mayer AD, et al. En block combined reduced-liver and small bowel transplants: From large donors to small children. Transplantation 2000;69: 555–9.

143. Fryer J, Pellar S, Ormond D, et al. Mortality in candidates waiting for combined liver-intestine transplants exceeds that for other candidates waiting for liver transplants. Liver Transpl 2003;9: 748–53.

144. Furukawa H, Manez R, Kusne S, et al. Cytomegalovirus disease in intestinal transplantation. Transpl P 1995;27:1357–8.

145. Eid AJ, Razonable RR. New developments in the management of cytomegalovirus infection after solid organ transplantation. Drugs 2010;70:965–81.

146. Kato T, Selvaggi G, Gaynor JJ, et al. Inclusion of donor colon and ileocecal valve in intestinal transplantation. Transplantation 2008;86:293–7.

147. Berney T, Kato T, Nishida S, et al. Portal versus systemic drainage of small bowel allografts: Comparative assessment of survival, function, rejection, and bacterial translocation. J Am Coll Surg 2002;195:804–13.

148. Ruiz P, Takahashi H, Delacruz V, et al. International grading scheme for acute cellular rejection in small-bowel transplantation: single-center experience. Transpl P 2010;42:47–53.

149. Shin CR, Nathan J, Alonso M, et al. Incidence of acute and chronic graft-versus-host disease and donor T-cell chimerism after small bowel or combined organ transplantation. J Pediatr Surg 2011;46:1732–8.

150. Potter DE, Holliday MA, Piel CF, et al. Treatment of end-stage renal disease in children: A 15-year experience. Kidney Int 1980;18:103–9.

151. Fine R. Renal Transplantation in Children. In: Morris P, editor. Kidney Transplantation: Principals and Practice. Orlando: Grune & Stratton; 1984. p. 509–46.

152. McEnery PT, Stablein DM, Arbus G, Tejani A. Renal transplantation in children. A report of the North American Pediatric Renal Transplant Cooperative Study. N Engl J Med 1992;326: 1727–32.

153. North American Pediatric Renal Transplant Cooperative Study. 2010 Annual Report.

154. Warady BA, Hebert D, Sullivan EK, et al. Renal transplantation, chronic dialysis, and chronic renal insufficiency in children and adolescents. The 1995 Annual Report of the North American Pediatric Renal Transplant Cooperative Study. Pediatr Nephrol 1997;11:49–64.

155. Hanna JD, Krieg RJ Jr, Scheinman JI, Chan JC. Effects of uremia on growth in children. Semin Nephrol 1996;16:230–41.

156. Benfield MR. Current status of kidney transplant: Update 2003. Pediatr Clin N Am 2003;50:1301–34.

157. Benfield MR, McDonald RA, Bartosh S, et al. Changing trends in pediatric transplantation: 2001 Annual Report of the North American Pediatric Renal Transplant Cooperative Study. Pediatr Transplant 2003;7:321–35.

158. Englund M, Berg U, Tyden G. A longitudinal study of children who received renal transplants 10–20 years ago. Transplantation 2003;76:311–18.

159. Fine RN. Growth following solid-organ transplantation. Pediatr Transplant 2002;6:47–52.

160. Grushkin CM, Fine RN. Growth in children following renal transplantation. Am J Dis Child 1973;125:514–56.

161. Rotundo A, Nevins TE, Lipton M, et al. Progressive encephalopathy in children with chronic renal insufficiency in infancy. Kidney Int 1982;21:486–91.

162. Najarian J, Ascher NL, Mauer SM. Kidney Transplantation. In: Welch K, Randolph J, Ravitch M, editors. Pediatric Surgery. Chicago: Year Book Medical; 1986. p. 360–73.

163. Turcotte J, Campbell DA, Dafoe D. Pediatric Renal Transplantation. In: Cerilli G, editor. Organ Transplantation and Replacement. Philadelphia: JB Lippincott; 1988. p. 349–60.

164. Ildstad ST, Tollerud DJ, Noseworthy J, et al. The influence of donor age on graft survival in renal transplantation. J Pediatr Surg 1990;25:134–9.

165. Ildstad ST, Tollerud DJ, Noseworthy J, et al. Renal transplantation in pediatric recipients. Transpl P 1989;21:1936–7.

166. Singh A, Stablein D, Tejani A. Risk factors for vascular thrombosis in pediatric renal transplantation: A special report of the North

American Pediatric Renal Transplant Cooperative Study. Transplantation 1997;63:1263–7.

167. Bereket G, Fine RN. Pediatric renal transplantation. Pediatr Clin N Am 1995;42:1603–28.

168. Mahmoud A, Said MH, Dawahra M, et al. Outcome of preemptive renal transplantation and pretransplantation dialysis in children. Pediatr Nephrol 1997;11:537–41.

169. Tejani A, Sullivan EK, Alexander S, et al. Posttransplant deaths and factors that influence the mortality rate in North American children. Transplantation 1994;57:547–53.

170. Sutherland DE. The case for pancreas transplantation. Diabetes Metab 1996;22:132–8.

171. Stratta RJ, Larsen JL, Cushing K. Pancreas transplantation for diabetes mellitus. Annu Rev Med 1995;46:281–98.

172. Bellin MD, Sutherland DE. Pediatric islet autotransplantation: Indication, technique, and outcome. Curr Diabetes Rep 2010; 10:326–31.

CHAPTER 46

LESIONS OF THE PANCREAS

John Wiersch • George K. Gittes

The pancreas originates during week 4 of gestation as dual evaginations from the foregut endoderm. The dorsal pancreatic bud gives rise to the body and tail of the pancreas, its minor duct (Santorini) and papilla, and the continuation of the major duct (Wirsung) into the body and tail. The ventral pancreatic bud arises from the biliary diverticulum and swings around the dorsal aspect of the duodenal anlage during gut rotation to give rise to the head of the pancreas as well as the proximal portion of Wirsung's duct (Fig. 46-1).[1]

The two pancreatic buds fuse to form one pancreas at approximately 7 weeks' gestation, although it appears that complete fusion of the two ducts to form the main pancreatic duct is delayed until the perinatal period.[2] The endocrine component of the pancreas, the islets of Langerhans, starts to differentiate before evagination of the pancreatic buds from the wall of the foregut. The islets comprise 10% of the pancreas during early embryonic and fetal life, but this contribution decreases to less than 1% in adulthood. Pancreatic acini begin to form at 12 weeks gestation and begin to accumulate organelles and zymogen granules at this stage, but do not secrete appreciable amounts of enzyme until birth.[1]

The pancreas is retroperitoneal and is light pink in children. The acini can be seen under low power loupe magnification, as can the septa dividing the lobulations. The head of the pancreas lies in the C-loop of the duodenum while the uncinate process, emanating from the posteromedial portion of the head, projects under the superior mesenteric artery (SMA) and vein. The neck of the pancreas is defined as that portion of the pancreas anterior to these vessels. The body and tail, to the left of these vessels, angle sharply towards the hilum of the spleen. The main pancreatic duct runs along the posterior aspect of the gland and curves downward in the head to run alongside the common bile duct, which runs in a groove posterior to the pancreas or within the substance of the posterior gland. The main pancreatic duct and common bile duct may fuse to form a 'common channel' before entry into the duodenum.

The pancreas is convex and its midportion is reflected over the anterior surface of the upper lumbar vertebrae and aorta. Its lateral aspects falls posteriorly toward each kidney (Fig. 46-2). The arterial supply of the pancreas is from the celiac and SMA, which form the pancreaticoduodenal arcade. The pancreas also has anastomoses from the splenic artery.[3]

CONGENITAL ANOMALIES

Ectopic pancreatic rests are frequently encountered along foregut derivatives such as stomach, duodenum, jejunum, and colon, but are also infrequently encountered in the thorax and other sites.[4-6] These lesions are found in approximately 2% of autopsy series and represent the most common anomaly of the gastric antrum. Moreover, they may cause gastric outlet obstruction.[7] Their origin is unknown, but may be the result of aberrant epithelial–mesenchymal interactions leading to the transdifferentiation of embryonic epithelium into pancreatic epithelium. Several studies have implicated defects in hedgehog signaling and Notch signaling as the cause of ectopic pancreatic rests.[8] Ectopic rests are typically asymptomatic and are encountered incidentally at laparotomy or during endoscopy. They can be identified as pancreatic tissue visually, because the surface has the same granular acinar appearance as the normal pancreas. These ectopic pancreatic rests usually do not become inflamed, possibly because they contain numerous small drainage ducts that usually do not obstruct; however, they can occasionally cause intestinal obstruction or bleeding. When encountered at laparotomy, ectopic rests should probably be excised, unless the excision would entail significant risk.

An annular pancreas is thought to result from faulty rotation of the ventral pancreatic bud in its course around the posterior aspect of the duodenal anlage. The duodenum is encircled and often obstructed by normal pancreatic tissue.[9] Abnormal expression patterns of endodermal hedgehog may be responsible for the formation of annular and ectopic pancreas.[8] Duodenal atresia and stenosis, intestinal malrotation, and trisomy 21 can often be found in combination with an annular pancreas.[10] The clinical significance relates primarily to intrinsic duodenal obstruction, typically with bilious vomiting. Radiographic studies may reveal the classic finding of the 'double-bubble' sign. Management consists of bypass of the obstructing lesion with a duodenoduodenostomy or gastrojejunostomy, depending on the anatomy. Resection or division of the annular pancreas should not be performed due to the variable and complex ductal drainage system. Occasionally, patients with complex ductal anatomy may require reoperation for pancreatobiliary anomalies not apparent at the time of the initial surgery.[11]

Cystic fibrosis (CF) is an autosomal recessive condition, seen primarily in Caucasians which occurs in about 1 of 2,500 births.[12] It is caused by mutations in the cystic fibrosis transmembrane conductance regulator (CFTR) gene that encodes a protein expressed on the apical membrane of exocrine epithelial cells. CF leads to significant pancreatic insufficiency. The pancreatic secretions generally have a reduced amount of bicarbonate, a lower pH, and a lower overall fluid volume. The inspissated secretions lead to blockage of the ducts with dilatation. This may lead to acinar cell degeneration, acute and chronic pancreatitis, and pancreatic fibrosis. The result

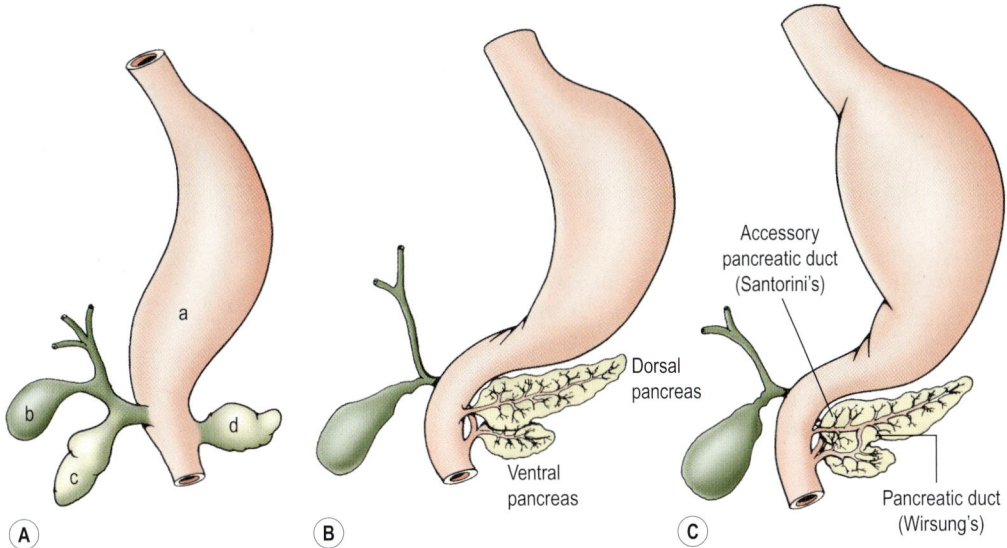

FIGURE 46-1 ■ Pancreatic embryology. **(A)** Stomach (a), gallbladder (b), and ventral (c) and dorsal (d) pancreatic buds develop separately at embryologic week 4. The pancreas develops as an evagination of the developing foregut. The dorsal bud evaginates directly off of the duodenal anlage. **(B)** The ventral bud evaginates from the biliary bud and then swings around to the left, with gut rotation occurring simultaneously. **(C)** The main pancreatic duct of Wirsung and the minor accessory duct of Santorini are shown.

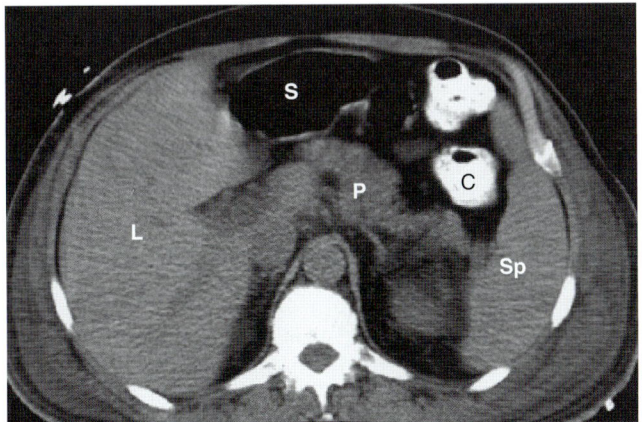

FIGURE 46-2 ■ CT scan showing the cross-sectional anatomy of the pancreas. The pancreas (P) lies convexly across the lumbar spine with the tail of the pancreas next to the spleen (Sp) and the hilum of the left kidney. The head of the pancreas lies to the right of the spine near the hilum of the right kidney. L, Liver; S, stomach; C, colon. (From Maher MM, Hahn PF, Gervais DA, et al. Portable abdominal CT: Analysis of quality and clinical impact in more than 100 consecutive cases. AJR Am J Roentgenol 2004;183:663–70.)

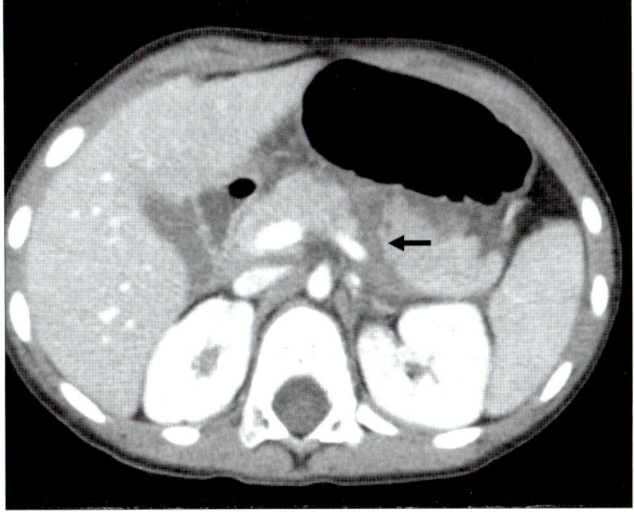

FIGURE 46-3 ■ This abdominal contrast-enhanced CT shows a complete transection (arrow) of the body of the pancreas following a bicycle handlebar injury to the epigastrium. The patient underwent laparoscopic distal pancreatectomy and recovered uneventfully.

is impaired digestion of fats and proteins from loss of these digestive enzymes.[13] See Chapter 32 for more information about CF.

PANCREATITIS

Acute Pancreatitis

Acute pancreatitis is an acute inflammation of the pancreas, varying in severity from mild abdominal pain to fulminant necrotizing pancreatitis and death. It has an incidence between 3.6 and 13.2 cases per 100,000 children. If episodes of acute inflammation completely resolve and then recur, it is termed acute recurrent pancreatitis. It is thought that complete interval resolution of morphology and function occurs between episodes, unlike in cases of chronic pancreatitis.[14]

The causes of acute pancreatitis include trauma, biliary tract stone disease, choledochal cyst, ductal developmental anomalies, drugs, metabolic derangements, and infections. Most commonly, the cause is not apparent and termed idiopathic. As the pancreas is fixed against the lumbar spine, trauma to the upper abdomen can fracture the pancreas or injure the major duct at that point (Fig. 46-3). Biliary stone disease, increasing in frequency in children, may lead to pancreatitis from transient pancreatic duct obstruction. Endoscopic retrograde cholangiopancreatography (ERCP) is safe and effective in children and is the preferred method for stone retrieval.[15] Drugs that are thought to induce pancreatitis include asparaginase and valproic acid.[16] Systemic illnesses and metabolic conditions, such as CF, Reye syndrome, Kawasaki disease, hyperlipidemias, and hypercalcemia as well as viral infections (e.g., coxsackievirus and rotavirus) and generalized bacterial sepsis, can also cause pancreatitis.[17]

Pancreas divisum is an anomaly of the pancreas present in 10% of the population and is thought to result from failure of the dorsal duct to fuse with the ventral duct. In pancreas divisum, the majority of exocrine pancreatic secretions, including those from the entire body and tail, must drain through the small minor duct of Santorini. The resulting relative obstruction may cause recurring episodes of pancreatitis. Symptomatic patients should undergo sphincteroplasty of the minor papilla. Endoscopic stenting, with or without sphincterotomy, is the preferred treatment, with operation reserved for recurrent cases. Choledochal cysts produce pancreatitis by pancreatic duct compression or bile reflux resulting from a long common biliary-pancreatic duct within the head of the pancreas. Other rare ductal anomalies may result in obstruction and recurring bouts of pancreatitis.[18]

Though acute pancreatitis has many etiologies, they all appear to share a common pathway of nonphysiologic calcium signaling in the pancreas, followed by the premature activation of acinar proenzymes. These enzymes, especially trypsin, lead to acinar cell injury and cytokine release. The cytokines, along with vascular dissemination of activated enzymes, free radical formation, and release of vasoactive substances, such as kallikreins and histamine, together mediate extrapancreatic inflammation.[19]

Diagnostic criteria for acute pancreatitis include at least two of the following: acute abdominal pain (especially in the epigastric region), serum amylase or lipase more than three times the upper limit of normal, and imaging findings characteristic or compatible with acute pancreatitis.[14] The abdomen is diffusely tender with signs of peritonitis, and distention occurs with a paucity of bowel sounds. In severe cases of necrotizing or hemorrhagic pancreatitis, hemorrhage may spread away from the pancreas along tissue planes, appearing as ecchymosis either in the flanks (Grey Turner's sign) or at the umbilicus (Cullen's sign) (Fig. 46-4). These ecchymoses generally take 1 to 2 days to develop.

Elevated amylase levels are helpful in the diagnosis, although a normal serum amylase level does not exclude pancreatitis. Hyperamylasemia may also be caused by salivary inflammation/trauma, intestinal disease (such as perforation, ischemia, necrosis, or inflammation), and macroamylasemia. Lipase has been suggested as an alternative marker, but can be falsely elevated in pancreatic cancer, macrolipasemia, renal insufficiency, cholecystitis, esophagitis, intestinal perforation, and hypertriglyceridemia. Elevated lipase tends to be more sensitive in infants and toddlers, and may also help differentiate pancreatic from salivary trauma. The degree of enzyme elevation does not correlate with disease severity.[19,20]

Imaging the abdomen is important as part of the evaluation of the patient with abdominal pain. In the patient

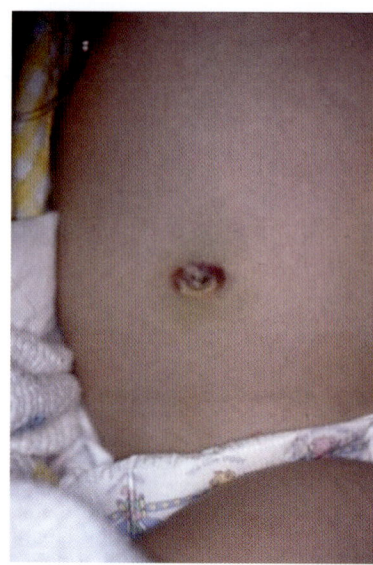

FIGURE 46-4 ■ Positive Cullen's sign, with periumbilical ecchymosis, in a patient with hemorrhagic pancreatitis.

with pancreatitis, plain abdominal radiographs may reveal an isolated loop of intestine in the vicinity of the inflamed pancreas, the so-called 'sentinel loop.' Pancreatic calcifications suggest chronic pancreatitis. Plain chest radiographs should be performed in all patients with acute pancreatitis to look for evidence of pleural effusion and pulmonary edema.

Abdominal ultrasonography (US) is useful in the evaluation of the patient with pancreatitis, but has limited applications. It is well established in the evaluation of biliary stone disease as the etiology for pancreatitis, and can detect choledochal cysts and pancreatic pseudocysts as well. Advanced techniques such as contrast-enhanced ultrasound and ultrasound elastography have also been shown to be useful in the diagnosis of pancreatitis and its complications, but their availability is limited to a few experienced centers.[21]

Abdominal computed tomography (CT) provides much better resolution of the pancreas than ultrasound. Its primary role is in the detection of early and late complications, such as pancreatic necrosis, pseudocysts, and fluid collections, and should be reserved for patients with more severe pathology, or recurrent symptomatology with an equivocal ultrasound. If necessary, CT can be combined with interventional procedures to drain fluid collections.[22]

Magnetic resonance cholangiopancreatography (MRCP) is a newer, noninvasive technique for evaluating the biliary tree and pancreatic duct (Fig. 46-5). It is the initial imaging study of choice for the evaluation of pancreatic ductal anatomy in children with recurrent or unexplained pancreatitis. Studies comparing MRCP and ERCP show high concordance in diagnoses. Its disadvantages are that it does not allow for therapeutic intervention (though it may direct the type of intervention necessary), its poor spatial resolution limits the visualization of ducts in smaller children, and it usually requires anesthesia in the pediatric age group.[21,23]

The most frequent indication for ERCP in children is in the diagnosis or treatment of acute, recurrent, or

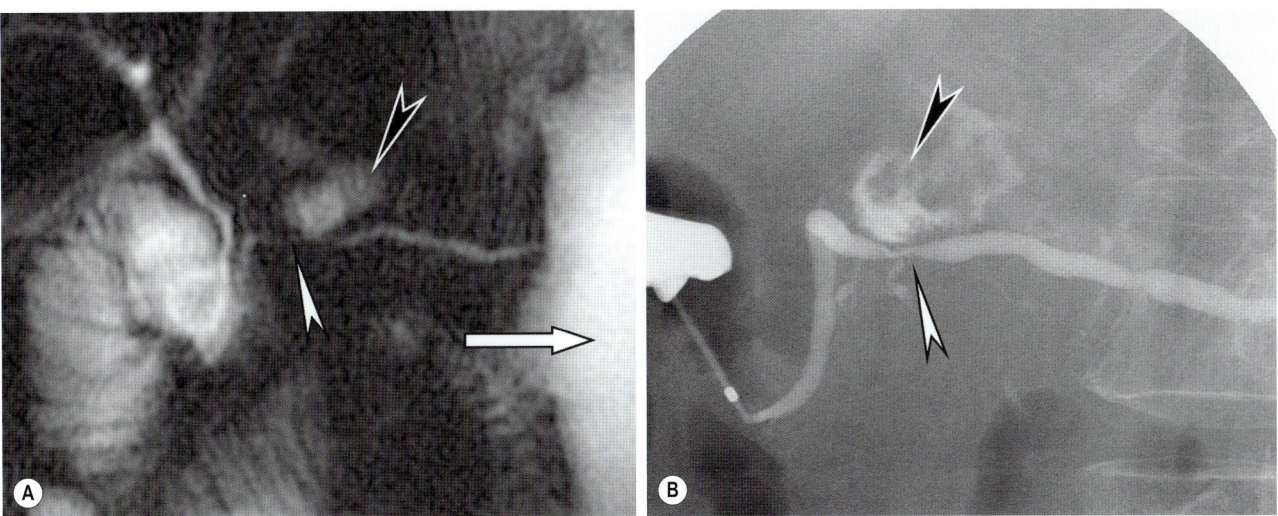

FIGURE 46-5 ■ **(A)** This secretin-enhanced MRCP was performed in a patient with pancreatic ductal stenosis. The white arrowhead shows stenosis of the main pancreatic duct at the neck along with diffuse ascites (white arrow). A fluid collection communicating with the duct is also seen (black arrowhead). **(B)** An ERCP in the same patient demonstrates the ductal stenosis (white arrowhead), distal duct dilation, and the communicating fluid collection (black arrowhead). (From Akisik MF, Sandrasegaran K, Aisen AA, et al. Dynamic secretin-enhanced MR cholangiopancreatography. Radiographics: A review publication of the Radiological Society of North America, Inc. 2006;26:665–77.)

chronic pancreatitis. A large single-institution retrospective study found a low rate of post-ERCP complications and a high therapeutic success rate.[15] ERCP was shown to be particularly useful in the diagnosis of recurrent pancreatitis, though in only 60% of patients an organic etiology was found. Sphincter of Oddi manometry was particularly useful in establishing a diagnosis when no anatomic abnormalities were present.

The treatment for pancreatitis has remained unchanged for decades. The mainstays of therapy are pain control, intravenous fluid resuscitation, pancreatic rest, and monitoring for complications. Fluid resuscitation and maintenance should be guided towards a goal urine output of 2 mL/kg/h measured by an indwelling urinary catheter. Because of circulating cytokines, activated digestive enzymes, and other pro-inflammatory molecules, extracellular fluid losses can be enormous. Constant monitoring is necessary to avoid the development of severe hypovolemia. Patients with severe acute pancreatitis may require nasogastric decompression. Most patients receive histamine-2 (H_2) receptor antagonists to reduce exposure of the duodenal secretin-producing cells to gastric acid, a potent stimulator of pancreatic secretion. This therapeutic regimen is logical but empirical, because no studies have shown improvement in outcomes with these interventions. The effectiveness of somatostatin in the treatment of pancreatitis is equivocal and probably serves more to mitigate complications of pancreatitis rather than to treat the disease itself. Further studies are needed to clearly define its role in both adults and children.[24]

Nutrition is critically important in patients with pancreatitis. The past decade has seen a paradigm shift in the nutritional management of patients with pancreatitis. Early nutrition, within the first 72 hours, is still recommended, however enteral nutrition (EN) has become the preferred method over total parenteral nutrition (TPN). Patients with mild to moderate cases of acute pancreatitis often resolve prior to requiring EN or TPN. More severe cases should be treated with EN via a nasojejunal tube, though studies have demonstrated tolerance of nasogastric feeding in severe pancreatitis as well. TPN use, especially early in the disease course during the peak inflammatory response, has been associated with increased length of stay and delayed advancement of diet. When EN is contraindicated, some advocate waiting as long as 5 days prior to starting TPN. Compared to TPN, EN has been shown to decrease length of stay, reduce the need for surgery, and reduce the risk of infection.[25] When restarting a diet, conservatively determined by resolution of symptoms, there appears to be no difference between clear liquid or solid food as the initial meal.[26] Unfortunately, these data come almost exclusively from the adult population as pediatric trials are lacking.[17,27]

Adequate analgesia is critical to minimizing the physiologic stress that develops from pain. While meperidine (Demerol) was once advocated because morphine was thought to cause spasm of the Sphincter of Oddi, no clinical trials have shown superiority of meperidine over other narcotic analgesics. Large doses of meperidine, however, are associated with the risk of seizure, euphoria, and drug interactions, suggesting other narcotics such as morphine and fentanyl may be safer alternatives. The diagnosis of pancreatitis must be certain prior to initiating treatment with high doses of narcotics as these may mask signs of serious nonpancreatic pathology, such as intestinal or gastric perforations.[28]

As pancreatitis progresses in severity, patients need to be monitored closely for signs of multisystem organ failure. Pleural effusions, pulmonary edema, and tense abdominal distention may lead to hypoxia requiring intubation and adult respiratory distress syndrome. Hypocalcemia, hypomagnesemia, anemia from hemorrhage, hyperglycemia, renal failure, and late sepsis can also be seen in these patients. Disagreement exists regarding the use of prophylactic antibiotics in severe cases of pancreatitis. The most recent adult data suggests a trend towards decreased mortality and infection with prophylactic antibiotics, but this study failed to reach statistical significance.[29] Imipenem is the antibiotic therapy of choice when necessary.

Operative exploration is usually not necessary in acute pancreatitis. However, exploration is needed in patients with infected necrotic pancreatitis or a pancreatic abscess. Infected pancreatic necrosis increases mortality significantly. Diagnosis is typically by CT pancreatography, with confirmation of infection by fine needle aspiration, clinical deterioration, or positive cultures. The latest adult data suggests that infected necrosis or peripancreatic abscesses are best treated in a stepwise manner from least to most invasive. When feasible, percutaneous drainage should be followed by minimally invasive necrosectomy if the patient fails to improve. Delayed operative therapy demonstrates improved mortality compared to primary necrosectomy.[30,31]

Pancreatic pseudocyst is a complication of trauma or pancreatitis that forms after injury to the pancreatic ductal system. The extravasated pancreatic enzymes and digested tissue are contained by the formation of a cavity composed from a fibroblastic reaction and inflammation that lacks an epithelial lining. The acute pseudocyst has an irregular wall on CT scan, is tender, and usually develops shortly after an episode of acute pancreatitis or trauma (Fig. 46-6). Chronic pseudocysts are usually spherical with a thick wall, and are commonly seen in patients with chronic pancreatitis. The distinction is important because half of acute pseudocysts resolve without treatment, while chronic pseudocysts rarely spontaneously resolve. An acute pseudocyst matures and forms a thick fibrous wall in four to six weeks, allowing for drainage. Those smaller than 5 cm in diameter usually spontaneously regress. When compared to those in adults, pseudocysts in children tend to resolve more frequently with medical therapy alone.[32] There are anecdotal reports of pseudocyst resolution in children after treatment with long-acting somatostatin analogs.[33]

The pancreatic pseudocysts that persist, or are symptomatic, require either a drainage procedure or excision. Endoscopic treatment, well established in adults, has been reported to be safe and efficacious in children as well.[34] This should only be performed at centers with sufficient experience with these techniques. Other options include laparoscopic transgastric and intragastric drainage either into the stomach or jejunum (Fig. 46-7). Percutaneous drainage is the preferred approach for infected pseudocysts because these cysts typically have thin, weak walls that are not amenable to internal drainage.

The three major complications of pancreatic pseudocysts are hemorrhage, rupture, and infection. Hemorrhage is the most serious complication and usually results from pressure and erosion of the cyst into a nearby visceral vessel. These patients require emergency angiography with embolization. Rupture or infection of a pseudocyst is uncommon. In both cases, external drainage is indicated.

Ascites in children usually follows trauma or pancreatic surgery.[35] Free fluid results from the uncontained leakage of a major pancreatic duct. Treatment initially consists of bowel rest with hyperalimentation and the use of long-acting somatostatin analogs. In many cases, the ascites resolves spontaneously with this treatment. When suspected, CT, ERCP, or MRCP should be performed to assess for duct injury. A growing body of evidence supports nonoperative management of pediatric pancreatic trauma even in the presence of ductal injury. When operative treatment is necessary, drainage alone may suffice. Distal duct injuries can be treated with distal resection. Proximal injuries require Roux-en-Y jejunal onlay anastomosis to preserve pancreatic tissue. Pseudocyst formation is common in this patient population.[36,37]

Pancreatic fistula can occur postoperatively. Most low-output fistulas close spontaneously but may drain for several months. Long-acting somatostatin analogs decrease fistula output and accelerate the rate of closure, but do not appear to induce closure of fistulas that would not otherwise have closed. Managing a pancreatic fistula centers around maintaining nutrition, with hyperalimentation necessary if enteral feeding increases fistula output, and ensuring the fistula tract does not become obstructed. Operative intervention with a Roux-en-Y jejunostomy anastomosed to the fistula site is usually curative if the fistula fails conservative management.[38]

Chronic Pancreatitis

Chronic pancreatitis is distinguished from acute pancreatitis by the irreversibility of the changes associated with the inflammation.[14] Chronic pancreatitis can be classified as either calcifying or noncalcifying. The calcifying form, most common in hereditary or idiopathic pancreatitis, is more prevalent than the obstructive form in children, and is associated with intraductal pancreatic stones, pseudocysts, and more aggressive scar formation. The obstructive type of chronic pancreatitis, which is associated with an anatomic or functional obstruction, is generally less severe with less scarring than calcifying pancreatitis. Single institutional experiences vary as to distributions in

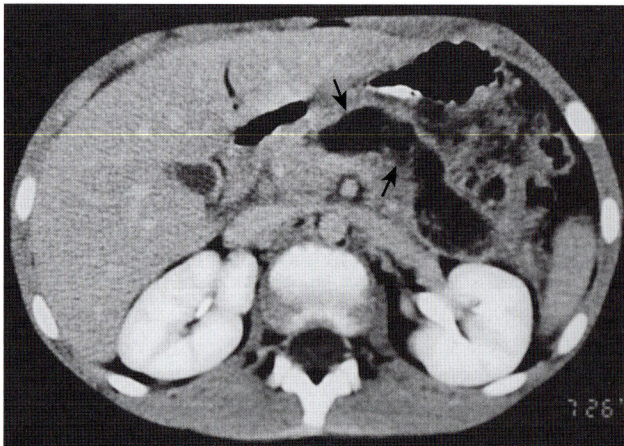

FIGURE 46-6 ■ CT scan of an acute pseudocyst in a patient after a severe motor vehicle accident. The wall (arrows) is irregular with nonloculated fluid inside.

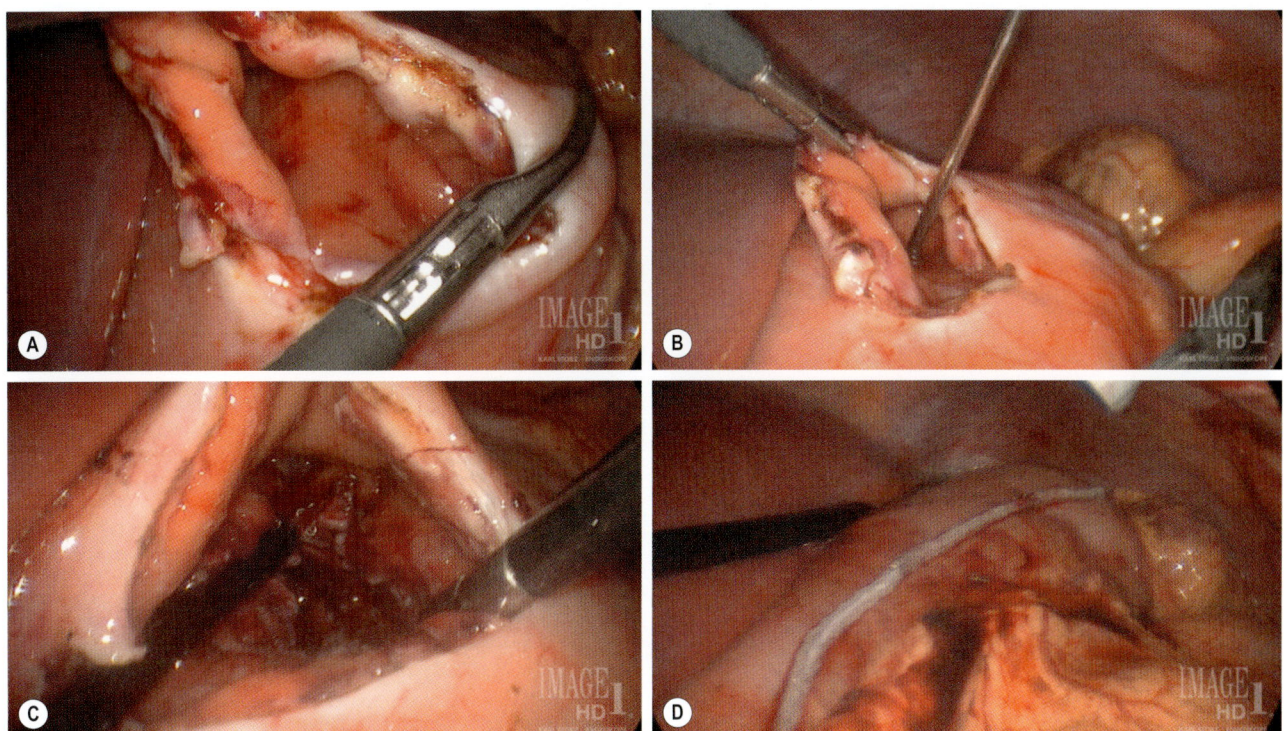

FIGURE 46-7 ■ This adolescent sustained blunt trauma from a motor vehicle accident which resulted in a pancreatic pseudocyst several weeks later. After six weeks, laparoscopic cyst gastrostomy was performed. **(A)** The stomach has been opened. **(B)** A needle is introduced into the pseudocyst through the posterior wall of the stomach. **(C)** The common wall between the pseudocyst and stomach has been excised and is opened widely for adequate drainage of the pseudocyst. **(D)** The resulting gastrotomy has been closed with an endoscopic stapler. The patient recovered uneventfully and has not developed any postoperative problems.

etiology, though the predominant causes are hereditary/genetic, obstructive, or idiopathic.[39,40]

The discovery of a genetic basis for certain forms of chronic pancreatitis represents a major breakthrough in our understanding of its pathogenesis. Current thinking is that familial pancreatitis results from a combination of environmental triggers, genetic susceptibility, and an inappropriate immune response leading to chronic inflammation and fibrosis. Hereditary pancreatitis, the most common genetic cause of pancreatitis, can result from abnormalities in the cationic trypsinogen gene *PRSS1*.[41] This autosomal dominant condition most commonly results from one of two mutations that either prevent degradation of prematurely activated trypsin or make trypsin resistant to inactivation. Penetrance in this condition is approximately 80%. Other gene mutations implicated in chronic pancreatitis are *SPINK1* and *CFTR*. Genetic testing is recommended for children with recurrent, idiopathic pancreatitis, with or without a family history of pancreatitis. Notably, patients with hereditary pancreatitis have a markedly increased risk of pancreatic cancer after age 50 years.

Obstructive pancreatitis is most often due to an anatomic or functional obstruction of the pancreatic duct. The most common anatomic causes are pancreas divisum followed by choledochal cysts. Uncertainty exists as to why a minority of patients with pancreas divisum develop chronic pancreatitis while most do not. The literature suggests that potential causes are the anatomic variant, structural narrowing of the minor papilla, sphincter of Oddi dysfunction, or the relatively high association with *CFTR* mutations.[18] Many patients with ductal dilatation and anatomic or functional obstruction clearly improve with endoscopic sphincterotomy and/or stents. Pancreatic dyskinesia, though not well studied in children, may be improved by endoscopic sphincterotomy and sometimes temporary stent placement.[42] For those in whom endoscopic treatment is not feasible or fails, individualized surgical treatment is reasonable based on the patient's ductal anatomy, level of obstruction, and severity of pancreatic fibrosis.

Chronic pancreatitis can manifest with a characteristic pain, diminished pancreatic function, and radiographic abnormalities. Increased stool fat, diabetes, and steatorrhea are signs of pancreatic insufficiency. Frequently on a CT scan, the pancreas has microcalcifications throughout the parenchyma and calcified stones in the duct (Fig. 46-8). Additionally, pancreatic pseudocysts or inflammation may be seen on the CT scan. ERCP or MRCP can evaluate the ductal anatomy and can identify anatomic causes of chronic pancreatitis. Only ERCP provides a means for evaluating sphincter pressure measurements for functional obstruction.[42]

Therapy for chronic pancreatitis is directed toward palliation of symptoms. Initial management for acute exacerbations is pain control and hydration. Steatorrhea indicates the need for pancreatic enzyme replacement. In general, these patients respond better with small, frequent meals. The diabetes that results from chronic pancreatitis tends to be unusually brittle, with a propensity

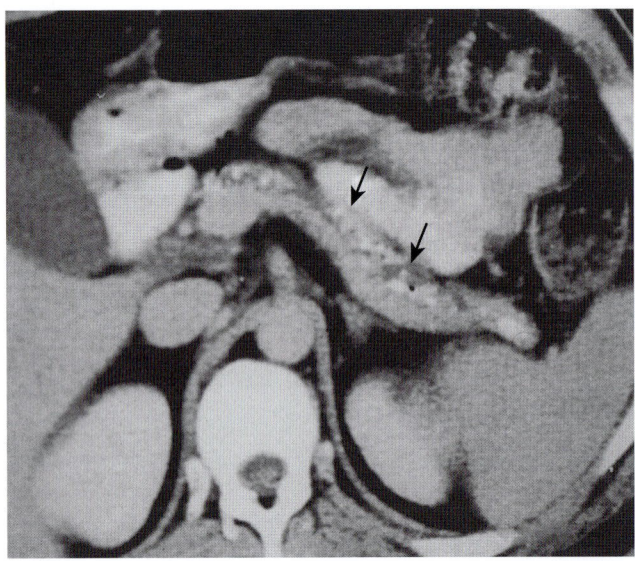

FIGURE 46-8 ■ CT scan of a pancreas with chronic calcifying pancreatitis. A dilated duct can be seen within the pancreas, further supporting the diagnosis of chronic pancreatitis. Calcified stones (arrows) can be seen in the dilated duct.

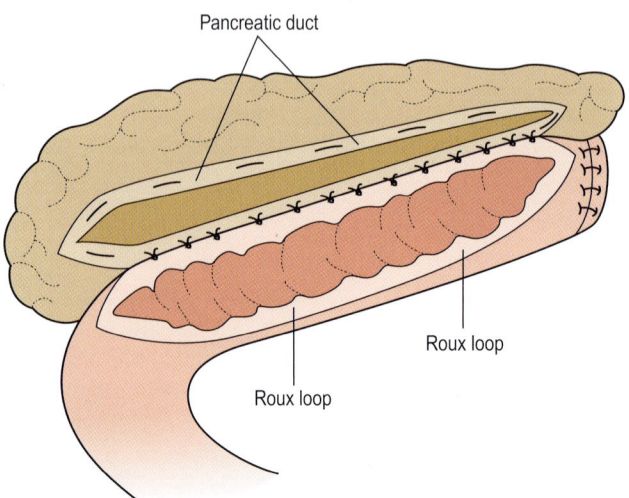

FIGURE 46-9 ■ Modified Puestow procedure. The pancreatic duct is opened longitudinally and a side-to-side anastomosis to a Roux loop of jejunum is performed. (Adapted from Mayo-Smith WW, Iannitti DA, Dupuy DE. Intraoperative sonographically guided wire cannulation of the pancreatic duct for patients undergoing a Puestow procedure. AJR Am J Roentgenol 2000;175:1639–40.)

for severe hypoglycemic episodes after even low doses of insulin. This hypersensitivity to insulin may be due to the loss of entire islets, which includes the glucagon-producing alpha cells that normally oppose the glucose-lowering effect of insulin.

In patients with chronic pancreatitis who have severe, intractable pain, ERCP or MRCP may help locate correctable problems such as large stones or a stricture with distal duct dilatation. Surgical options in chronic pancreatitis include sphincteroplasty, excision of localized pancreatitis, subtotal pancreatectomy, lateral pancreaticojejunostomy (modified Puestow procedure), and the duodenum or pylorus-preserving Whipple. Individualization of the operative approach and maximization of pancreatic ductal drainage are key. Patients failing more conservative surgical management may require a more definitive procedure to achieve symptomatic relief.[43] Although the operative results in patients with hereditary pancreatitis are generally disappointing, evidence exists that complicated patients treated with a modified Puestow procedure may experience an improved quality of life with subsequent improvement in pancreatic function and nutritional status (Fig. 46-9).[44] Unlike adults with hereditary pancreatitis, some reversal of the steatorrhea may be seen in children.

FUNCTIONAL PANCREATIC DISORDERS

The causes of persistent hypoglycemia in children vary greatly with age. In newborns and young infants, the major causes are: (1) congenital hyperinsulinism of infancy, previously called nesidioblastosis; (2) a lack of substrate for gluconeogenesis (e.g., glycogen storage disease); and (3) inadequate gluconeogenic hormones (e.g., hypothyroidism or growth hormone deficiency). In children with the onset of hypoglycemia after 1 year of

age, the causes are different, with insulinoma being the most common.

Congenital Hyperinsulinism

Nesidioblastosis, the original term for what is now called congenital hyperinsulinism of infancy (CHI), comes from the Greek *nesidio*, meaning 'island,' and *blast*, meaning 'new formation.' Nesidioblasts were originally thought to be progenitor cells in the wall of the pancreatic ducts which overproliferate in patients with this condition.[45] With the advent of genetic analysis, this pathogenesis was proven to be incorrect.

Mutations in seven genes are currently known to lead to CHI, though roughly half of cases are caused by genetic malformations not yet understood. Initially discovered was the loss of functioned mutations in the SUR1 and Kir6.2 components of the ATP-sensitive potassium channel (KATP) found in the cell membrane of the pancreatic β-cell. These mutations either impair the ability of Mg-adenosine diphosphate (ADP) to stimulate channel activity or affect the expression of the KATP channels at the surface membrane, resulting in continuous depolarization of the β-cell membrane and dysregulated insulin secretion.[46] Heterozygous gain-of-function mutations in *GULD1*, the mitochondrial gene encoding glutamate dehydrogenase, leads to CHI caused by insensitivity of the enzyme to inhibition by guanosine-5′-triphosphate. This mutation results in a milder form of CHI, which may be diagnosed later in childhood, and is associated with hyperammonemia and occasionally epilepsy. Heterozygous loss-of-function mutations in *HNF4A*, an islet transcription factor gene, are also associated with CHI through unknown mechanisms. More rare are cases of CHI caused by mutations in glucokinase (GCK), hydroxyacyl-coenzyme A dehydrogenase (HADH), and the solute carrier SLC16A1.[47]

CHI occurs in a focal and diffuse type, the differentiation of which is critical for operative management. However, the clinical presentation is identical. Patients with *SUR1* mutations often have the focal type. The focal type is actually a focal adenomatous hyperplasia, different from an adenoma. Histologically, it is seen as a confluence of hyperplastic but otherwise normal-appearing islets. There is little insulin present within the lesion due to excess secretion, while uninvolved islets outside are small with high insulin content. The diffuse type is macroscopically normal, but careful evaluation of the islets reveals enlarged β-cells with abnormally large nuclei, a large Golgi apparatus, and weak insulin staining due to hypersecretion.[48]

CHI patients typically develop hypoglycemia shortly after birth, though it may present at a later age. Infants with CHI are often macrosomic. Symptoms may be subtle, such as lethargy and irritability, or severe with apnea, seizures, and coma. Simultaneous insulin and glucose measurements show a high ratio of insulin to glucose, keeping in mind that insulin levels may be normal, but inappropriate in the presence of hypoglycemia. These patients differ from insulinoma patients, who usually have high absolute insulin levels. Another powerful indicator of CHI is a glucose requirement greater than 8 mg/kg/min.[49] Owing to the much higher incidence of insulinoma, patients older than 1 year at the onset of hypoglycemia should be evaluated for both conditions.

Stabilization of the CHI patient includes frequent intermittent or continuous feeding, with the addition of intravenous glucose as needed. Central venous access is advised because adequate venous access is lifesaving and high concentrations of glucose infusion may be necessary. Maintaining normoglycemia is key to preventing potentially disabling hypoglycemic brain injury. Intramuscular glucagon can be used as a temporizing measure until definitive venous access is obtained.

Treatment of CHI begins with medical management. Diazoxide remains a mainstay of therapy. Diazoxide binds the SUR1 component of the KATP channel and maintains it in a persistently open state, preventing insulin secretion. Patients with diazoxide-sensitive CHI who can tolerate fasting can be managed medically until they outgrow their condition. Those unresponsive to diazoxide should be managed with frequent feedings, glucose infusions, and somatostatin analogs. Somatostatin analogs inhibit pancreatic insulin secretion and can be administered subcutaneously either intermittently or continuously by a pump. Somatostatin analogs are associated with gallstones and biliary sludge, and have been implicated in cases of necrotizing enterocolitis.[50] Medical failure to control hypoglycemia necessitates surgical intervention.[49]

Distinguishing diffuse versus focal-type CHI is critical for operative planning. The recent development of an ^{18}F-DOPA PET-CT scanner has replaced pancreatic venous sampling as the optimal method for delineating focal versus diffuse disease with a sensitivity of 94% and specificity of 100% (Fig. 46-10).[51] Intraoperative ultrasound can provide additional anatomic detail to help avoid injury to the biliary tree.[52] For the focal type, resection of the hypermetabolic focus is curative. Focal lesions in the head may require duodenum-preserving pancreatic head resection and distal pancreaticojejunostomy while distal lesions are excised via spleen-preserving distal pancreatectomy. In patients with diffuse disease, a near-total pancreatectomy is needed, leaving only a rim of pancreatic tissue along the common bile duct (Fig. 46-11). The laparoscopic approach for both procedures has been reported but data are limited.[53,54] Operative complications include bile duct injury, pancreatic insufficiency,

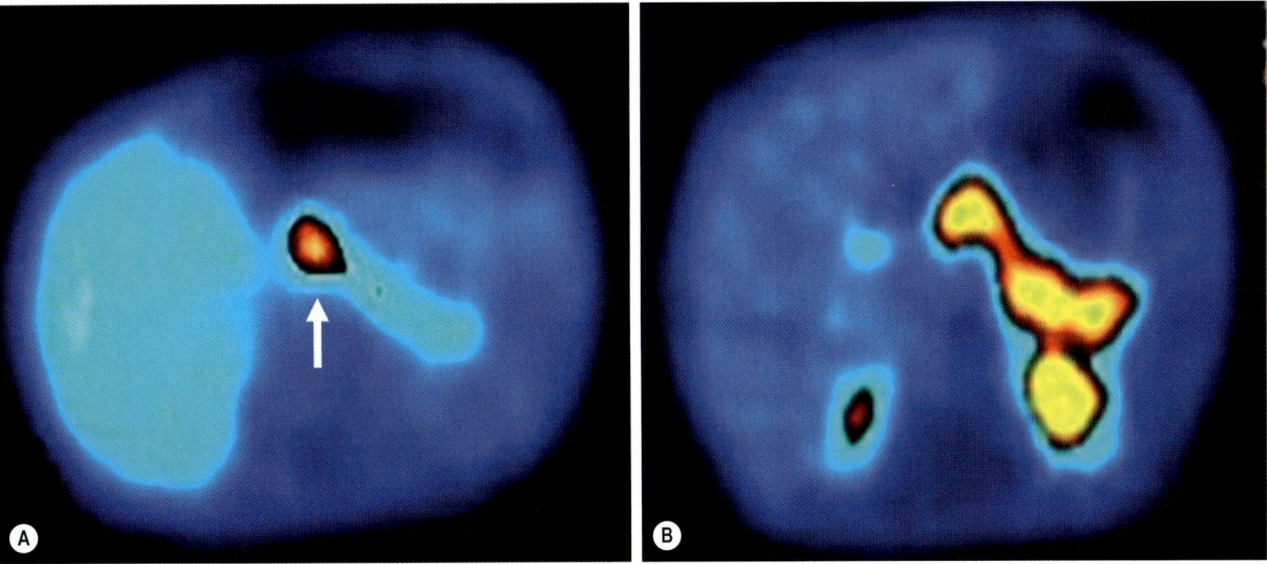

FIGURE 46-10 ■ ^{18}F-DOPA PET-CT scans of two patients with congenital hyperinsulinism of infancy. **(A)** A focal lesion (arrow) is detected in the head of the pancreas. **(B)** The more diffuse uptake of the tracer along the entirety of the pancreas indicates the diffuse type of this condition in this patient. (From Arnoux JB, Verkarre V, Saint-Martin C, et al. Congenital hyperinsulinism: Current trends in diagnosis and therapy. Orphanet Journal of Rare Diseases 2011;6:63.)

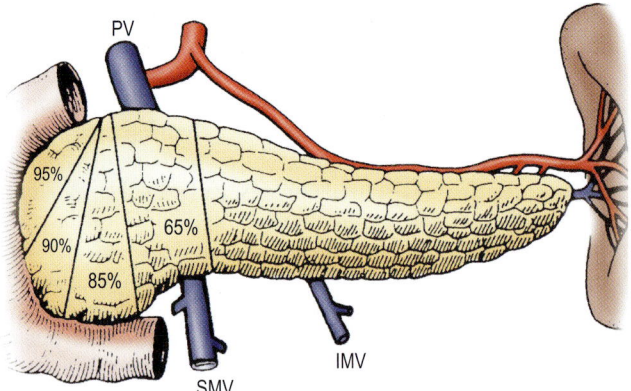

FIGURE 46-11 ■ Various degrees of pancreatectomy may be indicated for persistent hyperinsulinemic hypoglycemia of infancy. Typically, a 95% pancreatectomy, as shown here, leaves behind a cuff of pancreas along the C-loop of the duodenum. IMV, inferior mesenteric vein; PV, portal vein; SA, splenic artery; SMV, superior mesenteric vein; SV, splenic vein.

and the need for repeat pancreatic resection due to persistent hypoglycemia.[55]

Alternate forms of hyperinsulinemic hypoglycemia can arise secondary to maternal diabetes, birth asphyxia, or intrauterine growth retardation (IUGR). In these patients, the condition is transient, resolving for most patients within several days. A subgroup of patients with IUGR and prenatal asphyxia will have a prolonged condition that requires diazoxide for several months prior to resolution. Approximately 50% of children with Beckwith–Wiedemann syndrome have a CHI-like condition that tends to resolve spontaneously, but 5% will eventually require pancreatectomy.[49]

The long-term outlook for these patients depends primarily on the age at onset which reflects severity of disease, and on an expeditious diagnosis because a late diagnosis results in a higher incidence of neurologic sequelae.[56] Most patients seem to 'grow out of the disease' after several years, implying diminished activity of the beta cells. Near-total pancreatectomy in one series was associated with a 91% incidence of insulin-dependent diabetes by age 14, while no patient with focal resection required long-term insulin therapy, emphasizing the need for a conservative operative approach when possible.[57]

Glycogen Storage Disease

Glycogen storage disease type Ia (GSD-Ia) and Ib classically appear as severe hypoglycemia in infants caused by the inability to dephosphorylate hepatic glycogen subunits into glucose. GSD-Ia is caused by inactivating mutations of the glucose-6-phosphatase enzyme itself, while GSD-Ib results from inactivating mutations of the glucose-6-phosphate transporter. Hypoglycemia becomes apparent when the time between feedings increases and the liver fails to generate glucose from glycogen stores. It is clinically diagnosed by hypoglycemia, hypoinsulinemia, hepatomegaly, nephromegaly, ketosis, and hyperlipidemia. Central venous access is required for continuous infusion of highly concentrated glucose. Survivors into

adulthood have an increased incidence of hepatic adenoma after age 25 and have a 10% risk of malignant transformation. Liver transplantation ultimately becomes necessary in these patients.[58]

PANCREATIC TUMORS AND CYSTS

Pancreatic Endocrine Tumors

The only pancreatic endocrine tumors seen in infants and children are insulinomas, gastrinomas, and VIPomas. VIPoma is a tumor of vasoactive intestinal peptide (VIP) producing cells and only case reports exist in children.

Insulinoma is the most common of the three, though is still quite rare amongst pediatric tumors in general.[59] Only 10% of insulinomas are malignant, and these tend to spread to the liver and peripancreatic lymph nodes. Insulinomas cause symptoms of hypoglycemia, including dizziness, headaches, confusion, sweating, and seizures. The classic Whipple's triad was described in patients with insulinoma and consists of the following: symptoms of hypoglycemia with fasting, glucose levels less than half of normal when fasting, and relief of symptoms with glucose administration. Patients are typically in their adolescence, though younger children have been described with insulinoma. The lesions are usually solitary, except in multiple endocrine neoplasia type I (MEN I) in which multiple insulinomas may be found.[60]

The gold standard test for insulinoma is the 72-hour fast, though studies have shown that a positive result is achieved in 80% and 90% of patients with insulinoma after a shorter 24-hour or 48-hour fast, respectively. While fasting, periodic blood glucose levels are obtained. When the patient's blood glucose falls below 50 mg/dL and symptoms are present, blood is drawn for plasma glucose, C-peptide, proinsulin, insulin, β-hydroxybutarate, and sulfonylureas. Administration of exogenous insulin, followed by measurement of the C-peptide level, can be suggestive of an insulinoma, but is not completely reliable. Measuring the insulin : glucose ratio is no longer needed.[61]

Preoperative localization is challenging, but can be extremely helpful. Extrapancreatic insulinomas are rare. Most experts advocate for both transabdominal ultrasound and CT for initial localization, which identifies more than half of tumors. Centers experienced with endoscopic ultrasound also have reported good success in detecting insulinomas,[62] but expertise is not widely available. MRI is most useful for detecting liver metastases. If noninvasive studies fail to identify the tumor, intraarterial calcium stimulation via a catheter in several visceral arteries with parallel venous sampling from the right hepatic vein has been reported to regionally localize insulinomas in 80–94% of cases.[63] Intraoperative ultrasound is strongly advocated for identification of adjacent biliary and vascular structures, and as a method of last resort if nonoperative localization fails.[60,61]

All patients with insulinoma should undergo resection. Insulinomas are pink, firm, encapsulated, and are usually amenable to enucleation. In most cases, through preoperative and intraoperative analysis, the tumors can be localized, but in patients in whom they cannot be localized, blind distal pancreatic resection is no longer advised. The distinction between benign and malignant lesions is difficult, and is based on tumor size (<2 cm tend to be benign) and the presence of metastases. Insulinomas that are hard, cause puckering of surrounding tissues, appear infiltrating, or cause distal pancreatic duct dilation should be assumed malignant, and resected with a margin instead of enucleated. Malignant tumors can be treated with chemotherapy, biotherapy (such as octreotide), hepatic artery embolization/chemoembolization, radiation therapy, or radiofrequency ablation.[60]

Fetal gastrin-producing cells in the pancreas are believed to give rise to pancreatic gastrinoma. In the fetus, the primary source of gastrin is the pancreas. After birth, the gastric antrum becomes the principal source. Zollinger–Ellison syndrome (ZES) consists of gastric hypersecretion with severe peptic ulcer disease and a gastrin-producing tumor, classically in the pancreas. ZES may occur as part of the MEN I syndrome or sporadically. Gastrinomas are now understood to be frequently malignant, especially with spread to the liver, and their removal is strongly advocated.[64,65]

The diagnosis of gastrinoma is based on hypergastrinemia and gastric hypersecretion. Fasting gastrin levels are usually elevated, but can be normal. Patients suspected of having ZES should undergo a secretin stimulation test, which is considered positive if the gastrin level increases by 200 pg/mL or more. Localization can be challenging because the tumors are often small and may be extrapancreatic, but CT, MRI, endoscopic ultrasound, and [111]Indium octreotide scintigraphy have been utilized to localize the tumors. Extrapancreatic tumors are often found in the duodenal wall.

Medically, patients should initially be treated with omeprazole to control peptic ulcer disease and prevent bleeding. All disease should be excised if possible to control symptoms and help prevent metastases. Patients cured by resection should be followed closely as recurrence is common. Medical treatment for unresectable disease includes proton pump inhibitors and octreotide. Tumor debulking in unresectable cases is recommended to improve the patient's quality of life and increase the life expectancy.[65] Chemotherapy has been utilized in a few cases with good results reported.[66] There is a report of a patient with a multiple gastrinomas managed medically who survived 26 years before succumbing to unrelated causes.[67]

Non-Neoplastic Cysts

Although most cystic lesions of the pancreas are pseudocysts and are acquired, congenital cysts may be seen at an early age as a symptomatic mass with compression of surrounding structures. Alternatively, these congenital cysts may be noted incidentally on physical examination or radiographic studies. Congenital cysts contain cloudy, straw-colored fluid. The cysts are most often found in the distal pancreas and are amenable to local resection with a rim of normal pancreas. Lesions in the pancreatic head should be internally drained with a Roux-en-Y cystjejunostomy.[68]

Congenital duplications of the foregut may also present as pancreatic cysts. They have a gastric or intestinal mucosal lining and maintain pancreatic ductal communication. Gastric acid secretion from the cyst may cause episodes of pancreatitis. Surgical resection is necessary, either in the form of enucleation, distal pancreatectomy, or even pancreaticoduodenectomy.[69]

Acquired non-neoplastic cysts of the pancreas are called retention cysts, which appear to result from obstruction of the smaller pancreatic ducts. The preoperative distinction of a retention cyst from other types of cysts or pseudocysts may be difficult, but is supported by finding a small cystic lesion in communication with the pancreatic duct that has a proximal stricture. These can be excised if symptomatic, or otherwise observed. However, they are often confused with neoplastic cysts and are resected for this reason.[70]

Pancreatic Exocrine Tumors

The pancreatic exocrine system includes the pancreatic ducts, centroacinar cells, and acini. Tumors from this system include pseudopapillary tumors, ductal adenocarcinomas, acinar cell carcinomas, or pancreatoblastomas. Cystic tumors of the pancreas, including serous and mucinous cystadenomas and cystadenocarcinoma, are well described in adults, but are exceedingly rare in the pediatric population. Several case reports exist of serous and mucinous cystadenomas, but one review suggests that no confirmed reports of cystadenocarcinoma in children exist in the literature.[59] Management of serous cystadenoma is debated based on its benign nature, but excision appears curative.

Adenocarcinoma/Pancreatoblastoma

Exocrine pancreatic cancers account for roughly half of pancreatic neoplasms in children. While ductal adenocarcinoma is most common in adults, its embryonic counterpart pancreatoblastoma is more common in children. Pancreatoblastoma is believed to result from the persistence of embryonic pancreatic progenitor cells beyond the eighth week of gestation. It tends to be diagnosed in early childhood and is more common in boys and those of Asian descent. An allelic loss on 11p is often associated and suggests a similar pathogenesis with Beckwith–Wiedemann syndrome and other embryonic tumors. A recent large multicenter review demonstrated that the tumor distribution was homogenous throughout the pancreas, most were >5 cm at presentation, and over half had distant metastases.[71] Elevation of serum alpha-fetoprotein was an inconsistent feature. The prognosis is relatively good with complete resection and with appropriate neoadjuvant and/or adjuvant chemotherapy and radiation therapy. Relapse is common, so continued monitoring is essential.[72]

Acinar cell carcinoma and ductal adenocarcinoma are less common pancreatic exocrine tumors. Ductal adenocarcinoma is infrequently reported in the pediatric literature and no definitive recommendations are possible.[73] Acinar cell carcinoma is comparatively more common. Complete resection for both tumor types appears

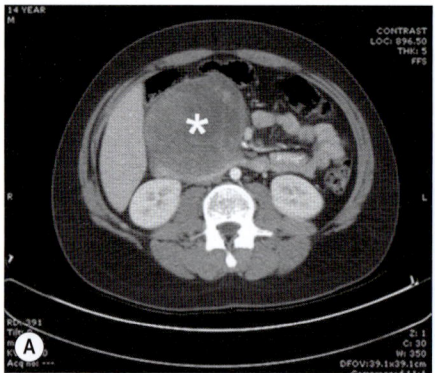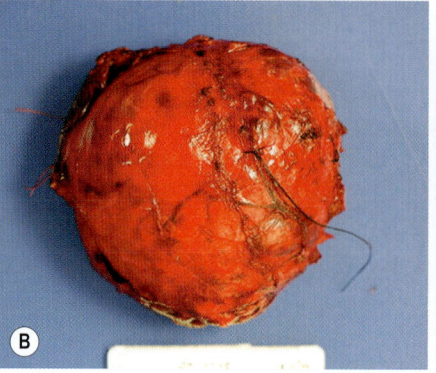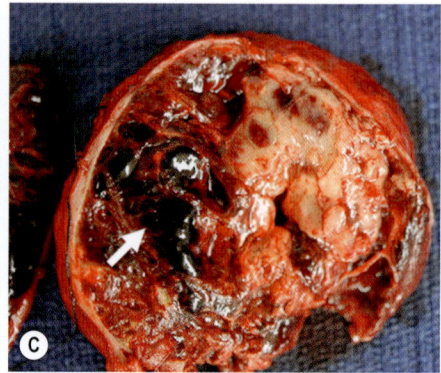

FIGURE 46-12 ■ This solid pseudopapillary tumor was found in a 14-year-old boy. **(A)** CT scan of the abdomen demonstrates a large, heterogeneous mass (asterisk) in the head of the pancreas. **(B)** The tumor is seen at excision. Note that the tumor appears encapsulated and well circumscribed. **(C)** Cut section of the mass demonstrates solid and cystic regions as well as an area of hemorrhagic necrosis (arrow). (From Speer AL, Barthel ER, Patel MM, et al. Solid pseudopapillary tumor of the pancreas: A single-institution 20-year series of pediatric patients. J Pediatr Surg 2012;47:1217–22.)

necessary with appropriate provision of neoadjuvant or adjuvant chemotherapy based on pre-treatment staging. Long-term survival improves with an earlier stage at presentation.[74,75]

Occurring slightly less frequently than pancreatoblastoma is the solid pseudopapillary tumor, also known as a papillary-cystic tumor or Frantz tumor. It has a female preponderance and is derived from exocrine cells, but without acinar or ductal structures. Presenting symptoms often include a palpable abdominal mass and abdominal pain. These tumors can be very large at the time of diagnosis (Fig. 46-12).[76] They are very slow growing, and there are reports of patients surviving 20 years after diagnosis without treatment.[77] While rarely metastatic, excision of regional and distal metastases greatly improves survival. Even with its indolent nature, an aggressive approach with complete resection is recommended as one retrospective study of patients with incomplete resections showed poor long-term survival.[78]

REFERENCES

1. Gittes GK. Developmental biology of the pancreas: A comprehensive review. Dev Biol 2009;326:4–35.
2. Dawson W, Langman J. An anatomical-radiological study on the pancreatic duct pattern in man. Anat Record 1961;139:59–68.
3. Bertelli E, Di Gregorio F, Bertelli L, et al. The arterial blood supply of the pancreas: A review I. The superior pancreaticoduodenal and the anterior superior pancreaticoduodenal arteries. An anatomical and radiological study. Surg Radiol Anat 1995;17:97–106.
4. Nakajima H, Kambayashi M, Okubo H, et al. Annular pancreas accompanied by an ectopic pancreas in the adult: A case report. Endoscopy 1995;27:713.
5. Heller RS, Tsugu H, Nabeshima K, et al. Intracranial ectopic pancreatic tissue. Islets 2010;2:65–71.
6. Tilson MD, Touloukian RJ. Mediastinal enteric sequestration with aberrant pancreas: A formes frustes of the intralobar sequestration. Ann Surg 1972;176:669–71.
7. Ozcan C, Celik A, Guclu C, et al. A rare cause of gastric outlet obstruction in the newborn: Pyloric ectopic pancreas. J Pediatr Surg 2002;37:119–20.
8. van den Brink GR. Hedgehog signaling in development and homeostasis of the gastrointestinal tract. Physiol Rev 2007;87:1343–75.
9. Skandalakis JE, Gray SW. Embryology for surgeons: The embryological basis for the treatment of congenital anomalies. 2nd ed. Baltimore: Williams & Wilkins; 1994. xx, 1101 p.
10. Sencan A, Mir E, Gunsar C, et al. Symptomatic annular pancreas in newborns. Med Sci Mont 2002;8:CR434–7.
11. Urushihara N, Fukumoto K, Fukuzawa H, et al. Recurrent pancreatitis caused by pancreatobiliary anomalies in children with annular pancreas. J Pediatr Surg 2010;45:741–6.
12. Naruse S, Kitagawa M, Ishiguro H, et al. Cystic fibrosis and related diseases of the pancreas. Best Pract Res Cl Ga 2002;16:511–26.
13. Taylor CJ, Aswani N. The pancreas in cystic fibrosis. Paediatr Respir Rev 2002;3:77–81.
14. Morinville VD, Husain SZ, Bai H, et al. Definitions of pediatric pancreatitis and survey of current clinical practices: Report from INSPPIRE (International Study Group Of Pediatric Pancreatitis: In search for a cure). J Pediatr Gastroenterol Nutr 2012;55:261–5.
15. Otto AK, Neal MD, Slivka AN, et al. An appraisal of endoscopic retrograde cholangiopancreatography (ERCP) for pancreaticobiliary disease in children: Our institutional experience in 231 cases. Surg Endosc 2011;25:2536–40.
16. Trivedi CD, Pitchumoni CS. Drug-induced pancreatitis: An update. J Clin Gastroenterol 2005;39:709–16.
17. Lowe ME, Greer JB. Pancreatitis in children and adolescents. Curr Gastroenterol Rep 2008;10:128–35.
18. Schneider L, Muller E, Hinz U, et al. Pancreas divisum: A differentiated surgical approach in symptomatic patients. World J Surg 2011;35:1360–6.
19. Bai HX, Lowe ME, Husain SZ. What have we learned about acute pancreatitis in children? J Pediatr Gastroenterol Nutr 2011;52:262–70.
20. Herman R, Guire KE, Burd RS, et al. Utility of amylase and lipase as predictors of grade of injury or outcomes in pediatric patients with pancreatic trauma. J Pediatr Surg 2011;46:923–6.
21. Darge K, Anupindi S. Pancreatitis and the role of ultrasound, MRCP and ERCP. Pediatr Radiol 2009;39(Suppl 2):S153–7.
22. Kim DH, Pickhardt PJ. Radiologic assessment of acute and chronic pancreatitis. Surg Clin N Am 2007;87:1341–58.
23. Neblett WW 3rd, O'Neill JA Jr. Surgical management of recurrent pancreatitis in children with pancreas divisum. Ann Surg 2000;231:899–908.
24. Li J, Wang R, Tang C. Somatostatin and octreotide on the treatment of acute pancreatitis—basic and clinical studies for three decades. Curr Pharm Design 2011;17(16):1594–601.
25. Marick PE, Zaloga GP. Meta-analysis of parenteral nutrition versus enteral nutirion in patients with acute pancreatitis. BMJ 2004;328:1407–12.
26. Moraes JM, Felga GE, Chebli LA, et al. A full solid diet as the initial meal in mild acute pancreatitis is safe and result in a shorter length of hospitalization: Results from a prospective, randomized, controlled, double-blind clinical trial. J Clin Gastroenterol 2010;44:517–22.
27. McClave SA, Chang WK, Dhaliwal R, et al. Nutrition support in acute pancreatitis: A systematic review of the literature. JPEN-Parenter Enter 2006;30:143–56.
28. Thompson DR. Narcotic analgesic effects on the sphincter of Oddi: A review of the data and therapeutic implications in treating pancreatitis. Am J Gastroenterol 2001;96:1266–72.

29. Villatoro E, Mulla M, Larvin M. Antibiotic therapy for prophylaxis against infection of pancreatic necrosis in acute pancreatitis. Cochrane Database Syst Rev 2010:CD002941.
30. Beger HG, Rau B, Mayer J, Pralle U. Natural course of acute pancreatitis. World J Surg 1997;21:130–5.
31. van Santvoort HC, Bakker OJ, Bollen TL, et al. A conservative and minimally invasive approach to necrotizing pancreatitis improves outcome. Gastroenterol 2011;141:1254–63.
32. Kisra M, Ettayebi F, Benhammou M. Pseudocysts of the pancreas in children in Morocco. J Pediatr Surg 1999;34:1327–9.
33. Wensil AM, Balasubramanian SA, Bell TL. Resolution of a post-traumatic pancreatic pseudocyst with octreotide acetate in a pediatric patient. Pharmacotherapy 2011;31:924.
34. Sharma SS, Maharshi S. Endoscopic management of pancreatic pseudocyst in children-a long-term follow-up. J Pediatr Surg 2008;43:1636–9.
35. D'Cruz AJ, Kamath PS, Ramachandra C, et al. Pancreatic ascites in children. Acta Paediatr Jpn 1995;37:630–3.
36. de Blaauw I, Winkelhorst JT, Rieu PN, et al. Pancreatic injury in children: Good outcome of nonoperative treatment. J Pediatr Surg 2008;43:1640–3.
37. Juric I, Pogorelic Z, Biocic M, et al. Management of blunt pancreatic trauma in children. Surg Today 2009;39:115–19.
38. Butturini G, Daskalaki D, Molinari E, et al. Pancreatic fistula: Definition and current problems. J Hepato-Biliary-Pan 2008;15:247–51.
39. Clifton MS, Pelayo JC, Cortes RA, et al. Surgical treatment of childhood recurrent pancreatitis. J Pediatr Surg 2007;42:1203–7.
40. Lucidi V, Alghisi F, Dall'Oglio L, et al. The etiology of acute recurrent pancreatitis in children: A challenge for pediatricians. Pancreas 2011;40:517–21.
41. Kandula L, Whitcomb DC, Lowe ME. Genetic issues in pediatric pancreatitis. Curr Gastroenterol Rep 2006;8:248–53.
42. Halata MS, Berezin SH. Biliary dyskinesia in the pediatric patient. Curr Gastroenterol Rep 2008;10:332–8.
43. Chromik AM, Seelig MH, Saewe B, et al. Tailored resective pancreatic surgery for pediatric patients with chronic pancreatitis. J Pediatr Surg 2008;43:634–43.
44. DuBay D, Sandler A, Kimura K, et al. The modified Puestow procedure for complicated hereditary pancreatitis in children. J Pediatr Surg 2000;35:343–8.
45. Laidlaw GF. Nesidioblastoma, the islet tumor of the pancreas. Am J Pathol 1938;14:125–34 5.
46. Saint-Martin C, Arnoux JB, de Lonlay P, et al. KATP channel mutations in congenital hyperinsulinism. Semin Pediatr Surg 2011;20:18–22.
47. Flanagan SE, Kapoor RR, Hussain K. Genetics of congenital hyperinsulinemic hypoglycemia. Semin Pediatr Surg 2011;20:13–17.
48. Rahier J, Guiot Y, Sempoux C. Morphologic analysis of focal and diffuse forms of congenital hyperinsulinism. Semin Pediatr Surg 2011;20:3–12.
49. Kapoor RR, Flanagan SE, James C, et al. Hyperinsulinaemic hypoglycaemia. Arch Dis Child 2009;94:450–7.
50. Laje P, Halaby L, Adzick NS, et al. Necrotizing enterocolitis in neonates receiving octreotide for the management of congenital hyperinsulinism. Pediatr Diabetes 2010;11:142–7.
51. Mohnike W, Barthlen W, Mohnike K, et al. Positron emission tomography/computed tomography diagnostics by means of fluorine-18-L-dihydroxyphenylalanine in congenital hyperinsulinism. Semin Pediatr Surg 2011;20:23–7.
52. von Rohden L, Mohnike K, Mau H, et al. Visualization of the focus in congenital hyperinsulinism by intraoperative sonography. Semin Pediatr Surg 2011;20:28–31.
53. Al-Shanafey S, Habib Z, Al Nassar S. Laparoscopic pancreatectomy for persistent hyperinsulinemic hypoglycemia of infancy. J Pediatr Surg 2009;44:134–8.
54. Bax KN, van der Zee DC. The laparoscopic approach toward hyperinsulinism in children. Sem Pediatr Surg 2007;16:245–51.
55. Pierro A, Nah SA. Surgical management of congenital hyperinsulinism of infancy. Semin Pediatr Surg 2011;20:50–3.
56. Leibowitz G, Glaser B, Higazi AA, et al. Hyperinsulinemic hypoglycemia of infancy (nesidioblastosis) in clinical remission: High incidence of diabetes mellitus and persistent beta-cell dysfunction at long-term follow-up. J Clin Endocr Metab 1995;80:386–92.
57. Beltrand J, Caquard M, Arnoux JB, et al. Glucose metabolism in 105 children and adolescents after pancreatectomy for congenital hyperinsulinism. Diabetes Care 2012;35:198–203.
58. Chou JY, Jun HS, Mansfield BC. Glycogen storage disease type I and G6Pase-beta deficiency: Etiology and therapy. Nat Rev Endocrinol 2010;6:676–88.
59. Shorter NA, Glick RD, Klimstra DS, et al. Malignant pancreatic tumors in childhood and adolescence: The Memorial Sloan-Kettering experience, 1967 to present. J Pediatr Surg 2002;37:887–92.
60. Mathur A, Gorden P, Libutti SK. Insulinoma. Surg Clin N Am 2009;89:1105–21.
61. Grant CS. Insulinoma. Best Pract Res Cl Ga 2005;19:783–98.
62. Patel KK, Kim MK. Neuroendocrine tumors of the pancreas: Endoscopic diagnosis. Curr Opin Gastroent 2008;24:638–42.
63. Guettier JM, Kam A, Chang R, et al. Localization of insulinomas to regions of the pancreas by intraarterial calcium stimulation: The NIH experience. J Clin Endocrinol Metab 2009;94:1074–80.
64. Jensen RT. Gastrointestinal endocrine tumours. Gastrinoma. Bailliere Clin Gastr 1996;10:603–43.
65. Schettini ST, Ribeiro RC, Facchin CG, et al. Gastrinoma in childhood: Case report and update on diagnosis and treatment. Eur J Pediatr Surg 2009;19:38–40.
66. Ohshio G, Hosotani R, Imamura M, et al. Gastrinoma with multiple liver metastases: Effectiveness of dacarbazine (DTIC) therapy. J Hepatobiliary Pancreat Surg 1998;5:339–43.
67. Quatrini M, Castoldi L, Rossi G, et al. A follow-up study of patients with Zollinger-Ellison syndrome in the period 1966–2002: Effects of surgical and medical treatments on long-term survival. J Clin Gastroenterol 2005;39:376–80.
68. Castellani C, Zeder SL, Spuller E, et al. Neonatal congenital pancreatic cyst: Diagnosis and management. J Pediatr Surg 2009;44:e1–4.
69. Fujishiro J, Kaneko M, Urita Y, et al. Enteric duplication cyst of the pancreas with duplicated pancreatic duct. J Pediatr Surg 2011;46:e13–16.
70. Goh BK, Tan YM, Chung YF, et al. Non-neoplastic cystic and cystic-like lesions of the pancreas: May mimic pancreatic cystic neoplasms. ANZ J Surg 2006;76:325–31.
71. Bien E, Godzinski J, Dall'igna P, et al. Pancreatoblastoma: A report from the European cooperative study group for paediatric rare tumours (EXPeRT). Eur J Cancer 2011;47:2347–52.
72. Lee YJ, Hah JO. Long-term survival of pancreatoblastoma in children. J Pediat Hematol Onc 2007;29:845–7.
73. Luttges J, Stigge C, Pacena M, et al. Rare ductal adenocarcinoma of the pancreas in patients younger than age 40 years. Cancer 2004;100:173–82.
74. Brecht IB, Schneider DT, Kloppel G, et al. Malignant pancreatic tumors in children and young adults: Evaluation of 228 patients identified through the Surveillance, Epidemiology, and End Result (SEER) database. Klinische Padiatrie 2011;223:341–5.
75. Ellerkamp V, Warmann SW, Vorwerk P, et al. Exocrine pancreatic tumors in childhood in Germany. Pediatric Blood Cancer 2012;58:366–71.
76. Speer AL, Barthel ER, Patel MM, et al. Solid pseudopapillary tumor of the pancreas: A single-institution 20-year series of pediatric patients. J Pediatr Surg 2012;47:1217–22.
77. Soloni P, Cecchetto G, Dall'igna P, et al. Management of unresectable solid papillary cystic tumor of the pancreas. A case report and literature review. J Pediatr Surg 2010;45:e1–6.
78. Campanile M, Nicolas A, LeBel S, et al. Frantz's tumor: Is mutilating surgery always justified in young patients? Surg Oncol 2011;20:121–5.

CHAPTER 47

SPLENIC CONDITIONS

Frederick J. Rescorla

The essential role of the spleen in the defense against bacterial organisms is well documented. King and Schumacher first described the susceptibility of splenectomized infants to infection in 1952.[1] The immunologic role of the spleen led pediatric surgeons to initiate a nonoperative approach to splenic injuries in children which has evolved into the preferred method for treating children and also adults.[2] Currently, the primary role of splenic surgery is in the management of hematologic disorders. The most significant change in management has been the introduction of laparoscopic splenectomy in adults by Delaitre and Maignien[3] and subsequently in children by Tulman and Holcomb.[4]

EMBRYOLOGY, ANATOMY AND PHYSIOLOGY

The splenic primordium develops as a mesenchymal bulge in the dorsal mesogastrium between the stomach and the pancreas, initially observed at the 8–10 mm embryo stage. A true epithelium is noted at the 10–12 mm stage as sinusoids communicate with capillaries. The spleen produces white and red cells by the fourth month of fetal life, although this function ceases later in gestation. The anatomic arrangement of the spleen is consistent with the various functions of the spleen. The splenic artery branches into segmental vessels, which further branch into trabecular arteries. After further bifurcations, small arteries enter the white pulp, which is composed of lymphocytes and macrophages arranged as a germinal center around the central artery. The central artery delivers particulate material into the white pulp, an arrangement that may facilitate antibody formation in response to particulate antigens.[5–8] The red pulp consists of the endothelial cords of Billroth, which receive the blood after it passes through the white pulp. The red pulp destroys old and defective cells. The spleen also removes Howell–Jolly bodies (nuclear remnants), Heinz bodies (denatured hemoglobin), and Pappenheimer bodies (iron granules). These particles are noted on peripheral smear after splenectomy. The immune response occurs in the white pulp as antigens come in contact with macrophages and helper T-cells. T-cells initiate cytokine synthesis, and activated T-cells circulate to modulate the response. A humoral response occurs as macrophages and helper T-cells come in contact with antigens.[9]

Splenic function also involves removal of particulate matter as well as production of nonspecific opsonins, which further activate the complement system. In addition, the spleen serves as a biologic filter. If little antibody is available for opsonization of bacteria, the spleen assumes a greater role. This may be a factor in the age-related differences in postsplenectomy infections in young children who lack an adequate antibody response.[6] The spleen also serves as a reservoir for platelets and factor VIII.

ANATOMIC ABNORMALITIES

Asplenia and Polysplenia

Asplenia is often noted with complex congenital heart disease as well as bilateral 'right-sidedness' such as bilateral three-lobed lungs and right-sided stomach and central liver.[10] Intestinal malrotation has also been observed with asplenia.[11] These infants are at risk for overwhelming infection and should receive antibiotics for prophylaxis.

Polysplenia usually consists of a cluster of very small splenic masses and is often found with biliary atresia. Other associated conditions include a preduodenal portal vein, situs inversus, malrotation, and cardiac defects.[10] These children have adequate splenic immune function.

Wandering Spleen

This condition is characterized by a lack of ligamentous attachments to the diaphragm, colon, and retroperitoneum, resulting in a mobile spleen. This is likely due to failure of development of the splenic ligaments from the dorsal mesentery.[12] Children can present with an abdominal mass and episodic pain, but also with torsion and infarction.[13,14] Pancreatitis has also been noted as a presenting sign.[15] Splenopexy is the preferred method of treatment and can be performed with placement of the spleen into a mesh basket, suture splenopexy, colonic displacement with gastropexy, placement in an omental basket, or placement in an extraperitoneal pocket.[16–20] The laparoscopic approach is the preferred technique, and the use of an absorbable or nonabsorbable mesh with fixation in the left upper quadrant is demonstrated in Figure 47-1.[21,22] Placement of the spleen in an extraperitoneal pocket is seen in Figure 47-2. Torsion with infarction requires splenectomy. Cases of chronic torsion have also been reported with massive splenomegaly which may necessitate splenectomy.[23]

Accessory Spleens

Accessory spleens have been noted in 15–30% of children, with a large series noting a 19% rate.[21] Accessory spleens likely originate from mesenchymal remnants that fail to fuse with the main splenic mass, with most (75%) located near the splenic hilum (Fig. 47-3). Other locations that must be evaluated during surgery include the lesser sac along the splenic vessels, omentum, and retroperitoneum. Eighty-six per cent of accessory spleens are single, 11% have two, and 3% have three or more.[24,25] A missed accessory spleen at the time of planned total splenectomy can lead to recurrence of the primary disease process, which in cases of immune thrombocytopenic purpura (ITP) is early and with hereditary spherocytosis (HS) is later.[26–28]

Splenic Gonadal Fusion

This condition in which the left gonad and the spleen are attached is a result of early fusion between the two structures prior to descent of the testes.[29] The remnant can be a continuous band (see Fig 50-6) or discontinuous with splenic tissue attached to the gonad. A splenic remnant has also been noted in the left scrotum as an accessory splenic remnant type of abnormality.[30]

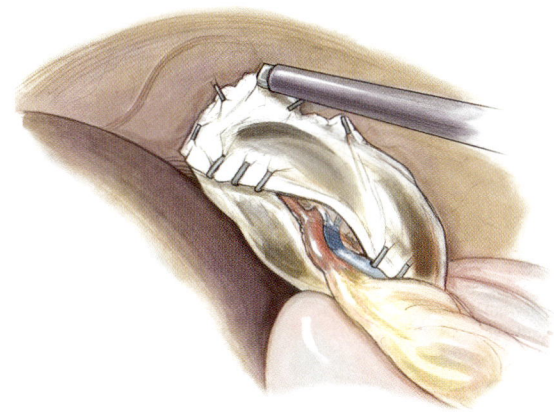

FIGURE 47-1 ■ Laparoscopic splenopexy with placement of the spleen between two sheets of absorbable mesh with fixation in the left upper quadrant. (© IUSM Visual Media.)

Splenic Cysts

Cysts of the spleen are most frequently primary splenic cysts containing an epithelial lining and are also referred to as epithelial or epidermoid cysts (Fig. 47-4). Posttraumatic pseudocysts are occasionally seen. Inclusion of surface mesothelium into the splenic parenchyma is the most likely etiology of epithelial cysts. They may present with symptoms related to their size with gastric compression or pain, an abdominal mass, rupture, or infection with abscess.[31,32] Simple cysts less than 5 cm can be observed, but cysts that are enlarging, symptomatic, or larger than 5 cm require treatment. Most symptomatic cysts are larger than 8 cm.[31] Percutaneous aspiration and sclerosis utilizing alcohol or other agents have been reported with variable success.[33,34]

Marsupialization is commonly performed but has been associated with a high recurrence rate if an adequate amount of cyst wall is not removed (Fig. 47-5).[35] In addition, a high recurrence rate with laparoscopic partial excision has also been observed.[36,37] However, others have had good success with this technique, and many also recommend partial splenectomy associated with cyst resection.[38,39] Our group has reported good results with partial splenectomy, emphasizing resection of a margin of normal spleen so that the cut surfaces cannot oppose which might lead to recurrence.[21] Other techniques involve lining the cyst with Surgicel (Ethicon, Inc., Somerville, NJ) and omentopexy.[40]

INDICATIONS FOR SPLENECTOMY

Hereditary Spherocytosis

HS, an autosomal dominant condition, is the most common inherited red cell disorder among Northern European descendants, with approximately 25% of affected children representing new mutations. Defects in red cell proteins ankyrin or spectrin result in poorly deformable spherocytes. Most affected children have

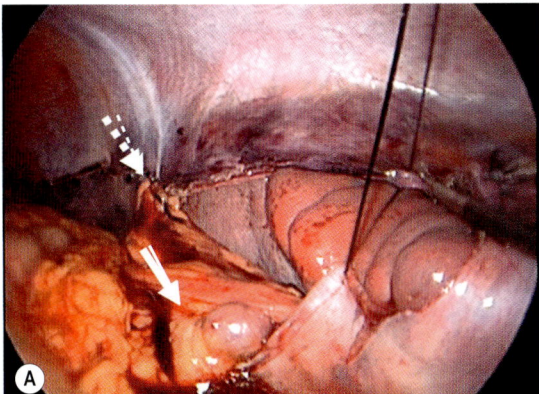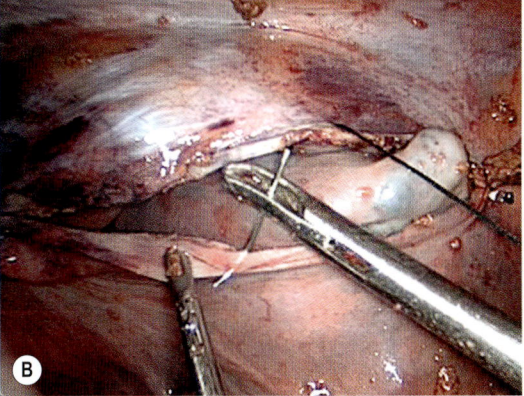

FIGURE 47-2 ■ **(A)** The upper pole of the spleen was placed in the retroperitoneal pouch, and the upper aspect of the pouch (dotted arrow) was closed with interrupted sutures. Note the splenic vessels (solid arrow) coursing into the spleen. A generous opening was left in the pouch for these vessels so that the vessels would not be compressed by closure of the pouch. **(B)** One of the interrupted silk sutures is being placed to approximate the peritoneal flaps over the spleen. At this point, most of the spleen has been placed into the extraperitoneal pouch. (From Upadhyaya P, St. Peter SD, Holcomb GW III. Laparoscopic splenopexy and cystectomy for an enlarged wandering spleen and splenic cyst. J Pediatr Surg 2007;42:E23–7. Reprinted with permission.)

anemia, an elevated reticulocyte count, and a mild elevation in bilirubin concentration. The degree of hemolysis can vary, with some only having a mild anemia. Spherocytes on peripheral smear along with a positive osmotic fragility test confirms the diagnosis. Affected children may develop an aplastic crisis associated with parvovirus B19 infection with suppression of bone marrow red cell production and ongoing splenic red cell destruction.[41] Splenectomy is usually performed for moderate-to-severe anemia. If possible, splenectomy is delayed until 5 to 6

years of age to decrease the likelihood of overwhelming postsplenectomy infection (OPSI). Splenomegaly is common in these patients. Gallstones are also often found, and an ultrasound evaluation of the gallbladder should be performed before splenectomy. The presence of gallstones in children undergoing splenectomy has been noted in 27% of those younger than age 10 years compared with 56% in children 10 years of age or older.[21]

Partial splenectomy is an attractive alternative to total splenectomy in an attempt to remove enough spleen to alleviate the anemia while preserving adequate spleen to prevent OPSI (Fig. 47-6). This may be particularly useful in young children requiring splenectomy, but the long-term results are not known.

Immune Thrombocytopenic Purpura

ITP occurs due to antiplatelet autoantibodies which subsequently are destroyed in the spleen. In most children, it is primary (idiopathic), whereas in some it may be secondary to lupus, human immunodeficiency virus, malignancy, or hepatitis C infection. Most children (80%) have acute ITP that resolves with simple observation or medical management. Most treatment plans target a decrease in platelet destruction. Management includes corticosteroids, which may have their effect by inhibiting the reticuloendothelial binding of platelet/antibody complexes; intravenous immunoglobulin (IVIG), which inhibits the Fc receptor binding of platelets by macrophages; or Rho(D) immunoglobulin in Rh-positive

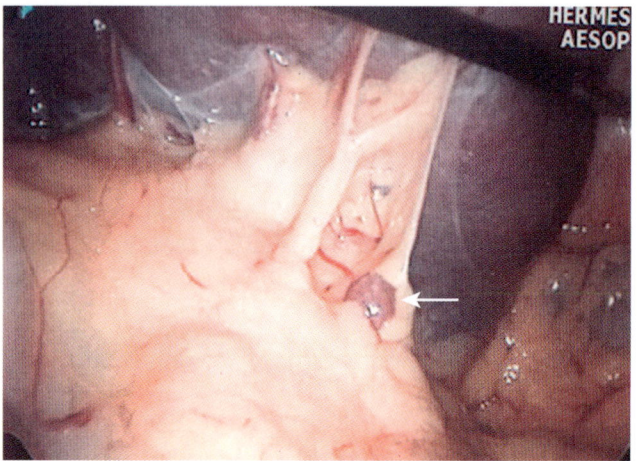

FIGURE 47-3 ■ An accessory spleen (arrow) is seen in the lienocolic ligament in this patient.

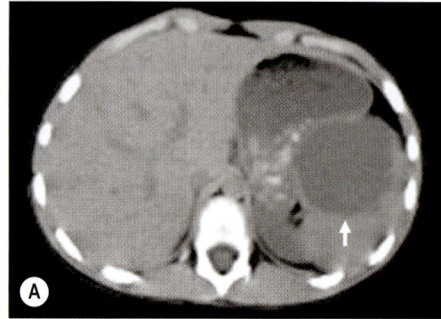
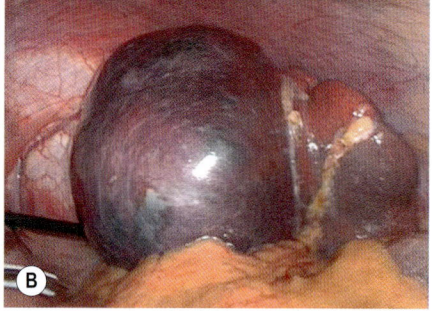

FIGURE 47-4 ■ **(A)** A large epithelial splenic cyst (arrow) is seen on the compsuted tomography scan. **(B)** At laparoscopy, the large cyst (seen in A) is seen to occupy most of the spleen.

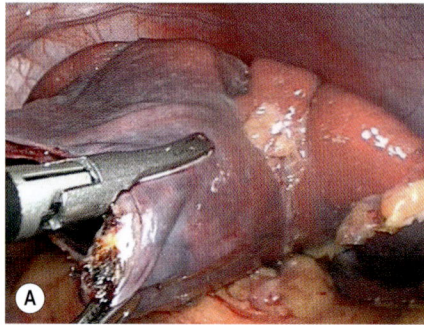
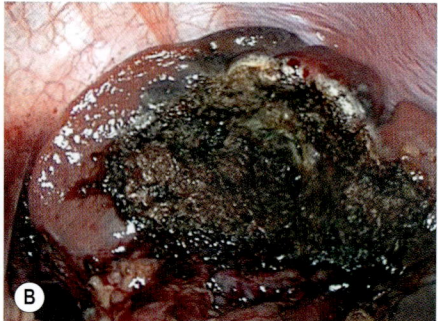

FIGURE 47-5 ■ **(A)** The wall of the large epithelial splenic cyst seen in Figure 47-4 is being excised. **(B)** The cyst was marsupialized and the remnant lining of the cyst was ablated with the argon beam coagulator.

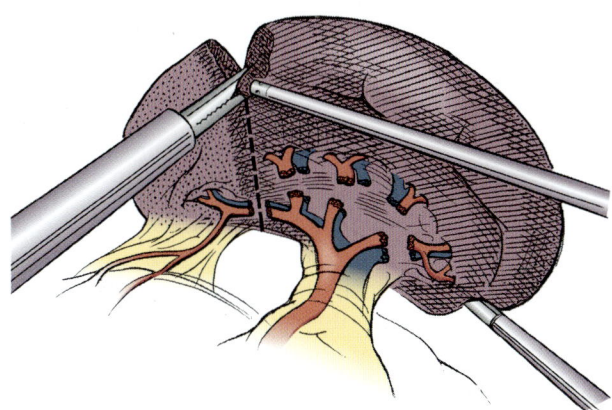

FIGURE 47-6 ■ Laparoscopic partial splenectomy with preservation of blood flow to the spleen through the most superior short gastric vessel is depicted. Note division of the parenchyma about 1 cm to the right of the devascularized margin. (© IUSM Visual Media.)

children, which bind red cells that then saturate the splenic receptors, allowing the platelets to avoid destruction.

Response to corticosteroids, IVIG, or both, have been thought to be excellent predictors of successful outcome with splenectomy.[42,43] However, two recent studies have failed to confirm this prior assumption. In a study of 19 children, Wood et al. failed to identify a positive correlation between preoperative medical treatment and response to splenectomy. In fact, they found an inverse relationship between the preoperative steroid response and response to splenectomy, with all nonresponders to steroids being complete responders to splenectomy.[44] In a similar study from our institution, 31 of 37 (84%) children with ITP had complete response to splenectomy, and 6 (16%) had partial response.[45] Of the eight with no response to steroids, six had a complete response and two had a partial response to splenectomy which suggests that failure to respond to steroids should not preclude splenectomy as definitive therapy.

Some children with ITP fail to respond to medical treatment, whereas others develop relapse when the treatment is stopped. In some of these patients, further therapy may include rituximab, a monoclonal antibody against CD20-positive B-cells. This depletes the B-cells and is somewhat of a 'medical splenectomy.' Other treatment modalities include azathioprine, cyclophosphamide, danazol, and mycophenolate mofetil.[46] Platelet production may be decreased in ITP. Thus, the use of thrombopoietic agents has emerged[46] and successful therapy with agents such as romiplostim (AMG 531, Amgen Inc., Thousand Oaks, CA) has been reported.[47] A recent follow-up report in adults noted that those treated with romiplostim (by weekly continuous infusion) had a higher rate of platelet response and a lower incidence of splenectomy than those treated with standard medical therapy.[48]

Children with thrombocytopenia for longer than six months are considered to have chronic ITP and are candidates for splenectomy. The response to splenectomy has been excellent in children who have responded to medical management. In adults, the response is not as

high. Accessory spleens or residual splenic tissue has been identified in up to 50% of adult patients with ITP, thus emphasizing both the importance of accessory spleen detection at exploration as well as the need to avoid parenchymal disruption.[26]

Sickle Cell Disease

Sickle cell disease (SCD) results from an amino acid substitution in the β-chain of normal hemoglobin A, which results in hemoglobin S. Children may be homozygous (SCD) or have less severe heterozygous types such as sickle-C or sickle-thalassemia. These red blood cells become rigid as they pass through the hypoxic environment of the spleen, leading to splenic sequestration. Although autoinfarction and atrophy lead to a functional asplenic state in most children, some develop symptomatic sequestration. If the sequestration is severe, these children develop anemia and splenomegaly with associated thrombocytopenia known as acute splenic sequestration crisis. Due to the associated morbidity and mortality, severe or recurrent episodes merit consideration for splenectomy.

A recent report of 53 children with SCD less than 4 years of age at the time of splenectomy found that 5.7% died during the 15 year study with one (1.8%) dying of OPSI.[49] The authors concluded that it is reasonable to perform a splenectomy around age 2 years if a child with SCD has had a serious episode of sequestration.

Thalassemia

The thalassemias are characterized by abnormal production of α- or β-chains of hemoglobin. Thalassemia major (β-thalassemia) is associated with the most severe clinical anemia among this group. Splenomegaly causes further red cell sequestration and need for transfusion. Total or partial splenectomy has been performed to decrease the need for transfusions in children with severe anemia.

Gaucher Disease

Gaucher disease is characterized by a deficiency of the enzyme β-glucocerebrosidase, resulting in excessive glucocerebroside in the macrophages of the spleen, liver, bone marrow, and lungs. Splenomegaly may be severe, and both partial and total splenectomy have been utilized to alleviate the symptomatic hypersplenism and to decrease destruction of the red blood cells, leukocytes, and platelets.[50] However, massive bleeding and death has been reported several months postoperatively in a child with Gaucher disease who underwent partial splenectomy.[51]

SPLENECTOMY

Open Splenectomy

The open technique through a left upper quadrant incision is usually reserved for massive splenomegaly. The initial division of the splenorenal, splenocolic, and splenophrenic ligaments allows the spleen to be mobilized from the left upper quadrant and out of the abdominal cavity. The short gastric vessels are divided initially, followed by the hilar vessels. A careful search must be undertaken for accessory spleens. A lateral muscle-splitting approach has been reported with a 2.7-day length of stay which is comparable to some early laparoscopic series but longer than more recent series.[21,52,53]

Laparoscopic Splenectomy

Laparoscopic splenectomy has evolved over the past 15 to 20 years to become the preferred approach for splenectomy.[3,4] Less pain, shorter hospitalization, faster return to regular activities, and smaller scars are the main advantages over open splenectomy. However, it is associated with a longer operative time and can be difficult in patients with splenomegaly. The main technical advances have been the result of smaller instrumentation and advanced energy sources such as the Harmonic Scalpel (Ethicon Endosurgery Inc, Cincinnati, OH) and Ligasure (Valley Lab, Tyco Healthcare Group, Boulder, CO). At our institution, we primarily utilize the Ligasure because it allows division of vessels up to 7 mm.

The most significant initial concern for the laparoscopic approach was related to accessory spleen detection. However, in adult studies and comparison pediatric series, similar rates of accessory spleen detection at laparoscopic and open splenectomy have been noted.[26,27,53–56] For the laparoscopic operation, most surgeons utilize a lateral approach with slight elevation of the left flank. One technique to improve the ease of port placement is to have the patient's left side initially elevated approximately 45° rather than the true lateral position. The operating table is then tilted to the patient's left to achieve a flat position for the port placement and then is tilted to the patient's right to achieve a lateral position for the procedure (Fig. 47-7). The surgeon and assistant stand on the patient's

right. In young children and patients with small spleens, the upper midline instruments (3 mm) can be inserted without cannulas because these instruments are not removed during the procedure (Fig. 47-8). The first assistant holds the two upper midline instruments to provide elevation of the spleen and traction on surrounding tissues. The surgeon holds the camera (5 mm, 30–45° telescope) in the left hand and the energy source in the right hand.

Initially, the splenocolic ligament is divided with the energy device, allowing the splenic flexure to fall away from the spleen. The inferior portion of the gastrosplenic ligament is divided, and the surgeon works in a cephalad direction dividing the short gastric vessels and opening the lesser sac (Fig. 47-9). The most superior short gastric vessels are often very short, and care must be taken to avoid injury to the stomach or diaphragm. This is often the most difficult part of the procedure. The lesser sac should be inspected for the presence of accessory spleens. The splenophrenic ligament is divided to fully mobilize the upper pole. At this point, the hilum can be approached. It is often easiest to divide the splenorenal ligament because this allows the option to use the endovascular stapler on the hilum. In the early era of laparoscopic splenectomy, clips were applied to individual hilar vessels with division using endoscopic scissors. Most surgeons now use an endoscopic stapler which has the disadvantage of requiring a 12 mm port (Fig. 47-10). Proximity of the hilum and pancreas is the main issue in terms of positioning the stapler. Pancreatitis and pancreatic fistula have been reported, although many reports have confirmed the safety of this technique.[57–60] The Ligasure has limited lateral thermal spread (<2 mm) and is relatively easy to use for dissection and ligation of the hilar vessels.[61]

One study comparing the endoscopic stapler to the Ligasure demonstrated safety and efficiency of both with a lower blood loss and conversion rate with the

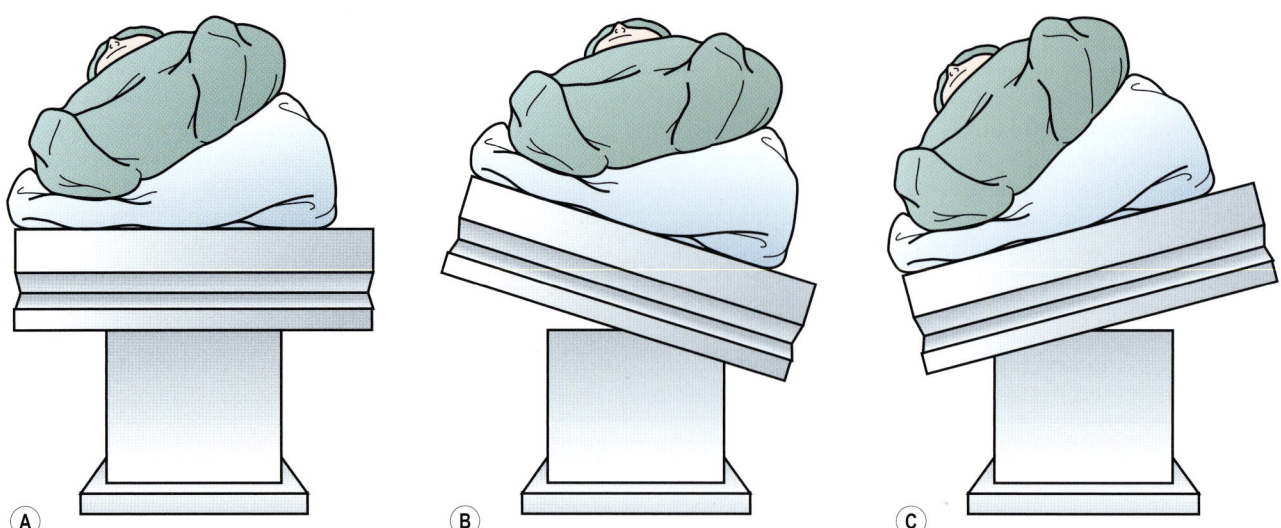

FIGURE 47-7 ■ **(A)** Initial positioning of the patient before any movement of the table. **(B)** The table has been tilted to the patient's left to obtain a near supine position of the patient for port placement. **(C)** The table is then rotated back to the patient's right to achieve a right lateral decubitus position for the operation. (From Rescorla FJ. Laparoscopic splenectomy. In: Holcomb GW III, Georgeson KE, Rothenberg SS, editors. Atlas of Pediatric Laparoscopy and Thoracoscopy. Philadelphia: Elsevier; 2008. p. 121–6. Reprinted with permission.)

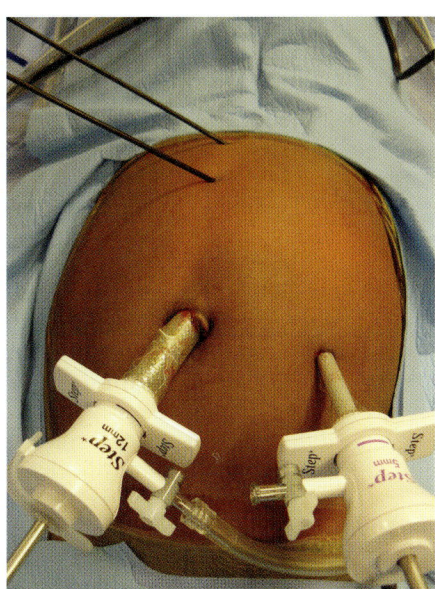

FIGURE 47-8 ■ Placement in a child of 3 mm midline instruments without the use of cannulas. The umbilical port is 12 mm, and the left lower quadrant port is 5 mm.

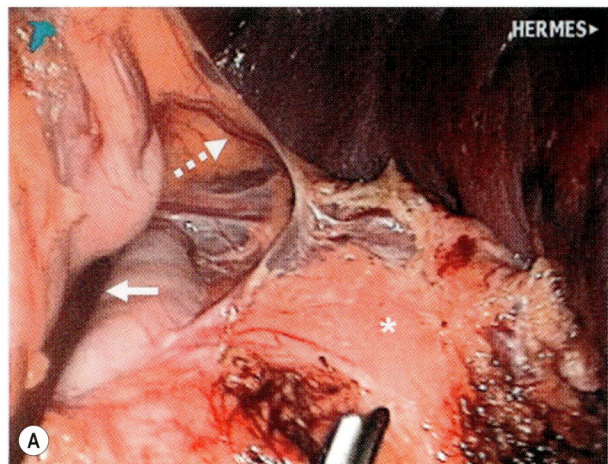

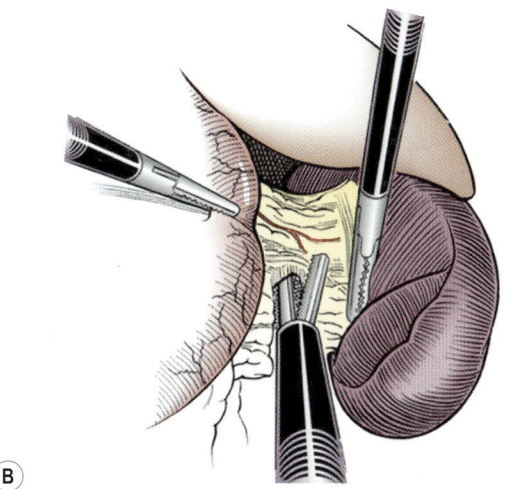

FIGURE 47-9 ■ After division of the short gastric vessels using the ultrasonic scalpel, the lesser sac is entered. In the operative photograph, the stomach is being retracted by the assistant's instrument (solid arrow). The ultrasonic scalpel, at the bottom of the photograph, is approaching one of the intact short gastric vessels (dotted arrow). The pancreas is marked with an asterisk. (From Rescorla FJ. Laparoscopic splenectomy. In: Holcomb GW III, Georgeson KE, Rothenberg SS, editors. Atlas of Pediatric Laparoscopy and Thoracoscopy. Philadelphia: Elsevier; 2008. p. 121–6. Reprinted with permission.)

Ligasure.[62] We utilize the Ligasure to ligate and divide the individual hilar vessels, usually with one application on the pancreas side without division and a second cautery toward the spleen with division.

The Endocatch II (Covidien, Norwalk, CT) can be inserted through a 15 mm umbilical port with the telescope moved to the left lower quadrant site. If a 12 mm port has been placed in the umbilicus, it can be removed and the bag can be introduced directly into the abdominal cavity. This bag has a 13 cm diameter opening with a 23 cm depth and can accommodate most spleens in children. A smaller bag can be used for smaller spleens. The neck of the bag is delivered through the umbilical incision, and either a finger or ring forceps is introduced to disrupt the capsule and morcellate the spleen (Fig. 47-11). Use of an ultrasonic morcellator and liposuction has been reported, but are not routinely used.[63]

These basic techniques are also utilized for treatment of splenic cysts and a wandering spleen. The laparoscopic approach is usually not applicable for traumatic splenic injuries because children who require operation are usually very unstable and unstable conditions require rapid control of bleeding. However, one report described laparoscopic splenectomy after splenic artery embolization in a 15-year-old girl with a traumatic injury.[64]

Single-port access splenectomy has been reported utilizing either a multi-instrument port or with separate umbilical fascial incisions after raising skin flaps.[65–68] A standard laparoscopic splenectomy can be performed although some surgeons have recommended avoiding large patients with splenomegaly, and some have extended the umbilical incision to remove the spleen intact which appears to diminish the benefit of the laparoscopic approach.[65,66] Several authors have utilized standard laparoscopic instruments without the use of roticulating graspers.[67,68]

Partial Splenectomy

Concerns about postsplenectomy infection have led to the concept of partial splenectomy. This is primarily utilized in children with HS but has also been utilized with Gaucher disease, hypersplenism with cystic fibrosis, splenic hamartomas, and splenic cysts.[50,69,70] Partial splenectomy generally involves removal of 85–95% of the enlarged spleen with preservation of approximately 25% of the normal splenic size. In this approach, the remnant spleen is supplied by one or two short gastric vessels with division of all of the hilar vessels (see Fig. 47-6). An alternative approach, depending on the anatomy of the segmental vessels, is to leave the uppermost segmental vessel as the only blood supply. Although historically most partial splenectomies have been performed through an open technique, the laparoscopic approach is gaining popularity.[21,71,72]

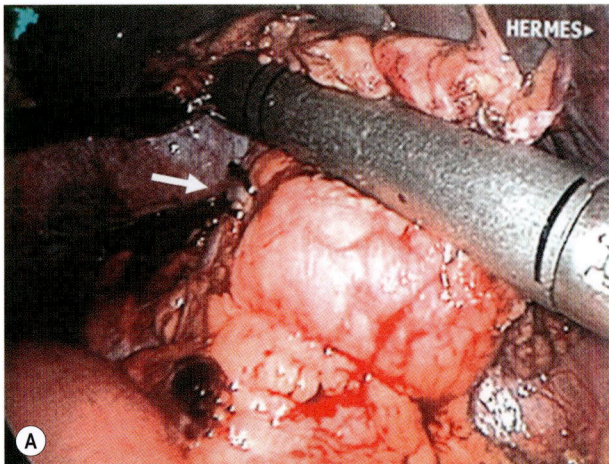

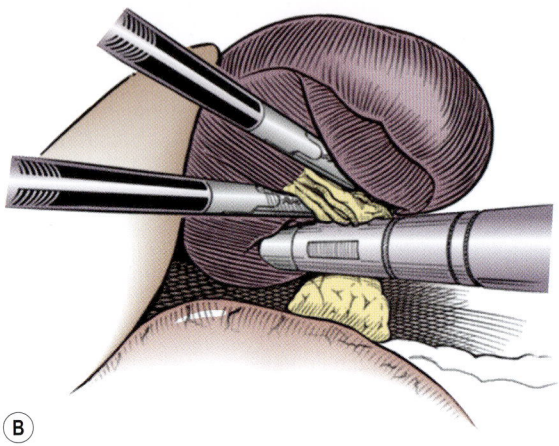

FIGURE 47-10 ■ Once the spleen has been mobilized and is attached only through the hilar vessels, the camera is rotated to the left lower quadrant port and the stapler is introduced through the umbilical port. It is then placed across the hilar vessels, taking care not to incorporate a portion of the pancreas in the tissue to be divided. In the operative photograph, note that the splenic artery has been ligated with clips (arrow) before hilar division because the spleen was extremely large. (From Rescorla FJ. Laparoscopic splenectomy. In: Holcomb GW III, Georgeson KE, Rothenberg SS, editors. Atlas of Pediatric Laparoscopy and Thoracoscopy. Philadelphia: Elsevier; 2008. p. 121–6. Reprinted with permission.)

The splenic parenchyma can be divided with a stapler, cautery, or energy device. Our group has reported 12 laparoscopic partial splenectomies.[21] In all cases, a combination of Ligasure and cautery were utilized, often with a topical agent placed over the cut surface. After devascularization, a clear line of demarcation is usually noted. We divide the spleen 1 cm onto the ischemic side to minimize bleeding. We currently use cautery to divide the splenic parenchyma and then apply a topical hemostatic agent and omentum to the exposed parenchyma. The upper splenorenal and splenophrenic ligaments are left to avoid torsion. Another report of seven laparoscopic partial splenectomies described using the ultrasonic scalpel for parenchymal division and complete mobilization of the spleen.[73] The authors then performed a splenopexy to prevent torsion. We have occasionally sutured the remaining parenchyma to the lateral abdominal wall superiorly near the diaphragm when the vascular anatomy required preservation of the lower pole vasculature rather than the upper pole.

Several series have noted an increase in red cell half-life, higher hemoglobin levels, and lower reticulocyte and bilirubin levels after partial splenectomy for spherocytosis.[71,74] The lack of Howell–Jolly bodies on peripheral smear and a decreased number of pitted red cells is evidence of preservation of splenic phagocytic function. Normal levels of IgM- and IgG-specific antibody titers after *Streptococcus pneumoniae* have also been observed. Splenic regeneration occurs in all patients although the degree of regrowth does not correlate with hemolysis.[72] The development of cholelithiasis after partial splenectomy varies from 7–22%, indicating ongoing hemolysis. Moreover, the need for subsequent total splenectomy has been reported.[71,75] Rice and colleagues have popularized this procedure and summarized their experience in 29 children undergoing partial splenectomy.[72] They noted decreased transfusion requirements, elimination of splenic sequestration, higher hematocrits, and lower reticulocyte counts and bilirubin levels. A recent multi-institutional study of 62 children with HS undergoing partial splenectomy noted a mean hemoglobin increase of 3.0 ± 1.4 g/dL and reticulocyte count decrease of $6.6 \pm 6.6\%$ at one year.[76] An alternative technique has been described that leaves a 10 cm³ remnant as a small cylinder supplied by one vessel.[77]

Another recent report of nine children undergoing laparoscopic partial splenectomy (10–30% remnant) observed improved hemoglobin levels (12.9 g/dL vs 10.9 g/dL) and decreased reticulocyte counts.[78] A second multicenter series of 11 partial splenectomies noted no need for subsequent total splenectomy with an average follow-up of 19 months (range, 4–53 months).[73] A recent comparative study found that laparoscopic partial splenectomy patients had more pain and a longer hospitalization than open partial splenectomy.[79] We have also noted an increased hospitalization with laparoscopic partial splenectomy (2.3 days) compared with an open operation (1.2 days).[80]

COMPLICATIONS AND CONTROVERSIES WITH LAPAROSCOPIC SPLENECTOMY

Accessory Spleen Detection

The identification of residual splenic function in up to 50% of selected adults after laparoscopic splenectomy has led to concern about the ability to adequately detect accessory spleens at laparoscopy.[26] Parenchymal injury at the time of laparoscopic splenectomy has also been associated with a higher rate of residual splenic function.[26,27] Although preoperative computed tomography and splenic scintigraphy have been used to identify accessory spleens preoperatively, most surgeons have abandoned this approach.[81]

There are reports of equivalent detection rates of accessory spleens with laparoscopy.[26,82] In reviewing several comparative pediatric series, accessory spleens were found in 20.3% of patients undergoing an open splenectomy and 20.2% at laparoscopy.[53–56] Our report of

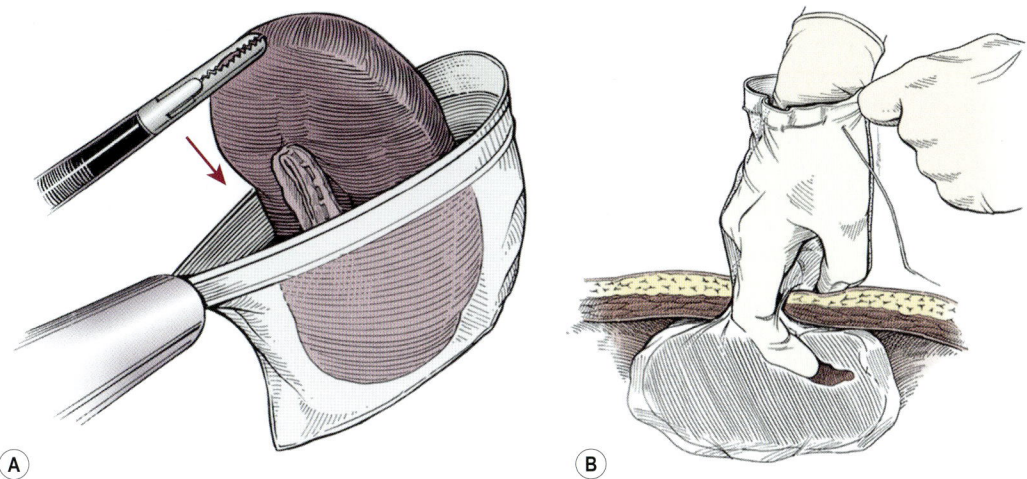

FIGURE 47-11 ■ **(A)** After complete mobilization, the spleen is dropped into an endoscopic retrieval bag. **(B)** The neck of the bag is then exteriorized through the umbilicus, and the surgeon's finger is used to fracture the splenic capsule. A combination of ring forceps and the surgeon's finger is then used to remove the splenic fragments. (From Rescorla FJ. Laparoscopic splenectomy. In: Holcomb GW III, Georgeson KE, Rothenberg SS, editors. Atlas of Pediatric Laparoscopy and Thoracoscopy. Philadelphia: Elsevier; 2008. p. 121–6. Reprinted with permission.)

over 200 laparoscopic splenectomies noted accessory spleens in 19%, and follow-up evaluation of over 300 laparoscopic splenectomies has confirmed this rate.[21] Laparoscopic removal of missed accessory spleens has been reported with good success; however, the efficacy of accessory splenectomy in improving ITP ranges from 26–75%.[83,84]

Splenomegaly

Splenomegaly in children is usually due to HS. The optimal management of children with splenomegaly is controversial as most articles come from the adult literature. The benefits of the laparoscopic technique have been demonstrated in adults with spleens between 15–25 cm.[85] Hand-assisted procedures have been utilized in adults with massive splenomegaly (700 g to >3 kg). In one report, a 7 cm right subcostal incision was used for hand access and also the retrieval site for a bowel bag with the spleen.[86] In this report, the conversion rate was only 2.3%; however, 5% required reoperation for bleeding. The hand-assisted laparoscopic technique compared to an open approach in patients with splenomegaly (>20 cm) has resulted in less blood loss and shorter length of stay.[87]

A recent study in adults with massive splenomegaly (craniocaudad length ≥17 cm or weight ≥600 g) and supramassive splenomegaly (craniocaudad length ≥22 cm or weight ≥1600 g) comparing laparoscopic to open splenectomy found lower blood loss and shorter length of stay with the laparoscopic approach.[88] This was accomplished at the expense of longer operative times and a 25% conversion rate, most frequently due to uncontrolled bleeding. Malignancy was the cause of the massive splenomegaly in the supramassive group, which is rare in children. The authors concluded that the laparoscopic approach was better than the open operation for massive splenomegaly, and at least comparable to hand-assisted laparoscopic splenectomy.

Conversion to Open Splenectomy

Splenomegaly and bleeding are the main reasons for conversion and has been reported in 1.3–2.8% of patients.[54,81,89,90] A relatively recent multicenter report of 159 laparoscopic splenectomies found a conversion rate of 5% with bleeding the most common reason.[91] This high conversion rate may have been due to surgeon experience as these data came from four centers over a ten-year time period. The largest pediatric series documented a 1.7% rate.[21] Higher conversion rates have been noted with larger spleens, less surgeon experience, and obese patients.[92] A large multicenter Italian registry study of 676 patients undergoing laparoscopic splenectomy found that body mass index and hematologic malignancy were independent predictors for intraoperative complications and conversion to an open splenectomy.[93] Their overall conversion rate was 5.8%. Complications occurred in 17% with bleeding in 4.5% and splenic/portal vein thrombosis in 2.1%.

Operative Time

The laparoscopic approach has uniformly been associated with somewhat longer operative times than open splenectomy.[53–56] A large series over 10 years noted a decrease in operative time from a mean of 110 ± 36 minutes in the early period to 86 ± 35 minutes in the later period as experience was gained.[21] This operative time is compared with 83 minutes for open splenectomy in a previous report from the same institution.[56]

Postoperative Hospitalization

Comparative studies in children have consistently demonstrated a lower duration of hospitalization with the laparoscopic approach compared with the open technique, ranging from 2.5–4.9 days for the open operation and 1.3–3.6 days for the laparoscopic approach.[21,54,55] Our series of over 200 cases noted the postoperative hospitalization to vary by diagnosis with HS at 1.23 days, ITP at 1.20 days, and SCD at 2.37 days.[21] An Italian single-institution series of 33 children (2000–2005) undergoing splenectomy (19 laparoscopic, 14 open) noted a shorter hospitalization (5.5 ± 2.9 versus 8.7 ± 4.8) in the laparoscopic cohort but still considerably longer than contemporary studies in the USA.[94] The increased length of stay in patients with SCD is secondary to the higher incidence of complications in this subgroup of patients, such as acute chest syndrome. Other retrospective series have confirmed the role of laparoscopy in children with SCD, noting a shorter hospitalization with the laparoscopic approach without an increase in postoperative pain or acute chest syndrome compared with open splenectomy.[95,96] Splenomegaly itself, which is common in HS, does not appear to affect the postoperative hospitalization. An unreported benefit of the shorter hospitalization after each operation is the effect on the parent's return to work. One study noted children return to full activity faster with laparoscopy compared with open splenectomy.[97]

Complications

Most pediatric series have had relatively few complications with the laparoscopic technique. A meta-analysis of adult and pediatric studies reported between 1991 and 2002 noted a complication rate of 15.5% for laparoscopic and 26.6% for open splenectomy ($p < 0.0001$).[98] The laparoscopic group had fewer pulmonary, wound, and infectious complications but more hemorrhagic complications when conversions for bleeding were included. A large adult comparative study noted equivalent grade I and II complications (minor, potentially life threatening) but higher grade III and IV (residual or lasting disability, death) with the open approach compared with laparoscopy.[99] Symptomatic splenosis has been reported in ITP due to rupture of an Endocatch II bag with thrombocytopenia occurring 13 months after the initial laparoscopic splenectomy.[100] Our review of over 200 pediatric laparoscopic splenectomies found an overall complication rate of 11% with no wound infections or deaths.[21] Postoperative ileus, acute chest syndrome, and bleeding requiring transfusion were the most common complications. The complication rate was 22% among the children with SCD and only 8.3% among those with other conditions ($p = 0.0083$). This report documented one (0.5%) symptomatic portal vein thrombosis.

Splenic vein or portal vein thrombosis is a rare complication after splenectomy but may be more common than is clinically appreciated, and is particularly common in patients with splenomegaly.[101,102] A small adult study identified a 50% incidence of portal or splenic vein thrombosis, with splenic weight the strongest predictor of thrombosis.[103] Another prospective study in adults identified an incidence of 4.79%, and noted spleen weight over 650 g and a platelet count over 650,000/mm³ to be associated with this complication.[104] A retrospective evaluation of splenic weight and portal vein thrombosis noted rates of 14%, 40%, 45%, and 71% for weights 700 g–1 kg, 1–2 kg, 2–3 kg, and >3 kg, respectively.[86] Despite early

anticoagulation, 13% of the entire group progressed to complete thrombosis. A prospective series in children noted an incidence of 5.88% with the same risk factors.[105] Of the patients with total splenic vein thrombosis, over 50% were symptomatic with fever and abdominal pain, emphasizing the need to evaluate for this condition in patients with these symptoms. Most authors recommend treatment with antithrombotic and antiplatelet therapy.

Postsplenectomy Sepsis

OPSI was initially reported by King and Shumacker in a group of five infants undergoing splenectomy for HS.[1] The actual risk of OPSI is difficult to determine because most of the data was accumulated before the routine use of preoperative vaccinations. Data from the 1990s note the rate of OPSI between 0.13–8.1% in children and adolescents less than 15 years of age compared with 0.28–1.9% in adults.[106–108] Most authors quote the current OPSI rate between 3.5–4.4%.[75,107,108] Some have also noted a higher mortality in children younger than 4 years of age (8.1%) compared with a lower rate (3.3%) in older children.[106–108] Most deaths occur within four years of splenectomy.[109,110] The causative organism is likely *Streptococcus pneumoniae* which has been found in 50–90% of all infections.[111,112] *Pneumococcus* is responsible for 60% of all fatal infections, followed by *Haemophilus influenzae*, meningococcus, and Group A *Streptococcus*.[113] Vaccinations have been shown to decrease the risk of bacteremia.[113,114]

A single-institution study compared two time periods.[107] The first one was prior to immunizations and antibiotics. The second era (with a 70% immunization rate and 100% antibiotic prophylaxis rate) noted a decrease in OPSI (6% to 3.8%) and mortality (3.9% to 0.9%). This study found age to be important as the rate of infection was 13.8% for those children younger than 6 years of age compared with 0.5% in older children. Although older studies noted mortality rates of 50% with OPSI, more recent studies have a rate of around 10%.[107,115,116]

Routine immunization against *S. pneumoniae*, *H. influenzae*, and meningococcus as well as postoperative antibiotics prophylaxis (usually penicillin) is recommended by most authors. Although the optimal length of antibiotic prophylaxis is unclear, the highest rate of OPSI appears to occur within the first 2 years. An adult study of sepsis in patients splenectomized as children noted an estimated frequency of late postsplenectomy infections of 0.69 and deaths at 0.46 per 1,000 patient years.[117] Of interest, one of the surviving patients had low antibody levels against pneumococcal serotypes despite pneumococcal meningitis and subsequent vaccinations, suggesting that nonresponders may be at increased risk for OPSI.

REFERENCES

1. King H, Shumacker HB Jr. Splenic studies: I. Susceptibility to infection after splenectomy performed in infancy. Ann Surg 1952:136:239–42.
2. Douglas GJ, Simpson JS. The conservative management of splenic trauma. J Pediatr Surg 1971:6:565–70.
3. Delaitre B, Maignien B. Splenectomy by the coelioscopic approach: Report of a case. Presse Med 1991;20:2263.

4. Tulman S, Holcomb GW III, Karamanoukian HL, et al. Pediatric laparoscopic splenectomy. J Pediatr Surg 1993;26:689–92.

5. Nossal GJV, Austin CM, Pye J, et al. Antigens in immunity: XII. Antigen trapping in the spleen. Int Arch Allergy Appl Immunol 1966;29:368–83.

6. Pearson HA. The spleen and disturbances of splenic function. In: Nathan DG, Orkin SH, editors. Hematology of Infancy and Childhood, vol. II. 5th ed. Philadelphia: WB Saunders; 1998. p. 1051–68.

7. Rowley DA. The effect of splenectomy on the formation of circulating antibody in the adult male albino rat. J Immunol 1950;64:289.

8. Rowley DA. The formation of circulating antibody in the splenectomized human being following intravenous injection of heterologous erythrocytes. J Immunol 1950;65:515.

9. Meyer AA. Spleen. In: Greenfield LJ, Mulholland MW, Oldham KT, et al, editors. Surgery. 2nd ed. Philadelphia: Lippincott-Raven; 1997. p. 1262–81.

10. Anderson C, Devine WA, Anderson RH, et al. Abnormalities of the spleen in relation to congenital malformations of the heart: A survey of necropsy findings in children. Br Heart J 1990;63: 122–8.

11. Tu ST, Wu JM, Yeh BH, et al. Intestinal obstruction in asplenia syndrome: Report of three cases. Acta Paediatr Sin 1994;35: 70–7.

12. Skandalakis LJ, Gray SW, Ricketts R, et al. The spleen. In: Skandalakis JE, Gray SW, editors. Embryology for Surgeons. 2nd ed. Baltimore: Williams & Wilkins; 1994. p. 334–65.

13. Greig JD, Sweet EM, Drainer IK. Splenic torsion in a wandering spleen, presenting as an acute abdominal mass. J Pediatr Surg 1994;29:571–2.

14. Schmidt SP, Andrews HG, White JJ. The splenic snood: An improved approach for the management of the wandering spleen. J Pediatr Surg 1992;27:1043–4.

15. Lebron R, Self M, Mangram A, et al. Wandering spleen presenting as recurrent pancreatitis. J Soc Laparoendosc Surg 2008; 12:310–13.

16. Allen KB, Andrews G. Pediatric wandering spleen—the case for splenopexy: Review of 35 reported cases in the literature. J Pediatr Surg 1989;24:432–5.

17. Lacreuse I, Moog R, Kauffmann I, et al. Laparoscopic splenopexy for wandering spleen in a child. J Laparoendosc Adv Surg Tech 2007;17:255–7.

18. Caracicolo F, Bonatti PC, Castruci G, et al. Wandering spleen: Treatment with colonic displacement. J R Coll Surg Edinb 1986;31:242–4.

19. Stringel G, Soucy P, Mercer S. Torsion of the wandering spleen: Splenectomy or splenopexy? J Pediatr Surg 1982;17: 373–5.

20. Upadhyaya P, St Peter SD, Holcomb GW III. Laparoscopic splenopexy and cystectomy for an enlarged wandering spleen and splenic cyst. J Pediatr Surg 2007;42:E23–7.

21. Rescorla FJ, West KW, Engum SA, et al. Laparoscopic splenic procedures in children: Experience in 231 children. Ann Surg 2007;246:683–8.

22. Palanivelu C, Rangarajan M, Senthilkumar DR, et al. Laparoscopic mesh splenopexy (sandwich technique) for wandering spleen. J Soc Laparoendosc Surg 2007;11:246–51.

23. Misawa T, Yoshida K, Shiba H, et al. Wandering spleen with chronic torsion. Am J Surg 2008;195:504–5.

24. Halpert B, Alden ZA. Accessory spleens in or at the tail of the pancreas. Arch Pathol 1964;77:652.

25. Halpert B, Gyorkey F. Lesions observed in accessory spleens of 311 patients. Am J Clin Pathol 1959;32:165.

26. Gigot JF, Jamar F, Ferrant A, et al. Inadequate detection of accessory spleens and splenosis with laparoscopic splenectomy: A shortcoming of the laparoscopic approach in hematologic diseases. Surg Endosc 1998;12:101–6.

27. Targarona EM, Espert JJ, Balagué C, et al. Residual splenic function after laparoscopic splenectomy: A clinical concern. Arch Surg 1998;133:56–60.

28. Crawford DL, Pickens PV, Moore JT. Hypertrophied splenic remnants in hereditary spherocytosis. Contemp Surg 1998;53:103–4.

29. Putschar WGJ, Manion WC. Splenic-gonadal fusion. Am J Pathol 1986;32:15.

30. Emmett JM, Dreyfuss ML. Accessory spleen in the scrotum: Review of literature on ectopic spleens and their associated surgical significance. Ann Surg 1943;117:754.

31. Tsakayannis DE, Mitchell K, Kozakewich HPW, et al. Splenic preservation in the management of splenic epidermoid cysts in children. J Pediatr Surg 1995;30:1468–70.

32. Rathaus V, Zissin R, Goldberg E. Spontaneous rupture of an epidermoid cyst of the spleen: Preoperative ultrasonographic diagnosis. J Clin Ultrasound 1991;19:235–7.

33. Akhan O, Baykan Z, Oguzkurta L, et al. Percutaneous treatment of a congenital splenic cyst with alcohol: A new therapeutic approach. Eur Radiol 1997;7:1067–70.

34. Moir C, Guttman F, Jequier S, et al. Splenic cysts: Aspiration, sclerosis, or resection. J Pediatr Surg 1989;24:646–8.

35. Morgenstern L. Nonparasitic splenic cysts: Pathogenesis, classification, and treatment. J Am Coll Surg 2002;194:306–14.

36. Fisher JC, Gurung B, Cowles RA. Recurrence after laparoscopic excision of nonparasitic splenic cysts. J Pediatr Surg 2008;43: 1644–8.

37. Schier F, Waag KL, Ure B. Laparoscopic unroofing of splenic cysts results in a high rate of recurrences. J Pediatr Surg 2007;42:1860–3.

38. Fan H, Zhang D, Zhao, X, et al. Laparoscopic partial splenectomy for large splenic epidermoid cyst. Chin Med J 2011;124:1751–3.

39. Keckler SJ, Peter SD, Tsao K, et al. Laparoscopic excision of splenic cysts: A comparison to the open approach. Eur J Pediatr Surg 2010;20:287–9.

40. McColl RJ, Hochman DJ, Sample C. Laparoscopic management of splenic cysts: Marsupialization, cavity lining with surgicel and omentectomy to prevent recurrence. Surg Laparosc Endosc Percutan Tech 2007;17:455–8.

41. Young NS, Brown KE. Parvovirus B19. N Engl J Med 2004;350:2006–7.

42. Davis PW, Williams DA, Shamberger RC. Immune thrombocytopenia: Surgical therapy and predictors of response. J Pediatr Surg 1991;26:407–13.

43. Holt D, Brown J, Terrill K, et al. Response to intravenous immunoglobulin predicts splenectomy response in children with immune thrombocytopenic purpura. Pediatrics 2003;111:87–9.

44. Hood JH, Partrick DA, Hays T, et al. Predicting response to splenectomy in children with immune thrombocytopenic purpura. J Pediatr Surg 2010;45:140–4.

45. Hollander LL, Leys CM, Weil BR, et al. Predictive value of response to steroid therapy on response to splenectomy in children with immune thrombocytopenic purpura. Surgery 2011;150: 643–8.

46. Bromberg ME. Immune thrombocytopenic purpura-the changing therapeutic landscape. N Engl J Med 2006;355:1643–5.

47. Bussel JB, Kluter DJ, Phil D, et al. AMG 531, a thrombopoiesis-stimulating protein, for chronic ITP. N Engl J Med 2006;355: 1672–81.

48. Kuter DJ, Phil D, Rummel M, et al. Romiplostim or standard care in patients with immune thrombocytopenia. NEJM 2010;363: 1889–961.

49. Lesher AP, Kalpatthi R, Glenn JB, et al. Outcome of splenectomy in children younger than 4 years with sickle cell disease. J Pediatr Surg 2009;44:1134–8.

50. Fonkalsrud EW, Philippart M, Feig S. Ninety-five percent splenectomy for massive splenomegaly: A new surgical approach. J Pediatr Surg 1990;25:267–9.

51. Holcomb GW III, Greene HL. Fetal intra-abdominal hemorrhage following partial splenectomy for Gaucher's disease. J Pediatr Surg 1993;18:1572–4.

52. Geiger JD, Dinh VV, Teitelbaum DH, et al. The lateral approach for open splenectomy. J Pediatr Surg 1998;33:1153–6.

53. Farah RA, Rogers ZR, Thompson RW, et al. Comparison of laparoscopic and open splenectomy in children with hematologic disorders. J Pediatr 1997;131:41–6.

54. Minkes RK, Lagzdins M, Langer JC. Laparoscopic versus open splenectomy in children. J Pediatr Surg 2000;35:699–701.

55. Reddy VS, Phan HH, O'Neill JA, et al. Laparoscopic versus open splenectomy in the pediatric population: A contemporary single-center experience. Am Surg 2001;67:859–63.

56. Rescorla FJ, Breitfeld PP, West KW, et al. A case-controlled comparison of open laparoscopic splenectomy in children. Surgery 1996;124:670–6.

57. Misawa T, Yoshida K, Iida T, et al. Minimizing intraoperative bleeding using a vessel sealing system and splenic hilum hanging maneuver in laparoscopic splenectomy. J Hepatobiliary Pancreat Surg 2009;16:786–91.

58. Gelmini R, Romano F, Quaranta N, et al. Sutureless and stapleless laparoscopic splenectomy using radiofrequency: LigaSure device. Surg Endosc 2006;20:991–4.

59. Kennedy JS, Stranahan PL, Taylor KD, et al. High burst strength, feedback controlled bipolar vessel sealing. Surg Endosc 1998;12:876–8.

60. Vecchio R, Marchese S, Swehli E, et al. Splenic hilum management during laparoscopic splenectomy. J Laparoendosc Adv Surg Tech 2011;21:717–20.

61. Machado NO, Kindy NA, Chopra PJ. Laparoscopic splenectomy using LigaSure. JSLS 2010;14:547–52.

62. Romano F, Gelmini R, Caprotti R, et al. Laparoscopic splenectomy: Ligasure versus EndoGIA: A comparative study. J Laparoendosc Adv Surg Tech 2007;17:763–7.

63. Lai PB, Leung KL, Ho WS, et al. The use of liposucker for spleen retrieval after laparoscopic splenectomy. Surg Laparosc Endosc Percutan Tech 2000;10:39–40.

64. Ransom KJ, Kavic MS. Laparoscopic splenectomy following embolization for blunt trauma. J Soc Laparoendosc Surg 2008; 12:202–5.

65. Malladi P, Hungness E, Nagle A. Single access laparoscopic splenectomy. JSLS 2009;13:601–4.

66. Rottman SJ, Podolsky ER, Kim E, et al. Single port access (SPA) splenectomy. JSLS 2010;14:48–52.

67. Hansen EN, Muensterer OJ. Single incision laparoscopic splenectomy in a 5-year-old with hereditary spherocytosis. JSLS 2010; 14:286–8.

68. Colon MJ, Telem D, Chan E, et al. Laparoendoscopic single site (LESS) splenectomy with a conventional laparoscope and instruments. JSLS 2011;15:384–6.

69. Thalhammer GH, Eber E, Uranus S, et al. Partial splenectomy in cystic fibrosis patients with hypersplenism. Arch Dis Child 2003;88:143–6.

70. Havlik RJ, Touloukian RJ, Markowitz RI, et al. Partial splenectomy for symptomatic splenic hamartoma. J Pediatr Surg 1990;25:1273–5.

71. Rice HE, Oldham KT, Hillery CA, et al. Clinical and hematologic benefits of partial splenectomy for congenital hemolytic anemias in children. Ann Surg 2003;237:281–8.

72. Diesen DL, Zimmerman SA, Thornburg CD, et al. Partial splenectomy for children with congenital hemolytic anemia and massive splenomegaly. J Pediatr Surg 2008;43:466–72.

73. Héry G, Becmeur F, Méfat L, et al. Laparoscopic partial splenectomy: Indications and results of a multicenter retrospective study. Surg Endosc 2008;22:45–9.

74. Bader-Meunier B, Gauthier F, Archambaud F, et al. Long-term evaluation of the beneficial effect of subtotal splenectomy for management of hereditary spherocytosis. Blood 2001;97:399–403.

75. de Buys Roessingh AS, de Lagausie P, Rohrlich P, et al. Follow-up of partial splenectomy in children with hereditary spherocytosis. J Pediatr Surg 2002;37:1459–63.

76. Buesing KL, Tracy ET, Kiernan C, et al. Partial splenectomy for hereditary spherocytosis: A multi-institutional review. J Pediatr Surg 2011;46:178–83.

77. Stoehr GA, Stauffer UG, Eber SW. Near-total splenectomy: A new technique for the management of hereditary spherocytosis. Ann Surg 2005;241:40–7.

78. Slater BJ, Chan FP, Davis K, et al. Institutional experience with laparoscopic partial splenectomy for hereditary spherocytosis. J Pediatr Surg 2010;45:1682–6.

79. Morinis J, Dutta S, Blanchette V, et al. Laparoscopic partial vs. total splenectomy in children with hereditary spherocytosis. J Pediatr Surg 2008;43:1649–52.

80. Seims AD, Croop JM, Rescorla FJ. Efficacy of laparoscopic partial splenectomy in the management of hereditary spherocytosis: An institutional review. Poster presentation at American Society of Pediatric Hematology Oncology, Baltimore, MD, 2011.

81. Esposito C, Schaarschmidt K, Settimi A, et al. Experience with laparoscopic splenectomy. J Pediatr Surg 2001;36:309–11.

82. Katkhouda N, Hurwitz MB, Rivera RT, et al. Laparoscopic splenectomy: Outcome and efficacy in 103 consecutive patients. Ann Surg 1998;228:568–78.

83. Szold A, Kamat M, Nadu A, et al. Laparoscopic accessory splenectomy for recurrent idiopathic thrombocytopenic purpura and hemolytic anemia. Surg Endosc 2000;14:761–3.

84. Choi YU, Dominguez EP, Sherman V, et al. Laparoscopic accessory splenectomy for recurrent idiopathic thrombocytopenic purpura. J Soc Laparoendosc Surg 2008;12:314–17.

85. Feldman LS, Demyttenaere SV, Polyhronopoulos GN, et al. Refining the selection criteria for laparoscopic versus open splenectomy for splenomegaly. J Laparoendosc Adv Surg Tech 2008;16:13–19.

86. Pietrabissa A, Morelli L, Peri A, et al. Laparoscopic treatment of splenomegaly: A case for hand-assisted laparoscopic surgery. Arch Surg 2011;146:818–23.

87. Swanson TW, Meneghetti AT, Sampath S, et al. Hand-assisted laparoscopic splenectomy versus open splenectomy for massive splenomegaly: 20-year experience at a Canadian centre. Can J Surg 2011;54:189–93.

88. Koshenkov VP, Nemeth ZH, Carter MS. Laparoscopic splenectomy: Outcome and efficacy for massive and supramassive spleens. Am J Surg 2012;203:517–22.

89. Rescorla FJ, Engum SA, West KW, et al. Laparoscopic splenectomy has become the gold standard in children. Am Surg 2002;68:297–302.

90. Terrosu G, Baccarani U, Bresadola V, et al. The impact of splenic weight on laparoscopic splenectomy for splenomegaly. Surg Endosc 2002;16:103–7.

91. Murawski M, Patkowski D, Korlacki W, et al. Laparoscopic splenectomy in children-a multicenter experience. J Pediatr Surg 2008;43:951–4.

92. Park AE, Birgisson G, Mastrangela MJ, et al. Laparoscopic splenectomy: Outcomes and lessons learned from over 200 cases. Surgery 2000;128:660–6.

93. Casaccia M, Torelli P, Pasa A, et al. Putative predictive parameters for the outcome of laparoscopic splenectomy. Ann Surg 2010; 251:287–91.

94. Mattioli G, Avanzini S, Prato AP, et al. Spleen surgery in pediatric age: Seven-year unicenter experience. J Laparoendosc Adv Surg Tech 2009;19:437–41.

95. Goers T, Panepinto J, DeBaun M, et al. Laparoscopic versus open abdominal surgery in children with sickle cell disease is associated with a shorter hospital stay. Pediatr Blood Cancer 2008;50:603–6.

96. Alwabari A, Parida L, Al-Salem AH. Laparoscopic splenectomy and/or cholecystectomy for children with sickle cell disease. Pediatr Surg Int 2009;25:417–21.

97. Waldhausen JHT, Tapper D. Is pediatric laparoscopic splenectomy safe and cost effective? Arch Surg 1997;132:822–4.

98. Winslow ER, Brunt LM. Perioperative outcomes of laparoscopic versus open splenectomy: A meta-analysis with an emphasis on complications. Surgery 2003;134:647–53.

99. Friedman RL, Hiatt JR, Korman JL, et al. Laparoscopic or open splenectomy for hematologic disease: Which approach is superior? J Am Coll Surg 1997;185:49–54.

100. Lansdale N, Marven S, Welch J, et al. Intra-abdominal splenosis following laparoscopic splenectomy causing recurrence in a child with chronic immune thrombocytopenic purpura. J Laparoendosc Adv Surg Tech 2007;17:387–91.

101. Pietrabissa A, Moretto C, Antonelli G, et al. Thombosis in the portal venous system after elective laparoscopic splenectomy. Surg Endosc 2004;18:1140–3.

102. Winslow ER, Brunt LM, Drebin JA, et al. Portal vein thrombosis after splenectomy. Am J Surg 2002;184:631–6.

103. Ikeda M, Sekimoto M, Takiguchi S, et al. Total splenic vein thrombosis after laparoscopic splenectomy: A possible candidate for treatment. Am J Surg 2007;193:21–5.

104. Stamou KM, Toutouzas KG, Kekis PB, et al. Prospective study of the incidence and risk factors of postsplenectomy thrombosis of the portal, mesenteric, and splenic veins. Arch Surg 2006;141: 663–9.

105. Soyer T, Ciftci AO, Tanyel FC, et al. Portal vein thrombosis after splenectomy in pediatric hematologic disease: Risk factors, clinical features, and outcome. J Pediatr Surg 2006;41:1899–902.

106. Lynch AM, Kapila R. Overwhelming postsplenectomy infection. Infect Dis Clin North Am 1996:4:693–707.

107. Jugenburg M, Haddock G, Freedman MH, et al. The morbidity and mortality of pediatric splenectomy: Does prophylaxis make a difference? J Pediatr Surg 1999;34:1064–7.

108. Meekes I, van der Staak, van Oostrom C. Results of splenectomy performed on a group of 91 children. Eur J Pediatr Surg 1995;5:19–22.
109. Eraklis AJ, Kewy SV, Diamond LK. Hazard of overwhelming infection after splenectomy in childhood. N Engl J Med 1967;276:1225–9.
110. Horan M, Colebatch JH. Relation between splenectomy and subsequent infection. Arch Dis Child 1962;37:398–414.
111. Ellison EC, Fabri PJ. Complications of splenectomy. Surg Clin North Am 1983;63:1313–30.
112. Styrt B. Infection associated with asplenia: Risks, mechanisms, and prevention. Am J Med 1990;88:33–42.
113. Holdsworth RJ, Irving AD, Cuschieri A. Postsplenectomy sepsis and its mortality rate: Actual versus perceived risks. Br J Surg 1991;78:1031–8.
114. Ejstrud P, Kristensen B, Hansen JB, et al. Risk and patterns of bacteraemia after splenectomy: A population-based study. Scand J Infect Dis 2000;32:521.
115. Bridgen ML. Overwhelming post-splenectomy infection-still a problem. West J Med 1992;157:440–3.
116. Bridgen ML, Pattullo AL. Prevention and management of overwhelming postsplenectomy infection-an update. Crit Care Med 1999;27:836–42.
117. Eber SW, Langendorfer CM, Ditzig M, et al. Frequency of very late fatal sepsis after splenectomy for hereditary spherocytosis: Impact of insufficient antibody response to pneumococcal infection. Ann Hematol 1999;78:524–8.

CHAPTER 48

CONGENITAL ABDOMINAL WALL DEFECTS

Saleem Islam

Abdominal wall defects are divided into omphalocele and gastroschisis. While often considered together, they are distinct and separate entities. Differences between gastroschisis and omphalocele are illustrated in Figure 48-1 and summarized in Table 48-1.

EMBRYOLOGY AND ETIOLOGY

The abdominal wall forms during the fourth week of gestation when differential growth of the embryo causes infolding in the craniocaudal and mediolateral directions. During the sixth week, rapid intestinal and liver growth leads to herniation of the midgut into the umbilical cord. Elongation and rotation of the midgut occurs over the ensuing four weeks. By week 10, the midgut returns to the abdominal cavity where the first, second, and third portions of the duodenum and the ascending and descending colon assume their fixed, retroperitoneal positions.

The current understanding of the etiology for an omphalocele suggests that this defect is not from a failure in body wall closure or migration. Rather, since the umbilical cord is attached to the sac, it is thought that an omphalocele develops due to a failure of the viscera to return to the abdominal cavity. Other intra-abdominal viscera including liver, bladder, stomach, ovary, and testis can also be found in the omphalocele sac. The sac consists of the covering layers of the umbilical cord and includes amnion, Wharton's jelly, and peritoneum. The location of the defect is in the mid-abdominal or central region, but may occur in the epigastric or hypogastric regions as well.

The etiology for gastroschisis is less clear. One theory suggests that gastroschisis results from failure of the mesoderm to form in the anterior abdominal wall. Currently, the ventral body folds theory, which suggests failure of migration of the lateral folds (more frequent on the right side), is most widely accepted.[1] This implies a gastroschisis develops early in gestation and prior to development of an omphalocele. Due to the increasing incidence of gastroschisis, there are a number of possible causative factors including tobacco, certain environmental exposures, lower maternal age and low socioeconomic status, all suggested by epidemiologic studies, but not proven.[1-4]

GASTROSCHISIS

Prenatal Management and Diagnosis

Gastroschisis occurs in 1 in 4,000 live births.[5] An increased incidence in mothers younger than 21 years of age has been widely documented.[6] There has also been a significant worldwide increase in the incidence of gastroschisis in all age groups over the past two decades.[7] Preterm delivery is more frequent in infants with gastroschisis, with an incidence of 28% compared with only 6% in babies without an abdominal wall defect.[8]

The majority of pregnancies complicated by gastroschisis are diagnosed sonographically by 20 weeks' gestation.[2,3] Often an ultrasound (US) evaluation is performed because of an abnormal maternal serum α-fetoprotein (AFP) level, which is universally elevated in the presence of gastroschisis.[9,10] Detection of bowel loops freely floating in the amniotic fluid and a defect in the abdominal wall to the right of a normal umbilical cord are diagnostic of gastroschisis. Intrauterine growth retardation (IUGR) has been noted in a large number of these fetuses as well.[11]

Some authors advocate selective preterm delivery based on the finding of bowel distention and thickening on prenatal ultrasound.[12] Dilated fetal bowel has been shown to correlate with a worse outcome, including fetal distress and demise in some series, but not in others.[13] One problem with using bowel dilatation to predict outcome is the lack of a definition of 'dilated,' with ranges from 7 to 25 mm being considered abnormal.[14,15] Moreover, there is also variability in the part of the intestine that is being measured. Studies in animal models have shown that the duration of amniotic fluid exposure is correlated with the degree of the inflammatory peel and intestinal dysmotility.[16-19] Efforts to reduce this exposure by either amniotic fluid exchange or intrauterine furosemide treatment, which induces fetal diuresis, have shown to be beneficial in animals.[19-22] These studies spurred early human trials with amniotic fluid exchange in Paris and Italy, but these trials have proven inconclusive.[20,23]

Concomitant bowel atresia is the most common associated anomaly in patients with gastroschisis, with rates ranging from 6.9–28% in several series (Table 48-2).[24,25] A recent literature review noted associated anomalies in the cardiac, pulmonary, nervous, musculoskeletal, genitourinary systems, as well as chromosomal abnormalities in babies with gastroschisis.[33]

Perinatal Care

The optimal mode and timing of delivery for a fetus with gastroschisis has been debated for many years.

TABLE 48-1 Differentiating Characteristics between Gastroschisis and Omphalocele

Characteristic	Omphalocele	Gastroschisis
Herniated viscera	Bowel ± liver	Bowel only
Sac	Present	Absent
Associated anomalies	Common (50%)	Uncommon (<10%)
Location of defect	Umbilicus	Right of umbilicus
Mode of delivery	Vaginal/cesarean	Vaginal
Surgical management	Nonurgent	Urgent
Prognostic factors	Associated anomalies	Condition of bowel

Proponents of routine cesarean delivery (C-section) argue that the process of vaginal birth results in injury or increased risks for infection and sepsis.[34] However, the literature suggests that both vaginal delivery and C-section are safe.[35,36] A recent meta-analysis failed to demonstrate a difference in outcomes for infants delivered either vaginally or by C-section.[37] Therefore, the delivery method should be at the discretion of the obstetrician and the mother, with C-section reserved for obstetric indications or fetal distress.

Preterm delivery of the fetus with gastroschisis has been advocated to limit exposure of the bowel to the amniotic fluid.[12] Interleukin-6, interleukin-8, and ferritin are elevated in the amniotic fluid in fetuses with gastroschisis when compared with controls.[18,38] Damage to the pacemaker cells and nerve plexi may contribute to the profound dysmotility and malabsorption seen in these infants.[39] Early delivery may mitigate these effects, but the literature is mixed.[12] A randomized trial from the UK found no benefit after induced early delivery with the only trends being an improvement in length of hospitalization and earlier initiation of feeding.[40] Another study demonstrated that birth weight less than 2 kg was associated with increased morbidity.[41] Currently available

TABLE 48-2 Treatment Options in Patients with Gastroschisis and Intestinal Atresia

Study	Number of Patients	Drop in	Anastomosis	Stoma
Amoury et al. 1977[26]	6	–	3	3
Pokorny et al. 1981[27]	5	1	–	4
Gornall 1989[28]	5	1	3	1
Shah and Woolley 1991[29]	4	3	–	1
Hoehner et al. 1998[30]	13	–	8	5
Fleet and de la Hunt 2000[31]	10	6	–	4
Emil et al. 2012[32]	8	7	–	1

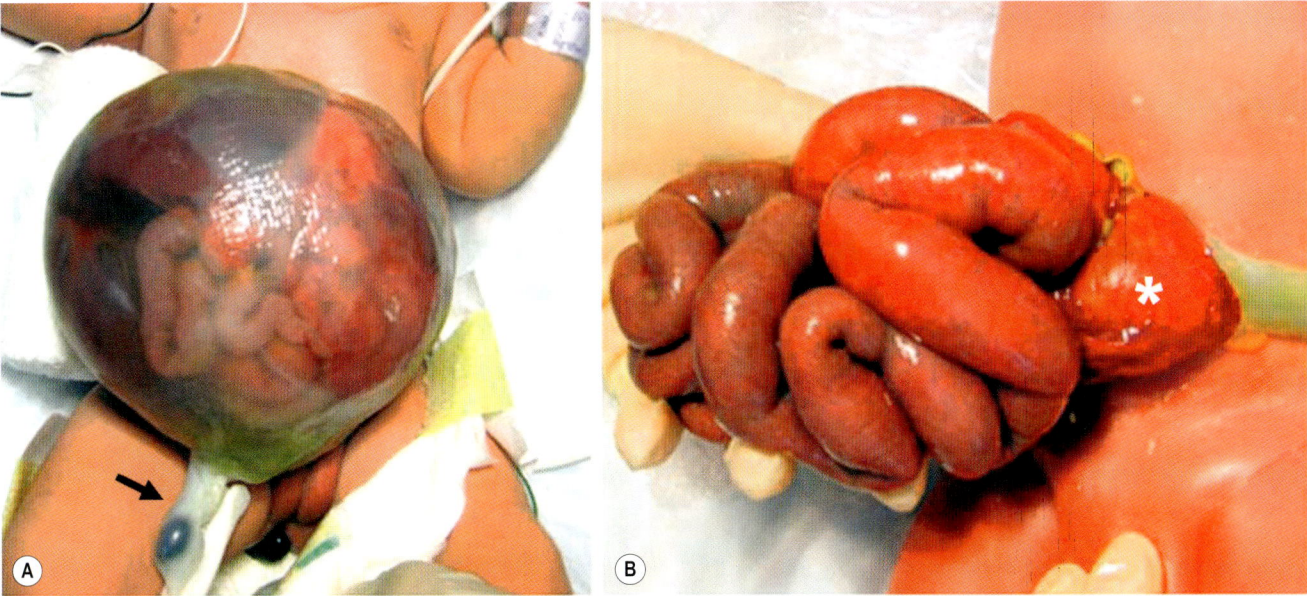

FIGURE 48-1 ■ These two photographs nicely depict the differences between an omphalocele and gastroschisis. **(A)** In an omphalocele both the liver and bowel can be herniated. A sac is always present and the umbilical cord (arrow) inserts onto the sac. Moreover, this is always a midline defect. **(B)** With a gastroschisis, the liver is never herniated and a sac is absent. The location of the fascial defect is to the right of the umbilicus, and the umbilical cord is attached to the umbilicus. In addition to the large and small intestine, the stomach (asterisk) can sometimes be herniated as well.

evidence does not support elective preterm delivery for gastroschisis.[42]

Neonatal Resuscitation and Management

Neonates with gastroschisis have significant evaporative water losses from the open abdominal cavity and exposed bowel. Appropriate intravenous access should be obtained and fluid resuscitation initiated after birth. Nasogastric (NG) decompression is important to prevent further gastric and intestinal distention. Routine endotracheal intubation is not necessary. The bowel should be wrapped in warm saline-soaked gauze and placed in a central position on the abdominal wall. The neonate should be positioned on the right side to prevent kinking of the mesentery with resultant bowel ischemia. The bowel should be wrapped with plastic wrap or the infant placed partially in a plastic bag to reduce evaporative losses and improve temperature homeostasis (Fig. 48-2). Although gastroschisis most often is an isolated anomaly, thorough examination of the neonate is important. In addition, the bowel must be carefully examined for intestinal atresia, necrosis, or perforation (Fig. 48-3). Recent evidence suggests that excess fluid resuscitation is detrimental and results in edema, an increase in time to closure, and an increased risk of abdominal compartment syndrome.[43]

Surgical Management

The primary goal is to return the viscera to the abdominal cavity while minimizing the risk of damage due to trauma or increased intra-abdominal pressure. The two most commonly used treatment options are placement of a silo followed by serial reductions and delayed closure, or attempted primary closure.[44] The timing and location of surgical intervention is also controversial.[45] In all cases, inspection of the bowel for obstructing bands, perforation, or atresia must be undertaken. Bands crossing the bowel loops should be lysed before silo placement or primary abdominal closure to avoid subsequent intestinal obstruction.

Primary Closure

Historically, urgent primary closure of gastroschisis was advocated in all cases. This approach is still commonly practiced in neonates in whom reduction of the herniated viscera appears possible.[46] Attempted primary closure has traditionally been performed in the operating room, but some authors have advocated primary closure at the bedside without general anesthesia.[47–49] Some surgeons prefer to close the skin only and leave the fascia separated. Others have described the use of the umbilicus as an allograft.[50,51] Prosthetic options for fascial closure include nonabsorbable mesh or bioprosthetic materials such as porcine small intestinal submucosa mesh.[52] In the past, most surgeons have excised the umbilicus during closure. However, preservation of the umbilicus has been shown to lead to an excellent cosmetic result (Fig. 48-4).[53,54]

Intra-abdominal pressure approximated from either the bladder pressure or stomach pressure can be used to

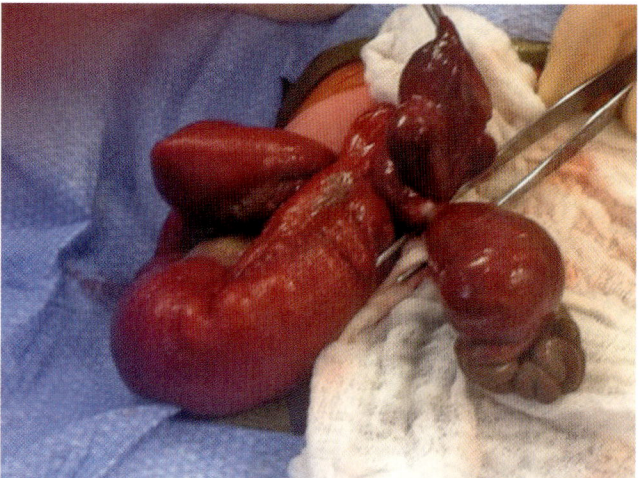

FIGURE 48-3 ■ This baby was born with gastroschisis and intestinal atresia. Note the atretic intestinal segment is being lifted up by the forceps. A silo was created and the baby underwent exploration and uneventful repair of the atresia at six weeks of age.

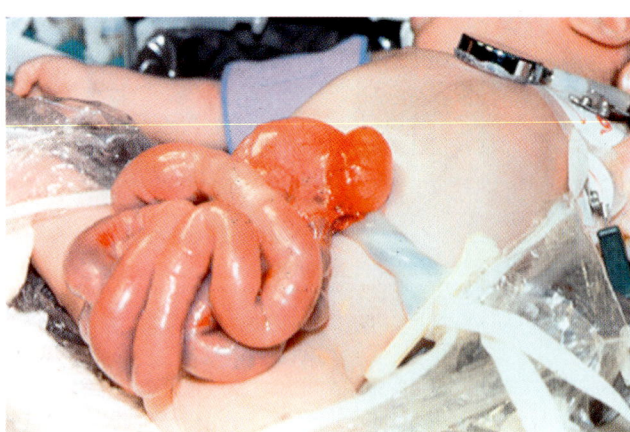

FIGURE 48-2 ■ Photograph of a neonate with gastroschisis who has been transported wrapped with a bowel bag. The bag has been untied to allow inspection of the herniated bowel.

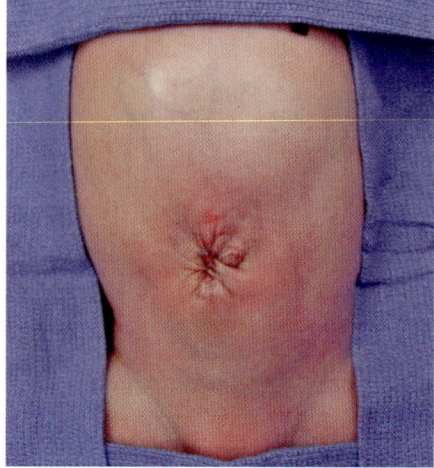

FIGURE 48-4 ■ An excellent cosmetic result after gastroschisis repair in which the umbilicus was preserved.

guide the surgeon during reduction.[55] Pressures higher than 10–15 mmHg are often associated with decreased renal and intestinal perfusion, and a silo or patch may be needed.[56] Pressures higher than 20 mmHg can lead to renal failure and bowel ischemia.[57] Similarly, an increase in central venous pressure greater than 4 mmHg has been correlated with the need for silo placement or patch closure.[58] Splanchnic perfusion pressure, the difference between mean arterial pressure and intra-abdominal pressure, has also been used to guide the reduction. A splanchnic perfusion pressure less than 44 mmHg implies a decrease in intestinal blood flow.[59]

Staged Closure

In the mid-1990s, a prefabricated silo was developed with a circular spring that is positioned under the fascial opening, without the need for sutures or general anesthesia.[60] This has made it possible to insert the silo in the delivery room or at the bedside (Fig. 48-5). After placement, the bowel is reduced daily into the abdominal cavity as the silo is shortened by sequential ligation. When the contents are entirely reduced, fascial and skin closure are performed. This process usually takes between one and 14 days with the majority being ready within a week, depending on the condition of the bowel and the infant.

Definitive closure in the operating room consists of raising small skin flaps around the fascial defect followed by fascial closure in a horizontal or vertical direction. Closure of the skin in a transverse direction creates a 'keyhole' appearance with a horizontal scar to the right of the umbilicus. This is why some surgeons advocate a vertical closure to allow for a central umbilicus. Also, a purse-string skin closure around the umbilicus can be

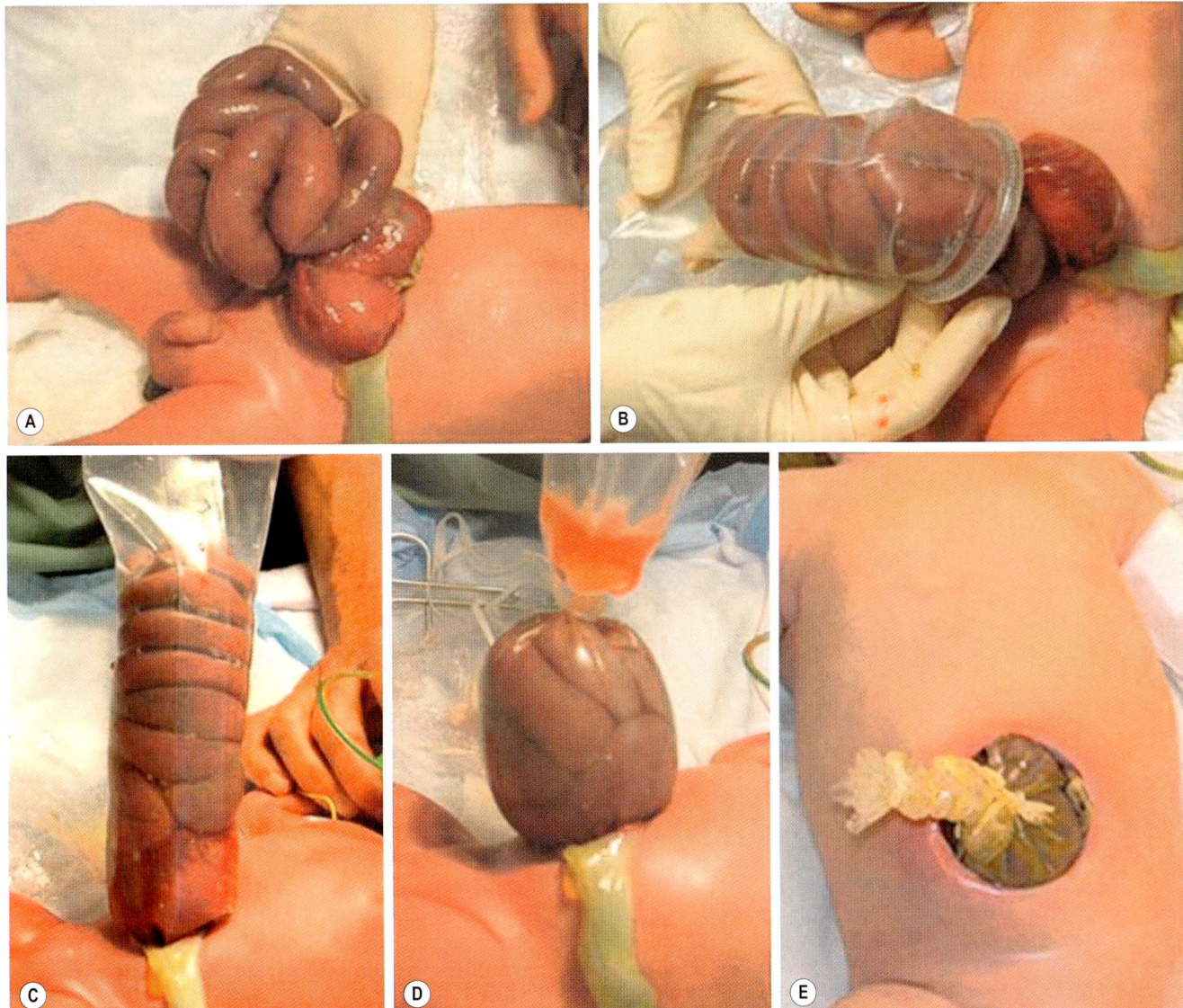

FIGURE 48-5 ■ The use of a spring-loaded prefabricated silo is shown in these photographs. **(A)** The gastroschisis defect is seen. **(B)** An appropriate-sized spring-loaded silo is then placed over the eviscerated intestine. **(C)** The ring of the silo has been positioned under the fascial defect and attached to an overhead support to keep the bowel from torquing, which may result in intestinal ischemia. **(D)** Gradual reduction of the silo is performed. **(E)** Finally, the bowel has been completely returned to the abdominal cavity and the neonate is ready for transport to the operating room for closure of the fascia and skin.

performed to create a circular scar for improved cosmesis. Recently, the 'plastic closure' method has been described in which the umbilical cord is tailored to fill the gastroschisis defect and is then covered with an adhesive dressing.[61,62] If the umbilical cord is not salvageable, the bowel can be covered with the dressing. Ingrowth of granulation tissue and epithelialization occurs over time. With this technique, an operation and general anesthesia can be avoided in many infants. Residual ventral hernia rates are reported to be 60–84%, the majority of which close spontaneously.[54]

The routine use of a preformed silo has increasingly come into favor, with the theory being that avoidance of high intra-abdominal pressure will avoid ischemic injury to the viscera and allow earlier extubation.[60,63] One study reported fewer days on mechanical ventilation for patients undergoing silo reduction when compared to primary closure.[47] However, there was no difference in time to full feeds or days on parenteral nutrition. Two reports noted a similar time to full enteral feedings but found that primary closure was associated with higher mean airway pressures, oxygen requirement, vasopressor requirement, and decreased urine output.[64,65] However, other reviews have suggested that the trend to use a silo instead of immediate closure may have swung too far.[66,67] Also, recent data from the Canadian Pediatric Surgeons Network (CAPSNet) database showed that infants who are able to undergo primary closure require less parenteral nutrition and hospitalization when compared with those who required staged reduction and repair.[68] An attempt at a prospective randomized multicenter trial looking at silo vs. attempted primary closure that centered on ventilator days did not meet accrual targets and failed to show any significant difference.[69] A similar trial has begun in the U.K.[70] Current data suggests that there is no significant difference in outcome with either approach (silo vs. immediate closure) for patients with uncomplicated gastroschisis.

Management of Associated Intestinal Atresia

Up to 10% of neonates with gastroschisis have an associated atresia, most commonly jejunal or ileal. In a database review of 4,344 infants with gastroschisis, a 5% incidence of small bowel atresia and a 2% incidence of large bowel atresia was noted.[24] These atresias can be treated at the time of abdominal wall closure with resection and primary anastomosis in cases where there is minimal inflammatory peel. If the condition of the bowel makes primary anastomosis inadvisable, the bowel is reduced with the atresia intact and repair is undertaken four to six weeks after the initial abdominal wall closure.[71] Some surgeons have chosen to create a stoma, particularly in the case of a distal atresia, to allow for enteral feeding while awaiting repair.[72] If perforation is found, the perforated segment can be resected and a primary anastomosis performed if the inflammation is minimal (Fig. 48-6). Alternatively, an ostomy can be created followed by ostomy closure at a later date.[73] There is no consensus about the optimal management for these complicated problems (see Table 48-2). Patients with an atresia are considered to be

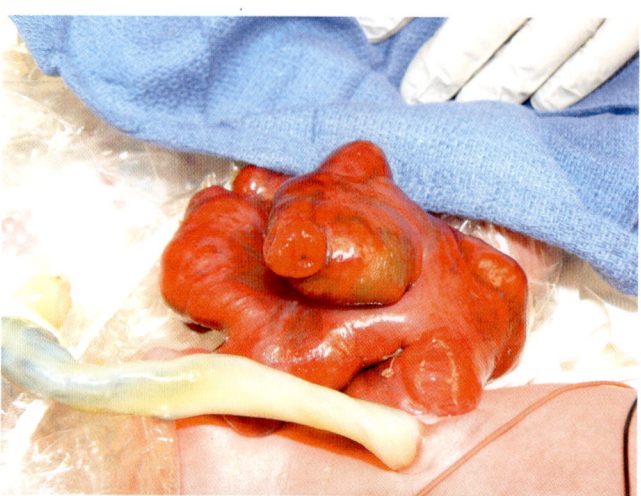

FIGURE 48-6 ■ This newborn presented with gastroschisis and intestinal perforation. Note the two lumens in the exposed segment of intestine. Because there was not significant inflammation, this perforation was closed primarily and the bowel was placed in a silo. The baby recovered uneventfully.

'complex' to differentiate them from the patients without any such association (simple). Most authors note worse outcomes with complex cases.[24,70,74]

An intestinal atresia should be differentiated from 'vanishing bowel' in infants with gastroschisis. This condition is usually associated with a very small abdominal wall defect and is characterized by necrosis and disappearance of some or all of the intestine (Fig. 48-7). Although this is a rare finding, it usually results in short bowel syndrome.[75,76]

Postoperative Course

Gastroschisis is associated with abnormal intestinal motility and nutrient absorption, both of which gradually improve in most patients. Introduction of enteral feeding is often delayed for weeks while awaiting return of bowel function. During this waiting period, nasogastric decompression and parenteral nutrition is required. When bowel activity occurs, enteral feeds can be started and slowly advanced. Because progression to full enteral feeding can take weeks, central venous access is important. Early oral stimulation is recommended to prevent loss of the sucking reflex.

Prokinetic medication may be helpful. In a rabbit model of gastroschisis, cisapride improved contractility of newborn intestine whereas erythromycin improved motility in control adult tissue only.[77] However, a randomized controlled trial of erythromycin versus placebo found that enterally administered erythromycin did not improve time to achieve full enteral feedings.[78] A similar randomized trial examining the use of cisapride in postoperative neonates, most of whom had gastroschisis, showed a beneficial effect, but this drug is not available in the USA.[79]

Long-Term Outcomes

Long-term outcomes for patients born with gastroschisis are generally excellent. The presence of complex disease

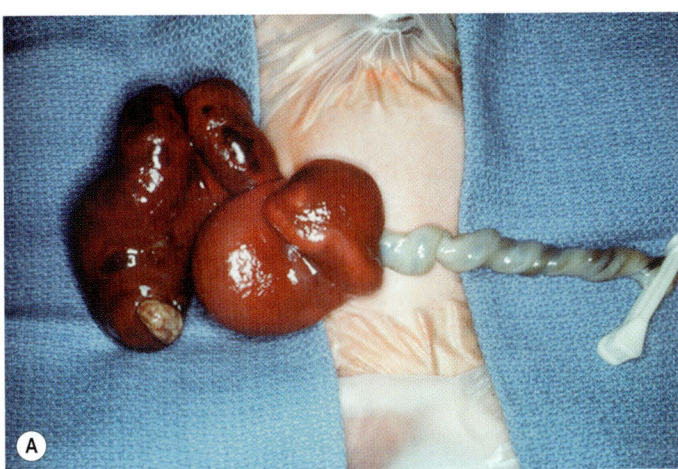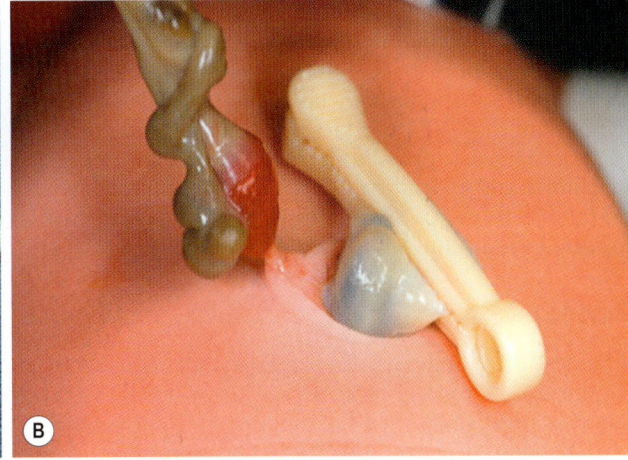

FIGURE 48-7 ■ These two photographs show different neonates with the prenatal diagnosis of gastroschisis. In each instance, the herniated intestine has died. At exploration, each patient was found to have short bowel syndrome due to very little small intestine.

is the most important prognostic determinant for a poor outcome.[80,81] A number of authors have attempted to stratify patients with gastroschisis according to risk.[82] A recent population-based cohort study from the UK with 301 patients noted that babies with complex gastroschisis took a median of 21 days longer to reach full enteral feedings, had a longer total parenteral nutrition (TPN) use, and had almost 2 months longer length of hospitalization.[70] In addition, they were twice as likely to develop intestinal failure and six times more likely to develop liver disease. Another study noted an increased incidence of central venous catheter-related sepsis, a longer time to full enteral feeding, and a longer hospital stay in infants with gastroschisis complicated by atresia or necrotic bowel.[83] Gastroschisis is the most common reason for intestinal transplantation.[84] The ability to risk-stratify gastroschisis patients with respect to increased morbidity and mortality has utility in counseling families, predicting hospital utilization, and identifying a group of patients who would benefit from further strategies to improve outcomes.

Necrotizing enterocolitis (NEC) has been found in full-term infants with gastroschisis in higher than expected frequencies (up to 18.5%).[85] Significant bowel loss from NEC can predispose to short bowel syndrome and its associated hepatic and infectious complications. On the other hand, another group found that the clinical course of babies with gastroschisis who developed NEC often had an uncomplicated course.[86] There is a report suggesting that infants with gastroschisis who were fed breast milk had a lower incidence of NEC than those fed with formula.[87]

Most gastroschisis patients have some degree of intestinal nonrotation. This is typically not repaired at the time of closure and does not have the same incidence of midgut volvulus as other causes of malrotation. However, the parents should be cautioned regarding bilious emesis and instructed to take urgent action if that occurs.

Cryptorchidism is associated with gastroschisis in 15–30% of cases.[88–90] Several retrospective analyses have shown that placement of the herniated testis into the abdominal cavity will result in normal testicular descent into the scrotum in most cases.[88] Most centers recommend allowing a year for spontaneous descent and then performing an orchiopexy if needed.[89]

If the umbilicus is sacrificed during the repair of the gastroschisis defect, up to 60% of children report psychosocial stress from not having an umbilicus.[91]

OMPHALOCELE

Prenatal Diagnosis And Management

Elevation of maternal serum AFP is also present in many pregnancies complicated by omphalocele, although not as commonly as with gastroschisis. The diagnosis of omphalocele can be made by two-dimensional ultrasound at the time of the normal 18-week ultrasound evaluation for dates. Early first trimester detection is possible if three-dimensional ultrasound is utilized.[92] The incidence of omphalocele seen at 14–18 weeks is as high as 1 in 1,100, but the incidence at birth drops to 1 in 4,000–6,000.[93] Thus there is a considerable 'hidden' mortality for a fetus with an omphalocele. One review noted that requests for termination of pregnancy in omphalocele cases were as high as 83%.[94]

Ultrasound evaluation is very useful for the detection of associated anomalies in these infants. This is important as an isolated omphalocele has a survival rate of over 90%, but is reduced with other defects.[93] Prenatal ultrasound and karyotyping are able to identify only 60–70% of the associated defects that are found postnatally.[94] One study that reviewed associated defects in omphalocele infants noted anomalies that involved every organ system, while another study found that only 14% of omphaloceles were truly isolated anomalies.[33,93] Prenatal screening in an infant with an omphalocele requires a detailed evaluation of the cardiac (14–47% incidence of anomalies) and central nervous (3–33% anomalies) systems as severe defects may lead to a discussion about termination of the pregnancy.[26] Recently, there has been some attention towards developing a reliable sonographic predictor of postnatal morbidity and survival.[95–97] Unfortunately, the prenatal finding of a 'giant' omphalocele has not been accurate in predicting outcomes. Investigators have studied ratios between the greatest omphalocele diameter compared to abdominal circumference (O/AC), the femur length (O/FL), and the head circumference (O/HC), and have attempted to correlate that with postnatal morbidity and mortality.[98,99] Of these variables, the most useful may be the O/HC.[98] Prospective studies are needed to assess the usefulness of this information.

Perinatal Care

The route of delivery of infants with an omphalocele should be dictated by obstetric considerations as C-section has not been shown to be superior.[100] Pregnancies are usually allowed to come to term, and spontaneous labor and vaginal delivery is preferred. However, despite the lack of data, many neonates with giant omphaloceles are delivered by C-section because of the fear of liver injury.

Neonatal Resuscitation And Management

After delivery, a thorough search for associated anomalies is important. All neonates should undergo an echocardiographic evaluation. Renal abnormalities can be detected by abdominal ultrasound. Neonatal hypoglycemia should alert the practitioner to the possibility of Beckwith–Weidemann syndrome. Blood samples for genetic evaluation should be obtained as well.

In preparing infants with omphalocele for transport, risks arising from associated anomalies should be specifically addressed. Infants with an omphalocele do not have as significant fluid and temperature losses as those with gastroschisis, but these losses are higher than those with an intact abdominal wall. The sac itself can be covered with saline-soaked gauze and an impervious dressing to minimize these losses. An NG tube should be inserted and placed to suction.

In some cases, the omphalocele sac may have ruptured either prenatally, during delivery, or postnatally (Fig. 48-8). A large, prenatally ruptured omphalocele is a

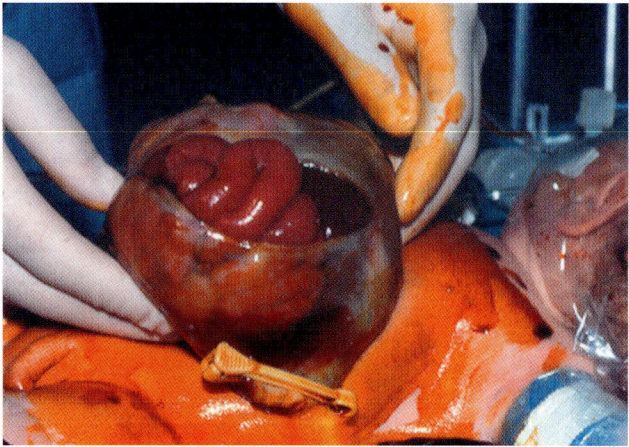

FIGURE 48-8 ■ This neonate was born with an omphalocele that ruptured during delivery. Thus, immediate management was needed. The sac was removed and a silo was created.

special situation that represents one of the most difficult problems in pediatric surgery. The goal is to cover the exposed abdominal viscera, which can be challenging. There is one small series that has good outcomes in terms of survival, but there was a high incidence of intestinal fistulas, sepsis, and pulmonary hypoplasia.[101]

Surgical Management

There are a large variety of repairs described as a 'one size fits all' option does not exist. In a recent survey, authors of reports from 1967–2009 discussing closure of 'giant' omphaloceles were asked to see if they were still using the same approach, or whether they had modified their techniques.[102] Interestingly, 42% of the authors no longer use the approach that they favored in their original article. They concluded that there is currently no completely accepted technique to treat 'giant' omphaloceles, and two methods are used the most: staged closure or delayed closure. Also, defining a giant defect is variable as some surgeons use size alone, others consider the presence or absence of the liver, while others use an estimate of the amount of intestinal contents, and still others have used a combination of the amount of liver and intestine in the sac. This lack of an accepted definition has resulted in an inability to arrive at a consensus for management.[44]

Immediate Primary Closure

Treatment options in infants with omphalocele depend on the size of the defect, the baby's gestational age, and the presence of associated anomalies. Defects that are less than 1.5 cm in diameter are referred to as hernia of the cord and are repaired shortly after birth without any issues as long as there are no associated anomalies.[103] The defects that are larger, but still easy to close without much loss of abdominal domain can also be closed soon after birth. Primary closure consists of excision of the sac and closure of the fascia and skin over the abdominal contents. It is not unusual for an omphalomesenteric duct remnant to be associated with a small omphalocele (Fig. 48-9). When dealing with a medium-sized omphalocele, care must be taken when excising the portion of the sac covering the liver, because the hepatic veins are located just under the epithelium/sac interface in the midline and can be injured. The sac is often adherent to the liver and significant hemorrhage can result from tears in the Glissen capsule. Therefore, it is usually best to leave part of the sac on the liver. The inferior portion of the sac covering the bladder can be quite thin, and excision of the sac in this area can lead to bladder injury as well. The intra-abdominal pressure can be elevated during reduction, leading to abdominal compartment syndrome.

There are a number of reports of primary closure of a 'giant' omphalocele shortly after birth with good results. In a report from London, 12 of 24 babies with a large defect had an immediate repair without any mortality. Compared to the other cases, these patients had a shorter ventilator requirement and time to full feeding.[79] However, this trial was not prospective and there was significant selection bias with using immediate repair for the full-term and normal birth weight neonates.

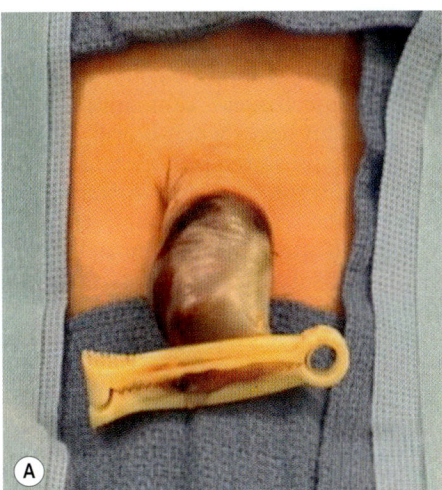
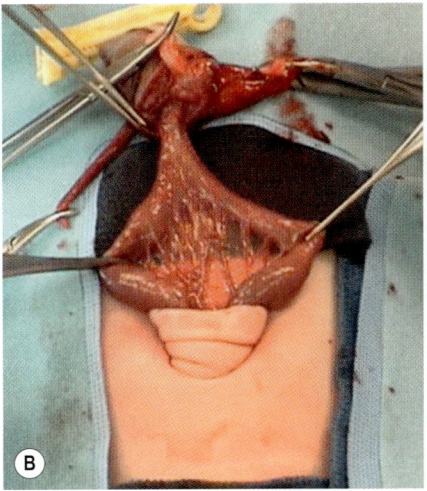
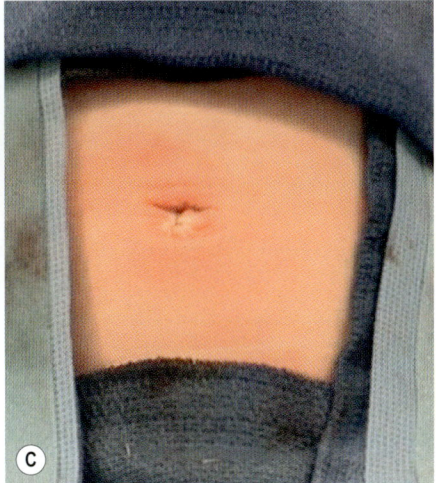

FIGURE 48-9 ■ **(A, B)** In patients with small omphaloceles, it is not unusual for an omphalomesenteric duct remnant to be found. **(C)** The diverticulum was excised primarily and the fascia and skin closed. This neonate recovered uneventfully.

Staged Neonatal Closure

In many cases, the loss of domain in the peritoneal cavity prevents primary closure without an undue increase in intra-abdominal pressure (Fig. 48-10). Multiple methods have been proposed to obtain primary abdominal wall closure in these babies.

Staged closure in the neonatal period involves the use of different techniques. These can be classified into methods that utilize the existing amnion sac with serial inversion, and those in which the sac is excised and replaced with mesh and then closed over time. Amnion inversion allows gradual reduction of the sac followed by sac excision and primary or mesh closure.[104,105] Methods involving primary repair with mesh require removal of the amnion sac with the mesh used to bridge the fascial gap followed by skin closure. Repeated procedures to excise central portions of the mesh may eventually allow native fascial closure, or mesh may be left in situ with skin over it.[44] Some authors have advocated the use of biologic mesh that allows vascular and tissue ingrowth.[106] Vacuum-assisted closure of these defects has also been described as has a novel external skin closure system.[101,107] There are many different techniques because no one method is uniformly applicable or successful.

Delayed Staged Closure

Historically, children with large omphaloceles were managed using skin flaps that were mobilized to cover the exposed viscera, leaving a large ventral hernia that could, hopefully, be closed later. In 1967, Schuster first described the use of a silastic 'silo' to allow staged reduction for children with an omphalocele.[108] With this method, the omphalocele sac is excised and the silastic sheeting is sewn to the rectus fascia. Alternatively, the silo can be sewn to the full thickness of the abdominal wall. In our experience, the use of preformed spring-loaded silos is usually unsuccessful in babies with omphalocele as the relatively large size of the defect allows the silo to become easily displaced. Serial reductions, similar to that for gastroschisis, are performed on a once- to twice-daily schedule until definitive closure can be obtained. If the fascial edges cannot be approximated in a reasonable time period, prosthetic closure can be utilized.

Scarification Treatment

Nonoperative techniques have in common the use of an agent that allows an eschar to develop over the intact amnion sac. This eschar epithelializes over time, leaving a ventral hernia that will likely require repair later in life. This approach is employed when the surgeon considers the defect too large to allow for a safe primary repair, or if the neonate has significant cardiac or respiratory issues. This is not a new concept, having evolved from the time of Dr Robert Gross who described using skin flaps in 1948.[109] The primary concern in a baby with a large omphalocele is that an initial repair will result in potential life-threatening abdominal compartment syndrome or the inability to provide skin coverage. Initial reports described mercurochrome, alcohol, and silver nitrate as the eschar-producing agents, which were very effective, but were associated with toxicity (Fig. 48-11).[110–112]

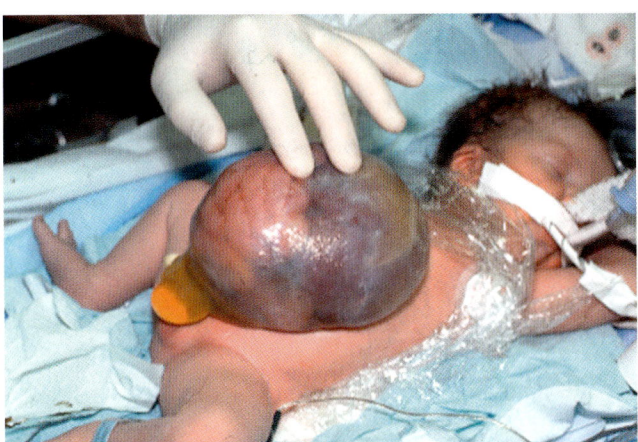

FIGURE 48-10 ■ This neonate was born with a large omphalocele. As is evident, the abdominal cavity is quite small. Primary closure is not possible in such a patient.

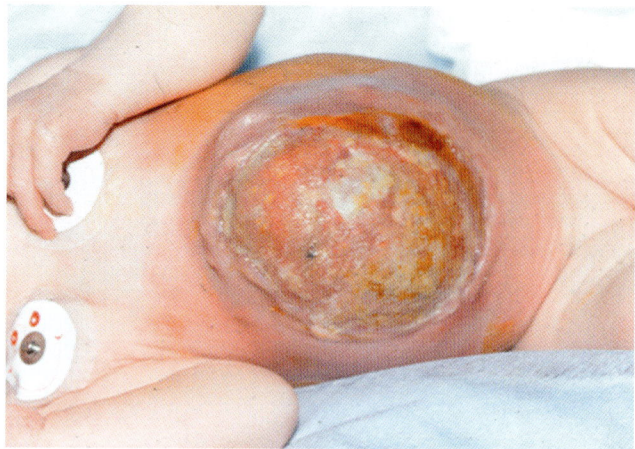

FIGURE 48-11 ■ An infant with a large omphalocele that was treated by scarification using mercurochrome. Note the intense inflammation on the abdominal wall surrounding the scarred sac. Reports of death due to mercury poisoning led to abandonment of this method.

Subsequently there have been reports of a number of substances including silver sulfadiazine, povidone-iodine solution, silver-impregnated dressings, neomycin, and polymixin/bacitracin ointments.[113] The eschar and epithelialization may take 4-10 weeks. There are also reports that combine the use of an agent listed above with compression dressing, which helps in sequentially reducing the contents into the abdomen and facilitates subsequent closure. Rarely, operative closure may not be needed as the defect contracts and closes similar to an umbilical hernia. However, most patients will eventually require closure of a ventral hernia between 1 and 5 years of age (Fig. 48-12).[114] The ventral hernia repair is performed using a variety of techniques: primary fascial closure, autologous repair with component separation, or mesh repair.[115] Although all may be successful, the number of patients in each report is small and failures are rarely reported. In some cases, innovative techniques have been utilized to recreate the abdominal domain including the use of tissue expanders (Fig. 48-13).[116] While the initial reports of the staged Gross operation had significant mortality and morbidity, current results are better.[114]

Postoperative Course

If primary closure has been accomplished, the majority of patients will require mechanical ventilation for a number of days. Feeding can begin when bowel activity resumes. Antibiotics are administered postoperatively for 48 hours unless there are signs of wound infection, in which case they are continued. If a ventral hernia develops, repair may be possible after age one year or later.

The method used for closure (primary *vs.* staged with delayed primary closure or mesh) has not been shown to affect length of hospitalization likely because the patient numbers are very small.[117] The time to enteral feeding may be shorter with primary closure, though this likely reflects a more favorable defect. In a review of treatment of omphaloceles at one institution, the authors reported a 12% incidence of complications of increased intra-abdominal pressure after closure, including acute hepatic congestion requiring reoperation, renal failure requiring dialysis, and bowel infarction.[118] In this retrospective review, wound complications including skin and fascial dehiscence occurred in up to 25% of patients undergoing primary closure.

Long-Term Outcomes

A number of long-term medical problems develop in patients with large omphaloceles.[119–121] These include gastroesophageal reflux (GERD), pulmonary insufficiency, recurrent lung infections or asthma, and feeding difficulty with failure to thrive.[122] In 23 patients with omphalocele, 43% were found to have GERD by esophageal biopsy or pH monitoring. Patients younger than 2 years had an increased rate of reflux compared with those older than two years of age.[123] Patients with large defects also had an increased incidence of reflux. In this study, only one child required a fundoplication, suggesting that reflux improves as the child ages.

Feeding difficulties can occur in up to 60% of infants with a giant omphalocele.[115] Many of these children require a gastrostomy for feeding. These difficulties seem to resolve by childhood, with height and weight measurements becoming similar to their peer group. The respiratory insufficiency associated with giant omphaloceles may be secondary to abnormal thoracic development with a

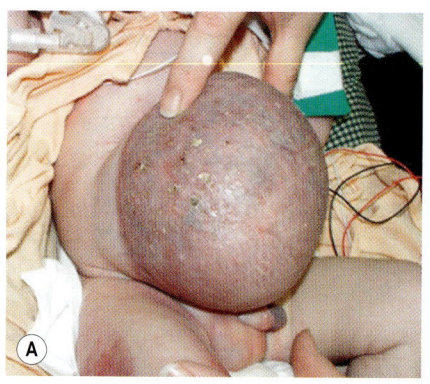
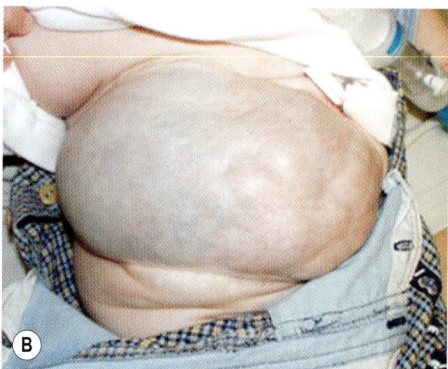
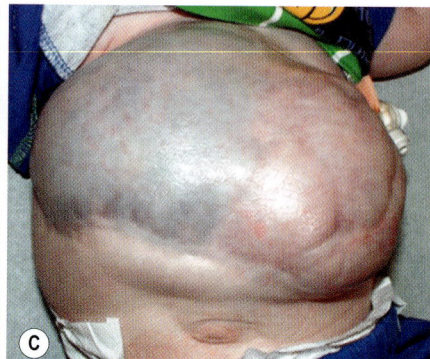

FIGURE 48-12 ■ This baby presented with a large omphalocele and multiple medical problems, including significant lung disease. **(A)** Initial management was with compression therapy. Subsequently, skin grafts were placed. **(B)** The baby is seen at 9-months-old and again at **(C)** 2-years-old. The baby underwent several operations to repair the large ventral hernia.

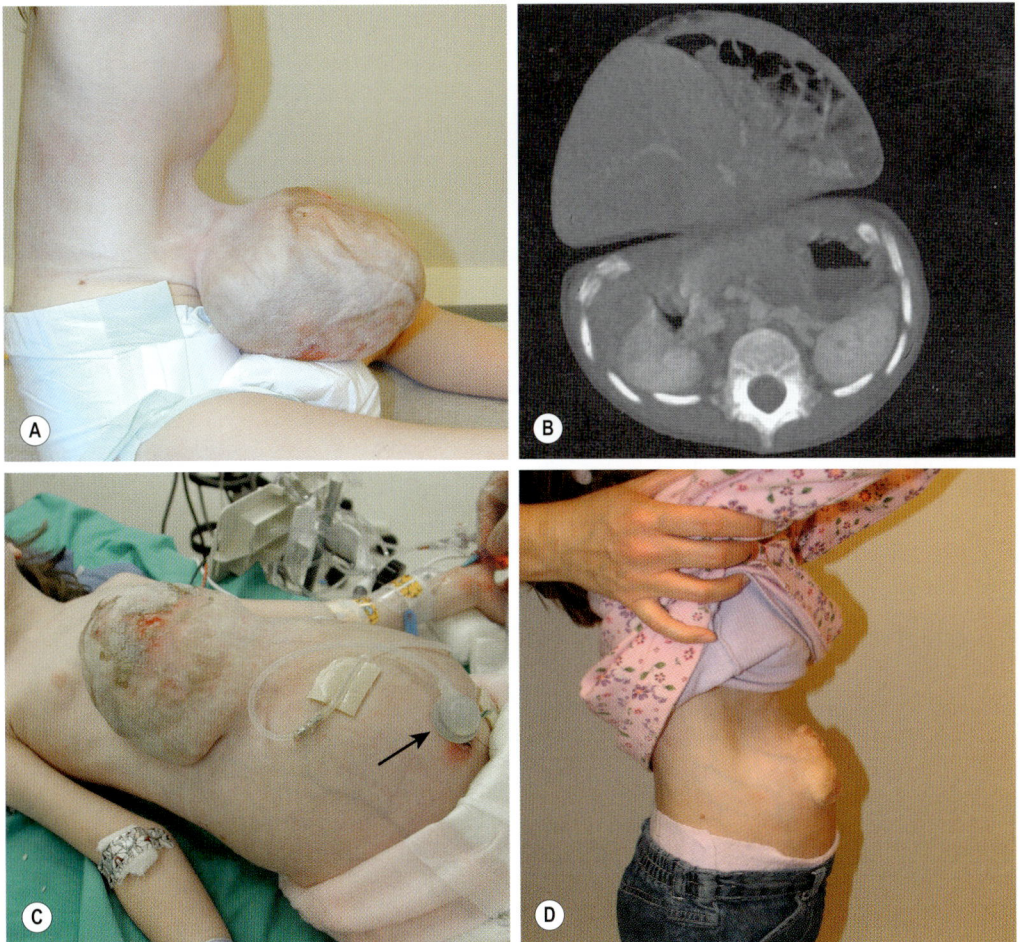

FIGURE 48-13 ■ A 4-year-old girl was born with a number of anomalies including a diaphragmatic hernia, pulmonary hypoplasia and pulmonary hypertension, atrial septal defect, and a large omphalocele. She underwent repair of the diaphragmatic hernia shortly after birth, but no attempt was made to repair the large omphalocele because of its massive size and the disproportion between the extraperitoneal viscera and the peritoneal cavity. **(A, B)** At 4 years old, she was found to have loss of abdominal domain, a narrow neck to the omphalocele sac, and most of the viscera in the sac. **(C)** She underwent placement of an intraperitoneal tissue expander in the pelvis. As an outpatient, the tissue expander was gradually filled to 900 mL of volume, through a catheter emanating from the expander (arrow). Over time, it was possible to expand the peritoneal cavity to the point that the abdominal muscles and fascia could be approximated. However, a biosynthetic patch was needed to complete the fascial closure. **(D)** She has recovered uneventfully and has a very reasonable appearing abdomen. (A and B reprinted with permission from Foglia R, Kane A, Becker D, et al. Management of giant omphalocele with rapid creation of abdominal domain. J Pediatr Surg 2006;41:704–9. Photos courtesy of Dr. Robert Foglia.)

narrow thorax and small lung area leading to pulmonary hypoplasia.[124] The cause of this hypoplasia is unclear as it has been noted in omphaloceles of varying size, but appears more common in the larger defects. Also, it may be associated with poor intrauterine diaphragmatic motion and altered chest wall development. Prolonged respiratory difficulties can occur in up to 20% of infants with giant omphaloceles, leading to increased time of mechanical ventilation and the need for supplemental oxygen during the neonatal period. Some neonates may require a tracheostomy.[125,126] Interestingly, in a study looking at the long-term cardiopulmonary consequences of large abdominal wall defects, lung volumes and oxygen consumption were found to be normal.[127]

Many of the intra-abdominal organs in infants with omphalocele will be abnormally positioned. The liver sits in a medial position with the hepatic veins in variable locations. The stomach is also usually in the middle of the abdomen, with a longitudinal rather than a horizontal orientation.

REFERENCES

1. Feldkamp ML, Carey JC, Sadler TW. Development of gastroschisis: Review of hypotheses, a novel hypothesis, and implications for research. Am J Med Genet A 2007;143:639–52.
2. Feldkamp ML, Carmichael SL, Shaw GM, et al. Maternal nutrition and gastroschisis: Findings from the National Birth Defects Prevention Study. Am J Obstet Gynecol 2011;204:404.
3. Feldkamp ML, Alder SC, Carey JC. A case control population-based study investigating smoking as a risk factor for gastroschisis in Utah, 1997–2005. Birth Defects Res A Clin Mol Teratol 2008;82:768–75.
4. Browne ML, Hoyt AT, Feldkamp ML, et al. Maternal caffeine intake and risk of selected birth defects in the National Birth Defects Prevention Study. Birth Defects Res A Clin Mol Teratol 2011;91:93–101.
5. Baird PA, MacDonald EC. An epidemiologic study of congenital malformations of the anterior abdominal wall in more than half a

million consecutive live births. Am J Hum Genet 1981;33: 470–8.

6. Forrester MB, Merz RD. Impact of demographic factors on prenatal diagnosis and elective pregnancy termination because of abdominal wall defects, Hawaii, 1986–1997. Fetal Diagn Ther 1999;14:206–11.

7. Castilla EE, Mastroiacovo P, Orioli IM. Gastroschisis: International epidemiology and public health perspectives. Am J Med Genet C Semin Med Genet 2008;148:162–79.

8. Lausman AY, Langer JC, Tai M, et al. Gastroschisis: What is the average gestational age of spontaneous delivery? J Pediatr Surg 2007;42:1816–21.

9. Cerekja A, Piazze J, Cozzi D. Early prenatal sonographic diagnosis of gastroschisis. J Clin Ultrasound 2012 ;40:526–8.

10. David AL, Tan A, Curry J. Gastroschisis: Sonographic diagnosis, associations, management and outcome. Prenat Diagn 2008;28: 633–44.

11. Juhasz-Boss I, Goelz R, Solomayer EF, et al. Fetal and neonatal outcome in patients with anterior abdominal wall defects (gastroschisis and omphalocele). J Perinat Med 2012;40:85–90.

12. Moir CR, Ramsey PS, Ogburn PL, et al. A prospective trial of elective preterm delivery for fetal gastroschisis. Am J Perinatol 2004;21:289–94.

13. Mills JA, Lin Y, Macnab YC, et al. Perinatal predictors of outcome in gastroschisis. J Perinatol 2010;30:809–13.

14. Alsulyman OM, Monteiro H, Ouzounian JG, et al. Clinical significance of prenatal ultrasonographic intestinal dilatation in fetuses with gastroschisis. Am J Obstet Gynecol 1996;175: 982–4.

15. Piper HG, Jaksic T. The impact of prenatal bowel dilation on clinical outcomes in neonates with gastroschisis. J Pediatr Surg 2006;41:897–900.

16. Langer JC, Longaker MT, Crombleholme TM, , et al. Etiology of intestinal damage in gastroschisis. I: Effects of amniotic fluid exposure and bowel constriction in a fetal lamb model. J Pediatr Surg 1989;24:992–7.

17. Olguner M, Akgur FM, Api A, et al. The effects of intraamniotic human neonatal urine and meconium on the intestines of the chick embryo with gastroschisis. J Pediatr Surg 2000;35:458–61.

18. Caglar M, Hakguder G, Ates O, et al. Amniotic fluid ferritin as a marker of intestinal damage in gastroschisis: A time course experimental study. J Pediatr Surg 2007;42:1710–15.

19. Hakguder G, Ates O, Olguner M, et al. Induction of fetal diuresis with intraamniotic furosemide increases the clearance of intraamniotic substances: An alternative therapy aimed at reducing intraamniotic meconium concentration. J Pediatr Surg 2002;37: 1337–42.

20. Marder AL, Moise K Jr, Chuang A, et al. Amnioexchange for the treatment of gastroschisis–an in vitro study to determine the volume and number of exchanges needed. Fetal Diagn Ther 2008;23:95–9.

21. Luton D, Guibourdenche J, Vuillard E, et al. Prenatal management of gastroschisis: The place of the amnioexchange procedure. Clin Perinatol 2003;30:551–72.

22. Hakguder G, Olguner M, Gurel D, et al. Induction of fetal diuresis with intraamniotic furosemide injection reduces intestinal damage in a rat model of gastroschisis. Eur J Pediatr Surg 2011;21:183–7.

23. Midrio P, Stefanutti G, Mussap M, et al. Amnioexchange for fetuses with gastroschisis: Is it effective? J Pediatr Surg 2007;42:777–82.

24. Arnold MA, Chang DC, Nabaweesi R, et al. Risk stratification of 4344 patients with gastroschisis into simple and complex categories. J Pediatr Surg 2007;42:1520–5.

25. Dixon JC, Penman DM, Soothill PW. The influence of bowel atresia in gastroschisis on fetal growth, cardiotocograph abnormalities and amniotic fluid staining. BJOG 2000;107:472–5.

26. Amoury RA, Ashcraft KW, Holder TM. Gastroschisis complicated by intestinal atresia. Surgery 1977;82:373–81.

27. Pokorny WJ, Harberg FJ, McGill CW. Gastroschisis complicated by intestinal atresia. J Pediatr Surg 1981;16:261–3.

28. Gornall P. Management of intestinal atresia complicating gastroschisis. J Pediatr Surg 1989;24:522–4.

29. Shah R., Woolley MM. Gastroschisis and intestinal atresia. J Pediatr Surg 1991;26:788–90.

30. Hoehner JC, Ein SH, Kim PC. Management of gastroschisis with concomitant jejuno-ileal atresia. J Pediatr Surg 1998;33:885–8.

31. Fleet MS, de la Hunt MN. Intestinal atresia with gastroschisis: A selective approach to management. J Pediatr Surg 2000;35: 1323–5.

32. Emil S, Canvasser N, Chen T, et al. Contemporary 2 year outcomes of complex gastroschisis. J Pediatr Surg 2012;47:1521–8.

33. Frolov P, Alali J, Klein MD. Clinical risk factors for gastroschisis and omphalocele in humans: A review of the literature. Pediatr Surg Int 2010;26:1135–48.

34. Snyder CL, St Peter SD. Trends in mode of delivery for gastroschisis infants. Am J Perinatol 2005;22:391–6.

35. Salihu HM, Emusu D, Aliyu ZY, et al. Mode of delivery and neonatal survival of infants with isolated gastroschisis. Obstet Gynecol 2004;104:678–83.

36. Puligandla PS, Janvier A, Flageole H, et al. Routine cesarean delivery does not improve the outcome of infants with gastroschisis. J Pediatr Surg 2004;39:742–5.

37. Segel SY, Marder SJ, Parry S, et al. Fetal abdominal wall defects and mode of delivery: A systematic review. Obstet Gynecol 2001;98:867–73.

38. Guibourdenche J, Berrebi D, Vuillard E, et al. Biochemical investigations of bowel inflammation in gastroschisis. Pediatr Res 2006;60:565–8.

39. Vargun R, Aktug T, Heper A, et al. Effects of intrauterine treatment on interstitial cells of Cajal in gastroschisis. J Pediatr Surg 2007;42:783–7.

40. Logghe HL, Mason GC, Thornton JG, et al. A randomized controlled trial of elective preterm delivery of fetuses with gastroschisis. J Pediatr Surg 2005;40:1726–31.

41. Charlesworth P, Njere I, Allotey J, et al. Postnatal outcome in gastroschisis: Effect of birth weight and gestational age. J Pediatr Surg 2007;42:815–18.

42. Maramreddy H, Fisher J, Slim M, et al. Delivery of gastroschisis patients before 37 weeks of gestation is associated with increased morbidities. J Pediatr Surg 2009;44:1360–6.

43. Jansen LA, Safavi A, Lin Y, et al. Preclosure fluid resuscitation influences outcome in gastroschisis. Am J Perinatol 2012;29: 307–12.

44. Mortellaro VE, St Peter SD, Fike FB, et al. Review of the evidence on the closure of abdominal wall defects. Pediatr Surg Int 2011;27:391–7.

45. Aldrink JH, Caniano DA, Nwomeh BC. Variability in gastroschisis management: A survey of North American pediatric surgery training programs. J Surg Res 2012;176:159–63.

46. Alali JS, Tander B, Malleis J, et al. Factors affecting the outcome in patients with gastroschisis: How important is immediate repair? Eur J Pediatr Surg 2011;21:99–102.

47. Owen A, Marven S, Jackson L, et al. Experience of bedside preformed silo staged reduction and closure for gastroschisis. J Pediatr Surg 2006;41:1830–5.

48. Hassan SF, Pimpalwar A. Primary suture-less closure of gastroschisis using negative pressure dressing (wound vacuum). Eur J Pediatr Surg 2011;21:287–91.

49. Bianchi A, Dickson AP. Elective delayed reduction and no anesthesia: 'minimal intervention management' for gastroschisis. J Pediatr Surg 1998;33:1338–40.

50. Wesson DE, Baesl TJ. Repair of gastroschisis with preservation of the umbilicus. J Pediatr Surg 1986;21:764–5.

51. Houben CH, Patel S. Gastroschisis closure: A technique for improved cosmetic repair. Pediatr Surg Int 2008;24:1057–60.

52. Hernandez Siverio N, M López-Tomassetti Fernández E, Mario Troyano Luque J. Gastroschisis: Primary closure using umbilical cord strengthened by a polypropylene mesh. J Perinat Med 2007;35:249–51.

53. Uceda J. Umbilical preservation in gastroschisis. J Pediatr Surg 1996;31:1367–8.

54. Bonnard A, Zamakhshary M, de Silva N, et al. Non-operative management of gastroschisis: A case-matched study. Pediatr Surg Int 2008;24:767–71.

55. Olesevich M, Alexander F, Khan M, Cotman K. Gastroschisis revisited: Role of intraoperative measurement of abdominal pressure. J Pediatr Surg 2005;40:789–92.

56. Lacey SR, Carris LA, Beyer AJ 3rd, et al. Bladder pressure monitoring significantly enhances care of infants with abdominal wall

defects: A prospective clinical study. J Pediatr Surg 1993;28: 1370–4.

57. Ein SH, Superina R, Bagwell C, et al. Ischemic bowel after primary closure for gastroschisis. J Pediatr Surg 1988;23: 728–30.
58. Yaster M, Scherer TL, Stone MM, et al. Prediction of successful primary closure of congenital abdominal wall defects using intra-operative measurements. J Pediatr Surg 1989;24:1217–20.
59. McGuigan RM, Mullenix PS, Vegunta R, et al. Splanchnic perfusion pressure: A better predictor of safe primary closure than intraabdominal pressure in neonatal gastroschisis. J Pediatr Surg 2006;41:901–4.
60. Kidd JN Jr, Jackson RJ, Smith SD, et al. Evolution of staged versus primary closure of gastroschisis. Ann Surg 2003;237:759–64.
61. Sandler A, Lawrence J, Meehan J, et al. A "plastic" sutureless abdominal wall closure in gastroschisis. J Pediatr Surg 2004;39: 738–41.
62. Orion KC, Krein M, Liao J, et al. Outcomes of plastic closure in gastroschisis. Surgery 2011;150:177–1785.
63. Jensen AR, Waldhausen JH, Kim SS. The use of a spring-loaded silo for gastroschisis: Impact on practice patterns and outcomes. Arch Surg 2009;144:516–19.
64. Chiu B, Lopoo J, Hoover JD, et al. Closing arguments for gastroschisis: Management with silo reduction. J Perinat Med 2006;34:243–5.
65. Schlatter M, Norris K, Uitvlugt N, et al. Improved outcomes in the treatment of gastroschisis using a preformed silo and delayed repair approach. J Pediatr Surg 2003;38:459–64.
66. Banyard D, Ramones T, Phillips SE, et al. Method to our madness: An 18-year retrospective analysis on gastroschisis closure. J Pediatr Surg 2010;45:579–84.
67. Weil BR, Leys CM, Rescorla FJ. The jury is still out: Changes in gastroschisis management over the last decade are associated with both benefits and shortcomings. J Pediatr Surg 2012;47:119–24.
68. Weinsheimer RL, Yanchar NL, Bouchard SB, et al. Gastroschisis closure–does method really matter? J Pediatr Surg 2008;43: 874–8.
69. Pastor AC, Phillips JD, Fenton SJ, et al. Routine use of a SILASTIC spring-loaded silo for infants with gastroschisis: A multicenter randomized controlled trial. J Pediatr Surg 2008;43:1807–12.
70. Bradnock TJ, Marven S, Owen A, et al. Gastroschisis: One year outcomes from national cohort study. BMJ 2011;343.
71. Fleet MS, de la Hunt MN. Intestinal atresia with gastroschisis: A selective approach to management. J Pediatr Surg 2000;35: 1323–5.
72. Phillips JD, Raval MV, Redden C, et al. Gastroschisis, atresia, dysmotility: Surgical treatment strategies for a distinct clinical entity. J Pediatr Surg 2008;43:2208–12.
73. Kronfli R, Bradnock TJ, Sabharwal A. Intestinal atresia in association with gastroschisis: A 26-year review. Pediatr Surg Int 2010;26:891–4.
74. Vachharajani AJ, Dillon PA, Mathur AM. Outcomes in neonatal gastroschisis: An institutional experience. Am J Perinatol 2007;24:461–5.
75. Houben C, Davenport M, Ade-Ajayi N, et al. Closing gastroschisis: Diagnosis, management, and outcomes. J Pediatr Surg 2009;44:343–7.
76. Barsoom MJ, Prabulos A, Rodis JF, et al. Vanishing gastroschisis and short-bowel syndrome. Obstet Gynecol 2000;96:818–19.
77. Langer JC, Bramlett G. Effect of prokinetic agents on ileal contractility in a rabbit model of gastroschisis. J Pediatr Surg 1997;32:605–8.
78. Curry JI, Lander AD, Stringer MD. A multicenter, randomized, double-blind, placebo-controlled trial of the prokinetic agent erythromycin in the postoperative recovery of infants with gastroschisis. J Pediatr Surg 2004;39:565–9.
79. Rijhwani A, Davenport M, Dawrant M, et al. Definitive surgical management of antenatally diagnosed exomphalos. J Pediatr Surg 2004;40:516–22.
80. Arnold MA, Chang DC, Nabaweesi R, et al. Development and validation of a risk stratification index to predict death in gastroschisis. J Pediatr Surg 2007;42:950–5.
81. Kassa AM, Lilja HE. Predictors of postnatal outcome in neonates with gastroschisis. J Pediatr Surg 2011;46:2108–14.
82. Molik KA, Gingalewski CA, West KW, et al. Gastroschisis: A plea for risk categorization. J Pediatr Surg 2001;36:51–5.
83. Lao OB, Larison C, Garrison MM, et al. Outcomes in neonates with gastroschisis in USA children's hospitals. Am J Perinatol 2010;27:97–101.
84. Wada M, Kato T, Hayashi Y, et al. Intestinal transplantation for short bowel syndrome secondary to gastroschisis. J Pediatr Surg 2006;41:1841–5.
85. Oldham KT, Coran AG, Drongowski RA, et al. The development of necrotizing enterocolitis following repair of gastroschisis: A surprisingly high incidence. J Pediatr Surg 1988;23:945–9.
86. Kurbegov AC, Sondheimer JM. Pneumatosis intestinalis in non-neonatal pediatric patients. Pediatrics 2001;108:402–6.
87. Jayanthi S, Seymour P, Puntis JW, et al. Necrotizing enterocolitis after gastroschisis repair: A preventable complication? J Pediatr Surg 1998;33:705–7.
88. Lawson A, de La Hunt MN. Gastroschisis and undescended testis. J Pediatr Surg 2001;36:366–7.
89. Hill SJ, Durham MM. Management of cryptorchidism and gastroschisis. J Pediatr Surg 2011;46:1798–803.
90. Berger AP, Hager J. Management of neonates with large abdominal wall defects and undescended testis. Urology 2006;68:175–8.
91. Davies BW, Stringer MD. The survivors of gastroschisis. Arch Dis Child 1997;77:158–60.
92. Solerte L. Three-dimensional multiplanar ultrasound in a limb-body wall complex fetus: Clinical evidence for counseling. J Matern Fetal Neonatal Med 2006;19:109–12.
93. Brantberg A, Blaas HG, Haugen SE, et al. Characteristics and outcome of 90 cases of fetal omphalocele. Ultrasound Obstet Gynecol 2005;26:527–37.
94. Cohen-Overbeek TE, Tong WH, Hatzmann TR, et al. Omphalocele: Comparison of outcome following prenatal or postnatal diagnosis. Ultrasound Obstet Gynecol 2010;36:687–92.
95. Nicholas SS, Stamilio DM, Dicke JM, et al. Predicting adverse neonatal outcomes in fetuses with abdominal wall defects using prenatal risk factors. Am J Obstet Gynecol 2009;201:383.
96. Kamata S, Usui N, Sawai T, et al. Prenatal detection of pulmonary hypoplasia in giant omphalocele. Pediatr Surg Int 2008;24: 107–11.
97. Hidaka N, Murata M, Yumoto Y, et al. Characteristics and perinatal course of prenatally diagnosed fetal abdominal wall defects managed in a tertiary center in Japan. J Obstet Gynaecol Res 2009;35:40–7.
98. Montero FJ, Simpson LL, Brady PC, et al. Fetal omphalocele ratios predict outcomes in prenatally diagnosed omphalocele. Am J Obstet Gynecol 2011;205:284.
99. Kleinrouweler CE, Kuijper CF, van Zalen-Sprock MM, et al. Characteristics and outcome and the omphalocele circumference/abdominal circumference ratio in prenatally diagnosed fetal omphalocele. Fetal Diagn Ther 2011;30:60–9.
100. Lurie S, Sherman D, Bukovsky I. Omphalocele delivery enigma: The best mode of delivery still remains dubious. Eur J Obstet Gynecol Reprod Biol 1999;82:19–22.
101. Baird R, Gholoum S, Laberge JM, Puligandla P. Management of a giant omphalocele with an external skin closure system. J Pediatr Surg 2010;45:E17–20.
102. van Eijck FC, Aronson DA, Hoogeveen YL, et al. Past and current surgical treatment of giant omphalocele: Outcome of a questionnaire sent to authors. J Pediatr Surg 2011;46:482–8.
103. Islam S. Clinical care outcomes in abdominal wall defects. Curr Opin Pediatr 2008;20:305–10.
104. Delorimier AA, Adzick NS, Harrison MR. Amnion inversion in the treatment of giant omphalocele. J Pediatr Surg 1991;26: 804–7.
105. Yokomori K, Ohkura M, Kitano Y, et al. Advantages and pitfalls of amnion inversion repair for the treatment of large unruptured omphalocele: Results of 22 cases. J Pediatr Surg 1992;27:882–4.
106. Alaish SM, Strauch ED. The use of Alloderm in the closure of a giant omphalocele. J Pediatr Surg 2006;41:e37–9.
107. Kilbride KE, Cooney DR, Custer MD. Vacuum-assisted closure: A new method for treating patients with giant omphalocele. J Pediatr Surg 2006;41:212–15.
108. Brown AL II, Roty AR Jr, Kilway JB. Increased survival with new techniques in treatment of gastroschisis. Am Surg 1978;44: 417–20.

109. Gross RE. A new method for surgical treatment of a large ompha-locele. Surgery 1948;24:277–92.

110. Mullins ME, Horowitz BZ. Iatrogenic neonatal mercury poisoning from Mercurochrome treatment of a large omphalocele. Clin Pediatr 1999;38:111–12.

111. Festen C, Severijnen RS, vd Staak FH. Nonsurgical (conservative) treatment of giant omphalocele. A report of 10 cases. Clin Pediatr 1987;26:35–9.

112. Whitehouse JS, Gourlay DM, Masonbrink AR, et al. Conservative management of giant omphalocele with topical povidone-iodine and its effect on thyroid function. J Pediatr Surg 2010;45:1192–7.

113. Almond S, Reyna R, Barganski N, et al. Nonoperative management of a giant omphalocele using a silver impregnated hydrofiber dressing: A case report. J Pediatr Surg 2010;45:1546–9.

114. Lee SL, Beyer TD, Kim SS, et al. Initial nonoperative management and delayed closure for treatment of giant omphaloceles. J Pediatr Surg 2006;41:1846–9.

115. van Eijck FC, de Blaauw I, Bleichrodt RP, et al. Closure of giant omphaloceles by the abdominal wall component separation technique in infants. J Pediatr Surg 2008;43:246–50.

116. De Ugarte DA, Asch MJ, Hedrick MH, et al. The use of tissue expanders in the closure of a giant omphalocele. J Pediatr Surg 2004;39:613–15.

117. Islam S. Advances in surgery for abdominal wall defects: Gastroschisis and omphalocele. Clin Perinatol 2012;39:375–86.

118. Maksoud-Filho JG, Tannuri U, da Silva MM, et al. The outcome of newborns with abdominal wall defects according to the method of abdominal closure: The experience of a single center. Pediatr Surg Int 2006;22:503–7.

119. Dunn JCY, Fonkalsrud EW. Improved survival of infants with omphalocele. Am J Surg 1997;173:284–7.

120. Wilson RD, Biard JM, Johnson MP, et al. Giant omphalocele: Prenatal diagnosis, short, and long-term outcomes. Am J Hum Genet 2003;73:594.

121. Lakasing L, Cicero S, Davenport M, et al. Current outcome of antenatally diagnosed exomphalos: An 11 year review. J Pediatr Surg 2006;41:1403–6.

122. Biard JM, Wilson RD, Johnson MP, et al. Prenatally diagnosed giant omphaloceles: Short- and long-term outcomes. Prenat Diagn 2004;24:434–9.

123. Koivusalo A, Rintala R, Lindahl H. Gastroesophageal reflux in children with a congenital abdominal wall defect. J Pediatr Surg 1999;34:1127–9.

124. Argyle JC. Pulmonary hypoplasia in infants with giant abdominal wall defects. Pediatr Pathol 1989;9:43–55.

125. Hershenson MB, Brouillette RT, Klemka L, et al. Respiratory insufficiency in newborns with abdominal wall defects. J Pediatr Surg 1985;20:348–53.

126. Edwards EA, Broome S, Green S, et al. Long-term respiratory support in children with giant omphalocele. Anaesth Intensive Care 2007;35:94–8.

127. Zaccara A, Iacobelli BD, Calzolari A, et al. Cardiopulmonary performances in young children and adolescents born with large abdominal wall defects. J Pediatr Surg 2003;38:478–81.

CHAPTER 49

UMBILICAL AND OTHER ABDOMINAL WALL HERNIAS

Thomas R. Weber

UMBILICAL HERNIA

Umbilical hernia is a common disorder in children that pediatric and general surgeons are frequently asked to evaluate and treat. Although the fascial defect is present at birth, unlike other hernias of childhood, an umbilical hernia may resolve without the need for an operation. An understanding of the embryology, anatomy, incidence, natural history, and complications is important to any surgeon managing umbilical hernias in children.

Anatomy

After birth, closure of the umbilical ring is the result of complex interactions of lateral body wall folding in a medial direction, fusion of the rectus abdominis muscles into the linea alba, and umbilical orifice contraction which is aided by elastic fibers from the obliterated umbilical arteries. Fibrous proliferation of surrounding lateral connective tissue plates and mechanical stress from rectus muscle tension may also help with natural closure. Failure of these closure processes results in umbilical hernia. The hernia sac is peritoneum, which is usually very adherent to the dermis of the umbilical skin. The actual fascial defect can range from several millimeters to 5 cm or more in diameter. The extent of skin protrusion is not always indicative of the size of the fascia defect. Frequently, small defects can result in alarmingly large proboscis-like protrusions (Fig. 49-1). Thus, it is important to palpate the actual fascia defect by reducing the hernia to assess whether operative or nonoperative treatment is appropriate.

Incidence

The incidence of umbilical hernia in the general population varies with age, race, gestational age, and coexisting disorders. In the USA, the incidence in African-American children from birth to 1-year-old ranges from 25–58%, whereas Caucasian children in the same age group have an incidence of 2–18.5%.[1,2] Premature and low birth weight infants have a higher incidence than full-term infants.[3] Infants with certain other conditions, such as Beckwith–Wiedemann syndrome, Hurler syndrome, various trisomy conditions (trisomy 13, 18, and 21), and congenital hypothyroidism, also have an increased incidence as do children requiring peritoneal dialysis.[4,5]

Treatment

For many years, it has been known that umbilical hernias will close spontaneously. It seems very safe to observe the hernia until ages 3 to 4 years to allow closure to occur. Pressure dressings and other devices to keep the hernia reduced do not enhance the closure process and may result in skin irritation and breakdown. Although dated, a number of studies in both Caucasian and African-American populations showed spontaneous resolution rates of 83–95% by 6 years of age.[6–10] Another study found that 50% of hernias still present at age 4 to 5 years will close by age 11 years.[9] One study suggests that hernias with fascial defects greater than 1.5 cm are unlikely to close by age 6 years, whereas other series conclude that even large defects will spontaneously resolve without operation.[8,11,12] The primary danger associated with observation therapy is the possibility of incarceration or strangulation. Studies have shown these complications to be quite rare, with an incidence of less than 0.2%.[8,12,13] Patients with small fascial defects (0.5–1.5 cm in diameter) appear more prone to incarceration.[14]

The operative closure of an umbilical hernia is generally straightforward, and can usually be completed as an outpatient procedure. Methods used commonly in the adult, such as prosthetic placement, are almost never needed in the child. The most common method of repair is shown in Figs 49-2 and 49-3. A small transverse infraumbilical incision is made, usually placed in the redundant skin, which is inverted at the conclusion of the procedure, thereby hiding the incision. The hernia sac is identified and dissected free from the dermis underlying the umbilical cicatrix. The author's preference is excision of the sac to the fascial edges, although other surgeons prefer a more limited excision of the sac or inversion of the sac through the fascial opening. Interrupted sutures of nonabsorbable or long-lasting absorbable sutures are placed and tied, closing the fascial defect in a transverse direction. The author leaves the needle attached to the central fascial suture, which is then used to tack the underside of the umbilical skin to the fascia. The skin incision is closed with an absorbable subcuticular suture, and a dressing is applied. Many surgeons use a pressure dressing to help prevent the development of hematoma and keep the umbilical skin inverted, but this type of dressing may not be necessary.[15]

Excision of the redundant skin is usually not performed because it tends to return to a normal appearance after the

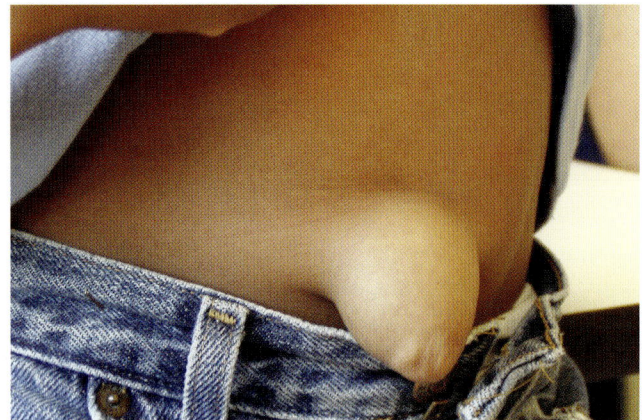

FIGURE 49-1 ■ This 5-year-old child has a large proboscis-like umbilical hernia.

hernia is repaired. This can take up to 12 months to occur, and the family should be reassured appropriately. If the umbilicus fails to return to an acceptable appearance after one to two years, there are a number of techniques described to restore it to a more normal configuration.[16–18]

There are a few complications of umbilical hernia repair and include seroma or hematoma formation. These are usually self-limited and resolve spontaneously. Wound infections can generally be managed with local care and antibiotics, whereas a recurrent hernia, occurring in less than 1%, requires reoperation.[14]

EPIGASTRIC HERNIA

Hernias of the abdominal wall through the midline linea alba, also termed epigastric hernias, are common in the pediatric age group. These hernias present as small masses, usually with incarcerated properitoneal fat, between the umbilicus and xiphoid process (Fig. 49-4). An epigastric hernia should not be confused with diastasis recti, which is generalized weakness in the linea alba from umbilicus to xiphoid, and virtually always resolves by age 10 years. Incarcerated epigastric hernias can be painful. These hernias can also be multiple and associated with an umbilical hernia. Epigastric hernias do not resolve and should be repaired.

A small midline incision over the hernia is generally used, with suture repair of the defect after the contents (properitoneal fat) are reduced or excised. The site of the hernia should always be marked before general anesthesia because the defect may be difficult to find after muscle relaxation. Recurrence is not common.

SPIGELIAN HERNIA

Spigelian hernias are quite rare in children and can be difficult to detect and diagnose. The actual defect occurs at the intersection of the linea semicircularis, linea semilunaris, and the lateral border of the rectus abdominis muscle. It usually involves absence or attenuation of the transversus abdominis and internal oblique muscles. These hernias are more frequently found in girls and

more commonly occur on the right side below the umbilicus.[19] They are also occasionally associated with skeletal abnormalities.[20] Pain in the area with a feeling of fullness or an actual mass are the most common symptoms. Ultrasonography may aid in the diagnosis. In select cases, computed tomography may be needed.

Repair consists of a transverse incision over the defect with excision of the sac and closure of the defect. Frequently, the sac is found below the external oblique muscle and may require mesh if the defect is large. A tension-free closure is important to prevent recurrence in this area that has a high level of muscle tension.

LUMBAR HERNIA

Lumbar hernias are usually visible shortly after birth as a bulge in the area bordered by the 12th rib, sacrospinalis

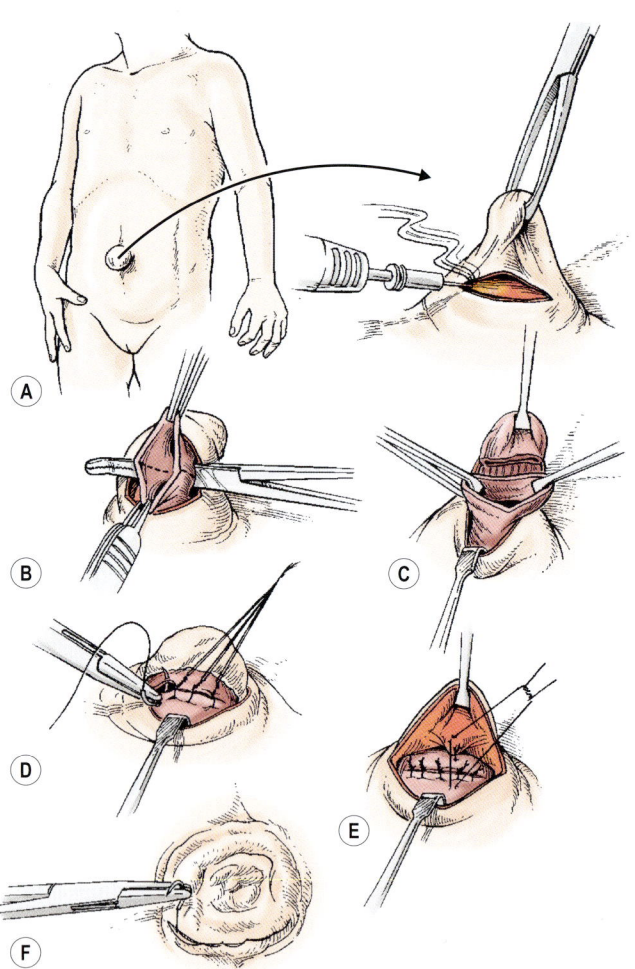

FIGURE 49-2 ■ The technique for operative repair for an umbilical hernia. **(A)** An infraumbilical skin crease incision is made. **(B)** The hernia sac is opened, leaving a portion of the sac attached to the umbilical skin for ease of subsequent umbilicoplasty. **(C)** The umbilical sac has been completely divided and excised to strong fascia. **(D)** The fascial defect is closed in a transverse fashion with interrupted, simple nonabsorbable sutures. **(E)** The remaining umbilical sac, which is attached to the umbilical skin, is secured to the fascia with interrupted, absorbable sutures. **(F)** The skin incision is closed with a subcuticular suture.

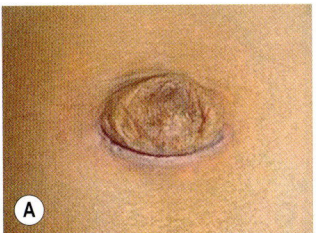 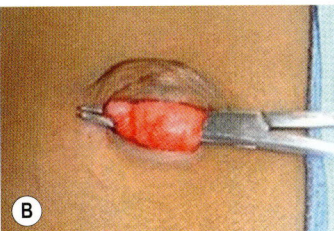 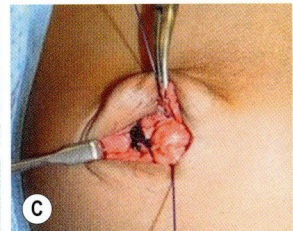 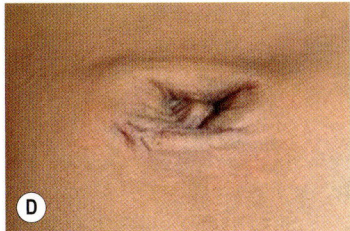

FIGURE 49-3 ■ The steps depicted in the operative diagram in Figure 49-2 are shown. **(A)** An infraumbilical incision is made. **(B)** The umbilical hernia sac has been encircled with a hemostat. **(C)** The umbilical hernia sac is excised, and transverse closure of the fascial defect is accomplished with interrupted long-lasting absorbable sutures. **(D)** The umbilicus has been tacked to the fascial closure, and the skin is approximated with a subcuticular closure.

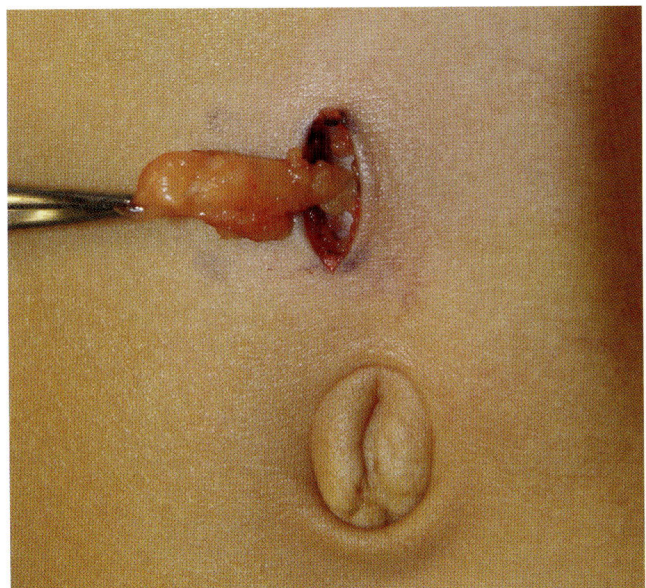

FIGURE 49-4 ■ At the time of epigastric hernia repair, this operative photograph shows herniation of properitoneal fat through a small fascial defect in the linea alba.

muscle, and internal oblique muscle. Occasionally, they extend inferiorly to the iliac crest. These hernias tend to develop at the site of penetration of the intercostal nerves and vessels, or of the ilioinguinal, iliohypogastric, and lumbar nerves. The bulge is usually properitoneal fat. Therefore, the physical findings include a soft mass that is easily reducible. Although frequently asymptomatic, repair is advisable because the defect never resolves spontaneously and incarceration is possible.

Repair sometimes requires prosthetic reinforcement of the fascia or muscle closure because the tissue available for repair is usually thin and weak. I prefer using absorbable mesh in the growing child that will not cause scoliosis later. Recurrence is not uncommon and several operations may be needed. Bilateral lumbar hernias can

be corrected with either staged or simultaneous closures, depending on the surgeon's and family's preferences.

REFERENCES

1. Crump EP. Umbilical hernia: Occurrence of the infantile type in Negro infants and children. J Pediatr 1952;40:214–33.
2. Evans AG. The comparative incidence of umbilical hernia in colored and white infants. J Natl Med Assoc 1940;33:158–60.
3. Vohr BR, Rosenfield AG, Oh W. Umbilical hernia in the low-birth weight infant (less than 1500 gm). J Pediatr 1977;90:807–8.
4. Jones KL. Abdominal wall. In: Jones KL, editor. Smith's Recognizable Patterns of Human Malformation. 4th ed. Philadelphia: WB Saunders; 1988. p. P753–754.
5. Tank EW, Hatch DA. Hernias complicating chronic ambulatory peritoneal dialysis in children. J Pediatr Surg 1986;21:41–2.
6. Woods GE. Some observations on umbilical hernias in infants. Arch Dis Child 1953;28:450–62.
7. Heifitz CJ, Bilsel ZE, Gans WW. Observations on the disappearance of umbilical hernias of infancy and childhood. Surg Gynecol Obstet 1963;116:467–73.
8. Walker SH. The natural history of umbilical hernia. Clin Pediatr 1967;6:29–32.
9. Hall DE, Roberts KB, Charney E. Umbilical hernia: What happens after age 5 years? J Pediatr 1981;98:415–17.
10. Sibley WL, Lynn HE, Harris LE. A twenty-five year study of infantile umbilical hernia. Surgery 1964;55:462–8.
11. Blumberg NA. Infantile umbilical hernia. Surg Gynecol Obstet 1980;150:187–92.
12. Halpern LJ. Spontaneous healing of umbilical hernias. JAMA 1962;182:851–2.
13. Mestal AL, Burns H. Incarcerated and strangulated umbilical hernias in infants and children. Clin Pediatr 1963;2:368–70.
14. Lassaletta L, Fonkalsrud EW, Tovar JA, et al. The management of umbilical hernia in infancy and childhood. J Pediatr Surg 1975;10:405–9.
15. Merci J. Umbilical hernia repair in children: Is pressure dressing necessary? Pediatr Surg Int 2006;22:446–8.
16. Jamra F. Reconstruction of umbilicus by a double V-Y procedure. Plast Reconstr Surg 1979;64:106–10.
17. Reyna T, Hllis H, Smith S. Surgical management of proboscoid hernia. J Pediatr Surg 1978;22:911–2.
18. Koshy C, Taams K. Umbilicoplasty. Plast Reconstr Surg 1999;104:1203–4.
19. Spangen L. Spigelian hernia. Surg Clin North Am 1984;64:351–66.
20. Asku B, Temizoz O, Inan M, et al. Bilateral Spigelian concomitant with multiple skeletal anomalies and fibular aplasia in a child. Eur J Pediatr Surg 2008;18:205–8.

SECTION V

INGUINAL REGION AND SCROTUM

CHAPTER 50

INGUINAL HERNIAS AND HYDROCELES

Jason D. Fraser • Charles L. Snyder

Inguinal hernia repair is one of the most common operations performed by pediatric surgeons, and consultations for an inguinal hernia are among the most frequent reasons for pediatric surgical referral. An inguinal hernia in a child usually refers to an indirect inguinal hernia but much less frequently may include a femoral hernia or a direct inguinal hernia.

HISTORY

The term hernia comes from the Greek 'hernios', meaning offshoot or bud. Inguinal hernias were described in the Ebers Papyrus in 1552 BC,[1] and were found in Egyptian mummies. Celsus is thought to have performed hernia repairs in 50 AD. Galen (b. 129 AD) described the processus vaginalis, defined hernias as a rupture of the peritoneum, and advised surgical repair.[2] Ambrose Paré advocated repair of inguinal hernias in childhood in the 16th century, and condemned concomitant castration.[1] In 1807, Cooper identified the transversalis fascia and the ligament associated with his name. In 1817, Cloquet observed that the processus vaginalis is often patent at birth and described femoral hernias.[3,4] Marcy reported high ligation of the hernia sac in 1871.[5] In 1877, von Czerny first described narrowing the inguinal canal and tightening the external inguinal ring,[6,7] followed by Bassini's description of internal inguinal ring tightening and reinforcement of the posterior canal in 1887.[8] Gross reported a 0.45% recurrence rate in a large series of inguinal hernia repairs (3,874 children) in 1953.[9]

INCIDENCE

Approximately 1–5% of all children will develop an inguinal hernia and a positive family history is found in about 10%.[10] There is an increased incidence in twins, more frequently in male twins.[11] In a series of 6,361 pediatric herniorrhaphies performed by a single surgeon, the male-to-female ratio was 5 to 1, and right-sided hernias were twice as common as those on the left.[12] The mean age at diagnosis was 3.3 years.

The incidence of an inguinal hernia varies directly with the degree of prematurity. The overall incidence of inguinal hernia in premature infants is estimated to be 10–30%, whereas term newborns have a rate of 3–5%.[13–15] The incidence by gender is closer to 1:1 in premature infants. Comorbidities such as chronic lung disease associated with prematurity may play a role in the development of an inguinal hernia.

ASSOCIATIONS

Cystic Fibrosis

Patients with cystic fibrosis have an increased risk of an inguinal hernia, with an incidence as high as 15%.[16] This heightened risk may be due to elevated intra-abdominal pressure from respiratory symptoms, but developmental and/or embryologic factors may also play a role because the risk of a hernia is also increased in unaffected siblings and parents.

Hydrocephalus

Ventriculoperitoneal shunts (VPS) are associated with an increased incidence of an inguinal hernia as well as increased chance of bilaterality, incarceration, and recurrence.[17] In a series of 430 children who underwent placement of a VPS, 15% developed a hernia.[18] Bilaterality was common; it occurred in nearly 50% in boys and approximately 25% of girls. Hydroceles occurred in another 6%. A large series of children with shunts found that inguinal hernias were more likely to develop in neonates than in older children and were more common in boys than in girls. The average time from placement of a VPS to hernia repair was approximately one year.[19]

Peritoneal Dialysis

As with VPS, patients on long-term peritoneal dialysis also have an increased risk of an inguinal hernia. Some authors even advocate searching for a patent processus during insertion of the dialysis catheter (either radiographically or via laparoscopy), and closing the sac at that time.[20]

Other

Other entities associated with an increased incidence of an inguinal hernia include cryptorchidism, abdominal wall defects, connective tissue disorders (Ehlers–Danlos syndrome), mucopolysaccharidoses (Hunter or Hurler syndrome), ascites, congenital hip dislocation, and meningomyelocele.

EMBRYOLOGY AND ANATOMY

The inguinal canal is a six-sided cylinder. The cephalad opening is the internal inguinal ring and the caudal border is the external inguinal ring. The cephalad aspect is bordered by the internal oblique, transversus abdominis, and medial external oblique fibers. The floor is formed by the transversalis fascia and the 'conjoint tendon.' The anterior roof is created primarily by the aponeurosis of the external oblique. The inferior wall is composed by the inguinal ligament, lacunar ligament (medial third), and iliopubic tract (lateral third). Contents include the ilioinguinal nerve (exiting through the external inguinal ring) and in males, the spermatic cord. In females, it also contains the round ligament.[21]

The processus vaginalis is a peritoneal diverticulum extending through the internal inguinal ring into the inguinal canal. It can be seen by 3 months of fetal life.[22] The somatic base of this diverticulum is the transversalis portion of the endoabdominal fascia. The gonads form on the anteromedial nephrogenic ridges in the retroperitoneum during the 5th week of gestation. The gonads are attached to the scrotum by the gubernaculum in the male and to the labia via the round ligament in the female. Gonadal descent begins by 3 months' gestation, and the testis reaches the internal inguinal ring by about 7 months. Descent of the testis is thought to be directed in the abdominal phase by insulin-like 3 protein, a product of the Leydig cells, and directed in the second phase by androgens and release of calcitonin gene-related peptide (CGRP) from the genitofemoral nerve (via fetal androgen release).[23,24] CGRP appears to mediate closure of the patent processus vaginalis (PPV), although this process is not completely understood.[24]

The testis begins to descend down the canal by the seventh month of fetal life preceded and guided by the processus vaginalis.[22,24,25] The processus, which is located anterior and medial to the cord structures, gradually obliterates, and the scrotal portion forms the tunica vaginalis. The female anlage of the processus vaginalis is the canal of Nuck, a structure that leads to the labia majora. This also closes by about 7 months of fetal life, and ovarian descent is arrested in the pelvis.[22] The precise incidence of PPV in newborns is unknown and depends on gender and gestational age. It is estimated to be 40–60%, but may be lower or higher.[26] However, at autopsy, only 5% of adults have a PPV.[22] PPVs can still close after birth, but this is felt less likely to occur with increasing age. It is failure of the PPV to close that results

in an indirect inguinal hernia. As mentioned, the factors driving PPV closure are incompletely understood. Intra-abdominal pressure probably plays a role because disorders with increased abdominal pressure/fluid (e.g., ascites, VPS) are associated with an increased incidence of indirect inguinal hernias and an increased incidence of bilaterality.[17] Indirect inguinal hernias are more common on the right. The various clinical findings related to the processus vaginalis are illustrated in Figure 50-1.

The layers of the abdominal wall contribute to the layers of the testis and spermatic cord as the gonad descends. The internal spermatic fascia is a continuation of the transversalis fascia, the cremaster muscle derives from the internal oblique, and the external spermatic fascia originates from the external oblique aponeurosis. The processus vaginalis envelops the testis as the visceral and parietal layers of the tunica vaginalis.[22]

CLINICAL PRESENTATION

Most hernias are asymptomatic except for inguinal bulging with straining. They are often found by the parents or pediatrician on routine physical examination. The diagnosis is clinical and rests squarely on the history and physical examination. Maneuvers such as having the child raise the head while supine or 'blowing up a balloon' with a thumb in the mouth may be helpful in small children. Standing the child upright may also help demonstrate the hernia. The differential diagnosis includes a retractile testis, lymphadenopathy, hydrocele, and prepubertal fat.

A common occurrence is a normal examination in combination with a suggestive history. Cell phone picture documentation by the parents has become commonplace. A good history is acceptable as an indication for operation. False-negative explorations are rare. In the previously mentioned series of 6,361 hernia repairs by a single surgeon (definitive inguinal hernia on examination was the indication for operation), there was only one false-negative exploration (0.02%).[12]

Children are often referred for inguinal pain in the absence of any history of bulging or swelling, often with

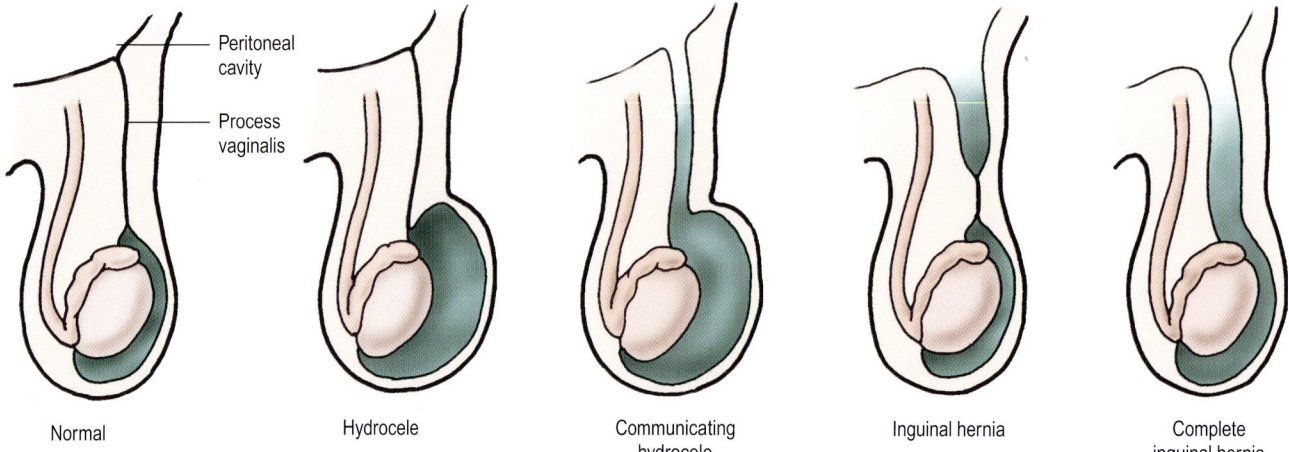

Peritoneal cavity

Process vaginalis

Normal　　　Hydrocele　　　Communicating hydrocele　　　Inguinal hernia　　　Complete inguinal hernia

FIGURE 50-1 ■ From left, configurations of hydrocele and hernia in relation to patency of the processus vaginalis.

a normal physical examination. Other sources such as musculoskeletal strain, gastrointestinal, or genitourinary abnormalities should be excluded before operative intervention. Diagnostic transumbilical laparoscopy is useful in a small subset with equivocal examinations or persistent symptoms and no other apparent cause.

Ancillary findings such as a 'silk glove sign' (feeling the thickened peritoneum of the patent processus as the cord is palpated) or examination under anesthesia are of variable reliability.[27,28] Radiologic diagnostic aids are not generally necessary or helpful. Ultrasonography (US) can be used to identify a PPV indirectly via widening of the internal inguinal ring (more than 4–5 mm is positive), but the technique is highly operator dependent and not widely used in children.[29,30] It is not generally necessary to restrict an asymptomatic child's activities until repair is scheduled, but prompt repair may decrease interim incarceration, particularly in the very young.

Sometimes an incidental PPV is discovered in a child undergoing operation for an unrelated problem. A common scenario is finding a unilateral or bilateral PPV during the course of a laparoscopic appendectomy, or other operation. It is probably best not to perform a PPV repair in that setting as the patient is not symptomatic. The child and the family should be informed of the findings and instructed to watch for symptoms.

Hydrocele

The management of asymptomatic hydroceles in infants is somewhat controversial. There is general agreement that a noncommunicating, asymptomatic hydrocele in an infant should simply be followed. One recent study found that 89% of 121 infants who were followed resolved by 1 year of age.[31] The duration of observation varies by surgeon, with most recommending operation by one or two years of age if the hydrocele fails to resolve or if a clinical hernia is apparent.[20,32]

Expectant management has been extended by some authors to infants with communicating hydroceles (and therefore PPVs). In a 2010 report, in 110 infant boys with an apparent communicating hydrocele, 63% had complete resolution without operation by a mean age of nearly one year.[33] Interim incarceration did not occur in this series.

Many authors recommend operation for an infant with a giant hydrocele, although the definition is subjective and variable. Most surgeons also repair hydroceles of the cord.[34]

Excision of the hydrocele sac is not necessary. The fluid should be evacuated, and the distal sac is opened widely. Large or thick sacs may be everted behind the cord (Bottle procedure).[35]

Hydroceles in adolescents are often a complication of varicocelectomy. A de novo hydrocele in this age group may represent an inguinal hernia or simply an idiopathic hydrocele. A thorough history and physical examination to exclude communication hernia should be performed. Also, an ultrasound (particularly if the testis is not palpable, since a reactive hydrocele accompanies about 15% of testicular tumors) should be obtained. A trans-scrotal hydrocelectomy is appropriate in adolescents in the absence of signs of hernia or tumor. Otherwise an inguinal approach is best.[36] Transumbilical diagnostic laparoscopy for evaluation for a PPV is a good option in equivocal cases.

An abdominoscrotal hydrocele is an hourglass-shaped collection with both an inguinoscrotal and abdominal component. A combined inguinal and laparoscopic approach may be helpful.[37]

Incarceration

The incidence of hernia incarceration is variable and ranges from 12–17%.[12,38,39] Younger age and prematurity are risk factors for incarceration.[40] The mean age of patients with incarceration is significantly lower than that of those who undergo elective repair.[12,41]

Symptoms of incarceration are frequently manifested as a fussy or inconsolable infant with intermittent abdominal pain and vomiting. A tender and sometimes erythematous irreducible mass is noted in the groin. Abdominal distention is a late sign, as are bloody stools. Peritoneal signs indicate strangulation. Incarceration may be the presenting sign of the hernia, especially in an infant. It can be difficult to distinguish a hydrocele of the cord from an incarcerated hernia. A happy infant with no tenderness suggests the former diagnosis, but if several examiners have vigorously attempted to reduce the hydrocele, the distinction can be difficult and ultrasound may be helpful.

It has been stated that gangrenous bowel cannot be reduced, but exceptions make this a dangerous rule to rely on. The presence of peritonitis or septic shock is an absolute contraindication to attempted reduction. Symptoms of bowel obstruction are a relative contraindication. Monitored conscious sedation is used after intravenous access and rehydration. Firm and continuous pressure is applied around the incarceration. Successful reduction is usually confirmed by a sudden 'pop' of the contents back into the peritoneal cavity. Questionable or incomplete reductions should be explored. Reduction en masse, in which the hernia contents are reduced into the peritoneal cavity but the bowel remains incarcerated internally in the hernia sac, is a very rare occurrence but the surgeon should be aware of this possibility.

Once an incarcerated hernia is reduced, a delay of 24 to 48 hours to allow resolution of edema is reasonable. Reliability of the family as well as clinical (very difficult reduction) and geographic considerations may dictate the need for admission and observation before definitive repair. Overall, 90–95% of incarcerated hernias can be successfully reduced.[42] In one report, only 8% required emergency operation out of 743 incarcerated hernias.[12] Two children required bowel resection.

Urgent operation is necessary if reduction fails. The hernia may reduce with induction of general anesthesia. If so, the hernia sac should be opened and inspected. The presence of enteric contents or bloody fluid mandates either open exploration via separate incision or La Roque maneuver (incision in the transversalis fascia through the same inguinal skin incision) or, more commonly, laparoscopic evaluation. It may be necessary to open the internal inguinal ring laterally to reduce the bowel. Some surgeons approach an incarcerated hernia by transumbilical laparoscopy to both reduce the hernia and evaluate the bowel.[43,44] There is some evidence that the laparoscopic approach is associated with fewer complications.[45]

Intestinal injury requiring treatment is rare (1% to 2%), even with incarceration.[12] The hernia sac is often quite edematous and friable, and repair of the hernia can be quite difficult. The risk of recurrence is significantly increased. We do not routinely employ laparoscopy looking for a contralateral PPV in patients with incarceration.

The testis on the incarcerated side is often edematous and somewhat cyanotic. Unless the gonad is frankly necrotic, it should be preserved. The parents of any boy with an incarcerated hernia should be counseled about the possibility of testicular loss or atrophy, but the incidence of this complication is only 2–3%.[42,46] Incarceration of an ovary in a hernia sac may not always impair its blood supply, but most pediatric surgeons will promptly (but not emergently) repair the hernia in a girl even with an asymptomatic, nontender incarcerated ovary.[47]

MANAGEMENT

Anesthesia

There are no good data comparing regional to general anesthesia for pediatric inguinal hernia repair. A 2003 Cochrane meta-analysis of available data regarding this issue in premature infants concluded: 'There is no reliable evidence from the trials reviewed concerning the effect of spinal as compared to general anesthesia on the incidence of postoperative apnea, bradycardia, or oxygen desaturation in ex-preterm infants undergoing herniorrhaphy.'[48]

Overnight hospitalization is not necessary after inguinal hernia repair for healthy children or term infants. However, the risk of postoperative apnea and bradycardia is increased in premature infants and overnight monitoring may be necessary. The postconceptual age (gestational age plus chronologic age) is commonly used to decide which infants require overnight admission. Several studies have addressed this issue.[49,50] A review of 127 premature infants admitted after inguinal hernia repair found a incidence of apnea of about 5%, and attempted to identify factors associated with a higher risk (history of prior apnea, lower gestational age and birth weight, comorbidities).[50] A less than 1% risk of postoperative apnea was found in former premature infants greater than 56 weeks postconceptual age in a comprehensive analysis of eight prospective studies.[51] Sixty weeks postconceptual age is widely used as a cut-off for admission (although there is substantial institutional variability). However, a more recent retrospective review at our hospital demonstrated a low incidence of adverse events after 50 weeks postconceptual age.[52]

Timing

As premature infants have an increased incidence of an inguinal hernia, this is a common diagnosis in the neonatal intensive care unit. The incidence of bowel incarceration in premature infants is significantly increased (three times in one large series).[12] Many institutions use 2 kg as a lower limit for repair in asymptomatic and otherwise relatively healthy newborns. We usually repair the hernia before discharge to avoid the need for readmission for herniorrhaphy and to decrease the risk of incarceration.[46,53–55] However, this depends on other comorbidities. One recent study compared repair before discharge or as an outpatient, and found an increased length of hospitalization in the former group (largely from respiratory complications) and a low incidence of incarceration in the latter group.[56] However, others have found that in-house repair is preferable due to a lower incarceration rate after discharge.[57,58]

Open Repair Technique

Pediatric indirect inguinal hernias are usually repaired through an inguinal crease incision by incising the external oblique aponeurosis to the internal inguinal ring. After the ilioinguinal nerve is identified, the anteromedial hernia sac is grasped and the vas and vessels (in the usual male hernia) are pushed away from the sac (Fig. 50-2A). The sac is clamped and divided (Fig. 50-2B). A high ligation is performed after the sac is opened and inspected. If contralateral laparoscopic evaluation is performed, a small cannula can be gently advanced through the opened sac (Fig. 50-2C). A 70°, 2.7 mm telescope allows examination of the contralateral side (Figs 50-3 and 50-4).

There is an uncommon but disturbing incidence of late inguinal abscess formation related to the use of silk suture material for ligation of the sac.[59,60] For this reason, we now prefer absorbable sutures. The sac may be twisted before ligation, but too much twisting may draw the vas and cord structures into the base of the sac where they risk being inadvertently ligated. Removing the distal sac may increase the risk of injury to the cord structures and the testis, and is not necessary. Distal hydroceles should be opened widely and drained. It is important to ensure that the testis is in the scrotum at the conclusion of the procedure to avoid iatrogenic cryptorchidism.

Sliding hernias are uncommon but are more frequent in females, with an incidence as high as 20–40%. A fallopian tube or ovary may be involved. The bladder may constitute the medial wall of the sac in infants.[61] The appendix (Amyand's hernia) may form a sliding component on the right. More distal ligation of the sac with proximal purse-string inversion is our preferred management technique for sliding inguinal hernias.[62]

Mesh or prosthetic materials are almost never required in children. One exception may be recurrent hernias in children with connective tissue disorders or mucopolysaccharidoses.

Laparoscopic Repair Technique

An accurate description of the current state of pediatric laparoscopic inguinal hernia repair is a moving target. In 2002, Schier and colleagues reported a large series of 933 laparoscopic inguinal hernia repairs in children with a

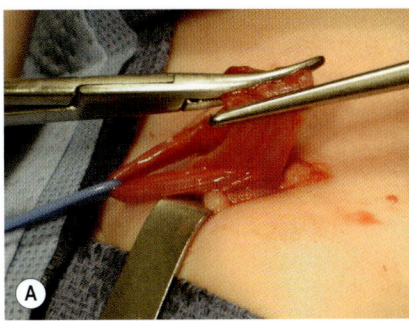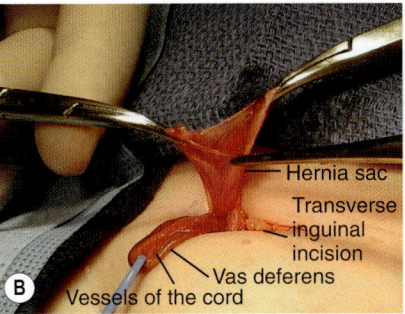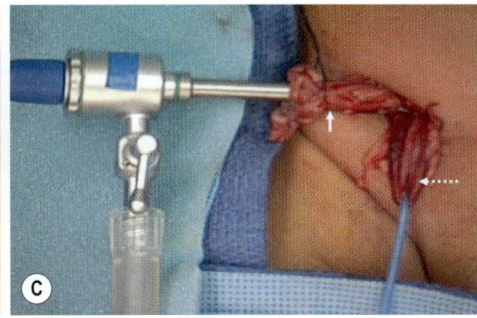

FIGURE 50-2 ■ **(A)** After a right inguinal incision in an infant boy, the sac has been separated from the vas and vessels by grasping the sac and 'teasing' the cord structures away. The hernia sac, located anteromedial to the cord, has been carefully separated from the vas and vessels (vessel loop) and is clamped in preparation for division of the sac. **(B)** In preparation for diagnostic laparoscopy to evaluate the contralateral internal ring, the sac is opened. A vessel loop is around the cord structures. **(C)** A cannula has been introduced into the opened hernia sac and the sac has been tied (solid arrow) to keep the abdomen insufflated. The cord structures (dotted arrow) are retracted with the vessel loop.

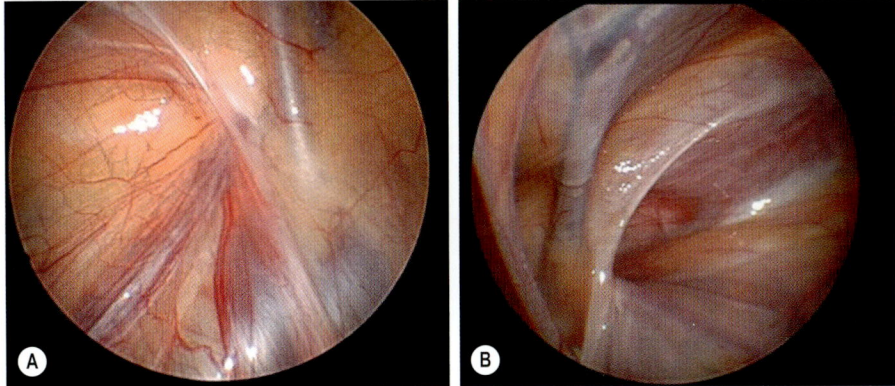

FIGURE 50-3 ■ Laparoscopic evaluation of the contralateral inguinal region is used by many pediatric surgeons. **(A)** A view of the left internal ring shows the inverted 'V' of the laterally located gonadal vessels and the medial vas. At the apex of the 'V,' the left internal inguinal ring is completely closed. **(B)** A right-patent process vaginalis is seen in a 7-year-old with a known left inguinal hernia.

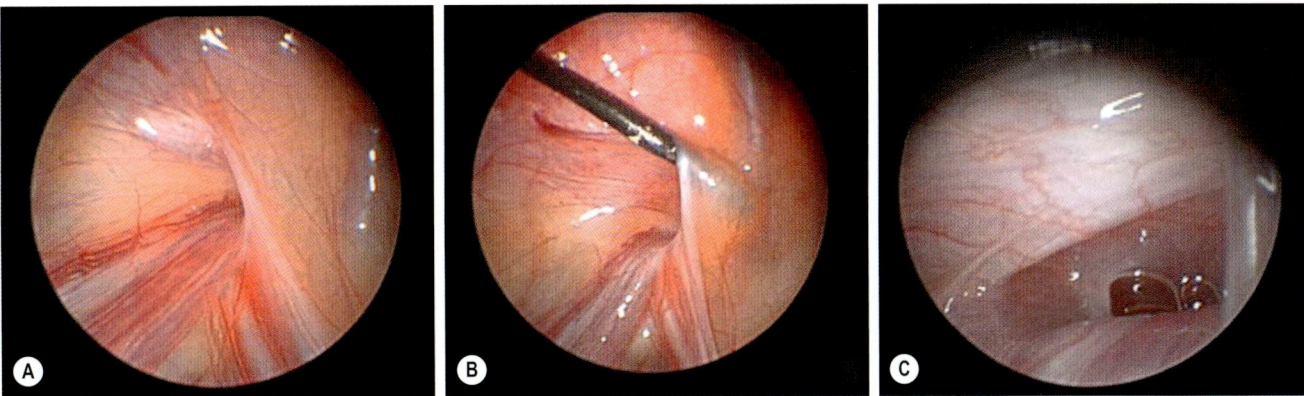

FIGURE 50-4 ■ **(A)** In a small percentage of cases, a veil of peritoneum will cover the contralateral internal ring and obscure the laparoscopic findings such that the surgeon is not completely certain whether a contralateral patent processus vaginalis (CPPV) is present. In this situation, a technique has been reported to retract the veil of tissue. **(B)** A silver probe is introduced in the contralateral lower abdomen/flank and used to retract the veil medially so that the 70-degree telescope can then look down the possible CPPV. **(C)** In this patient, a significant CPPV was visualized once the veil of peritoneum was retracted medially. (Adapted from Geiger JD. Selective laparoscopic probing for a contralateral patent processus vaginalis reduces the need for a contralateral exploration in inconclusive cases. J Pediatr Surg 2000;35:1151–4.)

mean age of 3.2 years and a recurrence rate of 3.4%.[63] Other reports followed with a similarly increased recurrence rate compared to open repairs.[64] However, in the last few years, there have been several large series of laparoscopic inguinal hernia repairs in infants and children with low recurrence and complication rates.[65–69]

A recent meta-analysis of three randomized controlled trials and four observational studies compared 1,543 laparoscopic repairs to 657 open repairs and found no difference in recurrence, a decreased incidence of metachronous hernia with laparoscopy, and decreased operative time for bilateral repairs done laparoscopically.[65] Another 2011 meta-analysis of 2,699 children found no statistically significant difference in recurrence rates, but an increased operative time with laparoscopic unilateral repair.[66] The authors confirmed the decreased incidence of metachronous hernia in the laparoscopic group. Improvement in laparoscopic recurrence rates appears to be due to various technical modifications of the procedure. Generally, it appears that extracorporeal knot-tying yields superior results. Several recent large series have reported recurrence rates less than 0.5%.[67–69]

Contralateral Evaluation

Contralateral exploration for unilateral inguinal hernia in children has a long and controversial history. Meta-, cost-, and decision-tree analyses have all been performed.[70–74] Routine contralateral open exploration is probably not justified. Surveys of pediatric surgeons have demonstrated a decrease in the practice of routine contralateral exploration over time, while laparoscopic evaluation of the contralateral side via the ipsilateral hernia opening has grown in popularity.[75,76]

Incidence of PPV

Diagnostic laparoscopy in children with a unilateral hernia allows identification of a contralateral PPV (see Figs 50-3 and 50-4), with the caveat that (1) some PPVs will not develop into clinically symptomatic hernias and (2) it may be difficult to distinguish a peritoneal fold from a true PPV. This technique was initially described in the early 1990s by Lobe and Holcomb.[77,78]

The mean additional operating time is minimal in most reports (four to five minutes).[79] There is some economic justification for this approach as well,[71,80] although not all other reports agree.[80] The reported incidence of PPV in unilateral hernia repairs has varied, but is typically 25–40%.

In a 2011 review of 684 children, contralateral laparoscopic evaluation was positive in 32% of right-sided and 42% of left-sided hernias.[81] A similar report of 1,001 children found a 24% incidence of PPV, decreasing with age and male gender.[79] A contralateral PPV was found in 38% of 453 children, decreasing with age.[82] Younger age, female gender, and a left-sided unilateral hernia have been used as selection criteria, while some authors argue for routine diagnostic contralateral laparoscopy in all children.[81–83]

Contralateral laparoscopic evaluation is impossible in about 5% of children, usually due to a very small hernia sac, or simply poor visualization.[28] Contralateral hernias after successful but negative contralateral evaluation been reported in 1.6–2.5% of patients.[81,84]

Incidence of Metachronous Hernia

Many reports have addressed the incidence of a contralateral clinical hernia after unilateral repair, and most have documented a 6–10% incidence.[74,85–88] Left-sided initial hernias may be associated with an increased risk of a symptomatic contralateral hernia. Younger patient age and prematurity have also been identified as markers for an increased risk of metachronous hernia.

A 2007 meta-analysis of 49 papers with data on 22,846 children found an overall incidence of 7.2%, with no gender difference.[89] However, a left-sided inguinal hernia had a significantly higher risk than right-sided (10.2% vs 6.3%). A prospective study of 548 patients followed for a mean of two years found that 8.8% developed a contralateral hernia, with an average interval of six months. The incidence was higher in younger infants, premature infants, and females.[90] An older meta-analysis of 15,310 patients from several studies found a 7% incidence of a metachronous hernia.[72] A prospective study in which 222 children with unilateral hernia underwent laparoscopy, and 67 clinically followed without repair of an incidental PPV noted that 6.8% developed a metachronous hernia.[91] MacGregor et al. followed 160 children under age 10 years who underwent a unilateral inguinal hernia repair over a 32-year period. Ninety-six percent were followed for a mean of 20 years. Over this time, 29% developed a symptomatic contralateral inguinal hernia. Interestingly, the authors did not recommend routine contralateral exploration due to its risks (in the open era).[92]

Pain Management

A randomized prospective trial of local instillation of long-acting analgesics (e.g., bupivacaine) versus caudal block for postoperative pain control in infants and children after inguinal hernia repair demonstrated no significant difference in pain control.[93] Instillation of local anesthetics into the wound ('splash technique') is effective as well. Ilioinguinal nerve block was also shown to provide better analgesia than transverse abdominis plane block in a prospective randomized trial.[94]

COMPLICATIONS

Recurrence

The risk of recurrence after an elective inguinal hernia repair is less than 1% in several large series.[12,95] It is higher in premature infants, in children with incarcerated hernias, and those with associated diseases (e.g., connective tissue disorder, VPS).[17,95] Recurrence rates can be as high as 50% in children with connective tissues disorders and mucopolysaccharidoses. A recurrent hernia even can be the presenting symptom in these diseases.[95] Recurrence rates may also be higher in teenagers.[12]

Injury to the Spermatic Cord or Testis

Injury to the spermatic cord or testis is a rare occurrence in elective hernia repairs, with an incidence of approximately 1 in 1,000.[12] The true incidence may be underestimated since instrument manipulation of the cord causes microscopic injury and scarring in animal models.[96,97] A recognized injury to the vas should be managed by immediate repair with fine (8-0) suture under magnification, and the family should be informed of the event. In institutions in which hernia sacs are routinely examined by a pathologist, mesonephric or adrenal rests are occasionally seen, but do not indicate injury to the vas. A review of 7,314 male pediatric hernia specimens over a 14-year period at a major children's hospital found either vas deferens or epididymis in 0.53% of specimens.[98] Recent reviews of the subject have concluded that routine histologic examination of male hernia sacs is not necessary.[99,100] Testicular atrophy from vascular injury during routine inguinal hernia repair is also uncommon.

Other Complications

In a recent retrospective review of 268 patients less than 2 years of age (98 of whom were premature), prematurity was a marker for an increased risk of complications following inguinal hernia repair (28% vs 12% in term infants).[58]

Infection occurs in 1–3% of cases, and postoperative hematoma has a similarly low incidence. Persistent hydrocele can occur, particularly if a very large hydrocele was present preoperatively. It is important to educate the family about this possibility before repair. Most postoperative hydroceles can be observed for six to 12 months. If they do not resolve, aspiration may be tried once or twice. In our experience, aspiration is not usually permanently successful. Persistent non-resolving hydroceles may require transumbilical diagnostic laparoscopy to exclude a recurrent hernia. In the absence of recurrence, a transcrotal exploration and obliteration of the hydrocele sac is usually effective.

Chronic pain after herniorrhaphy, although seen in adults, is uncommon in children. However, one recent review of 651 adults who had undergone inguinal hernia repair before age five years found that 13.5% of

the patients reported occasional mild groin pain, usually related to physical activity (pain was frequent or moderate in only 2%).[101]

Loss of domain due to a huge hernia is another problem more frequently seen in adults, but it can occur in infants or children and may require staged repair or other measures.[102] Iatrogenic cryptorchidism from failure to replace the testis in normal anatomic position is a rare occurrence (<1%). Bladder injury in infants in whom the medial wall of the sac contains urinary bladder is also a rare complication.[103]

Mortality directly related to inguinal hernia or its repair is exceedingly rare (<1%).

SPECIAL ISSUES

Direct Inguinal Hernia

Direct inguinal hernias are very unusual in children, even older teenagers.[104] However, the incidence was as high as 4% in one laparoscopic series.[105] Some recurrences after indirect inguinal hernia repair are direct inguinal hernias. Direct inguinal hernias in children are managed as standard 'adult' inguinal hernia repairs. Our preference is for a McVay repair (approximation of the transversalis aponeurotic arch and internal oblique aponeurosis to the anterior ileopubic tract and shelving edge of the inguinal ligament). Laparoscopic repair is another option.

Femoral Hernia

Femoral hernias are relatively equally distributed by gender,[106,107] but are much less common than indirect inguinal hernias. In two combined series of over 10,000 patients, 0.2% of hernias were femoral.[104,108] Most (two-thirds) are not suspected before operation (Fig. 50-5).[104,107] A mass below the inguinal ligament should alert the clinician to this possibility. Femoral hernias are bilateral in 10 to 20%. Recurrence is increased after femoral hernia repair compared with indirect inguinal herniorrhaphy.[106] McVay repair has been the standard technique for repair, but laparoscopic and mesh-plug repairs have been used as well.[109,110]

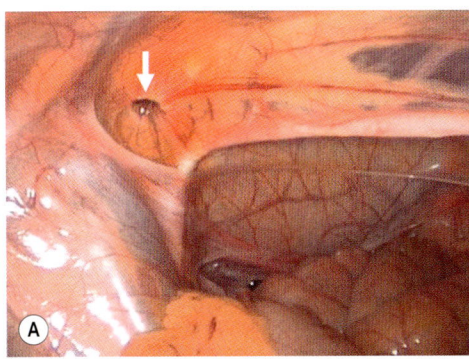 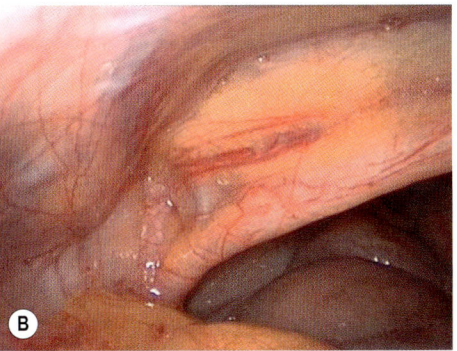

FIGURE 50-5 ■ This young girl presented with symptoms suggestive, but not conclusive, of a left femoral hernia. Therefore, diagnostic laparoscopy was performed through the umbilicus to confirm the diagnosis prior to an inguinal approach and a McVay repair. **(A)** The internal opening (arrow) to the femoral hernia is seen. **(B)** After the McVay repair, the femoral defect is closed.

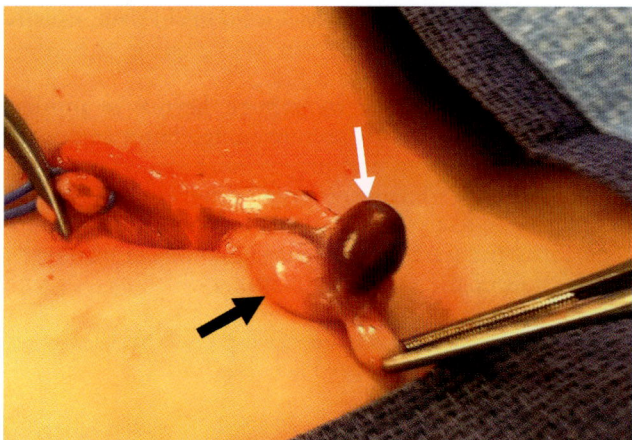

FIGURE 50-6 ■ Rarely, sphenogonadal fusion is found at the time of inguinal hernia repair. The splenic remnant (white arrow) and testis (black arrow) are fused. The splenic tissue was safely excised.

Absent or Atrophic Vas

Occasionally, a small or absent vas is found during inguinal hernia repair. Renal ultrasound is necessary because of associated ipsilateral renal agenesis.[111,112] This should also prompt a workup for cystic fibrosis. Congenital absence (bilateral or unilateral) of the vas is a heterogeneous disorder, largely due to mutations in the cystic fibrosis gene. Differing genotypes are noted with congenital absence of the vas as an isolated entity versus congenital absence of the vas in association with renal anomalies.[113]

Disorders of Sexual Differentiation

The finding of a testis during repair of a female hernia should raise the suspicion of congenital androgen insensitivity syndrome (CAIS) or true hermaphroditism.[114] As many as 1% of female infants with inguinal hernias will have CAIS.[115] Bilateral hernias in girls are not associated with a higher risk of CAIS than is a unilateral hernia. Conversely, as many as 75% of CAIS patients present with a hernia.

At the time of hernia repair (or later as a separate procedure), laparoscopy is a good way to evaluate for the presence or absence of the fallopian tube, ovary, and uterus. The gonad should be sampled. Some advocate rectal examination to palpate the uterus. Vaginoscopy is another option. In the presence of CAIS, an absent cervix will be found, and vaginal length is shortened in this syndrome.[115] Karyotyping and pelvic ultrasound should also be performed. Eventual gonadectomy will be necessary, although the optimal timing is controversial.

Other

Incidentally discovered yellow nodules along the spermatic cord or testis are due to adrenal rests. In one study, the incidence was 1.7% in 1,862 pediatric hernia repairs.[116] These should be removed if possible. Splenogonadal fusion is a very rare entity that may be difficult to distinguish preoperatively from a testicular neoplasm (Fig. 50-6). Frozen section confirmation usually allows gonadal preservation.

REFERENCES

1. Lau WY. History of treatment of groin hernia. World J Surg [Internet] 2002;26(6):748–59. Available from: http://www.springerlink.com/index/10.1007/s00268-002-6297-5.
2. Lascaratos JG, Tsiamis C, Kostakis A. Surgery for inguinal hernia in Byzantine Times (A.D. 324-1453): First Scientific Descriptions. World J Surg 2003;27:1165–9.
3. Cloquet's hernia (www.whonamedit.com) [Internet]. whonamedit.com. [cited 2012 Jun. 21]. Available from: http://www.whonamedit.com/synd.cfm/2654.html.
4. Cloquet J. Recherches Anatomiques sur les Hernies de l'Abdomen. Paris; 1817.
5. Marcy H. A new use of carbolized cat gut ligatures. Boston Med Surg J 1871;85:315–16.
6. Czerny Von V. Studien zur Radikalbehandlung der Hernien. Wien Med Wochenschr 1877;27:497–528–554–578.
7. Sachs M, Damm M, Encke A. Historical evolution of inguinal hernia repair. World J Surg 1997;21:218–23.
8. Bassini E. Nuovo Metodo Operativo per la Cura dell'Ernia Inguinale. R Stabilimento Prosperini; 1889.
9. Gross RE. Inguinal Hernia. The Surgery of Infancy and Childhood. Philadelphia: W.B. Saunders; 1953. p. 449–62.
10. Bronsther B, Abrams MW, Elboim C. Inguinal hernias in children–a study of 1,000 cases and a review of the literature. J Am Med Womens Assoc 1972;27:522–5.
11. Bakwin H. Indirect inguinal hernia in twins. J Pediatr Surg 1971;6:165–8.
12. Ein SH, Njere I, Ein A. Six thousand three hundred sixty-one pediatric inguinal hernias: A 35-year review. J Pediatr Surg 2006;1:980–6.
13. Harper RG, Garcia A, Sia C. Inguinal hernia: A common problem of premature infants weighing 1,000 grams or less at birth. Pediatrics 1975;56:112–15.
14. Kumar VHS, Clive J, Rosenkrantz TS, et al. Inguinal hernia in preterm infants. Pediatr Surg Int 2002;18:147–52.
15. Grosfeld JL. Current concepts in inguinal hernia in infants and children. World J Surg 1989;13:506–15.
16. Holsclaw DS, Shwachman H. Increased incidence of inguinal hernia, hydrocele, and undescended testicle in males with cystic fibrosis. Pediatrics 1971;48:442–5.
17. Celik A, Ergün O, Arda MS, et al. The incidence of inguinal complications after ventriculoperitoneal shunt for hydrocephalus. Childs Nerv Syst 2005;21:44–7.
18. Clarnette TD, Lam SK, Hutson JM. Ventriculo-peritoneal shunts in children reveal the natural history of closure of the processus vaginalis. J Pediatr Surg 1998;33:413–16.
19. Wu JC, Chen YC, Liu L, et al. Younger boys have a higher risk of inguinal hernia after Ventriculo-Peritoneal Shunt: A 13-year nationwide cohort study. JACS 2012;214:845–51.
20. Glick PL, Boulanger SC. Inguinal Hernias and Hydroceles. In: Coran AG, Adzick NS, Krummel T, et al, editors. Pediatric Surgery. 7th ed. Philadelphia: Elsevier/Saunders; 2012.
21. Ilioinguinal nerve [Internet]. en.wikipedia.org. [cited 2012 Jun. 27]. Available from: http://en.wikipedia.org/wiki/Ilioinguinal_nerve.
22. Gray SW, Skandalakis JE. Embryology for surgeons. 2nd ed. Baltimore: Williams & Wilkins; 1994. p. 540–93.
23. Lie G, Hutson JM. The role of cremaster muscle in testicular descent in humans and animal models. Pediatr Surg Int 2011;27:1255–65.
24. Clarnette TD, Hutson JM. The genitofemoral nerve may link testicular inguinoscrotal descent with congenital inguinal hernia. Aust N Z J Surg 1996;66:612–17.
25. Heyns CF. The gubernaculum during testicular descent in the human fetus. J Anat 1987;153:93–112.
26. Rowe MI, Copelson LW, Clatworthy HW. The patent processus vaginalis and the inguinal hernia. J Pediatr Surg 1969;4:102–7.
27. Luo C-C, Chao H-C. Prevention of unnecessary contralateral exploration using the silk glove sign (SGS) in pediatric patients with unilateral inguinal hernia. Eur J Pediatr 2006;166:667–9.

28. Valusek PA, Spilde TL, Ostlie DJ, et al. Laparoscopic evaluation for contralateral patent processus vaginalis in children with unilateral inguinal hernia. J Laparoendosc Adv Surg Tech A 2006;166:650–3.

29. Chen KC, Chu CC, Chou TY, et al. Ultrasonography for inguinal hernias in boys. J Pediatr Surg 1998;33:1784–7.

30. Erez I, Rathause V, Vacian I, et al. Preoperative ultrasound and intraoperative findings of inguinal hernias in children: A prospective study of 642 children. J Pediatr Surg 2002;37:865–8.

31. Naji H, Ingolfsson I, Isacson D, et al. Decision making in the management of hydroceles in infants and children. Eur J Pediatr 2012;171:807–10.

32. Lau ST, Lee Y-H, Caty MG. Current management of hernias and hydroceles. Sem Pediatr Surg 2007;16:50–7.

33. Koski M, Makari J, Adams M. Infant communicating hydroceles–do they need immediate repair or might some clinically resolve? J Pediatr Surg 2010;45:590–3.

34. Chang Y-T, Lee J-Y, Wang J-Y, et al. Hydrocele of the spermatic cord in infants and children: Its particular characteristics. Urology 2010;76:82–6.

35. Andrews EW. The "Bottle Operation" method for the radical cure of hydrocele. Ann Surg 1907;46:915–18.

36. Wilson J, Aaronson D, Schrader R. Hydrocele in the pediatric patient: Inguinal or scrotal approach? J Urol 2008;180:1427–727.

37. Martin K, Emil S, Laberge J-M. The value of laparoscopy in the management of abdominoscrotal hydroceles. J Laparoendosc Adv Surg Tech A 2012;22:419–21.

38. Stephens BJ, Rice WT, Koucky CJ, et al. Optimal timing of elective indirect inguinal hernia repair in healthy children: Clinical considerations for improved outcome. World J Surg 1992;16:952–6.

39. Rowe MI, Clatworthy HW. Incarcerated and strangulated hernias in children. A statistical study of high-risk factors. Arch Surg 1970;101:136–9.

40. Palmer BV. Incarcerated inguinal hernia in children. Ann R Coll Surg Engl 1978;60:121–4.

41. Stylianos S, Jacir NN, Harris BH. Incarceration of inguinal hernia in infants prior to elective repair. J Pediatr Surg 1993;28:582–3.

42. Puri P, Guiney EJ, O'Donnell B. Inguinal hernia in infants: The fate of the testis following incarceration. J Pediatr Surg 1984;19:44–6.

43. Shalaby R, Shams AM, Mohamed S, et al. Two-trocar needle-scopic approach to incarcerated inguinal hernia in children. J Pediatr Surg 2007;42:1259–62.

44. Takehara H, Hanaoka J, Arakawa Y. Laparoscopic strategy for inguinal ovarian hernias in children: When to operate for irreducible ovary. J Laparoendosc Adv Surg Tech A 2009;19:S129–S131.

45. Nah SA, Giacomello L, Eaton S, et al. Surgical repair of incarcerated inguinal hernia in children: Laparoscopic or open? Eur J Pediatr Surg 2011;21:8–11.

46. Nagraj S, Sinha S, Grant H, et al. The incidence of complications following primary inguinal herniotomy in babies weighing 5 kg or less. Pediatr Surg Int 2006;22:500–2.

47. Levitt MA, Ferraraccio D, Arbesman MC, et al. Variability of inguinal hernia surgical technique: A survey of North American pediatric surgeons. J Pediatr Surg 2002;37:745–51.

48. Craven PD, Badawi N, Henderson-Smart DJ, et al. Regional (spinal, epidural, caudal) versus general anaesthesia in preterm infants undergoing inguinal herniorrhaphy in early infancy. Cochrane Database Syst Rev 2003;(3):CD003669.

49. Coté CJ, Zaslavsky A, Downes JJ, et al. Postoperative apnea in former preterm infants after inguinal herniorrhaphy. A combined analysis. Anesthesiology 1995;82:809–22.

50. Murphy JJ, Swanson T, Ansermino M, et al. The frequency of apneas in premature infants after inguinal hernia repair: Do they need overnight monitoring in the intensive care unit? J Pediatr Surg 2008;43:865–8.

51. Malviya S, Swartz J, Lerman J. Are all preterm infants younger than 60 weeks postconceptual age at risk for postanesthetic apnea? Anesthesiology 1993;78:1076–81.

52. Laituri CA, Garey CL, Pieters BJ, et al. Overnight observation in former premature infants undergoing inguinal hernia repair. J Pediatr Surg 2012;47:217–20.

53. Misra D. Inguinal hernias in premature babies: Wait or operate? Acta Paediatr 2001;90:370–1.

54. Lautz TB, Raval MV, Reynolds M. Does timing matter? A national perspective on the risk of incarceration in premature neonates with inguinal hernia. J Pediatr 2011;158:573–7.

55. Miller GG, McDonald SE, Milbrandt K, et al. Risk of incarceration of inguinal hernia among infants and young children awaiting elective surgery. CMAJ 2008;179:1001–5.

56. Lee SL, Gleason JM, Sydorak RM. A critical review of premature infants with inguinal hernias: Optimal timing of repair, incarceration risk, and postoperative apnea. J Pediatr Surg 2011;46:217–20.

57. Vaos G, Gardikis S, Kambouri K, et al. Optimal timing for repair of an inguinal hernia in premature infants. Pediatr Surg Int 2010;26:379–85.

58. Gholoum S, Baird R, Laberge J-M, et al. Incarceration rates in pediatric inguinal hernia: Do not trust the coding. J Pediatr Surg 2010;45:1007–11.

59. Calkins CM, St Peter SD, Balcom A, et al. Late abscess formation following indirect hernia repair utilizing silk suture. Pediatr Surg Int 2007;23:349–52.

60. Nagar H. Stitch granulomas following inguinal herniotomy: A 10-year review. J Pediatr Surg 1993;28:1505–7.

61. Redman JF, Jacks DW, O'Donnell PD. Cystectomy: A catastrophic complication of herniorrhaphy. J Urol 1985;133:97–8.

62. Bevan A. Sliding inguinal hernia of the ascending colon and cecum, the descending colon, sigmoid, and the bladder. Ann Surg 1930;92:792–4.

63. Schier F, Montupet P, Esposito C. Laparoscopic inguinal herniorrhaphy in children: A three-center experience with 933 repairs. J Pediatr Surg 2002;37:395–7.

64. Schier F. Laparoscopic inguinal hernia repair-A prospective personal series of 542 children. J Pediatr Surg 2006;41:1081–4.

65. Yang C, Zhang H, Pu J, et al. Laparoscopic vs open herniorrhaphy in the management of pediatric inguinal hernia: A systemic review and meta-analysis. J Pediatr Surg 2011;46:1824–34.

66. Alzahem A. Laparoscopic versus open inguinal herniotomy in infants and children: A meta-analysis. Pediatr Surg Int 2011;27:605–12.

67. Tam YH, Lee KH, Sihoe JDY, et al. Laparoscopic hernia repair in children by the hook method: A single-center series of 433 consecutive patients. J Pediatr Surg 2009;44:1502–5.

68. Endo M, Watanabe T, Nakano M, et al. Laparoscopic completely extraperitoneal repair of inguinal hernia in children: A single-institute experience with 1,257 repairs compared with cut-down herniorrhaphy. Surg Endosc 2009;23:1706–12.

69. Chen K, Xiang G, Wang H, et al. Towards a near-zero recurrence rate in laparoscopic inguinal hernia repair for pediatric patients. J Laparoendosc Adv Surg Tech A 2011;21:445–8.

70. Burd RS, Heffington SH, Teague JL. The optimal approach for management of metachronous hernias in children: A decision analysis. J Pediatr Surg 2001;36:1190–5.

71. Miltenburg DM, Nuchtern JG, Jaksic T, et al. Laparoscopic evaluation of the pediatric inguinal hernia–A meta-analysis. J Pediatr Surg 1998;33:874–9.

72. Miltenburg DM, Nuchtern JG, Jaksic T, et al. Meta-analysis of the risk of metachronous hernia in infants and children. Am J Surg 1991;174:741–4.

73. Muensterer OJ, Woller T, Metzger R, et al. [The economics of contralateral laparoscopic inguinal hernia exploration: Cost calculation of herniotomy in infants.]. Chirurg 2008;79:1065–71.

74. Nataraja RM, Mahomed AA. Systematic review for paediatric metachronous contralateral inguinal hernia: A decreasing concern. Pediatr Surg Int 2011;27:953–61.

75. Antonoff MB, Kreykes NS, Saltzman DA, et al. American Academy of Pediatrics Section on Surgery hernia survey revisited. J Pediatr Surg 2005;40:1009–14.

76. Wiener ES, Touloukian RJ, Rodgers BM, et al. Hernia survey of the Section on Surgery of the American Academy of Pediatrics. J Pediatr Surg 1996;31:1166–9.

77. Lobe TE, Schropp KP. Inguinal hernias in pediatrics: Initial experience with laparoscopic inguinal exploration of the asymptomatic contralateral side. J Laparoendosc Surg 1992;2:135–40.

78. Holcomb GW III, Brock JW, Morgan WM. Laparoscopic evaluation for a contralateral patent processus vaginalis. J Pediatr Surg 1994;29:970–3.

79. Saad S, Mansson J, Saad A, et al. Ten-year review of groin laparoscopy in 1001 pediatric patients with clinical unilateral inguinal hernia: An improved technique with transhernia multiple-channel scope. J Pediatr Surg 2011;46:1011–14.

80. Lee SL, Sydorak RM, Lau ST. Laparoscopic contralateral groin exploration: Is it cost effective? J Pediatr Surg 2010;45:793–5.

81. Draus JM, Kamel S, Seims A, et al. The role of laparoscopic evaluation to detect a contralateral defect at initial presentation for inguinal hernia repair. Am Surg 2011;77:1463–6.

82. Lazar DA, Lee TC, Almulhim SI, et al. Transinguinal laparoscopic exploration for identification of contralateral inguinal hernias in pediatric patients. J Pediatr Surg 2011;46:2349–52.

83. Yerkes EB, Brock JW, Holcomb GW III, et al. Laparoscopic evaluation for a contralateral patent processus vaginalis: Part III. Urology 1998;51:480–3.

84. Juang D, Garey CL, Ostlie DJ, et al. Contralateral inguinal hernia after negative laparoscopic evaluation: A rare but real phenomenon. J Laparoendosc Adv Surg Tech A 2012;22:200–2.

85. Chertin B, De Caluwé D, Gajaharan M, et al. Is contralateral exploration necessary in girls with unilateral inguinal hernia? J Pediatr Surg 2003;38:756–7.

86. Shabbir J, Moore A, O'Sullivan JB, et al. Contralateral groin exploration is not justified in infants with a unilateral inguinal hernia. Ir J Med Sci 2003;172:18–19.

87. Ballantyne A, Jawaheer G, Munro FD. Contralateral groin exploration is not justified in infants with a unilateral inguinal hernia. Br J Surg 2001;88:720–3.

88. Given JP, Rubin SZ. Occurrence of contralateral inguinal hernia following unilateral repair in a pediatric hospital. J Pediatr Surg 1989;24:963–5.

89. Ron O, Eaton S, Pierro A. Systematic review of the risk of developing a metachronous contralateral inguinal hernia in children. Br J Surg 2007;94:804–11.

90. Tackett LD, Breuer CK, Luks FI, et al. Incidence of contralateral inguinal hernia: A prospective analysis. J Pediatr Surg 1999;34:684–7.

91. Maddox MM, Smith DP. A long-term prospective analysis of pediatric unilateral inguinal hernias: Should laparoscopy or anything else influence the management of the contralateral side? J Pediatr Urol 2008;4:141–5.

92. McGregor DB, Halverson K, McVay CB. The unilateral pediatric inguinal hernia: Should the contralateral side by explored? J Pediatr Surg 1980;15:313–17.

93. Machotta A, Risse A, Bercker S, et al. Comparison between instillation of bupivacaine versus caudal analgesia for postoperative analgesia following inguinal herniotomy in children. Paediatr Anaesth 2003;13:397–402.

94. Fredrickson MJ, Paine C, Hamill J. Improved analgesia with the ilioinguinal block compared to the transverse abdominis plane block after pediatric inguinal hernia surgery: A prospective randomized trial. Pediatr Anaesth 2010;20:1022–7.

95. Grosfeld JL, Minnick K, Shedd F, et al. Inguinal hernia in children: Factors affecting recurrence in 62 cases. J Pediatr Surg 1991;26:283–7.

96. Shandling B, Janik JS. The vulnerability of the vas deferens. J Pediatr Surg 1981;16:461–4.

97. Abasiyanik A, Güvenc H, Yavuzer D, et al. The effect of iatrogenic vas deferens injury on fertility in an experimental rat model. J Pediatr Surg 1997;32:1144–6.

98. Steigman CK, Sotelo-Avila C, Weber TR. The incidence of spermatic cord structures in inguinal hernia sacs from male children. Am J Surg Pathol 1999;23:880–5.

99. Miller GG, McDonald SE, Milbrandt K, et al. Routine pathological evaluation of tissue from inguinal hernias in children is unnecessary. Can J Surg 2003;46:117–19.

100. Kim B, Leonard MP, Bass J, et al. Analysis of the clinical significance and cost associated with the routine pathological analysis of pediatric inguinal hernia sacs. J Urol 2011;186:1620–4.

101. Aasvang EK, Kehlet H. Chronic pain after childhood groin hernia repair. J Pediatr Surg 2007;42:1403–8.

102. Khozeimeh N, Henry MCW, Gingalewski CA, et al. Management of congenital giant inguinal scrotal hernias in the newborn. Hernia 2011 (EPUB).

103. Aloi IP, Lais A, Caione P. Bladder injuries following inguinal canal surgery in infants. Pediatr Surg Int 2010;26:1207–10.

104. Fonkalsrud EW, Delorimier A, Clatworthy HW. Femoral and direct inguinal hernias in infants and children. JAMA 1965;192:597–9.

105. Gorsler CM, Schier F. Laparoscopic herniorrhaphy in children. Surg Endosc 2003;17:571–3.

106. De Caluwé D, Chertin B, Puri P. Childhood femoral hernia: A commonly misdiagnosed condition. Pediatr Surg Int 2003;19:608–9.

107. Al-Shanafey S, Giacomantonio M. Femoral hernia in children. J Pediatr Surg 1999;34:1104–6.

108. Burke J. Femoral hernia in childhood. Ann Surg 1967;166:287–9.

109. Adibe OO, Hansen EN, Seifarth FG, et al. Laparoscopic-assisted repair of femoral hernias in children. J Laparoendosc Adv Surg Tech A 2009;19:691–4.

110. Matthyssens LEM, Philippe P. A new minimally invasive technique for the repair of femoral hernia in children: About 13 laparoscopic repairs in 10 patients. J Pediatr Surg 2009;44:967–71.

111. Lukash F, Zwiren GT, Andrews HG. Significance of absent vas deferens at hernia repair in infants and children. J Pediatr Surg 1975;10:765–9.

112. Schlegel PN, Shin D, Goldstein M. Urogenital anomalies in men with congenital absence of the vas deferens. J Urol 1996;155:1644–8.

113. Casals T, Bassas L, Egozcue S, et al. Heterogeneity for mutations in the CFTR gene and clinical correlations in patients with congenital absence of the vas deferens. Hum Reprod 2000;15:1476–83.

114. Hughes IA, Davies JD, Bunch TI, et al. Androgen insensitivity syndrome. Lancet 2012;380:1419–28.

115. Hurme T, Lahdes-Vasama T, Makela E, et al. Clinical findings in prepubertal girls with inguinal hernia with special reference to the diagnosis of androgen insensitivity syndrome. Scand J Urol Nephrol 2009;43:42–6.

116. Ketata S, Ketata H, Sahnoun A, et al. Ectopic adrenal cortex tissue: An incidental finding during inguinoscrotal operations in pediatric patients. Urol Int 2008;81:316–19.

CHAPTER 51

UNDESCENDED TESTES AND TESTICULAR TUMORS

J. Joy Lee • Linda M. Dairiki Shortliffe

UNDESCENDED TESTES

Normal testicular descent relies on a complex interplay of numerous factors. Any deviation from the normal process can result in a cryptorchid or undescended testis (UDT) (Fig. 51-1). UDT is a common abnormality that carries fertility and malignancy implications.

Embryology

Testicular development and descent depend on a coordinated interaction among endocrine, paracrine, growth, and mechanical factors. Bipotential gonadal tissue located on the embryo's genital ridge begins differentiation into a testis during weeks 6 and 7 under the effects of the testis-determining SRY gene. Sertoli cells begin to produce Müllerian inhibitory factor (MIF) soon thereafter, causing regression of all Müllerian duct structures except for the remnant appendix testis and prostatic utricle. By week 9, Leydig cells produce testosterone and stimulate development of Wolffian structures, including the epididymis and vas deferens. The testis resides in the abdomen near the internal ring until descent through the inguinal canal at the beginning of the third trimester.

Two important hormones in testicular descent are insulin-like factor 3 (INSL3) and testosterone, both secreted by the testis, while two important anatomic players are the gubernaculum testis and the cranial suspensory ligament (CSL). The gubernaculum is thought to help anchor the testis near the internal inguinal ring as the kidney migrates cephalad. Androgens prompt the involution of the CSL, allowing for eventual downward migration of the testicle.[1] In humans, the frequency of UDT is increased in boys with diseases that affect androgen secretion or function.[2,3] When anti-androgens are given to pregnant rats, the rate of UDT in male offspring is 50%.[4,5] Estradiol downregulates INSL3 in experimental models, and maternal exposure to estrogens such as diethystilbesterol (DES) has also been associated with cryptorchidism.[6,7]

Under the influence of INSL3, the gubernaculum undergoes two phases: outgrowth and regression.[8,9] Outgrowth refers to rapid swelling by the gubernaculum, thereby dilating the inguinal canal and creating a pathway for descent. Mice with homozygous mutant INSL3 have been found to have poorly developed gubernacula and intra-abdominal testes.[10] Next, during regression, the gubernaculum undergoes cellular remodeling and becomes a fibrous structure.[11] It is believed that

intra-abdominal pressure then causes protrusion of the processus vaginalis through the internal inguinal ring, transmitting pressure to the gubernaculum and initiating testicular descent. However, the gubernaculum is not directly attached to the scrotum during inguinal passage, and does not act as a pulley. Transit through the inguinal canal is relatively rapid, starting around week 22 and typically completed after week 27.[12,13]

Other potential mediators of descent include MIF, by causing resorption of Müllerian structures and clearing anatomic roadblocks to descent, and calcitonin gene-related peptide (CGRP).[9] While research in rats has implicated CGRP in contraction of cremasteric muscle fibers and subsequent gubernacular and testicular descent,[14,15] in humans the cremaster is distinct from the gubernaculum.[12,16] In addition, growth factors such as epidermal growth factor act on the placenta to enhance gonadotropin release, which stimulates secretion of descendin, a growth factor for gubernacular development.[8]

Epididymal anomalies are found in up to 50% of men with UDT.[17,18] Some investigators postulate that the gubernaculum facilitates epididymal descent, indirectly guiding the testis into the scrotum.[19] Others believe that an abnormality of paracrine function is responsible for both epididymal anomalies and UDT, but that epididymal abnormalities are not causal.[1]

Classification

Variability in nomenclature regarding UDT has led to ambiguity in the literature and difficulty comparing treatment results. The clearest classification divides testes into palpable and nonpalpable.[20] The distinction can be blurred, however, as when a previously palpable testis falls back into the abdomen through the open ring, or an intra-abdominal 'peeping' testis can be felt at the upper inguinal canal. A retractile testis is a normally descended testis that retracts into the inguinal canal as a result of cremasteric contraction; it is not an UDT. Though retractile testes do not require operative repair, in some series as many as one-third become ascending UDTs, suggesting either an initial difficult diagnosis or suboptimal attachment within the scrotum that changes position of the testis with growth of the child.[21]

A true UDT has halted somewhere along the normal path of descent from abdomen to distal to the inguinal ring. An ectopic UDT is one that has deviated from the path of normal descent and can be found in the inguinal

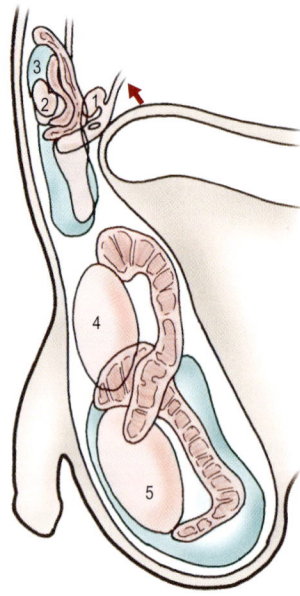

FIGURE 51-1 ■ Testicular descent in males: 1, 90 mm crown–rump length (CRL) (12–24 weeks of gestational age); 2, 125 mm CRL (15–17 weeks); 3, 230 mm CRL (24–26 weeks); 4, 280 mm CRL (28-30 weeks); 5, at term. The convoluted structure is the epididymis. (Adapted from Hadziselimovic F. Embryology of testicular descent and maldescent. In: Hadziselimovic F, editor. Cryptorchidism: Management and Implications. New York: Springer-Verlag; 1983. p. 23.)

region, perineum, femoral canal, penopubic area, or even contralateral hemiscrotum. Ascending or acquired UDT refers to a testis that was previously descended on examination, but at a later time can no longer be brought down into the scrotum. While an association between retractile testes and secondary testicular ascent has been identified, a link between rate of height growth and ascended testes suggests that the ability to reach the scrotum changes with a child's growth.[22,23] Acquired UDT may also be iatrogenic, as when a previously descended testis becomes trapped in scar tissue cephalad to the scrotum after inguinal surgery.

A nonpalpable testis may be simply intra-abdominal some of the time, or truly vanished due to intrauterine or perinatal torsion. This condition is known as monorchia, or anorchia if both testes are absent.

Incidence

UDT occurs in approximately 3% of term male infants and in up to 33–45% of premature and/or birth weight <2.5 kg male infants.[24] The majority of testes descend within the first 6 to 12 months such that at 1 year, the incidence is down to 1%. Testicular descent after 1 year is unlikely.[25] However, 2–3% of boys in the USA, and up to 5.3% in some European series, undergo orchiopexy for UDT.[26,27] This discrepancy between higher orchiopexy rates and actual incidence of the disease is thought to lie partially in misdiagnosis between retractile testes, but also from acquired UDT. The overall rate of secondary testicular ascent has been reported between 2–45%.[28,29]

Series documenting the location of a UDT find that two-thirds to three-quarters of cases are palpable, usually within the inguinal canal or distal to the external ring.[30,31] Anomalies associated with UDT include a patent processus vaginalis and epididymal abnormalities. Specific syndromes with higher rates of UDT include prune-belly syndrome, gastroschisis, bladder exstrophy, Prader–Willi, Kallman, Noonan, testicular dysgenesis and androgen insensitivity syndromes.[22]

Diagnosis

Given the historic variability in the definition of what constitutes an UDT, it is not surprising that confusion exists in the primary care setting as well. A careful history and physical examination is thus paramount.

The patient should be examined in a warm room in both supine and frog-legged sitting position. The scrotum is observed for hypoplasia and examined for the presence of either testis. In cases of monorchia, the solitary testis may be compensatorily hypertrophied. The first maneuver to locate the testis is to walk the fingers from the iliac crest along the inguinal canal towards the scrotum, pushing subcutaneous structures toward the scrotum. The scrotum should not be palpated prior to this maneuver as it may activate the cremasteric reflex, thus retracting the testis. Lubricating gel or soap may help reduce friction. Gentle mid-abdominal pressure may help push the testis into the inguinal canal. A cross-legged sitting or squatting position may also help identify the testis. It can be particularly challenging to obtain an accurate exam on a ticklish or obese boy. Approximately 18% of nonpalpable testes are subsequently palpated when examined under anesthesia in the operating room.[30,31]

On examination, both retractile testes and low UDTs may be manipulated into the scrotum. Once in scrotal position, the retractile testis appears to remain in place, whereas the low UDT does not. The ipsilateral hemiscrotum is fully developed with a retractile testis, whereas it may be underdeveloped in a UDT.

If neither testis is palpable, anorchia, androgen insensitivity syndrome, or a chromosomal abnormality must be differentiated from bilateral UDT. If the baseline follicle-stimulating hormone (FSH) level is elevated (three standard deviations above the mean) in a boy younger than 9 years, anorchia is likely and no further evaluation is recommended. If baseline luteinizing hormone (LH) and FSH levels are normal and human chorionic gonadotropic (hCG) stimulation results in an appropriate elevation of testosterone, functioning testicular tissue is likely to be present and the patient should undergo exploration. However, if the testosterone level does not increase appropriately, nonfunctional testicular tissue may still be present and exploration should still be performed. The hCG stimulation test does not distinguish between normal nonpalpable testes and functioning testicular remnants.[32]

Radiographic imaging is rarely helpful in locating a UDT and is not recommended routinely. Multiple studies have shown that the experienced surgeon/examiner has a higher sensitivity in locating the UDT than does ultrasonography (US), computed tomography (CT), or magnetic resonance imaging (MRI), especially because the sensitivity of imaging is poor in detection of soft tissue masses less than 1 cm.[33] In unusual situations of bilateral nonpalpable testes, MRI with gadolinium may be useful for detecting abdominal testes because testicular tissue is particularly bright on MRI.[34,35]

While easy to perform with minimal risk, ultrasound has low accuracy with a sensitivity of 45% and specificity of 78%, and adds unnecessary cost.[36,37] In one series, ultrasound incorrectly indicated UDT for 48% of patients when the testis was retractile.[38] In summary, negative imaging is not diagnostic of testicular absence.

Fertility

A UDT and, to a lesser degree, its contralateral descended mate have been demonstrated to be histologically abnormal by investigators who performed bilateral testes biopsies at the time of orchiopexy.[39,40] Clinically, patients with a history of UDT exhibit subnormal semen analyses.[41] Early studies showed fertility to be related to the position of the UDT; men with abdominal or canalicular testes had lower fertility than those with inguinal testes (83.3% vs 90%).[42,43] Despite these findings, the infertility rate of men with a history of unilateral UDT is equivalent to that of the normal population (10%).[43,44,45] However, men with bilateral UDT have paternity rates of 50–65% even if corrected early, and thus are six times more likely to be infertile relative to their normal counterparts.[46,47]

Mechanisms of infertility in UDT appear to be associated with effects on Sertoli and Leydig cells, as well as Wolffian duct abnormalities (vasal and epididymal), which may further inhibit transport of already insufficient sperm.[22] Elevated testicular temperature in a UDT results in immaturity of Sertoli cells in monkeys.[22] A blunted normal testosterone surge at 60 to 90 days postnatally results in a lack of Leydig cell proliferation and delay in transformation of gonocytes to adult dark spermatogonia on histopathology.[48] An experimental rat model has demonstrated preservation of germ cell number and spermatogenesis in rats undergoing early orchiopexy for UDT versus germ cell apoptosis in untreated rats.[49] Furthermore, delayed orchiopexy at 3 years versus 9 months resulted in impaired testicular catch-up growth in boys.[50]

A clinical trial of neoadjuvant LH-releasing hormone (LHRH) in young boys undergoing orchiopexy appeared to improve the fertility index (spermatogonia/tubule) in treated versus untreated boys, though these results need confirmation.[51] A similar prospective randomized trial on neoadjuvant gonadotropin-releasing hormone therapy prior to orchiopexy also found an improvement in the mean fertility index compared to the untreated group.[52] Neoadjuvant therapy prior to 24 months achieved the best results.

Risk of Malignancy

UDT appears to be associated with a two- to eightfold increased risk of malignancy.[25,53] The risk of malignancy arising from a UDT varies with location, e.g., 1% with inguinal and 5% with abdominal testes.[54,55] Cancers arising in testes that remain in the abdomen are most frequently seminomas (74%).[56,57] In contrast, malignancies arising after successful orchiopexy, regardless of original location, are most frequently nonseminomatous germ cell tumors (63%).[58,59]

Among men with testicular cancer, up to 10% have a history of UDT.[60] There are two competing theories regarding this increased risk. First, the 'position theory' implicates the carcinogenic potential of the altered micro- and macro-environment of the UDT. If true, then the timing of correction could potentially lessen or negate the development of malignancy. A 2007 epidemiologic study examining 16,983 Swedish men who underwent correction of a UDT showed that those having orchiopexy before age 13 had a 2.23 relative risk of developing cancer.[61] Those boys having surgery at 13 years or older had a relative risk of 5.40 (compared with normal men). An additional meta-analysis showed that orchiopexy after 10 years of age compared with before 10 was associated with six times the risk of malignancy.[62] The association of orchiopexy with a decrease in cancer risk has not been demonstrated prospectively. Nevertheless, orchiopexy facilitates subsequent testicular examination and cancer detection.

The alternate 'common cause' or 'testicular dysgenesis' theory posits that the malignancy risk may be due to an underlying genetic or hormonal etiology that predisposes to both cryptorchidism and testicular cancer.[63] In patients with a UDT, 15–20% of testicular tumors arise in the normally descended contralateral testis. In other words, the normally descended testis still carries an increased relative risk of 1.7.[64] The incidence of carcinoma in situ (CIS) is 2–4% in men with cryptorchidism compared with less than 1% in non-affected men. In the postpubertal male, CIS progresses to invasive germ cell tumors in 50% of cases within 5 years.[65] However, the natural history of CIS diagnosed in a young child at the time of orchiopexy is less clear. It has been recommended that these patients undergo repeated biopsies after puberty.[66]

Management and Treatment

Indications and Timing

Guidelines (AAP 1996 and EAU 2012) recommend that orchiopexy in otherwise healthy males be performed by 12–18 months of age, as the UDT is unlikely to descend after 12 months of age.[67,68] Despite this recommendation, many children are referred after age 2 years. In one review of over 28,000 children with UDT in the Pediatric Health Information System database, only 18% underwent operation by 1 year of age, and 43% by 2 years of age. Black and Hispanic boys less commonly underwent orchiopexy by age 2 years, regardless of payer group and socioeconomic status.[69] Repair may be undertaken even earlier if a symptomatic hernia is present. The risk of general anesthesia after 6 months is acceptably low in hospitals with dedicated pediatric anesthesiologists. In addition to the evidence that early scrotal placement may affect the risk of malignancy and infertility, treatment of a UDT also reduces the risk of torsion, facilitates testicular examination, improves the endocrine function of the testis, and creates a normal-appearing scrotum.

Hormonal Treatment

The value of hormonal therapy in the treatment of UDT is controversial. Buserelin, an LHRH agonist, is frequently used to treat UDT in Europe.[70] The highest success rates have been observed in cases where the testis is at or distal to the external inguinal ring.[71,72] Some authors recommend low-dose hCG therapy, regardless of the operative plan to restore a normal endocrine milieu and enhance germ cell maturation, particularly in bilateral UDT.[73] Trials combining buserelin and hCG have yielded success rates in the range of 60%, but orchiopexy is still required in 40% of patients.[74,75] Buserelin has not been approved for this use by the USA Food and Drug Administration, but as noted above, clinical trials of LHRH used in a neoadjuvant fashion in young boys undergoing orchiopexy suggest that it may improve fertility.[51]

Orchiopexy

The operative approach for UDT depends on whether the testis is palpable (Fig. 51-2). It is important to re-examine the patient under anesthesia because up to 18% of nonpalpable testes may become palpable on examination under anesthesia.[76] Unilateral and bilateral palpable UDT are managed similarly. Routine biopsy of

the testis at the time of surgery is not recommended, but may provide prognostic information regarding fertility.[77]

For the unilateral palpable UDT that presents after puberty, orchiopexy is preferred. If orchiopexy is difficult and a normal contralateral testis is present, or if the UDT is abnormally soft and small, then an orchiectomy should be performed. Likewise, orchiectomy is the treatment of choice for the postpubertal, unilateral intra-abdominal UDT because of the increased cancer risk. Laparoscopic orchiectomy is ideal in this setting.[78] In uncommon cases such as postpubertal males with significant anesthetic risks, or males older than 50, observation is an acceptable alternative to operation.[56]

Palpable Undescended Testes: Unilateral or Bilateral

The mainstay of therapy for the palpable UDT is orchiopexy with creation of a subdartos pouch.[79,80] This may be performed through a standard two-incision (inguinal and scrotal) approach, or a single-incision high scrotal approach.[81,82] With the standard inguinal approach, the success rate is as high as 95%.[83] Similar success rates have been reported for the high scrotal approach.[81,84] With both techniques, scrotal fixation is achieved by scarring of the everted tunica vaginalis to the surrounding tissues.[85] Placement of sutures in the tunica albuginea for fixation is generally discouraged because it causes significant testicular inflammation, increases infertility risk, and may damage intratesticular vessels.[86,87] Associated findings

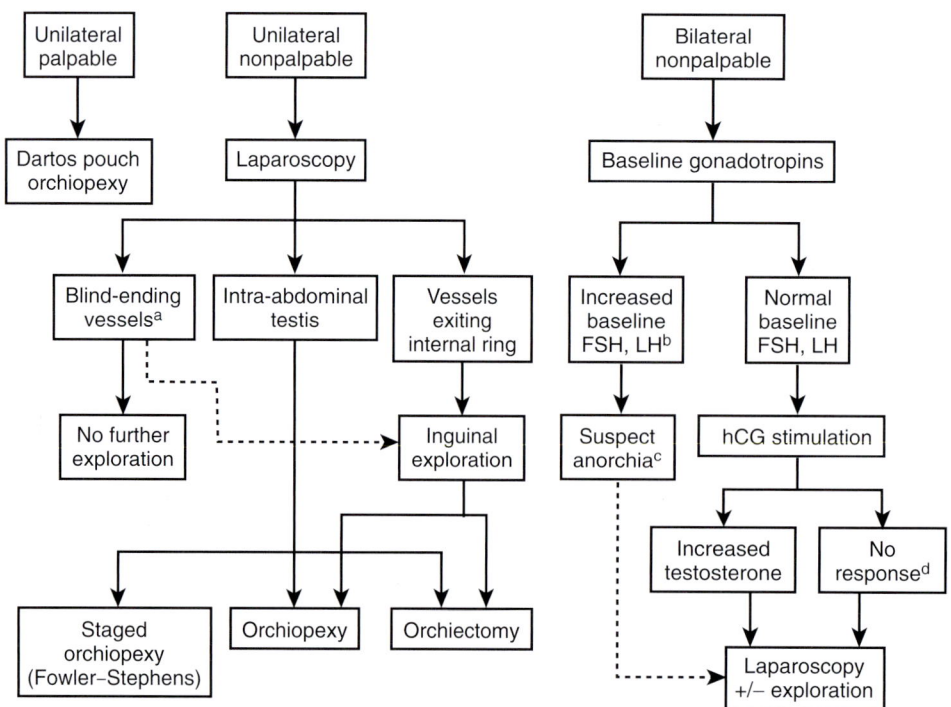

FIGURE 51-2 ■ Management algorithm for undescended testis. FSH, follicle-stimulating hormone; LH, luteinizing hormone; hCG, human chorionic gonadotropin. (a) If blind-ending vessels are unequivocally identified, then there is no need for further exploration. (b) Baseline FSH and LH levels are elevated if values are 3 SD above the mean. (c) Increased suspicion of anorchia with elevated baseline FSH and LH levels; however, exploration is still warranted. (d) Testicular remnant tissue may be present despite a negative hCG stimulation test; therefore, exploration for testicular remnant tissue should still be performed.

such as an open processus vaginalis or hernia should be repaired.

A standard inguinal approach to orchiopexy with a subdartos pouch is depicted in Figure 51-3. The operation is usually performed as an outpatient procedure under general anesthesia. The patient is supine. Intraoperative administration of an ilioinguinal nerve block with bupivacaine provides excellent postoperative analgesia. An incision is made along one of the Langer lines over the internal ring. The external oblique aponeurosis is incised in the direction of its fibers, avoiding injury to the ilioinguinal nerve. Once located, the testis and spermatic cord are freed from the canal and any cremasteric and ectopic gubernacular attachments. The tunica vaginalis is then dissected off the vas deferens and spermatic vessels. The proximal sac is twisted, doubly suture ligated, and amputated. Retroperitoneal dissection through the internal ring may provide additional cord length for the testis to reach the scrotum.

A tunnel is created from the inguinal canal into the scrotum by using a finger or a large clamp. A subdartos pouch is created by placing the finger through the tunnel, bluntly developing a space in a dependent portion of the scrotum, making a 1.5 cm incision in the skin over the finger, and creating a pouch using a hemostat inserted just under the skin to spread both superiorly and inferiorly. A clamp is carefully passed through this scrotal incision up into the inguinal canal and the adventitial tissue around the testis is secured, taking care not to grasp the testis or vas deferens. The testis is thereby delivered into the dartos pouch, and a suture is used to narrow the neck of the pouch to prevent testicular retraction. Testis measurements and biopsy may be performed at this time. The scrotal skin incision is closed with absorbable suture. The external oblique aponeurosis is reapproximated to restore the inguinal canal. The skin and subcuticular tissue are closed with subcuticular stitches. A skin sealant is useful, especially for boys in diapers.

The patient is seen in clinic after a few weeks for a wound check and again several months later for testicular examination, instruction on testicular self-examination, and repeat counseling on fertility and cancer risk. Final position and condition of the testis should be noted. Although rare, complications include atrophy and retraction. A single scrotal incision technique has also been applied to orchiopexy, with similar success rates and shorter operative times, but one group demonstrated an increased 3% risk of postoperative hernia with this approach.[81,88]

Nonpalpable Undescended Testes: Unilateral or Bilateral

For a unilateral UDT that is not palpable under anesthesia, initial management may be either through diagnostic laparoscopy or inguinal exploration. In the last decade, laparoscopy has become the preferred approach.[89]

If the surgeon decides to first perform inguinal exploration and no testis or remnant is identified, then diagnostic laparoscopy or laparotomy may still be needed to ensure the testis is not in an intra-abdominal location. In one retrospective review of 215 nonpalpable testes, only

34% were located distal to the internal ring, and an initial inguinal incision would have provided suboptimal exposure for the remaining 66%.[90]

The surgeon may begin with diagnostic laparoscopy through an umbilical port (Fig. 51-4).[91] If the vessels appear atretic or 'blind ending' as they exit the abdomen, some have recommended no further exploration, though this is controversial. If the testicular vessels are seen exiting the internal ring, a laparoscopic inguinal exploration is performed if the ring is open, or an open inguinal exploration if the ring is closed (Fig. 51-5).[89] Orchiopexy is performed if a viable testis is found. If the vessels end blindly in the inguinal canal, the tip of the vessels can be sent for pathologic examination. Remnants of testicular tissue or hemosiderin and calcifications are indicative of probable perinatal torsion and testicular resorption.

If diagnostic laparoscopy reveals a viable intra-abdominal testis, several options are available depending on its location. A recent review concluded that while there is not an optimal surgical technique for an intra-abdominal testis, preservation of the spermatic vessels is preferable.[89] If the gonadal vessels are long enough to allow for tension-free mobilization of the testis into the scrotum, orchiopexy may be performed open or laparoscopically depending on surgeon preference (Fig. 51-6). This is often feasible when the testis lies caudal to the iliac vessels.[78]

When the gonadal vessels are too short, there are various options. Open or laparoscopic exploration can be performed. The cord structures are mobilized cephalad towards their origin, freed from the posterior peritoneum, and the testicle brought into the scrotum. A neoinguinal ring may be created medial to the median umbilical ligament to shorten the path for scrotalization of the testis (Prentiss maneuver). Most series indicate a 95–100% success rate, defined as lack of atrophy and a normal scrotal position, with single-stage laparoscopic orchiopexy.[89] A staged orchiopexy can also be performed in which the high abdominal testis with its cord structures is first mobilized as low as possible. Six to 12 months later, it is mobilized into the scrotum. The advantage of this approach lies in preservation of both primary and collateral blood supply. However, during the second stage, injury may occur to the vascular supply and/or vas deferens because of scarring to surrounding tissues.

Alternately, in the setting of a short spermatic cord, a first stage Fowler–Stephens orchiopexy can be performed, typically laparoscopically.[92] The Fowler–Stephens orchiopexy involves clipping the spermatic vessels, which makes the testis dependent on the vasal and cremasteric vessels for viability.[93,94] For this reason, the Fowler–Stephens approach is not a good option after prior inguinal exploration because this secondary vascular supply to the testis may have been compromised. A delay of six months is recommended before stage 2 to allow development of collateral circulation. During the second stage, the spermatic vessels are then divided between the clips, and the testis located into the scrotum. The success rate in modern single-center case series with follow-up longer than 3 years exceeds 90%.[95–97] However, a higher failure rate was observed with a single-stage

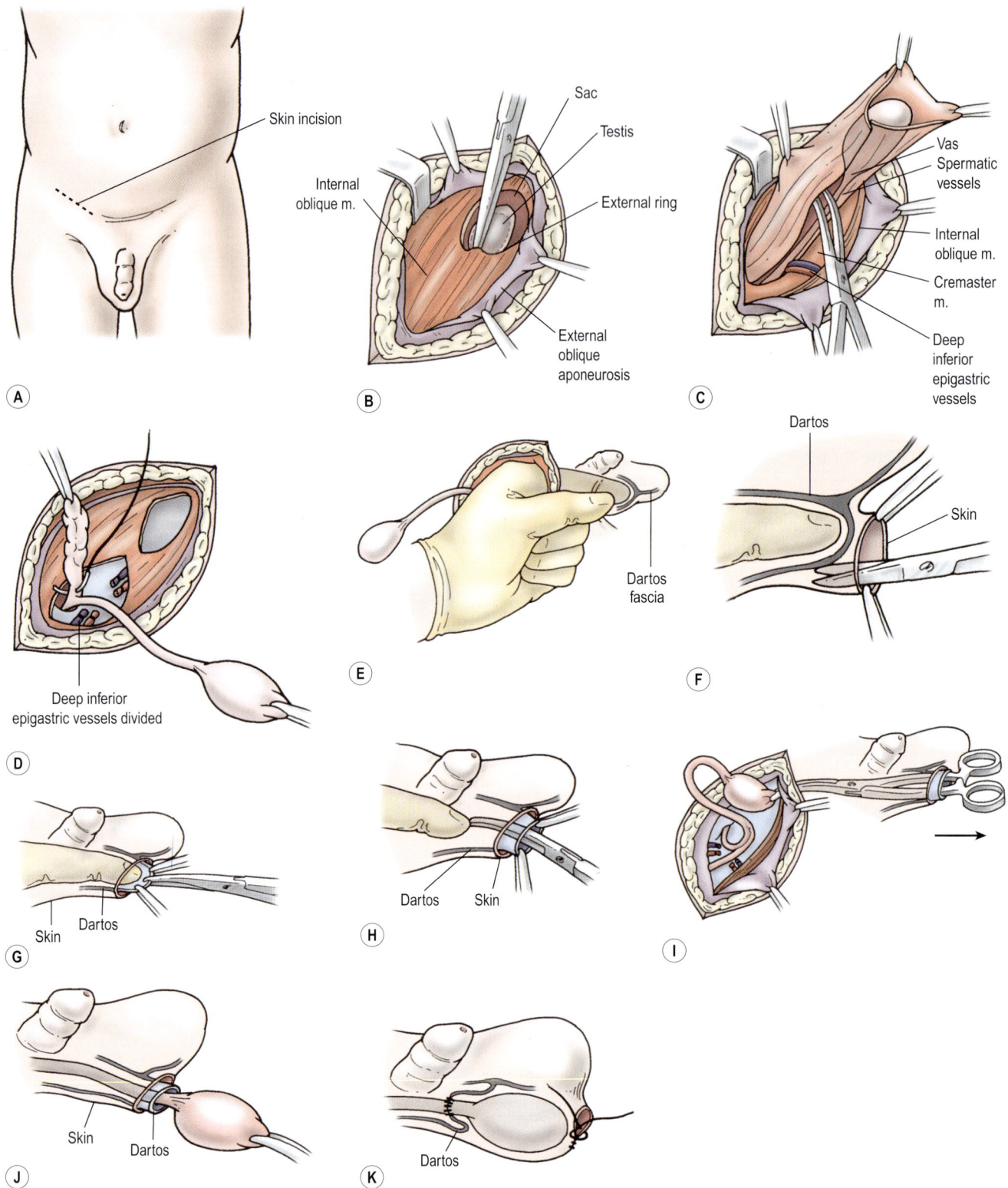

FIGURE 51-3 ■ Standard inguinal orchiopexy approach. **(A)** Transverse skin incision. **(B)** External oblique aponeurosis is opened in the directions of its fibers, with care taken to avoid the ilioinguinal nerve. **(C)** The testis is delivered, and the patent processus vaginalis is opened distally near the testis. **(D)** The processus vaginalis (or indirect hernia sac) is separated from the cord structures and ligated at the internal ring. Adequate cord length is usually obtained by retroperitoneal dissection of the cord contents. If additional length is required, the inferior epigastric vessels may be ligated (Prentiss maneuver), permitting medialization of the cord. **(E)** A finger is passed inferiorly into the scrotum to aid in creation of the dartos pouch. **(F–H)** Dartos pouch creation and passage of a clamp through the scrotum into the inguinal canal. **(I)** Adventitial tissue of the testis is grasped with the clamp. **(J)** The testis is brought into the dartos pouch. **(K)** Dartos fascia and skin are closed. (From Ellis DG. Undescended testes. In: Ashcraft KW, editor. Pediatric Urology. Philadelphia: WB Saunders; 1990. p. 423.)

Fowler–Stephens orchiopexy, and caution is advised with this approach.

Other options for operative management of high intra-abdominal testes include microvascular orchiopexy (autotransplantation). This technique is infrequently used as it requires special instrumentation, microsurgical skill, and sometimes an unexpected need for a second microvascular surgeon. An 83–96% success rate in experienced hands has been reported.[89]

If the testis is atrophic, whether found in the abdomen or inguinal canal, a laparoscopic or open orchiectomy is recommended, respectively. Debate exists regarding the role of contralateral fixation in cases of monorchism because of differing assumptions related to potential torsion. This largely remains the surgeon's preference.

Boys with bilateral nonpalpable UDT usually have genetic, endocrinologic, or imaging evaluation indicating the presence or absence of testicular tissue (i.e., hormonal evaluation confirming testosterone production). If laparoscopy reveals only one viable testicle, the child is managed as in the situation with unilateral, nonpalpable UDT. However, if bilateral viable testes are found, management may depend on the ease of orchiopexy. If difficult, one side may be fixed first, with the contralateral side fixed six to 12 months later. This allows the practitioner to assess the outcome of the first side prior to operating on the contralateral testis.[89]

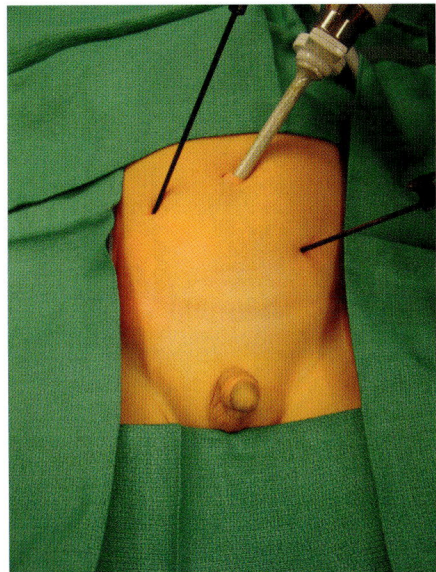

FIGURE 51-4 ■ After diagnostic laparoscopy through a 5 mm umbilical cannula, if ligation and division of the testicular vessels are required, two accessory 3 mm instruments are introduced into the abdominal cavity using the stab incision technique. The surgeon should stand on the side opposite the nonpalpable testis. (From Holcomb GW III. Laparoscopic orchiopexy. In: Holcomb GW III, Georgeson KE, Rothenberg SS, editors. Atlas of Pediatric Laparoscopy and Thoracoscopy. Philadelphia: Elsevier; 2008. p. 144–8.)

Secondary or Iatrogenic Undescended Testis

Secondary UDT is an uncommon complication of inguinal hernia repair, orchiopexy, or hydrocelectomy. Surgical technique differs from that of primary repair because scarring from the previous procedure makes cord dissection difficult with risk of vascular or vasal injury. Cartwright and associates described a technique for reoperative orchiopexy in which the entire cord and scar is mobilized en bloc along with a strip of external oblique aponeurosis.[98] The testis/cord/aponeurosis complex is dissected together superior to the internal ring where the aponeurosis is then cut and dissection continued above the area of previous scar into the retroperitoneum to allow more extended mobilization. If more length is necessary, division of the inferior epigastric vessels allows the cord to be displaced medially.

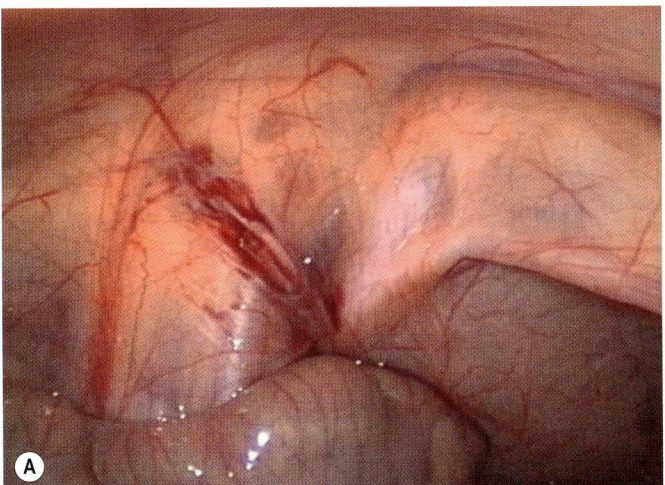 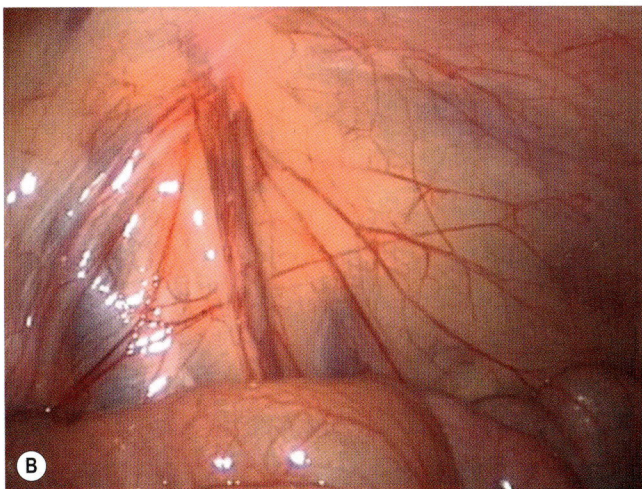

FIGURE 51-5 ■ (A) The vas deferens and testicular vessels in this patient end blindly in the retroperitoneum. The internal ring is closed. In this very unusual situation, inguinal exploration is not necessary. (B) In the more common scenario, the testicular vessels and vas deferens are seen to enter the inguinal canal. There is no evidence for a patent processus vaginalis. The vessels and vas deferens appear to be of relatively normal caliber. In this situation, inguinal exploration is necessary. (From Holcomb GW III. Laparoscopic orchiopexy. In: Holcomb GW III, Georgeson KE, Rothenberg SS, editors. Atlas of Pediatric Laparoscopy and Thoracoscopy. Philadelphia: Elsevier; 2008. p. 144–8.)

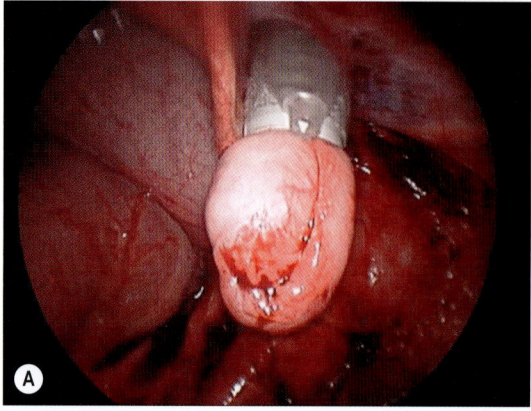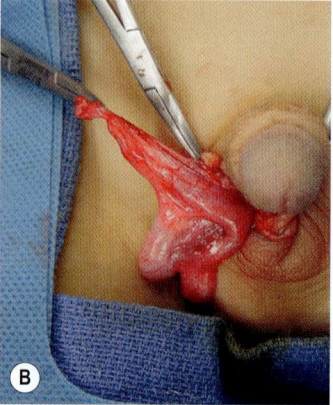

FIGURE 51-6 ■ **(A)** After intra-abdominal mobilization of the testis, the gubernaculum has been grasped with forceps inserted through a 10 mm cannula that has been introduced through the scrotal incision, over the pubic tubercle and into the abdomen. The testis is then withdrawn into the cannula. Often, it is not possible to place the testis entirely into the 10 mm port. **(B)** The testis is delivered over the pubic tubercle and into the right hemiscrotum. (From Holcomb GW III. Laparoscopic orchiopexy. In: Holcomb GW III, Georgeson KE, Rothenberg SS, editors. Atlas of Pediatric Laparoscopy and Thoracoscopy. Philadelphia: Elsevier; 2008. p. 144–8.)

TESTICULAR CANCER

Testicular cancer is uncommon in children, accounting for 1% to 2% of all pediatric solid tumors. The peak incidence of pediatric testicular tumors occurs between ages 12 to 24 months, followed by a second small peak during puberty. Prepubertal boys have a much larger percentage of benign-behaving testicular lesions than postpubertal and adult males.[99,100] Management of testicular tumors in prepubertal boys thus differs from postpubertal boys and adults as curative treatment may be partial or radical orchiectomy. These cancers generally respond well to chemotherapy, and retroperitoneal lymph node dissection (RPLND) is relatively rare.[101] Germ cell tumors comprise 65–85% of pediatric testicular tumors. Tumor registries have reported that greater than 60% of tumors were yolk sac (YST) and approximately 20% were teratomas (Table 51-1).[55,102] Males with gonadal dysgenesis, disorders of sexual development, and hypovirilization have an increased incidence of gonadal tumors.

TABLE 51-1 Primary Testes Tumor Types in 395 Boys Under 12 Years of Age

Tumor type	Frequency (%)
Yolk sac	62
Teratoma	23
Stromal (unspecified)	4
Epidermoid cyst	3
Juvenile granulosa cell	3
Sertoli cell	3
Leydig cell	1
Gonadoblastoma	1

Data from the Prepubertal Testis Tumor Registry established by the Urology Section of the American Academy of Pediatrics. Of 513 patients entered, 395 testicular tumors were found in children younger than 12 years of age.
Adapted from Ross JH, Rybicki L, Kay R. Clinical behavior and a contemporary management algorithm for prepubertal testis tumors: a summary of the Prepubertal Testis Tumor Registry. J Urol 2002;168(4 Pt 2):1675–8; discussion 1678–9.

Presentation and Diagnosis

A testicular tumor typically presents as a painless scrotal mass. A history of trauma is often given and may be the event that brings attention to the scrotal mass. Sometimes, a tumor arising in a UDT may cause torsion and present as acute abdominal pain. Malignancy typically is nontender, does not transilluminate, and is associated with a normal urinalysis. An associated hydrocele in 15–20% of patients may impede adequate testicular examination.[101] Hormonally active tumors may cause precocious puberty. As part of the initial evaluation for a testicular mass, color Doppler testicular ultrasound and serum tumor markers (α-fetoprotein (AFP), β-hCG) should be obtained. Ultrasound is nearly 100% sensitive.[101]

Though not pathognomonic, anechoic cystic lesions usually suggest benign disease. Internal calcifications and a mass with 'onion-skin' alternating hypo- and hyperechoic lesions suggests an epidermoid cyst.[103] These findings may be useful in preoperative planning for testis-sparing surgery. Serum tumor marker levels are valuable not only in the diagnosis, but also follow-up of testicular malignancy. AFP is a glycoprotein produced by the fetal yolk sac, liver, and gastrointestinal tract. It is elevated in a variety of benign and malignant diseases, including YSTs of the testis. The half-life of AFP is approximately 5.5 days, and the normal adult level of less than 10 ng/mL is not achieved until around 10 months of age (Fig. 51-7).[104] β-hCG is a glycoprotein produced by embryonal carcinomas and mixed teratomas. Its half-life is approximately 24 hours, and is normally not detected in significant amounts in boys (<5 IU/L).

Once the diagnosis of high-risk testicular cancer is made histologically, CT can be used to evaluate metastatic disease. CT has largely supplanted RPLND for the purposes of staging; however, it carries a 15% to 20% false-negative rate.[105] MRI also has been used, and it is probable that MRI will replace CT in children for diagnosis and follow-up due to the high ionizing radiation of CT and risk of future malignancy.[106] Prepubertal testis tumors are staged using the Children's Oncology Group staging system (Table 51-2).

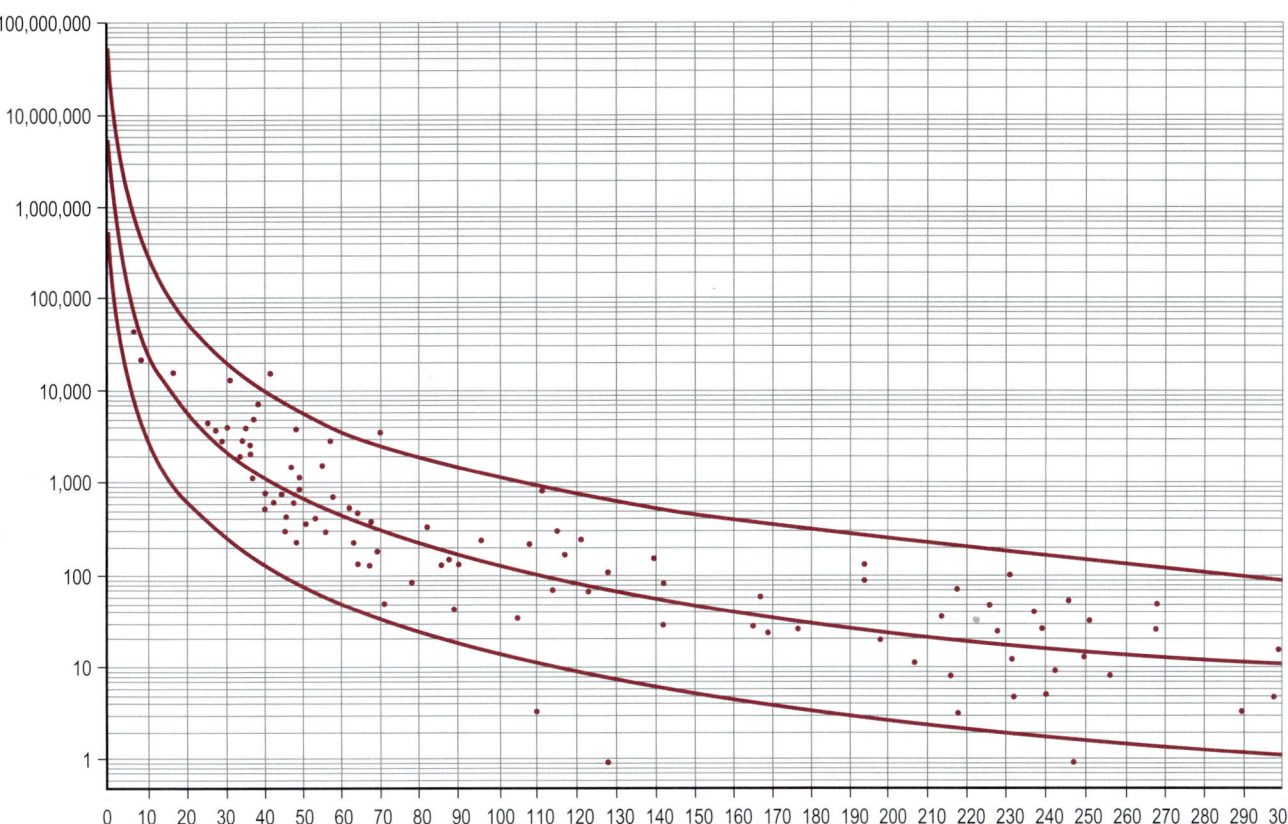

FIGURE 51-7 ■ This graph displays the normal ranges of serum α-fetoprotein (AFP) in early infancy. The AFP levels in nanograms per milliliter are on the *y*-axis and age in days is on the *x*-axis. The normal range for AFP may be estimated by the middle regression line. The two flanking lines represent the 95% confidence interval. (From Ohama K, Nagase H, Ogino K, et al. Alpha-fetoprotein (AFP) levels in normal children. Eur J Pediatr Surg 1997;7:267–9.)

TABLE 51-2	Children's Oncology Group Staging System for Testicular Cancer

Stage	Features
I	Limited to testis
	Completely resected by high inguinal orchiectomy
	No clinical, radiographic, or histologic evidence of disease beyond the testes
	Patients with normal or unknown tumor markers at diagnosis must have a negative ipsilateral retroperitoneal node sampling to confirm Stage 1 disease
II	Trans-scrotal biopsy or orchiectomy
	Microscopic disease in scrotum or high in spermatic cord (>5 cm from proximal end)
	Failure of tumor markers to normalize or decrease with an appropriate half-life
III	Retroperitoneal lymph node involvement
	No visceral or extra-abdominal involvement
IV	Distant metastases

Adapted from Hayes-Lattin B, Nichols CR. Testicular cancer: a prototypic tumor of young adults. Semin Oncol 2009;36(5):432–8.

Carcinoma in Situ

CIS of the testis is a premalignant lesion. Testicular cancer is reported to develop in at least 50% of testes known to harbor CIS.[65] CIS is seen in patients with UDT and intersex disorders, conditions that are known to carry a higher risk of testicular cancer than that in the general population.[107] Testicular microlithiasis is associated with an increased risk of CIS as well as testicular germ cell tumors, but its presence in a testis is not considered pre-malignant. Rather, it seems to be a marker of increased risk of cancer in infertile men with atrophic testes or those with known testis cancer and microlithiasis in the contralateral testis.[51,108] CIS is stimulated by endocrinologic changes during puberty. However, the natural history of CIS in prepubertal testes is less clear. When testicular biopsy at the time of orchiopexy is performed, CIS is seen in 0.36–0.45% of cases.[77,109] The prevalence of CIS in adult men with a history of UDT is 2–4%.[65,66] If CIS is identified in the prepubertal testis, it is typically managed with annual testicular examinations and testicular ultrasound. In postpubertal men, some clinicians recommend that these patients undergo biopsy of the contralateral testis and unilateral orchiectomy. If biopsy of the remaining testis also reveals CIS, they recommend 18–20 Gy of radiation treatment.[110]

Germ Cell Tumors

Yolk Sac Tumors

YSTs are also known as endodermal sinus tumors, embryonal adenocarcinomas, orchidoblastomas, or Teillum's tumors.[111] Most occur within the first 2 years of life.

Grossly, YSTs are firm and yellow/white. Microscopically, they are characterized by Schiller–Duval bodies and stain for AFP.[112,113]

Contrary to the behavior of embryonal carcinoma in adults, YST (which is histologically similar) in children has a more indolent course and spreads hematogenously. Approximately 95% of YSTs are confined to the testis, and metastases to the retroperitoneum are uncommon (5%).[100] The lungs are the most common site of distant metastasis, and retroperitoneal metastases are seen only 5% of the time.[101] The 5-year survival for YST approaches 99%.

The standard diagnostic and therapeutic procedure for YST is radical inguinal orchiectomy, and this alone is usually curative in children. To minimize the risk of metastases during manipulation, the spermatic cord is clamped or ligated immediately on entry into the inguinal canal.

Staging of YST requires abdominopelvic CT and chest radiography (CXR), histologic examination of the radical orchiectomy specimen, and determination of serum tumor markers. Stage I tumors are limited to the testis, and thus are usually cured by radical inguinal orchiectomy.[114] Tumor markers are measured monthly and CXRs obtained every 2 months for the first 2 years. Abdominopelvic CT or MRI scans are obtained every 3 months for the first year and every 6 months for the second year. After 2 years without recurrence, follow-up may be extended to every 6 months or yearly.[112]

Traditionally, RPLND was recommended for boys with unknown or normal markers at diagnosis to confirm stage I disease. Although confirmatory RPLND may still be considered, it is used less often because stage 1 YST has a high likelihood of stage 1 presentation (85%), as propensity for hematogenous spread to the lungs, and because RPLND has a high complication rate in children. The risk of recurrence is approximately 20% and almost always can be salvaged with chemotherapy.[101]

Stage II disease includes those tumors with residual disease in the scrotum or high proximal cord, node involvement on imaging, or persistent elevation of tumor markers after orchiectomy. Tumors diagnosed and treated with trans-scrotal orchiectomy also should be considered stage II because transscrotal resection alters the normal lymphatic drainage of the tumor. Lymphatic drainage of the testis is to the retroperitoneal nodes, whereas the scrotum drains to the inguinal nodes. Ipsilateral hemiscrotectomy can also be considered. All patients with stage II disease should receive combination chemotherapy with cisplatin, etoposide, and bleomycin (PEB).[101] Due to significant ototoxicity and nephrotoxicity with cisplatin, the UK Children's Cancer Study Group substituted carboplatin for cisplatin, and were able to maintain a 100% event-free survival at 5 years.[115] Patients with a persistent mass or elevated AFP after chemotherapy should undergo RPLND.

Stage III disease includes retroperitoneal spread (lymph node >4 cm) seen on imaging studies. Biopsy is used to confirm suspected nodal metastases, such as with lymph nodes >2 cm on CT. Metastasis beyond the retroperitoneum or to any viscera defines stage IV disease. For both stage III and stage IV disease, chemotherapy follows

the same protocols as for stage II disease, followed by RPLND. The overall survival approaches 100%.[100]

Teratoma

Teratomas account for 40% of testicular tumors in prepubertal children. Histologically, teratomas are composed of all three layers of embryonic tissue: ectoderm, endoderm, and mesoderm. Grossly, they may contain differentiated tissue such as cartilage, muscle, bone, and fat; a cystic component also may be present. Before puberty, they follow a benign course and can be cured with testis-sparing surgery.[116,117] Long-term mean follow-up of 7 years has demonstrated no tumor recurrence in the ipsilateral or contralateral gonad with a testis-sparing approach.[117] Also, no radiographic follow-up has been recommended for prepubertal patients who undergo partial orchiectomy.[101] If one accepts the dysplasia theory, however, whether benign or malignant, one might consider that a unilateral testicular tumor may pose an increased risk for the contralateral testis. On the other hand, when a child is seen at or after puberty, radical inguinal orchiectomy is indicated because the teratoma can follow a malignant postpubertal course.[101]

The enucleated tumor should always be sent for frozen section examination. If immature elements or pubertal changes are seen, radical orchiectomy should be performed. Overall disease-free survival after orchiectomy is excellent.[118] An elevated AFP or focus of YST may indicate potential recurrence. These patients can then be salvaged with platinum-based chemotherapy with 5-year survival rates in excess of 90%.[119]

Epidermoid cysts comprise about 15% of pediatric testis tumors, and as monodermal teratomas, follow a benign course. As such, a testis-sparing approach can be taken.[101]

Mixed Germ Cell Tumor

Teratocarcinoma, or mixed germ cell tumor, accounts for 20% of pediatric germ cell tumors. Teratocarcinoma is more commonly seen in an operatively corrected UDT and may contain any mixture of YST, embryonal carcinoma, choriocarcinoma, and seminoma.[120] Eighty per cent of teratocarcinomas are confined to the testis at presentation. Foci of choriocarcinoma confer a poorer prognosis. RPLND is usually performed even for stage I disease, and higher-stage disease is treated with chemotherapy similar to those used for adults.

Seminoma

Seminoma is rare in children, but is the most common tumor in an uncorrected abdominal UDT. Seminoma is treated with radical orchiectomy and retroperitoneal radiation.[121]

Nongerm Cell Tumors (Gonadal Stromal Tumors)

Leydig cell tumors are one of the most common nongerm cell tumors (NGCTs). The peak incidence in boys occurs from ages 5 to 9 years.[101,122] The clinical triad includes a unilateral testicular mass (90–93%), precocious puberty, and elevated 17-ketosteroid levels. As these tumors produce testosterone and occasionally other androgens, roughly 20% of patients may have signs of precocious puberty and gynecomastia.[123] Precocious puberty may also be caused by pituitary lesions, Leydig cell hyperplasia, and congenital adrenal hyperplasia so the pituitary/adrenal axis must be evaluated by assaying 17-ketosteroids, FSH, LH, and performing a dexamethasone suppression test. Reinke crystals on histologic examination are pathognomonic for this tumor and can be found in 35–40% of all patients.[124] When diagnosed preoperatively, testis-sparing enucleation may be considered because these tumors tend to follow a benign course.[125]

The granulosa cell tumor also has a benign course and can be managed with testis-sparing surgery. This tumor should be suspected in neonates with scrotal swelling, normal age-adjusted AFP levels, and a complex, cystic, multiseptated, hypoechoic mass on testicular ultrasound.[126]

The Sertoli cell tumor is a rare form of NGCT. A small percentage of patients have gynecomastia, though these are typically not as hormonally active as Leydig cell tumors.[127] The clinical course is usually benign in children under 5, and tumors can be managed with testis-sparing surgery. Older children, however, should have a metastatic evaluation with imaging.[101]

Gonadoblastoma is a form of NGCT usually associated with intersex disorders, occurring in dysgenetic gonads. The patients are typically 46XY phenotypic females (testicular feminization) with intra-abdominal testes who undergo virilization at puberty. Up to one-third of patients have bilateral gonadal lesions. The germ cell component of these tumors carries a 10% risk of malignant degeneration. Early gonadectomy is recommended, especially if the patient is raised as a female.[128,129] Patients with mixed gonadal dysgenesis raised as males should have streak gonads and UDTs removed, though some suggest that scrotal testes can be preserved since they are less prone to malignancy and can be surveyed more easily.

Testicular Microlithiasis

Lastly, testicular microlithiasis may be seen in conjunction with testicular tumors (seen synchronously in 15–46% of patients), but is also seen incidentally in 5% of healthy young men. While the risk of testicular microlithiasis in children for the development of cancer is not well studied and reported numbers are small, there appear to be low-risk and high-risk individuals. Boys who have (1) atrophic or dystrophic testes; (2) known chromosomal abnormalities; (3) contralateral testis cancer, and possibly (4) history of UDT need closer follow-up with routine serial examination and scrotal ultrasound.[130] Education about testicular self-examination is important for these patients.

REFERENCES

1. Husmann DA, Levy JB. Current concepts in the pathophysiology of testicular undescent. Urology 1995;46:267–76.
2. Bardin CW, Ross GT, Rifkind AB, et al. Studies of the pituitary-Leydig cell axis in young men with hypogonadotropic hypogonadism and hyposmia: Comparison with normal men, prepubertal boys, and hypopituitary patients. J Clin Invest 1969;48:2046–56.
3. Santen RJ, Paulsen CA. Hypogonadotropic eunuchoidism. II. Gonadal responsiveness to exogenous gonadotropins. J Clin Endocrinol Metab 1973;36:55–63.
4. Husmann DA, McPhaul MJ. Time-specific androgen blockade with flutamide inhibits testicular descent in the rat. Endocrinology 1991;129:1409–16.
5. Spencer JR, Torrado T, Sanchez RS, et al. Effects of flutamide and finasteride on rat testicular descent. Endocrinology 1991;129:741–8.
6. Emmen JM, McLuskey A, Adham IM, et al. Involvement of insulin-like factor 3 (Insl3) in diethylstilbestrol-induced cryptorchidism. Endocrinology 2000;141:846–9.
7. Nef S, Shipman T, Parada LF. A molecular basis for estrogen-induced cryptorchidism. Dev Biol 2000;15(224):354–61.
8. Fentener van Vlissingen JM, van Zoelen EJ, Ursem PJ, et al. In vitro model of the first phase of testicular descent: identification of a low molecular weight factor from fetal testis involved in proliferation of gubernaculum testis cells and distinct from specified polypeptide growth factors and fetal gonadal hormones. Endocrinology 1988;123:2868–77.
9. Heyns CF, Hutson JM. Historical review of theories on testicular descent. J Urol 1995;153:754–67.
10. Nef S, Parada LF. Cryptorchidism in mice mutant for Insl3. Nat Genet 1999;22:295–9.
11. Costa WS, Sampaio FJB, Favorito LA, et al. Testicular migration: Remodeling of connective tissue and muscle cells in human gubernaculum testis. J Urol 2002;167:2171–6.
12. Heyns CF. The gubernaculum during testicular descent in the human fetus. J Anat 1987;153:93–112.
13. Barteczko KJ, Jacob MI. The testicular descent in human. Origin, development and fate of the gubernaculum Hunteri, processus vaginalis peritonei, and gonadal ligaments. Adv Anat Embryol Cell Biol 2000;156:III–X, 1–98.
14. Goh DW, Momose Y, Middlesworth W, et al. The relationship among calcitonin gene-related peptide, androgens and gubernacular development in 3 animal models of cryptorchidism. J Urol 1993;150:574–6.
15. Park WH, Hutson JM. The gubernaculum shows rhythmic contractility and active movement during testicular descent. J Pediatr Surg 1991;26:615–17.
16. Hutson JM, Nation T, Balic A, et al. The role of the gubernaculum in the descent and undescent of the testis. Ther Adv Urol 2009;1:115–21.
17. Elder JS. Epididymal anomalies associated with hydrocele/hernia and cryptorchidism: Implications regarding testicular descent. J Urol 1992;148:624–6.
18. Gill B, Kogan S, Starr S, et al. Significance of epididymal and ductal anomalies associated with testicular maldescent. J Urol 1989;142:556–8.
19. Hadziselimovic F, Herzog B. The development and descent of the epididymis. Eur J Pediatr 1993;152(Suppl 2):S6–9.
20. Kaplan GW. Nomenclature of cryptorchidism. Eur J Pediatr 1993;152(Suppl 2):S17–19.
21. Agarwal PK, Diaz M, Elder JS. Retractile testis–is it really a normal variant? J Urol 2006;175:1496–9.
22. Singh R, Hamada AJ, Bukavina L, et al. Physical deformities relevant to male infertility. Nat Rev Urol 2012;9:156–74.
23. Stec AA, Thomas JC, DeMarco RT, et al. Incidence of testicular ascent in boys with retractile testes. J Urol 2007;178:1722–5.
24. Sijstermans K, Hack WWM, Meijer RW, et al. The frequency of undescended testis from birth to adulthood: A review. Int J Androl 2008;31:1–11.
25. Pohl H. The location and fate of the cryptorchid and impalpable testes. Dialogues in Pediatric Urology. Pearl River, NY: William J. Miller Associates; 1997. p. 3–4.
26. Capello SA, Giorgi LJ Jr, Kogan BA. Orchiopexy practice patterns in New York State from 1984 to 2002. J Urol 2006;176:1180–3.
27. Hack WWM, Meijer RW, Van Der Voort-Doedens LM, et al. Previous testicular position in boys referred for an undescended testis: Further explanation of the late orchidopexy enigma? BJU Int 2003;92:293–6.

28. Barthold JS, González R. The epidemiology of congenital cryptorchidism, testicular ascent and orchiopexy. J Urol 2003; 170:2396–401.

29. Guven A, Kogan BA. Undescended testis in older boys: Further evidence that ascending testes are common. J Pediatr Surg 2008;43:1700–4.

30. Docimo SG. The results of surgical therapy for cryptorchidism: A literature review and analysis. J Urol 1995;154:1148–52.

31. Kirsch AJ, Escala J, Duckett JW, et al. Surgical management of the nonpalpable testis: The Children's Hospital of Philadelphia experience. J Urol 1998;159:1340–3.

32. Jarow JP, Berkovitz GD, Migeon CJ, et al. Elevation of serum gonadotropins establishes the diagnosis of anorchism in prepubertal boys with bilateral cryptorchidism. J Urol 1986;136:277–9.

33. Esposito C, Cardona R, Centonze A, et al. Impact of laparoscopy on the management of an unusual case of nonpalpable testis in an adult patient. Surg Endosc 2003;17:1324.

34. De Filippo RE, Barthold JS, González R. The application of magnetic resonance imaging for the preoperative localization of nonpalpable testis in obese children: An alternative to laparoscopy. J Urol 2000;164:154–5.

35. Landa HM, Gylys-Morin V, Mattrey RF, et al. Magnetic resonance imaging of the cryptorchid testis. Eur J Pediatr 1987;146(Suppl 2):S16–17.

36. Elder JS. Ultrasonography is unnecessary in evaluating boys with a nonpalpable testis. Pediatrics 2002;110:748–51.

37. Tasian GE, Copp HL, Baskin LS. Diagnostic imaging in cryptorchidism: Utility, indications, and effectiveness. J Pediatr Surg 2011;46:2406–13.

38. Snodgrass W, Bush N, Holzer M, et al. Current referral patterns and means to improve accuracy in diagnosis of undescended testis. Pediatrics 2011;127:e382–8.

39. Huff DS, Hadziselimovic F, Snyder HM 3rd, et al. Histologic maldevelopment of unilaterally cryptorchid testes and their descended partners. Eur J Pediatr 1993;152(Suppl 2):S11–14.

40. Rusnack SL, Wu H-Y, Huff DS, et al. Testis histopathology in boys with cryptorchidism correlates with future fertility potential. J Urol 2003;169:659–62.

41. Puri P, O'Donnell B. Semen analysis of patients who had orchidopexy at or after seven years of age. Lancet 1988;5(2):1051–2.

42. Lee PA, Coughlin MT, Bellinger MF. Paternity and hormone levels after unilateral cryptorchidism: association with pretreatment testicular location. J Urol 2000;164:1697–701.

43. Lee PA. Fertility in cryptorchidism. Does treatment make a difference? Endocrinol Metab Clin North Am 1993;22:479–90.

44. Chilvers C, Dudley NE, Gough MH, et al. Undescended testis: The effect of treatment on subsequent risk of subfertility and malignancy. J Pediatr Surg 1986;21:691–6.

45. Lee PA, Coughlin MT. The single testis: paternity after presentation as unilateral cryptorchidism. J Urol 2002;168:1680–3.

46. Lee PA, Coughlin MT. Fertility after bilateral cryptorchidism. Evaluation by paternity, hormone, and semen data. Horm Res 2001;55:28–32.

47. Lee PA, O'Leary LA, Songer NJ, et al. Paternity after bilateral cryptorchidism. A controlled study. Arch Pediatr Adolesc Med 1997;151:260–3.

48. Hadziselimovic F, Thommen L, Girard J, et al. The significance of postnatal gonadotropin surge for testicular development in normal and cryptorchid testes. J Urol 1986;136(1 Pt 2):274–6.

49. Mizuno K, Hayashi Y, Kojima Y, et al. Early orchiopexy improves subsequent testicular development and spermatogenesis in the experimental cryptorchid rat model. J Urol 2008;179:1195–9.

50. Kollin C, Karpe B, Hesser U, et al. Surgical treatment of unilaterally undescended testes: Testicular growth after randomization to orchiopexy at age 9 months or 3 years. J Urol 2007;178:1589–93.

51. Jaganathan K, Ahmed S, Henderson A, et al. Current management strategies for testicular microlithiasis. Nat Clin Pract Urol 2007;4:492–7.

52. Schwentner C, Oswald J, Kreczy A, et al. Neoadjuvant gonadotropin-releasing hormone therapy before surgery may improve the fertility index in undescended testes: A prospective randomized trial. J Urol 2005;173:974–7.

53. Herrinton LJ, Zhao W, Husson G. Management of cryptorchism and risk of testicular cancer. Am J Epidemiol 2003;1(157):602–5.

54. Li FP, Fraumeni JF. Testicular cancers in children: Epidemiologic characteristics. J Natl Cancer Inst 1972;48:1575–81.

55. Ross JH, Rybicki L, Kay R. Clinical behavior and a contemporary management algorithm for prepubertal testis tumors: A summary of the Prepubertal Testis Tumor Registry. J Urol 2002;168:1675–9.

56. Wood HM, Elder JS. Cryptorchidism and testicular cancer: Separating fact from fiction. J Urol 2009;181:452–61.

57. Raja MA, Oliver RT, Badenoch D, et al. Orchidopexy and transformation of seminoma to non-seminoma. Lancet 1992;339:930.

58. Halme A, Kellokumpu-Lehtinen P, Lehtonen T, et al. Morphology of testicular germ cell tumours in treated and untreated cryptorchidism. Br J Urol 1989;64:78–83.

59. Jones BJ, Thornhill JA, O'Donnell B, et al. Influence of prior orchiopexy on stage and prognosis of testicular cancer. Eur Urol 1991;19:201–3.

60. Pike MC, Chilvers C, Peckham MJ. Effect of age at orchidopexy on risk of testicular cancer. Lancet 1986;31(1):1246–8.

61. Pettersson A, Richiardi L, Nordenskjold A, et al. Age at surgery for undescended testis and risk of testicular cancer. N Engl J Med 2007;3(356):1835–41.

62. Walsh TJ, Dall'Era MA, Croughan MS, et al. Prepubertal orchiopexy for cryptorchidism may be associated with lower risk of testicular cancer. J Urol 2007;178:1440–6.

63. Asklund C, Jørgensen N, Kold Jensen T, et al. Biology and epidemiology of testicular dysgenesis syndrome. BJU Int 2004; 93(Suppl 3):6–11.

64. Akre O, Pettersson A, Richiardi L. Risk of contralateral testicular cancer among men with unilaterally undescended testis: a meta-analysis. Int J Cancer 2009;1(124):687–9.

65. Dieckmann KP, Skakkebaek NE. Carcinoma in situ of the testis: Review of biological and clinical features. Int J Cancer 1999;10(83):815–22.

66. Giwercman A, Müller J, Skakkebaek NE. Cryptorchidism and testicular neoplasia. Horm Res 1988;30:157–63.

67. Timing of elective surgery on the genitalia of male children with particular reference to the risks, benefits, and psychological effects of surgery and anesthesia. American Academy of Pediatrics. Pediatrics 1996;97:590–4.

68. Tekgul S. Guidelines on Paediatric Urology. European Association of Urology; 2012.

69. Kokorowski PJ, Routh JC, Graham DA, et al. Variations in timing of surgery among boys who underwent orchiopexy for cryptorchidism. Pediatrics 2010;126:e576–82.

70. Bica DT, Hadziselimovic F. Buserelin treatment of cryptorchidism: A randomized, double-blind, placebo-controlled study. J Urol 1992;148:617–21.

71. Hadziselimovic; F, Huff D, Duckett J, et al. Long-term effect of luteinizing hormone-releasing hormone analogue (buserelin) on cryptorchid testes. J Urol 1987;138:1043–5.

72. Lala R, Matarazzo P, Chiabotto P, et al. Early hormonal and surgical treatment of cryptorchidism. J Urol 1997;157:1898–901.

73. Lala R, Matarazzo P, Chiabotto P, et al. Combined therapy with LHRH and HCG in cryptorchid infants. Eur J Pediatr 1993;152(Suppl 2):S31–3.

74. Giannopoulos MF, Vlachakis IG, Charissis GC. 13 Years' experience with the combined hormonal therapy of cryptorchidism. Horm Res 2001;55:33–7.

75. Waldschmidt J, Doede T, Vygen I. The results of 9 years of experience with a combined treatment with LH-RH and HCG for cryptorchidism. Eur J Pediatr 1993;152(Suppl 2):S34–6.

76. Elder JS. Why do our colleagues still image for cryptorchidism? Ignoring the evidence. J Urol 2011;185:1566–7.

77. Hadziselimovic; F, Hecker E, Herzog B. The value of testicular biopsy in cryptorchidism. Urol Res 1984;12:171–4.

78. Esposito C, Damiano R, Gonzalez Sabin MA, et al. Laparoscopy-assisted orchidopexy: An ideal treatment for children with intra-abdominal testes. J Endourol 2002;16:659–62.

79. Benson CD, Lotfi MW. The pouch technique in the surgical correction of cryptorchidism in infants and children. Surgery 1967;62:967–73.

80. Koop CE. Technique of herniorrhaphy and orchiopexy. Birth Defects Orig Artic Ser 1977;13:293–303.

81. Bassel YS, Scherz HC, Kirsch AJ. Scrotal incision orchiopexy for undescended testes with or without a patent processus vaginalis. J Urol 2007;177:1516–18.

82. Rajfer J. Technique of orchiopexy. Urol Clin North Am 1982; 9(3):421–7.

83. Saw KC, Eardley I, Dennis MJ, et al. Surgical outcome of orchiopexy. I. Previously unoperated testes. Br J Urol 1992;70:90–4.

84. Dayanc M, Kibar Y, Irkilata HC, et al. Long-term outcome of scrotal incision orchiopexy for undescended testis. Urology 2007;70(4):786–9.

85. Redman JF, Barthold JS. A technique for atraumatic scrotal pouch orchiopexy in the management of testicular torsion. J Urol 1995;154:1511–12.

86. Coughlin MT, Bellinger MF, LaPorte RE, et al. Testicular suture: A significant risk factor for infertility among formerly cryptorchid men. J Pediatr Surg 1998;33:1790–3.

87. Bellinger MF, Abromowitz H, Brantley S, et al. Orchiopexy: An experimental study of the effect of surgical technique on testicular histology. J Urol 1989;142:553–5.

88. Al-Mandil M, Khoury AE, El-Hout Y, et al. Potential complications with the prescrotal approach for the palpable undescended testis? A comparison of single prescrotal incision to the traditional inguinal approach. J Urol 2008;180:686–9.

89. Esposito C, Caldamone AA, Settimi A, et al. Management of boys with nonpalpable undescended testis. Nat Clin Pract Urol 2008;5:252–60.

90. Cisek LJ, Peters CA, Atala A, et al. Current findings in diagnostic laparoscopic evaluation of the nonpalpable testis. J Urol 1998; 160:1145–50.

91. Merguerian PA, Mevorach RA, Shortliffe LD, et al. Laparoscopy for the evaluation and management of the nonpalpable testicle. Urology 1998;51:3–6.

92. Lindgren BW, Franco I, Blick S, et al. Laparoscopic Fowler-Stephens orchiopexy for the high abdominal testis. J Urol 1999;162(3 Pt 2):990–4.

93. Fowler R, Stephens FD. The role of testicular vascular anatomy in the salvage of high undescended testes. Aust N Z J Surg 1959;29:92–106.

94. Law GS, Pérez LM, Joseph DB. Two-stage Fowler-Stephens orchiopexy with laparoscopic clipping of the spermatic vessels. J Urol 1997;158:1205–7.

95. Chang B, Palmer LS, Franco I. Laparoscopic orchidopexy: A review of a large clinical series. BJU Int 2001;87(6):490–3.

96. Radmayr C, Oswald J, Schwentner C, et al. Long-term outcome of laparoscopically managed nonpalpable testes. J Urol 2003; 170:2409–11.

97. Baker LA, Docimo SG, Surer I, et al. A multi-institutional analysis of laparoscopic orchidopexy. BJU Int 2001;87(6):484–9.

98. Cartwright PC, Velagapudi S, Snyder HM 3rd, et al. A surgical approach to reoperative orchiopexy. J Urol 1993;149:817–18.

99. Pohl HG, Shukla AR, Metcalf PD, et al. Prepubertal testis tumors: Actual prevalence rate of histological types. J Urol 2004;172: 2370–2.

100. Wu HY, Snyder HM 3rd. Pediatric urologic oncology: Bladder, prostate, testis. Urol Clin North Am 2004;31:619–27, xi.

101. Agarwal PK, Palmer JS. Testicular and paratesticular neoplasms in prepubertal males. J Urol 2006;176:875–81.

102. Walsh TJ, Grady RW, Porter MP, et al. Incidence of testicular germ cell cancers in USA children: SEER program experience 1973 to 2000. Urology 2006;68:402–5.

103. Langer JE, Ramchandani P, Siegelman ES, et al. Epidermoid cysts of the testicle: Sonographic and MR imaging features. AJR Am J Roentgenol 1999;173:1295–9.

104. Ohama K, Nagase H, Ogino K, et al. Alpha-fetoprotein (AFP) levels in normal children. Eur J Pediatr Surg 1997;7:267–9.

105. Pizzocaro G, Zanoni F, Salvioni R, et al. Difficulties of a surveillance study omitting retroperitoneal lymphadenectomy in clinical stage I nonseminomatous germ cell tumors of the testis. J Urol 1987;138:1393–6.

106. Cho J-H, Chang J-C, Park B-H, et al. Sonographic and MR imaging findings of testicular epidermoid cysts. AJR Am J Roentgenol 2002;178:743–8.

107. Wallace TM, Levin HS. Mixed gonadal dysgenesis. A review of 15 patients reporting single cases of malignant intratubular germ cell neoplasia of the testis, endometrial adenocarcinoma, and a complex vascular anomaly. Arch Pathol Lab Med 1990;14: 679–88.

108. van Casteren NJ, Looijenga LHJ, Dohle GR. Testicular microlithiasis and carcinoma in situ overview and proposed clinical guideline. Int J Androl 2009;32:279–87.

109. Cortes D, Thorup JM, Visfeldt J. Cryptorchidism: aspects of fertility and neoplasms. A study including data of 1,335 consecutive boys who underwent testicular biopsy simultaneously with surgery for cryptorchidism. Horm Res 2001;55:21–7.

110. Heidenreich A, Moul JW. Contralateral testicular biopsy procedure in patients with unilateral testis cancer: Is it indicated? Semin Urol Oncol 2002;20:234–8.

111. Kay R. Prepubertal Testicular Tumor Registry. J Urol 1993;150: 671–4.

112. Wu HY, Snyder HM. Advances in Pediatric Urologic Oncology. AUA Update Series XXII 2003.

113. Wold LE, Kramer SA, Farrow GM. Testicular yolk sac and embryonal carcinomas in pediatric patients: Comparative immunohistochemical and clinicopathologic study. Am J Clin Pathol 1984;81:427–35.

114. Hayes-Lattin B, Nichols CR. Testicular cancer: A prototypic tumor of young adults. Semin Oncol 2009;36:432–8.

115. Mann JR, Raafat F, Robinson K, et al. The United Kingdom Children's Cancer Study Group's second germ cell tumor study: Carboplatin, etoposide, and bleomycin are effective treatment for children with malignant extracranial germ cell tumors, with acceptable toxicity. J Clin Oncol 2000;15(18):3809–18.

116. Rushton HG, Belman AB, Sesterhenn I, et al. Testicular sparing surgery for prepubertal teratoma of the testis: A clinical and pathological study. J Urol 1990;144:726–30.

117. Shukla AR, Woodard C, Carr MC, et al. Experience with testis sparing surgery for testicular teratoma. J Urol 2004;171:161–3.

118. Marina NM, Cushing B, Giller R, et al. Complete surgical excision is effective treatment for children with immature teratomas with or without malignant elements: A Pediatric Oncology Group/Children's Cancer Group Intergroup Study. J Clin Oncol 1999;17:2137–43.

119. Mann JR, Gray ES, Thornton C, et al. Mature and immature extracranial teratomas in children: The UK Children's Cancer Study Group Experience. J Clin Oncol 2008;20(26):3590–7.

120. Batata MA, Whitmore WF Jr, Chu FC, et al. Cryptorchidism and testicular cancer. J Urol 1980;124:382–7.

121. Perry C, Servadio C. Seminoma in childhood. J Urol 1980;124: 932–3.

122. Coppes MJ, Rackley R, Kay R. Primary testicular and paratesticular tumors of childhood. Med Pediatr Oncol 1994;22:329–40.

123. Cheville JC, Sebo TJ, Lager DJ, et al. Leydig cell tumor of the testis: A clinicopathologic, DNA content, and MIB-1 comparison of nonmetastasizing and metastasizing tumors. Am J Surg Pathol 1998;22:1361–7.

124. Jain M, Aiyer HM, Bajaj P, et al. Intracytoplasmic and intranuclear Reinke's crystals in a testicular Leydig-cell tumor diagnosed by fine-needle aspiration cytology: A case report with review of the literature. Diagn Cytopathol 2001;25:162–4.

125. Henderson CG, Ahmed AA, Sesterhenn I, et al. Enucleation for prepubertal Leydig cell tumor. J Urol 2006;176:703–5.

126. Shukla AR, Huff DS, Canning DA, et al. Juvenile granulosa cell tumor of the testis: Contemporary clinical management and pathological diagnosis. J Urol 2004;171:1900–2.

127. Gabrilove JL, Freiberg EK, Leiter E, et al. Feminizing and nonfeminizing Sertoli cell tumors. J Urol 1980;124:757–67.

128. Gourlay WA, Johnson HW, Pantzar JT, et al. Gonadal tumors in disorders of sexual differentiation. Urology 1994;43:537–40.

129. Olsen MM, Caldamone AA, Jackson CL, et al. Gonadoblastoma in infancy: Indications for early gonadectomy in 46XY gonadal dysgenesis. J Pediatr Surg 1988;23:270–1.

130. Dagash H, Mackinnon EA. Testicular microlithiasis: What does it mean clinically? BJU Int 2007;99:157–60.

CHAPTER 52

THE ACUTE SCROTUM

John M. Gatti • Janine Pettiford

The term *acute scrotum* is defined as acute scrotal pain with or without swelling and erythema. Early recognition and prompt management are imperative because of the possibility of testicular torsion as the etiology with permanent ischemic damage to the testis. Box 52-1 lists the differential diagnoses for the acute scrotum. Although most conditions are nonemergent, prompt differentiation between testicular torsion and other causes is critical. Age at presentation is important because torsion of the appendix testis/epididymis is most common in prepubertal boys, whereas testicular torsion more commonly presents in neonates and adolescents.[1-3]

TESTICULAR TORSION

Torsion of the testis results from twisting of the spermatic cord which compromises the testicular vasculature and results in infarction. Even if the testis is not removed, the consequent ischemic damage can affect testicular morphology and fertility. There appears to be a 4-8-hour window before significant damage occurs once torsion develops.[4] Table 52-1 shows that the probability of testicular salvage declines significantly beyond six hours. Emergency exploration is indicated even beyond this window because testicular viability is difficult to predict.[5]

Two types of torsion occur: intravaginal and extravaginal. Intravaginal torsion is more common in children and adolescents (compared to neonates), and occurs when the spermatic cord twists within the tunica vaginalis (Fig. 52-1). Intravaginal torsion develops because of abnormal fixation of the testis and epididymis within the tunica vaginalis. Normally, the tunica will invest the epididymis and posterior surface of the testis, fixing it to the scrotum with a vertical lie. Abnormal fixation occurs when the tunica vaginalis attaches more proximally on the spermatic cord, creating a long mesorchium around which the testis can twist. The testis will then lie horizontally and the pendulous testis is predisposed to twisting with leg movement or cremasteric contraction. This anatomic variant is classically described as the 'bell-clapper' deformity and has an incidence as high as 12% in cadaveric studies. Often, it is found in the contralateral scrotum as well.[6]

Extravaginal torsion occurs perinatally when the spermatic cord twists proximal to the tunica vaginalis (Fig. 52-2). During testicular descent into the scrotum, the tunica vaginalis is not firmly fixed to the scrotum, allowing the tunica and testis to spin on the vascular pedicle.

Testicular torsion typically occurs before age 3 years or after puberty. It is less common in prepubertal boys and after age 25 years. Patients present with the sudden onset of severe, unilateral pain in the testis, lower thigh, or lower abdomen, often associated with nausea and vomiting. Episodes of intermittent testicular pain may precede the acute presentation, suggesting prior incomplete torsion with spontaneous detorsion. Physical examination may reveal an enlarged testis that is retracted up toward the inguinal region with a transverse orientation and an anteriorly located epididymis. However, it is usually difficult to obtain a good exam because of the scrotal pain and tenderness. In contrast, focal tenderness at the superior pole of the testis or along the epididymis is often found with a torsed appendix testis or epididymitis (Fig. 52-3). Depending on the duration of torsion, the hemiscrotum can show varying degrees of swelling and erythema, which may obliterate landmarks and make the examination more difficult. The cremasteric reflex is often absent with testicular torsion, but a positive reflex does not reliably exclude it.[7-9]

The diagnosis of testicular torsion is usually clinically apparent and managed by immediate scrotal exploration. When torsion is difficult to diagnosis, other studies may be beneficial. A urinalysis revealing pyuria and bacteriuria is more indicative of infectious epididymitis/orchitis, but can also be found with torsion. High-resolution ultrasonography (US) with color flow Doppler and radionuclide imaging allows determination of testicular blood flow. Ultrasound is more commonly used because it allows determination of the blood flow, is less time consuming, is more readily available, and does not expose the patient to ionizing radiation.[10,11] In experienced hands, color flow Doppler ultrasound imaging has a sensitivity of 89.9%, a specificity of 98.8%, and a false-positive rate of 1%.[12] Also, Doppler ultrasound may detect coiling of the spermatic cord, indicating torsion, even with normal blood flow within the testis.[13] Ultrasound should only be used when the diagnosis is equivocal because imaging studies will only delay scrotal exploration.

If testicular torsion is suspected but a delay to the operating room is unavoidable, manual detorsion can be attempted. Detorsion is performed with a medial to lateral, 'open book' rotation because this will be the correct direction in two-thirds of patients.[14] If successful, the testis will drop lower in the scrotum and the patient will report sudden pain relief. If the initial attempt is not successful, an attempt in the reverse direction may be warranted.[15] Although these maneuvers may decrease the degree of ischemia, prompt exploration and fixation remain mandatory because the detorsion may not be complete and torsion can reoccur.

Exploration is typically performed using a median raphe scrotal incision. The symptomatic hemiscrotum is entered and the testis delivered, detorsed, and placed in

BOX 52-1	Differential Diagnoses of the Acute Scrotum

Torsion of the testis
Torsion of the appendix testis/epididymis
Epididymitis/orchitis
Hernia/hydrocele
Trauma/sexual abuse
Tumor
Idiopathic scrotal edema (dermatitis, insect bite)
Cellulitis
Vasculitis (Henoch–Schönlein purpura)

TABLE 52-1   Duration of Torsion and Testicular Salvage Rates

Duration of Torsion (Hours)	Testicular Salvage (%)
<6	85–97
6–12	55–85
12–24	20–80
>24	<10

Data from Smith-Harrison L, Koontz WW Jr. Torsion of the testis: Changing concepts. In: Ball TP Jr, Novicki DE, Barrett DM, et al, editors. AUA Update Series, vol. 9 (lesson 32). Houston: American Urological Association Office of Education; 1990.

warm, moist sponges while the contralateral hemiscrotum is explored. The unaffected testis should be fixed to the scrotal wall with nonabsorbable suture in at least three points. Excluding the tunica vaginalis allows better fixation of the testis to the scrotum.[16,17] Attention is then turned back to the affected testis. If the testis is clearly nonviable, it should be removed to avoid potential damage to the contralateral testis from the formation of antisperm antibodies. If the torsed testis becomes reperfused or is bleeding from the cut surface, it should be fixed in the

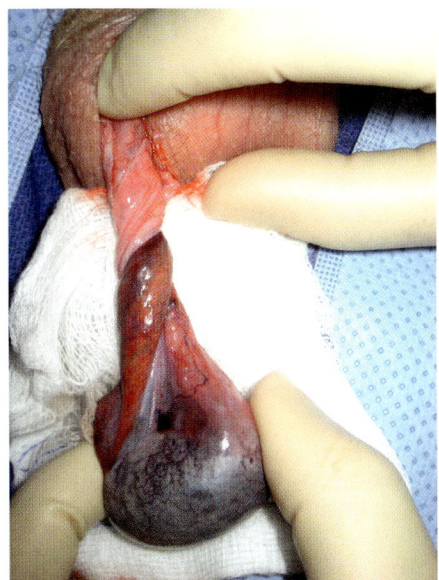

FIGURE 52-1 ■ Bell-clapper deformity. The tunica vaginalis inserts very high on the spermatic cord, which predisposes to testicular torsion.

same fashion as the contralateral testis. Bilateral fixation reduces the probability of torsion in the future, but cases of torsion after fixation have been described.[18] Therefore, any patient with symptoms of testicular torsion should be evaluated and managed appropriately, regardless if previous fixation was performed.

Intermittent Testicular Pain

Intermittent testicular pain is not uncommon in adolescent males, and may represent intermittent torsion with spontaneous resolution.[19] This diagnosis should be strongly considered in patients with significant testicular pain that has resolved, especially if there have been multiple episodes. This suspicion is reinforced if the testis has a transverse orientation or excess mobility. The diagnosis could be confirmed with Doppler ultrasound while symptomatic. If clinical concern remains despite a normal physical examination, elective scrotal exploration looking for a 'bell-clapper' deformity may be warranted.

Perinatal Testicular Torsion

The term *perinatal torsion* involves both prenatal and postnatal events with most (75%) occurring prenatally.[20] Distinguishing between the two types can be difficult, but knowing the difference affects the timing of operation. Prenatal torsion presents as a hard, nontender scrotal mass noted at birth, usually with underlying dark skin discoloration and fixation of the skin to the mass. These findings suggest testicular infarction secondary to a prior torsion. Postnatal torsion presents as an acutely inflamed scrotum with erythema and tenderness (see Fig. 52-2). The scrotum is often reported as normal at delivery, suggesting an acute postnatal event. This diagnosis requires emergent exploration with detorsion and bilateral fixation.

The timing of exploration for prenatal torsion has been controversial. Some surgeons believe exploration is not indicated because of negligible salvage rates and increased neonatal anesthetic risks.[21] However, this approach is challenged by reports of asynchronous torsion with loss of the remaining contralateral testis.[22–24] Furthermore, if the torsion were to happen at or just prior to delivery, testicular salvage may be possible. One series of 30 neonates with torsion who were explored within 6 hours of birth found two testes that could be salvaged and demonstrated normal growth 1 year later.[25] Therefore, many surgeons have become more aggressive with earlier exploration of these infarcted testes to fix the contralateral side and prevent the potential for bilateral torsion.

Although a testicular teratoma or a hernia sac filled with meconium or blood can mimic prenatal torsion, our practice has been early exploration. Postnatal torsion clearly mandates emergent exploration because salvage rates have been reported as high as 40–50%, which is similar to torsion later in life.[26] Scrotal exploration is performed through an inguinal incision because a testicular tumor may actually be present and a scrotal incision could lead to spread to the inguinal nodes.[27,28] Contralateral exploration is accomplished through a transverse scrotal incision, with placement of the testis in a dartos

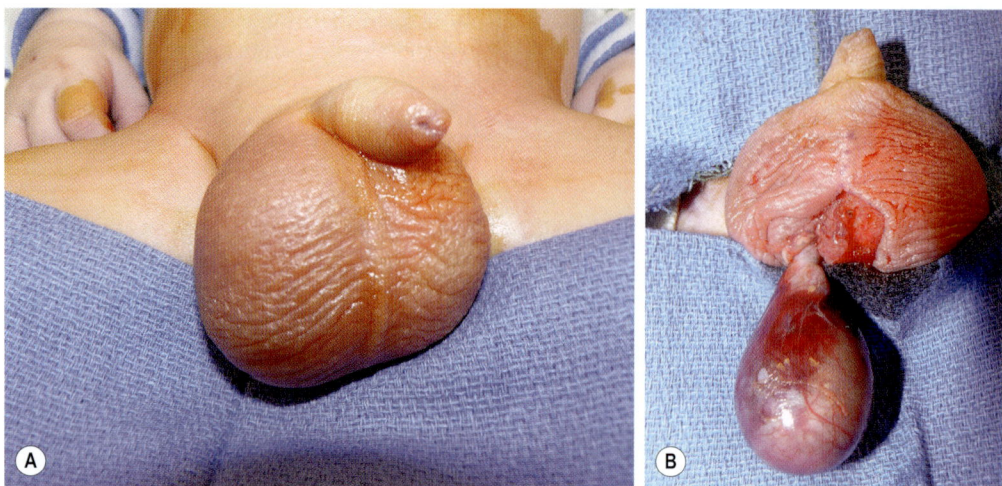

FIGURE 52-2 ■ **(A)** Shortly after birth, this newborn was found to have an enlarged and erythematous right hemiscrotum. It was unclear whether or not the right hemiscrotum was enlarged at birth. The baby underwent scrotal exploration through a median raphe incision and was found to have an extravaginal testicular torsion. **(B)** With this anomaly, the testis lies within the tunica vaginalis and the entire complex has twisted. An alternative approach would be to explore this child through an inguinal approach due to concerns about a possible testicular tumor.

pouch between the external spermatic fascia of the scrotum and the dartos fascia. This technique is less traumatic to the small, delicate neonatal gonad and provides similar fixation to using sutures.[16,17]

CONDITIONS MIMICKING TESTICULAR TORSION

Torsion of Testicular Appendages

Torsion of the appendix testis or appendix epididymis is the most common cause of an acute scrotum and is frequently misdiagnosed as acute epididymitis or

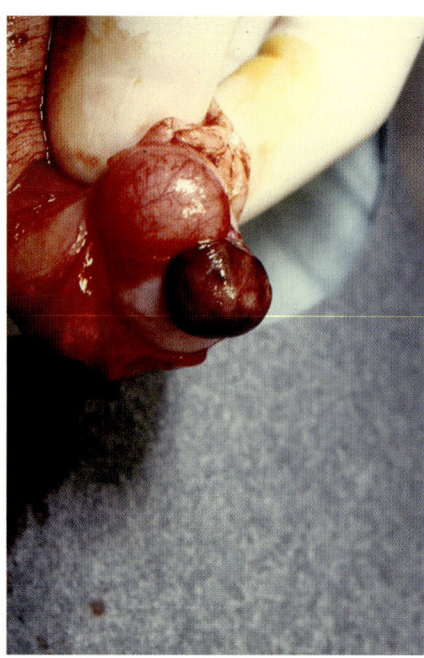

FIGURE 52-3 ■ A torsed and gangrenous appendix testis is shown. This is the cause of the 'blue dot' sign.

epididymo-orchitis. The testicular appendage represents a vestigial remnant of the Müllerian duct, and the epididymal appendage is of Wolffian duct origin. Torsion of these appendages occurs most commonly between ages 7 and 10 years. It is hypothesized that a prepubertal hormonal boost stimulates these structures, producing an increase in size and making them susceptible to twisting.[29]

Patients with appendage torsion present with sudden onset of pain and nausea. Results of the urinalysis are usually normal. The appendage can usually be palpated and is exquisitely and focally tender. The examiner may be able to elicit differential tenderness between the upper and lower poles of the affected testis. Classically called the 'blue dot' sign, the inflamed and ischemic appendage may be seen through the scrotal skin as a subtle blue-colored mass (see Fig. 52-3).[30] As inflammation increases, the epididymis, testis, and scrotal tissues become edematous and erythematous, and the diagnosis becomes more difficult. Ultrasound early in the presentation demonstrates a discrete appendage. However, later, it may only show increased blood flow to the adjacent epididymis and testis or, possibly, a reactive hydrocele, resulting in the misdiagnosis of acute epididymitis or epididymo-orchitis.[31]

Torsion of these appendages is self-limited and is best treated with nonsteroidal anti-inflammatory medications and comfort measures such as restricted activity and warm compresses. The pain resolves as the appendage infarcts and necroses, and may become a calcified free body within the tunica vaginalis.

Appendage torsion can occur at five anatomic sites: appendix testis, appendix epididymis, paradidymis/organ of Giraldes, and superior and inferior vas aberrans of Haller (Fig. 52-4).[32–34] Exploration is indicated when the diagnosis is unclear or when the symptoms are prolonged and fail to resolve spontaneously. The torsed appendage can be easily excised through a small scrotal incision with immediate symptom relief.

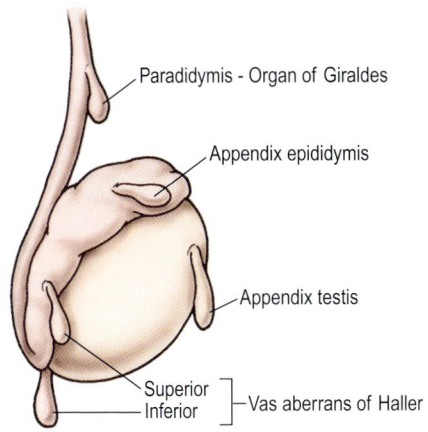

Paradidymis - Organ of Giraldes

Appendix epididymis

Appendix testis

Superior
Inferior   Vas aberrans of Haller

FIGURE 52-4 ■ Testicular appendages. (From Rolnick D, Kawanoue S, Szanto P, et al. Anatomic incidence of testicular appendages. J Urol 1968;100:755–6.)

Epididymitis

True bacterial epididymitis is rare in children, accounting for 10% to 15% of patients with an acute scrotum. The bacterial infection extends from the bladder and urethra to the epididymis in a retrograde direction via the ejaculatory ducts and can be associated with a clinical urinary tract infection or urethritis. The scrotal pain and swelling typically have a slow onset, worsening over days rather than hours. Examination reveals induration, swelling, and tenderness of the hemiscrotum. A positive urinalysis and culture, or urethral swab in sexually active adolescents suggests the diagnosis. *Neisseria gonorrhoeae* and *Chlamydia* are classically found in sexually active boys, but common urinary pathogens, including coliforms and *Mycoplasma* species, are more likely in younger children. When studies suggest a bacterial infection, appropriate antibiotic therapy is initiated and adjusted according to the culture results. If acute epididymitis is found on scrotal exploration, cultures should be obtained, but the contralateral side should not be opened to avoid spreading the infection. As with any urinary tract infection in a boy, a renal bladder sonogram and voiding cystourethrogram should be obtained after the infection has resolved. Vesicoureteric reflux is the most common finding, but an ectopic ureter (to the vas, ejaculatory duct, or seminal vesicle), ejaculatory duct obstruction, or urethral valves can also be found.

Viral infections are believed to be a common cause for acute epididymitis, but are usually diagnosed presumptively. Mumps orchitis is rare and occurs in approximately one-third of infected postpubertal boys.[35] Adenovirus, enterovirus, influenza, and parainfluenza virus infections have also been found. Management is supportive, antibiotics are not indicated, and the pain is generally self-limited.

Idiopathic Scrotal Edema

Scrotal swelling of unknown etiology is termed *idiopathic scrotal edema* and usually affects boys between the ages of 5 to 9 years. The syndrome is characterized by the insidious onset of swelling and erythema that typically begins in the perineum or inguinal region, and spreads to the hemiscrotum. Pruritus can occur, but the testis is not tender and ultrasound shows normal testicular blood flow. Contact dermatitis, insect bites, and minor trauma are often misdiagnosed as the etiology. Evaluation should seek to exclude cellulitis from an adjacent infection (inguinal, perirectal, or urethral). Treatment is with antihistamines or topical corticosteroids. If cellulitis is a concern, oral antibiotics can be administered.[36]

Henoch–Schönlein Purpura

Henoch–Schönlein purpura is a vasculitic syndrome that can involve the skin, joints, and gastrointestinal and genitourinary systems. Up to one-third of patients develop pain, erythema, and swelling of the scrotum and spermatic cord, most commonly in boys younger than 7 years of age. Doppler ultrasound demonstrates normal blood flow to the testis. Patients can also experience skin purpura, joint pain, and hematuria. Supportive measures are typically adequate, although systemic corticosteroids may be helpful.[37,38] Despite the rarity of coincident diagnoses, patients with Henoch–Schönlein purpura and testicular torsion have been described.[39]

TESTICULAR TRAUMA

Testicular trauma in children is rare. The diagnosis is made by taking a complete history, and paying close attention to factors suggesting sexual abuse. The injured testis is swollen and is markedly tender. Often there is swelling and bruising of the scrotum. The most common injury is a hematoma of the testis. Ultrasound should be obtained to evaluate for rupture of the tunica albuginea, which is an indication for operative repair. Repair is particularly important in postpubertal boys because of the potential for autoimmune injury to the contralateral testis. A large hematoma in the space between the tunica vaginalis and the tunica albuginea should be evacuated to avoid pressure necrosis of the testis. Epididymal injuries can occur, including disruption of the epididymis from the testis, with a poor outcome even after repair.

OTHER CONDITIONS

Other causes of the acute scrotum include an incarcerated inguinal hernia, hydrocele, voiding dysfunction, and neoplasia. Testicular tumors can occur in the neonatal period and early childhood, although they are usually not associated with pain or scrotal wall changes. They are usually firm on examination and should be further evaluated with ultrasound. Management is tailored to the diagnosis. See Chapter 51 for more information about testicular tumors.

REFERENCES

1. Sheldon CA. Undescended testis and testicular torsion. Surg Clin North Am 1985;65:1303–29.
2. Clift VL, Hutson JM. The acute scrotum in childhood. Pediatr Surg Int 1989;4:185–8.

3. Murphy JP, Gatti JM. Current management of the acute scrotum. Semin Pediatr Surg 2007;16:58–63.
4. Bartsch G, Frank S, Marberger H, et al. Testicular torsion: Late results with special regard to fertility and endocrine function. J Urol 1980;124:375–8.
5. Bentley DF, Ricchiuti DJ, Nasrallah PF, et al. Spermatic cord torsion with preserved testis perfusion: Initial anatomical considerations. J Urol 2004;172:2373–6.
6. Caesar RE, Kaplan GW. Incidence of the bell-clapper deformity in an autopsy series. Urology 2004;44:114–16.
7. Cifti AO, Senocak ME, Tanyel FC, et al. Clinical predictors for differential diagnosis of acute scrotum. Eur J Pediatr Surg 2004; 14:333–8.
8. Nelson CP, Williams JF, Bloom DA. The cremasteric reflex: A useful but imperfect sign in testicular torsion. J Pediatr Surg 2003;38:1248–9.
9. Rabinowitz R. The importance of the cremasteric reflex in acute scrotal swelling in children. J Urol 1984;132:89–90.
10. Nussbaum Blask AR, Bulas D, Shalaby-Rana E, et al. Color Doppler sonography and scintigraphy of the testis: A prospective, comparative analysis in children with acute scrotal pain. Pediatr Emerg Care 2002;18:67–71.
11. Wu HC, Sun SS, Kao A, et al. Comparison of radionuclide imaging and ultrasonography in the differentiation of acute testicular torsion and inflammatory testicular disease. Clin Nucl Med 2002;27:490–3.
12. Baker LA, Sigman D, Matthews RI, et al. An analysis of clinical outcomes using color Doppler testicular ultrasound for testicular torsion. Pediatrics 2000;105:604–7.
13. Karmazyn B, Steinberg R, Kornreich L, et al. Clinical and sonographic criteria of acute scrotum in children: A retrospective study of 172 boys. Pediatr Radiol 2005;35:302–10.
14. Kiesling VJ Jr, Schroeder DE, Pauljev P, et al. Spermatic cord block and manual reduction: Primary treatment for spermatic cord torsion. J Urol 1984;132:921–3.
15. Sessions AE, Rabinowitz R, Hulbert WC, et al. Testicular torsion: Direction, degree, duration, and disinformation. J Urol 2003;169: 663–5.
16. Bellinger MF, Abromowitz H, Brantley S, et al. Orchiopexy: An experimental study of the effect of surgical technique on testicular histology. J Urol 1989;142:553–5.
17. Rodriguez LE, Kaplan GW. An experimental study of methods to produce intrascrotal testicular fixation. J Urol 1988;139:565–7.
18. Mor Y, Pinthus JH, Nadu A, et al. Testicular fixation following torsion of the spermatic cord—does it guarantee prevention of recurrent torsion events? J Urol 2006;175:171–3.
19. Stillwell TJ, Kramer SA. Intermittent testicular torsion. Pediatrics 1986;77:908–11.
20. Das S, Singer A. Controversies of perinatal torsion of the spermatic cord: A review, survey and recommendations. J Urol 1990;143: 231–3.
21. Stone KT, Kass EJ, Cacciarelli AA, et al. Management of suspected antenatal torsion: What is the best strategy? J Urol 1995;153: 782–4.
22. Olguner M, Akgur FM, Aktug T, et al. Bilateral asynchronous perinatal testicular torsion: A case report. J Pediatr Surg 2000;35:1348–9.
23. Sorenson MD, Galansky SH, Striegl AM, et al. Prenatal bilateral extravaginal testicular torsion: A case presentation. Pediatr Surg Int 2004;20:892–3.
24. Ahmed SJ, Kaplan GW, DeCambre ME. Perinatal testicular torsion: Preoperative radiological findings and the argument for urgent surgical exploration. J Pediatr Surg 2008;43:1563–5.
25. Pinto KJ, Noe HN, Jerkins GR. Management of neonatal testicular torsion. J Urol 1997;158:1196–7.
26. Sorenson MD, Galansky SH, Striegl AM, et al. Perinatal extravaginal torsion of the testis in the first month of life is a salvageable event. Urology 2003;62:132–4.
27. Lusiri A, Vogler C, Steinhardt G, et al. Neonatal cystic testicular gonadoblastoma: Sonographic and pathologic findings. J Ultrasound Med 1991;10:59–61.
28. Masterson JS, McCullough AR, Smith RR, et al. Neonatal gonadal stromal tumor of the testis: Limitations of tumor markers. J Urol 1985;134:558–9.
29. Samnakay N, Cohen RJ, Orford J, et al. Androgen and oestrogen receptor status of the human appendix testis. Pediatr Surg Int 2003; 19:520–4.
30. Dresner ML. Torsed appendage. Diagnosis and management: Blue dot sign. Urology 1973;1:63–6.
31. Karmazyn B, Steinberg R, Livne P, et al. Duplex sonographic findings in children with torsion of the testicular appendages: Overlap with epididymitis and epididymo-orchitis. J Pediatr Surg 2006;41: 500–4.
32. Rolnick D, Kawanoue S, Szanto P, et al. Anatomical incidence of testicular appendages. J Urol 1968;100:755–6.
33. Orazi C, Fariello G, Malena S, et al. Torsion of paradidymis or Giraldes' organ: An uncommon cause of acute scrotum in pediatric age group. J Clin Ultrasound 1989;17:598–601.
34. Ballesteros Sampol JJ, Munne A, Bosch A. A vas aberrans torsion. Br J Urol 1986;58:97.
35. Beard CM, Benson RC Jr, Kelalis PP, et al. The incidence and outcome of mumps orchitis in Rochester, Minnesota, 1935 to 1974. Mayo Clin Proc 1977;52:3–7.
36. Rabinowitz R, Hulbert WC Jr. Acute scrotal swelling. Urol Clin North Am 1995;22:101–5.
37. Clark WR, Kramer SA. Henoch–Schönlein purpura and the acute scrotum. J Pediatr Surg 1986;21:991–2.
38. Soreide K. Surgical management of nonrenal genitourinary manifestations in children with Henoch–Schönlein purpura. J Pediatr Surg 2005;40:1243–7.
39. Loh HS, Jalan OM. Testicular torsion in Henoch-Schönlein syndrome. BMJ 1974;2:96–7.

CHAPTER 53

Developmental and Positional Anomalies of the Kidneys

Hsi-Yang Wu • Howard M. Snyder III

Anomalies of renal formation and position result in interesting radiographs, but their clinical importance lies in their associated anomalies. For example, the multicystic dysplastic kidney often involutes, yet the initial evaluation aims to determine that the contralateral kidney is not a risk from vesicoureteral reflux (VUR) or ureteropelvic junction (UPJ) obstruction. While no therapy is needed for unilateral renal agenesis, the link between a solitary kidney and the VACTERL (vertebral, anal, cardiac, tracheoesophageal fistula, renal, limb) and Mayer–Rokitansky (vaginal agenesis) syndromes is the main reason for further evaluation. Hydronephrosis is often seen in abnormalities of position and rotation, but does not necessarily mean that obstruction is present. Therefore, anomalies of renal formation and position often pose more of a diagnostic problem than a surgical one.

RENAL EMBRYOLOGY

The pronephros, which has no adult function, induces the mesonephros to differentiate into the mesonephric duct during the fourth to eighth week of fetal life. The mesonephric duct is the basis of the Wolffian system, which develops into the seminal vesicles, vas deferens, epididymis, and efferent ductules of the testis in boys, and the epoophoron and paraophoron (vestigial remnants between the fallopian tube and ovary) in girls. Between weeks 9 and 12, the ureteric bud branches off the mesonephric duct, contacts the metanephric blastema bud, and induces the entire collecting system of ureter, renal pelvis, calyx, and collecting tubules. The kidney develops via induction of the metanephric blastema by the ureteric bud into Bowman's capsule, the convoluted tubules, and the loop of Henle.[1] Figure 53-1 illustrates the progression of development from pronephros, to mesonephros, to metanephros.

The kidneys begin at the upper sacral level with the renal pelvis facing anteriorly. The kidneys ascend either because the lumbar and sacral regions grow faster than the cervical and thoracic regions between 4 to 8 weeks, or because there is active migration. As the kidneys ascend, the renal pelvis rotates medially by 90°, leading to the normal configuration of the renal pelvis lying medial to the parenchyma. During this time, the blood supply shifts from inferior branches of the aorta to more cephalad branches, with the final renal artery being located at about L2. Failure of normal ascent leads to the persistence of a low-lying blood supply.[1]

RENAL DYSPLASIA AND HYPOPLASIA

Since the development of the kidney depends on proper interaction between the ureteric bud and the metanephric blastema, it should not be surprising that an abnormality in the location of the ureteral orifice is associated with abnormally induced renal tissue.[2] Examination of the thickness of the renal parenchyma and number of glomeruli associated with normal and ectopic ureters in fetal specimens suggests that it is the initial interaction between bud and blastema, rather than subsequent obstruction or VUR, that determines if normal renal tissue will develop.[2] Figure 53-2 shows how a ureter which arises in the proper trigonal location (A, E, F) is associated with normal renal parenchyma whereas a ureter arising from a more cranial location (B, C, D) or caudal location (G, H) is associated with progressively less normal renal parenchyma.

Renal dysplasia and hypoplasia can be considered errors in renal induction. Figure 53-3 shows varying changes from agenesis to dysplasia and hypoplasia of the kidney. Although dysplasia is technically a histologic term, it refers to kidneys which contain primitive tubules either focally or diffusely. These ducts are lined by epithelium and surrounded by swirls of primitive collagen. No treatment is necessary for the dysplastic kidney, but there is an increased risk of reflux in the contralateral kidney.[3] Hypoplastic kidneys are small, normal kidneys with a decreased number of nephrons. Dysplasia can also occur in hypoplastic kidneys. While secondary hypoplasia can occur due to infection or obstruction, two types of hypoplastic kidneys are clinically important: the oligomeganephronic type, and the Ask–Upmark kidney. In oligomeganephronia, there is a decrease in the number of nephrons with an associated hypertrophy of the ones which are present. Patients present with polyuria and failure to concentrate their urine, but no hypertension. Imaging with ultrasound (US) reveals small kidneys. Medical management with protein restriction, and high fluid and salt intake is initiated. Once the glomerular filtration rate drops significantly, dialysis is required.[4] The Ask–Upmark kidney was initially felt to be a developmental problem, but is now believed to represent reflux nephropathy. The key finding is a small kidney with segmental hypoplasia, probably secondary to ascending pyelonephritis. VUR and hypertension are usually present. Most patients are over 10 years of age with a 2:1 female:male ratio. If the disease is unilateral, nephrectomy may cure the hypertension. Bilateral disease is managed medically.[5]

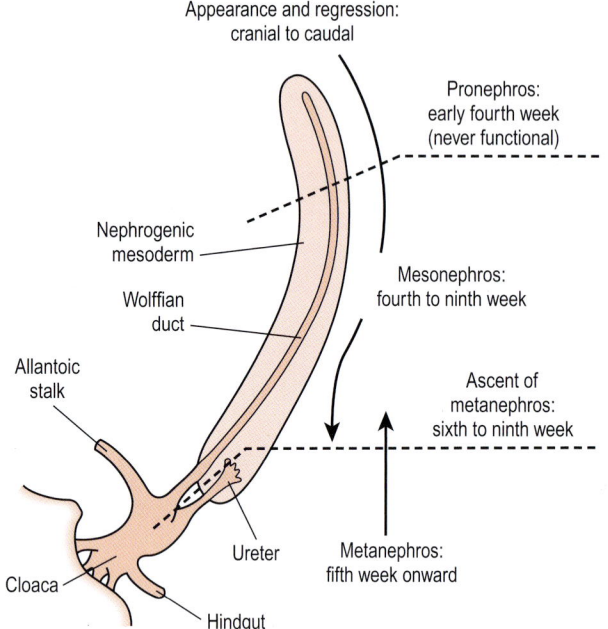

Appearance and regression:
cranial to caudal

Pronephros:
early fourth week
(never functional)

Nephrogenic
mesoderm

Wolffian
duct

Mesonephros:
fourth to ninth week

Allantoic
stalk

Ascent of
metanephros:
sixth to ninth week

Ureter

Metanephros:
fifth week onward

Cloaca

Hindgut

FIGURE 53-1 ■ Development of the kidney. (Redrawn from Gray SW, Skandalakis JE. Embryology for Surgeons. Philadelphia: WB Saunders; 1972. p. 444.)

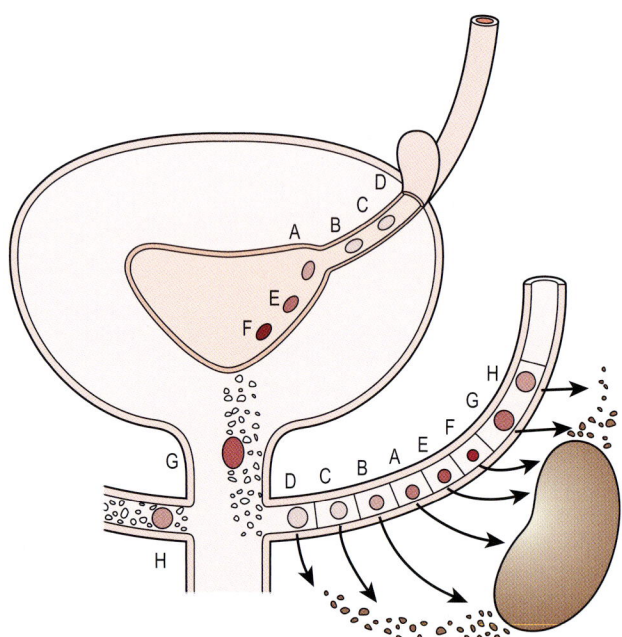

FIGURE 53-2 ■ Relation of ureteral orifice location and associated metanephric tissue. (Redrawn from Mackie GG, Stephens FD. Duplex kidneys: A correlation of renal dysplasia with position of the ureteral orifice. J Urol 1975;114:274–80.)

RENAL AGENESIS

Absence of a kidney may be due to abnormal induction of the metanephric blastema or involution of a multicystic dysplastic kidney. The presence or absence of the ureter is helpful in suggesting the cause of the renal agenesis. Absence of a hemitrigone implies that the ureteral bud failed to form properly. A normal trigone with some evidence of a ureter leading to a nubbin suggests involution of a multicystic dysplastic kidney.

Unilateral renal agenesis occurs in 1 : 1,000 live births with a 2 : 1 male predominance.[6,7] Unilateral renal agenesis can result in compensatory hypertrophy of the contralateral kidney. The left kidney is more likely to be affected in unilateral renal agenesis.[8] Since unilateral renal agenesis is asymptomatic and eventual renal function is normal, the diagnosis is usually made on prenatal ultrasound, or it is incidentally found during imaging for other abdominal symptoms. Sometimes it can be suspected on plain abdominal films if the colon is medially deviated at the splenic or hepatic flexures.[9] These patients should consider obtaining a medical alert bracelet so that in case of traumatic injury, the solitary kidney is not inadvertently removed.

In a newborn with the prenatal diagnosis of unilateral renal agenesis, physical examination at the time of birth should be focused on detecting the anomalies present in the VACTERL association (Box 53-1).[10] A voiding cystourethrogram (VCUG) should also be obtained since approximately 30% of VACTERL patients with unilateral renal agenesis will have VUR in the contralateral kidney.[10]

Males with unilateral renal agenesis are at risk for abnormal Wolffian structures. The vas and seminal vesicle may be absent (or the seminal vesicle may be present as a cyst), but the ipsilateral testis will be normal. Since the seminal vesicle develops as a separate bud from the Wolffian duct at 12 weeks, it can be present in cases of unilateral renal agenesis due to regression of a multicystic dysplastic kidney. Seminal vesicle cysts which are causing symptomatic obstruction are usually removed via a transvesical approach. Conversely, if a vas is found to be abnormal or absent during a hernia repair or orchiopexy, the kidneys should be evaluated postoperatively with an ultrasound.

Females with unilateral renal agenesis should have their genital anatomy evaluated since up to 30% will have an abnormality of the Müllerian duct due to the

---

BOX 53-1	**Associated Findings in Patients with Unilateral Renal Agenesis**

- VACTERL evaluation
- 30% will have VUR in contralateral kidney

MALES

- Can have abnormal ipsilateral Wolffian structures (vas deferens, seminal vesicle)
- Testes are normal

FEMALES

- Can have abnormal ipsilateral Müllerian structures (uterus, fallopian tubes, upper vagina—Mayer–Rokitansky syndrome)
- Ovaries are normal

VACTERL, vertebral, anorectal, cardiac, tracheoesophageal, renal, limb; VUR, vesicoureteral reflux.

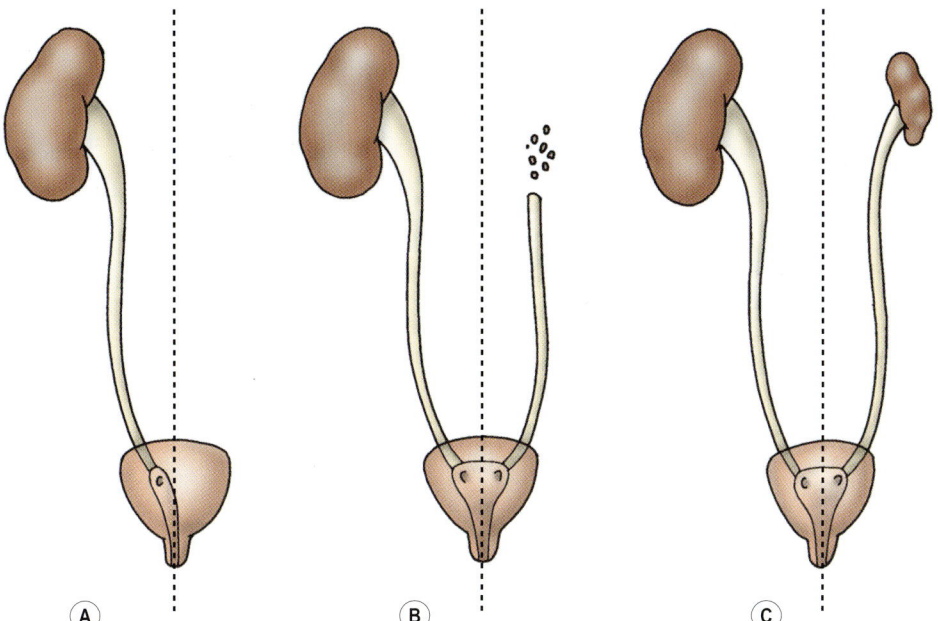

FIGURE 53-3 ■ Renal **(A)** agenesis, **(B)** dysplasia, and **(C)** hypoplasia. (Redrawn from Gray SW, Skandalakis JE. Embryology for Surgeons. Philadelphia: WB Saunders; 1972. p. 455.)

Mayer–Rokitansky syndrome (Müllerian, uterine, upper vaginal duplications with or without obstruction, or vaginal agenesis).[11,12] The abnormal induction of the mesonephric duct is believed to cause partial or complete nonunion of the paired Müllerian ducts.[13] Conversely, 40% of patients with abnormalities of the Müllerian organs will have unilateral renal agenesis or ectopia.[14] In patients with duplicated vaginas and unilateral vaginal agenesis, the side without a vagina is also the side without a kidney.[13]

If the diagnosis of Mayer–Rokitansky is not made prenatally, the patients can present either as infants with hydrocolpos, or as adolescents with lower abdominal pain after the onset of menses due to an obstructed vagina or uterus (with or without duplication). Magnetic resonance imaging (MRI) is useful in delineating the pelvic anatomy in these cases. In vaginal agenesis, the vagina is only present as a shallow pouch. There is a wide variety of abnormalities of the vagina, uterus, and fallopian tubes (Fig. 53-4), but the ovaries are embryologically normal.

Bilateral renal agenesis occurs in 1:4,800 live births, and has a 3:1 male predominance.[15] Infants affected with bilateral renal agenesis present with oligohydramnios, pulmonary hypoplasia, Potter's facies (low-set ears, broad flat nose, a prominent skin fold beginning over the eye and running to the cheek), and the great majority die soon after birth from their pulmonary hypoplasia. The renal arteries and ureters are usually absent, and the bladder is underdeveloped. The vas is usually present, but female genital structures are usually abnormal.[16,17] The adrenals are usually present but appear round, instead of flattened, due to the lack of compression by the kidneys.[15] Prenatal diagnosis is useful in determining that heroic efforts at extracorporeal membrane oxygenation or hemodialysis are not indicated after delivery.

SUPERNUMERARY KIDNEY

This is a rare condition in which a completely separate kidney is found in addition to two normally positioned kidneys. The additional kidney has its own blood supply and parenchyma, and usually is found caudal to the normal kidney. It is usually smaller than the normally positioned kidney. This additional kidney represents abnormal induction of metanephric blastema by an abnormally directed ureteric bud, either as a separate ureteral bud from the mesonephric duct, or as part of a 'Y' duplication. If the supernumerary kidney is located cranial to the normal kidney, the ureter is usually completely separate and may enter the bladder ectopically. Presumably this is a result of a completely separate ureteral bud inducing the metanephric blastema and migrating very low on the mesonephric duct, separate from the normally positioned kidney.[18,19] If the ureter ends ectopically, it may present as incontinence in a girl, or as infection in a poorly functioning renal unit. The diagnosis can be difficult.[20] Stone disease and hydronephrosis can be found in up to 50% of patients. Treatment should be reserved for these problems as the presence of a supernumerary kidney itself is not worrisome.[19] Like other ectopic kidneys, these kidneys may be more subject to trauma, so a medical alert bracelet may be helpful.

RENAL ECTOPIA

Failure of rotation, while not strictly ectopia, usually results in a kidney in which the renal pelvis is anteriorly directed. In the unusual situation in which hyper-rotation occurs, the renal pelvis can actually point posteriorly.

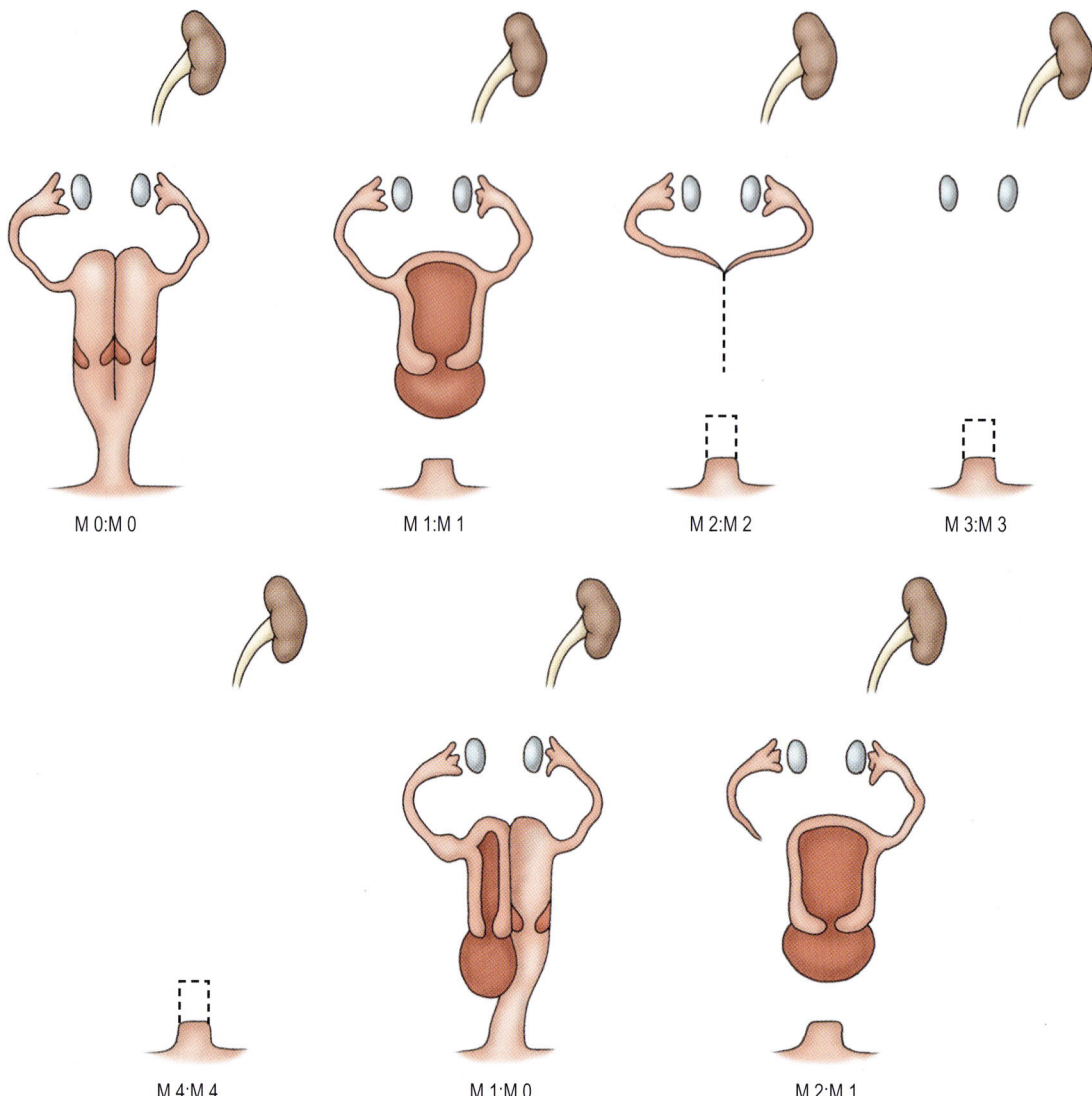

FIGURE 53-4 ■ Variations in Müllerian anatomy in Mayer–Rokitansky syndrome. M0, Right or left vagina and uterus, or duplex vagina and uterus with partial or complex septum. M1, Partial or complete absence of vagina. M2, Absence of vagina and uterus. M3, Absence of vagina, uterus, and fallopian tube. M4, Absence of vagina, uterus, fallopian tube, and ovary. (Redrawn from Tarry WR, Duckett JW, Stephens FD. The Mayer-Rokitansky syndrome: Pathogenesis, classification and management. J Urol 1989;136:648–52.)

The renal vessels are normally positioned. The renal pelvis and calyces will often appear abnormal on an intravenous urogram due to their unusual orientation. With oblique views the anatomy can be established, and does not usually require repair, even in poorly functioning units. One method to localize even poorly functioning ectopic renal tissue is with a nuclear medicine study. There are two technical factors to be considered in interpreting renal scans in ectopic kidneys. First, the radionuclide in the bladder can overlap a pelvic kidney so a catheter may need to be inserted for the study. Second, the pelvic kidney is located further anterior than orthotopic kidneys, and the function may be artificially lowered by the distance of the kidney from the camera. Placing the patient prone may result in a more accurate assessment. Magnetic resonance urography (MRU) is another emerging technique for localizing ectopic renal units.

Simple ectopia results in a kidney which is located anywhere from the pelvis to the diaphragm. The incidence is 1:1,000 live births with a 3:2 male predominance.[21] The contralateral kidney often also has a rotational abnormality or ectopia. The development of the ipsilateral adrenal gland is unaffected. A 'thoracic kidney' is actually subdiaphragmatic, although it may lie in the chest through a focal eventration of the diaphragm. It is not associated with a true congenital diaphragmatic hernia.[22] An ectopic 'abdominal kidney' is above the iliac crest, the 'lumbar kidney' is anterior to the iliac vessels at the sacral promontory, and the 'pelvic kidney' is below the aortic bifurcation and opposite the sacrum. All of these ectopic kidneys are more susceptible to trauma since they are not as well protected by the lower rib cage and are anterior in position. It may be advisable for these patients to avoid contact sports in which there is a risk of abdominal trauma.

Most ectopic kidneys are asymptomatic and are detected either on prenatal ultrasound or incidentally on other imaging studies. Ectopic kidneys are at higher risk for UPJ obstruction, VUR, and stone formation. The anatomy can include an extrarenal pelvis and infundibulum, and a high insertion of the ureter into the pelvis. This anatomical arrangement can mimic a UPJ obstruction so careful evaluation is necessary to avoid unnecessary surgery.[23] More than half will have a dilated renal pelvis. Of these, half are due to obstruction, 25% are due to reflux, and 25% are merely dilated without UPJ obstruction.[24] For repair of UPJ obstruction with a high insertion of the ureter, a side to side ureteropyelostomy or ureterocalycostomy to a dilated lower pole calyx is sometimes required to obtain dependent drainage.

While endoscopic techniques for treatment of UPJ obstruction have been used in children,[25] the presence of anomalous vessels suggests that either an open or laparoscopic approach would be safer than endoscopic incision of a UPJ obstruction in an ectopic kidney. The advent of computed tomography (CT) angiography and MRU has made the assessment of anomalous vessels in ectopic or horseshoe kidneys easier and less invasive.

FUSION DEFECTS

Horseshoe Kidney

A horseshoe kidney is found in 1:400 live births, and has a 2:1 male predominance.[26] The kidney is usually lower than normal, since the lower poles fuse in the midline and drape anteriorly over the spine. The isthmus can be fibrotic or contain parenchyma. This anomaly is believed to occur between 4 to 6 weeks of life, since the orientation of the renal pelvis is anterior. It is proposed that as the kidneys 'hurdle' the iliac vessels during ascent, they come into contact at the lower pole and fuse (Fig. 53-5). Other variations of upper pole and mid-pole contact are possible, but much less common than the usual lower pole fusion. The kidney is usually low due to its inability to ascend past the inferior mesenteric artery. Each renal moiety retains its ureter, which is draped over the isthmus. The renal pelvis is usually anterior. The arterial supply varies from the normal single vessel to each moiety to vessels arising from any conceivable nearby blood supply. Horseshoe kidneys are more commonly found in patients with sacral agenesis, high cloacas, and Turner syndrome (45,XO gonadal dysgenesis).[27] They are associated with a higher risk of renal cell carcinoma and Wilms tumor.[28–30] The presence of a Wilms tumor in a horseshoe kidney was not suspected preoperatively in 13/41 patients despite imaging studies.[30]

One-third of patients with horseshoe kidney have no symptoms. The patients with symptoms often complain of vague abdominal or back pain. 10% have ureteral duplication, 50% have VUR, and 33% have UPJ obstruction.[27,31,32] Repair of UPJ obstruction in a horseshoe kidney requires placement of the anastomosis to avoid a secondary kinking at the UPJ. Division of the isthmus is not required. Treatment of kidney stones in horseshoe kidneys can be accomplished by extracorporeal shock wave lithotripsy, ureteroscopy, or percutaneous nephrolithotomy. Percutaneous approaches are sometimes difficult as the kidneys do not reside next to the body wall, making access to the collecting system difficult. However, percutaneous approaches result in a higher stone-free

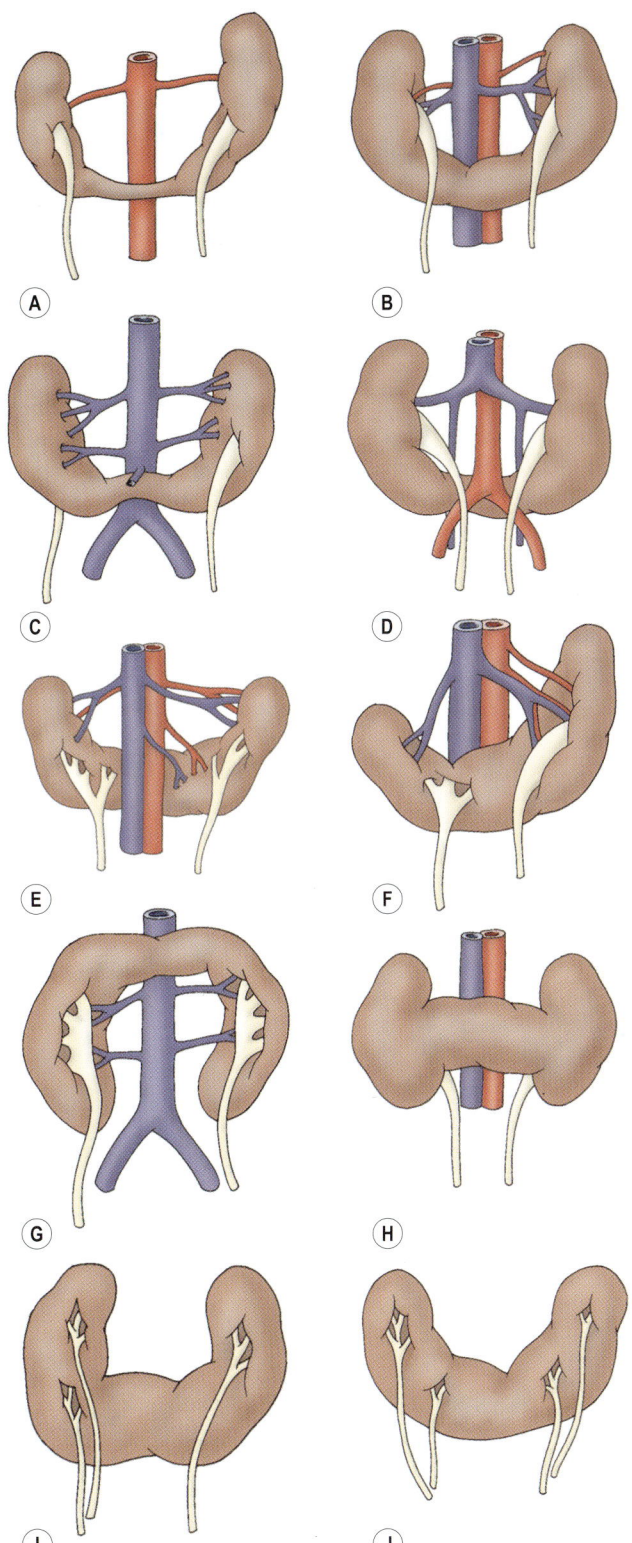

FIGURE 53-5 ■ Variations of horseshoe kidney. (Redrawn from Banjamin JA, Schullian DM. Observations of kidneys with horseshoe configuration: The contribution of Leonardo Botallo. J Hist Med Allied Sci 1950;5:315, after Gutierrez, 1931.)

rate than ureteroscopy or shock wave lithotripsy.[33,34] Although there is no increase in the rate of metabolic abnormalities in patients with horseshoe kidneys and kidney stones, suggesting that stasis in an extrarenal pelvis contributes to the formation of kidney stones,[35] patients with a horseshoe kidney and kidney stones are more likely to have hypocitraturia than other patients with kidney stones.[36]

Cross-fused Renal Ectopia

This anomaly is more common than crossed, non-fused renal ectopia and is more common in boys. The lower pole of one kidney crosses the midline to fuse with an orthotopically placed contralateral kidney. Usually the left kidney crosses the midline. Presumably during ascent, the left kidney encounters a roadblock, rotates, and fuses with the lower pole of the right kidney. The ureters insert in the normal position in the bladder. This has been described as an S- or L-shaped kidney. Diagnosis can be made using intravenous pyelogram (IVP), CT, or MRU. Solitary crossed ectopia (unilateral renal agenesis, contralateral kidney crossed to opposite side) is a rare finding. Multicystic dysplasia, obstruction, and VUR can be found in the ectopic kidney.

CYSTIC RENAL DISEASE AND CYSTIC TUMORS

Autosomal Recessive Polycystic Kidney Disease (ARPKD)

This disease was formerly called infantile polycystic kidney disease, which is inaccurate since it can present in older patients. While it occurs in 1:40,000 live births, many patients die soon afterwards. The kidneys are bilaterally enlarged, with very small cysts radially oriented throughout parenchyma (Fig. 53-6). The cysts represent dilated collecting tubules. Periportal hepatic fibrosis also occurs in varying degrees, and can lead to portal hypertension. The hepatic involvement appears to be inversely proportional to the renal involvement. The disease has been classified into four forms.[37] The severe perinatal form (>90% renal involvement) leads to death by six weeks from pulmonary hypoplasia. The neonatal form (60% renal involvement) is usually lethal by one year. The infantile form (25% renal involvement) results in hepatosplenomegaly, with survival up to 10 years. The juvenile form (<10% renal involvement) has severe periportal fibrosis. Some patients survive up to 15 years, but the development of portal hypertension is usually lethal. Since this is an autosomal recessive disease, family screening should be undertaken to determine which siblings are carriers.

A prenatal ultrasound showing bilaterally enlarged echogenic kidneys suggests ARPKD. The IVP or CT shows a classic striated 'sunburst' pattern. Unfortunately, the prognosis is poor for the perinatal or neonatal forms of ARPKD. The patients who survive the neonatal period seem to do well with some degree of renal insufficiency. Eventually, dialysis is usually required. In older patients, the kidneys become smaller as renal failure develops. The overall treatment for ARPKD is supportive, with renal transplantation being the ultimate therapy.

Autosomal Dominant Polycystic Kidney Disease (ADPKD)

While ADPKD tends to clinically present in the third to fifth decade, it has been diagnosed in the ultrasound era in asymptomatic children as well. The cysts in ADPKD are different in configuration, being few and scattered in

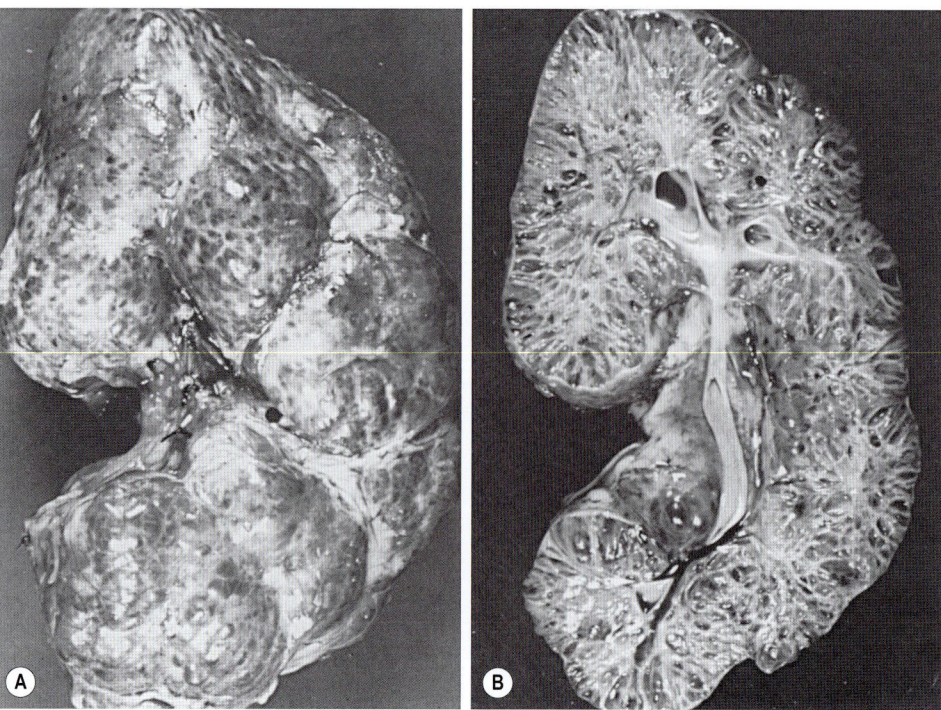

FIGURE 53-6 ■ Gross pathology of autosomal recessive polycystic kidney disease.

distinction to those seen in ARPKD. This condition occurs in 1:500 patients.[38] Patients usually present with flank pain, hematuria, hypertension, and possibly renal failure, if there are extensive bilateral cysts. Neonates can present with renal enlargement, although children from affected families who are screened usually only have a few cysts. Failure to see cysts on screening ultrasound in a child at risk for ARPKD does not exclude the disease since the cysts can develop later in life. Linkage analysis of the loci on chromosome 4 and 16 is more sensitive.[39] The cysts are located throughout the cortex and medulla, although the fetal form seems to affect the glomeruli predominantly. Hepatic involvement is limited to biliary cysts. Associated findings include cysts in the spleen, pancreas, and lungs, mitral valve prolapse, colon diverticuli, and berry aneurysms of the circle of Willis.

Hypertension is commonly found in these children, and may be part of the presentation. Renal failure in childhood is very rare. Periodic evaluation of blood pressure and proteinuria during childhood is recommended.[40,41] Unlike ARPKD, there is no increased risk of renal cell carcinoma. Renal transplant candidates can obtain organs from family members who have been screened for the disease.

Multicystic Dysplastic Kidney (MCDK)

The multicystic dysplastic kidney is believed to be caused by severe early ureteral obstruction or a failure in ureteric bud-metanephric blastema induction.[42,43] The main differential diagnosis is severe hydronephrosis due to UPJ obstruction. Radiographically, this occurs when the peripheral cysts surround a dominant central cyst mimicking the renal pelvis ('hydronephrotic' form of MCDK). The classic ultrasound appearance shows cysts randomly distributed throughout the kidney without a dominant medial cyst or evidence of communication between cysts. The parenchyma, if present, has abnormal echogenicity and is seen between the cysts, instead of being arranged on their periphery. A renal scan will show no function in a MCDK. The affected area may be the upper pole of a duplicated collecting system, or one-half of a horseshoe kidney.

The MCDK is the most common renal cystic mass in the newborn. Currently, most are detected on prenatal ultrasound. Bilateral forms are not compatible with life. Postnatal evaluation consists of a VCUG to look for VUR in the contralateral kidney, which is found 30% of the time.[44] If there is significant hydronephrosis (caliectasis) in the contralateral kidney (this occurs 12% of the time), then a diuretic renal scan may be necessary. Contralateral UPJ obstruction or VUR is more likely with a smaller MCDK or a lower ureteral atresia ipsilateral to the MCDK.[45,46] There are reports of malignancy arising from a MCDK, although it is unclear whether the affected kidneys were truly MCDK.[47] Hypertension has also been reported in association with MCDK, although resection is not always curative, and the rate does not appear to be any higher than the general population.[48]

MCDK usually involute, but they can occasionally grow.[48] The follow-up is repeat imaging with ultrasound every six months for the first two years of life. It is not usually feasible to monitor a patient indefinitely for a MCDK. We have taken an operative approach at 18 to 24 months of life if the MCDK is not involuting, or if parenchyma remains visible on the ultrasound. Although the indications are controversial, the kidney can be removed at that age via laparoscopy or a small incision as an outpatient procedure (Fig. 53-7). Occasionally, the MCDK can involute prenatally, leaving a ureter with a small nubbin of tissue in the renal fossa. These were previously called 'aplastic kidneys,' but are now felt to represent the remnants of a MCDK.

Cystic Nephroma

Formerly called a 'multilocular cyst,' this is a well demarcated tumor of cysts with an overall round configuration, lined with epithelium and septae which contain tubules.[49] It is considered to be the benign end of a spectrum progressing from cystic Wilms tumor, cystic partially differentiated nephroblastoma, to cystic nephroma. It usually is found in boys under age 4 (male:female ratio 2:1) or women over 30 (female:male ratio 8:1). It is rarely bilateral and is cured by partial nephrectomy, shelling out the tumor by following the plane of the pseudocapsule. There is a risk of sarcomatous degeneration in adults if it is not removed.[50]

Cystic Partially Differentiated Nephroblastoma

This lesion was formerly called a multilocular cystic nephroma. It is radiologically identical to the cystic nephroma, and can only be diagnosed pathologically. The

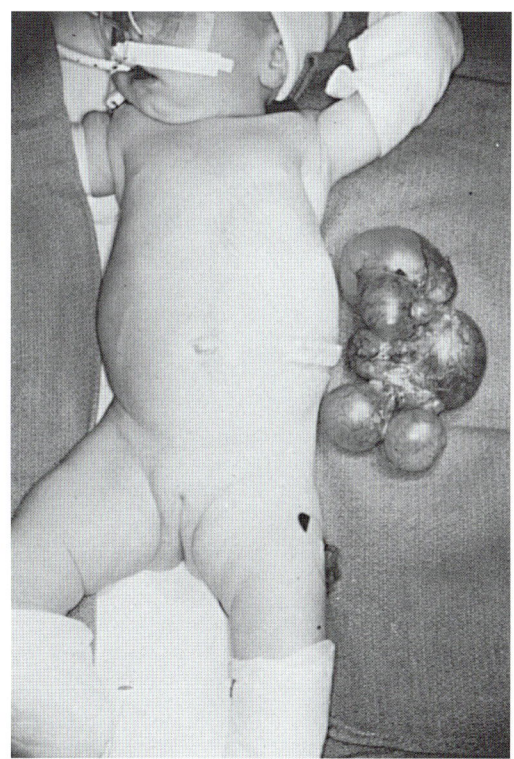

FIGURE 53-7 ■ Resected multicystic dysplastic kidney.

majority of patients are boys less than 2 years old, or women in their third to fourth decade. A classic (but not diagnostic) radiologic finding is herniation of a parenchymal mass into the renal pelvis.[22] The tumor is usually well circumscribed. Hemorrhage and calcification are usually absent. Pathologically, it differs from the cystic nephroma in that there is blastema found in the septations.

Patients usually present with an asymptomatic flank mass, and occasionally hematuria. Operative treatment consists of partial nephrectomy as for cystic nephroma, since the tumors rarely recur and are not multifocal. No chemotherapy is required for stage I (limited to capsule, fully resected) tumors. Although experience is limited, stage II (outside renal capsule but fully resected) are usually treated with vincristine, dactinomycin, and doxorubicin. Four year survival for both stages is 100%.[51,52]

Simple Cysts and Calyceal Diverticuli

The simple renal cyst on ultrasound has the following characteristics: distinct wall, no internal echoes, and posterior enhancement. If these criteria are not met, a CT scan is obtained to confirm that the fluid does not enhance. The differential diagnosis is a calyceal diverticulum or hydrocalyx, both of which communicate with the collecting system, and in which the fluid should enhance on either IVP or CT. Ultrasound is able to detect milk of calcium layering within a diverticulum. Calyceal diverticuli require treatment when they harbor stones or infection. In the IVP era, 40% of calyceal diverticuli were felt to be symptomatic.[53] In the ultrasound era, with its greater number of incidental findings, it is not clear how often calyceal diverticuli require treatment. Minimally invasive approaches such as percutaneous, laparoscopic, and ureteroscopic ablation appear to be equally successful.[54]

Simple cysts reside in the cortex and are lined by simple columnar epithelium. They can grow, resorb, or remain the same size. They are usually asymptomatic and are found incidentally. Once they are found, the authors usually follow with ultrasound at 3 to 6 month intervals to determine if the cyst is growing. The underlying concern is whether or not this cyst is the first sign of ADPKD. A family history of renal cystic disease, renal failure, or death in the neonatal period from unknown causes should be sought. Biopsy to rule out tumor, followed by drainage, or unroofing should only be undertaken if the cyst characteristics are other than those listed for a simple cyst, or if the cyst becomes symptomatic due to obstruction of an infundibulum or the UPJ. Minimally invasive approaches such as percutaneous puncture with instillation of sclerosing agents (absolute alcohol, bismuth, povidone-iodine[55]) or laparoscopic decortication[56] may shift the threshold for treatment of large asymptomatic simple cysts.

REFERENCES

1. Gray SW, Skandalakis JE. The kidney and ureter. In: Embryology for Surgeons. Philadelphia: WB Saunders; 1972. p. 443–518.
2. Mackie GG, Stephens FD. Duplex kidneys: A correlation of renal dysplasia with position of the ureteral orifice. J Urol 1975;114:274–80.
3. Atiyeh B, Husmann D, Baum M. Contralateral renal abnormalities in multicystic-dysplastic kidney disease. J Pediatr 1992;121:65–7.
4. Royer P, Habib R, Broyer M, et al. L'Hypoplasie renale bilaterale congenitale avec reduction du nombre et hypertrophie des nephrons chez l'enfant. Ann Pediatr (Paris) 1962;38:133–46.
5. Arant BS Jr, Sotelo-Avila C, Bernstein J. Segmental "hypoplasia" of the kidney (Ask-Upmark). J Pediatr 1979;95:931–9.
6. Doroshow LW, Abeshouse BS. Congenital unilateral solitary kidney: Report of 37 cases and a review of the literature. Urol Surv 1961;11:219–29.
7. Sheih CP, Hung CS, Wei CF, et al. Cystic dilatations within the pelvis in patients with ipsilateral renal agenesis or dysplasia. J Urol 1990;144:324–7.
8. Kohn G, Borns PF. The association of bilateral and unilateral renal aplasia in the same family. J Pediatr 1973;83:95–7.
9. Mascatello V, Lebowitz RL. Malposition of the colon in left renal agenesis and ectopia. Radiology 1976;120:371–6.
10. Kolon TF, Gray CL, Sutherland RW, et al. Upper urinary tract manifestations of the VACTERL association. J Urol 2000;163:1949–51.
11. Downs RA, Lane JW, Burns E. Solitary pelvic kidney. Its clinical implications. Urology 1973;1:51–6.
12. Thompson DP, Lynn HB. Genital anomalies associated with solitary kidney. Mayo Clin Proc 1966;41:538–48.
13. Tarry WF, Duckett JW, Stephens FD. The Mayer-Rokitansky syndrome: Pathogenesis, classification, and management. J Urol 1986;136:648–52.
14. Griffin JE, Edwards C, Madden JD, et al. Congenital absence of the vagina. The Mayer-Rokitansky-Kuster-Hauser syndrome. Ann Internal Med 1976;85:224–36.
15. Potter EL. Bilateral absence of ureters and kidneys: A report of 50 cases. Obstet Gynecol 1965;25:3–12.
16. Ashley DJ, Mostofi FK. Renal agenesis and dysgenesis. J Urol 1960;83:211–30.
17. Carpentier PJ, Potter EL. Nuclear sex and genital malformation in 48 cases of renal agenesis, with especial reference to nonspecific female pseudoheramphroditism. Am J Obstet Gynecol 1959;78:235–58.
18. Geisinger JG. Supernumerary kidney. J Urol 1937;38:331.
19. N'Guessan G, Stephens FD. Supernumerary kidney. J Urol 1983;130:649–53.
20. Weiss JP, Duckett JW, Snyder HM. Single unilateral vaginal ectopic ureter: Is it really a rarity? J Urol 1984;132:1177–9.
21. Malek, RS, Kelalis, PP, Burke EC. Ectopic kidney in children and frequency of association with other malformations. Mayo Clinic Proc 1971;46:461–7.
22. Zagoria RL, Tung GA. The kidney and retroperitoneum: Anatomy and congenital anomalies. In: Zagoria RL, editor. Genitourinary Radiology: The Requisites. St. Louis: Mosby; 1997. p. 51–79.
23. Dretler SP, Pfister R, Hendren WH. Extrarenal calyces in the ectopic kidney. J Urol 1970;103:406–10.
24. Gleason PE, Kelalis PP, Husmann DA, et al. Hydronephrosis in renal ectopia: Incidence, etiology, and significance. J Urol 1994;151:1660–1.
25. Jabbour ME, Goldfischer ER, Stravodimos KG, et al. Endopyelotomy for horseshoe and ectopic kidneys. J Urol 1998;160:694–7.
26. Dees J. Clinical importance of congenital anomalies of upper urinary tract. J Urol 1941;46:659.
27. Boatman DL, Kolln CP, Flocks RH. Congenital anomalies associated with horseshoe kidneys. J Urol 1972;107:205–7.
28. Buntley D. Malignancy associated with horseshoe kidney. Urology 1976;8:146–8.
29. Hohenfellner M, Schultz-Lampel D, Lempel A, et al. Tumor in the horseshoe kidney: Clinical implications and review of embryogenesis. J Urol 1992;147:1098–102.
30. Neville H, Ritchey ML, Shamberger RC, et al. The occurrence of Wilms' tumor in horseshoe kidneys: A report from the National Wilms' Tumor Study Group (NWTSG). J Pediatr Surg 2002;37:1134–7.
31. Segura JW, Kelalis PP, Burke EC. Horseshoe kidney in children. J Urol 1972;108:333–6.
32. Whitehouse GH. Some urographic aspects of horseshoe kidney anomaly – a review of 59 cases. Clin Radiol 1975;26:107–14.
33. Yohannes P, Smith AD. The endourological management of complications associated with horseshoe kidney. J Urol 2002;168:5–8.

34. Miller NL, Matlaga BR, Handa SE, et al. The presence of horseshoe kidney does not affect the outcome of percutaneous nephrolithotomy. J Endourol 2008;22:1219–25.

35. Evans WP, Resnick MI. Horseshoe kidney and urolithiasis. J Urol 1981;125:620–1.

36. Raj GV, Auge BK, Assimos D, et al. Metabolic abnormalities associated with renal calculi in patients with horseshoe kidney. J Endourol 2004;12:157–61.

37. Blyth H, Ockenden BG. Polycystic disease of kidney and liver presenting in childhood. J Med Genet 1971;8:257–84.

38. Gabow PA. Autosomal dominant polycystic kidney disease. N Engl J Med 1993;329:332–42.

39. Gabow PA, Kimberling WJ, Strain JD, et al. Utility of ultrasonography in the diagnosis of autosomal dominant polycystic kidney disease in children. J Am Soc Nephrol 1997;8:105–10.

40. Ravine D, Walker RG, Gibson RN, et al. Treatable complications in undiagnosed cases of autosomal dominant polycystic kidney disease. Lancet 1991;337:127–9.

41. Zerres K, Rudnik-Schoneborn S, Deget F. Routine examination of children at risk of autosomal dominant polycystic kidney disease. Lancet 1992;339:1356–7.

42. Beck AD. The effect of intra-uterine urinary obstruction upon the development of the fetal kidney. J Urol 1971;105:784–9.

43. Osathanondh V, Potter EL. Pathogenesis of polycystic kidneys: Historical survey. Arch Pathol 1964;77:459–65.

44. Flack CE, Bellinger, MF. The multicystic dysplastic kidney and contralateral vesicoureteral reflux: protection of the solitary kidney. J Urol 1993;150:1873–4.

45. Cendron J, Gubler JP, Valayer J, et al. Dysplasie multikystique du rein chez enfant. A propos de 45 observations. J Urol Nephrol (Paris) 1973;79:773–99.

46. Cendron J, Kiriakos S. Rein multikystique. J Urol Nephrol (Paris) 1976,82(S2):322–33.

47. Beckwith JB. Comment, Wilms' tumor and multicystic dysplastic kidney disease. J Urol 1997;158:2259–60.

48. Wacksman J, Phipps L. Report of the multicystic kidney registry: Preliminary findings. J Urol 1993;150:1870–2.

49. Joshi VV, Beckwith JB. Multilocular cyst of the kidney (cystic nephroma) and cystic, partially differentiated nephroblastoma. Terminology and criteria for diagnosis. Cancer 1989;64:466–79.

50. Castillo OA, Boyle ET Jr, Kramer SA. Multilocular cysts of the kidney. A study of 29 patients and review of literature. Urology 1991;37:156–62.

51. Blakely ML, Shamberger RC, Norkool P, et al. Outcome of children with cystic partially differentiated nephroblastoma treated with and without chemotherapy. J Pediatr Surg 2003;38:897–900.

52. Luithle T, Szavay P, Furtwangler R, et al. Treatment of cystic nephroma and cystic partially differentiated nephroblastoma – A report from SIOP/GPOH study group. J Urol 2007;177:294–6.

53. Timmons JW Jr, Malek RS, Hattery RR, et al. Caliceal diverticulum. J Urol 1975;114:6–9.

54. Canales B, Monga M. Surgical management of the calyceal diverticulum. Curr Opin Urol 2003;13:255–60.

55. Phelan M, Zajko A, Hrebinko RL. Preliminary results of percutaneous treatment of renal cysts with povidone-iodine sclerosis. Urology 1999;53:816–17.

56. Lifson BJ, Teichman JM, Hulbert JC. Role and long-term results of laparoscopic decortication in solitary cystic and autosomal dominant polycystic kidney disease. J Urol 1998;159:702–6.

CHAPTER 54

URETERAL OBSTRUCTION AND MALFORMATIONS

Erica J. Traxel • Douglas E. Coplen

Hydronephrosis and ureteral malformations are among the most common anomalies in the urinary tract in children. Most are now detected prenatally. Urinary tract dilation is present in 1 in 100 fetuses, but significant uropathy is found in only 1 in 500[1,2] (Fig. 54-1).

URETEROPELVIC JUNCTION OBSTRUCTION IN CHILDREN

With ureteropelvic junction (UPJ) obstruction, there is inadequate drainage of urine from the renal pelvis, resulting in hydrostatic distention of the pelvis and intrarenal calyces. The combination of increased intrapelvic pressure and urine stasis in the collecting ducts results in progressive damage to the kidney.

Historically, the incidence of UPJ obstruction has been estimated at 1 in 5,000 live births. However, with the advent of antenatal ultrasonography (US), the prevalence of dilation has been found to be much higher. Retrospective reviews show that although the incidence of detected dilation has increased, the actual number of operations for UPJ obstruction has been relatively constant at 1:1,250 births.[3,4] UPJ obstruction is more common in boys (2:1), and two-thirds occur on the left side. Bilateral dilation occurs in 5–10% of patients, and is much more frequently seen in younger children. Bilateral obstruction is much less common.[5]

Etiology

During development of the upper ureter, the lumen of the ureteral bud solidifies with ureteral lengthening and later recanalization.[6] Failure to recanalize adequately is thought to be the cause of most intrinsic UPJ obstructions. Other causes of intrinsic UPJ obstruction include ureteral valves, polyps, and leiomyomas.[7]

The most common observation is ureteral narrowing of a variable length that joins the renal pelvis above the expected dependent position.[8] At low volume, peristaltic waves of urine cross the UPJ. However, as the flow increases beyond a threshold, the renal pelvis dilates.[9] The dilated pelvis may functionally kink the ureter further, increasing the pelvic pressure. In 20–30% of patients, the ureter is draped over a lower-pole vessel, producing an extrinsic UPJ obstruction. In most situations, there is also a coexisting luminal narrowing of the ureter.[10]

Histologic evaluation reveals a decrease or complete absence of smooth muscle fibers at the UPJ.[11] Electron microscopy may show an increase in collagen deposition between the muscle fibers that is most likely a response to the obstruction as opposed to the cause.[12] Fibrosis and interruption of the smooth muscle continuity block transmission of the peristaltic wave, while defective innervation also may play a role.[13] UPJ obstruction also can be secondary, i.e., related to other ureteral pathology. It can be found in conjunction with high-grade vesicoureteral reflux (VUR), after cutaneous ureterostomy, and after decompression of the dilated urinary tract. VUR is present in 14% of patients with UPJ obstruction (Fig. 54-2).[14,15]

Clinical Presentation

Most renal dilation and obstruction are detected prenatally. Less frequently, it is detected because of an abdominal mass, urinary tract infection (UTI), or associated with other congenital anomalies (i.e., VACTERL syndrome). In older children, vague, poorly localized, cyclic or acute abdominal pain associated with nausea is common (Fig. 54-3). Some of these children are initially seen by gastroenterologists. The cause for the intermittent obstruction is unclear, but renal function is almost always preserved. Hematuria after minor trauma or vigorous exercise may be a presenting feature, most likely secondary to rupture of mucosal vessels in the dilated collecting system.[5]

Diagnosis

When the antenatal diagnosis of UPJ obstruction is made, the initial postpartum evaluation should be performed at 10 to 14 days of life to avoid false-negative studies resulting from the transitional nephrology of the newborn. Bilateral dilation is rarely associated with significant enough obstruction to cause oligohydramnios and warrant antenatal intervention. Ultrasound confirms the presence of pelvic and calyceal dilation, with variable thinning of the renal parenchyma. The Society for Fetal Urology (SFU) classification is typically used to describe the degree of dilation (Fig. 54-4).[16] The presence of corticomedullary junctions is indicative of preserved function.[15] Ultrasound is used to evaluate the contralateral kidney, the bladder, and the distal ipsilateral ureter to avoid confusion with a ureterovesical junction (UVJ) obstruction, but it does not provide functional information.

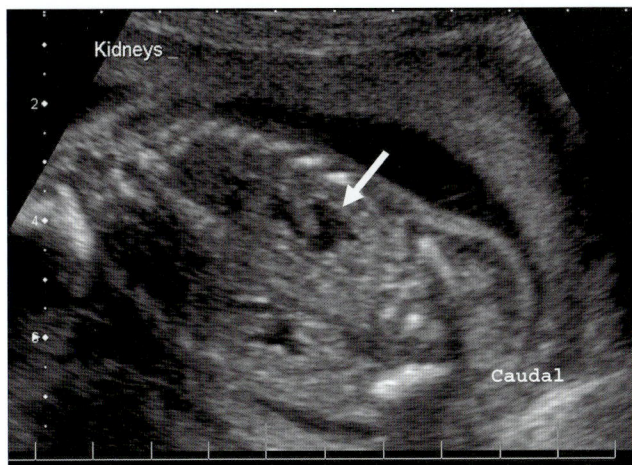

FIGURE 54-1 ■ Normal kidneys are typically identifiable by 18 weeks in all fetuses. Dilated kidneys can be seen as early as 12–14 weeks of gestation. The arrow demonstrates left-sided caliectasis on a coronal fetal image.

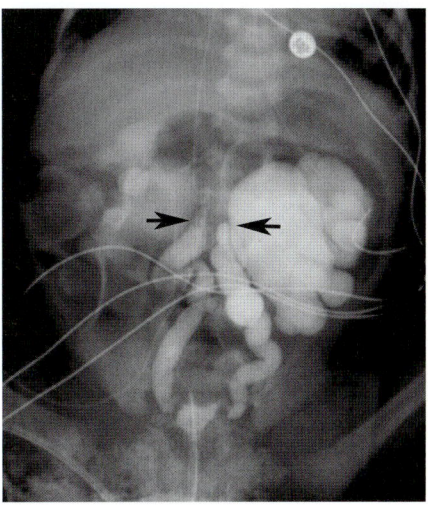

FIGURE 54-2 ■ This cystogram shows marked bilateral reflux in an infant with bilateral UPJ configuration (black arrows).

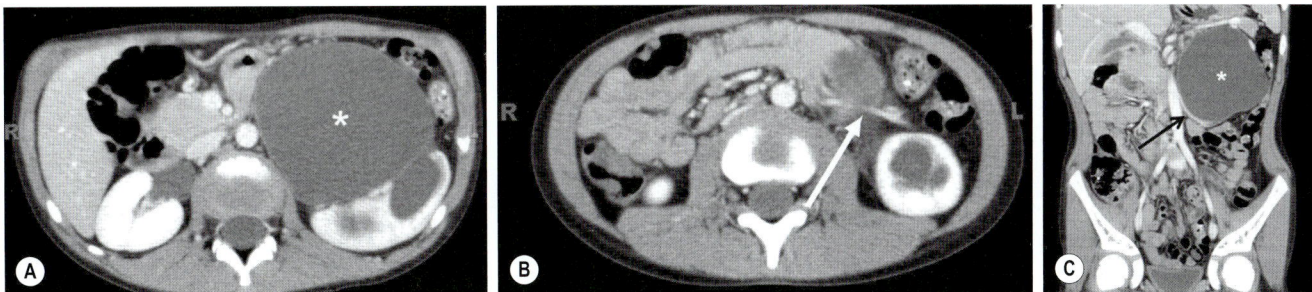

FIGURE 54-3 ■ This CT scan was obtained for evaluation of severe abdominal pain. **(A)** Axial view shows marked dilation of the left renal pelvis (asterisk) with preserved renal parenchyma. **(B, C)** A lower pole crossing vessel is seen (arrow).

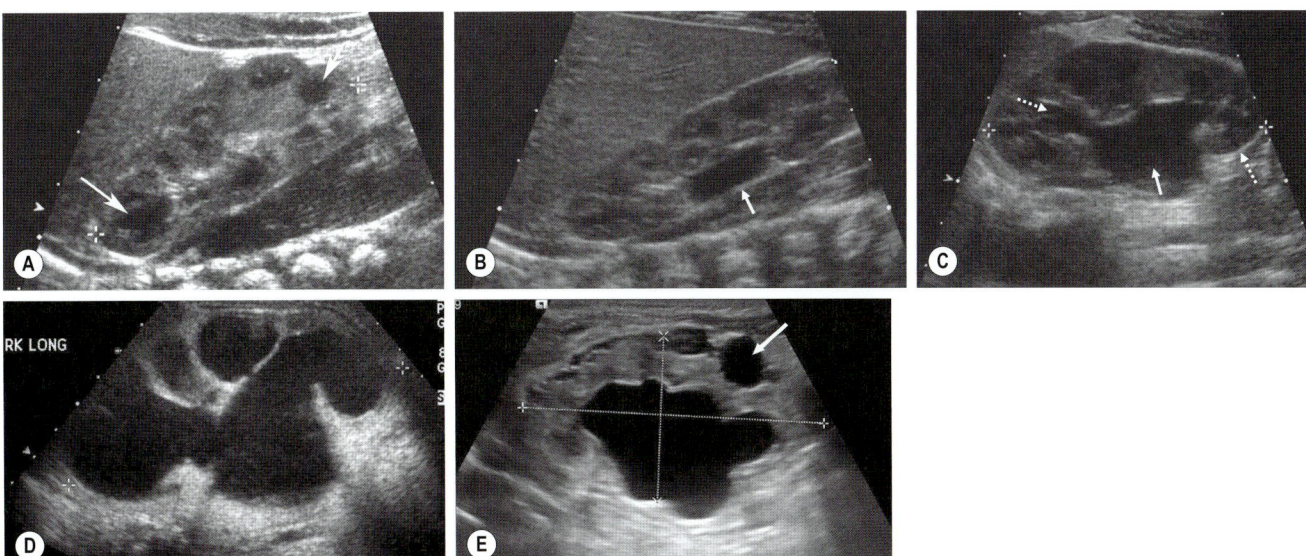

FIGURE 54-4 ■ These neonatal ultrasound images come from infants with a history of prenatally detected renal dilation. **(A)** This ultrasound is normal for comparison purposes. There are dark renal pyramids (arrow) and no renal pelvic dilation. **(B)** This image shows isolated renal pelvic dilation (arrow) (SFU grade I). **(C)** This image shows dilation of the renal pelvis (solid arrow) and upper and lower-pole calyces (dotted arrows) (SFU grade II). **(D)** Calyceal dilation and cortical thinning are seen (SFU grade IV). **(E)** Hydronephrosis with peripheral cysts (arrow) indicating dysplasia is seen. This kidney had no function on renal scan.

In the past, routine antibiotic prophylaxis was utilized in all infants with prenatal dilation but the risk of UTI is very small in the absence of reflux.[17] A voiding cystourethrogram (VCUG) was previously recommended in all patients being evaluated for UPJ obstruction. VUR increases the chance that infection will occur, even in a partially obstructed system. Between 5–30% of infants with prenatally detected dilation will have reflux, and the majority will spontaneously resolve without an infection.[15] Children with isolated pyelectasis and no ureteral dilation have a very low incidence of reflux and do not need a screening VCUG.

The diuretic isotopic renogram is very useful for evaluating hydronephrosis, differential renal function, and renal drainage (Fig. 54-5). In this study, the transit of an injected radioisotope through the urinary tract is monitored by a gamma camera. The early uptake (first 1 to 2 minutes) of the tracer indicates the split renal function, while the washout, augmented by the administration of a diuretic, is evaluated and plotted by a computer to demonstrate drainage.[18–20] The study is obtained with either ⁹⁹ᵐTc-mercaptoacetyltriglycine (⁹⁹ᵐTc-MAG3), whose clearance is predominantly via proximal tubular secretion, or with technetium-99m-labeled diethylenetriamine pentaacetic acid (⁹⁹ᵐTc-DTPA), whose renal clearance is by glomerular filtration. ⁹⁹ᵐTc-MAG3 is more efficiently excreted than ⁹⁹ᵐTc-DTPA and gives better images, particularly in patients with impaired renal function.[19,20]

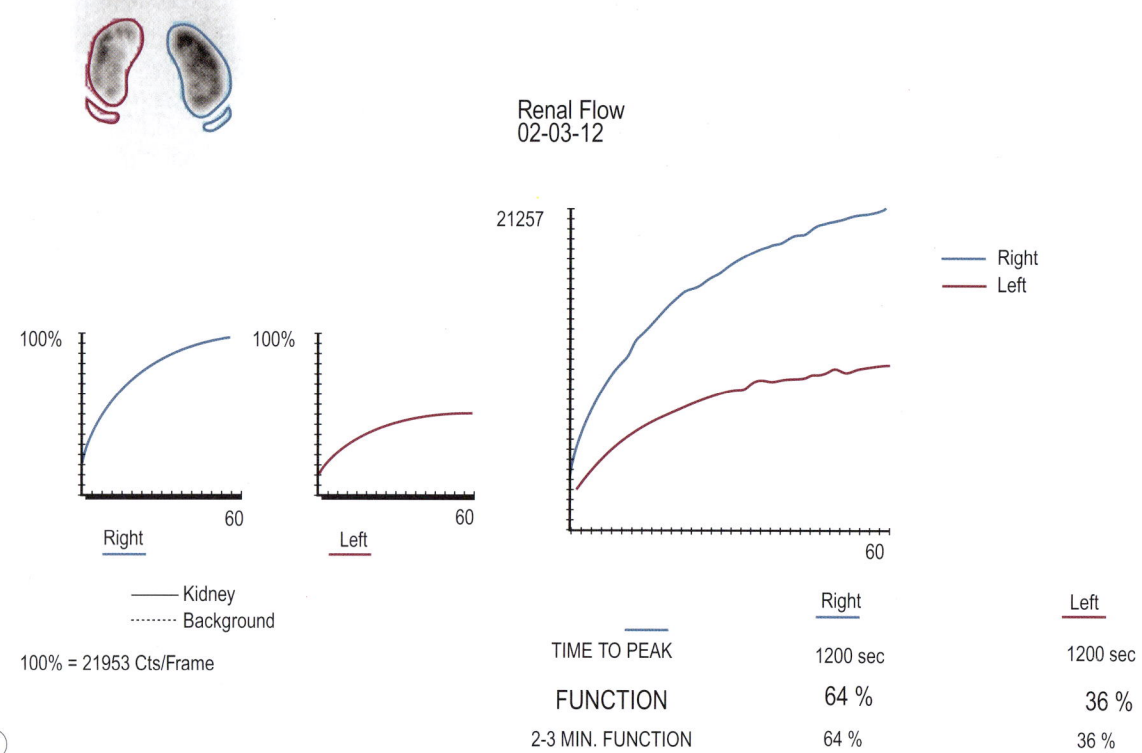

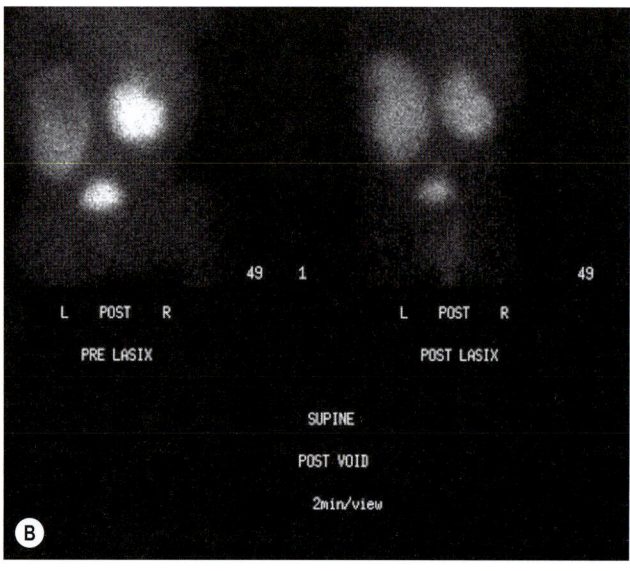

FIGURE 54-5 ■ Renal scan in the evaluation of prenatally identified hydronephrosis. The ultrasound study showed diffuse caliectesis and pelvic dilation consistent with UPJ obstruction. **(A)** The dilated left kidney has reduced function. **(B)** Lasix should be administered once the renal pelvis is completely distended. In this case, it appears there is further accumulation (increased counts) after Lasix administration. Observation was chosen because the dilation was predominantly extrarenal, the kidneys were not palpable even after Lasix administration, and concern that the drainage time was perhaps falsely elevated. One year later, the renal dilation was markedly improved.

The technique for diuretic renography is standardized.[20] Patients should be hydrated intravenously (15 mL/kg) 15 minutes before injection of the radionuclide. An indwelling catheter maintains an empty bladder and monitors urine output. The diuretic (1 mg/kg furosemide, up to 40 mg) is not administered until the activity peaks in the hydronephrotic kidney and renal pelvis. The tracer activity is then monitored for an additional 30 minutes, and a quantitative analysis is performed. Historically, persistence of more than 50% of the tracer in the renal pelvis 20 minutes after diuretic administration ($t_{1/2} > 20$) is diagnostic of obstruction, although the applicability of this threshold in pediatric patients is debatable. False-positive results may occur when the immature neonatal kidney fails to respond to diuretic, when the diuretic is administered prior to maximal renal pelvic distension, when the patient is dehydrated, when the bladder is distended, or when the pelvis is significantly dilated.

Magnetic resonance urography (MRU) can be used at any age. T_2-weighted images are independent of renal function, and hydronephrosis is readily detected. The anatomic images are excellent (Fig. 54-6). Enhanced MR images with gadolinium can give information regarding differential function if one kidney is anatomically and functionally normal.[21]

Rarely, when imaging is equivocal, invasive pressure flow studies may be indicated.[22] These tests assume that obstruction produces a constant restriction to outflow that necessitates elevated pressure to transport urine at high flow rates. However, not all obstructions are constant. If the obstruction is intrinsic, a linear relationship exists between pressure and flow. However, in some cases, the results reflect only the response of the renal pelvis to distention and may be positive in the absence of obstruction. These studies require general anesthesia in children and have limited applicability.

Retrograde urography at the time of operative correction is helpful if uncertainty exists regarding the site of obstruction. This is rarely required because a well-performed ultrasound evaluation and radionuclide study will exclude distal obstruction.[23] As there are risks with using instruments in the infant male urethra and the ureteral orifice, these retrograde studies are not usually performed.

Management

Indications for Intervention

Intermittent obstruction and pain are probably the most reliable indication for operation. Diminished function, delayed drainage, progression of pelvic and calyceal dilation on ultrasound, and loss of renal function are all potential indicators of obstruction. Randomization to operative and observational arms is complicated by a difficult decision that a parent has to make for the asymptomatic child.[24] The morphologic appearance of a dilated renal pelvis on excretory urography or ultrasound is not a good indication for operation because many of these findings will resolve without the need for operation (see Fig. 54-5).[25] Neonatal hydronephrosis can often be explained by physiologic polyuria and natural kinks and folds in the ureter.

The ongoing debate in the management of neonatal UPJ obstruction centers on the definition of significant obstruction. Diuretic renography has limitations in the neonate, although using the 'well-tempered' approach increases its value.[20] The standard half-time of 20 minutes for obstruction in the neonate is misleading in many cases.

Differential renal function or individual kidney uptake is the most useful information obtained during renography.[24–26] An indication for operation is diminished renal function in the presence of an obstructive pattern on renography. The threshold is arbitrary, but most surgeons believe that less than 35–40% function in the hydronephrotic kidney warrants correction. However, one series of patients with dilated kidneys and no more than 25% total renal function were found to improve to more than 40% of total function in all cases without operative correction.[25] Long-term studies of kidneys with greater than 40% function have shown that fewer than 15–20% will require operation for diminishing function, UTIs, or unexplained abdominal pain.[26,27] Some of these kidneys will regain some of the lost function.

The concern with an observational approach is that delaying correction until there is measurable deterioration of renal function is not optimal. In the past, urinary stasis (infection, calculi, hypertension, and pain) was the indication for correction. Whether more emphasis should be placed on stasis and less emphasis on differential renal function is an unanswered question. Pyeloplasty can be safely performed in the infant. Early intervention eliminates the indefinite period of surveillance. The decision to follow neonates nonoperatively requires vigilance and parental cooperation to avoid complications.

If the child is initially seen with acute pain or infection, it is advisable to wait one to two weeks to allow the inflammation to resolve. Percutaneous drainage or stent placement for sepsis is rarely required preoperatively. It

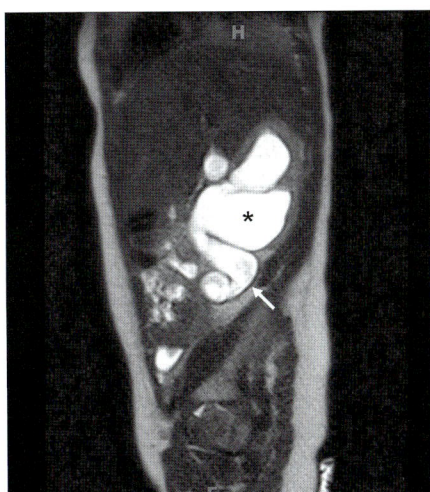

FIGURE 54-6 ■ In this 6-month-old infant, an ultrasound showed a dilated ureter below the kidney, but not at the level of the bladder. This coronal image shows marked dilation of the proximal ureter (arrow) and pelvis (asterisk) due to a proximal ureteral valve.

should be avoided in the absence of infection because of the inflammation that develops from a tube in the renal pelvis. Exploration of a poorly functioning kidney requires assessment of the renal parenchyma. If the parenchyma is grossly dysplastic or frozen-section analysis shows only dysplasia, then nephrectomy should be performed. No test accurately predicts recovery of function. Thus, nephrectomy is rarely performed in the infant with UPJ obstruction.

Operative Techniques

A dismembered pyeloplasty is the preferred technique to correct UPJ obstruction (Fig. 54-7). A successful outcome is achieved with construction of a funnel-shaped, dependent UPJ complex. The renal pelvis and upper ureter are mobilized and the ureter is divided just below the obstructed segment. It is spatulated on its lateral border through the aperistaltic segment. Usually, it is necessary to resect some of the renal pelvis to avoid postoperative obstruction. If this segment is particularly long, a flap of renal pelvis can be created. Foley YV-plasty and the Culp spiral flap were designed to maintain the continuity of the ureter and the pelvis.[28,29] These techniques are used in unusual cases of malrotation, fusion anomalies, or long, stenotic segments.

The anastomosis is performed with 6-0 polydioxanone or 6-0 polyglycolic acid. The anastomosis begins at the most dependent portion of the pyeloplasty with placement of interrupted everting sutures that do not bunch the tissues and cause obstruction. After the anastomosis to the dependent portion of the pelvis is completed, the remainder of the ureter and pelvis can be approximated with continuous suture, taking care to irrigate any clots from the pelvis before the closure is completed. It is not necessary to pass a catheter distally into the bladder because preoperative studies should have excluded a distal obstruction.

Pyeloplasties are frequently performed without diversion so it is important to be as gentle as possible.[30] Excessive handling of the pelvis and ureter increases edema. A stent is typically left in place after a laparoscopic repair. Even if leakage from the anastomosis occurs, a satisfactory outcome can usually be expected. A Penrose drain is

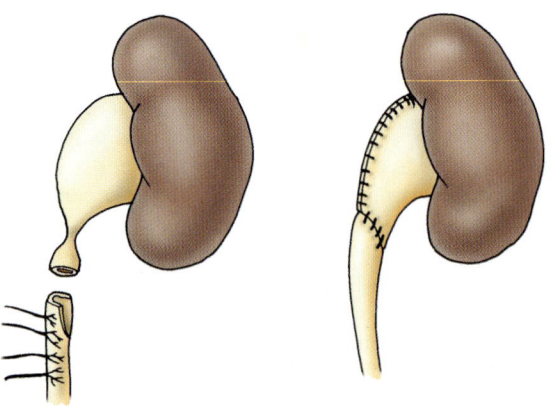

FIGURE 54-7 ■ Dismembered pyeloplasty showing reduction of the renal pelvis and spatulation of the ureter (see the text).

left near the anastomosis and can usually be removed within 48 hours. If drainage is prolonged, the child can be discharged with the drain in place. Renal drainage is indicated in solitary kidneys or when simultaneous bilateral pyeloplasties are performed. In reoperation, it is technically more difficult to achieve a watertight anastomosis and internal drainage (stent, nephrostomy or nephrostent) is indicated.

Extrinsic UPJ obstruction associated with an aberrant lower-pole vessel requires division of the ureter at the UPJ and performance of a standard dismembered pyeloplasty after transposing the ureter to a nonobstructed position. This is preferable to laparoscopic transposition of the crossing vessel. In the case of an intrarenal pelvis or when significant scarring is found at reoperation, a ureterocalicostomy is a useful technique.[31] A portion of the lower pole should be resected to prevent a postoperative stricture. The ureter is spatulated and then anastomosed to the exposed calyx in the lower pole.

The open approach still has a role in infants and young children. Laparoscopic pyeloplasty has been performed in all ages and the age of the patient is inversely related to benefits of decreased pain and convalescence.[32] Open pyeloplasty can be performed through a flank, anterior extraperitoneal approach, or posterior lumbotomy approach. The anterior approach involves a transverse incision from the edge of the rectus to the tip of the 12th rib.[33] The retroperitoneum is entered and the UPJ is exposed, with the kidney left in situ. In infants, this is a muscle-splitting incision with low morbidity. The posterior lumbotomy also can be easily performed in infancy and provides direct access to the UPJ.[34] The kidney does not require mobilization, and the ureter and renal pelvis can usually be delivered into the incision. In bilateral cases, the child does not need to be repositioned. The lumbotomy approach should not be used with a malrotated kidney or a kidney that has an intrarenal pelvis. An anterior or flank approach is always preferred for reoperation although laparoscopy and endopyelotomy have largely replaced open re-operative pyeloplasty.[35]

Endoscopic approaches (endopyelotomy) for UPJ obstruction were popularized in the 1980s and 1990s, but have been replaced by laparoscopic approaches.[36,37] Endopyelotomy successfully relieves primary UPJ obstruction in 70% of children.[38] As the success pales in comparison to pyeloplasty, it is not routinely utilized for primary repair. Endopyelotomy clearly has a role in recurrent UPJ obstruction, in which the success rate is >95%.[38] Depending on the age of the patient and the size of the ureter, this can be performed in either an antegrade or retrograde fashion (Fig. 54-8).

The first laparoscopic pyeloplasty in a child was reported in 1995 by Peters.[39] The first series was published by Tan in 1999.[40] Laparoscopic pyeloplasty has been reported in children as young as 2 months.[41] The introduction of robotic surgery with articulating instruments and three-dimensional visualization has made intracorporeal suturing easier and more precise. The success rate with minimally invasive techniques is equivalent to open pyeloplasty.[42,43] The benefits of laparoscopic and robotic surgery over an open approach may include a decreased length of hospitalization, decreased analgesic

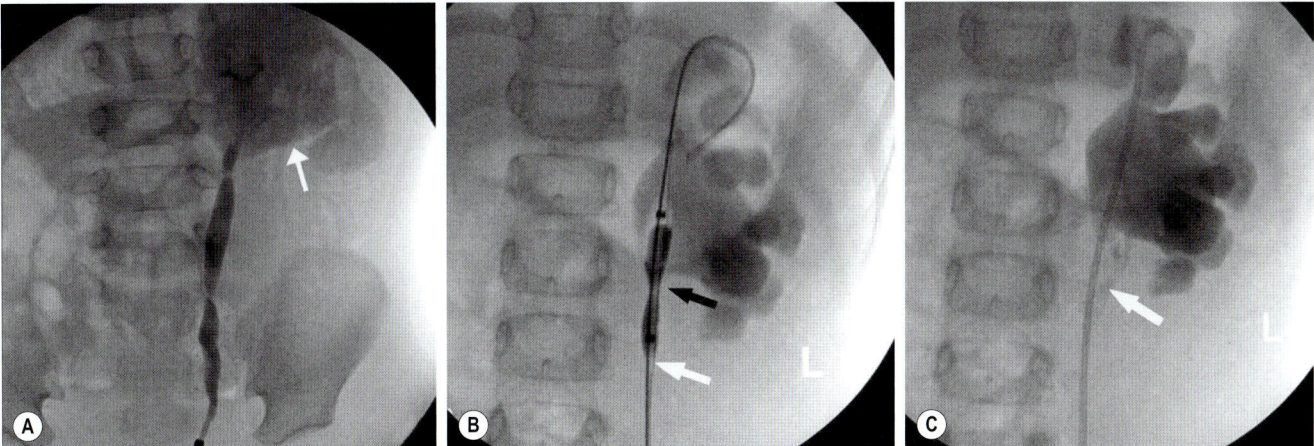

FIGURE 54-8 ■ Retrograde endopyelotomy. Sixteen-month-old infant with persistent hydronephrosis and preserved function, but no washout on renal scan 6 months after undergoing a dismembered pyeloplasty. **(A)** The retrograde pyelogram shows a UPJ configuration with dilute contrast in a dilated renal pelvis (arrow). **(B)** A balloon catheter is passed retrograde and inflated. The black arrow shows the narrowing (waist) and the white arrow demonstrates the cutting wire that is positioned laterally. **(C)** An indwelling stent is positioned after the endopyelotomy is performed. The white arrow points out the extravasation that is indicative of an appropriate depth of incision.

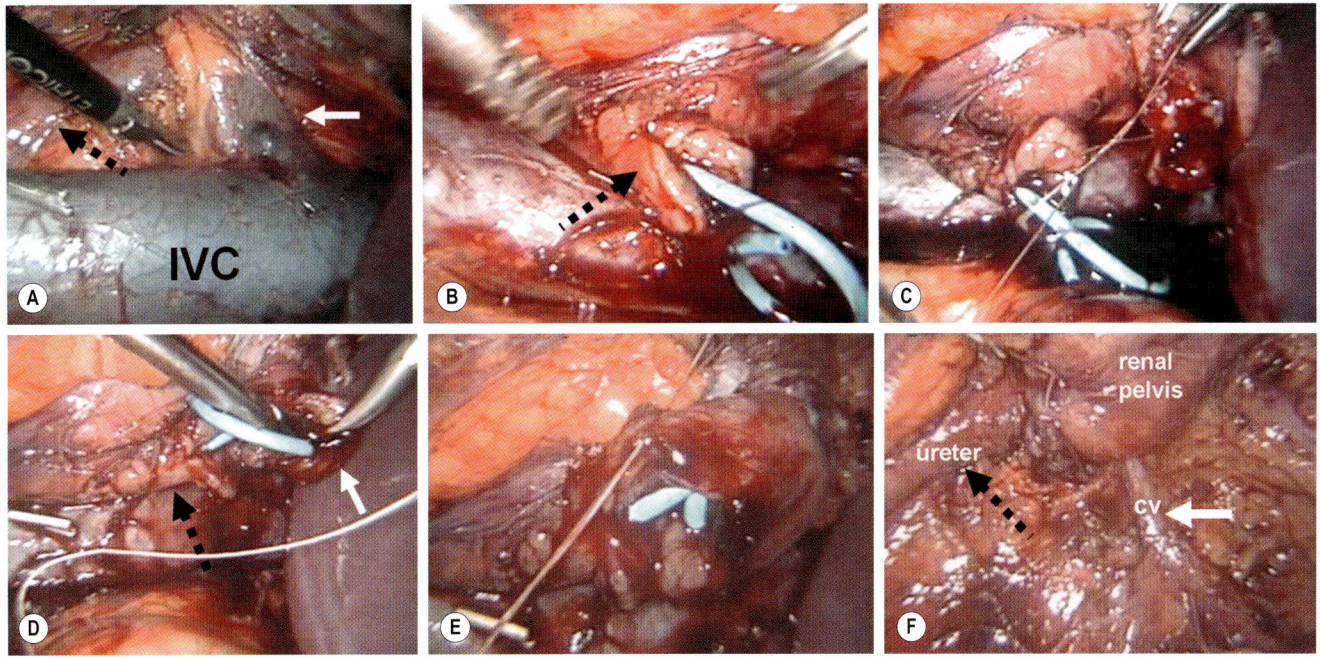

FIGURE 54-9 ■ Laparoscopic pyeloplasty. **(A)** Transperitoneal view of crossing vessel (solid white arrow) that is causing intermittent obstruction of the ureter (dotted black arrow). IVC, inferior vena cava. **(B)** The ureteropelvic junction has been transected and the ureter spatulated (arrow), and a double J stent has been positioned in the bladder and out the proximal ureter. This can be accomplished via a retrograde or antegrade approach. **(C)** The posterior anastomosis between the renal pelvis and ureter is being performed. **(D)** The proximal end of the stent is inserted into the renal pelvis (solid white arrow). The ureter is marked with the dotted black arrow. **(E)** The anterior anastomosis is being performed. **(F)** The completed anastomosis is seen with the crossing vessel (white arrow, CV) now located posterior to the pyeloplasty. Again, the ureter is marked with the dotted black arrow. (Images courtesy of R. Sherburne Figenshau, MD.)

requirements, improved cosmesis, and quicker return to normal activity.[42]

Laparoscopic pyeloplasties are mostly performed using the Anderson–Hynes dismembered technique (Fig. 54-9). This can be performed through either a transperitoneal or retroperitoneal approach using a similar technique once access and exposure are obtained. With both transabdominal and retroperitoneal approaches, the child is placed in a flank or modified flank position.

UPJ Obstruction in a Duplex Kidney

In a duplex kidney, the lower pole is most commonly affected because the upper pole lacks a true pelvis.[44]

Ultrasound may not be reliable for diagnosis because the duplex nature of the kidney may not be identified. A pyelogram or renogram will show a small nonobstructed upper segment.

The anatomy of the duplication dictates the operation. If the ureter is incompletely duplicated and a long lower-pole ureteral segment is found, a standard dismembered pyeloplasty can be performed. If a high bifurcation with a short distal segment is present, then the end of the renal pelvis can be anastomosed to the side of the upper-pole ureter. The appropriate technique can be determined after the kidney and pelvis are exposed.

Surgical Results and Complications

The results of operative correction have been uniformly successful when performed at children's hospitals.[27,30,55] The rate of recurrent UPJ obstruction is less than 1%, and the nephrectomy rate is less than 2%. The most common early complications are prolonged urinary extravasation and delayed drainage through the anastomosis. If a significant leak develops, either a stent or a percutaneous nephrostomy tube can be inserted. Once diversion is instituted, the leak will usually cease within 48 hours. Late scarring at the anastomotic site is common, but rarely occurs due to a leak.

Delayed opening of the anastomosis is seen most commonly when a nephrostomy tube is used. When this occurs, patience is important because 80% of these will open within three months. Secondary obstruction or failure of the primary procedure occurs due to scarring or fibrosis, a nondependent anastomosis, ureteral angulation secondary to renal malrotation, or ureteral narrowing distal to the anastomosis.

A functional assessment of the anastomosis should be obtained two to three months after the operation. Further evaluation is recommended 12 to 24 months after surgery. Problems are uncommon after this time in the absence of symptoms.

URETERAL ABNORMALITIES

Ureteral development begins during the fourth week of gestation when the ureteral bud arises from the mesonephric duct.[45] The bud elongates cephalad, and forms the ureter, renal pelvis, calyces, and collecting tubules. The distal end of the mesonephric duct from the ureteral bud to the vesicourethral tract is called the common excretory duct and expands in trumpet fashion into the bladder and urethra to form half of the trigone. The attachment of the ureter to the mesonephric duct switches from a posterior to an anterolateral location. With expansion and absorption of the common excretory duct into the urinary tract, the orifices of the ureteral bud and mesonephric duct become independent and move away and settle in the bladder and urethra, respectively.

Alterations in bud number, position, and time of development result in anomalies. VUR results from caudal displacement of the ureteral bud, whereas ureteral ectopia and obstruction result from cranial displacement. Renal development and dysplasia are related to the ureteral orifice location.[46]

Ureteral Duplication

Duplication is the most common ureteral anomaly. Both sides are equally affected, and girls are affected twice as often as boys. The autopsy incidence is approximately 1%, but the incidence was 2–4% in clinical series in which pyelograms were obtained for urinary symptoms.[45,46] Many of the duplicated units show congenital dysplasia (scarring) and hydronephrosis. There is an increased incidence of infection because both VUR and obstruction are much more common in duplicated systems.[45]

A partial or complete duplication of the ureter occurs when a single bud branches prematurely or when two ureteral buds arise from the mesonephric duct. A bifid renal pelvis is the highest level of bifurcation and occurs in 10% of the population. Other incomplete duplications occur throughout the ureter (Fig. 54-10). An inverted-Y

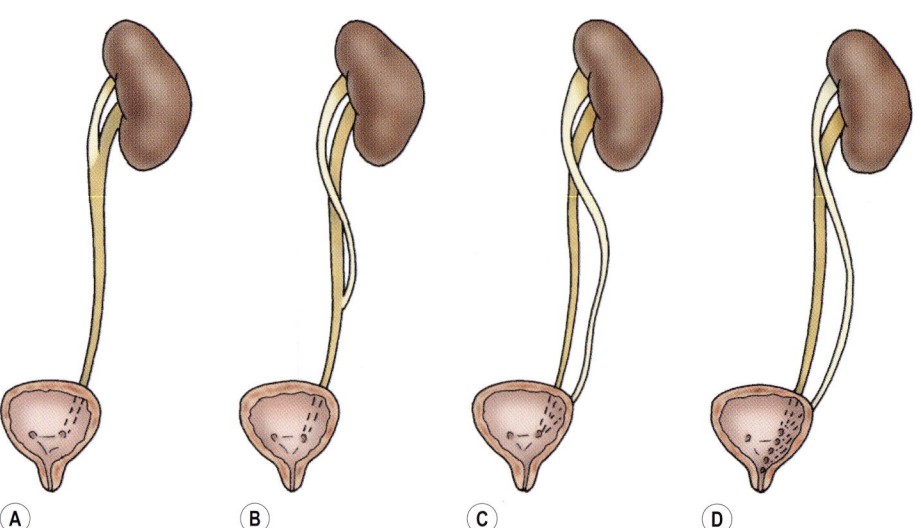

FIGURE 54-10 ■ Types of duplication. **(A)** Bifid pelvis. **(B)** 'Y' ureter. **(C)** 'V' ureter. **(D)** Complete duplication with various ectopic orifices.

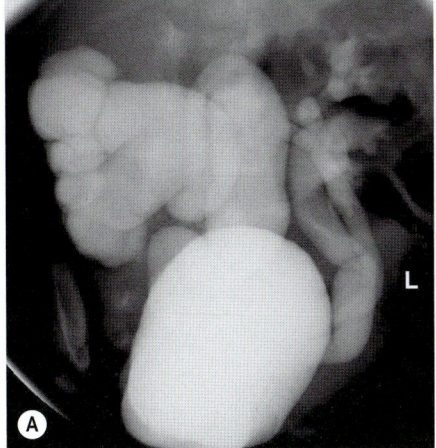
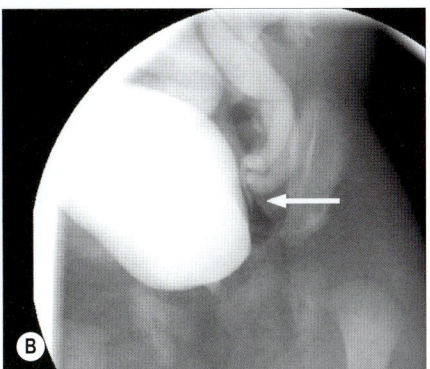

FIGURE 54-11 ■ Ureteral duplication and reflux. **(A)** This VCUG shows massive reflux into the lower pole of a duplex right kidney. There is also reflux into both moieties on the left. **(B)** Lateral oblique views show that the two left ureters join (arrow) just outside the bladder

ureter is the rarest of all branching anomalies.[47] This is presumably the result of separate ureteral buds that fuse before entering the metanephros.

In complete duplications, reflux into the lower renal moiety is the most common cause of renal disease. The more caudal ureteral bud ends up laterally and cranially deviated in the bladder and has a shorter intramural tunnel. The upper-pole ureter enters the bladder adjacent or distal to the lower ureter, as defined by the Weigert–Meyer law.[48] Reflux is identified in up to two-thirds of children with duplicated systems that develop infection.[49] Reflux may occur into the upper-pole ureter if the ureteral orifices are immediately adjacent or if the upper ureter is distally located at the level of the bladder neck without any submucosal support (Fig. 54-11).

The treatment of VUR in duplicated ureters follows the same principles as that in a single system. Initial treatment includes preventive antibiotics and radiographic monitoring. Low grades of VUR are associated with the same rate of spontaneous resolution as a single system. The distal ureters share a common vascular supply so reimplantation involves mobilization and reimplantation of the common sheath.[50] If an associated lower-pole UPJ obstruction is noted, ipsilateral end-to-side pyeloureterostomy is an effective management for both obstruction and reflux.[51] Even if significant scarring is present in the lower pole, reimplantation is usually effective unless major ureteral dilation is present. In the latter case, lower-pole nephroureterectomy may be needed.

Ureteral Triplication

This is one of the rarest anomalies of the upper urinary tract and results from either several ureteral buds or early branching. In most cases, all three ureters drain into a single orifice.[52] Triplication presents with incontinence, infection, and symptoms of obstruction, and is associated with both ectopia and ureteroceles.[53,54] Ureteral quadruplication has also been described.[55]

Retrocaval Ureter

The retrocaval or circumcaval ureter is a right ureter that passes behind the vena cava (Fig. 54-12).[56] This is the result of a developmental error in the formation of the

vena cava. The supracardinal vein (vena cava) lies dorsal to the developing ureter, whereas subcardinal veins lie ventral to the ureter. If the subcardinal vein persists as the vena cava, the ureter passes behind the vena cava and anterior to the iliac vein. If both veins persist, the ureter passes between the duplicated vena cava.[57]

Symptoms are related to chronic ureteral obstruction and infection, and rarely occur in children.[58] The radiographic appearance depends on the level of obstruction. The more common distal obstruction appears as a 'reversed J' on intravenous pyelogram. Less commonly, the ureter crosses at the level of the UPJ. Both of these can be confused with UPJ obstruction and should be suspected when pyelectasis and dilation of the upper third of the ureter are seen.

Treatment is required only when significant obstruction or symptoms are present. Reconstruction is essentially a dismembered ureteroplasty with division of the ureter and anastomosis anterior to the vena cava. The other option is division and reconstruction of the vena cava, which is more problematic.

Megaureter

Megaureter is not a diagnosis, but a descriptive term for a dilated ureter. Normal ureteral diameter in children is rarely greater than 5 mm. Ureters greater than 7 mm are

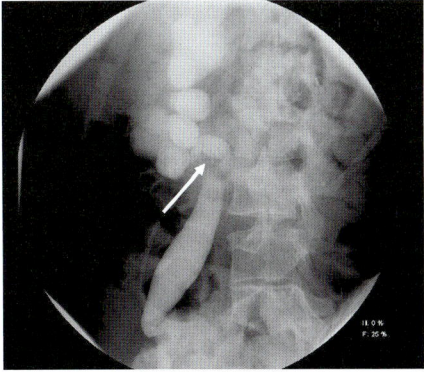

FIGURE 54-12 ■ Retrocaval ureter. A retrograde pyelogram shows reverse J-hooking of the ureter (arrow) as it passes behind the inferior vena cava. Note that the ureteral caliber is the same proximally and distally which indicates no obstruction.

considered megaureters.[59] The ultrasound appearance of the dilated and tortuous ureter is usually striking (Fig. 54-13). Pelvicalyceal dilation and parenchymal scarring or thinning depend on the primary disease process. Megaureter is the second most common urinary tract abnormality detected prenatally.[2] Infection and intermittent abdominal pain can also be presenting symptoms.[60]

Primary obstructive megaureter is most commonly caused by a distal adynamic ureteral segment, but ureteral valves[60] and ectopic ureteral insertion can also cause obstruction. Proximal smooth muscle hypertrophy and hyperplasia are seen. A normal caliber catheter will usually pass through the distal 3–4 mm segment, but the peristaltic wave does not propel urine across this area. This absent peristalsis is not a result of a ganglionic abnormality as seen in megacolon.[61] The distal ureter may exhibit a variety of histologic abnormalities, but the common finding is a disruption of muscular continuity that prevents propulsion of urine.[11,62]

These anomalies can be classified as nonobstructed, refluxing, and obstructed.[60] Some ureters also have reflux and simultaneous obstruction. Standard imaging allows classification and appropriate management. The diagnosis of a nonobstructed, nonrefluxing megaureter is one of exclusion and is made only when the secondary causes of megaureter have been excluded and diagnostic tests do not show obstruction. Box 54-1 gives clinical examples of each classification. Any normal ureter will dilate if the volume of urine exceeds emptying capacity. Moreover, bacterial endotoxins and infection alone can cause dilation that will resolve after treatment of the infection.[63,64]

Ultrasound almost always distinguishes megaureters from UPJ obstruction. The degree of distal ureteral dilation is often much more pronounced than the degree of renal pelvic dilation or caliectasis. A VCUG should be obtained in all patients. If significant reflux is found, delayed drainage films must be obtained to exclude simultaneous obstruction with a normal caliber distal ureteral segment. In a partially obstructed system, the contrast density in the ureter is decreased because of dilution related to stasis in the ureter (see Fig. 54-13).

Diuretic renography is used to assess function and drainage. The markedly dilated ureter can be a significant

---

BOX 54-1   Classification of Megaureter

REFLUXING MEGAURETER

   Primary (congenital reflux)
   Secondary (urethral valves, neurogenic bladder)

OBSTRUCTED MEGAURETER

   Primary (adynamic segment)
   Secondary (urethral obstruction, extrinsic mass, or tumor)

NONREFLUXING, NONOBSTRUCTED MEGAURETER

   Primary (idiopathic, physiologically insignificant adynamic segment)
   Secondary (polyuria, infection, postoperative residual dilation)

Modified from Khoury A, Bagli DJ. Reflux and megaureter. In: Wein AJ, Kavoussi LR, Novick AC, et al, editors. Campbell-Walsh Urology. 9th ed. Philadelphia: WB Saunders; 2007. p. 3468.

---

source of stasis, and determination of drainage half-time can be difficult. Diuretic administration must be delayed because the system is so capacious and may take 60 to 90 minutes to fill.

Treatment

Nonoperative management is based on clearance half-time and relative renal function of the hydronephrotic and contralateral kidneys. If observation is chosen, suppressive antibiotics are recommended and the child is followed with serial ultrasound and/or renal scans. Neonatal megaureter with obstruction found by renography, but with preserved function can be safely observed. Most ureters will become radiographically normal over time.[65–68] Operative correction for decreasing function or recurring infections will be needed in only 10–25% of patients by age 7 years. Evidence of delayed obstruction after normalization of radiographs has not been seen in these children.

Ureteral tapering with preservation of the ureteral blood supply was popularized in the early 1970s.[69] A longitudinal segment of ureter is excised and then closed

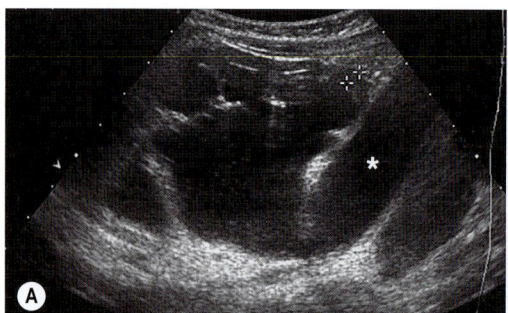
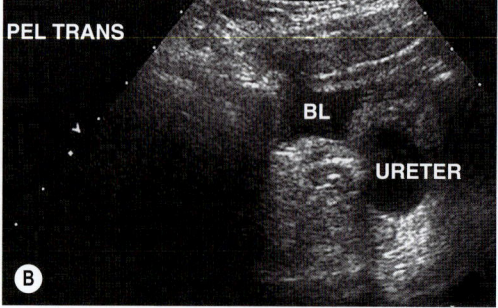
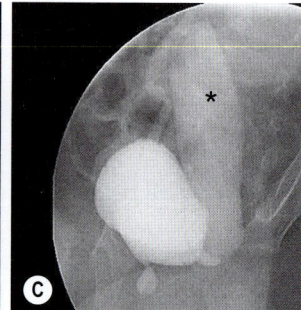

FIGURE 54-13 ■ This patient has congenital megaureter. **(A)** Renal ultrasound image shows diffuse caliectasis and cortical thinning with a markedly dilated left ureter (asterisk). **(B)** Ultrasound image of the bladder confirms the markedly dilated ureter adjacent to the bladder (BL). A MAG-3 scan was performed and showed preserved renal function on the left side. **(C)** The voiding cystourethrogram shows reflux into the markedly dilated left ureter (asterisk). Note that the contrast agent in the ureter is diluted (compared with the bladder), which is indicative of partial obstruction on that side.

over a 10–12 French catheter. When the ureter is tunneled submucosally, the suture line is positioned against the detrusor to decrease the chance of fistula. Initial repairs involved tailoring the entire ureter, but this was found to be unnecessary because the upper ureteral tortuosity and dilatation often disappears after tapering the distal ureter.[70] Ureteral folding techniques have been popularized because they theoretically decrease the risk of ischemic injury while achieving the decreased intraluminal diameter necessary for a successful reimplant.[71,72] However, the increased bulk is technically a problem in infant bladders. Although dissection is usually both intravesical and extravesical, extravesical reimplants alone have been described and may have lower morbidity.[73] A vesicopsoas hitch is a useful adjunct that helps achieve a longer submucosal tunnel length without risking ureteral kinking, although excisional tailoring usually eliminates this need. A nonrefluxing, nonobstructed reimplantation can be achieved in most patients with megaureters.[72,74] Recognized complications include persistent obstruction, reflux, and urinary extravasation. Most of these can be managed nonoperatively with drainage. Lower grades of postoperative VUR will often resolve.

When indicated, primary reconstruction is preferred, but temporary cutaneous diversion may be beneficial in a neonate or infant in whom the chance of successful reimplantation of a bulky ureter into a small bladder is diminished. Diversion may decrease the ureteral diameter and decrease the need for tailoring at the time of reimplantation. An end-cutaneous ureterostomy is preferred because a high diversion may require two or more procedures for correction.

Balloon dilation and stenting have been described in older children (mean 3 years) with a success rate greater than 95%.[75,76] This approach should definitely be considered in older children because of the marked decrease in morbidity associated with a completely endoscopic approach.

Ectopic Ureter

An ectopic ureter is defined as one that does not drain on the trigone, but at the bladder neck or more caudally. Embryologically, this results from a cranial insertion of the ureteral bud on the mesonephric duct that allows distal migration with the mesonephric duct as it is absorbed into the urogenital sinus.[77]

The incidence of ureteral ectopia is approximately 1 in 2000.[46] Eighty per cent of ectopic ureters are reported in association with a duplicated renal system. As clinical problems are more common in girls with ectopia, only 15% of ectopic ureters have been reported in boys.[46,77] Ectopia is bilateral 20% of the time.[46] Single ectopic ureters are rare but are more common in boys.[78]

Ectopic Ureter in Girls

The fundamental difference between ureteral ectopia in boys and girls arises from ureteral insertion distal to the continence mechanism in girls (Fig. 54-14). Approximately one-third of ureters open at the level of the bladder neck, one third are in the vestibule around the

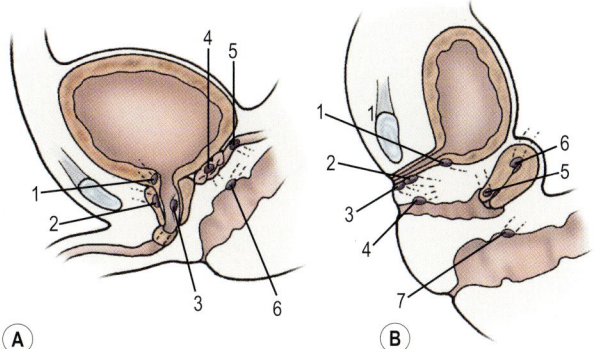

FIGURE 54-14 ■ **(A)** Ureteral ectopia in a boy. Possible sites are above the external sphincter (1–3), or into the seminal vesicle (4,5), or anorectal (6). **(B)** Ureteral ectopia in a girl may be located at the bladder neck (1), or beyond the continence mechanism in the urethra (2), or on the perineum (3). Uterine or vaginal insertion (4–6) may also cause incontinence. Anorectal insertion (7) can also occur.

urethral opening, and the remainder empty into the vagina, uterus, or cervix. All of these insertions are along the course of the mesonephric duct remnant (Gartner's duct).

Fifty per cent of affected girls initially have continuous urinary incontinence despite what appears to be a normal voiding pattern.[46,77] If the system is markedly hydronephrotic and functions poorly, urine leakage may occur only in the upright position and may be confused with stress incontinence. Persistent foul-smelling vaginal discharge can suggest an ectopic ureter. When the ectopic ureter is present in the urethra or the bladder neck, both obstruction and reflux are frequently found.

The diagnosis of an ectopic ureter may be obvious or can be difficult. When the distal end exits in the vagina, cervix or uterus, the kidney may not visualize on ultrasound if the renal moiety is small and atrophic, and not associated with hydronephrosis. Often significant hydronephrosis is found in the upper pole of a duplicated system and the ultrasound image may show a dilated ectopic ureter behind the bladder. However, the upper pole may also be a small remnant (Fig. 54-15). A scan using dimercaptosuccinic acid (DMSA) is a good test for localizing a small ectopic kidney when an orthotopic kidney is not identified on standard imaging and there is a high suspicion of an ectopic ureter in the vagina, cervix or uterus. As long as there is some dilation, MRU may be the most precise method for making this diagnosis.[79] A VCUG should be obtained to exclude occult reflux.[80]

The diagnosis is confirmed with physical examination, panendoscopy, and retrograde pyelography. Dyes that stain urine may have a role. Urine in the bladder changes color, whereas the poorly concentrated urine is evident as persistent clear leakage. Meticulous examination of the area around the urethral meatus and vagina will often reveal an asymmetry or bead of fluid coming from an opening that can be probed and injected in retrograde fashion (see Fig. 54-15). Vaginoscopy with attention to the superior lateral aspect of the vagina may reveal a large ectopic orifice.

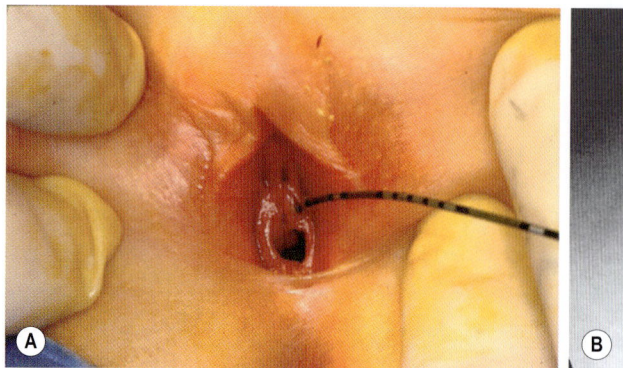
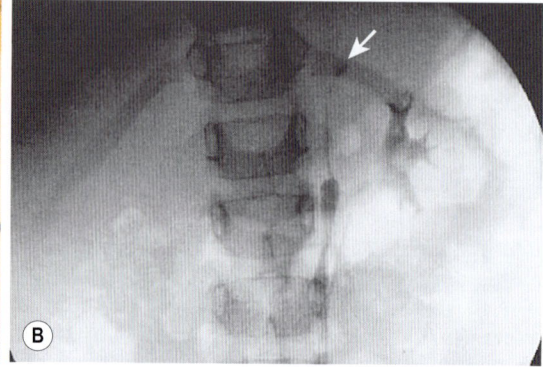

FIGURE 54-15 ■ This 3-year-old girl had continuous urinary incontinence despite a normal voiding pattern. The renal ultrasound image was essentially normal on both sides with no evidence of hydronephrosis or an echogenic upper pole. **(A)** A ureteral catheter has been inserted into an ectopic left ureter. **(B)** The retrograde ureterogram shows a very small upper left ureter and a small cystic calyx (arrow) in the left upper pole medial to the lower-pole collecting system that was opacified through an orifice on the trigone. The patient was continent after a laparoscopic left upper pole partial nephroureterectomy.

Ectopic Ureter in Boys

The most common sites of ectopic ureteral insertion in boys are the posterior urethra (40–50%) and the seminal vesicle (20–60%), depending on the age at presentation.[81] Symptoms in boys may not occur until after the onset of sexual activity and include prostatitis, seminal vesiculitis, or an infected seminal vesical cyst causing painful bowel movements. The genital insertion accounts for the common presentation with epididymitis. He may have postvoid dribbling secondary to pooling of urine in the prostatic urethra, but incontinence is never as pronounced as in a female.

Ectopic ureters in the boy are more commonly obstructed and hydronephrotic so ultrasound is often more useful. If the ectopic insertion site is outside the urethra, it is rarely identified on endoscopy.

Management of Ectopic Ureters

Operative treatment is dependent on the associated renal parenchyma.[82,83] Single-system ectopic ureters that enter the genital system usually have poor function, and nephroureterectomy is appropriate. When the ectopic ureter is associated with duplication, the function in the upper pole is usually poor, and an open or laparoscopic partial nephroureterectomy has historically been the most common approach. The distal ureter can be left open. A ureteroureterostomy can be performed proximally or distally as well. The dilated upper pole is diverted into the normal caliber lower pole system. There are potential concerns regarding the size discrepancy of the ureters and injury to the recipient ureter, but large series show excellent success with a very low complication rate.[84] This approach avoids potential injury to the lower pole of the kidney and can be performed through a small inguinal incision[85] or laparoscopically.[86] The obstruction, dilation, and incontinence usually resolve following ureteroureterostomy. Even if the upper pole is poorly functioning, it should not cause significant long-term problems. A common sheath ureteral reimplantation can be performed with tailoring of the ureter in the upper pole, but the increased morbidity and complication rate associated with ureteral tapering limit the utility of this approach.

The distal ureteral stump rarely causes a problem in genital ectopia. However, if urethral or bladder neck insertion of the ectopic ureter and reflux into the ureter is identified preoperatively, excision of the distal stump is important, but can be tedious.[83] If the plane of dissection is kept immediately adjacent to the ureter behind the bladder, the bladder neck and sphincter should not be damaged. A transvesical approach can also be useful and aids in exposure of the urethral insertion. In a postpubertal girl, access to the urethra can be performed transvaginally as well.

Bilateral Single Ectopic Ureters

This is a rare finding in which the altered ureteral embryologic development is associated with failure of normal bladder neck development.[87] Genital and anal anomalies are commonly present. In girls, the ureter inserts into the distal urethra. They are usually initially seen with infection or are noted to have continuous urinary leakage. The bladder is usually poorly developed because it has never stored urine. Boys have somewhat larger bladders because some urine will have entered it. However, because the bladder neck is not formed normally, they also have some degree of urinary incontinence.

The child who is incontinent with bilateral single ectopic ureters presents a major reconstructive challenge that may require ureteral reimplantation, bladder neck reconstruction, and bladder augmentation if the bladder capacity is insufficient.

URETEROCELES

Ureteroceles are cystic dilatations of the terminal, intravesical ureter that usually have a stenotic orifice.[46] In children, ureteroceles are most commonly associated with the upper pole of a duplex system (80%) and an ectopic orifice (60%) in the urethra. In adults, they are usually part of a completely intravesical single system. Ureteroceles occur four to seven times more frequently in girls and are more common in whites. Bilateral ureteroceles are found 10% of the time.

A single embryologic theory does not explain all ureteroceles. Historically, a persistent membrane (Chwalla's) at the junction of the Wolffian duct and urogenital sinus was theorized to cause a ureterocele.[88] It is more likely that a ureterocele is the result of an abnormal induction of the trigone and distal ureter by many of the genes and growth factors that are important in renal and ureteral growth and development. Gross inspection of the intravesical portion of ureteroceles shows deficiencies in the trigonal musculature of patients with ureteroceles that are not present in in ectopic ureters without ureterocele formation. This results in a pseudodiverticulum (ureterocele eversion) and reflux into laterally displaced, poorly supported ureters. This is further supported by the clinical observation of multicystic dysplasia and the absence of hydronephrosis in association with a ureterocele.[89]

The classification of ureteroceles can be confusing. The current recommended nomenclature classifies ureteroceles as either intravesical (entirely within the bladder) or ectopic (some portion is situated permanently at the bladder neck or in the urethra).[90]

Presentation and Diagnosis

Most ureteroceles are identified prenatally although 10–15% still present postnatally due to infection.[91–93] The obstructed renal unit may be palpable, but most have no clinically apparent abnormality. Bladder outlet obstruction is rare because most ureteroceles decompress during micturition, but the most common cause of urethral obstruction in girls is urethral prolapse of a ureterocele (Fig. 54-16).

Abdominal ultrasound reveals a well-defined cystic intravesical mass that is associated within the posterior bladder wall (Fig. 54-17). This can be followed to a dilated ureter in the pelvis and to upper-pole hydroureteronephrosis in a duplicated system. The thickness and echogenicity of the renal parenchyma are often consistent with dysplasia and poor function. A VCUG typically shows ipsilateral lower pole or contralateral reflux.[94]

During cystoscopy, the bladder should be examined when it is full and also completely empty because compressible ureteroceles may not be evident in a full bladder or may appear as a bladder diverticulum. The dilated lower end of an ectopic ureter or megaureter may

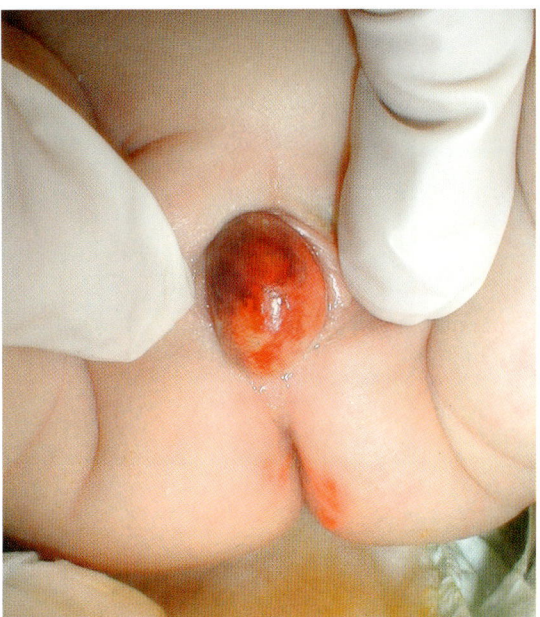

FIGURE 54-16 ■ This 2-week-old baby presented with sepsis and was found to have this prolapsing ectopic ureterocele. The ureterocele was aspirated with return of purulent debris and underwent prompt decompression. Recovery was uneventful.

elevate the trigone, creating the cystoscopic, radiographic, and ultrasound appearance of a ureterocele, a so-called pseudoureterocele.[95]

Treatment

The goals for ureterocele management include control of infection, preservation of renal function, protection of normal ipsilateral and contralateral units, and continence. There is a subset of ureteroceles associated with multicystic dysplasia, no hydroureter, and no reflux. The multicystic moiety usually involutes and the ureterocele rarely causes symptoms and can be observed.[89] Up to 10–15% of prenatally identified ureteroceles have these clinical findings. Neonates given suppressive antibiotics rarely develop a febrile UTI.[92,93] If significant hydroureteronephrosis is found, it is assumed that there is significant urinary tract obstruction and antibiotics should be initiated.

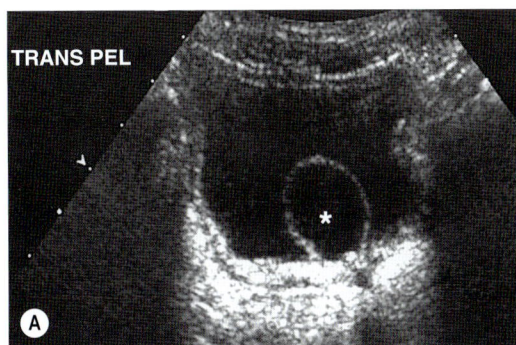
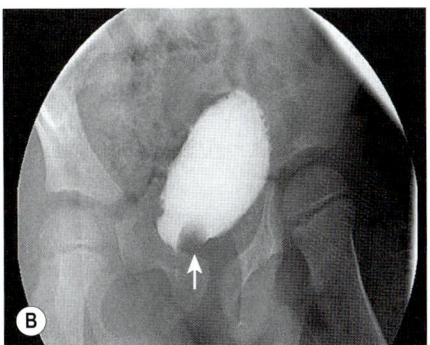

FIGURE 54-17 ■ **(A)** Ultrasound image of the bladder demonstrates a ureterocele (asterisk). **(B)** The ureterocele appears as a nonopacified filling defect (arrow) at the base of the bladder on the cystogram.

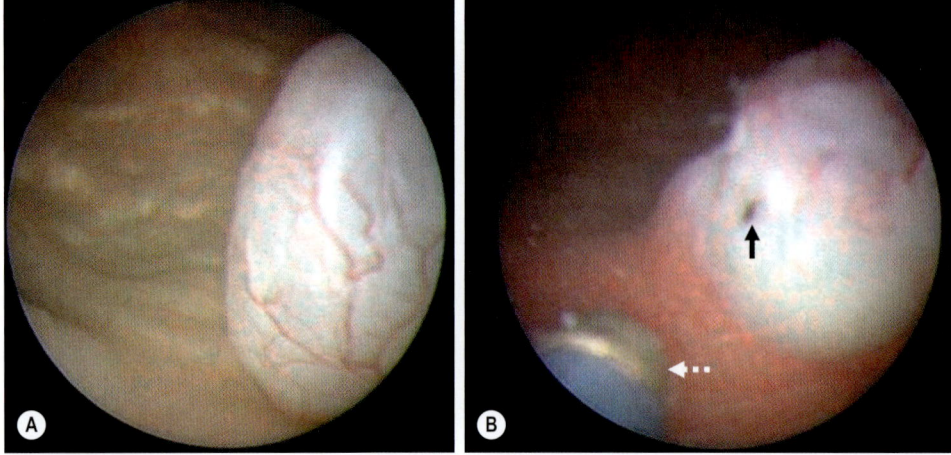

FIGURE 54-18 ■ **(A)** This intravesical ureterocele was found at cystoscopy. **(B)** The ureterocele was punctured (black arrow) and decompressed using a 3 French electrode (white arrow).

The usual treatment of duplex ectopic ureteroceles has been upper-pole heminephrectomy through a separate flank incision, ureterocele excision, and ipsilateral lower-pole ureteral reimplant via a lower incision. The bladder-level operation may require repair of a sizable defect in the bladder base and tapering or plication of the lower ureter. The distal extent of the ureterocele can often be dissected through the bladder neck. Incomplete excision may result in an obstructing urethral flap. Also, resection of the entire ureterocele risks damaging the continence mechanisms of the bladder neck. Experienced surgeons report excellent results with low rates of reoperation (<10%) and low complication rates (<10%).[96–98] These approaches assume that ureterocele excision is an essential component of management. However, because the distal ureter and bladder defect may not cause symptoms after decompression, an absolute indication to proceed with a simultaneous bladder operation is rarely present. In older children, when absence of function is noted on the affected side (upper and lower pole), nephroureterectomy is the preferred option.

Another option is upper-pole partial nephroureterectomy that avoids bladder-level reconstruction and its potential risks.[91,99] Nearly all of the ureter can be removed either through a flank incision or laparoscopically. The need for subsequent bladder-level excision and reconstruction varies between 10–62%, and is largely dependent on the presence of reflux.[91,93,99]

Most partial nephrectomy specimens show dysplasia, but some show only inflammatory and obstructive changes.[99,100] In patients with preserved function, a pyeloureterostomy or ureteroureterostomy (high or low) may be performed, along with distal ureterectomy and ureterocele decompression.[82]

Ureterocele incision is the least invasive technique for upper pole preservation (Fig. 54-18). Using a 3 French Bugbee electrode to incise the ureterocele just above the bladder neck is the recommended approach because reflux does not always develop (see Fig. 54-18).[92] Endoscopic incision successfully decompresses the ureterocele most of the time.[92,100–103] It is the definitive procedure in more than 90% of infants with intravesical ureteroceles.

However, subsequent reconstructive surgery may be needed in 50–90% of patients with ectopic ureteroceles. Reflux into the ureterocele moiety is the most common indication for reconstruction in these infants. Previous decompression of the system makes this reconstruction easier.[93] For an infected system, 'unroofing' of the ureterocele is advocated only as an initial drainage procedure prior to the definitive operation because it invariably results in reflux.[103,104]

Ureterocele incision should probably be the initial procedure in most neonates because reflux into the lower-pole moiety is usually present (>50%). Even when ultrasound shows little renal parenchyma in the upper pole of a duplex system, incision can be performed. The decompressed system may not require further treatment if iatrogenic upper-pole reflux does not develop. In older children, incision is the preferred option when functioning renal parenchyma is found, the ureterocele is intravesical, or the kidney is drained by a single system.

Single-system ureteroceles are more commonly seen in older children and adults, and are associated with better function and less hydronephrosis than is found in duplex kidneys. Most often, they are incidental findings that do not require treatment. Antenatally detected single-system ureteroceles may not show significant obstruction on a furosemide washout renal scan. Clinically, these behave like nonobstructed megaureters and can be safely followed with preventive antibiotics. If treatment is required, endoscopic incision is effective most of the time.

REFERENCES

1. Dicke JM, Blanco VM, Yan Y, et al. The type and frequency of fetal renal disorders and management of renal pelvis dilation. J Ultrasound Med 2006;25:973–7.
2. Lee RS, Cendron M, Kinnamon DD, et al. Antenatal hydronephrosis as a predictor of postnatal outcome: A meta-analysis. Pediatrics 2006;118:586–93.
3. Hubert KC, Palmer JS. Current diagnosis and management of fetal genitourinary abnormalities. Urol Clin North Am 2007;34:89–101.
4. Capello SA, Kogan BA, Giorgi LJ, et al. Prenatal ultrasound has led to earlier detection and repair of ureteropelvic junction obstruction. J Urol 2005;174:1425–8.

5. Carr MC, El-Ghoneimi A. Anomalies and surgery of the uretero-pelvic junction in children. In: Wein AJ, Kavoussi LR, Novick AC, editors. Campbell-Walsh Urology. 9th ed. Philadelphia: WB Saunders; 2007. p. 3359–82.

6. Ruano-Gil D, Coca-Payeras A, Tejedo-Mateu A. Obstruction and normal recanalization of the ureter in the human embryo: Its relation to congenital ureteric obstruction. Eur Urol 1975;1: 287–93.

7. Arams HJ, Buchbinder ME, Sutton AP. Benign ureteral lesions: Rare causes of hydronephrosis in children. Urology 1977;9: 517–20.

8. Stephens FD. Ureterovascular hydronephrosis and the 'aberrant' renal vessels. J Urol 1982;128:984–7.

9. Koff SA, Hayden LJ, Cirulli C, et al. Pathophysiology of UPJ obstruction: Experimental and clinical observations. J Urol 1986; 136:336–8.

10. Starr NT, Maizels M, Chou P, et al. Microanatomy and mor-phometry of the hydronephrotic 'obstructed' renal pelvis in asymptomatic infants. J Urol 1992;148:519–24.

11. Hanna MK, Jeffs RD, Sturgess JM, et al. Ureteral structure and ultrastructure: II. Congenital UPJ obstruction and primary obstructive megaureter. J Urol 1976;116:725–30.

12. Kjurhuus JC, Nerstrom B, Gyrd-Hansen N, et al. Experimental hydronephrosis: An electrophysiologic investigation before and after release of obstruction. Acta Chir Scand Suppl 1976;472:1728.

13. Wang Y, Puri P, Hassan J, et al. Abnormal innervation and altered nerve growth factor messenger ribonucleic acid expression in ure-teropelvic junction obstruction. J Urol 1995;154:679–83.

14. Hollowell JG, Altman HG, Snyder HM III, et al. Coexisting UPJ obstruction and vesicoureteral reflux: Diagnostic and therapeutic implications. J Urol 1989;142:490–3.

15. Coplen DE, Austin PF, Yan Y, et al. Correlation of prenatal and postnatal ultrasound findings with the incidence of vesicoureteral reflux in children with fetal renal pelvic dilatation. J Urol 2008;180:1631–4.

16. Nguyen HT, Herndon CD, Cooper C, et al. The Society for Fetal Urology consensus statement on the evaluation and management of antenatal hydronephrosis. Journal of Pediatric Urology 2010;6:212–31.

17. Islek A, Güven AG, Koyun M, et al. Probability of urinary tract infection in infants with ureteropelvic junction obstruction: Is antibiotic prophylaxis really needed? Pediatric Nephrology 2011;(26):1837–41.

18. Heyman S, Duckett JW. Extraction factor: An estimate of single kidney function in children during routine radionucleotide renog-raphy with 99m technetium diethylenetriamine pentaacetic acid. J Urol 1988;140:780–3.

19. Chung S, Majd M, Rushton HG, et al. Diuretic renography in the evaluation of neonatal hydronephrosis: Is it reliable? J Urol 1993;150:765–8.

20. Conway JJ. 'Well-tempered' diuresis renography: Its historical development, physiological and technical pitfalls and standardized technique protocol. Semin Nucl Med 1992;22:74–84.

21. Grattan-Smith JD, Little SB, Jones RA. MR urography evaluation of obstructive uropathy. Pediatric Radiology 2008;38(Suppl 1): S49–69.

22. Veenboer PW, de Jong TP. Antegrade pressure measurement as a tool in modern pediatric urology. World J Urol 2011;29:737–41.

23. Rushton HG. Pediatric pyeloplasty: Is routine retrograde pyelog-raphy necessary? J Urol 1994;152:604–6.

24. Palmer LS, Maizels M, Cartwright PC, et al. Surgery versus observation for managing obstructive grade 3 to 4 unilateral hydronephrosis: A report from the Society for Fetal Urology. J Urol 1988;159:222–8.

25. Ulman I, Jayanthi VR, Koff SA. The long-term follow-up of newborns with severe unilateral hydronephrosis initially treated nonoperatively. J Urol 2000;164:1101–5.

26. Yiee J, Wilcox D. Management of fetal hydronephrosis. Pediatr Nephrol 2008;23:347–53.

27. Cartwright PC, Duckett JW, Keating MA, et al. managing appar-ent ureteropelvic junction obstruction in the newborn. J Urol 1992;148:122–4.

28. Foley FE. A new plastic operation for stricture at the UPJ: Report of 20 cases. J Urol 1937;38:643.

29. Culp OS, DeWeerd JH. Pelvic flap operation for certain types of ureteropelvic obstruction. Mayo Clin Proc 1951;26:483–8.

30. Austin PF, Cain MP, Rink RC. Nephrostomy tube drainage with pyeloplasty: Is it necessarily a bad choice? J Urol 2001;57: 338–41.

31. Casale P, Mucksavage P, Resnick M, et al. Robotic ureterocalicos-tomy in the pediatric population. J Urol 2008;180-2643-8.

32. Tanaka ST, Grantham JA, Thomas JC, et al. A comparison of open vs. laparoscopic pediatric pyeloplasty using the pediatric health information system database-do benefits of laparoscopic approach recede at younger ages. Journal of Urology 2008;180:1479–85.

33. Duckett JW, Gibbons MD, Cromie WJ. An anterior extraperito-neal muscle-splitting approach for pediatric renal surgery. J Urol 1980;123:79–80.

34. Orland SM, Snyder HM, Duckett JW. The dorsal lumbotomy incision in pediatric urological surgery. J Urol 1987;138:963–6.

35. Lindgren BW, Hagerty J, Meyer T, et al. Robot-Assisted laparo-scopic reoperative repair for failed pyeloplasty in children: Safe and highly effective treatment option. J Urology 2012;188: 932–8.

36. Nakada SY, Johnson M. Ureteropelvic junction obstruction: Retrograde endopyelotomy. Urol Clin North Am 2000;27: 677–84.

37. Streem SB. Percutaneous endopyelotomy. Urol Clin North Am 2000;27:685–93.

38. Kim EH, Tanagho YS, Traxel EJ, et al. Endopyelotomy for pedi-atric ureteropelvic junction obstruction. A review of our 25-year experience. J Urol 2012;188: in press October 2012.

39. Peters CA, Schlussel RN, Retik AB. Pediatric laparoscopic dis-membered pyeloplasty. J Urol 1995;153:1962–5.

40. Tan HL. Laparoscopic Anderson-Hynes dismembered pyelo-plasty in children. J Urol 1999;162:1045–8.

41. Cascio S, Tien A, Chee W. Laparoscopic dismembered pyelo-plasty in children younger than 2 years. J Urol 2007;177:335–8.

42. Minnillo BJ, Cruz JA, Sayao RH, et al. Long-term experience and outcomes of robotic assisted laparoscopic pyeloplasty in children and young adults. J Urology 2011;185:1455–60.

43. Lam PN, Wong C, Mulholland TL, et al. Pediatric laparoscopic pyeloplasty: 4-year experience. J Endourol 2007;21:1467–71.

44. Ossandon F, Androulakakis P, Ransley PG. Surgical problems in pelviureteric junction obstruction of the lower pole moiety in incomplete duplex systems. J Urol 1981;125:871–2.

45. Mackie GG, Awang H, Stephens FD. The ureteric orifice: The embryologic key to radiologic status of the kidneys. J Pediatr Surg 1975;10:473–81.

46. Schlussel RN, Retik AB. Ectopic ureter, ureterocele and other anomalies of the ureter. In: Wein AJ, Kavoussi LR, Novick AC, et al, editors. Campbell-Walsh Urology. 9th ed. Philadelphia: WB Saunders; 2007. p. 3383–7.

47. Klauber GT, Reid EC. Inverted Y reduplication of the ureter. J Urol 1972;107:362–4.

48. Meyer R. Normal and abnormal development of the ureter in the human embryo: A mechanistic consideration. Anat Rec 1946; 96:355.

49. Fehrenbaker LG, Kelalis PP, Stickler GB. Vesicoureteral reflux and ureteral duplication in children. J Urol 1972;107:862–4.

50. Barrett DM, Malek RS, Kelalis PP. Problems and solutions in surgical treatment of 100 consecutive ureteral duplications in chil-dren. J Urol 1975;114:126–30.

51. Shelfo SW, Keller MS, Weiss RM. Ipsilateral pyeloureterostomy for managing lower-pole reflux with associated ureteropelvic junc-tion obstruction in duplex systems. J Urol 1997;157:1420–2.

52. Kohri K, Nagai N, Kaneko S, et al. Bilateral trifid ureters associ-ated with fused kidney, ureterovesical stenosis, left cryptorchidism and angioma of the bladder. J Urol 1978;120:249–50.

53. Zaontz MR, Maizels M. Type I ureteral triplication: An extension of the Weigert-Meyer law. J Urol 1985;134:949–50.

54. Finkel LI, Watts FB, Cobrett DP. Ureteral triplication with a ureterocele. Pediatr Radiol 1983;13:346–8.

55. Soderdahl DW, Shiraki IW, Schamber DT. Bilateral ureteral quadruplication. J Urol 1976;116:255–6.

56. Considine J. Retrocaval ureter. Br J Urol 1966;38:412–23.

57. Hollinshead WH. Anatomy for Surgeons, vol 2. 3rd ed. Philadel-phia: Harper & Row; 1982.

58. Zhang XD, Hou SK, Zhu JH, et al. Diagnosis and treatment of retrocaval ureter. Eur Urol 1990;18:207–10.

59. Hellstrom M, Hjalmas K, Jacobsson B, et al. Normal ureteral diameter in infancy and childhood. Acta Radiol 1985;26:433–9.

60. Khoury AE, Bagli DJ. Reflux and megaureter. In: Kavoussi LR, Novick AC, Partin AW, et al, editors. Campbell-Walsh Urology. 9th ed. Philadelphia: WB Saunders; 2007. p. 3423–81.

61. Leibowitz S, Bodian M. A study of the vesical ganglia in children and their relationship to the megaureter megacystis syndrome and Hirschsprung's disease. J Clin Pathol 1963;16:342–50.

62. Tanagho EA. Embryologic basis for lower ureteral anomalies: A hypothesis. Urology 1976;7:451–64.

63. Boyd SD, Raz S, Ehrlich RM. Diabetes insipidus and nonobstructive dilation of urinary tract. Urology 1980;16:266–9.

64. Kass EJ, Silver TM, Konnak JW, et al. The urographic findings in acute pyelonephritis: Non-obstructive hydronephrosis. J Urol 1976;116:544–6.

65. Mollard P, Foray P, De Godoy JL, et al. Management of primary obstructive megaureter without reflux in neonates. Eur Urol 1993;24:505–10.

66. Cozzi F, Madonna L, Maggi E, et al. Management of primary megaureter in infancy. J Pediatr Surg 1993;28:1031–3.

67. Keating MA, Escala J, Snyder HM, et al. Changing concepts in management of primary obstructive megaureter. J Urol 1989;142:636–40.

68. Baskin LS, Zderic SA, Snyder HM, et al. Primary dilated megaureter: Long-term follow-up. J Urol 1994;152:618–21.

69. Hendren WH. Operative repair of megaureter in children. J Urol 1969;101:491–507.

70. Hendren WH. Commentary: Surgery of megaureter. In: Whitehead D, Leiter E, editors. Current Operative Urology. Philadelphia: Harper & Row; 1984. p. 473–82.

71. Fretz PC, Austin JC, Cooper CS. Long-term outcome analysis of Starr plication for primary obstructive megaureters. J Urol 2004;172:703–5.

72. Perdzynski W, Kalicinski ZH. Long-term results after megaureter folding in children. J Pediatr Surg 1996;31:1211–17.

73. McLorie GA, Jayanthi VR, Kinahan TJ, et al. A modified extravesical technique for megaureter repair. Br J Urol 1994;74:715–19.

74. Peters CA, Mandell J, Lebowitz RL, et al. Congenital obstructed megaureters in early infancy: Diagnosis and treatment. J Urol 1989;142:641–5.

75. Christman MS, Kasturi S, Lambert SM, et al. Endoscopic management and the role of double stenting for primary obstructive megaureters. J Urol 2012;187:1018–22.

76. Garcia-Aparicio L, Rodo J, Krauel L, et al. High pressure balloon dilation of the ureterovesical junction—first line approach to treat primary obstructive megaureter? J Urol 2012;187:1834–8.

77. Schulman CC. Les implantations ectopiques de l'uretère. Acta Urol Belg 1972;40:201–478.

78. Johnston JH, Davenport TJ. The single ectopic ureter. Br J Urol 1969;41:428–33.

79. Kreissl MC, Lorenz R, Ohnheiser G, et al. Dystopic dysplastic kidney with ectopic ureter: Improved localization by fusion of MR urography and (99m)Tc-DMSA SPECT datasets. Pediatr Radiol 2008;38:241–4.

80. Wyly JB, Lebowitz RL. Refluxing urethral ectopic ureters: Diagnosis by the cyclic voiding cystourethrogram. AJR Am J Roentgenol 1984;142:1263–7.

81. Berrocal T, Lopez-Pereira P, Arjonilla A, et al. Anomalies of the distal ureter, bladder, and urethra in children: Embryologic, radiologic, and pathologic features. Radiographics 2002;22:1139–64.

82. Lashley DB, McAleer IM, Kaplan GW. Ipsilateral ureteroureterostomy for the treatment of vesicoureteral reflux or obstruction associated with complete duplication. J Urol 2001;165:552–4.

83. Plaire JC, Pope JC, Kropp BP, et al. Management of ectopic ureters: Experience with upper tract approach. J Urol 1997;158:1245–7.

84. Lashley DB, McAleer IM, Kaplan GW. Ipsilateral ureteroureterostomy for the treatment of vesicoureteral reflux or obstruction associated with complete ureteral duplication. J Urol 2001;165:552–4.

85. Prieto J, Ziada A, Baker L, Snodgrass W. Ureteroureterostomy via inguinal incision for ectopic ureters and ureteroceles without ipsilateral lower pole reflux. J Urol 2009;181:1844–8.

86. Storm DW, Modi A, Jayanthi VR. Laparoscopic ipsilateral ureteroureterostomy in the management of ureteral ectopia in infants and children. J Pediatr Urol 2011;7:529–33.

87. Noseworthy J, Persky L. Spectrum of bilateral ureteral ectopia. Urology 1982;19:489–94.

88. Chwalla R. The process of formation of cystic dilations of the vesical end of the ureter and of diverticula at the ureteral ostium. Urol Cutan Rev 1927;31:499.

89. Coplen DE, Austin PF. Outcome of prenatally detected ureteroceles associated with multicystic dysplasia. J Urol 2004;172:1662–5.

90. Glassberg KI, Braren V, Duckett JW, et al. Suggested terminology for duplex systems, ectopic ureters and ureteroceles. J Urol 1984;132:1153–4.

91. Caldamone AA, Snyder HM, Duckett JW. Ureteroceles in children: Follow-up of management with upper tract approach. J Urol 1984;131:1130–2.

92. Cooper CS, Passerini-Glazel G, Hutcheson JC, et al. Long-term follow-up of endoscopic incision of ureteroceles: Intravesical versus extravesical. J Urol 2000;164:1097–100.

93. Husmann DA, Ewalt DH, Glenski WJ, et al. Ureterocele associated with ureteral duplication and nonfunctioning upper pole segment: Management by partial nephroureterectomy alone. J Urol 1995;154:723–6.

94. Sen S, Beasley SW, Ahmed S, et al. Renal function and vesicoureteric reflux in children with ureteroceles. Pediatr Surg Int 1992;7:192–4.

95. Sumfest JM, Burns MW, Mitchell ME. Pseudoureterocele: Potential for misdiagnosis of an ectopic ureter as a ureterocele. Br J Urol 1995;75:401–5.

96. Coplen DE, Barthold JS. Controversies in the management of ectopic ureteroceles. Urology 2000;56:665–8.

97. Scherz HC, Kaplan GW, Packer MG, et al. Ectopic ureteroceles: Surgical management with preservation of continence: Review of 60 cases. J Urol 1989;142:538–41.

98. Shekarriz B, Upadhyay J, Fleming P, et al. Long-term outcome based on the initial surgical approach to ureterocele. J Urol 1999;162:1072–6.

99. Rickwood AM, Reiner I, Jones M, et al. Current management of duplex-system ureteroceles: Experience with 41 patients. Br J Urol 1992;70:196–200.

100. Tank ES. Experience with endoscopic incision and open unroofing of ureteroceles. J Urol 1986;136:241–2.

101. Hagg MJ, Mourachov PV, Snyder HM, et al. The modern endoscopic approach to ureterocele. J Urol 2000;163:940–3.

102. Husmann D, Strand B, Ewalt D, et al. Management of ectopic ureterocele associated with renal duplication: A comparison of partial nephrectomy and endoscopic decompression. J Urol 1999;162:1406–9.

103. Monfort G, Guys JM, Coquet M, et al. Surgical management of duplex ureteroceles. J Pediatr Surg 1992;27:634–8.

104. Snyder HM, Johnston JH. Orthotopic ureteroceles in children. J Urol 1978;119:543–6.

CHAPTER 55

URINARY TRACT INFECTIONS AND VESICOURETERAL REFLUX

W. Robert DeFoor, Jr. • Eugene Minevich • Curtis A. Sheldon

URINARY TRACT INFECTIONS

Urinary tract infections (UTIs) are a common and significant source of morbidity in children. By 7 years of age, approximately 8% of girls and 2% of boys will have had at least one UTI.[1,2] Children who have had at least one UTI are at risk for having a recurrence.[3] The long-term sequelae include renal scarring, hypertension, chronic renal insufficiency, and pregnancy-related complications. Predisposing risk factors for UTIs include renal and bladder structural abnormalities as well as functional bladder and bowel dysfunction.[4] Pediatric UTIs constitute a significant health burden and has been estimated to result in at least 13,000 hospital admissions with inpatient costs exceeding $180 million per year.[5]

Diagnosis

Localized clinical signs and symptoms are important clues in the diagnosis, but they are age dependent. Combinations of findings can be more useful than individual ones in identifying affected children.[6] For example, neonates rarely present with symptoms specific to the urinary tract. Nonspecific symptoms of lethargy, irritability, temperature instability, anorexia, emesis, or jaundice predominate. Bacteremia is common with neonatal UTI, and a urine culture is an important aspect in the evaluation of neonatal sepsis.[7] Confirmation of a UTI by microscopic examination and quantitative culture of a properly collected specimen is important. Older infants may present with nonspecific abdominal discomfort, emesis, diarrhea, poor weight gain including failure to thrive, and fever. Malodorous or cloudy urine may be reported by the parents.

Older children frequently present with dysuria and urinary frequency, urgency, and enuresis. Table 55-1 outlines the incidence of UTI symptoms as a function of age.[8,9] As the symptoms can sometimes be obscure, it is important that care providers have a high index of suspicion in ill-appearing children. An unexplained high fever in an infant or toddler should prompt the clinician to obtain a urine sample.

Analysis of a properly collected urine sample is the cornerstone in the diagnosis of UTI.[10] Errors in diagnosis most commonly result from failure to confirm a clinically suspected UTI by culture, or by reliance on a specimen that has been inadequately collected or mishandled. Specimens may be obtained by bag collection, clean catch, urethral catheterization, and suprapubic aspiration. Although invasive, urethral catheterization (or suprapubic aspiration) clearly offers the lowest risk of false-positive results.[11] The results of a bag specimen or clean-catch specimen in a non-toilet-trained child are helpful only if negative.[12] Bag specimens can be useful in an infant with a history of UTIs or structural abnormalities in whom a fever is present, but the suspicion for a UTI is otherwise low. Positive findings should be confirmed using a catheter or aspiration specimen unless the clinical presentation and laboratory findings are unequivocal. The accuracy of positive findings from a bag specimen in an infant has been estimated at 7.5%,[13] whereas those of the midstream clean catch specimen varies with age: 42% under 18 months of age and 71% from 3 to 12 years of age.[14] Specimens should be either analyzed and plated immediately, or placed on ice to minimize bacterial multiplication prior to testing.

The accepted gold standard for diagnosis remains the quantitative urine culture. The historically accepted criterion for diagnosis is greater than 10^5 colony-forming units per milliliter of a single bacterial species. The accuracy of such a positive finding on culture is estimated at 80% (single specimen) and 96% (confirmed by second culture).[15] Table 55-2 outlines the probability of infection as a function of colony count and methods of collection that are used in children.[16] One must avoid applying these criteria too strictly. The colony count varies as a function of hydration (dilution) and urinary frequency (bacterial multiplication time). One study of six untreated children with proven bacteriuria found colony counts to vary from 10^3 to 10^8 over a 24-hour period.[17]

Although clearly the most accurate laboratory test, urine culture results cannot provide an immediate diagnosis. As a result, initial treatment is generally guided by the urinalysis. Microscopic evaluation of a urine specimen should be done immediately on collection. This practice minimizes misleading ex vivo bacterial multiplication and deterioration of cellular elements. The identification of bacteria in an unspun urine specimen is very suggestive of significant bacteriuria.[17] Pyuria (more than 10 leukocytes/mm³) is suggestive,[18] but may also be seen in vaginitis, dehydration, calculi, trauma, chemical irritation, gastroenteritis, and viral immunization. Urinary Gram stain has been found to be reliable in detecting UTIs in young infants.[19]

A popular and indirect measurement of bacteriuria employs nitrite and leukocyte esterase analysis. Nitrate, normally present in urine, is converted to nitrite in the presence of bacteria. A positive nitrite reaction is indicative of bacteria with specificity and a positive predictive

TABLE 55-1 Presenting Symptoms in 200 Children with Urinary Tract Infection as a Function of Age

Symptom	Age			
	0–1 MONTHS	1–24 MONTHS	2–5 YEARS	5–12 YEARS
Failure to thrive, poor feeding	53%	36%	7%	0
Jaundice	44%	0	0	0
Screaming, irritability	0	13%	7%	0
Foul-smelling, cloudy urine	0	9%	13%	0
Diarrhea	18%	16%	0	0
Vomiting	24%	29%	16%	3%
Fever	11%	38%	57%	50%
Convulsions	2%	7%	9%	5%
Hematuria	0	7%	16%	6%
Frequency, dysuria	0	4%	34%	41%
Enuresis	0	0	27%	29%
Abdominal pain	0	0	23%	44%
Loin pain	0	0	0	12%
Male-to-female ratio	1:2	1:13	1:10	1:10

From Smellie JM, Hodson CJ, Edwards D, et al. Clinical and radiological features of urinary tract infection in childhood. BMJ 1964;2:1222; Bickerton MW, Duckett JW. Urinary tract infections in pediatric patients. AUA Update Service, Lesson 26, 1985;4:4.

TABLE 55-2 Criteria for Diagnosis of Urinary Tract Infections

Method of Collection	Colony Count (Pure Culture)	Probability of Infection
Suprapubic aspiration	Gram-negative bacilli: any number	>99%
	Gram-positive cocci: a few thousand	>99%
Catheterization	>10^5	95%
	10^4–10^5	Likely
	10^3–10^4	Suggestive
	<10^3	Unlikely
Clean voided (male)	>10^5	Likely
Clean voided (female)	Three specimens >10^5	95%
	Two specimens >10^5	90%
	One specimen >10^5	80%

Modified from Hellerstein S. Recurrent urinary tract infection in children. Pediatr Infect Dis 1982;1:275.

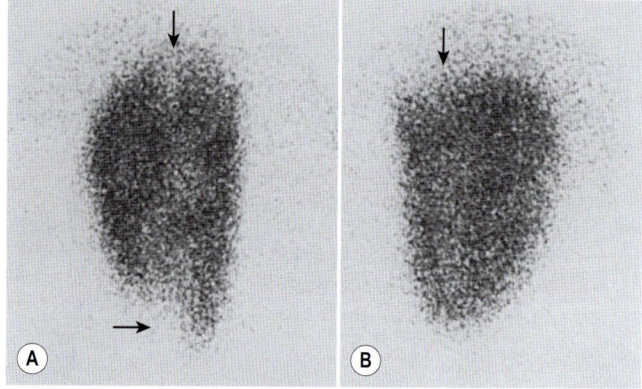

FIGURE 55-1 ■ Technetium-99m dimercaptosuccinic acid (DMSA) scan. **(A)** The magnified view of the left kidney, seen by using a pinhole collimator, demonstrates defects in both poles that extend deep into the renal parenchyma (arrows), suggestive of acute pyelonephritis. **(B)** The right kidney has an upper pole defect (arrow) that may represent either acute or chronic pyelonephritis. (Courtesy of Michael J. Gelfand, MD.)

value approaching 100%.[20] The nitrate-to-nitrite reaction requires a relatively long incubation period. Thus, urinary frequency and hydration may produce a false-negative result. Inadequate dietary nitrate and infection caused by nitrite-negative organisms may also cause false-negative reactions.[21] The combination of nitrite and leukocyte esterase is more sensitive and specific than either alone.[22] Overall, the combination of dipstick analysis and microscopic examination for bacteria have a sensitivity and negative predictive value approaching 100%.[20]

Classification

Classification of UTIs helps to determine the need for hospital admission and parenteral antibiotic therapy as opposed to outpatient oral antibiotic therapy. An attempt is made to distinguish between upper tract (pyelonephritis) and lower tract infections (cystitis). Fever, flank pain, and/or tenderness, and leukocytosis suggest pyelonephritis, and require antibiotics to minimize the risk of renal injury.

Laboratory studies designed to distinguish a lower tract from an upper tract UTI include antibody-coated bacteria assay, β_2-microglobulin excretion, antibodies to Tamm–Horsfall protein, and urinary lactic dehydrogenase assay and procalcitonin.[23,24] These tests are not sufficiently reliable for routine clinical use and thus are not typically employed. Direct culture by ureteral catheterization or percutaneous puncture is reliable, although cumbersome, and represents an option in complicated clinical situations. A quite useful study for localizing infection to the kidney is a radioisotope renal cortical scan (e.g., technetium-99m dimercaptosuccinic acid) during the initial presentation of the patient with a documented infection (Fig. 55-1).

Another important consideration regarding classification is the distinction between re-infection and persistent infection. Re-infection with a new organism is very common. Persistent UTI with the same organism, although less common, is important as it implies either an ineffective antimicrobial therapy or a structural abnormality, such as a urinary tract calculus or ureteral obstruction.

Epidemiology

Figure 55-2 outlines the age- and gender-related incidence of UTIs. At all ages, with the exception of the neonatal period, the incidence of UTI is greater in females than in males. In both males and females, the incidence increases with advanced age. Although the male has one early peak in the newborn period, the female has two peaks, one at 3 to 6 years, and the other at the onset of sexual activity. The actual incidence of infection as a function of age and gender is difficult to determine from the literature. Table 55-3 summarizes the available data.[16]

Pathophysiology

Host Factors

The establishment of clinical infection and its consequent injury to the urinary tract results from a complex interplay between host resistance and bacterial virulence. As a general rule, UTI-causing organisms originate from the feces of their host. Conceptually, four levels of defense are identifiable: periurethral, bladder, ureterovesical junction, and renal papillae.[9] These concepts are illustrated in Figure 55-3.

Bacteria generally possess an ability to adhere to vaginal mucosal cells in order to readily establish infection.[25] The resultant periurethral colonization then allows replication and migration, which ultimately lead to transurethral invasion to the bladder. Healthy girls have low bacterial colonizations of the periurethral region. Girls prone to UTIs experience greater colonization, especially prior to a new episode of UTI. Moreover, the cultured organism from the introital region belongs to the same strain as that from the urine during the UTI that ensues. Periurethral bacterial colonization is correspondingly low in UTI patients after resolution of recurrent UTIs.[26] A similar mechanism may apply to bacterial adherence in the prepuce of males.[27] This may explain why 92% of male infants less than 6 months old with a UTI are uncircumcised.[28]

A number of bladder defense mechanisms help maintain sterile urine. The most critical is the act of regular and complete voiding. The healthy bladder is capable of eliminating 99% of instilled bacteria and leaves a small residual urine that minimizes the inoculum at the onset of the following cycle.[29] High intravesical pressure may also potentiate infection in children. In the absence of an elevated residual urine, uninhibited bladder contractions are associated with an increased risk of recurrent UTI, which may be lessened by anticholinergic therapy.[30] Dysfunctional elimination syndrome with abnormal voiding habits and constipation can affect the development of UTI as well.[31] The acidic pH of urine, as well as its osmolality, further discourages bacterial growth.[32] The uroepithelial cells of healthy individuals suppress bacterial growth and are capable of killing bacteria. The uroepithelial cells secrete a mucopolysaccharide substance that, upon coating the surface of the uroepithelium, provides an additional barrier to uroepithelial adherence.[29] Glycosaminoglycans are continuously shed and thus function to entrap and eliminate bacteria.

TABLE 55-3	Incidence of Urinary Tract Infection as a Function of Age, Gender and Presence of Symptoms			
Age	**Symptomatic**		**Asymptomatic**	
	MALE	FEMALE	MALE	FEMALE
Newborn	0.15%		1.0–1.4%[a]	
Preschool	0.7%	2.8%	0.2%	0.8%
School age			0.03%	1.0–2.0%

[a]2.4–3.4% in premature infants.
Data compiled from multiple sources by Hellerstein S. Recurrent urinary tract infections in children. Pediatr Infect Dis 1982;1:271.

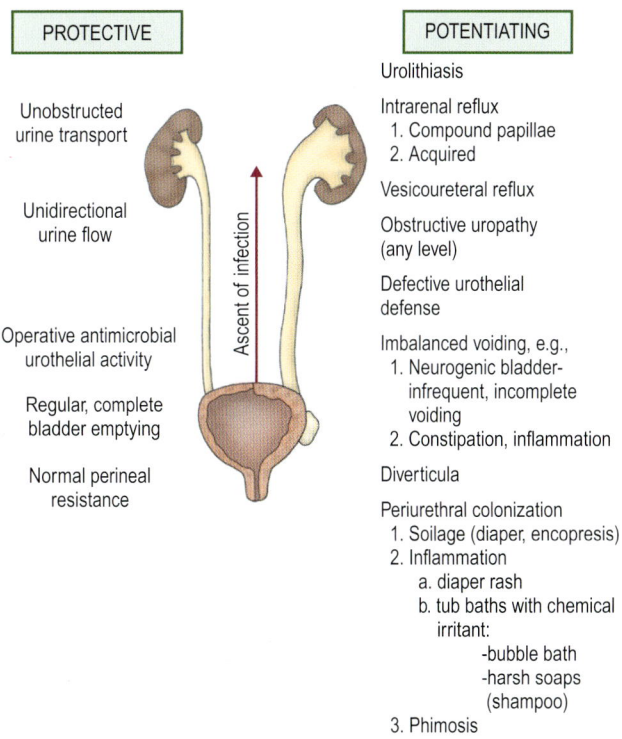

PROTECTIVE	POTENTIATING
Unobstructed urine transport	Urolithiasis
	Intrarenal reflux 1. Compound papillae 2. Acquired
Unidirectional urine flow	Vesicoureteral reflux
	Obstructive uropathy (any level)
Operative antimicrobial urothelial activity	Defective urothelial defense
	Imbalanced voiding, e.g., 1. Neurogenic bladder-infrequent, incomplete voiding 2. Constipation, inflammation
Regular, complete bladder emptying	Diverticula

Normal perineal resistance	Periurethral colonization
	1. Soilage (diaper, encopresis)
	2. Inflammation
	  a. diaper rash
	  b. tub baths with chemical irritant:
	    -bubble bath
	    -harsh soaps (shampoo)
	3. Phimosis

FIGURE 55-3 ■ Host factors that protect the urinary tract from infection and abnormalities that potentiate the establishment of invasive bacterial infection.

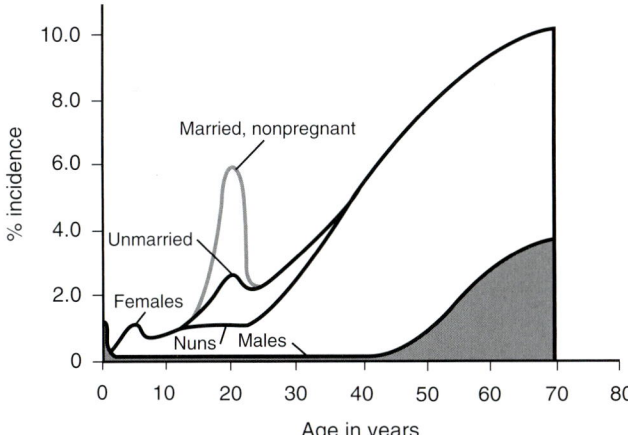

FIGURE 55-2 ■ The age and gender distribution of urinary tract infection incidence. (From Devine CJ, Stecker JF. Urology in Practice. Boston: Little, Brown; 1978. p. 444.)

Abnormalities at the ureterovesical junction (UVJ) and altered ureteral peristalsis may allow vesicoureteral reflux (VUR), which potentiates but is not always necessary for upper tract invasion. Distortion of the pyramids allows renal parenchymal invasion, which results in irreversible renal injury. The anatomy of the renal papillae usually prevents intrarenal reflux (Fig. 55-4).[9] Structural abnormalities that potentiate infection include phimosis, obstructive uropathy at any level (e.g., ureteropelvic and UVJ obstructions, posterior urethral valves [PUV]), VUR, bladder diverticula, urinary calculi or foreign bodies, and the renal papillary anatomy.

Bacterial Factors

Several bacterial factors may potentiate a UTI and are outlined in Box 55-1.[9,33] O antigens are lipopolysaccharides that are part of the cell wall. They are thought to be responsible for many of the systemic symptoms associated with infection. Of the more than 150 strains of *Escherichia coli* identified by O antigens, nine are responsible for the majority of UTIs.

K antigens are also polysaccharides, and their presence on Gram negative bacterial capsules is considered to be an important virulence factor. They are thought to protect against phagocytosis, to inhibit the induction of a specific immune response, and to facilitate bacterial adhesion. Bacterial strains causing UTI exhibit considerably more K antigen than those isolated from the feces. Urease, a virulence factor especially prominent with Proteus species, allows the breakdown of urea to ammonium. This process alkalinizes the urine and facilitates stone formation. Such bacteria are generally incorporated into the stone structure, making eradication extremely difficult. Mannose-resistant pili are important adherence factors. They promote adherence to uroepithelial cells as well as renal epithelial cells. This factor appears to counter the normal cleansing action of urine flow and allows tissue invasion and bacterial proliferation. That these factors truly are associated with virulence is shown in Figure 55-5.

Increasingly invasive urinary infections are associated with bacteria with a high number of virulence factors. Figure 55-6 demonstrates the pathophysiologic changes of renal injury that can occur in the absence of significant host factors. Colonization of the feces with a virulent organism allows periurethral colonization and ultimately

bladder entry. Uroepithelial adherence promotes bacterial proliferation and tissue invasion. This series of events is facilitated by the presence of one or more host factors (see Fig. 55-3).

Investigation

Rationale for Radiographic Imaging

Although many patients with UTI do not develop serious illness, the pediatric caregiver must be cognizant of several important risks. Urinary abnormalities are found in approximately 50% of children up to the age of 12 years who present with UTI.[34] VUR is found in up to

BOX 55-1	Bacterial Factors Potentiating Infection

O antigens (lipopolysaccharides)
  Primarily O_1, O_2, O_4, O_6, O_7, O_{11}, O_{18}, O_{35}, O_{75}
  Responsible for systemic reactions (e.g., fever, shock)
K antigens
  Primarily K_1, K_5
  Adhesive properties
  Low immunogenicity
H antigens (flagella)
  Bacterial locomotion
  Chemotaxis
Hemolysins (bacterial enzymes)
  Tissue damage
  Facilitates bacterial growth
Urease
  Alkalinizes urine
  Facilitates stone formation
P fimbriae—adherence
  Mannose sensitive (MS)
  Mannose resistant (MR)

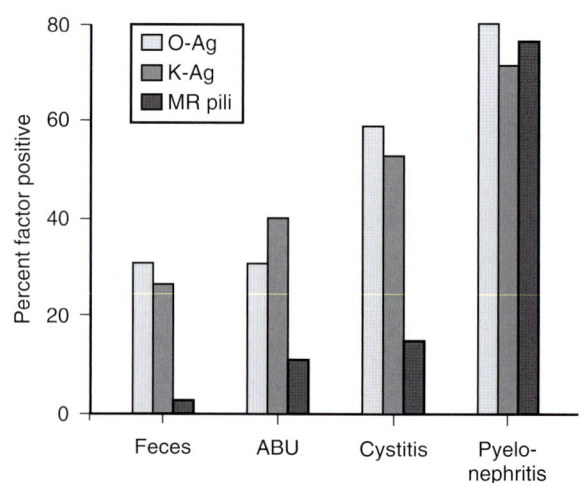

FIGURE 55-5 ■ Presence of bacterial virulence factors as a function of the clinical setting. More invasive infections are associated with a high incidence of virulence factors, implicating these factors in pathogenesis. MR, mannose resistant; Ag, antigen; ABU, asymptomatic bacteriuria. (From Mannhardt W, Schofer O, Schulte-Wisserman H. Pathogenic factors in recurrent urinary tract infection and renal scar formation in children. Eur J Pediatr 1986;145:330.)

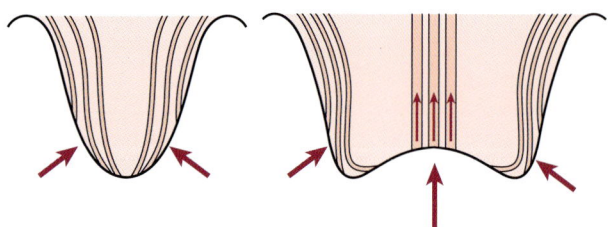

FIGURE 55-4 ■ The normal oblique insertion of the collecting ducts onto the surface of simple papillae prevent intrarenal reflux (*left*). Collecting duct insertion onto the surface of compound papillae may allow intrarenal reflux (*right*). (From Ransley PG. Intrarenal reflux: Anatomic, dynamic and radiological studies. Urol Res 1977;5:61.)

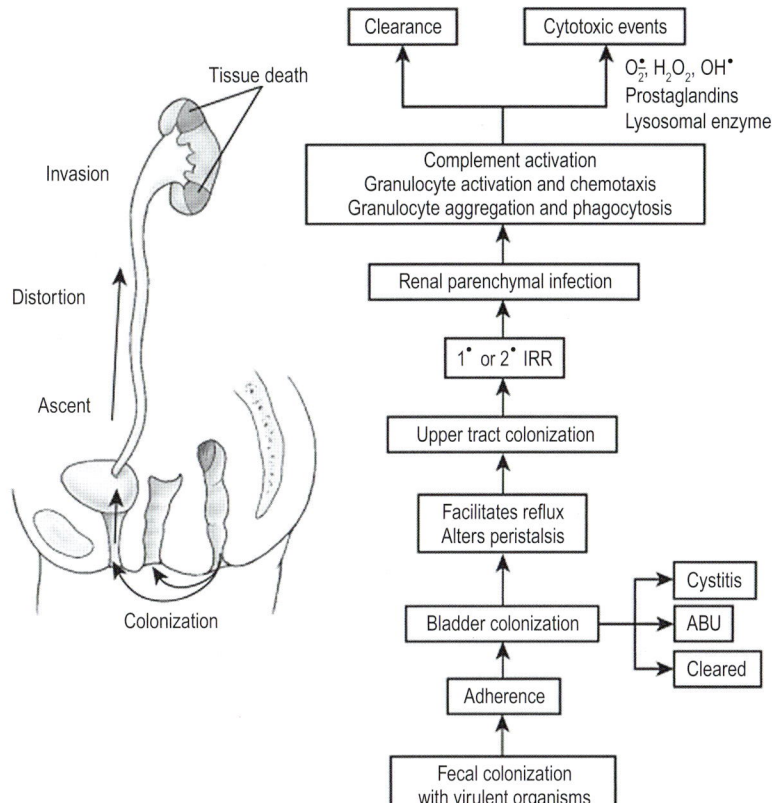

FIGURE 55-6 ■ The pathogenesis of destructive infection is shown. The process is facilitated by, but does not require, defects in the host protective factors outlined in Fig. 55-3. IRR, intrarenal reflux; ABU, asymptomatic bacteriuria.

35% and obstructive lesions in 8%. Nonobstructive, nonrefluxing lesions are found in 7%.

While renal scars develop in about 13% of girls and 5% of boys with unspecified infection,[35] they develop in up to 43% of kidneys involved in acute pyelonephritis.[36] A recent meta-analysis assessing the prevalence of renal scarring in children after an initial episode of UTI found that 57% had acute renal cortical changes consistent with pyelonephritis in the acute phase and 15% had evidence of renal scarring on the follow-up Tc-99m dimercaptosuccinic acid (DMSA) scan.[37] Pyelonephritic scarring is responsible for 11% of childhood hypertension cases[38] and a majority of cases of severe hypertension.[39] Although hypertension is most common with bilateral scarring, it is also seen with unilateral scarring.[40] Pyelonephritic scarring is also an important cause of end-stage renal failure in childhood and may require specific pretransplantation treatment, especially if associated with reflux.[41] Additionally, approximately 50% of patients will suffer from recurrent UTI.[33]

Current Controversies

The standard of care for many years has been to perform imaging studies in children to assess for structural abnormalities that might lead to recurrent UTIs and renal scarring. It was felt that not only infants[42] but older children, particularly males, should be investigated after the initial infection.[43] Several evidence-based guidelines have been published over the years.[44] Controversy persists, however, with many researchers proposing even less aggressive approaches to the child with a UTI. Recent published guidelines from the American Academy of Pediatrics recommends deferring a voiding cystourethrography (VCUG) until after the second documented UTI in children ages 2 to 24 months if the ultrasound (US) is normal and the child has a complete clinical response to treatment.[45] The urologic community has significant concerns about the paradigm shift made in these guidelines and the methodology employed in the meta-analysis upon which these recommendations were based.[46]

Imaging Studies

The initial radiographic evaluation ideally includes a fluoroscopic VCUG to precisely grade vesicoureteral reflux and assess for bladder and urethral abnormalities. Follow-up studies in females can be adequately performed with a radionuclear cystogram (RNC) that allows a somewhat lower radiation exposure to the ovaries. The exception is the girl with neurogenic bladder, ectopic ureter, bladder diverticulum, or ureterocele documented by ultrasound or previous cystograms. Radionuclide scanning using DMSA is readily available and can be used to diagnose acute pyelonephritis,[47] detect renal scarring, and assess differential renal function.[48]

Treatment

Acute Phase

The treatment of an acute UTI is dependent on the clinical presentation. Ill-appearing children with pyelonephritis should be treated immediately and aggressively with broad-spectrum antimicrobial therapy and intravenous hydration. Initial empiric therapy should be initiated with broad-spectrum parenteral antibiotics until cultures return. Prompt, effective treatment is the most important factor in preventing permanent renal injury.[49] Further therapy is dictated by culture and sensitivity findings. Indications for inpatient parenteral antibiotic therapy include very young age (<3 months), unusual or multi-resistant pathogens, persistent vomiting, concern for compliance with treatment, and/or significant urinary tract anomalies.

Once clinically stabilized and afebrile for 24–48 hours, patients with pyelonephritis and sensitive organisms may complete the course of parenteral culture-specific antibiotics on an outpatient basis, via a peripherally inserted central catheter (PICC) and a home-based nursing service. Some studies have shown that initial parenteral therapy followed by oral antibiotics can be as effective as a prolonged course of intravenous therapy in preventing renal scarring.[50,51] Patients with obstruction or renal abscess who do not become afebrile or have persistent severe symptoms require repeat upper tract imaging. An abscess or obstructed kidney may require percutaneous, or very rarely, open drainage.

Initial empiric therapy in less toxic appearing children without vomiting can be performed with oral broad-spectrum antibiotics (e.g., cephalosporins) after obtaining a reliable urine culture. Short treatment courses appear to be insufficient for treatment of childhood UTI.[52] Therefore, we prefer a 7–10-day course dictated by culture and sensitivity results.[53] Retention by the toilet-trained patient due to fear of voiding or dysuria may be managed with phenazopyridine (Pyridium) and hydration, and allowing the child to void while sitting in a tub of warm clear bath water.

Prophylactic Antibiotics

Patients who have recurrent UTIs or those who are managed nonoperatively for VUR are often treated with long-term suppressive antibiotics. It is unclear whether the benefit outweighs the risks, particularly in low-grade VUR without nephropathy.[45,54] The urothelial injury from an infection takes several months to fully recover. As a result, irritative voiding symptoms, such as dysuria, incontinence, and frequency, may persist despite the finding of sterile urine. A propensity for re-infection also exists.

Patients without obvious urinary tract structural abnormalities should be evaluated for functional bowel and bladder dysfunction. Regular and complete elimination is mandatory to diminish the risk of recurrence. Along with aggressive treatment of constipation and voiding dysfunction, three months of antibiotic suppression therapy may help to break the cycle. Table 55-4 outlines the characteristics of the drugs that are most commonly used for suppression.

VESICOURETERAL REFLUX

VUR refers to the retrograde passage of urine from the bladder into the ureter. Although VUR was first discovered in the late 1800s, its clinical importance has only been recognized in the last five decades. Hutch's studies, reported in the 1950s, demonstrated the pathophysiologic changes with VUR in children.[55] These reports and Hodson's observations in 1959 regarding the association between VUR, UTI, and pyelonephritic scarring set the stage for the modern era of reflux management.[56]

Although most commonly diagnosed during the evaluation for UTI, VUR may also be discovered during evaluations for hypertension, proteinuria, voiding dysfunction, or chronic renal insufficiency. In addition, VUR has been identified in asymptomatic patients with prenatally-detected hydronephrosis as well as through sibling screening.[57]

TABLE 55-4   **Characteristics of Commonly used Urosuppressive Antibiotics**

Drug	Therapeutic Dose	Suppressive Dose	Route of Administration	Comments
Nitrofurantoin	2 mg/kg PO qd	1 mg/kg PO qd	Suspension (5 mg/mL) Capsule (25, 50 mg)	Avoid in patients <1 month of age Not effective if CrCl <40 mL/min Nausea common with suspension; sprinkling macrocrystals may avoid this
Trimethoprim-sulfamethoxazole	4 mg/kg trimethoprim + 20 mg/kg sulfamethoxazole PO bid	2 mg/kg trimethoprim + 10 mg/kg sulfamethoxazole PO qd	Suspension (8 mg trimethoprim + 40 mg sulfamethoxazole per mL) Tablet (80 mg trimethoprim, 400 mg sulfamethoxazole)	Avoid in patients <2 months of age Contraindicated with hyperbilirubinemia May cause blood dyscrasias and Stevens–Johnson syndrome
Trimethoprim (Primsol)	5 mg/kg PO bid	2 mg PO qd	Oral solution 50 mg/5 mL	Avoid in patients <2 months of age
Amoxicillin	10 mg/kg PO tid	10 mg/kg PO qd	Suspension (25, 50 mg/mL) Drops (50 mg/mL)	Good alternative for neonates
Cephalexin	25 mg/kg PO bid	5–10 mg/kg qd	Suspension (125 mg/5 mL or 250 mg/5 mL)	Alternative for neonates

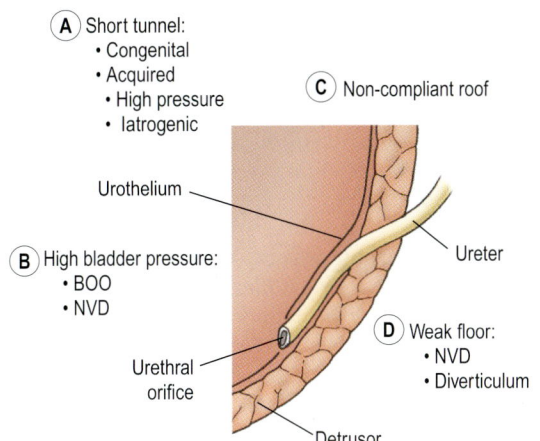

FIGURE 55-7 ■ Components of the competent ureterovesical junction. Those abnormalities most often implicated in the etiology of vesicoureteral reflux are outlined. BOO, bladder outlet obstruction; NVD, neurovesical dysfunction.

Pathophysiology

Figure 55-7 depicts the various anatomic components of the competent UVJ as well as the abnormalities most often implicated in the genesis of VUR. The normal UVJ is characterized by an oblique entry of the ureter into the bladder and a length of submucosal ureter providing a high ratio of tunnel length to ureteral diameter. This anatomic configuration provides a predominantly passive valve mechanism.[58,59] As the bladder fills and the intravesical pressure rises, the resulting bladder wall tension is applied to the roof of the ureteral tunnel. This results in a compression of the ureter which prevents retrograde passage of urine. Intermittent increases in bladder pressure, such as the act of voiding, upright posture, activity, and coughing, are met with an equal and immediate increase in resistance to retrograde urine flow. This effect is supplemented by the active effects of ureterotrigonal muscle contraction and ureteral peristalsis.[59,60]

Ureters with marginal tunnels can be made to reflux during infection due to UVJ distortion, loss of compliance of the valve roof, and intravesical hypertension. Excessively high intravesical pressure in neurovesical dysfunction (NVD) or bladder outlet obstruction (BOO) may also potentiate reflux as may a structurally weak detrusor floor (e.g., diverticulum or ureterocele). As the submucosal ureter tends to lengthen with age, the ratio of tunnel length to ureteral diameter increases, and the propensity for reflux may disappear.[58,59]

Of critical importance is the concept of intrarenal reflux (IRR), which has been demonstrated clinically[61] as well as experimentally.[62] The usually oblique entry of the papillary ducts onto the surface of simple papillae inhibits IRR. In contrast, the papillary duct entrance onto compound papillae facilitates IRR (see Fig. 55-4). The critical pressure for IRR is considered to be about 35 mmHg in compound papillae.[62,63] Experimentally, this same pressure may cause scar formation in the absence of infection.[62,64] When occurring intravesically, this pressure has been associated with an increased risk of renal deterioration. Higher pressure is thought to be necessary to induce IRR in simple papillae. The combination of infection and IRR is particularly devastating. Focal scarring appears to result from the difference in susceptibility of the renal papillae to IRR. The polar distribution of compound papillae corresponds closely to the predominant occurrence of renal scarring in the upper and lower poles of the kidney.

Classification

Many attempts at classification of VUR have been advanced. Reflux has been described as low pressure (occurring during the filling phase of the VCUG) or high pressure (occurring only during voiding). Reflux due to a congenitally deficient UVJ is referred to as *primary* reflux, whereas that due to a BOO or neurogenic bladder is referred to as *secondary* reflux. Further classification includes simple reflux and complex reflux. Complex reflux includes the refluxing megaureter, the refluxing duplicated ureter, the refluxing ureter associated with a diverticulum or ureterocele, and the occasional refluxing ureter associated with ipsilateral ureteropelvic or ureterovesical obstruction.

The most clinically pertinent classification systems, however, have attempted to quantitate the degree of reflux. At the present time, VUR is graded from I to V according to the international classification system diagrammed in Figure 55-8.[65] This classification system is based not only on the proximal extent of retrograde urine flow and ureteral and pelvic dilatation, but also on the resultant anatomy of the calyceal fornices. This system is currently universally accepted and used extensively in the literature.

Grade I VUR refers to the visualization of a nondilated ureter only, whereas grade II VUR refers to visualization of a nondilated renal pelvis and calyceal system in addition to the ureter. Grade III reflux involves mild to moderate dilatation or ureteral tortuosity with mild to moderate dilatation of the renal pelvis and calyces. The fornices, however, remain sharp or only minimally blunted. Once the forniceal angle is completely blunted, grade IV reflux has developed. Papillary impressions in the majority of calyces can still be appreciated. Loss of the papillary impressions along with increased dilatation and tortuosity is referred to as grade V reflux.

Epidemiology

The incidence of VUR in otherwise normal children is thought to be quite low.[66] A much higher incidence of VUR, between 30–40%, is reported in patients undergoing evaluation for UTI.[67–70] It is important to note that the incidence rises as age decreases.[71] Thus, the infant who is most vulnerable to the combination of UTI and VUR is precisely the pediatric patient in whom this combination is most likely to occur.

Although females account for the majority of reflux patients, a few important characteristics of males with VUR require comment. Although males account for approximately 14% of patients with VUR,[72] an increased incidence of VUR (30%) is found in those males presenting with UTI.[69] Boys with VUR tend to present at a

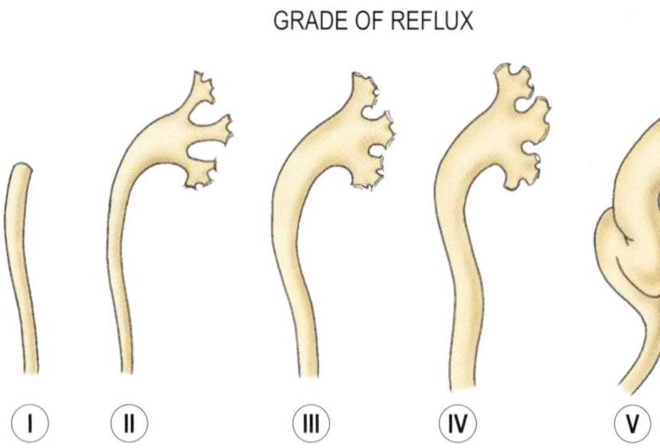

GRADE OF REFLUX

FIGURE 55-8 ■ The international grading system for vesicoureteral reflux. See text for description. (From The International Reflux Committee. Medical versus surgical treatment of primary vesicoureteral reflux. Pediatrics 1987;67:396.)

relatively young age (25% under 3 months) and younger children tend to have the more severe degrees of reflux.[72]

Multiple studies have documented a significant risk of VUR in family members of patients with reflux. The reported risk of sibling reflux ranges from 27–34%,[73–75] while as much as 66% of offspring of women with reflux also have VUR.[76] As a result of these studies, it has been suggested that siblings, especially those under 2 years of age, should have a screening investigation.[56,73,76] Another option is to perform a renal and bladder ultrasound in younger siblings and defer the VCUG if the ultrasound is normal, unless they have a documented UTI.

A particularly important subset of patients with reflux includes those who have secondary reflux. Most have NVD or BOO as the primary disease. Many patients, however, have reflux not because of increased bladder pressure alone, but rather because UVJ deficiency is associated with other congenital anomalies, such as imperforate anus,[77] ureterocele,[78] and bladder exstrophy. Although many patients with PUV have reflux due to or exacerbated by high intravesical pressure, as demonstrated by VUR resolution after valve ablation or vesicostomy, the incidence of VUR in PUV patients is only approximately 50%. Many have congenitally abnormal ureteral insertions.[79]

Although a significant incidence of NVD exists in patients with imperforate anus, this is not a prerequisite for VUR.[80] The diagnosis of VUR in imperforate anus thus assumes a critical importance to the pediatric surgeon. Not only may the association of NVD potentiate increased severity of reflux and the development of infection, the presence of a rectourethral or rectovesical fistula provides the opportunity for severe urinary contamination. Consequently, we believe that the patient with a rectovesical or rectourethral fistula should be managed with a completely diverting colostomy rather than a loop.

In addition to these structural associations, important functional associations are found as well, including florid NVD, as seen in myelodysplasia,[81] and a variety of more subtle voiding disturbances.[82–84] A particularly important subset of VUR patients are those who have uninhibited detrusor contractions (UDCs). Three important components of maturation are found with successful toilet training: (1) growth in bladder volume; (2) development of volitional control over the striated muscle sphincter; and

(3) control over bladder smooth muscle. Delay in this maturation leads to UDCs. Many children with reflux and recurrent UTI have UDCs. Such involuntary or uninhibited bladder contractions are not caused by neurologic disease. Intense voluntary constriction of the striated sphincter occurs in an attempt to ensure continence and results in excessively high intravesical pressures. Pressures often exceeding 150 cmH$_2$O have been observed resulting in intravesical distortions, such as diverticula, saccules, trabeculations, and abnormal ureteral orifices.[85] Reflux occurred in almost half of the children studied with UDC and UTI.

Thus, all patients with VUR should be screened for frequency, urgency, and incontinence, which suggest UDC's and voiding dysfunction. Vincent's curtsy, a squatting maneuver spontaneously employed to prevent incontinence, is particularly suggestive.[84] That these UDCs may cause reflux is suggested by an enhanced resolution of reflux with anticholinergic drug therapy. Equally important is the potential for UDCs to cause a false-negative cystogram.

Diagnostic Evaluation

VUR is diagnosed with a cyclic voiding cystourethrogram (VCUG), with either radiopaque contrast medium or radioisotope.[86,87] Body temperature contrast material, which is not excessively concentrated, is instilled into the bladder through a small catheter by gravity with modest pressure in a non-anesthetized child.

Imaging of the upper urinary tract (kidneys and ureters) is extremely important and may be accomplished by ultrasound and/or isotope renography. Both may detect scarring, but isotope renography is particularly sensitive and also defines the split differential function in the case of a small kidney. Ultrasound is helpful in quantitating renal growth and dilatation of the renal pelvis and/or ureters. Bladder views are important to obtain to check for bladder wall thickening, diverticula, distal ureteral dilatation, ureteroceles, and bladder emptying.

Patients with frequency, urgency, incontinence, and Vincent's curtsy should also be considered for noninvasive urodynamic studies including a uroflow and perineal electromyogram with a postvoid residual. A filling cystometrogram is indicated to follow neurovesical dysfunction or in those who have failed therapy. The presence of UDCs or detrusor-sphincter dyssynergia should be resolved before consideration is given to an antireflux operation. Although not formally described in the literature, our impression is that intervention in an unstable bladder is likely to result in a failed repair.

Natural History

The natural history of VUR is extremely variable, and ranges from spontaneous resolution without nephropathy to clinically silent scar formation to recurrent pyelonephritis with hypertension and end-stage renal disease (ESRD). Numerous factors may contribute to the potential for resolution, including the patient's age, the grade of reflux, the appearance of the ureteral orifice, the length of the ureteral submucosal tunnel, and the

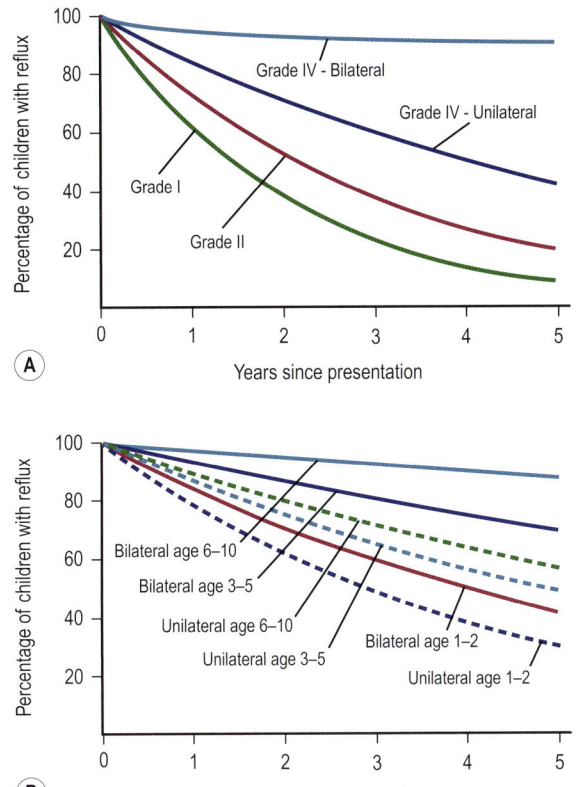

FIGURE 55-9 ■ **(A)** Percentage chance of reflux persistence, grades I, II, and IV, for 1 to 5 years after presentation. **(B)** Percentage chance of reflux persistence by age at presentation, grade III, for 1 to 5 years after presentation. (From Elder JS, Peters CA, Arant BS, et al. Report on the Management of Primary Vesicoureteral Reflux in Children. Baltimore: American Urological Association; 1997.)

intravesical dynamics. The American Urological Association Pediatric Vesicoureteral Reflux Guidelines Panel in 1997 analyzed 26 reports comprising 1,987 patients with conservative follow-up, to estimate the probability of reflux resolution (Fig. 55-9).[88] In general, a lower reflux grade correlated with a better chance of spontaneous resolution.

Younger children are thought to have better prognoses for resolution of VUR, particularly infant males in the first year of life. This may be due to a heightened degree of trigonal growth, but the diminishing prominence of UDCs with age is also likely. Spontaneous resolution is relatively independent of grade in secondary reflux, implicating management of primary bladder dysfunction as the primary prognostic variable (Fig. 55-10).[89]

Renal injury due to VUR may take the form of focal scarring, generalized scarring with atrophy, and failure of renal growth.[90] As a result, kidneys drained by refluxing ureters should be observed not only for scarring but also for renal growth with serial upper tract imaging by ultrasound.[91] Reflux-induced renal injury is usually a result of the association of VUR with UTI.[92] It has been generally considered that such injury is most likely in children under the age of 2 years.[71] It is now clear, however, that the risk of renal injury from VUR extends well beyond this age.[70,92–94] Reflux can also cause renal injury in the absence of UTI because of the pressure effects from

NVD and BOO. The ability of high intravesical pressure, when associated with VUR, to cause renal injury has been confirmed experimentally.[95]

Significant renal injury in the absence of BOO, NVD, and UTI can be found in infants.[96,97] The ureteral bud theory postulates that VUR associated with displacement of the ureteral orifice is associated with anomalies of renal differentiation.[98] Such ureters probably do not arise from the appropriate segment of the Wolffian duct and consequently make ectopic contact with the nephrogenic cord, resulting in abnormal renal development. Although this mechanism may be present in some patients, it is now clear that congenital VUR-associated renal injury in the absence of BOO, NVD, and UTI may occur in the presence of a normally positioned ureteral orifice.[99] This finding implies that pressure from in utero VUR may injure the developing kidney.

In a longitudinal study of 923 children, high-pressure bladder dynamics, severity of reflux, and frequency of UTIs were the chief contributing factors in the development of new scars or the worsening of old scars.[94] Children with low-grade VUR were relatively unlikely to develop progressive renal injury when compared with those children with grades IV and V reflux. A similar relationship is seen in infants and children with secondary reflux. When monitoring these patients for progression of renal injury as an indicator of success of a therapeutic regimen, one must be cognizant of the fact that sonographic evidence of new renal injury may take several months to become apparent.

There is little consensus regarding the long-term sequelae of minor renal scars detected by high-resolution renal cortical scans. However, in a small number of patients, a spectrum of symptomatic nephropathy exists, most notably renal parenchymal hypertension and ESRD. The significance and predominance of reflux nephropathy (RN) as a cause of renal parenchymal hypertension has been reviewed.[100] Approximately 30–65% of

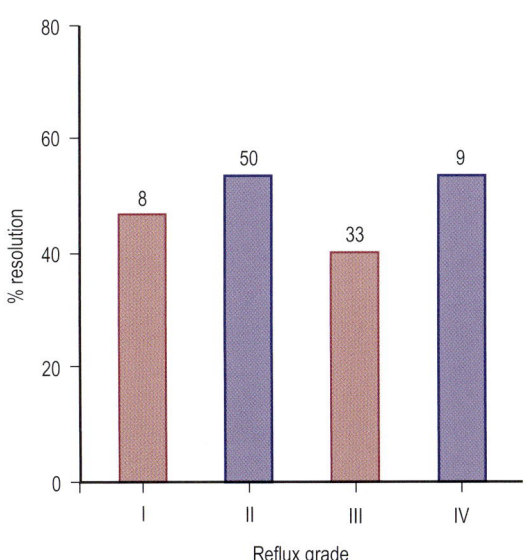

FIGURE 55-10 ■ The rate of spontaneous resolution of secondary vesicoureteral reflux as a function of reflux grade. (From Cohen RA, Roston MG, Belman AB, et al. Renal scarring and vesicoureteral reflux in children with myelodysplasia. J Urol 1990;144:541.)

childhood hypertension is associated with RN. RN is an important cause of end-stage renal failure in children and adults.[101–103] The 2008 report of the North American Pediatric Renal Trials and Collaborative Studies (NAPRTCS) lists reflux nephropathy as being the primary diagnosis in 5% of 9854 children who received transplants over the previous 20 years.[2]

Some patients so affected may not have had an evident prior infection or will have the first recognized infection at or near the time of diagnosis of ESRD.[101] As histologic evidence of chronic pyelonephritis is found, preceding infection is likely, underscoring the silent progressive nature of RN and the need for meticulous long-term follow-up of children with VUR. Glomerular lesions play an important role in the progression of RN. There is a clear association between RN, 'heavy' proteinuria, and glomerular lesions that resemble focal segmental glomerulosclerosis.[104] Although the mechanisms of this disease remain uncertain, immunologic injury, macromolecular trapping with mesangial injury, vascular alterations with hypertension, and glomerular hyperfiltration have been implicated. The latter theory of glomerular hyperfiltration is presently favored.

Treatment

Nonoperative management of VUR (Box 55-2) is successful in most patients. Such management may be considered in four stages: (1) diagnostic evaluation; (2) avoidance of infection; (3) voiding dysfunction treatment; and (4) active surveillance. Diagnostic evaluation has been previously reviewed. However, it is important to stress that the exclusion and treatment of voiding dysfunction and BOO is imperative. Patients with problematic uninhibited detrusor contraction can be managed with low-dose anticholinergic medication, such as oxybutynin hydrochloride. Side effects are manageable and include constipation and facial flushing/dry mouth. Voiding dysfunction with retentive characteristics may require timed/double voiding, alpha blockers, biofeedback, and in severe cases, intermittent catheterization (IC). Secondary reflux from neurovesical dysfunction often requires aggressive bladder management with IC and anti-cholinergics.

Good hydration, perineal hygiene, and bowel management are crucial and apply to all patients. With the exception of the asymptomatic toilet-trained child with low-grade reflux and normal kidneys, most children will benefit from low-dose continuous suppressive antibiotics (Table 55-4). It is important to remember that the prophylactic dose is approximately one-quarter the dose to treat an acute infection. Although generally well tolerated and having been a common practice for decades, the long-term implications of chronic antimicrobial suppression remain incompletely investigated and are actively debated.[4,45,105] Currently a prospective, multicenter, double-blind, placebo-controlled clinical trial of 600 patients funded by the National Institutes of Health is underway called the Randomized Intervention for Children with Vesicoureteral Reflux (RIVUR study).[106] This may help further define the role of antibiotic prophylaxis in the management of VUR. Until more evidence-based guidelines are published, the clinician must use caution in treating children with risk factors for recurrent UTI and renal scarring, including VUR.

Once a nonoperative regimen is selected, the patient is committed to long-term, strict surveillance. Renal imaging is performed every six to 12 months, depending on the age at diagnosis and the stability of the disease. Attention is directed at both renal growth as well as the detection of focal scarring. Voiding cystourethrography is generally performed no more often than once a year. The child's growth, renal function, and blood pressure

---

BOX 55-2   General Guidelines for the Nonoperative Management of Vesicoureteral Reflux

TREATMENT

Hydration Hygiene
  Perineal hygiene
  Avoid:
    Harsh soaps during tub baths
    Bubble baths
    Shampoos
Bowel management
  Avoid constipation
  Treat encopresis
Suppressive antibiotics
Observation without antibiotics
Anticholinergics, spasmolytics

SURVEILLANCE

Urine culture
  Monthly for 3 months after last UTI
  Thereafter, every 2 to 3 months
Renal imaging every 6 to 12 months
  Renal size (ultrasound, IVU)
  Focal scarring (renal scan, IVU)
Voiding cystourethrography (yearly)
  Radiographic VCUG
    Initial (male, female suspected NVD)
    Follow-up (NVD)
  Isotope VCUG
    Routine surveillance
Record growth yearly (height, weight)
Blood pressure
  Routine (yearly)
  Renal scarring (quarterly)
Renal function tests
  BUN, creatinine (yearly if bilateral RN)
GFR estimated (yearly if azotemic)

$$\frac{\text{Height (cm)} \times 0.55}{\text{Serum creatinine}} = \text{GFR (mL/min/1.73 m}^2)$$

Maximum urine osmolality (yearly if bilateral RN)
Cystoscopy
  Done at time of antireflux surgery; otherwise rarely necessary
Urodynamic evaluation
  History of voiding dysfunction

BUN, blood urea nitrogen; GFR, glomerular filtration rate; IVU, intravenous urogram; NVD, neurovesical dysfunction; RN, reflux nephropathy; UTI, urinary tract infection; VCUG, voiding cystourethrogram.

are monitored. The role of urodynamics has been previously outlined. Cystoscopy is rarely necessary except at the time of antireflux surgery when it is performed to exclude urothelial inflammation and to confirm the position and number of ureteral orifices.

While the decision to perform antireflux surgery must be carefully individualized, absolute indications for surgical correction of VUR include (1) progressive renal injury; (2) documented failure of renal growth; (3) breakthrough pyelonephritis; and (4) intolerance or noncompliance with antibiotic suppression. Other relative indications for correction of VUR are high grade (IV–V) reflux in young children after a year of conservative follow-up, pubertal age with nephropathy at diagnosis, parental preference, and failure to spontaneously resolve with watchful waiting.

The American Urological Association (AUA) Pediatric Vesicoureteral Reflux Guidelines Panel published their recommendations for management of VUR in children in 1997 and updated their guidelines in 2010. For VUR in an infant diagnosed after a febrile UTI or found to be high grade (III–V), then continuous antibiotic prophylaxis is still recommended. It is also recommended for an older child (>1 year of age) with recurrent febrile UTI, bowel/bladder dysfunction, and/or renal cortical anomalies. For asymptomatic older children with normal kidneys, suppression is an option. Breakthrough UTI management guidelines are summarized in Table 55-5.[4,88] There is little solid evidence or consensus about the management of VUR in older school-age patients or about the length of time that the clinician should observe nonoperatively before recommending surgery. The actual decision must be carefully individualized after a thorough discussion of all the treatment options with the parents.

The established principles of successful ureteral reimplantation include: (1) adequate ureteral exposure and mobilization; 2) meticulous preservation of the blood supply; and (3) creation of a valvular mechanism whose submucosal tunnel length to ureteral diameter ratio

exceeds 4:1. These goals can be attained by a variety of procedures, most commonly via an open Pfannensteil approach but also laparoscopically and robotic-assisted (Fig. 55-11).

Important differences exist between these operative procedures. Variables include (1) presence or absence of a ureteral anastomosis; (2) need for detrusor closure; (3) transgression of urothelium; and (4) whether the neo-hiatus is fashioned by an appropriately sized detrusor incision or by the closure of the detrusor around the ureter. Performance of a ureteral anastomosis increases the risk of postoperative obstruction, whereas the need for detrusor closure increases the risk of diverticula. Table 55-6 outlines the specific advantages and disadvantages of some representative procedures. Three of the most commonly employed operations for the treatment of primary VUR are diagramed in Figures 55-12 to 55-14.

In general, excellent results are nearly uniformly attainable with an open approach and early reports of robotic-assisted laparoscopic outcomes are encouraging.[107] A meta-analysis in 1997 of 86 reports, including 6472 patients (8563 ureters), found overall success for an open ureteral reimplantation to be 96%.[88] Success was achieved in 99% with grade I, 99.1% with grade II, 98.3% with grade III, 98.5% with grade IV and 80.7% in grade V.

At our institution, we prefer the extravesical detrusor-rhaphy approach (see Fig. 55-12).[108–110] Because the lumen of the bladder is not entered, there is no postoperative hematuria, with minimal bladder spasms and a short hospitalization. The absence of a uretero-vesical anastomosis decreases the risk of postoperative obstruction. No ureteral stents, suprapubic catheters, or perivesical drains are needed. The urethral catheter is removed on the first day after unilateral surgery and the second day following bilateral reimplantation. Once the patient voids, he/she is discharged on oral antibiotics for 1 week, then is placed back on suppression for 3 months.

Postoperative analgesia can be maintained with either an indwelling or single-shot epidural placed at the time of surgery, or infiltration of local anesthesia in the incision supplemented by intravenous narcotics as needed. The majority of children are discharged home simply on oral acetaminophen alone. Postoperative imaging includes a renal and bladder ultrasound at 2 weeks, 3 months, 12 months, and 24 months after the procedure. A VCUG is not typically obtained in an asymptomatic patient due to the high success rate of the procedure.

The four major principles of a successful extravesical detrusorrhaphy are: (1) complete mobilization of the ureter from the peritoneal reflection to the UVJ, leaving a wide sheath of its peri-adventitial blood supply; (2) distal fixation of the ureter with long-acting absorbable sutures; (3) wide mobilization of the detrusor muscle flaps to enable firm approximation of the detrusor over the ureter; and (4) development of a sufficient tunnel length. The use of the extravesical detrusorrhaphy has been successfully expanded to include a tapered excisional megaureter repair,[109] reimplantation of the ureters associated with paraureteral Hutch diverticula,[111] as well as correction of VUR associated with duplicated collecting systems.[112]

Complications of ureteral reimplantation are rare.[88,113] The most common complication is de novo contralateral

TABLE 55-5	Breakthrough UTI Management According to the 2010 American Urological Association Guidelines
Clinical Scenario	**Recommendation (R)/ Option (O)**
Symptomatic BT-UTI	R: Change of therapy guided by scenario
Patient on CAP with febrile BT-UTI	R: Consider open or endoscopic surgical intervention
Patient on CAP with single febrile BT-UTI without evidence of existing or new renal cortical abnormalities	O: Change to alternative antibiotics is an option before surgical intervention
Patient not on CAP with febrile UTI	R: Initiation of CAP
Patient not on CAP with afebrile UTI	R: Initiation of CAP
All patients with BT-UTI	O: Open or endoscopic surgical intervention

BT, breakthrough; CAP, continuous antibiotic prophylaxis.
Adapted from Peters CA, Skoog SJ, Arant BS Jr, et al. Summary of the AUA guideline on management of primary vesicoureteral reflux in children. J Urol 2010;184:1134.

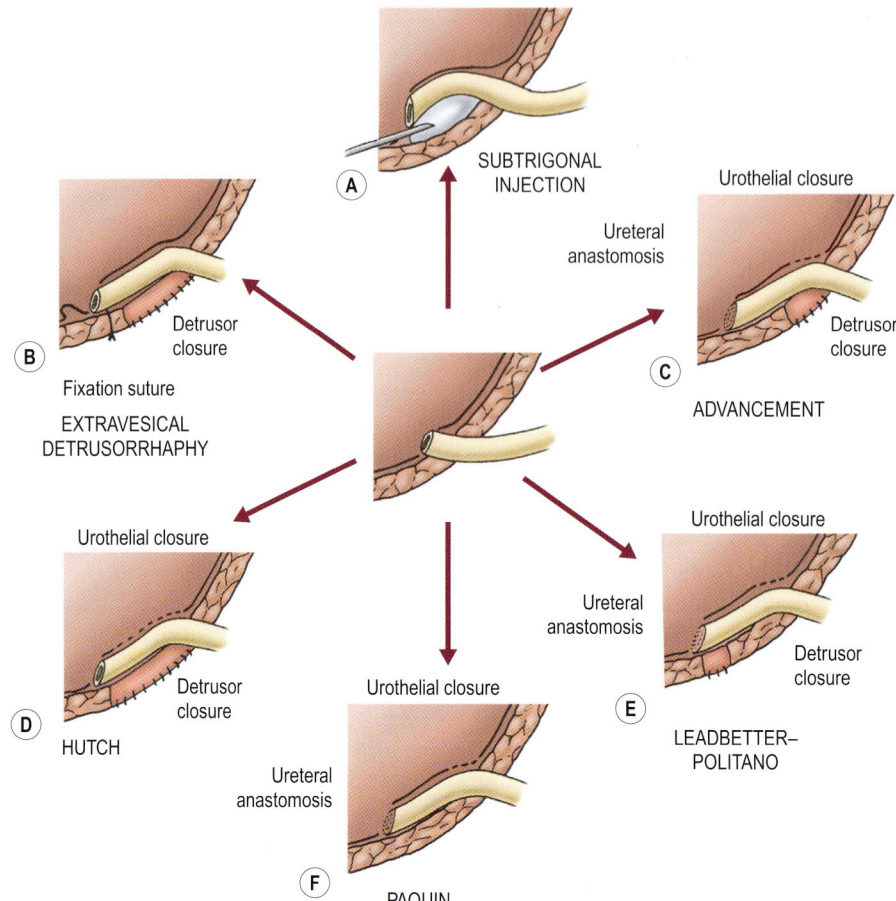

FIGURE 55-11 ■ Conceptual comparison of techniques to correct reflux. A common theme is the achievement of a long length of intravesical ureter based on a strong detrusor floor and covered with compressible urothelium.

TABLE 55-6	Specific Advantages and Disadvantages of Commonly Performed Antireflux Procedures	
Procedure	**Advantages**	**Disadvantages**
Subtrigonal injection	Endoscopic procedure	Material injected: Teflon—migration, granuloma formation Collagen—uncertain durability
Extravesical detrusorrhaphy	Bladder never opened No hematuria No ureteral anastomosis Minimal bladder spasms Endoscopically accessible ureteral orifices	
Advancement	Avoids complications of neohiatus formation in Leadbetter–Politano reimplantation	
Cohen (transtrigonal)		Transtrigonal: difficult to access ureter endoscopically
Glenn–Anderson		Glenn–Anderson: limited length of tunnel achievable
Hutch	No ureteral anastomosis Good alternative with large associated congenital diverticulum	
Leadbetter–Politano	Excellent ureteral tunnel dimensions with endoscopically accessible ureteral orifices	Risk of ureteral obstruction Risk of sigmoid colon injury with left reimplantation
Paquin	Versatility, extremely useful during complex reconstructive procedures	

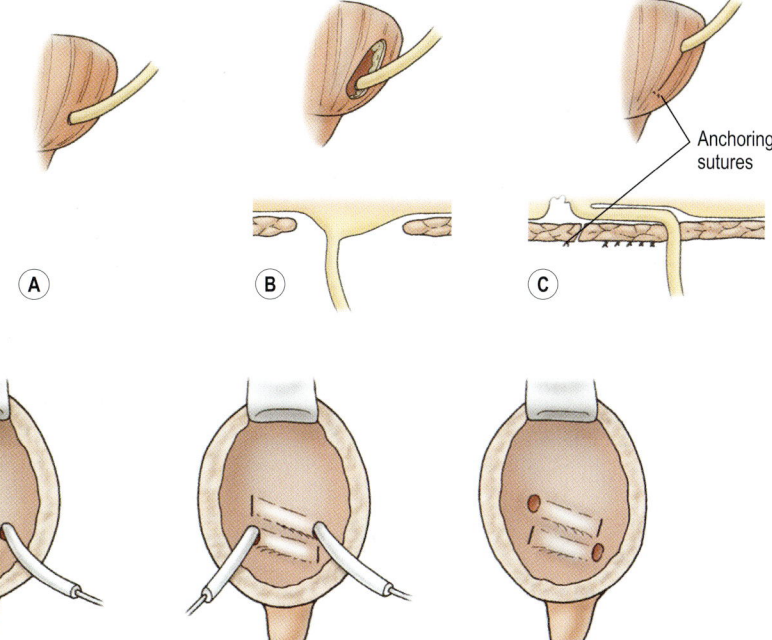

FIGURE 55-12 ■ The extravesical detrusorrhaphy antireflux technique conceptually viewed from behind the bladder. **(A)** The detrusor is incised. **(B)** The dissection is continued until the plane between urothelium and muscle has been developed. **(C)** The ureter is advanced and fixed into position with anchoring sutures. The detrusor is closed.

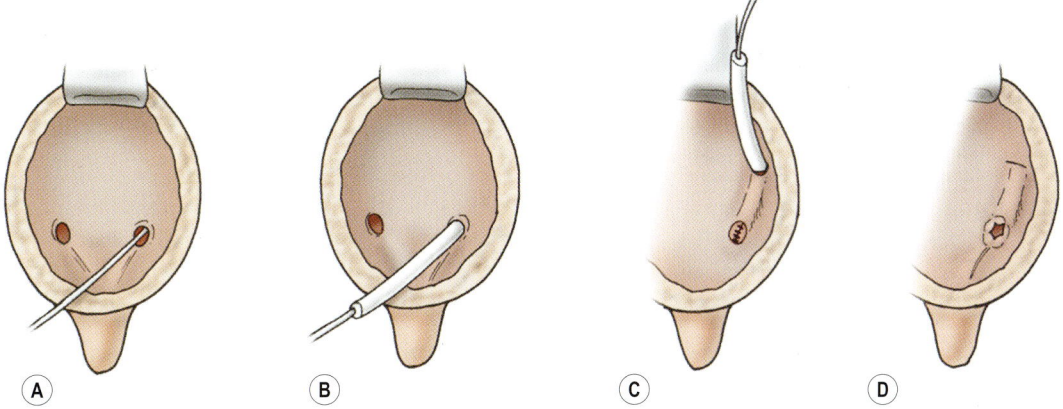

FIGURE 55-13 ■ The Cohen cross-trigonal ureteral reimplantation. **(A)** The ureter is intubated and the mucosa is incised circumferentially around the ureteral orifice. **(B)** The ureters are dissected from the muscular attachments and mobilized until free within the retroperitoneum. **(C)** Cross-trigonal tunnels are created by scissor dissection. **(D)** The ureteral anastomoses are completed.

FIGURE 55-14 ■ The Leadbetter–Politano ureteral reimplantation. **(A)** The ureter is intubated. **(B)** The ureter is mobilized. The hiatus is dilated, and the retroperitoneal ureter is mobilized. Under direct vision the peritoneum is reflected from the outer surface of the bladder. **(C)** The neohiatus is created, and the ureter is internalized into the bladder. The tunnel is created by scissor dissection, and the original hiatus is closed. **(D)** The ureteral anastomosis is completed.

reflux,[114] while the most common technical complications are ureteral obstruction, persistent reflux, and diverticula formation. Persistent reflux may be caused by an insufficient tunnel length to ureteral diameter ratio. However, the greatest risk for postoperative reflux is related to the high-pressure voiding dynamics due to uninhibited bladder contraction, detrusor sphincter dyssnergia, and/or urinary retention. Ureteral obstruction may be due to ureteral kinking (at the neohiatus or obliterated umbilical artery), an excessively high placed neohiatus, construction of a tight neohiatus, twisting, anastomotic stricture, devascularization, and tight tunnel.

With attention directed toward the avoidance of technical complications and the selection of a procedure associated with the lowest complication rate, ureteral reimplantation remains a safe and highly successful operation. The extravesical approach for bilateral ureteral reimplantation has been questioned because of a reportedly high incidence of postoperative urinary retention.[115] In our experience with a large group of patients, we have found acceptable rates of temporary incomplete bladder emptying (4%) which is transient and has minimal morbidity.[116] Risk factors appear to be infants under age one and girls with large, thin-walled bladders and preexisting retentive voiding dysfunction.

In 1984, a minimally invasive endoscopic procedure for the correction of VUR was reported (Fig. 55-15). This suburethral transurethral injection (STING) utilized polytetrafluoroethylene (Teflon) and has been used successfully outside the USA for many years.[117]

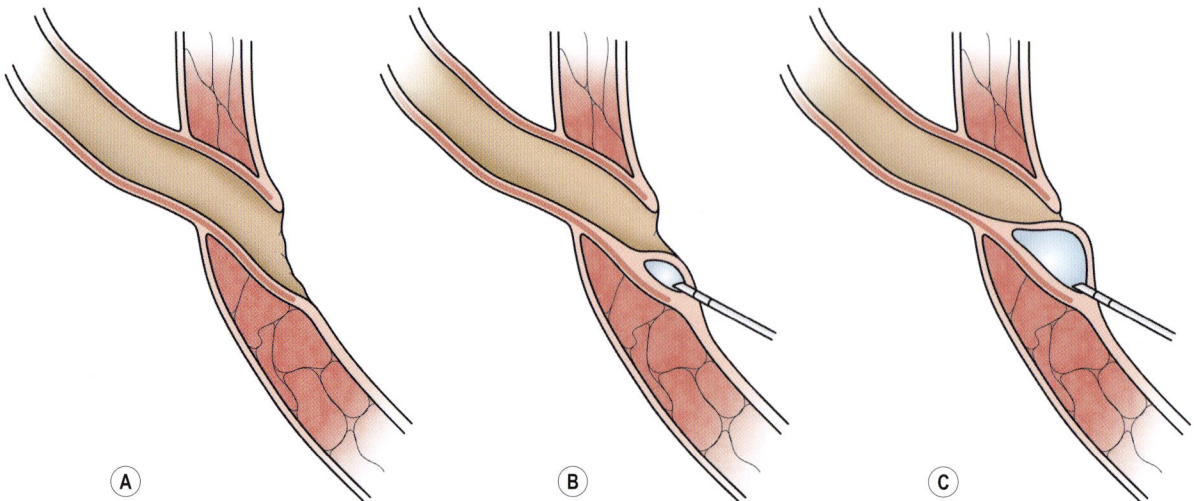

FIGURE 55-15 ■ Technique of subureteric transurethral injection of dextranomer/hyaluronic acid copolymer (STING procedure). (Figure used with permission from the Salix Corporation®, Raleigh, NC, USA.)

Many different injectable materials have subsequently been investigated and reported.[118–120] This ambulatory procedure performed under a brief general anesthetic has low morbidity and children may return to full activity as soon as the next day. The initial success rates were promising; however, they did not quite match those of ureteral reimplantation.[121]

In 2001, the Food and Drug Administration approved dextranomer/hyaluronic acid copolymer (Deflux) as the first injectable substance indicated in the USA for grades I–IV vesicoureteral reflux.[122] This substance is biodegradable, has no immunogenic properties, and does not seem to have potential for malignant transformation. Results vary, but most studies show success rates of around 70–80% for abolishing reflux.[122–125] Higher success rates with larger injected volumes and multiple injection sites have been reported.[126] Long-term reflux resolution rates appear to be stable, but recurrence has been found a year after the procedure.[127]

Other complications such as ureteral obstruction appear to be very low. Dysuria, gross hematuria, and urinary frequency occasionally occur, but are self-limiting. Flank pain and fever are rare. In our institution, a VCUG and renal ultrasound are obtained 3 months after the procedure, but the cystogram is not subsequently repeated if the patient remains asymptomatic off antibiotic prophylaxis. Patients having a febrile UTI after an apparently successful procedure should be re-investigated with a VCUG to assess for recurrent reflux.[128]

REFERENCES

1. Hellstrom A, Hanson E, Hansson S, et al. Association between urinary symptoms at 7 years old and previous urinary tract infection. Arch Dis Child 1991;66:232–4.
2. Montini G, Tullus K, Hewitt I. Febrile urinary tract infections in children. N Engl J Med 2011;365:239–50.
3. Panaretto K, Craig J, Knight J, et al. Risk factors for recurrent urinary tract infection in preschool children. J Paediatr Child Health 1999;35:454–9.
4. Peters CA, Skoog SJ, Arant BS Jr, et al. Summary of the AUA Guideline on Management of Primary Vesicoureteral Reflux in Children. J Urol 2010;184:1134–44.
5. Freedman AL. Urologic diseases in North America Project: Trends in resource utilization for urinary tract infections in children. J Urol 2005;173:949–54.
6. Shaikh N, Morone NE, Lopez J, et al. Does this child have a urinary tract infection? JAMA 2007;298:2895–904.
7. Hoberman A, Chao HP, Keller DM, et al. Prevalence of urinary tract infection in febrile infants. J Pediatr 1993;123:17–23.
8. Smellie J, Hodson C, Edwards D, et al. Clinical and radiological features of urinary infection in childhood. Br Med J 1964; 14(5419):1222–6.
9. Bickerton MW, Duckett JW. Urinary tract infections in pediatric patients. AUA update series 1985;4.
10. Liao JC, Churchill BM. Pediatric urine testing. Pediatr Clin North Am 2001;48:1425–40.
11. Pollack CV Jr, Pollack ES, Andrew ME. Suprapubic bladder aspiration versus urethral catheterization in ill infants: Success, efficiency and complication rates. Ann Emerg Med 1994;23:225–30.
12. Li PS, Ma LC, Wong SN. Is bag urine culture useful in monitoring urinary tract infection in infants? J Paediatr Child Health 2002;38:377–81.
13. Edelmann CM, Ogw JE, Fine BP, et al. The prevalence of bacteriuria in full-term and premature newborn infants. J Pediat 1973;82:125–32.
14. Aronson AS, Gustafson B, Svenningsen NW. Combined suprapubic aspiration and clean voided urine examination in infants and children. Acta Paediatr Scand 1973;62:396–400.
15. Iravani A. Treatment of urinary tract infections in young women. AUA update series 1993;12.
16. Hellerstein S. Recurrent urinary tract infections in children. Pediatr Infect Dis 1982;1:271–81.
17. Pryles CV, Lustik B. Laboratory diagnosis of urinary tract infection. Pediatr Clin North Am 1971;18:233.
18. Hoberman A, Wald ER, Reynolds EA, et al. Pyuria and bacteriuria in urine specimens obtained by catheter from young children with fever. J Pediatr 1994;124:513–19.
19. Gorelick MH, Shaw KN. Screening tests for urinary tract infection in children: A meta-analysis. Pediatrics 1999;104:e54.
20. Lohr JA, Portilla MG, Geuder TG, et al. Making a presumptive diagnosis of urinary tract infection by using a urinalysis performed in on-site laboratory. J Pediatr 1993;122:22–5.
21. Durbin WA, Peters G. Management of urinary tract infections in infants and children. Pediatr Infect Dis 1984;3:564–74.
22. Liptak GS, Campbell J, Stewart R, et al. Screening for urinary tract infection in children with neurogenic bladders. Am J Physical Med & Rehab 1993;72:122–6.
23. Sheldon CA, Gonzalez R. Differentiation of upper and lower urinary tract infections: How and when? Med Clin North Am 1984;68:321–33.
24. Pecile P, Romanello C. Procalcitonin and pyelonephritis in children. Curr Opin Infect Dis 2007;20:83–7.

25. Fowler J, Stamey T. Studies of introital colonization in women with recurrent urinary infections. VII. The role of bacterial adherence. J Urol 1977;117:472–6.

26. Stamey TA, Mihara G. Studies of introital colonization in women with recurrent urinary tract infection. VI. Analysis of segmented leukocytes in vaginal vestibule in relation to enterobacterial colonization. J Urol 1976;116:72–3.

27. Roberts JA. Pathogenesis of nonobstructive urinary tract infections in children. J Urol 1990;144:475–80.

28. Rushton HG, Majd M. Pyelonephritis in male infants: How important is the foreskin? J Urol 1992;148:733–8.

29. Parsons CL, Greenspan C, Mullholland SG. The primary antibacterial defense mechanism of the bladder. Invest Urol 1975;13:72–8.

30. Koff SA, Murtagh DS. The uninhibited bladder in children: Effect of treatment on recurrence of urinary infection and on vesicoureteral reflux resolution. J Urol 1983;130:1138–41.

31. Koff SA, Wagner TT, Jayanthi VR. The relationship among dysfunctional elimination syndromes, primary vesicoureteral reflux and urinary tract infections in children. J Urol 1998;160:1019–22.

32. Asscher AW, Sussman M, Waters WE, et al. Urine as a medium for bacterial growth. Lancet 1966;2:1037–41.

33. Mannhardt W, Schofer O, Schulte-Wiserman H. Pathogenic factors in recurrent urinary tract infection and renal scar formation in children. Eur J Pediatr 1986;145:330–6.

34. Smellie J, Normand I. Urinary tract infection: Clinical aspects. In: Johnston JH, Williams DI, editors. Paediatric Urology. London: Butterworths; 1982. p. 95.

35. Hanson L. Prognostic indicators in childhood urinary infection. Kidney Int 1982;21:659–67.

36. Rushton HG, Majd M, Jantausch B, et al. Renal scarring following reflux and nonreflux pyelonephritis in children: Evaluation with 99 mtechnetium-dimercaptosuccinic acid scintigraphy. J Urol 1992;147:1327–32.

37. Shaikh N, Ewing AL, Bhatnagar S, et al. Risk of renal scarring in children with a first urinary tract infection: A systematic review. Pediatrics 2010;126:1084–91.

38. Wallace D, Rothwell D, Williams D. The long term follow up of surgically treated vesicoureteral reflux. Br J Urol 1978;50:479–84.

39. Still J, Cottom D. Severe hypertension in childhood. Arch Dis Child 1967;42:34–9.

40. Scott J. Hypertension, reflux and renal scarring. In: Johnston JH, editor. Management of Vesicoureteral Reflux. Baltimore: Wiliams and Wilkins; 1984. p. 60.

41. Sheldon CA, Geary DF, Shely EA, et al. Surgical consideration in childhood end-stage renal disease. Pediatr Clin North Am 1987;34:1187–207.

42. Cascio S, Chertin B, Yoneda A, et al. Acute renal damage in infants after first urinary tract infection. Pediatr Nephrol 2002;17:503–5.

43. Chon CH, Lai FC, Shortliffe LM. Pediatric urinary tract infections. Pediatr Clin North Am 2001;48:1441–59.

44. UTI Guideline Team C. Evidence-based care guideline for medical management of first urinary tract infection in children 12 years of age or less. (Cincinnati Children's Hospital Medical Center) Guidelines 2006;7:1–23.

45. Roberts KB. Urinary tract infection: clinical practice guideline for the diagnosis and management of the initial UTI in febrile infants and children 2 to 24 months. Pediatrics 2011;128:595–610.

46. Wan J, Skoog SJ, Hulbert WC, et al. Section on Urology response to new guidelines for the diagnosis and management of UTI. Pediatrics 2012;129:e1051–3.

47. Craig JC, Wheeler DM, Irwig L, et al. How accurate is dimercaptosuccinic acid scintigraphy for the diagnosis of acute pyelonephritis? A meta-analysis of experimental studies. J Nucl Med 2000;41:986–93.

48. Kogan BA, Kay R, Wasnick RJ, et al. 99mTc-DMSA scanning to diagnose pyelonephritic scarring in children. Urology 1983;21:641–4.

49. Hiraoka M, Hashimoto G, Tsuchida S, et al. Early treatment of urinary infection prevents renal damage on cortical scintigraphy. Pediatr Nephrol 2003;18:115–18.

50. Hoberman A, Wald ER, Hickey RW, et al. Oral versus initial intravenous therapy for urinary tract infections in young febrile children. Pediatrics 1999;104:79–86.

51. Montini G, Toffolo A, Zucchetta P, et al. Antibiotic treatment for pyelonephritis in children: Multicentre randomised controlled non-inferiority trial. BMJ 2007;335:386.

52. Johnson CE, Maslow JN, Fattlar DC, et al. The role of bacterial adhesions in the outcome of childhood urinary tract infections. Amer J Dis Children 1993;147:1090–3.

53. Keren R, Chan E. A meta-analysis of randomized, controlled trials comparing short- and long-course antibiotic therapy for urinary tract infections in children. Pediatrics 2002;109:E70–0.

54. Mattoo TK. Evidence for and against urinary prophylaxis in vesicoureteral reflux. Pediatr Nephrol 2010;25:2379–82.

55. Hutch JA, Bunge RG, Flocks RH. Vesicoureteral reflux in children. J Urol 1955;74:607–20.

56. Hodson CJ, Edwards D. Chronic pyelonephritis and vesicoureteric reflux. Clin Radiol 1960;11:219–31.

57. Noe HN. The current status of screening for vesicoureteral reflux. Pediatr Nephrol 1995;9:638–41.

58. King LR, Kazmi SO, Belman AB. Natural history of vesicoureteral reflux: Outcome of a trial of nonoperative therapy. Urol Clin North Am 1974;1:441–55.

59. Stephens FD, Lenaghan D. Anatomical basis and dynamics of vesicoureteral reflux. J Urol 1962;87:669–80.

60. Eckman H, Jacobsson B, Kock NG, et al. High diuresis: A factor in preventing vesicoureteral reflux. J Urol 1966;95:511–15.

61. Rolleston GL, Maling TM, Hodson CJ. Intrarenal reflux and the scarred kidney. Arch Dis Child 1974;49:531–9.

62. Hodson CJ, Maling TM, McManamon PH, et al. The pathogenesis of reflux nephropathy. Br J Radiol (suppl) 1975;(Suppl. 13):1–26.

63. Thomsen H, Talner LB, Higgins CB. Intrarenal backflow during retrograde pyelography with graded intrapelvic pressure. A radiologic study. Invest Radiol 1982;17:593–603.

64. Hodson CJ, Twohill SA. The time factor in the development of sterile reflux scarring following high pressure vesicoureteral reflux. Contr Nephrol 1984;39:358–69.

65. Medical versus surgical treatment of primary vesicoureteral reflux: Report of the International Reflux Study Committee. Pediatrics 1981;67:392–400.

66. Arant BS Jr. Vesicoureteric reflux and renal injury. Am J Kid Dis 1991;17:49–511.

67. Mattoo TK. Vesicoureteral reflux and reflux nephropathy. Adv Chronic Kidney Dis 2011;18:348–54.

68. Bourchier D, Abbott GD, Maling TM. Radiological abnormalities in infants with urinary tract infections. Arch Dis Child 1984;59:620–4.

69. Sargent MA, Stringer DA. Voiding cystourethrography in children with urinary tract infection: The frequency of vesicoureteric reflux is independent of the specialty of the physician requesting the study. AJR 164 1995;164:1237–41.

70. Benador D, Benador N, Slosman D, et al. Are younger children at highest risk of renal sequelae after pyelonephritis? Lancet 1997;349:17–19.

71. Ditchfield M, deCampo, JF, Nolan TM, et al. Risk factors in the developement of early renal cortical defects in children with urinary tract infection. AJR 1994;162:1393–7.

72. Deckter RM, Roth DR, Gonzales ET. Vesicoureteral reflux in boys. J Urol 1988;40:1089–91.

73. Noe HN. The long-term results of prospective sibling reflux screening. J Urol 1992;148:1739–42.

74. Wan J, Greenfield SP, Ng M, et al. Sibling reflux: A dual center retrospective study. J Urol 1996;156:677–9.

75. Chertin B, Puri P. Familial vesicoureteral reflux. J Urol 2003;169:1804–8.

76. Noe HN, Wyatt RJ, Peeden JN Jr, et al. The transmission of vesicoureteral reflux from parent to child. J Urol 1992;148:1869–71.

77. McLorie GA, Sheldon CA, Fleisher M, et al. The genitourinary system in patients with imperforate anus. J Pediatr Surg 1987;22:1100–4.

78. DeFoor W, Minevich E, Tackett L, et al. Ectopic ureterocele: clinical application of classification based on renal unit jeopardy. J Urol 2003;169:1092–4.

79. Henneberry MD, Stephens FD. Renal hypoplasia and dysplasia in infants with posterior urethral valves. J Urol 1980;123:912–15.

80. Sheldon CA, Cormier M, Crone K, et al. Occult neurovesical dysfunction in children with imperforate anus. J Pediatr Surg 1991;26:49–54.

81. Agarwal SK, Khoury AE, Abramson RP, et al. Outcome analysis of vesicoureteral reflux in children with myelodysplasia. J Urol 1997;157:980–2.

82. Koff SA. Relationship between dysfunctional voiding and reflux. J Urol 1992;148:1703–5.

83. Chandra M, Maddix H, McVicar M. Transient urodynamic dysfunction of infancy: Relationship to urinary tract infections and vesicoureteral reflux. J Urol 1996;155:673–7.

84. van Gool JD, Hjalmas K, Tamminen-Mobius T, et al. Historical clues to the complex of dysfunctional voiding, urinary tract infection and vesicoureteral reflux. The International Study in Children. J Urol 1992;148:1699–702.

85. Koff SA, Lapides J, Piazza DH. Association of urinary tract infections and reflux with uninhibited bladder contractions and voluntary sphincteric obstruction. J Urol 1979;122:373–6.

86. Paltiel HJ, Rupich RC, Kiruluta HG. Enhanced detection of vesicoureteral reflux in infants and children with use of cyclic voiding cystourethrography. Radiology 1992;184:753–5.

87. Lebowitz RL. The detection and characterization of vesicoureteral reflux in child. J Urol 1992;148:1640–2.

88. Elder JS, Peters CA, Arant BS Jr, et al. Pediatric Vesicoureteral Reflux Guidelines Panel summary report on the management of primary vesicoureteral reflux in children. J Urol 1997;157:1846–51.

89. Cohen RA, Rushton HG, Belman AB, et al. Renal scarring and vesicoureteral reflux in children with myelodysplasia. J Urol 1990;144:541–4; discussion 545.

90. Smellie JM, Normand ICS. Reflux nephropathy in childhood. In: Hodson J, Kincaid-Smith P, editors. Reflux Nephropathy. New York: Masson; 1979. p. 14.

91. Claesson I, Jacobsson B, Olsson T, et al. Assessment of renal parenchymal thickness in normal children. Acta Radiol Diagn 1981;22:305–14.

92. Smellie JM, Ransley PG, Normand ICS, et al. Development of new renal scars: A collaborative study. Br Med J 1985;290:1957–60.

93. McLorie GA, McKenna PH, Jumper BM, et al. High grade vesicoureteral reflux: Analysis of observational therapy. J Urol 1990;144:537–40.

94. Shimada K, Matsui T, Ogino T, et al. Renal growth and progression of reflux nephropathy in children with vesicoureteral reflux. J Urol 1988;140:1097–100.

95. Ransley PG, Risdon RA. Reflux and renal scarring. Br J Radiol Suppl 1978;14:1.

96. Yeung CK, Godley ML, Dhillon HK, et al. The characteristics of primary vesico-ureteric reflux in male and female infants with pre-natal hydronephrosis. Br J Urol 1997;80:319–27.

97. Marra G, Barbieri G, Dell'Agnola CA, et al. Congenital renal damage associated with primary vesicoureteral reflux detected prenatally in male infants. J Pediatrics 1994;124:726–30.

98. Makie GG, Stephens FD. Duplex kidneys: A correlation of renal dysplasia with position of the ureteral orifice. J Urol 1975;114:274–80.

99. Najmaldin A, Burge DM, Atwell JD. Reflux nephropathy secondary to intrauterine reflux. J Pediatr Surg 1990;25:387–90.

100. Cortez J, Sheldon CA. Focal and diffuse renal parenchymal lesions associated with hypertension: the urologic surgeon's approach to evaluation and managemen. In: Loggie J, editor. Pediatric and Adolescent Hypertension. Cambridge: Blackwell Scientific; 1991. p. 217.

101. Salvatierra O, Kountz SL, Belzer FO. Primary vesicoureteral reflux and end-stage renal disease. JAMA 1973;226:1454–6.

102. McEnery PT, Alexander SR, Sullivan K, et al. Renal transplantation in children and adolescents: The 1992 annual report of the North American pediatric Renal Transplant Cooperative Study. Ped Nephr 1993;7:711–20.

103. Avner ED, Chavers B, Sullivan K, et al. Renal transplantation and chronic dialysis in children and adolescents: The 1993 annual report of the North American Pediatric Renal Transplant Cooperative Study. Pediatr Nephrol 1995;9:61–73.

104. Hinchliffe SA, Kreczy A, Ciftci AO, et al. Focal and segmental glomerulosclerosis in children with reflux nephropathy. Ped Pathology 1994;14:327–38.

105. Williams GJ, Wei L, Lee A, et al. Long-term antibiotics for preventing recurrent urinary tract infection in children. Cochrane Database Syst Rev 2006;3:CD001534.

106. Mathews R, Carpenter M, Chesney R, et al. Controversies in the management of vesicoureteral reflux: The rationale for the RIVUR study. J Pediatr Urol 2009;5:336–41.

107. Casale P, Kojima Y. Robotic-assisted laparoscopic surgery in pediatric urology: an update. Scand J Surg 2009;98:110–19.

108. Zaontz MR, Maizels M, Sugar EC, et al. Detrusorrhaphy: Extravesical ureteral advancement to correct vesicoureteral reflux in children. J Urol 1987;138:947–9.

109. Wacksman J, Gilbert A, Sheldon CA. Results of the renewed extravesical reimplant for surgical correction of vesicoureteral reflux. J Urol 1992;148:359–61.

110. Minevich E, Sheldon CA. Extravesical detrusorrhaphy (ureteroneocystostomy). AUA Updates XX, 2001.

111. Jayanthi VR, McLorie GA, Khoury AE, et al. Extravesical detrusorrhaphy for refluxing ureters associated with paraureteral diverticula. Urology 1995;45:664–6.

112. Minevich E, Tackett L, Wacksman J, et al. Extravesical common sheath detrusorrhaphy (ureteroneocystotomy) and reflux in duplicated collecting systems. J Urol 2002;167:288–90.

113. Gibbons MD, Gonzales ET. Complications of antireflux surgery. Urol Clin North Am 1983;10:489–501.

114. Minevich E, Wacksman J, Lewis AG, et al. Incidence of contralateral vesicoureteral reflux following unilateral extravesical detrusorrhaphy (ureteroneocystostomy). J Urol 1998;159:2126–8.

115. Fung LC, McLorie GA, Jain U, et al. Voiding efficiency after ureteral reimplantation: A comparison of extravesical and intravesical techniques. J Urol 1995;153:1972–5.

116. Minevich E, Aronoff D, Wacksman J, et al. Voiding dysfunction after bilateral extravesical detrusorrhaphy. J Urol 1998;160:1004–6.

117. O'Donnell B, Puri P. Treatment of vesicoureteric reflux by endoscopic injection of Teflon. Br Med J (Clin Res Ed) 1984;289:7–9.

118. Leonard MP, Canning DA, Peters CA, et al. Endoscopic injection of glutaraldehyde cross-linked bovine dermal collagen for correction of vesicoureteral reflux. J Urol 1991;145:115–19.

119. Smith DP, Kaplan WE, Oyasu R. Evaluation of polydimethylsiloxane as an alternative in the endoscopic treatment of vesicoureteral reflux. J Urol 1994;152:1221–4.

120. Diamond DA, Caldamone AA. Endoscopic correction of vesicoureteral reflux in children using autologous chondrocytes: Preliminary results. J Urol 1999;162:1185–8.

121. Chertin B, Kocherov S. Long-term results of endoscopic treatment of vesicoureteric reflux with different tissue-augmenting substances. J Pediatr Urol 2010;6:251–6.

122. Elder JS, Diaz M, Caldamone AA, et al. Endoscopic therapy for vesicoureteral reflux: A meta-analysis. I. Reflux resolution and urinary tract infection. J Urol 2006;175:716–22.

123. Higham-Kessler J, Reinert SE, Snodgrass WT, et al. A review of failures of endoscopic treatment of vesicoureteral reflux with dextranomer microspheres. J Urol 2007;177:710–14.

124. Yucel S, Gupta A, Snodgrass W. Multivariate analysis of factors predicting success with dextranomer/hyaluronic acid injection for vesicoureteral reflux. J Urol 2007;177:1505–9.

125. Kirsch AJ, Perez-Brayfield M, Smith EA, et al. The modified sting procedure to correct vesicoureteral reflux: Improved results with submucosal implantation within the intramural ureter. J Urol 2004;171:2413–16.

126. Kalisvaart JF, Scherz HC, Cuda S, et al. Intermediate to long-term follow-up indicates low risk of recurrence after Double HIT endoscopic treatment for primary vesico-ureteral reflux. J Pediatr Urol 2012;8:359–65.

127. Lee, EK, Murphy JP, Gatti JM, et al. Long term follow-up of Dextranomer/Hyaluronic acid for reflux: Late failure warrants continued follow-up. J. Urol 2009;181:1869–75.

128. Traxel E, DeFoor W, Reddy P, et al. Risk factors for urinary tract infection after dextranomer/hyaluronic acid endoscopic injection. J Urol 2009;182:1708–12.

CHAPTER 56

BLADDER AND URETHRA

Patrick C. Cartwright • Brent W. Snow • M. Chad Wallis

The bladder and urethra normally function as a coordinated unit to store and discharge urine from the body. Both structural and functional disorders of the bladder or urethra may be responsible for bleeding, incontinence, infection, discomfort, pain, and obstruction that can cause upper tract deterioration to the point of compromising renal function. This chapter focuses on the major diseases and dysfunctional conditions of the bladder and urethra as a unit and the management of such problems.

The bladder and upper urethra are composed of bundles of smooth muscle fibers arranged in a reticular lattice, the outermost bundles being more circular and the inner bundles more longitudinal in orientation at the bladder neck.[1] The smooth muscle bundles blend into the striated muscle of the external urethral sphincter, which is derived from the pelvic diaphragm. The bladder is lined by transitional epithelium, which is sensitive to irritants such as bacterial toxins and various urinary crystals. The urethra and trigone are especially sensitive, and the presence of any irritant in these areas can create significant discomfort.

Proper function of the lower urinary tract depends on intact autonomic and somatic nervous innervation. The detrusor muscle of the bladder is innervated by both sympathetic and parasympathetic fibers. Storage functions are mediated by the sympathetic component, which arises from spinal levels T10–L1. The chemical mediator of this process is norepinephrine, which acts on β-adrenergic receptors in the fundus of the bladder and causes muscle relaxation for low-pressure storage of urine. The same sympathetic stimulus acts on the β-adrenergic receptors of the trigone, bladder neck, and proximal urethra to increase internal sphincter activity and promote continence during urine storage by maintaining outlet resistance. The external urinary sphincter, innervated by the pudendal nerve, progressively increases its tone as the bladder fills, providing additional resistance. As the child develops, the external sphincter may be consciously contracted at times of urgency or stress to prevent the unwanted passage of urine. Properly coordinated function of the external urinary sphincter relies on an intact sacral reflex arc which should be well developed in normal infants, but is variably functional in infants with spinal cord abnormalities or pelvic lesions.[2,3]

The sensation of bladder fullness initiates a response in toilet-trained children that causes them to discharge their urine. When ready, the parasympathetic nervous system, via acetylcholine, causes cholinergic fibers of the detrusor to contract, resulting in a widened and shortened proximal urethra, eliminating its resistance to outflow. With relaxation of the volitional external sphincter, the bladder empties by sustained and complete contraction of the detrusor, leaving a residual urine volume of less than 5 mL.

Spinal pathways connect the sacral micturition center with three areas in the brain stem, collectively referred to as the pontine micturition center.[4] This center functions to inhibit urination during storage and to produce external sphincter relaxation during the voiding phase. Above this level are areas of cerebral cortex which oversee and modulate the autonomic process. It is the mature, integrated function of all these components that produces urinary continence.

Toilet training is, in large part, a learned phenomenon. It requires adequate recognition by the brain that micturition would be socially unacceptable in a given situation. With maturation, the bladder gains capacity, allowing for longer intervals between voiding. The approximate bladder volume in ounces may be estimated in a child as age in years plus 2. It may also be calculated by a more precise formula if needed.[5] Infants void 20 times per day, which decreases to about ten times per day by age 3 years.[6] The child also learns to resist the urge to void by voluntary contraction of the external sphincter until the detrusor contraction passes and the bladder once again relaxes. Thus, toilet training depends on the development of voluntary detrusor sphincter dyssynergia (DSD), which at times is dysfunctional.[7] Finally, full bladder control relies on the child developing volitional control over the spinal micturition reflex to be able to initiate or inhibit detrusor contractions. Most children attain day and night continence by 4 years of age.

Urinary incontinence may be in part due to immaturity of the bladder and its nervous system connections. The usual sequence of bladder development is linked to bowel development and is as follows: (1) control of bowel at night; (2) control of bowel during the day; (3) control of bladder during the day; and (4) control of bladder at night.

CHILDHOOD INCONTINENCE

Incontinence is the term used for the unintentional loss of urine after toilet training is achieved. The following definitions are clinically useful:[8]

Enuresis or nocturnal enuresis: intermittent incontinence while sleeping

Primary nocturnal enuresis: never been continent at night

Secondary nocturnal enuresis: nighttime incontinence following a dry period of at least 6 months.

Daytime incontinence: daytime wetting after toilet training

Stress incontinence: urine leakage due to physically stressful activities such as coughing.

Urge incontinence: unintentional loss of urine when bladder urgency occurs.

The discussion of incontinence is divided into sections on nocturnal enuresis and daytime incontinence, realizing that some children have both. The current recommendation for children with nocturnal enuresis and daytime incontinence is to focus on daytime treatment first followed by nocturnal enuresis therapy.

Nocturnal Enuresis

About 15–20% of children at 5 years of age continue to have bed wetting.[9–13] As so many children still wet at night before this age, it is considered within the range of normal and not termed nocturnal enuresis. After age 5, night wetting resolves at the rate of about 15% each year. By age 15 years, it has resolved in 99% of children.[13]

Etiology

Children with monosymptomatic nocturnal enuresis are, in general, physically and emotionally similar to their peers. The difference lies in their inability to awaken during sleep when their bladder is full or contracts. The etiology of this disorder is likely complex and several factors should be considered.

Genetic. Family history is significant. If both the parents had enuresis, 77% of their offspring will as well. If one parent was affected, 44% of the offspring are affected. If neither parent has a history, only 15% of their children have this problem.[12,14]

Psychological. Psychological stress can induce nocturnal enuresis in certain children. Secondary nocturnal enuresis often raises this concern. Common factors include divorce, changing homes, birth of a new sibling, trouble at school, or just starting school.

Developmental. As children grow, bladder capacity increases significantly each year at a proportion greater than urine volume produced.[11,15,16] Volitional control over bladder and sphincter also may mature at variable rates and may be related to subtle delays in perceptual abilities or fine motor skills.[17]

Urodynamic. Studies show that enuretic episodes occur when the bladder is full, and they simulate normal awake voiding.[16] Although nocturnal enuretic patients have more nighttime unstable bladder contractions, these are at low pressure and do not cause leakage.

Night wetting appears to occur in three ways: wetting associated with significant restlessness and visceral and somatic activity (deep respirations), wetting with a quick contraction and minimal movement, and wetting with no central nervous system response (parasomnia).

Sleep Disorders. Parents of children with nocturnal enuresis are generally convinced that these children sleep deeply and are difficult to arouse. However, this is probably not true. Enuretic patients sleep no more deeply than age-matched controls, wet in all stages of sleep, and show no different awakening patterns. Wetting episodes occur as the bladder fills throughout the night.[18]

Antidiuretic Hormone. Antidiuretic hormone (ADH) is released from the pituitary in a circadian rhythm so that levels are higher at night and thus diminish urine output. Some children may undersecrete ADH at night resulting in bed wetting.[19–22] Although some patients follow this pattern, others do not; the altered circadian patterns appear to normalize with maturation.[23]

Evaluation

The screening evaluation should include a history, physical examination, and urinalysis. If these are normal, then no other testing is needed because organic disease rarely causes monosymptomatic nocturnal enuresis. Any associated anomaly or problem such as urinary tract infection (UTI), sacral anomalies, or complex enuresis patterns warrant medical imaging.

Treatment

The treating physician should recognize enuresis as a symptom and not a disease. Realizing that there may be more than one cause permits the physician to consider more than one treatment option. Specific treatment is generally discouraged before the age of 7 years. Certain measures are sensible in all nocturnal enuretic patients: void just before getting into bed, avoid huge fluid loads during the evening hours, and avoid caffeine after 3:00 pm.

Enuretic Alarms. Wetting alarms are devices that fit in the underwear of the patients. When moistened, an alarm is sounded. This type of conditioning therapy requires a motivated patient and parents. A variety of products are available with either an audio alarm, a vibrating alarm, or both. In our experience, the best alarm is simply one that is easy to set up and is able to wake the child. The parent may need to help arouse the child, take him or her to the bathroom, and reset the alarm. This may occur multiple times each night, particularly at the onset of therapy. In two studies, wetting alarms were shown to give the best long-term results when compared with other treatments.[24,25] The length of treatment to achieve dryness varied between 18 nights and 2.5 months. Relapse may occur in 20–30% of treated children, but re-treatment can be successful.[25]

Medications. Imipramine, a tricyclic antidepressant, has been used for many years. The exact mechanism of action is unknown. Initial success has been reported in the 50% range. However, a recent review showed only a 20% success with a relapse rate of 96%.[26] Clinical practice reveals that the longer the initial treatment, the more benefit before the effect wanes. It is suggested that the medication be weaned slowly rather than stopped abruptly.

Side effects include anxiety, insomnia, dry mouth, nausea, and personality changes. An overdose can cause fatal cardiac arrhythmias.[27] Therefore, medication safety in the home is important. Imipramine may improve response rates to the enuretic alarm.

Desmopressin is an analog of ADH that mimics its urine-concentrating activity without the vasopressor effect.[28] The effect is dose dependent, usually requiring 20– 40 μg/day for success.

Complete dryness rates may be highest in patients with a strong family history of success. Efficacy and safety have been demonstrated in a number of studies, but long-term success remains lower than with alarm systems.[28–30] Desmopressin may occasionally have side effects, including electrolyte changes, nasal irritation, and headaches. Desmopressin is available as a nasal spray. However, this route is not approved for treating nocturnal enuresis due to a higher incidence of hyponatremia. Parents should be warned to avoid over-hydration to prevent this side effect.

Oxybutynin is the most common drug used for enuresis. It is effective when day and nighttime wetting occur in the same patient, but has no benefit over placebo when nighttime wetting is the only symptom.[31]

General Approach. Although many parents consider bed wetting a problem, they often do not consider it significant enough to treat, especially when medications are being considered. If therapy is desired, it is often most reasonable to begin with an enuretic alarm. This has the highest response rate, no side effects, and the lowest relapse rate. Combination therapy with imipramine may be considered when the alarm is not successful. If desmopressin has proved effective in a specific patient, the patient and family may choose to keep it available and use it only on specific nights when dryness is especially desired (e.g., sleepovers, campouts). Some patients do not respond to therapy, and time, reassurance, and a caring approach are all that can be offered.

Daytime Incontinence

The patient history is of paramount importance in sorting out the various categories of daytime incontinence.[32,33] The physical examination and evaluation should always assess for an abdominal mass or tenderness, distended bladder, normal genitalia, signs of spina bifida occulta, perineal sensation, sacral reflexes, gait, lower extremity reflexes, and urinalysis. Radiographic evaluation, usually voiding cystourethrogram (VCUG) and renal ultrasonography (US), are important in patients with UTI or complex incontinence patterns.

Bladder Instability

Bladder instability is by far the most common diagnosis in children with persistent daytime wetting.[34] These children are usually toilet trained, but later develop increasing 'accidents' associated with urgency. They describe not knowing that the bladder contraction was coming. They dash to the bathroom or try to 'hold it in.' Boys grab and compress the penis, and girls often cross their legs and dance around or squat with the heel compressed over the perineum (Vincent curtsy). In our experience, children with hyperactivity disorders or a willful disposition appear prone to this pattern.

Urodynamic studies demonstrate significant unstable (unwanted) contractions during bladder filling that cause leakage before sphincter contraction (or posturing) can control it. Because these unstable contractions or spasms occur frequently during the day, there develops a retentive pattern of using the external sphincter to 'hold on.' When these children do get to the bathroom and try to void, the sphincter relaxes poorly or only intermittently, resulting in stop-and-go voiding, difficulty initiating a urinary stream, straining, and poor emptying which is described by the term *voiding dysfunction* (VD). The elevated pressure during voiding and the poor emptying may result in secondary vesicoureteral reflux (VUR) and UTI. Finally, the overactivity of the urinary sphincter may carry over to the anal sphincter, making stool retention and encopresis commonly associated findings.

Treatment. Effective treatment rests on managing all aspects of this condition simultaneously. Constipation is treated with fiber or laxatives, and mineral oil after initial bowel clean-out. Recurring UTIs are managed with prophylactic antibiotics. Bladder instability is treated with timed voiding at frequent intervals (an alarm watch for the child is helpful) and anticholinergics such as oxybutynin or tolterodine.[35–37]

Biofeedback has gained in popularity for treatment of the VD. Electrodes placed on the perineum near the genitourinary diaphragm can be attached to monitors, an audio signal, or a computer display so the children can learn to relax their external sphincter voluntarily, resulting in better voiding coordination.[38–40] The process typically requires four to eight weekly visits, with follow-up as needed.

Neuromodulation has been used mainly in adults who have a refractory overactive bladder; however, there has been recent use in children. Transcutaneous electrical nerve stimulation (TENS) has been popular because of its non-invasive nature, though it requires numerous sessions. The TENS unit is thought to inhibit bladder activity via the pudendal–pelvic nerve reflex. Initial studies show promise with improvements ranging from 73–100% in small series.[41,42]

Initial success with any treatment is often followed by later relapse. If initial treatment is unsuccessful, it may be successful if re-tried later. Patients older than 8 years who fail treatment should be considered for urodynamic testing. Secondary VUR usually resolves (80%) as bladder function improves.[43] The unstable bladder of childhood is usually age limited.

Isolated Frequency Syndrome

A separate, and much less common, group of children present with acute onset of urinary frequency. They appear healthy, are normal on examination, and have normal urinalysis and culture. They do not have true urgency or any wetting, but feel that they must urinate frequently, sometimes every 5 to 10 minutes. They void a very small amount each time. Most sleep through the

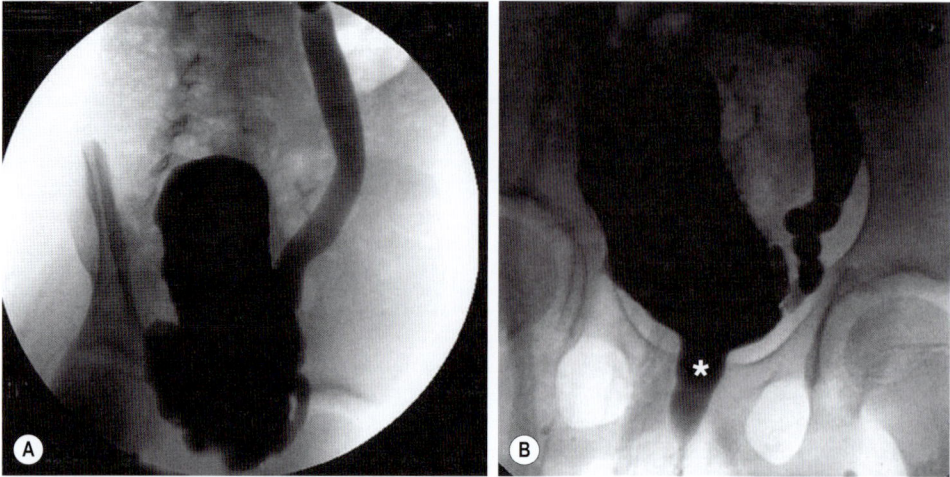

FIGURE 56-1 ■ **(A)** This cystogram shows the typical findings in a patient with Hinman syndrome: trabeculated bladder and severe reflux. **(B)** This voiding study in the same patient demonstrates dilation of the posterior urethra (asterisk) as a result of chronic contraction of the external sphincter during voiding.

night and void a large amount on awakening. The pattern may come and go over weeks or months.

The cause is unclear but is related to emotional stress in many cases. Careful assessment is crucial, and reassurance to parent and child is paramount. Sometimes, setting an alarm to progressively lengthen voiding intervals with a reward for success is helpful. This condition is benign and self-limited, although it may persist intermittently for months. Anticholinergics have no benefit, and further evaluation is not needed.

Infrequent Voider/Underactive Bladder

On the other end of the voiding spectrum are those children who void only once or twice daily and may not urinate until afternoon after waking in the morning.[44] These children have developed urinary retentive behavior without any bladder instability and have dilated, high-capacity, low-pressure bladders.[45] Some show an aversion to bathrooms or exhibit excessive neatness, whereas many others appear reasonably adjusted. They may be somewhat prone to UTI and stress incontinence.

It is important to exclude a neurologic cause and a structural obstruction to emptying. Ultrasound can demonstrate good emptying if performed before and after voiding. A timed voiding regimen is usually required to get these children to urinate regularly if problems are occurring. This pattern tends to improve with age.

Continuous Incontinence

Patients who present with total incontinence and constant dribbling have a higher probability of urinary tract anomaly pathology, and require radiographic and possibly urodynamic evaluation.

Hinman Syndrome

A small number of children demonstrate persistent incontinence, repeated febrile UTI, VUR, high bladder storage pressures, and very poor emptying.[46] This appears to be a deeply ingrained 'learned' disorder of severe voluntary DSD. In these patients, the urinary tract has the appearance of a patient with a neurogenic bladder. There is hydronephrosis, a trabeculated bladder, reflux, and sometimes progressive loss of renal function (Fig. 56–1).

Aggressive therapy with prophylactic antibiotics, anticholinergics, alpha blockers, urodynamic biofeedback training, timed voiding, or clean intermittent catheterization (CIC) may be required.[47,48] Some recalcitrant cases may require bladder diversion or augmentation to avoid renal failure. As with many 'functional' disorders, the severity of Hinman syndrome tends to wane with maturation, but progressive deterioration may not permit the surgeon to wait.

NEUROGENIC BLADDER

True neurogenic dysfunction of the bladder in childhood results from acquired or congenital lesions that affect bladder innervation. Acquired lesions may occur from trauma to the brain, spinal cord, or pelvic nerves, or as a result of tumor, infection, or vascular lesions affecting these same structures. Congenital lesions include spina bifida and other neural tube defects (most common), degenerative neuromuscular disorders, cerebral palsy, tethered cord, sacral agenesis, and other causes.[49]

The most practical way to classify neurogenic bladder abnormalities is by a simple functional system: failure to store, failure to empty, or a combination of both.[50] Failure to store urine may be caused by the detrusor muscle itself or by the bladder outlet. Detrusor hyperactivity or poor compliance causes elevated bladder pressures and incontinence on this basis. An incompetent bladder neck or urethral sphincter mechanism can be the outlet cause of failure to store urine even if storage pressures are reasonable. Failure to empty can be secondary to the hypotonic, neurogenic bladder which may not generate enough pressure to empty, or increased outlet resistance secondary to striated or smooth muscle sphincter dyssynergia. This classification helps to base treatment on urodynamic data.

Myelomeningocele

The most common cause of neurogenic bladder in childhood are neural tube defects, which range from occult spinal dysraphism to myelomeningocele.[51,52] Myelomeningocele is most common, reported in about 1 in 1,000 live births with notable geographic variations.[53,54] The etiology is multifactorial, with a clear familial association (2–5% sibling risk) and evidence that periconceptual folic acid supplementation (0.4 mg/day) reduces the risk by 60–80%.[55] Improved treatment for the neurosurgical aspects of this lesion since the late 1970s has increased the survival rate. Ninety per cent of newborns with myelomeningocele have normal upper tracts. However, if the bladder is not treated, at least half of these patients show signs of upper tract deterioration or reflux within five years.[56] Therefore, early urologic evaluation and continued follow-up is critical in these patients.[57,58]

Evaluation of the Newborn with Myelomeningocele

Fetal closure of myelomeningocele has been evaluated in a multi-institutional randomized controlled trial.[59] The results showed ventriculoperitoneal shunting was reduced by 50% at 12 months of age as was improved psychomotor development and motor function in children who underwent fetal repair. However, fetal intervention was associated with increased maternal and fetal risks. Unfortunately, there is still limited long-term data to demonstrate improved bowel or bladder function for these patients.[60]

Generally, the newborn with myelomeningocele has had a thorough neurologic assessment, closure of the lumbar defect, and possibly even ventriculoperitoneal shunting before any evaluation of the urinary tract. The level of the bony defect does not predict the functional cord level because the spinal cord lesion may be partial and patchy. Before discharge, renal and bladder ultrasound should be performed to evaluate parenchymal quality, the presence of hydronephrosis, and the size and function of the bladder. A small number of these patients have an abnormal ultrasound. In such cases, VCUG and possibly a renal scan should be performed. If the ultrasound is normal, other studies can probably be delayed a few months. About 3–5% of these patients have VUR in the newborn period. The incidence of VUR increases with time, particularly in patients with untreated DSD or detrusor hyperactivity.[49] Antibiotic prophylaxis is important and serum creatinine should be followed during the initial hospitalization. After closure of the defect, postvoid residuals should be measured before discharge from the hospital. CIC is begun if the residual urine is consistently greater than 15 ml. Crede's maneuver should be avoided because it is ineffective in emptying the bladder and magnifies the detrimental effects of high intravesical pressure if DSD or VUR are present.

Newborn urodynamic (UD) evaluation has been shown to have prognostic value in determining bladder function. Bladder pressures higher than 40 cmH$_2$O at the point of urinary leakage and those with DSD are much more likely to show upper tract deterioration or VUR.[58] Other factors known to indicate bladder 'hostility' include hyperreflexic contractions and high storage pressures.[61] Therefore, early UD evaluation (typically by 12 weeks of age) is essential to determine the frequency of follow-up studies and the timing of initiation of bladder therapy programs.

Childhood Management

Periodic reassessment of the anatomy and function of the urinary tract in patients with a neurogenic bladder is key because the clinical and UD picture may change with growth and spinal cord tethering.[62] Initiation of a bladder management program is generally undertaken when there is worsening bladder 'hostility,' VUR, hydronephrosis, or infection. If the urinary tract is stable, such management may be delayed until social continence is desired.

The cornerstone of treatment programs for neurogenic bladder is CIC. Popularized in the early 1970s, CIC has revolutionized the treatment program for these children.[62] The purpose of CIC is to provide periodic low-pressure emptying of the bladder, which can prevent or improve deterioration of the upper tracts.[63,64] In younger children, this task is performed by the caretaker. As children become older and more responsible, they can assume this task.

CIC is associated with a high incidence of bacteriuria, varying greatly in different series.[65,66] Bacteriuria is eventually found at least 60% of cases within one year, often with one or two symptomatic episodes per year.[67] In patients with no VUR and with normal intravesical pressure, asymptomatic bacteriuria appears to have little clinical significance. However, in patients with high storage pressures and/or VUR, the likelihood for upper tract infection increases significantly.[67] Infection with urea-splitting organisms (usually *Proteus* species) increases the potential for struvite stone formation.

Pharmacologic therapy for neurogenic bladder coupled with CIC is aimed at decreasing the pressures in the hypertonic, noncompliant bladder or increasing bladder outlet resistance to aid in obtaining continence. Anticholinergic drugs, such as oxybutynin, propantheline, or tolterodine, can be used to lower bladder storage pressures by blocking hypertonic detrusor activity.[68] Imipramine may also be useful alone or in combination with the anticholinergic agents because it can both relax the detrusor and tighten the outlet. Inadequate vesical outlet resistance may also respond to α-adrenergic medications, such as pseudoephedrine. Often, the combination of anticholinergics, α-agonists, and CIC is required to gain adequate continence. Side effects of the anticholinergics may sometimes limit their use. Tolterodine and extended release oxybutynin are purported to cause fewer side effects than other anticholinergics. Instillation of oxybutynin directly into the bladder can lessen the side effects and still maintain a therapeutic response. Also, the recently developed oxybutynin cutaneous patch may offer improved treatment for these patients.[69] Finally, cystoscopic injection of botulinum toxin type A received USA Food and Drug Administration approval in 2011 for detrusor overactivity in adults. Botox therapy has been applied to children with neurogenic bladder in an effort to decrease bladder pressures and increase compliance; however, data remains limited to small case series in children.[70,71] The effects of the injection are short term and repeated injections are required.

Urodynamic assessment may be elaborate in certain situations, but is usually a simple measurement of the pressure–volume relationship of the bladder during filling. It is performed using a double-lumen catheter in the bladder and involves simultaneous assessment of external sphincter function with a perineal electrode. It also can be performed with contrast material and monitored fluoroscopically to add information. Evaluation of bladder compliance, hyperreflexic contractions, leak-point pressure, stress leak-point pressure, and sphincter dyssynergia can be extremely helpful in choosing among treatment options. Figure 56-2 demonstrates the effect of anticholinergics in shifting the pressure–volume curve to the right and thus permitting the bladder to store more urine at any given pressure. Figure 56-3 shows the effect of α-adrenergic agonists on raising the leak-point pressure and thus improving continence.

It is crucial to understand that when bladder pressures remain greater than 35–40 cmH$_2$O, ureteral peristalsis does not effectively empty the upper tracts, and hydronephrosis and renal insufficiency eventually result. Thus, coupling UD data with a particular patient's estimated (or measured) hourly output permits the clinician to decide what CIC interval would keep bladder pressures in a safe range. Medications can then be adjusted to extend CIC intervals, achieve dryness, and avoid the development or progression of hydronephrosis.

In children with high bladder storage pressures and deterioration of the upper tracts that cannot be managed by CIC and pharmacologic therapy, temporary diversion with cutaneous vesicostomy may be necessary.[72,73] Protection of the upper urinary tracts from high bladder pressures is thus accomplished until such time that other treatments can be effective. We reserve this treatment for infants who have serious deterioration of the upper tract and those who, for social, medical, or anatomic reasons, cannot be managed with the other aforementioned forms of medical treatment. As an alternative, some advocate urethral dilation in girls to diminish the leak-point pressure. Surprisingly, relatively long-term benefit has been found.[74]

Surgical Treatment

Although most patients with neurogenic bladder can be managed adequately without operation, those with VUR, a poorly compliant bladder that is not responsive to medical therapy, or refractory incontinence may benefit.

Treatment of VUR in the neurogenic bladder is much the same as that for the normal bladder.[75] It is imperative that the bladder is adequately treated for poor compliance and hyperreflexia (CIC and anticholinergics) before and after operation to diminish the risk of recurrence.[76]

In some cases, bladder augmentation may be required. Bladder augmentation is designed to create a reservoir with good compliance and adequate capacity to store urine until it can be emptied by CIC at socially appropriate intervals. Detubularized segments of large or small bowel employed as a patch on the widely opened bladder (enterocystoplasty) are current popular techniques for augmentation (Fig. 56-4). Another approach is gastrocystoplasty, which was used in the 1990s, but has since fallen out of favor.[77,78] Its advantages over enterocystoplasty include a decrease in mucus formation, a possible decrease in infection, and maintenance of electrolyte balance in patients with renal insufficiency. Unfortunately, the hematuria–dysuria syndrome may affect up to one-third of patients, which limits its applicability.[79] This problem and other complications of enterocystoplasty—metabolic derangements secondary to the absorption of urine by the gastrointestinal (GI) tract, excessive mucus production, stone formation and even an increased risk of bladder cancer—have led to a search for other approaches.

Bladder autoaugmentation or detrusorectomy is an alternative augmenting technique that may prove useful in selected patients (Figs 56-5 and 56-6).[80] This approach involves removal of the detrusor muscle over the superior portion of the bladder, leaving the underlying bladder mucosa intact. This creates a large compliant surface, essentially a large diverticulum, which decreases bladder pressures and increases bladder capacity at the time of filling. The advantage of this technique is that the bladder epithelium is preserved and not replaced with gastrointestinal epithelium as in bowel augmentation,

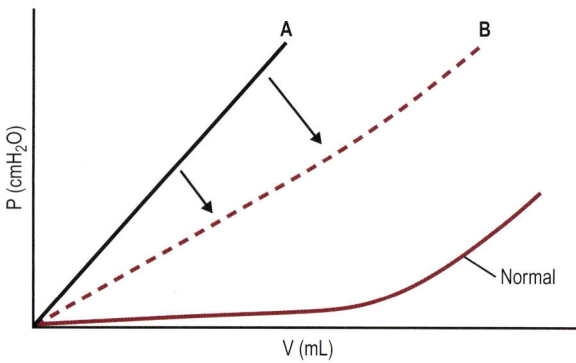

FIGURE 56-2 ■ Bladder filling pressure-volume curve in a patient with a neurogenic bladder. Note the shift of the curve to the right (A to B) when anticholinergics relax the detrusor, allowing lower pressure at any given volume.

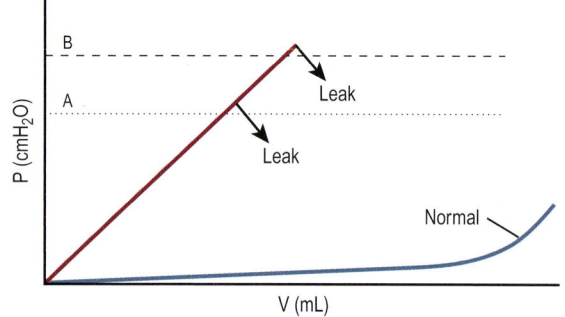

FIGURE 56-3 ■ Bladder filling pressure-volume curve demonstrating a higher leak-point pressure (from A to B), sometimes achieved with α-adrenergic agents such as pseudoephedrine and imipramine. The effect is to decrease incontinence at lower pressures.

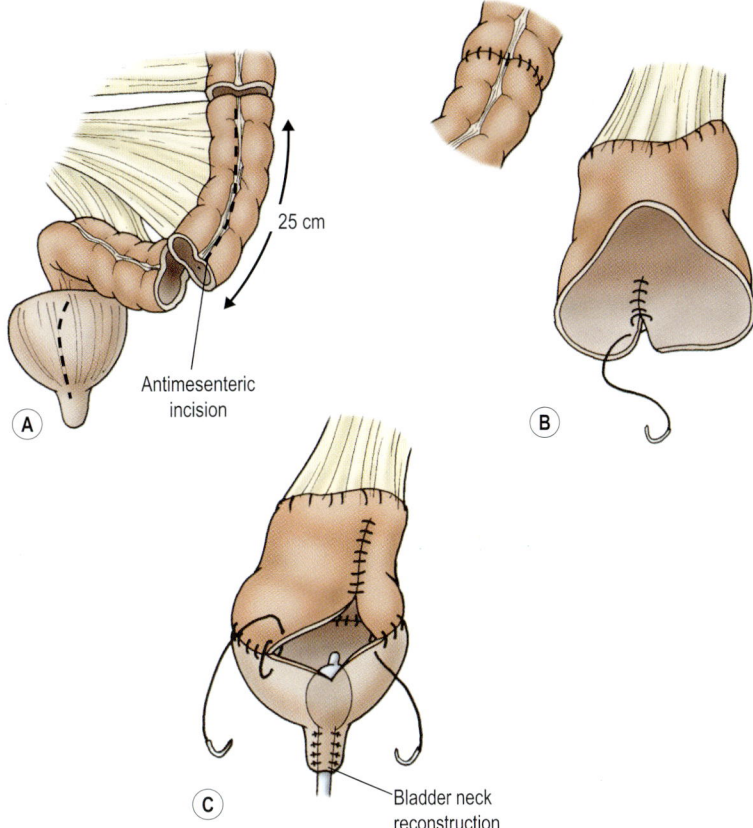

25 cm

Antimesenteric
incision

Bladder neck
reconstruction

FIGURE 56-4 ■ Bladder enlargement by enterocysto-plasty (sigmoid) and bladder neck reconstruction. Enterocystoplasty enlarges the bladder nicely but has significant potential complications, including occasional perforation, which may present as acute abdominal pain.

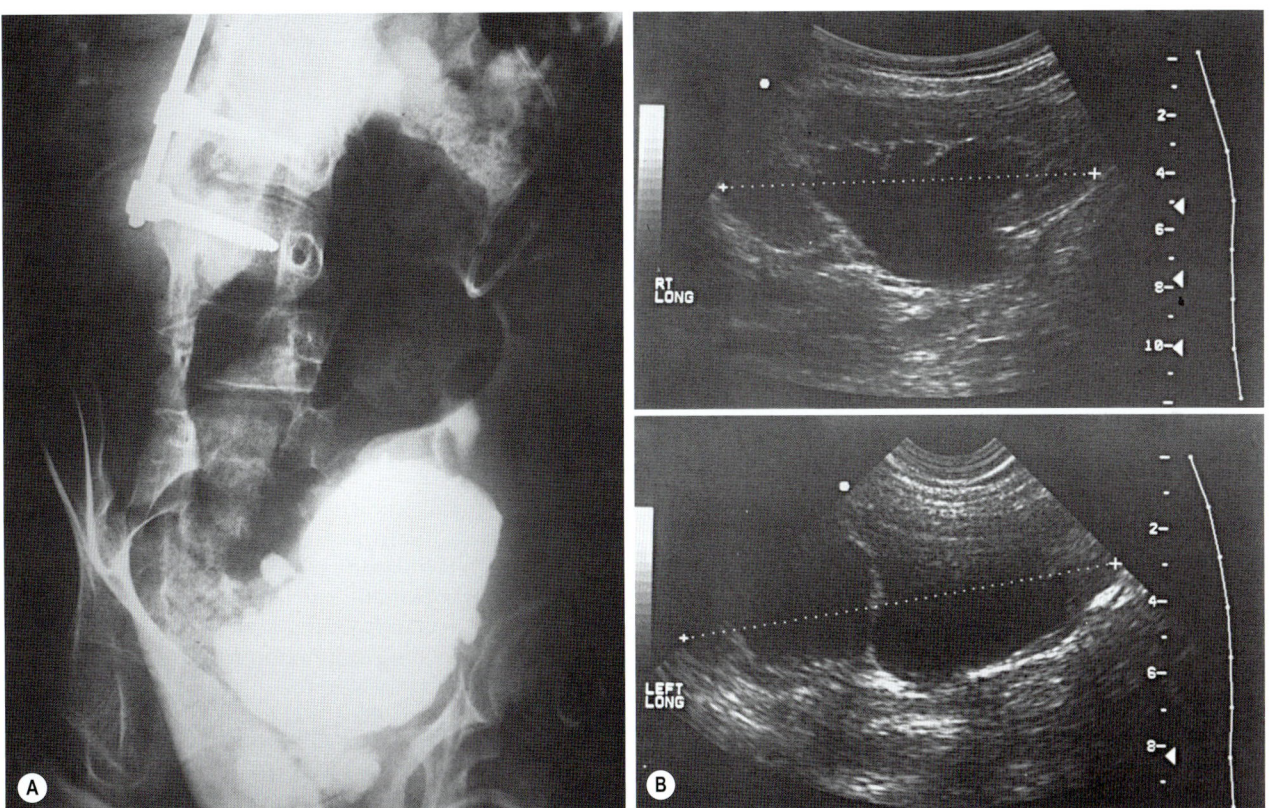

FIGURE 56-5 ■ **(A)** Radiographic and **(B)** ultrasonographic images of a patient with spina bifida showing a small, poorly compliant bladder and worsening hydronephrosis.

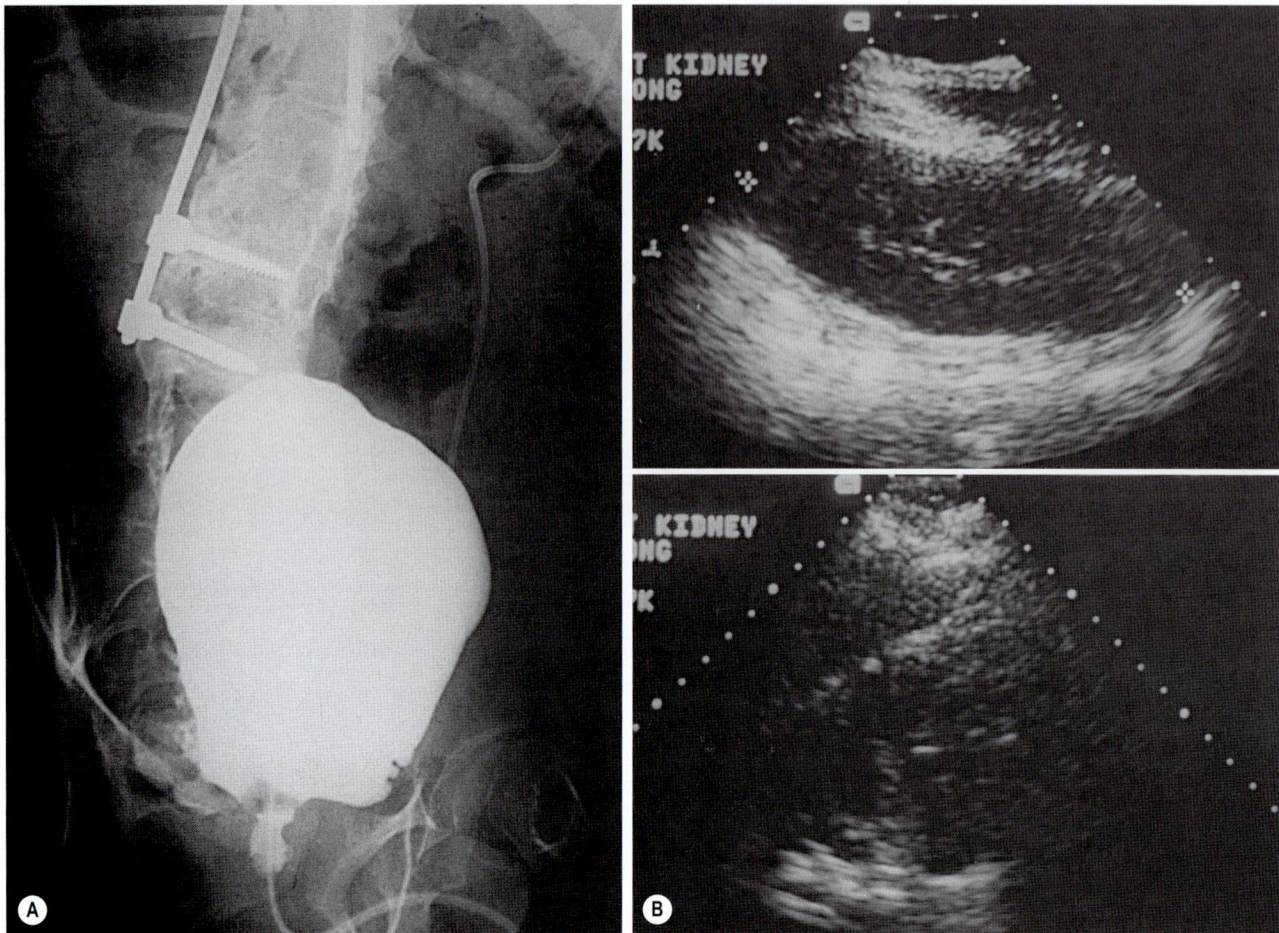

FIGURE 56-6 ■ **(A)** Radiographic and **(B)** ultrasonographic images in the patient shown in Fig. 56-5 after bladder autoaugmentation, demonstrating improved bladder capacity and better compliance, which resulted in continence and diminished hydronephrosis.

thus eliminating the problems associated with the secretory and absorptive functions of bowel mucosa. Long-term follow-up data on large numbers of children are lacking, but this technique appears to be a viable alternative for use in bladders with reasonable capacity and mainly poor compliance.[81] The concept has been extended to create 'composite' bladders by placing demucosalized bowel or stomach patches over the urothelial bulge created in autoaugmentation.[82,83] This concept of urothelial preservation during augmentation is carried forward by current innovative approaches to replace bladder wall with biodegradable scaffolds, typically seeded with urothelial and detrusor smooth muscle cells.[84]

Persistent incontinence, despite adequate treatment of the bladder to lower pressures and increase compliance, may require bladder outlet repair to increase resistance. The Young–Dees technique, which lengthens the urethra by infolding and tubularizing the trigone of the bladder, still has some advocates.[85] Kropp's procedure uses a tubularized anterior bladder strip reimplanted in the submucosa of the trigone to gain continence by a flap valve mechanism.[86] Continence is commonly achieved, but catheterization is sometimes difficult.[87] Pippi Salle's procedure creates a similar (but easier to catheterize) flap valve by onlaying an anterior bladder wall flap onto a posterior incised strip up the middle of the trigone.[88] Owing to the lack of a pop-off mechanism in both these procedures, if the bladder becomes overfilled, there is an increased potential for bladder rupture or for upper tract deterioration if high bladder pressure develops.

One of the more popular forms of increasing urethral resistance in a neurogenic bladder is by a bladder neck fascial sling.[89–93] This procedure has many advocates and involves securing a rectus fascial strip (or other material) around the bladder neck and suspending it from the anterior rectus fascia or pubis. This elevates and compresses the urethra to increase outlet resistance.

The artificial urinary sphincter is a fluid-filled pressurized cuff around the urethra or bladder neck, which can be deflated by a pump-reservoir device that permits the urethra to open and the bladder to drain (Fig. 56-7). The artificial urinary sphincter can also be used in higher-pressure bladders in conjunction with bladder augmentation.[94] The main disadvantage is that it is a mechanical device that can erode into the urethra and malfunction over time. If the device is in situ long enough, it will eventually need revision. For this reason, we prefer to use autologous tissue techniques in children, when possible.

The periurethral injection of dextranomer/ hyaluronic acid copolymer (Deflux™), Teflon, or

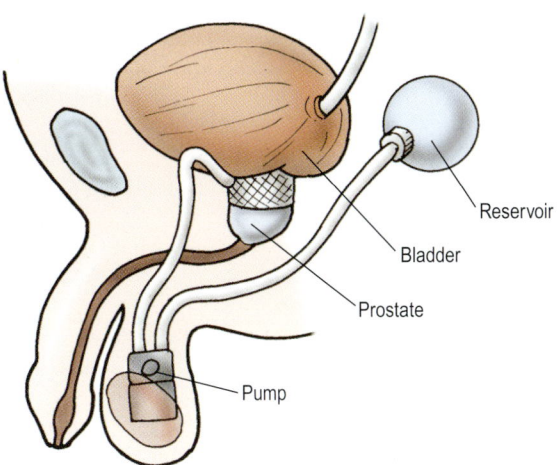

FIGURE 56-7 ■ Typical artificial urinary sphincter. The scrotal pump moves fluid from the cuff to the reservoir to permit bladder emptying.

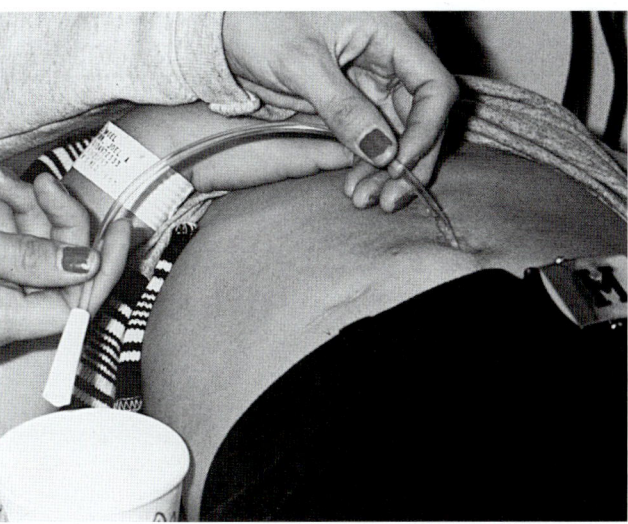

FIGURE 56-8 ■ Umbilical positioning of an appendicovesicostomy permits easy access for clean intermittent catheterization. Some patients can remain in their wheelchairs and drain the bladder into the toilet through a catheter extender.

polydimethysiloxane represents a simple, safe technique for enhancing urethral resistance in selected patients with poor intrinsic sphincter tone. It appears to be most applicable in patients requiring only a minimal increase in stress leak-point pressure. Long-term success is unlikely, and the usefulness of this approach in children is questionable.[95,96]

With all procedures to enhance resistance at the bladder outlet, it is crucial that the storage pressures of the bladder are considered simultaneously. When the bladder outlet is tightened but the bladder is unable to store increasing volumes at low pressure, hydronephrosis or VUR results. When the surgeon is considering bladder outlet reconstruction, it may be necessary to occlude the bladder neck with a urinary catheter balloon during preoperative UD assessment to determine bladder capacity and the storage pressures to determine whether augmentation is also needed.

One beneficial adjunct in patients unable to self-catheterize their urethra (e.g., owing to spinal deformity, discomfort, or false passage) is the creation of a continent catheterizable stoma. This can be performed using the appendix or another small tubularized structure implanted into the bladder and anastomosed to the skin (Mitrofanoff principle).[97,98] The implanted conduit can be hidden at the base of the umbilicus (Fig. 56-8)[99] and CIC carried out using it. Alternatively, the appendix may be left in continuity with the cecum and brought to the skin as a catheterizable channel for irrigation/enemas for the neurogenic colon. In this circumstance, a small segment of ileum can be fashioned as a catheterizable Monti–Yang stoma.[100] This concept has been a great adjunct to simplify catheterization for wheelchair-bound patients.

Cutaneous urinary diversion by ileal or colon conduit, or by cutaneous ureterostomy, is considered a last resort in these children. Long-term deterioration of the upper tracts is well documented in refluxing ileal conduits.[101] Some protection of the upper tracts is afforded by a nonrefluxing colon conduit, but the success rate beyond two decades is uncertain.[102] All reasonable efforts should be made to maintain ureteral drainage into the bladder.

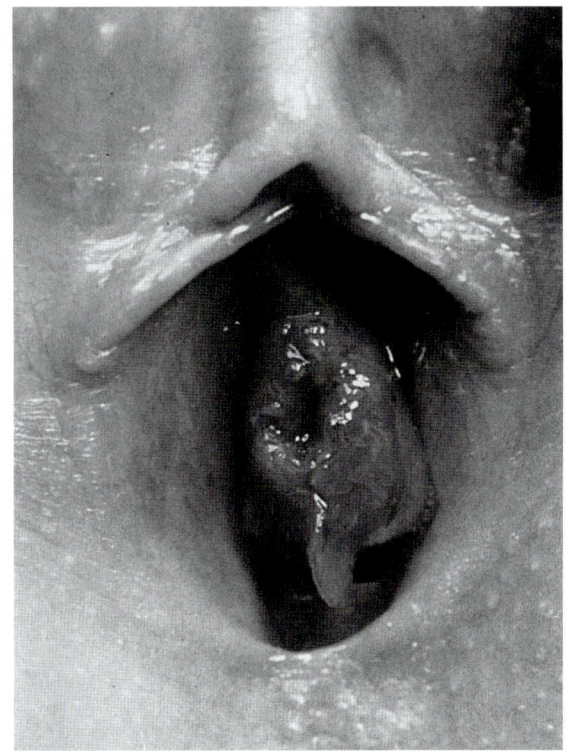

FIGURE 56-9 ■ Urethral prolapse is usually seen as a circumferential, purplish bulge at the meatus.

URETHRAL DISORDERS

Urethral Prolapse

Urethral prolapse occurs in girls at a mean age of 5 years, with those of African descent being particularly prone to this problem.[103] These patients present with dysuria, blood spotting on the underwear, and a bulging concentric purplish ring of prolapsed tissue at the urethral meatus (Fig. 56-9). Mild prolapse can be treated with an antibiotic ointment or estrogen cream applied to the area several times a day along with Sitz baths. There are times when a catheter is needed temporarily. In persistent cases, excision of the prolapsing tissue with reanastomosis of the skin edges is curative. Simple ligation of the prolapsing urethral epithelium over a Foley catheter is another described option. The prolapsed epithelium necroses and sloughs.

Meatal Stenosis

Meatal stenosis is the narrowing of the male urinary meatus following circumcision. It is thought to result from exposure and irritation of the meatus in the diaper.[104,105] For reasons that are uncertain, the stenosis is always on the ventral aspect of the meatus, causing dorsal deflection of the urinary stream that is forceful. It is important for the physician to not only examine the meatus but also watch the child void. If the stream is not narrow in caliber or is not dorsally deflected, then the meatal stenosis is not significant enough to require treatment. Occasionally, voiding causes the web to tear, resulting in dysuria or a drop of blood after urination. Some boys will have ongoing inflammation around the meatus which will respond to topical steroid application (betamethasone 0.05 %).

Meatotomy may be necessary and can be performed under general anesthesia or as an office procedure. Lidocaine/prilocaine (EMLA) cream can be applied topically, covered with a bio-occlusive dressing, and left for one hour before meatotomy with oral midazolam for sedation in selected patients. This can lead to a painless office procedure.[104] Once the glans is anesthetized, the ventral web is clamped with a hemostat and left for one minute for hemostasis. The ventral web is then incised one-half the distance to the coronal margin. Parents spread the meatus and apply ointment several times daily for 2–3 weeks. Meatal stenosis rarely recurs. Imaging studies and cystoscopy are not needed.

Megalourethra

Megalourethra is a rare genital anomaly, causing a deformed and elongated penis, that occurs in either a fusiform or scaphoid form (Fig. 56-10). These two forms differ in embryology and appearance. Megalourethra is seen more commonly in patients with prune-belly syndrome and has been reported in association with the VATER (vertebral defects, anorectal atresia, tracheoesophageal fistula, and renal dysplasia) syndrome.[105]

The less severe and most common form is the scaphoid variety, in which spongiosal tissue fails to invest the urethra.[106] The more severe fusiform variety is caused by failure of the penile mesoderm to form spongiosal tissue or corpora cavernosa within the penis.[107] It has been found in patients with prune-belly syndrome, stillborn fetuses, and patients with cloacal anomalies.[108,109] Associated urologic anomalies have been described, including megacystis, reflux, bladder diverticula, and renal dysplasia.[108] Upper tract assessment is indicated in all cases. Repair of the megalourethra relies on hypospadias techniques that tailor the urethra to a more normal size.

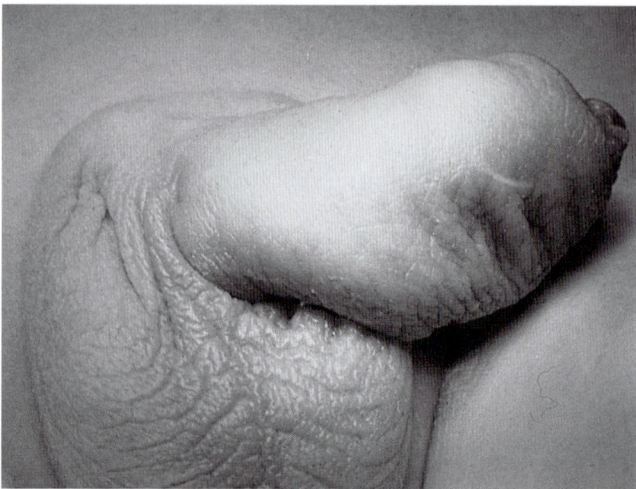

FIGURE 56-10 ■ A scaphoid megalourethra is seen in a boy with prune-belly syndrome.

Urethral Duplication

Urethral duplications occur in varied forms and can be broadly classified as dorsal or ventral to the normal meatus.[110–113] The duplication may be complete, but incomplete forms predominate. Occasionally, side-by-side duplications occur, usually associated with a duplicated phallus and bladder. Most commonly, the two channels form in the sagittal plane. The urethral channel closest to the rectum is generally the more functional conduit, having more normal spongiosal tissue and sphincter mechanism.[113] The more dorsal urethra is often small and poorly developed, and will commonly be in an epispadiac position and associated with dorsal chordee. Partial duplications that course along the penile urethra have been called Y-type duplications.[114] When the duplicated opening is in the perineum, it has been termed an H-type duplication.[115]

Treatment of urethral duplications must be individualized. When only a minor septum is present, cystoscopic division of the septum may be successful. Traditionally, with more significant duplications, efforts have been made to lengthen the ventrally-placed urethra to the tip of the penis using various hypospadias reconstruction techniques. Progressive dilation of the dorsal urethral channel to make it functional has also been advocated.[116]

Congenital Urethral Fistula

A urethral fistula can develop in the anterior urethra with incomplete development of the spongiosum, permitting a small diverticulum to form that ruptures antenatally.[117] These are uncommon and difficult to repair due to the lack of spongiosal tissue around the fistula.

Urethral Strictures and Stenosis

Most urethral strictures are acquired. Trauma, inflammatory conditions, and instrumentation by medical personnel are common causes. Congenital urethral stenosis is

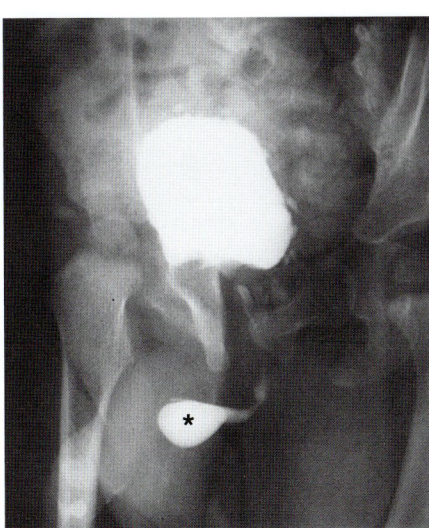

FIGURE 56-11 ■ This voiding cystogram shows an anterior urethral diverticulum (asterisk) that functions as a valve, causing outflow obstruction. Note the bladder trabeculation.

rare and generally focal. These stenoses are usually in the bulbar urethra, within the area of embryologic joining of the bulbous urethra which arises from genital folds and the posterior membranous urethra which arises from the urogenital sinus. If this junction is misaligned or incompletely canalized, a focal stricture may develop.[117]

Both of these entities can be treated with an internal urethrotomy, resection and end-to-end anastomosis, or pedicle flap/free graft urethroplasty. One report suggests a single internal urethrotomy for short strictures followed by an open repair for failures may be the best approach.[118]

Urethral Atresia

In order to be compatible with life, a patent urachus must be present when urethral atresia develops. Reconstruction can be difficult, and a vesicostomy followed by creation of a catheterizable stoma may be the best alternative.[98]

Urethral Diverticulum or Anterior Urethral Valve

A urethral diverticulum can occur ventrally when the spongiosum is absent or is thinned. The distal lip of the diverticulum functionally serves as an anterior urethral valve, blocking the urinary stream as it flows antegrade (Fig. 56-11). The diverticulum progressively fills during urination and further compresses the urethra. This valve effect can cause marked proximal dilation.[119–121] In some cases, there is a diverticulum with a narrow neck that does not function as a valve. Such a diverticulum may allow urinary stasis and can be a site of urethral infection.

The diagnosis is made either by urethrogram or cystoscopy. Treatment is accomplished by endoscopic incision in the distal lip of the neck of the diverticulum or, if more pronounced, by open excision and closure of the urethral defect.[122]

Cystic Cowper's Gland Ducts

Cowper's glands are a pair of small glands located within the urogenital membrane. The ducts from these glands course distally and enter the ventral wall of the proximal bulbar urethra. These are analogous to the female Bartholin's gland. Occasionally, these ducts become occluded, producing bulbar urethral filling defects and, occasionally, obstruction.[123] Cystoscopically, this appears to be a thin membrane over a fluid-filled cyst, sometimes called a syringocele.[124] If contrast enters a Cowper's duct, tubular channels can be seen coursing parallel to the bulbar urethra. Treatment of Cowper's duct cysts is endoscopic unroofing, but is not necessary unless there are clinical symptoms.

REFERENCES

1. Yeung CK, Sihoe JD. Non-neuropathic dysfunction of the lower urinary tract in children. In: Wein AJ, Kavoussi LR, Novick AC, et al, editors. Campbell's Urology. Philadelphia: Elsevier Saunders; 2012. p. 3411–230.
2. McGuire E, Woodside JR, Borden TA, et al. Prognostic value of urodynamic testing in myelodysplastic patients. J Urol 1981; 126:205–9.
3. Wan J, Park JM. Neurologic control of storage and voiding. In: Docimo SG, Canning DA, Khoury AE, editors. Clinical Pediatric Urology. UK: Informa Healthcare; 2007. p. 765–80.
4. Zderic S, Chacko S, DiSanto ME, et al. Voiding function: Relevant anatomy, physiology, pharmacology, and molecular aspects. In: Gillenwater JY, Grayhack J, Howards SS, et al, editors. Adult and Pediatric Urology. Philadelphia: Lippincott Williams & Wilkins; 2002. p. 1061–216.
5. Kaefer M, ZurakowskiD, Bauer SB, et al. Estimating normal bladder capacity in children. J Urol 1997;158:2261–4.
6. Goellner M, Ziegler EE, Fomon SJ. Urination during the first three years of life. Nephon 1981;28:174–8.
7. Allen T, Kaplan WE, Kroovand RL. Sphincter dysynergia. Dialog Pediatr Urol 1979;2:1–8.
8. Neveus T, von Gontard A, Hoebeke P, et al. Standardization of terminology of lower urinary tract function in children and adolescents: Report from the standardization committee of the International Children's Continence Society. J Urol 2006; 176:314–24.
9. Miller F. Children who wet the bed. In: Kolvin I, McKeith R, Meadow SR, editors. Bladder Control and Enuresis. London: W Heinemann Medical Books Ltd.; 1973. p. 47–52.
10. Tietjen D, Husmann DA. Nocturnal enuresis. A guide to evaluation and treatment. Mayo Clin Proc 1996;71:857–62.
11. Yeung CK. Nocturnal enuresis (bedwetting). Curr Opin Urol 2003;13:337–43.
12. von Gontard A, Heron J, Joinson C. Family history of nocturnal enuresis and urinary incontinence: Results from a large epidemiological study. J Urol 2011;185:2303–6.
13. Forsythe W, Redmond A. Enuresis in spontaneous cure rate: Study of 1,129 enuretics. Arch Dis Child 1974;49:259–63.
14. Bakwin H. The genetics of enuresis. In: Kolvin I, MacKeith R, Meadow S, editors. Bladder Control and Enuresis. London: WP Heinemann Medical Books Ltd.; 1973. p. 73–7.
15. Norgaard J. Urodynamics in enuresis 1: Reservoir function pressure-flow study. Neurourol Urodyn 1989;8:199–211.
16. Norgaard J. Pathophysiology of nocturnal enuresis. Scand J Urol Nephrol Suppl 1991;140:1–35.
17. Jarvelin M. Developmental history and neurological findings in enuretic children. Dev Med Child Neurol 1989;31:728–36.
18. Norgaard J, Hansen J, Nielsen J, et al. Simultaneous registration of sleep stages and bladder activity in enuresis. Urology 1985; 26:316–19.
19. Norgaard J, Pedersen E, Djurhuus J. Diurinal antidiuretic – Hormone levels in enuretics. J Urol 1985;134:1029–31.
20. Puri VN. Urinary levels of antidiuretic hormone in nocturnal enuresis. Indian Pediatrics 1980;17:675–6.

21. Rushton H, Belman AB, Zaontz MR, et al. The influence of small functional bladder capacity and other predictors on the response to desmopressin the management of monosymptomactic nocturnal enuresis. J Urol 1996;156:651–5.

22. Eller D, Austin PF, Tanguay S, et al. Daytime functional bladder capacity as a predictor of response to desmopressin in monosymptomatic nocturnal enureseis. Eur Urol 1998;33:25–9.

23. Hansen M, Rettig S, Siggaared C, et al. Intra-individual variability in nighttime urine production and functional bladder capacity estimated by home recordings in patient with nocturnal enuresis. J Urol 2001;166:2452–5.

24. Monda J, Husmann D. Primary nocturnal enuresis: A comparison among observation, Imipramine, Desmopressin Acetate and bedwetting alarm systems. J Urol 1995;154:745–8.

25. Glazener CM, Evans JHC, Peto RE. Alarm interventions for nocturnal enuresis in children. Cochrane Data Syst Rev 2005;(2):Art. No.: CD002911.

26. Glazener CM, Evans JHC, Peto R. Tricyclic and related drugs for nocturnal enuresis in children. Cochrane Data Syst Rev 2003;(Issue 3):Art. No.: CD002117.

27. Blackwell B, Currah J. The psychoparmacology of nocturnal enuresis. In: Kolvin I, MacKeith R, Meadow S, editors. Bladder Control and Enuresis. London: W Heinemann Medical Books Ltd; 1973. p. 231–57.

28. Klauber G. Clinical efficacy and safety of desmopressin in the treatment of nocturnal enuresis. J Pediatr 1989;114:719–22.

29. Rittig SM, Knudsen U, Sorensen S, et al. Desmopressin and nocturnal enuresis: Proceedings of an internal symposium. In: Meadow S, editors. London: Horus Medical Publications, England; 1989. p. 43–54.

30. Zong H, Yang C, Peng X, et al. Efficacy and safety of desmopressin for treatment of nocturia: A systematic review and meta-analysis of double-blinded trials. Int Urol Nephrol 2011;44:377–84.

31. Robson W. Diurnal enuresis. Pediatr Review 1997;18:407–12.

32. MacKeith R, Meadow S, Turner R. How children become dry. In: Kolvin I, MacKeith R, Meadow S, editors. Bladder Control and Enuresis. Philadelphia: LB Lippincott Co.; 1973. p. 3–21.

33. Bernard-Bonnin A. Diurnal enuresis in childhood. Canad Fam Physician 2000;46:1109–15.

34. Fernandes E, Veraier R, Gonzalez R. The unstable bladder in children. J Pediatr 1991;118:831–7.

35. ReinbergY, Crocker J, Wolpert J, et al. Therapeutic efficacy of extended release oxybutynin chloride and immediate release and long-acting tolterodine tartrate in children with diurnal urinary incontinence. J Urol 2003;169:317–19.

36. Munding M, Wessells H, Thornberry B, et al. Use of tolterodine in children with dysfunctional voiding: an initial report. J Urol 2001;165:926–8.

37. Goessl C, Sauter T, Michael T, et al. Efficacy and tolerability of tolterodine in children with detrusor hyperreflexia. Urology 2000;55:414–18.

38. Herndon CD, Decambre M, McKenna PH. Interactive computer games for treatment of pelvic floor dysfunction. J Urol 2001;166:1893–8.

39. McKenna PH, Herndon CD, Connery S, et al. Pelvic floor muscle retraining for pediatric voiding dysfunction using interactive computer games. J Urol 1999;162:1056–62.

40. Koenig JF, McKenna PH. Biofeedback therapy for dysfunctional voiding in children. Curr Urol Rep 2011;12:144–52.

41. Lordelo P, Teles A, Veiga ML, et al. Transcutaneous electrical nerve stimulation in children with overactive bladder: A randomized clinical trial. J Urol 2010;184:683–19.

42. DeGennaro M, Capitanucci ML, Mosiello G, et al. Current state of nerve stimulation technique for lower tract dysfunction in children. J Urol 2011;185:157–1577.

43. Koff S, Murtagh DS. The uninhibited bladder in children: Effect of treatment on recurrence of urinary infection and vesico-ureteral reflux. J Urol 1983;130:1158–60.

44. DeLuca F, Swenson O, Fisher JH, et al. The dysfunctional "lazy" bladder syndrome in children. Arch Dis Child 1962;37:197–223.

45. Bloom D, Seeley WW, Ritchey ML, et al. Toliet habits and continence in children: An opportunity sampling in search of normal parameters. J Urol 1993;149:1087–90.

46. Hinman F. Non-neurogenic neurogenic bladder (the Hinman syndrome) fifteen years later. J Urol 1986;136:769–75.

47. Austin P, Homsy YL, Masel JL, et al. Alpha-adrenegic blockage in children with neuropathic and non-neuropathic voiding dysfunction. J Urol 1999;162:1064–7.

48. Austin P. The role of alpha blockers in children with dysfunctional voiding. Scientific World Journal 2009;9:880–3.

49. Bauer S. Neurogenic voiding dysfunction and non-surgical management. In: Docimo SG, Canning DA, Houry AE, editors. Clinical Pediatric Urology. UK: Informa Healthcare; 2007. p. 781–818.

50. Steers W, Barrett DM, Wein AJ. Voiding dysfunction: diagnosis, classification and management. In: Gillenwater JY, Grayhack JT, Howards SS, et al, editors. Adult and Pediatric Urology. Philadelphia: Lippincott Williams & Wilkins; 2002. p. 1115–216.

51. Mandell J, Bauer SB, Hallett M, et al. Occult spinal Dysraphism: A rare but detectable cause of voiding dysfunction. Urol Clin North Am 1980;7:349–56.

52. Kaplan W. Management of myelomeningocele. Urol Clin North Am 1985;12:93–101.

53. MacLellan DL, Bauer SB. Infection of the lower urinary tract. In Wein AJ, Kavoussi LR, Novick AC, et al, editors. Campbell's Urology. Philadelphia: Elsevier Saunders; 2012. p. 2193–216.

54. Bauer S, Joseph DB. Management of the obstructed urinary tract associated with neurogenic bladder dysfunction. Urol Clin North Am 1990;17:395–406.

55. Weler M, Shapiro S, Mitchell AA. Periconceptual folic acid exposure and risk of occult neural tube defects. JAMA 1993;269:1257–63.

56. Bauer S, Hallett M, Khoshbin S, et al. Predictive value of urodynamic evaluation in newborns with myelodysplasia. JAMA 1984;252:650–2.

57. Wang S, McGuire EJ, Bloom DA. A bladder pressure management system for myelodysplasia: Clinical outcome. J Urol 1988;140:1499–502.

58. Galloway N, Mekras JA, Helms M, et al. An objective score to predict upper tract deterioration in myelodysplasia. J Urol 1991;145:535–7.

59. Adzick NS, Thom EA, Spong CY, et al. A randomized trial of prenatal versus postnatal repair of myelomeningocele. N Engl J Med 2011;364:993–1004

60. Carr MC. Fetal myelomeningocele repair: Urologic aspects. Curr Opin Urol 2007;17:257–61.

61. Tarcan R, Bauer S, Olmedo E, et al. Long-term follow up of newborns with myelodysplasia and normal urodynamic findings: Is it necessary? J Urol 2001;165:564–7.

62. Lapides J, Diokno AC, Silber SJ, et al. Clean intermittent self-catheterization in the treatment of urinary tract disease. J Urol 1971;107:458–62.

63. Klose A, Sackett CK, Mesrobian H. Management of children with myelodysplasia: Urologic alternatives. J Urol 1990;144:1446–9.

64. Joseph D, Bauser SB, Colodny AH, et al. Clean intermittent catheterization of infants with neurogenic bladder. Pediatrics 1989;84:78–82.

65. Cass A. Urinary tract complications in myelomeningocele patients. J Urol 1976;115:102–4.

66. Plunkett J, Braren V. Clean intermittent catheterization in children. J Urol 1979;121:469–71.

67. Klauber G, Sant GR. Complications of intermittent catheterization. Urol Clin North Am 1983;10:557–62.

68. Abrams P. Tolterodine, a new antimuscarinic agent: As effective but better tolerated than oxybutynin in patients with an overactive bladder. Br J Urol 1998;81:801–10.

69. Dmochowski R, Davila G, Zinner N, et al. Efficacy and safety of transdermal oxybutynin in patients with urge and mixed urinary incontinence. J Urol 2002;168:580–6.

70. Schulte-Baukloh H, Knispel HH, Stolze T, et al. Repeated botulinum-A toxin injections in treatment of children with neurogenic detrusor overactivity. Urology 2006;66:865–70.

71. Patel AK, Patterson JM, Chapple CR. Botulinum toxin injections for neurogenic and idiopathic detrusor overactivity: A critical analysis of results. Eur Urol 2006;50:684–709.

72. Duckett JJ. Cutaneous vesicostomy in childhood. Urol Clin North Am 1974;1:485–95.

73. Mandell J, Bauer SB, Colodny AH, et al. Cutaneous vesicostomy in infancy. J Urol 1981;126:92–3.

74. Bloom D, Knechtel JM, McGuire EJ. Urethral dilation improve bladder compliance in children with myelomeningocele and high leak point pressures. J Urol 1990;144:430–3.

75. Jeffs R, Jonas P, Schillinger JF. Surgical correction of vesicoureteral reflux in children with neurogenic bladder. J Urol 1976;114:449–51.

76. Agarwal S, McLorie GA, Grewal D, et al. Urodynamic correlates of resolution of reflux in myelomeningocele patients. J Urol 1997;158:580–2.

77. Adams M, Mitchell ME, Rink RC. Gastrocystoplasty: An alternative solution to the problem of urological reconstruction in the severely compromised patient. J Urol 1988;140:1152–6.

78. Adams M, Bihrle R, Rink RC. The use of stomach in urologic reconstruction. AUA Update Series 1995;14:218–23.

79. Nguyen D, Bain MA, Salmonson KL, et al. The syndrome of dysuria and hematuria in pediatric urinary reconstruction with stomach. J Urol 1993;150:707–9.

80. Cartwright P, Snow BW. Bladder augmentation: Early clinical experience. J Urol 1989;142:595–8.

81. Snow B, Cartwright PC. Bladder augmentation. Urol Clin North Am 1996;23:323–31.

82. Gonzalez R, Buson H, Reid C, et al. Seromuscular colocystoplasty lined with ureothelium: Experience with 16 patients. Urology 1994;45:124–9.

83. Dewan P, Byard R. Autoaugmentation gastrocystoplasty in a sheep model. Br J Urol 1993;72:56–9.

84. Atala A, Bauer SB, Soker S, et al. Tissue-engineered autologous bladders for patients needing cystoplasty. Lancet 2006;367:1241–6.

85. Reda E. The use of the Young-Dee Leadbetter procedure. Dialog Pediatr Urol 1991;14:7–8.

86. Kropp K, Angwafo FF. Urethral lengthening and reimplantation for neurogenic incontinence in children. J Urol 1986;135:533–6.

87. Kropp K. Management of urethral incompetence in the patient with neurogenic bladder. Dialo Pediatr Urol 1991;14:6–7.

88. Salle J, McLorie GA, Bagli DJ, et al. Urethral lengthening with anterior bladder wall flap (Pippi Salle procedure): Modification and extended indications of the technique. J Urol 1997;158:585–90.

89. McGuire J, Lytton B. Pubovaginal sling procedure for stress incontinence. J Urol 1978;119:82–4.

90. Bauer S, Peters CA, Colodny AH, et al. The use of rectus fascia to manage urinary incontinence. J Urol 1989;142:516–19.

91. McGuire E, Wang C, Usitalo H, et al. Modified pubovaginal sling in girls with myelodysplasia. J Urol 1986;135:94–6.

92. Elder J. Periurethral and puboprostatic sling repair for incontinence in patients with myelodysplasia. J Urol 1990;144:434–7.

93. Norbeck J, McGuire EJ. The use of pubovaginal and puboprostatic slings. Dialogs Pediatr Urol 1991;14:3–4.

94. Gonzalez R, Nguyen DH, Koleilat N, et al. Compatibility of enterocystoplasty and the artificial urinary sphincter. J Urol 1989;152:502–4.

95. Dyer L, Franco I, Firlit CT, et al. Endoscopic injection of bulking agents in children with incontinence: Dextranomer/hyaluronic acid copolymer versus polytetrafluroethylene. J Urol 2007;178:1628–31.

96. Lottmann HB, Margaryan M, Lortat-Jacob S, et al. Long-term effects of dextranomer endoscopic injections for the treatment of urinary incontinence: An update of a prospective study of 61 patients. J Urol 2006;176:1762–6.

97. Mitrofanoff P. Cystostomie continente trans-appendiculaire dans le traitement des vessies neurolgigues. Chir Pediatr 1980;21:297–301.

98. Cain M, Casale A, King S, et al. Appendicovesicostomy and newer alternatives for Mitrofanoff procedure: Results in the last 100 patients at Riley's Children's Hospital. J Urol 1999;162:1749–52.

99. Keating M, Rink RC, Adams MC. Appendicovesicostomy: A useful adjunct to continent reconstruction of the bladder. J Urol 1993;149:1091–4.

100. Monti P, Lava R, Dutra M, et al. Newer techniques for construction of efferent conduits based on mitrofanoff principle. Urology 1997;49:112–15

101. Cass A, Luxenberg M, Gleich P, et al. A 22 year follow up of ileal conduits in children with a neurogenic bladder. J Urol 1984;132:529–31.

102. Husmann D, McLorie GA, Churchill BM. Nonrefluxing colonic conduits: A long-term life table analysis. J Urol 1989;142:1201–5.

103. Brown M, Cartwright P, Snow B. Common office problems in pediatric urology and gynecology. In: Pediatri Clin North Am. Philadelphia: WB Saunders; 1997. p. 10911–1115.

104. Cartwright P, Snow B, McNees D. Office meatotomy utilizing EMLA cream as the anesthetic. J Urol 1996;156:857–9.

105. Fernbach S. Urethral abnormalities in male neonates with VATER association. AJR Am J Roentgenol 1991;156:137–40.

106. Stephens F, Smith ED, Huston JM. Congenital intrinsic lesions of the anterior urethra. In: Congenital Anomalies of the Urinary and Genital Tracts. Oxford, England: Isis Media; 1996. p. 119–24.

107. Dorairajan T. Defects of spongy tissue and congenital diverticuli of the penile urethra. Aus NZJ Surg 1963;32:209–14.

108. Hudson RG, Skoog SJ. Prune-Belly Syndrome. In: Docimo SG, Canning DA, Khoury AE, editors. Clinical Pediatric Urology. UK: Informa Healthcare; 2007. p. 1081–114.

109. Shrom S, Cromie W, Duckett J, et al. Megalourethra. Urology 1981;17:152–6.

110. Gross R, Moore T. Duplication of the urethra. Arch Surg 1950;60:749.

111. Das S, Brosman S. Duplication of the male urethra. J Urol 1977;117:452–4.

112. Woodhouse C, Williams D. Duplications of the lower urinary tract in children. Br J Urol 1979;51:461–87.

113. Salle J, Sibai H, Rosenstein D, et al. Urethral duplication in the male: Review of 16 cases. J Urol 2000;163:1936–8.

114. Williams D, Bloomberg S. Bifid urethra with three anal accessory tract (Y Duplication). Br J Urol 1976;197;47:877–82.

115. Stephens F, Donnellan W. H-Type urethral anal fistula. J Pediatr Surg 1977;12:95–102.

116. Passerini-Glazal G, Araguna F, Chiozza L. P.A.D.U.A. (Posterior augmentation by dilating the urethra anterior). Procedure of choice for treatment of severe urethral hypoplasia. J Urol 1988;140:1247–9.

117. Duckett J, Snow B. Disorders of the urethra and penis. In: Walsh P, Gittes R, Perlmutter A, Stamey T, editors. Campbell's Urology. Philadelphia: WB Saunders Co.; 1986. p. 2014–15.

118. Hsaio K, Baez-Trinidad L, Lendvay T, et al. Direct vision internal urethrotomy for the treatment of pediatric urethral strictures: Analysis of 50 patients. J Urol 2003;170:052.955.

119. Firlit C, King L. Anterior urethral valves in children. J Urol 1972;108:972–5.

120. Rudhe U, Ericsson N. Congenital urethral diverticuli. Ann Radiol 1970;13:289.

121. Williams D, Retik A. Congenital valves and diverticuli of the anterior urethra. Br J Urol 1969;41:228–34.

122. Firlit R, Firlit C, King L. Obstruction anterior urethral valves in children. J Urol 1978;119:819–21.

123. Colodny A, Lebowitz R. Lesions of Cowper's ducts and gland in infants and children. Urology 1978;11:321–5.

124. Maizel S, Stephens F, King L, et al. Cowper's syringocele: A classification of dilatations of Cowper's gland duct based upon clinical characteristics of eight boys. J Urol 1983;129:111–14.

CHAPTER 57

POSTERIOR URETHRAL VALVES

Jack S. Elder • Ellen Shapiro

Posterior urethral valves (PUV) are the most common cause of bladder outlet obstruction in boys, with an incidence of 1 in 5,000 to 8,000 male births.[1] Although the majority of boys with PUV are diagnosed antenatally, approximately one-third will be diagnosed during childhood or adolescence. PUV is the most common obstructive cause of end-stage renal disease (ESRD) in children, and is the etiology for approximately 35% of children who require renal transplantation.[2]

EMBRYOLOGY AND ANATOMY

At 5 to 6 weeks' gestation, the orifice of the mesonephric duct migrates from an anterolateral position in the cloaca to Müller's tubercle on the posterior wall of the urogenital sinus, occurring simultaneously with division of the cloaca. Remnants of the mesonephric duct normally remain as small distinct, paired lateral folds termed the inferior urethral crest and plicae colliculi. When the insertion of the mesonephric ducts into the cloaca is too anterior, normal migration of the ducts is impeded, and the ducts fuse anteriorly, resulting in abnormal ridges, which become the PUV. A smaller aperture between the leaflets causes more obstruction than those with a larger aperture and a less prominent anterior component.[3]

Three distinct types of PUV have been described. Type I is an obstructing membrane that radiates distally and anteriorly from the verumontanum toward the membranous urethra, fusing in the midline. Approximately 95% of PUV are type I, in which the valves are thought to be a single membranous structure with the opening positioned posteriorly near the verumontanum. Type III appears as a membranous diaphragm with a central opening at the verumontanum. The obstructing tissue also has been termed a congenital obstructing posterior urethral membrane.[4] It is thought that instrumentation with a urethral catheter might disrupt the posterior aspect of the membrane, resulting in the appearance of a type I valve. Type II valves are prominent longitudinal folds of hypertrophied smooth muscle that radiate cranially from the verumontanum to the posterolateral bladder neck, but these are nonobstructive and clinically insignificant.

ANTENATAL DIAGNOSIS, MANAGEMENT, AND OUTCOMES

About 10% of antenatally diagnosed obstructive uropathy is due to PUV, and approximately two thirds of PUV are diagnosed antenatally. Typical findings on ultrasound

(US) include bilateral hydroureteronephrosis, a distended bladder, and a dilated prostatic urethra, called a 'keyhole' sign.[5] Discrete focal cysts in the renal parenchyma are diagnostic of renal dysplasia. Amniotic fluid volume is variable. Those with normal or slightly reduced amniotic fluid have a better prognosis. In contrast, oligohydramnios suggests significant obstructive uropathy, and pulmonary hypoplasia secondary to renal dysplasia is common. Oligohydramnios prevents normal lung development in utero. Pathologically, this process results in reduced branching of the bronchial tree and reduced numbers and size of alveoli.

The gestational age at which hydronephrosis is recognized influences prognosis. In one study, fetuses with normal appearing renal anatomy before 24 weeks were more likely to have normal renal function than were those with hydronephrosis before 24 weeks.[6] One meta-analysis showed the best predictive value for postnatal renal function was the appearance of the fetal renal cortex.[7] A more recent study showed that ultrasound parameters alone are not able to predict postnatal renal function.[8] Prune-belly syndrome, urethral atresia, and bilateral high-grade vesicoureteral reflux (VUR) can have a similar prenatal sonographic appearance to PUV. Collectively, bladder outlet obstruction found prenatally can result in a significant (57%) incidence of renal failure by 2 years of age.[9]

In the fetus with suspected PUV and normal amniotic fluid volume, serial fetal sonograms are necessary to monitor the status of the hydronephrosis and amniotic fluid volume. If oligohydramnios develops, bladder drainage may help restore the amniotic fluid and allow normal pulmonary development. Before any intervention, a karyotype should be obtained to confirm the male gender and to detect chromosomal abnormalities, which occur in about 12%.[10] Fetal renal function is assessed with serial urinary electrolytes and β_2-microglobulin levels. Normally, fetal urine is hypotonic (favorable prognosis), with sodium less than 100 mEq/L, chloride less than 90 mEq/L, osmolality less than 210 mEq/L, and β_2-microglobulin levels less than 6 mg/L.[5] Elevated fetal urine electrolytes and β_2-microglobulin levels are an indication of irreversible renal dysfunction. Sequential bladder aspiration every 48 to 72 hours should be performed because the initial urine sample may be stagnant and fresh urine more accurately reflects the function of the fetal kidneys.[11,12]

If fetal urine is hypotonic, and oligohydramnios is present, then fetal intervention to restore the amniotic fluid volume should be considered, with the goal of preventing life-threatening pulmonary hypoplasia. This procedure has been performed in the first trimester,[13] although the majority of fetuses are diagnosed and treated in the second trimester. If the gestational age of the fetus is ≥32 weeks, early delivery is advisable. If the fetus is <32 weeks' gestation, however, the urine may be diverted into the amniotic fluid with a percutaneously placed vesicoamniotic shunt (VAS). In a recent meta-analysis, antenatal bladder drainage appears to improve perinatal survival and relieve bladder outlet obstruction, especially in those fetuses with poor prognostic criteria.[14] To date, there is no evidence that drainage of the obstructed fetal bladder will improve renal or bladder function.

In theory, VAS does not allow the bladder to cycle. Consequently, when counseling expectant parents, they need to understand that their newborn may have limited renal function or ESRD, even if the drainage procedure is successful. VAS can have complications in up to 45%.[5,15] The shunts become obstructed or displaced in 25% of cases, necessitating additional procedures that increase morbidity to the mother and fetus, and there is a 5% procedure-related chance of fetal loss. In addition, omental or bowel herniation through the fetal abdominal wall can occur.

Despite adequate bladder drainage, renal function may be so limited that the amniotic fluid volume remains low. In one study of high-risk fetuses identified in the first trimester with severe bilateral hydroureteronephrosis, bladder distention, and oligohydramnios managed with a VAS, a 60% overall survival rate and a 33% incidence of renal failure were found.[16] In a review of 14 fetuses with proven PUV and favorable fetal urinary electrolytes undergoing VAS at a mean gestational age of 22.5 weeks, six deaths occurred before term delivery. Of the surviving eight neonates, three had ESRD, and the other five had an elevated serum creatinine.[17] In a more optimistic study of 20 boys with 'lower urinary tract obstruction' managed by VAS, the overall 1-year survival was 91%. In this study, the mean birth weight was 2574 g, 40% had acceptable renal function, 20% had mild renal insufficiency, and 30% required dialysis.[18] Of this group, seven had PUV and seven had prune-belly syndrome, a nonobstructive condition. This lack of evidence regarding fetal drainage is the impetus for the study on Percutaneous Shunting in Lower Urinary Tract Obstruction (PLUTO) trial, which is an international randomized controlled trial comparing the effect of VAS versus no intervention. This study is evaluating prenatal and perinatal mortality, renal function, and other variables.[19]

Fetal ultrasound is useful in the diagnosis of lower urinary tract obstruction (LUTO). Sonographic features of LUTO include bilateral hydronephrosis, a thick wall dilated bladder, and dilated upper urethra. Unfortunately, there are a number of etiologies for this sonographic appearance, including urethral atresia, prune-belly syndrome, as well as PUV. The first two causes would not necessarily be an indication for either VAS or in utero endoscopic ablation. Percutaneous endoscopic ablation is now being performed in a few centers in the USA.[20–22] One meta-analysis showed a perinatal survival advantage using endoscopic ablation compared to observation, but there was no significant improvement in survival with ablation when compared to VAS.[23] Two small studies

have evaluated the role of fetal cystoscopy to improve the accuracy of the prenatal ultrasound findings regarding a definite etiology.[24,25] In addition, if PUV is identified at cystoscopy, then ablation can be considered.

CLINICAL PRESENTATION

Neonates with PUV not diagnosed prenatally can present with symptoms of delayed voiding or a reduced urinary stream.[15] Also, respiratory distress secondary to pulmonary hypoplasia may be the primary manifestation of PUV. Other postnatal signs and symptoms include an abdominal mass, failure to thrive, lethargy, poor feeding, urinary tract infection (UTI), and urinary ascites. Physical examination in the newborn typically discloses a palpable walnut-sized bladder, secondary to the hypertrophic detrusor muscle. Urinary ascites can result in significant abdominal distention. Older boys can have persistent diurnal incontinence or abdominal distention.

RADIOGRAPHIC EVALUATION

Significant bilateral hydroureteronephrosis and a thick-walled, distended bladder are seen on ultrasound. Corticomedullary differentiation is a favorable prognostic sign regarding renal function (Fig. 57-1). Conversely, echogenic kidneys or subcortical cysts and the loss of corticomedullary differentiation are unfavorable signs. Suprapubic or perineal ultrasound may demonstrate a dilated prostatic urethra, which is pathognomonic for PUV.

The voiding cystourethrogram (VCUG) is the only radiographic study that definitively establishes the diagnosis of PUV (Fig. 57-2). The valves appear as a defined lucency in the distal prostatic urethra. The posterior urethra is dilated and elongated. The bladder is

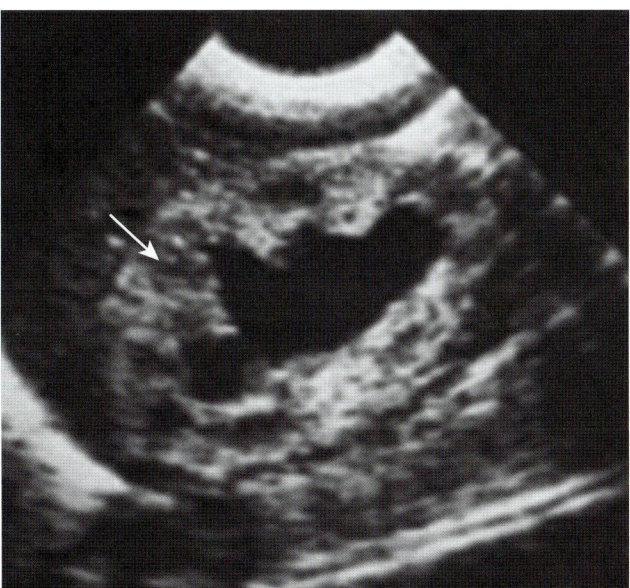

FIGURE 57-1 ■ This renal sonogram demonstrates a hydronephrotic kidney with intact corticomedullary junction (arrow) in an infant with posterior urethral valves.

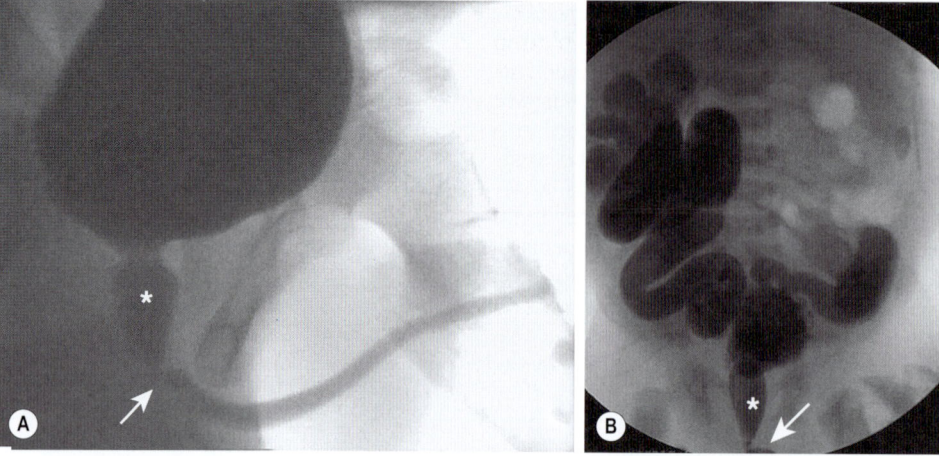

FIGURE 57-2 ■ These two voiding cystourethrograms show varying degrees of obstruction from posterior urethral valves. In both studies the location of the valves is marked with an arrow and the posterior urethra is identified with an asterisk. **(A)** There is no evidence of vesicoureteral reflux. **(B)** There is massive, bilateral grade V reflux.

trabeculated due to muscular hypertrophy with a clear delineation of the bladder neck. Unilateral VUR is present in 25% and bilateral VUR in 25% of infants with PUV.

Renal nuclear scintigraphy with a technetium-99m–labeled dimercaptosuccinic acid (^{99m}Tc-DMSA) is performed if imaging studies show thin or abnormal parenchyma in either kidney on ultrasound and/or high-grade VUR. The study should be delayed until 6 to 8 weeks of age to allow maturation of renal function. This study is effective in establishing baseline differential renal function. However, if renal function is poor, visualization of the kidneys will be suboptimal. An alternative to renal scintigraphy is dynamic contrast-enhanced magnetic resonance urography (MRU). This study provides high-resolution renal images and assessment of differential renal function, but requires an anesthetic.[26]

INITIAL MANAGEMENT

The initial treatment of neonates suspected of having PUV is to decompress the bladder with a 5 French or 8 French feeding tube. The catheter can be difficult to pass because of the valvular obstruction as well as the significant dilation of the prostatic urethra and hypertrophy of the bladder neck. The catheter tends to coil in the prostatic urethra. A Coudé tip catheter may help overcome this problem. Ultrasound can confirm placement of the catheter within the bladder. Insertion of a Foley catheter is discouraged because the inflated balloon can obstruct the ureteral orifices when the thick-walled bladder is decompressed, and can cause bladder spasm that obstruct the intramural ureters.

Amoxicillin or cephalexin prophylaxis should be initiated. Electrolytes, BUN (blood urea nitrogen), creatinine, and fluid status should be monitored carefully. The serum creatinine concentration at birth reflects maternal renal function. With satisfactory newborn renal function, the creatinine value should gradually decrease to 0.3–0.4 mg/dL. However, with limited renal function, the creatinine will remain the same or increase, even with

bladder decompression. Metabolic acidosis and hyperkalemia are common complications if renal function is impaired. Consultation with a pediatric nephrologist is invaluable because renal tubular acidosis (RTA), renal insufficiency, ESRD, and somatic growth abnormalities are common and need long-term monitoring. Neonates with respiratory distress may require immediate pulmonary resuscitation with endotracheal intubation and positive-pressure ventilation. If urinary ascites is present, paracentesis may be necessary to correct the fluid and electrolyte imbalance.

Primary Valve Ablation

Endoscopic valve ablation is performed after the neonate is stabilized. Well-lubricated infant urethral sounds should be passed to gently dilate the meatus and glandular urethra. The neonatal male urethra usually accepts a 9.5 French endoscope. Overly aggressive dilation of the urethra in order to pass a larger endoscope may lead to urethral trauma with subsequent stricture formation, and should be avoided. Vigorous dilation may also result in iatrogenic hypospadias due to splitting of the glans to the subcoronal level.[27]

An 8 French or 9.5 French cystoscope typically is used with a Bugbee electrode on low cutting current inserted through the operating channel. The valve leaflets should be incised using a low cutting current at the 5 and 7 o'clock positions (Fig. 57-3). Incision at the 12 o'clock position, where the valve leaflets fuse, also may be helpful. An alternative technique employs the Nd : YAG laser.[28] In a premature or small neonate, a cystoscope as small as 6.9 French can be used, although visualization of the PUV may be suboptimal. If urethral bleeding develops, coagulation should be performed carefully because injury to the urethra can occur with overzealous cautery. Following valve ablation, a pediatric feeding tube is left for one to two days.

A VCUG and renal ultrasound should be obtained two to four weeks after ablation to confirm satisfactory valve disruption and assess the upper urinary tracts. In addition, renal function should be monitored carefully. Valve ablation is successful in more than 90% of patients. The most common complication is incomplete valve ablation in which case repeat cystoscopy and valve incision is necessary. Urethral stricture is uncommon if small endoscopes are used.

Temporary Urinary Diversion

An alternative to primary valve ablation is cutaneous vesicostomy (Fig. 57-4). This approach is appropriate in a

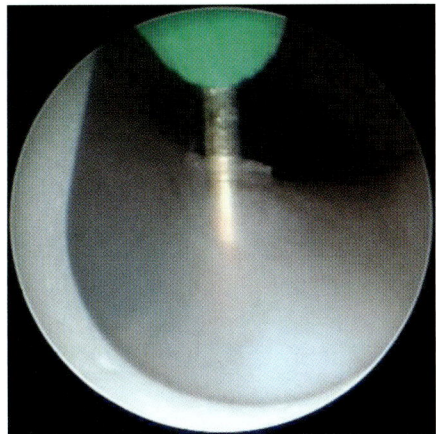

FIGURE 57-3 ■ This cystoscopic view shows valve ablation with an electrode placed through the operating channel of the cystoscope.

small or premature neonate when the pediatric cystoscope is too large for the urethra or if severe hydroureteronephrosis, urinary ascites, or high-grade VUR and poor renal function are present. In these cases, optimal upper urinary tract drainage is necessary to maintain existing renal function. The most popular technique was described by Blocksom and popularized by Duckett.[29] A small transverse incision is performed midway between the umbilicus and pubic symphysis, and the dome of the bladder is brought to the skin. The vesicostomy should calibrate to 24–26 French to avoid stenosis. Daily dilation of the stoma with a plastic medicine dropper helps prevent stomal contraction. The vesicostomy allows urine to drain directly into the diaper, obviating the need for a collection device. Complications include stomal stenosis, if the stomal size is less than 24–26 French, and prolapse, if the anterior wall of the bladder is exteriorized rather than the bladder dome.

Valve ablation should not be performed at the time of vesicostomy because the urethra will remain dry and stricture is likely. A vesicostomy allows the bladder to cycle and grow at low pressures, and does not reduce bladder capacity. These neonates should be maintained on antibiotic prophylaxis.

In the past, after insertion of a urinary catheter into the bladder, proximal diversion with cutaneous pyelostomy or cutaneous ureterostomy was advocated for neonates and infants with severe hydronephrosis and a persistently elevated creatinine.[30] Theoretically, proximal diversion provides better renal drainage than a

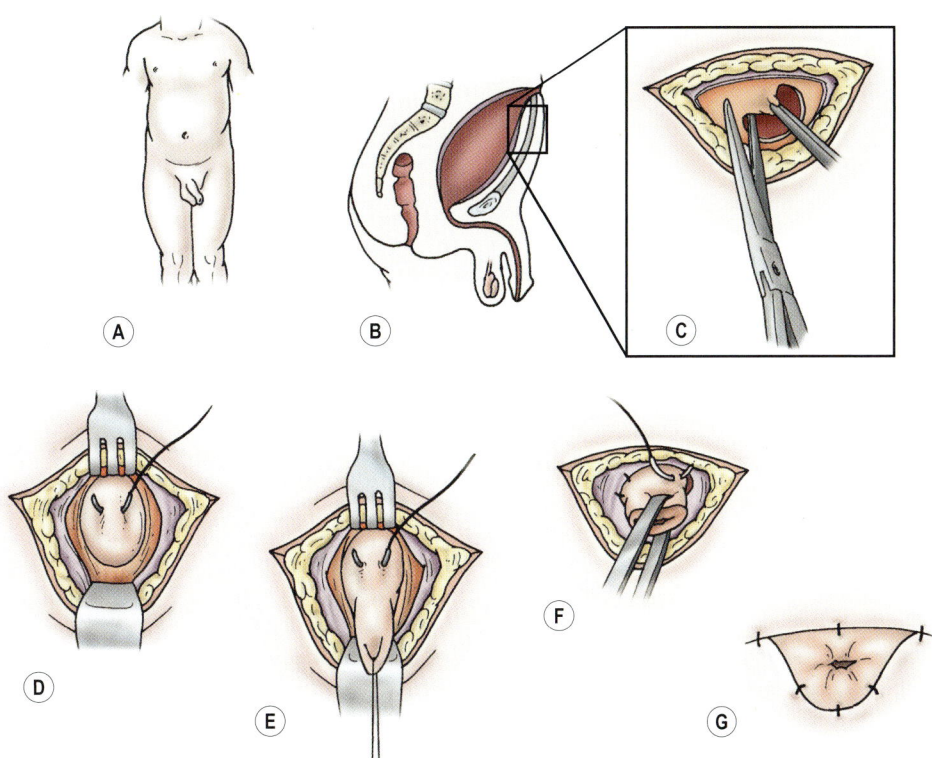

FIGURE 57-4 ■ Technique of cutaneous vesicostomy. **(A–C)** Transverse incision is made midway between the umbilicus and pubic symphysis. **(D,E)** Traction sutures are placed through the bladder, and it is mobilized superiorly to the dome of the bladder. **(F)** The detrusor should be fixed to the rectus fascia. The bladder is opened, and the mucosa is sutured to the skin. **(G)** Completed vesicostomy should be calibrated to 24 French.

vesicostomy, particularly with ureterovesical obstruction, and optimizes the potential for renal function and somatic growth. However, proximal drainage has not been shown to prevent ESRD because at least 85% of these patients have renal dysplasia.[31] In addition, by diverting the urine away from the bladder, regular cyclical bladder filling and contraction does not occur which results in a smaller, less compliant bladder.[32]

Currently, proximal diversion is reserved for the rare case in which valve ablation or vesicostomy fails to improve upper tract drainage. When needed, the preferred method of proximal diversion is the Sober-en-T ureterostomy in which the proximal ureter is divided and exteriorized on the abdominal wall (Fig. 57-5). The proximal end of the distal ureteral segment is then anastomosed to the renal pelvis. The advantage of this form of diversion is that it allows urine to drain into the bladder, thereby maintaining bladder cycling, while providing good upper tract drainage.[33] In one retrospective study of 36 boys who underwent bilateral Sober ureterostomies, the mean duration of diversion was 55 months.[34] Bladder compliance was normal in 69%, and bladder capacity was normal in 80%.

Rupture of the renal fornix with urinary extravasation and transudation into the peritoneum occurs in 5% to 15% of neonates with PUV.[35,36] Some infants develop a perirenal urinoma, whereas others have urinary ascites (Fig. 57-6). The differential renal function of kidneys with urinoma vs. those without is similar. However, with urinary ascites, significant electrolyte abnormalities can result from urinary reabsorption, and respiratory compromise may also occur from the abdominal distention.

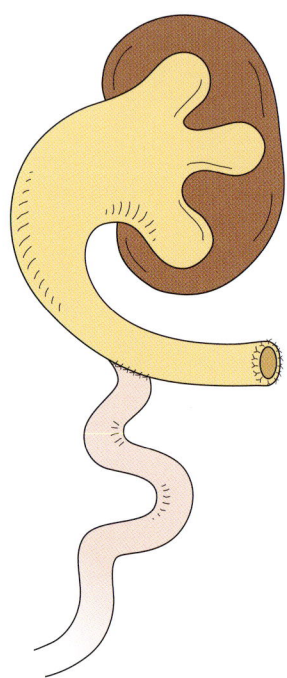

FIGURE 57-5 ■ This diagram describes the Sober-en-T cutaneous ureterostomy, which is the authors' preferred method for proximal diversion in patients with posterior urethral valves. The proximal ureter is divided and exteriorized on the abdominal wall. The proximal end of the distal ureteral segment is then anastomosed to the renal pelvis.

Evaluation for extravasation begins with ultrasound, VCUG, and renal scintigraphy. The early uptake phase of a ^{99m}Tc-MAG3 renal scan often demonstrates which kidney is involved. Inserting a 5 French or 8 French feeding tube into the bladder may decompress the bladder and upper urinary tract sufficiently that the forniceal extravasation stops. Percutaneous drainage is needed if the extravasation and the serum creatinine continue to increase, or respiratory compromise, infection, hypertension, or significant parenchymal compression develop. If extravasation persists, insertion of a percutaneous nephrostomy often solves the problem. Unfortunately, with forniceal extravasation, typically the renal pelvis is decompressed, making it difficult to insert the nephrostomy tube. In these cases, a drain can be inserted into the urinoma. Occasionally, exploration through a small flank incision may be necessary. In most cases, the kidney is intact. A cutaneous pyelostomy or ureterostomy is rarely necessary. However, in most cases, mobilizing the kidney, separating it from the adjacent peritoneum, and leaving a drain in the retroperitoneum will allow the leak to resolve, provided lower tract decompression has been achieved.

Follow-up After Initial Therapy

Antibiotic prophylaxis should be continued until the upper tract dilation improves, which may take several years if VUR persists. Most infants benefit from combined urologic and nephrologic care starting at birth. Common clinical problems include significant polyuria secondary to an inability of the kidneys to concentrate urine, metabolic acidosis (which may complicate somatic growth), renal insufficiency with hypocalcemia and hyperphosphatemia, and hypertension. If the patient remains clinically well with good somatic growth, periodic follow-up with ultrasound, electrolyte measurements, BUN and creatinine, urinalysis, and blood pressure evaluations will ensure satisfactory growth and development.

Early treatment with anticholinergic therapy (oxybutynin) may also be beneficial. In a nonrandomized study of infants with PUV, treatment with oxybutynin for two years resulted in significant reduction in high voiding pressures and significant improvement in bladder capacity.[37]

Prognosis After Initial Therapy

The prognosis for satisfactory renal function can be predicted from several factors. A serum creatinine concentration less than 0.8 mg/dL one month after initial treatment, or at age 1 year, is associated with favorable renal function.[38] Others have shown that the serum creatinine level after four to five days of catheter drainage is also predictive of long-term renal function ultimately.[39] Visualization of the corticomedullary junction differentiation on renal ultrasound is also associated with a favorable outcome (see Fig. 57-1).[40] This radiologic finding may not be present on the initial ultrasound, but may become apparent during the first few months of life. Achieving diurnal continence by the age of 5 years indicates that minimal or no bladder dysfunction is present and is also a favorable finding.[41] Another good prognostic

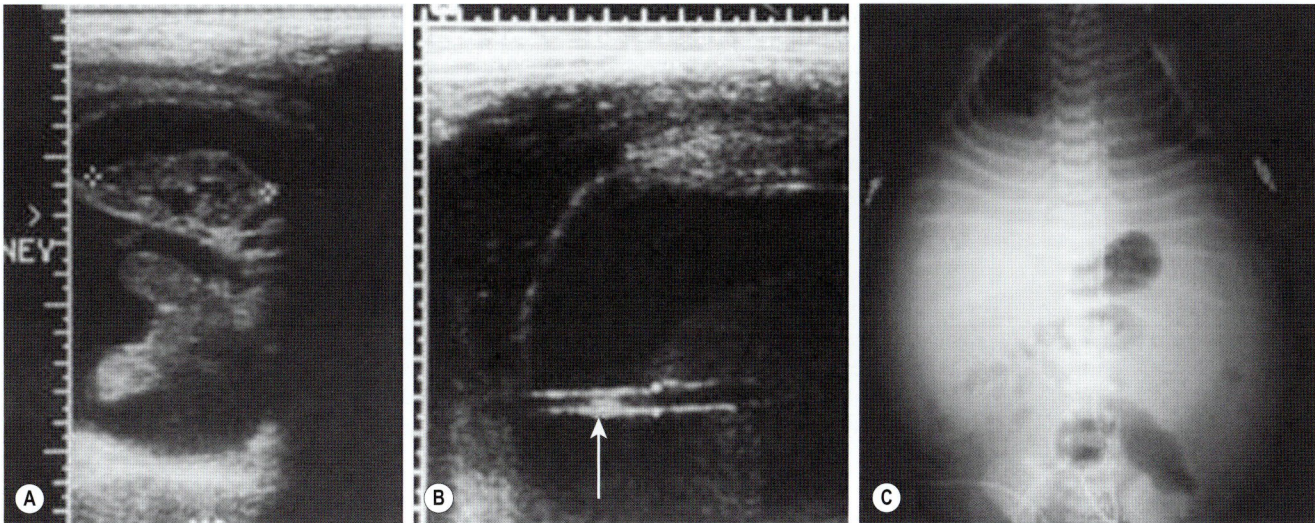

FIGURE 57-6 ■ Posterior urethral valves and ascites. **(A)** Prenatal ultrasound image demonstrating a perirenal urinoma around the right kidney, which is not hydronephrotic. **(B)** Prenatal ultrasound image showing ascites and stretched umbilical vessels (arrow). **(C)** Plain radiograph of the abdomen in a neonate with a distended abdomen from urinary ascites.

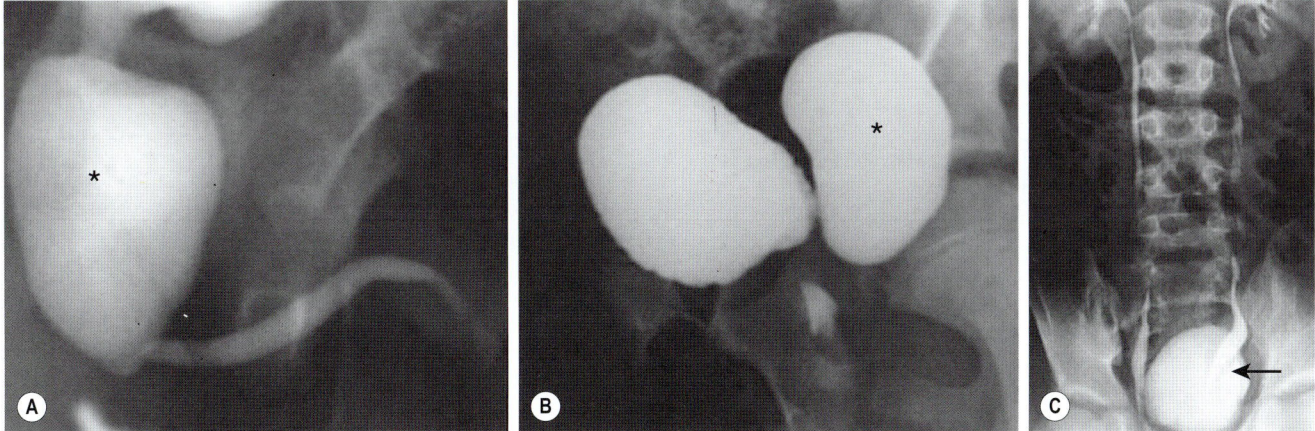

FIGURE 57-7 ■ The VURD syndrome. A 7-year-old boy was found to have posterior urethral valves and a bladder diverticulum. **(A)** The voiding cystourethrogram demonstrates a large, dilated posterior urethra (asterisk) secondary to the valves. **(B)** The lateral view of this study shows a trabeculated bladder with a large bladder diverticulum (asterisk). **(C)** The excretory urogram shows normal upper urinary tracts and deviation (arrow) of the distal left ureter due to the large bladder diverticulum. This boy underwent endoscopic valve ablation, excision of the bladder diverticulum, and left ureteroneocystostomy.

feature is the presence of a pressure pop-off mechanism such as massive VUR into a nonfunctioning kidney (termed the VURD syndrome: valves, unilateral reflux, dysplasia), urinary ascites, or a large bladder diverticulum (Fig. 57-7).[42] The concept is that the high intravesical pressure is dissipated, allowing more normal renal development. Although short-term studies have suggested that these mechanisms allow more normal renal development, at age 8 to 10 years only 30% of boys with the VURD syndrome have a normal serum creatinine.[43] One important favorable prognostic sign is the normal appearance of the contralateral kidney at diagnosis. Such patients had no UTIs or incontinence with long-term follow-up.[44] Finally, absence of reflux on the initial VCUG is also a favorable sign.

Adverse prognostic factors include bilateral VUR, persistence of the serum creatinine higher than 1.0 mg/dL after initial therapy,[45] identification of small subcapsular renal cysts (indicative of renal dysplasia), increased renal echogenicity,[46] and loss of corticomedully differentiation.[46] In addition, failure to achieve diurnal continence is an indication of bladder instability and detrusor sphincter dyssynergia (DSD), which can result in elevated upper urinary tract pressures and a gradual deterioration in renal function.

Review of studies of long-term renal function is difficult because of variable follow-up among study patients. In one report of 27 boys diagnosed between 1956 and 1970 with a 31- to 44-year follow-up, 18% died at an early age and 11% were lost to follow-up.[47] Of the remaining surviving men, 32% were uremic, 21% had moderate renal insufficiency, and 40% had signs of bladder dysfunction. This historical study does not reflect the impact of early diagnosis with prenatal ultrasound and lower tract pharmacotherapy. For example, in a more recent study of 79 cases of PUV prenatally diagnosed between 1987 and 2004, 65 were live births managed with primary valve ablation. In follow-up, only 17% had renal failure and 76% of toilet-trained men were completely continent.[48] Early gestational age at diagnosis and the presence of oligohydramnios were negative prognostic factors.

A contemporary retrospective study of 260 boys with PUV from 1992–2008 showed risk factors for progression to ESRD include nadir serum creatinine greater than 1.0 mg/dL, bilateral grade III or higher reflux at diagnosis, recurrent febrile UTIs, and severe bladder dysfunction. About 12% of these boys progressed to ESRD at a mean age of 11 years (range 5–16 years). Nadir serum creatinine and bladder dysfunction were found to be independent risk factors predictive of ultimate progression to ESRD.[49] Another recent study confirmed the high prognostic value of an elevated creatinine after primary valve ablation.[50]

LATE DIAGNOSIS

Although late presentation of PUV has been thought to be a more benign entity, studies over the past 15 years have shown that this may not be true. In a study of 47 patients, age 5–35 years, found to have PUV postnatally, common presenting symptoms were daytime incontinence (60%), UTI (40%), and voiding pain (13%).[51] Hydronephrosis was found in 40% and VUR in 33%. Serum creatinine was elevated in 35% and 10% had ESRD. If a VCUG had been performed only in those with hydronephrosis, an abnormal ultrasound, or a UTI, 30% of PUVs would not have been diagnosed.

A recent study evaluated the impact of the timing of diagnosis on long-term outcome in 52 patients with PUV who were diagnosed between 1994 and 2008.[52] Thirty-nine boys were diagnosed by 1 year of age and 13 were diagnosed after 1 year. There was no statistical difference between groups in the rate of ESRD at a mean of 7.2 years following valve ablation. In the early diagnosis group, 10% required renal transplant, while no patient in the late diagnosis group developed ESRD, suggesting a lower risk of long-term renal insufficiency. Chronic renal failure (CRF) occurred in 52% with early diagnosis who had abnormal renal parenchyma while CRF developed in 33% in the late diagnosis group who had normal appearing kidneys.

A retrospective review was performed on 141 boys with PUV that presented after birth.[53] Most (90%) patients were born after 1990 with a mean age of 46 months. The most common symptoms were UTI (28%) and voiding complaints (50%). In long-term follow-up, 12 patients (9%) had chronic renal disease. Five of the 12 had chronic disease at initial presentation without improvement following treatment, and seven of 12 developed chronic kidney disease 5 to 23 years after diagnosis. Disease progression was associated with bilateral hydronephrosis, increased severity of hydronephrosis, and bilateral VUR.

VESICOSTOMY CLOSURE

In those boys requiring early vesicostomy, the decision to close the vesicostomy should be made carefully. If febrile UTIs are noted with the vesicostomy, closure may be helpful because it will reduce the risk of bacterial contamination of the urinary tract. In other patients, closure may be necessary as a prerequisite to renal transplantation. In most cases, vesicostomy closure is performed after the upper urinary tracts have stabilized and the child is large enough to undergo simultaneous valve ablation, generally between ages 1 and 3 years. Preoperatively, a cystogram using a Foley catheter, introduced via the vesicostomy with the balloon inflated to avoid leakage of contrast, is performed to assess whether significant VUR is present and to evaluate the appearance of the bladder. If significant VUR is seen and the child is quite young, it is usually safe to close the vesicostomy at the time of valve ablation and delay reflux correction until the child is older and the bladder is larger. Anticholinergic medication is useful as long as the bladder is emptying. Following closure of the vesicostomy, the upper tracts should be monitored for worsening hydronephrosis, incomplete bladder emptying, and a significant change in serum creatinine.

VESICOURETERAL REFLUX

At the initial presentation of PUV, VUR is present in approximately 50% of boys. Half of these boys will have bilateral VUR and half unilateral. After valve ablation, nearly all patients will show improvement in reflux grade at 1 year.[32,54] Another 25% will develop spontaneous VUR. However, in these patients VUR may not resolve for as long as 3 years after initial treatment, and resolution of high-grade VUR is unlikely.[55] Antibiotic prophylaxis is continued, and periodic upper tract imaging and cystography should be performed. Renal deterioration without infection may be a sign of bladder dysfunction. Lower tract evaluation with videourodynamics is important.

VUR should be corrected if breakthrough infections occur or if it remains high grade. The efficacy of endoscopic subureteric injection therapy has not been proved, but its use remains an option. Most pediatric urologists are adept at performing ureteral reimplantation, but reimplanting thick, dilated ureters into the abnormal bladder can be challenging. A 15–30% complication rate has been reported, most often persistent reflux or ureteral obstruction.[56,57] If bilateral high-grade VUR is found, a transureteroureterostomy can be performed in conjunction with a single, long, tapered reimplant and a psoas hitch. However, if the single reimplanted ureter becomes obstructed, the upper tracts may deteriorate rapidly. If unilateral high-grade reflux into a kidney with reasonable function occurs, transureteroureterostomy into the non-refluxing ureter is an option.

In boys with unilateral VUR into a dysplastic kidney, a nephrectomy should be performed at some point. The ureter should be removed unless the bladder is small and/or poorly compliant. In this case, an ureterocystoplasty can be considered (Fig. 57-8). Postoperatively, the remaining kidney should be monitored carefully for the development of hydronephrosis because the pressure 'pop-off' mechanism has been removed.

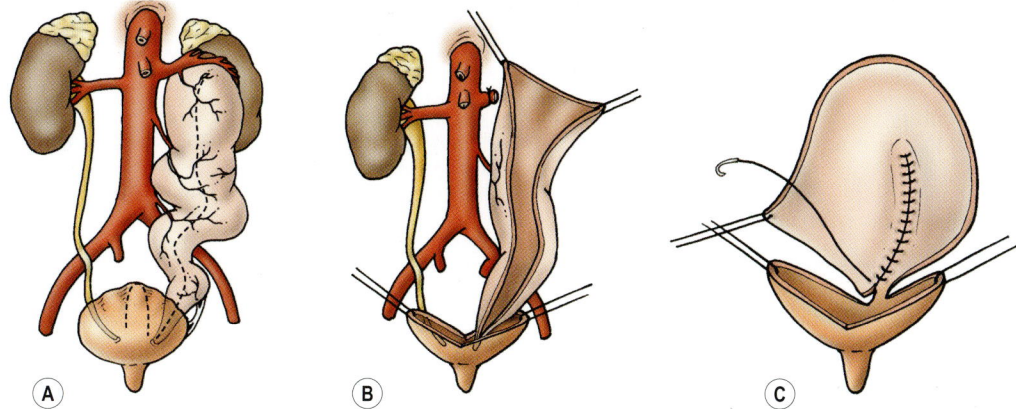

FIGURE 57-8 ■ Technique of ureterocystoplasty. **(A)** Left nonfunctional kidney and ureter are exposed. **(B)** After the left kidney is removed, the ureter is spatulated medially. **(C)** Left ureter is folded into a 'U' and sutured to opened bladder.

BLADDER DYSFUNCTION AFTER INITIAL THERAPY

The prognosis for boys with PUV depends on the status of the kidneys and the bladder at the time of diagnosis, and the method of bladder management as the child grows. In as many as 40% with PUV, ESRD or chronic renal insufficiency develops, and the vast majority of these boys have voiding dysfunction.[41] Many boys with PUV have a spectrum of urodynamic abnormalities that change over time as they age. For example, in a study of 16 prepubertal boys with PUV who were seen before age 1 year and observed from ages 4 to 14 years, initial bladder overactivity was observed.[58] Over time, however, the overactivity improved and the bladder capacity increased. Adolescent boys had a high-capacity bladder with low contractility and incomplete emptying. Other groups have reported similar findings.[59,60]

The bladder abnormalities seen in boys with PUV are manifested as incontinence and/or persistent hydronephrosis. Boys with significant urodynamic abnormalities most likely will develop severe renal functional impairment.[61] The cause of the bladder dysfunction is not completely understood, but experimental evidence suggests that fetal urethral obstruction causes irreversible changes in the smooth muscle cells of the bladder[62] and results in deposition of type III collagen in the bladder wall. In a study of fetuses with PUV, a greater than twofold increase in bladder wall thickness was demonstrated when compared to normal controls.[63]

As many as 50% of boys with PUV have ongoing daytime incontinence into late childhood.[41] Significant urodynamic abnormalities may persist following relief of the bladder outlet obstruction. Several potential causes for urinary incontinence are known in boys with PUV,[18,56] including the following:

1. Detrusor abnormalities such as (a) an overactive bladder secondary to uninhibited detrusor contractions, (b) overflow incontinence, (c) poor compliance, and (d) myogenic failure
2. High-pressure voiding secondary to incomplete valve ablation

3. DSD in which the sphincter muscle fails to relax during bladder contraction
4. Polyuria secondary to a concentrating defect as a result of long-standing obstructive uropathy that causes renal tubular damage
5. Valve bladder, which is a bladder with poor compliance resulting from fibrosis secondary to long-standing obstruction.[64–66] This clinical situation can cause secondary ureteral obstruction with worsening hydronephrosis if the bladder pressure is greater than 35 cmH$_2$O pressure (Table 57-1).

Consequently, long-term therapy for the boy with PUV includes management of the bladder as well as attention to renal function.[67–73] See Chapter 56 for more information about management of bladder dysfunction.

LONG-TERM RISK OF END-STAGE RENAL DISEASE

A recent study from Finland reported outcomes in 193/200 males with PUV from 1953 to 2003 with only seven patients lost to follow-up.[74] With a median age of 31 years (range 6–69 years), 22.8% had progressed to ESRD. The lifetime risk of ESRD in this cohort was 28.5%. The time to progression to ESRD correlated with the lowest serum creatinine value during the first postoperative year. An increased risk of ESRD was associated with early presentation, pneumothorax, bilateral VUR, and recurrent UTI following valve ablation. No patient progressed to ESRD after their mid 30s. In another series, one-third developed ESRD.[41] In a smaller series, 54% developed ESRD.[75] With improved neonatal care and management of ESRD in newborns, it is likely that the risk of ESRD will decrease.

RENAL TRANSPLANTATION

In many cases, impaired renal function can be stabilized during childhood. However, during adolescence, there may be insufficient renal reserve, and dialysis or renal

TABLE 57-1 **Pathophysiologic Changes in the Valve Bladder Syndrome**

Organ	Pathologic Process	Clinical Effect
Kidney	Dysplasia, renal tubular dysfunction	Poor renal function; polyuria
	Urine concentrating defect (polyuria)	Rapid filling of bladder, causing persistent hydroureteronephrosis and incontinence
	Renal tubular acidosis	Impaired somatic growth, bone demineralization
Ureters	Dilated with poor peristalsis	Large dead space
		Increased risk of urinary tract infection
	Fibrosis secondary to previous surgical procedures or infection	Poor drainage of upper tract
		Possible obstruction after ureteral reimplantation
Bladder	Poor compliance; small volume	High bladder pressure most of the time
	Reduced sensation to high pressure	Progressive renal functional damage
	Myogenic failure	Progressive renal and bladder damage
Bladder neck	Hypertrophy	Poor bladder emptying
		Voiding dysfunction
		Incontinence

From Close CE. The valve bladder. In: Gillenwater JY, Grayhack JT, Howards SS, et al, editors. Adult and Pediatric Urology. 4th ed. Philadelphia: Lippincott Williams & Wilkins; 2002. p. 2311–18.

transplantation becomes necessary. Retrospective studies of boys with PUV undergoing renal transplantation have suggested that the valve bladder may have a detrimental effect on graft survival. For example, in an older study, a significantly worse 5-year graft survival was noted for patients undergoing transplantation for ESRD due to PUV than was found in patients with nonobstructive abnormalities.[76] More recent studies, however, have demonstrated no difference in graft survival or serum creatinine levels between boys with PUV and children with nonobstructive causes of renal failure.[77–80] These results may reflect more effective treatment of the valve bladder in the recent past.

ADULT SEXUAL FUNCTION AND FERTILITY

Few long-term studies have evaluated the reproductive status of men who were born with PUV. Theoretically, prostate function might be affected because of elevated urethral pressure during embryonic development and ongoing voiding dysfunction. In addition, some boys with PUV have reflux into the seminal vesicles and ejaculatory ducts as well as a history of cryptorchidism, which might contribute to impaired fertility. In a recent report, sexual function was assessed using the International Index of Erectile Function.[81] There were 67 men with PUV and 102 age-matched controls with a mean age of 38 years in both groups. Increasing age was the only risk factor for developing erectile dysfunction. Only one of 61 (2%) sexually active men could not ejaculate. In this series, there was no increase in ejaculatory problems in those men who had undergone both PUV ablation and bladder neck incision, which was commonly performed several decades ago. Almost half of the men had children and four of seven with a renal transplant had children. Paternity rates were similar to the general Finnish population. Eight (12%) men had attempted to father children without success.

In another Finnish study, 68 men with PUV and 272 controls with a median age of 38.5 years responded to the Danish Prostatic Symptom Score.[82] Mild hesitancy, weak stream, incomplete bladder emptying, and straining were twice as common in patients with PUV than controls. The prevalence of lower urinary tract symptoms (LUTS) was increased about twofold in PUV men when compared to controls. Most of the study group reported little to no symptoms. Infrequently, pyospermia and reduced sperm counts were noted in men with a history of PUV and severe LUTS. Azoospermia was uncommon, but when observed, it was usually related to CRF. Another study of 16 men treated for PUV in infancy reported that sexual function and voiding symptoms were normal, and their semen analysis was adequate for fertility.[83]

REFERENCES

1. Malin G, Tonks A, Morris R, et al. Congenital lower urinary tract obstruction: A population-based epidemiological study. BJOG 2012, Epub ahead of print.
2. Penna FJ, Elder JS. CKD and bladder problems in children. Adv Chronic Kidney Dis 2011;18:362–9.
3. Krishnan A, de Souza A, Konijeti R, et al. The anatomy and embryology of posterior urethral valves. J Urol 2006;175:1214–20.
4. Dewan PA, Zappala PG, Ransley PG, et al. Endoscopic reappraisal of the morphology of congenital obstruction of the posterior urethra. Br J Urol 1992;70:439–44.
5. Elder JS. Management of antenatal hydronephrosis. In: Puri P, editor. Newborn Surgery. 3rd ed. London: Hodder-Arnold; 2011. p. 856–71.
6. Hutton KA, Thomas DF, Arthur RJ, et al. Prenatally detected posterior urethral valves: Is gestational age at detection a predictor of outcome? J Urol 1994;152:698–701.
7. Morris RK, Malin GL, Khan KS, et al. Antenatal ultrasound to predict postnatal renal function in congenital lower urinary tract obstruction: Systematic review of test accuracy. BJOG 2009;116:1290–9.
8. Bernardes LS, Salomon R, Aksnes G, et al. Ultrasound evaluation of prognosis in fetuses with posterior urethral valves. J Ped Surg 2011;46:1412–18.
9. Anumba DO, Scott JE, Plant ND, et al. Diagnosis and outcome of fetal lower urinary tract obstruction in the northern region of England. Prenat Diagn 2005;25:7–13.
10. Elder JS, Duckett JW, Snyder HM. Intervention for fetal obstructive uropathy: Has it been effective? Lancet 1987;2:1007–10.
11. Johnson MP, Bukowski TP, Reitleman C, et al. In-utero surgical treatment of fetal obstructive uropathy: A new comprehensive approach to identify appropriate candidates for vesicoamniotic shunt therapy. Am J Obstet Gynecol 1994;170:1770–9.

12. Johnson MP, Corsi P, Bradfield W, et al. Sequential urinalysis improves evaluation of fetal renal function in obstructive uropathy. Am J Obstet Gynecol 1995;173:59–65.

13. Kim SK, Won HS, Shim JY, et al. Successful vesicoamniotic shunting of posterior urethral valves in the first trimester of pregnancy. Ultrasound Obstet Gynecol 2005;26:666–8.

14. Morris RK, Malin GL, Khan KS, et al. Systematic review of the effectiveness of antenatal intervention for the treatment of congenital lower urinary tract obstruction. BJOG 2010;17:382–90.

15. Cendron M, Elder JS. Perinatal urology. In: Gillenwater JY, Grayhack JT, Howards SS, Mitchell M, editors. Adult and Pediatric Urology. 4th ed. Philadelphia: Lippincott Williams & Wilkins; 2002. p. 2041–127.

16. Freedman AL, Bukowski TP, Smith CA, et al. Fetal therapy for obstructive uropathy: Specific outcomes diagnosis. J Urol 1996;156: 720–4.

17. Holmes N, Harrison MR, Baskin LS. Fetal surgery for posterior urethral valves: Long-term postnatal outcomes. Pediatrics 2001; 108:e1–7.

18. Biard JM, Johnson MP, Carr MC, et al. Long-term outcomes in children treated by prenatal vesicoamniotic shunting for lower urinary tract obstruction. Obstet Gynecol 2005;106:503–8.

19. Morris RK, Kilby MD. An overview of the literature on congenital lower urinary tract obstruction and introduction to the PLUTO trial: Percutaneous shunting in lower urinary tract obstruction. Aust NZJ Obstet Gynecol 2009;49:6–10.

20. Quintero RA, Romero R, Johnson MP, et al. In-utero percutaneous cystoscopy in the management of fetal lower obstructive uropathy. Lancet 1995;346:537–40.

21. Quintero RA, Shukla AR, Homsy YL, et al. Successful in-utero endoscopic ablation of posterior urethral valves: A new dimension in fetal urology. Urology 2000;55:774.

22. Clifton MS, Harrison MR, Ball R, et al. Fetoscopic transuterine release of posterior urethral valves: A new technique. Fetal Diagn Ther 2008;23:89–94.

23. Morris RK, Kilby MD. Long-term renal and neurodevelopmental outcome in infants with LUTO, with and without fetal intervention. Early Hum Dev 2011;87:607–10.

24. Welsh A, Agarwal S, Kumar S, et al. Fetal cystoscopy in the management of fetal obstructive uropathy: Experience in a single European centre. Prenat Diagn 2003;30:1033–41.

25. Ruano R. Fetal surgery for severe lower urinary tract obstruction. Prenat Diagn 2011;31:661–74.

26. McMann LP, Kirsch AJ, Scherz HC, et al. Magnetic resonance urography in the evaluation of prenatally diagnosed hydronephrosis and renal dysgenesis. J Urol 2006;176:1786–92.

27. Shapiro E, Elder JS. Complications of surgery for posterior urethral valves. In Taneja SS, Smith RB, Ehrlich RM, editors. Complications of Urologic Surgery. 4th ed. Philadelphia: WB Saunders; 2010. p. 669–83.

28. Bhatnagar V, Agarwala S, Lal R, et al. Fulguration of posterior urethral valves using the Nd:YAG laser. Pediatr Surg Int 2000; 16:69–71.

29. Duckett JW Jr. Cutaneous vesicostomy in childhood: The Blocksom technique. Urol Clin North Am 1974;1:485–95.

30. Krueger RP, Hardy BE, Churchill BM. Growth in boys with posterior urethral valves: Primary valve resection vs. upper tract diversion. Urol Clin North Am 1980;7:265–72.

31. Tietjen DN, Gloor JM, Husmann DA. Proximal urinary diversion in the management of posterior urethral valves: Is it necessary? J Urol 1997;158:1008–10.

32. Close CE, Carr MC, Burns MW, et al. Lower urinary tract changes after early valve ablation in neonates and infants: Is early diversion warranted? J Urol 1997;157:984–8.

33. Liard A, Seguier-Liqszyc E, Mitrofanoff P. Temporary high diversion for posterior urethral valves. J Urol 2000;164:145–8.

34. Ghanem MA, Nijman RJ. Long-term followup of bilateral high (sober) urinary diversion in patients with posterior urethral valves and its effect on bladder function. J Urol 2005;173:1721–4.

35. Patil KK, Wilcox DT, Samuel M, et al. Management of urinary extravasation in 18 boys with posterior urethral valves. J Urol 2003;169:1508–11.

36. Hekkila J, Taskinen S, Rintala R. Urinomas associated with posterior urethral valves. J Urol 2008;180:1476–8.

37. Casey JT, Hagerty JA, Maizels M, et al. Early administration of oxybutynin improves bladder function and clinical outsomes in newborns with posterior urethral valves. J Urol 2012, Epub ahead of print.

38. Smith GH, Canning DA, Schulman SL, et al. The long-term outcome of posterior urethral valves treated with primary valve ablation and observation. J Urol 1996;155:1730–4.

39. Denes ED, Barthold JS, Gonzalez R. Early prognostic value of serum creatinine levels in children with posterior urethral valves. J Urol 1997;157:1441–3.

40. Hulbert WC, Rosenberg HK, Cartwright PC, et al. The predictive value of ultrasonography in evaluation of infants with posterior urethral valves. J Urol 1992;148:122–4.

41. Parkhouse HF, Barratt TM, Dillon MJ, et al. Long-term outcome of boys with posterior urethral valves. Br J Urol 1988;16:59–62.

42. Kaefer M, Keating MA, Adams MC, et al. Posterior urethral valves, pressure pop offs and bladder function. J Urol 1995;154:708–11.

43. Cuckow PM, Dinneen MD, Risdon RA, et al. Long-term renal function in the posterior urethral valves, unilateral reflux and renal dysplasia syndrome. J Urol 1997;158:1004–7.

44. Narasimhan KL, Mahajan JK, Kaur B, et al. The vesicoureteral reflux dysplasia syndrome in patients with posterior urethral valves. J Urol 2005;174:1433–5.

45. DeFoor W, Clark C, Jackson E, et al. Risk factors for end stage renal disease in children with posterior urethral valves. J Urol 2008;180:1705–8.

46. Duel BP, Mogbo K, Barthold JS, et al. Prognostic value of initial renal ultrasound in patients with posterior urethral valves. J Urol 1998;160:1198–200.

47. Holmdahl G, Sillen U. Boys with posterior urethral valves: Outcome concerning renal function, bladder function and paternity at ages 31 to 44 years. J Urol 2005;174:1031–4.

48. Sarhan O, Zaccaria I, Macher MA, et al. Long-term outcome of prenatally detected posterior urethral valves: Single center study of 65 cases managed by primary valve ablation. J Urol 2008;179: 307–12.

49. Ansari MS, Surdas R, Farai S, et al. Renal function reserve in children with posterior urethral valve- a novel test to predict long-term outcome. J Urol 2011;185:2329–33.

50. Sarhan OM, El-Ghoneimi AA, Helmy TE, et al. Posterior urethral valves: Multivariate analysis of factors affecting the final renal outcome. J Urol 2011;185:2491–5.

51. Bomalaski MD, Anema JG, Coplen DE, et al. Delayed presentation of posterior urethral valves: A not so benign condition. J Urol 1999; 162:2130–2.

52. Kibar Y, Ashley RA, Roth CC, et al. Timing of posterior urethral valve diagnosis and its impact on clinical outcome. J Ped Urol 2011;7:538–42.

53. Engel DL, Pope JC IV, Adams MC, et al. Risk factors associated with chronic kidney disease in patient with posterior urethral valves without prenatal hydronephrosis. J Urol 2011;185:2502–8.

54. Priti K, Rao KL, Menon P, et al. Posterior urethral valves: Incidence and progress of vesicoureteric reflux after primary fulguration. Pediatr Surg Int 2004;20:136–9.

55. Hassan JM, Pope JC IV, Brock JW III, et al. Vesicoureteral reflux in patients with posterior urethral valves. J Urol 2003;170: 1677–80.

56. Warshaw BL, Hymes LC, Trulock TS, et al. Prognostic features in infants with obstructive uropathy due to posterior urethral valves. J Urol 1985;133:240–3.

57. El-Sherbiny MT, Hafez AT, Ghoneim MA, et al. Ureteroneocystostomy in children with posterior urethral valves: Indications and outcome. J Urol 2002;168:1836–40.

58. Holmdahl G, Sillén U, Hanson E, et al. Bladder dysfunction in boys with posterior urethral valves before and after puberty. J Urol 1996;155:694–8.

59. De Gennaro M, Capitanucci ML, Mosiello G, et al. The changing urodynamic pattern from infancy to adolescence in boys with posterior urethral valves. Br J Urol 2000;85:1104–8.

60. Emir H, Eroglu E, Tekant G, et al. Urodynamic findings of posterior urethral valve patients. Eur J Pediatr Surg 2002;12:38–41.

61. Ghanem MA, Wolffenbuttel KP, de Vylder A, et al. Long term bladder dysfunction and renal function in boys with posterior urethral valves based on urodynamic findings. J Urol 2004;171: 2409–12.

62. Karim OM, Cendron M, Mostwin JL, et al. Developmental alterations in the fetal lamb bladder subjected to partial urethral obstruction in-utero. J Urol 1993;150:1060–3.

63. Freedman AL, Qureshi F, Shapiro E, et al. Smooth muscle development in the obstructed fetal bladder. Urology 1997;49:104–7.

64. Mitchell ME. Persistent ureteral dilatation following valve resection. Dial Pediatr Urol 1982;5:8–10.

65. Close CE. The valve bladder. In: Gillenwater JY, Grayhack JT, Howards SS, editors. Adult and Pediatric Urology. 4th ed. Philadelphia: Lippincott Williams & Wilkins; 2002. p. 2311–18.

66. Donohoe JM, Weinstein RP, Combs AJ, et al. When can persistent hydroureteronephrosis in posterior urethral valve disease be considered residual stretching? J Urol 2004;172:706–11.

67. Glassberg KL. The valve bladder syndrome: 20 years later. J Urol 2001;166:1406–14.

68. Capitanucci M, Marciano A, Zaccara A, et al. Long-term bladder function followup in boys with posterior urethral valves: Comparison of noninvasive vs invasive urodynamic studies. J Urol 2012; 188:953–7.

69. Cain MP, Wu SD, Austin PF, et al. Alpha blocker therapy for children with dysfunctional voiding and urinary retention. J Urol 2003;1770:1514–15.

70. Koff SA, Mutabagani KH, Jayanthi VR. The valve bladder syndrome: Pathophysiology and treatment with nocturnal bladder emptying. J Urol 2002;167:291–7.

71. Montane B, Abitbol C, Seeherunvong W, et al. Beneficial effects of continuous overnight catheter drainage in children with polyuric renal failure. BJU Int 2003;92:447–51.

72. Johal NS, Hamid R, Aslam Z, et al. Ureterocystoplasty: Long-term functional results. J Urol 2008;179:2373–5.

73. Austin PF, Lockhart JL, Bissada NK, et al. Multi-institutional experience with the gastrointestinal composite reservoir. J Urol 2001; 165:2018–21.

74. Hekkila J, Holmberg C, Kyllonen L, et al. Long-term risk of end stage renal disease in patients with posterior urethral valves. J Urol 2011;186:2392–6.

75. Caione P, Nappo SG. Posterior urethral valves: Long-term outcome. Pediatr Surg Int 2011;27:1027–35.

76. Reinberg Y, Gonzalez R, Fryd D. The outcome of renal transplantation on children with posterior urethral valves. J Urol 1988;140:1491–3.

77. Indudhara R, Joseph DB, Perez LM, et al. Renal transplantation in children with posterior urethral valves revisited: A 10-year follow-up. J Urol 1998;160:1201–3.

78. DeFoor W, Tackett L, Minevich E, et al. Successful renal transplantation in children with posterior urethral valves. J Urol 2003; 170:2402–4.

79. Fine MS, Smith KM, Shrivastava D, et al. Posterior urethral valve treatments and outcomes in children receiving kidney transplants. J Urol 2011;185:2507–11.

80. Kamal MM, El-Hefnawy AS, Soliman S, et al. Impact of posterior urethral valves on pediatric renal transplantation: A single-center comparative study of 297 cases. Pediatr Transplantation 2011;15: 482–97.

81. Taskinen S, Heikkilä J, Santtila P, et al. Posterior urethral valves and adult sexual function. BJU Int 2012;110:E392–6.

82. Tikkinen KA, Heikkila J, Rintala RJ, et al. Lower urinary tract symptoms in adults treated for posterior urethral valves in childhood: Matched cohort study. J Urol 2011;186:660–6.

83. Lopez Pereira R, Miguel M, Martinez Urrutia MJ, et al. Long-term bladder function, fertility and sexual function in patients with posterior urethral valves treated in infancy. J Ped Urol 2011; Epub ahead of print.

CHAPTER 58

BLADDER AND CLOACAL EXSTROPHY

Michael E. Mitchell • Richard Grady

The exstrophic anomalies, often referred to as the exstrophy–epispadias complex,[1] are considered a spectrum of embryological abnormalities including:

- Epispadias—the least severe anomaly, in which the urethra is a partial or complete open plate on the dorsal surface of the phallus
- Classic bladder exstrophy (BE)—the most common of these anomalies, in which the bladder is an open plate on the lower abdomen and always includes epispadias
- Cloacal exstrophy (CE)—the bladder and the ileocecal junction of the bowel are an open plate on the lower abdomen. This condition, commonly associated with other defects, is also known as the omphalocele/exstrophy/imperforate anus/spinal defect (OEIS) complex
- Exstrophy variants—partial manifestations are seen of the above anomalies, and commonly lack symmetry in the sagittal plane.

BLADDER EXSTROPHY

Classic BE occurs in one per 10,000–50,000 live births,[2,3] with a male to female ratio of 3–6 : 1.[4,5] CE is even more rare with an incidence of 1 in 200,000–400,000,[6] but is more common when stillborns are included in the data (1 in 10,000 to 1 in 50,000).[7] The natural history of BE is well known; the anomaly is nonlethal although it is associated with significant morbidity. Since the 19th century, various efforts to manage BE have been described. As the condition is rare, these approaches were empiric and usually unsuccessful. Until the 20th century, there was no effective surgical technique.

BE results from an anterior herniation of the developing bladder and urethra with subsequent herniation of posterior developing structures, preventing the normal development of the lower abdominal wall and anterior fusion of the pelvis. The result is a flattened pelvis with wide diastasis of the symphysis pubis. This anomaly has been described as 'if one blade of a pair of scissors were passed through the urethra of a normal person; the other blade were used to cut through the skin, abdominal wall, anterior wall of the bladder and urethra, and the symphysis pubis; and the cut edges were then folded laterally as if the pages of a book were being opened' (Fig. 58-1).[8] Children with BE typically have an anteriorly located anus. Also, the female genital anatomy is altered with a more vertically oriented vaginal opening following repair and a wider and shorter vagina than normal. The anterior component of the penis is also foreshortened in males compared to the general population. Classic BE,

however, is rarely associated with other organ system malformation.

Diagnosis

BE can be diagnosed antenatally, although many affected fetuses are not identified before birth.[9] Ultrasound (US) can reliably detect BE before the twentieth week of gestation.[10,11] Absence of the bladder is the hallmark. Other ultrasound findings include:

- A semisolid mass protruding from the abdominal wall[12]
- A lower abdominal protrusion
- An anteriorly displaced scrotum with a small phallus in male fetuses
- Normal kidneys in association with a low-set umbilical cord[13]
- An abnormal iliac crest widening.[10]

Subtle findings such as low umbilical cord insertion and the location of the genitalia will only be seen if the fetus is examined in a sagittal alignment with the spine.[14] As exstrophy affects the external genitalia, the diagnosis is easier to make in males than females. Iliac crest widening can also be seen during the routine prenatal evaluation of the lumbosacral spine to evaluate for myelomeningocele. The iliac angle will be about 110° rather than the usual 90°.[14] Since urine production is normal in these fetuses, amniotic fluid levels are normal.

Prenatal diagnosis allows for prenatal counseling, optimal perinatal management, and the chance to be delivered near a pediatric center trained to treat these babies. This counseling should include the expertise of an experienced pediatric urologist or surgeon. The overall prognosis for these children can be good if treated at medical centers with experience with this disorder.[15]

In many areas of the developing world, early treatment remains problematic due to the lack of healthcare infrastructure and resources to care for these patients. Management of these patients often includes significantly delayed time to closure and adds another level of challenge to achieve optimum outcomes in this patient group. A recent overview from South Africa highlighted this problem: 58% of the patients presented in a delayed fashion and mortality rates approached 42% due to concomitant medical conditions and poor primary health care.[16]

Pathogenesis

In the prescientific era, the cause of BE was attributed to trauma to the unborn child causing ulceration of the abdominal wall and subsequent bladder herniation.

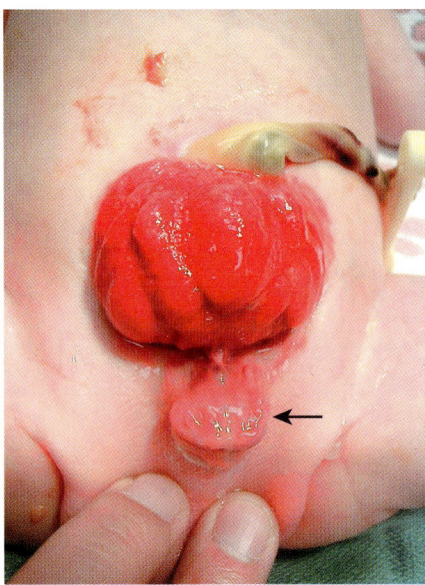

FIGURE 58-1 ■ Bladder exstrophy in a male. The urethral mucosa is marked with the arrow. The corporeal bodies lie posterior to the urethral mucosa.

Today, we know that the developing human embryo does not normally pass through a stage that corresponds to exstrophy. This knowledge excludes arrested development and implicates an error in embryogenesis involving the cloacal membrane.[17] This membrane serves to separate the coelomic cavity from the amniotic space in early development and can be identified by two to three weeks of gestation. By the fourth gestational week, it forms the ventral wall of the urogenital sinus with the unfused primordia of the genital tubercles sitting cephalad and lateral to it. With further development, the primordia grow and fuse in the midline, and mesoderm grows toward the midline creating an infra-umbilical abdominal wall. Simultaneously, the urorectal septum develops medially and caudally to separate the cloaca into the urogenital sinus and rectum.[18]

One theory suggests a persistent cloacal membrane during fetal development.[19] Persistence of this membrane could create a wedge effect that keeps the medially encroaching mesoderm from fusing in the midline.[17] To further study this hypothesis, an animal model of CE was created using the developing chick embryo. By placing a plastic graft in the region of the tail bud, it was found that CE resulted, perhaps due to persistence of the cloacal membrane.[17]

Other experimental models implicate the cloacal membrane as well, but postulate that early disruption, rather than persistence, causes exstrophy. Another model of CE in the developing chick embryo, created by using a CO_2 laser to create an early dehiscence in the tail bud caudal to the omphalomesenteric vessels, suggests that exstrophy may result from failure of the mesodermal ingrowth between the ectoderm and endoderm of the cloacal membrane which then later ruptures. It is hypothesized that such an event could be caused by early hypoxemic infarction in the region of the tail bud with subsequent cellular loss of the mesoderm followed

by herniation of the developing bladder or cloaca.[20] This type of ischemic injury has been implicated as the cause of gastroschisis and could explain the spectrum of the exstrophy/epispadias complex. Another possible mechanism resulting in a similar pathophysiology could be a defect in a genetic switch which results in premature senescence of the infra-umbilical membrane (analogous to an ischemic injury). This mechanism would imply an epigenetic basis for exstrophy.

Other proposed theories include caudal displacement of the paired primordia of the genital tubercles. Exstrophy is postulated to occur by this mechanism when the primordia of the genital tubercles fuse caudal to their usual location relative to where the urorectal fold divides the cloaca into the urogenital sinus and rectum.[21] This theory readily explains the spectrum of variation seen in the exstrophy. However, it fails to explain the higher incidence of exstrophy compared to epispadias.[8]

A relatively new maldevelopment theory for CE is based on a suramin-exposed chick model.[22] When chick embryos were examined at one or two days after pericardial injection of suramin, about 8% were noted to have a midline infra-umbilical opening into the cloaca and allantois, abnormal leg bud abduction, hypoplastic tail and allantois, a broad infra-umbilical pelvic region, and large aneurysmal dilation of the paired dorsal aorta at the level of the leg buds. The aortic dilation is transient, resolving on the second or third day after drug exposure.. These authors implicate the aneurysmal paired dorsal aorta as the primary defects leading to CE in this animal model. Pelvic maldevelopment has also been implicated in the pathogenesis of exstrophy and explains both the bony abnormalities as well as soft tissue anomalies.[23]

The chick model to study BE has inherent limitations. Unlike primates, chickens possess a cloaca; thus this precludes the creation of BE versus CE. Other animal models to study BE have been difficult to create. In an exstrophy sheep model, a significant increase in the ratio of collagen-to-smooth muscle was noted in exstrophic versus normal control bladders ($P < 0.05$). These histological changes are similar in part to changes seen in human BE specimens.[24,25]

To date, the underlying cause of human exstrophy remains in question perhaps secondary to environmental exposure, an infectious pathogen, or other causes in genetically susceptible individuals. In fact, epidemiologic studies implicate a role for inherited susceptibility. As a result of the associated physical anomalies with this condition, patients with BE often have to overcome significant obstacles to reproduce. Men may need to resort to assisted reproductive techniques because of difficulty with sexual intercourse and ejaculation.[26,27] Women with exstrophy are prone to uterine prolapse and miscarriage. Difficulty with conception and pregnancy are still a problem today despite in vitro fertilization and careful obstetric care.[28,29] These issues combined may explain, in part, why familial patterns of inheritance of exstrophy–epispadias complex are noted infrequently. To date, 37 familial cases of BE have been reported, the most recent of which describes a mother and son with BE.[30] Five cases of an affected parent–child pair have also been described.[30–32] Another 18 cases with BE have been found

TABLE 58-1 Goals of Reconstruction

Primary Goals	Secondary Goals
Preservation of kidney function	Minimization of urinary tract infections
Urinary continence	Adequate pelvic floor support
Low pressure urine storage reservoir	Minimization of the risk for malignancy associated with the urinary tract
Volitional voiding	Minimization of the risk for urinary calculi
Functionally and cosmetically acceptable external genitalia	Adequate abdominal wall fascia

in twins.[30] However, in a study population of greater than six million births and 208 reported cases of exstrophy, no case had a positive family history for this anomaly.[33]

Current counseling recommendations about the risk of recurrence in a sibling of a patient with exstrophy cite an estimate of about 1% and a 1:70 chance of transmission to the progeny of an affected parent.[31] A Florida population-based study found multiple births had a 46% increased risk of birth defects, with BE being the fifth highest adjusted relative risk.[34] These findings support a multifactorial etiology with evidence for genetic predisposition. More recently, an epidemiologic survey of families with BE found no link between exstrophy and parental age, maternal reproductive history, or periconceptional maternal exposure to alcohol, drugs, chemical noxae, radiation, or infections. Periconceptional maternal exposure to smoking was noted to be significantly more common in patients with CE.[35]

Principles of Reconstruction

Modern objectives for exstrophy reconstruction are placed broadly into primary and secondary goals (Table 58-1).

While these goals are straightforward and often interconnected, their successful achievement can be elusive. Many of the secondary goals address complications that can arise from operations used to treat exstrophy. The goals have expanded since the first operations were attempted in the 19th century. These objectives address the primary pathophysiology of exstrophy and the problems associated with its management (Table 58-2).

Natural History and Early Attempts at Treatment

Children with BE can survive untreated and some untreated patients with BE have lived into their eighth decade.[36] However, significant morbidity exists if these exstrophic conditions are left untreated, including total urinary incontinence, bladder and kidney infections, skin breakdown, and tumor development in the bladder plate. The surrounding skin around the exposed bladder is often inflamed secondary to urine contact dermatitis, loss of skin integrity from constant wetness, and secondary

infection. Untreated inguinal hernias can be life-threatening and organ prolapse is especially challenging to manage later. In addition, these patients are often social pariahs because of odor and hygiene problems. In contrast, when these patients receive effective surgical and medical treatment, they can lead productive, healthy lives with manageable morbidity.

The morbidity associated with untreated BE led physicians to develop empiric operative approaches for this anomaly such as urinary reconstructive or diversion procedures. Initial efforts were directed at partial reconstruction of the abdominal wall to allow the application of a urinary receptacle to collect urine. Others performed urinary diversion through the creation of a ureterosigmoid fistula. Early results were poor.[27] These early efforts were undertaken without an understanding of urinary tract and bladder physiology, or how these operations would affect urine storage and emptying, kidney function, electrolyte homeostasis, the propensity for urinary tract infection, or urinary calculus formation.

Current Operative Approaches

A wide range of operations have been performed to repair BE and can be grouped as: (1) urinary diversion; or (2) anatomic reconstruction. Surgeon preference and experience, patient anatomy, previous operations, timing of reconstruction, availability of tertiary care facilities, and access to medical care and resources all play a role in which operative procedure is chosen for a particular patient.

Urinary Diversion

Urinary diversion is not commonly used in the USA or most parts of Europe; this approach has been abandoned

TABLE 58-2 Primary Pathophysiology of Bladder Exstrophy and Complications that Occur in Relation to its Management

Primary Pathophysiology (If Untreated)	Complications (Associated with Management of Exstrophy)
Malignancy (related to chronic exposure of the bladder plate)	Malignancy (related to the use of intestine in bladder reconstruction)
Pyelonephritis	Pyelonephritis
Kidney stones	Kidney and bladder stones
Total urinary incontinence	Stress or urge urinary incontinence
Chronic bladder irritation	Hydronephrosis
Pelvic floor insufficiency	Cystocele, uterine prolapse
Abnormal hip dynamics, back pain	Abnormal hip dynamics, back pain
Symphyseal diastasis, pelvic flattening	Urinary outlet obstruction
Abdominal wall defect	Absent umbilicus
Ventral and inguinal hernias	Incisional hernias
Severe penile shortening with dorsal chordee	Inadequate phallus in males with subsequent social and psychological sequelae

in favor of an anatomically based approach. However, continent urinary diversion techniques can produce a more consistent degree of urinary continence with less intervention than that achieved with anatomic reconstruction.[37] Some urodynamic studies demonstrate low urine flow rates and poor contractility and continence in patients following primary bladder repair.[38,39]

Internal or incontinent urinary diversion avoids the potential complications associated with functional reconstruction such as urinary retention and subsequent kidney damage, and potential later dependence on clean intermittent catheterization (CIC) to empty the bladder. Advocates of early urinary diversion also cite a decreased risk of epididymitis and obstruction of the vas deferens by the creation of a receptacle with a suprapubic window at the level of the prostatic urethra.[40] Diversion can also be combined with cosmetic and functional reconstructive procedures for the external genitalia. Because of the difficulties encountered with functional bladder reconstruction, advocates of early urinary diversion argue that their approach achieves the primary goals with fewer operations and higher success rates than are achieved with bladder closure and urethral reconstruction.

Urinary diversion is also useful to achieve urinary continence in patients who have failed multiple attempts at anatomic reconstruction. Also, urinary diversion may be best for patients with bladder plates deemed too small to close. However, because we cannot accurately predict which bladder plates will increase significantly in size after primary closure, we do not use this as criteria for primary diversion and do not divert the urine primarily in young BE patients.

Given the successes of urinary diversion, why abandon it? Long-term complications associated with ureterosigmoidostomy (USO) are significant and include hyperchloremic metabolic acidosis, chronic pyelonephritis, bladder calculi, and a 250- to 300-fold increased risk of adenocarcinoma developing at the anastomosis.[41–43] As a result of these complications, USO was subsequently replaced by incontinent urinary diversions such as colonic and ileal conduits. A significant disadvantage to these conduits is the incontinent abdominal stoma that is associated with them.

The Mainz II pouch and the Sigma pouch represent significant improvements to the USO.[44–46] These rectal reservoirs permit urinary continence without reliance on CIC. In one study, renal preservation rates in children treated primarily with a urinary rectal reservoir (Mainz II pouch) approach 92% with continence rates up to 97%.[37] The Heitz–Boyer–Hovelaque procedure involves isolation of a rectal segment for ureteral implantation followed by posterior sagittal pull-through of the sigmoid colon through the anal sphincter. A small series using this approach reported continence rates of 95% with an acceptable complication rate.[47] Complications of this form of diversion include fecal-urinary incontinence in patients with impaired anorectal sphincter control. Metabolic electrolyte imbalances can be treated with frequent emptying of the rectal reservoir that reduces the contact time between urine and the absorptive rectal mucosa along with oral bicarbonate replacement. The significant risk of malignancy also remains a concern. Various modifications of the rectal reservoir to prevent admixture of feces and urine may decrease the incidence of adenocarcinoma if the risk is due to conversion of urinary nitrates into carcinogenic nitrites by fecal bacteria.[48] Long-term results are not yet available. Techniques for constructing urinary diversions are listed in Table 58-3.

As a result of these complications with urinary diversion, and even though anatomic reconstruction may produce less consistent results, anatomic resconstruction has become the standard approach when possible.

Anatomic Reconstruction

The first efforts at anatomic reconstruction for BE were unsuccessful, but set the stage for the current anatomic approach. In 1881, Trendelenberg described an exstrophy closure emphasizing the importance of pubic re-approximation in front of the reconstructed bladder in order to achieve continence and prevent dehiscence.[49] However, because of discouraging results, anatomic reconstruction was largely replaced by urinary diversion in the early part of the 20th century. During this time there were scattered published reports of successful outcomes.[50–53] However, several large series of patients who underwent single-stage anatomic reconstruction in the 1960s and 1970s reported continence rates of only 10–30%.[54–59] Renal damage was as high as 90% in these series, generally because of bladder outlet obstruction.[54]

As a result of these complications and the low rate of urinary continence with single-stage approaches, reconstructive efforts were subsequently modified toward staged bladder reconstruction, an approach pioneered in the 1970s, and further refined to what is now known as the modern staged repair of exstrophy (MSRE).[60–62]

TABLE 58-3 Surgical Options for Urinary Diversion

External Diversion (Continent Urinary Reservoir)	Internal Diversion (Rectal Sphincter–Based Continence)	Incontinent Diversions
Indiana pouch (cecal reservoir with ileal catheterizable channel)	Sigma pouch	Ileal conduit
Mainz pouch	Ghoneim reservoir	Colon conduit
Penn pouch (ileocecal reservoir with appendiceal catheterizable channel)	Gersuny	Ileocecal conduit
Kock pouch	Heitz–Boyer–Hovelacque	
	Rectal bladder with proximal colostomy	
	Ureterosigmoidostomy	
	Ileocecal ureterosigmoidostomy	

Recent advances in single-stage reconstruction for BE have been advocated and complete primary repair for exstrophy (CPRE) has gained favor.[63]

The primary goal of these approaches is to reconstruct and achieve anatomic and functional normalcy with minimal operative morbidity. In the subsequent section, two currently popular surgical techniques, the CPRE and the MSRE, are detailed. Closure of the female with BE is similar in the CPRE and MSRE methods with the end result being closure of the bladder, urethra, and abdominal wall. The main difference is a more aggressive mobilization of the vagina and urethral plate into the pelvic diaphragm in the CPRE technique. In contrast, closure of the male with BE is quite different in the CPRE and MSRE techniques. The CPRE closes and repositions the bladder and entire urethra at one stage. In contrast, the MSRE closes and repositions the bladder and posterior urethra at the first stage with the remainder of the urethra closed at a later stage.

Preoperative Care

After delivery, to reduce trauma to the bladder plate, the umbilical cord should be ligated with silk suture rather than a plastic or metal clamp. A hydrated gel dressing or plastic wrap can be used to protect the exposed bladder from superficial trauma. Dressings should be changed daily, and the bladder should be irrigated with normal saline with each diaper change. A humidified air incubator may also minimize bladder injury.[64]

Intravenous antibiotic therapy in the pre- and postoperative period is used to decrease the risk for infection following reconstruction. Preoperative ultrasound is helpful to evaluate the kidneys and to establish a baseline examination for later ultrasound studies. Preoperative spinal ultrasound examination should be considered if sacral dimpling or other signs of spina bifida occulta are noted on physical examination.

Operative Considerations

Ideally, the primary BE closure is performed in the newborn period. If the bladder template is amenable, early closure has several advantages. Early closure initiates the road toward anatomic normalcy as well as decreasing bladder exposure which can lead to histological changes such as acute and chronic inflammation, squamous metaplasia, cystitis glandularis and cystitis cystica, and muscular fibrosis which may adversely impact bladder capacity and compliance.[65] Electron microscopy studies have shown that the newborn exstrophy bladder is 'immature' when compared to control newborns,[66] and has fewer small nerve fibers,[67] less smooth muscle, and a threefold increase in type III collagen content.[68] While it is unclear whether these changes are part of the primary pathology or secondary to the lack of bladder cycling in utero, it is conceivable that early closure could 'mature' the bladder by restoring bladder cycling. Similarly, another study verified the importance of immediate postnatal exstrophy closure as infants closed before 7 days of age required fewer bladder augmentations to achieve eventual continence.[69]

Assessment of the adequacy of the bladder template is subjective. Even a small bladder template, if distensible and contractile, can enlarge to a useful size once closed. However, if the bladder template appears too small and stiff on initial assessment, some surgeons choose to defer early operation and re-evaluate the bladder at 4–6 months of age under anesthesia.[70] If the bladder continues to appear inadequate for closure, a nonrefluxing colon conduit can be created in combination with an abdominal wall closure and epispadias repair. At a later age this can be converted to a continent diversion or anastomosed to the rectosigmoid.

During general anesthesia, nitrous oxide should be avoided during primary closure as it can cause bowel distension, which decreases exposure during the operation and may increase the risk of wound dehiscence. Some advocate postoperative nasogastric tube drainage to decrease abdominal distension although we do not routinely use it.[71] We prefer an epidural catheter to reduce the inhaled anesthetic requirement during the operation. Tunneling the epidural may reduce the risk of infection if it is left in for prolonged periods after repair.[72]

For patients older than 3 days, or newborns with a wide pubic diastasis, we perform anterior iliac osteotomies. Osteotomies are recommended in most patients unless the pelvis is very pliable. Osteotomies assist closure and enhance anterior pelvic floor support, which may improve future urinary continence.[60,73]

Factors that appear to be important in the perioperative period include:

- Use of osteotomies in many cases to decrease the tension on the repair, especially if the repair is performed >72 hours after birth
- Ureteral stenting and bladder drainage catheters placed intraoperatively to divert the urine in the postoperative period
- Avoidance of abdominal distension
- Use of intraoperative antibiotics.[74,75]

Complete Primary Repair for Exstrophy

CPRE is best performed in the newborn period. Primary reconstruction in the newborn period is technically easier than in an older child. If one considers that the stimulus for bladder development is dependent on bladder cycling, then early closure offers this advantage. The bony pelvis is pliable in the newborn period so that osteotomies may not be needed in some cases, especially if closure can be performed within the first 72 hours of life.

Clinical experience in babies with posterior urethral valves suggests that early restoration of nonobstructive emptying and filling of the bladder allows the bladder to regain some of its normal physiologic and developmental potential.[76] This implies that the bladder progresses through developmental milestones in the first few months of life. Precedence for this form of organ development is found in the brain with the acquisition of language and visual perception, and this is also true for skeletal and neuromuscular development. Finally, early bladder reconstruction creates a more normal appearing baby, which may foster improved bonding between the parents and infant.

In the CPRE (or Mitchell) technique,[63] the bladder, bladder neck, and urethra are relocated posteriorly within the pelvis. This shift positions the proximal urethra within the pelvic diaphragm in an anatomically more normal position to maximize the effect of the pelvic muscles and support structures needed for urinary continence. Posterior location of the bladder neck and urethra also facilitates reapproximation of the pubic symphysis which, in turn, helps prevent anterior migration of the urethra and bladder neck, and provides a more anatomically normal pelvic diaphragm.

Total penile disassembly reduces anterior tension on the urethra because the urethra is separated from its attachments to the underlying corporal bodies. These attachments otherwise pull the urethral plate anteriorly and prevent posterior placement of the proximal urethra and bladder neck in the pelvis. Reducing this tension theoretically decreases the risk of bladder dehiscence and also temporarily reduces the dorsal tension on the corporal bodies that may contribute to dorsal chordee in males. Combining the epispadias repair with primary closure allows for the most important advantage of primary closure which is division of the intersymphyseal ligament or band located posterior to the urethra in these patients.

Closure in the newborn period optimizes the chance for early bladder cycling and may aid in bladder development. It may obviate the need for a multi-staged repair of the exstrophied bladder including further bladder neck reconstruction (BNR), bladder augmentation, and penile reconstructive surgery. The principles of this operation are also useful in some reoperations or delayed repairs for exstrophy.

CPRE Technique: Boys. After sterile preparation and draping, the lines of dissection are marked (Fig. 58-2). When marking these lines, it is important to exclude dysplastic tissue at the edges of the exstrophic bladder and bladder neck. This is particularly important at the bladder neck where remaining dysplastic tissue may impair later bladder neck function. Catheters (3–5 French) are placed into both ureters and sutured with 5-0

chromic suture. Bladder polyps should be removed prior to beginning the dissection as these can act as space-occupying lesions after the bladder is reconstructed. Initial dissection begins superiorly and proceeds inferiorly to separate the bladder from the adjacent skin and fascia since it is usually easiest to identify tissue planes in these areas. The umbilical vessels are ligated as the umbilicus will be moved superiorly to a more anatomically normal location, and will be later used as the location to exteriorize the suprapubic (SP) catheter.

Penile/Urethral Dissection. Traction sutures are placed into each hemiglans of the penis to aid in dissection. These sutures will rotate to a parallel vertical orientation because the corporal bodies will naturally rotate medially after they are separated from the urethral wedge (urethral plate plus underlying corpora spongiosa). We begin the penile dissection along the ventral aspect of the penis with a circumscribing incision (Fig. 58-3A). This step precedes dissection of the urethral wedge from the corporal bodies because it is easier to identify the plane of dissection ventrally above Buck's fascia. Buck's fascia is deficient or absent around the corpora spongiosum. As the dissection progresses medially to separate the urethra from the corpora cavernosa, it is important to realize that the plane shifts subtly from above Buck's fascia to just above the tunica albuginea. Failure to adjust the plane of dissection will carry the dissection into the corpora spongiosa which will result in excessive, difficult-to-control bleeding during the deep ventral dissection of the urethral wedge from the corporal bodies.

Shallow incisions are made laterally along the dorsal aspect of the urethra to begin the urethral dissection. Sharp dissection is used to develop the plane between the urethral wedge and the corporal bodies. Careful dissection will preserve urethral width and length. This is particularly important since the urethra is often too short to reach the glans penis once the bladder has been relocated into the pelvis.

Careful lateral dissection of the penile shaft skin and dartos fascia from the corporal bodies will avoid damaging the laterally located neurovascular bundles on the corpora of the epispadic penis. The lateral dissection on

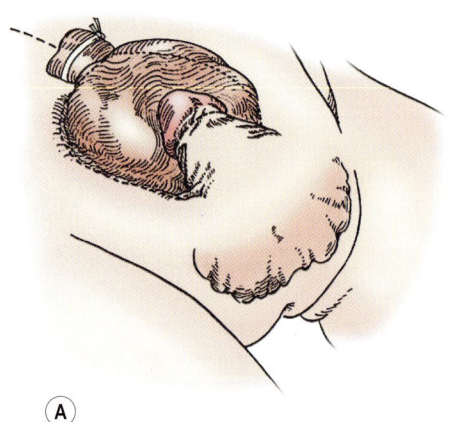

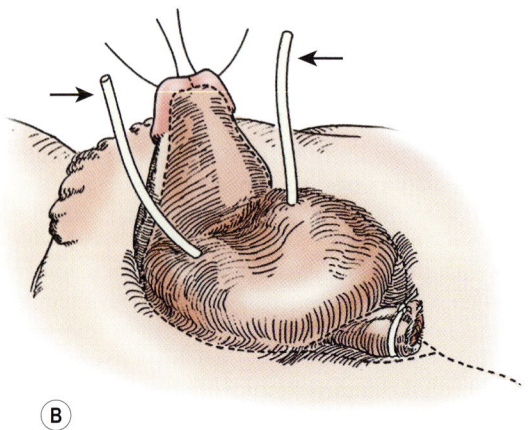

(A)   (B)

FIGURE 58-2 ■ In a male undergoing complete primary repair for bladder exstrophy, the outlines of the planes of dissection are seen in these drawings. **(A)** Ventral view. **(B)** Dorsal view. The ureteral stents are marked with arrows.

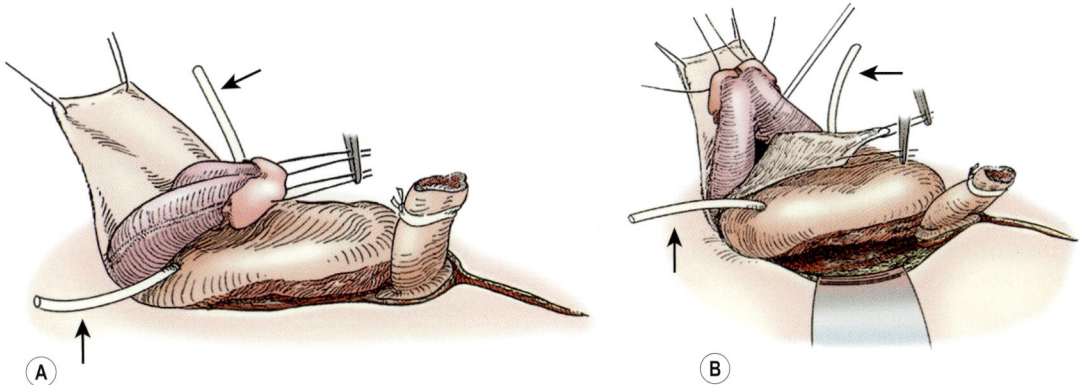

FIGURE 58-3 ■ These two diagrams show early portions of the ventral subcoronal and corporeal dissection. **(A)** Initiation of the subcoronal dissection is seen. This is typically the easiest plane to initiate dissection. **(B)** Corporeal dissection proximally and dorsally is shown. Initiation of corporeal separation is easiest to establish proximally. Note the ureteral catheters (arrows), which have been introduced into the ureteral orifices.

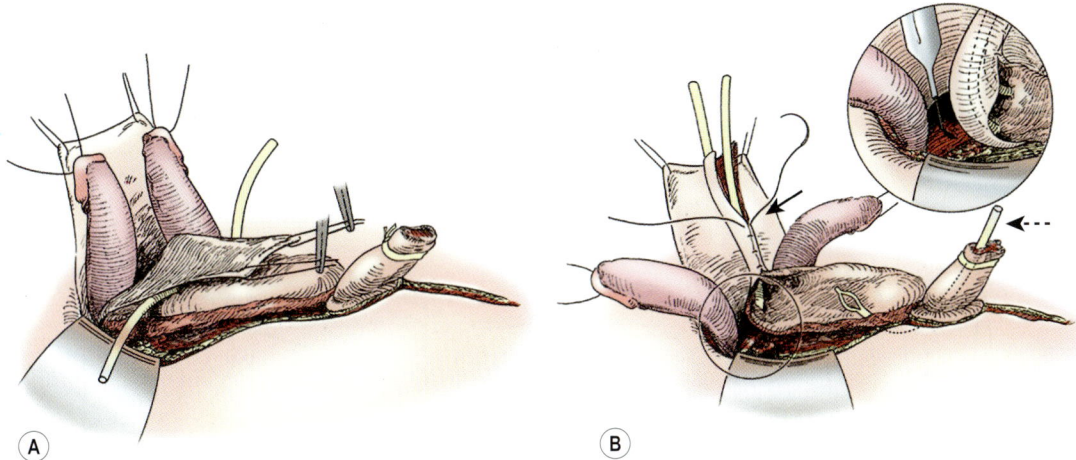

FIGURE 58-4 ■ **(A)** Separation of corporeal bodies and urethra. **(B)** Deep pelvic dissection. Note the division of the intersymphyseal band (inset) is critical to allowing placement of the bladder in the pelvis. Also note the tubularization of the neourethra over the urethral catheter (solid arrow) and the suprapubic tube in the still-open bladder (dotted arrow).

the penis should be superficial to Buck's fascia because of the lateral location of the neurovascular bundles in the epispadic penis.

Complete Penile Disassembly and Deep Dissection. Once a plane is established between the penis and the urethral wedge, the penis may be disassembled into three components: the right and left corporeal bodies with their respective hemiglans, and the urethral wedge.[77] This is performed in order to provide exposure to the intersymphyseal band and to allow adequate proximal dissection. We have found the easiest plane of dissection to completely isolate the corporeal bodies is proximal and ventral. The plane of dissection should be carried out at the level of the tunica albuginea on the corpora (Fig. 58-3B). After a plane is established between the urethral wedge and the corporeal bodies, this dissection is carried distally to separate the three components from each other (Fig. 58-4A). Complete separation of the corporeal bodies increases exposure to the pelvic diaphragm for deeper dissection. The corporeal bodies can be completely separated from each other since they are nourished via a separate blood supply. It is important to keep the underlying corpora spongiosa with the urethra as the vasculature to the

urethra is based on this corporal tissue (which should appear wedge-shaped after its dissection from the adjacent corpora cavernosa). The urethral/corpora spongiosa component will later be tubularized and placed ventral to the corporal bodies. Para-exstrophy skin flaps should not be made with this technique because creating these flaps may injure the blood supply to the distal urethra. As the bladder and urethra are located posteriorly in the pelvis as a unit (with a common blood supply), division of the urethral wedge is counter-intuitive to the intent of the repair.

In some cases, a male infant with a wide symphaseal diastasis and short urethral plate will be left with a hypospadias that will require later repair. Likewise, in patients with less symphysis separation and a longer segment of distal corporal midline connection, the urethra and corporal bodies do not always have to be completely separated distally. In such cases, the urethra is long enough and the bladder mobile enough to preserve the connection between them while still effectively carrying out the deep pelvic dissection that is integral to this repair.

After separating the components distally, the urethral dissection is carried proximally to the bladder neck.

Exposure to the pelvic diaphragm is optimized by complete proximal separation of the urethra and corporal bodies (Fig. 58-4B). This creates the exposure to perform the deep incision of the intersymphyseal band (the condensation of anterior pelvic fascia and ligaments) which is necessary to move the bladder and urethra posteriorly (Fig. 58-5). When dissecting the urethral wedge from the corporal bodies medially, the dissection plane is along the tunica albuginea of the corpora cavernosa. This medial dissection should be carried down through the intersymphyseal band.

With a deep incision of the intersymphyseal band posterior and lateral to each side of the urethral wedge, the bladder and bladder neck can be moved to a posterior position in the pelvis. This dissection should be carried

until the pelvic floor musculature becomes visible and the future bladder neck and proximal urethra lie deep in the pelvis with little anterior tension. Failure to adequately dissect the bladder and urethral wedge from these surrounding structures will prevent posterior movement of the bladder in the pelvis and will create anterior tension along the urethral plate, all of which can lead to failure of the closure (Fig. 58-5).

Primary Closure. Once the above steps are completed, the bladder closure and urethral tubularization can be initiated. This portion of the repair is straightforward and anatomic (Fig. 58-6A). To provide urinary drainage, an SP tube is used. The bladder is closed in three layers with monofilament absorbable suture. The urethra is tubularized using a two-layer running closure

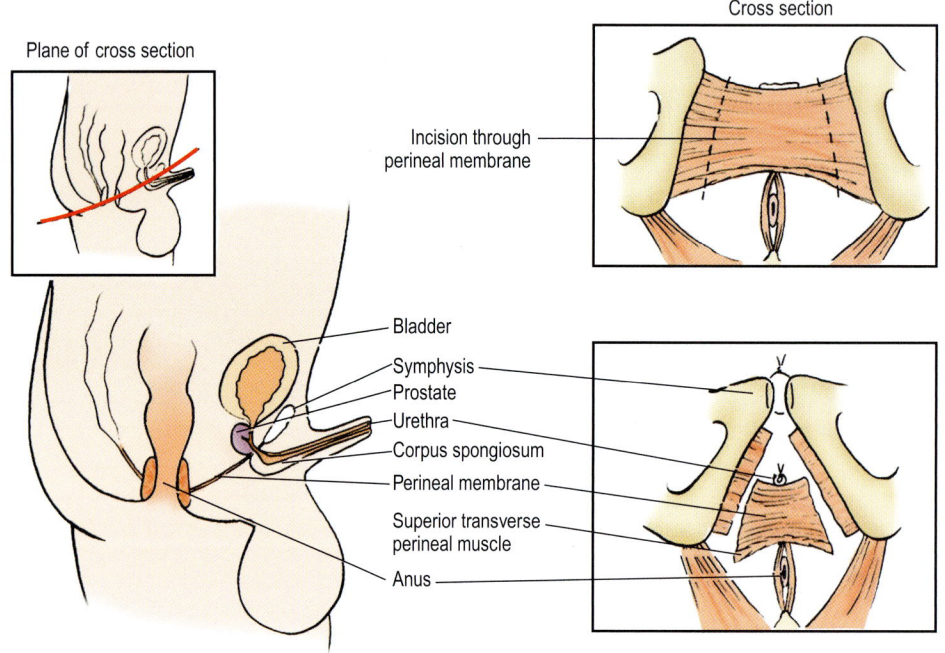

FIGURE 58-5 ■ Cross-sectional view of repair of bladder exstrophy in a male.

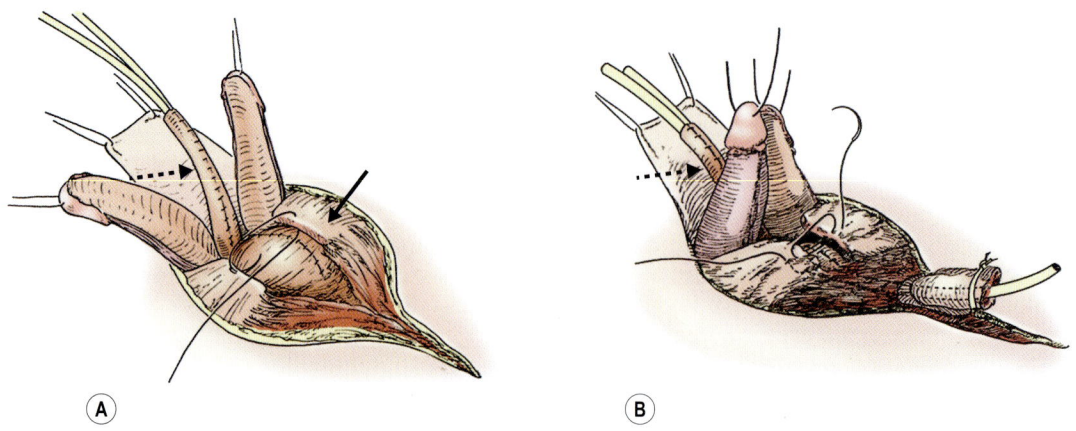

FIGURE 58-6 ■ Once the intersymphyseal band is adequately incised and the bladder and urethral wedge are dissected from the surrounding tissues, bladder repair and urethral tubularization can be performed. **(A)** The bladder is being closed in three layers using monofilament absorbable suture (solid arrow). The urethra has been tubularized using a two-layer running closure with monofilament and braided absorbable suture (dotted arrow). **(B)** This schematic depicts closure of the pubic symphysis with two number 1 polydioxanone interrupted sutures placed in a figure-of-eight fashion. The knots are placed anteriorly to prevent suture erosion into the neck of the bladder. The urethra (dotted arrow) has been placed ventral to the corpora.

with monofilament and braided absorbable suture. Because of the previous deep dissection, we can now position the tubularized urethra ventral to the corpora without tension. If the urethra cannot be positioned ventrally without creating tension and restricting the urine flow, it may be necessary to more aggressively incise the intersymphyseal band and pelvic diaphragm.

The pubic symphysis is reapproximated using two large polydiaxanone (PDS) interrupted sutures (Fig. 58-6B). Knots are left anteriorly to prevent erosion into the bladder neck. The rectus fascia is reapproximated using an interrupted or running 2-0 PDS. We also place interrupted 6-0 PDS sutures along the distal dorsal aspect of the corporal bodies to reapproximate them. Penile skin coverage is achieved with either a primary dorsal closure or reversed Byars flaps if needed. The skin covering the abdominal wall is reapproximated using a two-layer closure with absorbable monofilament suture.

The corporal bodies will rotate medially with symphasis closure. This rotation will assist in correcting the dorsal penile deflection and can be readily appreciated by observing the new vertical lie of the previously horizontally placed traction sutures on the glans. Occasionally, significant discrepancies in the lengths of the dorsal and ventral corpora will require a dermal graft to correct the resulting chordee.

If there is adequate urethral length, the urethra may be brought up to each hemiglans ventrally to create an orthotopic meatus. The glans is reconstructed using interrupted mattress sutures of PDS followed by horizontal mattress sutures of 7-0 monofilament suture to reapproximate the epithelium. The neourethra is matured with 7-0 polyglycolate suture. When needed, glans tissue reduction may also be performed to create a conical appearing glans and to eliminate the furrow between the two halves of the glans. Tacking sutures are placed ventrally and dorsally to prevent penile shaft skin from riding over the corporal bodies and 'burying' the penis.

The urethra lacks enough length to reach the glans in about half the cases. In this situation, it is matured along the ventral aspect of the penis to create a hypospadias (Fig. 58-7). Redundant shaft skin can be left ventrally in these patients to assist in later penile reconstruction.

CPRE Technique: Girls. The principles of the single-stage technique are similar in boys and girls (Fig. 58-8). The planned lines of incision are marked with the bladder neck, urethra, and vagina mobilized as a unit (Fig. 58-9). The appropriate plane of dissection is found anteriorly along the medial aspect of the glans clitoris and proceeds posteriorly along the lateral aspect of the vaginal vault (Fig. 58-10A). The vagina is mobilized with the urethra and bladder neck. Dissection along the vaginal wall extends laterally. Insertion of a hemostat in the vaginal vault will help with retraction to identify the plane of dissection. The urethra and bladder neck should not be dissected from the anterior vaginal wall as this dissection will compromise the vascular supply to the urethra. During the posterior–lateral dissection, the intersymphyseal band will be encountered and should be incised deeply to allow the urethra and bladder neck to be located posteriorly. The posterior limit of the dissection is the

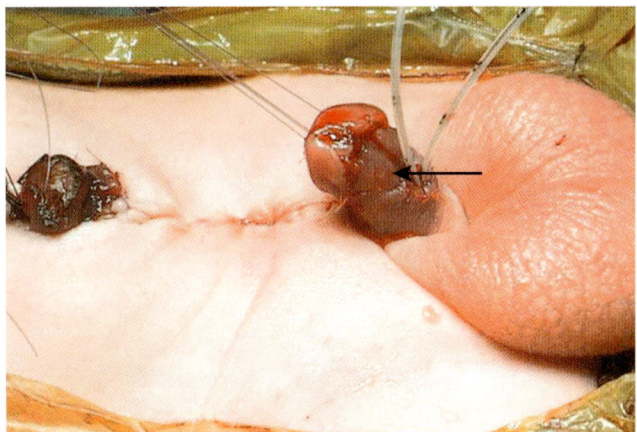

FIGURE 58-7 ■ If the urethra does not have adequate length to reach the glans (which occurs in about half of the cases), it is matured along the ventral aspect of the penis to create a hypospadias (arrow), as seen in this operative photograph. The hypospadias will be corrected at a later date.

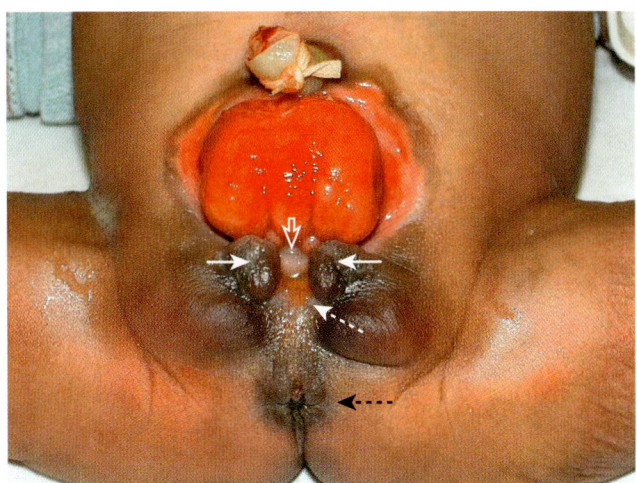

FIGURE 58-8 ■ Bladder exstrophy in a female infant. The epispadial urethra is marked with an open white arrow. The bifid clitoris is marked with solid white arrows, and the vagina is marked with a dotted white arrow. The anus is noted with a dotted black arrow.

pelvic floor musculature, and the bladder, bladder neck, and urethra are able to be moved into the pelvis without tension.

Following adequate dissection, the vagina, urethra, and bladder neck are moved posteriorly using a Y–V plasty if the vagina is anteriorly located. The bladder neck is lengthened by making proximal parallel incisions in the bladder to define the proximal urethra and these incisions are extended to the trigone. The urethra and bladder neck are then tubularized in two layers with absorbable suture (Fig. 58-10B). The lengthening of the proximal urethra to form the bladder neck is critical. Two 3 French ureteral catheters are left in place. Prior to the urethral closure, we place a suprapubic tube for postoperative drainage. The pubis symphysis is reapproximated using two large PDS sutures (Fig. 58-11A). Iliac osteotomies may be necessary when a wide pubic diastasis prevents a low-tension reapproximation of the pubic symphysis, or if the patient is older than 72 hours. The rectus fascia can

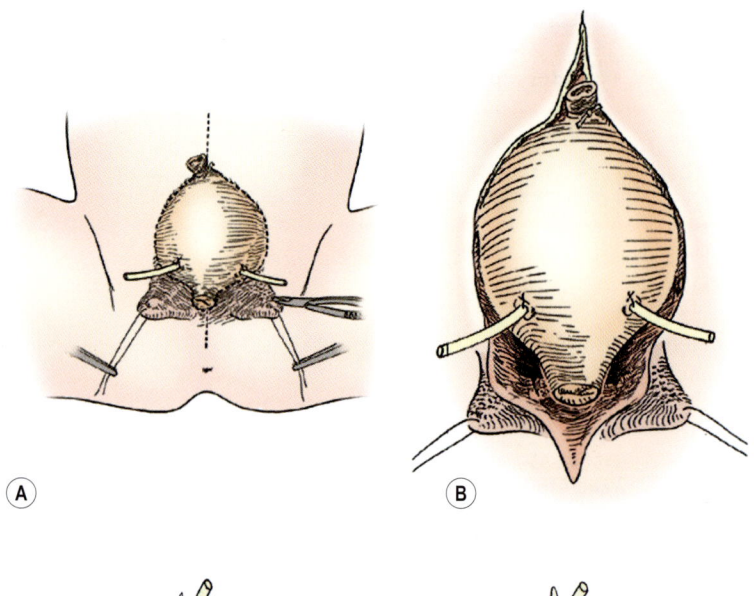

(A) (B)

FIGURE 58-9 ■ In a female infant, the bladder neck, urethra, and vagina are mobilized as a unit. **(A)** The lines of incision are seen. **(B)** The dissection is carried down dividing the intersymphyseal band (arrows). Note the ureteral catheters in both drawings.

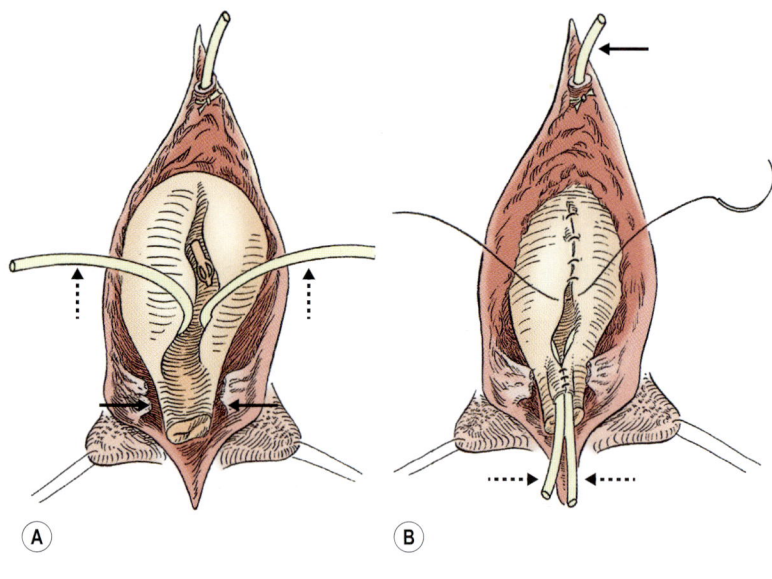

(A) (B)

FIGURE 58-10 ■ **(A)** The appropriate plane of dissection is found anteriorly along the medial aspect of the glans clitoris and proceeds posteriorly along the lateral aspect of the vaginal vault. The vagina is mobilized with the urethra and bladder neck (solid arrows). **(B)** The bladder and urethra are closed in multiple layers, and the suprapubic tube (arrow) is brought out superiorly. Note the ureteral catheters (dotted arrows) in both drawings.

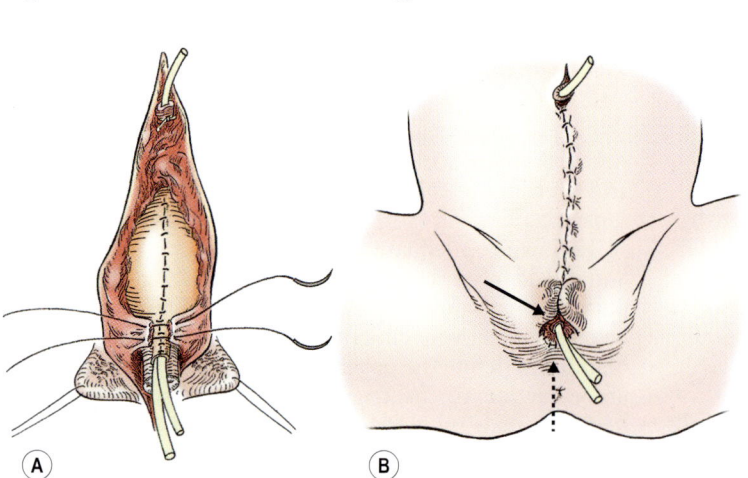

(A) (B)

FIGURE 58-11 ■ **(A)** Pelvic positioning of the bladder and vagina and closure of the pubic symphysis with figure-of-eight No. 1 polydioxanone sutures. **(B)** Repair of the vaginal introitus (solid arrow) is depicted. The labia majora are advanced posteriorly to the perineum at this time (dotted arrow).

then be closed in the midline. We mature the neourethra with 5-0 polyglycolate sutures and reapproximate the bifid clitoris with 7-0 PDS by denuding each half medially. The labia majora should be advanced to the perineum at this time as well (Fig. 58-11B). A Z-plasty technique aids in skin closure. A monsplasty provides a

satisfactory aesthetic result to the introital area and can be performed at the time of the primary repair.[78]

Other Primary Reconstructive Techniques. Other approaches for primary BE repair include the radical soft tissue mobilization technique (Kelly technique) which has been used at some institutions for decades. This approach avoids the need for osteotomies as the periosteum is mobilized to allow the soft tissues of the bladder, bladder neck and urethra to be reconstructed in the midline. In a recent study, long-term continence rates were reported at 70% for complete or partial urinary control.[79] Over half did not require bladder augmentation or CIC. Prolapse rates may be lower in adult females closed in this fashion. The abdominal wall was perceived as abnormal in adults repaired with this technique. Others have also reported successful short-term outcomes with the use of this approach. Complications such as bladder neck-cutaneous fistulas and penile loss have been described.[80]

Delayed Primary Closure. Several recent studies have advocated for delayed primary closure, especially in regard to the CPRE approach. Proponents of delayed repair argue that it is safer for the child, allows a more coordinated surgical effort, and allows an elective operation so that the most expert team of clinicians and personnel are available.[81] Others have shown it is possible to wait months after birth.[82] Another group used the delay to stimulate the penis with testosterone with the goal of reducing the chance for glans injury, and reported good short-term outcomes with this approach in six patients.[83] The successful use of a delayed closure approach is predicated on adequate protection of the exposed tissue. One series showed that the CPRE technique can be used in delayed or previous failed exstrophy closures.[84] Another study found an increased cost of as much as 50% with delayed closure.[85] Long-term outcomes will take years to mature.

Modern Staged Repair of Exstrophy

A staged approach for exstrophy repair developed in response to high rates of renal damage seen in single-stage approaches in the 1970s. The sequence for staged reconstruction initially consisted of bladder and posterior urethral closure at birth, BNR at 2–3 years of life, and epispadias repair later.[86] This sequence later shifted when bladder capacity was noted to increase with added resistance from early epispadias repair.[87] Currently, as described by the Johns Hopkins group, MSRE consists of bladder and posterior urethral closure at birth or soon thereafter (stage 1), epispadias repair at 6–12 months of life (stage 2), and BNR when the bladder capacity is adequate and the child is showing interest in toilet training (usually at 4–5 years of life) (stage 3).[88] Occasionally, epispadias repair and BNR ± ureteral reimplantation can be combined.[89,90]

MSRE Stage 1: Initial Early Bladder Exstrophy Closure. In the first stage of this repair, the objectives include: (1) closure and repositioning of the bladder and urethra (posterior urethra in males and entire urethra in females) inside the pelvic ring; and (2) approximation of the pelvic ring with closure of the abdominal wall. In male patients, at the end of stage 1, this repair ideally produces a result that mimics complete epispadias with incontinence and balanced posterior outlet resistance stimulating bladder growth while preserving renal function.

Male MSRE Bladder and Posterior Urethral Closure Technique. In MSRE stage 1 in the male child, ureteral catheters are inserted and secured. A traction suture is placed in the glans penis. The posterior urethra is developed by incising a 2 cm wide strip of mucosa from the distal trigone to below the distal verumontanum. Initial dissection begins at the umbilicus and is continued circumferentially, incising around the bladder plate. The two umbilical arteries are ligated and divided. The underlying detrusor muscle is mobilized from the rectus sheath to expose the peritoneum. The peritoneum is dissected off the dome of the bladder to allow deep pelvic placement of the bladder. Extraperitoneal dissection lateral to the bladder exposes the retroperitoneal space, and allows the dissection in the correct plane at the level of the bladder neck. At this level, the rectus fascia meets the pubis and the urogenital diaphragm fibers meet the posterior urethra/bladder neck. The urogenital diaphragm fibers and the intersymphyseal band must be completely taken down from the pubic subperiosteum to the pelvic floor on each side, or the posterior urethra and bladder cannot be recessed deep into the pelvis.

At this point, the posterior urethra is assessed. If the child has severe dorsal chordee and a short urethra that inhibits attempts at penile lengthening, an incision in the urethral plate may be necessary, but only after extensive mobilization of the bladder and prostatic plate from the rectus fascia, the pubic bones, and the inferior ramus of the pubis. After complete division of the urogenital diaphragm from the posterior urethra/bladder neck area, the prostatic urethra can be displaced into the pelvis. Lack of an adequate urethral plate length can be managed by dividing the prostatic plate distal to the verumontanum in a V-shaped fashion. After corporal mobilization and midline reapproximation, the penile urethral plate is fashioned from a lateral rotational flap which is generated after a single lateral incision into the paraexstrophy skin. Paraexstrophy skin flaps should be used with great caution because of a high complication rate.[55,91,92]

The corporal bodies are not approximated at this time since this will be performed after the urethra has been transposed beneath the corpora at the time of epispadias closure. An adequate dissection can be assessed by compressing a sound on the posterior urethra while manually approximating the pelvis.

After an SP tube has been placed, the umbilicus is excised and the bladder is closed in the midline in multiple layers with a running 2-0 polyglycolate suture. The posterior urethra is also closed onto the base of the penis, sizing it to accept a 12- to 14 French sound. It is important to perform a horizontal mattress closure of the pubic bones with heavy suture, and place the knot on the anterior surface of the pubis. Once the suture is placed but not tied, three sterile personnel are used to approximate the pubic symphysis. One individual applies pressure over each greater trochanter to push the pubic rami to the midline. A second individual depresses the posterior urethra and bladder neck. The third individual ties the suture. If the rectus fascia is strong, a second suture is placed just above the symphysis. The abdominal wall, subcutaneous tissues, and skin are then closed in multiple layers with construction of a neoumbilicus at or above the level of the iliac crests.

Female MSRE Bladder and Posterior Urethral Closure Technique.

In stage 1 of the MSRE in the female child, the technique of bladder, pelvic ring, and abdominal wall closure are identical to that described for the male. However, the female closure differs from the male closure in that the female urethra is completely reconstructed at stage 1.[1,93] The incision in the urethral plate mucosa is 2 cm wide, traversing from the distal trigone to the vaginal orifice, in the female. Paraexstrophy skin flaps are not necessary in females.[94] The medial aspect of each hemiclitoris is deepithelialized to permit approximation of the two glans clitori and reconstruction of the mons. The bladder and female urethra are closed in two layers with polyglycolate suture and the pubic bones, abdominal wall, subcutaneous tissue, and skin are closed as outlined in the male. The monsplasty and genitoplasty are then performed.

Postoperative Care of Stage 1 MSRE.

An adequate urethral caliber and minimal post-void residuals are assessed prior to removal of the SP tube at four weeks. The status of the upper tracts is assessed prior to discharge and is followed by ultrasound in 3 months and then every 6 months to 1 year. Antibiotic vesicoureteral reflux (VUR) prophylaxis is also given. Increasing hydronephrosis, worsening VUR, retained urine in the bladder, and recurrent urinary infections should prompt further evaluation for suture erosion or outlet obstruction. Between the ages of 1 to 3 years, yearly cystograms under anesthesia are performed to assess the degree of reflux, and more importantly, to assess the bladder capacity (ideally 60–85 mL at this age).

MSRE Stage 2: Epispadias Repair.

Epispadias repair is now typically performed at 12 to 18 months of age via the modified Cantwell–Ransley technique. The goals of epispadias repair include a straight penis and urethra, easy urethral catheterization, normal erectile function, and a cosmetically satisfactory phallus. These goals allow the patient to stand while voiding and to have intromission during intercourse.

Preoperative Considerations.

Prior to performing the epispadias repair, several surgeons have described topical or intramuscular testosterone to increase the size of the phallus and the phallic skin.[71,95] Intramuscular testosterone enanthate in oil (2 mg/kg) can be administered at five and two weeks prior to epispadias closure. Penile lengthening can usually be achieved at this time by division of all remnants of the suspensory ligament and scar tissue as well as further release of the crura from the inferior pubic rami. In some cases, further urethral lengthening may require free skin grafts, buccal mucosal grafts, ureteral grafts, or pedicle skin flaps. These same maneuvers can be used to repair the scarred or stenosed posterior urethra as well.

The Modified Cantwell–Ransley Technique.

Cantwell first described mobilization of the urethra and moving it ventrally for epispadias repair in the late nineteenth century. The technique has subsequently been modified.[92,96] To begin this procedure, a stay suture is placed into the glans. A reverse MAGPI or IPGAM procedure at the distal urethral plate allows advancement of the urethral meatus onto the glans. Skin incisions are then made on the lateral edges of the urethral plate and around the epispadic meatus. This plate is dissected from the corporal bodies to the level of the glans distally and to the prostatic urethra proximally. Glans wings should be developed distally as well. The corporal bodies are then separated from each other to allow medial rotation. The urethra is then tubularized over a 6 or 8 French urethral catheter using running 6-0 absorbable suture. The corporal bodies are rotated over the urethra and reapproximated using interrupted 5-0 absorbable suture. Cavernocavernosotomies may be performed prior to reapproximating the corporal bodies to help correct persistent chordee. These are performed at the point of maximal angulation. The neurovascular bundles may require mobilization to avoid injuring them if cavernosotomies are performed. The glans wings are then closed over the urethra using interrupted 5-0 absorbable suture. The penile shaft skin can be trimmed and tailored to cover the penis using interrupted 5-0 or 6-0 absorbable sutures. Z-plasties at the level of the pubis may decrease the chance of a dorsal retractile scar at the base of the penis. Postoperative care includes bladder antispasmodics, broad-spectrum antibiotics, and removal of the urethral catheter at two weeks. In the event of a significantly delayed primary closure or failure of an initial bladder closure, a simultaneous closure of the exstrophy bladder and the epispadias can be performed.

Bladder Neck Reconstruction.

In incontinent children after CPRE or MSRE, a continence procedure is appropriate when (1) the urethra is stricture-free and capable of catheterization if necessary; (2) under anesthesia, the bladder capacity has achieved a minimum volume of 60–85 mL; and (3) the child is mature enough to participate in the postoperative voiding program.[97] This is typically around 4–5 years of age at the earliest. Cystoscopy and gravity cystography are helpful for providing information regarding bladder capacity and the status of any previous repairs. Advocates of the staged reconstruction approach emphasize the importance of achieving adequate bladder capacity prior to performing BNR. A bladder capacity less than 60 mL under anesthesia or during urodynamic evaluation reduces the likelihood of continence after BNR. BNR requires an adequate bladder capacity because some volume is lost during construction of the bladder neck. Factors that increase the potential for the bladder to achieve an adequate capacity prior to BNR include:

- Avoidance of urinary tract infections
- Complete bladder emptying with institution of CIC if bladder emptying is incomplete
- Epispadias repair
- Avoidance of bladder prolapse.

Preoperative urodynamic evaluation should be considered because it allows detection of detrusor hyperactivity or atony as well as assessment of functional bladder capacity and leak point pressures. However, the urethra in these patients may be difficult to catheterize. In these situations, a urodynamic catheter can be placed suprapubically at the time of the cystourethroscopic examination and can be used later that day for the urodynamic evaluation.

Ureteroneocystostomy may be required at the time of BNR to correct VUR and to relocate the ureters away from the lower bladder where the bladder neck will be constructed. Although the Cohen technique is often employed, others have described a cephalotrigonal technique which is particularly applicable to exstrophy patients because of the angle of ureteral entry into the bladder.[98] The Marshall–Marchetti–Kranz (MMK) bladder neck suspension, or a bladder neck wrap using rectus or gracilis muscle or fascia, may be combined with BNR as well. Osteotomies may also be necessary to stabilize the intersymphyseal bar and improve continence at the time of BNR.

The following section describes the most commonly employed BNR techniques, including the modified Young–Dees–Leadbetter (YDL) and the Mitchell repairs.

MSRE Stage 3: Modified YDL-BNR. The modified YDL-BNR and the transtrigonal/cephalotrigonal bilateral ureteral reimplantation are the techniques employed in the MSRE Stage 3.[98,99] The combined thoughts of several surgeons spanning an 80-year period has led to the modern YDL-BNR.[97] To perform a modified YDL procedure, the bladder neck is extensively dissected and a vertical cystotomy is made. Occasionally, a portion of the intersymphyseal band needs to be divided completely for visualization. After transtrigonal/cephalotrigonal bilateral ureteral reimplantation, a strip of bladder mucosa, approximately 1.5–1.8 cm wide and 3–4 cm, long is generated, and the lateral bladder triangles are demucosalized. Use of an epinephrine-soaked sponge during this dissection aids in hemostasis. The bladder neck may be funneled further with small vertical incisions along the cut edge of the lateral bladder walls. The neourethra is tubularized over an 8 French catheter using interrupted or running polyglycolate suture (4-0 or 5-0). The two triangular regions of demucosalized detrusor muscle are then closed over the mucosal tube in a two-layer 'vest over pants' double-breasted technique using 3-0 polyglycolic acid suture. This reinforces the neobladder neck, decreases the risk of fistula, and augments the outlet resistance.[100] The sutures in the third layer are not cut since they are used in the subsequent MMK bladder neck suspension.[97]

Some surgeons recommend avoidance of a urethral catheter in the postoperative period because of concerns that it may later adversely affect urinary continence. Therefore, urinary drainage is achieved by using bilateral ureteral catheters and SP tube drainage. Ureteral stents are removed around two to three weeks, and voiding trials begin in the third week. The urethra is calibrated with a soft 8 French catheter, and voiding trials are begun with the SP tube in place after the urine has been sterilized. If no urine is passed, cystoscopy and urethral stenting may be required for a short period of time. A bladder readjustment period may span several months before day and subsequently night continence is achieved.

BNR: The Mitchell Repair. This repair employs a modification of the YDL technique described previously.[99] In this modification, a full-thickness incision is made in the anterior urethra and parallel incisions are extended cephalad to define the proximal urethral plate

and bladder neck. After cross trigonal ureteral reimplantation, the urethral strip is tubularized in two layers using absorbable or monocryl suture (4-0 or 5-0) over an 8 to 10 French urethral catheter, depending on the size of the patient. The bladder may be closed in continuity with the urethral closure. This procedure effectively narrows and lengthens the proximal urethra. It also moves the anterior fibrotic tissue at the level of the original bladder neck to a more cephalad position, away from the new bladder neck. This anterior redundant tissue can be used as a fibromuscular flap to encircle and support the new bladder neck. If a fibromuscular bladder wrap is not possible, then a fascial sling or wrap may be performed following the bladder and urethral closure.

Postoperatively, urine drains through a combination of ureteral stents through the urethra and an SP tube. The ureteral catheters are removed 7–10 days later. The SP tube remains for at least 3 weeks. Voiding trials are performed with measurement of post-void residual urine volumes to assess for urinary retention before removing the SP tube. As with any BNR procedure (without augmentation), several months of adjustment will be required before the patient develops adequate bladder awareness, capacity, and control to achieve urinary continence.

Occasionally, trigonal tubularization must be combined with bladder augmentation because of a small bladder capacity. Most BNRs decrease bladder capacity since the bladder is used to create the continence mechanism.[101] The stomach offers the best potential to preserve spontaneous volitional voiding in this group, but places these children at risk of hematuria–dysuria syndrome which can be especially troubling in patients with persistent urinary incontinence and normal sensory innervation.[102] Other intestinal segments may also be used depending on surgeon preference. If augmentation is needed and if the urethra is difficult to catheterize, appendicovesicostomy or another form of the Mitrofanoff operation is also performed because of the likelihood that they will require CIC to empty the bladder after BNR and augmentation.

Outcomes

Exstrophy

Complications can occur with any initial BE repair. The most commonly reported complication is an urethrocutaneous fistula (at the penopubic angle dorsally) in males. These fistulas may close spontaneously. They may initially be managed conservatively with urinary diversion via catheter drainage. If the fistula does not close, the bladder and urethra should be examined cystoscopically for the possibility of obstruction at the bladder neck or urethra. Complete breakdown of the bladder and abdominal wall closure is uncommon today, and usually reflects significant postoperative infection or a technical error in closure.

If a child develops chronic bladder and kidney infections following BE closure, he or she should be evaluated for possible outlet obstruction. Early intervention with CIC for several months will often protect the patient during this period. We routinely maintain our patients on suppressive antibiotic therapy because of the high incidence of VUR.

In the long term, patients are also concerned with issues of fertility. For men, fertility may be compromised as a consequence of dissection needed in the region of the bladder neck and posterior urethra. The vas deferens and ejaculatory ducts are normal at birth. Most men can experience orgasm, but some cannot effectively ejaculate. Intracystoplasmic sperm injection can be useful in this setting. Women with BE can become pregnant, but are prone to develop uterine prolapse, especially after delivery. The prolapse is thought to be due to further stress and damage to the already abnormal pelvic musculature.

Epispadias

The urethrocutaneous fistula rate varies widely from 5–40%. In one study, complications were more common in those patients who underwent epispadius repair at the same time as BE closure versus an isolated epispadias repair.[103] Other complications include atrophy of the corpora cavernosa and urethra. These complications can occur if the vascular supply to the corporal bodies or urethral wedge is damaged during dissection or during closure.[104] Similar complications have been found following the initial stage of a staged reconstruction as well as after the use of the complete penile disassembly technique.[105] In experienced hands, these complications are unusual and underscore the importance of involving surgeons experienced in the management of these patients.

Bladder Neck Reconstruction

After BNR, a good outcome is defined as a dry interval >2–3 hours accompanied by spontaneous voiding without catheterization. YDL-BNR and its variants have yielded urinary continence rates of 30% to 80% for patients with BE.[99,106–108] Many factors influence these outcomes. An initial failed bladder closure or prior failed BNR reduces the chance for achieving subsequent urinary continence.[109] A preoperative bladder capacity of >85 mL portends a greater continence rate after YDL-BNR.[110] Use of osteotomies and patient immobilization in the postoperative period increases the success of bladder closure and subsequent continence. Delayed bladder closure increases the likelihood of the eventual need for bladder augmentation due to inadequate bladder capacity that, in turn, reduces the chance for volitional voiding. One long-term study found that eight of 13 patients with an initially successful bladder closure and BNR required further surgery in their second decade of life because of poorly compliant, low-capacity bladders that caused urinary incontinence.[111]

Adjunctive Aspects of the Repair

Indirect inguinal hernias are commonly associated with BE in both male and female patients.[112,113] They arise as a consequence of enlarged internal and external inguinal rings combined with compromised fascial support and lack of obliquity of the inguinal canal.[114] In one study 56% of classic male exstrophy patients and 15% of classic female exstrophy patients developed inguinal hernias over a 10-year period.[64] The authors recommended these hernias be repaired at the time of primary bladder closure to prevent incarceration.

Due to the high incidence of VUR, we prescribe low-dose suppressive antibiotics for all newborns after bladder closure. This is continued until the VUR is corrected or resolves spontaneously. Some surgeons perform neoureterocystotomies at the time of initial closure. The success of this approach has not been reported.

Osteotomies

Approximation of the open pelvic ring eases abdominal wall closure, diminishes the rate of bladder and abdominal wall dehiscence,[74,115] allows the construction of an intrapelvic urethra, and reapproximates the pelvic floor musculature likely contributing to long-term continence.[60,115] Therefore, pelvic ring reapproximation is useful at the initial bladder closure or at later stages of reconstruction. If the pelvis is not sufficiently malleable, osteotomies are performed.

Osteotomies offer several advantages to the anatomic approach to BE closure including: (1) optimizing pubic symphysis apposition, diminishing tension on the fascial repair; (2) optimizing anatomic placement of the bladder, bladder neck, and urethra in the pelvis; (3) improving the reapproximation of the corporal and clitoral bodies; and (4) possibly decreasing the chance for later uterine prolapse.

The need for osteotomies is typically assessed under general anesthesia. Indications include patients more than 72 hours old, newborns with a wide pubic diastasis, newborns with CE, and patients who have had a previously failed closure. Osteotomies are usually performed at the same setting as bladder closure to help secure the closure. Although classic exstrophy represents a spectrum of pelvic abnormalities, it has been our impression that osteotomies improve the potential for successful repair and the potential for voiding with continence. Therefore, osteotomies are routinely performed in our primary exstrophy closures.

Several operative approaches are available. Posterior iliac osteotomies are performed with the patient in a prone position, after which the patient is then repositioned for the bladder closure. Increased blood loss and occasional malunion of the ileum have led to the pursuit of other approaches. Anterior iliac osteotomies offer the advantage of not having to turn the patient. Compared to posterior iliac osteotomies, an anterior approach also has been shown to result in less blood loss and better apposition and mobility of the pubic rami. Anterior approaches include an anterior diagonal technique or a combination of bilateral combined anterior innominate and vertical iliac osteotomies which have had excellent initial and long-term results compared to anterior iliac osteotomies alone in some series.[73,116] Both osteotomies can be performed through the same anterior skin incision on each side and with minimal blood loss and 4% complication rate.[117,118] A diagonal mid-iliac osteotomy performed through the same incision as the exstrophy closure has also been described.[119] Division of the superior pubic ramus is not as effective as the other methods described, but can be used in the newborn period.[120,121]

After the primary reconstructive procedure for exstrophy, the patient must be immobilized to decrease lateral stresses on the closure. Choice of immobilization remains controversial with a variety of techniques available. Current options include: (1) Bryant's traction; (2) use of an external fixator; (3) spica casting; and (4) mummy or mermaid wrapping. The most important variable with these techniques is familiarity of the user as they all have learning curves. We prefer a spica cast for 3 weeks to prevent external hip rotation and optimize pubic apposition. It can facilitate early discharge and home care (Fig. 58-12). Modified Buck's traction has also been used by many groups with success. A posterior lightweight splint can be used in newborns when the child is out of traction to maintain hip adduction. We have stopped using Buck's traction because spica casts are easier for the families at home. External fixation devices have also been used with success.[116] Fixator pins for these devices should be cleaned several times a day to reduce infection. Internal fixation may be necessary in older patients. Femoral nerve palsy is a possible complication with fixation which must be monitored and can be reduced by gradually tightening the fixator.

To avoid osteotomies, a technique has been developed that secures the pubic symphyseal closure with deeply placed polyglycolate sutures through the bone followed by placement of a miniature metal plate which may be removed later. Initial results are promising.[122] Osteotomies are not usually needed with the Kelly technique.[79]

Long-Term Considerations

Psychosocial Concerns

Children with exstrophy can experience marked difficulty in the development of their psychosocial identity.

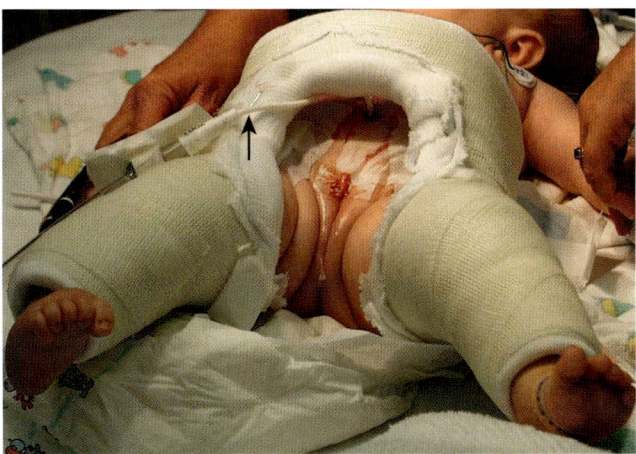

FIGURE 58-12 ■ In order to immobilize the patient to decrease lateral stresses on the closure after the primary reconstructive procedure, a number of immobilization techniques are possible. This photograph shows a spica cast that was applied to prevent external hip rotation and optimize pubic apposition in the early postoperative period. Note the suprapubic bladder catheter (arrow).

Adolescent males with exstrophy are psychosexually delayed for 2 to 4 years compared to their peers, and teenage girls with exstrophy struggle with sexual self-esteem issues such as body image and genital perception/appearance.[123] We recommend regular assessment of social development in this patient group including psychiatric evaluation and parental education.[124] Assessment can begin as early as 12 to 18 months of age and then as needed. Evaluation and intervention is also useful prior to reconstructive procedures. In these patients, anxiety and even suicidal ideation is greater than the general population.[125] Fortunately, adolescents with exstrophy are resilient and often develop creative strategies for coping with the chronic aspects of their condition.[126] Most adolescents with exstrophy express a strong desire to be normal and resent arrangements that emphasize their differences.[127]

Sexual Function

Although sexual function is of little relevance to the newborn or prepubertal child born with exstrophy, it is an issue of considerable importance to the parents of the child who will worry and wonder what future sexual function their children will experience, and also for the adolescents with exstrophy for whom sexual function or the potential for sexual function is an area of focus. Erectile function and sensation is usually intact for most male BE patients.[128,129] However, persistent or recurrent chordee and small penile size can create difficulty in achieving intercourse for some males.[129] Libido is usually present with or without operative correction. Studies of adult men with exstrophy have found that approximately one-third choose not to or cannot engage in intercourse.[130] In one series, 33 of 43 BE patients were married or living with a partner. Sexual counseling in these patients is important because of the difficulties they may encounter.

Exceedingly small penile size can severely limit the potential of some men to have sexual intercourse. In this setting, reconstruction with a radial forearm flap to construct a penis analogue has shown an improved quality of life.[131]

Ejaculation is often possible despite the extensive reconstructive procedures that are performed. However, seminal emission may be slow and continue several hours after orgasm. Sperm quality and quantity is often diminished which may be due to partial obstruction after surgery, epididymitis, or recurrent urinary infections. In one series, 63% had antegrade ejaculation.[132] Long-term studies in adults with BE found that a minority were able to conceive without assisted reproductive techniques.[130,133,134]

For women with exstrophy, sexual intercourse is possible and sexual function is often intact.[128] In one series, 14 of 23 patients were able to have typical intercourse.[135] Narrowing at the vaginal introitus can be problematic. This can be addressed with serial calibration and dilation as a first option, or with vaginal advancement skin flaps as another option. Fertility is unimpaired in female patients with BE. However, prolapse occurs more commonly because of the lack of pelvic floor support structures and bed-rest may be necessary in the later stages of pregnancy. Pregnancy in these patients is considered a high risk event.[28,136] Pregnancy complications such as hydronephrosis and bacteriuira are common, and may necessitate antimicrobial prophylaxis.[137] Cesarean section is the recommended mode of delivery as vaginal delivery can be problematic.[138] Vaginal and uterine prolapse is more common in women with BE and treatment occurs at a younger age than in the general population.[139]

CLOACAL EXSTROPHY

Although CE has been recognized for several hundred years, Spencer was the first surgeon to report successful repair and survival in 1965.[140] Mortality rates of CE infants remained high for years following this initial success. Affected infants routinely died of malnutrition and sepsis. With continuing improvement in total parenteral nutrition and neonatal management, mortality rates currently are less than 10%.[141] Quality of life issues are now paramount in this patient group.

The bladder plate associated with CE is divided in half by the hindgut plate, which represents the development anomaly of the colon that occurs with CE. Ileum enters and intussuscepts into the middle of the hindgut creating the 'trunk of an elephant's face' appearance with appendiceal appendages located laterally to give the impression of 'tusks on the face of the elephant' (Fig. 58-13).[142]

With CE, the bladder neck and external urethral sphincter are not fully developed due to the failed development of the bladder and urethral remnant located on the anterior and dorsal surfaces of the body wall and penis respectively. However, because innervation to these structures may be intact, anatomic closure theoretically offers the possibility of achieving urinary continence. The urethral plate is characteristically short as well.

Associated Anomalies

Renal anomalies are much more common in CE than with BE. They include anomalies in locations such as a pelvic kidney or crossed fused renal ectopia. Horseshoe kidneys, renal agenesis, and ureteropelvic junction obstruction are also found.

In CE, the penis is often separated into two hemiphalluses due to the wide pubic diastasis. This can make reconstructive efforts technically more challenging if a male phenotype is preserved. Cryptorchidism is the rule with CE. For girls, in addition to the genital pathology described previously with BE, uterus didelphys and other fusion anomalies of the Müllerian duct structures are seen in up to two-thirds of CE females. Vaginal agenesis occurs in one-third of CE females.

In addition to the typical exstrophy of the hindgut, ileal intussusception and the exposed appendices, other associated intestinal abnormalities include imperforate anus, foreshortening of the midgut, bowel duplication, malrotation, intestinal atresia, and Meckel's diverticulum.

In addition to the features seen with BE, up to one-half of patients with CE can have other skeletal abnormalities. These anomalies include congenital hip dislocation, talipes equinovarus, and a variety of limb deficiencies.[143]

The fascial anomalies associated with CE include those previously described for BE. In addition, omphaloceles are often found as well.[144,145] The omphalocele can be repaired during the initial bladder closure if it is small. If the omphalocele is large, it may require closure with the reapproximated bladder halves acting as a silo to reduce the intra-abdominal pressure. Alternatively, the omphalocele can be treated with antiseptic paint to promote epithelialization. The intra-abdominal pressure following omphalocele closure determines whether we can proceed with primary bladder closure at the same time or whether bladder closure is performed later. Too aggressive an attempt at one-stage CE repair can lead to organ ischemia from the increased intra-abdominal pressure. On the other hand, rupture of an omphalocele clearly requires immediate attention and takes priority over other considerations.

Neurologic involvement of the lower spinal cord is reported to occur in 50–100% of patients.[144,146,147] Most patients have lumbar or sacral cord involvement, but

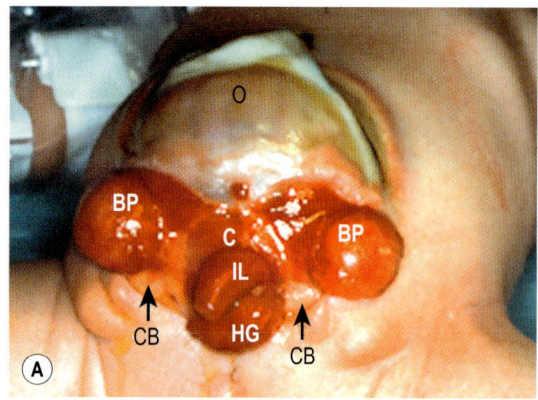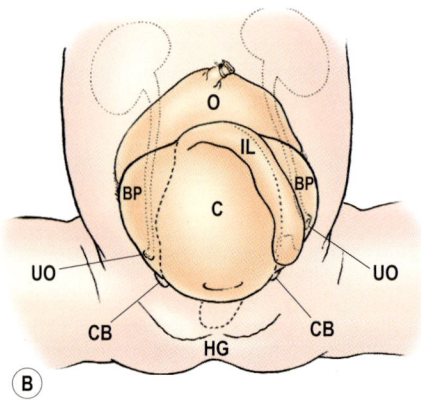

FIGURE 58-13 ■ Photograph and schematic drawing of a neonate with cloacal exstrophy. BP, bladder plate; C, cecal plate; CB, corporeal body; HG, hindgut; IL, ileum; O, omphalocele; UO, ureteral orifice.

thoracic level myelodysplasia has also been reported.[144] CE management must be coordinated with closure of the neural tube defect.

Perioperative Management

CE patients are best managed by an experienced team of pediatric urologists, surgeons, orthopedists, gastroenterologists, endocrinologists and neurosurgeons. Advances in neonatal care, intravenous nutrition, and the operative approach have markedly reduced the mortality and morbidity of this condition. Nonetheless, the management remains challenging.

In the neonatal period, the bladder and hindgut plate should be covered (plastic wrap or Vigilon®) to protect the exposed structures. Similar to BE, the umbilical cord is ligated with a suture to prevent an umbilical clamp from abrading the bladder or hindgut plate. Antibiotic prophylaxis should be administered because of the high incidence of renal abnormalities.

Preoperative studies include ultrasound, abdominal films and karyotyping. Sonographic examination allows the evaluation of the upper urinary tracts, internal genital structures, and spinal cord. Because of the associated genital anomalies, accurately identifying the gender may be difficult, and karyotyping is helpful to define the chromosomal sex in unclear situations.

Cloacal Exstrophy Closure Techniques

Each CE patient is unique, requiring an individualized operative plan. In general, this plan would include: (1) closure of the omphalocele with reapproximation of the posterior bladder halves, tubularization of the cecum and incorporation of the hindgut into the gastrointestinal tract (functionally this creates the anatomy of classic BE); and (2) repair of the exstrophic bladder and genitalia. If the baby is medically stable, the initial reconstructive procedures can be performed within the first 72 hours of life, thus taking advantage of the pliable bony pelvis if closure of the entire defect is possible. However, in up to 75% of these children, spina bifida is present and may need urgent closure, delaying the ventral abdominal wall closure. Also, the omphalocele, seen in almost 90% of the patients,[148] may require immediate care to prevent rupture. The size of the omphalocele, the size of the hindgut plate and bladder plates, the extent of the pubic diastasis, and the extent of comorbidities largely dictate the timing and staging of the initial closure. If the large omphalocele cannot be closed because of increased abdominal pressure, a silo can be placed or a biosynthetic patch used to bridge the abdominal wall fascial defect.

In the past, an ileostomy was routinely performed, but the metabolic consequences can be significant. Currently, management decisions focus around the use of the exstrophic cecal plate and the terminal blind-ending hindgut. The cecal plate can be retained in the bladder closure as a bladder augmentation or can be separated from the bladder plates and used in the gastrointestinal tract (Fig. 58-14A). However, to improve bowel length and water resorption, most feel the cecal plate should be tubularized, making the terminal ileum, cecum, and the

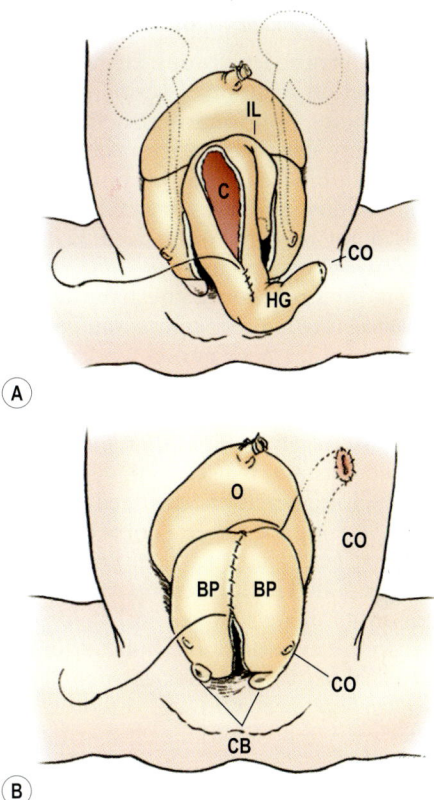

FIGURE 58-14 ■ (A) Depiction of removal and tubularization of the cecal plate. **(B)** Reapproximation of the bladder plates. BP, bladder plate; C, cecum; CB, corporeal body; CO, colostomy site; HG, hindgut; IL, ileum; O, omphalocele; UO, ureteral orifice.

blind-ending hindgut all in continuity. The hindgut segment can then be exteriorized as a colostomy.

In some cases, there are hindgut duplications. No segment of bowel should be discarded unless absolutely unusable, since it might be useful at some time for the bowel, bladder or vaginal reconstruction. Similarly, appendiceal segments should be preserved for possible use in reconstruction of the urinary tract. Because of altered innervation to the pelvis, not all patients with CE are candidates for an anal pull-through procedure. The best candidates are children with an anocutaneous fistula and preserved innervation.

At initial repair, ureteral catheters are positioned in the ureteral orifices and secured with 5-0 chromic suture. For the omphalocele repair, the dissection begins superiorly. Next, the umbilical vessels are ligated and the bladder plates separated from the adjacent skin as described in the CPRE and MSRE techniques. The medial cecal hindgut plate is separated from the paired, separated bladder plates, and tubularized. The bladder halves are then reapproximated in the midline (Fig. 58-14B). Inguinal hernias should be repaired if found. Bladder repair can be performed if the intra-abdominal pressure remains low after omphalocele closure. This is determined clinically by assessing a change in ventilatory parameters. A one-stage CE closure, including closure of the omphalocele, cecal plate tubularization and hindgut terminal colostomy, bladder and urethral closure, reconstruction of the external genitalia and osteotomies, should be performed only under optimal anatomical conditions. The decision to proceed with one-stage closure versus staged reconstruction spanning a period of months must be weighed carefully. Following tight closure, increased abdominal pressure can cause organ ischemia, excessive tension on the midline closure, or compromised lower extremity blood flow. If necessary, CE repair can be staged at this point by converting the CE into a classic BE. A colostomy is then created.

If staging is indicated, once the baby has recovered sufficiently to tolerate another operation, reconstruction of the bladder, bladder neck and genitalia is performed using either the CPRE or MSRE approach.[149]

Osteotomies are almost always necessary to assist in closure and posterior positioning of the urinary tract, given the pubic diastasis is usually more severe than in BE. Prior to the initial incision, the need for osteotomies is assessed by watching for ischemia of the lower extremities and external genitalia with reapproximation of the pubic symphysis. The Hopkins group recommends bilateral anterior innominate and vertical iliac osteotomies with gradual approximation of the bones over one to two weeks via external fixture and interfragmentary pins.[150,151] The Seattle group prefers iliac osteotomies. Other authors prefer to avoid osteotomies because they believe that osteotomies make the abdominal closure more difficult,[152] but this has not been our experience. Fewer wound dehiscences and abdominal wall hernias have been reported with osteotomies.[151]

Secondary procedures may be required on the urinary tract to achieve continence, including BNR, bladder neck closure, bladder augmentation with stomach, ileum or hindgut, and creation of a continent catheterizable stoma.[144,153–156] As most of these children will need CIC to achieve dryness, urinary reconstruction must be individualized to meet their needs.

Gender of Rearing

Gender assignment for patients with CE is currently debated both by the medical profession and by the lay public. Traditionally, male patients underwent gender conversion in infancy because of concerns that the small, paired male hemi-phalluses were inadequate in size. This approach was supported by anecdotal data of unsatisfied patients following genital reconstruction.[144] However, these observations, in conjunction with the prevailing notion that humans are gender neutral at birth and can undergo gender conversion safely in infancy, have recently come into question.[157] Gender identity now appears to be a much more complex issue than previously imagined.

Currently we reconstruct males with CE as males whenever technically possible. Many gender assigned individuals will later identify themselves in a male gender role in adolescence and adulthood.[157] Technically, however, reconstruction of external male genitalia in these patients can be quite challenging. The wide pubic diastasis and small phallic size add to the technical difficulty because it is more difficult to join the two phallic halves in the midline. In some cases, if one phallic half is diminutive, the small one is removed, and the reconstruction is performed using only the larger half.

Female genital reconstruction is complex as well. In genetic females, complete Müllerian and vaginal duplication often leads to attempted midline reapproximation. However, if one system appears more substantial, excision of the lesser unit may be prudent. In genetic males raised as female, neovaginal reconstruction is typically delayed and may require use of a hindgut segment or perineal skin.

Gastrointestinal Reconstruction

Short-gut syndrome is usually present at birth in babies with CE, even those with a normal length of bowel. The effects of malabsorption and fluid loss appear to be most clinically significant early in life.[158] Many such children require parenteral nutritional support in early infancy.[159,160] As a result of this problem, we feel the hindgut should be constructed and placed in continuity with the intestine during the initial operation. This may improve intestinal absorption and nutrition, and will also preserve intestinal tissue that can be used in later reconstruction of the urinary tract or vagina if needed.

REFERENCES

1. Gearhart JP. The exstrophy-epispadias complex in the new millennium–science, practice and policy. J Urol 1999;162:1421–3.
2. Lattimer JK, Smith MK. Exstrophy closure: A followup on 70 cases. J Urol 1966;95:356–9.
3. Engel RM. Exstrophy of the bladder and associated anomalies. Birth Defects Orig Artic Ser 1974;10:146–9.
4. Epidemiology of bladder exstrophy and epispadias: A communication from the International Clearinghouse for Birth Defects Monitoring Systems. Teratology 1987;36:221–7.
5. Ives E, Coffey R, Carter CO. A family study of bladder exstrophy. J Med Genet 1980;17:139–41.
6. Ziegler M, Duckett JW, Howell JG. Cloacal exstrophy. In: Welch J, editor. Pediatric Surgery. Chicago: Year Book Publishers; 1986.
7. Keppler-Noreuil KM. OEIS complex (omphalocele-exstrophy-imperforate anus-spinal defects): A review of 14 cases. Am J Med Genet 2001;99:271–9.
8. Brock J III, O'Neill J Jr. Bladder exstrophy. In: O'Neill J Jr, editor. Pediatric Surgery. Philadelphia: Lippincott; 1998. p. 1709–32.
9. Skari H, Bjornland K, Bjornstad-Ostensen A, et al. Consequences of prenatal ultrasound diagnosis: A preliminary report on neonates with congenital malformations. Acta Obstet Gynecol Scand 1998;77:635–42.
10. Gearhart JP, Ben-Chaim J, Jeffs RD, et al. Criteria for the prenatal diagnosis of classic bladder exstrophy. Obstet Gynecol 1995;85:961–4.
11. Mirk P, Calisti A, Fileni A. Prenatal sonographic diagnosis of bladder extrophy. J Ultrasound Med 1986;5:291–3.
12. Barth RA, Filly RA, Sondheimer FK. Prenatal sonographic findings in bladder exstrophy. J Ultrasound Med 1990;9:359–61.
13. Jaffe R, Schoenfeld A, Ovadia J. Sonographic findings in the prenatal diagnosis of bladder exstrophy. Am J Obstet Gynecol 1990;162:675–8.
14. Lee EH, Shim JY. New sonographic finding for the prenatal diagnosis of bladder exstrophy: A case report. Ultrasound Obstet Gynecol 2003;21:498–500.
15. Cacciari A, Pilu GL, Modenti M, et al. Prenatal diagnosis of bladder exstrophy: What counseling? J Urol 1999;161:259–62.
16. Wiersma R. Overview of bladder exstrophy: A third world perspective. J Pediatr Surg 2008;43:1520–3.
17. Muecke EC. The Role of the Cloacal Membrane in Exstrophy: The First Successful Experimental Study. J Urol 1964;92:659–67.

18. Klimberg I. The Development of Voiding Control. AUA Update Series 1988;7:162–7.

19. Marshall FF. Embryology of the lower genitourinary tract. Urol Clin North Am 1978;5:3–15.

20. Thomalla JV, Rudolph RA, Rink RC, et al. Induction of cloacal exstrophy in the chick embryo using the CO2 laser. J Urol 1985;134:991–5.

21. Patten BM, Barry A. The genesis of exstrophy of the bladder and epispadias. Am J Anat 1952;90:35–57.

22. Manner J, Kluth D. A chicken model to study the embryology of cloacal exstrophy. J Pediatr Surg 2003;38:678–81.

23. Beaudoin S, Barbet P, Bargy F. Pelvic development in the rabbit embryo: implications in the organogenesis of bladder exstrophy. Anat Embryol (Berl) 2004;208:425–30.

24. Slaughenhoupt BL, Mathews RI, Peppas DS, et al. A large animal model of bladder exstrophy: Observations of bladder smooth muscle and collagen content. J Urol 1999;162:2119–22.

25. Slaughenhoupt BL, Chen CJ, Gearhart JP. Creation of a model of bladder exstrophy in the fetal lamb. J Urol 1996;156:816–18.

26. Verpoest W, Platteau P, Van Steirteghem A, et al. Pregnancy in a couple with a male partner born with severe bladder exstrophy. Reprod Biomed Online 2004;8:240–2.

27. Gross SD. A Practical Treatise on the Diseases, Injuries, and Malformations of the Urinary Bladder, the Prostate Gland, and the Urethra. 3rd ed. Philadelphia: Henry C. Lea; 1876.

28. Burbige KA, Hensel TW, Chambers WJ, et al. Pregnancy and sexual function in women with bladder exstrophy. Urology 1986;28:12–14.

29. Mathews R, Gan M, Gearhart JP. Urogynaecological and obstetric issues in women with the exstrophy-epispadias complex. BJU Int 2003;91:845–9.

30. Froster UG, Heinritz W, Bennek J, et al. Another case of autosomal dominant exstrophy of the bladder. Prenat Diagn 2004;24:375–7.

31. Messelink EJ, Aronson DC, Knuist M, et al. Four cases of bladder exstrophy in two families. J Med Genet 1994;31:490–2.

32. Shapiro E, Lepor H, Jeffs RD. The inheritance of the exstrophy-epispadias complex. J Urol 1984;132:308–10.

33. Paidas MJ, Crombleholme TM, Robertson FM. Prenatal diagnosis and management of the fetus with an abdominal wall defect. Semin Perinatol 1994;18:196–214.

34. Tang Y, Ma CX, Cui W, et al. The risk of birth defects in multiple births: A population-based study. Matern Child Health J 2006;10:75–81.

35. Gambhir L, Höller T, Müller M, et al. Epidemiological survey of 214 families with bladder exstrophy-epispadias complex. J Urol 2008;179:1539–43.

36. O'Kane HO, Megaw JM. Carcinoma in the exstrophic bladder. Br J Surg 1968;55:631–5.

37. Hohenfellner R, Stein R. Primary urinary diversion in patients with bladder exstrophy. Urology 1996;48:28–830.

38. Hollowell JG, Hill PD, Duffy PG, et al. Lower urinary tract function after exstrophy closure. Pediatr Nephrol 1992;6:428–32.

39. Nisonson I, Lattimer JK. How well can the exstrophied bladder work? J Urol 1972;107:664–6.

40. Stein R, Fisch M, Stöckle M, et al. Colonic conduit in children: Protection of the upper urinary tract 16 years later? J Urol 1996;156:1146–50.

41. Husmann DA, Rathbun SR. Long-term follow up of enteric bladder augmentations: The risk for malignancy. J Pediatr Urol 2008;4:381–6.

42. Vemulakonda VM, Lendvay TS, Shnorhavorian M, et al. Metastatic adenocarcinoma after augmentation gastrocystoplasty. J Urol 2008;179:1094–7.

43. Husmann DA, Spence HM. Current status of tumor of the bowel following ureterosigmoidostomy: A review. J Urol 1990;144:607–10.

44. Fisch M, Wammack R, Hohenfellner R. The sigma rectum pouch (Mainz pouch II). World J Urol 1996;14:68–72.

45. Hohenfellner R. Continent urinary diversion in childhood: European experience. Scand J Urol Nephrol Suppl 1992;142:82–5.

46. Ghoneim MA. The modified rectal bladder: A bladder substitute controlled by the anal sphincter. Scand J Urol Nephrol Suppl 1992;142:89–91.

47. Tacciuoli M, Laurenti C, Racheli T. Sixteen years' experience with the Heitz Boyer-Hovelacque procedure for exstrophy of the bladder. Br J Urol 1977;49:385–90.

48. Crissey MM, Steele GD, Gittes RF. Rat model for carcinogenesis in ureterosigmoidostomy. Science 1980;207:1079–80.

49. Trendelenberg F. The treatment of ectopia vesicae. Ann Surg 1906;44:981–9.

50. Ansell JS. Surgical treatment of exstrophy of the bladder with emphasis on neonatal primary closure: Personal experience with 28 consecutive cases treated at the University of Washington hospitals from 1962 to 1977: Techniques and results. J Urol 1979;121:650–3.

51. Young H. Exstrophy of the bladder: The first case in which a normal bladder and urinary control have been obtained by plastic operations. Surg Gynecol Obstet 1942;74:729–37.

52. Montagnani CA. One stage functional reconstruction of exstrophied bladder: Report of two cases with six-year follow-up. Z Kinderchir 1982;37:23–7.

53. Fuchs J, Gluer S, Mildenberger H. One-stage reconstruction of bladder exstrophy. Eur J Pediatr Surg 1996;6:212–15.

54. King L, Wendel E. Primary cystectomy and permanent urinary diversion in the treatment of exstrophy of the urinary bladder. In: Scott JR, Gordon H, Carlton C, Beach PD, editor. Current Controversies in Urologic management. Philadelphia: WB Saunders Co; 1972. p. 242–50.

55. Johnston JH, Kogan SJ. The exstrophic anomalies and their surgical reconstruction. Curr Probl Surg 1974;1–39.

56. Williams DI, Keeton JE. Further progress with reconstruction of the exstrophied bladder. Br J Surg 1973;60:203–7.

57. Megall, M, Lattimer JK. Review of the management of 140 cases of exstrophy of the bladder. J Urol 1973;109:246–8.

58. Engel RM. Bladder exstrophy: Vesicoplasty or urinary diversion? Urology 1973;2:20–4.

59. Ezell WW, Carlson HE. A realistic look at exstrophy of the bladder. Br J Urol 1970;42:197–202.

60. Aadalen RJ, O'Phelan EH, Chisholm TC, et al. Exstrophy of the bladder: Long-term results of bilateral posterior iliac osteotomies and two-stage anatomic repair. Clin Orthop Relat Res 1980;151:193–200.

61. Jeffs RD. Functional closure of bladder exstrophy. Birth Defects Orig Artic Ser 1977;13:171–3.

62. Saltzman B, Mininberg DT, Muecke EC. Exstrophy of bladder: Evolution of management. Urology 1985;26:383–8.

63. Grady RW, Mitchell ME. Complete primary repair of exstrophy. J Urol 1999;162:1415–20.

64. Churchill B, Merguerian PA, Khoury AE, et al. Bladder exstrophy and epispadias. In: O'Donnel B, Koff S, editor. Pediatric Urology. Oxford, England: Reed Elsevier; 1997. p. 495–508.

65. Gearhart JP, Jeffs RD. Bladder exstrophy: Increase in capacity following epispadias repair. J Urol 1989;142:525–6.

66. Mathews R, Gosling JA, Gearhart JP. Ultrastructure of the bladder in classic exstrophy: Correlation with development of continence. J Urol 2004;172:1446–9.

67. Mathews R, Willis M, Perlman E, et al. Neural innervation of the newborn exstrophic bladder: An immunohistochemical study. J Urol 1999;162:506–8.

68. Lee BR, Perlman EJ, Partin AW, et al. Evaluation of smooth muscle and collagen subtypes in normal newborns and those with bladder exstrophy. J Urol 1996;156:2034–6.

69. McMahon DR, Cain MP, Husmann DA, et al. Vesical neck reconstruction in patients with the exstrophy-epispadias complex. J Urol 1996;155:1411–13.

70. Dodson JL, Surer I, Baker LA, et al. The newborn exstrophy bladder inadequate for primary closure: evaluation, management and outcome. J Urol 2001;165:1656–9.

71. Gearhart JP. Bladder exstrophy: Staged reconstruction. Curr Opin Urol 1999;9:499–506.

72. Kost-Byerly S, Jackson EV, Yaster M, et al. Perioperative anesthetic and analgesic management of newborn bladder exstrophy repair. J Pediatr Urol 2008;4:280–5.

73. Gearhart JP, Forschner DC, Jeffs RD, et al. A combined vertical and horizontal pelvic osteotomy approach for primary and secondary repair of bladder exstrophy. J Urol 1996;155:689–93.

74. Husmann DA, McLorie GA, Churchill BM. Closure of the exstrophic bladder: An evaluation of the factors leading to its

success and its importance on urinary continence. J Urol 1989;142:522–4.

75. Gearhart JP, Peppas DS, Jeffs DS. The failed exstrophy closure: Strategy for management. Br J Urol 1993;71:217–20.

76. Close CE, Carr MC, Burns MW, et al. Lower urinary tract changes after early valve ablation in neonates and infants: Is early diversion warranted? J Urol 1997;157:984–8.

77. Mitchell ME, Bagli DJ. Complete penile disassembly for epispadias repair: The Mitchell technique. J Urol 1996;155: 300–4.

78. Cook AJ, Farhat WA, Cartwright LM, et al. Simplified mons plasty: A new technique to improve cosmesis in females with the exstrophy-epispadias complex. J Urol 2005;173:2117–20.

79. Jarzebowski AC, McMullin ND, Grover SR, et al. The Kelly technique of bladder exstrophy repair: Continence, cosmesis and pelvic organ prolapse outcomes. J Urol 2009;182:1802–6.

80. Berrettini A, Castagnetti M, Rigamonti W. Radical soft tissue mobilization and reconstruction (Kelly procedure) for bladder extrophy [correction of exstrophy] repair in males: Initial experience with nine cases. Pediatr Surg Int 2009;25:427–31.

81. Canning D. Vesical Exstrophy Complete primary closure commentary. In: Hinman JaLBF, editor. Hinman's Atlas of Pediatric Urologic Surgery. Philadelphia, PA: Saunders Elsevier; 2009. p. 388.

82. Baradaran N, Stec AA, Schaeffer AJ, et al. Delayed primary closure of bladder exstrophy: Immediate postoperative management leading to successful outcomes. Urology 2012;79:415–19.

83. Zaccara A, Stec AA, Schaeffer AJ, et al. Delayed complete repair of exstrophy with testosterone treatment: An alternative to avoid glans complications? Pediatr Surg Int 2011;27:417–21.

84. Hafez AT, De Gennaro M, Di Lazzaro A, et al. Complete primary repair of bladder exstrophy in children presenting late and those with failed initial closure: single center experience. J Urol 2005;174:1549–52.

85. Nelson CP, North AC, Ward MK, et al. Economic impact of failed or delayed primary repair of bladder exstrophy: Differences in cost of hospitalization. J Urol 2008;179:680–3.

86. Jeffs RD. Exstrophy and cloacal exstrophy. Urol Clin North Am 1978;5:127–40.

87. Gearhart JP, Jeffs RD. State-of-the-art reconstructive surgery for bladder exstrophy at the Johns Hopkins Hospital. Am J Dis Child 1989;143:1475–8.

88. Baker LA, Gearhart JP. The staged approach to bladder exstrophy closure and the role of osteotomies. World J Urol 1998;16:205–11.

89. Baka-Jakubiak M. Combined bladder neck, urethral and penile reconstruction in boys with the exstrophy-epispadias complex. BJU Int 2000;86:513–18.

90. Baird AD, Mathews RI, Gearhart JP. The use of combined bladder and epispadias repair in boys with classic bladder exstrophy: Outcomes, complications and consequences. J Urol 2005;174: 1421–4.

91. Duckett JW. Use of paraexstrophy skin pedicle grafts for correction of exstrophy and epispadias repair. Birth Defects Orig Artic Ser 1977;13:175–9.

92. Gearhart JP, Sciortino C, Ben-Chaim J, et al. The Cantwell-Ransley epispadias repair in exstrophy and epispadias: Lessons learned. Urology 1995;46:92–5.

93. Gearhart JP, Ben-Chaim J, Sciortino C, et al. The multiple reoperative bladder exstrophy closure: What affects the potential of the bladder? Urology 1996;47:240–3.

94. Ben-Chaim J, Jeffs RD, Gearhart JP. Loss of urethrovaginal septum as a complication of exstrophy closure in girls. Eur Urol 1998;33:206–8.

95. Perović S, Scepanović D, Sremcević D, et al. Epispadias surgery–Belgrade experience. Br J Urol 1992;70:674–7.

96. Borzi PA, Thomas DF. Cantwell-Ransley epispadias repair in male epispadias and bladder exstrophy. J Urol 1994;151: 457–9.

97. Ferrer FA, Tadros YE, Gearhart J. Modified Young-Dees-Leadbetter bladder neck reconstruction: New concepts about old ideas. Urology 2001;58:791–6.

98. Canning DA, Gearhart JP, Peppas DS, et al. The cephalotrigonal reimplant in bladder neck reconstruction for patients with exstrophy or epispadias. J Urol 1993;150:156–8.

99. Jones JA, Mitchell ME, Rink RC. Improved results using a modification of the Young-Dees-Leadbetter bladder neck repair. Br J Urol 1993;71:555–61.

100. Ben-Chaim J, Gearhart JP. Current management of bladder exstrophy. Tech Urol 1996;2:2–33.

101. Mansi M, Ahmed S. Young-Dees-Leadbetter bladder neck reconstruction for sphincteric urinary incontinence: The value of augmentation cystoplasty. Scand J Urol Nephrol 1993;27:509–17.

102. Ganesan GS, Nguyen DH, Adams MC, et al. Lower urinary tract reconstruction using stomach and the artificial sphincter. J Urol 1993;149:1107–9.

103. Lottmann HB, Yaqouti M, Melin Y. Male epispadias repair: Surgical and functional results with the Cantwell-Ransley procedure in 40 patients. J Urol 1999;162:1176–80.

104. Gearhart JP. Complete repair of bladder exstrophy in the newborn: Complications and management. J Urol 2001;165:2431–3.

105. Gearhart JP, Mathews R. Penile reconstruction combined with bladder closure in the management of classic bladder exstrophy: Illustration of technique. Urology 2000;55:764–70.

106. Mollard P. [Bladder and urethral reconstruction for bladder exstrophy]. Bull Soc Sci Med Grand Duche Luxemb 1987;124(Spec No):225–30.

107. Surer I, Baker LA, Jeffs RD, et al. Modified Young-Dees-Leadbetter bladder neck reconstruction in patients with successful primary bladder closure elsewhere: A single institution experience. J Urol 2001;165:2438–40.

108. Shaw MB, Rink RC, Kaefer M, et al. Continence and classic bladder exstrophy treated with staged repair. J Urol 2004;172:1450–3.

109. Gearhart JP, Canning DA, Peppas DS, et al. Techniques to create continence in the failed bladder exstrophy closure patient. J Urol 1993;150:441–3.

110. Chan DY, Jeffs RD, Gearhart JP. Determinants of continence in the bladder exstrophy population: predictors of success? Urology 2001;57:774–7.

111. Woodhouse CR, Redgrave NG. Late failure of the reconstructed exstrophy bladder. Br J Urol 1996;77:590–2.

112. Stringer MD, Duffy PG, Ransley, PG. Inguinal hernias associated with bladder exstrophy. Br J Urol 1994;73:308–9.

113. Connolly JA, Peppas DS, Jeffs RD, et al. Prevalence and repair of inguinal hernias in children with bladder exstrophy. J Urol 1995;154:1900–1.

114. Husmann DA, McLorie GA, CHurchill BM, et al. Inguinal pathology and its association with classical bladder exstrophy. J Pediatr Surg 1990;25:332–4.

115. Oesterling JE, Jeffs RD. The importance of a successful initial bladder closure in the surgical management of classical bladder exstrophy: Analysis of 144 patients treated at the Johns Hopkins Hospital between 1975 and 1985. J Urol 1987;137:258–62.

116. Sponseller PD, Jani MM, Jeffs RD, et al. Anterior innominate osteotomy in repair of bladder exstrophy. J Bone Joint Surg Am 2001;83:184–93.

117. Okubadejo GO, Sponseller PD, Gearhart JP. Complications in orthopedic management of exstrophy. J Pediatr Orthop 2003;23:522–8.

118. Sponseller PD, Gearhart JP, Jeffs RD. Anterior innominate osteotomies for failure or late closure of bladder exstrophy. J Urol 1991;146:137–40.

119. McKenna PH, Khoury AE, McLorie GA, et al. Iliac osteotomy: A model to compare the options in bladder and cloacal exstrophy reconstruction. J Urol 1994;151:182–7.

120. Schmidt AH, Keenen TL, Tank ES, et al. Pelvic osteotomy for bladder exstrophy. J Pediatr Orthop 1993;13:214–19.

121. Frey P. Bilateral anterior pubic osteotomy in bladder exstrophy closure. J Urol 1996;156:812–15.

122. Kajbafzadeh AM, Tajik P. A novel technique for approximation of the symphysis pubis in bladder exstrophy without pelvic osteotomy. J Urol 2006;175:692–8.

123. Lee C, Reutter HM, Grässer MF, et al. Gender-associated differences in the psychosocial and developmental outcome in patients affected with the bladder exstrophy-epispadias complex. BJU Int 2006;97:49–353.

124. Reiner WG, Gearhart JP, Jeffs R. Psychosexual dysfunction in males with genital anomalies: Late adolescence, Tanner stages IV to VI. J Am Acad Child Adolesc Psychiatry 1999;38:865–72.

125. Reiner WG, Gearhart JP, Kropp B. Suicide and suicidal ideation in classic exstrophy. J Urol 2008;180:1661–4.

126. Wilson CJ, Pistrang N, Woodhouse CR, et al. The psychosocial impact of bladder exstrophy in adolescence. J Adolesc Health 2007;41:504–8.

127. Wilson C, Christie D, Woodhouse CR. The ambitions of adolescents born with exstrophy: a structured survey. BJU Int 2004; 94:607–12.

128. Woodhouse CR, Ransley PG, Williams DI. The patient with exstrophy in adult life. Br J Urol 1983;55:632–5.

129. Woodhouse CR. The management of erectile deformity in adults with exstrophy and epispadias. J Urol 1986;135:932–5.

130. Gobet R, Weber D, Horst M, et al. Long-term followup (37 to 69 years) in patients with bladder exstrophy treated with ureterosigmoidostomy: Psychosocial and psychosexual outcomes. J Urol 2009;182:1819–23.

131. Ricketts S, Hunter-Smith DJ, Coombs CJ. Quality of life after penile reconstruction using the radial forearm flap in adult bladder exstrophy patients - technique and outcomes. ANZ J Surg 2011;81:52–5.

132. Ben-Chaim J, Jeffs RD, Reiner WG, et al. The outcome of patients with classic bladder exstrophy in adult life. J Urol 1996; 155:1251–2.

133. Gambhir L, Reutter H, Ludwig M. Successful assisted reproduction in adult males with bladder extrophy-epispadias complex. Eur J Obstet Gynecol Reprod Biol 2008;139:259–60.

134. D'Hauwers KW, Feitz WF, Kremer JA. Bladder exstrophy and male fertility: pregnancies after ICSI with ejaculated or epididymal sperm. Fertil Steril 2008;89:387–9.

135. Woodhouse CR, Hinsch R. The anatomy and reconstruction of the adult female genitalia in classical exstrophy. Br J Urol 1997;79: 618–22.

136. Woodhouse CR. The gynaecology of exstrophy. BJU Int 1999; 83:34–8.

137. Ebert AK, Falkert A, Hofstädter A, et al. Pregnancy management in women within the bladder-exstrophy-epispadias complex (BEEC) after continent urinary diversion. Arch Gynecol Obstet 2011;284:1043–6.

138. Nikolov A, Markov P, Chanachev S. [Pregnancy and delivery in patients with surgically corrected congenital extrophy of the bladder, through the operations of the continent urinary derivation]. Akush Ginekol (Sofiia) 2011;50:60–3.

139. Rose CH, Rowe TF, Cox SM, et al. Uterine prolapse associated with bladder exstrophy: surgical management and subsequent pregnancy. J Matern Fetal Med 2000;9:150–2.

140. Spencer R. Exstrophia Splanchnica (Exstrophy of the Cloaca). Surgery 1965;57:751–66.

141. Davidoff AM, Hebra A, Balmer D, et al. Management of the gastrointestinal tract and nutrition in patients with cloacal exstrophy. J Pediatr Surg 1996;31:771–3.

142. Warren B. Exstrophy of the Cloaca. In: Ashcraft K, Holder T, editor. Pediatric Surgery. Philadelphia: W.B. Saunders Co.; 1993. p. 402–12.

143. Sponseller PD, Bisson LJ, Gearhart JP, et al. The anatomy of the pelvis in the exstrophy complex. J Bone Joint Surg Am 1995;77: 177–89.

144. Lund DP, Hendren WH. Cloacal exstrophy: Experience with 20 cases. J Pediatr Surg 1993;28:1360–9.

145. Hesser JW, Murata Y, Swalwell CI. Exstrophy of cloaca with omphalocele: Two cases. Am J Obstet Gynecol 1984;150: 1004–6.

146. Howell C, Caldamone A, Snyder H, et al. Optimal management of cloacal exstrophy. J Pediatr Surg 1983;18:365–9.

147. Hurwitz RS, Manzoni GA, Ransley PG, et al. Cloacal exstrophy: A report of 34 cases. J Urol 1987;138:1060–4.

148. Diamond DA, Jeffs RD. Cloacal exstrophy: A 22-year experience. J Urol 1985;133:779–82.

149. Lee RS, Grady R, Joyner B, et al. Can a complete primary repair approach be applied to cloacal exstrophy? J Urol 2006;176: 2643–8.

150. Silver RI, Sponseller PD, Gearhart JP. Staged closure of the pelvis in cloacal exstrophy: first description of a new approach. J Urol 1999;161:263–6.

151. Ben-Chaim J, Peppas DS, Spnseller PD, et al. Applications of osteotomy in the cloacal exstrophy patient. J Urol 1995;154: 865–7.

152. Husmann DA, Vandersteen DR, McLorie GA, et al. Urinary continence after staged bladder reconstruction for cloacal exstrophy: The effect of coexisting neurological abnormalities on urinary continence. J Urol 1999;161:1598–602.

153. Gearhart JP, Mathews R, Taylor S, et al. Combined bladder closure and epispadias repair in the reconstruction of bladder exstrophy. J Urol 1998;160:1182–90.

154. Mathews R, Jeffs RD, Reiner WG, et al. Cloacal exstrophy–improving the quality of life: The Johns Hopkins experience. J Urol 1998;160:2452–6.

155. Gearhart JP, Jeffs RD. Techniques to create urinary continence in the cloacal exstrophy patient. J Urol 1991;146:616–18.

156. Mitchell ME, Brito CG, Rink RC. Cloacal exstrophy reconstruction for urinary continence. J Urol 1990;144:554–8.

157. Reiner WG, Gearhart JP. Discordant sexual identity in some genetic males with cloacal exstrophy assigned to female sex at birth. N Engl J Med 2004;350:333–41.

158. Husmann DA, McLorie GA, Churchill BM, et al. Management of the hindgut in cloacal exstrophy: Terminal ileostomy versus colostomy. J Pediatr Surg 1988;23:1107–13.

159. Georgeson KE, Breaux CW Jr. Outcome and intestinal adaptation in neonatal short-bowel syndrome. J Pediatr Surg 1992;27: 344–50.

160. Figueroa-Colon R, Harris PR, Birdsong E, et al. Impact of intestinal lengthening on the nutritional outcome for children with short bowel syndrome. J Pediatr Surg 1996;31:912–16.

CHAPTER 59

HYPOSPADIAS

J. Patrick Murphy

Hypospadias is a developmental anomaly characterized by a urethral meatus that opens onto the ventral surface of the penis, proximal to the end of the glans. The meatus may be located anywhere along the shaft of the penis from the glans to the perineum.

Chordee, which is ventral curvature of the penis, has an inconsistent association with hypospadias. The degree of chordee is ultimately more significant in the surgical treatment of hypospadias than is the initial location of the meatus. A subcoronal hypospadias with little or no chordee is much less complicated to repair than is one with significant chordee and insufficient ventral skin. For this reason, when discussing the degrees of hypospadias, it is more appropriate to use the clinically relevant and common classification system that refers to the meatal location after the chordee has been released (Box 59-1).[1]

EMBRYOLOGY

Normal phallic development occurs in weeks 7 to 14 of gestation. By 6 weeks of gestation, the genital tubercle is formed anterior to the urogenital sinus. In the next week, two genital folds form caudad to the tubercle and a urethral plate develops between them. Under the influence of testosterone from the fetal testes, which begins to be produced at about 8 weeks of gestation, the inner genital folds fuse medially to create a tube that communicates with the urogenital sinus and runs distally to end at the base of the glans. The formation of the penile urethra is thus generally completed by the end of the first trimester.[2]

Classically, the glanular urethra is thought to form as an ectodermal ingrowth on the glans. This ingrowth deepens to meet the distal urethra that has formed from the closure of the endodermal genital folds. The capacious junction of these two structures is the fossa navicularis.[3] Recently, this theory has been challenged by the endodermal ingrowth theory. It suggests that the entire urethra forms from the urogenital sinus, which is endoderm. This endoderm differentiates into stratified squamous epithelium.[4] The formation of the glanular urethra is the last step in the formation of the completed urethra. This sequence probably accounts for the predominance of glanular and coronal hypospadias.

Dorsal to the developing urethra, the paired corporeal bodies develop from mesenchymal tissue. These are the major erectile tissue components and are invested by the tunica albuginea. Mesenchyme also forms Buck's fascia, the dartos fascia, and corpus spongiosum.

The corpus spongiosum is the supportive erectile tissue that normally surrounds the urethra and communicates with the erectile tissue of the glans. Buck's fascia is the deep layer of fascia that surrounds the corporeal bodies and invests the spongiosum. The dorsal neurovascular bundles are deep to this layer. Superficial to this layer is the dartos fascia, which is the loose subcutaneous layer that contains the superficial veins and lymphatics. These structures form subsequent to completion of the urethra by medial fusion of the outer genital folds, proceeding from the proximal to the distal aspect of the penis. This development accounts for how a fully formed urethra can have a poorly formed spongiosum with thin overlying skin and ventral tethering, despite the meatus being located at the tip of the glans. Finally, the prepuce is formed, originating at the coronal sulcus. It gradually encloses the glans circumferentially.

Arrested development of the urethra may leave the meatus located anywhere along the ventral surface of the penis. Typically, this leads to foreshortening of the ventral aspect of the penis distal to the meatus and failure of the prepuce to form circumferentially. However, in the megameatus form of hypospadias, the prepuce may form normally.

HISTORICAL PERSPECTIVE

The first description of hypospadias and its operative correction was reported in the 1st and 2nd centuries by the Alexandrian surgeons Heliodorus and Antyllus. They described the defect of hypospadias and its relation to problems with urination and ineffective coitus. They further described a surgical treatment consisting of amputation of the glans distal to the hypospadiac meatus.[5,6]

Little progress was made in the surgical treatment of hypospadias until the 19th century, when two Americans, Mettauer and Bush, described using a trocar to establish a channel from the meatus to the glans. Dieffenbach also described a similar technique in the 1830s. None of these methods was very successful.[5]

In 1874, Theophile Anger reported the successful repair of a penoscrotal hypospadias using the technique described in 1869 by Thiersch for the repair of epispadias in which lateral skin flaps were tubularized to form the neourethra. Anger's report initiated the modern era of hypospadias surgery characterized by the use of local skin flaps.[7,8] Duplay soon described his two-stage technique.[6] In the first stage, the chordee was released; in the second stage, a ventral midline strip of skin was covered by

BOX 59-1	Hypospadias Classification According to Meatal Location after Release of Chordee

ANTERIOR (65–70% OF CASES)
   Glanular
   Coronal
   Distal penile shaft

MIDDLE (10–15% OF CASES)
   Middle penile shaft

POSTERIOR (20% OF CASES)
   Proximal penile shaft
   Penoscrotal
   Scrotal
   Perineal

closure of the lateral penile skin flaps in the midline. Duplay did not believe that it was necessary to form the urethral tube completely because he thought that epithelialization would occur even if an incomplete tube was buried under the lateral skin flaps. Browne used this concept in his well-known 'buried strip' technique, which was widely used in the early 1950s.[9]

In the late 1800s, various surgeons reported on penile, scrotal, and preputial flap techniques for multistage procedures. Several of them used the technique of burying the penis in the scrotum to obtain skin coverage, similar to the technique described by Cecil and Cuip in the late 1950s.[10] In 1913, Edmonds was the first to describe the transfer of preputial skin to the ventrum of the penis at the time of release of chordee. At a second stage, the Duplay tube was created to complete the urethral closure. Byars popularized this two-stage technique in the early 1950s.[11] Smith further improved the outcomes by denuding the epithelium of one of the lateral skin flaps to give a 'pants-over-vest' closure to reduce the risk of fistula formation.[12] Belt devised another preputial transfer, two-stage procedure that was popularized by Fuqua in the 1960s.[13]

Nove-Josserand, in 1897, was the first to report the use of a free, split-thickness skin graft in an attempt to repair hypospadias.[14] Over the next 20 years, various other tissues were used as free grafts, including saphenous vein, ureter, and appendix, with varying success. McCormack used a free, full-thickness skin graft in a two-stage repair.[15] In 1941, Humby described a one-stage approach using the full thickness of the foreskin.[16] Devine and Horton later popularized this free preputial graft technique with very good results.[17]

In 1947, Memmelaar described the use of bladder mucosa as a free graft technique in a one-stage repair.[18] In 1955, Marshall and Spellman used bladder mucosa in a two-stage technique.[19] Urologists in China also experienced good success with a primary repair using bladder mucosa. This technique was developed independently during the period of scientific and cultural isolation in China.[20] Buccal mucosa from the lip was employed for urethral reconstruction in 1941 by Humby[16] and has recently gained renewed attention as a free graft technique.[21]

Improvement in preputial and meatal-based vascularized flaps over the last 30 to 40 years have greatly advanced hypospadias repair. Through contributions of surgeons such as Mathieu, Barcat,[1] Mustardé,[22] Broadbent,[23] Hodgson,[24] Horton and Devine,[17] Standoli,[25] and Duckett,[26] the single-stage repair of even the most severe forms of hypospadias has become commonplace.

CLINICAL ASPECTS

Incidence

The incidence of hypospadias has been estimated between 0.8 and 8.2 per 1,000 live male births.[27] The wide variation probably represents some geographic and racial differences, but of more significance is the exclusion of the more minor degrees of hypospadias in some reports. If all degrees of hypospadias, even the most minor, are included, then the incidence is probably 1 in 125 live male births.[28] With the most quoted figure of 1 per 250 live male births, it can be assumed that more than 6,000 boys are born with hypospadias each year in the USA.[29]

Etiology

A defect in the androgen stimulation of the developing penis, which precludes complete formation of the urethra and its surrounding structures, is the ultimate cause of hypospadias. This defect can occur from deficient androgen production by the testes and placenta, from failure of testosterone to convert to dihydrotestosterone by the 5α-reductase enzyme, or from deficient androgen receptors in the penis. Various disorders of sexual differentiation (DSD) can cause deficiencies at any point along the androgen-stimulation axis. These are discussed in Chapter 62.

The origin of hypospadias not associated with DSD is unclear. An endocrine cause has been implicated in some reports that show a diminished response to human chorionic gonadotropin (hCG) in some patients with hypospadias, suggesting delayed maturation of the hypothalamic–pituitary axis.[30,31] Other reports have described an increased incidence of hypospadias in monozygotic twins, suggesting an insufficient amount of hCG production by the single placenta to accommodate the two male fetuses.[32]

Environmental causes also have been implicated. A higher incidence of hypospadias has been noted in winter conceptions.[32] A weak association between hypospadias and the maternal ingestion of progestin-like agents has also been noted.[33,34] No association has been found between hypospadias and oral contraceptive use before or during early pregnancy.[35]

Genetic factors in the etiology of hypospadias are implicated by the higher incidence of this anomaly in first-degree relatives of hypospadiac patients.[27,34,36] In one study that evaluated 307 families, the risk of hypospadias in a second male sibling was 12%. If the index child and his father were affected, the risk for a second sibling increased to 26%. If the index child and a second-degree relative (rather than the father) were affected, the risk of the sibling being affected was only 19%.[36] This pattern suggests a multifactorial mode of inheritance, with these families having a higher than average number of influential genes for creation of hypospadias.[36] A combination of the endocrine, environmental, and genetic factors likely determines the potential for developing the hypospadias complex in any one individual.[31,32]

Anatomy of the Defect

The clinical significance of hypospadias is related to several factors. The abnormal location of the meatus and the tendency toward meatal stenosis result in a ventrally deflected and splayed stream. This fact makes the stream difficult to control and often makes it difficult for the patient to void while standing. The ventral curvature associated with chordee can lead to painful erections, especially with severe chordee. Impaired copulation and thus inadequate insemination is a further consequence of significant chordee. In addition, the unusual cosmetic appearance associated with the hooded foreskin, flattened glans, and ventral skin deficiency frequently has an adverse effect on the psychosexual development of the adolescent with hypospadias.[37-41] All of these factors are evidence that early surgical correction should be offered to all boys with hypospadias, regardless of the severity of the defect.

The distal form of hypospadias is the most common (see Box 59-1). Frequently, little or no associated chordee is present (Fig. 59-1). The size of the meatus and the quality of the surrounding supportive tissue as well as the configuration of the glans are variable, and ultimately determine the appropriate operative technique. Well-formed, mobile perimeatal skin and a deep ventral glans groove may allow development of perimeatal flaps to create the urethra (Fig. 59-2). In contrast, atrophic and immobile skin around the meatus may require tissue transfer from the preputium to form the neourethra.

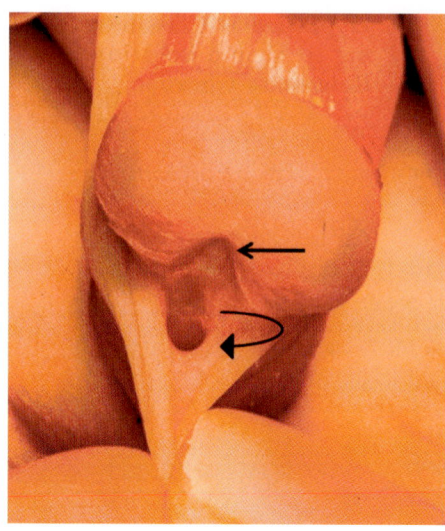

FIGURE 59-2 ■ Patulous, subcoronal meatus (curved arrow) with mobile perimeatal skin and deep ventral glans groove (straight arrow). This is a good variant for a meatal-based flap procedure, glans approximation (GAP), or tubularized incised urethral plate (TIP) repair.

An unusual variant of the distal hypospadias is the large wide-mouthed meatus with a circumferential foreskin (the megameatus/intact prepuce variant) (Fig. 59-3).[42] Owing to the intact prepuce, this variant is often not identified until a circumcision has been performed. If clinicians discover hypospadias during circumcision, they should stop and preserve the foreskin, even if the dorsal slit has been created.

At times, the distally located meatus may be associated with significant chordee, sometimes of a severe degree (Fig. 59-4). The release of the chordee places the meatus in a much more proximal location, requiring more complicated transfers of tissue to bridge the gap between the proximal meatus and the tip of the glans.

When the meatus is located on the penile shaft, the character of the urethral plate (midline ventral shaft skin distal to the meatus) is important in determining what type of repair is possible. A well-developed and elastic urethral plate suggests minimal, if any, distal ventral curvature (Fig. 59-5). However, a thin atrophic urethral plate heralds a significant chordee. The proximal supportive tissue of the urethra also is important. If there is a lack of spongiosum proximal to the hypospadiac meatus, this portion of the native urethra is not substantial enough to use in the repair (Fig. 59-6). Therefore, the neourethra must be constructed from the point of adequate spongiosum.

The position of the meatus at the penoscrotal, scrotal, or perineal location is usually associated with severe chordee, which requires chordee release and an extensive urethroplasty (Fig. 59-7). This type is usually more predictable in the preoperative period as to the choice of technique than are some of the more distal types previously discussed.

Other anatomic elements of the anomaly that are important include penile torsion, glans tilt, penoscrotal transposition, and chordee without hypospadias. These are discussed more completely later.

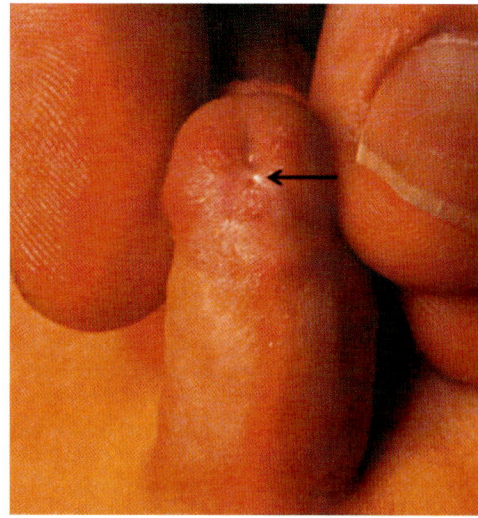

FIGURE 59-1 ■ Distal hypospadias with a stenotic meatus (arrow) located on the glans with no chordee. This patient is a good candidate for a meatal advancement and glanuloplasty (MAGPI) procedure or a tubularized incised urethral plate (TIP) operation.

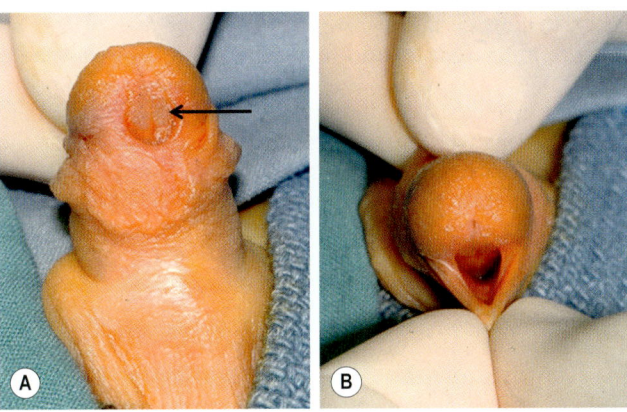

FIGURE 59-3 ■ **(A)** Previously circumcised penis with megameatus (arrow) and intact circumferential prepuce. **(B)** Large widemouthed meatus in the same penis as shown in (A).

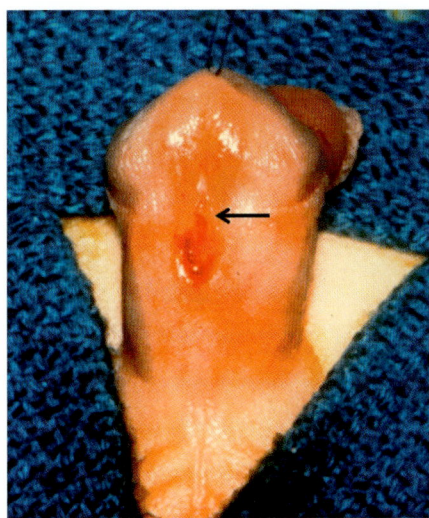

FIGURE 59-5 ■ Midshaft hypospadias with elastic, well-developed urethral plate distal to the meatus (arrow). No significant chordee is present. This is a good variant for an onlay island flap procedure or possibly a tubularized incised urethral plate operation.

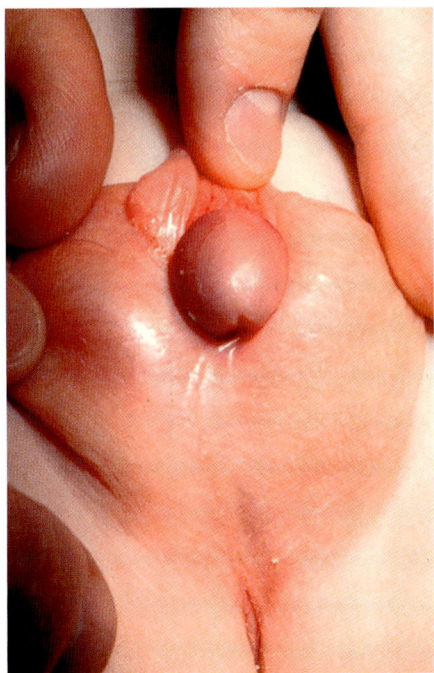

FIGURE 59-4 ■ Scrotal hypospadias with severe chordee and marked penoscrotal transposition is seen in this infant.

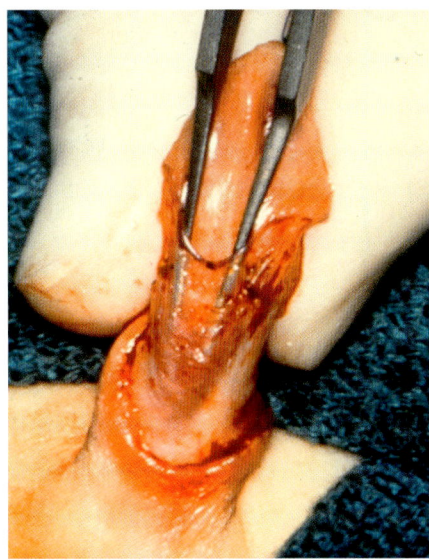

FIGURE 59-6 ■ Midshaft hypospadias with a lack of spongiosum support proximal to the meatus. The urethra should be opened back to an area of good spongiosum support at the penoscrotal junction.

Associated Anomalies

Inguinal hernia and undescended testes are the most common anomalies associated with hypospadias. They occur in 7–13% of patients with a greater incidence when the meatus is more proximal.[43–45] An enlarged prostatic utricle also is more common in posterior hypospadias, with an incidence of about 11%.[44] Infection is the most common complication of a utricle, but surgical excision is rarely necessary.[46] Several reports have emphasized significantly high numbers of upper urinary tract anomalies associated with hypospadias,[47–50] suggesting that routine upper tract screening is necessary. However, when the association is studied selectively, it is evident that the types of hypospadias at risk for significant upper tract anomalies are the penoscrotal and perineal forms, and those associated with other organ system

abnormalities.[43,45] When one, two, or three other organ system abnormalities also occur, the incidence of significant upper tract anomalies is 7%, 13%, and 37%, respectively. Associated myelomeningocele and imperforate anus carry a 33% and 46% incidence, respectively, of upper urinary tract malformations. In isolated posterior hypospadias, the incidence of associated upper tract anomalies is 5%.[45]

In middle and distal hypospadias, when not associated with other organ system anomalies, the incidence is similar to that in the general population.[43,45,51] Therefore, it is recommended that screening for upper urinary tract abnormalities by voiding cystourethrogram and renal ultrasonography be performed in patients with

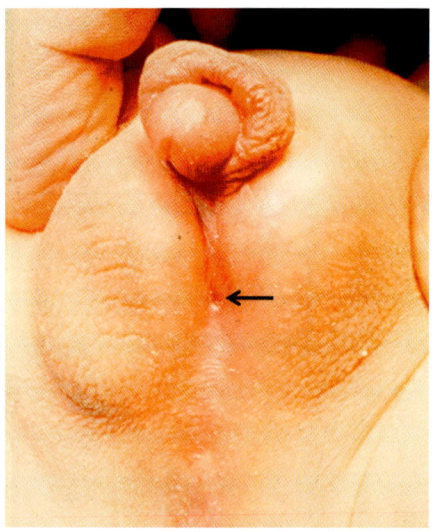

FIGURE 59-7 ■ Perineal/scrotal hypospadias (arrow) with severe chordee and a bifid scrotum.

penoscrotal and perineal forms of hypospadias, and in those with anomalies associated with at least one additional organ system. Screening should also be done in patients with other known indications, such as a history of urinary tract infection, upper or lower tract obstructive symptoms, hematuria, and in those boys having a strong family history of urinary tract abnormalities.[52]

DSD are also potentially associated with hypospadias. This association is rare in the routine forms of hypospadias. Failure of testicular descent, micropenis, penoscrotal transposition (see Fig. 59-4), or bifid scrotum (see Fig. 59-7) when associated with hypospadias, are all signs of potential DSD and warrant evaluation with karyotype screening.[27,53,54]

TREATMENT

The advent of safe anesthesia, fine suture material, delicate instruments, and good optical magnification has allowed virtually all types of hypospadias to be repaired in infancy. Generally, the repair is done on an outpatient basis. To deny a child the benefit of repair because the defect is 'too mild' or the risk of complication is 'too high' is inappropriate. The chance to make the phallus as normal as possible should be offered to all children, regardless of the severity of the defects.

Age at Repair

The technical advances over the past few decades have made it possible to repair hypospadias in the first 6 months of life in most patients.[55-57] Some surgeons have suggested delaying repair until after the child is age 2 years.[52,58-60] However, most surgeons who deal routinely with hypospadias prefer to perform the repair when the patient is 6 to 12 months old.[53,54,56,57,61,62] One study compared the emotional, psychosexual, cognitive, and operative risks for hypospadias. The 'optimal window' recommended for repair was age 6 to 15 months.[63] There

is also evidence that healing may be better with decreased inflammatory factors and less scarring in the less than 6 month age group.[62] Unless other health or social problems require delay, we believe the ideal time to complete penile reconstruction in the pediatric patient is about age 5 to 6 months.[64] The anesthetic risk is low and, at this age, postoperative care is much easier for the parents than it is when the child is a toddler.

Objectives of Repair

The objectives of hypospadias correction are divided into the following categories:
1. Complete straightening of the penis
2. Locating the meatus at the tip of the glans
3. Forming a symmetric, conically shaped glans
4. Constructing a neourethra uniform in caliber
5. Completing a satisfactory cosmetic skin coverage.

If these objectives can all be attained, the ultimate goal of forming a 'normal' penis for the child with hypospadias can be accomplished.

Straightening

Curvature of the penis is difficult to judge, at times, in the preoperative period. Artificial erection, by injecting physiologic saline in the corpora at the time of operation allows determination of the exact degree of curvature.[65] This curvature may be caused only by ventral skin or subcutaneous tissue tethering, which is corrected with the release of the skin and dartos layer.[66,67] Infrequently, the curvature may be secondary to true fibrous chordee, which requires division of the urethral plate and excision of the fibrous tissue down to the tunica albuginea.

Sometimes, even after extensive ventral dissection of chordee tissue, a repeated artificial erection still reveals the presence of significant ventral curvature. This finding is usually secondary to the uncommon problem of corporal body disproportion which is caused by a true deficiency of ventral corporal development. This problem can be corrected by making a releasing incision in the ventral tunica albuginea and inserting either a dermal or a tunica vaginalis patch to expand the deficient ventral surface.[68,69] Others have suggested the use of small intestinal submucosa as an off-the-shelf substitute for the autologous grafts.[70] Another technique is to excise wedges of tunica albuginea dorsally with transverse closure to shorten this dorsal surface and straighten the penis.[71,72] Other surgeons have had success with dorsal plication without excision of tunica albuginea.[73,74] Anatomic studies suggest that this plication should be done in the midline dorsally.[75] Still others advocate corporal rotation dorsally with or without penile disassembly to correct severe chordee.[76,77]

Axial rotation of the penis, or penile torsion, is another aspect of penis straightening that must be managed. This problem can generally be corrected by releasing the dartos layer as far proximal as possible on the penile shaft. This allows the ventral shaft to rotate back to the midline and corrects the torsion. Chordee or torsion can also occur without hypospadias (Fig. 59-8). The management of these boys encompasses the same spectrum of approaches as for hypospadias.[78,79]

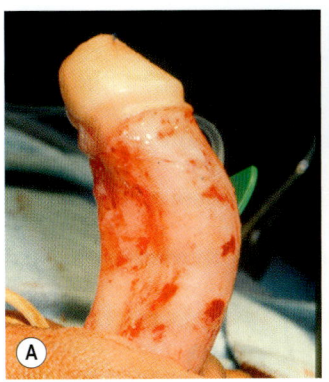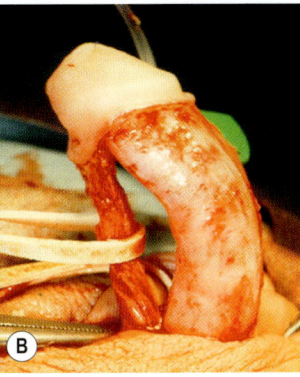

FIGURE 59-8 ■ **(A)** Chordee without hypospadias. The meatus is located at the tip of the glans with marked ventral curvature. **(B)** Fibrous ventral tissue is all released. The urethra is mobilized, but curvature persists, indicating corporeal body disproportion. This requires a ventral patch or dorsal plication (see text).

Locating the Meatus

Locating the meatus at the tip of the glans has not always been standard in hypospadias repair. Historically, the risk of complications was thought to be too great to recommend procedures that would locate the meatus beyond the subcoronal area. Multistage repairs popular in the 1950s and 1960s were designed to attain only a subcoronal location of the meatus. Operative techniques since then have improved sufficiently so that glans-channeling and glans-splitting maneuvers are used with minimal complications, making the distal tip meatus possible.

In glanular and subcoronal variants, the configuration of the meatus is the factor that determines what technique is used to move the meatus distally on the glans. Meatoplasty with or without dorsal advancement, distal urethral mobilization and tubularization, or meatal-based flaps are the methods selected in most cases of distal hypospadias.[80,81] In the more proximal forms, creating the neourethra with local vascularized skin flaps or free grafts allows positioning the urethra at the end of the penis. Alternatively, glans channeling or glans splitting allows creation of the meatus at the tip of the glans.[1,17,22,26,82,83]

Glans Shape

Creation of a symmetric, conically shaped glans is the objective of the glansplasty component of the repair. Approximating the lateral glanular tissue in the midline ventrally over a meatoplasty or meatal advancement corrects the flattened glans appearance to the more anatomically normal, conically shaped glans. Similarly, approximation of well-developed glans wings to the midline over a neourethra in a split glans restores the glans to its normal conical shape.

Urethral Construction

Formation of the neourethra can be accomplished with local skin flaps, various types of free grafts, or vascularized pedicle flaps. Local skin flaps can be formed from in situ skin or dorsal skin transferred to the ventrum in a previous stage. In either case, it is important to avoid making these flaps too narrow or thin because their vascular supply can be compromised. The hypospadiac urethral plate has been shown in histologic studies to consist of epithelium covering well-vascularized connective tissue without fibrosis.[84] This information supports the clinical findings that urethral plate preservation is helpful for successful urethroplasty. Free grafts depend on an adequately vascularized bed for survival. Therefore, they should not be placed in a scarred channel. Well-vascularized subcutaneous tissue and skin must cover them to allow adequate neovascularization and survival of the graft.[17]

Mobilized vascularized flaps of preputium have a more reliable blood supply than do free grafts. Therefore, if they are available, these flaps are the choice of most surgeons.[24,26,83,85] They may be used as patches onto a strip of native urethral plate to complete the urethra, or they may be tubularized and used as bridges over the gap between a proximal native urethra and the end of the glans.[26,86] A watertight closure of the well-vascularized neourethra is formed, with care being taken to make it uniform in caliber and of appropriate size for the age of the child. This closure helps avoid stricture and the formation of saccules, diverticula, and fistulas.

Cosmesis

Creating cosmetically appealing, well-vascularized skin coverage of the penile shaft after urethroplasty can sometimes be challenging. Transfer of vascularized dorsal preputial skin to the ventrum can be accomplished in several ways.

Buttonholes of the dorsal skin allow the penis to come through this defect, draping the distal preputium over the ventral surface of the penis.[19] This maneuver has the advantage of transferring well-vascularized skin over the repair, but it is not as appealing cosmetically.

A more satisfactory method of transferring skin to the ventrum is splitting the dorsal skin in the midline longitudinally and advancing the flaps around on either side to meet in the ventral midline. This technique allows a midline ventral closure, which simulates the median raphe. Moreover, it allows a subcoronal closure to the preputial skin circumferentially, which simulates the suture lines of a standard circumcision.[87,88] Another adjunct is to advance lateral flaps of inner preputial skin from each side to the ventral midline of the penis at the time of glansplasty or closure of glans wings.[89] Approximating these flaps in the midline gives the appearance of an intact circumferential preputial collar, further enhancing the potential for an anatomically normal skin closure (see Fig. 59-13).

Some patients, particularly those in European countries, prefer the appearance of a noncircumcised penis. In distal repairs, reconstruction of the preputium for a noncircumcised appearance can be accomplished in select cases.[90] Correction of the more significant degrees of penoscrotal transposition is often necessary to avoid the feminizing appearance. In some cases, this step can be done at the time of the original repair. However, when using vascularized pedicle flaps for the repair, it is usually safer to correct significant penoscrotal transposition with rotational flaps at a later time.[91–94]

OPERATIVE APPROACHES

Due to the wide variation in the anatomic presentation of hypospadias, no single urethroplasty is applicable for every patient. At times, a final decision regarding the degree of curvature and the ultimate location of the meatus cannot be made until the operation has started and an artificial erection is performed. The surgeon who repairs hypospadias must be adaptable and experienced to deal with all variants of the defect. Versatility and experience with all options of surgical treatment are the keys to successful management. By recognizing the sometimes subtle nuances of meatal variation, glans configuration, and curvature character, the experienced surgeon can choose the optimal technique (Fig. 59-9).

Anterior Variants

Some glanular variants are amenable to the meatal advancement and glansplasty (MAGPI) repair (Fig. 59-10).[95] A stenotic meatus with good mobility of the urethra and a fairly shallow ventral glanular groove are the anatomic characteristics best suited for the MAGPI. A wide-mouthed meatus is not amenable to the MAGPI repair. The meatal-based flap repair may be used effectively in this situation, assuming no chordee is present and mobile, well-vascularized skin exists proximal to the meatus (Fig. 59-11).[96,97] This repair works well when

there is a moderately deep ventral groove, allowing the urethra to be placed deep in the glans and a conically shaped glans to be created after closure of the glans wings. The glans approximation procedure is useful when a wide-mouthed proximal glanular meatus exists with a very deep groove (Figs 59-12 and 59-13).[98] The pyramid procedure is well suited for the fish-mouth type of meatus seen in the megameatus/intact prepuce variant.[42] These repairs give a very good cosmetic result when performed in the proper situation.

The tubularized incised plate urethroplasty (TIP) is a modification of the Thiersch–Duplay tubularization, which involves a deep longitudinal incision of the urethral plate in the midline (Fig. 59-14). This allows the lateral skin flaps to be mobilized and closed in the midline without tension. This procedure also allows repair of the wide-mouthed meatus variant with a flat, shallow ventral groove without the need for additional flaps.[99] The TIP urethroplasty has gained wide acceptance in the last 20 years. Its durability and long-term success have been demonstrated even in the more proximal variants.[100–102]

Middle Variants

The amount of ventral curvature generally dictates the type of repair in middle- and distal-shaft hypospadias. When no significant chordee is present, the TIP repair can frequently be performed. Another approach is the onlay island flap technique (Fig. 59-15).[86] This procedure involves mobilizing an inner preputial flap on its pedicle and rotating it ventrally to lay on the well-developed ventral urethral plate to complete the tubularization of

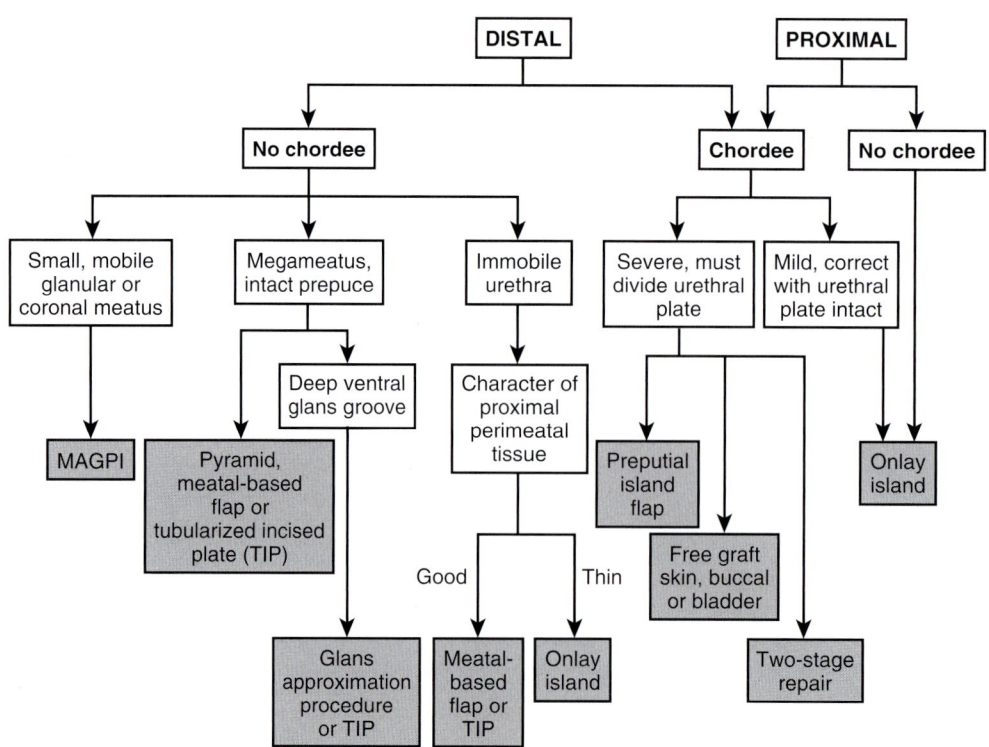

FIGURE 59-9 ■ Flow diagram for types of repair in variants of hypospadias. MAGPI, meatal advancement and glansplasty. TIP, tubularized incised plate urethroplasty.

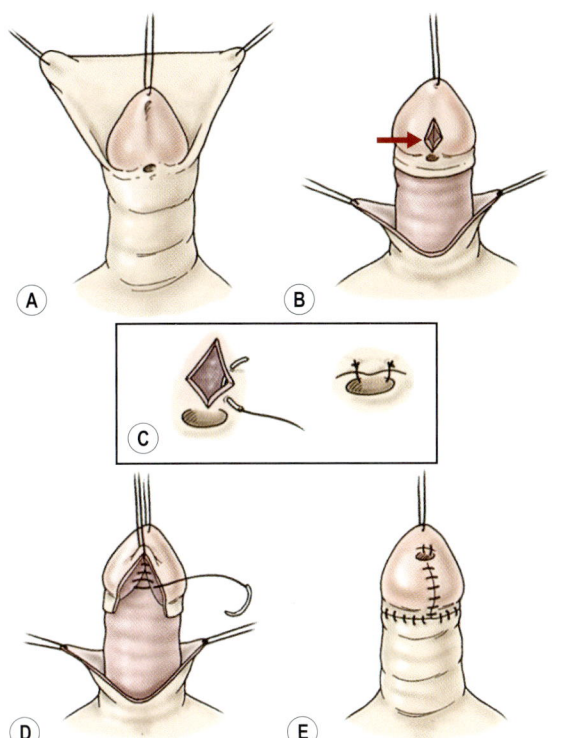

FIGURE 59-10 ■ Meatal advancement and glansplasty. **(A)** Circumferential subcoronal incision to deglove the penile shaft skin. **(B)** Longitudinal incision through the ventral groove of glans (arrow). **(C)** Transverse closure of glans groove incision to advance dorsal urethral plate and to open stenotic meatus. **(D)** Glans tissue approximated ventrally in the midline to restore conical configuration to glans. **(E)** Completion of the skin closure.

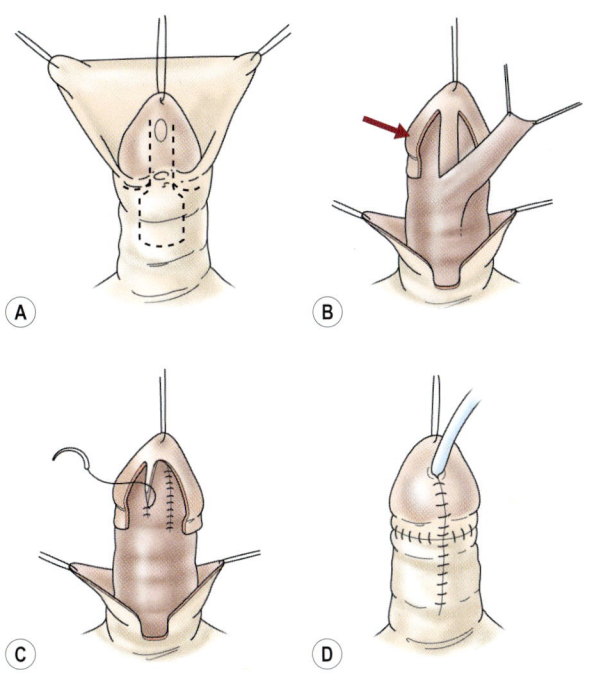

FIGURE 59-11 ■ Meatal-based flap repair. **(A)** Parallel incisions along ventral groove distal to the meatus and formation of meatal-based flap proximal to meatus. **(B)** Glans wings developed on either side of the urethral plate (arrow) to close over the neourethra later. Meatal-based flap is mobilized distally maintaining good vascular and tissue support. **(C)** Flap is anastomosed to bilateral edges of the urethral plate to form neourethra. **(D)** Glans wings are closed over the neourethra in the midline, giving conical glans configuration. Penile shaft is covered with dorsal foreskin advanced ventrally.

the neourethra. This technique is applicable to many forms of penile shaft hypospadias.

In milder degrees of chordee, the curvature can be corrected without dividing the urethral plate by incising tethering bands lateral to the urethral plate or by dorsal plication techniques.[74,75] This allows either the onlay island flap technique or TIP to be used instead of the tubularized pedicle flap or free graft, which have a higher incidence of complications.[54] If significant chordee is present, division of the urethral plate may be necessary. This moves the meatus more proximal and requires treatment as described for proximal variants.

Proximal Variants

Many of the scrotal and perineal forms of hypospadias are associated with significant chordee, which requires division of the urethral plate, and results in a gap between the proximal native urethra and the tip of the glans. This gap can be corrected during staged procedures in which coverage of the ventral penile shaft is attained by rotation of dorsal flaps to the ventrum, with later tubularization to form the neourethra (Fig. 59-16).

Another method is the tubularized free graft anastomosed to the native urethra proximally and extended to the end of the glans by a tunneling or splitting technique. The most commonly used free grafts are full-thickness skin, bladder mucosa, or buccal mucosa. Preputial skin is

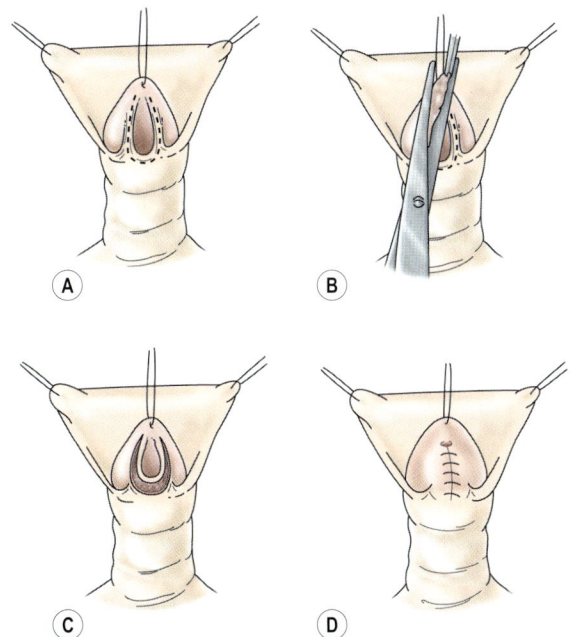

FIGURE 59-12 ■ Glans approximation procedure. **(A)** Deep ventral groove and patulous, coronal meatus with outline of proposed incision. **(B)** Skin is excised along previously marked U-shaped line. **(C)** De-epithelialized glans with the urethral plate intact. **(D)** Two-layer closure of the glanular urethra with glans skin still open. (From Zaontz MR. The GAP [glans approximation procedure] for glandular/coronal hypospadias. J Urol 1989;141:359–61.)

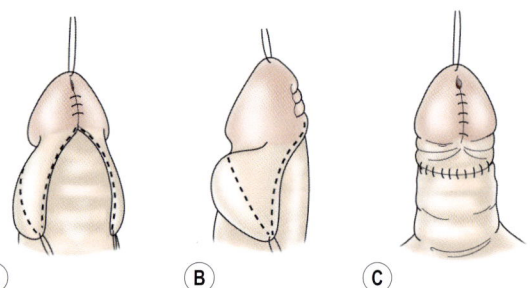

FIGURE 59-13 ■ **(A)** Glanular skin approximated and lateral wings of inner preputial skin outlined. **(B)** Lateral view of outline for preputial collar. **(C)** Lateral preputial wings closed in midline to give circumferential preputial collar. (From Zaontz MR. The GAP [glans approximation procedure] for glanular/coronal hypospadias. J Urol 1989;141:359–61.)

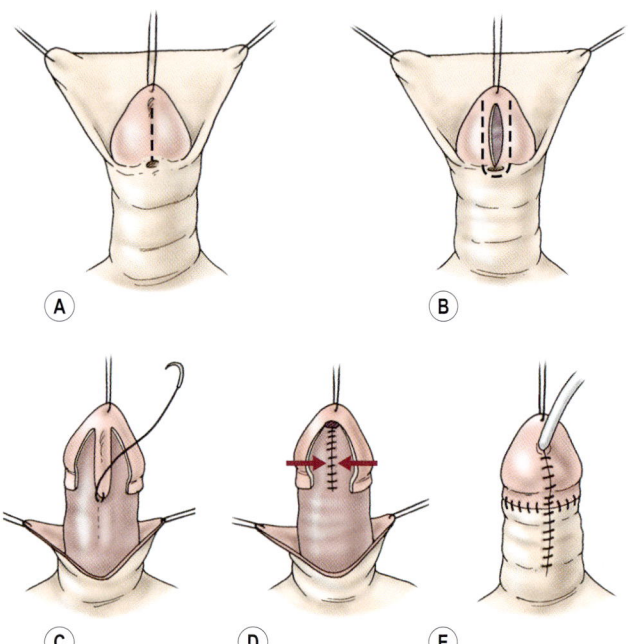

FIGURE 59-14 ■ Tubularized incised urethral plate (TIP) technique. **(A)** Urethral plate is incised longitudinally. **(B)** Glans incisions are made longitudinally, wide enough to leave two strips of epithelium for 10 French size neourethra. **(C)** Neourethra is tubularized in the midline with multiple layers and dartos flap to reinforce. **(D)** Glans wings are closed in the midline. **(E)** Skin closure is completed and the urethral stent is placed (optional).

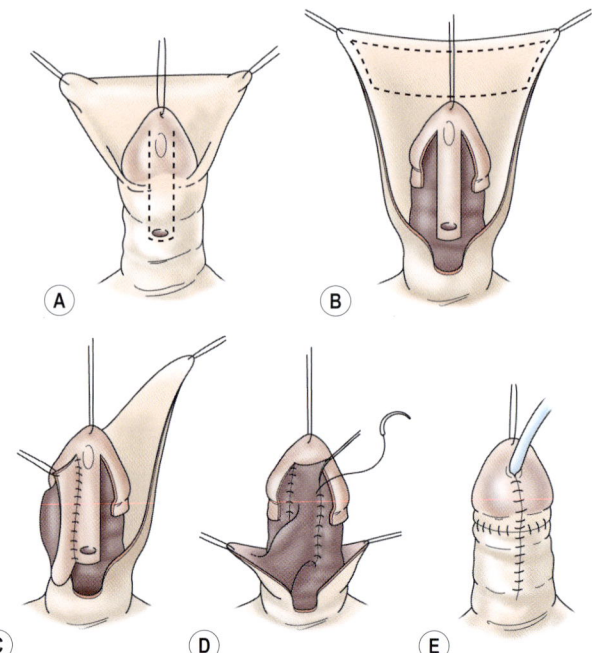

FIGURE 59-15 ■ Onlay island flap repair. **(A)** Outline of incisions along the well-developed urethral plate with no chordee. **(B)** Mobilization of glans wings and shaft skin with urethral plate intact distal to meatus. Outline of inner preputial island flap that will be transposed ventrally for onlay completion of neourethra. **(C)** Island flap transposed ventrally on pedicle. The first part of the anastomosis is completed. **(D)** Remainder of anastomosis to complete neourethra to tip of glans. **(E)** Glans wings are approximated over the neourethra in the ventral midline. The penile shaft is covered with the ventral advancement of dorsal foreskin.

The preputial vascularized tube graft can then be used to bridge the remaining distance to the end of the penis.[53]

In some cases, the penile shaft may be deficient enough to cause concern about ventral coverage after formation of the neourethra. The double-face island flap can solve this problem.[24] This technique leaves some of the outer preputial skin attached to the pedicle after tubularizing the inner preputial layer. This outer preputium is transferred to the ventrum with the pedicle and supplies skin coverage to the ventral shaft. However, the complications associated with the double-face island flap are numerous, and it has few advocates.[55]

The author prefers the transverse island flap in a one-stage procedure in most cases of proximal hypospadias with chordee.[106] In the rare case in which the skin deficiency is so severe that a vascularized pedicle cannot be used or in which the chordee is so severe that a dermal or tunica vaginalis graft is required to correct disproportion, a two-stage repair may be better.[107–109]

Technical Perspectives

Optical Magnification

Most surgeons agree that optical magnification is indispensable in hypospadias surgery. Standard operating loupes, ranging from 2.5× power to 4.5×, are generally thought to be ideal for the magnification needed for this

much preferred to extragenital skin.[17,103] If genital skin is not available, buccal mucosa may be the next best tissue.[21,104,105] Vascularized flaps are a more physiologically sound alternative to free grafts. The transverse inner preputial island flap that is tubularized and transposed ventrally to form the neourethra is the preferred vascularized flap (Fig. 59-17).[106] In contrast to free grafts, it provides good preputial skin with a reliable blood supply that does not rely on neovascularization for healing of the neourethra. Occasionally, the length of the prepuce alone may not be adequate to bridge the defect to a very proximal meatus. In this case, the shiny nonhair-bearing skin around the meatus can be tubularized (Fig. 59-18), moving the proximal urethra to the penoscrotal junction.

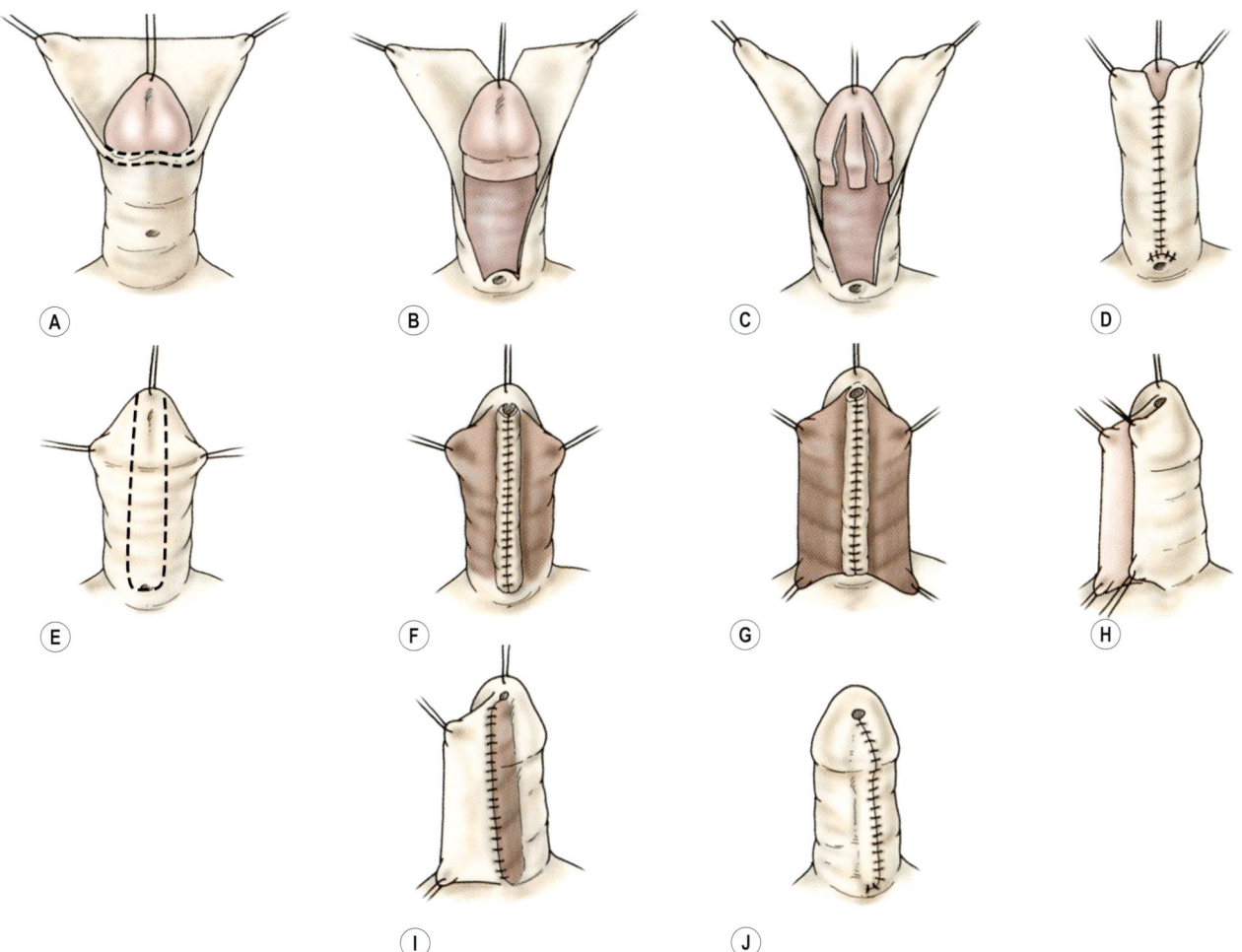

FIGURE 59-16 ■ Two-stage Durham Smith repair. **(A)** Release of chordee. **(B)** Splitting of dorsal preputium. **(C)** Denuded ventral glans before transposing preputial skin to ventrum. **(D)** Transposition of dorsal foreskin to ventrum completes the first stage. **(E)** U-shaped incision around the meatus and out onto glans. **(F)** Tubularization of Duplay-type tube to form the neourethra. **(G)** Second layer of soft tissue to reinforce suture line. **(H–J)** Overlapping skin closure with de-epithelialization of inner flap gives a 'double-breasted' closure of the skin. (Redrawn from Belman AB. Urethra. In: Kelalis PP, King LR, Belman AB, editors. Clinical Pediatric Urology. 2nd ed. Philadelphia: WB Saunders; 1985.)

type of surgery. Some surgeons advocate the use of the operating microscope and suggest an improved outcome.[110] However, most surgeons do not believe this degree of magnification is necessary. The microscope may be overly cumbersome for the small improvement in visualization it may provide.[111]

Sutures and Instruments

Fine absorbable suture is used by most surgeons to close the neourethra. Polyglycolic or polyglactin material is probably the most common suture choice. Some surgeons prefer the longer-lasting polydioxanone suture, but increased rates of stricture have been reported.[110,112] Permanent sutures of nylon or polypropylene, in a continuous stitch that is pulled out 10 to 14 days after surgery, are favored by some surgeons.[12,56]

The type of optical magnification also determines the size of the suture. Generally, 6-0 or 7-0 suture is preferred. With the microscope, 8-0 or 9-0 may be used. Skin closure is usually accomplished with either fine

chromic (6-0 or 7-0) or plain catgut suture. Small suture-sinus tracts may occur along these suture lines as they dissolve. I have used a subcuticular closure with either 6-0 chromic or polydioxanone for the past 10 years and have mostly eliminated the problem of these suture-sinus tracts.

The delicate instruments of ophthalmologic surgery are well designed for the precise tissue handling required in hypospadias repair. Small, single-toothed forceps or fine skin hooks allow tissue handling with minimal trauma. Standard microscopic tools are necessary for those who prefer the microscope over loupe magnification.

Urinary Diversion

The goal of the surgeon in any urinary diversion procedure in hypospadias repair is to protect the neourethra from the urinary stream during the initial healing phase. In theory, this diversion should decrease the complication rate, particularly fistula formation. The more traditional perineal urethrostomy and suprapubic cystostomy are

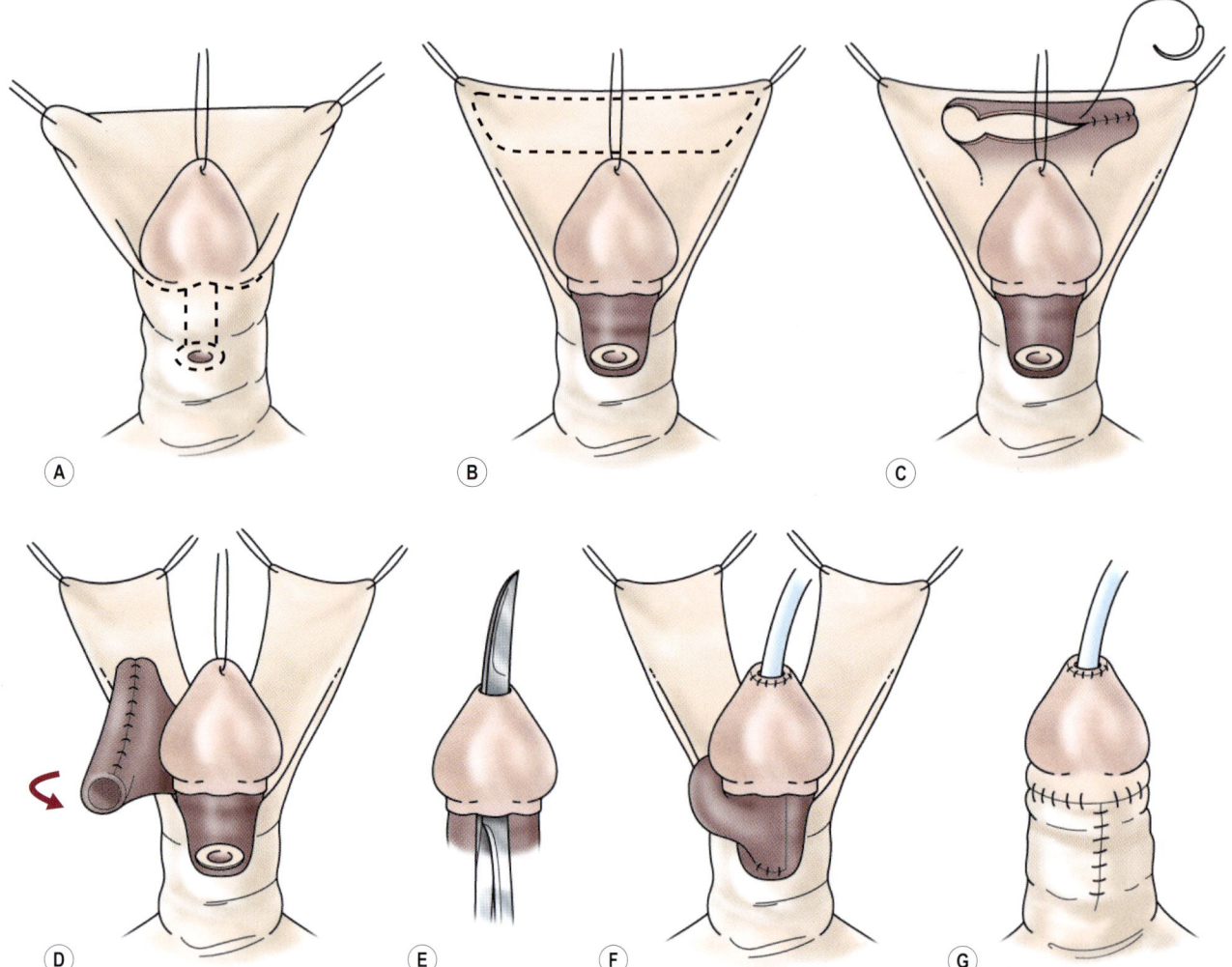

FIGURE 59-17 ■ Transverse preputial island flap tube repair. **(A)** Release of chordee and degloving of penile shaft skin. **(B)** Outline of inner preputial island flap. **(C)** Tubularization of inner preputial island flap. **(D)** Transposition of the tubularized island flap to the ventrum, maintaining pedicle blood supply. **(E)** Creation of a channel through glans tissue with sharp incisional and excisional technique. **(F)** Island tube anastomosed to proximal native urethra, brought through glans channel and anastomosed to epithelium at tip of glans. **(G)** Penile shaft covered with dorsal foreskin advanced ventrally. Skin closure is completed.

uncomfortable and cumbersome to manage in the postoperative period. Small indwelling 6-8 French polymeric silicone (Silastic) tubes left through the repair and into the bladder allow drainage of the urine into the diaper in infants (Fig. 59-19).[111] This technique greatly facilitates the outpatient care of these patients. These stents are well tolerated by the babies. Problems with the stents becoming plugged or dislodged are uncommon.

Some surgeons favor a stent that traverses the repair but is not indwelling in the bladder.[110] The patient is allowed to void, but the stent protects the repair. The author prefers the indwelling bladder stent, left for 5 to 14 days, depending on the complexity of the repair. In older children who will not tolerate wearing a diaper, a 6 to 8 French Foley catheter may be used in the simpler distal repairs and a suprapubic cystostomy can be performed in the more complex repairs. Suprapubic drainage should be used in complex reoperations or in any repairs requiring a free graft. Studies have suggested that diversion is not required for simpler distal

procedures, such as MAGPI, meatal-based flap, or distal Duplay tubes. Straightforward repairs of small fistulas can also be accomplished without diversion.[112-114]

Dressings

Hypospadias dressings should apply enough gentle pressure on the penis to help with hemostasis and to decrease edema, without compromising the vascularity of the repair. Various dressings accomplish this purpose. Common dressings include transparent adhesive dressings wrapped around the penis or fixed to the abdominal wall in a sandwich-like fashion (see Fig. 59-19). A DuoDerm (ConvaTec, Skillman, NJ) dressing can be applied around the penis as an alternative to using a transparent adhesive dressing.[110] Two prospective studies have shown that the type of dressing does not influence healing or complication rates.[115,116] I have continued to use a transparent dressing against the abdominal wall for its hemostatic effect in the first 12-24 postoperative hours.

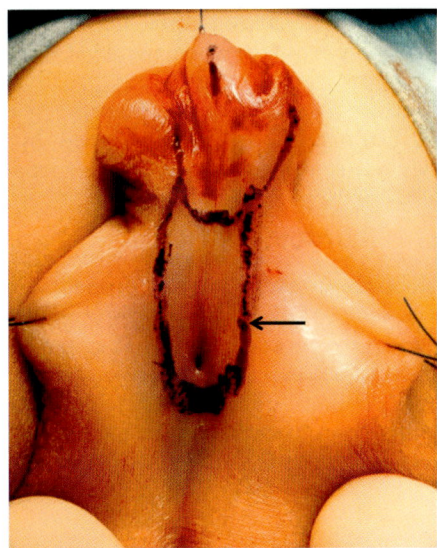

FIGURE 59-18 ■ Outline of nonhair-bearing skin distal to scrotal meatus (arrow) that will be tubularized to move the meatus to the penoscrotal junction. Island flap tube will complete the repair to the end of the glans.

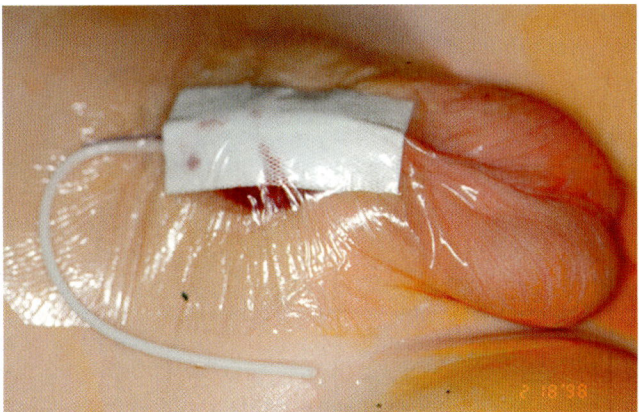

FIGURE 59-19 ■ Occlusive dressing of transparent adhesive material in sandwich fashion on the abdominal wall, with a 6 French soft polymeric silicone (Silastic) indwelling tube inserted for bladder drainage.

Analgesia

Postoperative pain is generally controlled with oral analgesics. Bladder spasms caused by indwelling catheters can be managed with propantheline bromide and opium suppositories or by oral oxybutynin. A dorsal penile nerve block performed intraoperatively with bupivacaine can help control postoperative pain.[117]

A caudal block is my preferred method for postoperative pain control. In most cases, the patients are comfortable for the entire day and evening of surgery, and are easily cared for at home with oral analgesia.[118]

COMPLICATIONS

The type and incidence of complications vary with the particular form of repair. Attention to detail and meticulous technique are imperative to reduce complications to

a minimum. The following is a discussion of some of the general complications that can occur with all types of repair.

Bleeding

Intraoperative bleeding can, at times, be troublesome. However, with the judicious use of the point tip cautery, it can generally be kept to a minimum. Tourniquets or cutaneous infiltrations with dilute concentrations of epinephrine can be helpful, but they should not replace careful technique. Postoperative bleeding is generally prevented by mildly compressive dressings. Subcutaneous hematomas may occur but generally do not need to be drained.

Infection

Wound infection is a rare problem in hypospadias repair, especially in the prepubertal patient. As long as good viability of tissue is maintained, infection should be a minor problem. Perioperative antibiotic prophylaxis is favored by some surgeons.[119] This is probably a reasonable precaution in an extensive repair, especially in the postpubertal patient. Urinary suppression with oral antibiotics is recommended with indwelling catheters that are open to drainage in the diaper.[68,120,121]

Devitalized Skin Flaps

If sloughing of the skin coverage occurs, it is usually on the ventral surface of the penis where dorsal skin has been transposed. When the devascularized skin is over a well-vascularized bed of tissue, such as with a pedicle flap, primary healing generally occurs without sequelae. If the slough is over poorly vascularized tissue, such as a free graft, breakdown of the repair can occur. Careful attention to transposing well-vascularized tissue for coverage of the neourethra is critical to avoid this problem.

Fistulas

A urethrocutaneous fistula is the most commonly reported complication of hypospadias surgery. It results from failure of healing at some point along the neourethral suture line and can range in size from pinpoint to large enough for all urine to exit at this site. Fistulas also may be associated with distal stenosis or stricture. Occasionally, small fistulas seen in the early postoperative period may close spontaneously. Operative closure should be postponed until complete tissue healing has occurred, which requires at least 6 months.[122,123] A small fistula may be closed by local excision of the fistula tract followed by closure of the urethral epithelium with fine absorbable suture. Approximating several layers of well-vascularized subcutaneous tissue over this closure is important to prevent recurrence. Urinary diversion is usually not necessary in small fistula repairs. Larger fistulas may require more complicated closures, with mobilization of tissue flaps or advancement of skin flaps to ensure an adequate amount of well-vascularized tissue for a multilayered closure.[122-124] Urinary diversion is often necessary with more complicated closures.

Strictures

Narrowing of the neourethra can occur anywhere along its course. However, the most common sites of stricture formation are at the meatus and at the proximal anastomosis. Most cases of meatal narrowing can be managed as an office procedure by gentle dilation in the first few postoperative weeks. Occasionally, meatotomy or meatoplasty is needed, especially when associated with a proximal fistula or neourethral diverticulum. More proximal strictures can generally be managed with dilation or an internal urethrotomy performed under vision.[125] However, in recurrences or long strictures, open urethroplasty may be needed, with excision of the stricture and a primary urethral anastomosis or patch graft urethroplasty.[122,123,125,126]

Diverticulum

Saccular dilation of the neourethra may result from distal stenosis causing progressive dilation, contained urinary extravasation from the breakdown of the repair, or initial creation of an oversized segment of the neourethra. Classic bulging of the urethra ventrally with voiding is evident with the development of a significant diverticulum (Fig. 59-20). Urinary stasis with chronic inflammation is common. Obstruction can result from kinking of the urethra when the diverticulum distends with voiding. Repair requires excision of the redundant neourethra with primary closure to restore a uniform caliber to the urethra.[127] Special attention should be paid to any narrowing of the distal neourethra as well.

Retrusive Meatus

Retraction of the meatus from its original position at the tip of the glans to a proximal glanular or subcoronal position can occur with any repair. A retrusive meatus is caused by the failure of the glansplasty closure or the

breakdown of devascularized distal neourethra. Retraction is a common problem when the MAGPI procedure is used in patients whose meatus is too proximal or when too much tension is placed on the glansplasty closure.[128] Correction can usually be accomplished by a repeat glansplasty, TIP, or a meatal-based flap procedure.[122,128]

Persistent Chordee

Residual ventral curvature after hypospadias repair can be a troublesome problem. It is usually related to inadequate release of chordee at the original procedure. Increased ventral curvature occurring as the penis grows is at least a theoretical possibility. The artificial erection has made this complication much less common. Treatment of the problem is similar to the treatment of chordee without hypospadias. Degloving of the penis and takedown of any ventral tethering tissue is accomplished by using the artificial erection technique to guide dissection. Dorsal plication, ventral excision with patching, and division of the urethra may all be necessary.[123,129]

Recurrent Multiple Complications

Patients with recurrent multiple complications generally have experienced multiple failed repairs that have resulted in a combination of severe complications. Extensive fibrosis of the urethra with fistulas, strictures, diverticula, and residual chordee may be present. The successful outcome of further repair depends on thorough evaluation of each complication and the use of all the techniques available to the surgeon experienced in hypospadias repair. If tissue is available, vascularized flaps or staging procedures are preferable to free grafts in a scarred phallus.[130] If a free graft is necessary, it is important to obtain the most vascularized bed possible in which to place the graft. Buccal mucosa is probably the best tissue for a free graft in this type of situation.[21,54,123] In patients with severe scarring and ventral skin loss, a split-thickness skin graft may be used for ventral coverage. This tissue may then be tubularized at a second stage.[131]

Sexual Function

Long-term results of hypospadias repair with regard to erectile function, ejaculation, and fertility are not available for the children who have undergone repairs at a younger age over the past decade. Historically, sexual difficulties after hypospadias repair have been reported. These were thought to be secondary to psychosexual factors related to surgery in childhood rather than to anatomic problems.[39,41] Fertility has been assessed by semen analysis in patients after hypospadias repair.[38] Higher rates of oligospermia are reported. These lower sperm counts generally occur in patients with associated anomalies such as cryptorchidism, chromosome abnormalities, varicoceles, or torsion. In a patient with an anatomically successful hypospadias repair and no associated anomalies that might affect fertility, a high potential for fertility and an adequate sexual function are expected.[39,132] Only close observation of children as they enter

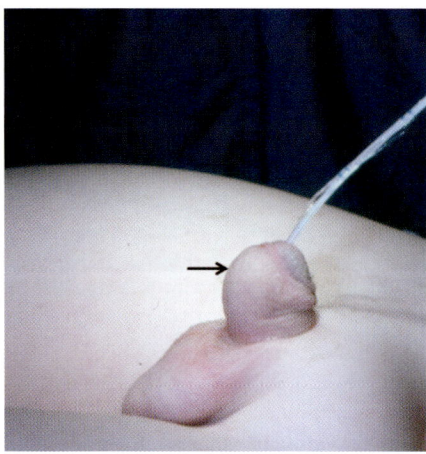

FIGURE 59-20 ■ A neourethral diverticulum is seen to be bulging ventrally (arrow) with voiding.

adulthood will reveal the true incidence of sexual dysfunction and fertility problems.

RESULTS

Complication rates in hypospadias repairs tend to be more frequent and more significant the more proximal the defect. Distal repairs with MAGPI, glans approximation procedure (GAP), TIP, and meatal-based flap have overall rates of about 1–5%.[97,98,100,112,128,133–137] Fistulas are most common, with meatal stenosis being a little more likely to occur in TIP repairs.[135]

The proximal repairs have higher rates of fistulas, strictures, and urethral diverticuli. The formation of a diverticulum is directly related to distal narrowing. Therefore, it is important to avoid being too aggressive with the glansplasty in the proximal repairs to avoid narrowing the distal urethra. Overall, complication rates in proximal repairs are 10–50%.[20,74,137–147]

In postpubertal patients, the complication rates are significantly higher, which reinforces the concept of performing hypospadias repairs early in life.[138]

REFERENCES

1. Barcat J. Current concepts of treatment. In: Horton CE editor. Plastic and Reconstructive Surgery of the Genital Area. Boston: Little, Brown; 1973. p. 249–63.
2. Bellinger MF. Embryology of the male external genitalia. Urol Clin North Am 1981;8:375–82.
3. Sommer JJ, Stephens FD. Dorsal urethral diverticulum of the fossa navicularis: Symptoms, diagnosis and treatment. J Urol 1980;124:94–7.
4. Kurzrock EA, Baskin LS, Cunha GR. Ontogeny of the male urethra: theory of endodermal differentiation. Differentiation 1999;64:115–22.
5. Rogers DO. History of external genital surgery. In: Horton CE editor. Plastic and Reconstructive Surgery of the Genital Area. Boston: Little, Brown; 1973. p. 3–47.
6. Horton CE, Devine CJ, Baran N. Pictorial history of hypospadias repair techniques. In Horton CE editor. Plastic and Reconstructive Surgery of the Genital Area. Boston: Little, Brown; 1973. p. 237–43.
7. Bachus LH, de Felice CA. Hypospadias, then and now. Plast Reconstr Surg 1960;25:146–60.
8. Creevy CD. The correction of hypospadias: A review. Urol Surv 1958;8:2–47.
9. Browne D. An operation for hypospadias. Proc R Soc Med 1949;41:466–8.
10. Cuip OS. Hypospadias with and without chordee. In: Horton CE editor. Plastic and Reconstructive Surgery of the Genital Area. Boston: Little, Brown; 1973. p. 315–20.
11. Byars LT. A technique for consistently satisfactory repair of hypospadias. Surg Gynecol Obstet 1955;100:184–90.
12. Smith ED. Durham Smith repair of hypospadias. Urol Clin North Am 1981;8:451–5.
13. Fuqua F. Renaissance of urethroplasty: The Belt technique of hypospadias repair. J Urol 1971;106:782–5.
14. Coleman JW, McGovern JH, Marshall VF. The bladder mucosal graft technique for hypospadias repair. Urol Clin North Am 1981;8:457–62.
15. McCormack RM. Simultaneous chordee repair and urethral reconstruction for hypospadias: Experimental and clinical studies. Plast Reconstr Surg 1954;13:257.
16. Humby G. A one-stage operation for hypospadias. Br J Surg 1941;29:84–92.
17. Devine CJ Jr, Horton DE. Hypospadias repair. J Urol 1972;85:166–72.
18. Memmelaar J. Use of bladder mucosa in a one-stage repair of hypospadias. J Urol 1947;58:68–73.
19. Marshall VF, Spellman RM. Construction of a urethra in hypospadias using vesicle mucosal grafts. J Urol 1955;73:335–42.
20. Chu LiZhong, Zheng Yu-Hen, Sheh Ya-Xiong, et al. One-stage urethroplasty for hypospadias using a tube constructed with bladder mucosa: A new procedure. Urol Clin North Am 1981;8:463–70.
21. Duckett JW, Coplen D, Ewalt D, et al. Buccal mucosal urethral replacement. J Urol 1995;153:1660–3.
22. Mustardé JC. One-stage correction of distal hypospadias and other people's fistulae. Br J Plast Surg 1965;18:413–22.
23. Broadbent TR, Woolf RM, Tosku E. Hypospadias: One-stage repair. Plast Reconstr Surg 1961;27:154–9.
24. Hodgson NB. Use of vascularized flaps in hypospadias repair. Urol Clin North Am 1981;8:471–81.
25. Standoli L. One-stage repair of hypospadias: Preputial island flap technique. Ann Plast Surg 1982;9:81–8.
26. Duckett JW. The island flap technique for hypospadias repair. Urol Clin North Am 1981;8:513–19.
27. Sweet RA, Schrott HG, Kurland R, et al. Study of the incidence of hypospadias in Rochester, Minnesota, 1940–1970, and a case control comparison of possible etiologic factors. Mayo Clin Proc 1974;49:52–8.
28. Duckett JW. Hypospadias. Pediatr Rev 1989;11:37–42.
29. Paulozzi LJ, Erickson JD, Jackson RJ. Hypospadias trends in two ultrasound surveillance systems. Pediatrics 1997;100:831–4.
30. Wang MH, Baskin LS. Endocrine disruptors, genital development, and hypospadias. J Androl 2008;19:499–505.
31. Kalfa N, Philibert P, Sultan C. Is hypospadias a genetic, endocrine, or environmental disease, or still an unexplained malformation? Int J Androl 2009;32:187–97.
32. Vander Zander LF, van Rooij IA, Feitz WF, et al. Aetiology of hypospadias: A systematic review of genes and environment. Human Reprod Update 2012;19:260–83.
33. Mau G. Progestins during pregnancy and hypospadias. Teratology 1981;24:285–7.
34. Avellan L. The incidence of hypospadias in Sweden. Scand J Plast Reconstr Surg 1975;9:129–39.
35. Kallen B, Mastroiacovo P, Lancaster PA, et al. Oral contraceptives in the etiology of isolated hypospadias. Contraception 1991;44:173–82.
36. Bauer SB, Retik AB, Colodny AH. Genetic aspects of hypospadias. Urol Clin North Am 1981;8:559–64.
37. Moriya K, Kakizaki H, Tanaka H, et al. Long-term cosmetic and sexual outcome of hypospadias surgery: Norm related study in adolescence. J Urol 2006;176:1889–92.
38. Moriya K, Kakizaki H, Tanaka H, et al. Long-term patient reported outcome of urinary symptoms after hypospadias surgery: Norm related study in adolescents. J Urol 2007;178:1659–62.
39. Rynja SP, deJong TP, Bosch JL. Functional, cosmetic and psychosexual in adult men who underwent hypospadias correction in childhood. J Pediatr Urol 2011;7:504–15.
40. Svensson J, Berg R, Berg G. Operated hypospadias: Late follow-up: Social, sexual and psychological adaptation. J Pediatr Surg 1981;16:134–5.
41. Berg R, Berg G. Penile malformation, gender identity and sexual orientation. Acta Psychiatr Scand 1983;68:154–66.
42. Duckett JW, Keating MA. Technical challenge of the megameatus intact prepuce hypospadias variant: The pyramid procedure. J Urol 1989;141:1407–9.
43. Cerasaro TS, Brock WA, Kaplan GW. Upper urinary tract anomalies associated with congenital hypospadias: Is screening necessary? J Urol 1986;135:537–58.
44. Friedman T, Shalom A, Hoshen G, et al. Detection and incidence of anomalies associated with hypospadias. Pediatr Nephrol 2008;23:1809–16.
45. Khuri FJ, Hardy BE, Churchill BM. Urologic anomalies associated with hypospadias. Urol Clin North Am 1981;8:565–71.
46. Ritchey ML, Benson RC, Kramer SA, et al. Management of müllerian duct remnants in the male patient. J Urol 1988;140:795–9.
47. Fallon B, Devine CJ Jr, Horton CE. Congenital anomalies associated with hypospadias. J Urol 1976;116:585–6.
48. Lutzker LG, Kogan SJ, Levitt SB. Is routine IV urography indicated in patients with hypospadias? Pediatrics 1977;59:630–3.
49. Kennedy PA. Hypospadias: A twenty-year review of 489 cases. J Urol 1961;85:814–17.

50. Neyman MA, Schirmer HKA. Urinary tract evaluation in hypospadias. J Urol 1965;94:439.
51. McArdle R, Lebowitz R. Uncomplicated hypospadias and anomalies of the upper urinary tract: Need for screening? Urology 1975;5:712–16.
52. Smith DS. Hypospadias. In: Ashcraft KW, editor. Pediatric Urology. Philadelphia: WB Saunders; 1990. p. 353–95.
53. Sheldon CA, Duckett JW. Hypospadias. Pediatr Clin North Am 1987;34:1259–72.
54. Keating MA, Duckett JW. Recent advances in the repair of hypospadias. Surg Ann 1990;22:405–25.
55. Wacksman J. Results of early hypospadias surgery using optical magnification. J Urol 1984;13:516–17.
56. Belman AB, Kass EJ. Hypospadias repair in children less than 1 year old. J Urol 1982;128:1273–4.
57. Perlmutter AE, Morabito R, Tarry WF. Impact of patient age on distal hypospadias repair: A surgical perspective. Urology 2006;68:648–51.
58. Kelalis PP, Bunge R, Barkin M, et al. The timing of elective surgery on the genitalia of male children with particular reference to undescended testes and hypospadias. Pediatrics 1975;56:479–83.
59. Smith DS. Timing of surgery in hypospadias repair. Aust N Z J Surg 1983;53:396–7.
60. Winslow BH, Horton CE. Hypospadias. Semin Urol 1987;5:236–42.
61. Mackay A. Hypospadias repair under the age of 1 year. Aust N Z J Surg 1983;53:449–52.
62. Bermudez DM, Canning DA, Liechty KW. Age and proinflammatory cytokine production: Wound-healing implications for scar formation and the timing of genital surgery in boys. J Pediatric Urol 2011;7:324–31.
63. Schultz JR, Klykylo WM, Wacksman J. Timing of elective hypospadias repair in children. Pediatrics 1983;71:342–51.
64. Kass EJ, Jogan SJ, Manley CB, et al. Timing of elective surgery on the genitalia of male children with particular reference to the risks, benefits and psychological effects of surgery and anesthesia. Pediatrics 1996;97:590–4.
65. Gittes RF, McClaughlin AP. Injection technique to induce penile erection. Urology 1974;4:473–5.
66. Allen TD, Spence HM. The surgical treatment of coronal hypospadias and related problems. J Urol 1968;100:504–8.
67. Devine CJ, Horton CE. Chordee without hypospadias. J Urol 1973;110:264–71.
68. Leslie JA, Cain MP, Kaefer M, et al. Corporeal grafting for severe hypospadias: A single institution experience with three techniques. J Urol 2008;180:1749–52.
69. Braga LH, Pippi Salle JL, Dave S, et al. Outcome analysis of severe chordee correction using tunica vaginalis as a flap in boys with proximal hypospadias. J Urol 2007;178:1693–7.
70. Weiser AC, Franco I, Herz DB, et al. Single layered small intestinal submucosa is the repair of severe chordee and complicated hypospadias. J Urol 2003;170:1593–5.
71. Nesbit RM. Congenital curvature of the phallus: Report of three cases with description of corrective operation. J Urol 1965;93:230–4.
72. Livne PM, Gibbons MD, Gonzales EI. Correction of disproportion of corpora cavernosa as cause of chordee in hypospadias. Urology 1983;22:608–10.
73. Hollowell JG, Keating MA, Snyder HM, et al. Preservation of the urethral plate in hypospadias repair: Extended applications and further experience with the onlay island flap urethroplasty. J Urol 1990;143:98–101.
74. Baskin L, Duckett JW. Dorsal tunica albuginea plication (TAP) for hypospadias curvature. J Urol 1994;151:1668–71.
75. Baskins LS, Erol A, Li YW. Anatomy of the neurovascular bundle: Is safe mobilization possible? J Urol 2000;164:977–80.
76. Decter RM. Chordee correction by corporal rotation: The split and roll technique. J Urol 1999;162:1152–5.
77. Perovic SC, Djordjevic ML. A new approach in hypospadias repair. World J Urol 1998;16:195–9.
78. Hurwitz RS, Devine CJ, Horton CE, et al. Chordee without hypospadias. Dialog Pediatr Urol 1986;9:1–8.
79. Donnahoo KK, Cain MP, Pope JC, et al. Etiology, management and surgical complications of congenital chordee without hypospadias. J Urol 1998;160:1120–2.
80. Gibbons MD, Gonzales ET. The subcoronal meatus. J Urol 1983;130:739–42.
81. Gibbons MD. Nuances of distal hypospadias. Urol Clin North Am 1985;12:169–74.
82. Hendren WH. The Belt-Fuqua technique for repair of hypospadias. Urol Clin North Am 1981;8:431–50.
83. Standoli L. Vascularized urethroplasty flaps: The use of vascularized flaps of preputial and penopreputial skin for urethral reconstruction in hypospadias. Clin Plast Surg 1980;15:355–70.
84. Snodgrass W, Patterson K, Plaire JC, et al. Histology of the urethral plate: Implications for hypospadias repair. J Urol 2000;164:988–90.
85. Shapiro SR, Zaontz MR, Scherz HC. Hypospadias repair: Update and controversies, part 1. Dialog Pediatr Urol 1990;13:1–8.
86. Elder JS, Duckett JW, Snyder HM. Onlay island flap in the repair of mid and distal penile hypospadias without chordee. J Urol 1987;138:376–9.
87. Sadove RC, Horton CE, McRoberts JW. The new era of hypospadias surgery. Clin Plast Surg 1988;15:341–54.
88. Snodgrass W, Decter RM, Roth DR, et al. Management of the penile shaft skin in hypospadias repair: Alternative to Byar's flaps. J Pediatr Surg 1988;23:181–2.
89. Firlit CF. The mucosal collar in hypospadias surgery. J Urol 1987;137:80–2.
90. Snodgrass WT, Koyle MA, Baskin LS, et al. Foreskin preservation in penile surgery. J Urol 2006;176:711–14.
91. Nonomura K, Koyanagi T, Imanaka K, et al. One-stage total repair of severe hypospadias with scrotal transposition: Experience in 18 cases. J Pediatr Surg 1988;23:177–80.
92. Glenn JF, Anderson EE. Surgical correction of incomplete penoscrotal transposition. J Urol 1973;110:603–5.
93. Ehrlich RM, Scardino PT. Simultaneous surgical correction of scrotal transposition and perineal hypospadias. Urol Clin North Am 1981;8:531–7.
94. Ehrlich RM, Scardino PT. Surgical corrections of scrotal transposition and perineal hypospadias. J Pediatr Surg 1982;17:175–7.
95. Duckett JW. MAGPI (meatoplasty and glanuloplasty). Urol Clin North Am 1981;8:513–19.
96. Mathieu P. Traitement en un temps de l'hypospadias balanique et juxtabalanique. J Chir 1932;39:481.
97. Wacksman J. Modification of the one-stage flip flap procedure to repair distal penile hypospadias. Urol Clin North Am 1981;8:527–30.
98. Zaontz MR. The gap (glans approximation procedure) for glanular/coronal hypospadias. J Urol 1989;141:359–61.
99. Snodgrass W. Tubularized incised plate urethroplasty for distal hypospadias. J Urol 1994;151:464–5.
100. Snodgrass W, Koyle M, Manzoni G. Tubularized incised plate hypospadias repair: Results of a multicenter experience. J Urol 1996;156:839–41.
101. Snodgrass W. Does tubularized incised plate hypospadias repair create neourethral strictures? J Urol 1999;162:1159–61.
102. Cheng EY, Vemulapalli SN, Kropp BP. Snodgrass hypospadias repair with vascularized dartos flap: The perfect repair for virgin cases of hypospadias? J Urol 2002;168:1723–6.
103. Hendren WH, Horton CE Jr. Experience with one-stage repair of hypospadias and chordee using free graft of prepuce. J Urol 1988;140:1250–64.
104. Koyle MA, Ehrlich RM. The bladder mucosa graft for urethral reconstruction. J Urol 1987;138:1093–5.
105. Dessanti A, Iannuccelli M, Ginesu G, et al. Reconstruction of hypospadias and epispadias with buccal mucosa free graft as primary surgery: More than 10 years of experience. J Urol 2003;170:1600–2.
106. Duckett JW. Transverse preputial island flap technique for repair of severe hypospadias. Urol Clin North Am 1980;7:423.
107. Gershbaum MD, Stock JA, Hanna MK. A case for 2-stage repair of perineoscrotal hypospadias with severe chordee. J Urol 2002;168:1727–9.
108. Greenfield SP, Sadler BT, Wan J. Two stage repair for severe hypospadias. J Urol 1994;152:498–501.
109. Retik AB, Bauer SB, Mandell J, et al. Management of severe hypospadias with two-stage repair. J Urol 1994;152:749–51.

110. Shapiro SR, Wacksman J, Koyle MA, et al. Hypospadias repair: Update and controversies, part 2. Dialog Pediatr Urol 1990;13:1–8.

111. Duckett JW. Hypospadias. J Urol [discussion] 1986;136:272.

112. DiSandro M, Palmer JM. Stricture incidence related to suture material in hypospadias surgery. J Pediatr Surg 1996;31:881–4.

113. Hakim S, Merguerian PA, Rabonowitz R. Outcome analysis of the modified Mathieu hypospadias repair: Comparison of stented and unstented repairs. J Urol 1996;156:836–8.

114. Steckler RE, Zaontz MR. Stent-free Thiersch-Duplay hypospadias repair with the Snodgrass modification. J Urol 1997;158:1178–80.

115. McLorie GA, Joyner BD, Bagli DJ, et al. A prospective randomized clinical trial to evaluate methods of postoperative care in hypospadias. Pediatrics 1999;104:813A.

116. VanSavage JG, Palanca LG, Slaughenhoupt BL. A prospective randomized trial of dressing versus no dressing for hypospadias repair. J Urol 2000;164:981–3.

117. Goulding FJ. Penile block for postoperative pain relief in penile surgery. J Urol 1981;126:337.

118. Thies KC, Driessen J, KHO HG, et al. Longer than expected-duration of caudal analgesia with two different doses of levobupivicaine in children undergoing hypospadias repair. J Pediatr Urol 2010;6:585–8.

119. Duckett JW, Kaplan GW, Woodard JR. Panel: Complications of hypospadias repair. Urol Clin North Am 1980;7:443–54.

120. Sugar EC, Firlit CF. Urinary prophylaxis and postoperative care of children at home with an indwelling catheter after hypospadias repair. Urology 1988;32:418–20.

121. Shohet I, Alagam M, Shafir R, et al. Postoperative catheterization and prophylactic antimicrobials in children with hypospadias. Urology 1983;22:391–3.

122. Horton CE Jr, Horton CE. Complications of hypospadias surgery. Clin Plast Surg 1988;15:371–9.

123. Retik AB, Keating MA, Mandell J. Complications of hypospadias surgery. Urol Clin North Am 1988;15:223–36.

124. Zagula EM, Braren V. Management of urethrocutaneous fistulas following hypospadias repair. J Urol 1983;130:743–5.

125. Gargolla PC, Cai AW, Borer JG, et al. Management of recurrent urethral strictures after hypospadias repair: is there a role for repeat dilation or endoscopic incision? J Pediatr Urol 2011;7:34–8.

126. Scherz HC, Kaplan GW, Packer MG, et al. Post-hypospadias repair urethral strictures: A review of 30 cases. J Urol 1988;140:1253–5.

127. Zaontz MR, Kaplan WE, Maizels M. Surgical correction of anterior urethral diverticula after hypospadias repair in children. Urology 1989;33:40–2.

128. Issa MM, Gearhart JP. The failed MAGPI: Management and prevention. Br J Urol 1989;64:169–71.

129. Vandersteen DR, Hussman DA. Late onset recurrent penile chordee after successful correction at hypospadias repair. J Urol 1998;160:1131–3.

130. Sheldon CA, Essig KA. Surgical strategies in the reconstruction of the failed hypospadias: Advantages and versatility of vascular based graft/flap techniques [abstract 250]: American Urological Association Meeting. J Urol 1990;143:251A.

131. Ehrlich RM, Alter G. Split-thickness skin graft urethroplasty and tunica vaginalis flaps for failed hypospadias repairs. J Urol 1996;155:131–4.

132. Subanj TB, Perovic SV, Milcevic RM, et al. Sexual behavior and sexual function of adults after hypospadias surgery: A comparative study. J Urol 2004;171:1876–9.

133. Duckett JW, Snyder HM. Meatal advancement and glanuloplasty hypospadias repair after 1000 cases: Avoidance of meatal stenosis and regression. J Urol 1992;147:665–9.

134. Retik AB, Mandell J, Bauer SB, et al. Meatal-based hypospadias repair with the use of a dorsal subcutaneous flap to prevent urethrocutaneous fistula. J Urol 1994;152:1229–31.

135. Braga LH, Lorenzo AJ, Pippi Salle JL. Tubularized incised plate urethroplasty for distal hypospadias: a literature review. Indian J Urol 2008;24:219–25.

136. Wilkinson DJ, Farrelly P, Kenny SE. Outcomes in distal hypospadias: A systematic review of the Mathieu and tabularized incised pate repairs. J Pediatr Urol 2012;8:307–12.

137. Jayanthi VR. The modified Snodgrass hypospadias repair: Techniques and results. Urology 2 1983;1:30–5.

138. Ching CB, Wood HM, Ross JH, et al. The Cleveland Clinic experience with adult hypospadias patients undergoing repair: Their presentation and a new classification system. BJU Int 2011;107:1142–6.

139. Hanna MK. Single-stage hypospadias repair: Techniques and results. Urology 1983;21:30–5.

140. Hendren WH, Horton CE. Experience with one-stage repair of hypospadias and chordee using free graft of prepuce. J Urol 1988;140:1259–64.

141. Robert PE, Perlmutter AD, Reitelman C. Experience with 81, one-stage hypospadias/chordee repairs with free graft urethroplasties. J Urol 1990;144:526–9.

142. Stock JA, Cortez J, Scherz HC, et al. The management of proximal hypospadias using a one-stage hypospadias repair with a preputial free graft for neourethral construction and a preputial pedicle flap for ventral skin coverage. J Urol 1994;152:2335–7.

143. Fichtner J, Fisch M, Filipas D, et al. Refinements in buccal mucosal graft urethroplasty for hypospadias repair. World J Urol 1998;16:192–4.

144. Carr MC. Buccal mucosa grafts: Long-term follow up. Dialog Pediatr Urol 2002;25:5–6.

145. Hensle TW, Kearney MC, Bingham JB. Buccal mucosa grafts for hypospadias surgery: Long-term results. J Urol 2002;168:1734–7.

146. Braga LH, Pippi Salle JL, Lorenzo AJ, et al. Comparative analysis of tubularized incised plate versus onlay island flap urethroplasty for penoscrotal hypospadias. J Urol 2007;178:1451–6.

147. Snodgrass W, Yucei S. Tubularized incised plate for mid shaft and proximal hypospadias repair. J Urol 2007;177:698–702.

CHAPTER 60

CIRCUMCISION

Oliver B. Lao • Stephen C. Raynor

Circumcision (removal of the redundant prepuce) is one of the most frequently performed surgical procedures in the world. There is a wide variability in the rate of circumcision among different populations. A lack of consensus regarding the function of the foreskin and uncertainty regarding the benefits of circumcision has led to controversy regarding the appropriateness of elective circumcision. The most recent policy statement from the American Academy of Pediatrics (AAP) states 'the health benefits of newborn male circumcision outweigh the risks and the procedure's benefits justify access to this procedure for those families who choose it'.[1]

Circumcision has been practiced since ancient times. A common reason for elective circumcision centers on religious beliefs. The Bible declares circumcision to be the sign of the covenant between God and the people of Israel.[2] In the Muslim faith, circumcision is recommended, but not obligatory.[3] Circumcision is common in the USA, areas of Africa, Australian aborigines, and portions of the Middle East.[4,5] In contrast, routine circumcision is rarely performed in Europe, Asia, and Central and South America.[4] This variation in incidence likely reflects religious and cultural differences.

THE PREPUCE

The prepuce is the anatomical covering of the glans. Contributing to the debate concerning the appropriateness of routine circumcision is a poor understanding of its function. The prepuce is specialized junctional mucocutaneous tissue that has both somatosensory and autonomic innervation. Innervation of the prepuce differs from the glans, which is innervated by free nerve endings with protopathic sensitivity. As a result of these differences, the inner mucosa of the prepuce is felt to be a part of penile erogenous tissue.[6] Given the possible relationship between the prepuce and sexual satisfaction, studies have looked into outcomes following circumcision.

Problems with sexual dysfunction (inability to ejaculate, lacking interest, premature ejaculation, pain during sex, not enjoying sex) appear to be slightly more prevalent among uncircumcised men.[7] For sexually active adult males undergoing circumcision, there does not appear to be any adverse, clinically important effects on sexual function or satisfaction.[8–11] Other studies, however, have shown difficulty with sexual enjoyment, erectile function, and a decrease in masturbatory pleasure following circumcision.[11,12] These mixed results hold true for homosexual men as well.[13] The effects on female partners of adult males who are circumcised are similarly mixed. Some report dyspareunia, orgasm difficulties, and

incomplete needs fulfillment, while others report no significant problems at all.[14,15]

MEDICAL INDICATIONS

The inability to retract the foreskin of a newborn is the result of incomplete keratinization of the glans and is not pathologic. Phimosis is the inability to retract the foreskin. True phimosis is associated with a white, scarred preputial orifice, most common just before puberty, and is an indication for circumcision.[16] Balanitis xerotica obliterans is a ring-like distal sclerosis of the prepuce with whitish discoloration or plaque formation that may involve the prepuce, glans, or urethral meatus, and is also an indication for circumcision.[17] Paraphimosis occurs when the foreskin has been retracted behind the corona and is unable to be brought back over the glans. This is also an indication for circumcision, though ardent opponents of circumcision would offer preputial stretching, plasty, or topical steroid creams as alternative therapy.[18–21] Balanitis is an infection of the glans, and posthitis is an infection of the prepuce. Recurrent infection with scarring of the prepuce is also an indication for circumcision.[5,22]

ROUTINE CIRCUMCISION AT BIRTH

The appropriateness of routine circumcision of healthy newborn males is an emotional and contentious issue. Underlying the argument is a poor understanding as to the function of the prepuce.[23] Opponents have presented circumcision as a symbol of the 'therapeutic state',[24] a mutilating procedure,[25] and have questioned the ethics and legality of newborn circumcision, especially with respect to human rights considerations and the notion of respect for bodily integrity.[26,27] Opponents have also cited an association between circumcision and subsequently developing poor breastfeeding outcomes, delayed cognitive abilities, and neonatal jaundice. However, these concerns have not been substantiated.[28,29] One urologic study among children without urinary complaints did find a relationship between circumcision and meatal stenosis.[30]

Circumcision is performed on the eighth day in the Jewish faith, traditionally by a mohel, a member of the faith trained in circumcision. In Islamic countries, circumcision is considered traditional but not obligatory, with a wide variability in age at circumcision.[3,31]

Proponents for routine newborn circumcision generally cite three advantages: prevention of urinary tract infections,[32] prevention of sexually transmitted disease, and prevention of cancer, both penile and prostate.

As rates of circumcision have diminished in the USA, reports have appeared showing an increased rate of urinary tract infections (UTIs) in uncircumcised infants with a male predominance in infants younger than 3 months of age.[33] A disproportionate number were uncircumcised. A large retrospective analysis of infants from military families suggested that uncircumcised infants have a 12-fold increased risk for UTI compared with circumcised infants.[34-36] A prospective study found a reduced incidence of asymptomatic UTI in circumcised children.[37] Finally, there is a tenfold increase in the cost of managing UTIs in uncircumcised compared to circumcised infants.[38]

An increased incidence of infection in uncircumcised children is believed to be secondary to adherence of pathogenic bacteria to the prepuce and may also hold true for young adults.[39,40] Proponents point to the 10% incidence of concurrent bacteremias and long-term sequelae of renal scarring after infection.[41] Critics have countered that these studies are retrospective analyses and that other studies associate genitourinary infection with circumcised children.[42-44] Additionally, they argue that colonization of the prepuce by nonmaternal uropathic bacteria could be prevented by strict rooming-in with the mother.[45]

There are many studies examining the relationship between circumcision and sexually transmitted diseases (STDs).[46] The benefits of circumcision relative to STDs are a strong factor in the support of circumcision in the new AAP statement. Studies have shown that uncircumcised individuals have an increased risk of acquiring Human immunodeficiency virus (HIV), human papillomavirus (HPV), and genital herpes.[47-50] However, other studies have found little support for or have refuted these findings altogether.[7,51,52] There is also evidence that circumcision is associated with a decreased risk of cervical cancer in women.[48] It is possible that the protective effect of circumcision against STDs may differ between developed and developing nations with poor hygiene.[51] Possible mechanisms for differing rates of STDs in relation to circumcision status include a more easily traumatized mucosa and epithelium of the uncircumcised phallus, the foreskin environment being more conducive to pathogens, or nonspecific balanitis in uncircumcised men predisposing to certain STDs. Behavior and sexual practice still represent the greatest risk factors in STD transmission.[48]

Epidemiological studies of HIV and acquired immune deficiency syndrome (AIDS) have raised another argument for prophylactic circumcision. There is a substantial amount of evidence linking uncircumcised men with an increased risk of HIV infection that is independent of the increased risk of genital ulcers in uncircumcised men.[53] In Africa, there is an increased rate of HIV/AIDS observed in areas with low circumcision rates.[54] A meta-analysis from Africa concluded that there was enough evidence that circumcision was associated with reduced HIV infection rates to consider male circumcision as a strategy to reduce HIV transmission.[45] Three randomized trials in Africa showed an estimated 50–60% reduction in the relative risk of HIV infection with circumcision.[54,55] Similar findings have been noted in the USA, with

uncircumcised homosexual men having a twofold increase in the risk of HIV infection.[56,57] An uncircumcised male partner also appears to be associated with an increased risk of transmission of HIV to heterosexual contacts.[58] The most recent Cochrane reviews cite a protective association between circumcision and HIV acquisition, and recommend routine circumcision among heterosexual men while stopping short of recommending the same in homosexual men.[59,60]

Circumcision may act as a protective measure against cancer, both prostate and invasive penile. It is believed that these cancers have infectious etiologies and that rationale underlies the reasoning that circumcision before first sexual intercourse may be associated with a decreased risk of prostate cancer.[61] The uncircumcised state has been strongly associated with invasive penile cancer in multiple case series, especially given its strong association with HPV.[53,62] The incidence of penile cancer in the USA is approximately one case per 100,000, with nearly all cases occurring in uncircumcised men.[63,64] The protective effect against penile cancer is diminished or lost when circumcision is performed after the newborn period.[5,64,65] Other factors associated with invasive penile cancer include smoking, a history of genital warts, penile rash or tears, multiple sexual partners, and poor penile hygiene.[53,65] Critics cite equally low rates of penile cancer in developed countries with low circumcision rates and feel that the incidence of penile cancer does not justify routine neonatal circumcision.[43,62]

There is no definitive answer to the question of the appropriateness of routine newborn circumcision. Current studies do not provide conclusive evidence definitively for or against routine newborn circumcision. Males not circumcised at birth have between a 2–10% likelihood of needing circumcision.[21,25] A longitudinal study comparing circumcised with uncircumcised males showed a higher risk of penile 'problems' in infancy in the circumcised group.[66] However, there was a higher rate of 'problems' in the uncircumcised group after infancy. By 8 years, the uncircumcised group had experienced 50% more penile 'problems.'

The previous circumcision policy statement from the AAP in 1999 acknowledged the potential medical benefits of newborn male circumcision, but did not recommend routine neonatal circumcision.[53] The 2012 statement states that the preventive health benefits outweigh the risks of the procedure, recommending access to the procedure but stopping short of recommending routine circumcision.[1] In the USA, the parental decision for newborn circumcision seems to be based more on social than medical reasons.[67]

SURGICAL TECHNIQUE

Circumcision has been practiced for centuries. Common to all methods, the goal is removal of an adequate amount of prepuce to uncover the glans, treat or prevent phimosis, and eliminate the possibility of paraphimosis. Whichever method is chosen, the surgeon must be familiar with and adept at the technique with a resultant low complication rate.[1] Informed consent should always be obtained.[68]

Newborn Circumcision

Circumcision is the most frequently performed male operation in the USA, with 64% of newborn males infants circumcised in 1995.[53] Newborn circumcision is most frequently performed with a device, which may be a shield, used in traditional Jewish circumcision, a Mogen clamp, a Gomco clamp, or a Plastibell.[4] Prior to the procedure, the penis should be inspected for any contraindication to circumcision including a short or small phallus, hypospadias, chordee with no hypospadias, hooded prepuce, dorsal penile cutaneous hump, penile curvature or torsion, penoscrotal fusion, or large inguinal hernias or hydroceles that engulf the penis.[69]

There is agreement for the need for adequate analgesia as studies have shown infants circumcised without analgesia have a stronger pain response to vaccination at 4 and 6 months of age as compared to those receiving analgesics.[70] Another study, looking at pain in relation to timing, recommended circumcision before 8 days of age.[71] Effective relief of circumcision pain has been found with acetaminophen, topical lidocaine–procaine cream, and local nerve blocks.[72-75] One study showed a subcutaneous ring block with 1% lidocaine without epinephrine to be the most effective pain relief.[53] Sucrose on a pacifier can also provide added pain control.[76]

Even though many circumcisions are performed outside the operating room, antisepsis is critical as infection is a serious potential complication. In performing a Gomco circumcision, the field is sterilely prepped, and adhesions between the glans and inner surface of the prepuce are bluntly separated. The extent of foreskin to be excised is marked with a pen or a crush of the dorsal prepuce with a straight clamp. A dorsal slit allows the appropriate-sized bell to be placed over the glans, inside the prepuce (Fig. 60-1). The bell and foreskin are then brought through the opening in the clamp, placed in the yoke, and then tightened. The excess foreskin distal to the base of the clamp is then excised after waiting for several minutes. Electrocautery should never be used because of transmission of the electrical current to the penis. The bell is released and removed, taking care not to disrupt the weld between the shaft skin and the remnant of the inner surface of the prepuce.

A Plastibell allows strangulation of the distal foreskin, with a resulting slough of the tissue. After sterile prep and dorsal slit, the appropriate-sized Plastibell is placed over the glans inside the prepuce (Fig. 60-2). A string is

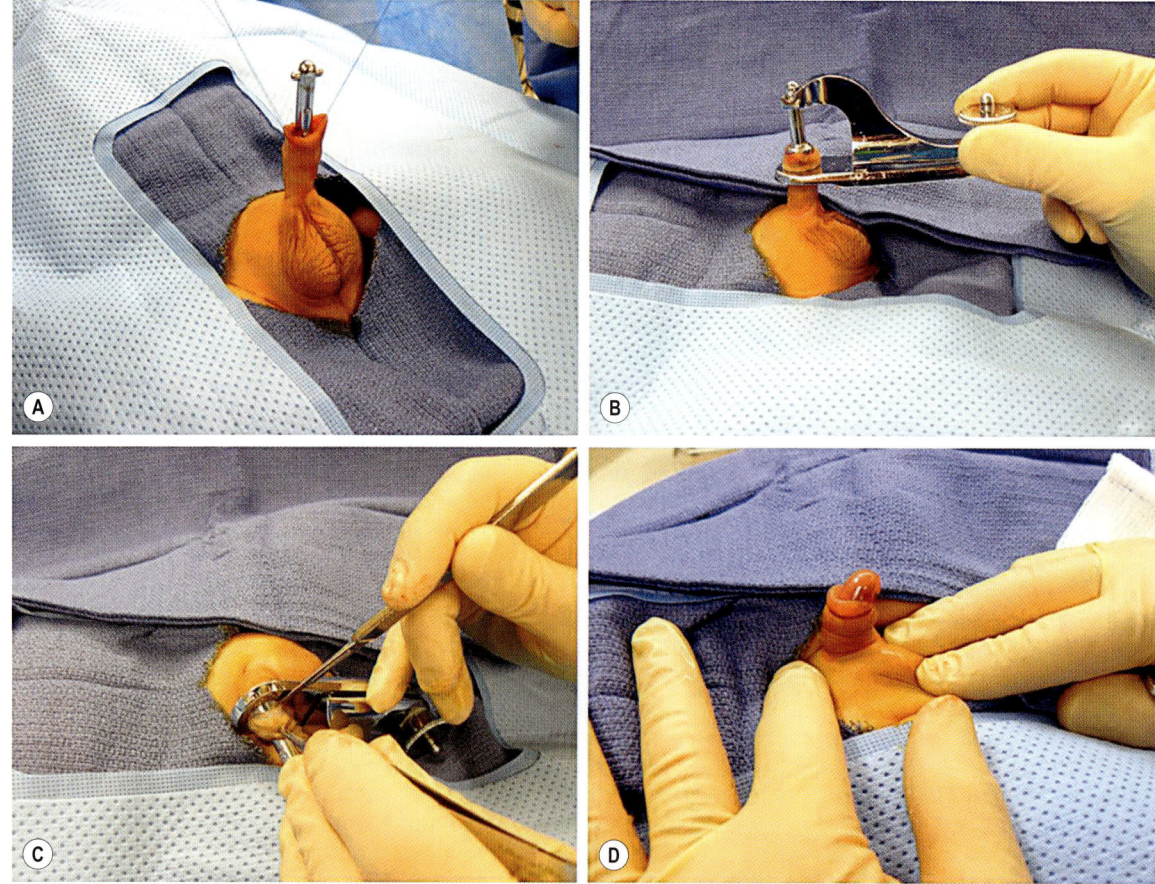

FIGURE 60-1 ■ The Gomco technique. **(A)** A short dorsal slit has been performed to allow an appropriate-sized bell to be placed over the glans and inside the prepuce. **(B)** Next, the prepuce to be excised along with the bell have been brought through the opening in the base of the clamp and placed in the yoke. **(C)** The yoke has then been tightened to coapt the skin edges. After waiting for 5 to 7 minutes, the excess prepuce is excised. Electrocautery must never be used to excise the foreskin because transmission of electrical current to the shaft of the penis will occur. **(D)** The bell has been released, and the circumcision is completed.

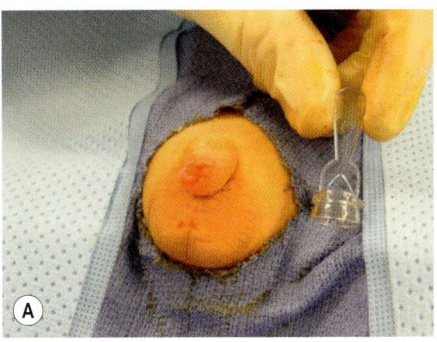 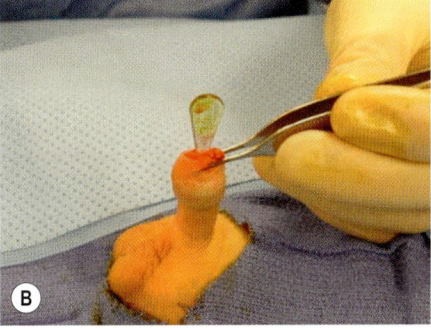 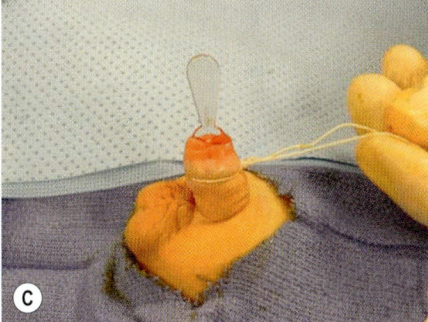

FIGURE 60-2 ■ Similar to the Gomco technique, in the Plastibell technique, adhesions between the glans and inner surface of the prepuce are bluntly separated. **(A)** An appropriate-size Plastibell has been selected. **(B)** The Plastibell is placed over the glans inside the prepuce. **(C)** A string is then tied around the prepuce and positioned in the groove of the bell. The excess foreskin is trimmed and the handle is broken off the bell. The foreskin remnant and bell are expected to slough in one to two weeks.

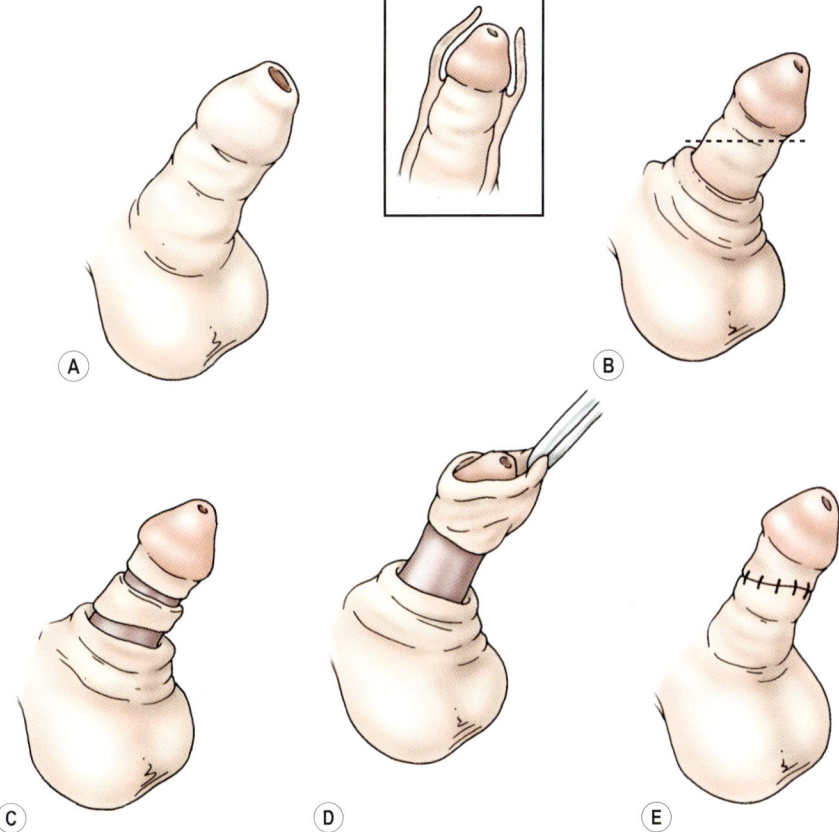

FIGURE 60-3 ■ **(A)** For a freehand circumcision, the initial incision is made in the shaft skin, leaving more skin ventrally. **(B)** A second incision is then made in the subcoronal sulcus **(C)**, leaving a generous cuff. The inset shows the amount of foreskin to be excised. **(D)** The isolated foreskin is then excised, and the shaft skin is sutured to the subcoronal skin **(E)**.

then tied around the prepuce, and positioned over a groove in the bell. The excess foreskin is trimmed and the handle is broken off the bell. The distal foreskin remnant and ring typically slough off in seven to 14 days.

Revision Circumcision

Following recovery from any of the above procedures, there may be redundancy or asymmetry of residual preputial skin that may not meet the cosmetic expectations of the family.[77] In situations where the family feels the redundant, residual prepuce is unsightly, or with a postoperative phimosis, they may seek an opinion regarding revision. As with primary circumcision, there is controversy surrounding the medical necessity and ethics of revision.[78]

One study reported 46 revisions where the indications were primarily preputial redundancy, residual cicatrix, preputial-glandular bridges, a sebaceous cyst and urethrocutaneous fistula.[79] Two other reported studies of circumcision revision both reported using the freehand or sleeve technique, with the most common indication being residual or redundant preputial skin.[79–81]

Freehand Circumcision

In older patients, circumcision is usually performed in the operating room and devices are less often used. As stated above, in cases of circumcision revision, the freehand technique is the preferred method. As shown in Figure 60-3, after prepping the field, any remaining adhesions between the glans and foreskin are bluntly lysed.

After marking the subcoronal sulcus, the foreskin is incised along the base of the glans with the foreskin in its normal position. Less skin is excised from the ventral surface. Dissection is carried down to Buck's fascia. The prepuce is then retracted and an incision made in the subcoronal sulcus, leaving a generous cuff of subcoronal skin. Injury to the urethra must be avoided ventrally. The collar of foreskin that is isolated is excised and electrocautery is used to obtain hemostasis. The shaft skin is approximated to the subcoronal skin using absorbable sutures.

COMPLICATIONS

When performed by experienced hands under sterile conditions, circumcision has a low complication rate between 2–10%.[62] Bleeding and infection are the most frequent complications and are generally minor.[1] Although adhesions between the foreskin remnant and the glans are common, most will resolve with time.[82] However, serious problems can result, including necrotizing fasciitis, sepsis, Fournier's gangrene, and meningitis.[5] Other complications include skin bridges, inclusion cysts, iatrogenic hypospadias or epispadias, partial glans amputation, and catastrophic loss of the penis when electrocautery is used with a metal device. There can be excision of too much or too little of the foreskin, with resultant postoperative phimosis or concealed penis. As described above, revision may sometimes be necessary later in childhood.[81]

REFERENCES

1. Circumcision Policy. Statement. Pediatrics 2012;130:585–6.
2. The Holy Bible. King James ed.
3. Rizvi SA, Naqvi SA, Hussain M, et al. Religious circumcision: A Muslim view. BJU Int 1999;83(Suppl. 1):13–16.
4. Holman JR, Lewis EL, Ringler RL. Neonatal circumcision techniques. Am Fam Physician 1995;52:511–18, 519–20.
5. Niku SD, Stock JA, Kaplan GW. Neonatal circumcision. Urol Clin North Am 1995;22:57–65.
6. Cold CJ, Taylor JR. The prepuce. BJU Int 1999;83(Suppl. 1): 34–44.
7. Laumann EO, Masi CM, Zuckerman EW. Circumcision in the United States. Prevalence, prophylactic effects, and sexual practice. JAMA 1997;277:1052–7.
8. Collins S, Upshaw J, Rutchik S, et al. Effects of circumcision on male sexual function: Debunking a myth? J Urol 2002;167: 2111–12.
9. Senkul T, Iser IC, Sen B, et al. Circumcision in adults: Effect on sexual function. Urology 2004;63:155–8.
10. Kigozi G, Watya S, Polis CB, et al. The effect of male circumcision on sexual satisfaction and function, results from a randomized trial of male circumcision for human immunodeficiency virus prevention, Rakai, Uganda. BJU Int 2008;101:65–70.
11. Fink KS, Carson CC, DeVellis RF. Adult circumcision outcomes study: Effect on erectile function, penile sensitivity, sexual activity and satisfaction. J Urol 2002;167:2113–16.
12. Kim D, Pang MG. The effect of male circumcision on sexuality. BJU Int 2007;99:619–22.
13. Mao L, Templeton DJ, Crawford J, et al. Does circumcision make a difference to the sexual experience of gay men? Findings from the Health in Men (HIM) cohort. J Sex Med 2008;5: 2557–61.
14. Kigozi G, Lukabwe I, Kagaayi J, et al. Sexual satisfaction of women partners of circumcised men in a randomized trial of male circumcision in Rakai, Uganda. BJU Int 2009;104:1698–701.
15. Frisch M, Lindholm M, Gronbaek M. Male circumcision and sexual function in men and women: A survey-based, cross-sectional study in Denmark. Int J Epidemiol 2011;40:1367–81.
16. Rickwood AM. Medical indications for circumcision. BJU Int 1999;83(Suppl. 1):45–51.
17. Gargollo PC, Kozakewich HP, Bauer SB, et al. Balanitis xerotica obliterans in boys. J Urol 2005;174(4 Pt 1):1409–12.
18. Cooper GG, Thomson GJ, Raine PA. Therapeutic retraction of the foreskin in childhood. Br Med J (Clin Res Ed) 1983; 286(6360):186–7.
19. Cuckow PM, Rix G, Mouriquand PD. Preputial plasty: A good alternative to circumcision. J Pediatr Surg 1994;29:561–3.
20. Holmlund DE. Dorsal incision of the prepuce and skin closure with Dexon in patients with phimosis. Scand J Urol Nephrol 1973;7: 97–9.
21. Lerman SE, Liao JC. Neonatal circumcision. Pediatr Clin North Am 2001;48:1539–57.
22. Escala JM, Rickwood AM. Balanitis. Br J Urol 1989;63:196–7.
23. Taylor JR, Lockwood AP, Taylor AJ. The prepuce: Specialized mucosa of the penis and its loss to circumcision. Br J Urol 1996;77:291–5.
24. Szasz T. Routine neonatal circumcision: Symbol of the birth of the therapeutic state. J Med Philos 1996;21:137–48.
25. Weiss GN, Weiss EB. A perspective on controversies over neonatal circumcision. Clin Pediatr (Phila) 1994;33:726–30.
26. Van Howe RS, Svoboda JS, Dwyer JG, et al. Involuntary circumcision: The legal issues. BJU Int 1999;83(Suppl. 1):63–73.
27. Dekkers W. Routine (non-religious) neonatal circumcision and bodily integrity: A transatlantic dialogue. Kennedy Inst Ethics J 2009;19:125–46.
28. Fergusson DM, Boden JM, Horwood LJ. Neonatal circumcision: Effects on breastfeeding and outcomes associated with breastfeeding. J Paediatr Child Health 2008;44:44–9.
29. Eroglu E, Balci S, Ozkan H, et al. Does circumcision increase neonatal jaundice? Acta Paediatr 2008;97:1192–3.
30. Joudi M, Fathi M, Hiradfar M. Incidence of asymptomatic meatal stenosis in children following neonatal circumcision. J Pediatr Urol 2011;7:526–8.
31. Sari N, Buyukunal SN, Zulfikar B. Circumcision ceremonies at the Ottoman palace. J Pediatr Surg 1996;31:920–4.
32. Mendez-Gallart R, Estevez E, Bautista A, et al. Bipolar scissors circumcision is a safe, fast, and bloodless procedure in children. J Pediatr Surg 2009;44:2048–53.
33. Ginsburg CM, McCracken GH Jr. Urinary tract infections in young infants. Pediatrics 1982;69:409–12.
34. Wiswell TE, Enzenauer RW, Holton ME, et al. Declining frequency of circumcision: Implications for changes in the absolute incidence and male to female sex ratio of urinary tract infections in early infancy. Pediatrics 1987;79:338–42.
35. Wiswell TE, Geschke DW. Risks from circumcision during the first month of life compared with those for uncircumcised boys. Pediatrics 1989;83:1011–15.
36. Wiswell TE, Hachey WE. Urinary tract infections and the uncircumcised state: An update. Clin Pediatr (Phila) 1993;32: 130–4.
37. Simforoosh N, Tabibi A, Khalili SA, et al. Neonatal circumcision reduces the incidence of asymptomatic urinary tract infection: A large prospective study with long-term follow up using Plastibell. J Pediatr Urol 2012;8:320323—Epub 2010.
38. Schoen EJ, Colby CJ, Ray GT. Newborn circumcision decreases incidence and costs of urinary tract infections during the first year of life. Pediatrics 2000;105(4 Pt 1):789–93.
39. Roberts JA. Norwich-Eaton lectureship. Pathogenesis of nonobstructive urinary tract infections in children. J Urol 1990;144(2 Pt 2):475–80.
40. Spach DH, Stapleton AE, Stamm WE. Lack of circumcision increases the risk of urinary tract infection in young men. JAMA 1992;267:679–81.
41. Wiswell TE. The prepuce, urinary tract infections, and the consequences. Pediatrics 2000;105(4 Pt 1):860–2.
42. American Academy of Pediatrics. Report of the Task Force on Circumcision. Pediatrics 1989;84:388–91.
43. Poland RL. The question of routine neonatal circumcision. N Engl J Med 1990;322:1312–15.

44. Prais D, Shoov-Furman R, Amir J. Is ritual circumcision a risk factor for neonatal urinary tract infections? Arch Dis Child 2009;94:191–4.

45. Winberg J, Bollgren I, Gothefors L, et al. The prepuce: A mistake of nature? Lancet 1989;1(8638):598–9.

46. Tobian AA, Serwadda D, Quinn TC, et al. Male circumcision for the prevention of HSV-2 and HPV infections and syphilis. N Engl J Med 2009;360:1298–309.

47. Castellsague X, Bosch FX, Munoz N, et al. Male circumcision, penile human papillomavirus infection, and cervical cancer in female partners. N Engl J Med 2002;346:1105–12.

48. Cook LS, Koutsky LA, Holmes KK. Circumcision and sexually transmitted diseases. Am J Public Health 1994;84:197–201.

49. Parker SW, Stewart AJ, Wren MN, et al. Circumcision and sexually transmissible disease. Med J Aust 1983;2:288–90.

50. Tobian AA, Gray RH, Quinn TC. Male circumcision for the prevention of acquisition and transmission of sexually transmitted infections: The case for neonatal circumcision. Arch Pediatr Adolesc Med 2010;164:78–84.

51. Donovan B, Bassett I, Bodsworth NJ. Male circumcision and common sexually transmissible diseases in a developed nation setting. Genitourin Med 1994;70:317–20.

52. Dickson NP, van Roode T, Herbison P, et al. Circumcision and risk of sexually transmitted infections in a birth cohort. J Pediatr 2008;152:383–7.

53. Circumcision policy statement. American Academy of Pediatrics. Task Force on Circumcision. Pediatrics 1999;103:686–93.

54. Moses S, Plummer FA, Bradley JE, et al. The association between lack of male circumcision and risk for HIV infection: A review of the epidemiological data. Sex Transm Dis 1994;21:201–10.

55. Vardi Y, Sadeghi-Nejad H, Pollack S, et al. Male circumcision and HIV prevention. J Sex Med 2007;4(4 Pt 1):838–43.

56. Kreiss JK, Hopkins SG. The association between circumcision status and human immunodeficiency virus infection among homosexual men. J Infect Dis 1993;168:1404–8.

57. Xu X, Patel DA, Dalton VK, et al. Can routine neonatal circumcision help prevent human immunodeficiency virus transmission in the United States? Am J Mens Health 2009;3:79–84.

58. McCarthy KH, Studd JW, Johnson MA. Heterosexual transmission of human immunodeficiency virus. Br J Hosp Med 1992;48:404–9.

59. Siegfried N, Muller M, Deeks JJ, et al. Male circumcision for prevention of heterosexual acquisition of HIV in men. Cochrane Database Syst Rev 2009:CD003362.

60. Wiysonge CS, Kongnyuy EJ, Shey M, et al. Male circumcision for prevention of homosexual acquisition of HIV in men. Cochrane Database Syst Rev 2011:CD007496.

61. Wright JL, Lin DW, Stanford JL. Circumcision and the risk of prostate cancer. Cancer 2012;118:4437–43.

62. Neonatal circumcision revisited. Fetus and Newborn Committee, Canadian Paediatric Society. CMAJ 1996;154:769–80.

63. Schoen EJ, Fischell AA. Dorsal penile nerve block for circumcision. JAMA 1989;261:701–2.

64. Schoen EJ. The relationship between circumcision and cancer of the penis. CA Cancer J Clin 1991;41:306–9.

65. Maden C, Sherman KJ, Beckmann AM, et al. History of circumcision, medical conditions, and sexual activity and risk of penile cancer. J Natl Cancer Inst 1993;85:19–24.

66. Fergusson DM, Lawton JM, Shannon FT. Neonatal circumcision and penile problems: An 8-year longitudinal study. Pediatrics 1988;81:537–41.

67. Brown MS, Brown CA. Circumcision decision: Prominence of social concerns. Pediatrics 1987;80:215–19.

68. Christakis DA, Harvey E, Zerr DM, et al. A trade-off analysis of routine newborn circumcision. Pediatrics 2000;105(1 Pt 3):246–9.

69. Redman JF, Elser JM. Neonatal circumcision: Anatomic contraindications. J Ark Med Soc 1997;94:73–5.

70. Taddio A, Katz J, Ilersich AL, et al. Effect of neonatal circumcision on pain response during subsequent routine vaccination. Lancet 1997;349(9052):599–603.

71. Banieghbal B. Optimal time for neonatal circumcision: An observation-based study. J Pediatr Urol 2009;5:359–62.

72. Howard CR, Howard FM, Weitzman ML. Acetaminophen analgesia in neonatal circumcision: The effect on pain. Pediatrics 1994; 93:641–6.

73. Lenhart JG, Lenhart NM, Reid A, et al. Local anesthesia for circumcision: Which technique is most effective? J Am Board Fam Pract 1997;10:13–19.

74. Serour F, Cohen A, Mandelberg A, et al. Dorsal penile nerve block in children undergoing circumcision in a day-care surgery. Can J Anaesth 1996;43:954–8.

75. Taddio A, Stevens B, Craig K, et al. Efficacy and safety of lidocaine-prilocaine cream for pain during circumcision. N Engl J Med 1997;336:1197–201.

76. Herschel M, Khoshnood B, Ellman C, et al. Neonatal circumcision. Randomized trial of a sucrose pacifier for pain control. Arch Pediatr Adolesc Med 1998;152:279–84.

77. Kaplan GW. Complications of circumcision. Urol Clin North Am 1983;10:543–9.

78. Fleiss PM. Re: Circumcision revision in prepubertal boys: Analysis of a 2-year experience and description of a technique. J Urol 1995;154:1143–4.

79. Redman JF. Circumcision revision in prepubertal boys: Analysis of a 2-year experience and description of a technique. J Urol 1995;153:180–2.

80. Al-Ghazo MA, Banihani KE. Circumcision revision in male children. Int Braz J Urol 2006;32:454–8.

81. Brisson PA, Patel HI, Feins NR. Revision of circumcision in children: Report of 56 cases. J Pediatr Surg 2002;37:1343–6.

82. Ponsky LE, Ross JH, Knipper N, et al. Penile adhesions after neonatal circumcision. J Urol 2000;164:495–6.

CHAPTER 61

PRUNE-BELLY SYNDROME

Heidi A. Stephany • John W. Brock III • Romano T. DeMarco

Frohlich first reported a neonate born with congenital absence of his abdominal musculature in 1839 and Parker later described the accompanying genitourinary tract abnormalities of hydroureteronephrosis, megacystis, and undescended testes (UDT).[1,2] Combined, this triad comprises the condition known as 'prune-belly syndrome' (PBS), which was coined by Osler in 1901 (Fig. 61-1).[3] Eagle and Barrett reviewed this rare, congenital syndrome and detailed the characteristic features that includes congenital absence or deficiency of the abdominal wall musculature, urinary tract abnormalities including a large hypotonic bladder (megacystis), dilated ureters, dilated prostatic urethra, and bilateral UDT.[4] In addition, other anomalies, such as cardiac, pulmonary, gastrointestinal, renal and orthopedic can also be present.[5] In an effort to quell the negative connotation that may be associated with this terminology, various other labels have been used, including Eagle–Barrett syndrome, triad syndrome, and abdominal musculature deficiency (AMD) syndrome.[5-7] Despite the good intentions of the new nomenclature, the most widely accepted designation has remained 'prune-belly syndrome.'

The incidence of PBS is approximately 3.8 per 100,000 live births based on data from the Kids' Inpatient Database.[8] Of those affected, nearly 50% are white, 30% black, and 10% Hispanic. Children with incomplete forms of the condition may present with the typical abdominal wall changes, but no urologic or testicular manifestations. Using strict criteria for the definition of PBS, which includes cryptorchidism, all patients must be male. Female patients, however, with characteristic abdominal wall and urologic findings, make up a small proportion of patients with an incomplete form of PBS.[9,10]

GENETICS

Genetic factors may play a role, yet no specific gene defect for PBS has been identified. Hepatocyte-nuclear factor-1β (HNF1β), a transcription factor responsible for regulating gene expression necessary for mesodermal and endodermal development, has recently become a gene of interest. Two case reports of PBS with interstitial deletions in chromosome 17q12 encompassing HNF1β have been described.[11,12] However, recently, 32 patients with PBS were screened for the presence of HNF1β mutations and only 1 (3%) was found to have a mutation.[13]

A study evaluating consanguineous union of parents with two male offspring found to have PBS and three with posterior urethral valves point to two loci, 1q and 11p, with likely only one being the causative gene.[14] Sporadic cases of PBS have also been associated with other chromosomal abnormalities, including Turner syndrome and trisomies 13 and 18.[15-18]

EMBRYOLOGY

The etiology for PBS is unclear. While there is no consensus, various hypotheses have been proposed to explain the usual constellation of findings. The most widely accepted mechanism is early urethral obstruction during gestation, leading to a massively distended bladder and ureters.[19] This obstruction may be anatomic,[20] but others have proposed a functional cause, potentially related to hypoplasia of the prostate.[21] Regardless whether if it is functional or anatomic, the urethral obstruction with ensuing bladder distension is thought to lead to the classic abdominal wall muscle and skin changes. In addition, the high grade urethral obstruction and secondary bladder changes can lead to renal dysplasia with oligohydramnios and the subsequent pulmonary dysplasia that is seen in many PBS children. Finally, to account for the cryptorchidism, it is suggested that the distended bladder prevents the normal descent of the testes, thus explaining their intra-abdominal position.

Another reasonable hypothesis involves a primary mesenchymal defect early in embryogenesis that leads to incomplete differentiation or failure of migration of the lateral mesoderm. The failure of migration of the lateral mesoderm explains the typical abdominal wall appearance, but does not account for the genitourinary and testicular abnormalities.[22] It is suggested that not only is there a defect in the lateral plate mesoderm, but there is also a defect within the intermediate plate mesoderm, which would then affect embryogenesis of the paramesonephric and mesonephric ducts.[23]

CLINICAL FEATURES

Genitourinary Anomalies

Bladder

The bladder is usually very large and irregular with a patent urachus identified in approximately 25% of patients.[4] PBS patients typically have a compliant bladder with a very large capacity and smooth wall that has an increased ratio of collagen to muscle fibers. Because of these findings, a delay in the first sensation to void is often seen.[24] In some patients with severe muscle loss, the bladder will bulge and give the impression of a pseudo-diverticulum most commonly seen at the dome of the

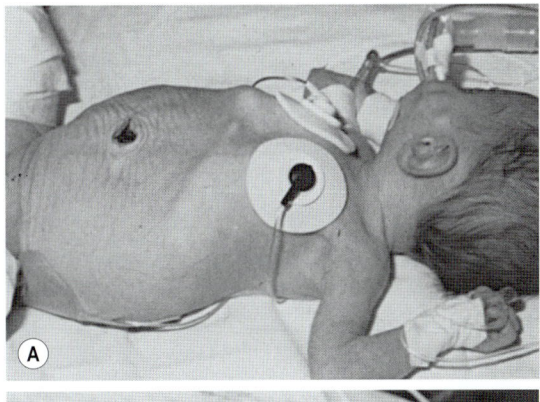
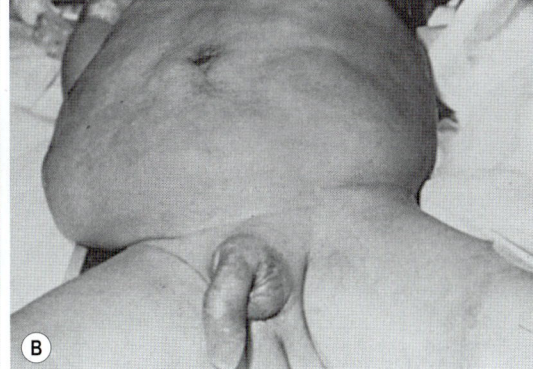
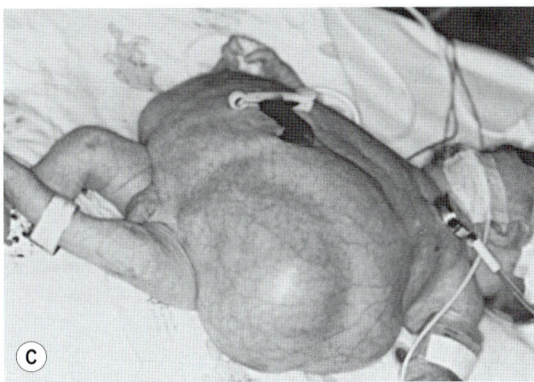

FIGURE 61-1 ■ Variable degrees of abdominal wall laxity can be seen in patients with PBS. (A) Subtle wrinkling in a less severely affected infant. (B) Typical appearance. (C) Severely affected neonate. (Courtesy of D. M. Joseph, MD.)

bladder.[7] The trigone is typically enlarged with displaced ureteral orifices laterally and superiorly, which likely contributes to the high incidence of vesicoureteral reflux (VUR).[5,7] A poorly defined bladder neck opens into a dilated prostatic urethra. Many patients will void efficiently, but this can vary and some believe a relative outlet resistance exists. Regardless, PBS patients should be followed closely as their ability to empty can deteriorate.[25]

Ureters

The ureteral orifices are displaced laterally and superiorly, and typically are dilated and tortuous, particularly distally where the smooth muscle is not as normal compared to the proximal ureter (Fig. 61-2). The degree of ureteral pathology can vary and may even be segmental.[26] Collagen fibers and connective tissue have been found to be abundant between muscle bundles containing few muscle cells. Thus, there is poor contractility of the ureter and the propulsion of urine is hindered, resulting in upper tract stasis.[27,28] With the bladder and ureteral abnormalities, it is no surprise that approximately 75% of patients will have VUR (Fig. 61-3).[29] It is rare, however, for PBS patients to have ureteral obstructions.[30]

Kidneys

Renal abnormalities span a large spectrum ranging from completely normal to severe dysplasia. Of those with dysplasia, one kidney may be affected with a normal contralateral kidney.[31] The mechanism for the renal abnormalities is uncertain but possibilities include bladder outlet obstruction and abnormal ureteral bud–metanephric blastema interaction.[32]

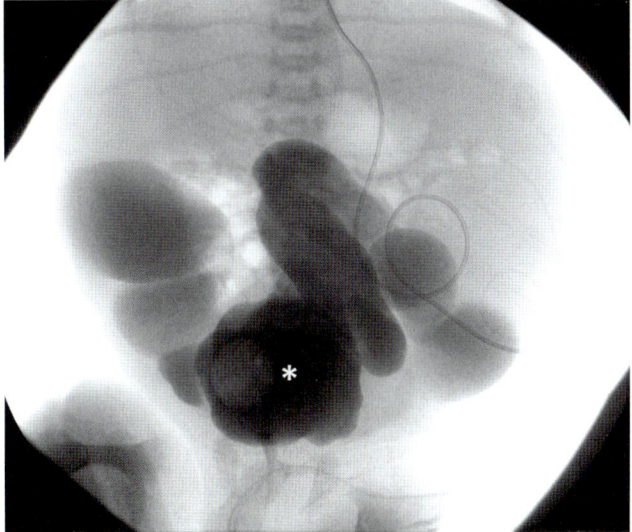

FIGURE 61-2 ■ This voiding cystourethrogram in a patient with PBS shows large, dilated distal ureters. The bladder is marked with an asterisk.

Hydronephrosis is typically seen and can be quite variable in spite of severe ureteral and renal pelvic distension. Most hydronephrosis is nonobstructive in nature, and the degree of hydroureteronephrosis does not directly correlate with the amount of parenchymal injury.[30,32]

Posterior Urethral, Prostate and Accessory Sex Organs

The extremely dilated posterior urethra seen in PBS children is thought to be secondary to generalized hypoplasia of the prostate epithelium with replacement of the normal

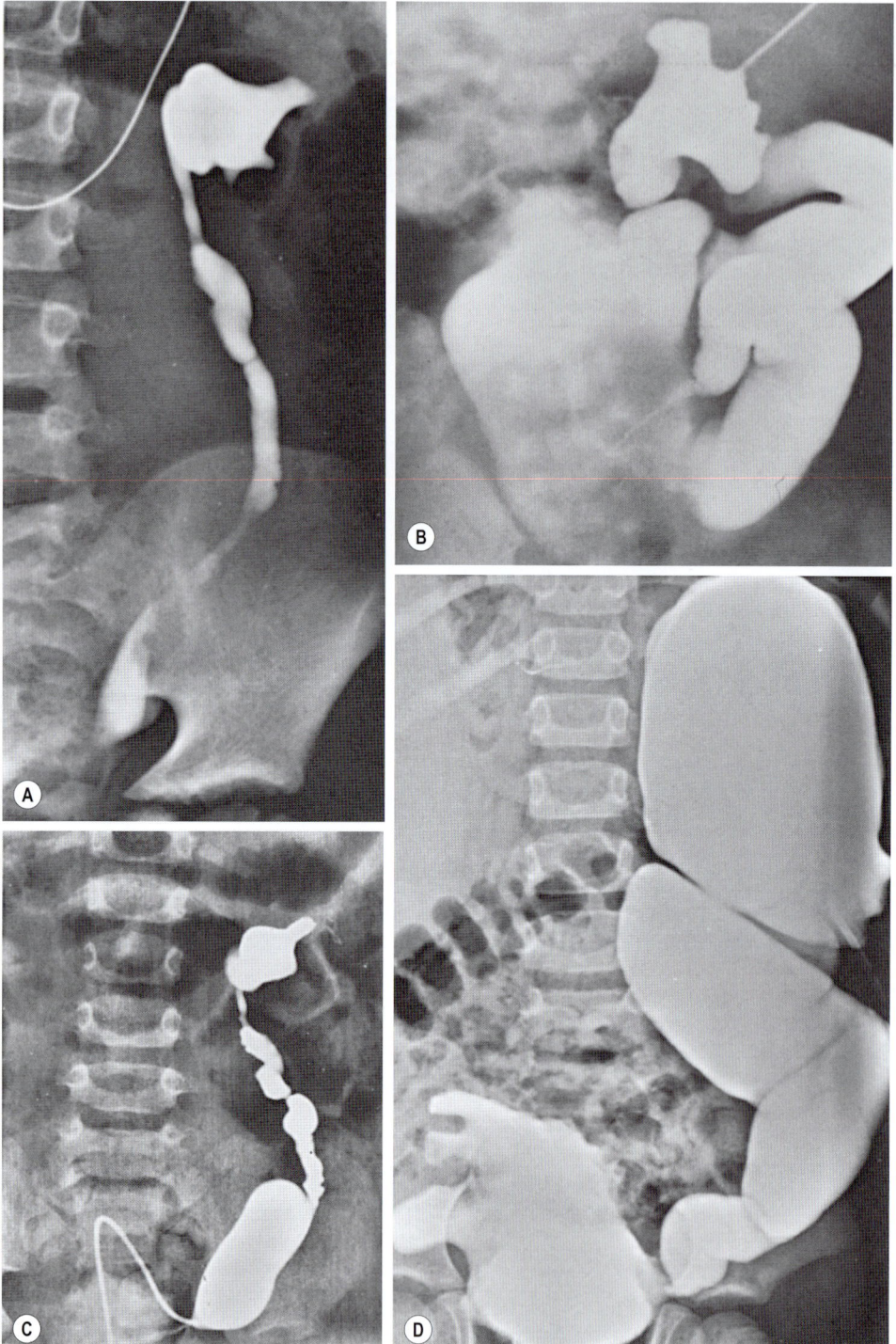

FIGURE 61-3 ■ Variable degrees of dilation and dysmorphism of the upper urinary tract are seen in PBS. **(A)** Dysmorphic renal pelvis with mild ureteral dilation. **(B)** Calyceal clubbing and a tortuous 'wandering' ureter. **(C)** Dysmorphic pelvis with exaggerated dilation of the distal ureteral spindle. **(D)** Bizarre appearance of the collecting system as well as the bladder.

smooth muscle anteriorly with connective tissue. While obstructive lesions are rare in the distal posterior urethra,[29,33] several investigators have described valve-like obstructive tissue in this location.[34–36]

The prostate appears widened secondary to the loss of smooth muscle support. One theory supporting this finding is an abnormal epithelial–mesenchymal interaction (Fig. 61-4).[20,37] Ejaculatory failure can result from this lack of normal prostatic parenchyma. Some patients may have retrograde ejaculation due to an incompetent bladder neck.[34,38]

The vas and seminal vesicles are typically affected, with atresia commonly present. However, some patients present with dilation of both of these structures.[23]

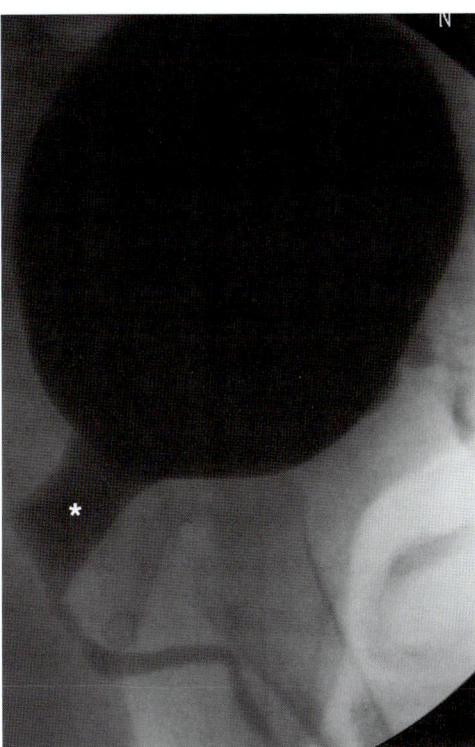

FIGURE 61-4 ■ Posterior urethral dilation (asterisk) is often found in children with PBS. This dilation is similar to that seen in boys with posterior urethral valves.

Anterior Urethra

Typically the anterior urethra is normal. However, atresia of the bulbar or membranous urethra has been reported, occurring in 18% of patients in one review.[39]

PBS is also associated with two variations of megalourethra.[40] The scaphoid megalourethra, the most common and less severe form, is associated with a deficiency of the spongiosum and preservation of the normal glans and corporal bodies (Fig. 61-5). The fusiform type has a deficiency of not only the spongiosum, but also of the corpus cavernosum.[41] With voiding, the entire phallus enlarges in patients with the fusiform variety, while those children with the scaphoid form only have dilation of the anterior urethra.

Testes

Most children have bilateral intra-abdominal testes which are commonly found near the ureterovesical junction. More proximal locations have also been described.[5,7] Data have varied regarding testicular histology in patients with PBS. Some reports have described normal testicular histology and other series have found diminished spermatogonia with Leydig cell hyperplasia when compared to normal controls, suggesting the testicular findings are caused by more than the cryptorchid state.[7,42] Regardless of the histological findings, azospermia is the rule in adult PBS patients, with no reported cases of a natural paternity from patients with PBS.[43]

Extragenitourinary Anomalies

Abdominal Wall

The most characteristic clinical finding in PBS patients is the wrinkled and floppy appearance to the abdominal wall with bulging flanks and creased skin in the newborn. As patients age and the amount of cutaneous abdominal adipose tissue increases, a more potbelly appearance is noted. The degree of the 'pruned' appearance and deficiency of the abdominal wall musculature can vary significantly (see Figure 61-1). While rarely completely absent, the medial and inferior aspects of the abdominal wall are most severely involved, with normal or near-normal abdominal wall at the periphery.[30,44] The most affected individual muscle is the transversus abdominis followed in decreasing frequency by the rectus abdominis inferior to the umbilicus, internal oblique, external oblique, and superior aspect of the rectus.[29] While the innervation of the abdominal muscle appears unaffected, microscopy has found variations in or decreased muscle fiber size, excessive collagen accumulation, and myofilamentous disarray and loss.[45]

Cardiac

Cardiac anomalies are present in approximately 10% of affected children. The most common findings include patent ductus arteriosus, atrial and ventricular septal defects, and tetralogy of Fallot.[46,47]

Pulmonary

Pulmonary issues are common and typically related to the degree of renal dysplasia and oligohydramnios. Neonates

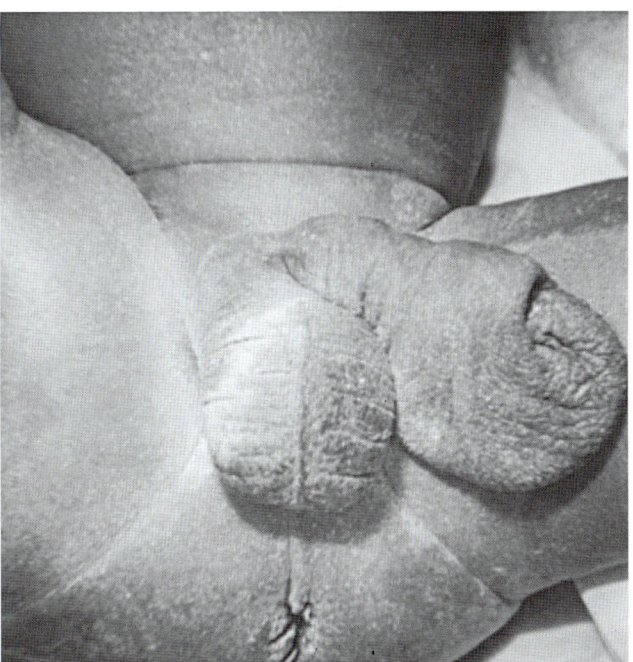

FIGURE 61-5 ■ Gross appearance of scaphoid megalourethra in a child with PBS.

exhibiting pulmonary distress should be presumed to have pulmonary hypoplasia and hyaline membrane disease. These children are also at increased risk for both pneumonia and spontaneous pneumothorax which is not necessarily related to the degree of hypoplasia.[48] Older patients may be found to have significant restrictive lung disease thought to be related to musculoskeletal abnormalities rather than parenchymal lung disease.[49]

Gastrointestinal

The most common gastrointestinal anomaly is intestinal malrotation.[29] This is thought to be due to an incomplete rotation of the midgut leading to a narrow mesentery.[50] Other intestinal abnormalities include persistent cloaca, gastroschisis, omphalocele, imperforate anus, colonic atresia, volvulus, and anorectal malformation.[50–53] A similar condition to PBS, known as megacystis-microcolon-intestinal hypoperistalsis syndrome (MMIHS), presents with a functional obstruction of the gastrointestinal tract with malrotation, microcolon, and a large non-obstructed bladder. Some have postulated a common pathogenesis, and a very rare case of both MMIHS and PBS has been reported.[54,55] Chronic constipation can be a life-long issue and is believed to be due to lack of intra-abdominal pressure from the lax abdominal wall.

Musculoskeletal

Musculoskeletal abnormalities are common, occurring in approximately 50% of children.[56–58] The most common orthopedic deformity is clubfoot, with an incidence of at least 25%, and nearly 50% are affected bilaterally.[58] Other findings include congenital scoliosis, talipes equinovarus, and pectus excavatum.[56,58] The specific mechanism leading to the orthopedic issues is unknown, but it is postulated to be secondary to in utero compression and oligohydramnios.[59]

CLINICAL PRESENTATION

Antenatal Diagnosis and Management

Patients with PBS present antenatally similarly to those patients with posterior urethral valves or other causes of bladder outlet obstruction. The typical antenatal ultrasound findings include bilateral hydroureteronephrosis, a distended bladder, and an irregular abdominal wall circumference.[60] These findings are not specific for PBS, but should be included in the differential diagnosis. The classic findings are typically seen early in the third trimester, but there have been reports of diagnosis as early as 11 weeks.[61,62]

In utero intervention has been proposed in patients with severe lower urinary tract obstruction meeting certain criteria, including favorable urine biochemistries. One review identified the amniotic fluid volume and renal parenchymal appearance to be the most specific in defining prognosis for early intervention.[63] More recently, perinatal survival in 300 fetuses was improved by prenatal bladder drainage in patients with severe bladder

| BOX 61-1 | Classification System for Prune-Belly Syndrome |

CATEGORY 1

Pulmonary hypoplasia and/or pneumothorax
Oligohydramnios
Renal dysplasia
Urethral atresia
Clubfeet

CATEGORY 2

Typical physical features
Renal dysplasia common but less severe than category 1
No pulmonary hypoplasia
Can progress to renal failure

CATEGORY 3

Incomplete or mild physical features
No renal dysplasia
No pulmonary dysplasia
Stable renal function

obstruction.[64] However, even with bladder drainage, there was no guarantee of good postnatal renal function. Fetal interventions, listed in order of increasing complexity, include vesicocentesis, vesico-amniotic shunting, and fetal cystoscopy.[65] Each therapeutic option has risks to both the fetus and mother. One case study reported the viable birth of a child with unfavorable prognostic findings after 32 vesicocenteses and amnioinfusion procedures.[66] Currently, it is the rare patient with PBS who would be considered a candidate for antenatal therapy as most of these pregnancies are carried to term.[67]

Neonatal Presentation

The classical appearance of a wrinkled abdominal wall in a newborn usually suggests the diagnosis. If one also has nonpalpable testes, the triad is nearly complete. If significant oligohydramnios is present, then limb abnormalities and pulmonary/chest anomalies may also be found.

The initial management entails a rapid and complete evaluation of all organ systems. A three-category classification system has been described by Woodward to aid clinicians in regards to the prognosis of children with PBS (Box 61-1).

The pulmonary and cardiac systems, if involved, are the first concern in these children. Initial urologic care includes a physical exam paying particular attention to the abdomen and assessing for kidney and bladder enlargement. Urethral atresia needs to be excluded as prompt intervention is required for bladder obstruction. Initial assessment of renal function is important, but early postnatal creatinine levels are most reflective of the mother. Therefore, electrolyte and creatinine trends are more predictive of long-term function. A nadir creatinine of >0.7 mg/dL in a term infant is a poor prognostic sign noted by several groups.[68,69]

Once stable, renal and bladder ultrasound is recommended to assess the renal parenchyma and degree of upper and lower tract dilation. Voiding cystourethrography is performed to assess bladder emptying, the bladder outlet, and VUR. Nuclear renography is typically performed at 4–6 weeks of age to assess renal function and obstruction.

MANAGEMENT

Controversy exists regarding the optimal treatment for the PBS patient. It is important that the pulmonary function is stable prior to operative intervention. Aggressive management of the urinary tract abnormalities has been advocated by some and historically was performed in the neonatal period. This approach usually entails ureteral tailoring and reimplantation with reduction cystoplasty in hopes of eliminating obstruction and correcting VUR.

A more conservative approach with close surveillance and aggressive medical management means surgical intervention is only needed in those patients with recurrent or persistent infections, or proven obstruction. Some studies have shown that patients can be maintained free of urinary tract infection (UTI), without worsening of their bladder dynamics and renal function, using this approach.[70,71] The argument for a more minimalistic approach is based on the fact that surgery has not been shown to slow progression of renal dysfunction, particularly in children with severe renal dysplasia.

The goal of both approaches is to keep the child free of UTI. Acquired renal scarring secondary to pyelonephritis is a common problem in children with PBS.[28] Antibiotic prophylaxis is recommended in all neonates, regardless of VUR status. Particular attention to urinary stasis, either at the bladder level or more proximally, is important.

SURGICAL MANAGEMENT

The operative management of the PBS patient focuses on three systems: the genitourinary system, the UDT, and the abdominal wall.

Genitourinary System

Urinary diversion may be a necessary temporary procedure in the setting of bladder outlet obstruction. The Blocksom technique (as modified by Duckett) is the preferred approach with special attention to creating a capacious stoma.[72] If a large diverticulum is encountered during creation of the vesicostomy, it should be excised.

Rarely, either upper or lower ureteral obstruction or stasis may necessitate more proximal diversion. A cutaneous pyelostomy is preferred as it provides the best form of upper tract drainage. Percutaneous nephrostomy tubes can be inserted for temporary drainage.

An internal urethrotomy may be needed in the older child with increased bladder outlet resistance clinically manifesting as poor bladder emptying and a large postvoid residual. An improvement in urinary flow rates and the overall radiographic appearance, along with lower postvoid residual urine, have been found following urethrotomy.[70]

Megalourethra is best treated with penile degloving, excision of the redundant urethra, and urethral tailoring and reconstruction. Urethral atresia requires immediate management in the neonatal period with a temporary cutaneous vesicostomy. Achieving a functional urethra usually requires a formal urethroplasty involving complex skin flaps and/or grafts. Progressive dilation of the hypoplastic urethra has been reported as an alternative approach.[73]

Poor bladder contractility and incomplete emptying is common. A spectrum of approaches can be tried to reduce the bladder size and create a more normal, spherical-shaped bladder including excision of the urachal diverticulum, complex reconstructive operations involving detrusor plication, or the creation of overlapping bladder flaps.[74,75] While early postoperative results seemed to be encouraging, long-term results have noted recurrence of a large bladder capacity and poor emptying.[74] Currently reduction cystoplasty is performed at the time of ureteral reconstruction and is rarely performed as a primary procedure. Options to improve bladder emptying include clean intermittent catheterization via the urethra or a continent catheterizable channel.

Ureteral tailoring and reimplantation are usually undertaken in those children with recurrent UTI. Routine and early postnatal ureteral reconstruction has generally been abandoned. The severity of VUR and ureteral distension are not indicators for reconstruction. Meticulous ureteral dissection is required and typically the distal, redundant, and ectatic ureter is discarded. Reimplantation into a large, floppy bladder can be challenging and fixation with a psoas hitch may be required to prevent angulation of the ureter.

Orchiopexy

The timing of orchiopexy is dependent on the child's overall health and the need for transscrotal positioning of the UDT at a young age. In the healthy child, bilateral orchiopexy is typically performed via a transabdominal approach around 6 months of age. Those infants requiring other procedures earlier in life can have the orchiopexies performed at the same time. The flaccid abdomen allows for excellent exposure and ligation of the internal spermatic vessels is usually not required for children less than two years of age.[76] In older children or those with high intra-abdominal testes, a primary or staged Fowler–Stephens approach may be needed. With the recent advancements in laparoscopy, this approach is promising, particularly in older children and those not requiring other concomitant surgery.[77,78] Reports of laparoscopic orchidopexy in PBS patients highlight technical considerations due to the floppy nature of the abdominal wall, including the use of smaller incisions, suture fixation of ports, and higher gas flow rates.[79,80]

Abdominoplasty

The management of the abdominal wall in children with PBS is determined by the severity of the condition. In children with very mild degrees of deformity, observation is usually preferred with some children having spontaneous improvement in their appearance. In those with more significant degrees of abdominal wall laxity, abdominoplasty is usually recommended as the cosmetic and psychological benefit is believed to outweigh the risks of the operation. Pulmonary, bladder, and bowel function following abdominoplasty may be improved, but is not well substantiated.[56,81] The timing of the abdominoplasty is dictated by the child's general health and need for future reconstructive operations. Children as young as 6 months have undergone abdominal wall reconstruction at the same setting as orchiopexy or bladder reconstruction.

Several methods and modifications have been described for abdominal wall reconstruction. Popular techniques include those described by Monfort[82] or Ehrlich.[83] The Ehrlich technique utilizes a transabdominal approach through a vertical midline incision with preservation of the umbilicus on a vascular pedicle via the inferior epigastric artery.[84] The skin and subcutaneous tissues are then elevated off the underlying fascia and muscle, with a pants over vest buttressing of the more normal lateral fascia and abdominal muscle. The excess abdominal skin is then removed and reapproximated longitudinally in the midline (Fig. 61-6).

Monfort's technique also employs a vertical incision. However, his modification uses an elliptically oriented incision as a means of excising the redundant skin. The incision usually extends from the tip of the xyphoid down to the pubis. A second elliptical incision is then made around the umbilicus for its preservation. Similar to the Ehrlich technique, the skin is dissected off the fascia and muscle laterally, at least to the anterior axillary line. However, the Monfort procedure includes the use of vertical relaxing fascial incisions lateral to the superior epigastric arteries, allowing mobilization of the lateral fascial flaps over a central fascial bridge. Durable functional results have been reported with this approach as well (Fig. 61-7).[82,85]

Others have described alternative techniques for abdominal wall reconstruction which include extraperitoneal dissection, fascial folding, or laparoscopic-assisted approaches.[86–88] Ehrlich et al. recently reported their long-term results with a mean follow-up of 20.4 years and found no major complications and satisfaction with the cosmetic appearance.[89]

Renal Transplant

Close follow-up and monitoring of renal function is essential in patients with PBS. Approximately 30% of patients presenting with renal insufficiency will develop chronic renal failure during childhood or in their adolescent years.[90,91] The timing of lower urinary tract reconstruction and renal transplantation has been debated. Some advocate urinary reconstruction prior to renal transplantation so that the immunosuppressive therapy does not impair healing.[92]

CONCLUSIONS

The outlook for children born with PBS has improved dramatically over the last several decades due to the advances in antenatal and neonatal care. A better understanding of the disease has led to improved medical management with appropriate and, often limited, surgical intervention.

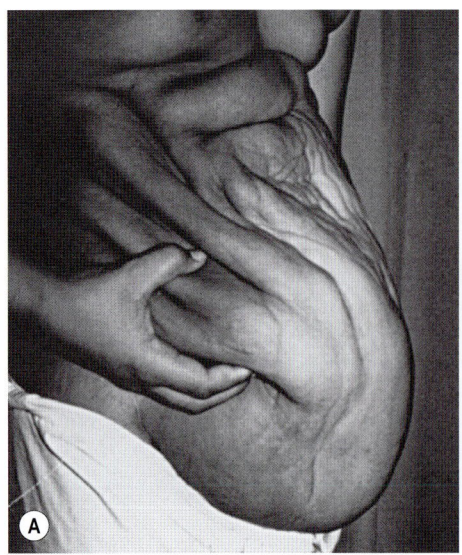
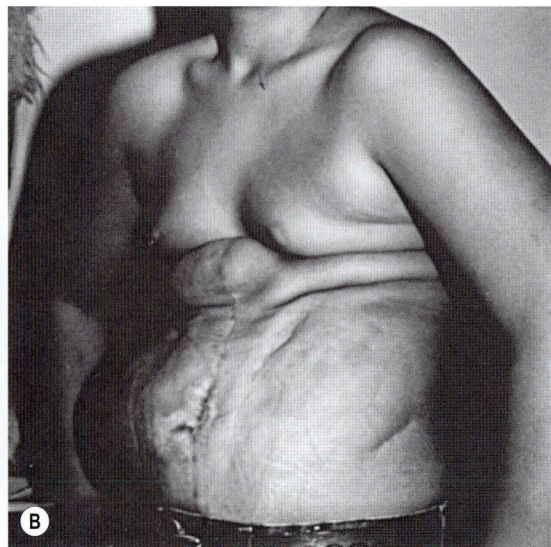

FIGURE 61-6 ■ The Ehrlich technique was used in this patient. **(A)** The preoperative appearance of the abdominal wall; **(B)** the postoperative view.

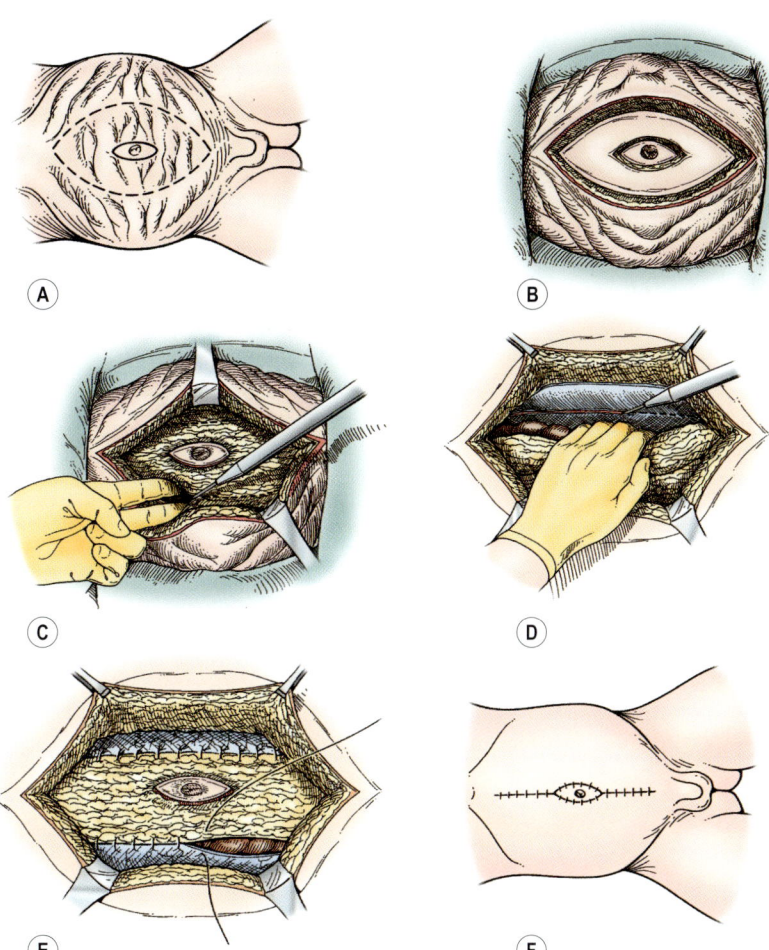

FIGURE 61-7 ■ The Monfort abdominoplasty is depicted. **(A)** Skin incisions circumscribe the umbilicus and define areas of adjacent abdominal wall redundancy to be removed. **(B)** Excision of skin (epidermis and dermis alone) by using electrocautery. **(C)** Abdominal wall central plate is incised at the lateral borders of the rectus muscle on either side, creating a central musculofascial plate. **(D)** The parietal peritoneum overlying the lateral abdominal wall musculature is scored with electrocautery. **(E)** Edges of the central plate are sutured along the scored line. **(F)** Excess skin is removed, and the midline approximation envelops the previously isolated umbilicus.

REFERENCES

1. Frohlich F. Der Mangel der Muskein, insbesondere der Seiten-bauchmuskein. Wurzburg: CA Surn; 1839.
2. Parker R. Absence of abdominal muscles in an infant. Lancet 1894;1:1252.
3. Osler W. Congenital absence of the abdominal muscles with distended and hypertrophied urinary bladder. Bull Johns Hopkins Hosp 1901;12:331.
4. Eagle J, Barrett G. Congenital deficiency of abdominal musculature with associated genitourinary abnormalities: A syndrome: Report of nine cases. Pediatrics 1950;6:721–36.
5. Williams DI, Burkholder GV. The prune-belly syndrome. J Urol 1967;98:244–51.
6. Welch KJ, Kraney GP. Abdominal musculature deficiency syndrome prune-belly. J Urol 1974;111:693–700.
7. Nunn IN, Stephens FD. The triad syndrome: A composite anomaly of the abdominal wall, urinary system and testes. J Urol 1961; 86:782–94.
8. Routh JC, Huang L, Retik AB, et al. Contemporary epidemiology and characterization of newborn males with prune-belly syndrome. Urology 2010;76:44.
9. Austin JC, Canning DA, Johnson MP, et al. Vesicoamniotic shunt in a female fetus with the prune-belly syndrome. J Urol 2001; 166:2382.
10. Reinberg Y, Shapiro E, Manivel JC, et al. Prune-belly syndrome in females: A triad of abdominal musculature deficiency and anomalies of the urinary and genital systems. J Pediatr 1991;118:395–8.
11. Murray PJ, Thomas K, Mulgrew CJ, et al. Whole gene deletion of the hepatocyte nuclear factor-1b gene in a patient with the prune-belly syndrome. Nephrol Dial Transplant 2008;23:2414–15.
12. Haeri S, Devers PL, Kaiser-Rogers KA, et al. Deletion of hepatocyte nuclear factor-1-beta in an infant with prune-belly syndrome. Am J Perinatol 2010;2 7:559–63.
13. Granberg CF, Harrison SM, Dajusta D, et al. Genetic basis of prune-belly syndrome: Screening for HNF1β gene. J Urol 2012;187:272–8.
14. Weber S, Mir S, Schlingmann KP, et al. Gene locus ambiguity in posterior urethral valves/prune-belly syndrome. Pediatr Nephrol 2005;20:1036–42.
15. Lubinsky M, Koyle K, Trunca C. The association of 'prune-belly' with Turner's syndrome. Am J Dis Child 1980;134:1171–2.
16. Beckmann H, Rehder H, Rauskolb R. Prune-belly sequence associated with trisomy 13. Am J Med Genet 1984;19:603–4.
17. Frydman M, Magenis RE, Mohandas TK, et al. Chromosome abnormalities in infants with prune-belly anomaly: Association with trisomy 18. Am J Med Genet 1983;15:145–8.
18. Kupferman JC, Druschel CM, Kupchik GS. Increased prevalence of renal and urinary tract anomalies in children with Down syndrome. Pediatrics 2009;124:e615–21.
19. Popek EJ, Tyson RW, Miller GJ, et al. Prostate development in prune-belly syndrome (PBS) and posterior urethral valves (PUV): Etiology of PBS–lower urinary tract obstruction or primary mesenchymal defect? Pediatr Pathol 1991;11:1–29.
20. Pagon RA, Smith DW, Shepard TH. Urethral obstruction malformation complex: A cause of abdominal muscle deficiency and the 'prune-belly'. J Pediatr 1979;94:900–6.
21. Moerman P, Fryns JP, Goddeeris P, et al. Pathogenesis of the prune-belly syndrome: A functional urethral obstruction caused by prostatic hypoplasia. Pediatrics 1984;73:470–5.
22. Straub E, Spranger J. Etiology and pathogenesis of the prune-belly syndrome. Kidney Int 1981;20:695–9.

23. Stephens FD, Gupta D. Pathogenesis of the prune-belly syndrome. J Urol 1994;152:2328–31.

24. Workman SJ, Kogan BA. Fetal bladder histology in posterior urethral valves and the prune-belly syndrome. J Urol 1990;144:337–9.

25. Kinahan TJ, Churchill BM, McLorie GA, et al. The efficiency of bladder emptying in the prune-belly syndrome. J Urol 1992;148:600–3.

26. Ehrlich RM, Brown WJ. Ultrastructural anatomic observations of the ureter in the prune-belly syndrome. Birth Defects Orig Artic Ser 1977;13:101–3.

27. Gearhart JP, Lee BR, Partin AW, et al. A quantitative histological evaluation of the dilated ureter of childhood. II: Ectopia, posterior urethral valves and the prune-belly syndrome. J Urol 1995;153:172–6.

28. Woodard JR, Zucker I. Current management of the dilated urinary tract in prune-belly syndrome. Urol Clin North Am 1990;17:407–18.

29. Berdon WE, Baker DH, Wigger HJ, et al. The radiologic and pathologic spectrum of the prune-belly syndrome. The importance of urethral obstruction in prognosis. Radiol Clin North Am 1977;15:83–92.

30. Manivel JC, Pettinato G, Reinbert Y, et al. Prune-belly syndrome: Clinicopathologic study of 29 cases. Pediatr Pathol 1989;9:691–711.

31. Schwarz RD, Stephens FD, Cussen LJ. The pathogenesis of renal dysplasia. I. Quantification of hypoplasia and dysplasia. Invest Urol 1981;19:94–6.

32. Woodard JR, Parrott TS. Reconstruction of the urinary tract in prune-belly uropathy. J Urol 1978;119:824–8.

33. Hoagland MH, Hutchins GM. Obstructive lesions of the lower urinary tract in the prune-belly syndrome. Arch Pathol Lab Med 1987;111:154–6.

34. Volmar KE, Fritsch MK, Perlman EJ, et al. Patterns of congenital lower urinary tract obstructive uropathy: Relation to abnormal prostate and bladder development and the prune-belly syndrome. Pediatr Dev Pathol 2001;4:467–72.

35. Nouaili EB, Chaouachi S, Nouira F, et al. Concordant posterior urethral valves in male monochorionic twins with secondary prune-belly syndrome. Tunis Med 2008;86:1086–8.

36. Weber S, Mir S, Schlingmann KP, et al. Gene locus ambiguity in posterior urethral valves/prune-belly syndrome. Pediatr Nephrol 2005;20:1036–42.

37. Deklerk DP, Scott WW. Prostatic maldevelopment in the prune-belly syndrome: A defect in prostatic stromal-epithelial interaction. J Urol 1978;120:341–4.

38. Woodhouse CR, Snyder HM 3rd. Testicular and sexual function in adults with prune-belly syndrome. J Urol 1985;133:607–9.

39. Reinberg Y, Chelimsky G, Gonzalez R. Urethral atresia and the prune-belly syndrome. Report of 6 cases. Br J Urol 1993;72:112–14.

40. Shrom SH, Cromie WJ, Duckett JW Jr. Megalourethra. Urology 1981;17:152–6.

41. Mortensen PH, Johnson HW, Coleman GU, et al. Megalourethra. J Urol 1985;134:358–61.

42. Orvis BR, Bottles K, Kogan BA. Testicular histology in fetuses with the prune-belly syndrome and posterior urethral valves. J Urol 1988;139:335–7.

43. Kolettis PN, Ross JH, Kay R, et al. Sperm retrieval and intracytoplasmic sperm injection in patients with prune-belly syndrome. Fertil Steril 1999;72:948–9.

44. Mininberg DT, Montoya F, Okada K, et al. Subcellular muscle studies in the prune-belly syndrome. J Urol 1973;109:524–6.

45. Afifi AK, Rebeiz J, Mire J, et al. The myopathology of the Prune-belly syndrome. J Neurol Sci 1972;15:153–65.

46. Adebonojo FO. Dysplasia of the anterior abdominal musculature with multiple congenital anomalies. Prune-belly or triad syndrome. J Natl Med Assoc 1973;65:327–33.

47. Yoshida M, Matsumura M, Shintaku Y, et al. Prenatally diagnosed female prune-belly syndrome associated with tetralogy of Fallot. Gynecol Obstet Invest 1995;39:141–4.

48. Geary DJ, MacLusky IB, Churchill BM. A broader spectrum of abnormalities in the prune-belly syndrome. J Urol 1986;135:324–6.

49. Crompton CH, MacLusky IB, Geary DF. Respiratory function in the prune-belly syndrome. Arch Dis Child 1993;68:505–6.

50. Wright JR Jr, Barth RF, Neff JC, et al. Gastrointestinal malformations associated with prune-belly syndrome: Three cases and a review of the literature. Pediatr Pathol 1986;5:421–48.

51. Morgan CL Jr, Grossman H, Novak R. Imperforate anus and colon calcification in association with the prune-belly syndrome. Pediatr Radiol 1978;7:19–21.

52. Mahajan JK, Ojha S, Rao KL. Prune-belly syndrome with anorectal malformation. Eur J Pediatr Surg 2004;14:351–4.

53. Giuliani S, Vendryes C, Malhotra A, et al. Prune-belly syndrome associated with cloacal anomaly, patent urachal remnant, and omphalocele in a female infant. J Pediatr Surg 2010;45:e39–42.

54. Oliveira G, Boechat MI, Ferreira MA. Megacystis-microcolon-intestinal hypoperistalsis syndrome in a newborn girl whose brother had prune-belly syndrome: Common pathogenesis? Pediatr Radiol 1983;13:294–6.

55. Levin TL, Soghier L, Blitman NM, et al. Megacystis-microcolon-intestinal hypoperistalsis and prune-belly: Overlapping syndromes. Pediatr Radiol 2004;34:995–8.

56. Woodard JR. Lessons learned in 3 decades of managing the prune-belly syndrome. J Urol 1998;159:1680.

57. Brinker MR, Palutsis RS, Sarwark JF. The orthopaedic manifestations of prune-belly (Eagle-Barrett) syndrome. J Bone Joint Surg Am 1995;77:251–7.

58. Loder RT, Guiboux JP, Bloom DA, et al. Musculoskeletal aspects of prune-belly syndrome. Description and pathogenesis. Am J Dis Child 1992;146:1224–9.

59. Green NE, Lowery ER, Thomas R. Orthopaedic aspects of prune-belly syndrome. J Pediatr Orthop 1993;13:496–501.

60. Shih WJ, Greenbaum LD, Baro C. In utero sonogram in prune-belly syndrome. Urology 1982;20:102–5.

61. Yamamoto H, Nishikawa S, Hayashi T, et al. Antenatal diagnosis of prune-belly syndrome at 11 weeks of gestation. J Obstet Gynaecol Res 2001;27:37–40.

62. Shimizu T, Ihara Y, Yomura W, et al. Antenatal diagnosis of prune-belly syndrome. Arch Gynecol Obstet 1992;251:211–14.

63. Morris RK, Malin GL, Khan KS, et al. Antenatal ultrasound to predict postnatal renal function in congenital lower urinary tract obstruction: Systematic review of test accuracy. BJOG 2009;116:1290–9.

64. Morris RK, Malin GL, Khan KS, et al. Systematic review of the effectiveness of antenatal intervention for the treatment of congenital lower urinary tract obstruction. BJOG 2010;117:382–90.

65. Ruano R. Fetal surgery for severe lower urinary tract obstruction. Prenat Diagn 2011;31:667–74.

66. Galati V, Beeson JH, Confer SD, et al. A favorable outcome following 32 vesicocentesis and amnioinfusion procedures in a fetus with severe prune-belly syndrome. J Pediatr Urol 2008;4:170–2.

67. Freedman AL, Bukowski TP, Smith CA, et al. Fetal therapy for obstructive uropathy: Diagnosis specific outcomes. J Urol 1996;156:20–723.

68. Noh PH, Cooper CS, Winkler AC, et al. Prognostic factors for long-term renal function in boys with the prune-belly syndrome. J Urol 1999;162:1399–401.

69. Reinberg Y, Manivel JC, Pettinato G, et al. Development of renal failure in children with the prune-belly syndrome. J Urol 1991;145:1017–19.

70. Woodhouse CR, Kellett MJ, Williams DI. Minimal surgical interference in the prune-belly syndrome. Br J Urol 1979;51:475–80.

71. Texter JH Jr, Koontz WW Jr. Dilation of the urethra in males. J Fam Pract 1980;11:111–17.

72. Duckett JW Jr. Cutaneous vesicostomy in childhood. The Blocksom technique. Urol Clin North Am 1974;1:485–95.

73. Passerini-Glazel G, Araguna F, Chiozza L, et al. The P.A.D.U.A. (progressive augmentation by dilating the urethra anterior) procedure for the treatment of severe urethral hypoplasia. J Urol 1988;140:1247–9.

74. Bukowski TP, Perlmutter AD. Reduction cystoplasty in the prune-belly syndrome: A long-term followup. J Urol 1994;152:2113–16.

75. Perlmutter AD. Reduction cystoplasty in prune-belly syndrome. J Urol 1976;116:356–62.

76. Fallat ME, Skoog SJ, Belman AB, et al. The prune-belly syndrome: A comprehensive approach to management. J Urol 1989;142:802–5.

77. Docimo SG, Moore RG, Adams J, et al. Laparoscopic orchiopexy for the high palpable undescended testis: Preliminary experience. J Urol 1995;154:1513–15.

78. Patil KK, Duffy PG, Woodhouse CR, et al. Long-term outcome of Fowler-Stephens orchiopexy in boys with prune-belly syndrome. J Urol 2004;171:1666–9.

79. Philip J, Mullassery D, Craigie RJ, et al. Laparoscopic orchidopexy in boys with prune-belly syndrome—outcome and technical considerations. J Endourol 2011;25:1115–17.

80. Saxena AK, Brinkmann OA. Unique features of prune-belly syndrome in laparoscopic surgery. J Am Coll Surg 2007;205:217–21.

81. Smith CA, Smith EA, Parrott TS, et al. Voiding function in patients with the prune-belly syndrome after Monfort abdominoplasty. J Urol 1998;159:1675–9.

82. Monfort G, Guys JM, Bocciardi A, et al. A novel technique for reconstruction of the abdominal wall in the prune-belly syndrome. J Urol 1991;146:639–40.

83. Ehrlich RM, Lesavoy MA, Fine RN. Total abdominal wall reconstruction in the prune-belly syndrome. J Urol 1986;136:282–5.

84. Ehrlich RM, Lesavoy MA. Umbilicus preservation with total abdominal wall reconstruction in prune-belly syndrome. Urology 1993;41:231–2.

85. Parrott TS, Woodard JR. The Monfort operation for abdominal wall reconstruction in the prune-belly syndrome. J Urol 1992;148:688–90.

86. Furness PD 3rd, Cheng EY, Franco I, et al. The prune-belly syndrome: A new and simplified technique of abdominal wall reconstruction. J Urol 1998;160:1195–7.

87. Franco I. Laparoscopic assisted modification of the firlit abdominal wall plication. J Urol 2005;174:280–3.

88. Levine E, Taub PJ, Franco I. Laparoscopic assisted abdominal wall reconstruction in prune-belly syndrome. Ann Plast Surg 2007; 58:162–5.

89. Lesavoy MA, Chang EI, Suliman A, et al. Long-term follow-up of total abdominal wall reconstruction for prune-belly syndrome. Plast Reconstr Surg 2012;129:104e–109e.

90. Fontaine E, Salomon L, Gagnadoux MF, et al. Long-term results of renal transplantation in children with the prune-belly syndrome. J Urol 1997;158:892–4.

91. Reinberg Y, Manivel JC, Fryd D, et al. The outcome of renal transplantation in children with the prune-belly syndrome. J Urol 1989;142:1541–2.

92. Djakovic N, Wagener N, Adams J, et al. Intestinal reconstruction of the lower urinary tract as a prerequisite for renal transplantation. BJU Int 2009;103:1555–60.

CHAPTER 62

DISORDERS OF SEXUAL DIFFERENTIATION

John M. Gatti

Disorders of sexual differentiation (DSD) are among the most fascinating conditions confronting the pediatric urologist and surgeon. Our understanding of these conditions and their causes continues to evolve, but gender assignment and the timing of reconstruction remain controversial.

NORMAL GENDER AND SEXUAL DIFFERENTIATION

The most commonly accepted paradigm, described by Jost, involves a stepwise process to gender and sexual development.[1] The primary determinant is the chromosomal gender, which is established at fertilization when the sperm provides an X or Y chromosome to the ovum's X chromosome. Chromosomal gender determines gonadal gender, with XX resulting in ovarian development and XY resulting in testicular formation. Finally, the gonadal function determines the phenotypic gender. Although this paradigm is a helpful cascade to explain gender development, the simple Y = male, no Y = female equations are not always valid.

The testis determining factor (TDF) is located on the short arm of the Y chromosome near the centromere at the distal aspect of the Y-unique region.[2] TDF is a 35 kb pair sequence on the 11.3 sub-band of the gender-determining region of the Y chromosome (SRY). Interestingly, SRY appears to be expressed by the somatic cells from the urogenital ridge and not from germ cells.

Many other genes play a role in gender development. Despite the presence of a functional SRY gene, the absence of the SOX9 gene results in a female phenotype in the majority of chromosomal males.[3,4] The Wilms tumor gene (WT1) appears to play a key role not only in renal development, but also in testicular development. Early alteration of WT1 function results in testicular agenesis and later dysfunction results in aberrant testicular development (streak gonad or dysgerminomas). This tumor suppressor gene has been implicated in Denys–Drash syndrome involving testicular (mixed gonadal dysgenesis) and renal (Wilms tumor) abnormalities.[5,6]

Fushi–Tarzu factor-1 (FTZ-F1) exerts its effect on gonadal development through its regulation of steroidogenic factor-1 (SF-1). The SF1 gene is involved with steroid hormone production and the production of Müllerian-inhibiting substance (MIS) by the Sertoli cells of the testis that causes regression of the Müllerian ductal system. Although FTZ-F1 and SF-1 are also expressed in ovarian tissues, the timing and intensity of their effect are critical for normal gonadal development.[5,7]

Finally, the lack of an SRY gene alone does not impart normal female phenotypic and gonadal development. The DAX1 gene appears to be essential for the development of the ovary. The DAX1 gene product appears to compete with the SRY gene product for a steroidogenic regulatory protein (StAR). A dosage-sensitive element is also important. Normally, the single SRY gene has a greater impact than a single DAX1 gene and causes upregulation of StAR. However, in those chromosomal abnormalities in which more than one DAX1 gene is present, downregulation of StAR occurs, testicular development is inhibited, and ovarian development is promoted. As in the case of Turner syndrome, these primordial ovaries develop into streak gonads. Likely, other genes are also important for normal ovarian development.[8–10]

Development of the internal ductal structures is dependent on hormone secretion by the developing gonads (Table 62-1). In the absence of functioning testicular tissue, the female internal Müllerian duct structures develop. The presence of a functioning testis results in male internal Wolffian duct development. This differentiation is mediated by the production of testosterone from the testis. Testosterone promotes Wolffian duct development along with MIS, which results in regression of the Müllerian duct structures. This is a paracrine effect and therefore results in gonad specific ipsilateral ductal differentiation. This effect is likely dependent on high concentrations of androgen produced by the physically proximate gonad. Decreased levels of MIS by an abnormal testis or streak gonad result in ipsilateral Müllerian development. This occurs despite regression of the Müllerian ducts on the contralateral side with normal testicular MIS production. Conversely, systemic administration of androgen does not result in male ductal development in a female fetus.

Produced by Sertoli cells, MIS functions as a suppressor of Müllerian duct development and is a specific marker for functioning testicular tissue in infancy. In its absence, the Müllerian structures develop. The concentration and timing of MIS secretion appear to be critical. Normally, secretion occurs during week 7 of gestation. By week 9, the Müllerian ducts become insensitive to MIS.[9]

External genital development follows a similar path (Fig. 62-1). In the absence of the testosterone metabolite dihydrotestosterone (DHT), the external genitalia

TABLE 62-1	Derivation of the Urogenital System		
Wolffian Duct (Mesonephric Duct)	**Urogenital Sinus**	**Müllerian Duct (Paramesonephric Duct)**	
Male			
Epididymis	Bladder	Appendix testis	
Vas deferens	Prostate	Prostatic utricle	
Seminal vesicles			
Female			
Epoöphoron	Bladder	Vagina (upper third)	
Gartner's ducts	Distal vagina	Uterus	
		Fallopian tubes	

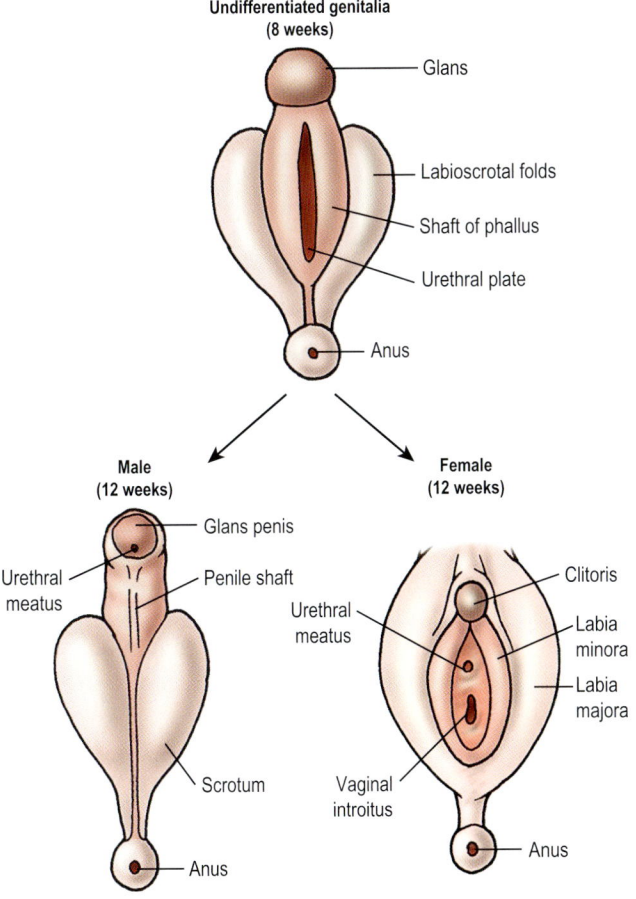

FIGURE 62-1 ■ Differentiation of the external genitalia.

develop into the female phenotype. The male and female phenotypes are identical until week 7. In the male, testosterone production by the testicular Leydig cells surges at 7 weeks and remains elevated until week 14 of gestation. Testosterone is converted to DHT by 5α-reductase in the tissues of the genital skin and urogenital sinus. The testosterone-binding receptor has much higher affinity for DHT than testosterone and serves to amplify the effect of testosterone on the developing external genitalia. In the absence of 5α-reductase, the internal Wolffian ducts are preserved, but the external structures are feminized.

After birth, neonatal testosterone levels in a male surge in response to the loss of feedback inhibition by maternal estrogens and the subsequent rise in neonatal luteinizing hormone (LH). Testosterone levels peak around the second to third month of life. By 6 months, levels remain identical in males and females until puberty. Androgen imprinting may occur on susceptible tissues, including genital organs and sensitive tissues in the brain related to male-type behaviors and gender orientation. This early exposure may determine how these tissues respond to subsequent androgen exposure during puberty and adulthood.

ABERRANT GENDER DEVELOPMENT

Incidence

In the Americas and Western Europe, congenital adrenal hyperplasia (CAH) is the most common cause of neonatal ambiguous genitalia, accounting for approximately 70% of cases.[11,12] The overall incidence is approximately 1 in 15,000 live births. The rate is much higher in stillborns and in certain regional populations (Yupic Eskimos and the people of La Réunion, France).[13] In the United States, mixed gonadal dysgenesis is the next most common intersex disorder, with ovotesticular DSD (true hermaphroditism) being the third most common.

Classification

Until recently, the most commonly used classification system was the one proposed by Allen in 1976 and was based primarily on gonadal histology.[14] This system categorized the most common DSD well, but did not accommodate less common syndromes easily. Also, the older 'hermaphrodite' terminology has become offensive to some. A newer classification released by the International Consensus Conference on Intersex has largely replaced Allen's system. This newer system incorporates an evolving understanding of the molecular basis of these disorders and replaces more offensive gender-based labels. The new terminology is used primarily in this text.[15]

46,XX DSD (Female Pseudohermaphrodite)

The majority of neonates with external genital ambiguity fall into this category. All patients have a 46,XX genotype and exclusively ovarian tissue in nonpalpable gonads. Simplistically, the cause of the gender ambiguity is an excess of androgen. More than 95% are due to CAH, with the remainder due to maternal androgen exposure. These patients have a normal female Müllerian ductal system with an upper vagina, uterus, and fallopian tubes (see Table 62-1). They also have normal regression of the Wolffian ducts. The level of virilization is largely dependent on the timing and magnitude of androgen exposure to the external genitalia. The phenotype can range from mild clitoromegaly to a normal male appearance.

Virilization in CAH is due to the inability of the adrenal gland to form cortisol. The precursors above the enzymatic defect are shunted into the mineralocorticoid or sex-steroid pathways. Also, the end products generally have some, albeit weak, glucocorticoid function. The lack of cortisol for negative feedback inhibition of adrenocorticotropic hormone (ACTH) production by the pituitary leaves this pathway unchecked. Excess androgen is produced and is responsible for the virilization. The corticosteroid synthetic and alternative pathways are shown in Figure 62-2. The most common form of CAH is 21-hydroxylase deficiency (21-OHD), which accounts for more than 90% of CAH.[16] 21-OHD has been mapped to the short arm of chromosome 6. The variable location of the adrenal defect and relative function of the gene results in salt-wasting and nonsalt-wasting forms.[17-19] Type 1 results in virilization but no salt wasting. The gene defect affects only the fasciculata zone of the adrenal, resulting in blocking cortisol production. However, the gene is normally expressed in the glomerulosa zone with preservation of mineralocorticoid production. In type 2, also called the classic type, the gene abnormality affects both adrenal zones. Salt wasting results in dehydration or vascular collapse, and hyperkalemia develops because of the block in mineralocorticoid production.

11β-Hydroxylase deficiency (type 3) is a less common cause of CAH. This gene has been mapped to the long arm of chromosome 8. This abnormality results in virilization associated with hypertension due to the synthetic block being below deoxycorticosterone (DOC). DOC has potent mineralocorticoid function resulting in sodium resorption, fluid overload, hypertension, and hypokalemic acidosis.

Finally, 3β-hydroxylase deficiency (type 4) is a rare form of CAH. It results in severe salt wasting, and survival is unusual. It is the only type of CAH to occur in both genders.

Virilization of the female fetus can be caused by exogenous androgen exposure from the mother. This occurs primarily with the use of progesterone, commonly used as an adjunct to assist with fertility and in-vitro fertilization. Endogenous androgen exposure due to virilizing maternal ovarian tumors also has been reported, but these tumors are usually virilizing to the mother with the fetus being unaffected.[20]

Diagnosis

The diagnosis of CAH is based on the previously described clinical and electrolyte abnormalities in addition to elevated 17-hydroxyprogesterone levels. DOC and deoxycortisol levels also aid in determining which enzymatic defect is present. The physical examination is notable for the absence of palpable gonads, the presence of a cervix on rectal examination, and bronzing of the skin. Palpation of a gonad virtually excludes the diagnosis of 46,XX DSD. The genitogram and an ultrasound (US) study mirror these findings, revealing Müllerian structures with a variable-length urogenital sinus.

Treatment

As all forms of CAH are inherited in an autosomal recessive manner, genetic counseling is recommended. Families with a history of CAH should consider maternal treatment with dexamethasone before week 10 of gestation to eliminate or improve the level of fetal virilization.[21] Postnatally, cortisol replacement with hydrocortisone is the mainstay of therapy, with the addition of fluorohydrocortisone if salt wasting is present. Supportive management of fluid and electrolyte abnormalities is best provided in a neonatal intensive care unit.

With regard to gender identity, the vast majority of patients with CAH identify as female and gender assignment is generally female given the 46,XX karyotype. The ovaries are normal and have fertility potential.[22] Surgical reconstruction requires a feminizing genitoplasty, and involves clitoroplasty, monsplasty, and vaginoplasty.

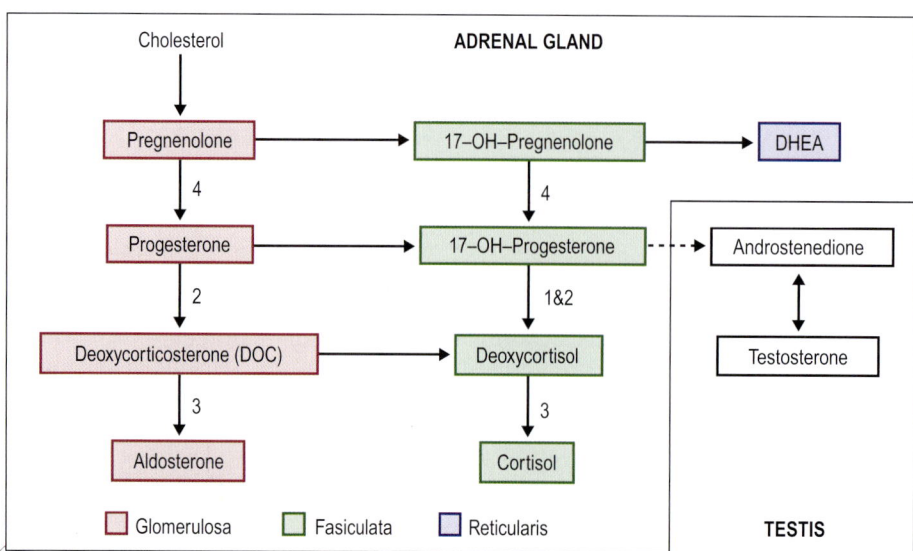

FIGURE 62-2 ■ Pathways of steroid biosynthesis. The numbers correspond to CAH type and the location of the enzyme defect (see the text).

46,XY DSD (Male Pseudohermaphrodite)

This group is the most heterogeneous in the new classification system. All patients have a 46,XY genotype and testicular tissue only. The gonads are sometimes palpable. The condition can be simplistically thought of as a deficit of either production or reception of androgen.

The androgen deficit may result from a defect in synthesis. Several rare adrenal enzyme deficiencies have been implicated, including 3β-hydroxylase, 17α-hydroxylase, and 20,22-desmolase. All are involved in the steps from cholesterol to androstenedione and testosterone, and are associated with severe CAH and often death. 3β-Hydroxylase and 20,22-desmolase deficiencies are associated with cortisol and aldosterone deficits with hyponatremia, hyperkalemia, and metabolic acidosis. In 17α-hydroxylase deficiency, mineralocorticoid production is preserved, resulting in excess salt and water retention, hypertension, and hypokalemia. In the male, the phenotype is variable, ranging from the appearance of a proximal hypospadias with cryptorchidism to that of a phenotypic female with a blind-ending vagina.

Defects in 17,20-desmolase and 17β-hydroxysteroid oxidoreductase act at the testicular level to convert androstenedione to testosterone. Because the adrenal is unaffected, CAH does not occur. The phenotype can be quite variable, but those with complete feminization can escape detection at birth and be reared as female. Progressive virilization is related to excess gonadotropin production at puberty, which may partially compensate for the lack of testosterone synthesis. Phallic growth and the development of male secondary sex characteristics create a conundrum with regard to gender reassignment when the diagnosis is made later in life.[23]

Despite adequate production of androgen, receptor defects can render cells blind to the virilizing effects of the hormone. The phenotype is variable and depends on the degree of insensitivity of the receptor for androgen.

The extreme is normal female external genitalia resulting from complete androgen insensitivity syndrome (CAIS, also termed testicular feminization). The incidence of this syndrome is approximately 1 in 40,000. It usually results from a point mutation in the androgen receptor gene, located on the X chromosome.[24,25]

Receptor defects seen in CAIS result in normal female external genitalia and a blind-ending vagina. Testes are present but may be nonpalpable. MIS production is intact, so no Müllerian ductal structures are present. These patients usually are initially seen at puberty with amenorrhea, but can be encountered earlier with the finding of a testis at the time of inguinal hernia repair.

Partial androgen insensitivity is associated with a large spectrum of phenotypic variation (e.g., Gilbert–Dreyfus, Lub, and Reifenstein syndromes). It can be a sporadic or inherited condition, and gender assignment and treatment are individualized.[26]

Testosterone is converted to DHT by 5α-reductase, type 2. DHT is a much more potent androgen with regard to virilization of the external genitalia and prostate. The phenotype is ambiguous, but virilization occurs at puberty related to the increased testosterone production and peripheral conversion by nongenital 5α-reductase, type 1. Unfortunately, the virilization is incomplete, and a small phallus and infertility are likely.

Diagnosis

Metabolically, the diagnosis of CAH is made similarly to the 46,XX DSD patient, noting excess steroid levels above the enzymatic block and elevated levels of ACTH. The physical examination confirms absence of a cervix on rectal examination, and bronzing of the skin may be present. Palpation of a cryptorchid or descended testis is possible. The genitogram and ultrasound mirror these findings, but a prominent utricle may be present that lacks a cervical impression at its apex. In CAIS, testosterone levels are elevated postpubertally, but the diagnosis in the prepubertal child may require human chorionic gonadotropin (hCG) stimulation and genital skin fibroblast androgen receptor studies. Receptor assays can delineate a quantitative versus qualitative receptor defect. LH levels are elevated, related to the loss of testosterone feedback inhibition, which requires normal receptor hormone interaction. 5α-reductase deficiency is confirmed by an elevated testosterone-to-DHT ratio and an abnormal 5α-reductase type 2 gene.[27]

Treatment

In CAIS, the gender assignment is always female. CAIS patients who are assigned as female in infancy later identify themselves as female.[28] Because the androgen receptor defect is ubiquitous, virilization of the brain does not occur. Orchiectomy is required, given the risk of malignant degeneration, but is often deferred until after puberty.[29] The testis synthesizes estradiol, facilitating feminine development at puberty. Orchiectomy before puberty necessitates hormone replacement for normal pubertal development.

Gender assignment in partial androgen insensitivity syndrome (PAIS) is largely based on the response of the external genitalia to exogenous testosterone. A significant virilization response argues for the male gender. If there is no response, the female gender is favored. This subgroup is the most variable and has the least consensus with regard to gender assignment. There are reports of gender reassignment at puberty.[30,31] Dissatisfaction with the gender of rearing occurs in approximately 25% of PAIS patients, whether raised male or female.[32] In 5α-reductase deficiency syndrome, the brain is normally virilized and these individuals identify with the male gender. Thus, male gender assignment is recommended.[33]

Müllerian-Inhibitory Substance Deficiency (Hernia Uterine Inguinale)

MIS is produced by the Sertoli cells in the testis and causes regression of the Müllerian ductal structures. In this rare syndrome of abnormal MIS production or MIS-receptor abnormality, Wolffian ductal development is unimpaired, but the Müllerian ducts also persist. Because the infant has a normal male phenotype, this syndrome is rarely encountered in the neonatal period. The most common presentation to the surgeon is that of finding a fallopian tube adjacent to an undescended testis in the hernia sac at the time of orchiopexy.[34]

If this scenario is encountered, a biopsy of the gonad should be performed, the hernia should be repaired, and all structures left intact until completion of a full evaluation with karyotype and MIS levels. Apparent males can also present with bilateral nonpalpable testes, and Müllerian structures are found at laparoscopy (Fig. 62-3). Abnormal MIS-receptor gene assays also can be helpful for verifying the diagnosis in those with a normal MIS level. Subsequent management is primarily orchiopexy. This, however, can be difficult because the vas deferens can be closely adherent or ectopic to the fallopian tube or uterus. Excision of discordant ductal structures may be attempted, but given the relatively low risk associated with leaving these structures, the risk of damage to the vas during this dissection outweighs the benefit of removal. Despite normal testosterone levels, the patient often has impaired spermatogenesis.[35–37]

Leydig Cell Abnormalities

As the Leydig cell is responsible for testosterone production in the testes, impaired testosterone production can also manifest from Leydig cell hypoplasia, agenesis, or abnormal Leydig cell gonadotropin receptors. These disorders are rare. Although the karyotype is 46,XY, the phenotype tends to be female, with a blind-ending vaginal pouch and absence of internal Müllerian structures. These patients usually are seen initially around puberty with amenorrhea and, therefore, are reared as female. Management is similar to that for CAIS, with orchiectomy and estrogen replacement.[38,39]

Ovotesticular DSD (True Hermaphrodite)

Ovotesticular DSD exists when both ovarian and testicular tissue are present. The gonadal configuration also can be quite variable, with the ovary/ovotestis combination being most common in the United States, but any combination can occur. Ovotestes are usually polar with an ovary at one end and a testis at the other, but the distribution can be longitudinal, requiring deep longitudinal biopsy to sample the gonad adequately. Because of the paracrine effect of the gonad, the ipsilateral internal duct structures correlate with the type of gonad present. Ovotestes are associated with a variable duct structure, but usually fallopian tubes prevail. A decisively Müllerian or Wolffian duct structure is usually found rather than an ipsilateral combination.[40]

Ovotesticular DSD can be associated with a variety of karyotypes, with 46,XX being the most common, but different chromosomal content has been correlated with different races. It is thought that a translocation of the *SRY* gene or associated genes to an X chromosome or autosome explains the development of testicular tissue in the 46,XX karyotype. It is more difficult to explain ovarian tissue in a patient with a 46,XY karyotype. Likely, key genes in ovarian development are present, but undetected to complement the normal X chromosomal content. An unappreciated mosaicism could also have occurred.

The phenotype covers the entire spectrum, with ambiguity and asymmetry the rule, but with a tendency toward masculinization. Although it is unusual for ovaries to be found in the labioscrotum, testes and ovotestes are often palpable. Fertility has been described in those raised as female, but testicular fibrosis makes this unlikely in those raised as male.[25,41]

Diagnosis

The diagnosis of ovotesticular DSD is suggested by a mosaic karyotype or ductal structures, but is confirmed by the presence of ovarian and testicular tissue on biopsy.

Treatment

Gender assignment in ovotesticular DSD is quite variable and should be based on the functional potential of the phenotype. In either case, the discordant gonads should be removed early in life. Retained testicular tissue will cause virilization in the female. In males, the testicular tissue is preserved and orchiopexy is performed. A 1–10% incidence of testicular tumors are found in males, predominantly gonadoblastomas and dysgerminomas, so long-term surveillance is needed.[42] Hypospadias repair also is required in the male, and feminizing genitoplasty is performed in the female. Males tend to require

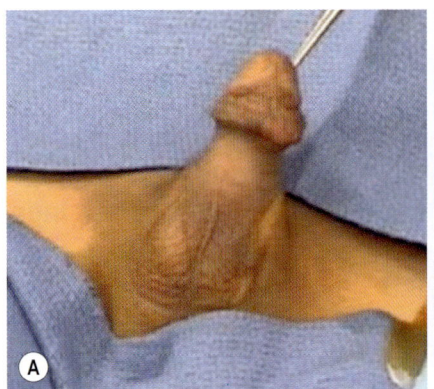 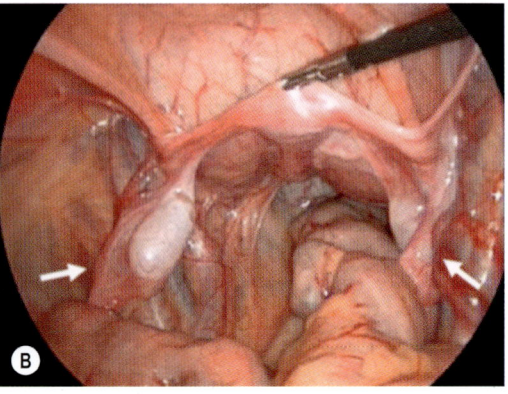

FIGURE 62-3 ■ A 2-year-old boy presented with nonpalpable testes. A karyotype showed XY. **(A)** External genitalia were male. **(B)** Laparoscopy revealed bilateral gonads that were testes on longitudinal biopsy. Müllerian structures (arrows) were also seen. Note the rudimentary uterus (being held by the grasping forceps). This patient had abnormal MIS-receptor function.

hormonal replacement because of the progressive testicular fibrosis, but females usually do not. Fertility is possible in those raised as female. Females should, however, be screened for testosterone levels, which can signal inadequate resection of testicular tissue.[43]

Mixed Gonadal Dysgenesis

Mixed gonadal dysgenesis (MGD) is the second most common form of neonatal ambiguous genitalia. The patient will have a testis on one side and a streak gonad on the other, characterized microscopically by normal ovarian stroma without oocytes (Fig. 62-4). The internal duct structure mirrors the ipsilateral gonad, with the streak associated with a fallopian tube and uterus resulting from the lack of MIS. The karyotype is generally a mosaic of 45,XO/46,XY, and the stigmata of Turner syndrome are variably present. The phenotype is ambiguous, but masculinized, and the testis may be descended, but more commonly is not.[44]

The risk of a gonadal tumor, usually gonadoblastoma, is as high as 20%, and tumors can develop in either the testis or streak gonad.[45] An increased risk of Wilms tumor also is present in MGD. The Denys–Drash syndrome occurs in approximately 5% of patients with MGD and is classically described as ambiguous genitalia, Wilms tumor, and glomerulopathy, which is often associated with hypertension.[46]

Diagnosis

The diagnosis is suggested by the physical stigmata of Turner syndrome on examination (webbed neck, shield chest) and 45,XO/46,XY karyotype. The finding of a testis and streak gonad, however, confirms the diagnosis.

Treatment

The majority of patients with MGD have been raised as female because of the short stature conferred by Turner syndrome and the malignant risk of the retained testis. Females undergo early gonadectomy and feminizing genitoplasty. Males require early excision of the streak

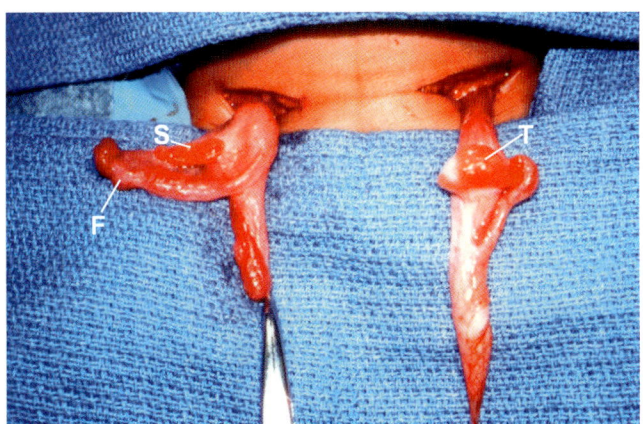

FIGURE 62-4 ■ Mixed gonadal dysgenesis. The left testis was descended, and the right streak gonad was intra-abdominal. T, testis; F, fallopian tube; S, streak gonad. (Photo taken from foot of table.)

gonad, orchiopexy or orchiectomy, and hypospadias repair. Infertility is the rule despite adequate testicular endocrine function. Because of the increasing awareness regarding testosterone imprinting on the brain, more masculinized patients are being raised as male. If individuals are raised as male, close surveillance of the testis is necessary, unless elective orchiectomy and hormone replacement are chosen. Testicular biopsy at the time of puberty to exclude dysgenetic elements is generally recommended.[42] If carcinoma in situ is identified, low-dose radiation therapy is curative.

Pure Gonadal Dysgenesis

Pure gonadal dysgenesis (PGD) is characterized by streak gonads bilaterally. The external phenotype and internal duct structures are female. These patients generally are seen at puberty with primary amenorrhea. The chromosomal makeup is classically 46,XX. PGD is an autosomally recessive trait, so genetic counseling is warranted. This implies that the condition can be caused by abnormalities in the X chromosome or supporting autosomal genes involved in gender differentiation. The gonads do not carry risk of malignant degeneration.

Other conditions are also closely related to bilateral streak gonads. The chromosomal makeup is quite variable and can be 46,XY (XY sex reversal, Swyer syndrome, or male Turner syndrome), 45,XO, or a mosaic. Variants with a Y chromosome differ in that they carry a high rate of malignancy in the retained streak gonads. The phenotype is as described earlier, but these patients may be first seen in infancy with gonadoblastomas or dysgerminomas, or with germ cell tumors that become more common in adolescence. The stigmata of Turner syndrome are often present. Multiple chromosomal deletions and mutations have been described causing this syndrome.

Diagnosis

The finding of a female external phenotype and an internal duct structure with bilateral streak gonads confirms the diagnosis. Follicle-stimulating hormone and LH levels are generally elevated, and estrogen and testosterone levels are decreased. The diagnosis may be suggested by the physical stigmata of Turner syndrome on examination.

Treatment

With the presence of a Y chromosome, gonadectomy should be performed, given the high incidence of malignancy. In classic 46,XX PGD, the gonads can be left in situ because there is no malignant potential. In either case, hormonal replacement at puberty is required because the streak gonads provide no endocrine function.

Other Syndromes of Aberrant Sexual Differentiation

Several syndromes worth mentioning do not neatly fit into the described classification systems.

Vanishing testis syndrome is characterized by a 46,XY karyotype, but absent testes bilaterally. This generally results in virilization to the point of normal external genitalia and internal duct structure, but absent testes. The testes were thought to have produced androgen at some point, resulting in masculinization, but subsequently vanished related to torsion or regression. Patients are generally raised as boys, and hormonal supplementation at puberty is required.[47]

Klinefelter syndrome is characterized by a male karyotype containing two or more X chromosomes (47,XXY, 48,XXXY, etc.). Although phenotypically male prepubertally, these patients acquire abnormal male secondary sexual characteristics (tall stature with disproportionately long legs, sparse facial hair, decreased muscle mass, and a feminine fat distribution) and infertility. The testes are small and hard, with decreased androgen production and elevated estradiol levels related to primary hypergonadotropic hypogonadism. Gynecomastia often occurs with an increased risk of breast cancer.[48] Fertility has been reported but requires assisted means, such as intracytoplasmic sperm injection.[49]

46,XX Testicular DSD (XX sex reversal) is characterized by a male phenotype with a 46,XX karyotype. Most commonly, this occurs from translocation of Y chromosomal material to the X chromosome, but it also can occur from mutation of the X chromosome or from mosaicism. The phenotype and management are similar to those of Klinefelter syndrome, with the exception of shorter stature.[50]

Mayer–Rokitansky–Küster–Hauser syndrome is characterized by a 46,XX karyotype with normal female external genitalia but a short, blind-ending vagina. Normal ovaries and fallopian tubes are present, but the uterus is generally rudimentary. Patients are seen initially with primary amenorrhea, but may have cyclical pain related to functioning endometrium. Treatment is geared toward vaginal reconstruction to allow menses or intercourse, or both.[51]

EVALUATION OF THE NEWBORN WITH AMBIGUOUS GENITALIA

The diagnosis of ambiguous genitalia is extremely disconcerting to the family and should be addressed as a medical emergency. Usually, genital ambiguity is obvious, but the finding of any degree of hypospadias, particularly in association with a nonpalpable testis, merits a DSD evaluation. In this population, a high rate of intersex conditions is found despite the absence of classic ambiguity.[52] Table 62-2 indicates other abnormal physical examination findings that warrant consideration for DSD. The family history may reveal maternal hormone exposure, previous fetal death, or a history of genital ambiguity.

The physical examination should focus on the genitalia. Assessment for palpable gonads is important, because a palpable gonad represents a testis or ovotestis and rules out 46,XX DSD, in which only ovaries are present, or PGD, in which only streak gonads are present. If both gonads are palpable, this generally indicates 46,XY DSD.

TABLE 62-2 **Physical Examination Findings that Warrant Consideration for DSD**

Apparent Female	Unsure	Apparent Male
Clitoral hypertrophy	Ambiguous	Impalpable testes
Fused labia		Severe hypospadias
Palpable gonad		Hypospadias and cryptorchidism

One palpable gonad is generally associated with MGD or ovotesticular DSD. Phallic stretched length, clitoral size, and the position of the urogenital sinus should be noted. A rectal examination may reveal a palpable uterus. The physical examination should include assessment for the stigmata of Turner syndrome associated with MGD and PGD. Bronzing of the areola or scrotum can suggest elevated ACTH production in CAH.

The initial metabolic evaluation should include a karyotype or fluorescent in situ hybridization to identify X and Y chromosomes. 17-OH progesterone levels should be obtained after 3 or 4 days of life, by which time spurious elevations resulting from the stress related to birth have subsided. Electrolyte levels should be monitored closely in the interim to identify salt wasting with CAH. Testosterone and DHT levels are important for evaluating 5α-reductase deficiency. An elevated LH level and a low MIS level suggest testis dysgenesis or absence. ACTH or hCG stimulation tests can be performed but are more controversial.[34] Genetic testing for nearly all known defective genes is now available, but the list is extensive and nondirected testing is not cost effective.[53]

Early imaging studies include pelvic ultrasound, which should identify a uterus if one is present. Although a gonad may be seen, ultrasound is not useful in differentiating a testis, ovotestis, or ovary. A genitogram performed by retrograde contrast injection into the urogenital sinus is helpful in identifying the level of confluence of a vagina and urethra and its relation to the urethral sphincter (Figs 62-5 and 62-6).

Gonadal biopsy is often required for diagnostic purposes, but the diagnosis of CAH can be made by metabolic evaluation alone. Endoscopy is not usually required for diagnosis, but is essential in characterizing the internal duct structure, level of confluence of the urogenital sinus, and planning for and performing the reconstructive procedures.[25]

A gender-assignment team should include a pediatric urologist/surgeon, endocrinologist, geneticist, neonatologist, psychologist, and social worker who together evaluate all newborns with ambiguous genitalia. This information is synthesized by the team and presented to the parents in a combined care conference. The goals of gender assignment and management should include preservation of sexual function and any reproductive potential with the least number of operations, appropriate gender appearance with a stable gender identity, and psychosocial well-being.[54]

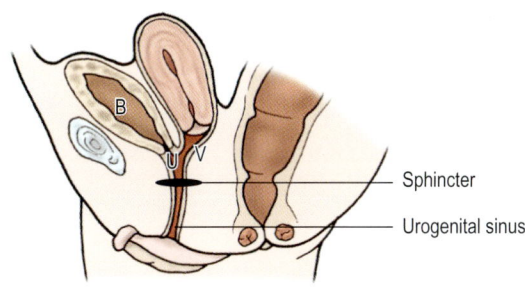

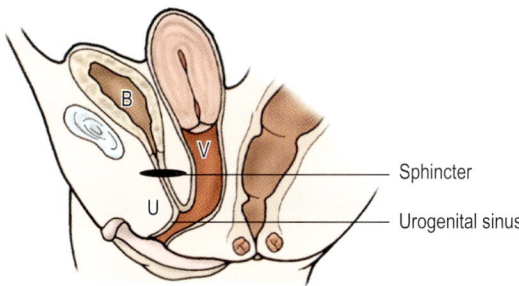

FIGURE 62-5 ■ High versus low urogenital confluence. B, Bladder; U, urethra; V, vagina.

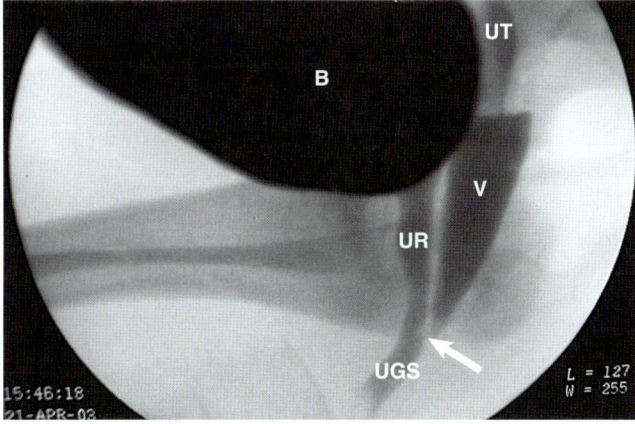

FIGURE 62-6 ■ Genitogram, lower confluence. White arrow, level of the confluence of urethra and vagina to become the urogenital sinus. B, Bladder; UT, uterus; V, vagina; UR, urethra; UGS, urogenital sinus.

RECONSTRUCTIVE GENITAL SURGICAL PROCEDURES

Controversies and Considerations

For more than 20 years, largely based on the work of John Money and the 'John/Joan Case,' the overwhelming bias was that gender identity was largely inducible and loosely dependent on chromosomal constitution.[55] The focus was on one of two twin boys who was reassigned to the female gender early in life after a demasculinizing circumcision injury. The child reportedly developed normally from a psychosocial standpoint and adapted well to life as a girl. Only with extended follow-up into adulthood was it discovered that the individual converted back

to the male gender after severe dissatisfaction with a female identity (including attempted suicide).[56] This rattled the fundamental concepts on which gender assignment had been based for decades and brought to the forefront a tremendous controversy regarding the appropriate management of children with ambiguous genitalia and gender reassignment.

As reconstruction is rarely done in response to any life-threatening issues, support groups for individuals with DSD have advocated delaying any reconstruction until the child can express his or her wishes regarding gender assignment.[57] Although this would decrease the likelihood of a mismatch between physical and psychological gender, the period of genital ambiguity could be quite challenging for child and family in our society. Despite the controversy, the International Consensus Panel on Intersex stated that the evidence is currently insufficient to abandon the practice of early genital reconstruction.[15] However, this must be discussed thoroughly with the family before embarking on any reconstructive operations.

In general, if genital reconstruction is thought to be appropriate, it is planned in the first 3 to 6 months of life. For feminizing reconstruction, the vaginal tissue is thicker as a result of maternal hormonal influence and the distance from the vagina to perineum is shorter at this age. Because parents have a great degree of anxiety surrounding the gender of their child, earlier repair may help reduce this anxiety and encourage parent/child bonding.[58]

Male Gender Assignment

Reconstructive efforts for the male gender of rearing include orchiopexy or orchiectomy, when appropriate, and hypospadias repair. These techniques are described elsewhere in this book. It bears mentioning again that orchiopexy may be extremely difficult because the vas deferens can be closely adherent to Müllerian duct remnants, such as a fallopian tube or uterus. A portion of these structures may be left in situ if the risk of damage to the vas deferens or testicular vasculature is significant, but this adherence may severely limit mobility of the testis and preclude orchiopexy. Methods of total penile reconstruction in cases of aphallia, demasculinizing penile trauma, or female-to-male gender reassignment by using local skin flaps, a radial forearm flap, or osteocutaneous fibula flap have been described with reasonable success.[59-61]

Female Gender Assignment

Feminizing genitoplasty includes three major components: monsplasty, clitoroplasty, and vaginoplasty (Figs 62-7 and 62-8). The timing of the vaginoplasty depends on the level of confluence of the urogenital sinus. For a low confluence, the vaginoplasty is performed in the neonatal period with the monsplasty and clitoroplasty. Even with a high confluence, the vaginoplasty can be performed with the monsplasty and clitoroplasty in the newborn. However, because vaginal dilation is often necessary after repair, it may better to defer the vaginoplasty

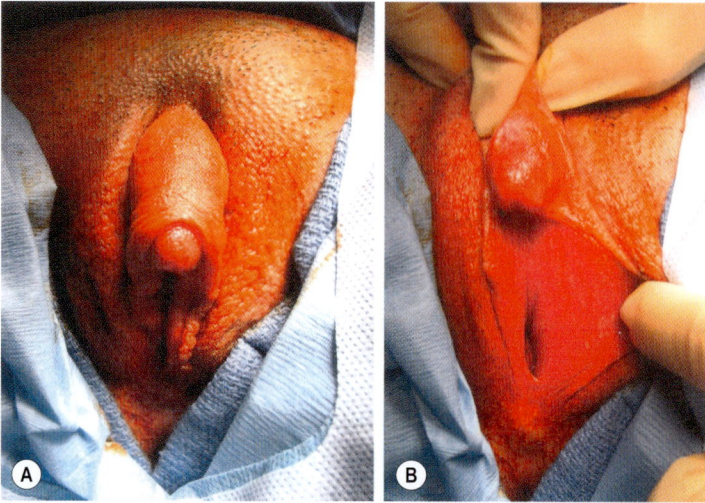

FIGURE 62-7 ■ Ambiguous genitalia. The patient has congenital adrenal hyperplasia, 21-hydroxylase deficiency.

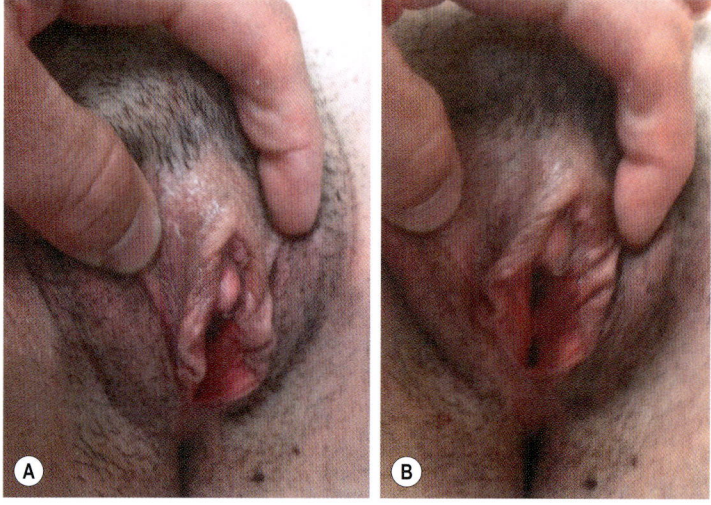

FIGURE 62-8 ■ Same patient as in Figure 63-7. Appearance of genitalia six months after undergoing a feminizing genitoplasty.

until the patient is peripubertal and more capable and interested in this requirement. Cystoscopy is invaluable for this assessment. We generally insert a Fogarty balloon catheter in the vagina and a catheter in the urethra and bladder to define the confluence during the dissection.

The procedure is initiated by placing a traction suture in the glans. A dorsolateral circumcising incision is made, leaving a 4–5 mm distal preputial cuff, much like is done in a hypospadias repair. The lateral borders of the mucosalized plate are incised, taking this back adjacent to the urogenital sinus. The shaft of the phallus is then degloved of skin superficial to Buck's fascia. Fascial incisions are then made lateral to the neurovascular bundles. A plane is created just beneath Buck's fascia from the level just proximal to the glans back to the pubic symphysis. The mucosalized plate is elevated on the ventrum and preserved to fill naturally the void between the urethral meatus and clitoris. The dorsal pedicles, including the neurovascular bundles, are preserved. The base of the corporeal bodies are suture ligated at the level of the pubic symphysis, and the distal corporeal tissue is excised.

An alternative technique preserving the corporeal bodies has been described to maintain the potential for reversibility, but long-term functional outcome is pending.[62]

No clitoral reduction is performed to avoid nerve injury. It can be recessed and has a quite normal appearance in adulthood.[63] The clitoris is anchored to the corporal stumps to secure its position, being sure not to compromise the dorsal neurovascular pedicle.

A posterior inverted U-shaped flap is then made from the level of the ischial tuberosities to just posterior to the urogenital meatus. For a very low confluence, dissection is carried along the posterior aspect of the urogenital sinus to the level of the confluence, the posterior wall is incised until the vaginal introitus is normal in caliber, and the U-flap is advanced to complete the posterior vaginal wall (Fig. 62-9). With higher confluences, total urogenital mobilization is favored.[64–66]

For total urogenital mobilization, the urogenital sinus is incised circumferentially and mobilized as one unit to the level of the confluence (Fig. 62-10). At this point, the vagina can be carefully separated from the urethra under

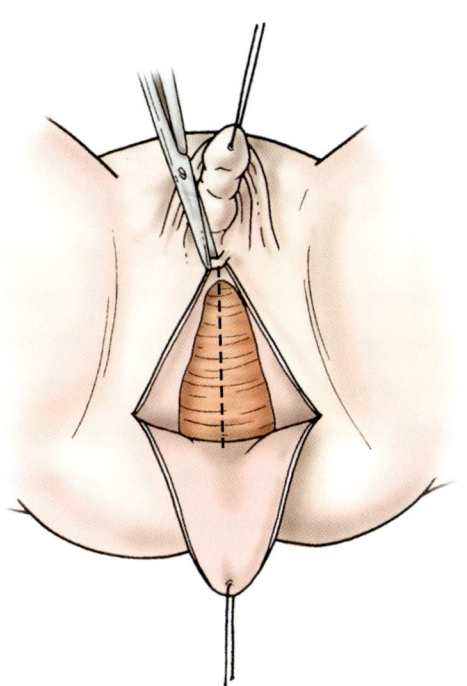

FIGURE 62-9 ■ Vaginal cutback procedure for the low urogenital confluence.

direct vision and the defect in the urethra is closed. The urogenital sinus can be incised in the ventral and dorsal midline and rotated posterolaterally to lengthen the distal vagina. Using this technique, a long distance to the perineum can be bridged.

Total urogenital mobilization is attractive as one can approach even the high urogenital confluences in the neonatal period without vaginal substitution or grafting, but the family must be appropriately cautioned. Although early results are favorable, descent of the bladder neck is counterintuitive when considering our knowledge of adult female stress incontinence and long-term continence could be an issue. To complete the monsplasty, the dorsal phallic shaft skin is incised vertically, a preputial hood is formed for the clitoris, and the majority of this tissue is used to construct the labia minor with V-shaped advancement flaps (Fig. 62-11). Other techniques for the high urogenital sinus include a posterior approach that requires incising the rectum and an anterior transvesical approach.[67,68]

In some patients with a high urogenital confluence, vaginal reconstruction is delayed until the peripubertal period, just before menarche. The techniques described are still used, but in some patients, especially those who

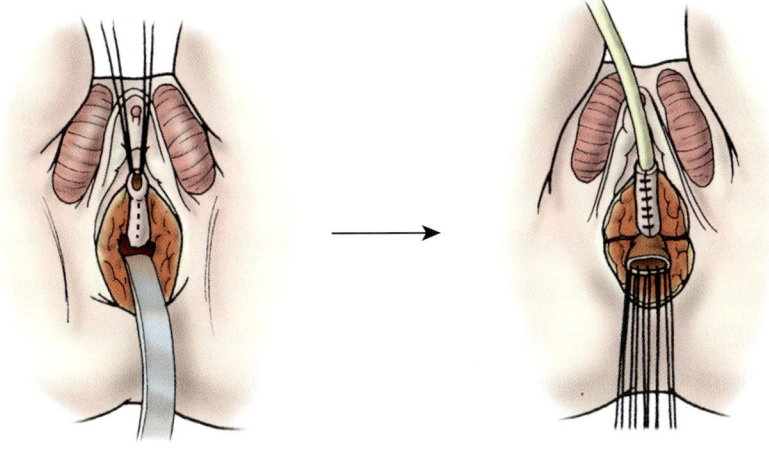

FIGURE 62-10 ■ Total urogenital mobilization. The urogenital sinus is mobilized as a unit, bringing the confluence toward the perineum. Once visualized, the vagina is then detached and the urethral defect is closed.

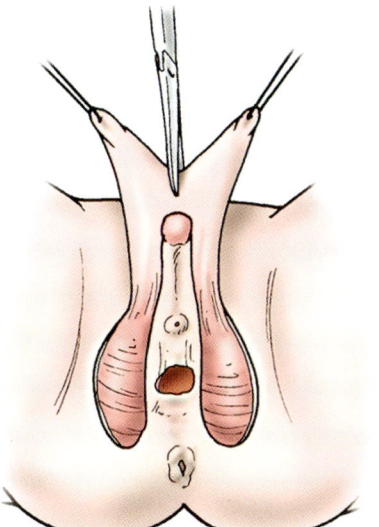

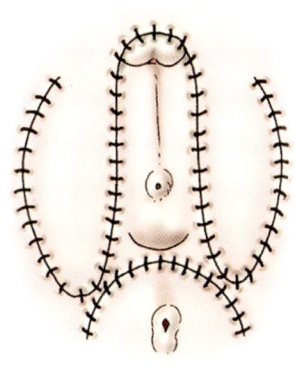

FIGURE 62-11 ■ Monsplasty. Dorsal shaft skin is degloved from the phallus and incised. These flaps are then advanced to become the labia minora. (Shown before and after excision of the corporeal tissues and clitoropexy.)

are obese, these methods are insufficient. In such cases, vaginal substitution with a colonic segment is preferred, but ileal substitutions and split-thickness skin grafts also have been used. The benefit of vascularized bowel substitution is less vaginal stenosis and the natural formation of lubricating mucus, but this may require wearing a pad if there is excessive mucus production. Colonic segments appear to have a lower rate of stenosis than do ileal segments.[69] Conversely, skin grafts have a tendency to become stenotic and may require frequent dilation and revision, but long-term satisfaction also has been reported.[70] The barrier function to sexually transmitted diseases is likely superior with skin grafts when compared with intestine.[71] If a rudimentary vagina or depression exists, sequential dilation with the technique described by Frank and modified to a dilating seat by Ingram may be successful.[72,73]

REFERENCES

1. Jost A, Vigier B, Prepin J, et al. Studies on sex differentiation in mammals. Recent Prog Horm Res 1973;29:1–41.
2. Lukusa T, Fryns JP, van der Berghe H. The role of the Y-chromosome in sex determination. Genet Couns 1992;3:1–11.
3. Clarkson MJ, Harley VR. Sex with two SOX on: SRY and SOX9 in testis development. Trends Endocrinol Metab 2002;13: 106–11.
4. Moog U, Jansen NJ, Scherer G, et al. Acampomelic campomelic syndrome. Am J Med Genet 2001;104:239–45.
5. Parker KL, Schimmer BP, Schedl A. Genes essential for early events in gonadal development. EXS 2001:11–24.
6. Schedl A, Hastie N. Multiple roles for the Wilms' tumour suppressor gene, WT1 in genitourinary development. Mol Cell Endocrinol 1998;140:65–9.
7. Nordqvist K. Sex differentiation—gonadogenesis and novel genes. Int J Dev Biol 1995;39:727–36.
8. Goodfellow PN, Camerino G. DAX-1, an 'antitestis' gene. Cell Mol Life Sci 1999;55:857–63.
9. Taguchi O, Cunha GR, Lawrence WD, et al. Timing and irreversibility of Mullerian duct inhibition in the embryonic reproductive tract of the human male. Dev Biol 1984;106:394–8.
10. Tajima K, Dantes A, Yao Z, et al. Down-regulation of steroidogenic response to gonadotropins in human and rat preovulatory granulosa cells involves mitogen-activated protein kinase activation and modulation of DAX-1 and steroidogenic factor-1. J Clin Endocrinol Metab 2003;88:2288–99.
11. Menon PS, Harinarayan CV, Forest MG. Congenital adrenal hyperplasia due to 11 beta-hydroxylase deficiency. Indian Pediatr 1992;29:98–103.
12. Pellerin D, Nihoul-Fekete C, Lortat-Jacob S. [Surgery of sexual ambiguity: Experience of 298 cases]. Bull Acad Natl Med 1989; 173:555–62.
13. Pang SY, Wallace MA, Hofman L, et al. Worldwide experience in newborn screening for classical congenital adrenal hyperplasia due to 21-hydroxylase deficiency. Pediatrics 1988;81:866–74.
14. Allen TD. Disorders of sexual differentiation. Urology 1976; 7:1–32.
15. Lee PA, Houk CP, Ahmed SF, et al. Consensus statement on management of intersex disorders. International Consensus Conference on Intersex. Pediatrics 2006;118:e488–500.
16. Dacou-Voutetakis C, Maniati-Christidi M, Dracopoulou-Vabouli M. Genetic aspects of congenital adrenal hyperplasia. J Pediatr Endocrinol Metab 2001;14:1303–8
17. Reindollar RH, Tho SP, McDonough PG. Abnormalities of sexual differentiation: Evaluation and management. Clin Obstet Gynecol 1987;30:697–713.
18. Laue L, Rennert OM. Congenital adrenal hyperplasia: molecular genetics and alternative approaches to treatment. Adv Pediatr 1995;42:113–43.
19. Wilson RC, Mercado AB, Cheng KC, et al. Steroid 21-hydroxylase deficiency: Genotype may not predict phenotype. J Clin Endocrinol Metab 1995;80:2322–9.
20. Calaf J, Prats J, Esteban-Altirriba J. Female pseudohermaphroditism caused by maternal hyperandrogenism. In: J M-M, editor. Intersexual States: Disorders of Sex Differentiation. Barcelona: Ediciones Doyma; 1994. p. 187–97.
21. Trautman PD, Meyer-Bahlburg HF, Postelnek J, et al. Mothers' reactions to prenatal diagnostic procedures and dexamethasone treatment of congenital adrenal hyperplasia. J Psychosom Obstet Gynaecol 1996;17:175–81.
22. Berenbaum SA, Bailey JM. Effects on gender identity of prenatal androgens and genital appearance: Evidence from girls with congenital adrenal hyperplasia. J Clin Endocrinol Metab 2003; 88:1102–6.
23. Saez JM, De Peretti E, Morera AM, et al. Familial male pseudohermaphroditism with gynecomastia due to a testicular 17-ketosteroid reductase defect. I. Studies in vivo. J Clin Endocrinol Metab 1971;32:604–10.
24. Quigley CA, De Bellis A, Marschke KB, et al. Androgen receptor defects: Historical, clinical, and molecular perspectives. Endocr Rev 1995;16:271–321.
25. Diamond DA. Sexual differentiation: Normal and abnormal. In: Walsh PC, Retik AB, Vaughn ED Jr, Wein AJ, editors. Campbell's Urology. 8th ed. Philadelphia: WB Saunders; 2002 pp. 2395–427.
26. Batch JA, Davies HR, Evans BA, et al. Phenotypic variation and detection of carrier status in the partial androgen insensitivity syndrome. Arch Dis Child 1993;68:453–7.
27. Barthold J, Gonzalez R. Intersex states. In: Gonzales E, Bauer SB, editor. Pediatric urology practice. Philadelphia: Lippincott Williams & Wilkins; 1999. p. 547.
28. Mazur T. Gender dysphoria and gender change in androgen insensitivity or micropenis. Arch Sex Behav 2005;34:411–21.
29. Muller J, Skakkebaek NE. Testicular carcinoma in situ in children with the androgen insensitivity (testicular feminisation) syndrome. Br Med J (Clin Res Ed) 1984;288:1419–20.
30. Rosler A, Kohn G. Male pseudohermaphroditism due to 17 beta-hydroxysteroid dehydrogenase deficiency: Studies on the natural history of the defect and effect of androgens on gender role. J Steroid Biochem 1983;19:663–74.
31. Imperato-McGinley J, Peterson RE, Gautier T, et al. Androgens and the evolution of male-gender identity among male pseudohermaphrodites with 5alpha-reductase deficiency. N Engl J Med 1979;300:1233–7.
32. Migeon CJ, Wisniewski AB, Gearhart JP, et al. Ambiguous genitalia with perineoscrotal hypospadias in 46,XY individuals: Long-term medical, surgical, and psychosexual outcome. Pediatrics 2002; 110:e31.
33. Wilson JD. Syndromes of androgen resistance. Biol Reprod 1992;46:168–73.
34. Huseman DA. The genitalia intersex. 4th ed. In: Gillenwater JY, Grayhack JT, Howards SS, Mitchell ME, editor. Philadelphia: Lippincott Williams & Wilkins; 2002.
35. Loeff DS, Imbeaud S, Reyes HM, et al. Surgical and genetic aspects of persistent mullerian duct syndrome. J Pediatr Surg 1994;29: 61–5.
36. Fernandes ET, Hollabaugh RS, Young JA, et al. Persistent mullerian duct syndrome. Urology 1990;36:516–18.
37. Gustafson ML, Lee MM, Asmundson L, et al. Mullerian inhibiting substance in the diagnosis and management of intersex and gonadal abnormalities. J Pediatr Surg 1993;28:439–44.
38. Eil C, Austin RM, Sesterhenn I, et al. Leydig cell hypoplasia causing male pseudohermaphroditism: Diagnosis 13 years after prepubertal castration. J Clin Endocrinol Metab 1984;58:441–8.
39. Lee PA, Rock JA, Brown TR, et al. Leydig cell hypofunction resulting in male pseudohermaphroditism. Fertil Steril 1982; 37:675–9.
40. Berkovitz GD, Fechner PY, Zacur HW, et al. Clinical and pathologic spectrum of 46,XY gonadal dysgenesis: Its relevance to the understanding of sex differentiation. Medicine (Baltimore) 1991;70: 375–83.
41. Walker AM, Walker JL, Adams S, et al. True hermaphroditism. J Paediatr Child Health 2000;36:69–73.
42. Verp MS, Simpson JL. Abnormal sexual differentiation and neoplasia. Cancer Genet Cytogenet 1987;25:191–218.
43. Hadjiathanasiou CG, Brauner R, Lortat-Jacob S, et al. True hermaphroditism: Genetic variants and clinical management. J Pediatr 1994;125:738–44.

44. Davidoff F, Federman DD. Mixed gonadal dysgenesis. Pediatrics 1973;52:725–42.
45. Robboy SJ, Miller T, Donahoe PK, et al. Dysgenesis of testicular and streak gonads in the syndrome of mixed gonadal dysgenesis: Perspective derived from a clinicopathologic analysis of twenty-one cases. Hum Pathol 1982;13:700–16.
46. Drash A, Sherman F, Hartmann WH, Blizzard RM. A syndrome of pseudohermaphroditism, Wilms' tumor, hypertension, and degenerative renal disease. J Pediatr 1970;76:585–93.
47. Edman CD, Winters AJ, Porter JC, et al. Embryonic testicular regression. A clinical spectrum of XY agonadal individuals. Obstet Gynecol 1977;49:208–17.
48. Klinefelter H Jr, Reifenstein E Jr, Albright F. Syndrome characterized by gynecomastia, aspermatogensis, without a-Leydigism and increased excretion of follicle stimulating hormone. J Clin Endocrinol Metab 1942;2:615.
49. Kitamura M, Matsumiya K, Koga M, et al. Ejaculated spermatozoa in patients with non-mosaic Klinefelter's syndrome. Int J Urol 2000;7:88–92.
50. Van Dyke DC, Hanson JW, Moore JW, et al. Clinical management issues in males with sex chromosomal mosaicism and discordant phenotype/sex chromosomal patterns. Clin Pediatr 1991;30: 15–21.
51. Griffin JE, Edwards C, Madden JD, et al. Congenital absence of the vagina. The Mayer-Rokitansky-Kuster-Hauser syndrome. Ann Intern Med 1976;85:224–36.
52. Kaefer M, Diamond D, Hendren WH, et al. The incidence of intersexuality in children with cryptorchidism and hypospadias: Stratification based on gonadal palpability and meatal position. J Urol 1999;162:1003–6.
53. Achermann JC, Ozisik G, Meeks JJ. Genetic causes of human reproductive disease. J Clin Endocrinol Metab 2002;87:2447–54.
54. Meyer-Bahlburg HF. Gender assignment and reassignment in intersexuality: Controversies, data, and guidelines for research. Adv Exp Med Biol 2002;511:199–223.
55. Money J. Ablatio penis: Normal male infant sex-reassigned as a girl. Arch Sex Behav 1975;4:65–71.
56. Diamond M, Sigmundson HK. Sex reassignment at birth. Long-term review and clinical implications. Arch Pediatr Adolesc Med 1997;151:298–304.
57. Recommendations for Treatment: Intersex infants and children. Intersex Society of North America; 1995.
58. Hensle TW, Bingham J. Feminizing genitoplasty. Adv Exp Med Biol 2002;511:251–65.
59. Jordan GH. Total phallic construction, option to gender reassignment. Adv Exp Med Biol 2002;511:275–80.
60. Sadove RC, Sengezer M, McRoberts JW, et al. One-stage total penile reconstruction with a free sensate osteocutaneous fibula flap. Plast Reconstr Surg 1993;92:1314–23.
61. De Castro R, Merlini E, Rigamonti W, et al. Phalloplasty and urethroplasty in children with penile agenesis: Preliminary report. J Urol 2007;177:1112–16.
62. Pippi Salle JL, Braga LP, Macedo N, et al. Corporeal sparing dismembered clitoroplasty: An alternative technique for feminizing genitoplasty. J Urol 2007;178:1796–800.
63. Minto CL, Liao LM, Woodhouse CR, et al. The effect of clitoral surgery on sexual outcome in individuals who have intersex conditions with ambiguous genitalia: A cross-sectional study. Lancet 2003;361:1252–7.
64. Pena A. Total urogenital mobilization–an easier way to repair cloacas. J Pediatr Surg 1997;32:263–7.
65. Rink RC, Pope JC, Kropp BP, et al. Reconstruction of the high urogenital sinus: Early perineal prone approach without division of the rectum. J Urol 1997;158:1293–7.
66. Rink RC, Adams MC. Feminizing genitoplasty: State of the art. World J Urol 1998;16:212–18.
67. Pena A, Filmer B, Bonilla E, et al. Transanorectal approach for the treatment of urogenital sinus: Preliminary report. J Pediatr Surg 1992;27:681–5.
68. Passerini-Glazel G. A new 1-stage procedure for clitorovaginoplasty in severely masculinized female pseudohermaphrodites. J Urol 1989;142:565–8.
69. Hensle TW, Dean GE. Vaginal replacement in children. J Urol 1992;148:677–9.
70. Martinez-Mora J, Isnard R, Castellvi A, et al. Neovagina in vaginal agenesis: Surgical methods and long-term results. J Pediatr Surg 1992;27:10–14.
71. Rink R, Kaefer M. Surgical management of intersexuality, cloacal malformations, and other abnormalities of the genitalia in girls. In: Walsh PC, Retk AB, Vaughn ED, Wein AJ, editors. Campbell's Urology. 8th ed. Philadelphia: WB Saunders; 2002. p. 2428–68.
72. Frank R. The formation of an artificial vagina without operation. Am J Obstet Gynecol 1938;35:1053.
73. Ingram JM. The bicycle seat stool in the treatment of vaginal agenesis and stenosis: A preliminary report. Am J Obstet Gynecol 1981;140:867–73.

CHAPTER 63

RENOVASCULAR HYPERTENSION

James A. O'Neill, Jr.

In 1934, Goldblatt and coworkers described the association between coarctation of the aorta and renal artery stenosis with hypertension.[1] However, it was not until the 1960s that activation of the renin–angiotensin system, which leads to the release of renin and the production of angiotensin II, was found to be the mechanism for the hypertension (Fig. 63-1). Subsequently, it has been shown that diminished renal perfusion pressure has direct effects on sodium excretion, sympathetic nerve activity, nitric oxide production, and intrarenal prostaglandin concentrations, resulting in renovascular hypertension.[2] Other studies have demonstrated different fractional angiotensin elevation patterns in children with renovascular hypertension as compared with essential hypertension.[3]

The incidence of hypertension in children in all age groups is 2–10%, with the higher figure representative of adolescence. However, because blood pressure is not routinely measured in infants and younger children, the diagnosis of hypertension is often delayed. Table 63-1 lists the common causes of hypertension in children according to the organ system involved. This chapter will focus on renovascular causes of hypertension, most of which are correctable.

The natural history of progressive, untreated renovascular hypertension often results in the development of renovascular lesions in sites other than those originally identified. The progressive nature of this disorder is the best justification for an aggressive approach for correction. Also, sustained and malignant forms of hypertension may result in left-sided heart failure, chronic renal failure based on chronic ischemic nephropathy, and stroke.

Essential hypertension is the most common cause (60%) of hypertension between birth and 20 years of age. However, the incidence of correctable hypertension is very high in patients younger than 15 years. In previous studies by our group, the incidence of correctable hypertension in the birth to 5-year age group was around 80%; in the 6- to 10-year age group, 45%; and in the 11- to 15-year and 16- to 20-year age groups, 20%.[4] Although a variety of causes were identified, the vast majority were renovascular. Renovascular disease comprises 8–10% of all forms of hypertension in children, while it is 1% of all forms in adults. Additionally, long-term follow-up of patients with renovascular hypertension clearly indicates that patients who have had successful repair of their lesions have sustained results and longer survival than those who do not. Moreover, the younger the patient, the better the result.[5] Such studies support an aggressive approach to correction of identified renovascular lesions in young patients.

ETIOLOGY

Renovascular hypertension may be congenital or acquired. Congenital causes include arterial hypoplasia or aplasia; neurofibromatosis and tuberous sclerosis tumors involving the renal artery; and Williams syndrome, which includes manifestations of supravalvular aortic stenosis, peripheral vascular stenosis particularly in the subclavian and renal arteries, mid-aortic narrowing, hypercalcemia, and elfin facies.[6] The most common acquired forms of renovascular hypertension are fibromuscular dysplasia (FMD), which involves one or both renal arteries, or a more generalized type of disease, such as Takayasu arteritis and subisthmic abdominal coarctation, now referred to as the mid-aortic syndrome.[7,8] Stenoses of visceral arteries such as the superior mesenteric and celiac arteries are also common in mid-aortic syndrome.[7] Other less common forms of acquired renovascular hypertension are renal artery trauma or thrombosis, thrombosis secondary to antithrombin deficiency, Kawasaki disease, and an anastomotic stenosis in renal transplants.[9]

Overall, the vast majority of children with renovascular hypertension have FMD. Presentation of newborns with aortic and arterial aplasia and hypoplasia suggest a congenital origin. In young adults, FMD appears to have an acquired pattern and may have a genetic basis in the syndromes mentioned above.[6] The majority of patients initially present at several years of age, usually with an active inflammatory phase followed by a quiescent phase of arteritis.[4,7] Although it was initially thought that FMD might be an autoimmune disease, relatively recent evidence suggests that T-cell-based immune mechanisms, macrophages, and antigen-presenting cells are mainly responsible for renovascular arteritis, and a variety of other arteritides as well.[10] The histology of the vascular lesion seen in the renal artery and aorta reveals medial and perimedial fibroplasia, which has inherent implications about approaches to treatment, particularly angioplasty. Although FMD is a systemic, occlusive arteriopathy that may involve the entire abdominal aorta and its branches, the renal arteries are the predominant vessels involved.[11]

CLINICAL PRESENTATION

Children with renovascular hypertension generally come to attention in one of two ways. Approximately 70% of patients are asymptomatic and are identified when they have their blood pressure taken during a routine evaluation. It is usually not known how long the hypertension

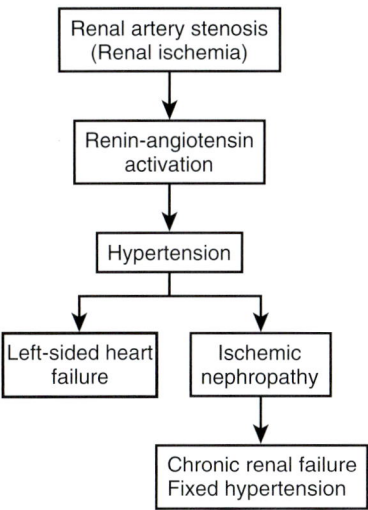

FIGURE 63-1 ■ The consequences of renal ischemia from renal artery disease are depicted.

TABLE 63-1	**Causes of Hypertension in Children**
Essential Hypertension	**Causes**
Renal	Glomerulonephritis, pyelonephritis, renal hypoplasia, polycystic kidney, Wilms tumor, neuroblastoma, arteritis, aneurysms, trauma
Cardiovascular	Aortic coarctation, Takayasu arteritis, neurofibromatosis, tuberous sclerosis, renovascular stenosis, collagen vascular disease
Central nervous system	Encephalitis, intracranial mass with increased pressure, dysautonomia
Endocrine	Pheochromocytoma, aldosteronoma, adrenogenital syndrome, Cushing syndrome
Secondary hypertension	Lead and mercury poisoning, glucocorticoid drugs, oral contraceptives

has been present. Repeated measurements verify the chronic nature of this problem, which leads to diagnostic evaluation. Approximately one-half of these asymptomatic patients will be found to have correctable hypertension. The remaining 30% of children are symptomatic with headaches, vision problems, encephalopathy, congestive heart failure, oliguric renal failure, and, occasionally, leg claudication. Physical findings may indicate the presence of heart failure with enlargement of the liver and heart, as well as retinopathy and retinal hemorrhage. In cases of mid-aortic syndrome, peripheral pulses and blood pressure may be diminished in the lower extremities. Although an abdominal bruit could probably be heard in the majority of instances of renal artery stenosis, it is not commonly found until a diagnosis is suspected.

In contrast to a young female predominance in adults with FMD, gender incidence is equal in children. Both renal arteries are involved in approximately 70% of patients. In occasional patients with unilateral lesions, FMD may develop in the opposite renal artery years later.

Renovascular causes of hypertension are more common in children younger than 10 years, as evidenced by an average age of 7 years in one of our studies.[5] In infants and toddlers, malignant forms of hypertension with encephalopathy and retinopathy are more likely to develop than in older children.

DIAGNOSIS

Before any invasive diagnostic studies are undertaken, clinical manifestations of severe hypertension such as headache, irritability, abdominal pain, heart failure, and seizures should be controlled with medications.

Laboratory Studies

Renovascular hypertension cannot be diagnosed by any specific laboratory study. Most laboratory studies are performed to document the patient's clinical status and renal function. Erythrocyte sedimentation rate (ESR) is important to assess whether the patient is in the inflammatory or the quiescent phase of arteritis. Urinary catecholamines are evaluated to exclude pheochromocytoma and other common endocrine causes, particularly in patients with manifestations of neurofibromatosis. (The author has not found plasma renin or provocative studies like captopril-stimulated renin studies to be helpful in young children.) Technetium-labeled pentetic acid (DTPA) radionuclide fractional-flow studies may indicate unilateral renovascular disease, but they are not useful when bilateral disease is present. Captopril renography has the same limitation.

Imaging

Although a number of imaging studies exist, currently it seems best to perform aortography and selective arteriography in all children with significant hypertension. Minimal complications have been encountered with these studies, even in very small patients. With appropriate hydration, even patients with some degree of oliguric renal failure can undergo aortography and selective arteriography by using CO_2 or low-osmolar or noniodinated contrast agents in limited amounts. For patients with a distal or intrarenal vascular stenosis, nitroglycerin-enhanced selective studies promote the identification of segmental areas of ischemia in the involved kidney. Angiography may also facilitate endoluminal procedures when feasible.

Duplex color-coded Doppler ultrasonography (US) is capable of demonstrating the renal arteries, as well as measuring flow velocity as an index of the degree of stenosis. However, Doppler ultrasound studies, whether performed preoperatively or postoperatively for follow-up, have limitations in terms of demonstrating precise anatomic detail, particularly in small vessels. The same is true of captopril scintigraphy and contrast-enhanced ultrasound. Magnetic resonance angiography (MRA) and computed tomographic angiography (CTA) are capable of demonstrating the renal arteries and the aorta and its branches better than Doppler ultrasound, but there are resolution issues in small subjects.[12,13] MRA is less accurate than CTA, and the volume of contrast material for CTA is often the same as with aortography with selective angiography, so no advantage accrues from the standpoint of nephrotoxicity. If one takes the point of view that the prime purpose of an imaging study is to select the most suitable therapeutic method, aortography with selective arteriography is the most definitive study and the one most capable of demonstrating precise anatomic detail (Fig. 63-2). Doppler ultrasound, MRA, and CTA are now considered best as screening or follow-up studies in children.

The diagnostic approach to children, who usually have bilateral renal artery stenosis associated with FMD, is simpler than the workup in adults who primarily have atherosclerotic lesions. Consequently, many of the non-invasive tests designed for adults with renovascular hypertension are not useful in children. For example, in an adult study, it was found that the preoperative calculation of a high renal resistance-index value derived by Doppler ultrasound is a predictor of the lack of success of operative correction of renal artery stenosis.[13] However, because successful revascularization in children routinely results in alleviation of hypertension, such studies are not relevant. The same is true for renal vein renin studies because renal artery stenosis in children with hypertension is always significant. Conversely, renal vein renin studies may be useful in determining the significance of distal stenoses or aneurysms of renal artery branches, or postoperative anastomotic stenoses.

As FMD is a systemic, occlusive arteriopathy, it is necessary to survey the entire lower thoracic and abdominal aorta to delineate those patients who not only have renal artery stenosis but also the mid-aortic syndrome, visceral artery stenosis, or other forms of renovascular hypertension.[7,11,14] Thus, full angiography is needed to delineate all diseased vessels so that an appropriate single-stage operation can be performed. It is interesting to note that hypertensive children who have renal artery stenosis, without co-morbid conditions, usually have a single, focal branch artery lesion.[12]

TREATMENT

Medical Treatment

Antihypertensive medications are needed to control blood pressure before undertaking any invasive procedure, including arteriography. Drug therapy is not an alternative to operative correction, but an integral part of patient management, preoperatively, intraoperatively, and postoperatively. Most patients referred for surgical or interventional treatment have severe hypertension with symptoms that are most effectively managed with intravenous drugs. Once the hypertension is controlled, the patient can gradually be transitioned to oral medications including diuretics, calcium-channel blockers, beta and alpha blockers, converting enzyme inhibitors, and angiotension II receptor antagonists. In severe cases, nitroprusside may be required as the initial treatment. Either concurrently or sequentially, intravenous labetalol or nifedipine, or both, are useful drugs. The same three medications are utilized in postoperative management if hypertension is exacerbated as a consequence of temporary ischemia associated with revascularization procedures. For long-term and outpatient treatment, propranolol, atenolol, minoxidil, and oral diuretics in various combinations are often used. Angiotensin-converting enzyme (ACE) inhibitors such as captopril and ramipril are very effective antihypertensive drugs, but they must be used with great caution in patients with renovascular hypertension because of the potential for drug-induced renal ischemia and possible oliguric renal failure.[5,15] Thus, if a decision is made to use ACE inhibitor medication, renal function must be monitored closely.

Another consideration related to the use of medical therapy is in the management of infants with severe hypertension related to renal artery stenosis. In these instances, because of the great risk for thrombosis with repair of tiny vessels, it may be best to administer antihypertensive drugs until the renal arteries are close to adult size, if possible (ages 5 to 8 years). After revascularization, it may take up to 6 to 12 months for the hypertension to resolve or improve during which time the antihypertensive drugs must be weaned gradually.

Interventional Procedures

Balloon angioplasty with and without stenting has been the subject of many reports with atherosclerotic disease as well as with FMD.[16,17] The results in patients with FMD have been more favorable in instances in which the orifice of the renal artery is not involved. Balloon dilation for orifice lesions has generally resulted in short-term improvement only. Experience reported in children with balloon angioplasty indicates that balloon dilation of orifice lesions is as ineffective as it is in adults. However, it is very successful in providing long-term relief from

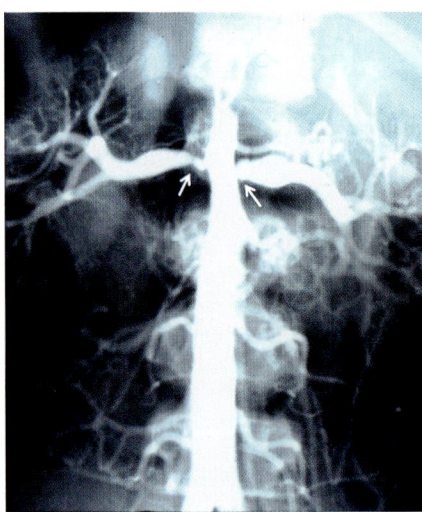

FIGURE 63-2 ■ The aortogram performed on a 6-year-old boy with severe hypertension demonstrates bilateral orificial narrowing of the renal arteries (arrows) with post-stenotic dilatation and some degree of associated aortic narrowing (mid-aortic syndrome). He was treated with aorto-aortic bypass and bilateral renal artery bypasses, and is normotensive 19 years later.

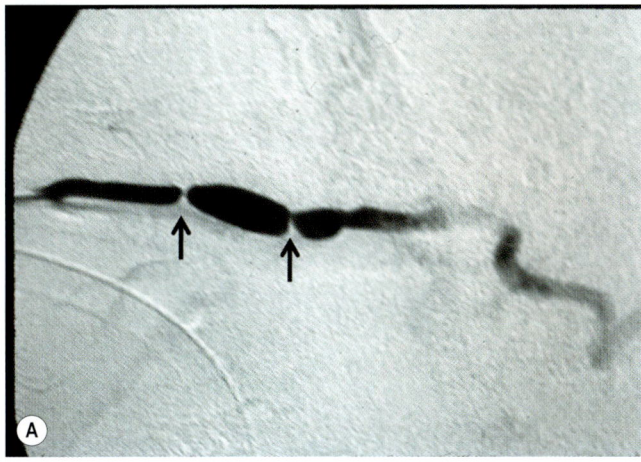

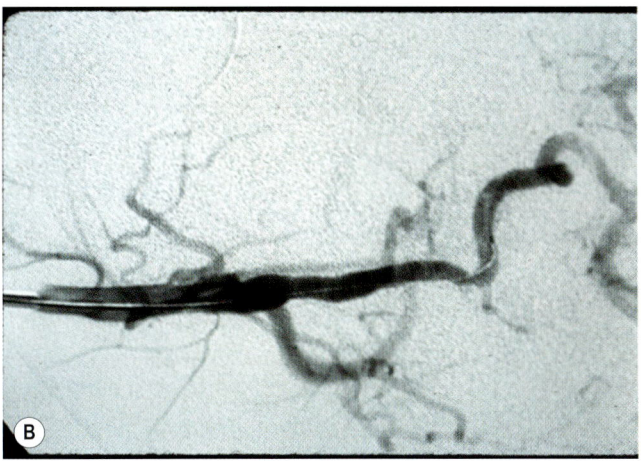

FIGURE 63-3 ■ **(A)** This selective left renal arteriogram shows typical findings (arrows) of FMD distal to the aortic orifice. **(B)** The artery is normal-sized following balloon angioplasty of the distal stenoses. Note the catheter in the renal artery.

stenosis of the main renal artery or its branches (Fig 63-3).[18–20]

Nonetheless, there are a number of reports in the interventional radiology literature that promote percutaneous transluminal angioplasty (PTA) for children with all forms of renal artery stenosis, and even describe the placement of stents in very small children. Unfortunately, very few of these reports describe long-term outcomes. Tobin and colleagues have recently proposed cutting balloon angioplasty in children with resistant renal artery stenosis, although that technique may carry a higher complication rate than surgical repair.[21] In one long-term follow-up report by Shroff and coworkers, PTA and stenting in a series of 33 children with a mean age of 10 years was associated with a high rate of re-stenosis, one procedure-related death, and a number of complications.[17] McTaggart and colleagues reported that PTA was ineffective for patients with neurofibromatosis lesions of the renal artery because of the fibrotic nature of the disease.[19] Lacombe and Ricco emphasize that when patients sustain complications of PTA such as dissection, rupture, or thrombosis, operative repair may then be difficult.[22] Due to the relatively greater degree of fibroplasia seen in children with FMD, it is not surprising that PTA

is associated with a much greater incidence of intimal dissection and thrombosis in children who most often have lesions at the ostia. Due to ongoing growth and young age, there is a reluctance to insert stents into these lesions after balloon dilation as stents may induce intimal hyperplasia or create obstruction as the child grows. However, dissolvable stents may prove useful in the future in some children.

In the rare instance of distal segmental renal artery lesions resulting in segmental renal infarction, interventional infusion of ethanol for ablation may be curative as an alternative to segmental resection.

Surgical Treatment

Effective operative management for renovascular hypertension in children is preferable to nonsurgical treatment. The method selected must be based on the etiology and distribution of the lesions causing the stenosis.[23,24]

Nephrectomy and partial nephrectomy should be avoided unless no other choice is available. For example, it may be necessary to perform nephrectomy in infants with uncontrollable hypertension who have unilateral renal involvement, particularly when severe hypoplasia is found. Partial nephrectomy has been used primarily in those instances of renal atrophy with diffuse vascular involvement, or when the vessels are too small for successful reconstruction. However, it is also reasonable to attempt revascularization because partial or total nephrectomy is available as a last resort if the vascular repair fails. Additionally, because FMD may involve the opposite kidney many years later, nephrectomy is undesirable if revascularization is possible.

Although children with FMD have a predominance of ostial lesions, sufficient involvement of the wall of the artery may exist such that the extent of the lesion is greater than what might be apparent on the arteriogram. Thus, patch angioplasty is only rarely effective. Reimplantation of the renal artery into another site on the aorta is the most effective approach, but its success depends on the aortic wall being normal where the new orifice is to be created and on sufficient renal artery length to reach without tension. Although autotransplantation is an alternative under these circumstances, it is more complicated because both arterial and venous anastomoses are needed. Reimplantation is contraindicated in patients with mid-aortic syndrome in which the aortic wall is involved with FMD. Also, direct anastomosis to the aorta is not an option for patients with branch vessel lesions, which must be treated with balloon dilatation, bypass, or partial nephrectomy for distally located lesions. It is unfortunate that reimplantation is usually not possible in this group of patients because it provides the best and most durable results.[5]

Due to the complicating factors mentioned previously, aortorenal bypass is usually the best option for revascularization. Bypass from the aorta to the side of the renal artery distal to the stenosis was often used in the past. More recently, division of the diseased artery from the aorta and an end-to-end anastomosis between the bypass graft and the distal renal artery has been preferred. Depending on the size of the anastomosis, either a continuous suture technique which is interrupted several times, or an interrupted suture technique for the anastomosis is appropriate. The anastomosis of the bypass graft to the aorta can usually be performed with a continuous suture that is interrupted at least three times. The opening in the aortic wall is made with an appropriate-sized punch instrument rather than a simple incision. A 6-0 polypropylene suture is commonly used for the aorta-to-graft anastomosis, and 7-0 polypropylene can be used for the distal graft-to-renal artery anastomosis. In instances of mid-aortic syndrome in which such severe coarctation exists that an aorto-aortic bypass is needed, the renal bypass grafts may be taken off the aortic bypass graft. The patient should be heparinized in the standard fashion during aortic clamping.

Some debate exists regarding the best choice of aortorenal bypass grafts. In adults, Gore-Tex (W.L. Gore & Associates, Elkton, MD) grafts are frequently used. However, thrombosis occurs more commonly in prosthetic grafts than with autogenous material. There is little debate that the best choice for bypass in children is autogenous hypogastric artery, provided that it is not involved with FMD and that a sufficient length of artery can be harvested for the bypass. Additionally, because 70% of patients have simultaneous bilateral renal artery stenosis, this would require both hypogastric arteries to be harvested. Certainly some concern exists about taking both hypogastric arteries in children, although the exact risks of impotence and incontinence are not known. Due to these potential complications, the hypogastric artery is not an option for many patients. Therefore, the next best option, and the one most frequently used today for aortorenal bypass in small patients, is the saphenous vein. Because of the risk of aneurysmal dilatation in as many as 40% of patients who have such grafts placed in the visceral location, a procedure to cover the saphenous vein bypass grafts with a loose mandrill of Dacron mesh has been effective over the long term.[18,20,25]

Another debated issue relates to a subset of patients with mid-aortic syndrome who have varying degrees of narrowing of the superior mesenteric and celiac arteries.[7,8,25,26] A few scattered reports of patients with visceral artery stenosis who were initially seen with severe intermittent abdominal pain or intestinal infarction are available. However, in contrast to adults with lesions of this nature, most children are not symptomatic. In children with signs or symptoms related to superior mesenteric or celiac narrowing, a revascularization procedure by either direct reimplantation or bypass grafting can be performed. There is no consensus about whether asymptomatic children with marked visceral artery stenosis should have preemptive repair. Certainly, concomitant visceral artery bypass carries a high risk in a patient who is already having a bilateral renal artery bypass procedure, and possibly a simultaneous aorto-aortic bypass. Generally selective treatment of symptomatic patients with splanchnic artery occlusive disease is favored.[7,24,25] As the overwhelming majority of patients with lesions of this nature are asymptomatic and have a remarkable amount of collateral circulation demonstrable on aortography, visceral artery revascularization in asymptomatic patients is not routinely performed (Fig. 63-4). Observation for as long as

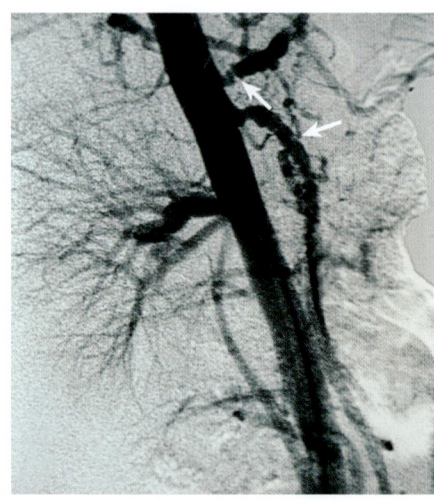

FIGURE 63-4 ■ This angiogram in a 7-year-old girl shows FMD changes in the celiac and superior mesenteric arteries (arrows). The patient has remained asymptomatic due to extensive collaterals from the inferior mesenteric artery via the arc of Riolan.

30 years has found that these patients have remained well, supporting a conservative approach.[5]

COMPLICATIONS AND OUTCOMES

A number of long-term follow-up studies of children who have had surgical repair for renovascular hypertension and its variants report a high degree of success and durable results, with cure rates ranging from 66–80%, improvement rates of 18–22%, and rare failures, with no mortality.[5,11,20,25] Additionally, no patients developed renal failure, and those who had preoperative oliguric renal failure invariably returned to normal after revascularization. Intraoperative renal thrombosis, embolization during the procedure, and intraoperative and postoperative hemorrhage were not reported. Postoperative graft thrombosis occurs in fewer than 5% of renal repairs. In cases where graft thrombosis is encountered, an immediate reoperation with thrombectomy and anastomotic revision, if necessary, is preferred over the use of thrombolytic agents. Late thrombosis can occur, but the incidence is less in children than in adults because of the absence of atherosclerosis. In patients who have late thrombosis, repeat bypass grafting is preferable, but often partial or total nephrectomy is required. It is important to monitor the patient's blood pressure indefinitely in follow-up because recurrence of hypertension usually indicates a problem with the vascular reconstruction or recurrent disease. Iliorenal bypass has been used in selected high-risk patients as a remedial operation with good results.[27]

Postoperative Imaging

Recurrent hypertension after revascularization procedures is due to either recurrent FMD or an anastomotic stenosis. As with renal transplant arterial stenosis, balloon dilatation has been an effective treatment approach. For follow-up, it is best to have the family monitor the child's blood pressure frequently at home with at least 6-month follow-up visits initially. The patient's blood pressure should remain normal, even with exercise. Some patients may require medication to keep their blood pressure within the normal range. In the asymptomatic patient, noninvasive imaging such as CTA or MRA is suggested every 5 years, with definitive selective angiography performed if these studies suggest abnormal findings.

Even when complicated, complete revascularization can be performed at a single operation and results are excellent. Whether patients have aortorenal bypass to either one or both kidneys, or a simultaneous aorto-aortic bypass procedure, 80% of children have been cured of their hypertension without the need for medications and 18% are markedly improved, needing minimal antihypertensive medications.[5,7] Only about 2% of patients are unchanged after operation. In the absence of a demonstrated vascular lesion, these patients probably have sustained hypertension because of ischemic nephrosclerosis.

REFERENCES

1. Goldblatt H, Lynch J, Hanzel RF, et al. Studies on experimental hypertension: Production of persistent elevation of systolic blood pressure by means of renal ischemia. J Exp Med 1934;59:347–9.
2. Safian RD, Textor SC. Renal artery stenosis. N Engl J Med 2001;334:431–42.
3. Simoes E, Silva AC, Diniz JS, et al. The renin-angiotensin system in childhood hypertension: Selective increase in angiotensin (1–7) in essential hypertension. J Pediatr 2004;145:93–8.
4. Foster JH, Pettinger WA, Oates JA, et al. Malignant hypertension secondary to renal artery stenosis in children. Ann Surg 1966;164:700–13.
5. O'Neill JA. Long-term outcome with surgical treatment of renovascular hypertension. J Pediatr Surg 1998;33:106–11.
6. Morris CA. Williams Syndrome. In: Pagon RA, Bird TD, Colan CR, et al, editors. Gene Reviews, (internet). Seattle: University of Washington; 2006.
7. O'Neill JA, Berkowitz H, Fellows KJ, et al. Mid-aortic syndrome and hypertension in childhood. J Pediatr Surg 1995;30:164–72.
8. Connolly JE, Wilson SE, Lawrence PL, et al. Middle aortic syndrome: Distal thoracic and abdominal coarctation, a disorder with multiple etiologies. J Am Coll Surg 2002;194:774–81.
9. Miura K, Takahashi T, Takahashi I, et al. Renovascular hypertension due to antithrombin deficiency in childhood. Pediatr Nephrol 2004;19:1294–6.
10. Johnson SL, Lock RJ, Gompels MM. Takayasu arteritis: A review. J Clin Pathol 2002;55:481–6.
11. Piercy KT, Hundley JC, Stafford JM, et al. Renovascular disease in children and adolescents. J Vasc Surg 2005;41:973–82.
12. Vo NJ, Hammelman BD, Rocadio JM, et al. Anatomic distribution of renal artery stenosis in children: Implications for imaging. Pediatr Radiol 2006;36:1032–6.
13. Radermacher J, Chavan A, Bleck J, et al. Use of Doppler ultrasonography to predict the outcome of therapy for renal artery stenosis. N Engl J Med 2001;344:410–17.
14. Upchurch GR, Henke PK, Eagleton MJ, et al. Pediatric splanchnic arterial occlusive disease: Clinical relevance and operative treatment. J Vasc Surg 2002;35:860–7.
15. Hricick DE, Bronning PJ, Kopelman R, et al. Captopril-induced functional renal insufficiency in patients with bilateral renal stenosis or renal artery stenosis in a solitary kidney. N Engl J Med 1983;308:373–6.
16. Marshalleck F. Pediatric arterial interventions. Tech Vasc Interventional Rad 2010;13:238–43
17. Shroff R, Roebuck DJ, Gordon I, et al. Angioplasty for renovascular hypertension in children: 20-year experience. Pediatrics 2006;118:268–75.
18. Berkowitz HD, O'Neill JA. Renovascular hypertension in children. J Vasc Surg 1989;9:46–55.
19. McTaggart SJ, Gulati S, Walker RG, et al. Evaluation and long-term outcome of pediatric renovascular hypertension. Pediatr Nephrol 2000;14:1022–9.
20. Lacombe M. Role of surgery in the treatment of renovascular hypertension in the child. Bull Acad Natl Med 2003;187:1081–93.
21. Tobin RB, Pelchovitz OJ, Baskin KM, et al. Cutting balloon angioplasty in children with resistant renal artery stenosis. J Vasc Interv Radiol 2007;18:663–9.
22. Lacombe M, Ricco JB. Surgical revascularization after complicated or failed percutaneous transluminal renal angioplasty. J Vasc Surg 2006;44:537–44.
23. Barral X, de Latour B, Vola M, et al. Surgery of the abdominal aorta and its branches in children: Late follow-up. J Vasc Surg 2006;43:1138–44.
24. O'Neill JA. Anomalies of the aorta and branches. In: Mulliken JB, Burrows PE, Fishman SJ, editor. Vascular Anomalies: Hemangiomas and Malformations. NY: Oxford Univ Press; 2012. in press.
25. Stanley JC, Criado E, Upchurch GR, et al. Pediatric renovascular hypertension: 132 primary and 30 secondary operations in 97 children. J Vasc Surg 2006;44:1219–28.
26. Delis KT, Gloviczki P. Middle aortic syndrome: From presentation to contemporary open surgical and endovascular treatment. Perspect Vasc Surg Endovasc Ther 2005;17:187–203.
27. Grigoryants V, Henke PK, Watson NC, et al. Iliorenal bypass: Indications and outcomes following 41 reconstructions. Ann Vasc Surg 2007;21:1–9.

NEOPLASMS

CHAPTER 64

PRINCIPLES OF ADJUVANT THERAPY IN CHILDHOOD CANCER

Daniel von Allmen

HISTORICAL OVERVIEW

Early strides in improving oncologic outcomes through the use of single chemotherapeutic agents were first reported by Farber in 1948[1] and Li in 1956.[2] As additional chemotherapeutic agents were developed, they were combined in multidrug regimens that demonstrated both significantly improved response rates and response duration.[3,4] By the late 1970s, multimodal therapy was shown to improve cure rates in children with Wilms tumor[5] and was being adopted for the treatment of rhabdomyosarcoma, Ewing sarcoma, lymphoma, and other solid tumors.[6] The close collaboration of multidisciplinary cooperative groups and the development of improved supportive care measures added impetus to progress. During the 1990s, dose-intensive chemotherapy programs were shown to be successful in improving outcome for patients with Burkitt lymphoma, neuroblastoma, and other advanced-stage solid tumors.[7–9] In addition, improvements in outcome were achieved either by alternating effective groups of chemotherapeutic agents to overcome or prevent resistance,[10] or by administering agents by continuous infusion rather than bolus.[11]

By 2001, noncytotoxic biologic therapies (e.g., signal transduction inhibitors, various tissue growth factor receptor inhibitors, antiangiogenesis agents, tumor-targeted antibodies, and adoptive immunotherapy techniques) were developed to target specific biologic pathways.[12] In addition, improvements in radiation therapy have led to the development of intraoperative radiation therapy and radiosurgery techniques. Collectively, these advancements have resulted in the continually increasing survival of children with solid tumors and a profound improvement in their quality of life.

The aim of this chapter is to present the key aspects of contemporary multimodal therapy, touching on treatment rationales, the impact of tumor biology on specific treatment approaches, and future trends.

INCIDENCE AND SURVIVAL RATES

Although childhood cancers account for only 2% of all reported cancer cases in the general population, they account for 10% of all deaths in children.[13] On average, 1 to 2 of every 10,000 children in the USA develop cancer each year.[14] The distribution of the types of cancer in childhood is different than in adults. Whereas most cancers in adults have an epithelial cell origin, <10% of childhood cancers fall into this category.

The incidence of specific cancers varies by age, gender, and race. Overall, however, it rose from 11.5 cases per 100,000 children in 1975 to 14.8 per 100,000 in 2004.[14] The peak incidence (>200 cases per million) is in children younger than 2 years of age. The incidence then decreases to a low of 82.5 cases per million by age 9 years, at which point it begins to rise again through adolescence. In children younger than age 2, central nervous system malignancies, neuroblastoma, acute myeloid leukemia (AML), Wilms tumor, and retinoblastoma account for the majority of diagnoses. In children 2 to 4 years of age, acute lymphoblastic leukemia (ALL) is the most common childhood cancer. After age 9 years, the incidence of Hodgkin disease, osteosarcoma, and Ewing sarcoma begins to increase sharply.[13]

Over the past several decades, the mortality from childhood cancers has declined dramatically (40%),[15] while the 5-year survival rate has risen from 58% in 1975–1977 to close to 80% in 1996–2003.[14]

TUMOR PATHOLOGY AND CHEMOTHERAPEUTIC REGIMENS

Although the spectrum of malignancies in children is more limited than that in adults, the exact diagnosis is often more difficult to establish due to the common histologic appearance of small round blue cells. As these primitive malignancies often lack morphologically distinguishing characteristics, Ewing sarcoma, neuroblastoma, lymphoma, small-cell osteosarcoma, and primitive neuroectodermal tumors may appear quite similar by light microscopy. Given that chemotherapy regimens must be carefully tailored to each specific tumor type, pediatric subspecialists have continued to better define prognostic subgroups for many tumors. These subgroups help to determine the best therapy and the dose intensity required for optimal outcomes. The initial step in the accurate diagnosis of a tumor is the availability of adequate tissue with which to make the diagnosis. The quality and quantity of this tissue should be discussed with the surgeon, the pathologist, and the pediatric oncologist before the procedure to ensure the proper handling of the specimen (e.g., the need for fresh tissue, frozen samples, and fixed specimens for histologic and biologic diagnostic use). Whereas light microscopy remains the primary tool of pathologists, immunohistology, electron microscopy, DNA content of tumor, cytogenetic abnormalities, and specific tumor gene expression are now used to determine specific tumor subgroups.

TUMOR BIOLOGY

Genetic alterations within a single cell, such as the activation of an oncogene or the loss of a tumor suppressor gene, can lead to the accumulation of cells lacking the ability to respond to growth-regulating signals and the subsequent development of cancer.

Understanding normal cell growth and regulation is a prerequisite to understanding both the genetic basis for the development of childhood cancer and the mechanisms of action of chemotherapeutic agents designed to kill rapidly proliferating cancer cells (Fig. 64-1). Normal cell growth occurs by the regulated progression of the cell through the cell cycle of DNA replication and mitosis. This cycle is separated by two intervening growth phases, referred to as G_1 and G_2. Cells can temporarily leave the cell cycle and enter a resting state referred to as G_0. They are programmed to proceed through the cell cycle by a series of external and internal stimuli. Binding of proteins (growth factors) to cell surface receptors stimulates a cascade of cytoplasmic signaling proteins (membrane kinases and signal transducers) that carries the stimuli to the nucleus. Other proteins (transcription factors) then bind to the DNA, resulting in the expression of growth-regulating genes. When functioning normally, these genes promote or prevent cell division, direct the cell to differentiate, or initiate apoptosis, the process of programmed cell death.

Alterations in one or several of these signaling proteins can lead to the unregulated cell growth characteristics of cancer cells. Oncogenes result from mutation or overexpression of the normal growth-promoting proto-oncogenes. Tumor suppressor genes are normally present in cells and function as negative regulators to slow the process of proliferation and allow time for cellular repair. When oncogenes become activated or tumor suppressor gene function is lost, cells lose their ability to respond to the usual regulatory protein stimuli and proliferate rapidly. Rapid cell proliferation leads to accumulation of more genetic defects, activation of additional oncogenes, and loss of more negative regulators as the cells become increasingly more malignant. Through the study of chromosomal aberrations, more than 100 oncogenes and 25 tumor suppressor genes have now been identified.

CANCER CYTOGENETICS

With the discovery of chromosomal banding techniques in the 1970s, cancer cytogeneticists were able to identify sub-chromosomal deletions, inversions, and translocations occurring in cancer cells. Investigation of these aberrant regions led to the identification of oncogenes and tumor suppressor genes, a process that continues today.

The presence of consistent cytogenetic abnormalities associated with a specific childhood leukemia or solid tumor is useful in both cancer diagnosis and prognosis. Specific cytogenetic aberrations have been identified in rhabdomyosarcoma, Ewing sarcoma, synovial sarcoma, germ cell tumors, medulloblastoma, neuroblastoma,

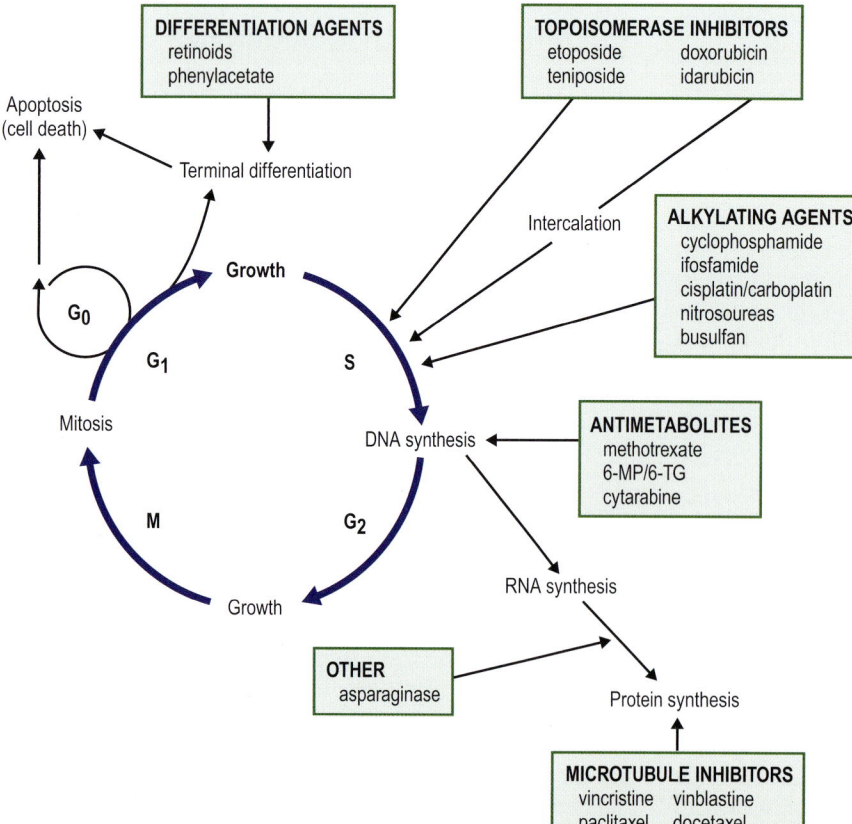

FIGURE 64-1 ■ The cell cycle. Normal cell growth proceeds through DNA replication (S) and mitosis (M), separated by two growth phases (G_1 and G_2). Cells leave the cell cycle to enter a resting phase (G_0) to differentiate or to die. Chemotherapy agents act at specific sites along the cell cycle, as indicated. (Adapted from Balis FRM, Holcenberg JS, Poplack DG. General principles of chemotherapy. In Pizzo P, Poplack D, editors. Principles and Practice of Pediatric Oncology. 3rd ed. Philadelphia: Lippincott-Raven; 1997. p. 219.)

retinoblastoma, and Wilms tumor.[16] Chromosomal aberrations can also be helpful in predicting prognosis. For example, the finding of a chromosome 1q deletion, the presence of double-minute chromatin bodies, or the presence of homogeneous staining regions in neuroblastoma confer a poor prognosis.[17]

The treatment of Wilms tumor based on risk stratification determined by multiple tumor characteristics that impact prognosis (including loss of heterozygosity at 1p and 16q) is a topic of ongoing study. In the future, specific tumors may be identified by a specific 'fingerprint' determined by microarray analysis that can simultaneously analyze expression of thousands of genes on a single chip.[18] The ability to tailor therapy to individual patients based on the genetic characteristics of their particular tumor is quickly becoming a reality.

CLINCIAL TRIALS

The goal of chemotherapy in children is to maximize tumor kill while maintaining acceptable side effects. Clinical trials have led to the development of combination chemotherapy regimens for most childhood cancers. Adjuvant therapy (initiated after local control measures) has remained the mainstay of treatment, though neoadjuvant chemotherapy (initiated before definitive local control measures) has proved to be effective in patients with metastatic disease as well as in those with large primary tumors. In the latter clinical setting, chemotherapy is used to decrease the size of the tumor, making it more amenable to complete resection.

The first step in the clinical development of an anticancer agent is to define a tolerable dose. Phase I clinical trials are designed as dose-escalation studies to determine the maximally tolerated dose of a new drug given as a single agent. In a phase II trial, a consistent dose of the agent is tested for efficacy in a variety of tumor types to establish the spectrum of activity of the agent. Once an agent has demonstrated activity toward a specific cancer, this agent is tested for efficacy when combined with other known active agents for that tumor system.

Standard therapy for a specific tumor type is established through phase III clinical trials. These trials use a prospective randomized design to compare two chemotherapy combinations. At the conclusion of the trial, the chemotherapy regimen with the greatest efficacy and the least toxicity is selected as the standard regimen for that tumor. Subsequent phase III trials compare new regimens with this newly established standard. It is through the development of phase I through III clinical trials within national cooperative groups that treatment advances are made.

Combination chemotherapy remains the mainstay of treatment. The likelihood of cure is maximized when all available active agents are administered simultaneously after local control measures have been undertaken and the tumor burden is as low as possible.[19] This approach has led to increased survival rates in children with neuroblastoma, Ewing sarcoma, anaplastic Wilms tumor, and osteosarcoma.

ADJUVANT AND NEOADJUVANT CHEMOTHERAPY

The use of adjuvant chemotherapy is supported by the finding that less than 20% of sarcoma and lymphoma patients with initially nonmetastatic solid tumors can be cured by operative or radiation therapy alone or combined.[20] Tumor recurrence is generally at a distant site, lending support to the hypothesis that micrometastatic disease exists at the time of presentation for most patients with clinically nonmetastatic disease. As many as 40% of patients with Wilms tumor can be cured with resection or radiation therapy alone. However, survival increases to 90% with the addition of combination chemotherapy.[21]

As the goal of adjuvant chemotherapy is to prevent the growth of metastatic disease, it is vital that chemotherapy begins as soon as possible after local control measures are employed. For this reason, most current chemotherapy protocols for childhood solid tumors advise that chemotherapy is initiated within 2 weeks of operation.[22] In children with Wilms tumor, rapid assessment of tumor biology and risk stratification is important for determining the appropriate chemotherapy regimen.

Neoadjuvant chemotherapy has become standard in the treatment of Ewing sarcoma and osteosarcoma, and has the theoretical advantage of minimizing resistance to chemotherapy.[10,23,24] Delayed surgical intervention may allow a more complete or less morbid resection, as well as histologic assessment of tumor responsiveness to the chemotherapy agents. Neoadjuvant chemotherapy is beneficial only in tumors for which a known highly effective combination chemotherapy program limits the risk of tumor progression at the primary site. For example, diagnostic biopsy followed by neoadjuvant chemotherapy and delayed resection of the primary tumor for complex neuroblastoma reduces the operative complication rate without compromising survival.[25]

DOSE INTENSITY AND DURATION OF CHEMOTHERAPY

Advances in supportive care have enabled increased dose intensity of active chemotherapy agents in pediatric clinical trials. These advances decrease or minimize the toxic effects of higher-dose chemotherapy on normal tissues. The use of cytokines (granulocyte colony-stimulating factor [G-CSF] and interleukin-11 [IL-11]) to speed recovery of white blood cells and platelets,[26,27] and the use of cardioprotectant agents to allow use of a higher cumulative dose of doxorubicin have helped in the development of new dose-intensive therapy for solid tumors.[28] Similarly, progress in bone marrow and stem cell transplantation have allowed dose intensities to be pushed to the upper limits.[29–32]

The positive impact of increasing the dose intensity on improving response rate and survival has been demonstrated for Burkitt lymphoma, osteosarcoma, Ewing sarcoma, testicular cancer, and advanced ovarian cancer.[7–9,33–36] The duration of chemotherapy programs for most pediatric solid tumors has been 1 year. However, as the dose intensity of chemotherapy programs has increased, the duration of therapy has concomitantly decreased. This downward trend is likely to continue.

CHEMOTHERAPEUTIC AGENTS

Chemotherapy drugs are divided into classes by their mechanism of action. These classes include alkylating agents (cisplatin and its analogs), antimetabolites, topoisomerase inhibitors, antimicrotubule agents, differentiation agents, miscellaneous nonclassified agents, and biologic agents. Understanding the mechanism of action for each of these agents helps in establishing combination therapies with synergistic antitumor effects. The most common agents from each class, their mechanism of action, common side effects, and tumors in which they are active are listed in Table 64-1.

ACUTE CHEMOTHERAPY TOXICITY AND SUPPORTIVE CARE

Most acute toxicities in childhood solid tumor therapy are reversible. Because toxicity is greatest in normal cells that have the highest rate of turnover, normal bone marrow cells, mucosal lining cells, liver cells, and hair cells are frequently affected. The most common side effects from combination chemotherapy include nausea and vomiting, myelosuppression, hair loss, mucositis, diarrhea, liver function abnormalities, and allergic reactions.

Myelosuppression is an expected side effect of almost all treatment protocols for solid tumors. Transfusions of packed cells and platelets are frequently needed. Of greatest concern is the risk of severe life-threatening bacterial or fungal infections that occur during episodes of neutropenia. In dose-intensive regimens, more than 75% of chemotherapy courses result in hospitalization for fever, with the incidence of bacteremia ranging from 10–20% per course.[37]

Several chemotherapeutic agents have specific toxicities. For example, vincristine and doxorubicin are vesicants and can cause severe skin and tissue necrosis if the drug extravasates into the subcutaneous tissue. Because doxorubicin and related anthracyclines have cumulative cardiotoxic effects, the total lifetime anthracycline dose must be limited for each patient to minimize the risk of developing congestive heart failure. Cisplatin has toxic renal effects and is often combined with another nephrotoxic agent, ifosfamide, in the treatment of osteosarcoma and neuroblastoma. Cisplatin also can cause hearing loss, especially in patients who receive high doses. Vincristine and vinblastine can cause cumulative peripheral neuropathies, and drug doses frequently must be altered to prevent significant morbidity. All of these toxicities must be considered when designing therapeutic programs.

Success in improving treatment outcomes is partially attributed to advances in supportive care. The routine use of hematopoietic growth factors, specifically G-CSF,

results in more rapid granulocyte recovery and shorter hospitalizations for fever and neutropenia.[26] In addition, IL-11 enhances platelet recovery, decreases the depth of the platelet nadir, and decreases platelet transfusion requirements.[27,38,39] It is well tolerated and is beneficial in combination regimens that induce severe thrombocytopenia.[40,41]

The gastrointestinal tract is injured by cytarabine, anthracyclines, and high-dose methotrexate; however, the folate derivative Leucovorin can be given to rescue normal mucosal and bone marrow cells from the effects of the latter. No rescue is known for the mucositis and diarrhea which occur with other agents. In addition to enhancing platelet production, IL-11 may help speed recovery from gastrointestinal injury after chemotherapy.[42]

Renal toxicity can occur from the use of cisplatin, ifosfamide, and high-dose methotrexate. Cisplatin causes renal tubular damage, leading to elevation of levels of blood urea nitrogen and creatinine; this effect is generally reversible. Both ifosfamide and cisplatin cause renal electrolyte wasting in which hypokalemia, hypocalcemia, hypophosphatemia, and hypomagnesemia can occur. Renal injury from these agents can be improved by hyperhydration and forced diuresis. Mesna can prevent hemorrhagic cystitis resulting from cyclophosphamide and ifosfamide by binding to the bladder-toxic acrolein metabolites.[40]

Additionally, a recent study demonstrates that amifostine administered prior to and during cisplatin infusion significantly reduces the risk of severe ototoxicity in children with average risk medulloblastoma who are undergoing treatment with dose-intense chemotherapy.[43]

TARGETING BIOLOGIC PATHWAYS

Over the past several decades, many of the key genetic events that control carcinogenesis have been identified. More recently, progress has been made in the development of agents designed to target specific biologic pathways. These agents include signal transduction inhibitors (tissue growth factor receptor inhibitors, antiangiogenesis agents, and biologic response modifiers), individual cytokines, tumor-targeted antibody therapies, and adoptive immunotherapy techniques. The development of these agents differs from the development of agents used in standard cytotoxic therapy. Whereas standard phase I studies for cytotoxic agents are designed to define the maximal tolerated dose, in biologic targeted therapy the optimal therapeutic dose is well below the maximal tolerated dose. The challenge in evaluating these newer agents is how to select the optimal dose and schedule, combine tumor-targeted agents with classic cytotoxic therapy, and validate the intended effect on the selected target for these biologic compounds designed to treat minimal residual disease.

Signal Transduction Inhibitors

Cellular signaling is a basic biologic function of all normal cells. Signaling can be extracellular (e.g., growth factor

TABLE 64-1 Chemotherapeutic Agents

Class of Agent	Mechanism of Action	Antitumor Activity	Acute Toxicities
Alkylating Agents			
Mustards			
Nitrogen mustard	Alkylation, DNA crosslinking	Hodgkin disease	Myelo, N/V, A, mucositis, phlebitis, vesicant
Melphalan	Alkylation, DNA crosslinking	Rhabdo; for BMT: Ewing, NB	Myelo, mucositis, N/V, A, VOD (HD)
Cyclophosphamide	(Prodrug) alkylation, DNA crosslinking	Rhabdo; Wilms; NB; Ewing	Myelo, immuno, N/V, A, cystitis, SIADH, cardiac (HD), lung (HD), VOD (HD)
Ifosfamide	Alkylation, DNA crosslinking	Ewing; rhabdo; osteosarcoma; NB	Myelo, N/V, A, hepatic, renal, cystitis, neuro
Busulfan	Alkylation, DNA crosslinking	Leukemia	Myelo, skin, lung, A
NITROSOUREAS			
BCNU	DNA crosslinking	CNS tumors; lymphoma	Myelo, N/V, A, lung, renal
CCNU	DNA crosslinking	CNS tumors; lymphoma	Myelo, N/V, A, lung, renal
TETRAZINES			
Dacarbazine (DTIC)	DNA methylation	Hodgkin; sarcomas; NB	Myelo, hepatic, flu-like illness, N/V, A
Temozolomide	DNA crosslinking	Brain tumors	Myelo, N/V, diarrhea, constipation, rash, lethargy, hepatic
Other Alkylators			
Thiotepa	Alkylation, DNA crosslinking	CNS tumors; for BMT: sarcomas, NB	Myelo, N/V, A, diarrhea, mucositis, skin, VOD (HD)
Procarbazine	(Prodrug) methylation; free radical formation	Hodgkin; CNS tumors	Myelo, N/V, rash, allergy, mucositis
Platinum Agents			
Cisplatin	DNA/platinum adduct formation; DNA crosslinking	Osteosarcoma; NB; hepatoblastoma; germ cell tumors; CNS tumors	N/V (severe), A, myelo, renal, neuro, mucositis, ototoxicity
Carboplatin	DNA/platinum adduct formation; DNA crosslinking	NB; CNS tumors; retinoblastoma; sarcomas in HD	Myelo, N/V (mild), renal and ototoxicity rare
Antimetabolites			
Methotrexate	Inhibitor of dihydrofolate reductase; interferes with folate metabolism	Leukemia; lymphoma; osteosarcoma in HD	Myelo, rash, mucositis, hepatic, renal (HD)
5-Fluorouracil	(Prodrug) inhibits thymidine synthesis	Hepatoblastoma; carcinomas	Myelo, N/V, mucositis, diarrhea, hyperpigmentation, neuro
Cytarabine	(Prodrug) incorporated into DNA; inhibits DNA replication	Leukemia; lymphoma	Myelo, malaise, N/V, mucositis, diarrhea, neuro (HD), eye (HD), skin (HD)
6-Mercaptopurine, 6-Thioguanine	(Prodrugs) inhibit purine synthesis	Leukemia	Myelo, N/V, hepatic, mucositis
Gemcitabine	Inhibitor of DNA synthesis	Hodgkin disease, in phase II testing for leukemia	Myelo, rash, fluid retention, hepatic, N/V
Topoisomerase Inhibitors			
Epipodophyllotoxins			
Etoposide	Non-DNA-binding topoisomerase II inhibitor; stabilizes DNA double-strand breaks	NB; Ewing; rhabdo; germ cell; leukemia; CNS tumors; lymphoma	Myelo, N/V, rash, allergy, low BP, A, mucositis, hepatic (HD)
Tenoposide	Same as etoposide	NB; leukemia	Myelo, N/V, rash, allergy, low BP, A, mucositis, hepatic (HD)
Anthracyclines			
Doxorubicin	DNA intercalation; free radical formation; topoisomerase II inhibitor	Wilms; Ewing; NB; lymphoma; leukemia	Myelo, N/V, A, mucositis, diarrhea, phlebitis, vesicant, hepatic, cardiac
Daunorubicin	Same as doxorubicin	Leukemia; lymphoma	Myelo, N/V, A, mucositis, diarrhea, phlebitis, vesicant, hepatic, cardiac
Dactinomycin	Same as doxorubicin	Wilms; rhabdo; Ewing	Myelo, N/V, A, mucositis, hepatic, vesicant
Bleomycin	DNA intercalation; free radical formation	Germ cell; Hodgkin; lymphoma	Myelo, skin, allergy, mucositis, lung

Continued

TABLE 64-1   **Chemotherapeutic Agents—cont'd**

Class of Agent	Mechanism of Action	Antitumor Activity	Acute Toxicities
Camptothecin Analogs			
Topotecan	Topoisomerase I inhibitor	Rhabdo, neuroblastoma	Myelo, N/V, A, mucositis, diarrhea, hepatic
Irinotecan	Topoisomerase I inhibitor	In phase II testing for rhabdo	Diarrhea, myelo, N/V, hepatic
Antimicrotubule Agents ***Vinca Alkaloids***			
Vincristine	Binds tubulin; prevents microtubule formation; blocks mitosis	Sarcomas; leukemia; Hodgkin; constipation, neuro, vesicant, Wilms; lymphoma	SIADH
Vinblastine	Same as vincristine	Hodgkin; germ cell	Myelo, mucositis, vesicant
Taxanes			
Paclitaxel (Taxol)	Binds microtubules; blocks microtubule depolymerization; blocks mitosis	Ovarian carcinoma	Myelo, A, mucositis, paresthesias, hypersensitivity
Docetaxel (Taxotere)	Same as paclitaxel	In phase II testing for sarcomas and other solid tumors	Myelo, A, skin, hypersensitivity, fluid retention, paresthesias, mucositis
Differentiation Agents ***Retinoids***			
Cis-retinoic acid	Binds to retinoic acid receptor; induces differentiation	NB	Skin, mucositis, eye, pseudotumor, hepatic, electrolyte
All-*trans*-retinoic acid	Same as *cis*-retinoic acid	APML; in phase II testing for Wilms	Skin, mucositis, eye, pseudotumor, hepatic, electrolyte
Fenretinide	Still being investigated; induces cell death, not differentiation	Phase II testing for NB	Dry skin/lips, loss of night vision, increased triglycerides, hepatic, N/V
Miscellaneous Nonclassified			
Corticosteroids	Lympholysis; multiple other effects not well classified	Leukemia (ALL); lymphoma	Weight gain, high BP, high glucose, mood change, many others
L-Asparaginase, PEG-asparaginase	Asparagine depletion; inhibition of protein synthesis	Leukemia (ALL); lymphoma	Anorexia, hepatic, pancreatitis, coagulopathy, neuro

A, alopecia; ALL, acute lymphoblastic leukemia; APML, acute promyelocytic leukemia; BMT, bone marrow transplant; BP, blood pressure; CNS tumors, central nervous system tumors; HD, high dose; myelo, myelosuppression; NB, neuroblastoma; neuro, neurologic toxicity; N/V, nausea and vomiting; PEG, polyethylene glycol; rhabdo, rhabdomyosarcoma; SIADH, syndrome of inappropriate antidiuretic hormone; VOD, veno-occlusive disease.

Data from Balis FM, Holcenberg JS, Poplack DG. General principles of chemotherapy. In: Pizzo P, Poplack D, editors. Principles and Practice of Pediatric Oncology. 3rd ed. Philadelphia: Lippincott-Raven; 1997. p. 215–72; Ratain M, Teicher B, O'Dwyer P, et al. Pharmacology of cancer chemotherapy. In: DeVita V, Hellman S, Rosenberg S, editors. Cancer: Principles and Practice of Oncology. Philadelphia: Lippincott-Raven; 1997. p. 375–85; Dorr R, Von Hoff D. Drug monographs. In: Dorr R, Von Hoff D, editors. Cancer Chemotherapy Handbook. Norwalk, CT: Appleton & Lange; 1994. p. 129.

receptor tyrosine kinase) or through multiple intracellular effector and survival pathways (e.g., RAS, RAF, TP53, BCL-2). Cancer cells differ from normal cells as they are associated with chromosomal mutations. These mutations result in cancer cells being dependent on several hyperactive signaling pathways. The rationale behind signal transduction therapy is that blocking the hyperactive pathways induces cancer cell apoptosis. By contrast, normal cells have redundant signaling pathways that protect them against cell death. Multiple new signal transduction inhibitors are in development.[44,45]

Biologic Response Modifiers

The goal of biologic response modifiers is to stimulate the immune system to help eradicate tumors. The human immune system is designed to identify and destroy foreign cells. One of the mysteries of oncology is why a patient's immune system is often unable to eliminate malignant cells. The development of biologic response modifiers is a relatively new branch of cancer therapy. It is designed to enhance or stimulate the natural products of the immune system (lymphocytes, antibodies, and cytokines) to better recognize and destroy cancer cells.

T-lymphocytes directly interact with specific cell surface antigens on a target cell, causing cell lysis through cytotoxic granule release or programmed cell death. These cytotoxic lymphocytes are involved with the killing of tumor cells. To initiate this response, antigens must be presented to the T cell by antigen-presenting cells (APCs) that express the antigens bound to major histocompatibility complex proteins in the presence of stimulatory cytokines. Cytokines or interleukins (e.g., IL-2, interferon-α, tumor necrosis factor) are proteins produced by helper T-lymphocytes and monocytes that help recruit other effector cells, including APCs, as well as regulate antibody production. The effector cells of the immune system (e.g., granulocytes, monocytes, macrophages, eosinophils, dendritic cells) can become tumor selective when activated by a specific antibody, a process called antibody-dependent cell-mediated cytotoxicity.

Immunotherapy with biologic response modifiers takes advantage of all these immune functions. The goal of this therapy is to improve the immunogenicity of a tumor and allow it to be recognized and targeted for destruction by the immune system. Immunotherapy can be divided into two major categories: adoptive immunotherapy and tumor-targeted antibody therapy.

Adoptive Immunotherapy

Adoptive immunotherapy involves the use of tumor vaccines made from autologous or allogeneic tumor-associated antigens. Specific purified tumor antigens can be made more immunogenic by attachment to carrier proteins (adjuvants). Clinical trials using this type of tumor vaccine have been performed primarily in melanoma patients.[46] Other forms of immunotherapy involve the use of cytokine infusions such as interferon-α, IL-2, and tumor necrosis factor to stimulate immune reaction against tumor cells.[47]

Tumor-Targeted Antibody Therapy

Passive immunity involves the use of monoclonal antibodies (mAbs) or cytotoxic effector cells produced in vitro and infused into the patient. mAbs have been tested in patients with neuroblastoma. A drawback of murine mAb therapy is that when these antibodies are repeatedly infused into humans, most patients will ultimately produce a human/anti-mouse antibody, which renders further antibody treatment useless.

Chimeric human/mouse antibodies have been produced that decrease the risk of human/anti-mouse antibody generation.[48] Recombinant chimeric antibodies are produced by linking the constant region of human antibodies to the variable combining region of a mouse mAb. These chimeric antibodies have been successfully used in the treatment of children with high-risk neuroblastoma.[49]

Although this field of targeted biologic therapy is still in its infancy, the future looks bright for the continued development of new targeted therapies. These therapies are the outgrowth of the rapid advances being made in the understanding of cellular signaling pathways and immune mechanisms.

LOCAL TUMOR CONTROL

As metastatic disease in young patients is more readily eradicated than in adults, control of local disease is critical to favorable outcomes in children. Advances in techniques used to obtain local control (other than complete surgical excision) are continually changing as new technology offers more and more opportunity to effectively treat disease locally while minimizing morbidity.

Radiation Oncology

Given the important role played by radiation therapy in the treatment of numerous pediatric tumors, it is important for clinicians to understand its biologic principles. Radiation impacts tumor growth through two primary mechanisms of action. Radiation can have a direct impact on the cellular DNA, resulting in impaired cell division. Alternatively, it can result in the production of reactive free radicals that indirectly damage genetic material and interfere with the reproductive capacity of normal or malignant tissues. In most cases, the radiation effect is through production of these free radicals.

The sensitivity of normal and malignant cells to radiation varies widely between cell populations. Ionizing radiation initially results in sublethal damage to cells. The therapeutic effect of radiation therapy exploits the differences between the ability of a normal cell to repair this sublethal damage and the slower response of radiosensitive tumor cells. Fractionated dosing allows normal cells to recover while having a cumulative effect on tumor cells. The effect of ionizing radiation on tumors depends on the number of actively reproducing cells at the time of exposure and the length of the cellular regeneration cycle. As most of the damage is indirect and focused on reproduction, malignant lesions usually show a delayed effect to radiation therapy. The tumor may begin to shrink or eventually disappear weeks to months after treatment.

Acute reactions to ionizing radiation depend on the balance between replication and cell death. These reactions are affected by increased intervals between dose fractions that allow enhanced cellular repopulation. The radiation fraction size has a small impact on what volume of cells are immediately destroyed. Conversely, the long-term effects of therapy depend primarily on the total exposure dose and the size of each treatment fraction. The therapeutic ratio may be enhanced by exploiting the difference between the early and late radiation effects. Techniques can be used to reduce the late effects by lowering the dose per fraction and increasing the number of fractions delivered over the conventional treatment time.

Radiation therapy may be combined with operation in a strategic manner to deliver the highest effective dose to a well-defined site while minimizing the dose to surrounding normal structures.[50] Preoperative radiation may permit a smaller treatment area because the operative bed has not been manipulated. In larger tumors, preoperative radiation may reduce the lesion volume sufficiently to allow a subsequent resection. In addition, potential tumor seeding during operative removal may be reduced because cells that may be surgically disseminated have been rendered incapable of reproducing. On the other hand, preoperative radiation may delay the surgical procedure and alter the staging information obtained at operation.

For these reasons, many combined strategies use postoperative radiation, which allows the treatment fields and doses to be determined after operative resection and histologic assessment.[51] Higher doses can be delivered postoperatively once the target volumes have been more accurately defined. Doses to the periphery of the tumor can be fine-tuned, depending on the presence of gross, microscopic, or no residual disease. However, postoperative delivery may require a wider treatment area after extensive surgical manipulation.

Soft tissue sarcoma provides a model for the adjunctive role of radiation therapy. Resection is the primary method of obtaining local control; however, radiation therapy can be effective when clear margins are not possible.[52] Combined therapy has resulted in dramatically improved survival.[53] In extremity lesions, radiation also allows more conservative resection with limb sparing. Although local tumor control rates of 75–98% have been achieved with limb salvage rates greater than 80%, wound complications occur in as many as 40% of patients. Neoadjuvant radiation at more modest doses (30 Gy total) has decreased the complication rate while maintaining excellent (>95%) five-year local control, and ultimately, limb salvage.[52] Postoperative adjuvant radiation therapy also may be advantageous.[54]

Several aspects of radiation treatment in pediatric patients warrant special consideration. Attention should be paid to immobilizing or sedating children so that ionizing doses can be targeted to the desired area without inappropriate exposure of surrounding tissues. Pediatric radiation oncologists may use lower treatment doses and accept a higher recurrence rate to ensure lower toxicity, especially in important developing organs such as the brain. The normal tolerance of organs or tissues may be adversely affected when chemotherapeutic agents are also used. The long-term effects of combined-modality therapy must be considered in regard to musculoskeletal and dental tissues, central nervous system (CNS) and neuropsychological sequelae, and endocrine and gonadal dysfunction, as well as direct effects on the heart, lungs, or kidneys.[55] The following sections describe techniques that allow safe, efficacious doses of radiation to be delivered, often in combination with surgical excision, to produce the maximal therapeutic benefit.

Brachytherapy

Brachytherapy is radiation treatment in which the ionizing source is in contact with the lesion, usually within the primary tumor. Catheters are placed in the tumor during surgery and may be loaded with temporary or permanent implant sources. Remote afterloading decreases radiation exposure to personnel and family members, and can be performed in the patient's room or on an outpatient basis. Low-dose-rate sources such as cesium provide about 1 cGy/min, whereas high-dose-rate sources such as iridium provide about 100 cGy/min.

As interstitial implants allow continuous-dose delivery over a much shorter time, they offer a radiobiologic advantage in high-grade tumors with rapid cell growth kinetics. Close cooperation between surgeon and radiation oncologist during the implant procedure is critical to ensure the most effective mapping of the tumor bed target.

Children with soft tissue sarcomas can benefit from specialized radiation treatment strategies. For children who have microscopic residual disease after operation, radiation provides excellent local tumor control.[56] High-dose-rate brachytherapy can be delivered in only a few minutes, which is particularly helpful in young children. In contrast, low-dose-rate brachytherapy provided by low energy source techniques requires sedation, immobilization, long exposure times, and hospitalization. The short therapy duration associated with high-dose-rate therapy also allows rapid reinstitution of chemotherapy. Morbidity is usually related to skin or mucosal reactions, which may progress as a 'recall' phenomenon in patients treated with radiosensitizing agents such as anthracyclines.[57] Brachytherapy, alone or in combination with external-beam irradiation, has been shown to provide a high rate of local tumor control in pediatric soft tissue sarcomas.[58-60]

Intraoperative Radiation

Intraoperative radiation therapy (IORT) allows the radiation dose to be directly applied to the target area while shielding adjacent structures. Whenever disease remains in surgically inaccessible areas, IORT may be an effective adjunct. Phase I and II studies have demonstrated that IORT can be performed safely in children.[61] It is used for patients in whom unresectable disease is present at diagnosis or for delayed primary or second-look procedures, residual lesions, or local tumor recurrence.

In children with retroperitoneal tumors, IORT may, however, lead to urologic complications. In a study reported in 1990, 3 of 6 patients treated with IORT and external-beam therapy required intervention for fibrotic ureteral strictures or renal artery stenosis; in two cases, the injured structures were within the supplemental external-beam treatment field. Also, neuropathies developed in two other patients. Nevertheless, all patients were survivors for up to 42 months' follow-up.[62] In a later study, the complications were minimized through more extensive dissection of normal structures and avoidance of overlapping radiation fields.[63]

Intensity-Modulated Radiation Therapy

Techniques continue to evolve to improve the impact of radiation therapy on tumor response while minimizing the dose of radiation imparted to surrounding normal tissues. Stereotactic radiation therapy is sometimes used for CNS tumors.[64-67] Imaging systems, treatment-planning software, and delivery systems have undergone dramatic advancements that allow sophisticated delivery of more precise courses of radiation. Intensity-modulated radiation therapy (IMRT) is an advanced form of three-dimensional conformal therapy that uses non-uniform radiation beam intensities determined by using various computer-based optimization techniques. Experience with IMRT in children is growing. Reports of mixed tumor cases, including pediatric patients, suggest that IMRT will be effective in reducing treatment-related morbidity and allow dose escalation to the target volume.[68,69] Significant reductions in radiation exposure to critical structures has been shown for intracranial, cervical, and abdominopelvic lesions.[70]

Proton Therapy

The driving principle in the evolution of radiation therapy techniques is to provide high doses of radiation to the tumor mass while reducing the dose delivered to surrounding tissues susceptible to the early and late complications associated with ionizing radiation. Proton therapy relies on the same mechanism of action as other forms of radiation therapy, but takes advantage of the physical properties of the energy transfer achieved to increase the precision of the radiation doses delivered. The physics of proton therapy result in less energy deposited in the tissue between the skin and the tumor, and increased energy delivered to the tumor when compared to photon therapy. This yields a biological effectiveness 10% greater than photons at the tumor site and the potential for significantly less impact on the surrounding tissue.

Proton therapy is very costly and there are currently fewer than 50 centers in the world capable of providing this treatment. Although most patients who have undergone therapy to date are adults, limited experience with pediatric CNS tumors and sarcomas has been reported.[71,72] Researchers at the Massachusetts General Hospital have described 30 patients with Ewing sarcoma who received proton therapy as a component of multimodal management. Three-year local control in 86% of patients was achieved with few adverse events.[71] The utility of proton therapy in other childhood tumors, including neuroblastoma and rhabdomyosarcoma, is also being explored.[72]

INNOVATIVE ADJUNCTIVE TECHNIQUES

Radiofrequency Ablation

Radiofrequency ablation (RFA) is a technique that applies thermal energy via a probe that results in coagulation necrosis of the target tissue. The technique involves image-guided application of the probe, primarily using ultrasound. The probe can be introduced percutaneously, laparoscopically, or via an open exposure. In adults, the most common applications are for primary or metastatic hepatic lesions, renal tumors, and pulmonary lesions.[73–77] Treatment of pediatric tumors with RFA is largely anecdotal. A small series reported the use of percutaneous RFA on fetuses with sacrococcygeal teratoma, but found a 50% fetal mortality rate.[78] Another report described severe soft tissue injury and sciatic nerve destruction at birth in an infant treated prenatally.[79]

Transcatheter Arterial Chemoembolization

Transcatheter arterial chemoembolization (TACE) is a technique used to directly instill chemotherapeutic agents into a tumor, thereby minimizing systemic toxicity. TACE is most commonly used in the management of liver lesions, taking advantage of the preferential arterial blood supply to these tumors.[80,81]

Although the pediatric experience with TACE is limited, there is some evidence to support its efficacy.[82,83] In one series, a suspension of cisplatin, doxorubicin, and mitomycin-C mixed with bovine collagen and radiopaque contrast material was used in 11 children with unresectable or recurrent lesions.[82] Six hepatoblastoma patients had an initial partial response, as measured by imaging and α-fetoprotein levels. Of these patients, three underwent subsequent surgical resection; one had progressive disease and died, and two survived for more than 15 months. The other three patients eventually also died of known progressive disease. In three children with hepatocellular carcinoma, one underwent surgical resection and was a long-term survivor for more than 65 months, one was alive with disease for more than 36 months, and one died of progressive liver failure with no evidence of malignancy. In another relatively recent report documenting the outcomes of 16 infants and children with unresectable hepatoblastoma, Li et al reported that TACE facilitated safe and complete surgical resection in 12 cases.[83] Three patients underwent partial resection. One patient underwent successful orthotopic liver transplantation after receiving TACE therapy.

Overall, chemoembolization is feasible in young patients and is associated with tolerable toxicity. This option represents a possible therapeutic alternative in persistent, unresectable, or recurrent hepatoblastoma, or in nonmetastatic hepatocellular carcinoma. Its use has also been proposed in unresectable Wilms tumor.[84]

Sentinel Lymph Node Biopsy

The utility of sentinel lymph node biopsy in children is evolving. Although it is standard practice for patients with intermediate thickness melanomas,[85] its value in soft tissue sarcomas remains unclear.[86,87]

The initial draining lymph node (sentinel node) is predictive of regional nodal metastases in a variety of tumors.[88] It is most commonly used to predict nodal status of patients with melanoma or breast cancer. In most cases, a combination of technetium-labeled sulfur colloid with either Lymphazurin or methylene blue dye is used to localize the sentinel node. Preoperative lymphoscintigraphy provides information regarding the location of the primary lymph node draining the tumor site. Lymphatic mapping is accomplished by injecting the technetium-labeled sulfur colloid at the primary tumor site. The affected region is then imaged to identify the sentinel lymph node. Just before incision, the blue dye is injected at the primary tumor site and a gamma probe is used to identify areas of high counts. The underlying tissue is then examined for lymph nodes containing the blue dye. The lymph nodes are removed and sent for histopathologic examination. If the sentinel node shows no evidence of metastases, the related regional lymphatic bed is highly likely to be tumor free. In these patients, the morbidity of lymphadenectomy can be avoided.

LATE EFFECTS OF CANCER THERAPY

According to the most recent National Cancer Institute statistics: (1) there are more than 328,000 survivors of childhood cancer in the USA and (2) 1 in 900 adults is now a cancer survivor.[89] The remarkable increase in survival has created a new and growing population who are at increased risk for late adverse effects of treatment and a diminished quality of life. All aspects of combined-modality therapy can contribute to the late effects. A number of chemotherapy agents have been associated with late toxicities. In addition, radiation therapy can significantly inhibit further growth of bone, muscle, heart, and kidney within the radiation field, and also can affect fertility.

Tissues with the highest cell-turnover rate are generally the most susceptible to the acute toxicities of chemotherapy, whereas tissues that replicate slowly or that can no longer regenerate may be susceptible to the late effects of therapy. Children are more susceptible to certain late effects of therapy than are adults because their tissues are still growing. Damage to these tissues may affect growth, fertility, and neuropsychological development.

Growth retardation is a late effect unique to children. The degree of impairment depends on the dose of chemotherapy or radiation and the age of the child at the time of therapy. The younger the child is at the time of the insult, the more severe the sequelae. More than 50% of childhood brain tumor patients treated with 3000 cGy or more to the whole brain will have severe growth retardation, with adult height being lower than the 5th percentile.[90] Cranial irradiation can lead to growth hormone deficiency, which results in poor linear growth, unless growth hormone replacement is given. In addition, patients who have received total-body irradiation or spinal radiation may not be able to achieve their full height potential because the irradiated bones have limited growth potential, even with growth hormone stimulation.[91]

Adjuvant therapy can also cause musculoskeletal problems, including scoliosis, avascular necrosis, osteoporosis, and atrophy or hypoplasia of tissues. Radiation to the head and neck results in hypoplasia of the jaw, orbit, or neck, with associated atrophy of the soft tissues. Associated endocrine, dental, and psychological consequences can occur.[92] Osteoporosis occurs as a result of corticosteroid treatment and from high-dose irradiation, as used for sarcomas.

Specific organs are often affected by chemotherapy. Heart, liver, lung, thyroid, and gonadal function are often impaired. Gonadal dysfunction (azoospermia, amenorrhea) frequently results from alkylator treatment. Therapy with mechlorethamine, vincristine, prednisone, and procarbazine has resulted in azoospermia in 80–100% of all male patients.[93] Combination chemotherapy programs for childhood Hodgkin disease have been adjusted to replace mechlorethamine with cyclophosphamide and eliminate dacarbazine from standard treatments in an attempt to decrease the infertility risk. It should be noted that the children of childhood cancer survivors are not at an increased risk for congenital anomalies.[94]

Cardiotoxicity from anthracycline antibiotics has been a problem in the treatment of Ewing sarcoma, osteosarcoma, and lymphomas. However, the use of continuous infusion anthracycline can decrease the risk of cardiac muscle damage and subsequent congestive heart failure.[95] Another strategy is the use of dexrazoxane to prevent anthracycline-induced cardiotoxicity.[28] Survivors of childhood brain tumor therapy treated with a combination of chemotherapy, irradiation, and surgery had a significantly increased risk of stroke, blood clots, and angina-like symptoms compared with their siblings.[96]

Pulmonary toxicity is a source of significant late toxicity of cancer therapy. Many alkylating agents and radiation therapy contribute to pulmonary fibrosis, resulting in decreased lung volume, lung compliance, and diffusing capacity. Nitrosoureas and bleomycin are the most common agents to cause pulmonary fibrosis.

Other significant organ-related late effects include chronic renal insufficiency from cisplatin therapy, chronic cystitis from cyclophosphamide or ifosfamide treatment, and prolonged hypogammaglobulinemia and T-lymphocyte dysfunction after multiple high-dose alkylators for bone marrow transplant.[97]

The most significant late effect of cancer therapy is the risk of secondary malignancy. This risk is highest in patients who have received both chemotherapy and radiation therapy. In 2001, Neglia and colleagues reported that the estimated cumulative incidence of all subsequent malignant neoplasms in a cohort of 13,581 childhood cancer survivors was 3.2% at 20 years after the primary diagnosis.[98] Hodgkin disease survivors have the highest secondary malignancy rates. Breast cancer is the most common solid tumor, with an estimated actuarial incidence in women of 35% by age 40 years. These patients are also at risk of developing leukemia, non-Hodgkin lymphoma, and thyroid carcinoma.[99] In survivors of childhood Hodgkin disease, the cumulative estimated incidence of second malignancies at 30 years ranges from 18% to 31%.[100,101] Patients who have received additional multimodality therapy for recurrent Hodgkin disease have the highest risk of second tumors. Patients with soft tissue sarcomas, retinoblastoma, and Ewing sarcoma who receive high-dose radiation to the primary lesion are at increased risk for secondary osteosarcoma within the radiation field.[102] Etoposide has been recognized as causing secondary AML.

REFERENCES

1. Farber S, Diamond LK. Temporary remissions in acute leukemia in children produced by folic acid antagonist, 4-aminopteroyl-glutamic acid (aminopterin). N Engl J Med 1948;238:787–93.
2. Li MC, Hertz R, Spencer D, et al. Effect of methotrexate upon choriocarcinoma and chorioadenoma. Proc Soc Exp Biol Med 1956;93:361–6.
3. Frei E III, Freireich EJ, Gehan E, et al. Studies of sequential and combination antimetabolite therapy in acute leukemia: 6-Mercaptopurine and methotrexate. Blood 1961;18:431–54.
4. Green DM, Jaffe N. Wilms' tumor: Model of a curable pediatric malignant solid tumor. Cancer Treat Rev 1978;5:143–72.
5. D'Angio GJ, Evans AE, Breslow N, et al. The treatment of Wilms' tumor: Results of the National Wilms' Tumor Study. Cancer 1976;38:647.
6. Link MP, Goorin AM, Miser AW, et al. The effect of adjuvant chemotherapy on relapse-free survival in patients with osteosarcoma of the extremity. N Engl J Med 1986;314:1600–6.
7. Schwenn MR, Blattner SR, Lynch E, et al. HiC-COM: A 2-month intensive chemotherapy regimen for children with stage III and IV Burkitt's lymphoma and B-cell acute lymphoblastic leukemia. J Clin Oncol 1991;9:133–8.
8. Cheung NK, Heller G. Chemotherapy dose intensity correlates strongly with response, median survival and median progression-free survival in metastatic neuroblastoma. J Clin Oncol 1991;9:1050–8.
9. Antman K, Ayash L, Elias A, et al. A phase II study of high dose cyclophosphamide, thiotepa, and carboplatin with autologous

marrow support in women with measurable advanced breast cancer responding to standard therapy. J Clin Oncol 1992;10:102–10.

10. Grier H, Krailo M, Link M, et al. Improved outcome in non-metastatic Ewing's sarcoma and PNET of bone with the addition of ifosfamide and etoposide to vincristine, Adriamycin, cyclophosphamide, and actinomycin: A Children's Cancer Group and Pediatric Oncology Group report. J Clin Oncol 1994;13(Suppl):421.

11. Clark PI, Slevin ML, Joel SP, et al. A randomized trial of two etoposide schedules in small-cell lung cancer: The influence of pharmacokinetics on efficacy and toxicity. J Clin Oncol 1994;12:1427–35.

12. Worth L, Jeha S, Kleinerman E. Biologic response modifiers in pediatric cancer. Hematol Oncol Clin North Am 2001;5:723–40.

13. Parker SL, Tong T, Bolden S, et al. Cancer statistics, 1997. CA Cancer J Clin 1997;47:5–27.

14. National Cancer Institute fact sheet [Internet]. Available at: http://www.cancer.gov/cancertopics/factsheet/Sites-Types/childhood.

15. Gloeckler Ries LA, Percy CL, Bunin GR. SEER Pediatric Monograph. Available at http://seer.cancer.gov/publications/childhood/introduction.

16. Kreissman SG. Molecular genetics: Toward an understanding of childhood cancer. Semin Pediatr Surg 1993;2:2–10.

17. Brodeur GM. Neuroblastoma: Clinical applications of molecular parameters. Brain Pathol 1990;1:47–54.

18. MacGregor PF. Gene expression in cancer: The application of microarrays. Expert Rev Mol Diagn 2003;3:185–200.

19. Goldie JH, Coldman AJ. A mathematic model for relating the drug sensitivity of tumors to the spontaneous mutation rate. Cancer Treat Rep 1979;63:1727–31.

20. Balis FM, Holcenberg JS, Poplack DG. General principles of chemotherapy. In: Pizzo P, Poplack D, editors. Principles and practice of pediatric oncology. 3rd ed. Philadelphia: Lippincott-Raven; 1997.

21. D'Angio GJ, Evans AE, Breslow N, et al. The treatment of Wilms' tumor: Results of the National Wilms' Tumor Study. Cancer 1976;38:633–46.

22. Green DM, Breslow NE, Evans I, et al. The effect of chemotherapy dose intensity on the hematological toxicity of treatment for Wilms' tumor: A report from the National Wilms' Tumor Study. Am J Pediatr Hematol Oncol 1994;16:207–12.

23. Picci P, Rougraff BT, Bacci G, et al. Prognostic significance of histopathologic response to chemotherapy in nonmetastatic Ewing's sarcoma of the extremities. J Clin Oncol 1993;11:1763–9.

24. Provisor AJ, Ettinger LJ, Nachman JB, et al. Treatment of non-metastatic osteosarcoma of the extremity with preoperative and postoperative chemotherapy: A report from the Children's Cancer Group. J Clin Oncol 1997;5:76–84.

25. Shamberger RC, Allarde-Segundo A, Kozakewich HP, et al. Surgical management of stage III and IV neuroblastoma: Resection before or after chemotherapy? J Pediatr Surg 1991;26:1113–18.

26. Householder SE, Rackoff W, Goldman J, et al. A case-control retrospective study of the efficacy of granulocyte colony stimulating factor in children with neuroblastoma. Am J Pediatr Hematol Oncol 1994;16:132–7.

27. Tepler I, Elias L, Smith JW, et al. A randomized placebo-controlled trial of recombinant human interleukin-11 in cancer patients with severe thrombocytopenia due to chemotherapy. Blood 1996;87:3607–14.

28. Lipshultz SE. Dexrazoxane for protection against cardiotoxic effects of anthracyclines in children. J Clin Oncol 1996;14:328–31.

29. Strother D, Ashley D, Kellie SJ, et al. Feasibility of four consecutive high-dose chemotherapy cycles with stem-cell rescue for patients with newly diagnosed medulloblastoma or supratentorial primitive neuroectodermal tumor after craniospinal radiotherapy: Results of a collaborative study. J Clin Oncol 2001;19:2696–704.

30. Welte K, Reiter A, Mempel K, et al. A randomized phase-III study of the efficacy of granulocyte colony-stimulating factor in children with high-risk acute lymphoblastic leukemia. Berlin-Frankfurt-Munster Study Group. Blood 1996;87:3143–50.

31. Burdach SE, Müschenich M, Josephs W, et al. Granulocyte-macrophage-colony stimulating factor for prevention of neutropenia and infections in children and adolescents with solid tumors.

Results of a prospective randomized study. Cancer 1995;76:510–16.

32. Hawkins DS, Felgenhauer J, Park J, et al. Peripheral blood stem cell support reduces the toxicity of intensive chemotherapy for children and adolescents with metastatic sarcomas. Cancer 2002;95:1354–65.

33. Frei E, Canellos GP. Dose: A critical factor in cancer chemotherapy. Am J Med 1980;69:585–94.

34. Broun R, Nichols CR, Kneebone P, et al. Long-term outcome of patients with relapsed and refractory germ cell tumors treated with high-dose chemotherapy and autologous bone marrow rescue. Ann Intern Med 1992;117:124–8.

35. Smith MA, Ungerleider RS, Horowitz ME, et al. Influence of doxorubicin dose intensity on response and outcome for patients with osteogenic sarcoma and Ewing's sarcoma. J Natl Cancer Inst 1991;83:1460–70.

36. Kaye SB, Lewis CR, Dave J, et al. A randomized study of two doses of cisplatin and cyclophosphamide in epithelial ovarian cancer. Lancet 1992;340:329–33.

37. Kreissman SG, Rackoff W, Lee M, et al. High dose cyclophosphamide with carboplatin: A tolerable regimen suitable for dose intensification in children with solid tumors. J Pediatr Hematol Oncol 1997;19:309–12.

38. Gordon MS, McCaskill-Stevens WJ, Battiato LA, et al. A phase I trial of recombinant human interleukin 11 (Neumega rgIL-11 growth factor) in women with breast cancer receiving chemotherapy. Blood 1996;87:3615–24.

39. Ali-Nazir A, Davenport G, Reaman G, et al. A phase I/II trial of rhIL-11 following ifosfamide, carboplatin, and etoposide (ICE) chemotherapy in pediatric patients with solid tumors or lymphoma. J Clin Oncol 1996;15(Suppl):274.

40. Shaw IC, Graham MI. Mesna: A short review. Cancer Treat Rev 1987;14:67–86.

41. Moritz T, MacKay W, Glassner B, et al. Retrovirus-mediated expression of DNA repair protein in bone marrow protects hematopoietic cells from nitrosourea-induced toxicity in vitro and in vivo. Cancer Res 1995;55:2608–14.

42. Sonis S, Muska A, O'Brien J, et al. Alterations in the frequency, severity, and duration of chemotherapy induced mucositis in hamsters by interleukin-11. Eur J Cancer 1995;31:261–6.

43. Fouladi M, Chintagumpala M, Ashley D, et al. Amifostine protects against cisplatin-induced ototoxicity in children with average-risk medulloblastoma. J Clin Oncol 2008;26:3749–55.

44. Corey SJ. Targeted therapy: for kids, too. Review. Pediatr Blood Cancer 2005;45:623–34.

45. Levitzki A, Klein S. Signal transduction therapy of cancer. Mol Aspects Med 2010;31:287–329.

46. Restifo NP, Snzol M. Cancer vaccines. In: DeVita VT, Hellman S, Rosenberg SA, editors. Cancer: Principles and Practice of Oncology. 5th ed. Philadelphia: Lippincott-Raven; 1997. p. 3033.

47. Rosenberg SA. Principles of cancer management: Biologic therapy. In: DeVita VT, Hellman S, Rosenberg SA, editors. Cancer: Principles and Practice of Oncology. 5th ed. Philadelphia: Lippincott-Raven; 1997. p. 364.

48. Frost JD, Hank JA, Reahman GH, et al. A phase I/IB trial of murine monoclonal anti-GD2 antibody 14. G2a plus interleukin-2 in children with refractory neuroblastoma: A report of the Children's Cancer Group. Cancer 1997;80:317–33.

49. Yu AL, Gilman AL, Ozkaynak MF, et al. Anti-GD2 antibody with GM-CSF, interleukin-2, and isotretinoin for neuroblastoma. N Engl J Med 2010;363:1324–34.

50. Eisbruch A, Lichter AS. What a surgeon needs to know about radiation. Ann Surg Oncol 1997;4:516–22.

51. Liu L, Glicksman AS. The role of radiation in the management of soft tissue sarcoma. Med Health RI 1997;80:32–6.

52. Temple WJ, Temple CLF, Arthur K, et al. Prospective cohort study of neoadjuvant treatment in conservative surgery of soft tissue sarcomas. Ann Surg Oncol 1997;4:586–90.

53. Marcus KC, Grier HE, Shamberger RC, et al. Childhood soft tissue sarcoma: A 20-year experience. J Pediatr 1997;131:603–7.

54. Lindberg RD, Martin RG, Romsdahl MM, et al. Conservative surgery and postoperative radiotherapy in 300 adults with soft-tissue sarcomas. Cancer 1981;47:2391–7.

55. Fryer CJH. Principles of pediatric radiation oncology. In: Holland JF, Frei E, Bast RC, editors. Cancer Medicine. 4th ed. Baltimore: Williams & Wilkins; 1996. p. 2899–905.

56. Donaldson S, Breneman J, Asmar L, et al. Hyperfractionated radiation in children with rhabdomyosarcoma. Results of an intergroup rhabdomyosarcoma pilot study. Int J Radiat Oncol Biol Phys 1995;32:903–11.

57. Nag S, Grecula J, Ruymann FB. Aggressive chemotherapy, organ-preserving surgery, and high-dose-rate remote brachytherapy in the treatment of rhabdomyosarcoma in infants and young children. Cancer 1993;72:2769–76.

58. Nag S, Olson T, Ruymann F, et al. High-dose-rate brachytherapy in childhood sarcomas: A local control strategy preserving bone growth and function. Med Pediatr Oncol 1995;25:463–9.

59. Nag S, Martinez-Monge R, Ruyman F, et al. Innovation in the management of soft tissue sarcomas in infants and young children: High dose brachytherapy. J Clin Oncol 1997;15:3075–84.

60. Merchant TE, Parsh N, del Valle PL, et al. Brachytherapy for pediatric soft-tissue sarcoma. Int J Radiat Oncol Biol Phys 2000;46:427–32.

61. Zelefsky MJ, LaQuaglia MP, Ghavimi F, et al. Preliminary results of phase I/II study of high-dose-rate intraoperative radiation therapy for pediatric tumors. J Surg Oncol 1996;62:267–72.

62. Ritchey ML, Gunderson LL, Smithson WA, et al. Pediatric urologic complications with intraoperative radiation therapy. J Urol 1990;143:89–91.

63. Haase GM, Meagher D Jr, McNeely LK, et al. Electron beam intraoperative radiation therapy for pediatric neoplasms. Cancer 1994;74:740–7.

64. Mehta MP. The physical, biologic, and clinical basis of radiosurgery. Curr Probl Cancer 1995;19:265–329.

65. Shaw E, Scott C, Souhami L, et al. Radiosurgery for the treatment of previously irradiated recurrent primary brain tumors and brain metastases: Initial analysis of Radiation Therapy Oncology Group protocol (RTOG) 9005. Int J Radiat Oncol Biol Phys 1994;30:166.

66. Smyth MD, Sneed PK, Ciricillo SF, et al. Stereotactic radiosurgery for pediatric intracranial arteriovenous malformations: The University of California at San Francisco experience. J Neurosurg 2002;97:48–55.

67. Shrieve DC, Alexander E, Wen PY, et al. Comparison of stereotactic radiosurgery and brachytherapy in the treatment of recurrent glioblastoma multiforme. Neurosurg 1995;36:275–84.

68. Teh BS, Mai WY, Grant WH, et al. Intensity modulated radiotherapy (IMRT) decreases treatment-related morbidity and potentially enhances tumor control. Cancer Invest 2002;20:437–51.

69. Swift P. Novel techniques in the delivery of radiation in pediatric oncology. Pediatr Clin North Am 2002;9:1107–29.

70. Bhatnagar A, Deutsch M. The role for intensity modulated radiation therapy (IMRT) in pediatric population. Technol Cancer Res Treat 2006;5:591–5.

71. Merchant TE. Proton beam therapy in pediatric oncology. Cancer J 2009;15:298–305.

72. Cotter SE, McBride SM, Yock TI. Proton radiation for solid tumors of childhood. Technol Cancer ResTreat 2012;11:267–77.

73. Curley SA. Radiofrequency ablation of malignant liver tumors. Ann Surg Oncol 2003;10:338–47.

74. Scaife CL, Curley SA. Complication, local recurrence, and survival rates after radiofrequency ablation for hepatic malignancies. Surg Oncol Clin North Am 2003;12:243–55.

75. Mayo-Smith WW, Dupuy DE, Parikh PM, et al. Image-guided percutaneous radiofrequency ablation of solid renal masses: Techniques and outcomes of 38 treatment sessions in 32 consecutive patients. AJR Am J Roentgenol 2003;180:1503–8.

76. Farrell MA, Charboneau WJ, DiMarco DS, et al. Image-guided radiofrequency ablation of solid renal tumors. Am J Roentgenol 2003;180:1509–13.

77. Herrera LJ, Fernando HC, Perry Y, et al. Radiofrequency ablation of pulmonary malignant tumors in non-surgical candidates. J Thorac Cardiovasc Surg 2003;125:929–37.

78. Paek BW, Jennings RW, Harrison MR, et al. Radiofrequency ablation of human fetal sacrococcygeal teratoma. Am J Obstet Gynecol 2001;184:503–7.

79. Ibrahim D, Ho E, Scherl LA, et al. Newborn with an open posterior hip dislocation and sciatic nerve injury after intrauterine radiofrequency ablation of a sacrococcygeal teratoma. J Pediatr Surg 2003;38:248–50.

80. Gunvén P. Liver embolizations in oncology: A review. Part I. (chemo)embolizations. Med Oncol 2008;25:1–11.

81. Bittles MA, Hoffer FA. Interventional radiology and the care of the pediatric oncology patient. Surg Oncol 2007;16:229–33.

82. Malogolowkin MH, Stanley P, Steele DA, et al. Feasibility and toxicity of chemoembolization for children with liver tumors. J Clin Oncol 2000;18:1279–84.

83. Li J, Chu J, Yang J, et al. Preoperative transcatheter selective arterial chemoembolization in treatment of unresectable hepatoblastoma in infants and children. Cardiovasc Intervent Radiol 2008;31:1117–23.

84. Li M, Zhou Y, Huang Y, et al. A retrospective study of the preoperative treatment of advanced Wilms tumor in children with chemotherapy versus transcatheter arterial chemoembolization alone or combined with short-term chemotherapy. J Vasc Interv Radiol 2011;22:279–86.

85. Topar G, Zelger B. Assessment of value of the sentinel lymph node biopsy in melanoma in children and adolescents and applicability of subcutaneous infusion anesthesia. J Pediatr Surg 2007;42:1716–20.

86. DeCorti F, Dall'Igna P, Bisogno G, et al. Sentinel node biopsy in pediatric soft tissue sarcomas of extremities. Pediatr Blood Cancer 2009;52:51–4.

87. Pacella SJ, Lowe L, Bradford C, et al. The utility of sentinel lymph node biopsy in head and neck melanoma in the pediatric population. Plast Reconstr Surg 2003;112:1257–65.

88. Morton DL, Wend D, Wong JH, et al. Technical details of intraoperative lymphatic mapping for early stage melanoma. Arch Surg 1992;127:392–9.

89. Mariotto AB, Rowland JH, Yabroff KR, et al. Long-term survivors of childhood cancers in the United States. Cancer Epidemiol Biomarkers Prev 2009;18:1033–40.

90. Oberfield SE, Allen JC, Pollack J, et al. A long-term endocrine sequelae after treatment of medulloblastoma: Prospective study of growth and thyroid function. J Pediatr 1986;108:219–23.

91. Huma Z, Boulad F, Black P, et al. Growth in children after bone marrow transplantation for acute leukemia. Blood 1995;86:819–24.

92. Larson DL, Kroll S, Jaffe N, et al. Long-term effects of radiotherapy in childhood and adolescence. Am J Surg 1990;160:348–50.

93. Whitehead E, Shalet SM, Morris-Jones PH, et al. Gonadal function after combination chemotherapy for Hodgkin's disease in childhood. Arch Dis Child 1982;57:287–91.

94. Green DM, Zevon MA, Lowrie G, et al. Congenital anomalies in children of patients who received chemotherapy for cancer in childhood or adolescence. N Engl J Med 1991;325:141–6.

95. Legha SS, Benjamin RS, Mackay B, et al. Reduction of doxorubicin cardiotoxicity by prolonged continuous infusion. Ann Intern Med 1982;96:133–9.

96. Gurney J, Kaden-Lottick N, Packer R, et al. Endocrine and cardiovascular late effects among adult survivors of childhood brain tumors: Childhood Cancer Survivors Study. Cancer 2003;97:663–73.

97. Blatt J, Copeland DR, Bleyer WA. Late effects of childhood cancer and its treatment. In: Pizzo PA, Poplack DG, editors. Principles and Practice of Pediatric Oncology. 3rd ed. Philadelphia: Lippincott-Raven; 1997. p. 1303.

98. Neglia JP, Friedman DL, Yasui Y, et al. Second malignant neoplasms in five-year survivors of childhood cancer; childhood cancer survivor study. J Natl Cancer Inst 2001;93:618–29.

99. Bhatia S, Robison LL, Oberlin O, et al. Breast cancer and other second neoplasm after childhood Hodgkin's disease. N Engl J Med 1996;334:745–51.

100. Jenkin D, Greenberg M, Fitzgerald A. Second malignant tumours in childhood Hodgkin's disease. Med Pediatr Oncol 1996;26:373–9.

101. Sankila R, Garwicz S, Olsen JH, et al. Risk of subsequent malignant neoplasms among 1,641 Hodgkin's disease patients diagnosed in childhood and adolescence: A population-based cohort study in the five Nordic countries. J Clin Oncol 1996;14:1442–6.

102. Smith MB, Xue H, Strong L, et al. Forty year experience with second malignancies after treatment of childhood cancer: Analysis of outcome following the development of the second malignancy. J Pediatr Surg 1993;28:1342–8.

CHAPTER 65

RENAL TUMORS

Peter F. Ehrlich • Robert C. Shamberger

Renal tumors are the second most common abdominal tumor seen in infants and children behind neuroblastoma. They represent a wide spectrum from benign to extremely malignant tumors (Box 65-1). These tumors include: Wilms tumor (WT) (also referred to as nephroblastoma or renal embryoma), renal cell carcinoma (RCC), clear cell sarcoma of the kidney (CCSK), rhabdoid tumor of the kidney (RTK), congenital mesoblastic nephroma (CMN), cystic renal tumor, and angiomyolipoma. Advances in the management of these tumors have been significant over the past six decades since Sidney Farber first administered dactinomycin (Actinomycin D) for advanced-stage WTs.[1] Multidisciplinary and multi-institutional prospective randomized cooperative group trials in both North America and Europe by the Children's Oncology Group (COG-formerly the National Wilms Tumor Study Group [NWTSG]) and the Société Internationale d'Oncologie Pédiatrique (SIOP) have produced a large body of evidence-based knowledge to establish the optimal risk-based treatments (Table 65-1). The goal of this chapter is to describe the early history of WT, followed by a discussion of the etiologic factors in renal tumor formation, molecular genetics, pathologic subtypes and premalignant syndromes, and current treatment algorithms for children.

WILMS TUMOR

History

The first descriptions of WT have been variably attributed to either Rance in 1814 or Wilms in 1899.[2-4] The first known specimen of this tumor was preserved by the British surgeon John Hunter between 1763 and 1793.[5] This specimen of a bilateral tumor in a young infant remains in the Hunterian Museum of the Royal College of Surgeons in London. Carl Max Wilhelm Wilms was a German pathologist and surgeon. Wilms' name became indelibly linked to this tumor in children after publication of his comprehensive monograph in 1899 titled 'Die Mischgeschwülste der Niere' which described seven children with nephroblastoma as part of a monograph on 'mixed tumors of the kidney'.[3,4] In it he proposed that tumor cells originate during the development of the embryo. The first successful nephrectomy was probably performed by Thomas Jessop at the General Infirmary in Leeds, England on the 7th of June, 1877 on a 2-year-old child with hematuria and a tumor of the kidney.[6,7]

Resection was recognized early as an effective treatment for WT and remains as the cornerstone of all therapies. However, at the beginning of the 20th century,

survival was approximately 5% and operative mortality was high. In 1916 radiation therapy was added as an adjuvant therapy by Friedlander.[8] In the 1930s, Ladd and Gross described the principles of operative therapy for WT, including transperitoneal exposure and early ligation of the renal pedicle.[7,9] They stressed the need to remove the perirenal fat to resect lymphatic extensions and to avoid rupture of the renal capsule, principles we continue to follow today. From 1931 to 1939, survival from resection alone, involving ligation of the renal pedicle before removal, was 32% at the Children's Hospital in Boston.[1,10] Gross and Neuhauser later proposed the routine addition of abdominal radiation to WT therapy and reported an estimated 47% cure.[11] Thus in 1940,[1] most patients began to receive postoperative irradiation to the renal fossa. This decreased the local recurrence rate, but did not significantly affect the incidence of pulmonary metastases or improve the long-term survival. Under Gross's tutelage, pediatric surgeons in North America generally performed primary resection of WT, while in Europe, the Paris school led by Schweisguth and Bamberger reported early success with preoperative irradiation, establishing a precedent for initial adjuvant therapy.[12]

WT was the first malignancy in which the importance of adjuvant treatment was recognized. This principle was espoused by Sidney Farber decades before it would be applied to other pediatric and adult solid tumors.[1] The concept of adjuvant therapy 'was based upon the supposition that in the children with WT who died, the tumor must have metastasized already at the time of discovery of the primary tumor', although no evidence of spread was available. Dactinomycin was the first active agent identified for the treatment of WT. Of the 53 patients who had no demonstrable metastases on admission treated with combined regimen of operation, local radiation, and dactinomycin from 1957 to 1964, an 89% 2-year disease-free survival was reported,[1] a very reasonable rate of survival even today. In patients with metastases identified at presentation, 18 of 31 (58%) were alive and free of disease more than 2 years later. In the early 1960s, vincristine sulfate was identified as an active agent against WT and was added to the standard therapy.[13]

Epidemiology

WT is the most frequent tumor of the kidney in infants and children. Its incidence is 7.6 cases for every million children younger than 15 years, or one case per 10,000 infants.[14] This translates into 600 to 650 cases a year in North America. It is less common in East Asian populations than in white children, but is more frequent in black

Wilms tumor (favorable, unfavorable)
Renal cell carcinoma
Renal tumors associated with TFE3 or TFEB translocations
Clear cell sarcoma
Malignant rhabdoid tumor of the kidney
Renal cell sarcoma
Renal adenocarcinoma
Ossifying renal tumor of infancy
Renal medullary carcinoma
Renal neurogenic tumor
Renal teratoma
Metanephric tumor (adenoma, stromal tumor, adenofibroma)
Mesoblastic nephroma
Angiolipoma
Cystic nephroma or partially cystic nephroma
Diffuse hyperblastic perilobar nephroblastomatosis
Nephrogenic rest

children.[15,16] The mean age at diagnosis is 36 months, with most children presenting between the ages of 12 and 48 months. Tumors tend to occur earlier in boys than girls. WT incidence decreases over the age of 10 and is less common under 6 months of age. However, it still constitutes 20% of all renal tumors in children less than 6 months. Bilateral Wilms tumors (BWT) occur in 4–13% of patients.[15,17]

WT occurs in several well-described syndromes. These comprise about 10% of all WT cases, and include sporadic aniridia, isolated hemihypertrophy, the Denys–Drash syndrome (nephropathy, renal failure, male pseudohermaphroditism, and WT), genital anomalies, Beckwith–Wiedemann syndrome (BWS; visceromegaly, macroglossia, omphalocele, and hyperinsulinemic hypoglycemia in infancy), and the WAGR complex (WT with aniridia, genitourinary malformations, and mental retardation). These congenital syndromes have helped identify the genetic and etiological mechanisms inherent in developing a WT. For example, children with WAGR syndrome, which is associated with a chromosomal defect in 11p13, are at a 30% higher risk of developing WT than a normal child. Aniridia is usually diagnosed at birth and helps identify these children.[18] BWS is a second common syndrome associated with WT. BWS affects 1 in 14,000 children. These children are at an increased risk of several types of embryonal tumors, including WT. The most frequently observed tumors in BWS are WT and hepatoblastoma, which comprise 43% and 12% of reported associated cancers, respectively.[19,20] The risk for malignant development is greatest in the first decade of life. Three large studies of children with BWS reported tumor frequencies of 7.1% (13/183), 7.5% (29/388), and 14% (22/159).[19,21–23]

Molecular Genetics of Wilms Tumor

WT is an embryonal tumor that was originally thought to fit the model proposed by Knudson's 'two-hit'

hypothesis for cancer development.[24] However, the genesis of WT has been shown to be far more complex. Multiple mutated WT genes have been identified as well as areas of loss of genetic material and allelic uniqueness (loss of heterozygosity) that are important to tumor development. A few of these genetic anomalies have been evaluated in clinical trials to assess their prognostic significance and are now being used in conjunction with traditional factors, such as stage, to determine the intensity of therapy.[19,25] A detailed discussion of all the genetic anomalies associated with WT is beyond the scope of this chapter; however, a summary of the key genes and genetic anomalies is presented in Table 65-2.

TP53

TP53 mutations in WT are almost exclusively found in tumors with anaplastic histology. Seventy-five per cent of anaplastic WT have *p53* mutations.[26,27] Interestingly, some tumors can contain both anaplastic and favorable histology. Studies in these tumors demonstrate that the *p53* mutation is found only in the areas of anaplasia and not in the area of favorable histology.[26] This implies that *p53* mutations may be essential for anaplastic progression.

CTNNB1

CTNNB1 plays a central role in the Wnt signal transduction pathway. The Wnt signaling pathway describes a network of proteins known for their roles in embryogenesis and cancer. Deregulation of *CTNNB1* has been linked to several malignancies. *CTNNB1* mutations have been reported to occur in 15% of WT.[28,29] The mutations resulted in areas of phosphorylation and degradation of beta catenin, which is highly correlated with *WT1* mutation and the *WTX* gene.

WTX

The *WTX* gene (also known as *AMER1* for adenomatous polyposis coli (APC) membrane recruitment 1) was found to be mutated in 15 of 51 (29%) WT tested, making it the most common known gene mutation in WT.[30] Localization of *WTX* on the X-chromosome results in complete inactivation by a single mutational event in males, and in females if the active X-chromosome is affected. The exact clinical impact of *WTX* on WT development remains to be defined.

WT1 (11p13)

WT1 gene was the first gene to be linked with WT development. Evidence suggests that *WT1* may act as a tumor suppressor gene or oncogene and is located at chromosome 11p13.[31,32] Wild-type *WT1* is important for normal cell development and survival. *WT1* is involved in cell growth, differentiation, and apoptosis.[33] Patients heterozygous for *WT1* germline mutations are predisposed to WT, and *WT1* is inactivated in tumors. This implies the loss of *WT1* function is associated with enhanced cell viability and/or proliferation. Ablation of

TABLE 65-1 **Summary of the Important Information Learned from Various Wilms Tumor Studies**

Study	Key Study Conclusions
NWTS-1	Anaplasia established as the most important factor in patient outcomes
	Vincristine and dactinomycin in combination are more effective than alone for stage II and III tumors.
	RT provided no survival advantage in children younger than 24 months with stage I favorable-histology tumors who also received 15 months of dactinomycin.
	Stage III tumors with a confined spill did not require whole abdominal RT, but had comparable outcomes with flank radiation.[123,127]
NWTS-2	Six months of vincristine and dactinomycin is equal to 15 months in children with favorable histology
	In children with stage II, III, IV tumors, doxorubicin improved RFS.
	Confirmed that RT can be avoided in all children with stage I WT if they received vincristine and dactinomycin
	Established that delaying RT longer than 10 to 14 days after resection was associated with a higher incidence of abdominal relapse, particularly among patients with unfavorable-histology tumors
NWTS-3	First study to stratify children by histology and grade
	Children with stage I tumors, with an 11-week regimen using vincristine and dactinomycin only, had a 4-year RFS and OS of 89.0% and 95.6%, respectively
	The addition of doxorubicin to the treatment of children with stage III tumors improved survival
	No benefit was found with the addition of doxorubicin or RT for children with stage II tumors
	No benefit was found with the addition of cyclophosphamide to the treatment of children with stage IV tumors.
	In stages II–IV unfavorable histology tumors, the addition of cyclophosphamide to three drug regimen improved survival for diffuse anaplasia (but not focal)
	10 Gy abdominal radiation was equal to 20 Gy. This was an important finding because it eliminated the need for an age-adjusted dose schedule, and significantly reduced the recommended dose of RT and its early and late toxicities.
	Anaplastic tumors tend to be more resistant to chemotherapy, and are also resistant to RT
NWTS-4	Analysis from early NWTS-1 to NWTS-4 studies identified a group of patients whose excellent outcomes were unaffected by chemotherapy. These children were less than 2 years of age, had tumors that weighed less than 550 g, and were stage I with favorable histology
	Addressed dose intensification and also evaluated the use of two time intervals for the administration of chemotherapy: a short course (18 to 26 weeks, depending on the regimen and stage) versus a long course (54 to 66 weeks)
	Key findings included discovery that the pulse-intensive regimens produced less hematologic toxicity than the standard regimens, and 6 months of chemotherapy is as good 15 months chemotherapy
	Patients with CCSK were treated with vincristine, dactinomycin and doxorubicin. OS improved on NWTS-4 compared to NWTS-3 (OS 83% versus 66.9% at 8 years, P < 0.01)
	An increased incidence of local recurrence was seen in NWTS-4 children in whom biopsy of lymph nodes was not performed, particularly in stage I cases
	Children with intravascular extension into the intrahepatic vena cava have reduced morbidity if treated with preoperative chemotherapy
NWTS-5	Outcomes for patients with LOH at 1p and 16q were at least 10% worse than those without LOH (Fig. 65-1)
	First study with specific relapse protocols
	EFS and OS of patients with Stage I and II relapse at 4 years was 71.1% and 81.8%, respectively
	EFS and OS of patients with Stage III and IV relapse at four years was 42.3% and 48.0%, respectively
	Therapy for stage I focal and diffuse anaplasia with only EE-4A is inadequate
	10 Gy abdominal radiation for Stage II and III AH is inadequate.
	Regimen I improved survival for all patients with CCSK
SIOP-1	Preoperative RT can reduce intraoperative rupture
SIOP-6	Pretreatment with chemotherapy almost always reduces the bulk of the tumor
SIOP-9	Pretreatment of chemotherapy results in a different histology compared to those who do not undergo neoadjuvant therapy
	Randomization between 4 and 8 weeks of preoperative chemotherapy with dactinomycin and vincristine did not decrease the incidence of tumor rupture nor did it result in more tumors being downstaged
	Tumor size decreased by more than half in 52% of the cases. During the second 4 weeks of therapy, there was another 50% reduction in 33% of the cases
	Patients were spared whole lung RT if they rapidly responded to three drug chemotherapy by 6 weeks. The five-year RFS for stage IV patients receiving preoperative chemotherapy alone was 62.5%
SIOP 2001	First study allowed NSS for unilateral polar or peripherally noninfiltrating tumors
	NSS was able to be performed in 3% of patients
	After NSS, 65% had positive margins mandating intensified therapy
	The five-year OS and EFS survival after NSS was 98.4 (95% CI: 95.3–100.0) and 92.5 (95% CI: 86.9–98), respectively

AH, anaplastic histology; CCSK, clear cell sarcoma of the kidney; EE–4A, actinomycin and dactinomycin; EFS, event-free survival; LOH, loss of heterozygosity; NSS, nephron-sparing surgery; NWTS, National Wilms Tumor Study; OS, overall survival; RFS, relapse-free survival; RT, radiation therapy; SIOP, Société Internationale d'Oncologie Pédiatrique.

WT1 at the initial stages of kidney development results in apoptosis and renal agenesis, indicating that it has a crucial role in maintaining cell viability. In some leukemias, the increased expression of *WT1* compared with normal bone marrow cells, along with some reports of *WT1* expression being a marker of poor prognosis, suggest that *WT1* functions as an oncogene.[26] By contrast, observations of *WT1* inactivating mutations in leukemias suggest it functions as a tumor suppressor gene. It should be emphasized that children with

TABLE 65-2   Summary of the Molecular Genetic Properties

Gene	Location	Type of Mutation	Frequency	Germline or Somatic?	Tumor Zygosity	Predicted Effect
WT1	11.13	Whole or partial gene deletion, insertion, nonsense and missense	~20%	Both	Predominantly homozygous	Inactivation of protein
WT2	11p15.5	Genetic imprinting	?	Both	Heterozygous	Abnormally high levels of IGF2 mRNA
WTX	Xq11.1	Whole or partial gene deletion and nonsense	~20%	Somatic only	Heterozygous and hemizygous	Inactivation of protein
CTNNB1	3p21	Inframe deletions and missense	~15%	Somatic only	Heterozygous	Stabilization of protein
TP53	Xq11.1	Missense	~5%	Both	Heterozygous and homozygous	Inactivation of protein

congenital syndromes and WT make up a very small proportion of the total WT population. However, loss of heterozygosity (LOH) is seen in 30–40% of WT patients in the region of *WT1*. Based on this observation, it would be expected that many patients with sporadic WT would have a mutation in the *WT1* gene. Surprisingly, the incidence of mutations of *WT1* associated with WT in the sporadic form of the disease is low (10–20%).[34,35]

WT2 (11p15.5)

This second WT gene location was identified by linkage analysis in children with BWS. This site is not a single gene, but contains several genes that may play a role in tumor development. In patients with BWS, it was found that uniformly the maternal allele of 11.15 was lost. The process which causes this is termed genomic imprinting, whereby one allele is imprinted, in a parental-specific manner, to be functionally inactive.

Loss of Heterozygosity

LOH refers to loss of genetic material and allelic uniqueness. A major aim of the fifth National Wilms Tumor Study (NWTS-5) was to determine if tumor-specific LOH for chromosomes 11p, 1p, or 16q was associated with an adverse prognosis for children with favorable-histology (FH) WT, a finding suggested in earlier retrospective studies.[25,36,37] The results of NWTS-5 demonstrated that outcomes for patients with LOH at 1p and 16q were at least 10% worse than those without LOH (Fig. 65-1). These findings were used as determinants for the intensity of therapy on the current COG renal tumor studies.

Pathologic Precursors: Nephrogenic Rests, Nephroblastomatosis, and Multicystic Dysplastic Kidneys

Nephrogenesis in the normal kidney is usually complete by 34 to 36 weeks gestation. The presence of nephrogenic rests (NRs; persistent metanephric tissue in the kidney after the 36th week of gestation) has been associated with the occurrence of WT. NR are considered precursor lesions to WT. However, only a small number

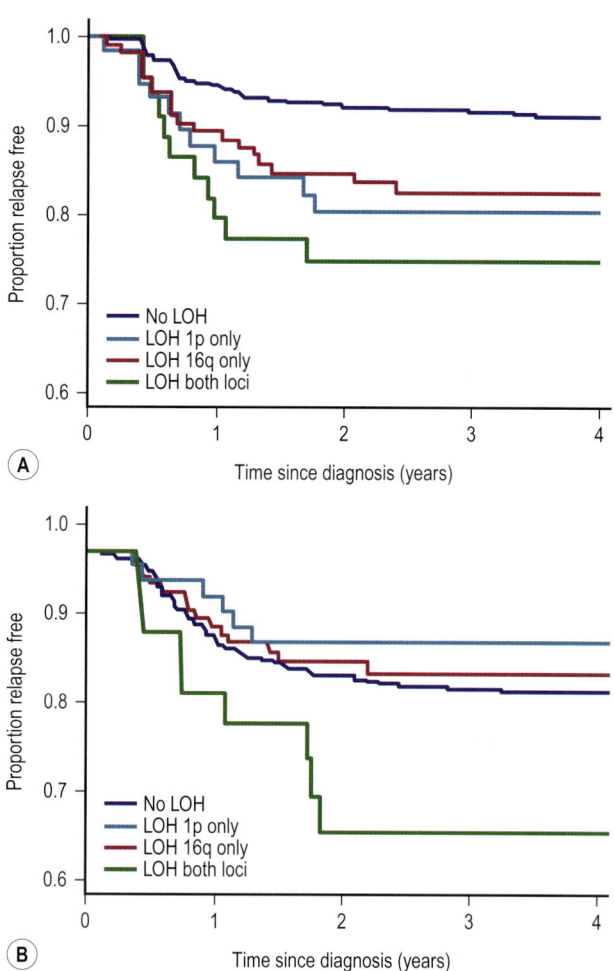

FIGURE 65-1 ■ **(A)** Relapse-free survival with loss of heterozygosity (LOH) at chromosomes 1p and 16q for patients with stage I/II Wilms tumor of favorable histology. **(B)** Relapse-free survival for patients with stage III/IV Wilms tumor with favorable histology and LOH at chromosome 1p and 16q. (From Grundy PE, Breslow N, Li S. Loss of heterozygosity for chromosomes 1p and 16q is an adverse prognostic factor in favorable-histology Wilms' tumor: A report from the National Wilms' Tumor Study Group. J Clin Oncol 2005;23:7312–21, with permission from the American Society of Clinical Oncology.)

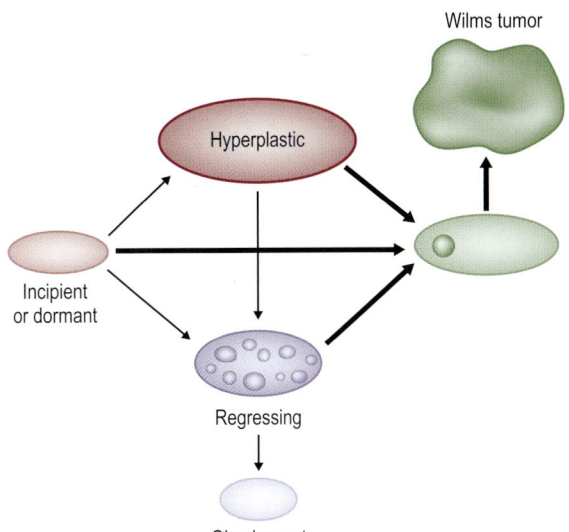

Wilms tumor

Hyperplastic

Incipient
or dormant

Regressing

Obsolescent

FIGURE 65-2 ■ Diagrammatic depiction of nephrogenic rests and their classification. Thick arrows indicate tumor induction. (From Beckwith JB. Precursor lesions of Wilms' tumor: Clinical and biological implications. Med Pediatr Oncol 1993;21:158–68.)

develop clonal transformation resulting in the development of WT. The presence of multiple or diffuse NRs is termed nephroblastomatosis.

These NRs may occur in a perilobar (PLNRs) or intralobar (ILNRs) location, and may be single or multiple (Fig. 65-2). In children with aniridia or the Denys–Drash syndrome, the lesions are primarily ILNRs, whereas children with hemihypertrophy or the BWS have predominantly PLNRs (Table 65-3).[38] NRs may be further classified by their growth phase, which has been separated into three phases; (1) incipient or dormant nephrogenic rests which show few well-formed tubular structures, but no evidence of proliferation and no mitoses; (2) hyperplastic nephrogenic rests which are composed of epithelial elements with nodular expansive growth; and (3) sclerosing rests which consist of stromal and epithelial elements with few blastemal nephrogenic elements. Most NRs are dormant or in the sclerosing phase, and the majority will spontaneously resolve. Hyperplastic NR can produce masses as large as conventional WT and can present a diagnostic dilemma. NRs are rare in the general population. In an autopsy series of infants younger than 3 months, nine of 1,035 infants

(0.87%) had PLNRs, while ILNRs occurred in only 2 of 2000 cases (0.1%).[39]

Pathologic distinction between NR and WT can be very difficult. In fact, it may be impossible to distinguish a hyperplastic NR from a WT based on an incisional or needle biopsy specimen that does not include the margin between the NR and the remaining kidney.[38,40] Most hyperplastic nodules lack a pseudocapsule at their periphery, whereas most WTs will have one. Thus, if the biopsy specimen does not contain the lesion and its margin, it will be difficult to differentiate between these two lesions. In these situations, the current recommendation is to use the term 'nephrogenic process, consistent with a WT or a nephrogenic rest'.[40,41] This is one reason that it is recommended to avoid percutaneous biopsies in children with renal masses.

The incidence of NRs is about 100 times greater than that of WT (1/10,000 infants). In a review of cases of WT reported in the NWTS-4, 41% of the unilateral WTs were associated with NRs, whereas in children with synchronous bilateral WT, the incidence of NRs was 99%.[38] These were primarily PLNRs. A child with a WT and NRs in the resected specimen is at increased risk of developing a metachronous tumor in the contralateral kidney.[42] In a child under one year of age, this risk is very significant, and these children need to be followed very carefully with sequential ultrasound (US) examinations. It is very difficult to diagnose NRs on imaging. Although magnetic resonance imaging (MRI) may be helpful, there is no gold standard.

Diffuse hyperplastic perilobar nephroblastomatosis (DHPLN) is a unique category of nephroblastomatosis in which the rests form a thick rind around the periphery of the kidney. Infants with DHPLN may initially present with large unilateral or bilateral flank masses (Fig. 65-3). A characteristic radiographic finding is massively enlarged kidneys that maintain their normal configuration and lack evidence of necrosis. As with the isolated NRs, proliferation of the thin rind of NRs on the periphery of the kidney will preserve the normal configuration of the kidney, but result in marked enlargement of its size. This is in contrast to WT, in which the normal renal configuration and collecting system are generally distorted. The optimal diagnosis and management of a child with DHPLN is unclear. In a 2006 study of 52 children and 33 cases of DHPLN, histologic examination alone was unable to establish a diagnosis in 21 children that underwent biopsy at the time of initial presentation.[41] In the

TABLE 65-3 Association of Nephrogenic Rests with Wilms Tumor Predisposition Syndromes and Congenital Anomalies

Clinical Phenotype	+ ILNR − PLNR	− ILNR + PLNR	+ ILNR + PLNR	− ILNR − PLNR
Denys–Drash	59%	0%	4%	37%
WAGR	73%	4%	4%	18%
Beckwith–Wiedemann	18%	35%	27%	20%
Male genitourinary anomalies	43%	9%	5%	44%

ILNR, intralobar nephrogenic rests; PLNR, perilobar nephrogenic rests; +, present; −, absent.
From Breslow NE, Beckwith JB, Perlman EJ, et al. Age distributions, birth weights, nephrogenic rests, and heterogeneity in the pathogenesis of Wilms tumor. Pediatr Blood Cancer 2006;47:260–7.

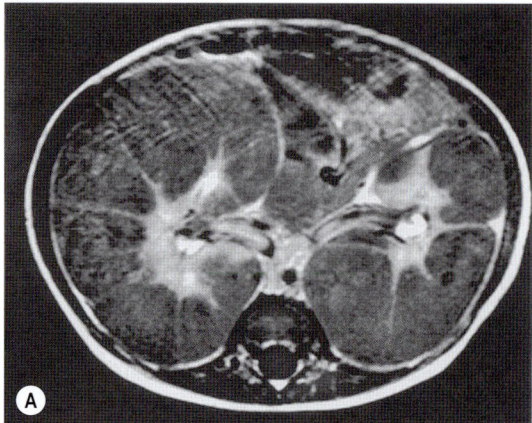
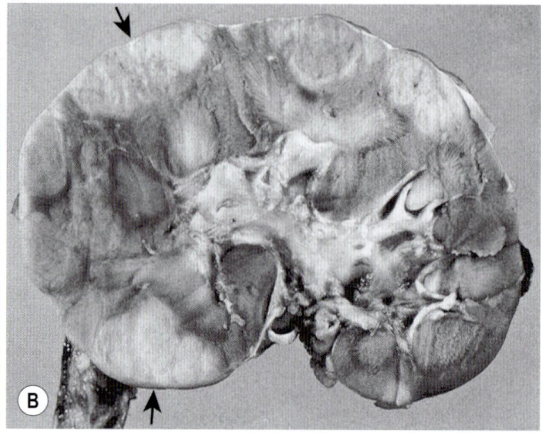

FIGURE 65-3 ■ **(A)** MR image of a 10-month-old infant who presented with large bilateral flank masses demonstrates a picture characteristic of diffuse hyperplastic perilobar nephroblastomatosis (DHPLN) with extensive involvement of the entire cortex of the kidney with no evidence of necrosis and general preservation of the shape of the kidney. **(B)** A resected kidney with a similar pattern of DHPLN reveals extensive involvement of the periphery of the cortex by severely hypertrophied nephrogenic rests (arrows). Resection of such kidneys should be avoided because, in most cases, the hypertrophy will resolve and the kidney will have excellent preservation of its function. (B courtesy of J. B. Beckwith, by permission.)

same study, 24 children developed WT during long-term follow-up with eight being anaplastic. Thirteen had single tumors and 11 were multiple. Treatment was variable and included surgery, radiation and chemotherapy, or expectant observation. The three patients who received no therapy developed WT 10 months after diagnosis. Chemotherapy may decrease the proliferative element in NRs, but it is unclear whether it prevents the development of malignancy. A current COG study includes a treatment protocol to address some of the questions with respect to DHPLN and its optimal therapy.

An increased risk of WT arising in multicystic dysplastic kidneys has been suggested. This is primarily based on case reports and all children have been under the age of four. In contrast, a report describing 1041 infants and children with multicystic dysplastic kidneys found no case associated with a WT.[43] The authors concluded that routine prophylactic nephrectomy was not needed in children with multicystic dysplastic kidneys. Furthermore, a review of the NWTS pathology files identified only three cases of dysplastic kidneys in more than 7,000 children with WT over a 26-year interval.[44] Thus, prophylactic nephrectomy in children with multicystic dysplastic kidney for malignancy is not justified. However, screening ultrasound in these children until age 4 is suggested.[43,44]

Pathology

WTs are currently divided into those with 'favorable' histology and those with 'unfavorable' histology. Unfavorable histology proved to be the most important factor in patient outcome in NWTS-1, a finding that has remained consistent through the current trials.[5,45] Fortunately, favorable histology comprises 90% of the tumors. These tumors are the 'classic WT' consisting of three elements: blastemal, stromal, and epithelial tubules (Fig. 65-4). Tumors contain various proportions of each of these elements. Triphasic are the most characteristic, but biphasic and monophasic lesions also occur.[46] The

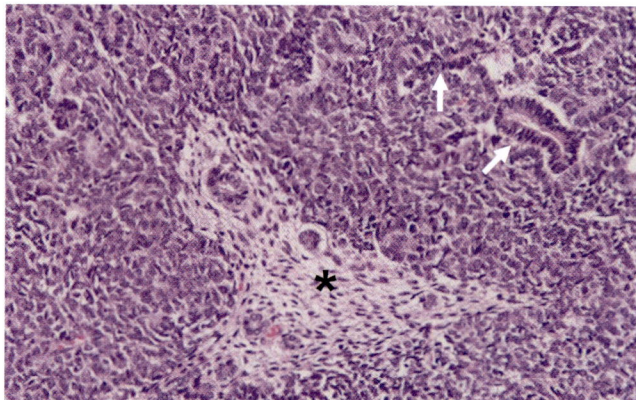

FIGURE 65-4 ■ The classic 'triphasic' histologic pattern (blastemal, epithelial, and mesenchymal derivatives) of a Wilms tumor is seen on this H&E slide. There is a predominance of small undifferentiated blastemal cells in the image that surround a few neoplastic duct and tubular epithelial structures (solid arrows). In the center is an island (asterisk) of spindle-shaped fibroblastic mesenchymal cells that surround a few tubules. The neoplastic cells in the image lack the requisite features of an anaplastic variant (see Fig. 65-5).

proportion of these three elements in WTs have been studied, but have not been shown to predict outcomes. Under the current treatment protocols, they are not utilized to determine therapy.[46,47] Abnormal mucinous or squamous epithelium, skeletal muscle, cartilage, osteoid, or fat are less frequent elements found in WT.[5]

Unfavorable tumors are those with focal or diffuse anaplasia.[5,48,49] Anaplasia is defined by multipolar polyploid mitotic figures, marked nuclear enlargement (giant nuclei with diameters at least three times those of adjacent cells), and hyperchromasia (Fig. 65-5).[50] Determining whether a tumor has diffuse or focal anaplasia is important for prognosis and therapy.[48] Focal anaplasia is defined as the presence of one or a few sharply localized regions of anaplasia within a primary tumor, the majority of which contains no nuclear atypia. Tumor designated

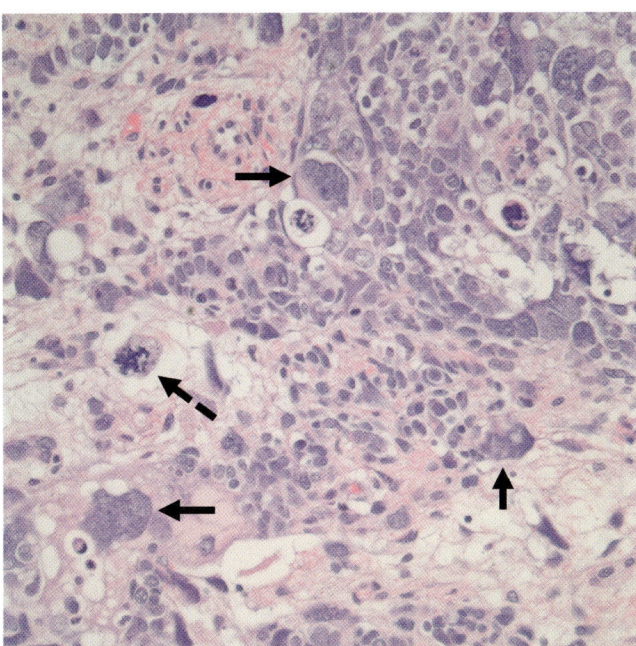

FIGURE 65-5 ■ Salient features of the anaplastic Wilms' tumor variant with H&E staining. Anaplasia is defined by three requisite criteria that are all depicted in the image: atypical mitotic figures (dotted arrow) (often tripolar or multipolar); nuclear enlargement (solid arrows) to greater than three times the size of resident cell nuclei of the same type; and nuclear hyperchromicity present in some of the cells. Enlargement and hyperchromicity reflect the fact that anaplastic Wilms tumors contain nearly twice the amount of DNA as normal cells with duplication of many whole chromosomes in each cell.

as diffuse anaplasia must have at least one of the following four criteria: anaplastic cells outside of the kidney, presence of anaplasia in a random kidney biopsy, anaplasia in more than one region of the kidney, or anaplasia in one region with extreme nuclear pleomorphism in another site. Anaplasia occurs primarily in children older than 2 years. In NWTS-1, 66.7% of patients with anaplasia experienced relapse and 58.3% died of their tumor.[45] Of note, there was a higher frequency of relapse and death in the 'diffuse' subgroup. Additionally, anaplasia in extrarenal tumor sites and a predominantly blastemal tumor pattern were both adverse prognostic factors.[50] Moreover, anaplasia is a marker of resistance to therapy, not of aggressive behavior.[46,47,50] *TP53* deletion on chromosome 17 has been associated with anaplasia. However, a recent study demonstrated recurrent anaplasia-specific genomic loss and under-expression in several additional regions, most strikingly 4q and 14q, suggesting anaplasia is not linked solely to deletions of chromosome 17, but is associated with loss at multiple loci.[51]

CCSK and malignant RTK were grouped in the initial NWTSG studies with the unfavorable histology WT. They are now considered distinct entities from WT, based on their pathologic appearance, biologic behavior, and response to different therapies.[52,53] CCSK is a highly malignant tumor with an unusual proclivity for bony metastasis. It generally appears as a large unifocal and unilateral tumor with a homogeneous mucoid, tan, or gray/tan cut surface, often with foci of necrosis or prominent cysts.[52] This tumor invades and surrounds the renal parenchyma rather than compresses the margin into a pseudocapsule as is seen in a WT. Its classic appearance is that of a deceptively bland tumor with uniform oval nuclei with a delicate chromatin pattern, a prominent nuclear membrane, and sparse, poorly stained vacuolated 'water-clear' cytoplasm with indistinct cell membranes. Although the cells generally appear in cords or nests divided by an arborizing network of vessels and supporting spindle cell septa, there are variations and nine major histologic patterns have been identified.[52,53] Recently, a translocation t(10;17) and deletion (14q) have also been described in CCSK, suggesting that they may play a role in its pathogenesis.[54] The cell of origin of this tumor is not known. In addition to osseous metastases, CCSKs also have a significant incidence of metastases to the brain. Long-term follow-up is important as one report found 30% of the relapses occur more than two years after diagnosis.[55]

Malignant RTK occur in young infants with a median age of 11 months.[56] Most (85%) cases occur within the first two years of life. It is the most aggressive and lethal of all pediatric renal tumors, and fortunately only accounts for 2% of renal tumors. Grossly these tumors are unencapsulated and invasive with characteristic involvement of the perihilar renal parenchyma. Histologically, RTKs are characterized by monomorphous, discohesive, rounded to polygonal cells with acidophilic cytoplasm and eccentric nuclei containing prominent large 'owl eye' nucleoli reminiscent of skeletal muscle, but lacking its cytoplasmic striations, ultrastructural features, and immunochemical markers.[57] A large periodic acid–Schiff (PAS)-positive hyaline cytoplasmic inclusion occurs in a variable population of tumor cells and is a hallmark of this tumor.[58] Ultrastructural examination reveals parallel cytoplasmic filamentous inclusions packed in concentric whorled arrays, a distinctive feature of this tumor, which suggests a neuroectodermal origin. The tumor tends to infiltrate the adjacent renal parenchyma rather than to compress it. These tumors are notable for the occurrence of a second primary tumor in the midline of the brain, resembling medulloblastoma.[59] A consistent deletion (22q11-12) has been described in both renal and extrarenal rhabdoid tumors.[60,61] These deletions delineate an area of overlap at the site of the hSNF5/INI1 gene, and tumors have biallelic alterations or deletions of this gene.[62–64] For all renal tumors except RTK, immunohistochemical staining for the wild type INI-1 protein shows nuclear positivity. In renal and extra renal rhabdoid tumors, this is absent.[64]

Staging

Two principal staging systems are used for children with WT (Table 65-4). The COG system is based on pretreatment findings prior to administration of chemotherapy or radiotherapy. Patients are given a local stage and a disease stage. The local stage defines the extent of abdominal disease, while the disease stage considers both the local extent of disease and distant metastasis. Both factors determine therapy with the use of local radiation therapy to the tumor bed based on the local stage, and

TABLE 65-4   COG and SIOP Wilms Tumor Staging Systems

Stage	Criteria
COG Staging System	
I	The tumor is limited to the kidney and has been completely resected
	The tumor was not ruptured or biopsied prior to removal
	No penetration of the renal capsule or involvement of renal sinus vessels
II	The tumor extends beyond the capsule of the kidney but was completely resected with no evidence of tumor at or beyond the margins of resection
	There is penetration of the renal capsule or invasion of the renal sinus vessels
III	Gross or microscopic residual tumor remains postoperatively, including inoperable tumor, positive surgical margins, tumor spillage, regional lymph node metastases, positive peritoneal cytology, or transected tumor thrombus
	The tumor was ruptured or biopsied prior to removal
IV	Hematogenous metastases or lymph node metastases outside the abdomen, e.g., lung, liver, bone, brain
V	Bilateral renal involvement is present at diagnosis and each side may be considered to have a 'local' stage
SIOP Staging System	
I	The tumor is limited to the kidney or surrounded with a fibrous pseudocapsule if outside the normal contours of the kidney
	The renal capsule or pseudocapsule may be infiltrated with the tumor, but it does not reach the outer surface, and it is completely resected
	The tumor may be protruding (bulging) into the renal pelvis and dipping into the ureter, but it is not infiltrating their walls
	The vessels of the renal sinus are not involved. Intrarenal vessels may be involved
II	The tumor extends beyond the kidney or penetrates through the renal capsule and/or fibrous pseudocapsule into the perirenal fat, but is completely resected
	The tumor infiltrates the renal sinus and/or invades blood and lymphatic vessels outside the renal parenchyma, but it is completely resected
	The tumor infiltrates adjacent organs or vena cava, but is completely resected
	The tumor has been surgically biopsied (wedge biopsy) prior to preoperative chemotherapy or surgery
III	Incomplete excision of the tumor, which extends beyond resection margins (gross or microscopic tumor remains postoperatively)
	Any abdominal lymph nodes are involved. Tumor rupture before or during surgery (irrespective of other criteria for staging)
	The tumor has penetrated the peritoneal surface. Tumor implants are found on the peritoneal surface
	Tumor thrombi are present at resection margins of vessels, or ureter is transected or removed piecemeal by surgeon
IV	Hematogenous metastases (lung, liver, bone, brain, etc.) or lymph node metastases outside the abdominopelvic region
V	Bilateral renal tumors at diagnosis. Each side has to be substaged according to above classifications

the intensity of chemotherapy based on the disease stage.[65]

SIOP protocols generally recommend chemotherapy followed by nephrectomy, with surgicopathologic staging occurring at the time of nephrectomy. The SIOP classification was revised in 2010 based on a review of the histologic appearance of the tumors at resection (post neoadjuvant chemotherapy) and the corresponding outcomes.[66,67] Tumors are now classified on SIOP protocols as completely necrotic (low-risk tumor), blastemal (high-risk tumor), and other histology (intermediate-risk tumors).

Prognostic Factors

The current prognostic factors used in COG trials are histology, stage, age, tumor weight, response to therapy and LOH at 1p and 16q. The two most important factors continue to be the histology and the stage of the tumor.[25,68,69] The details and prognostic significance of tumor pathology has been previously discussed in the Pathology section. The tumor stage is determined by the results of the imaging studies, the findings at operation, and the histological findings.

Analysis from early NWTS studies identified a group of patients whose excellent outcomes were unaffected by chemotherapy. These children were less than 2 years of age, had tumors that weighed less than 550 g, and were stage I with favorable histology. The treatment for children with these characteristics in the current protocol is operative resection alone. Ongoing studies are examining various molecular markers to determine if this risk category can be better defined.

Rapid response to chemotherapy is a prognostic category that is being evaluated in patients who present with stage IV disease due to lung metastasis. The goal in these patients is to avoid lung radiation. Response to therapy is also being assessed in BWTs. Also, LOH at both 1p and 16q is now being used for determination of therapy in the current COG renal tumor studies.[25]

Clinical Presentation and Diagnosis

The differential diagnosis for a malignant abdominal mass in a child includes WT, neuroblastoma, hepatoblastoma, rhabdomyosarcoma and lymphoma. WT is often noted during a bath or by the pediatrician at a routine visit. This is in marked contrast to neuroblastoma, which

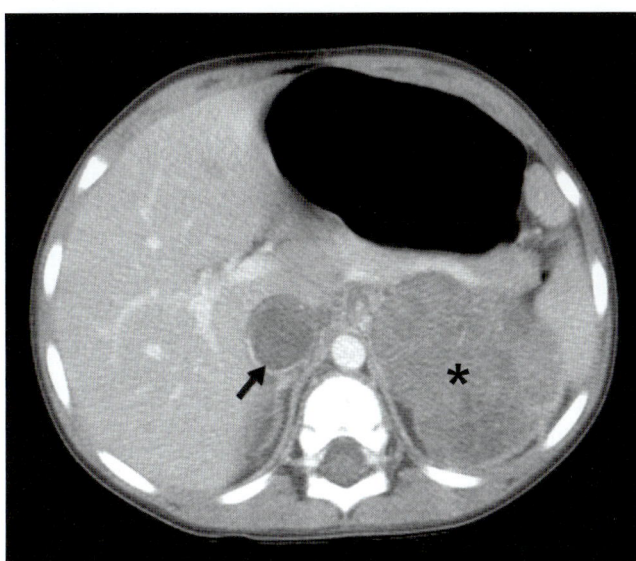

FIGURE 65-6 ■ A transverse cut of a CT scan demonstrating a left Wilms tumor (asterisk) that extends into the inferior vena cava (arrow).

that allow accurate diagnosis. Intra-abdominal staging has been difficult to assess radiographically unless extensive lymph node involvement or intrahepatic metastases are present. A recent study by Khanna and associates, using the COG database of 3,000 cases, found the preoperative imaging sensitivity and specificity of ultrasound in detecting WT rupture to be 53.7% and 88.4%, respectively, compared to the findings at operation.[74] The common sites of metastatic spread are the lungs and the liver; hence CT scans of the chest should be included in the staging studies.

Treatment

The treatment for WT includes operation, chemotherapy, and in some cases, radiation therapy (RT). In the past decade, as a result of excellent outcomes and a greater appreciation for the long-term late effects, adjuvant therapy has been avoided in a small proportion of children with an extremely low-risk of local recurrence and metastasis. In other protocols, treatment reductions are now being explored as well.

Surgery

Surgical Details

The essential tasks that are required of the surgeon, irrespective of when the WT resection occurs, are: (1) safe resection of the tumor; (2) accurate staging of the tumor; (3) avoidance of complications that 'upstage' the tumor (rupture or unnecessary biopsy); and (4) accurate documentation of the operative findings and details of the procedure in the operative notes. Tumor spill, failure to biopsy lymph nodes (for both unilateral and bilateral tumors), incomplete tumor removal, failure to assess for extrarenal tumor extension, and operative complications will adversely impact patient survival.[75–77]

is seen in the same age group, but frequently presents with pain, often from osseous metastasis. WT also may be associated with hematuria (gross in 18.2% and microscopic in 24.5% of patients), but with a much lower frequency than is seen with RCC.[16] Twenty to 25% of patients present with hypertension, and 10% with fever. Occasionally, a child may have abdominal trauma and demonstrate pain out of proportion to what is expected, and an abdominal mass is found that cannot be attributed to the trauma.

Radiographic imaging is performed to determine the anatomic location and extent of the mass. WT can extend into the renal vein (11% of cases) or the vena cava (4% of cases) (Fig. 65-6).[70,71] Embolization of a caval thrombus to the pulmonary artery can be lethal, and the presence of a thrombus must be identified preoperatively to prevent this occurrence. Ultrasound has been the recommended screening study for an abdominal mass to determine its site of origin and to assess for possible intravascular or ureteral extension. However, a 2012 COG study demonstrated computed tomography (CT) can accurately identify cavo-atrial tumor thrombus as well.[72] Routine Doppler ultrasound evaluation, after CT has already been performed, may not be needed. A CT/MRI scan of the abdomen will confirm a renal origin to the mass, and whether there are bilateral tumors. Historically, bilateral renal explorations were recommended by NWTSG protocols because early generations of CT scans missed 7–10% of bilateral lesions. However, with new helical CT scans only 0.25% of bilateral tumors are missed.[73] Based on these results, bilateral exploration is not recommended on current protocols from the COG.

A neuroblastoma will generally indent the kidney whereas WTs arise from within the kidney and distort its internal configuration. Also, a thin lip of renal parenchyma can often be seen extending over the neoplasm in a WT, known as the claw sign (Fig. 65-7). Unfortunately, there are no characteristic radiographic findings of WTs

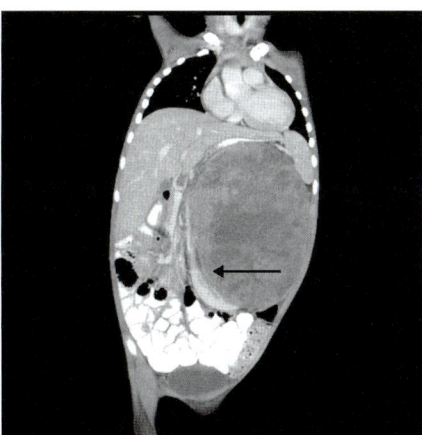

FIGURE 65-7 ■ CT scan of a 4-year-old boy found on routine physical examination demonstrating a very large left renal tumor and the classic 'claw sign' of a Wilms tumor that occurs with extension of the thin lip of renal parenchyma (arrow) over the tumor.

Although WTs are usually initially seen as a large mass, most are resectable (Fig. 65-8). Renal tumors should be excised through an adequate subcostal or thoracoabdominal incision. Struggling through an inadequate incision will often result in tumor rupture, which increases both the stage of the tumor and the risk for intra-abdominal recurrence.[77] A flank incision should not be used for resection of pediatric renal tumors because of the limited exposure it provides. Initial exploration of the abdomen includes inspection for hepatic metastases or intraperitoneal spread. The vena cava, if it is accessible, should be palpated to assess for intravascular extension of tumor. The colon is then mobilized off the anterior aspect of the kidney and the renal mass. Although early descriptions of the operative technique recommended initial control of the renal hilum, this is often not feasible with extremely large tumors and must await mobilization of the mass to allow safe exposure of the hilum. Premature attempts at vascular control, particularly for left-sided tumors, may result in ligation of the superior mesenteric artery.[78] The renal mass should not be biopsied unless the decision is made to not proceed with a complete resection. Biopsy will produce contamination of the peritoneum and increase the tumor stage to stage III.

Biopsy of lymph nodes in the renal hilum and along the vena cava and aorta is critical for adequate staging. Even in children with stage IV disease, local staging is vital because it will determine whether abdominal radiation therapy is used in children treated on COG protocols. Studies have demonstrated that the surgeon's gross evaluation and assessment of lymph nodes does not reliably correspond with the histologic involvement of tumor in the nodes, with false-negative and false-positive rates of 31.3% and 18.1%, respectively.[79] An increased incidence of local recurrence was seen in NWTS-4 children in whom biopsy of lymph nodes was not performed,

particularly in stage I cases.[77] This suggests that under treatment of local disease in these children, due to inadequate staging, resulted in an increased frequency of local recurrence. Although grossly involved lymph nodes are generally resected, an extensive retroperitoneal lymph node resection has not been demonstrated to improve local control.[80] There has recently been increased interest in determining the extent of node dissection required for both WT and other renal tumors, although to date the data are inconclusive and retrospective.[81,82] As the tumor is being mobilized, the ureter is palpated for tumor and is resected close to the bladder. Gross hematuria in children with WT is infrequent, but its occurrence suggests involvement of the renal pelvis with possible extension down into the ureter.[83] Cystoscopy should be considered in these children to identify bladder involvement to avoid transection of the tumor thrombus during division of the ureter. Complete resection of the ureteral extension prevents this finding from increasing the local stage of the tumor. If the tumor involves the upper pole of the kidney, the adrenal gland is generally resected to provide adequate margins around the tumor. With lower-pole lesions, the adrenal gland may be preserved.

The factors associated with an increased risk of local recurrence include stage III disease, unfavorable histology, failure to biopsy the lymph nodes, and tumor rupture during operation.[77] Tumor rupture and biopsy of the lymph nodes are the factors that the surgeon can impact. Multiple regression analysis adjusting for the combined effects of histology, lymph node involvement, and age reveal that tumor spillage remained significant and was greatest in children with stage II disease who received less intensive therapy. Most tumor ruptures occur during mobilization of the posterior aspects of the tumor where it is adherent to the diaphragm. This can be best prevented by the use of an adequate incision for exposure and resection of a segment of the adherent diaphragm if necessary. In a review of 2,000 cases of WT, size of tumor greater than 15 cm was the most significant risk for tumor rupture.[84] Tumor rupture/spillage results in a stage III classification which results in additional chemotherapy and RT in a child who otherwise might have stage II disease.

'Spill' refers to a break in the tumor capsule during resection whether accidental, unavoidable, or by design. Spill is also considered to have occurred if the tumor is transected when the renal vein or ureter is divided. In COG protocols, a preoperative or intraoperative biopsy (needle or open) are stage III criteria. This is not true for patients on SIOP protocols where fine needle or Tru-cut biopsies are stage II criteria and incisional biopsies mean stage III. 'Rupture' refers to either the spontaneous or post-traumatic rupture of the tumor preoperatively with the result that tumor cells are disseminated throughout the peritoneal or retroperitoneal space.[85] Blood in the peritoneal cavity may be a sign of rupture. When found, a thorough examination of the tumor surface is mandated. Rupture is also considered to have occurred if the tumor penetrates the renal capsule, with tumor extending into the peritoneal cavity. When encountered, all of these situations make the child stage III (COG and SIOP) and must be carefully documented in the operative note.

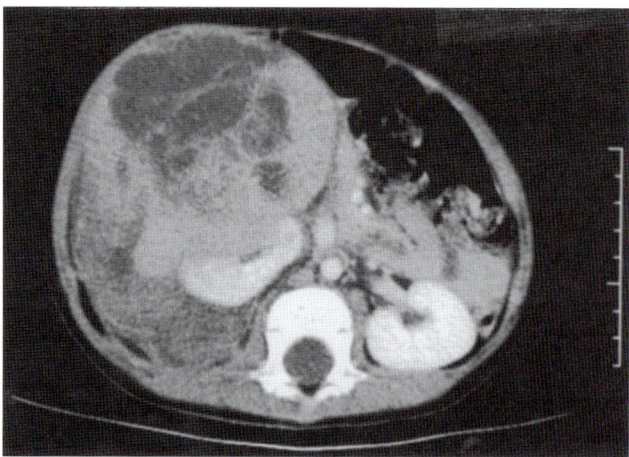

FIGURE 65-8 ■ CT scan of a 3-year-old boy who presented with a history of abdominal pain, fever, and a right flank mass. The tumor is very large with extension outside the renal capsule into the retroperitoneal tissues posterior to the kidney. Despite its size, this lesion was able to be completely resected. Lymph nodes and specimen margins were negative for tumor. This tumor was therefore stage II, and the infant was able to avoid both anthracycline therapy and abdominal irradiation because of the complete resection.

Resection of adjacent organs (liver, spleen, or pancreas) or resection of massive WT are discouraged because such extensive resections are associated with a significant increase in surgical complications.[76,86] In this situation the surgeon should only sample the primary tumor.

Prior to operation, coagulation studies should be obtained because acquired von Willebrand disease (vWD) has been reported in WT and other malignancies.[87,88] A single prospective study of 50 WT patients found the incidence of acquired vWD was 8%.[88] However, the true incidence and prevalence is unknown. Historically, when coagulation abnormalities were identified, they were felt to be clinically insignificant.[89] However, reports of profuse intraoperative bleeding (despite normalization of FVIII, vWF activity, and antigen level prior to operation) that only stopped after ligation of the renal vessels have contradicted this assumption.[89,90] Once the renal vessels were ligated, all abnormal bleeding stopped. The mechanism of acquired vWD in WT is unknown.[91,92] In all cases where bleeding occurred, the child had a prolonged PT and PTT. Correction of these abnormalities is important. The observation that bleeding stopped when the renal vessels were ligated suggests that preoperative embolization should be considered as a management strategy.

Surgical Complications

The complications detailed in the NWTS-4 study have also been assessed.[76] In this study, surgeons were discouraged from performing extensive operations involving resection of adjacent organs or massive tumors. Complications occurred in 12.7% of a random sample of 534 of the 3335 patients treated in this study. Again, intestinal obstruction was the most frequent complication (5.1%), followed by extensive hemorrhage (1.9%), wound infection (1.9%), and vascular injury (1.5%). The factors associated with an increased risk of complications were assessed. Intravascular tumor extension into the inferior vena cava (IVC) or atrium, and nephrectomy performed through a flank or paramedian incision were both significant factors. Tumor diameter of 10 cm or larger also was associated with increased complications. Finally, the risk of complications was increased if the resection was performed by a general surgeon rather than a pediatric surgeon or pediatric urologist. In a study involving 598 patients registered on SIOP-9, a complication rate of 8% was reported. These patients were pretreated with vincristine, dactinomycin, and epirubicin or doxorubicin before nephrectomy.[93] The most frequent events were small bowel obstruction (3.7%) and tumor rupture (2.8%).

Unresectable Tumors

In some cases, tumor biopsy and biopsy of the regional lymph nodes should be performed, followed by administration of chemotherapy before a second attempt at resection.

The current guidelines for an unresectable tumor are: (1) when there is extension of tumor thrombus into the IVC above the level of the hepatic veins; (2) the tumor involves contiguous structures whereby the only means of removing the kidney tumor requires removal of the other structures (e.g., spleen, pancreas, colon, but excluding the adrenal gland and diaphragm); (3) bilateral tumors; (4) tumor in a solitary kidney; or (5) if there is pulmonary compromise due to extensive pulmonary metastases. SIOP studies have shown that pretreatment with chemotherapy almost always reduces the bulk of the tumor.[93,94] This makes tumor removal easier, and may reduce the incidence of operative complications.

Intravascular Extension

Identification of vascular extension by preoperative radiographic studies (see Fig. 65-6) or during exploration is critical to avoid a tumor embolus during mobilization of the kidney. The presence of intravascular extension does not affect the prognosis of the tumor as long as it is successfully resected.[95] Initially, intravascular extension was managed with removal of the tumor thrombus from the renal vein or IVC using cardiopulmonary bypass if necessary. However, this strategy has been found to have significant complications (70%).[96,97] A review of all of the children treated on the NWTS-4 protocol described 165 of 2731 patients with intravascular extension into the IVC (134 patients) or atrium (31 patients).[95] Sixty-nine of these patients received preoperative chemotherapy (55 with IVC extension and 14 with atrial extension). Five complications were encountered during preoperative chemotherapy, including tumor embolism and tumor progression in one patient each, and three patients developed adult respiratory distress syndrome, one of whom died. Intravascular extension of the tumor regressed in 39 of 49 children with comparable pre- and post-therapy radiographic studies, including regression in seven of 12 in whom the tumor regressed from an atrial location, avoiding the need for cardiopulmonary bypass. A high incidence of operative complications occurred in these patients, with 36.7% in the children with atrial extension and 17.2% in those with IVC involvement. The frequency of operative complications was 26% in the primary resection group versus 13.2% in children with preoperative therapy. When all the complications were considered, including those that occurred during preoperative chemotherapy (one of these five patients also had a surgical complication), the incidence of complications among those receiving preoperative therapy was not statistically different from the incidence among those who underwent initial resection. However, the most severe complications occurred in the primary resection group. Also, preoperative therapy was found to facilitate surgical resection by decreasing the extent of the tumor thrombus.

Management of Tumor Extension in the Ureter

Extension of WT into the ureter is a rare event which can be difficult to detect with preoperative imaging. In NWTS-5, the incidence of ureteral extension was 2%. However, preoperative imaging detected the ureteral involvement in only 30%.[83] Clinical findings of ureteral involvement may include gross hematuria, passage of tissue per urethra, hydronephrosis, and a urethral mass. If these findings are encountered, ureteral involvement should be suspected. Cystoscopy with a retrograde ureterogram may aid in the preoperative evaluation. When encountered or suspected, the ureter with tumor extension should be resected with clear margins.

Horseshoe Kidney, Single Kidney and Nonfunctioning Kidney

Children with a tumor in a horseshoe kidney should be treated as having a unilateral tumor, not a bilateral tumor. The blood supply to horseshoe kidneys is quite variable as is the location of the ureters which should be delineated prior to surgery.[98] The side of the kidney containing the tumor, the isthmus, and the ipsilateral ureter are resected and the lymph nodes are sampled for staging. Children with a single kidney, or a situation where a tumor occurs in one kidney but the second kidney is nonfunctioning, should be managed using a renal-sparing approach with preoperative chemotherapy to facilitate preservation of renal tissue.

Resection Alone for Very Low Risk Wilms Tumor (VLRWT)

The outcomes of children younger than 2 years with stage I tumor specimens weighing less than 550 g registered in the NWTSG studies were reviewed. Adjuvant therapy made little apparent impact on their survival which exceeded 90%.[99] In a prospective pilot study at Children's Hospital in Boston, eight children meeting these criteria were followed without adjuvant therapy.[100] In seven of eight, there was no recurrence. In one child, a metachronous tumor was cured by resection and chemotherapy.

One treatment arm of NWTS-5 was a trial of operation only for children with these VLRWTs.[101] Seventy-five infants were enrolled. In three infants, a metachronous, contralateral WT developed, and eight patients experienced relapse 0.3 to 1.05 years after diagnosis. The sites of relapse were pulmonary (five cases) and the operative bed (three cases). The 2-year disease-free survival, including both relapse and metachronous tumors, was 86.5%, and the two-year survival rate was 100%, with a median follow-up of 2.84 years. The 2-year disease-free survival, excluding metachronous contralateral WT, was 89.2%, and the 2-year cumulative risk of metachronous contralateral WT was 3.1%. The stopping rules for the study required closure after these 75 infants were enrolled. A recent long-term follow-up study was reported on this surgery-only cohort as well as the children entered on the protocol that eventually were treated with vincristine and actinomycin D (EE-4A).[102] With a median follow-up of 8.2 years, the estimated 5-year event-free survival (EFS) for surgery-only was 84%; for the EE-4A patients it was 97% ($P = 0.002$). One death was observed in each group. The estimated 5-year overall survival (OS) was 98% for surgery-only and 99% for EE-4A ($P = 0.70$). The surgery-only EFS was lower than EE-4A, consistent with the earlier report. The salvage rate for the surgery-only cohort exceeded that seen with children who had

received two-drug chemotherapy. Thus, 85% of the infants avoided any chemotherapy, while those who did receive it for relapse, were treated with three agents, vincristine, actinomycin D and doxorubicin (DD-4A), resulting in an OS equivalent to the group which received chemotherapy.

A recent biological study looking at the surgery-only arm in NWTS-5 found that a *WT1* mutation and 11p15 LOH were associated with relapse in the patients with VLRWTs who did not receive chemotherapy.[103] 11p15 LOH was identified in 19 (41%) of 46 evaluable VLRWTs and was significantly associated with relapse ($P < 0.001$). A *WT1* mutation was identified in nine (20%) of 45 evaluable VLRWTs and was significantly associated with relapse ($P = 0.004$); All nine cases also had 11p15 LOH. A current study in COG is assessing this cohort again and is evaluating biological markers for this very low-risk group.

Neonatal Wilms Tumor

Neonatal renal lesions are rare and include benign and malignant tumors.[104,105] In the perinatal period, CMN accounts for greater than 50% of the renal tumors followed in rank by WT, RTK, and CCSK. Of note, after 3 months of age, CMN accounts for less than 10%. In a 2008 report, 210 renal tumors diagnosed prenatally ($n = 47$) and at birth ($n = 163$) were evaluated.[105] The cohort consisted of four main tumors: CMN (139 cases or 66%), WT (41 or 20%), RTK (23 or 11%), and CCSK (7 or 3%). A recent international retrospective study of 750 neonatal renal tumors in children less than 7 months of age found that 63.4% were WT.[104] Eighty-two per cent of these were stage I/II. In contrast, RTK presented with advanced disease (53% stage III/IV). Outcomes paralleled older children with excellent results for neonates with WT (5-year OS of 93.4%) and poor outcome for RTK (5-year OS of 16.4%).

Extrarenal Wilms Tumor

An extrarenal site of primary WT is uncommon. These extrarenal tumors behave identically to tumors arising within the kidney and should be treated both locally and systemically based on the same criteria.[106,107] Common sites of occurrence of extrarenal WT include the retroperitoneum, inguinal canal, scrotum, and vagina. Less common sites are the uterus, cervix, ovary, and the presacral space.

Chemotherapy

WT was the first malignant pediatric solid tumor with a demonstrated response to dactinomycin.[1] Many additional effective agents have been subsequently identified including vincristine, doxorubicin, cyclophosphamide, ifosfamide, and etoposide. Today the backbone of all WT chemotherapeutic regimens continues to be dactinomycin and vincristine, and they remain the sole chemotherapy for patients with stage I and II tumors.

NWTS-1 and 2 established the main chemotherapeutic regimen for stage I WT. NWTS-3 and NWTS-4 were the first studies to prospectively evaluate the benefit of additional/different chemotherapy for these tumors.[108] Key results from NWTS-3 were: (1) children with stage I tumors, with an 11-week regimen composed of vincristine and dactinomycin only, had a 4-year relapse-free survival (RFS) and OS of 89.0% and 95.6%; (2) the addition of doxorubicin to the treatment of children with stage III tumors improved survival; (3) no benefit was found with the addition of doxorubicin or radiation therapy for children with stage II tumors; and (4) no benefit from the addition of cyclophosphamide to the treatment of children with stage IV tumors.[109] A follow-up analysis of doxorubicin for stage III patients demonstrated an increase in the 8-year EFS and OS of randomized patients who received doxorubicin, dactinomycin, and vincristine (84% and 89%) when compared with those who received dactinomycin and vincristine alone (74% and 83%).[110]

NWTS-4 addressed dose intensification and also evaluated the use of two time intervals for the administration of chemotherapy: a short course (18 to 26 weeks, depending on the regimen and stage) versus a long course (54 to 66 weeks). Key findings were that the pulse-intensive regimens produced less hematologic toxicity than the standard regimens, allowing greater dose intensity with comparable outcomes.[108,111] The second randomization demonstrated no benefit in any of the stages for the long interval of therapy compared with the short interval. In NWTS-4, the 4-year EFS and OS averaged 90% for patients with favorable histology.[108,112]

NWTS-5 focused on evaluating biological markers of prognosis, developing more effective therapy for recurrent disease, and reducing therapy in children with low-risk tumors. Patients with LOH at both 1p and 16q had EFS and OS which were 10% worse than those in patients without LOH (see Fig. 65-1). In the current COG protocols, children with LOH at these sites will receive more intensive therapy; children with stage I or II will receive three drug therapy with DD-4A and children with stage III and IV will receive regimen M (Table 65-5).

NWTS-5 had specific relapse protocols for children with stage I and II, as well as stage III and IV disease. Fifty-eight children with initial stage I and II disease experienced relapse after treatment with EE-4A.[113] Their relapse therapy included alternating courses of vincristine, doxorubicin, cyclophosphamide, and etoposide, along with surgery if feasible, and RT. After this specified relapse therapy, EFS at 4 years was 71.1% and OS was 81.8%. The lung was the only site of relapse in 31 children. Those with only pulmonary relapse had similar EFS (67.8%) and OS (81.0%). Sixty patients with stage III and IV disease relapsed after initial therapy with DD-4A and radiation.[114] Their relapse therapy included alternating cycles of cyclophosphamide/etoposide and carboplatin/etoposide along with surgery and RT. After therapy, EFS in these patients at 4 years was 42.3% and OS was 48.0%. The lung was the sole site of relapse in 33 patients with an EFS of 48.9% and OS of 52.8%. At present, there is no open relapse study in SIOP or COG. The current COG chemotherapeutic regimens are shown in Table 65-5.

TABLE 65-5 COG Chemotherapy Regimens for Unilateral Wilms Tumor

Regimen	Agents
EE-4A	Vincristine and dactinomycin
DD-4A	Vincristine, dactinomycin, doxorubicin, plus RT
Regimen I	Vincristine, dactinomycin, doxorubicin, cyclophosphamide, and etoposide, plus RT
Regimen M	Vincristine, dactinomycin, doxorubicin, cyclophosphamide, and etoposide, plus RT
Revised UH-1	Vincristine, dactinomycin, doxorubicin, cyclophosphamide, carboplatin, etoposide, plus RT
Revised UH2	Vincristine, dactinomycin, doxorubicin, cyclophosphamide, carboplatin, etoposide, irinotecan, plus RT
Vincristine/irinotecan Window therapy	Vincristine and irinotecan in conjunction with revised UH-1 or revised UH-2 depending on response

COG, Children's Oncology Group; RT, radiation therapy.

Treatment of children with diffuse anaplastic tumors remains a challenge. NWTS-3 and NWTS-4 studies demonstrated that children with focal anaplasia had an excellent outcome when treated with vincristine, doxorubicin, and dactinomycin.[49] In NWTS-5, in order to reduce toxicity, patients with focal anaplasia or diffuse stage I were treated with EE-4A. Unfortunately, the four-year EFS and OS estimates for stage I (focal or diffuse) anaplastic WT were lower than in previous studies (EFS 69.5% and OS 82.6%). Thus, therapy with EE-4A above is inadequate. In NWTS-5, children with stage II to IV diffuse anaplastic WT were treated with alternating courses of vincristine, doxorubicin, and cyclophosphamide, and cyclophosphamide and etoposide (regimen I). The four-year EFS estimates for stages II-IV diffuse anaplastic WT in NWTS-5 were 82.6%, 64.7%, and 33.3%, respectively, with similar OS.[47]

The chemotherapy treatment for CCSK on NWTS-1 to NWTS-3 was the same as for WT and the outcomes were poor (OS 66.9% at 8 years).[115] In NWTS-4, patients with CCSK were treated with vincristine, dactinomycin, and doxorubicin, and were randomized to standard (ST) versus pulse-intensive (PI) chemotherapy and short-duration versus long-duration chemotherapy. OS improved on NWTS-4 compared to NWTS-3 (OS 83% versus 66.9% at 8 years, $P < 0.01$).[115] To further improve survival, patients on NWTS-5 with CCSK were treated using regimen I, because etoposide and cyclophosphamide were active against CCSK in preclinical models.[116] Four-year OS for stage I patients was 100%. Stage II, III, and IV had 4-year OS of 88.9%, 94.8% and 41.7%, respectively. LOH was not found in patients with CCSK and is not predictive of outcomes. In the current COG study, children with stage I disease will continue to be treated with regimen I, but will not receive RT. In order to improve survival for children with higher stage disease, they will be treated with the more intensive revised UH-1 (see Table 65-5).

The rhabdoid tumors have remained the most resistant of all pediatric renal tumors. An analysis of 142 children treated on NWTS-1 to NWTS-5 showed an OS of 23.2% at four years.[117] Survival was stage dependent and children with stage I/II disease had a 41.8% 4-year survival, while children with stage III, IV, or V tumors had a 15.9% four-year survival. Survival was also clearly related to the age at presentation. The 4-year survival was worst for those between birth and 5 months of age at diagnosis (8.8%) and best for those older than 2 years of age (41.1%). NWTS-5 used an intensive therapy with carboplatin, etoposide, and cyclophosphamide, and showed no significant improvement. Children with RTK on the current COG study are treated using revised UH-1 if they are stage I-IV after operation and have no measurable disease. If they have measureable disease (stage III, IV), they will receive a vincristine/irinotecan 'window,' followed by revised UH-2 if they have a clinical response. The rational for this treatment strategy was based on reviewing the outcomes from the IRS studies and several case reports that documented the successful treatment of advanced or metastatic RTK.[118–120]

Pretreatment Prior to Surgery

SIOP has promoted the use of preoperative treatment of children with WT with RT or chemotherapy since the early 1970s. The major driving force for the use of preoperative therapy by SIOP was the high rate of tumor rupture at operation that occurred in their early series during which patients did not receive preliminary treatment. The rupture rate decreased from 33% (20 of 60) to 4% (3 of 72) with preoperative abdominal irradiation (20 Gy) in the first randomized SIOP study of renal tumors (SIOP-1).[121] It must be noted, however, that 33% is an extremely high rupture rate. In addition, survival was not improved by the decrease in operative rupture, and the incidence of local recurrence was not reported. It is difficult to compare rupture rates between SIOP and COG as the definition of what is a rupture differs between the two groups. SIOP reported an intraoperative rupture rate of less than 8%.[122] The most recent COG data from 2012 reports an intraoperative rupture rate of 9.8%.[84]

Histologic confirmation of the diagnosis before therapy is not routinely performed in SIOP protocols. This approach has several risks. One is the potential for administration of chemotherapy for benign disease. Second, modification of tumor histology by the chemotherapy may occur. Third, staging information may be lost. Fourth, a malignant RTK or CCSK, if present, will not respond to standard therapies. NWTSG and SIOP studies have demonstrated a 7.6–9.9% rate of benign or altered malignant diagnosis in children with a prenephrectomy diagnosis of WT.[123,124] The United Kingdom Children's Cancer Study Group (UKCCSG) identified 12% of cases that were clinically and radiographically consistent with WT, but had other diagnoses established by biopsy.[125] For SIOP-9 inappropriate preoperative therapy was given to 5.5% of the patients, including 1.6% with benign lesions or malignant lesions not expected to respond to the therapy, including neuroblastoma, lymphoma, RTK, and RCC.

Tumors that are treated with chemotherapy before resection differ in their histopathological findings from tumors resected primarily. The SIOP risk classification uses these histological findings as prognostic indicators to determine further therapies. Low-risk tumors are those that are completely necrotic following preoperative chemotherapy. Intermediate-risk tumors include all histologies other than completely necrotic, rhabdoid, anaplastic or blastemal (less than 66%) dominant. High-risk tumors are those with diffuse anaplasia, rhabdoid, and blastemal dominance (greater than 66%) after chemotherapy.

In the SIOP-9 study, the most common subtype of tumors resected without neoadjuvant chemotherapy was triphasic mixed histology (45.1%), followed by blastemal (39.4%) and epithelial dominant (15.5%), whereas in tumors that received preoperative chemotherapy, the most common histology was regressive (37.6%), followed by mixed (29.4%), stromal (14%), blastemal (9.3%) and epithelial predominant (3.1%). 6.6% of tumors were completely necrotic.[67,126]

In the SIOP-9 study, a randomization was performed between 4 and 8 weeks of preoperative therapy with dactinomycin and vincristine to determine whether the additional 4 weeks of therapy produced a larger proportion of stage I tumors.[93] No advantage was seen from the extended therapy in terms of staging at resection between the 4-week and 8-week courses (stage I,64% versus 62%) or the incidence of tumor rupture (1% vs 3%). For all cases, tumor size decreased by more than half in 52% of the cases. During the second 4 weeks of therapy, there was another 50% reduction in 33% of the cases.

Radiotherapy

The three principle fields for RT for renal tumors are whole abdominal, flank, and lung (metastatic lung disease). Favorable histology tumors are generally very radiosensitive. Current guidelines for radiation therapy in the North American protocols are based on the results of prior cooperative group studies. In 1950, Gross demonstrated that postoperative RT could improve survival to 47%.[11] NWTS-1 concluded that RT provided no survival advantage in children younger than 24 months with stage I FH tumors who also received 15 months of dactinomycin. NWTS-1 also showed that stage III tumors with a confined spill did not require whole abdominal RT, but had comparable outcomes with flank radiation.[123,127] Currently, whole abdominal radiation is only used in three instances: (1) peritoneal seeding; (2) preoperative tumor rupture;, and (3) an intraoperative spill that is widespread in the opinion of the operating surgeon.

NWTS-2 confirmed that RT could be avoided in all children with stage I WT if they received vincristine and dactinomycin.[128] NWTS-2 also established that delaying RT longer than 10 to 14 days after resection was associated with a higher incidence of abdominal relapse, particularly among patients with unfavorable-histology tumors and a small radiation field.[123,127,129] A recent review from NWTS-3 and -4 data confirmed this finding.[130]

NWTS-3 demonstrated that RT could be avoided in children with stage II tumors who received vincristine and dactinomycin, and showed that children with stage III favorable histology tumors who received 10.8 Gy radiotherapy, vincristine, dactinomycin, and doxorubicin had similar tumor control to those who received 20 Gy with vincristine and dactinomycin. This was an important finding, because it eliminated the need for an age-adjusted dose schedule, and significantly reduced the recommended dose of radiation and its subsequent early and late toxicity. Anaplastic tumors tend to be more resistant to chemotherapy, and are also resistant to RT. NWTS-5 did not give RT for stage I anaplastic histology(AH) tumors. However, patients with AH stage II and III tumors in NWTS-5 did receive 10 Gy in conjunction with nephrectomy and chemotherapy. The outcomes for both of these treatment strategies were suboptimal as described above. Fifty per cent of stage III recurrences were local, suggesting that the dose of 10 Gy was not adequate.

Regarding liver metastases, only those that are unresectable at diagnosis are radiated. The treatment portal includes that portion of the liver involved on CT or MRI studies. The whole liver is treated in children with diffuse hepatic metastases.

The management of pulmonary disease in children with WT has become more complicated. The use of CT scans instead of chest radiographs to establish the presence of pulmonary metastasis has resulted in more lesions being identified—not all of which may be cancer.[131] Complicating the possibility of unnecessary radiation is the fact that radiation therapy is a major cause of long-term morbidity, particularly to the lung and heart, producing myocardial injury, pulmonary fibrosis and second malignancy.[132–134] From NWTS-5, the 5-year EFS (95% CI) for stage IV category was: lung only 76% (72–80%); liver and lung 70% (57–80%).[135]

The current COG protocol has made significant changes with regard to patients with pulmonary disease. First, lesions seen by CT scan will be considered pulmonary metastasis unless biopsy proven not to be metastatic disease. Second, in an attempt to spare pulmonary radiation in those children who appear to have responsive disease, children will not receive radiation therapy if the pulmonary lesions radiographically resolve by CT scan after six weeks of chemotherapy. This second change was based on several observations. In SIOP-9, patients were spared whole lung radiation therapy if they rapidly responded to three drug chemotherapy by 6 weeks. The five-year RFS for stage IV patients receiving preoperative chemotherapy was 62.5%.[136] A COG study of patients with pulmonary lesions detected by CT only (as opposed to CT and chest radiograph), and treated with only two chemotherapeutic agents, showed an inferior outcome compared to those treated with three drugs, irrespective of whether or not they received pulmonary RT.[135] The results of these studies have been controversial. The UKCCSG-Wilms Tumor Study 1 followed a similar protocol, yet their six-year EFS was only 50%.[137] In the second UKCCSG-Wilms tumor study (UKWT2), the majority of children with lung metastases received whole lung irradiation (WLI), and the 4-year survival rate improved to 75%.[138]

Bilateral Wilms Tumor

BWT occurs in 4–13% of patients.[17,69,139,140] The EFS and OS in children with bilateral tumors have been lower than those with unilateral tumors. In NWTS-5, the four-year OS was 80.8% for a child with favorable histology and 43.8% for a child with anaplastic histology.[47] SIOP-9 reported 28 children with BWT, all treated with individualized preoperative therapy.[136] Overall survival at 5 years was 85.1% (95% CI: 71.6–98.6%), and RFS was 80.5% (95% CI: 65.2– 95.8%).[136]

COG initiated the first cooperative group trial of BWT in 2009. Reviews of patients treated prior to this time revealed that in addition to poor outcomes, children with BWT had significantly higher rates of renal failure and underwent prolonged chemotherapy regimens compared to those with unilateral tumors. BWT was the greatest risk factor for renal failure (16.4% for NWTS-1 and -2, 9.9% for NWTS-3, and 3.8% for NWTS-4).[141] Other risk factors identified were: Denys–Drash syndrome, metachronous tumor, progressive disease requiring bilateral nephrectomies, and radiation nephritis. Breslow reported the 20-year end-stage renal disease (ESRD) outcomes in children treated for WT.[142] The major risk factors he identified for renal failure were BWT, Denys–Drash and WAGR, and congenital genitourinary anomalies (hypospadias or cryptorchidism).

Two studies highlight the issue of prolonged chemotherapy in patients with BWT. One study found 38 of 188 patients with BWT had progressive or nonresponsive disease (PNRD).[143] Patients with PNRD fell into two categories. The first category included patients with anaplastic tumors that were not sensitive to the administered therapy (four patients). Due to this lack of response to therapy once the diagnosis of anaplasia is made, a complete resection is needed.[47,144–146] The second category included patients who had tumors with very mature rhabdomyomatous or differentiated stromal elements (14 patients) or with complete necrosis. These patients had good outcomes and are best served with resection. In the other 20 patients, 12 weeks of chemotherapy did not result in any tumor shrinkage. Another study evaluated the histological changes in BWT that did not respond to chemotherapy, and the relationship between these changes and prognosis.[147] The results mirrored those of the NWTS study. The findings of these two reports emphasize that in cases of bilateral lesions that do not respond radiographically to therapy, it is critical to establish whether this is due to anaplasia or a mature histology.

How long to treat a child who has BWT with chemotherapy before intervening surgically remains an important consideration. In SIOP-9, patients with unilateral tumors were randomized to receive either 4 or 8 weeks of dactinomycin and vincristine preoperatively. On average, a 48% and 62% reduction in tumor volume was seen at four and eight weeks, respectively.[93,148] A review by the German Pediatric Hematology Group (GPOH) looking at patients with BWT reported that maximum tumor shrinkage occurred in the first 12 weeks of chemotherapy.[149]

The two principal aims of the current COG study for BWT are to improve four-year EFS and prevent complete removal of at least one kidney in 50% of patients. This is a response-based protocol starting with chemotherapy followed by evaluation at 6 and 12 weeks with definitive operative therapy in all patients by 12 weeks. For most patients with BWT, the initial regimen is an intensive combination of three drugs (vincristine, actinomycin D and doxorubicin) based on regimens used with good results and minimal toxicities by both SIOP and the UKCCSG WT Group.[150] This regimen was chosen to provide enhanced therapy for possible stage III disease. Additionally, it was elected to intensify the chemotherapy rather than administer radiotherapy, which would increase the development of radiation nephritis and loss of renal function in the remaining kidney. Finally, a more intensive therapy was selected to avoid the use of sequential regimens of increasing intensity, thereby delaying resection of tumors which was identified in the review of the prior cohort of NWTS-4 BWT patients.

Health Consequences for Survivors

WT treatment impacts general health, renal function, pregnancy, cardiac function, thoracic function, and the occurrence of second malignancies.[134,151–153] Table 65-6 shows the causes of early and late mortality in a cohort of 10,000 children diagnosed with WT.[151]

General Health

Chronic health conditions, health status, health care utilization, socioeconomic status, subsequent malignant neoplasms, and mortality of 1,256 WT survivors (1970–1986) were compared to the USA population, and a sibling cohort (n = 4023) in an effort to determine the long-term effects of WT on survivors (Fig. 65-9).[154] The cumulative incidence of all and severe chronic health

TABLE 65-6	Causes of Early and Late Mortality in Children Diagnosed with Wilms' Tumor (n = 11,157)	
	Number of Deaths	
Cause of Death	LESS THAN 5 YEARS AFTER DIAGNOSIS (n = 6185)	LONGER THAN 5 YEARS AFTER DIAGNOSIS (n = 4972)
Original cancer	771	64
Subsequent malignant neoplasm	11	27
Cardiac	6	14
End-stage renal disease	5	13
Pulmonary	0	3
External	7	16

From Cotton CA, Peterson S, Norkool PA, et al. Early and late mortality after diagnosis of Wilms' tumor. J Clin Oncol 2009;27:1304–9.

conditions was 65.4% and 24.2%, respectively, at 25 years. WT survivors reported a more adverse general health status than the sibling group. However, mental health status, socioeconomic outcome, and health care utilization were similar.

Renal Function

Factors that contribute to renal failure include intrinsic progressive renal disease, inadequate renal parenchyma after one or more tumor resections, nephrotoxic effects of chemotherapy and radiation, and the potential for hyperfiltration injury to the remaining renal parenchyma. Breslow reported the 20-year ESRD outcomes in children treated for WT in 2005.[142] The major risk factors identified for renal failure were BWT and congenital syndromes. However, for a standard unilateral nonsyndromic WT patient, the risk of renal failure at 20 years was very low (0.6%).

Although transplantation is an option for children with renal failure, the current recommendations are to wait 2 years before considering a transplant.[155]

Pregnancy

The National Wilms Tumor Long-Term Follow-Up Study evaluated 700 maternal/offspring pairs.[156] Hypertension complicating pregnancy (P < 0.001), or threatened labor (P = 0.002) and malposition of fetus (P = 0.04) were more frequent among irradiated women and were related to radiation therapy dose.

Secondary Malignancies

An international cohort of 13,351 children with WT diagnosed before 15 years of age from 1960 to 2004 was established to determine the risk of second malignant neoplasms.[134] One hundred and seventy-four solid tumors and 28 leukemias were found in 195 people. The age-specific incidence of secondary solid tumors increased

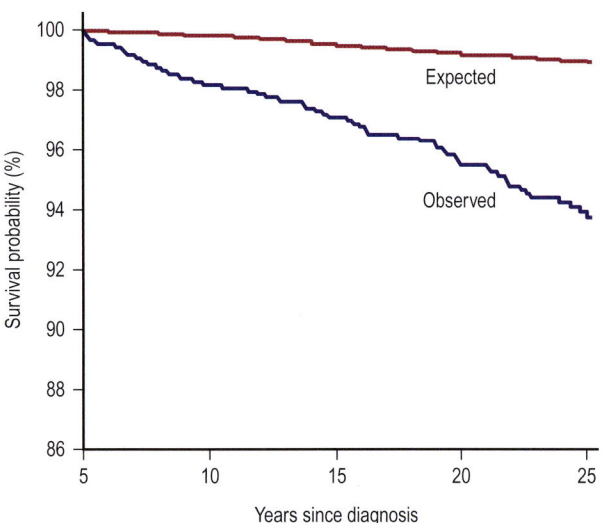

FIGURE 65-9 ■ Graph of observed vs expected mortality in a 25 year follow-up of children with Wilms tumor. (Permission from Termuhlen AM, Tersak JM, Liu Q, et al. Twenty-five year follow-up of childhood Wilms tumor: A report from the Childhood Cancer Survivor Study. Pediatr Blood Cancer 2011;57(7):1210–16.)

from approximately one case per 1,000 person years at age 15 to five cases per 1,000 person years at age 40. The cumulative incidence of solid tumors at age 40 was 6.7%. In those patients where WT was diagnosed after 1980, there was a lower age-specific incidence rate for second tumors compared to those treated before 1980. Paradoxically, the incidence of leukemia was higher in those diagnosed after 1990 (Fig. 65-10). This may be due to the decreasing use of radiation therapy and increasing the intensity of chemotherapy in modern protocols for treatment of WT.

Congestive Heart Failure

The relative risk of congestive heart failure was found to be increased in females (RR = 4.5; $P = 0.004$), and related to the cumulative doxorubicin dose (RR = 3.2/100 mg/m^2; $P < 0.001$), lung irradiation (RR = 1.6 for every/10 Gy; $P = 0.037$), and left abdominal irradiation (RR = 1.8/10 Gy; $P = 0.013$).[157] The cumulative risk of congestive heart failure was 4.4% 20 years after initial treatment with doxorubicin, and 17.4% 20 years after treatment with doxorubicin for a first or subsequent relapse. Preliminary results suggest that cardiotoxicity is lower with current radiation doses, but patients still have a substantial life-time risk of developing cardiac disease.[151,158]

Thoracic

The late effects of pulmonary radiation include pneumonitis, restrictive lung disease, scoliosis, kyphosis, reduced lung capacity, and secondary tumors. In girls, breast hypoplasia and cancer have also been described.[132,133] Paulino and his associates reported on the late complications of pulmonary RT in 55 long-term survivors of WT.[132] Two-thirds of the patients had at least one complication. Forty-three percent had scoliosis or kyphosis

and 10% developed benign chest tumors (osteochondromas). Secondary tumors were noted in three patients within the lung field (two osteogenic sarcomas of the rib and one breast cancer), and all succumbed to these tumors. Pulmonary function was examined in another study.[133] Subjectively, 63% percent of patients had mild to moderate exercise intolerance. Objective measurement of vital capacity and total lung capacity was decreased compared to age and height predicted values in patients. All females had breast hypoplasia.

Current Children's Oncology Group Renal Tumor Studies

Since 2006, five renal tumor studies have opened and are currently accruing patients. One is a classification and banking study into which all patients must enroll. If eligible, the patient is then assigned to one of four therapeutic studies. The primary or secondary specific aims of these trials that impact surgery are as follows:

ARENO3B2: Renal Tumors Classification, Biology, and Banking Study

The aims of this study that impact surgeons are to ensure that patients are properly placed in therapeutic trials, and ensure appropriateness of the operative procedures as well as the radiological and pathological classification of the tumors. Two other relevant study aims are radiological in nature. The first is looking at the sensitivity and specificity of CT scanning in determining vascular involvement and the second is evaluating the sensitivity and specificity of CT and MRI in diagnosing NRs. This study will also maintain a biological tumor bank for further research

ARENO532: Treatment for Very Low and Standard Risk Favorable Histology Wilms Tumor

An aim of this study is to demonstrate that very low-risk WT patients who undergo the appropriate operation can be treated by operation alone.

ARENO533: Treatment of Newly Diagnosed Higher Risk Favorable Histology Wilms Tumors

One aim of this study is to identify a population of patients with pulmonary disease who can be spared lung radiation. During various treatment stages, surgeons may be asked to biopsy lung lesions to determine whether or not there is malignancy in the lung lesion(s).

ARENO321: Treatment in High-Risk Renal Tumors

The aims of this study concern chemotherapy and radiotherapy intensification for specific high-risk tumors such as RTK and RCC. There are no surgical specific aims in this study. However, observational data are being collected on children with RCC.

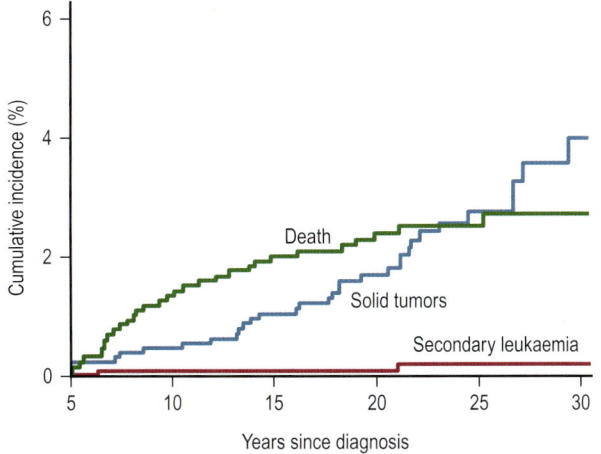

FIGURE 65-10 ■ Cumulative incidence of second malignancies in childhood survivors of Wilms tumor. (Permission from Termuhlen AM, Tersak JM, Liu Q, et al. Twenty-five year follow-up of childhood Wilms tumor: A report from the Childhood Cancer Survivor Study. Pediatr Blood Cancer 2011;57(7):1210–16.)

ARENO534: Treatment for Patients with Bilateral, Multicentric, or Bilaterally Predisposed Unilateral Wilms Tumor

This study has surgical aims that focus on renal-sparing surgery: (1) to improve 4-year EFS to 73% for patients with BWT; (2) to prevent complete removal of at least one kidney in 50% of patients with BWT by using prenephrectomy three-drug chemotherapy induction with vincristine, dactinomycin and doxorubicin; (3) to have 75% of children with BWT undergo definitive operation by 12 weeks after initiation of chemotherapy; (4) to evaluate the efficacy of chemotherapy in preserving renal units in children with diffuse DHPLN and in preventing WT development; and (5) to facilitate partial nephrectomy in lieu of nephrectomy in 25% of children with unilateral tumors and aniridia, BWS, hemihypertrophy, or other overgrowth syndromes, by using prenephrectomy chemotherapy.

RENAL CELL CARCINOMA

Children with RCC are generally older than those with WT.[159] RCC in children displays gross and histological features similar to those seen in adults. Clinical stage at the time of diagnosis is the most important prognostic factor, and the identification of renal vascular invasion does not appear to be an adverse predictor. Radical nephrectomy and regional lymphadenectomy have been the primary modality for cure, and children with distant spread have a grave prognosis. In a study of 22 children, the mean age at presentation with RCC was 14 years.[159] Overall survival was much worse than for WT, with a five-year survival of only 30%. Analysis of multiple factors including age, tumor size, location, and histology failed to demonstrate predictors of survival. Only stage and complete tumor resection were meaningful prognostic factors. In another study, survival was 60% in children with complete resection of the primary tumor and zero in those with only partial resection.[160] Survival was also stage dependent: 92.5% for stage I, 84.5% for stage II, 72.7% for stage III, and 12.7% for stage IV. It should be noted, however, that those with positive nodes but no distant metastasis had survival rates three times that of adult historical controls. RCC is remarkably resistant to chemotherapy, preventing cure in most children with metastatic disease.[161] Ten to 20% of patients have nodal involvement identified at operation, but lack evidence of distant metastatic disease. No benefit has been found for adjuvant therapy in children.[160]

Nephron-sparing resection has been used in adults with small polar lesions in whom no evidence of a multicentric tumor is found. In these selected cases with tumors smaller than 4 cm and a normal contralateral kidney, the risk of local recurrence is reported to be 2% or less, which is comparable to the frequency of metachronous recurrence in the contralateral kidney after unilateral radical nephrectomy.[161]

The development of late recurrences long after nephrectomy, prolonged stability of disease in the absence of systemic therapy, and rare cases of spontaneous regression of tumors have led to an interest in immunotherapy comparable to that used for melanoma. Trials of immunomodulating therapy with interferon-alpha and interleukin-2 have demonstrated efficacy in some studies, but maintenance of a durable cure has been elusive.[162] In contrast, a trial of 294 patients with advanced-stage RCC randomized to receive placebo or nine months of subcutaneous lymphoblastoid interferon demonstrated similar recurrence rates between the two groups and worse survival for the treatment group.[163] With the significant toxicity involved with immunotherapy, demonstration of improved survival in randomized trials will be required before this can be adopted as standard therapy.

MESOBLASTIC NEPHROMA

Congenital mesoblastic nephroma, also referred to as fetal renal hamartoma or leiomyomatous hamartoma, is the most common renal tumor identified in the neonatal period. Although initially diagnosed and treated as a congenital Wilms tumor, mesoblastic nephroma was defined as a distinct entity in 1967.[164] Mesoblastic nephromas are found most frequently in the neonatal period as a palpable flank mass which can be massive. Additional symptoms seen at presentation include hematuria, hypertension, vomiting, and jaundice.[165]

Mesoblastic nephroma accounted for 2.8% of 1,905 renal tumors submitted to the early NWTSG studies. Grossly, these tumors have a homogeneous rubbery appearance resembling a uterine fibroid in color and consistency (Fig. 65-11). Microscopically they are composed of sheets of fibrous or mesenchymal stroma, within which bizarre and dysplastic tubules and glomeruli are irregularly scattered.[166] The tumor can invade intact renal parenchyma, and extrarenal infiltration into the perihilar connective tissues is common. The histologic subtypes of this tumor include classic type (24% of cases), cellular type (66%), and mixed type (10%). The pluripotency of

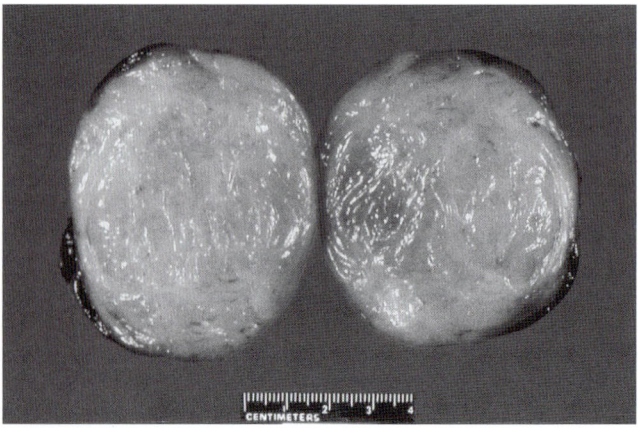

FIGURE 65-11 ■ Cross section of a mesoblastic nephroma identified in an infant on a neonatal examination. Note the rubbery appearance of this tumor, which resembles a fibroid tumor of the uterus with a very thin margin of normal renal parenchyma around the periphery.

these tumors is revealed by their differentiation into angiomatoid patterns, cartilaginous nests, and their elicitation of intratumoral hematopoiesis in addition to the tiny nephroblastic epithelial foci.

A characteristic chromosomal translocation, (t12;15) (p13;q25), has been recently found.[167] It results in fusion of the *ETV6* (also known as *TEL*) gene from 12p13 with the *NRTK3* neurotrophin-3 receptor gene (also known as *TRKC*) from 15q25.27,29 This fusion results in a chimeric RNA, which is characteristic of both infantile fibrosarcoma and the cellular variant of CMN. This may be helpful in differentiating the cellular variant from other lesions that must be considered in the differential diagnosis, including CCSK and RTK. It also suggests a close relation between infantile fibrosarcoma and the cellular variant of mesoblastic nephroma.

This generally benign tumor usually can be cured with nephrectomy alone. This should include generous margins around the tumor to avoid local recurrence. Particular attention should be paid to the medial aspect of the kidney, including the hilum and great vessels, because of the tumor's proclivity to have extensions into these perirenal soft tissues. Several children have been reported with local recurrence or metastases to the brain, bones, lungs, and heart.[168–170] The histology in some cases has revealed an unusual degree of mesenchymal cell immaturity and hypercellularity, suggesting a more aggressive tumor. This also supports the concept that mesoblastic nephroma cannot be considered a simple hamartoma and that complete nephrectomy with negative margins is critical in all cases.[166]

In a series of 51 children with mesoblastic nephroma identified in the NWTSG series, eight had local extension and ten had tumor spillage during resection.[165] The use of adjuvant therapy in these cases depended on the era in which the children were treated. Twenty-three infants treated after 1978 underwent resection alone. Prior to 1978, 24 underwent an operation and chemotherapy, and before 1976, four children also received irradiation. Survival was excellent in this entire group with only one child dying of sepsis during chemotherapy. One child's tumor recurred at 6 months despite receiving dactinomycin and vincristine. The tumor was re-excised, and the child was treated with cyclophosphamide and doxorubicin and remained without disease 18 months later.

A SIOP report of 29 children with CMN confirmed the early age at which this tumor is seen.[171] Only five infants were older than 4 months at presentation in the series. Interestingly, treatment of a neonate with an extensively infiltrating tumor with eight weekly courses of vincristine before resection has been reported.[172] Shrinkage of the tumor occurred with this treatment, facilitating its eventual resection and cure.

Beckwith reported the largest cohort of children with recurrent or metastatic lesions from his large collected series.[173] Twenty-four patients with an aggressive tumor were seen in a series of 330 mesoblastic nephromas. Of these 24 cases, eight had metastatic disease, 17 had relapse in the peritoneum or retroperitoneum, and six infants have died of persistent disease. Recurrences developed in children after initial chemotherapy or radiation, which suggests that conventional adjuvant therapy may not decrease the incidence of recurrence. Histologic criteria were not helpful in predicting outcome. Beckwith supports aggressive surgical attempts to remove all gross tumor.[173] He also stresses the need for close monitoring for one year after resection because relapse in 23 of the 24 cases was apparent within 11 months of resection. Ultrasound of the local site is adequate, and scans for metastatic disease are unrewarding.

CYSTIC NEPHROMA

Cystic nephroma is indistinguishable grossly and radiographically from its malignant neoplastic 'cousins,' cystic partially differentiated nephroblastoma (CPDN) and cystic nephroblastoma. All lesions are composed of purely cystic masses characterized by multiple thin-walled septations (Fig. 65-12). In cystic nephroma, the septations are lined by flattened, cuboidal, or hobnail epithelium, and are composed entirely of differentiated tissues without blastemal or other embryonal elements that are the distinguishing characteristics of CPDN.[174] Although the term multilocular cyst of the kidney has been used, cystic nephroma is preferred because the lesion appears to be neoplastic rather than congenital. In the cystic nephroblastoma or cystic WT, solid nodules on the septa of blastemal or embryonal elements are characteristic of WT. An unexplained synchronous occurrence has been reported between cystic nephroma and pleuropulmonary blastoma.[175,176]

These lesions should not be confused with cystic CCSK, cystic CMN, or multicystic dysplastic kidney.[177] Cystic nephroma, CPDN, and cystic nephroblastoma can

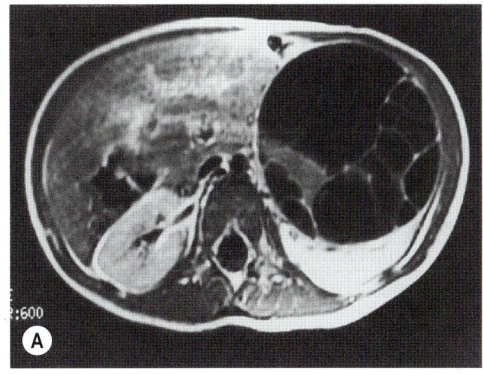
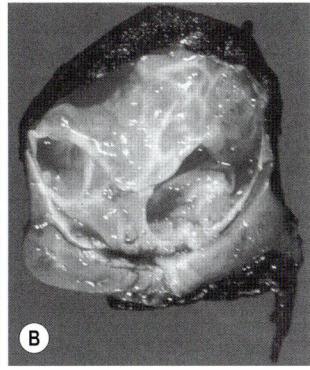

FIGURE 65-12 ■ **(A)** MR image obtained in a 2-year-old infant with an asymptomatic left flank mass. Note the multilocular cystic mass extending out from the normal renal tissue posteriorly. **(B)** Cross section of the tumor and kidney reveals thin-walled septa within the mass. Histologic examination of this tumor revealed a cystic partially differentiated nephroblastoma.

be distinguished from multicystic dysplastic kidney because the former are confined to only a portion of the kidney with normal renal parenchyma being identified, whereas the cystic changes of multicystic dysplastic kidney almost always involve the entire kidney due to the fact that it develops early in gestation from urinary traction obstruction. Contralateral renal anomalies are frequent in dysplastic kidneys, including ureteropelvic junction obstruction and reflux. A multicystic dysplastic kidney is often identified antenatally or in the neonatal period, whereas the other lesions occur later.

Generally, nephrectomy will be curative in both cystic nephroma and CPDN. Twenty-three children with these cystic lesions were identified in the NWTSG series: 5 with cystic nephroma and 18 with CPDN.[178] Only one patient with CPDN had local recurrence, and no distant metastases were found. A more recent review of the GPOH and SIOP files of the CPDN cases has again confirmed that primary resection appears to be adequate for all lesions removed intact.[179] In cases in which the lesion is isolated to one pole of the kidney, a partial nephrectomy can be considered. However, it must be remembered that these tumors can resemble cystic variants of CCSK, which carries an entirely different prognosis.[180–182]

OSSIFYING RENAL TUMOR OF INFANCY

Ossifying renal tumor of infancy is a relatively rare tumor occurring entirely in infancy. In many cases, children with this lesion initially have gross hematuria, although a palpable mass may be present.[183] These lesions are attached to a renal papilla, but are seen primarily within the lumen of the calyx and may extend into the renal pelvis. They have been confused occasionally with staghorn calculi. Histologically, they contain osteoid, osteoblastic cells, and spindle cells. Their true histogenesis has not been established, although it has been suggested that they represent hyperplastic ILNRs. Metastasis or local spread of these tumors has not been reported. Renal-sparing procedures may be reasonable, although this may not result in significant ipsilateral renal function.[184,185]

REFERENCES

1. Farber S. Chemotherapy in the treatment of leukemia and Wilms' tumor. JAMA 1966;198:826–36.
2. Rance T. Case of fungus hematodes of the kidneys. Med Phys J 1814;32:19.
3. wilms M. Diagnostischer und therapeutischer Werth der Lumbalpunction. Druckbestimmung mit Quicksilvermanometer. Munch Med Wochenschr 1897;3:53–7.
4. Wilms M. Die Mischgeschwülste der Niere. Leipzig: Verlag von Arthur Georgi; 1899.
5. Beckwith JB. Wilms' tumor and other renal tumors of childhood: A selective review from the National Wilms' Tumor Study Pathology Center. Hum Pathol 1983;14:481–92.
6. Willets IE. Jessop and the Wilms Tumor. J Pediatr Surg 2003;38:1496–8.
7. Gross RE. Embryoma of the Kidney (Wilms Tumor). In: Gross RE, editor. The surgery of infancy and childhood. Philadelphia, WB Saunders; 1953. p. 588–605.
8. Friedlander A. Sarcoma of the kidney treated by roetgen ray. Am J Dis Child 1916;12:328–31.
9. Ladd WE. Embryoma Of The Kidney (Wilms' Tumor). Ann Surg 1938;108:885–902.
10. Mukherjee S. The Emperor of All Maladies: A Biography of Cancer. New York: Scribner; 2010.
11. Gross RE, Neuhauser EB. Treatment of mixed tumors of the kidney in childhood. Pediatrics 1950;6:843–52.
12. Schweisguth O, Bamberger J. Le nephroblastome de l'enfant. Ann Chir Infant 1963;4:335–54.
13. Sutow W. Vincristine (Leurocristine) sulfate in the treatment of children with metastatic Wilms' tumor. Pediatrics 1963;32:880–7.
14. Bersntein L, Linet M, Smith MA, et al. Renal Tumors. Bethesda: National Cancer Institute, SEER Program; 1999. Report No.: 99-4649.
15. Breslow N, Olshan A, Beckwith JB, et al. Epidemiology of Wilms tumor. Med Pediatr Oncol 1993;21:172–81.
16. Green DM. The diagnosis and management of Wilms' tumor. Pediatr Clin North Am 1985;32:735–54.
17. Coppes MJ, de Kraker J, van Dijken PJ. Bilateral Wilms' tumor: Long-term survival and some epidemiological features. J Clin Oncol 1989;7:310–15.
18. Breslow N, Norris N, Norkool P, et al. Characteristics and outcomes of children with the Wilms tumor-Aniridia syndrome: A report from the National Wilms Tumor Study Group. J Clin Oncol 2003;21:4579–85.
19. Debaun MR, Tucker MA. Risk of cancer during the first four years of life in the children from the Beckwith-Wiedemann syndrome registry. J Pediatr 1998;132:398–400.
20. Rao A, Rothman J., Nichols KE. Genetic testing and tumor surveillance for children with cancer predisposition syndromes. Curr Opin Pediatr 2008;20:1–7.
21. Tan Ty, Armour DJ. Tumour surveillance in Beckwith-Wiedemann syndrome and hemihyperplasia: A critical review of the evidence and suggested guidelines for local practice. J Paediatr Child Health 2006;42:486–90.
22. Wiedemann HR, Wiedemann H-R. Tumours and hemihypertrophy associated with Wiedemann-Beckwith syndrome [Letter]. Eur J Pediat 1983;141:129.
23. Goldman M, Smith A, Shuman C, et al. Renal abnormalities in Beckwith-Wiedemann syndrome are associated with 11p15.5 uniparental disomy. J Am Soc Nephrol 2002;13:2077–84.
24. Knudson AG, Strong LC. Mutation and Cancer: A model for Wilms' tumor of the kidney. J Nat Cancer Inst 1972;48:313–24.
25. Grundy PE, Breslow N, Li S, et al. Loss of heterozygosity for chromosomes 1p and 16q is an adverse prognostic factor in favorable-histology Wilms tumor: A report from the National Wilms Tumor Study Group. J Clin Oncol 2005;23:7312–21.
26. Huff V. Wilms' tumours: About tumour suppressor genes, an oncogene and a chameleon gene. Nat Rev Cancer 2011;11:111–21.
27. Malkin D, Li FP, Strong LC, et al. Germ line p53 mutations in a familial syndrome of breast cancer, sarcomas, and other neoplasms. Science 1990;250:1233–8.
28. Maiti S, Alam R, Amos CI, et al. Frequent association of beta-catenin and WT1 mutations in Wilms tumors. Cancer Res 2000;60:6288–92.
29. Koesters R, Ridder R, Kopp-Schneider A, et al. Mutational activation of the beta-catenin proto-oncogene is a common event in the development of Wilms tumors. Cancer Res 1999;59:3880–2.
30. Rivera MN, Kim WJ, Wells J, et al. An X chromosome gene, WTX, is commonly inactivated in Wilms tumor. Science 2007;315:642–5.
31. Call KM, Glaser T, Ito CY, et al. Isolation and characterization of a zinc finger polypeptide gene at the human chromosome 11 Wilms tumor locus. Cell 1990;60:509–20. Ref Type: Internet Communication.
32. Yang Y, Han Y, Sauez Saiz F, et al. A tumor suppressor and oncogene: The WT1 story. Leukemia 2007;21:868–76.
33. Rainer S, Johnson LA, Dobry CJ, et al. Relaxation of imprinted genes in human cancer. Nature 1993;362:747–9.
34. Little MH, Wells C. A clinical overview of WT1 gene mutations. Hum Mutat 1997;9:209–25.
35. Fukuzawa R, Heathcott RW, More HE, et al. Sequential WT1 and CTNNB1 mutations and alterations of beta-catenin localisation in intralobar nephrogenic rests and associated Wilms tumours: Two case studies. J Clin Pathol 2007;60:1013–16.

36. Grundy PE, Koufos A, Morgan K, et al. Familial predisposition to Wilms' tumour does not map to the short arm of chromosome 11. Nature 1988;336:374–6.

37. Rahman N, Arbour L, Tonin P, et al. Evidence for a familial Wilms' tumour gene (FWT1) on chromosome 17q12-q21. Nat Genet 1996;13:461–3.

38. Beckwith JB, Kiviai NB, Bonadio JF. Nephrogenic rests, nephroblastomatosis and the pathogenesis of Wilms tumor. Pediatr Pathol 1990;10:1–36.

39. Bennington J, Beckwith J. Tumor of the kidney, renal pelvis and ureter. In: Armed Forces Institute of Pathology; Atlas of Tumor Pathology. Washington DC: AFIP; 1975. p. 31–91.

40. Perlman EJ. Pediatric renal tumors: Practical updates for the pathologist. Pediatr Dev Pathol 2005;8:320–38.

41. Perlman EJ, Faria P, Soares A, et al. Hyperplastic perilobar nephroblastomatosis: Long term survival in 52 patients. Pediatr Blood Cancer 2006;46:203–21.

42. Coppes MJ, Beckwith JB, Ritchey ML, et al. Factors affecting the risk of contralateral Wilms tumor development (A report from the national Wilms tumor study group). Cancer 1999;85:1616–25.

43. Cambio A, Evans C, Kurzrock E. Non-surgical management of multicystic dysplastic kidney. BJU Int 2008;101:804–8.

44. Narchi H, Narchi H. Risk of Wilms' tumour with multicystic kidney disease: A systematic review. Arch Dis Child 2005;90:147–9.

45. Beckwith JB, Palmer NF. Histopathology and prognosis of Wilms tumors: Results from the First National Wilms' Tumor Study. Cancer Genet Cytogenet 1978;41:1937–48.

46. Murphy WM, Grignon DJ, Perlman EJ. Tumors of the kidney, bladder and related urinary structures. AFIP 2004.

47. Dome JS, Cotton CA, Perlman EJ. Treatment of anaplastic histology Wilms' tumor: Results from the fifth National Wilms' Tumor Study. J Clin Oncol 2006;24:2352–8.

48. Faria P, Beckwith JB, Mishra K, et al. Focal versus diffuse anaplasia in Wilms tumor - New definitions with prognostic significance. Am J Surg Pathol 1996;20:920.

49. Green DM, Beckwith JB, Breslow N, et al. Treatment of children with stages II to IV anaplastic Wilms Tumor: A report from the National Wilms' Tumor Study Group. J Clin Oncol 1994;12:2126–31.

50. Zuppan CW, Beckwith JB, Luckey DW. Anaplasia in unilateral Wilms tumor. A report from the National Wilms Tumor Study Pathology Center. Hum Path 1988 2010;19:1199–209.

51. Williams RD, Al-Saadi R, Natrajan R, et al. Molecular profiling reveals frequent gain of MYCN and anaplasia-specific loss of 4q and 14q in Wilms tumor. Genes Chromosomes Cancer 2011;50:982–95.

52. Marsden HB, Lawler W, Kumar PM, et al. Bone metastasizing renal tumor of childhood: Morphological and clinical features, and differences from Wilms' tumor. Cancer 1978;42:1922–8.

53. Argani P, Perlman EJ, Breslow N, et al. Clear cell sarcoma of the kidney: A review of 351 cases from the National Wilms' Tumour Study Pathology Center. Am J Surg Pathol 2000;24:4–18.

54. Brownlee NA, Perkins LA, Stewart W. Recurring translocation (10;17) and deletion (14q) in clear cell sarcoma of the kidney. Arch Pathol Lab Med 2007;131:446–51.

55. Kusumakumary P, Chellam VG, Rojymon J, et al. Late recurrence of clear cell sarcoma of the kidney. Med Pediatr Oncol 1997;28:355–7.

56. Weeks DA, Beckwith JB, Mierau GW, et al. Rhabdoid tumor of kidney: A report of 111 cases from the National Wilms' Tumor Study Pathology Center. Am J Surg Pathol 1989;13:439–58.

57. Argani P, Hawkins A, Griffin CA, et al. A distinctive pediatric renal neoplasm characterized by epithelioid morphology, basement membrane production, focal HMB45 immunoreactivity, and t(6;11)(p21.1;q12) chromosome translocation. Am J Pathol 2001;158:2089–96.

58. Hass JE, Palmer NF, Weinberg AG. Ultrastructure of malignant rhabdoid tumor of the kidney: A distinctive renal tumor of children. Hum Pathol 1981;12:646–57.

59. Bonnin JM, Rubenstein IJ, Palmer NF, et al. The association of embryonal tumors originating in the kidney and the brain. Cancer 1984;54:2137–46.

60. Perlman EJ, Ali SZ, Robinson R, et al. Infantile extrarenal rhabdoid tumor. Pediatr Dev Pathol 1998;1:149–52.

61. Schofield DE, Beckwith JB, Sklar J. Loss of heterozygosity at chromosome regions 22q11-12 and 11p15.5 in renal rhabdoid tumors. Genes Chromosomes Cancer 1996;15:10–17.

62. Versteege I, Sevenet N, Lange J, et al. Truncating mutations of hSNF5/INI1 in aggressive paediatric cancer. Nature 1998;394:203–6.

63. Biegel JA, Zhou J, Rorke L, et al. Germ-line and acquired mutations of INI1 in atypical teratoid and rhabdoid tumors. Cancer 2012;59:74–9.

64. Hoot AC, Russo P, Judkins AR, et al. Immunohistochemical analysis of hSNF5/INI1 distinguishes renal and extra-renal malignant rhabdoid tumors from other pediatric soft tissue tumors. Am J Surg Pathol 2004;28:1485–91.

65. Grundy PE, Dome JD, Perlman EJ, et al. Renal Tumors Classification, Biology, and Banking Study. https://members childrensoncologygroup org/Prot/AREN03B2/AREN03B2DOC pdf 2006.

66. Vujanic G, Sandstedt B, Harms D. Revised International Society of Paediatric Oncology (SIOP)Working Classification of Renal Tumors of Childhood. Med Pediatr Oncol 2002;38:79–82.

67. Vujanic G, Sandstedt B. The pathology of Wilms' tumour (nephroblastoma): The International Society of Paediatric Oncology approach. J Clin Pathol 2010;63:102–9.

68. Grundy PE, Perlman EJ, Ehrlich PF, et al. Current issues in Wilms tumor management . Cur Prob Cancer 2005;29:221–60.

69. Kalapurakal JA, Dome JS, Perlman EJ, et al. Management of Wilms' tumour: Current practice and future goals. Lancet Oncol 2004;5:37–46.

70. Breslow N, Olshan A, Beckwith JB, et al. Epidemiology of Wilms tumor. Med Pediatr Oncol 1993;21:172–81.

71. Dome JD, Perlman EJ, Ritchey ML, et al. Renal tumours. In: Pizzo PA, Poplack DG, editors. Principles and Practice of Pediatric Oncology. 5th ed. Philadelphia: Lippincott Williams and Wilkins; 2006. p. 905–32.

72. Khanna G, Rosen N, Anderson J, et al. Evaluation of diagnostic performance of CT for detection of tumor thrombus in children with Wilms tumor: A report from the Children's Oncology Group. Pediatr Blood Cancer 2012;58:551–5.

73. Ritchey ML, Shamberger RC, Hamilton TE, et al. Fate of bilateral renal lesions missed on preoperative imaging: A report from the National Wilms Tumor Study Group. J Urol 2005;174:1519–21.

74. Khanna G, Naranjo A, Hoffer F, et al. Detection of preoperative Wilms tumor rupture with CT: a report from the Children's Oncology Group. Radiology 2013;266(2):610–17. doi: 10.1148/radiol.12120670. Epub 2012 Nov 28.

75. Ehrlich PF, Ritchey ML, Hamilton TE, et al. Quality assessment for Wilms' tumor: A report from the National Wilms' Tumor Study-5. J Pediatr Surg 2005;40:208–12.

76. Ritchey ML, Shamberger RC, Haase G, et al. Surgical complications after primary nephrectomy for Wilms' tumor: Report from the National Wilms' Tumor Study Group. J Am Col Surg 2001;192:63–8.

77. Shamberger RC, Guthrie KA, Ritchey ML, et al. Surgery related factors and local recurrence of Wilms tumor in the national Wilms tumor study 4. Ann Surg 1999;229:292–7.

78. Ritchey ML, Lally KP, Haase GM, et al. Superior mesenteric artery injury during nephrectomy for Wilms' tumor. J Pediatr Surg 1992;27:612–15.

79. Othersen HB, Delorimier A, Hrabovsky E, et al. Surgical evaluation of lymph node metastases in Wilms tumor. J Pediatr Surg 1990;25:330–1.

80. D'Angio GJ, Evans AE, Breslow N. The Treatment of Wilms' Tumor: Results of the Second National Wilms' Tumor Study. Am Cancer Soc 1981;4:2302–10.

81. Kieran K, Anderson J, Dome JS, et al. Lymph node involvement in Wilms tumor: Results from National Wilms Tumor Studies 4 and 5. J Pediatr Surg 2012;47:700–6.

82. Ehrlich PF, Dome JS, Shamberger RC, et al. Clinico-pathologic Findings predictive of relapse in children with Stage III Favorable Histology Wilms Tumor: The importance of lymph nodes. Pediatr Blood Cancer 2010;55:794.

83. Ritchey ML, Daley S, Shamberger RC, et al. Ureteral extension in Wilms' tumor: A report from the National Wilms' Tumor Study Group (NWTSG). J Pediatr Surg 2008;43:1625–9.

84. Gow K, Barnhart DC, Hamilton TE, et al. Primary nephrectomy and intraoperative tumor spill: Report from the Children's Oncology Group (COG) Renal Tumors Committee. J Pediatr Surg 2012. In Press.

85. Grundy PE, Dome JS, Ehrlich PF. Renal tumors classification, biology and banking studies. https://members childrensoncologygroup org/Prot/AREN03B2/AREN03B2DOC pdf 2007. p. 18–33.

86. Ehrlich PF, Ferrer F, Ritchey ML, et al. Hepatic metastasis at diagnosis in patients with Wilms tumor is not an independent adverse prognostic factor for stage IV Wilms tumor. A report from the childrens oncology group/national wilms tumor study group. Ann Surg 2009;250:642–8.

87. Elli M, Pinarli FG, Dagdemir A. Acquired von Willebrand syndrome in a patient with Ewing sarcoma. Pediatr Hematol Oncol 2006;23:111–14.

88. Coppes MJ, Zandvoort SW, Sparling CR. Acquired von Willebrand disease in Wilms' tumor patients. J Clin Oncol 1992;10:422–7.

89. Scott JP, Mongomery RR, Tubergen DG, et al. Acquired von Willebrand's disease in association with Wilm's tumor: Regression following treatment. Blood 1981;58:665–9.

90. Baxter PA, Nutchtern JG, Guillerman RP, et al. Acquired von Willebrand Syndrome and Wilms Tumor: Not Always Benign. Pediatr Blood Cancer 2009;52:392–428.

91. Bracey AW, Wu AH, Aceves J, et al. Platelet dysfunction associated with Wilms tumor and hyaluronic acid. Am J Hematol 1987;24:247–57.

92. Michiels JJ, Budde U, van der Planken M, et al. Acquired von Willebrand syndromes: Clinical features, aetiology, pathophysiology, classification and management. Best Pract Res Clin Haematol 2001;14:401–36.

93. Tournade MF, Com-Nougue C, de Kraker J, et al. Optimal duration of preoperative chemotherapy in unilateral non metastatic Wilms tumor in children older then six months. Results of the ninth International Society of Pediatric Oncology tumor trial. J Clin Oncol 2001;19:488–500.

94. Tournade MF, Com-Nougue C, Voute PA, et al. Results of the sixth International Society of Pediatric Oncology Wilms' tumor trial and study: A risk-adapted therapeutic approach in Wilms' tumor. J Clin Oncol 1993;11:1014–23.

95. Shamberger RC, Ritchey ML, Haase G, et al. Intravascular extension of Wilms tumor. Ann Surg 2001;234:116–21.

96. Lall A, Pritchard-Jones K, Walker J, et al. Wilms' tumor with intracaval thrombus in the UK Children's Cancer Study Group UKW3 trial. J Pediatr Surg 2006;41:382–7.

97. Nakayama D.K, Norkool P, Delorimier A, et al. Intracardiac extension of Wilms' tumor: A report of the National Wilms' Tumor Study. Ann Surg 1986;204:693–7.

98. Ritchey ML. Renal sparing surgery for Wilms tumor. J Urol 2005;174:1172–3.

99. Green DM, Breslow N, Beckwith JB, et al. Treatment outcomes in patients less than 2 years of age with small, stage I, favorable-histology Wilms' tumors: A report from the National Wilms' Tumor Study. J Clin Oncol 1993;11:91–5.

100. Larsen E, Perez- Atayde A, Green DM, et al. Surgery only for the treatment of patients with stage I (Cassady) Wilms' tumor. Cancer 1990;66:264–6.

101. Green DM, Breslow N, Beckwith JB, et al. Treatment with nephrectomy only for small, stage I/favorable histology Wilms' tumor: A report from the National Wilms' Tumor Study Group. J Clin Oncol 2001;19:3719–24.

102. Shamberger RC, Anderson J, Breslow N, et al. Long-term outcomes for infants with very low risk Wilms tumor treated with surgery alone in National Wilms Tumor Study-5. Ann Surg 2010;251:555–8.

103. Sredni ST, Gadd S, Huang CC. Subsets of very low risk Wilms tumor show distinctive gene expression, histologic, and clinical features. Clin Cancer Res 2009;15:6800–9.

104. van den Heuvel-Eibrink MM, Grundy PE, Graf N, et al. Characteristics and survival of 750 children diagnosed with a renal tumor in the first seven months of life: A collaborative study by the SIOP/GPOH/SFOP, NWTSG, and UKCCSG Wilms tumor study groups. Pediatr Blood Cancer 2008;50:1130–4.

105. Isaacs H. Fetal and neonatal renal tumors. J Pediatr Surg 2008;43:1587–95.

106. Andrews PE, Kelalis P, Haase G. Extrarenal Wilms' tumor: Results of the National Wilms' Tumor Study. J Pediatr Surg 1992;27:1181–4.

107. Coppes MJ, Wilson PC, Weitzman S. Extrarenal Wilms' tumor: Staging, treatment, and prognosis. J Clin Oncol 1991;9:167–74.

108. Green DM, Breslow N, Beckwith JB. Comparison between single-dose and divided-dose administration of dactinomycin and doxorubicin for patients with Wilms' tumor: A report from the National Wilms' tumor study group. J Clin Oncol 1998;16:237–45.

109. D'Angio GJ, Breslow N, Beckwith JB, et al. Treatment of Wilms' Tumor. Results of the Third National Wilms' Tumor Study. Cancer 1989;64:360.

110. Breslow N, Ou SS, Beckwith JB, et al. Doxorubicin for favorable histology, Stage II-III Wilms tumor - Results from the National Wilms Tumor Studies. Cancer 2004;101:1072–80.

111. Green DM, Breslow N, Evans I, et al. The effect of chemotherapy dose intensity on the hematological toxicity of the treatment for Wilms' tumor. A report of the National Wilms Tumor Study. Am J Pediatr Hematol Oncol 1994;16:207–12.

112. Green DM, Breslow N, Beckwith JB, et al. Effect of duration of treatment on treatment outcome and cost of treatment for Wilms tumor: A report from the National Wilms Tumor Study Group. J Clin Oncol 1998;16:3744–51.

113. Green DM, Cotton CA, Malogolowkin M, et al. Treatment of Wilms tumor relapsing after initial treatment with vincristine snd actinomycin D: A report form the National Wilms Tumor Study. Pediatr Blood Cancer 2007;48:493–9.

114. Malogolowkin M, Cotton CA, Green DM, et al. Treatment of Wilms tumor relapsing after initial treatment with vincristine, actinomycin D, and doxorubicin. A report from the National Wilms Tumor Study Group. Pediatr Blood Cancer 2008;50:236–41.

115. Seibel NL, Breslow N, Beckwith JB, et al. Effect of duration of treatment on treatment outcome for patients with clear-cell sarcoma of the kidney: A report from the National Wilms' Tumor Study Group. J Clin Oncol 2004;22:468–73.

116. Abu-Ghosh AM. Ifosfamide, carboplatin and etoposide in children with poor risk relapsed Wilms' tumor: A Children's Cancer Group report. Ann Oncol 2002;13:460.

117. Tomlinson GE, Breslow NE, Dome J, et al. Rhabdoid tumor of the kidney in the National Wilms' Tumor Study: Age at diagnosis as a prognostic factor. J Clin Oncol 2005;23:7641–5.

118. Waldron PE, Rodgers BM, Kelly MD, et al. Successful treatment of a patient with stage IV rhabdoid tumor of the kidney: Case report and review. J Pediatr Hematol Oncol 1999;21:53–7.

119. Wagner L, Hill DA, Fuller C, et al. Treatment of metastatic rhabdoid tumor of the kidney. J Pediatr Hematol Oncol 2002;24:385–8.

120. Gururangan S, Bowman LC, Parham DM, et al. Primary extracranial rhabdoid tumors. Cancer Genet Cytogenet 1993;71:2653–9.

121. Lemerle J, Voute PA, Tournade MF, et al. Preoperative versus postoperative radiotherapy, single versus multiple courses of actinomycin D, in the treatment of Wilms' tumor: Preliminary results of a controlled clinical trial conducted by the International Society of Paediatric Oncology. Cancer 1976;38:647–54.

122. Godzinski J, Tournade MF, deKraker J, et al. Rarity of surgical complications after postchemotherapy nephrectomy for nephroblastoma. Experience of the International Society of Paediatric Oncology-Trial and Study 'SIOP-9'. International Society of Paediatric Oncology Nephroblastoma Trial and Study Committee. Eur J Pediatr Surg 1998;8:83–6.

123. D'Angio GJ, Evans AE, Breslow N, et al. The treatment of Wilms' tumor: Results of the National Wilms' Tumor Study. Cancer 1976;38:633–46.

124. Zoeller G, Pekrun A, Lakomek M, et al. Wilms tumor: The problem of diagnostic accuracy in children undergoing preoperative chemotherapy without histological tumor verification. J Urol 1994;151:169–71.

125. Vujanic G, Kelsey A, Mitchell C, et al. The role of biopsy in the diagnosis of renal tumors of childhood: Results of the UKCCSG Wilms' tumor study 3. Med Pediatr Oncol 2003;40:18–22.

126. Weirich A, Leuschner I, Harms D, et al. Clinical impact of histologic subtypes in localized non-anaplastic nephroblastomatreated according to the trial and study SIOP-9/GPOH. Ann Oncol 2001;12:311–19.

127. D'Angio GJ, Tefft M, Breslow N, Meyer JA. Radiation therapy of Wilms' tumor: Results according to dose, field, post-operative timing and histology. Int J Radiat Oncol Biol Phys 1978;4:769–80.

128. Thomas PRM, Tefft M, Farewell VT, et al. Abdominal relapses in irradiated second National Wilms' Tumor Study patients. J Clin Oncol 1984;2:1098–101.

129. Thomas PRM, Tefft M, Compaan PJ, et al. Results of two radiotherapy randomizations in the Third National Wilms' Tumor Study (NWTS-3). Cancer 1991;68:1703–7.

130. Kalapurakal JA, Li SM, Breslow N, et al. Influence of radiation therapy delay on abdominal tumor recurrence in patients with favorable histology Wilms' tumor treated on NWTS-3 and NWTS-4: A report from the National Wilms' Tumor Study Group. Int J Radiat Oncol Biol Phys 2003;57:495–9.

131. Green DM. Use of chest computed tomography for staging and treatment of Wilms' tumor in children. J Clin Oncol 2002;20:2763–4.

132. Paulino AC, Wen BC, Brown CK, et al. Late effects in children treated with radiation therapy for Wilms tumor. Int J Rad Oncol 2000;46:1239–46.

133. Attard-Montalto SP, Kingston JE, Eden OB, Plowman PN. Late follow-up of lung function after whole lung irradiation for Wilms tumor. Br J Radiol 1992;65:1114–18.

134. Breslow N, Lange JM, Friedman DL, et al. Secondary malignant neoplasms after Wilms tumor: An international collaborative study. Int J Cancer 2009;127:657–66.

135. Grundy PE, Green DM, Dirks A, et al. Clinical significance of pulmonary nodules detected by CT and Not CXR in patients treated for favorable histology Wilms tumor on national Wilms tumor studies-4 and -5: A report from the Children's Oncology Group. Med Pediatr Oncol 2003;41:251.

136. Weirich A, Ludwig R, Graf N. Survival in nephroblastoma treated according to the trial and study SIOP-9/GPOH with respect to relapse and morbidity. Ann Oncol 2004;15:808–20.

137. Prichard J, Imeson J, Barnes J, et al. Results of the United Kingdoms children's cancer study group first Wilms tumor study. J Clin Oncol 1995;13:124–33.

138. Mitchell C, Jones PM, Kelsey A, et al. The treatment of Wilms' tumour: Results of the United Kingdom Children's Cancer Study Group (UKCCSG) second Wilms' tumour study. Br J Cancer 2000;83:602–8.

139. Petruzzi MJ, Green DM. Wilms tumor. Pediatr Clin North Am 1997;44:939–52.

140. Ritchey ML. Renal sparing surgery for children with bilateral Wilms tumor. Cancer 2008;112:1877–8.

141. Ritchey ML, Green DM, Thomas PRM. Renal failure in Wilms tumor patients: A report from the National Wilms Tumor Study Group. Med Pediatr Oncol 1996;26:75–80.

142. Breslow N, Collins AJ, Ritchey ML, et al. End stage renal failure in patients with Wilms tumor: Results from the national Wilms tumor study group and the United States renal data system. J Urol 2005;174:1972–5.

143. Shamberger RC, Haase GM, Argani P. Bilateral Wilms' tumors with progressive or nonresponsive disease. J Pediatr Surg 2006;41:642–57.

144. Green DM, Beckwith JB, Breslow N, et al. Treatment of children with stages II to IV anaplastic Wilms Tumor: A report from the National Wilms' Tumor Study Group. J Clin Oncol 1994;12:2126–31.

145. Hamilton TE, Green DM, Perlman EJ, et al. Bilateral Wilms' tumor with anaplasia: Lessons from the National Wilms' Tumor Study. J Pediatr Surg 2006;41:1641–4.

146. Kumar R, Fitzgerald R, Breatnach F. Conservative surgical managment of bilateral Wilms tumor: Results of the United Kingdom children's cancer study group. J Urol 1998;160:1450–3.

147. Anderson J, Slater O, McHugh K, et al. Response without shrinkage in Bilateral Wilms Tumor: Significance of Rhabdomyomatous Histology. J Pediatr Hem Oncol 2002;24:31–4.

148. Graf N, Tournade MF, de Kraker J. The role of preoperative chemotherapy in the management of Wilms tumor. The SIOP studies. Urol Clin North Am 2000;27:443–54.

149. Graf N. 2010. Unpublished Work.

150. Ritchey ML. 2010. Unpublished Work.

151. Cotton CA, Peterson SS, Norkool PA. Early and late mortality after diagnosis of Wilms tumor. J Clin Oncol 2009;27:1304–9.

152. Green DM, Grigoriev YA, Nan B, et al. Congestive heart failure after treatment for Wilms' tumor: A report from the National Wilms' Tumor Study group. J Clin Oncol 2001;19:1926–34.

153. van Dijk IW, Oldenburger F, Cardous-Ubbink MC. Evaluation of late adverse events in long-term Wilms' Tumor survivors. Int J Radiat Oncol Biol Phys 2010;78:370–8.

154. Termuhlen AM, Tersak JM, Liu Q, et al. Twenty-five year follow-up of childhood Wilms tumor: A report from the Childhood Cancer Survivor Study. Pediatr Blood Cancer 2011;57:1210–16.

155. Grigoriev Y, Lange J, Peterson SM, et al. Treatments and outcomes for end-stage renal disease following Wilms tumor. Pediatr Nephrol 2012;27:1325–33.

156. Green DM, Lange JM, Peabody EM. Pregnancy Outcome after treatment for Wilms Tumor: A report from the National Wilms Tumor Long-Term Follow-Up Study. J Clin Oncol 2010;28:2824–30.

157. Green DM, Grigoriev YA, Nan B, et al. Correction to 'Congestive heart failure after treatment for Wilms' tumor'. J Clin Oncol 2003;21:2447–8.

158. Pein F, Sakiroglu O, Dahan M, et al. Cardiac abnormalities 15 years and more after adriamycin therapy in 229 childhood survivors of a solid tumour at the Institut Gustave Roussy. Br J Cancer 2004;91:37–44.

159. Aronson DC, Medary I, Findlay JL. Renal cell carcinoma in childhood and adolescence: A retrospective survey for prognostic factors in 22 cases. J Pediatr Surg 1996;31:183–6.

160. Geller JI, Dome JS. Local lymph node involvement does not predict poor outcome in pediatric renal cell carcinoma. Cancer 2004;101:1575–83.

161. Motzer RJ, Bander NH, Nanus DM. Renal-cell carcinoma. N Engl J Med 1996;335:865–75.

162. Fyfe G, Fisher RI, Rosenberg SA, et al. Results of treatment of 255 patients with metastatic renal cell carcinoma who received high-dose recombinant interleukin-2 therapy. J Clin Oncol 1995;13:688–96.

163. Messing EM, Manola J, Wilding G, et al. Phase III study of interferon alfa-NL as adjuvant treatment for resectable renal cell carcinoma: An Eastern Cooperative Oncology Group/Intergroup trial. J Clin Oncol 2003;21:1214–22.

164. Bolande RP, Brough AJ, Izant RJ. Congenital mesoblastic nephroma of infancy. A report of eight cases and the relationship to Wilms' tumor. Pediatrics 1967;40:272–8.

165. Howell CG, Othersen HB, Kiviat NE, et al. Therapy and outcome in 51 children with mesoblastic nephroma: A report of the National Wilms' Tumor Study. J Pediatr Surg 1982;17:826–31.

166. Bolande RP. Congenital and infantile neoplasia of the kidney. Lancet 1974;2:1497–9.

167. Argani P, Fritsch M, Kadkol SS, et al. Detection of the ETV6-NTRK3 chimeric RNA of infantile fibrosarcoma/cellular congenital mesoblastic nephroma in paraffin-embedded tissue: Application to challenging pediatric renal stromal. Mod Pathol 2000;13:29–36.

168. Beckwith JB. Mesenchymal renal neoplasms of infancy revisited. J Pediatr Surg 1974;9:803–5.

169. Heidelberger KP, Ritchey ML, Dauser RC, et al. Congenital mesoblastic nephroma metastatic to the brain. Cancer 1993;72:2499–502.

170. Vujanic G, Delemarre JF, Moeslichan S, et al. Mesoblastic nephroma metastatic to the lungs and heart–another face of this peculiar lesion: Case report and review of the literature. Pediatre Pathol 1993;13:143–53.

171. Sandstedt B, Delamarre JFM, Krul EJ, et al. Mesoblastic nephromas: A study of 29 tumours from the SIOP nephroblastoma file. Histopathology 1985;9:741–50.

172. Chan KL, Chan KW, Lee CW. Preoperative chemotherapy for mesoblastic nephroma. Med Pediatr Oncol 1995;24:271–3.

173. Beckwith JB. Reply. Pediatre Pathol 1993;13:886–7.

174. Agrons GA, Wagner BJ, Davidson AJ, et al. Multilocular cystic renal tumor in children: Radiologic-pathologic correlation. Radiographics 1995;15:653–69.

175. Delanhunt B, Thomson K, Ferguson A. Familial cystic nephroma and pleuro-pulmonary blastoma. Cancer 1993;71:1338–42.

176. Ishida Y, Kato K, Kigasawa H, et al. Synchronous occurrence of pleuropulmonary blastoma and cystic nephroma: Possible genetic link in cystic lesions of the lung and the kidney. Med Pediatr Oncol 2000;35:85–7.

177. Joshi VV, Beckwith JB. Multilocular cyst of the kidney (cystic nephroma) and cystic, partially differentiated nephroblastoma. Terminology and criteria for diagnosis. Cancer 1989; 64:466–79.

178. Blakely ML, Shamberger RC, Norkool P, et al. Outcome of children with cystic partially differentiated nephroblastoma treated with or without chemotherapy. J Pediatr Surg 2003;38:897–900.

179. Luithle T, Szavay P, Furtwängler R, et al. Treatment of cystic nephroma and cystic partially differentiated nephroblastoma–a report from the SIOP/GPOH study group. J Urol 2007;177:294–6.

180. Beckwith JB. The John Lattimer lecture: Wilms' tumor and other renal tumors of childhood: An update. J Urol 1986;136:320–4.

181. Steif W, Gassner I, Janetschek G, et al. Partial nephrectomy in a cystic partially differentiated nephroblastoma. Med Pediatr Oncol 1997;28:416–19.

182. Sacher P, Willi U, Niggli F, et al. Cystic nephroma: A rare benign renal tumor. Pediatr Surg Int 1998;13:197–9.

183. Mushtaq I, Carachi R, Roy G, et al. Childhood renal tumours with intravascular extension. Br J Urol 1996;78:772–6.

184. Vazquez JL, Barnewolt CE, Shamberger RC. Ossifying renal tumor of infancy presenting as a palpable abdominal mass. Pediatr Radiol 1998;28:454–7.

185. Steffens J, Kraus J, Misho B, et al. Ossifying renal tumor of infancy. J Urol 1993;149:1080–1.

CHAPTER 66

Neuroblastoma

Andrew M. Davidoff

Neuroblastoma is the most common solid extracranial malignancy of childhood and the most common malignant tumor in infants.[1] The overall incidence of neuroblastoma is 1 per 100,000 children in the USA, thereby comprising 7–10% of all malignancies diagnosed in patients younger than 15 years of age. Yet neuroblastoma is responsible for approximately 15% of all pediatric cancer deaths.[2] Neuroblastoma is a heterogeneous disease; tumors can spontaneously regress or mature, or display a very aggressive, malignant phenotype.[3] Because of these unique characteristics, neuroblastoma has been of great interest to both clinicians and basic science researchers. Progress in molecular and cellular biology in the past 30 years has contributed greatly to a better understanding of this disease. Unfortunately, this progress has not significantly altered the clinical outcome for patients with advanced-stage neuroblastoma. Although the prognosis for these patients has improved in the past three decades, the long-term outcome remains very poor.

The etiology of neuroblastoma is currently unknown, and no environmental factors have been convincingly linked to its development. The disease generally occurs sporadically, but familial neuroblastoma occurs in about 2% of the cases. The substantial biologic and clinical heterogeneity is also observed in familial cases.[4] The germline mutation associated with hereditary neuroblastoma has been identified: activating mutations in the tyrosine kinase domain of the anaplastic lymphoma kinase (*ALK*) oncogene on the short arm of chromosome 2 (2p23).[5] These mutations can also be somatically acquired, although the prevalence of ALK activation in sporadic neuroblastoma remains to be determined.

The treatment of neuroblastoma requires a multidisciplinary approach. Although resection may be the only therapy required for patients at 'low-risk' for disease recurrence, the surgeon provides but one element of the modern multimodal treatment of children with 'high-risk' disease. Oncologists, radiation therapists, and bone marrow transplantation (BMT) specialists are among the other important members of the pediatric oncology team. The therapy for patients with neuroblastoma, as for children with other malignancies, is generally driven by clinical research protocols. Many of these protocols are sponsored by the Children's Oncology Group (COG) or by the larger children's hospitals.

PATHOLOGY

Neuroblastoma is an embryonal tumor of the sympathetic nervous system. These tumors arise during fetal or early postnatal life from sympathetic cells (sympathogonia) derived from the neural crest. Therefore, tumors can originate anywhere along the path which neural crest cells migrate, including the adrenal medulla, paraspinal sympathetic ganglia, and sympathetic paraganglia such as the organ of Zuckerkandl. The German pathologist Rudolph Virchow is generally credited with being the first to describe the histologic appearance of what is now known as neuroblastoma in his 1864 article entitled, 'Hyperplasia of the pineal and suprarenal glands'.[6] The first to use the term 'neuroblastoma' was James Homer Wright in 1910 who described the classic appearance of rosettes of tumor cells around central neural fibrils.[7] He also noted the association between the common sites of tumor development and the pattern of migration of primitive neural cells.

As one of the 'small, round blue cell' tumors of infancy and childhood, neuroblastoma, particularly when undifferentiated, must be distinguished from other neoplasms in this group (Ewing sarcoma family of tumors [ESFT], non-Hodgkin lymphoma, and rhabdomyosarcoma). Neuroblastoma can be distinguished histologically by the presence of neuritic processes (neuropil) and Homer Wright rosettes (neuroblasts surrounding eosinophilic neuropil). Scattered ganglion cells or immature chromaffin cells can also be seen. The appearance of the tumor cells may vary from undifferentiated cells to fully mature ganglion cells. In addition, neuroblastomas have variable degrees of Schwannian cell stroma, reactive non-neoplastic tissue recruited by the tumor cells. This stroma is intermixed, to a greater or lesser degree, as wavy bundles and sheets of spindle cells and produces antiproliferative and differentiation-inducing factors that are crucial to neuronal differentiation.[8,9] In addition, the Schwannian stroma appears to produce a variety of antiangiogenic factors, including pigment epithelium derived factor (PEDF)[10] and secreted protein acidic and rich in cysteine (SPARC).[11] Histopathologic variables among neuroblastic tumors include the degree of differentiation, maturation, lymphoid infiltration, calcification, anaplasia, necrosis, mitotic activity, neurofibrillary material (neuropil), and the presence of multinucleate cells. Finally, immunohistochemical analysis usually generates positive staining when antibodies to neuroblastoma-specific antigens such as synaptophysin, neuron-specific enolase, and chromogranin are used, and is negative when antibodies to actin, desmin, cytokeritin, leukocyte common antigen, vimentin, and CD99 are used.

Neuroblastoma is characterized by several unique clinical behaviors, including the secretion of catecholamine products and the potential to regress or mature, either spontaneously or in response to treatment. Small nodules of primitive neuroblasts are routinely found in the developing adrenal gland, even during the early postnatal period. Beckwith and Perrin described microscopic nodules that they termed 'neuroblastoma in situ' in the adrenals of infants undergoing autopsy following death from non-malignancy related causes.[12] The incidence of this finding was more than 200-fold greater than the clinical incidence of neuroblastoma, which suggests that perhaps many neuroblastomas spontaneously regress or mature into lesions that never become clinically apparent. The process of involution is well described during embryonic life, especially in the developing central and peripheral nervous systems. Although initially thought to be mediated by the immune system, the process of involution may be the result of the withdrawal of neurotrophic maintenance factors such as nerve growth factor (NGF). Clinically apparent neuroblastoma can also regress or spontaneously mature, but the mechanism remains unknown.

Histopathologic Classification

In 1984, Shimada and colleagues first developed an age-linked classification system of neuroblastic tumors based on tumor morphology in which neuroblastomas were divided into two prognostic subgroups, favorable histology and unfavorable histology.[13] In 1999, the International Neuroblastoma Pathology Classification (INPC) was devised, and then modified in 2003, and is an adaptation of the original Shimada system.[14,15] The INPC is based mainly on morphologic changes associated with the maturational sequence of neuroblastic tumors. It remains an age-linked classification that depends on the differentiation grade of the neuroblasts, the cellular turnover index (mitosis-karyorrhexis index [MKI]), and the presence or absence of Schwannian stroma. The INPC classifies neuroblastic tumors into three morphologic categories: neuroblastoma, ganglioneuroblastoma, and ganglioneuroma (Fig. 66-1).

Neuroblastomas are, by definition, Schwannian stroma poor (<50% of the tumor tissue) and can be subtyped as undifferentiated, poorly differentiated, or differentiating. Undifferentiated requires supplemental diagnostic methods such as immunohistochemistry, electron microscopy, or cytogenetics. Moreover, neuropil is not present. In poorly differentiated, <5% of tumor cells have features of differentiation, and neuropil is present. Differentiating tumors demonstrate >5% of tumor cells differentiating toward ganglion cells. To classify a cell as a differentiating neuroblast, there must be synchronous differentiation of the nucleus and eosinophilic cytoplasm.[14]

Additional factors that contribute to the prognostic distinction of stroma-poor neuroblastic tumors (neuroblastoma) as favorable or unfavorable subtypes include the MKI, which is defined as the number of tumor cells in mitosis or karyorrhexis per 5000 neuroblastic cells (i.e., low MKI, <100 cells; intermediate, 100–200 cells; high, >200 cells), and the patient's age (<1.5 years, 1.5-5 years, >5 years) (Table 66-1). It has been hypothesized that neuroblastic cells with maturational potential require a latent period before demonstrating histologic evidence of differentiation. Therefore, there is a certain allowance for mitotic and karyorrhectic activities of neuroblastic cells in tumors in infants and younger children.[16]

The importance of this histopathologic classification was confirmed in a large, retrospective analysis reported by Shimada et al.[17] The INPC classification of tumor histology provided independent prognostic information where tumors of favorable histology had a 90.8% probability of 5-year event-free survival [EFS] compared to 31.2% EFS for tumors of unfavorable histology. More recently, the INPC classification has been shown to add independent prognostic information beyond the prognostic contribution of age.[18] Therefore, histopathology remains in the current multifactorial risk stratification for patients with neuroblastoma. This determination is particularly important in patients with *MYCN* non-amplified tumors who are older than 18 months and have stage 3 disease, or 12 to 18 months of age and have stage 4 disease, or have 4S disease. As the histopathologic pattern within a tumor can be heterogeneous, it is recommended that representative sections from at least 1 cm³ of viable, non-necrotic tissue be analyzed to determine histopathologic classification. The prognostic value of assessing the histopathology of a neuroblastoma after chemotherapy or radiation therapy has not been validated.

Stroma-rich neuroblastic tumors are classified as either ganglioneuroblastomas or ganglioneuromas. Ganglioneuroblastomas contain cells that are transitioning toward differentiation but are not completely differentiated/mature. Also, <50% of the total volume is made up of neuroblastic cells. Ganglioneuroblastomas can be further divided into 'intermixed' and 'nodular' subtypes, depending on the distribution of the neuroblastic cells. The distinction is important because of the significantly worse prognosis associated with the latter subtype, in which the neuroblastic clones that comprise grossly distinct nodules appear to be responsible for the aggressive phenotype for this subtype.[16] Ganglioneuromas contain either maturing or mature cells, and lack any neuroblastomatous component. Most stroma-rich tumors (ganglioneuroblastoma, *intermixed* and ganglioneuroma, *maturing* subtype) are classified as 'favorable' by the INPC. However, the pathologic/prognostic classification of the ganglioneuroblastoma, *nodular* subtype is based on the morphologic evaluation of the neuroblastomatous nodule(s), and can, therefore, be unfavorable. Tumors that fit the criteria for ganglioneuroma, *mature* subtype, with abundant Schwannian stroma and fully mature ganglion cells, in the absence of neuroblasts, are considered benign, and are generally not considered for enrolment in protocols for neuroblastic tumors. Despite this, ganglioneuromas can be quite large and infiltrative, and attempts at removal can be associated with significant complications. In addition, survival does not seem to be influenced by extent of resection.[19] Therefore, aggressive attempts at resection of ganglioneuromas are not recommended.

MOLECULAR BIOLOGY

Advances in molecular biology research in the past three decades have resulted in an increased understanding of the genetic events in the pathogenesis and progression of many human malignancies, including those of childhood.

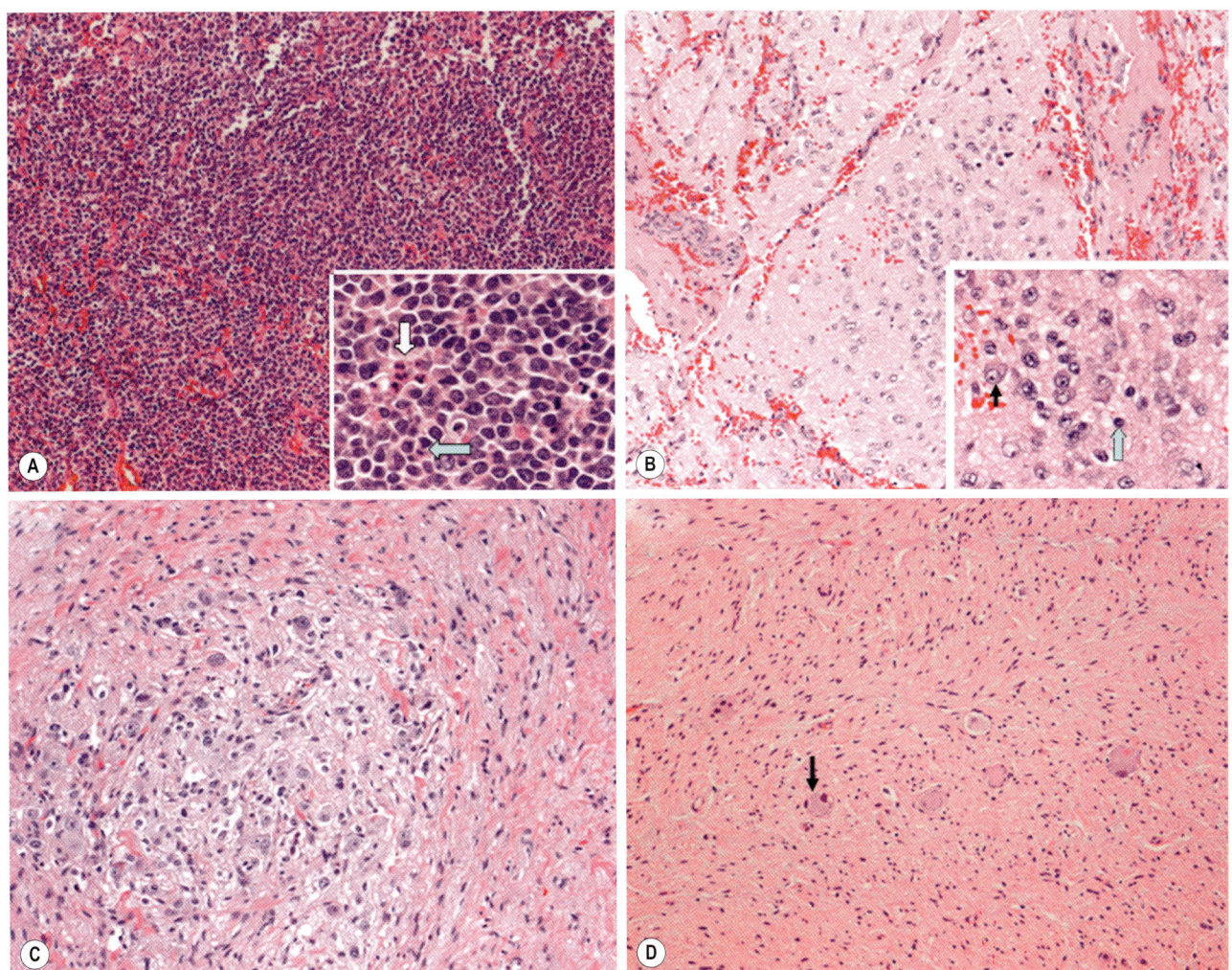

FIGURE 66-1 ■ Histologic appearance of neuroblastic tumors. **(A)** An undifferentiated neuroblastoma with high MKI (10×). A clump of karyorrhectic tumor cells (white arrow) and a tumor cell undergoing mitosis (open arrow) are shown in the insert (60×). **(B)** A differentiating neuroblastoma, with low MKI (10×). A primitive neuroblast (gray arrow) and a differentiating tumor cell (black arrow), with features of differentiation in both the nucleus and cytoplasm, are shown in the insert (60×). Abundant neuropil is also seen. **(C)** A stroma-rich ganglioneuroblastoma with infrequent neuroblasts intermixed within abundant Schwannian stroma and ganglion cells (10×). **(D)** A stroma-rich ganglioneuroma. Ganglion cells are seen (arrow) (10×). Infiltrating lymphoid cells are also seen but no neuroblasts are present. (Courtesy of Jesse Jenkins MD and Christine Fuller MD, St. Jude Children's Research Hospital, Memphis TN. Reprinted from Neuroblastoma, Davidoff AM. In Oldham KT, Colombani PM, Foglia RP, et al, editors. Principles and Practice of Pediatric Surgery. Philadelphia: Lippincott, Williams & Wilkins; 2005.)

Neuroblastoma, in particular, has served as a model for a molecular approach to treating patients with cancer, highlighting the utility of genetic analysis for diagnosis, risk stratification, and treatment planning. Chromosomal structural changes play a role in neuroblastoma, particularly those that result in the loss of tumor suppressors, or gain of oncogenes, gene amplification, and activating or inactivating mutations of relevant genes or their regulatory elements. The end result of alterations in these genetic elements, regardless of their specific mechanisms, is the disruption of the normal balance between cell proliferation and cell death.

DNA Content

Normal human cells contain two copies of each of 23 chromosomes; thus, a normal diploid cell has 46

chromosomes. The majority (55%) of primary neuroblastomas are triploid or 'near-triploid/hyperdiploid' and contain between 58 and 80 chromosomes; the remainder (45%) are either 'near-diploid' (35–57 chromosomes) or 'near-tetraploid' (81–103 chromosomes).[20] The 'DNA index' of a tumor is the ratio of the number of chromosomes present to a diploid number of chromosome (i.e., 46). Therefore, diploid cells have a DNA index of 1.0, whereas near-triploid cells have a DNA index ranging from 1.26 to 1.76. Neuroblastomas that are near-diploid or near-tetraploid usually have structural genetic abnormalities, most frequently chromosome 1p deletion and *MYCN* amplification. Near-triploid or hyperdiploid tumors are characterized by almost three complete haploid sets of chromosomes with few structural abnormalities. Importantly, patients with near-triploid tumors typically have favorable clinical and biologic prognostic

TABLE 66-1 Prognostic Evaluation of Neuroblastic Tumors According to the International Neuroblastoma Pathology Classification

International Neuroblastoma Pathology Classification		Prognostic Group
NEUROBLASTOMA	**SCHWANNIAN STROMA POOR**	
<1.5 years	Poorly differentiated or differentiating, and low or intermediate MKI tumor	Favorable
1.5–5 years	Differentiating and low MKI tumor	
<1.5 years	(a) Undifferentiated tumor or (b) high MKI tumor	Unfavorable
1.5–5 years	(a) Undifferentiated or poorly differentiated tumor, or (b) intermediate or high MKI tumor	
≥5 years	All tumors	
Ganglioneuroblastoma, intermixed	Schwannian stroma rich	Favorable
Ganglioneuroblastoma, nodular	Composite schwannian stroma rich/stroma-dominant and stroma poor	Unfavorable or favorable (based on nodule histology)
Ganglioneuroma	Schwannian stroma-dominant	Favorable
Maturing		
Mature		

MKI, mitosis-karyorrhexis index.
Adapted from Shimada H, Ambros IM, Dehner LP, et al. The International NB Pathology Classification (the Shimada System). Cancer 1999;86:364–72.

factors and excellent survival rates, as compared with those patients who have near-diploid or near-tetraploid tumors.[21] This association is most important for infants with advanced disease as the prognostic significance of tumor ploidy appears to be lost in patients older than 2 years.[22] Currently, ploidy only potentially impacts the risk group assessment of infants age 12–18 months with metastatic disease and infants with 4S disease in the COG risk stratification schema.

Amplification of *MYCN*

Investigation of the molecular biology of neuroblastoma began with the cytogenetic characterization of tumor-derived cell lines. These studies showed the frequent presence of extrachromosomal double-minute chromatin bodies (DMs) and chromosomally integrated homogeneously staining regions (HSRs) characteristic of gene amplification (Fig. 66-2).[23] Since that time, it has been shown that the amplified region was derived from the distal short arm of chromosome 2 (2p24) and contained the *MYCN* proto-oncogene. *MYCN* encodes a 64 kDa nuclear phosphoprotein that forms a transcriptional complex by associating with other nuclear proteins expressed in the developing nervous system and other tissues.[24] Enforced expression of *MYCN* increases the rates of DNA synthesis and cell proliferation, and shortens the G_1 phase of the cell cycle.[25] *MYCN* can also function as a classic dominant oncogene that cooperates with activated *ras* to transform normal cells.[26] Targeted expression of *MYCN* in transgenic mice results in the development of neuroblastomas.[27] This activity is potentiated when combined with mutations in *ALK*.[28]

Overall, approximately 25% of primary neuroblastomas in children have *MYCN* amplification, with *MYCN* amplification being present in 40% with advanced disease but only 5–10% with low-stage disease.[29] The copy number, which can range from 5- to 500-fold

amplification, is usually consistent among primary and metastatic sites and at different times during tumor evolution and treatment.[30] This finding suggests that *MYCN* amplification is an early event in the pathogenesis of neuroblastoma. Amplification of *MYCN* is associated with advanced stages of disease, rapid tumor progression, and poor outcome; therefore, it is a powerful prognostic indicator of tumor behavior.[29,31] Amplification can be detected either by routine metaphase cytogenetics or fluorescent in situ hybridization (FISH), and current therapeutic neuroblastoma protocols have incorporated the presence or absence of *MYCN* amplification into their risk stratification schema.

Chromosomal Changes

Also noted on early karyotype analyses of neuroblastoma-derived cell lines were frequent deletions of the short arm of chromosome 1.[32] Deletions of genetic material in tumors suggest the presence (and subsequent loss) of a tumor suppressor gene. Although no individual tumor suppressor gene has been confirmed on chromosome 1p, recent data have identified *CHD5* as a strong candidate for the tumor suppressor gene that is deleted from 1p36.31 in neuroblastoma.[33] Functional confirmation of the presence of a 1p tumor suppressor gene came from the demonstration that transfection of chromosome 1p into a neuroblastoma cell line resulted in morphologic changes and ultimately cell senescence.[34] Approximately 20–35% of primary neuroblastomas exhibit 1p deletion, as determined by FISH, with the smallest common region of loss located within region 1p36.[35] About 70% of advanced-stage neuroblastomas have 1p deletions.[36] Molecular studies have shown that there is a strong correlation between 1p deletion and *MYCN* amplification and other high-risk features such as age older than 1 year and advanced-stage disease.[35] One recent study has demonstrated that 1p deletions are independently

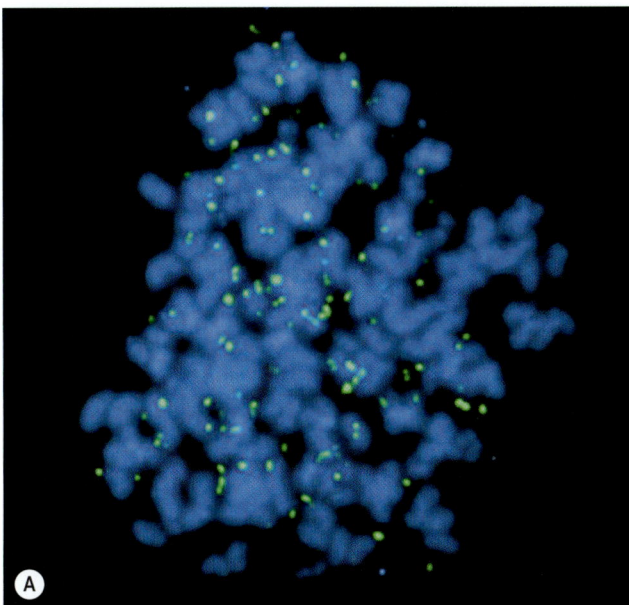

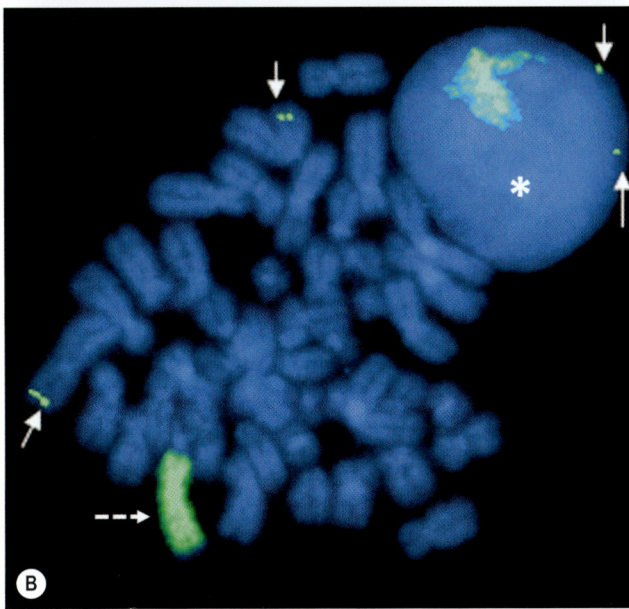

FIGURE 66-2 ■ FISH analysis of a neuroblastoma. **(A)** Chromosomes in metaphase. The bright spots are double-minute chromatin bodies. **(B)** The metaphase chromosomes are again seen. An intact interphase nucleus is marked with an *asterisk*. The normal two copies of the *MYCN* gene are marked with *solid arrows*. Homogeneously staining regions (HSRs) are also seen. One is seen in the interphase nucleus, and the other is marked with a *dotted arrow*. (Courtesy of Marc Valentine, St. Jude Children's Research Hospital, Memphis, TN.)

associated with a worse outcome in patients with neuroblastoma.[37]

Deletion of the long arm of chromosome 11 (11q) also appears to be common in neuroblastoma, being present in about 40% of cases. Unbalanced deletion of 11q (loss with either retention or gain of 11p material) is inversely related to *MYCN* amplification,[37,38] yet is strongly associated with other high-risk features. Recently, Attiyeh et al., on behalf of COG, showed in a large cohort of patients that unbalanced deletion of 11q and 1p36 were independently associated with a worse outcome in patients with neuroblastoma.[39] Therefore, the duration of treatment for children with intermediate-risk neuroblastoma on the recent COG study was based, in part, on the 1p and 11q allelic status of the tumor.

Mutations

An example of proto-oncogene activation by point mutation involves the tyrosine kinase receptor, ALK, on the short arm of chromosome 2 (2p23). Receptor tyrosine kinases (RTK) are high-affinity cell surface receptors for many growth factors, cytokines, and hormones. When activated through ligand binding, these proteins mediate phosphorylation of tyrosine on target molecules or substrates, resulting in intracellular signaling and, ultimately, the regulation of normal cellular processes. Mutation of RTK's can lead to constitutive activation of the signaling pathway in the absence of ligand. Recently, activating mutations of *ALK* have been shown to be the germline abnormality associated with hereditary neuroblastoma.[40] These mutations can also be somatically acquired, as can amplification of the gene, although the prevalence of ALK activation in sporadic neuroblastoma is not known.[41] Activated ALK has proven to be a targetable abnormality in neuroblastoma, with drugs such as crizotinib, an anti-ALK antibody, showing efficacy.[42] Further studies have identified loss-of-function mutations in the homeobox gene *PHOXB2* on 4p13 that are also associated with familial neuroblastoma, particularly when occurring together with Hirschsprung disease and/or central hypoventilation.[43]

Recently, inactivating mutations of *ATRX*, a transcriptional regulator that is part of a multiprotein complex that plays a role in regulating chromatin remodeling, nucleosome assembly, and telomere maintenance, have been found in neuroblastoma, particularly high-stage tumors in older patients.[44] *ATRX* mutations appear to be loss-of-function mutations associated with an absence of the ATRX protein in the nucleus, and with long telomeres. How these alterations lead to lengthened telomeres is uncertain. These results may provide a molecular marker and potential therapeutic target for neuroblastoma among adolescents and young adults. It may also delineate the subset of children with neuroblastoma who have a chronic but progressive clinical course when receiving standard therapeutic approaches and who may benefit from a different treatment strategy.

Other Molecular Abnormalities

Neurotrophins and their tyrosine kinase receptors are important in the development of the sympathetic nervous system and have been implicated in the pathogenesis of neuroblastoma. Three receptor-ligand pairs have been identified: TrkA, the primary receptor for NGF; TrkB, the primary receptor of brain-derived neurotrophic factor (BDNF); and TrkC, the receptor for neurotrophin-3 (NT-3).[45] TrkA appears to mediate differentiation of developing neurons or neuroblastoma in the presence of NGF ligand, and apoptosis in the absence of NGF.[46] High TrkA expression is associated with favorable tumor biology and good outcome[47] and is inversely correlated with *MYCN* amplification.[48] Conversely, the TrkB/BDNF pathway appears to promote neuroblastoma survival through autocrine or paracrine signaling, especially in *MYCN*-amplified tumors.[49] TrkB is expressed in about 40% of neuroblastomas, usually advanced-stage disease. TrkC is expressed in approximately 25% of neuroblastomas and is strongly associated with TrkA expression.[50]

Other molecular abnormalities frequently detected in neuroblastoma include inactivation of caspase 8, expression of CD44, and overexpression of multidrug resistance genes. Studies have demonstrated inactivation of caspase 8, a component of the Fas death-signaling complex, in *MYCN*-amplified neuroblastomas.[51] It has been proposed that inactivation of caspase 8 renders tumor cells resistant to apoptotic signals. CD44 is a cell surface glycoprotein that appears to play a role in tumor cell adhesion.[52] In neuroblastomas, CD44 expression is inversely correlated with *MYCN* amplification and is undetectable in most disseminated neuroblastomas.[53] Multidrug resistance-associated protein (MRP) is an efflux pump whose expression in neuroblastoma appears to be correlated with *MYCN* amplification and poor prognosis.[54,55] The presence of MRP may explain the common clinical situation in which neuroblastomas initially respond well to chemotherapy but subsequently become resistant.

Genome-Wide Association Studies

Recently, microarray technologies have generated extensive amounts of data that have aided in identifying genomic (DNA) and transcriptomic (RNA) abnormalities associated with neuroblastoma. In addition, these abnormalities have been shown to have significant predictive power when anticipating outcome for these patients.[56,57] Many of these findings were generated by large scale genome-wide association studies (GWAS). This is a technique whereby all or most of the genes of patients with neuroblastoma are analyzed to find differences with the population as a whole, looking for variations that are associated with the development and aggressiveness of neuroblastoma. The causal relationship between the DNA variant associated with the cancer is uncertain but an excessive inheritance of risk variants has been postulated to increase susceptibility to the disease. Several GWAS studies have been performed in patients with neuroblastoma and have identified a number of such genetic risk variants.[58] These observations suggest that developmental childhood cancers are likely influenced by common DNA variations, leading to the development of a putative genetic model.[58] Recent data suggest that the higher prevalence of high-risk disease in Black and Native American patients with neuroblastoma may be associated with certain genetic variants found more commonly in these ethnic groups.[59]

One such type of variation is a single-nucleotide polymorphism (SNP) in which there is a variation in the DNA sequence for a single nucleotide between children with neuroblastoma and those without neuroblastoma, and with varying degrees of tumor phenotype. Another type of variation is copy number variation (CNV) which is an alteration of the DNA resulting in an abnormal number of copies of one or more sections of the DNA. CNVs correspond to relatively large regions of the genome that have been deleted or duplicated.

One method for detecting CNVs is by comparative genomic hybridization (CGH). Early CGH studies showed that gain of genetic material on the long arm of chromosome 17 (17q) is perhaps the most common genetic abnormality in neuroblastomas, occurring in approximately 75% of primary tumors.[60] It is unclear at this time how extra copies of 17q contribute to the malignant phenotype of neuroblastoma and which gene(s) on 17q are the critical ones. Nevertheless, gain of chromosome 17q is strongly associated with other known prognostic factors, but it may also be a powerful predictor of adverse outcome.[61] More recently, GWAS studies have shown that inherited CNV at chromosome 1q21.1 is associated with neuroblastoma, implicating a neuroblastoma breakpoint family gene in early neuroblastoma genesis.[62]

Other studies have revealed that common genetic variation at chromosome bands 6p22[63] and 2q35[64] are associated with susceptibility to high-risk neuroblastoma, providing the first evidence that childhood cancers can also arise from complex interactions of polymorphic variants. More recently, a GWAS study has identified common polymorphisms including germline SNP risk alleles and somatic copy number gain, resulting in increased expression of the cysteine-rich transcriptional regulator LIM domain only 1 (LMO1) at 11p15.4. These have been shown to be strongly associated with susceptibility to developing neuroblastoma, and often are associated with advanced disease and poor survival.[65]

Finally, whole-genome sequencing of tumors, made possible recently by significant advances in technology, has been performed to investigate the genetic landscape of a variety of pediatric tumors.[66] Initially it was felt that early alterations of genes such as *MYCN* may underlie the rapid acquisition of cooperating mutations in key cancer pathways through chromosome instability. However, few recurring amino acid changes have been detected in neuroblastoma specimens, suggesting that the tumor genomes were more stable than previously believed.[44,67] Also, unlike the genetic landscape, the epigenetic profiles showed profound changes which suggests that epigenetic changes may have a more dominant role in pediatric tumorigenesis.

CLINICAL PRESENTATION

Patients with neuroblastoma usually present with signs and symptoms that reflect the primary site and extent of disease, although localized disease is often asymptomatic. As 75% of neuroblastoma occurs in the abdominal cavity, an abdominal mass detected on physical examination is a common clinical feature, as is the complaint of abdominal pain. Other primary sites of neuroblastoma include the posterior mediastinum (20%), the cervical region (1%), and the pelvis (4%) (organ of Zuckerkandel) (Fig. 66-3). Respiratory distress or dysphagia may be a reflection of a thoracic tumor. Altered defecation or urination may be caused by mechanical compression from a pelvic tumor

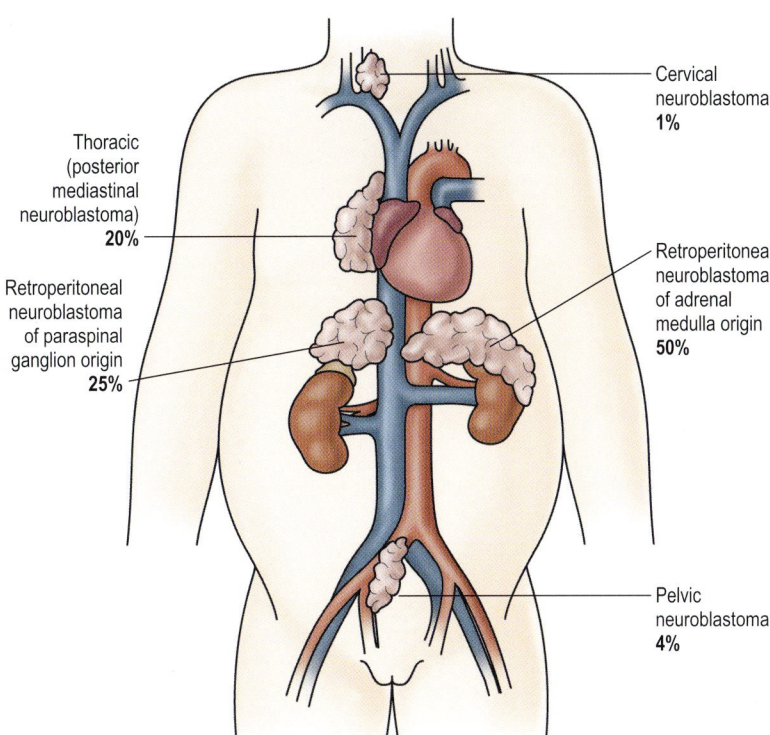

Cervical
neuroblastoma
1%

Thoracic
(posterior
mediastinal
neuroblastoma)
20%

Retroperitoneal
neuroblastoma
of paraspinal
ganglion origin
25%

Retroperitoneal
neuroblastoma
of adrenal
medulla origin
50%

Pelvic
neuroblastoma
4%

FIGURE 66-3 ■ Primary sites for neuroblastoma are depicted in this anatomic drawing. (Reprinted from Davidoff AM. Neuroblastoma. In: Oldham KT, Colombani PM, Foglia RP, et al, editors. Principles and Practice of Pediatric Surgery. Philadelphia: Lippincott Williams & Wilkins; 2005.)

or by spinal cord compression by a paraspinal tumor. Spinal cord compression may also present as an altered gait. A tumor in the neck or upper thorax can produce Horner syndrome (ptosis, miosis, and anhydrosis), enophthalmos, and heterochromia of the iris. Acute cerebellar ataxia has also been observed, characterized by the dancing-eye syndrome, which includes opsoclonus, myoclonus, and chaotic nystagmus. Two-thirds of these cases occur in infants with mediastinal primary tumors.[68,69] Additional signs and symptoms that reflect excessive catecholamine or vasoactive intestinal polypeptide (VIP) secretion include diarrhea, weight loss, and hypertension.

More than 40% of patients have metastatic disease at diagnosis. These patients are often quite ill and have systemic symptoms caused by widespread disease. Neuroblastoma in older patients has a pattern of metastatic disease in which metastases to the bone marrow, lymph nodes, and bone predominate. The frequency of involvement of distant sites is shown in Table 66-2. These metastases may manifest as bone pain from cortical metastases or anemia from marrow infiltration. The brain, spinal cord, heart, and lungs are rare sites of metastases, except with end-stage disease. Metastatic disease may be also associated with darkened eyes, referred to as 'raccoon eyes,' as a result of retroorbital venous plexus spread (Fig. 66-4A). This is an ominous physical sign, as is the presence of a limp in children without a history of head or extremity trauma. Infants with metastatic neuroblastoma can have stage 4S disease, which, by definition, is a localized primary tumor in patients younger than 1 year, with dissemination limited to skin, liver, or bone marrow (<10% of nucleated cells). These patients may present with 'blueberry muffin' cutaneous lesions (Fig. 66-4B),

respiratory distress secondary to massive hepatomegaly, and anemia secondary to bone marrow disease. The diagnosis of neuroblastoma is generally made by histopathologic evaluation of primary or metastatic tumor tissue, or by the demonstration of tumor cells in the bone marrow together with elevated levels of urinary catecholamines.

Laboratory Findings

Lactate Dehydrogenase

Despite its lack of specificity, serum lactate dehydrogenase (LDH) can have great prognostic significance. High serum levels of LDH reflect high proliferative activity or large tumor burden, and an LDH level higher than 1500 IU/L appears to be associated with a poor prognosis.[70,71] Thus, LDH can be used to monitor disease activity or the response to therapy.

Ferritin

High levels of serum ferritin (>150 ng/mL) may also reflect a large tumor burden or rapid tumor progression. Elevated serum ferritin is often seen in advanced-stage neuroblastomas and indicates a poor prognosis.[72] Levels often return to normal during clinical remission.

Neuron-Specific Enolase

Neuron-specific enolase (NSE) is another useful prognostic marker of advanced-stage neuroblastoma. The incidence of elevated NSE levels increases with stage.[73] A serum level of NSE >100 ng/mL is associated with a poor outcome. NSE has been reported to correlate with

TABLE 66-2 **Sites of Metastases at Diagnosis for Patients with Evans Stage IV-S and Stage IV**

	Stage IV–S (%)	Stage IV <1 Year (%)	Stage IV ≥1 Year (%)	Total (%)
Bone marrow	34.6	57.1	81.3	70.5
Bone	0	48.9	68.2	55.7
Lymph node	8.6	28.6	35.7	30.9
Liver	80.2	53.4	12.9	29.6
Intracranial/orbit	0	25.6	19.6	18.2
Adrenal	6.2	13.5	6.0	7.6
Skin	13.6	8.3	0.9	4.0
Pleura	0	4.5	3.7	3.4
Lung	0	2.3	4.1	3.2
Peritoneum	0	3.8	2.1	2.2
Other	0	3.8	1.6	1.9
Central nervous system	0	0	0.9	0.6

Adapted from Dubois SG, Kalika Y, Lukens JN, et al. Metastatic sites in stage IV and IVS neuroblastoma correlate with age, tumor biology, and survival. Pediatr Hematol Oncol 1999;21:181–9.

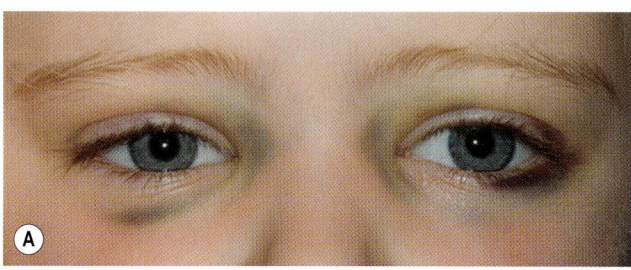

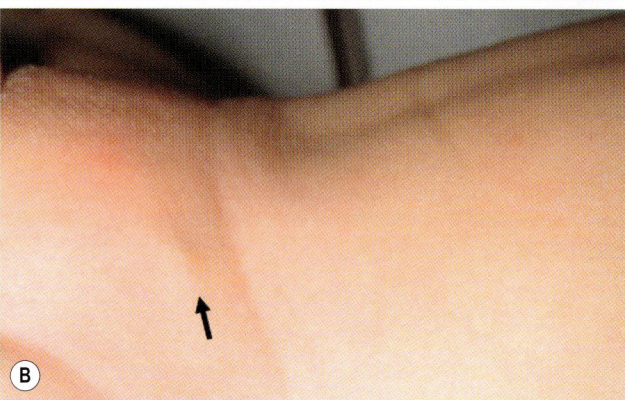

FIGURE 66-4 ■ Clinical evidence of metastatic neuroblastoma. **(A)** 'Raccoon eyes,' characteristic of metastatic neuroblastoma in the posterior orbital venous plexus, are seen in a child with stage IV disease. **(B)** 'Blueberry muffin' spot (arrow) in the skin, characteristic of metastatic neuroblastoma, is seen in the suprapubic region of an infant with a 4S neuroblastoma. (Courtesy of Stephen Shochat, MD, St. Jude Children's Research Hospital, Memphis, TN).

tumor burden, suggesting its reliability as a marker of disease course.[74]

Catecholamine Metabolites

Neuroblastoma is characterized by the relatively unique capacity for secretion of catecholamine products, the metabolites of which can be detected in the urine of more than 90% of patients with neuroblastoma. Thus, a urine specimen is of clinical value in diagnosing neuroblastoma and determining the response to therapy. Documentation of elevated urinary catecholamines is required if the diagnosis of neuroblastoma is being made solely by the identification of neuroblasts in the bone marrow. Urinary levels of these two catabolites can also be used as markers of tumor progression or relapse, and serve as a surrogate prognostic indicator. Random urine samples are preferable to 24-hour urine estimations for younger children.[75]

Diagnostic Imaging

Standard Radiographs

Chest radiography can be a useful tool for demonstrating the presence of a posterior mediastinal mass, which in a child is usually a thoracic neuroblastoma. A Pediatric Oncology Group (POG) study demonstrated that a mediastinal mass was discovered on incidental chest radiographs in almost half of patients with thoracic neuroblastoma who had symptoms seemingly unrelated to their tumors.[76] Abdominal radiography is less often the modality by which a neuroblastoma is discovered; however, as many as half of abdominal neuroblastomas are detectable as a mass with fine calcification.

Ultrasonography

Although ultrasonography (US) is the modality most often used during the initial assessment of a suspected abdominal mass, its sensitivity and accuracy are less than that of computed tomography (CT) or magnetic resonance imaging (MRI) for diagnosing neuoblastoma.[77] These latter modalities are generally used after screening with ultrasound to assist in generating a differential diagnosis and for further anatomic definition once the presence of a mass has been confirmed.

Computed Tomography

CT can demonstrate calcification in almost 85% of neuroblastomas, and intraspinal extension of the tumor can be determined on contrast-enhanced CT.[78] Overall, contrast-enhanced CT has been reported to be 82%

accurate in defining neuroblastoma extent, with the accuracy increasing to nearly 97% when performed with a bone scan.[79] Although some consider CT to have been supplanted by MRI, others still consider it to be the image modality of choice for patients with neuroblastoma, especially when used in conjunction with bone scintigraphy.[80]

Magnetic Resonance Imaging

MRI is becoming the most useful and most sensitive imaging modality for the diagnosis and staging of neuroblastoma.[77,81] MRI appears to be more accurate than CT for detection of stage 4 disease. The sensitivity of MRI is 83%, and that of CT is 43%, and the specificity of MRI is 97%, and that of CT is 88%.[81] Metastases to the bone and bone marrow, in particular, are better detected by MRI, as is intraspinal tumor extension (Fig. 66-5).[81] When considering skeletal metastases alone, MRI and bone scan have been shown to be equivalent.[81] Encasement of major vessels can be better defined by MRI than CT, especially with the use of MR angiography

(see Fig. 66-5). MRI in the coronal plane is suitable for routine assessment of the whole body from the neck to the pelvis. Evaluating the utility of whole-body MRI, perhaps performed in conjunction with a functional imaging study such as positron-emission tomography (PET), is being considered for future clinical staging studies. CT and MRI are not very accurate for staging localized disease; however, the sensitivity of T1- and T2-weighted MRIs is 100% for detecting neuroblastomas in infants identified by mass screening.[65]

Metaiodobenzylguanidine Imaging

Metaiodobenzylguanidine (MIBG) is transported to and stored in the chromaffin cells in the same way as norepinephrine. The MIBG scintiscan is the preferred imaging study for evaluating the bone and bone marrow involvement by neuroblastoma (Fig. 66-6), having largely replaced technetium-99m methylene diphosphonate (^{99m}Tc-MDP) bone scans, which are generally inferior to MIBG in detecting skeletal or extraskeletal involvement. In addition, monitoring MDP-avid neuroblastomas by

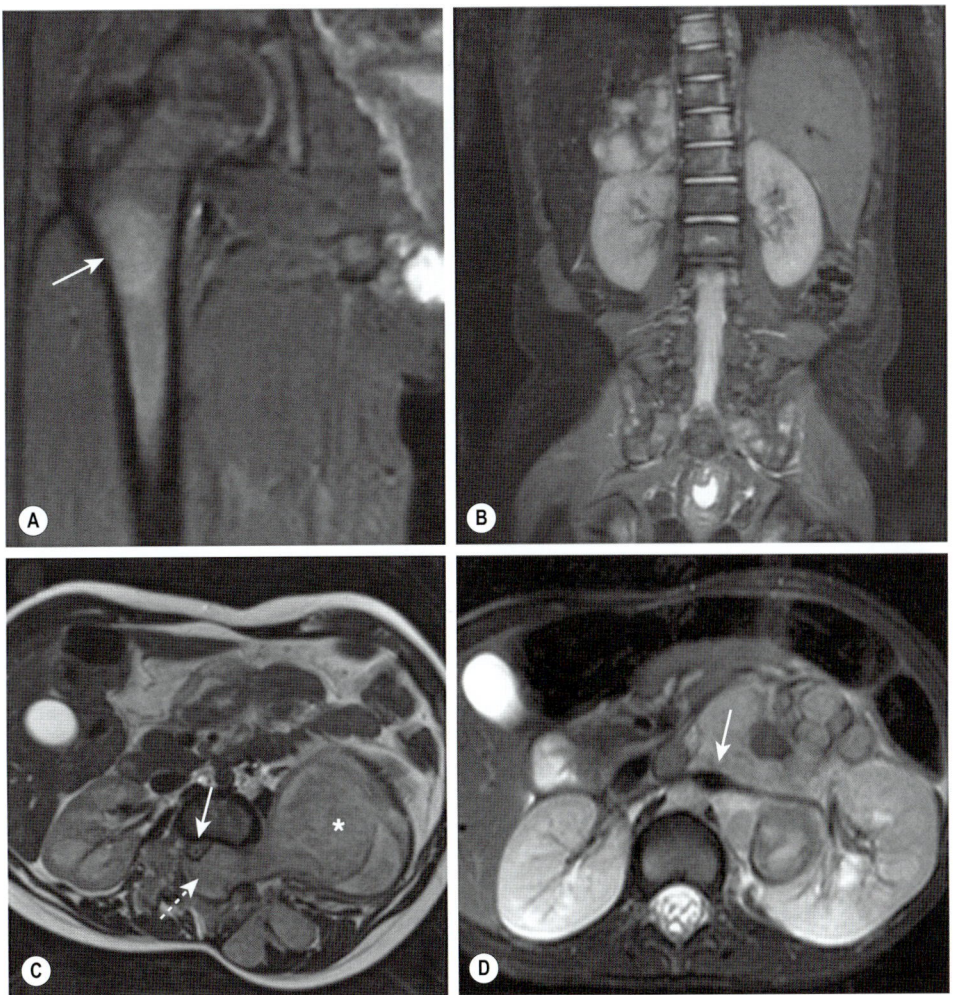

FIGURE 66-5 ■ These MR images highlight several characteristics of high-risk neuroblastoma. **(A)** Bone metastasis in femur (arrow). **(B)** Bone marrow metastases in the vertebral bodies. **(C)** Intraspinal tumor extension (dotted arrow). Note displacement of spinal cord (solid arrow) from a large tumor (asterisk). **(D)** Encasement of major intra-abdominal vessels (arrow points to the aorta and left renal artery).

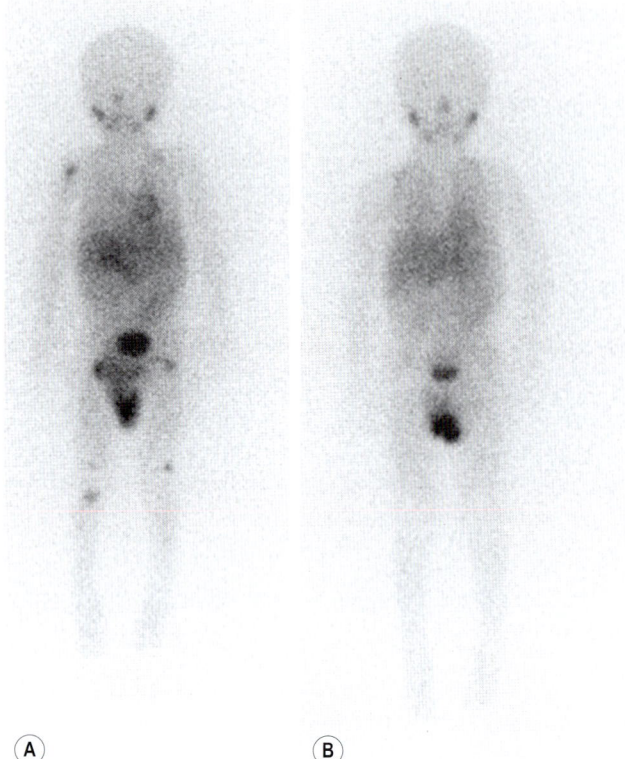

FIGURE 66-6 ■ Imaging of neuroblastoma with MIBG scintigraphy. **(A)** Scan obtained at presentation of a patient with metastatic neuroblastoma. There is diffusely abnormal activity throughout much of the skeleton including the proximal right humerus, both proximal and distal femurs, and the proximal right tibia. There is also a focus of activity in the right upper retroperitoneum at the site of the primary tumor. **(B)** Scan obtained of the same patient after completion of therapy shows no scintigraphic evidence of MIBG-avid neuroblastoma.

bone scintigraphy often results in false-positive imaging for months after tumor remission. Thus, ^{99m}Tc-MDP bone scanning is a second choice if MIBG imaging is not available or does not visualize known disease.[82,83] Iodine-131 (^{131}I) or iodine-123 (^{123}I) can be used to label MIBG. ^{123}I-MIBG supplies a reduced absorbed radiation dose and superior spatial resolution.[84] The reported sensitivity of MIBG in the detection of neuroblastomas with metastases to the bone and bone marrow is 82%, and the specificity is 91%.[85] Primary tumors and lymph node metastases are also detectable. MIBG can demonstrate more sites of tumor involvement in bone and bone marrow than either bone scintigraphy or standard radiography.[85] However, false-negative MIBG scans have been seen in cases in which the bone scintigraphy was positive.[83]

Bone Marrow Examination

Marrow biopsy is a routine method for detecting bone marrow involvement. Both aspiration and trephine biopsy should be performed, although the latter has better diagnostic value. To collect more accurate information, taking specimens from multiple sites is recommended. Immunohistochemical staining with antibodies

such as anti-ganglioside G_{D2}, S-100, NSE, and ferritin is also useful for reducing the number of false-negative cases.[86] Because biopsy is invasive and painful, noninvasive alternatives are being tested. Studies have suggested the superiority of MR imaging[87] and MIBG scintigraphy[88] over bone marrow biopsy in detecting bone marrow infiltration by neuroblastoma; however, the specificity of these modalities requires further evaluation.

Differential Diagnosis

Making a correct diagnosis of neuroblastoma can be difficult, because patients present with such diverse symptoms. For example, acute cerebellar ataxia with opsoclonus-myoclonus can be mistaken for a primary neurologic disease. Widespread bone involvement may resemble non-neoplastic bone disease such as osteomyelitis or rheumatoid arthritis, or be associated with systemic inflammatory changes. Symptoms referable to VIP secretion such as diarrhea can be misinterpreted as symptoms of an enteric infection or inflammatory bowel disease. Histologically, undifferentiated, small blue round cell neuroblastomas may be hard to distinguish from rhabdomyosarcoma, primitive neuroectodermal tumors, ESFT, or non-Hodgkin lymphoma. Use of a panel of specific antibodies, as mentioned previously, can facilitate histologic differentiation.[87]

Tumor Staging

International criteria for a common neuroblastoma staging system were first described in 1988, and subsequently revised in 1993.[89] The International Neuroblastoma Staging System (INSS) is a surgicopathologic staging system that depends on the completeness of resection of the primary tumor, assessment of ipsilateral and contralateral lymph nodes, and the relation of the primary tumor to the midline (Table 66-3). Evaluation of the primary tumor and involvement of metastatic sites in the INSS system depends largely on imaging studies (CT or MRI) although involvement of the bone marrow continues to be an important component. MIBG scanning is also recommended as part of the initial evaluation of new patients and, subsequently, for monitoring tumor response to therapy.

Although INSS has been shown to have prognostic relevance, there have been some difficulties with its widespread use. The expertise and aggressiveness of the surgeon influence tumor stage, lymph node sampling is done erratically, and patients who are simply observed without surgery cannot be appropriately staged. Therefore, a uniform, pretreatment staging system that could be used easily throughout the world, and subject to real-time central review, was sought. Montclair et al, on behalf of the International Neuroblastoma Risk Group (INRG), proposed a new staging system in 2009 based on tumor imaging rather than the extent of surgical resection.[90] In this staging system, localized tumors are staged based on the absence (L1) or presence (L2) of one or more of 20 image-defined risk factors (IDRFs). Previously, Cecchetto et al. had reported that the presence of one or more of these image-defined surgical risk factors was associated with a lower complete resection rate and a greater risk of surgery-related complications when attempting an initial resection of a localized neuroblastoma.[91]

Metastatic tumors are defined as stage M. Stage MS, similar to INSS stage 4S, refers to disease with metastases limited to skin, liver and bone marrow (less than 10% involvement) in children less than 18 months of age at diagnosis, although the INSS 4S age cut-off is 12 months. These young patients can have L1 or L2 primary tumors. The IDRFs are listed in Box 66-1 and generally reflect encasement of vital structures, primarily vessels and nerves, as determined by diagnostic imaging studies. Absence of these factors had previously been shown to be associated with safe, complete tumor resection.[91] In a review of 661 patients in the INRG database, Monclair et al. found that INRG staging had prognostic significance.[90] Patients with stage L1 disease had a significantly greater 5-year EFS than those with stage L2 disease (90% ± 3% vs 78% ± 4%, $p = 0.001$). Although INSS is currently still the staging system used for COG patients, the

---

BOX 66-1 Image-Defined Risk Factors for Primary Resection of Localized Neuroblastoma

Neck
1. Tumor encasing major vessel(s) (e.g., carotid artery, vertebral artery, internal jugular vein)
2. Tumor extending to base of skull
3. Tumor compressing the trachea
4. Tumor encasing the brachial plexus

Thorax
1. Tumor encasing major vessel(s) (e.g., subclavian vessels, aorta, superior vena cava)
2. Tumor compressing the trachea or principal bronchi
3. Lower mediastinal tumor, infiltrating the costovertebral junction between T9 and T12 (may involve the artery of Adamkiewicz supplying the lower spinal cord)

Abdomen
1. Tumor infiltrating the porta hepatis and/or the hepatoduodenal ligament
2. Tumor encasing the origin of the celiac axis and/or the superior mesenteric artery
3. Tumor invading one or both renal pedicles
4. Tumor encasing the aorta and/or vena cava
5. Tumor encasing the iliac vessels
6. Pelvic tumor crossing the sciatic notch

Dumbbell tumors with symptoms of spinal cord compression: Any location

Infiltration of adjacent organs/structures: Diaphragm, kidney, liver, duodenopancreatic block, and mesentery

Adapted from Cecchetto G, Mosseri V, DeBernardi B, et al. Surgical risk factors in primary surgery for localized neuroblastoma: The LNESG1 study of the European International Society of Pediatric Oncology NB Group. J Clin Oncol 2005;23:8483–9.

TABLE 66-3 International Neuroblastoma Staging System Criteria

Stage	Definition
1	Localized tumor with complete gross excision, with or without microscopic residual disease; representative ipsilateral lymph nodes negative for tumor microscopically (nodes attached to and removed with the primary tumor may be positive)
2A	Localized tumor with incomplete gross excision; representative ipsilateral nonadherent lymph nodes negative for tumor microscopically
2B 3	Localized tumor with or without complete gross excision, with ipsilateral nonadherent lymph nodes positive for tumor. Enlarged contralateral lymph nodes must be negative microscopically
	Unresectable unilateral tumor infiltrating across the midline,[a] with or without regional lymph node involvement *or* Localized unilateral tumor with contralateral regional lymph node involvement *or* Midline tumor with bilateral extension by infiltration (unresectable) or by lymph node involvement
4	Any primary tumor with dissemination to distant lymph nodes, bone, bone marrow, liver, skin, or other organs (except as defined for stage 4S).
4S	Localized primary tumor (as defined for stage 1, 2A, or 2B), with dissemination limited to skin, liver, and bone marrow[b] (limited to infants younger than 1 year old)

[a]The midline is defined as the vertebral column. Tumors originating on one side and crossing the midline must infiltrate to or beyond the opposite side of the vertebral column.

[b]Marrow involvement in stage 4S should be minimal (i.e., <10% of total nucleated cells identified as malignant on bone marrow biopsy or on marrow aspirate). More extensive marrow involvement would be considered to be stage 4. The metaiodobenzylguanidine scan (if performed) should be negative in the marrow.

INRG stage assignment is being collected prospectively on all patients for subsequent evaluation.

BIOLOGICALLY BASED RISK GROUPS AND THERAPY

As previously mentioned, one of the notable characteristics of neuroblastoma is the substantial heterogeneity of the disease, which ranges from spontaneous regression or maturation, even without therapy, to a highly malignant, aggressive phenotype that is poorly responsive to current intensive, multimodal therapy. Increasing evidence indicates that the biologic and molecular features of neuroblastoma are highly predictive of clinical behavior. Therefore, neuroblastoma has served as a paradigm for phenotypic risk assessment and treatment assignment whereby those at high risk for disease relapse are given intensive multimodal therapy. Those at low risk for relapse can have treatment intensity diminished in an attempt to avoid therapy-associated toxicity, while still achieving a high rate of cure. The predictive value of these biologic factors is important not only for the oncologist when considering appropriate chemotherapy, but also for the surgeon when considering the timing and extent of an operative resection in a child with neuroblastoma.

Current treatment of children with neuroblastoma is based not only on stage but also on risk stratification that takes into account clinical and biologic variables predictive of relapse. The most important clinical variables appear to be age at the time of diagnosis, with 18 months as the cut-off, and stage at diagnosis.[92-94] The most powerful biologic factors at this time appear to be *MYCN* status and histopathologic classification.[17,29,31]

In addition, other biologic and molecular variables continue to be evaluated and two, the allelic status at chromosomes 1p36 and 11q23, may influence the duration of therapy for certain patients. Taken together, these variables currently define the COG risk stratification (Table 66-4). On the basis of these clinical and biological variables, infants and children with neuroblastoma are categorized into three risk groups predictive of relapse: low, intermediate, and high risk. The probability of prolonged disease-free survival for patients in each group is >95%, >90%, and <30%, respectively. Other factors are still being evaluated and may help further refine risk assessment in the future. These factors are currently being refined and augmented by analyses performed by the INRG task force. This group, which initially convened in 2004, is composed of investigators from the major pediatric cancer cooperative groups throughout the world. The main objective of this task force is to develop a consensus approach to pretreatment risk stratification for children with neuroblastoma.

Proposed INRG Risk Stratification

In an effort to establish an international consensus on pretreatment risk stratification, the INRG task force developed the INRG Classification System based on an analysis of 8800 patients treated for neuroblastoma between 1990 and 2002. They used survival tree regression analyses with EFS as the primary endpoint to test the prognostic significance of 13 potentially prognostic factors.[95] The analyses determined that seven of these prognostic variables could define 16 different pretreatment risk groups (Table 66-5). These risk groups could then be divided into four categories based on expected five-year event-free survival: very low (>85% EFS, 28.2% of patients), low (>75 to ≤85% EFS, 26.8% of patients), intermediate (≥50 to 75% EFS, 9.0% of patients) and high (<50% EFS, 36.1% of patients) risk.[96] These factors are being prospectively collected on all neuroblastoma patients with the hope that these homogeneous cohorts will facilitate future comparisons of risk-based trials performed throughout the world. Of note, analysis of the prognostic importance of histopathology has been confounded by the inclusion of age, itself an independent prognostic factor, in the past. Therefore, in the INRG classification, schema tumor differentiation and MKI are separated for risk stratification.

Low-Risk Disease

Resection is currently the only therapy given to patients with low-risk disease, based on the prior experiences of each of the legacy groups (POG and Children's Cancer Group [CCG]). The POG 8104 study found that 2-year survival was 89% for patients with POG stage A (INSS stage 1) disease, despite microscopic residual disease, when patients were treated with operation alone.[96,97] In a similar cohort of patients, the CCG 3881 study found 3-year EFS and overall survival to be 94% and 99%, respectively, for patients with Evans stage I disease.[98] That study also found that although patients with Evans stage II disease (similar to INSS 2A/2B) had a three-year

---

TABLE 66-4   Children's Oncology Group Risk Stratification for Children with Neuroblastoma

Risk Stratification	INSS Stage	Age	Biology
Low			
Group 1	1	Any	Any
	2A/2B (>50% resected)	Any	*MYCN*-NA, any histology/ploidy
	4S	<365 days	*MYCN*-NA, FH, DI > 1
Intermediate			
Group 2	2A/2B (<50% resected or biopsy only)	Birth-12 years	*MYCN*-NA, any histology/ploidy[a]
	3	<365 days	*MYCN*-NA, FH, DI > 1[a]
	3	>365 days to 12 years	*MYCN*-NA, FH[a]
	4S (symptomatic)	<365 days	*MYCN*-NA, FH, DI > 1[a]
Group 3	3	<365 days	*MYCN*-NA, either UH or DI = 1[a]
	4	<365 days	*MYCN*-NA, FH, DI >1[a]
	4S	<365 days	*MYCN*-NA, either UH or DI = 1[a]; or unknown biology
Group 4	4	<365 days	*MYCN*-NA, either DI = 1 or UH
	3	365 to <547 days	*MYCN*-NA, UH, any ploidy
	4	365 to <547 days	*MYCN*-NA, FH, DI >1
High			
	2A/2B, 3, 4, 4S	Any	*MYCN*-amplified, any histology/ploidy
	3	≥547 days	*MYCN*-NA, UH, any ploidy
	4	365 to > 547 days	*MYCN*-NA, UH or DI = 1
	4	>547 days	Any

[a]If tumor contains chromosomal 1p LOH or unbalanced 11q LOH, or if data are missing, treatment assignment is upgraded to next group.
MYCN-NA, *MYCN* not amplified; FH, favorable histology; UH, unfavorable histology; DI, DNA index.

TABLE 66-5 International Neuroblastoma Risk Group (INRG) Pretreatment Classification

INRG Stage	Age (Months)	Histologic Category	Grade of Tumor Differentiation	MYCN	11q Aberration	Ploidy	Pretreatment Risk Group
L1/L2		GN maturing; GNB intermixed					A Very low
L1		Any, except		NA			B Very low
		GN maturing or GNB intermixed		Amp			K High
L2	<18	Any, except		NA	No		D Low
		GN maturing or GNB intermixed			Yes		G Intermediate
	>18	GNB nodular neuroblastoma	Differentiating	NA	No		E Low
					Yes		H Intermediate
			Poorly differentiated or undifferentiated	NA			
				Amp			N High
M	<18			NA		Hyperdiploid	F Low
	<12			NA		Diploid	I Intermediate
	12 to <18			NA		Diploid	J Intermediate
	<18			Amp			Q High
	>18						P High
MS	<18			NA	No		C Very low
					Yes		Q High
							R High

Amp, amplified; GN, ganglioneuroma; GNB, ganglioneuroblastoma; NA, not amplified.
Adapted from Cohn SL, Pearson AD, London WB, et al. The International Neuroblastoma Risk Group (INRG) classification system: An INRG Task Force report. J Clin Oncol 2009;27:289–97.

EFS of 81% irrespective of the extent of surgical resection and subsequent treatment, the overall survival for these patients was 99%.[98] This finding suggests that even if these patients experience disease relapse, most can be salvaged with additional therapy. Therefore, neither adjuvant chemotherapy nor radiation therapy appears to be necessary for the initial management of most patients with low-risk disease.

On the basis of these data, a COG study (P9641), was conducted from 1998–2006 to evaluate primary surgical therapy for biologically defined low-risk neuroblastoma. The overall strategy of this study was to treat patients with low-risk neuroblastoma with resection and supportive care only. Adjuvant therapy was given only when less than 50% of the tumor was resected or when symptoms that were life- or organ-threatening developed. A probability of 3-year survival more than 95% was predicted for these patients with low-risk disease. The results from this study were published recently and showed excellent survival rates in asymptomatic, low-risk patients with stage 2A/B neuroblastoma after operation alone and that the immediate use of chemotherapy could be restricted to a minority of patients with symptomatic low-risk disease.[99] Patients with stage 2B disease who were older or had diploid or unfavorable histology tumors fared worse.

Intermediate-Risk Disease

COG study (A3961) was conducted from 1998–2006 to further refine therapy for patients with intermediate-risk disease. The overriding aim of this study was to maintain or improve survival while minimizing both acute and long-term morbidity in patients with intermediate-risk neuroblastoma. Patients received four of the most active agents against neuroblastoma: cyclophosphamide, doxorubicin, carboplatin, and etoposide, given for either four cycles (favorable biology) or eight cycles (unfavorable biology); cycles were given every 3 weeks. Radiation therapy was not used unless there was progressive disease or an unresectable primary tumor with unfavorable prognostic features at the end of chemotherapy. The outcome after reduced chemotherapy for intermediate-risk neuroblastoma was published recently.[100] The 3-year overall survival for the entire group was 96%. Survival was 98% for those with favorable biologic features and 93% for those with unfavorable features.

The most recent COG protocol (ANBL0531) sought to further refine the minimal therapy needed to achieve these excellent outcomes for patients with intermediate-risk neuroblastoma. The results have not yet been published. As such, many patients, as defined by favorable clinical and biologic factors, received a further reduction in therapy. However, those patients in whom there was loss of heterozygosity (LOH, i.e., loss of one of two normally paired chromosomal regions) at chromosome 1p or 11q (unbalanced) were not eligible for this dose reduction, as these findings have been shown to be independently associated with decreased progression-free survival in patients with low- and intermediate-risk disease.[37] Patients received cycles of cyclophosphamide, doxorubicin, carboplatin, and etoposide every three weeks. The duration of therapy (i.e., the number of cycles) depended upon which of three intermediate-risk groups a patient was enrolled. Group stratification again was based on clinical and biologic risk factors.

The overall surgical goal in intermediate-risk patients is to perform the most complete tumor resection possible, consistent with preservation of full organ and neurologic function. This may necessitate leaving residual disease adherent to critical structures. If a primary tumor is judged by the surgeon to be unresectable, a diagnostic biopsy is generally obtained and chemotherapy initiated. Delayed operation is performed after the prescribed number of cycles, as dictated by the group assignment. A reduction in surgical therapy is being considered for infants with 4S disease as it is no longer required that they undergo resection of their primary tumor. In addition, if they are too unstable at presentation, it is no longer required that they undergo an initial biopsy.

Radiation is administered only to symptomatic intermediate-risk patients when there is a risk of organ impairment due to tumor bulk not responding to initial chemotherapy. Although rare, this will most often be encountered in infants with 4S disease and patients with epidural disease and symptoms of spinal cord compression.

Patients >12 years of age with localized tumors have an indolent clinical course, but ultimately have an unfavorable outcome, and are being considered for more intensive therapy.[101,102]

High-risk Disease

For patients with advanced neuroblastoma, chemotherapy has been the mainstay of multimodality treatment. Neuroblastoma is generally a chemotherapy-sensitive tumor, and multiagent chemotherapy is usually effective in achieving at least a partial response in older children with disseminated disease. However, this approach rarely is curative. The vast majority of these patients ultimately succumb to chemotherapy-resistant disease, despite the use of increasingly intensive chemotherapy.

The general approach to treating patients with high-risk neuroblastoma has included intensive induction chemotherapy, myeloablative consolidation therapy with stem cell rescue, and targeted therapy for minimal residual disease. Stem cell harvest is typically performed after the first two cycles of induction therapy, and resection of the primary tumor and bulky metastatic sites is attempted after the fifth cycle (Fig. 66-7). The CCG-3891 protocol enrolled patients with high-risk neuroblastoma between 1991 and 1996 and was designed to assess whether myeloablative therapy, in conjunction with autologous BMT, improved EFS when compared with chemotherapy alone, and whether subsequent treatment with 13-*cis*-retinoic acid would further improve EFS.[103] The results from this double-randomization study demonstrated that the three-year EFS was significantly better in patients who underwent BMT during the first randomization (34%) than in those who did not (22%; $p = 0.034$). In the second randomization, those who received 13-*cis*-retinoic acid after BMT experienced a significantly better three-year EFS (46%) than those who did not receive the retinoid (29%, $p = 0.027$). Unfortunately, the long-term survival advantage for these patients is becoming less apparent. Nevertheless, autologous stem cell transplantation and 13-*cis*-retinoic acid are now part of most current high-risk neuroblastoma protocols.

The recently concluded COG high-risk neuroblastoma protocol (ANB0532) had as its primary goal to test whether further intensification of myeloablative therapy would improve the cure rate. Randomization to either one myeloablative consolidation with a carboplatin/etoposide/melphalan preparative regimen or two myeloablative consolidations, in which the initial regimen included thiotepa and cyclophosphamide, occurred at the completion of induction chemotherapy. Another aim of this study was to determine whether additional radiation therapy delivered to gross residual disease improved local control. Four to 6 weeks after stem cell transplantation, radiation therapy was administered to the region of the primary tumor site, including involved adjacent lymph

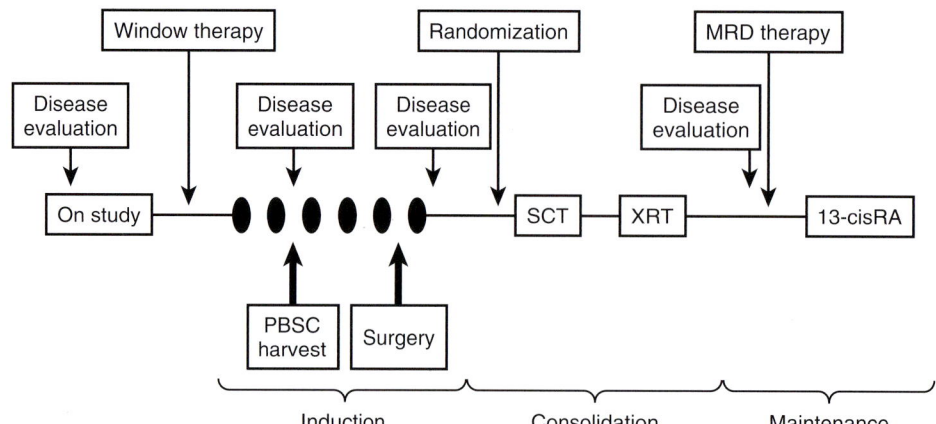

FIGURE 66-7 ■ General schema of multimodal therapy for treating children with high-risk neuroblastoma. Variations include the testing of new drugs or combinations during 'window therapy,' the use of different 'induction' regimens, randomizing patients to receive different consolidation therapy, and testing different approaches for treating minimal residual disease. Patients generally undergo PBSC harvest after two cycles of induction therapy and undergo delayed resection of the primary tumor (and locoregional disease) after five cycles of induction therapy. SCT, stem cell transplant; XRT, radiation therapy; MRD, minimal residual disease; RA, retinoic acid; PBSC, peripheral blood stem cell.

nodes. The target volume was the area of residual disease, which was determined radiographically, after induction chemotherapy but prior to delayed surgical resection, with an additional 1.5 cm margin added, even if a complete resection was ultimately achieved. Sites of persistent active metastatic disease prior to stem cell transplantation were irradiated at the same time and with the same dose as the primary site. Those patients whose primary site achieved a complete response at the end of induction therapy received 21.6 Gy to the site of primary locoregional disease while areas with gross residual disease were treated with an additional boost of 14.4 Gy (36 Gy total).

The third primary aim of ANB0532 was to test the use of a dose-intensive topotecan-containing induction regimen, substituting two cycles of dose-intensive cyclophosphamide and topotecan for the first two cycles of induction used on A3973. Secondary surgical objectives embedded in this protocol included: (1) To determine if resection completeness is predictive of local control rate or EFS. (2) To prospectively describe the complications related to efforts at local control. (3) To describe the neurologic outcomes in patients with paraspinal primary tumors.

Recurrent High-Risk Neuroblastoma

Patients with recurrent high-risk neuroblastoma have a uniformly dismal outcome. Several phase I and II trials are currently open and are testing new treatment strategies for these patients. However, although a few patients with relatively limited initial disease can be cured with salvage therapies at the time of relapse, for most stage 4 patients, disease recurrence portends a dismal outlook (<5% survival). Radiation therapy can be used for the treatment of refractory sites of metastatic disease and for palliation of painful sites of metastatic disease, with some success in providing pain relief and disease control.[104]

SURGERY FOR NEUROBLASTOMA

Complete resection of a tumor offers definitive therapy with a generally excellent outcome for most patients with localized neuroblastomas. However, the benefit of complete tumor removal may be overestimated because of the possibility that localized neuroblastomas may undergo spontaneous maturation or even regression. The role of surgery is even less clear in the curative treatment of patients with high-risk neuroblastomas.[105] Unfortunately, more than half of patients with neuroblastoma present with advanced local or metastatic disease, which requires intensive multimodal therapy in addition to surgery. It is crucial that surgeons consider the heterogeneous nature of neuroblastoma, and the molecular and biologic characteristics associated with good or bad prognoses when determining the role of surgery for any specific case.

Localized Tumors

Most localized neuroblastomas have favorable biologic features and are successfully treated with excision alone.[97,106–109] In addition, studies suggest that a subset of localized tumors will spontaneously regress, and that these patients can be observed without any treatment.[110–113] Local recurrences, while they rarely occur, can generally be managed surgically.[114] Thus, complete resection of a localized neuroblastoma may be the only therapy required for some patients.[115] Regardless of the presence of microscopic or even gross residual disease with positive ipsilateral lymph nodes, no further therapy is given to patients with low-risk disease. Therefore, all patients with INSS stage 1 tumors, stage 2A/2B tumors without *MYCN* amplification (and >50% resection), or stage 3 tumors of the midline that undergo gross total resection with negative lymph node are treated with resection alone.

In most instances, performing a biopsy before resection is unnecessary in patients with localized tumors that are likely to be neuroblastoma, appear to be easily resectable, and have had a negative metastatic workup, especially for those whose primary site is thoracic since patients with low-risk disease will not receive adjuvant therapy. Even for patients with intermediate- or high-risk disease who will receive adjuvant chemotherapy, earlier removal of bulky disease may be feasible and potentially decrease the likelihood of developing drug-resistant tumor clones.[116] However, primary resection in these patients should be done only if it can clearly be accomplished safely, without injury to adjacent organs or blood vessels and without delaying the initiation of chemotherapy. In all cases, if there is any question of resectability, pre-resection risk determination should be performed, as this may influence the operative plan. Assessment of the *MYCN* status can be performed on a minimal amount of tumor tissue, including tumor cells in the bone marrow. *MYC*-amplified tumors, unless stage 1, are all high risk. To determine the histopathologic status, COG currently requires 1 cm³ of tissue. Therefore, an open or laparoscopic biopsy is recommended, as opposed to a percutaneous core biopsy, which generally provides smaller samples.

Locoregional Disease in Patients with Metastatic Disease

More than 80% of patients who are older than 1 year of age and have metastatic neuroblastoma will have tumor in the bone marrow.[117] The presence of disseminated neuroblastoma is often suggested by a patient's ill appearance, anemia, 'raccoon eyes,' bone pain, or a limp, and can be confirmed by finding neuroblasts in the bone marrow. Therefore, most of these patients can have the diagnosis of neuroblastoma confirmed by bone marrow aspirate/biopsy and the demonstration of elevated catecholamines in the urine. A biopsy of the tumor is only required if there is no involvement of the bone marrow, if the histopathology of the tumor is important in determining the risk classification, or to obtain sufficient tissue to support biologic studies. Most patients with disseminated disease should receive neoadjuvant chemotherapy prior to attempted resection of the primary tumor and locoregional lymphadenopathy.

Delayed Surgical Resection of Locoregional Disease

The role of surgery in the management of children with high-risk neuroblastoma is controversial. Several reports have suggested that patients with INSS stage 3 or 4 disease who undergo gross total resection of their primary tumor and locoregional disease experience improved local tumor control and increased overall survival.[118–120] However, other reports have not confirmed these observations.[121–123] LaQuaglia et al. reported that the outcome for patients with stage 4 disease who were older than 1 year at the time of diagnosis was improved with gross total resection of the primary tumor, though the influence of resection was not independent of chemotherapy intensity.[124] A more recent paper from the same group provided further data suggesting that local control and overall survival are correlated with gross total resection of the primary tumor in high-risk neuroblastoma.[120] Similarly, Haase et al.[125] supported the use of aggressive resection for patients with metastatic disease in an attempt to improve outcome, and Grosfeld et al.[126] found improved survival in patients with metastatic disease who underwent complete resection of the primary tumor during delayed second-look procedures. Finally, a large meta-analysis of the outcomes for patients with stage 3 and 4 disease, and a review of the impact of the extent of primary site resection on EFS, overall survival, and local recurrence in high-risk neuroblastoma for patients treated on A3973 suggested that ≥90% resection is associated with a significant decrease in local recurrence, with a slight but sustained improvement in both EFS and overall survival, although this was not statistically significant.[127,128]

In contrast, several studies have found that the extent of resection does not affect the final outcome.[122,129] One study found that the extent of surgical resection affected only certain subgroups of patients with high-risk disease.[121] In addition, substantial complication rates have been reported after aggressive attempts at removing all gross tumor from the retroperitoneum.[130] Another study noted that the outcome for patients with stage 4 neuroblastoma depended more on the biologic characteristics of the tumor than on the extent of surgical resection.[131] This conclusion is further highlighted by the results of the CCG 3881 study which showed that, at least in infants with stage 4 disease and single-copy *MYCN* tumors, survival was excellent, regardless of whether gross total resection (3-year EFS, 91%) or incomplete resection (3-year EFS, 94%) was performed.[132] However, survival was poor if the tumor was *MYCN* amplified regardless of the extent of resection; 3-year EFS after total resection was 14%, and 3-year EFS after incomplete resection was 10% ($p = 0.18$). Although the role of cytoreduction is unclear, resection of as much gross tumor as possible in patients who receive autologous or allogeneic BMT in combination with high-dose chemotherapy and total-body irradiation (TBI) may be of some benefit.[133]

Despite the uncertainty about the role of surgery, the COG recommends attempting gross total resection of the primary tumor and locoregional disease in patients with high-risk neuroblastoma. Most children undergo delayed operation after the completion of the fifth cycle of induction chemotherapy, even though reduction in tumor volume plateaus after the second or third cycle of chemotherapy.[134] Other groups are performing surgery as soon as locoregional disease appears to be resectable on imaging studies.[135] Although initial resection is often not appropriate for patients with neuroblastoma, the principle of resection at the earliest feasible time should be considered. Because no prospective, randomized studies have been performed, the influence of the extent of operative resection is unknown. However, in considering aggressive resection, the risks involved, including vascular injury and significant bleeding, kidney or bowel infarction, infection, delay in chemotherapy, and long-term complications such as renal atrophy and diarrhea, need to be weighed carefully against the uncertain benefits of extensive surgery. Certainly removal of kidneys or other organs is to be avoided as this may hinder or delay the ability to give potentially effective chemotherapy.

The age of the patient and the tumor biology are of critical importance when planning resection. For example, survival of infants with stage 4, single-copy *MYCN* disease is greater than 93%, regardless of the extent of surgical resection of locoregional disease.[132] This favorable outcome for patients with stage 4, single-copy *MYCN* disease probably includes patients up to 18 months of age if the tumor's Shimada histology is also favorable. Clearly, the excellent prognosis for these patients should not be jeopardized by overly aggressive surgery. The extent of surgery also did not appear to significantly affect the survival of infants with *MYCN*-amplified tumors in this nonrandomized trial as survival was very poor (<15%). Perhaps infants with stage 4 disease and *MYCN*-amplified tumors would benefit from more aggressive attempts at complete resection, despite the attendant risks, given that current adjuvant therapy is unlikely to cure them.

Surgery for Recurrent Disease

Surgery may have a limited role in the management of patients with relapsed neuroblastoma where the recurrence has been documented to be localized and refractory to available chemotherapeutic agents.

Operative Principles

More than half of neuroblastomas arise in the abdominal cavity. Tumor size, the extent of vascular encasement, and exact tumor location should be considered in selecting the approach for a retroperitoneal neuroblastoma. Options available for the abdominal incision include a transverse incision, bilateral subcostal (Chevron) incisions, or a midline incision. A transthoracic (intercostal), transdiaphragmatic extension can be added to either incision if needed. The tumor and adjacent lymphadenopathy should be carefully exposed to determine the relation between the tumor and normal organs and vessels. If encasement of major vessels such as the aorta, vena cava, or their branches is found, tumor dissection must be performed to free the vessels completely. Use of the Cavitron (Cavitron Corporation, Stamford, CT, USA) ultrasonic aspirator in selected patients may allow for better tumor dissection from the major vessels, with less blood loss and fewer complications.[136] Use of the argon beam coagulator and lasers also helps to achieve complete or near-complete resection, and reduces operative complications.[125,136]

A detailed description of extensive surgical resection is available.[122] Briefly, the major points include: (1) approach the operation as a vascular-type operation in which identification and skeletonization of the major intra-abdominal vessels is critical. If encasement of major vessels such as the aorta, vena cava, or their branches is found, tumor dissection must be performed to free the vessels completely. Generally tumor can be separated from the vessel by dissecting in a subadventitial plane. (2) The tumor should be removed piecemeal. In particular, undue torque on the renal artery in an effort to clear tumor from behind the renal hilum in one piece may result in injury to the intima of the artery with vessel spasm and/or thrombosis, leading to renal ischemia. (3) Dissection commences distal to the lower edge of the tumor, generally along the common or external iliac artery, and proceeds proximally to encounter the tumor along the aorta identifying the major arterial branches (and left renal vein). With deliberate dissection of the tumor from the mesenteric and renal vessels, injury to the liver, bowel, spleen and kidneys can be avoided (Fig. 66-8) although this frequently results in piecemeal division and excision of the tumor. (4) Right-sided tumors are managed similarly and are generally less complicated unless intimately involved with the structures of the porta hepatis.

Pelvic tumors may involve the sacral plexus in addition to the iliac vessels. Thoracic tumors are usually more easily cleared from the vascular structures, but often extend into the intervertebral foramina. Extraction of tumor from this location is of uncertain benefit and can be associated with significant complications. A standard posterolateral thoracotomy can be used to expose tumors of the posterior mediastinum, and cervical incisions can be used to approach tumors of the neck. A laparoscopic or thoracoscopic approach may be used for resection of selected neuroblastomas in the abdomen and thorax.[137,138]

Operative Complications

Due to the extensive surgery often required, intraoperative and postoperative complications are not uncommon.[139–142] As many as 80% of patients will experience significant blood loss that requires transfusion either in the operating room or in the early postoperative period. Up to 10% will suffer an injury to a major vascular structure (aorta, vena cava, or renal vessels). Injury to other viscera (stomach, bowel, liver, spleen, or kidney) occurs in approximately 5% of cases. On occasion, this necessitates removal of the injured organ, with the kidney being the most common. Postoperative complications are variable. Wound complications occur is 1–5%, as does postoperative bowel obstruction. In addition, hypertension, chyle leak into the thorax or abdomen, pleural effusion, infection and sepsis, diarrhea, and the need for prolonged total parenteral nutrition have been known to occur. Rarely, a patient will have to be emergently re-explored for postoperative hemorrhage or bowel obstruction.

SPECIAL MANAGEMENT SITUATIONS

Screening for Neuroblastoma

Because the two most important clinical variables for predicting outcome in patients with neuroblastoma are tumor stage and patient age at the time of diagnosis, it was hypothesized that earlier detection of neuroblastoma through mass population screening might significantly impact neuroblastoma-associated mortality. In the 1980s in Japan, mass screening of neuroblastoma was performed in infants by quantitating urinary vanillyl mandelic acid (VMA) and homovanillic acid (HVA). Initially, this mass screening showed very encouraging results.[143] However, subsequent population-based studies with concurrent control groups performed in Germany and North America found that although the incidence of

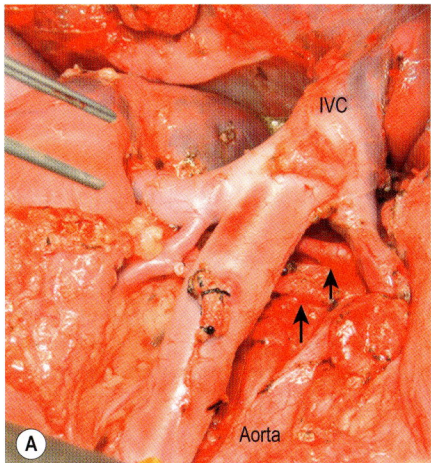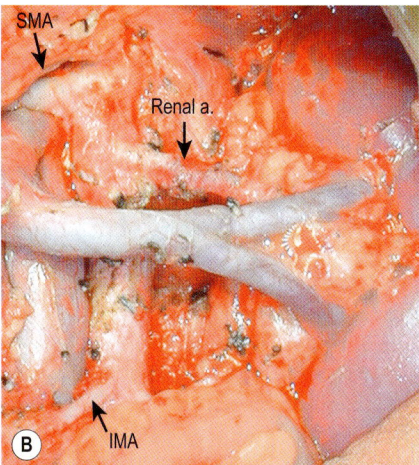

FIGURE 66-8 ■ Intraoperative photographs after resection of retroperitoneal neuroblastomas. **(A)** Right-sided dissection: note the presence of two right renal arteries coming from the aorta (arrows). **(B)** Left-sided dissection: seen are the skeletonized aorta, mesenteric arteries, and left renal artery and vein. IVC, inferior vena cava; SMA, superior mesenteric artery; IMA, inferior mesenteric artery.

neuroblastoma increased, the additional cases were largely early stage, favorable biology, low-risk tumors.[144,145] Because the overall mortality of patients with neuroblastoma was not affected, mass screening most likely detected tumors that would have undergone spontaneous regression and not been detected clinically. Thus, there currently appears to be no role for screening infants for neuroblastoma.

Small, localized neuroblastomas in young infants tend to regress spontaneously. Based on this observation, the COG protocol, ANBLOOP2, included an arm of expectant observation for patients with these lesions to further define their natural history. This study was designed to prove the hypothesis that close biochemical and sonographic observation could be safely applied in infants with small adrenal masses. Resection was reserved for those rare cases in which there was evidence of continued growth. To be eligible, infants with an adrenal mass had to be <6 months of age when the mass was first identified; the mass must be <16 mL in volume, if solid, or <65 mL if at least 25% cystic; and disease must be limited to the adrenal gland. The results from this study were published recently and confirmed that expectant observation of infants with small adrenal masses led to excellent three-year EFS (97.7 ± 2.3%) and 100% overall survival while avoiding operative intervention in >80% of patients.[146]

Stage 4S Neuroblastoma

In 1971, D'Angio, Evans, and Koop reported a number of patients with a 'special' variant of metastatic neuroblastoma, termed IVS (now referred to as 4S).[147] These patients were infants who typically had a single, small primary tumor, but had extensive metastatic disease in the liver, skin nodules ('blueberry muffin' lesions), and small amounts of disease in the bone marrow (<10% of the mononuclear cells). Patients with 4S neuroblastoma were quite remarkable because the large amount of disease generally underwent spontaneous regression, even without treatment, and the infants ultimately had no evidence of disease.

Only supportive therapy has been recommended for this stage of neuroblastoma because of the high incidence of spontaneous regression and the good prognosis.[148] Most of these patients have a tumor with favorable biology (single-copy MYCN, favorable Shimada histology, and DNA index >1). Therefore, they are assigned to the low-risk classification and receive no therapy. However, despite the generally benign course of their malignancy, these infants can die of complications caused by the initial bulk of their disease. Limited chemotherapy, local irradiation, or minimal resection can be used to treat infants with life-threatening symptoms of hepatomegaly. Creation of a Silastic pouch may be needed for those with significant hepatomegaly that causes either respiratory compromise secondary to diaphragmatic elevation or obstruction of the inferior vena cava. This procedure may help to avoid life-threatening events until shrinkage of the liver is achieved by either spontaneous regression or therapy. The rare infant with 4S disease and either unfavorable Shimada histology or a DNA index of 1 (or if the biology is not known) will be treated as intermediate-risk disease. Those with 4S disease that is MYCN amplified will be treated as high-risk disease.

Intraspinal Extension of Neuroblastoma

In a subset of patients with paraspinal neuroblastoma, tumor growth may extend into the spinal canal ('dumbbell' tumors). If neurologic symptoms result, urgent treatment is required to prevent permanent injury caused by compression of the cord. Each of the three main therapeutic modalities (surgery, radiation, and chemotherapy) has been used. A POG report showed similar rates of neurologic recovery in patients treated with surgery or chemotherapy, but significant orthopedic sequelae were seen more commonly in patients undergoing operation.[149] Although chemotherapy is probably considered most appropriate for the initial management of these patients, improvements in neurosurgical techniques, including the use of laminotomy instead of laminectomy to access the intraspinal tumor, may allow reconsideration about the optimal approach, especially in patients with acutely progressive symptoms.

The appropriate approach for patients with asymptomatic intraspinal tumor extension is also uncertain. For patients with low- or intermediate-risk disease, the risks of attempting to remove the intraspinal component of a paraspinal tumor probably outweigh the benefits. This situation most commonly arises in patients with thoracic primary tumors. The intrathoracic component is resected, and gross residual disease remains in the spinal canal. Care should be taken to minimize operative complications such as leakage of cerebrospinal fluid or uncontrollable intraspinal bleeding. As residual foraminal disease rarely grows to a symptom-developing size, the importance of conservative therapy in this circumstance should be emphasized. In the absence of metastatic disease or unfavorable tumor biology, these patients will be classified as stage 2A/B, low risk, and have a very favorable prognosis with no further therapy. For patients with high-risk disease, the importance of resecting gross intraspinal disease is uncertain.

Opsoclonus–Myoclonus Syndrome

The opsoclonus–myoclonus syndrome (OMS) consists of myoclonic jerks and random eye movements or progressive cerebellar ataxia. OMS occurs in as many as 4% of patients, usually infants with thoracic primary tumors. Although the exact etiology of this syndrome is not known, the presence of cross-reactive autoantibodies to neural antigens in some of these patients suggests that it is it mediated by the immune system.[150] Although patients generally have a good prognosis with regard to their tumor, neurologic symptoms often persist after successful removal of the tumor and can be debilitating.[68,69] Some symptomatic relief can be attained by high doses of corticosteroids or adrenocorticotropic hormones. Studies have suggested that chemotherapy or intravenous IgG therapy (or both) may improve the long-term neurologic outcome for these patients.[151,152] COG is currently testing this approach in a prospective clinical trial.

NEW TREATMENT STRATEGIES

Differentiating Agents

Retinoids are vitamin A derivatives of 13-*cis*-retinoic acid. Retinoids decrease the proliferation and expression of *MYCN* of neuroblastoma cell lines in vitro and induce morphologic differentiation.[153-156] Due to these attractive characteristics and the observation that resistance to chemotherapy does not result in resistance to 13-*cis*-retinoic acid, retinoids have been tested clinically. The CCG 3891 clinical trial randomized patients with high-risk neuroblastoma treated using chemotherapy or autologous BMT into two groups that received either 13-*cis*-retinoic acid for 6 months or no further therapy.[103] The 3-year EFS of patients who received 13-*cis*-retinoic acid (46%) was significantly higher than that of patients who received no further therapy (29%; $p = 0.027$) and was independent of the initial randomization to either chemotherapy or autologous BMT. Thus, currently, all patients with high-risk neuroblastoma receive oral 13-*cis*-retinoic acid twice daily for 2 weeks and are then off therapy for 2 weeks. This treatment is continued for six cycles (6 months total). Some intermediate-risk patients also receive 13-*cis*-retinoic acid.

Immunotherapy

Neuroblastoma cells are sensitive to antibody-dependent cell-mediated cytotoxicity and complement-dependent cytotoxicity.[157] Immunotherapy using anti-ganglioside antibodies targeting G_{D2}, the predominant antigen in neuroblastoma cells, appears to be a promising approach for the treatment of advanced neuroblastoma. As the induction of antibody-dependent cell-mediated cytotoxicity with anti-ganglioside G_{D2} antibodies is enhanced by cytokines such as GM-CSF[158] and IL-2,[159] a phase III trial was conducted to determine whether treatment with ch14.18 and cytokines (GM-CSF and IL-2) together with 13-*cis*-retinoic acid improves EFS and overall survival after autologous BMT, as compared to treatment with 13-*cis*-retinoic acid alone in patients with high-risk neuroblastoma. The study was stopped early because immunotherapy was superior to standard therapy (2-year EFS: 66% vs 46%, $p = 0.01$ and 2-year OS: 86% vs 75%, $p = 0.02$).[160] Current trials are investigating the safety and efficacy of a ch14.18-Il-2 fusion protein, given with GM-CSF and isotretinoin.

MIBG Therapy

Refractory neuroblastoma has been treated with ^{131}I-MIBG because it is readily taken-up by the tumor cells.[161] In an investigation of patients with advanced chemoresistant neuroblastomas, response rates approached 33%.[162] Studies further suggest that this treatment can be used as front-line therapy, followed by chemotherapy, without significant hematologic toxicity.[163] ^{125}I-MIBG may be an even better treatment option for neuroblastomas with micrometastases or bone marrow infiltration, and is being tested for the treatment of patients with 'ultra high-risk' neuroblastoma (expected survival of less than 15%).[164]

Targeted Therapy

As more information regarding diagnostically and prognostically useful genetic markers of neuroblastoma become available, therapeutic strategies will change accordingly. In addition, molecular profiling will lead to new drug development designed to induce differentiation of tumor cells, block dysregulated growth pathways, or reactivate silenced apoptotic pathways. One of the most exciting prospects for improving the therapeutic index, as well as overcoming the problem of tumor resistance to therapy, involves targeted therapy.

ALK Inhibition

Constitutive activation of the ALK receptor tyrosine kinase by mutation or translocation appears to contribute to the malignant phenotype of neuroblastoma. The orally bioavailable small molecule inhibitor of *ALK*, PF-02341066, is currently being tested in a COG phase I/II trial of relapsed/refractory solid tumors.

TRK Inhibition

As previously described, neurotrophins and their tyrosine kinase receptors are important in the development of the sympathetic nervous system and have been implicated in the pathogenesis of neuroblastoma. Studies are ongoing to test agonists of TrkA in an attempt to induce cellular differentiation. Conversely, blocking the BDNF/TrkB signaling pathway with Trk-specific tyrosine kinase inhibitors, such as CEP-751, may induce apoptosis by blocking crucial survival pathways.[49,165-167]

Epigenetic Targeting

The hallmark of cancer is dysregulated gene expression. However, not only do genetic factors influence gene expression but epigenetic factors do as well. Epigenetic alterations are defined as those heritable changes in gene expression that do not result from direct changes in DNA sequence. Mechanisms of epigenetic regulation most commonly include DNA methylation and modification of histones.

Genome-wide DNA methylation analysis of neuroblastic tumors revealed that hypermethylation events are extensive and contribute to the clinicopathologic features of these tumors.[168] Promoter methylation resulting in silencing of caspase 8, a protein involved in apoptosis, for example, likely contributes to the pathogenesis of *MYCN*-amplified neuroblastoma.[169]

Histones are the proteins that give structure to DNA. Both histones and DNA form the major components of chromatin. Alterations in histones can mediate changes in chromatin structure. The compacted form of DNA, termed heterochromatin, is largely inaccessible to transcription factors and, therefore, genes in the affected regions are silent. Other modifications of histones can cause DNA to take a more open or extended configuration (euchromatin), allowing for gene transcription. Histones can be modified by a number of different processes including methylation and acetylation, mediated by histone acetyl transferases and deacetylases, and histone methyltransferases. Each of these processes alters histone function, which, in turn alters the structure of chromatin and, therefore, the accessibility of DNA to transcription factors. Inhibiting the histone-mediated epigenetic processes that silence tumor suppressors in neuroblastoma is currently being tested in clinical trials.

Future Approaches

As more information regarding diagnostically and prognostically useful genetic markers for neuroblastoma become available, therapeutic strategies will change and ultimately lead to individualized treatment regimens based on the molecular biologic profile of a patient's tumor.

REFERENCES

1. Brodeur GM, Castleberry RP. Neuroblastoma. In: Pizzo PA, Poplack DG, editors. In Principles and Practice of Pediatric Oncology. Philadelphia: J. B. Lippincott; 1993.
2. Young JL Jr, Ries LG, Silverberg E, et al. Cancer incidence, survival, and mortality for children younger than age 15 years. Cancer 1986;58:598–602.
3. Brodeur GM, Nakagawara A. Molecular basis of clinical heterogeneity in neuroblastoma. Am J Pediatr Hematol Oncol 1992;14:111–16.
4. Maris JM, Tonini GP. Genetics of familial neuroblastoma. In: Brodeur GM, Sawada T, Tsudhica T, et al, editors. Neuroblastoma. 1st ed. Amsterdam: Elsevier Science; 2000. p. 125–35.
5. Mosse YP, Laudenslager M, Longo L, et al. Identification of ALK as a major familial neuroblastoma predisposition gene. Nature 2008;455:930–5.
6. Virchow R. Hyperplasie der Zirbel und der Nebenniern. In: Die Krankhaften Geschwulste, Vol 2 August Hirshwald. Berlin: 1865. p. 149–50.
7. Wright JH. Neurocytoma or neuroblastoma, a kind of tumor not generally recognized. J Exp Med 1910;12:556–61.
8. Ambros IM, Zellner A, Roald B, et al. Role of ploidy, chromosome 1p, and Schwann cells in the maturation of neuroblastoma. N Engl J Med 1996;334:1505–11.
9. Ambros IM, Zellner A, Stock C, et al. Proof of the reactive nature of the Schwann cell in neuroblastoma and its clinical implications. Prog Clin Biol Res 1994;385:331–7.
10. Crawford SE, Stellmach V, Ranalli M, et al. Pigment epithelium-derived factor (PEDF) in neuroblastoma: A multifunctional mediator of Schwann cell antitumor activity. J Cell Sci 2001;114:4421–8.
11. Chlenski A, Liu S, Crawford SE, et al. SPARC is a key Schwannian-derived inhibitor controlling neuroblastoma tumor angiogenesis. Cancer Res 2002;62:7357–63.
12. Beckwith JB, Perrin EV. In situ neuroblastoma: A contribution to the natural history of neural crest tumors. Am J Pathol 1963;43:1089.
13. Shimada H, Chatten J, Newton WA Jr, et al. Histopathologic prognostic factors in neuroblastic tumors: Definition of subtypes of ganglioneuroblastoma and an age-linked classification of neuroblastomas. J Natl Cancer Inst 1984;73:405–16.
14. Shimada H, Ambros IM, Dehner L, et al. Terminology and morphologic criteria of neuroblastic tumors: Recommendations by the International Neuroblastoma Pathology Committee. Cancer 1999;86:349–63.
15. Peuchmaur M, d'Amore ES, Joshi VV, et al. Revision of the International Neuroblastoma Pathology Classification: Confirmation of favorable and unfavorable prognostic subsets in ganglioneuroblastoma, nodular. Cancer 2003;98:2274–81.
16. Shimada H, Ambros IM, Dehner LP, et al. The International Neuroblastoma Pathology Classification (the Shimada system). Cancer 1999;86:364–72.
17. Shimada H, Umehara S, Monobe Y, et al. International neuroblastoma pathology classification for prognostic evaluation of patients with peripheral neuroblastic tumors: A report from the Children's Cancer Group. Cancer 2001;92:2451–61.
18. Sano H, Bonadio J, Gerbing RB, et al. International neuroblastoma pathology classification adds independent prognostic information beyond the prognostic contribution of age. Eur J Cancer 2006;42:1113–19.
19. De BB, Gambini C, Haupt R, et al. Retrospective study of childhood ganglioneuroma. J Clin Oncol 2008;26:1710–16.
20. Kaneko Y, Kanda N, Maseki N, et al. Different karyotypic patterns in early and advanced stage neuroblastomas. Cancer Res 1987;47:311–18.
21. Look AT, Hayes FA, Nitschke R, et al. Cellular DNA content as a predictor of response to chemotherapy in infants with unresectable neuroblastoma. N Engl J Med 1984;311:231–5.
22. Bowman LC, Castleberry RP, Cantor A, et al. Genetic staging of unresectable or metastatic neuroblastoma in infants: A Pediatric Oncology Group study. J Natl Cancer Inst 1997;89:373–80.
23. Schwab M, Alitalo K, Klempnauer KH, et al. Amplified DNA with limited homology to myc cellular oncogene is shared by human neuroblastoma cell lines and a neuroblastoma tumour. Nature 1983;305:245–8.
24. Kohl NE, Kanda N, Schreck RR, et al. Transposition and amplification of oncogene-related sequences in human neuroblastomas. Cell 1983;35:359–67.
25. Lutz W, Stohr M, Schurmann J, et al. Conditional expression of N-myc in human neuroblastoma cells increases expression of alpha-prothymosin and ornithine decarboxylase and accelerates progression into S-phase early after mitogenic stimulation of quiescent cells. Oncogene 1996;13:803–12.
26. Yancopoulos GD, Nisen PD, Tesfaye A, et al. N-myc can cooperate with ras to transform normal cells in culture. Proc Natl Acad Sci U S A 1985;82:5455–9.
27. Weiss WA, Aldape K, Mohapatra G, et al. Targeted expression of MYCN causes neuroblastoma in transgenic mice. EMBO J 1997;16:2985–95.
28. Berry T, Luther W, Bhatnagar N, et al. The ALK(F1174L) mutation potentiates the oncogenic activity of MYCN in neuroblastoma. Cancer Cell 2012;22:117–30.
29. Brodeur GM, Seeger RC, Schwab M, et al. Amplification of N-myc in untreated human neuroblastomas correlates with advanced disease stage. Science 1984;224:1121–4.
30. Brodeur GM, Hayes FA, Green AA, et al. Consistent N-myc copy number in simultaneous or consecutive neuroblastoma samples from sixty individual patients. Cancer Res 1987;47:4248–53.
31. Seeger RC, Brodeur GM, Sather H, et al. Association of multiple copies of the N-myc oncogene with rapid progression of neuroblastomas. N Engl J Med 1985;313:1111–16.
32. Brodeur GM, Sekhon G, Goldstein MN. Chromosomal aberrations in human neuroblastomas. Cancer 1977;40:2256–63.
33. Fujita T, Igarashi J, Okawa ER, et al. CHD5, a tumor suppressor gene deleted from 1p36.31 in neuroblastomas. J Natl Cancer Inst 2008;100:940–9.
34. Bader SA, Fasching C, Brodeur GM, et al. Dissociation of suppression of tumorigenicity and differentiation in vitro effected by transfer of single human chromosomes into human neuroblastoma cells. Cell Growth Differ 1991;2:245–55.
35. Fong CT, Dracopoli NC, White PS, et al. Loss of heterozygosity for the short arm of chromosome 1 in human neuroblastomas: Correlation with N-myc amplification. Proc Natl Acad Sci U S A 1989;86:3753–7.
36. Gilbert F, Feder M, Balaban G, et al. Human neuroblastomas and abnormalities of chromosomes 1 and 17. Cancer Res 1984;44:5444–9.
37. Attiyeh EF, London WB, Mosse YP, et al. Chromosome 1p and 11q deletions and outcome in neuroblastoma. N Engl J Med 2005;353:2243–53.
38. Takayama H, Suzuki T, Mugishima H, et al. Deletion mapping of chromosomes 14q and 1p in human neuroblastoma. Oncogene 1992;7:1185–9.
39. Attiyeh EF, London WB, Mosse YP, et al. Chromosome 1p and 11q deletions and outcome in neuroblastoma. N Engl J Med 2005;353:2243–53.

40. Mosse YP, Laudenslager M, Longo L, et al. Identification of ALK as a major familial neuroblastoma predisposition gene. Nature 2008;455:930–5.

41. Caren H, Abel F, Kogner P, et al. High incidence of DNA mutations and gene amplifications of the ALK gene in advanced sporadic neuroblastoma tumours. Biochem J 2008;416:153–9.

42. Carpenter EL, Mosse YP. Targeting ALK in neuroblastoma-preclinical and clinical advancements. Nat Rev Clin Oncol 2012;9:391–9.

43. Mosse YP, Laudenslager M, Khazi D, et al. Germline PHOX2B mutation in hereditary neuroblastoma. Am J Hum Genet 2004;75:727–30.

44. Cheung NK, Zhang J, Lu C, et al. Association of age at diagnosis and genetic mutations in patients with neuroblastoma. JAMA 2012;307:1062–71.

45. Barbacid M. Neurotrophic factors and their receptors. Curr Opin Cell Biol 1995;7:148–55.

46. Levi-Montalcini R. The nerve growth factor 35 years later. Science 1987;237:1154–62.

47. Nakagawara A, Arima-Nakagawara M, Scavarda NJ, et al. Association between high levels of expression of the TRK gene and favorable outcome in human neuroblastoma. N Engl J Med 1993;328:847–54.

48. Nakagawara A, Arima M, Azar CG, et al. Inverse relationship between trk expression and N-myc amplification in human neuroblastomas. Cancer Res 1992;52:1364–8.

49. Nakagawara A, Azar C, Scavarda N. Expression and function of TRK-B and BDNF in human neuroblastomas. Mol Cell Biol 1994;14:759–67.

50. Svensson T, Ryden M, Schilling FH, et al. Coexpression of mRNA for the full-length neurotrophin receptor trk-C and trk-A in favourable neuroblastoma. Eur J Cancer 1997;33:2058–63.

51. Teitz T, Wei T, Valentine MB, et al. Caspase 8 is deleted or silenced preferentially in childhood neuroblastomas with amplification of MYCN. Nat Med 2000;6:529–35.

52. Gunthert U, Hofmann M, Rudy W, et al. A new variant of glycoprotein CD44 confers metastatic potential to rat carcinoma cells. Cell 1991;65:13–24.

53. Combaret V, Gross N, Lasset C, et al. Clinical relevance of CD44 cell-surface expression and N-myc gene amplification in a multicentric analysis of 121 pediatric neuroblastomas. J Clin Oncol 1996;14:25–34.

54. Bradshaw DM, Arceci RJ. Clinical relevance of transmembrane drug efflux as a mechanism of multidrug resistance. J Clin Oncol 1998;16:3674–90.

55. Norris MD, Bordow SB, Marshall GM, et al. Expression of the gene for multidrug-resistance-associated protein and outcome in patients with neuroblastoma. N Engl J Med 1996;334:231–8.

56. Oberthuer A, Berthold F, Warnat P, et al. Customized oligonucleotide microarray gene expression-based classification of neuroblastoma patients outperforms current clinical risk stratification. J Clin Oncol 2006;24:5070–8.

57. Janoueix-Lerosey I, Schleiermacher G, Michels E, et al. Overall genomic pattern is a predictor of outcome in neuroblastoma. J Clin Oncol 2009;27:1026–33.

58. Maris JM. Recent advances in neuroblastoma. N Engl J Med 2010;362:2202–11.

59. Henderson TO, Bhatia S, Pinto N, et al. Racial and ethnic disparities in risk and survival in children with neuroblastoma: A Children's Oncology Group study. J Clin Oncol 2011;29:76–82.

60. Vandesompele J, Van Roy N, Van Gele M, et al. Genetic heterogeneity of neuroblastoma studied by comparative genomic hybridization. Genes Chromosomes. Cancer 1998;23:141–52.

61. Bown N, Cotterill S, Lastowska M, et al. Gain of chromosome arm 17q and adverse outcome in patients with neuroblastoma. N Engl J Med 1999;340:1954–61.

62. Diskin SJ, Hou C, Glessner JT, et al. Copy number variation at 1q21.1 associated with neuroblastoma. Nature 2009;459:987–91.

63. Maris JM, Mosse YP, Bradfield JP, et al. Chromosome 6p22 locus associated with clinically aggressive neuroblastoma. N Engl J Med 2008;358:2585–93.

64. Capasso M, Devoto M, Hou C, et al. Common variations in BARD1 influence susceptibility to high-risk neuroblastoma. Nat Genet 2009;41:718–23.

65. Wang K, Diskin SJ, Zhang H, et al. Integrative genomics identifies LMO1 as a neuroblastoma oncogene. Nature 2011;469:216–20.

66. Downing JR, Wilson RK, Zhang J, et al. The pediatric cancer genome project. Nat Genet 2012;44:619–22.

67. Molenaar JJ, Koster J, Zwijnenburg DA, et al. Sequencing of neuroblastoma identifies chromothripsis and defects in neuritogenesis genes. Nature 2012;483:589–93.

68. Russo C, Cohn SL, Petruzzi MJ, et al. Long-term neurologic outcome in children with opsoclonus-myoclonus associated with neuroblastoma: A report from the Pediatric Oncology Group. Med Pediatr Oncol 1997;28:284–8.

69. Rudnick E, Khakoo Y, Antunes NL, et al. Opsoclonus-myoclonus-ataxia syndrome in neuroblastoma: Clinical outcome and antineuronal antibodies-a report from the Children's Cancer Group Study. Med Pediatr Oncol 2001;36:612–22.

70. Berthold F, Kassenbohmer R, Zieschang J. Multivariate evaluation of prognostic factors in localized neuroblastoma. Am J Pediatr Hematol Oncol 1994;16:107–15.

71. Joshi VV, Cantor AB, Brodeur GM, et al. Correlation between morphologic and other prognostic markers of neuroblastoma. A study of histologic grade, DNA index, N-myc gene copy number, and lactic dehydrogenase in patients in the Pediatric Oncology Group. Cancer 1993;71:3173–81.

72. Silber JH, Evans AE, Fridman M. Models to predict outcome from childhood neuroblastoma: The role of serum ferritin and tumor histology. Cancer Res 1991;51:1426–33.

73. Berthold F, Engelhardt-Fahrner U, Schneider A, et al. Age dependence and prognostic impact of neuron specific enolase (NSE) in children with neuroblastoma. In Vivo 1991;5:245–7.

74. Tsuchida Y, Honna T, Iwanaka T, et al. Serial determination of serum neuron-specific enolase in patients with neuroblastoma and other pediatric tumors. J Pediatr Surg 1987;22:419–24.

75. Fitzgibbon MC, Tormey WP. Paediatric reference ranges for urinary catecholamines/metabolites and their relevance in neuroblastoma diagnosis. Ann Clin Biochem 1994;31(Pt 1):1–11.

76. Adams GA, Shochat SJ, Smith EI, et al. Thoracic neuroblastoma: A Pediatric Oncology Group study. J Pediatr Surg 1993;28:372–7.

77. Tanabe M, Yoshida H, Ohnuma N, et al. Imaging of neuroblastoma in patients identified by mass screening using urinary catecholamine metabolites. J Pediatr Surg 1993;28:617–21.

78. Ng YY, Kingston JE. The role of radiology in the staging of neuroblastoma. Clin Radiol 1993;47:226–35.

79. Stark DD, Moss AA, Brasch RC, et al. Neuroblastoma: Diagnostic imaging and staging. Radiology 1983;148:101–5.

80. Cheung NK, Kushner BH. Should we replace bone scintigraphy plus CT with MR imaging for staging of neuroblastoma? Radiology 2003;226:286–7.

81. Siegel MJ, Ishwaran H, Fletcher BD, et al. Staging of neuroblastoma at imaging: Report of the radiology diagnostic oncology group. Radiology 2002;223:168–75.

82. Brodeur GM, Pritchard J, Berthold F, et al. Revisions of the international criteria for neuroblastoma diagnosis, staging, and response to treatment. J Clin Oncol 1993;11:1466–77.

83. Turba E, Fagioli G, Mancini AF, et al. Evaluation of stage 4 neuroblastoma patients by means of MIBG and 99mTc-MDP scintigraphy. J Nucl Biol Med 1993;37:107–14.

84. Paltiel HJ, Gelfand MJ, Elgazzar AH, et al. Neural crest tumors: I-123 MIBG imaging in children. Radiology 1994;190:117–21.

85. Gelfand MJ. Meta-iodobenzylguanidine in children. Semin Nucl Med 1993;23:231–42.

86. Wirnsberger GH, Becker H, Ziervogel K, et al. Diagnostic immunohistochemistry of neuroblastic tumors. Am J Surg Pathol 1992;16:49–57.

87. Corbett R, Olliff J, Fairley N, et al. A prospective comparison between magnetic resonance imaging, meta-iodobenzylguanidine scintigraphy and marrow histology/cytology in neuroblastoma. Eur J Cancer 1991;27:1560–4.

88. Osmanagaoglu K, Lippens M, Benoit Y, et al. A comparison of iodine-123 meta-iodobenzylguanidine scintigraphy and single bone marrow aspiration biopsy in the diagnosis and follow-up of 26 children with neuroblastoma. Eur J Nucl Med 1993;20:1154–11560.

89. Brodeur GM, Pritchard J, Berthold F, et al. Revisions of the international criteria for neuroblastoma diagnosis, staging, and response to treatment. J Clin Oncol 1993;11:1466–77.

90. Monclair T, Brodeur GM, Ambros PF, et al. The International Neuroblastoma Risk Group (INRG) staging system: An INRG Task Force report. J Clin Oncol 2009;27:298–303.

91. Cecchetto G, Mosseri V, De Bernardi B, et al. Surgical risk factors in primary surgery for localized neuroblastoma: The LNESG1 study of the European International Society of Pediatric Oncology Neuroblastoma Group. J Clin Oncol 2005;23:8483–9.

92. Moroz V, Machin D, Faldum A, et al. Changes over three decades in outcome and the prognostic influence of age-at-diagnosis in young patients with neuroblastoma: A report from the International Neuroblastoma Risk Group Project. Eur J Cancer 2011; 47:561–71.

93. London WB, Castleberry RP, Matthay KK, et al. Evidence for an age cutoff greater than 365 days for neuroblastoma risk group stratification in the Children's Oncology Group. J Clin Oncol 2005;23:6459–65.

94. Evans AE, D'Angio GJ, Propert K, et al. Prognostic factor in neuroblastoma. Cancer 1987;59:1853–9.

95. Cohn SL, Pearson AD, London WB, et al. The International Neuroblastoma Risk Group (INRG) classification system: An INRG Task Force report. J Clin Oncol 2009;27:289–97.

96. Alvarado CS, London WB, Look AT, et al. Natural history and biology of stage A neuroblastoma: A Pediatric Oncology Group Study. J Pediatr Hematol Oncol 2000;22:197–205.

97. Nitschke R, Smith EI, Shochat S, et al. Localized neuroblastoma treated by surgery: A Pediatric Oncology Group Study. J Clin Oncol 1988;6:1271–9.

98. Matthay KK, Lukens J, Haase GM, et al. Outcome and prognostic factors for 1008 children with neuroblastoma treated from 1989-1995 on Children's Cancer Group (CCG) protocols. Advances in Neuroblastoma Research. Philadelphia: 1996.

99. Strother DR, London WB, Schmidt ML, et al. Outcome after surgery alone or with restricted use of chemotherapy for patients with low-risk neuroblastoma: results of Children's Oncology Group study P9641. J Clin Oncol 2012;30:1842–8.

100. Baker DL, Schmidt ML, Cohn SL, et al. Outcome after reduced chemotherapy for intermediate-risk neuroblastoma. N Engl J Med 2010;363:1313–23.

101. Gaspar N, Hartmann O, Munzer C, et al. Neuroblastoma in adolescents. Cancer 2003;98:349–55.

102. Franks LM, Bollen A, Seeger RC, et al. Neuroblastoma in adults and adolescents: An indolent course with poor survival. Cancer 1997;79:2028–35.

103. Matthay KK, Villablanca JG, Seeger RC, et al. Treatment of high-risk neuroblastoma with intensive chemotherapy, radiotherapy, autologous bone marrow transplantation, and 13-cis-retinoic acid. Children's Cancer Group. N Engl J Med 1999;341:1165–73.

104. Paulino AC. Palliative radiotherapy in children with neuroblastoma. Pediatr Hematol Oncol 2003;20:111–17.

105. Ziegler MM. Pediatric surgical oncology. Curr Opin Pediatr 1990;2:580.

106. Perez CA, Matthay KK, Atkinson JB, et al. Biologic variables in the outcome of stages I and II neuroblastoma treated with surgery as primary therapy: A children's cancer group study. J Clin Oncol 2000;18:18–26.

107. Kushner BH, Cheung NK, LaQuaglia MP, et al. International neuroblastoma staging system stage 1 neuroblastoma: A prospective study and literature review. J Clin Oncol 1996;14:2174–80.

108. Evans AE, Silber JH, Shpilsky A, et al. Successful management of low-stage neuroblastoma without adjuvant therapies: A comparison of two decades, 1972 through 1981 and 1982 through 1992, in a single institution. J Clin Oncol 1996;14:2504–10.

109. Berthold F, Treuner J, Brandeis WE, et al. [Neuroblastoma study NBL 79 of the German Society for Pediatric Oncology. Report after 2 years]. Klin Padiatr 1982;194:262–9.

110. Yamamoto K, Hanada R, Kikuchi A, et al. Spontaneous regression of localized neuroblastoma detected by mass screening. J Clin Oncol 1998;16:1265–9.

111. Suita S, Zaizen Y, Sera Y, et al. Mass screening for neuroblastoma: quo vadis? A 9-year experience from the Pediatric Oncology Study Group of the Kyushu area in Japan. J Pediatr Surg 1996;31:555–8.

112. Nishihira H, Toyoda Y, Tanaka Y, et al. Natural course of neuroblastoma detected by mass screening: A 5-year prospective study at a single institution. J Clin Oncol 2000;18:3012–17.

113. Oue T, Inoue M, Yoneda A, et al. Profile of neuroblastoma detected by mass screening, resected after observation without treatment: Results of the Wait and See pilot study. J Pediatr Surg 2005;40:359–63.

114. Maris JM, Hogarty MD, Bagatell R, et al. Neuroblastoma. Lancet 2007;369:2106–20.

115. Nitschke R, Smith EI, Shochat S, et al. Localized neuroblastoma treated by surgery: A Pediatric Oncology Group Study. J Clin Oncol 1988;6:1271–9.

116. Davidoff AM, Corey BL, Hoffer FA, et al. Radiographic assessment of resectability of locoregional disease in children with high-risk neuroblastoma during neoadjuvant chemotherapy. Pediatr Blood Cancer 2005;44:158–62.

117. DuBois SG, Kalika Y, Lukens JN, et al. Metastatic sites in stage IV and IVS neuroblastoma correlate with age, tumor biology, and survival. J Pediatr Hematol Oncol 1999;21:181–9.

118. Haase GM, Wong KY, deLorimier AA, et al. Improvement in survival after excision of primary tumor in stage III neuroblastoma. J Pediatr Surg 1989;24:194–200.

119. Adkins ES, Sawin R, Gerbing RB, et al. Efficacy of complete resection for high-risk neuroblastoma: A Children's Cancer Group study. J Pediatr Surg 2004;39:931–6.

120. La Quaglia MP, Kushner BH, Su W, et al. The impact of gross total resection on local control and survival in high-risk neuroblastoma. J Pediatr Surg 2004;39:412–17.

121. von Schweinitz D, Hero B, Berthold F. The impact of surgical radicality on outcome in childhood neuroblastoma. Eur J Pediatr Surg 2002;12:402–9.

122. Kiely EM. The surgical challenge of neuroblastoma. J Pediatr Surg 1994;29:128–33.

123. Kuroda T, Saeki M, Honna T, et al. Clinical significance of intensive surgery with intraoperative radiation for advanced neuroblastoma: Does it really make sense? J Pediatr Surg 2003;38:1735–8.

124. La Quaglia MP, Kushner BH, Heller G, et al. Stage 4 neuroblastoma diagnosed at more than 1 year of age: Gross total resection and clinical outcome. J Pediatr Surg 1994;29:1162–5.

125. Haase G, O'Leary M, Ramsay N, et al. Aggressive surgery combined with intensive chemotherapy improves survival in poor-risk neuroblastoma. J Pediatr Surg 1991;26:1119–23.

126. Grosfeld JL, Baehner RL. Neuroblastoma: An analysis of 160 cases. World J Surgery 1980;4:29–38.

127. LaQuaglia MP, von Allmen D, Davidoff A, et al. A comprehensive review of the role of primary tumor resection in stages 3 and 4 neuroblastoma. Presented at the Advances in Neuroblastoma Research Conference, Chiba, Japan, May 2008.

128. LaQuaglia MP, Davidoff A, London W, et al. The impact of the extent of primary site resection on event-free survival, overall survival, and local recurrence in high-risk neuroblastoma. A report from the Children's Oncology Group A3973 Study. Presented at the Advances in Neuroblastoma Research Conference, Chiba, Japan, May 2008.

129. Castel V, Tovar JA, Costa E, et al. The role of surgery in stage IV neuroblastoma. J Pediatr Surg 2002;37:1574–8.

130. Azizkhan RG, Shaw A, Chandler JG. Surgical complications of neuroblastoma resection. Surgery 1985;97:514–17.

131. Shorter NA, Davidoff AM, Evans AE, et al. The role of surgery in the management of stage IV neuroblastoma: A single institution study. Med Pediatr Oncol 1995;24:287–91.

132. Schmidt ML, Lukens JN, Seeger RC, et al. Biologic factors determine prognosis in infants with stage IV neuroblastoma: A prospective Children's Cancer Group study. J Clin Oncol 2000;18:1260–8.

133. Azizkhan R, Haase G. Current biologic and therapeutic implications in the surgery of neuroblastoma. Semin Surg Oncol 1993;9:493–501.

134. Medary I, Aronson D, Cheung NK, et al. Kinetics of primary tumor regression with chemotherapy: Implications for the timing of surgery. Ann Surg Oncol 1996;3:521–5.

135. Davidoff AM, Corey BL, Hoffer FA, et al. Radiographic assessment of resectability of locoregional disease in children with high-risk neuroblastoma during neoadjuvant chemotherapy. Medical and Pediatric Oncology 2003; In press.

136. Loo R, Applebaum H, Takasugi J, et al. Resection of advanced stage neuroblastoma with the cavitron ultrasonic surgical aspirator. J Pediatr Surg 1988;23:1135–8.

137. Iwanaka T, Arai M, Ito M, et al. Surgical treatment for abdominal neuroblastoma in the laparoscopic era. Surg Endosc 2001;15:751–4.

138. Lobe TE. The applications of laparoscopy and lasers in pediatric surgery. Surg Annu 1993;25(Pt 1):175–91.

139. Losty P, Quinn F, Breatnach F, et al. Neuroblastoma–a surgical perspective. Eur J Surg Oncol 1993;19:33–6.

140. Azizkhan RG, Shaw A, Chandler JG. Surgical complications of neuroblastoma resection. Surgery 1985;97:514–17.

141. Berthold F, Utsch S, Holschneider AM. The impact of preoperative chemotherapy on resectability of primary tumour and complication rate in metastatic neuroblastoma. Z Kinderchir 1989;44:21–4.

142. Kiely EM. Radical surgery for abdominal neuroblastoma. Semin Surg Oncol 1993;9:489–92.

143. Sawada T. Past and future of neuroblastoma screening in Japan. Am J Pediatr Hematol Oncol 1992;14:320–6.

144. Schilling FH, Spix C, Berthold F, et al. Neuroblastoma screening at one year of age. N Engl J Med 2002;346:1047–53.

145. Woods WG, Gao RN, Shuster JJ, et al. Screening of infants and mortality due to neuroblastoma. N Engl J Med 2002;346:1041–6.

146. Nuchtern JG, London WB, Barnewolt CE, et al. A prospective study of expectant observation as primary therapy for neuroblastoma in young infants: A Children's Oncology Group study. Ann Surg 2012;In Press.

147. D'Angio GJ, Evans AE, Koop CE. Special pattern of widespread neuroblastoma with a favourable prognosis. Lancet 1971;1:1046–9.

148. Nickerson HJ, Matthay KK, Seeger RC, et al. Favorable biology and outcome of stage IV-S neuroblastoma with supportive care or minimal therapy: A Children's Cancer Group study. J Clin Oncols 2000;18:477–86.

149. Katzenstein HM, Kent PM, London WB, et al. Treatment and outcome of 83 children with intraspinal neuroblastoma: The Pediatric Oncology Group experience. J Clin Oncol 2001;19:1047–55.

150. Antunes NL, Khakoo Y, Matthay KK, et al. Antineuronal antibodies in patients with neuroblastoma and paraneoplastic opsoclonus-myoclonus. J Pediatr Hematol Oncol 2000;22:315–20.

151. Veneselli E, Conte M, Biancheri R, et al. Effect of steroid and high-dose immunoglobulin therapy on opsoclonus-myoclonus syndrome occurring in neuroblastoma. Med Pediatr Oncol 1998;30:15–17.

152. Borgna-Pignatti C, Balter R, Marradi P, et al. Treatment with intravenously administered immunoglobulins of the neuroblastoma-associated opsoclonus-myoclonus. J Pediatr 1996;129:179–80.

153. Reynolds CP, Kane DJ, Einhorn PA, et al. Response of neuroblastoma to retinoic acid in vitro and in vivo. Prog Clin Biol Res 1991;366:203–11.

154. Reynolds CP, Schindler P, Jones D, et al. Comparisons of 13-cisretinoic acid to trans-retronic acid using human neuroblastoma cell lines. In: Evans AE, Biedler JL, Brodeur G, et al, editors. Advances in Neuroblastoma Research 4. New York: Wiley; 1994. p. 237–44.

155. Sidell N, Altman A, Haussler MR, et al. Effects of retinoic acid (RA) on the growth and phenotypic expression of several human neuroblastoma cell lines. Exp Cell Res 1983;148:21–30.

156. Thiele CJ, Reynolds CP, Israel MA. Decreased expression of N-myc precedes retinoic acid-induced morphological differentiation of human neuroblastoma. Nature 1985;313:404–6.

157. Cheung NK. Immunotherapy. Neuroblastoma as a model. Pediatr Clin North Am 1991;38:425–41.

158. Ozkaynak MF, Sondel PM, Krailo MD, et al. Phase I study of chimeric human/murine anti-ganglioside G(D2) monoclonal antibody (ch14.18) with granulocyte-macrophage colony-stimulating factor in children with neuroblastoma immediately after hematopoietic stem-cell transplantation: A Children's Cancer Group Study. J Clin Oncol 2000;18:4077–85.

159. Hank JA, Surfus J, Gan J, et al. Treatment of neuroblastoma patients with antiganglioside GD2 antibody plus interleukin-2 induces antibody-dependent cellular cytotoxicity against neuroblastoma detected in vitro. J Immunother 1994;15:29–37.

160. Yu AL, Gilman AL, Ozkaynak MF, et al. Anti-GD2 antibody with GM-CSF, interleukin-2, and isotretinoin for neuroblastoma. N Engl J Med 2010;363:1324–34.

161. Gelfand MJ. Meta-iodobenzylguanidine in children. Semin Nucl Med 1993;23:231–42.

162. Lashford LS, Lewis IJ, Fielding SL, et al. Phase I/II study of iodine 131 metaiodobenzylguanidine in chemoresistant neuroblastoma: A United Kingdom Children's Cancer Study Group investigation. J Clin Oncol 1992;10:1889–96.

163. Haase GM, Meagher DP Jr, McNeely LK, et al. Electron beam intraoperative radiation therapy for pediatric neoplasms. Cancer 1994;74:740–7.

164. Hoefnagel CA, Smets L, Voute PA, et al. Iodine-125-MIBG therapy for neuroblastoma. J Nucl Med 1991;32:361–2.

165. Evans AE, Kisselbach KD, Yamashiro DJ, et al. Antitumor activity of CEP-751 (KT-6587) on human neuroblastoma and medulloblastoma xenografts. Clin Cancer Res 1999;5:3594–602.

166. Acheson A, Conover JC, Fandl JP, et al. A BDNF autocrine loop in adult sensory neurons prevents cell death. Nature 1995;374:450–3.

167. Matsumoto K, Wada RK, Yamashiro JM, et al. Expression of brain-derived neurotrophic factor and p145TrkB affects survival, differentiation, and invasiveness of human neuroblastoma cells. Cancer Res 1995;55:1798–806.

168. Buckley PG, Das S, Bryan K, et al. Genome-wide DNA methylation analysis of neuroblastic tumors reveals clinically relevant epigenetic events and large-scale epigenomic alterations localized to telomeric regions. Int J Cancer 2011;128:2296–305.

169. Teitz T, Wei T, Valentine MB, et al. Caspase 8 is deleted or silenced preferentially in childhood neuroblastomas with amplification of MYCN. Nat Med 2000;6:529–35.

CHAPTER 67

LESIONS OF THE LIVER

Walter S. Andrews • Richard J. Hendrickson

Hepatic tumors in children are relatively rare. The most common malignant hepatic neoplasms are not primary tumors, but rather metastatic lesions such as Wilms tumor, lymphoma, and neuroblastoma.[1] Primary liver tumors comprise between 1–4% of all solid tumors in children. Malignant hepatic tumors occur at a rate of about 1 to 1.5 per million children per year.[1,2] However, ten primary liver masses occur with some frequency in the pediatric age group Five of these occur only in children: infantile hepatic hemangiomas, hepatoblastoma, mesenchymal hamartoma, rhabdomyosarcoma of the biliary tract, and undifferentiated embryonal sarcoma (Table 67-1). The age distribution for hepatic masses is distinctive, with hepatoblastoma and infantile hepatic hemangioma occurring most commonly in the first two years of life, and hepatocellular carcinoma and focal nodular hyperplasia occurring most commonly after age 5 years (Table 67-2).[1]

Couinaud's elegant description of the segmental anatomy of the liver has allowed hepatic operations to evolve to a level at which they can be performed with an acceptable morbidity and mortality (Fig. 67-1).[3,4] The cumulative experience with hepatic resection and hepatic transplantation has allowed the development of techniques for both subsegmental and multisegmental resections of the liver in children. With the continued expansion of knowledge about these tumors, reasonable surgical and medical management plans can be devised.[5]

BENIGN HEPATIC TUMORS

Infantile Hepatic Hemangiomas

Incidence

Infantile hepatic hemangioma (IHH) is the most common benign solid hepatic tumor in children, comprising about 16% of all pediatric liver tumors.[1] It also is the most common liver tumor in the first year of life. Almost all children with IHH are seen initially before age 6 months, and the majority are encountered in the first 2 months.[6,7] Historically, a slight female predominance has been found, but this finding has not been uniformly seen.[8]

Clinical Presentation

IHHs can be either single lesions that can expand to a massive size or a multinodular infiltrative mass. Occasionally these lesions are asymptomatic and present as an abdominal mass or abdominal distention. Hepatic hemangiomas can also be found in association with congenital syndromes such as Osler–Weber–Rendu, Klippel–Trénaunay–Weber, and Ehlers–Danlos. IHH has also been reported in association with Beckwith–Wiedemann syndrome, diaphragmatic hernia, trisomy 21, transposition of the great arteries, and extranumerary digits.[9,10]

Infants with IHH can present with significant symptoms including hepatomegaly, high-output congestive heart failure, respiratory distress, and anemia. Occasionally these infants present with the Kasabach–Merritt syndrome that is characterized by acute thrombocytopenia, a microangiopathic hemolytic anemia, and a consumptive coagulopathy.[11] This syndrome can be life threatening and requires aggressive supportive treatment, as well as treatment of the hemangioma itself. Fortunately, the Kasabach–Merritt syndrome occurs infrequently and is usually associated with IHH that have rapid growth to a diameter of 5 cm or more. No cases have been reported in association with smaller tumors.[12]

The Boston Children's Hospital Vascular Anomalies Center has recently made a proposal to classify IHH as either focal, multifocal, or diffuse.[13] Focal lesions tend to be asymptomatic, are rarely associated with cutaneous hemangiomas, and often are identified on prenatal ultrasound (US). Focal lesions can have high-flow shunts and can have an associated low grade anemia or thrombocytopenia. Multifocal lesions also can be asymptomatic. They are often found on visceral imaging that is performed when evaluating patients with multiple cutaneous hemangiomas. These extrahepatic hemangiomas can occur at multiple distant sites including the skin (45%), lung (10%), pancreas, lymph nodes, and bone.[14,15] Some of these multifocal IHH lesions, however, are associated with high-output cardiac failure from either intralesional or portovenous shunting. The diffuse lesions present with near total replacement of the hepatic parenchyma with multiple hemangiomas which can result in massive hepatomegaly, abdominal compartment syndrome, or significant respiratory compromise. This lesion is often associated with severe hypothyroidism due to the overproduction of type III iodothronine deiodinase.[16,17] The hypothyroidism can be severe enough to cause low-output cardiac failure or significant mental retardation. Interestingly, there has not been a patient reported with diffuse IHH who has developed high-output cardiac failure. Other symptoms that can occur in patients with IHH include jaundice, failure to thrive, respiratory difficulties, or poor feeding. Historically, as many as 50–60% of infants with IHH have symptoms of congestive heart failure that seems to be age related.[18,19] Neonates with a focal hemangioma tend to present with high-output heart failure at birth, whereas infants with multifocal lesions

TABLE 67-1 **Hepatic Tumors in Pediatric Patients, Birth to 2 Years (AFIP 1970–1999)**

Type of Tumor	Number	%
Hepatoblastoma	124	43.5
Infantile hemangioendothelioma	103	36.1
Mesenchymal hamartoma	38	13.3
Nodular regenerative hyperplasia	6	2.1
Hepatocellular carcinoma	4	1.4
Angiosarcoma	4	1.4
Focal nodular hyperplasia	3	1.1
Undifferentiated embryonal sarcoma	3	1.1
Hepatocellular adenoma	0	0
Embryonal rhabdomyosarcoma	0	0
TOTAL	**285**	**100.0**

Reprinted from Stocker JT. Hepatic tumors in children. In: Suchy FJ, Sokol RJ, Balistreri WF, editors. Liver Disease in Children. 2nd ed. Philadelphia: Lippincott Williams & Wilkins; 2001. p. 915.

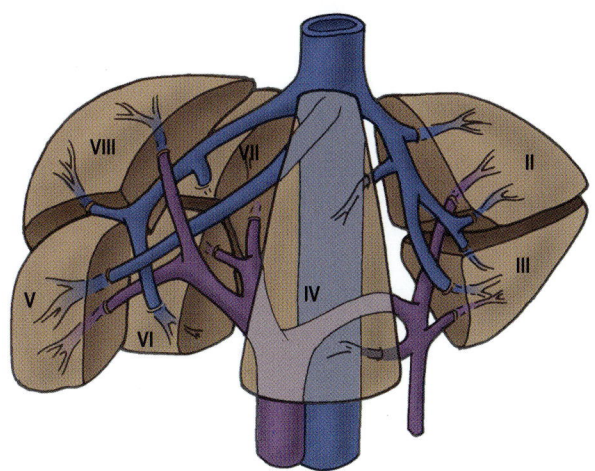

FIGURE 67-1 ■ The segmental hepatic anatomy as defined by Couinaud. A comprehensive understanding of the hepatic segmental division is necessary for successful hepatic resection. (From Couinaud C. Surgical anatomy of the liver: Several new aspects. Chirurgie 1986;112:337–42; Couinaud C. The anatomy of the liver. Ann Ital Chir 1992;63:693–7.)

TABLE 67-2 **Hepatic Tumors in Pediatric Patients, 5 to 20 Years (AFIP 1970–1999)**

Type of Tumor	Number	%
Hepatocelluar carcinoma	96	36.6
Focal nodular hyperplasia	40	15.3
Undifferentiated embryonal sarcoma	39	14.9
Nodular regenerative hyperplasia	26	9.9
Hepatocellular adenoma	22	8.4
Hepatoblastoma	22	8.4
Angiosarcoma	6	2.3
Mesenchymal hamartoma	5	1.9
Infantile hemangioendothelioma	4	1.5
Embryonal rhabdomyosarcoma	2	0.8
TOTAL	**262**	**100.0**

Reprinted from Stocker JT. Hepatic tumors in children. In: Suchy FJ, Sokol RJ, Balistreri WF, editors. Liver Disease in Children. 2nd ed. Philadelphia: Lippincott Williams & Wilkins; 2001.

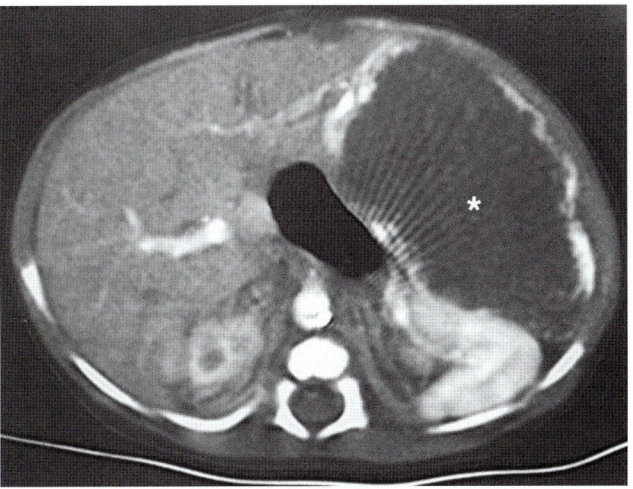

FIGURE 67-2 ■ CT scan after intravenous administration of a contrast agent shows a large hemangioendothelioma (asterisk) with peripheral enhancement in the left lateral segment.

tend to present with heart failure between the ages of 1 and 16 weeks.

In patients with IHH, the hepatic transaminase levels and occasionally the α-fetoprotein (AFP) level can be elevated. The cause of this AFP elevation is unclear. Moreover, an elevated AFP level in neonates must be interpreted with some caution. The AFP level is normally elevated in neonates and it does not decrease to adult levels until about 6 months of age.[15] When there is a significant elevation of the AFP level, however, hepatoblastoma must be excluded by either imaging studies or biopsy of the lesion.[20]

A significant incidence of placental abnormalities has recently been reported in very low birth weight infants (<1500 g) who present with infantile hemangiomas.[21] These researchers discovered a variety of anomalies that could potentially lead to the shedding of placental cells into the fetal circulation. If fetal hypoxic stress is also present, these placental cells could be exposed to an increased level of angiogenic factors that could then lead to increased endothelial cell or placental cell proliferation in the postnatal period with the subsequent development of an IHH.

Imaging

The ultrasound evaluation of IHH can be highly variable. Solitary lesions can have a heterogeneous echogenicity, and the Doppler spectral analysis can show a variety of flow patterns. Multifocal lesions, however, tend to be more uniform in their appearance and are seen as echolucent nodules associated with a high-flow vessel.[22] On computed tomography (CT) with intravenous contrast, classically the lesions either enhance diffusely or show rim enhancement that is followed by gradual filling of the center of the lesion (Fig. 67-2).[19,23,24] In one series, the

CT enhancement pattern was correlated to the size of the lesions. Lesions less than 1 cm enhanced homogeneously in the arterial phase. Lesions greater than 2 cm demonstrated peripheral rim enhancement and those in between 1–2 cm showed a mixed enhancement pattern in the arterial phase (Fig. 67-3).[25] Unfortunately, this 'classic' enhancement pattern is not always present in IHH which can make the radiologic diagnosis difficult.

Magnetic resonance imaging (MRI) is emerging as the single most useful modality to show both the location of the hemangioma and its flow pattern and structure.[26,27] The addition of intravenous gadolinium and a gradient-recalled-echo sequence to the MRI enhances its utility.

Focal lesions on MRI are well defined and hypointense to the liver on T_1 images and hyperintense on T_2-weighted images. Gadolinium demonstrates peripheral enhancement with variable central enhancement that is related to the amount of hemorrhage or thrombosis that is present in the lesion. Multifocal and diffuse lesions tend to show similar MRI findings except that there are multiple lesions present. Recently, however, there has been a case report of a hypervascular hepatoblastoma that had an MRI pattern that was identical to a hemangioendothelioma.[28] Therefore, again, radiology alone cannot reliably distinguish between benign and malignant lesions.

IHH also has been seen in conjunction with both focal nodular hyperplasia and hepatic mesenchymal hamartoma.[29,30] These associations are important to remember during the radiologic evaluation of a child with multiple hepatic masses.

Histology

Microscopically, the histologic pattern has been divided into type 1 and type 2 lesions. A type 1 lesion consists of a single layer or, occasionally, several layers of flat endothelial cells on a supporting fibrous stroma.[31] In a type 2 lesion (20% of cases), the endothelial cells are pleomorphic, larger, and more hyperchromatic than those seen in type 1 tumors. Also, there are poorly formed vascular spaces that often show tufting or branching. It is thought that the histologic picture of the type 2 lesion is more characteristic of a rapidly proliferating process. The histological differentiation between a type 2 lesion and an angiosarcoma can be difficult.[14,32] The addition of a histologic stain for the marker Glut 1 can be helpful in making the diagnosis of IHH.[9] Focal lesions do not stain positive for Glut 1, while multifocal lesions will be positive for this marker.[33,34] Well-preserved bile ducts can frequently be seen near the periphery of a type 1 lesion, whereas bile ducts are absent in a type 2 lesion.

Treatment

The life cycle of infantile cutaneous hemangiomas is divided into three stages. The first starts usually after birth and is a characterized by a rapid growth phase that lasts about 9 to 12 months. In the second phase, the hemangioma begins the process of involution. This process can take anywhere between 5 and 7 years. The last phase is the involuted phase where the hemangioma is permanently replaced by fibrofatty tissue.[13] Hepatic hemangiomas also tend to follow a similar life cycle. The therapy for IHH depends on the severity of the presenting symptoms and the size of the mass(es).

Asymptomatic lesions are monitored, and no specific therapy is instituted until symptoms occur.[11,35] As part of the evaluation of the asymptomatic patient with multifocal hemangiomas, imaging studies of the brain and chest should also be performed to make sure there are no associated intracranial or pulmonary lesions. In addition, all patients with multifocal lesions should be screened for hypothyroidism. Focal IHH are felt to follow a unique clinical course that is similar to the clinical course of a cutaneous rapidly involuting congenital hemangioma where involution is seen by 12 to 14 months of age.[36]

Infants who present with congestive heart failure, coagulopathy, or respiratory compromise require intervention. Mortality rates in these patients have been reported to range from 17–35%, with some reports of death in as many as 90% of those who are severely

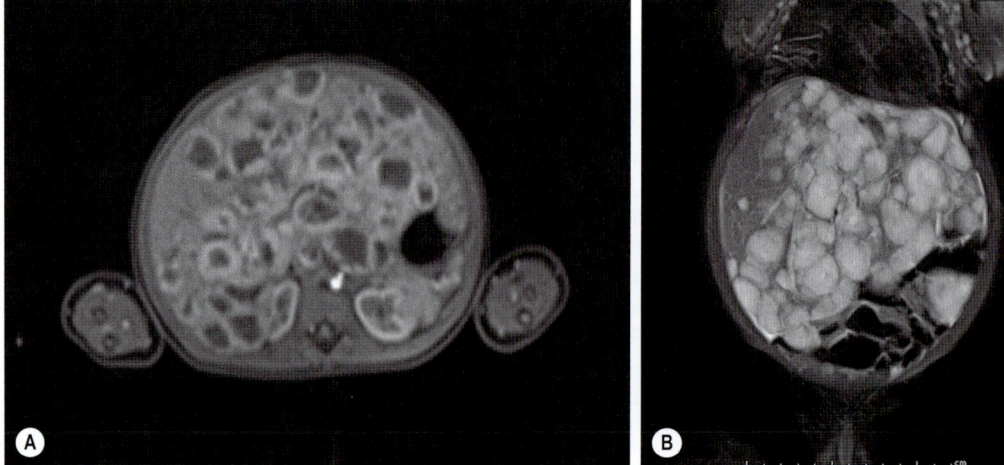

FIGURE 67-3 ■ Infantile hepatic hemangioma: diffuse form. **(A)** An MRI in the arterial phase showing rim enhancement of the hemangiomas after injection with gadoxetate disodium (Eovist). **(B)** The T_2-weighted image showing the same liver that is filled with hemangiomas.

symptomatic.[37–39] Risk factors for death include congestive heart failure, jaundice, multiple tumor nodules, and the histologic absence of cavernous differentiation.

In patients with congestive heart failure, stabilization is initiated with digoxin and diuretics. Supportive measures may be necessary in patients with respiratory compromise either from the high-output cardiac failure or from restriction of diaphragmatic movement by the abdominal mass. Coagulation factors can be administered if a coagulopathy is present.

If there is hemodynamic instability, respiratory compromise, or coagulopathy, then therapy directed toward the hemangioma is needed. The usual initial treatment for a symptomatic lesion is prednisone or prednisolone at a dose of 2–3 mg/kg/day. The symptomatic response rate to corticosteroids is reported to be about 45%.[40,41] If steroids are ineffective, then some IHHs have shown a response to vincristine at a weekly dose of 1–2 mg/m[2] for two weeks.[12] Labreze et al. have reported on the use of propranolol (2 mg/kg/day) for the treatment of severe infantile capillary hemangiomas with excellent results.[42] Marsciani et al. have successfully used the combination of propranolol (1 mg/kg/day followed by 2 mg/kg/day) and steroids in the treatment of a 2-month-old child with diffuse IHH.[43] They noted a dramatic decrease in liver size only one week after the addition of the propranolol. Another agent that has been reported to be possibly effective in IHH is curcumin, which is derived from the spice tumeric. Curcumin has antiangiogenic activity and has been tested with some success in a variety of tumors.[44] Hassell et al. described its apparent successful use in a 6 month old with a multifocal IHH.[45]

Resection should be considered if the hemangioma is confined to a single lobe. In this situation, a survival rate of 92% has been reported, even if the clinical situation is complicated by congestive heart failure.[32,46] However, some authors feel that resection is rarely needed if both pharmacotherapy and embolization are aggressively pursued.[13]

Embolization is an important part of the therapy of symptomatic hemangiomas.[47,48] In order to decrease the chance of the IHH recurring, it is important that both the arterial and portal vascular supply to the IHH are occluded as distally as possible.[11,19] After successful embolization, a rapid improvement in the clinical course usually occurs within five days. However, there may not be any associated change in the size of the hemangioma itself.[47,48] Embolization should be considered early in the treatment course in those infants who are in significant cardiac failure. Unfortunately, embolization has not been helpful in infants with diffuse disease because of the absence of significant shunting.

Finally, in infants in whom other modes of treatment have failed, liver transplantation has been used successfully for severe congestive heart failure or unremitting coagulopathy (or both).[49] The infants that will most commonly need to be considered for a liver transplant will be those who have the diffuse IHH subtype. Infants who experience rapid clinical deterioration in the postnatal period have a high mortality after liver transplantation so careful consideration needs to be given to their candidacy.[50]

The Vascular Anomalies Center at Boston Children's Hospital has suggested a treatment algorithm for IHH.[13] All asymptomatic lesions should be monitored with ultrasound until resolution. Symptomatic lesions should be treated with steroids. If there is no response, then the hemangioma should be embolized. Infants with diffuse disease should have a TSH checked and be started on steroids. If abdominal compartment syndrome is present, then the infant needs to be evaluated for a liver transplant in case there is no response to steroids.

Malignant transformation of an IHH to an angiosarcoma has been reported in older children.[18,51] For this reason, patients who are asymptomatic or who become asymptomatic after therapy must be monitored for complete anatomic resolution of their hemangioma. Resection of any residual lesion should be strongly considered.

Mesenchymal Hamartoma

Incidence

Mesenchymal hamartoma is reported to be the third most common hepatic tumor and the second most common benign tumor in children.[1] Of all benign hepatic lesions, mesenchymal hamartomas account for between 18–29% of these tumors.[52,53]

Epidemiology

The reasons for the development of a mesenchymal hamartoma are unclear. One theory is that it results from abnormal development of the primitive mesenchyme, which appears to occur at the level of the hepatic ductal plate, causing abnormal bile ducts.[54] This concept is supported by the histologic finding of a combination of cystic, anaplastic, and proliferating bile ducts, as well as the presence of multiple portal vein branches, within the tumor. It is postulated that the tumor then develops a cystic component as a result of obstruction and dilatation of lymphatics or from occluded bile ducts (or both). The tumor enlarges during infancy as the cystic areas increase in size. Most of the proliferative growth appears to occur before or just after birth because no observable mesenchymal mitotic activity is visible on histologic sections of the tumor.[55]

A second theory is that the lesions are reactive rather than developmental.[56] It is hypothesized that an abnormal blood supply to an otherwise normal hepatic parenchyma causes ischemic necrosis, leading to reactive cystic changes within that portion of the liver. This theory is supported by the findings that hamartomas often have a necrotic center, are often attached to the liver by only a thin pedicle, and rarely are found centrally in the liver.

The third theory suggests that a mesenchymal hamartoma is a proliferative lesion. This theory is supported by several findings. Increased fibroblast growth factor-2 (FGF-2) staining has been noted in the proliferating hepatic stellate cells adjacent to the mesenchymal hamartoma.[57] Both the stellate cells in the liver and the spindle cells in the mesenchymal hamartoma tissue strongly express molecules of the FGF-receptor family. It is

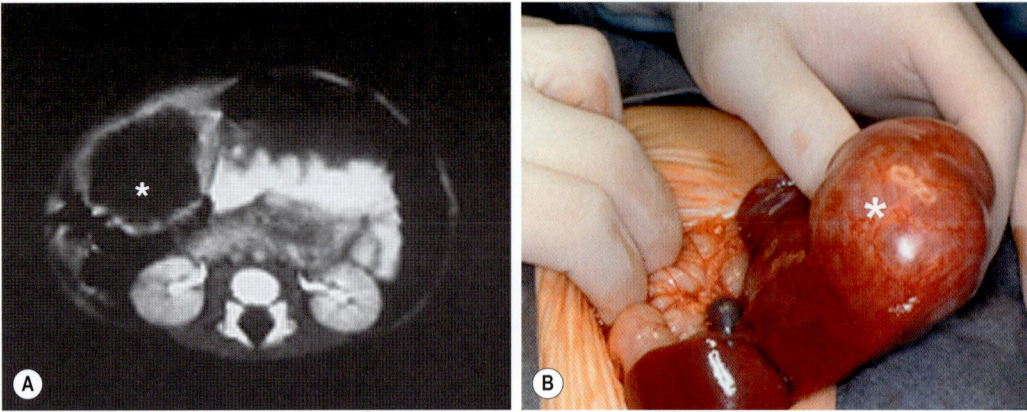

FIGURE 67-4 ■ This young child presented with a palpable right upper abdominal mass. **(A)** CT scan shows an anechoic mass (asterisk) in the periphery of the liver. **(B)** At operation, the mass (asterisk) was found to be pedunculated and emanating from the right lobe of the liver. This hamartoma was easily removed.

speculated that a local increase of FGF-2 secretion could stimulate the growth of the spindle cells to form the mesenchymal hamartoma. FGF-2 also is a potent angiogenic factor that could contribute to the intense vascularization seen within some of these lesions. A recent study has identified that the spindle cells that make up the predominant cell line in a mesenchymal hamartoma appear to be derived from hepatic stellate cells.[58] A possible genetic cause for these abnormalities has been proposed as well. Cytogenetic studies of these tumors have documented several abnormalities including translocation/deletion of chromosome19q13 or the loss of heterozygosity due to multiple monosomies. The resulting dysregulated imprinting may be an additional cause for a mesenchymal hamartoma.[59–63]

Clinical Presentation

The widespread use of prenatal imaging has led to the detection of hepatic masses before birth.[15] Cases of hepatic mesenchymal hamartoma that were diagnosed prenatally have been described.[64,65] One of the unique characteristics of a prenatal mesenchymal hamartoma is that it can be solid as well as cystic. Unfortunately, the prognosis for these antenatally diagnosed neonates is often poor with a reported mortality rate of 29%.[66] This mortality is related to: (1) the development of congestive heart failure from compression of the inferior vena cava or the umbilical vein by the tumor mass; or (2) the development of hydrops that can occur from fluid losses into cysts or decreased albumin production by the liver. Thus, it may be best to deliver these fetuses before fetal hydrops develops.[65] Another series reported the use of repeated intrauterine aspiration of the cysts until the infants could be delivered and definitive treatment initiated.[67] While this therapy is appealing, there currently is insufficient evidence to recommend its widespread use.[66]

In the neonate, these lesions can have a varying presentation. High-output cardiac failure, pulmonary hypertension, and disseminated intravascular coagulopathy have been reported in neonates with highly vascular mesenchymal hamartomas.[68–70] Respiratory distress secondary to a large hepatic mass impinging on the diaphragm

has also been described.[65] Unfortunately, the prognosis for infants with a perinatal diagnosis is also poor with a reported mortality of 35%.[66]

The presentation of a mesenchymal hamartoma in the older child is usually that of progressive abdominal distention or an abdominal mass (or both). There is a significant right-sided predilection for these masses, and they tend to be somewhat more common in males.[1] Occasionally, the associated symptoms of nausea and vomiting can occur that are secondary to the compression of the stomach and intestine by the expanding mass.

On physical examination, abdominal distention or a palpable abdominal mass is most common. The mass tends to be nontender and fixed. Laboratory studies almost always are normal, including liver function studies. The AFP level can be moderately elevated and it returns to normal after resection. However, it is important to remember that patients have been treated with chemotherapy for hepatoblastoma until a tumor biopsy was performed and a mesenchymal hamartoma was subsequently diagnosed.[71,72]

Imaging

CT, ultrasound, and MRI have all been used for diagnosis. On CT and ultrasound, a multiseptated, multicystic, anechoic mass is usually located either in the periphery or scattered throughout the liver.[73,74] Occasionally the mass is pedunculated. Calcification within the tumor is unusual, but has been reported so the presence of calcifications within a tumor does not exclude a mesenchymal hamartoma.[75,76] MR angiography has proven useful both in the diagnosis and planning of resection.[77,78] The finding of a small round hyperechoic parietal nodule on ultrasound is usually highly sensitive for making the diagnosis.[79]

Histology

Mesenchymal hamartomas typically are large, well-circumscribed tumors that measure at least 8–10 cm in diameter (Fig. 67-4). Seventy-five per cent of these tumors occur in the right lobe of the liver, and only 3% are seen in both lobes of the liver. On cut section, multiple cysts can measure from a few millimeters to 15 cm in diameter. These cysts are filled with either serous or viscous fluid separated by loose fibrous and myxoid tissue (Fig. 67-5). The surrounding tissue is yellow-tan to brown and is loose to moderately dense.

Microscopically, the tissue consists of a mixture of bile ducts, liver cell cysts, and mesenchyme. The cysts may be dilated bile ducts, dilated lymphatics, or amorphous cysts surrounded by mesenchyme. In older patients, the cysts may be lined with cuboidal epithelium (Fig. 67-6). Elongated or tortuous bile ducts surrounded by connective tissue are unevenly distributed throughout the mesenchyme. Typically the hepatocytes appear normal, and they are not a predominant part of the pathologic process. The bile ducts in the periphery of the lesion seem to be undergoing active proliferation.[1]

Despite the fact that the majority of these tumors are localized, there have been reports of these tumors being multifocal.[63] This may account for the occasional recurrences that are seen after resection of the primary tumor.

Treatment

Various management strategies have been used for these lesions. Because they are sometimes encapsulated,

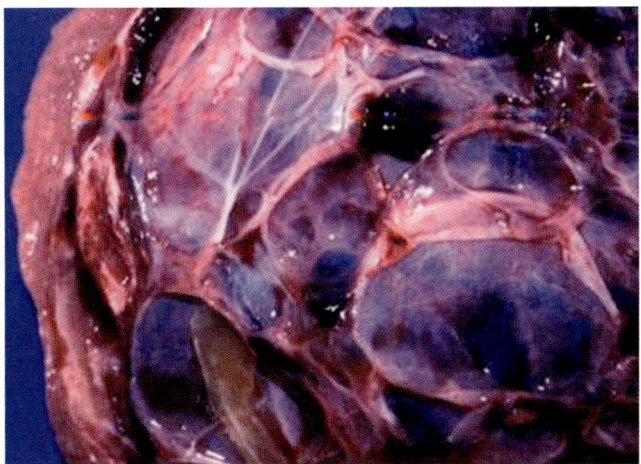

FIGURE 67-5 ■ Cut surface of a mesenchymal hamartoma showing multiple cysts.

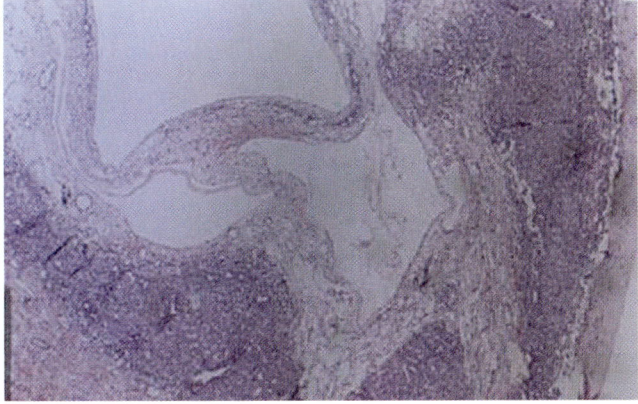

FIGURE 67-6 ■ Light microscopy of mesenchymal hamartoma showing a cyst lined with cuboidal epithelium.

enucleation may be possible. Very large, bilobar tumors that are not amenable to resection can be marsupialized into the peritoneal cavity, but recurrence after marsupialization can occur. If marsupialization is performed or the resection is incomplete, careful, long-term follow-up is important because of the risk of recurrence or the development of undifferentiated embryonal sarcoma.[80] Complete excision of the lesion with a margin of normal liver is curative (including the use of liver transplantation for large, bilobar lesions) and is the recommended therapy.[81,82] For massive lesions with multiple cysts, one group reported the use of ultrasound-guided, intraoperative aspiration of the cysts.[83] This technique substantially reduced the size of the mass and made the resection much easier. Spontaneous involution of these lesions has been reported, but is unusual.[84]

There is now strong evidence that an undifferentiated embryonal sarcoma of the liver can develop within a preexisting mesenchymal hamartoma.[63,85-88] This association has occurred both synchronously and metachronously. The evidence for a direct link between a mesenchymal hamartoma and an undifferentiated embryonal hepatic sarcoma comes from the simultaneous finding of both tumors arising within the same mass. Moreover, aneuploidy and similar chromosomal abnormalities involving chromosome 19q13 have been reported in both a hepatic mesenchymal hamartoma and an undifferentiated embryonal sarcoma.[60,61,89,90]

Focal Nodular Hyperplasia

Incidence

Focal nodular hyperplasia (FNH) accounts for about 10% of the hepatic tumors in children.[1] The reported age range is between 7 months and 16 years, with a mean of 7 years, and there is a slight female predominance.[91] The majority of these tumors are discovered incidentally.[91,92] The most common symptom is abdominal pain, but some patients describe decreased appetite, an abdominal mass, weight loss, or a combination. Hepatomegaly is a common finding, and liver function abnormalities are often present.

FNH has been seen in association with a variety of different conditions and situations, including previous liver trauma, other liver tumors, hemochromatosis, Klinefelter syndrome, the use of itraconazole, after a successful Kasai procedure, after liver transplantation, and with cigarette smoking.[93-100]

The etiology of FNH is not certain, but the evidence suggests that it may be a congenital vascular abnormality. These lesions have a single feeding artery and there is an absence of bile ducts or veins in the lesion. The large artery causes a hyperperfused area of the parenchyma with subsequent growth of the liver tissue around the artery.[101] In addition, FNH has been associated with other vascular lesions such as hemangiomas, arteriovenous malformations, and hereditary hemorrhagic telangiectasia.[102,103] Further evidence that FNH is a reactive lesion secondary to vascular anomalies comes from a study in which an increase in the angiopoietin ratio (ANGPT1/ANGPT2) was seen.[104] The *ANGPT1* and *ANGPT2* genes are necessary for normal vascular development. In FNH, an overexpression of the *ANGPT1* gene and an absence of the antagonistic *ANGPT2* gene lead to uncontrolled and disorganized vascular development. Although it is not clear that this is the exact pathogenesis of FNH, it certainly suggests that this genetic imbalance may play a causative role. FNH can also develop from an acquired abnormality of the hepatic vasculature. Thrombosis of either a hepatic artery or portal venous branch can initially cause ischemia of a portion of the liver followed by recannulation and reperfusion, which leads to hepatocyte proliferation.[105]

Controversy exists about the relation between oral contraceptive use and the development of FNH. In a case–control study, it was noted that neither menstrual nor reproductive factors correlated with FNH risk. However, oral contraceptive use was a significant risk factor in the development of FNH.[99] As the use of oral contraceptives also appears to be associated with hepatocellular adenomas, a history of oral contraceptive use does not help in distinguishing between these two entities.[99]

In children, an association has been noted between the congenital absence of the portal vein (Abernathy syndrome) and FNH.[106–108] In addition, these patients have an increased incidence of other solid tumors such as hepatoblastoma, hepatocellular carcinoma, and hepatocellular adenoma.[109,110] FNH also has been seen, albeit less frequently than hepatocellular adenoma, in patients with glycogen storage disease (GSD) type 1.[108]

Over the last six years there has been an increasing awareness of the occurrence of FNH in oncologic patients who have completed their therapy. The reported incidence of FNH in the general pediatric population is 0.02% but is 0.45% in the postoncology treatment population.[111] As opposed to nononcologic patients where the FNH is usually solitary, post-treatment oncologic patients frequently have multiple FNHs. The cause of these post oncologic FNHs is not known, but is felt to be secondary to alterations in liver perfusion that occur as the result of the chemotherapy or radiation that these patients receive.[105,112] The development of hepatic mass(es) in an oncology patient leads to a diagnostic dilemma between an FNH or a recurrent tumor. One of the higher risk groups for developing an FNH after therapy are patients who were treated for neruoblastoma.[111–116] There also seems to be an increase in the development of FNHs in children who have received a hematopoietic stem cell transplant.[117–119] Therefore, a liver lesion that occurs after treatment of a previous cancer does not always mean that there has been a recurrence of the primary tumor. A biopsy of the lesion should always be done before the initiation of further therapy.[120]

Imaging

The diagnosis of FNH often requires the use of multiple different imaging modalities. On CT, the classic findings are early enhancement of the lesion and the presence of a central scar (Fig. 67-7).[121] Unfortunately, this pathognomonic association is not often seen.[122,123] Additional imaging modalities include single-photon emission radionuclide scans with either radiolabeled sulfur colloid or

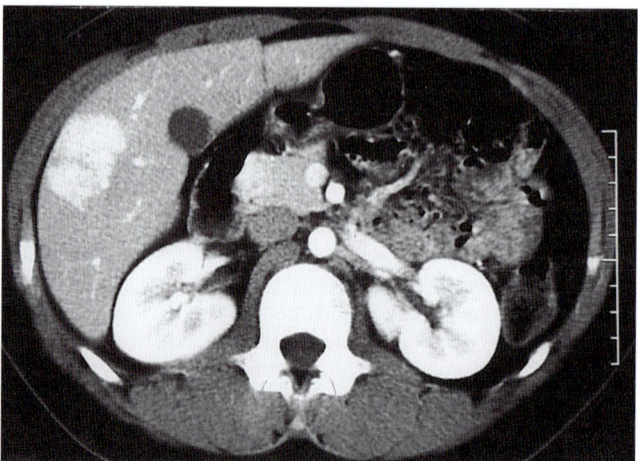

FIGURE 67-7 ■ CT scan after intravenous administration of a contrast agent shows an early enhancing lesion in the right lobe with hypodense central scar consistent with focal nodular hyperplasia.

hepatobiliary iminodiacetic acid (HIDA) imaging. These studies usually demonstrate hypervascularization, increased tumor tracer uptake, and a central cold area.[124–126] Technetium-99m sulfur colloid scanning can also be useful in distinguishing between FNH and a hepatic adenoma. FNH lesions take up the tracer because the Kupffer cells in the FNH take up the colloid but hepatic adenomas do not take up tracer because they lack Kupffer cells.[127] MRI also has been useful when coupled with either gadolinium enhancement or the use of liver-specific contrast agents such as mangafodipir trisodium or iron oxide. During the arterial phase of dynamic contrast enhancement, an FNH will demonstrate distinct hypervascularity.[128] These contrast agents can also help diagnose an FNH by allowing better identification of the central scar.[129,130]

Histology

FNH classically is characterized by nodular architecture, a central or eccentric scar containing malformed vessels that resemble an arteriovenous malformation, and a variable amount of bile duct proliferation (Figs 67-8 and 67-9).[131,132] FNHs always occur in the setting of a noncirrhotic liver.

Histologically, the classic form of FNH with a central scar accounts for about 80% of the lesions. Twenty per cent are nonclassic where the FNH lacks either the nodular architecture or the presence of the malformed blood vessels. These nonclassic lesions are subdivided into three histologic categories: the telangiectatic form, the mixed hyperplastic form, and the adenomatous form.[133] These nonclassic categories always lack a macroscopic scar and all three forms can be difficult to distinguish from and may be related to a hepatocellular adenoma.[134] Immunohistochemical staining for cytokeratins 7 and 19 along with staining for neuronal cell adhesion molecule (CD56) has shown to be very helpful in distinguishing between FNH and hepatocellular

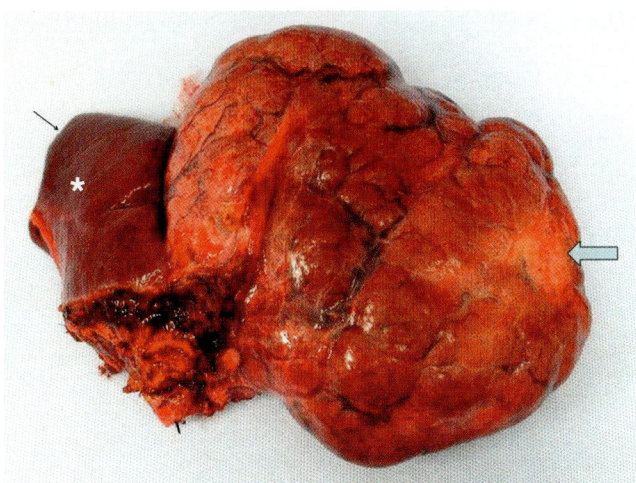

FIGURE 67-8 ■ A large focal nodular hyperplasia lesion was resected. External scarring (arrow) is seen in the lesion. An asterisk marks normal liver.

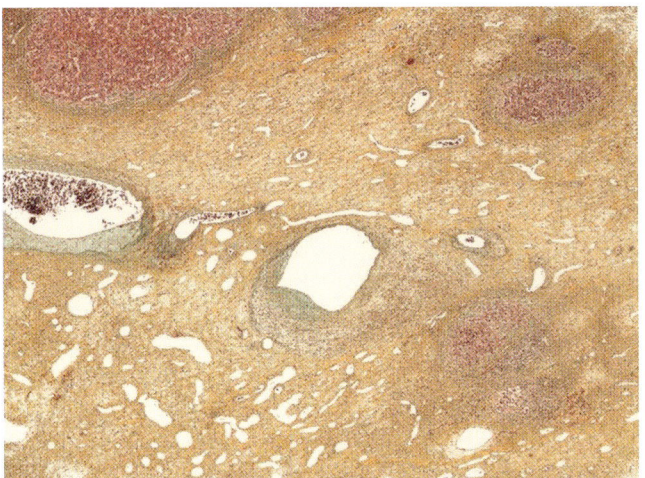

FIGURE 67-9 ■ Light microscopy of a focal nodular hyperplasia showing a central scar containing abnormal blood vessels.

adenoma.[134] Hepatocellular adenomas have been reported to be present in association with FNH in about 4% of the cases.[131]

Recently, there has been a case report of what appears to be malignant transformation of an FNH to a fibrolamellar hepatocellular carcinoma.[135] Also, FNH has been reported to occur in association with a well-differentiated fibrolamellar hepatocellular carcinoma.[135,136] This observation is important to remember in patients who have multiple hepatic nodules.[137,138]

Treatment

The treatment of FNH depends on the clinical situation. If the diagnosis is certain, and the patient is asymptomatic, the consensus is that these patients can be followed with serial ultrasound to ensure that no progression of the lesion occurs.[91,122] Percutaneous biopsy can be helpful in the diagnosis.[139] However, if the patient is symptomatic, if the lesion is greater than 5 cm, if progression of the mass is seen, or if the diagnosis is unclear, then a biopsy or a resection of the lesion is recommended.[140–143]

Due to the association of FNH with hepatocellular carcinoma, patients who are expectantly managed must have serial evaluations to ensure that no progression occurs. Moreover, they need to be monitored for the development of other hepatic lesions.

Several reports have noted a 40–50% regression rate in cases of FNH that have been monitored.[144,145] In the pediatric population, the true incidence of regression is not known due to the lack of long-term follow-up studies; however, it may be much lower than in the adult population.[143] Regression of FNH is more likely if the use of oral contraceptives ceases.[146,147]

In two symptomatic patients in whom the FNH was in an area that was thought to be difficult for resection, arterial embolization either with Lipiodol and absorbable gelatin foam (Gelfoam) or iodized oil and polyvinyl alcohol resulted in a significant regression in the size of the mass.[148–150]

Hepatocellular Adenoma

Incidence

Hepatocellular adenoma is a very rare hepatic tumor in children, comprising only about 4% of all solid liver tumors.[1] It is most commonly seen in women in their 20s and is associated with the use of oral contraceptives.

Clinical Presentation

In children, these lesions are often asymptomatic and are discovered during evaluation for other problems. Occasionally, they can produce intermittent abdominal pain and rarely can spontaneously rupture resulting in hemoperitoneum and the clinical signs of acute volume depletion.

Imaging

Hepatic adenomas are solitary lesions in most cases, but occasionally two to three adenomas can be seen in one patient.[149,151,152] On ultrasound, these lesions can have a variable appearance, depending on the tumor composition. They can have a hyperechoic, hypoechoic, or a mixed echoic pattern depending on whether it is a simple adenoma, an adenoma with fatty metamorphosis, or an adenoma with hemorrhagic necrosis.[149]

On CT, the adenoma can either be isoattenuating relative to the normal liver or hyperattenuating (due to the presence of fat). They are usually sharply marginated and nonlobular, but can be encapsulated or calcified in some patients.[153] Hyperattenuated areas often correspond to areas of recent hemorrhage. On CT scan with intravenous contrast, a hypodense discrete lesion will show either arterial-phase enhancement or peripheral enhancement secondary to large subcapsular feeding vessels.[154]

On MRI, these lesions are either hypo- to hyperintense on T_1-weighted images with uniform signal loss on out of phase T_1-weighted views. On T_2 images, the lesions are isointense to slightly hyperintense and gadolinium enhancement is maximal during the arterial phase with rapid fading.[154] The finding of central hemorrhage or necrosis on CT scan helps differentiate hepatocellular adenoma from FNH.

Associated Conditions

Hepatocellular adenomas were extremely rare prior to 1960, which corresponds to the year in which oral contraceptives were first introduced.[155] In women who have never used oral contraceptives, the annual incidence of hepatic adenoma is estimated to be about one per million. The duration of oral contraceptive use is directly related to the risk of developing a hepatic adenoma. The use of contraceptives for 5 to 7 years carries a fivefold increased risk, and use for 9 or more years has a 25-fold increased risk.[156–158]

Hepatocellular adenomas also have been associated with galactosemia, hypothyroidism, polycythemia, diabetes, Fanconi anemia, polycystic ovary syndrome, and the use of anabolic steroids.[159–162]

Hepatocellular adenomas are a significant complication in patients with type 1A GSD from their teenage years into adulthood.[163,164] The estimated prevalence of adenomas in these patients is close to 50%.[165,166] The pathogenesis of adenoma development is poorly understood in this group, but may be related in part to the tightness of the metabolic control.[167] These adenomas are often multiple rather than solitary lesions. Unfortunately, in this patient population, hepatocellular carcinoma can occur in association with hepatocellular adenomas. The youngest reported patient with GSD was 6 years old at the time of the diagnosis of hepatocellular carcinoma.[168] In several series, hepatocellular carcinoma has been found to develop in up to 18% of patients with a hepatocellular adenoma.[169–173] Direct evidence for malignant transformation of a hepatocellular adenoma into a carcinoma has been confirmed with the reporting of a hepatocellular carcinoma within a hepatic adenoma in patients with GSD.[174] Abnormalities in chromosome 6 have been also been identified in type 1A GSD adenomas and similar chromosome 6 alterations have been identified in hepatocellular carcinomas, suggesting a possible genetic link between these two diagnoses.[175]

Adenomatosis (the occurrence of more than ten simultaneous adenomas) is a rare disorder, with 38 cases reported in the literature through 2000.[176] There is a massive form, characterized by multiple nodules measuring between 2–10 cm, and the multifocal form, in which most lesions are smaller than 1 cm, with only a few larger than 4 cm.[177] Oral contraceptive use has been seen in about half of the female patients. Interestingly, diabetes and hepatic steatosis has been noted in these patients, but it is not clear if there is a causative relation.[177,178] Adenomatosis has also been reported in patients seven to nine years after a Fontan procedure.[179]

Histology

Hepatocellular adenomas histologically consist of large plates or cords of cells that resemble normal hepatocytes. These plates are separated by dilated vascular sinusoids, which are equivalent to thin-walled capillaries perfused by arterial pressure. Adenomas do not have a portal

venous supply and are fed solely by peripheral arterial vessels that account for the hypervascular nature of these lesions. Kupffer cells are found in reduced numbers and have little or no function. The absence of bile ducts serves as a key histologic feature that helps distinguish the hepatocellular adenoma from FNH. Lipid accumulation is responsible for the characteristic yellow appearance on the cut surface.[1]

The exact reason for their development is unclear. Two reports have cited the mutations of the Wnt/β-catenin pathway in patients with hepatocellular adenoma.[180,181] This pathway mutation has been identified in many hepatocellular neoplasms, although its direct contribution to carcinogenesis is not completely understood. A second mutation has been found in the *HNF1A* gene that leads to the downregulation of hepatocyte nuclear factor-1α. This downregulation has been linked to the development of hepatic steatosis and hepatic adenomas.[182] The significance of these findings in hepatocellular adenoma is also unknown.

Hepatocellular adenomas may be asymptomatic, but also can be the site of hemorrhage. Larger lesions are more likely to bleed than are smaller lesions. Contained hemorrhage may result in rapid enlargement of the adenoma, but rupture with intraperitoneal hemorrhage can occur if the lesion is near the liver surfaces. The patient may show signs of blood loss and/or peritonitis.

Treatment

The treatment approach for these lesions depends on a variety of factors. In patients who are receiving oral contraceptives or androgenic steroid therapy, the first step should be withdrawal of these medications. Multiple case reports mention regression of the adenomas after withdrawal of these compounds. However, in other multiple reports, withdrawal of these agents has resulted in persistence of the adenoma.[183–185] If discontinuation is not effective, then the adenoma should be resected. This removes the potential for future hemorrhage or malignant degeneration (10% of lesions).[186] If the adenoma is larger than 5 cm or if the diagnosis of the hepatic lesion is uncertain, then excision is recommended.[187,188]

For patients with ruptured hepatocellular adenomas, the current suggested therapy in the hemodynamically stable patient is nonoperative monitoring and hemodynamic support. Once the hemorrhage has resolved and the patient has recovered, elective resection can be performed. In patients who continue to bleed actively, hepatic arterial embolization should be performed. This not only stops the hemorrhage but also can decrease the size of the adenoma.[189] After resolution of the hemorrhage, resection is indicated. This management plan results in a decrease in size of the lesion and allows a more limited hepatic resection under controlled conditions.[190,191]

In patients with type 1 GSD in whom multiple adenomas develop, hepatic transplantation should be considered because of the significant probability of the development of a concurrent hepatocellular carcinoma. Liver transplantation not only corrects the potential hemorrhagic problem, but also removes the potential for cancer development.

MALIGNANT HEPATIC TUMORS

Hepatoblastoma

Most hepatoblastomas develop before age 3 years, with a median age of about 18 months.[192] About 4% are present at the time of birth; 69% are present by the end of two years, and 90% develop by the end of 5 years. Only 3% of cases are noted in children older than 15 years.[193] A definite male predominance (1.7 : 1) is seen.[5]

Epidemiology

Hepatoblastomas are associated with a variety of clinical conditions, syndromes, and malformations (Box 67-1). Beckwith–Wiedemann syndrome is associated most commonly with Wilms tumor, but other tumors such as hepatoblastomas, gonadoblastomas, and adrenal carcinomas are also seen.[194,195] The association with hepatoblastoma is so strong that patients with Beckwith–Wiedemann syndrome must be monitored with serial AFP levels every three months until the age of 4 years and an abdominal ultrasound every three months until they reach age 8 years.[195–197] Screening studies for hepatoblastoma are also recommended in patients with familial adenomatous polyposis. These patients should be screened for the APC tumor/suppressor gene. If this gene is present, then these patients are at increased risk for developing hepatoblastoma.[198,199]

Another interesting association exists between hepatoblastoma and extreme prematurity (<1000 g). In the Japanese Children's Cancer Registry (JCCR), it was noted that hepatoblastomas accounted for 58% of the malignancies diagnosed in extremely low birth weight children.[200] In recent epidemiologic studies, several factors were associated with an increased risk for the development of neonatal hepatoblastoma, including birth weight less than 1000 g, maternal age younger than 20 years, use of infertility treatment, maternal smoking, and a higher pre-pregnancy body mass index (BMI of 25–29).[201,202] The time from birth to onset of hepatoblastoma in this population ranges from six months to six years.[203] Unfortunately, the tumors that occurred in this group grew rapidly and had an unfavorable biologic behavior.[204] Although the etiology for the predilection of hepatoblastomas to develop in very low birth weight infants is not

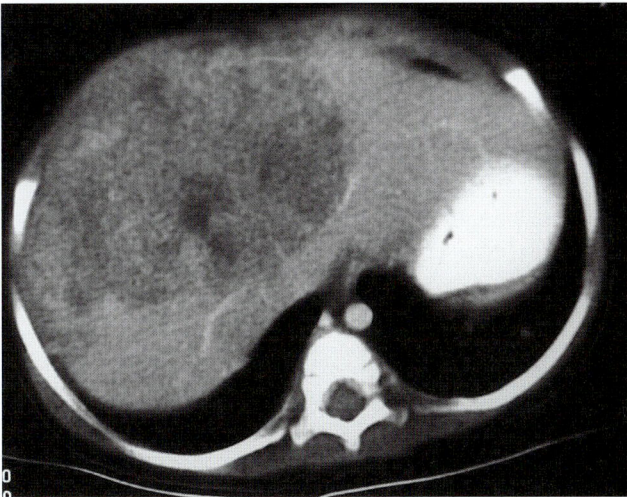

FIGURE 67-10 ■ CT scan after intravenous administration of a contrast agent shows a large right lobe hepatoblastoma extending into the left lateral segment.

known, oxygen therapy, furosemide use, and failure of the infant to grow appropriately were noted to be risk factors.[204] The highest correlation was with the duration of oxygen therapy. The risk of hepatoblastoma increased by 20% if oxygen therapy was continued for 30 days, and the risk increased by 100% in children who were treated with oxygen for four months.

Cysteine has also been implicated as a contributing factor. Cysteine is an amino acid that is necessary for the production of glutathione and taurine, both of which are intracellular antioxidants. In premature infant livers, there appears to be impaired production of cysteine.[205] Due to the complexities in treating 'micropremies' through their first few months, multiple other interventions could influence the development of a hepatoblastoma.

Histology

Hepatoblastomas tend to be unifocal lesions in most cases. Fifty per cent are isolated to the right lobe, 15% are in the left lobe, and 27% are centrally located to involve both lobes (Fig. 67-10).

Histologically, the tumor can be divided into six different subtypes (Figs 67-11 and 67-12) based on light microscopy (Box 67-2). A correlation between clinical outcome and the histologic subtypes has been suggested. The pure fetal subtype appears to be associated with the better prognosis, whereas the small cell undifferentiated subtype appears to have a very poor prognosis.[206–209] In several other studies, chemotherapy was initiated before surgical intervention and likely altered the accuracy of histologic definition of the resected tumor, making it difficult to correlate histology and outcome.[210]

Biology and Cytogenetics

Thrombocytosis is common in patients with hepatoblastoma. This may be related to increased thrombopoietin levels, which have been reported in hepatoblastoma cell extracts.[210] Elevated interleukin-1b levels also have been

BOX 67-1	Conditions Associated with Hepatoblastoma

Beckwith–Wiedemann syndrome
Budd–Chiari syndrome
Gardner syndrome
Hemihypertrophy
Heterozygous α1-antitrypsin deficiency
Isosexual precocity
Polyposis coli families
Trisomy 18
Type 1a glycogen storage disease
Very low birth weight

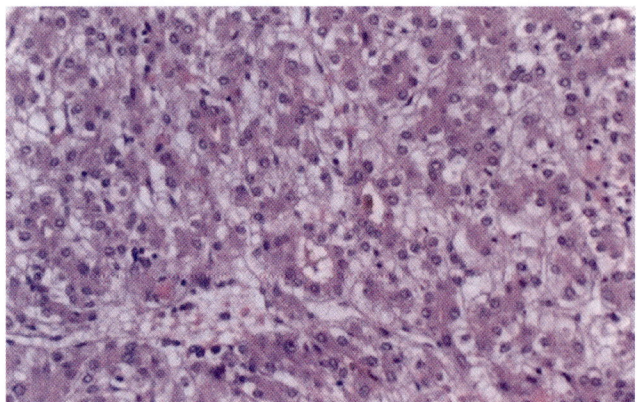

FIGURE 67-11 ■ Histology of a pure fetal hepatoblastoma. Note the hepatocytes have clear glycogen-rich cytoplasm and small, regular nuclei.

noted in hepatoblastoma cell lines.[211] This results in an increased production of interleukin-6, which is known to stimulate thrombopoiesis and thrombocytosis.[212]

Chromosomal abnormalities have been documented in patients with hepatoblastoma.[213] The most common defects have been trisomy of chromosomes 20, 2, or 8, or a combination of these. Trisomy 18 also has been found.[214] However, to date, no correlation has been noted between these cytogenetic abnormalities and either clinical outcome or tumor biology.

An association between hepatoblastoma and the APC gene was noted in patients with familial adenomatous polyposis and Gardner syndrome.[212,215] A recent study found an association between the activation of the Wnt/β-catenin signaling pathway and the development of carcinogenesis in hepatoblastoma and hepatocellular carcinoma.[216]

Clinical Presentation

Patients with hepatoblastoma are most commonly seen with an asymptomatic right upper abdominal mass that is noted incidentally by either a parent or the pediatrician. Rarely these patients have tumor rupture, followed by significant hemorrhage and hypovolemia.

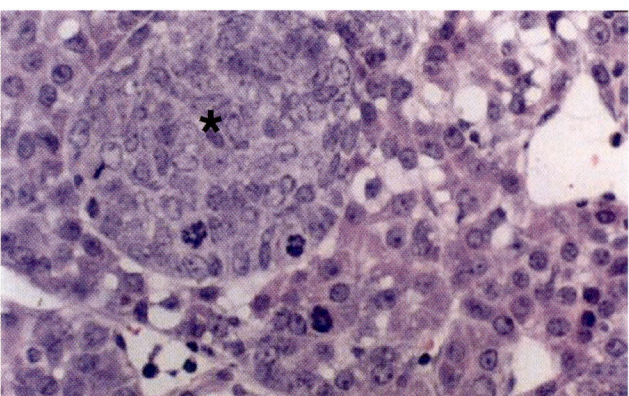

FIGURE 67-12 ■ Histology of a hepatoblastoma with mixed fetal and embryonal elements. Note the large solid nest (asterisk) of poorly defferentiating cells (embryonal components). In contrast, note the surrounding trabeculae of the differentiating fetal hepatoblasts.

BOX 67-2	Histologic Subtypes of Hepatoblastoma

Pure fetal
Embryonal
Macrotrabecular
Small cell undifferentiated
Mixed epithelial and mesenchymal pattern
   With teratoid features
   Without teratoid features

Sexual precocity may be a presenting feature with hepatoblastoma, secondary to the tumor producing human chorionic gonadotropin. With large tumors, it is not unusual to see anorexia and failure to thrive. These lesions can become very large (15 cm) and can extend across the midline or down into the pelvis.

Imaging

The first diagnostic test is usually an ultrasound. This usually differentiates between a renal and hepatic mass. An abdominal CT scan is then usually performed. In half of patients, calcification is noted within the mass.[217] Spiral CT with an intravenous bolus of a contrast agent not only is helpful in the diagnosis, but also is useful in the staging of the tumor and in determining its resectability. With three-dimensional reconstruction, the location of the mass with respect to the vena cava, the hepatic veins, and the portal venous system can often be precisely delineated (Fig. 67-13). MRI is becoming an increasingly helpful modality for determining the relation of the tumor to the hepatic anatomy and in differentiating hepatoblastomas from other childhood hepatic tumors.[218] However, no current noninvasive study can always differentiate between a benign or malignant liver lesion.[28] If there is any concern about the diagnosis, a biopsy should be performed.

Laboratory Studies

Anemia and thrombocytosis (platelet count >500,000/mm^3) are often found in patients with hepatoblastoma.[219] However, the hallmark of hepatoblastoma is an elevated AFP level, which occurs in up to 90% of patients.[220] The serum levels of AFP can sometimes exceed 1 million ng/mL. This can lead to the 'hook' effect in which the initially reported AFP level can be low despite the actual level being very high. If the lesion is suspicious for hepatoblastoma, a request should be made to dilute the AFP sample before retesting.[221] Serum AFP has a half-life of between 4 and 9 days, and the levels usually decrease to normal by 4 to 8 weeks after complete removal of the tumor.[222] It is important to remember that neonates normally have an elevated AFP level (25–50,000 ng/mL) at birth that does not decrease to 'adult' levels until age 6 months.[15] This becomes important when evaluating a neonate with a hepatic mass or when monitoring the AFP after liver resection in a neonate or infant.

AFP also has been useful for monitoring purposes. In one case report, a radioimmunodetection method was

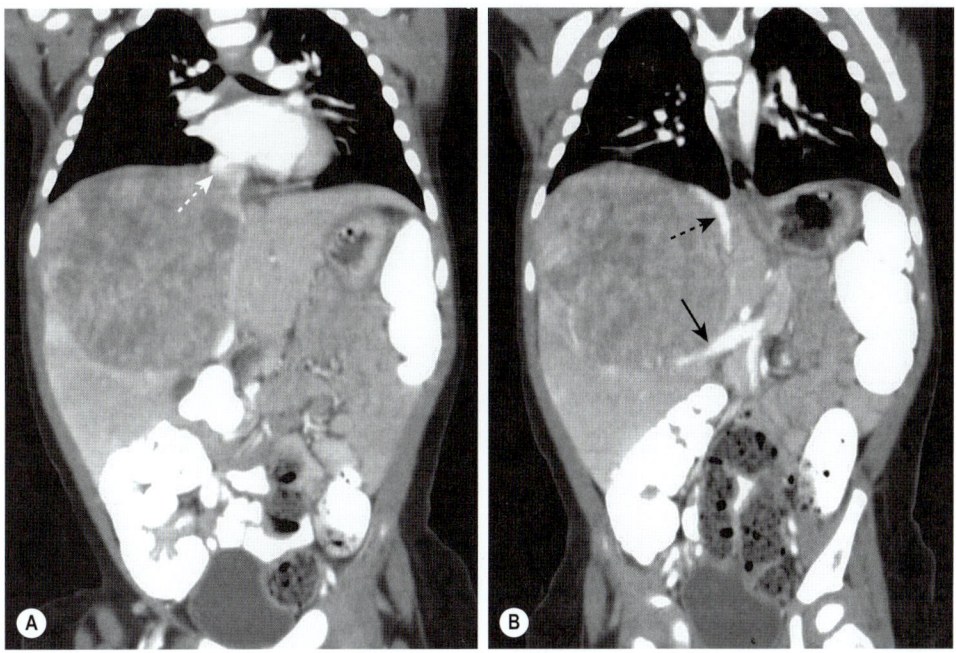

FIGURE 67-13 ■ **(A)** This CT scan obtained after intravenous administration of a contrast agent in a 1-year-old child shows a large mass in the right hepatic lobe. On other images, the mass appears to invade or compress the medial segment of the left lobe. The middle hepatic vein (dotted arrow) is being compressed by the tumor. **(B)** The inferior vena cava (dotted arrow) is being displaced medially and anteriorly by the mass, and the portal vein (solid arrow) is markedly displaced inferiorly.

used (technetium-labeled mouse antihuman monoclonal antibody to AFP).[223] After an initial decline in the AFP following liver resection, it began to increase, and an anti-AFP nuclear medicine study accurately located an active tumor in the remaining liver.

Recently, a new marker has been found for hepatoblastoma. Glypican 3 (GPC3) has been detected in hepatic stem cells and has been identified as being expressed by fetal, embryonal, and small cell undifferentiated hepatoblastomas. This marker is also shed by the tumor cells and has the potential to be used as a serum marker for hepatoblastoma.[224]

Staging

Two staging systems are currently used. In the USA, a combined histologic and surgical staging system is used by the Children's Oncology Group (COG) (Table 67-3).[225] This tumor staging system is self-explanatory and is based on information gathered before any chemotherapy is started. The second staging system, used by the International Society of Pediatric Oncology (SIOP), is based on the radiologic location of the tumor before treatment and is called the PRETEXT (Pretreatment Extent of Disease) Grouping System (Fig. 67-14).[226] Both of these staging systems are currently being used in ongoing studies so patient groups can be compared across different study groups.

In the PRETEXT system, the liver is divided into four sections: the anterior and posterior sectors on the right, and the medial and lateral sectors on the left. Therefore, based on the extent of the tumor, the patient is classified as follows: PRETEXT 1, with three adjoining sectors free (tumor in only one sector); PRETEXT 2, with two

TABLE 67-3 Children's Oncology Group Staging System and Outcomes

Stage	Description	Five-Year Survival
I	Complete resection, clear margin, pure fetal histology	100%
IU	Complete resection, clear margin, unfavorable histology	98%
II	Gross total resection with microscopic residual or perioperative rupture	100%
III	Unresectable or resection with gross residual or lymph node involvement	69%
IV	Metastatic disease	37%

From Ortega J, Siegel S. Biological markers in pediatric cancer. In: Pizzo P, Poplack D, editors. Principles and Practice of Pediatric Oncology. Philadelphia: Lippincott; 1989. p. 149–62, with permission.

adjoining sectors free (two sectors involved); PRETEXT 3, in which only one sector is free or a total of three nonadjoining sectors are involved (tumor involves two or three sectors); and PRETEXT 4, in which no sector is free (tumor in all four sectors). It also takes into account hepatic vein or portal vein involvement, if extrahepatic spread has occurred (enlargement of the hilar lymph nodes), or if metastases are found. Both staging systems have been shown to have direct correlations with patient survival (Table 67-4).

In addition to the staging systems, in upcoming protocols, the patients will also be stratified according to risk. In the COG staging system, low-risk patients will be

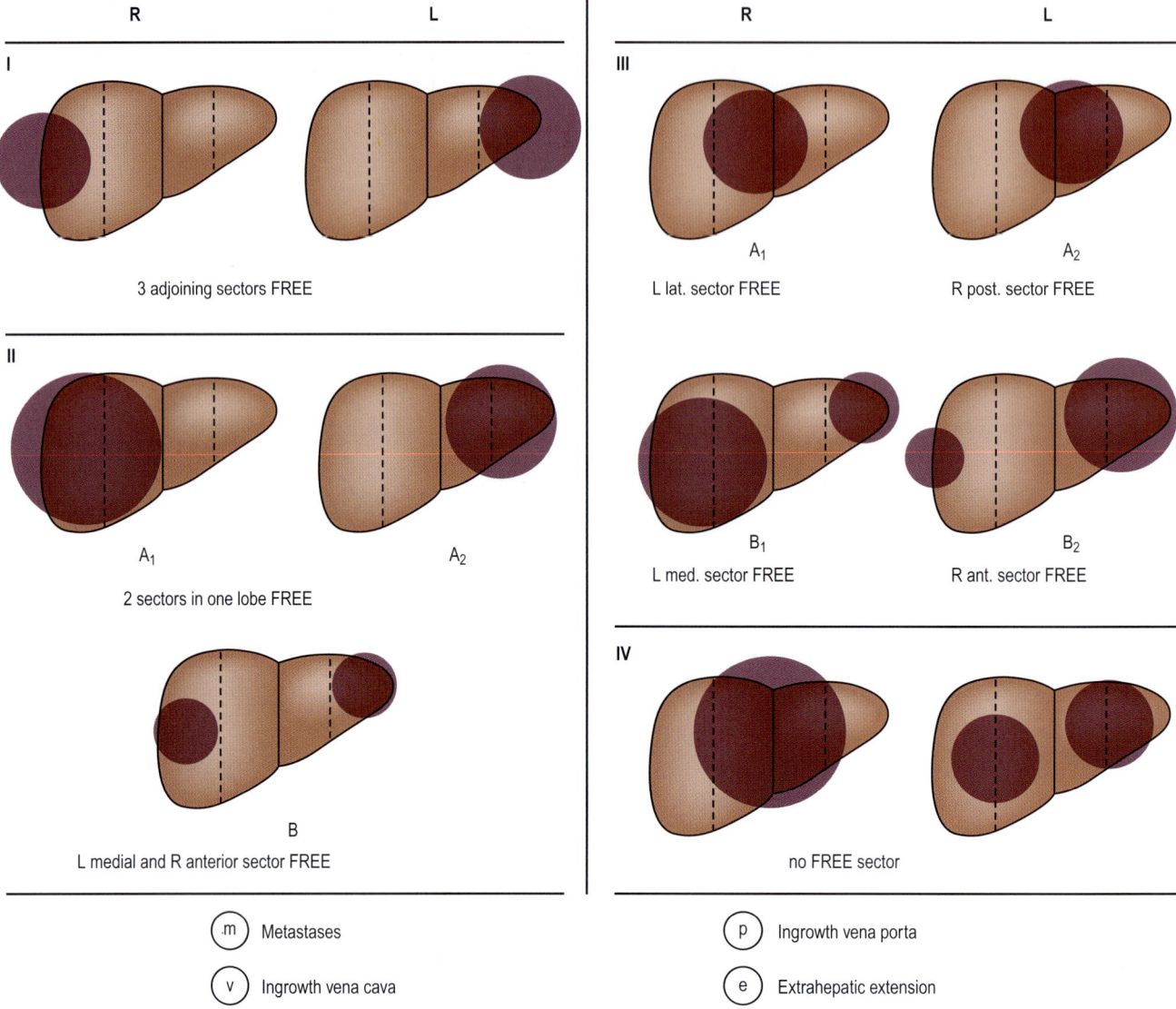

R   L

I

3 adjoining sectors FREE

II

A₁   A₂

2 sectors in one lobe FREE

B

L medial and R anterior sector FREE

R   L

III

A₁
L lat. sector FREE   A₂
R post. sector FREE

B₁
L med. sector FREE   B₂
R ant. sector FREE

IV

no FREE sector

ⓜ Metastases

ⓥ Ingrowth vena cava

ⓟ Ingrowth vena porta

ⓔ Extrahepatic extension

FIGURE 67-14 ■ PRETEXT (Pretreatment Extent of Disease) staging system. Stage is determined by the number of liver sectors free of tumor.

TABLE 67-4 SIOP PRETEXT Staging and Outcome

Stage	Five-Year Survival
I	100%
II	91%
III	68%
IV	57%

SIOP, International Society of Pediatric Oncology.
From Brown J, Perilongo G, Shafford E, et al. Pretreatment prognostic factors for children with hepatoblastoma: Results from the International Society of Pediatric Oncology (SIOP) Study SIOPEL 1. Eur J Cancer 2000;36:1418–25.

stage I/II without unfavorable biologic features, intermediate-risk patients will be stage III or stage I/II with small cell undifferentiated histology, and high-risk patients will be stage IV or stage I, II, III with an AFP less than 100 ng/mL at diagnosis. In the SIOPEL studies, the patients are stratified into standard risk (PRETEXT I, II, III) or high risk (PRETEXT IV or any tumor with metastases, vena cava or portal vein invasion, contiguous extrahepatic disease, or tumors with an AFP <100 ng/mL at presentation).[227]

Treatment

The treatment of hepatoblastoma requires a multidisciplinary approach. Except on very rare occasions, chemotherapy alone is unable to eradicate the tumor. The only chance for a long-term cure is complete resection of the primary tumor. This goal can be achieved by the use of either traditional hepatic resections (right lobectomy: segments 5–8; left lobectomy: segments 2–4; or left lateral segmentectomy: segments 2–3) or extended resections (right trisegmentectomy: segments 4–8; or left trisegmentectomies: segments 2–4, 5, 8). The resection can be performed using either open or laparoscopic techniques. There have been several case reports and two large series of laparoscopic liver resections in adults for both benign and malignant disease.[228–231] The outcomes of these laparoscopic series have been identical to the results of resections by an open approach.

The resection should be planned so that there is an anticipated margin of normal liver around the tumor. Fortunately, this margin does not need to be large (2–3 mm).[232] If it is doubtful that the tumor can be resected with a clear margin, then the patient should undergo preoperative chemotherapy to try to reduce the size of the tumor to the point where complete resection is possible. In several studies, only between 30% and 50% of the patients were able to undergo either a complete or gross total resection of the tumor at the initial procedure.[233,234] In the COG trials, only 23% of the patients initially presented with stage I or stage II disease.[235]

If a difficult liver resection is elected, the conundrum exists as to what to do if the resection is unsuccessful and microscopic residual disease is left after a resection. The data from the COG studies, SIOPEL-1 and SIOPEL-2, indicate that microscopic residual disease after resection can be successfully treated with additional chemotherapy.[208,236,237] On the other hand, several series have reported that the most common reason for tumor recurrence is either a gross or microscopically incomplete resection.[238–241] If local recurrence of the tumor occurs, the prognosis is poor.[222,242,243] 'Rescue' transplantation for local recurrence results in a survival rate of only 30%.[244] This would suggest that there must be multiple, yet to be defined, variables that determine if microscopic disease can be eradicated or if it will result in recurrent disease. In any case, there must be careful thought before undertaking a 'difficult' liver resection when the possibility exists of leaving residual disease versus referring the patient directly for liver transplant evaluation.

If chemotherapy is necessary, it should be noted that there are two distinct approaches to its utilization in the treatment of hepatoblastoma. The COG approach is based on the premise that all patients who present with hepatoblastoma should be evaluated for a primary resection. If this is not possible, then the patient receives chemotherapy with the goal of shrinking the tumor to the point where it is resectable. The intent of this approach is to limit the patient's exposure to chemotherapeutic drugs that carry significant side effects including renal, cardiac, and ototoxicity. The SIOP approach is fundamentally different in that all their patients receive chemotherapy before any consideration for resection. The logic behind this approach is that chemotherapy will provide multiple benefits, such as shrinking the tumor, thereby potentially decreasing the size and risks of hepatic resection, decreasing the viability of the tumor prior to surgical manipulation, and decreasing the vascularity of the tumor. The SIOP group uses the PRETEXT staging system, but the correlation between survival and PRETEXT stage is based on the fact that all PRETEXT staged tumors (regardless of stage) have received chemotherapy. It should be noted that neither approach has been proved to be superior to the other in multiple, multicenter trials.

Multiple chemotherapy regimens have been evaluated for hepatoblastoma.[225,245] The most active chemotherapy agent for hepatoblastoma is cisplatin. This drug is then combined with either vincristine, doxorubicin, or 5-fluorouracil, and used in either an adjuvant or neoadjuvant fashion. The current recommended COG chemotherapy regimen for initially unresectable hepatoblastoma is doxorubicin, cisplatin, 5-fluorouracil, and vincristine.[246] In the patients who have had complete resection of their tumor (without preoperative chemotherapy), either four to six postoperative courses of chemotherapy are given. In those children in whom the liver tumor was deemed unresectable at the initial operation (stage III disease), two rounds of chemotherapy are initially given, followed by repeat imaging.

If the tumor appears resectable, then resection should be done at this time. If the tumor is not resectable, then the patient undergoes an additional two rounds of chemotherapy. In addition, the patient also needs to be referred to a center where there is the option for transplantation. If after the additional two rounds of chemotherapy the tumor is resectable (total of four rounds), then resection is performed (Fig. 67-15). With chemotherapy and delayed or second-look surgery, the resection rate has been reported to increase to between 69% and 98% (Fig. 67-16).[5,247–249] In patients with stage IV disease (initially unresectable), only 40% of these tumors were rendered resectable after four rounds of chemotherapy. If the tumor is still unresectable, the patient needs to be evaluated and listed for a liver transplant.

Current United Network Organ Sharing (UNOS) policy allows hepatoblastoma patients to be listed as status 1B in order to maximize their chance of being transplanted within one month of listing. Preferably the

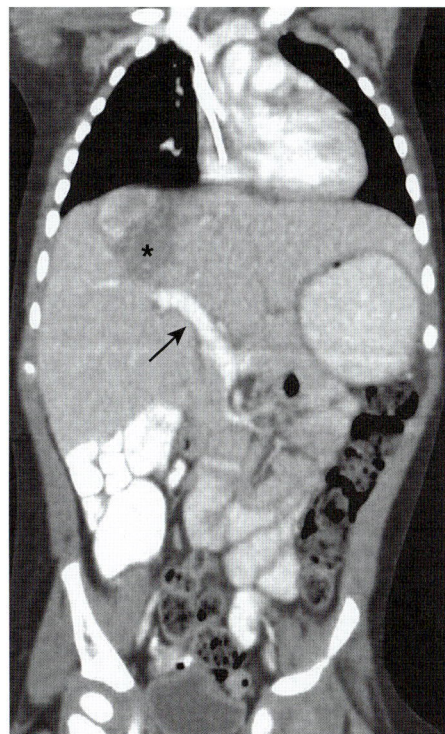

FIGURE 67-15 ■ After four cycles of chemotherapy, the CT scan showed marked diminution in the size of the mass (asterisk). Note the portal vein (solid arrow) has returned to its normal anatomic position. Compare with the prechemotherapy CT scan seen in Figure 67-13.

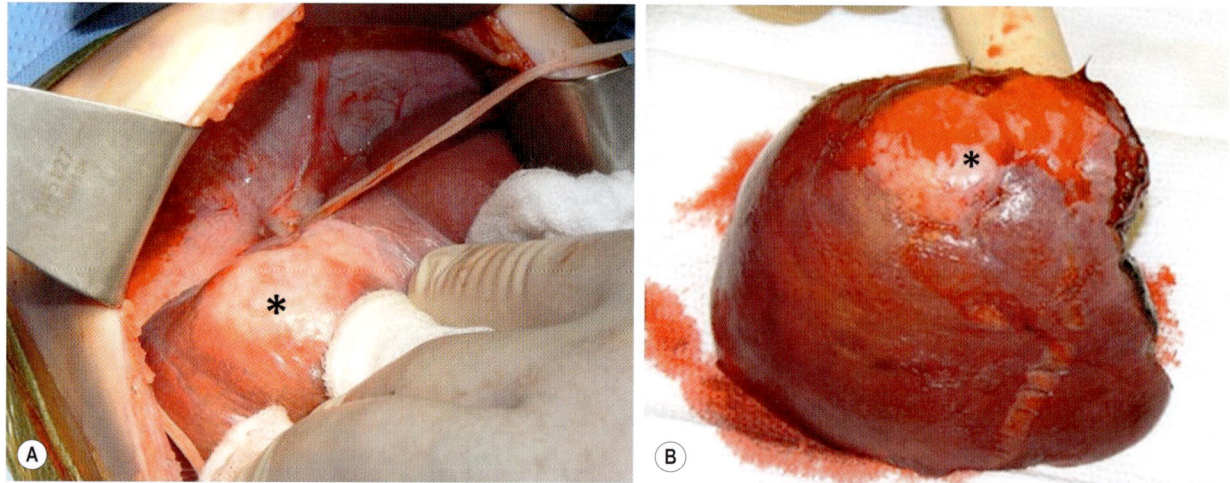

FIGURE 67-16 ■ Operative findings of the patient whose CT scans are seen in Figures 67-13 and 67-15. **(A)** An umbilical tape has been used to encircle the middle hepatic vein. Note the residual tumor (asterisk) in the cephalad portion of the right hepatic lobe. **(B)** The right hepatic lobe containing the lesion (asterisk) is seen. It was possible to obtain a normal margin of liver in the left lobe, but a trisegmentectomy was needed.

time between the last round of chemotherapy and transplantation should be less than four weeks because it is now known that up to 80% of hepatoblastomas will develop drug resistance after four to five courses of chemotherapy.[248,250] After transplant, the patient receives a final two rounds of chemotherapy.

Some newer chemotherapy agents have been investigated for hepatoblastoma. Topotecan inhibits growth and neovascularization in a mouse model.[251] In addition, the suppressive effects of the topotecan lasted several weeks after discontinuation of the agent. Irinotecan appears to have some promise in salvaging patients who have recurrent disease. This drug could potentially be added to front-line chemotherapy regimens.[252] High-dose chemotherapy with stem cell rescue has been attempted but has not been successful.

Another approach to the unresectable hepatoblastoma is the use of preoperative chemoembolization. In one study, transarterial catheterization with selective tumor chemoembolization was able to shrink the tumor by an average of 26%, which allowed subsequent complete tumor resection in every case.[253] Interestingly, the surgical specimens showed only minimally viable or no viable tumor. It was postulated that this technique may be useful not only as a therapeutic modality for unresectable hepatoblastomas but also potentially for resectable tumors that could be made minimally viable to nonviable before surgical intervention.[254]

Another therapeutic dilemma occurs in the child first seen with a ruptured tumor. In one review, all three patients who survived the initial rupture had no evidence of recurrent disease, with a mean survival of 36 months.[255] Even though tumor rupture and peritoneal soiling occurred, no peritoneal growths were subsequently identified in any patient.

Outcome

Patient-outcome studies have been based on histologic type, the extent of the original tumor, or tumor response to chemotherapy.[206] Several studies have shown a good outcome with fetal histology and with complete resection of the tumor.[51,194,209,256,257] All the studies that have consistently shown a good outcome based on fetal histology have limited this diagnosis to tumors with a mitotic activity less than two per ten high-power fields. Conversely, several studies have consistently reported a poor outcome for those patients who have small cell undifferentiated hepatoblastoma.[207] Except for these data, no consistent correlation has been found with any of the other histologic patterns and patient outcomes.

The AFP level also has been found to have both prognostic and therapeutic implications. Patients with an AFP level less than 100 ng/mL or greater than 1 million ng/mL have a worse prognosis.[258] The low AFP group comprised patients with small cell undifferentiated tumors, suggesting that a low AFP level could be related to a very primitive and poorly differentiated tumor that was unable to make AFP.[259] Patients who had a slow decline in their AFP levels, either after resection or chemotherapy, had a worse long-term prognosis than did those who had an early, very rapid decline (>99% drop in AFP levels).[260]

The best survival rate in patients with hepatoblastoma is for those tumors with pure fetal histology. A recent COG study demonstrated that after complete surgical resection of a stage I tumor with pure fetal histology, the patient can be carefully monitored with no further therapy.[261] However, if an area of undifferentiated small cell histology is noted within an otherwise pure fetal histology tumor, then aggressive chemotherapy should be instituted.[207]

In another COG study, the 3-year event free survival (EFS) was 90% for stage I/II tumors, 50% for stage III tumors, and only 20% for stage IV tumors.[262] The European SIOPEL-2 study reported that the 3-year survival for standard risk tumors was 90% and was 50% for high-risk tumors. These data compare favorably with those of a large German series that noted an EFS of 100% for stage I, 80% for stage II, and 68% for stage III disease.[249]

None of the patients with stage IV disease in the German trial survived. In another prospective study, the German group showed that the important prognostic factors for survival appeared to be the tumor growth pattern, vascular invasion, and serum AFP levels.[257,263]

As the patients in the high-risk PRETEXT or COG trials have poor outcomes despite a complete surgical resection, additional or different chemotherapy regimens are necessary to improve patient survival in these groups.[257] Currently there are ongoing studies that are evaluating the possibility of modifying different cellular or gene targets in hepatoblastoma cells that will make them more susceptible to chemotherapy.[264]

There are several treatment options currently under clinical evaluation by COG. For more information on ongoing studies, please check the COG website (www.childrensoncologygroup.org).

Transplantation

Once a patient has completed four rounds of chemotherapy, a decision is made to either perform a resection with the goal of complete tumor excision or to refer the patient for liver transplantation. Several characteristics of hepatoblastoma have recently been reported as indicators of unresectability. Patients with these indicators are possible candidates for liver transplantation. Patients who were younger than 3 years of age at presentation tend to respond better to chemotherapy with greater reductions in tumor size when compared with older children.[265] Bilobar, multifocal tumors at presentation are candidates for transplantation because, despite apparent radiologic clearing of a lobe after chemotherapy, microscopic disease can persist in the liver leading to later recurrent disease.[236,266,267] Patients who present with low AFP levels (<100 ng/mL) tend not to respond to chemotherapy, so they should be considered for either upfront resection or transplantation. Patients who have tumor extension into the inferior vena cava, all three hepatic veins, or the bifurcation of the portal vein are unlikely to sufficiently shrink their tumor with chemotherapy to allow a complete resection and therefore should be considered as possible candidates for transplantation.[244]

Orthotopic liver transplantation is a successful treatment for unresectable hepatoblastoma.[268] A recurrence-free survival rate of between 79% and 92% has been reported.[244,269,270] In several series, an important prognostic factor that predicted good results after transplantation was a good initial response to chemotherapy. In one series, only 60% of the patients who were poor responders are currently alive, with a follow-up of less than 1 year.[269] As mentioned previously, liver transplantation for local tumor recurrence after resection is associated with a post-transplant recurrence rate of 30%.

Although two post-transplant rounds of chemotherapy are currently utilized, one multicenter review noted no significant difference in survival rates between those patients who received chemotherapy (77%) versus those who did not (70%).[241,271–273]

Patients with extrahepatic metastases found on initial evaluation can be successfully treated with liver transplantation if the metastatic disease is eradicated before the transplant. Hepatoblastoma commonly metastasizes to the lungs, and lung metastases are often present at diagnosis. Because this tumor tends to be chemoresponsive, these metastases will often disappear after the first several rounds of chemotherapy. If the pulmonary metastases do not resolve, then current data would suggest that these patients should undergo a metastasectomy for any remaining disease, either before or shortly after hepatic resection, and before consideration for transplantation. This approach has been successful in increasing patient survival.[274,275] Unfortunately the data on resection of pulmonary recurrences are less optimistic. There may be a role for resection of late pulmonary metastasis in patients who presented with stage I disease. However, pulmonary relapse in stage III and IV disease portends a poor prognosis that is not changed by lung resection.

Undifferentiated Embryonal Sarcoma

Incidence

Undifferentiated embryonal sarcoma of the liver makes up about 7% of the solid liver tumors in children.[1] Unfortunately, this is a very malignant tumor with a poor outcome.

Clinical Presentation

Undifferentiated embryonal sarcoma most commonly affects children between the ages of 6 and 10 years, but has been reported in a child as young as 19 months.[276] A slight male predominance has been noted. The most common clinical presentation is either right upper quadrant or epigastric pain with or without a palpable abdominal mass. Occasionally, marked hepatomegaly is seen without a definite mass. Rarely, this tumor can even masquerade as a hepatic abscess or infection.[277] Other nonspecific presenting complaints can include vomiting, anorexia, and lethargy. Laboratory studies, including AFP level, are usually normal.

Imaging

On ultrasound examination, the lesion appears predominantly solid.[278] However, on CT and MRI, the lesion appears cystic without any significant solid component (Fig. 67-17). This same type of disparity has been reported only in Wilms' tumor metastatic to the liver. Thus, it appears that such a discrepancy between the two imaging techniques would be highly suggestive of an undifferentiated embryonal sarcoma.

Histology

Undifferentiated embryonal sarcoma is a neoplasm with a very primitive mesenchymal phenotype. These tumors tend to occur predominantly in the right lobe of the liver and to be large, with an average diameter of 14–21 cm.[278] In cross section, the tumors are often variegated, with white mucoid or gelatinous areas alternating with other areas of tumor necrosis and hemorrhage (Fig. 67-18).

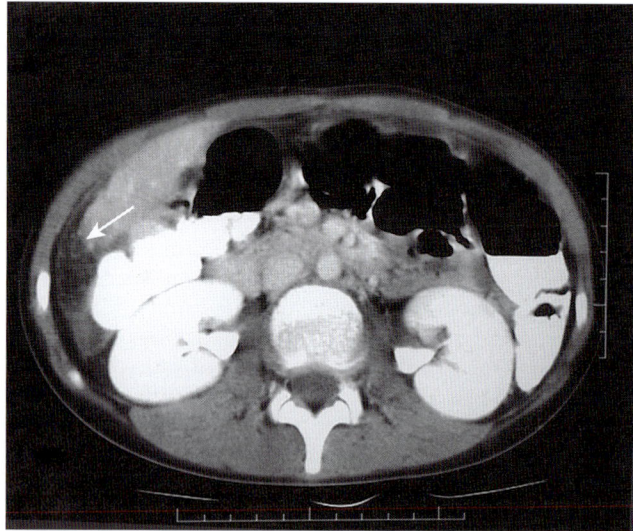

FIGURE 67-17 ■ CT scan of an undifferentiated embryonal sarcoma after intravenous administration of a contrast agent shows a hypodense area (arrow) in the right lobe of the liver.

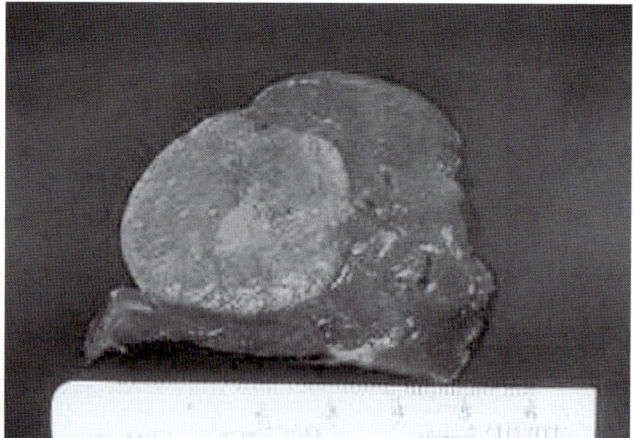

FIGURE 67-18 ■ Note the variegated appearance on cut section of an undifferentiated embryonal sarcoma.

The tumor typically is well demarcated from the adjacent liver by a compressed, fibrous pseudocapsule.[276]

On microscopic section, these tumors are composed of medium to large spindle- to stellate-type cells in a variable amount of myxoid stroma (Fig. 67-19). The cells are usually densely arranged in a myxomatous background. In the periphery, entrapped bile ducts or hepatic cords have been noted.[4,276] Mitoses are frequent and usually bizarre.

No characteristic immunohistochemical stain pattern has been identified for embryonal sarcoma.[279] The only consistent cell markers have been vimentin and the 'histiocytic' determinants α1-antitrypsin and α-antichymotrypsin.[280,281]

In a cytogenetic study, extensive chromosomal rearrangements were noted to be very similar to other soft tissue sarcomas such as leiomyosarcoma, osteosarcoma, and malignant fibrous histiocytoma.[282] In only a few cytometric studies, the tumors have ranged from diploid to tetraploid to aneuploid.[283,284]

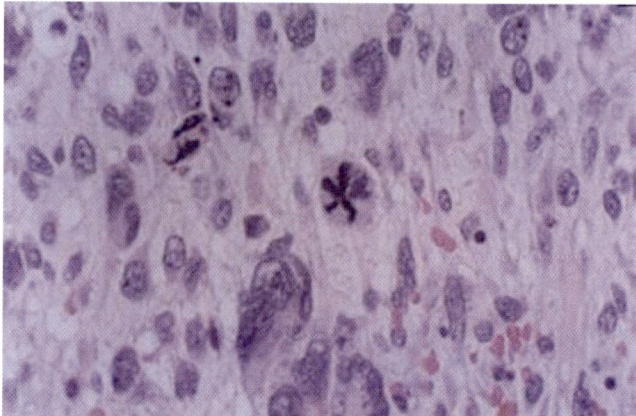

FIGURE 67-19 ■ Histology of undifferentiated embryonal sarcoma shows large spindle cells with multiple mitoses.

Treatment

In addition to the highly suggestive radiologic findings, these patients can be diagnosed by fine needle aspiration. Two separate reports have noted that the cytologic features of undifferentiated embryonal sarcoma are distinctive and different from other childhood tumors.[285,286]

The initial experience with undifferentiated embryonal sarcoma of the liver was poor. In a review of patients treated from 1950 to 1988, only 37% of the patients were noted to survive.[284] This tumor usually proves fatal because of massive upper abdominal growth with secondary involvement of the diaphragm, stomach, abdominal wall, ribs, or pancreas rather than by metastases. Occasionally, intra-abdominal dissemination of the tumor can occur, causing diffuse matting of the small bowel. Pulmonary and pleural metastases have been noted but are much less common than the secondary involvement of the extrahepatic tissue by direct extension.[276]

The only chance for cure is radical excision.[287,288] Unfortunately, despite complete resection of the tumor, many patients have recurrent disease, which suggests the need for postoperative chemotherapy.[289]

The chemotherapy regimens that have been used are based on nonrhabdomyosarcomatous soft tissue sarcoma-type protocols.[290] With these regimens, survival rates have improved to 66%, because these tumors are very chemotherapy sensitive.[291,292] This finding has led to the use of preoperative chemotherapy to shrink an unresectable tumor to a size at which a radical hepatic resection is possible.[293] This is similar to the approach used to manage an initially nonresectable hepatoblastoma.

With the ongoing improvement in chemotherapy regimens for sarcomas, the previously bleak outlook for this tumor is now much more optimistic. The use of an aggressive chemotherapy regimen, along with complete resection of the primary tumor, has resulted in a 37% survival rate in patients whose tumors initially presented as free intraperitoneal rupture.[292]

Moreover, a prospective series from the Italian and German Soft Tissue Sarcoma Cooperative Groups reported a protocol that included surgery or biopsy followed by neoadjuvant chemotherapy for four cycles. This was followed by second-look surgery to try to remove residual tumor followed by additional chemotherapy. In their series, ten of 17 patients survived with complete remission.[294]

In patients in whom complete resection of the tumor is not possible despite chemotherapy, liver transplantation has been advocated as another possible means for complete excision.[295,296] This aggressive approach is reasonable because these tumors are sensitive to chemotherapy.

Hepatocellular Carcinoma

Hepatocellular carcinoma (HCC) is a relatively rare, highly malignant tumor that is more commonly seen in adults than in children. It is the second most common pediatric liver tumor, occurring about 19% of the time, but it still comprises less than 1% of all pediatric cancers.[297] Its peak incidence is between 10 and 15 years, and it is more common in boys.[298]

The predisposing factors for HCC are distinctly different between children and adults. In adults, cirrhosis seems to be the primary etiology. The cirrhosis is usually seen in patients with either hepatitis B, hepatitis C, genetic hemochromatosis, alcohol-related cirrhosis, or cirrhosis due to primary biliary cirrhosis. In a recent review, it was noted that patients in these groups were at a significantly increased risk for developing HCC.[299] Hepatic ultrasound and serum AFP evaluations every 6 months were recommended in these populations to detect this tumor at an early stage.

In contrast, cirrhosis is often not part of the antecedent process in children. Moreover, a previous congenital or acquired disorder of the liver may be found (Box 67-3).[300] HCC in children has been associated with a variety of metabolic, familial, and infectious disorders. Some of these metabolic disorders include tyrosinemia,

α1-antitrypsin deficiency, and hemochromatosis.[301] Patients with tyrosinemia seem to be at a particularly high risk for development of HCC. Because of this high prevalence rate, it has been suggested that liver transplantation be performed in this population before age 2 years.[302,303] HCC also has been seen in patients with type 1 GSD. Most hepatic masses that develop in this population are hepatic adenomas, but carcinomas do present a real risk in this group[304] A variety of other noncirrhotic liver diseases also have been associated with HCC, including familial polyposis, Gardner syndrome, Sotos syndrome, Blum syndrome, neurofibromatosis, Abernathy malformation, methotrexate therapy, and neonatal hepatitis. There is also an association with parenteral nutrition.[305–310]

Congenital and infectious disorders also are associated with this tumor, including extrahepatic biliary atresia, congenital hepatic fibrosis, Alagille syndrome, persistent familial intrahepatic cholestasis (PFIC),[311] hepatitis B, and hepatitis C. In areas where hepatitis B is endemic, it ranks fifth in the causes of childhood malignancies and outnumbers hepatoblastoma by 3 : 1.[312] The importance of hepatitis B and the subsequent development of HCC in children is highlighted by the aggressive hepatitis B vaccination program that began in 1984 in Taiwan.[313] When the mortality from liver carcinoma in the group from birth to age 9 years was compared between the years 1984 and 1993, a substantial and statistically significant decrease in the mortality was seen by 1993. Similar results have been found in Gambia and the USA.[313] Hepatitis C also has been linked to the development of hepatocellular carcinoma.[314] In contrast to hepatitis B, the cirrhosis and the subsequent development of HCC in the hepatitis C population usually takes several decades to develop.[315]

Of particular interest is the association between HCC and biliary atresia.[298,316] In a review, except for one patient first seen at age 5 months, all the other patients were older than 2 years with a mean of age 7.5 years when the HCC was discovered. These tumors were found either at autopsy or incidentally at the time of liver transplantation for biliary atresia. In those patients in whom HCC was identified at the time of transplantation, all of these patients are alive and well after transplant. This association between HCC and biliary atresia, or any other disease that leads to hepatic cirrhosis, suggests that a routine screening protocol every 6 months with hepatic ultrasound and AFP levels is warranted.[317]

Clinical Presentation

Most patients are initially seen with either an abdominal mass or abdominal pain. Other associated symptoms include nausea and vomiting, anorexia, malaise, and a significant weight loss. As many as 10% are seen initially with tumor rupture and hemoperitoneum.[318] More than one-third of HCCs appear as multiple nodules rather than a single tumor.[319]

Laboratory studies can show mild elevations in the serum glutamic oxaloacetic transaminase (SGOT) and lactic dehydrogenase (LDH) levels. The AFP is elevated in about 85% of patients but can be normal or only mildly elevated with the fibrolamellar variant.[318, 320] An elevated

BOX 67-3	**Conditions Associated with Hepatocellular Carcinoma in Children**

α1-Antitrypsin deficiency
Anomalies of abdominal venous drainage (Abernathy syndrome)
Alagille syndrome
Biliary atresia
Congenital hepatic fibrosis
Familial hepatocellular carcinoma
Familial polyposis
Focal nodular hyperplasia of the liver
Gardner syndrome
Hepatic adenoma
Hepatitis B infection
Hepatitis C infection
Hereditary tyrosinemia
Hyperalimentation
Progressive familial intrahepatic cholestasis
Methotrexate therapy
Oral contraceptives
Glycogen storage disease - types I and III
Wilms tumor
Wilson disease

AFP is associated with an increased risk for recurrence after resection and therefore reflects a worse prognosis.[321,322]

Imaging

CT and MRI are both helpful for delineating the mass and for determining resectability. With the advent of spiral CT with intravenous bolus contrast administration, the hepatic veins and portal venous system can be well delineated, and any tumor involvement can be adequately assessed. The American Association for the Study of Liver Diseases has published criteria for the noninvasive diagnosis of HCC. In nodules less than 2 cm in diameter in cirrhotic livers, the diagnosis of HCC can be made without biopsy of the lesion if two coincidental dynamic imaging studies (e.g., CT/MRI) reveal arterial-phase hypervascularity followed by wash-out in the portal venous phase.[323] The fibrolamellar variant is notable as a hypodense, single or multilobed mass on CT that tends to be hypervascular as well as sometimes showing a central scar.[324] This appearance could easily be confused with FNH, and care must be taken to distinguish between these two lesions.

Histology

HCC can vary in size from 2–25 cm, and the surrounding liver can exhibit either micro- or macronodular cirrhosis in up to 60% of cases (Figs 67-20 and 67-21).[1] Microscopically, trabeculae that are two to ten cell layers in thickness are seen with the larger trabeculae sometimes displaying central necrosis. The individual cells are usually larger than normal hepatocytes, with nuclear hypochromasia and frequent and bizarre mitosis (Fig. 67-22). Vascular invasion may be prominent. Tumors less than 2 cm generally are well differentiated. Over time, as the tumor grows, the original tumor cells are replaced by poorly differentiated cell clones.[325] Moreover, as the tumor enlarges, its blood supply becomes more dependent on newly formed arterial vessels and less dependent on the portal circulation. This imbalance between the hepatic arterial and portal venous supply leads to the hypervascular pattern that is the radiologic hallmark for HCC.

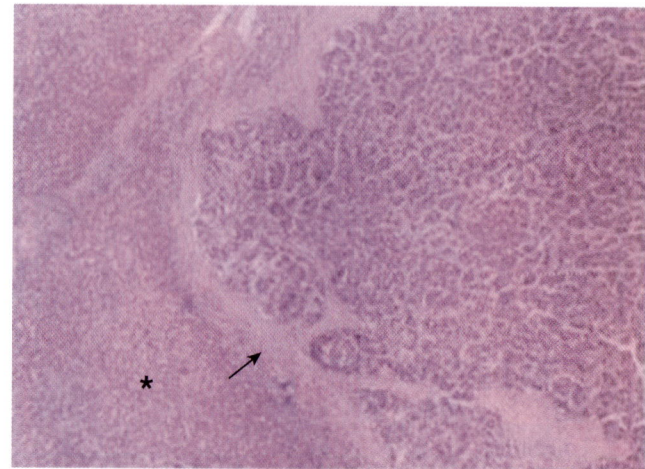

FIGURE 67-21 ■ This histologic photomicrograph shows hepatocellular carcinoma with surrounding cirrhosis (arrow) and uninvolved liver (asterisk).

In the fibrolamellar variant, the hepatocytes are large, deeply eosinophilic, and embedded within a lamellar fibrosis. Clusters of cells are often separated by broad bands of laminated collagen.[1,326] The presence of large amounts of fibrosis alone is not sufficient in itself for the diagnosis of fibrolamellar carcinoma.[327]

Treatment

The treatment of HCC for stages I and II is complete surgical resection followed by chemotherapy. A COG study in 2002 reported that seven of eight patients with stage I disease survived after adjuvant cisplatin-based chemotherapy.[328] Moreover, it has been postulated that routine use of chemotherapy with cisplatin and doxorubicin may benefit children with completely resected HCC.[5,329]

Unfortunately, primary resection is not always possible because either the tumor is bilobar or the tumor is associated with cirrhosis. Because of the cirrhosis, concern may exist that the hepatic resection might leave the patient with insufficient functioning parenchyma.

In one pediatric report of 49 children, resection was possible in only 10%. Only two patients lived for more

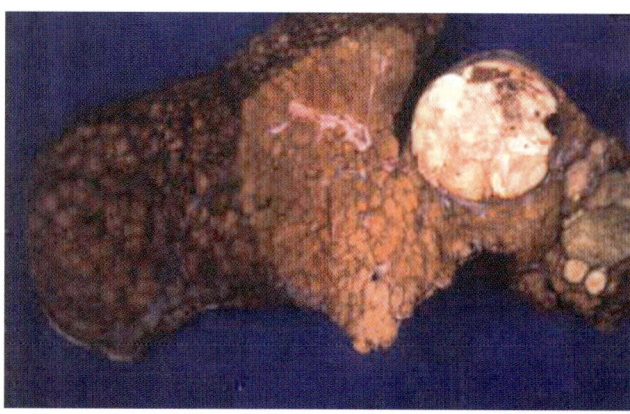

FIGURE 67-20 ■ Hepatocellular carcinoma in the setting of cirrhosis.

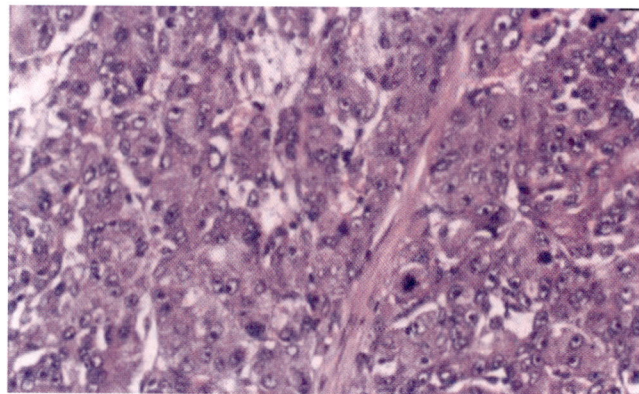

FIGURE 67-22 ■ Histology of a hepatocellular carcinoma demonstrating enlarged hepatocytes and nuclear hypochromasia.

than 2 years.[312] If a complete, microscopically free, radical resection is possible, the prognosis can be good, with an 80–90% survival.[330] Unfortunately, the overall cure rate for this tumor in children is a dismal 15%. In the adult population, 3-year survival rates between 34–57% have been reported.[331,332] Multiple studies have looked at prognostic factors that influence outcome and recurrence after resection for HCC. Multiple staging systems have been proposed based on multivariant analyses of various prognostic factors. Three factors that have been repeatedly associated with improved survival and decreased recurrence rates are small tumor size (<2 cm), the number of tumor nodules, and a histologic increase in tumor microvascular density. These findings are highly predictive of tumor relapse after resection.[333] Unfortunately, it is rare to see patients initially with all three favorable variables. In most series, the tumors are usually larger than 5 cm in diameter at presentation.[331,334]

An important variant that should be mentioned is the fibrolamellar type. Only in the 1980s did this variant become established as a histologic and clinically distinct entity.[335] This lesion is characterized by relatively slow growth and occurs almost exclusively in a noncirrhotic liver.[326] The fibrolamellar variant usually occurs in adolescents and young adults, with a peak incidence in the second decade of life.[336,337] It accounts for between 16–50% of HCC diagnosed in patients younger than 21 years of age.[338] In contrast to conventional HCC, fibrolamellar carcinoma is not associated with risk factors such as cirrhosis or chronic hepatitis B infection.[339,340] However, an association does exist between FNH and the fibrolamellar variant.

Radiologically, the fibrolamellar variant is often hypodense on noncontrast CT and can show variable perfusion, including hypervascularity, on contrast CT. In addition, a central hypodense or hypervascular area can be seen that can mimic a central scar.[341] This can create confusion between the diagnosis of the fibrolamellar variant and FNH. MRI may be helpful in distinguishing between these two diagnoses.[342] The results after resection for fibrolamellar carcinoma in adults are very good, with 50% 5-year survivals. However, after apparent curative resections, recurrences or metastases can occur after very long disease-free intervals.[343,344] Unfortunately when the fibrolamellar variant was examined in children, there was no survival benefit to this diagnosis.[262]

Transplantation for Hepatocellular Carcinoma

Liver transplantation has been used as curative therapy for HCC.[272,345] The early experience of liver transplantation in adults for HCC was discouraging.[346] However, in a review of 344 patients who underwent liver transplantation for HCC (excluding the fibrolamellar type), three factors were associated with tumor-free survival: a unilobar tumor, a tumor smaller than 2 cm, and the absence of vascular invasion.[347] Two different pretransplant selection criteria are currently being utilized in adults (Table 67-5).

The Milan criteria are widely recognized as excellent predictors of a low recurrence rate after transplantation.[348] These criteria, however, have not been verified in

TABLE 67-5 Milan and UCSF Transplant Criteria for Hepatocellular Carcinoma

	Milan Criteria	UCSF Criteria
Single tumor maximum diameter	≤5.0 cm	≤6.5 cm
Maximum number	3	3
Largest tumor size	≤3.0 cm	≤4.5 cm
Total tumor size	NA	≤8.0 cm

NA, not applicable; UCSF, University of California at San Francisco.

the pediatric population, and their applicability in children is unclear.[349] As HCC can be a rapidly growing tumor, it is common for the tumor to exceed these criteria by the time an organ becomes available and the patient is no longer a candidate for transplant. The University of California at San Francisco criteria are an attempt to allow an increased pretransplant tumor burden and still have a low post-transplant recurrence rate. Several studies have supported this hypothesis.[350,351]

Two absolute contraindications to transplantation for HCC in children are extrahepatic spread and macroscopic vascular invasion.[272] The SIOPEL-1 study reported no long-term survivors among those who failed to respond to chemotherapy.[352] Therefore, the lack of response to preoperative chemotherapy is a relative contraindication to transplantation. Despite these possible limitations, liver transplantation in children for HCC has a very good five-year survival rate between 63–89%.[272,353] Both adult and child patients are given additional points in the UNOS matching system so they can be transplanted before the tumor progresses.

Interestingly, in contrast to patients with hepatoblastoma, several studies have shown that liver transplantation is an appropriate salvage procedure for patients with HCC who experience a recurrence after a resection. Their post-transplant survival is comparable to that of patients who underwent primary transplantation for HCC.[354,355]

Postresection chemotherapy has been uniformly ineffective in preventing or treating recurrences in the Pediatric Oncology Group (POG), SIOPEL, and German studies.[328,352,356,357] New chemotherapeutic approaches are needed for this tumor, and currently studies are planned that will combine chemotherapeutic agents with antiangiogenic agents. However, in two small series, chemotherapy was given to children with unresectable HCC before transplant. Eighty per cent of these children had a dramatic decrease in their tumor size.[297,358] At the time of transplant, all tumors still had viable cells but only one patient after transplant had a recurrence and subsequently died.

Patients who are not surgical or transplant candidates, patients who demonstrate recurrences, or patients who are on the transplant list and their tumors have grown to the point that they exceed the Milan criteria can potentially benefit from several nonsurgical strategies, including percutaneous ethanol injection, radiofrequency ablation, or chemoembolization of the tumor.[359] All of these therapies have proved efficacious in decreasing or eradicating localized tumors, treating recurrent tumors, or shrinking tumors so that the patient again falls within the transplant criteria.[360] These therapies also improved survival with this tumor, but unfortunately, none has been proved to be curative.[299]

A catastrophic presentation of HCC is spontaneous rupture. These patients present with acute right upper quadrant pain and hypovolemic shock. The diagnosis can be made with ultrasound or abdominal CT. In the hemodynamically stable patient, the treatment is conservative with correction of volume status and correction of any coagulopathy. Then a careful assessment of the tumor needs to be made with the goal of primary resection of the tumor. If the patient is unstable, then transarterial embolization of the tumor should be performed to control the hemorrhage. After the patient's condition has stabilized, he or she needs to be evaluated for a resection.[361]

The outcome for patients with HCC, regardless of the treatment modality, is still not as good as the outcome for hepatoblastoma. Further improvements in survival for HCC will come from advances in chemotherapy regimens that will prevent tumor recurrences.

Rhabdomyosarcoma of the Biliary Tree

Incidence and Clinical Presentation

Even though rhabdomyosarcoma is the most common sarcoma in children, it accounts for only 1% of all liver tumors and only 0.8% of all rhabdomyosarcomas in children.[1,362] Hepatobiliary rhabdomyosarcoma tends to be a disease of the young, with a median age of 3 years. It is rarely seen in children older than 15 years.[363,364] This tumor most commonly arises in the intrahepatic biliary system and then extends into the liver parenchyma. It also has been reported to arise from a variety of other sites, including an intrahepatic cyst, the gallbladder, the cystic duct, the ampulla of Vater, a choledochal cyst, and the hepatic parenchyma itself.[363–369]

As it arises most commonly from the bile ducts, the most common presenting symptom is jaundice. The median tumor diameter at diagnosis is 8 cm. Therefore an abdominal mass is a common finding.[362]

Laboratory Findings and Differential Diagnosis

As jaundice is a common presenting symptom, elevated direct bilirubin, alkaline phosphatase, and γ-glutamyltransferase (GGT) levels are common. The differential diagnosis for an intraductal lesion in a child includes either an inflammatory pseudotumor or a cholangiocarcinoma, but these are extraordinarily rare.[370] If the rhabdomyosarcoma is a predominantly hepatic mass with minimal bile duct involvement, then the differential diagnosis would be more dependent on the patient's age, as noted in previous sections.

The pathology of the intraductal lesions is similar to that of rhabdomyosarcoma at extrabiliary sites. The intraductal tumor is usually either the botryoid or embryonal subtype, unless the lesion involves predominantly the hepatic parenchyma, in which the alveolar subtype predominates.[371]

Imaging

Multiple imaging modalities have been useful for diagnosis. Ultrasound typically reveals biliary dilatation and possibly a mass in the biliary system. Larger lesions may have cystic areas within them, possibly reflecting areas of partial tumor necrosis (Fig. 67-23).[217] CT will often show an intraductal mass in association with areas of low attenuation within the tumor. MRI may have an advantage over CT in that not only can it show the anatomic source and location of the mass but, with the advent of MR cholangiography, also can evaluate the bile ducts by demonstrating biliary dilatation and intraductal irregularity.[372] Percutaneous transhepatic cholangiography (PTC)

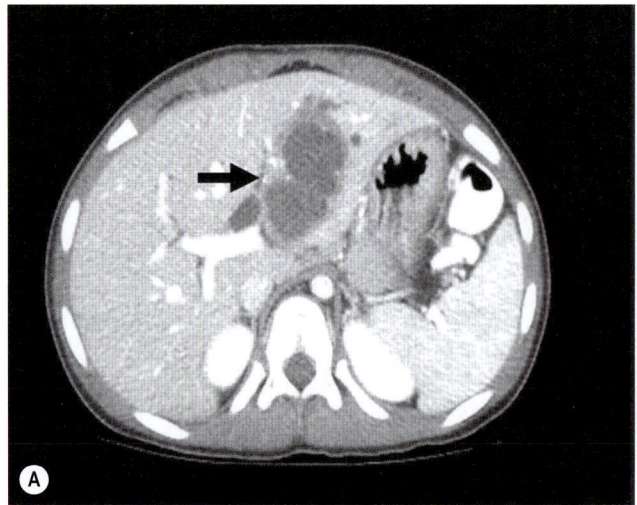
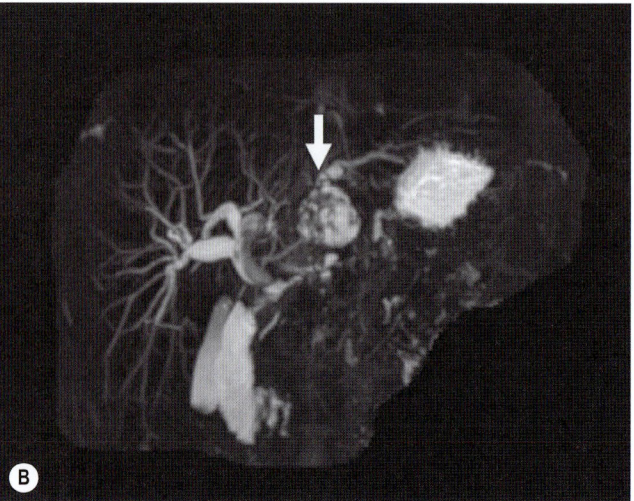

FIGURE 67-23 ■ This child was found to have a rhabdomyosarcoma of the left biliary system. **(A)** CT scan; **(B)** magnetic resonance cholangiopancreatography. The arrows point to the tumor in each study.

also can be useful in patients who have a dilated biliary system. PTC can demonstrate multiple filling defects that correspond to the intraductal tumor.[373] PTC also has the advantage of providing external drainage of the biliary system in those patients with obstructive jaundice.

Treatment and Prognosis

The best treatment for biliary rhabdomyosarcoma is a multidisciplinary approach using operation, chemotherapy, and, potentially, radiation therapy. Unfortunately, resection alone is not usually possible because of spread of the tumor into the liver parenchyma or direct local extension into the duodenum, stomach, or pancreas. It is common to find lymphatic spread at the initial operation. Because of these problems, adequate resection is usually possible in only 20–40% of the patients.[362-364] In patients in whom primary resection is not possible, the initial approach should be biopsy and lymph node sampling, followed by standard rhabdomyosarcoma chemotherapy protocols and a second-look procedure. In a study of biliary rhabdomyosarcoma that used this multimodality approach, four of ten children remained disease free after a mean of four years.[362]

REFERENCES

1. Stocker JT. Hepatic Tumors in Children. In: Suchy FJ, Sokol RJ, Balistreri WF, editors. Liver Disease in Children. 2nd ed. Philadelphia: Lippincott Williams & Wilkins; 2001. p. 915.
2. Silverberg E. Cancer statistics. 1986. CA Cancer J Clin 1986;36:9–25.
3. Couinaud C. Surgical anatomy of the liver. Several new aspects. Chirurgie 1986;112:337–42.
4. Couinaud C. The anatomy of the liver. Ann Ital Chir 1992;63:693–7.
5. Exelby PR, Filler RM, Grosfeld JL. Liver tumors in children in the particular reference to hepatoblastoma and hepatocellular carcinoma: American Academy of Pediatrics Surgical Section Survey–1974. J Pediatr Surg 1975;10:329–37.
6. Boon LM, Burrows PE, Paltiel HJ, et al. Hepatic vascular anomalies in infancy: A twenty-seven-year experience. J Pediatr 1996;129:346–54.
7. Iyer CP, Stanley P, Mahour GH. Hepatic hemangiomas in infants and children: A review of 30 cases. Am Surg 1996;62:356–60.
8. Chen CC, Kong MS, Yang CP, et al. Hepatic hemangioendothelioma in children: Analysis of thirteen cases. Acta Paediatr Taiwan 2003;44:8–13.
9. Drut RM, Drut R. Extracutaneous infantile haemangioma is also Glut1 positive. J Clin Pathol 2004;57:1197–200.
10. Riley MR, Garcia MG, Cox KL, et al. Hepatic infantile hemangioendothelioma with unusual manifestations. J Pediatr Gastroenterol Nutr 2006;42:109–13.
11. Burrows PE, Dubois J, Kassarjian A. Pediatric hepatic vascular anomalies. Pediatr Radiol 2001;31:533–45.
12. Perez J, Pardo J, Gomez C. Vincristine–an effective treatment of corticoid-resistant life-threatening infantile hemangiomas. Acta Oncol 2002;41:197–9.
13. Christison-Lagay ER, Burrows PE, Alomari A, et al. Hepatic hemangiomas: Subtype classification and development of a clinical practice algorithm and registry. J Pediatr Surg 2007;42:62–8.
14. Selby DM, Stocker JT, Waclawiw MA, et al. Infantile hemangioendothelioma of the liver. Hepatology 1994;20:39–45.
15. Novaks D, Suchy FL, Balistreri W. Disorders of the liver and biliary system relevant to clinical practice. In Feigin RD, DeAngelis CD, Douglas Jones M, editors. Oski's Principles and Practice of Pediatrics. Philadelphia: JB Lippincott; 1990. p. 1746–77.
16. Huang SA, Tu HM, Harney JW, et al. Severe hypothyroidism caused by type 3 iodothyronine deiodinase in infantile hemangiomas. N Engl J Med 2000;343:185–9.
17. Mason KP, Koka BV, Eldredge EA, et al. Perioperative considerations in a hypothyroid infant with hepatic haemangioma. Paediatr Anaesth 2001;11:228–32.
18. Daller JA, Bueno J, Gutierrez J, et al. Hepatic hemangioendothelioma: Clinical experience and management strategy. J Pediatr Surg 1999;34:98–106.
19. Holcomb GW 3rd, O'Neill JA Jr, Mahboubi S, et al. Experience with hepatic hemangioendothelioma in infancy and childhood. J Pediatr Surg 1988;23:661–6.
20. Sari N, Yalcin B, Akyuz C, et al. Infantile hepatic hemangioendothelioma with elevated serum alpha-fetoprotein. Pediatr Hematol Oncol 2006;23:639–47.
21. Lopez Gutierrez JC, Avila LF, Sosa G, et al. Placental anomalies in children with infantile hemangioma. Pediatr Dermatol 2007;24:353–5.
22. Paltiel HJ, Patriquin HB, Keller MS, et al. Infantile hepatic hemangioma: Doppler ultrasound. Radiology 1992;182:735–42.
23. Keslar PJ, Buck JL, Selby DM. From the archives of the AFIP. Infantile hemangioendothelioma of the liver revisited. Radiographics 1993;13:657–70.
24. Horton KM, Bluemke DA, Hruban RH, et al. CT and MR imaging of benign hepatic and biliary tumors. Radiographics 1999;19:431–51.
25. Feng ST, Chan T, Ching AS, et al. CT and MR imaging characteristics of infantile hepatic hemangioendothelioma. Eur J Radiol 2010;76:e24–9.
26. Chung T, Hoffer FA, Burrows PE, et al. MR imaging of hepatic hemangiomas of infancy and changes seen with interferon alpha-2a treatment. Pediatr Radiol 1996;26:341–8.
27. Mortele KJ, Mergo PJ, Urrutia M, et al. Dynamic gadolinium-enhanced MR findings in infantile hepatic hemangioendothelioma. J Comput Assist Tomogr 1998;22:714–17.
28. Lu M, Greer ML. Hypervascular multifocal hepatoblastoma: Dynamic gadolinium-enhanced MRI findings indistinguishable from infantile hemangioendothelioma. Pediatr Radiol 2007;37:587–91.
29. Vilgrain V, Uzan F, Brancatelli G, et al. Prevalence of hepatic hemangioma in patients with focal nodular hyperplasia: MR imaging analysis. Radiology 2003;229:75–9.
30. Behr GG, Fishman SJ, Caty MG, et al. Hepatic mesenchymal hamartoma and infantile hemangioma: A rare association. J Pediatr Surg 2012;47:448–52.
31. Dehner LP, Ishak KG. Vascular tumors of the liver in infants and children. A study of 30 cases and review of the literature. Arch Pathol 1971;92:101–11.
32. Becker JM, Heitler MS. Hepatic hemangioendotheliomas in infancy. Surg Gynecol Obstet 1989;168:189–200.
33. Mo JQ, Dimashkieh HH, Bove KE. GLUT1 endothelial reactivity distinguishes hepatic infantile hemangioma from congenital hepatic vascular malformation with associated capillary proliferation. Hum Pathol 2004;35:200–9.
34. Hernández F, Navarro M, Encinas JL, et al. The role of GLUT1 immunostaining in the diagnosis and classification of liver vascular tumors in children. J Pediatr Surg 2005;40:801–4.
35. Prokurat A, Kluge P, Chrupek M, et al. Hemangioma of the liver in children: Proliferating vascular tumor or congenital vascular malformation? Med Pediatr Oncol 2002;39:524–9.
36. Mulliken JB, Enjolras O. Congenital hemangiomas and infantile hemangioma: Missing links. J Am Acad Dermatol 2004;50:875–82.
37. Woltering MC, Robben S, Egeler RM. Hepatic hemangioendothelioma of infancy: Treatment with interferon alpha. J Pediatr Gastroenterol Nutr 1997;24:348–51.
38. Wong DC, Masel JP. Infantile hepatic haemangioendothelioma. Australas Radiol 1995;39:140–4.
39. Davenport M, Hansen L, Heaton ND, et al. Hemangioendothelioma of the liver in infants. J Pediatr Surg 1995;30:44–8.
40. Samuel M, Spitz L. Infantile hepatic hemangioendothelioma: The role of surgery. J Pediatr Surg 1995;30:1425–9.
41. Wu TJ, Teng RJ, Tsou Yau KI. Hepatic hemangioendothelioma: Successful treatment with steroid in a very-low-birth-weight infant. Zhonghua Min Guo Xiao Er Ke Yi Xue Hui Za Zhi 1996;37:56–8.
42. Léauté-Labrèze C, Dumas de la Roque E, Hubiche T, et al. Propranolol for severe hemangiomas of infancy. N Engl J Med 2008;358(24):2649–51.

43. Marsciani A, Pericoli R, Alaggio R, et al. Massive response of severe infantile hepatic hemangioma to propanolol. Pediatr Blood Cancer 2010;54:176.

44. Sharma RA, Euden SA, Platton SL, et al. Phase I clinical trial of oral curcumin: Biomarkers of systemic activity and compliance. Clin Cancer Res 2004;10:6847–54.

45. Hassell LA, Roanh le D. Potential response to curcumin in infantile hemangioendothelioma of the liver. Pediatr Blood Cancer 2010;55:377–9.

46. Isaacs H Jr. Fetal and neonatal hepatic tumors. J Pediatr Surg 2007;42:1797–803.

47. Kullendorff CM, Cwikiel W, Sandstrom S. Embolization of hepatic hemangiomas in infants. Eur J Pediatr Surg 2002;12:348–52.

48. Warmann S, Bertram H, Kardorff R, et al. Interventional treatment of infantile hepatic hemangioendothelioma. J Pediatr Surg 2003;38:1177–81.

49. Achilleos OA, Buist LJ, Kelly DA, et al. Unresectable hepatic tumors in childhood and the role of liver transplantation. J Pediatr Surg 1996;31:1563–7.

50. Grabhorn E, Richter A, Fischer L, et al. Neonates with severe infantile hepatic hemangioendothelioma: Limitations of liver transplantation. Pediatr Transplant 2009;13:560–4.

51. Weinberg AG, Finegold MJ. Primary hepatic tumors of childhood. Hum Pathol 1983;14:512–37.

52. Luks FI, Yazbeck S, Brandt ML, et al. Benign liver tumors in children: A 25-year experience. J Pediatr Surg 1991;26:1326–30.

53. Ehren H, Mahour GH, Isaacs H Jr. Benign liver tumors in infancy and childhood. Report of 48 cases. Am J Surg 1983;145:325–9.

54. Caty MG, Shamberger RC. Abdominal tumors in infancy and childhood. Pediatr Clin North Am 1993;40:1253–71.

55. Stocker JT, Ishak KG. Mesenchymal hamartoma of the liver: Report of 30 cases and review of the literature. Pediatr Pathol 1983;1:245–67.

56. Helal A, Nolan M, Bower R, et al. Pathological case of the month. Mesenchymal hamartoma of the liver. Arch Pediatr Adolesc Med 1995;149:315–16.

57. von Schweinitz D, Dammeier BG, Gluer S. Mesenchymal hamartoma of the liver–New insight into histogenesis. J Pediatr Surg 1999;34:1269–71.

58. Shintaku M, Watanabe K. Mesenchymal hamartoma of the liver: A proliferative lesion of possible hepatic stellate cell (Ito cell) origin. Pathol Res Pract 2010;206:532–6.

59. Reed RC, Kapur RP. Hepatic mesenchymal hamartoma: A disorder of imprinting. Pediatr Dev Pathol 2008;11:264–5.

60. Mascarello JT, Krous HF. Second report of a translocation involving 19q13.4 in a mesenchymal hamartoma of the liver. Cancer Genet Cytogenet 1992;58:141–2.

61. Speleman F, De Telder V, De Potter KR, et al. Cytogenetic analysis of a mesenchymal hamartoma of the liver. Cancer Genet Cytogenet 1989;40:29–32.

62. Otal TM, Hendricks JB, Pharis P, et al. Mesenchymal hamartoma of the liver. DNA flow cytometric analysis of eight cases. Cancer 1994;74:1237–42.

63. Stringer MD, Alizai NK. Mesenchymal hamartoma of the liver: A systematic review. J Pediatr Surg 2005;40:1681–90.

64. Kamata S, Nose K, Sawai T, et al. Fetal mesenchymal hamartoma of the liver: Report of a case. J Pediatr Surg 2003;38:639–41.

65. Dickinson JE, Knowles S, Phillips JM. Prenatal diagnosis of hepatic mesenchymal hamartoma. Prenat Diagn 1999;19:81–4.

66. Cornette J, Festen S, van den Hoonaard TL, et al. Mesenchymal hamartoma of the liver: A benign tumor with deceptive prognosis in the perinatal period. Case report and review of the literature. Fetal Diagn Ther 2009;25:196–202.

67. Tsao K, Hirose S, Sydorak R, et al. Fetal therapy for giant hepatic cysts. J Pediatr Surg 2002;37:E31.

68. Balmer B, Le Coultre C, Feldges A, et al. Mesenchymal liver hamartoma in a newborn; case report. Eur J Pediatr Surg 1996;6:303–5.

69. Ros PR, Goodman ZD, Ishak KG, et al. Mesenchymal hamartoma of the liver: Radiologic-pathologic correlation. Radiology 1986;158:619–24.

70. Wan P, Susman J, Kandel J, et al. Neonatal hepatic mesenchymal hamartoma causing cardiac failure and disseminated intravascular coagulopathy. Am J Perinatol 2009;26:601–4.

71. Justrabo E, Martin L, Yaziji N, et al. Hepatic mesenchymal hamartoma in children. Immunohistochemical, ultrastructural and flow cytometric case study. Gastroenterol Clin Biol 1998;22:964–8.

72. Unal E, Koksal Y, Akcoren Z, et al. Mesenchymal hamartoma of the liver mimicking hepatoblastoma. J Pediatr Hematol Oncol 2008;30:458–60.

73. Raffensperger JG, Gonzalez-Crussi F, Skeehan T. Mesenchymal hamartoma of the liver. J Pediatr Surg 1983;18:585–7.

74. Ito H, Kishikawa T, Toda T, et al. Hepatic mesenchymal hamartoma of an infant. J Pediatr Surg 1984;19:315–17.

75. Abramson SJ, Lack EE, Teele RL. Benign vascular tumors of the liver in infants: Sonographic appearance. AJR Am J Roentgenol 1982;138:629–32.

76. Steiner MA, Giles HW. Mesenchymal hamartoma of the liver demonstrating peripheral calcification in a 12-year-old boy. Pediatr Radiol 2008;38:1232–4.

77. Ye BB, Hu B, Wang LJ, et al. Mesenchymal hamartoma of liver: Magnetic resonance imaging and histopathologic correlation. World J Gastroenterol 2005;11:5807–10.

78. Moore M, Anupindi SA, Mattei P, et al. Mesenchymal cystic hamartoma of the liver: MR imaging with pathologic correlation. J Radiol Case Rep 2009;3:22–6.

79. Koumanidou C, Vakaki M, Papadaki M, et al. New sonographic appearance of hepatic mesenchymal hamartoma in childhood. J Clin Ultrasound 1999;27:164–7.

80. Shehata BM, Gupta NA, Katzenstein HM, et al. Undifferentiated embryonal sarcoma of the liver is associated with mesenchymal hamartoma and multiple chromosomal abnormalities: A review of eleven cases. Pediatr Dev Pathol 2011;14:111–16.

81. Sharif K, Ramani P, Lochbuhler H, et al. Recurrent mesenchymal hamartoma associated with 19q translocation. A call for more radical surgical resection. Eur J Pediatr Surg 2006;16:64–7.

82. Karpelowsky JS, Pansini A, Lazarus C, et al. Difficulties in the management of mesenchymal hamartomas. Pediatr Surg Int 2008;24:1171–5.

83. Anil G, Fortier M, Low Y. Cystic hepatic mesenchymal hamartoma: The role of radiology in diagnosis and perioperative management. Br J Radiol 2011;84:e91–94.

84. Barnhart DC, Hirschl RB, Garver KA, et al. Conservative management of mesenchymal hamartoma of the liver. J Pediatr Surg 1997;32:1495–8.

85. de Chadarevian JP, Pawel BR, Faerber EN, et al. Undifferentiated (embryonal) sarcoma arising in conjunction with mesenchymal hamartoma of the liver. Mod Pathol 1994;7:490–3.

86. O'Sullivan MJ, Swanson PE, Knoll J, et al. Undifferentiated embryonal sarcoma with unusual features arising within mesenchymal hamartoma of the liver: Report of a case and review of the literature. Pediatr Dev Pathol 2001;4:482–9.

87. Ramanujam TM, Ramesh JC, Goh DW, et al. Malignant transformation of mesenchymal hamartoma of the liver: Case report and review of the literature. J Pediatr Surg 1999;34:1684–6.

88. Millard J, Fraser N, Stewart RJ. Mesenchymal hamartoma of the liver: Is biopsy always necessary? Pediatr Surg Int 2006;22:622–5.

89. Rajaram V, Knezevich S, Bove KE, et al. DNA sequence of the translocation breakpoints in undifferentiated embryonal sarcoma arising in mesenchymal hamartoma of the liver harboring the t(11;19)(q11;q13.4) translocation. Genes Chromosomes Cancer 2007;46:508–13.

90. Talmon GA, Cohen SM. Mesenchymal hamartoma of the liver with an interstitial deletion involving chromosome band 19q13.4: A theory as to pathogenesis? Arch Pathol Lab Med 2006;130:1216–18.

91. Reymond D, Plaschkes J, Luthy AR, et al. Focal nodular hyperplasia of the liver in children: Review of follow-up and outcome. J Pediatr Surg 1995;30:1590–3.

92. Stocker JT, Ishak KG. Focal nodular hyperplasia of the liver: A study of 21 pediatric cases. Cancer 1981;48:336–45.

93. Okugawa Y, Uchida K, Inoue M, et al. Focal nodular hyperplasia in biliary atresia patient after Kasai hepatic portoenterostomy. Pediatr Surg Int 2008;24:609–12.

94. Ra SH, Kaplan JB, Lassman CR. Focal nodular hyperplasia after orthotopic liver transplantation. Liver Transpl 2010;16:98–103.

95. Savoye-Collet C, Herve S, Koning E, et al. Focal nodular hyperplasia occurring after blunt abdominal trauma. Eur J Gastroenterol Hepatol 2002;14:329–30.
96. Iordanidis F, Hytiroglou P, Drevelegas A, et al. A 25-year-old man with a large hepatic tumor and multiple nodular lesions. Semin Liver Dis 2002;22:97–102.
97. Hohler T, Lohse AW, Schirmacher P. Progressive focal nodular hyperplasia of the liver in a patient with genetic hemochromatosis–growth promotion by iron overload? Dig Dis Sci 2000;45:587–90.
98. Santarelli L, Gabrielli M, Orefice R, et al. Association between Klinefelter syndrome and focal nodular hyperplasia. J Clin Gastroenterol 2003;37:189–91.
99. Scalori A, Tavani A, Gallus S, et al. Risk factors for focal nodular hyperplasia of the liver: An Italian case-control study. Am J Gastroenterol 2002;97:2371–3.
100. Wolf R, Wolf D, Kuperman S. Focal nodular hyperplasia of the liver after intraconazole treatment. J Clin Gastroenterol 2001;33:418–20.
101. Knowles DM, Wolff M. Focal nodular hyperplasia of the liver: A clinicopathologic study and review of the literature. Hum Pathol 1976;7:533–45.
102. Mathieu D, Zafrani ES, Anglade MC, et al. Association of focal nodular hyperplasia and hepatic hemangioma. Gastroenterology 1989;97:154–7.
103. Buscarini E, Danesino C, Plauchu H, et al. High prevalence of hepatic focal nodular hyperplasia in subjects with hereditary hemorrhagic telangiectasia. Ultrasound Med Biol 2004;30:1089–97.
104. Paradis V, Bieche I, Dargere D, et al. A quantitative gene expression study suggests a role for angiopoietins in focal nodular hyperplasia. Gastroenterology 2003;124:651–9.
105. Kumagai H, Masuda T, Oikawa H, et al. Focal nodular hyperplasia of the liver: Direct evidence of circulatory disturbances. J Gastroenterol Hepatol 2000;15:1344–7.
106. Kinjo T, Aoki H, Sunagawa H, et al. Congenital absence of the portal vein associated with focal nodular hyperplasia of the liver and congenital choledochal cyst: A case report. J Pediatr Surg 2001;36:622–5.
107. Altavilla G, Guariso G. Focal nodular hyperplasia of the liver associated with portal vein agenesis: A morphological and immunohistochemical study of one case and review of the literature. Adv Clin Path 1999;3:139–45.
108. Tanaka Y, Takayanagi M, Shiratori Y, et al. Congenital absence of portal vein with multiple hyperplastic nodular lesions in the liver. J Gastroenterol 2003;38:288–94.
109. Osorio MJ, Bonow A, Bond GJ, et al. Abernethy malformation complicated by hepatopulmonary syndrome and a liver mass successfully treated by liver transplantation. Pediatr Transplant 2011;15:E149–51.
110. Lisovsky M, Konstas AA, Misdraji J. Congenital extrahepatic portosystemic shunts (Abernethy malformation): A histopathologic evaluation. Am J Surg Pathol 2011;35:1381–90.
111. Bouyn CI, Leclere J, Raimondo G, et al. Hepatic focal nodular hyperplasia in children previously treated for a solid tumor. Incidence, risk factors, and outcome. Cancer 2003;97:3107–13.
112. Towbin AJ, Luo GG, Yin H, et al. Focal nodular hyperplasia in children, adolescents, and young adults. Pediatr Radiol 2011;41:341–9.
113. Benz-Bohm G, Hero B, Gossmann A, et al. Focal nodular hyperplasia of the liver in longterm survivors of neuroblastoma: How much diagnostic imaging is necessary? Eur J Radiol 2010;74:e1–5.
114. Gutweiler JR, Yu DC, Kim HB, et al. Hepatoblastoma presenting with focal nodular hyperplasia after treatment of neuroblastoma. J Pediatr Surg 2008;43:2297–300.
115. Gobbi D, Dall'Igna P, Messina C, et al. Focal nodular hyperplasia in pediatric patients with and without oncologic history. Pediatr Blood Cancer 2010. 551420–422.
116. Sugito K, Uekusa S, Kawashima H, et al. The clinical course in pediatric solid tumor patients with focal nodular hyperplasia of the liver. Int J Clin Oncol 2011;16:482–7.
117. Sudour H, Mainard L, Baumann C, et al. Focal nodular hyperplasia of the liver following hematopoietic SCT. Bone Marrow Transplant 2009;43:127–32.
118. Anderson L, Gregg D, Margolis D, et al. Focal nodular hyperplasia in pediatric allogeneic hematopoietic cell transplant: Case series. Bone Marrow Transplant 2010;45:1357–9.
119. Masetti R, Biagi C, Kleinschmidt K, et al. Focal nodular hyperplasia of the liver after intensive treatment for pediatric cancer: Is hematopoietic stem cell transplantation a risk factor? Eur J Pediatr 2011;170:807–12.
120. Citak EC, Karadeniz C, Oguz A, et al. Nodular regenerative hyperplasia and focal nodular hyperplasia of the liver mimicking hepatic metastasis in children with solid tumors and a review of literature. Pediatr Hematol Oncol 2007;24:281–9.
121. Cheon JE, Kim WS, Kim IO, et al. Radiological features of focal nodular hyperplasia of the liver in children. Pediatr Radiol 1998;28:878–83.
122. Somech R, Brazowski E, Kesller A, et al. Focal nodular hyperplasia in children. J Pediatr Gastroenterol Nutr 2001;32:480–3.
123. Bioulac-Sage P, Balabaud C, Wanless IR. Diagnosis of focal nodular hyperplasia: Not so easy. Am J Surg Pathol 2001;25:1322–5.
124. Huang YE, Wang PW, Huang HH, et al. A central scar in hepatic focal nodular hyperplasia detected on liver SPECT imaging. Clin Nucl Med 2001;26:367–9.
125. Swingle CA, Fajman WA, Alazraki N. Early enhancing lesion seen on computed tomography consistent with focal nodular hyperplasia. Clin Nucl Med 2003;28:134–5.
126. Steiner D, Klett R, Puille M, et al. Diagnosis of focal nodular hyperplasia with hepatobiliary scintigraphy using a modified SPECT technique. Clin Nucl Med 2003;28:136–7.
127. Casillas VJ, Amendola MA, Gascue A, et al. Imaging of nontraumatic hemorrhagic hepatic lesions. Radiographics 2000;20:367–78.
128. Marin D, Brancatelli G, Federle MP, et al. Focal nodular hyperplasia: Typical and atypical MRI findings with emphasis on the use of contrast media. Clin Radiol 2008;63:577–85.
129. Ba-Ssalamah A, Schima W, Schmook MT, et al. Atypical focal nodular hyperplasia of the liver: Imaging features of nonspecific and liver-specific MR contrast agents. AJR Am J Roentgenol 2002;179:1447–56.
130. Asbach P, Klessen C, Koch M, et al. Magnetic resonance imaging findings of atypical focal nodular hyperplasia of the liver. Clin Imaging 2007;31:244–52.
131. Nguyen BN, Flejou JF, Terris B, et al. Focal nodular hyperplasia of the liver: A comprehensive pathologic study of 305 lesions and recognition of new histologic forms. Am J Surg Pathol 1999;23:1441–54.
132. Bioulac-Sage P, Rebouissou S, Thomas C, et al. Hepatocellular adenoma subtype classification using molecular markers and immunohistochemistry. Hepatology 2007;46:740–8.
133. Wanless IR, Albrecht S, Bilbao J, et al. Multiple focal nodular hyperplasia of the liver associated with vascular malformations of various organs and neoplasia of the brain: A new syndrome. Mod Pathol 1989;2:456–62.
134. Ahmad I, Iyer A, Marginean CE, et al. Diagnostic use of cytokeratins, CD34, and neuronal cell adhesion molecule staining in focal nodular hyperplasia and hepatic adenoma. Hum Pathol 2009;40:726–34.
135. Petsas T, Tsamandas A, Tsota I, et al. A case of hepatocellular carcinoma arising within large focal nodular hyperplasia with review of the literature. World J Gastroenterol 2006;12:6567–71.
136. Langrehr JM, Pfitzmann R, Hermann M, et al. Hepatocellular carcinoma in association with hepatic focal nodular hyperplasia. Acta Radiol 2006;47:340–4.
137. Saul SH, Titelbaum DS, Gansler TS, et al. The fibrolamellar variant of hepatocellular carcinoma. Its association with focal nodular hyperplasia. Cancer 1987;60:3049–55.
138. Saxena R, Humphreys S, Williams R, et al. Nodular hyperplasia surrounding fibrolamellar carcinoma: A zone of arterialized liver parenchyma. Histopathology 1994;25:275–8.
139. Fabre A, Audet P, Vilgrain V, et al. Histologic scoring of liver biopsy in focal nodular hyperplasia with atypical presentation. Hepatology 2002;35:414–20.
140. Li T, Qin LX, Ji Y, et al. Atypical hepatic focal nodular hyperplasia presenting as acute abdomen and misdiagnosed as hepatocellular carcinoma. Hepatol Res 2007;37:1100–5.
141. Okada T, Sasaki F, Kamiyama T, et al. Management and algorithm for focal nodular hyperplasia of the liver in children. Eur J Pediatr Surg 2006;16:235–40.

142. Yang Y, Fu S, Li A, et al. Management and surgical treatment for focal nodular hyperplasia in children. Pediatr Surg Int 2008; 24:699–703.

143. Lautz T, Tantemsapya N, Dzakovic A, et al. Focal nodular hyperplasia in children: Clinical features and current management practice. J Pediatr Surg 2010;45:1797–803.

144. Pain JA, Gimson AE, Williams R, et al. Focal nodular hyperplasia of the liver: Results of treatment and options in management. Gut 1991;32:524–7.

145. Di Stasi M, Caturelli E, De Sio I, et al. Natural history of focal nodular hyperplasia of the liver: An ultrasound study. J Clin Ultrasound 1996;24:345–50.

146. Ohmoto K, Honda T, Hirokawa M, et al. Spontaneous regression of focal nodular hyperplasia of the liver. J Gastroenterol 2002;37:849–53.

147. Leconte I, Van Beers BE, Lacrosse M, et al. Focal nodular hyperplasia: Natural course observed with CT and MRI. J Comput Assist Tomogr 2000;24:61–6.

148. Geschwind JF, Degli MS, Morris JM, et al. Re: Treatment of focal nodular hyperplasia with selective transcatheter arterial embolization using iodized oil and polyvinyl alcohol. Cardiovasc Intervent Radiol 2002;25:340–1.

149. Hung CH, Changchien CS, Lu SN, et al. Sonographic features of hepatic adenomas with pathologic correlation. Abdom Imaging 2001;26:500–6.

150. Wilhelm L, Albrecht L, Kirsch M, et al. Preoperative application of selective angiographic embolization in the treatment of focal nodular hyperplasia. Surg Laparosc Endosc Percutan Tech 2006;16:177–81.

151. Ichikawa T, Federle MP, Grazioli L, et al. Hepatocellular adenoma: Multiphasic CT and histopathologic findings in 25 patients. Radiology 2000;214:861–8.

152. Paulson EK, McClellan JS, Washington K, et al. Hepatic adenoma: MR characteristics and correlation with pathologic findings. AJR Am J Roentgenol 1994;163:113–16.

153. Grazioli L, Federle MP, Brancatelli G, et al. Hepatic adenomas: Imaging and pathologic findings. Radiographics 2001;21: 877–94.

154. Das CJ, Dhingra S, Gupta AK, et al. Imaging of paediatric liver tumours with pathological correlation. Clin Radiol 2009;64: 1015–25.

155. Edmonson HA. Atlas of Tumor Pathology: Tumors of the liver and intrahepatic bile ducts. Washington, D.C.: Armed Forces Institute of Pathology; 1958.

156. Lizardi-Cervera J, Cuellar-Gamboa L, Motola-Kuba D. Focal nodular hyperplasia and hepatic adenoms: A review. Ann Hepatol 2006;5:206–11.

157. Giannitrapani L, Soresi M, La Spada E, et al. Sex hormones and risk of liver tumor. Ann N Y Acad Sci 2006;1089: 228–36.

158. Reddy KR, Schiff ER. Approach to a liver mass. Semin Liver Dis 1993;13:423–35.

159. Bagia S, Hewitt PM, Morris DL. Anabolic steroid-induced hepatic adenomas with spontaneous haemorrhage in a body-builder. Aust N Z J Surg 2000;70:686–7.

160. Toso C, Rubbia-Brandt L, Negro F, et al. Hepatocellular adenoma and polycystic ovary syndrome. Liver Int 2003;23: 35–7.

161. Adusumilli PS, Lee B, Parekh K, et al. Hemoperitoneum from spontaneous rupture of a liver cell adenoma in a male with hyperthyroidism. Am Surg 2002;68:582–3.

162. Marie-Cardine A, Schneider P, Greene V, et al. Erythrocytosis in a child with a hepatic adenoma. Med Pediatr Oncol 2001;36: 659–61.

163. Howell RR, Stevenson RE, Ben-Menachem Y, et al. Hepatic adenomata with type 1 glycogen storage disease. JAMA 1976;236: 1481–4.

164. Coire CI, Qizilbash AH, Castelli MF. Hepatic adenomata in type Ia glycogen storage disease. Arch Pathol Lab Med 1987;111: 166–9.

165. Mason HH, Andersen DH. Glycogen disease of the liver (von Gierke's disease) with hepatomata; case report with metabolic studies. Pediatrics 1955;16:785–800.

166. Zangeneh F, Limbeck GA, Brown BI, et al. Hepatorenal glycogenosis (type I glycogenosis) and carcinoma of the liver. J Pediatr 1969;74:73–83.

167. Wang DQ, Fiske LM, Carreras CT, et al. Natural history of hepatocellular adenoma formation in glycogen storage disease type I. J Pediatr 2011;159:442–6.

168. Fraumeni JF Jr, Miller RW, Hill JA. Primary carcinoma of the liver in childhood: An epidemiologic study. J Natl Cancer Inst 1968;40:1087–99.

169. Nakamura T, Tamakoshi K, Kitagawa M, et al. A case of hepatocellular carcinoma in type I a glycogen storage disease. Nihon Shokakibyo Gakkai Zasshi 1997;94:866–70.

170. Labrune P, Trioche P, Duvaltier I, et al. Hepatocellular adenomas in glycogen storage disease type I and III: A series of 43 patients and review of the literature. J Pediatr Gastroenterol Nutr 1997;24:276–9.

171. Kerlin P, Davis GL, McGill DB, et al. Hepatic adenoma and focal nodular hyperplasia: Clinical, pathologic, and radiologic features. Gastroenterology 1983;84(5 Pt 1):994–1002.

172. Foster JH, Berman MM. The malignant transformation of liver cell adenomas. Arch Surg 1994;129:712–17.

173. Tao LC. Oral contraceptive-associated liver cell adenoma and hepatocellular carcinoma. Cytomorphology and mechanism of malignant transformation. Cancer 1991;68:341–7.

174. Micchelli ST, Vivekanandan P, Boitnott JK, et al. Malignant transformation of hepatic adenomas. Mod Pathol 2008;21: 491–7.

175. Kishnani PS, Chuang TP, Bali D, et al. Chromosomal and genetic alterations in human hepatocellular adenomas associated with type Ia glycogen storage disease. Hum Mol Genet 2009;18: 4781–90.

176. Chiche L, Dao T, Salame E, et al. Liver adenomatosis: Reappraisal, diagnosis, and surgical management: eight new cases and review of the literature. Ann Surg 2000;231:74–81.

177. Musthafa CP, Chettupuzha AP, Syed AA, et al. Liver adenomatosis. Indian J Gastroenterol 2003;22:30–1.

178. Vetelainen R, Erdogan D, de Graaf W, et al. Liver adenomatosis: Re-evaluation of aetiology and management. Liver Int 2008; 28:499–508.

179. Babaoglu K, Binnetoglu FK, Aydoğan A, et al. Hepatic adenomatosis in a 7-year-old child treated earlier with a Fontan procedure. Pediatr Cardiol 2010;31:861–4.

180. Takayasu H, Motoi T, Kanamori Y, et al. Two case reports of childhood liver cell adenomas harboring beta-catenin abnormalities. Hum Pathol 2002;33:852–5.

181. Chen YW, Jeng YM, Yeh SH, et al. P53 gene and Wnt signaling in benign neoplasms: Beta-catenin mutations in hepatic adenoma but not in focal nodular hyperplasia. Hepatology 2002;36(4 Pt 1):927–35.

182. Rebouissou S, Bioulac-Sage P, Zucman-Rossi J. Molecular pathogenesis of focal nodular hyperplasia and hepatocellular adenoma. J Hepatol 2008;48:163–70.

183. Aseni P, Sansalone CV, Sammartino C, et al. Rapid disappearance of hepatic adenoma after contraceptive withdrawal. J Clin Gastroenterol 2001;33:234–6.

184. Steinbrecher UP, Lisbona R, Huang SN, et al. Complete regression of hepatocellular adenoma after withdrawal of oral contraceptives. Dig Dis Sci 1981;26:1045–50.

185. Ramseur WL, Cooper MR. Asymptomatic liver cell adenomas. Another case of resolution after discontinuation of oral contraceptive use. JAMA 1978;239:1647–8.

186. Barthelmes L, Tait IS. Liver cell adenoma and liver cell adenomatosis. HPB (Oxford) 2005;7:186–96.

187. Ault GT, Wren SM, Ralls PW, et al. Selective management of hepatic adenomas. Am Surg 1996;62:825–9.

188. Leese T, Farges O, Bismuth H. Liver cell adenomas. A 12-year surgical experience from a specialist hepato-biliary unit. Ann Surg 1988;208:558–64.

189. Stoot JH, van der Linden E, Terpstra OT, et al. Life-saving therapy for haemorrhaging liver adenomas using selective arterial embolization. Br J Surg 2007;94:1249–53.

190. Terkivatan T, de Wilt JH, de Man RA, et al. Treatment of ruptured hepatocellular adenoma. Br J Surg 2001;88: 207–9.

191. Heeringa B, Sardi A. Bleeding hepatic adenoma: Expectant treatment to limit the extent of liver resection. Am Surg 2001; 67:927–9.

192. Ross JA. Hepatoblastoma and birth weight: Too little, too big, or just right? J Pediatr 1997;130:516–17.

193. Stocker J, Conran R, Selby D. Tumor and Pseudo Tumors of the Liver. London: Chapman & Hall; 1998.
194. Lack EE, Neave C, Vawter GF. Hepatoblastoma. A clinical and pathologic study of 54 cases. Am J Surg Pathol 1982;6:693–705.
195. Martelli C, Blandamura S, Massaro S, et al. A case study of Beckwith-Wiedemann syndrome associated with hepatoblastoma. Clin Exp Obstet Gynecol 1993;20:82–7.
196. McNeil DE, Brown M, Ching A, et al. Screening for Wilms tumor and hepatoblastoma in children with Beckwith-Wiedemann syndromes: A cost-effective model. Med Pediatr Oncol 2001;37:349–56.
197. Tan TY, Amor DJ. Tumour surveillance in Beckwith-Wiedemann syndrome and hemihyperplasia: A critical review of the evidence and suggested guidelines for local practice. J Paediatr Child Health 2006;42:486–90.
198. Aretz S, Koch A, Uhlhaas S, et al. Should children at risk for familial adenomatous polyposis be screened for hepatoblastoma and children with apparently sporadic hepatoblastoma be screened for APC germline mutations? Pediatr Blood Cancer 2006;47:811–18.
199. Hirschman BA, Pollock BH, Tomlinson GE. The spectrum of APC mutations in children with hepatoblastoma from familial adenomatous polyposis kindreds. J Pediatr 2005;147:263–6.
200. Ikeda H, Matsuyama S, Tanimura M. Association between hepatoblastoma and very low birth weight: A trend or a chance? J Pediatr 1997;130:557–60.
201. McLaughlin CC, Baptiste MS, Schymura MJ, et al. Maternal and infant birth characteristics and hepatoblastoma. Am J Epidemiol 2006;163:818–28.
202. Reynolds P, Urayama KY, Von Behren J, et al. Birth characteristics and hepatoblastoma risk in young children. Cancer 2004;100:1070–6.
203. Ikeda H, Hachitanda Y, Tanimura M, et al. Development of unfavorable hepatoblastoma in children of very low birth weight: Results of a surgical and pathologic review. Cancer 1998;82:1789–96.
204. Maruyama K, Ikeda H, Koizumi T, et al. Case-control study of perinatal factors and hepatoblastoma in children with an extremely low birthweight. Pediatr Int 2000;42:492–8.
205. Shew SB, Keshen TH, Jahoor F, et al. Assessment of cysteine synthesis in very low-birth weight neonates using a 13C6 glucose tracer. J Pediatr Surg 2005;40:52–6.
206. Rowland JM. Hepatoblastoma: assessment of criteria for histologic classification. Med Pediatr Oncol 2002;39:478–83.
207. Haas JE, Feusner JH, Finegold MJ. Small cell undifferentiated histology in hepatoblastoma may be unfavorable. Cancer 2001;92:3130–4.
208. Stringer MD, Hennayake S, Howard ER, et al. Improved outcome for children with hepatoblastoma. Br J Surg 1995;82:386–91.
209. Haas JE, Muczynski KA, Krailo M, et al. Histopathology and prognosis in childhood hepatoblastoma and hepatocarcinoma. Cancer 1989;64:1082–95.
210. Nickerson HJ, Silberman TL, McDonald TP. Hepatoblastoma, thrombocytosis, and increased thrombopoietin. Cancer 1980;45:315–17.
211. von Schweinitz D, Hadam MR, Welte K, et al. Production of interleukin-1 beta and interleukin-6 in hepatoblastoma. Int J Cancer 1993;53:728–34.
212. Oda H, Imai Y, Nakatsuru Y, et al. Somatic mutations of the APC gene in sporadic hepatoblastomas. Cancer Res 1996;56:3320–3.
213. Surace C, Leszl A, Perilongo G, et al. Fluorescent in situ hybridization (FISH) reveals frequent and recurrent numerical and structural abnormalities in hepatoblastoma with no informative karyotype. Med Pediatr Oncol 2002;39:536–9.
214. Maruyama K, Ikeda H, Koizumi T. Hepatoblastoma associated with trisomy 18 syndrome: A case report and a review of the literature. Pediatr Int 2001;43:302–5.
215. Giardiello FM, Petersen GM, Brensinger JD, et al. Hepatoblastoma and APC gene mutation in familial adenomatous polyposis. Gut 1996;39:867–9.
216. Yamaoka H, Ohtsu K, Sueda T, et al. Diagnostic and prognostic impact of beta-catenin alterations in pediatric liver tumors. Oncol Rep 2006;15:551–6.
217. Miller JH, Greenspan BS. Integrated imaging of hepatic tumors in childhood. Part I: Malignant lesions (primary and metastatic). Radiology 1985;154:83–90.
218. Powers C, Ros PR, Stoupis C, et al. Primary liver neoplasms: MR imaging with pathologic correlation. Radiographics 1994;14:459–82.
219. Shafford EA, Pritchard J. Extreme thrombocytosis as a diagnostic clue to hepatoblastoma. Arch Dis Child 1993;69:171.
220. Stocker J, Conran R. Hepatoblastoma. New York: Churchill Livingstone; 1997.
221. Jassam N, Jones CM, Briscoe T, et al. The hook effect: A need for constant vigilance. Ann Clin Biochem 2006;43(Pt 4):314–17.
222. Ortega J, Siegel S. Biological Markers in Pediatric Cancer. Philadelphia: JB Lippincott; 1989.
223. Kairemo KJ, Lindahl H, Merenmies J, et al. Anti-alpha-fetoprotein imaging is useful for staging hepatoblastoma. Transplantation 2002;73:1151–4.
224. Zynger DL, Gupta A, Luan C, et al. Expression of glypican 3 in hepatoblastoma: An immunohistochemical study of 65 cases. Hum Pathol 2008;39:224–30.
225. Stringer MD. Liver tumors. Semin Pediatr Surg 2000;9:196–208.
226. MacKinlay GA, Pritchard J. A common language for childhood liver tumors. Pediatr Surg Int 1992;7:325–6.
227. Roebuck DJ, Aronson D, Clapuyt P, et al. 2005 PRETEXT: A revised staging system for primary malignant liver tumours of childhood developed by the SIOPEL group. Pediatr Radiol 2007;37:123–32.
228. Cho JY, Han HS, Yoon YS, et al. Experiences of laparoscopic liver resection including lesions in the posterosuperior segments of the liver. Surg Endosc 2008;22:2344–9.
229. Koffron AJ, Auffenberg G, Kung R, et al. Evaluation of 300 minimally invasive liver resections at a single institution: Less is more. Ann Surg 2007;246:385–94.
230. Yoon YS, Han HS, Choi YS, et al. Total laparoscopic left lateral sectionectomy performed in a child with benign liver mass. J Pediatr Surg 2006;41:e25–28.
231. Dutta S, Nehra D, Woo R, et al. Laparoscopic resection of a benign liver tumor in a child. J Pediatr Surg 2007;42:1141–5.
232. Dicken BJ, Bigam DL, Lees GM. Association between surgical margins and long-term outcome in advanced hepatoblastoma. J Pediatr Surg 2004;39:721–5.
233. Ortega JA, Douglass EC, Feusner JH, et al. Randomized comparison of cisplatin/vincristine/fluorouracil and cisplatin/continuous infusion doxorubicin for treatment of pediatric hepatoblastoma: A report from the Children's Cancer Group and the Pediatric Oncology Grou. J Clin Oncol 2000;18:2665–75.
234. Carceller A, Blanchard H, Champagne J, et al. Surgical resection and chemotherapy improve survival rate for patients with hepatoblastoma. J Pediatr Surg 2001;36:755–9.
235. Katzenstein HM, Krailo M, Malogolowkin MH, et al. Biology and treatment of children with all stages of hepatoblastoma: COG proposal AHEP-0731, submitted to CTEP and NCI, 2007.
236. Perilongo G, Shafford E, Maibach R, et al. Risk-adapted treatment for childhood hepatoblastoma. final report of the second study of the International Society of Paediatric Oncology–SIOPEL 2. Eur J Cancer 2004;40:411–21.
237. Schnater JM, Aronson DC, Plaschkes J, et al. Surgical view of the treatment of patients with hepatoblastoma: Results from the first prospective trial of the International Society of Pediatric Oncology Liver Tumor Study Grou. Cancer 2002;94:1111–20.
238. Casas-Melley AT, Malatack J, Consolini D, et al. Successful liver transplant for unresectable hepatoblastoma. J Pediatr Surg 2007;42:184–7.
239. Chen LE, Shepherd RW, Nadler ML, et al. Liver transplantation and chemotherapy in children with unresectable primary hepatic malignancies: Development of a management algorithm. J Pediatr Gastroenterol Nutr 2006;43:487–93.
240. Ang JP, Heath JA, Donath S, et al. Treatment outcomes for hepatoblastoma: An institution's experience over two decades. Pediatr Surg Int 2007;23:103–9.
241. Tiao GM, Bobey N, Allen S, et al. The current management of hepatoblastoma: A combination of chemotherapy, conventional resection, and liver transplantation. J Pediatr 2005;146:204–11.
242. Raney B. Hepatoblastoma in children: A review. J Pediatr Hematol Oncol 1997;19:418–22.
243. Feusner JH, Krailo MD, Haas JE, et al. Treatment of pulmonary metastases of initial stage I hepatoblastoma in childhood. Report from the Childrens Cancer Group. Cancer 1993;71:859–64.

244. Otte JB, de Ville de Goyet J. The contribution of transplantation to the treatment of liver tumors in children. Semin Pediatr Surg 2005;14:233–8.

245. Perilongo G, Shafford EA. Liver tumours. Eur J Cancer 1999;35:953–9.

246. Malogolowkin MH, Katzenstein H, Krailo MD, et al. Intensified platinum therapy is an ineffective strategy for improving outcome in pediatric patients with advanced hepatoblastoma. J Clin Oncol 2006;24:2879–84.

247. Brown J, Perilongo G, Shafford E, et al. Pretreatment prognostic factors for children with hepatoblastoma– results from the International Society of Paediatric Oncology (SIOP) study SIOPEL 1. Eur J Cancer 2000;36:1418–25.

248. von Schweinitz D, Byrd DJ, Hecker H, et al. Efficiency and toxicity of ifosfamide, cisplatin and doxorubicin in the treatment of childhood hepatoblastoma. Study Committee of the Cooperative Paediatric Liver Tumour Study HB89 of the German Society for Paediatric Oncology and Haematology. Eur J Cancer 1997;33:1243–9.

249. von Schweinitz D, Burger D, Bode U, et al. Results of the HB-89 Study in treatment of malignant epithelial liver tumors in childhood and concept of a new HB-94 protocol. Klin Padiatr 1994;206:282–8.

250. Stringer MD. The role of liver transplantation in the management of paediatric liver tumours. Ann R Coll Surg Engl 2007;89:1 2–21.

251. McCrudden KW, Yokoi A, Thosani A, et al. Topotecan is antiangiogenic in experimental hepatoblastoma. J Pediatr Surg 2002;37:857–61.

252. Katzenstein HM, Rigsby C, Shaw PH, et al. Novel therapeutic approaches in the treatment of children with hepatoblastoma. J Pediatr Hematol Oncol 2002;24(9):751–5.

253. Tashjian DB, Moriarty KP, Courtney RA, et al. Preoperative chemoembolization for unresectable hepatoblastoma. Pediatr Surg Int 2002;18:187–9.

254. Xuewu J, Jianhong L, Xianliang H, et al. Combined treatment of hepatoblastoma with transcatheter arterial chemoembolization and surgery. Pediatr Hematol Oncol 2006;23:1–9.

255. Chan KL, Fan ST, Tam PK, et al. Management of spontaneously ruptured hepatoblastoma in infancy. Med Pediatr Oncol 2002;38:137–8.

256. Kasai M, Watanabe I. Histologic classification of liver-cell carcinoma in infancy and childhood and its clinical evaluation. A study of 70 cases collected in Japan. Cancer 1970;25:551–63.

257. von Schweinitz D, Hecker H, Schmidt-von-Arndt G, Harms D. Prognostic factors and staging systems in childhood hepatoblastoma. Int J Cancer 1997;74(6):593–9.

258. von Schweinitz D, Hecker H, Schmidt-von-Arndt G, et al. Complete resection before development of drug resistance is essential for survival from advanced hepatoblastoma–a report from the German Cooperative Pediatric Liver Tumor Study HB-89. J Pediatr Surg 1995;30:845–52.

259. De Ioris M, Brugieres L, Zimmermann A, et al. Hepatoblastoma with a low serum alpha-fetoprotein level at diagnosis: The SIOPEL group experience. Eur J Cancer 2008;44:545–50.

260. Van Tornout JM, Buckley JD, Quinn JJ, et al. Timing and magnitude of decline in alpha-fetoprotein levels in treated children with unresectable or metastatic hepatoblastoma are predictors of outcome: A report from the Children's Cancer Group. J Clin Oncol 1997;15:1190–7.

261. Malogolowkin MH, Katzenstein HM, Meyers RL, et al. Complete surgical resection is curative for children with hepatoblastoma with pure fetal histology: A report from the Children's Oncology Group. J Clin Oncol 2011;29:3301–6.

262. Malogolowkin MH, Katzenstein HM, Krailo M, et al. Redefining the role of doxorubicin for the treatment of children with hepatoblastoma. J Clin Oncol 2008;26:2379–83.

263. von Schweinitz D. Identification of risk groups in hepatoblastoma–another step in optimising therapy. Eur J Cancer 2000;36:1343–6.

264. Warmann SW, Fuchs J. Drug resistance in hepatoblastoma. Curr Pharm Biotechnol 2007;8:93–7.

265. D'Antiga L, Vallortigara F, Cillo U, et al. Features predicting unresectability in hepatoblastoma. Cancer 2007;110:1050–8.

266. Dall'Igna P, Cecchetto G, Toffolutti T, et al. Multifocal hepatoblastoma: Is there a place for partial hepatectomy? Med Pediatr Oncol 2003;40:113–17.

267. Czauderna P, Otte JB, Aronson DC, et al. Guidelines for surgical treatment of hepatoblastoma in the modern era–recommendations from the Childhood Liver Tumour Strategy Group of the International Society of Paediatric Oncology (SIOPEL). Eur J Cancer 2005;41:1031–6.

268. Tagge EP, Tagge DU, Reyes J, et al. Resection, including transplantation, for hepatoblastoma and hepatocellular carcinoma: Impact on survival. J Pediatr Surg 1992;27:292–7.

269. Pimpalwar AP, Sharif K, Ramani P, et al. Strategy for hepatoblastoma management: Transplant versus nontransplant surgery. J Pediatr Surg 2002;37:240–5.

270. Srinivasan P, McCall J, Pritchard J, et al. Orthotopic liver transplantation for unresectable hepatoblastoma. Transplantation 2002;74:652–5.

271. Otte JB, Pritchard J, Aronson DC, et al. Liver transplantation for hepatoblastoma: Results from the International Society of Pediatric Oncology (SIOP) study SIOPEL-1 and review of the world experience. Pediatr Blood Cancer 2004;42:74–83.

272. Reyes JD, Carr B, Dvorchik I, et al. Liver transplantation and chemotherapy for hepatoblastoma and hepatocellular cancer in childhood and adolescence. J Pediatr 2000;136:795–804.

273. Molmenti EP, Wilkinson K, Molmenti H, et al. Treatment of unresectable hepatoblastoma with liver transplantation in the pediatric population. Am J Transplant 2002;2:535–8.

274. Meyers RL, Katzenstein HM, Krailo M, et al. Surgical resection of pulmonary metastatic lesions in children with hepatoblastoma. J Pediatr Surg 2007;42:2050–6.

275. Hacker FM, von Schweinitz D, Gambazzi F. The relevance of surgical therapy for bilateral and/or multiple pulmonary metastases in children. Eur J Pediatr Surg 2007;17:84–9.

276. Lack EE, Schloo BL, Azumi N, et al. Undifferentiated (embryonal) sarcoma of the liver. Clinical and pathologic study of 16 cases with emphasis on immunohistochemical features. Am J Surg Pathol 1991;15:1–16.

277. Aoyama C, Hachitanda Y, Sato JK, et al. Undifferentiated (embryonal) sarcoma of the liver. A tumor of uncertain histogenesis showing divergent differentiation. Am J Surg Pathol 1991;15:615–24.

278. Buetow PC, Buck JL, Pantongrag-Brown L, et al. Undifferentiated (embryonal) sarcoma of the liver: Pathologic basis of imaging findings in 28 cases. Radiology 1997;203:779–83.

279. Kiani B, Ferrell LD, Qualman S, et al. Immunohistochemical analysis of embryonal sarcoma of the liver. Appl Immunohistochem Mol Morphol 2006;14:193–7.

280. Abramowsky CR, Cebelin M, Choudhury A, et al. Undifferentiated (embryonal) sarcoma of the liver with alpha-1-antitrypsin deposits: Immunohistochemical and ultrastructural studies. Cancer 1980;45:3108–13.

281. Keating S, Taylor GP. Undifferentiated (embryonal) sarcoma of the liver: Ultrastructural and immunohistochemical similarities with malignant fibrous histiocytoma. Hum Pathol 1985;16:693–9.

282. Iliszko M, Czauderna P, Babinska M, et al. Cytogenetic findings in an embryonal sarcoma of the liver. Cancer Genet Cytogenet 1998;102:142–4.

283. Cho HS, Park YN, Lyu CJ, et al. Embryonal sarcoma of the liver: Multiple recurrences and histologic dedifferentiation. Med Pediatr Oncol 1999;32(5):386–8.

284. Leuschner I, Schmidt D, Harms D. Undifferentiated sarcoma of the liver in childhood: Morphology, flow cytometry, and literature review. Hum Pathol 1990;21:68–76.

285. Pollono DG, Drut R. Undifferentiated (embryonal) sarcoma of the liver: Fine-needle aspiration cytology and preoperative chemotherapy as an approach to diagnosis and initial treatment. A case report. Diagn Cytopathol 1998;19:102–6.

286. Krishnamurthy SC, Datta S, Jambhekar NA. Fine needle aspiration cytology of undifferentiated (embryonal) sarcoma of the liver: A case report. Acta Cytol 1996;40:567–70.

287. Newman KD, Schisgall R, Reaman G, et al. Malignant mesenchymoma of the liver in children. J Pediatr Surg 1989;24:781–3.

288. Harris MB, Shen S, Weiner MA, et al. Treatment of primary undifferentiated sarcoma of the liver with surgery and chemotherapy. Cancer 1984;54:2859–62.

289. Walker NI, Horn MJ, Strong RW, et al. Undifferentiated (embryonal) sarcoma of the liver. Pathologic findings and long-term survival after complete surgical resection. Cancer 1992;69:52–9.

290. Nicol K, Savell V, Moore J, et al. Distinguishing undifferentiated embryonal sarcoma of the liver from biliary tract rhabdomyosarcoma: A Children's Oncology Group study. Pediatr Dev Pathol 2007;10:89–97.

291. Urban CE, Mache CJ, Schwinger W, et al. Undifferentiated (embryonal) sarcoma of the liver in childhood. Successful combined-modality therapy in four patients. Cancer 1993;72: 2511–16.

292. Uchiyama M, Iwafuchi M, Yagi M, et al. Treatment of ruptured undifferentiated sarcoma of the liver in children: A report of two cases and review of the literature. J Hepatobiliary Pancreat Surg 2001;8:87–91.

293. Baron PW, Majlessipour F, Bedros AA, et al. Undifferentiated embryonal sarcoma of the liver successfully treated with chemotherapy and liver resection. J Gastrointest Surg 2007;11: 73–5.

294. Bisogno G, Pilz T, Perilongo G, et al. Undifferentiated sarcoma of the liver in childhood: A curable disease. Cancer 2002;94:252–7.

295. Okajima H, Ohya Y, Lee KJ, et al. Management of undifferentiated sarcoma of the liver including living donor liver transplantation as a backup procedure. J Pediatr Surg 2009;44:e33–38.

296. Kelly MJ, Martin L, Alonso M, et al. Liver transplant for relapsed undifferentiated embryonal sarcoma in a young child. J Pediatr Surg 2009;44:e1–3.

297. Broughan TA, Esquivel CO, Vogt DP, et al. Pretransplant chemotherapy in pediatric hepatocellular carcinoma. J Pediatr Surg 1994;29:1319–22.

298. Esquivel CO, Gutierrez C, Cox KL, et al. Hepatocellular carcinoma and liver cell dysplasia in children with chronic liver disease. J Pediatr Surg 1994;29:1465–9.

299. Ryder SD. Guidelines for the diagnosis and treatment of hepatocellular carcinoma (HCC) in adults. Gut 2003;52(Suppl 3): iii1–8.

300. Stocker J. Hepatic Tumors. New York: Taylor & Francis; 1990.

301. M R, Gatzimos CD. Primary carcinoma of the liver in infants and children. Cancer 1957;10:678–86.

302. Manowski Z, Silver MM, Roberts EA, et al. Liver cell dysplasia and early liver transplantation in hereditary tyrosinemia. Mod Pathol 1990;3:694–701.

303. Kvittingen EA. Tyrosinaemia–treatment and outcome. J Inherit Metab Dis 1995;18:375–9.

304. Fink AS, Appelman HD, Thompson NW. Hemorrhage into a hepatic adenoma and type Ia glycogen storage disease: A case report and review of the literature. Surgery 1985;97:117–24.

305. Gruner BA, DeNapoli TS, Andrews W, et al. Hepatocellular carcinoma in children associated with Gardner syndrome or familial adenomatous polyposis. J Pediatr Hematol Oncol 1998; 20:274–8.

306. Sugarman GI. Heuser ET and Reed WB: A case of cerebral gigantism and hepatocarcinoma. Am J Dis Child 1977;131: 631–3.

307. Jain D, Hui P, McNamara J, Schwartz D, et al. Bloom syndrome in sibs: First reports of hepatocellular carcinoma and Wilms tumor with documented anaplasia and nephrogenic rests. Pediatr Dev Pathol 2001;4(6):585–9.

308. Ettinger LJ, Freeman AI. Hepatoma in a child with neurofibromatosis. Am J Dis Child 1979;133:528–31.

309. Ruymann FB, Mosijczuk AD, Sayers RJ. Hepatoma in a child with methotrexate-induced hepatic fibrosis. JAMA 1977;238(24): 2631–3.

310. Moore L, Bourne AJ, Moore DJ, et al. Hepatocellular carcinoma following neonatal hepatitis. Pediatr Pathol Lab Med 1997;17:601–10.

311. Bekassy AN, Garwicz S, Wiebe T, et al. Hepatocellular carcinoma associated with arteriohepatic dysplasia in a 4-year-old girl. Med Pediatr Oncol 1992;20:78–83.

312. Ni YH, Chang MH, Hsu HY, et al. Hepatocellular carcinoma in childhood. Clinical manifestations and prognosis. Cancer 1991;68: 1737–41.

313. Lee CL, Ko YC. Hepatitis B vaccination and hepatocellular carcinoma in Taiwan. Pediatrics 1997;99:351–3.

314. Yu MW, Chen CJ. Hepatitis B and C viruses in the development of hepatocellular carcinoma. Crit Rev Oncol Hematol 1994;17: 71–91.

315. Strickland DK, Jenkins JJ, Hudson MM. Hepatitis C infection and hepatocellular carcinoma after treatment of childhood cancer. J Pediatr Hematol Oncol 2001;23:527–9.

316. Kohno M, Kitatani H, Wada H, et al. Hepatocellular carcinoma complicating biliary cirrhosis caused by biliary atresia: Report of a case. J Pediatr Surg 1995;30:1713–16.

317. Wang JD, Chang TK, Chen HC, et al. Pediatric liver tumors: Initial presentation, image finding and outcome. Pediatr Int 2007;49:491–6.

318. Brower S, Hoff P, Jones D, et al. Pancreatic Cancer, Hepatobiliary Cancer, and Neuroendocrine Cancers of the GI Tract. Huntington; 1998.

319. Bolondi L. Screening for hepatocellular carcinoma in cirrhosis. J Hepatol 2003;39(6):1076–84.

320. Berman MA, Burnham JA, Sheahan DG. Fibrolamellar carcinoma of the liver: An immunohistochemical study of nineteen cases and a review of the literature. Hum Pathol 1988;19:784–94.

321. Kumada T, Nakano S, Takeda I, et al. Patterns of recurrence after initial treatment in patients with small hepatocellular carcinoma. Hepatology 1997;25:87–92.

322. A new prognostic system for hepatocellular carcinoma: A retrospective study of 435 patients: The Cancer of the Liver Italian Program (CLIP) investigators. Hepatology 1998;28:751–5.

323. Bruix J, Sherman M. Management of hepatocellular carcinoma. Hepatology 2005;42:1208–36.

324. Soyer P, Roche A, Levesque M, et al. CT of fibrolamellar hepatocellular carcinoma. J Comput Assist Tomogr 1991;15: 533–8.

325. Trevisani F, Cantarini MC, Wands JR, et al. Recent advances in the natural history of hepatocellular carcinoma. Carcinogenesis 2008;29(7):1299–305.

326. Debray D, Pariente D, Fabre M, et al. Fibrolamellar hepatocellular carcinoma: Report of a case mimicking a liver abscess. J Pediatr Gastroenterol Nutr 1994;19:468–72.

327. El-Gazzaz G, Wong W, El-Hadary MK, et al. Outcome of liver resection and transplantation for fibrolamellar hepatocellular carcinoma. Transpl Int 2000;13(Suppl 1):S406–409.

328. Katzenstein HM, Krailo MD, Malogolowkin MH, et al. Hepatocellular carcinoma in children and adolescents: Results from the Pediatric Oncology Group and the Children's Cancer Group intergroup study. J Clin Oncol 2002;20:2789–97.

329. Czauderna P, Mackinlay G, Perilongo G, et al. Hepatocellular carcinoma in children: Results of the first prospective study of the International Society of Pediatric Oncology group. J Clin Oncol 2002;20:2798–804.

330. von Schweinitz D. Management of liver tumors in childhood. Semin Pediatr Surg 2006;15:17–24.

331. Lau H, Fan ST, Ng IO, et al. Long term prognosis after hepatectomy for hepatocellular carcinoma: A survival analysis of 204 consecutive patients. Cancer 1998;83:2302–11.

332. Arii S, Okamoto E, Imamura M. Registries in Japan: Current status of hepatocellular carcinoma in Japan. Liver Cancer Study Group of Japan. Semin Surg Oncol 1996;12:204–11.

333. Poon RT, Ng IO, Lau C, et al. Tumor microvessel density as a predictor of recurrence after resection of hepatocellular carcinoma: A prospective study. J Clin Oncol 2002;20:1775–85.

334. Izumi R, Shimizu K, Ii T, et al. Prognostic factors of hepatocellular carcinoma in patients undergoing hepatic resection. Gastroenterology 1994;106:720–7.

335. Craig JR, Peters RL, Edmondson HA, et al. Fibrolamellar carcinoma of the liver: A tumor of adolescents and young adults with distinctive clinico-pathologic features. Cancer 1980;46: 372–9.

336. Farhi DC, Shikes RH, Murari PJ, et al. Hepatocellular carcinoma in young people. Cancer 1983;52:1516–25.

337. Nagorney DM, Adson MA, Weiland LH, et al. Fibrolamellar hepatoma. Am J Surg 1985;149:113–19.

338. Lack EE, Neave C, Vawter GF. Hepatocellular carcinoma. Review of 32 cases in childhood and adolescence. Cancer 1983;52: 1510–15.

339. Friedman AC, Lichtenstein JE, Goodman Z, et al. Fibrolamellar hepatocellular carcinoma. Radiology 1985;157:583–7.

340. Paradinas FJ, Melia WM, Wilkinson ML, et al. High serum vitamin B12 binding capacity as a marker of the fibrolamellar variant of hepatocellular carcinoma. Br Med J (Clin Res Ed) 1982;285:840–2.

341. Brandt DJ, Johnson CD, Stephens DH, et al. Imaging of fibrolamellar hepatocellular carcinoma. AJR Am J Roentgenol 1988;151:295–9.

342. Titelbaum DS, Hatabu H, Schiebler ML, et al. Fibrolamellar hepatocellular carcinoma: MR appearance. J Comput Assist Tomogr 1988;12:588–91.

343. Ang PT, Evans H, Pazdur R. Fibrolamellar hepatocellular carcinoma. Therapeutic implications of a ten-year disease-free interval. Am J Clin Oncol 1991;14:175–8.

344. O'Grady JG, Polson RJ, Rolles K, et al. Liver transplantation for malignant disease. Results in 93 consecutive patients. Ann Surg 1988;207:373–9.

345. Bilik R, Superina R. Transplantation for unresectable liver tumors in children. Transplant Proc 1997;29:2834–5.

346. Iwatsuki S, Gordon RD, Shaw BW Jr, Starzl TE. Role of liver transplantation in cancer therapy. Ann Surg 1985;202: 401–7.

347. Iwatsuki S, Dvorchik I, Marsh JW, et al. Liver transplantation for hepatocellular carcinoma: A proposal of a prognostic scoring system. J Am Coll Surg 2000;191:389–94.

348. Mazzaferro V, Regalia E, Doci R, et al. Liver transplantation for the treatment of small hepatocellular carcinomas in patients with cirrhosis. N Engl J Med 1996;334:693–9.

349. Beaunoyer M, Vanatta JM, Ogihara M, et al. Outcomes of transplantation in children with primary hepatic malignancy. Pediatr Transplant 2007;11:655–60.

350. Yao FY, Ferrell L, Bass NM, et al. Liver transplantation for hepatocellular carcinoma: Expansion of the tumor size limits does not adversely impact survival. Hepatology 2001;33: 1394–403.

351. Leung JY, Zhu AX, Gordon FD, et al. Liver transplantation outcomes for early-stage hepatocellular carcinoma: Results of a multicenter study. Liver Transpl 2004;10:1343–54.

352. Czauderna P, Mackinlay G, Perilongo G, et al. Hepatocellular carcinoma in children: Results of the first prospective study of the International Society of Pediatric Oncology grou. J Clin Oncol 2002;20:2798–804.

353. Austin MT, Leys CM, Feurer ID, et al. Liver transplantation for childhood hepatic malignancy: A review of the United Network for Organ Sharing (UNOS) database. J Pediatr Surg 2006;41: 182–6.

354. Lau WY, Lai EC. Hepatocellular carcinoma: Current management and recent advances. Hepatobiliary Pancreat Dis Int 2008;7: 237–57.

355. Scatton O, Zalinski S, Terris B, et al. Hepatocellular carcinoma developed on compensated cirrhosis: Resection as a selection tool for liver transplantation. Liver Transpl 2008;14:779–88.

356. Von Schweinitz D, et al. Treatment of liver tumors in chldren, in Liver Tumors: Current and Emerging Therapies. In: Clavien PA, Fong Y, Lyerly HK, editors. Boston: Jones and Barlett; 2004. p. 409–26.

357. Katzenstein HM, Krailo MD, Malogolowkin MH, et al. Fibrolamellar hepatocellular carcinoma in children and adolescents. Cancer 2003;97:2006–12.

358. Ahn SI, Seo JM, Shin SH, et al. Hepatocellular carcinoma with lung metastasis in a 9-year-old-boy. J Pediatr Surg 2001;36: 1599–601.

359. Yeh CN, Chen MF, Jeng LB. Resection of peritoneal implantation from hepatocellular carcinoma. Ann Surg Oncol 2002;9:863–8.

360. Salmi A, Turrini R, Lanzani G, et al. Long-term effectiveness of radiofrequency ablation for hepatocellular carcinoma of 3.5 cm or less. Hepatogastroenterology 2008;55:191–6.

361. Wang B, Lu Y, Zhang XF, et al. Management of spontaneous rupture of hepatocellular carcinoma. ANZ J Surg 2008;78: 501–3.

362. Ruymann FB, Raney RB Jr, Crist WM, et al. Rhabdomyosarcoma of the biliary tree in childhood. A report from the Intergroup Rhabdomyosarcoma Study. Cancer 1985;56:575–81.

363. Pollono DG, Tomarchio S, Berghoff R, et al. Rhabdomyosarcoma of extrahepatic biliary tree: Initial treatment with chemotherapy and conservative surgery. Med Pediatr Oncol 1998;30:290–3.

364. Sanz N, de Mingo L, Florez F, et al. Rhabdomyosarcoma of the biliary tree. Pediatr Surg Int 1997;12:200–1.

365. Schweizer PSM, Wehrmann M. Major resection for embryonal rhabdomyosarcoma of the biliary tree. Pediatr Surg Int 1994: 268–73.

366. Mihara S, Matsumoto H, Tokunaga F, et al. Botryoid rhabdomyosarcoma of the gallbladder in a child. Cancer 1982;49:812–18.

367. Horowitz ME, Etcubanas E, Webber BL, et al. Hepatic undifferentiated (embryonal) sarcoma and rhabdomyosarcoma in children. Results of therapy. Cancer 1987;59:396–402.

368. Isaacson C. Embryonal rhabdomyosarcoma of the ampulla of Vater. Cancer 1978;41:365–8.

369. Patil KK, Omojola MF, Khurana P, et al. Embryonal rhabdomyosarcoma within a choledochal cyst. Can Assoc Radiol J 1992;43:145–8.

370. Haith EE, Kepes JJ, Holder TM. Inflammatory pseudotumor involving the common bile duct of a six-year-old boy: Successful pancreaticoduodenectomy. Surgery 1964;56:436–41.

371. Huang FC, Eng HL, Chen CL, et al. Primary pleomorphic rhabdomyosarcoma of the liver: A case report. Hepatogastroenterology 2003;50:73–6.

372. Hirohashi S, Hirohashi R, Uchida H, et al. Pancreatitis: Evaluation with MR cholangiopancreatography in children. Radiology 1997;203:411–15.

373. Friedburg H, Kauffmann GW, Bohm N, et al. Sonographic and computed tomographic features of embryonal rhabdomyosarcoma of the biliary tract. Pediatr Radiol 1984;14:436–8.

CHAPTER 68

TERATOMAS, DERMOIDS, AND OTHER SOFT TISSUE TUMORS

Jean-Martin Laberge • Pramod S. Puligandla • Kenneth Shaw

TERATOMAS

Teratomas are generally divided into gonadal and extragonadal types. This chapter focuses on those in extragonadal locations, the most common being sacrococcygeal teratomas (SCT).

Embryology and Pathology

Teratoma, from the Greek *teratos* ('of the monster') and *onkoma* ('swelling'), is a term first applied by Virchow in 1869 to 'sacrococcygeal growths'.[1] Teratomas are composed of multiple tissues foreign to the organ or site from which they arise.[2] Although teratomas are sometimes defined as having three embryonic layers (endoderm, mesoderm, and ectoderm), recent classifications also include monodermal types.[2,3]

Teratomas are thought by some to arise from totipotent primordial germ cells.[3] These cells develop among the endodermal cells of the yolk sac near the origin of the allantois and migrate to the gonadal ridges during weeks 4 and 5 of gestation (Fig. 68-1).[4] Some cells may miss their target destination and give rise to a teratoma anywhere from the brain to the coccygeal area, usually in the midline. Another theory has teratomas arising from remnants of the primitive streak or primitive node.[4–6] During week 3 of development, midline cells at the caudal end of the embryo divide rapidly and, in a process called gastrulation, give rise to all three cell layers of the embryo (Fig. 68-2).[4] By the end of week 3, the primitive streak shortens and disappears. This theory explains the more common occurrence of teratomas in the sacrococcygeal region. With either theory, the totipotent cells could give rise to monoclonal neoplasms. Evidence shows that, whereas immature teratomas may be monoclonal, mature teratomas can be polyclonal, more like a hamartoma than a neoplasm.[7] This finding is compatible with the third theory that teratomas are a form of incomplete twinning.[2,3]

The primordial germ cell is the principal but probably not the exclusive progenitor of a teratoma. The recent trend is to include teratomas under the classification of germ cell tumors.[2,3,5] This histologic classification also includes germinomas (formerly dysgerminomas), embryonal carcinomas, yolk sac tumors (YST), choriocarcinomas, gonadoblastomas, and mixed germ cell tumors. Gonadal and extragonadal teratomas may have a different origin, explaining the different behavior according to tumor site.

Teratomas are fascinating tumors owing to the diversity of tissues they may contain and the varying degree of organization of these tissues. Many tumors contain skin elements, neural tissue, teeth, fat, cartilage, and intestinal mucosa, often with normal ganglion cells. These tissues are usually present as disorganized islands of cells with cystic spaces. The tumor sometimes consists of more organized tissue, such as small bowel, limbs, and even a beating heart. These have been called fetiform teratomas (Fig. 68-3).[2,3,5,8,9] When the mass includes vertebrae or notochord and a high degree of structural organization, the term fetus in fetu is used. This is viewed by some as a variant of conjoined twinning but is classified as a teratoma by others, owing to the absence of a recognizable umbilical cord in its vascular pedicle.[3,10] Whether teratomas are at one end of a spectrum that includes fetus in fetu, parasitic twins, conjoined twins, and normal twins is the subject of controversy. One certainly cannot dismiss the many reports of teratomas associated with fetus in fetu in the same patient and with a twin pregnancy.[2,3,11–13]

The overall tissue architecture is variable in teratomas. Moreover, a spectrum of cellular differentiation exists. Most benign teratomas are composed of mature cells, but 20–25% also contain immature elements, most often neuroepithelium. However, the degree of histologic immaturity is of proven prognostic significance only in ovarian teratomas.[3,14] Even this concept is being questioned, since one large cooperative study demonstrated that overlooked microscopic foci of YST, rather than the grade of immaturity, was more predictive of recurrence.[15] In neonatal teratoma, immature tissue is considered normal and without any influence on prognosis.[2,5,16] Spontaneous maturation of malignant tumors has been reported after partial excision of giant SCTs in two fetuses at 23 and 27 weeks of gestation.[17]

Teratomas may also contain or develop foci of malignancy. A malignant germ cell tumor may be found in sites typical for teratomas, such as the mediastinum or sacrococcygeal area. Whether the lesion was malignant from the onset or the malignant cells destroyed and replaced the benign teratoma component is often difficult to ascertain. The most common malignant component within a teratoma is a YST (formerly also called 'endodermal sinus tumor'). Other malignant germ cell tumors can occur, and, rarely, malignancy in other tissues composing the teratoma, such as neuroblastoma,[18,19] squamous cell carcinoma,[20] carcinoid,[21] and others, can develop. Malignancy at birth is uncommon but increases

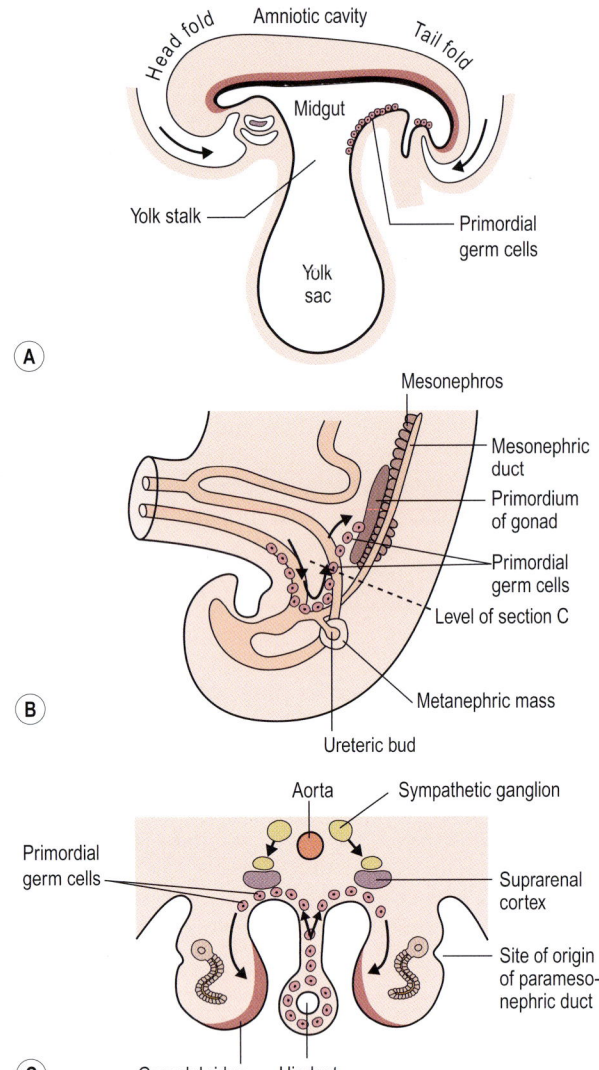

FIGURE 68-1 ■ Commonly cited theory on the origin of teratomas. **(A)** Drawing of embryo during week 4 (longitudinal section), showing primordial germ cells at the base of the yolk sac. **(B, C)** During week 5, these cells migrate toward the gonadal ridges. According to this theory, some cells could miss their intended destination. (Modified from Moore KL, Persaud TVN. The Developing Human. Philadelphia: WB Saunders; 1993. p. 71, 181.)

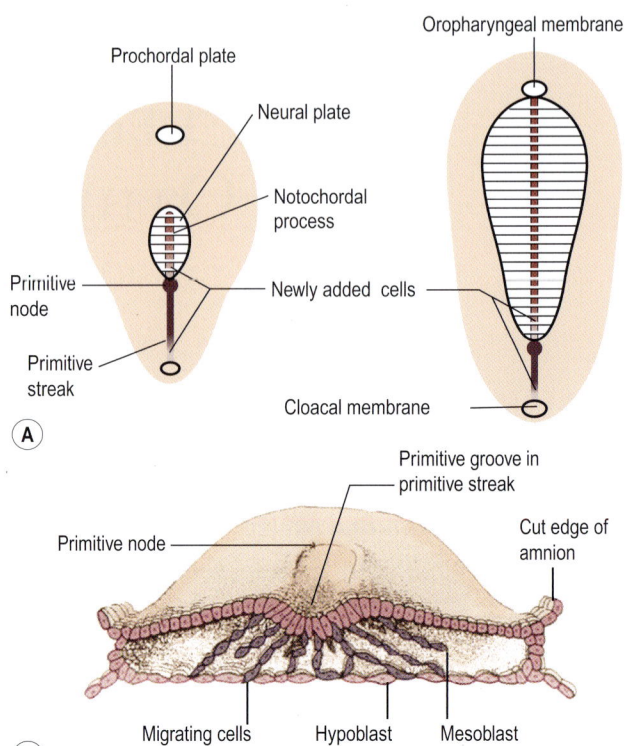

FIGURE 68-2 ■ Alternate theory on embryogenesis of teratomas. **(A)** Sketches of dorsal views of the embryonic disk on days 17 and 18, showing the primitive streak and primitive node. **(B)** Drawing of a transverse cut of the embryonic disk during week 3. This shows that cells from the primitive streak migrate to form the mesoblast (the origin of all mesenchymal tissues) and also displace the hypoblast to form the endoderm. Hence, remnants of these pluripotent primitive streak cells could give rise to teratomas and could account for the more frequent sacrococcygeal location. (From Moore KL, Persaud TVN. The Developing Human. Philadelphia: WB Saunders; 1993. p. 55–6.)

with age and with incomplete resection. An apparently mature teratoma may recur several months or years after resection as a malignant YST, illustrating the difficulties in histologic sampling of large tumors and the need for close follow-up.[2,5]

Most YSTs and some embryonal carcinomas secrete α-fetoprotein (AFP), which can be measured in the serum and demonstrated in the cells by immunohistochemistry.[22] This marker is particularly useful for assessing the presence of residual or recurrent disease. AFP levels are normally very high in neonates and decrease with time.[22,23] The postoperative half-life is about six days. Persistently high levels may be an indication for the need for further surgical procedures or chemotherapy. Other markers that may be elevated are β-human chorionic gonadotropin (β-hCG), produced by choriocarcinomas, and, rarely, carcinoembryonic antigen. CA 125 was also found helpful in the follow-up of patients with SCTs, but not CA 19–9.[24] Secretion of β-hCG by the tumor may be sufficient to cause precocious puberty.[25]

The genetic basis of teratomas is not yet understood. Most germ cell tumors appear to have an amplification, or isochromosome, in a region of the short arm of chromosome 12, designated i(12p).[3,26] This has been well described in adults but was not confirmed in one pediatric series in which deletions on chromosomes 1 and 6 were found instead.[27] Similarly, oncogenes and tumor suppressor genes did not appear to correlate with prognosis in one study.[28] *MYCN* gene amplification was present in immature teratomas, but absent in mature teratomas in another report.[29] *BAX* mutation and overexpression correlated with survival in another study of childhood germ cell tumors.[30] The clinical usefulness of these findings remains unclear.

Associated Anomalies

Teratomas are usually isolated lesions. A well-recognized association is the Currarino triad of anorectal malformation, sacral anomaly, and a presacral mass.[31,32] The presacral mass is usually a teratoma or an anterior meningocele. However, hamartomas, duplication cysts,

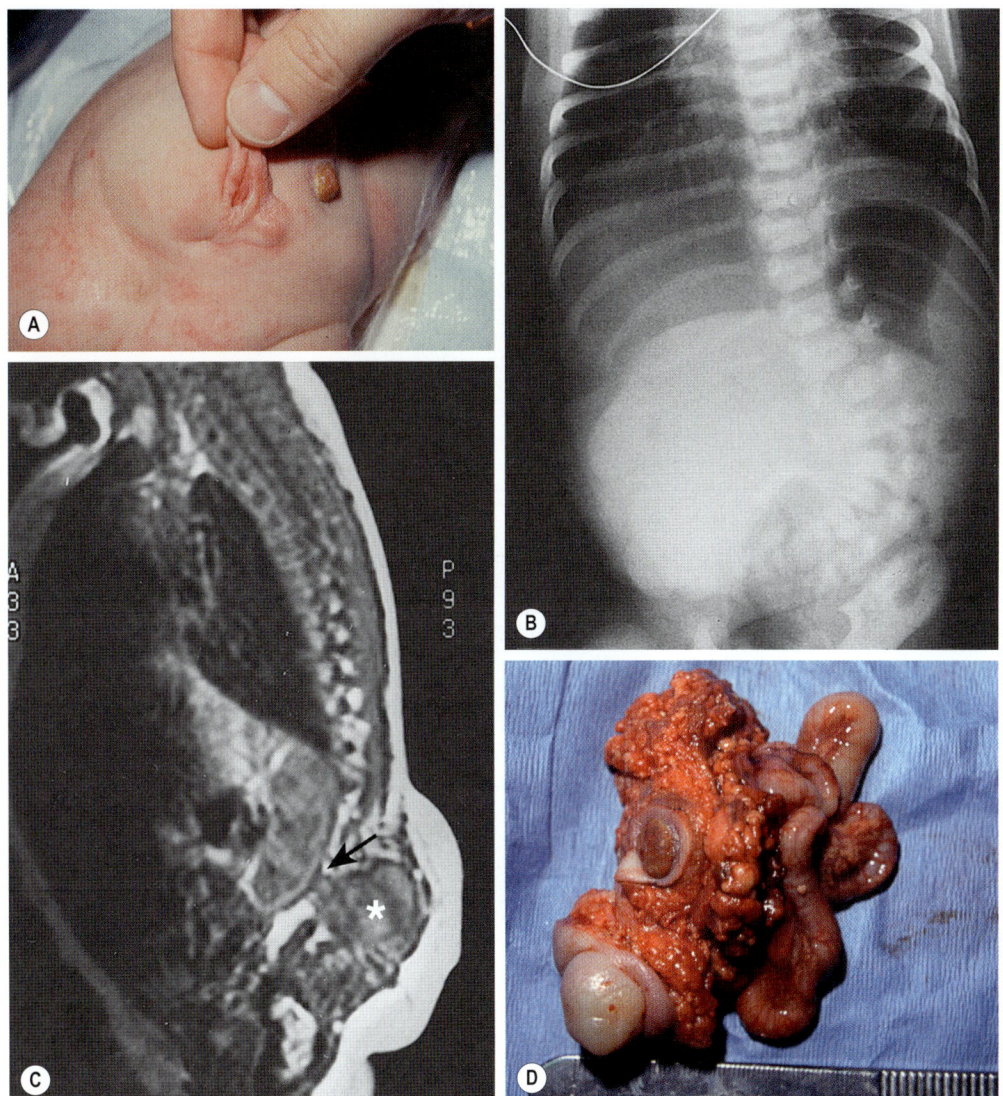

FIGURE 68-3 ■ **(A)** This child had a large fluctuant lumbar mass at birth. The patient is prone with the head at the top of the photograph. A family history of myelomeningocele existed in a great aunt. She also had an atrophic right leg with neurologic impairment below the L3 root and clubbing of the right foot. Note the ulcerated, arachnoid-looking area cranially and the pedunculated skin caudally, which had the appearance of a vulva and was oozing serous fluid. **(B)** Plain radiograph shows a severe lumbosacral scoliosis with vertebral anomalies. CT confirmed the vertebral anomalies with spina bifida and demonstrated a pattern of intestine with inspissated or calcified meconium in the teratoma. **(C)** MR image reveals that the mass (asterisk) extended into the retroperitoneum, where it was contiguous with the lower pole of the right kidney (arrow). **(D)** At operation, normal-looking blind bowel loops were found deep to the vulva-like structure. Part of the mass extended along the spinal cord, which required dissection and untethering by a neurosurgeon. The pathologic diagnosis was a mature fetiform teratoma that contained, among many other things, two adrenals, two ovaries, renal tissue with some glomeruli and tubules, bone with bone marrow, and portions of stomach and small and large bowel. The child recovered well neurologically but required spinal instrumentation owing to progressive scoliosis at age 2 years.

and dermoid cysts have been described, as have combinations of these lesions.

An extensive review of the English and German literature found 51 cases of infants with the Currarino triad and highlighted several important facts.[33] Twenty per cent of patients were older than 12 years at the time of diagnosis, yet no reports of malignancy were found. This contrasts to a 75% malignancy rate in patients older than 1 year who had the usual SCT.[34] However, a subsequent case report described a malignant recurrence that resulted in the patient's demise at 4 years of age despite chemotherapy.[35] Since then, more reports of malignant transformation of a presacral teratoma in the context of the

Currarino triad have appeared, and the risk of malignant transformation has been estimated at 1%.[36,37] This can occur well into adulthood.[38] Hence, one should not dismiss the presacral mass as always being benign in these patients. The female preponderance for patients with this triad is 1.5 : 1, which is less than the 3 : 1 ratio noted in isolated SCTs. A familial predisposition is noted in 57% of cases and has an autosomal dominant inheritance pattern.[39] Although all variants of anorectal malformations have been described, by far the most common is anal or anorectal stenosis. In one report, this triad was present in 38% of all patients with anorectal stenosis and in 1.6% of patients with low imperforate anus.[40]

Anal anomalies also have been reported in conjunction with a presacral mass, but in the absence of sacral defects. Hirschsprung disease has been incorrectly diagnosed in some cases,[41,42] indicating the need to eliminate the presence of a presacral mass by digital rectal examination, by a metal sound when the anus is too tight, or by imaging studies. In the screening of family members, normal plain radiographs of the sacrum are not adequate, because a presacral mass may exist in the absence of a bony defect.[43] The low incidence of malignancy has led one author to conclude that the presacral lesion in this context is a hamartoma rather than a teratoma.[44] This is supported by the demonstration of deletions or mutations of the homeobox gene *HLXB9*, located at 7q36, in several affected families.[45] In two families where one member had died from a malignant neuroendocrine tumor originating from a presacral teratoma, the diagnosis of Currarino syndrome was made through identification of a *HLXB9* mutation.[36,38]

The mutated gene has recently been renamed 'motor neuron and pancreas homeobox 1 (MNX1).'[45a] Urogenital anomalies, such as hypospadias, vesicoureteral reflux, vaginal or uterine duplications, and other anomalies are associated with teratomas.[32,34,46,47] Congenital dislocation of the hip has been found in 7% of patients with SCTs which can lead to late orthopedic sequelae.[48] Vertebral anomalies can also be found (see Fig 68-3). Central nervous system lesions, such as anencephaly, trigonocephaly, Dandy–Walker malformations, spina bifida, and myelomeningocele can occur as well.[2,3,49,50] Another peculiar association with SCTs is a family history of twins in as many as 10% of the patients.[39,51,52] Although not confirmed in all series, this finding, combined with reports of simultaneous twin pregnancy or sequential familial occurrences of fetus in fetu and teratoma, supports the theory that teratomas may be just one end of the spectrum of conjoint twinning.[2,3,9]

Klinefelter syndrome is strongly associated with mediastinal teratoma[50,53] and has been reported in patients with intracranial[54] and retroperitoneal tumors.[55] It is estimated that 8% of male patients with primary mediastinal germ cell tumors have Klinefelter syndrome, which is 50 times the expected frequency.[53] These tumors are often malignant, are of the choriocarcinoma type, secrete β-hCG, and produce precocious puberty. Histiocytosis and leukemia are also associated with mediastinal teratoma, both with and without Klinefelter syndrome.[56–58] Other hematologic malignancies, such Hodgkin disease, occur rarely.[59]

The following rare associations have been reported, most often with nonsacrococcygeal lesions: trisomy 13, trisomy 21, Morgagni hernia, congenital heart defects, Beckwith–Wiedemann syndrome, pterygium, cleft lip and palate, and rare syndromes, such as Proteus and Schinzel-Giedion syndromes.[49,50,60–64]

Diagnosis and Management by Tumor Site

Sacrococcygeal Teratoma

SCTs account for 35–60% of teratomas (gonadal included) in large series (Table 68-1).[65–67] This is the most common

TABLE 68-1	Relative Frequency of Teratomas by Site	
Site	**Number of Cases (%)**
Sacrococcygeal	290 (45)
Gonadal:	
Ovary	176 (27)
Testis	31 (5)
Mediastinal	41 (6)
Central nervous system	30 (5)
Retroperitoneal	28 (4)
Cervical	20 (3)
Head	20 (3)
Gastric	3 (<1)
Hepatic	2 (<1)
Pericardial	1 (<1)
Umbilical cord	1 (<1)
Total	**643 (100)**

Data are from five series of teratomas in children.
Modified from Dehner LP. Gonadal and extragonadal germ cell neoplasms: Teratomas in childhood. In: Finegold M, editor. Pathology of Neoplasia in Children and Adolescents. Philadelphia: WB Saunders; 1986. p. 282–312.

tumor in the newborn, even when stillbirths are considered.[49] The estimated incidence is 1 per 35,000 to 40,000 live births.[3,16]

Diagnosis. In countries where prenatal ultrasonography (US) is not readily available, most SCTs are seen as a visible mass at birth, making the diagnosis obvious (Fig. 68-4). Prenatal diagnosis has important implications and will be discussed further.

There is an unexplained female preponderance of 3 : 1.[34,65,67] The main differential diagnosis is meningocele.

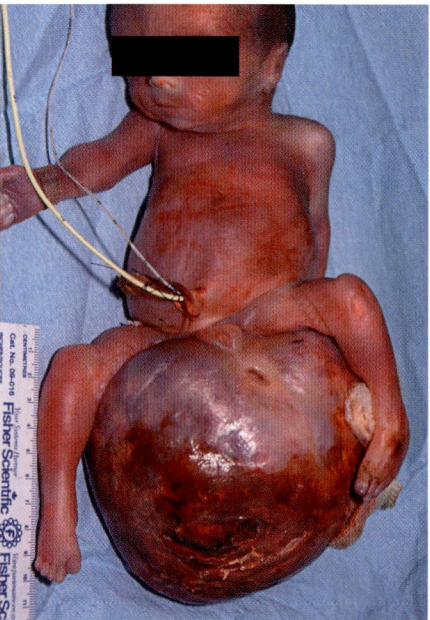

FIGURE 68-4 ■ This infant was diagnosed with a large sacrococcygeal teratoma in utero. Within days, premature labor occurred, prompting cesarian delivery at 25 weeks gestation. The baby died despite resuscitation attempts.

Typically, meningoceles occur cephalad to the sacrum and are covered by dura, but sometimes they are covered by skin. Examination of the child reveals bulging of the fontanelle with gentle pressure on a sacral meningocele, helping to establish the diagnosis before plain radiography, ultrasound, and magnetic resonance imaging (MRI) confirms it. The co-existence of meningocele with teratoma is well recognized in the familial form, but these are usually presacral. Rarely, a typical exophytic teratoma may have an intradural extension.[68,69] Other lesions in the differential diagnosis of neonatal sacrococcygeal masses include lymphangiomas, lipomas, tail-like remnants (Fig. 68-5), meconium pseudocysts, rectal duplications, and several other rare conditions.[34,70-73]

Although many neonates with SCTs do not have symptoms, some require intensive care because of prematurity, high-output cardiac failure, disseminated intravascular coagulation, and tumor rupture or bleeding within the tumor.[74-78] Lethal hyperkalemia from tumor necrosis has also been described.[79] Lesions with a large intrapelvic component may cause urinary obstruction.[78,80] Besides looking for signs of a myelomeningocele, the physical examination should always include a rectal examination to evaluate for an intrapelvic component. The most helpful imaging studies consist of plain anteroposterior and lateral radiographs of the pelvis and spine, looking for calcifications in the tumor and for spinal defects, and ultrasound of the abdomen, pelvis, and spine. Further preoperative studies are unnecessary in most newborns.

The diagnosis of purely intrapelvic teratomas is often delayed.[34] Children develop constipation, urinary retention, an abdominal mass, or symptoms of malignancy, such as failure to thrive. Age is a predictor of malignancy in patients with testicular, mediastinal, and SCTs.[2] The risk of malignancy is less than 10% at birth, but rises to more than 75% after age 1 year for SCTs, with the exception of familial presacral teratomas. The risk of malignancy also is high for incompletely excised lesions.

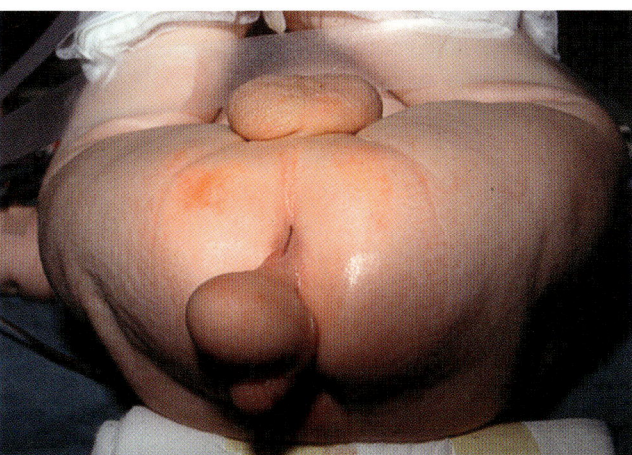

FIGURE 68-5 ■ This patient had a scrotum-like perianal mass with anal stenosis at birth. An anoplasty was done with removal of the mass, which was not attached to the coccyx. Pathology showed only fibroadipose tissue with smooth muscle, vascular structures, and cartilage, consistent with a hamartomatous process or caudal vestige (also called a tail remnant).

Complete excision of the tumor should be carried out as soon as the neonate is stable enough to undergo the operation. Serum markers should be determined before the operation for later comparison.

In recent decades, the diagnosis has often been made on prenatal ultrasound, especially when this examination is routinely performed in the second trimester. The site of the lesion, its complex appearance, and intrapelvic extension, with or without urinary tract obstruction, are easily recognized. Although most small teratomas do not adversely affect the fetus, the presence of a large solid vascular tumor is associated with a significant mortality rate, both in utero and perinatally.[75,76,78,81-83] Perinatal mortality is usually related to prematurity or tumor rupture with exsanguination (or both). Premature delivery may occur spontaneously from polyhydramnios or may be induced urgently because of fetal distress or maternal pre-eclampsia.

Repeated ultrasound assessment of tumor size is important because the fetus should be delivered by cesarean section if the tumor is larger than 5 cm or larger than the fetal biparietal diameter.[84] Dystocia during vaginal delivery is associated with tumor rupture and hemorrhage, and is an avoidable obstetric complication. The options in managing unexpected cases with dystocia include emergency cesarean completion of the partially delivered fetus, who has been intubated and ventilated after vaginal presentation of the head.[84]

Polyhydramnios with larger tumors may lead to premature labor; amnioreduction is often required to decrease uterine irritability.[78,83] Tumors that are larger than the fetal biparietal diameter at diagnosis, or that grow faster than the fetus or grow faster than 150 mL/week, are associated with a poor prognosis.[82,85] As the tumor enlarges, the fetus may develop placentomegaly or hydrops, caused by high-output cardiac failure from vascular shunting within the tumor, with fetal anemia from intratumoral bleeding also playing a role. This is a harbinger of impending fetal death and should lead to urgent cesarean delivery, especially when the maternal mirror syndrome has developed.[86] Open fetal surgical excision/debulking is one option in fetuses considered too premature to deliver. It has been performed with success in three of eight cases in one center and in three of four cases in another.[76,87] Interestingly, there were no cases of fetal resection in the latter center in a more recent cohort of 23 fetuses with SCT, emphasizing that the indications for such a procedure are limited.[82]

As a result of the maternal and fetal risks, less invasive therapeutic options have been sought. Successful intrauterine endoscopic laser ablation of the large feeding arteries has been described.[88] There have been several other reports, a few with good outcomes, but some with poor outcomes often related to severe fetal anemia and cardiac failure.[78,89,90] Alcohol injection has also been used.[78] Attempts at interrupting the high vascular flow have also been described by using radiofrequency ablation, with two survivors in the first four attempts.[91] One survivor had significant perineal damage.[92] As the technology has improved, there seems to be a renewed interest in this approach.[93-95] However, it remains unclear when early delivery is preferable to intervention in utero

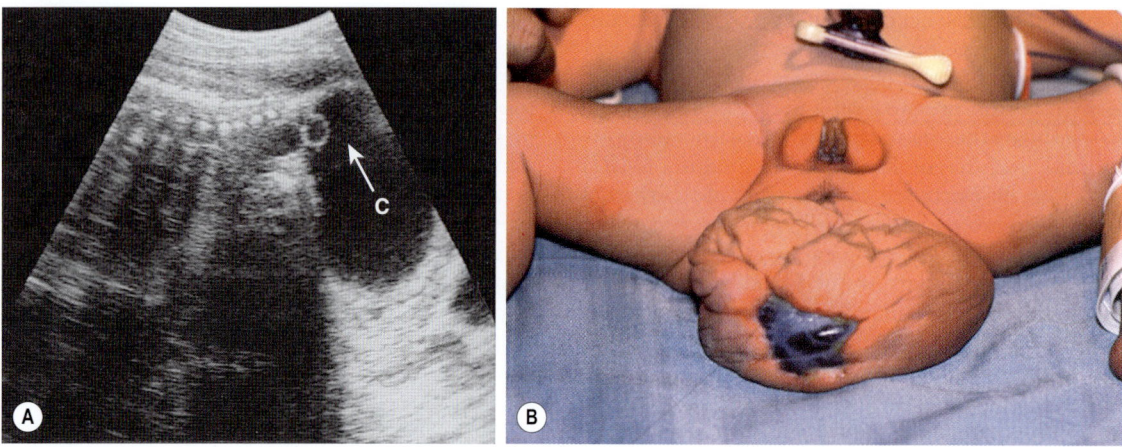

FIGURE 68-6 ■ **(A)** Ultrasound image of a female fetus at 38 weeks of gestation, showing a large cystic mass (C) attached to the coccyx, with tiny cysts anterior to the sacrum (arrow). An ultrasound evaluation at 18 weeks was normal. The cyst was gradually enlarging from an initial diameter of 9.5 cm at 31 weeks of gestation. The cyst was aspirated for 650 mL of fluid, permitting external rotation from breech to the vertex position. Two days later, when labor was induced, another 200 mL of fluid was removed to permit an uncomplicated vaginal delivery. **(B)** Twenty-four hours postnatally, the lesion remained floppy with an area of skin ulceration, likely a consequence of excessive in utero distention. A mature cystic teratoma was confirmed histologically.

in fetuses with early hydrops and placentomegaly. Some advocate a fetal operation before 30 weeks of gestation,[82] with the same group recently suggesting early delivery in selected fetuses after 27 weeks of gestation.[96] Others have reported survival after emergency delivery as early as 26 weeks of gestation.[97] The EXIT procedure (ex utero intrapartum treatment) has been used as an adjunct to allow safer resection of a ruptured teratoma in a 27 week gestation fetus, but long-term neurological sequelae were noted.[96]

Purely cystic teratomas occur in 10–15% of cases. Prenatal diagnosis allows percutaneous aspiration to facilitate delivery (Fig. 68-6), to decrease uterine irritability, or to prevent tumor rupture at delivery.[76,78,81,98,99] In another report, prenatal decompression using a cyst-amniotic shunt was successfully performed to relieve the obstructive uropathy caused by the cystic teratoma.[100] Fetal MRI is a useful adjunct to the prenatal evaluation, providing additional information that aids in counseling and preoperative planning.[101] It also helps in the differential diagnosis when the teratoma is entirely presacral.[102]

Operative Approach. Adequate intravenous access, preferably in the upper extremities, and the availability of blood products should be ascertained before starting the operation, especially with large tumors.

For most tumors, the major component is extrapelvic and the patient is placed in the prone position. If a significant intrapelvic or intra-abdominal component is present, or if the tumor is highly vascular and bleeding within the tumor is suspected, it may be wise to begin with a laparotomy or laparoscopy (see above). Generally, most resections can be achieved completely in the prone position, especially if the internal portion is cystic (Fig. 68-7).[78] When in doubt, a safe approach is to prepare the skin from the lower chest to the toes, allowing the infant to be turned to the supine position without having to re-drape. Vaseline packing in the rectum facilitates

its identification throughout the procedure. En bloc excision, including the coccyx, is preferable. Failure to remove the coccyx is associated with a high recurrence rate.[2,3,103] An acceptable gluteal crease and perineum is formed by the appropriate positioning of the perianal musculature. The use of plastic surgical principles to close the skin improves the cosmetic appearance of the scar (see Fig. 68-7, inset).[104]

Although the chevron incision has been used by most surgeons, a vertical incision is sometimes advantageous. It is preferred for smaller teratomas because it leaves a nearly normal-looking median raphe (Fig. 68-8). Resection of the excess skin at the closure gives an optimal cosmetic result. Others have reported using this approach for large tumors as well.[105]

Several techniques have been described to help in the management of giant SCTs. These include intraoperative snaring of the aorta,[77] laparoscopic division of the median sacral artery,[106,107] the use of extracorporeal membrane oxygenation and hypothermic perfusion,[108] devascularization and staged resection,[97,109] and preoperative embolization with or without radiofrequency ablation.[110,111] Autologous cord blood transfusion is another useful adjunct.[112]

Prognosis. Fetuses with an SCT diagnosed in utero have a survival rate in excess of 90% if the tumor is small and discovered by routine prenatal ultrasound. If a complicated pregnancy is the indication for ultrasound evaluation, the mortality increases to 60%. Nearly 100% of patients die when hydrops or placentomegaly develop.[76,78,81,113] Dystocia or tumor rupture during delivery are likely underreported as a cause of mortality.[83,114] In one series, 10% of babies died during transfer, all before the widespread use of antenatal ultrasound.[115] In a report describing 24 patients with a SCT diagnosed on routine obstetric ultrasound, 3 were aborted electively, four died in utero at 20 to 27 weeks of gestation, and three died of tumor rupture during delivery at 29 to 35

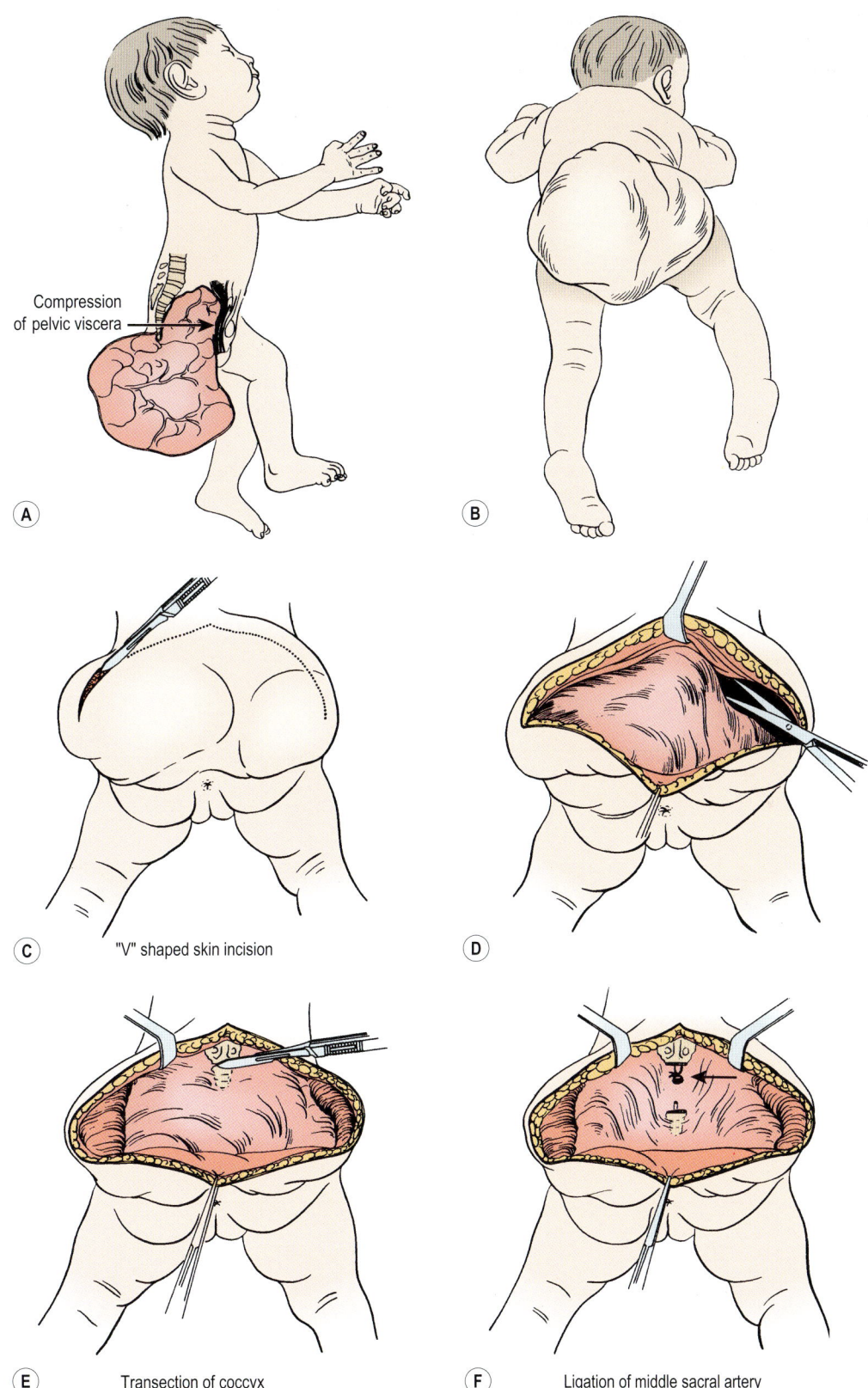

Compression of pelvic viscera

(A)

(B)

(C) "V" shaped skin incision

(D)

(E) Transection of coccyx

(F) Ligation of middle sacral artery

FIGURE 68-7 ■ **(A)** The teratomatous attachment may compress the rectum, vagina, and bladder anteriorly. **(B)** The patient is placed on the operating table in a prone jackknife position, with general endotracheal anesthesia. An appropriate intravenous cannula should be placed in an arm vein. **(C)** The incision is an inverted V-shape to allow excision of the tumor and to facilitate an eventually satisfactory cosmetic closure. The amount of skin excised is dependent on the size and shape of the tumor. **(D)** The tumor is dissected from the gluteus maximus muscle. **(E)** The coccyx is transected and removed in continuity with the tumor. **(F)** The middle sacral artery is the major blood supply to the tumor and is ligated (arrow) after transection of the coccyx.

Continued

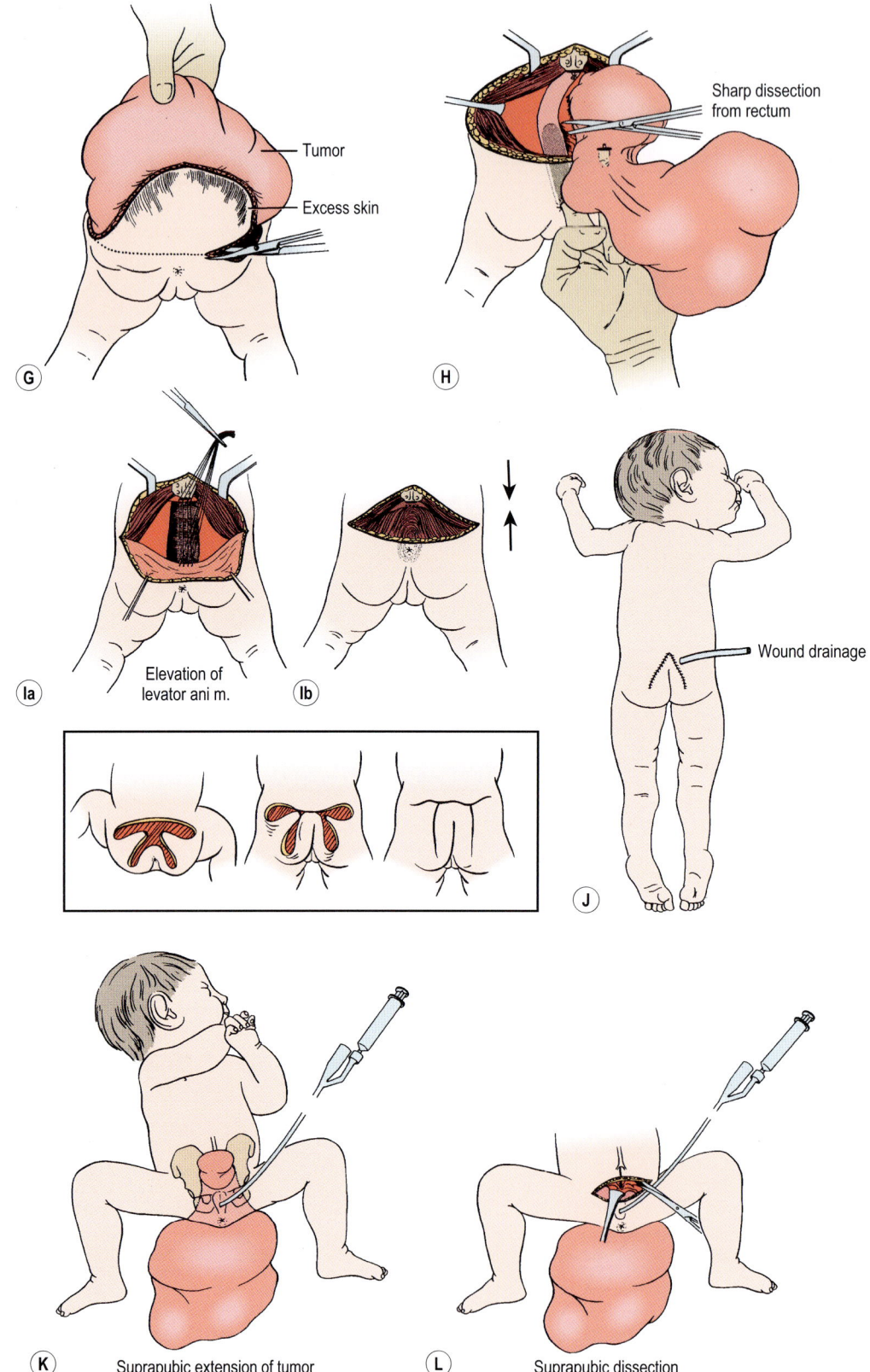

FIGURE 68-7, Cont'd ■ **(G)** Excess skin is excised to facilitate closure. **(H)** As the tumor is adherent to the rectum, sharp dissection can be directed by placing a finger in the rectum. **(I)** Placement of sutures between the anal sphincter and the presacral fascia (a). When the sutures are tied, the anal sphincter is pulled upward to the sacrum to form a gluteal crease (b). **(J)** A drain is left in the surgical site for drainage of postoperative serosanguineous fluid. Inset, Recently described technique for closure after excision of large teratomas. Using plastic surgery principles, this avoids 'dog ears' and places the scars along natural skin lines for a much-improved long-term cosmetic result. **(K)** If the tumor extends through the bony pelvis into the retroperitoneum, a urinary bladder catheter is inserted to facilitate suprapubic dissection. **(L)** Lower abdominal transverse incision allows interruption of the middle sacral artery and dissection of the tumor from the sacrum and pelvis, which is eventually removed from the perineum. (Inset redrawn from Fishman SJ, Jennings RW, Johnson SM, et al. Contouring buttock reconstruction after sacrococcygeal teratoma resection. J Pediatr Surg 2004;39:439–41; with permission.)

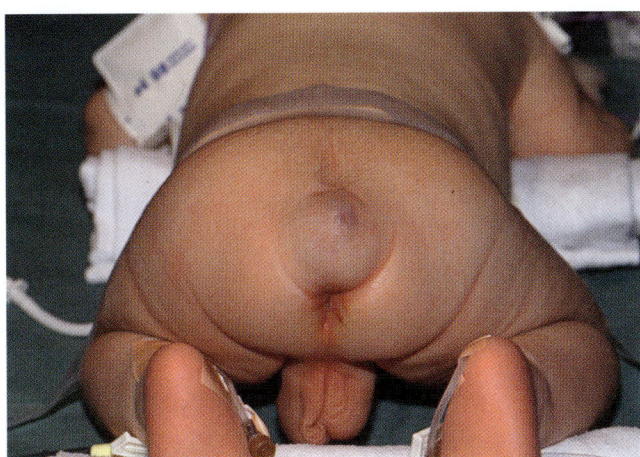

FIGURE 68-8 ■ Smaller cystic teratoma at age 1 month, initially mistaken for a hemangioma owing to its soft compressible nature and bluish skin discoloration. This tumor lends itself well to a longitudinal elliptical excision with midline closure, as in a posterior sagittal anorectoplasty.

weeks of gestation (one after vaginal and two after cesarean delivery).[75] The incidence of placentomegaly (none), hydrops (5%), and polyhydramnios (19%) was lower than in series in which ultrasound was performed for an obstetric reason.[76,84,116] Tumor size, vascularity, and content were used to develop a prognostic classification from a cohort of 44 fetal SCTs.[117] Fifty per cent of infants with tumors 10 cm or greater that were highly vascular or fast growing died, whereas none died if these features were absent or if the tumor was predominantly cystic. Recently, a growth rate >150 mL/week was found to be associated with an increased risk of perinatal mortality.[82] A vena cava diameter ≥6 mm and cardiac output ≥600 mL/kg/min have also been used to detect high-output cardiac failure in the early stages.[82] Another prognostic classification involves the ratio of solid tumor volume over the head volume.[118] In a series of 28 cases, none of the fetuses with STV/HV ratio <1 died, while 61% with a ratio >1 died. The same center has also reported risk stratification based on fetal echocardiographic findings.[119] Finally, the ratio of tumor volume over fetal weight was found to be an early prognostic marker.[120]

In the absence of severe prematurity and perinatal complications, the prognosis is dependent on the presence of malignancy and is therefore related to age at operation and completeness of resection.[121,122] When the tumor is benign and completely excised, recurrence is low, unless the tumor is large and mostly solid.[123] The recurrent tumor may be benign or malignant, and benign metastatic tissue may become evident in lymph nodes.[124] Although immature or fetal elements in gonadal teratomas are associated with a higher risk of aggressive behavior, this is not considered true for SCTs.[2,5,16] However, a multicenter study identified immature histology, in addition to malignancy and incomplete resection, as risk factors for recurrence.[122] Although malignant recurrence of a 'benign' teratoma may be as high as 10–15%,[6,122] the original benign diagnosis may have been due to sampling error,[15] an undetected residual microscopic focus of malignant tumor,[125] or secondary to incomplete coccygectomy at the initial operation.[35] Patients whose tumors

are resected after the newborn period have a higher risk of malignant recurrence, especially when an elevated AFP level is present at diagnosis. The elevated AFP likely signifies the presence of malignancy in the original tumor.[15,126] It is important to monitor all patients by physical examination, including rectal examination and serum markers (AFP and CA 125), every two or three months for at least 3 years because most recurrences occur within three years of operation.[24,127]

Recurrent disease is usually local, but metastases to inguinal nodes, lung, liver, brain, and peritoneum can occur, including pseudomyxoma peritonei.[128] The prognosis of a malignant tumor or a malignant recurrence was dismal until the advent of platinum-based chemotherapy.[125] Survival rates of 80–90% are now achieved, even in the presence of metastatic disease, but the risk of late recurrences or second malignancies persists.[129–131] Older patients presenting with large malignant tumors usually undergo biopsy followed by chemotherapy before resection is attempted to avoid sacrificing vital structures.[16,130,132]

A Children's Cancer Group (CCG) review illustrates the shift in mortality causes, from late diagnosis/malignancy to perinatal events.[129] The mortality was 10% in 126 patients treated in 15 institutions from 1972 to 1994. Three patients died of severe associated anomalies. Two died of hemorrhagic shock postoperatively and six due to combinations of severe prematurity, birth asphyxia due to failed vaginal delivery, or preoperative tumor rupture. Death from a metastatic YST occurred in one patient. A second patient with metastatic disease was lost to follow-up and is presumed dead. Thus, only two deaths occurred from malignancy, despite a total of 20 YSTs (13 malignant at initial operation, seven malignant recurrences after resection of 'benign' teratomas). Owing to the effectiveness of current chemotherapy in treating recurrent disease, as well as its toxicity in young infants, it appears that a completely excised malignant YST does not require adjuvant therapy. These patients should be closely monitored clinically and with serial AFP measurements.[133] Similar encouraging results have been found in the German Cooperative Studies.[134]

In the current era of the rather routine use of ultrasound in pregnancy, the prognosis for patients with an SCT is not dependent on Altman's classification[34] but rather on tumor size, physiologic consequences, histology, and associated anomalies. The prognosis of malignant tumors depends on tumor type, stage, location, and patient age.[129] Functional results in survivors have been reported as excellent in most series.[78,135,136] However, several reports draw attention to fecal and urinary continence problems, as well as lower limb weakness.[121,137–141] Some of these problems are clearly related to associated anomalies,[115] the need for reoperation,[142] or to the presence of large presacral or intra-abdominal tumors,[80,135] but they can occur after excision of purely extrapelvic benign tumors. A good outcome requires meticulous dissection along the tumor capsule, preservation and reconstruction of muscular structures, and long-term follow-up. One group advocates earlier cesarean delivery to minimize urologic sequelae in patients with large tumors causing urinary tract dilatation.[139] Others have placed vesico-amniotic shunts in such cases with good outcomes.[78,100] Urodynamic studies and surveillance ultrasound are now being performed more regularly in some centers.[143] Patients with Currarino syndrome, who often have a tethered cord in addition to the presacral tumor, appear to have an increased risk of bladder and bowel dysfunction.[144,145] A poor cosmetic result was noted in more than half of the patients in another review.[146] These authors advocate early assessment of bladder, anorectal, and sexual function along with cosmetic results within a structured oncology follow-up program. The technique described by the Boston Children's group is a major step to improve cosmesis (see Fig. 68-7),[104] while others favor a sagittal incision.[105]

Thoracic Teratomas

The anterior mediastinum is the most common site of thoracic teratomas, which account for 7–10% of all teratomas (see Table 68-1).[2,3]

Mediastinal Teratomas. Mediastinal teratomas are diagnosed from the fetal period to adolescence and even adulthood.[2,147–149] Most are located in the anterior mediastinum, but a few have been described in the posterior mediastinum, some with epidural extension.[150–152] In infants, respiratory distress is a common presenting manifestation,[153] but in older children the teratoma is often an incidental finding on chest radiograph (Fig. 68-9).[2] Any patient with a mediastinal mass that presents with orthopnea or a reduction in the tracheal cross-sectional diameter of greater than 50% on axial imaging is at a significant risk for airway collapse during general anesthesia.[154] In these cases, procedures using local or regional anesthesia may be required to obtain a confirmatory diagnosis. Mediastinal teratomas may be first seen as a chest wall tumor and may even erode through the skin. They also can erode into a bronchus, with hemoptysis as the initial manifestation,[155] or rupture into the pleural cavity.[156] Secondary pericardial effusion and tamponade

have also been described.[157] A strong association has been found with Klinefelter syndrome. In these cases, choriocarcinoma in the teratoma often leads to precocious puberty (see under Associated Anomalies).[2,25,58] Mediastinal germ cell tumors have also been observed concurrently or after treatment for hematologic malignancies such as Langerhan's cell histiocytosis and hemophagocytic syndrome.[57,158,159] Histologically, the presence of immature tissue does not affect the prognosis in children younger than 15 years. After age 15, mediastinal teratomas have a high incidence of malignant behavior, which is usually indicated by elevated levels of AFP or β-hCG, or both.[149] For those with malignancy, YST is most prevalent in girls and young boys while mixed histology prevails in over 50% of older adolescent males.[160]

Tumors should be excised through either a median sternotomy or a thoracotomy.[16,161] Smaller tumors may be approached through an anterior mediastinotomy (see Fig. 68-9) or by thoracoscopy,[162] although tumor seeding is a concern with the latter. Complete resection is the goal, but often these masses are too large at presentation and require initial biopsy followed by chemotherapy.[16,163,164] During chemotherapy, attention should be paid to the 'growing teratoma syndrome' that occurs when the benign elements within a germ cell tumor continue to grow.[165] A Pediatric Oncology Group (POG) and Children Cancer Group (CCG) intergroup study involving 38 patients demonstrated that primary resection could be achieved in 14 patients.[160] In another 18, chemotherapy reduced tumor size in 57% while the remainder were stable or increased in size. All patients with residual disease underwent successful postchemotherapy resection. The overall survival for malignant mediastinal germ cell tumors was 71% which is less than for other extragonadal sites. The prognosis is best for young children with YSTs and worst in older adolescents with mixed germ cell histology.[149,160] In a recent series from Memorial Sloan-Kettering Cancer Center, normalization or reduction in preoperative tumor markers was the strongest predictor of increased survival.[161]

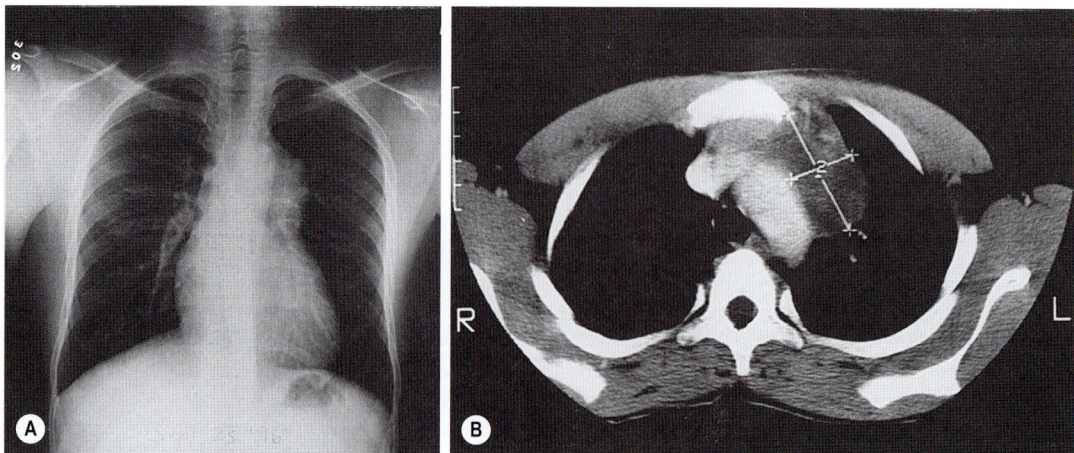

FIGURE 68-9 ■ **(A)** A 13-year-old African boy has an asymptomatic anterior mediastinal mass that was discovered on routine immigration chest radiograph. **(B)** The CT scan shows a heterogeneous mass adjacent to the aorta, suggestive of a neoplasm (thymoma or lymphoma). During consideration of a fine-needle aspiration biopsy, ultrasonography was done and suggested the presence of cysts with debris (not shown). MRI (not shown) confirmed the presence of the cystic components as well as fat. A mature teratoma was excised through a small left anterior mediastinotomy, removing the left second costal cartilage.

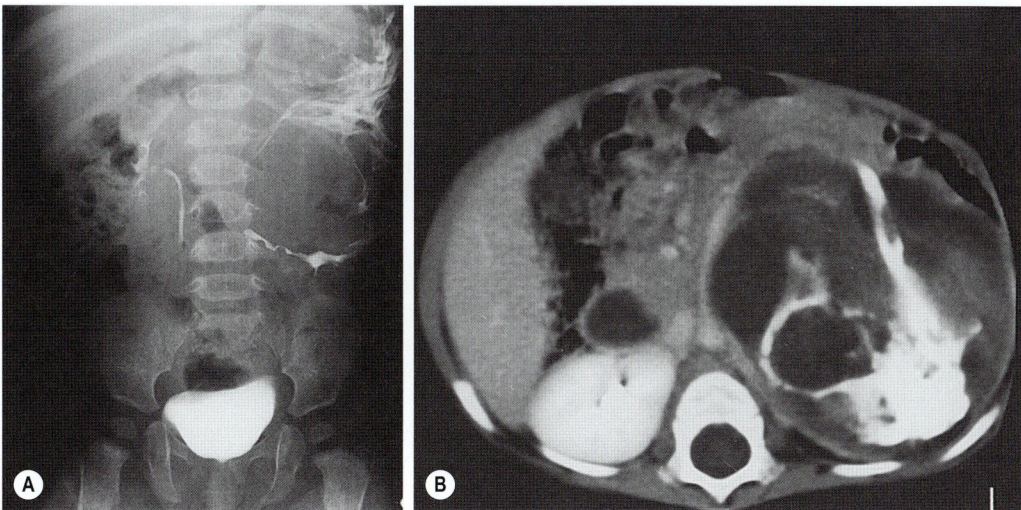

FIGURE 68-10 ■ This 7-month-old girl was found to have an abdominal mass on physical examination. **(A)** Plain radiograph films showed a large calcified left upper quadrant mass, which can be seen to displace the kidney inferiorly after injection of intravenous contrast. Ultrasonography (not shown) revealed multiple cystic areas. **(B)** This was confirmed by CT, which also revealed areas of fat density, making teratoma much more likely than neuroblastoma. The mature teratoma contained all types of cerebral and cerebellar tissues; respiratory, transitional, and squamous epithelium; sebaceous and salivary glands; smooth muscle; cartilage; and fat. Serum markers were normal.

Intrapericardial Teratomas. Intrapericardial teratomas are most commonly seen in the newborn period or in utero, with evidence of cardiorespiratory distress secondary to pericardial effusions or nonimmune fetal hydrops resulting from cardiac compression.[2,3,166] While a fetal diagnosis allows for early postnatal treatment in most newborns, it may also offer an opportunity for antenatal interventions such as fetal pericardiocentesis.[167] Early delivery for emergency surgical excision should be considered if the baby develops signs of cardiac tamponade.[168] Intrapericardial teratomas are also the leading cause of massive pericardial effusion in the neonate and any delays in diagnosis could be fatal.[3,169] In older infants, it may present with respiratory distress or poor feeding. Ultrasound imaging usually demonstrates a cystic or solid teratoma located anterior to the right atrium and ventricle with attachments to the great vessels (see Fig. 25-4).[170] The tumor may also be found incidentally on chest radiographs performed for other reasons. The only treatment option for this lesion is excision. On histologic examination, these teratomas are usually composed of mature tissue with or without neuroglial elements.[2,3]

Intracardiac Teratomas. Intracardiac teratomas are rare and arise from the atrium or ventricle. Many can be cured by resection.[171]

Pulmonary Teratomas. Few cases of intrapulmonary teratoma have been described.[172] Symptoms include trichoptysis or hemoptysis. Lobectomy is the usual treatment.

Abdominal Teratomas

The most frequent abdominal teratomas are the gonadal teratomas, which are discussed in other chapters.

Retroperitoneal Teratomas. Retroperitoneal teratomas occur outside the pelvis, often in a suprarenal location. They represent about 4% of all childhood teratomas, and 75% occur in children younger than 5 years.[3,173] They occur twice as frequently in females and may have an association with Klinefelter syndrome.[16,55] While more than 90% are benign, up to one-quarter may be malignant when diagnosed in the first month of life.[174] Usually the tumor is discovered as an abdominal mass that compresses the gastrointestinal tract, causing symptoms such as vomiting, difficulty feeding and constipation.[163] Presentation with an acute abdomen from infection has also been described.[175] Abdominal radiographs may show calcifications or bony structures within the tumor (Fig. 68-10). ultrasound, CT scan, or MRI, and the assessment of serum markers are the essential aspects of preoperative evaluation. Operative excision is usually straightforward,[176,177] but occasionally the tumor may encase major vessels, making resection difficult.[178] Malignant lesions present as bulky masses that are not easily resectable.[163] In a POG/CCG intergroup study involving 25 patients, only five could be resected primarily.[179] The remainder underwent initial biopsy and platinum-based chemotherapy, of which four did not require further surgery. The remaining patients in this series underwent total or partial resection with a 6-year event-free survival of over 80% and an overall survival close to 90%. The retroperitoneum is also the most common site for the fetus in fetu malformations and intermediate fetiform teratomas.[2,3,180,181]

Gastric Teratomas. Gastric teratomas are rare lesions seen most commonly in infant boys.[2,182] They account for 1% of all teratomas. Clinically, the tumors present with hematemesis or vomiting due to gastric-outlet obstruction in the postnatal period, but rapid growth in utero has also been described leading to fetal distress and emergency cesarean delivery.[183] A palpable mass is common. The tumor is usually an exophytic mass in the lesser curvature or posterior wall of the stomach, but the whole stomach may be involved. Most gastric teratomas are benign with mature and immature elements, most frequently containing neuroglial tissue. Benign peritoneal gliomatosis has been found incidentally in hernia sacs after resection of a gastric teratoma as an infant, illustrating the unusual behavior of some of these tumors.[184] Excision is curative. Recurrence and malignancy are rare, despite local infiltration or nodal metastasis.[182,185] Periodic follow-up including AFP measurements is nevertheless important.[186]

Others. Other rare sites of abdominal teratomas include liver, gallbladder, pancreas, kidney, intestine, bladder, prostate, uterus, mesentery, omentum, abdominal wall and diaphragm.[2,3,187–192]

Head and Neck Teratomas

More than 10% of teratomas in children originate from the neck, head, and central nervous system.[2,3,193,194] Many of these tumors are now diagnosed with prenatal ultrasound (Fig. 68-11). They are associated with an increased incidence of stillbirth, especially in the absence of prenatal diagnosis.[174,195]

Cervical Teratomas. Cervical teratomas represent up to 8% of all teratomas.[18,195] These tumors are initially seen as a partly or completely cystic neck mass. Large teratomas often lead to severe polyhydramnios, presumably because of esophageal compression; in turn, this may

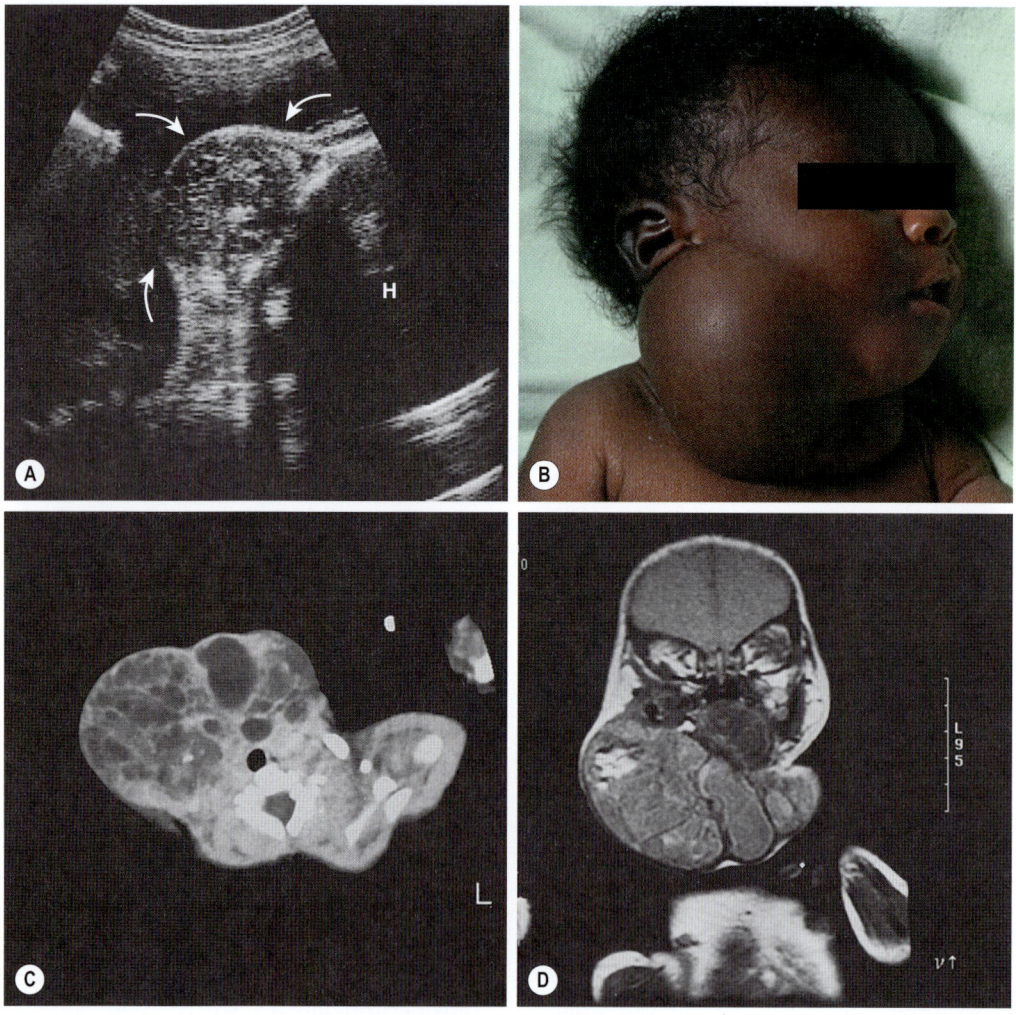

FIGURE 68-11 ■ **(A)** Fetal ultrasound image at 34 weeks of gestation shows a 7 cm cervical mass of mixed echogenicity, containing blood flow by Doppler (arrows point to the mass; H, head). **(B)** After birth by cesarean section, the neonate had only mild tachypnea despite the large right cervical mass extending to the left side. Parts of the mass transilluminated, suggesting the diagnosis of a lymphangioma. **(C)** CT scan of the lower cervical area shows an intact trachea and multiple cysts in the mass. **(D)** MRI confirmed the presence of fat, which appears bright on T_1-weighted images as well as on the proton density–weighted imaging sequence shown here. At operation, the mass appeared to originate from the right lobe of the thyroid gland. It contained epithelium-lined cysts, cartilage, bone, glandular tissue, and complex papillary structures. A predominance of neuroepithelial tissue was found with a few small areas of immature, neuroblastoma-like tissue. Preoperative vanillylmandelic acid levels were normal. The patient required postoperative thyroid hormone supplementation because of subclinical hypothyroidism (elevated thyroid-stimulating hormone with normal thyroxine and triiodothyronine levels).

lead to premature labor. Serial amnioreduction may be required to prevent this complication (see Fig. 68-12). Tracheal deviation and/or obstruction may also be identified on prenatal imaging studies such as fetal MRI,[196] thus necessitating a strategy to secure the airway immediately after birth. Indeed, death may result in the inability to intubate a severely compressed or deviated trachea.[18,197] Predictors of airway obstruction based on prenatal ultrasound have also been identified, including the presence of polyhydramnios, a presumptive diagnosis of teratoma as well as a tracheoesophageal displacement index greater than 12.[198] Prenatal diagnosis permits cesarean section and the establishment of an airway by the surgical team before the cord is clamped.[197] Refinements of this technique (EXIT procedure) have been well documented in a series of 87 infants from Children's Hospital of Philadelphia, of whom 17 had giant cervical teratomas.[199] Extension of tumor to the mediastinum or displacement of the trachea and carina may cause pulmonary hypoplasia, which increases respiratory morbidity and mortality.[200] The tumor is usually well defined and may contain calcifications. The differential diagnosis includes cervical lymphangioma, congenital goiter, foregut duplication cyst, branchial cleft cyst, or rarely cystic neuroblastoma (Fig. 68-12).[166,169] Postnatal investigations should include plain radiographs, ultrasound, and a measurement of AFP and β-hCG, as well as urinary catecholamine metabolites. CT and MRI may be useful adjuncts to establish the diagnosis and to define anatomic relationships.

Complete excision is accomplished through a wide collar incision. The tumor is usually not difficult to separate from the strap muscles and the fascial planes, but the pretracheal fascia is sometimes very adherent. Often, the site of origin cannot be identified, yet in many instances, the tumor is firmly attached to and appears to originate from the thyroid gland. A thyroid lobectomy should be performed in these cases. In other instances, the tumor is adherent to the pharynx. In these cases, meticulous dissection and pharyngotomy, if necessary, are important to prevent tumor recurrence. Giant teratomas may distort the anatomy, leading to permanent sequelae. Generally, the tumor is composed of both mature and immature neuroglial tissue, but cartilage and bronchial epithelium are not uncommon.[18,201] In 35% of cases, the tumor contains thyroid tissue, and hypothyroidism is a well-known postoperative complication.[202] Cervical teratomas are usually benign, but malignancy has been reported, even in infants. A report from the CCG showed that 20% of tumors clearly contained malignant elements, most often neuroblastoma, but also teratocarcinoma, neuroblastoma-like tumor, and neuroectodermal tumor.[18] Complete excision in the newborn period results in a survival rate of 80–90%. As for teratomas in other sites, one newborn was reported with a benign thyroid teratoma accompanied by neuroglial tissue deposits in cervical nodes.[203] A prognostic classification for cervical teratomas takes into account birth status, age at diagnosis, and presence of respiratory distress.[201] In neonates without respiratory distress, the mortality rate was 2.7%, compared with 43.4% in those with respiratory compromise. Prenatal diagnosis and delivery using the EXIT procedure can undoubtedly increase survival.[199]

Thyroid teratomas may be present in older children and adults, and are often malignant in the latter.[204,205] Spindle epithelial tumor with thymus-like elements (SETTLE) is a malignant thyroid neoplasm that can sometimes be confused with thyroid teratomas due to their spindle cell and epithelial components.[206] These unique neoplasms have a propensity for delayed metastases, particularly to the lungs, kidney, mediastinum, lymph nodes, liver and vertebrae. Adjuvant chemotherapy and radiotherapy do not seem to have a significant impact on overall outcome for metastatic disease. In these cases, survival is poor.[206]

Craniofacial Teratomas. Craniofacial teratomas include a spectrum of lesions that may be life-threatening.

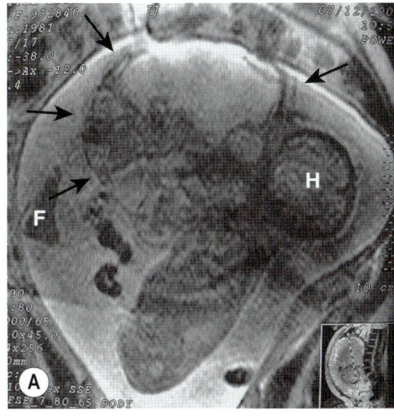
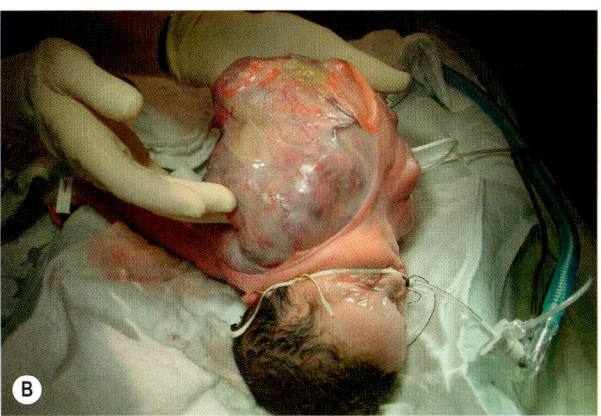

FIGURE 68-12 ■ **(A)** A fetus has a giant cervical teratoma which is seen on magnetic resonance imaging at 30 weeks of gestation. The lesion was first diagnosed on routine ultrasonography at 18 weeks and grew much faster than the fetus. Several amnioreductions were required because of polyhydramnios, and an EXIT procedure was performed at 34 weeks of gestation (H, head; F, foot; arrows outline the tumor). **(B)** After securing the airway during the EXIT procedure and stabilizing the neonate, resection was completed successfully. During resection, it was found that the left carotid artery and jugular vein entered the tumor. The left vagus nerve (hence the left recurrent nerve) was never seen, and the left glossopharyngeal nerve also was sacrificed. The tumor originated from the left pharyngeal wall. Including the fluid within the cystic parts, the teratoma weighed 1.4 kg, and the neonate weighed 1.6 kg postoperatively.

Epignathus. Epignathus is a term used to describe teratomas protruding from the mouth (Fig. 68-13). These tumors arise from the soft or hard palate in the region of Rathke's pouch.[207,208] They generally fill the oral cavity and extend out through the mouth. They can prevent fetal swallowing, which leads to polyhydramnios. An EXIT procedure may be required.[209] Surgical excision is mandatory. These lesions are usually benign, and recurrence is rare. A high degree of organization often gives them the appearance of a parasitic fetus. Prenatally, the differential diagnosis includes a large epulis, a benign lesion which will be discussed further in this chapter.[210]

Nasopharyngeal Teratomas. Nasopharyngeal teratomas arise from the posterior aspect of the nasopharynx.[211] Large tumors can interfere with fetal swallowing and produce polyhydramnios, cause severe respiratory distress at birth, and lead to stillbirth.[2] Most pharyngeal teratomas are benign, and the treatment is excision.

Oropharyngeal Teratomas. Oropharyngeal teratomas represent 2% of all teratomas.[212] These tumors can originate from the tongue, sinuses, mandible, and tonsils. Airway compromise requires immediate care at the time of delivery. For oro- and nasopharyngeal teratomas, the EXIT procedure may be indicated when a large tumor detected prenatally appears to obstruct the airway.[213] Most tumors are benign, and recurrence is uncommon after complete resection. Separate tumors may occur in the same infant, and intracranial extension has been described.[214]

Other Sites. Craniofacial teratomas can be found in the orbit, the middle ear, and skull.[215,216] Intracranial teratomas account for only 2–4% of all teratomas, but represent nearly 50% of brain tumors in the first two months of life.[2,3] Most are benign in neonates but can be malignant in older children and young adults, and are often unresectable.[217,218] These teratomas can appear in utero and cause massive hydrocephalus. Perinatal mortality is high, with only a 6% survival when diagnosed in the fetus or newborn.[3,219] The pineal gland is the most common site of origin, but intracranial teratomas can be seen in different areas, such as the hypothalamus, ventricles, cavernous sinus, cerebellum, and suprasellar region.[218,220] Pineal gland teratomas can secrete enough β-hCG to cause precocious puberty.[2,219]

Miscellaneous Sites

Teratomas have been reported in other sites, such as skin, parotid, vulva, perianal region well away from the coccyx, spinal canal, umbilical cord (possibly associated with omphalocele), and placenta.[2,3,221–224] Some of the spinal teratomas are now considered to be enterogenous cysts.[225]

DERMOID, EPIDERMOID, AND RELATED CYSTS

Dermoid Cysts

Dermoid cysts are congenital cysts that are lined by skin with fully mature pilosebaceous structures.[226] They are the result of sequestration of skin along lines of embryonic closure. Typical locations are under the lateral part of the eyebrow, the scalp, the glabella, the tip of the nose, and the orbit. The head and neck are the sites of predilection, but these lesions have been described in other midline sites, including the sacral area, perineal raphe, scrotum, and presternal area. The so-called dermoids of the ovary are, in fact, cystic teratomas and are discussed in Chapter 74.

Dermoids are usually round, soft, and often fixed to deep tissues or to bone. They usually present as a painless mass of 1–2 cm in diameter but can grow up to 4 cm or more if untreated. Some are associated with a sinus tract, especially those on the nose. This site is also typical for intracranial extension and a familial occurrence.[227] Dermoids in the head area are usually deep to muscles and often cause an indentation in the outer table of the skull. They can even erode through both bony tables and extend intracranially. A skull radiograph may show the defect, but it may be normal if the cyst is situated over a fontanelle or

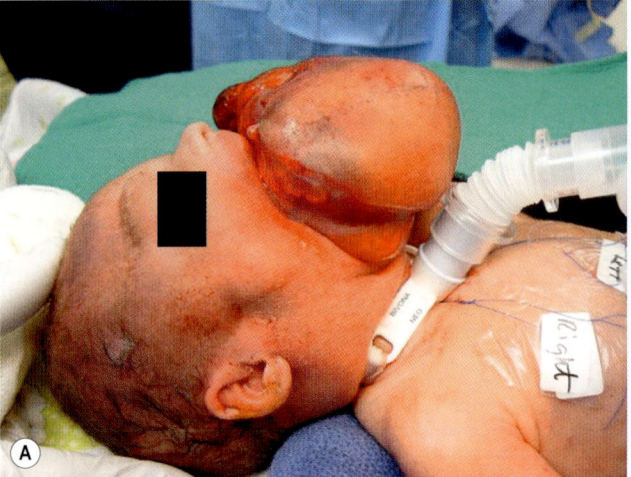
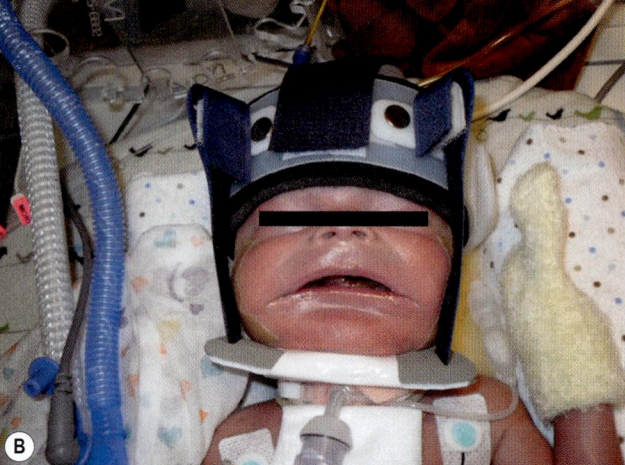

FIGURE 68-13 ■ On prenatal ultrasound, this baby was found to have a large epignathus and was born via an EXIT approach. **(A)** A tracheostomy was performed during the EXIT procedure. **(B)** The epignathus has been excised and the baby is in a mandibular molding device to help re-shape the mandible which was splayed out due to the large intraoral mass.

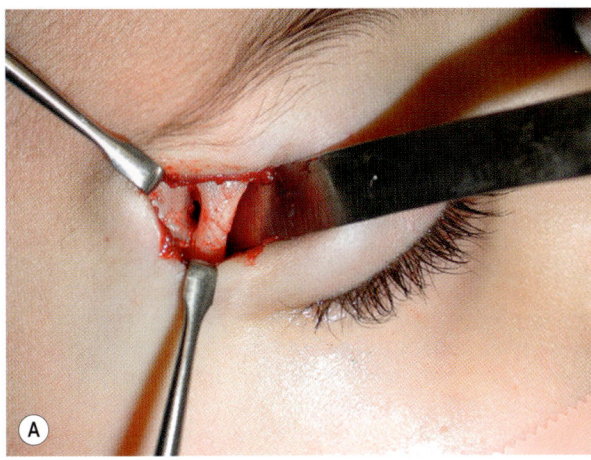
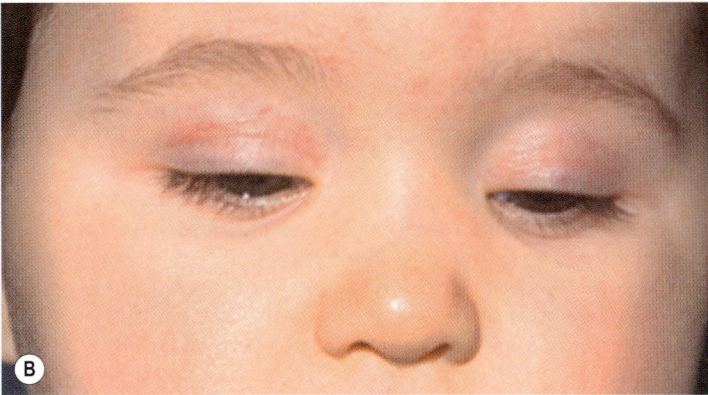

FIGURE 68-14 ■ Two different infants with right supraorbital dermoid cysts, for which a palpebral skin incision was used for excision. This approach requires a slightly longer incision and retraction, but the scar is almost invisible. **(A)** In this patient the approach was ideal since the cyst had eroded into the orbit (courtesy of Patricia Bortoluzzi, MD). **(B)** A different patient shown at one month follow-up; the scar is invisible when the eyes are open.

an unfused suture. Further imaging is essential in those cases, and neurosurgical consultation is advisable.

Dermoids deep to the lateral part of the eyebrow are usually approached through an incision just above the eyebrow because an incision within the eyebrow leaves a more visible scar. Very good cosmetic results are achieved long-term.[228] We have been impressed with an alternative incision through the palpebral crease.[229,230] This requires a slightly longer incision and more retraction but leaves an invisible scar. This approach also has the advantage of allowing access to the orbit for the rare cases in which the cyst penetrates through the orbital bone in a dumb-bell fashion (Fig. 68-14).[229] Another alternative is an endoscopic approach through a scalp incision.[231] This approach requires special instruments, is more indirect, and the scar posterior to the hairline may become visible later in life in balding males.

Dermoids in the cervical area are usually midline, mostly suprahyoid or submental. Because they are deep within muscles, they tend to move with swallowing, just as thyroglossal duct cysts do. On ultrasound, they usually appear echogenic and are often misinterpreted as being solid rather than cystic. They can be differentiated intra-operatively by their yellowish appearance and their soft, buttery content with sebaceous material and hair (Fig. 68-15). This appearance alleviates the need for a hyoidectomy.

Dermoid cysts should be excised because they tend to grow and may rupture or become infected, resulting in a more difficult excision and a higher risk of recurrence.

Epidermal Cysts

Epidermal or epidermoid cysts have a wall composed of true epidermis, as seen on the skin surface and in the infundibulum of hair follicles (hence, they also are called infundibular cysts).[226] They do not contain pilosebaceous units or hair. Some have a congenital origin like dermoid cysts, whereas others are acquired, either spontaneously arising from hair follicles or secondary to trauma with implantation of epidermis into the dermis or subcutaneous tissue.

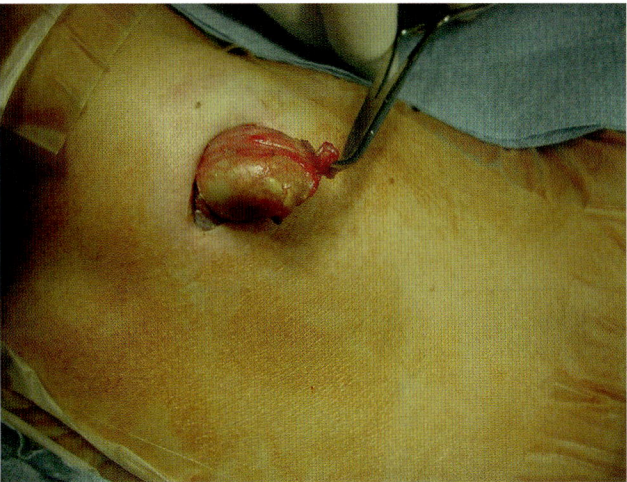

FIGURE 68-15 ■ Dermoid cysts in the cervical region are found in the midline. They are usually suprahyoid or submental. This operative photograph shows a midline cervical dermoid cyst with its characteristic yellowish appearance. The head is to the left. The cyst consists of a soft, buttery, cheesy content with sebaceous material. Preoperatively, these lesions are usually confused with a thyroglossal duct cyst. However, removal of the hyoid bone is not needed if a dermoid cyst is found.

Epidermal cysts are slow growing and are formed by the desquamation of epithelial cells. They are round, intradermal, or subcutaneous lesions that stop growing after having reached 1–5 cm in diameter. They occur most commonly on the face, scalp, neck, and trunk (i.e., hair-bearing areas). They may be associated with a small sinus tract or dimpling of the skin. In the neck and infra-clavicular area, they may be confused with branchial cleft remnants. Preauricular sinuses and cysts are often considered epidermal cysts. Epidermoid cysts of the spleen are discussed in Chapter 47.

Some patients may have more than one cyst, but the presence of multiple cysts, especially on the scalp and face, should raise the possibility of Gardner syndrome.[226,232,233]

Treatment is excision, which often can be achieved under local anesthesia, even in young children.

Preauricular cysts are better excised under general anesthesia, owing to their deep attachment to the helix cartilage.[234] Spontaneous rupture of any epidermal cyst leads to an intense foreign-body reaction, and the child presents with an abscess-like mass. This may require incision and drainage but often can be treated with antibiotics and local warm compresses. This mode of presentation increases the risk of cyst recurrence after excision, and often results in a wider scar than would have occurred with earlier excision. Infection of the cyst also may be caused by bacteria tracking along the small sinus tract that is sometimes present. These lesions rarely degenerate to epidermoid or basal cell carcinomas.[233] The treatment of small preauricular sinuses is controversial as they may remain asymptomatic, but generally excision is recommended with a palpable cyst or discharge of material from the sinus tract.

Epidermoid cysts of the skull and central nervous system share some similarities with dermoids, but they usually become symptomatic at an older age, between 20 and 40 years. Most are thought to have a congenital origin, although iatrogenic and inflammatory mechanisms are likely for intraspinal epidermoids (caused by multiple lumbar punctures, especially when using a needle without stylet) and middle ear epidermoids (cholesteatomas), respectively.

Trichilemmal Cysts

Trichilemmal cysts, also called pilar or sebaceous cysts, are thought to arise from hair follicles.[226] Most are acquired and appear in adulthood. They often show an autosomal dominant inheritance pattern and are solitary in only 30% of the cases. Some authors classify these as epidermal cysts that occur on the scalp.[233]

SOFT TISSUE AND NERVE TUMORS

Numerous soft tissue tumors have been described in children and are of mainly ectodermal and mesodermal origin. Some of these neoplasms are classified in Table 68-2. Only those soft tissue tumors likely to be encountered by pediatric surgeons are discussed here. More extensive discussions of soft tissue tumors are available.[235] Many benign soft tissue tumors are cutaneous or subcutaneous and are amenable to excision under local anesthesia.

Epidermal and Adnexal Tumors

Pyogenic Granulomas

Pyogenic granulomas (also known as lobular capillary hemangiomas) are solitary polypoid capillary lesions often associated with trauma or local irritation. They are commonly found on the skin as red, raised, occasionally bleeding lesions or in the mouth in association with pregnancy.[236] They are usually treated with topical silver nitrate or liquid nitrogen or ligature of the polyp neck. Rarely, excision or electrocautery is needed.

Warts

Warts are uncommon before age 4 years but are a common pediatric complaint. Various subtypes of human papillomavirus affect different body areas. Verrucae spread through families, sports teams, and schoolmates, and are most common on the hands and feet. Topical treatment includes salicylic or trichloroacetic acid, liquid nitrogen, or fine-tip electrocautery. A Cochrane review on topical treatment suggested cryotherapy may be only equivalent to older remedies.[237] Excision is occasionally required.

Condylomata acuminata occur in the perineal skin and suggest, but do not prove, child sexual abuse. The virus may be transmitted by hand contact during diaper changes in infants or acquired at birth during vaginal delivery, but the lesions may take months to develop. One study suggested that sexual abuse is an unlikely source of transmission in children younger than 3 years if no other signs of abuse are found.[238] These lesions have a core of connective tissue covered in epithelium, occurring as solitary or cauliflower-like lesions. Spontaneous regression is known, but topical podophyllin may be required. Some cases may need cauterization under general anesthesia as a

TABLE 68-2	Simplified Classification of Soft Tissue Tumors That Occur in Children	
Tissue	**Benign**	**Malignant**
Ectoderm		
Skin	Epidermoid and dermoid cysts, nevus sebaceous	Epidermoid cancer (squamous cell carcinoma)
Adnexae	Hidradenoma	Adenocarcinoma
	Calcifying epithelioma (pilomatrixoma)	
Melanocytes	Nevus	Malignant melanoma
Nerve tissue	Neurofibroma, schwannoma	Malignant peripheral nerve sheath tumor
Mesoderm		
Undifferentiated	Myxoma	Undifferentiated sarcoma
Fibrous tissue	Myofibroma, fibromatosis, keloid	Fibrosarcoma
Vascular tissue	Hemangioma, lymphangioma, glomus	Hemangioendothelioma, angiosarcoma
Adipose tissue	Lipoma, lipoblastoma	Liposarcoma
Muscle	Rhabdomyoma	Rhabdomyosarcoma
Synovial tissue	Giant cell tumor of tendon sheath, ganglion cyst, synovial cyst	Synovial sarcoma

thorough rectoscopic and vaginoscopic assessment can also be performed.

Calcifying Epithelioma of Malherbe

The calcifying epithelioma of Malherbe or pilomatrixoma is a solitary benign calcifying tumor of hair follicles. This is one of the most common acquired soft tissue lesions in children. Clinically, a circumscribed, firm, intracutaneous or subcutaneous nodule is palpable, with occasional yellowish or bluish coloration (Fig. 68-16).[227] These lesions are most common before age 20 years, and 60–70% are found in the head and neck region.[236] Extremities are also common locations, followed by the trunk. Most are smaller than 1 cm, although lesions up to 4 cm have been reported.[239] Only 2–3% are multiple, and in such cases there may be a familial predisposition and an association with Gardner syndrome.[227] They are more common than sebaceous cysts in younger patients. Local excision is curative.

Malignant Epithelial Tumors

Malignant epithelial tumors are rare in children. General treatment principles include wide local excision and radiation therapy for certain high-risk tumors.[240] The basal cell nevus syndrome, also known as Gorlin syndrome, is an autosomal dominant disease with basal cell lesions of the eyes, nose, and cheeks in association with anomalies of the mouth, skin, skeleton, central nervous system, eyes, and genitals.[241] These patients may have concomitant xeroderma pigmentosum. Epidermoid cancers in pediatric transplant recipients also have been reported.[242]

Tumors of Nerve Tissue

Neurofibromas

A neurofibroma is a benign neoplasm of Schwann cells, usually of peripheral nerves. When multiple, or associated with multiple café-au-lait skin lesions, it suggests the presence of neurofibromatosis type 1 (NF-1) or von Recklinghausen disease, an autosomal dominant disorder due to a mutation of the *NF-1* gene on chromosome 17.[243] Diagnosis may be delayed but affected probands can be diagnosed early by genetic testing or in utero by ultrasound.[244] Mucosal neurofibromas are associated with MEN 2B.[245] The NF-2 genetic anomaly occurs on chromosome 22 and is associated with bilateral acoustic neuromas. NF-1 has several clinical forms summarized in Table 68-3. NF-1 and NF-2 are compared in Table 68-4.[243] About half of the cases of NF-1 represent de novo mutations.[246]

Operative management is not curative of this genetic disorder and these children optimally have multidisciplinary approach to their care. NF 1 patients may have additional functional and cognitive disabilities requiring screening[247] and benefit from parent support groups (such as http://www.nfmidatlantic.org).

Highly aggressive sarcomas may develop and new symptoms require appropriate imaging using ultrasound, CT, or MRI. NF-1 patients have a 7–12% lifetime incidence of malignant peripheral nerve sheath tumors (MPNST), often arising from plexiform neurofibromas.[248] Malignant transformation may be heralded by pain, rapid growth, and new neurologic deficits in a previously stable lesion.[249] MRI criteria for malignancy

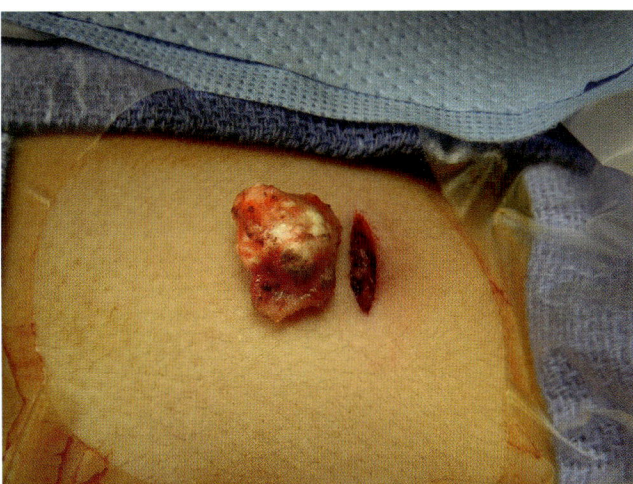

FIGURE 68-16 ■ This operative photograph shows a pilomatrixoma (calcifying epithelioma of Malherbe). These lesions are circumscribed, are firm, and have a distinctive 'knobby' appearance. Once removed, they are seen to have a yellowish content. Most of these lesions are found in the head and neck region.

TABLE 68-3	Clinical Patterns in Neurofibromatosis
Clinical Pattern	**Description**
Fibroma molluscum	Hundreds or thousands of pedunculated nodules; number makes resection impractical
Plexiform neurofibroma	Occur usually in the face and scalp, causing bony deformity by pressure erosion; resections for cosmesis may be repeated because curative resection is rare
Elephantiasis nervorum	With neurofibromas of the extremities, these cause greatly thickened skin simulating limb hypertrophy; resection is done to manage disfigurement
Thoracic neurofibroma	May have intraspinal extension (dumbbell tumor); has a high incidence of malignancy
Visceral neurofibroma	May affect intestine, kidney, and bladder because of the presence of associated nerves; when large, neurofibrosarcoma incidence increases
Skeletal syndromes	Include kyphoscoliosis, pseudarthrosis of tibia and ulna
Cranial syndromes	Meningiomas, gliomas, and optic gliomas have been reported
Endocrine syndromes	Sexual precocity, medullary thyroid carcinoma, and pheochromocytoma have been reported
Cardiovascular syndromes	Heart is rarely involved, but coarctation of the aorta and renal artery lesions have been reported

TABLE 68-4   **Comparison of Neurofibromatosis Types 1 and 2**

	Neurofibromatosis Type 1 (NF-1)	Neurofibromatosis Type 2 (NF-2)
Synonyms	Peripheral NF von Recklinghausen neurofibromatosis	Central NF Bilateral acoustic neuroma
Frequency	1:3500	1:25,000
Inheritance	Autosomal dominant	Autosomal dominant
Penetrance	High	High
% Sporadic	30–50%	50%
% Mosaic	>4%	17–28%
Gene	NF-1	NF-2
Chromosome	17q11.2	22q12.2
Associated tumors	Neurofibroma Optic and brain gliomas Malignant peripheral nerve sheath tumors	Bilateral vestibular schwannomas Meningiomas Schwannomas

Modified from Curatolo P, Riva D. Neurocutaneous syndromes in children. Montrouge. France: John Libbey Eurotext; 2006. p. 170.

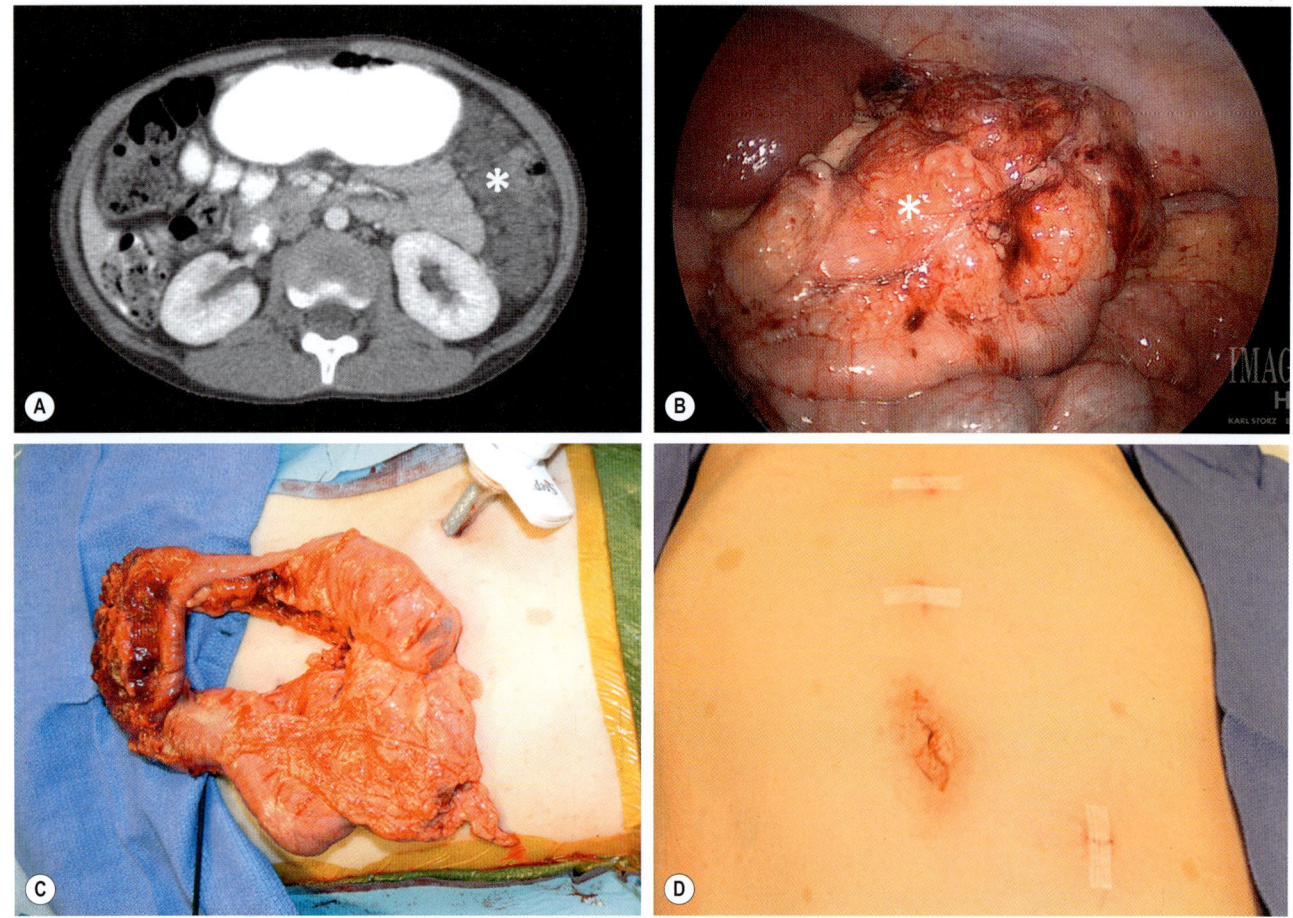

FIGURE 68-17 ■ **(A)** This 8-year-old child with NF-1 has developed abdominal pain and a large neurofibroma (asterisk) is seen in the left abdomen on the CT scan. **(B)** At laparoscopy, the mass (asterisk) is also visualized and involves the transverse mesocolon. **(C)** The transverse colon and mass were mobilized and were then exteriorized by enlarging the umbilical incision. The mass was very adherent to the transverse colon and colon resection was also required. **(D)** The port sites used for the laparoscopic-assisted operation are seen. Note the café-au-lait spots on the abdominal wall.

include large size (median 14.5 cm), central necrosis, peripheral enhancement, and perilesional edema-like zone.[250] Other reports also suggest of a positive role for PET scans in identifying malignancy.[246,251]

Where symptoms warrant, excision or debulking remain the mainstay for treatment of benign disease (Figs 68-17 and 68-18) while novel therapies are being explored, including rapamycin and antiangiogenic drugs.[246] MPNSTs are highly malignant, especially in the context of NF-1; standard of care consists of wide surgical excision followed by radiotherapy. The tumors are usually chemoresistant, metastases are common, and five-year survival has been reported at 28–33%.[252,253] The Children's Tumor Foundation (www.ctf.org) is currently

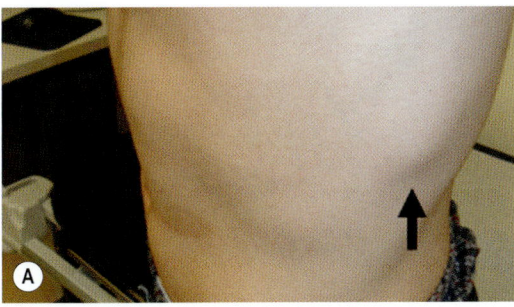
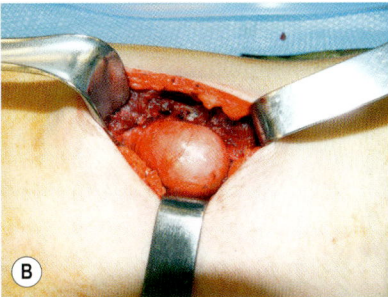
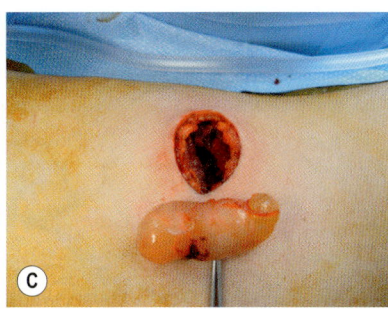

FIGURE 68-18 ■ This 15-year-old has been followed for several years and has previously required excision of a large lumbar neurofibroma which was causing discomfort. **(A)** This neurofibroma located between the ninth and tenth ribs (arrow) was causing significant pain. **(B)** Note the café-au-lait spot on the skin on the left abdominal wall. The lesion is seen through the left transverse chest wall incision. **(D)** The lesion is visualized following its complete excision.

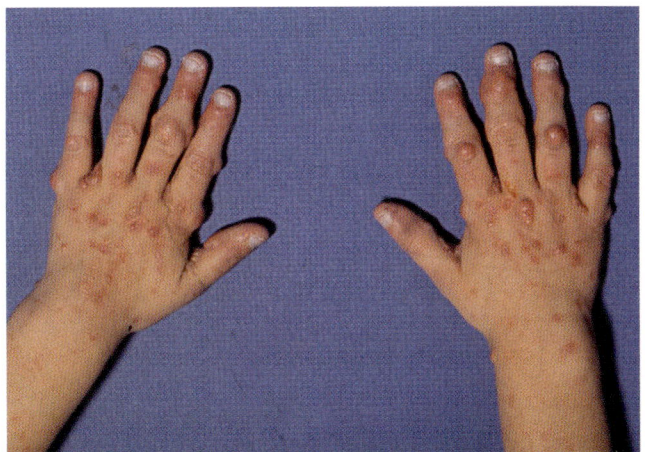

FIGURE 68-19 ■ Multiple xanthomas are seen on the hands of a child with Alagille syndrome.

sponsoring drug trials and encouraging networking between NF clinics.

Xanthomas

A xanthoma is a tumor of lipid-laden histiocytes or foam cells forming yellowish skin nodules.[254] It may be due to uncontrolled diabetes mellitus or biliary tract obstruction, which unbalances triglyceride and cholesterol metabolism, leading to lipid accumulation in histiocytes. Xanthomas are typical features of Alagille syndrome (syndromic paucity of bile ducts) and familial hypercholesterolemia (Fig. 68-19). Correcting the underlying disorder reverses these lesions, but excisional biopsy may be indicated for bothersome lesions or for diagnostic purposes.

Tumors of Mesoderm

Myxomas

A myxoma is a benign primitive connective tissue cell and stroma tumor resembling mesenchyme. It occurs mainly in the heart, producing symptoms by obstructing normal blood flow, and is removed using cardiopulmonary bypass.[255] Cutaneous and other sites are uncommon in children. They may be associated with the Carney complex.[235,255]

Fibrous Tissue Tumors

Nodular Fasciitis

Nodular fasciitis is the most common fibrous tissue tumor in all age groups. It is a self-limiting reactive process. These tumors may be subcutaneous, intramuscular, or fascial in location and are commonly found in the head and neck of children.[256] Half of cases are associated with discomfort, and 40% of lesions occur in patients younger than 20 years.[257] Excisional biopsy is necessary to differentiate these rapidly growing lesions from malignancy. Recurrence is rare.

Myofibromas/myofibromatosis

This category represents the most common fibrous tumor of childhood. Most present as a solitary skin nodule involving the head and neck, trunk or extremity, but they can involve bone or internal organs.[257,258] Spontaneous regression is possible. Infantile myofibromatosis (formerly called congenital fibromatosis) usually is first seen in infancy with multiple firm rubbery masses in the soft tissues, generally in the lower extremities and head and neck. Multifocal superficial lesions have a good prognosis, but a generalized form with visceral lesions (1–2% of cases) is often lethal due to pulmonary lesions.[257]

Fibrosarcomas

Fibrosarcomas include several specific entities, among which congenital infantile fibrosarcoma, presenting in the first two years of life as a large superficial or visceral mass (Fig. 68-20), and adult-type fibrosarcoma, which has a less favorable prognosis.[258] The infantile type is treated with complete excision, preceded by low-dose chemotherapy if necessary to avoid mutilating surgery. Cytogenetic studies are often required to separate the two entities and differentiate the congenital type from infantile myofibromatosis.[257,259]

Congenital Epulis

Congenital epulis is a benign granular cell tumor occurring almost exclusively in girls. It can be detected on prenatal ultrasound.[210] It originates from the gingival mucosa and averages 1–2 cm in diameter. Larger masses

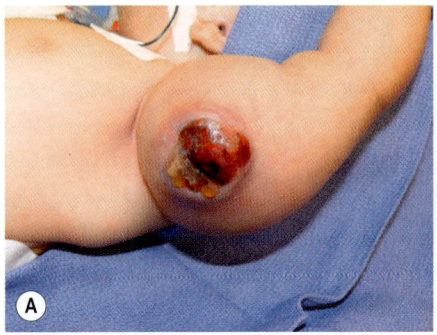 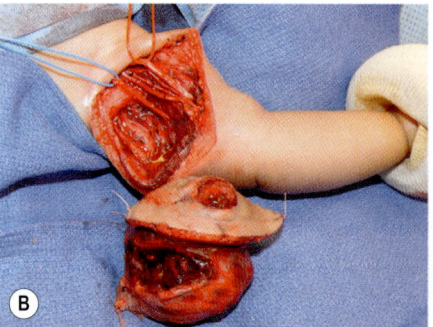 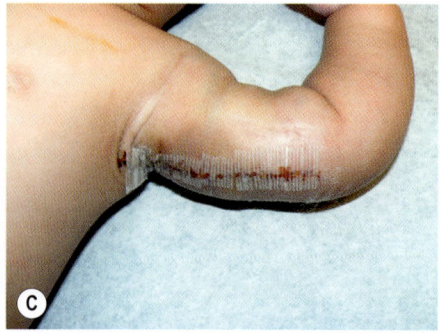

FIGURE 68-20 ■ **(A)** This 4-week-old baby was initially seen with a large mass in his left arm which had become ulcerated. **(B)** The baby underwent excision of the lesion with sparing of the underlying neurovascular structures. **(C)** The postoperative appearance. This patient has recovered uneventfully and remains disease free after 4 years. The lesion was an infantile fibrosarcoma.

could be confused with epignathus (see Fig. 68-13). Its exact nature is not clear.[260] Some classify it under tumors of peripheral nerves, whereas others consider it a fibrous tumor, hence the synonym granular cell fibroblastoma. Spontaneous regression is possible,[261] and simple excision is curative.

Keloid

A keloid is a sharply elevated, irregularly shaped, progressively enlarging scar caused by excessive collagen in the dermis during connective tissue re-modeling. Unlike the hypertrophic scar (which does not progress), a keloid extends beyond the wound and may recur after excision. Treatment with intradermal injection of corticosteroids, silicone pressure garments (as used for burn patients), pulsed dye laser, and cryosurgery may be attempted. Rarely, judicious excision with radiation therapy may be used.[233] Keloids developing after minor procedures are common. Their incidence is higher in blacks, but they can occur in any racial group. Patients prone to keloids are advised to avoid body piercing and tattooing.

Desmoid Tumors

Desmoid tumors are part of a broad group of benign fibroblastic proliferations called fibromatoses, which include palmar and plantar fibromatoses as well as fibromatosis colli (congenital torticollis). Desmoid tumors can be found in extra-abdominal, intra-abdominal, and retroperitoneal locations.[235,257] They are not encapsulated and are locally invasive, although they do not metastasize. An association with Gardner syndrome or familial adenomatous polyposis syndrome occurs in 10–15% and similar mutations of the *APC* gene can be demonstrated.[262]

First line therapy is complete surgical excision, but when they arise from the mesentery or retroperitoneum, complete resection may not be possible without risking damage to splanchnic vessels. High-dose radiation therapy or interstitial brachytherapy may be considered for residual tumor.[263] Antihormonal therapy (tamoxifen), nonsteroidal anti-inflammatory drugs (indomethacin and sulindac), and various chemotherapy protocols have been used in recurrent and inoperable tumors with positive, but variable results.[262] Because of the unpredictable

behavior of desmoid tumors, some advocate a conservative approach in selected patients.[264] Nonsteroidal anti-inflammatory medications are often used as first line therapy for unresectable asymptomatic disease, and chemotherapy is indicated for rapidly growing or life-threatening tumors.[262]

Adipose Tissue Tumors

A lipoma is a benign, soft, rubbery, encapsulated tumor of adipose tissue composed of mature fat cells occurring on the trunk, neck, and forearms. In one review of adipose tumors, lipomas represented 94%; lipoblastoma, 4.7%; and liposarcoma, 1.3%.[257] All are slow-growing tumors. Diagnosed often before age 3 years, lipoblastoma may be superficial and well encapsulated, or it may be deep and infiltrative. Definitive treatment of adipose tumors is complete resection. Chemotherapy may play a role in treating residual liposarcoma. Local recurrence rates for lipoblastoma and liposarcoma are 10% to 20%. Characterized by a myxoid stroma, embryonal lipoblasts, and mature fat cells, the myxoid variant of liposarcoma is similar histologically to lipoblastoma. Tumor karyotyping may be useful in differentiating these adipose tumors.[265]

Tumors of Synovial Tissue

Synovial Cysts

Synovial cysts or ganglion cysts arise from joints or tendon sheaths, resulting in firm 0.5–2 cm, mucin-filled lesions with a fibrous capsule. They are most common on the hand, especially on the dorsum of the wrist, but also occur on the ankle, foot, and popliteal fossa (where they are called Baker's cysts).

Pathology texts separate synovial cysts that have a true synovial lining (e.g., Baker's cysts) from ganglia, which are thought to be degenerative and are without a synovial lining. Symptoms of pain and weakness can occur, but most children present with an asymptomatic mass. Spontaneous resolution of all types of synovial cysts and ganglia is common in children. Surgical treatment is reserved for patients with persistently symptomatic lesions.[266] Traumatic disruption ('strike it with the family Bible') or corticosteroid injection should be discouraged because of the high recurrence rate and associated pain. The use of nonsteroidal anti-inflammatory agents, coupled with rest or wrist splinting, is usually sufficient if the cyst causes transient discomfort. Ultrasound examination may useful in the evaluation of Baker's cysts, especially in the context of juvenile arthritis.[267]

REFERENCES

1. Virchow R. Ueber Die Sakralgeschwulst Des Schliewener Kindes. Klin Wschr 1869;46:132.
2. Dehner LP. Gonadal and extragonadal germ cell neoplasms: Teratomas in childhood. In: Finegold M, editor. Pathology of Neoplasia in Children and Adolescents. Philadelphia: W B Saunders; 1986. p. 282–312.
3. Isaacs H. Germ cell tumors. In: Isaacs H, editor. Tumors of the Fetus and Newborn. Philadelphia: W B Saunders; 1997. p. 15–38.
4. Moore KL, Persaud TVN. The Developing Human: Clinically Oriented Embryology. 8th ed. Philadelphia: WB Saunders Elsevier; 2008.
5. Isaacs H. Tumors. In: Gilbert-Barness A, editor. Potter's Pathology of the Fetus and Infant. Philadelphia: Mosby Elsevier; 2007. p. 1677–709.
6. Bale PM. Sacrococcygeal developmental abnormalities and tumors in children. Perspect Pediatr Pathol 1984;8:9–56.
7. Sinnock KL, Perez-Atayde AR, Boynton KA, et al. Clonal analysis of sacrococcygeal 'teratomas'. Pediatr Pathol Lab Med 1996;16:865–75.
8. Chadha R, Bagga D, Malhotra CJ, et al. Accessory limb attached to the back. J Pediatr Surg 1993;28:1615–17.
9. de Lagausie P, de Napoli Cocci S, Stempfle N, et al. Highly differentiated teratoma and fetus-in-fetu: A single pathology? J Pediatr Surg 1997;32:115–16.
10. Heifetz SA, Alrabeeah A, Brown BS, et al. Fetus in fetu: A fetiform teratoma. Pediatr Pathol 1988;8:215–26.
11. Hanquinet S, Damry N, Heimann P, et al. Association of a fetus in fetu and two teratomas: Ultrasound and MRI. Pediatr Radiol 1997;27:336–8.
12. Drut RM, Drut R, Fontana A, et al. Mature presacral sacrococcygeal teratoma associated with a sacral 'epignathus'. Pediatr Pathol 1992;12:99–103.
13. Parizek J, Nemecek S, Pospisilova B, et al. Mature sacrococcygeal teratoma containing the lower half of a human body. Childs Nerv Syst 1992;8:108–10.
14. Kooijman CD. Immature teratomas in children. Histopathology 1988;12:491–502.
15. Heifetz SA, Cushing B, Giller R, et al. Immature teratomas in children: Pathologic considerations: A report from the combined Pediatric Oncology Group/Children's Cancer Group. Am J Surg Pathol 1998;22:1115–24.
16. Rescorla FJ. Pediatric germ cell tumors. Semin Pediatr Surg 2012;21:51–60.
17. Graf JL, Housely HT, Albanese CT, et al. A surprising histological evolution of preterm sacrococcygeal teratoma. J Pediatr Surg 1998;33:177–9.
18. Azizkhan RG, Haase GM, Applebaum H, et al. Diagnosis, management, and outcome of cervicofacial teratomas in neonates: A Childrens Cancer Group study. J Pediatr Surg 1995;30:312–16.
19. Unal E, Koksal Y, Toy H, et al. Neuroblastoma arising from an unresected sacrococcygeal teratoma in a child. J Pediatr Hematol Oncol 2010;32:233.
20. Hijiya N, Horikawa R, Matsushita T, et al. Malignant mediastinal germ-cell tumors in childhood: A report of two cases achieving long-term disease-free survival. Am J Pediatr Hematol Oncol 1989;11:437–40.
21. Stringer DA, Sprigg A, Kerrigan D, et al. Malignant carcinoid within a recurrent sacrococcygeal teratoma in childhood. Can Assoc Radiol J 1990;41:105–7.
22. Tsuchida Y, Endo Y, Saito S, et al. Evaluation of alpha-fetoprotein in early infancy. J Pediatr Surg 1978;13:155–62.
23. Wu JT, Book L, Sudar K. Serum alpha fetoprotein (AFP) levels in normal infants. Pediatr Res 1981;15:50–2.
24. Pauniaho SL, Tatti O, Lahdenne P, et al. Tumor markers AFP, CA 125, and CA 19-9 in the long-term follow-up of

25. sacrococcygeal teratomas in infancy and childhood. Tumour Biol 2010;31:261–5.
25. Volkl TM, Langer T, Aigner T, et al. Klinefelter syndrome and mediastinal germ cell tumors. Am J Med Genet A 2006;140:471–81.
26. Rodriguez E, Reuter VE, Mies C, et al. Abnormalities of 2q: A common genetic link between rhabdomyosarcoma and hepatoblastoma? Genes Chromosomes Cancer 1991;3:122–7.
27. Perlman EJ, Cushing B, Hawkins E, et al. Cytogenetic analysis of childhood endodermal sinus tumors: A Pediatric Oncology Group study. Pediatr Pathol 1994;14:695–708.
28. Kruslin B, Hrascan R, Manojlovic S, et al. Oncoproteins and tumor suppressor proteins in congenital sacrococcygeal teratomas. Pediatr Pathol Lab Med 1997;17:43–52.
29. Ishiwata I, Ishiwata C, Soma M, et al. N-myc gene amplification and neuron specific enolase production in immature teratomas. Virchows Arch A Pathol Anat Histopathol 1991;418:333–8.
30. Addeo R, Crisci S, D'Angelo V, et al. Bax mutation and overexpression inversely correlate with immature phenotype and prognosis of childhood germ cell tumors. Oncol Rep 2007;17:1155–61.
31. Currarino G, Coln D, Votteler T. Triad of anorectal, sacral, and presacral anomalies. AJR Am J Roentgenol 1981;137:395–8.
32. Ng WT, Ng TK, Cheng PW. Sacrococcygeal teratoma and anorectal malformation. Aust N Z J Surg 1997;67:218–20.
33. Tsuchida Y, Watanasupt W, Nakajo T. Anorectal malformations associated with a presacral tumor and sacral defect. Pediatr Surg Int 1989;4:398–402.
34. Altman RP, Randolph JG, Lilly JR. Sacrococcygeal teratoma: American Academy of Pediatrics Surgical Section Survey-1973. J Pediatr Surg 1974;9:389–98.
35. Tander B, Baskin D, Bulut M. A case of incomplete Currarino triad with malignant transformation. Pediatr Surg Int 1999;15:409–10.
36. Urioste M, Garcia-Andrade MdC, Valle L, et al. Malignant degeneration of presacral teratoma in the Currarino anomaly. Am J Med Genet A 2004;128A:299–304.
37. Sen G, Sebire NJ, Olsen O, et al. Familial Currarino syndrome presenting with peripheral primitive neuroectodermal tumour arising with a sacral teratoma. Pediatr Blood Cancer 2008;50:172–5.
38. Ciotti P, Mandich P, Bellone E, et al. Currarino syndrome with pelvic neuroendocrine tumor diagnosed by post-mortem genetic analysis of tissue specimens. Am J Med Genet A 2011;155A:2750–3.
39. Ashcraft KW, Holder TM. Hereditary presacral teratoma. J Pediatr Surg 1974;9:691–7.
40. Lee SC, Chun YS, Jung SE, et al. Currarino triad: Anorectal malformation, sacral bony abnormality, and presacral mass–a review of 11 cases. J Pediatr Surg 1997;32:58–61.
41. Shija JK. Anorectal malformation presenting as Hirschsprung's disease: A case report. East Afr Med J 1995;72:130–1.
42. Sonnino RE, Chou S, Guttman FM. Hereditary sacrococcygeal teratomas. J Pediatr Surg 1989;24:1074–5.
43. Singh SJ, Rao P, Stockton V, et al. Familial presacral masses: Screening pitfalls. J Pediatr Surg 2001;36:1841–4.
44. Weinberg AG. 'Teratomas' in the Currarino triad: A misnomer. Pediatr Dev Pathol 2000;3:110–11.
45. Ross AJ, Ruiz-Perez V, Wang Y, et al. A homeobox gene, HLXB9, is the major locus for dominantly inherited sacral agenesis. Nat Genet 1998;20:358–61.
45a. Zu S, Winberg J, Arnberg F, et al. Mutation analysis of the motor neuron and pancreas homeobox 1 (MNX1, former HLXB9) gene in Swedish patients with Currarino syndrome. J Pediatr Surg 2011;46:1390–5.
46. Subbarao P, Bhatnagar V, Mitra DK. The association of sacrococcygeal teratoma with high anorectal and genital malformations. Aust N Z J Surg 1994;64:214–15.
47. Shalaby MS, O'Toole S, Driver C, et al. Urogenital anomalies in girls with sacrococcygeal teratoma: A commonly missed association. J Pediatr Surg 2012;47:371–4.
48. Lahdenne P, Heikinheimo M, Jaaskelainen J, et al. Vertebral abnormalities associated with congenital sacrococcygeal teratomas. J Pediatr Orthop 1991;11:603–7.
49. Werb P, Scurry J, Ostor A, et al. Survey of congenital tumors in perinatal necropsies. Pathology 1992;24:247–53.

50. Lakhoo K. Neonatal teratomas. Early Hum Dev 2010;86: 643–7.
51. Rowe MI, O'Neill JA, Grosfeld JL, et al. Teratomas and germ cell tumors. In: Rowe MI, O'Neill JA, Grosfeld JL, et al, editors. Essentials of Pediatric Surgery. St-Louis: CV Mosby; 1995. p. 296–305.
52. Gross RW, Clatworthy HW Jr, Meeker IA Jr. Sacrococcygeal teratomas in infants and children; A report of 40 cases. Surg Gynecol Obstet 1951;92:341–54.
53. Hasle H, Jacobsen BB, Asschenfeldt P, et al. Mediastinal germ cell tumour associated with Klinefelter syndrome. A report of case and review of the literature. Eur J Pediatr 1992;151:735–9.
54. Casalone R, Righi R, Granata P, et al. Cerebral germ cell tumor and XXY karyotype. Cancer Genet Cytogenet 1994;74:25–9.
55. Czauderna P, Stoba C, Wysocka B, et al. Association of Klinefelter syndrome and abdominal teratoma: A case report. J Pediatr Surg 1998;33:774–5.
56. Zon R, Orazi A, Neiman RS, et al. Benign hematologic neoplasm associated with mediastinal mature teratoma in a patient with Klinefelter's syndrome: A case report. Med Pediatr Oncol 1994;23: 376–9.
57. Sasou S, Nakamura SI, Habano W, et al. True malignant histiocytosis developed during chemotherapy for mediastinal immature teratoma. Hum Pathol 1996;27:1099–103.
58. Hiramatsu H, Morishima T, Nakanishi H, et al. Successful treatment of a patient with Klinefelter's syndrome complicated by mediastinal germ cell tumor and AML (M7). Bone Marrow Transplant 2008;41:907–8.
59. Zambudio AR, Lanzas JT, Calvo MJ, et al. Mediastinal cystic teratoma associated with a Hodgkin's lymphoma. Eur J Cardiothorac Surg 2001;20:650–1.
60. Dische MR, Gardner HA. Mixed teratoid tumors of the liver and neck in trisomy 13. Am J Clin Pathol 1978;69:631–7.
61. Quah BS, Menon BS. Down syndrome associated with a retroperitoneal teratoma and Morgagni hernia. Clin Genet 1996;50: 232–4.
62. Falik-Borenstein TC, Korenberg JR, Davos I, et al. Congenital gastric teratoma in Wiedemann-Beckwith syndrome. Am J Med Genet 1991;38:52–7.
63. Zachariou Z, Krug M, Benz G, et al. Proteus syndrome associated with a sacrococcygeal teratoma; A rare combination. Eur J Pediatr Surg 1996;6:249–51.
64. Robin NH, Grace K, DeSouza TG, et al. New finding of Schinzel-Giedion syndrome: A case with a malignant sacrococcygeal teratoma. Am J Med Genet 1993;47:852–6.
65. Billmire DF, Grosfeld JL. Teratomas in childhood: Analysis of 142 cases. J Pediatr Surg 1986;21:548–51.
66. Schropp KP, Lobe TE, Rao B, et al. Sacrococcygeal teratoma: The experience of four decades. J Pediatr Surg 1992;27:1075–8.
67. Isaacs H Jr. Perinatal (fetal and neonatal) germ cell tumors. J Pediatr Surg 2004;39:1003–13.
68. Powell RW, Weber ED, Manci EA. Intradural extension of a sacrococcygeal teratoma. J Pediatr Surg 1993;28:770–2.
69. Kunisaki SM, Maher CO, Powelson I, et al. Benign sacrococcygeal teratoma with spinal canal invasion and paraplegia. J Pediatr Surg 2011;46:e1–4.
70. West DK, Touloukian RJ. Meconium pseudocyst presenting as a buttock mass. J Pediatr Surg 1988;23:864–5.
71. York DG, Wolfe H, von Allmen D. Fetal abdomino-perineal lymphangioma: Differential diagnosis and management. Prenat Diagn 2006;26:692–5.
72. Lu T, Zhao GP, Wang K, et al. An unusual case of tubular rectal duplication mimicking teratoma recurrence and review of the literature. European Journal of Radiology Extra 2010;73:e17–e19.
73. Al-Salem AH. Congenital-infantile fibrosarcoma masquerading as sacrococcygeal teratoma. J Pediatr Surg 2011;46:2177–80.
74. Murphy JJ, Blair GK, Fraser GC. Coagulopathy associated with large sacrococcygeal teratomas. J Pediatr Surg 1992;27: 1308–10.
75. Holterman AX, Filiatrault D, Lallier M, et al. The natural history of sacrococcygeal teratomas diagnosed through routine obstetric sonogram: A single institution experience. J Pediatr Surg 1998;33: 899–903.
76. Hedrick HL, Flake AW, Crombleholme TM, et al. Sacrococcygeal teratoma: Prenatal assessment, fetal intervention, and outcome. J Pediatr Surg 2004;39:430–8.
77. Angel CA, Murillo C, Mayhew J. Experience with vascular control before excision of giant, highly vascular sacrococcygeal teratomas in neonates. J Pediatr Surg 1998;33:1840–2.
78. Makin EC, Hyett J, Ade-Ajayi N, et al. Outcome of antenatally diagnosed sacrococcygeal teratomas: Single-center experience (1993-2004). J Pediatr Surg 2006;41:388–93.
79. Jona JZ. Progressive tumor necrosis and lethal hyperkalemia in a neonate with sacrococcygeal teratoma (SCT). J Perinatol 1999; 19:538–40.
80. Le LD, Alam S, Lim FY, et al. Prenatal and postnatal urologic complications of sacrococcygeal teratomas. J Pediatr Surg 2011;46:1186–90.
81. Brace V, Grant SR, Brackley KJ, et al. Prenatal diagnosis and outcome in sacrococcygeal teratomas: A review of cases between 1992 and 1998. Prenat Diagn 2000;20:51–5.
82. Wilson RD, Hedrick H, Flake AW, et al. Sacrococcygeal teratomas: Prenatal surveillance, growth and pregnancy outcome. Fetal Diagn Ther 2009;25:15–20.
83. Usui N, Kitano Y, Sago H, et al. Outcomes of prenatally diagnosed sacrococcygeal teratomas: The results of a Japanese nationwide survey. J Pediatr Surg 2012;47:441–7.
84. Flake AW. Fetal sacrococcygeal teratoma. Semin Pediatr Surg 1993;2:113–20.
85. Veschambre P, Wartanian R, Lebouvier B, et al. Facteurs pronostiques anténatals des tératomes sacro-coccygiens. Rev Fr Gynecol Obstet 1993;88:325–30.
86. Finamore PS, Kontopoulos E, Price M, et al. Mirror syndrome associated with sacrococcygeal teratoma: A case report. J Reprod Med 2007;52:225–7.
87. Heerema-McKenney A, Harrison MR, Bratton B, et al. Congenital teratoma: A clinicopathologic study of 22 fetal and neonatal tumors. Am J Surg Pathol 2005;29:29.
88. Hecher K, Hackeloer BJ. Intrauterine endoscopic laser surgery for fetal sacrococcygeal teratoma. Lancet 1996;347:470.
89. Ding J, Chen Q, Stone P. Percutaneous laser photocoagulation of tumour vessels for the treatment of a rapidly growing sacrococcygeal teratoma in an extremely premature fetus. J Matern Fetal Neonatal Med 2010;23:1516.
90. Ruano R, Duarte S, Zugaib M. Percutaneous laser ablation of sacrococcygeal teratoma in a hydropic fetus with severe heart failure–Too late for a surgical procedure? Fetal Diagn Ther 2009;25:26–30.
91. Paek BW, Jennings RW, Harrison MR, et al. Radiofrequency ablation of human fetal sacrococcygeal teratoma. Am J Obstet Gynecol 2001;184:503–7.
92. Ibrahim D, Ho E, Scherl SA, et al. Newborn with an open posterior hip dislocation and sciatic nerve injury after intrauterine radiofrequency ablation of a sacrococcygeal teratoma. J Pediatr Surg 2003;38:248–50.
93. Ryan G, Beecroft R, Finan E, et al. P27. 10: Successful fetal therapy for massive fetal sacrococcygeal teratoma (SCT) using radio frequency ablation (RFA). Ultrasound Obstet Gynecol 2010;36:275.
94. Kim J, Won H, Shim J, et al. P27. 09: Prenatal diagnosis of type II sacrococcygeal teratoma and its management in-utero using percutaneous radiofrequency ablation (RFA): Case report. Ultrasound Obstet Gynecol 2010;36:275.
95. Lee MY, Won HS, Hyun MK, et al. Perinatal outcome of sacrococcygeal teratoma. Prenat Diagn 2011;31:1217–21.
96. Roybal JL, Moldenhauer JS, Khalek N, et al. Early delivery as an alternative management strategy for selected high-risk fetal sacrococcygeal teratomas. J Pediatr Surg 2011;46: 1325–32.
97. Robertson FM, Crombleholme TM, Frantz ID 3rd, et al. Devascularization and staged resection of giant sacrococcygeal teratoma in the premature infant. J Pediatr Surg 1995;30:309–11.
98. Kay S, Khalife S, Laberge JM, et al. Prenatal percutaneous needle drainage of cystic sacrococcygeal teratomas. J Pediatr Surg 1999;34:1148–51.
99. Stefanovic V, Halmesmäki E. Peripartum ultrasound-guided drainage of cystic fetal sacrococcygeal teratoma for the prevention of the labor dystocia: A report of two cases. Am J Perinatol Rep 2011;1:87–90.
100. Jouannic JM, Dommergues M, Auber F, et al. Successful intrauterine shunting of a sacrococcygeal teratoma (SCT) causing fetal bladder obstruction. Prenat Diagn 2001;21:824–6.

101. Danzer E, Hubbard AM, Hedrick HL, et al. Diagnosis and characterization of fetal sacrococcygeal teratoma with prenatal MRI. AJR Am J Roentgenol 2006;187:W350–6.

102. Garel C, Mizouni L, Menez F, et al. Prenatal diagnosis of a cystic type IV sacrococcygeal teratoma mimicking a cloacal anomaly: Contribution of MR. Prenat Diagn 2005;25:216–19.

103. De Backer A, Madern GC, Hakvoort-Cammel FGAJ, et al. Study of the factors associated with recurrence in children with sacrococcygeal teratoma. J Pediatr Surg 2006;41:173–81.

104. Fishman SJ, Jennings RW, Johnson SM, et al. Contouring buttock reconstruction after sacrococcygeal teratoma resection. J Pediatr Surg 2004;39:439–41.

105. Jan IA, Khan EA, Yasmeen N, et al. Posterior sagittal approach for resection of sacrococcygeal teratomas. Pediatr Surg Int 2011; 27:545–8.

106. Bax N, van der Zee DC. The laparoscopic approach to sacrococcygeal teratomas. Surg Endosc 2004;18:128–30.

107. Solari V, Jawaid W, Jesudason EC. Enhancing safety of laparoscopic vascular control for neonatal sacrococcygeal teratoma. J Pediatr Surg 2011;46:e5.

108. Lund DP, Soriano SG, Fauza D, et al. Resection of a massive sacrococcygeal teratoma using hypothermic hypoperfusion: A novel use of extracorporeal membrane oxygenation. J Pediatr Surg 1995;30:1557–9.

109. Smithers CJ, Javid PJ, Turner CG, et al. Damage control operation for massive sacrococcygeal teratoma. J Pediatr Surg 2011;46: 566–9.

110. Cowles RA, Stolar CJ, Kandel JJ, et al. Preoperative angiography with embolization and radiofrequency ablation as novel adjuncts to safe surgical resection of a large, vascular sacrococcygeal teratoma. Pediatr Surg Int 2006;22:554–6.

111. Lahdes-Vasama TT, Korhonen PH, Seppanen JM, et al. Preoperative embolization of giant sacrococcygeal teratoma in a premature newborn. J Pediatr Surg 2011;46:e5–8.

112. Hosono S, Mugishima H, Nakano Y, et al. Autologous cord blood transfusion in an infant with a huge sacrococcygeal teratoma. J Neonatal Perinatal Med 2004;32:187–9.

113. Gucciardo L, Uyttebroek A, De Wever I, et al. Prenatal assessment and management of sacrococcygeal teratoma. Prenat Diagn 2011;31:678–88.

114. Hoehn T, Krause MF, Wilhelm C, et al. Fatal rupture of a sacrococcygeal teratoma during delivery. J Perinatol 1999;19:596–8.

115. Shanbhogue LKR, Bianchi A, Doig CM, et al. Management of benign sacrococcygeal teratoma: Reducing mortality and morbidity. Pediatr Surg Int 1990;5:41–4.

116. Chisholm CA, Heider AL, Kuller JA, et al. Prenatal diagnosis and perinatal management of fetal sacrococcygeal teratoma. Am J Perinatol 1999;16(1):47–50. Epub 1999/06/11.

117. Benachi A, Durin L, Maurer SV, et al. Prenatally diagnosed sacrococcygeal teratoma: A prognostic classification. J Pediatr Surg 2006;41:1517–21.

118. Sy ED, Filly RA, Cheong ML, et al. Prognostic role of tumor-head volume ratio in fetal sacrococcygeal teratoma. Fetal Diagn Ther 2009;26:75–80.

119. Byrne FA, Lee H, Kipps AK, et al. Echocardiographic risk stratification of fetuses with sacrococcygeal teratoma and twin-reversed arterial perfusion. Fetal Diagn Ther 2011;30:280–6.

120. Rodriguez MA, Cass DL, Lazar DA, et al. Tumor volume to fetal weight ratio as an early prognostic classification for fetal sacrococcygeal teratoma. J Pediatr Surg 2011;46:1182–5.

121. Schmidt B, Haberlik A, Uray E, et al. Sacrococcygeal teratoma: Clinical course and prognosis with a special view to long-term functional results. Pediatr Surg Int 1999;15:573–6.

122. Derikx JP, De Backer A, van de Schoot L, et al. Factors associated with recurrence and metastasis in sacrococcygeal teratoma. Br J Surg 2006;93:1543–8.

123. Bilik R, Shandling B, Pope M, et al. Malignant benign neonatal sacrococcygeal teratoma. J Pediatr Surg 1993;28:1158–60.

124. Ouimet A, Russo P. Fetus in fetu or not? J Pediatr Surg 1989;24:926–7.

125. Gilcrease MZ, Brandt ML, Hawkins EP. Yolk sac tumor identified at autopsy after surgical excision of immature sacrococcygeal teratoma. J Pediatr Surg 1995;30:875–7.

126. Malogolowkin MH, Ortega JA, Krailo M, et al. Immature teratomas: Identification of patients at risk for malignant recurrence. J Natl Cancer Inst 1989;81:870–4.

127. Hawkins E, Issacs H, Cushing B, et al. Occult malignancy in neonatal sacrococcygeal teratomas. A report from a Combined Pediatric Oncology Group and Children's Cancer Group study. Am J Pediatr Hematol Oncol 1993;15:406–9.

128. McKenney JK, Longacre TA. Low-grade mucinous epithelial neoplasm (intestinal type) arising in a mature sacrococcygeal teratoma with late recurrence as pseudomyxoma peritonei. Hum Pathol 2008;39:629–32.

129. Rescorla FJ, Sawin RS, Coran AG, et al. Long-term outcome for infants and children with sacrococcygeal teratoma: A report from the Childrens Cancer Group. J Pediatr Surg 1998;33:171–6.

130. Gobel U, Schneider DT, Calaminus G, et al. Multimodal treatment of malignant sacrococcygeal germ cell tumors: A prospective analysis of 66 patients of the German cooperative protocols MAKEI 83/86 and 89. J Clin Oncol 2001;19:1943–50.

131. Rescorla F, Billmire D, Stolar C, et al. The effect of cisplatin dose and surgical resection in children with malignant germ cell tumors at the sacrococcygeal region: A pediatric intergroup trial (POG 9049/CCG 8882). J Pediatr Surg 2001;36:12–17.

132. Khalil BA, Aziz A, Kapur P, et al. Long-term outcomes of surgery for malignant sacrococcygeal teratoma: 20-year experience of a regional UK centre. Pediatr Surg Int 2009;25:247–50.

133. Marina NM, Cushing B, Giller R, et al. Complete surgical excision is effective treatment for children with immature teratomas with or without malignant elements: A Pediatric Oncology Group/Children's Cancer Group Intergroup Study. J Clin Oncol 1999;17:2137–43.

134. Gobel U, Calaminus G, Schneider DT, et al. The malignant potential of teratomas in infancy and childhood: The MAKEI experiences in non-testicular teratoma and implications for a new protocol. Klinische Padiatrie 2006;218:309–14.

135. Draper H, Chitayat D, Ein SH, et al. Long-term functional results following resection of neonatal sacrococcygeal teratoma. Pediatr Surg Int 2009;25:243–6.

136. Cozzi F, Schiavetti A, Zani A, et al. The functional sequelae of sacrococcygeal teratoma: A longitudinal and cross-sectional follow-up study. J Pediatr Surg 2008;43:658–61.

137. Malone PS, Spitz L, Kiely EM, et al. The functional sequelae of sacrococcygeal teratoma. J Pediatr Surg 1990;25:679–80.

138. Havranek P, Hedlund H, Rubenson A, et al. Sacrococcygeal teratoma in Sweden between 1978 and 1989: Long-term functional results. J Pediatr Surg 1992;27:916–18.

139. Uchiyama M, Iwafuchi M, Naitoh M, et al. Sacrococcygeal teratoma: A series of 19 cases with long-term follow-up. Eur J Pediatr Surg [et al] = Zeitschrift fur Kinderchirurgie 1999;9: 158–62.

140. Derikx JP, De Backer A, van de Schoot L, et al. Long-term functional sequelae of sacrococcygeal teratoma: A national study in The Netherlands. J Pediatr Surg 2007;42:1122–6.

141. Gabra HO, Jesudason EC, McDowell HP, et al. Sacrococcygeal teratoma–a 25-year experience in a UK regional center. J Pediatr Surg 2006;41:1513–16.

142. Berger M, Heinrich M, Lacher M, et al. Postoperative bladder and rectal function in children with sacrococcygeal teratoma. Pediatr Blood Cancer 2011;56:397–402.

143. Tailor J, Roy PG, Hitchcock R, et al. Long-term functional outcome of sacrococcygeal teratoma in a UK regional center (1993 to 2006). J Pediatr Hematol Oncol 2009;31:183.

144. Lee NG, Gana R, Borer JG, et al. Urodynamic findings in patients with Currarino syndrome. J Urol 2012;187:2195–200.

145. Yoshida A, Maoate K, Blakelock R, et al. Long-term functional outcomes in children with Currarino syndrome. Pediatr Surg Int 2010;26:677–81.

146. Bittmann S, Bittmann V. Surgical experience and cosmetic outcomes in children with sacrococcygeal teratoma. Curr Surg 2006;63:51–4.

147. Avci A, Eren S. Life-threatening giant mediastinal cystic teratoma in a 4-month-old male baby. Gen Thorac Cardiovasc Surg 2009;57:389–91.

148. Takayasu H, Kitano Y, Kuroda T, et al. Successful management of a large fetal mediastinal teratoma complicated by hydrops fetalis. J Pediatr Surg 2010;45:e21–4.

149. Schneider DT, Calaminus G, Reinhard H, et al. Primary mediastinal germ cell tumors in children and adolescents: Results of the German cooperative protocols MAKEI 83/86, 89, and 96. Clin Oncol 2000;18:832–9.

150. Magu S, Rattan KN, Mishra DS. Posterior mediastinal teratomas. Indian J Pediatr 2000;67:236–40.

151. Kaneko M, Ohkawa H, Iwakawa M, et al. Extensive epidural teratoma in early infancy treated by multi-stage surgery. Pediatr Surg Int 1999;15:280–3.

152. Hari S, Kumar J, Kumar A, et al. Posterior mediastinal teratoma. Intern Med J 2008;38:448–9.

153. Kuroiwa M, Suzuki N, Takahashi A, et al. Life-threatening mediastinal teratoma in a neonate. Pediatr Surg Int 2001;17:235–8.

154. Perger L, Lee EY, Shamberger RC. Management of children and adolescents with a critical airway due to compression by an anterior mediastinal mass. J Pediatr Surg 2008;43:1990–7.

155. Nenna R, Papoff P, Moretti C, et al. What could hemoptysis hide in an otherwise healthy child? Pediatr Pulmonol 2011;46:1146–8.

156. Miyazawa M, Yoshida K, Komatsu K, et al. Mediastinal mature teratoma with rupture into pleural cavity due to blunt trauma. Ann Thorac Surg 2012;93:990–2.

157. Revere DJ, Makaryus AN, Bonaros EP Jr, et al. Chylopericardium presenting as cardiac tamponade secondary to an anterior mediastinal cystic teratoma. Tex Heart Inst J 2007;34:379–82.

158. Chaudary IU, Bojal SA, Attia A, et al. Mediastinal endodermal sinus tumor associated with fatal hemophagocytic syndrome. Hematol Oncol Stem Cell Ther 2011;4:138–41.

159. Urban C, Lackner H, Schwinger W, et al. Fatal hemophagocytic syndrome as initial manifestation of a mediastinal germ cell tumor. Med Pediatr Oncol 2003;40:247–9.

160. Billmire D, Vinocur C, Rescorla F, et al. Malignant mediastinal germ cell tumors: An intergroup study. J Pediatr Surg 2001;36:18–24.

161. Sarkaria IS, Bains MS, Sood S, et al. Resection of primary mediastinal non-seminomatous germ cell tumors: A 28-year experience at Memorial Sloan-Kettering Cancer Center. J Thorac Oncol 2011;6:1236–41.

162. Nakajima K, Fukuzawa M, Minami M, et al. Videothoracoscopic resection of anterior mediastinal teratoma in a child. Report of a case. Surg Endosc 1998;12:54–6.

163. Billmire DF. Malignant germ cell tumors in childhood. Semin Pediatr Surg 2006;15:30–6.

164. Zamboni M, Lannes DC, Cordeiro Pde B, et al. Transthoracic biopsy with core cutting needle (Trucut) for the diagnosis of mediastinal tumors. Rev Port Pneumol 2009;15:589–95.

165. Logothetis CJ, Samuels ML, Trindade A, et al. The growing teratoma syndrome. Cancer 1982;50:1629–35.

166. Liddle AD, Anderson DR, Mishra PK. Intrapericardial teratoma presenting in fetal life: Intrauterine diagnosis and neonatal management. Congenit Heart Dis 2008;3(6):449–51.

167. Goldberg SP, Boston US, Turpin DA, et al. Surgical management of intrapericardial teratoma in the fetus. J Pediatr 2010;156:848–9.

168. Tollens T, Casselman F, Devlieger H, et al. Fetal cardiac tamponade due to an intrapericardial teratoma. Ann Thorac Surg 1998;66:559–60.

169. Pratt JW, Cohen DM, Mutabagani KH, et al. Neonatal intrapericardial teratomas: Clinical and surgical considerations. Cardiol Young 2000;10:27–31.

170. Sumner TE, Crowe JE, Klein A, et al. Intrapericardial teratoma in infancy. Pediatr Radiol 1980;10(1):51–3. Epub 1980/09/01.

171. Gunther T, Schreiber C, Noebauer C, et al. Treatment strategies for pediatric patients with primary cardiac and pericardial tumors: A 30-year review. Pediatr Cardiol 2008;29:1071–6.

172. Rana SS, Swami N, Mehta S, et al. Intrapulmonary teratoma: An exceptional disease. Ann Thorac Surg 2007;83:1194–6.

173. Horton Z, Schlatter M, Schultz S. Pediatric germ cell tumors. Surg Oncol 2007;16:205–13.

174. Barksdale EM Jr, Obokhare I. Teratomas in infants and children. Curr Opin Pediatr 2009;21:344.

175. Nguyen CT, Kratovil T, Edwards MJ. Retroperitoneal teratoma presenting as an abscess in childhood. J Pediatr Surg 2007;42:E21–3.

176. Luo CC, Huang CS, Chu SM, et al. Retroperitoneal teratomas in infancy and childhood. Pediatr Surg Int 2005;21:536–40.

177. Chaudhary A, Misra S, Wakhlu A, et al. Retroperitoneal teratomas in children. Indian J Pediatr 2006;73:221–3.

178. Jones NM, Kiely EM. Retroperitoneal teratomas-potential for surgical misadventure. J Pediatr Surg 2008;43:184–7.

179. Billmire D, Vinocur C, Rescorla F, et al. Malignant retroperitoneal and abdominal germ cell tumors: An intergroup study. J Pediatr Surg 2003;38:315–18.

180. Federici S, Prestipino M, Domenichelli V, et al. Fetus in fetu: Report of an additional, well-developed case. Pediatr Surg Int 2001;17:483–5.

181. Khadaroo RG, Evans MG, Honore LH, et al. Fetus-in-fetu presenting as cystic meconium peritonitis: Diagnosis, pathology, and surgical management. J Pediatr Surg 2000;35:721–3.

182. Gupta DK, Srinivas M, Dave S, et al. Gastric teratoma in children. Pediatr Surg Int 2000;16:329–32.

183. Jeong HC, Cha SJ, Kim GJ. Rapidly grown congenital fetal immature gastric teratoma causing severe neonatal respiratory distress. J Obstet Gynaecol Res 2012;38:449–51.

184. Yeo DM, Lim GY, Lee YS, et al. Gliomatosis peritonei of the scrotal sac associated with an immature gastric teratoma. Pediatr Radiol 2010;40:1288–92.

185. Saha M. Malignant gastric teratoma: Report of two cases from a single center. Pediatr Surg Int 2010;26:931–4.

186. Ukiyama E, Endo M, Yoshida F, et al. Recurrent yolk sac tumor following resection of a neonatal immature gastric teratoma. Pediatr Surg Int 2005;21:585–8.

187. Shah RS, Kaddu SJ, Kirtane JM. Benign mature teratoma of the large bowel: A case report. J Pediatr Surg 1996;31:701–2.

188. Cakmak O, Senel E, Erdogan D, et al. Ileal teratoma with multiple congenital anomalies. J Pediatr Surg 2000;35:1370–1.

189. Torikai M, Tahara H, Kaji T, et al. Immature teratoma of gallbladder associated with gliomatosis peritonei, a case report. J Pediatr Surg 2007;42:E25–7.

190. Rivkine E, Goasguen N, Chelbi E, et al. [Cystic teratoma of the pancreas]. Gastroenterol Clin Biol 2007;31:1016–19. Teratome kystique du pancreas.

191. Yoshida A, Murabayashi N, Shiozaki T, et al. Case of mature cystic teratoma of the greater omentum misdiagnosed as ovarian cyst. J Obstet Gynaecol Res 2005;31:399–403.

192. Ariizumi T, Ogose A, Hotta T, et al. Cystic teratoma of the diaphragm which mimicked soft tissue lipoma. Skeletal Radiol 2007;36:991–4.

193. Filston HC. Hemangiomas, cystic hygromas, and teratomas of the head and neck. Semin Pediatr Surg 1994;3:147–59.

194. Kountakis SE, Minotti AM, Maillard A, et al. Teratomas of the head and neck. Am J Otolaryngol 1994;15:292–6.

195. Garmel SH, Crombleholme TM, Semple JP, et al. Prenatal diagnosis and management of fetal tumors. Semin Perinatol 1994;18:350–65.

196. Figueiredo G, Pinto PS, Graham EM, et al. Congenital giant cervical teratoma: Pre- and postnatal imaging. Fetal Diagn Ther 2010;27:231–2.

197. Langer JC, Tabb T, Thompson P, et al. Management of prenatally diagnosed tracheal obstruction: Access to the airway in-utero prior to delivery. Fetal Diagn Ther 1992;7:12–16.

198. Lazar DA, Cassady CI, Olutoye OO, et al. Tracheoesophageal displacement index and predictors of airway obstruction for fetuses with neck masses. J Pediatr Surg 2012;47:46–50.

199. Laje P, Johnson MP, Howell LJ, et al. Ex utero intrapartum treatment in the management of giant cervical teratomas. J Pediatr Surg 2012;47:1208–16.

200. Liechty KW, Hedrick HL, Hubbard AM, et al. Severe pulmonary hypoplasia associated with giant cervical teratomas. J Pediatr Surg 2006;41:230–3.

201. Jordan RB, Gauderer MW. Cervical teratomas: An analysis. Literature review and proposed classification. J Pediatr Surg 1988;23:583–91.

202. Martino F, Avila LF, Encinas JL, et al. Teratomas of the neck and mediastinum in children. Pediatr Surg Int 2006;22:627–34.

203. Keen CE, Said AJ, Agrawal M, et al. Congenital thyroid teratoma: A case with persistent neuroglial involvement of cervical lymph nodes. Pediatr Dev Pathol 1998;1:322–7.

204. Craver RD, Lipscomb JT, Suskind D, et al. Malignant teratoma of the thyroid with primitive neuroepithelial and mesenchymal sarcomatous components. Ann Diagn Pathol 2001;5:285–92.

205. Thompson LD, Rosai J, Heffess CS. Primary thyroid teratomas: A clinicopathologic study of 30 cases. Cancer 2000;88:1149–58.

206. Grushka JR, Ryckman J, Mueller C, et al. Spindle epithelial tumor with thymus-like elements of the thyroid: A multi-institutional case series and review of the literature. J Pediatr Surg 2009;44: 944–8.

207. Oliveira-Filho AG, Carvalho MH, Bustorff-Silva JM, et al. Epignathus: Report of a case with successful outcome. J Pediatr Surg 1998;33:520–1.

208. Wilson JW, Gehweiler JA. Teratoma of the face associated with a patent canal extending into the cranial cavity (Rathke's pouch) in a three-week-old child. J Pediatr Surg 1970;5:349–59.

209. Chung JH, Farinelli CK, Porto M, et al. Fetal epignathus: The case of an early EXIT (ex utero intrapartum treatment). Obstet Gynecol 2012;119:466–70.

210. Kovacs L, Volpe C, Laberge JM, et al. Gingival mass in a newborn infant diagnosed in-utero. J Pediatr 2002;141:837.

211. Maartens IA, Wassenberg T, Halbertsma FJ, et al. Neonatal airway obstruction caused by rapidly growing nasopharyngeal teratoma. Acta Paediatr (Oslo, Norway: 1992) 2009;98:1852–4.

212. Sauter ER, Diaz JH, Arensman RM, et al. The perioperative management of neonates with congenital oropharyngeal teratomas. J Pediatr Surg 1990;25:925–8.

213. Morof D, Levine D, Grable I, et al. Oropharyngeal teratoma: Prenatal diagnosis and assessment using sonography, MRI, and CT with management by ex utero intrapartum treatment procedure. AJR Am J Roentgenol 2004;183:493–6.

214. Jarrahy R, Cha ST, Mathiasen RA, et al. Congenital teratoma of the oropharyngeal cavity with intracranial extension: Case report and literature review. J Craniofac Surg 2000;11:106–12.

215. Lee GA, Sullivan TJ, Tsikleas GP, et al. Congenital orbital teratoma. Aust N Z J Ophthalmol 1997;25:63–6.

216. Roncaroli F, Scheithauer BW, Pires MM, et al. Mature teratoma of the middle ear. Otol Neurotol 2001;22:76–8.

217. Washburne JF, Magann EF, Chauhan SP, et al. Massive congenital intracranial teratoma with skull rupture at delivery. Am J Obstet Gynecol 1995;173:226–8.

218. Hunt SJ, Johnson PC, Coons SW, et al. Neonatal intracranial teratomas. Surg Neurol 1990;34:336–42.

219. Chien YH, Tsao PN, Lee WT, et al. Congenital intracranial teratoma. Pediatr Neurol 2000;22:72–4.

220. Sawamura Y, Kato T, Ikeda J, et al. Teratomas of the central nervous system: Treatment considerations based on 34 cases. J Neurosurg 1998;89:728–37.

221. Jona JZ. Congenital anorectal teratoma: Report of a case. J Pediatr Surg 1996;31:709–10.

222. Kreczy A, Alge A, Menardi G, et al. Teratoma of the umbilical cord. Case report with review of the literature. Arch Pathol Lab Med 1994;118:934–7.

223. Pirodda A, Ferri GG, Truzzi M, et al. Benign cystic teratoma of the parotid gland. Otolaryngol Head Neck Surg 2001;125: 429–30.

224. Cakmak M, Savas C, Ozbasar D, et al. Congenital vulvar teratoma in a newborn. J Pediatr Surg 2001;36:620–1.

225. Daszkiewicz P, Roszkowski M, Przasnek S, et al. Teratoma or enterogenous cyst? The histopathological and clinical dilemma in co-existing occult neural tube dysraphism. Folia Neuropathol 2006;44:24–33.

226. Kirkham N. Tumors and cysts of the epidermis. In: Elder DE, Elenitsas R, Johnson BL, et al, editors. Lever's Histopathology of the Skin. 10th ed. Philadelphia: Lippincott Williams&Wilkins; 2011.

227. Li WY, Reinisch JF. Cysts, pits, and tumors. Plast Reconstr Surg 2009;124:106e.

228. Gur E, Drielsma R, Thomson HG. Angular dermoid cysts in the endoscopic era: Retrospective analysis of aesthetic results using the direct, classic method. Plast Reconstr Surg 2004;113: 1324.

229. Ruszkowski A, Caouette-Laberge L, Bortoluzzi P, et al. Superior eyelid incision: An alternative approach for frontozygomatic dermoid cyst excision. Ann Plast Surg 2000;44:591.

230. Cozzi DA, Mele E, d'Ambrosio G, et al. The eyelid crease approach to angular dermoid cysts in pediatric general surgery. J Pediatr Surg 2008;43:1502–6.

231. Dutta S, Lorenz HP, Albanese CT. Endoscopic excision of benign forehead masses: A novel approach for pediatric general surgeons. J Pediatr Surg 2006;41:1874–8.

232. Vijay K, Choudhary AK. Multiple scalp epidermoid cysts in a child with Gardner syndrome. Pediatr Radiol 2010;40:S172.

233. Paller ASMAJ. Cutaneous tumors and tumor syndromes. In: Paller ASMAJ, editor. Hurwitz Clinical Pediatric Dermatology. 3rd ed. Philadelphia: Elsevier Saunders; 2006. p. 205–55.

234. Ban R, Shinohara H, Matsuo K, et al. Limited distribution of gravitation abscess caused by infected preauricular sinus depends on anatomical structure. Eur J Plast Surg 2008;31:59–63.

235. Weiss SWGJR. Enzinger and Weiss's Soft Tissue Tumors. 5th ed. Philadelphia: Mosby Elsevier; 2008.

236. Reddy VB, Husain AN. The skin. In: Stocker JT, Dehner LP, Husain AN, editor. Pediatric Pathology. 3rd ed. Philadelphia: Wolters Kluwer Lippincott Williams&Wilkins; 2011. p. 1105–46.

237. Gibbs S, Harvey I. Topical treatments for cutaneous warts. Cochrane Database Syst Rev 2006:CD001781.

238. Cohen BA, Honig P, Androphy E. Anogenital warts in children. Clinical and virologic evaluation for sexual abuse. Arch Dermatol 1990;126:1575–80.

239. Schlechter R, Hartsough NA, Guttman FM. Multiple pilomatricomas (calcifying epitheliomas of Malherbe). Pediatr Dermatol 1984;2:23–5.

240. Lee EH, Levine VJ, Nehal KS. Cutaneous Squamous Cell Carcinoma. In: Alam M, editor. Evidence-Based Procedural Dermatology. New York NY: Springer; 2012, p. 57–74.

241. Tom WL, Hurley MY, Oliver DS, et al. Features of basal cell carcinomas in basal cell nevus syndrome. Am J Med Genet A 2011;155A:2098–104.

242. Chow CW, Tabrizi SN, Tiedemann K, et al. Squamous cell carcinomas in children and young adults: A new wave of a very rare tumor? J Pediatr Surg 2007;42:2035–9.

243. Curatolo P, Riva D. Neurocutaneous syndromes in children. Montrouge, France: John Libbey Eurotext; 2006.

244. Friedman JM, Birch PH. Type 1 neurofibromatosis: A descriptive analysis of the disorder in 1,728 patients. Am J Med Genet 1997;70:138–43.

245. Pujol RM, Matias-Guiu X, Miralles J, et al. Multiple idiopathic mucosal neuromas: A minor form of multiple endocrine neoplasia type 2B or a new entity? J Am Acad Dermatol 1997;37:349–52.

246. Williams VC, Lucas J, Babcock MA, et al. Neurofibromatosis type 1 revisited. Pediatrics 2009;123:124–33.

247. Gilboa Y, Rosenblum S, Fattal-Valevski A, et al. Application of the International Classification of Functioning, Disability and Health in children with neurofibromatosis type 1: A review. Dev Med Child Neurol 2010;52:612–19.

248. Ferner RE. Neurofibromatosis 1. Eur J Hum Genet 2007;15: 131–8.

249. Ferner RE, Huson SM, Thomas N, et al. Guidelines for the diagnosis and management of individuals with neurofibromatosis 1. J Med Genet 2007;44:81–8.

250. Wasa J, Nishida Y, Tsukushi S, et al. MRI features in the differentiation of malignant peripheral nerve sheath tumors and neurofibromas. AJR Am J Roentgenol 2010;194:1568–74.

251. Bredella MA, Torriani M, Hornicek F, et al. Value of PET in the assessment of patients with neurofibromatosis type 1. AJR Am J Roentgenol 2007;189:928–35.

252. Ferrari A, Bisogno G, Macaluso A, et al. Soft-tissue sarcomas in children and adolescents with neurofibromatosis type 1. Cancer 2007;109:1406–12.

253. Porter D, Prasad V, Foster L, et al. Survival in malignant peripheral nerve sheath tumours: A comparison between sporadic and neurofibromatosis type 1-associated tumours. Sarcoma 2009;2009: 756395.

254. Weiss SWGJR. Benign fibrohistiocytic tumors. In: Weiss SWGJR, editor. Enzinger and Weiss's Soft Tissue Tumors. 5th ed. Philadelphia: Mosby Elsevier; 2008. p. 331–70.

255. Bielefeld KJ, Moller JH. Cardiac tumors in infants and children: study of 120 operated patients. Pediatr Cardiol 2012:1–4.

256. Weiss SWGJR. Benign fibroblastic/myofibroblastic proliferations. In: Weiss SWGJR, editor. Enzinger and Weiss's Soft Tissue Tumors. 5th ed. Philadelphia: Mosby Elsevier; 2008. p. 175–225.

257. Dehner LP. Soft tissue. In: Stocker JT, Dehner LP, Husain AN, editor. Pediatric Pathology. 3rd ed. Philadelphia: Wolters Kluwer/Lippincott Williams&Wilkins; 2011. p. 1040–104.

258. Weiss SW. Fibrous tumors of infancy and childhood. In: Enzinger FM, Weiss SW, editor. Soft Tissue Tumors. 5th ed. Philadelphia: Mosby Elsevier; 2008. p. 257–302.

259. Triche TJHJ, Sorensen PHB. Diagnostic Pathology of Pediatric Malignancies. In: Pizzo PAPDG, editor. Principles and Practice of Pediatric Oncology. 6th ed. Philadelphia: Wolters Kluwer Health/Lippincott Williams & Wilkins; 2011.

260. Childers ELB, Fanburg-Smith JC. Congenital epulis of the newborn: 10 new cases of a rare oral tumor. Ann Diagn Pathol 2011;15:157–61.

261. Sakai VT, Oliveira TM, Silva TC, et al. Complete spontaneous regression of congenital epulis in a baby by 8 months of age. Int J Paediatr Dent 2007;17:309–12.

262. Kasper B, Ströbel P, Hohenberger P. Desmoid tumors: Clinical features and treatment options for advanced disease. Oncologist 2011;16:682–93.

263. Jabbari S, Andolino D, Weinberg V, et al. Successful treatment of high risk and recurrent pediatric desmoids using radiation as a component of multimodality therapy. Int J Radiat Oncol Biol Phys 2009;75:177–82.

264. Stoeckle E, Coindre J, Longy M, et al. A critical analysis of treatment strategies in desmoid tumours: A review of a series of 106 cases. Eur J Surg Oncol 2009;35:129–34.

265. Miller GG, Yanchar NL, Magee JF, et al. Lipoblastoma and liposarcoma in children: An analysis of 9 cases and a review of the literature. Can J Surg 1998;41:455–8.

266. Cypel TKS, Mrad A, Somers G, et al. Ganglion cyst in children: Reviewing treatment and recurrence rates. Can J Plast Surg 2011;19:53–5.

267. Alessi S, Depaoli R, Canepari M, et al. Baker's cyst in pediatric patients: Ultrasonographic characteristics. J Ultrasound 2012; 15:76–81.

CHAPTER 69

LYMPHOMAS

Karen B. Lewing • Alan S. Gamis

Lymphomas are a result of chromosomal alterations resulting in the uncontrolled growth of cells of lymphoid origin. Among all ages, lymphomas constitute just 5% of all cancers diagnosed annually in the USA. In children, however, this percentage increases to 8%.[1] Combined, Hodgkin and non-Hodgkin lymphoma are the second most common childhood solid tumors (behind brain tumors and ahead of soft tissue sarcomas and neuroblastoma).

Lymphomas have classically been divided into two distinct groups: Hodgkin disease (HD) and non-Hodgkin lymphoma (NHL). In 2001, HD was designated Hodgkin lymphoma (HL) by the World Health Organization (WHO) lymphoma classification system.[2] HL and NHL have a relatively similar prevalence among children and young adults, but NHL becomes significantly more common after 40 years of age (Fig. 69-1). Typically, patients with both HL and NHL are initially seen with enlarged lymph nodes and may have systemic symptoms of fever, fatigue and/or extralymphatic spread. However, these two types of lymphoma also have clear differences. HL usually is seen as an indolent process, whereas NHL is most often seen in children with a rapid onset of symptoms. Due to this propensity for rapid growth, children with NHL often have associated anatomic and metabolic co-morbidities to such a degree that their recognition and need for treatment constitutes a medical emergency. With HL, treatment is based primarily on staging and less on histologic subtype. In contrast, the current treatment of NHL depends on the histologic and immunophenotypic subtypes in addition to stage.

These two lymphomas are truly a study of contrasts. This is no more evident than in the evolution of their therapy. For years, HL has been one of the most curable cancers. Now, with markedly improved treatment protocols, NHL has a nearly equivalent cure rate.[3] Children under 15 years of age had 5-year relative survival rates of 96% for HL and 86% for NHL from 2001–2007, up from 81% and 43%, respectively, from 1975–1977.[1] Owing to the historic high survival rate with HL, its therapy has focused on a reduction in intensity. In contrast, because of its previously poor prognosis, NHL therapy has focused on intensification of therapy. The use of higher doses of chemotherapy over a short period (as compared with prior methods) has resulted in the dramatic improvement in cure and response of NHL.

In considering the surgeon's role in the treatment for childhood lymphomas, there are no real differences between the two types of lymphomas. However, in contrast to other solid tumors of childhood, in which initial resection of the tumor is important, the primary role of the surgeon in the initial management of lymphomas is to ensure the rapid attainment of adequate and properly preserved biopsy material to allow the pathologist the opportunity to make the diagnosis of the specific type and subtype of lymphoma. Except for select situations, resection at the time of presentation is not part of the current management of lymphomas.

HODGKIN LYMPHOMA

Thomas Hodgkin, in his classic thesis in 1832, described the gross necropsy examinations of seven patients.[4] He noted the association of generalized lymphadenopathy and splenomegaly in six patients without evidence of infection or inflammation. Histologic descriptions of the Reed–Sternberg (RS) cell, the pathognomonic multinucleated giant cell, did not occur until after the turn of the century.[5,6] Even though the etiology was unclear, therapeutic interventions began soon after the discovery of X-rays. More successful application of radiation therapy awaited the description of the disease's propensity for contiguous spread. With this knowledge, application of radiation to the involved and adjacent nodal areas (extended-field technique) resulted in improvements in survival in the late 1930s.[7] In the early 1960s, due to limitations in the radiologic techniques of that era, the practice of systematic laparotomy, splenectomy, and celiac node and liver biopsy at the time of initial presentation was developed for the purpose of staging and for targeted therapy.[8] This has properly been described as the model for the careful staging of cancer as a required prerequisite to the design of therapy, which is a hallmark of oncologic practice today.[9,10]

During this same time, combination chemotherapy entered into the treatment armamentarium, and remission and cure rates markedly improved. These improvements have made HL one of the most curable cancers today, with a five-year survival of 96% for pediatric patients diagnosed between 2002 and 2008.[11] With this high expectation for cure, attention over the past decade has focused on reducing the long-term sequelae of treatment. To this end, chemotherapy has evolved from an adjunctive role to a primary one, with the hope of eliminating the need for irradiation (and its attendant sequelae) altogether. When irradiation is needed, if used in combination with chemotherapy, the focus has been to reduce the size of the fields (from extended to involved) and the doses used. The two classic chemotherapy combinations (MOPP: nitrogen mustard, vincristine [Oncovin], procarbazine, prednisone; and ABVD: doxorubicin [Adriamycin], bleomycin, vinblastine, dacarbazine) have evolved. Hybrids of these

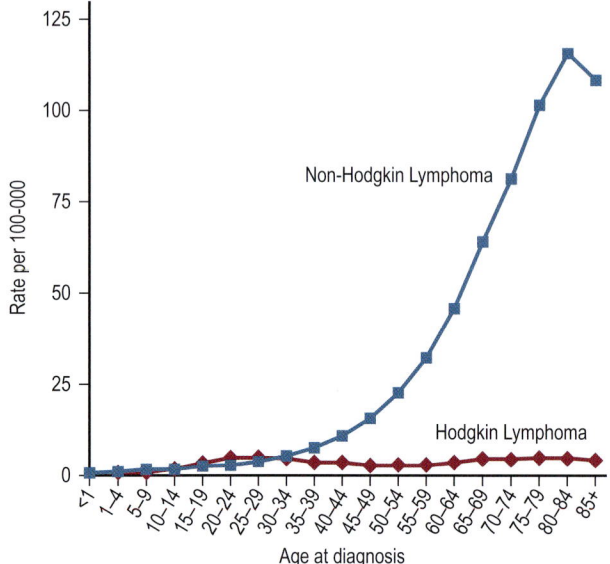

FIGURE 69-1 ■ Age-specific incidence rates per 100,000 population for Hodgkin lymphoma and non-Hodgkin lymphoma from 2000–2009. (Howlader N, Noone AM, Krapcho M, et al, editors. SEER Cancer Statistics Review, 1975–2009 (Vintage 2009 Populations). Bethesda, MD: National Cancer Institute. http://seer.cancer.gov/csr/1975_2009_pops09/, based on November 2011 SEER data submission, posted to the SEER web site, 2012)

combinations are now being utilized to reduce the toxicity to the patient.

Incidence and Epidemiology

It is estimated that 9,060 individuals will be diagnosed with HL in the USA each year, accounting for just 0.6% of all cancers and only 11% of all lymphomas.[1] However, in children, it is the sixth most common type of cancer, with approximately 400 children diagnosed annually.[1,12] This constitutes 4% of all childhood cases of cancer and approximately half of all childhood cases of lymphoma.[1] HL has an incidence of 3.2 cases/100,000 teens aged 15–19 years.[13] A bimodal distribution exists when considering all ages, but in children alone, a gradual trend is seen of increasing incidence with increasing age. HL is exceedingly rare in children younger than age 2 years and peaks in the adolescent years.[14] Beyond age 11 years, it is the most common of the two types of lymphoma and accounts for about 15% of all cancer in young adults ages 15 to 24 years.[13] A slight male predominance (1.3:1)[11] is noted, but in the youngest children, the male-to-female ratio is much larger (12–19:1).[15]

Monozygotic twins of HL patients have been found to be at greater risk of developing HL than are dizygotic twins, strongly implicating genetics as a principal risk factor.[16] In young adults, an increased risk of HL is found with higher socioeconomic status.[17] Young adults with HL come from smaller families, have fewer infectious exposures as young children, and/or have later exposure to infections than do control populations.[17,18] This correlates closely with socioeconomic status and implicates delayed exposure to infections as a principal risk factor.

Most likely, a combination of genetic risk and infectious exposure predisposes a young adult to HL.

Immunodeficiency may be the link between these two risk factors, at least in a subgroup of HL patients. HL is more prevalent in human immunodeficiency virus (HIV)-infected patients.[19–21] Also, patients with HL have a higher incidence of cellular immunodeficiency at the time of diagnosis.[22] Etiologic theories encompass these two risk factors and focus primarily on the Epstein–Barr virus (EBV). Genomic material from EBV has been found in the RS cells in up to 79% of HL cases.[23–25] A higher risk of HL has been noted in individuals with a history of infectious mononucleosis[26–28] and with previously high titers to EBV.[29] One hypothesis that incorporates these factors suggests the following sequence: (1) a genetic, iatrogenic, or viral immunosuppression; (2) subsequently or coincidentally, an EBV infection or oncogenetic rearrangement in a lymphoid precursor cell; (3) further genetic alterations; followed by (4) clonal expansion of lymphoid cells with morphologic features of RS cells; finally resulting in (5) the clinical syndrome known as HL, diagnosed by the presence of RS cells.[30]

Classification and Histologic Subtyping

The diagnosis of classical HL requires the dual finding of the diagnostic Hodgkin and RS cells (HRS cells) plus a reactive cellular background.[31] The RS cell is a large cell (15–45 mm) with an 'owl's eye' appearance (Fig. 69-2). It has a multilobed nucleus (or is multinucleated), each with a prominent eosinophilic nucleolus surrounded by a clear zone (halo) and an intensely stained nuclear membrane. The 'owl's eye' appearance is the result of a bilobed nucleus. The RS cell often makes up no more than 2% of the involved cells. Hodgkin cells are the mononuclear variant of RS cells. The cellular background is a reactive, pleomorphic mixture of inflammatory cells

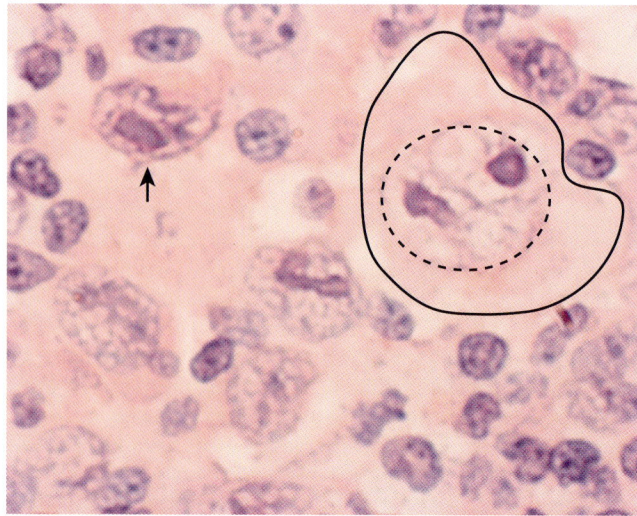

FIGURE 69-2 ■ This photograph depicts a RS cell, which is pathognomonic for HD. On the right side of the slide, the large nucleolus is outlined by the dotted circle and the entire cell is outlined by the solid line. Note the relatively pale nuclear chromatin. The nucleolus has the appearance of an 'owl's eye' from which it receives its name. The arrow points to a mononuclear variant of the RS cell, which has reticulated nuclear chromatin surrounding an almost rectangular macronucleus.

including reactive lymphocytes, histiocytes, plasma cells, eosinophils, neutrophils, and fibroblasts, with varying degrees of fibrosis and sclerosis. The HRS cell is a clonal, neoplastic cell seen in classical HL and is thought to induce the reactive background through the abundant release of various cytokines.[32] HRS cells typically are CD15 and CD30 positive and negative for CD45 and B-lineage antigens.[33] In contrast, the nodular lymphocyte predominant (LP) HL cells (popcorn cells) are usually positive for B-lineage antigens, CD15 and CD30 expressions are lacking, and the immunoglobulin genes are expressed.[33]

For histologic typing, the Rye classification was commonly used for three decades but has been supplanted by the WHO classification. The 2008 WHO classification lists two main types of HL: classical HL and nodular LP. Classical HL is further divided into four subtypes by morphology. These subtypes include nodular sclerosis (NS, the most common), mixed cellularity (MC), lymphocyte-rich (LRHL), and lymphocyte-depleted (LDHL).[34] The NS subtype is seen in 40% of younger patients and 70% of adolescents.[35] It is characterized by tumor nodules surrounded by broad sclerotic bands arising from a thickened fibrotic capsule.[31] This subtype has a strong predilection for involving the lower cervical, supraclavicular, and mediastinal lymph nodes. The MC subtype is found in 30% of cases and has an increased incidence in younger children.[15] HRS cells are typically increased in number. The lymph node architecture is often completely effaced by the HRS cells and their surrounding reactive cells. This subtype often is first seen with advanced, widely disseminated disease in extranodal sites. In addition to its relatively common incidence among all HL patients, it is the most common histologic type seen in HIV-infected patients.[21]

From 2001 to 2009, the National Cancer Institute (NCI)-sponsored SEER data revealed the following 5-year survival rates for patients age 0–19 years: LRHL 100%; NS 95.7%; MC 92%; and nodular LP 100% (Table 69-1). In patients of all ages, the 5-year survival rate for LDHL was 58%.[11] Reports have shown that LPHL has a better prognosis and needs markedly reduced

therapy to achieve cure.[36,37] This differentiation of therapeutic response between LPHL and the other classic HL histologic types appears to validate the distinction observed in the immunophenotyped RS cells.[38] The worse outcome of the MC and LDHL types may reflect their typically higher stage at diagnosis.

Clinical Presentation

Classically, children with HL present with painless enlarged lymph nodes, typically in the cervical or supraclavicular nodal groups (see Table 69-1). Nodes are often described as rubbery and fixed. They may be either single or matted with other nodes. Occasionally, because of rapid growth, tenderness may develop. Tumor lysis syndrome, a result of rapid and extensive tumor growth and a common complication in children with NHL, is rarely seen in children with HL.

HL tends to spread in a contiguous manner. Therefore, at presentation, one must examine carefully the nodal groups adjacent to the initially identified nodes. More than 90% of patients have involvement of either the cervical or mediastinal nodal groups (or both).[39] Interestingly, HL tends to spread from the cervical nodes of one side of the neck to the mediastinum before it spreads to the contralateral cervical nodes. When laparotomy was included in the staging process (which is no longer routinely performed), the spleen was noted to be involved in 27% of patients.[39] When evaluating the histologic subtypes and patterns of initial involvement, the MC and LD subtypes of HL have more widespread involvement than do the NS or LP HL subtypes (see Table 69-1).

Mediastinal disease, in addition to a predilection for certain histologic subtypes, is most common in girls older than 12 years, and in those with constitutional symptoms (also known as B symptoms).[40] Mediastinal disease may appear with significant respiratory compromise due to compression of the trachea, carina, (or both), including the major bronchi.[41] These patients may have dyspnea on exertion or at rest, persistent cough, or stridor. They may have recently been treated for presumed asthma or bronchiolitis, without radiographic imaging. Patients with this

---

TABLE 69-1 Hodgkin Lymphoma: Sites of Involvement at the Time of Initial Diagnosis

Histologic Subtype	Incidence (% of Patients Age 0–19 Years Diagnosed with HL in 2001–2009[a])	Five-Year Relative Survival Rate SEER 2001–2009	Typical Presentation
Nodular LP	5%	100%	Localized disease
Classical NS	73%	95.7%	Lower cervical, supraclavicular, and mediastinal nodes
Classical MC	7%	92%	Often advanced disease and extranodal involvement
Classical LD	0%	N/A	Rare in children, common in HIV-infected patients, widespread disease with bone and bone marrow involvement
Classical LR	2%	100%	Localized disease

[a]Eleven per cent of patients were classified as NOS (not otherwise specified) and are not included in the histologic subtypes listed above.
LP, lymphocyte predominant; NS, nodular sclerosis; MC, mixed cellularity; LD, lymphocyte depleted; LR, lymphocyte rich.
Data from Howlader N, Noone AM, Krapcho M, et al, editors. SEER Cancer Statistics Review, 1975–2009 (Vintage 2009 Populations). Bethesda, MD: National Cancer Institute. http://seer.cancer.gov/csr/1975_2009_pops09/, based on November 2011 SEER data submission, posted to the SEER web site, 2012.

presentation may have a history of orthopnea and are most comfortable in an upright forward-leaning position to relieve the pressure on the airway (from the anterior mediastinal mass). The physician must be vigilant for mediastinal disease because it can be silent until a patient is sedated for a radiologic or surgical procedure. These patients may prove impossible to ventilate, even with intubation, because of distal tracheal or bronchial obstruction. It is imperative that all patients with suspected lymphoma (HL or NHL) have a chest radiograph or chest CT scan before any sedation or procedure. Signs of superior vena caval obstruction, including edema and cyanosis of the face and jugular venous distention, may also be present. Extralymphatic involvement can include the liver (the most common extralymphatic organ involved), lungs, bone, bone marrow, and skin, among other sites. Whereas bone marrow involvement is present in only 4–14% of patients overall, among those patients with stage IV disease it occurs one-third of the time.[42]

Most patients have no systemic symptoms at the time of initial diagnosis. About one-quarter of patients will have one or more B symptoms, defined as weight loss of more than 10% in the previous 6 months, unexplained recurrent fevers greater than 38°C, or drenching night sweats.[39] Pruritus, fatigue, and anorexia are other nonspecific symptoms seen in HL patients. Laboratory findings at diagnosis are nonspecific and typically are indicative of an inflammatory process. The erythrocyte sedimentation rate (ESR), serum copper, and ferritin levels are frequently elevated and may be useful later as monitors for relapse. A high ferritin (>142 ng/mL) level or increased ESR (>50) has been associated with a worse prognosis.[43,44] The lactate dehydrogenase (LDH) may be elevated as well. Although not common, leukopenia may be indicative of bone marrow involvement.[42]

Diagnosis

The diagnostic evaluation should include a physical examination and laboratory and radiologic studies (Box 69-1). The physical examination should be directed to the obviously involved nodal groups and also to adjacent groups, keeping in mind the natural history of HL and its propensity for contiguous spread. More than four involved nodal groups in stage II patients is associated with a worse prognosis.[45] Bulky disease (nodes or nodal aggregates >10 cm and/or mediastinal tumor width more than one-third of intrathoracic width on a posteroanterior chest radiograph or CT) is associated with a worse outcome in low-stage patients, and necessitates additional therapy to achieve equivalent outcomes.[46–48] Auscultation of the airway, palpation of the abdomen, and examination of distant nodal groups are all critical as well.

Laboratory examination should include full blood cell counts and chemistries, including hepatic function tests, LDH, and ESR. Serum copper and ferritin levels also should be obtained. However, no clinical findings are pathognomonic for HL. Ultimately, the diagnosis awaits the biopsy of involved sites, most commonly an excised lymph node. The surgeon's goal is to biopsy the most accessible nodal region to obtain adequate tissue for diagnosis. Open excision of the largest lymph node is

---

BOX 69-1	Hodgkin Lymphoma: Diagnostic and Staging Evaluation at Presentation

Complete physical examination with documentation of involved nodal groups (including measurements of nodes), and involved extralymphatic organs
Complete blood cell count, chemistry panel including hepatic function tests, erythrocyte sedimentation rate, copper, ferritin, lactate dehydrogenase
Chest radiography to evaluate for possible mediastinal disease and airway compression
CT scans of areas identified on physical examination (also include chest, neck, abdomen and pelvis)
PET-FDG imaging
Gallium scan if PET is not available
Bone scan
Excisional biopsy of node
Bone marrow biopsies and aspirates (bilateral)
Staging laparotomy/laparoscopy (mandatory if considering radiation therapy alone) with splenectomy, nodal sampling, and wedge biopsies of hepatic lobes

CT, computed tomography; FDG, ^{18}flurodeoxyglucose; PET, positron emission tomography.

---

preferred because fine-needle aspirations generally do not provide adequate tissue. Excisional biopsy is where the diagnosis is made, based on the pathognomonic finding of HRS cells within a reactive cellular background. For cytogenetic and molecular genetic evaluations, it is imperative that all tissues are placed in a sterile container for fresh samples. Formalin should not be used. For patients critically ill at diagnosis, such as those with severe airway obstruction, diagnosis by alternative methods may need to be considered. These include nodal biopsy with local anesthesia alone, CT-guided percutaneous needle biopsy of the mass, aspiration of a pleural effusion, or a bone marrow biopsy and aspirate.

Staging

Further evaluation of a patient with HL is required to determine the extent of disease at diagnosis and thus the stage of disease (Table 69-2). The common staging system for HL was adopted in 1971.[49] This system is based on the observation of contiguous nodal spread in HL. Patients are further divided into asymptomatic (A) and symptomatic (B) subcategories. This subclassification for symptomatic patients is based on the findings of a worse prognosis for B patients and the need for a systemic therapy approach (i.e., chemotherapy in addition to radiation). This likely reflects the finding that patients with B symptoms are more likely to have distant, widespread disease when histologically staged.[50]

For HL, the decision for the type and intensity of therapy rests on the staging results. Traditionally, two methods of staging were used in HL patients: clinical and histologic. In the past, all patients underwent both methods. Clinical staging includes physical, laboratory, and radiologic evaluations. Histologic staging requires a staging laparotomy with splenectomy, nodal sampling, and wedge biopsies of both hepatic lobes. Radiologic evaluations continue to evolve. Lymphangiograms, once

TABLE 69-2 **Ann Arbor Staging Classification for Hodgkin Lymphoma**

Stage	Definition
I	Involvement of a single lymph node region (I) or of a single extralymphatic organ or site (IE)
II	Involvement of two or more lymph node regions on the same side of the diaphragm (II) or localized involvement of an extralymphatic organ or site and its regional lymph node(s) with involvement of one or more lymph node regions on the same side of the diaphragm (IIE)
III	Involvement of lymph node regions on both sides of the diaphragm (III), which may be accompanied by involvement of the spleen (IIIS) or by localized involvement of an extralymphatic organ or site (IIIE) or both (IIISE)
IV	Disseminated (multifocal) involvement of one or more extralymphatic organs or tissues with or without associated lymph node involvement or isolated extralymphatic organ involvement with distant (nonregional) nodal involvement

a critical component of staging in HL, have been supplanted by more modern and less invasive imaging modalities. CT examination is used most frequently.[51] For those who will be treated by irradiation alone, accurate assessment of abdominal disease is critical. Staging laparotomy with splenectomy, nodal sampling, and wedge biopsies of both hepatic lobes has been shown to increase the stage of disease in up to 35% of patients initially evaluated with CT (i.e., the difference between clinical and histologic staging).[52,53] This would seem to indicate that abdominal exploration is important. However, with the use of systemic chemotherapy and the de-emphasis on irradiation, this discrepancy between clinical and histologic staging no longer appears to have a significant impact on treatment or outcome.[54,55]

For the majority of children with HL, staging is based on clinical criteria. Laparotomy (or laparoscopy) is not encouraged or recommended. However, abdominal staging should continue to be used in patients destined to be treated with irradiation alone (although this is now rare in children) because abdominal disease would have a significant impact on planned therapy.[56] Staging laparotomy (or laparoscopy) with splenectomy is not without its risks. There are the typical postoperative complications of abdominal surgery. Moreover, with splenectomy, there is a lifelong risk of overwhelming sepsis with encapsulated organisms and these patients require lifelong antibiotic prophylaxis.[57] An increased risk of secondary leukemia also exists in those HL patients treated with chemotherapy who have undergone splenectomy (5.9%) compared with those who have not (0.7%) as part of their staging procedure.[58–60]

Nuclear medicine scans are another modality used for staging HL patients. ^{18}flurodeoxyglocose (FDG) imaging has gradually supplanted gallium scans. Fluorodeoxyglucose-labeled positron emission tomography (FDG-PET) has been found to be more sensitive and specific than either gallium or CT.[61–64] Similar to gallium scanning, it leads to a higher staging in a significant

percentage of patients. FDG-PET during and after therapy has been highly predictive of patient outcome[65,66] and helps to differentiate residual scar tissue from residual lymphoma,[67] although false-positive findings with inflammatory conditions have been reported.[66] In children, it is important also to recognize the phenomena of thymic rebound after therapy. This may result in both an enlarging mediastinal mass on CT and a positive nuclear medicine scan. An experienced radiologist will recognize this phenomenon by its timing (within the first 6 months after therapy has been completed) and by the normal (although enlarged) homogeneous appearance of the thymic tissue. However, false-negative interpretations can occur. Thus, close follow-up of these patients is critical. Finally, the bone marrow examination continues to be important, regardless of planned methods of therapy, because its involvement would upgrade the patient's disease to stage IV status and necessitate more intensive chemotherapy.

Treatment

Principles of Therapy

Prior to treatment, children with HL are placed in risk groups that are based on clinical staging, presence or absence of bulky disease, and systemic 'B' symptoms. Different cooperative groups have used various methods of risk stratification. The Children's Oncology Group (COG) defines low-risk disease as stage IA or IIA with no bulky disease and no extranodal extension. High-risk patients are those with stage IIIB or IVB, and intermediate risk includes the remaining patients that are not low or high risk.

Several strategies have been effective in the treatment of HL. These include radiation therapy alone, combinations of irradiation and chemotherapy, and, most recently, chemotherapy without radiation. For children in particular, four principles guide modern HL therapy. For those with early or low-stage HL (I to III), reduction of therapy duration and intensity to reduce long-term sequelae (while maintaining the current high cure rates) is a central principle in today's regimens. In concert with this, the reduction and eventual elimination of irradiation as a method of therapy in children with early or low-stage HL is important. The third and most recent principle is response-based therapy. This reduces therapy for those who do not require additional doses by adjusting or eliminating anticipated cycles of chemotherapy based on the tumor's response to the initial courses of therapy. Fourth, for those with advanced-stage HL (stage IV), intensification of therapy and identification of new and more effective regimens to increase relapse-free survival is needed.

Finally, advances in pediatric oncology have been substantial, primarily owing to patients being managed on protocols through the international cooperative groups. Children, including adolescents, diagnosed with HL should be referred to, and their treatment coordinated through, one of the many centers associated with these groups. These children, through participation in the clinical trials, receive the most advanced and effective therapy available today.

Principles of Radiation Therapy in the Treatment of Hodgkin Lymphoma

Despite the goal of eliminating radiation from the therapeutic regimens for children with early stage HL, it must be recognized that HL is a very radiosensitive neoplasm. A long record of efficacy exists, using radiation either alone or in combination with chemotherapy for this neoplasm. Radiation therapy has traditionally been given to the sites of disease and contiguous, clinically uninvolved, areas. This is known as extended-field irradiation. More recently, involved-field irradiation has become more widely used. This is a more attractive option when combined with chemotherapy. In children, involved-field irradiation has been shown to provide excellent local control (97%).[68] A study from Germany found that not only were the remission rate and disease-free survival (DFS) no different between involved-field and extended-field irradiation, but the side effects (leukopenia, thrombocytopenia, nausea, gastrointestinal toxicity, and pharyngeal toxicity) were significantly reduced when using only involved-field irradiation.[69]

The use of radiation therapy alone remains an option for therapy in adults with low-stage (I to III) HL because it allows them the opportunity to avoid the toxicity associated with chemotherapy.[70-73] Even if relapse occurs in those treated with radiation only, the ability to salvage a long-term cure does not appear to be compromised by delaying the use of chemotherapy until the first relapse.

The severe and lifelong side effects of irradiation (cosmetic defects, growth retardation, endocrinologic sequelae, and secondary malignancy) on a growing and developing child are a compelling reason to look for alternative methods. Appreciation for these long-term effects has led to a gradual reduction in the dose and in the size of the field treated. More recently, the focus has been to eliminate irradiation in subsets of children with HL. Trials of patients with stage IA and IIA HL as well as nonbulky disease (low-risk HL) are underway to evaluate whether radiation can be eliminated after three cycles of a more intensively timed chemotherapy regimen.

Currently, however, combined-modality therapy remains the standard of care for children and adolescents with HL.[74]

Principles of Chemotherapy

Chemotherapy is the therapeutic backbone for children with both early and advanced-stage HL. A large number of chemotherapy combinations have been used for HL. Historically, two regimens have been the most widely and effectively used for patients with early stage HL. MOPP or ABVD was administered over a 12-month period and resulted in excellent outcomes.[75,76] However, these combinations have significant long-term sequelae when administered in full doses for a year. The recognition that successful treatment with chemotherapy for children with HL would have significant impact on their quality of life and ultimate survival has led to newer combinations of chemotherapy. In general, these regimens have been variations of MOPP and ABVD. These hybrids have either replaced those agents having the worst sequelae (e.g., cyclophosphamide for nitrogen mustard) or have involved the originals being given at significantly lower doses, or both.

Newer regimens in low-stage patients have been examined with lower-dose alkylating agents, which are the causes of the majority of the long-term sequelae seen in these patients.[77] In addition, the number of cycles or overall duration has been significantly decreased as well.[48,78] Typically, a complete therapeutic protocol currently is given over 3 to 6 months. Radiation therapy sometimes remains a part of these regimens, although it is given at lower doses and encompasses smaller fields. In some studies, the chemotherapy regimens that have been given without irradiation have produced equivalent results to regimens with irradiation in patients with low-stage disease.[79-81] For those with high-risk HL, therapeutic regimens that are response-based and intensifying in both dose and timing are showing improved outcomes over the traditional regimens, with DFS now in excess of 90%.[82]

Stage, Histology, and Response-Based Therapy

Until recently, therapy for HL was primarily dictated by the stage at which the child was first seen. Now histology and response to therapy are added to the equation.[36,83] Those with LPHL histology and low-stage disease may be considered for further reductions in chemotherapy. If the disease is completely resected via an excisional biopsy, no further treatment may be needed. In a European study of 58 children with low-stage LPHL treated with surgery alone, outcomes were good with 67% progression free survival (PFS) for those who achieved a complete response (CR) with surgery only, and with an overall survival (OS) rate of 100%.[84] A COG clinical trial is attempting to confirm the results of smaller studies showing favorable outcomes with resection alone in stage I patients with LPHL, a single involved lymph node, and a complete resection. Many regimens now incorporate this concept into their design, with fewer cycles of chemotherapy or elimination of irradiation for those with early CRs.

Currently, blood or marrow stem cell transplantation is reserved for those patients whose disease is refractory to systemic chemotherapy or who have experienced relapse. Recent trials have shown that regardless of the duration of initial remission, those who are treated with high-dose chemotherapy and stem cell rescue have less treatment failure than do those treated with conventional chemotherapy.[85,86] Autologous stem cell transplant (ASCT) has become the standard of care for relapsed HL.[87]

Promising new therapies are being investigated, including brentuximab (SGN-35), a monoclonal antibody to CD-30 that has been linked to an antitubulin agent. In a study of 42 relapsed HL patients, 15 patients had objective responses with nine CRs.[88] Other novel, targeted therapies are being studied, including rituximab, an anti-CD 20 antibody; Bortezomib, a reversible proteosome inhibitor; and histone deacetylase inhibitors.[87]

Results

Most patients treated with combinations of chemotherapy and radiation enter into CR (>90%).[89,90] Many patients, especially those with the NS subtype, may have persistent adenopathy or mediastinal enlargement for months or years after therapy. Although most prove to be cured, close follow-up is necessary. For those who do not enter remission with today's front-line chemotherapy/irradiation combinations, the prognosis is poor. Therapeutic intensification with subsequent stem cell transplant will likely be needed.[86,91]

For low-risk patients, combined-modality (chemotherapy and radiation) therapy typically results in greater than 90% five-year DFS and OS rates. For intermediate risk patients, greater than 80% 5-year EFS rates are found. For high-risk patients, significant advances have been made, with EFS and OS greater that 90% in relatively recent trials.[82,92,93]

Early Complications

Early complications of therapy are due to either the tumor itself or the therapy. All patients suspected of having a lymphoma should have an immediate chest radiograph or CT scan to determine whether a mediastinal mass is present. Therapy with chemotherapy (preferable in children) or irradiation is effective in the immediate relief of these symptoms. Complications from splenectomy can occur due to overwhelming sepsis from encapsulated organisms. This risk is increased because of the myelosuppression and immunocompromising effects of chemotherapy. Fever in the neutropenic patient necessitates hospitalization and intravenous antibiotic therapy. Bone marrow suppression may require transfusions of either red cells or platelets. Specific chemotherapy agents may have immediate complications. These include nausea and vomiting, restrictive pulmonary disease (bleomycin, irradiation), extravasation burns (nitrogen mustard, vincristine, vinblastine, doxorubicin [Adriamycin]), and chemical phlebitis (nitrogen mustard, vinblastine, DTIC). To alleviate these risks, right atrial catheters are often placed. This also reduces the discomfort of repeated venipuncture required throughout the duration of treatment.

Long-Term Sequelae

The concern over long-term sequelae guides much of modern therapy for HL, both in adults and particularly in children. These sequelae result from both radiation therapy and chemotherapy.[94,95] The long-term sequelae of irradiation in growing children are the overriding reason for the efforts to reduce or eliminate it from therapeutic regimens. Bone irradiation may result in shortening of the clavicles in those patients receiving mantle radiation or a shortened height in those receiving radiation to the spine.[96] Radiation to the neck often results in permanent hypothyroidism[97] and increases the risk of thyroid cancer.[98,99] If radiation is to be given to the pelvis of a female patient, consideration should be given to positioning the ovaries away from the field of irradiation.[100]

Second malignancies are a major concern after therapy for HL.[101-103] The most frequent cause of death in long-term survivors of HL is a second malignancy.[104] The relative risk of a second malignancy in HL patients has been estimated to be five- to 11-fold that of the general population.[102,105] This represents a 15- to 25-year actuarial risk of 7% to 23%.[102,105-107] Second malignancies are more prevalent in those with HL treated before age 21 years than in the older age groups for all tumors except lung cancer.[102] These second cancers include leukemia and solid tumors. The risk of leukemia seems primarily related to the type of chemotherapy used,[105,108] with a cumulative incidence of 3.3%, with a plateau after about ten years. However, one study found a decrease in secondary leukemia among those treated with the newer hybrid regimens.[107] This likely is a result of the reduction in nitrogen mustard and procarbazine (in MOPP) doses, the principal culprits in the development of secondary leukemia.[109,110] Patients treated with ABVD do not have an increased risk of leukemia. The reduction in the incidence of leukemia may be a result of the decreasing use of splenectomy for staging as this operation has been shown to increase the risk of leukemia in HL patients treated with chemotherapy.[109,111]

Solid tumors, including those of lung, stomach, melanoma, bone, and soft tissue, have accounted for most of the second malignancies, with a cumulative incidence of 13–22% at 15 to 25 years. No plateau has been appreciated.[102,105,106] This risk in HL survivors has not decreased when cohorts treated in the 1960s are compared with those in the 1980s.[102] This increased risk of solid tumors is related primarily to irradiation,[112,113] with some added risk when subsequent chemotherapy is used in relapse patients.[114] It has been recognized that radiation exposure to the breast tissue in adult women has resulted in a fourfold increase in rates of subsequent breast cancer,[115-118] whereas the risk of subsequent breast cancer is increased by 39-fold if the breasts are irradiated during adolescence.[119] For an adolescent, this increases the probability of developing breast cancer between the ages of 20 and 30 years from 0.04% to 1.6%[120] and may be as high as 35% by age 40 years. Other long-term sequelae include cardiac complications secondary to mantle irradiation and/or the use of doxorubicin (Adriamycin in ABVD regimens) that affect up to 13% of patients.[121,122]

NON-HODGKIN LYMPHOMA

In contrast to the similarities between adult and pediatric HL, the types of NHL that occur in adults and children, their presentation, their treatment, and their outcome are dramatically different. Most adults with NHL have low- or intermediate-grade lymphomas. In contrast, children with these types of lymphomas are exceedingly rare. Instead, virtually all children with NHL have one of four high-grade, diffuse types: Burkitt lymphoma (BL, formerly small, noncleaved cell lymphoma [SNCCL]), lymphoblastic lymphoma (formerly precursor T-cell lymphoblastic lymphoma [T-LL]), diffuse large B-cell lymphoma (DLBCL), or anaplastic large cell lymphoma

(ALCL). Most patients present with advanced or disseminated disease (stages III and IV).

These lymphomas typically appear as a rapidly expanding mass with a short symptomatic history. This propensity for rapid growth makes the diagnostic evaluation in a child with suspected NHL a medical urgency, if not emergency. Of all the childhood tumors, NHL has the greatest chance of presenting with complications. Anatomic impingement of adjacent structures (mediastinal tumors on the trachea and bronchi, nasopharyngeal tumors on the orbits, bowel obstruction with or without intussusception) and metabolic derangements due to tumor lysis (before and after therapy is initiated) are not infrequent results of its very rapid growth. Better management of the initial anatomic and metabolic complications, improved methods of determining the subtypes of NHL (perhaps the most important reason for improved survival), and better chemotherapy combinations (more intensive, yet shorter) have brought the most dramatic improvements in DFS and OS for children with NHL over the past several decades.[123] Five-year relative survival (adjusted for normal life expectancy) was 86% for patients diagnosed with NHL from 2001 to 2007.[1] Between 1975 and 2006, a 75% decline in mortality was seen in children with NHL.[124] In addition to more intense therapy of shorter duration, the other major change in therapy for children with NHL is the virtual elimination of radiation from treatment regimens. This should reduce the long-term sequelae that would have otherwise resulted. For the surgeon seeing the child with suspected lymphoma, rapid evaluation and proper handling of biopsy material will have dramatic beneficial effects on the outcomes.

Incidence and Epidemiology

NHL accounts for 4% of all cancers in adult and pediatric patients. It is estimated that 70,130 men and women will be diagnosed with NHL in the USA in 2012.[11] In children (ages 0 to 14 years), NHL patients accounted for 4% of childhood cancers[1] and approximately 50% of all lymphomas.[1] The annual incidence is 1.3 cases/100,000 children ages 10–14 and 1.8 cases/100,000 children ages 15–19 years.[11] Before age 11 years, it is the most common of the two types of lymphoma. A high male-to-female ratio of 3.0 is found,[11] making it the most disproportionately occurring tumor between the two genders during childhood. This large difference is found in all ages of childhood. The age distribution demonstrates two small peaks in incidence from 6 to 7 years and between 12 and 14 years (see Fig. 69-1). The 6- and 7-year-olds overwhelmingly have BL, and the teenagers typically have T-LL.

NHL of B-cell origin, either BL or DLBCL, occurs more often in patients with prior EBV exposure, in individuals with a history of immune suppression, and in equatorial Africa.[125–127] It is known that in patients with an iatrogenic (e.g., post-transplant, immunosuppressive therapy) or acquired immunodeficiency, congenital-EBV infection has an etiologic role in either the development or the predisposition to B-cell NHL.[128,129] Correlations have been made between the viral load and the risk of post-transplant lymphoproliferative disorders (PTLDs).[130–132] Patients at greatest risk for PTLDs are those in whom their primary infection with EBV occurs within the first 3 to 4 months after transplantation. For T-LL or ALCL, no such etiologic correlations have been found.

Classification

Over the years, several classification schemes have been used.[133] The Revised European American Lymphoma Classification is the basis for the WHO classification that was updated in 2008.[34] Childhood NHL primarily consists of four major subtypes in the WHO system: (1) BL/leukemia and Burkitt-like (mature B-cell neoplasms accounting for 39% of NHL patients[3]); (2) lymphoblastic lymphoma (28%[3]); (3) DLBCL; and (4) ALCL. DLBCL and ALCL were previously lumped together as large cell lymphomas and comprised about one-third of the NHL of childhood. With the separation of these two entities, the cases previously identified as large cell lymphoma are now divided almost equally between DLBCL and ALCL.[134] The first two classifications are part of the 'small, round, blue cell tumors,' which presents the pathologist with the challenge of proper identification. To differentiate these from the other three classic small round blue cell tumors (neuroblastoma, rhabdomyosarcoma, and Ewing sarcoma) requires the presence of the immunocytochemical marker leukocyte common antigen CD45 (LCA), which is absent in the other tumor cell types.

BL has classically been divided into Burkitt and non-Burkitt (Burkitt-like in the REAL classification) subtypes. These are of a mature B-cell origin, with flow cytometric immunophenotyping revealing the presence of surface immunoglobulin IgM, CD10, CD19, CD20, CD22, CD79a, and human leukocyte antigen (HLA)-DR antigens. The histologic appearance of these two types differs in the degree of pleomorphism, with Burkitt being more uniform appearing than non-Burkitt. Although a distinction has been made for years between Burkitt and non-Burkitt subtypes of diffuse SNCCL lymphomas, no clinical differences are found between these two subtypes.[135] Histologically, the cells of BL are medium sized with round nuclei containing two to five nucleoli, abundant basophilic cytoplasm, and cytoplasmic lipid vacuoles. Owing to its extreme rates of proliferation and spontaneous cell death, a number of macrophages are seen within this monomorphic field, consuming the dying cells and giving rise to the classic 'starry sky' appearance of BL.[136]

Lymphoblastic lymphomas (LL) are distinguished by round or convoluted nuclei, finely dispersed chromatin, inconspicuous nucleoli, and scant cytoplasm. In the vast majority of these tumors, flow cytometry reveals the presence of the T-cell markers CD3 and CD7, with variable positivity for CD2 and CD5. These cells are typically Tdt positive, whereas BLs are Tdt negative. This subtype is classified as a precursor T-cell LL in the WHO classification. A small number of LL cases are B-cell precursor and express pre–B-cell antigen profiles.[134]

Large cell lymphomas are a heterogeneous group of neoplasms. Histologically, approximately half are immunoblastic, 40% are large noncleaved cell, and fewer than 5% are large cleaved cell.[137] Flow cytometry shows relatively equal frequencies of B- or T-cell origin (36% and 33%, respectively) with 30% indeterminate.[138,139] A unique subset, identified by the immunophenotype CD30+ (the antigen identified by the Ki-1 monoclonal antibody),[140] is recognized morphologically by its anaplastic characteristics, including very large cells with abundant cytoplasm, atypical lobulated nuclei, and prominent nucleoli. These cells exhibit a cohesive pattern with lymph node sinusoidal invasion. In the WHO classification, this is referred to as ALCL. In the past, this subtype has also been referred to as malignant histiocytosis. The majority (60%) of these children have a T-cell immunophenotype.[138,141] Although it was originally thought to be uncommon in children, this subtype accounts for 40–50% of the large cell lymphoma cases.[138,139,142,143]

Clinical Presentation

By Initial Site of Disease

Overall, unlike those with HL and adult NHL, children with NHL are often initially seen with extranodal disease and typically have disease that spreads by routes other than contiguous nodal pathways. In children, the abdomen is the originating site of disease in 31%, the mediastinum in 27%, and the head and neck in 29%.[3] Other sites include peripheral nodes, bone, and skin. Most abdominal disease primary lesions are due to BL, whereas most mediastinal/intrathoracic primary lesions are due to LL. Disease that occurs primarily in the peripheral nodes and bones is often due to large cell lymphomas, and skin involvement is primarily associated with the Ki-1+ large cell lymphoma subtype (ALCL).[139,144,145] Correlating with this distribution and the known age peaks of the two types of small cell lymphomas, abdominal primary lesions occur more often in children younger than 10 years, whereas mediastinal primary lesions are more likely to occur in adolescents.

Children with abdominal primary lesions may present with nausea, vomiting, abdominal pain, and changes in bowel habits. On physical examination, they may be found to have an abdominal mass in any of the quadrants. Also, they may present with an acute abdomen due to either intussusception (typically due to infiltration of Peyer's patches) (Fig. 69-3) or small bowel obstruction, perforation of an involved bowel wall, or an ileocecal mass mimicking acute appendicitis.[146]

A child older than age 5 years with an intussusception must strongly be considered to have NHL until proven otherwise. Moreover, NHL should always be part of one's differential diagnosis when faced with a 5- to 10-year-old child with an abdominal mass. Radiographic evaluation with either CT or ultrasound typically reveals a homogeneous mass with or without evidence of central necrosis, arising either from the retroperitoneum or from the bowel wall. Accompanying adenopathy and metastatic dissemination to the liver and spleen is often seen. The bowel loops may simply be shifted away from the mass or may show evidence of intussusception or obstruction (or both).

Children with mediastinal primary lesions may have minimal symptoms, such as a mild cough or audible wheeze, or can have impending airway obstruction. These latter patients can also have significant engorgement of the vasculature in the head, face, and upper thorax because of superior vena cava compression. Thrombosis may be present in these vessels as well. Often these patients will assume a forward-leaning position and cannot tolerate being placed in the supine position because of the anterior mediastinal mass. The patient's history may reveal orthopnea as well as shortness of breath and dyspnea on exertion. The recent onset of asthma symptoms is not uncommon. Shortness of breath also may be due to pleural effusions. A chest radiograph or chest CT scan is an essential component of the patient's initial evaluation before sedation or any procedure (Fig. 69-4). Chest radiography and chest CT will reveal the widened mediastinum with often dramatic narrowing of

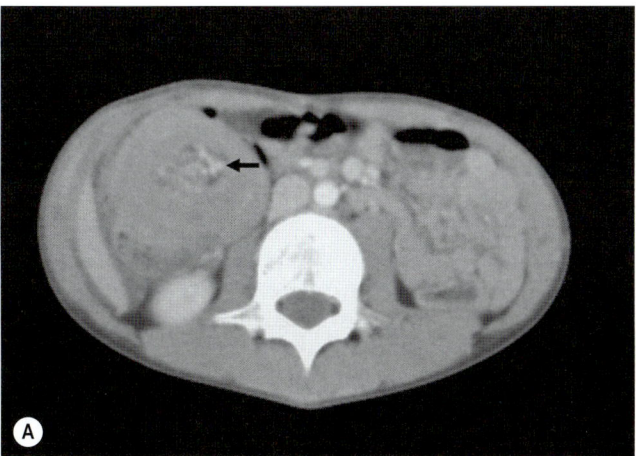
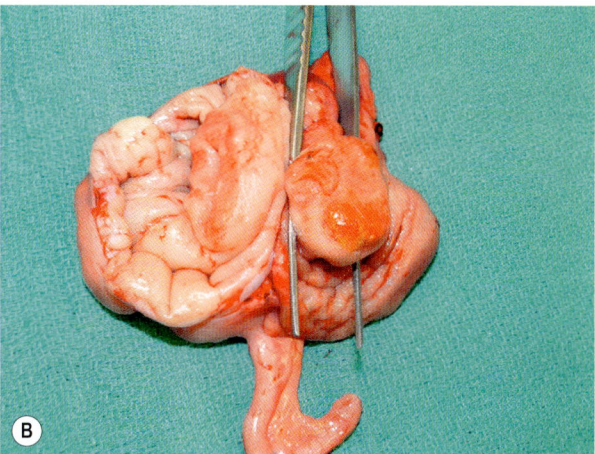

FIGURE 69-3 ■ This 12-year-old child presented with abdominal pain, nausea, and vomiting. An abdominal mass was palpable in the right abdomen. (A) The CT scan shows a large ileocolic intussusception in the right mid-abdomen. The mesenteric vessels within the intussusceptum are marked with the arrow. The lead point for this intussusception was a non-Hodgkin lymphoma. (B) The resected specimen shows a lymphoma in the small bowel which led to the intussusception.

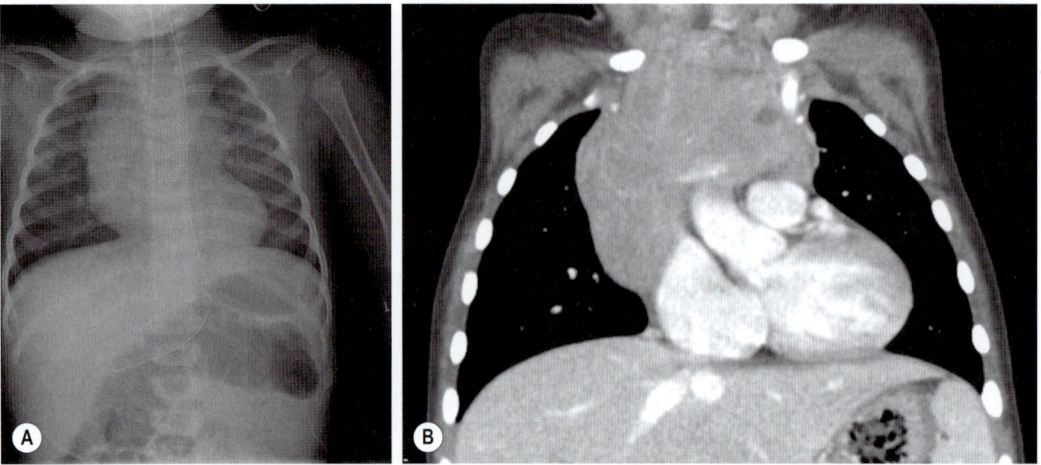

FIGURE 69-4 ■ This 17-month-old boy had a 1-month history of stridor and several episodes of perioral cyanosis when he was fussy. The patient was seen in an emergency room where the **(A)** chest radiograph showed a large anterior mediastinal mass. **(B)** A contrasted CT scan showed the large heterogeneous, noncalcified mediastinal mass which extends across the anterior mediastinum. The mass encases and abuts, but does not occlude, the left subclavian and innominate veins. The mass measures 4.6 cm × 6.8 cm × 6.5 cm. On another view, the distal trachea was seen to narrow to 2 mm in AP diameter just proximal to the carina. Bone marrow examination and lumbar puncture were normal. CT-guided biopsy of the mediastinal mass yielded NHL. This infant responded nicely to chemotherapy and has completely recovered.

the trachea and bronchi. Pericardial effusions are often present and may be seen on CT, magnetic resonance imaging (MRI), or echocardiography.[147]

Patients with head and neck lymphomas may have a history of rapidly progressive adenopathy, recent onset of snoring at night, mouth breathing, halitosis, epistaxis, proptosis or periorbital edema, diplopia, extraocular muscle paralysis due to entrapment, cranial nerve paralysis, sudden blindness, or a combination of these symptoms. Physical examination of the nares, oral cavity, and extraocular movements is important and may reveal signs not appreciated as abnormal by the child. The presence of asymmetric and painless tonsillar hypertrophy should also alert the clinician to the possibility of NHL.[148]

Evaluation with CT often reveals a homogeneous mass that may show destruction of the adjacent bony structures. Bone NHL primary disease is usually seen as lytic lesions found on radiographs obtained for various reasons, including localized tenderness.[149–151] Skin lesions are typically ulcerative and fail to heal, but also may be completely subcutaneous.[144] Patients with central nervous system (CNS) involvement may be asymptomatic, have seizures, or have signs and symptoms related to tumor infiltration in the brain.

Laboratory findings at the time of diagnosis are dependent on the amount of tumor present (regardless of the histologic subtype). Generally, patients will have an elevated ESR or C-reactive protein (CRP) level. Those with large tumor burdens typically have high LDH levels as an indicator of tumor lysis risk,[152,153] disease regression, and disease progression. The degree of LDH elevation has been used as an adverse prognostic factor.[3,154,155] For those with a high tumor burden at presentation, laboratory signs of tumor lysis will also include elevated uric acid, phosphorus, and potassium levels along with a low calcium level. Some patients may already be in renal failure at the time of presentation or have an elevated creatinine.[152,153] Hematologic values are

nonspecific, and the presence of cytopenias should raise the suspicion of marrow involvement. Cerebrospinal fluid (CSF) pleocytosis may or may not be present in those with CNS involvement.

More than 60% of patients have advanced or disseminated (stages III and IV) disease at diagnosis.[3,156] Bone marrow metastasis is defined as greater than 5% but less than 25% involvement. Patients with more than 25% disease in the bone marrow are classified as having leukemia. Fourteen per cent of patients initially have some bone marrow involvement, and 3% have CNS involvement.[3]

By Histologic Subtype

BL was first described by the surgeon Denis Burkitt in Uganda, where he identified the common finding of enormous involvement of the nodes around the jaw.[157] Later, it was determined that, although this was a common presentation of those patients with endemic Burkitt (African) lymphoma, those with sporadic Burkitt (American) lymphoma more typically had presentation of disease either in the abdomen or the nasopharynx.[158] Patients with endemic BL have accompanying abdominal disease in roughly half the cases, and patients with sporadic BL have jaw involvement 15–20% of the time.[159] Patients with sporadic BL have a higher incidence of bone marrow involvement (21% vs 7%) but lower CNS dissemination (11% vs 17%). Approximately two thirds of BL patients will have disseminated or advanced disease (defined as stages III and IV) at diagnosis.[160]

T-LL patients most often are adolescents with supradiaphragmatic disease, affecting either the intrathoracic region or the head and neck. Disseminated disease is present in nearly 90% of T-LL patients at diagnosis.[160] In T-LL patients, involvement of the bone marrow has been found in approximately one fourth of children, and CNS disease is present in fewer than 10%.[160]

ALCL patients may present with disease in all sites but there is a higher prevalence than the other two subtypes for skin, bone, and peripheral nodes.[144,151,161] ALCL is found in two distinct clinical forms: primary cutaneous ALCL and primary systemic ALCL (as fevers and weight loss, and in advanced stage).[134] Disseminated disease in ALCL patients is present at diagnosis in up to 65% of patients.[160] Involvement of the bone marrow or CNS in ALCL patients is rare. DLBCL may present as a mediastinal primary lesion or as nodal or extranodal disease, most commonly in the abdomen or head and neck.[134]

In Immunodeficient Patients

For patients with congenital or acquired immunodeficiency, NHL presentation will vary from polyclonal plasmacytic hyperplasia, most often localized in nasopharyngeal nodes or tonsils, to a clonal polymorphic lymphoma slowly arising in the lymph nodes or extranodal sites, to widely disseminated, rapidly progressive immunoblastic lymphoma.[162,163] Symptoms may be nonspecific, with fever and malaise. Hepatosplenomegaly and lymphadenopathy may be presenting signs. Gastrointestinal symptoms of longer than 14 days duration with anorexia, weight loss, and diarrhea should raise suspicion for this condition.[132] NHL has become more common with the use of very potent antirejection drugs after solid organ or bone marrow transplantation. Involvement of the transplanted organ is not unusual.[132,164]

Diagnosis

Children initially suspected of having NHL should be evaluated immediately because of the high risk of either metabolic or anatomic complications before therapy begins. The rapid growth of these tumors may create a life-threatening complication overnight in a child who seemed relatively healthy the previous day (Box 69-2).

BOX 69-2	**Non-Hodgkin Lymphoma: Diagnostic and Staging Evaluation at Presentation**

Complete physical examination with documentation of involved nodal groups (including measurements of nodes) and involved extralymphatic organs

Complete blood cell count, chemistry panel (including hepatic and renal function tests), erythrocyte sedimentation rate, lactate dehydrogenase

Chest radiography to evaluate for mediastinal disease and airway compression

CT scans of areas identified on physical examination (also include chest, neck, and abdomen)

Bone scan

Gallium scan

Excisional biopsy of node or mass with samples sent for routine pathology, molecular genetics, cytogenetics, and flow cytometry

Bone marrow biopsies and aspirates (bilateral)

Lumbar puncture with CSF analysis of cytocentrifuged sample

CT, computed tomography; CSF, cerebrospinal fluid.

No clinical findings are pathognomonic for NHL. Ultimately, the diagnosis awaits the biopsy of involved sites, most commonly an excised lymph node or percutaneous needle biopsy. Fine needle aspirations do not provide enough tissue for the necessary subtyping, which is performed with flow cytometry, molecular genetics, and cytogenetics. It is critical for the excised tissue to be delivered quickly as a fresh specimen for processing.

Similar to HL, for patients critically ill at diagnosis, such as those with severe airway obstruction, diagnosis by alternative methods may be required. NHL is a systemic disease that requires chemotherapy so debulking operations or attempts at local control are not necessary. The one exception in which initial total resection may be considered are those patients with an abdominal mass in whom bowel resection is already required because of perforation or obstruction. In this case, total resection of the tumor should be considered. In this setting, resection reduces the stage of the patient's disease, improves survival, and reduces the amount of therapy required.[165] For all other patients, resection of the mass provides no improvement in staging or long-term cure, and delays the time to initiation of chemotherapy. It should be remembered that most patients have disseminated disease at presentation. Also, it is important to note that with chemotherapy alone, more than 90% will achieve a complete remission.

Once NHL is suspected, a concerted and well-conceived plan of evaluation is important to achieve a diagnosis as quickly as possible. This should include laboratory examination to evaluate tumor burden and presence or risk of tumor lysis syndrome. The radiographic evaluation in these patients is extremely important.[51] No procedures or sedation should be attempted until a mediastinal mass has been excluded. To identify the extent of disease, CTs of the neck, chest, abdomen, and pelvis are required. An examination of the head, either CT or MRI, should be obtained in those patients with CNS symptoms, with CSF pleocytosis, or in whom the primary lesions are parameningeal based. Bone scans should typically be obtained. [18]FDG-PET or gallium scans are currently recommended. [18]FDG-PET scans have gradually replaced gallium scans and are now considered an essential tool in the initial evaluation of patients with NHL. Advantages of PET over gallium include same-day imaging, improved resolution, and a higher target-to-background ratio.[166] Diagnostic PET scans are reliable (greater than 90% positive) in patients with DLBCL. Studies of patients with HL and NHL have found PET to be superior to gallium for diagnosing disease sites.[66] Also, PET has been shown to be more sensitive than CT or gallium scans in staging NHL.[167] PET may be fused with CT for improved imaging. PET is also an important component in evaluating response to treatment.

Histologic evaluation of the biopsy material should include general histochemical techniques to confirm the lymphoma and its subtype. Additional tests include flow cytometric analysis of cell-surface markers to determine the immunophenotype of the lymphoma, cytogenetic evaluation for diagnostic translocations, fluorescent in situ hybridization (FISH), and DNA analysis using either Southern blotting or the polymerase chain reaction

(PCR) for detection of the pathognomonic oncogenes (gene rearrangements), even in the absence of identifiable cytogenetic translocations.[168] Examination of markers in tumor cells for EBV is important in the evaluation of PTLDs. Therapy differences between the subtypes of lymphoma are such that assignment to the wrong subtype due to a lack of adequate diagnostic material will adversely affect the chance of cure. These evaluations may be performed with biopsy material from any involved site, including the primary mass, enlarged lymph nodes, effusions, and bone marrow. Gene expression profiling, which uses DNA microarrays, has been shown to categorize patients further into specific histologic and genetic subsets of lymphoma, with much greater predictability of the clinical outcome.[169] This technique has revolutionized diagnostic and prognostic characterization for NHL.

Completing the diagnostic protocol is the determination of whether or not there is CNS or bone marrow dissemination. Lumbar puncture for cytocentrifuged CSF analysis should be performed in all patients. However, in those with localized abdominal BL, and those with large cell lymphoma, the benefit gained from this is arguable because of the low incidence of CNS disease in these subpopulations. Bone marrow evaluation should include bilateral iliac crest biopsies and aspirates.

Staging

Once the diagnosis of NHL is made, staging permits determination of the extent of disease at presentation. This provides direction in monitoring disease response to therapy. In contrast to HL, relapse does not necessarily occur at the site of initial or previous disease in NHL. Thus, this initial staging should not limit the extent of monitoring for relapse after therapy is completed.

Staging is important in the determination of therapeutic planning. The most widely used staging schema today is the St. Jude's or Murphy system (Table 69-3).[170] This is an adaptation of the Ann Arbor scheme and is applicable to all types of childhood NHL. It divides patients into localized (stage I or II) and disseminated or advanced (stage III or IV) disease. Involvement of the CNS or bone marrow immediately places the patient in the stage IV category. Patients with more than 25% bone marrow involvement are, by definition, diagnosed with leukemia rather than with lymphoma. These include B-cell or Burkitt leukemia (L3 leukemia morphologic classification) and T-cell leukemia. The former patients are treated on B-cell NHL protocols with much better results than previously obtained on acute lymphoblastic leukemia (ALL) regimens. Many of the B-cell NHL protocol results reported in the literature include these patients in their stage IV populations. The T-cell leukemia patients remain on ALL protocols, but many similarities exist between these protocols and those used in T-LL therapy.

Prognostic Risk Factors

When all patients are treated similarly, the stage of the lymphoma at diagnosis is a strong predictor of outcome.[3] Prediction of a patient's eventual outcome stratifies

TABLE 69-3	St. Jude's (Murphy) Staging System for Childhood Non-Hodgkin's Lymphoma
Stage	**Definition**
I	Single tumor (extranodal) or single anatomic area (nodal), excluding mediastinum or abdomen
II	Single tumor (extranodal) with regional node involvement On same side of diaphragm: (a) Two or more nodal areas (b) Two single (extranodal) tumors with or without regional node involvement Primary gastrointestinal tract tumor (usually ileocecal) with or without associated mesenteric node involvement, grossly completely resected
III	On both sides of diaphragm: (a) Two single tumors (extranodal) (b) Two or more nodal areas All primary intrathoracic tumors (mediastinal, pleural, thymic) All extensive primary intra-abdominal disease; unresectable All primary paraspinal or epidural tumors regardless of other sites
IV	Any of the above with initial CNS or bone marrow involvement (<25%)

CNS, central nervous system.

patients at high risk for relapse to more intensive or novel therapies and patients at low risk to shorter, more moderate therapies. Many prognostic factors have been evaluated over the years. All prognostic factors are dependent on the therapy subsequently given.[3] It has been definitively shown that histology-based therapy is of critical importance in the successful outcome of these patients.[156]

CNS involvement in both SNCCL and LL patients has predictably worse outcomes.[156] In patients with BL, the adverse effect of CNS disease on outcome has, in some studies, been more attributable to tumor burden at diagnosis than to the presence of CNS disease alone (i.e., those with greater tumor burden are more likely to have CNS disease).[171] Patients with BL older than 15 years of age have a worse prognosis than patients younger than 15 years old. An LDH greater than 500 IU/L also predicts a worse outcome for patients with BL.[172]

Treatment

Therapy for childhood NHL has evolved over the past several decades, and is based on the knowledge that this tumor is extremely chemosensitive. For BL and large cell lymphoma, the duration of therapy has become shorter as it became apparent that most, if not all, patients were experiencing relapse within the first 6 to 8 months of therapy.[160,173] Despite reducing therapy to 6 months or less, no increase in relapse has been seen. Relapses for the most part have occurred within the first 6 to 8 months after diagnosis and virtually all have occurred within the first 2 years.[154–156,173,174] Therapy for BL has shown a clear improvement as methotrexate and cytarabine doses have been increased. These two agents, in addition to cyclophosphamide, vincristine, doxorubicin (Adriamycin), and prednisone (and etoposide for the stage IV patients), now play a critical role in the successful outcome of these children.[160,165,174,175] The addition of radiation has not shown improvements in DFS or OS.[142,144,176] The addition of rituximab (an anti-CD20 monoclonal antibody) is currently being studied.

For T-LL, the duration of therapy has been decreased to two years. The most effective regimens for LL have been ones similar to the intensive T-cell ALL protocols in current use. For patients with LL, irradiation to areas of bulky disease has been eliminated. However, for those patients with LL and CNS disease at diagnosis, irradiation remains an important part of their therapy. For ALCL patients, the use of T-cell regimens without much CNS-directed therapy has been efficacious.

Several additional points deserve mention. The use of corticosteroids should be avoided until the diagnosis is made. Steroids can induce rapid necrosis in the lymphoma, making subtype determination difficult if not impossible, and potentially jeopardizing the patient's outcome. However, once adequate tissue has been obtained, chemotherapy including corticosteroids is an excellent method for rapid reduction of a life-threatening mass. Because of the extreme sensitivity of NHL, one can anticipate rapid reduction of tumor size once therapy is initiated. Radiation therapy is not necessary. It is not unusual to have symptoms completely resolve within 24 hours and have patients in complete radiographic remission within seven days. Many protocols now call for a period of reduced-dose chemotherapy for the first week to obtain a more controlled tumor reduction because of the severe tumor lysis that can accompany more rapid, therapy-induced necrosis.

NHL in immunodeficient individuals is most often a B-cell lymphoma, either small or large cell. Therapy for these patients has typically been directed toward these histologic types. For patients with ongoing iatrogenic immune suppression, a reduction in the immunosuppressive agent, with or without acyclovir, may be adequate to induce a remission in up to 75% of cases.[132,177] In the past few years, for resistant disease, new methods using monoclonal antibody therapy, primarily rituximab, have been used with promising results alone, but these antibodies are most efficacious when combined with chemotherapy.[178]

Results

When reviewing the outcomes of children treated for NHL, it is quickly apparent that considerable improvement in DFS and OS has occurred over the past several decades.[3] Today, typically 90–100% of patients will achieve complete remission.[142,173,179] Five-year relative survival rates for children ages birth to 19 years, and diagnosed between 1996 and 2004, were 83.3%.[13]

Patients with localized disease have an overall excellent prognosis, regardless of histologic subtype, with DFS typically exceeding 90–95%. BL patients with advanced disease have experienced DFS exceeding 80% in the recent trials. Patients with LL with disseminated disease are not faring as well, but DFS for these patients

is exceeding 65–70% in most trials. Overall, when they occur, treatment failures typically happen within the first two years after diagnosis. Patients with BL who experience relapse primarily do so within the first 6 to 8 months. LL patients will have an occasional late failure after two years, although even in this group of patients the vast majority of failures will occur early.[179] The prognosis for patients with DLBCL is excellent with three-year EFS of ≥90% in a recent trial.[180] Patients with advanced-stage ALCL have 2-year EFS of approximately 70%.[181]

Early Complications

Depending on the tumor burden at diagnosis, patients may initially have a constellation of significant metabolic derangements known as tumor lysis syndrome.[152,153] These problems include hyperuricemia, hyperphosphatemia, hyperkalemia, and hypocalcemia. Recognition of this syndrome is critical to prevent life-threatening complications, including acute renal failure. Without treatment, the incidence of acute renal failure may be as high as 30%.[182] Tumor lysis syndrome is the result of the rapid turnover of cells within the tumor. The fraction of tumor cells in S phase at any given time can approach 27% in some patients.[183] These tumors have a high degree of spontaneous lysis at the time of diagnosis because they rapidly outgrow their blood supply. Any manipulation, including transfusion or operation, may induce a sudden worsening of this syndrome.

Therapy is primarily based on preventing hyperuricemia. For those at high risk, determined by the presence of an elevated LDH, creatinine, or uric acid value, intervention is important. For most patients with little or no elevation in these values, adequate hydration (>3000 mL/m^2/day) and pH monitoring (maintain between 7.0 and 7.5) is adequate, along with the initiation of allopurinol to reduce the production of uric acid through inhibition of xanthine oxidase.[184] Rasburicase cleaves uric acid into allantoin, a soluble by-product. This agent, administered daily for one to five days, dramatically reduces measurable uric acid levels to immeasurable levels, thus allowing the clinician to focus on prevention or treatment of hyperphosphatemia, which requires maintaining acidic urine.[185,186] Despite these measures, it may be necessary to place patients on dialysis either to treat oliguria/anuria or to prevent it in the presence of rapidly increasing uric acid, phosphorus (typically >10 mg/dL), or potassium (>7.5 mEq/L) levels.[160,187] In an effort to avoid this complication, an initial low-dose therapy (usually 1 week) to more slowly reduce the tumor burden is used in some treatment regimens.

As a result of the much more myelosuppressive protocols required in NHL therapy, infection is a much greater risk for NHL patients as compared with HL patients.[156] In one recent study, 63% of the deaths were due to infection. Most patients require transfusion support during treatment because of the myelosuppression. The chemotherapy itself may cause acute complications, including severe chemical burns due to extravasation of certain vesicant agents (vincristine, anthracyclines). As most children require the placement of right atrial catheters to facilitate their therapy, thrombosis of this area and the surrounding vasculature has become more frequent.[188] Mucositis is seen in a significant number of patients during therapy for Burkitt lymphoma as well.

Long-Term Sequelae

As long-term survival has improved, the concern over lifelong sequelae has increased in these patients. With current therapy, these complications include cardiac toxicity,[122] infertility as a result of the alkylating agents used,[189] and secondary leukemias due to epipodophyllotoxins (etoposide, tenoposide) and the alkylating agents used in the NHL regimens.[190] The risk for developing cardiac toxicity is related to several factors, including the irradiation dose, cumulative anthracycline dose, and age at exposure. Patients are at an increased risk for anthracycline-related cardiomyopathy if they are female, have received doses greater than 200–300 mg/m^2, and were younger when given anthracyclines.[191]

REFERENCES

1. Siegel R, Naishadham D, Jemal A. Cancer Statistics, 2012. CA Cancer J Clin 2012;62:10–29.
2. In: Jaffe ES, Harris NL, Stein H, et al, editors. World Health Organization Classification of Tumours: Pathology and Genetics of Tumours of Haematopoietic and Lymphoid Tissues. Lyon: IARC Press; 2001.
3. Murphy SB, Fairclough DL, Hutchison RE, et al. Non-Hodgkin's lymphomas of childhood: An analysis of the histology, staging, and response to treatment of 338 cases at a single institution. J Clin Oncol 1989;7:186–93.
4. Hodgkin T. On some morbid appearances of the absorbent glands and spleen. Med Chirurg Trans 1832;17:68–114.
5. Sternberg C. Uber eine eigenartige unter dem Bilde der Pseudoleukaemie verlaufende Tuberculose des lymphatischen Apparetes. Z Heilkd 1898;19:21–92.
6. Reed D. On the pathological changes in Hodgkin's disease: With especial reference to its relation to tuberculosis. Johns Hopkins Hosp Rep 1902;10:133–96.
7. Gilbert R. Radiotherapy in Hodgkin's disease. AJR Am J Roentgenol 1939;41:198–240.
8. Kaplan HS, Rosenberg SA. The management of Hodgkin's disease. Cancer 1975;36:796–803.
9. Hellman S. Thomas Hodgkin and Hodgkin's disease: Two paradigms appropriate to medicine today. JAMA 1991;265:1007–10.
10. Zantinga AR, Coppes MJ. Thomas Hodgkin (1798–1866): Pathologist, social scientist, and philanthropist. Med Pediatr Oncol 1996;27:122–7.
11. Howlader N, Noone AM, Krapcho M, et al, editors. SEER Cancer Statistics Review, 1975–2009 (Vintage 2009 Populations). Bethesda, MD: National Cancer Institute. http://seer.cancer.gov/csr/1975_2009_pops09/, based on November 2011 SEER data submission, posted to the SEER web site, 2012.
12. American Cancer Society. Cancer Facts and Figures 2007. Atlanta: American Cancer Society; 2007.
13. Ries LAG, Melbert D, Krapcho M, et al, editors. SEER Cancer Statistics Review, 1975–2005. Bethesda, MD: National Cancer Institute. Based on November 2007 SEER data submission, posted to the SEER website, 2008. Available at http//seer.cancer.gov/csr/1975_2005/
14. Gurney JG, Severson RK, Davis S, et al. Incidence of cancer in children in the United States. Cancer 1995;75:2186–95.
15. Kung FH. Hodgkin's disease in children 4 years of age or younger. Cancer 1991;67:1428–30.
16. Mack TM, Cozen W, Shibata DK, et al. Concordance for Hodgkin's disease in identical twins suggesting genetic susceptibility to the young-adult form of the disease. N Engl J Med 1995;332:413–18.
17. Grufferman S, Delzell E. Epidemiology of Hodgkin's disease. Epidemiol Rev 1984;6:76–106.
18. Gutensohn N, Cole P. Childhood social environment and Hodgkin's disease. N Engl J Med 1981;304:135–40.
19. Reynolds P, Sunders LD, Layefsky ME, et al. The spectrum of acquired immunodeficiency syndrome (AIDS)—associated malignancies in San Francisco, 1980–1987. Am J Epidemiol 1993;137:19–30.
20. Hessol NA, Katz MH, Liu JY, et al. Increased incidence of Hodgkin disease in homosexual men with HIV infection. Ann Intern Med 1992;117:309–11.
21. Volberding P, Baker K, Levine A. Human immunodeficiency virus hematology. Hematology Am Soc Hematol Educ Program 2003;294–313.
22. Riggs S, Hagemeister FB. Immunodeficiency states: A predisposition to lymphoma. In: Fuller LM, Hagemeister FB, Sullivan M, editors. Hodgkin's Disease and Non-Hodgkin's Lymphomas in Adults and Children. New York: Raven; 1988. p. 451.
23. Ambinder RF, Browning PJ, Lorenzana I, et al. Epstein-Barr virus and childhood Hodgkin's disease in Honduras and the United States. Blood 1993;81:462–7.
24. Herbst H, Steinbrecher E, Niedobitek G, et al. Distribution and phenotype of Epstein-Barr virus–harboring cells in Hodgkin's disease. Blood 1992;80:484–91.
25. Knecht H, Odermatt B, Bachmann E, et al. Frequent detection of Epstein-Barr virus DNA by the polymerase chain reaction in lymph node biopsies from patients with Hodgkin's disease without genomic evidence of B- or T-cell clonality. Blood 1991;78:760–7.
26. Rosdahl N, Larsen SO, Clemmesen J. Hodgkin's disease in patients with previous infectious mononucleosis: 30 years' experience. BMJ 1974;2:253–6.
27. Hjalgrim H, Askling J, Sorenson P, et al. Risk of Hodgkin's disease and other cancers after infectious mononucleosis. J Natl Cancer Inst 2000;92:1522–8.
28. Hjalgrim H, Askling J, Rostgaard K, et al. Characteristics of Hodgkin's lymphoma after infectious mononucleosis. N Engl J Med 2003;349:1324–32.
29. Evans AS, Gutensohn NM. A population-based case-control study of EBV and other viral antibodies among persons with Hodgkin's disease and their siblings. Int J Cancer 1984;34:149–57.
30. Haluska FG, Brufsky AM, Canellos GP. The cellular biology of the Reed-Sternberg cell. Blood 1994;84:1005–19.
31. Lukes RJ, Butler JJ. The pathology and nomenclature of Hodgkin's disease. Cancer Res 1966;26:1063–83.
32. Gruss HJ, Pinto A, Duyster J, et al. Hodgkin's disease: A tumor with disturbed immunological pathways. Immunol Today 1997;18:156–63.
33. Hudson MM, Onciu M, Donaldson SS. Hodgkin lymphoma. In: Pizzo PA, Poplack DG, editors. Principles and Practice of Pediatric Oncology. 5th ed. Philadelphia: Lippincott Williams & Wilkins; 2006. p. 695–721.
34. Swerdlow SH, Campo E, Harris NL, et al. WHO Classification of Tumours of Haematopoietic and Lymphoid Tissues. 4th ed. Lyon, France: IARC Press; 2008.
35. Donaldson SS, Link MP. Childhood lymphomas: Hodgkin's disease and non-Hodgkin's lymphoma. In: Moosa AR, Robson MC, Schimpff SC, editors. Comprehensive Textbook of Oncology. Baltimore: Williams & Wilkins; 1986. p. 1161.
36. Murphy S, Morgan E, Katzenstein H, et al. Results of little or no treatment for lymphocyte-predominant Hodgkin's disease in children and adolescents. Am J Pediatr Hematol Oncol 2003;25:684–7.
37. Pellegrino B, Terrier-Lacombe M, Oberlin O, et al. Lymphocyte-predominant Hodgkin's lymphoma in children: Therapeutic abstention after initial lymph node resection: A study of the French Society of Pediatric Oncology. J Clin Oncol 2003;21:2948–52.
38. Stein H, Diehl V, Marafioti T, et al. The nature of Reed-Sternberg cells, lymphocytic and histiocytic cells and their molecular biology in Hodgkin's disease. In: Mauch PM, Armitage JO, Diehl V, et al, editors. Hodgkin's disease. Philadelphia: Lippincott Williams & Wilkins; 1999. p. 121.
39. Mauch PM, Kalish LA, Kadin M, et al. Patterns of Hodgkin disease: Implications for etiology and pathogenesis. Cancer 1993;71:2062–71.

40. Maity A, Goldwein JW, Lange B, et al. Mediastinal masses in children with Hodgkin's disease. Cancer 1992;69:2755–60.
41. Jeffery GM, Mead GM, Whitehouse JM. Life-threatening airway obstruction at the presentation of Hodgkin's disease. Cancer 1991;67:506–10.
42. Munker R, Hasenclaver D, Brosteanu O, et al. Bone marrow involvement in Hodgkin's disease: An analysis of 135 consecutive cases. J Clin Oncol 1995;13:403–9.
43. Hann HL, Lange B, Stahlhut MW, et al. Prognostic importance of serum transferrin and ferritin in childhood Hodgkin's disease. Cancer 1990;66:313–16.
44. Tubiana M, Henry-Arnar M, Burgers MV, et al. Prognostic significance of erythrocyte sedimentation rate in clinical stages I-II of Hodgkin's disease. J Clin Oncol 1984;2:194–200.
45. Cosset J, Henry Amar M, Meerwadt J, et al. The EORTC trials for limited stage Hodgkin's disease. Eur J Cancer 1992;28A:1847–50.
46. Longo D, Russo A, Duffey P, et al. Treatment of advanced stage massive mediastinal Hodgkin's disease: The case for combined modality therapy. J Clin Oncol 1991;9:227–35.
47. Maity A, Goldwein J, Lange B, et al. Mediastinal mass in children with Hodgkin's disease. Cancer 1992;69:2755–60.
48. Vecchi V, Pileri S, Burnelli R, et al. Treatment of pediatric Hodgkin's disease tailored to stage, mediastinal mass, and age. Cancer 1993;72:2049–57.
49. Carbone PP, Kaplan HS, Husshoff K, et al. Report of the committee on Hodgkin's disease staging classification. Cancer Res 1971;31:1860–1.
50. Mauch P, Larson D, Osteen R, et al. Prognostic factors for positive surgical staging in patients with Hodgkin's disease. J Clin Oncol 1990;8:257–65.
51. Castellino RA. Diagnostic imaging evaluation of Hodgkin's disease and non-Hodgkin's lymphoma. Cancer 1991;67:1177–80.
52. Muraji T, Hays DM, Siegel SE, et al. Evaluation of the surgical aspects of staging laparotomy for Hodgkin's disease in children. J Pediatr Surg 1982;17:843–8.
53. Mendenhall NP, Cantor AB, Williams JL, et al. With modern imaging techniques, is staging laparotomy necessary in pediatric Hodgkin's disease? A Pediatric Oncology Group Study. J Clin Oncol 1993;11:2218–25.
54. Gomez GA, Reese PA, Nava H, et al. Staging laparotomy and splenectomy in early Hodgkin's disease: No therapeutic benefit. Am J Med 1984;77:205–10.
55. Jenkin D, Chan H, Freedman M, et al. Hodgkin's disease in children: Treatment results with MOPP and low-dose, extended field irradiation. Ca Treatment Rep 1982;66:949–59.
56. Russel KJ, Donaldson SS, Cox RS, et al. Childhood Hodgkin's disease: Patterns of relapse. J Clin Oncol 1984;2:80–7.
57. American Academy of Pediatrics, Committee on Infectious Diseases. Visual Red Book on CD-ROM, 2001 Update. Elk Grove Village, IL: American Academy of Pediatrics; 2001.
58. Kaldor JM, Day NE, Clarke EA, et al. Leukemia following Hodgkin's disease. N Engl J Med 1990;322:7–13.
59. Tura S, Fiacchini M, Zinzani PL, et al. Splenectomy and the increasing risk of secondary acute leukemia in Hodgkin's disease. J Clin Oncol 1993;11:925–30.
60. Dietrich PY, Henry-Amar M, Cosset JM, et al. Second primary cancers in patients continuously disease-free from Hodgkin's disease: A protective role for the spleen? Blood 1994;84:1209–15.
61. Kostakoglu L, Leonard J, Kuji I, et al. Comparison of fluorine-18 fluorodeoxyglucose positron emission tomography and Ga-67 scintigraphy in evaluation of lymphoma. Cancer 2002;94:879–88.
62. Wirth A, Seymour J, Hicks R, et al. Fluorine-18 fluorodeoxyglucose positron emission tomography, gallium-67 scintigraphy, and conventional staging for Hodgkin's disease and non-Hodgkin's lymphoma. Am J Med 2002;112:262–8.
63. Shen Y, Kao A, Yen R. Comparison of 18F-fluoro-2-deoxyglucose positron emission tomography and gallium-67 citrate scintigraphy for detecting malignant lymphoma. Oncol Rep 2002;9:321–5.
64. Buchmann I, Reinhardt M, Elsner K. 2-(Fluorine-18)fluoro-2-deoxy-d-glucose positron emission tomography in the detection and staging of malignant lymphoma: A bicenter trial. Cancer 2001;91:889–99.
65. Kostakoglu L, Coleman M, Leonard J, et al. PET predicts prognosis after 1 cycle of chemotherapy in aggressive lymphoma and Hodgkin's disease. J Nucl Med 2002;43:1018–27.
66. Friedberg J, Chengazi V. PET scans in the staging of lymphoma: Current status. Oncologist 2003;8:438–47.
67. Weihrauch M, Re D, Scheidhauer K, et al. Thoracic positron emission tomography using 18F-fluorodeoxyglucose for the evaluation of residual mediastinal Hodgkin disease. Blood 2001;98:2930–4.
68. Donaldson SS, Link MP. Combined modality treatment with low-dose radiation and MOPP chemotherapy for children with Hodgkin's disease. J Clin Oncol 1987;5:742–9.
69. Engert A, Schiller P, Josting A, et al. Involved-field radiotherapy is equally effective and less toxic compared with extended-field radiotherapy after four cycles of chemotherapy in patients with early-stage unfavorable Hodgkin's lymphoma: Results of the HD8 trial of the German Hodgkin's Lymphoma Study Group. J Clin Oncol 2003;21:3601–8.
70. Sears JD, Greven KM, Ferree CR, et al. Definitive irradiation in the treatment of Hodgkin's disease. Cancer 1997;79:145–51.
71. Mauch PM, Canellos GP, Shulman LN, et al. Mantle irradiation alone for selected patients with laparotomy-staged IA to IIA Hodgkin's disease: Preliminary results of a prospective trial. J Clin Oncol 1995;13:947–52.
72. Wasserman TH, Trenkner DA, Fineberg B, et al. Cure of early-stage Hodgkin's disease with subtotal nodal irradiation. Cancer 1991;68:1208–15.
73. Donaldson SS, Whitaker SJ, Plowman PN, et al. Stage I-II pediatric Hodgkin's disease: Long-term follow-up demonstrates equivalent survival rates following different management schemes. J Clin Oncol 1990;8:1128–37.
74. Nachman J, Sposto R, Herzog P, et al. Randomized comparison of low-dose involved-field radiotherapy and no radiotherapy for children with Hodgkin's disease who achieve a complete response to chemotherapy. J Clin Oncol 2002;20:3765–71.
75. Devita VT, Serpick A, Carbone PP. Combination chemotherapy in the treatment of advanced Hodgkin's disease. Ann Intern Med 1970;73:881–95.
76. Bonnadonna G, Zucali R, Monfardini S, et al. Combination chemotherapy of Hodgkin's disease with Adriamycin, bleomycin, vinblastine, and imidazole carboxamide versus MOPP. Cancer 1975;36:252–9.
77. Donaldson S, Link M, Weinstein H, et al. Final results of a prospective clinical trial with VAMP and low-dose involved-field radiation for children with low risk Hodgkin's disease. J Clin Oncol 2007;25:332–7.
78. Hutchinson R, Fryer C, Krailo M, et al. Comparison of MOPP/ABVD with ABVD/XRT for treatment of advanced Hodgkin's disease in children (CCG-521). Proc ASCO 1992;11:340.
79. Ekert H, Waters K, Smith P, et al. Treatment with MOPP or CHLVPP chemotherapy only for all stages of childhood Hodgkin's disease. J Clin Oncol 1988;6:1845–50.
80. Ekert H, Fox L, Dalla-Pozzo K, et al. A pilot study of EVAP/ABV chemotherapy in 25 newly diagnosed children with Hodgkin's disease. Br J Cancer 1993;67:159–62.
81. Behrendt H, Brinkhuis M, Van Leeuwen EF. Treatment of childhood Hodgkin's disease with ABVD without radiotherapy. Med Pediatr Oncol 1996;26:244–8.
82. Kelly KM, Sposto R, Hutchinson R, et al. BEACOPP chemotherapy is a highly effective regimen in children and adolescents with high risk Hodgkin lymphoma: A report from the Children's Oncology Group CCG-59704 clinical trial. Blood 2011;117:2596–603.
83. Weiner MA, Leventhal B, Brecher ML, et al. Randomized study of intensive MOPP-ABVD with or without low-dose-nodal radiation therapy in the treatment of stages IIB, IIIA2, IIIB, and IV Hodgkin's disease in pediatric patients: A Pediatric Oncology Group study [see comments]. J Clin Oncol 1997;15:2769–79.
84. Mauz-Korholz C, Gorde-Grosjean S, Hasenclever D, et al. Resection alone in 58 children with limited stage, lymphocyte-predominant Hodgkin lymphoma-experience from the European network group on pediatric Hodgkin lymphoma. Cancer 2007;110(1):179–85.
85. Friedman DI, Wolden S, Constine L, et al. AHOD0031: A Phase III study of dose-intensive therapy for intermediate risk Hodgkin Lymphoma: A report from the Children's Oncology Group. 53rd

American Society of Hematology Annual Meeting 2010; Abstract #766.

86. Schmitz N, Pfistner B, Sextro M, et al. Aggressive conventional chemotherapy compared with high-dose chemotherapy with autologous haematopoietic stem-cell transplantation for relapsed chemosensitive Hodgkin's disease: A randomized trial. Lancet 2002;359:2065–71.

87. Freed J, Kelly KM. Current approaches to the management of pediatric Hodgkin Lymphoma. Pediatr Drugs 2010;12(2):85–98.

88. Younes A, Bartlett NL, Leonard JP, et al. Brentuximab vedotin (SGN-35) for relapsed CD30-positive lymphomas. N Engl J Med 2010;363:1812–21.

89. Oberlin O, Leverger G, Pacquement H, et al. Low-dose radiation therapy and reduced chemotherapy in childhood Hodgkin's disease: The experience of the French Society of Pediatric Oncology. J Clin Oncol 1992;10:1602–8.

90. Hunger SP, Link MP, Donaldson SS. ABVD/MOPP and low-dose involved-field radiotherapy in pediatric Hodgkin's disease: The Stanford experience. J Clin Oncol 1994;12:2160–6.

91. Bonfante V, Santoro A, Viviani S, et al. Outcome of patients with Hodgkin's disease failing after primary MOPP-ABVD. J Clin Oncol 1997;15:528–34.

92. Diehl V, Franklin J, Pfreundschuh M, et al. Standard and increased-dose BEACOPP chemotherapy compared with COPP-ABVD for advanced Hodgkin's disease. N Engl J Med 2003; 348:2386–95.

93. Sieber M, Bredenfeld H, Josting A, et al. 14-day variant of the bleomycin, etoposide, doxorubicin, cyclophosphamide, vincristine, procarbazine, and prednisone regimen in advanced-stage Hodgkin's lymphoma: Results of a pilot study of the German Hodgkin's Lymphoma Study Group. J Clin Oncol 2003;21: 1734–9.

94. Bookman MA, Longo DL, Young RC. Late complications of curative treatment in Hodgkin's disease. JAMA 1988;260:680–3.

95. Aleman B, van den Belt-Dusebout AW, Klokman WJ, et al. Long-term cause-specific mortality of patients treated for Hodgkin's disease. J Clin Oncol 2003;21:3431–9.

96. Willman KY, Cox RS, Donaldson SS. Radiation induced height impairment in pediatric Hodgkin's disease. Int J Radiat Oncol Biol Phys 1994;28:85–92.

97. Constine LS, Donaldson SS, McDougall JR, et al. Thyroid dysfunction after radiotherapy in children with Hodgkin's disease. Cancer 1984;53:878–83.

98. McHenry C, Jarosz H, Calandra D, et al. Thyroid neoplasia following radiation therapy for Hodgkin's lymphoma. Arch Surg 1987;122:684–6.

99. Sankila R, Garwicz S, Olsen JH, et al. Risk of subsequent malignant neoplasms among 1641 Hodgkin's disease patients diagnosed in childhood and adolescence: A population-based cohort study in the five Nordic countries. J Clin Oncol 1996;14:1442–6.

100. Thibaud E, Ramirez M, Brauner R, et al. Preservation of ovarian function by ovarian transposition performed before pelvic irradiation during childhood. J Pediatr 1992;121:880–4.

101. Bhatia S, Robison LL, Oberlin O, et al. Breast cancer and other second neoplasms after childhood Hodgkin's disease. N Engl J Med 1996;334:745–51.

102. Dores G, Metayer C, Curtis R, et al. Second malignant neoplasms among long-term survivors of Hodgkin's disease: A population-based evaluation over 25 years. J Clin Oncol 2002;20:3484–94.

103. Longo D. Radiation therapy in the treatment of Hodgkin's disease: Do you see what I see? J Natl Cancer Inst 2003;95: 928–9.

104. Hoppe RT. Hodgkin's disease: Complications of therapy and excess mortality. Ann Oncol 1997;8(Suppl. 1):S115–18.

105. Tucker MA, Coleman CN, Cox RS, et al. Risk of second cancers after treatment for Hodgkin's disease. N Engl J Med 1988;318:76–81.

106. Cimino G, Papa G, Tura S, et al. Second primary cancer following Hodgkin's disease: Updated results of an Italian multicentric study. J Clin Oncol 1991;9:432–7.

107. Van Leeuwen FE, Klokman WJ, Hagenbeek A, et al. Second cancer risk following Hodgkin's disease: A 20-year follow-up study. J Clin Oncol 1994;12:312–25.

108. Kaldor JM, Day NE, Clarke EA, et al. Leukemia following Hodgkin's disease. N Engl J Med 1990;322:7–13.

109. Tura S, Fiacchini M, Zinzani PL, et al. Splenectomy and the increasing risk of secondary acute leukemia in Hodgkin's disease. J Clin Oncol 1993;11:925–30.

110. Van Leeuwen FE, Chorus AM, van den Belt-Dusebout AW, et al. Leukemia risk following Hodgkin's disease: Relation to cumulative dose of alkylating agents, treatment with teniposide combinations, number of episodes of chemotherapy, and bone marrow damage. J Clin Oncol 1994;12:1063–73.

111. Dietrich PY, Henry-Amar M, Cosset JM, et al. Second primary cancers in patients continuously disease-free from Hodgkin's disease: A protective role for the spleen? Blood 1994;84: 1209–15.

112. Biovin JF, O'Brien K. Solid cancer risk after treatment of Hodgkin's disease. Cancer 1988;61:2541–6.

113. Salloum E, Doria R, Shubert W, et al. Second solid tumors in patients with Hodgkin's disease cured after radiation or chemotherapy plus adjuvant low-dose radiation. J Clin Oncol 1996;14: 2435–43.

114. Doria R, Holford T, Farber LR, et al. Second solid malignancies after combined modality therapy for Hodgkin's disease. J Clin Oncol 1995;13:2016–22.

115. Curtis RE, Boice JD Jr. Second cancers after radiotherapy for Hodgkin's disease. N Engl J Med 1988;319:244–5.

116. Prior P, Pope DJ. Hodgkin's disease: Subsequent primary cancers in relation to treatment. Br J Cancer 1988;58:512–17.

117. Kaldor JM, Day NE, Band P, et al. Second malignancies following testicular cancer, ovarian cancer, and Hodgkin's disease: An international collaborative study among cancer registries. Int J Cancer 1987;39:571–85.

118. Wahner-Roedler D, Nelson D, Croghan I, et al. Risk of breast cancer and breast cancer characteristics in woman treated with supradiaphragmatic radiation for Hodgkin lymphoma: Mayo Clinic experience. Mayo Clin Proc 2003;78:708–15.

119. Hancock SL, Horning SJ, Hoppe RT. Breast cancer after the treatment of Hodgkin's disease [abstract]. Int J Radiat Oncol Biol Phys 1991;21:157.

120. Shapiro CL, Mauch PM. Radiation-associated breast cancer after Hodgkin's disease: Risks and screening in perspective. J Clin Oncol 1992;10:1662–5.

121. Hancock SL, Tucker MA, Hoppe RT. Factors affecting late mortality from heart disease after treatment of Hodgkin's disease. JAMA 1993;270:1949–55.

122. Steinherz LJ, Steinherz PG, Tan CT, et al. Cardiac toxicity 4 to 20 years after completing anthracycline therapy. JAMA 1991;266:1672–7.

123. Novakovic B. USA childhood cancer survival, 1973–1987. Med Pediatr Oncol 1994;23:480–6.

124. Smith MA, Seibel NL, Altekruse SF, et al. Outcomes for children and adolescents with cancer: Challenges for the twenty-first century. J Clin Oncol 2010;28:2625–34.

125. Magrath IT. The pathogenesis of Burkitt's lymphoma. Recent Adv Cancer Res 1990;55:133–270.

126. Hanto DW, Frizzera G, Gajl-Peczalska KJ. Epstein-Barr virus, immunodeficiency, and B cell lymphoproliferation. Transplantation 1985;39:461–72.

127. Cohen JI. Epstein-Barr virus lymphoproliferative disease associated with acquired immune deficiency. Medicine 1991;70: 137–60.

128. Shibata D, Weiss LM, Nathwani BN, et al. Epstein-Barr virus in benign lymph node biopsies from individuals infected with the human immunodeficiency virus is associated with concurrent or subsequent development of non-Hodgkin's lymphoma. Blood 1991;77:1527–33.

129. Neri A, Barriga F, Inghirami G, et al. Epstein-Barr virus infection precedes clonal expansion in Burkitt's and acquired immunodeficiency syndrome-associated lymphomas. Blood 1991;77:1092–5.

130. Savoie A, Perpete C, Carpentier L, et al. Direct correlation between the load of Epstein-Barr virus-infected lymphocytes in the peripheral blood of pediatric transplant patients and risk of lymphoproliferative disease. Blood 1994;83:2715–22.

131. Rooney CM, Loftin SK, Holladay HS, et al. Early identification of Epstein-Barr virus-associated post-transplantation lymphoproliferative disease. Br J Haematol 1995;89:98–103.

132. Holmes R, Sokol R. Epstein-Barr virus and post-transplant lymphoproliferative disease. Pediatr Transplant 2002;6:456–64.

133. Sreenan JJ, Tubbs RR. The influence of immunology and genetics on lymphoma classification: A historical perspective. Ca Invest 1996;14:572–88.

134. Link MP, Weinstein HJ. Malignant Non-Hodgkin lymphomas in children. In: Pizzo PA, Poplack DG, editors. Principles and Practice of Pediatric Oncology. 5th ed. Philadelphia: Lippincott Williams & Wilkins; 2006. p. 722–47.

135. Hutchison RE, Murphy SB, Fairclough DL, et al. Diffuse small noncleaved cell lymphoma in children: Burkitt's versus non-Burkitt's types. Cancer 1989;64:23–8.

136. Harris NL, Jaffe ES, Stein H, et al. A revised European-American classification of lymphoid neoplasms: A proposal from the International Lymphoma Study Group. Blood 1994;84:1361–92.

137. Nathwani BN, Griffith RC, Kelly DR, et al. A morphologic study of childhood lymphoma of the diffuse 'histiocytic' type: The pediatric oncology experience. Cancer 1987;59:1138–42.

138. Hutchison RE, Berard CW, Shuster JJ, et al. B-cell lineage confers favorable outcome among children and adolescents with large-cell lymphoma: A Pediatric Oncology Group study. J Clin Oncol 1995;13:2023–32.

139. Sandland JT, Pui CH, Santana VM, et al. Clinical features and treatment outcome for children with CD30+ large-cell non-Hodgkin's lymphoma. J Clin Oncol 1994;12:895–8.

140. Falini B, Pileri S, Pizzolo G, et al. CD30 (Ki-1) molecule: A new cytokine receptor of the tumor necrosis factor receptor superfamily as a tool for diagnosis and immunotherapy. Blood 1995;85:1–14.

141. Fillipa DA, Ladanyi M, Wollner N, et al. CD30 (Ki-1)-positive malignant lymphomas: Clinical, immunophenotypic, histologic, and genetic characteristics and differences with Hodgkin's disease. Blood 1996;87:2905–17.

142. Reiter A, Schrappe M, Tiemann M, et al. Successful treatment strategy for Ki-1 anaplastic large-cell lymphoma of childhood: A prospective analysis of 62 patients enrolled in three consecutive Berlin-Frankfurt-Munster Group studies. J Clin Oncol 1994;12:899–908.

143. Kaden ME. Ki-1/CD30+ (anaplastic) large-cell lymphoma: Maturation of a clinicopathologic entity with prospects of effective therapy. J Clin Oncol 1994;12:884–7.

144. Kadin ME, Sako D, Berliner N, et al. Childhood Ki-1 lymphoma presenting with skin lesions and peripheral lymphadenopathy. Blood 1986;68:1042–9.

145. Howat AJ, Thomas H, Waters KD, et al. Malignant lymphoma of bone in children. Cancer 1987;59:335–9.

146. Meyers PA, Potter VP, Wolner N, et al. Bowel perforation during initial treatment of childhood non-Hodgkin's lymphoma. Cancer 1985;56:259–61.

147. Tesoro-Tess JD, Biasi S, Balzarini L, et al. Heart involvement in lymphomas. Cancer 1993;72:2484–90.

148. Ridgway D, Wolff LJ, Neerhout RC, et al. Unsuspected non-Hodgkin's lymphoma of the tonsils and adenoids in children. Pediatrics 1987;79:399–402.

149. Ghelman B. Radiology of bone tumors. Orthop Clin North Am 1989;20:287–312.

150. Clayton F, Butler JJ, Ayala AG, et al. Non-Hodgkin's lymphoma in bone. Cancer 1987;60:2494–501.

151. Wollner N, Lane JM, Marcove RC, et al. Primary skeletal non-Hodgkin's lymphoma in the pediatric age group. Med Pediatr Oncol 1992;20:506–13.

152. Tsokos GC, Balow JE, Spiegel RJ, et al. Renal and metabolic complications of undifferentiated and lymphoblastic lymphomas. Medicine 1981;60:218–29.

153. Hande KR, Garrow GC. Acute tumor lysis syndrome in patients with high-grade non-Hodgkin's lymphoma. Am J Med 1993;94:133–9.

154. Finlay JL, Anderson JR, Cecalupo AJ, et al. Disseminated nonlymphoblastic lymphoma of childhood: A Children's Cancer Group study, CCG-552. Med Pediatr Oncol 1994;23:453–63.

155. Schwenn MR, Blattner SR, Lynch SR, et al. hic-COM: A 2-month intensive chemotherapy regimen for children with stage III and IV Burkitt's lymphoma and B-cell acute lymphoblastic leukemia. J Clin Oncol 1991;9:133–8.

156. Anderson JR, Jenkin RDT, Wilson JF, et al. Long-term follow-up of patients treated with COMP or LSA2L2 therapy for childhood

157. Burkitt D. A sarcoma involving the jaws in African children. Br J Surg 1958;46:218–23.

158. Shad A, Magrath I. Malignant non-Hodgkin's lymphomas in children. In: Pizzo PA, Poplack DG, editors. Principles and Practice of Pediatric Oncology. 3rd ed. Philadelphia: Lippincott-Raven; 1997. p. 545–87.

159. Sariban E, Donahue A, Magrath IT. Jaw involvement in American Burkitt's lymphoma. Cancer 1984;53:141–6.

160. Reiter A, Schrappe M, Parwaresch R, et al. Non-Hodgkin's lymphomas of childhood and adolescence: Results of a treatment stratified for biologic subtypes and stage: A report of the Berlin-Frankfurt-Munster Group. J Clin Oncol 1995;13:359–72.

161. Stein H, Foss H, Durkop H, et al. CD30+ anaplastic large cell lymphoma: A review of its histopathologic, genetic, and clinical features. Blood 2000;96:3681–95.

162. Levine AM. Acquired immunodeficiency syndrome-related lymphoma. Blood 1992;80:8–20.

163. Knowles DM, Cesarman E, Chadburn A, et al. Correlative morphologic and molecular genetic analysis demonstrates three distinct categories of post-transplantation lymphoproliferative disorders. Blood 1995;85:552–65.

164. Ho M. Risk factors and pathogenesis of post-transplant lymphoproliferative disorders. Transplant Proc 1995;27:38–40.

165. Reiter A, Zimmerman W, Zimmerman M, et al. The role of initial laparotomy and second look surgery in the treatment of abdominal B-cell non-Hodgkin's lymphoma of childhood: A report of the BFM group. Eur J Pediatr Surg 1994;4:74–81.

166. Palestro CJ, Rini JN, Tomas MB. Lymphoma. In: Charron M, editor. Practical Pediatric PET Imaging. New York: Springer; 2006. p. 220–42.

167. Hernandez-Pampaloni M, Takalkar A, Yu JQ, et al. F-18 FDG-PET imaging and correlation with CT in staging and follow-up of pediatric lymphomas. Pediatr Radiol 2006;36:524–31.

168. Downing JR, Shurtleff SA, Zielenska M, et al. Molecular detection of the (2;5) translocation of non-Hodgkin's lymphoma by reverse transcriptase-polymerase chain reaction. Blood 1995;85:3416–22.

169. Staudt L. Molecular diagnosis of the hematologic cancers. N Engl J Med 2003;348:1777–85.

170. Murphy SB. Classification, staging and end results of treatment of childhood non-Hodgkin's lymphomas: Dissimilarities from lymphomas in adults. Semin Oncol 1980;7:332–9.

171. Haddy TB, Adde MA, Magrath IT. CNS involvement in small noncleaved cell lymphoma: Is CNS disease per se a poor prognostic sign? J Clin Oncol 1991;9:1973–82.

172. Cairo MS, Sposto R, Perkins SL, et al. Burkitt's and Burkitt-like lymphoma in children and adolescents: A review of the Children's Cancer Group experience. Br J Haematol 2003;120:660–70.

173. Meadows AT, Sposto R, Jenkin RD, et al. Similar efficacy of 6 and 18 months of therapy with four drugs (COMP) for localized non-Hodgkin's lymphoma of children: A report from the Children's Cancer Study Group. J Clin Oncol 1989;7:92–9.

174. Patte C, Philip T, Rodary C, et al. High survival rate in advanced-stage B-cell lymphomas and leukemias without CNS involvement with a short intensive polychemotherapy: Results from the French Pediatric Oncology Society of a randomized trial of 216 children. J Clin Oncol 1991;9:123–32.

175. Bowman WP, Shuster JJ, Cook B, et al. Improved survival for children with B-cell acute lymphoblastic leukemia and stage IV small noncleaved-cell lymphoma: A Pediatric Oncology Group study. J Clin Oncol 1996;14:1252–61.

176. Sullivan MP, Ramirez I. Curability of Burkitt's lymphoma with high-dose cyclophosphamide, high-dose methotrexate therapy and intrathecal chemoprophylaxis. J Clin Oncol 1985;3:627–36.

177. Swinnen LJ, Mullen GM, Carr TJ, et al. Aggressive treatment for postcardiac transplant lymphoproliferation. Blood 1995;86:3333–40.

178. Orjuela M, Gross T, Cheung Y, et al. A pilot study of chemoimmunotherapy (cyclophosphamide, prednisone, and rituximab) in patients with post-transplant lymphoproliferative disorder following solid organ transplantation. Clin Cancer Res 2003;9:3945S–52S.

non-Hodgkin's lymphoma: A report of CCG-551 from the Children's Cancer Group. J Clin Oncol 1993;11:1024–32.

179. Link MP, Donaldson SS, Berard CW, et al. Results of treatment of childhood localized non-Hodgkin's lymphoma with combination chemotherapy with or without radiotherapy. N Engl J Med 1990;322:1169–74.

180. Oschlies I, Klapper W, Zimmermann M, et al. Diffuse large B-cell lymphoma in pediatric patients belongs predominantly to the germinal-center type B-cell lymphomas: Clinicopathologic analysis of cases included in the German BFM (Berlin-Frankfurt-Münster) Multicenter Trial. Blood 2006;107:4047–52.

181. Le Deley MC, Rosolen A, Reiter A, et al. The impact of the association of vinblastine during induction chemotherapy and as maintenance treatment in children and adolescents with high-risk anaplastic large cell lymphoma: Results of a randomized trial of the EICNHL Group. Blood 2008;112:577 abstr.

182. Cohen LF, Balow JE, Magrath IT, et al. Acute tumor lysis syndrome: A review of 37 patients with Burkitt's lymphoma. Am J Med 1980;68:486–91.

183. Murphy SB, Melvin SL, Mauer AM, et al. Correlation of tumor cell kinetic studies with surface marker results in childhood non-Hodgkin's lymphoma. Cancer Res 1979;39:1534–8.

184. Smalley R, Guaspari A, Haase-Statz S, et al. Allopurinol: Intravenous use for prevention and treatment of hyperuricemia. J Clin Oncol 2000;18:1758–63.

185. Pui C, Mahmoud H, Wiley J, et al. Recombinant urate oxidase for the prophylaxis or treatment of hyperuricemia in patients with leukemia or lymphoma. J Clin Oncol 2001;19:697–704.

186. Goldman S, Holcenberg J, Finklestein J, et al. A randomized comparison between rasburicase and allopurinol in children with lymphoma or leukemia at high risk for tumor lysis. Blood 2001;97:2998–3003.

187. Allegretta GJ, Weisman SJ, Altman AJ. Oncologic emergencies I: Metabolic and space-occupying consequences of cancer and cancer treatment. Pediatr Clin North Am 1985;32:601–11.

188. Korones DN, Buzzard CJ, Asselin BL. Right atrial thrombi in children with cancer and indwelling catheters. J Pediatr 1996;128:841–6.

189. Pryzant RM, Meistrich ML, Wilson G, et al. Long-term reduction in sperm count after chemotherapy with and without radiation therapy for non-Hodgkin's lymphomas. J Clin Oncol 1993;11:239–47.

190. Sandoval C, Pui CH, Bowman LC, et al. Secondary acute myeloid leukemia in children previously treated with alkylating agents, intercalating topoisomerase II inhibitors, and irradiation. J Clin Oncol 1993;11:1039–45.

191. Friedman DL, Meadows AT. Late effects following lymphoma treatment. In: Weinstein HJ, Hudson MM, Link MP, editors. Pediatric Lymphomas. Berlin: Springer; 2007. p. 259–80.

CHAPTER 70

RHABDOMYOSARCOMA

Shauna M. Levy • Robert A. Hetz • Phillip A. Letourneau • Richard J. Andrassy

Rhabdomyosarcoma (RMS) is a soft tissue tumor originating from immature mesenchymal cells that form any tissue except bone. It is the most common soft tissue sarcoma in children and adolescents, accounting for approximately 50% of soft tissue sarcomas. The overall survival (OS) of RMS patients has improved to 71% as a result of the Intergroup Rhabdomyosarcoma Study Group (IRSG; established in 1972), which is now continued by the Children's Oncology Group Soft Tissue Sarcoma (COG-STS) committee.[1,2]

RMS is the third most common childhood extracranial solid tumor, after neuroblastoma and Wilms tumor.[3] Approximately 350 new cases of RMS are diagnosed annually in the USA, corresponding to an incidence of 4.5 cases per million children aged 20 years or younger.[4,5] RMS has a bimodal distribution with approximately 65% of cases occurring in children <6 years and the remaining cases developing in children aged 10–18 years.[6] More than 80% of cases are diagnosed before the age of 14 years.[7] Outcomes are worse in adolescents who usually present with alveolar RMS, lymph node involvement, delay in diagnosis, and metastases.[8] Poor outcomes are also seen in infants usually due to failure to achieve adequate local control.[9]

Approximately one-third of RMS occurs in the head and neck (including parameningeal locations). Genitourinary locations are found in 22–31% of cases; trunk and extremities are the next most common sites.[1,5]

RMS is classified as a small, round, blue cell tumor of childhood, a category including neuroblastoma, Ewing sarcoma, small cell osteogenic sarcoma, non-Hodgkin lymphoma, and leukemia. Six major pathologic subtypes of RMS are outlined by the International Classification of RMS in order of decreasing 5-year survival: (1) embryonal (botryoid); (2) embryonal (spindle cell); (3) embryonal, not otherwise specified (NOS); (4) alveolar, NOS or solid variant; (5) anaplasia, diffuse; and (6) undifferentiated sarcoma.[10] Botryoid RMS is associated with a superior 5-year survival rate of 95% and most commonly occurs in the bladder or vagina in infants and young children, and in the nasopharynx in older children.[11] Spindle cell RMS is commonly found in the paratesticular area, head and neck, extremities, or orbit.[12] Embryonal and embryonal variants account for approximately 60–70% of all pediatric RMS cases in younger patients.[5,11,13,14] Alveolar, anaplastic, and undifferentiated variants of RMS account for approximately 35% of all new cases, and generally have the worst prognosis. The incidence of alveolar RMS is increasing with an annual per cent change (APC) of 4.09%.[5] The alveolar subtype is seen more commonly in older patients.[11] A 'solid alveolar' variant lacks the characteristic alveolar septations but

behaves similarly to the alveolar subtype.[15] The prognostic value of each specific histologic subtype has varied somewhat in different studies.[14–16] However, in IRS-IV, 3-year failure-free survival (FFS) was 83% for embryonal, 66% for alveolar, 55% for undifferentiated, and 66% for unclassified sarcoma ($P < 0.001$).[1]

STAGING

Two classification schemes have been used to categorize RMS. The clinical grouping system was devised by the IRSG and is a surgicopathologic system based on the initial operative assessment (Table 70-1).[11] Stratification of survival was based on the ability for complete resection; thus, an initial surgical approach was required, which varied by institution.[13] Clinical grouping has consistently been an independent prognostic indicator as shown in Figure 70-1.

The second classification scheme is a pretreatment staging system based on the tumor/node/metastasis (TNM) system, which was introduced by the COG-STS committee (Table 70-2).[17] The system includes primary tumor site, lymph node involvement, distant metastatic disease, and size. Favorable primary sites include the orbit, eyelid, other nonparameningeal head/neck sites, and nonbladder, nonprostate genitourinary structures. Unfavorable primary sites include extremities (including buttock), trunk, retroperitoneum, perineum, urinary bladder and prostate, and cranial parameningeal sites. IRS-IV was the first study to use this staging system to classify patients prospectively. FFS data for patients with local or regional tumors, according to stage, are shown in Figure 70-2. For these tumors, pretreatment staging is a more accurate predictor of outcome than the clinical grouping classification system.

MOLECULAR BIOLOGY

Characterization of RMS tumors utilizing specific molecular fingerprints is important in establishing a diagnosis in select cases. Additionally, specific molecular markers offer promise as prognostic indicators, and identification of specific molecular pathways offers potential therapeutic targets.

Mutations in certain tumor suppressor genes, including *TP53*, predispose individuals to RMS. Patients with Li–Fraumeni syndrome and neurofibromatosis type 1 are more likely to develop RMS, and approximately 10% of patients with RMS have one of these syndromes.[18,19]

TABLE 70-1	Intergroup Rhabdomyosarcoma Study Group Clinical Grouping Classification of Rhabdomysarcoma		
Clinical Group		**Extent of Disease**	
	TUMOR	RESECTABILITY/MARGINS	LYMPH NODE STATUS
1	Localized	Complete resection Negative margins	Negative Confined to tissue of origin
1a	Localized	Complete resection Negative margins	Negative Not confined to tissue of origin
2a	Localized	Complete gross resection Microscopically positive margins	Negative
2b	Localized	Complete gross resection Microscopically positive margins	Positive regional nodes
2c	Localized	Complete gross resection Positive margins	Positive regional nodes
3a	Localized/locally extensive	Residual disease after biopsy only	
3b	Localized/locally extensive	Residual disease after debulking of >50% tumor	
4	Distant metastasis		

From Qualman SJ, Coffin CM, Newton WA, et al. Intergroup Rhabdomyosarcoma Study: Update for pathologists. Pediatr Dev Pathol 1998;1:550–61.

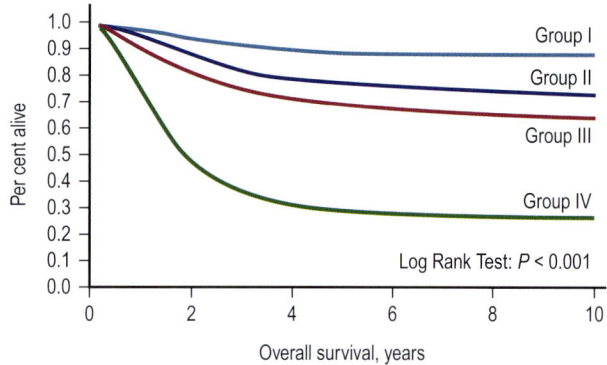

FIGURE 70-1 ■ Overall survival according to clinical group assignment (Intergroup Rhabdomyosarcoma Study [IRS] I to IV). Survival of patients treated on IRS-I, IRS-II, IRS-III/IV-P (IV pilot), and IRS-IV by clinical group at diagnosis is shown. A significant difference is seen in outcome by the extent of initial surgical resection, with the best outcome among the patients with completely resected tumors (group I), followed by those with microscopic residual (group II) and gross residual (group III) disease. Patients with metastatic disease (group IV) at diagnosis fare poorly. (Anderson JR. Personal communication, 2000; from Pizzo PA, Poplack DG, editors. Principles and Practice of Pediatric Oncology. 4th ed. Philadelphia: Lippincott Williams & Wilkins; 2002.)

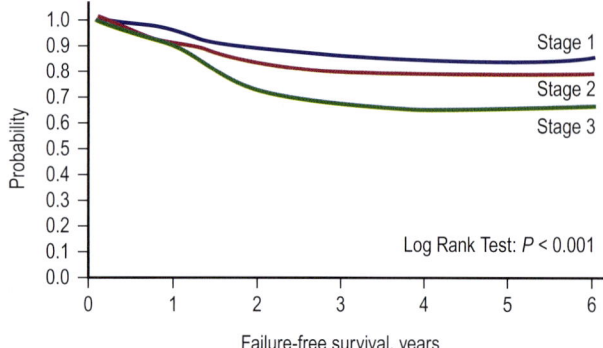

FIGURE 70-2 ■ Failure-free survival for nonmetastatic disease patients according to staging classification in Intergroup Rhabdomyosarcoma Study-IV.

Embryonal RMS is characterized by loss of heterozygosity (LOH) with loss of maternal genetic information and duplication of paternal genetic information at the 11p15 locus.[20] This genetic locus is the site of the insulin-like growth factor-2 (*IGF-2*) gene and LOH results in overexpression, which can lead to RMS through several different possible pathways.[13,18] The etiology of RMS can also be linked to the loss of 9q22, which corresponds to a tumor suppressor gene in embryonal RMS patients.[20]

In approximately 70% of alveolar RMS, a common translocation between chromosomes 2 and 13, t(2;13) (q35;q14), is present.[21] This translocation usually involves the *PAX3* gene that regulates transcription driving neuromuscular development and the *FOXO1* gene that is involved in the differentiation process of myoblasts.[22] Less commonly, the translocation involves the PAX7 gene located at 1p36 to the same location on chromosome 13.[23] *PAX3/FOXO1* expression can increase *IGF-2* expression and an IGF-binding protein, providing a common pathway for both embryonal and alveolar RMS. These known molecular disturbances are now being adopted and studied clinically. Several studies have demonstrated a worse prognosis with the presence of a *PAX3/FOXO1* fusion gene in alveolar subtypes of RMS, and an improved prognosis with *PAX7/FOXO1*.[18,24,25] Additionally, the t(2;13) translocation has been shown to characterize alveolar RMS with a poor prognosis, whereas the t(1;13) translocation is associated with improved outcome.[26] The *ELMO1* gene has been implicated in alveolar RMS metastasis.[27] Another recent study has correlated a 34-metagene with COG risk classification groups.[28] The exact molecular pathway leading to the development of alveolar RMS potentially caused or exacerbated by these translocations remains to be found.

CLINICAL PRESENTATION

The clinical presentation of RMS is variable and depends largely on tumor site, patient age, and the presence of

TABLE 70-2 **Rhabdomyosarcoma Tumor/Node/Metastasis (TNM) Pretreatment Staging Classification**

TNM Stage	Sites	Tumor[a]	Size[b]	Node[c]	Metastasis[d]
Stage 1	Orbit Head and neck (excluding parameningeal) Genitourinary: nonbladder/ prostate	T1 or T2	a or b	N0 or N1 or Nx	M0
Stage 2	Bladder/prostate Extremity Head and neck Parameningeal Other (includes trunk, retroperitoneum, etc.)	T1 or T2	a	N0 or Nx	M0
Stage 3	Bladder/prostate Extremity Head and neck parameningeal Other (includes trunk, retroperitoneum, etc.)	T1 or T2	a b	N1 N0 or N1 or Nx	M0 M0
Stage 4	All	T1 or T2	a or b	N0 or N1	M1

[a]Tumor: T1, confined to anatomic site of origin. T2, extension and/or fixation to surrounding tissue.
[b]a, <5 cm in diameter; b, ≥5 cm in diameter.
[c]Regional nodes: N0, regional nodes not clinically involved; N1, regional nodes clinically involved by neoplasm; Nx, clinical status of regional nodes unknown (especially sites that preclude lymph node evaluation).
[d]Metastasis: M0, no distant metastases present; M1, distant metastases.

distant metastases. Most symptoms are secondary to the local mass effect. RMSs involving the head and neck region including orbits, parameningeal tissues (middle ear, nasal cavity, paranasal sinuses, nasopharynx, and infratemporal fossa), and nonparameningeal tissues (scalp, face, oral cavity, oropharynx, hypopharynx and neck) are most commonly embryonal subtype and rarely involve regional lymph nodes. Symptoms can include proptosis, ophthalmoplegia, nasal/sinus obstruction with or without discharge, cranial nerve palsies, meningeal symptoms, or a painless, enlarging mass. Paratesticular RMS may present as a painless swelling in the scrotum or inguinal canal, and have a high rate of lymph node spread to the retroperitoneum.

Tumors involving the bladder, urinary tract, or prostate can cause obstruction, hematuria, constipation, and/or urinary frequency. Vaginal tumors are more common in very young patients and may present as vaginal bleeding, discharge, or a mass. Tumors involving the uterus more commonly present in older girls with extensive tumor at diagnosis. RMSs involving the extremity usually present as a mass, tend to be more aggressive, and most are alveolar subtype. They have an approximately 50% incidence of regional lymph node involvement and around 15% of patients present with metastatic disease. Presentation in the neonate is extremely rare with most babies having the embryonal/botryoid/undifferentiated subtypes (0.4%).[14,29-34]

DIAGNOSIS

The diagnosis of RMS may be suspected clinically, but needs to be confirmed by biopsy. Depending on location, this may require endoscopy, needle biopsy, or excisional/incisional biopsies. Biopsy incisions should be made so that complete excision is possible if a subsequent wide local excision is necessary. Prior to the definitive operation, a full evaluation including imaging, laboratory studies, and bone marrow evaluation should be performed (Box 70-1).[7]

> **BOX 70-1** **Preoperative Treatment/Evaluation of Pediatric Rhabdomyosarcoma**
>
> - History/physical examination
> - Measurement of lesion (physical or imaging)
> - Complete blood cell count with differential and platelets
> - Urinalysis
> - Electrolytes, creatinine, calcium, and phosphorus
> - Liver function tests (alkaline phosphatase, lactate dehydrogenase, bilirubin, and transaminases)
> - Bone marrow biopsy/aspirate
> - Chest radiograph
> - MRI/CT of primary lesion
> - CT of chest
> - MRI/CT of head (for head tumors)
> - Bone scintigraphy
> - Cerebrospinal fluid cytology (for parameningeal tumors)
> - Electrocardiography or echocardiography (selective)

SURGICAL TREATMENT

Primary Resection

Prognosis in rhabdomyosarcoma patients is linked to the amount of residual disease present after resection (see Fig. 70-1). Complete tumor resection, with no microscopic residual disease, offers the best chance for cure. However, in many sites such as the orbit, bladder, prostate, vagina, uterus, complete tumor resection is not feasible while still preserving function of vital organs and avoiding a mutilating procedure. Over the last 35 years, organ salvage rates have increased without adversely affecting OS. The operative approach depends on the primary tumor site, size, presence or absence of lymph node involvement, and distant metastases. These decisions must be made in the context of a multidisciplinary team, including the surgeon, oncologist, pediatric radiologist, and radiotherapist to allow optimal patient care. A tissue biopsy and biologic studies are recommended for definitive diagnosis if resection of the primary tumor site with negative margins is not possible.

Primary Re-excision

Primary re-excision (PRE) of a tumor includes any repeat attempt at complete resection before the initiation of any other form of therapy. As with the primary tumor resection, PRE is performed to allow a clinical group I classification without sacrificing vital structures or organs causing impaired function or poor cosmesis. PRE is recommended in patients whose initial resection had positive or unknown margin status, or was performed for presumed benign disease. If not feasible, reliance on adjuvant irradiation and chemotherapy is advisable. PRE has been shown to improve survival by converting a significant proportion of patients from group IIa to group I in patients with extremity tumors and perineal RMS.[17,35,36] The Italian Cooperative Study Group concluded that PRE is the treatment of choice for children with RMS and nonrhabdomyosarcoma soft tissue sarcoma (NRSTS) who are age 3 years or younger and cannot receive radiation therapy (RT). It is also preferred for paratesticular sites as well.[35] PRE and postoperative irradiation showed equivalent results in achieving local control in extremity and trunk sites. PRE was not effective for tumors >5 cm.

Lymph Node Evaluation

RMS frequently spreads to regional lymph nodes early in the disease and lymph node involvement significantly worsens the prognosis. However, involved nodes can go undetected by sophisticated imaging techniques. Any clinically or radiographically suspicious lymph node requires histologic confirmation. It is important to determine regional lymph node status to determine if more aggressive treatments such as RT are needed. Pediatric surgeons may be asked to evaluate the regional lymph node status, but lymphadenectomy serves a diagnostic purpose only.[7]

Specific recommendations regarding regional lymph node evaluation will be reviewed according to the specific site. However, in general, it is recommended that RMS patients with primary tumors of the extremity, primary tumors of the perineum, and paratesticular tumors in children older than 10 years old undergo operative evaluation of regional lymph node status even if there is no clinically apparent disease.[19,37] If disease is found, then distal lymph nodes should be sampled to determine metastatic disease.[19] Additionally, during the course of tumor resection for genitourinary and retroperitoneal tumors, lymph node sampling should be performed if feasible.

Lymphatic mapping with sentinel lymph node biopsy may allow adequate staging while limiting operative morbidity.[37,38] Most experience with this technique has been gained with extremity and truncal tumors, and with adult breast cancer and melanoma.[19] Typically, lymphoscintigraphic mapping is performed before the planned operation. Intraoperatively, vital blue dye is injected at the primary tumor site and a detector is used to identify the sentinel lymph node. Through a small incision and limited dissection, a blue sentinel lymph node(s) with evidence of the radioactive tracer is excised. These techniques often limit the extent and morbidity of the operation when compared with formal lymph node dissection as was previously performed.

Second-Look Operations

At the initial operation, the size, invasion, or location of RMS tumors frequently prohibits complete resection to achieve group I or II status. In IRS-IV, among all patients without metastatic disease ($n = 883$), 62% were classified as group III.[1] After intensive multiagent chemotherapy with or without irradiation, these patients usually benefit from a second-look operation. Clinical and radiographic assessments are often inaccurate. The goals of the second-look operation are to remove residual tumor and determine response prior to additional therapy. This approach has been shown to improve patient survival and/or to classify patients as complete responders.[19,39,40] Alternatively, a negative biopsy (i.e., no tumor) at second-look operation does not exclude or diminish the possibility of recurrence.[39,41]

Surgical Treatment for Recurrent Disease

Despite the successes of primary therapy for RMS, survival after relapse remains very poor. Approximately 30% of RMS patients will experience relapse, and between 50% and 95% of these will die of progressive disease.[42] Results from the Cooperative Weichteilsarkom Studiengruppe identified certain factors that may predict relapse including increased age (>10 years), histology (alveolar), tumor size (>5 cm), tumor site, stage after surgery, and lack of RT.[43]

In a large review of relapsed RMS patients, 95% of all failures occurred within 3 years from treatment initiation.[42] Patterns of relapse were as follows: local, 35%; regional, 16%; distant, 41%; and unknown, 8%. Overall, the median survival time from first recurrence or progression was 0.8 year, and the estimated 5-year survival after recurrence was 17%. Higher survival postrelapse was associated with botryoid histology and initial clinical group I assignment. For embryonal RMS, local recurrence predicted improved survival compared to those patients with regional or distant recurrences. Factors associated with a better prognosis with recurrent disease include embryonal/botryoid histology, stage or group I disease, and relapse >1 year after completing primary therapy.[7,44] RMS patients with local relapse compose a very challenging patient population, and the results of repeated attempts at surgical resection are not fully known. Many RMS patients with locally recurrent disease are those with primary tumors of the extremities, pelvis, retroperitoneum, and other sites at which repeated operations are difficult, and often mutilating.

The IRSG recommends that patients with locally recurrent disease be treated according to risk stratification. For more favorably rated relapse patients, intensive multiagent chemotherapy followed by RT and/or surgical treatment, and for less favorably rated patients, initial dose-intensified chemotherapy and maintenance therapy or experimental therapies may be offered.[42] In a smaller study of RMS and NRSTS patients with first relapse (*n* = 44), repeat resection appeared to improve survival with embryonal RMS, but not with alveolar RMS or other soft tissue sarcoma histologic subtypes.[45] A retrospective review of patients treated at MD Anderson Cancer Center for recurrent RMS over an 11-year period (*n* = 32) demonstrated a 37% disease-free survival with a mean follow-up period of 4.9 years.[46] Morbidity was 35%, and 52% of the operations were considered aggressive. Several factors prevalent in survivors included embryonal/botryoid histology and RMS of vaginal/paratesticular origin. Factors associated with those who died included alveolar histology and extremity and bladder/prostate disease.

Surgical Treatment for Metastatic Rhabdomyosarcoma

Approximately 30% of RMS patients present with distant metastatic disease, most commonly involving lung (39%), bone marrow (32%), lymph nodes (30%), or bones (27%).[5,47] Patients with distant metastatic disease have a median survival of 20 months. The OS at 5, 15, and 30 years is 33%, 29%, and 23%, respectively, and FFS is <30%.[2,5] Operation combined with neoadjuvant or adjuvant RT improves survival by 20 months, and significantly increases 5-year survival compared to operation or RT alone.[5]

In the IRS-IV patient cohort, 24% had metastases isolated to the lung.[47] Most patients underwent a diagnostic biopsy followed by intensive salvage multimodality therapy. There was no difference in survival between patients who underwent operation with histologic confirmation of lung metastases and those diagnosed only by imaging. The value of aggressive resection of RMS pulmonary metastases remains unclear as opposed to other soft tissue sarcomas in children and adults where aggressive resection of isolated pulmonary metastases is thought to be beneficial for longer survival.[47,48]

SITE-SPECIFIC SURGICAL GUIDELINES

Head/Neck Tumors

Nonparameningeal orbital and other head and neck RMS tumors are considered favorable sites and are classified as stage 1, regardless of size or nodal status. Operative management for orbital and other head and neck RMS tumors is largely restricted to biopsy followed by adjuvant chemotherapy and RT (Fig. 70-3). Parameningeal tumors have slightly worse prognosis due to the presence of abundant lymphatics and a delay in diagnosis because of the hidden tumor. Previously, mutilating operations were performed. However, with more effective systemic therapy, these operations are rarely needed. Metastatic disease to regional nodes is present in <3% of cases.[30] Unless there is clinical evidence of lymph node involvement, routine nodal sampling is not warranted. An aggressive operative approach may be justified with recurrent disease. Additionally, surgical intervention may be warranted when

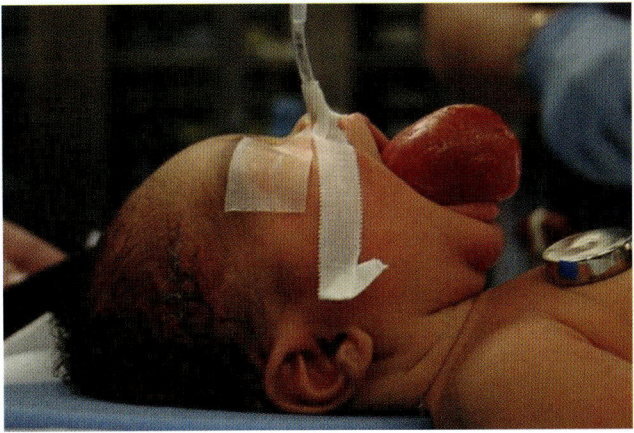

FIGURE 70-3 ■ This neonate was born with this large tongue mass. Biopsy showed it to be a rhabdomyosarcoma. Tracheostomy was done to protect his airway, and gastrostomy was performed for enteral alimentation. The patient has required numerous debulking procedures in addition to chemotherapy.

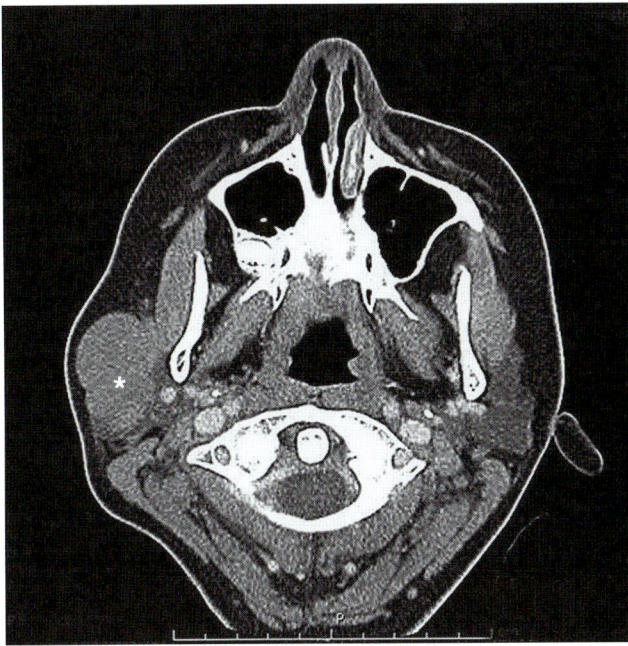

FIGURE 70-4 ■ A 13-year-old child presented with a large right parotid mass. The CT scan shows the large mass (asterisk) in the right parotid gland. The patient underwent total parotidectomy and tolerated the operation well. However, metastatic disease subsequently developed.

there is evidence of persistent disease after adjuvant therapy. These tumors are optimally managed by oncologic otolaryngologists and neurosurgeons. Superficial lesions such as parotid tumors and small eyelid lesions may benefit from primary resection especially when wide surgical excision is feasible (Fig. 70-4).

Tumors of the Extremities

Extremity RMS constitutes 15–20% of all pediatric RMS, with the median age of 6 years.[19,47,49] Extremity tumors are considered to be an unfavorable site, and 71% have alveolar histology. Initial staging of extremity RMS begins at stage 2, but can be upstaged based on size, nodal involvement, and metastasis (see Table 70-2). Evaluation of extremity RMS starts with careful physical examination and is followed by computed tomography (CT) to evaluate for bony erosion and magnetic resonance imaging (MRI) to determine tumor size and involvement of surrounding structures.[50] F-fluorodeoxyglucose positron emission tomography (FDG-PET) is also helpful for clinically negative nodes or distant metastases that are equivocal by conventional CT or MRI.[51]

The operative goal for primary extremity tumors <5 cm is to obtain circumferential disease-free margins while preserving form and function. In one study, FFS and OS were not affected by utilizing conservative surgery and adjuvant RT versus primary amputation in RMS of the hands and feet.[52] The required resection margin is unclear based on current evidence, but a 5 mm circumferential margin is currently recommended.[50] Moreover, there is no clear evidence that a larger margin decreases the chance of recurrence. After distortion of the tissues associated with resection and histopathologic processing, the actual margin measured in pathology is usually smaller.[53] Unfortunately, complete resection with negative margins is rarely achieved in extremity RMS patients.[14] Removal of tumor in a piecemeal fashion is considered group II even if the surgeon is confident all tumor is removed. When gross or microscopic tumor is left in the tumor bed, titanium clips should be placed to aid in RT and possible re-excision.[50]

For patients with larger tumors, or those in unfavorable anatomic sites involving neurovascular beds, an initial incisional biopsy is recommended. The biopsy incision should be oriented longitudinally along the long axis of the limb so that it does not interfere with a later attempt at resection. Definitive diagnosis and adequate tissue for biological studies is best obtained with an incisional biopsy rather than fine-needle or cone biopsies. After intensive multiagent chemotherapy and possibly RT, a second-look operation can be planned to resect residual disease.

A high rate of regional lymph node involvement is found with extremity RMS. Lymph node disease status is a critical component of the preoperative staging classification scheme (see Table 70-2) and has a direct impact on the plan of care. Therefore, evaluation of the regional lymph drainage basin is mandatory, regardless of clinical node status.[19] In IRS-IV (n = 139), 37% of all extremity RMS patients had positive regional lymph nodes. Positive regional lymph nodes were found in 50% of the patients who underwent surgical evaluation (n = 76). An additional 13 patients had regional node disease diagnosed by imaging alone. Among patients with a negative clinical and radiologic examination, 17% had positive nodes found on biopsy.[14] These findings imply that some patients with negative imaging who did not undergo lymph node biopsy probably had undetected positive lymph nodes. Undetected positive nodal disease will lead to inaccurate staging and perhaps less than optimal treatment. However, complete nodal dissection offers no survival benefit and discovery of a positive node does not warrant nodal dissection. Sentinel node biopsy is a viable option for the evaluation of the draining nodal basin.[38,54,55]

If the nodal basin is found to harbor a positive node, more proximal nodal evaluation is warranted to exclude in-transit disease to further clarify tumor stage and group.[52]

Survival with multimodality therapy now approaches 75%, with a significantly lower rate for patients with nodal disease.[19] As reviewed previously, for extremity RMS with microscopically positive or indeterminant margins, or after an initial resection was performed for presumed benign disease, PRE is recommended and has been shown to improve survival.[36]

Genitourinary Tumors

Within the genitourinary system, RMS can arise from the vagina, vulva, uterus, paratesticular region, prostate, or bladder. Rarely, the kidney or ureter may be involved. In the IRS-IV study, genitourinary RMS accounted for 12% of all patients and >30% of nonmetastatic tumor patients.[47] Bladder/prostate genitourinary primary tumors were most common.

Bladder/Prostate Tumors

RMS of the bladder and prostate occur in 2% and 4%, respectively.[5] Ultrasound is usually performed at initial diagnosis, and serial CT or MRI are used to track the efficacy of primary chemotherapy.[53] Secondary to the tumor location, the initial operative approach is usually limited to biopsy, which can usually be obtained using endoscopy. However, the surgeon should be aware of the amount of tissue taken for biopsy as the endoscopic biopsy forceps take very small samples. Also, artifact from using cautery can mimic a spindle cell appearance or destroy the entire sample. Open biopsy is performed when endoscopy is not possible. Pelvic and retroperitoneal lymph nodes also should be sampled for disease in these patients. Internal ureteral stents and/or percutaneous nephrostomy tubes may be necessary with urinary obstruction. Suprapubic catheters are not advised secondary to the risk of seeding the tract with tumor.[53] Historically, aggressive initial resection was performed with good local control rates, but with significant morbidity and low bladder salvage rates. Survival has improved significantly since the IRSG trials, and bladder salvage is now the primary goal in these patients. However, complete resection may be feasible when the primary tumor involves only the dome of the bladder. Most bladder and prostate tumors are treated with chemotherapy and RT, followed by a more limited and conservative resection.[56] More aggressive tumor resection including anterior or total pelvic exenteration may be indicated to achieve local control if the tumor fails to respond to primary chemotherapy. The rate of exenterative cystectomy with current treatment is approximately 30% (Figs 70-5 and 70-6).[57-59] Many patients will develop bladder dysfunction even with bladder salvage.[19]

Vagina, Vulva, or Uterus

Tumors of the female genitourinary tract are considered a favorable site (stage 1). They have a 5-year OS >80%

and comprise 3.5% all RMS tumors with half originating in the vagina. They are typically embryonal or botryoid histologic subtype (Fig. 70-7) and lymph node involvement is uncommon.[60] Management begins with a biopsy, often transvaginally, and relies on effective chemotherapy such as systemic high dose cyclophosphamide as primary treatment. There is no role for initial aggressive resection such as vaginectomy or hysterectomy.[61] Some physicians recommend avoidance of RT in group II and III vaginal RMS in patients <24 months old due to the high morbidity associated with external beam radiation.[62] These patients are followed with routine abdominal and pelvic MRI to document tumor response.[63,64] A second-look operation with cystoscopy and re-biopsy is common. As with other pelvic RMS, relapsed or persistent disease in the vagina, vulva, and uterus is associated with a very poor outcome. In such cases, aggressive attempts at local control, including RT, partial or total vaginectomy, hysterectomy, or pelvic exenteration, are all viable options.

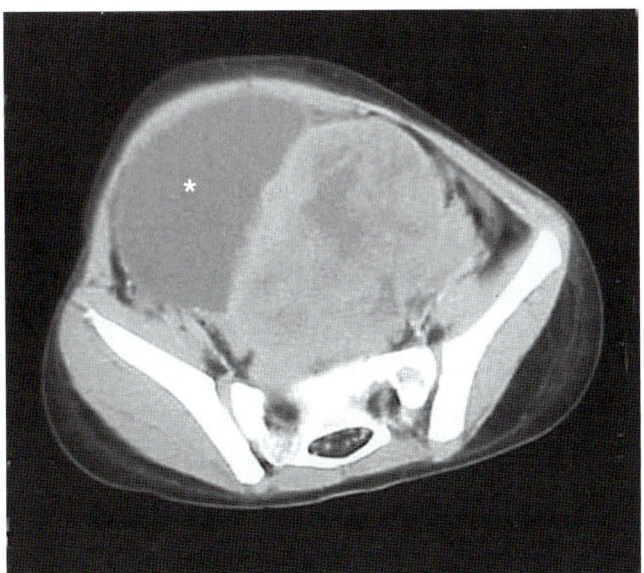

FIGURE 70-5 ■ This CT scan shows a large mass emanating from the pelvis. Biopsy confirmed this mass to be a rhabdomyosarcoma. The bladder has been marked with an asterisk.

Unless there is direct involvement of the ovary by advanced/recurrent disease, there is no role for oophorectomy.

Paratesticular Tumors

Paratesticular RMS is considered a favorable site, with all paratesticular patients classified preoperatively as having stage 1 disease regardless of tumor size, invasiveness, or lymph node status. The overall FFS rate for paratesticular RMS is > 80%, and is 90% in patients younger than 10 years old.[1]

The recommended initial operative approach for paratesticular tumors is radical orchiectomy with proximal ligation of the spermatic cord at the internal inguinal ring via an inguinal incision. A trans-scrotal incision for biopsy or resection is contraindicated. If done, a subsequent hemiscrotectomy may be required to resect the contaminated tumor bed. Meticulous operative technique is extremely important. Tumor spillage upstages patients to clinical group IIa regardless of the completeness of resection.[65] When paratesticular tumors are fixed to the scrotal skin or invade the overlying scrotal skin, hemiscrotectomy is indicated. With this approach, 90% to 95% of patients are able to have complete resection (groups I or II).[37]

Paratesticular RMS has a high incidence (~30%) of spread to the retroperitoneal lymph nodes (RPLNs). Therefore, careful evaluation of these nodes is an important part of the staging workup for these patients. All patients should have thin-cut (3.8–5.0 mm) abdominal and pelvic CT scans to assess the retroperitoneum. The treatment guidelines vary by age since the outcome and the frequency of RPLN positivity with paratesticular RMS is partially age dependent. For patients younger than 10 years who are clinical group I, and do not have lymph node enlargement on CT scan, RPLN dissection or sampling is not recommended. These patients are followed with CT scans every 3 months. Suggestive or positive CT scans should prompt ipsilateral retroperitoneal node dissection with further therapy depending on the histologic findings. For all patients 10 years or older, or with tumor >5 cm, ipsilateral RPLN dissection

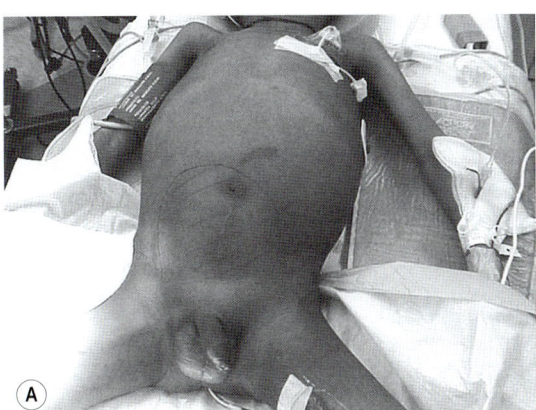
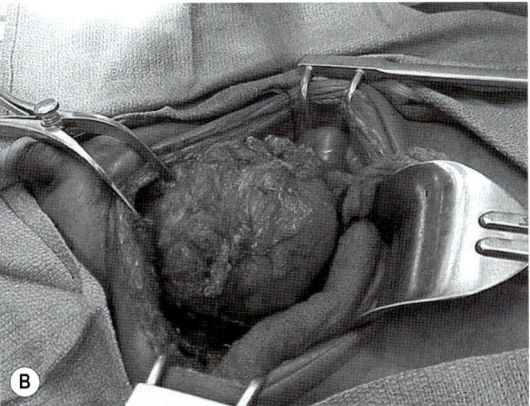

FIGURE 70-6 ■ **(A)** The patient presented with lower abdominal distention and a large mass that was palpable. **(B)** The mass (visualized in the operative photograph) was not responsive to chemotherapy, and an attempt at complete resection was made. Most, but not all, of the mass could be excised. The patient eventually died of metastatic disease. This patient's CT scan is seen in Figure 70-5.

is recommended up to the level of the renal hilum. A systematic approach is used to remove lymph nodes from the internal inguinal ring, along the iliac vessels and aorta, up to the renal hilum. Positive suprarenal nodes are considered metastatic. Thus, patients are considered group IV.[50] RPLN dissection is associated with significant morbidity, including loss of ejaculatory function and lower extremity lymphedema. Thus, risk-based guidelines are used to limit unnecessary patient morbidity secondary to RPLN dissection.[66] However, involved lymph nodes are missed in 15–20% of patients by CT scan, and a high index of suspicion is necessary.[14,17,29]

Other Sites

RMS occurring in other sites is rare. Primary tumors arising in the thorax, abdomen, pelvis, and perineum were found in only 12% of all IRS-IV patients.[47] Truncal RMS tumors usually have an alveolar subtype. Primary resection is preferred in truncal tumors <5 cm when a negative operative margin can be realistically anticipated. For larger primary tumors, initial incisional biopsy is preferred. Additionally, postoperative reconstructive

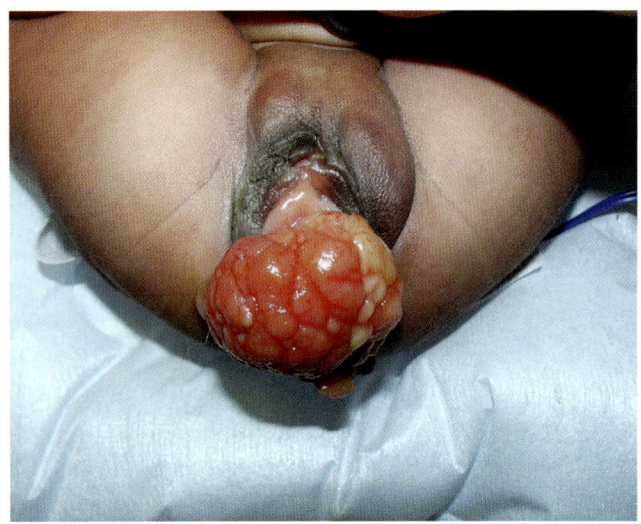

FIGURE 70-7 ■ This neonate was born with this protruding mass from her vagina. Biopsy of the mass showed rhabdomyosarcoma. She underwent chemotherapy and has recovered uneventfully. Rhabdomyosarcoma of the vagina has been termed *sarcoma botryoides*.

procedures may be necessary, especially with larger tumors, using prosthetic meshes or myocutaneous flaps.[19] Paraspinal masses need to be differentiated from extraosseous Ewing's sarcoma. No data are available from which to make definitive guidelines regarding regional lymph node evaluation. For many truncal lesions, the primary lymphatic drainage basin can be equivocal and preoperative lymphoscintigraphy may be helpful.

Retroperitoneal and nongenitourinary pelvic tumors can be difficult to manage because of their relatively hidden location and subsequent late presentation. More than 90% present with large invasive tumors as clinical group III or IV.[67] These patients generally undergo initial biopsy, aggressive multiple-agent chemotherapy, RT, and second-look operation, if indicated. The role for debulking large retroperitoneal or nongenitourinary pelvic tumors is unclear. However, data have demonstrated survival benefit in a subset of patients who underwent debulking.[68,69]

Biliary RMS generally has a good prognosis without the need for aggressive resection. Most patients have botryoid RMS that responds well to chemotherapy. Biopsy followed by neoadjuvant chemotherapy frequently results in resolution of symptoms, including jaundice. Operative intervention is fraught with complications, including the inability to resect all disease in most cases and infections associated with external biliary drains.[50,70]

Perineal and perianal RMSs also are sites that have an overall poor outcome partially due to late presentation.[71] More than one-third of patients are seen initially with presumed benign disease (usually infections).[47] Improved survival is associated with tumors <5 cm, low clinical group and stage, negative nodes, and age younger than 10 years. Outcomes are not related to the tumor histology in this site.[50] PRE frequently lowers the clinical group assignment, which improves outcome. From 1972 to 1997, 71 patients had perineal and perianal tumors, with a five-year FFS rate of 45%. In this group, 46% of patients had regional lymph node involvement with five-year OS of 33% and 71% for N1 and N0 respectively.[17]

CURRENT/FUTURE RESEARCH

Data from IRS-III and IRS-IV were used to develop the risk stratification groupings used for IRS-V and current studies (Table 70-3). Low-risk patients are estimated to

TABLE 70-3 Intergroup Rhabdomyosarcoma Study Group Studies Based on Risk-Based Protocol Assignment

Risk	Five-year FFS[a]	Stage	Group	Histology	Current Study
Low, subset A	90%	1 or 2	I or II	Embryonal	ARST0331
		1	III orbit	Embryonal	
Low, subset B	87%	1	III nonorbit	Embryonal	ARST0331
		3	I or II	Embryonal	
Intermediate	65–73%	2 or 3	III	Embryonal	ARST0531
		1, 2, or 3	I, II, or III	Alveolar	
High	<30%	4	IV	Embryonal or Alveolar	ARST08P1

[a]Data from IRS-III and IRS-IV.
FFS, Failure-free survival; IRS, Intergroup Rhabdomyosarcoma Study.

have three-year FFS rates of 88%.[72] The low-risk patient group is broken down into subset A with a 90% FFS and subset B with an 87% FFS. This subgroup is limited to patients with localized embryonal, botryoid, or spindle cell tumors. Patients receive either VAC (vincristine, actinomycin D, cyclophosphamide) or VA (vincristine, actinomycin D) chemotherapy and RT to residual tumor after resection. Current research (ARST0331) is focused on reducing the dose and subsequent systemic side effects of cyclophosphamide therapy while evaluating the impact on survival.[2]

Intermediate-risk patients have a predicted FFS rate of 65–73% and include those with localized alveolar or undifferentiated sarcoma, stages 1 to 3, or embryonal RMS stages 2 and 3 with gross residual disease, or stage 4 embryonal RMS patients younger than 10 years old. In IRS-V, these patients were randomized to VAC and RT or VAC alternating with vincristine, topotecan, and cyclophosphamide and RT, but there was no survival benefit seen.[2] Multiple chemotherapy regimens were evaluated with other IRS studies and vincristine with irinotecan (VI) showed the best response rate. Thus, in the most recent trial (ARST0531), patients are being randomized to either VAC or VAC alternating with VI.[2]

High-risk patients have a 3-year FFS of <30% and include stage 4 or group IV alveolar or undifferentiated tumors and embryonal RMS patients older than 10 years old. These patients receive chemotherapy with irinotecan followed by VAC and RT. For patients responding to irinotecan, treatment continues with four additional cycles of irinotecan and vincristine, in addition to VAC. Current research (ARST08P1) is designed to evaluate whether or not the addition of cixutumumab and/or temozolomide to the current chemotherapeutic regimen will improve outcomes.[2]

An important component of ongoing IRS studies is the investigation of the biology of these tumors. Success hinges on full participation by pediatric surgeons and oncologists. All newly diagnosed or relapsed RMS patients should be considered for enrollment in ongoing biology study protocols. The surgeon should facilitate the submission of fresh tumor specimens as well as peripheral blood and bone marrow when indicated so that continued improvements in the care of these children can be realized.

REFERENCES

1. Crist WM, Anderson JR, Meza JL, et al. Intergroup rhabdomyosarcoma study-IV: Results for patients with nonmetastatic disease. J Clin Oncol 2001;19:3091–102.
2. Malempati S, Hawkins DS. Rhabdomyosarcoma: Review of the Children's Oncology Group (COG) soft-tissue Sarcoma committee experience and rationale for current COG studies. Pediatr Blood Cancer 2012;59:5–10.
3. Kramer S, Meadows AT, Jarrett P, et al. Incidence of childhood cancer: Experience of a decade in a population-based registry. J Natl Cancer Inst 1983;70:49–55.
4. Gurney JG, Young JL Jr, Roffers SD, et al. Soft tissue sarcomas. In: Ries LAG, Smith MA, Gurney JG, et al, editors. Cancer Incidence and Survival among Children and Adolescents: United States SEER Program 1975–1995. Bethesda, MD: National Cancer Institute, SEER Program; 1999.
5. Perez EA, Kassira N, Cheung MC, et al. Rhabdomyosarcoma in children: A SEER population based study. J Surg Res 2011; 170(2):e243–51.
6. Dagher R, Helman L. Rhabdomyosarcoma: An overview. Oncologist 1999;4:34–44.
7. Rodeberg D, Paidas C. Childhood rhabdomyosarcoma. Semin Pediatr Surg 2006;15:57–62.
8. Bisogno G, Compostella A, Ferrari A, et al. Rhabdomyosarcoma in adolescents: A report from the AIEOP Soft Tissue Sarcoma Committee. Cancer 2012;118:821–7.
9. Malempati S, Rodeberg DA, Donaldson SS, et al. Rhabdomyosarcoma in infants younger than 1 year: A report from the Children's Oncology Group. Cancer 2011;117:3493–501.
10. Newton WA Jr, Soule EH, Hamoudi AB, et al. Histopathology of childhood sarcomas, Intergroup Rhabdomyosarcoma Studies I and II: Clinicopathologic correlation. J Clin Oncol 1988;6:67–75.
11. Qualman SJ, Coffin CM, Newton WA, et al. Intergroup Rhabdomyosarcoma Study: Update for pathologists. Pediatr Dev Pathol 1998;1:550–61.
12. Leuschner I, Newton WA Jr, Schmidt D, et al. Spindle cell variants of embryonal rhabdomyosarcoma in the paratesticular region. A report of the Intergroup Rhabdomyosarcoma Study. Am J Surg Pathol 1993;17:221–30.
13. Wexler LH, Crist LM, Helman LJ. Rhabdomyosarcoma and the undifferentiated sarcomas. In: Pizzo PA, Poplack DG, editors. Principles and Practice of Pediatric Oncology. 4th ed. Philadelphia: Lippincott Williams & Wilkins; 2002. p. 939–71.
14. Neville HL, Andrassy RJ, Lobe TE, et al. Preoperative staging, prognostic factors, and outcome for extremity rhabdomyosarcoma: A preliminary report from the Intergroup Rhabdomyosarcoma Study IV (1991–1997). J Pediatr Surg 2000;35:317–21.
15. Tsokos M, Webber BL, Parham DM, et al. Rhabdomyosarcoma. A new classification scheme related to prognosis. Arch Pathol Lab Med 1992;116:847–55.
16. Kodet R, Newton WA Jr, Hamoudi AB, et al. Orbital rhabdomyosarcomas and related tumors in childhood: Relationship of morphology to prognosis–an Intergroup Rhabdomyosarcoma study. Med Pediatr Oncol 1997;29:51–60.
17. Blakely ML, Andrassy RJ, Raney RB, et al. Prognostic factors and surgical treatment guidelines for children with rhabdomyosarcoma of the perineum or anus: A report of Intergroup Rhabdomyosarcoma Studies I through IV, 1972 through 1997. J Pediatr Surg 2003;38:347–53.
18. Slater O, Shipley J. Clinical relevance of molecular genetics to paediatric sarcomas. J Clin Pathol 2007;60:1187–94.
19. Leaphart C, Rodeberg D. Pediatric surgical oncology: Management of rhabdomyosarcoma. Surg Oncol 2007;16:173–85.
20. Bridge JA, Liu J, Weibolt V, et al. Novel genomic imbalances in embryonal rhabdomyosarcoma revealed by comparative genomic hybridization and fluorescence in situ hybridization: An intergroup rhabdomyosarcoma study. Genes Chromosomes Cancer 2000; 27:337–44.
21. Turc-Carel C, Lizard-Nacol S, Justrabo E, et al. Consistent chromosomal translocation in alveolar rhabdomyosarcoma. Cancer Genet Cytogenet 1986;19:361–2.
22. Shapiro DN, Sublett JE, Li B, et al. Fusion of PAX3 to a member of the forkhead family of transcription factors in human alveolar rhabdomyosarcoma. Cancer Res 1993;53:5108–12.
23. Davis RJ, D'Cruz CM, Lovell MA, et al. Fusion of PAX7 to FKHR by the variant t(1;13)(p36;q14) translocation in alveolar rhabdomyosarcoma. Cancer Res 1994;54:2869–72.
24. Khan J, Bittner ML, Saal LH, et al. cDNA microarrays detect activation of a myogenic transcription program by the PAX3-FKHR fusion oncogene. Proc Natl Acad Sci U S A 1999;96: 13264–9.
25. Duan F, Smith LM, Gustafson DM, et al. Genomic and clinical analysis of fusion gene amplification in rhabdomyosarcoma: A report from the Children's Oncology Group. Genes Chromosomes Cancer 2012;51:662–74.
26. Kelly KM, Womer RB, Sorensen PH, et al. Common and variant gene fusions predict distinct clinical phenotypes in rhabdomyosarcoma. J Clin Oncol 1997;15:1831–6.
27. Rapa E, Hill SK, Morten KJ, et al. The over-expression of cell migratory genes in alveolar rhabdomyosarcoma could contribute to metastatic spread. Clin Exp Metastasis 2012;29:419–29.
28. Davicioni E, Anderson MJ, Buckley JD, et al. Gene expression profiling for survival prediction in pediatric rhabdomyosarcomas: A report from the children's oncology group. J Clin Oncol 2010; 28:1240–6.

29. Wiener ES, Anderson JR, Ojimba JI, et al. Controversies in the management of paratesticular rhabdomyosarcoma: Is staging retroperitoneal lymph node dissection necessary for adolescents with resected paratesticular rhabdomyosarcoma? Semin Pediatr Surg 2001;10:146–52.

30. Crist W, Gehan EA, Ragab AH, et al. The Third Intergroup Rhabdomyosarcoma Study. J Clinl Oncol 1995;13:610–30.

31. Raney RB Jr. Rhabdomyosarcoma and related tumors of the head and neck in childhood. In: Maurer HM, Ruymann FB, Pochedly C, editors. Rhabdomyosarcoma and Related Tumors in Children and Adolescents. Boca Raton, FL: CRC; 1991.

32. Raney RB Jr, Tefft M, Newton WA, et al. Improved prognosis with intensive treatment of children with cranial soft tissue sarcomas arising in nonorbital parameningeal sites. A report from the Intergroup Rhabdomyosarcoma Study. Cancer 1987;59:147–55.

33. Rodeberg D, Arndt C, Breneman J, et al. Characteristics and outcomes of rhabdomyosarcoma patients with isolated lung metastases from IRS-IV. J Pediatr Surg 2005;40:256–62.

34. Lobe TE, Wiener ES, Hays DM, et al. Neonatal rhabdomyosarcoma: The IRS experience. J Pediatr Surg 1994;29:1167–70.

35. Cecchetto G, Carli M, Sotti G, et al. Importance of local treatment in pediatric soft tissue sarcomas with microscopic residual after primary surgery: Results of the Italian Cooperative Study RMS-88. Med Pediatr Oncol 2000;34:97–101.

36. Hays DM, Lawrence W Jr, Wharam M, et al. Primary reexcision for patients with 'microscopic residual' tumor following initial excision of sarcomas of trunk and extremity sites. J Pediatr Surg 1989;24:5–10.

37. Wiener ES, Lawrence W, Hays D, et al. Retroperitoneal node biopsy in paratesticular rhabdomyosarcoma. J Pediatr Surg 1994;29:171–7.

38. Neville HL, Andrassy RJ, Lally KP, et al. Lymphatic mapping with sentinel node biopsy in pediatric patients. J Pediatr Surg 2000;35:961–4.

39. Hays DM, Raney RB, Crist WM, et al. Secondary surgical procedures to evaluate primary tumor status in patients with chemotherapy-responsive stage III and IV sarcomas: A report from the Intergroup Rhabdomyosarcoma Study. J Pediatr Surg 1990;25:1100–5.

40. Schalow EL, Broecker BH. Role of surgery in children with rhabdomyosarcoma. Med Pediatr Oncol 2003;41:1–6.

41. Godzinski J, Flamant F, Rey A, et al. Value of postchemotherapy bioptical verification of complete clinical remission in previously incompletely resected (stage I and II pT3) malignant mesenchymal tumors in children: International Society of Pediatric Oncology 1984 Malignant Mesenchymal Tumors Study. Med Pediatr Oncol 1994;22:22–6.

42. Pappo AS, Anderson JR, Crist WM, et al. Survival after relapse in children and adolescents with rhabdomyosarcoma: A report from the Intergroup Rhabdomyosarcoma Study Group. J Clin Oncol 1999;17:3487–93.

43. Dantonello TM, Int-Veen C, Winkler P, et al. Initial patient characteristics can predict pattern and risk of relapse in localized rhabdomyosarcoma. J Clin Oncol 2008;26:406–13.

44. Mattke AC, Bailey EJ, Schuck A, et al. Does the time-point of relapse influence outcome in pediatric rhabdomyosarcomas? Pediatr Blood Cancer 2009;52:772–6.

45. Klingebiel T, Pertl U, Hess CF, et al. Treatment of children with relapsed soft tissue sarcoma: Report of the German CESS/CWS REZ 91 trial. Med Pediatr Oncol 1998;30:269–75.

46. Hayes-Jordan A, Doherty DK, West SD, et al. Outcome after surgical resection of recurrent rhabdomyosarcoma. J Pediatr Surg 2006;41:633–8.

47. Breneman JC, Lyden E, Pappo AS, et al. Prognostic factors and clinical outcomes in children and adolescents with metastatic rhabdomyosarcoma–a report from the Intergroup Rhabdomyosarcoma Study IV. J Clin Oncol 2003;21:78–84.

48. Hacker FM, von Schweinitz D, Gambazzi F. The relevance of surgical therapy for bilateral and/or multiple pulmonary metastases in children. Eur J Pediatr Surg 2007;17:84–9.

49. Sultan I, Qaddoumi I, Yaser S, et al. Comparing adult and pediatric rhabdomyosarcoma in the surveillance, epidemiology and end results program, 1973 to 2005: An analysis of 2,600 patients. J Clin Oncol 2009;27:3391–7.

50. Dasgupta R, Rodeberg DA. Update on rhabdomyosarcoma. Semin Pediatr Surg 2012;21:68–78.

51. Kumar R, Shandal V, Shamim SA, et al. Clinical applications of PET and PET/CT in pediatric malignancies. Expert Rev Anticancer Ther 2010;10:755–68.

52. La TH, Wolden SL, Su Z, et al. Local therapy for rhabdomyosarcoma of the hands and feet: Is amputation necessary? A report from the Children's Oncology Group. Int J Radiat Oncol Biol Phys 2011;80:206–12.

53. Ferrer FA, Isakoff M, Koyle MA. Bladder/prostate rhabdomyosarcoma: Past, present and future. J Urol 2006;176:1283–91.

54. Gow KW, Rapkin LB, Olson TA, et al. Sentinel lymph node biopsy in the pediatric population. J Pediatr Surg 2008;43:2193–8.

55. De Corti F, Dall'Igna P, Bisogno G, et al. Sentinel node biopsy in pediatric soft tissue sarcomas of extremities. Pediatr Blood Cancer 2009;52:51–4.

56. Lobe TE, Wiener E, Andrassy RJ, et al. The argument for conservative, delayed surgery in the management of prostatic rhabdomyosarcoma. J Pediatr Surg 1996;31:1084–7.

57. Corpron CA, Andrassy RJ, Hays DM, et al. Conservative management of uterine pediatric rhabdomyosarcoma: A report from the Intergroup Rhabdomyosarcoma Study III and IV pilot. J Pediatr Surg 1995;30:942–4.

58. Hays DM, Lawrence W Jr, Crist WM, et al. Partial cystectomy in the management of rhabdomyosarcoma of the bladder: A report from the Intergroup Rhabdomyosarcoma Study. J Pediatr Surg 1990;25:719–23.

59. Hays DM, Raney RB, Ragab A, et al. Retention of functional bladders among patients with vesicle/prostatic sarcomas in the intergroup rhabdomyosarcoma studies (IRS) (1978–1990) [Abstract]. Med Pediatr Oncol 1991:423.

60. Arndt CA, Donaldson SS, Anderson JR, et al. What constitutes optimal therapy for patients with rhabdomyosarcoma of the female genital tract? Cancer 2001;91:2454–68.

61. Andrassy RJ, Wiener ES, Raney RB, et al. Progress in the surgical management of vaginal rhabdomyosarcoma: A 25-year review from the Intergroup Rhabdomyosarcoma Study Group. J Pediatr Surg 1999;34:731–4.

62. Walterhouse DO, Meza JL, Breneman JC, et al. Local control and outcome in children with localized vaginal rhabdomyosarcoma: A report from the Soft Tissue Sarcoma committee of the Children's Oncology Group. Pediatr Blood Cancer 2011;57:76–83.

63. Fletcher BD, Kaste SC. Magnetic resonance imaging for diagnosis and follow-up of genitourinary, pelvic, and perineal rhabdomyosarcoma. Urol Radiol 1992;14:263–72.

64. Finelli A, Babyn P, Lorie GA, et al. The use of magnetic resonance imaging in the diagnosis and followup of pediatric pelvic rhabdomyosarcoma. J Urol 2000;163:1952–3.

65. Hamilton CR, Pinkerton R, Horwich A. The management of paratesticular rhabdomyosarcoma. Clin Radiol 1989;40:314–17.

66. Heyn R, Raney RB Jr, Hays DM, et al. Late effects of therapy in patients with paratesticular rhabdomyosarcoma. Intergroup Rhabdomyosarcoma Study Committee. J Clin Oncol 1992;10:614–23.

67. Blakely ML, Spurbeck WW, Pappo AS, et al. The impact of margin of resection on outcome in pediatric nonrhabdomyosarcoma soft tissue sarcoma. J Pediatr Surg 1999;34:672–5.

68. Blakely ML, Lobe TE, Anderson JR, et al. Does debulking improve survival rate in advanced-stage retroperitoneal embryonal rhabdomyosarcoma? J Pediatr Surg 1999;34:736–41.

69. Raney RB, Stoner JA, Walterhouse DO, et al. Results of treatment of fifty-six patients with localized retroperitoneal and pelvic rhabdomyosarcoma: A report from The Intergroup Rhabdomyosarcoma Study-IV, 1991–1997. Pediatr Blood Cancer 2004;42:618–25.

70. Spunt SL, Lobe TE, Pappo AS, et al. Aggressive surgery is unwarranted for biliary tract rhabdomyosarcoma. J Pediatr Surg 2000;35:309–16.

71. Hill DA, Dehner LP, Gow KW, et al. Perianal rhabdomyosarcoma presenting as a perirectal abscess: A report of 11 cases. J Pediatr Surg 2002;37:576–81.

72. Raney RB, Anderson JR, Barr FG, et al. Rhabdomyosarcoma and undifferentiated sarcoma in the first two decades of life: A selective review of intergroup rhabdomyosarcoma study group experience and rationale for Intergroup Rhabdomyosarcoma Study V. J Pediatr Hematol Oncol 2001;23:215–20.

SECTION VIII

SKIN AND SOFT TISSUE DISEASES

CHAPTER 71

NEVUS AND MELANOMA

Arlet G. Kurkchubasche • Thomas F. Tracy, Jr.

Pigmented skin lesions comprise a significant portion of the clinical experience of pediatric surgeons. This chapter attempts to provide a basis for understanding the nomenclature of pigmented skin lesions, their biologic behavior, and their potential for malignancy. Unfortunately, skin lesions in children are often evaluated based on the adult perspective and this can lead to an excessive number of unnecessary operations. Those lesions mimicking cutaneous melanoma, particularly the atypical spitzoid lesions and melanoma proper, are discussed in the context of their evaluation and management in infants and children.

TERMINOLOGY AND CLASSIFICATION OF SKIN LESIONS

The terminology used for pigmented and nonpigmented cutaneous lesions is often confusing with multiple designations. The correct dermatologic terms are essential for clear communication (Table 71-1). An understanding of the epithelial embryology, anatomy, and physiology is also important for the clinical identification and correct classification of these lesions. As a reference, Figures 71-1 and 71-2 depict the basic anatomy of the dermis and epidermis.

Anatomy of the Dermis and Epidermis

The skin is a morphologically and functionally complex tissue providing protection against physical elements by its anatomic structure and potential for immune responsiveness. The outermost layer is the stratum corneum or horny layer, which is composed of devitalized keratinocytes (see Fig 71-1). While the dermal layer is a derivative of the paraxial mesoderm, embryologically the epidermis is of ectodermal origin.

The basal layer of the epidermis is the site of mitotic activity leading to the proliferation of keratinocytes. This basal layer consists of columnar cells anchored to the basement membrane via hemidesmosomes and anchored to the dermis via penetrating fibrils (see Fig. 71-1). Interspersed between the basal cells reside melanocytes that are dendritic cells and are the source of melanin (see Fig. 71-2). Melanocytes are not secured via desmosomes or tonofilaments. Functional units (epidermal melanin units) are composed of a melanocyte and the keratinocytes to which it is responsible for the transfer of melanin. Melanosomes are the cytoplasmic organelles that result from the fusion of vesicles containing tyrosinase and vesicles containing the structural melanosomal proteins, both

of which are generated by the melanocyte's endoplasmic reticulum. Differential skin pigmentation amongst individuals results from the variable production of melanosomes, their content and rate of degradation, and not on numbers of melanocytes. The absence of tyrosinase prevents formation of melanosomes and results in albinism. The melanosomes migrate from the perinuclear area along microtubules to the dendritic tips where these are phagocytized by the keratinocyte. As the squamous cells differentiate, the melanosomes are degraded by lysosomal enzymes.

The more superficial layer of dermis is the papillary dermis, which interacts with the epidermis via a basement membrane and sends interdigitating papillary and neurovascular structures to support the epidermis. The appendages to the skin, the hair follicles, sweat, sebaceous and apocrine glands, originate in the dermis. The fibroblast-derived matrix of collagen and elastin reside primarily in the deeper, reticular dermis.

CLASSIFICATION OF NEVI

The term nevus indicates a proliferation of cells within the tissue of origin. The classification of nevi is descriptive and can contain multiple dimensions (cell of origin, location within dermis and epidermis, congenital, and acquired) that are not necessarily mutually exclusive, but can add to confusion. A precise classification should help the clinician to correctly identify lesions that require vigilance as opposed to those that are clearly benign.

The most definitive classification is according to the cell of origin, and results in stratification between melanocytic and nonmelanocytic lesions. The melanocyte is a dendritic cell and neural crest derivative (Fig. 71-3). During development, the melanocyte precursors (melanoblasts) migrate to the dermis, hair follicles, leptomeninges, uveal tract, and retina. After the eighth week of development, they migrate from the dermis to the epidermis. Melanocytic nevi are derived from melanocytes or their precursors, and distinguish themselves by virtue of (1) the absence of dendrites; (2) the clustering of cells; (3) their variable location within the dermis and epidermis; and (4) their variable content of melanin (Table 71-2).

Nonmelanocytic nevi are generally derived from keratinocytes and are also referred to as epidermal nevi. They can be primarily keratinocytic or organoid, indicating their origins from the accessory structures of the skin. Pigmentation associated with a nevus does not serve to distinguish between melanocytic and nonmelanocytic nevi.

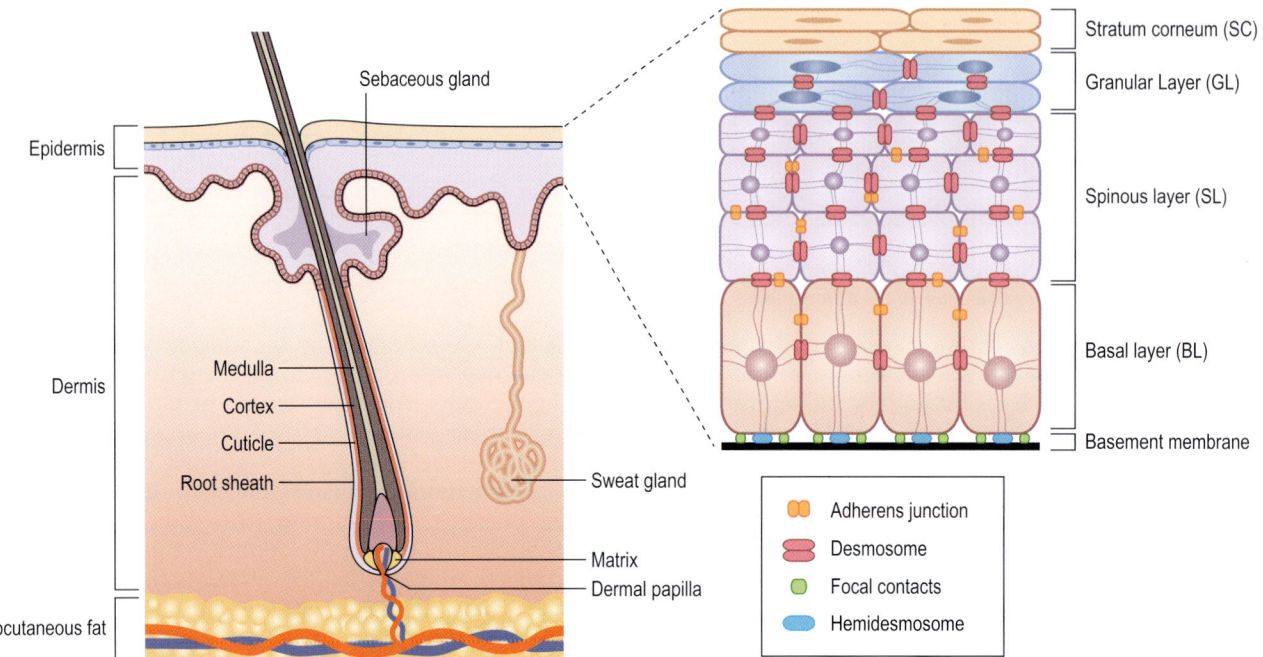

FIGURE 71-1 ■ Structural organization of the epidermis and dermis. (Redrawn from Fuchs E, Raghavan S. Getting under the skin of epidermal morphogenesis. Nat Rev Genet 2002;3:199–209.)

TABLE 71-1	**Glossary for Skin Lesions**
Term	**Definition**
Nevus	Proliferation of cells within their tissue of origin
Macule	Circumscribed, pigmented lesion, less than 5 mm in diameter without elevation or depression from the surrounding skin
Patch	Lesion with larger area of involvement without palpable characteristics
Papules	Solid elevated lesions less than 5 mm in diameter and plaques are raised lesions larger than 5 mm
Nodules	Lesions that arise from the dermis or subcutaneous tissues
Dermal melanoses	Pigmented lesions resulting from the deposit of melanin in melanophages, free melanin in the dermis or in dermal melanocytes
Melanocytosis	Lesion associated with increased number of melanocytes

The principal location of the nevus in the skin serves as a second potential descriptor. In contrast to the non-melanocytic epidermal nevus, melanocytic nevi can be situated: (1) at the junction of the epidermis/dermis (junctional); (2) involve both regions (compound); or (3) be confined to the dermis (dermal). These are generic histological terms and do not imply biologic behavior.

The third dimension is related to the time of appearance. Melanocytic nevi can be classified according to whether or not they involve disorders of (1) melanocyte migration or (2) proliferation. These lesions are most

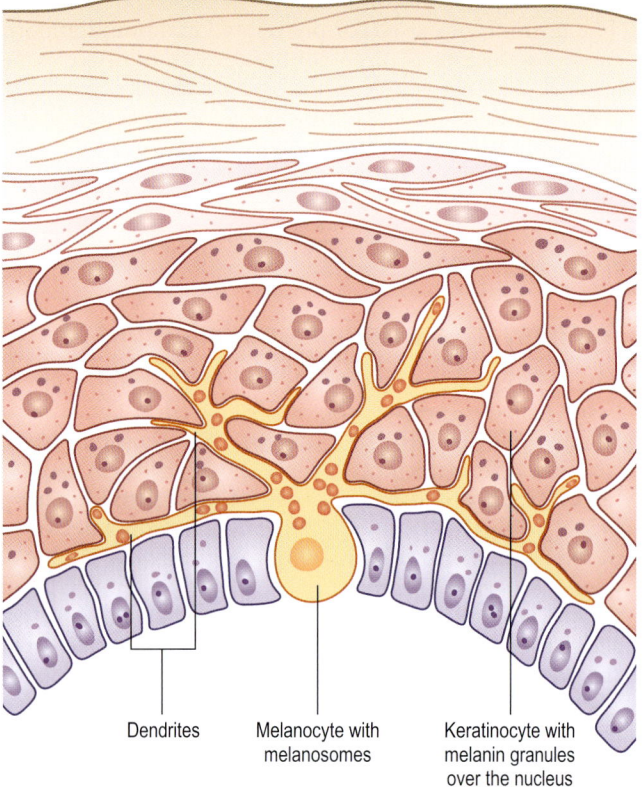

FIGURE 71-2 ■ The melanocyte rests within the basal layer of the epidermis and is associated with a group of keratinocytes to which it delivers the melanosomes. (Redrawn from Gray J. The World of Skin Care. Available at http://www.pg.com/science/skincare/Skin_tws_16.htm.)

TABLE 71-2   **Clinical and Histologic Features of Melanocytic Nevi**

	Junctional	Compound	Dermal
Histologic location	Junction of epidermis and dermis	Involving both dermis and junctional region	Involving dermis only[a]
Configuration	Flat, round to oval, symmetric	Raised, becomes more elevated with age	Protuberant, dome shaped, pedunculated
Surface	Smooth, hairless	Smooth to verrucous, may have hair	Smooth to verrucous
Pigmentation	Uniform dark brown to black	Flesh colored or brown, may have uniform distribution of darker spots, may develop halo	Flesh colored, tan to pink, may have halo or telangiectases

[a]Only in the presence of ulceration or reticular dermal invasion.

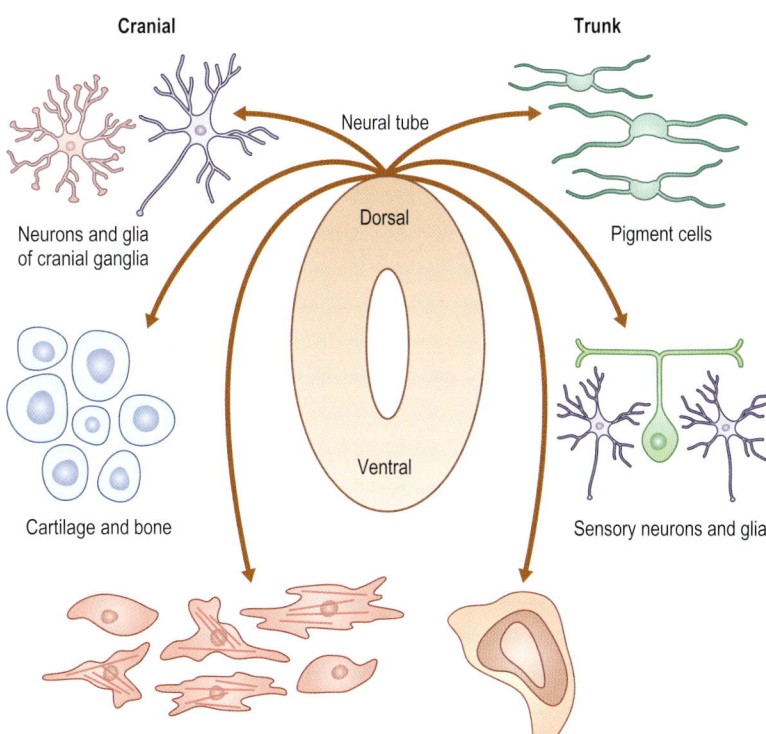

FIGURE 71-3 ■ The neural crest derivation of these dendritic cells explains the association of melanocytic disorders with CNS, bony, and ophthalmic disorders. (Redrawn from www.nature.com/nrg/journal/v3/n6/images/nrg819-i1.jpg.)

commonly categorized based on age at presentation as either congenital or acquired (Fig. 71-4) Congenital melanocytic nevi (CMN) result from failure of embryologic migration of the melanocyte precursors and form hamartomatous lesions evident at birth, which may evolve over time. In addition, congenital nevi can occasionally present after birth up to age 6 months. Failure of migration also results in a variety of dermal melanoses, some of which are encountered most frequently as the 'Mongolian' spot over the dorsal sacral region of infants. In contrast to the congenital nevi, acquired nevi are proliferative lesions and represent benign neoplasms of the skin that are located within the epidermis, dermis, or both. Acquired melanocytic nevi are the result of benign proliferative disorders of nevi that have a tendency to increase in number during childhood, adolescence and early adulthood, but then spontaneously regress with age. Based on more specific clinical characteristics, including total numbers of lesions, family history, and specific appearance, subsets of nevi can be identified that will have unique risks related to melanoma.

Many of these nevi are sufficiently clinically distinct to retain specific descriptive or eponymous names. These warrant individual discussion since it is their features that may prompt referral for biopsy to exclude malignancy. Examples of these lesions include the blue nevus, Spitz nevus, and halo nevus.

NONMELANOCYTIC NEVI

Epidermal nevi are skin lesions not associated with proliferation of melanocytes. Instead, these represent proliferations of ectodermal origin that are classified based on their hyperplastic element. Keratinocytic lesions involve the epidermal layer only, whereas the organoid lesions involve the sebaceous, apocrine, eccrine, and follicular structures. These epidermal nevi are clinically distinct and appear as raised, pigmented, velvety to wart-like proliferations of the dermis along dermatomal distributions. Lesions are usually apparent in infancy, but some may appear in later childhood. The incidence in newborns is

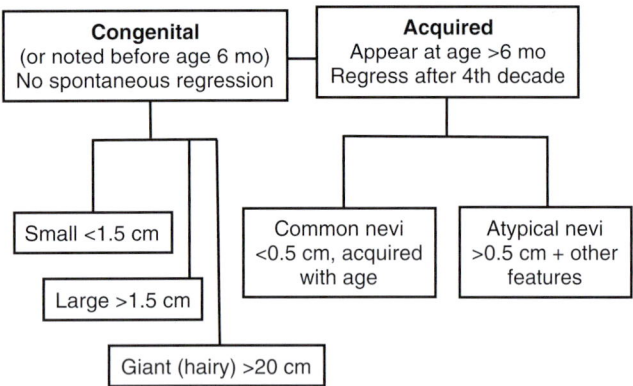

FIGURE 71-4 ■ Pigmented lesions are classified based on their age at appearance and further stratified by size and other physical features to yield two subsets that require close monitoring of the patient for the development of melanoma.

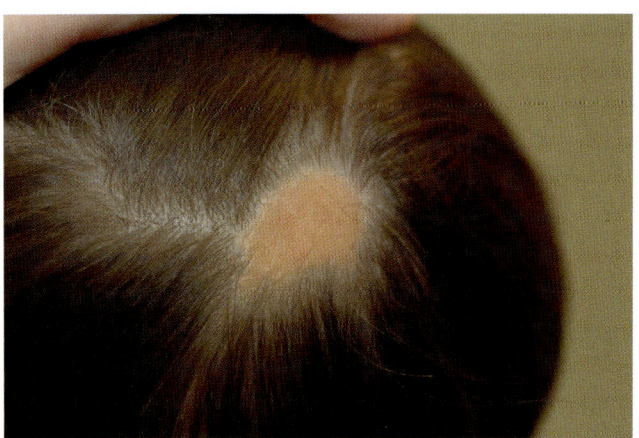

FIGURE 71-5 ■ This young child has the classic appearance of a nevus sebaceous, which is a solitary yellow-orange plaque on the scalp. These lesions are well circumscribed, hairless, oval to round, and usually less than 2–3 cm in diameter.

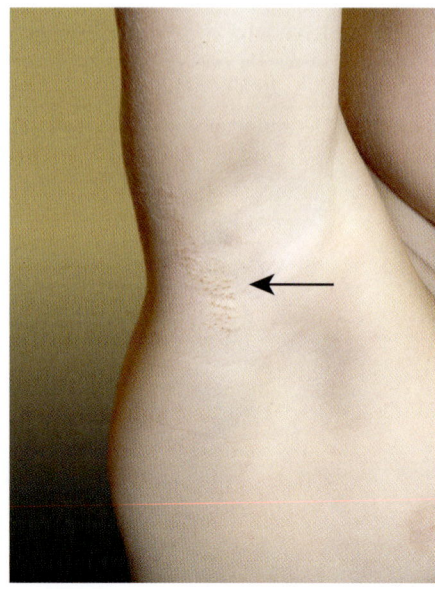

FIGURE 71-6 ■ In the right axilla of this 5-year-old is a nevus comedonicus (arrow). This lesion is a well-circumscribed plaque that is composed of keratin-plugged hair follicles. It was present at birth and has been slowly enlarging.

less than 1%. The most common sites involved are the scalp, face, trunk, and proximal extremities. Often a hairless patch is noted on the scalp or a raised linear yellow-tan to orange plaque is evident on the face or trunk during infancy. With age and the hormonal changes during puberty, these lesions change in appearance and become verrucous or develop more coarse hair growth. These progressive changes are what initiate the request for excision, along with the concern for potential malignant degeneration after puberty.

A number of syndromes are associated with these epidermal nevi, particularly when they are large or extensive. The epidermal nevus syndromes typically involve abnormalities of the central nervous system (CNS), ocular system, and skeletal system. While the classification of these lesions and syndromes is based on clinical findings, advances in molecular biology suggest that these disorders are based on genomic mosaicism and future biologic classification will become possible.[1] The common variants of epidermal nevi include the (1) nevus sebaceous (Fig. 71-5) that represent 50% of the epidermal nevi; (2) keratinocytic nevi; (3) nevus comedonicus (Fig. 71-6); (4), inflammatory linear verrucous nevus; (5) linear Cowden nevus; and (6) Becker's nevus (pigmented hairy epidermal

nevus). Table 71-3 summarizes their clinical and histological features.

These lesions are associated with a risk for transformation. The most common association is between nevus sebaceous and basal cell carcinoma (BCC), and this risk of transformation is believed to be based on shared deletions within the PTCH tumor suppressor gene. This natural history has formed the basis for current recommendations for excision prior to adolescence. A recent review by Rosen et al. suggests that the incidence of carcinoma may be less than previously reported as the demographic features of prior reports focused on predominantly adult populations.[2] In this study, the mean age was 7.2 years (range 0.3–54 years). Six hundred fifty-one epidermal lesions in 631 patients were evaluated for the presence of a second intralesional diagnosis. Five patients had BCC (0.8%) and 1.1% had syringocystadenoma papilliferum. The mean age of BCC diagnosis was 12.5 years (range 9.7–17.4 years). On the basis of this finding of occasional prepubertal malignant degeneration, the authors advise individual counseling with patients and their families, informing them of the extent of resection and reconstruction techniques that may be required. The scalp pliability of the young child may also offer advantages and opportunities that must be taken into consideration when cosmetic concerns outweigh the concerns for malignant transformation. Certainly there is no scientific basis for suggesting an intervention to avoid malignant degeneration in infancy and early childhood.

MELANOCYTIC NEVI

Congenital Nevi

CMN are pigmented lesions of variable size that develop during the first few months of life. They are the

TABLE 71-3   Characteristics of Epidermal Nevus Variants

Primary Name	Other Names	Cutaneous Features	Histologic Features	Other Features or Associations
Linear sebaceous nevus (LSN)	Nevus sebaceous, organoid nevus, Jadassohn nevus, phakomatosis	Yellowish orange plaque, affects scalp and face, hairless, 2–3 cm diameter	Epidermal, follicular, sebaceous and apocrine abnormalities	Epidermal nevus syndrome with seizures, CNS and ocular anomalies
Linear nevus comedonicus (NC)	Comedone nevus, nevus follicularis	Firm dark papules that look like comedones in linear pattern	Keratin-plugged hair follicles	Cataracts, variable CNS and bony defects (e.g., scoliosis, fused vertebrae, spina bifida occulta, absent fifth finger)
Linear epidermal nevus (LEN)	Nonorganoid epidermal nevus	Verrucous, nonerythematous, nonpruritic hyperkeratosis	Keratinocytic changes only	Significant involvement of other organ systems, neurodevelopmental delay, seizures, movement disorders
Inflammatory linear verrucous epidermal nevus (ILVEN)	Psoriasiform hyperplasia	Linear persistent pruritic plaque, usually on limb, tends to coalesce as linear formation	Inflammatory infiltrate, hyperkeratosis	Pruritic, female predominance 4:1, uncommon musculoskeletal associations
Linear Cowden nevus	Nonorganoid epidermal nevus	Thick linear lesion	Papillomatous	Cowden disease (germline PTEN mutation)

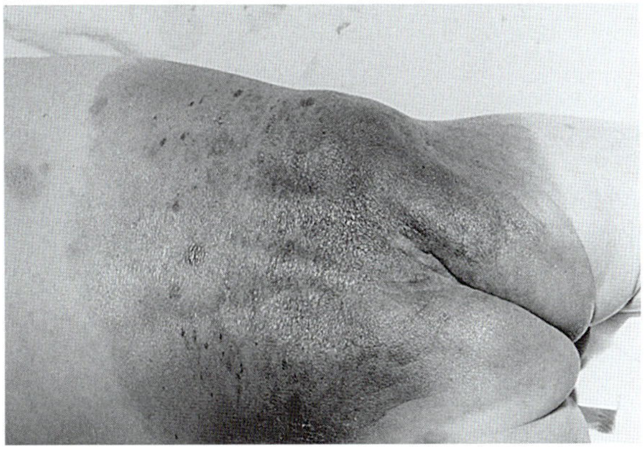

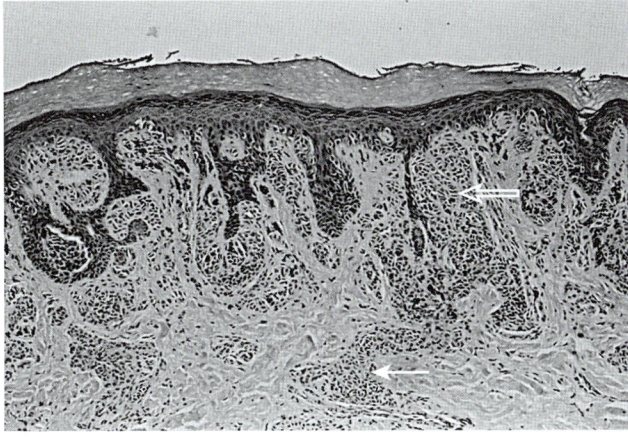

FIGURE 71-7 ■ Giant congenital melanocytic nevus (garment nevus) of the back and buttock in a neonate.

FIGURE 71-8 ■ Congenital melanocytic nevus is characterized by nevus cells extending from the dermal–epidermal junction (open arrow) along skin appendage structures into the deep dermis (solid arrow).

consequence of failure of melanocytic migration into the epidermis. These lesions grow proportionally with the infant and are generally categorized as small (<1.5 cm), medium (1.5–20 cm), and large (>20 cm). Those especially large lesions (>40 cm) are also referred to as a garment nevus, giant hairy nevus, or bathing trunk nevus since they tend to cover large truncal areas in confluence (Fig. 71-7). Although the pigmentation and surface are initially uniform and flat, the lesions evolve into thick, dark, and often hair-covered lesions. Histologically, the melanocytic cells in congenital nevi are located deeper than in acquired nevi (Fig. 71-8). The absence of superficial involvement may explain why transformation is often not noticed until late in its development. The incidence of transformation is greatest in the large or giant congenital nevi, and low in small to medium size lesions. The size of the congenital nevus therefore becomes the key element in discussing management.

Excision of small and medium CMN can be delayed or avoided in favor of lifelong observation. The estimated lifetime risk of melanoma in these lesions is estimated at 1%, and most occur after puberty. Biopsy may be of value in stratifying the risk of malignant degeneration. If histological examination shows the more superficial variant, continued observation is warranted, since any transformation is likely to be associated with epidermal changes that will be apparent on close follow-up or self-examination. If the histological variant demonstrates deep melanocytes, then prophylactic excision is recommended.

The management of large or giant CMN is more controversial. The melanoma risk for these lesions is increased and estimated to be 5–10% over a lifetime with 50% of this risk during the first five years of life.[3,4] The highest risk lesions are associated with the nevus that is situated over the posterior trunk, greater than 40 cm in maximal dimension, and associated with satellite nevi. Melanoma in these patients can arise from the deep dermal layer or even originate from sites distant from the skin such as the CNS (2.3% in one study[5]) or retroperitoneum.[4] These patients are also at risk for neurocutaneous melanosis (7% in one study[5]) and CNS malformations such as Dandy–Walker malformation, defects of the vertebra, skull, and intraspinal lipomas. Screening MRI of the brain and spinal cord is recommended during first six months of life in these patients.[5] Conversely, two-thirds of patients with neurocutaneous melanosis have giant CMN and the others have multiple nongiant lesions. The prognosis for patients with symptomatic neurocutaneous melanosis is extremely poor even in the absence of malignancy.[6] The increased routine surveillance with MRI during infancy for children with large CMN has identified those with asymptomatic CNS involvement, and hopefully will impact the care and outcome of these patients in a positive manner. These patients are also at risk for other soft tissue malignancies such as rhabdomyosarcoma[7] or neurofibrosarcoma (peripheral nerve sheath tumor).

Since operative resection of these extensive lesions is often not feasible and never completely eliminates the risk for melanoma, these patients need close medical surveillance. Areas of epidermal change within the nevus should be biopsied. However, caution must be exercised in interpreting the histological results, since the proliferative nodules may resemble melanoma, but behave in a benign manner.[8] Features useful in differentiating a cellular nodule from melanoma include: (1) lack of high grade uniform cellular atypia; (2) lack of necrosis within the nodule; (3) rarity of mitoses: (4) evidence of maturation; (5) lack of pagetoid spread; and (6) no destructive expansile growth.[9]

When operative intervention is needed, collaboration with colleagues with added expertise in the use of tissue expanders, rotational flaps, and skin grafting may be helpful. In one study, the mean age for intervention was 5.1 years and took an average 1.3 years to complete resection and reconstruction in these patients with large and giant CMN.[10] While the authors expressed a preference for earlier intervention, they acknowledged that the average age of the patients referred to them was 4.7 years, and many had already undergone an operative procedure. Over half of the cohort required more than one operative intervention and 22 of 40 patients needed skin grafts. Also, 18 patients benefitted from tissue expanders and autologous cultured skin replacements.

Acquired Nevi

Acquired nevi are benign neoplasms of the skin which appear after 6 months of age and persist through the fourth decade, after which many disappear. They are most frequently located on sun-exposed areas and are rare on the breast or buttock. Common to all these acquired nevi is that they are less than 6–8 mm in diameter, symmetric in shape, have a homogeneous surface and even pigmentation, and have a regular outline with a sharply demarcated border. On close inspection, they may have some pigmentary stippling.

Histologically, these acquired melanocytic nevi are divided into subtypes based on the location of the nests of nevus cells, and this feature corresponds with certain clinical findings (see Table 71-2). Junctional nevi tend to be flat with brown/black pigmentation and the nevus cells are located at the dermal–epidermal junction. When the nevus cells extend from the junction into the dermis, the lesion is described as a compound nevus. Clinically, this corresponds to a lesion that is slightly raised and pigmented brown/black. When the nevus cells migrate completely into the dermis, the lesion is an intradermal nevus, which is raised and typically not pigmented. In general, the deeper the nests of nevus cells, the more raised and less pigmented the lesion. (i.e., dark flat lesions vs raised tan lesions). The temporal evolutionary path of nevi was originally described by Stegmaier and explains the clinical observations of progressive change within individual nevi or their resolution.[11] Newer nevi tend to be small and flat (junctional), and either develop a raised profile or disappear with time as a consequence of fibrosis. In one study, when the nevi on adolescents were followed over a 4-year period, there was a net increase of 50% in total number of nevi, despite a complete regression in 15%.[12] This demonstrates the potential for active turnover in individual patients. Freckling and lighter colored skin are associated with increased numbers of nevi. In darker skinned individuals, nevi also develop, but are usually found on the palms and soles, unlike in the more fair complexioned individuals.

Sun exposure during childhood, especially when it is intense, intermittent, and not necessarily associated with sunburn, is a promoter for nevus development, and is the major environmental factor associated with the risk of melanoma. Recent evidence suggests that sunscreen use has led to a false sense of security in that it provides incomplete protection to UV rays.[13] Sunscreen alone does not provide sufficient protection. Public health education must focus on the avoidance of midday sun and the use of physical barriers such as UV protectant clothing and hats.[13–16]

The role for excision of these acquired nevi is limited when they are clearly defined by their age at presentation and the features described in Table 71-2. The natural evolution and changes in these common lesions should not be mistaken for malignant progression.

Atypical Nevi

Atypical nevi, previously referred to as dysplastic nevi or Clark's nevi, are common lesions found in 5% of the population, and may occur either sporadically or in a familial pattern (Fig. 71-9). The onset of their first appearance is usually during adolescence on the sun-exposed areas of skin, and they continue to increase in number and size with age. Unlike the common acquired nevi, these lesions are usually larger than 5 mm (up to 15 mm), and have an irregular surface ranging from completely flat to flat with a raised center resembling a fried egg. The pigmentation usually is dark and irregular, and the border of the lesion is often irregular as well. These lesions are most common in persons with light skin and hair color. Ultraviolet light has been implicated in the transformation of melanocytes in these nevi.

When a patient has multiple atypical nevi or moles, they may be diagnosed with the atypical mole syndrome. While it can be normal to have up to 10 to 20 nevi, people with this syndrome may have in excess of 100 moles. Individuals with 50–100 nevi and one or more first- or second-degree relatives with melanoma are considered to have the familial atypical mole and melanoma (FAMM) syndrome that identifies them at significantly increased risk (approaching 100%) for the development of melanoma. It is important to note that the melanoma may arise de novo on any part of the body and not necessarily from a preexisting atypical lesion. Simple excision of an atypical nevus therefore does not obviate the patient from close dermatologic follow-up. In families with the FAMM syndrome, nevi arising on the scalp can be an early predictor for this syndrome, although the scalp nevus itself may involute with time. In these individuals, the nevi tend to be similar in appearance, the corollary being that a new nevus that varies in appearance or location should be regarded with suspicion. The ability of clinical health care providers as well as nonclinicians to identify the 'ugly duckling' has been found to be reliable.[17] Routine surveillance examinations with photo documentation are recommended with dermoscopic (epiluminescence microscopy) evaluation of those nevi undergoing significant change. Dermoscopy has been shown to improve sensitivity and specificity with regard to detecting melanoma.[18]

Atypical nevi are not necessarily removed to confirm the histological pattern of atypia, but should be biopsied when melanoma is suspected. The biopsy should encompass a 1–2 mm rim of normal tissue and be sufficiently deep to allow to assess the depth of invasion in the event that melanoma is identified. The original designation of dysplastic nevus has been replaced with the term atypical nevus, and the pathologic description currently should use the term 'nevus with architectural disorder' and indicate the extent of cytologic atypia. The concordance between clinically atypical nevi and the histological findings of dysplasia is poor. These lesions are at the heart of

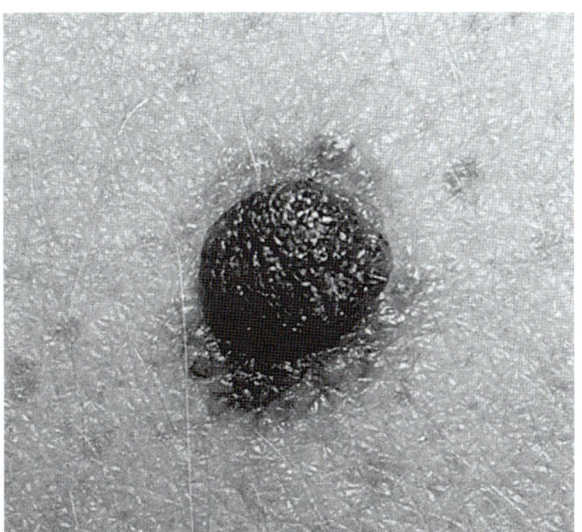

FIGURE 71-9 ■ Clark's nevus (dysplastic nevus) with 'fried egg' appearance.

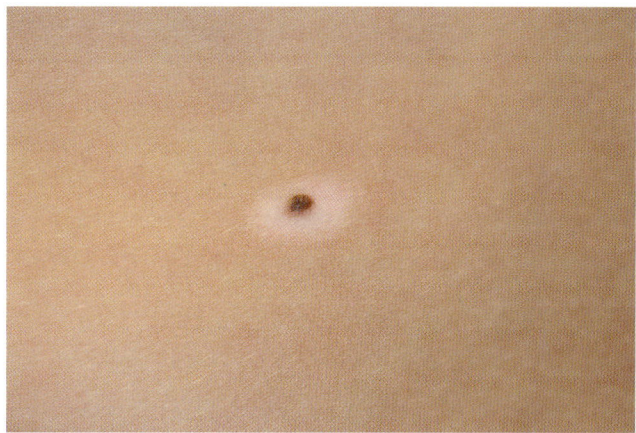

FIGURE 71-10 ■ The classic appearance of a halo nevus. These small pigmented lesions are surrounded by a rim of hypopigmentation. They are typically seen in adolescents and are most commonly located over the trunk, especially on the back. Treatment is usually not needed unless the pigmented portion of the halo nevus appears atypical. In that case, excision of the entire lesion, including the halo, is recommended.

much of the unfortunate controversy and misinformation that surrounds patients and referring physicians with terms and descriptions of atypia and dysplasia. These descriptive features have led to inappropriate re-excision of some lesions, and have even prompted sentinel lymph node biopsies for a completely benign process. Expert dermatopathologic review is essential for achieving the best care.

Specific Congenital or Acquired Melanocytic Lesions Requiring Distinction from Melanoma

Several melanocytic nevi are discussed separately due to their unique features, which frequently prompt their evaluation for malignancy. These lesions can be congenital or acquired, and are described in terms of their junctional, compound, or dermal location (Table 71-4). A recent review by Schaffer provides some practical advice regarding these specific lesions.[13]

Halo nevi (Sutton's nevi) are unique lesions which appear between 6–15 years of age, and are typically located on the trunk or extremities. They appear as round or oval lesions, with a central area of pigmentation that may be tan to brown in color, and are surrounded by a rim of depigmentation (Fig. 71-10). Histologically, the central nevus is usually a compound or dermal nevus surrounded by a uniform infiltrate of T-lymphocytes. Pigmentation can be intermittent. Excision is limited to those that develop atypical characteristics within the pigmented part. There is no association with malignancy. These nevi cause clinical suspicion only because regressing melanoma may be gray or white.

A blue nevus is a benign proliferation of dendritic dermal melanocytes. Its etiology is attributed to a dermal arrest in embryonic migration of neural crest melanocytes that fail to reach the epidermis and thus create a hamartoma. This is a lesion with a large amount of pigment within the dermis, resulting in absorption of

TABLE 71-4   General Guidelines for Excision of Congenital and Acquired Lesions

Type of Lesion	Age at Presentation, Site	Configuration, Size, Surface	Pigmentation	Biopsy Indication
Common acquired	After age 6 months	Small (<5 mm) flat	Brown-black	None
Atypical nevus	Usually adolescence; sun-exposed areas	Irregular, 5–15 mm Uneven, maculopapular 'fried egg'	Uneven, dark	Acute change[a]
Blue nevus	Any time; on scalp, dorsum of hands/feet	Nodular, <5 mm smooth	Dark gray to blue-black	None
Cellular blue nevus	Scalp, sacrum, buttock, face	5–15 mm	Dark gray to blue-black	Acute change[a]
Spitz nevus	Face, lower extremities	Dome shaped, 5–15 mm, smooth to warty	Light tan to pink, telangiectasia	Acute change[a]
Halo nevus	6–15 years; back	Central nevus with halo of depigmentation, flat to slightly raised	Area of depigmentation	Acute change in center of lesion[a]
Becker's nevus	Adolescent male; shoulder	Variable shape, flat	Brown macule or patch of hair	Acute change[a]

[a]Based on clinical behavior.

longer wavelengths of light and scattering of blue light known as the Tyndall effect. Two variants of blue nevi are distinguished based on their size: (1) the common blue nevus is usually less than 5 mm; and (2) the cellular blue nevus measures 1–3 cm.

The common blue nevus appears in adolescence and is most often located on the head and neck, the sacrum, and the dorsal aspect of the hands and feet. Given their dermal location, these lesions are usually nodular, and can be mistaken for nodular melanoma, except that there will be no precedent history of rapid growth. Dermatoscopy shows a uniform blue-gray pigment profile that helps distinguish the blue nevus from melanoma.

The cellular blue nevus usually presents on the scalp, buttock, sacrum, and face. It may be congenital or acquired. Histologically, it is located within the deep (reticular) dermis, and is a well-demarcated nodule. Cellular lesions may have occasional mitoses, but significant atypia and necrosis are absent. A potential for malignant degeneration exists only in these cellular lesions, and is clinically heralded by increase in size and ulceration.

The presence of multiple blue nevi should prompt consideration for the Carney complex of myxomas, spotty pigmentation, and endocrine neoplasias. The persistence of extensive dermal melanoses such as those found in Mongolian spots, especially when in a ventral distribution, should prompt evaluation for lysosomal storage diseases such as Hurler syndrome and GM1 gangliosidosis.

Spitz nevi are raised, often light or nonpigmented lesions (light tan-red or reddish-brown) that appear dome-shaped with either a smooth or a verrucous surface (Fig. 71-11). Histologically, these lesions are compound nevi, although pure junctional and pure dermal variants exist as well. Dermatoscopic examination shows a starburst pattern (Fig. 71-12). These lesions tend to occur on the face or lower extremities, and measure 0.3–1.5 cm in diameter. There is a slight female preponderance with 50% of these occurring in children under 10 years of age and 70% under 20 years of age. The increased red coloration is due in part to increased vascularity, with

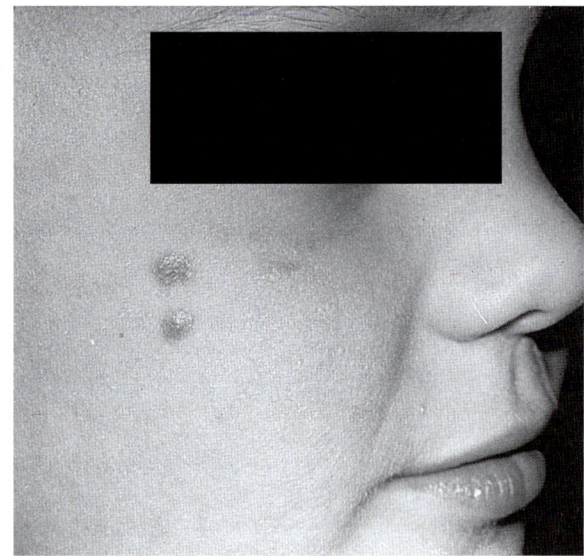

FIGURE 71-11 ■ Two Spitz nevi on the face.

telangiectasia in the superficial dermis. The vascular surface features explain why these lesions are more prone to bleeding with minimal trauma.

The pigmented variant of the Spitz nevus is known as a nevus of Reed, and typically occurs on the leg of a young woman. The appearance of Spitz nevi may be quite sudden, prompting the concern for potential melanoma. Spitz nevi were previously classified as 'benign juvenile melanoma,' a misnomer which was responsible for the misconception that pediatric melanoma was less aggressive than the adult melanoma counterpart. Most Spitz nevi are completely benign; however, atypical clinical features such as a diameter greater than 1 cm, asymmetry, or ulceration should prompt complete excision. Most often, a young patient who has undergone a shave biopsy is referred for complete excision of the lesion so that it may be fully evaluated by a dermatopathologist. One must remember that one pitfall of a shave biopsy is that the most atypical portion of the lesion is examined

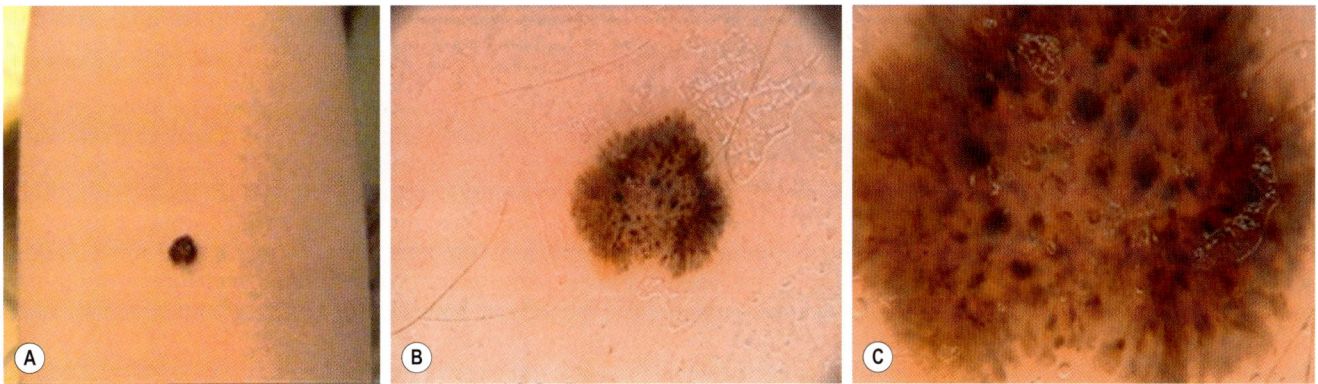

FIGURE 71-12 ■ This patient has a Spitz nevus on her arm. Dermatoscopic examination shows a classic starburst pattern. (Photographs courtesy of Dr. Eric Ehrsam. Reprinted with permission.)

and may incorrectly reflect the overall nature of the lesion. There is a spectrum of lesions from the benign Spitz nevus to the spitzoid melanoma. Those intermediate lesions with atypical histologic features have become the center of much controversy, and are often referred to as melanocytic or spitzoid tumor of uncertain malignant potential.

The clinical features of Spitz nevi can be complex, but they generally are reassuring when the lesion is uniform and symmetric. Histologically, the junctional nests of melanocytes have few or no mitoses. The nevus includes spindle cells and large epithelioid cells in variable architectural arrangements. Multinucleated cells may be present, but should not exhibit much pleomorphism. Nucleoli are often prominent and rounded. Some of these features in another clinical context could be reminiscent of melanoma, which requires that these lesions be evaluated by dermatopathologists with significant experience in all of the elements of this variant. Those Spitz lesions with unusual histological features should be excised completely.

In approximately 10% of all cases, histological features within these lesions do not permit distinction between a Spitz nevus and a spitzoid melanoma. These atypical Spitz nevi then become diagnostic and treatment dilemmas. In these complicated instances, one might consider the safest approach would be to treat the lesion as a melanoma equivalent of the same depth. Berk et al. have reviewed the Stanford experience regarding these lesions.[19] Although some surgeons have advocated for sentinel lymph node biopsy (SLNB) as a supplemental tool for categorizing the histologically indeterminate lesion, this approach has been strongly criticized as being unnecessarily invasive for the limited information gained. In the limited numbers of patients who underwent SLNB and were then treated with completion lymph node dissection (CLND) and chemotherapy, there was no disease recurrence.[20] Also, the current biologic and clinical evidence indicates that the presence of melanocytic lymphoid infiltrate does not predict clinical behavior, and may not even identify metastases or even malignancy as it does for melanoma.[21]

Several authors have recently reported their experience in the management of these confounding lesions. In a meta-analysis of 10 recently published series, 175 patients underwent SLNB and 67 were found to have positive SLN status (38%).[22] However, this relatively high incidence of SLN positivity does not provide the prognostic information that it does for adult melanoma, and seriously questions the overall utility of SLNB. This is further emphasized by Ghazi et al., who found that on a median follow-up of 56 months, 90% of their patients are free of recurrence.[23] They suggest that therapeutic SLND should be limited to those patients with clinically palpable nodes, and patients who have positive SLN should simply be monitored with ultrasound (US) for recurrence or progression rather than being subjected to CLND. Another group reported on their patients treated without SLNB. Twenty-nine patients underwent resection of the primary lesion, and with a mean follow-up of 8.4 years (range 3.5–15.8 years), 14 had no recurrence.[24] An additional 10 patients had a shorter duration of follow-up (mean 2.8 years), and had no evidence of recurrence. Their recommendation for these atypical spitzoid tumors is excision with clear margins and careful clinical follow-up.

The nevus of Ito and nevus of Ota are congenital dermal melanocytic disorders that develop because of incomplete migration of melanocytes resulting in a hamartomatous lesion. These lesions are most commonly found in Asian populations. In the case of the nevus of Ota, the lesion appears along the distribution of the ophthalmic and maxillary branches of the trigeminal nerve on the face, and is evident as a blue-gray patch. These nevi may also involve the ocular and mucosal surfaces. The nevus of Ito involves pigmentation over the shoulder area and is often associated with a nevus of Ota. The pigmentation becomes more prominent with age and may be amenable to laser therapy.[25] Melanoma has been reported to arise infrequently in the nevus of Ota, but the association with glaucoma is important and should lead to ophthalmologic referral.[26]

Nevi Occurring at Special Sites

A number of nevi occur at sites that have been particularly concerning for melanoma. They are now referred to as 'lesions with site-related atypia that must be distinguished from their malignant counterpart'.[27] Atypical scalp nevi are a frequent cause for referral for excisional biopsy on the basis that they may be difficult to follow. They can also be markers for patients with the FAMM syndrome or dysplastic nevus syndrome. A recent observational study of 44 scalp lesions documented that they are morphologically active lesions during the childhood years, and suggested that the same principles for excision should apply as for other atypical nevi.[28]

Acral nevi are found on the palms and soles. Although they may exhibit linear streaks, they must be viewed with suspicion if they have mottled pigmentation and are greater than 7 mm.[29] Longitudinal melanonychia are pigmented streaks emanating from the nail matrix and can be a normal variant that is most frequently seen in darker skinned individuals. Dark bands and those lesions that are wider than 6 mm, or associated with nail dystrophy, or extending beyond the nail fold, should be biopsied to exclude melanoma.[30,31] On mucosal surfaces, distinction must be made between labial melanotic macules which are benign lesions on the lower lip of women that resemble freckles but do not darken with sun exposure, and more concerning lesions in the oral cavity.[32] In young women presenting with melanotic lesions over the vulvar area, it is important not to overtreat these generally benign lesions.[33]

PRACTICAL CONSIDERATIONS FOR EXCISION OR BIOPSY OF MELANOCYTIC LESIONS

The many major and minor differences in the clinical and pathologic features for the benign lesions discussed thus far have led to confusion about the role for excision of these lesions in infants and children. Pressure for excision from families and pediatricians can be significant and is often based on important but vague family histories of 'skin cancer.' Once referred to a pediatric surgeon, many patients and families expect that an excision will be performed rather than considering the office visit to be the start of what may be a period of observation and collaborative consultation with dermatologists and other physicians. Prior to the referral, the patients are often not informed about the relative risks and benefits of excision for a young patient who may require anesthesia or conscious sedation. Scarring is unpredictable and excision should not occur in the case of a benign lesion that does not have cosmetic consequences and has no future potential for transformation. The natural evolution of acquired lesions and the changes that occur with age, puberty, and exposure to UV radiation need to be considered, and clinical judgment and experience should guide decisions for resection. Scalp pliability and the tolerance for suture or staple removal from large scalp excisions need to be considered, and might lead to a delay in resection of larger lesions such as nevus sebaceous until around puberty. On the other hand, one cannot overlook the dangers of transformation during the first 5 years in infants with giant CMN. Staged resections and tension-relieving techniques must be factored as well as the use of techniques, such as tissue expansion and rotational flaps, for the best functional outcome and cosmesis.

Therefore, we have established general guidelines for excision of congenital and acquired lesions.

The Spitz nevi are often the most worrisome lesions because they can rapidly progress, and resemble a nodular melanoma. These temporal and physical characteristics along with their variable coloration often prompt biopsy. A shave biopsy demonstrating epithelioid and spindle features with or without atypia are common reasons for referral for complete excision with a 2 mm margin. Expert pathologic review must be available to differentiate them from melanoma and to avoid unnecessary SLNB in young patients.

PEDIATRIC MELANOMA

Melanoma remains a rare cancer in childhood, with children representing less than 2% of all patients with melanoma.[34] There has been a worldwide doubling in the number of melanoma cases in adults over a period of 25 years with age-standardized incidences now at 15 per 100,000/year and 22 per 100,000/year in men and women, respectively.[35] Pediatric melanoma has become more prevalent, but the rate of increase is not as dramatic and primarily affects the postpubertal age group. Current estimates show an annual incidence of 0.8/million in the first decade of life. Melanoma becomes an increasingly prevalent neoplasm with age. In patients cohorted by age <15years, 15–19 years and 20–24 years, melanoma contributes to 1%, 7% and 12%, respectively, of all malignancies in each category.[36] The highest rates are reported from Australia and New Zealand where melanoma affects 30/million in the 10–14 year age group.[37] Regardless of geographic factors, these data are indicative of a dramatic increase in the lifetime risk of cutaneous melanoma for children born today (1/58 as compared to 1/250 in 1980).[38]

Fortunately, there has also been a leveling off in the mortality associated with melanoma. The identification of patients at risk has allowed for improved surveillance. This has presumably resulted in improved early detection, with 90% of new diagnoses involving thin, less than 1 mm melanomas. Some of this improvement in early diagnosis can be linked to the use of dermoscopy[39] and computer-based dermoscopy in differentiating between small melanomas and atypical moles.[40]

The known melanoma risk factors are both environmental as well as heritable. Although melanoma is not limited to Caucasians, evidence has shown that the melanoma risk is associated with fair complexion, the presence of freckles and moles, and intermittent intense sun exposure, even in the absence of severe sunburns. While patients with large CMN are at risk early in life, those patients with the atypical mole syndrome and FAMM syndrome must undergo careful clinical surveillance at all ages. The most important factor for the development of melanoma is the presence of melanocytic nevi, with an eightfold increase in relative risk for those with greater than 100 moles.[35] If a person has five or more atypical nevi, he/she has a nearly 50-fold risk of developing melanoma. If a family history of melanoma is present, the incidence approaches 100%. Recent studies based on genetic analysis of families with mutations in the melanoma predisposition gene CDKN2A suggest that the FAMM syndrome has a 70% lifetime penetrance of melanoma with sun exposure. Mutations in the melanocortin-1 receptor further impact the development of melanoma.[41,42]

It is critical to understand that most (80%) lesions arise de novo and not from preexisting lesions. For example, in a series of 33 prepubertal patients with melanoma, seven cases arose from nongiant CMN, two from an acquired nevus, and 24 (73%) de novo.[34] Whereas genetic factors and pigment traits contribute to the development of nevi, the only controllable factor for melanoma is the cumulative environmental effects of sun exposure. These sun factors are best limited with physical barriers such as clothing and hats, and avoidance of the midday sun. The use of sunscreen appears to be principally effective in preventing sunburn. Blistering sunburns during childhood and adolescence have been implicated in the development of melanoma.[15]

The demographics of pediatric cutaneous melanoma are well described in an extensive review that compares their experience with 137 patients to other published series.[43] The authors found that gender neither predisposed nor conferred a measurable survival advantage for melanoma. As noted earlier, the incidence escalates with age and the relevant cutoff appears to be the transition between prepubertal and pubertal patients, which normative data suggests is around 10 years of age. Postpubertal patients have a higher mortality from melanoma. The rate in 15–19-year-olds is estimated to be eight- to 18-fold higher when compared to their younger counterparts. Site of involvement is variably reported as extremities > trunk > head and neck. It is not clear that this has prognostic implications, except that head and neck lesions are perhaps more difficult to treat, which has given them the reputation for a less favorable prognosis.

The extent of disease is localized in most pediatric patients (>80%), while 10–15% may have nodal involvement, and 1–3% will present with metastases to distant sites including lung, liver, LN, subcutaneous tissues, and brain.[44]

Specific Predisposing Conditions for Pediatric Melanoma

The diagnosis of melanoma is made in children in several discrete clinical contexts. Congenital melanoma is the least common, and is associated with transplacental transmission. It also may arise from a primary cutaneous lesion. The appearance of any rapidly growing, ulcerating, or bleeding lesion in the newborn should be evaluated promptly. However, the incidence of this clinical scenario is so low that projections about outcome are difficult to estimate, but the prognosis is generally poor. Confounding variables include reports of spontaneous regression and the presence of micrometastases that do not appear to correlate with survival.[8,45]

Melanoma associated with CMN has been well described and presents a unique set of clinical issues (Fig. 71-13). The lifetime risk for development of melanoma in patients with CMN is variably estimated between

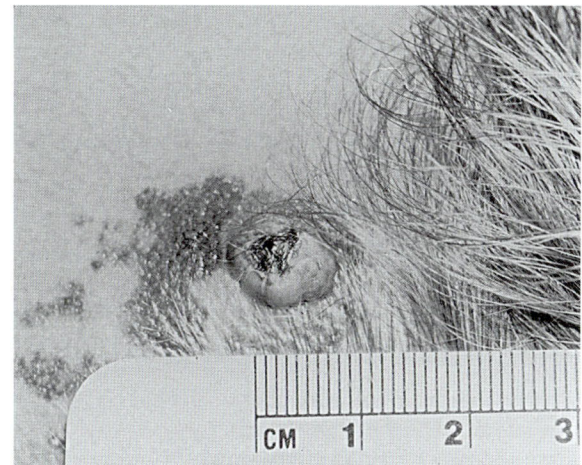

FIGURE 71-13 ■ Congenital melanocytic nevus of the scalp with a melanoma arising from it (raised centrally pigmented lesion).

5–40%.[46] More conservative estimates indicate a 5–10% lifetime risk, with half of this risk distributed within the first five years of life.[3,47] Two recent prospective studies of patients with giant CMN showed the incidence of melanoma during the first five years of life was between 3.3–4.5%.[48,49] Those patients with a posterior axial location and numerous satellite lesions have the greatest risk as compared to those with lesions restricted to the head and extremities.[13]

These tumors may originate from deep dermal sites and are often not visually apparent. Despite the sometimes ominous appearance of the satellite lesions, these have not been documented as the primary site for melanoma. Proliferative nodules within giant CMN often raise the specter of malignancy, but numerous authors caution against hasty conclusions in this clinical scenario.[8,50] Neurocutaneous melanosis occurs in conjunction with large CMN and is the most common cause for nonepithelial melanoma. Although techniques for resection and reconstruction have improved such that disfigurement can often be avoided, these remain challenging operations. Moreover, there is no assurance in alleviating this risk for nonepithelial melanoma despite full-thickness removal of the CMN. In contrast, the smallest (less than 1.5 cm) CMN lesions are not associated with any increased risk for melanoma. It is within the intermediate group that little data exist to help guide management. At Massachusetts General Hospital, CMN lesions up to 5 cm have not been associated with melanoma in patients under 20 years of age.[46] Illig et al. reported melanoma arising in CMN lesions less than 10 cm only after 18 years of age.[51] Rhodes and Melski calculated a lifetime risk of 2.5–5.0% in persons with small CMN living to 60 years of age.[52]

While large and perhaps some intermediate-sized CMN help identify patients at risk for the development of melanoma, radical excisional therapy can be tempered by the recognition that cautious observation and selective biopsy can be an alternative therapy, especially since the melanoma can arise from sites other than the CMN. When resection is considered, preoperative planning allows for the optimal use of reconstructive techniques including skin and tissue expanders and a variety of rotational flaps or free tissue transfers in addition to skin grafts.

Other conditions predisposing to melanoma include patients with xeroderma pigmentosum in whom the inability to repair UV induced DNA damage results in a 2000-fold increased risk of skin cancer.[53] Patients with genetic immunodeficiency syndromes are reported to have a three- to sixfold increased risk.[54] Children on chemotherapy for childhood malignancies or children undergoing solid organ transplantation experience an increase in total nevi counts as well as the induction of atypical nevi.[55] Although neonatal phototherapy for hyperbilirubinemia has been demonstrated to induce an increased number of nevi, it is uncertain whether this will escalate the risk for future melanoma.[56] Unfortunately, it is important to remember that 60–80% of malignant melanoma in patients under 20 years of age occurs in the absence of known cutaneous risk factors.[54]

Diagnosis

The difficulty in making the diagnosis of melanoma during childhood relates to a number of variables. The natural evolution of congenital and acquired nevi during childhood and adolescence often limits the effectiveness of adult data. Also, there is limited value to the mnemonic ABCDE (*a*symmetry, *b*order irregularity, *c*olor variegation, lesion *d*iameter greater than 6 mm and *e*volution) (Fig. 71-14) for a pigmented lesion since variegations and irregular shape are frequently associated with an atypical nevus. Specifically, the physical characteristics of giant CMN that predispose to melanoma arise in the deep dermal layers and extend within the deep subcutaneous tissues, rather than becoming apparent externally. Consequently, childhood melanoma may present in a markedly different manner from its adult counterpart. Recent growth, ulceration, or bleeding may be the most frequent presenting features. In contrast to the adult experience with thin (less than 1 mm) melanomas, pediatric melanomas are typically greater than 1.5 mm in thickness. This

may be due to delays in diagnosis, a deeper origin within a CMN, and a higher incidence of nodular melanomas in children.[38] In one series of melanoma in children, the most common presenting symptoms were recent growth, pain, ulceration, itching, bleeding, and change in color in the lesion.[57] In the 13 patients, three had lesions that resembled pyogenic granuloma. Only one patient presented with evidence of metastatic disease. Eleven of 13 were nodular and only two were superficial spreading. The mean tumor thickness was 3.2 mm in this series.

In a series in children under age 12 years, the clinical parameters that favored melanoma were a rapid increase in size (55% of patients), bleeding (35%), or color change (23%) of a nodular lesion.[54] Less frequent signs or symptoms included a subcutaneous mass (6%), pruritis (15%), and enlargement of a regional LN (7%). In 7% of the patients where a melanoma developed in association with a preexisting nevus, the patients had no clinical symptoms.

A study of 33 prepubertal patients attempted to delineate the clinical features and outcomes of pediatric melanoma.[31] In this series, the sites of origin were most frequently the extremity (*n* = 15), trunk (*n* = 10), and head or neck (*n* = 8). Interestingly, 14 of 28 patients had amelanotic lesions and the majority of lesions were raised and resembled pyogenic granuloma.[34] Superficial spreading (*n* = 15) and the nodular melanoma subtypes (*n* = 9) were the most common lesions. The median lesional thickness was 2.5 mm.

The consistently thicker lesions in childhood melanoma suggest either a delay in diagnosis or reflect biologic characteristics such as the propensity for nodular melanoma and for lesions to arise from the deep dermal layers. Unfortunately, these lesions may be misdiagnosed initially. Only their sudden appearance and rapid growth over a few months may prompt biopsy. Therefore, despite the infrequency of this diagnosis, the clinician must consider melanoma in the differential diagnosis of cutaneous lesions in children.

The roles of clinical dermatoscopy, computer dermatoscopy (digital epiluminesence microscopy), and ultrasound imaging of the skin have been described for monitoring high risk adult patients.[39,58–60] However, there are no current reports focusing on children.

SURGICAL MANAGEMENT OF THE LESION SUSPECTED TO BE MELANOMA

Once a decision has been made to evaluate a cutaneous lesion for possible malignancy, the aim is to accomplish this with the least negative impact on function and cosmesis. The clinical scenarios most often encountered are: (1) a primary referral for excision of a suspicious lesion; (2) re-excision of a lesion that was previously incompletely excised and showed atypia; and (3) re-excision of a lesion with dysplastic and potentially malignant features.

In these instances, most young children benefit from an excision under general anesthesia which allows the surgeon to focus on a full-thickness biopsy with an adequate margin. When the lesion is being excised for the

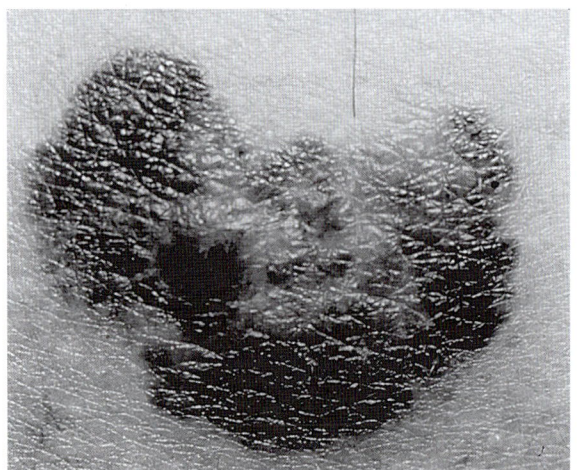

FIGURE 71-14 ■ This malignant melanoma demonstrates some of the classic ABCD features for melanoma: *a*symmetry, *b*order irregularity, *c*olor variegation, and *d*iameter greater than 6 mm.

first time or re-excised for atypia, it is reasonable to target a 1–2 mm circumferential margin. However, there are no prospective data to provide evidence-based recommendations. In the setting of dysplastic changes or frank malignancy, the parameters set forth by the American Joint Committee on Cancer (AJCC) for melanoma should guide the resection based on the Breslow stage and Clark's level (Table 71-5). A shave biopsy of such a lesion may not provide sufficient data and excision with an adequate 1–2 cm margin is recommended. It is in these settings that a discussion must be held with the family regarding the option for proceeding with SLNB under the same anesthetic, if appropriate.

It is important to assess the potential for primary closure after excision at the time of the preoperative visit. Lesions over joints, on the distal extremities, and on the face require consideration of more advanced techniques such as tension-relieving plasties, skin grafts, and rotational flaps. Despite the anxiety about a potential tumor, parents must understand that healing and scarring can be unpredictable. The best results for achieving adequate margins are obtained by marking and measuring the margins along the periphery of the lesion while it is in situ. The orientation of the incision depends on the location of the lesion and its relationship to Langer lines. Consideration should be given to the potential need for re-excision as well. Sharp excision of the marked skin perimeter limits coagulation artifact and hemostasis can rapidly be achieved along the retained skin border. The deeper tissues can be excised with electrocautery to limit bleeding. Any suspicious lesion should be marked for orientation in the event that re-excision becomes necessary. Specimens should be submitted for permanent section as frozen section has no role in this setting. Techniques for skin closure require consideration of the physical characteristics of the incision as well as on the tolerance of the child for suture removal. The use of long-acting local anesthetic agents such as bupivacaine should be encouraged for postoperative analgesia in combination with appropriate oral medications. With more extensive resections or resections across joints, immobilizing splints may be needed.

In the presence of established malignancy, a re-excision with margins may be needed. In the more common scenario of the histologic diagnosis of an atypical nevus with dysplasia, the likelihood of malignant degeneration is low, and a conservative re-excision is advised. This topic is most controversial in the context of Spitz nevi with

cellular atypia. While most Spitz nevi can be histologically identified as benign lesions, many show atypical features that complicate their differentiation from melanoma. One set of authors have offered a well-designed proposal for the evaluation of pediatric patients with spitzoid melanocytic tumors where there is diagnostic controversy.[61] A recent publication affirms that SLNB, when applied to atypical melanocytic neoplasms, shows a 30% (seven of 24 patients) incidence of positivity in the absence of further LN involvement on CLND and no progression of disease.[62] While SLNB has been proposed as a means for differentiation between a benign and malignant lesion, it has limited effectiveness since the presence of melanocytic cells within a sentinel lymph node does not necessarily indicate the presence of a metastasis. The features of the melanocytic cell and its location within the lymph node may indicate that these are benign nodal melanocytes that arrived at draining nodes by lymphatic migration or formed in the nodes during development. However, even the presence of 'metastatic' cells in the sentinel lymph node does not appear to have the same biologic effect as they would in melanoma as the frequency of recurrent disease is virtually absent in the scenario of Spitz nevi with cellular atypia.

The collective experience from cancer centers offering SNLB for spitzoid melanocytic tumors have shown that the rates of 'positive nodes' range from 29–50%. A recent review indicated that 78% of the patients (*n* = 205) underwent SLNB and that 62 (39%) were found to have micrometastases, which then prompted >90% of these patients to undergo CLND with only 10% having additional positive nodes.[20] There have been no reported deaths of LN positive pediatric patients with primary Spitz tumors.

If controversy persists, then fluorescence in situ hybridization (FISH) or comparative genomic hybridization should be performed, and may lead to results that favor either a nevus or a melanoma.[63-66] At the same time, it is important to remember the lack of correlation with survival for indeterminate melanocytic lesions based on SLNB. There will always be a few cases where the long-term follow-up will be the most important concern, recalling that nodal melanocytes may not resolve the question for the family. The best clinical course is to avoid the trap to perform SLNB or falsely offer it as a clinical advantage in these difficult cases. In the absence of a clinical trial, the therapeutic role of SLNB in this population of patients with atypical spitzoid tumors is debatable.[67]

Management of Histologically Confirmed Melanoma

Staging and treatment protocols of histologically confirmed melanoma are derived from the adult literature. The recommendations for extent of re-excision are based on the thickness of the tumor and generally requires a 0.5 cm margin for in situ lesions, a margin of 1 cm for lesions up to 2 mm, and 2 cm margins for lesions greater than 2 mm in thickness. SLNB is advised for lesions thicker than 1mm or those between 0.76 mm and 1 mm

---

TABLE 71-5 American Joint Committee on Cancer Guidelines for Surgical Management of Melanoma

Lesion Depth	Margin (cm)	Sentinel Node Dissection
In situ	0.5	
<1 mm	1.0	
0.76–1.0 mm[a]	1.0	+
1–2 mm	1.0–2.0	+
>2 mm	2.0	+

[a]Only in the presence of ulceration or reticular dermal invasion.

with ulceration or reticular dermal invasion (see Table 71-5). The new AJCC staging system is primarily based on: (1) Breslow tumor thickness with 1 mm, 2 mm and 4 mm indicating the current cutoffs for thin, intermediate, and thick lesions; and (2) histological features such as ulceration which is perhaps most important in the intermediate thickness group. Clarke's levels are only taken into account in thin melanomas. Lymph node involvement is stratified by the number of nodes involved, and whether microscopic or macroscopic metastases are present. Finally, three subgroups of distant metastases are distinguished: (1) skin and soft tissue; (2) lung; (3) other visceral organs. Patients with visceral metastases have the worst prognosis. In this new classification, the serum LDH is used to further stratify risk. If elevation of the LDH is verified in the presence of either skin, soft tissue, or lung metastases, the prognosis is equivalent to that in patients with visceral metastases.[68]

The standard imaging techniques used to identify potential metastatic disease sites include computed tomography (CT), magnetic resonance imaging and positron emission tomography (PET). PET-CT has been approved for this use as it has been demonstrated to be particularly helpful in identifying developing metastases.[69] The limitations in PET scanning continue to relate to the size of the lesion, such that it cannot compete with lymph node biopsy for nonpalpable lymph nodes.[70]

The Role of SLNB

In adult melanoma therapy, SLNB has become a mandatory procedure in the current AJCC staging system to detect lymph node micrometastases. With a positive SLNB, the recommendation is to proceed with a CLND. A negative SLNB, however, does not guarantee lack of distant spread. It is evident that this algorithm protects against early locoregional recurrences, but does not have an impact on overall survival. These protocols have been applied to pediatric patients with melanoma and atypical melanocytic tumors. In one review, 20 patients under 21 years of age underwent SLNB for melanoma or atypical nevi.[71] No complications occurred as a result of the SLNB, and results showed that positivity correlated with tumor thickness. Five of 15 patients with melanoma had a positive SLNB as did three of five with melanocytic proliferation. Seven of eight patients underwent CLND (one patient with blue nevus did not). Complications such as lymphedema and wound infection occurred with the completion lymphadenectomy in four patients. When this was further explored in a subsequent study, the investigators found a higher incidence of positive SLNB in a group of patients younger than 20 years with either melanoma or melanocytic lesions (40%) as compared to a group of adults (18%).[72] None of the pediatric patients with a positive SLNB recurred while 25% of the adults did.

More recent series further document that positive SLNB is associated with a 10–15% of positive CLND and that the breakpoint in prognostic value appears to lie at puberty, with a higher incidence of SNLB in those <10years of age, but a worse prognosis for the older cohort.[43,73–75] These series and others suggest that while SLNB is feasible, it may not be of sufficient value or

benefit to the patient.[76] As in adults, SLNB provides prognostic value, but does not affect outcomes. Also, there is no survival benefit to immediate CLND vs. observation, and the morbidity of this second procedure must be considered carefully. The biological differences between pre-pubescent and older patients based on tumor thickness must somehow be related in part to local conditions including a relative difference in skin thickness, altered dermal immune reactivity, and perhaps altered lymphatic drainage thresholds.

Adjuvant therapies include chemotherapy, radiation therapy, and immunotherapy.[77] Despite the encouraging reports from the mid-1980s, the use of cytotoxic agents has a limited role in current adjuvant therapy. Combination protocols using cyclophosphamide, vincristine, and dactinomycin, or single agent dacarbazine and isolated regional perfusion with melphalan, were also reported to be effective, but did not provide for improved long-term outcomes. Radiation therapy has limited applicability and is primarily reserved for palliation. Most active trials and current research focus on immunomodulating agents, such as interleukin 2 (IL-2) and interferon alpha (IFN-α2b). In limited series, these agents have shown the ability to induce partial and even total remission.[77] The use of high dose IFN-α is limited to patients with high risk, resected tumors and involvement of the nodal basin. It appears that the early use of IFN-α contributes to improved relapse-free survival in these patients.[36] There have been conflicting reports about pediatric patients being able to tolerate high-dose interferon regimens. In one series, no dose reduction was necessary,[78] but was needed in 50% of patients in another series.[79] Vaccines have also been tried and consist of either polyvalent vaccines or defined melanoma antigens such as the ganglioside GM2, which is the most immunogenic ganglioside expressed on melanoma cells. More recent reports on the use of heat shock proteins as vehicles for the vaccines have been encouraging.[38,80] Further advances in our understanding of the germline and somatic mutations in melanoma are potential new therapeutic targets.[81]

OUTCOME AND PROGNOSIS

Statistics for pediatric specific studies on melanoma are limited. The most recent focused report from the National Cancer Institute (NCI) Surveillance, Epidemiology and End Results (SEER) database indicated that patients under 20 had an overall 5-year survival of 93.6%. The hazard ratio of death from melanoma increased for male gender, increased age, and more advanced disease as well as for location other than trunk or extremity.[82] This compares favorably with an older review which showed overall 5-year survival rates at 34% for stage 4 patients and as high as 90% for stage 1 and 2 patients.[83] The most important prognostic parameters remain thickness of tumor and the clinical stage of disease. There appears to be a biologic difference in prepubertal children as compared to adolescents, particularly when evaluating positive SLN status and tumor thickness, although this does not translate into a difference in overall survival and event-free survival.[43,84]

Postoperative follow-up is best performed under strict guidelines. Risk-adapted, scheduled follow-up examinations in the German protocols have been validated for 3-monthly intervals during the first 5 years and every 6 months for the next 5 years.[35] With this, 83% of all recurrences were identified on screening rather than by the patient (17%). Fifty per cent were detected sufficiently early that complete excision was possible. These authors further stratified risk by indicating that patients with thin melanoma lesions could undergo surveillance by physical examination rather than a technology-based system every 6 months. Those with lesions greater than 1mm thick should undergo lymph node ultrasound and determination of the S100 tumor marker protein.

Melanoma remains a challenge for diagnosis and treatment. With a concerted effort to study new modalities in the context of clinical trials, more advances in treatment will hopefully lead to improved outcomes for this rare, and sometimes lethal, cancer.

REFERENCES

1. Sugarman JL. Epidermal nevus syndromes. Semin Cutan Med Surg 2007;26:221–30.
2. Rosen H, Schmidt B, Lan HP, et al. Management of nevus sebaceous and the risk of basal cell carcinoma: An 18 year review. Pediatr Dermatol 2009;26:676–81.
3. Marghoob AA, Schoenbach SP, Kopf AW, et al. Large congenital melanocytic nevi and the risk for the development of malignant melanoma. A prospective study. Arch Dermatol 1996;132: 170–5.
4. Arneja JS, Gosain AK. Giant congenital melanocytic nevi. Plast Reconstr Surg 2007;120:26e–40e.
5. Ramaswamy V, Delaney H, Haque S, et al. Spectrum of central nervous system abnormalities in neurocutaneous melanocytosis. Dev Med Child Neurol 2012;54:563–8.
6. Di Rocco F, Sabatino G, Koutzoglou M, et al. Neurocutaneous melanosis. Childs Nerv Syst 2004;20:23–8.
7. Ilyas EN, Goldsmith K, Lintner R, et al. Rhabdomyosarcoma arising in a giant congenital melanocytic nevus. Cutis 2004;73: 39–43.
8. Leech SN, Bell H, Leonard N, et al. Neonatal giant congenital nevi with proliferative nodules: A clinicopathologic study and literature review of neonatal melanoma. Arch Dermatol 2004;140: 83–8.
9. Xu X, Bellucci KS, Elenitsas R, et al. Cellular nodules in congenital pattern nevi. J Cutan Pathol 2004;31:153–9.
10. Warner PM, Yakuboff KP, Kagan RJ, et al. An 18 year experience in the management of congenital nevomelanocytic nevi. Ann Plast Surg 2008;60:283–7.
11. Stegmaier OC. Natural regression of the melanocytic nevus. J Invest Dermatol 1959;32:413–21.
12. Siskind V, Darlington S, Green L, Green A. Evolution of melanocytic nevi on the faces and necks of adolescents: A 4-year longitudinal study. J Invest Dermatol 2002;118:500–4.
13. Schaffer JV. Pigmented lesions in children: When to worry. Curr Opin Pediatr 2007;19:430–40.
14. Harrison SL, Buettner PG, Maclennan R. The north Queensland 'sun-safe clothing' study: Design and baseline results of a randomized trial to determine the effectiveness of sun-protective clothing in preventing melanocytic nevi. Am J Epidemiol 2005 15; 161:536–45.
15. Holman CD, Armstrong BK. Cutaneous malignant melanoma and indicators of total accumulated exposure to the sun: An analysis separating histogenetic types. J Natl Cancer Inst 1984;73: 75–82.
16. Oliveria SA, Saraiya M, Geller AC, et al. Sun exposure and risk of melanoma. Arch Dis Child 2006;91:131–8.
17. Scope A, Dusza SW, Halpern AC, et al. The 'ugly duckling' sign: Agreement between observers. Arch Dermatol 2008;144:58–64.
18. Heliasos E, Kerner M, Jaimes N, et al. Dermoscopy for the pediatric dermatologist: Part III: Dermoscopy for melanocytic lesions. Pediatr Dermatol 2012;1–12. Epub ahead of print.
19. Berk DR, LaBuz E, Dadras SS, et al. Melanoma and melanocytic tumors of uncertain malignant potential in children and young adults- the Stanford experience 1995-2008. Pediatr Dermatol 2012;27:244–54.
20. Hill SJ, Delman KA. Pediatric melanomas and the atypical spitzoid melanocytic neoplasms. Am J Surg 2012;203:761–7.
21. Dahlstrom JE, Scolyer RA, Thompson JF, et al. Spitz naevus: Diagnostic problems and their management implications. Pathology 2004;36:452–7.
22. Luo S, Sepehr A, Tsao H. Spitz nevi and other spitzoid neoplasms. J AM Acad Dermatol 2011;65:1087–92.
23. Ghazi B, Carlson GW, Murray DR, et al. Utility of lymph node assessment for atypical melanocytic neoplasms. Ann Surg Oncol 2010;17:2471–5.
24. Cerrato F, Wallins JS, Webb ML, et al. Outcomes in pediatric atypical spitz tumors treated without sentinel lymph node biopsy. Pediatr Dermatol 2012;29:448–53.
25. Ferguson RE Jr, Vasconez HC. Laser treatment of congenital nevi. J Craniofac Surg 2005;16:908–14.
26. Harrison-Balestra C, Gugic D, Vincek V. Clinically distinct form of acquired dermal melanocytosis with review of published work. J Dermatol 2007;34:178–82.
27. Hosler GA, Moresi JM, Barrett TL. Nevi with site-related atypia: A review of melanocytic nevi with atypical histologic features based on anatomic site. J Cutan Pathol 2008;35:889–98.
28. Gupta M, Berk DR, Gray C, et al. Morphologic features and natural history of scalp nevi in children. Arch Dermatol 2010;146:506–11.
29. Saida T, Miyazaki A, Oguchi S, et al. Significance of dermoscopic patterns in detecting malignant melanoma on acral volar skin: Results of a multicenter study in Japan. Arch Dermatol 2004; 140:1233–8.
30. Braun RP, Baran R, Le Gal FA, et al. Diagnosis and management of nail pigmentations. J Am Acad Dermatol 2007;56:835–47.
31. Iorizzo M, Tosti A, Di Chiacchio N, et al. Nail melanoma in children: Differential diagnosis and management. Dermatol Surg 2008;34:974–8.
32. Buchner A, Merrell PW, Carpenter WM. Relative frequency of solitary melanocytic lesions of the oral mucosa. J Oral Pathol Med 2004;33:550–7.
33. Gleason BC, Hirsch MS, Nucci MR, et al. Atypical genital nevi. A clinicopathologic analysis of 56 cases. Am J Surg Pathol 2008;32: 51–7.
34. Ferrari A, Bono A, Baldi M, et al. Does melanoma behave differently in younger children than in adults? A retrospective study of 33 cases of childhood melanoma from a single institution. Pediatrics 2005;115:649–54.
35. Garbe C, Eigentler TK. Diagnosis and treatment of cutaneous melanoma: State of the art 2006. Melanoma Res 2007;17:117–27.
36. Neier M, Pappo A, Navid F. Management of melanomas in children and young adults. J Pediatr Hematol Oncol 2012;34:S51–4.
37. Whiteman D, Valery P, McWhirter W, et al. Incidence of cutaneous childhood melanoma in Queensland, Australia. Int J Cancer 1995;63:765–8.
38. Huynh PM, Grant-Kels JM, Grin CM. Childhood melanoma: Update and treatment. Int J Dermatol 2005;44:715–23.
39. Massone C, Di Stefani A, Soyer HP. Dermoscopy for skin cancer detection. Curr Opin Oncol 2005;17:147–53.
40. Friedman RJ, Gutkowicz-Krusin D, Farber MJ, et al. The diagnostic performance of expert dermoscopists vs. a computer-vision system on small-diameter melanomas. Arch Dermatol 2008;144: 476–82.
41. Bishop JN, Harland M, Randerson-Moor J, et al. Management of familial melanoma. Lancet Oncol 2007;8:46–54.
42. Pho L, Grossman D, Leachman SA. Melanoma genetics: A review of genetic factors and clinical phenotypes in familial melanoma. Curr Opin Oncol 2006;18:173–9.
43. Paradela A, Fonseca E, Pita-Fernandez S, et al. Prognostic factors for melanoma in children and adolescents. Cancer 2010;116: 4334–44.
44. Neier M, Pappo A, Navid F. Management of melanomas in children and young adults. J Pediatr Hematol Oncol 2012;34:S51–4.

45. Downard CD, Rapkin LB, Gow KW. Melanoma in children and adolescents. Surg Oncol 2007;16:215–20.
46. Tannous ZS, Mihm MC Jr, Sober AJ, et al. Congenital melanocytic nevi: Clinical and histopathologic features, risk of melanoma, and clinical management. J Am Acad Dermatol 2005;52:197–203.
47. Krengel S, Hauschild A, Schafer T. Melanoma risk in congenital melanocytic naevi: A systematic review. Br J Dermatol 2006;155:1–8.
48. Ruiz-Maldonado R, Tamayo L, Laterza AM, et al. Giant pigmented nevi: Clinical, histopathologic and therapeutic considerations. J Pediatr 1992;120:906–11.
49. Marghoob AA, Schoenbach SP,Kopf AW, et al. Large congenital melanocytic nevi and the risk for development of malignant melanoma. A prospective study. Arch Dermatol 1996;132:170–5.
50. Herron MD, Vanderhooft SL, Smock K, et al. Proliferative nodules in congenital melanocytic nevi: A clinicopathologic and immuno-histochemical analysis. Am J Surg Pathol 2004;28:1017–25.
51. Illig LF, Weidner M, Hundeiker H, et al. Congenital nevi less than or equal to 10 cm as precursors to melanoma. 52 cases, a review, and a new conception Arch Dermatol 1985;121:1274–81.
52. Rhodes AR, Melski JW. Small congenital nevocellular nevi and the risk of cutaneous melanoma. J Pediatr 1982;100:219–24.
53. Kraemer KH, Lee MM, Scotto J. Xeroderma pigmentosum: Cutaneous, ocular, and neurologic abnormalities in 830 published cases. Arch Dermatol 1987;123:241–50.
54. Ruiz-Maldonado R, Orozco-Covarrubias ML. Malignant melanoma in children. A review. Arch Dermatol 1997;133:363–71.
55. Baird EA, McHenry PM, MacKie RM. Effect of maintenance chemotherapy in childhood on numbers of melanocytic naevi. Br Med J 1992;305:799–801.
56. Matichard E, Le Henanff A, Sanders A, et al. Effect of neonatal phototherapy on melanocytic nevus count in children. Arch Dermatol 2006;142:1599–604.
57. Jafarian F, Powell J, Kokta V, et al. Malignant melanoma in childhood and adolescence: Report of 13 cases. J Am Acad Dermatol 2005;53:816–22.
58. Robinson JK, Nickoloff BJ. Digital epiluminescence microscopy monitoring of high-risk patients. Arch Dermatol 2004;140:49–56.
59. Massone C, Wurm EM, Hofmann-Wellenhof R, et al. Teledermatology: An update. Semin Cutan Med Surg 2008;27:101–5.
60. Banky JP, Kelly JW, English DR, et al. Incidence of new and changed nevi and melanomas detected using baseline images and dermoscopy in patients at high risk for melanoma. Arch Dermatol 2005;141:998–1006.
61. Busam KJ, Pulitzer M. Sentinel lymph node biopsy for patients with diagnostically controversial spitzoid melanocytic tumors? Adv Anat Pathol 2008;15:253–62.
62. Mills OL, Marzban S, Zagar JS, et al. Sentinel lymph node biopsy in atypical melanocytic neoplasms in childhood: A single institution experience in 24 patients. J Cutan Pathol 2012;39:331–6.
63. Takata M, Lin J, Takayanagi S, et al. Genetic and epigenetic alterations in the differential diagnosis of malignant melanoma and spitzoid lesion. Br J Dermatol 2007;156:1287–94.
64. Tom WL, Hsu JW, Eichenfield LF, et al. Pediatric 'STUMP' lesions: Evaluation and management of difficult atypical spitzoid lesions in children. J Am Acad Dermatol 2011;64:559–72.
65. Raskin L, Ludgate M, Iyer RK, et al. Copy number variations and clinical outcome in atypical spitz tumors. Am J Surg Pathol 2011;35:243–52.
66. Ali L, Helm T, Cheney R, et al. Correlating array comparative genomic hybridization findings with histology and outcome in spitzoid melanocytic neoplasms. Int J Clin Exp Pathol 2010;3:593–9.
67. Sepehr A, Chao E, Trefrey B, et al. Longterm outcome of Spitz-type melanocytic tumors. Arch Dermatol 2011;147:1173–9.
68. Balch CM, Buzaid AC, Soong SJ, et al. Final version of the American Joint Committee On Cancer staging system for cutaneous melanoma. J Clin Oncol 2001;19:3635–48.
69. Been LB, Suurmeijer AJ, Cobben DC, et al. [18F]FLT-PET in oncology: Current status and opportunities. Eur J Nucl Med Mol Imaging 2004;31:1659–72.
70. Kumar R, Alavi A. Clinical applications of fluorodeoxyglucose–positron emission tomography in the management of malignant melanoma. Curr Opin Oncol 2005;17:154–9.
71. Roaten JB, Partrick DA, Pearlman N, et al. Sentinel lymph node biopsy for melanoma and other melanocytic tumors in adolescents. J Pediatr Surg 2005;40:232–5.
72. Roaten JB, Partrick DA, Bensard D, et al. Survival in sentinel lymph node-positive pediatric melanoma. J Pediatr Surg 2005;40:988–92.
73. Howman-Giles R, Shaw HM, Scolyer RA, et al. Sentinel lymph node biopsy in pediatric and adolescent cutaneous melanoma patients. Ann Surg Oncol 2010;17:138–43.
74. Han D, Zager JS, Han G, et al. The unique clinical charactcristics of melanoma diagnosed in children. Ann Surg Oncol 2012;19:3888–95.
75. Mu E, Lange JR, Strouse JJ. Comparison of the use and results of sentinel lymph node biopsy in children and young adults with melanoma. Cancer 2012;118:2700–7.
76. Butter A, Hui T, Chapdelaine J, et al. Melanoma in children and the use of sentinel lymph node biopsy. J Pediatr Surg 2005;40:797–800.
77. Ascierto PA, Scala S, Ottaiano A, et al. Adjuvant treatment of malignant melanoma: Where are we? Crit Rev Oncol Hematol 2006;57:45–52.
78. Chao MM, Schwartz JL, Wechsler DS, et al. High-risk surgically resected pediatric melanoma and adjuvant interferon therapy. Pediatr Blood Cancer 2005;44:441–8.
79. Shah NC, Gerstle JT, Stuart M, et al. Use of sentinel lymph node biopsy and high-dose interferon in pediatric patients with high-risk melanoma: The Hospital for Sick Children experience. J Pediatr Hematol Oncol 2006;28:496–500.
80. Ralph SJ. An update on malignant melanoma vaccine research: Insights into mechanisms for improving the design and potency of melanoma therapeutic vaccines. Am J Clin Dermatol 2007;8:123–41.
81. Kirkwood JM, Jukic D, Averbrook BJ, et al. Melanoma in pediatric, adolescent and young adult patients. Semin Oncol 2009;36:419–31.
82. Strouse JJ, Fears TR, Tucker MA, et al. Pediatric melanoma: Risk factor and survival analysis of the surveillance, epidemiology and end results database. J Clin Oncol 2005 20;23:4735–41.
83. Tate PS, Ronan SG, Feucht KA, et al. Melanoma in childhood and adolescence: Clinical and pathological features of 48 cases. J Pediatr Surg 1993;28:217–22.
84. Moore-Olufema S, Herzog C, Warneke C, et al. Outcomes in pediatric melanoma comparing prepubertal to adolescent pediatric patients. Ann Surg 2011;253:1211–15.

CHAPTER 72

Vascular and Lymphatic Anomalies

Kirsty L. Rialon • Steven J. Fishman

Vascular anomalies are broadly divided into two groups based on biologic and clinical behavior: vascular tumors and vascular malformations.[1] Vascular tumors are true neoplasms that arise from cellular hyperplasia. In contrast, vascular malformations are congenital lesions originating from errors of embryonic development and exhibit normal endothelial cell turnover.[1] Historically, the field of vascular anomalies has been hindered by a myriad of confusing and misused terminology and nomenclature. This, along with the rarity and often complex nature of some of these disorders, has combined to make diagnosis and treatment of vascular anomalies difficult. However, the last several decades have brought better insight and understanding into the field of vascular anomalies, with improved knowledge of blood vessel angiogenesis and the development of a more logical classification system.

CLASSIFICATION

In 1996, the International Society of the Study of Vascular Anomalies formally accepted the biological classification system in use today (Table 72-1).[2,3] This system divides these anomalies into vascular tumors and vascular malformations based on physical characteristics, natural history, and cellular features. Examples of vascular tumors are infantile hemangioma (IH), kaposiform hemangioendothelioma (KHE), and tufted angioma (TA). Vascular malformations can be divided based on vascular channel type (capillary, lymphatic, venous, arterial, or combined) or by flow (slow or fast). Examples of slow-flow lesions are capillary malformations (CM), lymphatic malformations (LM), and venous malformations (VM). Fast-flow lesions include arteriovenous fistulas (AVF) and arteriovenous malformations (AVM).

NOMENCLATURE

Though now more clear, the nomenclature and classification of vascular anomalies have historically been confusing, with the same or similar terms used to describe vastly different lesions. The various vascular anomalies often have a similar appearance whether involving the skin, mucosa, or viscera. They are flat or raised lesions that can have pink, red, purple, or blue coloration. For centuries, these cutaneous vascular nevi were named based on resemblance to common foods such as 'cherry', 'strawberry', or 'port-wine stain.' The term 'nevus' refers to any generic circumscribed lesion of the skin, especially if colored by hyperpigmentation or increased vascularity.

In the 19th century, Virchow first described the histologic features of vascular nevi.[4] He initiated the term 'angioma', which became the default term to describe all such nevi regardless of natural history or other clinical features. He also labeled the IH 'angioma simplex', a lesion that has been historically referred to as 'capillary hemangioma' and 'strawberry hemangioma.' Virchow's 'angioma cavernosum' was used to label two distinct lesions, IH (when located deep to the skin) and VM, because both have similar appearance on physical examination. 'Angioma racemosum' was Virchow's designation for what today is termed an arteriovenous malformation and which has previously been called an 'arteriovenous hemangioma.'

Wegener, a student of Virchow, described the histology of LMs, which he called 'lymphangiomas.'[5] The classic term 'cystic hygroma', referring to LM, unfortunately also continues to have common usage. Thus, both the terms cystic hygroma and lymphangioma should be abandoned in favor of LM (macrocystic and microcystic, respectively). The problems with this jumble of descriptive and histologic terms are obvious. The same lesion can often have several different names, and simultaneously, the same name can refer to several different lesions. For example, the term 'hemangioma', combined with descriptive modifiers such as 'strawberry', 'cavernous', and 'lympho-', is used to describe tumors, birthmarks, and vascular malformations alike. Vascular anomalies with quite distinct features, whether congenital or acquired, or whether they spontaneously regress or progress over time, become lumped under the umbrella term 'hemangioma.' These faulty designations lead to improper diagnosis and treatment for patients as well as leading to misguided interdisciplinary communication and research efforts.

VASCULAR TUMORS

Infantile Hemangioma

IH are the most common tumor of infancy. They occur in about 4% of infants, though early studies were as high as 10%, probably due to the inclusion of other vascular lesions.[6] The incidence is higher in premature infants, Caucasians, and females (by a 3 to 5 : 1 ratio).[6,7] Advanced maternal age, multiple gestations, and placental abnormalities are also risk factors.[8] IH have a unique and

TABLE 72-1 Classification of Vascular Anomalies

Vascular Tumors	Slow-Flow Vascular Malformations	Fast-Flow Vascular Malformations	Combined Vascular Malformations
Hemangioma Kaposiform hemangioendothelioma (KHE) Tufted angioma (TA)	Capillary malformation (CM) Venous malformation (VM) Lymphatic malformation (LM)	Arteriovenous fistula (AVF) Arteriovenous malformation (AVM)	Klippel–Trénaunay syndrome, a capillary lymphaticovenous malformation (CLVM) Parkes–Weber syndrome, a capillary arteriovenous malformation (CAVM)

characteristic life cycle consisting of three phases: proliferative, involuting, and involuted.

Pathophysiology

The precise etiology of IH remains unknown. Viral causes have been speculated, but none elucidated. Some studies suggest that they arise from the clonal expansion of endothelial stem/progenitor cells, the source of which is unclear.[9–11] One report concluded these cells arise from a population of resident angioblasts, arrested in an early stage of vascular development.[12] As hemangiomas are more common in females, estrogen, which has a stimulatory effect on endothelial cells, may factor in the development of these lesions. Its receptors are present on endothelial cells and elevated levels of estradiol have been found in infants with hemangiomas.[13,14]

The expression of placental markers (including CD 32, Fcγ-RIIb, glucose transporter 1 [GLUT-1], indoleamine deoxygenase [IDO], insulin growth factor 2 [IGF-2] Lewis Y antigen, merosin, type II 17-hydroxysteroid dehydrogenase [17HSDβ2], tissue factor pathway inhibitor 2 [TFPI-2], and type III iodothyronine deoidinase) by hemangioma endothelial cells suggests a placental origin.[15–21] GLUT-1, an erythrocyte type glucose transporter, is a specific marker for endothelial cells of hemangiomas, but is not found in other vascular anomalies.[15] The placental cells may arrive at fetal tissue following local placental disruption as an embolic nidus though the permissive right to left shunt of fetal circulation. This may occur during chorionic villus sampling or placental complications such as pre-eclampsia and placenta previa, which have shown to be predisposing factors for hemangiomas.[8,22,23]

The dysregulation of angiogenesis can be seen during the proliferation and involution of hemangiomas, and is suspected to be a cause of the disease. IH in the proliferative phase express high levels of fibroblast growth factor (FGF), TIE-2, angiopoietins, matrix metalloproteinases (MMPs) and vascular endothelial growth factor A (VEGF-A) and its receptor (VEGFR), all of which play critical roles in the formation of blood vessels during and after embryogenesis.[24–30] The tumor during this phase is composed of plump, rapidly dividing endothelial cells forming a mass of sinusoidal vascular channels. Enlarged feeding arteries and draining veins often vascularize the tumor. Markers for mature endothelium, CD-31 and von Willebrand factor, are present on these neoplastic endothelial cells. Involuted hemangiomas express normal levels of these factors, but elevated levels of tissue inhibitor of TIMP1, a metalloproteinase that inhibits new blood vessel formation, and interferon-β.[28,29] The endothelial cells of the tumor flatten as apoptosis progresses, the vascular channels dilate, and the tumor assumes a lobular architecture with replacement by fibrofatty stroma.[31] All that remains in the involuted phase is a residuum of fibrofatty tissue with tiny capillaries and mildly dilated draining vessels.

Clinical Features

IH are not fully developed at birth and first appear in the neonatal period with a median age of onset of 2 weeks. A premonitory cutaneous sign may be present at birth in 30–50% of cases.[1] They are most often cutaneous (80%) and have an anatomic predilection for the head and neck region (60%). They occur in the trunk and extremities 25% and 15% of the time, respectively.[2] Internal and visceral lesions are uncommon. Up to 20% of patients can have multiple lesions, and these cases are most likely to have internal involvement affecting organs such as the liver and gastrointestinal (GI) tract.[1]

The proliferative phase of IH is marked by rapid growth for the first six to eight months that typically plateaus by age 10–12 months. Tumors that involve the superficial dermis present as a red, raised lesion (Fig. 72-1A). Superficial tumors that are larger or that exhibit more rapid growth can occasionally cause ulceration of the skin with bleeding. Tumors in the lower dermis, subcutaneous tissue, or muscle appear bluish in color with slightly raised overlying skin (previously incorrectly termed 'cavernous' hemangiomas). With experience, history and physical examination can establish an accurate diagnosis for most of these tumors. The involuting phase of hemangiomas occurs from age 1 to 7 years during which time the tumor slowly regresses, although it may grow in proportion with the child. This phase is notable for fading color of the tumor from crimson to a dull purple, accompanied by a deflation of the tumor mass (Fig. 72-1B).[1] The skin may become pale, usually in the center of the tumor first, spreading outwards. Fifty per cent of tumors have completed involution by 5 years of age, and 70% by age 7 years. There is continued gradual improvement in these aspects until the regression is entirely complete by age 10–12 years.[32] In the final involuted phase of the tumor, 50% of patients have nearly normal skin in the area of the prior lesion. Patients with larger tumors can have lax or redundant skin and yellowish discoloration. Scars will persist if parts of the tumor were previously ulcerated.[1]

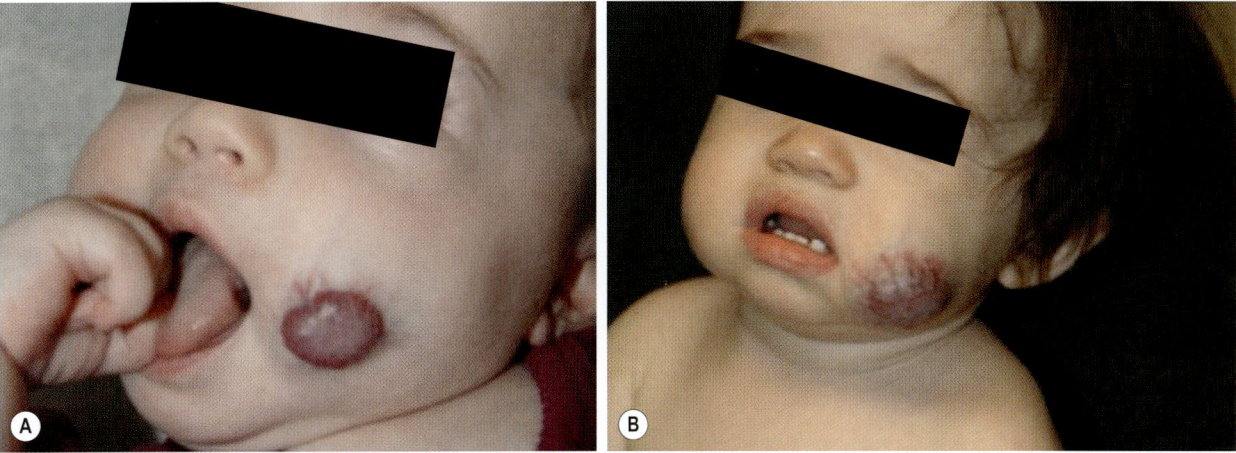

FIGURE 72-1 ■ **(A)** This infant has an infantile hemangioma that is in the proliferative phase. This hemangioma was not present at birth but was noted at several weeks of age. **(B)** This hemangioma is in its involuting phase.

The differential diagnosis of cutaneous hemangiomas consists primarily of other vascular anomalies. CM that involves the skin can be mistaken for superficial hemangiomas, or vice versa. Deeper hemangiomas can be confused for VM or LM as all can appear as bluish masses through the skin. Hemangiomas with fast-flow vascularity of the parenchyma could be confused for AVM, but the age of onset and history generally distinguishes the two. Congenital hemangiomas, discussed in a later section, may be misdiagnosed as vascular malformations, which are congenital by definition. Pyogenic granulomas may be differentiated from hemangiomas by their rare appearance before six months (mean age is 6 to 7 years), and their frequent association with minor trauma.[33,34] Other tumors such as TA, hemangiopericytoma, and fibrosarcoma can also be confused.[35]

The primary local complications that can occur with cutaneous hemangiomas are ulceration, bleeding, and pain. Hemangiomas are rarely life-threatening, but complications can be anticipated by recognition of the anatomic distribution of the lesion.[36] Lesions in the cervicofacial region can lead to airway obstruction as they grow during the proliferative phase. Very large hemangiomas, notably in the liver, can lead to high-output congestive heart failure (secondary to fast-flow and vascular shunting within the tumor), hypothyroidism, and abdominal compartment syndrome. Facial lesions involving the eyelid, nose, lip, or ear can result in tissue destruction with cosmetic consequences. Periorbital and eyelid hemangiomas can cause visual axis obstruction, leading to deprivation amblyopia (Fig. 72-2). Alternatively, distortion of the cornea can cause astigmatic amblyopia. GI hemangiomas are very rare, but may manifest with GI bleeding.

Associated Congenital Anomalies

IH are rarely associated with other anomalies. However, a few such anomalies have been described, more commonly with larger and midline hemangiomas. Cervicothoracic hemangiomas can be seen in conjunction with sternal nonunion.[37] Tumors of the lumbosacral area have

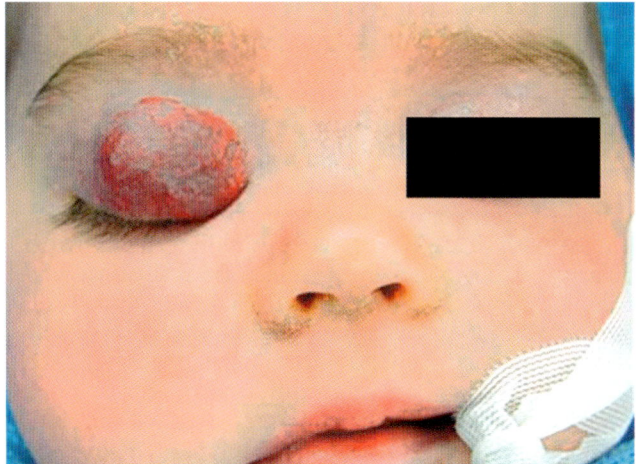

FIGURE 72-2 ■ Periorbital and eyelid hemangiomas, such as seen in this photograph, can cause visual axis obstruction and can lead to deprivation amblyopia.

been noted to occur along with spinal dysraphism abnormalities such as meningocele and tethered spinal cord.[38,39] Hemangiomas of the pelvis and perineum have been found in association with urogenital and anorectal anomalies. PHACES association describes hemangiomas associated with congenital ocular abnormalities such as microophthalmia, cataracts, optic nerve hypoplasia, posterior fossa cystic malformations, hypoplasia or absence of carotid and vertebral vessels, as well as malformation of the aortic arch (Fig 72-3).[40,41] Females are affected in 90% of cases. These patients are at risk for stroke in the neonatal period and migraines in older ages.

Other Manifestations

The presence of multiple disseminated hemangiomas is termed hemangiomatosis. The cutaneous tumors are usually tiny (<5 mm) and dome-like. When five or more lesions are present, occult visceral lesions, most commonly in the liver, may also be present (Fig. 72-4). Screening patients with ultrasound (US) and/or magnetic

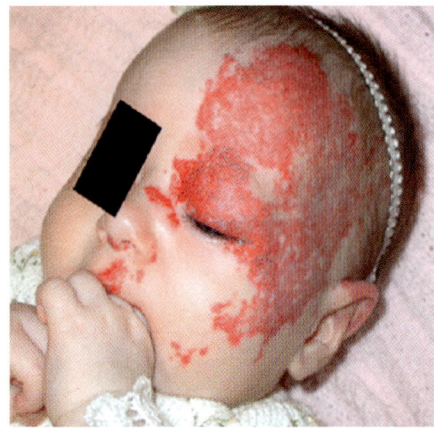

FIGURE 72-3 ■ This infant has the PHACES association with congenital ocular abnormalities as well as vascular anomalies.

resonance imaging (MRI) may be indicated for these patients.

Imaging

Proper radiologic diagnosis of vascular anomalies is dependent on specific expertise and clinical experience with the radiologic features of these lesions.[42] Ultrasound and MRI are the most useful imaging modalities. Ultrasound of proliferative phase hemangiomas demonstrates a mass with dense parenchyma exhibiting fast-flow vascularity.[43,44] This distinguishes deep IH from VM, which exhibit slow-flow vascularity and larger blood-filled spaces. MRI of proliferating hemangiomas shows a lobulated solid mass of intermediate intensity with T_1 spin-echo sequences, and moderate hyperintensity on T_2 spin-echo. Flow voids that represent fast flow and shunting are seen in and around the tumor. During the involuting phase, MRI demonstrates decreased flow voids and vascularity, with the mass taking on a more lobular and fatty appearance.[45]

Treatment

The majority of IH do not require any specific treatment other than observation and reassurance of the parents.[46] Even tumors that exhibit rapid growth or fiery red skin will spontaneously regress and leave behind little to no evidence of their presence. However, regular follow-up is important as the potential complications have few prognostic indicators. Serial photographs are very helpful in documenting progression and subsequent improvement. Reasons for treatment or referral to a vascular anomalies specialist or center include dangerous locations (impinging on a vital structure such as the airway or eye), unusually large size or rapid growth, and local or endangering complications (skin ulceration or high-output heart failure).

Hemangiomas exhibiting the above risk factors or complications should be considered for treatment. Since hemangiomas are tumors of pure angiogenesis, pharmacologic therapy involves angiogenesis inhibition. Systemic corticosteroids, which inhibit the expression of VEGF-A by hemangioma-derived stem cells and thus angiogenesis, were first line therapy for decades.[47–49] Oral prednisone is given at a dose of 2–3 mg/kg/day. Doses up to 5 mg/kg/day have been used for life-threatening complications of large hemangiomas causing airway obstruction or heart failure. The overall response rate is 80–90% with initial improvement in the color and tension of the mass usually noted within one week. The steroids are maintained with a very gradual taper every two to four weeks with the goal of discontinuation around age 10–11 months. Live vaccines such as polio, measles, mumps, rubella, and varicella should be withheld while children are taking prednisone. Hemangiomas will have rebound growth if steroids are tapered or stopped too quickly. Return to the initial dosage and slower tapering will usually treat this problem. Potential complications of steroid use in infants and children include impaired growth and weight gain in about one-third of cases. Almost all children will have 'catch up' growth and return to pretreatment growth curves by age 14–24 months.[50] Cushingoid facies occur in almost all patients and normalizes upon tapering. In rare circumstances, steroids may induce hypertension or hypertrophic cardiomyopathy, both of which are indications to wean or change therapy.[50]

Intralesional corticosteroids are used for small cutaneous hemangiomas that cause local deformity or ulceration, especially for lesions of the eyelid, nose, cheek, or lip.[51] A total of three to five injections are typically given at intervals of six to eight weeks at a dose of 3–5 mg/kg/injection.[52] The response rate approaches that of systemic steroids. Subcutaneous atrophy is a potential complication of steroid injection, but is usually temporary. There have been reported cases of blindness following intralesional steroid injection for periorbital hemangiomas.[53] This is presumed to be secondary to particle embolization into the retinal artery through feeding vessels.

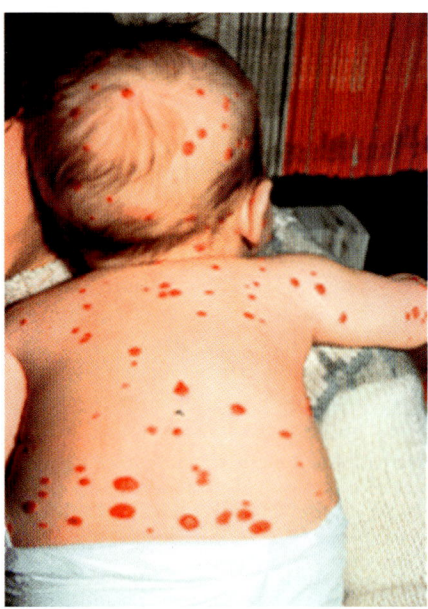

FIGURE 72-4 ■ This baby has hemangiomatosis. When multiple cutaneous lesions are found, occult visceral lesions, most commonly in the liver, may also be present. Screening for visceral hemangiomas with ultrasound may be indicated in these patients.

Manual compression around the periphery of the tumor is recommended during injection to minimize embolization through draining veins.

Propranolol, a nonselective beta blocker, has recently been recognized as an important treatment option for hemangiomas and in most centers has become first line pharmacotherapy. A child with a nasal capillary hemangioma treated with propranolol for steroid-induced cardiomyopathy had regression of his lesion.[54] This revelation led to the publication of several more studies supporting this finding.[55–58] Propranolol is given orally at 2–3 mg/kg/day, in two or three divided doses, and discontinued following regression of the lesion.[55,59] Treatment often leads to a consistent, rapid, therapeutic effect with softening of the lesion on palpation and color shift from intense red to purple.[55] Propranolol is well tolerated but can cause rare side effects such as bradycardia, gastroesophageal reflux, hypoglycemia, hypotension, rash, somnolence, and wheezing.[55,56,58–61] Several mechanisms of action have been proposed.[62] Propranolol inhibits β-adrenoreceptors, which are activated by adrenaline, causing vasoconstriction of capillaries supplying the hemangioma.[63,64] This likely leads to the visible changes in color and palpable softening. Blockage of β-adrenoreceptors also results in decreased expression of VEGF and MMPs, thereby inhibiting angiogenesis, and induces apoptosis in endothelial cells.[65,66]

Recombinant interferon was once considered as a second line agent, but has fallen out of favor except in very limited circumstances.[67–71] A small subset of patients (5–12%) may develop a severe complication known as spastic diplegia.[72,73] Spasticity usually resolves if the drug is terminated quickly. Children receiving IFN should be followed carefully by a neurologist. Though experience is limited, low-dose, high frequency anti-angiogenic regimens using vincristine can be effective.[74] The use of interferon and vincristine has waned since the introduction of propranolol therapy.

Although attractive in concept, laser therapy is not often beneficial for IHs, except for a few specific indications.[75] The flash lamp pulse-dye laser penetrates the dermis to a depth of only 0.75–1.2 mm. Most cutaneous hemangiomas are deeper than this, and therefore not affected by laser treatment. Additionally, laser therapy carries risks of scarring, skin hypopigmentation, and ulceration, which may lead to a poor result compared to observation alone. One instance in which the laser is advantageous is the treatment of telangiectasias that often remain in the involuted phase of hemangioma. The use of endoscopic continuous wave carbon dioxide laser has been shown to be a good strategy for controlling proliferative phase hemangiomas in the unilateral subglottic location.[76] Lastly, intralesional photocoagulation with bare fiber Nd:YAG laser can be useful for hemangiomas in certain locations, such as the upper eyelid when visual obstruction is a concern.

Indications for resection of IH vary with patient age. During the proliferative phase in infancy, well-localized or pedunculated tumors can be expeditiously resected with linear closure, especially for tumors complicated by bleeding and ulceration. Sites that are most amenable to resection are the scalp, trunk, and extremities. Other modalities to treat ulceration include wound care with dressing changes, topical antibiotics, and topical steroids, which can accelerate healing.[77] Tumors of the upper eyelid that obstruct vision and that do not respond to pharmacologic therapy may also require excision or debulking. Focal lesions of the GI tract with bleeding that fail medical management may require enterotomy and resection, or endoscopic band ligation. Diffuse, patchy involvement is the more common presentation of GI hemangiomas. Management is difficult but most lesions eventually involute and stop bleeding.[78] Preoperative localization with capsule endoscopy and/or intraoperative endoscopy may be necessary to identify lesions in the small bowel.[79]

During the involuting phase, resection may be needed for hemangiomas that are large and protuberant, and therefore likely to create excess and lax overlying skin.[80] Indications for resection include: (1) it is obvious that resection will be necessary sooner or later; (2) the surgical scar will be identical regardless of timing of operation; and (3) the surgical scar can easily be hidden. Lesions of the nose, eyelids, lips, and ears require special expertise. It is often preferable to perform the operation for the above indications during the preschool years before children become aware of and focus on body image differences that may lead to low self-esteem.

After complete involution of hemangioma, cosmetic distortion often becomes the primary indication for resection. Fibrofatty residuum and redundant skin can be excised in staged operations if necessary. Occasionally, extensive scarring from tissue destruction may necessitate reconstructive techniques.

Finally, for the difficult to treat and life-threatening large hemangiomas, especially in the liver, angiographic embolization may be required to manage high-output cardiac failure. Arterial catheterization in infants carries significant risks and should generally be limited to those situations with cardiac compromise in which there is the capacity and intent to perform simultaneous embolization. In these rare cases, anti-angiogenic pharmacotherapy remains the first line of therapy and should continue along with angiographic procedures. Repeat embolization procedures may be required. Success with embolization is dependent on occlusion of macrovascular shunts within the tumor rather than occlusion of feeding vessels.[81]

Congenital Hemangioma

Two types of rare congenital hemangiomas exist that are fully developed at birth and that do not usually exhibit postnatal tumor growth.[82] These have been termed rapidly involuting congenital hemangioma (RICH) and the noninvoluting congenital hemangioma (NICH) (Fig. 72-5). Lesions are solitary and affect both genders equally. Unlike IHs, they do not stain positive for GLUT-1.[83] The diagnosis is typically made on physical exam at birth, although some can be diagnosed prenatally as early as 12 weeks of gestation.[82] Most do not require therapy.

As opposed to IH, RICH is more common on the extremities. Also, RICH will spontaneously regress, much more quickly than IH, by 6 to 14 months; NICH

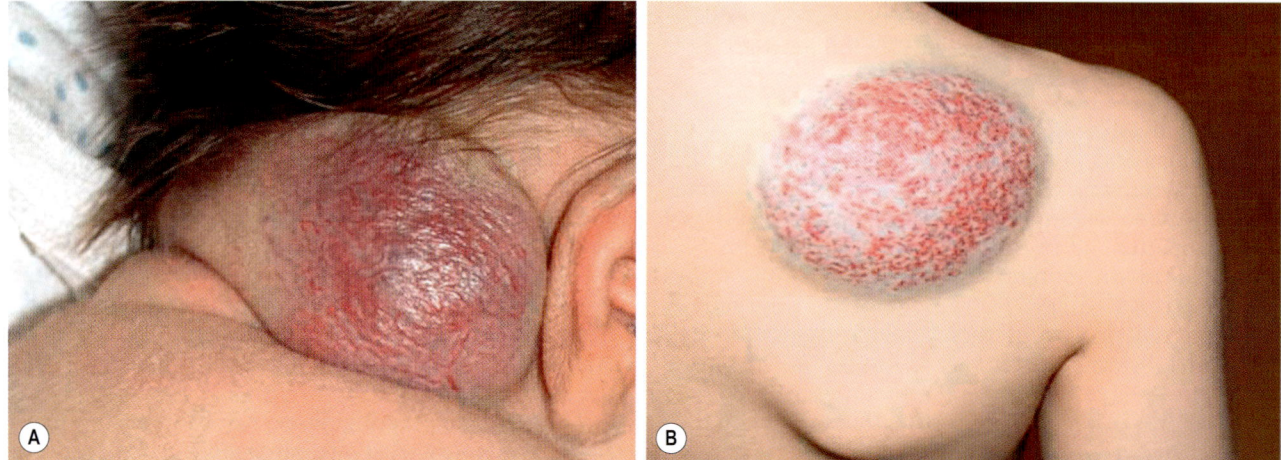

FIGURE 72-5 ■ These two patients are examples of rapid involuting congenital hemangiomas (RICH) and noninvoluting congenital hemangiomas (NICH). (A) The newborn baby has a RICH. This lesion was present at birth and will spontaneously regress, much more quickly than the typical infantile hemangioma. (B) This 9-year-old child has a NICH. This hemangioma has not resolved. If treatment is needed, arterial embolization may be beneficial as these lesions have significant flow to them.

do not involute and grow with the child.[82] RICH appear raised and violaceous, often with a central depression or scar, ulceration, telangiectasia, or surrounding pale rim.[82,83] MRI will show enhancing hyperintense masses, high-flow vessels within and adjacent to the mass, and the presence of vascular flow voids on T_2-weighted imaging.[83] NICH are well-circumscribed, plaque-like lesions, often with coarse telangiectasias, areas of pallor, or a white to bluish rim.[84] They appear on MRI as homogeneous lesions with isointense signal on T_1-weighted imaging and hyperintense on T2-weighted sequences. Both lesions are fast flow on Doppler ultrasound. If treatment is needed for NICH, arterial embolization may be beneficial as these lesions have significant flow to them. Operative excision is reserved for cases with equivocal diagnosis, poor cosmetic appearance, or for complications such as ulceration, bleeding, obstruction, or congestive heart failure.[83,85]

Hepatic Hemangioma

Hepatic hemangiomas (HH) in infants should be differentiated from 'hepatic hemangiomas' that present in adulthood.[85] Adult 'hepatic hemangiomas', which are sometimes called 'cavernous hemangiomas', are in fact VMs. In contrast, HH of infancy are true tumors and have a similar pattern of involution to cutaneous IH. Contrary to popular belief, not all liver hemangiomas are life-threatening. The classic triad of heart failure, anemia, and hepatomegaly is unusual, and most involute without long-term sequelae.

The majority of HH can be divided into three categories: focal, multifocal, and diffuse, each with distinct features (Fig. 72-6).[86] Focal HH are the hepatic equivalent of the cutaneous RICH, and also do not stain positive for GLUT-1. They are histologically distinct from the typical IH.[15,87] They are fully grown at birth and regress much faster than IH. Many focal lesions are detected antenatally on prenatal ultrasound, or are discovered as an abdominal mass in otherwise healthy infants.[88] They are usually asymptomatic, found in equal numbers in both genders, and rarely associated with cutaneous hemangiomas. Transient anemia and moderate thrombocytopenia, due to intralesional thrombosis, are observed in some infants and generally resolve spontaneously. This is in contradistinction to the profound thrombocytopenia seen with Kasabach–Merritt phenomenon (KMP). However, a subset of focal hepatic RICH-type

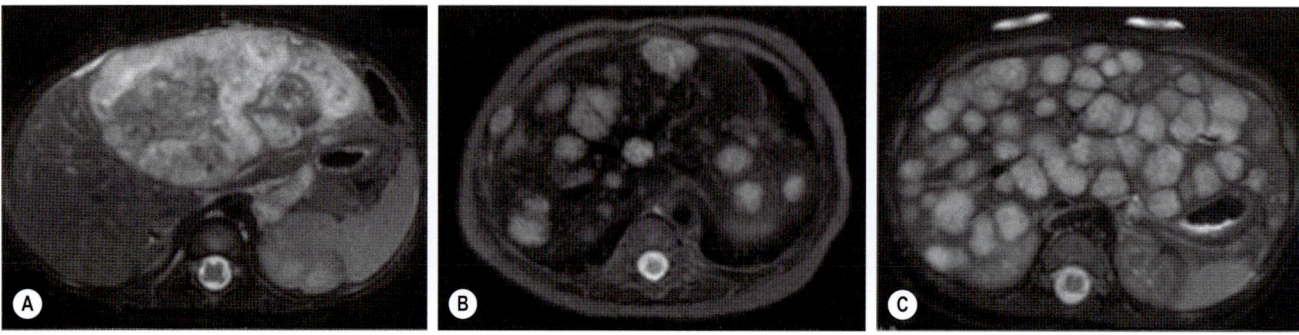

FIGURE 72-6 ■ Most hepatic hemangiomas can be divided into three categories: focal, multifocal, and diffuse. (A) A large focal hepatic hemangioma. (B) The scan depicts multifocal hepatic hemangiomas. (C) Diffuse hepatic hemangioma.

hemangiomas will have macrovascular shunts from the hepatic arteries and/or portal veins to the hepatic veins. These shunts can cause a large steal, accounting for blood-flow demands above and beyond the hypervascular tumor parenchyma, and can result in high-output cardiac failure. These shunts may close as the tumors involute. However, cardiac strain can often mandate interruption of the shunts via embolization. Steroids have been used for solitary focal hepatic lesions with in-utero cardiac failure/cardiomegaly.[88,89] However, these lesions may have undergone rapid spontaneous involution and the benefit of steroids remains unproven, though still should be attempted before employing more invasive therapies. Resection is rarely indicated.

Multifocal HH are true IH and biologically distinct from focal HH. They undergo involution similar to cutaneous IH and stain positive for GLUT-1.[87,90,91] They are more common in females and Caucasians.[92] Infants with multifocal lesions are typically born earlier and are asymptomatic, but are diagnosed later than focal lesions. These patients often have cutaneous IH and are identified following screening for visceral hemangiomas. Some of these patients will have hypothyroidism. Thus, a serum TSH should be checked in patients with multifocal disease. Infants who are asymptomatic should be observed; however, some can have high-output cardiac failure from macrovascular shunting. Treatment with steroids or propranolol can often close these shunts.[54,55] Embolization can be employed in those who fail medical therapy. Serial abdominal ultrasound should be performed in infants with multifocal HH until the lesions involute.

Diffuse HH are also true IH, but are far more serious lesions with a more difficult clinical course. Like multifocal lesions, diagnosis occurs in the weeks following birth. They are more common in Caucasians and females, are associated with cutaneous IH and follow a similar course of involution, and express GLUT-1.[92] These patients all develop severe hypothyroidism from high levels of type 3 iodothyronine deiodinase, which inactivates circulating thyroid hormones.[20] Aggressive exogenous thyroid hormone replacement is essential to prevent hypothyroid complications such as mental retardation and cardiac failure. Involution of the lesions will usually result in amelioration of the hypothyroidism.[93] These innumerable lesions often almost completely replace the normal hepatic parenchyma. Those with considerable disease may have respiratory compromise from compression of the diaphragm and thoracic cavity, but can also develop abdominal compartment syndrome and multisystem organ failure. Aggressive pharmacotherapy with propranolol, steroids, and occasionally low-dose vincristine is warranted in those with cardiac failure, hemodynamically significant shunting, or hypothyroidism to hasten involution.[55,86,94–96] Hepatic transplantation is the last resort for critically ill infants.[86]

The differential diagnosis of HH includes AVM and malignant tumors such as hepatoblastoma and metastatic neuroblastoma. The diagnosis is established by imaging with ultrasound, MRI, or CT scan. If the typical imaging patterns of one of the various HH types are not present, percutaneous biopsy may be needed to ensure a malignancy is not present.

Tufted Angioma and Kaposiform Hemangioendothelioma

These vascular tumors of childhood are more aggressive and invasive than IH. TA and KHE probably exist within the same spectrum as they share many overlapping clinical and histologic features.[21,97] Both tumors typically present at birth, although they occur postnatally as well. Males and females are affected equally. The tumors are unifocal and are most often located on the trunk, shoulder, thigh, or retroperitoneum. TA present as erythematous macules or plaques and histology reveals small tufts of capillaries.[97] KHE are more extensive tumors that present with deep, red-purple skin discoloration and overlying and surrounding ecchymosis (Fig. 72-7). The natural history of these tumors is one of continued proliferation into early childhood followed by subsequent, but incomplete regression. These tumors usually persist, albeit in a smaller form.[98] Fortunately, they are usually asymptomatic in later stages, though may cause musculoskeletal pain. Histology of these lesions reveals infiltrating sheets of spindle-shaped endothelial cells in the form of irregular lobules, sheets, and lacy network.[99] Imaging of KHE depicts an enhancing lesion on MRI with poorly defined margins that extend across tissue planes. This is in contrast to IH, which are well-circumscribed and respective of tissue planes.

Kasabach–Merritt Phenomenon

KMP was first reported in 1940 in a case of profound thrombocytopenia, petechiae, and bleeding in conjunction with a 'giant hemangioma.'[100] As with many terms in the field of vascular anomalies, this term has been often misused in connection with coagulopathy and other vascular lesions, most prominently VM. However, the profound and persistent thrombocytopenia that occurs with KMP does not occur with either VM or IH. The only

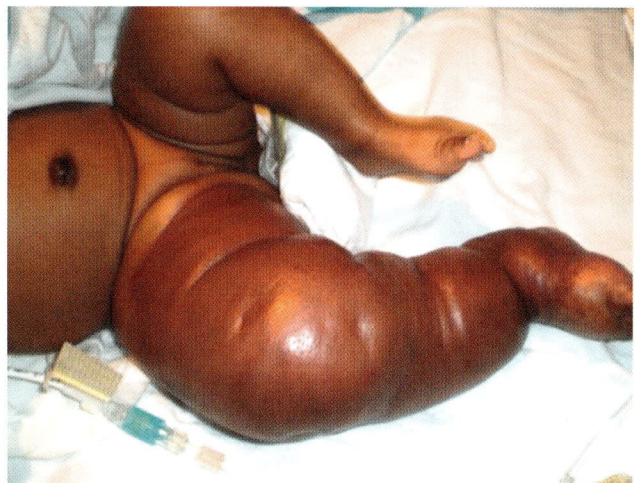

FIGURE 72-7 ■ This infant has a kaposiform hemangioendothelioma (KHE). KHE are more extensive tumors that present with deep, red-purple skin discoloration and overlying ecchymosis. These lesions usually regress later in childhood, although usually not completely.

known true associations are with TA and KHE.[99,101,102] The platelet count with KMP is typically under 10,000/μL, and may be associated with decreased fibrinogen levels, increased D-dimer, and mildly elevated partial prothrombin time (PT) and partial thromboplastin time (PTT). Bleeding can result from this platelet trapping coagulopathy at many sites, including intracranial, GI, peritoneal, pleural, and pulmonary. A microangiopathic hemolytic anemia is also present. Treatment for KHE with KMP is primarily medical as the tumor is usually too large and extensive to be resected. Corticosteroids and interferon-alfa have been effective in about 50% of cases; actinomycin, anti-platelet therapy, cyclophosphamide, doxorubicin, gemcitabine, propranolol, sirolimus, and vincristine have also been found to be beneficial in several case series, as single drugs or in combination, but none of these agents have been shown to be consistently successful.[103–111] Platelet transfusions are ineffective and should be avoided unless there is active bleeding. Additionally, heparin may stimulate tumor growth and worsens the thrombocytopenia of KMP and should likewise be avoided. Mortality rates with KHE and TA remain high at 20–30%. KHE not associated with KMP can be followed without treatment as long as the size and location of tumor are limited.

VASCULAR MALFORMATIONS

Vascular malformations are congenital lesions of vascular dysmorphogenesis that can be local or diffuse. The majority of vascular malformations are sporadic, though some rare varieties are familial.[112–114] They occur in 1.5% of the population.[115] Vascular malformations probably result from genetic mutations that lead to dysfunction in the regulation of endothelial proliferation and apoptosis, cellular differentiation, maturation, and cell-to-cell adhesions.[116]

Embryology and Development of the Vascular and Lymphatic Systems

The vascular system develops during embryogenesis through the processes of vasculogenesis, the formation of new vascular channels from mesodermally derived endothelial precursor cells (hemangioblasts), and angiogenesis, the formation of new blood vessels from preexisting blood vessels. The destiny of endothelial precursors to create different types of blood vessels appears to be imprinted early in embryogenesis by unique cell surface markers.[117] The differentiation of angioblasts into an early vascular plexus leads to the creation of primitive blood vessels.[118] Following formation of the primary vascular plexus, endothelial cells proliferate and sprout or split from their vessel of origin to form new capillaries. A process called 'pruning' then occurs, during which the vascular plexus is remodeled into a system with larger and smaller vessels. The signals for microvascular endothelial cells to proliferate and differentiate for vessel development are controlled by a number of growth factors and their receptors, including VEGF, basic fibroblast growth factor 2 (FGF-2), and angiopoietin 1 (Ang-1).[119]

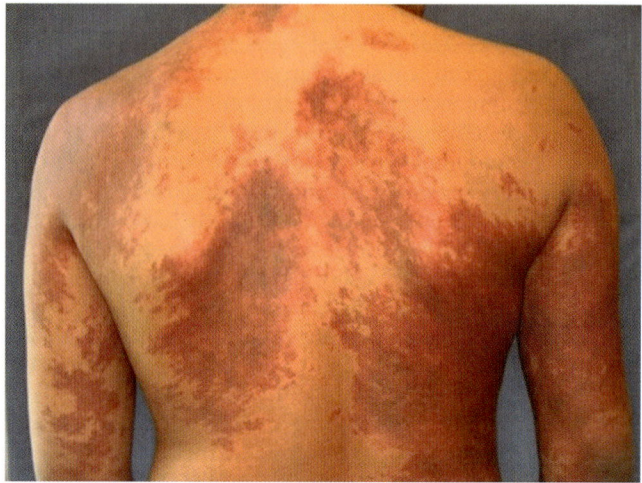

FIGURE 72-8 ■ This child has a capillary malformation. Such lesions were previously referred to as a port-wine stain.

The lymphatic system develops around midgestation after the blood vasculature forms, and is thought to derive from either venous endothelial cells or mesenchymal progenitor cells.[120–123] It is a one-way valve system that collects fluid and macromolecules from tissue. In 1902, Sabin described the prevailing model of lymphangiogenesis in which venous endothelial cells commit to become lymphatic endothelium and then migrate and proliferate to form lymph sacs.[122] These sacs then form a lymphatic plexus, which remodel and mature into the lymphatic vasculature.[120,123] Venous endothelial cells along the anterior cardinal vein capable of differentiating into lymphatic endothelial cells (LECs) begin to express lymphatic endothelial hyaluronan receptor-1 (LYVE-1) on embryonic day (E) 9, a marker specific for lymphatic endothelium.[120,123,124] A subgroup of endothelial cells on one side of the vein then begin to express prospero-related homeobox 1 (Prox-1).[125] This transcription factor is required for the maturation and differentiation of LECs.[125,126] VEGFR3, also known as Flt4, plays an important role in lymphatic development as well. VEGFR is expressed in both blood and lymphatic vasculature in early embryogenesis, but is restricted to mostly lymphatic vessels later in development[127–129] VEGFR3 knockout mice die on E9 with major venous anomalies before any lymphatic sprouting has occurred.[116] In contrast, transgenic mice that overexpress the ligand for VEGFR3 (VEGF-C) will develop distended lymphatic channels.[130]

Capillary Malformations

CM, previously referred to as 'port-wine stains', are present at birth as permanent flat, pink-red cutaneous lesions (Fig. 72-8). In the newborn nursery, CM can be confused with nevus flammeus neonatorum, commonly called 'angel's kiss' when located on the face, or 'stork bite' when in the posterior cervical location. However, these discolorations are due to transient dilations of dermal vessels and fade with time, whereas CM does not. CM occur with equal gender distribution in 0.3% of infants.[131] Multiple CM are rare. The majority of CM appear sporadically, but some familial forms exist that are inherited in an autosomally dominant fashion.[132] Capillary malformation–arteriovenous malformations (CM-AVM) are associated with mutations in *RASA1*, a gene coding for p120-RasGTPase.[133] Histologically, cutaneous CM consist of dilated capillary- to venule-sized vessels located in the superficial dermis, with a paucity of surrounding normal nerve fibers.[134] These abnormal vessels gradually dilate over time leading to darkening color and occasionally nodular ectasias. CM can also be found in complex-combined vascular malformations.

CM can be associated with underlying soft tissue and skeletal overgrowth, as well as other internal abnormalities. CM of the occiput can signal an underlying encephalocele or ectopic meninges. When located over the spine, underlying spinal dysraphism is a concern. Facial CM affecting the trigeminal dermatomes can be associated with ipsilateral ocular and leptomeningeal vascular anomalies in Sturge–Weber syndrome. Ocular lesions lead to increased risk for retinal detachment, glaucoma, and blindness. Leptomeningeal involvement can manifest with seizures, hemiplegia, and impaired motor and cognitive function. MRI reveals the CNS abnormalities showing pial vascular enhancement and gyriform calcifications.[135]

Treatment for CM is primarily related to cosmesis. Flash lamp pulse-dye laser therapy will cause photothermolysis and improve the appearance by lightening the color of the lesions in most (70%) patients.[136] Repeated treatments are usually needed and the timing of therapy remains controversial.[137] Treatment in infants less than six months of age has been shown to improve facial CM.[138] Ablative and orthopedic surgical procedures can be tailored to treat cosmetic and functional problems related to soft tissue and bony hypertrophy.

Cutis Marmorata Telangiectatica Congenita

Cutis marmorata telangiectatica congenita (CMTC) is an uncommon congenital vascular anomaly, first described in 1922, and characterized by a deep purple reticular vascular pattern.[139] Lesions are noted at birth or shortly after, and both genders are equally affected. CMTC can have a localized or generalized distribution; localized lesions are more common on the extremities.[140,141] Histopathology demonstrates dilated capillaries in the papillary dermis and proliferation of blood vessels in the reticular dermis.[142] Approximately 50% of cases are associated with other congenital anomalies. The most common is hypertrophy or atrophy of an involved extremity, but cardiovascular, craniofacial, cutaneous, neurologic, and skeletal abnormalities have also been described.[142–148] Partial regression of the capillary stains begins in the first year of life, but prominent dilated veins and discoloration often remain in adults.

Telangiectasias

Telangiectasias are tiny acquired vascular marks that can appear on children in the preschool and school-aged years, and are commonly known as 'spider nevus' or 'spider telangiectasias.' They may be present in nearly half of all children, with no preference for gender.[115]

Some may spontaneously disappear, but can be removed with pulsed-dye laser.

Hereditary hemorrhagic telangiectasia (HHT or Rendu–Osler–Weber disease) was the first vascular anomaly to be elucidated at a genetic level.[149] This autosomal dominant disease has five genetic types linked to mutations in genes coding for endoglin (an endothelial glycoprotein), activin receptor-like kinase 1, and Smad4, an intracellular signaling protein, all of which are involved in the binding and signaling of transforming growth factor-β.[150–153] Definite diagnosis of HHT is based on the presence of three of the following criteria: epistaxis, multiple telangiectasias (lips, oral cavity, fingers, nose), visceral lesions (GI, pulmonary, hepatic cerebral, or spinal AVMs), and family history (first degree relative with HHT).[154] Children often present with recurrent, spontaneous nosebleeds before school age. Telangiectasias of the skin and buccal mucosa present in the third decade of life. Chronic anemia from lower GI bleeds occurs in about one-third of patients.[155]

Lymphatic Malformations

Clinical Features

LM are usually noted at birth, but can manifest at any age or even be identified prenatally on fetal ultrasound.[156,157] The etiology of this anomaly is unknown. Lymphedema, a type of LM, does have heritable forms.[113] LM are classified as microcytic (diameter <1 cm), macrocystic (diameter >1 cm), or a combination thereof. These descriptions are also useful therapeutically as size determines whether or not the cystic cavity can be aspirated or compressed. Clinical presentation varies across a wide spectrum, from localized masses, to areas of diffuse infiltration, to chylous fluid accumulations in various body cavities.

The skin and soft tissues are most commonly affected, but LM can also involve the subcutaneous tissues, muscle, bone, and more rarely, internal organs such as the GI tract and lungs. As with CM, underlying localized soft tissue and skeletal hypertrophy is often associated with LM. LM appear as soft compressible masses, similarly to VM, and may have a bluish hue, although not to the same extent as VM (Fig. 72-9). LM appear histologically as thin-walled vascular channels lined by LECs, whose lumen can be empty or filled with a proteinaceous fluid containing macrophages and lymphocytes.[158] These cells stain positive for podoplanin (D2-40) and LYVE-1.[159] Involvement of the dermis may produce puckering of the skin or vesicles that weep clear yellowish fluid. Diffuse infiltration of the subcutaneous tissue can produce extensive lymphedema that also falls within the spectrum of LM. One unique factor among the vascular anomalies is that LMs are at risk for infection that can lead to cellulitis or even systemic illness. Similarly, infections located elsewhere in the body, or viral illnesses, can cause increased size and tension in the LM. The cystic components of LM are also subject to intralesional bleeding secondary to trauma or abnormal venous connections. The vesicles from cutaneous involvement can also leak thin sanguineous fluid or appear as red, purple, or black nodules.

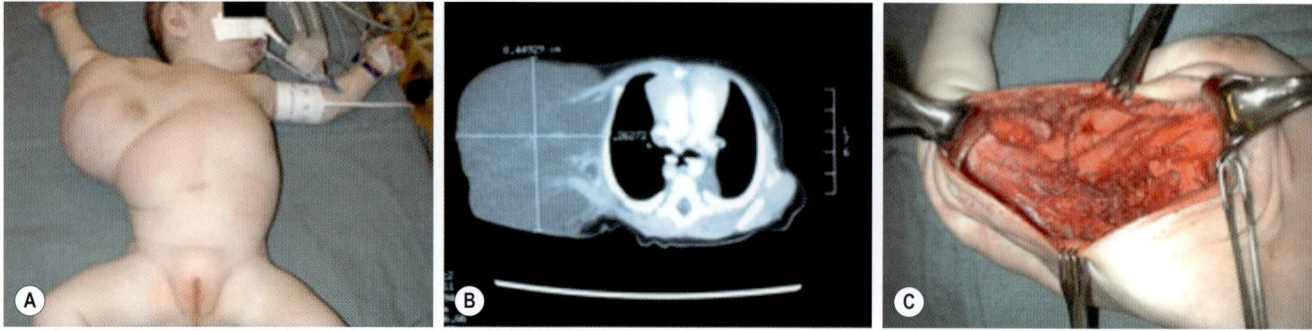

FIGURE 72-9 ■ This baby has a **(A)** large right axillary lymphatic malformation which is seen on the CT scan **(B)**. **(C)** This operative photograph shows the residual cavity after resection of the mass.

LM at various anatomic locations are prone to unique associated anomalies. Periorbital LM can lead to proptosis. Facial LM can cause the associated deformities of macrocheilia, macroglossia, and macromala. Overgrowth of the mandible, sometimes massive, can be seen with cervicofacial LM.[160] Congenital airway obstruction is rare but also possible (Fig. 72-10). Lesions of the tongue and floor of the mouth, on the other hand, may more commonly produce obstruction of the oropharynx. LM in the cervical and axillary regions can signal associated LM in the mediastinum. Anomalies of the central conducting lymphatic channels, the thoracic duct and cisterna chyli, can lead to very problematic and recurrent chylous effusions that affect the pleural, pericardial, and/or peritoneal cavities. In addition, LM of the GI tract can lead to loss of chyle and subsequent protein losing enteropathy. In the pelvis, associated problems include recurrent infection and bladder outlet obstruction. LM of the extremities are seen in conjunction with overgrowth and limb length discrepancy.

Gorham Syndrome

A rare but very difficult problem arises with Gorham syndrome, in which soft tissue and skeletal LM lead to progressive osteolysis and 'disappearing bone disease' (Fig. 72-11).[161] It presents most frequently in the second and third decades of life, and is seen slightly more often in males.[162,163] Presenting symptoms include pain, limping, extremity weakness, and spontaneous fractures, most commonly involving the shoulder, facial, spine, and pelvic bones.[164,165] The clinical course is variable, ranging from mild disability to paraplegia. On imaging, well-circumscribed intramedullary and subcortical lucencies resembling osteoporosis are seen early.[166] Biopsy typically demonstrates a matrix of thin-walled vessels lined with a single layer of endothelium surrounded by extensive fibrovascular connective tissue, but without signs of inflammation or malignancy.[164] A variety of treatments have been reported. Interferon alpha-2b is believed to have anti-angiogenic activity and has been shown to induce remission.[167,168] Bisphophonates can also stabilize disease, presumably by inhibition of osteoclasts.[169] The mTOR inhibitor rapamycin is currently under investigation and has been effective for treatment in children with refractory lymphatic anomalies.[170] Surgery, reserved for symptomatic lesions, involves resection of affected areas and reconstruction.

Lymphedema

Lymphedema, which occurs when protein-rich fluid leaks into the subcutaneous tissue, should be considered a type of LM. It can be inherited or acquired.[171] Milroy disease is an autosomal dominant, congenital lymphedema caused by a mutation in the *VEGR3* gene.[172,173] Bilateral, below-the-knee swelling is a consistent phenotypic feature of the disorder, and is usually present at birth. Cellulitis, dilated lower extremity veins, upslanting toenails, and papillomatosis are also present.[174] Males may often develop a hydrocele. In contrast, Meige disease and lymphedema-distichiasis syndrome (LD) present in puberty or later in adulthood with lymphedema. Both are autosomal dominant disorders. Meige disease is more common in females. No genetic cause has been found. LD patients can also present with distichiasis (double rows of eyelashes), varicose veins, ptosis, cleft palate, and cardiac abnormalities.[175] A mutation in the FOXC2 forkhead/winged-helix transcription factor, which plays a role in somite formation, is responsible for the disease.[176]

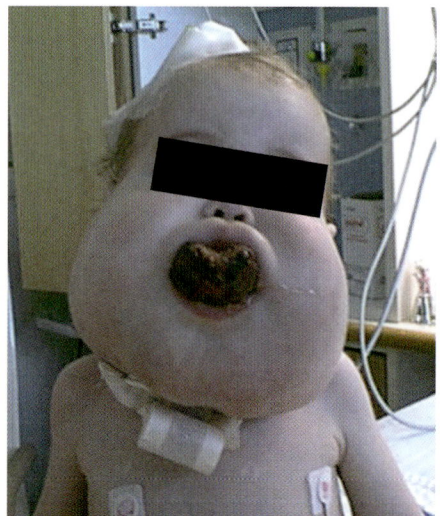

FIGURE 72-10 ■ This baby has undergone a tracheostomy due to oropharyngeal obstruction from this large cervicofacial lymphatic malformation.

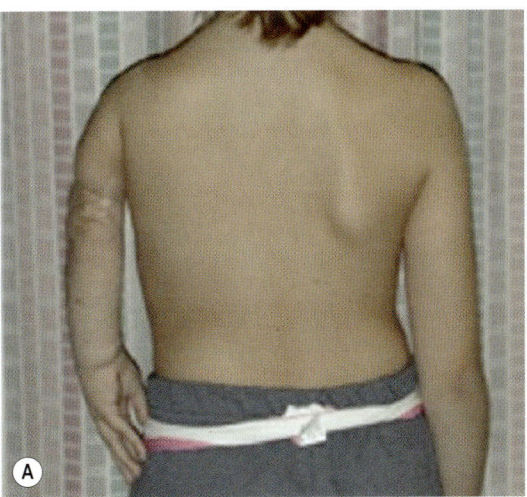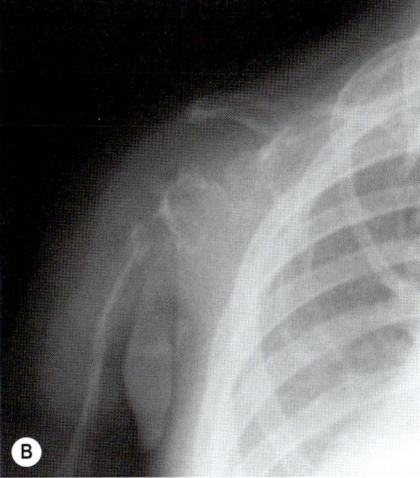

FIGURE 72-11 ■ This child has Gorham disease in which soft tissue and skeletal lymphatic malformations leads to progressive osteolysis. **(A)** Note the foreshortening of the left arm due to osteolysis of the left shoulder. **(B)** On the left upper extremity radiograph, note the loss of the humerus, clavicle, and shoulder joint.

Imaging

Well-localized and cystic LM are easily characterized by ultrasound and CT (see Fig. 72-9B). MRI, however, provides the most reliable diagnosis and is best for documenting the full extent of more complex LM as well as their macrocystic and microcystic components. LM are hyperintense on T_2 sequences because of their high water content. Within the cysts, fluid-fluid levels denote layering of protein and/or blood. Cystic rims and intralesional septae are highlighted by contrast enhancement. Adjacent enlarged or anomalous venous channels may be apparent as well. The differential diagnosis of these cystic lesions in the infant includes teratoma and infantile fibrosarcoma. For lymphatic anomalies of the thoracic duct and chylous effusions, contrast lymphangiography, although technically difficult to perform, can be helpful to identify the abnormal lymphatic channels or site of leakage.[177]

Treatment

The indications for LM treatment vary with the extent and location of the lesions.[178] Focal and macrocystic LM are amenable to ablation by both sclerotherapy and resection. In contrast, more diffuse and predominantly microcystic LM are difficult to eradicate by any method. For local intralesional bleeding that causes sudden enlargement of LM and pain, conservative management with rest and pain medications is sufficient. Similarly, the enlargement of LM that coincides with systemic viral or bacterial infections can be managed expectantly as it is usually harmless. On the other hand, bacterial infections presenting with cellulitis require treatment. Infected LM become tense and swollen producing erythema, pain, and toxicity; the incidence of this complication is around 15–20%. Treatment consists of systemic antibiotics; hospitalization for intravenous antibiotics is often necessary.

Indications for ablation or resection include recurrent complications with infection, cosmesis, deformity, dysfunction, and leakage into body cavities or from the skin.

Commonly used agents such as ethanol, sodium tetradecyl sulfate, and doxycycline produce scarring and collapse of the cysts. For simple, well-localized macrocystic LM, sclerotherapy can ameliorate most lesions. For more diffuse and complex LM, sclerotherapy procedures need to be staged and can lead to significant improvement. However, re-expansion of the lesions to some extent usually occurs. Weeping or bleeding from cutaneous vesicles can be controlled with local sclerotherapy or carbon dioxide laser, though leakage generally resumes in six to 24 months. Significant complications from sclerotherapy include injury to adjacent nerves, necrosis of overlying skin, and cardiotoxicity related to the overall dose.

Resection for complex LM can also be of significant benefit (see Fig. 72-9C), but staging is often needed.[179] The operations may be long and tedious, and often require meticulous dissection to preserve vital structures. General guidelines for resection are: (1) each operation should focus on a defined anatomic region, removing as much of the lesion as possible including neurovascular dissection, but without injuring vital structures; (2) limit blood loss to less than the patient's blood volume; and (3) prolonged closed-suction drainage of the resulting cavity is required. The recurrence rate following 'macroscopically complete excision' ranges from 15–40%. This recurrence is thought to be secondary to regrowth and re-expansion of unexcised lymphatic channels. Sclerotherapy of the residual cavity following excision may be helpful in this regard. Following resection, it is common for cutaneous vesicles to occur within the scar. These can be controlled to some extent by local intravesicular sclerotherapy or laser. Alternatively, additional staged excision, pulling uninvolved dermis over the resection bed, may prevent this annoying result.

Some other caveats about operation for LM are worthy of mention. Cervicofacial LM will often require staged orthognathic procedures to improve bite and speech impediments related to maxillary and mandibular overgrowth. Tracheostomy may be needed in cases of oropharyngeal and airway obstruction, and should precede attempts at sclerotherapy for cervicofacial LM. Reactive inflammatory swelling can be dramatic in the initial period following sclerotherapy, and can exacerbate partial oropharyngeal obstruction. Lesions of the cervical and axillary regions often involve the brachial plexus. The use of nerve stimulators is a useful adjunct to prevent injury in these cases. Resection of thoracic and mediastinal LM to treat recurrent pleural and pericardial effusions involves dissection and skeletonization of the great vessels, and vagus and phrenic nerves. For pelvic and anorectal LM, detailed knowledge of the anatomy of the ischiorectal fossa and sciatic nerve are important. Preoperative sclerotherapy is often useful as well to shrink lesions, but discernment is necessary as scarring can impede the preservation of important nerves. Lastly, for the specific type of cutaneous LM, 'lymphangioma circumscriptum', wide resection and closure, if necessary with split thickness skin grafts, can be curative. However, serial resections, allowing adjacent skin to grow, is generally preferable to grafting.

Venous Malformations

Clinical Features

VM, often mistermed 'cavernous hemangiomas', are slow-flow lesions consisting of venous channels that can develop anywhere in the body, most commonly in the skin and soft tissues. VM may be seen at birth or become apparent later, depending on the anatomic location. A wide spectrum of presentations is possible, including simple varicosities and ectasias, discreet spongy masses, and complex channels that can permeate any tissue or organ system. VMs are probably the most common of the vascular malformations, and are more likely to be multiple as well. They tend to slowly enlarge with normal growth of the patient, but can dilate and become symptomatic at any time. As with other VMs, the proportional growth that occurs may become exaggerated during puberty. On examination, these soft, bluish, compressible lesions can expand with dependent position and Valsalva maneuver (Fig. 72-12). Episodes of phlebothrombosis secondary to stasis may lead to acute pain and swelling. Phleboliths can be palpated in many VM. Associated local overgrowth and limb length discrepancy are not

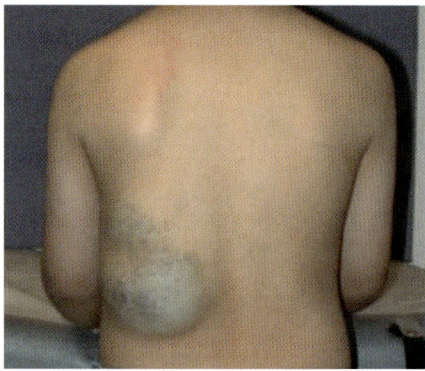

FIGURE 72-12 ■ This adolescent has a venous malformation in the subcutaneous tissues of his back. These soft, bluish, compressible lesions can expand with dependent position and during Valsalva maneuver.

uncommon. Involvement of bones and joints creates risk for pathologic fractures and hemarthroses, with subsequent arthritis.

Histologically, VM most often consist of sinusoidal vascular spaces with variable communication to adjacent veins. The dilated venous channels are thin walled, compared to normal veins, and smooth muscle actin staining reveals abnormal smooth muscle architecture that may be responsible for the gradual expansion seen over time with these lesions. Calcified phleboliths can be seen that provide evidence of prior clot formation within the VM. A variant of VM, glomovenous malformation (GVM, also incorrectly called 'glomangioma'), has the additional presence of ball-shaped glomus cells that line the vascular channels.

Approximately 90% of VM are sporadic; half of those result from a mutation in the vascular endothelial cell-specific receptor tyrosine kinase TIE-2 and its associated *TEK* gene.[180,181] The TIE-2 signaling pathways play an important role in angiogenic remodeling and vessel stabilization during development.[182] Cutaneomucosal venous malformations (VMCM), inherited through autosomal dominant transmission, are caused by a gain-of-function mutation in TIE-2 and represent 1–2% of VM.[181,183] GVM, also autosomal dominant, represents 5% of VM and results from loss-of-function mutations in glomulin, which affects vascular smooth muscle differentiation.[184]

VM of the GI tract are often multiple as well, and can affect every part from mouth to anus. They are more common in the left colon and rectum when associated with VM of the pelvis and perineum. GI bleeding, typically chronic in nature, can result. Blue rubber bleb nevus syndrome (or 'Bean syndrome') represents a specific rare disorder consisting of multifocal VM that affect the skin and GI tract primarily.[185] The skin lesions are unique in that they are often quite numerous and resemble tiny 'blue rubber nipples.' These skin lesions present diffusely and are classically seen on the palms and soles of the feet (Fig. 72-13). As with other GI VM, chronic bleeding, and intussusception can result. Diagnosis of GI VM is generally based on endoscopy. Patients with rectal VM can have associated ectatic mesenteric veins and are at risk for developing portomesenteric venous thrombosis.[186]

Large VM can also be complicated by localized intravascular coagulopathy caused by stasis and stagnation of blood within the malformation, leading to consumption of coagulation factors. The clotting profile consists of prolonged prothrombin time, decreased fibrinogen, and elevated D-dimers. The PTT is often normal. Thrombocytopenia can occur with a typical platelet range of less than 100,000/μL. The distinction between this coagulopathy and KMP is important. Lesions causing KMP are treated with anti-angiogenic agents, while VM will not respond to pharmacotherapy.

Imaging

Radiologic modalities useful for the diagnosis of VM include ultrasound, MRI, and venography. MRI is most informative and demonstrates hyperintense lesions with T_2 sequences. Contrast enhancement of the vascular

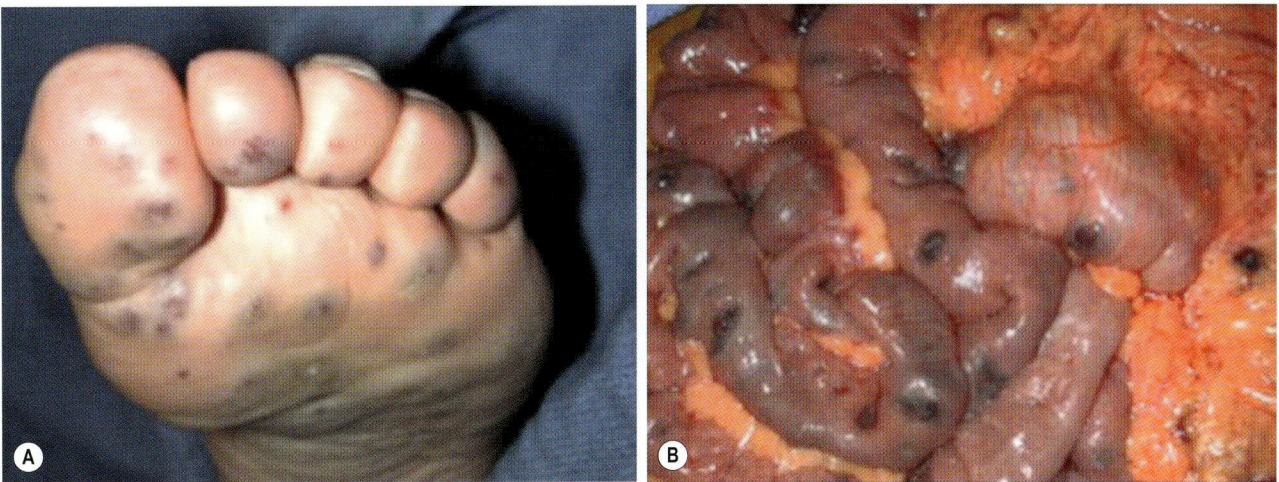

FIGURE 72-13 ■ Blue rubber bleb nevus syndrome. **(A)** Classic cutaneous venous malformations are seen on the sole of the foot. **(B)** Venous malformations of the small intestine and colon were found at operation.

spaces distinguishes VM from LM, as does the presence of pathognomonic phleboliths. Intralesional bleeding within LM can represent an exception to this rule. In contrast to AVM, VM do not demonstrate evidence of arterial flow on MRI.

Treatment

Indications for treatment include appearance, pain, functional impairment, and bleeding. Unfortunately, cure for VM, as with LM, is difficult to achieve for all but the most localized, and therefore less problematic lesions. For extensive VM of the extremities, conservative management with the use of graded compression stockings can achieve significant improvement in size and symptoms. Patient satisfaction with this treatment depends on a proper customized fit, but can be elusive, especially for children and teenagers. In order to prevent phlebothrombosis of VM with resultant pain and swelling, low-dose aspirin may be beneficial.

Intralesional sclerotherapy is the mainstay of treatment for most VM.[187] Sclerosing agents, most commonly ethanol and sodium tetradecyl sulfate, cause direct endothelial damage, thrombosis, and scarring. For small VM, the injection process is similar to that for simple varicosities. Larger lesions are accessed by direct puncture and the therapeutic agents are injected under fluoroscopy, with the use of tourniquets and compression of venous drainage to prevent systemic administration of the sclerosants. General anesthesia is required in most instances. Staged therapy and occasional embolization of large venous channels are useful for more complex VM. The more complex lesions are best treated by a skilled interventional radiologist who has experience with vascular anomalies.

VM have a propensity for recanalization and re-enlargement. Cure with sclerotherapy is rare. Given that recurrence is so prevalent, results from treatment are often stated in terms of patient satisfaction with decreased pain and appearance. Resection is typically reserved for well-localized lesions, but is marked by procedural morbidity and recurrence, especially for complex VM. Preoperative sclerotherapy is recommended preceding operations for extensive VM to shrink the lesion and decrease bleeding during the resection.

Unifocal GI lesions can be excised. Diffuse colorectal malformations causing significant bleeding may be treated by colectomy, anorectal mucosectomy, and colo-anal pull-through.[188] For multifocal VM in the blue rubber bleb nevus syndrome, complete resection of all lesions, combined with endoscopy of the entire GI tract at the time of operation, provides the only chance for possible cure. Bowel resection for these lesions is rarely indicated. Rather, wedge excision and polypectomy by intussusception of successive lengths of intestine are the preferred methods of resection.[189]

Arteriovenous Malformations

Clinical Features

AVM are fast-flow vascular malformations characterized by abnormal connections or shunts between feeding arteries and draining veins, without an intervening capillary bed. These shunts define the nidus of the malformation. Lesions tend to be localized, but can be extensive as well. AVM are one of the most common vascular anomalies that occur in the central nervous system and are more frequent than extracranial AVM. A clinical staging system was developed to describe the natural history of progression (Table 72-2).[190] At birth, they appear as a pink cutaneous blemish that can be confused with both CM and the premonitory sign of an IH. The fast flow through the shunt becomes more evident in childhood and adolescence as the lesion expands and develops into a mass.[191] Lesions will feel warm to the touch, often with a bruit or thrill. With continued expansion, they become more red and prominent. Puberty, pregnancy, or local trauma tends to trigger more rapid expansion. Skin ischemia can develop from expansion or local steal phenomenon, leading to pain, ulceration, and bleeding (Fig. 72-14). Large AVM can cause high-output cardiac failure.

TABLE 72-2	Schobinger Clinical Staging System for Arteriovenous Malformations
Stage	**Clinical Findings**
I (quiescent)	Pink to bluish stain, cutaneous warmth, and arteriovenous shunting by Doppler ultrasound imaging
II (expanding)	Same as stage I, plus enlargement, pulsation, thrill, bruit, and tortuous and tense veins
III (destructive)	Same as stage II, plus skin ulceration, bleeding, persistent pain, or tissue necrosis
IV (decompensating)	Same as stage III, plus cardiac failure

Most AVM are sporadic, but heritable forms exist. Mutations in RASA1 cause the autosomal dominant disorder CM-AVM.[133] The CM are multifocal, small, round-to-oval, pinkish-to-red lesions, and are usually randomly distributed. They can be associated with an AVM or arteriovenous fistula.[192]

Imaging

Ultrasound and Doppler imaging can elucidate the fast flow of these lesions and distinguish them from VM. On CT, dilated feeding arteries and veins are seen as areas of contrast enhancement. MRI and MRA are the most useful modalities to demonstrate the full extent of lesions. They appear as signal flow voids (black tubular structures) on MRI, or areas of contrast enhancement (white tubular structures) on MRA. Superselective angiography can clearly identify the nidus when treatment is planned.

Treatment

The majority of AVM require treatment because of continued expansion, which can lead to local tissue ischemia and pain.[190,193] The mainstays of treatment are angiographic embolization alone or in combination with excision. Local recurrence following early intervention can complicate future procedures. Very well-localized stage I AVM may be amenable to excision. Intervention is often delayed until symptoms (focal pain, ulceration, and bleeding) develop which is indicative of stage III. Treatment during infancy is indicated in cases of heart failure. The proximal feeding arteries should not be embolized or ligated during treatment as they provide the only avenue by which to reach the nidus of the AVM for subsequent embolization. The nidus will recruit other nearby arteries after the primary feeding vessels are occluded, and the AVM will recur and continue to enlarge.

Embolization should be directed to the nidus itself and the arteriovenous fistulae at the epicenter of the lesion. Direct puncture sclerotherapy of the AVM nidus can be an adjunct to embolization, especially when the feeding arteries are too tortuous or have been previously ligated. Retrograde transvenous embolization is often the best strategy for AVM with few venous outflow channels. Repeated and staged embolization procedures are typically necessary for these lesions, but often only provide temporary improvement. The quantity and microscopic nature of the arteriovenous fistulae that comprise the nidus of the AVM make it difficult to achieve complete occlusion of these microscopic shunts. Nonetheless, patients often have significant improvement in their symptoms, and cures with embolization alone have occurred.

The preferred treatment strategy for AVM typically consists of resection carried out two to three days following preoperative embolization of the nidus. Angiographic embolization facilitates the operation by decreasing bleeding, but does not decrease the extent of tissue to be resected. Whenever possible, the goal should be complete excision of the lesion. Both the nidus of the AVM and the involved skin should be removed. The most important factor for success is the extent of resection. Review of radiologic imaging, including the earliest available MRI scans and angiograms before any other treatment, is necessary. Intraoperatively, observation of the pattern of bleeding at the resection margins can also guide the extent of excision, as can intraoperative frozen section analysis. Primary closure is sometimes not possible without tissue transfer techniques. Vacuum-assisted closure devices can also be useful in areas with large soft tissue loss that precludes linear closure. The best results are seen with an AVM that is well localized. Yet, even in these cases, it is prudent to follow these patients for years to evaluate for recurrence. Unfortunately, most AVM are extensive and often not amenable to an operative approach. For these difficult lesions, embolization is used for palliation. For difficult AVM of the extremities, if distal in location, amputation becomes an option.

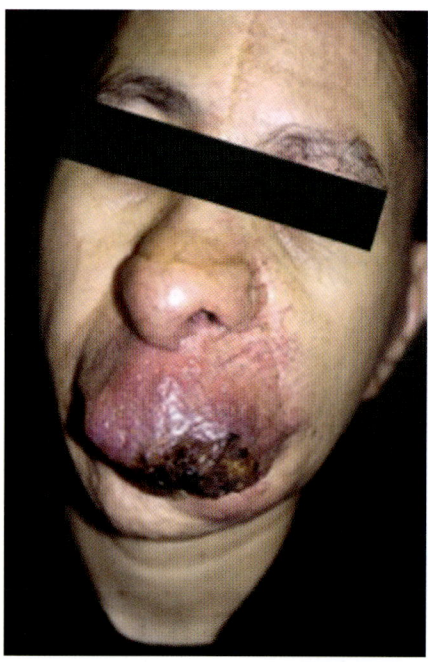

FIGURE 72-14 ■ A facial arteriovenous malformation (stage III) with ulceration of the skin is seen in this patient.

COMBINED VASCULAR MALFORMATIONS

As with other vascular malformation, combined malformations are classified as either slow-flow or fast flow. Generally, these more complex disorders are associated with soft tissue and skeletal overgrowth. They tend to be named for the person or persons who first described them. However, these eponyms often create confusion because of misuse. Therefore, it is preferred to use the anatomic terms that best describe the anomalous vascular channels that are present.

Klippel–Trenaunay Syndrome

Klippel–Trenaunay syndrome, or KT, is a slow-flow combined vascular malformation involving abnormal capillaries, lymphatics, and veins.[194-196] This capillary-lymphatico-venous malformation (CLVM) usually involves one or more extremities, most often a lower limb, and is associated with prominent soft tissue and bony hypertrophy (Fig. 72-15). This syndrome is sporadic and obvious at birth, with a wide range in severity. The CM component can be multiple, and typically presents as a large geographic pattern affecting the extremity, buttock, and trunk. It is macular at birth and develops lymphatic vesicles over time. The lymphatic anomalies have variable presentation including hypoplasia, lymphedema, and macrocystic LM, and are common in the buttock, pelvis, and perineum. Anomalous lateral superficial veins in the extremity, usually dilated with incompetent valves, are persistent embryonic vessels, the most common being the marginal vein of Servelle. There are anomalous deep system veins as well that may be hypoplastic or even absent. Thrombophlebitis of the anomalous veins occurs with a frequency of 20–45%, and pulmonary emboli are found in up to one-quarter of the patients.

Limb hypertrophy is also obvious at birth and tends to be progressive over time. Though the affected extremity is generally larger, it is occasionally shorter. With CLVM of the legs, pelvic involvement with LM and VM can also occur, but is often asymptomatic. Alternatively, problems with recurrent infections, hematuria, hematochezia, and bladder outlet obstruction may develop. With CLVM of the superior trunk and arms, the mediastinum or retropleural space can harbor the vascular malformation as well.

Imaging plays an important role in the evaluation of patients with KT. Plain films are used to serially document limb length discrepancies. MRI provides the foundation for describing the type and extent of each of the vascular malformation components. Hypertrophic fatty tissue is often seen in areas of overgrowth. A common pattern seen with LM of the lower extremity is macrocystic lesions in the pelvis and thigh, and microcystic LM affecting the abdominal wall, buttock, and distal extremity. These LM can be localized to the subcutaneous tissues or extend into the intramuscular compartments. Magnetic resonance venography can elucidate the anatomy of the deep system veins. Identification of a subcutaneous vein coursing along the lateral calf and thigh, the marginal vein of Servelle, is typical for KT.

Treatment for KT is often conservative. Symptoms of pain and deformity secondary to venous anomalies and oozing from the LM can often be improved with compression stockings. Alternatively, sclerotherapy can treat certain components of CLVM such as focal VM, macrocystic LM, and bleeding lymphatic vesicles. Recurrence after sclerotherapy however is often a problem. Endovenous laser ablation or resection can treat persistent embryonic veins, and veins with direct connections to the inferior vena cava or femoral or iliac veins, as these are at risk for causing pulmonary embolism (PE).

Operative therapies, mainly debulking procedures, can manage some of the specific problems encountered, primarily for overgrowth.[197] Staged contour resection can be used to treat areas of soft tissue overgrowth and lymphedema (Fig. 72-16).[198] It is critical to determine the location of the overgrowth, which can be either

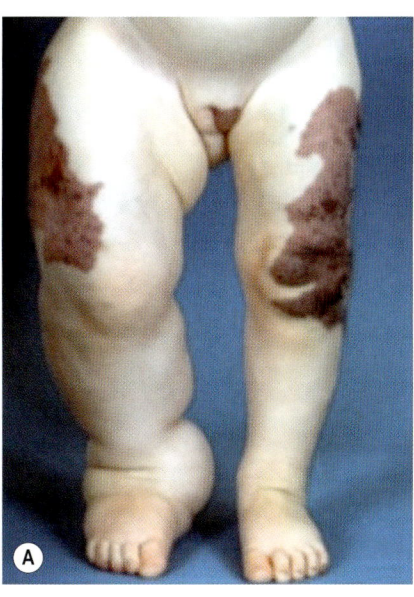
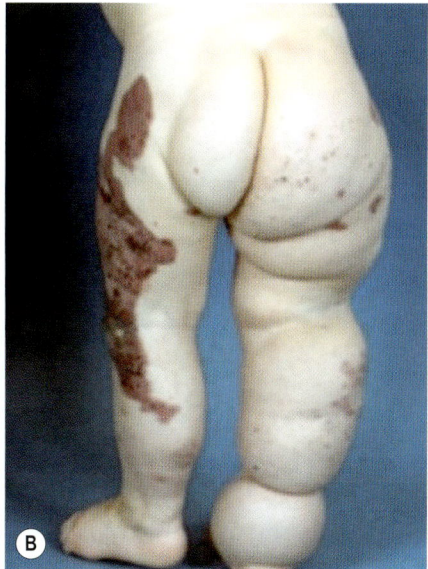

FIGURE 72-15 ■ This patient has Klippel-Trenaunay syndrome. This capillary-lymphatico-venous malformation usually involves one or more extremities, most often a lower limb, and is associated with prominent soft tissue and bony hypertrophy. The capillary malformation component typically presents as a large geographic pattern affecting the extremity, buttocks, and trunk.

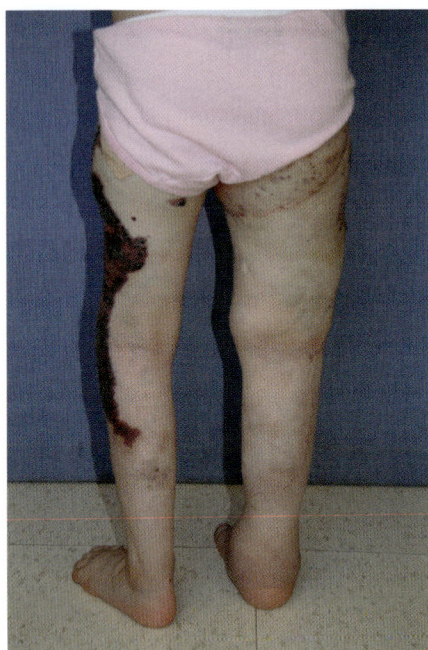

FIGURE 72-16 ■ This is a photograph of the same patient depicted in Figure 72-15. The patient is now older and has undergone staged debulking procedures for management of the soft tissue overgrowth and lymphedema in the right leg. Most of the capillary hemangioma component has also been excised.

extrafascial or intrafascial. Intrafascial overgrowth should not be debulked secondary to risk of injury to major neurovascular structures and immobility. Debulking of the trunk and thoracic wall is feasible, but excision of intrathoracic and mediastinal malformations should generally not be undertaken, especially if asymptomatic. Tissue with poor lymphatic drainage and altered circulation makes for poor tissue flaps, leading to delayed postoperative healing and protracted use of closed-suction drains. Perioperative management during significant resections should include consideration for anticoagulation and temporary inferior vena cava filter placement to help prevent deep venous thrombosis and PE.

Gross foot enlargement, which can impair ambulation and the ability to wear shoes, requires orthopedic corrective procedures and partial amputations to permit the use of regular or even custom footwear. Limb length discrepancy should be followed annually by an orthopedic surgeon to document and predict severity; differences less than 0.5 cm do not require therapy. Children with discrepancies greater than 1.5 cm should use shoe lifts to prevent limping and scoliosis. Epiphysiodesis of the distal femoral and/or proximal tibial growth plates are sometimes performed around the age of 11–12 years to correct overgrowth. Correction for arm length discrepancies is unnecessary. Resection of anomalous veins producing pain or potential sources of PE can be considered if too large for endovenous approaches.

CLOVES Syndrome

This syndrome is named for its phenotypic features: congenital lipomatous overgrowth, vascular malformations, epidermal nevi, seizures, scoliosis, and skeletal/spinal

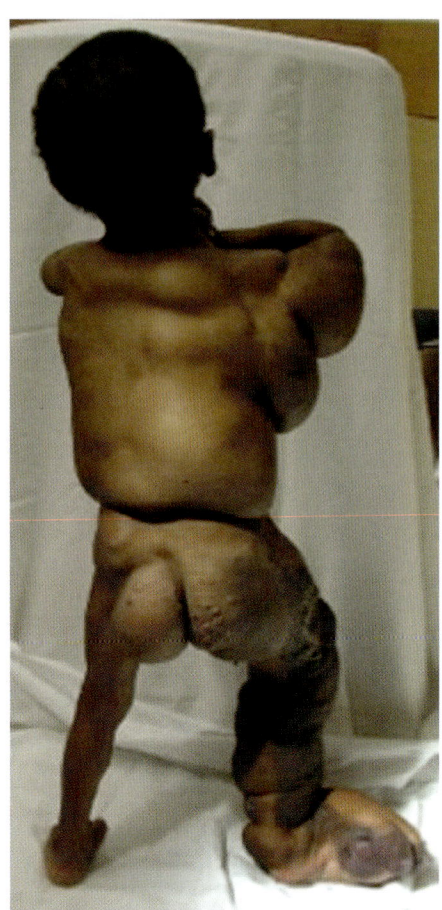

FIGURE 72-17 ■ This patient has CLOVES syndrome. Truncal lipomatous masses are present at birth often with an overlying capillary malformation. Musculoskeletal abnormalities usually involve extremities and include macrodactyly, wide triangular feet, or widened sandal gap. Both high-flow and low-flow venous malformations can also be found in this syndrome.

anomalies (Fig. 72-17).[199,200] It may be misdiagnosed as Proteus syndrome. Truncal lipomatous masses are present at birth, typically with an overlying capillary malformation, and may be identified on prenatal imaging.[201] The masses can extend into the mediastinum, pleural cavity, retroperitoneum, and paraspinal-intraspinal space. Both low-flow and high-flow vascular malformation are seen in CLOVES. Musculoskeletal abnormalities usually involve the extremities and include macrodactyly, large hands, wide triangular feet, or widened sandal gap.[199] Recently, mutations in *PIK3CA*, which encodes for a subunit of PI3K, have been identified as the cause of CLOVES.[202] Activation of PI3K eventually leads to phosphorylation of AKT, levels of which are increased by the PI3K mutations seen in CLOVES. Mutations in this gene have been shown to induce angiogenesis and malignant cell growth.[203]

Maffucci Syndrome

This syndrome consists of exophytic VM of the soft tissue and bones, bony exostoses, and endochondromas. This sporadic disorder is not usually evident at birth and can be uni- or bilateral. The bony lesions and endochondromas manifest first in childhood, while the venous anomalies appear later. Spindle cell hemangioendotheliomas commonly occur and denote reactive vascular proliferation within the preexisting VM, rather than true tumors.[204] The endochondromas can undergo malignant transformation in 20% to 30% of cases, leading to chondrosarcomas.[205] Two studies have recently identified somatic mosaic mutations in *IDH-1* and *IDH-2*, which code for different forms of the enzyme isocitrate dehydrogenase, as the cause of Maffucci syndrome.[206,207]

PTEN Hamartoma Tumor Syndrome

Bannayan–Riley–Ruvalcaba (BRRS) and Cowden syndromes (CS) are autosomal dominant disorders caused by mutations of the tumor-suppressor gene PTEN (phosphatase tensin homolog on chromosome 10), collectively termed PTEN hamartoma tumor syndrome.[208] BRRS is primarily an overgrowth syndrome that has vascular malformations as a minor component. The more prominent clinical features are macrocephaly, developmental delay, multiple lipomas, hamartomatous polyps of the ileum and colon, genital lentiginosis, and Hashimoto thyroiditis.[209] CS is characterized by mucocutaneous and papillomatous lesions, lipomas, hamartomatous intestinal lesions, and an increased risk for thyroid, breast, and endometrial cancer. Multifocal fast-flow vascular anomalies associated with ectopic fat are seen in about half of patients with PTEN mutations.[210] Macrocephalic patients with fast-flow vascular anomalies or multiple intracranial developmental venous anomalies should be tested for PTEN mutations.

Proteus Syndrome

Proteus syndrome is probably diagnosed more often than it actually occurs.[211] This overgrowth disorder is associated with activating mutations in the oncogene AKT-1 and is progressive over time.[212] Vascular, skeletal, and soft tissue anomalies tend to be asymmetrical and variably expressed. Common features include lipomas or lipomatosis, macrocephaly, and gigantism of the hands or feet (or both).

Parkes Weber Syndrome

Parkes Weber syndrome is a sporadic, combined fast-flow vascular malformation affecting the limb and trunk, with the lower extremity being the most common site.[213,214] Capillary arteriovenous fistulae (CAVF) and CM-AVM are combined with hypertrophy of the bone and muscle of the affected limb. CM-AVM is obvious at birth, appearing as overgrowth with a large geographic macular pink stain. In contrast to CLVM seen with KT syndrome, the limb hypertrophy is symmetrical along the length and substance of the extremity. The macular stain associated with CM-AVM has much greater cutaneous warmth than does typical CM. The finding of bruits or thrills on examination confirms the diagnosis. MRI demonstrates symmetric muscular and bony overgrowth, with generalized enlargement of the normal named arteries and veins within the affected limb. Angiography depicts the discrete arteriovenous fistulae. In rare cases, superselective embolization is used to occlude the arteriovenous shunts if symptoms of ischemia, pain, or high-output congestive heart failure occur.

INTERDISCIPLINARY VASCULAR ANOMALIES CENTER

The clarification of nomenclature and biologic classification of vascular anomalies has provided a useful clinical framework for the diagnosis and treatment of these lesions. Nevertheless, patients with vascular anomalies often provide complex exceptions to these designations. Lesions that are congenital malformations may not become apparent until adulthood, either due to anatomic location or progressive expansion over time. Neoplastic lesions, such as IH, often have a premonitory cutaneous sign at birth. Additionally, hemangiomas, when they have a significant fast-flow component, can be difficult to distinguish from AVM. VM can also at times exhibit enlargement and even endothelial hyperplasia triggered by clotting, ischemia, or partial resection, which leads to their propensity for recurrence after treatment. For these reasons, several regional and international centers have developed interdisciplinary vascular anomalies teams that serve as referral centers and which combine the medical, surgical, and radiologic expertise required to effectively diagnose and treat these often complex disorders. Guidelines have been established for referral to vascular anomalies centers.[215] Patients with unclear diagnoses, vascular malformation (except for CM), and rare vascular tumors should be referred to these centers for management and treatment.

REFERENCES

1. Mulliken JB, Fishman SJ, Burrows PE. Vascular anomalies. Curr Probl Surg 2000;37:517–84.
2. Finn MC, Glowacki J, Mulliken JB. Congenital vascular lesions: Clinical application of a new classification. J Pediatr Surg 1983; 18:894–900.
3. Mulliken JB, Glowacki J. Hemangiomas and vascular malformations in infants and children: A classification based on endothelial characteristics. Plast Reconstr Surg 1982;69:412–22.
4. Virchow R. Angioma in die krankhaften Geschwüstele, vol. 3. Berlin: Hirshwald; 1863.
5. Wegener G. Ueber lymphangiome. Arch Klin Chir 1877;20: 641–707.
6. Holmdahl K. Cutaneous hemangiomas in premature and mature infants. Acta Paediatri Scand 1955;44:370–9.
7. Amir J, Metzker A, Krikler R, et al. Strawberry hemangioma in preterm infants. Pediatr Dermatol 1986;3:331–2.
8. Haggstrom AN, Drolet BA, Baselga E, et al. Prospective study of infantile hemangiomas: Demographic, prenatal, and perinatal characteristics. J Pediatr 2007;150:291–4.
9. Smoller BR, Apfelberg DB. Infantile (juvenile) capillary hemangioma: A tumor of heterogeneous cellular elements. J Cutan Pathol 1993;20:330–6.
10. Khan ZA, Melero-Martin JM, Wu X, et al. Endothelial progenitor cells from infantile hemangioma and umbilical cord blood display unique cellular responses to endostatin. Blood 2006;108:915–21.
11. Boye E, Yu Y, Paranya G, et al. Clonality and altered behavior of endothelial cells from hemangiomas. J Clin Invest 2001;107: 745–52.
12. Dadras SS, North PE, Bertoncini J, et al. Infantile hemangiomas are arrested in an early developmental vascular differentiation state. Mod Pathol 2004;17:1068–79.

13. Lui W, Zhang S, Hu T, et al. Sex hormone receptors of hemangiomas in children. Chin Med J (Engl) 1997;110:349–51.

14. Sasaki GH, Pang CY, Wittliff JL. Pathogenesis and treatment of infant skin strawberry hemangiomas: Clinical and in vitro studies of hormonal effects. Plast Reconstr Surg 1984;73:359–70.

15. North PE, Waner M, Mizeracki A, et al. GLUT1: A newly discovered immunohistochemical marker for juvenile hemangiomas. Hum Pathol 2000;31:11–22.

16. Barnes CM, Huang S, Kaipainen A, et al. Evidence by molecular profiling for a placental origin of infantile hemangioma. Proc Natl Acad Sci U S A 2005;102:19097–102.

17. Ritter MR, Dorrell MI, Edmonds J, et al. Insulin-like growth factor 2 and potential regulators of hemangioma growth and involution identified by large-scale expression analysis. Proc Natl Acad Sci U S A 2002;99:7455–60.

18. Yu Y, Wylie-Sears J, Boscolo E, et al. Genomic imprinting of IGF2 is maintained in infantile hemangioma despite its high level of expression. Mol Med 2004;10:117–23.

19. Huang SA, Dorfman DM, Genest DR, et al. Type 3 iodothyronine deiodinase is highly expressed in the human uteroplacental unit and in fetal epithelium. J Clin Endocrinol Metab 2003;88:1384–8.

20. Huang SA, Tu HM, Harney JW, et al. Severe hypothyroidism caused by type 3 iodothyronine deiodinase in infantile hemangiomas. N Engl J Med 2000;343:185–9.

21. Ritter MR, Moreno SK, Dorrell MI, et al. Identifying potential regulators of infantile hemangioma progression through large-scale expression analysis: A possible role for the immune system and indoleamine 2,3 dioxygenase (IDO) during involution. Lymph Res Biol 2003;1:291–9.

22. Burton SK, Schulz CJ, Angle B, et al. An increased incidence of haemangiomas in infants born following chorionic villus sampling (CVS). Prenat Diagn 1995;15:209–14.

23. Kaplan P, Normandin JJ, Wilson GN, et al. Malformations and minor anomalies in children whose mothers had prenatal diagnosis: Comparison between CVS and amniocentesis. Am J Med Genet 1990;37:366–70.

24. Sato TN, Tozawa Y, Deutsch U, et al. Distinct roles of the receptor tyrosine kinases Tie-1 and Tie-2 in blood vessel formation. Nature 1995;376:70–4.

25. Suri C, Jones PF, Patan S, et al. Requisite role of angiopoietin-1, a ligand for the TIE2 receptor, during embryonic angiogenesis. Cell 1996;87:1171–80.

26. Maisonpierre PC, Suri C, Jones PF, et al. Angiopoietin-2, a natural antagonist for Tie2 that disrupts in vivo angiogenesis. Science 1997;277:55–60.

27. Roberts DM, Kearney JB, Johnson JH, et al. The vascular endothelial growth factor (VEGF) receptor Flt-1 (VEGFR-1) modulates Flk-1 (VEGFR-2) signaling during blood vessel formation. Am J Pathol 2004;164:1531–5.

28. Bielenberg DR, Bucana CD, Sanchez R, et al. Progressive growth of infantile cutaneous hemangiomas is directly correlated with hyperplasia and angiogensis of adjacent epidermis and inversely correlated with expression of the endogenous angiogenesis inhibitor, INF-beta. Int J Oncol 1999;14:401–8.

29. Takahashi K, Mulliken JB, Kozakewich HP, et al. Cellular markers that distinguish the phases of hemangioma during infancy and childhood. J Clin Invest 1994;93:2357–64.

30. Yu Y, Varughese J, Brown LF, et al. Increased Tie2 expression, enhanced response to angiopoietin-1, and dysregulated angiopoietin-2 expression in hemangioma-derived endothelial cells. Am J Pathol 2001;159:2271–80.

31. Razon MJ, Kraling BM, Mulliken JB, et al. Increased apoptosis coincides with onset of involution in infantile hemangioma. Microcirculation 1998;5:189–95.

32. Bowers RE, Graham EA, Tomlinson KM. The natural history of the strawberry nevus. Arch Dermatol 1960;82:667–80.

33. Patrice SJ, Wiss K, Mulliken JB. Pyogenic granuloma (lobular capillary hemangioma): A clinicopathologic study of 178 cases. Pediatr Dermatol 1991;8:267–76.

34. Kirschner RE, Low DW. Treatment of pyogenic granuloma by shave excision and laser photocoagulation. Plast Reconstr Surg 1999;104:1346–9.

35. Boon LM, Fishman SJ, Lund DP, et al. Congenital fibrosarcoma masquerading as congenital hemangioma: Report of two cases. J Pediatr Surg 1995;30:1378–81.

36. Enjolras O, Gelbert F. Superficial hemangiomas: Association and management. Pediatr Dermatol 1997;14:173–9.

37. Hersh JH, Waterfill D, Rutledge J, et al. Sternal malformatio/vascular dysplasia association. Am J Med Genet 1985;21:177–86.

38. Goldberg NS, Hebert AA, Esterly NB. Sacral hemangiomas and multiple congenital anomalies. Arch Dermatol 1986;122:684–7.

39. Albright AL, Gartner JC, Wiener ES. Lumbar cutaneous hemangiomas as indicators of tethered spinal cords. Pediatrics 1989;83:977–80.

40. Gorlin RJ, Kantaputra P, Aughton DJ, et al. Marked female predilection in some syndromes associated with facial hemangiomas. Am J Med Genet 1994;52:130–5.

41. Frieden IJ, Reese V, Cohen D. PHACE syndrome. The association of posterior fossa brain malformations, hemangiomas, arterial anomalies, coarctation of the aorta and cardiac defects, and eye abnormalities. Arch Dermatol 1996;132:307–11.

42. Burrows PE, Laor T, Paltiel H, et al. Diagnostic imaging in the evaluation of vascular birthmarks. Dermatol Clin 1998;16:455–88.

43. Dubois J, Patriquin HB, Garel L, et al. Soft-tissue hemangiomas in infants and children: Diagnosis using Doppler sonography. AJR Am J Roentgenol 1998;171:247–52.

44. Paltiel HJ, Burrows PE, Kozakewich HP, et al. Soft-tissue vascular anomalies: Utility of ultrasound for diagnosis. Radiology 2000;214:747–54.

45. Meyer JS, Hoffer FA, Barnes PD, et al. Biological classification of soft-tissue vascular anomalies: MR correlation. AJR Am J Roentgenol 1991;157:559–64.

46. Margileth AM, Museles M. Cutaneous hemangiomas in children. Diagnosis and conservative management. JAMA 1965;194:523–6.

47. Bennett ML, Fleischer ABJ, Chamlin SL, et al. Oral corticosteroid use is effective for cutaneous hemangiomas: An evidence-based evaluation. Arch Dermatol 2001;137:1208–13.

48. Greenberger S, Boscolo E, Adini I, et al. Corticosteroid suppression of VEGF-A in infantile hemangioma-derived stem cells. N Engl J Med 2010;362:1005–13.

49. Crum R, Szabo S, Folkman J. A new class of steroids inhibits angiogenesis in the presence of heparin or a heparin fragmnet. Science 1985;230:1375–8.

50. Boon LM, MacDonald DM, Mulliken JB. Complications of systemic corticosteroid therapy for problematic hemangiomas. Plast Reconstr Surg 1999;104:1616–23.

51. Sloan GM, Reinisch JF, Nichter LS, et al. Intralesional corticosteroid therapy for infantil hemangiomas. Plast Reconstr Surg 1989;83:459–67.

52. Marler JJ, Mulliken JB. Vascular Anomalies. 2nd ed. Philadephia: Elsevier; 2006.

53. Ruttum MS, Abrams GW, Harris GJ, et al. Bilateral retinal embolization associated with intralesional corticosteroid injection for capillary hemangioma of infancy. J Pediatr Ophthalmol Strabismus 1993;30:4–7.

54. Leute-Labreze C, Dumas de la Roque E, Hubiche T, et al. Propanolol for severe hemangiomas of infancy. N Engl J Med 2008;358:2649–51.

55. Sans V, de la Roque ED, Berge J, et al. Propanolol for severe infantile hemangiomas: Follow-up report. Pediatrics 2009;124:e423–31.

56. Buckmiller LM, Munson PD, Dyamenahalli U, et al. Propranolol for infantile hemangiomas: Early experience at a tertiary vascular anomalies center. Laryngoscope 2010;120:676–81.

57. Bigorre M, Van Kien AK, Valette H. Beta-blocking agent for treatment of infantile hemangioma. Plast Reconstr Surg 2009;123:195e–6e.

58. Bagazgoitia L, Torrelo A, Gutierrez JC, et al. Propranolol for infantile hemangiomas. Pediatr Dermatol 2011;28:108–14.

59. Cushing SL, Boucek RJ, Manning SC, et al. Initial experience with a multidisciplinary strategy for initiation of propranolol therapy for infantile hemangiomas. Otolaryngol Head Neck Surg 2011;144:78–84.

60. Holland KE, Frieden IJ, Frommelt PC, et al. Hypoglycemia in children taking propranolol for the treatment of infantile hemangioma. Arch Dermatol 2010;146:775–8.

61. Harrison DC, Meffin PJ, Winkle RA. Clinical pharmacokinetics of antiarrhythmic drugs. Prog Cardiovasc Dis 1977;20:217–42.

62. Storch CH, Hoeger PH. Propranolol for infantile haemangiomas: Insights into the molecular mechanisms of action. Br J Dermatol 2010;163:269–74.
63. Westfall TC, Westfall DP. Neurotransmission: The autonomic and somatic motor nervous system. 11th ed. New York: McGraw-Hill; 2006.
64. Guimaraes S, Moura D. Vascular adrenoceptors: An update. Pharmacol Rev 2001;53:319–56.
65. Sommers Smith SK, Smith DM. Beta blockade induces apoptosis in cultured capillary endothelial cells. In Vitro Cell Dev Biol Anim 2002;38:298–304.
66. Yang EV, Sood AK, Chen M, et al. Norepinephrine up-regulates the expression of vascular endothelial growth factor, matrix metalloproteinase (MMP)-2, and MMP-9 in nasopharyngeal carcinoma tumor cells. Cancer Res 2006;66:10357–64.
67. White CW, Wolf SJ, Korones DN, et al. Treatment of childhood angiomatous diseases with recombinant interferon alfa-2a. J Pediatr 1991;118:59–66.
68. Tamayo L, Ortiz DM, Orozco-Covarrubias L, et al. Therapeutic efficacy of interferon alfa-2b in infants with life-threatening giant hemangiomas. Arch Dermatol 1997;133:1567–71.
69. Ricketts RR, Hatley RM, Corden BJ, et al. Interferon-alpha-2a for the treatment of complex hemangiomas of infancy and childhood. Ann Surg 1994;219:605–12.
70. Greinwald JH Jr, Burke DK, Bonthius DJ, et al. An update on the treatment of hemangiomas in children with interferon alfa-2a. Arch Otolaryngol Head Neck Surg 1999;125:21–7.
71. Ezekowitz RA, Mulliken JB, Folkman J. Interferon alfa-2a therapy for life-threatening hemangiomas of infancy. N Engl J Med 1992;326:1456–63.
72. Barlow CF, Priebe CJ, Mulliken JB, et al. Spastic diplegia as a complication of interferon Alfa-2a treatment of hemangiomas of infancy. J Pediatr 1998;132:527–30.
73. Deb G, Jenkner A, Donfrancesco A. Spastic diplegia and interferon. J Pediatr 1999;134:382.
74. Perez J, Pardo J, Gomez C. Vincristine–an effective treatment of corticoid-resistant life-threatening infantile hemangiomas. Acta Oncol 2002;41:197–9.
75. Scheepers JH, Quaba AA. Does the pulsed tunable dye laser have a role in the management of infantile hemangiomas: Observations based on 3 years experience. Plast Reconstr Surg 1995;95:305–12.
76. Sie KC, McGill T, Healy GB. Subglottic hemangioma: Ten years' experience with the carbon dioxide laser. Ann Otol Rhinol Laryngol 1994;103:167–72.
77. Morelli JG, Tan OT, Yohn JJ, et al. Treatment of ulcerated hemangiomas infancy. Arch Pediatr Adolesc Med 1994;148:1104–5.
78. Fishman SJ, Fox VL. Visceral vascular anomalies. Gastrointest Endosc Clin N Am 2001;11:813–34.
79. Fishman SJ, Burrows PE, Leichtner AM, et al. Gastrointestinal manifestations of vascular anomlies in childhood: Varied etiologies require multiple therapeutic modalities. J Pediatr Surg 1998;33:1163–7.
80. Mulliken JB, Rogers GF, Marler JJ. Circular excision of hemangioma and purse-string closure: The smallest possible scar. Plast Reconstr Surg 2002;109:1544–54.
81. Enjolras O, Riche MC, Merland JJ, et al. Management of alarming hemangiomas in infancy: A review of 25 cases. Pediatrics 1990;85:491–8.
82. Boon LM, Enjolras O, Mulliken JB. Congenital hemangioma: Evidence of accelerated involution. J Pediatr 1996;128:329–35.
83. Berenguer B, Mulliken JB, Enjolras O, et al. Rapidly involuting congenital hemangioma: Clinical and histopathologic features. Pediatr Dev Pathol 2003;6:495–510.
84. Enjolras O, Mulliken JB, Boon LM, et al. Noninvoluting congenital hemangioma: A rare cutaneous vascular anomaly. Plast Reconstr Surg 2001;107:1647–54.
85. Boon LM, Burrows PE, Paltiel HJ, et al. Hepatic vascular anomalies in infancy: A twenty-seven-year experience. J Pediatr 1996;129:346–54.
86. Christison-Lagay ER, Burrows PE, Alomari A, et al. Hepatic hemangiomas: Subtype classification and development of a clinical practice algorithm and registry. J Pediatr Surg 2007;42:62–7.
87. Mo JQ, Dimashkieh HH, Bove KE. GLUT1 endothelial reactivity distinguishes hepatic infantile hemangioma from congenital hepatic vascular malformation with associated capillary proliferation. Hum Pathol 2004;35:200–9.
88. Morris J, Abbott J, Burrows P, et al. Antenatal diagnosis of fetal hepatic hemangioma treated with maternal corticosteroids. Obstet Gynecol 1999;94:813–15.
89. Mejides AA, Adra AM, O'Sullivan MJ, et al. Prenatal diagnosis and therapy for a fetal hepatic vascular malformation. Obstet Gynecol 1995;85:850–3.
90. Hernandez F, Navarro M, Encinas JL, et al. The role of GLUT1 immunostaining in the diagnosis and classification of liver vascular tumors in children. J Pediatr Surg 2005;40:801–4.
91. Drut RM, Drut R. Extracutaneous infantile haemangioma is also Glut1 positive. J Clin Pathol 2004;57:1197–200.
92. Kulungowski AM, Alomari AI, Chawla A, et al. Lessons from a liver hemangioma registry: Subtype classification. J Pediatr Surg 2012;47:165–70.
93. Konrad D, Ellis G, Perlman K. Spontaneous regression of severe acquired infantile hypothyroidism associated with multiple liver hemangiomas. Pediatrics 2003;112:1424–6.
94. Draper H, Diamond IR, Temple M, et al. Multimodal management of endangering hepatic hemangioma: Impact on tranplast avoidance: A descriptive case series. J Pediatr Surg 2008;43:120–5.
95. Dickie B, Dasgupta R, Nair R, et al. Spectrum of hepatic hemangiomas: Management and outcome. J Pediatr Surg 2009;44:125–33.
96. Perez-Valle S, Peinador M, Herraiz P, et al. Vincristine, an efficacious alternative for diffuse neonatal haemangiomatosis. Acta Paediatr 2010;99:311–15.
97. Jones EW, Orkin M. Tufted angioma (angioblastoma): A benign progressive angioma, not to be confused with Kaposi's sarcoma or low grade angiosarcoma. J Am Acad Dermatol 1989;20:214–25.
98. Enjolras O, Mulliken JB, Wassef M, et al. Residual lesions after Kasabach-Merritt phenomenon in 41 patients. J Am Acad Dermatol 2000;42:225–35.
99. Sarkar M, Mulliken JB, Kozakewich HP, et al. Thrombocytopenic coagulopathy (Kasabach-Merritt phenomenon) is associated with Kaposiform hemangioendothelioma and not with common infantile hemangioma. Plast Reconstr Surg 1997;100:1377–86.
100. Kasabach HH, Merritt KK. Capillary hemangioma with extensive purpura: A report of a case. Am J Dis Child 1940;59:1063–70.
101. Enjolras O, Wassef M, Mazoyer E, et al. Infants with Kasabach-Merritt syndrome do not have 'true' hemangiomas. J Pediatr 1997;130:631–40.
102. Zuckerberg LR, Nikoloff BJ, Weiss SW. Kaposiform hemangioendothelioma of infancy and childhood: An aggressive neoplasm associated with Kasabach-Merritt syndrome and lymphangiomatosis. Am J Surg Pathol 1993;17:321–8.
103. Vin-Christian K, McCalmont TH, Frieden IJ. Kaposiform hemangioendothelioma: An aggressive, locally invasive vascular tumor that can mimic hemangioma of infancy. Arch Dermatol 1997;133:1573–8.
104. Hu B, Lachman R, Phillips J, et al. Kasabach-Merritt syndrome-associated kaposiform hemangioendothelioma successfully treated with cyclophosphagmide, vincristine and actionmycin D. J Pediatr Hematol Oncol 1998;20:567–9.
105. Haisley-Royster C, Enjolras O, Frieden IJ, et al. Kasabach-merritt phenomenon: A retrospective study of treatment with vincristine. J Pediatr Hematol Oncol 2002;24:459–62.
106. Enjolras O, Wassef M, Dosquet C, et al. [Kasabach-Merritt syndrome on a congenital tufted angioma]. Ann Dermatol Venereol 1998;125:257–60.
107. Blatt J, Stavas J, Moats-Staats B, et al. Treatment of childhood kaposiform hemangioendothelioma with sirolimus. Pediatr Blood Cancer 15 2010;55:1396–8.
108. Chiu YE, Drolet BA, Blei F, et al. Variable response to propranolol treatment of kaposiform hemangioendothelioma, tufted angioma, and Kasabach-Merritt phenomenon. Pediatr Blood Cancer. Pediatr Blood Cancer 2012;59:934–8.
109. Adams DM. The nonsurgical management of vascular lesions. Facial Plast Surg Clin North Am 2001;9(4):601–8.
110. Hermans DJ, van Beynum IM, van der Vijver RJ, et al. Kaposiform hemangioendothelioma with Kasabach-Merritt syndrome: A new indication for propranolol treatment. J Pediatr Hematol Oncol 2011;33:e171–3.

111. Lopez V, Marti N, Pereda C, et al. Successful management of Kaposiform hemangioendothelioma with Kasabach-Merritt phenomenon using vincristine and ticlopidine. Pediatr Dermatol 2009;26:365–6.

112. Vikkula M, Boon LM, Mulliken JB, et al. Molecular basis of vascular anomalies. Trends Cardiovasc Med 1998;8:281–92.

113. Brouillard P, Vikkula M. Genetic causes of vascular malformations. Hum Mol Genet 2007;16(Spec No. 2):R140–9.

114. Limaye N, Boon LM, Vikkula M. From germline towards somatic mutations in the pathophysiology of vascular anomalies. Hum Mol Genet 2009;18:R65–74.

115. Christison-Lagay ER, Fishman SJ. Vascular anomalies. Surg Clin North Am 2006;86:393–425.

116. Dumont DJ, Fong GH, Puri MC, et al. Vascularization of the mouse embryo: A study of flk-1, tek, tie, and vascular endothelial growth factor expression during development. Dev Dyn 1995; 203:80–92.

117. Folkman J, D'Amore PA. Blood vessel formation: What is its molecular basis? Cell 1996;87:1153–5.

118. Risau W. Mechanisms of angiogenesis. Nature 1997;386:671–4.

119. Ramsauer M, D'Amore PA. Contextual role for angiopoietins and TGFbeta1 in blood vessel stabilization. J Cell Sci 2007;120: 1810–17.

120. Karpanen T, Alitalo K. Molecular biology and pathology of lymphangiogenesis. Annu Rev Pathol 2008;3:367–97.

121. Huntington GS, McClure CFW. The anatomy and development of the jugular lymph sac in the domestic cat (Felis domestica). Anat Rec 1908;2:1–19.

122. Sabin FR. The lymphatic system in human embryos, with a consideration of the morphology of the system as a whole. Am J Anat 1909;9:43–91.

123. Oliver G. Lymphatic vasculature development. Nat Rev Immunol 2004;4:35–45.

124. Banerji S, Ni J, Wang SX, et al. LYVE-1, a new homologue of the CD44 glycoprotein, is a lymph-specific receptor for hyaluronan. J Cell Biol 1999;144:789–801.

125. Wigle JT, Oliver G. Prox1 function is required for the development of the murine lymphatic system. Cell 1999;98:769–78.

126. Wigle JT, Harvey N, Detmar M, et al. An essential role for Prox1 in the induction of the lymphatic endothelial cell phenotype. EMBO J 2002;21:1505–13.

127. Karkkainen MJ, Alitalo K. Lymphatic endothelial regulation, lymphoedema, and lymph node metastasis. Semin Cell Dev Biol 2002;13:9–18.

128. Kaipainen A, Korhonen J, Mustonen T, et al. Expression of the fms-like tyrosine kinase 4 gene becomes restricted to lymphatic endothelium during development. Proc Natl Acad Sci U S A 1995;92:3566–70.

129. Dumont DJ, Jussila L, Taipale J, et al. Cardiovascular failure in mouse embryos deficient in VEGF receptor-3. Science 1998;282: 946–9.

130. Jeltsch M, Kaipainen A, Joukov V, et al. Hyperplasia of lymphatic vessels in VEGF-C transgenic mice. Science 1997;276:1423–5.

131. Jacobs AH, Walton RG. The incidence of birthmarks in the neonate. Pediatrics 1976;58:218–22.

132. Eerola I, Boon LM, Watanabe S, et al. Locus for susceptibility for familial capillary malformation ('port-wine stain') maps to 5q. Eur J Hum Genet 2002;10:375–80.

133. Eerola I, Boon LM, Mulliken JB, et al. Capillary malformation-arteriovenous malformation, a new clinical and genetic disorder caused by RASA1 mutations. Am J Hum Genet 2003;73: 1240–9.

134. Smoller BR, Rosen S. Port-wine stains. A disease of altered neural modulation of blood vessels? Arch Dermatol 1986;122: 177–9.

135. Enjolras O, Riche MC, Merland JJ. Facial port-wine stains and Sturge-Weber syndrome. Pediatrics 1985;76:48–51.

136. Tan OT, Sherwood K, Gilchrest BA. Treatment of children with port-wine stains using the flashlamp pumped tunable dye laser. N Engl J Med 1989;320:416–21.

137. van der Horst CM, Koster PH, de Borgie CA, et al. Effect of the timing of treatment of port-wine stains with the flash-lamp-pumped pulsed-dye laser. N Engl J Med 1998;338:1028–33.

138. Chapas AM, Eickhorst K, Geronemus RG. Efficacy of early treatment of facial port wine stains in newborns: A review of 49 cases. Lasers Surg Med 2007;39:563–8.

139. Van Lohuizen CHJ. Uber eine seltene angeborene Hautanomalie (cutis marmorata telangiectatica congenita). Acta Derm Venereol 1922;3:202–11.

140. Kienast AK, Hoeger PH. Cutis marmorata telangiectatica congenita: A prospective study of 27 cases and review of the literature with proposal of diagnostic criteria. Clin Exp Dermatol 2009;34:319–23.

141. Amitai DB, Fichman S, Merlob P, et al. Cutis marmorata telangiectatica congenita: Clinical findings in 85 patients. Pediatr Dermatol 2000;17:100–4.

142. Fujita M, Darmstadt GL, Dinulos JG. Cutis marmorata telangiectatica congenita with hemangiomatous histopathologic features. J Am Acad Dermatol 2003;48:950–4.

143. South DA, Jacobs AH. Cutis marmorata telangiectatica congenita (congenital generalized phlebectasia). J Pediatr 1978;93:944–9.

144. Requena L, Sangueza OP. Cutaneous vascular proliferation. Part II. Hyperplasias and benign neoplasms. J Am Acad Dermatol 1997;37:887–919.

145. Picascia DD, Esterly NB. Cutis marmorata telangiectatica congenita: Report of 22 cases. J Am Acad Dermatol 1989;20: 1098–104.

146. O'Toole EA, Deasy P, Watson R. Cutis marmorata telangiectatica congenita associated with a double aortic arch. Pediatr Dermatol 1995;12:348–50.

147. Devillers AC, de Waard-van der Spek FB, Oranje AP. Cutis marmorata telangiectatica congenita: Clinical features in 35 cases. Arch Dermatol 1999;135:34–8.

148. Vogel AM, Paltiel HJ, Kozakewich HP, et al. Iliac artery stenosis in a child with cutis marmorata telangiectatica congenita. J Pediatr Surg 2005;40:e9–12.

149. Guttmacher AE, Marchuk DA, White RI Jr. Hereditary hemorrhagic telangiectasia. N Engl J Med 1995;333:918–24.

150. McDonald J, Damjanovich K, Millson A, et al. Molecular diagnosis in hereditary hemorrhagic telangiectasia: Findings in a series tested simultaneously by sequencing and deletion/duplication analysis. Clin Genet 2011;79:335–44.

151. McAllister KA, Grogg KM, Johnson DW, et al. Endoglin, a TGF-beta binding protein of endothelial cells, is the gene for hereditary haemorrhagic telangiectasia type 1. Nat Genet 1994;8:345–51.

152. Johnson DW, Berg JN, Baldwin MA, et al. Mutations in the activin receptor-like kinase 1 gene in hereditary haemorrhagic telangiectasia type 2. Nat Genet 1996;13:189–95.

153. Gallione CJ, Repetto GM, Legius E, et al. A combined syndrome of juvenile polyposis and hereditary haemorrhagic telangiectasia associated with mutations in MADH4 (SMAD4). Lancet 2004; 363:852–9.

154. Shovlin CL, Guttmacher AE, Buscarini E, et al. Diagnostic criteria for hereditary hemorrhagic telangiectasia (Rendu-Osler-Weber syndrome). Am J Med Genet 2000;91(1):66–7.

155. Govani FS, Shovlin CL. Hereditary haemorrhagic telangiectasia: A clinical and scientific review. Eur J Hum Genet 2009;17: 860–71.

156. Marler JJ, Fishman SJ, Upton J, et al. Prenatal diagnosis of vascular anomalies. J Pediatr Surg 2002;37:318–26.

157. Gallagher PG, Mahoney MJ, Gosche JR. Cystic hygroma in the fetus and newborn. Semin Perinatol 1999;23:341–56.

158. Bruder E, Perez-Atayde AR, Jundt G, et al. Vascular lesions of bone in children, adolescents, and young adults. A clinicopathologic reappraisal and application of the ISSVA classification. Virchows Arch 2009;454:161–79.

159. Florez-Vargas A, Vargas SO, Debelenko LV, et al. Comparative analysis of D2-40 and LYVE-1 immunostaining in lymphatic malformations. Lymphology 2008;41:103–10.

160. Padwa BL, Hayward PG, Ferraro NF, et al. Cervicofacial lymphatic malformation: Clinical course, surgical intervention, and pathogenesis of skeletal hypertrophy. Plast Reconstr Surg 1995;95:951–60.

161. Gorham LW, Stout AP. Massive osteolysis (acute spontaneous absorption of bone, phantom bone, disappearing bone); Its relation to hemangiomatosis. J Bone Joint Surg Am 1955;37-A: 985–1004.

162. Pedicelli G, Mattia P, Zorzoli AA, et al. Gorham syndrome. JAMA 21 1984;252:1449–51.

163. Kulenkampff HA, Richter GM, Hasse WE, et al. Massive pelvic osteolysis in the Gorham-Stout syndrome. Int Orthop 1990;14: 361–6.

164. Venkatramani R, Ma NS, Pitukcheewanont P, et al. Gorham's disease and diffuse lymphangiomatosis in children and adolescents. Pediatr Blood Cancer 2011;56:667–70.

165. Papadakis SA, Khaldi L, Babourda EC, et al. Vanishing bone disease: Review and case reports. Orthopedics 2008;31:278.

166. Vinee P, Tanyu MO, Hauenstein KH, et al. CT and MRI of Gorham syndrome. J Comput Assist Tomogr 1994;18:985–9.

167. Takahashi A, Ogawa C, Kanazawa T, et al. Remission induced by interferon alfa in a patient with massive osteolysis and extension of lymph-hemangiomatosis: A severe case of Gorham-Stout syndrome. J Pediatr Surg 2005;40:E47–50.

168. Hagberg H, Lamberg K, Astrom G. Alpha-2b interferon and oral clodronate for Gorham's disease. Lancet 1997;350:1822–3.

169. Hammer F, Kenn W, Wesselmann U, et al. Gorham-Stout disease–stabilization during bisphosphonate treatment. J Bone Miner Res 2005;20:350–3.

170. Hammill AM, Wentzel M, Gupta A, et al. Sirolimus for the treatment of complicated vascular anomalies in children. Pediatr Blood Cancer 2011;57:1018–24.

171. Smeltzer DM, Stickler GB, Schirger A. Primary lymphedema in children and adolescents: A follow-up study and review. Pediatrics 1985;76:206–18.

172. Karkkainen MJ, Ferrell RE, Lawrence EC, et al. Missense mutations interfere with VEGFR-3 signalling in primary lymphoedema. Nat Genet 2000;25:153–9.

173. Irrthum A, Karkkainen MJ, Devriendt K, et al. Congenital hereditary lymphedema caused by a mutation that inactivated VEGR3 tyrosine kinase. Am J Hum Genet 2000;67:295–301.

174. Brice G, Child AH, Evans A, et al. Milroy disease and the VEGFR-3 mutation phenotype. J Med Genet 2005;42:98–102.

175. Brice G, Mansour S, Bell R, et al. Analysis of the phenotypic abnormalities in lymphoedema-distichiasis syndrome in 74 patients with FOXC2 mutations or linkage to 16q24. J Med Genet 2002;39:478–83.

176. Fang J, Dagenais SL, Erickson RP, et al. Mutations in FOXC2 (MFH-1), a forkhead family transcription factor, are responsible for the hereditary lymphedema-distichiasis syndrome. Am J Hum Genet 2000;67:1382–8.

177. Fishman SJ, Burrows PE, Upton J, et al. Life-threatening anomalies of the thoracic duct: Anatomic delineation dictates management. J Pediatr Surg 2001;36:1269–72.

178. Alqahtani A, Nguyen LT, Flageole H, et al. 25 years' experience with lymphangiomas in children. J Pediatr Surg 1999;34:1164–8.

179. Upton J, Coombs CJ, Mulliken JB, et al. Vascular malformations of the upper limb: A review of 270 patients. J Hand Surg Am 1999;24:1019–35.

180. Limaye N, Wouters V, Uebelhoer M, et al. Somatic mutations in angiopoietin receptor gene TEK cause solitary and multiple sporadic venous malformations. Nat Genet 2009;41:118–24.

181. Vikkula M, Boon LM, Carraway KL 3rd, et al. Vascular dysmorphogenesis caused by an activating mutation in the receptor tyrosine kinase TIE2. Cell 1996;87:1181–90.

182. Jones N, Iljin K, Dumont DJ, et al. Tie receptors: New modulators of angiogenic and lymphangiogenic responses. Nat Rev Mol Cell Biol 2001;2:257–67.

183. Calvert JT, Riney TJ, Kontos CD, et al. Allelic and locus heterogeneity in inherited venous malformations. Hum Mol Genet 1999;8:1279–89.

184. Brouillard P, Boon LM, Mulliken JB, et al. Mutations in a novel factor, glomulin, are responsible for glomuvenous malformations ('glomangiomas'). Am J Hum Genet 2002;70:866–74.

185. AP O. Blue rubber bleb nevus syndrome. Pediatr Dermatol 1986;3:304–10.

186. Kulungowski AM, Fox VL, Burrows PE, et al. Portomesenteric venous thrombosis associated with rectal venous malformations. J Pediatr Surg 2010;45:1221–7.

187. Berenguer B, Burrows PE, Zurakowski D, et al. Sclerotherapy of craniofacial venous malformations: Complications and results. Plast Reconstr Surg 1999;104:1–11.

188. Fishman SJ, Shamberger RC, Fox VL, et al. Endorectal pull-through abates gastrointestinal hemorrhage from colorectal venous malformations. J Pediatr Surg 2000;35:982–4.

189. Fishman SJ, Smithers CJ, Folkman J, et al. Blue rubber bleb nevus syndrome: Surgical eradication of gastrointestinal bleeding. Ann Surg 2005;241:523–8.

190. Kohout MP, Hansen M, Pribaz JJ, et al. Arteriovenous malformations of the head and neck: Natural history and management. Plast Reconstr Surg 1998;102:643–54.

191. Liu AS, Mulliken JB, Zurakowski D, et al. Extracranial arteriovenous malformations: Natural progression and recurrence after treatment. Plast Reconstr Surg 2010;125:1185–94.

192. Revencu N, Boon LM, Mulliken JB, et al. Parkes Weber syndrome, vein of Galen aneurysmal malformation, and other fast-flow vascular anomalies are caused by RASA1 mutations. Hum Mutat 2008;29:959–65.

193. Yakes WF, Rossi P, Odink H. How I do it. Arteriovenous malformation management. Cardiovasc Intervent Radiol 1996;19:65–71.

194. Cohen MM Jr. Klippel-Trenaunay syndrome. Am J Med Genet 2000;93:171–5.

195. Jacob AG, Driscoll DJ, Shaughnessy WJ, et al. Klippel-Trenaunay syndrome: Spectrum and management. Mayo Clin Proc 1998; 73:28–36.

196. Klippel M, Trenaunay P. Du naevus variqueux osteohypertrophique. Arch Gen Med (Paris) 1900;185:641–72.

197. Servelle M. Klippel and Trenaunay's syndrome. 768 operated cases. Ann Surg 1985;201:365–73.

198. Kulungowski AM, Fishman SJ. Management of combined vascular malformations. Clin Plast Surg 2011;38:107–20.

199. Alomari AI. Characterization of a distinct syndrome that associates complex truncal overgrowth, vascular, and acral anomalies: A descriptive study of 18 cases of CLOVES syndrome. Clin Dysmorphol 2009;18:1–7.

200. Sapp JC, Turner JT, van de Kamp JM, et al. Newly delineated syndrome of congenital lipomatous overgrowth, vascular malformations, and epidermal nevi (CLOVE syndrome) in seven patients. Am J Med Genet A 2007;143A:2944–58.

201. Fernandez-Pineda I, Fajardo M, Chaudry G, et al. Perinatal clinical and imaging features of CLOVES syndrome. Pediatr Radiol 2010;40:1436–9.

202. Kurek KC, Luks VL, Ayturk UM, et al. Somatic Mosaic Activating Mutations in PIK3CA Cause CLOVES Syndrome. Am J Hum Genet 2012;90:1108–15.

203. Bader AG, Kang S, Vogt PK. Cancer-specific mutations in PIK3CA are oncogenic in vivo. Proc Natl Acad Sci U S A 2006; 103:1475–9.

204. Perkins P, Weiss SW. Spindle cell hemangioendothelioma. An analysis of 78 cases with reassessment of its pathogenesis and biologic behavior. Am J Surg Pathol 1996;20:1196–204.

205. Sun TC, Swee RG, Shives TC, et al. Chondrosarcoma in Maffucci's syndrome. J Bone Joint Surg Am 1985;67:1214–19.

206. Amary MF, Damato S, Halai D, et al. Ollier disease and Maffucci syndrome are caused by somatic mosaic mutations of IDH1 and IDH2. Nat Genet 2011;43:1262–5.

207. Pansuriya TC, van Eijk R, d'Adamo P, et al. Somatic mosaic IDH1 and IDH2 mutations are associated with enchondroma and spindle cell hemangioma in Ollier disease and Maffucci syndrome. Nat Genet 2011;43:1256–61.

208. Cohen MM Jr. Bannayan-Riley-Ruvalcaba syndrome: Renaming three formerly recognized syndromes as one etiologic entity. Am J Med Genet 1990;35:291–2.

209. Parisi MA, Dinulos MB, Leppig KA, et al. The spectrum and evolution of phenotypic findings in PTEN mutation positive cases of Bannayan-Riley-Ruvalcaba syndrome. J Med Genet 2001;38: 52–8.

210. Tan WH, Baris HN, Burrows PE, et al. The spectrum of vascular anomalies in patients with PTEN mutations: Implications for diagnosis and management. J Med Genet 2007;44:594–602.

211. Biesecker LG, Happle R, Mulliken JB, et al. Proteus syndrome: Diagnostic criteria, differential diagnosis, and patient evaluation. Am J Med Genet 1999;84:389–95.

212. Lindhurst MJ, Sapp JC, Teer JK, et al. A mosaic activating mutation in AKT1 associated with the Proteus syndrome. N Engl J Med 2011;365:611–19.

213. Weber FP. Angioma formation in connection with hypertrophy of limbs and hemi-hypertrophy. Br J Dermatol Syph 1907; 19:231–5.

214. Weber FP. Haemangiectatic hypertrophy of limbs: Congenital phlebarteriectasis and so-called congenital varicose veins. Br J Dis Child 1918;15:13–17.

215. Greene AK, Liu AS, Mulliken JB, et al. Vascular anomalies in 5621 patients: guidelines for referral. J Pediatr Surg 2011;46:1784–9.

CHAPTER 73

HEAD AND NECK SINUSES AND MASSES

Jarod McAteer • John H.T. Waldhausen

Lesions of the head and neck in children can be subdivided by etiology as those resulting from infection, trauma, neoplasm, or those of congenital origin. The more common benign neoplasms including hemangiomas, lymphangiomas, and cystic hygromas are discussed in Chapter 72. Malignant neoplasms of childhood (e.g., neuroblastoma, lymphoma, and rhabdomyosarcoma), which occur as primary or metastatic masses in the head and neck, lesions of the thyroid and parathyroid, as well as traumatic injuries of the head and neck, also are discussed in other chapters. In this chapter, common congenital head and neck malformations are discussed, and inflammatory lesions are reviewed.

LESIONS OF EMBRYONIC ORIGIN

Congenital cysts and sinuses in the neck result from embryonic structures that have failed to mature or have persisted in an aberrant fashion.[1,2] Both diagnosis and therapy depend on a working knowledge of the embryologic origin and differentiation of the head and neck structures.[3,4] This knowledge is particularly important because complete resection of cartilaginous remnants, remnants of the branchial arch and cleft structures, and midline fusion abnormalities is needed to avoid recurrence. Congenital lesions of the head and neck, in descending order of frequency, are thyroglossal duct cysts, preauricular pits and sinuses, branchial cleft anomalies, dermoid cysts, and median cervical clefts.

Thyroglossal Duct Cyst

One of the most common lesions in the midline of the neck is the thyroglossal duct cyst. Thyroglossal duct remnants are found in 7% of the population and most are asymptomatic.[4,5] Although embryonic in origin, it is rare for these lesions to manifest in the newborn period.[1] More commonly, they are noted in preschool-age children.[1] Thyroglossal duct cysts also are common in young adults and, with the exception of thyroid goiter, are the most common midline neck mass.[6]

The embryogenesis of the thyroglossal duct is intimately involved with that of the thyroid gland, the hyoid bone, and the tongue.[7] The foramen cecum is the site of the development of the thyroid diverticulum. In the embryo, this structure develops caudal to the central tuberculum impar, which is one of the pharyngeal buds that leads to the formation of the tongue. As the tongue develops, the thyroid diverticulum descends into the neck, maintaining its connection to the foramen cecum.

The hyoid bone is developing from the second branchial arch at this time. The thyroid gland develops between weeks 4 and 7 of gestation and descends into its pretracheal position in the neck.[8] As a result of these multiple events occurring simultaneously, the thyroglossal duct may pass in front of or behind the hyoid bone, but most commonly, it passes through it. Normally, the duct disappears by the time the thyroid reaches its appropriate position by 5 to 8 weeks gestation.[5,9] Thyroglossal duct cysts never have a primary external opening because the embryologic thyroglossal tract never reaches the surface of the neck.[8] A cyst can be located anywhere along the migratory course of the thyroglossal tract if it fails to become obliterated (Fig. 73-1). Occasionally, the cysts attach to the pyramidal lobe or may be intrathyroidal.[10] Complete failure of migration of the thyroid results in a lingual thyroid, which develops beneath the foramen cecum at the base of the tongue.[11] In this instance, no thyroid tissue is found in the neck.

Two-thirds of thyroglossal duct anomalies are discovered within the first three decades of life.[5] Classically, the thyroglossal cysts are located in the midline at or just below the hyoid bone (Fig. 73-2). Suprahyoid thyroglossal cysts must be distinguished from submental dermoid cysts and from submental lymph nodes.[12] Rarely, the cysts are suprasternal in location. The initial sign is usually a painless mass in the midline of the neck, with 66% found adjacent to the hyoid bone.[9] On physical examination, the thyroglossal duct cyst is smooth, soft, and nontender. To distinguish this lesion from the more superficial dermoid cyst, one should palpate the lesion while the child sticks out his or her tongue. Owing to its attachment to the foramen cecum, the thyroglossal duct cyst usually moves cephalad when the tongue protrudes. This maneuver is more reliable than asking the child to swallow and determining whether the mass moves with swallowing. Owing to the communication to the mouth via the foramen cecum, thyroglossal cysts can become infected with oral flora. One-third of patients will present with a concurrent or prior infection, and one-quarter will present with a draining sinus from spontaneous or incisional drainage of an abscess.[9] Some patients may present with a foul taste in the mouth from spontaneous drainage of the cyst via the foramen cecum.

The preoperative evaluation for a patient with a suspected thyroglossal duct cyst includes a complete history and physical examination. Patients with findings concerning for hypothyroidism should undergo thyroid function testing and additional imaging to exclude median ectopic thyroid. The incidence of ectopic thyroid tissue in or near the duct is reported to be from 10–45%, and

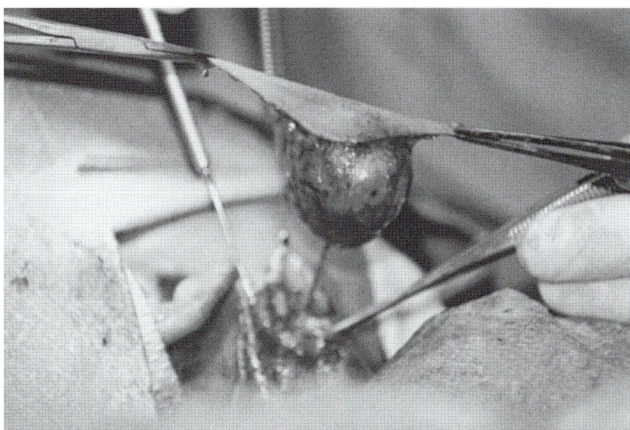

FIGURE 73-3 ■ Complete excision of a previously infected thyroglossal duct cyst. Surrounding skin was removed because of changes related to a previous infection. Note the well-defined tract leading toward the hyoid bone and the floor of the mouth. The operation was completed by excising the central portion of the hyoid bone and suture ligating the tract.

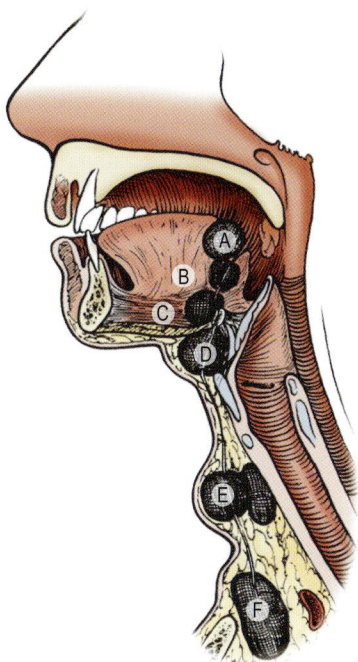

FIGURE 73-1 ■ Thyroglossal duct cysts can be located anywhere from the base of the tongue to behind the sternum. A and B, Lingual (rare); C and D, adjacent to hyoid bone (common); E and F, suprasternal fossa (rare). (From Welch KJ, Randolph JG, Ravitch MM, et al. editors. Pediatric Surgery. 4th ed. Chicago: Year Book Medical; 1986. p. 549.)

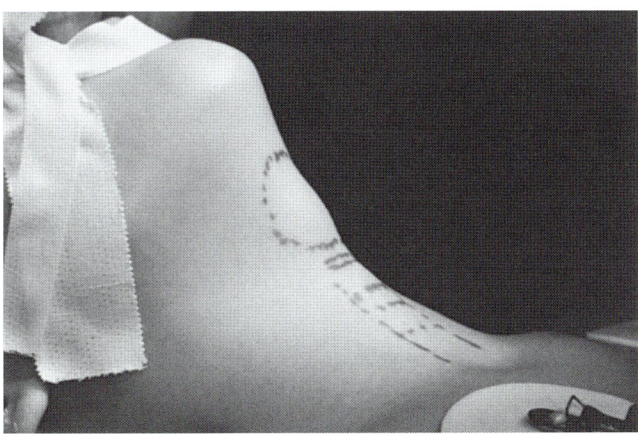

FIGURE 73-2 ■ A classic thyroglossal duct cyst located in the midline just below the hyoid bone. Markings on the neck represent the thyroid, cricoid and tracheal cartilages.

some clinicians have advocated preoperative thyroid scanning or ultrasound (US) to eliminate the possibility of an ectopic thyroid gland masquerading as a thyroglossal duct cyst.[13–17] Ultrasound appears to be very accurate and avoids the need for radiation and possible sedation in younger children.[16] Although ultrasound has been noted to have significant limitations in differentiating thyroglossal duct cysts from other midline neck masses, it can be useful in differentiating cysts and ectopic thyroid.[18] Ninety per cent of ectopic thyroid tissue lies at the base of the tongue, and thyroglossal duct cysts are rarely found there. Abnormal thyroid function tests, a suggestive history, or a solid mass on ultrasound should

prompt a preoperative thyroid scan to ensure the lesion is not the only thyroid gland present, which occurs in less than 1–2% of thyroglossal duct cysts.[9,15,19] If ectopic thyroid tissue is found, the management is controversial, but some clinicians suggest a trial of medical suppression to decrease the size of the mass.[19]

Elective surgical excision a of thyroglossal duct cyst is advised to avoid the complications of infection and the small risk (<1%) of cancer (papillary thyroid carcinoma) developing in the cyst.[15] The operation includes complete excision of the cyst and its tract upward to the base of the tongue (Fig. 73-3), and resection of the central portion of the hyoid bone as described by Sistrunk in 1920.[20–22] Several other studies have shown that multiple smaller tracts can connect through the hyoid bone to the floor of the mouth, requiring wide resection of tracts above the hyoid.[20–22] If these suprahyoid tracts remain, the incidence of recurrence increases.[23] The best chance for successful excision is adequate wide resection at the initial procedure.[24]

As with all neck surgery, the patient should be supine with the neck slightly hyperextended (Fig. 73-4). The thyroglossal cyst is exposed through a transverse incision. The cyst has a characteristic appearance, distinctly different from that of thyroid tissue. The dissection should continue cephalad to the hyoid, resecting a block of tissue along the tract. Transecting the hyoid is simplified by using angled scissors, similar to Potts scissors, or by using a side-cutting bone cutter. Alternatively, some advocate use of an ultrasonic osteotomy device to minimize trauma to surrounding soft tissues.[25] The base of the tract at the floor of the mouth is ligated with absorbable suture. The wings of the hyoid do not need to be approximated. The incision is closed in layers. If the floor of the mouth is entered inadvertently, this can be repaired with absorbable suture. The incision is copiously irrigated. Occasionally, the dissection may be made simpler by having the anesthesiologist place his or her finger at the base of the child's tongue to identify the cephalad extent of the dissection. With complete excision, including the central

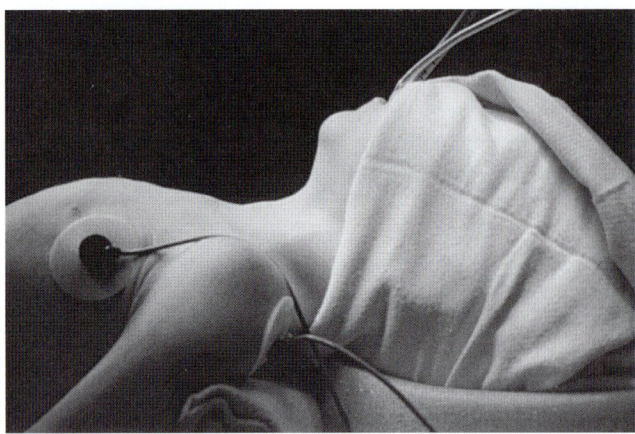

FIGURE 73-4 ■ Positioning a child for a cervical operation. Hyper-extension of the head with support under the shoulders and stabilization with a bean bag keeps the child in a stable position and facilitates exposure. The head of the bed should be elevated 30° to decrease venous pressure in the neck.

portion of the hyoid bone, the risk of recurrence is low, 2–5%.[5,9,23,26] Some authors advocate more extensive excision of the infrahyoid tissue as well as exposure of the posterior hyoid space, noting that extensive arborization of thyroglossal ducts exists at all levels, and residual ducts can result in recurrence. Recurrence rates in series employing these extended excisions range from 0–1.67%.[27,28] Risk factors for recurrence include simple cyst excision alone (recurrence rates of 38–70%), intraoperative cyst rupture, presence of a cutaneous component secondary to infection, and postoperative wound infections.[5,9,29] The cyst is usually connected to the foramen cecum by single or multiple tracts, which pass through the hyoid. Under histologic exam, the duct lining is stratified squamous epithelium or ciliated pseudostratified columnar epithelium, with associated mucus-secreting glands.[9] The cyst contains a characteristic glairy mucus.

Infected cysts or sinuses should be initially managed by treating the infection. The usual route of infection is via the mouth; thus the common organisms are *Haemophilus influenzae*, *Staphylococus aureus*, and *Staphylococcus epidermidis*.[9] Directed antibiotic therapy should be initiated. Needle aspiration may be required to decompress the cyst and allow for identification of the organism, but formal incision and drainage should be avoided. This may seed ductal cells outside of the cyst and increase recurrence rates.[9] If incision and drainage is required, the incision should be placed so that it can be completely excised during a formal Sistrunk procedure once the infection clears. Excision of acutely infected cysts should be avoided, as recurrence can occur in 25% of patients.[30] Three months should be allowed for inflammation to resolve prior to definitive operative treatment.

If a solid mass is found, it should be sent for frozen section to rule out median ectopic thyroid. If it is normal thyroid tissue and there is additional functional thyroid tissue in the normal location, a Sistrunk procedure with excision of the mass should be performed.[9] If there is no other thyroid tissue present, management is controversial. One option is to leave the tissue in situ or reposition it into the strap muscles. This is done to prevent the

patient from becoming permanently hypothyroid; however, most patients still require thyroid hormone therapy for hypothyroidism or to control the size of the ectopic thyroid. Due to this likely need for long-term therapy and possible malignant degeneration, some surgeons recommend completely excising the ectopic thyroid tissue regardless of the presence or absence of additional thyroid tissue.[9] If the mass is found to represent carcinoma, then management is dependent on the extent of disease. The vast majority of cases are papillary carcinoma. If confined to the cyst specimen, it can be adequately treated with a Sistrunk procedure alone.[31] More extensive cancers should undergo risk stratification and generally warrant total thyroidectomy and consideration of adjuvant therapy, including radioactive iodine in some cases.[32]

Remnants of Embryonic Branchial Apparatus

Branchial anomalies represent approximately 30% of congenital neck masses and can present as cysts, sinuses, or fistulae.[5,33] They are equally common in males and females and present in childhood or early adulthood.

During weeks 4 to 8 after fertilization, four pairs of well-developed ridges (branchial arches) dominate the lateral cervicofacial area of the human embryo.[34] These four pairs are accompanied by two rudimentary pairs, which are analogous to the gill apparatus of fish.[2,34] No true gill mechanisms are found in any stage of the human embryo. These pharyngeal arches and clefts are formed without a true connection between the outer ectodermal clefts and the inner endodermal pharyngeal pouches (Fig. 73-5). The mature structures of the head and neck are derivatives of several branchial arches and their intervening clefts.[34,35] The clefts and pouches are gradually obliterated by mesenchyme to form those structures. Branchial cleft anomalies result if that process is incomplete.[33]

Each arch transforms during gestation into a defined anatomic pattern. Understanding this pattern and its relationship to normal neck structures is key in the diagnosis and treatment of these anomalies. Each anomaly is classified by the cleft or pouch of origin which can be determined by the internal opening of the sinus as well as its relationship to nerves, arteries, and muscles. Careful attention to these relationships is necessary to prevent injury to surrounding tissues and ensure complete resection.[33] The embryology and anatomy for each cleft will be discussed later.

Branchial anomalies are lined with either respiratory or squamous epithelium; sinuses and fistulas usually the former and cysts the latter.[33] One can also see lymphoid tissue, sebaceous glands, salivary tissue or cholesterol crystals. Squamous cell cancer can be seen in adults, but it is rare and it can be difficult to distinguish a primary branchogenic anomaly from a metastatic lesion or an occult primary.[5]

Complete fistulas are more common than external sinuses. Both are more common than branchial cysts, at least during childhood.[36,37] In adults, cysts predominate.[36] By definition, all branchial remnants are truly congenital and are present at birth.[37,38] Cysts are remnants of sinuses

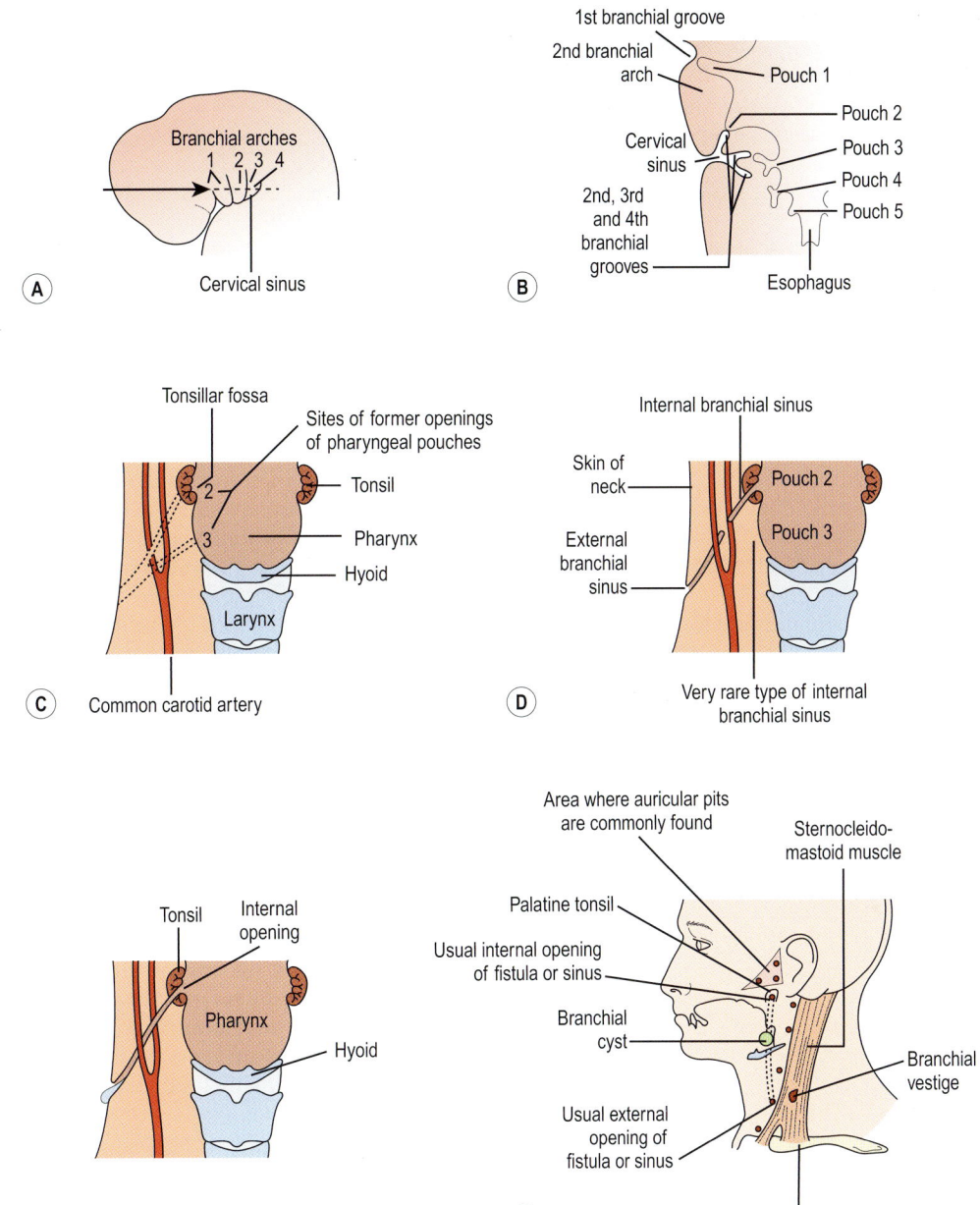

FIGURE 73-5 ■ **(A)** The head and neck region of a 5-week-old embryo. **(B)** Horizontal section through the embryo illustrating the relationship of the cervical sinus to the branchial arches and pharyngeal pouches. **(C)** The child's neck region, indicating the former sites of openings of the cervical sinus and the pharyngeal pouches. The dotted lines indicate possible courses of branchial fistulas. **(D)** The embryologic basis of various types of branchial sinuses. **(E)** A branchial fistula resulting from persistence of parts of the second branchial cleft and the second pharyngeal pouch. **(F)** Possible sites of branchial cysts and openings of branchial sinuses and fistulas. A branchial vestige also is illustrated. (From Moore KL. The Developing Human: Clinically Oriented Embryology. Philadelphia: WB Saunders; 1977.)

without an external opening and usually appear later in childhood than do sinuses, fistulas, and cartilaginous remnants, which appear in infancy.[5,38] Sinuses have the persistence of the external opening only, while fistulas involve the persistence of the branchial groove with breakdown of the branchial membrane.[5] Commonly, the tiny external opening of the fistula and the external sinuses remain unnoticed for some time. Spontaneous mucoid drainage from the ostium along the border of the sternocleidomastoid muscle (SCM) usually heralds its presence and initiates the parent's concern and the reason

for the child's referral. The first clinical presentation may be an infected mass as a result of the inability of the thick mucoid material to drain spontaneously. Infection is, however, less common in fistulas and external sinuses than in cysts.[1] The cutaneous openings are occasionally marked by skin tags or cartilaginous remnants. The tract itself may be palpable. A cordlike structure can sometimes be felt ascending in the neck by hyperextending the child's neck and making the skin taut. Compression along the tract may produce mucoid material exiting from the ostium.

The evaluation of these lesions starts with a thorough history and physical examination. Palpating the tract and observing the mucoid discharge can be confirmatory. Although colored dye or radiopaque material may be injected to delineate the tract, these manipulations generally are unnecessary. Upper endoscopy may be helpful to locate the pharyngeal opening. Both the pyriform sinus and tonsillar fossas should be examined. Cysts may be more difficult to diagnose. They lie deep to the skin along the anterior border of the SCM.[1] They can usually be distinguished from cystic hygromas, which are subcutaneous and can be transilluminated. Ultrasound, computed tomography (CT), and magnetic resonance imaging (MRI) can help define the lesion and may be helpful in narrowing the differential diagnosis, but CT is most often used and can demonstrate a fistula in two-thirds of cases.[39] Barium esophagram has 50–80% sensitivity for third and fourth branchial fistulas.[40] While fine needle aspiration is necessary in adults to exclude metastatic carcinoma, it is not necessary in children and incisional biopsy should be avoided.[33]

The goal of treating all congenital neck sinuses, cysts, and fistulas is usually complete excision, when no inflammation is present.[41] Timing of resection is controversial with some advocating for early resection to prevent infection while others wait until age 2 or 3 years.[33,42,43] As with thyroglossal duct cysts, if the lesion is infected at clinical presentation, antibiotic therapy and warm soaks to encourage spontaneous drainage of mucoid plugs should precede definitive excision. Approximately 20% of lesions will have been infected at least once prior to surgery.[42] Attempts at complete excision in an inflamed, infected field increase the risk of nerve injury and incomplete resection. Aspiration or limited incision and drainage (I&D) is sometimes necessary to resolve the infection. Complete surgical excision is delayed until the inflammation subsides and the surrounding skin is supple. Endoscopic cauterization of fourth branchial cleft sinuses has been described either at the time of initial abscess drainage or four to six weeks later. Recurrence with this technique seems unusual.[44]

Surgical resection is performed under general anesthesia with the positioning as shown in Figure 73-4. A small transverse elliptical incision is made around the external opening and deepened beneath the cervical fascia. The initial dissection is along the inferior border of the incision, so that the ascending tract is identified from below and not injured. Placement of a 2-0 or 3-0 monofilament suture or probe within the tract can facilitate dissection. Dissection proceeds cephalad, staying on the tract until visualization of the most superior portion of the tract becomes difficult. At this level, a second, more cephalad, parallel 'stair-step' incision or extension of the first incision may be necessary for adequate exposure. The tract is pulled through the second incision, and the dissection is continued cephalad between the bifurcation of the carotid artery to the point where the tract dives into the pharynx. The fistula is suture ligated with absorbable suture. The incision is closed in layers with absorbable sutures. No drains are needed if excision is complete. Recurrences are rare and imply that a portion of the epithelium-lined tract was overlooked. The incidence of recurrence is higher in patients with previously infected lesions. The specific embryology, anatomy, and treatment for each type will now be discussed.

First Cleft Anomalies

The first branchial arch forms the mandible and contributes to the maxillary process of the upper jaw.[35,38,45] Abnormal development of the first branchial arch results in a host of facial deformities, including cleft lip and palate, abnormal shape or contour of the external ear, and malformed internal ossicles.[35,38] The first branchial cleft contributes to the tympanic cavity, eustachian tube, middle ear cavity, and mastoid air cells. Microtia and aural atresia occur with failure of the first branchial cleft to develop.[34,35]

First branchial anomalies are rare and account for less than 1% of branchial cleft malformations.[33] Cysts are seen as swellings posterior or anterior to the ear or inferior to the earlobe in the submandibular region. External openings, if found, are located inferior to the mandible in a suprahyoid position. One-third open into the external auditory canal.[6] The tract may be intimately associated with, or course through, the parotid gland. This association and the proximity of cranial nerve VII make resection difficult, particularly in the younger patient who is likely to have a tract deep to the facial nerve.[39] First cleft anomalies are classified as type I or type II (Figs 73-6 and 73-7).[5,33] Type I remnants contain only ectoderm, course lateral to the facial nerve, and present as swellings near the ear. Type II lesions consist of both mesoderm and ectoderm, can contain cartilage, pass medial to the facial nerve, and present as swellings inferior to the angle of the mandible or anterior to the SCM in a preauricular, infra-auricular, or postauricular position. First branchial anomalies are more common in females than males and are often misdiagnosed leading to delay in excision.[46] Presentation can include cervical,

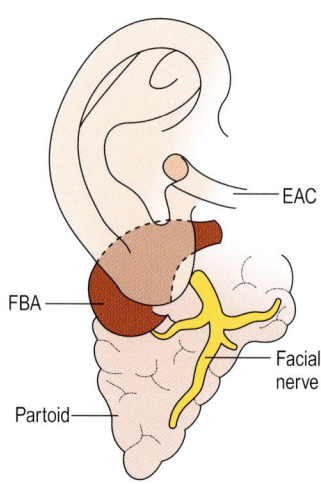

FIGURE 73-6 ■ Type I first branchial cleft anomaly (FBA). Note that the anomaly, located in the parotid gland, has no connection to the external auditory canal (EAC). (From Mukherji SK, Fatterpekar G, Castillo M, et al. Imaging of congenital anomalies of the branchial apparatus. Neuroimaging Clin North Am 2000; 10:75–93.)

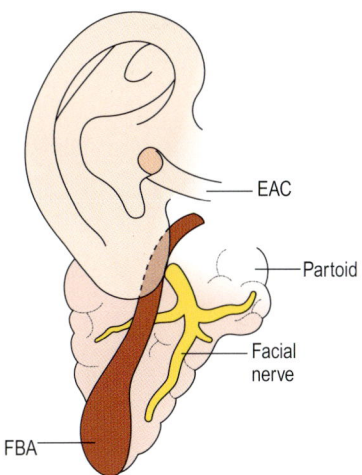

FIGURE 73-7 ■ Type II first branchial cleft anomaly (FBA). The anomaly connects with the external auditory canal (EAC) and extends deep into the parotid gland. (From Mukherji SK, Fatterpekar G, Castillo M, et al. Imaging of congenital anomalies of the branchial apparatus. Neuroimaging Clin North Am 2000;10:75–93.)

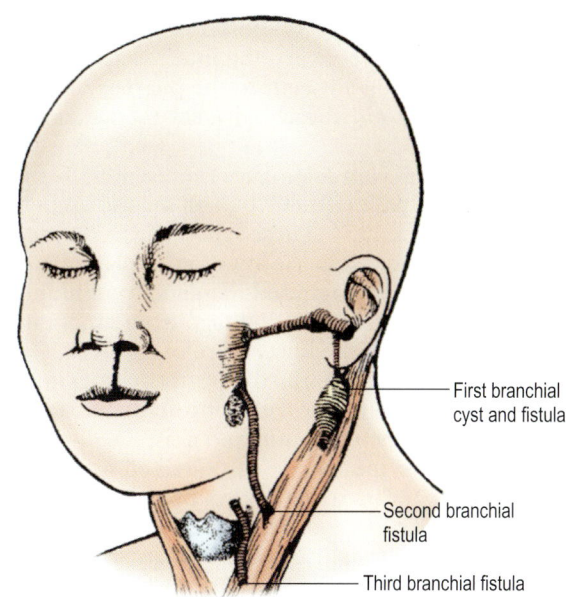

FIGURE 73-8 ■ A child with a cleft lip and remnants of the first three branchial systems. Note the important relation to the sternocleidomastoid muscle and the fistula's origin. (From Welch KJ, Randolph JG, Ravitch MM, et al. editors. Pediatric Surgery. 4th ed. Chicago: Year Book Medical; 1986. p. 543.)

parotid, or auricular signs. Cervical signs include drainage from a pit-like depression at the angle of the mandible. Parotid signs result from rapid enlargement due to inflammation. Auricular signs can consist of swelling or otorrhea.

Resection of first arch anomalies often requires at least partial facial nerve dissection and superficial parotidectomy. It is important to resect any involved skin or cartilage of the external auditory canal. If it extends medial to the tympanic membrane, a second procedure may be necessary to remove the medial component. Tracts that go to the middle ear are more likely to travel deep or split around the facial nerve.[46] A superficial parotidectomy incision allows good exposure and facial nerve monitoring may decrease the risk of nerve injury.[47] Another option is to open the fistula tract longitudinally and facilitate the dissection by visualizing it from the inside, but this approach requires microsurgical techniques.[48] In any case, identification of the nerve is essential, as the risk of temporary and permanent facial paralysis is significantly higher when the nerve is not identified.[49] Recurrence is common, and 2.4 procedures are required on average for complete resection.[50] Each repeat operation places the facial nerve at greater risk due to prior scarring, emphasizing the importance of complete resection at the first attempt.[33]

Second Cleft Anomalies

The second arch forms the hyoid bone and the cleft of the tonsillar fossa.[1,2] The second pouch gives rise to the tonsillar and supratonsillar fossa.[33] The external ostium of the second branchial cleft is along the anterior border of the SCM, generally at the junction of the lower and middle thirds.[36] Owing to its embryonic origin, the second cleft tract penetrates the platysma and cervical fascia to ascend along the carotid sheath to the level of the hyoid bone. Remnants may be found anywhere along this course. The residual tract turns medially between the branches of the carotid artery, behind the posterior belly

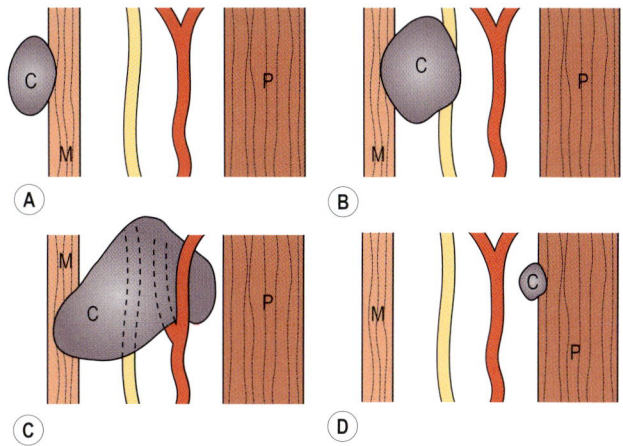

FIGURE 73-9 ■ Types I to IV second branchial cleft anomalies. **(A)** Type I: the cyst (C) is superficial to the sternocleidomastoid muscle (M). **(B)** Type II: the cyst is adjacent to the carotid sheath. **(C)** Type III: the cyst passes between the internal and external carotid arteries to the lateral wall of the pharynx (P). **(D)** Type IV: the cyst is deep to the carotid sheath abutting the pharynx. (From Mukherji SK, Fatterpekar G, Castillo M, et al. Imaging of congenital anomalies of the branchial apparatus. Neuroimaging Clin North Am 2000;10:75–93.)

of the digastric and stylohyoid muscles, and in front of the hypoglossal nerve to end in the tonsillar fossa[36] (Fig. 73-8). Although the internal opening can be anywhere in the nasopharynx or oropharynx, it is most commonly found in the tonsillar fossa. Figure 73-9 demonstrates the four types of second arch anomalies. Type I lies anterior to the SCM and does not come into contact with the carotid sheath. Type II is the most common, passing deep to the SCM and anterior or posterior to the carotid sheath. Type III passes between the internal and external carotid arteries, ending adjacent to the pharynx. Type IV is medial to the carotid sheath adjacent to the tonsillar fossa.

Second branchial cleft anomalies represent 95% of all branchial cleft anomalies. About 10% of second branchial remnants are bilateral.[36] These anomalies commonly present as a fistula or cyst in the lower, anterolateral neck. Fistulas are commonly diagnosed in infancy or childhood after presenting with chronic drainage from an opening anterior to the SCM in the lower third of the neck. Cysts usually present during the third to fifth decades of life with an acute increase in size following an upper respiratory infection.[5,33] When operating on a fistula, dissection of the tract follows the course as described above with care taken during the resection to protect the spinal accessory, hypoglossal, and vagus nerves. A finger or bougie in the oropharynx can help identify the opening in the tonsillar fossa and the tract must be carefully ligated at this entry point. An alternative to open resection of the fistula is a stripping technique utilizing a guidewire passed between the opening in the neck and the internal opening in the tonsillar fossa. There is, however, only limited experience with this technique, and the long-term recurrence risk is not known.[51] Second cleft cysts can be approached via a conventional cervical incision or a retroauricular hairline incision for improved cosmesis.[52] Endoscopic cyst resections have also been described and noted to have low recurrence rates, but the learning curve for such procedures may limit their widespread adoption.[53]

Third and Fourth Cleft Anomalies

Third and fourth branchial anomalies are rare. The third and fourth pouches form the pharynx below the hyoid bone. Thus these fistulas enter into the pyriform sinus. The third cleft migrates lower in the neck to form the inferior parathyroid glands and the thymus.[7,36] The descent of the fourth cleft stops higher in the neck to form the superior parathyroid glands. The fourth pouch has added significance in that its ventral portion develops into the ultimobranchial body, which contributes thyrocalcitonin-producing parafollicular cells to the thyroid gland.[7] It is unusual to find cysts and sinuses from the third branchial cleft.[2,35] When found, they are in the same area as those of the second cleft but ascend posterior to the carotid artery rather than through the bifurcation (Fig. 73-10).[35] The fistula pierces the thyrohyoid membrane and enters the pyriform sinus. Fourth branchial fistulae are difficult to differentiate from other associated anomalies. Fourth pouch cysts also are highly unusual and must be differentiated from laryngoceles. These tracts originate at the apex of the pyriform sinus, descend beneath the aortic arch, and then ascend anterior to the carotid artery to end in the vestigial cervical sinus of His (Fig. 73-11).[54] Other anomalies arising from the third and fourth branchial pouches may appear as cystic structures in the neck. Thymic cysts can occur as a result of incomplete degeneration of the thymal pharyngeal duct or of progressive cystic degeneration of epithelial remnants of

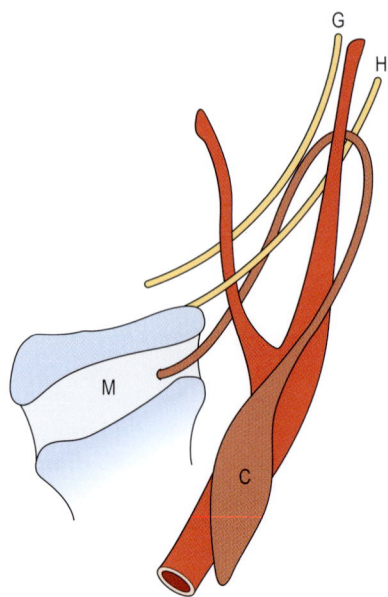

FIGURE 73-10 ■ Third branchial cleft anomaly. The cyst (C) is posterior to the sternocleidomastoid muscle, and the tract ascends posterior to the internal carotid artery. It then passes medially between the hypoglossal (H) and glossopharyngeal (G) nerves. It pierces the thyroid membrane (M) to enter the pyriform sinus. (From Mukherji SK, Fatterpekar G, Castillo M, et al. Imaging of congenital anomalies of the branchial apparatus. Neuroimaging Clin North Am 2000;10:75–93.)

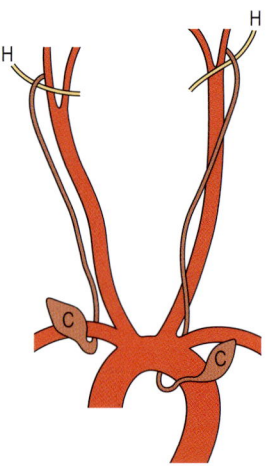

FIGURE 73-11 ■ Fourth branchial cleft anomaly. The cysts (C) are located anterior to the aortic arch on either side. The tract hooks either the subclavian artery or the aortic arch, depending on the side, and ascends to loop over the hypoglossal nerve (H). (From Mukherji SK, Fatterpekar G, Castillo M, et al. Imaging of congenital anomalies of the branchial apparatus. Neuroimaging Clin North Am 2000;10:75–93.)

Hassall corpuscles.[54] Most are found on the left side of the neck. Parathyroid cysts may be located anywhere around the thyroid gland or in the mediastinum. These are usually not associated with biochemical abnormalities, although reports of hyperparathyroidism secondary to functioning cysts have been seen. The etiology of these cysts is not clear, but they may be embryologic remnants of third and fourth branchial pouches, or may represent cystic degeneration of adenomas or gradual enlargement of microcysts.[54]

Both third and fourth cleft lesions can present at any age. In the neonate, both can present with tracheal compression or airway compromise due to rapid enlargement. Infectious complications are the most common presentation outside the neonatal period. A recent review found that 39% of third arch anomalies presented as neck abscesses and 33% as acute suppurative thyroiditis.[55] For fourth arch anomalies, 42% presented initially as abscesses and 45% as thyroiditis in one series.[56]

The operative approach for third and fourth arch anomalies is similar to the second arch, with a few notable exceptions. Endoscopy should be used to find the pyriform sinus entry point to allow cannulation of the tract to aid with dissection. Fourth arch anomaly resections require ipsilateral hemithyroidectomy for complete excision and partial resection of the thyroid cartilage may be necessary to expose the pyriform sinus.[57] In cases presenting with infection, antibiotics should be administered initially and operative excision delayed until the inflammation has resolved, which helps to decrease the risk of recurrent nerve injury.[56] For both third and fourth arch anomalies, children older than 8 years generally have fewer postoperative complications than younger patients. As such, it has been suggested that initial management in children older than 8 years should be excision of the fistula tract while management in younger children should begin with endoscopic cauterization of the internal fistula opening. While ipsilateral thyroidectomy appears to decrease recurrence rates for fourth arch fistulas, there is no role for this procedure in the management of third arch anomalies.[55,56]

Preauricular Pits, Sinuses, and Cysts

Preauricular pits, cysts, and sinuses are not of true branchial cleft origin.[58] They represent ectodermal inclusions, which are related to embryonic ectodermal mounds (auditory hillocks) that essentially form the auricles of the ear.[35,59] The sinuses are often short and end blindly. They never connect internally to the external auditory canal or eustachian tube, and they characteristically end in thin strands that blend with the periosteum of the external auditory canal.[58] Some authors propose that they are a marker of teratogenic exposure.[59] Preauricular cysts are located in the subcutaneous layer superficial to the parotid fascia, but may seem deeper if they become infected. The lining cells of these cysts and sinuses are stratified squamous epithelium. They do not contain hair-bearing follicles owing to their origin from the ectoderm associated with external ear formation.[41]

The estimated incidence of preauricular sinuses is 0.1–0.9% in the USA and as high as 4–10% in Africa.[59] Preauricular cysts and sinuses are commonly noted at birth, more commonly on the right side.[59] The parent may remark about the familial and bilateral nature of these lesions.[36] Although preauricular pits are associated with renal abnormalities in certain syndromes, renal ultrasound is generally indicated only in cases of multiple anomalies or a family history of such syndromes.[60] Excision of these preauricular sinuses is not needed unless

there is a history of drainage. Sinuses that drain are often connected to subcutaneous cysts that have an increased likelihood of staphylococcal infection. Ideally these lesions should be completely excised before becoming infected (Fig. 73-12). Prior infection increases the difficulty of complete surgical excision, which increases the risk of recurrence.

Complete surgical excision of the sinus tract and subcutaneous cyst to the level of the temporalis fascia is the treatment of choice in the uninfected draining sinus. It is important to avoid rupture of the sinus and to completely excise the sinus/cyst to decrease the risk of recurrence.[61] If infection supervenes, the lesion is treated with antibiotics and warm soaks to encourage drainage and control of the surrounding inflammation. Occasionally, as with infected branchial cysts, I&D or needle aspiration may be required to control the infection. Excision is often accomplished through an elliptic incision with a small, chevron skin flap surrounding the sinus. The cyst is then dissected from the subcutaneous tissue and removed in its entirety.[58] The cyst or sinus may have multiple branches, making complete resection difficult. Removal of a small bit of adjacent cartilage reduces the risk of missing one of these branching tracts.[59] The incidence of recurrence is as high as 42% owing to these multiple branches, and some clinicians have advocated an extended preauricular incision to enhance exposure.[61] Alternatively, extension of the elliptical excision superiorly allows removal of the subcutaneous tissue between the temporalis fascia and the helix perichondrium, which is the plane in which the sinus tracts exist. This facilitates complete excision without necessitating visualization of all the tracts, and has been noted to decrease recurrence rates.[62]

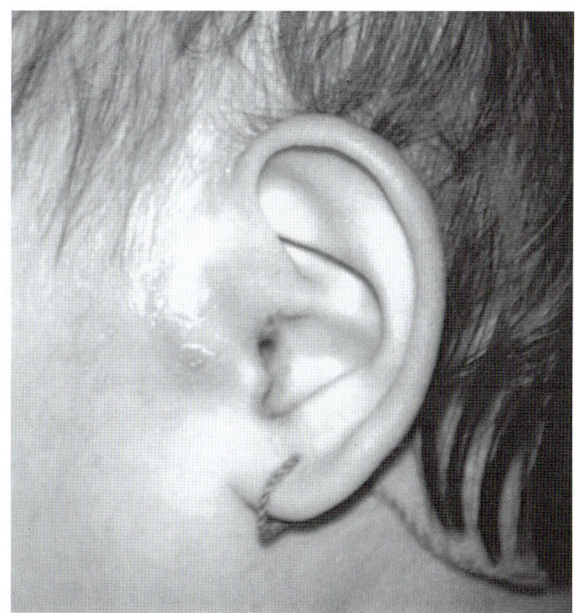

FIGURE 73-12 ■ An infected preauricular cyst. The pit anterior to the helix is difficult to see. Note the swelling and skin changes anterior to the tragus. Preauricular sinuses that drain sebaceous material should be excised electively. Warm compresses and antibiotics allowed the inflammation to diminish. The cyst and sinus were then completely excised.

Dermoid and Epidermoid Cysts

Dermoid cysts embryologically represent ectodermal elements that either were trapped beneath the skin along median or paramedian embryonic lines of fusion or failed to separate from the neural tube.[63–65] Dermoid cysts are differentiated from epidermoid cysts histologically by the accessory glandular structures found in dermoids.[63] Dermoid cysts contain sebaceous glands, hair follicles, connective tissues, and papillae.[63] Both contain sebaceous material within the cyst cavity.

Most dermoid or epidermoid cysts are diagnosed before the patient is 3 years of age.[5] The most common location for dermoid cysts in children is along the supraorbital palpebral ridge. This lesion commonly appears as a characteristic swelling in the corner of the eyebrow and is most commonly first noticed at birth or within the first 1 to 3 months of life. Although usually attached to the underlying bony fascia, this lesion is movable and nontender. Occasionally, the mass may be dumbbell shaped and penetrate through the orbital bone. Dermoid cysts may occur along the midline or in atypical locations such as the medial orbital wall, nose, floor of the mouth, or submental and submaxillary areas.[66] Midline dermoid cysts can be confused with midline thyroglossal duct cysts. Dermoid cysts, however, are more superficial and are usually mobile in the soft tissues, but do not move cephalad when the tongue protrudes as they lack a connecting tract to the hyoid bone. Nasal dermoid cysts may present as a cyst or sinus anywhere from the glabella to the base of the columella.[66] Any midline scalp lesion suspected of being a dermoid cyst should undergo preoperative radiographic evaluation to exclude intracranial extension. This is especially important for nasal dermoid cysts which have been reported to extend to the cribriform plate in 12–45% of cases.[66] Imaging is also recommended for orbital dermoids with palpably indistinct margins, as such lesions may require deep orbital dissection.[67] The best way to evaluate for deep extension of a midline lesion is controversial. Both CT and MRI may be used in a complementary fashion, with CT better evaluating bony abnormalities and MRI better defining soft tissue structures. Some clinicians argue that CT alone is adequate; however, false negatives have been reported.[66] Dermoids and epidermoid cysts gradually increase in size due to the accumulation of sebum.[65] Infection is rare, but the cysts can rupture resulting in granulomatous inflammation.[5,65] Fine needle aspirate may also be helpful in distinguishing an infected thyroglossal duct from a ruptured dermoid.[65]

Excision is the treatment of choice for all dermoid and epidermoid cysts, especially those which are symptomatic, enlarging, or have ruptured. This has been most commonly performed as an open operation, although increasing experience with removing these lesions is accruing by using endoscopic minimally invasive techniques.[68] Proponents of the open technique report good cosmetic results with minimal complications, while early reports using the endoscopic approach have reported a few partial facial nerve injuries especially early in the surgeon's learning curve.[69] Excellent cosmetic results have also been reported using an eyelid crease incision to excise angular dermoids.[70] It is important to completely remove the capsule and avoid intraoperative rupture to decrease the risk of recurrence. Infection is possible secondary to repeated local trauma. Malignant degeneration of dermoids also is possible but rare.[24] Complete surgical removal is curative.

Torticollis

Torticollis in childhood may be congenital or acquired. Congenital torticollis resulting from fibrosis and shortening in the SCM is the most common type.[71–73] The shortening of the SCM characteristically pulls the head and neck to the side of the lesion. The resulting 'mass' represents the fibrous tissue palpable within the muscle. The etiology of this 'fibrous tumor' is debatable.[72] The significant incidence of breech presentations and other abnormal obstetric positions has been used to support both the injury and tumor etiology. Those who favor tumor see the abnormal presentation as the result of the fixed abnormal head position, whereas those who favor trauma see the difficult extraction as the cause of injury.[72,74] No one theory completely explains this condition. The etiology of acquired torticollis includes cervical hemivertebrae and imbalance of the ocular muscles. In children in whom no identifiable muscular etiology is found, a high likelihood exists of Klippel–Feil anomalies or a neurologic disorder as the cause.[75] Acquired torticollis also should raise the suspicion of otolaryngologic infection, gastroesophageal reflux (Sandifer syndrome), or the possibility of a neoplastic condition as the underlying cause.[74,75]

Histologically, the basic abnormality in congenital torticollis is endomysial fibrosis—the deposition of collagen and fibroblasts around individual muscle fibers that undergo atrophy.[72] The sarcoplasmic nuclei are compacted to form 'muscle giant cells,' which appear to be multinucleated.[72] The severity and distribution of fibrosis differ widely from patient to patient. Some cases of fibrosis occur bilaterally. The fact that mature fibrous tissue is present even in the neonate suggests that the disease begins well before birth and is probably not due to a difficult delivery.

In a series of 100 infants with torticollis, 66% had a 'tumor' in the muscle, and the other 34% had fibrosis but no tumor.[26,76] A series of 1,086 cases from China noted only 42.7% with a tumor.[77] In the typical case, the mass is not found in the newborn period but is noted at the first 'well-baby' check-up, some 6 weeks after birth. The infant has the characteristic posture, with the face and chin rotated away from the affected side and the head tilted toward the ipsilateral shoulder (Fig. 73-13).[73] Acquired torticollis may develop at any age, and it is important to keep in mind the various causes of the acquired lesion. Its appearance depends on the severity of the lesion, the distribution of the fibrosis, and the child's growth pattern. With time, facial and cranial asymmetry develop, and a notable flattening of the facial structures on the side of the lesion occurs. This may become irreversible by age 12 years, although reports have described good results when the operative correction is performed after age 10.[78,79]

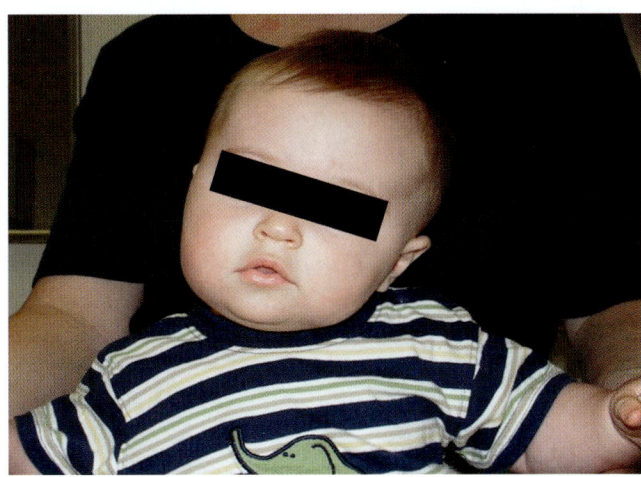

FIGURE 73-13 ■ This young child has left torticollis. He is sitting on his mother's lap. The face and chin are tilted away from the involved side and the head is tilted toward the ipsilateral shoulder.

Experience with this condition has shown that more than 90% of patients respond to nonoperative management.[77] The key to successful treatment is early recognition and prompt physical therapy.[71,80] The longer the shortening of the muscle persists, the more facial and cranial asymmetry develops, and the deeper the cervical tissues become involved in the process. The need for potential surgical intervention is associated with the severity of the rotational deficit, an older age at presentation, and the presence of 'tumor' rather than fibrosis without tumor.[77] Ultrasound may be used not only as a diagnostic tool but also to help determine which children may be more likely to need operative therapy. In another study from China, the cross-sectional as well as longitudinal extent of fibrosis in the SCM correlated well with the need for operation.[81]

In most instances, complete correction can be achieved by early range-of-motion and stretching exercises, and positional changes with the baby in the crib. The parents should be taught to perform these exercises with the baby several times each day. One parent holds the child's shoulder down against a firm surface, and the other rotates the head toward the opposite shoulder. When the child's head is rotated toward the opposite shoulder, the muscle is gently kneaded along its entire course. Often one parent can accomplish the stretching exercises by placing the baby on his or her lap, turning the baby's head, and gently extending the head and neck over the parent's knees. An additional maneuver is rearranging the baby's room, changing objects in the crib, and encouraging the baby to look toward the side opposite the involved muscle. One study showed a mean duration of 4.7 months for successful nonoperative resolution.[82] Some clinicians have used botulinum toxin injections in select patients who have failed to improve after six months of aggressive physical therapy, avoiding operation in 74–95% of patients.[83,84]

Some clinicians have suggested that the criterion for operation, regardless of age, is the development of facial hemihypoplasia.[80] In children with significant torticollis, facial hemihypoplasia is invariably present, not always

with a linear relation between the two conditions.[80] The muscle can be divided anywhere, but transection in the middle third, through a lateral collar incision, is the simplest and provides the most aesthetically acceptable scar.[80] Through this incision, one can divide the fascia colli of the neck, which is often tight and may need to be divided anteriorly as far as the midline and posteriorly to the anterior border of the trapezius. Intensive physiotherapy, including full rotation of the neck in both directions and full extension of the cervical spine, is instituted as soon as possible. For optimal results, application of a soft cervical collar for at least 3 months following fibrous band release is recommended.[85] Some authors advise delaying operative intervention until the patient is at least five years of age as studies have shown better long-term outcomes due to improved compliance with physical therapy and collar therapy in older children.[86]

INFLAMMATORY LESIONS

Enlarged cervical lymph nodes are by far the most common neck masses in childhood. In most instances, they are the result of nonspecific reactive hyperplasia.[1] The etiology is often viral or related to an upper respiratory tract or skin infection. In such cases, the adenitis resolves spontaneously. Most cases are first seen with enlarged nodes bilaterally. Because the anterior cervical nodes drain the mouth and pharynx, almost all upper respiratory and pharyngeal infections have some effect on the anterior cervical nodes. Enlarged cervical lymph nodes are frequently palpable in children between ages 2 and 10 years. Palpable nodes are uncommon in infants. A mass in a child younger than 2 years is more likely to be a cystic hygroma, thyroglossal duct cyst, dermoid cyst, or branchial cyst.[87]

As the head contains so many structures through which bacteria or viruses can enter the body, the cervical lymph nodes frequently become involved in many infections and inflammatory diseases. Cervical nodes also may be the first clinical manifestations of various tumors, particularly lymphomas.[1] The most frequent inflammatory lesion of the cervical lymph nodes is suppurative lymphadenitis (Fig. 73-14). Others of importance are cat-scratch disease, atypical mycobacterial lymphadenitis, and tuberculous lymphadenitis. Less common but important considerations in the differential diagnosis of cervical adenitis include Kawasaki disease and acquired immunodeficiency syndrome (AIDS).

Acute Suppurative Cervical Lymphadenitis

The most common cause of acute cervical lymphadenopathy is a bacterial infection arising in the oropharynx or elsewhere in the drainage area.[88] The most common organisms are penicillin-resistant *Staphylococcus aureus* and *Streptococcus pyogenes*, although cultures of the pus often yield a mixture of both or prove to be sterile.[88] *Staphylococcus* may be more prevalent in infants.[89] Anaerobes, although common in the oropharynx, are not common pathogens in cervical adenitis. Fever is variable

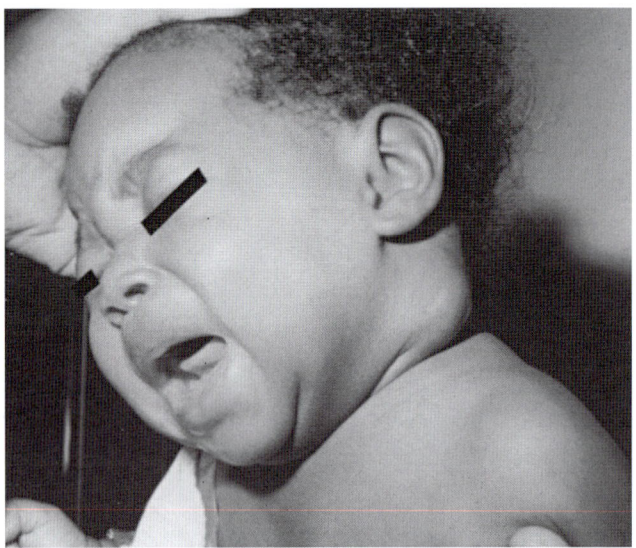

FIGURE 73-14 ■ Acute suppurative cervical adenitis. Skin is shiny and taut over the centralized abscess cavity.

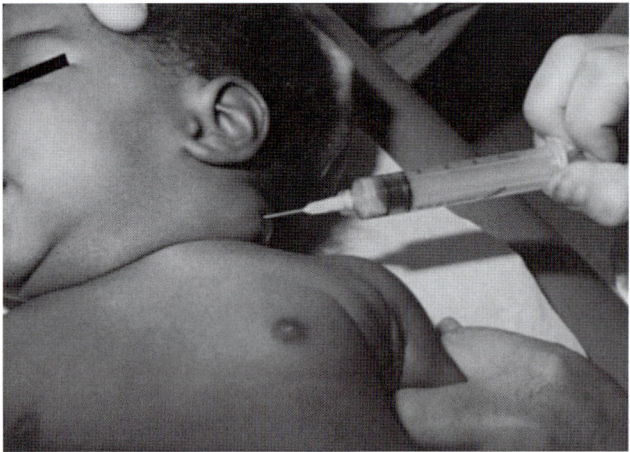

FIGURE 73-15 ■ Aspiration of purulent material confirms the diagnosis of suppurative lymphadenitis. Frequently, repeated aspirations may be necessary to remove the majority of debris and can often obviate the need for formal incision and drainage.

and usually mild. Initial treatment with antibiotics is often followed by resolution without suppuration. Without treatment, the node often enlarges and becomes fluctuant, eventually leading to thinning of the overlying skin and abscess formation. Needle aspiration can be both diagnostic and therapeutic. Aspiration of purulent material confirms the diagnosis. The material obtained can be cultured (Fig. 73-15). Frequently, needle aspiration and drainage of the purulent material coupled with judicious antibiotic therapy may alleviate the necessity of formal I&D. Occasionally, repeated aspirations may be necessary.

If the child appears toxic or is quite young, hospitalization and intravenous antibiotics, including a β-lactamase-resistant antibiotic, may be helpful, but formal I&D is often required. The node can be incised and the cavity packed loosely with a Penrose drain. The parent can be taught to irrigate through the Penrose drain, which

encourages drainage of the residual debris. Improvement is usually evident in two to three days, although antibiotic therapy should be continued for ten days. Complete resolution of the adenopathy may take weeks.

Chronic Lymphadenitis

Children occasionally have impressively enlarged nodes that do not seem to be acutely infected. The nodes are not as inflamed or as tender as those in acute bacterial adenitis. Moreover, progression to fluctuation is unlikely. The child with this type of lymphadenopathy must be evaluated for tuberculosis, atypical mycobacterial infection, and cat-scratch disease. Most children should receive a full 2-week course of an oral antistaphylococcal antibiotic. The same physician should examine the child on a number of occasions to assess the results of therapy. A single dominant lymph node present for longer than 6 to 8 weeks, which has not responded to appropriate antibiotic therapy, should be completely excised, fully cultured, and submitted for histologic examination to rule out the diagnosis of neoplasm. Nodes present in the supraclavicular space and posterior triangle tend to elicit more concern for malignancy than those found in the submandibular or anterior triangle.

Mycobacterial Lymphadenitis

The prevalence and the relative incidence of infections caused by different mycobacteria vary with the success of preventive health measures in particular populations.[90] Seventy to 95% of mycobacterial lymphadenitis in the United States is caused by nontuberculous strains, usually the atypical mycobacteria of the *Mycobacterium avium-intracellulare-scrofulaceum* (MAIS) complex.[90] Internationally adopted terminology (MAIS) defines this group of 10 to 15 mycobacteria, which produce a specific and localized form of lymphadenitis.[90] The portal of entry is primarily through the mucous membranes of the pharynx. Lymphadenitis resulting from infection with *M. tuberculosis* is thought to be an extension of a primary pulmonary infection and usually involves the supraclavicular nodes.[91] Infection with the atypical strains usually involves higher cervical nodes, most commonly the submandibular or submaxillary.[91] This finding is consistent with the etiology being a primary infection and not pulmonary disease. Infection is most commonly seen between ages 1 and 5 years; occurrence before age 1 year is rare. The disease involves unilateral nodes, and dissemination is rare. Atypical mycobacteria enter from the environment and are not contagious, although the reservoir may be the mouth and oropharynx of apparently healthy children.[89] Person-to-person spread of disease has not been documented, and isolation is not necessary.

Infection with atypical mycobacteria is generally limited to the lymph nodes, but fluctuance and spontaneous drainage occur in up to 50% of cases, with sinus tracts forming in up to 10%. The nodes are usually nontender. Spontaneous regression of atypical nodal infection may occur but is likely to lead to breakdown of the nodes and sinus or fistula formation. Children with tuberculous scrofula usually are symptomatic. Most have pulmonary tuberculosis when the diagnosis is made.[92] It is rare for the infection to progress from cervical adenopathy to pulmonary disease if the initial chest roentgenograms are clear. Degeneration of nodes with abscess and fistula formation is unusual.

In children, tuberculous or atypical mycobacterial lymphadenitis presents with a clinical picture of chronic lymph node hypertrophy.[93] Pulmonary tuberculosis on chest radiograph helps to identify the cause of the cervical swelling. Patients with MAIS usually have a normal chest roentgenogram. Skin testing helps differentiate these diseases. All children with tuberculosis should show positive test results to second-strength purified protein derivative (PPD). Children with atypical mycobacterial infection have either a negative or a doubtful skin test. If the initial PPD is inconclusive, second-strength PPD may help confirm the mycobacterial etiology. A history of familial exposure to tuberculosis should suggest tuberculosis as more likely than atypical mycobacteria. Final diagnosis may depend on culture results or histopathology after excision of the involved nodes.[94]

It is important to distinguish tuberculous from MAIS lymphadenitis because the treatment is significantly different. In tuberculous infections, antituberculous chemotherapy is required, usually resulting in marked resolution of the lymphadenopathy within a few months. Chemotherapy is continued for 2 years.[92] Surgical intervention in a human tuberculosis infection is confined to an excisional biopsy of a node, if the diagnosis cannot be made on other grounds. Most children with tuberculous lymphadenitis respond well to chemotherapy with standard drugs. Treatment of MAIS infections has been primarily surgical. Clarithromycin, ethambutol, and rifampicin may be used in patients whose lesions are too close to the facial nerve or other key structures, or for involvement of nodes deep to the SCM without overlying skin involvement.[95,96] Patients requiring operation need careful, thorough excision of all clinically involved nodes, sinus tracts, and overlying skin. This procedure should ideally be performed before extensive ulceration of the overlying skin occurs. Children with atypical mycobacterial infection respond well to complete surgical excision without additional drug therapy.

Cat-Scratch Disease

The incidence of cat-scratch disease varies greatly in different parts of the world. In developed countries, cat-scratch disease is the most common cause of nonbacterial chronic lymphadenopathy.[97] *Bartonella henselae*, a Gram-negative, rickettsial organism, is responsible for most cases of cat-scratch disease.[98] The disease is usually transmitted via a superficial wound caused by a cat, dog, or monkey. The healthy kitten is the most frequent vector. The disease begins as a superficial infection or pustule forming in 3 to 5 days and is followed by regional adenopathy in 1 to 2 weeks. Generally, only one node is involved. Nodal involvement corresponds to the inoculation site and the nodes that drain it. The axilla is the most commonly involved area.[1] The diagnosis can be made by a commercially available indirect fluorescent antibody test for detection of antibody or by polymerase chain reaction studies for *B. henselae* on a fine needle aspirate.[98] Complete excision of the involved node is recommended to confirm the diagnosis, if necessary. Patients usually have tender lymphadenopathy and few systemic symptoms. On rare occasion, complications include encephalitis, retinitis, and osteomyelitis. Treatment for cat-scratch disease is most often symptomatic as the disease is usually self-limited. Lymphadenopathy resolves spontaneously over a period of weeks to months with only occasional suppuration. Specific antimicrobial therapy against *B. henselae* has not proven efficacious, although it is susceptible to many common antibiotics. Azithromycin, rifampin, ciprofloxacin, and trimethorprim-sulfamethoxazole may be efficacious if antibiotics are needed.[99,100]

REFERENCES

1. Filston HC. Head and neck-sinuses and masses. In: Holder TM, Ashcraft KW, editors. Pediatric Surgery. Philadelphia: WB Saunders; 1980. p. 1062–79.
2. Gray SW, Skandalakis JE. The pharynx and its derivatives. In: Skandalakis JE, Gray SW, editors. Embryology for Surgeons: The Embryological Basis for the Treatment of Congenital Defects. Philadelphia: WB Saunders; 1972. p. 15–62.
3. Guarisco JL. Congenital head and neck masses in infants and children, Part II. Ear Nose Throat J 1991;70:75–82.
4. Telander RL, Deane SA. Thyroglossal and branchial cleft cysts and sinuses. Surg Clin North Am 1977;57:779–96.
5. Enepekides DJ. Management of congenital anomalies of the neck. Facial Plast Surg Clin North Am 2001;9:131–45.
6. Roback SA, Telander RL. Thyroglossal duct cysts and branchial cleft anomalies. Semin Pediatr Surg 1994;3:142–6.
7. Gray SW, Skandalakis JE, Akin JT Jr. Embryological considerations of thyroid surgery: Developmental anatomy of the thyroid, parathyroids, and the recurrent laryngeal nerve. Am Surg 1976;42:621–8.
8. Ward PA, Straham RW, Acquerelle M, et al. The many faces of cysts of the thyroglossal tract. Trans Am Acad Ophthalmol Otolaryngol 1970;74:310–16.
9. Folley DS, Fallat ME. Thyroglossal duct and other congenital midline cervical anomalies. Semin Pediatr Surg 2006;15:70–5.
10. Sonnino RE, Spigland N, Laberge JM, et al. Unusual patterns of congenital neck masses in children. J Pediatr Surg 1989;24:966–9.
11. Katz AD, Zager WT. The lingual thyroid. Arch Surg 1971;102:582–5.
12. Welch KJ, Tapper D, Vawter GP. Surgical treatment of thymic cysts and neoplasms in children. J Pediatr Surg 1979;14:691–8.
13. Strickland AL, Macfee JA, VanWyk JJ, et al. Ectopic thyroid glands simulating thyroglossal duct cysts. JAMA 1969;208:307–10.
14. Nanson EM. Salivary gland drainage into the thyroglossal duct. Surg Gynecol Obstet 1979;149:203–5.
15. Radkowski D, Arnold J, Healy GB, et al. Thyroglossal duct remnants: Preoperative evaluation and management. Arch Otolaryngol Head Neck Surg 1991;117:1378–81.
16. Gupta P, Maddalozzo J. Preoperative sonography in presumed thyroglossal duct cysts. Arch Otolaryngol 2001;127:200–2.
17. Kessler A, Eviatar E, Lapinsky J, et al. Thyroglossal duct cyst: Is thyroid scanning necessary in the preoperative evaluation? Israel Med J Assoc 2001;3:409–10.
18. Sidell DR, Shapiro NL. Diagnostic accuracy of ultrasonography for midline neck masses in children. Otolaryngol Head Neck Surg 2011;144:431–4.
19. Pinczower E, Crockett DM, Atkinson JB, et al. Preoperative thyroid scanning in presumed thyroglossal duct cysts. Arch Otolaryngol Head Neck Surg 1992;118:985–8.
20. Sistrunk WE. Technique of removal of cyst and sinuses of the thyroglossal duct. Surg Gynecol Obstet 1928;46:109–12.
21. Bennett KG, Organ CH Jr, Williams GR. Is the treatment for thyroglossal duct cysts too extensive? Am J Surg 1986;152:602–5.

22. Obiako MN. The Sistrunk operation for the treatment of thyroglossal cysts and sinuses. Ear Nose Throat J 1985;64:196–201.

23. Ein SH, Shandling B, Stephens CA, et al. Management of recurrent thyroglossal duct remnants. J Pediatr Surg 1984;19:437–9.

24. Hoffman MA, Schuster SR. Thyroglossal duct remnants in infants and children: Reevaluation of histopathology and methods for resection. Ann Otol Rhinol Laryngol 1988;97:483–6.

25. Salgarelli AC, Robiony M, Consolo U, et al. Piezosurgery to perform hyoid bone osteotomies in thyroglossal duct cyst surgery. J Craniofac Surg 2011;22:2272–4.

26. Mukel RA, Calcaterra TC. Management of recurrent thyroglossal duct cyst. Arch Otolaryngol 1983;109:34–6.

27. Ahmed J, Leong A, Jonas N, et al. The extended Sistrunk procedure for the management of thyroglossal duct cysts in children: How we do it. Clin Otolaryngol 2011;36:271–5.

28. Maddalozzo J, Alderfer J, Modi V. Posterior hyoid space as related to excision of the thyroglossal duct cyst. Laryngoscope 2010; 120:1773–8.

29. Ostlie DJ, Burjonrappa SC, Snyder CL, et al. Thyroglossal duct infections and surgical outcomes. J Pediatr Surg 2004;39: 396–9.

30. Kaselas C, Tsikopoulos G, Chortis C, et al. Thyroglossal duct cyst's inflammation. When do we operate? Pediatr Surg Int 2005;21:991–3.

31. Motamed M, McGlashan JA. Thyroglossal duct carcinoma. Curr Opin Otolaryngol Head Neck Surg 2004;12:106–9.

32. Forest VI, Murali R, Clark JR. Thyroglossal duct cyst carcinoma: Case series. J Otolaryngol Head Neck Surg 2011;40:151–6.

33. Waldhausen JHT. Branchial cleft and arch anomalies in children. Semin Pediatr Surg 2006;15:64–9.

34. Moore GW, Hutchins GM, O'Rahilly R. The estimated age of staged human embryos and early fetuses. Obstetrics 1982;139: 500–6.

35. Burge D, Middleton A. Persistent pharyngeal pouch derivatives in the neonate. J Pediatr Surg 1983;18:230–4.

36. Soper RT, Pringle KC. Cysts and sinuses of the neck. In: Welch K, et al. editors. Pediatric Surgery. 4th ed. Chicago: Year Book Medical; 1986. p. 539–51.

37. Frazer JE, Bertwistle AP. The nomenclature of disease states caused by certain vestigial structures in the neck. Br J Surg 1923;2:131–4.

38. Randall P, Royster HP. First branchial cleft anomalies. Plast Reconstr Surg 1963;31:497–501.

39. D'Souza AR, Uppal HS, De R, et al. Updating concepts of first branchial cleft defects: A literature review. Int J Pediatr Otolaryngol 2002;62:103–9.

40. Shrime M, Kacker A, Bent J, et al. Fourth branchial complex anomalies: A case series. Int J Pediatr Otolaryngol 2003;67: 1227–33.

41. Lee K, Klein TR. Surgery of cysts and tumors of the neck. In: Paparella MM, Shumrick DA, editors. Otolaryngology. Philadelphia: WB Saunders; 1973.

42. Roback SA, Telander RL. Thyroglossal duct cysts and branchial cleft anomalies. Semin Pediatr Surg 1994;3:142–6.

43. O'Mara W, Amedee R. Anomalies of the branchial apparatus. J La State Med Soc 1998;150:570–3.

44. Jordan JA, Graves JE, Manning SC, et al. Endoscopic cauterization for treatment of fourth branchial cleft sinuses. Arch Otolaryngol 1998;124:1021–4.

45. Gaisford JC, Anderson VS. First branchial cleft cysts and sinuses. Plast Reconstr Surg 1975;55:299–304.

46. Triglia JM, Nicollas R, Ducroz V, et al. First branchial cleft anomalies. Arch Otolaryngol Head Neck Surg 1998;124:291–5.

47. Bajaj Y, Tweedie D, Ifeacho S, et al. Surgical technique for excision of first branchial cleft anomalies: How we do it. Clin Otolaryngol 2011;36:371–4.

48. Chen Z, Wang Z, Dai C. An effective surgical technique for the excision of first branchial cleft fistula: Make-inside-exposed method by tract incision. Eur Arch Otorhinolaryngol 2010;267: 267–71.

49. D'Souza AR, Uppal HS, De R, et al. Updating concepts of first branchial cleft defects: A literature review. Int J Pediatr Otorhinolaryngol 2002;62:103–9.

50. Ford GR, Balakrishnan A, Evans JN, et al. Branchial cleft and pouch anomalies. J Laryngol Otol 1992;106:137–43.

51. Van Zele T, Katrien B, Philippe D, et al. Stripping of a fistula for complete second branchial cleft. J Plast Reconstr Aesthet Surg 2010;63:1052–4.

52. Roh JL, Yoon YH. Removal of pediatric branchial cleft cyst using a retroauricular hairline incision (RAHI) approach. Int J Pediatr Otorhinolaryngol 2008;72:1503–7.

53. Chen LS, Sun W, Wu PN, et al. Endoscope-assisted versus conventional second branchial cleft cyst resection. Surg Endosc 2012;26:1397–402.

54. Benson MT, Dalen K, Mancuso AA, et al. Congenital anomalies of the branchial apparatus: Embryology and pathologic anatomy. Radiographics 1992;12:943–60.

55. Nicoucar K, Giger R, Jaecklin T, et al. Management of congenital third branchial arch anomalies: A systematic review. Otolaryngol Head Neck Surg 2010;142:21–8.e2.

56. Nicoucar K, Giger R, Pope HG, et al. Management of congenital fourth branchial arch anomalies: A review and analysis of published cases. J Pediatr Surg 2009;44:1432–9.

57. Nicollas R, Ducroz V, Garabedian EN, et al. Fourth branchial pouch anomalies: A study of six cases and a review of the literature. Int J Pediatr Otorhinolaryngol 1998;44:5–10.

58. Singer R. A new technique for extirpation of preauricular cysts. Am J Surg 1966;111:291–5.

59. Scheinfeld NS, Silverberg NB, Weinberg JM, et al. The preauricular sinus: A review of its clinical presentation, treatment, and associated conditions. Ped Derm 2004;21:191–6.

60. Tan T, Constantinides H, Mitchell TE. The preauricular sinus: A review of its aetiology, clinical presentation and management. Int J Pediatr Otorhinolaryngol 2005;69:1469–74.

61. Currie AR, King WW, Vlantis AC, et al. Pitfalls in the management of preauricular sinuses. Br J Surg 1996;83:1722–4.

62. Leopardi G, Chiarella G, Conti S, et al. Surgical treatment of recurring preauricular sinus: supra-auricular approach. Acta Otorhinolaryngol Ital 2008;28:302–5.

63. Gold BC, Skeinkopf DE, Levy B. Dermoid, epidermoid and teratomatous cysts of the tongue and the floor of the mouth. J Oral Surg 1974;32:107–11.

64. Smirniotopoulos JG, Chiechi MV. Teratomas, dermoids, and epidermoids of the head and neck. Radiographics 1995;15:1437–55.

65. Acierno SP, Waldhausen JHT. Congenital cervical cysts, sinuses, and fistulae. Otolaryngol Clin N Am 2007;40:161–76.

66. Sreetharan V, Kangesu L, Sommerlad BC. Atypical congenital dermoids of the face: A 25-year experience. J Plast Reconstr Aesthet Surg 2006;60:1025–9.

67. Cavazza S, Laffi GL, Lodi L, et al. Orbital dermoid cyst of childhood: Clinical pathologic findings, classification and management. Int Ophthalmol 2011;31:93–7.

68. Huang MG, Cohen SR, Burstein FD, et al. Endoscopic pediatric plastic surgery. Ann Plast Surg 1997;38:1–8.

69. Gur E, Drielsma R, Thomson HG. Angular dermoid cysts in the endoscopic era: Retrospective analysis of aesthetic results using the direct, classic method. Plast Reconstr Surg 2004;113(5): 1324–9.

70. Cozzi DA, Mele E, d'Ambrosio G, et al. The eyelid crease approach to angular dermoid cysts in pediatric general surgery. J Pediatr Surg 2008;43:1502–6.

71. Jones PG. Torticollis. In: Welch KJ, editor. Pediatric Surgery. 4th ed. Chicago: Year Book Medical; 1986. p. 552–6.

72. Mickelson MR, Cooper RR, Ponseti IV. Ultrastructure of the sternocleidomastoid muscle in muscular torticollis. Clin Orthop 1975;110:11–18.

73. Dunn PM. Congenital postural deformities: Perinatal associations. Proc R Soc Med 1972;65:735–9.

74. Kahn ML, Davidson R, Drummond DS. Acquired torticollis in children. Orthop Rev 1991;20:667–74.

75. Bredenkamp JK, Maceri DR. Inflammatory torticollis in children. Arch Otolaryngol Head Neck Surg 1990;116:310–13.

76. Ling CM, Low YS. Sternomastoid tumor and muscular torticollis. J Bone Joint Surg Br 1969;41:432–7.

77. Cheng JC, Tang SP, Chen TM, et al. The clinical presentation and outcome of treatment of congenital muscular torticollis in infants–a study of 1,086 cases. J Pediatr Surg 2000;35:1091–6.

78. Yu SW, Wand NH, Chin LS, et al. Surgical correction of muscular torticollis in older children. Chung Hua I Hsueh Tsa Chih Taipei 1995;5:168–71.

79. Cheng JCY, Tang SP. Outcome of surgical treatment of congenital muscular torticollis. Clin Orthop 1999;362:190–200.

80. Soeur R. Treatment of congenital torticollis. J Bone Joint Surg 1940;38:35–40.

81. Lin JN, Chou ML. Ultrasonographic study of the sternocleido-mastoid muscle in the management of congenital muscular torticollis. J Pediatr Surg 1997;32:1648–51.

82. Emery C. The determinants of treatment duration for congenital muscular torticollis. Phys Ther 1994;74:921–9.

83. Oleszek JL, Chang N, et al. Botulinum toxin type A in the treatment of children with congenital muscular torticollis. Am J Phys Med Rehabil 2005;84(10):813–16.

84. Joyce MB, de Chalain TMB. Treatment of recalcitrant idiopathic muscular torticollis in infants with botulinum toxin type A. J Craniofacial Surg 2005;16(2):321–7.

85. Lee IJ, Lim SY, Song HS, et al. Complete tight fibrous band release and resection in congenital muscular torticollis. J Plast Reconstr Aesthet Surg 2010;63:947–53.

86. Shim JS, Jang HP. Operative treatment of congenital torticollis. J Bone Joint Surg Br 2008;90:934–9.

87. Jones PG. Glands of the neck. In: Welch K, editor. Pediatric Surgery. 4th ed. Chicago: Year Book Medical; 1986. p. 517–20.

88. Hieber JP, Davis AT. Staphylococcal cervical adenitis in young infants. Pediatrics 1976;57:424–6.

89. Bodenstein L, Altman RP. Cervical lymphadenitis in infants and children. Semin Pediatr Surg 1994;3:134–41.

90. Altman RP, Margeleth AM. Cervical lymphadenopathy from atypical mycobacteria: Diagnosis and surgical treatment. J Pediatr Surg 1975;10:419–22.

91. Belin RP, Richardson JD, Richardson DL, et al. Diagnosis and management of scrofula in children. J Pediatr Surg 1974;9:103–7.

92. Kent PC. Tuberculous lymphadenitis: Not a localized disease process. Am J Med Sci 1967;254:866–74.

93. Lincoln EM, Gilbert LA. Disease in children due to mycobacteria other than Mycobacterium tuberculosis. Am Rev Respir Dis 1972;105:683–90.

94. Pinder SE, Colville A. Mycobacterial cervical lymphadenitis in children: Can histological assessment help differentiate infections caused by non-tuberculous mycobacteria from Mycobacterium tuberculosis? Histopathology 1993;22:59–64.

95. Fraser L, Moore P, et al. Atypical mycobacterial infection of the head and neck in children: A five year retrospective review. Otolaryngol 2008;138:311–14.

96. Harris RL, Modayil P, Adam J, et al. Cervicofacial nontuberculous mycobacterium lymphadenitis in children: Is surgery always necessary? Int J Pediatr Otorhinolaryngol 2009;73:1297–301.

97. Carithers HA. Cat scratch skin test antigen: Purification by heating. Pediatrics 1977;60:928–9.

98. Scott MA, McCurley TL, Vnencak-Jones CL, et al. Cat scratch disease: Detection of Bartonella henselae DNA in archival biopsies from patients with clinically, serologically, and histologically defined disease. Am J Pathol 1996;149:2161–7.

99. Chia JKS, Nakate MM, Lami JLM, et al. Azithromycin for the treatment of cat-scratch disease. Clin Infectious Dis 1998;26:193–4.

100. Margileth AM. Antibiotic therapy for cat-scratch disease: Clinical study of therapeutic outcome in 268 patients and a review of the literature. Pediatr Infect Dis J 1992;11:474–8.

SPECIAL TOPICS

CHAPTER 74

PEDIATRIC AND ADOLESCENT GYNECOLOGY

Julie L. Strickland

From birth through adulthood, many gynecologic diseases mimic urologic or general surgical conditions. Surgeons who care for children must be equipped to diagnose and treat a variety of developmental and acquired disorders of the female genital tract. It is important to begin with an understanding of the normal anatomy and developmental changes. Knowledge of examination techniques in children is important to obtain diagnostic information. Common gynecologic problems found in children and adolescents will be reviewed.

NORMAL GENITAL ANATOMY

The genital tract undergoes visible morphologic changes from infancy through childhood and adolescence.[1,2] At birth, owing to the influence of maternal circulating estrogens, the labia majora are anteriorly placed and edematous. They are thickened and cover the introital opening. The clitoral proportion is also larger. The vestibule and hymen are pale and thickened, and can occlude visualization of the vaginal canal without manipulation. The vagina is rugated and moist, and vaginal secretions may be present. The cervix is visible, and the uterus may contain functioning endometrial tissue, which can result in estrogen-withdrawal bleeding in infancy.

During early childhood, the vulva remodels with thinning and attenuation of the labia majora and minora. The vestibule becomes erythematous with prominent vascular markings. It may now be unopposed by the labia, allowing for easy visualization of the vaginal orifice with minimal retraction. The hymen of a prepubescent female is normally easily visualized and is thin, often translucent, and inelastic. Normal variations in the shape and amount of hymenal tissue have been described (Fig. 74-1).[3–5] The vagina has an erythematous appearance without rugations. Normally, the pH is mildly basic and a mixture of bacterial flora is present. The cervix is flush with the vaginal vault and the uterine fundus is poorly developed, with no endometrial development.

With the onset of puberty, the vestibule begins to lose its erythematous appearance. The hymen thickens and becomes elastic and redundant.[6] The vagina grows in length and develops rugations. The cervix has a well-defined junction from the uterus, and the uterine fundus develops a rounded appearance. Endometrial tissue is present.

Follicular activity within the ovary, with small cyst formation, can be observed on imaging as early as 16 weeks of gestation.[7] Three to 5% of children have small incidental ovarian cysts detected on ultrasound (US).[8] Follicular growth followed by involution continue throughout childhood, with increased follicular activity and size coinciding with increasing age.[9] Ovarian volume and position change with age, with the ovaries being intra-abdominal in childhood and assuming a pelvic position at puberty.

GENITAL EXAMINATION

An adequate light source and proper positioning are usually all that are needed to accomplish an examination in a prepubertal child.[10] For visualization of the vulva, introital opening, and lower vagina, gentle downward traction on the labia in a lithotomy position is usually successful (Fig. 74-2). The knee–chest position may offer a clearer view of the hymen and lower vagina (Fig. 74-3).[11] A colposcope (or otoscope) may be helpful to see the detail of the vestuble and lower vagina.[12] The office use of vaginal speculums is discouraged in prepubertal children. When vaginal inspection is needed, it should be done using endoscopic instruments under sedation.[13,14] By gently occluding the vaginal orifice, the entire vaginal canal can be visualized with hydrodistention.[15] Speculum examinations of the vagina are usually well tolerated in postpubertal girls when a narrow-caliber straight blade speculum is gently inserted. Bimanual examinations can be accomplished through a rectal approach or, in adolescents, with a single digit inserted into the vaginal fornix. Imaging with abdominal ultrasound or, occasionally magnetic resonance imaging (MRI), is adjuvant to examination and provides additional information about the upper genital tract.[16]

Vulvar Abnormalities

Vulvar pruritus, pain, and discharge are common complaints in children. An etiology can be obtained in most cases with careful external inspection and, if necessary, blind vaginal cultures. Biopsy is seldom indicated. Most often, symptoms involve irritation or eruption of the vulvar skin related to hygiene or common skin conditions. Atopic or irritant dermatitis are the most common diagnoses.[17] Infections are associated with acute inflammation with mucosal erythema and the presence of a vaginal discharge.[18] Common respiratory pathogens such as *Streptococcus pyogenes* and *Haemophilus influenzae* may

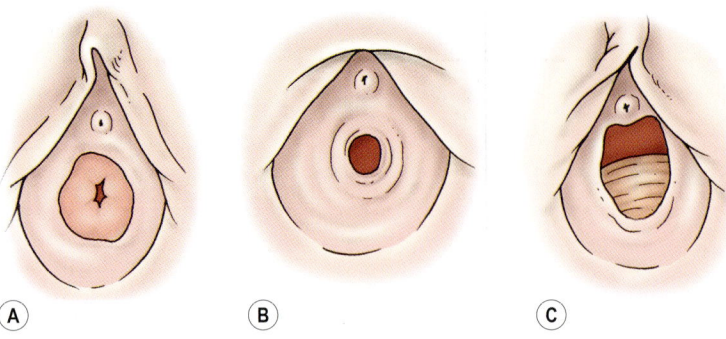

(A)   (B)   (C)

FIGURE 74-1 ■ Normal anatomic variations of the hymen. (Adapted from Pokorny SF, Stormer J. Atraumatic removal of secretions from the prepubertal vagina. Am J Obstet Gynecol 1987;156:581–3.)

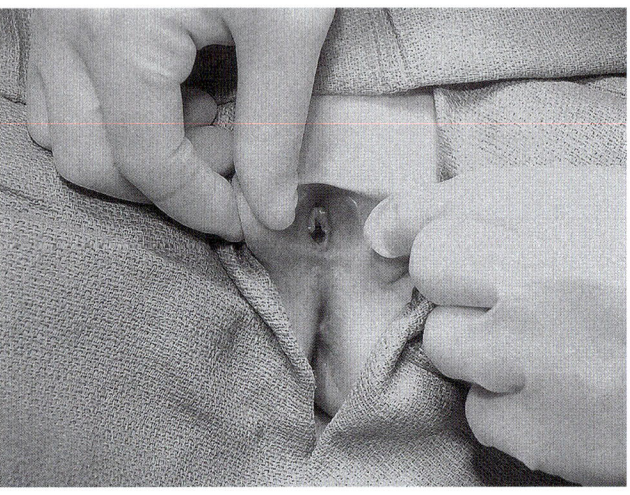

FIGURE 74-2 ■ Examination of the genitalia by labial traction. Gently grasping the posterior labia majora and pulling anteriorly and superiorly allows visualization of the genital structures.

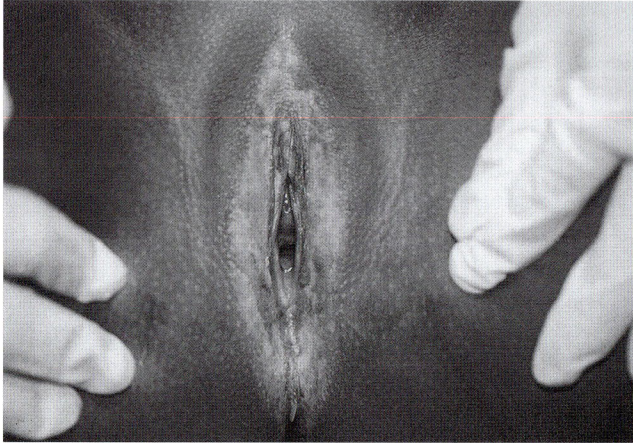

FIGURE 74-4 ■ Lichen sclerosis diagnosed in a 5-year-old. A sharp demarcation of hypopigmented, thin epithelium is seen. This lesion is often associated with fissures and purpura.

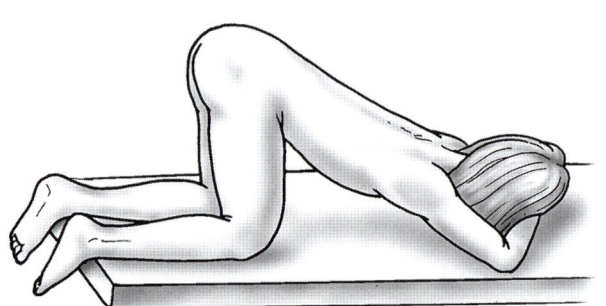

FIGURE 74-3 ■ Knee–chest positioning. The lower vagina and hymen can occasionally be viewed more successfully by using the knee–chest position.

occasionally cause acute genital symptoms.[19,20] When a bacterial infection is suspected, cultures of the vagina can be obtained by using moistened urethral swabs, feeding tubes, or catheters.

Recurrent or persistent vaginitis, despite treatment, should alert the clinician to the presence of a retained foreign body in the vagina. When a foreign body is suspected, vaginal lavage can be attempted in the office by using warm-water saline through a urinary catheter. Vaginoscopy under sedation may be necessary to retrieve the object.

Vulvar dermatoses can lead to acute vulvovaginal symptoms. Lichen sclerosis has the hallmark characteristic of a loss of skin markings with a sharply demarcated pale epithelial ring encircling the introitus, but sparing the vagina (Fig. 74-4). Signs of inflammation and trauma may be present, with purpura, fissures, and secondary infection associated with scratching. Principles of treatment include avoidance of irritation and loose clothing, mild soaps, and the generous use of emollients. Early treatment with ultrapotent corticosteroids may be effective in reducing symptoms of lichen sclerosis and minimizing long-term scarring. In 20% of patients, ultrapotent corticosteroids have been shown to reverse skin changes.[21] Tacrolimus has also been reported to offer similar benefit to pediatric patients.[22] Other dermatologic conditions such as psoriasis, eczema, and allergic dermatitis also may mimic vulvovaginitis.[19]

Labial adhesions occur frequently in prepubescent girls (Fig. 74-5). Adhesions are thought to occur because of irritation or trauma to the unestrogenized labia. Adhesions can be associated with urinary tract infections, perineal wetness, symptomatic vulvitis, and an inability to access the urethra. When symptomatic, preferred treatment has historically been estrogen-based cream applied under traction to the labia. Newer investigations suggest that betamethasone cream may have equal efficacy.[23,24] The need for adhesiolysis is low because of the efficacy of topical therapy, but may be necessary in both unusually dense adhesions or those that have required previous

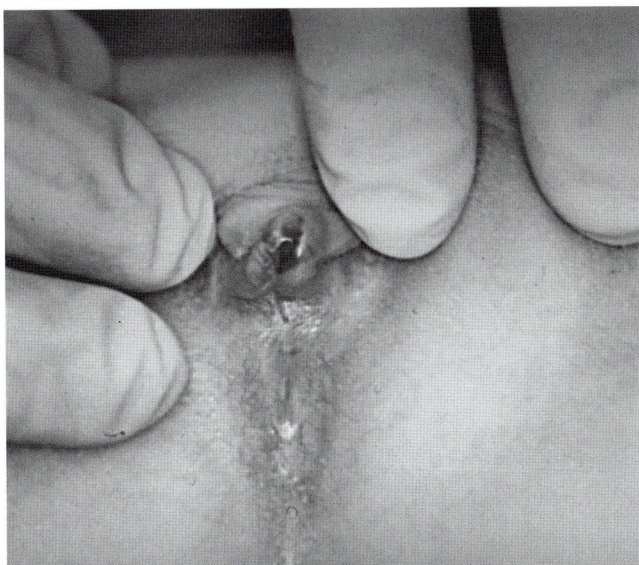

FIGURE 74-5 ■ A 2-year-old child with labial (minora) adhesions is seen.

BOX 74-1	**Causes of Genital Bleeding in Prepubescent Girls**

Genital trauma: Accidental, sexual abuse
Genitourinary: Urethral prolapse, urinary tract infections
Gastrointestinal: Inflammatory bowel disease, rectal fissure, hemorrhoids
Vulvovaginitis: Acute dermatitis, pinworms, β-hemolytic *Streptococcus*, *Shigella*
Foreign body
Vulvar dermatosis: Lichen sclerosis
Condylomata acuminata
Hemangiomas
Tumors
Malignant or benign endocrine abnormalities: isosexual precocious puberty, pseudoprecocious puberty, exogenous hormonal stimulation

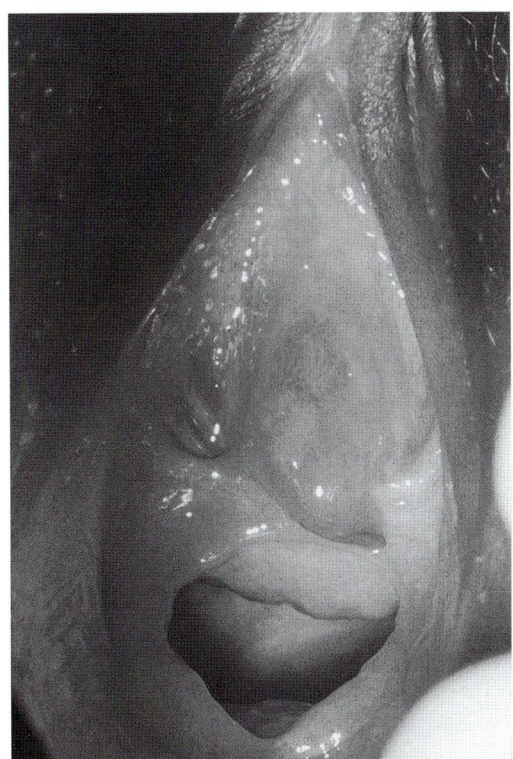

FIGURE 74-6 ■ Urethral prolapse was found in this 6-year-old child with a history of recurrent painless genital bleeding.

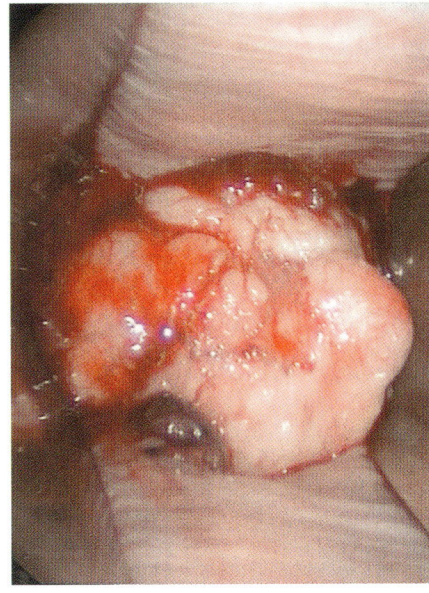

FIGURE 74-7 ■ A 12-year-old adolescent, presenting with refractory dysfunctional uterine bleeding, is diagnosed with a neuroendocrine tumor of the cervix at vaginoscopy.

separation. Manual separation of the adhesions without anesthesia should be avoided because of the discomfort and the high risk of recurrence. For thin adhesions, office separation using long acting local anesthetics, such as EMLA cream, is a reasonable option.[25]

Genital Bleeding

Bleeding from the genital area in a prepubescent child is always abnormal (Box 74-1). Bleeding is most commonly extragenital, resulting from hematuria, rectal fissures, and vulvar epithelial irritation. Prolapse of the urethra can occur and may be associated with bleeding or even gangrenous changes (Fig. 74-6). Topical treatment with estrogen-based cream usually relieves the symptoms. If symptoms persist, excision of the redundant tissue may be necessary.[26] Vaginal bleeding can be associated with precocious puberty or autonomous production, or with exogenous sources of hormonal stimulation. It is important to perform a detailed physical examination searching for evidence of breast development, estrogenization of

the genital tract, or the presence of an abdominal mass. In the absence of a satisfactory explanation for the source of bleeding, vaginoscopy should be performed to exclude a foreign body, trauma, infection or, rarely, primary and metastatic tumors of the lower genital canal (Fig. 74-7).

Acute genital bleeding in children requires immediate evaluation for the presence of serious injury or sexual abuse.[27] If the source of bleeding is not readily apparent, if the entire lesion cannot be identified, or if the patient is not tolerant of the examination, vaginoscopy under sedation is needed.[28,29] Straddle injuries are common during childhood from accidental falls onto blunt objects, resulting in soft tissue trauma from striking the perineum. Straddle injuries usually involve the mons, clitoris, and labia, sparing the vaginal ring or perineal body (Fig. 74-8). They may result in a hematoma, linear lacerations, or abrasions. Vulvar hematomas can be extensive but are more commonly self-limited. In the absence of acute ongoing hemorrhage, small or moderate hematomas can be managed conservatively with bed rest, ice, and pain control. Evacuation of extremely large hematomas causing distortion of the midline pelvic structures occasionally is necessary to facilitate recovery. Evacuation with debridement should be performed with the child under anesthesia by incising the medial mucosal surface and placing absorbable sutures for hemostasis and closure of dead space.

Penetrating injuries can occur through accidental impalements onto irregular objects, but the possibility of sexual abuse must always be considered (Figs 74-9 and 74-10). In the prepubertal child, lacerations involving or occurring above the hymenal ring require vaginoscopy under general anesthesia. Because of the inelasticity of the vaginal epithelium, penetrating injuries can result in disruption of the vagina, with possible internal hemorrhage and hematoma formation.[29] Injuries that cannot readily be explained by the history should be referred to child protection. Surgeons should familiarize themselves with the legal and social resources for sexual abuse and care that are available within their communities.

Introital masses in children occasionally come to the attention of surgeons. Masses of the introitus or vagina are most commonly epithelial inclusion cysts of the hymen or lower vagina, and often spontaneously resolve. There is a rare possibility of embryonic rhabdomyosarcoma, a malignant primary tumor that appears as indolent, grape-like masses protruding from the vagina (Fig. 74-11). Other possibilities include condylomata acuminata, ectopic ureter, or an obstructive vaginal anomaly.

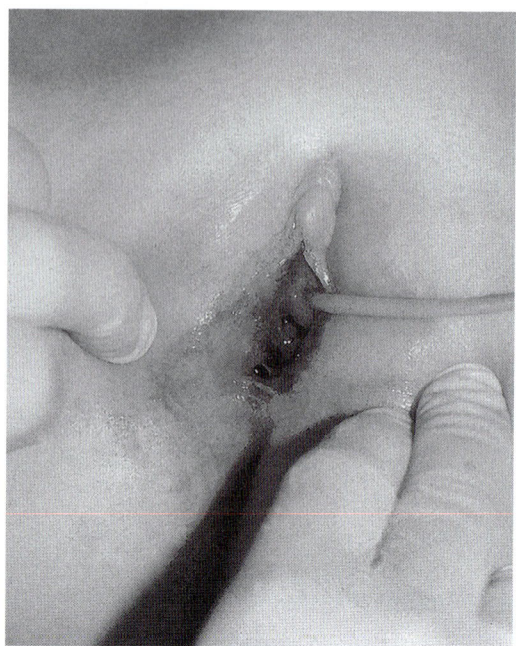

FIGURE 74-9 ■ A 9-year-old girl has a penetrating posterior vaginal injury sustained after falling onto an open cabinet. A urinary catheter has been inserted in the urethra.

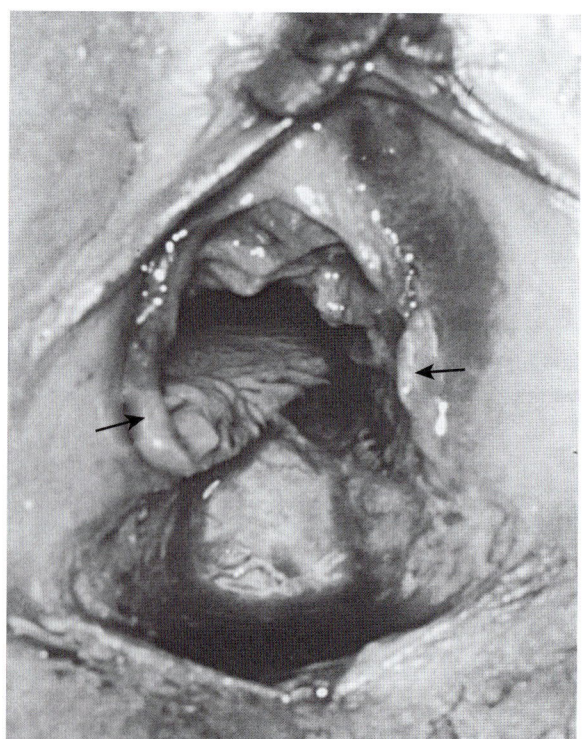

FIGURE 74-10 ■ An 8-year-old victim of acute sexual assault has small bowel herniating through the apex of the avulsed vagina. Note the abundant, although transected, amount of hymenal tissue (arrows) present, indicating that she had not had significant stretch trauma to her hymen before this episode of rape. (From Pokorny SF, Pokorny WJ, Kramer W. Acute genital injury in the prepubertal girl. Am J Obstet Gynecol 1992;166:1461–6.)

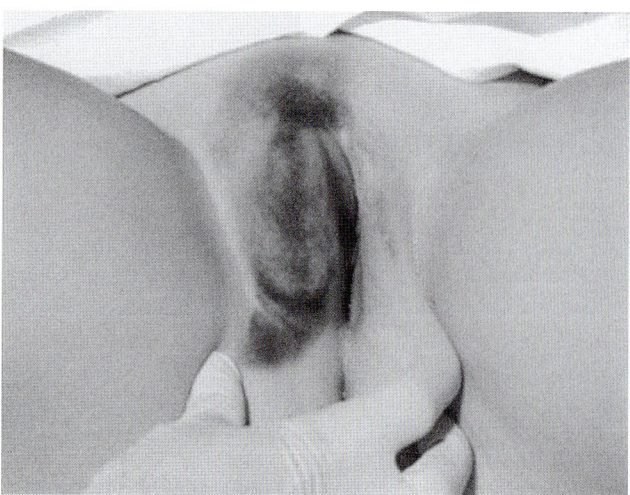

FIGURE 74-8 ■ An extensive vulvar hematoma is seen after a straddle injury. (Courtesy of Diane Merritt, MD.)

Occasionally, the Bartholin gland or periurethral gland may occlude or form an abscess, leading to an acquired lateral mass. Transperineal ultrasound can be helpful. In cases that are unclear, biopsy or excision (or both) may be necessary.

UTEROVAGINAL ANOMALIES

Developmental abnormalities causing agenesis or obstruction of the genital tract can present in childhood. These can be recognized in the newborn period, but the majority are diagnosed in adolescence with the lack of anticipated menses or with symptoms of obstruction.

Imperforate hymen is the most commonly diagnosed obstructive anomaly, but has an incidence of less than 1%.[30] It arises as an isolated anomaly from failure of canalization of the urogenital sinus. Symptoms typically are first noted during late puberty with cyclic pelvic pain and introital distention, associated with the absence of

menstruation. With the continued accumulation of menstrual blood, a pelvic mass and obstructive genitourinary or gastrointestinal symptoms may develop. Occasionally, newborns will present with mucous accumulation and an abdominal mass (Fig. 74-12). Transabdominal ultrasound reveals a dilated vaginal and uterine canal. If this is found during childhood and is asymptomatic, correction is usually deferred until the onset of puberty. Surgical excision of the hymen with evacuation of the retained menstrual fluid provides permanent relief (Fig. 74-13). An incision is made in the membrane inferior to the urethral meatus. After decompression, the individual flaps of tissue are then excised. The vaginal mucosa is sutured to the introital edge with interrupted absorbable sutures to avoid stenosis (Fig. 74-14). It is important to recognize

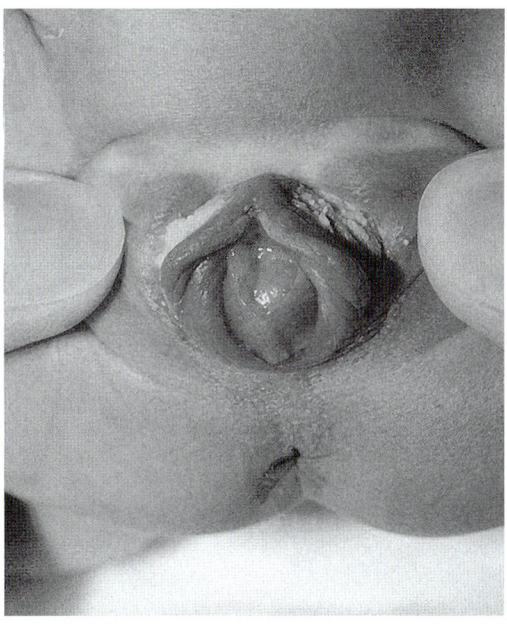

FIGURE 74-12 ■ Mucocolpos, leading to urinary obstruction in a 2-day-old infant.

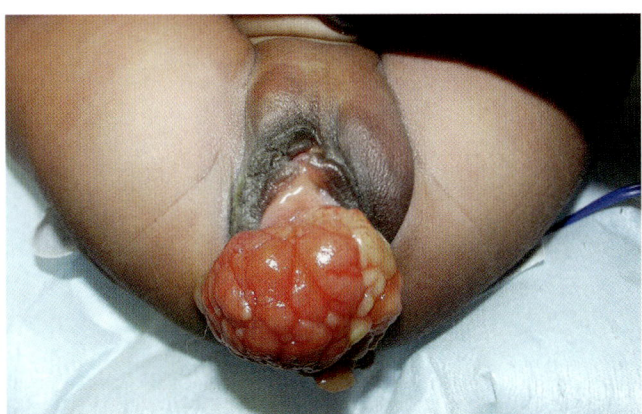

FIGURE 74-11 ■ This infant was found to have a mass protruding from her vagina which is an embryonic rhabdomyosarcoma (sarcoma botryoides). The mass was attached to the wall of the vagina and was able to be completely excised.

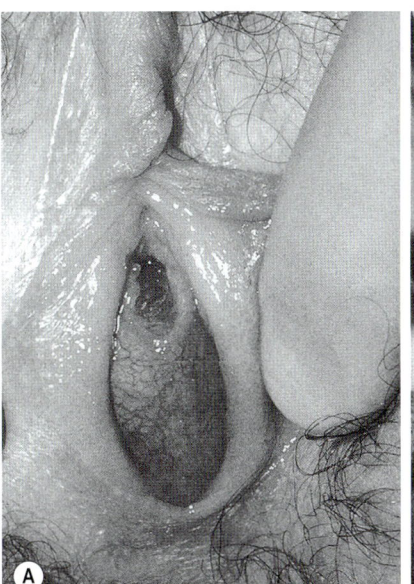
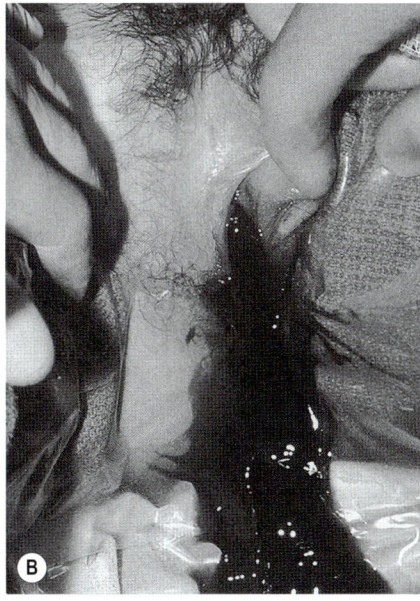

FIGURE 74-13 ■ (A) Imperforate hymen in a 12-year-old girl with a 6-month history of recurrent abdominal pain. (B) Evacuation of the menstrual obstruction at hymenotomy.

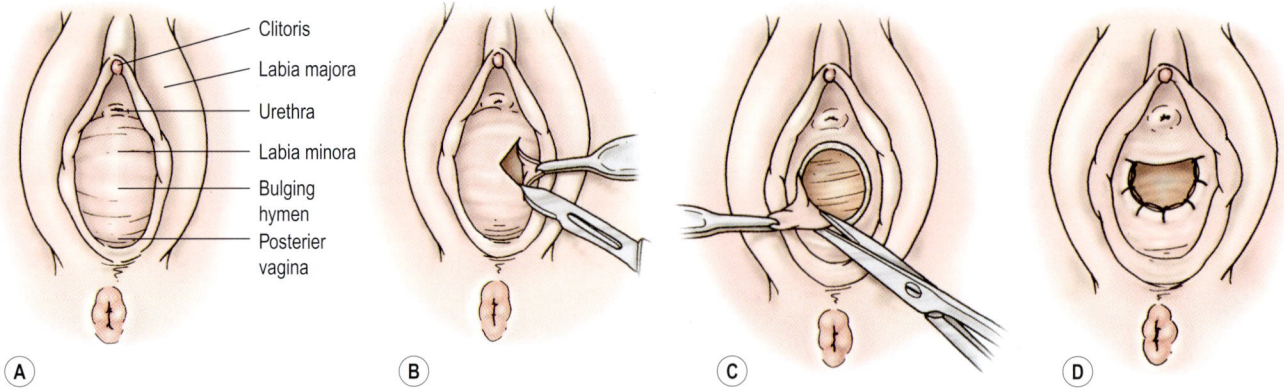

FIGURE 74-14 ■ **(A)** Imperforate hymen. **(B)** A cruciate incision is made in the apex of the hymen after identifying the outer hymenal borders. **(C)** The hymenal remnants are trimmed. **(D)** Interrupted sutures are utilized for hemostasis.

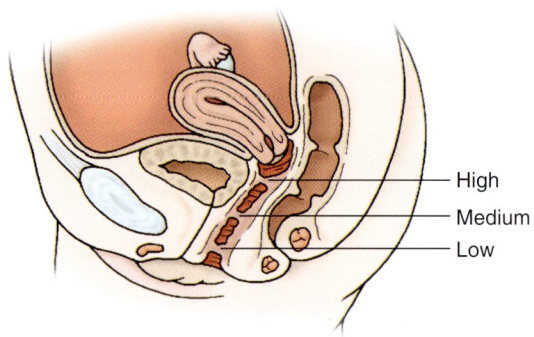

FIGURE 74-15 ■ The transverse vaginal septum is the result of failed unification or canalization of the urogenital sinus and the müllerian duct. It can arise anywhere in the vagina, but is most common in the upper vagina.

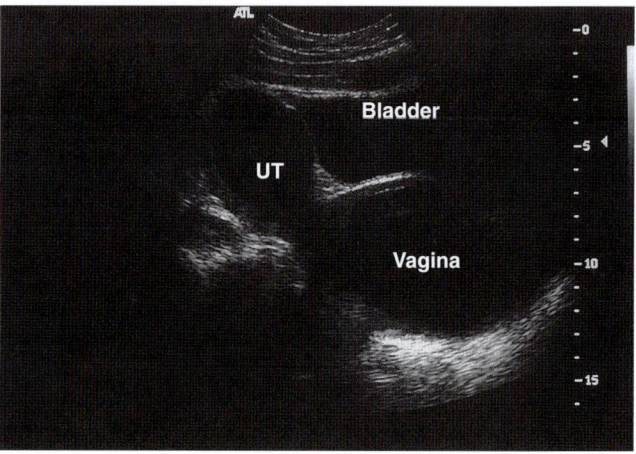

FIGURE 74-16 ■ A sonographic sagittal view of the pelvis of a 16-year-old girl with cervicovaginal agenesis and a resultant hematometra. Note the dilated vagina and uterus (UT).

that significant distention of the posterior vaginal wall may cause the hymenal membrane to be located in a more superior position. Needle aspiration without definitive surgical correction is contraindicated because of the possibility of bacterial seeding and the development of an abscess.

A transverse vaginal septum, either complete or partial, can be found at various levels of the vagina due to failure of unification of the urogenital sinus and the Müllerian ducts during embryogenesis (Fig. 74-15). As the introitus can appear normal, the diagnosis may be delayed. MRI or ultrasound are helpful in defining this anomaly and documenting the thickness of the septum prior to surgical exploration.[31] Operative correction entails excision of the septum with a mucosal anastomosis. A thick septum may require preoperative vaginal dilation, mobilization of the upper vagina, or occasionally a skin graft to maintain vaginal patency. Circumferential stenosis is common at the anastomotic site, particularly with high or thick septae. Vaginal dilation or stent placement may be necessary. Occasionally, a uterine duplication is associated with hypoplasia of one cervix and obstruction. This condition is treatable with laparoscopic hemihysterectomy of the affected side.[32] True cervicovaginal agenesis is rare and is associated with an obstructed uterine canal, the absence of a patent cervix, and agenesis of the upper

vagina (Fig. 74-16). This condition has a poor prognosis for reconstruction, with reports of significant morbidity from ascending infection and even death.[33] Hysterectomy is usually recommended, but creation of a vagino-uterine fistula has also been described.[34,35]

Occasionally, patients may be seen with a duplication of the uterus and cervix, and a unilateral obstructing longitudinal septum of the vagina. Associated ipsilateral renal agenesis or hypoplasia is commonly found.[36] Menstruation occurs from the nonobstructed side, so the diagnosis may be made well past menarche with pelvic ultrasound or MRI (Fig. 74-17).[31,37] Repair through a vaginal approach is performed at diagnosis, with complete excision of the vaginal septum.

Mayer–Rokitansky–Küster-Hauser syndrome was first described in 1961 and includes primary amenorrhea in women with normal secondary sexual characteristics, uterine hypoplasia, and congenital absence of the upper vagina.[38] The incidence is approximately 1 in 5000.[39] Renal and skeletal anomalies are commonly associated with this disorder. Although patients have primary amenorrhea, pubertal development and ovarian function are normal. The diagnosis can be made clinically on the basis of a normal phenotype, chromosomal analysis, and the

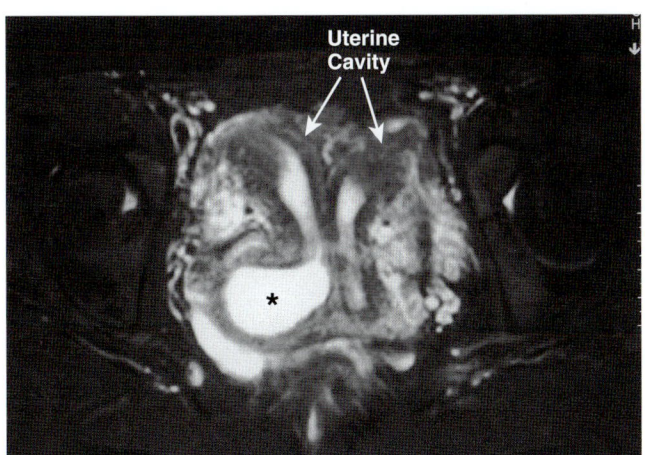

FIGURE 74-17 ■ MR image of a 16-year-old girl with a complete uterine duplication and a blind right hemivagina. Note the obstructed and dilated right hemivagina (asterisk) and the resultant right-sided hematocolpos and hematometra.

genital findings cited earlier. Management is centered on creation of an adequate vaginal pouch to allow normal sexual functioning. The use of Lucite dilators, first popularized in the 1930s, has provided a highly effective non-surgical alternative for many patients with vaginal agenesis (Fig. 74-18).[40,41] Through the use of successive pressure dilators introduced at the hymenal ring over a 2-3-month period, the vaginal vault can be lengthened and enhanced to provide adequate vaginal capacity. This approach has the advantage of being patient controlled and is associated with extremely low morbidity. Sexual satisfaction of young women treated with dilation has been shown to be comparable with the normal population.[42] In selected patients, operative creation of an artificial vagina may be needed.[43]

Many surgical options for vaginal substitution have been described, with the split-thickness skin graft vaginoplasty being advocated most often for patients with agenesis (Fig. 74-19).[44] Surgical outcomes and patient satisfaction remain high for this type of vaginoplasty

although risks and complications exist.[45] Other materials such as amnion, peritoneum, absorbable adhesion barriers (Interceed, Ethicon, Somerville, NJ), and buccal mucosa have been described as an alternative to skin grafting.[46,47] Novel laparoscopic techniques using these alternatives have also been reported including laparoscopic methods using advancement of the peritoneum or a transperitoneal pulley system to advance the neovagina.[48,49] The use of sigmoid bowel pedicles pulled to the introitus for vaginal creation is less commonly utilized for this problem, but also may be associated with good long-term results.[50,51]

ADNEXAL DISEASE

Ovarian cysts may develop at any time from fetal life to adulthood. Simple cysts in the neonate are generally follicular and originate from the influence of maternal estrogens. Complex masses in this age group may represent in utero or neonatal torsion with the risk of malignancy being very low.[52] Both simple and complex masses are likely to resolve without therapy, but operative intervention may be necessary for torsion, hemorrhage, or mass effect.[52] Percutaneous aspiration is indicated for cysts larger than 5 cm to minimize the risk of torsion.[53,54] Indications for operative intervention include the presence of a complex mass that fails to resolve in the neonatal period, the recurrence of a cyst after aspiration, the development of acute abdominal symptoms, or a combination. Treatment consists of laparoscopic fenestration of simple cysts or cystectomy.[55]

In childhood, small cysts representing follicular development and atresia are common and not pathologic.[8] Management of ovarian cysts in children is based on size, the presence of symptoms, and cyst composition. Worrisome findings include cysts larger than 5 cm, cysts with solid or complex internal echoes on ultrasound, and fixed masses accompanied by systemic symptoms of disease or precocious development.[56]

Occasionally, cysts may be associated with breast development or vaginal bleeding (Fig. 74-20). The diagnosis of an ovarian tumor must be considered in children, especially in those with a large, persistent complex mass that has solid components (Table 74-1). The most common ovarian tumor in children is a mature cystic teratoma, followed by stromal tumors.[57,58] Malignant tumors are rare, comprising less than 10% of all operatively treated masses.[57-59]

In prepubertal girls, operative exploration is needed for ovarian masses that are symptomatic or associated with worrisome radiologic signs. In the absence of malignancy, conservation of ovarian tissue should be attempted, whenever possible.

Ovarian cysts are extremely common in adolescence because of persistent anovulation or ovulatory dysfunction. They may be associated with rupture, pain, or hemorrhage (Fig. 74-21). A mass in the pelvis may be present, or the cyst may be found incidentally at the time of other studies. In adolescents, a variety of reproductive disorders such as endometriosis, pelvic inflammatory disease, disorders of the fallopian tube, congenital uterine

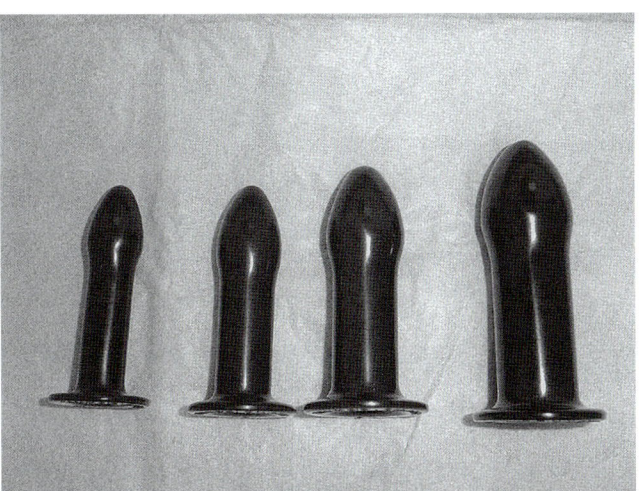

FIGURE 74-18 ■ Sequential vaginal dilators are often used to create a coital pouch in individuals with vaginal agenesis.

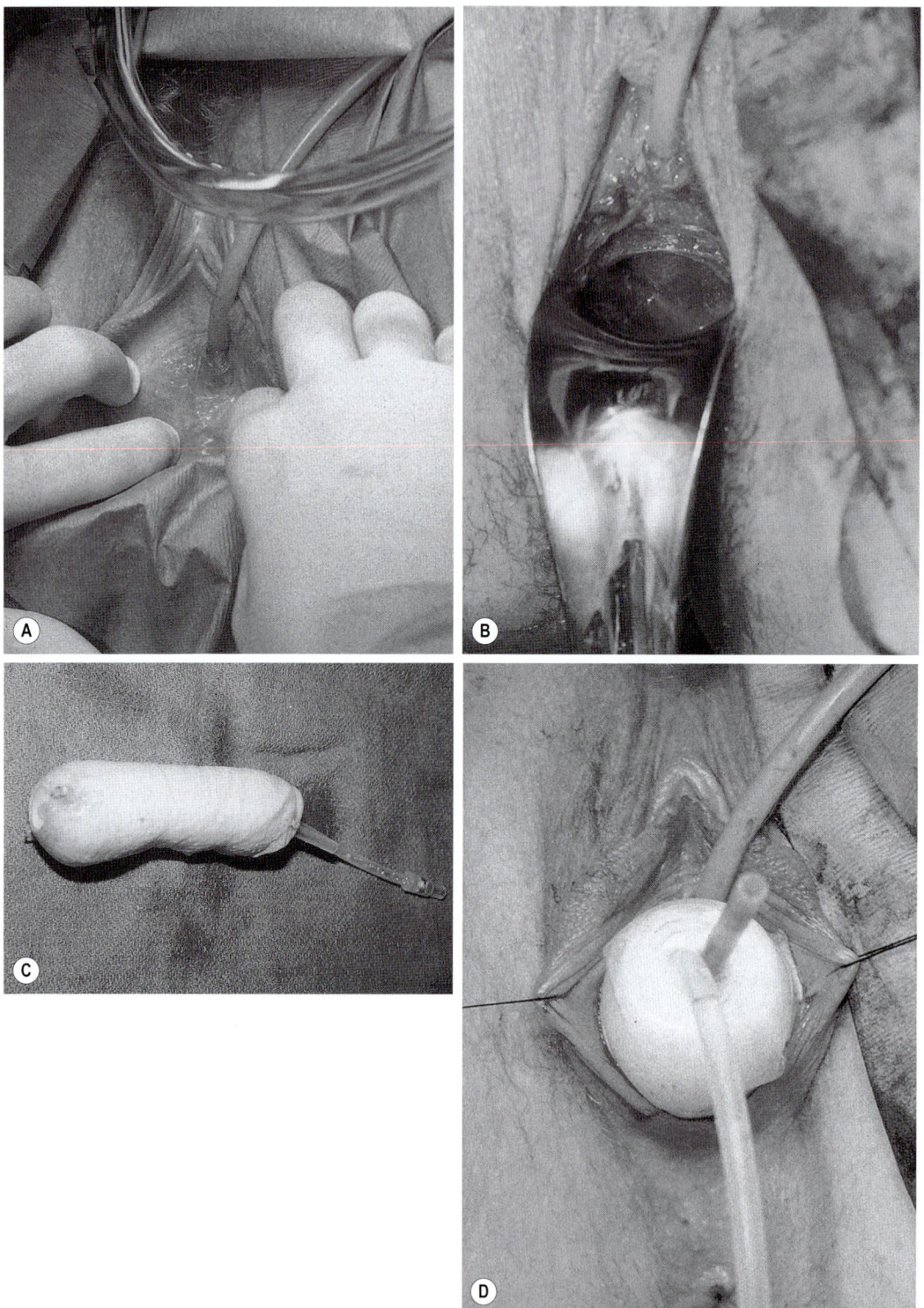

FIGURE 74-19 ■ Creation of a vaginal pouch by using a split-thickness free graft is shown. **(A)** The perineum of a patient with vaginal agenesis is seen. **(B)** A speculum has been introduced into the space that has been created between the urethra and rectum. **(C)** Covering of a vaginal mold with split-thickness grafted skin. **(D)** Placement of the mold into the space noted in (B).

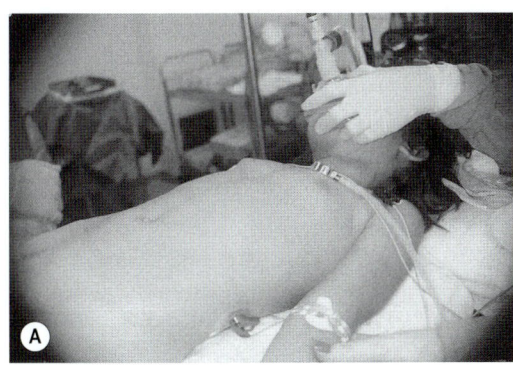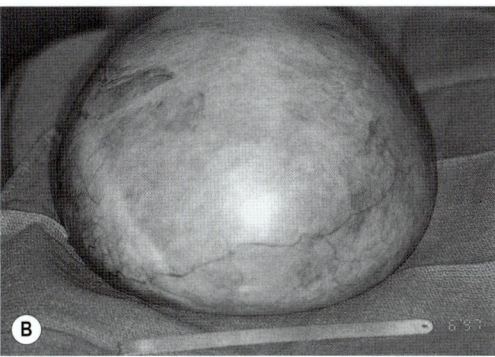

FIGURE 74-20 ■ **(A)** A 6-year-old girl presented with precocious puberty and a large pelvic mass. **(B)** An autonomously functioning ovarian serous cystadenoma was found. All pubertal signs regressed after its removal.

TABLE 74-1 Neoplasms in Female Children and Adolescents

Tumor Neoplasm	Appearance	Markers	Other Information
Teratoma (dermoid)	Irregular, cystic and solid; or primarily cystic	None	Most common germ cell tumor 6–8% malignant Malignant immature forms may be associated with other germ cell tumors
Dysgerminoma	Thick, white, opaque; cytologic reactivity with alkaline phosphatase	None	Inspect other ovary 15–20% bilateral, 95% cure (stage I) Chemotherapy for advanced disease
Endodermal sinus tumor (yolk sac tumor)	Solid and cystic Schiller–Duval bodies	AFP	Primarily unilateral Surgery and chemotherapy for all stages 15% survival after stage I
Embryonal carcinoma	Smooth with areas of hemorrhage and necrosis Schiller–Duval bodies	β-hCG	Usually part of a mixed germ cell tumor 60% endocrinologically active (precocious puberty) Surgery and chemotherapy for all stages (50% survival stage I)
Choriocarcinoma	Syncytiotrophoblasts and cytotrophoblasts	β-hCG	Rare primary tumor in pediatric age group; surgery and chemotherapy for all stages
Mixed germ cell tumor	Predominantly solid, or cystic and solid, depending on composition	AFP	Most commonly composed of dysgerminoma and endodermal sinus tumor
Sex cord stromal tumors	Granulosa–theca or Sertoli–Leydig cells	None	More common in younger patients Isosexual precocious puberty or androgenization
Juvenile granulosa–theca cell tumor	Very vascular	None	Malignancy related to percentage of granulosa cells Pure thecomas benign Surgery alone for stage I Surgery and chemotherapy for advanced disease
Sertoli–Leydig cell tumors (arrhenoblastoma)			Variable malignant potential
Epithelial tumors Serous cystadenoma	Predominantly cystic		Commonly large size May have borderline variants Low malignant potential
Mucinous cystadenoma	Predominantly cystic with septations		From coelomic epithelium
Serous or mucinous cystadenocarcinoma			Rare in children and adolescents
Miscellaneous tumors Polyembryoma	Tissues resemble embryos with all three germ cell types (amniotic cavity, yolk sac, placental primordia)		
Gonadoblastoma Mesothelioma Metastatic disease			Predominantly dysgenetic gonads

AFP, α-fetoprotein; β-hCG, human chorionic gonadotropin.
FROM BACON JL: Surgical treatment of adnexal pathology. In Hewitt G (ed): Operative Techniques in Gynecologic Surgery. Philadelphia, WB Saunders, 1999, vol 4, p 215.

anomalies, or disorders of pregnancy can have the appearance of ovarian cysts (Box 74-2). It is essential to elicit a full history, including the details of menstrual function and sexual activity. Pregnancy needs to be excluded, and the possibility of complications of a sexually transmitted infection considered. Ultrasound is very helpful in the management of ovarian cysts in adolescents.[60]

The conservative approach to the management of ovarian cysts in adolescents is based on the low rate of malignancy and the high rate of functional cysts or benign tumors. Observation is recommended as an initial therapy. Indications for operation include cysts larger than 10 cm, persistent complex masses, acute symptoms, or a high suspicion for malignancy. In the absence of findings suggestive of neoplasm, laparoscopy can be paired with cystectomy and ovarian conservation. Cystectomy is performed by incising the ovary on the antimesenteric portion of the ovary. Blunt dissection separates the cyst from the ovarian capsule, allowing the cyst wall to be removed in toto (Fig. 74-22). Electrocautery or sutures may be needed to obtain hemostasis. Closure of the cyst wall is not necessary. Although marked distortion of the ovarian capsule may occur, rapid involution develops. Studies have found laparoscopic removal of ovarian

teratomas to be safe, efficient, and without long-term sequelae, even in the presence of rupture and spillage (Fig. 74-23).[61,62] When malignancy is suspected, oophorectomy through a midline laparotomy incision allows proper staging with careful exploration, collection of pelvic cytology, and pelvic and periaortic lymph node sampling.

The ovaries or tubes may occasionally undergo torsion, with ischemia and ultimately necrosis of the adnexa, creating a surgical emergency (Fig. 74-24). Torsion of the ovary is recognized by the acute onset of pain, nausea, vomiting, and a pelvic mass. Ovarian torsion is classically associated with the presence of an ovarian cyst or tumor, but can occur in normal ovaries.[63] Doppler-enhanced

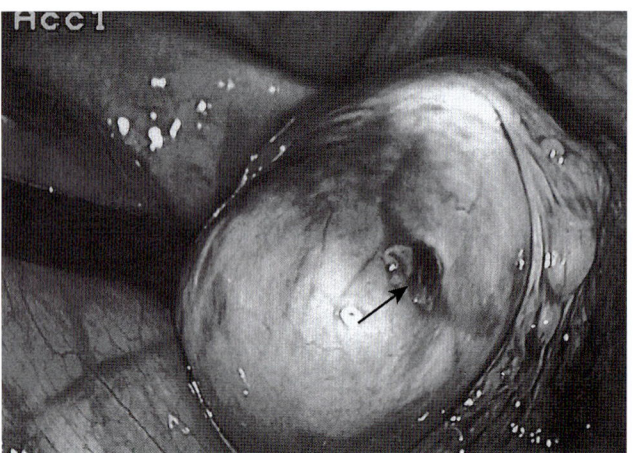

FIGURE 74-21 ■ A ruptured corpus luteum cyst in a 15-year-old girl with acute pelvic pain. The site of rupture is marked by the arrow.

BOX 74-2	**Etiology of Adnexal Masses in Adolescent Girls**

OVARIAN

  Follicular cyst
  Corpus luteum
  Endometrioma
  Ovarian torsion
  Benign or malignant neoplasm
    Fallopian tube
      Paraovarian cyst
      Ectopic pregnancy

UTERUS

  Uterine anomaly
    Pregnancy
    Myoma
  Gastrointestinal
    Abscess
    Appendicitis
    Inflammatory bowel disease
  Urinary
    Pelvic kidney
    Acute urinary retention
    Urachal cyst
  Neoplasms
    Sarcoma
    Lymphoma
    Teratoma
    Hemangioma

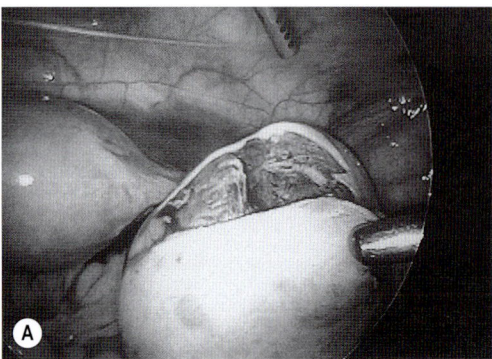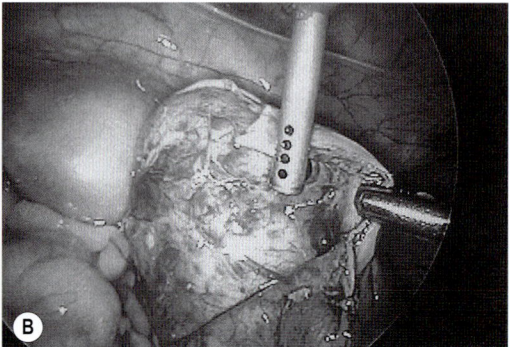

FIGURE 74-22 ■ Laparoscopic ovarian cystectomy. **(A)** An incision is made on the antimesenteric portion of the ovary. **(B)** The capsule is separated from the ovarian cyst with blunt and sharp dissection.

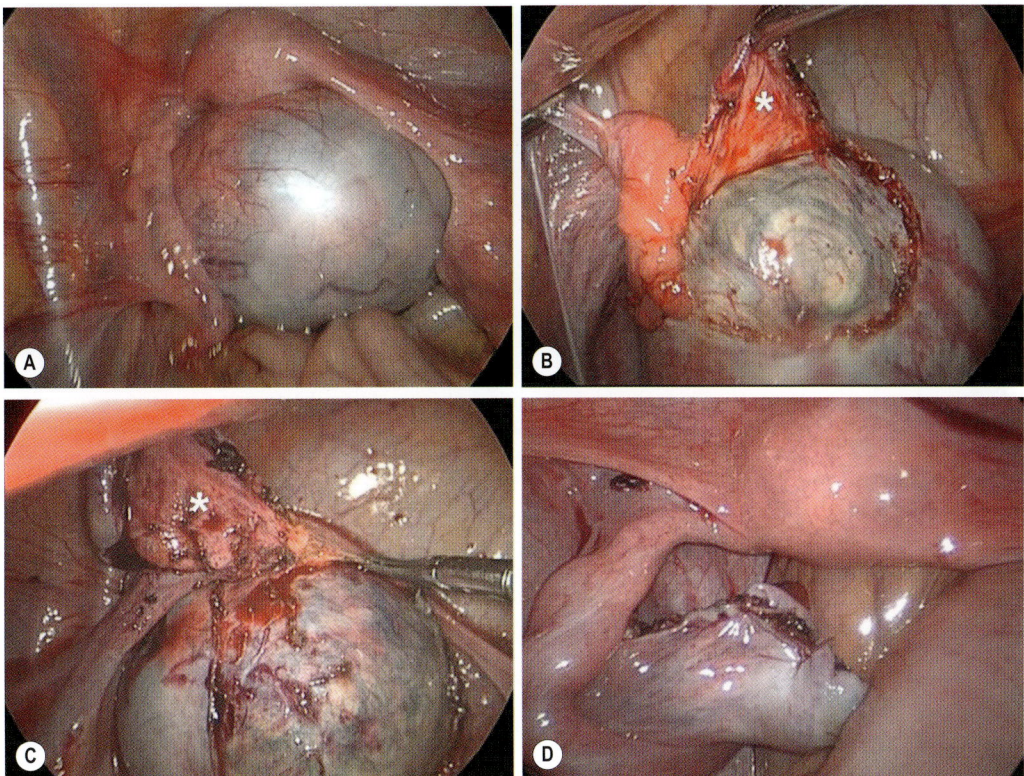

FIGURE 74-23 ■ A 14-year-old presented with abdominal pain. Ultrasonography and CT showed calcifications within this left ovarian mass **(A)**, indicating that it was a likely ovarian teratoma. **(B)** Laparoscopic excision of the teratoma was initiated by incising the outer layer and peeling back the normal ovarian parenchyma (asterisk). **(C)** The ovarian parenchyma (asterisk) has almost been completely stripped from the teratoma. **(D)** The ovarian parenchyma was approximated after excision of the mass. The teratoma was placed into an endoscopic retrieval bag and exteriorized through the umbilicus after some morcellation. Histologic examination showed it to be a benign teratoma.

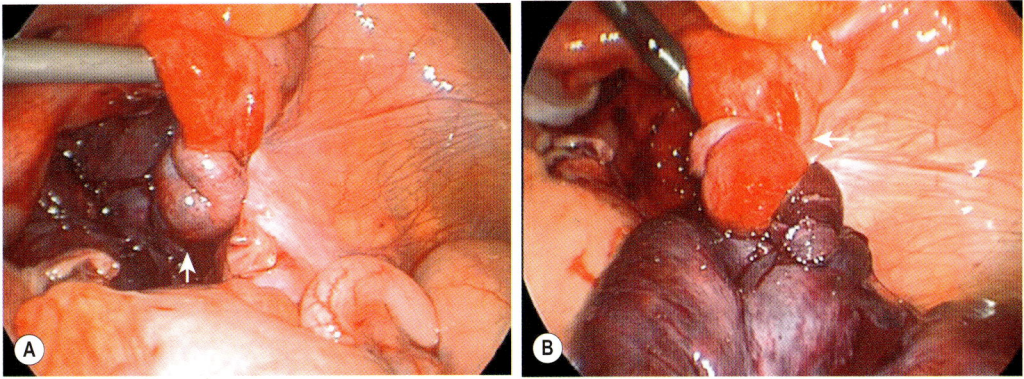

FIGURE 74-24 ■ Right ovarian torsion in a 14-year-old girl with acute abdominal pain **(A)**. The fallopian tube and ovarian vascular pedicle are twisted several times (arrow), resulting in acute venous congestion. **(B)** Untwisting the pedicle (arrow) allowed return of arterial flow and resolution of the venous congestion. Although the ovary appeared ischemic, it was not removed.

ultrasound demonstrating the absence of blood flow has historically been used to diagnose ovarian torsion, but has been shown to be less predictive than ovarian enlargement.[64,65] If a prompt diagnosis is made, the ovary may be salvaged with detorsion and cystectomy, even when it visually appears to have vascular compromise.[66] Oöphorectomy is reserved for necrotic ovaries. Oöphoropexy by side-wall fixation or shortening of the meso-ovarian ligament has been advocated by some to decrease the risk of subsequent contralateral torsion, although there is no evidence showing its efficacy.[66]

ENDOMETRIOSIS

Endometriosis refers to the presence of endometrial glands and functioning stroma outside the uterine lining. Traditionally, endometriosis has been thought to be a disease of women in their 20s and 30s, and is well described in the adolescent population with the exact prevalence unknown. As many as 75% of adolescent girls with medically refractory pelvic pain are found to have endometriosis at laparoscopy.[67] Although symptoms can suggest the

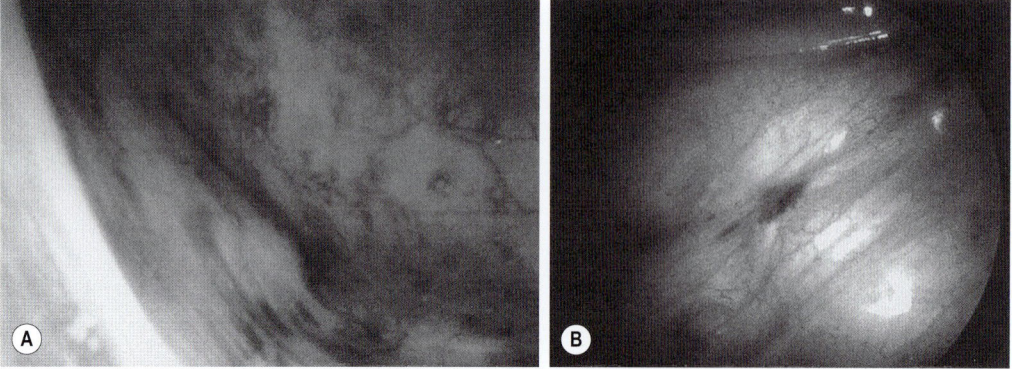

FIGURE 74-25 ■ **(A)** The peritoneal surface of a 14-year-old with endometriosis. Note the hypervascularity and subtle vesicular type lesions. **(B)** The peritoneal surface of a 17-year-old with endometriosis. Note the classic 'powder burn' appearance.

diagnosis, definitive diagnosis is made by laparoscopic visualization or biopsy (or both). Clear, vesicular-appearing lesions and low-stage disease are more common in adolescence, with more classic hemosiderin 'powder burn lesions' identified in older adults (Fig. 74-25).[68,69]

The treatment in adolescents is based on alleviation of symptoms and slowing the progression of disease. For patients undergoing an operation, removal of all visible lesions by resection or destruction should be performed. Menstrual suppression with oral contraceptives or progesterone-only medication (or both), along with non-steroidal anti-inflammatory agents, are the mainstays of therapy. Gonadotropin-releasing agonists may be used on a short-term basis as an adjuvant to operation, but carries the risk of a detrimental effect on bone density. This therapy should be used cautiously in younger adolescents. Likewise, newer therapies that control the symptoms of endometriosis, such as the Levonorgestrel IUS (Schering Health, Berlin-Wedding, Germany) and aromatase inhibitors, have not been studied in adolescents.[70,71] Noninterventional pain therapies may have a place in managing the chronic pain associated with endometriosis. The long-term outcomes, including infertility and chronic pain, in those diagnosed with endometriosis as adolescents is not well known.

REFERENCES

1. Huffman JW, Dewhurst CJ, Caparo VJ. Anatomy and physiology. The Gynecology of Childhood and Adolescence. 2nd ed. Philadelphia: WB Saunders; 1981. p. 24–69.
2. Siegfried EC, Frasier LD. The spectrum of anogenital diseases in children. In: Callen JP, editors. Current Problems in Dermatology. St. Louis: Mosby; 1997. p. 35–80.
3. Pokorny SF. Configuration of the prepubertal hymen. Am J Obstet Gynecol 1987;157:950–6.
4. McCann J, Wells R, Simon M, et al. Genital findings in prepubertal girls selected for nonabuse: A descriptive study. Pediatrics 1990; 86:428–39.
5. Berenson AB, Hegar AH, Hayes JM, et al. Appearance of the hymen in prepubertal girls. Pediatrics 1992;89:387–94.
6. Edgardh K, Ormstad K. The adolescent hymen. J Reprod Med 2002;47:710–14.
7. Peters H, Himelstein-Braw R, Faber M. The normal development of the ovary in childhood. Acta Endocrinol 1976;82:617–30.
8. Millar DM, Blake JM, Stringer DA, et al. Prepubertal ovarian cyst formation: 5 years' experience. Obstet Gynecol 1993;81: 434–7.
9. Himelstein-Braw R, Byskov AG, Peters H, et al. Follicular atresia in the infant human ovary. J Reprod Fertil 1976;46:55–9.
10. Hariston L. Physical examination of the prepubertal girl. Clin Obstet Gynecol 1997;40:127–34.
11. McCann J, Welis R, Simon M, et al. Comparison of genital examination techniques in prepubertal girls. Pediatrics 1990;85:182–7.
12. Mendriatta V. Office gynecologic evaluation of the pediatric patient: Indications, examination, and procedures. In: Hewett G, editor. Operative Techniques in Gynecologic Surgery. Philadelphia: WB Saunders; 1999. p. 164–75.
13. Golan A, Lurie S, Sagio R, et al. Continuous-flow vaginoscopy in children and adolescents. J Am Assoc Gynecol Laparosc 2000;7: 526–8.
14. Parker JD, Hibbert ML, Dainty LD, et al. Micro-hydrovaginoscopy in examining children. Obstet Gynecol 2000;96:772–4.
15. Nakhal RS, Wood D, Creighton SM. The role of examination under anesthesia (EUA) and vaginoscopy in pediatric and adolescent gynecology- a retrospective review. J Pediatr Adolesc Gynecol 2012;25:64–6.
16. Teele RL, Share JC. Ultrasonography of the female pelvis in childhood and adolescence. Radiol Clin North Am 1992; 30:743–58.
17. Fischer G, Rogers M. Vulvar disease in children: A clinical audit of 130 cases. Pediatr Dermatol 2000;17:1–6.
18. VanEyk N, Allen L, Giebrecht E, et al. Pediatric vulovaginal disorders: A diagnostic approach and review of the literature. J Obstet Gynecol Can 2009;31:850–62.
19. Straumanis JP, Bocchini JA. Group A beta-hemolytic streptococcal vulvovaginitis in prepubertal girls: A case report and review of the literature. Pediatr Infect Dis 1990;9:845–7.
20. Cox RA. Haemophilus influenzae: An underrated cause of vulvovaginitis in young girls. J Clin Pathol 1997;50:765–8.
21. Cooper SM, Gao XH, Powell JJ, et al. Does treatment of vulvar lichen sclerosis influence its prognosis? Arch Dermatol 2006;140: 702–6.
22. Matsumoto Y, Yamamoto T, Isobe T, et al. Successful treatment of vulvar lichen sclerosus in a child with low-concentration topical tacrolimus ointment. J Dermatol 2007;34:114–16.
23. Bacon JL. Prepubertal labial adhesions: Evaluation of a referral population. Am J Obstet Gynecol 2003;187:327–32.
24. Kumetz LM, Quint EH, Fisshea S, et al. Estrogen treatment success in recurrent and persistent labial agglutination. J Pediatr Adolesc Gynecol 2006;19:381–4.
25. Hoebeke P, Depauw P, Van Laecke E, et al. The use of EMLA cream as an anaesthetic for minor urological surgery in children. Acta Urol Belg 1997;65:25–8.
26. Holbrook C, Misra D. Surgical management of urethral prolapsed in girls: 13 years' experience. BJU 2012;110:132–4.
27. Scheidler MG, Schultz BL, Schall L, et al. Mechanisms of blunt perineal injury in female pediatric patients. J Pediatr Surg 2000; 35:1317–19.
28. Merritt DF. Genital trauma in children and adolescents. Clin Obstet Gynecol 2008;51:237–48.
29. Pokorny SF, Pokorny WJ, Kramer W. Acute genital injury in the prepubertal girl. Am J Obstet Gynecol 1992;166:1461–6.
30. Hager AH, Ticson L, Guerra L, et al. Appearance of the genitalia in girls selected for nonabuse: Review of hymenal morphology and nonspecific findings. J Pediatr Adolesc Gynecol 2002;15:27–35.

31. Lang IM, Babyn P, Oliver GD. MR imaging of paediatric uterovaginal anomalies. Pediatr Radiol 1999;29:163–70.
32. Lee CL, Wang CJ, Swei LD, et al. Laparoscopic hemi-hysterectomy in treatment of a didelphic uterus with a hypoplastic cervix and obstructed hemivagina. Hum Reprod 1999;14:1741–3.
33. Casey AC, Laufer MR. Cervical agenesis: Septic death after surgery. Obstet Gynecol 1997;90:706–7.
34. Rock JA, Schlaff WD, Jones HW Jr. The clinical management of congenital absence of the uterine cervix. Int J Gynaecol Obstet 1984;22:231–5.
35. Deffarges JV, Haddad B, Musset R, et al. Utero-vaginal anastomosis in women with uterine cervix atresia: Long-term follow-up and reproductive performance: A study of 18 cases. Hum Reprod 2001;16:1722–5.
36. Woolfe RB, Allen WM. Concomitant malformations: The frequency, simultaneous occurrence of congenital malformations of the reproductive and urinary tracts. Obstet Gynecol 1954;2: 236–65.
37. Fedele L, Ferrazzi E, Dorta M, et al. Ultrasonography in the differential diagnosis of double uteri. Fertil Steril 1988;50:361–4.
38. Hauser GA, Schreiner WE. Das Mayer–Rokitansky–Küster–Hauser syndrome. Schweiz Med Wochenschr 1961;91:381–4.
39. Evans TN, Poland ML, Boving RL. Vaginal malformations. Am J Obstet Gynecol 1981;141:910–20.
40. Frank RT. The formation of an artificial vagina without operation. Am J Obstet Gynecol 1938;35:1053–5.
41. Edmonds DK, Rose G, Lipton MG, et al. Das Mayer–Rokitansky–Küster–Hauser syndrome: A review of 245 consecutive cases managed by a multidisciplinary approach with vaginal dilators. Fertil Steril 2012;97:686–90.
42. Nadarajah S, Quek J, Rose GL, et al. Sexual function in women treated with dilators for vaginal agenesis. J Pediatr Adolesc Gynecol 2005;18:39–42.
43. Rock JA, Jones HW Jr. Construction of a neovagina for patients with a flat perineum. Am J Obstet Gynecol 1989;160:845–51.
44. Wiser WL, Bates W. Management of agenesis of the vagina. Surg Gynecol Obstet 1984;159:108–12.
45. Martinez-Mora J, Isnard R, Castellvi A, et al. Neovagina in vaginal agenesis: Surgical methods and long-term results. J Pediatr Surg 1992;27:10–4.
46. Morton KE, Dewhurst CJ. Human amnion in the treatment of vaginal malformations. Br J Obstet Gynaecol 1986;93:50–4.
47. Jackson ND, Rosenblatt PL. Use of intercede absorbable adhesion barrier for vaginoplasty. Obstet Gynecol 1994;84:1048–50.
48. Dietrich JE, Hertweck P, Traynor MP, et al. Laparoscopically assisted creation of a neovagina using the Louisville modification. Fertil Steril 2007;88:1431–4.
49. Darwish AM. A simplified novel laparoscopic formation of neovagina for cases of Mayer-Rokitansky-Küster-Hauser syndrome. Fertil Steril 2007;88:1427–30.
50. Kapoor R, Sharma DK, Singh KJ, et al. Sigmoid vaginoplasty: Long-term results. Urology 2006;67:1212–15.
51. Karateke A, Haliloglu B, Parlak O, et al. Intestinal vaginoplasty: Seven years experience of a tertiary center. Fertil Steril 2010; 94:2312–16.
52. Monnery-Noche ME, Auber F, Jouannic JM, et al. Fetal and neonatal ovarian cysts: Is surgery indicated? Prenat Diagn 2008;28: 15–20.
53. Shozu M, Akasofu K, Lika K, et al. Treatment of antenatally diagnosed fetal ovarian cysts by needle aspiration during the neonatal period. Arch Gynecol Obstet 1991;2149:103–6.
54. Kessler A, Nagar H, Graif M, et al. Percutaneous drainage as the treatment of choice for neonatal ovarian cysts. Pediatr Radiol 2006;37:330–2.
55. Esposito C, Garipoli V, Di Matteo G, et al. Laparoscopic management of ovarian cysts in newborns. Surg Endosc 1998;12:1152–4.
56. Meire HB, Farrord P, Guha T. Distinction of benign from malignant ovarian cysts by ultrasound. Br J Obstet Gynaecol 1978;85: 893–9.
57. Templeman C, Fallat ME, Blinchevsky A, et al. Noninflammatory ovarian masses in girls and young women. Obstet Gynecol 2000; 96:229–33.
58. De Silva KS, Kanumakala S, Grover SR, et al. Ovarian lesions in children and adolescence—an 11-year review. J Pediatr Endocrinol Metab 2004;17:951–7.
59. Quint EH, Smith YR. Ovarian surgery in premenarchal girls. J Pediatr Adolesc Gynecol 1999;12:27–30.
60. Wu A, Siegel MJ. Sonography of pelvic masses in children: Diagnostic predictability. AJR Am J Roentgenol 1987;147:1199–202.
61. Luxman D, Cohen J, David MP. Laparoscopic conservative removal of ovarian dermoid cysts. J Am Assoc Gynecol Laparosc 1996;3: 409–11.
62. Templeman CL, Hertweck SP, Scheetz JP, et al. The management of mature cystic teratomas in children and adolescents: A retrospective analysis. Hum Reprod 2000;15:2669–72.
63. Kokosa ER, Keller MS, Weber TR. Acute ovarian torsion in children. Am J Surg 2000;180:462–5.
64. Servaes S, Zurakowski D, Laufer MR, et al. Sonographic findings of ovarian torsion in children. Pediatr Radiol 2007;37:446–51.
65. Shadinger LL, Andreotti RF, Kurian RL. Preoperative sonographic and clinical characteristics as predictors of ovarian torsion. J Ultrasound Med 2008;27:7–13.
66. Dolgin SE, Lubin M, Shlasko E. Maximizing ovarian salvage when treating idiopathic adnexal torsion. J Pediatr Surg 2000;35: 624–8.
67. Laufer MR, Goitein L, Bush M, et al. Prevalence of endometriosis in adolescent girls with chronic pelvic pain not responding to conventional therapy. J Pediatr Adolesc Gynecol 1997;10:199–202.
68. Redwine DB. Age-related evolution in color appearance of endometriosis. Fertil Steril 1987;48:1062.
69. Martin DC, Hubert GD, Vander Zwagg R, et al. Laparoscopic appearance of peritoneal endometriosis. Fertil Steril 1989;51: 63–7.
70. Bahamondes L, Petta CA, Fernandes A, et al. Use of the levonorgestrel-releasing intrauterine system in women with endometriosis, chronic pelvic pain and dysmenorrhea. Contraception 2007;75:S134–9.
71. Patwardhan S, Nawathe A, Yates D, et al. Systematic review of the effects of aromatase inhibitors on pain associated with endometriosis. Br J Obstet Gynaecol 2008;115:818–22.

CHAPTER 75

BREAST DISEASE

Don K. Nakayama

DEVELOPMENT, ANATOMY, AND PHYSIOLOGY

The first step in development of the embryonic breast is the appearance of a pair of longitudinal streaks, which are ectodermal thickenings on the ventral surface of the embryonic torso called the primitive mammary ridges, and commonly known as the 'milk lines'.[1] Paired lens-shaped placodes appear as thickenings at specific locations along these milk lines. These placodes may be numerous in other mammals, but generally develop as a single pair in humans. Epithelial cells invaginate from the placode into the underlying mesenchyme to form the breast bud. A dense mesenchymal stroma then coalesces around the bud. At the final stage of embryogenesis, proliferating epithelial cells sprout from the mesenchyme into a fat pad that has developed beneath the dermis.

There is a rudimentary ductal tree with lactiferous ducts established by 16 weeks. These ducts eventually coalesce at the developing nipple. The areola is seen first at 20 to 24 weeks, and a true nipple has developed by the final trimester. During the final weeks of gestation, placental estrogens stimulate the breast buds in both genders to enlarge and create a true breast nodule, about 1 cm in size, at birth. The 'minipuberty of early infancy', a bimodal surge in hypothalamic–pituitary–gonadal axis activity that occurs after birth, may lead to persistent breast enlargement well into the first few months of life.[2] The fall of hormonal levels to baseline at around 6 months of age may stimulate prolactin secretion and the production of small amounts of milk ('witch's milk'). Throughout prepuberty, breast tissue is minimal and the nipple lies nearly flush with the skin in both boys and girls.

The onset of puberty is characterized by an increase in pulsatile secretion of gonadotropin-releasing hormone and gonadotropins that stimulate estrogen production by maturing ovarian follicles.[3] The onset of development of a mature breast, known as thelarche, results from estrogen-stimulated ductal development and site-specific adipose deposition. In the absence of significant levels of circulating estrogen, male adolescents fail to produce a significant breast mass. This is not the case in females where the normal stages of the female breast development have been defined by Marshall and Tanner (Table 75-1).[4]

PATHOPHYSIOLOGY

Benign female breast disease in children can be seen as an aberration of normal development and involution (ANDI).[5] ANDI links adult breast pathology to events in early breast development. Thus, many of the same disease processes observed in adults may be present in children. Fibroadenoma is a disorder of normal lobular development. Excessive stroma development results in juvenile hypertrophy. Benign conditions that result from ductal involution seen in older adults may be encountered during infancy, such as periductal mastitis, nipple discharge, and nipple retraction.

Breast cancer is extremely rare in children. When it is encountered, it is almost exclusively seen in late adolescence.[6] The study of early mammary development has importance because signals that control mammary gland embryogenesis and involution may be deregulated in breast cancer.[7]

DISORDERS OF DEVELOPMENT AND GROWTH

Neonatal Hypertrophy

The newborn breast bud may enlarge in response to newborn prolactin that rises from falling levels of maternal estrogen in the days after birth (Fig. 75-1).[8] These involute spontaneously within a few weeks without specific treatment.

Polythelia

Extra nipples, areolae, and occasionally, a true accessory breast, may develop anywhere along the milk line from axilla to pubis in about 5% of children. They are most commonly located on the chest wall below the actual breast (Fig. 75-2).[9] Unsightly polythelia should be excised.

Hypoplasia and Aplasia

Breast aplasia and hypoplasia may complicate Poland syndrome. Reconstruction of the chest wall and insertion of a breast prosthesis or breast reconstruction by a variety of flap techniques is usually indicated.[10]

Breast hypoplasia with an associated abnormality of pubertal development mandates an endocrinologic evaluation for ovarian failure, including gonadal dysgenesis, congenital adrenal hyperplasia, and varieties of disorders of sexual development.[3] Breast augmentation is an option for these patients.

Incisions during a central venous catheter or chest tube insertion, as well as drainage of a breast abscess, may interfere with later breast growth and development.[11]

TABLE 75-1	Normal Stages of Breast Development in Females
Stage	**Description**
Stage 1	Preadolescent: elevation of papilla only
Stage 2	Breast bud stage: elevation of breast and areola as a small mound, enlargement of areola diameter
Stage 3	Further enlargement of breast and areola, with no separation of their contours
Stage 4	Projection of areola and papilla to form a secondary mound above the level of the breast
Stage 5	Mature stage: Projection of papilla only, resulting from recession of the areola to the general contour of the breast

Data from Marshall WA, Tanner JM. Variations in pattern of pubertal changes in girls. Arch Dis Child 1969;44:291–303.

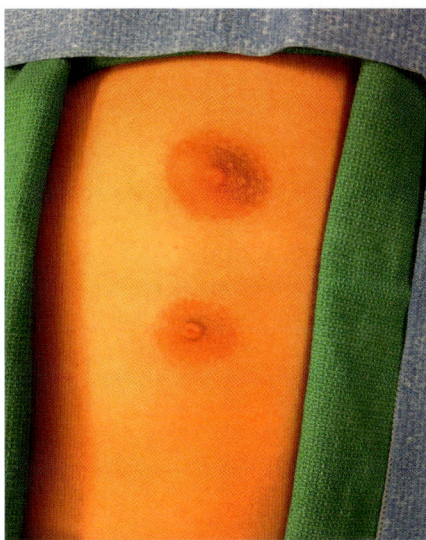

FIGURE 75-2 ■ This 6-year-old girl has polythelia. The accessory breast is inferior to the normal breast.

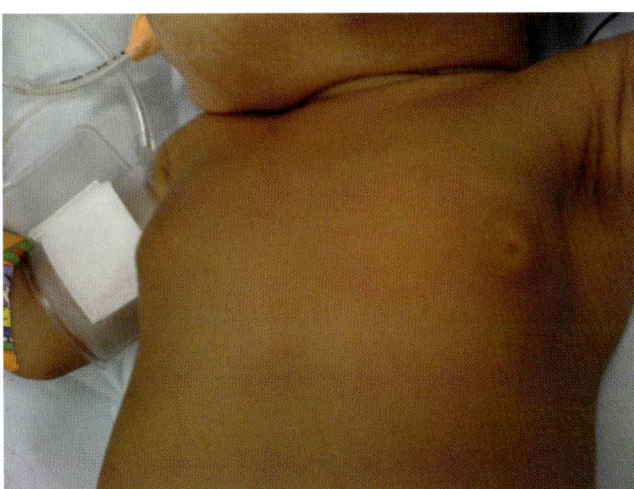

FIGURE 75-1 ■ This 3-month-old girl with neonatal hypertrophy is undergoing an operation for another indication. Breast enlargement in early infancy is normal and regresses without treatment.

Extreme care must be taken when placing these incisions, particularly in prematurely born infants in whom the breast bud may be barely visible.

Atrophy

Atrophy of the breast may result from weight loss from any cause. Hypothalamic suppression and hypoestrogenism may complicate eating disorders, further retarding breast growth.[12] In an otherwise well-nourished adolescent, breast atrophy should prompt a search for endocrine disorders that result in low estrogen or increased androgen.

Premature Thelarche

The differential diagnosis of breast enlargement in females is listed in Box 75-1. Breast development is defined as premature if it occurs before 6 years of age.[13] Premature thelarche is defined as isolated breast development without findings of puberty, such as pubic hair,

vaginal mucosal estrogenization, linear growth spurt, adult body odor, and pubertal behavioral changes. It is unilateral in 50% of cases, has a peak incidence between 6 months to 2 years, and resolves spontaneously in more than half of patients.

Premature thelarche can be distinguished from physiologic perinatal breast development and precocious puberty.[3] Precocious puberty is associated with two or more of the other features of puberty previously listed, and has a peak incidence between 5 and 8 years later than true premature thelarche. Gentle retraction of the labia allows inspection of the vaginal mucosa, which is reddish and delicate during its prepubertal state, and pink and thicker when estrogenized. About 20% of girls with premature thelarche proceed to develop precocious puberty.

Drugs, toxins. and environmental causes of premature thelarche should be considered.[14] A number of compounds have been implicated in the disorder, including xenoestrogens (compounds that bind to the estrogen receptor), phytoestrogens (compounds in plants), environmental toxins (pesticides, cosmetics, and packaging material), and estrogens in poultry, cosmetics, and hair products.

Hypertrophy

Virginal breast hypertrophy arises from exaggerated responses to pubertal hormonal fluxes. Both stroma and ducts are hypertrophic. Breast tissue and skin becomes ischemic and necrotic from the weight. Little experience is available with nonoperative treatment, although some improvement has been reported with tamoxifen.[15] Reduction mammoplasty is an appropriate procedure for virginal hypertrophy.[9] Continued breast growth may require repeated reductions.

Unilateral hypertrophy may produce breast asymmetry. Decisions regarding operation to correct the asymmetry require judgment as asymmetry is often seen between the two breasts. Ongoing breast growth may magnify the asymmetrical differences. Once Tanner stage 5 breast maturity is reached, equalization in the size of the breasts is reasonable with augmentation and reduction techniques.

Gynecomastia

Gynecomastia is the benign proliferation of glandular tissue of the male breast to the extent that it can be felt or seen as an enlarged breast (Fig. 75-3).[16] Male breast enlargement can occur physiologically in the neonate, adolescent, or elderly. Gynecomastia that occurs before puberty warrants an urgent referral to a pediatric endocrinologist. Up to 60% of boys exhibit physiologic or pubertal gynecomastia. Although its etiology is not fully known, one hypothesis is that the effects of testosterone lag behind the estrogen effects at the onset of puberty. However, careful assays have not detected significant hormonal differences in boys with and without gynecomastia. Pubertal gynecomastia first appears between 10 and 12 years of age, with the highest prevalence at 13 to 14 years, corresponding to Tanner stage 3 or 4 (see Table 75-1). Involution is generally complete at 16 to 17 years, but may persist longer in obese boys.

Pathologic gynecomastia results from conditions that cause imbalanced estrogen and androgen concentrations. Elevated estrogen levels occur in neoplasms that secrete the hormone or its precursors (e.g., testicular germ cell, Sertoli cell, and Leydig cell tumors) as well as adrenal neoplasms. Feminizing adrenal tumors are generally malignant. Increased aromatase conversion of androgens into active estrogen occurs in obesity and in infants with hepatocellular carcinoma. Decreased androgen levels or androgenic effects can result from gonadal failure that may be primary (e.g., Klinefelter syndrome, mumps orchitis, castration) or secondary (hypothalamic and pituitary disease). Serum levels of sex-hormone binding globulin affect the balance of free testosterone and estrogen. Displacement of androgens from their receptors by the many drugs associated with gynecomastia (Table 75-2) may result in unopposed estrogen effects in sex hormone-sensitive tissue, including the breast.

Early stages of gynecomastia may have active cellular activity, known as the proliferative or florid stage, with ductal epithelial proliferation, inflammatory infiltration, increased stromal fibroblasts, and enhanced vascularity. These events may also explain breast pain and tenderness associated with gynecomastia. These changes then subside and the stroma begins to undergo fibrosis and hyalinization. Clinical resolution of breast enlargement and pain occurs in less than a year in 85% of cases, a fact that must be considered when evaluating treatment options.

On palpation, true gynecomastia is a disc of rubbery tissue arising concentrically beneath and around the nipple and areola. This distinguishes it from pseudogynecomastia where adipose tissue beneath the breast causes prominence of the area under the true breast. A thorough history and physical examination, especially of the testes (with 6-month follow-up examinations), is sufficient in adolescent boys. As noted, pubertal gynecomastia generally resolves within one year. Gynecomastia occurring well before the onset of puberty, rapid increase in breast size, macrogynecomastia greater than 4 cm in diameter, and pubertal gynecomastia that persists longer than one year should lead to a directed endocrine and oncologic workup. Drugs and/or medications should be discontinued, if possible, and the patient should be re-examined in one month. Imaging of the testes and adrenals are mandatory if a tumor is suspected.

Indications for operation include severe pain, tenderness, or embarrassment sufficient to interfere with the patient's activities. Subcutaneous mastectomy through a periareolar incision and liposuction are both acceptable.[9,17] It has been suggested that histologic examination of excised breast tissue from adolescent boys may be

BOX 75-1	**Differential Diagnosis of Breast Hypertrophy**

Virginal hypertrophy
Inflammation
Giant fibroadenoma
Cystosarcoma phyllodes
Hormone-secreting tumors of the ovary, adrenal gland, or pituitary gland
Lymphoma
Sarcoma
Adenocarcinoma

From Samuelov R, Siplovich L. Juvenile gigantomastia. J Pediatr Surg 1988;23:1014–15, with permission.

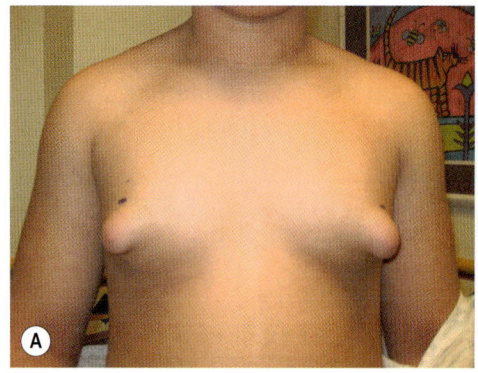
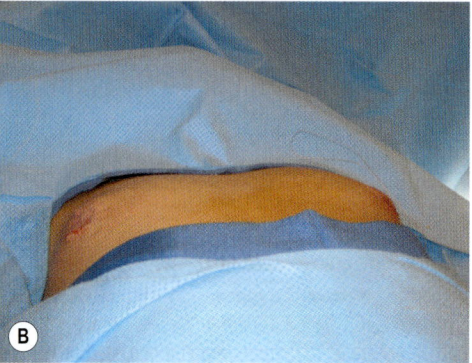

FIGURE 75-3 ■ **(A)** This teenager has gynecomastia, which was causing him discomfort as well as having negative psychosocial ramifications. **(B)** On the operating table, the enlarged breast tissue was removed and a nice cosmetic appearance achieved.

TABLE 75-2	Drugs Associated with Gynecomastia
Drug	**Examples**
Hormones	Androgens, anabolic steroids, estrogens, estrogen agonists and human chorionic gonadotropic
Antiandrogens/ inhibitors of androgen synthesis	Bicalutamide, flutamide, nilutamide, cyproterone and gonadotropin-releasing hormone agonists (leuprolide and goserelin)
Antibiotics	Metronidazole, ketoconazole, β-minocycline, isoniazid
Anti-ulcer	Cimetidine, ranitidine, omeprazole
Abuse	Alcohol, heroin, amphetamines
Chemotherapy	Methotrexate, alkylating agents, *Vinca* alkaloids, cyclophosphamide
Cardiovascular	Digoxin, furosemide, spironolactone, angiotensin-converting enzyme inhibitors (captopril and enalapril), calcium channel blockers (diltiazem, nifedipine, verapamil), reserpine, amiodarone, α-methyldopa, sprionolactone, and minoxidil
Psychiatric/neurologic	Anxiolytic agents (e.g., diazepam), tricyclic antidepressants, phenothiazines, haloperidol, phenytoin, risperidone, clonidine, selective serotonin reuptake inhibitors
Other	Antiretroviral therapy for HIV, metoclopramide, penicillamine, phenytoin, sulindac, cyclosporine

From Johnson RE, Murad MH. Gynecomastia: Pathophysiology, evaluation and management. Mayo Clin Proc 2009;84:1010–15. Reprinted with permission.

unnecessary because breast cancer has never been found in male children with gynecomastia.[18] However, a report of bilateral ductal carcinoma in gynecomastia specimens in three adolescent boys is concerning.[19] Assessment of the effectiveness of pharmacologic interventions in this population are problematic because so many cases resolve without therapy.

INFLAMMATORY LESIONS

Breast Trauma and Fat Necrosis

Fat necrosis, a benign condition that can mimic breast carcinoma, may develop in injured areas of the breast.[20] An area of fat necrosis may create a mass with features that suggest carcinoma: painless, firm, fixed, tethered and thickened skin, and spiculated calcifications on mammography. The rarity of malignancy in adolescent girls is reassuring, but biopsy may be necessary to exclude malignancy.

Mastitis and Abscess

Infections in the neonatal breast affect the breast before the ductal involution occurs later in infancy.[21] The peak incidence of neonatal infections is in the fourth and fifth weeks of life and affects girls more often than boys (3.5 to 1). *Staphylococcus* is the causative organism in more than 90% of cases. *Streptococcus*, *Salmonella*, and *Escherichia coli* have also been found. The skin and nipple are red with swelling and edema surrounding the area with simple mastitis (Fig. 75-4A). Fluctuance and deep discoloration suggest an abscess or extension of infection beneath the fascia. A small drop of pus may be expressed from the nipple due to insufficient drainage if an abscess is present. Fever, irritability, and refusal to feed may be present in 10–25% of patients. A quarter have pustular skin lesions elsewhere, usually in the inguinal region. Ultrasound (US) may be useful in diagnosis, distinguishing abscesses from inflammation.[22]

Mastitis in neonates generally responds to antibiotics and warm packs to the affected breast. Initial antibiotic therapy should cover methicillin-resistant *Staphylococcus aureus* (MRSA). Progression of inflammation while taking antibiotics suggests the presence of an abscess that requires incisional drainage (I & D), or an organism other than MRSA. When draining an abscess, it is important to avoid damage to the breast bud and its vascular supply as breast deformity later in adolescence may result. Needle aspiration is the recommended initial intervention, with repeated aspirations performed if the inflammatory signs improve. A true abscess may require I & D in an area away from the developing breast bud (Fig. 75-4B). One study documented a significant decrease in breast size relative to the opposite breast in two of five patients who required I & D of a breast abscess as a neonate.[23]

NIPPLE DISCHARGE

Galactorrhea

Galactorrhea is lactation not related to pregnancy.[24] The five etiologic groups are neurogenic, hypothalamic, endocrine, drug-induced, and idiopathic. Neurogenic causes result from local breast and nipple irritation and stimulation. Prolactinoma, the most common hypothalamic cause of galactorrhea in adults, is rare in childhood and adolescence.[25] Cessation of oral contraceptives, polycystic ovary, adrenal tumors, and gonadal tumors may cause galactorrhea in adolescents. Galactorrhea in boys is always abnormal and a prolactinoma is the most common cause.

Other Nipple Discharges

Nonmilky discharges include pus, cyst contents, and blood.[26] Serous drainage of brown to green fluid may indicate the presence of a communicating breast cyst, and is usually self-limited. Bloody drainage, a sign of cancer in adults, usually occurs from an intraductal papilloma or ductal ectasia in children and adolescents. Bloody nipple drainage should be cultured because it may be positive for *Staphylococcus* which should be treated if positive. Most causes of nipple discharge are self-limited and resolve spontaneously. Excision of the abnormal duct is indicated if drainage persists or recurs (Fig. 75-5).

Mastalgia

Although common in adults, breast pain (mastalgia) is poorly characterized and often underreported among young and adolescent girls.[27] Initial evaluation should focus on exclusion of masses and inflammatory causes. Pain is characterized as cyclic or noncyclic, which is an important distinction as cyclic pain is more likely to respond to therapy. Up to 22% of cyclic and 50% of noncyclic cases resolve without therapy in one year. Dietary interventions help, such as restriction of caffeine and other methylxanthines, and additional flaxseed products. Vitamin E and evening primrose oil have not shown clinical benefit. Tamoxifen, danazol, and topical nonsteroidal anti-inflammatory gels may improve symptoms.[27]

BREAST MASSES

Evaluation of Breast Masses

The age of the patient affects the differential diagnosis and the diagnostic approach for breast masses in children (Boxes 75-2 and 75-3). Patient age with a complete history and physical examination are sufficient to make the diagnosis in most cases. In a review of 374 breast specimens from patients aged 20 years and younger, the majority were identified as benign and fell into these three categories: fibroadenoma (44%), gynecomastia (22%), and juvenile hypertrophy (14%).[28] Twenty-two lesions were a variety of soft tissue tumors, including phyllodes tumor, granular cell tumor, neurofibroma, angiosarcoma, stromal sarcoma, metastatic alveolar rhabdomyosarcoma, giant cell fibroblastoma, and only one papillary carcinoma.

Traditional terms, such as fibrocystic disease, lack pathological and clinical precision. An accurate diagnosis based on histology defines the risk for malignancy so that appropriate interventions may be initiated.[29] Thus, evaluation of breast masses require imaging and tissue sampling.

Regarding diagnostic evaluation, multiple radiographic and interventional options are available. Ultrasound distinguishes cystic from solid masses. Diagnostic mammography and magnetic resonance imaging are not

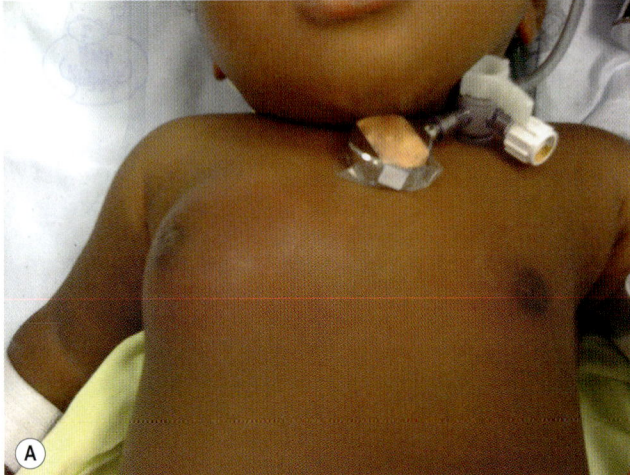
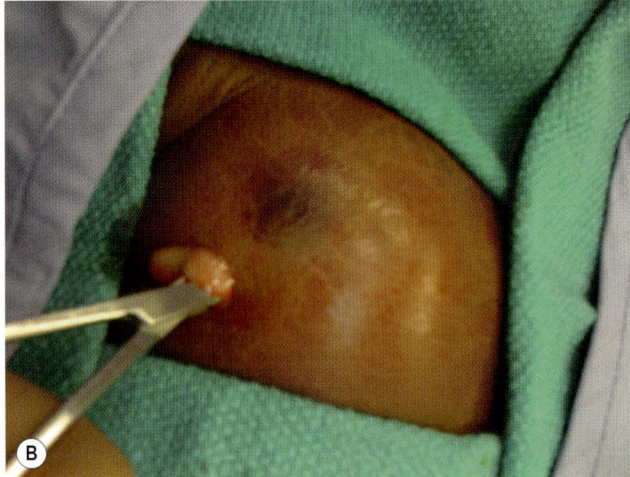

FIGURE 75-4 ■ **(A)** A breast abscess is seen in a one month-old girl with redness and induration surrounding the breast bud. **(B)** Incision and drainage was performed through a limited incision at the inferior aspect of the abscess to avoid injuring the breast tissue under the nipple.

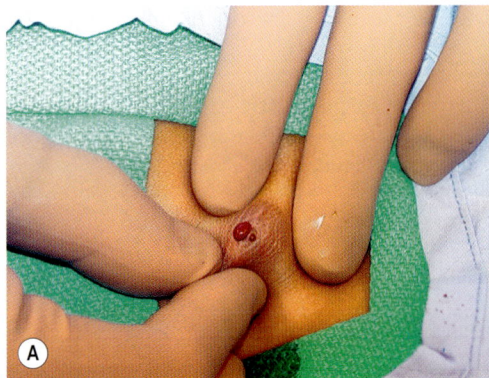
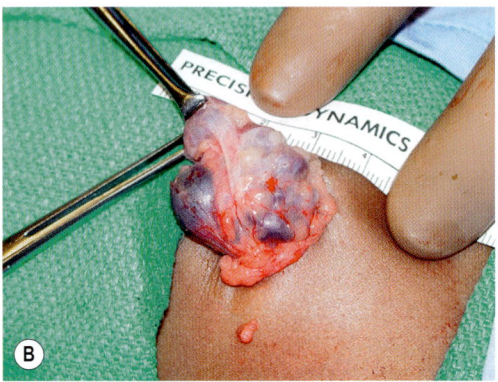

FIGURE 75-5 ■ **(A)** Bloody and green discharge from a 5-month-old boy is seen. **(B)** Multiple subareolar epithelial cysts, which were causing the drainage, were removed.

BOX 75-2   Breast Masses in Children

Physiologic
- Normal breast bud
- Premature thelarche

Pathologic
- Inflammatory
  - Mastitis
  - Breast abscess
  - Fibrosis
  - Fat necrosis
- Benign neoplasms
  - Hemangioma
  - Cyst
  - Lipoma
  - Papilloma
- Malignant neoplasms
  - Metastatic (e.g., rhabdomyosarcoma, lymphoma)
  - Secretory carcinoma

BOX 75-3   Breast Masses in Adolescents

Physiologic
- Thelarche
- Unilateral hypertrophy

Pathologic
- Inflammatory
  - Mastitis
  - Breast abscess
  - Fibrosis
  - Fat necrosis
- Benign neoplasms
  - Fibroadenoma
  - Phyllodes tumor
  - Cyst
  - Fibrocystic disease
  - Neurofibroma
- Malignant neoplasms
  - Primary breast cancer
  - Metastatic (e.g., lymphoma)

routinely used in adolescents. Fine needle aspiration (25 or 22 gauge) will empty simple cysts and sample sufficient numbers of cells to make the diagnosis of fibroadenoma and ductal hyperplasia.[30] Core needle biopsy (14 to 9 gauge) with vacuum or automated devices provides larger samples with architectural detail. Sonography locates deep and small lesions for needle biopsy if a mass is difficult to palpate. Unfortunately, small adolescent breasts may not accommodate a core biopsy needle, and open biopsy is occasionally necessary.

Recent clinical evidence indicates that breast self-examination does not affect breast cancer outcome, with one national task force recommending against it.[31] Individuals with an inherited predisposition to breast cancer should begin intensive monitoring between ages 20 and 25 years.[32]

Prepubertal Breast Masses

Prepubertal breast masses are nearly always benign. The most important diagnosis to consider is asynchronous thelarche, one breast bud appearing weeks to months ahead of the other. A breast bud is easily recognized as a disc of firm tissue beneath the areola. Biopsy is never indicated because of the possibility of iatrogenic amastia.

Benign Breast Disease

Pearlman classifies benign breast disease into three broad categories: nonproliferative disorders, proliferative disorders without atypia, and atypical hyperplasia.[29] Simple cysts, hyperplasia, and duct ectasia comprise the nonproliferatrive group. Fibroadenomas, papillomas, tubular adenomas, benign phyllodes tumors, and mild epithelial hyperplasia represent proliferative disorders without atypia. Atypical hyperplasias include moderate or florid hyperplasia and lobular carcinoma in-situ. The number of epithelial layers and degree that they fill the duct determine the difference between mild (four or fewer, do not fill the duct) and moderate or florid hyperplasia (more than four that often fill the duct). The three groups roughly parallel the relative risk for later development of breast cancer.[33] Nonproliferative disorders generally do not increase breast cancer risk while proliferative disorders without atypia have a small increase (relative risk, 1.5–2.0). Lesions with atypical hyperplasia pose a moderate risk of later development of cancer (>2.0). Benign breast disease encountered in adolescence is nearly always in the lower risk categories.

Juvenile papillomatosis is a rare variant of epithelial hyperplasia, with a histological appearance that would be considered premalignant in adults.[34] Histology includes ductal stasis and apocrine cysts that give it a descriptive pathological term, 'Swiss cheese disease'. Some patients develop breast cancer later in adulthood, and one-fourth have a family history of breast cancer.

Tubular adenomas have prominent adenosis-like epithelial proliferation with sparse intervening stroma.[35] They are generally seen in young women of childbearing age, and are rarely encountered in adolescents. Because they present as a well-circumscribed breast lump clinically indistinguishable from a fibroadenoma, these lesions require needle or excisional biopsy for tissue diagnosis.

Simple Cysts

Benign cysts can occur throughout childhood, however, they are commonly associated with thelarche.[36] They are soft and painless, range in size from 1–10 mm in diameter, and are not fixed to surrounding breast tissue. They are thought to arise when acini or terminal ductules dilate and untwist. Those close to the skin may appear blue-tinged. The columnar epithelium that lines simple cysts have apocrine-like features, and may form papillary tufts. The apocrine changes may represent metaplasia, but these cysts do not have an increased cancer risk if they are not associated with other proliferative lesions that have a higher risk. Needle aspiration will usually show serous or brown fluid, and results in complete resolution. Biopsy is required if the mass persists after aspiration.

FIBROEPITHELIAL TUMORS

Fibroadenomas

Fibroadenomas are the most common breast mass seen by pediatric surgeons.[28] Two variants, adult and juvenile, affect children. Adult fibroadenomas affect older adolescents and young women (Fig. 75-6). They may be multiple in 10–15% of cases. The mass is usually 1–2 cm in diameter, painless, distinct, rubbery, and mobile. A fibroadenoma does not have a true capsule, but rather a well-demarcated stromal interface where the tumor comes in contact with normal tissue. Areas of focal hemorrhage may be present, and lead to pain and rapid enlargement. Juvenile fibroadenomas affect younger adolescents around the time of puberty.[37] In contrast to an adult fibroadenoma, the juvenile variant tends to be much larger (average diameter 4 cm), and may cause considerable breast deformity. Microscopic examination reveals a rich cellular stroma and a prominent glandular epithelium.

Fibroadenomas are benign, but the adult variant is a long-term risk factor for breast cancer and can harbor a carcinoma.[34,38] Ductal carcinomas have not been reported in juvenile fibroadenomas; however, juvenile variants may be related to phyllodes tumors.

Fine-needle aspiration is useful in distinguishing fibroadenomas from carcinomas and phyllodes tumors. Differentiating fibroadenomas from other benign conditions is more difficult.[39] Fibroadenomas can be followed without operation if the lesion is less than 3 cm in diameter and exhibits the expected characteristic features: solitary, firm, rubbery, nontender, and well circumscribed.[40] The probability of disappearance of the mass is 0.46 at 5 years and 0.69 at 9 years.[41] Because of the rarity of breast cancer among adolescents, it is reasonable to wait a period of years to see whether a small lesion will disappear.

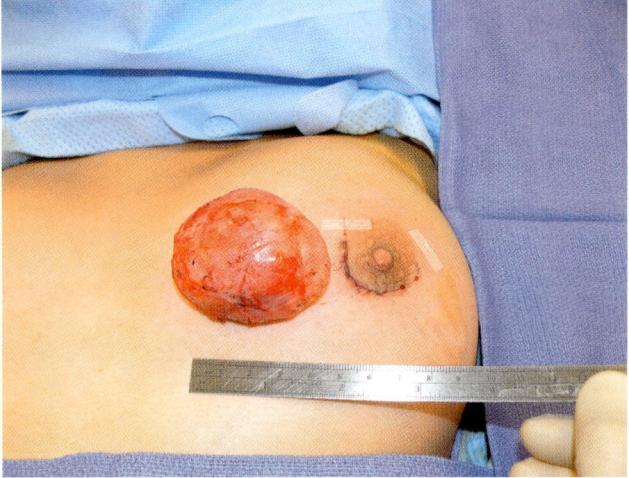

FIGURE 75-6 ■ This 16-year-old developed an enlarging, painful fibroadenoma in her left breast. The lesion measured 7 cm × 5 cm × 4 cm on ultrasound examination. She underwent excision of the medially placed lesion through a circumareolar incision and tolerated the operation well. The histologic examination returned a benign fibroadenoma. Her symptoms have resolved.

Fibroadenomas that are growing should be excised to avoid further enlargement and preserve the architecture of the remaining normal breast tissue. A periareolar incision gives a better cosmetic result at 6 months, but results in an increased incidence in loss of nipple sensation.[42] Recently, a minimally invasive approach to facilitate removal of a giant juvenile fibroadenoma has been described.[43] Rapid growth may lead to impressively large lesions that require complex reconstructive surgery.[9]

Phyllodes Tumors

Phyllodes tumors, formerly called cystosarcoma phyllodes, are rare fibroepithelial tumors that can be benign (with significant risk for local recurrence) or malignant (with rapidly growing metastases).[44] They can range in size from 1–40 cm. Only about 10% of phyllodes tumors occur in women younger than the age of 20 years. The clinical presentation is a rapidly growing breast mass larger than 6 cm. Like a fibroadenoma, a phyllodes tumor lacks a true capsule and appears well circumscribed. Features that distinguish it from a fibroadenoma are fibrous areas interspersed with soft fleshy areas, and cysts filled with clear or semisolid bloody fluid. There may be epithelial and stromal hyperplasia and areas of atypia, metaplasia, and malignancy. The mitotic activity in the stromal elements determines whether a phyllodes tumor is malignant (Fig. 75-7). Clonal activity from three patients in whom a phyllodes tumor of the breast developed after excision of a fibroadenoma suggests that the former developed from the latter.[45]

The mean age of these patients is in the fourth decade, about a decade older than that for an adult fibroadenoma (mean age, 28.5 years in fibroadenoma, 44 years in phyllodes tumor). A phyllodes tumor tends to be larger (>4 cm in diameter) compared to a fibroadenoma. On sonography, cysts within an otherwise solid mass are indicative of phyllodes tumor. Diagnosis using fine-needle aspiration centers on the detection of a dimorphic pattern of stromal elements and benign epithelial tissue. The diagnosis of phyllodes tumor can be made from a core needle biopsy specimens in most cases.[46] When the preoperative workup cannot distinguish between a fibroadenoma and a phyllodes tumor, excisional biopsy is indicated.

In cases in which the preoperative diagnosis is known, wide local excision with a 1 cm margin of normal breast tissue is recommended.[47] Tumors that extend to the pectoralis fascia require removal of the muscle adjacent to the tumor. If the diagnosis of phyllodes tumor is discovered only after histologic examination, most authors recommend re-excision of normal breast tissue because of the 20% risk of local recurrence. Malignant phyllodes tumors are treated with simple mastectomy. Lymph node dissection is not indicated as these tumors do not metastasize to lymph nodes.

Breast Cancer

Malignancy of the breast in children falls into three groups: primary malignancies, metastatic tumors that involve the breast, and second malignancies. Although extremely rare in children, breast cancer has been found

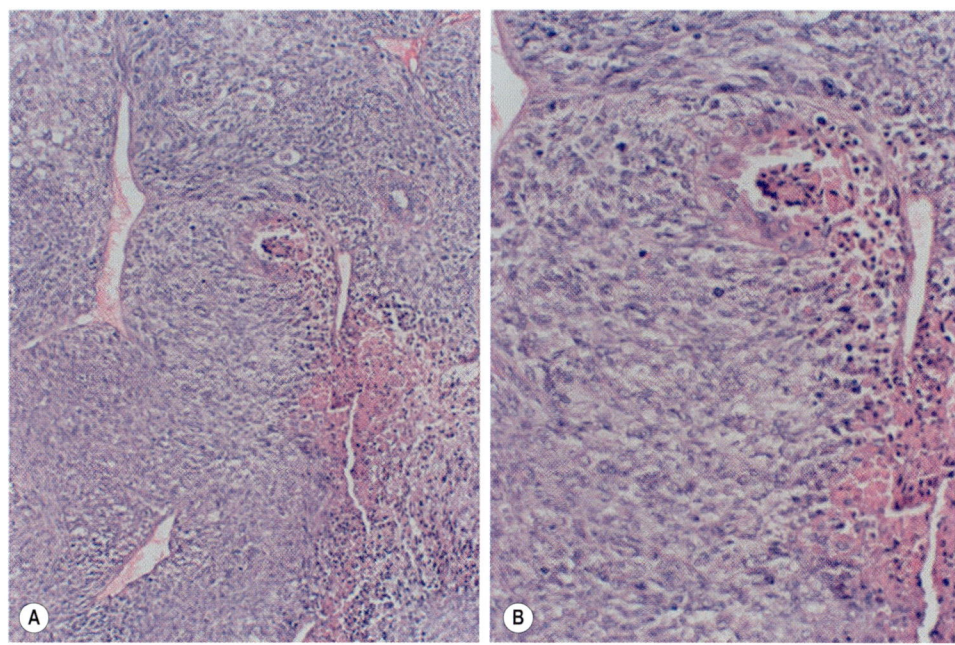

FIGURE 75-7 ■ A 16-year-old girl underwent resection of a malignant phyllodes tumor. **(A)** Photomicrograph shows an area of necrosis typical of rapidly growing neoplasms (×10). **(B)** A higher-power view shows stromal and epithelial atypia and numerous mitotic figures (×20). (Courtesy of Edgar Pierce, MD, and Earl Mullis, MD, Medical Center of Central Georgia.)

in both boys and girls under 5 years of age.[48] More than 90% of children are first seen with a breast mass. Nipple discharge can also be a presenting sign. Thus, a cytologic examination of the fluid is advised.

Secretory carcinoma is the primary malignancy that occurs most often in children.[49] Girls are affected five times more often than boys; however, the youngest patient reported is a 3-year-old boy.[50] It may appear as a benign nodule or group of nodules on ultrasound.[51] Clinically involved enlarged axillary lymph nodes are present in approximately 20% of cases. It has a low-grade clinical behavior with a good prognosis for long-term survival after simple mastectomy. Axillary node dissection is indicated if the nodes are clinically involved. Recurrence after lumpectomy has been described.[49-51] Long-term follow-up is imperative owing to the indolent nature of the disease and the risk for late recurrence.

Nonsecretory breast cancers are less common in children. A 40-year review of adolescent patients at the M.D. Anderson Cancer Center identified 10 patients with primary adenocarcinoma of the breast, four with malignant phyllodes tumors, and two with metastatic tumors.[6] Ages ranged from 13 to 19 years. Four patients had a positive family history for breast disease. The cases of adenocarcinoma probably represent the leading edge of the prevalence distribution for adult primary breast cancer and included the histologic types seen in primary breast cancers in mature women: invasive intraductal, invasive lobular, and signet ring cancers. The treatment regimen is the same as for adult primary breast cancer and is dictated by histology, stage, presence of hormone receptors, tumor markers, and patient menstrual status.

The breast has also been reported as the primary site for leukemia, lymphoma and rhabdomyosarcoma.[28,52] More commonly, it is the site of acute leukemic relapse.

Alveolar rhabdomyosarcoma appears to have a relative predilection for the breast, with 6% to 10% of cases metastasizing to the breast.[53] Other childhood tumors (retinoblastoma, osteosarcoma, neuroblastoma) may also metastasize to the breast.

REFERENCES

1. McKiernan J, Coyne J, Cahalane S. Histology of breast development in early life. Arch Dis Child 1988;63:136–9.
2. Kuiri-Hanninen T, Kallio S, Seuri R, et al. Postnatal developmental changes in the pituitary-ovarian axis in preterm and term infant girls. J Clin Endocrinol Metab 2011;96:3432–9.
3. Loomba-Albrecht LA, Styne DM. The physiology of puberty and its disorders. Pediatr Ann 2012;41:el–9.
4. Marshall WA, Tanner JM. Variations in pattern of pubertal changes in girls. Arch Dis Child 1969;44:291–303.
5. Hughes LE. Aberrations of normal development and involution (ANDI): An update. In: Mansell RE, editor. Recent Developments in the Study of Benign Breast Disease. London: Parthenon; 1994. p. 65–73.
6. Corpron CA, Black CT, Singletary SE, et al. Breast cancer in adolescent females. J Pediatr Surg 1995;30:322–4.
7. Cowin P, Wysolmerski J.. Molecular mechanisms guiding embryonic mammary gland development. Cold Spring Harb Perspect Biol 2010;2:a003251. Epub 2010 May 19.
8. Amer A, Fischer H. Images in clinical medicine. Neonatal breast enlargement. N Engl J Med 2009;360:1445.
9. van Aalst JA, Phillips JD, Sadove AM. Pediatric chest wall and breast deformities. Plast Reconstr Surg 2009;124:38e–49e.
10. Urschel HC Jr. Poland syndrome. Semin Thorac Cardiovasc Surg 2009;21:89–94.
11. Eidlitz-Markus T, Mukamel M, Haimi-Cohen Y, et al. Breast asymmetry during adolescence: Physiologic and non-physiologic causes. Isr Med Assoc J 2010;12:203–6.
12. Greydanus DE, Matytsina L, Gains M. Breast disorders in children and adolescents. Prim Care 2006;33:455–502.
13. Lee CT, Tung YC, Tsai WY. Premature thelarche in Taiwanese girls. J Pediatr Endocrinol Metab 2010;23:879–84.
14. Rudel RA, Fenton SE, Ackerman JM, et al. Environmental exposures and mammary gland development: State of the science, public

health implications, and research recommendations. Environ Health Perspect 2011;119:1053–61.

15. Hoppe IC, Patel PP, Singer-Granick CJ, Granick MS. Virginal mammary hypertrophy: Ameta-analysis and treatment algorithm. Plast Reconstr Surg 2011;127:2224–31.

16. Johnson RE, Murad MH. Gynecomastia: Pathophysiology, evaluation, and management. Mayo Clin Proc 2009;84:1010–15.

17. Hodgson EL, Fruhstorfer RH, Malata CM. Ultrasonic liposuction in the treatment of gynecomastia. Plast Reconstr Surg 2005;116: 646–53.

18. Koshy JC, Goldberg JS, Wolfswinkel EM, et al. Breast cancer incidence in adolescent males undergoing subcutaneous mastectomy for gynecomastia: Is pathologic examination justified? A retrospective and literature review. Plast Reconstr Surg 2011;127: 1–7.

19. Lemoine C, Mayer SK, Beaunoyer M, et al. Incidental finding of synchronous bilateral ductal carcinoma in situ associated with gynecomastia in a 15-year-old obese boy: Case report and review of the literature. J Pediatr Surg 2011;46:e17–20.

20. Taboada JL, Stephens TW, Krishnamurthy S, et al. The many faces of fat necrosis in the breast. Am J Roentgenol 2009;192: 815–25.

21. Stricker T, Navratil F, Sennhauser FH. Mastitis in early infancy. Acta Paediatr 2005;94:166–9.

22. Borders H, Mychaliska G, Gebarski KS. Sonographic features of neonatal mastitis and breast abscess. Pediatr Radiol 2009;39: 955–8.

23. Rudoy RC, Nelson JD. Breast abscess during the neonatal period. Am J Dis Child 1975;129:1031–4.

24. Hussain AN, Policarpio C, Vincent MT. Evaluating nipple discharge. Obstet Gyncol Surv 2006;61:278–83.

25. Richmond IL, Wilson CB. Pituitary adenomas in childhood and adolescence. J Neurosurg 1978;49:163–8.

26. Marshall PS, Duarte GM, Torresan RZ, Cabello C. Bloody nipple discharge in childhood. Breast J 2011;17:692–3.

27. Rosolowich V, Saettler E, Szuck B, et al. Mastalgia. J Obstet Gynaecol Can 2006;28:49–74.

28. Dehner LP, Hill DA, Deschryver K. Pathology of the breast in children, adolescents and young adults. Semin Diag Pathol 1999;16:235–47.

29. Pearlman MD, Griffin JL. Benign breast disease. Obstet Gynecol 2010;116:747–58.

30. Neal L, Tortorelli CL, Nassar A. Clinician's guide to imaging and pathologic findings in benign breast disease. Mayo Clin Proc 2010;85:274–9.

31. Gregory KD, Sawaya GF. Updated recommendations for breast cancer screening. Curr Opin Obstet Gynecol 2010;22:498–505.

32. Clark AS, Domchek SM. Clinical management of hereditary breast cancer syndromes. J Mammary Gland Biol Neoplasia 2011;16: 17–25.

33. Santen RJ, Mansel R. Benign breast disorders. N Engl J Med 2005; 353:275–85.

34. Gill J, Greenall M. Juvenile papillomatosis and breast cancer. J Surg Educ 2007;64:234–6.

35. Salemis NS, Gemenetzis G, Karagkiouzis G, et al. Tubular adenoma of the breast: A rare presentation and review of the literature. J Clin Med Res 2011;4:64–7.

36. Grobmyer SR, Copeland EM III, Simpson JF, Page DL. Benign, high-risk, and premalignant lesions of the breast. In: Bland KI, Copeland EM III, editors. The Breast, Edition 4. Philadelphia: Saunders; 2009.

37. Wechselberger G, Schoeller T, Piza-Katzer H. Juvenile fibroadenoma of the breast. Surgery 2002;132:106–7.

38. Ozzello L, Gump FE. The management of patients with carcinomas in fibroadenomatous tumors of the breast. Surg Gynecol Obstet 1985;160:99–104.

39. Alle KM, Moss J, Venegas RJ, et al. For debate: Conservative management of fibroadenoma of the breast. Br J Surg 1996;83: 992–3.

40. Jayasinghe Y, Simmons PS. Fibroadenomas in adolescence. Curr Opin Obstet Gynecol 2009;21:402–6.

41. Cant PJ, Madden MV, Coleman MG, et al. Nonoperative management of breast masses diagnosed as fibroadenoma. Br J Surg 1995;82:792–4.

42. Liu X-F, Zhang J-X, Zhou Q, et al. A clinical study on the resection of breast fibroadenoma using two types of incision. Scan J Surg 2011;100:147–52.

43. Cheng PJ, Vu LT, Cass DL, et al. Endoscopic specimen pouch technique for removal of giant fibroadenomas of the breast. J Pediatr Surg 2012;47:803–7.

44. Khosravi-Shahi P. Management of non metastatic phyllodes tumors of the breast: Review of the literature. Surg Oncol 2011;20: e143–8.

45. Noguchi S, Yokouchi H, Aihara T, et al. Progression of fibroadenoma to phyllodes tumor demonstrated by clonal analysis. Cancer 1995;76:1779–85.

46. Johnson NB, Collins LC. Update on percutaneous needle biopsy of nonmalignant breast lesions. Adv Anat Pathol 2009;16:183–95.

47. Chen W-H, Cheng S-P, Tzen C-Y, et al. Surgical treatment of phyllodes tumors of the breast: Retrospective review of 172 cases. J Surg Oncol 2005;91:185–94.

48. Rogers DA, Lobe TE, Rao RN, et al. Breast malignancy in children. J Pediatr Surg 1994;29:48–51.

49. Li D, Xiao X, Yang W, et al. Secretory breast carcinoma: A clinicopathological and immunophenotypic study of 15 cases with a review of the literature. Mod Pathol 2012;25:567–75.

50. Karl SR, Ballantine TV, Zaino R. Juvenile secretory carcinoma of the breast. J Pediatr Surg 1985;20:368–71.

51. Mun SH, Ko EY, Han BK, et al. Secretory carcinoma of the breast: Sonographic features. J Ultrasound Med 2008;27:947–54.

52. Pettinato G, Manivel JC, Kelly DR, et al. Lesions of the breast in children exclusive of typical fibroadenoma and gynecomastia. A clinicopathologic study of 113 cases. Pathol Annu 1989;24 Pt2: 296–328.

53. Hays DM, Donaldson SS, Shimada H, et al. Primary and metastatic rhabdomyosarcoma in the breast: Neoplasms of adolescent females, a report from the Intergroup Rhabdomyosarcoma Study. Med Pediatr Oncol 1997;29:181–9.

CHAPTER 76

ENDOCRINE DISORDERS AND TUMORS

Diana L. Diesen • **Michael A. Skinner**

THYROID GLAND

Diseases of the thyroid gland are uncommon conditions in children occurring in 37 of 1,000 school-aged children in the USA.[1] Most of these lesions are diffuse gland hypertrophy or simple goiters. Thyroiditis is the second most common abnormality, followed by thyroid nodules and functional disorders. The incidence of thyroid cancer is 0.54 per 100,000, though it is more common with multiple endocrine neoplasia (MEN) syndromes and radiation exposure.[2] Operative management plays a role in many of these conditions.

Embryology and Physiology

The thyroid gland arises as an out-pouching of the embryonic alimentary tract at about 24 days' gestation. It descends from the base of the tongue, ventral to the hyoid bone and larynx, to its final location by about seven weeks' gestation. Persistence of the thyroglossal diverticulum results in a pyramidal thyroid lobe. Accessory thyroid tissue can appear anywhere along its descent. Rarely, nondescent results in a lingual thyroid.

Histologically, by week 11 of gestation, colloid begins to form and thyroxine (T4) can be demonstrated in the embryo. Parafollicular cells, or C cells, arise from the ultimobranchial bodies found throughout the thyroid gland.

Thyroglobulin is recognized histologically as colloid. Thyroid hormone is synthesized at the interface between the follicular cell and thyroglobulin. The first step in thyroid synthesis is the iodination of tyrosine molecules, which are then coupled, and form the thyroid hormones thyroxine (T4) and triiodothyronine (T3). T4 and T3 are produced at a ratio of ~4:1. T3 is more potent than T4 on the target cell. Both T3 and T4 enter the target cell at which point all T4 is converted to T3. T3 then enters the nucleus of the target cell and the T3 molecule interacts with nuclear thyroid receptors. This receptor–T3 complex binds to DNA to regulate genetic transcription.[3] Thyroid hormone increases cellular oxygen consumption and basal metabolic rate, stimulates protein synthesis, and influences carbohydrate, lipid, and vitamin metabolism.

Production and secretion of T3 and T4 are stimulated by thyroid-stimulating hormone (TSH) secreted by the pituitary in response to thyrotropin-releasing hormone, which is released from the hypothalamus. Other peptides are present within the thyroid gland such as neuropeptide Y, substance P, cholecystokinin, and vasoactive intestinal peptide, which may assist in the production and secretion of thyroid hormones.

TSH usually is decreased in hyperthyroidism and elevated in hypothyroidism. The plasma free T4 level is a measure of biologically active thyroid hormone, unaffected by protein binding. Alternatively, when total plasma T3 and T4 are measured, it is necessary to consider the level of thyroid-binding globulin to estimate the level of unbound biologically active hormone.

Non-neoplastic Thyroid Conditions

Goiter and Thyroiditis

The causes of thyromegaly in one study are listed in Table 76-1.[4] Simple adolescent colloid goiters are the most common cause. Physiologically, diffuse thyroid enlargement may be due to a defect in hormone production, related to autoimmune diseases, or a response to an inflammatory condition. Goiters are classified as diffusely enlarged or nodular, and either toxic or euthyroid. Most goiters are euthyroid, and resection is rarely indicated.

The differential diagnosis for diffuse thyroid enlargement is seen in Box 76-1. Laboratory evaluation should begin with plasma free T4 and TSH levels. With a simple colloid goiter, the patient is euthyroid. Ultrasonography (US) or scintigraphy reveals uniform enlargement, and serum thyroid antibody titers are normal. The etiology of this condition may be an autoimmune process.[5] The natural history of colloid goiter is not well known, but one study of adolescents reported that nearly 60% of the glands were normal in size 20 years after diagnosis.[1] Exogenous thyroid hormone does not significantly improve resolution of the goiter. In rare cases, resection may be indicated because of size or the suspicion of neoplasia.

Chronic lymphocytic (Hashimoto) thyroiditis is another cause of diffuse thyroid enlargement, occurring most frequently in female adolescents. This condition is part of the spectrum of autoimmune thyroid disorders. It is thought CD4 T-cells are activated against thyroid antigens and recruit cytotoxic CD8 T-cells, which kill thyroid cells, leading to hypothyroidism.[6] Children are initially euthyroid and slowly progress to become hypothyroid. However, approximately 10% of children are hyperthyroid, a condition known as 'hashitoxicosis.' The thyroid gland is usually pebbly or granular, and may be mildly tender.

Ninety-five per cent of patients with Hashimoto thyroiditis have elevated antithyroid microsomal antibodies

TABLE 76-1 Etiology of Thyroid Gland Enlargement (n = 152 Children)

Diagnosis	Frequency (%)
Simple goiter	83
Chronic lymphocytic thyroiditis	12.5
Graves disease	2.5
Benign adenoma	1.5
Cyst	1

Adapted from Jaksic J, Dumic M, Filipovic B, et al. Thyroid disease in a school population with thyromegaly. Arch Dis Child 1994;70:103–6.

or antithyroid peroxidase antibodies. Plasma thyroid hormone levels are normal or low, and TSH levels are elevated in 70% of patients. Thyroid imaging is usually not necessary if clinical and laboratory findings are strongly suggestive of the diagnosis. The radionuclide scan usually shows patchy uptake of the tracer and may mimic the findings in Graves disease or multinodular goiter. The principal ultrasound finding is nonspecific, diffuse thyroid hypoechogenicity. Rarely, autoantibodies cannot be detected and fine needle aspiration is needed to confirm the diagnosis. In as many as one-third of adolescent patients, the thyroiditis resolves spontaneously with the gland becoming normal and the antibodies disappearing. Thus, expectant management should be considered. Exogenous thyroid hormone is administered in the hypothyroid patient. However, in euthyroid children, it is ineffective in reducing the size of the goiter.[7]

Subacute (de Quervain) thyroiditis, a viral inflammation of the thyroid gland, is unusual in children. The thyroid is swollen, painful, and tender. Mild thyrotoxicosis results from injury to the thyroid follicles, with release of thyroid hormone into the circulation. Serum T3 and T4 levels are elevated, and TSH is decreased. Because of thyroid follicular cell dysfunction, decreased radioactive iodine uptake occurs, a finding that distinguishes subacute thyroiditis from Graves disease. Histologically, granulomas and epithelioid cells may be seen. The treatment of subacute thyroiditis is symptomatic and generally consists of nonsteroidal anti-inflammatory agents or corticosteroids. The condition typically lasts 2 to 9 months, and complete recovery is common.

BOX 76-1 Differential Diagnosis of Diffuse Thyroid Enlargement (Goiter) in Children

Autoimmune mediated
  Chronic lymphocytic (Hashimoto) thyroiditis
  Graves disease
  Simple colloid goiter
Compensatory
  Iodine deficiency
  Medications
  Goitrogens
  Hormone or receptor defect
Inflammatory conditions
  Acute suppurative thyroiditis
  Subacute thyroiditis

Acute suppurative thyroiditis is a bacterial infection of the gland characterized by sepsis and an inflamed gland. Patients are usually euthyroid. Staphylococci or mixed aerobic and anaerobic flora are common causal agents. A congenital pharyngeal sinus tract may predispose the patient to infection. Management is intravenous antibiotics and abscess drainage, if necessary. The thyroid gland should recover completely.

Graves Disease

Graves disease, or diffuse toxic goiter, is the most common cause of hyperthyroidism in childhood. The condition is an autoimmune disease caused by IgG immunoglobulins directed against components of the thyroid plasma membrane, possibly including the TSH receptor. Graves disease occurs in girls five times more often than in boys, and the incidence increases throughout childhood, peaking in adolescences. Congenital Graves disease, resulting from the transplacental passage of maternal antibodies, occurs in about 1% of infants born to women with active Graves disease. The onset may be delayed until 2 to 3 weeks after birth.

TSH receptor antibodies are present in more than 95% of patients with active Graves disease, but the inciting event eliciting the antibody response against the TSH receptor is unknown. Infection may produce antibodies that react with the TSH receptor. These antibodies stimulate the thyroid follicles to increase iodide uptake and cyclic adenosine monophosphate production, and induce production and secretion of excess thyroid hormone. Scattered epidemiologic reports of disease clustering supports an infectious etiology for Graves disease.[8]

Usually, Graves disease develops over several months. Initial symptoms include nervousness, emotional changes, and declining school performance followed by weight loss, sweating, palpitations, heat intolerance, and general malaise. A smooth, firm, nontender goiter is present in most cases. A bruit may be heard on auscultation. Exophthalmos is unusual, but a conspicuous stare may be evident. Laboratory evaluation generally reveals elevated free T4 and decreased TSH levels. Ten to 20% of patients will have elevation of T3 only, a condition known as T3 toxicosis. The presence of TSH receptor antibodies definitively establishes the diagnosis of Graves disease.

Although basic pathogenesis of Graves disease is understood, there are no uniformly successful methods for correcting the immunologic defect. Thus, the treatment is palliative and designed to decrease production and secretion of thyroid hormone. The natural course of untreated Graves disease is unpredictable. In some patients, thyrotoxicosis may be persistent but variable in severity. In others, it may be cyclic, with exacerbations of varying degree and duration.

Current management includes antithyroid medications, ablation with radioactive ^{131}I, and resection.[9] In the USA, most pediatric endocrinologists initiate therapy with methimazole (MTH) or propylthiouracil (PPU) which reduce thyroid hormone production by inhibiting follicle cell organification of iodide and the coupling of iodotyrosines. PPU also inhibits peripheral conversion of T4 to T3, and may be the preferred agent if rapid alleviation of thyrotoxicosis is desired. Both medications possess some immunosuppressive activity as evident by a reduction in antithyroid antibodies. In most cases, MTH is preferred because of its increased potency, longer half-life, and associated improved compliance. The initial adolescent dose is 30 mg once daily, which is reduced if the patient is younger. When the patient becomes euthyroid, as determined by normal T3 and T4 levels, the daily dose of MTH should be reduced to 10 mg. T3 and T4 levels should be monitored. The thyroid gland decreases in size in one-half of patients. Thyroid enlargement with therapy signals either an intensification of the disease or hypothyroidism due to overtreatment.

Side effects of MTH include nausea, minor skin reactions, urticaria, arthralgias, arthritis, and fevers. The most serious reaction is an idiosyncratic agranulocytosis, occurring in less than 1% of patients. This can occur at any time during the treatment course or even during a second course of the drug. The most common symptom of agranulocytosis is pharyngitis with fever, for which the patient should seek medical attention. In most cases, the granulocyte count increases 2 to 3 weeks after stopping the drug, but fatal opportunistic infections rarely occur. Treatment with parenteral antibiotics during the recovery period is recommended.

When treating Graves disease, the goal is to allow natural resolution of the underlying autoimmune process. In general, disease remission rate is approximately 25% after two years of treatment, with a further 25% remission every two years.[10] The resolution rate decreases if TSH receptor antibodies persist during and after treatment. The addition of T4 to MTH has had variable results in reducing disease recurrence. However, the use of T4 cannot be recommended in children receiving antithyroid medications.

The thyroid gland must be ablated if resistance or severe reactions to the antithyroid medications develop. Both resection and ablation with radioactive ^{131}I have complications. The advantages of ^{131}I therapy include effectiveness, safety, ease of administration, and relatively low cost.[9] Even though the disease recurrence rate is low after ^{131}I treatment, patients risk long-term hypothyroidism. Concerns remain over the possibility of teratogenic or carcinogenic effects of ^{131}I in children and adolescents.[11]

Either a subtotal or total thyroidectomy is indicated for failure or refusal of medical management, or for airway symptoms (Fig. 76-1). Antithyroid medication should be administered to decrease T3 and T4 levels into the normal range before operation. Alternatively, β-blocking agents, such as propranolol, may be used to ameliorate the adrenergic symptoms of hyperthyroidism. In addition, Lugol's solution, five to ten drops per day, should be administered for 4 to 7 days before thyroidectomy to reduce the vascularity of the gland.

The incidence of hypothyroidism after subtotal thyroidectomy is variable (10–50%) and the hypothyroidism may be subclinical in up to 45% of children.[12] When abnormal TSH levels are considered, the incidence of hyperthyroidism or hypothyroidism is even higher. The rate of recurrent hyperthyroidism is approximately 15%. It is likely the relapse rate increases with time after operation because up to 30% of adult patients exhibit recurrent hyperthyroidism 25 years after their subtotal thyroidectomy.[13]

Hypothyroidism

Hypothyroidism may result from a defect anywhere in the hypothalamic–pituitary–thyroid axis and is rarely treated surgically. Approximately 90% of pediatric hypothyroidism is congenital, detected by neonatal screening programs, and results from dysgenesis of the thyroid gland. Two-thirds of these infants have a rudimentary gland, and complete absence of thyroid tissue is noted in the remainder. The rudimentary gland can be ectopic (e.g., the base of the tongue). Maternal thyroid hormone can prevent symptoms even with complete thyroid agenesis. Ectopic thyroid tissue can supply a sufficient amount of T4 for years, or may prove to be insufficient later in childhood.

Neoplastic Thyroid Conditions

Thyroid Nodules

Thyroid nodules are uncommon in children, but have a 20–25% incidence of malignancy.[14,15] Appropriate and prompt evaluation and management are important to decrease disease progression. Various pathology is noted

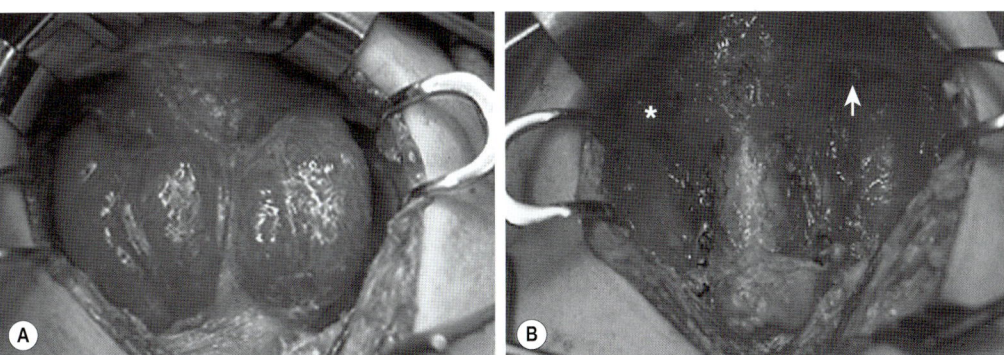

FIGURE 76-1 ■ This teenage girl developed Graves disease and her parents declined radioiodine treatment. **(A)** The diffusely enlarged, hyperemic thyroid gland is visualized. **(B)** The thyroid bed is seen after subtotal thyroidectomy. Each upper pole (asterisk, arrow) was left intact.

in children who undergo an operation for thyroid nodules (Table 76-2). Other diagnostic possibilities for thyroid nodules include cystic hygroma, thyroglossal duct remnant, and germ cell tumor.

Girls have twice the incidence of thyroid nodules as boys. Most patients are initially seen with an asymptomatic mass in the low anterior neck. It is impossible to differentiate benign from malignant lesions on clinical grounds, but a careful neck examination should be performed to determine characteristics of the lesions and presence of enlarged cervical lymph nodes. Thyroid imaging studies are unreliable in distinguishing benign from malignant nodules. However, if ultrasound reveals multiple nodules, the diagnosis of thyroiditis becomes more likely. Similarly, thyroid scintiscan is not a reliable diagnostic modality because malignant nodules may be either functioning or nonfunctioning. A therapeutic trial of exogenous thyroid hormone to induce nodule regression is not recommended for children.

As a result of the increased risk of malignancy in younger children, excision of thyroid nodules in prepubescent children is recommended. The natural history of benign lesions in younger children is unknown, and the safety of nonoperative treatment has not been demonstrated. Based on these data, the current recommendation for management of all thyroid nodules in children younger than age 13 is resection. Preoperative ultrasound and thyroid scintigraphy aid in determining the location.[14,16]

The adolescent spectrum of thyroid disease is similar to that of adults. Thus, fine-needle aspiration is acceptable in evaluating thyroid nodules in this population.[17,18] The incidence of malignancy in thyroid nodules in patients age 13 to 18 years is approximately 10%.[19] Benign nodules in adolescent patients can be followed with serial examinations and ultrasound. Exogenous thyroid hormone to suppress benign thyroid nodules has not been shown to alter their natural history. Excision

should be performed if the nodule is malignant, has indeterminate cytology, increasing size, compressive symptoms, or cosmetic concerns.[16] If a cystic thyroid lesion disappears after aspiration, excision can be deferred. If the lesion recurs, it should be removed. Even though cyst fluid can be sent for cytologic analysis, the sensitivity of this test for determining the presence of cancer in children is unknown. Lobectomy can be performed if malignancy is not confirmed preoperatively. If there is a family history, a radiation history, bilateral disease, atypia or suspicious histology, or the lesion is >4 cm, thyroidectomy is recommended.[16]

Thyroid Carcinoma

Ten per cent of malignant thyroid tumors occur in children, representing about 3% of all pediatric malignancies in the USA. The incidence of childhood thyroid malignancy has decreased in most parts of the world since the mid-1970s due to the reduced use of radiation to treat benign head and neck diseases. However, the incidence may be increasing, perhaps due to improved detection. Overall, mortality remains stable.[20]

Pediatric thyroid cancer is found more commonly in Caucasians (86%), adolescents (94%), and females (81%). At the time of diagnosis, thyroid cancer is limited to the thyroid gland (42%) or found in the regional lymph nodes (46%).[20] In comparison to adults, children with thyroid carcinoma present with more advanced-stage disease and a higher incidence of lymph node and pulmonary metastases, but have a lower mortality rate.[21] Compared to adolescents, prepubertal children have a greater degree of extrathyroid extension, lymph node involvement, and lung metastases at diagnosis.[22]

Exposure to radiation is a significant risk factor for developing thyroid cancer. A 62-fold increase in thyroid tumors was noted in the Republics of Belarus and Ukraine after the 1986 Chernobyl nuclear power plant catastrophe.[23] The tumors were particularly aggressive with increased tumor spread, local invasion, and nodal metastases. The use of radiation for diagnostic purposes has also been linked to increased childhood cancers. It is estimated computed tomography (CT) scans increase risk of malignancy as high as one fatal cancer per 1000 CT scans performed.[24,25]

Treatment of previous malignancies is another risk factor for thyroid carcinoma. Thyroid cancers constitute about 9% of second malignancies.[26] Hodgkin lymphoma is the most common malignancy associated with a subsequent thyroid cancer, followed by non-Hodgkin lymphoma, and leukemia.[27] Whereas most thyroid second neoplasms follow previous radiation exposure to the neck, alkylating agents also predispose to thyroid cancer. The mean age at diagnosis of thyroid second neoplasms is 20 years, demonstrating the importance of careful surveillance for second malignancies.

Various molecular biologic events may account for the disparity in behavior of the different histological subtypes of thyroid cancer.[28] *RAS* proto-oncogene mutations are found in about 20% of papillary tumors and 80% of follicular tumors.[29] Other studies report *RAS* is frequently activated in benign follicular adenomas, suggesting this

TABLE 76-2	**Diagnosis in 251 Pediatric Patients Treated for Thyroid Nodules**
Number that were malignant	42 (17%)
Histologic subtype:	
Papillary	29
Follicular	6
Mixed	2
Anaplastic	2
Medullary	2
Lymphoma	1
Number that were benign	209 (83%)
Diagnosis:	
Follicular adenoma	101
Thyroiditis	27
Thyroglossal cyst	5
Colloid nodule	59
Branchial cyst	12

Data from Desjardins JG, Khan AH, Montupet P, et al. Management of thyroid nodules in children: A 20-year experience. J Pediatr Surg 1987;22:736–9; Hung W, Anderson KD, Chandra RS, et al. Solitary thyroid nodules in 71 children and adolescents. J Pediatr Surg 1992;27:1407–9; Yip FWK, Reeve TS, Poole AG, et al. Thyroid nodules in childhood and adolescence. Aust N Z J Surg 1994;64:676–8.

TABLE 76-3 **Clinical Aspects of Differentiated Thyroid Cancer in Children from Seven Large Pediatric Series[133,134]**

	Clinical Series						
	A	B	C	D	E	F	G
Total number of patients	89	59	58	100	49	72	1753
Mean age (years)	12.8	NA	11.9	13.3	14.0	11	15.9
Girls (%)	81	66	69	71	69	71	81
Histology (number)							
Papillary	83	37	58	87	44	50	60
Follicular variant of papillary							23
Follicular	6	19	0	7	4	21	9.5
Medullary	0	1	0	0	1	0	5
Other	0	2	0	6	0	0	2.7
Metastasis (%)	88	50	90	71	73	75	54
Median follow-up (years)	NA	11	28	20	7.7	13	30
Cancer mortality rate (%)	2.2	3.4	3.4	0	2.0	17	10

NA, data not available.

Data from: A, Harness JA, Thompson NW, McLeod MK, et al. Differentiated thyroid carcinoma in children and adolescents. World J Surg 1992;16:547–5542; B, Samuel AM, Sharma SM. Differentiated thyroid carcinomas in children and adolescents. Cancer 1991;67:2186–90; C, Zimmerman D, Hay ID, Gough IR, et al. Papillary thyroid carcinoma in children and adults: Long-term follow-up of 1039 patients conservatively treated at one institution during three decades. Surgery 1988;104:1157–63; D, La Quaglia MP, Corbally MT, Heller G, et al. Recurrence and morbidity in differentiated thyroid carcinoma in children. Surgery 1998;104:1149–56; E, Ceccarelli C, Pacini F, Lippi F, et al. Thyroid cancer in children and adolescents. Surgery 1988;104:1143–8; F, Schlumberger M, De Vathaire F, Travagli JP, et al. Differentiated thyroid carcinoma in childhood: Long-term follow-up in 72 patients. J Clin Endocrinol Metab 1987;65:1088–94; G, Hogan A.R, Zhuge Y, Perez, EA, et al. Pediatric thyroid carcinoma: incidence and outcomes in 1753 patients. J Surg Res 2009;156:167–72.

genetic event occurs early in the transformation process.[30] An activating mutation of the *RET* proto-oncogene is found in about 35% of papillary thyroid cancers.[31] The *RET* protein is a receptor tyrosine-kinase molecule, which probably functions within the cell to regulate proliferation or differentiation. This protein may be responsible for the development of medullary thyroid carcinoma (MTC). Specific point mutations are associated with the MEN type 2 (MEN 2A, MEN 2B) syndromes and familial MTC (FMTC). In addition, as many as 40% of patients with sporadic MTCs possess *RET* mutations.[32]

Family history is an important factor in pediatric thyroid cancer. Patients with familial nonmedullary thyroid cancer have more aggressive tumors with increased rates of extrathyroid extension, lymph node metastases, and frequently show the phenomenon of 'anticipation' (earlier age at disease onset and increased severity in successive generations).[33]

Thyroid carcinoma usually presents clinically as a thyroid mass, sometimes with enlarged cervical lymph nodes. Regional lymph node metastases are present in three of four children when the disease is first detected (Table 76-3).[34,35] Diagnosis of thyroid carcinoma requires appropriate imaging and histological examination. Ultrasound is the diagnostic modality of choice for thyroid lesions with some authors creating Thyroid Imaging Reporting and Data System (TIRADS) to uniformly classify ultrasound characteristics of thyroid nodules.[36] In young children, excision is recommended for thyroid nodules after ultrasound evaluation of the thyroid and lymph node basin. In adolescents, ultrasound and ultrasound-guided fine needle aspiration (FNA) is recommended as these patients' course tends to most resemble adult thyroid disease. US-guided FNA is safe and effective in adolescents when done in experienced centers.[16–18,37] As

pulmonary metastases are frequent, a preoperative chest radiograph should be obtained in these patients.

Treatment for thyroid cancer in children is total or subtotal thyroidectomy. Thyroid cancer is bilateral in up to two-thirds of cases. Approximately 80% of tumors exhibit multifocality. While lobectomy with isthmus resection may be sufficient for isolated lesions, most pediatric surgeons believe total or near-total thyroidectomy should be performed.[38,39] No clinical trial has established whether total thyroidectomy, with lymph node dissection if the regional nodes are involved, is better than subtotal thyroidectomy.[40] Radioiodine ablative therapy is more effective after removal of the entire gland because functioning thyroid tissue takes up the radionuclide. Surgeons preferring a lesser resection believe differentiated thyroid carcinoma is an indolent disease, and that survival is not related to the extent of gland removal.[40,41]

If there is regional nodal metastases, a central or modified radial neck dissection is recommended. Prophylactic central node dissection is recommended for T3 or T4 papillary lesions.[16] In patients with locally advanced disease, it is imperative to remove as much of the thyroid gland as possible to allow subsequent radioiodine scanning and treatment if the tumor recurs.

Although complications occur less commonly in recent reports, the historical incidence of recurrent laryngeal nerve injury ranges from 0–24%, whereas permanent hypocalcemia occurs in 6–27% of patients undergoing total thyroidectomy.[42,43] During dissection, the laryngeal nerve should be identified and protected. When the tumor invades the laryngeal nerve, the nerve can be safely preserved without compromising survival through adjuvant therapy with ^{131}I irradiation to eradicate residual tumor.[44] The most reliable way to preserve parathyroid gland function is to identify and preserve the glands at the time of thyroidectomy (Fig. 76-2). If there is apparent devascularization, then one should autotransplant one or two of the glands into the sternocleidomastoid muscle or into the nondominant forearm.[45,46]

The incidence of pulmonary metastases in children at diagnosis is about 6%, but they rarely occur in the absence of significant cervical lymph node metastases.[41,47] Pulmonary metastases require treatment with radioiodine. Plain chest films demonstrate the pulmonary disease in only 60% of cases, making scanning with radioiodine necessary. The pulmonary scintiscan can be falsely negative if significant residual thyroid gland remains in the neck.[47]

In one study, overall survival in non-MTC was 98%.[21] A higher rate of recurrence was seen in children who did not receive postoperative ^{131}I than in those who did.[21] The time to first recurrence ranged from 8 months to 14.8 years (mean, 5.3 years), thereby emphasizing the importance of long-term follow-up. Prognostic factors associated with recurrence include younger age at diagnosis, histology, capsular or soft tissue invasion, positive margins, and tumor location at diagnosis (thyroid, lymph nodes, lung).[21,42] A whole-body ^{131}I scan should be performed approximately six weeks after the initial thyroid resection and followed by therapeutic doses of the radionuclide administered as necessary to ablate residual tissue and treat metastatic disease. Radioactive ablation (RAI) has been shown to decrease the risk of local recurrence, increase the sensitivity of subsequent diagnostic whole-body scans, and improve the utility of serum thyroglobulin as a marker for recurrent or residual disease during long-term follow-up.[38] RAI is recommended for all patients with known distant metastases, gross extrathyroidal extension, and primary tumor >4 cm. RAI is recommended for select patients with high risk features such as worrisome histologic subtypes, intrathyroidal vascular invasion, or gross/microscopic multifocal diseases. RAI is not recommended for lesions <1 cm.[16] The association of

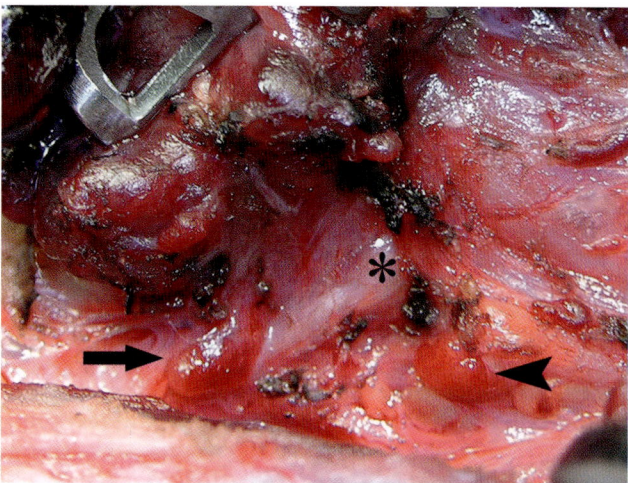

FIGURE 76-2 ■ The relationship of the parathyroid glands to the recurrent laryngeal nerve during prophylactic thyroidectomy for MEN type 2 is seen. The left recurrent laryngeal nerve is marked by an asterisk. The superior parathyroid gland (arrowhead) is typically located posterior to the nerve. The inferior parathyroid gland (arrow) is usually found anterior to the nerve.

radioactive iodine with second cancers has led to recommendations in the adult literature to avoid radioactive iodine in low risk patients.[48]

Follow-up for these patients should include physical examination, ultrasound, and thyroglobulin levels. Thyroglobulin can be a useful marker of residual or metastatic thyroid cancer. The plasma level of this protein should be measured yearly, and an elevated value should raise the suspicion of recurrent disease.[49] The diagnostic accuracy of this test is decreased in children with residual thyroid tissue or in those who are taking thyroid hormone supplementation. In a long-term study of patients with papillary thyroid cancer, up to 32% of patients had recurrent disease at 40 years follow-up, especially if unilateral lobectomy was performed, emphasizing the need for long-term follow-up.[50]

MTC accounts for approximately 5% of pediatric thyroid neoplasms. Arising from the parafollicular C cells, MTC may occur either sporadically or in association with MEN 2A, MEN 2B, or the FMTC syndrome. MTC is usually the first tumor to develop in MEN patients and is the most common cause of death in this group. The neoplasm is particularly virulent in patients with MEN 2B and can occur in infancy.[51]

As with other pediatric thyroid neoplasms, the clinical diagnosis of MTC, not associated with a known familial or MEN syndrome, is usually made only after metastatic spread of the tumor has occurred to the adjacent cervical lymph nodes or to distant sites.[52] Resection is the only effective treatment for MTC, underscoring the importance of early diagnosis and therapy before metastases occur.[53] For this reason, current management of MTC from MEN 2 and FMTC kindreds relies on the presymptomatic detection of the *RET* proto-oncogene mutation responsible for the disease. Prophylactic thyroidectomy in young asymptomatic children carrying a mutated allele of the *RET* proto-oncogene in MEN 2A kindreds has been demonstrated to prevent or cure MTC. In a study of 50 children and teenagers with the *RET* proto-oncogene mutation who underwent prophylactic thyroidectomy, 66% already had foci of MTC within the thyroid gland.[54] However, no child younger than 8 years of age was found to have metastatic disease at surgery. Moreover, when followed for 5 to 8 years, none had evidence of persistent or recurrent disease when screened by physical examination and plasma calcitonin levels obtained after calcium and pentagastrin stimulation. Based on this information, it is recommended that affected children with MEN 2A undergo total thyroidectomy at approximately age 5 years.[55-57]

Due to the increased virulence of MTC in children with MEN 2B, prophylactic thyroidectomy should be performed at approximately age 1 year. Total thyroidectomy is recommended because of the high incidence of bilateral disease.[58] Central lymph node dissection, with removal of lymph nodes medial to the carotid sheaths and between the hyoid bone and the sternum, is likely not necessary except in older children, or when gross lymphadenopathy is discovered at the time of prophylactic thyroidectomy. Early detection by DNA mutation analysis and early operative intervention result in a normal life expectancy.[59]

BOX 76-2 **Differential Diagnosis of Hypercalcemia in Childhood**

Elevated parathyroid hormone level
Primary hyperparathyroidism
Secondary hyperparathyroidism
Ectopic parathyroid hormone production
Hypervitaminosis D
Sarcoidosis
Subcutaneous fat necrosis
Familial hypocalciuric hypercalcemia
Idiopathic hypercalcemia of infancy
Thyrotoxicosis
Hypervitaminosis A
Hypophosphatasia
Prolonged immobilization
Thiazide diuretics

PARATHYROID GLANDS

Embryology and Physiology

Parathyroid glands begin to develop about week 5 of gestation when epithelium in the dorsal portions of the third and fourth pharyngeal pouches begins to proliferate. During week 6, the inferior parathyroid glands, associated with the third pair of pharyngeal pouches, migrate caudad with the thymic primordium and come to rest on the dorsal surface of the thyroid gland low in the neck. The superior parathyroid glands arise from the fourth pharyngeal pouches and come to rest cephalad to the other glands. Mobilization of calcium from the bones is stimulated by parathormone (PTH), a process that also requires vitamin D.

Hyperparathyroidism

PTH is secreted as an 84 amino acid residue protein, which is rapidly cleaved in the liver and kidney into carboxyl-terminal, amino-terminal, and mid-region fragments. The biologic activity of PTH resides in the amino-terminal segment, but the plasma level of this moiety is low, owing to its very short half-life in the circulation. The carboxyl-terminal fragment levels are 50- to 500-fold those of the amino-terminal fragment. Most clinical assays of PTH measure the carboxyl-terminal levels of the hormone. These assays are usually effective for the evaluation of hyperparathyroidism, but plasma levels of the carboxyl-terminal fragment may be selectively elevated if there is a component of renal failure. The laboratory hallmark of hyperparathyroidism is the finding of an inappropriately elevated plasma PTH level with hypercalcemia.

The differential diagnosis of hypercalcemia in childhood is shown in Box 76-2. Unlike hypercalcemia in adults, hypercalcemia in children is rarely related to a neoplasm. Rarely, pediatric tumors may secrete a parathyroid-related polypeptide that elevate serum calcium levels. Reported neoplasms producing PTH-like protein include malignant rhabdoid tumor, mesoblastic nephroma, rhabdomyosarcoma, neuroblastoma, and lymphoma. In these patients, the natural PTH level is usually normal or decreased.

Primary Hyperparathyroidism

Primary hyperparathyroidism in childhood typically results from a solitary hyperfunctioning adenoma and more rarely from diffuse hyperplasia of all four glands.[60] These lesions are often asymptomatic, but can present with urinary and bone tissue impairment.[61] Hyperparathyroidism resulting from hyperplasia in all four glands is a feature of MEN 1. Hyperparathyroidism develops in approximately 30% of MEN 2A patients by their second or third decade of life.[62] At the time of prophylactic thyroidectomy for MEN 2, the parathyroid glands can be identified and autotransplanted into the nondominant forearm.[45] If hyperparathyroidism develops, a portion of the heterotopic tissue can easily be removed from the forearm.

Primary hyperparathyroidism of infancy is a rare, often fatal, condition usually developing within the first 3 months of life.[63,64] Signs include hypotonicity, respiratory distress, failure to thrive, lethargy, and polyuria. The serum PTH level is always elevated, and diffuse parathyroid gland hyperplasia occurs. In about half of the cases, a familial component is found. Early recognition and treatment are essential for normal growth and development.

The management of primary hyperparathyroidism in children is surgical. A solitary hyperfunctioning adenoma accounts for the majority of primary hyperparathyroidism which is often treated safely and effectively with a unilateral neck exploration when preoperative studies demonstrate a single abnormal gland.[61,65] Unilateral neck exploration with focused evaluation and excision relies on accurate preoperative localization studies (ultrasound, sestamibi scans, ± CT/MRI) and rapid intraoperative PTH (IO-PTH) assays to confirm that the offending gland or glands are excised. ^{99m}Tc-sestamibi is avidly taken up by parathyroid tissue, especially adenomas (Fig. 76-3).[66] The sensitivity of detecting abnormal parathyroid glands by sestamibi scan alone is 87%; however, in conjunction with ultrasound, the sensitivity reaches 96%.[67,68] After excision of the abnormal parathyroid gland (Fig. 76-4), a baseline serum PTH level is obtained, followed by PTH levels drawn at 5 and 10 minutes. As the intact PTH half-life is only a few minutes, a greater than 50% drop in IO-PTH level within ten minutes signifies successful removal of the hyperfunctioning parathyroid tissue (Fig. 76-5).[69] In children, some surgeons feel that due to the rapid IO-PTH decline, the five minute time point is sufficient for determining if the resection is sufficient.[70] This approach had the advantage of limiting blood draws and operative time.

Neck exploration with evaluation of all four parathyroid glands is the standard parathyroid operation and should be employed if the patient has an inappropriate response to single gland excision, a single lesion is not identified, parathyroid gland hyperplasia, or suspected MEN. Surgical options for parathyroid gland hyperplasia involving all of the glands include either 3½ gland parathyroidectomy or total parathyroidectomy

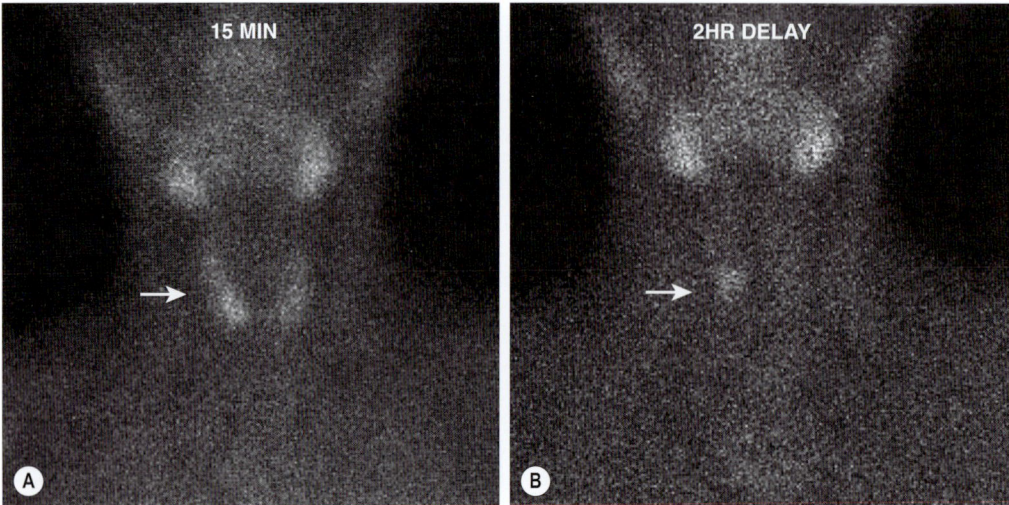

FIGURE 76-3 ■ Early and delayed ^{99m}Tc-sestamibi scintigraphy in a 12-year-old boy with primary hyperparathyroidism. **(A)** The image at 15 minutes demonstrates rapid uptake of the radioisotope by the thyroid gland (arrow). **(B)** The image at 2 hours reveals that the radioisotope has been washed out of the thyroid, but a focus persists (arrow) that is consistent with a right parathyroid adenoma.

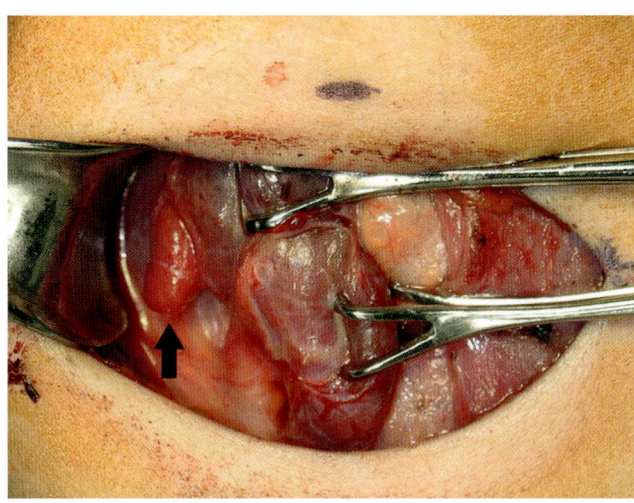

FIGURE 76-4 ■ This intraoperative photograph demonstrates an enlarged right superior parathyroid adenoma (arrow) during unilateral neck exploration that was directed by preoperative localizing studies.

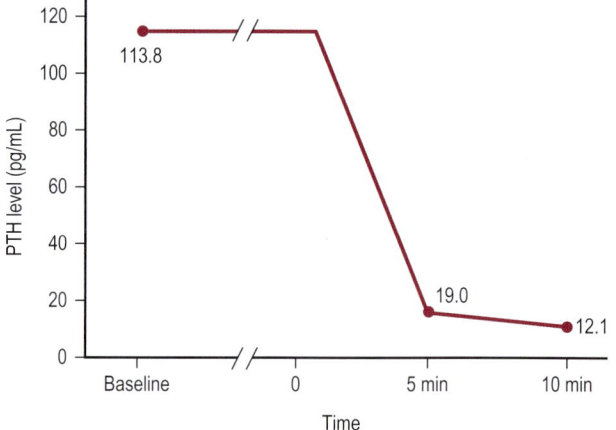

FIGURE 76-5 ■ A rapid intraoperative parathyroid hormone (IO-PTH) assay during unilateral focused parathyroidectomy is depicted. Baseline plasma PTH levels have been drawn. Time 0 represents the moment of resection of the hypersecreting parathyroid gland. PTH levels are drawn at 5 and 10 minutes. A 50% decline in PTH level from baseline at 10 minutes indicates that the offending parathyroid gland or glands have been removed.

with heterotopic autotransplantation of some parathyroid tissue back into the nondominant forearm.[63] The latter approach is safe in infants and children, and has the advantage of avoiding repeated neck exploration if hyperparathyroidism should recur.[45,57] Moreover, total parathyroidectomy with heterotopic autotransplantation results in improved survival in infants with severe hypercalcemia.[63] Patients with total parathyroidectomy and autotransplantation require a short period of vitamin D and calcium supplementation until heterotopic tissue begins to function.[45]

Familial Hypocalciuric Hypercalcemia

Familial hypocalciuric hypercalcemia is an inherited autosomal dominant disorder caused by a heterozygous mutation in the Ca^{2+}-sensing receptor gene.[71] It differs from primary hypoparathyroidism in that the PTH value is normal, but urinary excretion of calcium is low. Patients are usually asymptomatic with an elevated serum calcium level. The serum magnesium level also may be elevated. The parathyroid glands are normal, and usually there is no benefit to parathyroidectomy. If both parents are carriers, severe hypercalcemia may develop in the newborn. These neonates have inherited mutations in both copies of the Ca^{2+}-sensing receptor gene, and often have hyperplasia of all of their parathyroid glands. These infants benefit from parathyroidectomy with transplantation of one gland.

Secondary Hyperparathyroidism

Secondary hyperparathyroidism occurs in children with renal insufficiency or malabsorption. PTH production increases in response to decreased calcium levels. Affected patients typically respond to medical treatment designed to decrease intestinal phosphorus absorption. In rare cases, severe renal osteodystrophy develops, manifested by skeletal fractures and metastatic calcifications. Especially severe cases of secondary hyperparathyroidism may be candidates for total parathyroidectomy with autotransplantation.[60]

Tertiary Hyperparathyroidism

Tertiary hyperparathyroidism occurs when persistent hyperfunction of the parathyroid glands continues even after the inciting stimulus has been removed. This can be seen in chronic renal failure patients and secondary hyperparathyroidism patients who undergo renal transplantation. Tertiary hyperparathyroidism is commonly due to hyperplasia of all four glands. Children with this condition are candidates for total parathyroidectomy with autotransplantation.

ADRENAL GLANDS

Anatomy and Embryology

The primordial adrenal cortex arises from the coelomic mesoderm and becomes visible between weeks 4 and 6 of development. During embryogenesis, the fetal adrenal gland contains a permanent cortex, fetal cortex, and medulla. The fetal cortex, whose function is unknown, is responsible for the large size of the fetal adrenal gland, with the fetal adrenal gland being four times the size of the fetal kidney at the fourth month of gestation. The fetal cortex decreases in size within hours of birth and disappears by the first year of life. The cells of the permanent cortex are arranged into three separate zones: the zona glomerulosa, zona fasciculata, and zona reticularis. The zona glomerulosa gives rise to the narrowed zona fasciculata and reticularis of the adult cortex. The zona reticularis does not reach adult form until late childhood.[72]

The adrenal glands weigh 1 g at birth and grow to 4–5 g by late childhood. The mature adrenal gland measures 3–5 cm in length and 4–6 mm in thickness. Adrenal glands have a profuse arterial supply. One or more middle adrenal arteries arise from the aorta, six to eight superior adrenal arteries from the inferior phrenic artery, and one or more inferior adrenal arteries from the renal artery. Each adrenal gland is drained by a single large adrenal vein with the right adrenal vein draining into the inferior vena cava and the left adrenal vein draining into the left renal vein.

The adrenal gland is found in several anomalous locations. In adrenal heterotopia, the gland is situated in the normal location, but lies under the capsule of the kidney (adrenal–renal heterotopia) or capsule of the liver (adrenal–hepatic heterotopia). Extra-adrenal tissue (adrenal rest) may be located anywhere in the abdominal cavity, but usually is found along the anatomic derivatives of the urogenital ridge for the adrenal cortex and along the dorsal root ganglia for the medullary tissue. Accessory adrenal glands usually occur without a medullary subcomponent and have been found in 16% of autopsies.[73] Another 16% had complete accessory glands.

Physiology

The adrenal cortex produces three major hormones: aldosterone, cortisol, and androgens. The zona glomerulosa is exclusively responsible for the production of aldosterone because it lacks the enzyme 17α-hydroxylase, which is necessary to produce the precursors to cortisol and androgens. The zona fasciculata and zona reticularis together produce cortisol, androgens, and small amounts of estrogens. These areas lack the enzymes necessary to produce the precursors to aldosterone.

Aldosterone

Aldosterone regulates extracellular fluid volume, sodium, and potassium balance. Aldosterone is regulated by the renin-angiotensin system. Renin is secreted by juxtaglomerular cells in response to decreased pressure in renal afferent arterioles and by decreased plasma concentration detected by the macula densa. Renin converts angiotensinogen into angiotensin I, which is converted to angiotensin II by the angiotensin converting enzyme in the lung. Angiotensin II is a potent vasoconstrictor and directly stimulates the zona glomerulosa to release aldosterone. Aldosterone stimulates renal tubular reabsorption of sodium in exchange for potassium and hydrogen, thereby increasing renal fluid resorption and expanding intravascular volume.

Cortisol

The regulation of cortisol is controlled through cortisol-releasing factor (CRF) from the hypothalamus and subsequent stimulation of pituitary adrenocorticotropic hormone (ACTH). The neuroendocrine control of cortisol results in an early morning peak in the cortisol level and a nadir in late evening. Metabolic effects of cortisol include stimulation of hepatic gluconeogenesis, inhibition of protein synthesis, increased protein catabolism, and lipolysis of adipose tissue. Cortisol also causes a loss of collagen, inhibition of wound healing through decreased fibroblast activity, and induction of a negative calcium balance, leading to osteoporosis.

Androgens

Adrenal androgens include dehydroepiandrosterone (DHEA) and DHEA sulfate (DHEA-S). These hormones undergo peripheral conversion to the biologically active forms testosterone and dihydrotestosterone. In the normal male, adrenal androgens account for less than 5% of the circulating testosterone. Adrenal androgens become most clinically relevant with congenital adrenal hyperplasia (CAH), a group of autosomal recessive enzyme deficiencies that result in an accumulation of steroid precursors shuttled away from the synthesis of cortisol and/or aldosterone and into the pathway of androgens. Deficiency in the enzyme 21-hydroxylase accounts for over 90% of CAH.

Functional tumors
   Adrenal adenoma
   Adrenocortical carcinoma
   Pheochromocytoma
Nonfunctional tumors
   Neuroblastoma
   Adrenal cyst
   Hemangioma
   Leiomyoma
   Leiomyosarcoma
   Non-Hodgkin lymphoma
   Malignant melanoma
Metastatic disease to the adrenal gland
   Squamous cell carcinoma of the lung
   Hepatocellular carcinoma
   Breast cancer
Traumatic adrenal hemorrhage
   Neonatal child abuse

Adrenal Masses

The differential diagnosis of adrenal masses is listed in Box 76-3. Neuroblastoma accounts for more than 90% of adrenal masses. Adrenal masses are detected at a greater rate than previously described because of increased diagnostic testing for other conditions. The significance of such adrenal masses seen on CT is unknown in children. At autopsy, adrenal masses are detected in less than 1% of patients younger than age 30 years.[74] This incidence increases to 7% in patients older than 70 years. Follow-up of patients with nonfunctioning adrenal masses demonstrates that 5–25% enlarge by at least 1 cm, and the risk of malignancy is 1 in 1,000. Patients who have an incidentally discovered adrenal mass should undergo hormone evaluation, including a 1 mg dexamethasone suppression test, aldosterone levels, and measurement of plasma free metanephrines.[74] Surgical treatment is indicated for all functioning adrenal cortical tumors and pheochromocytoma. In children, most surgeons will resect adrenal tumors regardless of size; however, no clear evidence supports this management over conservative therapy, especially in lesions smaller than 3 cm (Fig. 76-6).[75,76]

Adrenal Cortex

Hypercortisolism (Cushing Syndrome)

Hypercortisolism, or Cushing syndrome, describes any form of glucocorticoid excess that can be caused by ACTH secreting pituitary adenomas, adrenal tumors including carcinoma and adenoma, ectopic ACTH syndrome, nodular adrenal hyperplasia, and ACTH-producing tumors (Box 76-4). Additionally, the administration of supraphysiologic quantities of ACTH or glucocorticoids can lead to iatrogenic Cushing syndrome, the most common cause of hypercortisolism in adults and children. Cushing disease is caused by a pituitary micro-adenoma or, more rarely, by a macroadenoma. It is the second most common cause of Cushing syndrome in children. Ectopic ACTH syndrome is rare in children, but has been reported in infants younger than 1 year. Tumors that can produce ACTH include pulmonary neoplasms, neuroblastomas, pancreatic islet cell carcinomas, thymomas, carcinoids, MTCs, and pheochromocytomas. In children, the most frequent cause of ectopic ACTH is a bronchial carcinoid. ACTH levels are usually ten to 100 times higher than those seen in Cushing disease. These markedly elevated levels of ACTH lead to hypokalemic alkalosis. Additionally, ACTH-independent multinodular adrenal hyperplasia is characterized by hypersecretion of both cortisol and adrenal androgens.

Hypercortisolism is more common in children than previously recognized. In Harvey Cushing's original description,[77] the patient was a 23-year-old woman whose clinical features indicated long-standing disease. In infants and children younger than 7 years, the most common cause of Cushing syndrome is an adrenal tumor (Fig. 76-7). In adults and children older than 7 years, adrenal hyperplasia secondary to hypersecretion of pituitary ACTH predominates.

Clinical features of Cushing syndrome can take five years or longer to develop. Thus, the classic Cushing appearance may not be seen in children. The most frequent and reliable findings with Cushing syndrome are weight gain and growth failure.[78] Specifically, any obese child who stops growing should be evaluated for Cushing syndrome.

The initial part of the work-up for Cushing syndrome is to screen for the syndrome followed by localization.[79] Screening for Cushing syndrome involves measuring the plasma cortisol at 8:00 am (normal levels, <14 mg/dL) and 6:00 pm (normal levels, <8 mg/dL) to coincide with the diurnal variation. The loss of diurnal rhythm is usually the earliest laboratory evidence of Cushing disease. A single measurement at midnight should be less than 2 mg/dL in normal patients and more than 2 mg/dL in Cushing disease.[80] The most sensitive screening test is the 24-hour urinary 17-hydroxycorticosteroid or free cortisol value, which is more than 150 mg/day in patients with Cushing

ACTH-dependent causes
   Cushing disease (pituitary adenoma)
   Ectopic ACTH production
   Small cell bronchogenic carcinoma
   Carcinoid tumors
   Pancreatic islet cell carcinoma
   Thymoma
   Medullary thyroid carcinoma
   Pheochromocytoma
ACTH-independent causes
   Adrenal adenoma
   Adrenocortical carcinoma
   Adrenal hyperplasia
   Administration of ACTH

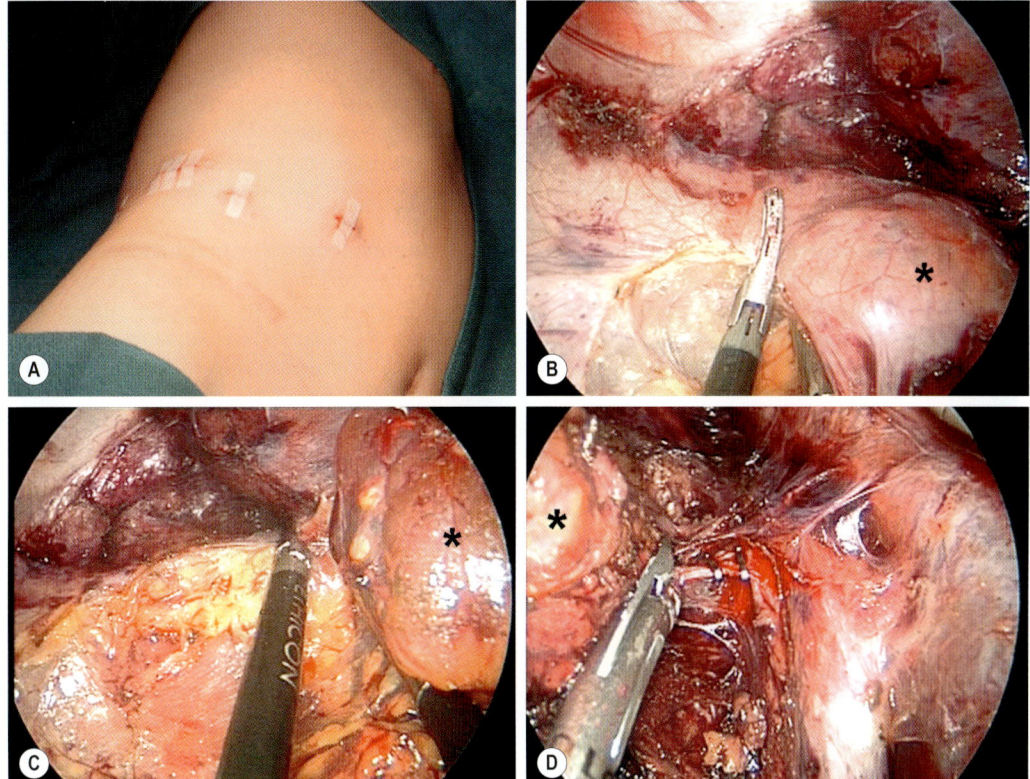

FIGURE 76-6 ■ This teenager was found to have a right adrenal mass measuring 4.5 cm in greatest dimension. Preoperative evaluation did not reveal evidence of a functioning tumor. **(A)** She was placed in the left lateral decubitus position for the laparoscopic right adrenalectomy. The incisions utilized for the operation are seen. **(B)** The harmonic scalpel is being used to free the tumor (asterisk) from the lateral surrounding tissue. **(C)** The tumor (asterisk) has been almost completely mobilized and the cephalad attachments are being lysed with the harmonic scalpel. **(D)** The tumor (asterisk) is being retracted laterally, and the right adrenal vein is being clipped with endoscopic clips. This tumor was excised uneventfully and was found to be a nonfunctioning adrenal adenoma. The patient was discharged on her first postoperative day.

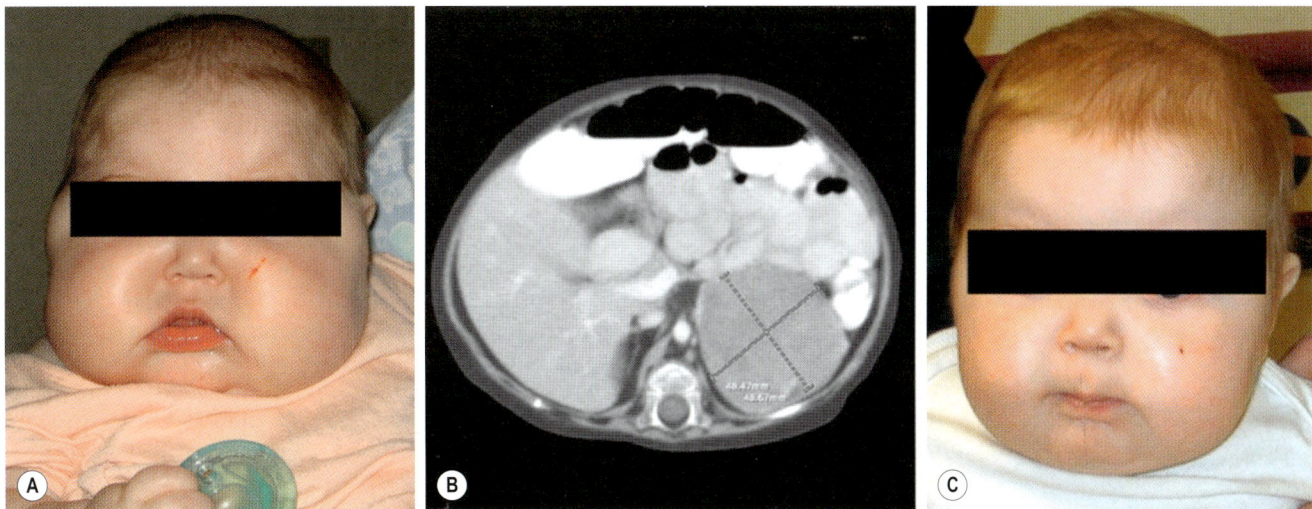

FIGURE 76-7 ■ This 8-month-old child was seen in the emergency department for progressive facial swelling. **(A)** Examination reveals cushingoid features with moon facies. In addition, she had generalized obesity. Her plasma cortisol level was elevated and her ACTH level was suppressed. **(B)** CT scan revealed a 4.3 cm × 4.8 × 4.8 cm left adrenal mass that was homogeneous and showed no evidence of invasion of adjacent structures. The infant subsequently underwent laparoscopic left adrenalectomy and was discharged on postoperative day 2. **(C)** At two-month follow-up, there is marked improvement in the physical manifestations of her Cushing syndrome. (From Kim E, Aguayo P, St. Peter SD, et al. Adrenocortical adenoma expressing glucocorticoid in an 8-month-old female. Eur J Pediatr Surg 2008;18:1–2. Reprinted with permission.)

syndrome. The overnight dexamethasone suppression test is performed by administering 1 mg of dexamethasone at 11:00 pm and measuring the plasma cortisol level the following morning at 8:00 am. In normal individuals, ACTH is suppressed and the cortisol level is decreased by 50% or more of baseline (<5 mg/dL). This dose of dexamethasone is insufficient to cause cortisol suppression in patients with Cushing syndrome.

Once Cushing syndrome is established, further tests determine the specific cause. The high-dose dexamethasone suppression test distinguishes pituitary causes from nonpituitary causes. An oral dose of 2 mg of dexamethasone is given every 6 hours for 48 hours (or 40 mg/kg/dose for infants). Urine is then collected for 24 hours to measure free cortisol and 17-hydroxysteroids. In patients with a pituitary neoplasm, the steroid excretion levels are suppressed to 50% of baseline. In patients with an adrenal adenoma, adrenocortical carcinoma, or most patients with tumors producing ACTH, levels are not suppressed. Plasma ACTH levels are generally low or normal with adrenal causes of hypercortisolism, modestly elevated with pituitary neoplasms, and extremely elevated with tumors producing ectopic ACTH.

Among children, 80–85% of those with Cushing disease have a surgically identifiable microadenoma[81] and transsphenoidal hypophysectomy is indicated. Twenty per cent of patients experience relapse after complete resection and manifest Cushing disease within 5 years. Alternate therapies include pituitary irradiation, adrenalectomy, and drugs inhibiting adrenal function. Of these alternate therapies, adrenalectomy is the preferred treatment when two transsphenoidal procedures fail. Mitotane, an adrenolytic agent, causes a chemical adrenalectomy, but has severe side effects, including nausea, anorexia, and vomiting.

Primary Hyperaldosteronism

Primary hyperaldosteronism is defined as excess production of aldosterone from the adrenal glands with consequent suppression of renin. An adrenal adenoma, or Conn syndrome, is the most common cause of primary hyperaldosteronism in adults, whereas adrenocortical hyperplasia is the most common cause in children.[82] Rarely, an adrenal carcinoma can present as primary hyperaldosteronism. Primary hyperaldosteronism is also seen in MEN1-related adrenal tumors.[83]

Signs and symptoms of primary hyperaldosteronism are nonspecific. Patients have hypertension, muscle weakness, polydipsia, and polyuria. Hyperaldosteronism increases total body sodium and consequently increases total body fluid. It is characterized by hypertension and hypokalemic alkalosis. The elevated aldosterone levels suppress renin and angiotensin.

The diagnosis should be entertained in any child with hypertension and hypokalemia. Initial screening involves checking the potassium level. Hypokalemia (<3.5 mEq/L) is consistent with primary hyperaldosteronism. The aldosterone level is elevated, the renin level is suppressed, and patients frequently have a metabolic alkalosis. If necessary, the diagnosis can be confirmed by performing a saline load challenge. In normal subjects, the saline

bolus should decrease plasma aldosterone levels below 6–8 ng/dL. Alternatively, an outpatient saline load test consists of administering a high-sodium diet for three to five days that fails to suppress aldosterone in patients with hyperaldosteronism. The serum aldosterone level should be determined in the morning before the patient has assumed an upright position.

After hyperaldosteronism is diagnosed, it is important to distinguish between an aldosterone-secreting adenoma or bilateral adrenal hyperplasia. A solitary adrenal mass greater than 1 cm with a normal-appearing contralateral gland on CT or MRI supports the diagnosis of an adenoma.[84] When imaging does not clearly demonstrate a solitary adrenal mass, selective adrenal vein sampling can differentiate unilateral versus bilateral aldosterone hypersecretion. Alternatively, some institutions utilize scintigraphy with ^{131}I-iodomethylnorcholesterol (NP-59), a cholesterol analog taken up as cholesterol in the steroidogenic pathway. Dexamethasone suppression of ACTH-dependent adrenocortical tissue is followed by NP-59 administration. An adenoma is suggested if asymmetric adrenal uptake occurs. Bilateral hyperplasia is suggested if the uptake is symmetric.

The treatment of a functioning adrenal adenoma is resection which can be performed laparoscopically.[85,86] The mortality rate following resection is less than 1%, with a cure rate of 75%. Treatment of patients with bilateral adrenal hyperplasia is with spironolactone.

Adrenocortical Carcinoma

Adrenocortical carcinoma is rare. National Cancer Institute's Surveillance, Epidemiology and End Results data indicate adrenocortical carcinoma represents 1.3% of all carcinomas in children and adolescents younger than 20 years of age in the USA, accounting for only 0.1% of all childhood malignancies.[87] There is a female-to-male ratio of 2 : 1 with half of these tumors occurring in patients <5 years of age. The tumors occur equally on the right and left sides, and are hormonally functional in 80–100% of patients. Around the world, there is geographic variability, with southern Brazil having a 15-fold greater incidence compared with other regions. This increased incidence has been attributed to a unique germline missense mutation.[88]

The etiology of adrenocortical carcinoma is unknown, but its association with several hereditary tumor syndromes gives insight into the molecular pathogenesis of this malignancy. Li–Fraumeni syndrome is an autosomal dominant familial disease characterized by the early onset of tumors, including sarcomas, osteosarcomas, breast and brain cancers, leukemia, and adrenocortical carcinoma. Germ line mutations in the *TP53* tumor suppressor gene on chromosome 17p13.1 are found in 70% of affected families.[89] These mutations have been found in 20–27% of sporadic cases of adrenocortical carcinomas. Beckwith–Wiedemann syndrome is a congenital overgrowth disorder where patients are predisposed to certain embryonal tumors such as Wilms tumor, hepatoblastoma, neuroblastoma, rhabdomyosarcoma, and adrenocortical carcinoma. Overexpression of insulin-like growth factor (IGF)-2 is believed to contribute to the tumorigenesis in

Beckwith–Wiedemann syndrome.[90] Several genetic alterations, such as loss of imprinting or loss of heterozygosity of the 11 p15 gene locus causing a strong IGF-2 overexpression, have been demonstrated in the majority of adrenocortical carcinomas.[88,91,92] Other hereditary syndromes associated with adrenocortical tumors include Carney complex, MEN 1, and congenital adrenal hyperplasia.[83] However, these adrenal tumors are mostly adenomas and rarely carcinoma.

The clinical presentation of adrenocortical carcinoma is usually associated with steroid overproduction. In contrast to adult tumors, most adrenocortical tumors are hormonally active. Virilization is the most frequent presenting feature (66%), whereas the remainder of children will be seen with Cushing syndrome symptoms.[93,94] Virilization is secondary to secretion of the adrenal androgens. Features include axillary and pubic hair, deepening of the voice, acne, rapid height growth, hirsutism, enlargement of the penis or clitoromegaly, and development of body odor. Feminization may occur in 2–25% of patients from an overproduction of estrogens, particularly estradiol.[95] Only about 5% of pediatric adrenocortical cancers produce no clinical evidence of hormone excess. Accordingly, these patients present with more advanced disease.

As most tumors present with virilization symptoms, evaluation includes measurements of plasma testosterone, and urinary and plasma DHEA and DHEA-S. Urinary 17-ketosteroids are also important because two-thirds of 17-ketosteroids are derived from adrenal androgens. Although the most specific assessment of adrenal androgen production is DHEA-S, 17-ketosteroids are more frequently elevated in malignant disease.[96] The clinical presentation of Cushing syndrome is confirmed by hypercortisolism and the loss of diurnal variation. Cortisol excess is determined by elevated plasma cortisol, urinary 17-hydroxycorticosteroids, and urinary free cortisol. Adrenal malignant disease generally causes markedly greater elevations of 17-hydroxycorticosteroids and plasma cortisol than is usually seen with functioning adenomas.

Radiographic studies should proceed concurrently with endocrine evaluation so surgical intervention is expedient. Ultrasound should be used initially for evaluating the adrenal region and for postoperative assessment of recurrence. Smaller lesions are smooth and homogeneous with no pattern of hyperechogenicity or hypoechogenicity. Larger lesions usually demonstrate a 'scar sign', radiating linear echoes representing an interphase between separate areas of necrosis, hemorrhage, and neoplasm.[97] CT detects tumors as small as 0.5 cm and can identify regional invasion or distant metastases in the liver, lung, or brain. MRI has an accuracy similar to CT with lesions larger than 1–2 cm.[98] Finally, adrenal scintigraphy using iodocholesterol-labeled analogs has shown promise in identifying and differentiating functional adrenal lesions.[99] Differentiation between hyperplasia, adenoma, and carcinoma is made possible by the inability of carcinoma to concentrate radionuclide. Bilateral symmetric images indicate hyperplasia, unilateral uptake suggests adenoma, and nonvisualization is suggestive of carcinoma.[100]

Resection offers the only chance for cure. If extensive disease is found at operation, wide en-bloc resection of the tumor, lymph nodes, and involved organs is indicated.[101] Higher-volume centers demonstrated improved outcomes with a lower recurrence rate and improved mean time to recurrence.[102] For less extensive disease, minimally invasive techniques for adrenalectomy have been advocated, although most authors cite invasive disease as a contraindication to laparoscopic resection.

Adjuvant therapy has marginal results.[103] Survival in patients undergoing adjuvant therapy with localized disease has been reported to be 5 years versus 2.3 years for patients who have tumor spread beyond the adrenal gland.[101] For patients who underwent further operations for recurrent disease, survival is extended 3.5 years. Pediatric series report the incidence of metastases at diagnosis between 5–64%.[89] Mitotane has been the most widely used chemotherapeutic agent. It is used for metastatic disease, for incompletely excised tumors, and for the hormonal effects from the tumors. In adults, tumor response rates to mitotane vary widely (10–60%),[89] with a mean response duration of only 10.2 months.[104] In the pediatric literature, tumor responses have been reported between 30–40%, though the benefit of adjuvant mitotane is controversial.[103,105,106] Additional regimens that have shown some promise include the combination of cisplatin, etoposide, and taxol. The role of radiation therapy has not been well established. In adults, adrenocortical carcinoma is thought to be radioresistant. However, some response has been noted in small series of children with metastatic disease.[95] In one report, radiation was used to shrink an unresectable tumor that was subsequently completely excised.[89]

Patients left untreated with adrenocortical carcinomas have a mean survival of 2.9 months.[107] These tumors are highly lethal, with nonfunctional tumors and delay in diagnosis leading to worse prognosis. The range of time from symptoms to diagnosis is 6–36 months.[89] The prognosis depends on the child's age and the resectability of the tumor. In one review of 55 children with adrenal carcinoma, the two-year survival rates were 82% for children <2 years and 29% for children >2 years. Survival rates were more than 67% if the tumors were completely excised, but no survivors were found after partial resection.[108]

Adrenal Medulla

Pheochromocytoma is a neuroendocrine tumor arising from neural crest–derived chromaffin cells in the adrenal medulla. During embryologic development, chromaffin cells migrate to the adrenal medulla and other areas such as the paraganglia of the carotid arteries, aortic arch, abdominal aorta, and thoracic sympathetic ganglia. Any of these nests of chromaffin cells have the potential to become a tumor, and are the cause of extra-adrenal pheochromocytoma, also termed paraganglioma. The adrenal gland accounts for 85% of all pheochromocytomas in adults. Children have a higher incidence of extra-adrenal pheochromocytoma (30%),[109] multifocal, and familial disease,[110] but a lower incidence of malignancy compared with adults.[111] As in adults, children present with signs and symptoms of catecholamine excess, including hypertension, headaches, sweating, visual complaints, nausea, vomiting, weight loss, polydipsia, and polyuria. Pheochromocytoma should be considered in any child with hypertension.[112]

The evaluation of pheochromocytoma includes biochemical studies to establish the diagnosis and radiologic imaging to localize the disease.[113] Current guidelines, based on the First International Symposium on Pheochromocytoma, recommends initial testing for pheochromocytoma including measurements of fractionated metanephrines (i.e., normetanephrine and metanephrine) in plasma, urine, or both.[114] Radiologic imaging options include MRI, CT, and [123]I- or ^{131}I-metaiodobenzylguanidine (MIBG) scanning. MRI has the highest sensitivity and is preferred over CT because of decreased radiation exposure.[110,115] Although not as sensitive, ^{131}I-MIBG scanning is the most specific imaging technique and is favored when recurrent or metastatic disease is suspected. Most paragangliomas are found in the abdomen and pelvis. When pheochromocytoma is suspected biochemically but not found by imaging, an intrathoracic or intracranial tumor should be suspected.

The perioperative management of patients with pheochromocytoma is critical to a successful outcome. These patients are in a hyperadrenergic state with a low intravascular volume. Catecholamine blockade and intravascular volume expansion are standard preoperative strategies. An α-adrenergic antagonist (e.g., phenoxybenzamine, prazosin, doxazosin, or terazosin) is started a minimum of two weeks before operation. β-adrenergic blockers may be used to treat tachycardia, but should not be used until adequate α blockade has been achieved due to risks of unopposed α-adrenergic stimulation with β-blockade alone. Alternatively, calcium channel blockers have been successfully utilized in the perioperative management of pheochromocytoma and may provide fewer fluctuations in blood pressure as well as cardioprotective effects.[111]

Historically, pheochromocytoma resection has been performed via an open approach. Even with appropriate preoperative preparation, intraoperative hypertensive and hypotensive episodes are common, and must be anticipated by the anesthesia and surgical team. At operation, it is important to ligate the adrenal vein early and to minimize handling the gland to limit catecholamine surges during the procedure. Laparoscopic transabdominal adrenalectomy has gained significant popularity and been validated for pheochromocytoma resections in adults.[116] Although the data in children are currently limited to small series, it appears equally safe and effective in experienced hands (Fig. 76-8).[85,86,117,118]

Up to 25% of pheochromocytomas are familial, and germline mutations in the following genes have been associated with pheochromocytoma: *VHL* (von Hippel–Lindau syndrome); *NF1* (von Recklinghausen neurofibromatosis type 1); *RET* (MEN 2A or 2B); *SDHD* and *SDHB* (familial paragangliomas associated with gene mutations of the mitochondrial succinate dehydrogenase family).[110,119] Pheochromocytomas are more frequently associated with MEN 2 syndromes in children than in adults. Also, pheochromocytomas associated with the MEN 2 syndrome are more likely to be bilateral and benign.

In familial pheochromocytoma such as in MEN 2 or VHL syndrome, bilateral tumors inevitably occur. Controversy exists over management of these patients. Bilateral adrenalectomy has been suggested, but predisposes these patients to significant morbidity secondary to corticosteroid replacement as well as complications of medication noncompliance, such as addisonian crises.[120] Cortical-sparing adrenalectomies have been proposed for patients with bilateral tumors and those at high risk for developing a metachronous contralateral lesion.[121]

For patients with metastatic disease, ^{131}I-MIBG scanning and chemotherapy may be effective. Current evidence supports high initial doses of ^{131}I-MIBG for all patients with metastatic lesions who have positive diagnostic ^{131}I-MIBG scans. With tumors responding symptomatically or hormonally to treatment, survival is 4.7 years after treatment.[122] Chemotherapy seems to have an additive effect with ^{131}I-MIBG scanning to increase survival in these patients.[123] Although serious toxicity may occur, the survival and response rates achieved with

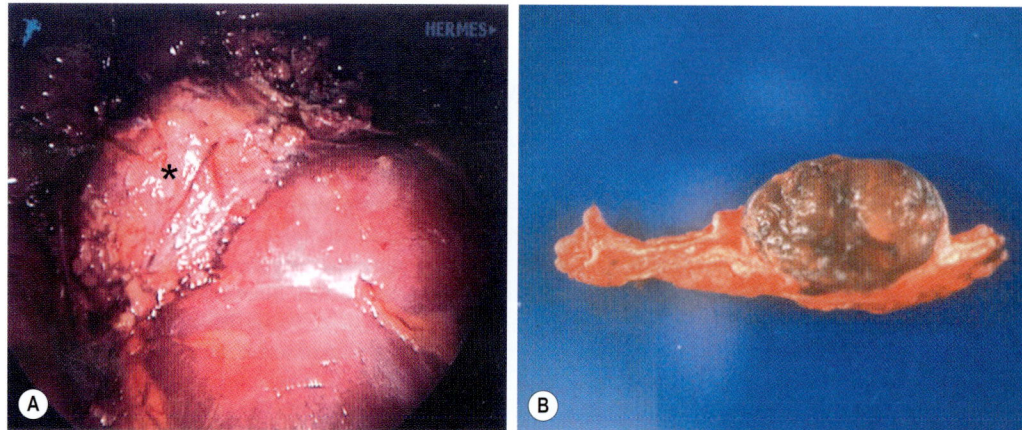

FIGURE 76-8 ■ A teenage boy was found to have marked hypertension and a pheochromocytoma after a metabolic evaluation. He underwent laparoscopic left adrenalectomy and tolerated the procedure nicely. **(A)** The pheochromocytoma (asterisk) is seen lying on the cephalad portion of the left kidney. The tumor was removed uneventfully. **(B)** On the cut section of the adrenal gland, the tumor can be seen to be nicely demarcated from the normal adrenal gland.

high-dose ^{131}I-MIBG suggest its utility in the management of selected patients with metastatic pheochromocytoma and paraganglioma.[124]

PRECOCIOUS PUBERTY

In boys, precocious puberty is defined as the development of secondary sexual characteristics before age 9 years. In girls, the development of breasts (thelarche) before age 7.5 years, the development of pubic hair (pubarche) before age 8.5 years, or the onset of menses (menarche) before age 9.5 years is considered precocious. Precocious puberty can be complete or incomplete.

True precocious puberty is due to premature maturation of the hypothalamic–pituitary axis and results in gonadal enlargement and premature development of secondary sexual characteristics. The secondary sexual characteristics developing in true precocious puberty are appropriate for the sex of the child and merely occur at a younger-than-appropriate age. In incomplete or pseudoprecocious puberty, only one secondary sexual characteristic develops prematurely. Moreover, it may or may not be appropriate for the patient's gender. Pseudoprecocious puberty is not due to pituitary gonadotropin secretion. Rather, it is due to production of human chorionic gonadotropin (hCG), luteinizing hormone (LH), follicle-stimulating hormone (FSH), androgens or estrogens, or it is due to stimulation of their receptors by some tumors.

Precocious Puberty in Girls

True precocious puberty, resulting from premature activation of the hypothalamic–pituitary axis, is idiopathic in most girls. The condition may be a normal variant simply at the younger age of a normal distribution curve. Neurogenic disturbances can cause true precocious puberty by interfering with inhibitory signals from the central nervous system to the hypothalamus, or by producing excitatory signals. Neurogenic disorders may include hydrocephalus, cerebral palsy, trauma, irradiation, chronic inflammatory disorders, or tumors, such as hypothalamic hamartomas or pineal tumors.

McCune–Albright syndrome is an interesting disorder causing either true precocious puberty or pseudoprecocious puberty. Patients have the classic triad of precocious puberty, café-au-lait nevi with irregular 'coast of Maine' borders, and polyostotic fibrous dysplasia. In these patients, autonomously functioning ovarian follicular cysts can develop, causing precocious puberty. Excess production of LH, FSH, or prolactin by pituitary adenomas also has been described. Other endocrine abnormalities including acromegaly, Cushing syndrome, and hyperthyroidism have been associated with this syndrome.[125]

Generally, incomplete precocious puberty is first seen as isolated premature breast development (thelarche) or premature growth of pubic hair (pubarche). Premature pubarche is caused by androgen excess. Isolated prepubertal menses is rare, and prepubertal vaginal bleeding is usually caused by a foreign body, sexual abuse, or tumors of the genital tract. Incomplete precocious puberty can be a normal variant or can be due to the production of hormones from neuroendocrine, adrenal, ovarian, or exogenous sources. In the Van Wyk–Grumbach syndrome, premature breast development is associated with hypothyroidism. Unlike most other causes of precocious puberty, growth is inhibited rather than stimulated. This syndrome may be due to the shared α-subunit of LH, FSH, or TSH. Tumors producing excess quantities of LH or hCG can cause virilization.

Precocious Puberty in Boys

As with girls, true precocious puberty in boys may be neurogenic, constitutional, or idiopathic. However, in boys, true precocious puberty is more often neurogenic than idiopathic.

The most common neurogenic tumor causing male precocious puberty is a hamartoma of the tuber cinereum. These hamartomas are ectopic hypothalamic tissue connected to the posterior hypothalamus. As they are nonprogressive tumors and in a surgically precarious location, they are generally treated with gonadotropin-releasing hormone (GnRH) agonists. Other disorders causing precocious puberty in boys are gliomas of the optic nerve or hypothalamus, astrocytomas, choriocarcinomas, meningiomas, rhabdomyosarcomas, neurofibrosarcomas, nonlymphocytic leukemia, ependymomas, neurofibromatosis type 1, and germinomas. Other space-occupying lesions or causes of increased intracranial pressure such as head trauma, suprasellar cysts, granulomas, brain irradiation, and hydrocephalus also can cause true precocious puberty. Some of these conditions can cause both precocious puberty and growth hormone deficiency. In these patients, the growth rate may appear normal because the testosterone stimulates growth and compensates for the deficiency of growth hormone. However, the degree of growth is inadequate for the degree of pubertal development.

Incomplete precocious puberty can be caused by autonomous production of androgens or hCG. In this condition, the testes are not enlarged as they are with true precocious puberty. As with girls, the McCune–Albright syndrome can cause either true or pseudoprecocious puberty. Tumors producing hCG such as teratomas, chorioepitheliomas, hepatomas, hepatoblastomas, or germinomas of the pineal gland may lead to Leydig cell stimulation. Testotoxicosis is an autosomal recessive disorder in which premature Leydig cell maturation causes incomplete precocious puberty. The etiology in some families is due to stimulation of the LH receptor and can cause the onset of precocious puberty at age 1 to 4 years. Ketoconazole, spironolactone, and testolactone are used to treat testotoxicosis.

Excess androgen production causing virilization can be caused by congenital adrenal hyperplasia, specifically the 21-hydroxylase or the 11-hydroxylase enzymatic defects. During embryonic development, adrenal rests may be left in the testes. In untreated adrenal hyperplasia, ACTH stimulation can cause enlargement of these adrenal rests and the secretion of androgens. These testes have an irregular appearance. Excess testosterone production also can be caused by interstitial cell tumors of the testes. Finally, exogenous administration of androgens or hCG (for treatment of undescended testes) can cause precocious puberty.

Evaluation

For both boys and girls, evaluation of precocious puberty begins with a thorough history and physical examination including height, weight, bone age, and growth curve evaluation. If the bone age and the height age correlate closely, it is likely the presenting symptom is an extreme variant of normal. The patient is evaluated in 6 months to verify the diagnosis. However, if the bone age is abnormally accelerated relative to the height age, further investigation is warranted. The Tanner stage should be carefully documented. In boys, the size and shape of the testes are of utmost importance. In true precocious puberty, the testes generally enlarge symmetrically, whereas asymmetric or nodular enlargement is noted with Leydig cell tumors or adrenal rests. Feminization in boys may appear as gynecomastia.

Serum estradiol, testosterone, and DHEA levels should be obtained. In girls, a vaginal smear for estrogen effect may be more sensitive than a serum estradiol level. Significantly elevated DHEA levels are typically seen in adrenal tumors. Evidence of association with other syndromes may warrant measuring other hormone levels, including prolactin, thyroid hormone, or cortisol. A GnRH test can be useful in determining whether the patient has complete or incomplete precocious puberty. Patients with true precocious puberty respond to GnRH with a typical pubertal pattern, whereas those with pseudoprecocious puberty have a minimal response to gonadotropin. Alternatively, a sleep-related increase in plasma LH levels can be diagnostic, but is more cumbersome to obtain. In patients with feminizing or masculinizing features, ultrasound is useful to locate abdominal or pelvic masses. MRI is recommended in patients with true precocious puberty to evaluate for intracranial lesions.

Treatment

In general, tumors causing precocious puberty should be removed if they are surgically accessible. There are a number of agents used to medically treat precocious puberty. True (gonadotropin-dependent) precocious puberty treatment is long-acting GnRH agonists. Although initially these agents stimulate gonadotropin secretion, ultimately, GnRH receptors are downregulated, and LH and FSH secretion is subsequently reduced. GnRH agonists include deslorelin, buserelin, nafarelin, leuprolide, and triptorelin.

Other medications are used in the medical treatment of incomplete precocious puberty. Medroxyprogesterone acetate, a progestational agent, can halt the progression of secondary sexual characteristic development and can prevent menstruation. Ketoconazole is an antifungal agent that also inhibits the synthesis of testosterone by blocking the conversion of 17-hydroxyprogesterone to androstenedione. Testolactone competitively inhibits the aromatase enzyme that converts androgens to estrogens. Androgen antagonists include cyproterone acetate and spironolactone.

CARCINOID TUMORS

Carcinoid tumors comprise less than 0.1% of tumors identified at one large pediatric cancer center,[126] though they account for 34% of the primary solid tumors of the colon and rectum.[127] These tumors arise from amine uptake and decarboxylation cells, and are usually classified according to their site of origin as foregut, midgut, or hindgut carcinoids.[128] Foregut tumors can arise in the bronchus, stomach, or duodenum. Midgut tumors account for 80% to 85% of carcinoid tumors. The majority of carcinoids arise from the appendix (46%), followed by the jejunum and ileum (28%). Hindgut tumors are most commonly located in the rectum (17%). Carcinoid tumors are also found in the biliary ductal system and in ovarian teratomas.

Most patients present with vague symptoms. Only 10% of patients have symptoms of carcinoid syndrome (flushing, diarrhea, abdominal pain, asthma, and right-sided cardiac valvular problems).[129] Carcinoids are detected incidentally in up to 60% of patients, usually after appendectomy for acute appendicitis.

Most children are seen with appendiceal carcinoids smaller than 2 cm (Fig. 76-9). These can be treated with

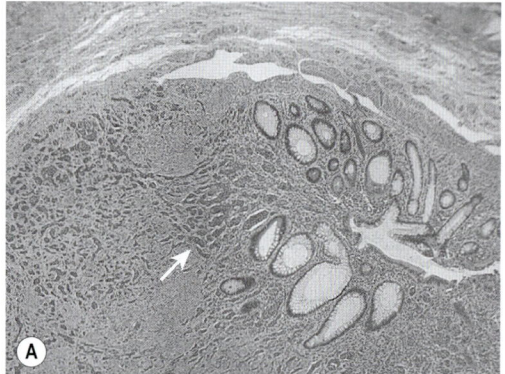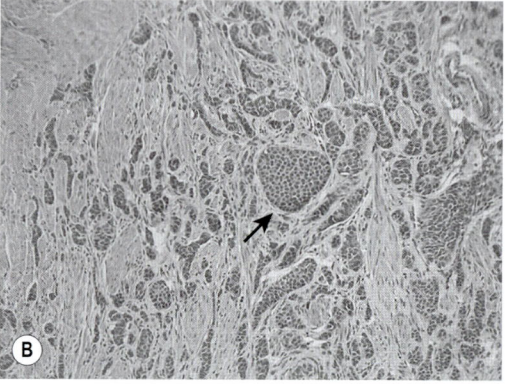

FIGURE 76-9 ■ These two histologic photomicrographs depict a carcinoid tumor of the appendix. **(A)** Lower-power view shows the nests of neuroendocrine cells (arrow) that are seen invading the muscularis mucosa. **(B)** Higher-power view shows the solid islands or nests (arrow) of uniform oval to polygonal cells with minimal pleomorphism. There are indistinct cellular borders and round uniform nucleoli with finely granular diffuse chromatin and inconspicuous nucleoli. Mitotic figures are rare.

simple appendectomy.[127]Right hemicolectomy is indicated for tumors larger than 2 cm, close to the cecum, or with mucin production. Metastases are rare, but regular follow-ups with measurement of serotonin and chromogranin A is important.[130] Treatment of metastatic disease includes hepatic chemoembolization and resection of isolated hepatic metastases. Long-acting octreotide or ^{131}I-MIBG is used for widely metastatic disease.[131]

Carcinoids are fairly indolent tumors. In one retrospective series of 40 children with appendiceal carcinoids, no recurrences or metastases were reported.[132] The site of origin has universally been shown to predict survival, with the appendix having the best survival and the midgut or hindgut having the worst.

The most common pulmonary tumor is the bronchial carcinoid. These most frequently appear with recurrent or persistent pneumonia secondary to bronchial obstruction from the tumor. Usually these tumors excrete low levels of serotonin. Children commonly present with wheezing, atelectasis, and weight loss. Also, they can have cough, pneumonitis, and hemoptysis, symptoms that are frequently seen in adults. Bronchial carcinoids can be diagnosed by bronchoscopy. They have a characteristic pink, friable, mulberry appearance. Due to this classic appearance and their propensity to bleed, biopsy is not recommended. If there is no evidence of lymph node involvement, segmental bronchial resection can be performed. However, lobectomy or pneumonectomy is often required for treatment. These tumors are radiosensitive and radiation therapy can be considered for unresectable disease. The prognosis after complete resection is excellent, with a 10-year survival rate of approximately 90%.[133,134]

REFERENCES

1. Rallison ML, Dobyns BM, Meikle AW, et al. Natural history of thyroid abnormalities: Prevalence, incidence, and regression of thyroid diseases in adolescents and young adults. Am J Med 1991;91:363–70.
2. Davies L, Welch HG. Increasing incidence of thyroid cancer in the United States, 1973–2002. JAMA 2006;295:2164–7.
3. Brent GA. The molecular basis of thyroid hormone action. N Engl J Med 1994;331:847–53.
4. Jaksic J, Dumic M, Filipovic B, et al. Thyroid diseases in a school population with thyromegaly. Arch Dis Child 1994;70:103–6.
5. Fisher DA, Pandian MR, Carlton E. Autoimmune thyroid disease: An expanding spectrum. Pediatr Clin North Am 1987;34:907–18.
6. Dayan CM, Daniels GH. Chronic autoimmune thyroiditis. N Engl J Med 1996;335:99–107.
7. Rother KI, Zimmerman D, Schwenk WF. Effect of thyroid hormone treatment on thyromegaly in children and adolescents with Hashimoto disease. J Pediatr 1994;124:599–601.
8. Phillips DI, Barker DJ, Rees Smith B, et al. The geographical distribution of thyrotoxicosis in England according to the presence or absence of TSH-receptor antibodies. Clin Endocrinol (Oxf) 1985;23:283–7.
9. Bahn RS, Burch HB, Cooper DS, et al. Hyperthyroidism and other causes of thyrotoxicosis: Management guidelines of the American Thyroid Association and American Association of Clinical Endocrinologists. Endocr Pract 2011;17:456–520.
10. Lippe BM, Landaw EM, Kaplan SA. Hyperthyroidism in children treated with long term medical therapy: Twenty-five percent remission every two years. J Clin Endocrinol Metab 1987;64:1241–5.
11. Lang BH, Wong IO, Wong KP, et al. Risk of second primary malignancy in differentiated thyroid carcinoma treated with radioactive iodine therapy. Surgery 2012;151:844–50.
12. Waldhausen JH. Controversies related to the medical and surgical management of hyperthyroidism in children. Semin Pediatr Surg 1997;6:121–7.
13. Franklyn JA. The management of hyperthyroidism. N Engl J Med 1994;330:1731–8.
14. Hung W, Anderson KD, Chandra RS, et al. Solitary thyroid nodules in 71 children and adolescents. J Pediatr Surg 1992;27:1407–9.
15. Desjardins JG, Khan AH, Montupet P, et al. Management of thyroid nodules in children: A 20-year experience. J Pediatr Surg 1987;22:736–9.
16. Cooper DS, Doherty GM, Haugen BR, et al. Revised American Thyroid Association management guidelines for patients with thyroid nodules and differentiated thyroid cancer. Thyroid 2009;19:1167–214.
17. Corrias A, Einaudi S, Chiorboli E, et al. Accuracy of fine needle aspiration biopsy of thyroid nodules in detecting malignancy in childhood: Comparison with conventional clinical, laboratory, and imaging approaches. J Clin Endocrinol Metab 2001;86:4644–8.
18. Izquierdo R, Shankar R, Kort K, et al. Ultrasound-guided fine-needle aspiration in the management of thyroid nodules in children and adolescents. Thyroid 2009;19:703–5.
19. Yip FW, Reeve TS, Poole AG, et al. Thyroid nodules in childhood and adolescence. Aust N Z J Surg 1994;64:676–8.
20. Hogan AR, Zhuge Y, Perez EA, et al. Pediatric thyroid carcinoma: Incidence and outcomes in 1753 patients. J Surg Res 2009;156:167–72.
21. Grigsby PW, Gal-or A, Michalski JM, et al. Childhood and adolescent thyroid carcinoma. Cancer 2002;95:724–9.
22. Lazar L, Lebenthal Y, Steinmetz A, et al. Differentiated thyroid carcinoma in pediatric patients: Comparison of presentation and course between pre-pubertal children and adolescents. J Pediatr 2009;154:708–14.
23. Nikiforov Y, Gnepp DR. Pediatric thyroid cancer after the Chernobyl disaster. Pathomorphologic study of 84 cases (1991-1992) from the Republic of Belarus. Cancer 1994;74:748–66.
24. Rice HE, Frush DP, Farmer D, et al. Review of radiation risks from computed tomography: Essentials for the pediatric surgeon. J Pediatr Surg 2007;42:603–7.
25. Pearce MS, Salotti JA, Little MP, et al. Radiation exposure from CT scans in childhood and subsequent risk of leukaemia and brain tumours: A retrospective cohort study. Lancet 2012;380:499–505.
26. Smith MB, Xue H, Strong L, et al. Forty-year experience with second malignancies after treatment of childhood cancer: Analysis of outcome following the development of the second malignancy. J Pediatr Surg 1993:1342–8.
27. Taylor AJ, Croft AP, Palace AM, et al. Risk of thyroid cancer in survivors of childhood cancer: Results from the British Childhood Cancer Survivor Study. Int J Cancer 2009;125:2400–5.
28. Diesen DL, Skinner MA. Pediatric thyroid cancer. Semin Pediatr Surg 2012;21:44–50.
29. Lemoine NR, Mayall ES, Wyllie FS, et al. Activated ras oncogenes in human thyroid cancers. Cancer Res 1988;48:4459–63.
30. Lemoine NR, Mayall ES, Wyllie FS, et al. High frequency of ras oncogene activation in all stages of human thyroid tumorigenesis. Oncogene 1989;4:159–64.
31. Bongarzone I, Butti MG, Coronelli S, et al. Frequent activation of ret protooncogene by fusion with a new activating gene in papillary thyroid carcinomas. Cancer Res 1994;54:2979–85.
32. Eng C, Smith DP, Mulligan LM, et al. Point mutation within the tyrosine kinase domain of the RET proto-oncogene in multiple endocrine neoplasia type 2B and related sporadic tumours. Hum Mol Genet 1994;3:237–41.
33. Bonora E, Tallini G, Romeo G. Genetic predisposition to familial nonmedullary thyroid cancer: An update of molecular findings and state-of-the-art studies. J Oncol 2010:385–6.
34. Scholz S, Smith JR, Chaignaud B, et al. Thyroid surgery at Children's Hospital Boston: A 35-year single-institution experience. J Pediatr Surg 2011;46:437–42.
35. Roy R, Kouniavsky G, Schneider E, et al. Predictive factors of malignancy in pediatric thyroid nodules. Surgery 2011;150:1228–33.
36. Horvath E, Majlis S, Rossi R, et al. An ultrasonogram reporting system for thyroid nodules stratifying cancer risk for clinical management. J Clin Endocrinol Metab 2009;94:1748–51.

37. Hung W. Solitary thyroid nodules in 93 children and adolescents. A 35-years experience. Horm Res 1999;52:15–18.

38. Hung W, Sarlis NJ. Current controversies in the management of pediatric patients with well-differentiated nonmedullary thyroid cancer: A review. Thyroid 2002;12:683–702.

39. Haveman JW, van Tol KM, Rouwe CW, et al. Surgical experience in children with differentiated thyroid carcinoma. Ann Surg Oncol 2003;10:15–20.

40. Enomoto Y, Enomoto K, Uchino S, et al. Clinical features, treatment, and long-term outcome of papillary thyroid cancer in children and adolescents without radiation exposure. World J Surg 2012;36:1241–6.

41. Zimmerman D, Hay ID, Gough IR, et al. Papillary thyroid carcinoma in children and adults: Long-term follow-up of 1039 patients conservatively treated at one institution during three decades. Surgery 1988;104:1157–66.

42. La Quaglia MP, Corbally MT, Heller G, et al. Recurrence and morbidity in differentiated thyroid carcinoma in children. Surgery 1988;104:1149–56.

43. de Roy van Zuidewijn DB, Songun I, Kievit J, et al. Complications of thyroid surgery. Ann Surg Oncol 1995;2:56–60.

44. Nishida T, Nakao K, Hamaji M, et al. Preservation of recurrent laryngeal nerve invaded by differentiated thyroid cancer. Ann Surg 1997;226:85–91.

45. Wells SA Jr, Farndon JR, Dale JK, et al. Long-term evaluation of patients with primary parathyroid hyperplasia managed by total parathyroidectomy and heterotopic autotransplantation. Ann Surg 1980;192:451–8.

46. Skinner MA, Norton JA, Moley JF, et al. Heterotopic autotransplantation of parathyroid tissue in children undergoing total thyroidectomy. J Pediatr Surg 1997;32:510–13.

47. Vassilopoulou-Sellin R, Klein MJ, Smith TH, et al. Pulmonary metastases in children and young adults with differentiated thyroid cancer. Cancer 1993;71:1348–52.

48. Iyer NG, Morris LG, Tuttle RM, et al. Rising incidence of second cancers in patients with low-risk (T1N0) thyroid cancer who receive radioactive iodine therapy. Cancer 2011;117:4439–46.

49. Kirk JM, Mort C, Grant DB, et al. The usefulness of serum thyroglobulin in the follow-up of differentiated thyroid carcinoma in children. Med Pediatr Oncol 1992;20:201–8.

50. Hay ID, Gonzalez-Losada T, Reinalda MS, et al. Long-term outcome in 215 children and adolescents with papillary thyroid cancer treated during 1940 through 2008. World J Surg 2010; 34:1192–202.

51. Samaan NA, Draznin MB, Halpin RE, et al. Multiple endocrine syndrome type IIb in early childhood. Cancer 1991;68:1832–4.

52. Gorlin JB, Sallan SE. Thyroid cancer in childhood. Endocrinol Metab Clin North Am 1990;19:649–62.

53. Kloos RT, Eng C, Evans DB, et al. Medullary thyroid cancer: Management guidelines of the American Thyroid Association. Thyroid 2009;19:565–612.

54. Skinner MA, Moley JA, Dilley WG, et al. Prophylactic thyroidectomy in multiple endocrine neoplasia type 2A. N Engl J Med 2005;353:1105–13.

55. Szinnai G, Meier C, Komminoth P, et al. Review of multiple endocrine neoplasia type 2A in children: Therapeutic results of early thyroidectomy and prognostic value of codon analysis. Pediatrics 2003;111:E132–9.

56. Wells SA Jr, Chi DD, Toshima K, et al. Predictive DNA testing and prophylactic thyroidectomy in patients at risk for multiple endocrine neoplasia type 2A. Ann Surg 1994;220:237–47.

57. Skinner MA, DeBenedetti MK, Moley JF, et al. Medullary thyroid carcinoma in children with multiple endocrine neoplasia types 2A and 2B. J Pediatr Surg 1996;31:177–81.

58. Telander RL, Zimmerman D, van Heerden JA, et al. Results of early thyroidectomy for medullary thyroid carcinoma in children with multiple endocrine neoplasia type 2. J Pediatr Surg 1986;21:1190–4.

59. Wiersinga WM. Thyroid cancer in children and adolescents–consequences in later life. J Pediatr Endocrinol Metab 2001;5:1289–96.

60. Ross AJ 3rd. Parathyroid surgery in children. Prog Pediatr Surg 1991;26:48–59.

61. Li CC, Yang C, Wang S, et al. A 10-year retrospective study of primary hyperparathyroidism in children. Exp Clin Endocrinol Diabetes 2012;120:229–33.

62. Howe JR, Norton JA, Wells SA Jr. Prevalence of pheochromocytoma and hyperparathyroidism in multiple endocrine neoplasia type 2A: Results of long-term follow-up. Surgery 1993;114:1070–7.

63. Ross AJ 3rd, Cooper A, Attie MF, et al. Primary hyperparathyroidism in infancy. J Pediatr Surg 1986;21:493–9.

64. Kulczycha H, Kaminski W, Wozniewicz B, et al. Primary hyperparathyroidism in infancy: Diagnostic and therapeutic difficulties. Klin Padiatr 1991;84:116–18.

65. Palazzo FF, Delbridge LW. Minimal-access/minimally invasive parathyroidectomy for primary hyperparathyroidism. Surg Clin North Am 2004;84:717–34.

66. Coakley AJ, Kettle AG, Wells CP, et al. 99Tcm sestamibi–a new agent for parathyroid imaging. Nucl Med Commun 1989;10:791–4.

67. McBiles M, Lambert AT, Cote MG, et al. Sestamibi parathyroid imaging. Semin Nucl Med 1995;25:221–34.

68. Arici C, Cheah WK, Ituarte PH, et al. Can localization studies be used to direct focused parathyroid operations? Surgery 2001;129:720–9.

69. Garner SC, Leight GS Jr. Initial experience with intraoperative PTH determinations in the surgical management of 130 consecutive cases of primary hyperparathyroidism. Surgery 1999;126:1132–7.

70. Burke JF, Scheider DF, Nichol PF, et al. Analysis of intraoperative parathyroid hormone levels in children: Does standard protocol apply? Presented at the 2012 AAP Meeting.

71. Pollak MR, Brown EM, Chou YH, et al. Mutations in the human Ca(2+)-sensing receptor gene cause familial hypocalciuric hypercalcemia and neonatal severe hyperparathyroidism. Cell 1993; 75:1297–303.

72. Sucheston ME, Cannon MS. Development of zonular patterns in the human adrenal gland. J Morphol 1968;126:477–91.

73. Graham LS. Celiac accessory adrenal glands. Cancer 1953;6:149–52.

74. Grumbach MM, Biller BM, Braunstein GD, et al. Management of the clinically inapparent adrenal mass ('incidentaloma'). Ann Intern Med 2003;138:424–9.

75. Masiakos PT, Gerstle JT, Cheang T, et al. Is surgery necessary for incidentally discovered adrenal masses in children? J Pediatr Surg 2004;39:754–8.

76. Stewart JN, Flageole H, Kavan P. A surgical approach to adrenocortical tumors in children: The mainstay of treatment. J Pediatr Surg 2004;39:759–63.

77. Cushing H. The basophil adenomas of the pituitary body and their clinical manifestations. Bull Johns Hopkins Hospital. 1932;50:137–95.

78. Devoe DJ, Miller WL, Conte FA, et al. Long-term outcome in children and adolescents after transsphenoidal surgery for Cushing's disease. J Clin Endocrinol Metab 1997;82:3196–202.

79. Nieman LK, Biller BM, Findling JW, et al. The diagnosis of Cushing's syndrome: An Endocrine Society Clinical Practice Guideline. J Clin Endocrinol Metab 2008;93:1526–40.

80. Newell-Price J, Trainer P, Besser M, et al. The diagnosis and differential diagnosis of Cushing's syndrome and pseudo-Cushing's states. Endocr Rev 1998;19:647–72.

81. Styne DM, Grumbach MM, Kaplan SL, et al. Treatment of Cushing's disease in childhood and adolescence by transsphenoidal microadenomectomy. N Engl J Med 1984;310:889–93.

82. Chudler RM, Kay R. Adrenocortical carcinoma in children. Urol Clin North Am 1989;16:469–79.

83. Gatta-Cherifi B, Chabre O, Murat A, et al. Adrenal involvement in MEN1. Analysis of 715 cases from the Groupe d'etude des Tumeurs Endocrines database. Eur J Endocrinol 2012;166:269–79.

84. Al Fehaily M, Duh QY. Clinical manifestation of aldosteronoma. Surg Clin North Am 2004;84:887–905.

85. IPEG guidelines for the surgical treatment of adrenal masses in children. J Laparoendosc Adv Surg Tech A 2010;20:vii–ix.

86. St Peter SD, Valusek PA, Hill S, et al. Laparoscopic adrenalectomy in children: A multicenter experience. J Laparoendosc Adv Surg Tech A 2011;21:647–9.

87. Bernstein L, Gurney JG. Carcinomas and other malignant epithelial neoplasms. In: Ries LAG, Smith MA, Gurney JG, et al, editors. Cancer and survival among children and adolescents:

United States SEER program 1975-1995. Bethesda, MD: 1999. p. 139–47.

88. Sutter JA, Grimberg A. Adrenocortical tumors and hyperplasias in childhood–etiology, genetics, clinical presentation and therapy. Pediatr Endocrinol Rev 2006;4:32–9.

89. Soon PS, McDonald KL, Robinson BG, Sidhu SB. Molecular markers and the pathogenesis of adrenocortical cancer. Oncologist 2008;13:548–61.

90. Liou LS, Kay R. Adrenocortical carcinoma in children. Review and recent innovations. Urol Clin North Am 2000;27:403–21.

91. Fottner C, Hoeflich A, Wolf E, et al. Role of the insulin-like growth factor system in adrenocortical growth control and carcinogenesis. Horm Metab Res 2004;36:397–405.

92. Ilvesmaki V, Kahri AI, Miettinen PJ, et al. Insulin-like growth factors (IGFs) and their receptors in adrenal tumors: High IGF-II expression in functional adrenocortical carcinomas. J Clin Endocrinol Metab 1993;77:852–8.

93. Michalkiewicz E, Sandrini R, Figueiredo B, et al. Clinical and outcome characteristics of children with adrenocortical tumors: A report from the International Pediatric Adrenocortical Tumor Registry. J Clin Oncol 2004;22:838–45.

94. Hayles AB, Hahn HB Jr, Sprague RG, et al. Hormone-secreting tumors of the adrenal cortex in children. Pediatrics 1966;37: 19–25.

95. Stewart DR, Jones PH, Jolleys A. Carcinoma of the adrenal gland in children. J Pediatr Surg 1974;9:59–67.

96. Neblett WW, Frexes-Steed M, Scott HW Jr. Experience with adrenocortical neoplasms in childhood. Am Surg 1987;53: 117–25.

97. Prando A, Wallace S, Marins JL, et al. Sonographic findings of adrenal cortical carcinomas in children. Pediatr Radiol 1990;20: 163–5.

98. Glazer GM. MR imaging of the liver, kidneys, and adrenal glands. Radiology 1988;166:303–12.

99. Gross MD, Shapiro B, Francis IR, et al. Scintigraphic evaluation of clinically silent adrenal masses. J Nucl Med 1994;35:1145–52.

100. Thrall JH, Freitas JE, Beierwaltes WH. Adrenal scintigraphy. Semin Nucl Med 1978;8:23–41.

101. Cohn K, Gottesman L, Brennan M. Adrenocortical carcinoma. Surgery 1986;100:1170–7.

102. Lombardi CP, Raffaelli M, Boniardi M, et al. Adrenocortical carcinoma: Effect of hospital volume on patient outcome. Langenbecks Arch Surg 2012;397:201–7.

103. Grubbs EG, Callender GG, Xing Y, et al. Recurrence of adrenal cortical carcinoma following resection: Surgery alone can achieve results equal to surgery plus mitotane. Ann Surg Oncol 2010; 17:263–70.

104. Hutter AM Jr, Kayhoe DE. Adrenal cortical carcinoma. Results of treatment with o,p'DDD in 138 patients. Am J Med 1966; 41:581–92.

105. Mayer SK, Oligny LL, Deal C, et al. Childhood adrenocortical tumors: Case series and reevaluation of prognosis–a 24-year experience. J Pediatr Surg 1997;32:911–15.

106. Teinturier C, Pauchard MS, Brugieres L, et al. Clinical and prognostic aspects of adrenocortical neoplasms in childhood. Med Pediatr Oncol 1999;32:106–11.

107. Macfarlane DA. Cancer of the adrenal cortex; the natural history, prognosis and treatment in a study of fifty-five cases. Ann R Coll Surg Engl 1958;23:155–86.

108. Sabbaga CC, Avilla SG, Schulz C, et al. Adrenocortical carcinoma in children: Clinical aspects and prognosis. J Pediatr Surg 1993;28:841–3.

109. Manger WM. An overview of pheochromocytoma: History, current concepts, vagaries, and diagnostic challenges. Ann N Y Acad Sci 2006;1073:1–20.

110. Lenders JW, Eisenhofer G, Mannelli M, et al. Phaeochromocytoma. Lancet 2005;366:665–75.

111. Ross JH. Pheochromocytoma. Special considerations in children. Urol Clin North Am 2000;27:393–402.

112. Januszewicz P, Wieteska-Klimczak A, Wyszynska T. Pheochromocytoma in children: Difficulties in diagnosis and localization. Clin Exp Hypertens A 1990;12:571–9.

113. Waguespack SG, Rich T, Grubbs E, et al. A current review of the etiology, diagnosis, and treatment of pediatric pheochromocytoma and paraganglioma. J Clin Endocrinol Metab 2010;95: 2023–37.

114. Pacak K, Eisenhofer G, Ahlman H, et al. Pheochromocytoma: Recommendations for clinical practice from the First International Symposium. October 2005. Nat Clin Pract Endocrinol Metab 2007;3:92–102.

115. Quint LE, Glazer GM, Francis IR, et al. Pheochromocytoma and paraganglioma: Comparison of MR imaging with CT and I-131 MIBG scintigraphy. Radiology 1987;165:89–93.

116. Kercher KW, Novitsky YW, Park A, et al. Laparoscopic curative resection of pheochromocytomas. Ann Surg 2005;241:919–26.

117. Miller KA, Albanese C, Harrison M, et al. Experience with laparoscopic adrenalectomy in pediatric patients. J Pediatr Surg 2002; 37:979–82.

118. Skarsgard ED, Albanese CT. The safety and efficacy of laparoscopic adrenalectomy in children. Arch Surg 2005;140:905–8.

119. Armstrong R, Sridhar M, Greenhalgh KL, et al. Phaeochromocytoma in children. Arch Dis Child 2008;93:899–904.

120. Caty MG, Coran AG, Geagen M. Current diagnosis and treatment of pheochromocytoma in children. Experience with 22 consecutive tumors in 14 patients. Arch Surg 1990;125:978–81.

121. Neumann HP, Bender BU, Reincke M, et al. Adrenal-sparing surgery for phaeochromocytoma. Br J Surg 1999;86:94–7.

122. Safford SD, Coleman RE, Gockerman JP, et al. Iodine -131 metaiodobenzylguanidine is an effective treatment for malignant pheochromocytoma and paraganglioma. Surgery 2003;134:956–62.

123. Sisson JC, Shapiro B, Shulkin BL, et al. Treatment of malignant pheochromocytomas with 131-I metaiodobenzylguanidine and chemotherapy. Am J Clin Oncol 1999;22:364–70.

124. Gonias S, Goldsby R, Matthay KK, et al. Phase II study of high-dose [131I]metaiodobenzylguanidine therapy for patients with metastatic pheochromocytoma and paraganglioma. J Clin Oncol 2009;27:4162–8.

125. Rosenfield RL. Puberty and its disorders in girls. Endocrinol Metab Clin North Am 1991;20:15–42.

126. Spunt SL, Pratt CB, Rao BN, et al. Childhood carcinoid tumors: The St Jude Children's Research Hospital experience. J Pediatr Surg 2000;35:1282–6.

127. Yang R, Cheung MC, Zhuge Y, et al. Primary solid tumors of the colon and rectum in the pediatric patient: A review of 270 cases. J Surg Res 2010;161:209–16.

128. Stinner B, Kisker O, Zielke A, et al. Surgical management for carcinoid tumors of small bowel, appendix, colon, and rectum. World J Surg 1996;20:183–8.

129. Onaitis MW, Kirshbom PM, Hayward TZ, Quayle FJ, et al. Gastrointestinal carcinoids: Characterization by site of origin and hormone production. Ann Surg 2000;232:549–56.

130. Doede T, Foss HD, Waldschmidt J. Carcinoid tumors of the appendix in children–epidemiology, clinical aspects and procedure. Eur J Pediatr Surg 2000;10:372–7.

131. Safford SD, Coleman RE, Gockerman JP, et al. Iodine-131 metaiodobenzylguanidine treatment for metastatic carcinoid. Results in 98 patients. Cancer 2004;101:1987–93.

132. Parkes SE, Muir KR, al Sheyyab M, et al. Carcinoid tumours of the appendix in children 1957-1986: Incidence, treatment and outcome. Br J Surg 1993;80:502–4.

133. Wang LT, Wilkins EW Jr, Bode HH. Bronchial carcinoid tumors in pediatric patients. Chest 1993;103:1426–8.

134. Hancock BJ, Di Lorenzo M, Youssef S, et al. Childhood primary pulmonary neoplasms. J Pediatr Surg 1993;28:1133–6.

CHAPTER 77

Bariatric Surgery in Adolescents

Sean J. Barnett • Thomas H. Inge

Childhood obesity continues to be an increasingly prevalent and progressive disease with limited treatment options. Not only have increasing numbers of children and adolescents been affected, but the average weight of obese children continues to soar. In the USA alone, it is estimated that approximately 4% (over 2 million children and teens) are extremely obese (BMI > 99th percentile).[1] Evidence from clinical trials show that behavioral weight management may have longer-lasting effects in younger children compared with adults, but good long-term outcomes are rare. These conventional treatment approaches are not effective for most who suffer with severe obesity,[2-5] leading to the consideration of surgical weight loss options for select adolescents. A number of important factors must be considered when contemplating bariatric operations in adolescents. Surgical weight loss results in significant improvement, if not resolution, of most obesity-related comorbidity in adults.[6] Short-term results suggest that this also is true for adolescents,[7-11] but little is known about long-term efficacy and potential adverse consequences to an adolescent with the lifelong restriction of calories and certain micronutrients. The issue of recidivism and the potential multigenerational consequences necessitate that considerable care and deliberation be applied to decision-making concerning surgical weight management in this population.

DEFINITIONS

Obesity specifically refers to the condition of having excess body fat. Measurement of body mass index (BMI) is a reasonably accurate method for predicting adiposity, is reproducible in the clinical setting, and can be used as a screening tool.[12-15] In children and adolescents, physiologic increases in adiposity, height, and weight during growth are expected. Given that childhood obesity is a global problem, it should be noted that there are ethnic and racial variations in onset, prevalence, and severity of the metabolic consequences of childhood obesity. Growth charts that are typically used to define obesity are age and gender specific.[16-18]

The terms overweight (BMI for age and gender >85th percentile), obese (BMI for age and gender >95th percentile), and extreme obesity (BMI for age and gender >99th percentile) have been used to refer to the increasing weight problem in children.[18-20] The 85th and 95th percentiles of BMI for age were chosen mainly because these percentile boundaries approximate the BMI in young adults of 25 kg/m^2 (overweight) and 30 kg/m^2 (obese), respectively. Whereas more than 32% of adults in the USA are obese, about 18% of children and adolescents are obese, a prevalence that has more than tripled in the past two decades.[1,21] Regarding extreme obesity, adolescent boys and most adolescent girls younger than age 18 with a BMI of 35 kg/m^2 are above the 99th BMI percentile.[1,18] Increasing metabolic risks associated with higher BMI for age, especially greater than or equal to the 99th BMI percentile, have been found when compared with lower levels of obesity.[1] In addition, because all children with a BMI above the 99th percentile become obese adults (BMI ≥30 kg/m^2) and because obese adults who were obese as children have more health complications and a higher mortality,[1,22,23] bariatric surgical procedures in the mature adolescent may be a reasonable option for weight reduction that may well reduce the risk of obesity-related morbidity and early mortality.[24]

CONSEQUENCES OF ADOLESCENT OBESITY

Adolescent obesity is a multifaceted disease with serious immediate, intermediate, and long-term consequences.[25,26] Critical periods exist between preconception and adolescence during which the risk of development of obesity is increased.[27] Important risk factors for childhood and adolescent obesity are (1) low birth weight;[28-31] (2) bottle feeding;[32,33] (3) early adiposity rebound;[34-38] (4) having a diabetic mother;[39,40] (5) puberty;[41-43] and (6) parental obesity.[44-47] Knowledge of these risk factors for adolescent obesity gives insight into the genetic and environmental factors that result in obesity. With few exceptions, little understanding exists about which risk factors portend the development of extreme obesity.[48-50]

Associated with the remarkable increase in the prevalence of pediatric obesity is a parallel increase in the severity of obesity and in obesity-related chronic diseases. These diseases have an onset at a younger age and carry an increased risk for adult morbidity and mortality.[51-55] Childhood obesity has adverse social and economic consequences.[56-58] Numerous comorbid conditions exist in childhood obesity, affecting every major organ system.

GUIDELINES FOR PERFORMING BARIATRIC SURGICAL PROCEDURES IN ADOLESCENCE

Patient Selection Criteria

National Institutes of Health (NIH) guidelines suggest that it is reasonable to consider weight loss surgery for adults with a BMI of 35 kg/m^2 or greater in the presence of severe obesity-related comorbidities (e.g., sleep apnea, diabetes, joint disease severe enough to require joint replacement) or a BMI of 40 kg/m^2 in the presence or absence of comorbidities.[59] Although these criteria have remained unchanged since 1991, investigators at several institutions have used lower BMI guidelines for studying the effect of weight loss surgery on adults without adverse consequences. Data support the use of lowered BMI guidelines for patients with severe comorbidities, such as type 2 diabetes, which are responsive to weight loss.[60]

Recently published best practice guidelines consider a BMI greater than or equal to 35 kg/m^2 with significant comorbidities or BMI of 40 kg/m^2 with other comorbidities as factors to be used in the selection of adolescents who are most likely to benefit from bariatric surgical procedures.[61] Physical maturity should be documented by either history and physical examination or radiographic study, thus generally limiting surgery to those individuals over the age of 12 years.

Specifically, when a teenager has reached physical maturity and has achieved a BMI greater than or equal to 35 kg/m^2 with serious obesity-related comorbidity, and surgical therapy will be predictably successful in reversing the obesity and comorbidity, it is reasonable to consider a surgical treatment before adulthood. This is the case for adolescents with type 2 diabetes mellitus, pseudotumor cerebri, sleep apnea (apnea–hypopnea index >15), and severe steatohepatitis. For adolescents with less severe comorbidities or risk factors for long-term diseases, for which there is no disadvantage of waiting until adulthood, it is recommended that a BMI of 40 kg/m^2 be used as a threshold for operative intervention. These comorbidities include, among others, mild obstructive sleep apnea syndrome (OSAS), hypertension, milder forms of obstructive sleep apnea (OSA), impaired quality of life, insulin resistance, glucose intolerance, or dyslipidemia.[61] Figure 77-1 outlines a suggested algorithm for management.

Bariatric Programs for Adolescents

For highly motivated adolescents with comorbid conditions (Box 77-1) who have been unsuccessful with prior dedicated attempts at weight loss (generally at least 6 months), bariatric surgery should be considered as a therapeutic option. Young patients being considered for

BOX 77-1	Obesity-Related Conditions that may Be Improved with Bariatric Surgical Procedures

SERIOUS CONDITIONS

Type 2 diabetes mellitus
Obstructive sleep apnea
Pseudotumor cerebri

LESS SERIOUS CONDITIONS

Hypertension
Dyslipidemias
Nonalcoholic steatohepatitis
Venous stasis disease
Significant impairment in activities of daily living
Intertriginous soft tissue infections
Stress urinary incontinence
Gastroesophageal reflux disease
Weight-related arthropathies that impair physical activity
Obesity-related psychosocial distress

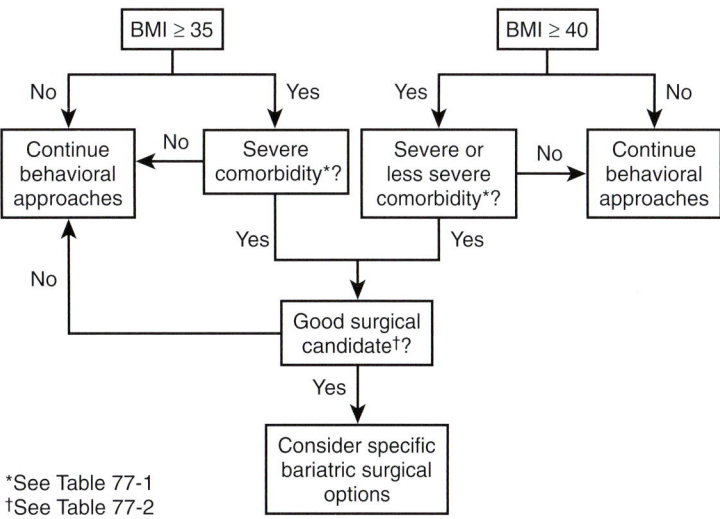

FIGURE 77-1 ■ Algorithm of management strategies for the severely obese adolescent.

*See Table 77-1
†See Table 77-2

bariatric surgical procedures should be referred to a specialized center with a multidisciplinary bariatric team with pediatric expertise. Such a team is equipped for the sometimes difficult patient selection decisions and can provide long-term follow-up and management of the unique challenges posed by the severely obese adolescent. Guidelines have been established by the American Society for Bariatric Surgery (ASBS) (www.asbs.org), and the American College of Surgeons (ACS) that define such teams to include specialists with expertise in obesity evaluation and management, psychology, nutrition, physical activity, and bariatric surgical treatment.[62] Depending on the individual needs of the adolescent patient, additional expertise in general pediatrics, adolescent medicine, endocrinology, pulmonology, gastroenterology, cardiology, orthopedics, and ethics should be readily available. At Cincinnati Children's Hospital, the patient review process is similar to that used in our multidisciplinary oncology and transplant programs.[63] This review by a panel of experts from various disciplines results in specific treatment recommendations for individual patients, including appropriateness and timing of possible operative intervention.

Factors Influencing Timing of Surgery

Physical Maturation

The timing for surgical treatment of extremely obese adolescents remains controversial and depends, in most cases, on the compelling health needs of the patient. However, certain physiologic factors must be considered in treatment planning. There is a theoretical concern about the impact of significant caloric restriction on the attainment of a genetically predetermined adult stature. Physiologic maturation is generally complete by sexual maturation (Tanner) stage 4.[64] Skeletal maturation (adult stature) is normally attained by the age of 13 to 14 years in girls and 15 to 16 years in boys.[65] Overweight children generally experience accelerated onset of puberty. As a result, they are likely to be taller and have advanced bone age compared with age-matched nonobese children.

If uncertainty exists about whether adult stature has been attained, skeletal maturation (bone age) can be objectively assessed with a radiograph of the hand and wrist.[66] If an individual has attained more than 95% of adult stature, it is unlikely that a bariatric procedure would significantly impair completion of linear growth.[67] For those who have not yet reached or nearly reached their predicted adult stature, one must balance the risks of growth delay due to caloric restriction against the potentially more significant risks of progression of obesity-related comorbid conditions if surgery is delayed.

Psychological Maturation

Adolescent psychological development also impacts the ability to participate in surgical decision-making and postoperative dietary compliance. Cognitive development refers to the development of the ability to think and reason. At any given age, adolescents are at varying stages of cognitive, psychosocial, and biologic maturity. The

BOX 77-2	Suggested Attributes of A 'Good' Adolescent Bariatric Candidate

- Patient is motivated and has good insight
- Patient has realistic expectations
- Family support and commitment are present
- Patient is compliant with health care commitments
- Family and patient understand that long-term lifestyle changes are needed
- Patient agrees to long-term follow-up
- Decisional capacity is present
- Weight loss attempts are well documented and at least temporarily successful
- No major psychiatric disorders are evident that may complicate postoperative regimen adherence
- No major conduct/behavioral problems are noted
- No substance abuse has occurred in the preceding year
- No plans for pregnancy are present in the upcoming two years

more mature adolescent who can reason and think abstractly is better able to consider the consequences of taking or not taking nutritional supplements or of following and adhering to the prescribed medical and nutritional regimens that are necessary for lifelong success (e.g., maintenance of weight loss and prevention of avoidable nutritional complications) after bariatric procedures.[68]

Before any decision for an operation is made, all candidates should undergo a comprehensive psychological evaluation.[69] Goals of this evaluation include:

- To determine the level of cognitive and psychosocial development, primarily to judge the extent to which the adolescent is capable of participating in the decision to proceed with the intervention
- To identify past and present psychiatric, emotional, behavioral, or eating disorders
- To define potential support for, or barriers to, regimen compliance, the family readiness for surgical treatment, and the required lifestyle changes (particularly if one or both parents are obese)
- To assess reasoning and problem-solving ability
- To assess whether reasonable outcome expectations exist
- To assess family unit stability and identify psychological stressors or conflicts within the family
- To determine whether the adolescent is autonomously motivated to consider bariatric surgical treatment or whether any element of coercion is present
- To assess weight-related quality of life status.

Unfortunately, no 'relative value scale' exists that would enable one to assign appropriate significance to the wealth of information (subjective and objective) obtained in the psychological evaluation. However, during a comprehensive assessment, we have found that a complete psychological assessment is very helpful for team decision-making and that generally good team agreement is reached about whether a particular patient has a majority (or conversely a minority) of the attributes of a good candidate for bariatric surgery (Box 77-2).

SURGICAL OPTIONS

In 1991, the NIH Bariatric Consensus Development Conference established parameters that led to a more uniform application of bariatric operations for adults. After that conference, an increase in the use of these procedures occurred. This conference concluded that, at that time, insufficient data existed to make recommendations about bariatric surgical treatment for patients younger than 18 years. Fortunately, outcome data are emerging for the adolescent age group, and adolescent bariatric research is now receiving some attention at the NIH. Indeed, multiple studies with an adolescent bariatric focus have now been funded by the National Institute of Diabetes and Digestive and Kidney Diseases to examine various outcomes of adolescent weight loss surgery. The largest and most comprehensive study to date, a multicenter research consortium called Teen-Longitudinal Assessment of Bariatric Surgery (TEEN-Labs), has been formed that includes investigators at Cincinnati Children's Hospital, Texas Children's Hospital, Children's Hospital of Alabama, Nationwide Children's Hospital, and the University of Pittsburgh. Recruitment for this study is now complete with the anticipation of numerous outcome papers to be published from the data set in the very near future. More information about this research consortium can be obtained on the website www.cchmc.org/teen-LABS.

Of the many procedures that have been advocated for weight loss, the operations that have been used primarily can be classified as either purely restrictive or a combination of restriction and malabsorption (Fig. 77-2). The laparoscopic adjustable gastric band (AGB) and laparoscopic vertical sleeve gastrectomy (LSG) are purely restrictive procedures, and the degree of weight loss with these operations in adults has generally been satisfactory. The LSG is a relatively new operation that produces significant initial weight loss with low operative risk in both adult[70,71] and pediatric studies.[72] Because it likely does not affect micronutrient absorption, it may be a safe alternative with fewer nutritional risks than Roux-en-Y gastric bypass (RYGB), and also may avoid device-related long-term risks inherent in the AGB procedure.

There are good reasons to think that adolescents may be better served by purely restrictive options such as the AGB[73] (Figs 77-3 and 77-4) or LSG[72] (Figs 77-5 and 77-6). Although nutritional deficiencies are not as likely to develop from the purely restrictive operations as compared with diversionary operations (gastric bypass, duodenal switch), these operations still impair overall energy intake significantly. This may lead to impaired intake of important vitamins and minerals if not adequately supplemented. With operations that do not transect the gastrointestinal tract, there is less risk and a reportedly lower mortality risk compared with gastric bypass.[74] A specific patient group for which one might suspect that a purely restrictive operation would be well suited is the younger adolescent, or even preadolescent, with a significant, progressive comorbid condition (e.g., type 2 diabetes, OSAS, or pseudotumor cerebri). However, these patients have the greatest potential for noncompliance with postoperative nutritional recommendations.

The AGB is not currently approved by the USA Food and Drug Administration (FDA) for patients younger than 18 years of age. A randomized control trial from Australia demonstrated a modest amount of weight loss at two years when compared to lifestyle intervention (BMI reduction of 28% vs 3%) but noted a high (33%) rate of reoperation.[75] The theoretical benefits of non-transectional operations are lost when considering LSG owing to the long staple line. Both the AGB and the LSG must be viewed as procedures with less than adequate long-term outcome data in the adolescent population. Any patient undergoing these operations must be carefully counseled about the unknown long-term efficacy. Clinical outcome data is currently being collected prospectively to enable objective assessment of efficacy and safety.

The RYGB (Figs 77-7 to 77-9) consists of both a restrictive pouch and a mildly malabsorptive component (the bypass of the stomach and duodenum). Moreover, it also offers an additional negative reinforcement of 'dumping syndrome' in some patients, providing excellent weight loss in adolescents and adults.[76] The partial biliopancreatic bypass with duodenal switch is primarily a malabsorptive procedure that results in good weight loss for adults with the highest classes of obesity (generally >60 kg/m² BMI), but with higher risks of operative complications and postoperative nutritional problems. Thus, the duodenal switch is not widely recommended for adolescents.

Regardless of the procedure used, surgeons and allied health personnel new to the field should, at a minimum, undergo a basic training course offered by one of the professional surgical organizations (ASBS, ACS, or the Society of American Gastrointestinal Endoscopic Surgeons). Before performing laparoscopic bariatric operations, surgeons must meet all local credentialing requirements for the performance of bariatric procedures and advanced laparoscopic operations. Credentialing guidelines for both open and laparoscopic bariatric procedures have been outlined previously.[77-81]

PERIOPERATIVE AND SURGICAL MANAGEMENT

Preoperative Education and Management

The multidisciplinary preoperative evaluation that leads to the decision to offer surgical treatment is followed by considerable patient and family preoperative education. It is important that this process is organized and not rushed because patients must comprehend a great deal of information about the postoperative anatomic and physiologic changes that impact success as well as the risks for the short- and long-term complications. This process generally lasts a minimum of 6 months. Patients may also benefit from discussion with others who have undergone surgical treatment. At our institution, we find that support groups involving the patient's own peers at various stages of the process provides the most benefit. In the weeks before the operation, a final outpatient visit for

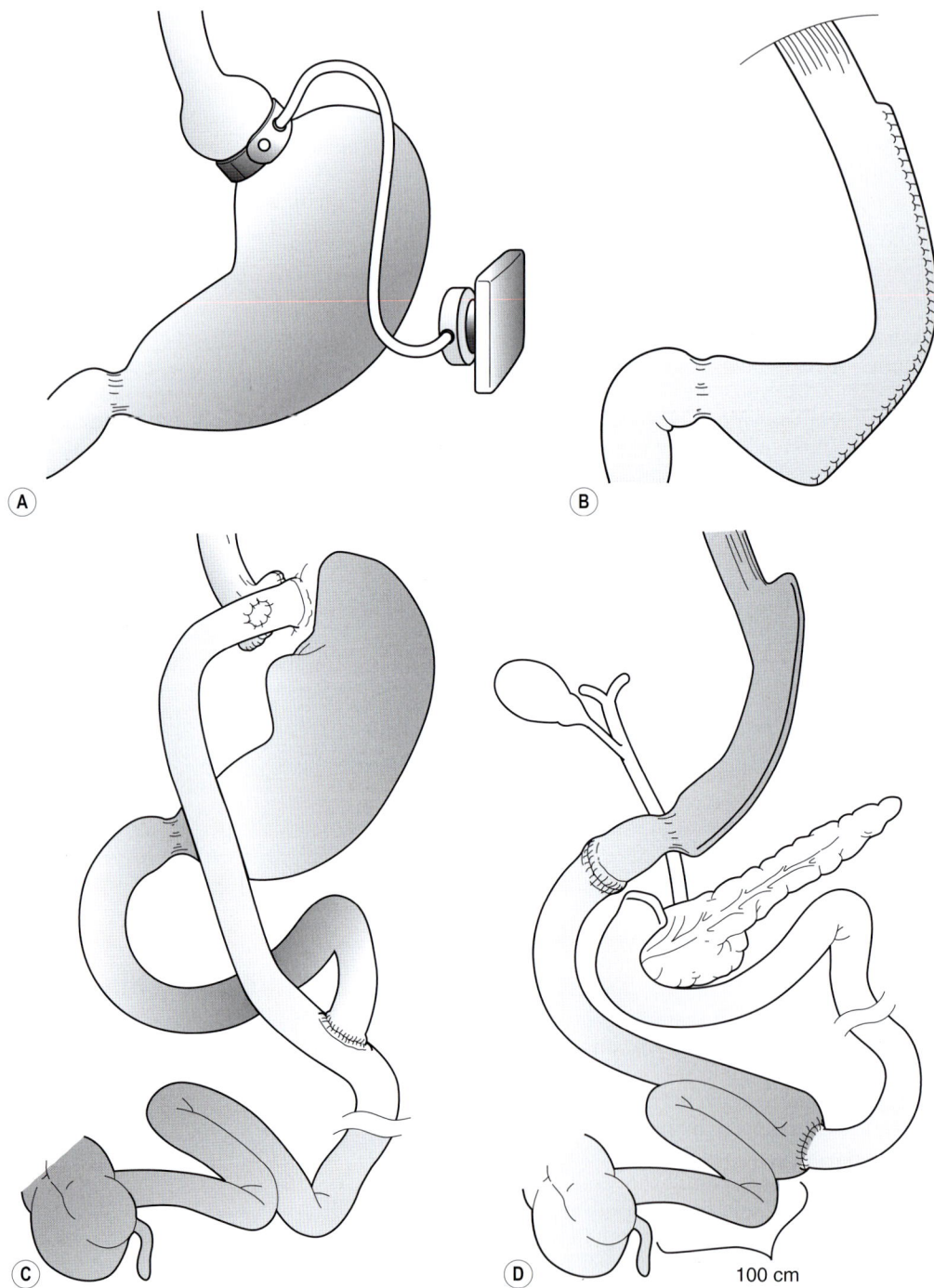

FIGURE 77-2 ■ Operative procedures for weight loss that are performed laparoscopically. **(A)** Adjustable gastric band (AGB). **(B)** Vertical sleeve gastrectomy (VSG). **(C)** Roux-en-Y gastric bypass (RYGB). **(D)** Duodenal switch operation.

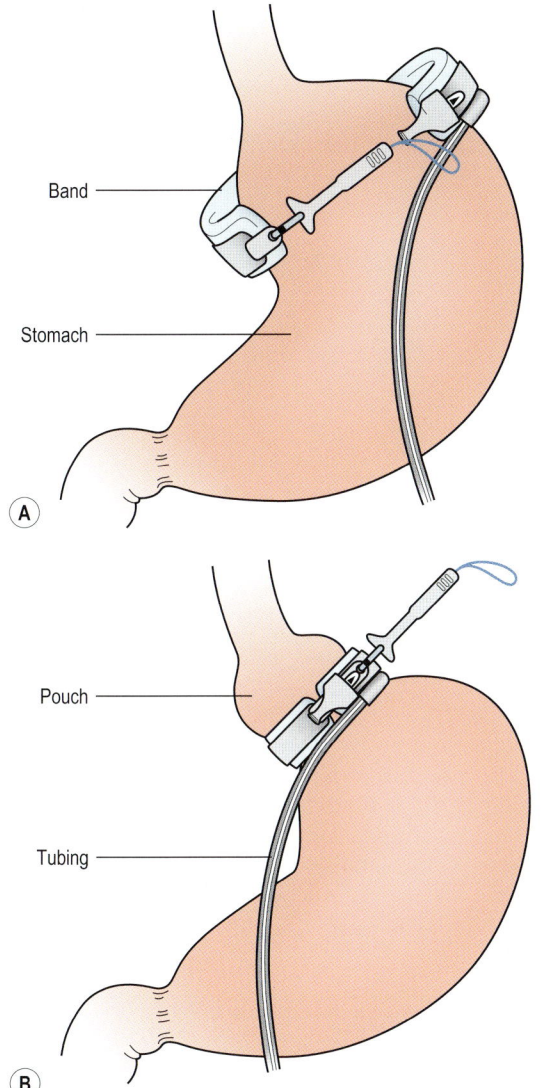

FIGURE 77-3 ■ **(A)** After careful dissection in the retrogastric space, the adjustable gastric band is pulled behind the stomach with a grasping instrument. **(B)** The instrument is then placed through the buckle, and the locking portion is grasped and pulled through the buckle and locked in place.

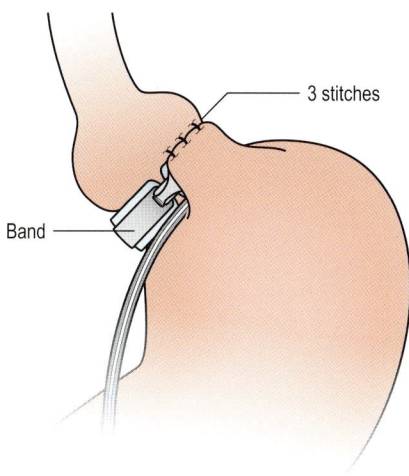

FIGURE 77-4 ■ Plication of the anterior wall of the stomach over the gastric band is accomplished with three or four sutures using 2-0 permanent suture. These sutures should be deep and full thickness. It is important to remove the orogastric tube before placement of these sutures so that the tube is not incorporated in these plication sutures.

anesthesiology consultation, final informed permission (consent) discussion, and final review of the postoperative regimen is scheduled.

During the evaluation of a potential surgical patient, studies include serum chemistry and liver profiles, lipid profile, complete blood cell count, hemoglobin A_{1C} level, fasting blood glucose levels, thyroid-stimulating hormone level, and *Helicobacter pylori* titers. If these titers are positive, a breath test is done to confirm or exclude active *H. pylori* infection. Formal esophagogastric duodenoscopy should be considered in those patients with significant gastroesophageal reflux disease symptoms, especially when considering LSG. An electrocardiogram can be obtained to screen for cardiac problems and dysrhythmias. For instance, prolonged QT syndrome exists in morbidly obese adolescent patients and may have been previously unrecognized. Because unrecognized sleep disorders are relatively prevalent in the severely obese, a complete sleep history is sought, including a history of snoring, irregular breathing, and increased daytime somnolence. A history suggestive of sleep apnea should prompt formal polysomnography. If the fasting glucose concentration is elevated, or if other symptoms of diabetes are found, patients should undergo a two hour glucose tolerance test to determine if more significant abnormalities of carbohydrate metabolism exist, including impaired glucose tolerance and type 2 diabetes.

Beginning a few days before the operation, the patients are limited to clear liquids. Low-molecular-weight heparin (40 mg injected subcutaneously) is administered in the preoperative holding area prior to surgery and continued twice daily postoperatively while in the hospital. A second-generation cephalosporin antibiotic (Cefoxitin) is administered within one hour of surgery. Sequential compression boots also are used intraoperatively and postoperatively. Most patients are candidates for laparoscopic procedures, although some of the heavier and centrally obese patients may present challenges, particularly in the early portion of a surgeon's learning curve.

General Aspects of Surgical Techniques for the Morbidly Obese

In general, an open laparotomy should be avoided in morbidly obese individuals due to difficulty with adequate visualization and the higher risk of wound complications. For initial abdominal access, we have found that a laparoscopically guided technique using a transparent, bladeless, 12 mm cannula is safe and effective. Alternatively, some surgeons prefer a blind puncture using the Veress needle in the left upper quadrant. To access the gastroesophageal junction for bariatric procedures, a wide variety of surgical instruments have been developed with the morbidly obese patient in mind. However, it

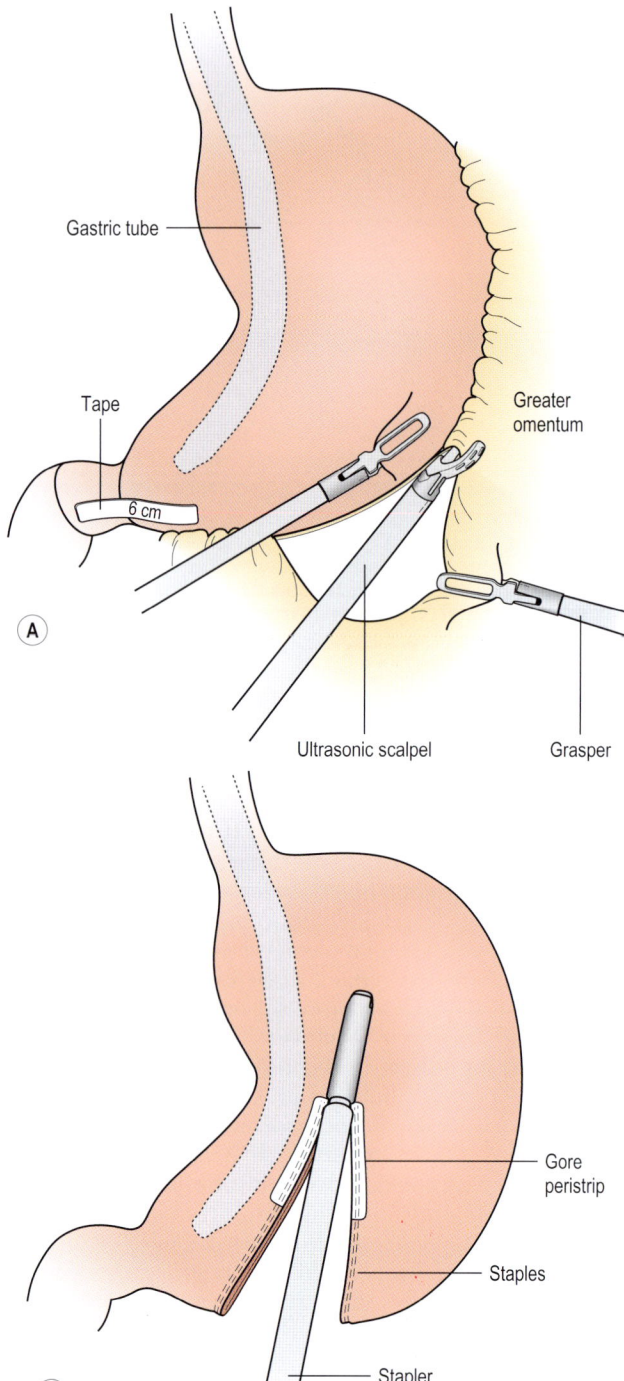

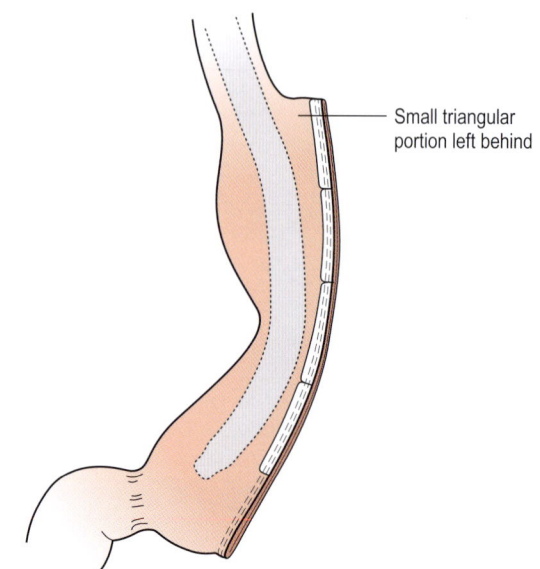

FIGURE 77-6 ■ The completed sleeve gastrectomy is seen. Note that a small triangle of stomach is left near the gastroesophageal junction to help prevent any inadvertent resection or encroachment on the esophagus.

FIGURE 77-5 ■ **(A)** For the LSG the greater omental attachments and the short gastric vessels are taken down along the entire extent of the greater curvature of the stomach using the ultrasonic scalpel. This dissection is started 6 cm from the end of the pylorus. **(B)** The endoscopic stapler, first using a green load and then a blue load, is used to ligate and divide the stomach. A 34 French bougie is inserted along the lesser curve of the stomach to act as a guide for resection.

should be noted that the majority of laparoscopic procedures in morbidly obese individuals can be efficiently and safely accomplished using standard adult 5 mm instrumentation. The details and nuances of the procedures used for adolescents can be obtained from a variety of excellent bariatric texts.[82,83]

POSTOPERATIVE MANAGEMENT

Postoperatively, the patients are placed in a monitored, nonintensive care unit setting, and maintenance fluids are administered based on lean body weight (typically 40–50% of actual weight). Early warning signs of complications include fever, tachycardia, tachypnea, increasing oxygen requirement, oliguria, hiccoughs, regurgitation, left shoulder pain, worsening abdominal pain, a feeling of anxiety, or an acute alteration in mental status. These signs warrant aggressive attention and appropriate investigation because they may signal a gastrointestinal leak, pulmonary embolus, bowel obstruction, or acute dilation and impending rupture of a bypassed gastric remnant. At our institution, a water-soluble upper gastrointestinal contrast study is obtained on postoperative day 1 for patients who have undergone RYGB, but not generally for LSG. After satisfactory passage of contrast is documented (RYGB) or on postoperative day number 1 (LSG), patients are begun on clear liquids and subsequently advanced to a high protein liquid diet for the first month after operation. Due to issues with nausea, especially in LSG, patients are aggressively treated with intravenous Ondansetron (4–8 mg per dose) and a scopolamine patch immediately postoperatively.

Bariatric operations reduce the intake and decrease the absorption of food rich in essential fatty acids, vitamins, and other specific nutrients, the long-term results of

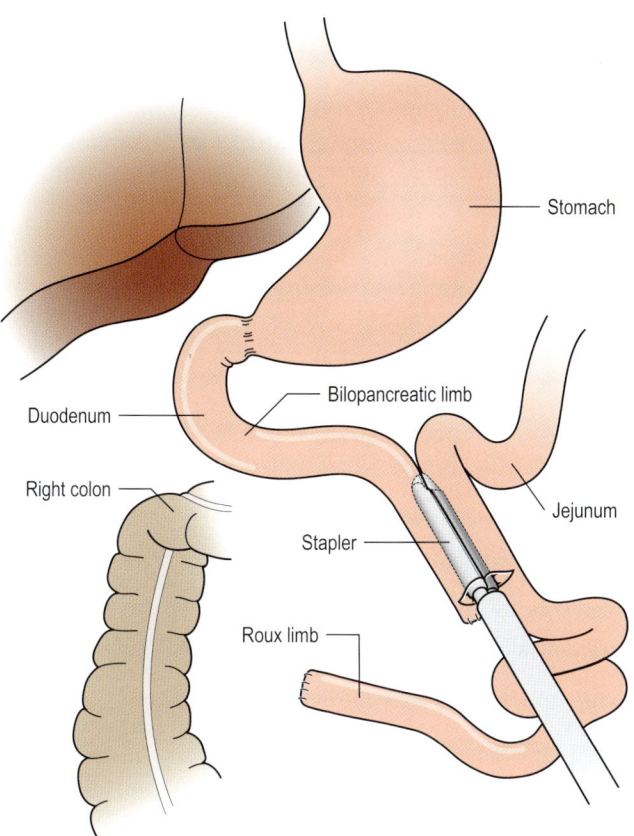

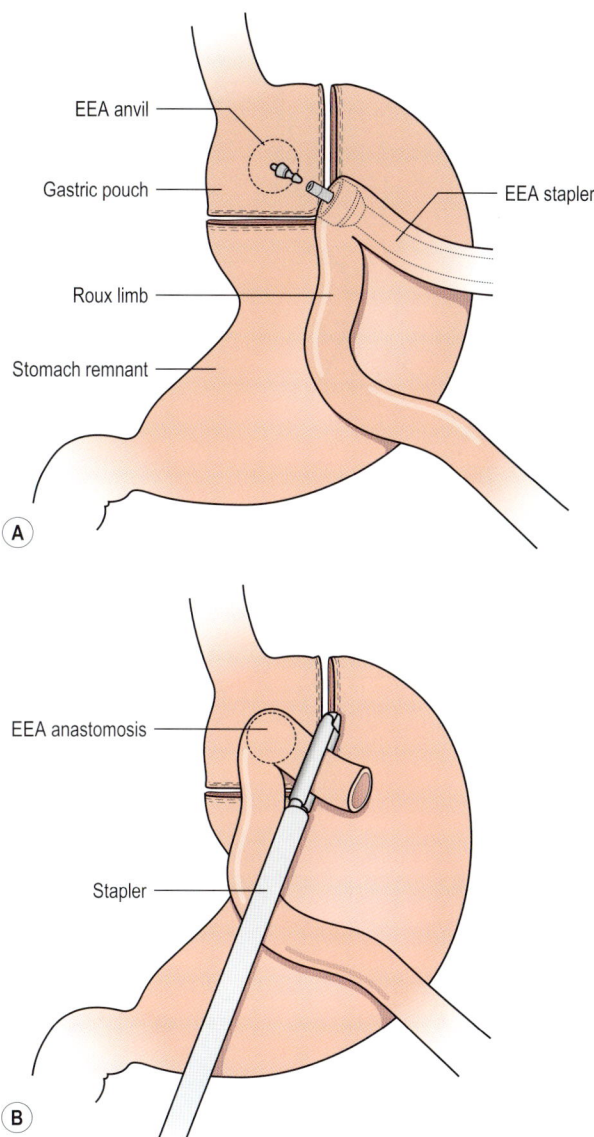

FIGURE 77-7 ■ For the RYGB, a jejunostomy is created with a linear stapler connecting a 50 cm bilopancreatic limb and 100–150 cm roux limb as shown. The mesenteric defect is then closed to prevent herniation of bowel through this space.

FIGURE 77-8 ■ **(A)** A 30 mL gastric pouch is created along the lesser curve of the stomach just beyond the gastroesophageal junction using a linear cutting stapler with the anvil of the 25 mm EEA stapler in place. The Roux limb is brought anterior to the colon and gastric remnant. The end of the Roux limb is then opened and the EEA stapler is introduced, extended, and then mated with the anvil as shown to perform the gastrojejunostomy. **(B)** The open end of the roux limb is then stapled closed, thus completing the gastrojejunostomy.

which are not well understood and are of legitimate concern. Poor nutrition during fetal development can result in a variety of adverse health outcomes, including future obesity, as suggested by the Dutch famine cohort.[28] Therefore, success in adolescent bariatric surgical treatment requires an expanded definition—not only sustained weight loss but also subsequent normal progression through the remainder of adolescence, adulthood, and eventually uncomplicated reproduction with normal offspring.

Nutritional and metabolic consequences of bariatric operations have been well delineated in adults[84–95] and adolescents.[96] To avoid nutritional complications, patients must adhere to procedure-specific guidelines for diet and vitamin/mineral supplementation. Restrictive procedures (including gastric bypass) essentially require a very low-calorie intake, thus requiring attention to an adequate (0.5 g/kg) daily protein intake to minimize lean mass loss during the rapid weight loss phase (generally the first postoperative year). Impaired absorption of iron, folate, calcium, and vitamin B12 may occur after gastric bypass.[87,96,97] Often obese adolescents will have vitamin deficiency even before operative intervention.[96,98] Even with postoperative supplementation, severe deficiencies can occur. Adolescence also may be a particular risk for thiamine deficiency.[99] In addition, poor postoperative compliance among adolescents who have undergone

bariatric operations has been reported.[100] As certain micronutrient deficiencies, such as folate and calcium, have established ramifications for the patient and potential offspring, both warrant special consideration.

Folate is a water-soluble B vitamin that is essential for growth, cell differentiation and embryonic morphogenesis, gene regulation, repair, and host defense.[101] Adequate maternal periconceptional folic acid consumption during critical periods of organ formation early in the first trimester may reduce the likelihood of fetal malformations, including neural tube defects and perinatal complications such as low birth weight, prematurity, and

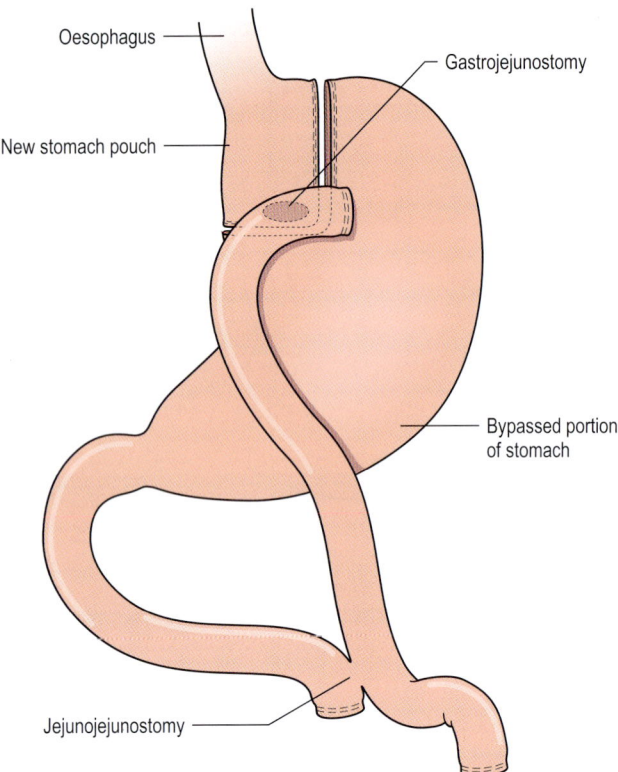

Oesophagus

Gastrojejunostomy

New stomach pouch

Bypassed portion of stomach

Jejunojejunostomy

FIGURE 77-9 ■ The Roux-en-Y gastric bypass consists of both a restrictive pouch size and a mildly malabsorptive component (the bypass of the stomach and duodenum). The gastric pouch is based on the lesser curve and is created using a 34 French orogastric tube as a guide. A 75–150 cm Roux limb is used in most patients.

placental abruption and infarction. This information is particularly relevant because the majority of adolescents seeking bariatric surgical treatment are girls, many of whom will want to be mothers. Thus, physicians caring for adolescents who undergo bariatric surgical procedures must stress the importance of daily folate and other B-complex vitamin intake. Moreover, patients should be monitored annually (and before planned conception) for serum vitamin levels, particularly when uncertainty about compliance exists.[101]

When compared to their obese counterparts, women who become pregnant after bariatric surgery appear to have improved fertility and lower maternal and neonatal complications.[102,103] There are no studies examining outcomes of pregnancy after bariatric operations in the adolescent population. However, unplanned adolescent pregnancy is a legitimate concern after massive weight loss.[104] We strongly recommend that all girls and caregivers are informed about increased fertility (a physiologic change due to increased insulin sensitivity) and the likelihood for increased risk-taking after surgical weight loss. These patients should be counseled to avoid pregnancy during the two-year period after operation and should be offered reliable contraception. The modern intrauterine devices are effective and safe, may be placed at the time of the bariatric operation, and are commonly used by our program.

Adolescence is a period of rapid skeletal mineral accretion and is, therefore, a window of opportunity to influence lifelong bone health, both positively and negatively. While obese adolescents have higher than average bone mineral density/content, they may well have less than normal bone mineral density and content for their weight. This may translate into greater risk for fractures.[105] Furthermore, impaired accretion of bone mineral content in adolescence increases the risk for osteoporosis and results in a two-fold greater risk of fracture in later life.[106] Given the impaired absorption of both vitamin D and calcium after bariatric surgical procedures and the large individual variation in bone accretion, it is essential to monitor closely the bone mineral density of adolescents undergoing bariatric procedures. Behavioral strategies can and should be used to encourage compliance with postoperative vitamin and mineral intake, which should positively influence nutritional outcomes after adolescent bariatric operations.[106]

Adolescent compliance may be enhanced by: (1) visual aids; (2) focus on immediate benefit from treatment; (3) participation in self-management; (4) self-monitoring; and (5) reinforcement (Box 77-3).[107] With the alterations in eating patterns required after bariatric surgical procedures, repetitive reinforcement is needed to facilitate the formation of lifelong health-promoting habits. The adolescent bariatric surgical program should build on the best practices of other adolescent disease-management programs. Success will be based on the premise that sustained weight control for the adolescent requires ongoing behavioral intervention, structured family involvement, and continued support.[106, 108–110]

LONG-TERM MANAGEMENT

Postoperative follow-up visits after adolescent bariatric operations are intensive but depend in part on the type of operation performed. For example, we see gastric bypass and sleeve gastrectomy patients at 2 weeks, 6

BOX 77-3 | **Strategies to Improve Postoperative Compliance**

- Rehearse the dietary regimen to enable preoperative problem identification and solving before the surgical intervention
- Use actual measuring cups, a food scale, and photographs of specific recommended food items to enhance the adolescent's ability to follow through with plans
- Provide the adolescent with a diet diary and exercise diary with form pages to fill out, and practice this preoperatively
- Provide a list of acceptable food items for every phase of the postoperative recovery (first week, second through fourth weeks, second through third months) including the caloric density and protein, carbohydrate, and fat content of the items to encourage label reading
- Provide a detailed listing of micronutritional supplements needed postoperatively, including why the supplement is needed and the potential consequences of not taking it

weeks, 3 months, 6 months, 12 months, 18 months, 24 months, and then annually following operation. Dietary advancement after the first month is a methodical process of introducing new items of gradually increasing complexity toward the goal of a well-balanced, small portion (approximately one cup per meal) diet, which includes the daily intake of 0.5–1 g of protein per kilogram of ideal weight. Nonsteroidal anti-inflammatory medications should be avoided to reduce the risk of intestinal ulceration and bleeding after gastric bypass. Ranitidine is often prescribed postoperatively and switched to a proton pump inhibitor if reflux symptoms persist. This is often seen following sleeve gastrectomy, but these patients can often be weaned off by 6 months. Postoperative vitamin and mineral supplementation typically consists of two pediatric chewable multivitamins, a calcium/vitamin D supplement, and an iron supplement for menstruating females (Table 77-1). Due to the severity of thiamine deficiency, additional B-complex vitamins beyond what is contained in multivitamin preparations should be given.[99] We routinely re-emphasize five basic 'rules' with each patient encounter: (1) eat protein first; (2) drink 64 to 96 ounces of water or sugar-free liquids daily; (3) do not snack between meals; (4) exercise 30 to 60 minutes per day; and (5) always remember vitamins and minerals.

Serum chemistries, complete blood cell count, and representative B-complex vitamin levels (e.g., B1, B12, folate) are obtained at 6 months and 12 months postoperatively, and then yearly. Body composition can be assessed preoperatively with either bioelectrical impedance or dual-energy X-ray absorptiometry (DEXA), and then on an annual basis after operation. DEXA not only allows for the measurement of the rate and relative amounts of fat and lean body mass loss, but also provides a quantitative assessment of bone mineral density changes.

OUTCOMES IN ADOLESCENTS

Results of RYGB have been retrospectively reviewed in small series of adolescents with generally satisfactory results.[76,111–121] However, a 14-year follow-up of a small cohort of nine patients demonstrating considerable late weight re-gain suggests that adolescents may require different selection criteria or postoperative management than adults to achieve optimal long-term weight loss outcomes.[7] A recent study from our institution demonstrated significant weight loss (decrease in BMI by 37% at one year) in patients following gastric bypass. It was noted that the timing of operation is an important consideration given that those patients with the highest BMI values, even with significant weight loss, still do not reach a nonobese nadir weight.[76]

Although the AGB is currently not approved by the FDA for adolescents younger than 18 years of age, there have been a few short-term studies. These studies show a modest amount of weight loss at 1 year, but long-term follow-up is lacking.[122–124] A randomized trial from Australia, discussed earlier, demonstrated a decrease in BMI by 28% at two years compared to 3% in those treated medically, but with a 33% re-operative rate.[75]

Results for adolescents undergoing sleeve gastrectomy are also scarce with one reasonable size study published to date.[72] This demonstrated comparable weight loss at 2 years to gastric bypass and an excellent safety profile. Although encouraging, more long-term studies are needed. The current TEEN-Labs trial hopes to answer many of the questions regarding all three operations while providing significant data in regards to the long-term weight loss and comorbidity reduction seen in these obese adolescents.

Supplement	Recommendation
Multivitamin (with folic acid)	One to two daily
Calcium citrate with vitamin D	1500–1800 mg/day
Vitamin D	1000 IU/day (if deficient preoperatively)
Vitamin B12	500 µg/day oral or 1000 µg/ month intramuscular
Elemental iron	65 mg elemental iron for menstruating females
Vitamin B1	Consider 50 mg daily in first 6 months
Vitamin A, K	Treat if symptomatic

TABLE 77-1 Recommended Nutritional Supplementation Following Weight Loss Surgery

Laboratories are checked at 6 months postoperatively and then yearly unless symptoms arise.
Adapted from Xanthakos SA. Nutritional deficiencies in obesity and after bariatric surgery. Pediatr Clin North Am 2009;56:1105–21.

REFERENCES

1. Freedman DS, Mei Z, Srinivasan SR, et al. Cardiovascular risk factors and excess adiposity among overweight children and adolescents: The Bogalusa Heart Study. J Pediatr 2007;150:12–17.
2. Epstein LH, Valoski A, Wing RR, et al. Ten-year follow-up of behavioral, family-based treatment for obese children. JAMA 1990;264:2519–23.
3. Yanovski JA. Intensive therapies for pediatric obesity. Pediatr Clin North Am 2001;48:1041–53.
4. Spear BA, Barlow SE, Ervin C, et al. Recommendations for treatment of child and adolescent overweight and obesity. Pediatrics 2007;120(Suppl 4):S254–88.
5. Hearnshaw C, Matyka K. Managing childhood obesity: When lifestyle change is not enough. Diabetes Obes Metab 2010; 12(11):947–57.
6. Wittgrove AC, Clark GW. Laparoscopic gastric bypass, Roux-en-Y in 500 patients: Technique and results, with 3–60 month follow-up. Obes Surg 2000;10:233–9.
7. Sugerman HJ, Sugerman EL, DeMaria EJ, et al. Bariatric surgery for severely obese adolescents. J Gastrointest Surg 2003;7:102–8.
8. Strauss RS, Bradley LJ, Brolin RE. Gastric bypass surgery in adolescents with morbid obesity. J Pediatr 2001;138:499–504.
9. Ippisch HM, Inge TH, Daniels SR, et al. Reversibility of cardiac abnormalities in morbidly obese adolescents. J Am Coll Cardiol 2008;51:1342–8.
10. Zeller MH, Noll JG, Long JD, Inge TH. Psychosocial functioning improves following adolescent bariatric surgery. Obesity 2009;17:985–90.
11. Inge TH, Miyano G, Bean J, et al. Reversal of type 2 diabetes mellitus and improvements in cardiovascular risk factors after surgical weight loss in adolescents. Pediatrics 2009;123:214–22.

12. Himes JH, Dietz WH. Guidelines for overweight in adolescent preventive services: Recommendations from an expert committee. The Expert Committee on Clinical Guidelines for Overweight in Adolescent Preventive Services. Am J Clin Nutr 1994;59: 307–16.

13. Daniels SR, Khoury PR, Morrison JA. The utility of body mass index as a measure of body fatness in children and adolescents: Differences by race and gender. Pediatrics 1997;99:804–7.

14. Pietrobelli A, Faith MS, Allison DB, et al. Body mass index as a measure of adiposity among children and adolescents: A validation study. J Pediatr 1998;132:204–10.

15. Dietz WH, Robinson TN. Use of the body mass index (BMI) as a measure of overweight in children and adolescents. J Pediatr 1998;132:191–3.

16. Cole TJ, Bellizzi MC, Flegal KM, et al. Establishing a standard definition for child overweight and obesity worldwide: International survey. BMJ 2000;320:1240–3.

17. Rolland-Cachera MF, Sempe M, Guilloud-Bataille M, et al. Adiposity indices in children. Am J Clin Nutr 1982;36: 178–84.

18. Flega KM, Wei R, Ogden CL, et al. Characterizing extreme values of body mass index-for-age by using the 2000 centers for disease control and prevention growth charts. Am J Clin Nutr 2009;90:1314–20.

19. Strauss RS, Pollack HA. Epidemic increase in childhood overweight, 1986–1998. JAMA 2001;286:2845–8.

20. Ogden CL, Flegal KM, Carroll MD, et al. Prevalence and trends in overweight among ultrasound children and adolescents, 1999–2000. JAMA 2002;288:1728–32.

21. Ogden CL, Carroll MD, Curtin LR, et al. Prevalence of overweight and obesity in the United States, 1999–2004. JAMA 2006;295:1549–55.

22. Whitaker RC, Wright JA, Pepe MS, et al. Predicting obesity in young adulthood from childhood and parental obesity. N Engl J Med 1997;337:869–73.

23. Vanhala M, Vanhala P, Kumpusalo E, et al. Relation between obesity from childhood to adulthood and the metabolic syndrome: Population-based study. BMJ 1998;317:319–20.

24. Inge TH. Bariatric surgery for morbidly obese adolescents: Is there a rationale for early intervention? Growth Horm IGF Res 2006;16:S15–9.

25. Must A, Strauss RS. Risks and consequences of childhood and adolescent obesity. Int J Obes Relat Metab Disord 1999;23: S2–11.

26. Nadler EP, Brotman LM, Miyoshi T, Fryer GE, Weitzman M. Morbidity in obese adolescents who meet the adult national institutes of health criteria for bariatric surgery. J Pediatr Surg 2009;44:1869–76.

27. Wahlqvist ML. Chronic disease prevention: A life-cycle approach which takes account of the environmental impact and opportunities of food, nutrition and public health policies—the rationale for an eco-nutritional disease nomenclature. Asia Pac J Clin Nutr 2002;11:S759–62.

28. Ravelli AC, van Der Meulen JH, Osmond C, et al. Obesity at the age of 50 y in men and women exposed to famine prenatally. Am J Clin Nutr 1999;70:811–6.

29. Parsons TJ, Power C, Logan S, et al. Childhood predictors of adult obesity: A systematic review. Int J Obes Relat Metab Disord 1999;23:S1–107.

30. Sorensen HT, Sabroe S, Rothman KJ, et al. Relation between weight and length at birth and body mass index in young adulthood: Cohort study. BMJ 1997;315:1137.

31. Wei JN, Li HY, Sung FC, et al. Birth weight correlates differently with cardiovascular risk factors in youth. Obesity (Silver Spring) 2007;15:1609–16.

32. Bergmann KE, Bergmann RL, Von Kries R, et al. Early determinants of childhood overweight and adiposity in a birth cohort study: Role of breast-feeding. Int J Obes Relat Metab Disord 2003;27:162–72.

33. Michels KB, Willett WC, Graubard BI, et al. A longitudinal study of infant feeding and obesity throughout life course. Int J Obes (Lond) 2007;31:1078–85.

34. He Q, Karlberg J. Probability of adult overweight and risk change during the BMI rebound period. Obes Res 2002;10: 135–40.

35. Cameron N, Demerath EW. Critical periods in human growth and their relationship to diseases of aging. Am J Phys Anthropol 2002;35:159–84.

36. Whitaker RC, Pepe MS, Wright JA, et al. Early adiposity rebound and the risk of adult obesity. Pediatrics 1998;101:E5.

37. Eriksson JG, Forsen T, Tuomilehto J, et al. Early adiposity rebound in childhood and risk of Type 2 diabetes in adult life. Diabetologia 2003;46:190–4.

38. Rolland-Cachera MF, Deheeger M, Bellisle F, et al. Adiposity rebound in children: A simple indicator for predicting obesity. Am J Clin Nutr 1984;39:129–35.

39. Silverman BL, Rizzo TA, Cho NH, et al. Long-term effects of the intrauterine environment. The Northwestern University Diabetes in Pregnancy Center. Diabetes Care 1998;21:B142–9.

40. Jouret B, Ahluwalia N, Cristini C, et al. Factors associated with overweight in preschool-age children in southwestern France. Am J Clin Nutr 2007;85:1643–9.

41. Caprio S. Insulin resistance in childhood obesity. J Pediatr Endocrinol Metab 2002;15:487–92.

42. Heald FP, Khan MA. Teenage obesity. Pediatr Clin North Am 1973;20:807–17.

43. Ong KK, Northstone K, Wells JC, et al. Earlier mother's age at menarche predicts rapid infancy growth and childhood obesity. PLoS Med 2007;4:e132.

44. Whitaker RC, Wright JA, Pepe MS, et al. Predicting obesity in young adulthood from childhood and parental obesity. N Engl J Med 1997;337:869–73.

45. Whitaker RC. Understanding the complex journey to obesity in early adulthood. Ann Intern Med 2002;136:923–5.

46. Durand EF, Logan C, Carruth A. Association of maternal obesity and childhood obesity: Implications for healthcare providers. J Community Health Nurs 2007;24:167–76.

47. Santiago S, Zazpe I, Cuervo M, Martinez JA. Perinatal and parental determinants of childhood overweight in 6–12 years old children. Nutr Hosp 2012;27:599–605.

48. Farooqi IS, O'Rahilly S. Recent advances in the genetics of severe childhood obesity. Arch Dis Child 2000;83:31–4.

49. Clement K, Boutin P, Froguel P. Genetics of obesity. Am J Pharmacogenomics 2002;2:177–87.

50. Haqq AM, Farooqi IS, O'Rahilly S, et al. Serum ghrelin levels are inversely correlated with body mass index, age, and insulin concentrations in normal children and are markedly increased in Prader-Willi syndrome. J Clin Endocrinol Metab 2003;88: 174–8.

51. Fontaine KR, Redden DT, Wang C, et al. Years of life lost due to obesity. JAMA 2003;289:187–93.

52. Must A, Jacques PF, Dallal GE, et al. Long-term morbidity and mortality of overweight adolescents: A follow-up of the Harvard Growth Study of 1922 to 1935. N Engl J Med 1992;327:1350–5.

53. Biro FM, Wien M. Childhood obesity and adult morbidities. Am J Clin Nutr 2010;91(Suppl.):S1499–505.

54. The N, Suchindran C, North KE, Popkin BM, Gordon-Larsen P. Association of adolescent obesity with risk of severe obesity in adulthood. JAMA 2010;304:2042–7.

55. Reilly JJ, Kelly J. Long-term impact of overweight and obesity in childhood and adolescence on morbidity and premature mortality in adulthood: Systematic review. Int J Obes (Lond) 2011;35(7): 891–8.

56. Strauss RS. Childhood obesity. Pediatr Clin North Am 2002; 49:175–201.

57. Gortmaker SL, Must A, Perrin JM, et al. Social and economic consequences of overweight in adolescence and young adulthood. N Engl J Med 1993;329:1008–12.

58. Wang G, Dietz WH. Economic burden of obesity in youths aged 6 to 17 years: 1979–1999. Pediatrics 2002;109:E81.

59. NIH conference: Gastrointestinal surgery for severe obesity. Consensus Development Conference Panel. Ann Intern Med 1991;115: 956–61.

60. O'Brien PE, Dixon JB, Laurie C, et al. Treatment of mild to moderate obesity with laparoscopic adjustable gastric banding or an intensive medical program: A randomized trial. Ann Intern Med 2006;144:625–33.

61. Pratt JS, Lenders CM, Dionne EA, et al. Best practice updates for pediatric/adolescent weight loss surgery. Obesity (Silver Spring) 2009;17(5):901–10.

62. Gastrointestinal surgery for severe obesity: National Institutes of Health Consensus Development Conference Statement. Am J Clin Nutr 1992;55:S615–19.

63. Inge TH, Garcia VF, Daniels SR, et al. A multidisciplinary approach to the adolescent bariatric surgical patient. J Pediatr Surg 2004;39:442–7.

64. Tanner JM. Growth at Adolescence. 2nd ed. Oxford: Blackwell Scientific Publications; 1962.

65. Marshall WA, Tanner JM. Variations in the pattern of pubertal changes in boys. Arch Dis Child 1970;45:13–23.

66. Greulich WW, Pyle SI. Radiographic Atlas of Skeletal Development of the Hand and Wrist. Palo Alto, CA: Stanford University Press; 1959.

67. Tanner JM. Assessment of Skeletal Maturity and Prediction of Adult Height (TW2 method). San Diego, CA: Academic Press; 1983.

68. Piaget J. The stages of the intellectual development of the child. Bull Menninger Clin 1962;26:120–8.

69. Greenberg I, Sogg S, Perna FM. Behavioral and psychological care in weight loss surgery: Best practice update. Obesity 2009; 17:880–4.

70. Aggarwal S, Kini SU, Herron DM. Laparoscopic sleeve gastrectomy for morbid obesity: A review. Surg Obes Relat Dis 2007;3: 189–94.

71. Cottam D, Qureshi FG, Mattar SG, et al. Laparoscopic sleeve gastrectomy as an initial weight-loss procedure for high-risk patients with morbid obesity. Surg Endosc 2006;20:859–63.

72. Alqahtani AR, Antonisamy B, Alamri H, et al. Laparoscopic sleeve gastrectomy in 108 obese children and adolescents aged 5 to 21 years. Ann Surg 2013;256:266–73.

73. Dolan K, Creighton L, Hopkins G, et al. Laparoscopic gastric banding in morbidly obese adolescents. Obes Surg 2003;13: 101–4.

74. Chapman A, Game P, O'Brien P, et al. Laparoscopic adjustable gastric banding for the treatment of obesity: A systematic literature review. Surgery 2004;135:326–51.

75. O'Brien PE, Sawyer SM, Laurie C, et al. Laparoscopic adjustable gastric banding in severely obese adolescents. JAMA 2010;303: 519–26.

76. Inge TH, Jenkins TM, Zeller M, et al. Baseline BMI is a strong predictor of nadir BMI after adolescent gastric bypass. J Pediatr 2010;156:103–8.

77. Martin LF, O'Leary JP. Standards of excellence for bariatric surgery: Great concept, but how? Obes Surg 1998;8:229–31.

78. Buchwald H. Mainstreaming bariatric surgery. Obes Surg 1999; 9:462–70.

79. Al-Saif O, Gallagher SF, Banasiak M, et al. Who should be doing laparoscopic bariatric surgery? Obes Surg 2003;13:82–7.

80. Guidelines for laparoscopic and open surgical treatment of morbid obesity: American Society for Bariatric Surgery and Society of American Gastrointestinal Endoscopic Surgeons. Obes Surg 2000;10:378–9.

81. Oria HE, Brolin RE. Performance standards in bariatric surgery. Eur J Gastroenterol Hepatol 1999;11:77–84.

82. Inge TH. Laparoscopic Roux-en-Y gastric bypass. In: Holcomb GW III, Georgeson KE, Rothenberg SS, editors. Atlas of Pediatric Laparoscopy and Thoracoscopy. Philadelphia: Elsevier; 2008. p. 181–7.

83. Barnett SJ, Inge TH. Bariatric surgery: Principles. In: Spitz L, Coran A, editors. Operative Pediatric Surgery. 7th ed. 2013.

84. Gollobin C, Marcus WY. Bariatric beriberi. Obes Surg 2002;12: 309–11.

85. Chaves LC, Faintuch J, Kahwage S, et al. A cluster of polyneuropathy and Wernicke-Korsakoff syndrome in a bariatric unit. Obes Surg 2002;12:328–34.

86. Amaral JF, Thompson WR, Caldwell MD, et al. Prospective hematologic evaluation of gastric exclusion surgery for morbid obesity. Ann Surg 1985;201:186–93.

87. Halverson JD. Vitamin and mineral deficiencies following obesity surgery. Gastroenterol Clin North Am 1987;16:307–15.

88. Halverson JD. Micronutrient deficiencies after gastric bypass for morbid obesity. Am Surg 1986;52:594–8.

89. MacLean LD, Rhode BM, Shizgal HM. Nutrition following gastric operations for morbid obesity. Ann Surg 1983; 198:347–55.

90. Mason EE. Starvation injury after gastric reduction for obesity. World J Surg 1998;22:1002–7.

91. Schilling RF, Gohdes PN, Hardie GH. Vitamin B12 deficiency after gastric bypass surgery for obesity. Ann Intern Med 1984;101: 501–2.

92. Boylan LM, Sugerman HJ, Driskell JA. Vitamin E, vitamin B-6, vitamin B-12, and folate status of gastric bypass surgery patients. J Am Diet Assoc 1988;88:579–85.

93. Lynch RJ, Eisenberg D, Bell RL. Metabolic consequences of bariatric surgery. J Clin Gastroenterol 2006;40:659–68.

94. Shikora SA, Kim JJ, Tarnoff ME. Nutrition and gastrointestinal complications of bariatric surgery. Nutr Clin Pract 2007;22: 29–40.

95. Tucker ON, Szomstein S, Rosenthal RJ. Nutritional consequences of weight-loss surgery. Med Clin North Am 2007;91:499–514.

96. Xanthakos SA. Nutritional deficiencies in obesity and after bariatric surgery. Pediatr Clin North Am 2009;56:1105–21.

97. Alvarez-Leite JI. Nutrient deficiencies secondary to bariatric surgery. Curr Opin Clin Nutr Metab Care 2004;7:569–75.

98. Carrodeguas L, Kaidar-Person O, Szomstein S, et al. Preoperative thiamine deficiency in obese population undergoing laparoscopic bariatric surgery. Surg Obes Relat Dis 2005;1: 517–22.

99. Towbin A, Inge TH, Garcia VF, et al. Beriberi after gastric bypass surgery in adolescence. J Pediatr 2004;145:263–7.

100. Rand CS, Macgregor AM. Adolescents having obesity surgery: A 6-year follow-up. South Med J 1994;87:1208–13.

101. Hall JG, Solehdin F. Folate and its various ramifications. Adv Pediatr 1998;45:1–35.

102. Guelinckx I, Devlieger R, Vansant G. Reproductive outcome after bariatric surgery: A critical review. Hum Reprod Update 2009;15: 189–201.

103. Maggard MA, Yermilov I. Pregnancy and fertility following bariatric surgery: A systematic review. JAMA 2008;300: 2286–96.

104. Roehrig HR, Xanthakos SA, Sweeney J, et al. Pregnancy after gastric bypass surgery in adolescents. Obes Surg 2007;17: 873–7.

105. Goulding A, Taylor RW, Jones IE, et al. Spinal overload: A concern for obese children and adolescents? Osteoporos Int 2002;13:835–40.

106. Wysocki T, Greco P, Harris MA, et al. Behavior therapy for families of adolescents with diabetes: Maintenance of treatment effects. Diabetes Care 2001;24:441–6.

107. In: Rapoff MA, et al, editors. Compliance with Pediatric Medical Regimens. New York: Raven Press; 1991.

108. Zeller MH, Guilfoyle SM, Reiter-Purtill J, et al. Adolescent bariatric surgery: Caregiver and family functioning across the first postoperative year. Surg Obes Relat Dis 2011;7:145–50.

109. Fielding D, Duff A. Compliance with treatment protocols: Interventions for children with chronic illness. Arch Dis Child 1999;80:196–200.

110. Rapoff MA. Assessing and enhancing adherence to medical regimens for juvenile rheumatoid arthritis. Pediatr Ann 2002;31: 373–9.

111. Jen HC, Rickard DG, Shew SB, et al. Trends and outcomes of adolescent bariatric surgery in California, 2005–2007. Pediatrics 2010;126:e746–53.

112. Breaux CW. Obesity surgery in children. Obes Surg 1995;5: 279–84.

113. Strauss RS, Bradley LJ, Brolin RE. Gastric bypass surgery in adolescents with morbid obesity. J Pediatr 2001;138:499–504.

114. Sugerman HJ, Sugerman EL, DeMaria EJ, et al. Bariatric surgery for severely obese adolescents. J Gastrointest Surg 2003;7: 102–7.

115. Greenstein RJ, Rabner JG. Is adolescent gastric-restrictive antiobesity surgery warranted? Obes Surg 1995;5:138–44.

116. Anderson AE, Soper RT, Scott DH. Gastric bypass for morbid obesity in children and adolescents. J Pediatr Surg 1980;15: 876–81.

117. Soper RT, Mason EE, Printen KJ, et al. Gastric bypass for morbid obesity in children and adolescents. J Pediatr Surg 1975;10: 51–8.

118. Rand CS, Macgregor AM. Adolescents having obesity surgery: A 6-year follow-up. South Med J 1994;87:1208–13.

119. Inge TH, Garcia V, Daniels S, et al. A multidisciplinary approach to the adolescent bariatric surgical patient. J Pediatr Surg 2004;39:442–7.

120. Lawson ML, Kirk S, Mitchell T, et al. One-year outcomes of Roux-en-Y gastric bypass for morbidly obese adolescents: A multicenter study from the Pediatric Bariatric Study Group. J Pediatr Surg 2006;41:137–43.

121. Barnett SJ, Stanley C, Hanlon M, et al. Long-term follow-up and the role of surgery in adolescents with morbid obesity. Surg Obes Relat Dis 2005;1:394–8.

122. Ananthapavan J, Moodie M, Haby M, et al. Assessing cost-effectiveness in obesity: Laparoscopic adjustable gastric banding for severely obese adolescents. Surg Obes Relat Dis 2010;6: 377–85.

123. Holterman AX, Browne A, Tussing L, et al. A prospective trial for laparoscopic adjustable gastric banding in morbidly obese adolescents: An interim report of weight loss, metabolic and quality of life outcomes. J Pediatr Surg 2010;45:74–8.

124. de la Cruz-Munoz N, Messiah SE, Cabrera JC, et al. Four-year weight outcomes of laparoscopic gastric bypass surgery and adjustable gastric banding among multiethnic adolescents. Surg Obes Relat Dis 2010;6:542–7.

CHAPTER 78

Evidence-Based Medicine

Shawn D. St. Peter

'In God we trust; all others must bring data.'
—W. EDWARDS DEMING, PHYSICIST AND QUALITY IMPROVEMENT PIONEER

Evidence-based medicine (EBM) is defined as the conscientious, explicit, and judicious use of the current best evidence in making decisions about the care of individual patients.[1] A simpler concept would be treating patients based on data rather than the surgeon's thoughts or beliefs. EBM represents the concept that medical practice can be largely dictated by evidence gained from the scientific method. Given that the practice of medicine has historically been based on knowledge handed down from mentor to apprentice, the concepts of EBM embody a new paradigm, replacing the traditional paradigm that was based on authority. In a global sense, it describes a methodology for evaluating the validity of clinical research and applying those results to the care of patients.

HISTORY

The initial groundwork forming the framework for EBM can be considered the earliest scientists who pursued explanatory truth instead of accepting beliefs. The process of discovering truth became replicable for aspiring scientists when the scientific method was developed. No one individual can be credited for creating the scientific method because it is the result of the progressive recognition for a natural process of acquiring facts. However, the earliest publication alluding to the steps of current scientific methodology may be found in Book of Optics published in 1021 by Ibn al-Haytham (Alhazen).[2] His investigations were based on experimental evidence. Furthermore, his experiments were systematic and repeatable as he demonstrated that rays of light are emitted from objects rather than from the eyes. In Western literature, Roger Bacon wrote about a repeating cycle of observation, hypothesis, and experimentation in the 1200s. Influenced by the contributions of many scientists and philosophers, Francis Bacon delineated a recognizable form of the scientific method in the 1620 publication of Novum Organum Scientificum.[3] He suggested that mastery of the world in which man lives is dependent on careful understanding. Moreover, this understanding is based entirely on the facts of this world and not, as the ancients portrayed it, in philosophy. Nearly 400 years later, we find ourselves coming to the same conclusions in the practice of medicine and surgery. We now understand that facts and truths transcend experience, and that facts about optimal care can be gained through experimentation more reliably than from beliefs generated through experience.

The establishment of the scientific method in the pursuit of proven truths was fundamental to the development of EBM as an entity. The current scientific method consists of several steps that are outlined in Box 78-1. However, the concepts of EBM are not simply encompassed by the application of these steps to attain facts, but also address the ability to understand the value of the results generated from experimentation. Under the auspices of EBM, investigators are burdened with the first five steps, from inquiry to experimentation, while all caregivers must develop a deep understanding of experimental methodology, analysis of data, and how conclusions are drawn to be able to place appropriate value on published studies to influence their practice.

The movement urging physicians to utilize proven facts in the development of decision-making algorithms began in 1972 with the publication of the revolutionary book Effectiveness and Efficiency: Random Reflections on Health Services.[4] The author, Archie Cochrane, a Scottish epidemiologist working in the UK National Health Service, has likely had the greatest influence on the development of an organized means of guiding care through data and results. The book demonstrates disdain for the scientific establishment, devalues expert opinion, and shows that physicians should systematically question what is the best care for the patient. Most impressively, Cochrane calls for an international registry of randomized controlled trials and for explicit quality criteria for appraising published research. At the time of his passing in 1988, these aspirations had not fully materialized. However, the field of medicine is fortunate that Cochrane's prophetic ideas have precipitated the maturation of centers of EBM research that make up the global not-for-profit organization called the Cochrane Collaboration. The product of this collaboration is The Cochrane Library, which is a collection of seven databases that contain high-quality, independent evidence to inform health care decision-making.[5] The most clinically utilized database is the Cochrane Database of Systematic Reviews containing reviews on the highest level of evidence on which to base clinical treatment decisions. There are now over 550,000 entries.

After Cochrane and other proponents of EBM showed the importance of comparative data, it took over a decade for the amorphous clouds of these concepts to solidify into tangible terms and usable methods. The methodology of

TABLE 78-1 **Levels of Evidence as Defined by the Oxford Centre for Evidence-Based Medicine**

Level	Type of Evidence
1a	Systematic review of randomized trials displaying homogeneity
1a–	Systematic review of randomized trials displaying worrisome heterogeneity
1b	Individual randomized controlled trials (with narrow confidence interval)
1b–	Individual randomized controlled trials (with a wide confidence interval)
1c	All or none randomized controlled trials
2a	Systematic reviews (with homogeneity) of cohort studies
2a–	Systematic reviews of cohort studies displaying worrisome heterogeneity
2b	Individual cohort study or low-quality randomized controlled trials (<80% follow-up)
2b–	Individual cohort study or low-quality randomized controlled trials (<80% follow-up/wide confidence interval)
2c	'Outcomes' research; ecological studies
3a	Systematic review (with homogeneity) of case-control studies
3a–	Systematic review of case-control studies with worrisome heterogeneity
3b	Individual case-control study
4	Case series (and poor quality cohort and case-control studies)
5	Expert opinion without explicit critical appraisal, or based on physiology, bench research, or 'first principles'

specifically qualifying data and judging the relative merits of available studies did not begin to appear in the literature until the early 1990s. In a paper published in 1990 by David Eddy on the role of guidelines in medical decision-making, the term evidence-based first appeared in the literature.[6] Much of the framework currently used to determine best available evidence was established by David Sackett and Gordon Guyatt at the McMaster University-based research group called the Evidence-Based Medicine Working Group. In 1992, JAMA published the group's landmark paper titled, 'Evidence-Based Medicine: A New Approach to Teaching the Practice of Medicine,' and the term evidence-based medicine was born.[7] A cementing moment in the paradigm shift occurred when the Centre for Evidence-Based Medicine was established in Oxford, England, in 1995 as the first of several centers. Over the past decade, centers or departments focusing on clinical research and EBM have been developed at universities and hospitals around the world, including our own (www.cmhclinicaltrials.com). EBM principles are now represented in the core curriculum that is integral to three of the six general competencies outlined by the Accreditation Council for Graduate Medical Education that oversees the accredited residency training programs in the United States. The concept of EBM is no longer a movement of progressive physicians, but rather a basic guiding principle of medical training and practice.

LEVELS OF EVIDENCE

Utilization of evidence in guiding health care decision-making requires an understanding of the merits of the evidence and the ability to decipher whether a given course of treatment has been proven superior. The quality of evidence specifically indicates the extent to which one can be confident that an estimate of effect is correct. Systems to stratify evidence by quality have been developed by several sources. Although there are specific differences in published rankings, the generally accepted levels in a broad sense are defined as follows:

Level 1—evidence is supported by prospective, randomized trials

Level 2—evidence is supported by cohort studies, outcomes data, or low-quality prospective trials

Level 3—evidence comprises case-control studies

Level 4—evidence is based on case series

Level 5—evidence is expert opinion or beliefs based on rational principles.

The quality of data that is conveyed within each level and study type is clearly a wide spectrum. The complete delineation in the levels of evidence as defined by the Oxford Centre for Evidence-Based Medicine is outlined in Table 78-1.

As can be seen by the levels listed in Table 78-1, the strength of evidence improves significantly by the application of prospective data collection. In clinical medicine, and particularly in the practice of surgery, many aspects of trial design are not feasible such as blinding, placebo treatments, independent follow-up evaluation, and others. However, if one accepts these limitations and conducts a trial with prospective evaluation, the results remain markedly more meaningful than a retrospective case-control comparative series that compares surgeons and/or timeframes against one another.

The review of several studies can gain strength over an individual study, which is valid in many models and fields of medicine. However, one should be cautioned about the real strengths of such a meta-analysis before considering it to have a high level of evidence. The strength of these combined reviews is derived from the strength of the individual trials providing the numbers for the analysis. In the best scenario, such a combined review is composed of multiple prospective trials with similar design that each compares the effect of two treatments on a specific outcome. However, in the field of pediatric surgery, multiple prospective trials with similar designs that address the same disease with the same interventions are nonexistent. Also, surgeons should not overvalue the influence of combined reviews derived from retrospective studies. Such reviews should be interpreted as a mosaic of the individual studies. Any attempt by authors to combine a number of retrospective studies to harness statistical power is fraught with hazard.

GRADES OF RECOMMENDATION

The quality of the evidence as defined in Tables 78-1 and 78-2 applies a score of strength for each individual contribution in the literature. However, on many topics, particularly common clinical scenarios, there is an abundance of published studies such that the appropriate care cannot be guided by a single study. The total body of available information places caregivers in the difficult position of evaluating the published principles from the multiple sources that make up practice guidelines. The caregiver applying these clinical practice guidelines and other recommendations needs to know how much confidence can be placed in the recommendations from a conglomerate of citations. Strength of recommendation scales were born from this need.[8-12] Given that the level of evidence indicates the extent to which one can be confident that an estimate of effect is correct, the strength or grade of recommendation indicates the extent to which one can be confident that adherence to the recommendation will do more good than harm.[13] As with the levels of evidence, there are multiple published grading scales. The grading format used by the Oxford Centre for Evidence-Based Medicine is outlined in Table 78-2.

The levels of evidence are more easily assessed because each contribution falls into a given level based on study design. However, establishing the grade of recommendation can be more complex given the fact that multiple levels of evidence from different timeframes invariably exist on any given clinical topic. This is further confusing because many disease processes have multiple outcome measures. Also, each treatment option can affect different outcomes in independent ways that must be balanced against the risk or toxicity of each treatment. A working group has outlined a process for establishing grade based on the following sequential steps:[14]

1. Assess the quality of evidence across studies for each important outcome

2. Decide which outcomes are critical to a decision
3. Judge the overall quality of evidence across these critical outcomes
4. Evaluate balance between benefits and harms
5. Levy the strength of the recommendation.

At this time, an accepted standard for respecting the level of evidence and assessing grades of recommendation is lacking in the pediatric surgery field.

LANDSCAPE OF PEDIATRIC SURGERY

Progress in the field of pediatric surgery regarding EBM has been hindered by its relatively young age and the small size of its membership. As opposed to our adult general surgery colleagues who operate on a foundation built through centuries of work, the first American textbook in pediatric surgery, Abdominal Surgery of Infancy and Childhood by Robert Gross and William Ladd, was published in 1941. These men trained the initial cohort of pediatric surgeons who then developed other training centers around the country. The total number of training sites has remained relatively small. As a result, the philosophies of only a few people have been taught to the entire practicing population of pediatric surgeons. The practice of pediatric surgery has generally progressed without extensive critical analysis. This phenomenon is pronounced in the pediatric surgery literature, which has been replete with retrospective case-control studies and case series (levels 3 and 4). There are few publications in the pediatric surgery literature that entail comparative analysis, and most of these are retrospective in nature.

The future of care being directed by comparative research is brightening. There has historically been a great focus on basic science research when resource allocation is considered. However, despite the fact that government funding for basic science has far exceeded clinical research, the impact on clinical care relative to the investment has been low. The National Institutes of Health (NIH) is beginning to place greater emphasis on comparative effectiveness research versus classic basic science investigations. The Obama administration has recently approved $400M of funds to the NIH, while the Agency for Healthcare Research and Quality (AHRQ) received $300M from the Recovery Act legislation in addition to $400M that can be used at the discretion of the Secretary of Health for comparativeness effectiveness research.[15] Comparative effective research is defined by AHRQ as research designed to inform health care decisions by providing evidence on the effectiveness, benefits, and harms of different treatment options. The evidence is generated from research studies that compare drugs, medical devices, tests, operations, or ways to deliver health care.

RETROSPECTIVE STUDIES

As our field is overly represented with retrospective comparisons, it is important to recognize the natural flaws introduced by retrospective analysis. At least one of two confounding factors is present when an institution reviews and compares different therapies retrospectively. When

TABLE 78-2	Grades of Recommendation as Defined by the Oxford Centre for Evidence-Based Medicine
Grade	**Level of Evidence**
A	Consistent level 1 studies
B	Consistent level 2 or 3 studies or extrapolations from level 1 studies
C	Level 4 studies or extrapolations from level 2 or 3 studies
D	Level 5 evidence or troublingly inconsistent or inconclusive studies of any level

an institution is concurrently using different treatment plans, usually the comparison between treatment plans also compares caregivers. The other possibility is that the center has changed treatment plans and then retrospectively investigates the effect of this change. Although this sounds attractive, it becomes a comparison between timeframes. Historical comparison groups are difficult to use with confidence because of the rapid ongoing changes in hospital systems. Many institutions have quality assurance programs that intend to make all patient care more consistent and efficient. Such change will impact outcomes regardless of the surgical treatment. A universal concern with retrospective studies is the assurance of reviewing the entire population and the entire dataset. It can be very difficult to accurately identify all the data desired when retrospectively collecting information. As a result, datasets are often incomplete, which decreases scientific confidence. Another issue, rarely acknowledged in retrospective studies, is the difficulty with capturing the entire population intended for study. There are many coding nuances within an institution that may exclude patients from lists when the database is searched by ICD-9 code. A specific type of patient, such as a treatment failure, can go undetected, because of being hidden under a different diagnosis code. This can create tremendous error in the published data.

CONSIDERATIONS FOR PROSPECTIVE TRIALS IN PEDIATRIC SURGERY

Although it is clear that prospective trials offer the highest scientific integrity and the best vehicle for determining superior efficacy among options, they have been underutilized in the field of surgery, and specifically, pediatric surgery. Critics have postulated that consented prospective trials would have a limited role in pediatric surgery because parents would be unwilling to enroll their children into such studies. Studies should not be conducted in any human population when there is substantial risk of harm balanced against questionable benefit. A well-designed study should offer patients the potential for a better outcome than the standard means of treatment outside the study. However, there is no example in the published literature to support the speculation that studies should not be attempted in children. Moreover, there are now several prospective, randomized trials being conducted and emerging in the pediatric surgery literature that would suggest otherwise.[16–24]

The specific details of trial development are beyond the scope of this chapter, but there are general considerations that can allow pediatric surgeons to identify situations for which a trial can be employed. Specifically, these include an understanding of equipoise or stepwise progression, the need for patient volume, an understanding of population characteristics, and the possibility of influencing practice habits.

Equipoise

There is usually a role for a trial when equipoise exists for the currently available therapeutic options. Equipoise is the assumption that two treatment plans are equal. Thus, the trial simply pits the two options head to head to identify which is superior. Each caregiver participating in a study does not need to possess true inherent equipoise without bias. Naturally, each practitioner will have biases and suppositions about which management strategy is superior, but there remains a role for a trial when each caregiver can honestly acknowledge that there is not enough evidence to prove his or her own thoughts are correct. The most obvious examples of the need for a trial are circumstances in which more than one management strategy is utilized in a given institution. This usually occurs due to caregiver bias. An example would be the use of irrigation during laparoscopic appendectomy for perforated appendicitis.[16] Most surgeons will believe in one or the other, but not both. Another would be tube thoracostomy and fibrinolysis versus thoracoscopic decortication for empyema.[17,18] If a given patient condition is treated by pathway A or B based simply on the caregivers who were on call and there is no evidence to support either pathway, then not only is there a role for a trial, but, in reality, there is an ethical need to conduct such a study to prevent the potential tragedy wherein half of the patients are receiving inferior care simply due to bias without evidence.[25]

The other natural situation for prospective evaluation is when caregivers want to simplify care, but that next step may be at the expense of increasing the chances of a negative outcome. For example, if a group would like to shorten the length of any therapy, then this is clearly advantageous to the patient unless there is a greater risk of a negative outcome. As caregivers we owe it to the patients to pursue courses of treatment that improve their care, but we cannot compromise the outcome. Parents would enjoy a shorter course of anal dilation after anoplasty for imperforate anus but not to the point that it results in a detectable increase in anal stricture. Also, caregivers contemplating fewer doses of antibiotics, shorter periods of observation for various injuries, or less invasive therapeutic options should introduce them under prospective evaluation to be sure the attenuation in care is not offset by higher negative event rates. Under this paradigm, once each study is complete, then a treatment protocol can exist that becomes simple to compare to the next advancement. Our colleagues in oncology understand this concept well. In the cooperative oncology groups, each treatment plan follows a protocol with known outcomes and is compared to a potentially better regimen. Under this plan, once survival for a given cancer becomes high enough, then stepwise progression focuses on minimizing toxicity or operative morbidity. The surgical fields have been less effective in advancing care using this model, largely due to the individual surgeon being unwilling to relinquish his or her independent thoughts.

Patient Volume

The conduction of a study requires adequate patient volume, which is not a concern for common conditions. However, acquisition of good evidence has long been difficult in pediatric surgery owing to the wide variety of individually rare conditions. When considering less common conditions, physicians often simply suggest expanding the number of institutions participating in a trial to overcome volume limitations. This is the common answer, but is difficult to implement because each additional institution will need to take on a significant workload. Moreover, not all surgeons at each institution will be invested in the study and therefore may not adhere to the study design. Also, depending on the nature of the study, not all surgeons may be able to offer treatment in both arms. For instance, one of the reasons that a prospective randomized trial failed in comparing open and minimally invasive approaches for cancer in the mid-1990s was because very few of the surgeons could perform the required minimally invasive surgical procedures.[26] It remains a fact that the integrity of the study will decrease with the addition of more institutions and more caregivers because it is less likely the protocols will be followed completely.

The lack of large volumes with certain conditions can be interpreted in a different and more pragmatic way for the practicing surgeon. Instead of focusing on the attainment of a large number of patients to try to detect a difference with strong statistical power, perhaps we should investigate more reasonable sample sizes to see if a larger difference can be detected. Why would we intentionally seek a larger difference when a smaller one might be detected in a larger study? For example, if a busy group of six surgeons were to conduct a study that enrolls over 5 years, and the study fails to detect a difference in any outcome parameter, even though the calculated power may be statistically small and unconvincing by traditional trial design, the number of patients treated by the group is the equivalent volume that an individual surgeon would treat over a 30-year career. Therefore, if the difference is small enough not to be evident over an individual surgeon's career, the surgeon should not be too concerned about the relevance of the variable studied and should focus on other treatment variables to improve patient outcome.

Population Characteristics

The most important consideration of the study population is the homogeneity of the disease. A study on two types of stomal takedown techniques would be difficult due to the large variations in reasons for stoma placement, the intestinal level of the stoma, the degree of expected adhesions, the integrity of the remaining bowel, the function of the anus, and so on. The population should provide enough patient-to-patient similarity that the outcome from one patient can be related to another.

Generalizability

A study is less useful when there are just a few surgeons who can use the results. This applies not only to technologies or techniques that very few centers can provide, but also to the development of the protocol. The protocol should attempt to assimilate real-world, typical practice problems without compromising structural integrity. If the protocol is overly strict, although it provides superior ability for detection of any differences, the results may not be applicable to the typical practice. Therefore,

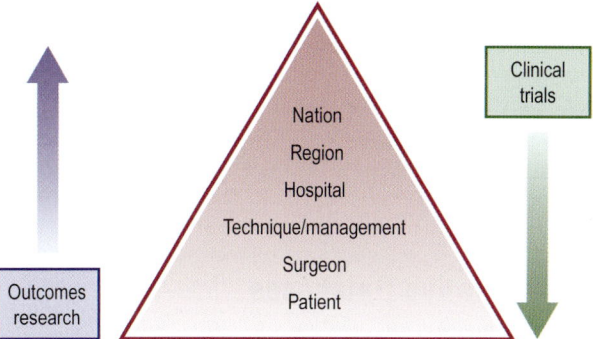

FIGURE 78-1 ■ This figure depicts the differing focus between outcomes research and clinical trials. Outcomes research provides a top down view with more strength at the top of the pyramid while clinical trials provide a more clear focus at the patient and management level.

the subsequent value of the study diminishes. Multicenter studies are felt to be more generalizable; however, with each additional center the study loses integrity as more protocol deviations can be expected. The study design therefore has to consider these competing forces and decide which is more important: answering the question or applying the question to the population.

Relevance

Before developing a project that will provide an answer, the question needs to be asked as to whether a problem exists in the first place. The important parameters for relevance are the event rate and the burden. While a powerful study could be done on two different methods of skin closure after an inguinal hernia repair, the event rate of infection or wound breakdown is so small that surgeons are not too concerned about this problem. The time required for skin closure is a minute or less regardless of technique. Moreover, when infection does occur, the wound is not large enough to create a clinically important problem. Therefore, the practicing surgeon is unlikely to alter his or her technical habits of hernia repair based on the results of such a study.

OUTCOMES RESEARCH

Outcomes research is the analysis of outcomes and their predictors at different levels in the health care delivery system.[27] The critical difference between clinical trials research and outcomes or database research is the scope of view as depicted in Figure 78-1.[28] Clinical trials set inclusion criteria to create a desired population most likely to answer the question of interest. Thus, the patients are defined from the outset. Outcomes research uses all patients in the database. Clinical trials control for patient differences by randomization. In outcomes research, however, one can control for differences only in the analysis models. While some may argue outcomes research provides a better answer that is generalizable to the practicing community, the inability to sort out patients with confounding variables makes outcomes research more practical in addressing national, regional, and hospital trends where the view of individual patient management becomes blurred. Clinical trials provide more a clear picture to answer specific management questions. However, outcomes research can be utilized to benchmark quality of care, compare therapeutic effectiveness, refine management strategies, provide patient education, and produce important marketing information.[28]

Administrative Databases

Administrative databases are typically large computerized data files compiled for billing purposes. The data is gathered by billing coders and not clinicians, and are mostly based on ICD-9 coding systems. The ICD-9 coding system has a separate diagnosis code as well as a separate procedure code. Of the administrative databases, the National Inpatient Sample (NIS) is the most generalized database.[29] There are other subspecialty databases publicly available for trauma, oncology, and transplant. The Kids' Inpatient Database (KID) is a weighted pediatrics sample that is an all-payer inpatient care database for children in the USA.[30] It is released every 3 years. The KID database is de-identified, but includes unique provider and hospital codes that allows for hospital-level analysis and can be linked to other databases containing other non-medical information. The Child Healthcare Corporation of America (CHCA) maintains the Pediatric Health Information Systems (PHIS) database which currently collects billing data from 44 tertiary referral children's hospitals in the USA.

There are disadvantages to these databases. They contain only inpatient data with limited clinical course information, limiting the ability to follow a patient's course upon discharge. Additionally, it can be difficult to determinate the timing of the diagnoses.[28]

Clinical Databases

Clinical databases, on the other hand, are populated through a clinician reviewer. The most well-known and utilized clinical database is the American College of Surgeons-National Surgical Quality Improvement Program (ACS-NSQIP).[31]

NSQIP is the first validated adjusted outcomes program to measure the quality of surgical care. It employs a prospective, peer control, validated database that provides 30-day risk-adjusted outcomes. Individual specialties categorized include general, vascular, cardiac, thoracic, neurosurgery, orthopedics, otolaryngology, gynecology, urology, and plastics.

In 2005, a children's NSQIP module was developed. The pediatric NSQIP module's starting algorithm section is 35 major cases every eight days on patients <18 years of age, rotating on each subsequent week day.[32] There are 121 data points from most surgical specialties within the pediatric module compared to 135 in the adult NSQIP. These include demographics, hospitalization characteristics, and complications with additional data points for neonates. Outcomes for both adult and pediatric NSQIP modules are assessed for 30 days following the procedure.

Adult and pediatric trauma patients are tracked by the National Trauma Data Bank (NTDB), which includes 900 trauma centers.[33] Adult and pediatric malignancies are maintained in the Surveillance, Epidemiology, and End Results (SEER) database, which is maintained by National Cancer Institute.[34] The SEER registries routinely collect data on patient demographics, primary tumor site, tumor morphology and stage at diagnosis, first course of treatment, and follow-up status. The mortality data reported by SEER is provided by the National Center for Health Statistics. The American College of Surgeons Committee on Cancer maintains the National Cancer Data Base (NCDB) containing adult and pediatric patients from 1,400 Commission-Accredited Cancer Programs following survival data until death.[35] The United Network for Organ Sharing (UNOS) database was established in 1996 by Congress to track every organ donation event in the USA along with long-term patient and graft survival.[36]

RESOURCES

The application of EBM practices requires a functional knowledge of how to identify, interpret, and implement the information available into care plans and practice guidelines. Although many institutions have entire departments focusing on EBM utilization, not all physicians have ready access to the information. In the field of surgery, there are many examples of heterogeneous care plans within institutions and group practices despite convincing, high-level evidence. Also, there are many reasons for these often conflicting care plans. One is that personal bias for some providers is stronger than their ability to interpret data. Thus, they continue working in their comfort zone and are skeptical of sound data. Some of these surgeons completed training in the apprentice era, and they have continued to follow what their chief told them. Also, some physicians who understand the

TABLE 78-3	Websites that Pertain to Evidence-Based Medicine
Name of Website	**Address**
The Cochrane Collaboration	www.cochrane.org
The Cochrane Library	www3.interscience.wiley.com
National Guideline Clearinghouse	www.guideline.gov
Centre for Evidence-Based Medicine	www.cebm.net
Berkeley Systematic Reviews Group	http://epi.berkeley.edu/
Clinical Evidence	www.clinicalevidence.org
Evidence-Based Medicine Resource Center	www.ebmny.org
Welch Medical Library	http://welch.jhmi.edu/welchone/
Prime Answers	www.primeanswers.org
Evidence-Based Practice Centers	www.ahrq.gov
PubMed	www.ncbi.nlm.nih.gov/entrez/query.fcgi?db=PubMed

principles of EBM simply do not have wide access to the evolving body of EBM. To overcome some of these hurdles, several web-based support sites have been developed for both EBM tutorial and review of available studies. A few examples are listed in Table 78-3.

REFERENCES

1. Sackett DL, Rosenberg WM, Gray JA, et al. Evidence based medicine: What it is and what it isn't. BMJ 1996;312:71–2.
2. Steffens BB. Ibn Al-Haytham: First Scientist. Greensboro, NC: Morgan Reynolds Publishing; 2006.
3. Bacon F. Novum Organum, 1620.
4. Cochrane AL. Effectiveness and Efficiency: Random Reflections on Health Services. London: Nuffield: Provincial Hospitals Trust; 1972.
5. www.cochrane.org and http://www3.interscience.wiley.com/cgi-bin/mrwhome/106568753/HOME.
6. Eddy DM. Practice policies: Where do they come from? JAMA 1990;263:1265–72.
7. Guyatt G, Cairns J, Churchill D, et al. (Evidence-Based Medicine Working Group): Evidence-based medicine: A new approach to teaching the practice of medicine. JAMA 1992;268:2420–5.
8. Harbour R, Miller J. A new system for grading recommendations in evidence based guidelines. BMJ 2001;323:334–6.
9. Atkins D, Briss PA, Eccles M, et al. GRADE Working Group. Systems for grading the quality of evidence and the strength of recommendations II: Pilot study of a new system. BMC Health Serv Res 2005;5:25–37.
10. West S, King V, Carey TS, et al. Systems to rate the strength of scientific evidence. Rockville, MD: Agency for Healthcare Research and Quality (AHRQ publication No. 02–E016); 2002. p. 51–63.
11. Jüni P, Altman DG, Egger M. Assessing the quality of randomised controlled trials. In: Egger M, Davey Smith G, Altman DG, editors. Systematic reviews in health care: Meta-analysis in context. London: BMJ Books; 2001. p. 87–121.
12. Zaza S, Wright-De A, Briss PA, et al. Data collection instrument and procedure for systematic reviews in the guide to community preventive services. Am J Prev Med 2000;18:44–74.
13. Atkins D, Best D, Briss PA. Grading quality of evidence and strength of recommendations. BMJ 2004;328:1490.
14. GRADE Working Group: David Atkins, Dana Best, Peter A Briss, Martin Eccles, Yngve Falck-Ytter, Signe Flottorp, Gordon H Guyatt, Robin T Harbour, Margaret C Haugh, David Henry, Suzanne Hill, Roman Jaeschke, Gillian Leng, Alessandro Liberati, Nicola Magrini, James Mason, Philippa Middleton, Jacek Mrukowicz, Dianne O'Connell, Andrew D Oxman, Bob Phillips, Holger J Schünemann, Tessa Tan-Torres Edejer, Helena Varonen, Gunn E Vist, John W Williams Jr, Stephanie Zaza.
15. Overview of the American Recovery and Reinvestment Act of 2009 (Recovery Act). Rockville, MD: Agency for Healthcare Research and Quality (AHRQ); 2010. http://www.ahrq.gov/fund/cefarraover.htm.
16. St. Peter SD, Adibe OO, Iqbal CW, et al. Irrigation versus suction alone during laparoscopic appendectomy for perforated appendicitis: A prospective randomized trial. Ann Surg 2012;256:581–5.
17. St. Peter SD, Tsao K, Spilde TL, et al. Thoracoscopic decortication versus tube thoracostomy with fibrinolysis for empyema in children: A prospective, randomized trial. J Pediatr Surg 2009;44:106–11.
18. Sonnappa S, Cohen G, Owens CM, et al. Comparison of urokinase and video-assisted thoracoscopic surgery for treatment of childhood empyema. Am J Respir Crit Care Med 2006;174:221–7.
19. Fraser JD, Aguayo P, Leys CM, et al. A complete course of intravenous antibiotics versus a combination of intravenous and oral antibiotics for perforated appendicitis in children: A prospective, randomized trial. J Pediatr Surg 2010;45:1198–202.
20. St. Peter SD, Tsao K, Spilde TL, et al. Single daily dosing ceftriaxone and Flagyl versus standard triple antibiotic regimen for perforated appendicitis in children: A prospective, randomized trial. J Pediatr Surg 2008;43:981–5.
21. St. Peter SD, Barnhart DC, Ostlie DJ, et al. Minimal versus extensive esophageal mobilization during laparoscopic fundoplication: A prospective randomized trial. J Pediatr Surg 2011;46:163–8.
22. Blakely ML, Williams R, Dassinger MS, et al. Early versus interval appendectomy for children with perforated appendicitis. Arch Surg 2011;146:660–5.
23. St. Peter SD, Weesner KA, Weissand EE, et al. Epidural versus patient controlled analgesia for pain control following pectus excavatum repair: A prospective, randomized trial. J Pediatr Surg 2012;47:148–53.
24. St. Peter SD, Adibe OO, Juang D, et al. Single incision versus standard laparoscopic 3 port appendectomy: A prospective, randomized trial. Ann Surg 2011;254:586–90.
25. Adibe OO, St. Peter SD. Ethical ramifications from the loss of equipoise and the necessity of randomized trials. Arch Surg In Press.
26. Ehrlich PF, Newman KD, Haase GM, et al. Lessons learned from a failed multi-institutional randomized controlled study. J Pediatr Surg 2002;37:431–6.
27. Outcomes Research. Fact Sheet. AHRQ Publication No. 00-P011. Rockville, MD: Agency for Healthcare Research and Quality; 2000. http://www.ahrq.gov/clinic/outfact.htm.
28. Abdullah F, Ortega G, Islam S, et al. Outcomes research in pediatric surgery. Part 1: Overview and resources. J Pediatr Surg 2011;46:221–5.
29. Overview of HCUP-SID Database. Healthcare Cost and Utilization Project (HCUP). Rockville, MD: Agency for Healthcare Research and Quality; 2010. www.hcupus.ahrq.gov/sidoverview.jsp.
30. Overview of HCUP-KID Database. Healthcare Cost and Utilization Project (HCUP). Rockville, MD: Agency for Healthcare Research and Quality; 2010. www.hcupus.ahrq.gov/kidoverview.jsp.
31. Overview of the American College of Surgeons National Surgical Quality Improvement Program. c2006 [cited 2010 Jul]. Available from: https://acsnsqip.org/main/about_overview.asp.
32. Overview of the American College of Surgeons National Surgical Quality Improvement Program- Pediatrics. c2009 [cited 2010 Jul 31]. Available from: http://www.pediatric.acsnsqip.org/default.aspx.
33. American College of Surgeons Committee on Trauma- Overview of the National Trauma Data Bank. c1996–2010 [updated 2010 April 20; cited 2010 Jul 31]. Available from: http://www.facs.org/trauma/ntdb/ntdbapp.html.
34. Overview of the Surveillance, Epidemiology, and End Results Data sets. [Updated 2010 April 14; cited 2010 Jul 31]. Available from: http://seer.cancer.gov/data/.
35. American College of Surgeons Commission on Cancer- Overview of the National Cancer Data Base. c2002–2010 [updated 2010 June 2; cited 2010 Jul 31]. Available from: http://www.facs.org/cancer/ncdb/index.html.
36. USA Department of Health and Human Services- Health Resources and Services Administration-Organ Procurement and Transplantation Network- Overview of the United Network for Organ Sharing. [Cited 2010 Jul 31]. Available from: http://optn.transplant.hrsa.gov/data/about/.

CHAPTER 79

TISSUE ENGINEERING

Daniel E. Levin • Martin A. Birchall • Tracy C. Grikscheit

Scientific progress has improved outcomes for patients with organ failure, but many of these therapies are temporary, expensive, and require specialized care. Historically, organ replacement has been managed with inexact tissue substitutions such as colon interposition for the esophagus, materials such as Dacron for vascular grafts, extracorporeal circuits that replace the missing organ function such as hemodialysis machines or ventilators, and organ transplantation. Each of these approaches has its own disadvantages. Tissue engineering is an ideal approach for replacing the critical organ or tissue that is lacking, perhaps with the patient's own cells.

In 1954, Dr Joseph Murray performed the first successful human kidney transplant, introducing the world to an entire new field of medicine.[1] Organ and tissue transplant is a remarkable and life-saving option for many patients. Nevertheless, it is limited by donor scarcity, need for lifelong immunosuppression, and the risk of infection and rejection.[2] For these reasons, tissue engineers are working toward developing methods of growing whole organs from a patient's own cells or banked lines of cells that can be used to replace diseased and damaged tissues.

By definition, a tissue-engineered organ must be capable of performing the key functions of the replaced organ or tissue. Also, it should be durable, self-repairing, and match the longevity of the patient. It should not require the sacrifice or prioritization of other organs as is the case for operations such as gastric pull-up, vein harvest, or a myocutaneous flap. Tissue engineering strategies often employ overlapping techniques that can be applied to a number of organ systems. These approaches include: (1) a progenitor cell source; (2) a biological or synthetic scaffold for in vivo implantation; and (3) a method of expanding cell mass via in vitro cell culture, bioreactor, or in vivo implantation. Figure 79-1 illustrates a common approach for cell isolation, seeding of a scaffold, and implantation into the host. This general concept has been adapted to multiple organ systems and animal models.

CELL SOURCE

Concurrent with the expansion of regenerative medicine and tissue engineering programs in the last decade, remarkable progress has been made in understanding stem and progenitor cells. Embryonic stem cells (ESC) are harvested from the inner cell mass of the blastocyst in embryos and are considered pluripotent cells, able to develop into any cell type except for the extra-embryonic tissues. This is advantageous because they are a potential source for any tissue in the body.[3] However, work performed with ESC, particularly human ESC, is subject to considerable scrutiny and ethical concerns. Moreover, ESC may possess tumorigenic potential.[4] Somatic or adult stem cells can be derived from the patient who requires the tissue-engineered organ, but lack totipotency. Instead, these cells are committed toward a particular lineage, but maintain the potential for self-renewal and possess multipotency, which is the ability to differentiate into multiple, but not all cell types.[3] For example, the intestinal stem cell is capable of self-renewal and producing all differentiated cells of the intestinal epithelium, but it usually does not differentiate into a hepatocyte. A central dogma is that once a cell has differentiated, it is committed to that cell line.

In 2006, a method of reprogramming somatic cells to a pluripotent state was developed.[5] These cells are termed induced pluripotent stem cells (iPSC). These cells overcome many of the ethical and immunologic concerns surrounding ESC; however, one disadvantage is that they maintain tumorigenic potential.[4] Many of the current techniques for reprogramming these cells require the introduction of oncogenic viral vectors, thereby limiting clinical application.[6] Additional sources of pluripotent cells include mesenchymal stem cells (MSC). MSC were initially described in 1968 as a population of bone marrow derived cells capable of osteogenic differentiation.[7] Since then, MSC capable of self-renewal and differentiation have also been isolated from adipose, skin, blood, synovial membrane and amniotic fluid, and other mesodermally derived tissues.[8]

SCAFFOLD

Many scaffold materials have been investigated for cell delivery. These can be divided into two broad categories: synthetic and biological. Both synthetic and biological scaffolds are designed to reproduce the properties of native mesenchymal support, sometimes with the associated extracellular matrix (ECM).

Synthetic scaffolds are designed to be porous enough to allow imbibition of nutrients until vasculogenesis and angiogenesis occurs, but also rigid enough to provide structural support. Frequently used materials include polyglycolic acid (PGA) and poly(L-lactic acid) (PLLA) that are biodegradable polymers designed to be hydrolyzed and absorbed by the recipient as the engineered product grows.[9] With advancements in the field of biomaterials, synthetic scaffolds have become increasingly

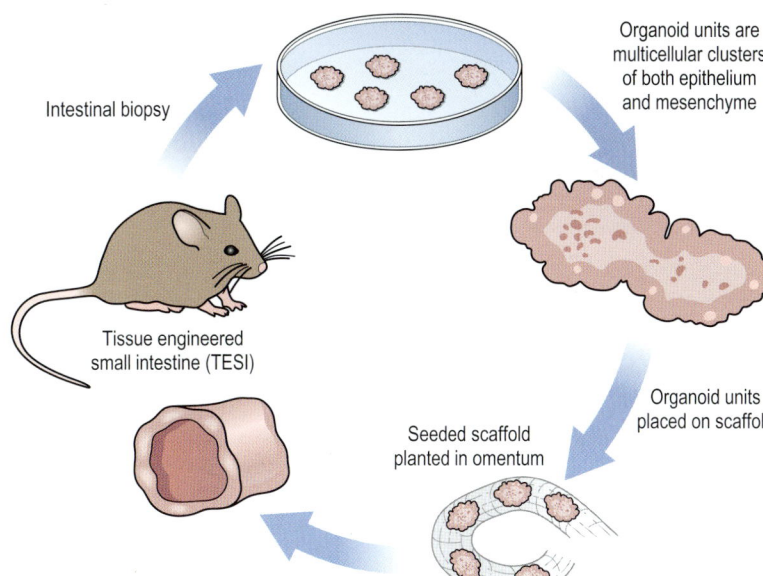

Intestinal biopsy

Organoid units are multicellular clusters of both epithelium and mesenchyme

Tissue engineered small intestine (TESI)

Organoid units placed on scaffold

Seeded scaffold planted in omentum

FIGURE 79-1 ■ A representative schematic of tissue-engineered technique. In the example above, murine tissue-engineered small intestine is generated. However similar techniques have been applied to many organ systems. Tissue is obtained for the isolation of a cellular source. These cells are used to seed a scaffold which is then implanted into a host. The tissue-engineered product is harvested after a period of growth.

complex. Polyhedral oliogmericsilsesquioxane bonded to poly-[carbonate-urea] urethane (POSS-PCU), for example, is biocompatible, nonreactive, nontoxic, and can be designed to fit the patient's needs. This scaffold has already been successfully used in a tracheobronchial transplant.[9] The structure of some commonly used synthetic scaffolds are demonstrated in Figure 79-2.

Biological scaffolds composed of naturally occurring macromolecules, in particular those that formulate the ECM, have also been described. These include porous collagen lattice, chitosan, glycosaminoglycans, silk fibroin, alginate, and starch.[10] More recently, in an attempt to create more complex biological scaffolds, researchers have turned toward decellularized extracellular matrices as a potential material. Decellularization is a process in which organs are treated with detergents and enzymes to remove nuclear, cytoplasmic, and antigenic material while leaving behind the ECM (Figure 79-3). This methodology preserves the macroscopic and microscopic architecture of the original tissue, including vascular inflow and outflow, facilitating future vascular anastomosis and circulation.[11] Subsequent recellularization is possible using an appropriate cell source.

CELL EXPANSION AND GROWTH

A bioengineered organ must be of sufficient size to adequately support function. Methods for culturing cells include one or more of the following techniques. Many scientists have designed artificial bioreactors that attempt to mimic many of the physiologic processes that occur in an organism. These include control of pH, oxygen tension, temperature, waste removal, and even the pulsatile flow of blood.[12] However, no bioreactor can fully recreate the complexity of a living animal. An alternative approach is to expand cells in vivo in what can be thought of as a living bioreactor. This has the advantage of encouraging the growth of blood vessels that will ultimately be needed to support the growing engineered

tissue and access to circulating factors that may be important for cell growth. A marked disadvantage is the unpredictable number of variables introduced by the host, which increases the challenge of deciphering the cellular and molecular mechanisms of growing the tissue-engineered organ. The greatest challenge facing most tissue engineers is expanding the volume of tissue growth to a clinically relevant size while maintaining specific tissue functions with this growth.

RESPIRATORY SYSTEM

Trachea and Bronchi

Tissue-engineered trachea is conceptualized for the replacement of long-segment tracheal defects. Primary disease of the trachea, such as tracheal agenesis, is rare with an incidence of less than 1 in 50,000 live births.[13] However, iatrogenic injury or malignant invasion may necessitate segmental resection. Primary repair is possible if the defect is less than 5 cm in adults and one-third the tracheal length in children.[14] Although an allograft transplant is possible, it is limited by the lack of a suitable vascular pedicle and the probable need for lifelong immunosuppression.[15] Prosthetic conduits have also been attempted. However, these are frequently complicated by product migration, infection, erosion, and disruption.[14]

Implantation of a tissue-engineered airway has been performed successfully in humans.[16] The human donor trachea was decellularized to remove all cells and major histocompatibility complex (MHC) antigens. The recipient's own epithelial cells and chondrocytes were then cultured and used to seed this biological scaffold. The bioengineered trachea was then anastomosed to replace the left main stem bronchus in a 30-year old woman with end-stage bronchomalacia. Follow-up 4 months later confirmed the patient was breathing normally without the need for immunosuppressive medications.

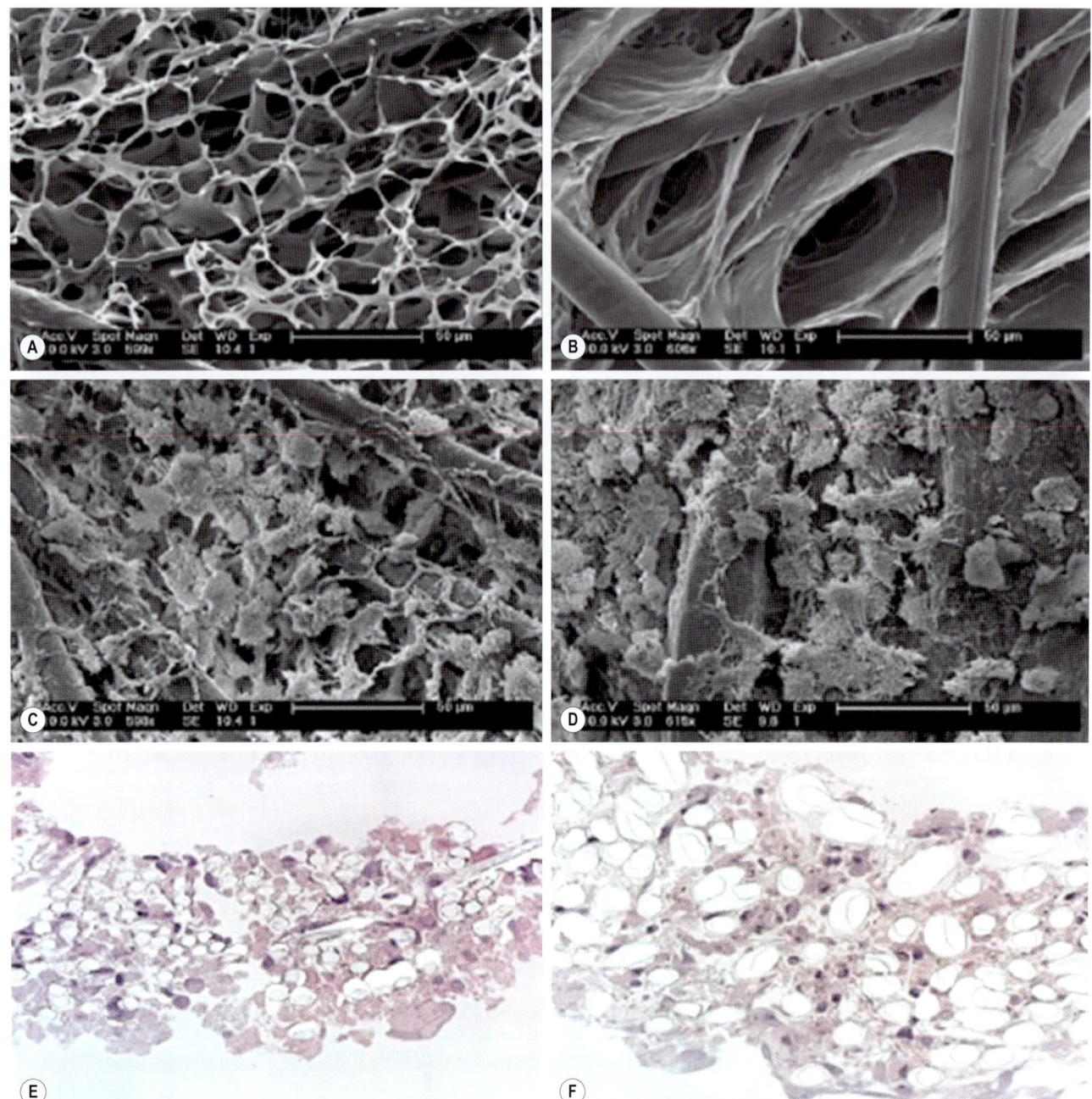

FIGURE 79-2 ■ Common synthetic scaffolds for in vivo tissue engineering. Highly porous structures are necessary to support tissue growth as demonstrated by scanning electron microscopy of **(A)** PGA-P(CL/LA) scaffold and **(B)** PLLA-P(CL/LA) scaffold. The scaffolds can be seeded with cells as demonstrated in **(C)** PGA-P(CL/LA) and **(D)** PLLA-P(CL/LA). These cells survive by imbibition until neovascularization occurs. The close approximation of cells and scaffold can be further demonstrated by staining with hematoxylin and eosin for both **(E)** PGA-P(CL/LA) and **(F)** PLLA-P(CL/LA) scaffolds. PGA, polyglycolic acid; PLLA, poly-L-lactic acid; P(CL/LA), copolymer sealant δ-caprolactone and L-lactide. (Adapted and reproduced with permission from Roh JD, Nelson GN, Brennan MP, et al. Small-diameter biodegradable scaffolds for functional vascular tissue engineering in the mouse model. Biomaterials 2008;29:1454–63.)

The first long-term follow-up for a tissue-engineered tracheal replacement in a child was published in 2012.[17] The authors reported the case of a 12-year-old boy born with long-segment tracheal stenosis and a pulmonary sling. After years of failed interventions, including multiple stainless steel expandable stents and emergent repair of an aortotracheal fistula, he was the recipient of a tissue-engineered trachea. Prior to the operation, MSC from the patient were isolated and a cadaveric donor trachea was decellularized. At the time of the operation, the decellularized scaffold was seeded with MSC and patches of tracheal epithelium, and anastomosed to replace a 7 cm segment of stenotic trachea. In addition, the scaffold was treated intraoperatively with erythropoietin, granulocyte colony-stimulating factor, and transforming growth factor beta (TGF-β). These factors serve to enhance angiogenesis, improve recruitment of MSC, and induce chondrogenesis, respectively. During the

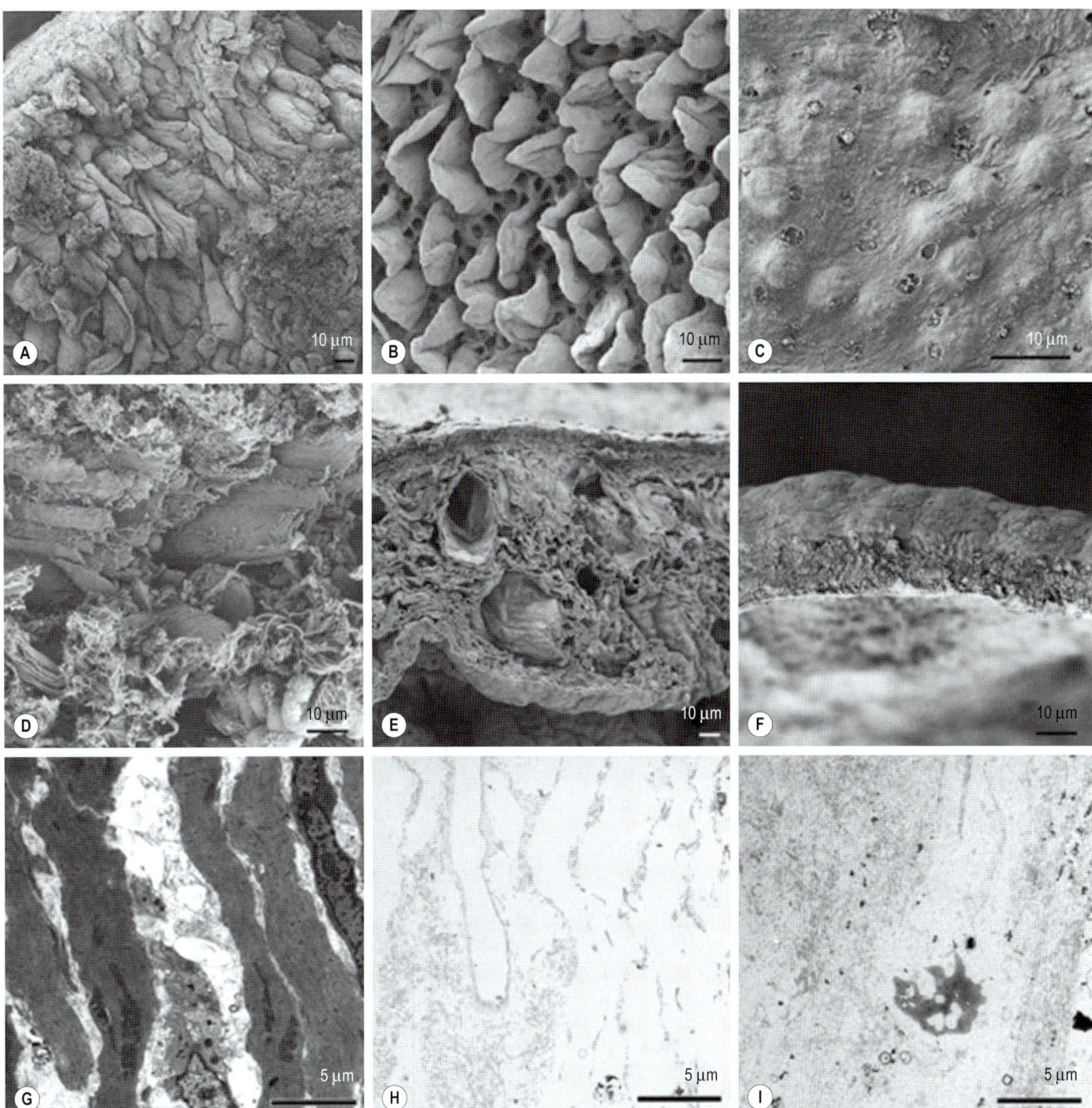

FIGURE 79-3 ■ Biological scaffolds derived from decellularized organs have been attempted. **(A)** Scanning electron microscopy (SEM) of native intestine. During decellurization, crypt/villus structure of the extracellular matrix (ECM) is preserved after **(B)** one cycle, but is lost **(C)** after four cycles. The collagen fiber network as it appears on SEM for **(D)** native intestine remains intact after **(E)** one cycle of decellurization, but is lost **(F)** after four cycles. A transmission electron micrograph (TEM) of **(G)** native intestine demonstrates normal cellularity. TEM confirms acellularity of the biological scaffold following **(H)** one and **(I)** four cycles of decellularization. (Adapted and reproduced with permission from Totonelli G, Maghsoudlou P, Garriboli M, et al. A rat decellularized small bowel scaffold that preserves villus-crypt architecture for intestinal regeneration. Biomaterials 2012;33:3401–12.)

immediate postoperative recovery, the child required stent placement. However, 2 years later, the child was breathing comfortably and had returned to school without the need for tracheal stenting. The graft had revascularized, demonstrating an epithelial lining, and appeared normal on computed tomography (CT) and ventilation-perfusion scan.

A limiting factor in the technique described above is the need for donor trachea that is subsequently decellularized. To avoid this need, synthetic scaffolds have also been used. In nonhuman studies, PGA was tubularized and coated with sheets of cultured MSC. MSC treated with glucocorticoids and TGF-β will differentiate along a chondrogenic lineage. These bioengineered, cartilaginous tubes closely resemble human trachea.[18] Other cell sources and scaffold materials have also been tried including sheep nasal chondrocytes on a PGA and silicon tube matrix, or human nasal chondrocytes on hydrogel and high-density polyethylene.[19,20] Although these methods are successful in generating a cartilaginous conduit, they have not been applied in humans.

Tissue-engineered lung parenchyma has posed a significantly greater challenge. Development of a tissue-engineered lung with fully differentiated pneumocytes and clara cells has not been achieved to date.[21] Current methods are unable deliver cells in the appropriate cellular distribution and architecture to participate in normal gas exchange.

CARDIOVASCULAR SYSTEM

Heart

The Centers for Disease Control (CDC) reports that 40,000 infants are born with congenital heart defects each year in the USA. Among adults, heart disease is the leading cause of death. The CDC estimates the annual financial burden of cardiovascular disease approximates $444 billion. Tissue engineering cardiac replacements such as myocardial tissue and heart valves may help alleviate some of these costs. Murine ESC can be expanded in culture and differentiated into cardiomyocytes.[22] Similar results have been shown with human cells.[23] Ethical concerns have limited the transition to human experiments prompting increased interest in iPSC[24] which can be driven towards a cardiac lineage after reprogramming.[24,25]

In 2001, implantation of autologous skeletal myoblasts into scar tissue was performed on a patient during coronary artery bypass grafting. Echocardiography performed five months after the operation demonstrated improved areas of myocardial contractility within the scar.[26] However, in a randomized placebo-controlled study performed on 94 patients, these results could not demonstrate an improvement in heart function, partly due to the development of arrhythmic areas.[27] Aiming to improve delivery and distribution of cells, laboratories are looking into seeding myoblasts on a polyurethane scaffold prior to implantation. In a rat model of myocardial infarction, such an approach prevented progression to heart failure more effectively than sham operation or unloaded scaffold implantation.[28]

Heart Valves

Nearly one-third of congenital heart defects involve the aortic or pulmonary valves, with current methods of valve replacement not providing optimal therapeutic solutions. Mechanical prosthetic valves are prone to thrombus and require long-term anticoagulation, increasing the risk of hemorrhage. Bovine and porcine bioprostheses may fail secondary to calcification or structural damage. All prosthetics valves can be complicated by infection or paravalvular leak. For the pediatric population, the failure of replacement valves to grow with the patient requires multiple operations into adulthood. Tissue-engineered heart valves (TEHV) offer the hypothetical advantage of autologous growth, self-repair, and remodeling with the patient.

Native heart valves have three layers, namely: fibrosa (interstitial cells and collagen), spongiosa (proteoglycans), and ventricularis (elastin sheets).[29] These valves possess remarkable mechanical durability, capable of opening and closing three billion times over a lifespan.[30] Decellularized porcine valves, fibrin, collagen-rich material, and PLLA have been used as scaffolds. Cells for TEHV have generally been applied by one of two methods: either directly seeded on the scaffold prior to in situ implantation, or subsequent attachment of endothelial cells from the blood stream after implantation of an empty scaffold. Bone marrow MSC, umbilical blood progenitor cells, and circulating endothelial progenitor cells have served as possible cell sources.

Expression of the glycoprotein antigen CD133 has been used as a marker for progenitor cells, and is important for the identification and isolation of hematopoietic stem cells.[31] Translation to human use has already been demonstrated. Dohmen et al produced TEHV by combining cadaveric human decellularized pulmonary heart valve scaffolds that were seeded with autologous vascular endothelial cells and were implanted into 11 patients.[32] At ten-year follow-up, all patients were alive with no regurgitation or accelerated velocities on transthoracic echocardiography and no structural defects on CT. These are encouraging results for the future of TEHV, but require additional validation prior to becoming standard of care.[33]

Blood Vessels

Vascular bypass is frequently needed as an organ preserving and life-saving operation. Autologous venous and arterial grafts are preferred over synthetic materials, but necessitate the sacrifice of the donor vessel.[34] Synthetic materials are prone to infection and maintain patency rates of only 38–49% at 5 years.[35] Similar to synthetic valves, synthetic blood vessels do not increase in size with a growing child. In the mid-1980s, Weinberg and Bell ushered in the dawn of tissue-engineered vascular grafts (TEVG; Fig. 79-4) when they seeded endothelial cells onto a scaffold made from bovine smooth muscle cells, cultured fibroblasts, and Dacron mesh.[36] Although these grafts failed at pressures greater than 180 mmHg, this research demonstrated that generation of a TEVG is possible. Standards for producing TEVG dictate that durable replacements should have a burst pressure greater than 2000 mmHg.[37,38] Since then, multiple scaffolds have been developed, including PGA and decellularized allograft vessels, that are capable of withstanding burst pressures upwards of 2100 mmHg.[34]

In 2001, the first TEVG was transplanted into a 4-year-old girl to replace her right intermediate pulmonary artery that had occluded following a Fontan procedure.[39] A peripheral vein was harvested providing cells for culture. Once cultured to 12×10^6, they were seeded on a 2 cm long polycaprolactone-polylactic acid and PGA scaffold. This group performed a similar procedure on

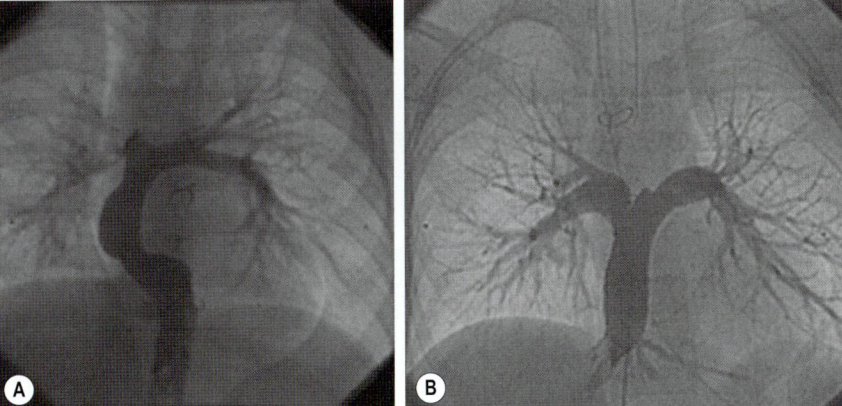

FIGURE 79-4 ■ Treatment of human disease with TEVG. Angiography confirms that there were no stenotic, aneurysmal, or calcified lesions at (**A**) 5 years and (**B**) 4 years post implantation for these two patients. (Adapted and reproduced with permission from Hibino N, McGillicuddy E, et al. Late-term results of tissue-engineered vascular grafts in humans. The Journal of Thoracic and Cardiovasc Surg 2010;139:431–6.)

two additional patients, before changing the cell source to aspirated bone marrow cells. At 5.5 years of follow-up, all 25 patients were alive and there was no evidence of aneurysm, rupture, infection, or calcification. Four patients were successfully treated percutaneously for stenosis, and one patient required anticoagulation for a partial thrombus.[40] Currently, another group of surgeons are conducting a phase I clinical trial for the implantation of TEVG.[41] Based on these results, it is possible that TEVG will become a component in the management algorithm for the routine treatment of vascular disease in the near future.

ALIMENTARY SYSTEM

Esophagus

Esophageal lengthening via mobilization, circular myotomy, or a staged approach may close gaps up to 3 cm in babies with isolated esophageal atresia. Beyond this distance, an esophageal replacement is often needed.[42] An adequate replacement conduit can be constructed via gastric pull-up or the interposition of colon or jejunum, but these approaches rely on prioritizing and sacrificing an area of the gastrointestinal tract.[43–45] Tissue-engineered esophagus (TEE) has been successful in rat and dog esophageal replacement models.[46,47] In dogs, an amniotic membrane was cultured with oral keratinocytes and fibroblasts. These cultured cells were fashioned into a tube on a PGA scaffold and implanted with smooth muscle tissue into the omentum of the host dog. Then, at 3 weeks, the TEE was transferred as a pedicle graft to close a 3 cm esophageal gap. More than a year later, dogs who underwent this operation were alive and healthy. Although peristalsis of the TEE segment was not evident on imaging, both solids and liquids were able to pass easily from mouth to stomach.

An earlier study in rats isolated esophageal organoid units (OU) for the production of TEE. OU are cellular constructs containing all cells necessary to generate full-thickness tissue such as progenitor cells, supportive mesenchymal cells, and differentiated epithelial cells. OUs were loaded onto a PGA/PLLA scaffold and implanted into the omentum of host rats. After 4 weeks of growth, the TEE was either harvested for histology or

anastomosed as an interposition graft ($n = 3$) or onlay patch ($n = 3$). Both the interposition and patch groups had one mortality and two survivors. The surviving animals in both groups gained weight and possessed a patent TEE when evaluated with fluoroscopy. Histologic evaluation confirmed the presence of a stratified squamous epithelial lining similar to native esophagus.[46]

A similar technique has been demonstrated in a sheep model. The omental implantation of ovine esophageal epithelial cells seeded onto a tube of collagen produced TEE with areas of normal appearing esophageal epithelium. During the proliferative phase, the lumen was maintained by a stent that was removed at harvest. These constructs also demonstrated vascular ingrowth, a necessary feature for successful in vivo tissue engineering.[48,49] A variety of cellular sources as well as synthetic and biological scaffold materials have been tested for TEE. In one study, various cell and scaffold arrangements were evaluated. It was found that human esophageal squamous cells and a porcine esophageal matrix scaffold grew TEE that most closely and reliably reproduced normal appearing esophageal morphology.[50]

Stomach

Conditions requiring total gastrectomy such as gastric volvulus with necrosis and gastric cancer are rare in children. However, among adults, gastric cancer is the second leading cause of cancer mortality in the world and a common indication for gastric resection.[51] For both adults and children requiring gastrectomy, subsequent esophagojejunostomy lacks the reservoir capacity and digestive physiology of native stomach. Tissue-engineered stomach (TES) is a promising means of restoring normal gastric function.

From outer wall to inner lining, the stomach is composed of a serosa, muscularis externa, submucosa, and mucosa. The mucosa contains gastric pits and glands. The glands are comprised of specialized epithelial cells including the parietal cell producing hydrochloric acid, chief cell producing pepsinogen, enteroendocrine cell producing hormones, G cell producing gastrin, and mucous neck cell producing mucus.

TES has been grown in a rat model with OUs. OUs were seeded onto a synthetic scaffold that was implanted into the omentum of the host animal. As the TES grew, the host animal hydrolyzed the scaffold. After 30 days of growth, the TES was a well-vascularized, muscular sphere with a mucosal lining similar to native stomach.[52,53]

In a study designed to test the function of rat TES, the construct was sutured in situ as a gastric replacement.[54] The control group underwent Roux-en-Y reconstruction. After 24 weeks, the TES and control groups survived without evidence of obstruction. On histologic evaluation, the harvested TES demonstrated smooth muscle-like layers with an epithelial lining containing parietal and G cells. Interestingly, the TES group was less anemic, which may have been secondary to increased production of intrinsic factor by the parietal cells in the TES. Of note, however, there was no difference between the two groups when comparing weight, total protein, or lipid profile. TES has been similarly generated in the mouse model. Transition to a mouse model may allow investigators to elucidate cellular and molecular mechanisms driving TES growth, and may reveal potential targets and improve tissue yield.[55]

Small Intestine

A leading cause of intestinal failure in children is short bowel syndrome (SBS).[56] SBS occurs when intestinal length is reduced to the point where the patient is unable to absorb sufficient nutrition, resulting in profound malnutrition, dehydration, and electrolyte derangements. Common causes of SBS in children include midgut volvulus, gastroschisis, and necrotizing enterocolitis (NEC).[57] Currently, SBS is treated with diet modification, total parenteral nutrition (TPN), medications to delay intestinal transit, and operation. Operative interventions include bowel elongation and intestinal transplant.[58] Outcomes from intestinal transplant have improved greatly, yet they are still limited by donor scarcity, lifelong immunosuppression, infection, and rejection.[59] Tissue-engineered small intestine (TESI) may be used at some point as an intestinal replacement for SBS. The success of TESI is dependent on the ability to develop normal small intestine structure and function.

The mucosa of the small intestine is arranged as finger-like projections known as villi and intervillus invaginations called crypts. The villi greatly increase the absorptive surface area of the small intestine. There are four main differentiated epithelial cells: enterocytes, goblet cells, enteroendocrine cells, and Paneth cells. The enterocyte is a simple columnar epithelial cell and is the predominant cell population in the villus. It is responsible for the absorption of water, ions, carbohydrates, peptides, lipids, and unconjugated bile salts.[60] Mucus secreted by goblet cells is necessary for lubrication and barrier defense.[61] Enteroendocrine cells produce over 30 hormones and peptides.[62] The remaining secretory cell, the Paneth cell, is located in the crypt and is interspersed with the crypt base columnar cell (CBCC). The Paneth cell secretes antimicrobial defensins[63] and has recently been shown to support the stem cell niche. Improved proliferation and differentiation were found when cultured intestinal stem cells (ISC) were paired with Paneth cells in comparison to ISC cultured in isolation. This appears related to the production of growth hormones acting via paracrine signaling between the adjacent Paneth cells and ISC.[64]

A population of stem cells, first described in the 1970s, is characteristically quiescent and located, on average, four cell positions from the crypt base and thought to be necessary in response to injury and healing.[65,66] Interestingly, the CBCC has recently been identified as a second population of ISC residing within the crypt base. These cells, marked by their expression of a G-protein, Lgr5, are rapidly cycling and capable of self-renewal and differentiation into all cell types.[67] The theory of two stem cell populations, a traditional quiescent population necessary for response to injury and a second population important for the rapid cellular turnover of intestinal homeostasis, is a fascinating new paradigm in the study of intestinal regeneration.[68]

All of the above cell types, as well as smooth muscle, vessels, and nerves are necessary for the normal structure and function of the small intestine. Within the field of intestinal regeneration, some investigators have focused on mechanisms of epithelial development and regeneration while others are committed to therapeutic translation, and have focused on the generation of full-thickness intestine. In an effort to refine studies in intestinal epithelial physiology, one group of investigators implanted collagen I matrix scaffolds with cultured human colonic fibroblasts and umblical vein endothelial cells grafted with human intestinal epithelial cells inside a rotating bioreactor.[69] In ten to 15 days, the system grew villus-like structures containing differentiated epithelial cells and components of intestinal microanatomy such as brush borders, tight junctions, and glucose transporters. Others have created a three-dimensional culture system for the study of intestinal drug transport across the gut-blood barrier.[70] Recently, iPSC that had been cultured in conditions mirroring embryronic development were driven to differentiate along intestinal lineages. This generated three-dimensional structures with crypt and villus-like architecture similar to intestinal morphology.[71] These in vitro systems are superior to traditional two-dimensional culture methods as they more closely approximate native intestine. For complete organ replacement, however, full-thickness TESI is needed.

Experiments designed to grow full-thickness intestine began in the late 1980s. The Vacanti group adapted a technique from Evans et al. for the isolation of intestinal OU, seeding a biodegradable polymer scaffold and implanting these constructs in host rats.[72,73] The resulting TESI demonstrated fully differentiated secretory and absorptive cells, as well as supportive mesenchyme and muscle. In an experiment aiming to investigate function, two groups were generated. The rat control group underwent a massive small bowel resection resembling SBS. The experimental group also underwent massive small bowel resection, with the TESI anastomosed in-line with the severely truncated intestine. Both groups initially lost weight. However, at 40 days, the TESI group had regained significantly more weight, reaching 98% of preoperative values. The TESI group also had normal B12 levels compared to low levels in the control group.

A current limitation in the transition of TESI to human therapy is the amount of intestine that can be

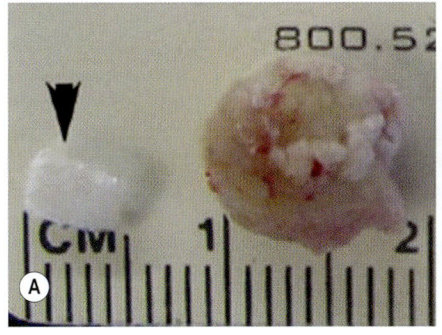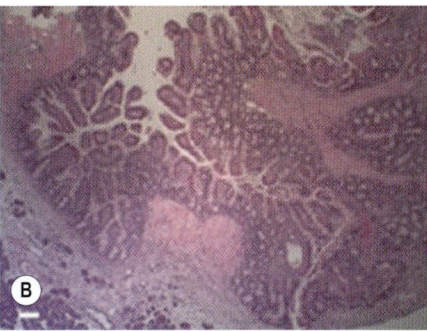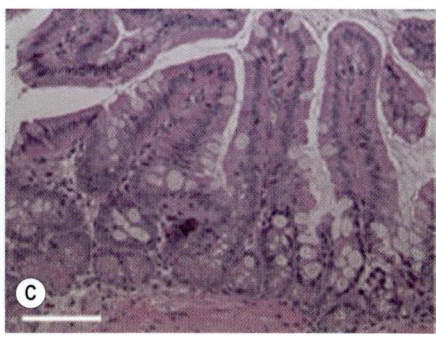

FIGURE 79-5 ■ Murine TESI. **(A)** An unseeded synthetic PGA scaffold tube sealed with PLLA and coated with collagen (arrowhead) adjacent to TESI explanted four weeks after omental implantation. **(B)** A 20 × magnification of TESI stained with H&E reveals an epithelium toward the lumen. **(C)** At 40 × magnification, TESI stained with H&E reveals a simple columnar epithelium arranged in crypts and villi. Additionally, goblet and Paneth cells appear in their normal position and distribution. Scale bar: 40 μM. TESI, tissue-engineered small intestine; PGA, polyglycolic acid; PLLA, poly-L-lactic acid; H&E, hematoxylin and eosin stain. (Adapted and reproduced with permission from Sala F, Matthews J, Speer A, et al. A multicellular approach forms a significant amount of tissue-engineered small intestine in the mouse. Tissue Eng 2011;17:1841–9.)

generated. The addition of growth factors to the PGA scaffold has resulted in a modest ability to increase TESI yield in comparison to TESI generated without growth factors. Holo-transferrin increased TESI surface area (9.11 ± 0.66 mm vs 3.01 ± 0.22 mm, $P < 0.01$) and glucagon-like peptide 2 increased the total number of TESI cysts (8.88 ± 0.46 vs 4.18 ± 0.25, $P < 0.01$).[74] To increase the amount of TESI that can be grown to a clinically relevant volume, investigators are looking at the cellular mechanisms responsible for TESI growth. The goal is to identify targets in the form of growth factors or improved donor populations that may be added to augment TESI growth. Studying TESI growth in the mouse, in which transgenic and molecular tools are available, may lead to identification of these targets.

TESI in a mouse model demonstrates normal appearing crypt and villus architecture (Fig. 79-5). In addition, it contains a fully differentiated epithelium with entero-cytes, goblet cells, enteroendocrine cells, Paneth cells, a smooth muscle layer as well as intestinal subepithelial myofibroblasts (ISEMF).[75] ISEMF are located immediately beneath the crypt and are thought to support the stem cell niche with an active role in injury and immune response.[76] Nerve components and blood vessels are also present, verifying the presence of all necessary cells required for normal structure and function.

Prior to human trials, it is necessary to establish the feasibility of generating autologous donor cells as would be expected in a sick neonate with NEC. These cells need to be harvested, prepared, loaded on a scaffold, and then implanted in a single operation. This has been performed in a Yorkshire swine model.[77]

LARGE INTESTINE AND ANUS

Infants and children with NEC, Hirschsprung disease, familial adenomatosis polyposis, or inflammatory bowel disease face specific morbidities associated with colon resection. Ileoanal anastomosis may be associated with diminished quality of life secondary to day or nighttime fecal incontinence, depression and anxiety, and dietary restrictions and daily requirement of antidiarrheal medication.[78,79] End ileostomy is complicated by skin irritation, poor adherence of the ostomy appliance, with leaking as well as a decreased quality of life.[80,81] Severe diarrhea causing dehydration is a frequent cause of readmission following creation of an ileostomy.[82] In addition, complete colectomy leads to malabsorption of bile acids secondary to loss of intestinal microbiota.[83]

Tissue-engineered colon (TEC) has been grown in a rat model and found to have normal appearing architecture. To assess function in a replacement model of TEC, two groups of rats were compared after undergoing colectomy with end ileostomy. The first group underwent an ileostomy to TEC anastomosis while the control group had the ileostomy. The rats with TEC demonstrated greater weight gain, increased stool transit time, less diarrhea, and improved bile acid absorption.[84]

Restoration of colonic absorption and normalization of the enterohepatic circulation and stool microbiota are key points required for translation of TEC to humans. Restitution of fecal continence requires a competent anal sphincter. Interventions designed to treat conditions such as imperforate anus or anal fissures may predispose patients to develop an incompetent anal sphincter. The anal sphincter may also be damaged or excised secondary to trauma or with abdominoperineal resection. In mice, smooth muscle cells have been harvested from the internal anal sphincter (IAS) and seeded onto a fibrin mold. When cultured, these cells naturally formed a ring that could be implanted subcutaneously into a host mouse.[85] Further testing revealed the bioengineered IAS could generate resting tonicity and was able to relax and contract with stimulation.[85,86] Additionally, fetal mouse enteric neurons have been cultured with human IAS smooth muscle and implanted into a murine host with preserved muscle and nerve function.[87] In the future, it may be possible to restore bowel continence and enhance the options for lower intestinal reconstruction with a bioengineered IAS. This has the potential to greatly improve the lives of many patients.

INTEGUMENTARY AND MUSCULOSKELETAL SYSTEM

Skin

Complex wound closure and treatment of severe burns pose significant challenges for plastic and reconstructive surgery. Adequate skin replacement has been sought since Reverdin first described the use of skin grafts in the late 19th century.[88] Skin grafts can provide adequate coverage, but they may also result in function limiting wound contracture. Also, cosmetic results are frequently suboptimal. Furthermore, the site for autologous donor skin is painful, has the potential to heal poorly, and may not be of sufficient surface area. These limitations may be overcome with tissue-engineered skin. Potential regenerative strategies can be divided into two groups. The first are biological substitutes that offer temporary wound coverage until patient skin appendages re-epithelialize the wound surface or a skin graft is placed. These include cadaveric skin, porcine xenograft, porcine small intestine submucosa, and cryopreserved amniotic membrane.

A second group involves tissue-engineered skin products that substitute epidermal, dermal, or both layers. There are a large number of commercially available products for the treatment of full and partial thickness burns and ulcers. Many of these are variable constructs of sheets of human fibroblasts and keratinocytes.[89] However, current Food and Drug Administration (FDA) approved bioengineered skin replacements are inadequate for treatment of many large wounds. Although these products may facilitate wound healing, they do not recreate normal skin architecture and frequently fail to revascularlize. Skin is deceptively complex and more than a simple watertight barrier of stratified epithelium. Hair follicles, sweat and sebaceous glands, dendritic cells, blood vessels, nerve, and stem cells all contribute to the normal function of skin. Over the last decade, scientists have sought to expand stem cells for skin regeneration.[90]

The addition of MSC to tissue-engineered skin has resulted in better keratinization, less wound contracture, and improved vascularization when grafted onto pigs.[91] Generating full-thickness tissue-engineered skin remains challenging. Preliminary success in a mouse model was achieved using adipose stem cells to regenerate the dermal layer upon which an epidermal layer can be reconstructed. This technique also permits manipulation of the adipogenic potential of these stromal cells, allowing for development of the hypodermis as well.[92] Skin substitutes, composed of cultured keratinocytes and fibroblasts, self-assemble into a stratified and cornified epithelium.[93] These self-assembled skin substitutes are the subject of a recently completed phase II trial evaluating their success in closing venous ulcers. The results of this trial have yet to be published.[94]

Bone

Large bone defects can result from trauma, cancer resections, and congenital defects. Infusion of aspirated bone marrow containing MSC has been used for the treatment of bony nonunion since the early 1990s.[95] It has recently been demonstrated that transplant of culture-expanded bone marrow cells (directed toward osteogenic lineage with dexamethasone treatment) and platelet-rich plasma can accelerate callus formation.[96] However, generation of a vascularized bone replacement remains a challenge. For repair of larger defects, cellular-seeded scaffolds may be needed. Quarto et al. reported the successful ex vivo expansion of osteoprogenitor cells, seeding of a hydroxyapatite scaffold, and in vivo implantation for the treatment of large bone defects. They reported three patients (defects ranging from 4–7 cm) who regained limb function up to 15 months later.[97] Over the last 10 years, a large variety of autologous cell sources and scaffold materials have been explored along with the use of bioreactors to improve in vitro growth.[98]

Tendons and Ligaments

Normal tendons and ligaments are composed of collagen I, fibroblasts and fibrocytes (ligament), or tenoblasts and tenocytes (tendon). Injury is common among athletes, the elderly, and working members of society. One's natural ability to regenerate these tissues is poor. Current management is stratified into either conservative or invasive approaches. Usual conservative therapy includes rest, ice packs, and anti-inflammatory medications or injections. Operative intervention may involve primary repair of an acute rupture, autograft from a patellar tendon, semitendinosus tendon or anterior cruciate ligament (ACL), allograft, or artificial prostheses.[99] Delayed healing, joint stiffness or instability, allograft rejection, and long-term failure frequently limit the therapeutic outcomes from these approaches.

Tissue engineering cell sources have included autologous tenocytes harvested from patellar or calcaneal tendon, cells removed from the tendon sheath, and dermis fibroblasts obtained from skin biopsy.[99] ACL-derived stem cells (LSC) can be induced to express type I collagen, type III collagen, fibronectin, and alpha-smooth muscle actin following exposure to TGF-β. This has promising applications as a future cell source for a bioengineered ligament.[100]

URINARY SYSTEM

Kidney

End-stage renal disease (ESRD) affects approximately 1200 children each year in the USA. Common etiologies include renal dysplasia, obstructive uropathy, and focal sclerosing glomerular nephritis.[101] ESRD treatment components include dialysis and transplantation.[102] Complications from dialysis as well as the shortcomings of allograft transplants could be avoided with a functioning tissue-engineered kidney. Bioengineered renal grafts have been created using decellularized rat kidney scaffolds that were injected with ESC ex vivo from the arterial and ureteral routes. These tissue-engineered kidneys were incubated in a perfusion bioreactor for 3 days prior to immunohistologic evaluation. Interestingly, despite not adding growth factors, the seeded cells expressed markers of renal differentiation such as pancytokeratin, Pax-2, and Ksp-Cadherin. These observations have implications not only for tissue engineering, but also in understanding the dynamic contributions the ECM may have on cellular differentiation.[103]

Similar experiments have been performed on a larger scale. Nakayama et al. layered Rhesus monkey fetal kidney tissue onto a decellularized kidney and demonstrated the feasibility of this technique to support the growth of renal tissue.[104] Further experiments will be required to verify this technique with postnatal tissue to avoid the ethical concerns and clinical limitations of a therapy requiring fetal tissue.

Urethra

For the repair of a long urethral stricture or large urethral defect, urethroplasty has been performed in rabbits using a tissue-engineered urethra to replace a 1 cm defect in the rabbit's native urethra.[105] Initially, bladder biopsies were performed to obtain cells for expansion. Following culture, the cells were seeded onto tubularized collagen. After one month, there was no evidence of urethral stricture. Histologic evaluation demonstrated smooth muscle and epithelial cells approximating normal architecture. Urethral repair with collagen matrix as well as acellular bladder matrix and demineralized bone matrix have both been successful in humans.[106,107]

In 2011, the results of urethral reconstructions with tissue-engineered urethra in five boys was reported.[108] These boys with urethral defects underwent muscle and urothelial cell biopsy. The cells were expanded in culture for three to six weeks, then seeded on a tubularized PGA scaffold, followed by implantation for urethral reconstruction. Two of the five boys required a second procedure to improve voluntary voiding. Median follow-up at 71 months showed all patients to have a patent urethra without radiographic or endoscopic evidence of stricture. These are encouraging results, but will require further validation in greater numbers prior to widespread acceptance. In addition, some researchers have expressed concern over the ability of urethra-like tissue to fully replace the hydrolyzed scaffold and for adequate neovascularization to occur.[109] However, if these limitations can be overcome, these techniques may become the preferred approach for treatment of large urethral defects.

Bladder

Replacement of the urinary bladder with intestinal segments can be problematic and synthetic materials frequently fail. As with other organ systems, cellular seeding onto scaffolds has been attempted and urothelial cells have often been chosen as the donor cells.[110,111] A human trial studied autologous urothelial and muscle cells expanded in culture and seeded onto a collagen and PGA sphere for patients with myelomeningocele and poor bladder function. The neobladder took 2 months to prepare prior to implantation and was transplanted into seven children (mean age 11 years). At 3.5 years follow-up,

the patients had improved urinary continence with a normal architecture on biopsy.[112] There was no evidence of renal failure, calculi, or abnormal mucous production. Long-term follow-up will be needed to validate the durability of these repairs.

HEPATOBILIARY SYSTEM

Liver

Biliary atresia is the most common indication for liver transplantation in children.[113] Other causes of liver failure include viral hepatitis, hepatotoxic medications, and metabolic disorders. Common regenerative strategies have been applied to tissue engineering of the liver, including hepatocyte growth on synthetic and biological scaffolds.[114] The in vitro metabolic function of human hepatocytes cultured in a spherical polyurethane foam was found to be improved in comparison to a monolayer culture. Ammonia removal and amino acid and bile acid metabolism was increased when the hepatocytes were cultured in the three-dimensional synthetic scaffold as opposed to routine monolayer culture.[115]

Unfortunately, the organized structure of the portal triad has not been created by means of tissue engineering as yet. Despite the fact that a tissue-engineered whole liver has not yet been developed, cultured hepatocytes have been used for developing bioartificial liver support systems. The blood of patients with liver failure is circulated through a device embedded with hepatocytes. This artificial hepatic support may be sufficient to bridge the gap to liver transplant or hepatic recovery. Currently, there are several clinical trials evaluating the safety and utility of these devices.[116]

Additionally, advances in liver stem cell research are likely to yield important advances in liver bioengineering. Hepatocyte-like cells have already been generated from growth factor treated ESC.[117] Ex vivo portal vein infusion of adult rat hepatocytes into a decellularized liver matrix generated liver grafts with cells capable of in vitro albumin secretion, urea synthesis, and cytochrome P450 expression.[118] Moreover, hepatocyte morphology and enzymatic function was maintained following in vivo transplantation of these grafts into recipient rats. Grafts were anastomosed to the renal vein and artery, and perfused for 8 hours before harvest and immunohistochemical analysis. This marked a critical first step toward establishing a three-dimensional, vascularized bioengineered liver graft for the treatment of hepatic failure.

Pancreas

Tissue-engineered pancreas would be an optimal treatment for type 1 diabetics. Regarding cell-based therapies, islet cell transplantation is possible and temporarily restores normoglycemia.[119] Unfortunately, this approach frequently fails over time and requires donor islet cells.[120] The generation of differentiated beta cells from progenitor cells may be possible in the future.[121] Kodama et al. dissociated rat pancreatic biopsies into single cells and seeded them onto PGA scaffolds, which were cultured in growth factor enriched media for 40 days prior to implantation into diabetic mice.[122] All mice that received transplanted tissue-engineered pancreas attained normoglycemia without insulin administration. Histologic staining demonstrated differentiated cells that could secrete insulin, somatostatin, and glucagon. These are encouraging results for the future of pancreatic tissue engineering.

REFERENCES

1. Merrill JP, Harrison JH, Murray J, et al. Successful homotransplantation of the kidney in an identical twin. Trans Am Clin Climatol Assoc 1956;67:166–73.
2. Ueno T, Fukuzawa M. Current status of intestinal transplantation. Surg Today 2010;40:1112–22.
3. Sylvester KG, Longaker MT. Stem cells: Review and update. Arch Surg 2004;139:93–9.
4. Ben-David U, Benvenisty N. The tumorigenicity of human embryonic and induced pluripotent stem cells. Nat Rev Cancer 2011;11:268–77.
5. Takahashi K, Yamanaka S. Induction of pluripotent stem cells from mouse embryonic and adult fibroblast cultures by defined factors. Cell 2006;126:663–76.
6. Li M, Chen M, Han W, et al. How far are induced pluripotent stem cells from the clinic? Ageing Res Rev 2010;9:257–64.
7. Friedenstein AJ, Petrakova KV, Kurolesova AI, et al. Heterotopic of bone marrow. Analysis of precursor cells for osteogenic and hematopoietic tissues. Transplantation 1968;6:230–47.
8. Keating A. Mesenchymal stromal cells: New directions. Cell Stem Cell 2012;10:709–16.
9. Jungebluth P, Alici E, Baiguera S, et al. Tracheobronchial transplantation with a stem-cell-seeded bioartificial nanocomposite: A proof-of-concept study. Lancet 2011;378:1997–2004.
10. Carletti E, Motta A, Migliaresi C. Scaffolds for tissue engineering and 3D cell culture. Methods Mol Biol 2011;695:17–39.
11. Badylak SF, Weiss DJ, Caplan A, et al. Engineered whole organs and complex tissues. Lancet 2012;379:943–52.
12. Mabvuure N, Hindocha S, Khan WS. The role of bioreactors in cartilage tissue engineering. Curr Stem Cell Res Ther 2012;7: 287–92.
13. Ergun S, Tewfik T, Daniel S. Tracheal agenesis: A rare but fatal congenital anomaly. Mcgill J Med 2011;13:10.
14. Grillo H. Tracheal replacement: A critical review. Ann Thorac Surg 2002;73:1995–2004.
15. Delaere P, Vranckx J, Verleden G, et al. Tracheal allotransplantation after withdrawal of immunosuppressive therapy. N Engl J Med 2010;362:138–45.
16. Macchiarini P, Jungebluth P, Go T, et al. Clinical transplantation of tissue-engineered airway. The Lancet 2008;372:2023–30.
17. Elliott MJ, De Coppi P, Speggiorin S, et al. Stem-cell-based, tissue engineered tracheal replacement in a child: A 2-year follow-up study. Lancet 2012;380:994–1000.
18. Liu L, Wu W, Tuo X, et al. Novel strategy to engineer trachea cartilage graft with marrow mesenchymal stem cell macroaggregate and hydrolyzable scaffold. Artificial Organs 2010;34: 426–33.
19. Ruszymah B, Chua K, Latif M, et al. Formation of in vivo tissue engineered human hyaline cartilage in the shape of a trachea with internal support. Int J Pediatr Otorhinolaryngol 2005;69: 1489–95.
20. Kojima K, Bonassar L, Ignotz R, et al. Comparison of tracheal and nasal chondrocytes for tissue engineering of the trachea. Ann Thorac Surg 2003;76:1884–8.
21. Song JJ, Ott HC. Bioartificial lung engineering. Am J Transplant 2012;12:283–8.
22. Yuasa S, Itabashi Y, Koshimizu U, et al. Transient inhibition of BMP signaling by Noggin induces cardiomyocyte differentiation of mouse embryonic stem cells. Nat Biotechnol 2005;23:607–11.
23. Mummery C, Ward-van Oostwaard D, Doevendans P, et al. Differentiation of human embryonic stem cells to cardiomyocytes: Role of coculture with visceral endoderm-like cells. Circulation 2003;107:2733–40.
24. Liau B, Zhang D, Bursac N. Functional cardiac tissue engineering. Regen Med 2012;7:187–206.
25. Mummery CL, Zhang J, Ng ES, et al. Differentiation of human embryonic stem cells and induced pluripotent stem cells to cardiomyocytes: A methods overview. Circ Res 2012;111:344–58.
26. Menasche P, Hagege AA, Scorsin M, et al. Myobast transplantation for heart failure. The Lancet 2001;357:279–80.
27. Menasché P, Alfieri O, Janssens S, et al. The myoblast autologous grafting in ischemic cardiomyopathy (MAGIC) trial: First randomized placebo-controlled study of myoblast transplantation. Circulation 2008;117:1189–200.
28. Siepe M, Giraud M-N, Pavlovic M, et al. Myoblast-seeded biodegradable scaffolds to prevent post-myocardial infarction evolution toward heart failure. J Thorac Cardiovasc Surg 2006;132:124–31.
29. Rippel RA, Ghanbari H, Seifalian AM. Tissue-Engineered heart valve: Future of cardiac surgery. World J Surg 2012;36:1581–91.
30. Schoen FJ. Heart valve tissue engineering: Quo vadis? Curr Opin Biotechnol 2011;22:698–705.
31. Yin AH, Miraglia S, Zanjani ED, et al. AC133, a novel marker for human hematopoietic stem and progenitor cells. Blood 1997;90:5002–12.
32. Dohmen PM, Lembcke A, Holinski S, et al. Ten years of clinical results with a tissue-engineered pulmonary valve. Ann Thorac Surg 2011;92:1308–14.
33. Mendelson K, Schoen FJ. Heart valve tissue engineering: Concepts, approaches, progress, and challenges. Ann Biomed Eng 2006;34:1799–819.
34. Orlando G, Wood KJ, De Coppi P, et al. Regenerative medicine as applied to general surgery. Ann Surg 2012;225:867–80.
35. Takagi H, Goto SN, Matsui M, et al. A contemporary metaanalysis of Dacron versus polytetrafluoroethylene grafts for femoropopliteal bypass grafting. J Vasc Surg 2010;52:232–6.
36. Weinberg C, Bell E. A blood vessel model constructed from collagen and cultured vascular cells. Science 1986;231:397–400.
37. Drilling S, Gaumer J, Lannutti J. Fabrication of burst pressure competent vascular grafts via electrospinning: Effects of microstructure. J Biomed Mater Res A 2009;88:923–34.
38. Niklason LE, Gao J, Abbott WM, et al. Functional arteries grown in vitro. Science 1999;284:489–93.
39. Shin'oka T, Imai Y, Ikada Y. Transplantation of tissue-engineered pulmonary artery. N Engl J Med 2001;344:532–3.
40. Hibino N, McGillicuddy E, Matsumura G, et al. Late-term results of tissue-engineered vascular grafts in humans. J Thorac Cardiovasc Surg 2010;139:431–6.
41. Breuer C. A pilot study investigating the clinical use of tissue engineered vascular grafts in congenital heart surgery. ClinicalTrialsgov. 2010: Phase 1; Identifier: NCT01034007.
42. Brown AK, Tam PK. Measurement of gap length in esophageal atresia: A simple predictor of outcome. J Am Coll Surg 1996;182:41–5.
43. Spitz L, Ruangtrakool R. Esophageal substitution. Semin Pediatr Surg 1998;7:130–3.
44. Cusick EL, Batchelor AA, Spicer RD. Development of a technique for jejunal interposition in long-gap esophageal atresia. J Pediatr Surg 1993;28:990–4.
45. Raffensperger JG, Luck SR, Reynolds M, et al. Intestinal bypass of the esophagus. J Pediatr Surg 1996;31:38–47.
46. Grikscheit T, Ochoa ER, Srinivasan A, et al. Tissue-engineered esophagus: Experimental substitution by onlay patch or interposition. J Thorac Cardiovasc Surg 2003;126:537–44.
47. Nakase Y, Nakamura T, Kin S, et al. Intrathoracic esophageal replacement by in situ tissue-engineered esophagus. J Thorac Cardiovasc Surg 2008;136:850–9.
48. Saxena A, Ainoedhofer H, Hollwarth M. Culture of Ovine Esohageal Eithelial Cells and In Vitro Esophagus Tissue Engineering. Tissue Eng: Part C 2010;16:109–14.
49. Saxena A, Baumgart H, Komann C, et al. Esophagus tissue engineering: In situ generation of rudimentary tubular vascularized esophageal conduit using the ovine model. J Pediatr Surg 2010;45:859–64.
50. Green N, Huang Q, Kahn L, et al. The development and characterization of an organotypic tissue-engineered human esophageal mucosal model. Tissue Eng: Part A 2010;16:1053–64.
51. Parkin D, Bray F, Ferlay J, et al. Global cancer statistics, 2002. CA Cancer J Clin 2005;55:74–108.

52. Maemura T, Shin M, Sato M, et al. A tissue-engineered stomach as a replacement of the native stomach. Transplantation 2003; 76:61–5.

53. Grikscheit T, Srinivasan A, Vacanti JP. Tissue-engineered stomach: A preliminary report of a versatile in vivo model with therapeutic potential. J Pediatr Surg 2003;38:1305–9.

54. Maemura T, Shin M, Kinoshita M, et al. A tissue-engineered stomach shows presence of proton pump and G-cells in a rat model, resulting in improved anemia following total gastrectomy. Artif Organs 2008;32:234–9.

55. Speer AL, Sala FG, Matthews JA, et al. Murine tissue-engineered stomach demonstrates epithelial differentiation. J Surg Res 2011;156:205–12.

56. Barclay AR, Beattie LM, Weaver LT, et al. Systematic review: Medical and nutritional interventions for the management of intestinal failure and its resultant complications in children. Aliment Pharmacol Ther 2011;33:175–84.

57. Miyasaka EA, Brown PI, Kadoura S, et al. The adolescent child with short bowel syndrome: New onset of failure to thrive and need for increased nutritional supplementation. J Pediatr Surg 2010;45:1280–6.

58. Misiakos E, Macheras A, Kapetanakis T, et al. Short bowel syndrome: Current medical and surgical trends. J Clin Gastroenterol 2007;41:5–18.

59. Kato T, Tzakis A, Selvaggi G, et al. Intestinal and multivisceral transplantation in children. Ann Surg 2006;243:764–6.

60. Thomson AB, Keelan M, Thiesen A, et al. Small bowel review: Normal physiology part 1. Dig Dis Sci 2001;46:2567–87.

61. Dharmani P, Srivastava V, Kissoon-Singh V, et al. Role of intestinal mucins in innate host defense mechanisms against pathogens. J Innate Immun 2009;1:123–35.

62. Ahlman H, Nilsson. The gut as the largest endocrine organ in the body. Ann Oncol 2001;12(Suppl 2):S63–8.

63. Sato T, van Es JH, Snippert H, et al. Paneth cells constitute the niche for Lgr5 stem cells in intestinal crypts. Nature 2011;469: 415–19.

64. Bevins CL. The Paneth cell and the innate immune response. Curr Opin Gastroenterol 2004;20:572–80.

65. Cheng H, Leblond C. Origin, differentiation and renewal of the four main epithelial cell types in the mouse small intestine. V. Unitarian theory of the origin of the four epithelial cell types. Am J Anat 1974;141:537–62.

66. Potten C, Gandara R, Mahida Y, et al. The stem cells of the small intestinal crypts: Where are they? Cell Prolif 2009;42: 731–50.

67. Barker N, van Es JH, Kuipers J, et al. Identification of stem cells in small intestine and colon by marker gene Lgr5. Nature 2007;449:1003–8.

68. Yan KS, Chia LA, Li X, et al. The intestinal stem cell markers Bmi1 and Lgr5 identify two functionally distinct populations. Proc Natl Acad Sci U S A 2012;109:466–71.

69. Salerno-Goncalves R, Fasano A, Sztein M. Engineering of a multicellular organotypic model of the human intestinal mucosa. Gastroenterology 2011;141:18–21.

70. Pusch J, Votteler M, Göhler S, et al. The physiological performance of a three-dimensional model that mimics the microenvironment of the small intestine. Biomaterials 2011;32:7469–78.

71. Spence JR, Mayhew CN, Rankin SA, et al. Directed differentiation of human pluripotent stem cells into intestinal tissue in vitro. Nature 2011;470:105–9.

72. Evans G, Flint N, Somers A, et al. The development of a method for the preparation of rat intestinal epithelial cell primary cultures. J Cell Sci 1992;101:219–31.

73. Choi RS, Vacanti JP. Preliminary studies of tissue-engineered intestine using isolated epithelial organoid units on tubular synthetic biodegradable scaffolds. Transplant Proc 1997;29:848–51.

74. Wulkersdorfer B, Kao KK, Agopian VG, et al. Growth factors adsorbed on polyglycolic acid mesh augment growth of bioengineered intestinal neomucosa. J Surg Res 2011;169:169–78.

75. Sala FG, Matthews JA, Speer AL, et al. A multicellular approach forms a significant amount of tissue-engineered small intestine in the mouse. Tissue Eng Part A 2011;17:1841–50.

76. Lahar N, Lei NY, Wang J, et al. Intestinal subepithelial myofibroblasts support in vitro and in vivo growth of human small intestinal epithelium. PLoS One 2011;6:e26898.

77. Sala FG, Kunisaki SM, Ochoa ER, et al. Tissue-engineered small intestine and stomach form from autologous tissue in a preclinical large animal model. J Surg Res 2009;156:205–12.

78. Durno CA, Wong J, Berk T, et al. Quality of life and functional outcome for individuals who underwent very early colectomy for familial adenomatous polyposis. Dis Colon Rectum 2012; 55:436–43.

79. You YN, Chua HK, Nelson H, et al. Segmental vs. extended colectomy: Measurable differences in morbidity, function, and quality of life. Dis Colon Rectum 2008;51:1036–43.

80. Formijne Jonkers HA, Draaisma WA, Roskott AM, et al. Early complications after stoma formation: A prospective cohort study in 100 patients with 1-year follow-up. Int J Colorectal Dis 2012;27:1095–9.

81. Karadağ A, Menteş BB, Uner A, et al. Impact of stomatherapy on quality of life in patients with permanent colostomies or ileostomies. Int J Colorectal Dis 2003;18:234–8.

82. Messaris E, Sehgal R, Deiling S, et al. Dehydration is the most common indication for readmission after diverting ileostomy creation. Dis Colon Rectum 2012;55:175–80.

83. Nissinen MJ, Gylling H, Järvinen HJ, et al. Ileal pouch-anal anastomosis, conventional ileostomy and ileorectal anastomosis modify cholesterol metabolism. Dig Dis Sci 2004;49:1444–53.

84. Grikscheit TC, Ochoa ER, Ramsanahie A, et al. Tissue-engineered large intestine resembles native colon with appropriate in vitro physiology and architecture. Ann Surg 2003;238:35–41.

85. Raghavan S, Miyasaka EA, Hashish M, et al. Successful implantation of physiologically functional bioengineered mouse internal anal sphincter. Am J Physiol Gastrointest Liver Physiol 2010;299: G430–9.

86. Hashish M, Raghavan S, Somara S, et al. Surgical implantation of a bioengineered internal anal sphincter. J Pediatr Surg 2010; 45:52–8.

87. Raghavan S, Gilmont RR, Miyasaka EA, et al. Successful implantation of bioengineered, intrinsically innervated, human internal anal sphincter. Gastroenterol 2011;141:310–19.

88. Priya SG, Jungvid H, Kumar A. Skin tissue engineering for tissue repair and regeneration. Tissue Eng: Part B 2008;14:105–18.

89. Auger F, Lacroix D, Germain L. Skin substitutes and wound healing. Skin Pharmacol Physiol 2009;22:94–102.

90. Cerqueira MT, Marques AP, Reis RL. Using stem cells in skin regeneration: Possibilities and reality. Stem Cells Dev 2012;21: 1201–14.

91. Liu P, Deng Z, Han S, et al. Tissue-engineered skin containing mesenchymal stem cells improves burn wounds. Artificial Organs 2008;32:925–31.

92. Trotteir V, Marceau-Fortier G, Germain L, et al. IFATS collection: Using human adipose-derived stem/stromal cells for the production of new skin substitutes. Stem Cells 2008;26: 2713–23.

93. Cvetkovska B, Islam N, Goulet F, et al. Identification of functional markers in a self-assembled skin substitute in vitro. In Vitro Cell Dev Biol Anim 2008;44:444–50.

94. Auger FA. Treatment of cutaneous ulcers with a novel biological dressing. ClinicalTrialsgov. 2012:ultrasound National Institutes of Health; Identifier NCT00207818.

95. Connolly J, Guse R, Tiedeman J, et al. Autologous marrow injection as a substitute for operative grafting of tibial nonunions. Clin Orthop Rel Res 1991;266:259–70.

96. Kitoh H, Kawasumi M, Kaneko H, et al. Differential effects of culture-expanded bone marrow cells on the regeneration of bone between the femoral and the tibial lengthenings. J Pediatr Orthop 2009;29:643–9.

97. Quarto R, Mastrogiacomo M, Cancedda R, et al. Repair of large bone defects with the use of autologous bone marrow stromal cells. N Eng J Med 2001;344:385–6.

98. Salter E, Goh B, Hung B, et al. Bone tissue engineering bioreactors: A role in the clinic? Tissue Eng: Part B 2012;18:62–75.

99. Rodrigues MT, Reis RL, Gomes ME. Engineering tendon and ligament tissues: Present developments towards successful clinical products. J Tissue Eng Regen Med 2012. [Epub ahead of print].

100. Cheng M-T, Liu C-L, Chen T-H, et al. Comparison of potentials between stem cells isolated from human anterior cruciate ligament and bone marrow for ligament tissue engineering. Tissue Eng: Part A 2010;16:2237–53.

101. Rilke RM, Elegies D. Pediatric end-stage renal disease; 2010 Atlas of End-Stage Renal Disease in the United States: http://www.usrds.org; 2010 [cited 2012 June 1].

102. Kanzelmeyer NK, Pape L. State of pediatric kidney transplantation in 2011. Minerva Pediatr 2012;64:205–11.

103. Ross EA, Williams MJ, Hamazaki T, et al. Embryonic stem cells proliferate and differentiate when seeded into kidney scaffolds. J Am Soc Nephrol 2009;20:2338–47.

104. Nakayama KH, Batchelder CA, Lee CI, et al. Decellularized rhesus monkey kidney as a three-dimensional scaffold for renal tissue engineering. Tissue Eng: Part A 2010;16:2207–16.

105. De Filippo R, Yoo J, Atala A. Urethral replacement using cel seeded tubularized collagen matrices. J Urol 2002;168:1789–92.

106. El-Kassaby A, Retik A, Yoo J. Urethral stricture matrix with an off-the shelf collagen matrix. J Urol 2003;169:170–3.

107. El-Kassaby A, AbouShwareb T, Atala A. Randomized comparative study between buccal mucosal and acellular bladder matrix grafts in comples anterior urethral strictures. J Urol 2008;179:1432–6.

108. Raya-Rivera A, Esquiliano DR, Yoo JJ, et al. Tissue-engineered autologous urethras for patients who need reconstruction: An observational study. Lancet 2011;377:1175–82.

109. Yang B, Peng B, Zheng J. Cell-based tissue-engineered urethras. Lancet 2011;378:568–9.

110. Atala A, Freeman M, Vacanti J, et al. Formation of urothelial structures consisting of rabbit and human urothelium and human bladder muscle. J Urol 1993;150:608–12.

111. Pariente J, Kim B, Atala A. In vitro biocompatability assessment of naturally derived and synthetic biomaterials using normal human urothelial cells. J Biomed Mat Res 2001;55:33–9.

112. Atala A, Bauer SB, Soker S, et al. Tissue-engineered autologous bladders for patients needing cystoplasty. The Lancet 2006;367:1241–5.

113. Santos JL, Choquette M, Bezerra JA. Cholestatic liver disease in children. Curr Gastroenterol Rep 2010;12:30–9.

114. Chistiakov DA. Liver regenerative medicine: Advances and challenges. Cells Tissues Organs 2012:1–22.

115. Yamashita Y, Shimada M, Tsujita E, et al. High metabolic function of primary human and porcine hepatocytes in a polyurethane foam/spheroid culture system in plasma from patients with fulminant hepatic failure. Cell Transplant 2002;11:379–84.

116. Rozga J, Malkowski P. Artificial liver support: Quo vadis? Ann Transplant 2010;15:92–101.

117. Imamura T, Cui L, Teng R, et al. Embryonic stem cell-derived embryoid bodies in three-dimensional culture systems form hepatocyte-like cells in vitro and in vivo. Tissue Eng 2004;10:1716–24.

118. Uygun BE, Soto-Gutierrez A, Yagi H, et al. Organ reengineering through development of a transplantable recellularized liver graft using decellularized liver matrix. Nat Med 2010;16:814–21.

119. Shapiro AM, Lakey JR, Ryan EA, et al. Islet transplantation in seven patients with type 1 diabetes mellitus using a glucocorticoid-free immunosuppressive regimen. N Engl J Med 2000;343:230–8.

120. Shapiro AM, Ricordi C, Hering BJ, et al. International trial of the Edmonton protocol for islet transplantation. N Engl J Med 2006;355:1318–30.

121. Hebrok M. Generating beta cells from stem cells-the story so far. Cold Spring Harb Perspect Med 2012;2:1–12.

122. Kodama S, Kojima K, Furuta S, et al. Engineering functional islets from cultured cells. Tissue Eng Part A 2009;15:3321–9.

CHAPTER 80

ETHICS IN PEDIATRIC SURGERY

Aviva L. Katz

Despite extensive training, many pediatric surgeons feel ill prepared in the area of medical ethics. The breadth of pediatric surgery from prenatal consultations to surgery in young adults across a wide range of diagnoses exposes the pediatric surgeon to a variety of ethical concerns. The practicing pediatric surgeon should be prepared to deal with the ethical issues that are integral to this broad spectrum of clinical encounters. Certainly no text or course of study could prepare one for each possible clinical scenario and its associated ethical issues. This chapter will provide a framework for understanding and addressing the ethical concerns that arise daily with patients and families. It is anticipated that this discussion will include some familiar as well as new perspectives on medical decision-making.

WHAT IS ETHICS?

In general, ethics is a term for understanding the moral life. In considering medical ethics, we most commonly think of normative ethics that attempts to define a set of general moral norms which can be broadly accepted as a guide to conduct. This can be an increasingly difficult task, especially in our multicultural society with a vast array of cultural and religious backgrounds, but the identification of a shared moral ground is critical to discussing and resolving difficult ethical issues. Practical or applied ethics refers to the application of these moral norms or ethical theories to the resolution of ethical dilemmas. This common morality contains moral norms, the core dimension of morality that binds all persons in a community, although they may come from diverse backgrounds. In this manner, the common morality can be seen as normative, describing and establishing moral standards and obligations for the broad community, with further moral virtues and obligations specific for physicians as described in a professional morality. These special role-related moral norms for medical professionals are rooted and developed from the common morality. True ethical dilemmas are difficult because the conflict is generally between moral principles pertinent to the problem at hand. A background in medical ethics provides the tools to balance these conflicting moral principles to reach an ethically acceptable solution.

FRAMEWORKS FOR MEDICAL ETHICS

A commonly utilized framework of moral principles reflecting the common morality is principle-based ethics as described by Beauchamp and Childress.[1] This account identifies four moral principles that can function as guidelines in considering options in patient care and professional behavior. These principles include respect for autonomy, nonmaleficence, beneficence, and justice. Nonmaleficence (avoiding harm) and beneficence (providing benefit and balancing benefit against harm) reflect values stated in the Hippocratic Oath. Historically, these values have been viewed as the physician's primary obligation, as suggested by the statement *primum non nocere*. Respect for autonomy is a more modern concept and is derived from Kantian moral philosophy. Key elements are liberty, defined as the capacity to live life according to one's own reasons and motives, and agency, defined as the rational capacity for intentional action. Although many pediatric patients lack the agency required to be truly autonomous, this framework remains important in resolving ethical dilemmas. The principle of justice can be understood as fairness. Justice can be viewed as equals being treated equally. Distributive justice is reflected by fair, equitable, and appropriate distribution of goods and risks, an important consideration in the use of human subjects in research.

While the principle-based approach to medical ethics has been widely utilized for several decades, other frameworks have been recently developed. There has been significant recent interest in virtue ethics. Virtue ethics can be derived from Aristotle's account of the virtues in the Nicomachean Ethics.[2] Virtues are understood as dispositions not only to act in a particular way, but also to feel in a particular way. Rather than focusing on the rightness or wrongness of action, virtue ethics focuses on the nature or character of the agent. In this manner, virtue ethics has contributed significantly to the current work on professionalism. Many professional codes stress the importance of these virtues, and the development of the moral character of the professional. Pellegrino has written extensively on the nature of medicine as a moral enterprise.[3] While not suggesting that virtue ethics can provide a foundation for all medical ethics, he is persuasive in suggesting that the physician's character and virtues are at the heart of moral choice and ethical actions. While this framework is helpful in teaching and evaluating professionalism, it clearly has limitations in addressing all the ethical concerns that may arise in a tertiary or quaternary children's hospital.

A relatively new framework for analysis of ethical concerns has been developed in significant part from feminist writings and theory. This framework is most commonly referred to as an ethics of care. Gilligan developed the theory that due to social roles and expectations, men and women develop different conceptions of moral problem solving.[4] Women more often take a contextual approach to what they view as conflicting responsibilities, while men may take a more formal or abstract approach to what may be seen as competing rights. This focus on relationships, interconnectedness, and caring contributes to the notion of caring as primary in the ethics of care. Rather than focusing on the protection of autonomy, an ethic of care provides an opportunity to assess the problem in terms of responsibilities within relationships. Rather than seeing autonomy in decision-making as an ideal, an ethic of care places the patient within a web of relationships, providing a very different orientation to the discussion of ethical concerns.

The development of this framework of caring provides another alternative to principle-based ethics in resolving ethical dilemmas. Although both are valid, an ethics of care helps more with the problems we face in pediatric surgery as all our patients reside within interdependent webs of relationships. Although an ethics of care is often portrayed as being in conflict with a principle-based ethical framework, these systems should be viewed as complementary to allow a more robust evaluation of moral problems in clinical care. A quote demonstrating this balance between these frameworks is provided by Dietrich Bonhoeffer: 'An essential perspective in assessing a moral question is the 'view from below' ... which is the perspective of 'those who suffer' and which those who seek to 'do justice to life in its entire dimension' can learn to appreciate.'[5]

With this background in ethical theory, several of the ethical issues faced by pediatric surgeons will be addressed.

ETHICAL ISSUES FOR THE PEDIATRIC SURGEON

Informed Consent and Assent

Although the need to obtain informed consent prior to proceeding with a procedure or operation is assumed to be a routine part of patient care, this is a relatively new concept when considering the scope of medical history. The current concept of informed consent has roots in both ethical theory and law, and the phrase 'informed consent' is adopted verbatim from an *amicus curiae* brief filed by the American College of Surgeons in Salgo vs Leland Stanford Jr University Board of Trustees in 1957: 'A physician violates his duty to his patient and subjects himself to liability if he withholds any facts which are necessary to form the basis of an intelligent consent ... In discussing the element of risk, a certain amount of discretion must be employed consistent with the full disclosure of facts necessary for an informed consent.'[6] The ethical roots of informed consent lie within the principle of autonomy.

In the practice of pediatric surgery, most discussions regarding the direction of care are three sided, and involve the physician, the patient, and the patient's surrogate(s). Most commonly, the parent(s) will act as the patient's surrogate decision-maker with the understanding that parents know their child's interests better than others, and will be deeply committed to pursuing care that fulfills their child's best interests. Additionally, there

is a general understanding of the importance of family autonomy and privacy, allowing medical decision-making within broad ethical boundaries that reflect family values. A parent's medical decision-making for their child can be framed as a responsibility, rather than a right, with the focus remaining on the child's best interests, rather than the parent's(s') assertion of autonomy. This focus may help to minimize conflict during the process of difficult medical decision-making. While other surrogates will be able to use substituted judgment in medical decision-making for adults who no longer have the capacity to consent for their own care, parental decision-making for the child is based on a broad vision of the best interest standard, incorporating the child's emotional, social, and medical concerns, as well as the interests of the child's family.

The elements associated with the process of informed consent are fairly constant, and help create a framework for our conversations with families and patients. Informed consent discussions must include:

- A provision of information: explanations in understandable, developmentally appropriate language about the nature of the illness or condition, the proposed diagnostic steps and/or treatments and the probability of their success, the existence and the nature of the risks and anticipated benefits, and the existence, potential benefits, and risks of potential alternative treatments, including the option of no treatment.
- An assessment of the understanding of this information
- An assessment of the capacity of the patient and surrogate to make the decisions necessary for care
- Assurance, as far as can be determined from ongoing discussions, that the patient and surrogate have the freedom to choose among the alternative treatments without undue influence or coercion, recognizing that we are all subject to subtle pressures in decision-making, and that medical decision-making cannot occur in isolation from other concerns and relationships.

These discussions regarding medical decision-making should be understood as a longitudinal process over time, recognizing that many decisions are made throughout the medical course as new information emerges.

An often overlooked, but important issue is the need for patient assent. The value of involving children and adolescents in their own medical decision-making is being increasingly recognized.[7] The respect owed children as medical decision-makers is dependent on several factors, including their cognitive abilities, maturity of judgment, and the general respect owed a moral agent. Although many minors reach the formal operational stage of cognitive development that allows abstract thinking by mid-adolescence, newer insight into brain structure and function demonstrates slower development of executive function and judgment.[8-10] Executive function is key to the ability to balance risks and benefits and plan for long-term goals, skills that are necessary for meaningful informed consent discussions. While this cognitive control system which promotes self-regulation and impulse control develops during young adulthood, reward seeking behavior is prominent during adolescence, resulting in the risky behavior often seen in this age group. There is increasing evidence that, in general, adolescents make decisions differently than adults, and this slow neuromaturation may limit the adolescent's medical decision-making ability, despite good cognitive skills.[11,12]

Despite these concerns, it is very important to include children and adolescents in discussions regarding their medical care. Assent from children as young as 7 years for medical and surgical interventions can foster moral growth and developing autonomy in young patients, contributing to empowerment and potentially even compliance with the treatment plan.[13] Assent includes helping the patient achieve a developmentally appropriate awareness of the nature of his/her condition, telling the patient what he/she can expect regarding tests and treatments, making an assessment of the patient's understanding of the situation, and soliciting an expression of the patient's willingness to accept the proposed care.

Throughout this process, it is very important that the child is not deceived. Although information should be provided, one should not attempt to solicit the child's assent if the treatment is required. Within these limitations, a child should still be given as much control over the actual treatments as possible. Dissent from the child should carry increased weight when the proposed intervention is not essential and/or can be deferred without substantial risk. In situations with a poor prognosis, and interventions associated with significant risk and discomfort, more consideration should be given to the adolescent's opportunity to provide assent or refusal.

There are special circumstances under which an adolescent can legally provide his/her own consent for health care. The opportunity for adolescents to legally consent generally involves health care issues related to sexual activity. While all states allow adolescents to consent for treatment for sexually transmitted infections, protection of the adolescent's confidentiality is less widespread. The majority of states allow at least some access to contraceptive services, but there can be great variation.[14] There is similar variability among the states regarding adolescents' access to mental health and substance abuse prevention and treatment services. These statutes do not reflect acceptance of the adolescent's decision-making skills. Rather, allowing adolescents the opportunity to access this care is a public health decision, recognizing the concern that adolescents may not seek care for these issues if they are required to involve their parents for consent.

Another area sometimes encountered by the pediatric surgeon is the issue of the adolescent parent. While there are significant limitations on the adolescent's legal right to consent for medical care, all states presume adolescent parents to be the appropriate surrogate decision-makers for their children, and allow them to give informed consent for their child's medical care. This right reflects the adolescent's status as a parent, rather than maturity of their decision-making abilities. At the same time, there is clearly significant concern in having an adolescent take responsibility for complex medical decision-making for their child while, in general, they are protected and guided in their own medical decision-making.

Withdrawing and Withholding Care

While decisions to withdraw or withhold care are extremely difficult for patients, families and care providers, most children who die in a hospital in the USA die following the withdrawal or withholding of clinical interventions.[15,16] Although many clinicians feel uncomfortable discontinuing life-sustaining treatments that are already in place, there is no true legal or ethical distinction between withholding a treatment and withdrawing a treatment. This is important as refusal to withdraw already existing interventions may have negative outcomes. In this situation, patients may be forced to endure continued treatment, with its associated discomfort, despite demonstration that it fails to provide the anticipated benefit. Additionally, concern regarding the withdrawal of previously instituted interventions may make the clinician reluctant to offer a trial of therapy that may provide benefit to the patient, due to the fear of being committed to the technology.

When discussing potential medical interventions with families and patients, it is important that the pediatric surgeon has an understanding of their goals of care. A discussion of the goals of care should have the family and patient contributing their understanding of their illness and their personal values. The surgeon should contribute information on the diagnosis, benefits, burdens of the proposed and alternative therapies, and anticipated prognosis. Discussions that proceed from an understanding of the overall goals of care are more likely to result in a thoughtful, coherent care plan as opposed to episodic discussions of individual interventions. The appropriateness of a medical intervention should not be assessed in a vacuum, but should be evaluated as to how it promotes the goals of care.

Adults with the capacity to make their own medical decisions have the opportunity to accept or refuse all medical interventions, including life-saving medical treatments (LSMT). Additionally, adults are encouraged to create documentation, with the assistance of their physicians and family, that clarifies their preferences regarding their care and choice of surrogate decision-maker in the event that they lose the capacity to make their own health care decisions. In this situation, the surrogate is expected to make medical decisions utilizing a substituted judgment standard: striving to make the same decisions that the patient would have made. Children and their parents are generally not offered such a robust autonomy, especially regarding medical decision-making surrounding LSMT. Parents are expected to approach medical decision-making for their children from a best interest standard. The best interest standard should be considered broadly and includes not only prolongation of life, but also improved quality of life, such as reduction of pain, ability to interact with others, and ability to participate in pleasurable activities. It is very important to recognize that quality of life should be assessed utilizing the patient and family's preferences and values.

Few adolescents are given the opportunity to discuss advance directives that would address their preferences for end of life care. This discussion, although difficult and requiring a great deal of sensitivity, may be appropriate for mature adolescents who have experienced a chronic illness and want to make their preferences known before further deterioration in their health prevents them from taking part in such discussions. In this situation, parents are able to utilize substituted judgment in making decisions regarding LSMT.

Similar to other medical interventions, decision-making surrounding LSMT should seek to balance the benefits and burdens associated with the proposed intervention(s), and their relationship to the overall goals of care. Although LSMT may provide for extension of length of life, this potential benefit must be considered in the light of associated burdens, especially if the prolongation of life results primarily in the continuation of biologic existence without consciousness. Burdens associated with LSMT may include intractable chronic pain, emotional suffering, repeated invasive procedures, prolonged hospitalizations, and the inability to interact with loved ones and participate in pleasurable activities.

Although Hippocrates is quoted as saying that physicians should 'refuse to treat those who are overmastered by their disease, realizing that in such cases medicine is powerless', this statement needs some clarification.[17] First, it is important to acknowledge the difficulty in determining that the patient has been 'overmastered by their disease'. Good ethics is often dependent on good facts. Second opinions or subspecialty consultation may be helpful. Most importantly, medicine should never be considered powerless in providing comfort. While LSMT may be withdrawn or withheld, care is never withdrawn, and comfort measures should be provided. The involvement of an integrated palliative care service is valuable in the transition of the goals to supportive care and comfort.

When consensus has been reached among the physicians, family, and when appropriate, the patient, that the burdens of LSMT outweigh their benefit, it is appropriate to proceed with withdrawal of these interventions, and focus attention on measures that will provide comfort to the patient and family. Many physicians are less familiar with the option of forgoing medically provided nutrition and hydration in children who may not require mechanical ventilation, but in whom a decision has been made to withdraw LSMT. The decision to withdraw or withhold medically provided fluid and nutrition is often controversial and uncomfortable, in large part due to the symbolism associated with feeding and nurturing infants and children. It is critical to distinguish between medically provided fluids and nutrition and feeding a child who is hungry and capable of eating. It has become clear both ethically and legally that the decision-making process surrounding medically provided fluid and nutrition is the same as for other medical interventions: it appears such care can be withheld when the physicians and family agree that the burdens of care outweigh the potential benefits.[18]

Medically provided fluids and nutrition are medical interventions with associated risks. These risks include, but are not limited to the potential for complications, the adverse effects of fluid overload including dyspnea and skin breakdown, systemic infection, and the need for frequent monitoring for fluid and electrolyte imbalance. Infants and children, in whom it may be reasonable to consider the withdrawal of medically provided fluids and nutrition, may include those in a persistent vegetative state and those with congenital central nervous system (CNS) malformations or perinatal CNS injury where a poor prognosis has been established and there is no capacity for conscious awareness or the ability to feed orally. Infants with a severe gastrointestinal injury or a disease that results in the destruction of a large portion of the small intestine, leading to total intestinal failure, are another population in whom the withdrawal of hydration and nutrition may be discussed. Although total parenteral nutrition may provide support for years, the associated morbidities, especially in the absence of any intestinal function, are significant, even in the current era of intestinal transplantation.

Difficult decisions are best made when there is consensus between the family, the patient when appropriate, and the health care providers. As with other LSMT, parents have the responsibility regarding medical decision-making, and they may choose to continue hydration and nutrition with the goal of continued survival. When a decision has been made to withdraw hydration and nutrition, it is important to involve the services of an integrated palliative care team to minimize suffering and provide comfort measures within a broader palliative care plan.

Issues Involved in Donation after Circulatory Determination of Death

The opportunity for organ recovery is one of the many issues that needs to be addressed with patients and families during discussions centered on end of life care. An opportunity to provide organs may offer comfort for a family grieving the death of their child. With increased social awareness, many adolescents have had an opportunity to consider this opportunity prior to their illness or injury, and may have shared their interest in being an organ donor.

The ethical issues related to organ transplantation are well described, and this discussion will focus on donation after circulatory determination of death (DCDD). DCDD serves at least two major purposes: to expand the pool of potential organ donors, and to provide an opportunity for families to proceed with organ donation in those situations where a decision has been made to withdraw LSMT but the child does not make the criteria for brain death. DCDD had been the initial form of deceased organ donation prior to the development of brain death criteria by an ad hoc committee at the Harvard Medical School in 1968.[19] With the publication of a 1981 report on a whole brain determination of death by the Presidential Commission,[20] and the passage of the Uniform Determination of Death act,[21] brain death became a widely accepted definition of death, and patients meeting these criteria became the most utilized source of organ donation, in significant part due to their physiologic stability providing improved organ function after transplantation.

Both the increasing disparity between the number of patients awaiting organ transplantation and the organs available for transplant, and an increased understanding of the need for broadened discussion regarding end of life care have increased attention on DCDD. This increased attention has resulted in regulatory policy regarding DCDD by both the Joint Commission and United Network for Organ Sharing (UNOS). The Joint Commission mandates that while hospitals may not offer DCDD, they must have policies that address it.[22] UNOS/OPTN requires that transplant hospitals must develop DCDD recovery protocols that include the model elements as developed by UNOS/OPTN.[23] It is therefore important that all health care providers, especially pediatric surgeons, develop a working knowledge of DCDD and its associated ethical concerns.

There is a significant difference between the recovery of organs from a patient who has met brain death criteria, and one for whom a decision has been made to proceed with DCDD. With controlled DCDD, the patient is generally brought to the operating room and all LSMT are removed, and the patient is monitored until asystole is documented. Most protocols require the use of an echocardiogram or central arterial tracing to confirm asystole. There is variation, generally between two and five minutes, in the length of time required following asystole for determination of death at which point the transplant team is allowed to proceed with organ recovery.

While it is important that families have the opportunity to proceed with DCDD if they wish, it is also important that there be no coercion or pressure applied to their decision. The decision to withdraw LSMT must be prior to and separate from any consideration of proceeding with DCDD. Sometimes, hospital policy on DCDD will include a mandatory ethics consult to allow for independent evaluation of separation of these two decisions, and to help ensure that the family is able to come to this decision without coercion. The goal is to avoid a decision to proceed with withdrawal of LSMT for the purpose of providing organs for recovery. It is ethically critical that the decision to proceed with withdrawal of LSMT is made to further the patient's best interests, because the interventions no longer provide benefit in the family's judgment, and not to serve a utilitarian goal of organ recovery.

Proceeding with DCDD is likely to alter the family's opportunity to be with the child at the time of death. Most often, the patient is moved to the operating room prior to the removal of LSMT to allow for rapid recovery of organs following determination of death. Although withdrawal of LSMT is deferred until the patient is moved to the operating room in the anticipation that asystole and death will occur shortly after, this is not entirely predictable. Most DCDD policies anticipate this problem, and limit the amount of time spent waiting for asystole following removal of LSMT to between 30 and 60 minutes. Families should be prepared for the potential that the patient will be returned to the intensive care unit (ICU), where comfort care will continue until death ensues.

There are additional ethical issues concerning DCDD that significantly impact the health care provider. The concept of DCDD, and the creation of a policy supporting its use, is dependent on a specific understanding and definition of death, which is not universally shared among physicians. Certainly a shorter period of observation following the onset of asystole may increase the concern as to whether the patient is dead prior to the organ recovery. These concerns are due to both the potential for autoresuscitation following the onset of asystole and the fear that the patient is actually in the process of dying, but is not yet dead. It is critical that the patient is dead prior to proceeding with organ recovery as cadaveric organ transplantation operates under the dead donor rule. This rule can be conceptualized two ways: organ recovery must not cause the donor's death, and the donor must be dead prior to proceeding with the recovery of organs.[24] Clearly, providing assurance that the donor is dead is critical to an ethical approach to organ recovery as it minimizes the risk of using patients as a means to an end, and it supports public trust in organ donation and transplantation. While there has been general acceptance by the Institute of Medicine, critical care societies, and UNOS/OPTN regarding the determination of death under DCDD criteria, individual practitioners may have valid concerns about this management. Hospitals should have a process that allows for individual practitioners to decline to support DCDD care, while still providing this service to families that request it.

A related ethical issue is the need for the physicians involved to avoid a conflict of interest in the patient's care. The attending physician for a patient undergoing removal of LSMT and proceeding with DCDD should not be involved in the organ recovery or transplantation. The transplant surgeons/organ recovery team should have no contact with the patient until after the determination of death. There are other interesting issues surrounding DCDD, including the place of extracorporeal membrane oxygenation (ECMO) in stabilization for DCDD, and social justice issues concerning uncontrolled DCDD, but these concerns go beyond the scope of this chapter.

Conscientious Objection

Conscientious objection among health care professionals has become the subject of increasing attention in the ethics literature as well as the courts and legislature. Conscientious objection refers to health care professionals who may object to or even refuse to provide an otherwise legally available medical treatment within the scope of their practice based on a moral objection to the treatment or procedure. Circumcision is an example in pediatric surgery that may raise concerns in the realm of conscientious objection. Circumcision is well within the scope of practice of the pediatric surgeon, yet there may be reasonable objection to performing circumcision without medical indication on infants and children too young to provide meaningful assent to the procedure. Decisions surrounding end of life care and the conflicts surrounding DCDD are other areas within pediatric surgery where issues of conscientious objection arise.

Conscientious objection is an interesting and important ethical dilemma, as it requires balancing the competing ethical claims of the physician and the patient. There are morally important reasons to protect the health care professional's exercise of conscience.[25] Requiring a health care professional to provide a therapy or perform a procedure that violates their conscience may undermine their sense of integrity and self-respect, and result in a negative effect on their professional persona. Protection of rights of conscience is important in allowing health care professionals to maintain a sense of self, and protects basic religious freedom by allowing the individual to live according to their innermost values.

Issues of conscientious objection reflect an objection based on personal or religious morality rather than commonly accepted professional ethics. While the practice of conscientious objection is important and legally protected, the patient's right to care must also be respected and protected. Conflicts occur when claims of conscientious objection interfere with access to medical care. Generally, claims of conscience, and refusal to provide a specific medical treatment or intervention, are acceptable as long as the patient is not put at risk and referral is made in a timely fashion to another skilled practitioner who will provide the contested care. A problem arises if the health care provider not only refuses to provide the morally objectionable care, but also refuses to refer the patient to another provider on the grounds of complicity. Complicity is concerned not only with the performance of an act, but also with the facilitation of another's performance of an act that one finds morally objectionable. This may seriously limit the patient's right to medical care.[26]

An understanding of informed consent is critical in considering the ethical conflicts raised by conscientious objection. Providing the information and counseling required for an informed consent is a basic professional ethical and legal requirement so that patients and their surrogates can make an informed judgment regarding their choice of care. This includes information on treatments that the health care practitioner does not provide and/or finds morally objectionable. Informed consent seeks in part to provide adequate information so that the patient and family can match treatment options with their own deeply held values, even if these differ from the health care provider's values. This opportunity is seriously compromised if the information provided is significantly filtered by the practitioner's values and nonmedical judgment.

The discussions surrounding informed consent should support and respect the autonomy of the patient and family, recognizing the diversity of backgrounds and values represented in the patient population. Physicians must understand the significant imbalance in power and knowledge between themselves and the patient. Patients should be able to expect a full disclosure from their physician about their diagnosis and all treatment options. Professional licensure defines a social role that includes special responsibilities. Licensure allows physicians as a professional society the right to regulate the training and education required for entrance into the profession. Licensure also allows physicians as a professional society a monopoly over the provision of medical services. This power and control comes with reciprocal responsibilities, which are voluntarily assumed when physicians enter the medical profession. These professional role expectations include activities that support the ethical principles of beneficence. As part of this professional obligation, it is expected that physicians will place the patient's needs

before their own, and these responsibilities must be considered in balancing the values and needs of the physician and patient. In an effort to balance these competing concerns, it is appropriate to respect a constrained right to conscientious objection, allowing the physician the right to decline to provide a morally objectionable medical intervention as long as information is provided about treatment options with a timely referral to another available skilled practitioner.

Clinical Research

All clinical research in the United States is guided by the principles expressed in the Belmont Report. The Belmont Report (the Ethical Principles and Guidelines for the Protection of Human Subjects of Research) was prepared by the National Commission for the Protection of Human Subjects of Biomedical and Behavioral Research and published in 1979.[27] This work was undertaken due to public outcry over well publicized ethical lapses in clinical research in the USA despite what should have been learned following the Nuremberg Doctors' Trial.[28] The report first distinguished between accepted clinical practice and research by clarifying that research describes an activity designed to test a hypothesis or contribute to general knowledge. In addition, the report also briefly addresses the issue of innovation, and distinguishes between clinical innovation and research, noting that major innovation should move towards formal research at an early stage. Unfortunately, this is the extent of discussion on innovation in the report, and more work needs to be done with innovation and the safety of patients and research subjects. The report clarifies that all activity considered research should undergo review for the protection of human subjects.

The report identifies three basic ethical principles that are particularly relevant to assessing research involving human subjects: respect for persons, beneficence, and justice. Respect for persons is reflected in the principle of autonomy. The principle of autonomy is demonstrated by respecting individuals as autonomous agents when they have the capacity to provide consent. The report discusses the need for protection of individuals who lack the capacity to function as autonomous agents, recognizing that this capacity may fluctuate over time. The principle of beneficence is incorporated in the obligation to maximize benefits and minimize possible harms. The report emphasizes that investigators should seek to design research protocols that will minimize risks to subjects while maximizing the benefit. The principle of justice reflects a fair distribution of both risks and benefits, with equals being treated equally. Care must be taken to insure that the burdens and risks of participating in research will be distributed fairly among the population.

The report then goes on to demonstrate the applicability of these general principles to the creation of guidelines for the protection of human research subjects. There is an extensive discussion of the need for informed consent, recognizing that this level of informed consent may need to go beyond the more standard consent obtained in the clinical setting. Additionally, the discussion of informed consent in the report strengthens the position of assent by older children and adults with limited capacity, giving these subjects the opportunity to decline to participate in research. This is a much stronger protection of the minor's right to assent to or decline an intervention than exists in the clinical realm. The requirement that the research protocol demonstrates a favorable risk-benefit analysis is seen as an example of the principle of beneficence. Finally, the principle of justice is manifest in the discussion on the selection of subjects. The report clearly discusses the concern regarding the involvement of vulnerable populations in research, and the risk of further burdening an already burdened class including children, prisoners, and the institutionalized mentally ill.

The USA Department of Health and Human Services (HHS) has applied the ethical principles detailed in the Belmont Report to the development of federal policy regarding the protection of human research subjects. This federal policy, HHS regulation 45 CFR 46, is known as the Common Rule as it is utilized by 15 different federal departments and agencies in guiding regulations regarding research.[29] This HHS regulation provides general guidelines regarding oversight for human subjects research including the responsibilities and membership of institutional review boards (IRB) and the requirements for informed consent. Subpart D of this regulation discusses the additional protections for children and the need to seek permission from the child's surrogate to allow their participation in research.

As a vulnerable population, the risks that children may be exposed to are more constrained than the adult population. Children may participate in research not involving greater than minimal risk, or greater than minimal risk, but presenting the prospect of direct benefit to the individual subject. Also, they may be recruited for research with greater than minimal risk and no prospect of direct benefit to individual subjects, but likely to yield generalizable knowledge about the subject's condition. Research protocols that do not fit any of these three categories, but which present an opportunity to understand, prevent or alleviate a serious problem affecting the welfare of children cannot be approved independently by a local IRB, but require review by a panel of experts at the federal level.

The determination of risk is an area where there may be valid disagreement between IRBs. Minimal risk means that the probability and magnitude of harm or discomfort anticipated in the research are not greater in and of themselves than those ordinarily encountered in daily life or during the performance of routine physical examinations and tests. This definition is most likely intentionally broad, allowing for local interpretation. While the rules are developed to protect the interests of the individual research subject, they place significant limitations on clinical research in children.

REFERENCES

1. Beauchamp TL, Childress JF. Principles of Biomedical Ethics. 5th ed. New York, NY: Oxford University Press; 2001.
2. Aristotle, translated by Thomson JAK. The Nicomachean Ethics (Books II through VI). Penguin Books; 2004.
3. Pellegrino ED, Thomasma DC. The Virtues in Medical Practice (Chapter 3). New York NY: Oxford University Press; 1993.
4. Gilligan C. In a Different Voice. Cambridge MA: Harvard University Press; 1982.
5. Bonhoeffer D. Dietrich Bonhoeffer Works, Volume 8: Letters and Papers from Prison. Augsburg Fortress; 2009.
6. Salgo v. Leland Stanford Jr. University Board of Trustees, 54 Cal. App 2d 560, 1957.
7. Levy MDL, Larcher V, Kurz R. Ethics Working Group of the CESP. Informed consent/assent in children: Statement of the Ethics Working Group of the Confederation of European Specialists in Pediatrics (CESP). Eur J Pediatr 2003;162:629–33.
8. Giedd J, Blumenthal J, Jeffries NO, et al. Brain development during childhood and adolescence: A longitudinal MRI study. Nature Neurosci 1999;2:861–3.
9. Sowell ER, Thompson PM, Holmes CJ, et al. In vivo evidence for post-adolescent brain maturation in frontal and striatal regions. Nature Neurosci 1999;2:859–61.
10. Giedd JN. The teen brain: Insights from neuroimaging. J Adolesc Health 2008;42:335–43.
11. Van Leijenhorst L, Gunther Moor B, Op de Macks ZA, et al. Adolescent risky decision-making: Neurocognitive development of reward and control regions. Neuroimage 2010;51:345–55.
12. Steinberg L. Cognitive and affective development in adolescence. Trends Cognit Sci 2005;9:69–74.
13. Waller B. Patient autonomy naturalized. Perspect Biol Med 2001;44:584–93.
14. Guttmacher Institute State Policies in Brief Minors' Access to Contraceptive Services. Accessed at http://www.guttmacher.org/statecenter/spibs/spib_MACS.pdf.
15. Carter BS, Howenstein M, Gilmer MJ, et al. Circumstances surrounding the deaths of hospitalized children: Opportunities for pediatric palliative care. Pediatrics 2004;114:e361–6.
16. Tan GH, Totapally BR, Torbati D, et al. End-of-life decisions and palliative care in a children's hospital. J Palliat Med 2006;9: 332–42.
17. Scannell K, Henry SC. Medical Futility. Permanente Journal 2002;6:52–4.
18. Diekema DS, Botkin JR. Forgoing medically provided nutrition and hydration in children. Pediatrics 2009;124:813–22.
19. Ad Hoc Committee of the Harvard Medical School to Examine the Definition of Brain Death: A definition of irreversible coma. JAMA 1968;205:337–40.
20. President's Commission for the Study of Ethical Problems in Medicine and Biomedical and Behavioral Research: A report on the medical, legal and ethical issues in the determination of death, 1981, accessed at http://bioethics.georgetown.edu/pcbe/reports/past_commissions/defining_death.pdf.
21. National Conference of commissioners on Uniform State Laws. Uniform Determination of Death Act, 1980. Accessed at http://www.uniformlaws.org/Act.aspx?title=Determination of Death Act.
22. Joint Commission on Accreditation of Healthcare Organizations. Revisions to standard LD.3.110. Jt Comm Perspect 2006;26:7.
23. Attachment III to Appendix B of the UNOS Bylaws: Model Elements for Controlled DCD Recovery Protocols 2007. Accessed at http://www.unos.org/docs/Appendix_B_AttachIII.pdf.; Appendix B to Bylaws – Criteria for Institutional Membership: Transplant Hospitals 2010. Accessed at http://www.unos.org/docs/Appendix_B_II.pdf.
24. Arnold RM, Youngener SJ. The dead donor rule: Should we stretch it, bend it, or abandon it? Kennedy Inst Ethics J 1993;3:263–78.
25. Wicclair MR. Conscientious objection in medicine. Bioethics 2000;14:205–27.
26. May T, Aulisio MP. Personal morality and professional obligations. Persp Biol Med 2009;52:30–8.
27. Ultrasound National Commission for the Protection of Human Subjects of Biomedical and Behavioral Research. The Belmont Report: Ethical principles and guidelines for the protection of human subjects of research. DHEW Publication no. (OS)78-0012-78-0014.
28. Annas GH, Grodin MA. The Nazi Doctors and the Nuremberg Code Human Rights in Human Experimentation. New York, NY: Oxford University Press; 1992.
29. Code of Federal Regulations Title 45 Public Welfare Department of Health and Human Services Part 46 Protection of Human Subjects 2009. Accessed at http://www.hhs.gov/ohrp/humansubjects/guidance/45cfr46.html.

Page numbers followed by 'f' indicate figures, 't' indicate tables, and 'b' indicate boxes.